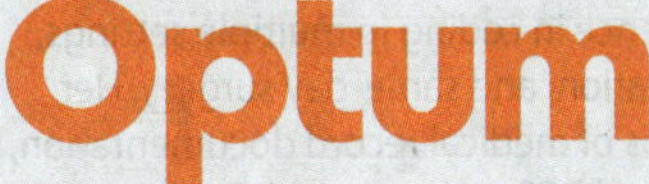

Professional

ICD-10-CM Professional for Hospitals

The complete official code set

Codes valid from October 1, 2022 through September 30, 2023

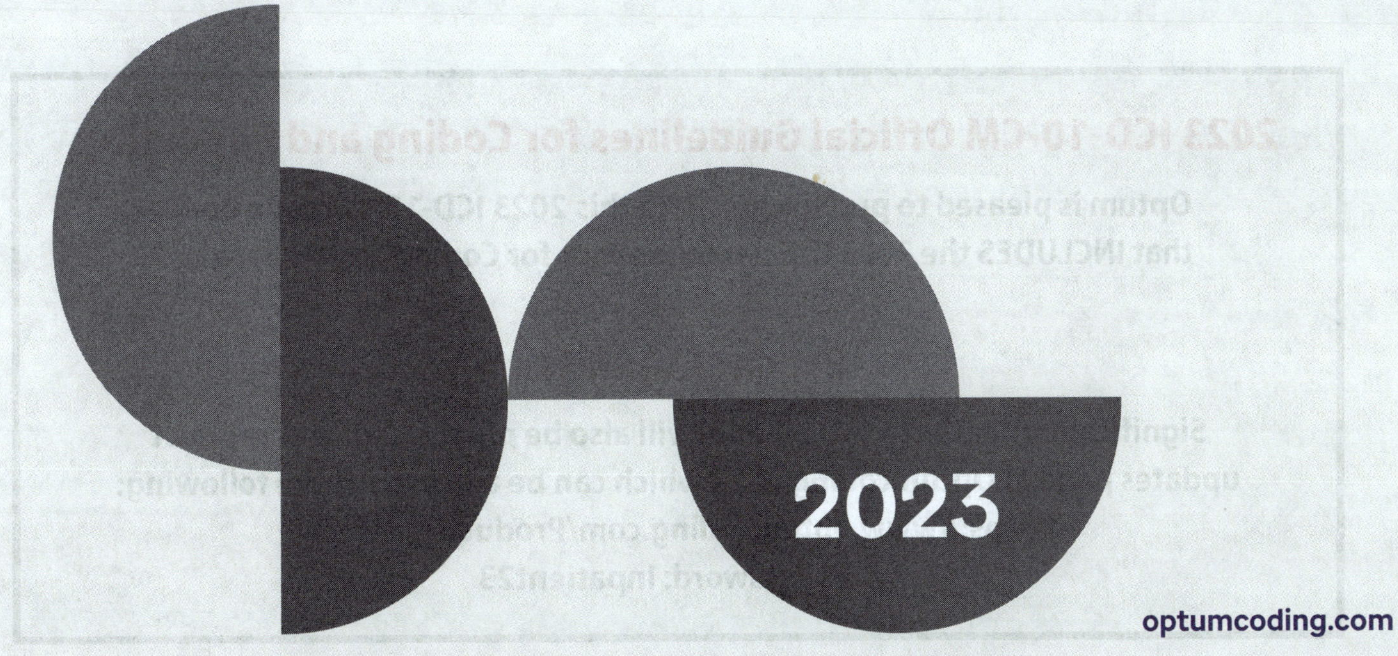

optumcoding.com

Publisher's Notice

The *ICD-10-CM Professional for Hospitals: The Complete Official Code Set* is designed to be an accurate and authoritative source regarding coding and every reasonable effort has been made to ensure accuracy and completeness of the content. However, Optum makes no guarantee, warranty, or representation that this publication is accurate, complete or without errors. It is understood that Optum is not rendering any legal or other professional services or advice in this publication and that Optum bears no liability for any results or consequences that may arise from the use of this book.

Acknowledgments

Marianne Randall, CPC, *Product Manager*
Anita Schmidt, BS, RHIA, AHIMA-approved ICD-10-CM/PCS Trainer, *Subject Matter Expert*
LaJuana Green, RHIA, CCS, *Subject Matter Expert*
Leanne Patterson, CPC, *Subject Matter Expert*
Jacqueline R. Petersen, BS, RHIA, CHDA, CPC, *Subject Matter Expert*
Stacy Perry, *Manager, Desktop Publishing*
Tracy Betzler, *Senior Desktop Publishing Specialist*
Hope M. Dunn, *Senior Desktop Publishing Specialist*
Katie Russell, *Desktop Publishing Specialist*
Kate Holden, *Editor*

Our Commitment to Accuracy

Optum is committed to producing accurate and reliable materials.

To report corrections, please email customerassistance@optum.com. You can also reach customer service by calling 1.800.464.3649, option 1.

Made in the USA
ISBN 978-1-62254-833-0

Anita Schmidt, BS, RHIA, AHIMA-approved ICD-10-CM/PCS Trainer

Ms. Schmidt has expertise in ICD-10-CM/PCS, DRG, and CPT with more than 15 years' experience in coding in multiple settings, including inpatient, observation, and same-day surgery. Her experience includes analysis of medical record documentation, assignment of ICD-10-CM and PCS codes, and DRG validation. She has conducted training for ICD-10-CM/PCS and electronic health record. She has also collaborated with clinical documentation specialists to identify documentation needs and potential areas for physician education. Most recently she has been developing content for resource and educational products related to ICD-10-CM, ICD-10-PCS, DRG, and CPT. Ms. Schmidt is an AHIMA-approved ICD-10-CM/PCS trainer and is an active member of the American Health Information Management Association (AHIMA) and the Minnesota Health Information Management Association.

LaJuana Green, RHIA, CCS

Ms. Green is a Registered Health Information Administrator with over 35 years of experience in multiple areas of information management. She has proven expertise in the analysis of medical record documentation, assignment of ICD-10-CM and PCS codes, DRG validation, and CPT code assignment in ambulatory surgery units and the hospital outpatient setting. Her experience includes serving as a director of a health information management department, clinical technical editing, new technology research and writing, medical record management, utilization review activities, quality assurance, tumor registry, medical library services, and chargemaster maintenance. Ms. Green is an active member of the American Health Information Management Association (AHIMA).

2023 ICD-10-CM Official Guidelines for Coding and Reporting

Optum is pleased to provide you with this 2023 ICD-10-CM code book that INCLUDES the 2023 Official Guidelines for Coding and Reporting.

Product Updates

Significant updates to this manual will also be provided on our product updates page at Optumcoding.com, which can be accessed at the following:
https://www.optumcoding.com/ProductUpdates/
Password: Inpatient23

Welcome to over 25 years of coding expertise

Every medical organization knows that medical documentation and coding accuracy are vital to the revenue cycle. As a leading health services business, Optum has proudly created industry-leading coding, billing and reimbursement solutions for more than 25 years. Serving the broad health market, including physicians, health care organizations, payers and government, we help health systems reduce costs and achieve timely and accurate revenue.

You'll find ICD-10-CM/PCS, CPT®, HCPCS, DRG, specialty and reference content across our full suite of medical coding, billing and reimbursement products. And to ensure you have expert insight and the right information at your fingertips, our subject matter experts have incorporated proprietary features into these resources. These include supplementary edits and notations, coding tips and tools, and appendixes — making each product comprehensive and easy to use. Think of it as coding resources built by coders, for coders like you.

Your coding, billing and reimbursement product team,

Ryan Nichole Greg LaJuana Anita Ken Denise Karen Leanne Jacqui Marianne Elizabeth Nann Debbie

Put Optum medical coding, billing and reimbursement content at your fingertips today. Choose what works for you.

- Publications (print and eBook)
- Online coding tools
- Data files
- Web services

Visit us at **optumcoding.com** to browse our products, or call us at 1-800-464-3649, option 1, for more information.

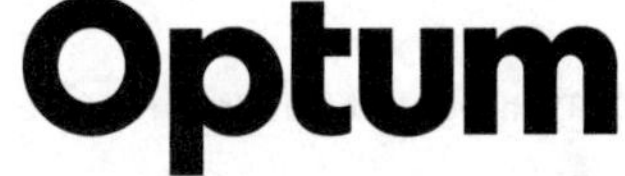

Contents

How to Use ICD-10-CM Professional for Hospitals 2023

Introduction

ICD-10-CM Professional for Hospitals: The Complete Official Code Set is your definitive coding resource, combining the work of the National Center for Health Statistics (NCHS), Centers for Medicare and Medicaid Services (CMS), American Hospital Association (AHA), and Optum experts to provide the information you need for coding accuracy.

The International Classification of Diseases, 10th Revision, Clinical Modification (ICD-10-CM), is an adaptation of ICD-10, copyrighted by the World Health Organization (WHO). The development and maintenance of this clinical modification (CM) is the responsibility of the NCHS as authorized by WHO. Any new concepts added to ICD-10-CM are based on an established update process through the collaboration of WHO's Update and Revision Committee and the ICD-10-CM Coordination and Maintenance Committee.

In addition to the ICD-10-CM classification, other official government source information has been included in this manual. Depending on the source, updates to information may be annual or quarterly. This manual provides the most current information that was available at the time of publication. For updates to the source documents that may have occurred after this manual was published, please refer to the following:

- **NCHS, International Classification of Diseases, Tenth Revision, Clinical Modification (ICD-10-CM)**

  https://www.cms.gov/medicare/icd-10/2023-icd-10-cm

- **CMS Inpatient Prospective Payment System Proposed Rule, FY2023**

  https://www.cms.gov/medicare/acute-inpatient-pps/fy-2023-ipps-proposed-rule-home-page

- **CMS Inpatient Prospective Payment System Proposed Rule, FY 2023 — Proposed, version 40, MS-DRG grouper software, Definitions Manual files and Medicare Code Editor (MCE) Files**

  https://www.cms.gov/Medicare/Medicare-Fee-for-Service-Payment/AcuteInpatientPPS/MS-DRG-Classifications-and-Software

- **CMS Risk Adjustment Model, version 24**

  https://www.cms.gov/Medicare/Health-Plans/MedicareAdvtgSpecRateStats/Risk-Adjustors.html

- **CMS Long-term Care Hospital Prospective Payment System Proposed Rule and Data Files, FY 2023**

  https://www.cms.gov/medicaremedicare-fee-service-paymentlongtermcarehospitalppsltchpps-regulations-and-notices/cms-1771-p

- **AHA Coding Clinics**

  https://www.codingclinicadvisor.com/

The official NCHS ICD-10-CM classification includes three main sections: the guidelines, the indexes, and the tabular list, all of which make up the bulk of this coding manual. To complement the classification, Optum's coding experts have incorporated Medicare-related coding edits and proprietary features, such as supplementary notations, coding tools, and appendixes, into a comprehensive and easy-to-use reference. This publication is organized as follows:

What's New for 2023

This section provides a high-level overview of the code changes made for FY 2023. The list of codes provided identifies new, revised, and deleted codes. Asterisked codes identify prior midyear changes that were made to the classification, effective April 1, 2022. All changes are based on an official addendum, provided by the National Center for Health Statistics (NCHS), the agency charged with maintaining and updating ICD-10-CM. NCHS is part of the Centers for Disease Control and Prevention (CDC).

Conversion Table

The conversion table was developed by National Center for Healthcare Statistics (NCHS) to help facilitate data retrieval as new codes are added to the ICD-10-CM classification. This table provides a crosswalk from each FY 2023 new code to the equivalent code(s) assigned, prior to October 1, 2022, for that diagnosis or condition. Asterisked codes identify prior midyear additions, effective April 1, 2022. For the full conversion table, refer to the Conversion Table zip file at https://www.cms.gov/medicare/icd-10/2023-icd-10-cm.

10 Steps to Correct Coding

This step-by-step tutorial walks the coder through the process of finding the correct code — from locating the code in the official indexes to verifying the code in the tabular section — while following applicable conventions, guidelines, and instructional notes. Specific examples are provided with detailed explanations of each coding step along with advice for proper sequencing.

Official ICD-10-CM Guidelines for Coding and Reporting

This section provides the full official conventions and guidelines regulating the appropriate assignment and reporting of ICD-10-CM codes. These conventions and guidelines are published by the U.S. Department of Health and Human Services (DHHS) and approved by the cooperating parties (American Health Information Management Association [AHIMA], National Center for Health Statistics [NCHS], Centers for Disease Control and Prevention [CDC], and the American Hospital Association [AHA]).

Indexes

Index to Diseases and Injuries

The Index to Diseases and Injuries is arranged in alphabetic order by terms specific to a disease, condition, illness, injury, eponym, or abbreviation as well as terms that describe circumstances other than a disease or injury that may require attention from a health care professional.

Neoplasm Table

The Neoplasm Table is arranged in alphabetic order by anatomical site. Codes are then listed in individual columns based upon the histological behavior (malignant, in situ, benign, uncertain, or unspecified) of the neoplasm.

Table of Drugs and Chemicals

The Table of Drugs and Chemicals is arranged in alphabetic order by the specific drug or chemical name. Codes are listed in individual columns based upon the associated intent (poisoning, adverse effect, or underdosing). **Note:** Drugs with an asterisk identify substances added to the table by Optum subject matter experts.

External Causes Index

The External Causes Index is arranged in alphabetic order by main terms that describe the cause, the intent, the place of occurrence, the activity, and the status of the patient at the time the injury occurred or health condition arose.

Index Notations

With

The word "with" or "in" should be interpreted to mean "associated with" or "due to." The classification presumes a causal relationship between the two conditions linked by these terms in the index. These conditions should be coded as related even in the absence of provider documentation explicitly linking them unless the documentation clearly states the conditions are unrelated or when another guideline specifically requires a documented linkage between two conditions (e.g., the sepsis guideline for "acute organ dysfunction that is not clearly associated with the sepsis"). For conditions not specifically linked by these relational terms in the classification or when a guideline requires explicit documentation of a linkage between two conditions, provider documentation must link the conditions to code them as related.

The word "with" in the index is sequenced immediately following the main term, not in alphabetical order.

> **Dermatopolymyositis** M33.9Ø
> with
> myopathy M33.92
> respiratory involvement M33.91
> specified organ involvement NEC M33.99
> amyopathic M33.93

See

When the instruction "see" follows a term in the index, it indicates that another term must be referenced to locate the correct code.

> **Hematoperitoneum** — *see* Hemoperitoneum

See Also

The instructional note "see also" simply provides alternative terms the coder may reference that may be useful in determining the correct code but are not necessary to follow if the main term supplies the appropriate code.

> **Hematinuria** — *see also* Hemaglobinuria
> malarial B5Ø.8

Default Codes

In the index, the default code is the code listed next to the main term and represents the condition most commonly associated with that main term. This code may be assigned when documentation does not support reporting a more specific code. Alternatively, it may provide an unspecified code for the condition.

> **Hemiatrophy** R68.89
> cerebellar G31.9
> face, facial, progressive (Romberg) G51.8
> tongue K14.8

Parentheses

Parentheses in the indexes enclose nonessential modifiers, supplementary words that may be present or absent in the statement of a disease without affecting the code.

> **Pseudomeningocele** (cerebral) (infective) (post-traumatic) G96.198
> postprocedural (spinal) G97.82

Brackets

ICD-10-CM has a coding convention addressing code assignment for manifestations that occur as a result of an underlying condition. This convention requires the underlying condition to be sequenced first, followed by the code or codes for the associated manifestation. In the index, italicized codes in brackets identify manifestation codes.

> **Polyneuropathy** (peripheral) G62.9
> alcoholic G62.1
> amyloid (Portuguese) E85.1 *[G63]*
> transthyretin-related (ATTR) familial E85.1 *[G63]*

Shaded Guides

Exclusive vertical shaded guides in the Index to Diseases and Injuries and External Causes Index help the user easily follow the indent levels for the subentries under a main term. Sequencing rules may apply depending on the level of indent for separate subentries.

> **Hemicrania**
> congenital malformation QØØ.Ø
> continua G44.51
> meaning migraine — *see also* Migraine G43.9Ø9
> paroxysmal G44.Ø39
> chronic G44.Ø49
> intractable G44.Ø41
> not intractable G44.Ø49
> episodic G44.Ø39
> intractable G44.Ø31
> not intractable G44.Ø39
> intractable G44.Ø31
> not intractable G44.Ø39

Following References

The Index to Diseases and Injuries includes "following" references to assist in locating out-of-sequence codes in the tabular list. Out-of-sequence codes contain an alphabetic character (letter) in the third- or fourth-character position. These codes are placed according to the classification rules — according to condition — not according to alphabetic or numeric sequencing rules.

> **Carcinoma** (malignant) — *see also* Neoplasm, by site, malignant
> neuroendocrine — *see also* Tumor, neuroendocrine
> high grade, any site C7A.1 (*following* C75)
> poorly differentiated, any site C7A.1 (*following* C75)

Additional Character Required

The Index to Diseases and Injuries, Neoplasm Table, and External Causes Index provide an icon after certain codes to signify to the user that additional characters are required to make the code valid. The tabular list should be consulted for appropriate character selection.

> **Fall, falling** (accidental) W19 ☑
> building W2Ø.1 ☑

Tabular List of Diseases

ICD-10-CM codes and descriptions are arranged numerically within the tabular list of diseases with 19 separate chapters providing codes associated with a particular body system or nature of injury or disease. There is also a chapter providing codes for external causes of an injury or health conditions, a chapter for codes that address encounters with healthcare facilities for circumstances other than a disease or injury, and finally a chapter for codes that capture special circumstances such as new diseases of uncertain etiology or emergency use codes.

Code and Code Descriptions

ICD-10-CM is an alphanumeric classification system that contains categories, subcategories, and valid codes. The first character is always a letter with any additional characters represented by either a letter or number. A three-character category without further subclassification is equivalent to a valid three-character code. Valid codes may be three, four, five, six, or seven characters in length, with each level of subdivision after a three-character category representing a subcategory. The final level of subdivision is a valid code.

Boldface

Boldface type is used for all codes and descriptions in the tabular list.

Italics

Italicized type is used to identify manifestation codes, those codes that should not be reported as first-listed diagnoses.

Deleted Text

~~Strikethrough~~ on a code and code description indicates a deletion from the classification for the current year.

Key Word

Green font is used throughout the Tabular List of Diseases to differentiate the key words that appear in similar code descriptions in a given category or subcategory. The key word convention is used only in those categories in which there are multiple codes with very similar descriptions with only a few words that differentiate them.

For example, refer to the list of codes below from category H55:

4th H55 Nystagmus and other irregular eye movements
5th H55.0 Nystagmus
H55.00 Unspecified nystagmus
H55.01 Congenital nystagmus
H55.02 Latent nystagmus
H55.03 Visual deprivation nystagmus
H55.04 Dissociated nystagmus
H55.09 Other forms of nystagmus

The portion of the code description that appears in **green font** in the tabular list helps the coder quickly identify the key terms and the correct code. This convention is especially useful when the codes describe laterality, such as the following codes from subcategory H40.22:

6th H40.22 Chronic angle-closure glaucoma
Chronic primary angle closure glaucoma
7th H40.221 Chronic angle-closure glaucoma, right eye
7th H40.222 Chronic angle-closure glaucoma, left eye
7th H40.223 Chronic angle-closure glaucoma, bilateral
7th H40.229 Chronic angle-closure glaucoma, unspecified eye

Tabular Notations

Official parenthetical notes as well as Optum's supplementary notations are provided at the chapter, code block, category, subcategory, and individual code level to help the user assign proper codes. The information in the notation can apply to one or more codes depending on where the citation is placed.

Official Notations

Includes Notes

The word INCLUDES appears immediately under certain categories to further define, clarify, or give examples of the content of a code category.

Inclusion Terms

Lists of inclusion terms are included under certain codes. These terms indicate some of the conditions for which that code number may be used. Inclusion terms may be synonyms with the code title, or, in the case of "other specified" codes, the terms may also provide a list of various conditions included within a classification code. The inclusion terms are not exhaustive. The index may provide additional terms that may also be assigned to a given code.

Excludes Notes

ICD-10-CM has two types of excludes notes. Each note has a different definition for use. However, they are similar in that they both indicate that codes excluded from each other are independent of each other.

Excludes 1

An EXCLUDES 1 note is a "pure" excludes. It means "NOT CODED HERE!" An Excludes 1 note indicates mutually exclusive codes: two conditions that cannot be reported together. An Excludes1 note indicates that the code excluded should never be used at the same time as the code above the Excludes1 note. An Excludes1 is used when two conditions cannot occur together, such as a congenital form versus an acquired form of the same condition.

An exception to the Excludes 1 definition is when the two conditions are unrelated to each other. If it is not clear whether the two conditions involving an Excludes 1 note are related or not, query the provider. For example, code F45.8 Other somatoform disorders, has an Excludes 1 note for "sleep related teeth grinding (G47.63)" because "teeth grinding" is an inclusion term under F45.8. Only one of these two codes should be assigned for teeth grinding. However, psychogenic dysmenorrhea is also an inclusion term under F45.8, and a patient could have both this condition and sleep-related teeth grinding. In this case, the two conditions are clearly unrelated to each other, so it would be appropriate to report F45.8 and G47.63 together.

Excludes 2

An EXCLUDES 2 note means "NOT INCLUDED HERE." An Excludes 2 note indicates that although the excluded condition is not part of the condition it is excluded from, a patient may have both conditions at the same time. Therefore, when an Excludes 2 note appears under a code, it may be acceptable to use both the code and the excluded code together if supported by the medical documentation.

Note

The term "NOTE" appears as an icon and precedes the instructional information. These notes function as alerts to highlight coding instructions within the text.

Code First/Use additional code

These instructional notes provide sequencing instruction. They may appear independently of each other or to designate certain etiology/manifestation paired codes. These instructions signal the coder that an additional code should be reported to provide a more complete picture of that diagnosis.

In etiology/manifestation coding, ICD-10-CM requires the underlying condition to be sequenced first, followed by the manifestation. In these situations, codes with "In diseases classified elsewhere" in the code description are never permitted as a first-listed or principal diagnosis code and must be sequenced following the underlying condition code.

Code Also

A "code also" note alerts the coder that more than one code may be required to fully describe the condition. The sequencing depends on the circumstances of the encounter. Factors that may determine sequencing include severity and reason for the encounter.

Revised Text

The revised text ▶◀ "bow ties" alert the user to changes in official notations for the current year. Revised text may include the following:

- A change in a current parenthetical description
- A change in the code(s) associated with a current parenthetical note
- A change in how a current parenthetical note is classified (e.g., an Excludes 1 note that changed to an Excludes 2 note)
- Addition of a new parenthetical note(s) to a code

Deleted Text

~~Strikethrough~~ on official notations indicate a deletion from the classification for the current year.

Optum Notations

AHA Coding Clinic Citations

Coding Clinics are official American Hospital Association (AHA) publications that provide coding advice specific to ICD-10-CM and ICD-10-PCS.

Coding Clinic citations included in this manual are current up to the second quarter of 2022.

These citations identify the year, quarter, and page number of one or more *Coding Clinic* publications that may have coding advice relevant to a particular code or group of codes. With the most current citation listed first, these notations are preceded by the symbol **AHA:** and appear in purple type.

> **I15.1 Hypertension secondary to other renal disorders**
> **AHA:** 2016, 3Q, 22

Definitions

Definitions explain a specific term, condition, or disease process in layman's terms. These notations are preceded by the symbol **DEF:** and appear in purple type.

> ✓5th **M51.4 Schmorl's nodes**
> **DEF:** Irregular bone defect in the margin of the vertebral body that causes herniation into the end plate of the vertebral body.

Coding Tips

The tips in the tabular list offer coding advice that is not readily available within the ICD-10-CM classification. It may relate official coding guidelines, indexing nuances, or advice from *AHA's Coding Clinic for ICD-10-CM/PCS*. These notations are preceded by the symbol **TIP:** and appear in brown type.

> ✓5th **B97.2 Coronavirus as the cause of diseases classified elsewhere**
> **TIP:** Do not report a code from this subcategory for COVID-19; refer to U07.1.

Icons

Note: The following icons are placed to the left of the code.

Changes to ICD-10-CM codes, since the last published edition of this manual, are highlighted in two ways:

The following green icons identify new or revised codes effective April 1, 2022:

- ● **New Code – Midyear**
- ▲ **Revised Code – Midyear**

The following black icons identify new or revised codes effective October 1, 2022:

- ● **New Code**
- ▲ **Revised Code**

✓ **Additional Characters Required**

- ✓4th This symbol indicates that the code requires a 4th character.
- ✓5th This symbol indicates that the code requires a 5th character.
- ✓6th This symbol indicates that the code requires a 6th character.
- ✓7th This symbol indicates that the code requires a 7th character.

> ✓5th **H60.3 Other infective otitis externa**
> ✓6th **H60.31 Diffuse otitis externa**
> **H60.311 Diffuse otitis externa, right ear**
> **H60.312 Diffuse otitis externa, left ear**
> **H60.313 Diffuse otitis externa, bilateral**
> **H60.319 Diffuse otitis externa, unspecified ear**

√x7th **Placeholder Alert**

This symbol indicates that the code requires a 7th character following the placeholder "X". Codes with fewer than six characters that require a 7th character must contain placeholder "X" to fill in the empty character(s).

> √x7th **T16.1 Foreign body in right ear**

This manual provides the most current information that was available at the time of publication. Except where otherwise noted, the icons and/or color bars reflect edits associated with the inpatient prospective payment system (IPPS). Because the fiscal 2023 IPPS final rule was not available at the time this book was printed, the edits in this manual are based on the proposed, version 40, MS-DRG grouper software, Definitions Manual files, and Medicare Code Editor (MCE) files, published with the fiscal 2023 IPPS proposed rule.

In an effort to provide the most current edit information, Optum has provided a searchable data file that includes the final edit designations for all ICD-10-CM codes based on the fiscal 2023 IPPS final rule official files, effective October 1, 2022. The edits included in the data file are as follows:

- Age
- Sex
- Hospital-acquired condition (HAC)
- CC
- MCC
- HIV
- Manifestation code
- Unacceptable principal diagnosis
- Questionable principal diagnosis
- Unspecified site

This data file can be accessed at the following:

https://www.optumcoding.com/ProductUpdates/
Title: "2023 ICD-10-CM for Hospital Edits Data File"
Password: Inpatient23

Note: The following icons are placed at the end of the code description.

Age Edits

N **Newborn Age: 0**
These diagnoses are intended for newborns and neonates and the patient's age must be 0 years.

N47.Ø Adherent prepuce, newborn N ♂

P **Pediatric Age: 0-17**
These diagnoses are intended for children and the patient's age must be between 0 and 17 years.

L21.1 Seborrheic infantile dermatitis P

M **Maternity Age: 9-64**
These diagnoses are intended for childbearing patients between the age of 9 and 64 years.

OØ2.9 Abnormal product of conception, unspecified M ♀

A **Adult Age: 15-124**
These diagnoses are intended for patients between the age of 15 and 124 years.

R54 Age-related physical debility A
Frailty
Old age
Senescence
Senile asthenia
Senile debility
EXCLUDES 1 *age-related cognitive decline (R41.81)*
sarcopenia (M62.84)
senile psychosis (FØ3)
senility NOS (R41.81)

Sex Edits

♂ **Male diagnosis only**

Q98.Ø Klinefelter syndrome karyotype 47, XXY ♂

♀ **Female diagnosis only**

N35.12 Postinfective urethral stricture, not elsewhere classified, female ♀

H1-H14 **Hospital Acquired Condition (HAC)**
These codes identify conditions that are high cost or high volume or both, are either a complication or comorbidity (CC) or major complication or comorbidity (MCC) that as a secondary diagnosis results in assignment of a case to a higher-paying MS-DRG. These conditions are reasonably preventable through the application of evidence-based guidelines. If the condition is not present on admission (meaning it developed during the hospital admission), the case will not group to the higher-paying MS-DRG based solely upon the reporting of the HAC code. Many of these HACs are conditional, and are based on reporting the specific diagnosis code(s) in combination with certain procedure codes.
Note: Hospital-acquired conditions do not impact MS-LTC-DRG assignment.

N15.1 Renal and perinephric abscess MCC H6

CC **CC Condition**
This symbol designates a complication or comorbidity diagnosis that may affect DRG assignment. A complication or comorbidity diagnosis, CC condition, is defined as a significant acute disease, a significant acute manifestation of a chronic disease, an advanced or end-stage chronic disease, or a chronic disease associated with systemic physiological decompensation and debility that have consistently greater impact on hospital resources.

G9Ø.59 Complex regional pain syndrome I of other specified site CC

MCC **MCC Condition**
This symbol designates a major complication or comorbidity diagnosis that may affect DRG assignment. An MCC condition meets the same criteria as a CC condition but is associated with a higher acuity level and hospital resource consumption is expected to be higher than that for a CC condition. There are fewer conditions that meet the criteria as an MCC than those for a CC condition.

✓7th **S35.238 Other injury of inferior mesenteric artery** MCC

Note: The assignment of an MS-DRG or MS-LTC-DRG often depends on the presence or absence of a secondary diagnosis code that is designated as an MCC or CC. However, in some instances the MCC or CC designation for that secondary diagnosis code is negated due to its relationship with the principal diagnosis; this is referred to as CC exclusion. The ICD-10 MS-DRG Definitions Manual included with the IPPS final rule provides a list of all principal diagnosis codes that would render ineffective the MCC/CC designation for a particular ICD-10-CM code when used as a secondary diagnosis. Optum has provided this CC exclusion list in an easily searchable data file, which can be accessed at the following:
https://www.optumcoding.com/ProductUpdates/
Title: "2023 ICD-10-CM for Hospitals CC Excludes Data File"
Password: Inpatient23

UNS **Unspecified Site**
Identifies codes that are considered an MCC or CC but lack specificity in regard to their anatomical location. The medical record documentation should be reviewed carefully, to ensure that no other code within the same category or subcategory can be assigned for greater specificity.

G81.ØØ Flaccid hemiplegia affecting unspecified side CC UNS HCC

UPD **Unacceptable Principal Diagnosis**
This symbol identifies codes that should not be assigned as principal diagnosis for *inpatient* admissions. Codes with an unacceptable principal diagnosis edit are considered supplementary — describing circumstances that influence an individual's health status or an additional code — identifying conditions that are not specific manifestations but may be due to an underlying cause.

✓7th **T48.5X5 Adverse effect of other anti-common-cold drugs** UPD

HIV **HIV-related Condition**
This symbol indicates that the condition is considered a major HIV-related diagnosis. When the condition is coded in combination with a diagnosis of human immunodeficiency virus (HIV), code B20, the case will move from MS-DRG/MS-LTC-DRG 977 to MS-DRGs/MS-LTC-DRGs 974-976.

G96.9 Disorder of central nervous system, unspecified HIV

HCC **CMS-HCC Condition**

Identify conditions that are considered a CMS-HCC (hierarchical condition category) diagnosis.

The HCC codes represented in this manual have been updated to reflect the 2023 Initial ICD-10-CM Mappings for CMS-HCC Model v24.

Note: Finalized ICD-10-CM-to-HCC mappings for CMS-HCC have been provided in an easily searchable data file that can be accessed at the following:

https://www.optumcoding.com/ProductUpdates/

Title: "2023 Final ICD-10-CM HCC Mappings Data File"

Password: Inpatient23

> **Y62.2 Failure of sterile precautions during kidney dialysis and other perfusion** HCC

Color Bars

Manifestation Code

Codes defined as manifestation codes appear in italic type, with a blue color bar over the code description. A manifestation cannot be reported as a first-listed code; it is sequenced as a secondary diagnosis with the underlying disease code listed first.

> *G32.89* ***Other specified degenerative disorders of nervous system in diseases classified elsewhere***
> Degenerative encephalopathy in diseases classified elsewhere

Questionable Admission Diagnoses

Questionable admission diagnoses will appear with a yellow color bar over the code description. These codes, although not unacceptable as a PDx, may be considered a "questionable admission" when used as PDx in an acute care hospital.

> **E66.09 Other obesity due to excess calories**

Wrong Procedure Performed Edit

An orange color bar over the code title indicates the Wrong Procedure Performed edit. This edit was created to identify cases in which wrong surgeries occurred. Any claim with a code from Y65.51-Y65.53 will be denied and returned to the provider. A surgical or other invasive procedure is considered to be a wrong procedure if one of the following is true:

- The procedure was performed on the wrong site.
- The procedure was performed on the wrong patient.
- The incorrect procedure was performed on a patient.

> **Y65.51 Performance of wrong procedure (operation) on correct patient**
> Wrong device implanted into correct surgical site
> EXCLUDES 1 *performance of correct procedure (operation) on wrong side or body part (Y65.53)*

Unspecified Diagnosis

Codes that appear with a gray color bar over the alphanumeric code identify unspecified diagnoses. These codes should be used in limited circumstances, when neither the diagnostic statement nor the documentation provides enough information to assign a more specific diagnosis code. The abbreviation NOS, "not otherwise specified," in the tabular list may be interpreted as "unspecified."

> **G03.9 Meningitis, unspecified** MCC
> Arachnoiditis (spinal) NOS

Footnotes

Certain codes in the tabular section have a numerical superscript located to the upper left of the code. This numerical superscript corresponds to a specific footnote description.

For example:

> [1] **R57.1 Hypovolemic shock** MCC HCC

For convenience, the footnote descriptions are provided on the front cover.

The following list also provides the footnote descriptions of all numerical superscripts found in the Tabular List of Diseases:

1. These codes are considered major complication/comorbidity (MCC) conditions only if the patient is discharged alive.
2. This condition is considered an MCC only when reported as an initial encounter for an open fracture (7th character B or C specific to category).
3. This condition is considered a CC only when reported as an initial encounter for a fracture (7th character A, B, or C specific to category) or a subsequent encounter for nonunion or malunion fracture (7th character K, M, N, P, Q, or R specific to category).
4. This condition is considered a CC only when reported as a subsequent encounter for a nonunion or malunion fracture (7th character K, M, N, P, Q, or R specific to category).
5. This condition is considered a CC only when reported as an initial encounter or subsequent encounter (7th character A or D).
6. This condition is considered an HCC when reported as initial encounter (7th character A, B, or C specific to category).
7. This condition is considered an HCC when reported as initial encounter (7th character A or B specific to category) or as a sequela.
8. This condition is considered an HCC when reported as a sequela.

Chapter-Level Notations

Chapter-Specific Guidelines with Coding Examples

Each chapter begins with the Official Guidelines for Coding and Reporting specific to that chapter, where provided. Coding examples specific to inpatient care settings have been provided to illustrate the coding and/or sequencing guidance in these guidelines.

Muscle and Tendon Table

ICD-10-CM categorizes certain muscles and tendons in the upper and lower extremities by their action (e.g., extension or flexion) as well as their anatomical location. The Muscle/Tendon table is provided at the beginning of chapter 13 and chapter 19 to help users when code selection depends on the action of the muscle and/or tendon.

Note: This table is not all-inclusive, and proper code assignment should be based on the provider's documentation.

Illustrations

This section includes illustrations of normal anatomy with ICD-10-CM-specific terminology.

What's New for 2023

Official Updates

A summary of changes to the official ICD-10-CM code set is provided below, identifying changes made for fiscal 2023, effective October 1, 2022, to September 30, 2023. Asterisked codes identify prior midyear changes that were made to the classification, effective April 1, 2022. All code changes were made by the agency charged with maintaining and updating the ICD-10-CM code set, the National Center for Health Statistics (NCHS), a section of the Centers for Disease Control and Prevention (CDC).

1179 New Codes

B37.31 B37.32 D59.30 D59.31 D59.32
D59.39 D68.00 D68.01 D68.020 D68.021
D68.022 D68.023 D68.029 D68.03 D68.04
D68.09 D75.821 D75.822 D75.828 D75.829
D75.84 D81.82 E34.30 E34.31 E34.321
E34.322 E34.328 E34.329 E34.39 E87.20
E87.21 E87.22 E87.29 F01.511 F01.518
F01.52 F01.53 F01.54 F01.A0 F01.A11
F01.A18 F01.A2 F01.A3 F01.A4 F01.B0
F01.B11 F01.B18 F01.B2 F01.B3 F01.B4
F01.C0 F01.C11 F01.C18 F01.C2 F01.C3
F01.C4 F02.811 F02.818 F02.82 F02.83
F02.84 F02.A0 F02.A11 F02.A18 F02.A2
F02.A3 F02.A4 F02.B0 F02.B11 F02.B18
F02.B2 F02.B3 F02.B4 F02.C0 F02.C11
F02.C18 F02.C2 F02.C3 F02.C4 F03.911
F03.918 F03.92 F03.93 F03.94 F03.A0
F03.A11 F03.A18 F03.A2 F03.A3 F03.A4
F03.B0 F03.B11 F03.B18 F03.B2 F03.B3
F03.B4 F03.C0 F03.C11 F03.C18 F03.C2
F03.C3 F03.C4 F06.70 F06.71 F10.90
F10.91 F11.91 F12.91 F13.91 F14.91
F15.91 F16.91 F18.91 F19.91 F43.81
F43.89 G71.031 G71.032 G71.033 G71.0340
G71.0341 G71.0342 G71.0349 G71.035 G71.038
G71.039 G90.A G93.31 G93.32 G93.39
I20.2 I25.112 I25.702 I25.712 I25.722
I25.732 I25.752 I25.762 I25.792 I31.31
I31.39 I34.81 I34.89 I47.20 I47.21
I47.29 I71.010 I71.011 I71.012 I71.019
I71.10 I71.11 I71.12 I71.13 I71.20
I71.21 I71.22 I71.23 I71.30 I71.31
I71.32 I71.33 I71.40 I71.41 I71.42
I71.43 I71.50 I71.51 I71.52 I71.60
I71.61 I71.62 I77.82 J95.87 K76.82
M51.A0 M51.A1 M51.A2 M51.A3 M51.A4
M51.A5 M62.5A0 M62.5A1 M62.5A2 M62.5A9
M93.004 M93.014 M93.024 M93.034 M93.041
M93.042 M93.043 M93.044 M93.051 M93.052
M93.053 M93.054 M93.061 M93.062 M93.063
M93.064 M93.071 M93.072 M93.073 M93.074
M96.A1 M96.A2 M96.A3 M96.A4 M96.A9
N14.11 N14.19 N76.82 N80.00 N80.01
N80.02 N80.03 N80.101 N80.102 N80.103
N80.109 N80.111 N80.112 N80.113 N80.119
N80.121 N80.122 N80.123 N80.129 N80.201
N80.202 N80.203 N80.209 N80.211 N80.212
N80.213 N80.219 N80.221 N80.222 N80.223
N80.229 N80.30 N80.311 N80.312 N80.319
N80.321 N80.322 N80.329 N80.331 N80.332
N80.333 N80.339 N80.341 N80.342 N80.343
N80.349 N80.351 N80.352 N80.353 N80.359
N80.361 N80.362 N80.363 N80.369 N80.371
N80.372 N80.373 N80.379 N80.381 N80.382
N80.383 N80.389 N80.391 N80.392 N80.399
N80.3A1 N80.3A2 N80.3A3 N80.3A9 N80.3B1
N80.3B2 N80.3B3 N80.3B9 N80.3C1 N80.3C2
N80.3C3 N80.3C9 N80.40 N80.41 N80.42
N80.50 N80.511 N80.512 N80.519 N80.521
N80.522 N80.529 N80.531 N80.532 N80.539
N80.541 N80.542 N80.549 N80.551 N80.552
N80.559 N80.561 N80.562 N80.569 N80.A0
N80.A1 N80.A2 N80.A41 N80.A42 N80.A43
N80.A49 N80.A51 N80.A52 N80.A53 N80.A59
N80.A61 N80.A62 N80.A63 N80.A69 N80.B1
N80.B2 N80.B31 N80.B32 N80.B39 N80.B4
N80.B5 N80.B6 N80.C0 N80.C10 N80.C11
N80.C19 N80.C2 N80.C3 N80.C4 N80.C9
N80.D0 N80.D1 N80.D2 N80.D3 N80.D4
N80.D5 N80.D6 N80.D9 N85.A O35.00X0
O35.00X1 O35.00X2 O35.00X3 O35.00X4 O35.00X5
O35.00X9 O35.01X0 O35.01X1 O35.01X2 O35.01X3
O35.01X4 O35.01X5 O35.01X9 O35.02X0 O35.02X1
O35.02X2 O35.02X3 O35.02X4 O35.02X5 O35.02X9
O35.03X0 O35.03X1 O35.03X2 O35.03X3 O35.03X4
O35.03X5 O35.03X9 O35.04X0 O35.04X1 O35.04X2
O35.04X3 O35.04X4 O35.04X5 O35.04X9 O35.05X0
O35.05X1 O35.05X2 O35.05X3 O35.05X4 O35.05X5
O35.05X9 O35.06X0 O35.06X1 O35.06X2 O35.06X3
O35.06X4 O35.06X5 O35.06X9 O35.07X0 O35.07X1
O35.07X2 O35.07X3 O35.07X4 O35.07X5 O35.07X9
O35.08X0 O35.08X1 O35.08X2 O35.08X3 O35.08X4
O35.08X5 O35.08X9 O35.09X0 O35.09X1 O35.09X2
O35.09X3 O35.09X4 O35.09X5 O35.09X9 O35.10X0
O35.10X1 O35.10X2 O35.10X3 O35.10X4 O35.10X5
O35.10X9 O35.11X0 O35.11X1 O35.11X2 O35.11X3
O35.11X4 O35.11X5 O35.11X9 O35.12X0 O35.12X1
O35.12X2 O35.12X3 O35.12X4 O35.12X5 O35.12X9
O35.13X0 O35.13X1 O35.13X2 O35.13X3 O35.13X4
O35.13X5 O35.13X9 O35.14X0 O35.14X1 O35.14X2
O35.14X3 O35.14X4 O35.14X5 O35.14X9 O35.15X0
O35.15X1 O35.15X2 O35.15X3 O35.15X4 O35.15X5
O35.15X9 O35.19X0 O35.19X1 O35.19X2 O35.19X3
O35.19X4 O35.19X5 O35.19X9 O35.AXX0 O35.AXX1
O35.AXX2 O35.AXX3 O35.AXX4 O35.AXX5 O35.AXX9
O35.BXX0 O35.BXX1 O35.BXX2 O35.BXX3 O35.BXX4
O35.BXX5 O35.BXX9 O35.CXX0 O35.CXX1 O35.CXX2
O35.CXX3 O35.CXX4 O35.CXX5 O35.CXX9 O35.DXX0
O35.DXX1 O35.DXX2 O35.DXX3 O35.DXX4 O35.DXX5
O35.DXX9 O35.EXX0 O35.EXX1 O35.EXX2 O35.EXX3
O35.EXX4 O35.EXX5 O35.EXX9 O35.FXX0 O35.FXX1
O35.FXX2 O35.FXX3 O35.FXX4 O35.FXX5 O35.FXX9
O35.GXX0 O35.GXX1 O35.GXX2 O35.GXX3 O35.GXX4
O35.GXX5 O35.GXX9 O35.HXX0 O35.HXX1 O35.HXX2
O35.HXX3 O35.HXX4 O35.HXX5 O35.HXX9 P28.30
P28.31 P28.32 P28.33 P28.39 P28.40
P28.41 P28.42 P28.43 P28.49 Q21.10
Q21.11 Q21.12 Q21.13 Q21.14 Q21.15
Q21.16 Q21.19 Q21.20 Q21.21 Q21.22
Q21.23 Q85.81 Q85.82 Q85.83 Q85.89
S06.0XAA S06.0XAD S06.0XAS S06.1XAA S06.1XAD
S06.1XAS S06.2XAA S06.2XAD S06.2XAS S06.30AA
S06.30AD S06.30AS S06.31AA S06.31AD S06.31AS
S06.32AA S06.32AD S06.32AS S06.33AA S06.33AD
S06.33AS S06.34AA S06.34AD S06.34AS S06.35AA
S06.35AD S06.35AS S06.36AA S06.36AD S06.36AS
S06.37AA S06.37AD S06.37AS S06.38AA S06.38AD
S06.38AS S06.4XAA S06.4XAD S06.4XAS S06.5XAA

SØ6.5XAD SØ6.5XAS SØ6.6XAA SØ6.6XAD SØ6.6XAS
SØ6.81AA SØ6.81AD SØ6.81AS SØ6.82AA SØ6.82AD
SØ6.82AS SØ6.89AA SØ6.89AD SØ6.89AS SØ6.8AØA
SØ6.8AØD SØ6.8AØS SØ6.8A1A SØ6.8A1D SØ6.8A1S
SØ6.8A2A SØ6.8A2D SØ6.8A2S SØ6.8A3A SØ6.8A3D
SØ6.8A3S SØ6.8A4A SØ6.8A4D SØ6.8A4S SØ6.8A5A
SØ6.8A5D SØ6.8A5S SØ6.8A6A SØ6.8A6D SØ6.8A6S
SØ6.8A7A SØ6.8A8A SØ6.8A9A SØ6.8A9D SØ6.8A9S
SØ6.8AAA SØ6.8AAD SØ6.8AAS SØ6.9XAA SØ6.9XAD
SØ6.9XAS T43.651A T43.651D T43.651S T43.652A
T43.652D T43.652S T43.653A T43.653D T43.653S
T43.654A T43.654D T43.654S T43.655A T43.655D
T43.655S T43.656A T43.656D T43.656S V2Ø.Ø1XA
V2Ø.Ø1XD V2Ø.Ø1XS V2Ø.Ø9XA V2Ø.Ø9XD V2Ø.Ø9XS
V2Ø.11XA V2Ø.11XD V2Ø.11XS V2Ø.19XA V2Ø.19XD
V2Ø.19XS V2Ø.21XA V2Ø.21XD V2Ø.21XS V2Ø.29XA
V2Ø.29XD V2Ø.29XS V2Ø.31XA V2Ø.31XD V2Ø.31XS
V2Ø.39XA V2Ø.39XD V2Ø.39XS V2Ø.41XA V2Ø.41XD
V2Ø.41XS V2Ø.49XA V2Ø.49XD V2Ø.49XS V2Ø.51XA
V2Ø.51XD V2Ø.51XS V2Ø.59XA V2Ø.59XD V2Ø.59XS
V2Ø.91XA V2Ø.91XD V2Ø.91XS V2Ø.99XA V2Ø.99XD
V2Ø.99XS V21.Ø1XA V21.Ø1XD V21.Ø1XS V21.Ø9XA
V21.Ø9XD V21.Ø9XS V21.11XA V21.11XD V21.11XS
V21.19XA V21.19XD V21.19XS V21.21XA V21.21XD
V21.21XS V21.29XA V21.29XD V21.29XS V21.31XA
V21.31XD V21.31XS V21.39XA V21.39XD V21.39XS
V21.41XA V21.41XD V21.41XS V21.49XA V21.49XD
V21.49XS V21.51XA V21.51XD V21.51XS V21.59XA
V21.59XD V21.59XS V21.91XA V21.91XD V21.91XS
V21.99XA V21.99XD V21.99XS V22.Ø1XA V22.Ø1XD
V22.Ø1XS V22.Ø9XA V22.Ø9XD V22.Ø9XS V22.11XA
V22.11XD V22.11XS V22.19XA V22.19XD V22.19XS
V22.21XA V22.21XD V22.21XS V22.29XA V22.29XD
V22.29XS V22.31XA V22.31XD V22.31XS V22.39XA
V22.39XD V22.39XS V22.41XA V22.41XD V22.41XS
V22.49XA V22.49XD V22.49XS V22.51XA V22.51XD
V22.51XS V22.59XA V22.59XD V22.59XS V22.91XA
V22.91XD V22.91XS V22.99XA V22.99XD V22.99XS
V23.Ø1XA V23.Ø1XD V23.Ø1XS V23.Ø9XA V23.Ø9XD
V23.Ø9XS V23.11XA V23.11XD V23.11XS V23.19XA
V23.19XD V23.19XS V23.21XA V23.21XD V23.21XS
V23.29XA V23.29XD V23.29XS V23.31XA V23.31XD
V23.31XS V23.39XA V23.39XD V23.39XS V23.41XA
V23.41XD V23.41XS V23.49XA V23.49XD V23.49XS
V23.51XA V23.51XD V23.51XS V23.59XA V23.59XD
V23.59XS V23.91XA V23.91XD V23.91XS V23.99XA
V23.99XD V23.99XS V24.Ø1XA V24.Ø1XD V24.Ø1XS
V24.Ø9XA V24.Ø9XD V24.Ø9XS V24.11XA V24.11XD
V24.11XS V24.19XA V24.19XD V24.19XS V24.21XA
V24.21XD V24.21XS V24.29XA V24.29XD V24.29XS
V24.31XA V24.31XD V24.31XS V24.39XA V24.39XD
V24.39XS V24.41XA V24.41XD V24.41XS V24.49XA
V24.49XD V24.49XS V24.51XA V24.51XD V24.51XS
V24.59XA V24.59XD V24.59XS V24.91XA V24.91XD
V24.91XS V24.99XA V24.99XD V24.99XS V25.Ø1XA
V25.Ø1XD V25.Ø1XS V25.Ø9XA V25.Ø9XD V25.Ø9XS
V25.11XA V25.11XD V25.11XS V25.19XA V25.19XD
V25.19XS V25.21XA V25.21XD V25.21XS V25.29XA
V25.29XD V25.29XS V25.31XA V25.31XD V25.31XS
V25.39XA V25.39XD V25.39XS V25.41XA V25.41XD
V25.41XS V25.49XA V25.49XD V25.49XS V25.51XA
V25.51XD V25.51XS V25.59XA V25.59XD V25.59XS
V25.91XA V25.91XD V25.91XS V25.99XA V25.99XD
V25.99XS V26.Ø1XA V26.Ø1XD V26.Ø1XS V26.Ø9XA
V26.Ø9XD V26.Ø9XS V26.11XA V26.11XD V26.11XS
V26.19XA V26.19XD V26.19XS V26.21XA V26.21XD
V26.21XS V26.29XA V26.29XD V26.29XS V26.31XA
V26.31XD V26.31XS V26.39XA V26.39XD V26.39XS
V26.41XA V26.41XD V26.41XS V26.49XA V26.49XD
V26.49XS V26.51XA V26.51XD V26.51XS V26.59XA
V26.59XD V26.59XS V26.91XA V26.91XD V26.91XS
V26.99XA V26.99XD V26.99XS V27.Ø1XA V27.Ø1XD
V27.Ø1XS V27.Ø9XA V27.Ø9XD V27.Ø9XS V27.11XA
V27.11XD V27.11XS V27.19XA V27.19XD V27.19XS
V27.21XA V27.21XD V27.21XS V27.29XA V27.29XD
V27.29XS V27.31XA V27.31XD V27.31XS V27.39XA
V27.39XD V27.39XS V27.41XA V27.41XD V27.41XS
V27.49XA V27.49XD V27.49XS V27.51XA V27.51XD
V27.51XS V27.59XA V27.59XD V27.59XS V27.91XA
V27.91XD V27.91XS V27.99XA V27.99XD V27.99XS
V28.Ø1XA V28.Ø1XD V28.Ø1XS V28.Ø9XA V28.Ø9XD
V28.Ø9XS V28.11XA V28.11XD V28.11XS V28.19XA
V28.19XD V28.19XS V28.21XA V28.21XD V28.21XS
V28.29XA V28.29XD V28.29XS V28.31XA V28.31XD
V28.31XS V28.39XA V28.39XD V28.39XS V28.41XA
V28.41XD V28.41XS V28.49XA V28.49XD V28.49XS
V28.51XA V28.51XD V28.51XS V28.59XA V28.59XD
V28.59XS V28.91XA V28.91XD V28.91XS V28.99XA
V28.99XD V28.99XS V29.ØØ1A V29.ØØ1D V29.ØØ1S
V29.ØØ8A V29.ØØ8D V29.ØØ8S V29.Ø91A V29.Ø91D
V29.Ø91S V29.Ø98A V29.Ø98D V29.Ø98S V29.1Ø1A
V29.1Ø1D V29.1Ø1S V29.1Ø8A V29.1Ø8D V29.1Ø8S
V29.191A V29.191D V29.191S V29.198A V29.198D
V29.198S V29.2Ø1A V29.2Ø1D V29.2Ø1S V29.2Ø8A
V29.2Ø8D V29.2Ø8S V29.291A V29.291D V29.291S
V29.298A V29.298D V29.298S V29.31XA V29.31XD
V29.31XS V29.39XA V29.39XD V29.39XS V29.4Ø1A
V29.4Ø1D V29.4Ø1S V29.4Ø8A V29.4Ø8D V29.4Ø8S
V29.491A V29.491D V29.491S V29.498A V29.498D
V29.498S V29.5Ø1A V29.5Ø1D V29.5Ø1S V29.5Ø8A
V29.5Ø8D V29.5Ø8S V29.591A V29.591D V29.591S
V29.598A V29.598D V29.598S V29.6Ø1A V29.6Ø1D
V29.6Ø1S V29.6Ø8A V29.6Ø8D V29.6Ø8S V29.691A
V29.691D V29.691S V29.698A V29.698D V29.698S
V29.811A V29.811D V29.811S V29.818A V29.818D
V29.818S V29.881A V29.881D V29.881S V29.888A
V29.888D V29.888S V29.91XA V29.91XD V29.91XS
V29.99XA V29.99XD V29.99XS W23.2XXA W23.2XXD
W23.2XXS ZØ3.83 *Z28.31Ø *Z28.311 *Z28.39
Z59.82 Z59.86 Z59.87 Z71.87 Z71.88
Z72.823 Z79.6Ø Z79.61 Z79.62Ø Z79.621
Z79.622 Z79.623 Z79.624 Z79.63Ø Z79.631
Z79.632 Z79.633 Z79.634 Z79.64 Z79.69
Z79.85 Z87.61 Z87.68 Z87.731 Z87.732
Z87.76Ø Z87.761 Z87.762 Z87.763 Z87.768
Z91.11Ø Z91.118 Z91.119 Z91.19Ø Z91.198
Z91.199 Z91.A1Ø Z91.A18 Z91.A2Ø Z91.A28
Z91.A3 Z91.A4 Z91.A5 Z91.A9

28 Revised Codes

Note: Each code is listed with its revised description only.

C84.4Ø Peripheral T-cell lymphoma, not elsewhere classified, unspecified site

C84.41 Peripheral T-cell lymphoma, not elsewhere classified, lymph nodes of head, face, and neck

C84.42 Peripheral T-cell lymphoma, not elsewhere classified, intrathoracic lymph nodes

C84.43 Peripheral T-cell lymphoma, not elsewhere classified, intra-abdominal lymph nodes

C84.44 Peripheral T-cell lymphoma, not elsewhere classified, lymph nodes of axilla and upper limb

C84.45 Peripheral T-cell lymphoma, not elsewhere classified, lymph nodes of inguinal region and lower limb

C84.46 Peripheral T-cell lymphoma, not elsewhere classified, intrapelvic lymph nodes

C84.47 Peripheral T-cell lymphoma, not elsewhere classified, spleen

C84.48 Peripheral T-cell lymphoma, not elsewhere classified, lymph nodes of multiple sites

C84.49 Peripheral T-cell lymphoma, not elsewhere classified, extranodal and solid organ sites

C94.6 Myelodysplastic disease, not elsewhere classified

FØ1.5Ø Vascular dementia, unspecified severity, without behavioral disturbance, psychotic disturbance, mood disturbance, and anxiety

FØ2.8Ø Dementia in other diseases classified elsewhere, unspecified severity, without behavioral disturbance, psychotic disturbance, mood disturbance, and anxiety

FØ3.9Ø Unspecified dementia, unspecified severity, without behavioral disturbance, psychotic disturbance, mood disturbance, and anxiety

G31.Ø9 Other frontotemporal neurocognitive disorder

G31.83 Neurocognitive disorder with Lewy bodies

G31.84 Mild cognitive impairment of uncertain or unknown etiology

K35.32 Acute appendicitis with perforation, localized peritonitis, and gangrene, without abscess

K35.33 Acute appendicitis with perforation, localized peritonitis, and gangrene, with abscess

M93.Ø11 Acute slipped upper femoral epiphysis, stable (nontraumatic), right hip

M93.Ø12 Acute slipped upper femoral epiphysis, stable (nontraumatic), left hip

M93.Ø13 Acute slipped upper femoral epiphysis, stable (nontraumatic), unspecified hip

M93.Ø21 Chronic slipped upper femoral epiphysis, stable (nontraumatic), right hip

M93.Ø22 Chronic slipped upper femoral epiphysis, stable (nontraumatic), left hip

M93.Ø23 Chronic slipped upper femoral epiphysis, stable (nontraumatic), unspecified hip

M93.Ø31 Acute on chronic slipped upper femoral epiphysis, stable (nontraumatic), right hip

M93.Ø32 Acute on chronic slipped upper femoral epiphysis, stable (nontraumatic), left hip

M93.Ø33 Acute on chronic slipped upper femoral epiphysis, stable (nontraumatic), unspecified hip

251 Deleted Codes

O35.ØXXØ O35.ØXX1 O35.ØXX2 O35.ØXX3 O35.ØXX4
O35.ØXX5 O35.ØXX9 O35.1XXØ O35.1XX1 O35.1XX2
O35.1XX3 O35.1XX4 O35.1XX5 O35.1XX9 V2Ø.ØXXA
V2Ø.ØXXD V2Ø.ØXXS V2Ø.1XXA V2Ø.1XXD V2Ø.1XXS
V2Ø.2XXA V2Ø.2XXD V2Ø.2XXS V2Ø.3XXA V2Ø.3XXD
V2Ø.3XXS V2Ø.4XXA V2Ø.4XXD V2Ø.4XXS V2Ø.5XXA
V2Ø.5XXD V2Ø.5XXS V2Ø.9XXA V2Ø.9XXD V2Ø.9XXS
V21.ØXXA V21.ØXXD V21.ØXXS V21.1XXA V21.1XXD
V21.1XXS V21.2XXA V21.2XXD V21.2XXS V21.3XXA
V21.3XXD V21.3XXS V21.4XXA V21.4XXD V21.4XXS
V21.5XXA V21.5XXD V21.5XXS V21.9XXA V21.9XXD
V21.9XXS V22.ØXXA V22.ØXXD V22.ØXXS V22.1XXA
V22.1XXD V22.1XXS V22.2XXA V22.2XXD V22.2XXS
V22.3XXA V22.3XXD V22.3XXS V22.4XXA V22.4XXD
V22.4XXS V22.5XXA V22.5XXD V22.5XXS V22.9XXA
V22.9XXD V22.9XXS V23.ØXXA V23.ØXXD V23.ØXXS
V23.1XXA V23.1XXD V23.1XXS V23.2XXA V23.2XXD
V23.2XXS V23.3XXA V23.3XXD V23.3XXS V23.4XXA
V23.4XXD V23.4XXS V23.5XXA V23.5XXD V23.5XXS
V23.9XXA V23.9XXD V23.9XXS V24.ØXXA V24.ØXXD
V24.ØXXS V24.1XXA V24.1XXD V24.1XXS V24.2XXA
V24.2XXD V24.2XXS V24.3XXA V24.3XXD V24.3XXS
V24.4XXA V24.4XXD V24.4XXS V24.5XXA V24.5XXD
V24.5XXS V24.9XXA V24.9XXD V24.9XXS V25.ØXXA
V25.ØXXD V25.ØXXS V25.1XXA V25.1XXD V25.1XXS
V25.2XXA V25.2XXD V25.2XXS V25.3XXA V25.3XXD
V25.3XXS V25.4XXA V25.4XXD V25.4XXS V25.5XXA
V25.5XXD V25.5XXS V25.9XXA V25.9XXD V25.9XXS
V26.ØXXA V26.ØXXD V26.ØXXS V26.1XXA V26.1XXD
V26.1XXS V26.2XXA V26.2XXD V26.2XXS V26.3XXA
V26.3XXD V26.3XXS V26.4XXA V26.4XXD V26.4XXS
V26.5XXA V26.5XXD V26.5XXS V26.9XXA V26.9XXD
V26.9XXS V27.ØXXA V27.ØXXD V27.ØXXS V27.1XXA
V27.1XXD V27.1XXS V27.2XXA V27.2XXD V27.2XXS
V27.3XXA V27.3XXD V27.3XXS V27.4XXA V27.4XXD
V27.4XXS V27.5XXA V27.5XXD V27.5XXS V27.9XXA
V27.9XXD V27.9XXS V28.ØXXA V28.ØXXD V28.ØXXS
V28.1XXA V28.1XXD V28.1XXS V28.2XXA V28.2XXD
V28.2XXS V28.3XXA V28.3XXD V28.3XXS V28.4XXA
V28.4XXD V28.4XXS V28.5XXA V28.5XXD V28.5XXS
V28.9XXA V28.9XXD V28.9XXS V29.ØØXA V29.ØØXD
V29.ØØXS V29.Ø9XA V29.Ø9XD V29.Ø9XS V29.1ØXA
V29.1ØXD V29.1ØXS V29.19XA V29.19XD V29.19XS
V29.2ØXA V29.2ØXD V29.2ØXS V29.29XA V29.29XD
V29.29XS V29.3XXA V29.3XXD V29.3XXS V29.4ØXA
V29.4ØXD V29.4ØXS V29.49XA V29.49XD V29.49XS
V29.5ØXA V29.5ØXD V29.5ØXS V29.59XA V29.59XD
V29.59XS V29.6ØXA V29.6ØXD V29.6ØXS V29.69XA
V29.69XD V29.69XS V29.81XA V29.81XD V29.81XS
V29.88XA V29.88XD V29.88XS V29.9XXA V29.9XXD
V29.9XXS

Proprietary Updates

The following proprietary features have also been added:

- New definitions that describe, in lay terms, a specific condition or disease process
- New coding tips that provide coding advice beyond the code classification
- Updated *AHA Coding Clinic* references through second quarter 2022

What's New for 2023

Conversion Table of ICD-10-CM Codes

The FY 2023 (October 1, 2022-September 30, 2023) Conversion Table for new ICD-10-CM codes is provided to assist users in data retrieval. For each new code the table shows its previously assigned code equivalent. Asterisks identify new codes added to the classification April 1, 2022.

Code Assignment Beginning 10/1/2022	Previous Code(s) Assignment
B37.31	B37.3
B37.32	B37.3
D59.30	D59.3
D59.31	D59.3
D59.32	D59.3
D59.39	D59.3
D68.00	D68.0
D68.01	D68.0
D68.020	D68.0
D68.021	D68.0
D68.022	D68.0
D68.023	D68.0
D68.029	D68.0
D68.03	D68.0
D68.04	D68.0
D68.09	D68.0
D75.821	D75.82
D75.822	D75.82
D75.828	D75.82
D75.829	D75.82
D75.84	D75.89
D81.82	D81.89
E34.30	E34.3
E34.31	E34.3
E34.321	E34.3
E34.322	E34.3
E34.328	E34.3
E34.329	E34.3
E34.39	E34.3
E87.20	E87.2
E87.21	E87.2
E87.22	E87.2
E87.29	E87.2
F01.511	F01.51
F01.518	F01.51
F01.52	F01.51
F01.53	F01.51
F01.54	F01.51
F01.A0	F01.50
F01.A11	F01.51
F01.A18	F01.51
F01.A2	F01.51
F01.A3	F01.51
F01.A4	F01.51
F01.B0	F01.50
F01.B11	F01.51
F01.B18	F01.51
F01.B2	F01.51
F01.B3	F01.51
F01.B4	F01.51
F01.C0	F01.50
F01.C11	F01.51
F01.C18	F01.51
F01.C2	F01.51
F01.C3	F01.51
F01.C4	F01.51
F02.811	F02.81
F02.818	F02.81
F02.82	F02.81
F02.83	F02.81
F02.84	F02.81
F02.A0	F02.80
F02.A11	F02.81
F02.A18	F02.81
F02.A2	F02.81
F02.A3	F02.81
F02.A4	F02.81
F02.B0	F02.80
F02.B11	F02.81
F02.B18	F02.81
F02.B2	F02.81
F02.B3	F02.81
F02.B4	F02.81
F02.C0	F02.80
F02.C11	F02.81
F02.C18	F02.81
F02.C2	F02.81
F02.C3	F02.81
F02.C4	F02.81
F03.911	F03.91
F03.918	F03.91
F03.92	F03.91
F03.93	F03.91
F03.94	F03.91
F03.A0	F03.90
F03.A11	F03.91
F03.A18	F03.91
F03.A2	F03.91
F03.A3	F03.91
F03.A4	F03.91
F03.B0	F03.90
F03.B11	F03.91
F03.B18	F03.91
F03.B2	F03.91
F03.B3	F03.91
F03.B4	F03.91
F03.C0	F03.90
F03.C11	F03.91
F03.C18	F03.91
F03.C2	F03.91
F03.C3	F03.91
F03.C4	F03.91
F06.70	G31.84
F06.71	G31.84
F10.90	Z72.89
F10.91	Z72.89
F11.91	F11.90
F12.91	F12.90
F13.91	F13.90
F14.91	F14.90
F15.91	F15.90
F16.91	F16.90
F18.91	F18.90
F19.91	F19.90
F43.81	F43.8
F43.89	F43.8
G71.031	G71.09
G71.032	G71.09
G71.033	G71.09
G71.0340	G71.09
G71.0341	G71.09
G71.0342	G71.09
G71.0349	G71.09
G71.035	G71.09
G71.038	G71.09
G71.039	G71.09
G90.A	I49.8
G93.31	G93.3
G93.32	G93.3; R53.82
G93.39	G93.3
I20.2	I20.0-I20.1; I20.8
I25.112	I25.110-I25.111; I25.118
I25.702	I25.700-I25.701; I25.708
I25.712	I25.710-I25.711; I25.718
I25.722	I25.720-I25.721; I25.728
I25.732	I25.730-I25.731; I25.738
I25.752	I25.750-I25.751; I25.758
I25.762	I25.760-I25.761; I25.768
I25.792	I25.790-I25.791; I25.798
I31.31	I31.3
I31.39	I31.3
I34.81	I34.8
I34.89	I34.8
I47.20	I47.2
I47.21	I47.2
I47.29	I47.2
I71.010	I71.01
I71.011	I71.01
I71.012	I71.01
I71.019	I71.01
I71.10	I71.1
I71.11	I71.1
I71.12	I71.1
I71.13	I71.1
I71.20	I71.2
I71.21	I71.2
I71.22	I71.2
I71.23	I71.2
I71.30	I71.3
I71.31	I71.3
I71.32	I71.3
I71.33	I71.3
I71.40	I71.4
I71.41	I71.4
I71.42	I71.4
I71.43	I71.4
I71.50	I71.5
I71.51	I71.5
I71.52	I71.5
I71.60	I71.6
I71.61	I71.6
I71.62	I71.6
I77.82	I77.89
J95.87	J95.89
K76.82	K72.90-K72.91
M51.A0	M51.86
M51.A1	M51.86
M51.A2	M51.86
M51.A3	M51.87
M51.A4	M51.87
M51.A5	M51.87
M62.5A0	M62.58
M62.5A1	M62.58
M62.5A2	M62.58
M62.5A9	M62.58
M93.004	M93.001 & M93.002
M93.014	M93.011 & M93.012
M93.024	M93.021 & M93.022
M93.034	M93.031 & M93.032
M93.041	M93.011
M93.042	M93.012
M93.043	M93.013
M93.044	M93.011 & M93.012
M93.051	M93.031
M93.052	M93.032
M93.053	M93.033
M93.054	M93.031 & M93.032
M93.061	M93.011
M93.062	M93.012
M93.063	M93.013
M93.064	M93.011 & M93.012
M93.071	M93.031
M93.072	M93.032
M93.073	M93.033
M93.074	M93.031 & M93.032
M96.A1	M96.89 & Y84.8
M96.A2	M96.89 & Y84.8
M96.A3	M96.89 & Y84.8
M96.A4	M96.89 & Y84.8
M96.A9	M96.89 & Y84.8
N14.11	N14.1
N14.19	N14.1
N76.82	N76.89
N80.00	N80.0
N80.01	N80.0
N80.02	N80.0
N80.03	N80.0
N80.101	N80.1
N80.102	N80.1
N80.103	N80.1
N80.109	N80.1
N80.111	N80.1
N80.112	N80.1
N80.113	N80.1
N80.119	N80.1
N80.121	N80.1
N80.122	N80.1
N80.123	N80.1
N80.129	N80.1
N80.201	N80.2
N80.202	N80.2
N80.203	N80.2
N80.209	N80.2
N80.211	N80.2
N80.212	N80.2
N80.213	N80.2
N80.219	N80.2
N80.221	N80.2
N80.222	N80.2
N80.223	N80.2
N80.229	N80.2
N80.30	N80.3
N80.311	N80.3
N80.312	N80.3
N80.319	N80.3
N80.321	N80.3
N80.322	N80.3
N80.329	N80.3
N80.331	N80.3
N80.332	N80.3
N80.333	N80.3
N80.339	N80.3
N80.341	N80.3
N80.342	N80.3
N80.343	N80.3
N80.349	N80.3
N80.351	N80.3
N80.352	N80.3
N80.353	N80.3
N80.359	N80.3
N80.361	N80.3
N80.362	N80.3
N80.363	N80.3
N80.369	N80.3
N80.371	N80.3
N80.372	N80.3
N80.373	N80.3
N80.379	N80.3
N80.381	N80.3
N80.382	N80.3
N80.383	N80.3
N80.389	N80.3
N80.3A1	N80.3
N80.3A2	N80.3
N80.3A3	N80.3
N80.3A9	N80.3
N80.3B1	N80.3
N80.3B2	N80.3
N80.3B3	N80.3
N80.3B9	N80.3
N80.3C1	N80.3
N80.3C2	N80.3
N80.3C3	N80.3
N80.3C9	N80.3
N80.391	N80.3
N80.392	N80.3
N80.399	N80.3
N80.40	N80.3
N80.41	N80.4
N80.42	N80.4
N80.50	N80.5
N80.511	N80.5
N80.512	N80.5
N80.519	N80.5
N80.521	N80.5
N80.522	N80.5
N80.529	N80.5
N80.531	N80.5
N80.532	N80.5
N80.539	N80.5

Code Assignment Beginning 10/1/2022	Previous Code(s) Assignment
N8Ø.541	N8Ø.5
N8Ø.542	N8Ø.5
N8Ø.549	N8Ø.5
N8Ø.551	N8Ø.5
N8Ø.552	N8Ø.5
N8Ø.559	N8Ø.5
N8Ø.561	N8Ø.5
N8Ø.562	N8Ø.5
N8Ø.569	N8Ø.5
N8Ø.AØ	N8Ø.8
N8Ø.A1	N8Ø.8
N8Ø.A2	N8Ø.8
N8Ø.A41	N8Ø.8
N8Ø.A42	N8Ø.8
N8Ø.A43	N8Ø.8
N8Ø.A49	N8Ø.8
N8Ø.A51	N8Ø.8
N8Ø.A52	N8Ø.8
N8Ø.A53	N8Ø.8
N8Ø.A59	N8Ø.8
N8Ø.A61	N8Ø.8
N8Ø.A62	N8Ø.8
N8Ø.A63	N8Ø.8
N8Ø.A69	N8Ø.8
N8Ø.B1	N8Ø.8
N8Ø.B2	N8Ø.8
N8Ø.B31	N8Ø.8
N8Ø.B32	N8Ø.8
N8Ø.B39	N8Ø.8
N8Ø.B4	N8Ø.8
N8Ø.B5	N8Ø.8
N8Ø.B6	N8Ø.8
N8Ø.CØ	N8Ø.8
N8Ø.C1Ø	N8Ø.8
N8Ø.C11	N8Ø.8
N8Ø.C19	N8Ø.8
N8Ø.C2	N8Ø.8
N8Ø.C3	N8Ø.8
N8Ø.C4	N8Ø.8
N8Ø.C9	N8Ø.8
N8Ø.DØ	N8Ø.8
N8Ø.D1	N8Ø.8
N8Ø.D2	N8Ø.8
N8Ø.D3	N8Ø.8
N8Ø.D4	N8Ø.8
N8Ø.D5	N8Ø.8
N8Ø.D6	N8Ø.8
N8Ø.D9	N8Ø.8
N85.A	N85.8
O35.ØØXØ	O35.ØXXØ
O35.ØØX1	O35.ØXX1
O35.ØØX2	O35.ØXX2
O35.ØØX3	O35.ØXX3
O35.ØØX4	O35.ØXX4
O35.ØØX5	O35.ØXX5
O35.ØØX9	O35.ØXX9
O35.Ø1XØ	O35.ØXXØ
O35.Ø1X1	O35.ØXX1
O35.Ø1X2	O35.ØXX2
O35.Ø1X3	O35.ØXX3
O35.Ø1X4	O35.ØXX4
O35.Ø1X5	O35.ØXX5
O35.Ø1X9	O35.ØXX9
O35.Ø2XØ	O35.ØXXØ
O35.Ø2X1	O35.ØXX1
O35.Ø2X2	O35.ØXX2
O35.Ø2X3	O35.ØXX3
O35.Ø2X4	O35.ØXX4
O35.Ø2X5	O35.ØXX5
O35.Ø2X9	O35.ØXX9
O35.Ø3XØ	O35.ØXXØ
O35.Ø3X1	O35.ØXX1
O35.Ø3X2	O35.ØXX2
O35.Ø3X3	O35.ØXX3
O35.Ø3X4	O35.ØXX4
O35.Ø3X5	O35.ØXX5
O35.Ø3X9	O35.ØXX9
O35.Ø4XØ	O35.ØXXØ
O35.Ø4X1	O35.ØXX1
O35.Ø4X2	O35.ØXX2
O35.Ø4X3	O35.ØXX3
O35.Ø4X4	O35.ØXX4
O35.Ø4X5	O35.ØXX5
O35.Ø4X9	O35.ØXX9
O35.Ø5XØ	O35.ØXXØ
O35.Ø5X1	O35.ØXX1
O35.Ø5X2	O35.ØXX2
O35.Ø5X3	O35.ØXX3
O35.Ø5X4	O35.ØXX4
O35.Ø5X5	O35.ØXX5
O35.Ø5X9	O35.ØXX9
O35.Ø6XØ	O35.ØXXØ
O35.Ø6X1	O35.ØXX1
O35.Ø6X2	O35.ØXX2
O35.Ø6X3	O35.ØXX3
O35.Ø6X4	O35.ØXX4
O35.Ø6X5	O35.ØXX5
O35.Ø6X9	O35.ØXX9
O35.Ø7XØ	O35.ØXXØ
O35.Ø7X1	O35.ØXX1
O35.Ø7X2	O35.ØXX2
O35.Ø7X3	O35.ØXX3
O35.Ø7X4	O35.ØXX4
O35.Ø7X5	O35.ØXX5
O35.Ø7X9	O35.ØXX9
O35.Ø8XØ	O35.ØXXØ
O35.Ø8X1	O35.ØXX1
O35.Ø8X2	O35.ØXX2
O35.Ø8X3	O35.ØXX3
O35.Ø8X4	O35.ØXX4
O35.Ø8X5	O35.ØXX5
O35.Ø8X9	O35.ØXX9
O35.Ø9XØ	O35.ØXXØ
O35.Ø9X1	O35.ØXX1
O35.Ø9X2	O35.ØXX2
O35.Ø9X3	O35.ØXX3
O35.Ø9X4	O35.ØXX4
O35.Ø9X5	O35.ØXX5
O35.Ø9X9	O35.ØXX9
O35.1ØXØ	O35.1XXØ
O35.1ØX1	O35.1XX1
O35.1ØX2	O35.1XX2
O35.1ØX3	O35.1XX3
O35.1ØX4	O35.1XX4
O35.1ØX5	O35.1XX5
O35.1ØX9	O35.1XX9
O35.11XØ	O35.1XXØ
O35.11X1	O35.1XX1
O35.11X2	O35.1XX2
O35.11X3	O35.1XX3
O35.11X4	O35.1XX4
O35.11X5	O35.1XX5
O35.11X9	O35.1XX9
O35.12XØ	O35.1XXØ
O35.12X1	O35.1XX1
O35.12X2	O35.1XX2
O35.12X3	O35.1XX3
O35.12X4	O35.1XX4
O35.12X5	O35.1XX5
O35.12X9	O35.1XX9
O35.13XØ	O35.1XXØ
O35.13X1	O35.1XX1
O35.13X2	O35.1XX2
O35.13X3	O35.1XX3
O35.13X4	O35.1XX4
O35.13X5	O35.1XX5
O35.13X9	O35.1XX9
O35.14XØ	O35.1XXØ
O35.14X1	O35.1XX1
O35.14X2	O35.1XX2
O35.14X3	O35.1XX3
O35.14X4	O35.1XX4
O35.14X5	O35.1XX5
O35.14X9	O35.1XX9
O35.15XØ	O35.1XXØ
O35.15X1	O35.1XX1
O35.15X2	O35.1XX2
O35.15X3	O35.1XX3
O35.15X4	O35.1XX4
O35.15X5	O35.1XX5
O35.15X9	O35.1XX9
O35.19XØ	O35.1XXØ
O35.19X1	O35.1XX1
O35.19X2	O35.1XX2
O35.19X3	O35.1XX3
O35.19X4	O35.1XX4
O35.19X5	O35.1XX5
O35.19X9	O35.1XX9
O35.AXXØ	O35.8XXØ
O35.AXX1	O35.8XX1
O35.AXX2	O35.8XX2
O35.AXX3	O35.8XX3
O35.AXX4	O35.8XX4
O35.AXX5	O35.8XX5
O35.AXX9	O35.8XX9
O35.BXXØ	O35.8XXØ
O35.BXX1	O35.8XX1
O35.BXX2	O35.8XX2
O35.BXX3	O35.8XX3
O35.BXX4	O35.8XX4
O35.BXX5	O35.8XX5
O35.BXX9	O35.8XX9
O35.CXXØ	O35.8XXØ
O35.CXX1	O35.8XX1
O35.CXX2	O35.8XX2
O35.CXX3	O35.8XX3
O35.CXX4	O35.8XX4
O35.CXX5	O35.8XX5
O35.CXX9	O35.8XX9
O35.DXXØ	O35.8XXØ
O35.DXX1	O35.8XX1
O35.DXX2	O35.8XX2
O35.DXX3	O35.8XX3
O35.DXX4	O35.8XX4
O35.DXX5	O35.8XX5
O35.DXX9	O35.8XX9
O35.EXXØ	O35.8XXØ
O35.EXX1	O35.8XX1
O35.EXX2	O35.8XX2
O35.EXX3	O35.8XX3
O35.EXX4	O35.8XX4
O35.EXX5	O35.8XX5
O35.EXX9	O35.8XX9
O35.FXXØ	O35.8XXØ
O35.FXX1	O35.8XX1
O35.FXX2	O35.8XX2
O35.FXX3	O35.8XX3
O35.FXX4	O35.8XX4
O35.FXX5	O35.8XX5
O35.FXX9	O35.8XX9
O35.GXXØ	O35.8XXØ
O35.GXX1	O35.8XX1
O35.GXX2	O35.8XX2
O35.GXX3	O35.8XX3
O35.GXX4	O35.8XX4
O35.GXX5	O35.8XX5
O35.GXX9	O35.8XX9
O35.HXXØ	O35.8XXØ
O35.HXX1	O35.8XX1
O35.HXX2	O35.8XX2
O35.HXX3	O35.8XX3
O35.HXX4	O35.8XX4
O35.HXX5	O35.8XX5
O35.HXX9	O35.8XX9
P28.3Ø	P28.3
P28.31	P28.3
P28.32	P28.3
P28.33	P28.3
P28.39	P28.3
P28.4Ø	P28.4
P28.41	P28.4
P28.42	P28.4
P28.43	P28.4
P28.49	P28.4
Q21.1Ø	Q21.1
Q21.11	Q21.1
Q21.12	Q21.1
Q21.13	Q21.1
Q21.14	Q21.1
Q21.15	Q21.1
Q21.16	Q21.1
Q21.19	Q21.1
Q21.2Ø	Q21.2
Q21.21	Q21.2
Q21.22	Q21.2
Q21.23	Q21.2
Q85.81	Q85.8
Q85.82	Q85.8
Q85.83	Q85.8
Q85.89	Q85.8
SØ6.ØXAA	SØ6.ØX9A
SØ6.ØXAD	SØ6.ØX9D
SØ6.ØXAS	SØ6.ØX9S
SØ6.1XAA	SØ6.1X9A
SØ6.1XAD	SØ6.1X9D
SØ6.1XAS	SØ6.1X9S
SØ6.2XAA	SØ6.2X9A
SØ6.2XAD	SØ6.2X9D
SØ6.2XAS	SØ6.2X9S
SØ6.3ØAA	SØ6.3Ø9A
SØ6.3ØAD	SØ6.3Ø9D
SØ6.3ØAS	SØ6.3Ø9S
SØ6.31AA	SØ6.319A
SØ6.31AD	SØ6.319D
SØ6.31AS	SØ6.319S
SØ6.32AA	SØ6.329A
SØ6.32AD	SØ6.329D
SØ6.32AS	SØ6.329S
SØ6.33AA	SØ6.339A
SØ6.33AD	SØ6.339D
SØ6.33AS	SØ6.339S
SØ6.34AA	SØ6.349A
SØ6.34AD	SØ6.349D
SØ6.34AS	SØ6.349S
SØ6.35AA	SØ6.359A
SØ6.35AD	SØ6.359D
SØ6.35AS	SØ6.359S
SØ6.36AA	SØ6.369A
SØ6.36AD	SØ6.369D
SØ6.36AS	SØ6.369S
SØ6.37AA	SØ6.379A
SØ6.37AD	SØ6.379D
SØ6.37AS	SØ6.379S
SØ6.38AA	SØ6.389A
SØ6.38AD	SØ6.389D
SØ6.38AS	SØ6.389S
SØ6.4XAA	SØ6.4X9A
SØ6.4XAD	SØ6.4X9D
SØ6.4XAS	SØ6.4X9S
SØ6.5XAA	SØ6.5X9A
SØ6.5XAD	SØ6.5X9D
SØ6.5XAS	SØ6.5X9S
SØ6.6XAA	SØ6.6X9A
SØ6.6XAD	SØ6.6X9D
SØ6.6XAS	SØ6.6X9S
SØ6.81AA	SØ6.819A
SØ6.81AD	SØ6.819D
SØ6.81AS	SØ6.819S
SØ6.82AA	SØ6.829A
SØ6.82AD	SØ6.829D
SØ6.82AS	SØ6.829S
SØ6.8AØA	SØ6.ØXØA
SØ6.8AØD	SØ6.ØXØD
SØ6.8AØS	SØ6.ØXØS
SØ6.8A1A	SØ6.ØX9A
SØ6.8A1D	SØ6.ØX9D
SØ6.8A1S	SØ6.ØX9S
SØ6.8A2A	SØ6.ØX9A
SØ6.8A2D	SØ6.ØX9D
SØ6.8A2S	SØ6.ØX9S
SØ6.8A3A	SØ6.ØX9A
SØ6.8A3D	SØ6.ØX9D
SØ6.8A3S	SØ6.ØX9S
SØ6.8A4A	SØ6.ØX9A
SØ6.8A4D	SØ6.ØX9D
SØ6.8A4S	SØ6.ØX9S
SØ6.8A5A	SØ6.ØX9A
SØ6.8A5D	SØ6.ØX9D
SØ6.8A5S	SØ6.ØX9S
SØ6.8A6A	SØ6.ØX9A
SØ6.8A6D	SØ6.ØX9D
SØ6.8A6S	SØ6.ØX9S
SØ6.8A7A	SØ6.ØX9A
SØ6.8A8A	SØ6.ØX9A
SØ6.8AAA	SØ6.ØX9A
SØ6.8AAD	SØ6.ØX9D
SØ6.8AAS	SØ6.ØX9S
SØ6.8A9A	SØ6.ØX9A
SØ6.8A9D	SØ6.ØX9D
SØ6.8A9S	SØ6.ØX9S
SØ6.89AA	SØ6.ØX9A
SØ6.89AD	SØ6.ØX9D
SØ6.89AS	SØ6.ØX9S
SØ6.9XAA	SØ6.9X9A
SØ6.9XAD	SØ6.9X9D
SØ6.9XAS	SØ6.9X9S
T43.651A	T43.621A
T43.651D	T43.621D
T43.651S	T43.621S
T43.652A	T43.622A
T43.652D	T43.621D
T43.652S	T43.621S
T43.653A	T43.623A
T43.653D	T43.623D
T43.653S	T43.623S
T43.654A	T43.624A
T43.654D	T43.624D
T43.654S	T43.624S
T43.655A	T43.625A
T43.655D	T43.625D
T43.655S	T43.625S
T43.656A	T43.626A
T43.656D	T43.626D
T43.656S	T43.626S

Code Assignment Beginning 10/1/2022	Previous Code(s) Assignment
V2Ø.Ø1XA	V2Ø.ØXXA
V2Ø.Ø1XD	V2Ø.ØXXD
V2Ø.Ø1XS	V2Ø.ØXXS
V2Ø.Ø9XA	V2Ø.ØXXA
V2Ø.Ø9XD	V2Ø.ØXXD
V2Ø.Ø9XS	V2Ø.ØXXS
V2Ø.11XA	V2Ø.1XXA
V2Ø.11XD	V2Ø.1XXD
V2Ø.11XS	V2Ø.1XXS
V2Ø.19XA	V2Ø.1XXA
V2Ø.19XD	V2Ø.1XXD
V2Ø.19XS	V2Ø.1XXS
V2Ø.21XA	V2Ø.2XXA
V2Ø.21XD	V2Ø.2XXD
V2Ø.21XS	V2Ø.2XXS
V2Ø.29XA	V2Ø.2XXA
V2Ø.29XD	V2Ø.2XXD
V2Ø.29XS	V2Ø.2XXS
V2Ø.31XA	V2Ø.3XXA
V2Ø.31XD	V2Ø.3XXD
V2Ø.31XS	V2Ø.3XXS
V2Ø.39XA	V2Ø.3XXA
V2Ø.39XD	V2Ø.3XXD
V2Ø.39XS	V2Ø.3XXS
V2Ø.41XA	V2Ø.4XXA
V2Ø.41XD	V2Ø.4XXD
V2Ø.41XS	V2Ø.4XXS
V2Ø.49XA	V2Ø.4XXA
V2Ø.49XD	V2Ø.4XXD
V2Ø.49XS	V2Ø.4XXS
V2Ø.51XA	V2Ø.5XXA
V2Ø.51XD	V2Ø.5XXD
V2Ø.51XS	V2Ø.5XXS
V2Ø.59XA	V2Ø.5XXA
V2Ø.59XD	V2Ø.5XXD
V2Ø.59XS	V2Ø.5XXS
V2Ø.91XA	V2Ø.9XXA
V2Ø.91XD	V2Ø.9XXD
V2Ø.91XS	V2Ø.9XXS
V2Ø.99XA	V2Ø.9XXA
V2Ø.99XD	V2Ø.9XXD
V2Ø.99XS	V2Ø.9XXS
V21.Ø1XA	V21.ØXXA
V21.Ø1XD	V21.ØXXD
V21.Ø1XS	V21.ØXXS
V21.Ø9XA	V21.ØXXA
V21.Ø9XD	V21.ØXXD
V21.Ø9XS	V21.ØXXS
V21.11XA	V21.1XXA
V21.11XD	V21.1XXD
V21.11XS	V21.1XXS
V21.19XA	V21.1XXA
V21.19XD	V21.1XXD
V21.19XS	V21.1XXS
V21.21XA	V21.2XXA
V21.21XD	V21.2XXD
V21.21XS	V21.2XXS
V21.29XA	V21.2XXA
V21.29XD	V21.2XXD

Code Assignment Beginning 10/1/2022	Previous Code(s) Assignment
V21.29XS	V21.2XXS
V21.31XA	V21.3XXA
V21.31XD	V21.3XXD
V21.31XS	V21.3XXS
V21.39XA	V21.3XXA
V21.39XD	V21.3XXD
V21.39XS	V21.3XXS
V21.41XA	V21.4XXA
V21.41XD	V21.4XXD
V21.41XS	V21.4XXS
V21.49XA	V21.4XXA
V21.49XD	V21.4XXD
V21.49XS	V21.4XXS
V21.51XA	V21.5XXA
V21.51XD	V21.5XXD
V21.51XS	V21.5XXS
V21.59XA	V21.5XXA
V21.59XD	V21.5XXD
V21.59XS	V21.5XXS
V21.91XA	V21.9XXA
V21.91XD	V21.9XXD
V21.91XS	V21.9XXS
V21.99XA	V21.9XXA
V21.99XD	V21.9XXD
V21.99XS	V21.9XXS
V22.Ø1XA	V22.ØXXA
V22.Ø1XD	V22.ØXXD
V22.Ø1XS	V22.ØXXS
V22.Ø9XA	V22.ØXXA
V22.Ø9XD	V22.ØXXD
V22.Ø9XS	V22.ØXXS
V22.11XA	V22.1XXA
V22.11XD	V22.1XXD
V22.11XS	V22.1XXS
V22.19XA	V22.1XXA
V22.19XD	V22.1XXD
V22.19XS	V22.1XXS
V22.21XA	V22.2XXA
V22.21XD	V22.2XXD
V22.21XS	V22.2XXS
V22.29XA	V22.2XXA
V22.29XD	V22.2XXD
V22.29XS	V22.2XXS
V22.31XA	V22.3XXA
V22.31XD	V22.3XXD
V22.31XS	V22.3XXS
V22.39XA	V22.3XXA
V22.39XD	V22.3XXD
V22.39XS	V22.3XXS
V22.41XA	V22.4XXA
V22.41XD	V22.4XXD
V22.41XS	V22.4XXS
V22.49XA	V22.4XXA
V22.49XD	V22.4XXD
V22.49XS	V22.4XXS
V22.51XA	V22.5XXA
V22.51XD	V22.5XXD
V22.51XS	V22.5XXS
V22.59XA	V22.5XXA

Code Assignment Beginning 10/1/2022	Previous Code(s) Assignment
V22.59XD	V22.5XXD
V22.59XS	V22.5XXS
V22.91XA	V22.9XXA
V22.91XD	V22.9XXD
V22.91XS	V22.9XXS
V22.99XA	V22.9XXA
V22.99XD	V22.9XXD
V22.99XS	V22.9XXS
V23.Ø1XA	V23.ØXXA
V23.Ø1XD	V23.ØXXD
V23.Ø1XS	V23.ØXXS
V23.Ø9XA	V23.ØXXA
V23.Ø9XD	V23.ØXXD
V23.Ø9XS	V23.ØXXS
V23.11XA	V23.1XXA
V23.11XD	V23.1XXD
V23.11XS	V23.1XXS
V23.19XA	V23.1XXA
V23.19XD	V23.1XXD
V23.19XS	V23.1XXS
V23.21XA	V23.2XXA
V23.21XD	V23.2XXD
V23.21XS	V23.2XXS
V23.29XA	V23.2XXA
V23.29XD	V23.2XXD
V23.29XS	V23.2XXS
V23.31XA	V23.3XXA
V23.31XD	V23.3XXD
V23.31XS	V23.3XXS
V23.39XA	V23.3XXA
V23.39XD	V23.3XXD
V23.39XS	V23.3XXS
V23.41XA	V23.4XXA
V23.41XD	V23.4XXD
V23.41XS	V23.4XXS
V23.49XA	V23.4XXA
V23.49XD	V23.4XXD
V23.49XS	V23.4XXS
V23.51XA	V23.5XXA
V23.51XD	V23.5XXD
V23.51XS	V23.5XXS
V23.59XA	V23.5XXA
V23.59XD	V23.5XXD
V23.59XS	V23.5XXS
V23.91XA	V23.9XXA
V23.91XD	V23.9XXD
V23.91XS	V23.9XXS
V23.99XA	V23.9XXA
V23.99XD	V23.9XXD
V23.99XS	V23.9XXS
V24.Ø1XA	V24.ØXXA
V24.Ø1XD	V24.ØXXD
V24.Ø1XS	V24.ØXXS
V24.Ø9XA	V24.ØXXA
V24.Ø9XD	V24.ØXXD
V24.Ø9XS	V24.ØXXS
V24.11XA	V24.1XXA
V24.11XD	V24.1XXD
V24.11XS	V24.1XXS

Code Assignment Beginning 10/1/2022	Previous Code(s) Assignment
V24.19XA	V24.1XXA
V24.19XD	V24.1XXD
V24.19XS	V24.1XXS
V24.21XA	V24.2XXA
V24.21XD	V24.2XXD
V24.21XS	V24.2XXS
V24.29XA	V24.2XXA
V24.29XD	V24.2XXD
V24.29XS	V24.2XXS
V24.31XA	V24.3XXA
V24.31XD	V24.3XXD
V24.31XS	V24.3XXS
V24.39XA	V24.3XXA
V24.39XD	V24.3XXD
V24.39XS	V24.3XXS
V24.41XA	V24.4XXA
V24.41XD	V24.4XXD
V24.41XS	V24.4XXS
V24.49XA	V24.4XXA
V24.49XD	V24.4XXD
V24.49XS	V24.4XXS
V24.51XA	V24.5XXA
V24.51XD	V24.5XXD
V24.51XS	V24.5XXS
V24.59XA	V24.5XXA
V24.59XD	V24.5XXD
V24.59XS	V24.5XXS
V24.91XA	V24.9XXA
V24.91XD	V24.9XXD
V24.91XS	V24.9XXS
V24.99XA	V24.9XXA
V24.99XD	V24.9XXD
V24.99XS	V24.9XXS
V25.Ø1XA	V25.ØXXA
V25.Ø1XD	V25.ØXXD
V25.Ø1XS	V25.ØXXS
V25.Ø9XA	V25.ØXXA
V25.Ø9XD	V25.ØXXD
V25.Ø9XS	V25.ØXXS
V25.11XA	V25.1XXA
V25.11XD	V25.1XXD
V25.11XS	V25.1XXS
V25.19XA	V25.1XXA
V25.19XD	V25.1XXD
V25.19XS	V25.1XXS
V25.21XA	V25.2XXA
V25.21XD	V25.2XXD
V25.21XS	V25.2XXS
V25.29XA	V25.2XXA
V25.29XD	V25.2XXD
V25.29XS	V25.2XXS
V25.31XA	V25.3XXA
V25.31XD	V25.3XXD
V25.31XS	V25.3XXS
V25.39XA	V25.3XXA
V25.39XD	V25.3XXD
V25.39XS	V25.3XXS
V25.41XA	V25.4XXA
V25.41XD	V25.4XXD

Code Assignment Beginning 10/1/2022	Previous Code(s) Assignment
V25.41XS	V25.4XXS
V25.49XA	V25.4XXA
V25.49XD	V25.4XXD
V25.49XS	V25.4XXS
V25.51XA	V25.5XXA
V25.51XD	V25.5XXD
V25.51XS	V25.5XXS
V25.59XA	V25.5XXA
V25.59XD	V25.5XXD
V25.59XS	V25.5XXS
V25.91XA	V25.9XXA
V25.91XD	V25.9XXD
V25.91XS	V25.9XXS
V25.99XA	V25.9XXA
V25.99XD	V25.9XXD
V25.99XS	V25.9XXS
V26.Ø1XA	V26.ØXXA
V26.Ø1XD	V26.ØXXD
V26.Ø1XS	V26.ØXXS
V26.Ø9XA	V26.ØXXA
V26.Ø9XD	V26.ØXXD
V26.Ø9XS	V26.ØXXS
V26.11XA	V26.1XXA
V26.11XD	V26.1XXD
V26.11XS	V26.1XXS
V26.19XA	V26.1XXA
V26.19XD	V26.1XXD
V26.19XS	V26.1XXS
V26.21XA	V26.2XXA
V26.21XD	V26.2XXD
V26.21XS	V26.2XXS
V26.29XA	V26.2XXA
V26.29XD	V26.2XXD
V26.29XS	V26.2XXS
V26.31XA	V26.3XXA
V26.31XD	V26.3XXD
V26.31XS	V26.3XXS
V26.39XA	V26.3XXA
V26.39XD	V26.3XXD
V26.39XS	V26.3XXS
V26.41XA	V26.4XXA
V26.41XD	V26.4XXD
V26.41XS	V26.4XXS
V26.49XA	V26.4XXA
V26.49XD	V26.4XXD
V26.49XS	V26.4XXS
V26.51XA	V26.5XXA
V26.51XD	V26.5XXD
V26.51XS	V26.5XXS
V26.59XA	V26.5XXA
V26.59XD	V26.5XXD
V26.59XS	V26.5XXS
V26.91XA	V26.9XXA
V26.91XD	V26.9XXD
V26.91XS	V26.9XXS
V26.99XA	V26.9XXA
V26.99XD	V26.9XXD
V26.99XS	V26.9XXS
V27.Ø1XA	V27.ØXXA

Code Assignment Beginning 10/1/2022	Previous Code(s) Assignment
V27.Ø1XD	V27.ØXXD
V27.Ø1XS	V27.ØXXS
V27.Ø9XA	V27.ØXXA
V27.Ø9XD	V27.ØXXD
V27.Ø9XS	V27.ØXXS
V27.11XA	V27.1XXA
V27.11XD	V27.1XXD
V27.11XS	V27.1XXS
V27.19XA	V27.1XXA
V27.19XD	V27.1XXD
V27.19XS	V27.1XXS
V27.21XA	V27.2XXA
V27.21XD	V27.2XXD
V27.21XS	V27.2XXS
V27.29XA	V27.2XXA
V27.29XD	V27.2XXD
V27.29XS	V27.2XXS
V27.31XA	V27.3XXA
V27.31XD	V27.3XXD
V27.31XS	V27.3XXS
V27.39XA	V27.3XXA
V27.39XD	V27.3XXD
V27.39XS	V27.3XXS
V27.41XA	V27.4XXA
V27.41XD	V27.4XXD
V27.41XS	V27.4XXS
V27.49XA	V27.4XXA
V27.49XD	V27.4XXD
V27.49XS	V27.4XXS
V27.51XA	V27.5XXA
V27.51XD	V27.5XXD
V27.51XS	V27.5XXS
V27.59XA	V27.5XXA
V27.59XD	V27.5XXD
V27.59XS	V27.5XXS
V27.91XA	V27.9XXA
V27.91XD	V27.9XXD
V27.91XS	V27.9XXS
V27.99XA	V27.9XXA
V27.99XD	V27.9XXD
V27.99XS	V27.9XXS
V28.Ø1XA	V28.ØXXA
V28.Ø1XD	V28.ØXXD
V28.Ø1XS	V28.ØXXS
V28.Ø9XA	V28.ØXXA
V28.Ø9XD	V28.ØXXD
V28.Ø9XS	V28.ØXXS
V28.11XA	V28.1XXA
V28.11XD	V28.1XXD
V28.11XS	V28.1XXS
V28.19XA	V28.1XXA
V28.19XD	V28.1XXD
V28.19XS	V28.1XXS
V28.21XA	V28.2XXA
V28.21XD	V28.2XXD
V28.21XS	V28.2XXS
V28.29XA	V28.2XXA
V28.29XD	V28.2XXD
V28.29XS	V28.2XXS

Code Assignment Beginning 10/1/2022	Previous Code(s) Assignment
V28.31XA	V28.3XXA
V28.31XD	V28.3XXD
V28.31XS	V28.3XXS
V28.39XA	V28.3XXA
V28.39XD	V28.3XXD
V28.39XS	V28.3XXS
V28.41XA	V28.4XXA
V28.41XD	V28.4XXD
V28.41XS	V28.4XXS
V28.49XA	V28.4XXA
V28.49XD	V28.4XXD
V28.49XS	V28.4XXS
V28.51XA	V28.5XXA
V28.51XD	V28.5XXD
V28.51XS	V28.5XXS
V28.59XA	V28.5XXA
V28.59XD	V28.5XXD
V28.59XS	V28.5XXS
V28.91XA	V28.9XXA
V28.91XD	V28.9XXD
V28.91XS	V28.9XXS
V28.99XA	V28.9XXA
V28.99XD	V28.9XXD
V28.99XS	V28.9XXS
V29.001A	V29.00XA
V29.001D	V29.00XD
V29.001S	V29.00XS
V29.008A	V29.00XA
V29.008D	V29.00XD
V29.008S	V29.00XS

Code Assignment Beginning 10/1/2022	Previous Code(s) Assignment
V29.091A	V29.09XA
V29.091D	V29.09XD
V29.091S	V29.09XS
V29.098A	V29.09XA
V29.098D	V29.09XD
V29.098S	V29.09XS
V29.101A	V29.10XA
V29.101D	V29.10XD
V29.101S	V29.10XS
V29.108A	V29.10XA
V29.108D	V29.10XD
V29.108S	V29.10XS
V29.191A	V29.19XA
V29.191D	V29.19XD
V29.191S	V29.19XS
V29.198A	V29.19XA
V29.198D	V29.19XD
V29.198S	V29.19XS
V29.201A	V29.20XA
V29.201D	V29.20XD
V29.201S	V29.20XS
V29.208A	V29.20XA
V29.208D	V29.20XD
V29.208S	V29.20XS
V29.291A	V29.29XA
V29.291D	V29.29XD
V29.291S	V29.29XS
V29.298A	V29.29XA
V29.298D	V29.29XD
V29.298S	V29.29XS

Code Assignment Beginning 10/1/2022	Previous Code(s) Assignment
V29.31XA	V29.3XXA
V29.31XD	V29.3XXD
V29.31XS	V29.3XXS
V29.39XA	V29.3XXA
V29.39XD	V29.3XXD
V29.39XS	V29.3XXS
V29.401A	V29.40XA
V29.401D	V29.40XD
V29.401S	V29.40XS
V29.408A	V29.40XA
V29.408D	V29.40XD
V29.408S	V29.40XS
V29.491A	V29.49XA
V29.491D	V29.49XD
V29.491S	V29.49XS
V29.498A	V29.49XA
V29.498D	V29.49XD
V29.498S	V29.49XS
V29.501A	V29.50XA
V29.501D	V29.50XD
V29.501S	V29.50XS
V29.508A	V29.50XA
V29.508D	V29.50XD
V29.508S	V29.50XS
V29.591A	V29.59XA
V29.591D	V29.59XD
V29.591S	V29.59XS
V29.598A	V29.59XA
V29.598D	V29.59XD
V29.598S	V29.59XS

Code Assignment Beginning 10/1/2022	Previous Code(s) Assignment
V29.601A	V29.60XA
V29.601D	V29.60XD
V29.601S	V29.60XS
V29.608A	V29.60XA
V29.608D	V29.60XD
V29.608S	V29.60XS
V29.691A	V29.69XA
V29.691D	V29.69XD
V29.691S	V29.69XS
V29.698A	V29.69XA
V29.698D	V29.69XD
V29.698S	V29.69XS
V29.811A	V29.80XA
V29.811D	V29.80XD
V29.811S	V29.80XS
V29.818A	V29.80XA
V29.818D	V29.80XD
V29.818S	V29.80XS
V29.881A	V29.89XA
V29.881D	V29.89XD
V29.881S	V29.89XS
V29.888A	V29.89XA
V29.888D	V29.89XD
V29.888S	V29.89XS
V29.91XA	V29.9XXA
V29.91XD	V29.9XXD
V29.91XS	V29.9XXS
V29.99XA	V29.9XXA
V29.99XD	V29.9XXD
V29.99XS	V29.9XXS

Code Assignment Beginning 10/1/2022	Previous Code(s) Assignment
W23.2XXA	W23.0XXA & W23.1XXA
W23.2XXD	W23.0XXD & W23.1XXD
W23.2XXS	W23.0XXS & W23.1XXS
Z03.83	Z03.89
*Z28.310	Z28.3
*Z28.311	Z28.3
*Z28.39	Z28.3
Z59.82	Z59.89
Z59.86	Z59.89
Z59.87	Z59.89
Z71.87	Z71.89
Z71.88	Z71.89
Z72.823	Z72.89
Z79.60	Z79.899
Z79.61	Z79.899
Z79.620	Z79.899
Z79.621	Z79.899
Z79.622	Z79.899
Z79.623	Z79.899
Z79.624	Z79.899
Z79.630	Z79.899
Z79.631	Z79.899
Z79.632	Z79.899
Z79.633	Z79.899
Z79.634	Z79.899
Z79.64	Z79.899

Code Assignment Beginning 10/1/2022	Previous Code(s) Assignment
Z79.69	Z79.899
Z79.85	Z79.899
Z87.61	Z87.898
Z87.68	Z87.898
Z87.731	Z87.738
Z87.732	Z87.738
Z87.760	Z87.76
Z87.761	Z87.76
Z87.762	Z87.76
Z87.763	Z87.76
Z87.768	Z87.76
Z91.110	Z91.11
Z91.118	Z91.11
Z91.119	Z91.11
Z91.190	Z91.19
Z91.198	Z91.19
Z91.199	Z91.19
Z91.A10	Z91.19
Z91.A18	Z91.19
Z91.A20	Z91.19
Z91.A28	Z91.19
Z91.A3	Z91.19
Z91.A4	Z91.19
Z91.A5	Z91.19
Z91.A9	Z91.19

10 Steps to Correct Coding

Follow the 10 steps below to correctly code encounters for health care services.

Step 1: Identify the reason for the visit or encounter (i.e., a sign, symptom, diagnosis and/or condition).
The medical record documentation should accurately reflect the patient's condition, using terminology that includes specific diagnoses and symptoms or clearly states the reasons for the encounter.

Choosing the main term that best describes the reason chiefly responsible for the service provided is the most important step in coding. If symptoms are present and documented but a definitive diagnosis has not yet been determined, code the symptoms. *For outpatient cases, do not code conditions that are referred to as "rule out," "suspected," "probable," or "questionable."* Diagnoses often are not established at the time of the initial encounter/visit and may require two or more visits to be established. Code only what is documented in the available outpatient records and only to the highest degree of certainty known at the time of the patient's visit. For inpatient medical records, uncertain diagnoses may be reported if documented at the time of discharge.

Step 2: After selecting the reason for the encounter, consult the alphabetic index.
The most critical rule is to begin code selection in the alphabetic index. Never turn first to the tabular list. The index provides cross-references, essential and nonessential modifiers, and other instructional notations that may not be found in the tabular list.

Step 3: Locate the main term entry.
The alphabetic index lists conditions, which may be expressed as nouns or eponyms, with critical use of adjectives. Some conditions known by several names have multiple main entries. Reasons for encounters may be located under general terms such as admission, encounter, and examination. Other general terms such as history, status (post), or presence (of) can be used to locate other factors influencing health.

Step 4: Scan subterm entries.
Scan the subterm entries, as appropriate, being sure to review continued lines and additional subterms that may appear in the next column or on the next page. Shaded vertical guidelines in the index indicate the indentation level for each subterm in relation to the main terms.

Step 5: Pay close attention to index instructions.

- Parentheses ( ) enclose nonessential modifiers, terms that are supplementary words or explanatory information that may or may not appear in the diagnostic statement and do not affect code selection.
- Brackets [ ] enclose manifestation codes that can be used only as secondary codes to the underlying condition code immediately preceding it. If used, manifestation codes must be reported with the appropriate etiology codes.
- Default codes are listed next to the main term and represent the condition most commonly associated with the main term or the unspecified code for the main term.
- *"See"* cross-references, identified by italicized type and "code by" cross-references indicate that another term *must be referenced* to locate the correct code.
- *"See also"* cross-references, identified by italicized type, provide alternative terms that may be useful to look up but *are not mandatory*.
- "Omit code" cross-references identify instances when a code is not applicable depending on the condition being coded.
- "With" subterms are listed out of alphabetic order and identify a presumed causal relationship between the two conditions they link.
- "Due to" subterms identify a relationship between the two conditions they link.
- "NEC," abbreviation for "not elsewhere classified," follows some main terms or subterms and indicates that there is no specific code for the condition even though the medical documentation may be very specific.
- "NOS," abbreviation for "not otherwise specified," follows some main terms or subterms and is the equivalent of unspecified; NOS signifies that the information in the medical record is insufficient for assigning a more specific code.
- *Following* references help coders locate alphanumeric codes that are out of sequence in the tabular section.
- Check-additional-character symbols flag codes that require additional characters to make the code valid; the characters available to complete the code should be verified in the tabular section.

Step 6: Choose a potential code and locate it in the tabular list.
To prevent coding errors, always use both the alphabetic index (to identify a code) and the tabular list (to verify a code), as the index does not include the important instructional notes found in the tabular list. An added benefit of using the tabular list, which groups like things together, is that while looking at one code in the list, a coder might see a more specific one that would have been missed had the coder relied solely on the alphabetic index. Additionally, many of the codes require a fourth, fifth, sixth, or seventh character to be valid, and many of these characters can be found only in the tabular list.

Step 7: Read all instructional material in the tabular section.
The coder must follow any Includes, Excludes 1 and Excludes 2 notes, and other instructional notes, such as "Code first" and "Use additional code," listed in the tabular list for the chapter, category, subcategory, and subclassification levels of code selection that direct the coder to use a different or additional code. Any codes in the tabular range AØØ.Ø- through T88.9- may be used to identify the diagnostic reason for the encounter. The tabular list encompasses many codes describing disease and injury classifications (e.g., infectious and parasitic diseases, neoplasms, symptoms, nervous and circulatory system, etc.).

Codes that describe symptoms and signs, as opposed to definitive diagnoses, should be reported when an established diagnosis has not been made (confirmed) by the physician. Chapter 18 of the ICD-10-CM code book, "Symptoms, Signs, and Abnormal Clinical and Laboratory Findings, Not Elsewhere Classified" (codes RØØ–R99), contains many, but not all, codes for symptoms.

ICD-10-CM classifies encounters with health care providers for circumstances other than a disease or injury in chapter 21, "Factors Influencing Health Status and Contact with Health Services" (codes ZØØ–Z99). Circumstances other than a disease or injury often are recorded as chiefly responsible for the encounter.

A code is invalid if it does not include the full number of characters (greatest level of specificity) required. Codes in ICD-10-CM can contain from three to seven alphanumeric characters. A three-character code is to be used only if the category is not further subdivided into four-, five-, six-, or seven-character codes. Placeholder character X is used as part of an alphanumeric code to allow for future expansion and as a placeholder for empty characters in a code that requires a seventh character but has no fourth, fifth, or sixth character. Note that certain categories require seventh characters that apply to all codes in that category. Always check the category level for applicable seventh characters for that category.

Step 8: Consult the official ICD-10-CM conventions and guidelines.

The *ICD-10-CM Official Guidelines for Coding and Reporting* govern the use of certain codes. These guidelines provide both general and chapter-specific coding guidance.

Step 9: Confirm and assign the code.

Having reviewed all relevant information concerning the possible code choices, assign the code that most completely describes the condition.

Repeat steps 1 through 9 for all additional documented conditions that meet the following criteria:

- They exist at the time of the visit *AND*
- They require or affect patient care, treatment, or management

Step 10: Sequence codes correctly.

Sequencing is the order in which the codes are listed on the claim. List first the ICD-10-CM code for the diagnosis, condition, problem, or other reason for the encounter/visit that is shown in the medical record to be chiefly responsible for the services provided. List additional codes that describe any coexisting conditions. Follow the official coding guidelines (see the guidelines, section II, "Selection of Principal Diagnosis"; section III, "Reporting Additional Diagnoses"; and section IV, "Diagnostic Coding and Reporting Guidelines for Outpatient Services") on proper sequencing of codes.

Coding Examples

Diagnosis: Anorexia

Step 1: The reason for the encounter was the condition, anorexia.

Step 2: Consult the alphabetic index.

Step 3: Locate the main term "Anorexia."

Step 4: Two possible subterms are available, "hysterical" and "nervosa." Neither is documented in this instance, however, so they cannot be used in code selection.

Step 5: The code listed next to the main term is called the default code selection. Because the two subentries (essential modifiers) do not apply in this instance, the default code (R63.Ø) should be used.

Step 6: Turn to code R63.Ø in the tabular list and read all instructional notes.

Step 7: The Excludes 1 note at code R63.Ø indicates that anorexia nervosa and loss of appetite determined to be of nonorganic origin should be reported with a code from chapter 5. The diagnostic statement does not describe the condition as anorexia nervosa, however, and does not indicate that the anorexia is of a nonorganic origin. There is no further division of the category past the fourth-character subcategory. Therefore, code R63.Ø is at the highest level of specificity.

Step 8: Review of official guideline I.C.18 indicates that a symptom code is appropriate when a more definitive diagnosis is not documented.

Step 9: The default code, R63.Ø Anorexia, is the correct code selection.

Repeat steps 1 through 9 for any concomitant diagnoses.

Step 10: Since anorexia is listed as the chief reason for the health care encounter, the first-listed, or principal, diagnosis is R63.Ø. Note that this is a chapter 18 symptom code but can be assigned for both inpatient and outpatient records since the provider did not establish a more definitive diagnosis, according to sections II.A and IV.D.

Diagnosis: Acute bronchitis

Step 1: The reason for the encounter was the condition, acute bronchitis.

Step 2: Consult the alphabetic index.

Step 3: Locate the main term "Bronchitis."

Step 4: There is a subterm for "acute or subacute." Additional subterms are not included in the diagnostic statement.

Step 5: Nonessential modifiers (with bronchospasm or obstruction) are terms that do not affect code assignment. Since no other subterms indented under "acute" apply here, the code listed next to this subentry—in this case J2Ø.9—should be chosen.

Step 6: Turn to code J2Ø.9 in the tabular list and read all instructional notes.

Step 7: The Includes note under category J2Ø lists alternative terms for acute bronchitis. Note that the list is not exhaustive but is only a representative selection of diagnoses that are included in the subcategory. The Excludes 1 note refers to category J4Ø for bronchitis and tracheobronchitis NOS. There are several conditions in the Excludes 2 notes that, if applicable, can be coded in addition to this code.

Note that the codes included in J2Ø represent acute bronchitis due to various infectious organisms that could be selected if identified in the documentation. In this case, the organism was not identified and there is no further division of the category past the fourth character subcategory. Therefore, code J2Ø.9 is at the highest level of specificity.

Step 8: Review of official guideline I.C.10 provides no additional information affecting the code selected.

Step 9: Assign code J2Ø.9 Acute bronchitis, unspecified.

Repeat steps 1 through 9 for any concomitant diagnoses.

Step 10: In the absence of additional diagnoses that may affect sequencing, code J2Ø.9 should be sequenced as the first-listed, or principal, diagnosis.

Diagnosis: Cerebellar ataxia in myxedema

Step 1: The reason for the encounter was the condition, cerebellar ataxia.

Step 2: Consult the alphabetic index.

Step 3: Locate the main term "Ataxia."

Step 4: Available subterms include "cerebellar (hereditary)," with additional indented subterms for "in" and "myxedema," all essential modifiers that are included in the diagnostic statement. Two codes are provided, EØ3.9 and G13.2, the latter of which is in brackets.

Step 5: Note the nonessential modifier (in parentheses) after the subterm cerebellar includes the term "hereditary." Because it is in parentheses, this term is not required in the diagnostic statement for this subentry to apply. The brackets around G13.2 identify this code as a manifestation of the condition described by code EØ3.9 and indicate that the two must be reported together and sequencing rules apply.

Step 6: Locate codes EØ3.9 and G13.2 in the tabular list, and read all instructional notes.

Step 7: For code EØ3.9, there are no instructional notes in the tabular list at the category EØ3 or code level that indicate that this condition should be coded elsewhere in the classification or that additional codes are required. Without further information from the diagnostic statement, myxedema, not otherwise specified (NOS), is appropriately reported with code EØ3.9 Hypothyroidism, unspecified, according to the inclusion term at this code.

Code G13.2 in the tabular list has an instructional note to "Code first underlying disease," which includes conditions found in category EØ3.-. Based on this note, codes EØ3.9 and G13.2 are to be coded together, with G13.2 listed only as a secondary diagnosis. This correlates with what the alphabetic index indicated. As there is no further division of codes in category G13 beyond the fourth character, G13.2 is at the highest level of specificity.

Step 8: Although there are some general conventions, such as how to interpret brackets in the alphabetic index, no chapter-specific guidelines apply to this coding scenario.

Step 9: Assign codes EØ3.9 Hypothyroidism, unspecified, and G13.2 Systemic atrophy primarily affecting the central nervous system in myxedema.

Repeat steps 1 through 9 for any concomitant diagnoses.

Step 10: Based on the alphabetic index and tabular instructional notations, code EØ3.9 should be sequenced as the first-listed, or principal, diagnosis followed by G13.2 as a secondary diagnosis.

Diagnosis: Decubitus ulcer of right elbow with skin loss and necrosis of subcutaneous tissue

Step 1: The reason for the encounter was the condition, decubitus ulcer.

Step 2: Consult the alphabetic index.

Step 3: Locate the main term "Ulcer."

Step 4: For the subterm "decubitus," there is no code provided or additional subterms indented, but a cross-reference is listed.

Step 5: The italicized cross-reference instructs the coder to "*see* Ulcer, pressure, by site."

Repeat steps 3 through 5 for the cross-reference:

Step 3: Locate the main term "Ulcer."

Step 4: Review the subentries for the subterm "pressure." The next level of indent lists either the site of the ulcer or the specific stage of the ulcer (stage 1–4, unstageable, and unspecified stages). The diagnostic statement provides the site, right elbow, and the extent of tissue damage (skin loss and necrosis of subcutaneous tissue) but does not specifically state that the ulcer is stage 1, stage 2, etc. Nonessential modifiers (in parentheses) at each stage include a description of the typical extent of damage at each stage. For example, stage 1 describes "pre-ulcer skin changes limited to persistent focal edema." Based on the documentation in the record, the coder can correlate the documentation to the nonessential modifiers and choose the specific stage from the index. The coder can also go directly to the body site, choosing the stage of the ulcer after reviewing the code options and instructional notations in the tabular list.

The diagnostic statement indicates that the extent of the damage to the elbow includes skin loss and necrosis of subcutaneous tissue, coinciding with the nonessential modifier next to the subentry "stage 3." The body site of elbow (L89.Ø-) is listed as another level of indent with other body sites.

Step 5: Note that code L89.Ø is followed by a dash and an additional-character-required icon, which indicate that more characters are needed to complete the code. From here, the tabular listing for L89.Ø- can be consulted.

Step 6: Locate code L89.Ø- in the tabular list and read all instructional notes.

Step 7: The tabular listing at category L89 has an Includes note for "decubitus ulcer," which confirms that category L89 is the appropriate category to represent what is documented in the diagnostic statement. Several Excludes 2 notes are also listed at the category level. Excludes 2 notes represent conditions that can occur concomitantly with the decubitus ulcer and can be coded in addition to code L89, if supported by the documentation.

The subcategory codes under L89.Ø indicate that the fifth character describes laterality. Locate the right elbow at subcategory L89.Ø1. See that an additional sixth character to specify the stage of the ulcer is now needed to complete the code. The stage can be determined either by the specific documentation of the stage (e.g., stage 1, stage 2) or, in this case, a description that matches one of the inclusion terms that follow each stage code. For example, the diagnostic description in this case of "skin loss and necrosis of the subcutaneous tissue" matches the inclusion term under L89.Ø13 Pressure ulcer of right elbow, stage 3. No additional characters are required because code L89.Ø13 is at its highest level of specificity.

Step 8: The official guidelines contain quite a bit of information relating to pressure ulcers in chapter-specific guideline I.C.12 as well as information in general guideline I.B.14. These and any other pertinent guidelines should be reviewed to ensure appropriate code assignment.

Step 9: Assign code L89.Ø13 Pressure ulcer of right elbow, stage 3.

Repeat steps 1 through 9 for any concomitant diagnoses.

Step 10: Since the decubitus ulcer is listed as the chief reason for the health care encounter, the first-listed, or principal, diagnosis is L89.Ø13. However, according to the code first instructional note at the L89 category level, gangrene (I96) would be sequenced before the pressure ulcer if it were documented.

Diagnosis: Emergency department visit for bimalleolar fracture of the right ankle due to trauma

Step 1: The reason for the encounter was the condition, bimalleolar fracture.

Step 2: Consult the alphabetic index.

Step 3: Locate the main term "Fracture." Note that many main terms represent fractures: "Fracture, burst," "Fracture, chronic," "Fracture, insufficiency," "Fracture, nontraumatic NEC," "Fracture, pathological," and "Fracture, traumatic." Since the diagnostic statement specifically states that this fracture was the result of trauma, the main term "Fracture, traumatic" should be used.

Step 4: Subterms that should be referenced are "ankle" and "bimalleolar (displaced)," which lists code S82.84-.

Step 5: A nonessential modifier (in parentheses) next to the term bimalleolar for "displaced" indicates that S82.84- is the default category unless the fracture is specifically identified as "nondisplaced."

Note that code S82.84- is followed by a dash and an additional-character icon, both of which indicate that more characters are required. From here, the tabular list can be consulted.

Step 6: Locate code S82.84- in the tabular list and read all instructional notes.

Step 7: The instructional notes at category S82 indicate that fractures not specified as displaced or nondisplaced default to displaced and that fractures not designated as open or closed default to closed. Additional instructional notes can be found at the category level but none pertain to the current scenario.

Read through the subcategory codes under S82.84, and note that the sixth character specifies displaced or nondisplaced and laterality. Based on the index nonessential modifier (displaced) and the code note at category S82, code selection should identify a displaced fracture of the right side. A displaced bimalleolar fracture of the right lower leg is coded to S82.841.

To complete the code, a seventh character must be assigned to identify the type of encounter (initial, subsequent, or sequela) and whether the fracture is open or closed. Most of the codes in category S82 require a seventh character represented in the list at the category level. However, it is important to note that some subcategories have their own specific set of seventh characters. In this instance, subcategory S82.84- does not have a unique set of seventh characters and the list provided at the category level should be used. Without documentation of the fracture being open, the tabular notation indicates that the default is closed. Character A, representing "initial encounter for closed fracture," listed in the box at the category level is the most appropriate option.

2023 ICD-10-CM Official Guidelines for Coding and Reporting

Narrative changes effective October 1, 2022 appear in **bold** text

Narrative changes effective April 1, 2022 appear in shaded text

Items underlined have been moved within the guidelines since the FY 2022 version

Italics are used to indicate revisions to heading changes

The Centers for Medicare and Medicaid Services (CMS) and the National Center for Health Statistics (NCHS), two departments within the U.S. Federal Government's Department of Health and Human Services (DHHS) provide the following guidelines for coding and reporting using the International Classification of Diseases, 10th Revision, Clinical Modification (ICD-10-CM). These guidelines should be used as a companion document to the official version of the ICD-10-CM as published on the NCHS website. The ICD-10-CM is a morbidity classification published by the United States for classifying diagnoses and reason for visits in all health care settings. The ICD-10-CM is based on the ICD-10, the statistical classification of disease published by the World Health Organization (WHO).

These guidelines have been approved by the four organizations that make up the Cooperating Parties for the ICD-10-CM: the American Hospital Association (AHA), the American Health Information Management Association (AHIMA), CMS, and NCHS.

These guidelines are a set of rules that have been developed to accompany and complement the official conventions and instructions provided within the ICD-10-CM itself. The instructions and conventions of the classification take precedence over guidelines. These guidelines are based on the coding and sequencing instructions in the Tabular List and Alphabetic Index of ICD-10-CM, but provide additional instruction. Adherence to these guidelines when assigning ICD-10-CM diagnosis codes is required under the Health Insurance Portability and Accountability Act (HIPAA). The diagnosis codes (Tabular List and Alphabetic Index) have been adopted under HIPAA for all healthcare settings. A joint effort between the healthcare provider and the coder is essential to achieve complete and accurate documentation, code assignment, and reporting of diagnoses and procedures. These guidelines have been developed to assist both the healthcare provider and the coder in identifying those diagnoses that are to be reported. The importance of consistent, complete documentation in the medical record cannot be overemphasized. Without such documentation accurate coding cannot be achieved. The entire record should be reviewed to determine the specific reason for the encounter and the conditions treated.

The term encounter is used for all settings, including hospital admissions. In the context of these guidelines, the term provider is used throughout the guidelines to mean physician or any qualified health care practitioner who is legally accountable for establishing the patient's diagnosis. Only this set of guidelines, approved by the Cooperating Parties, is official.

The guidelines are organized into sections. Section I includes the structure and conventions of the classification and general guidelines that apply to the entire classification, and chapter-specific guidelines that correspond to the chapters as they are arranged in the classification. Section II includes guidelines for selection of principal diagnosis for non-outpatient settings. Section III includes guidelines for reporting additional diagnoses in non-outpatient settings. Section IV is for outpatient coding and reporting. It is necessary to review all sections of the guidelines to fully understand all of the rules and instructions needed to code properly.

Section I. Conventions, general coding guidelines and chapter specific guidelines

The conventions, general guidelines and chapter-specific guidelines are applicable to all health care settings unless otherwise indicated. The conventions and instructions of the classification take precedence over guidelines.

A. Conventions for the ICD-10-CM

The conventions for the ICD-10-CM are the general rules for use of the classification independent of the guidelines. These conventions are incorporated within the Alphabetic Index and Tabular List of the ICD-10-CM as instructional notes.

1. The Alphabetic Index and Tabular List

The ICD-10-CM is divided into the Alphabetic Index, an alphabetical list of terms and their corresponding code, and the Tabular List, a structured list of codes divided into chapters based on body system or condition. The Alphabetic Index consists of the following parts: the Index of Diseases and Injury, the Index of External Causes of Injury, the Table of Neoplasms and the Table of Drugs and Chemicals.

See Section I.C.2. ***Neoplasms***

See Section I.C.19. Adverse effects, poisoning, underdosing and toxic effects

2. Format and Structure:

The ICD-10-CM Tabular List contains categories, subcategories and codes. Characters for categories, subcategories and codes may be either a letter or a number. All categories are 3 characters. A three-character category that has no further subdivision is equivalent to a code. Subcategories are either 4 or 5 characters. Codes may be 3, 4, 5, 6 or 7 characters. That is, each level of subdivision after a category is a subcategory. The final level of subdivision is a code. Codes that have applicable 7th characters are still referred to as codes, not subcategories. A code that has an applicable 7th character is considered invalid without the 7th character.

The ICD-10-CM uses an indented format for ease in reference.

3. Use of codes for reporting purposes

For reporting purposes only codes are permissible, not categories or subcategories, and any applicable 7th character is required.

4. Placeholder character

The ICD-10-CM utilizes a placeholder character "X". The "X" is used as a placeholder at certain codes to allow for future expansion. An example of this is at the poisoning, adverse effect and underdosing codes, categories T36-T5Ø. Where a placeholder exists, the X must be used in order for the code to be considered a valid code.

5. 7th Characters

Certain ICD-10-CM categories have applicable 7th characters. The applicable 7th character is required for all codes within the category, or as the notes in the Tabular List instruct. The 7th character must always be the 7th character in the data field. If a code that requires a 7th character is not 6 characters, a placeholder X must be used to fill in the empty characters.

6. Abbreviations

a. Alphabetic Index abbreviations

NEC "Not elsewhere classifiable"

This abbreviation in the Alphabetic Index represents "other specified." When a specific code is not available for a condition, the Alphabetic Index directs the coder to the "other specified" code in the Tabular List.

NOS "Not otherwise specified"

This abbreviation is the equivalent of unspecified.

b. Tabular List abbreviations

NEC "Not elsewhere classifiable"

This abbreviation in the Tabular List represents "other specified". When a specific code is not available for a condition, the Tabular List includes an NEC entry under a code to identify the code as the "other specified" code.

NOS "Not otherwise specified"

This abbreviation is the equivalent of unspecified.

7. Punctuation

[ ] Brackets are used in the Tabular List to enclose synonyms, alternative wording or explanatory phrases. Brackets are used in the Alphabetic Index to identify manifestation codes.

( ) Parentheses are used in both the Alphabetic Index and Tabular List to enclose supplementary words that may be present or absent in the statement of a disease or procedure without affecting the code number to which it is assigned. The terms within the parentheses are referred to as nonessential modifiers. The nonessential modifiers in the Alphabetic Index to Diseases apply to subterms following a main term except when a nonessential modifier and a subentry are mutually exclusive, the subentry takes precedence. For example, in the ICD-10-CM Alphabetic Index under the main term Enteritis, "acute" is a nonessential modifier and "chronic" is a subentry. In this case, the nonessential modifier "acute" does not apply to the subentry "chronic".

: Colons are used in the Tabular List after an incomplete term which needs one or more of the modifiers following the colon to make it assignable to a given category.

8. Use of "and".

See Section I.A.14. Use of the term "And"

9. Other and Unspecified codes

a. "Other" codes

Codes titled "other" or "other specified" are for use when the information in the medical record provides detail for which a specific code does not exist. Alphabetic Index entries with NEC in the line designate "other" codes in the Tabular List. These Alphabetic Index entries represent specific disease entities for which no specific code exists, so the term is included within an "other" code.

b. "Unspecified" codes

Codes titled "unspecified" are for use when the information in the medical record is insufficient to assign a more specific code. For those categories for which an unspecified code is not provided, the "other specified" code may represent both other and unspecified.

See Section I.B.18. Use of Signs/Symptom/Unspecified Codes

10. Includes Notes

This note appears immediately under a three-character code title to further define, or give examples of, the content of the category.

11. Inclusion terms

List of terms is included under some codes. These terms are the conditions for which that code is to be used. The terms may be synonyms of the code title, or, in the case of "other specified" codes, the terms are a list of the various conditions assigned to that code. The inclusion terms are not necessarily exhaustive. Additional terms found only in the Alphabetic Index may also be assigned to a code.

12. Excludes Notes

The ICD-10-CM has two types of excludes notes. Each type of note has a different definition for use, but they are all similar in that they indicate that codes excluded from each other are independent of each other.

a. Excludes1

A type 1 Excludes note is a pure excludes note. It means "NOT CODED HERE!" An Excludes1 note indicates that the code excluded should never be used at the same time as the code above the Excludes1 note. An Excludes1 is used when two conditions cannot occur together, such as a congenital form versus an acquired form of the same condition.

An exception to the Excludes1 definition is the circumstance when the two conditions are unrelated to each other. If it is not clear whether the two conditions involving an Excludes1 note are related or not, query the provider. For example, code F45.8, Other somatoform disorders, has an Excludes1 note for "sleep related teeth grinding (G47.63)," because "teeth grinding" is an inclusion term under F45.8. Only one of these two codes should be assigned for teeth grinding. However psychogenic dysmenorrhea is also an inclusion term under F45.8, and a patient could have both this condition and sleep related teeth grinding. In this case, the two conditions are clearly unrelated to each other, and so it would be appropriate to report F45.8 and G47.63 together.

b. Excludes2

A type 2 Excludes note represents "Not included here." An excludes2 note indicates that the condition excluded is not part of the condition represented by the code, but a patient may have both conditions at the same time. When an Excludes2 note appears under a code, it is acceptable to use both the code and the excluded code together, when appropriate.

13. Etiology/manifestation convention ("code first", "use additional code" and "in diseases classified elsewhere" notes)

Certain conditions have both an underlying etiology and multiple body system manifestations due to the underlying etiology. For such conditions, the ICD-10-CM has a coding convention that requires the underlying condition be sequenced first, if applicable, followed by the manifestation. Wherever such a combination exists, there is a "use additional code" note at the etiology code, and a "code first" note at the manifestation code. These instructional notes indicate the proper sequencing order of the codes, etiology followed by manifestation.

In most cases the manifestation codes will have in the code title, "in diseases classified elsewhere." Codes with this title are a component of the etiology/ manifestation convention. The code title indicates that it is a manifestation code. "In diseases classified elsewhere" codes are never permitted to be used as first listed or principal diagnosis codes. They must be used in conjunction with an underlying condition code and they must be listed following the underlying condition. See category F02, Dementia in other diseases classified elsewhere, for an example of this convention.

There are manifestation codes that do not have "in diseases classified elsewhere" in the title. For such codes, there is a "use additional code" note at the etiology code and a "code first" note at the manifestation code, and the rules for sequencing apply.

In addition to the notes in the Tabular List, these conditions also have a specific Alphabetic Index entry structure. In the Alphabetic Index both conditions are listed together with the etiology code first followed by the manifestation codes in brackets. The code in brackets is always to be sequenced second.

An example of the etiology/manifestation convention is dementia **with** Parkinson's disease. In the Alphabetic Index, code G20 is listed first, followed by code F02.80 or F02.81- in brackets. Code G20 represents the underlying etiology, Parkinson's disease, and must be sequenced first, whereas codes F02.80 and F02.81- represent the manifestation of dementia in diseases classified elsewhere, with or without behavioral disturbance.

"Code first" and "Use additional code" notes are also used as sequencing rules in the classification for certain codes that are not part of an etiology/ manifestation combination.

See Section I.B.7. Multiple coding for a single condition.

14. "And"

The word "and" should be interpreted to mean either "and" or "or" when it appears in a title.

For example, cases of "tuberculosis of bones", "tuberculosis of joints" and "tuberculosis of bones and joints" are classified to subcategory A18.0, Tuberculosis of bones and joints.

15. "With"

The word "with" or "in" should be interpreted to mean "associated with" or "due to" when it appears in a code title, the Alphabetic Index (either under a main term or subterm), or an instructional note in the Tabular List. The classification presumes a causal relationship between the two conditions linked by these terms in the Alphabetic Index or Tabular List. These conditions should be coded as related even in the absence of provider documentation explicitly linking them, unless the documentation clearly states the conditions are unrelated or when another guideline exists that specifically requires a documented linkage between two conditions (e.g., sepsis guideline for "acute organ dysfunction that is not clearly associated with the sepsis").

For conditions not specifically linked by these relational terms in the classification or when a guideline requires that a linkage between two conditions be explicitly documented, provider documentation must link the conditions in order to code them as related.

The word "with" in the Alphabetic Index is sequenced immediately following the main term or subterm, not in alphabetical order.

16. "See" and "See Also"

The "see" instruction following a main term in the Alphabetic Index indicates that another term should be referenced. It is necessary to go to the main term referenced with the "see" note to locate the correct code.

A "see also" instruction following a main term in the Alphabetic Index instructs that there is another main term that may also be referenced that may provide additional Alphabetic Index entries that may be useful. It is not necessary to follow the "see also" note when the original main term provides the necessary code.

17. "Code also" note

A "code also" note instructs that two codes may be required to fully describe a condition, but this note does not provide sequencing direction. The sequencing depends on the circumstances of the encounter.

18. Default codes

A code listed next to a main term in the ICD-10-CM Alphabetic Index is referred to as a default code. The default code represents that condition that is most commonly associated with the main term or is the unspecified code for the condition. If a condition is documented in a medical record (for example, appendicitis) without any additional information, such as acute or chronic, the default code should be assigned.

19. Code assignment and Clinical Criteria

The assignment of a diagnosis code is based on the provider's diagnostic statement that the condition exists. The provider's statement that the patient has a particular condition is sufficient. Code assignment is not based on clinical criteria used by the provider to establish the diagnosis. **If there is conflicting medical record documentation, query the provider.**

B. General Coding Guidelines

1. Locating a code in the ICD-10-CM

To select a code in the classification that corresponds to a diagnosis or reason for visit documented in a medical record, first locate the term in the Alphabetic Index, and then verify the code in the Tabular List. Read and be guided by instructional notations that appear in both the Alphabetic Index and the Tabular List.

It is essential to use both the Alphabetic Index and Tabular List when locating and assigning a code. The Alphabetic Index does not always provide the full code. Selection of the full code, including laterality and any applicable 7th character can only be done in the Tabular List. A dash (-) at the end of an Alphabetic Index entry indicates that additional characters are required. Even if a dash is not included at the Alphabetic Index entry, it is necessary to refer to the Tabular List to verify that no 7th character is required.

2. Level of Detail in Coding

Diagnosis codes are to be used and reported at their highest number of characters available and to the highest level of specificity documented in the medical record.

ICD-10-CM diagnosis codes are composed of codes with 3, 4, 5, 6 or 7 characters. Codes with three characters are included in ICD-10-CM as the heading of a category of codes that may be further subdivided by the use of fourth and/or fifth characters and/or sixth characters, which provide greater detail.

A three-character code is to be used only if it is not further subdivided. A code is invalid if it has not been coded to the full number of characters required for that code, including the 7th character, if applicable.

3. Code or codes from A00.0 through T88.9, Z00-Z99.8, U00-U85

The appropriate code or codes from A00.0 through T88.9, Z00-Z99.8, and U00-U85 must be used to identify diagnoses, symptoms, conditions, problems, complaints or other reason(s) for the encounter/visit.

4. Signs and symptoms

Codes that describe symptoms and signs, as opposed to diagnoses, are acceptable for reporting purposes when a related definitive diagnosis has not been established (confirmed) by the provider. Chapter 18 of ICD-10-CM, Symptoms, Signs, and Abnormal Clinical and Laboratory Findings, Not Elsewhere Classified (codes R00.0-R99) contains many, but not all, codes for symptoms.

See Section I.B.18. Use of Signs/Symptom/Unspecified Codes

5. Conditions that are an integral part of a disease process

Signs and symptoms that are associated routinely with a disease process should not be assigned as additional codes, unless otherwise instructed by the classification.

6. Conditions that are not an integral part of a disease process

Additional signs and symptoms that may not be associated routinely with a disease process should be coded when present.

7. Multiple coding for a single condition

In addition to the etiology/manifestation convention that requires two codes to fully describe a single condition that affects multiple body systems, there are other single conditions that also require more than one code. "Use additional code" notes are found in the Tabular List at codes that are not part of an etiology/manifestation pair where a secondary code is useful to fully describe a condition. The sequencing rule is the same as the etiology/manifestation pair, "use additional code" indicates that a secondary code should be added, if known.

For example, for bacterial infections that are not included in chapter 1, a secondary code from category B95, Streptococcus, Staphylococcus, and Enterococcus, as the cause of diseases classified elsewhere, or B96, Other bacterial agents as the cause of diseases classified elsewhere, may be required to identify the bacterial organism causing the infection. A "use additional code" note will normally be found at the infectious disease code, indicating a need for the organism code to be added as a secondary code.

"Code first" notes are also under certain codes that are not specifically manifestation codes but may be due to an underlying cause. When there is a "code first" note and an underlying condition is present, the underlying condition should be sequenced first, if known.

"Code, if applicable, any causal condition first" notes indicate that this code may be assigned as a principal diagnosis when the causal condition is unknown or not applicable. If a causal condition is known, then the code for that condition should be sequenced as the principal or first-listed diagnosis.

Multiple codes may be needed for sequela, complication codes and obstetric codes to more fully describe a condition. See the specific guidelines for these conditions for further instruction.

8. Acute and Chronic Conditions

If the same condition is described as both acute (subacute) and chronic, and separate subentries exist in the Alphabetic Index at the same indentation level, code both and sequence the acute (subacute) code first.

9. Combination Code

A combination code is a single code used to classify:

Two diagnoses, or

A diagnosis with an associated secondary process (manifestation)

A diagnosis with an associated complication

Combination codes are identified by referring to subterm entries in the Alphabetic Index and by reading the inclusion and exclusion notes in the Tabular List.

Assign only the combination code when that code fully identifies the diagnostic conditions involved or when the Alphabetic Index so directs. Multiple coding should not be used when the classification provides a combination code that clearly identifies all of the elements documented in the diagnosis. When the combination code lacks necessary specificity in describing the manifestation or complication, an additional code should be used as a secondary code.

10. Sequela (Late Effects)

A sequela is the residual effect (condition produced) after the acute phase of an illness or injury has terminated. There is no time limit on when a sequela code can be used. The residual may be apparent early, such as in cerebral infarction, or it may occur months or years later, such as that due to a previous injury. Examples of sequela include: scar formation resulting from a burn, deviated septum due to a nasal fracture, and infertility due to tubal occlusion from old tuberculosis. Coding of sequela generally requires two codes sequenced in the following order: the condition or nature of the sequela is sequenced first. The sequela code is sequenced second.

An exception to the above guidelines are those instances where the code for the sequela is followed by a manifestation code identified in the Tabular List and title, or the sequela code has been expanded (at the fourth, fifth or sixth character levels) to include the manifestation(s). The code for the acute phase of an illness or injury that led to the sequela is never used with a code for the late effect.

See Section I.C.9. Sequelae of cerebrovascular disease

See Section I.C.15. Sequelae of complication of pregnancy, childbirth and the puerperium

See Section I.C.19. Application of 7th characters for Chapter 19

11. Impending or Threatened Condition

Code any condition described at the time of discharge as “impending” or “threatened” as follows:

If it did occur, code as confirmed diagnosis.

If it did not occur, reference the Alphabetic Index to determine if the condition has a subentry term for “impending” or “threatened” and also reference main term entries for “Impending” and for “Threatened.”

If the subterms are listed, assign the given code.

If the subterms are not listed, code the existing underlying condition(s) and not the condition described as impending or threatened.

12. Reporting Same Diagnosis Code More than Once

Each unique ICD-10-CM diagnosis code may be reported only once for an encounter. This applies to bilateral conditions when there are no distinct codes identifying laterality or two different conditions classified to the same ICD-10-CM diagnosis code.

13. Laterality

Some ICD-10-CM codes indicate laterality, specifying whether the condition occurs on the left, right or is bilateral. If no bilateral code is provided and the condition is bilateral, assign separate codes for both the left and right side. If the side is not identified in the medical record, assign the code for the unspecified side.

When a patient has a bilateral condition and each side is treated during separate encounters, assign the “bilateral” code (as the condition still exists on both sides), including for the encounter to treat the first side. For the second encounter for treatment after one side has previously been treated and the condition no longer exists on that side, assign the appropriate unilateral code for the side where the condition still exists (e.g., cataract surgery performed on each eye in separate encounters). The bilateral code would not be assigned for the subsequent encounter, as the patient no longer has the condition in the previously-treated site. If the treatment on the first side did not completely resolve the condition, then the bilateral code would still be appropriate.

When laterality is not documented by the patient’s provider, code assignment for the affected side may be based on medical record documentation from other clinicians. If there is conflicting medical record documentation regarding the affected side, the patient’s attending provider should be queried for clarification. Codes for “unspecified” side should rarely be used, such as when the documentation in the record is insufficient to determine the affected side and it is not possible to obtain clarification.

14. Documentation by Clinicians Other than the Patient's Provider

Code assignment is based on the documentation by the patient's provider (i.e., physician or other qualified healthcare practitioner legally accountable for establishing the patient's diagnosis). There are a few exceptions when code assignment may be based on medical record documentation from clinicians who are not the patient’s provider (i.e., physician or other qualified healthcare practitioner legally accountable for establishing the patient’s diagnosis). In this context, “clinicians” other than the patient’s provider refer to healthcare professionals permitted, based on regulatory or accreditation requirements or internal hospital policies, to document in a patient’s official medical record.

These exceptions include codes for:

- Body Mass Index (BMI)
- Depth of non-pressure chronic ulcers
- Pressure ulcer stage
- Coma scale
- NIH stroke scale (NIHSS)
- Social determinants of health (SDOH)
- Laterality
- Blood alcohol level
- **Underimmunization status**

This information is typically, or may be, documented by other clinicians involved in the care of the patient (e.g., a dietitian often documents the BMI, a nurse often documents the pressure ulcer stages, and an emergency medical technician often documents the coma scale). However, the associated diagnosis (such as overweight, obesity, acute stroke, pressure ulcer, or a condition classifiable to category F1Ø, Alcohol related disorders) must be documented by the patient’s provider. If there is conflicting medical record documentation, either from the same clinician or different clinicians, the patient’s attending provider should be queried for clarification.

The BMI, coma scale, NIHSS, blood alcohol level codes, codes for social determinants of health **and underimmunization status** should only be reported as secondary diagnoses.

See Section I.C.21.c.17. for additional information regarding coding social determinants of health.

15. Syndromes

Follow the Alphabetic Index guidance when coding syndromes. In the absence of Alphabetic Index guidance, assign codes for the documented manifestations of the syndrome. Additional codes for manifestations that are not an integral part of the disease process may also be assigned when the condition does not have a unique code.

16. Documentation of Complications of Care

Code assignment is based on the provider’s documentation of the relationship between the condition and the care or procedure, unless otherwise instructed by the classification. The guideline extends to any complications of care, regardless of the chapter the code is located in. It is important to note that not all conditions that occur during or following medical care or surgery are classified as complications. There must be a cause-and-effect relationship between the care provided and the condition, and **the documentation must support that the condition is clinically significant. It is not necessary for the provider to explicitly document the term “complication.” For example, if the condition alters the course of the surgery as documented in the operative report, then it would be appropriate to report a complication code.** Query the provider for clarification **if the documentation is not clear as to the relationship between the condition and the care or procedure.**

17. Borderline Diagnosis

If the provider documents a “borderline” diagnosis at the time of discharge, the diagnosis is coded as confirmed, unless the classification provides a specific entry (e.g., borderline diabetes). If a borderline condition has a specific index entry in ICD-10-CM, it should be coded as such. Since borderline conditions are not uncertain diagnoses, no distinction is made between the care setting (inpatient versus outpatient). Whenever the documentation is unclear regarding a borderline condition, coders are encouraged to query for clarification.

18. Use of Sign/Symptom/Unspecified Codes

Sign/symptom and "unspecified" codes have acceptable, even necessary, uses. While specific diagnosis codes should be reported when they are supported by the available medical record documentation and clinical knowledge of the patient's health condition, there are instances when signs/symptoms or unspecified codes are the best choices for accurately reflecting the healthcare encounter. Each healthcare encounter should be coded to the level of certainty known for that encounter.

As stated in the introductory section of these official coding guidelines, a joint effort between the healthcare provider and the coder is essential to achieve complete and accurate documentation, code assignment, and reporting of diagnoses and procedures. The importance of consistent, complete documentation in the medical record cannot be overemphasized. Without such documentation accurate coding cannot be achieved. The entire record should be reviewed to determine the specific reason for the encounter and the conditions treated.

If a definitive diagnosis has not been established by the end of the encounter, it is appropriate to report codes for sign(s) and/or symptom(s) in lieu of a definitive diagnosis. When sufficient clinical information isn't known or available about a particular health condition to assign a more specific code, it is acceptable to report the appropriate "unspecified" code (e.g., a diagnosis of pneumonia has been determined, but not the specific type). Unspecified codes should be reported when they are the codes that most accurately reflect what is known about the patient's condition at the time of that particular encounter. It would be inappropriate to select a specific code that is not supported by the medical record documentation or conduct medically unnecessary diagnostic testing in order to determine a more specific code.

19. Coding for Healthcare Encounters in Hurricane Aftermath

a. Use of External Cause of Morbidity Codes

An external cause of morbidity code should be assigned to identify the cause of the injury(ies) incurred as a result of the hurricane. The use of external cause of morbidity codes is supplemental to the application of ICD-10-CM codes. External cause of morbidity codes are never to be recorded as a principal diagnosis (first-listed in non-inpatient settings). The appropriate injury code should be sequenced before any external cause codes. The external cause of morbidity codes capture how the injury or health condition happened (cause), the intent (unintentional or accidental; or intentional, such as suicide or assault), the place where the event occurred, the activity of the patient at the time of the event, and the person's status (e.g., civilian, military). They should not be assigned for encounters to treat hurricane victims' medical conditions when no injury, adverse effect or poisoning is involved. External cause of morbidity codes should be assigned for each encounter for care and treatment of the injury. External cause of morbidity codes may be assigned in all health care settings. For the purpose of capturing complete and accurate ICD-10-CM data in the aftermath of the hurricane, a healthcare setting should be considered as any location where medical care is provided by licensed healthcare professionals.

b. Sequencing of External Causes of Morbidity Codes

Codes for cataclysmic events, such as a hurricane, take priority over all other external cause codes except child and adult abuse and terrorism and should be sequenced before other external cause of injury codes. Assign as many external cause of morbidity codes as necessary to fully explain each cause. For example, if an injury occurs as a result of a building collapse during the hurricane, external cause codes for both the hurricane and the building collapse should be assigned, with the external causes code for hurricane being sequenced as the first external cause code. For injuries incurred as a direct result of the hurricane, assign the appropriate code(s) for the injuries, followed by the code X37.Ø-, Hurricane (with the appropriate 7th character), and any other applicable external cause of injury codes. Code X37.Ø- also should be assigned when an injury is incurred as a result of flooding caused by a levee breaking related to the hurricane. Code X38.-, Flood (with the appropriate 7th character), should be assigned when an injury is from flooding resulting directly from the storm. Code X36.Ø.-, Collapse of dam or man-made structure, should not be assigned when the cause of the collapse is due to the hurricane. Use of code X36.Ø- is limited to collapses of man-made structures due to earth surface movements, not due to storm surges directly from a hurricane.

c. Other External Causes of Morbidity Code Issues

For injuries that are not a direct result of the hurricane, such as an evacuee that has incurred an injury as a result of a motor vehicle accident, assign the appropriate external cause of morbidity code(s) to describe the cause of the injury, but do not assign code X37.Ø-, Hurricane. If it is not clear whether the injury was a direct result of the hurricane, assume the injury is due to the hurricane and assign code X37.Ø-, Hurricane, as well as any other applicable external cause of morbidity codes. In addition to code X37.Ø-, Hurricane, other possible applicable external cause of morbidity codes include:

X3Ø-, Exposure to excessive natural heat
X31-, Exposure to excessive natural cold
X38-, Flood

d. Use of Z codes

Z codes (other reasons for healthcare encounters) may be assigned as appropriate to further explain the reasons for presenting for healthcare services, including transfers between healthcare facilities, or provide additional information relevant to a patient encounter. The ICD-10-CM Official Guidelines for Coding and Reporting identify which codes maybe assigned as principal or first-listed diagnosis only, secondary diagnosis only, or principal/first-listed or secondary (depending on the circumstances). Possible applicable Z codes include:

Z59.Ø-, Homelessness
Z59.1, Inadequate housing
Z59.5, Extreme poverty
Z75.1, Person awaiting admission to adequate facility elsewhere
Z75.3, Unavailability and inaccessibility of health-care facilities
Z75.4, Unavailability and inaccessibility of other helping agencies
Z76.2, Encounter for health supervision and care of other healthy infant and child
Z99.12, Encounter for respirator [ventilator] dependence during power failure

The external cause of morbidity codes and the Z codes listed above are not an all-inclusive list. Other codes may be applicable to the encounter based upon the documentation. Assign as many codes as necessary to fully explain each healthcare encounter. Since patient history information may be very limited, use any available documentation to assign the appropriate external cause of morbidity and Z codes.

C. Chapter-Specific Coding Guidelines

In addition to general coding guidelines, there are guidelines for specific diagnoses and/or conditions in the classification. Unless otherwise indicated, these guidelines apply to all health care settings. Please refer to Section II for guidelines on the selection of principal diagnosis.

1. Chapter 1: Certain Infectious and Parasitic Diseases (AØØ-B99), UØ7.1, UØ9.9

a. Human Immunodeficiency Virus (HIV) Infections

1) Code only confirmed cases

Code only confirmed cases of HIV infection/illness. This is an exception to the hospital inpatient guideline Section II, H.

In this context, "confirmation" does not require documentation of positive serology or culture for HIV; the provider's diagnostic statement that the patient is HIV positive or has an HIV-related illness is sufficient.

2) Selection and sequencing of HIV codes

(a) Patient admitted for HIV-related condition

If a patient is admitted for an HIV-related condition, the principal diagnosis should be B2Ø, Human immunodeficiency virus [HIV] disease followed by additional diagnosis codes for all reported HIV-related conditions.

An exception to this guideline is if the reason for admission is hemolytic-uremic syndrome associated with HIV disease. Assign code D59.31, Infection-associated hemolytic-uremic syndrome, followed by code B2Ø, Human immunodeficiency virus [HIV] disease.

(b) Patient with HIV disease admitted for unrelated condition

If a patient with HIV disease is admitted for an unrelated condition (such as a traumatic injury), the code for the unrelated condition (e.g., the nature of injury code) should be the principal diagnosis. Other diagnoses would be B2Ø followed by additional diagnosis codes for all reported HIV-related conditions.

(c) Whether the patient is newly diagnosed

Whether the patient is newly diagnosed or has had previous admissions/encounters for HIV conditions is irrelevant to the sequencing decision.

(d) Asymptomatic human immunodeficiency virus

Z21, Asymptomatic human immunodeficiency virus [HIV] infection status, is to be applied when the patient without any documentation of symptoms is listed as being "HIV positive," "known HIV," "HIV test positive," or similar terminology. Do not use this code if the term "AIDS" or "HIV disease" is used or if the patient is treated for any HIV-related illness or is described as having any condition(s) resulting from his/her HIV positive status; use B2Ø in these cases.

(e) Patients with inconclusive HIV serology
Patients with inconclusive HIV serology, but no definitive diagnosis or manifestations of the illness, may be assigned code R75, Inconclusive laboratory evidence of human immunodeficiency virus [HIV].

(f) Previously diagnosed HIV-related illness
Patients with any known prior diagnosis of an HIV-related illness should be coded to B2Ø. Once a patient has developed an HIV-related illness, the patient should always be assigned code B2Ø on every subsequent admission/encounter. Patients previously diagnosed with any HIV illness (B2Ø) should never be assigned to R75 or Z21, Asymptomatic human immunodeficiency virus [HIV] infection status.

(g) HIV Infection in Pregnancy, Childbirth and the Puerperium
During pregnancy, childbirth or the puerperium, a patient admitted (or presenting for a health care encounter) because of an HIV-related illness should receive a principal diagnosis code of O98.7-, Human immunodeficiency [HIV] disease complicating pregnancy, childbirth and the puerperium, followed by B2Ø and the code(s) for the HIV-related illness(es). Codes from Chapter 15 always take sequencing priority.

Patients with asymptomatic HIV infection status admitted (or presenting for a health care encounter) during pregnancy, childbirth, or the puerperium should receive codes of O98.7- and Z21.

(h) Encounters for testing for HIV
If a patient is being seen to determine his/her HIV status, use code Z11.4, Encounter for screening for human immunodeficiency virus [HIV]. Use additional codes for any associated high-risk behavior, if applicable.

If a patient with signs or symptoms is being seen for HIV testing, code the signs and symptoms. An additional counseling code Z71.7, Human immunodeficiency virus [HIV] counseling, may be used if counseling is provided during the encounter for the test.

When a patient returns to be informed of his/her HIV test results and the test result is negative, use code Z71.7, Human immunodeficiency virus [HIV] counseling.

If the results are positive, see previous guidelines and assign codes as appropriate.

(i) HIV managed by antiretroviral medication
If a patient with documented HIV disease, **HIV-related illness or AIDS** is currently managed on antiretroviral medications, assign code B2Ø, Human immunodeficiency virus [HIV] disease. Code Z79.899, Other long term (current) drug therapy, may be assigned as an additional code to identify the long-term (current) use of antiretroviral medications.

b. Infectious agents as the cause of diseases classified to other chapters
Certain infections are classified in chapters other than Chapter 1 and no organism is identified as part of the infection code. In these instances, it is necessary to use an additional code from Chapter 1 to identify the organism. A code from category B95, Streptococcus, Staphylococcus, and Enterococcus as the cause of diseases classified to other chapters, B96, Other bacterial agents as the cause of diseases classified to other chapters, or B97, Viral agents as the cause of diseases classified to other chapters, is to be used as an additional code to identify the organism. An instructional note will be found at the infection code advising that an additional organism code is required.

c. Infections resistant to antibiotics
Many bacterial infections are resistant to current antibiotics. It is necessary to identify all infections documented as antibiotic resistant. Assign a code from category Z16, Resistance to antimicrobial drugs, following the infection code only if the infection code does not identify drug resistance.

d. Sepsis, Severe Sepsis, and Septic Shock Infections resistant to antibiotics

1) Coding of Sepsis and Severe Sepsis

(a) Sepsis
For a diagnosis of sepsis, assign the appropriate code for the underlying systemic infection. If the type of infection or causal organism is not further specified, assign code A41.9, Sepsis, unspecified organism.

A code from subcategory R65.2, Severe sepsis, should not be assigned unless severe sepsis or an associated acute organ dysfunction is documented.

(i) Negative or inconclusive blood cultures and sepsis
Negative or inconclusive blood cultures do not preclude a diagnosis of sepsis in patients with clinical evidence of the condition; however, the provider should be queried.

(ii) Urosepsis
The term urosepsis is a nonspecific term. It is not to be considered synonymous with sepsis. It has no default code in the Alphabetic Index. Should a provider use this term, he/she must be queried for clarification.

(iii) Sepsis with organ dysfunction
If a patient has sepsis and associated acute organ dysfunction or multiple organ dysfunction (MOD), follow the instructions for coding severe sepsis.

(iv) Acute organ dysfunction that is not clearly associated with the sepsis
If a patient has sepsis and an acute organ dysfunction, but the medical record documentation indicates that the acute organ dysfunction is related to a medical condition other than the sepsis, do not assign a code from subcategory R65.2, Severe sepsis. An acute organ dysfunction must be associated with the sepsis in order to assign the severe sepsis code. If the documentation is not clear as to whether an acute organ dysfunction is related to the sepsis or another medical condition, query the provider.

(b) Severe sepsis
The coding of severe sepsis requires a minimum of 2 codes: first a code for the underlying systemic infection, followed by a code from subcategory R65.2, Severe sepsis. If the causal organism is not documented, assign code A41.9, Sepsis, unspecified organism, for the infection. Additional code(s) for the associated acute organ dysfunction are also required.

Due to the complex nature of severe sepsis, some cases may require querying the provider prior to assignment of the codes.

2) Septic shock
Septic shock generally refers to circulatory failure associated with severe sepsis, and therefore, it represents a type of acute organ dysfunction.

For cases of septic shock, the code for the systemic infection should be sequenced first, followed by code R65.21, Severe sepsis with septic shock or code T81.12, Postprocedural septic shock.

Any additional codes for the other acute organ dysfunctions should also be assigned. As noted in the sequencing instructions in the Tabular List, the code for septic shock cannot be assigned as a principal diagnosis.

3) Sequencing of severe sepsis
If severe sepsis is present on admission, and meets the definition of principal diagnosis, the underlying systemic infection should be assigned as principal diagnosis followed by the appropriate code from subcategory R65.2 as required by the sequencing rules in the Tabular List. A code from subcategory R65.2 can never be assigned as a principal diagnosis.

When severe sepsis develops during an encounter (it was not present on admission), the underlying systemic infection and the appropriate code from subcategory R65.2 should be assigned as secondary diagnoses.

Severe sepsis may be present on admission, but the diagnosis may not be confirmed until sometime after admission. If the documentation is not clear whether severe sepsis was present on admission, the provider should be queried.

For infection-associated hemolytic-uremic syndrome with severe sepsis, see guideline I.C.1.d.9.

4) Sepsis or severe sepsis with a localized infection

If the reason for admission is sepsis or severe sepsis and a localized infection, such as pneumonia or cellulitis, a code(s) for the underlying systemic infection should be assigned first and the code for the localized infection should be assigned as a secondary diagnosis. If the patient has severe sepsis, a code from subcategory R65.2 should also be assigned as a secondary diagnosis. If the patient is admitted with a localized infection, such as pneumonia, and sepsis/severe sepsis doesn't develop until after admission, the localized infection should be assigned first, followed by the appropriate sepsis/severe sepsis codes.

For hemolytic-uremic syndrome associated with sepsis, see guideline I.C.1.d.9.

5) Sepsis due to a postprocedural infection

(a) Documentation of causal relationship

As with all postprocedural complications, code assignment is based on the provider's documentation of the relationship between the infection and the procedure.

(b) Sepsis due to a postprocedural infection

For infections following a procedure, a code from T81.4Ø, to T81.43 Infection following a procedure, or a code from O86.ØØ to O86.Ø3, Infection of obstetric surgical wound, that identifies the site of the infection should be coded first, if known. Assign an additional code for sepsis following a procedure (T81.44) or sepsis following an obstetrical procedure (O86.Ø4). Use an additional code to identify the infectious agent. If the patient has severe sepsis, the appropriate code from subcategory R65.2 should also be assigned with the additional code(s) for any acute organ dysfunction.

For infections following infusion, transfusion, therapeutic injection, or immunization, a code from subcategory T8Ø.2, Infections following infusion, transfusion, and therapeutic injection, or code T88.Ø-, Infection following immunization, should be coded first, followed by the code for the specific infection. If the patient has severe sepsis, the appropriate code from subcategory R65.2 should also be assigned, with the additional codes(s) for any acute organ dysfunction.

(c) Postprocedural infection and postprocedural septic shock

If a postprocedural infection has resulted in postprocedural septic shock, assign the codes indicated above for sepsis due to a postprocedural infection, followed by code T81.12-, Postprocedural septic shock. Do not assign code R65.21, Severe sepsis with septic shock. Additional code(s) should be assigned for any acute organ dysfunction.

6) Sepsis and severe sepsis associated with a noninfectious process (condition)

In some cases, a noninfectious process (condition) such as trauma, may lead to an infection which can result in sepsis or severe sepsis. If sepsis or severe sepsis is documented as associated with a noninfectious condition, such as a burn or serious injury, and this condition meets the definition for principal diagnosis, the code for the noninfectious condition should be sequenced first, followed by the code for the resulting infection. If severe sepsis is present, a code from subcategory R65.2 should also be assigned with any associated organ dysfunction(s) codes. It is not necessary to assign a code from subcategory R65.1, Systemic inflammatory response syndrome (SIRS) of non-infectious origin, for these cases.

If the infection meets the definition of principal diagnosis, it should be sequenced before the non-infectious condition. When both the associated non-infectious condition and the infection meet the definition of principal diagnosis, either may be assigned as principal diagnosis.

Only one code from category R65, Symptoms and signs specifically associated with systemic inflammation and infection, should be assigned. Therefore, when a non-infectious condition leads to an infection resulting in severe sepsis, assign the appropriate code from subcategory R65.2, Severe sepsis. Do not additionally assign a code from subcategory R65.1, Systemic inflammatory response syndrome (SIRS) of non-infectious origin.

See Section I.C.18. SIRS due to non-infectious process

7) Sepsis and septic shock complicating abortion, pregnancy, childbirth, and the puerperium

See Section I.C.15. Sepsis and septic shock complicating abortion, pregnancy, childbirth and the puerperium

8) Newborn sepsis

See Section I.C.16. f. Bacterial sepsis of Newborn

9) Hemolytic-uremic syndrome associated with sepsis

If the reason for admission is hemolytic-uremic syndrome that is associated with sepsis, assign code D59.31, Infection-associated hemolytic-uremic syndrome, as the principal diagnosis. Codes for the underlying systemic infection and any other conditions (such as severe sepsis) should be assigned as secondary diagnoses.

e. Methicillin Resistant Staphylococcus aureus (MRSA) Conditions

1) Selection and sequencing of MRSA codes

(a) Combination codes for MRSA infection

When a patient is diagnosed with an infection that is due to methicillin resistant *Staphylococcus aureus* (MRSA), and that infection has a combination code that includes the causal organism (e.g., sepsis, pneumonia) assign the appropriate combination code for the condition (e.g., code A41.Ø2, Sepsis due to Methicillin resistant Staphylococcus aureus or code J15.212, Pneumonia due to Methicillin resistant Staphylococcus aureus). Do not assign code B95.62, Methicillin resistant Staphylococcus aureus infection as the cause of diseases classified elsewhere, as an additional code, because the combination code includes the type of infection and the MRSA organism. Do not assign a code from subcategory Z16.11, Resistance to penicillins, as an additional diagnosis.

See Section C.1. for instructions on coding and sequencing of sepsis and severe sepsis.

(b) Other codes for MRSA infection

When there is documentation of a current infection (e.g., wound infection, stitch abscess, urinary tract infection) due to MRSA, and that infection does not have a combination code that includes the causal organism, assign the appropriate code to identify the condition along with code B95.62, Methicillin resistant Staphylococcus aureus infection as the cause of diseases classified elsewhere for the MRSA infection. Do not assign a code from subcategory Z16.11, Resistance to penicillins.

(c) Methicillin susceptible Staphylococcus aureus (MSSA) and MRSA colonization

The condition or state of being colonized or carrying MSSA or MRSA is called colonization or carriage, while an individual person is described as being colonized or being a carrier.

Colonization means that MSSA or MSRA is present on or in the body without necessarily causing illness. A positive MRSA colonization test might be documented by the provider as "MRSA screen positive" or "MRSA nasal swab positive".

Assign code Z22.322, Carrier or suspected carrier of Methicillin resistant Staphylococcus aureus, for patients documented as having MRSA colonization. Assign code Z22.321, Carrier or suspected carrier of Methicillin susceptible Staphylococcus aureus, for patients documented as having MSSA colonization. Colonization is not necessarily indicative of a disease process or as the cause of a specific condition the patient may have unless documented as such by the provider.

(d) MRSA colonization and infection

If a patient is documented as having both MRSA colonization and infection during a hospital admission, code Z22.322, Carrier or suspected carrier of Methicillin resistant Staphylococcus aureus, and a code for the MRSA infection may both be assigned.

f. Zika virus infections

1) Code only confirmed cases

Code only a confirmed diagnosis of Zika virus (A92.5, Zika virus disease) as documented by the provider. This is an exception to the hospital inpatient guideline Section II, H. In this context, "confirmation" does not require documentation of the type of test performed; the provider's diagnostic statement that the condition is confirmed is sufficient. This code should be assigned regardless of the stated mode of transmission.

If the provider documents "suspected", "possible" or "probable" Zika, do not assign code A92.5. Assign a code(s) explaining the reason for encounter (such as fever, rash, or joint pain) or Z2Ø.821, Contact with and (suspected) exposure to Zika virus.

g. Coronavirus infections

1) COVID-19 infection (infection due to SARS-CoV-2)

(a) Code only confirmed cases

Code only a confirmed diagnosis of the 2019 novel coronavirus disease (COVID-19) as documented by the provider, or documentation of a positive COVID-19 test result. For a confirmed diagnosis, assign code UØ7.1, COVID-19. This is an exception to the hospital inpatient guideline Section II, H. In this context, "confirmation" does not require documentation of a positive test result for COVID-19; the provider's documentation that the individual has COVID-19 is sufficient.

If the provider documents "suspected," "possible," "probable," or "inconclusive" COVID-19, do not assign code UØ7.1. Instead, code the signs and symptoms reported. See guideline I.C.1.g.1.g.

(b) Sequencing of codes

When COVID-19 meets the definition of principal diagnosis, code UØ7.1, COVID-19, should be sequenced first, followed by the appropriate codes for associated manifestations, except when another guideline requires that certain codes be sequenced first, such as obstetrics, sepsis, or transplant complications.

For a COVID-19 infection that progresses to sepsis, see Section I.C.1.d. Sepsis, Severe Sepsis, and Septic Shock

See Section I.C.15.s. for COVID-19 infection in pregnancy, childbirth, and the puerperium

See Section I.C.16.h. for COVID-19 infection in newborn

For a COVID-19 infection in a lung transplant patient, see Section I.C.19.g.3.a. Transplant complications other than kidney.

(c) Acute respiratory manifestations of COVID-19

When the reason for the encounter/admission is a respiratory manifestation of COVID-19, assign code UØ7.1, COVID-19, as the principal/first-listed diagnosis and assign code(s) for the respiratory manifestation(s) as additional diagnoses.

The following conditions are examples of common respiratory manifestations of COVID-19.

(i) Pneumonia

For a patient with pneumonia confirmed as due to COVID-19, assign codes UØ7.1, COVID-19, and J12.82, Pneumonia due to coronavirus disease 2019.

(ii) Acute bronchitis

For a patient with acute bronchitis confirmed as due to COVID-19, assign codes UØ7.1, and J2Ø.8, Acute bronchitis due to other specified organisms.

Bronchitis not otherwise specified (NOS) due to COVID-19 should be coded using code UØ7.1 and J4Ø, Bronchitis, not specified as acute or chronic.

(iii) Lower respiratory infection

If the COVID-19 is documented as being associated with a lower respiratory infection, not otherwise specified (NOS), or an acute respiratory infection, NOS, codes UØ7.1 and J22, Unspecified acute lower respiratory infection, should be assigned.

If the COVID-19 is documented as being associated with a respiratory infection, NOS, codes UØ7.1 and J98.8, Other specified respiratory disorders, should be assigned.

(iv) Acute respiratory distress syndrome

For acute respiratory distress syndrome (ARDS) due to COVID-19, assign codes UØ7.1, and J8Ø, Acute respiratory distress syndrome.

(v) Acute respiratory failure

For acute respiratory failure due to COVID-19, assign code UØ7.1, and code J96.Ø-, Acute respiratory failure.

(d) Non-respiratory manifestations of COVID-19

When the reason for the encounter/admission is a non-respiratory manifestation (e.g., viral enteritis) of COVID-19, assign code UØ7.1, COVID-19, as the principal/first-listed diagnosis and assign code(s) for the manifestation(s) as additional diagnoses.

(e) Exposure to COVID-19

For asymptomatic individuals with actual or suspected exposure to COVID-19, assign code Z2Ø.822, Contact with and (suspected) exposure to COVID-19.

For symptomatic individuals with actual or suspected exposure to COVID-19 and the infection has been ruled out, or test results are inconclusive or unknown, assign code Z2Ø.822, Contact with and (suspected) exposure to COVID-19. See guideline I.C.21.c.1, Contact/Exposure, for additional guidance regarding the use of category Z2Ø codes.

If COVID-19 is confirmed, see guideline I.C.1.g.1.a.

(f) Screening for COVID-19

During the COVID-19 pandemic, a screening code is generally not appropriate. Do not assign code Z11.52, Encounter for screening for COVID-19. For encounters for COVID-19 testing, including preoperative testing, code as exposure to COVID-19 (guideline I.C.1.g.1.e).

Coding guidance will be updated as new information concerning any changes in the pandemic status becomes available.

(g) Signs and symptoms without definitive diagnosis of COVID-19

For patients presenting with any signs/symptoms associated with COVID-19 (such as fever, etc.) but a definitive diagnosis has not been established, assign the appropriate code(s) for each of the presenting signs and symptoms such as:

- RØ5.1, Acute cough, or RØ5.9, Cough, unspecified
- RØ6.Ø2 Shortness of breath
- R5Ø.9 Fever, unspecified

If a patient with signs/symptoms associated with COVID-19 also has an actual or suspected contact with or exposure to COVID-19, assign Z2Ø.822, Contact with and (suspected) exposure to COVID-19, as an additional code.

(h) Asymptomatic individuals who test positive for COVID-19

For asymptomatic individuals who test positive for COVID-19, see guideline I.C.1.g.1.a. Although the individual is asymptomatic, the individual has tested positive and is considered to have the COVID-19 infection.

(i) Personal history of COVID-19

For patients with a history of COVID-19, assign code Z86.16, Personal history of COVID-19.

(j) Follow-up visits after COVID-19 infection has resolved

For individuals who previously had COVID-19, without residual symptom(s) or condition(s), and are being seen for follow-up evaluation, and COVID-19 test results are negative, assign codes ZØ9, Encounter for follow-up examination after completed treatment for conditions other than malignant neoplasm, and Z86.16, Personal history of COVID-19.

For follow-up visits for individuals with symptom(s) or condition(s) related to a previous COVID-19 infection, see guideline I.C.1.g.1.m.

See Section I.C.21.c.8, Factors influencing health states and contact with health services, Follow-up

(k) Encounter for antibody testing

For an encounter for antibody testing that is not being performed to confirm a current COVID-19 infection, nor is a follow-up test after resolution of COVID-19, assign ZØ1.84, Encounter for antibody response examination.

Follow the applicable guidelines above if the individual is being tested to confirm a current COVID-19 infection.

For follow-up testing after a COVID-19 infection, see guideline I.C.1.g.1.j.

(l) Multisystem Inflammatory Syndrome

For individuals with multisystem inflammatory syndrome (MIS) and COVID-19, assign code UØ7.1, COVID-19, as the principal/first-listed diagnosis and assign code M35.81, Multisystem inflammatory syndrome, as an additional diagnosis.

If an individual with a history of COVID-19 develops MIS, assign codes M35.81, Multisystem inflammatory syndrome, and UØ9.9, Post COVID-19 condition, unspecified.

If an individual with a known or suspected exposure to COVID-19, and no current COVID-19 infection or history of

COVID-19, develops MIS, assign codes M35.81, Multisystem inflammatory syndrome, and Z20.822, Contact with and (suspected) exposure to COVID-19.

Additional codes should be assigned for any associated complications of MIS.

(m) Post COVID-19 Condition

For sequela of COVID-19, or associated symptoms or conditions that develop following a previous COVID-19 infection, assign a code(s) for the specific symptom(s) or condition(s) related to the previous COVID-19 infection, if known, and code U09.9, Post COVID-19 condition, unspecified.

Code U09.9 should not be assigned for manifestations of an active (current) COVID-19 infection.

If a patient has a condition(s) associated with a previous COVID-19 infection and develops a new active (current) COVID-19 infection, code U09.9 may be assigned in conjunction with code U07.1, COVID-19, to identify that the patient also has a condition(s) associated with a previous COVID-19 infection. Code(s) for the specific condition(s) associated with the previous COVID-19 infection and code(s) for manifestation(s) of the new active (current) COVID-19 infection should also be assigned.

(n) Underimmunization for COVID-19 Status

Code Z28.310, Unvaccinated for COVID-19, may be assigned when the patient has not received **a** COVID-19 vaccine **of any type.** Code Z28.311, Partially vaccinated for COVID-19, may be assigned when the patient has **been partially vaccinated for COVID-19 as per the recommendations of** the Centers for Disease Control and Prevention (CDC) in place at the time of the encounter. For information, visit the CDC's website https://www.cdc.gov/coronavirus/2019-ncov/vaccines/.

See Section I.B.14. for underimmunization documentation by clinicians other than patient's provider.

2. Chapter 2: Neoplasms (C00-D49)

General Guidelines

Chapter 2 of the ICD-10-CM contains the codes for most benign and all malignant neoplasms. Certain benign neoplasms, such as prostatic adenomas, may be found in the specific body system chapters. To properly code a neoplasm, it is necessary to determine from the record if the neoplasm is benign, in-situ, malignant, or of uncertain histologic behavior. If malignant, any secondary (metastatic) sites should also be determined.

Primary malignant neoplasms overlapping site boundaries

A primary malignant neoplasm that overlaps two or more contiguous (next to each other) sites should be classified to the subcategory/code .8 ('overlapping lesion'), unless the combination is specifically indexed elsewhere. For multiple neoplasms of the same site that are not contiguous such as tumors in different quadrants of the same breast, codes for each site should be assigned.

Malignant neoplasm of ectopic tissue

Malignant neoplasms of ectopic tissue are to be coded to the site of origin mentioned, e.g., ectopic pancreatic malignant neoplasms involving the stomach are coded to malignant neoplasm of pancreas, unspecified (C25.9).

The neoplasm table in the Alphabetic Index should be referenced first. However, if the histological term is documented, that term should be referenced first, rather than going immediately to the Neoplasm Table, in order to determine which column in the Neoplasm Table is appropriate. For example, if the documentation indicates "adenoma," refer to the term in the Alphabetic Index to review the entries under this term and the instructional note to "see also neoplasm, by site, benign." The table provides the proper code based on the type of neoplasm and the site. It is important to select the proper column in the table that corresponds to the type of neoplasm. The Tabular List should then be referenced to verify that the correct code has been selected from the table and that a more specific site code does not exist.

See Section I.C.21. Factors influencing health status and contact with health services, Status, for information regarding Z15.0, codes for genetic susceptibility to cancer.

a. ***Admission/Encounter for treatment of primary site***

If the malignancy **is chiefly responsible for occasioning the patient admission/encounter and treatment is directed at the primary site**, designate the **primary** malignancy as the principal/**first-listed** diagnosis.

The only exception to this guideline is if the administration of chemotherapy, immunotherapy or external beam radiation therapy **is chiefly responsible for occasioning the admission/encounter. In that case**, assign the appropriate Z51.-- code as the first-listed or principal diagnosis, and the **underlying** diagnosis or problem for which the service is being performed as a secondary diagnosis.

b. ***Admission/Encounter for*** **treatment of secondary site**

When a patient is admitted because of a primary neoplasm with metastasis and treatment is directed toward the secondary site only, the secondary neoplasm is designated as the principal diagnosis even though the primary malignancy is still present.

c. Coding and sequencing of complications

Coding and sequencing of complications associated with the malignancies or with the therapy thereof are subject to the following guidelines:

1) Anemia associated with malignancy

When admission/encounter is for management of an anemia associated with the malignancy, and the treatment is only for anemia, the appropriate code for the malignancy is sequenced as the principal or first-listed diagnosis followed by the appropriate code for the anemia (such as code D63.0, Anemia in neoplastic disease).

2) Anemia associated with chemotherapy, immunotherapy and radiation therapy

When the admission/encounter is for management of an anemia associated with an adverse effect of the administration of chemotherapy or immunotherapy and the only treatment is for the anemia, the anemia code is sequenced first followed by the appropriate codes for the neoplasm and the adverse effect (T45.1X5-, Adverse effect of antineoplastic and immunosuppressive drugs).

When the admission/encounter is for management of an anemia associated with an adverse effect of radiotherapy, the anemia code should be sequenced first, followed by the appropriate neoplasm code and code Y84.2, Radiological procedure and radiotherapy as the cause of abnormal reaction of the patient, or of later complication, without mention of misadventure at the time of the procedure.

3) Management of dehydration due to the malignancy

When the admission/encounter is for management of dehydration due to the malignancy and only the dehydration is being treated (intravenous rehydration), the dehydration is sequenced first, followed by the code(s) for the malignancy.

4) Treatment of a complication resulting from a surgical procedure

When the admission/encounter is for treatment of a complication resulting from a surgical procedure, designate the complication as the principal or first-listed diagnosis if treatment is directed at resolving the complication.

d. Primary malignancy previously excised

When a primary malignancy has been previously excised or eradicated from its site and there is no further treatment directed to that site and there is no evidence of any existing primary malignancy at that site, a code from category Z85, Personal history of malignant neoplasm, should be used to indicate the former site of the malignancy. Any mention of extension, invasion, or metastasis to another site is coded as a secondary malignant neoplasm to that site. The secondary site may be the principal or first-listed diagnosis with the Z85 code used as a secondary code.

See section I.C.2.t. Secondary malignant neoplasm of lymphoid tissue.

e. Admissions/Encounters involving chemotherapy, immunotherapy and radiation therapy

1) Episode of care involves surgical removal of neoplasm

When an episode of care involves the surgical removal of a neoplasm, primary or secondary site, followed by adjunct chemotherapy or radiation treatment during the same episode of care, the code for the neoplasm should be assigned as principal or first-listed diagnosis.

2) Patient admission/encounter solely for administration of chemotherapy, immunotherapy and radiation therapy

If a patient admission/encounter is solely for the administration of chemotherapy, immunotherapy or external beam radiation therapy assign code Z51.0, Encounter for antineoplastic radiation therapy, or Z51.11, Encounter for antineoplastic chemotherapy, or Z51.12, Encounter for antineoplastic immunotherapy as the first-listed or principal diagnosis. If a patient receives more than one of these therapies during the same admission more than one of these codes may be assigned, in any sequence.

The malignancy for which the therapy is being administered should be assigned as a secondary diagnosis.

If a patient admission/encounter is for the insertion or implantation of radioactive elements (e.g., brachytherapy) the appropriate code for the malignancy is sequenced as the principal or first-listed diagnosis. Code Z51.Ø should not be assigned.

3) **Patient admitted for radiation therapy, chemotherapy or immunotherapy and develops complications**
When a patient is admitted for the purpose of external beam radiotherapy, immunotherapy or chemotherapy and develops complications such as uncontrolled nausea and vomiting or dehydration, the principal or first-listed diagnosis is Z51.Ø, Encounter for antineoplastic radiation therapy, or Z51.11, Encounter for antineoplastic chemotherapy, or Z51.12, Encounter for antineoplastic immunotherapy followed by any codes for the complications.

When a patient is admitted for the purpose of insertion or implantation of radioactive elements (e.g., brachytherapy) and develops complications such as uncontrolled nausea and vomiting or dehydration, the principal or first-listed diagnosis is the appropriate code for the malignancy followed by any codes for the complications.

f. **Admission/encounter to determine extent of malignancy**
When the reason for admission/encounter is to determine the extent of the malignancy, or for a procedure such as paracentesis or thoracentesis, the primary malignancy or appropriate metastatic site is designated as the principal or first-listed diagnosis, even though chemotherapy or radiotherapy is administered.

g. **Symptoms, signs, and abnormal findings listed in Chapter 18 associated with neoplasms**
Symptoms, signs, and ill-defined conditions listed in Chapter 18 characteristic of, or associated with, an existing primary or secondary site malignancy cannot be used to replace the malignancy as principal or first-listed diagnosis, regardless of the number of admissions or encounters for treatment and care of the neoplasm.

See section I.C.21. Factors influencing health status and contact with health services, Encounter for prophylactic organ removal.

h. **Admission/encounter for pain control/management**
See Section I.C.6. for information on coding admission/encounter for pain control/management.

i. **Malignancy in two or more noncontiguous sites**
A patient may have more than one malignant tumor in the same organ. These tumors may represent different primaries or metastatic disease, depending on the site. Should the documentation be unclear, the provider should be queried as to the status of each tumor so that the correct codes can be assigned.

j. **Disseminated malignant neoplasm, unspecified**
Code C8Ø.Ø, Disseminated malignant neoplasm, unspecified, is for use only in those cases where the patient has advanced metastatic disease and no known primary or secondary sites are specified. It should not be used in place of assigning codes for the primary site and all known secondary sites.

k. **Malignant neoplasm without specification of site**
Code C8Ø.1, Malignant (primary) neoplasm, unspecified, equates to Cancer, unspecified. This code should only be used when no determination can be made as to the primary site of a malignancy. This code should rarely be used in the inpatient setting.

l. **Sequencing of neoplasm codes**

1) **Encounter for treatment of primary malignancy**
If the reason for the encounter is for treatment of a primary malignancy, assign the malignancy as the principal/first-listed diagnosis. The primary site is to be sequenced first, followed by any metastatic sites.

2) **Encounter for treatment of secondary malignancy**
When an encounter is for a primary malignancy with metastasis and treatment is directed toward the metastatic (secondary) site(s) only, the metastatic site(s) is designated as the principal/first-listed diagnosis. The primary malignancy is coded as an additional code.

3) **Malignant neoplasm in a pregnant patient**
When a pregnant patient has a malignant neoplasm, a code from subcategory O9A.1-, Malignant neoplasm complicating pregnancy, childbirth, and the puerperium, should be sequenced first, followed by the appropriate code from Chapter 2 to indicate the type of neoplasm.

4) **Encounter for complication associated with a neoplasm**
When an encounter is for management of a complication associated with a neoplasm, such as dehydration, and the treatment is only for the complication, the complication is coded first, followed by the appropriate code(s) for the neoplasm.

The exception to this guideline is anemia. When the admission/encounter is for management of an anemia associated with the malignancy, and the treatment is only for anemia, the appropriate code for the malignancy is sequenced as the principal or first-listed diagnosis followed by code D63.Ø, Anemia in neoplastic disease.

5) **Complication from surgical procedure for treatment of a neoplasm**
When an encounter is for treatment of a complication resulting from a surgical procedure performed for the treatment of the neoplasm, designate the complication as the principal/first-listed diagnosis. See the guideline regarding the coding of a current malignancy versus personal history to determine if the code for the neoplasm should also be assigned.

6) **Pathologic fracture due to a neoplasm**
When an encounter is for a pathological fracture due to a neoplasm, and the focus of treatment is the fracture, a code from subcategory M84.5, Pathological fracture in neoplastic disease, should be sequenced first, followed by the code for the neoplasm.

If the focus of treatment is the neoplasm with an associated pathological fracture, the neoplasm code should be sequenced first, followed by a code from M84.5 for the pathological fracture.

m. **Current malignancy versus personal history of malignancy**
When a primary malignancy has been excised but further treatment, such as an additional surgery for the malignancy, radiation therapy or chemotherapy is directed to that site, the primary malignancy code should be used until treatment is completed.

When a primary malignancy has been previously excised or eradicated from its site, there is no further treatment (of the malignancy) directed to that site, and there is no evidence of any existing primary malignancy at that site, a code from category Z85, Personal history of malignant neoplasm, should be used to indicate the former site of the malignancy.

Codes from subcategories Z85.Ø – Z85.85 should only be assigned for the former site of a primary malignancy, not the site of a secondary malignancy. Code Z85.89 may be assigned for the former site(s) of either a primary or secondary malignancy.

See Section I.C.21. Factors influencing health status and contact with health services, History (of)

n. **Leukemia, Multiple Myeloma, and Malignant Plasma Cell Neoplasms in remission versus personal history**
The categories for leukemia, and category C9Ø, Multiple myeloma and malignant plasma cell neoplasms, have codes indicating whether or not the leukemia has achieved remission. There are also codes Z85.6, Personal history of leukemia, and Z85.79, Personal history of other malignant neoplasms of lymphoid, hematopoietic and related tissues. If the documentation is unclear as to whether the leukemia has achieved remission, the provider should be queried.

See Section I.C.21. Factors influencing health status and contact with health services, History (of)

o. **Aftercare following surgery for neoplasm**
See Section I.C.21. Factors influencing health status and contact with health services, Aftercare

p. **Follow-up care for completed treatment of a malignancy**
See Section I.C.21. Factors influencing health status and contact with health services, Follow-up

q. **Prophylactic organ removal for prevention of malignancy**
See Section I.C. 21, Factors influencing health status and contact with health services, Prophylactic organ removal

r. **Malignant neoplasm associated with transplanted organ**
A malignant neoplasm of a transplanted organ should be coded as a transplant complication. Assign first the appropriate code from category T86.-, Complications of transplanted organs and tissue, followed by code C8Ø.2, Malignant neoplasm associated with transplanted organ. Use an additional code for the specific malignancy.

s. Breast Implant Associated Anaplastic Large Cell Lymphoma

Breast implant associated anaplastic large cell lymphoma (BIA-ALCL) is a type of lymphoma that can develop around breast implants. Assign code C84.7A, Anaplastic large cell lymphoma, ALK-negative, breast, for BIA-ALCL. Do not assign a complication code from chapter 19.

t. Secondary malignant neoplasm of lymphoid tissue

When a malignant neoplasm of lymphoid tissue metastasizes beyond the lymph nodes, a code from categories C81-C85 with a final character "9" should be assigned identifying "extranodal and solid organ sites" rather than a code for the secondary neoplasm of the affected solid organ. For example, for metastasis of B-cell lymphoma to the lung, brain and left adrenal gland, assign code C83.39, Diffuse large B-cell lymphoma, extranodal and solid organ sites.

3. Chapter 3: Disease of the blood and blood-forming organs and certain disorders involving the immune mechanism (D5Ø-D89)

Reserved for future guideline expansion

4. Chapter 4: Endocrine, Nutritional, and Metabolic Diseases (EØØ-E89)

a. Diabetes mellitus

The diabetes mellitus codes are combination codes that include the type of diabetes mellitus, the body system affected, and the complications affecting that body system. As many codes within a particular category as are necessary to describe all of the complications of the disease may be used. They should be sequenced based on the reason for a particular encounter. Assign as many codes from categories EØ8 – E13 as needed to identify all of the associated conditions that the patient has.

1) Type of diabetes

The age of a patient is not the sole determining factor, though most type 1 diabetics develop the condition before reaching puberty. For this reason, type 1 diabetes mellitus is also referred to as juvenile diabetes.

2) Type of diabetes mellitus not documented

If the type of diabetes mellitus is not documented in the medical record the default is E11.-, Type 2 diabetes mellitus.

3) Diabetes mellitus and the use of insulin, oral hypoglycemics, and injectable non-insulin drugs

If the documentation in a medical record does not indicate the type of diabetes but does indicate that the patient uses insulin, code E11-, Type 2 diabetes mellitus, should be assigned. Additional code(s) should be assigned from category Z79 to identify the long-term (current) use of insulin, oral hypoglycemic drugs, or injectable non-insulin antidiabetic, as follows:

If the patient is treated with both oral **hypoglycemic drugs** and insulin, both code Z79.4, Long term (current) use of insulin, and code Z79.84, Long term (current) use of oral hypoglycemic drugs, should be assigned.

If the patient is treated with both insulin and an injectable non-insulin antidiabetic drug, assign codes Z79.4, Long term (current) use of insulin, and **Z79.85, Long-term (current) use of injectable non-insulin antidiabetic drugs.**

If the patient is treated with both oral hypoglycemic drugs and an injectable non-insulin antidiabetic drug, assign codes Z79.84, Long term (current) use of oral hypoglycemic drugs, and **Z79.85, Long-term (current) use of injectable non-insulin antidiabetic drugs.**

Code Z79.4 should not be assigned if insulin is given temporarily to bring a type 2 patient's blood sugar under control during an encounter.

4) Diabetes mellitus in pregnancy and gestational diabetes

See Section I.C.15. Diabetes mellitus in pregnancy.

See Section I.C.15. Gestational (pregnancy induced) diabetes

5) Complications due to insulin pump malfunction

(a) Underdose of insulin due to insulin pump failure

An underdose of insulin due to an insulin pump failure should be assigned to a code from subcategory T85.6, Mechanical complication of other specified internal and external prosthetic devices, implants and grafts, that specifies the type of pump malfunction, as the principal or first-listed code, followed by code T38.3X6-, Underdosing of insulin and oral hypoglycemic [antidiabetic] drugs. Additional codes for the type of diabetes mellitus and any associated complications due to the underdosing should also be assigned.

(b) Overdose of insulin due to insulin pump failure

The principal or first-listed code for an encounter due to an insulin pump malfunction resulting in an overdose of insulin, should also be T85.6-, Mechanical complication of other specified internal and external prosthetic devices, implants and grafts, followed by code T38.3X1-, Poisoning by insulin and oral hypoglycemic [antidiabetic] drugs, accidental (unintentional).

6) Secondary diabetes mellitus

Codes under categories EØ8, Diabetes mellitus due to underlying condition, EØ9, Drug or chemical induced diabetes mellitus, and E13, Other specified diabetes mellitus, identify complications/manifestations associated with secondary diabetes mellitus. Secondary diabetes is always caused by another condition or event (e.g., cystic fibrosis, malignant neoplasm of pancreas, pancreatectomy, adverse effect of drug, or poisoning).

(a) Secondary diabetes mellitus and the use of insulin, oral hypoglycemic drugs, or injectable non-insulin drugs

For patients with secondary diabetes mellitus who routinely use insulin, oral hypoglycemic drugs, or injectable non-insulin drugs, additional code(s) from category Z79 should be assigned to identify the long-term (current) use of insulin, oral hypoglycemic drugs, or non-injectable non-insulin drugs as follows:

If the patient is treated with both oral **hypoglycemic drugs** and insulin, both code Z79.4, Long term (current) use of insulin, and code Z79.84, Long term (current) use of oral hypoglycemic drugs, should be assigned.

If the patient is treated with both insulin and an injectable non-insulin antidiabetic drug, assign codes Z79.4, Long-term (current) use of insulin, and **Z79.85, Long-term (current) use of injectable non-insulin antidiabetic drugs.**

If the patient is treated with both oral hypoglycemic drugs and an injectable non-insulin antidiabetic drug, assign codes Z79.84, Long-term (current) use of oral hypoglycemic drugs, and **Z79.85, Long-term (current) use of injectable non-insulin antidiabetic drugs.**

Code Z79.4 should not be assigned if insulin is given temporarily to bring a secondary diabetic patient's blood sugar under control during an encounter.

(b) Assigning and sequencing secondary diabetes codes and its causes

The sequencing of the secondary diabetes codes in relationship to codes for the cause of the diabetes is based on the Tabular List instructions for categories EØ8, EØ9 and E13.

(i) Secondary diabetes mellitus due to pancreatectomy

For postpancreatectomy diabetes mellitus (lack of insulin due to the surgical removal of all or part of the pancreas), assign code E89.1, Postprocedural hypoinsulinemia.

Assign a code from category E13 and a code from subcategory Z9Ø.41, Acquired absence of pancreas, as additional codes.

(ii) Secondary diabetes due to drugs

Secondary diabetes may be caused by an adverse effect of correctly administered medications, poisoning or sequela of poisoning.

See section I.C.19.e. for coding of adverse effects and poisoning, and section I.C.20 for external cause code reporting.

5. Chapter 5: Mental, Behavioral and Neurodevelopmental disorders (FØ1-F99)

a. Pain disorders related to psychological factors

Assign code F45.41, for pain that is exclusively related to psychological disorders. As indicated by the Excludes 1 note under category G89, a code from category G89 should not be assigned with code F45.41.

Code F45.42, Pain disorders with related psychological factors, should be used with a code from category G89, Pain, not elsewhere classified, if there is documentation of a psychological component for a patient with acute or chronic pain.

See Section I.C.6. Pain

b. Mental and behavioral disorders due to psychoactive substance use

1) In Remission

Selection of codes **describing** "in remission" for categories F1Ø-F19, Mental and behavioral disorders due to psychoactive substance use (categories F1Ø-F19 with -.11, -.21, **-.91**) requires the provider's clinical judgment **and** are assigned only on the basis of provider documentation (as defined in the Official Guidelines for Coding and Reporting), unless otherwise instructed by the classification.

Mild substance use disorders in early or sustained remission are classified to the appropriate codes for substance abuse in remission, and moderate or severe substance use disorders in early or sustained remission are classified to the appropriate codes for substance dependence in remission.

2) Psychoactive Substance Use, Abuse and Dependence

When the provider documentation refers to use, abuse and dependence of the same substance (e.g. alcohol, opioid, cannabis, etc.), only one code should be assigned to identify the pattern of use based on the following hierarchy:

- If both use and abuse are documented, assign only the code for abuse
- If both abuse and dependence are documented, assign only the code for dependence
- If use, abuse and dependence are all documented, assign only the code for dependence
- If both use and dependence are documented, assign only the code for dependence.

3) Psychoactive Substance Use, Unspecified

As with all other unspecified diagnoses, the codes for unspecified psychoactive substance use (F1Ø.9-, F11.9-, F12.9-, F13.9-, F14.9-, F15.9-, F16.9-, F18.9-, F19.9-) should only be assigned based on provider documentation and when they meet the definition of a reportable diagnosis (see Section III, Reporting Additional Diagnoses). These codes are to be used only when the psychoactive substance use is associated with a substance related disorder (chapter 5 disorders such as sexual dysfunction, sleep disorder, or a mental or behavioral disorder) or medical condition, and such a relationship is documented by the provider.

4) Medical Conditions Due to Psychoactive Substance Use, Abuse and Dependence

Medical conditions due to substance use, abuse, and dependence are not classified as substance-induced disorders. Assign the diagnosis code for the medical condition as directed by the Alphabetical Index along with the appropriate psychoactive substance use, abuse or dependence code. For example, for alcoholic pancreatitis due to alcohol dependence, assign the appropriate code from subcategory K85.2, Alcohol induced acute pancreatitis, and the appropriate code from subcategory F1Ø.2, such as code F1Ø.2Ø, Alcohol dependence, uncomplicated. It would not be appropriate to assign code F1Ø.288, Alcohol dependence with other alcohol-induced disorder.

5) Blood Alcohol Level

A code from category Y9Ø, Evidence of alcohol involvement determined by blood alcohol level, may be assigned when this information is documented and the patient's provider has documented a condition classifiable to category F1Ø, Alcohol related disorders. The blood alcohol level does not need to be documented by the patient's provider in order for it to be coded.

See Section I.B.14. for blood alcohol level documentation by clinicians other than patient's provider.

c. Factitious Disorder

Factitious disorder imposed on self or Munchausen's syndrome is a disorder in which a person falsely reports or causes his or her own physical or psychological signs or symptoms. For patients with documented factitious disorder on self or Munchausen's syndrome, assign the appropriate code from subcategory F68.1-, Factitious disorder imposed on self.

Munchausen's syndrome by proxy (MSBP) is a disorder in which a caregiver (perpetrator) falsely reports or causes an illness or injury in another person (victim) under his or her care, such as a child, an elderly adult, or a person who has a disability. The condition is also referred to as "factitious disorder imposed on another" or "factitious disorder by proxy." The perpetrator, not the victim, receives this diagnosis. Assign code F68.A, Factitious disorder imposed on another, to the perpetrator's record. For the victim of a patient suffering from MSBP, assign the appropriate code from categories T74, Adult and child abuse, neglect and other maltreatment, confirmed, or T76, Adult and child abuse, neglect and other maltreatment, suspected.

See Section I.C.19.f. Adult and child abuse, neglect and other maltreatment

d. Dementia

The ICD-10-CM classifies dementia (categories FØ1, FØ2, and FØ3) on the basis of the etiology and severity (unspecified, mild, moderate or severe). Selection of the appropriate severity level requires the provider's clinical judgment and codes should be assigned only on the basis of provider documentation (as defined in the *Official Guidelines for Coding and Reporting*), unless otherwise instructed by the classification. If the documentation does not provide information about the severity of the dementia, assign the appropriate code for unspecified severity.

If a patient is admitted to an inpatient acute care hospital or other inpatient facility setting with dementia at one severity level and it progresses to a higher severity level, assign one code for the highest severity level reported during the stay.

6. Chapter 6: Diseases of the Nervous System (GØØ-G99)

a. Dominant/nondominant side

Codes from category G81, Hemiplegia and hemiparesis, and subcategories G83.1, Monoplegia of lower limb, G83.2, Monoplegia of upper limb, and G83.3, Monoplegia, unspecified, identify whether the dominant or nondominant side is affected. Should the affected side be documented, but not specified as dominant or nondominant, and the classification system does not indicate a default, code selection is as follows:

- For ambidextrous patients, the default should be dominant.
- If the left side is affected, the default is non-dominant.
- If the right side is affected, the default is dominant.

b. Pain - Category G89

1) General coding information

Codes in category G89, Pain, not elsewhere classified, may be used in conjunction with codes from other categories and chapters to provide more detail about acute or chronic pain and neoplasm-related pain, unless otherwise indicated below.

If the pain is not specified as acute or chronic, post-thoracotomy, postprocedural, or neoplasm-related, do not assign codes from category G89.

A code from category G89 should not be assigned if the underlying (definitive) diagnosis is known, unless the reason for the encounter is pain control/ management and not management of the underlying condition.

When an admission or encounter is for a procedure aimed at treating the underlying condition (e.g., spinal fusion, kyphoplasty), a code for the underlying condition (e.g., vertebral fracture, spinal stenosis) should be assigned as the principal diagnosis. No code from category G89 should be assigned.

(a) Category G89 Codes as Principal or First-Listed Diagnosis

Category G89 codes are acceptable as principal diagnosis or the first-listed code:

- When pain control or pain management is the reason for the admission/encounter (e.g., a patient with displaced intervertebral disc, nerve impingement and severe back pain presents for injection of steroid into the spinal canal). The underlying cause of the pain should be reported as an additional diagnosis, if known.
- When a patient is admitted for the insertion of a neurostimulator for pain control, assign the appropriate pain code as the principal or first-listed diagnosis. When an admission or encounter is for a procedure aimed at treating the underlying condition and a neurostimulator is inserted for pain control during the same admission/encounter, a code for the underlying condition should be assigned as the principal diagnosis and the appropriate pain code should be assigned as a secondary diagnosis.

(b) Use of Category G89 Codes in Conjunction with Site Specific Pain Codes

(i) Assigning Category G89 and Site-Specific Pain Codes

Codes from category G89 may be used in conjunction with codes that identify the site of pain (including codes from chapter 18) if the category G89 code provides additional information. For example, if the code describes the site of the pain, but does not fully describe whether the pain is acute or chronic, then both codes should be assigned.

(ii) Sequencing of Category G89 Codes with Site-Specific Pain Codes

The sequencing of category G89 codes with site-specific pain codes (including chapter 18 codes), is dependent on the circumstances of the encounter/admission as follows:

- If the encounter is for pain control or pain management, assign the code from category G89 followed by the code identifying the specific site of pain (e.g., encounter for pain management for acute neck pain from trauma is assigned code G89.11, Acute pain due to trauma, followed by code M54.2, Cervicalgia, to identify the site of pain).
- If the encounter is for any other reason except pain control or pain management, and a related definitive diagnosis has not been established (confirmed) by the provider, assign the code for the specific site of pain first, followed by the appropriate code from category G89.

2) Pain due to devices, implants and grafts

See Section I.C.19. Pain due to medical devices

3) Postoperative Pain

The provider's documentation should be used to guide the coding of postoperative pain, as well as *Section III. Reporting Additional Diagnoses* and *Section IV. Diagnostic Coding and Reporting in the Outpatient Setting.*

The default for post-thoracotomy and other postoperative pain not specified as acute or chronic is the code for the acute form.

Routine or expected postoperative pain immediately after surgery should not be coded.

(a) Postoperative pain not associated with specific postoperative complication

Postoperative pain not associated with a specific postoperative complication is assigned to the appropriate postoperative pain code in category G89.

(b) Postoperative pain associated with specific postoperative complication

Postoperative pain associated with a specific postoperative complication (such as painful wire sutures) is assigned to the appropriate code(s) found in Chapter 19, Injury, poisoning, and certain other consequences of external causes. If appropriate, use additional code(s) from category G89 to identify acute or chronic pain (G89.18 or G89.28).

4) Chronic pain

Chronic pain is classified to subcategory G89.2. There is no time frame defining when pain becomes chronic pain. The provider's documentation should be used to guide use of these codes.

5) Neoplasm Related Pain

Code G89.3 is assigned to pain documented as being related, associated or due to cancer, primary or secondary malignancy, or tumor. This code is assigned regardless of whether the pain is acute or chronic.

This code may be assigned as the principal or first-listed code when the stated reason for the admission/encounter is documented as pain control/pain management. The underlying neoplasm should be reported as an additional diagnosis.

When the reason for the admission/encounter is management of the neoplasm and the pain associated with the neoplasm is also documented, code G89.3 may be assigned as an additional diagnosis. It is not necessary to assign an additional code for the site of the pain.

See Section I.C.2. for instructions on the sequencing of neoplasms for all other stated reasons for the admission/encounter (except for pain control/pain management).

6) Chronic pain syndrome

Central pain syndrome (G89.Ø) and chronic pain syndrome (G89.4) are different than the term "chronic pain," and therefore codes should only be used when the provider has specifically documented this condition.

See Section I.C.5. Pain disorders related to psychological factors

7. Chapter 7: Diseases of the Eye and Adnexa (HØØ-H59)

a. Glaucoma

1) Assigning Glaucoma Codes

Assign as many codes from category H4Ø, Glaucoma, as needed to identify the type of glaucoma, the affected eye, and the glaucoma stage.

2) Bilateral glaucoma with same type and stage

When a patient has bilateral glaucoma and both eyes are documented as being the same type and stage, and there is a code for bilateral glaucoma, report only the code for the type of glaucoma, bilateral, with the seventh character for the stage.

When a patient has bilateral glaucoma and both eyes are documented as being the same type and stage, and the classification does not provide a code for bilateral glaucoma (i.e. subcategories H4Ø.1Ø, and H4Ø.2Ø) report only one code for the type of glaucoma with the appropriate seventh character for the stage.

3) Bilateral glaucoma stage with different types or stages

When a patient has bilateral glaucoma and each eye is documented as having a different type or stage, and the classification distinguishes laterality, assign the appropriate code for each eye rather than the code for bilateral glaucoma.

When a patient has bilateral glaucoma and each eye is documented as having a different type, and the classification does not distinguish laterality (i.e., subcategories H4Ø.1Ø, and H4Ø.2Ø), assign one code for each type of glaucoma with the appropriate seventh character for the stage.

When a patient has bilateral glaucoma and each eye is documented as having the same type, but different stage, and the classification does not distinguish laterality (i.e., subcategories H4Ø.1Ø and H4Ø.2Ø), assign a code for the type of glaucoma for each eye with the seventh character for the specific glaucoma stage documented for each eye.

4) Patient admitted with glaucoma and stage evolves during the admission

If a patient is admitted with glaucoma and the stage progresses during the admission, assign the code for highest stage documented.

5) Indeterminate stage glaucoma

Assignment of the seventh character "4" for "indeterminate stage" should be based on the clinical documentation. The seventh character "4" is used for glaucomas whose stage cannot be clinically determined. This seventh character should not be confused with the seventh character "Ø", unspecified, which should be assigned when there is no documentation regarding the stage of the glaucoma.

b. Blindness

If "blindness" or "low vision" of both eyes is documented but the visual impairment category is not documented, assign code H54.3, Unqualified visual loss, both eyes. If "blindness" or "low vision" in one eye is documented but the visual impairment category is not documented, assign a code from H54.6-, Unqualified visual loss, one eye. If "blindness" or "visual loss" is documented without any information about whether one or both eyes are affected, assign code H54.7, Unspecified visual loss.

8. Chapter 8: Diseases of the Ear and Mastoid Process (H6Ø-H95)

Reserved for future guideline expansion

9. Chapter 9: Diseases of the Circulatory System (IØØ-I99)

a. Hypertension

The classification presumes a causal relationship between hypertension and heart involvement and between hypertension and kidney involvement, as the two conditions are linked by the term "with" in the Alphabetic Index. These conditions should be coded as related even in the absence of provider documentation explicitly linking them, unless the documentation clearly states the conditions are unrelated.

For hypertension and conditions not specifically linked by relational terms such as "with," "associated with" or "due to" in the classification, provider documentation must link the conditions in order to code them as related.

1) Hypertension with Heart Disease

Hypertension with heart conditions classified to I5Ø.- or I51.4-I51.7, I51.89, I51.9, are assigned to a code from category I11, Hypertensive heart disease. Use additional code(s) from category I5Ø, Heart failure, to identify the type(s) of heart failure in those patients with heart failure.

The same heart conditions (I5Ø.-, I51.4-I51.7, I51.89, I51.9) with hypertension are coded separately if the provider has documented they are unrelated to the hypertension. Sequence according to the circumstances of the admission/encounter.

2) Hypertensive Chronic Kidney Disease

Assign codes from category I12, Hypertensive chronic kidney disease, when both hypertension and a condition classifiable to category N18, Chronic kidney disease (CKD), are present. CKD should not be coded as hypertensive if the provider indicates the CKD is not related to the hypertension.

The appropriate code from category N18 should be used as a secondary code with a code from category I12 to identify the stage of chronic kidney disease.

See Section I.C.14. Chronic kidney disease.

If a patient has hypertensive chronic kidney disease and acute renal failure, the acute renal failure should also be coded. Sequence according to the circumstances of the admission/encounter.

3) Hypertensive Heart and Chronic Kidney Disease

Assign codes from combination category I13, Hypertensive heart and chronic kidney disease, when there is hypertension with both heart and kidney involvement. If heart failure is present, assign an additional code from category I5Ø to identify the type of heart failure.

The appropriate code from category N18, Chronic kidney disease, should be used as a secondary code with a code from category I13 to identify the stage of chronic kidney disease.

See Section I.C.14. Chronic kidney disease.

The codes in category I13, Hypertensive heart and chronic kidney disease, are combination codes that include hypertension, heart disease and chronic kidney disease. The Includes note at I13 specifies that the conditions included at I11 and I12 are included together in I13. If a patient has hypertension, heart disease and chronic kidney disease, then a code from I13 should be used, not individual codes for hypertension, heart disease and chronic kidney disease, or codes from I11 or I12.

For patients with both acute renal failure and chronic kidney disease, the acute renal failure should also be coded. Sequence according to the circumstances of the admission/encounter.

4) Hypertensive Cerebrovascular Disease

For hypertensive cerebrovascular disease, first assign the appropriate code from categories I6Ø-I69, followed by the appropriate hypertension code.

5) Hypertensive Retinopathy

Subcategory H35.Ø, Background retinopathy and retinal vascular changes, should be used along with a code from categories I1Ø-I15, in the Hypertensive diseases section, to include the systemic hypertension. The sequencing is based on the reason for the encounter.

6) Hypertension, Secondary

Secondary hypertension is due to an underlying condition. Two codes are required: one to identify the underlying etiology and one from category I15 to identify the hypertension. Sequencing of codes is determined by the reason for admission/encounter.

7) Hypertension, Transient

Assign code RØ3.Ø, Elevated blood pressure reading without diagnosis of hypertension, unless patient has an established diagnosis of hypertension. Assign code O13.-, Gestational [pregnancy-induced] hypertension without significant proteinuria, or O14.-, Pre-eclampsia, for transient hypertension of pregnancy.

8) Hypertension, Controlled

This diagnostic statement usually refers to an existing state of hypertension under control by therapy. Assign the appropriate code from categories I1Ø-I15, Hypertensive diseases.

9) Hypertension, Uncontrolled

Uncontrolled hypertension may refer to untreated hypertension or hypertension not responding to current therapeutic regimen. In either case, assign the appropriate code from categories I1Ø-I15, Hypertensive diseases.

10) Hypertensive Crisis

Assign a code from category I16, Hypertensive crisis, for documented hypertensive urgency, hypertensive emergency or unspecified hypertensive crisis. Code also any identified hypertensive disease (I1Ø-I15). The sequencing is based on the reason for the encounter.

11) Pulmonary Hypertension

Pulmonary hypertension is classified to category I27, Other pulmonary heart diseases. For secondary pulmonary hypertension (I27.1, I27.2-), code also any associated conditions or adverse effects of drugs or toxins. The sequencing is based on the reason for the encounter, except for adverse effects of drugs (See Section I.C.19.e.).

b. Atherosclerotic Coronary Artery Disease and Angina

ICD-10-CM has combination codes for atherosclerotic heart disease with angina pectoris. The subcategories for these codes are I25.11, Atherosclerotic heart disease of native coronary artery with angina pectoris and I25.7, Atherosclerosis of coronary artery bypass graft(s) and coronary artery of transplanted heart with angina pectoris.

When using one of these combination codes it is not necessary to use an additional code for angina pectoris. A causal relationship can be assumed in a patient with both atherosclerosis and angina pectoris, unless the documentation indicates the angina is due to something other than the atherosclerosis.

If a patient with coronary artery disease is admitted due to an acute myocardial infarction (AMI), the AMI should be sequenced before the coronary artery disease.

See Section I.C.9. Acute myocardial infarction (AMI)

c. Intraoperative and Postprocedural Cerebrovascular Accident

Medical record documentation should clearly specify the cause-and-effect relationship between the medical intervention and the cerebrovascular accident in order to assign a code for intraoperative or postprocedural cerebrovascular accident.

Proper code assignment depends on whether it was an infarction or hemorrhage and whether it occurred intraoperatively or postoperatively. If it was a cerebral hemorrhage, code assignment depends on the type of procedure performed.

d. Sequelae of Cerebrovascular Disease

1) Category I69, Sequelae of Cerebrovascular disease

Category I69 is used to indicate conditions classifiable to categories I6Ø-I67 as the causes of sequela (neurologic deficits), themselves classified elsewhere. These "late effects" include neurologic deficits that persist after initial onset of conditions classifiable to categories I6Ø-I67. The neurologic deficits caused by cerebrovascular disease may be present from the onset or may arise at any time after the onset of the condition classifiable to categories I6Ø-I67.

Codes from category I69, Sequelae of cerebrovascular disease, that specify hemiplegia, hemiparesis and monoplegia identify whether the dominant or nondominant side is affected. Should the affected side be documented, but not specified as dominant or nondominant, and the classification system does not indicate a default, code selection is as follows:

- For ambidextrous patients, the default should be dominant.
- If the left side is affected, the default is non-dominant.
- If the right side is affected, the default is dominant.

2) Codes from category I69 with codes from I6Ø-I67

Codes from category I69 may be assigned on a health care record with codes from I6Ø-I67, if the patient has a current cerebrovascular disease and deficits from an old cerebrovascular disease.

3) Codes from category I69 and Personal history of transient ischemic attack (TIA) and cerebral infarction (Z86.73)

Codes from category I69 should not be assigned if the patient does not have neurologic deficits.

See Section I.C.21.4. History (of) for use of personal history codes

e. Acute myocardial infarction (AMI)

1) Type 1 ST elevation myocardial infarction (STEMI) and non-ST elevation myocardial infarction (NSTEMI)

The ICD-10-CM codes for type 1 acute myocardial infarction (AMI) identify the site, such as anterolateral wall or true posterior wall. Subcategories I21.Ø-I21.2 and code I21.3 are used for type 1 ST elevation myocardial infarction (STEMI). Code I21.4, Non-ST elevation (NSTEMI) myocardial infarction, is used for type 1 non-ST elevation myocardial infarction (NSTEMI) and nontransmural MIs.

If a type 1 NSTEMI evolves to STEMI, assign the STEMI code. If a type 1 STEMI converts to NSTEMI due to thrombolytic therapy, it is still coded as STEMI.

For encounters occurring while the myocardial infarction is equal to, or less than, four weeks old, including transfers to another acute setting or a postacute setting, and the myocardial infarction meets the definition for "other diagnoses" (see Section III, Reporting Additional Diagnoses), codes from category I21 may continue to be reported. For encounters after the 4-week time frame and the patient is still receiving care related to the myocardial infarction, the appropriate aftercare code should be assigned, rather than a code from category I21. For old or healed myocardial infarctions not requiring further care, code I25.2, Old myocardial infarction, may be assigned.

2) Acute myocardial infarction, unspecified

Code I21.9, Acute myocardial infarction, unspecified, is the default for unspecified acute myocardial infarction or unspecified type. If only type 1 STEMI or transmural MI without the site is documented, assign code I21.3, ST elevation (STEMI) myocardial infarction of unspecified site.

3) AMI documented as nontransmural or subendocardial but site provided

If an AMI is documented as nontransmural or subendocardial, but the site is provided, it is still coded as a subendocardial AMI.

See Section I.C.21.3. for information on coding status post administration of tPA in a different facility within the last 24 hours.

4) Subsequent acute myocardial infarction

A code from category I22, Subsequent ST elevation (STEMI) and non-ST elevation (NSTEMI) myocardial infarction, is to be used when a patient who has suffered a type 1 or unspecified AMI has a new AMI within the 4 week time frame of the initial AMI. A code from category I22 must be used in conjunction with a code from category I21. The sequencing of the I22 and I21 codes depends on the circumstances of the encounter.

Do not assign code I22 for subsequent myocardial infarctions other than type 1 or unspecified. For subsequent type 2 AMI assign only code I21.A1. For subsequent type 4 or type 5 AMI, assign only code I21.A9.

If a subsequent myocardial infarction of one type occurs within 4 weeks of a myocardial infarction of a different type, assign the appropriate codes from category I21 to identify each type. Do not assign a code from I22. Codes from category I22 should only be assigned if both the initial and subsequent myocardial infarctions are type 1 or unspecified.

5) Other Types of Myocardial Infarction

The ICD-10-CM provides codes for different types of myocardial infarction. Type 1 myocardial infarctions are assigned to codes I21.Ø-I21.4.

Type 2 myocardial infarction (myocardial infarction due to demand ischemia or secondary to ischemic imbalance) is assigned to code I21.A1, Myocardial infarction type 2 with the underlying cause coded first. Do not assign code I24.8, Other forms of acute ischemic heart disease, for the demand ischemia. If a type 2 AMI is described as NSTEMI or STEMI, only assign code I21.A1. Codes I21.Ø1-I21.4 should only be assigned for type 1 AMIs.

Acute myocardial infarctions type 3, 4a, 4b, 4c and 5 are assigned to code I21.A9, Other myocardial infarction type.

The "Code also" and "Code first" notes should be followed related to complications, and for coding of postprocedural myocardial infarctions during or following cardiac surgery.

10. Chapter 10: Diseases of the Respiratory System (JØØ-J99), UØ7.Ø

a. Chronic Obstructive Pulmonary Disease [COPD] and Asthma

1) Acute exacerbation of chronic obstructive bronchitis and asthma

The codes in categories J44 and J45 distinguish between uncomplicated cases and those in acute exacerbation. An acute exacerbation is a worsening or a decompensation of a chronic condition. An acute exacerbation is not equivalent to an infection superimposed on a chronic condition, though an exacerbation may be triggered by an infection.

b. Acute Respiratory Failure

1) Acute respiratory failure as principal diagnosis

A code from subcategory J96.Ø, Acute respiratory failure, or subcategory J96.2, Acute and chronic respiratory failure, may be assigned as a principal diagnosis when it is the condition established after study to be chiefly responsible for occasioning the admission to the hospital, and the selection is supported by the Alphabetic Index and Tabular List. However, chapter-specific coding guidelines (such as obstetrics, poisoning, HIV, newborn) that provide sequencing direction take precedence.

2) Acute respiratory failure as secondary diagnosis

Respiratory failure may be listed as a secondary diagnosis if it occurs after admission, or if it is present on admission, but does not meet the definition of principal diagnosis.

3) Sequencing of acute respiratory failure and another acute condition

When a patient is admitted with respiratory failure and another acute condition, (e.g., myocardial infarction, cerebrovascular accident, aspiration pneumonia), the principal diagnosis will not be the same in every situation. This applies whether the other acute condition is a respiratory or nonrespiratory condition. Selection of the principal diagnosis will be dependent on the circumstances of admission. If both the respiratory failure and the other acute condition are equally responsible for occasioning the admission to the hospital, and there are no chapter-specific sequencing rules, the guideline regarding two or more diagnoses that equally meet the definition for principal diagnosis (Section II, C.) may be applied in these situations.

If the documentation is not clear as to whether acute respiratory failure and another condition are equally responsible for occasioning the admission, query the provider for clarification.

c. Influenza due to certain identified influenza viruses

Code only confirmed cases of influenza due to certain identified influenza viruses (category JØ9), and due to other identified influenza virus (category J1Ø). This is an exception to the hospital inpatient guideline Section II, H. (Uncertain Diagnosis).

In this context, "confirmation" does not require documentation of positive laboratory testing specific for avian or other novel influenza A or other identified influenza virus. However, coding should be based on the provider's diagnostic statement that the patient has avian influenza, or other novel influenza A, for category JØ9, or has another particular identified strain of influenza, such as H1N1 or H3N2, but not identified as novel or variant, for category J1Ø.

If the provider records "suspected" or "possible" or "probable" avian influenza, or novel influenza, or other identified influenza, then the appropriate influenza code from category J11, Influenza due to unidentified influenza virus, should be assigned. A code from category JØ9, Influenza due to certain identified influenza viruses, should not be assigned nor should a code from category J1Ø, Influenza due to other identified influenza virus.

d. Ventilator associated Pneumonia

1) Documentation of Ventilator associated Pneumonia

As with all procedural or postprocedural complications, code assignment is based on the provider's documentation of the relationship between the condition and the procedure.

Code J95.851, Ventilator associated pneumonia, should be assigned only when the provider has documented ventilator associated pneumonia (VAP). An additional code to identify the organism (e.g., Pseudomonas aeruginosa, code B96.5) should also be assigned. Do not assign an additional code from categories J12-J18 to identify the type of pneumonia.

Code J95.851 should not be assigned for cases where the patient has pneumonia and is on a mechanical ventilator and the provider has not specifically stated that the pneumonia is ventilator-associated pneumonia. If the documentation is unclear as to whether the patient has a pneumonia that is a complication attributable to the mechanical ventilator, query the provider.

2) Ventilator associated Pneumonia Develops after Admission

A patient may be admitted with one type of pneumonia (e.g., code J13, Pneumonia due to Streptococcus pneumonia) and subsequently develop VAP. In this instance, the principal diagnosis would be the appropriate code from categories J12-J18 for the pneumonia diagnosed at the time of admission. Code J95.851, Ventilator associated pneumonia, would be assigned as an additional diagnosis when the provider has also documented the presence of ventilator associated pneumonia.

e. Vaping-related disorders

For patients presenting with condition(s) related to vaping, assign code U07.0, Vaping-related disorder, as the principal diagnosis. For lung injury due to vaping, assign only code U07.0. Assign additional codes for other manifestations, such as acute respiratory failure (subcategory J96.0-) or pneumonitis (code J68.0).

Associated respiratory signs and symptoms due to vaping, such as cough, shortness of breath, etc., are not coded separately, when a definitive diagnosis has been established. However, it would be appropriate to code separately any gastrointestinal symptoms, such as diarrhea and abdominal pain.

See Section I.C.1.g.1.c.i. for Pneumonia confirmed as due to COVID-19

11. Chapter 11: Diseases of the Digestive System (K00-K95)

Reserved for future guideline expansion

12. Chapter 12: Diseases of the Skin and Subcutaneous Tissue (L00-L99)

a. Pressure ulcer stage codes

1) Pressure ulcer stages

Codes in category L89, Pressure ulcer, identify the site and stage of the pressure ulcer.

The ICD-10-CM classifies pressure ulcer stages based on severity, which is designated by stages 1-4, deep tissue pressure injury, unspecified stage, and unstageable.

Assign as many codes from category L89 as needed to identify all the pressure ulcers the patient has, if applicable.

See Section I.B.14. for pressure ulcer stage documentation by clinicians other than patient's provider.

2) Unstageable pressure ulcers

Assignment of the code for unstageable pressure ulcer (L89.--0) should be based on the clinical documentation. These codes are used for pressure ulcers whose stage cannot be clinically determined (e.g., the ulcer is covered by eschar or has been treated with a skin or muscle graft). This code should not be confused with the codes for unspecified stage (L89.--9). When there is no documentation regarding the stage of the pressure ulcer, assign the appropriate code for unspecified stage (L89.-- 9).

If during an encounter, the stage of an unstageable pressure ulcer is revealed after debridement, assign only the code for the stage revealed following debridement.

3) Documented pressure ulcer stage

Assignment of the pressure ulcer stage code should be guided by clinical documentation of the stage or documentation of the terms found in the Alphabetic Index. For clinical terms describing the stage that are not found in the Alphabetic Index, and there is no documentation of the stage, the provider should be queried.

4) Patients admitted with pressure ulcers documented as healed

No code is assigned if the documentation states that the pressure ulcer is completely healed at the time of admission.

5) Pressure ulcers documented as healing

Pressure ulcers described as healing should be assigned the appropriate pressure ulcer stage code based on the documentation in the medical record. If the documentation does not provide information about the stage of the healing pressure ulcer, assign the appropriate code for unspecified stage.

If the documentation is unclear as to whether the patient has a current (new) pressure ulcer or if the patient is being treated for a healing pressure ulcer, query the provider.

For ulcers that were present on admission but healed at the time of discharge, assign the code for the site and stage of the pressure ulcer at the time of admission.

6) Patient admitted with pressure ulcer evolving into another stage during the admission

If a patient is admitted to an inpatient hospital with a pressure ulcer at one stage and it progresses to a higher stage, two separate codes should be assigned: one code for the site and stage of the ulcer on admission and a second code for the same ulcer site and the highest stage reported during the stay.

7) Pressure-induced deep tissue damage

For pressure-induced deep tissue damage or deep tissue pressure injury, assign only the appropriate code for pressure-induced deep tissue damage (L89.--6).

b. Non-Pressure Chronic Ulcers

1) Patients admitted with non-pressure ulcers documented as healed

No code is assigned if the documentation states that the non-pressure ulcer is completely healed at the time of admission.

2) Non-pressure ulcers documented as healing

Non-pressure ulcers described as healing should be assigned the appropriate non-pressure ulcer code based on the documentation in the medical record. If the documentation does not provide information about the severity of the healing non-pressure ulcer, assign the appropriate code for unspecified severity.

If the documentation is unclear as to whether the patient has a current (new) non-pressure ulcer or if the patient is being treated for a healing non-pressure ulcer, query the provider.

For ulcers that were present on admission but healed at the time of discharge, assign the code for the site and severity of the non-pressure ulcer at the time of admission.

3) Patient admitted with non-pressure ulcer that progresses to another severity level during the admission

If a patient is admitted to an inpatient hospital with a non-pressure ulcer at one severity level and it progresses to a higher severity level, two separate codes should be assigned: one code for the site and severity level of the ulcer on admission and a second code for the same ulcer site and the highest severity level reported during the stay.

See Section I.B.14. for pressure ulcer stage documentation by clinicians other than patient's provider

13. Chapter 13: Diseases of the Musculoskeletal System and Connective Tissue (M00-M99)

a. Site and laterality

Most of the codes within Chapter 13 have site and laterality designations. The site represents the bone, joint or the muscle involved. For some conditions where more than one bone, joint or muscle is usually involved, such as osteoarthritis, there is a "multiple sites" code available. For categories where no multiple site code is provided and more than one bone, joint or muscle is involved, multiple codes should be used to indicate the different sites involved.

1) Bone versus joint

For certain conditions, the bone may be affected at the upper or lower end, (e.g., avascular necrosis of bone, M87, Osteoporosis, M80, M81). Though the portion of the bone affected may be at the joint, the site designation will be the bone, not the joint.

b. Acute traumatic versus chronic or recurrent musculoskeletal conditions

Many musculoskeletal conditions are a result of previous injury or trauma to a site, or are recurrent conditions. Bone, joint or muscle conditions that are the result of a healed injury are usually found in chapter 13. Recurrent bone, joint or muscle conditions are also usually found in chapter 13. Any current, acute injury should be coded to the appropriate injury code from chapter 19. Chronic or recurrent conditions should generally be coded with a code from chapter 13. If it is difficult to determine from the documentation in the record which code is best to describe a condition, query the provider.

c. Coding of Pathologic Fractures

7th character A is for use as long as the patient is receiving active treatment for the fracture. While the patient may be seen by a new or different provider over the course of treatment for a pathological fracture, assignment of the 7th character is based on whether the patient is undergoing active treatment and not whether the provider is seeing the patient for the first time.

7th character D is to be used for encounters after the patient has completed active treatment for the fracture and is receiving routine care for the fracture during the healing or recovery phase. The other 7th characters, listed under each subcategory in the Tabular List, are to be used for subsequent encounters for treatment of problems associated with the healing, such as malunions, nonunions, and sequelae.

Care for complications of surgical treatment for fracture repairs during the healing or recovery phase should be coded with the appropriate complication codes.

See Section I.C.19. Coding of traumatic fractures.

d. Osteoporosis

Osteoporosis is a systemic condition, meaning that all bones of the musculoskeletal system are affected. Therefore, site is not a component of the codes under category M81, Osteoporosis without current pathological fracture. The site codes under category M8Ø, Osteoporosis with current pathological fracture, identify the site of the fracture, not the osteoporosis.

1) Osteoporosis without pathological fracture

Category M81, Osteoporosis without current pathological fracture, is for use for patients with osteoporosis who do not currently have a pathologic fracture due to the osteoporosis, even if they have had a fracture in the past. For patients with a history of osteoporosis fractures, status code Z87.31Ø, Personal history of (healed) osteoporosis fracture, should follow the code from M81.

2) Osteoporosis with current pathological fracture

Category M8Ø, Osteoporosis with current pathological fracture, is for patients who have a current pathologic fracture at the time of an encounter. The codes under M8Ø identify the site of the fracture. A code from category M8Ø, not a traumatic fracture code, should be used for any patient with known osteoporosis who suffers a fracture, even if the patient had a minor fall or trauma, if that fall or trauma would not usually break a normal, healthy bone.

e. Multisystem Inflammatory Syndrome

See Section I.C.1.g.1.l. for Multisystem Inflammatory Syndrome

14. Chapter 14: Diseases of Genitourinary System (NØØ-N99)

a. Chronic kidney disease

1) Stages of chronic kidney disease (CKD)

The ICD-10-CM classifies CKD based on severity. The severity of CKD is designated by stages 1-5. Stage 2, code N18.2, equates to mild CKD; stage 3, codes N18.3Ø-N18.32, equate to moderate CKD; and stage 4, code N18.4, equates to severe CKD. Code N18.6, End stage renal disease (ESRD), is assigned when the provider has documented end-stage renal disease (ESRD).

If both a stage of CKD and ESRD are documented, assign code N18.6 only.

2) Chronic kidney disease and kidney transplant status

Patients who have undergone kidney transplant may still have some form of chronic kidney disease (CKD) because the kidney transplant may not fully restore kidney function. Therefore, the presence of CKD alone does not constitute a transplant complication. Assign the appropriate N18 code for the patient's stage of CKD and code Z94.Ø, Kidney transplant status. If a transplant complication such as failure or rejection or other transplant complication is documented, see section I.C.19.g for information on coding complications of a kidney transplant. If the documentation is unclear as to whether the patient has a complication of the transplant, query the provider.

3) Chronic kidney disease with other conditions

Patients with CKD may also suffer from other serious conditions, most commonly diabetes mellitus and hypertension. The sequencing of the CKD code in relationship to codes for other contributing conditions is based on the conventions in the Tabular List.

See I.C.9. Hypertensive chronic kidney disease.

See I.C.19. Chronic kidney disease and kidney transplant complications.

15. Chapter 15: Pregnancy, Childbirth, and the Puerperium (OØØ-O9A)

a. General Rules for Obstetric Cases

1) Codes from chapter 15 and sequencing priority

Obstetric cases require codes from chapter 15, codes in the range OØØ-O9A, Pregnancy, Childbirth, and the Puerperium. Chapter 15 codes have sequencing priority over codes from other chapters. Additional codes from other chapters may be used in conjunction with chapter 15 codes to further specify conditions. Should the provider document that the pregnancy is incidental to the encounter, then code Z33.1, Pregnant state, incidental, should be used in place of any chapter 15 codes. It is the provider's responsibility to state that the condition being treated is not affecting the pregnancy.

2) Chapter 15 codes used only on the maternal record

Chapter 15 codes are to be used only on the maternal record, never on the record of the newborn.

3) Final character for trimester

The majority of codes in Chapter 15 have a final character indicating the trimester of pregnancy. The timeframes for the trimesters are indicated at the beginning of the chapter. If trimester is not a component of a code, it is because the condition always occurs in a specific trimester, or the concept of trimester of pregnancy is not applicable. Certain codes have characters for only certain trimesters because the condition does not occur in all trimesters, but it may occur in more than just one.

Assignment of the final character for trimester should be based on the provider's documentation of the trimester (or number of weeks) for the current admission/encounter. This applies to the assignment of trimester for pre-existing conditions as well as those that develop during or are due to the pregnancy. The provider's documentation of the number of weeks may be used to assign the appropriate code identifying the trimester.

Whenever delivery occurs during the current admission, and there is an "in childbirth" option for the obstetric complication being coded, the "in childbirth" code should be assigned. When the classification does not provide an obstetric code with an "in childbirth" option, it is appropriate to assign a code describing the current trimester.

4) Selection of trimester for inpatient admissions that encompass more than one trimester

In instances when a patient is admitted to a hospital for complications of pregnancy during one trimester and remains in the hospital into a subsequent trimester, the trimester character for the antepartum complication code should be assigned on the basis of the trimester when the complication developed, not the trimester of the discharge. If the condition developed prior to the current admission/encounter or represents a pre-existing condition, the trimester character for the trimester at the time of the admission/encounter should be assigned.

5) Unspecified trimester

Each category that includes codes for trimester has a code for "unspecified trimester." The "unspecified trimester" code should rarely be used, such as when the documentation in the record is insufficient to determine the trimester and it is not possible to obtain clarification.

6) 7th character for fetus identification

Where applicable, a 7th character is to be assigned for certain categories (O31, O32, O33.3-O33.6, O35, O36, O4Ø, O41, O6Ø.1, O6Ø.2, O64, and O69) to identify the fetus for which the complication code applies.

Assign 7th character "Ø":

- For single gestations

  When the documentation in the record is insufficient to determine the fetus affected and it is not possible to obtain clarification.

- When it is not possible to clinically determine which fetus is affected.

7) Completed weeks of gestation

In ICD-10-CM, "completed" weeks of gestation refers to full weeks. For example, if the provider documents gestation at 39 weeks and 6 days, the code for 39 weeks of gestation should be assigned, as the patient has not yet reached 40 completed weeks.

b. Selection of OB Principal or First-listed Diagnosis

1) Routine outpatient prenatal visits

For routine outpatient prenatal visits when no complications are present, a code from category Z34, Encounter for supervision of normal pregnancy, should be used as the first-listed diagnosis. These codes should not be used in conjunction with chapter 15 codes.

2) Supervision of High-Risk Pregnancy

Codes from category OØ9, Supervision of high-risk pregnancy, are intended for use only during the prenatal period. For complications during the labor or delivery episode as a result of a high-risk pregnancy, assign the applicable complication codes from Chapter 15. If there are no complications during the labor or delivery episode, assign code O8Ø, Encounter for full-term uncomplicated delivery.

For routine prenatal outpatient visits for patients with high-risk pregnancies, a code from category OØ9, Supervision of high-risk pregnancy, should be used as the first-listed diagnosis. Secondary chapter 15 codes may be used in conjunction with these codes if appropriate.

3) Episodes when no delivery occurs

In episodes when no delivery occurs, the principal diagnosis should correspond to the principal complication of the pregnancy which necessitated the encounter. Should more than one complication exist, all of which are treated or monitored, any of the complication codes may be sequenced first.

4) When a delivery occurs

When an obstetric patient is admitted and delivers during that admission, the condition that prompted the admission should be sequenced as the principal diagnosis. If multiple conditions prompted the admission, sequence the one most related to the delivery as the principal diagnosis. A code for any complication of the delivery should be assigned as an additional diagnosis. In cases of cesarean delivery, if the patient was admitted with a condition that resulted in the performance of a cesarean procedure, that condition should be selected as the principal diagnosis. If the reason for the admission was unrelated to the condition resulting in the cesarean delivery, the condition related to the reason for the admission should be selected as the principal diagnosis.

5) Outcome of delivery

A code from category Z37, Outcome of delivery, should be included on every maternal record when a delivery has occurred. These codes are not to be used on subsequent records or on the newborn record.

c. Pre-existing conditions versus conditions due to the pregnancy

Certain categories in Chapter 15 distinguish between conditions of the mother that existed prior to pregnancy (pre-existing) and those that are a direct result of pregnancy. When assigning codes from Chapter 15, it is important to assess if a condition was pre-existing prior to pregnancy or developed during or due to the pregnancy in order to assign the correct code.

Categories that do not distinguish between pre-existing and pregnancy-related conditions may be used for either. It is acceptable to use codes specifically for the puerperium with codes complicating pregnancy and childbirth if a condition arises postpartum during the delivery encounter.

d. Pre-existing hypertension in pregnancy

Category O1Ø, Pre-existing hypertension complicating pregnancy, childbirth and the puerperium, includes codes for hypertensive heart and hypertensive chronic kidney disease. When assigning one of the O1Ø codes that includes hypertensive heart disease or hypertensive chronic kidney disease, it is necessary to add a secondary code from the appropriate hypertension category to specify the type of heart failure or chronic kidney disease.

See Section I.C.9. Hypertension.

e. Fetal Conditions Affecting the Management of the Mother

1) Codes from categories O35 and O36

Codes from categories O35, Maternal care for known or suspected fetal abnormality and damage, and O36, Maternal care for other fetal problems, are assigned only when the fetal condition is actually responsible for modifying the management of the mother, i.e., by requiring diagnostic studies, additional observation, special care, or termination of pregnancy. The fact that the fetal condition exists does not justify assigning a code from this series to the mother's record.

2) In utero surgery

In cases when surgery is performed on the fetus, a diagnosis code from category O35, Maternal care for known or suspected fetal abnormality and damage, should be assigned identifying the fetal condition. Assign the appropriate procedure code for the procedure performed.

No code from Chapter 16, the perinatal codes, should be used on the mother's record to identify fetal conditions. Surgery performed in utero on a fetus is still to be coded as an obstetric encounter.

f. HIV Infection in Pregnancy, Childbirth and the Puerperium

During pregnancy, childbirth or the puerperium, a patient admitted because of an HIV-related illness should receive a principal diagnosis from subcategory O98.7-, Human immunodeficiency [HIV] disease complicating pregnancy, childbirth and the puerperium, followed by the code(s) for the HIV-related illness(es).

Patients with asymptomatic HIV infection status admitted during pregnancy, childbirth, or the puerperium should receive codes of O98.7- and Z21, Asymptomatic human immunodeficiency virus [HIV] infection status.

g. Diabetes mellitus in pregnancy

Diabetes mellitus is a significant complicating factor in pregnancy. Pregnant patients who are diabetic should be assigned a code from category O24, Diabetes mellitus in pregnancy, childbirth, and the puerperium, first, followed by the appropriate diabetes code(s) (EØ8-E13) from Chapter 4.

h. Long term use of insulin and oral hypoglycemics

See section I.C.4.a.3 for information on the long-term use of insulin and oral hypoglycemics.

i. Gestational (pregnancy induced) diabetes

Gestational (pregnancy induced) diabetes can occur during the second and third trimester of pregnancy in patients who were not diabetic prior to pregnancy. Gestational diabetes can cause complications in the pregnancy similar to those of pre-existing diabetes mellitus. It also puts the patient at greater risk of developing diabetes after the pregnancy.

Codes for gestational diabetes are in subcategory O24.4, Gestational diabetes mellitus. No other code from category O24, Diabetes mellitus in pregnancy, childbirth, and the puerperium, should be used with a code from O24.4.

The codes under subcategory O24.4 include diet controlled, insulin controlled, and controlled by oral hypoglycemic drugs. If a patient with gestational diabetes is treated with both diet and insulin, only the code for insulin-controlled is required. If a patient with gestational diabetes is treated with both diet and oral hypoglycemic medications, only the code for "controlled by oral hypoglycemic drugs" is required. Codes Z79.4, Long-term (current) use of insulin, Z79.84, Long-term (current) use of oral hypoglycemic drugs, **and Z79.85, Long-term (current) use of injectable non-insulin antidiabetic drugs,** should not be assigned with codes from subcategory O24.4.

An abnormal glucose tolerance in pregnancy is assigned a code from subcategory O99.81, Abnormal glucose complicating pregnancy, childbirth, and the puerperium.

j. Sepsis and septic shock complicating abortion, pregnancy, childbirth and the puerperium

When assigning a chapter 15 code for sepsis complicating abortion, pregnancy, childbirth, and the puerperium, a code for the specific type of infection should be assigned as an additional diagnosis. If severe sepsis is present, a code from subcategory R65.2, Severe sepsis, and code(s) for associated organ dysfunction(s) should also be assigned as additional diagnoses.

k. Puerperal sepsis

Code O85, Puerperal sepsis, should be assigned with a secondary code to identify the causal organism (e.g., for a bacterial infection, assign a code from category B95-B96, Bacterial infections in conditions classified elsewhere). A code from category A4Ø, Streptococcal sepsis, or A41, Other sepsis, should not be used for puerperal sepsis. If applicable, use additional codes to identify severe sepsis (R65.2-) and any associated acute organ dysfunction.

Code O85 should not be assigned for sepsis following an obstetrical procedure (See Section I.C.1.d.5.b., Sepsis due to a postprocedural infection).

l. Alcohol, tobacco and drug use during pregnancy, childbirth and the puerperium

1) Alcohol use during pregnancy, childbirth and the puerperium

Codes under subcategory O99.31, Alcohol use complicating pregnancy, childbirth, and the puerperium, should be assigned for any pregnancy case when a patient uses alcohol during the pregnancy or postpartum. A secondary code from category F1Ø, Alcohol related disorders, should also be assigned to identify manifestations of the alcohol use.

2) Tobacco use during pregnancy, childbirth and the puerperium

Codes under subcategory O99.33, Smoking (tobacco) complicating pregnancy, childbirth, and the puerperium, should be assigned for any pregnancy case when a patient uses any type of tobacco product during the pregnancy or postpartum.

A secondary code from category F17, Nicotine dependence, should also be assigned to identify the type of nicotine dependence.

3) Drug use during pregnancy, childbirth and the puerperium

Codes under subcategory O99.32, Drug use complicating pregnancy, childbirth, and the puerperium, should be assigned for any pregnancy case when a patient uses drugs during the pregnancy or postpartum. This can involve illegal drugs, or inappropriate use or abuse of prescription drugs. Secondary code(s) from categories F11-F16 and F18-F19 should also be assigned to identify manifestations of the drug use.

m. Poisoning, toxic effects, adverse effects and underdosing in a pregnant patient

A code from subcategory O9A.2, Injury, poisoning and certain other consequences of external causes complicating pregnancy, childbirth, and the puerperium, should be sequenced first, followed by the appropriate injury, poisoning, toxic effect, adverse effect or underdosing code, and then the additional code(s) that specifies the condition caused by the poisoning, toxic effect, adverse effect or underdosing.

See Section I.C.19. Adverse effects, poisoning, underdosing and toxic effects.

n. Normal Delivery, Code O8Ø

1) Encounter for full term uncomplicated delivery

Code O8Ø should be assigned when a patient is admitted for a full-term normal delivery and delivers a single, healthy infant without any complications antepartum, during the delivery, or postpartum during the delivery episode. Code O8Ø is always a principal diagnosis. It is not to be used if any other code from chapter 15 is needed to describe a current complication of the antenatal, delivery, or postnatal period. Additional codes from other chapters may be used with code O8Ø if they are not related to or are in any way complicating the pregnancy.

2) Uncomplicated delivery with resolved antepartum complication

Code O8Ø may be used if the patient had a complication at some point during the pregnancy, but the complication is not present at the time of the admission for delivery.

3) Outcome of delivery for O8Ø

Z37.Ø, Single live birth, is the only outcome of delivery code appropriate for use with O8Ø.

o. The Peripartum and Postpartum Periods

1) Peripartum and Postpartum periods

The postpartum period begins immediately after delivery and continues for six weeks following delivery. The peripartum period is defined as the last month of pregnancy to five months postpartum.

2) Peripartum and postpartum complication

A postpartum complication is any complication occurring within the six-week period.

3) Pregnancy-related complications after 6-week period

Chapter 15 codes may also be used to describe pregnancy-related complications after the peripartum or postpartum period if the provider documents that a condition is pregnancy related.

4) Admission for routine postpartum care following delivery outside hospital

When the mother delivers outside the hospital prior to admission and is admitted for routine postpartum care and no complications are noted, code Z39.Ø, Encounter for care and examination of mother immediately after delivery, should be assigned as the principal diagnosis.

5) Pregnancy associated cardiomyopathy

Pregnancy associated cardiomyopathy, code O9Ø.3, is unique in that it may be diagnosed in the third trimester of pregnancy but may continue to progress months after delivery. For this reason, it is referred to as peripartum cardiomyopathy. Code O9Ø.3 is only for use when the cardiomyopathy develops as a result of pregnancy in a patient who did not have pre-existing heart disease.

p. Code O94, Sequelae of complication of pregnancy, childbirth, and the puerperium

1) Code O94

Code O94, Sequelae of complication of pregnancy, childbirth, and the puerperium, is for use in those cases when an initial complication of a pregnancy develops a sequela or sequelae requiring care or treatment at a future date.

2) After the initial postpartum period

This code may be used at any time after the initial postpartum period.

3) Sequencing of Code O94

This code, like all sequela codes, is to be sequenced following the code describing the sequelae of the complication.

q. Termination of Pregnancy and Spontaneous abortions

1) Abortion with Liveborn Fetus

When an attempted termination of pregnancy results in a liveborn fetus, assign code Z33.2, Encounter for elective termination of pregnancy and a code from category Z37, Outcome of Delivery.

2) Retained Products of Conception following an abortion

Subsequent encounters for retained products of conception following a spontaneous abortion or elective termination of pregnancy, without complications are assigned OØ3.4, Incomplete spontaneous abortion without complication, or code OØ7.4, Failed attempted termination of pregnancy without complication. This advice is appropriate even when the patient was discharged previously with a discharge diagnosis of complete abortion. If the patient has a specific complication associated with the spontaneous abortion or elective termination of pregnancy in addition to retained products of conception, assign the appropriate complication code (e.g., OØ3.-, OØ4.-, OØ7.-) instead of code OØ3.4 or OØ7.4.

3) Complications leading to abortion

Codes from Chapter 15 may be used as additional codes to identify any documented complications of the pregnancy in conjunction with codes in categories in OØ4, OØ7 and OØ8.

4) Hemorrhage following elective abortion

For hemorrhage post elective abortion, assign code OØ4.6, Delayed or excessive hemorrhage following (induced) termination of pregnancy. Do not assign code O72.1, Other immediate postpartum hemorrhage, as this code should not be assigned for post abortion conditions. Do not assign code Z33.2, Encounter for elective termination of pregnancy, when the patient experiences a complication post elective abortion.

r. Abuse in a pregnant patient

For suspected or confirmed cases of abuse of a pregnant patient, a code(s) from subcategories O9A.3, Physical abuse complicating pregnancy, childbirth, and the puerperium, O9A.4, Sexual abuse complicating pregnancy, childbirth, and the puerperium, and O9A.5, Psychological abuse complicating pregnancy, childbirth, and the puerperium, should be sequenced first, followed by the appropriate codes (if applicable) to identify any associated current injury due to physical abuse, sexual abuse, and the perpetrator of abuse.

See Section I.C.19. Adult and child abuse, neglect and other maltreatment.

s. COVID-19 infection in pregnancy, childbirth, and the puerperium

During pregnancy, childbirth or the puerperium, when COVID-19 is the reason for admission/encounter , code O98.5-, Other viral diseases complicating pregnancy, childbirth and the puerperium, should be sequenced as the principal/first-listed diagnosis, and code UØ7.1, COVID-19, and the appropriate codes for associated manifestation(s) should be assigned as additional diagnoses. Codes from Chapter 15 always take sequencing priority.

If the reason for admission/encounter is unrelated to COVID-19 but the patient tests positive for COVID-19 during the admission/encounter, the appropriate code for the reason for admission/encounter should be sequenced as the principal/first-listed diagnosis, and codes O98.5- and UØ7.1, as well as the appropriate codes for associated COVID-19 manifestations, should be assigned as additional diagnoses.

16. Chapter 16: Certain Conditions Originating in the Perinatal Period (PØØ-P96)

For coding and reporting purposes the perinatal period is defined as before birth through the 28th day following birth. The following guidelines are provided for reporting purposes.

a. General Perinatal Rules

1) Use of Chapter 16 Codes

Codes in this chapter are never for use on the maternal record. Codes from Chapter 15, the obstetric chapter, are never permitted on the newborn record. Chapter 16 codes may be used throughout the life of the patient if the condition is still present.

2) Principal Diagnosis for Birth Record

When coding the birth episode in a newborn record, assign a code from category Z38, Liveborn infants according to place of birth and type of delivery, as the principal diagnosis. A code from category Z38 is assigned only once, to a newborn at the time of birth. If a newborn is transferred to another institution, a code from category Z38 should not be used at the receiving hospital.

A code from category Z38 is used only on the newborn record, not on the mother's record.

3) Use of Codes from other Chapters with Codes from Chapter 16

Codes from other chapters may be used with codes from chapter 16 if the codes from the other chapters provide more specific detail. Codes for signs and symptoms may be assigned when a definitive diagnosis has not been established. If the reason for the encounter is a perinatal condition, the code from chapter 16 should be sequenced first.

4) Use of Chapter 16 Codes after the Perinatal Period

Should a condition originate in the perinatal period, and continue throughout the life of the patient, the perinatal code should continue to be used regardless of the patient's age.

5) Birth process or community acquired conditions

If a newborn has a condition that may be either due to the birth process or community acquired and the documentation does not indicate which it is, the default is due to the birth process and the code from Chapter 16 should be used. If the condition is community-acquired, a code from Chapter 16 should not be assigned.

For COVID-19 infection in a newborn, see guideline I.C.16.h.

6) Code all clinically significant conditions

All clinically significant conditions noted on routine newborn examination should be coded. A condition is clinically significant if it requires:

- clinical evaluation; or
- therapeutic treatment; or
- diagnostic procedures; or
- extended length of hospital stay; or
- increased nursing care and/or monitoring; or
- has implications for future health care needs

Note: The perinatal guidelines listed above are the same as the general coding guidelines for "additional diagnoses," except for the final point regarding implications for future health care needs. Codes should be assigned for conditions that have been specified by the provider as having implications for future health care needs.

b. Observation and Evaluation of Newborns for Suspected Conditions not Found

1) Use of ZØ5 codes

Assign a code from category ZØ5, Observation and evaluation of newborn for suspected **diseases and** conditions ruled out, to identify those instances when a healthy newborn is evaluated for a suspected condition/**disease** that is determined after study not to be present. Do not use a code from category ZØ5 when the patient **is documented to have** signs or symptoms of a suspected problem; in such cases code the sign or symptom.

2) ZØ5 on other than the birth record

A code from category ZØ5 may also be assigned as a principal or first-listed code for readmissions or encounters when the code from category Z38 code no longer applies. Codes from category ZØ5 are for use only for healthy newborns and infants for which no condition after study is found to be present.

3) ZØ5 on a birth record

A code from category ZØ5 is to be used as a secondary code after the code from category Z38, Liveborn infants according to place of birth and type of delivery.

c. Coding Additional Perinatal Diagnoses

1) Assigning codes for conditions that require treatment

Assign codes for conditions that require treatment or further investigation, prolong the length of stay, or require resource utilization.

2) Codes for conditions specified as having implications for future health care needs

Assign codes for conditions that have been specified by the provider as having implications for future health care needs.

Note: This guideline should not be used for adult patients.

d. Prematurity and Fetal Growth Retardation

Providers utilize different criteria in determining prematurity. A code for prematurity should not be assigned unless it is documented. Assignment of codes in categories PØ5, Disorders of newborn related to slow fetal growth and fetal malnutrition, and PØ7, Disorders of newborn related to short gestation and low birth weight, not elsewhere classified, should be based on the recorded birth weight and estimated gestational age.

When both birth weight and gestational age are available, two codes from category PØ7 should be assigned, with the code for birth weight sequenced before the code for gestational age.

e. Low birth weight and immaturity status

Codes from category PØ7, Disorders of newborn related to short gestation and low birth weight, not elsewhere classified, are for use for a child or adult who was premature or had a low birth weight as a newborn and this is affecting the patient's current health status.

See Section I.C.21. Factors influencing health status and contact with health services, Status.

f. Bacterial Sepsis of Newborn

Category P36, Bacterial sepsis of newborn, includes congenital sepsis. If a perinate is documented as having sepsis without documentation of congenital or community acquired, the default is congenital and a code from category P36 should be assigned. If the P36 code includes the causal organism, an additional code from category B95, Streptococcus, Staphylococcus, and Enterococcus as the cause of diseases classified elsewhere, or B96, Other bacterial agents as the cause of diseases classified elsewhere, should not be assigned. If the P36 code does not include the causal organism, assign an additional code from category B96. If applicable, use additional codes to identify severe sepsis (R65.2-) and any associated acute organ dysfunction.

g. Stillbirth

Code P95, Stillbirth, is only for use in institutions that maintain separate records for stillbirths. No other code should be used with P95. Code P95 should not be used on the mother's record.

h. COVID-19 Infection in Newborn

For a newborn that tests positive for COVID-19, assign code UØ7.1, COVID-19, and the appropriate codes for associated manifestation(s) in neonates/newborns in the absence of documentation indicating a specific type of transmission. For a newborn that tests positive for COVID-19 and the provider documents the condition was contracted in utero or during the birth process, assign codes P35.8, Other congenital viral diseases, and UØ7.1, COVID-19. When coding the birth episode in a newborn record, the appropriate code from category Z38, Liveborn infants according to place of birth and type of delivery, should be assigned as the principal diagnosis.

17. Chapter 17: Congenital malformations, deformations, and chromosomal abnormalities (QØØ-Q99)

Assign an appropriate code(s) from categories QØØ-Q99, Congenital malformations, deformations, and chromosomal abnormalities when a malformation/deformation or chromosomal abnormality is documented. A malformation/deformation/or chromosomal abnormality may be the principal/first-listed diagnosis on a record or a secondary diagnosis.

When a malformation/deformation or chromosomal abnormality does not have a unique code assignment, assign additional code(s) for any manifestations that may be present.

When the code assignment specifically identifies the malformation/deformation or chromosomal abnormality, manifestations that are an inherent component of the anomaly should not be coded separately. Additional codes should be assigned for manifestations that are not an inherent component.

Codes from Chapter 17 may be used throughout the life of the patient. If a congenital malformation or deformity has been corrected, a personal history code should be used to identify the history of the malformation or deformity. Although present at birth, a malformation/deformation/or chromosomal abnormality may not be identified until later in life. Whenever the condition is diagnosed by the provider, it is appropriate to assign a code from codes QØØ-Q99. For the birth admission, the appropriate code from category Z38, Liveborn infants, according to place of birth and type of delivery, should be sequenced as the principal diagnosis, followed by any congenital anomaly codes, QØØ-Q99.

18. Chapter 18: Symptoms, signs, and abnormal clinical and laboratory findings, not elsewhere classified (RØØ-R99)

Chapter 18 includes symptoms, signs, abnormal results of clinical or other investigative procedures, and ill-defined conditions regarding which no diagnosis classifiable elsewhere is recorded. Signs and symptoms that point to a specific diagnosis have been assigned to a category in other chapters of the classification.

a. Use of symptom codes

Codes that describe symptoms and signs are acceptable for reporting purposes when a related definitive diagnosis has not been established (confirmed) by the provider.

b. Use of a symptom code with a definitive diagnosis code

Codes for signs and symptoms may be reported in addition to a related definitive diagnosis when the sign or symptom is not routinely associated with that diagnosis, such as the various signs and symptoms associated with complex syndromes. The definitive diagnosis code should be sequenced before the symptom code.

Signs or symptoms that are associated routinely with a disease process should not be assigned as additional codes, unless otherwise instructed by the classification.

c. Combination codes that include symptoms

ICD-10-CM contains a number of combination codes that identify both the definitive diagnosis and common symptoms of that diagnosis. When using one of these combination codes, an additional code should not be assigned for the symptom.

d. Repeated falls

Code R29.6, Repeated falls, is for use for encounters when a patient has recently fallen and the reason for the fall is being investigated.

Code Z91.81, History of falling, is for use when a patient has fallen in the past and is at risk for future falls. When appropriate, both codes R29.6 and Z91.81 may be assigned together.

e. Coma

Code R40.20, Unspecified coma, may be assigned in conjunction with codes for any medical condition.

Do not report codes for unspecified coma, individual or total Glasgow coma scale scores for a patient with a medically induced coma or a sedated patient.

1) Coma Scale

The coma scale codes (R40.21- to R40.24-) can be used in conjunction with traumatic brain injury codes. These codes are primarily for use by trauma registries, but they may be used in any setting where this information is collected. The coma scale codes should be sequenced after the diagnosis code(s).

These codes, one from each subcategory, are needed to complete the scale. The 7th character indicates when the scale was recorded. The 7th character should match for all three codes.

At a minimum, report the initial score documented on presentation at your facility. This may be a score from the emergency medicine technician (EMT) or in the emergency department. If desired, a facility may choose to capture multiple coma scale scores.

Assign code R40.24-, Glasgow coma scale, total score, when only the total score is documented in the medical record and not the individual score(s).

If multiple coma scores are captured within the first 24 hours after hospital admission, assign only the code for the score at the time of admission. ICD-10-CM does not classify coma scores that are reported after admission but less than 24 hours later.

See Section I.B.14. for coma scale documentation by clinicians other than patient's provider

f. Functional quadriplegia

GUIDELINE HAS BEEN DELETED EFFECTIVE OCTOBER 1, 2017

g. SIRS due to Non-Infectious Process

The systemic inflammatory response syndrome (SIRS) can develop as a result of certain non-infectious disease processes, such as trauma, malignant neoplasm, or pancreatitis. When SIRS is documented with a noninfectious condition, and no subsequent infection is documented, the code for the underlying condition, such as an injury, should be assigned, followed by code R65.10, Systemic inflammatory response syndrome (SIRS) of non-infectious origin without acute organ dysfunction, or code R65.11, Systemic inflammatory response syndrome (SIRS) of non-infectious origin with acute organ dysfunction. If an associated acute organ dysfunction is documented, the appropriate code(s) for the specific type of organ dysfunction(s) should be assigned in addition to code R65.11. If acute organ dysfunction is documented, but it cannot be determined if the acute organ dysfunction is associated with SIRS or due to another condition (e.g., directly due to the trauma), the provider should be queried.

h. Death NOS

Code R99, Ill-defined and unknown cause of mortality, is only for use in the very limited circumstance when a patient who has already died is brought into an emergency department or other healthcare facility and is pronounced dead upon arrival. It does not represent the discharge disposition of death.

i. NIHSS Stroke Scale

The NIH stroke scale (NIHSS) codes (R29.7- -) can be used in conjunction with acute stroke codes (I63) to identify the patient's neurological status and the severity of the stroke. The stroke scale codes should be sequenced after the acute stroke diagnosis code(s).

At a minimum, report the initial score documented. If desired, a facility may choose to capture multiple stroke scale scores.

See Section I.B.14. for NIHSS stroke scale documentation by clinicians other than patient's provider

19. Chapter 19: Injury, poisoning, and certain other consequences of external causes (S00-T88)

a. Application of 7th Characters in Chapter 19

Most categories in chapter 19 have a 7th character requirement for each applicable code. Most categories in this chapter have three 7th character values (with the exception of fractures): A, initial encounter, D, subsequent encounter and S, sequela. Categories for traumatic fractures have additional 7th character values. While the patient may be seen by a new or different provider over the course of treatment for an injury, assignment of the 7th character is based on whether the patient is undergoing active treatment and not whether the provider is seeing the patient for the first time.

For complication codes, active treatment refers to treatment for the condition described by the code, even though it may be related to an earlier precipitating problem. For example, code T84.50XA, Infection and inflammatory reaction due to unspecified internal joint prosthesis, initial encounter, is used when active treatment is provided for the infection, even though the condition relates to the prosthetic device, implant or graft that was placed at a previous encounter.

7th character "A", initial encounter is used for each encounter where the patient is receiving active treatment for the condition.

7th character "D" subsequent encounter is used for encounters after the patient has completed active treatment of the condition and is receiving routine care for the condition during the healing or recovery phase.

The aftercare Z codes should not be used for aftercare for conditions such as injuries or poisonings, where 7th characters are provided to identify subsequent care. For example, for aftercare of an injury, assign the acute injury code with the 7th character "D" (subsequent encounter).

7th character "S", sequela, is for use for complications or conditions that arise as a direct result of a condition, such as scar formation after a burn. The scars are sequelae of the burn. When using 7th character "S", it is necessary to use both the injury code that precipitated the sequela and the code for the sequela itself. The "S" is added only to the injury code, not the sequela code. The 7th character "S" identifies the injury responsible for the sequela. The specific type of sequela (e.g. scar) is sequenced first, followed by the injury code.

See Section I.B.10. Sequelae, (Late Effects)

b. Coding of Injuries

When coding injuries, assign separate codes for each injury unless a combination code is provided, in which case the combination code is assigned. Codes from category T07, Unspecified multiple injuries should not be assigned in the inpatient setting unless information for a more specific code is not available. Traumatic injury codes (S00-T14.9) are not to be used for normal, healing surgical wounds or to identify complications of surgical wounds.

The code for the most serious injury, as determined by the provider and the focus of treatment, is sequenced first.

1) Superficial injuries

Superficial injuries such as abrasions or contusions are not coded when associated with more severe injuries of the same site.

2) Primary injury with damage to nerves/blood vessels

When a primary injury results in minor damage to peripheral nerves or blood vessels, the primary injury is sequenced first with additional code(s) for injuries to nerves and spinal cord (such as category S04), and/or injury to blood vessels (such as category S15). When the primary injury is to the blood vessels or nerves, that injury should be sequenced first.

3) Iatrogenic injuries

Injury codes from Chapter 19 should not be assigned for injuries that occur during, or as a result of, a medical intervention. Assign the appropriate complication code(s).

c. Coding of Traumatic Fractures

The principles of multiple coding of injuries should be followed in coding fractures. Fractures of specified sites are coded individually by site in accordance with both the provisions within categories S02, S12, S22, S32, S42, S49, S52, S59, S62, S72, S79, S82, S89, S92 and the level of detail furnished by medical record content.

A fracture not indicated as open or closed should be coded to closed. A fracture not indicated whether displaced or not displaced should be coded to displaced.

More specific guidelines are as follows:

1) Initial vs. subsequent encounter for fractures

Traumatic fractures are coded using the appropriate 7th character for initial encounter (A, B, C) for each encounter where the patient is receiving active treatment for the fracture. The appropriate 7th character for initial encounter should also be assigned for a patient who delayed seeking treatment for the fracture or nonunion.

Fractures are coded using the appropriate 7th character for subsequent care for encounters after the patient has completed active treatment of the fracture and is receiving routine care for the fracture during the healing or recovery phase.

Care for complications of surgical treatment for fracture repairs during the healing or recovery phase should be coded with the appropriate complication codes.

Care of complications of fractures, such as malunion and nonunion, should be reported with the appropriate 7th character for subsequent care with nonunion (K, M, N,) or subsequent care with malunion (P, Q, R).

Malunion/nonunion: The appropriate 7th character for initial encounter should also be assigned for a patient who delayed seeking treatment for the fracture or nonunion.

The open fracture designations in the assignment of the 7th character for fractures of the forearm, femur and lower leg, including ankle are based on the Gustilo open fracture classification. When the Gustilo classification type is not specified for an open fracture, the 7th character for open fracture type I or II should be assigned (B, E, H, M, Q).

A code from category M8Ø, not a traumatic fracture code, should be used for any patient with known osteoporosis who suffers a fracture, even if the patient had a minor fall or trauma, if that fall or trauma would not usually break a normal, healthy bone.

See Section I.C.13. Osteoporosis.

The aftercare Z codes should not be used for aftercare for traumatic fractures. For aftercare of a traumatic fracture, assign the acute fracture code with the appropriate 7th character.

2) Multiple fractures sequencing

Multiple fractures are sequenced in accordance with the severity of the fracture.

3) Physeal fractures

For physeal fractures, assign only the code identifying the type of physeal fracture. Do not assign a separate code to identify the specific bone that is fractured.

d. Coding of Burns and Corrosions

The ICD-10-CM makes a distinction between burns and corrosions. The burn codes are for thermal burns, except sunburns, that come from a heat source, such as a fire or hot appliance. The burn codes are also for burns resulting from electricity and radiation. Corrosions are burns due to chemicals. The guidelines are the same for burns and corrosions.

Current burns (T2Ø-T25) are classified by depth, extent and by agent (X code). Burns are classified by depth as first degree (erythema), second degree (blistering), and third degree (full-thickness involvement). Burns of the eye and internal organs (T26-T28) are classified by site, but not by degree.

1) Sequencing of burn and related condition codes

Sequence first the code that reflects the highest degree of burn when more than one burn is present.

a. When the reason for the admission or encounter is for treatment of external multiple burns, sequence first the code that reflects the burn of the highest degree.

b. When a patient has both internal and external burns, the circumstances of admission govern the selection of the principal diagnosis or first-listed diagnosis.

c. When a patient is admitted for burn injuries and other related conditions such as smoke inhalation and/or respiratory failure, the circumstances of admission govern the selection of the principal or first-listed diagnosis.

2) Burns of the same anatomic site

Classify burns of the same anatomic site and on the same side but of different degrees to the subcategory identifying the highest degree recorded in the diagnosis (e.g., for second and third degree burns of right thigh, assign only code T24.311-).

3) Non-healing burns

Non-healing burns are coded as acute burns.

Necrosis of burned skin should be coded as a non-healed burn.

4) Infected burn

For any documented infected burn site, use an additional code for the infection.

5) Assign separate codes for each burn site

When coding burns, assign separate codes for each burn site. Category T3Ø, Burn and corrosion, body region unspecified is extremely vague and should rarely be used.

Codes for burns of "multiple sites" should only be assigned when the medical record documentation does not specify the individual sites.

6) Burns and corrosions classified according to extent of body surface involved

Assign codes from category T31, Burns classified according to extent of body surface involved, or T32, Corrosions classified according to extent of body surface involved, for acute burns or corrosions when the site of the burn or corrosion is not specified or when there is a need for additional data. It is advisable to use category T31 as additional coding when needed to provide data for evaluating burn mortality, such as that needed by burn units. It is also advisable to use category T31 as an additional code for reporting purposes when there is mention of a third-degree burn involving 20 percent or more of the body surface. Codes from categories T31 and T32 should not be used for sequelae of burns or corrosions.

Categories T31 and T32 are based on the classic "rule of nines" in estimating body surface involved: head and neck are assigned nine percent, each arm nine percent, each leg 18 percent, the anterior trunk 18 percent, posterior trunk 18 percent, and genitalia one percent. Providers may change these percentage assignments where necessary to accommodate infants and children who have proportionately larger heads than adults, and patients who have large buttocks, thighs, or abdomen that involve burns.

7) Encounters for treatment of sequela of burns

Encounters for the treatment of the late effects of burns or corrosions (i.e., scars or joint contractures) should be coded with a burn or corrosion code with the 7th character "S" for sequela.

8) Sequelae with a late effect code and current burn

When appropriate, both a code for a current burn or corrosion with 7th character "A" or "D" and a burn or corrosion code with 7th character "S" may be assigned on the same record (when both a current burn and sequelae of an old burn exist). Burns and corrosions do not heal at the same rate and a current healing wound may still exist with sequela of a healed burn or corrosion.

See Section I.B.10. Sequela (Late Effects)

9) Use of an external cause code with burns and corrosions

An external cause code should be used with burns and corrosions to identify the source and intent of the burn, as well as the place where it occurred.

e. Adverse Effects, Poisoning, Underdosing and Toxic Effects

Codes in categories T36-T65 are combination codes that include the substance that was taken as well as the intent. No additional external cause code is required for poisonings, toxic effects, adverse effects and underdosing codes.

1) Do not code directly from the Table of Drugs

Do not code directly from the Table of Drugs and Chemicals. Always refer back to the Tabular List.

2) Use as many codes as necessary to describe

Use as many codes as necessary to describe completely all drugs, medicinal or biological substances.

3) If the same code would describe the causative agent

If the same code would describe the causative agent for more than one adverse reaction, poisoning, toxic effect or underdosing, assign the code only once.

4) If two or more drugs, medicinal or biological substances

If two or more drugs, medicinal or biological substances are taken, code each individually unless a combination code is listed in the Table of Drugs and Chemicals.

If multiple unspecified drugs, medicinal or biological substances were taken, assign the appropriate code from subcategory

T5Ø.91, Poisoning by, adverse effect of and underdosing of multiple unspecified drugs, medicaments and biological substances.

5) The occurrence of drug toxicity is classified in ICD-10-CM as follows:

(a) Adverse Effect

When coding an adverse effect of a drug that has been correctly prescribed and properly administered, assign the appropriate code for the nature of the adverse effect followed by the appropriate code for the adverse effect of the drug (T36-T5Ø). The code for the drug should have a 5th or 6th character "5" (for example T36.ØX5-) Examples of the nature of an adverse effect are tachycardia, delirium, gastrointestinal hemorrhaging, vomiting, hypokalemia, hepatitis, renal failure, or respiratory failure.

(b) Poisoning

When coding a poisoning or reaction to the improper use of a medication (e.g., overdose, wrong substance given or taken in error, wrong route of administration), first assign the appropriate code from categories T36-T5Ø. The poisoning codes have an associated intent as their 5th or 6th character (accidental, intentional self-harm, assault and undetermined). If the intent of the poisoning is unknown or unspecified, code the intent as accidental intent. The undetermined intent is only for use if the documentation in the record specifies that the intent cannot be determined. Use additional code(s) for all manifestations of poisonings.

If there is also a diagnosis of abuse or dependence of the substance, the abuse or dependence is assigned as an additional code.

Examples of poisoning include:

(i) Error was made in drug prescription

Errors made in drug prescription or in the administration of the drug by provider, nurse, patient, or other person.

(ii) Overdose of a drug intentionally taken

If an overdose of a drug was intentionally taken or administered and resulted in drug toxicity, it would be coded as a poisoning.

(iii) Nonprescribed drug taken with correctly prescribed and properly administered drug

If a nonprescribed drug or medicinal agent was taken in combination with a correctly prescribed and properly administered drug, any drug toxicity or other reaction resulting from the interaction of the two drugs would be classified as a poisoning.

(iv) Interaction of drug(s) and alcohol

When a reaction results from the interaction of a drug(s) and alcohol, this would be classified as poisoning.

See Section I.C.4. if poisoning is the result of insulin pump malfunctions.

(c) Underdosing

Underdosing refers to taking less of a medication than is prescribed by a provider or a manufacturer's instruction. Discontinuing the use of a prescribed medication on the patient's own initiative (not directed by the patient's provider) is also classified as an underdosing. For underdosing, assign the code from categories T36-T5Ø (fifth or sixth character "6"). **Documentation of a change in the patient's condition is not required in order to assign an underdosing code. Documentation that the patient is taking less of a medication than is prescribed or discontinued the prescribed medication is sufficient for code assignment.**

Codes for underdosing should never be assigned as principal or first-listed codes. If a patient has a relapse or exacerbation of the medical condition for which the drug is prescribed because of the reduction in dose, then the medical condition itself should be coded.

Noncompliance (Z91.12-, Z91.13- and Z91.14-) or complication of care (Y63.6-Y63.9) codes are to be used with an underdosing code to indicate intent, if known.

(d) Toxic Effects

When a harmful substance is ingested or comes in contact with a person, this is classified as a toxic effect. The toxic effect codes are in categories T51-T65.

Toxic effect codes have an associated intent: accidental, intentional self-harm, assault and undetermined.

f. Adult and child abuse, neglect and other maltreatment

Sequence first the appropriate code from categories T74, Adult and child abuse, neglect and other maltreatment, confirmed, or T76, Adult and child abuse, neglect and other maltreatment, suspected, for abuse, neglect and other maltreatment, followed by any accompanying mental health or injury code(s).

If the documentation in the medical record states abuse or neglect, it is coded as confirmed (T74.-). It is coded as suspected if it is documented as suspected (T76.-).

For cases of confirmed abuse or neglect an external cause code from the assault section (X92-YØ9) should be added to identify the cause of any physical injuries. A perpetrator code (YØ7) should be added when the perpetrator of the abuse is known. For suspected cases of abuse or neglect, do not report external cause or perpetrator code.

If a suspected case of abuse, neglect or mistreatment is ruled out during an encounter code ZØ4.71, Encounter for examination and observation following alleged physical adult abuse, ruled out, or code ZØ4.72, Encounter for examination and observation following alleged child physical abuse, ruled out, should be used, not a code from T76.

If a suspected case of alleged rape or sexual abuse is ruled out during an encounter code ZØ4.41, Encounter for examination and observation following alleged adult rape or code ZØ4.42, Encounter for examination and observation following alleged child rape, should be used, not a code from T76.

If a suspected case of forced sexual exploitation or forced labor exploitation is ruled out during an encounter, code ZØ4.81, Encounter for examination and observation of victim following forced sexual exploitation, or code ZØ4.82, Encounter for examination and observation of victim following forced labor exploitation, should be used, not a code from T76.

See Section I.C.15. Abuse in a pregnant patient.

g. Complications of care

1) General guidelines for complications of care

(a) Documentation of complications of care

See Section I.B.16. for information on documentation of complications of care.

2) Pain due to medical devices

Pain associated with devices, implants or grafts left in a surgical site (for example painful hip prosthesis) is assigned to the appropriate code(s) found in Chapter 19, Injury, poisoning, and certain other consequences of external causes. Specific codes for pain due to medical devices are found in the T code section of the ICD-10-CM. Use additional code(s) from category G89 to identify acute or chronic pain due to presence of the device, implant or graft (G89.18 or G89.28).

3) Transplant complications

(a) Transplant complications other than kidney

Codes under category T86, Complications of transplanted organs and tissues, are for use for both complications and rejection of transplanted organs. A transplant complication code is only assigned if the complication affects the function of the transplanted organ. Two codes are required to fully describe a transplant complication: the appropriate code from category T86 and a secondary code that identifies the complication.

Pre-existing conditions or conditions that develop after the transplant are not coded as complications unless they affect the function of the transplanted organs.

See I.C.21. for transplant organ removal status

See I.C.2. for malignant neoplasm associated with transplanted organ.

(b) Kidney transplant complications

Patients who have undergone kidney transplant may still have some form of chronic kidney disease (CKD) because the kidney transplant may not fully restore kidney function. Code T86.1- should be assigned for documented complications of a kidney transplant, such as transplant failure or rejection or other transplant complication. Code T86.1- should not be assigned for post kidney transplant patients who have chronic kidney (CKD) unless a transplant complication such as transplant failure or rejection is documented. If the documentation is unclear as to whether the patient has a complication of the transplant, query the provider.

Conditions that affect the function of the transplanted kidney, other than CKD, should be assigned a code from subcategory T86.1, Complications of transplanted organ, Kidney, and a secondary code that identifies the complication.

For patients with CKD following a kidney transplant, but who do not have a complication such as failure or rejection, *see section I.C.14. Chronic kidney disease and kidney transplant status.*

4) Complication codes that include the external cause

As with certain other T codes, some of the complications of care codes have the external cause included in the code. The code includes the nature of the complication as well as the type of procedure that caused the complication. No external cause code indicating the type of procedure is necessary for these codes.

5) Complications of care codes within the body system chapters

Intraoperative and postprocedural complication codes are found within the body system chapters with codes specific to the organs and structures of that body system. These codes should be sequenced first, followed by a code(s) for the specific complication, if applicable.

Complication codes from the body system chapters should be assigned for intraoperative and postprocedural complications (e.g., the appropriate complication code from chapter 9 would be assigned for a vascular intraoperative or postprocedural complication) unless the complication is specifically indexed to a T code in chapter 19.

20. Chapter 20: External Causes of Morbidity (VØØ-Y99)

The external causes of morbidity codes should never be sequenced as the first-listed or principal diagnosis.

External cause codes are intended to provide data for injury research and evaluation of injury prevention strategies. These codes capture how the injury or health condition happened (cause), the intent (unintentional or accidental; or intentional, such as suicide or assault), the place where the event occurred the activity of the patient at the time of the event, and the person's status (e.g., civilian, military).

There is no national requirement for mandatory ICD-10-CM external cause code reporting. Unless a provider is subject to a state-based external cause code reporting mandate or these codes are required by a particular payer, reporting of ICD-10-CM codes in Chapter 20, External Causes of Morbidity, is not required. In the absence of a mandatory reporting requirement, providers are encouraged to voluntarily report external cause codes, as they provide valuable data for injury research and evaluation of injury prevention strategies.

a. General External Cause Coding Guidelines

1) Used with any code in the range of AØØ.Ø-T88.9, ZØØ-Z99

An external cause code may be used with any code in the range of AØØ.Ø-T88.9, ZØØ-Z99, classification that represents a health condition due to an external cause. Though they are most applicable to injuries, they are also valid for use with such things as infections or diseases due to an external source, and other health conditions, such as a heart attack that occurs during strenuous physical activity.

2) External cause code used for length of treatment

Assign the external cause code, with the appropriate 7th character (initial encounter, subsequent encounter or sequela) for each encounter for which the injury or condition is being treated.

Most categories in chapter 20 have a 7th character requirement for each applicable code. Most categories in this chapter have three 7th character values: A, initial encounter, D, subsequent encounter and S, sequela. While the patient may be seen by a new or different provider over the course of treatment for an injury or condition, assignment of the 7th character for external cause should match the 7th character of the code assigned for the associated injury or condition for the encounter.

3) Use the full range of external cause codes

Use the full range of external cause codes to completely describe the cause, the intent, the place of occurrence, and if applicable, the activity of the patient at the time of the event, and the patient's status, for all injuries, and other health conditions due to an external cause.

4) Assign as many external cause codes as necessary

Assign as many external cause codes as necessary to fully explain each cause. If only one external code can be recorded, assign the code most related to the principal diagnosis.

5) The selection of the appropriate external cause code

The selection of the appropriate external cause code is guided by the Alphabetic Index of External Causes and by Inclusion and Exclusion notes in the Tabular List.

6) External cause code can never be a principal diagnosis

An external cause code can never be a principal (first-listed) diagnosis.

7) Combination external cause codes

Certain of the external cause codes are combination codes that identify sequential events that result in an injury, such as a fall which results in striking against an object. The injury may be due to either event or both. The combination external cause code used should correspond to the sequence of events regardless of which caused the most serious injury.

8) No external cause code needed in certain circumstances

No external cause code from Chapter 20 is needed if the external cause and intent are included in a code from another chapter (e.g., T36.ØX1-, Poisoning by penicillins, accidental (unintentional)).

b. Place of Occurrence Guideline

Codes from category Y92, Place of occurrence of the external cause, are secondary codes for use after other external cause codes to identify the location of the patient at the time of injury or other condition.

Generally, a place of occurrence code is assigned only once, at the initial encounter for treatment. However, in the rare instance that a new injury occurs during hospitalization, an additional place of occurrence code may be assigned. No 7th characters are used for Y92.

Do not use place of occurrence code Y92.9 if the place is not stated or is not applicable.

c. Activity Code

Assign a code from category Y93, Activity code, to describe the activity of the patient at the time the injury or other health condition occurred.

An activity code is used only once, at the initial encounter for treatment. Only one code from Y93 should be recorded on a medical record.

The activity codes are not applicable to poisonings, adverse effects, misadventures or sequela.

Do not assign Y93.9, Unspecified activity, if the activity is not stated.

A code from category Y93 is appropriate for use with external cause and intent codes if identifying the activity provides additional information about the event.

d. Place of Occurrence, Activity, and Status Codes Used with other External Cause Code

When applicable, place of occurrence, activity, and external cause status codes are sequenced after the main external cause code(s). Regardless of the number of external cause codes assigned, generally there should be only one place of occurrence code, one activity code, and one external cause status code assigned to an encounter. However, in the rare instance that a new injury occurs during hospitalization, an additional place of occurrence code may be assigned.

e. If the Reporting Format Limits the Number of External Cause Codes

If the reporting format limits the number of external cause codes that can be used in reporting clinical data, report the code for the cause/intent most related to the principal diagnosis. If the format permits capture of additional external cause codes, the cause/intent, including medical misadventures, of the additional events should be reported rather than the codes for place, activity, or external status.

f. Multiple External Cause Coding Guidelines

More than one external cause code is required to fully describe the external cause of an illness or injury. The assignment of external cause codes should be sequenced in the following priority:

If two or more events cause separate injuries, an external cause code should be assigned for each cause. The first-listed external cause code will be selected in the following order:

External codes for child and adult abuse take priority over all other external cause codes.

See Section I.C.19., Child and Adult abuse guidelines.

External cause codes for terrorism events take priority over all other external cause codes except child and adult abuse.

External cause codes for cataclysmic events take priority over all other external cause codes except child and adult abuse and terrorism.

External cause codes for transport accidents take priority over all other external cause codes except cataclysmic events, child and adult abuse and terrorism.

Activity and external cause status codes are assigned following all causal (intent) external cause codes.

The first-listed external cause code should correspond to the cause of the most serious diagnosis due to an assault, accident, or self-harm, following the order of hierarchy listed above.

g. Child and Adult Abuse Guideline

Adult and child abuse, neglect and maltreatment are classified as assault. Any of the assault codes may be used to indicate the external cause of any injury resulting from the confirmed abuse.

For confirmed cases of abuse, neglect and maltreatment, when the perpetrator is known, a code from YØ7, Perpetrator of maltreatment and neglect, should accompany any other assault codes.

See Section I.C.19. Adult and child abuse, neglect and other maltreatment

h. Unknown or Undetermined Intent Guideline

If the intent (accident, self-harm, assault) of the cause of an injury or other condition is unknown or unspecified, code the intent as accidental intent. All transport accident categories assume accidental intent.

1) Use of undetermined intent

External cause codes for events of undetermined intent are only for use if the documentation in the record specifies that the intent cannot be determined.

i. Sequelae (Late Effects) of External Cause Guidelines

1) Sequelae external cause codes

Sequela are reported using the external cause code with the 7th character "S" for sequela. These codes should be used with any report of a late effect or sequela resulting from a previous injury.

See Section I.B.10. Sequela (Late Effects)

2) Sequela external cause code with a related current injury

A sequela external cause code should never be used with a related current nature of injury code.

3) Use of sequela external cause codes for subsequent visits

Use a late effect external cause code for subsequent visits when a late effect of the initial injury is being treated. Do not use a late effect external cause code for subsequent visits for follow-up care (e.g., to assess healing, to receive rehabilitative therapy) of the injury when no late effect of the injury has been documented.

j. Terrorism Guidelines

1) Cause of injury identified by the Federal Government (FBI) as terrorism

When the cause of an injury is identified by the Federal Government (FBI) as terrorism, the first-listed external cause code should be a code from category Y38, Terrorism. The definition of terrorism employed by the FBI is found at the inclusion note at the beginning of category Y38. Use additional code for place of occurrence (Y92.-). More than one Y38 code may be assigned if the injury is the result of more than one mechanism of terrorism.

2) Cause of an injury is suspected to be the result of terrorism

When the cause of an injury is suspected to be the result of terrorism a code from category Y38 should not be assigned. Suspected cases should be classified as assault.

3) Code Y38.9, Terrorism, secondary effects

Assign code Y38.9, Terrorism, secondary effects, for conditions occurring subsequent to the terrorist event. This code should not be assigned for conditions that are due to the initial terrorist act.

It is acceptable to assign code Y38.9 with another code from Y38 if there is an injury due to the initial terrorist event and an injury that is a subsequent result of the terrorist event.

k. External Cause Status

A code from category Y99, External cause status, should be assigned whenever any other external cause code is assigned for an encounter, including an Activity code, except for the events noted below. Assign a code from category Y99, External cause status, to indicate the work status of the person at the time the event occurred. The status code indicates whether the event occurred during military activity, whether a non-military person was at work, whether an individual including a student or volunteer was involved in a non-work activity at the time of the causal event.

A code from Y99, External cause status, should be assigned, when applicable, with other external cause codes, such as transport accidents and falls. The external cause status codes are not applicable to poisonings, adverse effects, misadventures or late effects.

Do not assign a code from category Y99 if no other external cause codes (cause, activity) are applicable for the encounter.

An external cause status code is used only once, at the initial encounter for treatment. Only one code from Y99 should be recorded on a medical record.

Do not assign code Y99.9, Unspecified external cause status, if the status is not stated.

21. Chapter 21: Factors influencing health status and contact with health services (ZØØ-Z99)

Note: The chapter specific guidelines provide additional information about the use of Z codes for specified encounters.

a. Use of Z Codes in Any Healthcare Setting

Z codes are for use in any healthcare setting. Z codes may be used as either a first-listed (principal diagnosis code in the inpatient setting) or secondary code, depending on the circumstances of the encounter. Certain Z codes may only be used as first-listed or principal diagnosis.

b. Z Codes Indicate a Reason for an Encounter or Provide Additional Information about a Patient Encounter

Z codes are not procedure codes. A corresponding procedure code must accompany a Z code to describe any procedure performed.

c. Categories of Z Codes

1) Contact/Exposure

Category Z2Ø indicates contact with, and suspected exposure to, communicable diseases. These codes are for patients who are suspected to have been exposed to a disease by close personal contact with an infected individual or are in an area where a disease is epidemic.

Category Z77, Other contact with and (suspected) exposures hazardous to health, indicates contact with and suspected exposures hazardous to health.

Contact/exposure codes may be used as a first-listed code to explain an encounter for testing, or, more commonly, as a secondary code to identify a potential risk.

2) Inoculations and vaccinations

Code Z23 is for encounters for inoculations and vaccinations. It indicates that a patient is being seen to receive a prophylactic inoculation against a disease. Procedure codes are required to identify the actual administration of the injection and the type(s) of immunizations given. Code Z23 may be used as a secondary code if the inoculation is given as a routine part of preventive health care, such as a well-baby visit.

3) Status

Status codes indicate that a patient is either a carrier of a disease or has the sequelae or residual of a past disease or condition. This includes such things as the presence of prosthetic or mechanical devices resulting from past treatment. A status code is informative, because the status may affect the course of treatment and its outcome. A status code is distinct from a history code. The history code indicates that the patient no longer has the condition.

A status code should not be used with a diagnosis code from one of the body system chapters, if the diagnosis code includes the information provided by the status code. For example, code Z94.1, Heart transplant status, should not be used with a code from subcategory T86.2, Complications of heart transplant. The status code does not provide additional information. The complication code indicates that the patient is a heart transplant patient.

For encounters for weaning from a mechanical ventilator, assign a code from subcategory J96.1, Chronic respiratory failure, followed by code Z99.11, Dependence on respirator [ventilator] status.

The status Z codes/categories are:

Z14 Genetic carrier

Genetic carrier status indicates that a person carries a gene, associated with a particular disease, which may be passed to offspring who may develop that disease. The person does not have the disease and is not at risk of developing the disease.

Z15 Genetic susceptibility to disease

Genetic susceptibility indicates that a person has a gene that increases the risk of that person developing the disease.

Codes from category Z15 should not be used as principal or first-listed codes. If the patient has the condition to which he/she is susceptible, and that condition is the reason for the encounter, the code for the current condition should be sequenced first. If the patient is being seen for follow-up after completed treatment for this condition, and the condition no longer exists, a follow-up code should be sequenced first, followed by the appropriate personal history and genetic susceptibility codes. If the purpose of the encounter is genetic counseling associated with procreative management, code Z31.5, Encounter for genetic counseling, should be assigned as the first-listed code, followed by a code from category Z15. Additional codes should be assigned for any applicable family or personal history.

Z16 Resistance to antimicrobial drugs
This code indicates that a patient has a condition that is resistant to antimicrobial drug treatment. Sequence the infection code first.

Z17 Estrogen receptor status

Z18 Retained foreign body fragments

Z19 Hormone sensitivity malignancy status

Z21 Asymptomatic HIV infection status
This code indicates that a patient has tested positive for HIV but has manifested no signs or symptoms of the disease.

Z22 Carrier of infectious disease
Carrier status indicates that a person harbors the specific organisms of a disease without manifest symptoms and is capable of transmitting the infection.

Z28.3 Underimmunization status
See Section I.B.14. for underimmunization documentation by clinicians other than the patient's provider.

Z33.1 Pregnant state, incidental
This code is a secondary code only for use when the pregnancy is in no way complicating the reason for visit. Otherwise, a code from the obstetric chapter is required.

Z66 Do not resuscitate
This code may be used when it is documented by the provider that a patient is on do not resuscitate status at any time during the stay.

Z67 Blood type

Z68 Body mass index (BMI)
BMI codes should only be assigned when there is an associated, reportable diagnosis (such as obesity). Do not assign BMI codes during pregnancy.
See Section I.B.14. for BMI documentation by clinicians other than the patient's provider.

Z74.Ø1 Bed confinement status

Z76.82 Awaiting organ transplant status

Z78 Other specified health status
Code Z78.1, Physical restraint status, may be used when it is documented by the provider that a patient has been put in restraints during the current encounter. Please note that this code should not be reported when it is documented by the provider that a patient is temporarily restrained during a procedure.

Z79 Long-term (current) drug therapy
Codes from this category indicate a patient's continuous use of a prescribed drug (including such things as aspirin therapy) for the long-term treatment of a condition or for prophylactic use. It is not for use for patients who have addictions to drugs. This subcategory is not for use of medications for detoxification or maintenance programs to prevent withdrawal symptoms (e.g., methadone maintenance for opiate dependence). Assign the appropriate code for the drug use, abuse, or dependence instead.
Assign a code from Z79 if the patient is receiving a medication for an extended period as a prophylactic measure (such as for the prevention of deep vein thrombosis) or as treatment of a chronic condition (such as arthritis) or a disease requiring a lengthy course of treatment (such as cancer). Do not assign a code from category Z79 for medication being administered for a brief period of time to treat an acute illness or injury (such as a course of antibiotics to treat acute bronchitis).

Z88 Allergy status to drugs, medicaments and biological substances
Except: Z88.9, Allergy status to unspecified drugs, medicaments and biological substances status

Z89 Acquired absence of limb

Z9Ø Acquired absence of organs, not elsewhere classified

Z91.Ø- Allergy status, other than to drugs and biological substances

Z92.82 Status post administration of tPA (rtPA) in a different facility within the last 24 hours prior to admission to a current facility
Assign code Z92.82, Status post administration of tPA (rtPA) in a different facility within the last 24 hours prior to admission to current facility, as a secondary diagnosis when a patient is received by transfer into a facility and documentation indicates they were administered tissue plasminogen activator (tPA) within the last 24 hours prior to admission to the current facility.
This guideline applies even if the patient is still receiving the tPA at the time they are received into the current facility.
The appropriate code for the condition for which the tPA was administered (such as cerebrovascular disease or myocardial infarction) should be assigned first.
Code Z92.82 is only applicable to the receiving facility record and not to the transferring facility record.

Z93 Artificial opening status

Z94 Transplanted organ and tissue status

Z95 Presence of cardiac and vascular implants and grafts

Z96 Presence of other functional implants

Z97 Presence of other devices

Z98 Other postprocedural states
Assign code Z98.85, Transplanted organ removal status, to indicate that a transplanted organ has been previously removed. This code should not be assigned for the encounter in which the transplanted organ is removed. The complication necessitating removal of the transplant organ should be assigned for that encounter.
See section I.C.19. for information on the coding of organ transplant complications.

Z99 Dependence on enabling machines and devices, not elsewhere classified
Note: Categories Z89-Z9Ø and Z93-Z99 are for use only if there are no complications or malfunctions of the organ or tissue replaced, the amputation site or the equipment on which the patient is dependent.

4) History (of)

There are two types of history Z codes, personal and family. Personal history codes explain a patient's past medical condition that no longer exists and is not receiving any treatment, but that has the potential for recurrence, and therefore may require continued monitoring.

Family history codes are for use when a patient has a family member(s) who has had a particular disease that causes the patient to be at higher risk of also contracting the disease.

Personal history codes may be used in conjunction with follow-up codes and family history codes may be used in conjunction with screening codes to explain the need for a test or procedure. History codes are also acceptable on any medical record regardless of the reason for visit. A history of an illness, even if no longer present, is important information that may alter the type of treatment ordered.

The reason for the encounter (for example, screening or counseling) should be sequenced first and the appropriate personal and/or family history code(s) should be assigned as additional diagnos(es).

The history Z code categories are:

Z8Ø Family history of primary malignant neoplasm

Z81 Family history of mental and behavioral disorders

Z82 Family history of certain disabilities and chronic diseases (leading to disablement)

Z83 Family history of other specific disorders

Z84 Family history of other conditions

Z85 Personal history of malignant neoplasm

Z86 Personal history of certain other diseases

Z87 Personal history of other diseases and conditions

Z91.4- Personal history of psychological trauma, not elsewhere classified

Z91.5- Personal history of self-harm

Z91.81 History of falling

Z91.82 Personal history of military deployment

Z92 Personal history of medical treatment
Except: Z92.Ø, Personal history of contraception
Except: Z92.82, Status post administration of tPA (rtPA) in a different facility within the last 24 hours prior to admission to a current facility

5) Screening

Screening is the testing for disease or disease precursors in seemingly well individuals so that early detection and treatment can be provided for those who test positive for the disease (e.g., screening mammogram).

The testing of a person to rule out or confirm a suspected diagnosis because the patient has some sign or symptom is a diagnostic examination, not a screening. In these cases, the sign or symptom is used to explain the reason for the test.

A screening code may be a first-listed code if the reason for the visit is specifically the screening exam. It may also be used as an additional code if the screening is done during an office visit for other health problems. A screening code is not necessary if the screening is inherent to a routine examination, such as a pap smear done during a routine pelvic examination.

Should a condition be discovered during the screening then the code for the condition may be assigned as an additional diagnosis.

The Z code indicates that a screening exam is planned. A procedure code is required to confirm that the screening was performed.

The screening Z codes/categories:

Z11 Encounter for screening for infectious and parasitic diseases

Z12 Encounter for screening for malignant neoplasms

Z13 Encounter for screening for other diseases and disorders
Except: Z13.9, Encounter for screening, unspecified

Z36 Encounter for antenatal screening for mother

6) Observation

There are three observation Z code categories. They are for use in very limited circumstances when a person is being observed for a suspected condition that is ruled out. The observation codes are not for use if an injury or illness or any signs or symptoms related to the suspected condition are present. In such cases the diagnosis/symptom code is used with the corresponding external cause code.

The observation codes are primarily to be used as a principal/first-listed diagnosis. An observation code may be assigned as a secondary diagnosis code when the patient is being observed for a condition that is ruled out and is unrelated to the principal/first-listed diagnosis. Also, when the principal diagnosis is required to be a code from category Z38, Liveborn infants according to place of birth and type of delivery, then a code from category ZØ5, Encounter for observation and evaluation of newborn for suspected diseases and conditions ruled out, is sequenced after the Z38 code. Additional codes may be used in addition to the observation code, but only if they are unrelated to the suspected condition being observed.

Codes from subcategory ZØ3.7, Encounter for suspected maternal and fetal conditions ruled out, may either be used as a first-listed or as an additional code assignment depending on the case. They are for use in very limited circumstances on a maternal record when an encounter is for a suspected maternal or fetal condition that is ruled out during that encounter (for example, a maternal or fetal condition may be suspected due to an abnormal test result). These codes should not be used when the condition is confirmed. In those cases, the confirmed condition should be coded. In addition, these codes are not for use if an illness or any signs or symptoms related to the suspected condition or problem are present. In such cases the diagnosis/symptom code is used.

Additional codes may be used in addition to the code from subcategory ZØ3.7, but only if they are unrelated to the suspected condition being evaluated.

Codes from subcategory ZØ3.7 may not be used for encounters for antenatal screening of mother. *See Section I.C.21. Screening.*

For encounters for suspected fetal condition that are inconclusive following testing and evaluation, assign the appropriate code from category O35, O36, O4Ø or O41.

The observation Z code categories:

ZØ3 Encounter for medical observation for suspected diseases and conditions ruled out

ZØ4 Encounter for examination and observation for other reasons Except: ZØ4.9, Encounter for examination and observation for unspecified reason

ZØ5 Encounter for observation and evaluation of newborn for suspected diseases and conditions ruled out

7) Aftercare

Aftercare visit codes cover situations when the initial treatment of a disease has been performed and the patient requires continued care during the healing or recovery phase, or for the long-term consequences of the disease. The aftercare Z code should not be used if treatment is directed at a current, acute disease. The diagnosis code is to be used in these cases. Exceptions to this rule are codes Z51.Ø, Encounter for antineoplastic radiation therapy, and codes from subcategory Z51.1, Encounter for antineoplastic chemotherapy and immunotherapy. These codes are to be first listed, followed by the diagnosis code when a patient's encounter is solely to receive radiation therapy, chemotherapy, or immunotherapy for the treatment of a neoplasm. If the reason for the encounter is more than one type of antineoplastic therapy, code Z51.Ø and a code from subcategory Z51.1 may be assigned together, in which case one of these codes would be reported as a secondary diagnosis.

The aftercare Z codes should also not be used for aftercare for injuries. For aftercare of an injury, assign the acute injury code with the appropriate 7th character (for subsequent encounter).

The aftercare codes are generally first listed to explain the specific reason for the encounter. An aftercare code may be used as an additional code when some type of aftercare is provided in addition to the reason for admission and no diagnosis code is applicable. An example of this would be the closure of a colostomy during an encounter for treatment of another condition.

Aftercare codes should be used in conjunction with other aftercare codes or diagnosis codes to provide better detail on the specifics of an aftercare encounter visit, unless otherwise directed by the classification. The sequencing of multiple aftercare codes depends on the circumstances of the encounter.

Certain aftercare Z code categories need a secondary diagnosis code to describe the resolving condition or sequelae. For others, the condition is included in the code title.

Additional Z code aftercare category terms include fitting and adjustment, and attention to artificial openings.

Status Z codes may be used with aftercare Z codes to indicate the nature of the aftercare. For example, code Z95.1, Presence of aortocoronary bypass graft, may be used with code Z48.812, Encounter for surgical aftercare following surgery on the circulatory system, to indicate the surgery for which the aftercare is being performed. A status code should not be used when the aftercare code indicates the type of status, such as using Z43.Ø, Encounter for attention to tracheostomy, with Z93.Ø, Tracheostomy status.

The aftercare Z category/codes:

Z42 Encounter for plastic and reconstructive surgery following medical procedure or healed injury

Z43 Encounter for attention to artificial openings

Z44 Encounter for fitting and adjustment of external prosthetic device

Z45 Encounter for adjustment and management of implanted device

Z46 Encounter for fitting and adjustment of other devices

Z47 Orthopedic aftercare

Z48 Encounter for other postprocedural aftercare

Z49 Encounter for care involving renal dialysis

Z51 Encounter for other aftercare and medical care

8) Follow-up

The follow-up codes are used to explain continuing surveillance following completed treatment of a disease, condition, or injury. They imply that the condition has been fully treated and no longer exists. They should not be confused with aftercare codes, or injury codes with a 7th character for subsequent encounter, that explain ongoing care of a healing condition or its sequelae. Follow-up codes may be used in conjunction with history codes to provide the full picture of the healed condition and its treatment. The follow-up code is sequenced first, followed by the history code.

A follow-up code may be used to explain multiple visits. Should a condition be found to have recurred on the follow-up visit, then the diagnosis code for the condition should be assigned in place of the follow-up code.

The follow-up Z code categories:

Z08 Encounter for follow-up examination after completed treatment for malignant neoplasm

Z09 Encounter for follow-up examination after completed treatment for conditions other than malignant neoplasm

Z39 Encounter for maternal postpartum care and examination

9) Donor

Codes in category Z52, Donors of organs and tissues, are used for living individuals who are donating blood or other body tissue. These codes are for individuals donating for others, as well as for self-donations. They are not used to identify cadaveric donations.

10) Counseling

Counseling Z codes are used when a patient or family member receives assistance in the aftermath of an illness or injury, or when support is required in coping with family or social problems.

The counseling Z codes/categories:

Z30.0- Encounter for general counseling and advice on contraception

Z31.5 Encounter for procreative genetic counseling

Z31.6- Encounter for general counseling and advice on procreation

Z32.2 Encounter for childbirth instruction

Z32.3 Encounter for childcare instruction

Z69 Encounter for mental health services for victim and perpetrator of abuse

Z70 Counseling related to sexual attitude, behavior and orientation

Z71 Persons encountering health services for other counseling and medical advice, not elsewhere classified

Note: Code Z71.84, Encounter for health counseling related to travel, is to be used for health risk and safety counseling for future travel purposes.

Code Z71.85, Encounter for immunization safety counseling, is to be used for counseling of the patient or caregiver regarding the safety of a vaccine. This code should not be used for the provision of general information regarding risks and potential side effects during routine encounters for the administration of vaccines.

Code Z71.87, Encounter for pediatric-to-adult transition counseling, should be assigned when pediatric-to-adult transition counseling is the sole reason for the encounter or when this counseling is provided in addition to other services, such as treatment of a chronic condition. If both transition counseling and treatment of a medical condition are provided during the same encounter, the code(s) for the medical condition(s) treated and code Z71.87 should be assigned, with sequencing depending on the circumstances of the encounter.

Z76.81 Expectant mother prebirth pediatrician visit

11) Encounters for Obstetrical and Reproductive Services

See Section I.C.15. Pregnancy, Childbirth, and the Puerperium, for further instruction on the use of these codes.

Z codes for pregnancy are for use in those circumstances when none of the problems or complications included in the codes from the Obstetrics chapter exist (a routine prenatal visit or postpartum care). Codes in category Z34, Encounter for supervision of normal pregnancy, are always first listed and are not to be used with any other code from the OB chapter.

Codes in category Z3A, Weeks of gestation, may be assigned to provide additional information about the pregnancy. Category Z3A codes should not be assigned for pregnancies with abortive outcomes (categories O00-O08), elective termination of pregnancy (code Z33.2), nor for postpartum conditions, as category Z3A is not applicable to these conditions. The date of the admission should be used to determine weeks of gestation for inpatient admissions that encompass more than one gestational week.

The outcome of delivery, category Z37, should be included on all maternal delivery records. It is always a secondary code.

Codes in category Z37 should not be used on the newborn record.

Z codes for family planning (contraceptive) or procreative management and counseling should be included on an obstetric record either during the pregnancy or the postpartum stage, if applicable.

Z codes/categories for obstetrical and reproductive services:

Z30 Encounter for contraceptive management

Z31 Encounter for procreative management

Z32.2 Encounter for childbirth instruction

Z32.3 Encounter for childcare instruction

Z33 Pregnant state

Z34 Encounter for supervision of normal pregnancy

Z36 Encounter for antenatal screening of mother

Z3A Weeks of gestation

Z37 Outcome of delivery

Z39 Encounter for maternal postpartum care and examination

Z76.81 Expectant mother prebirth pediatrician visit

12) Newborns and Infants

See Section I.C.16. Newborn (Perinatal) Guidelines, for further instruction on the use of these codes.

Newborn Z codes/categories:

Z76.1 Encounter for health supervision and care of foundling

Z00.1- Encounter for routine child health examination

Z38 Liveborn infants according to place of birth and type of delivery

13) Routine and Administrative Examinations

The Z codes allow for the description of encounters for routine examinations, such as, a general check-up, or, examinations for administrative purposes, such as, a pre-employment physical. The codes are not to be used if the examination is for diagnosis of a suspected condition or for treatment purposes. In such cases the diagnosis code is used. During a routine exam, should a diagnosis or condition be discovered, it should be coded as an additional code. Pre-existing and chronic conditions and history codes may also be included as additional codes as long as the examination is for administrative purposes and not focused on any particular condition.

Some of the codes for routine health examinations distinguish between "with" and "without" abnormal findings. Code assignment depends on the information that is known at the time the encounter is being coded. For example, if no abnormal findings were found during the examination, but the encounter is being coded before test results are back, it is acceptable to assign the code for "without abnormal findings." When assigning a code for "with abnormal findings," additional code(s) should be assigned to identify the specific abnormal finding(s).

Pre-operative examination and pre-procedural laboratory examination Z codes are for use only in those situations when a patient is being cleared for a procedure or surgery and no treatment is given.

The Z codes/categories for routine and administrative examinations:

Z00 Encounter for general examination without complaint, suspected or reported diagnosis

Z01 Encounter for other special examination without complaint, suspected or reported diagnosis

Z02 Encounter for administrative examination
Except: Z02.9, Encounter for administrative examinations, unspecified

Z32.0- Encounter for pregnancy test

14) Miscellaneous Z Codes

The miscellaneous Z codes capture a number of other health care encounters that do not fall into one of the other categories. Some of these codes identify the reason for the encounter; others are for use as additional codes that provide useful information on circumstances that may affect a patient's care and treatment.

Prophylactic Organ Removal

For encounters specifically for prophylactic removal of an organ (such as prophylactic removal of breasts due to a genetic susceptibility to cancer or a family history of cancer), the principal or first-listed code should be a code from category Z4Ø, Encounter for prophylactic surgery, followed by the appropriate codes to identify the associated risk factor (such as genetic susceptibility or family history).

If the patient has a malignancy of one site and is having prophylactic removal at another site to prevent either a new primary malignancy or metastatic disease, a code for the malignancy should also be assigned in addition to a code from subcategory Z4Ø.Ø, Encounter for prophylactic surgery for risk factors related to malignant neoplasms. A Z4Ø.Ø code should not be assigned if the patient is having organ removal for treatment of a malignancy, such as the removal of the testes for the treatment of prostate cancer.

Miscellaneous Z codes/categories:

Z28 Immunization not carried out
Except: Z28.3-, Underimmunization status

Z29 Encounter for other prophylactic measures

Z4Ø Encounter for prophylactic surgery

Z41 Encounter for procedures for purposes other than remedying health state
Except: Z41.9, Encounter for procedure for purposes other than remedying health state, unspecified

Z53 Persons encountering health services for specific procedures and treatment, not carried out

Z72 Problems related to lifestyle
Note: These codes should be assigned only when the documentation specifies that the patient has an associated problem

Z73 Problems related to life management difficulty
Note: These codes should be assigned only when the documentation specifies that the patient has an associated problem.

Z74 Problems related to care provider dependency
Except: Z74.Ø1, Bed confinement status

Z75 Problems related to medical facilities and other health care

Z76.Ø Encounter for issue of repeat prescription

Z76.3 Healthy person accompanying sick person

Z76.4 Other boarder to healthcare facility

Z76.5 Malingerer [conscious simulation]

Z91.1- Patient's noncompliance with medical treatment and regimen

Z91.83 Wandering in diseases classified elsewhere

Z91.84- Oral health risk factors

Z91.89 Other specified personal risk factors, not elsewhere classified

See Section I.B.14. for Z55-Z65 Persons with potential health hazards related to socioeconomic and psychosocial circumstances, documentation by clinicians other than the patient's provider

15) Nonspecific Z Codes

Certain Z codes are so non-specific, or potentially redundant with other codes in the classification, that there can be little justification for their use in the inpatient setting. Their use in the outpatient setting should be limited to those instances when there is no further documentation to permit more precise coding. Otherwise, any sign or symptom or any other reason for visit that is captured in another code should be used.

Nonspecific Z codes/categories:

ZØ2.9 Encounter for administrative examinations, unspecified

ZØ4.9 Encounter for examination and observation for unspecified reason

Z13.9 Encounter for screening, unspecified

Z41.9 Encounter for procedure for purposes other than remedying health state, unspecified

Z52.9 Donor of unspecified organ or tissue

Z86.59 Personal history of other mental and behavioral disorders

Z88.9 Allergy status to unspecified drugs, medicaments and biological substances status

Z92.Ø Personal history of contraception

16) Z Codes That May Only be Principal/First-Listed Diagnosis

The following Z codes/categories may only be reported as the principal/first-listed diagnosis, except when there are multiple encounters on the same day and the medical records for the encounters are combined:

ZØØ Encounter for general examination without complaint, suspected or reported diagnosis
Except: ZØØ.6

ZØ1 Encounter for other special examination without complaint, suspected or reported diagnosis

ZØ2 Encounter for administrative examination

ZØ4 Encounter for examination and observation for other reasons

Z33.2 Encounter for elective termination of pregnancy

Z31.81 Encounter for male factor infertility in female patient

Z31.83 Encounter for assisted reproductive fertility procedure cycle

Z31.84 Encounter for fertility preservation procedure

Z34 Encounter for supervision of normal pregnancy

Z39 Encounter for maternal postpartum care and examination

Z38 Liveborn infants according to place of birth and type of delivery

Z4Ø Encounter for prophylactic surgery

Z42 Encounter for plastic and reconstructive surgery following medical procedure or healed injury

Z51.Ø Encounter for antineoplastic radiation therapy

Z51.1- Encounter for antineoplastic chemotherapy and immunotherapy

Z52 Donors of organs and tissues
Except: Z52.9, Donor of unspecified organ or tissue

Z76.1 Encounter for health supervision and care of foundling

Z76.2 Encounter for health supervision and care of other healthy infant and child

Z99.12 Encounter for respirator [ventilator] dependence during power failure

17) Social Determinants of Health

Codes describing **problems or risk factors related to** social determinants of health (SDOH) should be assigned when this information is documented. **Assign as many SDOH codes as are necessary to describe all of the problems or risk factors. These codes should be assigned only when the documentation specifies that the patient has an associated problem or risk factor. For example, not every individual living alone would be assigned code Z6Ø.2, Problems related to living alone.**

For social determinants of health, such as information found in categories Z55-Z65, Persons with potential health hazards related to socioeconomic and psychosocial circumstances, code assignment may be based on medical record documentation from clinicians involved in the care of the patient who are not the patient's provider since this information represents social information, rather than medical diagnoses.

For example, coding professionals may utilize documentation of social information from social workers, community health workers, case managers, or nurses, if their documentation is included in the official medical record.

Patient self-reported documentation may be used to assign codes for social determinants of health, as long as the patient self-reported information is signed-off by and incorporated into the medical record by either a clinician or provider.

Social determinants of health codes are located primarily in these Z code categories:

Z55 Problems related to education and literacy

Z56 Problems related to employment and unemployment

Z57 Occupational exposure to risk factors

Z58 Problems related to physical environment

Z59 Problems related to housing and economic circumstances

Z6Ø Problems related to social environment

Z62 Problems related to upbringing

Z63 Other problems related to primary support group, including family circumstances

Z64 Problems related to certain psychosocial circumstances

Z65 Problems related to other psychosocial circumstances

See Section I.B.14. Documentation by Clinicians Other than the Patient's Provider.

22. **Chapter 22: Codes for Special Purposes (U00-U85)**
    U07.0 Vaping-related disorder (see Section I.C.10.e., Vaping-related disorders)
    U07.1 COVID-19 (see Section I.C.1.g.1., COVID-19 infection)
    U09.9 Post COVID-19 condition, unspecified (see Section I.C.1.g.1.m.)

Section II. Selection of Principal Diagnosis

The circumstances of inpatient admission always govern the selection of principal diagnosis. The principal diagnosis is defined in the Uniform Hospital Discharge Data Set (UHDDS) as "that condition established after study to be chiefly responsible for occasioning the admission of the patient to the hospital for care."

The UHDDS definitions are used by hospitals to report inpatient data elements in a standardized manner. These data elements and their definitions can be found in the July 31, 1985, Federal Register (Vol. 50, No, 147), pp. 31038-40.

Since that time, the application of the UHDDS definitions has been expanded to include all non-outpatient settings (acute care, short term, long term care and psychiatric hospitals; home health agencies; rehab facilities; nursing homes, etc.). The UHDDS definitions also apply to hospice services (all levels of care).

In determining principal diagnosis, coding conventions in the ICD-10-CM, the Tabular List and Alphabetic Index take precedence over these official coding guidelines.

(See Section I.A., Conventions for the ICD-10-CM)

The importance of consistent, complete documentation in the medical record cannot be overemphasized. Without such documentation the application of all coding guidelines is a difficult, if not impossible, task.

A. Codes for symptoms, signs, and ill-defined conditions
Codes for symptoms, signs, and ill-defined conditions from Chapter 18 are not to be used as principal diagnosis when a related definitive diagnosis has been established.

B. Two or more interrelated conditions, each potentially meeting the definition for principal diagnosis.
When there are two or more interrelated conditions (such as diseases in the same ICD-10-CM chapter or manifestations characteristically associated with a certain disease) potentially meeting the definition of principal diagnosis, either condition may be sequenced first, unless the circumstances of the admission, the therapy provided, the Tabular List, or the Alphabetic Index indicate otherwise.

C. Two or more diagnoses that equally meet the definition for principal diagnosis
In the unusual instance when two or more diagnoses equally meet the criteria for principal diagnosis as determined by the circumstances of admission, diagnostic workup and/or therapy provided, and the Alphabetic Index, Tabular List, or another coding guidelines does not provide sequencing direction, any one of the diagnoses may be sequenced first.

D. Two or more comparative or contrasting conditions
In those rare instances when two or more contrasting or comparative diagnoses are documented as "either/or" (or similar terminology), they are coded as if the diagnoses were confirmed and the diagnoses are sequenced according to the circumstances of the admission. If no further determination can be made as to which diagnosis should be principal, either diagnosis may be sequenced first.

E. A symptom(s) followed by contrasting/comparative diagnoses
GUIDELINE HAS BEEN DELETED EFFECTIVE OCTOBER 1, 2014

F. Original treatment plan not carried out
Sequence as the principal diagnosis the condition, which after study occasioned the admission to the hospital, even though treatment may not have been carried out due to unforeseen circumstances.

G. Complications of surgery and other medical care
When the admission is for treatment of a complication resulting from surgery or other medical care, the complication code is sequenced as the principal diagnosis. If the complication is classified to the T80-T88 series and the code lacks the necessary specificity in describing the complication, an additional code for the specific complication should be assigned.

H. Uncertain Diagnosis
If the diagnosis documented at the time of discharge is qualified as "probable," "suspected," "likely," "questionable," "possible," or "still to be ruled out," "compatible with," "consistent with," or other similar terms indicating uncertainty, code the condition as if it existed or was established. The bases for these guidelines are the diagnostic workup, arrangements for further workup or observation, and initial therapeutic approach that correspond most closely with the established diagnosis.

Note: This guideline is applicable only to inpatient admissions to short-term, acute, long-term care and psychiatric hospitals.

I. Admission from Observation Unit

1. **Admission Following Medical Observation**
   When a patient is admitted to an observation unit for a medical condition, which either worsens or does not improve, and is subsequently admitted as an inpatient of the same hospital for this same medical condition, the principal diagnosis would be the medical condition which led to the hospital admission.
2. **Admission Following Post-Operative Observation**
   When a patient is admitted to an observation unit to monitor a condition (or complication) that develops following outpatient surgery, and then is subsequently admitted as an inpatient of the same hospital, hospitals should apply the Uniform Hospital Discharge Data Set (UHDDS) definition of principal diagnosis as "that condition established after study to be chiefly responsible for occasioning the admission of the patient to the hospital for care."

J. Admission from Outpatient Surgery
When a patient receives surgery in the hospital's outpatient surgery department and is subsequently admitted for continuing inpatient care at the same hospital, the following guidelines should be followed in selecting the principal diagnosis for the inpatient admission:

- If the reason for the inpatient admission is a complication, assign the complication as the principal diagnosis.
- If no complication, or other condition, is documented as the reason for the inpatient admission, assign the reason for the outpatient surgery as the principal diagnosis.
- If the reason for the inpatient admission is another condition unrelated to the surgery, assign the unrelated condition as the principal diagnosis.

K. Admissions/Encounters for Rehabilitation
When the purpose for the admission/encounter is rehabilitation, sequence first the code for the condition for which the service is being performed. For example, for an admission/encounter for rehabilitation for right-sided dominant hemiplegia following a cerebrovascular infarction, report code I69.351, Hemiplegia and hemiparesis following cerebral infarction affecting right dominant side, as the first-listed or principal diagnosis.

If the condition for which the rehabilitation service is being provided is no longer present, report the appropriate aftercare code as the first-listed or principal diagnosis, unless the rehabilitation service is being provided following an injury. For rehabilitation services following active treatment of an injury, assign the injury code with the appropriate seventh character for subsequent encounter as the first-listed or principal diagnosis. For example, if a patient with severe degenerative osteoarthritis of the hip, underwent hip replacement and the current encounter/admission is for rehabilitation, report code Z47.1, Aftercare following joint replacement surgery, as the first-listed or principal diagnosis. If the patient requires rehabilitation post hip replacement for right intertrochanteric femur fracture, report code S72.141D, Displaced intertrochanteric fracture of right femur, subsequent encounter for closed fracture with routine healing, as the first-listed or principal diagnosis.

See Section I.C.21.c.7., Factors influencing health states and contact with health services, Aftercare.

See Section I.C.19.a., for additional information about the use of 7th characters for injury codes.

Section III. Reporting Additional Diagnoses

GENERAL RULES FOR OTHER (ADDITIONAL) DIAGNOSES

For reporting purposes, the definition for "other diagnoses" is interpreted as additional conditions that affect patient care in terms of requiring:

clinical evaluation; or

therapeutic treatment; or

diagnostic procedures; or

extended length of hospital stay; or

increased nursing care and/or monitoring.

The UHDDS item #11-b defines Other Diagnoses as "all conditions that coexist at the time of admission, that develop subsequently, or that affect the treatment received and/or the length of stay. Diagnoses that relate to an earlier episode which have no bearing on the current hospital stay are to be excluded." UHDDS definitions apply to inpatients in acute care, short-term, long term care and psychiatric hospital setting. The UHDDS definitions are used by acute care short-term hospitals to report inpatient data elements in a standardized manner. These data elements and their definitions can be found in the July 31, 1985, Federal Register (Vol. 50, No, 147), pp. 31038-40.

Since that time, the application of the UHDDS definitions has been expanded to include all non-outpatient settings (acute care, short term, long term care and psychiatric hospitals; home health agencies; rehab facilities; nursing homes, etc.). The UHDDS definitions also apply to hospice services (all levels of care).

The following guidelines are to be applied in designating "other diagnoses" when neither the Alphabetic Index nor the Tabular List in ICD-10-CM provide direction. The listing of the diagnoses in the patient record is the responsibility of the attending provider.

A. Previous conditions

If the provider has included a diagnosis in the final diagnostic statement, such as the discharge summary or the face sheet, it should ordinarily be coded. Some providers include in the diagnostic statement resolved conditions or diagnoses and status-post procedures from previous admissions that have no bearing on the current stay. Such conditions are not to be reported and are coded only if required by hospital policy.

However, history codes (categories Z8Ø-Z87) may be used as secondary codes if the historical condition or family history has an impact on current care or influences treatment.

B. Abnormal findings

Abnormal findings (laboratory, x-ray, pathologic, and other diagnostic results) are not coded and reported unless the provider indicates their clinical significance. If the findings are outside the normal range and the attending provider has ordered other tests to evaluate the condition or prescribed treatment, it is appropriate to ask the provider whether the abnormal finding should be added.

Please note: This differs from the coding practices in the outpatient setting for coding encounters for diagnostic tests that have been interpreted by a provider.

C. Uncertain Diagnosis

If the diagnosis documented at the time of discharge is qualified as "probable," "suspected," "likely," "questionable," "possible," or "still to be ruled out," "compatible with," "consistent with," or other similar terms indicating uncertainty, code the condition as if it existed or was established. The bases for these guidelines are the diagnostic workup, arrangements for further workup or observation, and initial therapeutic approach that correspond most closely with the established diagnosis.

Note: This guideline is applicable only to inpatient admissions to short-term, acute, long-term care and psychiatric hospitals.

Section IV. Diagnostic Coding and Reporting Guidelines for Outpatient Services

These coding guidelines for outpatient diagnoses have been approved for use by hospitals/ providers in coding and reporting hospital-based outpatient services and provider-based office visits. Guidelines in Section I, Conventions, general coding guidelines and chapter-specific guidelines, should also be applied for outpatient services and office visits.

Information about the use of certain abbreviations, punctuation, symbols, and other conventions used in the ICD-10-CM Tabular List (code numbers and titles), can be found in Section IA of these guidelines, under "Conventions Used in the Tabular List." Section I.B. contains general guidelines that apply to the entire classification. Section I.C. contains chapter-specific guidelines that correspond to the chapters as they are arranged in the classification. Information about the correct sequence to use in finding a code is also described in Section I.

The terms encounter and visit are often used interchangeably in describing outpatient service contacts and, therefore, appear together in these guidelines without distinguishing one from the other.

Though the conventions and general guidelines apply to all settings, coding guidelines for outpatient and provider reporting of diagnoses will vary in a number of instances from those for inpatient diagnoses, recognizing that:

The Uniform Hospital Discharge Data Set (UHDDS) definition of principal diagnosis does not apply to hospital-based outpatient services and provider-based office visits.

Coding guidelines for inconclusive diagnoses (probable, suspected, rule out, etc.) were developed for inpatient reporting and do not apply to outpatients.

A. Selection of first-listed condition

In the outpatient setting, the term first-listed diagnosis is used in lieu of principal diagnosis.

In determining the first-listed diagnosis the coding conventions of ICD-10-CM, as well as the general and disease specific guidelines take precedence over the outpatient guidelines.

Diagnoses often are not established at the time of the initial encounter/visit. It may take two or more visits before the diagnosis is confirmed.

The most critical rule involves beginning the search for the correct code assignment through the Alphabetic Index. Never begin searching initially in the Tabular List as this will lead to coding errors.

1. Outpatient Surgery

When a patient presents for outpatient surgery (same day surgery), code the reason for the surgery as the first-listed diagnosis (reason for the encounter), even if the surgery is not performed due to a contraindication.

2. Observation Stay

When a patient is admitted for observation for a medical condition, assign a code for the medical condition as the first-listed diagnosis.

When a patient presents for outpatient surgery and develops complications requiring admission to observation, code the reason for the surgery as the first reported diagnosis (reason for the encounter), followed by codes for the complications as secondary diagnoses.

B. Codes from AØØ.Ø through T88.9, ZØØ-Z99, UØØ-U85

The appropriate code(s) from AØØ.Ø through T88.9, ZØØ-Z99 and UØØ-U85 must be used to identify diagnoses, symptoms, conditions, problems, complaints, or other reason(s) for the encounter/visit.

C. Accurate reporting of ICD-10-CM diagnosis codes

For accurate reporting of ICD-10-CM diagnosis codes, the documentation should describe the patient's condition, using terminology which includes specific diagnoses as well as symptoms, problems, or reasons for the encounter. There are ICD-10-CM codes to describe all of these.

D. Codes that describe symptoms and signs

Codes that describe symptoms and signs, as opposed to diagnoses, are acceptable for reporting purposes when a diagnosis has not been established (confirmed) by the provider. Chapter 18 of ICD-10-CM, Symptoms, Signs, and Abnormal Clinical and Laboratory Findings Not Elsewhere Classified (codes RØØ-R99) contain many, but not all codes for symptoms.

E. Encounters for circumstances other than a disease or injury

ICD-10-CM provides codes to deal with encounters for circumstances other than a disease or injury. The Factors Influencing Health Status and Contact with Health Services codes (ZØØ-Z99) are provided to deal with occasions when circumstances other than a disease or injury are recorded as diagnosis or problems.

See Section I.C.21. Factors influencing health status and contact with health services.

F. Level of Detail in Coding

1. ICD-10-CM codes with 3, 4, 5, 6 or 7 characters

ICD-10-CM is composed of codes with 3, 4, 5, 6 or 7 characters. Codes with three characters are included in ICD-10-CM as the heading of a category of codes that may be further subdivided by the use of fourth, fifth, sixth or seventh characters to provide greater specificity.

2. Use of full number of characters required for a code

A three-character code is to be used only if it is not further subdivided. A code is invalid if it has not been coded to the full number of characters required for that code, including the 7th character, if applicable.

3. Highest level of specificity

Code to the highest level of specificity when supported by the medical record documentation.

G. ICD-10-CM code for the diagnosis, condition, problem, or other reason for encounter/visit

List first the ICD-10-CM code for the diagnosis, condition, problem, or other reason for encounter/visit shown in the medical record to be chiefly responsible for the services provided. List additional codes that describe any coexisting conditions. In some cases, the first-listed diagnosis may be a symptom when a diagnosis has not been established (confirmed) by the provider.

H. Uncertain diagnosis

Do not code diagnoses documented as "probable", "suspected," "questionable," "rule out," "compatible with," "consistent with," or "working diagnosis" or other similar terms indicating uncertainty. Rather, code the condition(s) to the highest degree of certainty for that encounter/visit, such as symptoms, signs, abnormal test results, or other reason for the visit.

Please note: This differs from the coding practices used by short-term, acute care, long-term care and psychiatric hospitals.

I. Chronic diseases

Chronic diseases treated on an ongoing basis may be coded and reported as many times as the patient receives treatment and care for the condition(s)

J. Code all documented conditions that coexist

Code all documented conditions that coexist at the time of the encounter/visit and that require or affect patient care, treatment or management. Do not code conditions that were previously treated and no longer exist. However, history codes (categories Z8Ø-Z87) may be used as secondary codes if the historical condition or family history has an impact on current care or influences treatment.

K. Patients receiving diagnostic services only

For patients receiving diagnostic services only during an encounter/visit, sequence first the diagnosis, condition, problem, or other reason for encounter/visit shown in the medical record to be chiefly responsible for the outpatient services provided during the encounter/visit. Codes for other diagnoses (e.g., chronic conditions) may be sequenced as additional diagnoses.

For encounters for routine laboratory/radiology testing in the absence of any signs, symptoms, or associated diagnosis, assign ZØ1.89, Encounter for other specified special examinations. If routine testing is performed during the same encounter as a test to evaluate a sign, symptom, or diagnosis, it is appropriate to assign both the Z code and the code describing the reason for the non-routine test.

For outpatient encounters for diagnostic tests that have been interpreted by a physician, and the final report is available at the time of coding, code any confirmed or definitive diagnosis(es) documented in the interpretation. Do not code related signs and symptoms as additional diagnoses.

Please note: This differs from the coding practice in the hospital inpatient setting regarding abnormal findings on test results.

L. Patients receiving therapeutic services only

For patients receiving therapeutic services only during an encounter/visit, sequence first the diagnosis, condition, problem, or other reason for encounter/visit shown in the medical record to be chiefly responsible for the outpatient services provided during the encounter/visit. Codes for other diagnoses (e.g., chronic conditions) may be sequenced as additional diagnoses.

The only exception to this rule is that when the primary reason for the admission/encounter is chemotherapy or radiation therapy, the appropriate Z code for the service is listed first, and the diagnosis or problem for which the service is being performed listed second.

M. Patients receiving preoperative evaluations only

For patients receiving preoperative evaluations only, sequence first a code from subcategory ZØ1.81, Encounter for pre-procedural examinations, to describe the pre-op consultations. Assign a code for the condition to describe the reason for the surgery as an additional diagnosis. Code also any findings related to the pre-op evaluation.

N. Ambulatory surgery

For ambulatory surgery, code the diagnosis for which the surgery was performed. If the postoperative diagnosis is known to be different from the preoperative diagnosis at the time the diagnosis is confirmed, select the postoperative diagnosis for coding, since it is the most definitive.

O. Routine outpatient prenatal visits

See Section I.C.15. Routine outpatient prenatal visits.

P. Encounters for general medical examinations with abnormal findings

The subcategories for encounters for general medical examinations, ZØØ.Ø- and encounter for routine child health examination, ZØØ.12-, provide codes for with and without abnormal findings. Should a general medical examination result in an abnormal finding, the code for general medical examination with abnormal finding should be assigned as the first-listed diagnosis. An examination with abnormal findings refers to a condition/diagnosis that is newly identified or a change in severity of a chronic condition (such as uncontrolled hypertension, or an acute exacerbation of chronic obstructive pulmonary disease) during a routine physical examination. A secondary code for the abnormal finding should also be coded.

Q. Encounters for routine health screenings

See Section I.C.21. Factors influencing health status and contact with health services, Screening

Appendix I. Present on Admission Reporting Guidelines

Introduction

These guidelines are to be used as a supplement to the *ICD-10-CM Official Guidelines for Coding and Reporting* to facilitate the assignment of the Present on Admission (POA) indicator for each diagnosis and external cause of injury code reported on claim forms (UB-04 and 837 Institutional).

These guidelines are not intended to replace any guidelines in the main body of the *ICD-10-CM Official Guidelines for Coding and Reporting*. The POA guidelines are not intended to provide guidance on when a condition should be coded, but rather, how to apply the POA indicator to the final set of diagnosis codes that have been assigned in accordance with Sections I, II, and III of the official coding guidelines. Subsequent to the assignment of the ICD-10-CM codes, the POA indicator should then be assigned to those conditions that have been coded.

As stated in the Introduction to the *ICD-10-CM Official Guidelines for Coding and Reporting*, a joint effort between the healthcare provider and the coder is essential to achieve complete and accurate documentation, code assignment, and reporting of diagnoses and procedures. The importance of consistent, complete documentation in the medical record cannot be overemphasized. Medical record documentation from any provider involved in the care and treatment of the patient may be used to support the determination of whether a condition was present on admission or not. In the context of the official coding guidelines, the term "provider" means a physician or any qualified healthcare practitioner who is legally accountable for establishing the patient's diagnosis.

These guidelines are not a substitute for the provider's clinical judgment as to the determination of whether a condition was/was not present on admission. The provider should be queried regarding issues related to the linking of signs/symptoms, timing of test results, and the timing of findings.

Please see the CDC website for the detailed list of ICD-10-CM codes that do not require the use of a POA indicator (https://www.cdc.gov/nchs/icd/icd10cm.htm). The codes and categories on this exempt list are for circumstances regarding the healthcare encounter or factors influencing health status that do not represent a current disease or injury or that describe conditions that are always present on admission.

General Reporting Requirements

All claims involving inpatient admissions to general acute care hospitals or other facilities that are subject to a law or regulation mandating collection of present on admission information.

Present on admission is defined as present at the time the order for inpatient admission occurs -- conditions that develop during an outpatient encounter, including emergency department, observation, or outpatient surgery, are considered as present on admission.

POA indicator is assigned to principal and secondary diagnoses (as defined in Section II of the Official Guidelines for Coding and Reporting) and the external cause of injury codes.

Issues related to inconsistent, missing, conflicting or unclear documentation must still be resolved by the provider.

If a condition would not be coded and reported based on UHDDS definitions and current official coding guidelines, then the POA indicator would not be reported.

Reporting Options

- Y – Yes
- N – No
- U – Unknown
- W – Clinically undetermined
- Unreported/Not used – (Exempt from POA reporting)

Reporting Definitions

- Y = present at the time of inpatient admission
- N = not present at the time of inpatient admission
- U = documentation is insufficient to determine if condition is present on admission
- W = provider is unable to clinically determine whether condition was present on admission or not

Timeframe for POA Identification and Documentation

There is no required timeframe as to when a provider (per the definition of "provider" used in these guidelines) must identify or document a condition to be present on admission. In some clinical situations, it may not be possible for a provider to make a definitive diagnosis (or a condition may not be recognized or reported by the patient) for a period of time after admission. In some cases, it may be several days before the provider arrives at a definitive diagnosis. This does not mean that the condition was not present on admission. Determination of whether the condition was present on admission or not will be based on the applicable POA guideline as identified in this document, or on the provider's best clinical judgment.

If at the time of code assignment the documentation is unclear as to whether a condition was present on admission or not, it is appropriate to query the provider for clarification.

Assigning the POA Indicator

Condition is on the "Exempt from Reporting" list

Leave the "present on admission" field blank if the condition is on the list of ICD-10-CM codes for which this field is not applicable. This is the only circumstance in which the field may be left blank.

POA Explicitly Documented

Assign Y for any condition the provider explicitly documents as being present on admission.

Assign N for any condition the provider explicitly documents as not present at the time of admission.

Conditions diagnosed prior to inpatient admission

Assign "Y" for conditions that were diagnosed prior to admission (example: hypertension, diabetes mellitus, asthma)

Conditions diagnosed during the admission but clearly present before admission

Assign "Y" for conditions diagnosed during the admission that were clearly present but not diagnosed until after admission occurred.

Diagnoses subsequently confirmed after admission are considered present on admission if at the time of admission they are documented as suspected, possible, rule out, differential diagnosis, or constitute an underlying cause of a symptom that is present at the time of admission.

Condition develops during outpatient encounter prior to inpatient admission

Assign Y for any condition that develops during an outpatient encounter prior to a written order for inpatient admission.

Documentation does not indicate whether condition was present on admission

Assign "U" when the medical record documentation is unclear as to whether the condition was present on admission. "U" should not be routinely assigned and used only in very limited circumstances. Coders are encouraged to query the providers when the documentation is unclear.

Documentation states that it cannot be determined whether the condition was or was not present on admission

Assign "W" when the medical record documentation indicates that it cannot be clinically determined whether or not the condition was present on admission.

Chronic condition with acute exacerbation during the admission

If a single code identifies both the chronic condition and the acute exacerbation, see POA guidelines pertaining to codes that contain multiple clinical concepts.

If a single code only identifies the chronic condition and not the acute exacerbation (e.g., acute exacerbation of chronic leukemia), assign "Y."

Conditions documented as possible, probable, suspected, or rule out at the time of discharge

If the final diagnosis contains a possible, probable, suspected, or rule out diagnosis, and this diagnosis was based on signs, symptoms or clinical findings suspected at the time of inpatient admission, assign "Y."

If the final diagnosis contains a possible, probable, suspected, or rule out diagnosis, and this diagnosis was based on signs, symptoms or clinical findings that were not present on admission, assign "N".

Conditions documented as impending or threatened at the time of discharge

If the final diagnosis contains an impending or threatened diagnosis, and this diagnosis is based on symptoms or clinical findings that were present on admission, assign "Y".

If the final diagnosis contains an impending or threatened diagnosis, and this diagnosis is based on symptoms or clinical findings that were not present on admission, assign "N".

Acute and Chronic Conditions

Assign "Y" for acute conditions that are present at time of admission and N for acute conditions that are not present at time of admission.

Assign "Y" for chronic conditions, even though the condition may not be diagnosed until after admission.

If a single code identifies both an acute and chronic condition, see the POA guidelines for codes that contain multiple clinical concepts.

Codes That Contain Multiple Clinical Concepts

Assign "N" if at least one of the clinical concepts included in the code was not present on admission (e.g., COPD with acute exacerbation and the exacerbation was not present on admission; gastric ulcer that does not start bleeding until after admission; asthma patient develops status asthmaticus after admission).

Assign "Y" if all of the clinical concepts included in the code were present on admission (e.g., duodenal ulcer that perforates prior to admission).

For infection codes that include the causal organism, assign "Y" if the infection (or signs of the infection) were present on admission, even though the culture results may not be known until after admission (e.g., patient is admitted with pneumonia and the provider documents Pseudomonas as the causal organism a few days later).

Same Diagnosis Code for Two or More Conditions

When the same ICD-10-CM diagnosis code applies to two or more conditions during the same encounter (e.g. two separate conditions classified to the same ICD-10-CM diagnosis code):

Assign "Y" if all conditions represented by the single ICD-10-CM code were present on admission (e.g. bilateral unspecified age-related cataracts).

Assign "N" if any of the conditions represented by the single ICD-10-CM code was not present on admission (e.g. traumatic secondary and recurrent hemorrhage and seroma is assigned to a single code T79.2, but only one of the conditions was present on admission).

Obstetrical conditions

Whether or not the patient delivers during the current hospitalization does not affect assignment of the POA indicator. The determining factor for POA assignment is whether the pregnancy complication or obstetrical condition described by the code was present at the time of admission or not.

If the pregnancy complication or obstetrical condition was present on admission (e.g., patient admitted in preterm labor), assign "Y".

If the pregnancy complication or obstetrical condition was not present on admission (e.g., 2nd degree laceration during delivery, postpartum hemorrhage that occurred during current hospitalization, fetal distress develops after admission), assign "N".

If the obstetrical code includes more than one diagnosis and any of the diagnoses identified by the code were not present on admission assign "N". (e.g., Category O11, Pre-existing hypertension with pre-eclampsia)

Perinatal conditions

Newborns are not considered to be admitted until after birth. Therefore, any condition present at birth or that developed in utero is considered present at admission and should be assigned "Y". This includes conditions that occur during delivery (e.g., injury during delivery, meconium aspiration, exposure to streptococcus B in the vaginal canal).

Congenital conditions and anomalies

Assign "Y" for congenital conditions and anomalies except for categories QØØ-Q99, Congenital anomalies, which are on the exempt list. Congenital conditions are always considered present on admission.

External cause of injury codes

Assign "Y" for any external cause code representing an external cause of morbidity that occurred prior to inpatient admission (e.g., patient fell out of bed at home, patient fell out of bed in emergency room prior to admission)

Assign "N" for any external cause code representing an external cause of morbidity that occurred during inpatient hospitalization (e.g., patient fell out of hospital bed during hospital stay, patient experienced an adverse reaction to a medication administered after inpatient admission).

ICD-10-CM Index to Diseases and Injuries

A

Aarskog's syndrome Q87.19
Abandonment — *see* Maltreatment
Abasia (-astasia) (hysterical) F44.4
Abderhalden-Kaufmann-Lignac syndrome (cystinosis) E72.Ø4
Abdomen, abdominal — *see also* condition
  muscle deficiency syndrome Q79.4
  angina K55.1
  acute R1Ø.Ø
Abdominalgia — *see* Pain, abdominal
Abduction contracture, hip or other joint — *see* Contraction, joint
Aberrant (congenital) — *see also* Malposition, congenital
  adrenal gland Q89.1
  artery (peripheral) Q27.8
    basilar NEC Q28.1
    cerebral Q28.3
    coronary Q24.5
    digestive system Q27.8
    eye Q15.8
    lower limb Q27.8
    precerebral Q28.1
    pulmonary Q25.79
    renal Q27.2
    retina Q14.1
    specified site NEC Q27.8
    subclavian Q27.8
    upper limb Q27.8
    vertebral Q28.1
  breast Q83.8
  endocrine gland NEC Q89.2
  hepatic duct Q44.5
  pancreas Q45.3
  parathyroid gland Q89.2
  pituitary gland Q89.2
  sebaceous glands, mucous membrane, mouth, congenital Q38.6
  spleen Q89.Ø9
  subclavian artery Q27.8
  thymus (gland) Q89.2
  thyroid gland Q89.2
  vein (peripheral) NEC Q27.8
    cerebral Q28.3
    digestive system Q27.8
    lower limb Q27.8
    precerebral Q28.1
    specified site NEC Q27.8
    upper limb Q27.8
Aberration
  distantial — *see* Disturbance, visual
  mental F99
Abetalipoproteinemia E78.6
Abiotrophy R68.89
Ablatio, ablation
  retinae — *see* Detachment, retina
Ablepharia, ablepharon Q1Ø.3
Abnormal, abnormality, abnormalities — *see also* Anomaly
  acid-base balance (mixed) E87.4
  albumin R77.Ø
  alphafetoprotein R77.2
  alveolar ridge KØ8.9
  anatomical relationship Q89.9
  apertures, congenital, diaphragm Q79.1
  atrial septal, specified NEC Q21.19
  auditory perception H93.29- ☑
    diplacusis — *see* Diplacusis
    hyperacusis — *see* Hyperacusis
    recruitment — *see* Recruitment, auditory
    threshold shift — *see* Shift, auditory threshold
  autosomes Q99.9
    fragile site Q95.5
  basal metabolic rate R94.8
  biosynthesis, testicular androgen E29.1
  bleeding time R79.1
  blood amino-acid level R79.83
  blood level (of)
    cobalt R79.Ø
    copper R79.Ø
    iron R79.Ø

Abnormal, abnormality, abnormalities — *continued*
  blood level — *continued*
    lithium R78.89
    magnesium R79.Ø
    mineral NEC R79.Ø
    zinc R79.Ø
  blood pressure
    elevated RØ3.Ø
    low reading (nonspecific) RØ3.1
  blood sugar R73.Ø9
  blood-gas level R79.81
  bowel sounds R19.15
    absent R19.11
    hyperactive R19.12
  brain scan R94.Ø2
  breathing RØ6.9
  caloric test R94.138
  cerebrospinal fluid R83.9
    cytology R83.6
    drug level R83.2
    enzyme level R83.Ø
    hormones R83.1
    immunology R83.4
    microbiology R83.5
    nonmedicinal level R83.3
    specified type NEC R83.8
  chemistry, blood R79.9
    C-reactive protein R79.82
    drugs — *see* Findings, abnormal, in blood
    gas level R79.81
    minerals R79.Ø
    pancytopenia D61.818
    PTT R79.1
    specified NEC R79.89
    toxins — *see* Findings, abnormal, in blood
  chest sounds (friction) (rales) RØ9.89
  chromosome, chromosomal Q99.9
    with more than three X chromosomes, female Q97.1
    analysis result R89.8
      bronchial washings R84.8
      cerebrospinal fluid R83.8
      cervix uteri NEC R87.89
      nasal secretions R84.8
      nipple discharge R89.8
      peritoneal fluid R85.89
      pleural fluid R84.8
      prostatic secretions R86.8
      saliva R85.89
      seminal fluid R86.8
      sputum R84.8
      synovial fluid R89.8
      throat scrapings R84.8
      vagina R87.89
      vulva R87.89
      wound secretions R89.8
    dicentric replacement Q93.2
    ring replacement Q93.2
    sex Q99.8
      female phenotype Q97.9
        specified NEC Q97.8
      male phenotype Q98.9
        specified NEC Q98.8
      structural male Q98.6
    specified NEC Q99.8
  clinical findings NEC R68.89
  coagulation D68.9
    newborn, transient P61.6
    profile R79.1
    time R79.1
  communication — *see* Fistula
  conjunctiva, vascular H11.41- ☑
  coronary artery Q24.5
  cortisol-binding globulin E27.8
  course, eustachian tube Q17.8
  creatinine clearance R94.4
  cytology
    anus R85.619
      atypical squamous cells cannot exclude high grade squamous intraepithelial lesion (ASC-H) R85.611
      atypical squamous cells of undetermined significance (ASC-US) R85.61Ø

Abnormal, abnormality, abnormalities — *continued*
  cytology — *continued*
    anus — *continued*
      cytologic evidence of malignancy R85.614
      high grade squamous intraepithelial lesion (HGSIL) R85.613
      human papillomavirus (HPV) DNA test
        high risk positive R85.81
        low risk postive R85.82
      inadequate smear R85.615
      low grade squamous intraepithelial lesion (LGSIL) R85.612
      satisfactory anal smear but lacking transformation zone R85.616
      specified NEC R85.618
      unsatisfactory smear R85.615
    female genital organs — *see* Abnormal, Papanicolaou (smear)
  dark adaptation curve H53.61
  dentofacial NEC — *see* Anomaly, dentofacial
  development, developmental Q89.9
    central nervous system QØ7.9
  diagnostic imaging
    abdomen, abdominal region NEC R93.5
    biliary tract R93.2
    bladder R93.41
    breast R92.8
    central nervous system NEC R9Ø.89
    cerebrovascular NEC R9Ø.89
    coronary circulation R93.1
    digestive tract NEC R93.3
    gastrointestinal (tract) R93.3
    genitourinary organs R93.89
    head R93.Ø
    heart R93.1
    intrathoracic organ NEC R93.89
    kidney R93.42- ☑
    limbs R93.6
    liver R93.2
    lung (field) R91.8
    musculoskeletal system NEC R93.7
    renal pelvis R93.41
    retroperitoneum R93.5
    site specified NEC R93.89
    skin and subcutaneous tissue R93.89
    skull R93.Ø
    testis R93.81- ☑
    ureter R93.41
    urinary organs specified NEC R93.49
  direction, teeth, fully erupted M26.3Ø
  ear ossicles, acquired NEC H74.39- ☑
    ankylosis — *see* Ankylosis, ear ossicles
    discontinuity — *see* Discontinuity, ossicles, ear
    partial loss — *see* Loss, ossicles, ear (partial)
  Ebstein Q22.5
  echocardiogram R93.1
  echoencephalogram R9Ø.81
  echogram — *see* Abnormal, diagnostic imaging
  electrocardiogram [ECG] [EKG] R94.31
  electroencephalogram [EEG] R94.Ø1
  electrolyte — *see* Imbalance, electrolyte
  electromyogram [EMG] R94.131
  electro-oculogram [EOG] R94.11Ø
  electrophysiological intracardiac studies R94.39
  electroretinogram [ERG] R94.111
  erythrocytes
    congenital, with perinatal jaundice D58.9
  feces (color) (contents) (mucus) R19.5
  finding — *see* Findings, abnormal, without diagnosis
  fluid
    amniotic — *see* Abnormal, specimen, specified
    cerebrospinal — *see* Abnormal, cerebrospinal fluid
    peritoneal — *see* Abnormal, specimen, digestive organs
    pleural — *see* Abnormal, specimen, respiratory organs
    synovial — *see* Abnormal, specimen, specified
    thorax (bronchial washings) (pleural fluid) — *see* Abnormal, specimen, respiratory organs
    vaginal — *see* Abnormal, specimen, female genital organs

Abnormal, abnormality, abnormalities — *continued*
- form
  - teeth KØØ.2
  - uterus — *see* Anomaly, uterus
- function studies
  - auditory R94.12Ø
  - bladder R94.8
  - brain R94.Ø9
  - cardiovascular R94.3Ø
  - ear R94.128
  - endocrine NEC R94.7
  - eye NEC R94.118
  - kidney R94.4
  - liver R94.5
  - nervous system
    - central NEC R94.Ø9
    - peripheral NEC R94.138
  - pancreas R94.8
  - placenta R94.8
  - pulmonary R94.2
  - special senses NEC R94.128
  - spleen R94.8
  - thyroid R94.6
  - vestibular R94.121
- gait — *see* Gait
  - hysterical F44.4
- gastrin secretion E16.4
- globulin R77.1
  - cortisol-binding E27.8
  - thyroid-binding EØ7.89
- glomerular, minor — *see also* NØØ-NØ7 with fourth character .Ø NØ5.Ø
- glucagon secretion E16.3
- glucose tolerance (test) (non-fasting) R73.Ø9
- gravitational (G) forces or states (effect of) T75.81 ☑
- hair (color) (shaft) L67.9
  - specified NEC L67.8
- hard tissue formation in pulp (dental) KØ4.3
- head movement R25.Ø
- heart
  - rate RØØ.9
    - specified NEC RØØ.8
  - shadow R93.1
  - sounds NEC RØ1.2
- hemoglobin (disease) — *see also* Disease, hemoglobin D58.2
  - trait — *see* Trait, hemoglobin, abnormal
- histology NEC R89.7
- immunological findings R89.4
  - in serum R76.9
    - specified NEC R76.8
- increase in appetite R63.2
- involuntary movement — *see* Abnormal, movement, involuntary
- jaw closure M26.51
- karyotype R89.8
- kidney function test R94.4
- knee jerk R29.2
- leukocyte (cell) (differential) NEC D72.9
- liver function test — *see also* Elevated, liver function, test R79.89
- loss of
  - height R29.89Ø
  - weight R63.4
- mammogram NEC R92.8
  - calcification (calculus) R92.1
  - microcalcification R92.Ø
- Mantoux test R76.11
- movement (disorder) — *see also* Disorder, movement
  - head R25.Ø
  - involuntary R25.9
    - fasciculation R25.3
    - of head R25.Ø
    - spasm R25.2
    - specified type NEC R25.8
    - tremor R25.1
- myoglobin (Aberdeen) (Annapolis) R89.7
- neonatal screening PØ9.9
  - for
    - congenital adrenal hyperplasia PØ9.2
    - congenital endocrine disease PØ9.2
    - congenital hematologic disorders PØ9.3
    - critical congenital heart disease PØ9.5
    - cystic fibrosis PØ9.4
    - hemoglobinothies PØ9.3
    - hypothyroidism PØ9.2
    - inborn errors of metabolism PØ9.1

Abnormal, abnormality, abnormalities — *continued*
- neonatal screening — *continued*
  - for — *continued*
    - neonatal hearing loss PØ9.6
    - red cell membrane defects PØ9.3
    - sickle cell PØ9.3
    - specified NEC PØ9.8
- oculomotor study R94.113
- palmar creases Q82.8
- Papanicolaou (smear)
  - anus R85.619
    - atypical squamous cells cannot exclude high grade squamous intraepithelial lesion (ASC-H) R85.611
    - atypical squamous cells of undetermined significance (ASC-US) R85.61Ø
    - cytologic evidence of malignancy R85.614
    - high grade squamous intraepithelial lesion (HGSIL) R85.613
    - human papillomavirus (HPV) DNA test
      - high risk positive R85.81
      - low risk postive R85.82
    - inadequate smear R85.615
    - low grade squamous intraepithelial lesion (LGSIL) R85.612
    - satisfactory anal smear but lacking transformation zone R85.616
    - specified NEC R85.618
    - unsatisfactory smear R85.615
  - bronchial washings R84.6
  - cerebrospinal fluid R83.6
  - cervix R87.619
    - atypical squamous cells cannot exclude high grade squamous intraepithelial lesion (ASC-H) R87.611
    - atypical squamous cells of undetermined significance (ASC-US) R87.61Ø
    - cytologic evidence of malignancy R87.614
    - high grade squamous intraepithelial lesion (HGSIL) R87.613
    - inadequate smear R87.615
    - low grade squamous intraepithelial lesion (LGSIL) R87.612
    - non-atypical endometrial cells R87.618
    - satisfactory cervical smear but lacking transformation zone R87.616
    - specified NEC R87.618
    - thin preparaton R87.619
    - unsatisfactory smear R87.615
  - nasal secretions R84.6
  - nipple discharge R89.6
  - peritoneal fluid R85.69
  - pleural fluid R84.6
  - prostatic secretions R86.6
  - saliva R85.69
  - seminal fluid R86.6
  - sites NEC R89.6
  - sputum R84.6
  - synovial fluid R89.6
  - throat scrapings R84.6
  - vagina R87.629
    - atypical squamous cells cannot exclude high grade squamous intraepithelial lesion (ASC-H) R87.621
    - atypical squamous cells of undetermined significance (ASC-US) R87.62Ø
    - cytologic evidence of malignancy R87.624
    - high grade squamous intraepithelial lesion (HGSIL) R87.623
    - inadequate smear R87.625
    - low grade squamous intraepithelial lesion (LGSIL) R87.622
    - specified NEC R87.628
    - thin preparation R87.629
    - unsatisfactory smear R87.625
  - vulva R87.69
  - wound secretions R89.6
- partial thromboplastin time (PTT) R79.1
- pelvis (bony) — *see* Deformity, pelvis
- percussion, chest (tympany) RØ9.89
- periods (grossly) — *see* Menstruation
- phonocardiogram R94.39
- plantar reflex R29.2
- plasma
  - protein R77.9
    - specified NEC R77.8
  - viscosity R7Ø.1
- pleural (folds) Q34.Ø

Abnormal, abnormality, abnormalities — *continued*
- posture R29.3
- product of conception OØ2.9
  - specified type NEC OØ2.89
- prothrombin time (PT) R79.1
- pulmonary
  - artery, congenital Q25.79
  - function, newborn P28.89
  - test results R94.2
- pulsations in neck RØØ.2
- pupillary H21.56- ☑
  - function (reaction) (reflex) — *see* Anomaly, pupil, function
- radiological examination — *see* Abnormal, diagnostic imaging
- red blood cell(s) (morphology) (volume) R71.8
- reflex — *see* Reflex
- renal function test R94.4
- response to nerve stimulation R94.13Ø
- retinal correspondence H53.31
- retinal function study R94.111
- rhythm, heart — *see also* Arrhythmia
- saliva — *see* Abnormal, specimen, digestive organs
- scan
  - kidney R94.4
  - liver R93.2
  - thyroid R94.6
- secretion
  - gastrin E16.4
  - glucagon E16.3
- semen, seminal fluid — *see* Abnormal, specimen, male genital organs
- serum level (of)
  - acid phosphatase R74.8
  - alkaline phosphatase R74.8
  - amylase R74.8
  - enzymes R74.9
    - specified NEC R74.8
  - lipase R74.8
  - triacylglycerol lipase R74.8
- shape
  - gravid uterus — *see* Anomaly, uterus
- sinus venosus Q21.16
- size, tooth, teeth KØØ.2
- spacing, tooth, teeth, fully erupted M26.3Ø
- specimen
  - digestive organs (peritoneal fluid) (saliva) R85.9
    - cytology R85.69
    - drug level R85.2
    - enzyme level R85.Ø
    - histology R85.7
    - hormones R85.1
    - immunology R85.4
    - microbiology R85.5
    - nonmedicinal level R85.3
    - specified type NEC R85.89
  - female genital organs (secretions) (smears) R87.9
    - cytology R87.69
      - cervix R87.619
        - human papillomavirus (HPV) DNA test
          - high risk positive R87.81Ø
          - low risk positive R87.82Ø
        - inadequate (unsatisfactory) smear R87.615
        - non-atypical endometrial cells R87.618
        - specified NEC R87.618
      - vagina R87.629
        - human papillomavirus (HPV) DNA test
          - high risk positive R87.811
          - low risk positive R87.821
        - inadequate (unsatisfactory) smear R87.625
      - vulva R87.69
    - drug level R87.2
    - enzyme level R87.Ø
    - histological R87.7
    - hormones R87.1
    - immunology R87.4
    - microbiology R87.5
    - nonmedicinal level R87.3
    - specified type NEC R87.89
  - male genital organs (prostatic secretions) (semen) R86.9
    - cytology R86.6
    - drug level R86.2
    - enzyme level R86.Ø
    - histological R86.7

Abrasion — *continued*
- arm (upper) S4Ø.81- ☑
- auditory canal — *see* Abrasion, ear
- auricle — *see* Abrasion, ear
- axilla — *see* Abrasion, arm
- back, lower S3Ø.81Ø ☑
- breast S2Ø.11- ☑
- brow SØØ.81 ☑
- buttock S3Ø.81Ø ☑
- calf — *see* Abrasion, leg
- canthus — *see* Abrasion, eyelid
- cheek SØØ.81 ☑
  - internal SØØ.512 ☑
- chest wall — *see* Abrasion, thorax
- chin SØØ.81 ☑
- clitoris S3Ø.814 ☑
- cornea SØ5.Ø- ☑
- costal region — *see* Abrasion, thorax
- dental KØ3.1
- digit(s)
  - foot — *see* Abrasion, toe
  - hand — *see* Abrasion, finger
- ear SØØ.41- ☑
- elbow S5Ø.31- ☑
- epididymis S3Ø.813 ☑
- epigastric region S3Ø.811 ☑
- epiglottis S1Ø.11 ☑
- esophagus (thoracic) S27.818 ☑
  - cervical S1Ø.11 ☑
- eyebrow — *see* Abrasion, eyelid
- eyelid SØØ.21- ☑
- face SØØ.81 ☑
- finger(s) S6Ø.41- ☑
  - index S6Ø.41- ☑
  - little S6Ø.41- ☑
  - middle S6Ø.41- ☑
  - ring S6Ø.41- ☑
- flank S3Ø.811 ☑
- foot (except toe(s) alone) S9Ø.81- ☑
  - toe — *see* Abrasion, toe
- forearm S5Ø.81- ☑
  - elbow only — *see* Abrasion, elbow
- forehead SØØ.81 ☑
- genital organs, external
  - female S3Ø.816 ☑
  - male S3Ø.815 ☑
- groin S3Ø.811 ☑
- gum SØØ.512 ☑
- hand S6Ø.51- ☑
- head SØØ.91 ☑
  - ear — *see* Abrasion, ear
  - eyelid — *see* Abrasion, eyelid
  - lip SØØ.511 ☑
  - nose SØØ.31 ☑
  - oral cavity SØØ.512 ☑
  - scalp SØØ.Ø1 ☑
  - specified site NEC SØØ.81 ☑
- heel — *see* Abrasion, foot
- hip S7Ø.21- ☑
- inguinal region S3Ø.811 ☑
- interscapular region S2Ø.419 ☑
- jaw SØØ.81 ☑
- knee S8Ø.21- ☑
- labium (majus) (minus) S3Ø.814 ☑
- larynx S1Ø.11 ☑
- leg (lower) S8Ø.81- ☑
  - knee — *see* Abrasion, knee
  - upper — *see* Abrasion, thigh
- lip SØØ.511 ☑
- lower back S3Ø.81Ø ☑
- lumbar region S3Ø.81Ø ☑
- malar region SØØ.81 ☑
- mammary — *see* Abrasion, breast
- mastoid region SØØ.81 ☑
- mouth SØØ.512 ☑
- nail
  - finger — *see* Abrasion, finger
  - toe — *see* Abrasion, toe
- nape S1Ø.81 ☑
- nasal SØØ.31 ☑
- neck S1Ø.91 ☑
  - specified site NEC S1Ø.81 ☑
  - throat S1Ø.11 ☑
- nose SØØ.31 ☑
- occipital region SØØ.Ø1 ☑
- oral cavity SØØ.512 ☑

Abrasion — *continued*
- orbital region — *see* Abrasion, eyelid
- palate SØØ.512 ☑
- palm — *see* Abrasion, hand
- parietal region SØØ.Ø1 ☑
- pelvis S3Ø.81Ø ☑
- penis S3Ø.812 ☑
- perineum
  - female S3Ø.814 ☑
  - male S3Ø.81Ø ☑
- periocular area — *see* Abrasion, eyelid
- phalanges
  - finger — *see* Abrasion, finger
  - toe — *see* Abrasion, toe
- pharynx S1Ø.11 ☑
- pinna — *see* Abrasion, ear
- popliteal space — *see* Abrasion, knee
- prepuce S3Ø.812 ☑
- pubic region S3Ø.81Ø ☑
- pudendum
  - female S3Ø.816 ☑
  - male S3Ø.815 ☑
- sacral region S3Ø.81Ø ☑
- scalp SØØ.Ø1 ☑
- scapular region — *see* Abrasion, shoulder
- scrotum S3Ø.813 ☑
- shin — *see* Abrasion, leg
- shoulder S4Ø.21- ☑
- skin NEC T14.8 ☑
- sternal region S2Ø.319 ☑
- submaxillary region SØØ.81 ☑
- submental region SØØ.81 ☑
- subungual
  - finger(s) — *see* Abrasion, finger
  - toe(s) — *see* Abrasion, toe
- supraclavicular fossa S1Ø.81 ☑
- supraorbital SØØ.81 ☑
- temple SØØ.81 ☑
- temporal region SØØ.81 ☑
- testis S3Ø.813 ☑
- thigh S7Ø.31- ☑
- thorax, thoracic (wall) S2Ø.91 ☑
  - back S2Ø.41- ☑
  - front S2Ø.31- ☑
- throat S1Ø.11 ☑
- thumb S6Ø.31- ☑
- toe(s) (lesser) S9Ø.416 ☑
  - great S9Ø.41- ☑
- tongue SØØ.512 ☑
- tooth, teeth (dentifrice) (habitual) (hard tissues) (occupational) (ritual) (traditional) KØ3.1
- trachea S1Ø.11 ☑
- tunica vaginalis S3Ø.813 ☑
- tympanum, tympanic membrane — *see* Abrasion, ear
- uvula SØØ.512 ☑
- vagina S3Ø.814 ☑
- vocal cords S1Ø.11 ☑
- vulva S3Ø.814 ☑
- wrist S6Ø.81- ☑

Abrism — *see* Poisoning, food, noxious, plant

Abruptio placentae O45.9- ☑
- with
  - afibrinogenemia O45.Ø1- ☑
  - coagulation defect O45.ØØ- ☑
    - specified NEC O45.Ø9- ☑
  - disseminated intravascular coagulation O45.Ø2- ☑
  - hypofibrinogenemia O45.Ø1- ☑
- specified NEC O45.8- ☑

Abruption, placenta — *see* Abruptio placentae

Abscess (connective tissue) (embolic) (fistulous) (infective) (metastatic) (multiple) (pernicious) (pyogenic) (septic) LØ2.91
- with
  - diverticular disease (intestine) K57.8Ø
    - with bleeding K57.81
    - large intestine K57.2Ø
      - with
        - bleeding K57.21
        - small intestine K57.4Ø
          - with bleeding K57.41
    - small intestine K57.ØØ
      - with
        - bleeding K57.Ø1
        - large intestine K57.4Ø
          - with bleeding K57.41

Abscess — *continued*
- with — *continued*
  - lymphangitis — *code by* site under Abscess
- abdomen, abdominal
  - cavity K65.1
  - wall LØ2.211
- abdominopelvic K65.1
- accessory sinus — *see* Sinusitis
- adrenal (capsule) (gland) E27.8
- alveolar KØ4.7
  - with sinus KØ4.6
- amebic AØ6.4
  - brain (and liver or lung abscess) AØ6.6
  - genitourinary tract AØ6.82
  - liver (without mention of brain or lung abscess) AØ6.4
  - lung (and liver) (without mention of brain abscess) AØ6.5
  - specified site NEC AØ6.89
  - spleen AØ6.89
- anerobic A48.Ø
- ankle — *see* Abscess, lower limb
- anorectal K61.2
- antecubital space — *see* Abscess, upper limb
- antrum (chronic) (Highmore) — *see* Sinusitis, maxillary
- anus K61.Ø
- apical (tooth) KØ4.7
  - with sinus (alveolar) KØ4.6
- appendix K35.33
- areola (acute) (chronic) (nonpuerperal) N61.1
  - puerperal, postpartum or gestational — *see* Infection, nipple
- arm (any part) — *see* Abscess, upper limb
- artery (wall) I77.89
- atheromatous I77.2
- auricle, ear — *see* Abscess, ear, external
- axilla (region) LØ2.41- ☑
  - lymph gland or node LØ4.2
- back (any part, except buttock) LØ2.212
- Bartholin's gland N75.1
  - with
    - abortion — *see* Abortion, by type complicated by, sepsis
    - ectopic or molar pregnancy OØ8.Ø
  - following ectopic or molar pregnancy OØ8.Ø
- Bezold's — *see* Mastoiditis, acute
- bilharziasis B65.1
- bladder (wall) — *see* Cystitis, specified type NEC
- bone (subperiosteal) — *see also* Osteomyelitis, specified type NEC
  - accessory sinus (chronic) — *see* Sinusitis
  - chronic or old — *see* Osteomyelitis, chronic
  - jaw (lower) (upper) M27.2
  - mastoid — *see* Mastoiditis, acute, subperiosteal
  - petrous — *see* Petrositis
  - spinal (tuberculous) A18.Ø1
    - nontuberculous — *see* Osteomyelitis, vertebra
- bowel K63.Ø
- brain (any part) (cystic) (otogenic) GØ6.Ø
  - amebic (with abscess of any other site) AØ6.6
  - gonococcal A54.82
  - pheomycotic (chromomycotic) B43.1
  - tuberculous A17.81
- breast (acute) (chronic) (nonpuerperal) N61.1
  - newborn P39.Ø
  - puerperal, postpartum, gestational — *see* Mastitis, obstetric, purulent
- broad ligament N73.2
  - acute N73.Ø
  - chronic N73.1
- Brodie's (localized) (chronic) M86.8X- ☑
- bronchi J98.Ø9
- buccal cavity K12.2
- bulbourethral gland N34.Ø
- bursa M71.ØØ
  - ankle M71.Ø7- ☑
  - elbow M71.Ø2- ☑
  - foot M71.Ø7- ☑
  - hand M71.Ø4- ☑
  - hip M71.Ø5- ☑
  - knee M71.Ø6- ☑
  - multiple sites M71.Ø9
  - pharyngeal J39.1
  - shoulder M71.Ø1- ☑
  - specified site NEC M71.Ø8
  - wrist M71.Ø3- ☑
- buttock LØ2.31
- canthus — *see* Blepharoconjunctivitis

Abscess — *continued*
- penis — *continued*
  - gonococcal (accessory gland) (periurethral) A54.1
- perianal K61.Ø
- periapical KØ4.7
  - with sinus (alveolar) KØ4.6
- periappendicular K35.33
- pericardial I3Ø.1
- pericecal K35.33
- pericemental — *see* Periodontitis, aggressive, localized
- pericholecystic — *see* Cholecystitis, acute
- pericoronal — *see* Periodontitis, aggressive, localized
- peridental — *see* Periodontitis, aggressive, localized
- perimetric — *see also* Disease, pelvis, inflammatory N73.2
- perinephric, perinephritic — *see* Abscess, kidney
- perineum, perineal (superficial) LØ2.215
  - urethra N34.Ø
- periodontal (parietal) — *see* Periodontitis, aggressive, localized
  - apical KØ4.7
- periosteum, periosteal — *see also* Osteomyelitis, specified type NEC
  - with osteomyelitis — *see also* Osteomyelitis, specified type NEC
    - acute — *see* Osteomyelitis, acute
    - chronic — *see* Osteomyelitis, chronic
- peripharyngeal J39.Ø
- peripleuritic J86.9
  - with fistula J86.Ø
- periprostatic N41.2
- perirectal K61.1
- perirenal (tissue) — *see* Abscess, kidney
- perisinuous (nose) — *see* Sinusitis
- peritoneum, peritoneal (perforated) (ruptured) K65.1
  - with appendicitis — *see also* Appendicitis K35.33
  - pelvic
    - female — *see* Peritonitis, pelvic, female
    - male K65.1
  - postoperative T81.43 ☑
  - puerperal, postpartum, childbirth O85
  - tuberculous A18.31
- peritonsillar J36
- perityphlic K35.33
- periureteral N28.89
- periurethral N34.Ø
  - gonococcal (accessory gland) (periurethral) A54.1
- periuterine — *see also* Disease, pelvis, inflammatory N73.2
- perivesical — *see* Cystitis, specified type NEC
- petrous bone — *see* Petrositis
- phagedenic NOS LØ2.91
  - chancroid A57
- pharynx, pharyngeal (lateral) J39.1
- pilonidal LØ5.Ø1
- pituitary (gland) E23.6
- pleura J86.9
  - with fistula J86.Ø
- popliteal — *see* Abscess, lower limb
- postcecal K35.33
- postlaryngeal J38.7
- postnasal J34.Ø
- postoperative (any site) — *see also* Infection, postoperative wound T81.49 ☑
  - retroperitoneal K68.11
- postpharyngeal J39.Ø
- posttonsillar J36
- post-typhoid AØ1.Ø9
- pouch of Douglas — *see* Peritonitis, pelvic, female
- premammary — *see* Abscess, breast
- prepatellar — *see* Abscess, lower limb
- presacral K68.19
- prostate N41.2
  - gonococcal (acute) (chronic) A54.22
- psoas muscle K68.12
- puerperal — *code by* site under Puerperal, abscess
- pulmonary — *see* Abscess, lung
- pulp, pulpal (dental) KØ4.Ø1
  - irreversible KØ4.Ø2
  - reversible KØ4.Ø1
- rectovaginal septum K63.Ø
- rectovesical — *see* Cystitis, specified type NEC
- rectum K61.1
- renal — *see* Abscess, kidney
- retina — *see* Inflammation, chorioretinal
- retrobulbar — *see* Abscess, orbit
- retrocecal K65.1
- retrolaryngeal J38.7

Abscess — *continued*
- retromammary — *see* Abscess, breast
- retroperitoneal NEC K68.19
  - postprocedural K68.11
- retropharyngeal J39.Ø
- retrouterine — *see* Peritonitis, pelvic, female
- retrovesical — *see* Cystitis, specified type NEC
- root, tooth KØ4.7
  - with sinus (alveolar) KØ4.6
- round ligament — *see also* Disease, pelvis, inflammatory N73.2
- rupture (spontaneous) NOS LØ2.91
- sacrum (tuberculous) A18.Ø1
  - nontuberculous M46.28
- salivary (duct) (gland) K11.3
- scalp (any part) LØ2.811
- scapular — *see* Osteomyelitis, specified type NEC
- sclera — *see* Scleritis
- scrofulous (tuberculous) A18.2
- scrotum N49.2
- seminal vesicle N49.Ø
- septal, dental KØ4.7
  - with sinus (alveolar) KØ4.6
- serous — *see* Periostitis
- shoulder (region) — *see* Abscess, upper limb
- sigmoid K63.Ø
- sinus (accessory) (chronic) (nasal) — *see also* Sinusitis
  - intracranial venous (any) GØ6.Ø
- Skene's duct or gland N34.Ø
- skin — *see* Abscess, by site
- specified site NEC LØ2.818
- spermatic cord N49.1
- sphenoidal (sinus) (chronic) J32.3
- spinal cord (any part) (staphylococcal) GØ6.1
  - tuberculous A17.81
- spine (column) (tuberculous) A18.Ø1
  - epidural GØ6.1
  - nontuberculous — *see* Osteomyelitis, vertebra
- spleen D73.3
  - amebic AØ6.89
- stitch T81.41 ☑
  - following an obstetrical procedure O86.Ø1
- subarachnoid GØ6.2
  - brain GØ6.Ø
  - spinal cord GØ6.1
- subareolar — *see* Abscess, breast
- subcecal K35.33
- subcutaneous — *see also* Abscess, by site
  - following procedure T81.41 ☑
    - obstetrical O86.Ø1
  - pheomycotic (chromomycotic) B43.2
- subdiaphragmatic K65.1
- subdural GØ6.2
  - brain GØ6.Ø
    - sequelae GØ9
  - spinal cord GØ6.1
- sub-fascial, following an obstetrical procedure O86.Ø2
- subgaleal LØ2.811
- subhepatic K65.1
- sublingual K12.2
  - gland K11.3
- submammary — *see* Abscess, breast
- submandibular (region) (space) (triangle) K12.2
  - gland K11.3
- submaxillary (region) LØ2.Ø1
  - gland K11.3
- submental LØ2.Ø1
  - gland K11.3
- subperiosteal — *see* Osteomyelitis, specified type NEC
- subphrenic K65.1
  - following an obstetrical procedure O86.Ø3
  - postoperative T81.43 ☑
- suburethral N34.Ø
- sudoriparous L75.8
- supraclavicular (fossa) — *see* Abscess, upper limb
- supralevator K61.5
- suprapelvic, acute N73.Ø
- suprarenal (capsule) (gland) E27.8
- sweat gland L74.8
- tear duct — *see* Inflammation, lacrimal, passages, acute
- temple LØ2.Ø1
- temporal region LØ2.Ø1
- temporosphenoidal GØ6.Ø
- tendon (sheath) M65.ØØ
  - ankle M65.Ø7- ☑
  - foot M65.Ø7- ☑
  - forearm M65.Ø3- ☑
  - hand M65.Ø4- ☑

Abscess — *continued*
- tendon — *continued*
  - lower leg M65.Ø6- ☑
  - pelvic region M65.Ø5- ☑
  - shoulder region M65.Ø1- ☑
  - specified site NEC M65.Ø8
  - thigh M65.Ø5- ☑
  - upper arm M65.Ø2- ☑
- testis N45.4
- thigh — *see* Abscess, lower limb
- thorax J86.9
  - with fistula J86.Ø
- throat J39.1
- thumb — *see also* Abscess, hand
  - nail — *see* Cellulitis, finger
- thymus (gland) E32.1
- thyroid (gland) EØ6.Ø
- toe (any) — *see also* Abscess, foot
  - nail — *see* Cellulitis, toe
- tongue (staphylococcal) K14.Ø
- tonsil(s) (lingual) J36
- tonsillopharyngeal J36
- tooth, teeth (root) KØ4.7
  - with sinus (alveolar) KØ4.6
  - supporting structures NEC — *see* Periodontitis, aggressive, localized
- trachea J39.8
- trunk LØ2.219
  - abdominal wall LØ2.211
  - back LØ2.212
  - chest wall LØ2.213
  - groin LØ2.214
  - perineum LØ2.215
  - umbilicus LØ2.216
- tubal — *see* Salpingitis
- tuberculous — *see* Tuberculosis, abscess
- tubo-ovarian — *see* Salpingo-oophoritis
- tunica vaginalis N49.1
- umbilicus LØ2.216
- upper
  - limb LØ2.41- ☑
  - respiratory J39.8
- urethral (gland) N34.Ø
- urinary N34.Ø
- uterus, uterine (wall) — *see also* Endometritis
  - ligament — *see also* Disease, pelvis, inflammatory N73.2
  - neck — *see* Cervicitis
- uvula K12.2
- vagina (wall) — *see* Vaginitis
- vaginorectal — *see* Vaginitis
- vas deferens N49.1
- vermiform appendix K35.33
- vertebra (column) (tuberculous) A18.Ø1
  - nontuberculous — *see* Osteomyelitis, vertebra
- vesical — *see* Cystitis, specified type NEC
- vesico-uterine pouch — *see* Peritonitis, pelvic, female
- vitreous (humor) — *see* Endophthalmitis, purulent
- vocal cord J38.3
- von Bezold's — *see* Mastoiditis, acute
- vulva N76.4
- vulvovaginal gland N75.1
- web space — *see* Abscess, hand
- wound T81.49 ☑
- wrist — *see* Abscess, upper limb

Absence (of) (organ or part) (complete or partial)
- adrenal (gland) (congenital) Q89.1
  - acquired E89.6
- albumin in blood E88.Ø9
- alimentary tract (congenital) Q45.8
  - upper Q4Ø.8
- alveolar process (acquired) — *see* Anomaly, alveolar
- ankle (acquired) Z89.44- ☑
- anus (congenital) Q42.3
  - with fistula Q42.2
- aorta (congenital) Q25.41
- appendix, congenital Q42.8
- arm (acquired) Z89.2Ø- ☑
  - above elbow Z89.22- ☑
    - congenital (with hand present) — *see* Agenesis, arm, with hand present
      - and hand — *see* Agenesis, forearm, and hand
  - below elbow Z89.21- ☑
    - congenital (with hand present) — *see* Agenesis, arm, with hand present
      - and hand — *see* Agenesis, forearm, and hand
  - congenital — *see* Defect, reduction, upper limb

Index

- **Absence** — *continued*
  - teeth, tooth — *continued*
    - acquired — *continued*
      - due to — *continued*
        - caries — *continued*
          - class IV KØ8.134
        - periodontal disease KØ8.129
          - class I KØ8.121
          - class II KØ8.122
          - class III KØ8.123
          - class IV KØ8.124
        - specified NEC KØ8.199
          - class I KØ8.191
          - class II KØ8.192
          - class III KØ8.193
          - class IV KØ8.194
        - trauma KØ8.119
          - class I KØ8.111
          - class II KØ8.112
          - class III KØ8.113
          - class IV KØ8.114
      - partial KØ8.4Ø9
        - class I KØ8.4Ø1
        - class II KØ8.4Ø2
        - class III KØ8.4Ø3
        - class IV KØ8.4Ø4
        - due to
          - caries KØ8.439
            - class I KØ8.431
            - class II KØ8.432
            - class III KØ8.433
            - class IV KØ8.434
          - periodontal disease KØ8.429
            - class I KØ8.421
            - class II KØ8.422
            - class III KØ8.423
            - class IV KØ8.424
          - specified NEC KØ8.499
            - class I KØ8.491
            - class II KØ8.492
            - class III KØ8.493
            - class IV KØ8.494
          - trauma KØ8.419
            - class I KØ8.411
            - class II KØ8.412
            - class III KØ8.413
            - class IV KØ8.414
  - tendon (congenital) Q79.8
  - testis (congenital) Q55.Ø
    - acquired Z9Ø.79
  - thumb (acquired) Z89.Ø1- ☑
    - congenital — *see* Agenesis, hand
  - thymus gland Q89.2
  - thyroid (gland) (acquired) E89.Ø
    - cartilage, congenital Q31.8
    - congenital EØ3.1
  - toe(s) (acquired) Z89.42- ☑
    - with foot — *see* Absence, foot and ankle
    - congenital — *see* Agenesis, foot
    - great Z89.41- ☑
  - tongue, congenital Q38.3
  - trachea (cartilage), congenital Q32.1
  - transverse aortic arch, congenital Q25.49
  - tricuspid valve Q22.4
  - umbilical artery, congenital Q27.Ø
  - upper arm and forearm with hand present, congenital — *see* Agenesis, arm, with hand present
  - ureter (congenital) Q62.4
    - acquired Z9Ø.6
  - urethra, congenital Q64.5
  - uterus (acquired) Z9Ø.71Ø
    - with cervix Z9Ø.71Ø
    - with remaining cervical stump Z9Ø.711
    - congenital Q51.Ø
  - uvula, congenital Q38.5
  - vagina, congenital Q52.Ø
  - vas deferens (congenital) Q55.4
    - acquired Z9Ø.79
  - vein (peripheral) congenital NEC Q27.8
    - cerebral Q28.3
    - digestive system Q27.8
    - great Q26.8
    - lower limb Q27.8
    - portal Q26.5
    - precerebral Q28.1
    - specified site NEC Q27.8
    - upper limb Q27.8
  - vena cava (inferior) (superior), congenital Q26.8
- **Absence** — *continued*
  - ventricular septum Q2Ø.4
  - vertebra, congenital Q76.49
  - von Willebrand factor, complete (near) — *see also* Disease, von Willebrand D68.Ø3
  - vulva, congenital Q52.71
  - wrist (acquired) Z89.12- ☑
- **Absorbent system disease** I87.8
- **Absorption**
  - carbohydrate, disturbance K9Ø.49
  - chemical — *see* Table of Drugs and Chemicals
    - through placenta (newborn) PØ4.9
      - environmental substance PØ4.6
      - nutritional substance PØ4.5
      - obstetric anesthetic or analgesic drug PØ4.Ø
  - drug NEC — *see* Table of Drugs and Chemicals
    - addictive
      - through placenta (newborn) — *see also* Newborn, affected by, maternal, use of PØ4.4Ø
        - cocaine PØ4.41
        - hallucinogens PØ4.42
        - specified drug NEC PØ4.49
    - medicinal
      - through placenta (newborn) PØ4.19
    - through placenta (newborn) PØ4.19
      - obstetric anesthetic or analgesic drug PØ4.Ø
  - fat, disturbance K9Ø.49
    - pancreatic K9Ø.3
  - noxious substance — *see* Table of Drugs and Chemicals
  - protein, disturbance K9Ø.49
  - starch, disturbance K9Ø.49
  - toxic substance — *see* Table of Drugs and Chemicals
  - uremic — *see* Uremia
- **Abstinence symptoms, syndrome**
  - alcohol F1Ø.239
    - with delirium F1Ø.231
  - cocaine F14.23
  - neonatal P96.1
  - nicotine — *see* Dependence, drug, nicotine, with, withdrawal
  - opioid F11.93
    - with dependence F11.23
  - psychoactive NEC F19.939
    - with
      - delirium F19.931
      - dependence F19.239
        - with
          - delirium F19.231
          - perceptual disturbance F19.232
        - uncomplicated F19.23Ø
      - perceptual disturbance F19.932
    - uncomplicated F19.93Ø
  - sedative F13.939
    - with
      - delirium F13.931
      - dependence F13.239
        - with
          - delirium F13.231
          - perceptual disturbance F13.232
        - uncomplicated F13.23Ø
      - perceptual disturbance F13.932
    - uncomplicated F13.93Ø
  - stimulant NEC F15.93
    - with dependence F15.23
- **Abulia** R68.89
- **Abulomania** F6Ø.7
- **Abuse**
  - adult — *see* Maltreatment, adult
    - as reason for
      - couple seeking advice (including offender) Z63.Ø
  - alcohol (non-dependent) F1Ø.1Ø
    - with
      - anxiety disorder F1Ø.18Ø
      - intoxication F1Ø.129
        - with delirium F1Ø.121
        - uncomplicated F1Ø.12Ø
      - mood disorder F1Ø.14
      - other specified disorder F1Ø.188
      - psychosis F1Ø.159
        - delusions F1Ø.15Ø
        - hallucinations F1Ø.151
      - sexual dysfunction F1Ø.181
      - sleep disorder F1Ø.182
      - unspecified disorder F1Ø.19
      - withdrawal F1Ø.139
        - with
          - perceptual disturbance F1Ø.132
          - delirium F1Ø.131
- **Abuse** — *continued*
  - alcohol — *continued*
    - with — *continued*
      - withdrawal — *continued*
        - uncomplicated F1Ø.13Ø
    - counseling and surveillance Z71.41
    - in remission (early) (sustained) F1Ø.11
  - amphetamine (or related substance) — *see also* Abuse, drug, stimulant NEC
    - stimulant NEC F15.1Ø
      - with
        - anxiety disorder F15.18Ø
        - intoxication F15.129
          - with
            - delirium F15.121
            - perceptual disturbance F15.122
        - withdrawal F15.13
  - analgesics (non-prescribed) (over the counter) F55.8
  - antacids F55.Ø
  - antidepressants — *see* Abuse, drug, psychoactive NEC
  - anxiolytic — *see* Abuse, drug, sedative
  - barbiturates — *see* Abuse, drug, sedative
  - caffeine — *see* Abuse, drug, stimulant NEC
  - cannabis, cannabinoids — *see* Abuse, drug, cannabis
  - child — *see* Maltreatment, child
  - cocaine — *see* Abuse, drug, cocaine
  - drug NEC (non-dependent) F19.1Ø
    - with sleep disorder F19.182
    - amphetamine type — *see* Abuse, drug, stimulant NEC
    - analgesics (non-prescribed) (over the counter) F55.8
    - antacids F55.Ø
    - antidepressants — *see* Abuse, drug, psychoactive NEC
    - anxiolytics — *see* Abuse, drug, sedative
    - barbiturates — *see* Abuse, drug, sedative
    - caffeine — *see* Abuse, drug, stimulant NEC
    - cannabis F12.1Ø
      - with
        - anxiety disorder F12.18Ø
        - intoxication F12.129
          - with
            - delirium F12.121
            - perceptual disturbance F12.122
          - uncomplicated F12.12Ø
        - other specified disorder F12.188
        - psychosis F12.159
          - delusions F12.15Ø
          - hallucinations F12.151
        - unspecified disorder F12.19
        - withdrawal F12.13
      - in remission (early) (sustained) F12.11
    - cocaine F14.1Ø
      - with
        - anxiety disorder F14.18Ø
        - intoxication F14.129
          - with
            - delirium F14.121
            - perceptual disturbance F14.122
          - uncomplicated F14.12Ø
        - mood disorder F14.14
        - other specified disorder F14.188
        - psychosis F14.159
          - delusions F14.15Ø
          - hallucinations F14.151
        - sexual dysfunction F14.181
        - sleep disorder F14.182
        - unspecified disorder F14.19
        - withdrawal F14.13
      - in remission (early) (sustained) F14.11
    - counseling and surveillance Z71.51
    - hallucinogen F16.1Ø
      - with
        - anxiety disorder F16.18Ø
        - flashbacks F16.183
        - intoxication F16.129
          - with
            - delirium F16.121
            - perceptual disturbance F16.122
          - uncomplicated F16.12Ø
        - mood disorder F16.14
        - other specified disorder F16.188
        - perception disorder, persisting F16.183
        - psychosis F16.159
          - delusions F16.15Ø
          - hallucinations F16.151
        - unspecified disorder F16.19
      - in remission (early) (sustained) F16.11

Absence — Abuse

- **Abuse** — *continued*
  - drug — *continued*
    - hashish — *see* Abuse, drug, cannabis
    - herbal or folk remedies F55.1
    - hormones F55.3
    - hypnotics — *see* Abuse, drug, sedative
    - in remission (early) (sustained) F19.11
    - inhalant F18.10
      - with
        - anxiety disorder F18.180
        - dementia, persisting F18.17
        - intoxication F18.129
          - with delirium F18.121
          - uncomplicated F18.120
        - mood disorder F18.14
        - other specified disorder F18.188
        - psychosis F18.159
          - delusions F18.150
          - hallucinations F18.151
        - unspecified disorder F18.19
      - in remission (early) (sustained) F18.11
    - laxatives F55.2
    - LSD — *see* Abuse, drug, hallucinogen
    - marihuana — *see* Abuse, drug, cannabis
    - morphine type (opioids) — *see* Abuse, drug, opioid
    - opioid F11.10
      - with
        - intoxication F11.129
          - with
            - delirium F11.121
            - perceptual disturbance F11.122
          - uncomplicated F11.120
        - mood disorder F11.14
        - other specified disorder F11.188
        - psychosis F11.159
          - delusions F11.150
          - hallucinations F11.151
        - sexual dysfunction F11.181
        - sleep disorder F11.182
        - unspecified disorder F11.19
        - withdrawal F11.13
      - in remission (early) (sustained) F11.11
    - PCP (phencyclidine) (or related substance) — *see* Abuse, drug, hallucinogen
    - psychoactive NEC F19.10
      - with
        - amnestic disorder F19.16
        - anxiety disorder F19.180
        - dementia F19.17
        - intoxication F19.129
          - with
            - delirium F19.121
            - perceptual disturbance F19.122
          - uncomplicated F19.120
        - mood disorder F19.14
        - other specified disorder F19.188
        - psychosis F19.159
          - delusions F19.150
          - hallucinations F19.151
        - sexual dysfunction F19.181
        - sleep disorder F19.182
        - unspecified disorder F19.19
        - withdrawal F19.139
          - with
            - perceptual disturbance F19.132
          - delirium F19.131
          - uncomplicated F19.130
    - sedative, hypnotic or anxiolytic F13.10
      - with
        - anxiety disorder F13.180
        - intoxication F13.129
          - with delirium F13.121
          - uncomplicated F13.120
        - mood disorder F13.14
        - other specified disorder F13.188
        - psychosis F13.159
          - delusions F13.150
          - hallucinations F13.151
        - sexual dysfunction F13.181
        - sleep disorder F13.182
        - unspecified disorder F13.19
        - withdrawal F13.139
          - with
            - perceptual disturbance F13.132
          - delirium F13.131
          - uncomplicated F13.130
      - in remission (early) (sustained) F13.11
    - solvent — *see* Abuse, drug, inhalant
- **Abuse** — *continued*
  - drug — *continued*
    - steroids F55.3
    - stimulant NEC F15.10
      - with
        - anxiety disorder F15.180
        - intoxication F15.129
          - with
            - delirium F15.121
            - perceptual disturbance F15.122
          - uncomplicated F15.120
        - mood disorder F15.14
        - other specified disorder F15.188
        - psychosis F15.159
          - delusions F15.150
          - hallucinations F15.151
        - sexual dysfunction F15.181
        - sleep disorder F15.182
        - unspecified disorder F15.19
        - withdrawal F15.13
      - in remission (early) (sustained) F15.11
    - tranquilizers — *see* Abuse, drug, sedative
    - vitamins F55.4
  - hallucinogens — *see* Abuse, drug, hallucinogen
  - hashish — *see* Abuse, drug, cannabis
  - herbal or folk remedies F55.1
  - hormones F55.3
  - hypnotic — *see* Abuse, drug, sedative
  - inhalant — *see* Abuse, drug, inhalant
  - laxatives F55.2
  - LSD — *see* Abuse, drug, hallucinogen
  - marihuana — *see* Abuse, drug, cannabis
  - morphine type (opioids) — *see* Abuse, drug, opioid
  - non-psychoactive substance NEC F55.8
    - antacids F55.0
    - folk remedies F55.1
    - herbal remedies F55.1
    - hormones F55.3
    - laxatives F55.2
    - steroids F55.3
    - vitamins F55.4
  - opioids — *see* Abuse, drug, opioid
  - PCP (phencyclidine) (or related substance) — *see* Abuse, drug, hallucinogen
  - physical (adult) (child) — *see* Maltreatment
  - psychoactive substance — *see* Abuse, drug, psychoactive NEC
  - psychological (adult) (child) — *see* Maltreatment
  - sedative — *see* Abuse, drug, sedative
  - sexual — *see* Maltreatment
  - solvent — *see* Abuse, drug, inhalant
  - steroids F55.3
  - vitamins F55.4
- **Acalculia** R48.8
  - developmental F81.2
- **Acanthamebiasis** (with) B60.10
  - conjunctiva B60.12
  - keratoconjunctivitis B60.13
  - meningoencephalitis B60.11
  - other specified B60.19
- **Acanthocephaliasis** B83.8
- **Acanthocheilonemiasis** B74.4
- **Acanthocytosis** E78.6
- **Acantholysis** L11.9
- **Acanthosis** (acquired) (nigricans) L83
  - benign Q82.8
  - congenital Q82.8
  - seborrheic L82.1
    - inflamed L82.0
  - tongue K14.3
- **Acapnia** E87.3
- **Acarbia** E87.29
- **Acardia, acardius** Q89.8
- **Acardiacus amorphus** Q89.8
- **Acardiotrophia** I51.4
- **Acariasis** B88.0
  - scabies B86
- **Acarodermatitis** (urticarioides) B88.0
- **Acarophobia** F40.218
- **Acatalasemia, acatalasia** E80.3
- **Acathisia** (drug induced) G25.71
- **Accelerated atrioventricular conduction** I45.6
- **Accentuation of personality traits** (type A) Z73.1
- **Accessory** (congenital)
  - adrenal gland Q89.1
  - anus Q43.4
  - appendix Q43.4
  - atrioventricular conduction I45.6
- **Accessory** — *continued*
  - auditory ossicles Q16.3
  - auricle (ear) Q17.0
  - biliary duct or passage Q44.5
  - bladder Q64.79
  - blood vessels NEC Q27.9
    - coronary Q24.5
  - bone NEC Q79.8
  - breast tissue, axilla Q83.1
  - carpal bones Q74.0
  - cecum Q43.4
  - chromosome(s) NEC (nonsex) Q92.9
    - with complex rearrangements NEC Q92.5
      - seen only at prometaphase Q92.8
    - 13 — *see* Trisomy, 13
    - 18 — *see* Trisomy, 18
    - 21 — *see* Trisomy, 21
    - partial Q92.9
    - sex
      - female phenotype Q97.8
  - coronary artery Q24.5
  - cusp(s), heart valve NEC Q24.8
    - pulmonary Q22.3
  - cystic duct Q44.5
  - digit(s) Q69.9
  - ear (auricle) (lobe) Q17.0
  - endocrine gland NEC Q89.2
  - eye muscle Q10.3
  - eyelid Q10.3
  - face bone(s) Q75.8
  - fallopian tube (fimbria) (ostium) Q50.6
  - finger(s) Q69.0
  - foreskin N47.8
  - frontonasal process Q75.8
  - gallbladder Q44.1
  - genital organ(s)
    - female Q52.8
      - external Q52.79
      - internal NEC Q52.8
    - male Q55.8
  - genitourinary organs NEC Q89.8
    - female Q52.8
    - male Q55.8
  - hallux Q69.2
  - heart Q24.8
    - valve NEC Q24.8
      - pulmonary Q22.3
  - hepatic ducts Q44.5
  - hymen Q52.4
  - intestine (large) (small) Q43.4
  - kidney Q63.0
  - lacrimal canal Q10.6
  - leaflet, heart valve NEC Q24.8
  - ligament, broad Q50.6
  - liver Q44.7
    - duct Q44.5
  - lobule (ear) Q17.0
  - lung (lobe) Q33.1
  - muscle Q79.8
  - navicular of carpus Q74.0
  - nervous system, part NEC Q07.8
  - nipple Q83.3
  - nose Q30.8
  - organ or site not listed — *see* Anomaly, by site
  - ovary Q50.31
  - oviduct Q50.6
  - pancreas Q45.3
  - parathyroid gland Q89.2
  - parotid gland (and duct) Q38.4
  - pituitary gland Q89.2
  - preauricular appendage Q17.0
  - prepuce N47.8
  - renal arteries (multiple) Q27.2
  - rib Q76.6
    - cervical Q76.5
  - roots (teeth) K00.2
  - salivary gland Q38.4
  - sesamoid bones Q74.8
    - foot Q74.2
    - hand Q74.0
  - skin tags Q82.8
  - spleen Q89.09
  - sternum Q76.7
  - submaxillary gland Q38.4
  - tarsal bones Q74.2
  - teeth, tooth K00.1
  - tendon Q79.8
  - thumb Q69.1
  - thymus gland Q89.2

Accessory — *continued*
- thyroid gland Q89.2
- toes Q69.2
- tongue Q38.3
- tooth, teeth KØØ.1
- tragus Q17.Ø
- ureter Q62.5
- urethra Q64.79
- urinary organ or tract NEC Q64.8
- uterus Q51.28
- vagina Q52.1Ø
- valve, heart NEC Q24.8
  - pulmonary Q22.3
- vertebra Q76.49
- vocal cords Q31.8
- vulva Q52.79

Accident
- birth — *see* Birth, injury
- cardiac — *see* Infarct, myocardium
- cerebral I63.9
- cerebrovascular (embolic) (ischemic) (thrombotic) I63.9
  - aborted I63.9
  - hemorrhagic — *see* Hemorrhage, intracranial, intracerebral
  - old (without sequelae) Z86.73
    - with sequelae (of) — *see* Sequelae, infarction, cerebral
- coronary — *see* Infarct, myocardium
- craniovascular I63.9
- vascular, brain I63.9

Accidental — *see* condition

Accommodation (disorder) — *see also* condition
- hysterical paralysis of F44.89
- insufficiency of H52.4
- paresis — *see* Paresis, of accommodation
- spasm — *see* Spasm, of accommodation

Accouchement — *see* Delivery

Accreta placenta O43.21- ☑

Accretio cordis (nonrheumatic) I31.Ø

Accretions, tooth, teeth KØ3.6

Acculturation difficulty Z6Ø.3

Accumulation secretion, prostate N42.89

Acephalia, acephalism, acephalus, acephaly QØØ.Ø

Acephalobrachia monster Q89.8

Acephalochirus monster Q89.8

Acephalogaster Q89.8

Acephalostomus monster Q89.8

Acephalothorax Q89.8

Acerophobia F4Ø.298

Acetonemia R79.89
- in Type 1 diabetes E1Ø.1Ø
  - with coma E1Ø.11

Acetonuria R82.4

Achalasia (cardia) (esophagus) K22.Ø
- congenital Q39.5
- pylorus Q4Ø.Ø
- sphincteral NEC K59.89

Ache(s) — *see* Pain

Acheilia Q38.6

Achillobursitis — *see* Tendinitis, Achilles

Achillodynia — *see* Tendinitis, Achilles

Achlorhydria, achlorhydric (neurogenic) K31.83
- anemia D5Ø.8
- diarrhea K31.83
- psychogenic F45.8
- secondary to vagotomy K91.1

Achluophobia F4Ø.228

Acholia K82.8

Acholuric jaundice (familial) (splenomegalic) — *see also* Spherocytosis
- acquired D59.8

Achondrogenesis Q77.Ø

Achondroplasia (osteosclerosis congenita) Q77.4

Achroma, cutis L8Ø

Achromat (ism), achromatopsia (acquired) (congenital) H53.51

Achromia, congenital — *see* Albinism

Achromia parasitica B36.Ø

Achylia gastrica K31.89
- psychogenic F45.8

Acid
- burn — *see* Corrosion
- deficiency
  - amide nicotinic E52
  - ascorbic E54
  - folic E53.8
  - nicotinic E52

Acid — *continued*
- deficiency — *continued*
  - pantothenic E53.8
- intoxication — *see also* Acidosis E87.29
- peptic disease K3Ø
- phosphatase deficiency E83.39
- stomach K3Ø
  - psychogenic F45.8

Acidemia — *see also* Acidosis E87.2Ø
- argininosuccinic E72.22
- isovaleric E71.11Ø
- metabolic (newborn) P19.9
  - first noted before onset of labor P19.Ø
  - first noted during labor P19.1
  - noted at birth P19.2
- methylmalonic E71.12Ø
- pipecolic E72.3
- propionic E71.121

Acidity, gastric (high) K3Ø
- psychogenic F45.8

Acidocytopenia — *see* Agranulocytosis

Acidocytosis D72.1Ø

Acidopenia — *see* Agranulocytosis

Acidosis (lactic) E87.2Ø
- in Type 1 diabetes E1Ø.1Ø
  - with coma E1Ø.11
- kidney, tubular N25.89
- lactic E87.2Ø
  - acute E87.21
  - chronic E87.22
- metabolic NEC E87.2Ø
  - with respiratory acidosis E87.4
  - acute E87.21
  - chronic E87.22
  - hyperchloremic, of newborn P74.421
  - late, of newborn P74.Ø
- mixed metabolic and respiratory, newborn P84
- newborn P84
- renal (hyperchloremic) (tubular) N25.89
- respiratory E87.29
  - acute J96.Ø2
  - chronic J96.12
  - complicated by
    - metabolic
      - acidosis E87.4
      - alkalosis E87.4
- specified NEC E87.29

Aciduria
- 4-hydroxybutyric E72.81
- argininosuccinic E72.22
- gamma-hydroxybutyric E72.81
- glutaric (type I) E72.3
  - type II E71.313
  - type III E71.5- ☑
- orotic (congenital) (hereditary) (pyrimidine deficiency) E79.8
  - anemia D53.Ø

Acladiosis (skin) B36.Ø

Aclasis, diaphyseal Q78.6

Acleistocardia Q21.19

Aclusion — *see* Anomaly, dentofacial, malocclusion

Acne L7Ø.9
- artificialis L7Ø.8
- atrophica L7Ø.2
- cachecticorum (Hebra) L7Ø.8
- conglobata L7Ø.1
- cystic L7Ø.Ø
- decalvans L66.2
- excoriée (des jeunes filles) L7Ø.5
- frontalis L7Ø.2
- indurata L7Ø.Ø
- infantile L7Ø.4
- keloid L73.Ø
- lupoid L7Ø.2
- necrotic, necrotica (miliaris) L7Ø.2
- neonatal L7Ø.4
- nodular L7Ø.Ø
- occupational L7Ø.8
- picker's L7Ø.5
- pustular L7Ø.Ø
- rodens L7Ø.2
- rosacea L71.9
- specified NEC L7Ø.8
- tropica L7Ø.3
- varioliformis L7Ø.2
- vulgaris L7Ø.Ø

Acnitis (primary) A18.4

Acosta's disease T7Ø.29 ☑

Acoustic — *see* condition

Acousticophobia F4Ø.298

ACPO (acute colonic pseudo-obstruction) K59.81

Acquired — *see also* condition
- immunodeficiency syndrome (AIDS) B2Ø

Acrania QØØ.Ø

Acroangiodermatitis I78.9

Acroasphyxia, chronic I73.89

Acrobystitis N47.7

Acrocephalopolysyndactyly Q87.Ø

Acrocephalosyndactyly Q87.Ø

Acrocephaly Q75.Ø

Acrochondrohyperplasia — *see* Syndrome, Marfan's

Acrocyanosis I73.89
- newborn P28.2
  - meaning transient blue hands and feet — *omit code*

Acrodermatitis L3Ø.8
- atrophicans (chronica) L9Ø.4
- continua (Hallopeau) L4Ø.2
- enteropathica (hereditary) E83.2
- Hallopeau's L4Ø.2
- infantile papular L44.4
- perstans L4Ø.2
- pustulosa continua L4Ø.2
- recalcitrant pustular L4Ø.2

Acrodynia — *see* Poisoning, mercury

Acromegaly, acromegalia E22.Ø

Acromelalgia I73.81

Acromicria, acromikria Q79.8

Acronyx L6Ø.Ø

Acropachy, thyroid — *see* Thyrotoxicosis

Acroparesthesia (simple) (vasomotor) I73.89

Acropathy, thyroid — *see* Thyrotoxicosis

Acrophobia F4Ø.241

Acroposthitis N47.7

Acroscleriasis, acroscleroderma, acrosclerosis — *see* Sclerosis, systemic

Acrosphacelus I96

Acrospiroma, eccrine — *see* Neoplasm, skin, benign

Acrostealgia — *see* Osteochondropathy

Acrotrophodynia — *see* Immersion

ACTH ectopic syndrome E24.3

Actinic — *see* condition

Actinobacillosis, actinobacillus A28.8
- mallei A24.Ø
- muris A25.1

Actinomyces israelii (infection) — *see* Actinomycosis

Actinomycetoma (foot) B47.1

Actinomycosis, actinomycotic A42.9
- with pneumonia A42.Ø
- abdominal A42.1
- cervicofacial A42.2
- cutaneous A42.89
- gastrointestinal A42.1
- pulmonary A42.Ø
- sepsis A42.7
- specified site NEC A42.89

Actinoneuritis G62.82

Action, heart
- disorder I49.9
- irregular I49.9
  - psychogenic F45.8

Activated protein C resistance D68.51

Activation
- mast cell (disorder) (syndrome) D89.4Ø
  - idiopathic D89.42
  - monoclonal D89.41
  - secondary D89.43
  - specified type NEC D89.49

Active — *see* condition

Acute — *see also* condition
- abdomen R1Ø.Ø
- gallbladder — *see* Cholecystitis, acute

Acyanotic heart disease (congenital) Q24.9

Acystia Q64.5

Adair-Dighton syndrome (brittle bones and blue sclera, deafness) Q78.Ø

Adamantinoblastoma — *see* Ameloblastoma

Adamantinoma — *see also* Cyst, calcifying odontogenic
- long bones C4Ø.9Ø
  - lower limb C4Ø.2- ☑
  - upper limb C4Ø.Ø- ☑
- malignant C41.1
  - jaw (bone) (lower) C41.1
    - upper C41.Ø
- tibial C4Ø.2- ☑

Adamantoblastoma — *see* Ameloblastoma

Index

Adenofibroma — *continued*
- specified site — *see* Neoplasm, benign, by site
- unspecified site D27.9

Adenofibrosis
- breast — *see* Fibroadenosis, breast
- endometrioid N8Ø.ØØ

Adenoiditis (chronic) J35.Ø2
- with tonsillitis J35.Ø3
- acute JØ3.9Ø
  - recurrent JØ3.91
  - specified organism NEC JØ3.8Ø
    - recurrent JØ3.81
  - staphylococcal JØ3.8Ø
    - recurrent JØ3.81
  - streptococcal JØ3.ØØ
    - recurrent JØ3.Ø1

Adenoids — *see* condition

Adenolipoma — *see* Neoplasm, benign, by site

Adenolipomatosis, Launois-Bensaude E88.89

Adenolymphoma
- specified site — *see* Neoplasm, benign, by site
- unspecified site D11.9

Adenoma — *see also* Neoplasm, benign, by site
- acidophil
  - specified site — *see* Neoplasm, benign, by site
  - unspecified site D35.2
- acidophil-basophil, mixed
  - specified site — *see* Neoplasm, benign, by site
  - unspecified site D35.2
- adrenal (cortical) D35.ØØ
  - clear cell D35.ØØ
  - compact cell D35.ØØ
  - glomerulosa cell D35.ØØ
  - heavily pigmented variant D35.ØØ
  - mixed cell D35.ØØ
- alpha-cell
  - pancreas D13.7
  - specified site NEC — *see* Neoplasm, benign, by site
  - unspecified site D13.7
- alveolar D14.3Ø
- apocrine
  - breast D24- ☑
  - specified site NEC — *see* Neoplasm, skin, benign, by site
  - unspecified site D23.9
- basal cell D11.9
- basophil
  - specified site — *see* Neoplasm, benign, by site
  - unspecified site D35.2
- basophil-acidophil, mixed
  - specified site — *see* Neoplasm, benign, by site
  - unspecified site D35.2
- beta-cell
  - pancreas D13.7
  - specified site NEC — *see* Neoplasm, benign, by site
  - unspecified site D13.7
- bile duct D13.4
  - common D13.5
  - extrahepatic D13.5
  - intrahepatic D13.4
  - specified site NEC — *see* Neoplasm, benign, by site
  - unspecified site D13.4
- black D35.ØØ
- bronchial D38.1
  - cylindroid type — *see* Neoplasm, lung, malignant
- ceruminous D23.2- ☑
- chief cell D35.1
- chromophobe
  - specified site — *see* Neoplasm, benign, by site
  - unspecified site D35.2
- colloid
  - specified site — *see* Neoplasm, benign, by site
  - unspecified site D34
- eccrine, papillary — *see* Neoplasm, skin, benign
- endocrine, multiple
  - single specified site — *see* Neoplasm, uncertain behavior, by site
  - two or more specified sites D44- ☑
  - unspecified site D44.9
- endometrioid — *see also* Neoplasm, benign
  - borderline malignancy — *see* Neoplasm, uncertain behavior, by site
- eosinophil
  - specified site — *see* Neoplasm, benign, by site
  - unspecified site D35.2
- fetal
  - specified site — *see* Neoplasm, benign, by site
  - unspecified site D34

Adenoma — *continued*
- follicular
  - specified site — *see* Neoplasm, benign, by site
  - unspecified site D34
- hepatocellular D13.4
- Hurthle cell D34
- islet cell
  - pancreas D13.7
  - specified site NEC — *see* Neoplasm, benign, by site
  - unspecified site D13.7
- liver cell D13.4
- macrofollicular
  - specified site — *see* Neoplasm, benign, by site
  - unspecified site D34
- malignant, malignum — *see* Neoplasm, malignant, by site
- microcystic
  - pancreas D13.6
  - specified site NEC — *see* Neoplasm, benign, by site
  - unspecified site D13.6
- microfollicular
  - specified site — *see* Neoplasm, benign, by site
  - unspecified site D34
- mucoid cell
  - specified site — *see* Neoplasm, benign, by site
  - unspecified site D35.2
- multiple endocrine
  - single specified site — *see* Neoplasm, uncertain behavior, by site
  - two or more specified sites D44- ☑
  - unspecified site D44.9
- nipple D24- ☑
- papillary — *see also* Neoplasm, benign, by site
  - eccrine — *see* Neoplasm, skin, benign, by site
- Pick's tubular
  - specified site — *see* Neoplasm, benign, by site
  - unspecified site
    - female D27.9
    - male D29.2Ø
- pleomorphic
  - carcinoma in — *see* Neoplasm, salivary gland, malignant
    - specified site — *see* Neoplasm, malignant, by site
    - unspecified site CØ8.9
- polypoid — *see also* Neoplasm, benign
  - adenocarcinoma in — *see* Neoplasm, malignant, by site
  - adenocarcinoma in situ — *see* Neoplasm, in situ, by site
- prostate — *see* Neoplasm, benign, prostate
- rete cell D29.2Ø
- sebaceous — *see* Neoplasm, skin, benign
- Sertoli cell
  - specified site — *see* Neoplasm, benign, by site
  - unspecified site
    - female D27.9
    - male D29.2Ø
- skin appendage — *see* Neoplasm, skin, benign
- sudoriferous gland — *see* Neoplasm, skin, benign
- sweat gland — *see* Neoplasm, skin, benign
- testicular
  - specified site — *see* Neoplasm, benign, by site
  - unspecified site
    - female D27.9
    - male D29.2Ø
- tubular — *see also* Neoplasm, benign, by site
  - adenocarcinoma in — *see* Neoplasm, malignant, by site
  - adenocarcinoma in situ — *see* Neoplasm, in situ, by site
  - Pick's
    - specified site — *see* Neoplasm, benign, by site
    - unspecified site
      - female D27.9
      - male D29.2Ø
- tubulovillous — *see also* Neoplasm, benign, by site
  - adenocarcinoma in — *see* Neoplasm, malignant, by site
  - adenocarcinoma in situ — *see* Neoplasm, in situ, by site
- villous — *see* Neoplasm, uncertain behavior, by site
  - adenocarcinoma in — *see* Neoplasm, malignant, by site
  - adenocarcinoma in situ — *see* Neoplasm, in situ, by site
- water-clear cell D35.1

Adenomatosis
- endocrine (multiple) E31.2Ø
  - single specified site — *see* Neoplasm, uncertain behavior, by site
- erosive of nipple D24- ☑
- pluriendocrine — *see* Adenomatosis, endocrine
- pulmonary D38.1
  - malignant — *see* Neoplasm, lung, malignant
- specified site — *see* Neoplasm, benign, by site
- unspecified site D12.6

Adenomatous
- goiter (nontoxic) EØ4.9
  - with hyperthyroidism — *see* Hyperthyroidism, with, goiter, nodular
  - toxic — *see* Hyperthyroidism, with, goiter, nodular

Adenomyoma — *see also* Neoplasm, benign, by site
- prostate — *see* Enlarged, prostate

Adenomyometritis N8Ø.ØØ

Adenomyosis (uterus) N8Ø.Ø3

Adenopathy (lymph gland) R59.9
- generalized R59.1
- inguinal R59.Ø
- localized R59.Ø
- mediastinal R59.Ø
- mesentery R59.Ø
- syphilitic (secondary) A51.49
- tracheobronchial R59.Ø
  - tuberculous A15.4
    - primary (progressive) A15.7
- tuberculous — *see also* Tuberculosis, lymph gland
  - tracheobronchial A15.4
    - primary (progressive) A15.7

Adenosalpingitis — *see* Salpingitis

Adenosarcoma — *see* Neoplasm, malignant, by site

Adenosclerosis I88.8

Adenosis (sclerosing) breast — *see* Fibroadenosis, breast

Adenovirus, as cause of disease classified elsewhere B97.Ø

Adentia (complete) (partial) — *see* Absence, teeth

Adherent — *see also* Adhesions
- labia (minora) N9Ø.89
- pericardium (nonrheumatic) I31.Ø
  - rheumatic IØ9.2
- placenta (with hemorrhage) O72.Ø
  - without hemorrhage O73.Ø
- prepuce, newborn N47.Ø
- scar (skin) L9Ø.5
- tendon in scar L9Ø.5

Adhesions, adhesive (postinfective) K66.Ø
- with intestinal obstruction K56.5Ø
  - complete K56.52
  - incomplete K56.51
  - partial K56.51
- abdominal (wall) — *see* Adhesions, peritoneum
- appendix K38.8
- bile duct (common) (hepatic) K83.8
- bladder (sphincter) N32.89
- bowel — *see* Adhesions, peritoneum
- cardiac I31.Ø
  - rheumatic IØ9.2
- cecum — *see* Adhesions, peritoneum
- cervicovaginal N88.1
  - congenital Q52.8
  - postpartal O9Ø.89
    - old N88.1
- cervix N88.1
- ciliary body NEC — *see* Adhesions, iris
- clitoris N9Ø.89
- colon — *see* Adhesions, peritoneum
- common duct K83.8
- congenital — *see also* Anomaly, by site
  - fingers — *see* Syndactylism, complex, fingers
  - omental, anomalous Q43.3
  - peritoneal Q43.3
  - tongue (to gum or roof of mouth) Q38.3
- conjunctiva (acquired) H11.21- ☑
  - congenital Q15.8
- cystic duct K82.8
- diaphragm — *see* Adhesions, peritoneum
- due to foreign body — *see* Foreign body
- duodenum — *see* Adhesions, peritoneum
- ear
  - middle H74.1- ☑
- epididymis N5Ø.89
- epidural — *see* Adhesions, meninges
- epiglottis J38.7
- eyelid HØ2.59
- female pelvis N73.6

Adenofibroma — Adhesions, adhesive

Adhesions, adhesive — *continued*
- gallbladder K82.8
- globe H44.89
- heart I31.Ø
  - rheumatic IØ9.2
- ileocecal (coil) — *see* Adhesions, peritoneum
- ileum — *see* Adhesions, peritoneum
- intestine — *see also* Adhesions, peritoneum
  - with obstruction K56.5Ø
    - complete K56.52
    - incomplete K56.51
    - partial K56.51
- intra-abdominal — *see* Adhesions, peritoneum
- iris H21.5Ø- ☑
  - anterior H21.51- ☑
  - goniosynechiae H21.52- ☑
  - posterior H21.54- ☑
  - to corneal graft T85.898 ☑
- joint — *see* Ankylosis
  - knee M23.8X ☑
  - temporomandibular M26.61- ☑
- labium (majus) (minus), congenital Q52.5
- liver — *see* Adhesions, peritoneum
- lung J98.4
- mediastinum J98.59
- meninges (cerebral) (spinal) G96.12
  - congenital QØ7.8
  - tuberculous (cerebral) (spinal) A17.Ø
- mesenteric — *see* Adhesions, peritoneum
- nasal (septum) (to turbinates) J34.89
- ocular muscle — *see* Strabismus, mechanical
- omentum — *see* Adhesions, peritoneum
- ovary N73.6
  - congenital (to cecum, kidney or omentum) Q5Ø.39
- paraovarian N73.6
- pelvic (peritoneal)
  - female N73.6
    - postprocedural N99.4
  - male — *see* Adhesions, peritoneum
  - postpartal (old) N73.6
  - tuberculous A18.17
- penis to scrotum (congenital) Q55.8
- periappendiceal — *see also* Adhesions, peritoneum
- pericardium (nonrheumatic) I31.Ø
  - focal I31.8
  - rheumatic IØ9.2
  - tuberculous A18.84
- pericholecystic K82.8
- perigastric — *see* Adhesions, peritoneum
- periovarian N73.6
- periprostatic N42.89
- perirectal — *see* Adhesions, peritoneum
- perirenal N28.89
- peritoneum, peritoneal (postinfective) K66.Ø
  - with obstruction (intestinal) K56.5Ø
    - complete K56.52
    - incomplete K56.51
    - partial K56.51
  - congenital Q43.3
  - pelvic, female N73.6
    - postprocedural N99.4
  - postpartal, pelvic N73.6
  - postprocedural K66.Ø
  - to uterus N73.6
- peritubal N73.6
- periureteral N28.89
- periuterine N73.6
- perivesical N32.89
- perivesicular (seminal vesicle) N5Ø.89
- pleura, pleuritic J94.8
  - tuberculous NEC A15.6
- pleuropericardial J94.8
- postoperative (gastrointestinal tract) K66.Ø
  - with obstruction — *see also* Obstruction, intestine, postoperative K91.3Ø
  - due to foreign body accidentally left in wound — *see* Foreign body, accidentally left during a procedure
  - pelvic peritoneal N99.4
  - urethra — *see* Stricture, urethra, postprocedural
  - vagina N99.2
- postpartal, old (vulva or perineum) N9Ø.89
- preputial, prepuce N47.5
- pulmonary J98.4
- pylorus — *see* Adhesions, peritoneum
- sciatic nerve — *see* Lesion, nerve, sciatic
- seminal vesicle N5Ø.89
- shoulder (joint) — *see* Capsulitis, adhesive

Adhesions, adhesive — *continued*
- sigmoid flexure — *see* Adhesions, peritoneum
- spermatic cord (acquired) N5Ø.89
  - congenital Q55.4
- spinal canal G96.12
- stomach — *see* Adhesions, peritoneum
- subscapular — *see* Capsulitis, adhesive
- temporomandibular M26.61- ☑
- tendinitis (*see also* Tenosynovitis, specified type NEC)
  - shoulder — *see* Capsulitis, adhesive
- testis N44.8
- tongue, congenital (to gum or roof of mouth) Q38.3
  - acquired K14.8
- trachea J39.8
- tubo-ovarian N73.6
- tunica vaginalis N44.8
- uterus N73.6
  - internal N85.6
  - to abdominal wall N73.6
- vagina (chronic) N89.5
  - postoperative N99.2
- vitreomacular H43.82- ☑
- vitreous H43.89
- vulva N9Ø.89

Adiaspiromycosis B48.8

Adie (-Holmes) **pupil or syndrome** — *see* Anomaly, pupil, function, tonic pupil

Adiponecrosis neonatorum P83.88

Adiposis — *see also* Obesity
- cerebralis E23.6
- dolorosa E88.2

Adiposity — *see also* Obesity
- heart — *see* Degeneration, myocardial
- localized E65

Adiposogenital dystrophy E23.6

Adjustment
- disorder — *see* Disorder, adjustment
- implanted device — *see* Encounter (for), adjustment (of)
- prosthesis, external — *see* Fitting
- reaction — *see* Disorder, adjustment

Administration of tPA (rtPA) in a different facility within the last 24 hours prior to admission to current facility Z92.82

Admission (for) — *see also* Encounter (for)
- adjustment (of)
  - artificial
    - arm Z44.ØØ- ☑
      - complete Z44.Ø1- ☑
      - partial Z44.Ø2- ☑
    - eye Z44.2 ☑
    - leg Z44.1Ø- ☑
      - complete Z44.11- ☑
      - partial Z44.12- ☑
  - brain neuropacemaker Z46.2
    - implanted Z45.42
  - breast
    - implant Z45.81 ☑
    - prosthesis (external) Z44.3 ☑
  - colostomy belt Z46.89
  - contact lenses Z46.Ø
  - cystostomy device Z46.6
  - dental prosthesis Z46.3
  - device NEC
    - abdominal Z46.89
    - implanted Z45.89
      - cardiac Z45.Ø9
        - defibrillator (with synchronous cardiac pacemaker) Z45.Ø2
        - pacemaker (cardiac resynchronization therapy (CRT-P)) Z45.Ø18
          - pulse generator Z45.Ø1Ø
        - resynchronization therapy defibrillator (CRT-D) Z45.Ø2
      - hearing device Z45.328
        - bone conduction Z45.32Ø
        - cochlear Z45.321
      - infusion pump Z45.1
      - nervous system Z45.49
        - CSF drainage Z45.41
        - hearing device — *see* Admission, adjustment, device, implanted, hearing device
        - neuropacemaker Z45.42
        - visual substitution Z45.31
      - specified NEC Z45.89
      - vascular access Z45.2
      - visual substitution Z45.31

Admission — *continued*
- adjustment — *continued*
  - device — *continued*
    - nervous system Z46.2
      - implanted — *see* Admission, adjustment, device, implanted, nervous system
    - orthodontic Z46.4
    - prosthetic Z44.9
      - arm — *see* Admission, adjustment, artificial, arm
      - breast Z44.3 ☑
      - dental Z46.3
      - eye Z44.2 ☑
      - leg — *see* Admission, adjustment, artificial, leg
      - specified type NEC Z44.8
    - substitution
      - auditory Z46.2
        - implanted — *see* Admission, adjustment, device, implanted, hearing device
      - nervous system Z46.2
        - implanted — *see* Admission, adjustment, device, implanted, nervous system
      - visual Z46.2
        - implanted Z45.31
    - urinary Z46.6
  - hearing aid Z46.1
    - implanted — *see* Admission, adjustment, device, implanted, hearing device
  - ileostomy device Z46.89
  - intestinal appliance or device NEC Z46.89
  - neuropacemaker (brain) (peripheral nerve) (spinal cord) Z46.2
    - implanted Z45.42
  - orthodontic device Z46.4
  - orthopedic (brace) (cast) (device) (shoes) Z46.89
  - pacemaker (cardiac resynchronization therapy (CRT-P))
    - cardiac Z45.Ø18
      - pulse generator Z45.Ø1Ø
    - nervous system Z46.2
      - implanted Z45.42
  - portacath (port-a-cath) Z45.2
  - prosthesis Z44.9
    - arm — *see* Admission, adjustment, artificial, arm
    - breast Z44.3 ☑
    - dental Z46.3
    - eye Z44.2 ☑
    - leg — *see* Admission, adjustment, artificial, leg
    - specified NEC Z44.8
  - spectacles Z46.Ø
- aftercare — *see also* Aftercare Z51.89
  - postpartum
    - immediately after delivery Z39.Ø
    - routine follow-up Z39.2
  - radiation therapy (antineoplastic) Z51.Ø
- attention to artificial opening (of) Z43.9
  - artificial vagina Z43.7
  - colostomy Z43.3
  - cystostomy Z43.5
  - enterostomy Z43.4
  - gastrostomy Z43.1
  - ileostomy Z43.2
  - jejunostomy Z43.4
  - nephrostomy Z43.6
  - specified site NEC Z43.8
    - intestinal tract Z43.4
    - urinary tract Z43.6
  - tracheostomy Z43.Ø
  - ureterostomy Z43.6
  - urethrostomy Z43.6
- breast augmentation or reduction Z41.1
- breast reconstruction following mastectomy Z42.1
- change of
  - dressing (nonsurgical) Z48.ØØ
  - neuropacemaker device (brain) (peripheral nerve) (spinal cord) Z46.2
    - implanted Z45.42
  - surgical dressing Z48.Ø1
- circumcision, ritual or routine (in absence of diagnosis) Z41.2
- clinical research investigation (control) (normal comparison) (participant) ZØØ.6
- contraceptive management Z3Ø.9
- cosmetic surgery NEC Z41.1
- counseling — *see also* Counseling
  - dietary Z71.3
  - gestational carrier Z31.7

- **Admission** — *continued*
  - counseling — *see also* Counseling — *continued*
    - HIV Z71.7
    - human immunodeficiency virus Z71.7
    - nonattending third party Z71.Ø
    - procreative management NEC Z31.69
  - delivery, full-term, uncomplicated O8Ø
    - cesarean, without indication O82
  - desensitization to allergens Z51.6
  - dietary surveillance and counseling Z71.3
  - ear piercing Z41.3
  - examination at health care facility (adult) — *see also* Examination ZØØ.ØØ
    - with abnormal findings ZØØ.Ø1
    - clinical research investigation (control) (normal comparison) (participant) ZØØ.6
    - dental ZØ1.2Ø
      - with abnormal findings ZØ1.21
    - donor (potential) ZØØ.5
    - ear ZØ1.1Ø
      - with abnormal findings NEC ZØ1.118
    - eye ZØ1.ØØ
      - with abnormal findings ZØ1.Ø1
      - following failed vision screening ZØ1.Ø2Ø
        - with abnormal findings ZØ1.Ø21
    - general, specified reason NEC ZØØ.8
    - hearing ZØ1.1Ø
      - with abnormal findings NEC ZØ1.118
      - infant or child (over 28 days old) ZØØ.129
        - with abnormal findings ZØØ.121
    - postpartum checkup Z39.2
    - psychiatric (general) ZØØ.8
      - requested by authority ZØ4.6
    - vision ZØ1.ØØ
      - with abnormal findings ZØ1.Ø1
      - following failed vision screening ZØ1.Ø2Ø
        - with abnormal findings ZØ1.Ø21
      - infant or child (over 28 days old) ZØØ.129
        - with abnormal findings ZØØ.121
  - fitting (of)
    - artificial
      - arm — *see* Admission, adjustment, artificial, arm
      - eye Z44.2 ☑
      - leg — *see* Admission, adjustment, artificial, leg
    - brain neuropacemaker Z46.2
      - implanted Z45.42
    - breast prosthesis (external) Z44.3 ☑
    - colostomy belt Z46.89
    - contact lenses Z46.Ø
    - cystostomy device Z46.6
    - dental prosthesis Z46.3
    - dentures Z46.3
    - device NEC
      - abdominal Z46.89
      - nervous system Z46.2
        - implanted — *see* Admission, adjustment, device, implanted, nervous system
      - orthodontic Z46.4
      - prosthetic Z44.9
        - breast Z44.3 ☑
        - dental Z46.3
        - eye Z44.2 ☑
      - substitution
        - auditory Z46.2
          - implanted — *see* Admission, adjustment, device, implanted, hearing device
        - nervous system Z46.2
          - implanted — *see* Admission, adjustment, device, implanted, nervous system
        - visual Z46.2
          - implanted Z45.31
    - hearing aid Z46.1
    - ileostomy device Z46.89
    - intestinal appliance or device NEC Z46.89
    - neuropacemaker (brain) (peripheral nerve) (spinal cord) Z46.2
      - implanted Z45.42
    - orthodontic device Z46.4
    - orthopedic device (brace) (cast) (shoes) Z46.89
    - prosthesis Z44.9
      - arm — *see* Admission, adjustment, artificial, arm
      - breast Z44.3 ☑
      - dental Z46.3
      - eye Z44.2 ☑
      - leg — *see* Admission, adjustment, artificial, leg
      - specified type NEC Z44.8
    - spectacles Z46.Ø
  - follow-up examination ZØ9
- **Admission** — *continued*
  - intrauterine device management Z3Ø.431
    - initial prescription Z3Ø.Ø14
  - mental health evaluation ZØØ.8
    - requested by authority ZØ4.6
  - observation — *see* Observation
  - Papanicolaou smear, cervix Z12.4
    - for suspected malignant neoplasm Z12.4
  - plastic and reconstructive surgery following medical procedure or healed injury NEC Z42.8
  - plastic surgery, cosmetic NEC Z41.1
  - postpartum observation
    - immediately after delivery Z39.Ø
    - routine follow-up Z39.2
  - poststerilization (for restoration) Z31.Ø
    - aftercare Z31.42
  - procreative management Z31.9
  - prophylactic (measure) — *see also* Encounter, prophylactic measures
    - organ removal Z4Ø.ØØ
      - breast Z4Ø.Ø1
      - fallopian tube(s) Z4Ø.Ø3
        - with ovary(s) Z4Ø.Ø2
      - ovary(s) Z4Ø.Ø2
      - specified organ NEC Z4Ø.Ø9
      - testes Z4Ø.Ø9
    - vaccination Z23
  - psychiatric examination (general) ZØØ.8
    - requested by authority ZØ4.6
  - radiation therapy (antineoplastic) Z51.Ø
  - reconstructive surgery following medical procedure or healed injury NEC Z42.8
  - removal of
    - cystostomy catheter Z43.5
    - drains Z48.Ø3
    - dressing (nonsurgical) Z48.ØØ
    - implantable subdermal contraceptive Z3Ø.46
    - intrauterine contraceptive device Z3Ø.432
    - neuropacemaker (brain) (peripheral nerve) (spinal cord) Z46.2
      - implanted Z45.42
    - staples Z48.Ø2
    - surgical dressing Z48.Ø1
    - sutures Z48.Ø2
    - ureteral stent Z46.6
  - respirator [ventilator] use during power failure Z99.12
  - restoration of organ continuity (poststerilization) Z31.Ø
    - aftercare Z31.42
  - sensitivity test — *see also* Test, skin
    - allergy NEC ZØ1.82
    - Mantoux Z11.1
  - tuboplasty following previous sterilization Z31.Ø
    - aftercare Z31.42
  - vasoplasty following previous sterilization Z31.Ø
    - aftercare Z31.42
  - vision examination ZØ1.ØØ
    - with abnormal findings ZØ1.Ø1
    - following failed vision screening ZØ1.Ø2Ø
      - with abnormal findings ZØ1.Ø21
    - infant or child (over 28 days old) ZØØ.129
      - with abnormal findings ZØØ.121
  - waiting period for admission to other facility Z75.1
- **Adnexitis** (suppurative) — *see* Salpingo-oophoritis
- **Adolescent X-linked adrenoleukodystrophy** E71.521
- **Adrenal** (gland) — *see* condition
- **Adrenalism, tuberculous** A18.7
- **Adrenalitis, adrenitis** E27.8
  - autoimmune E27.1
  - meningococcal, hemorrhagic A39.1
- **Adrenarche, premature** E27.Ø
- **Adrenocortical syndrome** — *see* Cushing's, syndrome
- **Adrenogenital syndrome** E25.9
  - acquired E25.8
  - congenital E25.Ø
  - salt loss E25.Ø
- **Adrenogenitalism, congenital** E25.Ø
- **Adrenoleukodystrophy** E71.529
  - neonatal E71.511
  - X-linked E71.529
    - Addison only phenotype E71.528
    - Addison-Schilder E71.528
    - adolescent E71.521
    - adrenomyeloneuropathy E71.522
    - childhood cerebral E71.52Ø
    - other specified E71.528
- **Adrenomyeloneuropathy** E71.522
- **Adventitious bursa** — *see* Bursopathy, specified type NEC
- **Adverse effect** — *see* Table of Drugs and Chemicals, categories T36-T5Ø, with 6th character 5
- **Advice** — *see* Counseling
- **Adynamia** (episodica) (hereditary) (periodic) G72.3
- **Aeration lung imperfect, newborn** — *see* Atelectasis
- **Aerobullosis** T7Ø.3 ☑
- **Aerocele** — *see* Embolism, air
- **Aerodermectasia**
  - subcutaneous (traumatic) T79.7 ☑
- **Aerodontalgia** T7Ø.29 ☑
- **Aeroembolism** T7Ø.3 ☑
- **Aerogenes capsulatus infection** A48.Ø
- **Aero-otitis media** T7Ø.Ø ☑
- **Aerophagy, aerophagia** (psychogenic) F45.8
- **Aerophobia** F4Ø.228
- **Aerosinusitis** T7Ø.1 ☑
- **Aerotitis** T7Ø.Ø ☑
- **Affection** — *see* Disease
- **Afibrinogenemia** — *see also* Defect, coagulation D68.8
  - acquired D65
  - congenital D68.2
  - following ectopic or molar pregnancy OØ8.1
  - in abortion — *see* Abortion, by type, complicated by, afibrinogenemia
  - puerperal O72.3
- **African**
  - sleeping sickness B56.9
  - tick fever A68.1
  - trypanosomiasis B56.9
    - gambian B56.Ø
    - rhodesian B56.1
- **Aftercare** — *see also* Care Z51.89
  - following surgery (for) (on)
    - amputation Z47.81
    - attention to
      - drains Z48.Ø3
      - dressings (nonsurgical) Z48.ØØ
        - surgical Z48.Ø1
      - sutures Z48.Ø2
    - circulatory system Z48.812
    - delayed (planned) wound closure Z48.1
    - digestive system Z48.815
    - explantation of joint prosthesis (staged procedure)
      - hip Z47.32
      - knee Z47.33
      - shoulder Z47.31
    - genitourinary system Z48.816
    - joint replacement Z47.1
    - neoplasm Z48.3
    - nervous system Z48.811
    - oral cavity Z48.814
    - organ transplant
      - bone marrow Z48.29Ø
      - heart Z48.21
      - heart-lung Z48.28Ø
      - kidney Z48.22
      - liver Z48.23
      - lung Z48.24
      - multiple organs NEC Z48.288
      - specified NEC Z48.298
    - orthopedic NEC Z47.89
    - planned wound closure Z48.1
    - removal of internal fixation device Z47.2
    - respiratory system Z48.813
    - scoliosis Z47.82
    - sense organs Z48.81Ø
    - skin and subcutaneous tissue Z48.817
    - specified body system
      - circulatory Z48.812
      - digestive Z48.815
      - genitourinary Z48.816
      - nervous Z48.811
      - oral cavity Z48.814
      - respiratory Z48.813
      - sense organs Z48.81Ø
      - skin and subcutaneous tissue Z48.817
      - teeth Z48.814
    - specified NEC Z48.89
    - spinal Z47.89
    - teeth Z48.814
  - fracture — *code to* fracture with seventh character D
  - involving
    - removal of
      - drains Z48.Ø3
      - dressings (nonsurgical) Z48.ØØ
      - staples Z48.Ø2
      - surgical dressings Z48.Ø1
      - sutures Z48.Ø2

- **Agranulocytosis** — *continued*
  - cytoreductive cancer chemotherapy sequela D7Ø.1
  - drug-induced D7Ø.2
    - due to cytoreductive cancer chemotherapy D7Ø.1
  - due to infection D7Ø.3
  - secondary D7Ø.4
    - drug-induced D7Ø.2
      - due to cytoreductive cancer chemotherapy D7Ø.1
- **Agraphia** (absolute) R48.8
  - with alexia R48.Ø
  - developmental F81.81
- **Ague** (dumb) — *see* Malaria
- **Agyria** QØ4.3
- **Ahumada-del Castillo syndrome** E23.Ø
- **Aichomophobia** F4Ø.298
- **AIDS** (related complex) B2Ø
- **Ailment heart** — *see* Disease, heart
- **Ailurophobia** F4Ø.218
- **AIN** — *see* Neoplasia, intraepithelial, anal
- **Ainhum** (disease) L94.6
- **AIPHI** (acute idiopathic pulmonary hemorrhage in infants (over 28 days old)) RØ4.81
- **Air**
  - anterior mediastinum J98.2
  - compressed, disease T7Ø.3 ☑
  - conditioner lung or pneumonitis J67.7
  - embolism (artery) (cerebral) (any site) T79.Ø ☑
    - with ectopic or molar pregnancy OØ8.2
    - due to implanted device NEC — *see* Complications, by site and type, specified NEC
    - following
      - abortion — *see* Abortion by type, complicated by, embolism
      - ectopic or molar pregnancy OØ8.2
      - infusion, therapeutic injection or transfusion T8Ø.Ø ☑
    - in pregnancy, childbirth or puerperium — *see* Embolism, obstetric
    - traumatic T79.Ø ☑
  - hunger, psychogenic F45.8
  - rarefied, effects of — *see* Effect, adverse, high altitude
  - sickness T75.3 ☑
- **Airplane sickness** T75.3 ☑
- **Akathisia** (drug-induced) (treatment-induced) G25.71
  - neuroleptic induced (acute) G25.71
  - tardive G25.71
- **Akinesia** R29.898
- **Akinetic mutism** R41.89
- **Akureyri's disease** G93.39
- **Alactasia, congenital** E73.Ø
- **Alagille's syndrome** Q44.7
- **Alastrim** BØ3
- **Albers-Schönberg syndrome** Q78.2
- **Albert's syndrome** — *see* Tendinitis, Achilles
- **Albinism, albino** E7Ø.3Ø
  - with hematologic abnormality E7Ø.339
    - Chédiak-Higashi syndrome E7Ø.33Ø
    - Hermansky-Pudlak syndrome E7Ø.331
    - other specified E7Ø.338
  - I E7Ø.32Ø
  - II E7Ø.321
  - ocular E7Ø.319
    - autosomal recessive E7Ø.311
    - other specified E7Ø.318
    - X-linked E7Ø.31Ø
  - oculocutaneous E7Ø.329
    - other specified E7Ø.328
    - tyrosinase (ty) negative E7Ø.32Ø
    - tyrosinase (ty) positive E7Ø.321
  - other specified E7Ø.39
- **Albinismus** E7Ø.3Ø
- **Albright** (-McCune)(-Sternberg) syndrome Q78.1
- **Albuminous** — *see* condition
- **Albuminuria, albuminuric** (acute) (chronic) (subacute) — *see also* Proteinuria R8Ø.9
  - complicating pregnancy — *see* Proteinuria, gestational
    - with
      - gestational hypertension — *see* Pre-eclampsia
      - pre-existing hypertension — *see* Hypertension, complicating pregnancy, pre-existing, with, pre-eclampsia
  - gestational — *see* Proteinuria, gestational
    - with
      - gestational hypertension — *see* Pre-eclampsia
      - pre-existing hypertension — *see* Hypertension, complicating pregnancy, pre-existing, with, pre-eclampsia
- **Albuminuria, albuminuric** — *continued*
  - orthostatic R8Ø.2
  - postural R8Ø.2
  - pre-eclamptic — *see* Pre-eclampsia
  - scarlatinal A38.8
- **Albuminurophobia** F4Ø.298
- **Alcaptonuria** E7Ø.29
- **Alcohol, alcoholic, alcohol-induced**
  - addiction (without remission) F1Ø.2Ø
    - with remission F1Ø.21
  - amnestic disorder, persisting F1Ø.96
    - with dependence F1Ø.26
  - anxiety disorder F1Ø.98Ø
  - bipolar and related disorder F1Ø.94
  - brain syndrome, chronic F1Ø.97
    - with dependence F1Ø.27
  - cardiopathy I42.6
  - counseling and surveillance Z71.41
    - family member Z71.42
  - delirium (acute) (tremens) (withdrawal) F1Ø.921
    - with intoxication F1Ø.921
    - in
      - abuse F1Ø.121
      - dependence F1Ø.221
    - dependence (acute) (tremens) (withdrawal) F1Ø.231
  - dementia F1Ø.97
    - with dependence F1Ø.27
  - depressive disorder F1Ø.94
  - deterioration F1Ø.97
    - with dependence F1Ø.27
  - hallucinosis (acute) F1Ø.951
    - in
      - abuse F1Ø.151
      - dependence F1Ø.251
  - insanity F1Ø.959
  - intoxication (acute) (without dependence) F1Ø.129
    - with
      - delirium F1Ø.121
      - dependence F1Ø.229
        - with delirium F1Ø.221
        - uncomplicated F1Ø.22Ø
    - uncomplicated F1Ø.12Ø
  - jealousy F1Ø.988
  - Korsakoff's, Korsakov's, Korsakow's F1Ø.26
  - liver K7Ø.9
    - acute — *see* Disease, liver, alcoholic, hepatitis
  - major neurocognitive disorder, amnestic-confabulatory type F1Ø.96
  - major neurocognitive disorder, nonamnestic-confabulatory type F1Ø.97
  - mania (acute) (chronic) F1Ø.959
  - mild neurocognitive disorder F1Ø.988
  - paranoia, paranoid (type) psychosis F1Ø.95Ø
  - pellagra E52
  - poisoning, accidental (acute) NEC — *see* Table of Drugs and Chemicals, alcohol, poisoning
  - psychosis — *see* Psychosis, alcoholic
  - psychotic disorder F1Ø.959
  - sexual dysfunction F1Ø.981
  - sleep disorder F1Ø.982
  - withdrawal (without convulsions) F1Ø.239
    - with delirium F1Ø.231
- **Alcoholism** (chronic) (without remission) F1Ø.2Ø
  - with
    - psychosis — *see* Psychosis, alcoholic
    - remission F1Ø.21
  - Korsakov's F1Ø.96
    - with dependence F1Ø.26
- **Alder** (-Reilly) **anomaly or syndrome** (leukocyte granulation) D72.Ø
- **Aldosteronism** E26.9
  - familial (type I) E26.Ø2
  - glucocorticoid-remediable E26.Ø2
  - primary (due to (bilateral) adrenal hyperplasia) E26.Ø9
  - primary NEC E26.Ø9
  - secondary E26.1
  - specified NEC E26.89
- **Aldosteronoma** D44.1Ø
- **Aldrich** (-Wiskott) **syndrome** (eczema-thrombocytopenia) D82.Ø
- **Alektorophobia** F4Ø.218
- **Aleppo boil** B55.1
- **Aleukemic** — *see* condition
- **Aleukia**
  - congenital D7Ø.Ø
  - hemorrhagica D61.9
    - congenital D61.Ø9
  - splenica D73.1
- **Alexia** R48.Ø
  - developmental F81.Ø
  - secondary to organic lesion R48.Ø
- **Algoneurodystrophy** M89.ØØ
  - ankle M89.Ø7- ☑
  - foot M89.Ø7- ☑
  - forearm M89.Ø3- ☑
  - hand M89.Ø4- ☑
  - lower leg M89.Ø6- ☑
  - multiple sites M89.Ø- ☑
  - shoulder M89.Ø1- ☑
  - specified site NEC M89.Ø8
  - thigh M89.Ø5- ☑
  - upper arm M89.Ø2- ☑
- **Algophobia** F4Ø.298
- **Alienation, mental** — *see* Psychosis
- **Alkalemia** E87.3
- **Alkalosis** E87.3
  - metabolic E87.3
    - with respiratory acidosis E87.4
    - of newborn P74.41
  - respiratory E87.3
- **Alkaptonuria** E7Ø.29
- **Allen-Masters syndrome** N83.8
- **Allergy, allergic** (reaction) (to) T78.4Ø ☑
  - air-borne substance NEC (rhinitis) J3Ø.89
  - alveolitis (extrinsic) J67.9
    - due to
      - Aspergillus clavatus J67.4
      - Cryptostroma corticale J67.6
      - organisms (fungal, thermophilic actinomycete) growing in ventilation (air conditioning) systems J67.7
    - specified type NEC J67.8
  - anaphylactic reaction or shock T78.2 ☑
  - angioneurotic edema T78.3 ☑
  - animal (dander) (epidermal) (hair) (rhinitis) J3Ø.81
  - bee sting (anaphylactic shock) — *see* Toxicity, venom, arthropod, bee
  - biological — *see* Allergy, drug
  - colitis — *see also* Colitis, allergic K52.29
  - dander (animal) (rhinitis) J3Ø.81
  - dandruff (rhinitis) J3Ø.81
  - dental restorative material (existing) KØ8.55
  - dermatitis — *see* Dermatitis, contact, allergic
  - diathesis — *see* History, allergy
  - drug, medicament & biological (any) (external) (internal) T78.4Ø ☑
    - correct substance properly administered — *see* Table of Drugs and Chemicals, by drug, adverse effect
    - wrong substance given or taken NEC (by accident) — *see* Table of Drugs and Chemicals, by drug, poisoning
  - due to pollen J3Ø.1
  - dust (house) (stock) (rhinitis) J3Ø.89
    - with asthma — *see* Asthma, allergic extrinsic
  - eczema — *see* Dermatitis, contact, allergic
  - epidermal (animal) (rhinitis) J3Ø.81
  - feathers (rhinitis) J3Ø.89
  - food (any) (ingested) NEC T78.1 ☑
    - anaphylactic shock — *see* Shock, anaphylactic, due to food
    - dermatitis — *see* Dermatitis, due to, food
    - dietary counseling and surveillance Z71.3
    - in contact with skin L23.6
    - rhinitis J3Ø.5
    - status (without reaction) Z91.Ø18
      - beef Z91.Ø14
      - eggs Z91.Ø12
      - lamb Z91.Ø14
      - mammalian meats Z91.Ø14
      - milk products Z91.Ø11
      - peanuts Z91.Ø1Ø
      - pork Z91.Ø14
      - red meats Z91.Ø14
      - seafood Z91.Ø13
      - specified NEC Z91.Ø18
  - gastrointestinal — *see also* specific type of allergic reaction
    - meaning colitis — *see also* Colitis, allergic K52.29
    - meaning gastroenteritis — *see also* Gastroenteritis, allergic K52.29
    - meaning other adverse food reaction not elsewhere classified T78.1 ☑
  - grain J3Ø.1
  - grass (hay fever) (pollen) J3Ø.1

- **Allergy, allergic** — *continued*
  - grass — *continued*
    - asthma — *see* Asthma, allergic extrinsic
  - hair (animal) (rhinitis) J3Ø.81
  - history (of) — *see* History, allergy
  - horse serum — *see* Allergy, serum
  - inhalant (rhinitis) J3Ø.89
    - pollen J3Ø.1
  - kapok (rhinitis) J3Ø.89
  - medicine — *see* Allergy, drug
  - milk protein — *see also* Allergy, food Z91.Ø11
    - anaphylactic reaction T78.Ø7 ☑
    - dermatitis L27.2
    - enterocolitis syndrome K52.21
    - enteropathy K52.22
    - gastroenteritis K52.29
    - gastroesophageal reflux — *see also* Reaction, adverse, food K21.9
      - with esophagitis (without bleeding) K21.ØØ
        - with bleeding K21.Ø1
    - proctocolitis K52.29
  - nasal, seasonal due to pollen J3Ø.1
  - pneumonia J82.89
  - pollen (any) (hay fever) J3Ø.1
    - asthma — *see* Asthma, allergic extrinsic
  - primrose J3Ø.1
  - primula J3Ø.1
  - proctocolitis K52.29
  - purpura D69.Ø
  - ragweed (hay fever) (pollen) J3Ø.1
    - asthma — *see* Asthma, allergic extrinsic
  - rose (pollen) J3Ø.1
  - seasonal NEC J3Ø.2
  - Senecio jacobae (pollen) J3Ø.1
  - serum — *see also* Reaction, serum T8Ø.69 ☑
    - anaphylactic shock T8Ø.59 ☑
  - shock (anaphylactic) T78.2 ☑
    - due to
      - administration of blood and blood products T8Ø.51 ☑
      - adverse effect of correct medicinal substance properly administered T88.6 ☑
      - immunization T8Ø.52 ☑
      - serum NEC T8Ø.59 ☑
      - vaccination T8Ø.52 ☑
  - specific NEC T78.49 ☑
  - tree (any) (hay fever) (pollen) J3Ø.1
    - asthma — *see* Asthma, allergic extrinsic
  - upper respiratory J3Ø.9
  - urticaria L5Ø.Ø
  - vaccine — *see* Allergy, serum
  - wheat — *see* Allergy, food
- **Allescheriasis** B48.2
- **Alligator skin disease** Q8Ø.9
- **Allocheiria, allochiria** R2Ø.8
- **Almeida's disease** — *see* Paracoccidioidomycosis
- **Alopecia** (hereditaria) (seborrheica) L65.9
  - androgenic L64.9
    - drug-induced L64.Ø
    - specified NEC L64.8
  - areata L63.9
    - ophiasis L63.2
    - specified NEC L63.8
    - totalis L63.Ø
    - universalis L63.1
  - cicatricial L66.9
    - specified NEC L66.8
  - circumscripta L63.9
  - congenital, congenitalis Q84.Ø
  - due to cytotoxic drugs NEC L65.8
  - mucinosa L65.2
  - postinfective NEC L65.8
  - postpartum L65.Ø
  - premature L64.8
  - specific (syphilitic) A51.32
  - specified NEC L65.8
  - syphilitic (secondary) A51.32
  - totalis (capitis) L63.Ø
  - universalis (entire body) L63.1
  - X-ray L58.1
- **Alpers' disease** G31.81
- **Alpine sickness** T7Ø.29 ☑
- **Alport syndrome** Q87.81
- **ALTE** (apparent life threatening event) **in newborn and infant** R68.13
- **Alteration** (of), **Altered**
  - awareness
    - transient R4Ø.4
- **Alteration** (of), **Altered** — *continued*
  - awareness — *continued*
    - unintended under general anesthesia, during procedure T88.53 ☑
  - mental status R41.82
  - pattern of family relationships affecting child Z62.898
  - sensation
    - following
      - cerebrovascular disease I69.998
        - cerebral infarction I69.398
        - intracerebral hemorrhage I69.198
        - nontraumatic intracranial hemorrhage NEC I69.298
        - specified disease NEC I69.898
        - subarachnoid hemorrhage I69.Ø98
- **Alternating** — *see* condition
- **Altitude, high** (effects) — *see* Effect, adverse, high altitude
- **Aluminosis** (of lung) J63.Ø
- **Alveolitis**
  - allergic (extrinsic) — *see* Pneumonitis, hypersensitivity
  - due to
    - Aspergillus clavatus J67.4
    - Cryptostroma corticale J67.6
  - fibrosing (cryptogenic) (idiopathic) J84.112
  - jaw M27.3
  - sicca dolorosa M27.3
- **Alveolus, alveolar** — *see* condition
- **Alymphocytosis** D72.81Ø
  - thymic (with immunodeficiency) D82.1
- **Alymphoplasia, thymic** D82.1
- **Alzheimer's disease or sclerosis** — *see* Disease, Alzheimer's
- **Amastia** (with nipple present) Q83.8
  - with absent nipple Q83.Ø
- **Amathophobia** F4Ø.228
- **Amaurosis** (acquired) (congenital) — *see also* Blindness
  - fugax G45.3
  - hysterical F44.6
  - Leber's congenital H35.5Ø
  - uremic — *see* Uremia
- **Amaurotic idiocy** (infantile) (juvenile) (late) E75.4
- **Amaxophobia** F4Ø.248
- **Ambiguous genitalia** Q56.4
- **Amblyopia** (congenital) (ex anopsia) (partial) (suppression) H53.ØØ- ☑
  - anisometropic — *see* Amblyopia, refractive
  - deprivation H53.Ø1- ☑
  - hysterical F44.6
  - nocturnal — *see also* Blindness, night
    - vitamin A deficiency E5Ø.5
  - refractive H53.Ø2- ☑
  - strabismic H53.Ø3- ☑
  - suspect H53.Ø4- ☑
  - tobacco H53.8
  - toxic NEC H53.8
  - uremic — *see* Uremia
- **Ameba, amebic** (histolytica) — *see also* Amebiasis
  - abscess (liver) AØ6.4
- **Amebiasis** AØ6.9
  - with abscess — *see* Abscess, amebic
  - acute AØ6.Ø
  - chronic (intestine) AØ6.1
    - with abscess — *see* Abscess, amebic
  - cutaneous AØ6.7
  - cutis AØ6.7
  - cystitis AØ6.81
  - genitourinary tract NEC AØ6.82
  - hepatic — *see* Abscess, liver, amebic
  - intestine AØ6.Ø
  - nondysenteric colitis AØ6.2
  - skin AØ6.7
  - specified site NEC AØ6.89
- **Ameboma** (of intestine) AØ6.3
- **Amelia** Q73.Ø
  - lower limb — *see* Agenesis, leg
  - upper limb — *see* Agenesis, arm
- **Ameloblastoma** — *see also* Cyst, calcifying odontogenic
  - long bones C4Ø.9- ☑
    - lower limb C4Ø.2- ☑
    - upper limb C4Ø.Ø- ☑
  - malignant C41.1
    - jaw (bone) (lower) C41.1
      - upper C41.Ø
  - tibial C4Ø.2- ☑
- **Amelogenesis imperfecta** KØØ.5
  - nonhereditaria (segmentalis) KØØ.4
- **Amenorrhea** N91.2
  - hyperhormonal E28.8
  - primary N91.Ø
  - secondary N91.1
- **Amentia** — *see* Disability, intellectual
  - Meynert's (nonalcoholic) FØ4
- **American**
  - leishmaniasis B55.2
  - mountain tick fever A93.2
- **Ametropia** — *see* Disorder, refraction
- **AMH** (asymptomatic microscopic hematuria) R31.21
- **Amianthosis** J61
- **Amimia** R48.8
- **Amino-acid disorder** E72.9
  - anemia D53.Ø
- **Aminoacidopathy** E72.9
- **Aminoaciduria** E72.9
- **Amnesia** R41.3
  - anterograde R41.1
  - auditory R48.8
  - dissociative F44.Ø
    - with dissociative fugue F44.1
  - hysterical F44.Ø
  - postictal in epilepsy — *see* Epilepsy
  - psychogenic F44.Ø
  - retrograde R41.2
  - transient global G45.4
- **Amnes(t)ic syndrome** (post-traumatic) FØ4
  - induced by
    - alcohol F1Ø.96
      - with dependence F1Ø.26
    - psychoactive NEC F19.96
      - with
        - abuse F19.16
        - dependence F19.26
    - sedative F13.96
      - with dependence F13.26
- **Amnion, amniotic** — *see* condition
- **Amnionitis** — *see* Pregnancy, complicated by
- **Amok** F68.8
- **Amoral traits** F6Ø.89
- **Amphetamine** (or other stimulant) **-induced**
  - anxiety disorder F15.98Ø
  - bipolar and related disorder F15.94
  - delirium F15.921
  - depressive disorder F15.94
  - obsessive-compulsive and related disorder F15.988
  - psychotic disorder F15.959
  - sexual dysfunction F15.981
  - sleep disorder F15.982
  - stimulant withdrawal F15.23
- **Ampulla**
  - lower esophagus K22.89
  - phrenic K22.89
- **Amputation** — *see also* Absence, by site, acquired
  - neuroma (postoperative) (traumatic) — *see* Complications, amputation stump, neuroma
  - stump (surgical)
    - abnormal, painful, or with complication (late) — *see* Complications, amputation stump
    - healed or old NOS Z89.9
  - traumatic (complete) (partial)
    - arm (upper) (complete) S48.91- ☑
      - at
        - elbow S58.Ø1- ☑
          - partial S58.Ø2- ☑
        - shoulder joint (complete) S48.Ø1- ☑
          - partial S48.Ø2- ☑
      - between
        - elbow and wrist (complete) S58.11- ☑
          - partial S58.12- ☑
        - shoulder and elbow (complete) S48.11- ☑
          - partial S48.12- ☑
      - partial S48.92- ☑
    - breast (complete) S28.21- ☑
      - partial S28.22- ☑
    - clitoris (complete) S38.211 ☑
      - partial S38.212 ☑
    - ear (complete) SØ8.11- ☑
      - partial SØ8.12- ☑
    - finger (complete) (metacarpophalangeal) S68.11- ☑
      - index S68.11- ☑
      - little S68.11- ☑
      - middle S68.11- ☑
      - partial S68.12- ☑
        - index S68.12- ☑
        - little S68.12- ☑

- **Amputation** — *continued*
  - traumatic — *continued*
    - finger — *continued*
      - partial — *continued*
        - middle S68.12- ☑
        - ring S68.12- ☑
      - ring S68.11- ☑
      - thumb — *see* Amputation, traumatic, thumb
      - transphalangeal (complete) S68.61- ☑
        - index S68.61- ☑
        - little S68.61- ☑
        - middle S68.61- ☑
        - partial S68.62- ☑
          - index S68.62- ☑
          - little S68.62- ☑
          - middle S68.62- ☑
          - ring S68.62- ☑
        - ring S68.61- ☑
    - foot (complete) S98.91- ☑
      - at ankle level S98.Ø1- ☑
        - partial S98.Ø2- ☑
      - midfoot S98.31- ☑
        - partial S98.32- ☑
      - partial S98.92- ☑
    - forearm (complete) S58.91- ☑
      - at elbow level (complete) S58.Ø1- ☑
        - partial S58.Ø2- ☑
      - between elbow and wrist (complete) S58.11- ☑
        - partial S58.12- ☑
      - partial S58.92- ☑
    - genital organ(s) (external)
      - female (complete) S38.211 ☑
        - partial S38.212 ☑
      - male
        - penis (complete) S38.221 ☑
          - partial S38.222 ☑
        - scrotum (complete) S38.231 ☑
          - partial S38.232 ☑
        - testes (complete) S38.231 ☑
          - partial S38.232 ☑
    - hand (complete) (wrist level) S68.41- ☑
      - finger(s) alone — *see* Amputation, traumatic, finger
      - partial S68.42- ☑
      - thumb alone — *see* Amputation, traumatic, thumb
      - transmetacarpal (complete) S68.71- ☑
        - partial S68.72- ☑
    - head
      - ear — *see* Amputation, traumatic, ear
      - nose (partial) SØ8.812 ☑
        - complete SØ8.811 ☑
      - part SØ8.89 ☑
      - scalp SØ8.Ø ☑
    - hip (and thigh) (complete) S78.91- ☑
      - at hip joint (complete) S78.Ø1- ☑
        - partial S78.Ø2- ☑
      - between hip and knee (complete) S78.11- ☑
        - partial S78.12- ☑
      - partial S78.92- ☑
    - labium (majus) (minus) (complete) S38.21- ☑
      - partial S38.21- ☑
    - leg (lower) S88.91- ☑
      - at knee level S88.Ø1- ☑
        - partial S88.Ø2- ☑
      - between knee and ankle S88.11- ☑
        - partial S88.12- ☑
      - partial S88.92- ☑
    - nose (partial) SØ8.812 ☑
      - complete SØ8.811 ☑
    - penis (complete) S38.221 ☑
      - partial S38.222 ☑
    - scrotum (complete) S38.231 ☑
      - partial S38.232 ☑
    - shoulder — *see* Amputation, traumatic, arm
      - at shoulder joint — *see* Amputation, traumatic, arm, at shoulder joint
    - testes (complete) S38.231 ☑
      - partial S38.232 ☑
    - thigh — *see* Amputation, traumatic, hip
    - thorax, part of S28.1 ☑
      - breast — *see* Amputation, traumatic, breast
    - thumb (complete) (metacarpophalangeal) S68.Ø1- ☑
      - partial S68.Ø2- ☑
      - transphalangeal (complete) S68.51- ☑

- **Amputation** — *continued*
  - traumatic — *continued*
    - thumb — *continued*
      - transphalangeal — *continued*
        - partial S68.52- ☑
    - toe (lesser) S98.13- ☑
      - great S98.11- ☑
        - partial S98.12- ☑
      - more than one S98.21- ☑
        - partial S98.22- ☑
      - partial S98.14- ☑
    - vulva (complete) S38.211 ☑
      - partial S38.212 ☑
- **Amputee** (bilateral) (old) Z89.9
- **Amsterdam dwarfism** Q87.19
- **Amusia** R48.8
  - developmental F8Ø.89
- **Amyelencephalus, amyelencephaly** QØØ.Ø
- **Amyelia** QØ6.Ø
- **Amygdalitis** — *see* Tonsillitis
- **Amygdalolith** J35.8
- **Amyloid heart** (disease) E85.4 *[I43]*
- **Amyloidosis** (generalized) (primary) E85.9
  - with lung involvement E85.4 *[J99]*
  - familial E85.2
  - genetic E85.2
  - heart E85.4 *[I43]*
  - hemodialysis-associated E85.3
  - light chain (AL) E85.81
  - liver E85.4 *[K77]*
  - localized E85.4
  - neuropathic heredofamilial E85.1
  - non-neuropathic heredofamilial E85.Ø
  - organ limited E85.4
  - Portuguese E85.1
  - pulmonary E85.4 *[J99]*
  - secondary systemic E85.3
  - senile systemic (SSA) E85.82
  - skin (lichen) (macular) E85.4 *[L99]*
  - specified NEC E85.89
  - subglottic E85.4 *[J99]*
  - wild-type transthyretin-related (ATTR) E85.82
- **Amylopectinosis** (brancher enzyme deficiency) E74.Ø3
- **Amylophagia** — *see* Pica
- **Amyoplasia congenita** Q79.8
- **Amyotonia** M62.89
  - congenita G7Ø.2
- **Amyotrophia, amyotrophy, amyotrophic** G71.8
  - congenita Q79.8
  - diabetic — *see* Diabetes, amyotrophy
  - lateral sclerosis G12.21
  - neuralgic G54.5
  - spinal progressive G12.25
- **Anacidity, gastric** K31.83
  - psychogenic F45.8
- **Anaerosis of newborn** P28.89
- **Analbuminemia** E88.Ø9
- **Analgesia** — *see* Anesthesia
- **Analphalipoproteinemia** E78.6
- **Anaphylactic**
  - purpura D69.Ø
  - shock or reaction — *see* Shock, anaphylactic
- **Anaphylactoid shock or reaction** — *see* Shock, anaphylactic
- **Anaphylactoid syndrome of pregnancy** O88.Ø1- ☑
- **Anaphylaxis** — *see* Shock, anaphylactic
- **Anaplasia cervix** — *see also* Dysplasia, cervix N87.9
- **Anaplasmosis** [A. phagocytophilum] (transfusion transmitted) A79.82
  - human A77.49
- **Anarthria** R47.1
- **Anasarca** R6Ø.1
  - cardiac — *see* Failure, heart, congestive
  - lung J18.2
  - newborn P83.2
  - nutritional E43
  - pulmonary J18.2
  - renal NØ4.9
- **Anastomosis**
  - aneurysmal — *see* Aneurysm
  - arteriovenous ruptured brain I6Ø.8
    - intracerebral I61.8
    - intraparenchymal I61.8
    - intraventricular I61.5
    - subarachnoid I6Ø.8
  - intestinal K63.89
    - complicated NEC K91.89

- **Anastomosis** — *continued*
  - intestinal — *continued*
    - complicated — *continued*
      - involving urinary tract N99.89
  - retinal and choroidal vessels (congenital) Q14.8
- **Anatomical narrow angle** H4Ø.Ø3- ☑
- **Ancylostoma, ancylostomiasis** (braziliense) (caninum) (ceylanicum) (duodenale) B76.Ø
  - Necator americanus B76.1
- **Andersen's disease** (glycogen storage) E74.Ø9
- **Anderson-Fabry disease** E75.21
- **Andes disease** T7Ø.29 ☑
- **Andrews' disease** (bacterid) LØ8.89
- **Androblastoma**
  - benign
    - specified site — *see* Neoplasm, benign, by site
    - unspecified site
      - female D27.9
      - male D29.2Ø
  - malignant
    - specified site — *see* Neoplasm, malignant, by site
    - unspecified site
      - female C56.9
      - male C62.9Ø
  - specified site — *see* Neoplasm, uncertain behavior, by site
  - tubular
    - with lipid storage
      - specified site — *see* Neoplasm, benign, by site
      - unspecified site
        - female D27.9
        - male D29.2Ø
    - specified site — *see* Neoplasm, benign, by site
    - unspecified site
      - female D27.9
      - male D29.2Ø
  - unspecified site
    - female D39.1Ø
    - male D4Ø.1Ø
- **Androgen insensitivity syndrome** — *see also* Syndrome, androgen insensitivity E34.5Ø
- **Androgen resistance syndrome** — *see also* Syndrome, androgen insensitivity E34.5Ø
- **Android pelvis** Q74.2
  - with disproportion (fetopelvic) O33.3 ☑
    - causing obstructed labor O65.3
- **Androphobia** F4Ø.29Ø
- **Anectasis, pulmonary** (newborn) — *see* Atelectasis
- **Anemia** (essential) (general) (hemoglobin deficiency) (infantile) (primary) (profound) D64.9
  - with (due to) (in)
    - disorder of
      - anaerobic glycolysis D55.29
      - pentose phosphate pathway D55.1
    - koilonychia D5Ø.9
  - achlorhydric D5Ø.8
  - achrestic D53.1
  - Addison (-Biermer) (pernicious) D51.Ø
  - agranulocytic — *see* Agranulocytosis
  - amino-acid-deficiency D53.Ø
  - aplastic D61.9
    - congenital D61.Ø9
    - drug-induced D61.1
    - due to
      - drugs D61.1
      - external agents NEC D61.2
      - infection D61.2
      - radiation D61.2
    - idiopathic D61.3
    - red cell (pure) D6Ø.9
      - chronic D6Ø.Ø
      - congenital D61.Ø1
      - specified type NEC D6Ø.8
      - transient D6Ø.1
    - specified type NEC D61.89
    - toxic D61.2
  - aregenerative
    - congenital D61.Ø9
  - asiderotic D5Ø.9
  - atypical (primary) D64.9
  - Baghdad spring D55.Ø
  - Balantidium coli AØ7.Ø
  - Biermer's (pernicious) D51.Ø
  - blood loss (chronic) D5Ø.Ø
    - acute D62
  - bothriocephalus B7Ø.Ø *[D63.8]*
  - brickmaker's B76.9 *[D63.8]*
  - cerebral I67.89

- **Aneurysm** — *continued*
  - carotid artery (common) (external) I72.Ø
    - internal (intracranial) I67.1
      - extracranial portion I72.Ø
    - ruptured into brain I6Ø.Ø- ☑
    - syphilitic A52.Ø9
      - intracranial A52.Ø5
  - cavernous sinus I67.1
    - arteriovenous (congenital) (nonruptured) Q28.3
      - ruptured I6Ø.8
  - celiac I72.8
  - central nervous system, syphilitic A52.Ø5
  - cerebral — *see* Aneurysm, brain
  - chest — *see* Aneurysm, thorax
  - circle of Willis I67.1
    - congenital Q28.3
      - ruptured I6Ø.6
    - ruptured I6Ø.6
  - common iliac artery I72.3
  - congenital (peripheral) Q27.8
    - aorta (root) (sinus) Q25.43
    - brain Q28.3
      - ruptured I6Ø.7
    - coronary Q24.5
    - digestive system Q27.8
    - lower limb Q27.8
    - pulmonary Q25.79
    - retina Q14.1
    - specified site NEC Q27.8
    - upper limb Q27.8
  - conjunctiva — *see* Abnormality, conjunctiva, vascular
  - conus arteriosus — *see* Aneurysm, heart
  - coronary (arteriosclerotic) (artery) I25.41
    - arteriovenous, congenital Q24.5
    - congenital Q24.5
    - ruptured — *see* Infarct, myocardium
    - syphilitic A52.Ø6
    - vein I25.89
  - cylindroid (aorta) I71.9
    - ruptured I71.8
    - syphilitic A52.Ø1
  - ductus arteriosus Q25.Ø
  - endocardial, infective (any valve) I33.Ø
  - femoral (artery) (ruptured) I72.4
  - gastroduodenal I72.8
  - gastroepiploic I72.8
  - heart (wall) (chronic or with a stated duration of over 4 weeks) I25.3
    - valve — *see* Endocarditis
  - hepatic I72.8
  - iliac (common) (artery) (ruptured) I72.3
  - infective I72.9
    - endocardial (any valve) I33.Ø
  - innominate (nonsyphilitic) I72.8
    - syphilitic A52.Ø9
  - interauricular septum — *see* Aneurysm, heart
  - interventricular septum — *see* Aneurysm, heart
  - intrathoracic (nonsyphilitic) — *see also* Aneurysm, aorta, thorax I71.2Ø
    - ruptured — *see also* Aneurysm, aorta, thorax, ruptured I71.1Ø
    - syphilitic A52.Ø1
  - lower limb I72.4
  - lung (pulmonary artery) I28.1
  - mediastinal (nonsyphilitic) I72.8
    - syphilitic A52.Ø9
  - miliary (congenital) I67.1
    - ruptured — *see* Hemorrhage, intracerebral, subarachnoid, intracranial
  - mitral (heart) (valve) I34.89
  - mural — *see* Aneurysm, heart
  - mycotic I72.9
    - endocardial (any valve) I33.Ø
    - ruptured, brain — *see* Hemorrhage, intracerebral, subarachnoid
  - myocardium — *see* Aneurysm, heart
  - neck I72.Ø
  - pancreaticoduodenal I72.8
  - patent ductus arteriosus Q25.Ø
  - peripheral NEC I72.8
    - congenital Q27.8
      - digestive system Q27.8
      - lower limb Q27.8
      - specified site NEC Q27.8
      - upper limb Q27.8
  - popliteal (artery) (ruptured) I72.4
  - precerebral
    - congenital (nonruptured) Q28.1

- **Aneurysm** — *continued*
  - precerebral — *continued*
    - specified site, NEC I72.5
  - pulmonary I28.1
    - arteriovenous Q25.72
      - acquired I28.Ø
    - syphilitic A52.Ø9
    - valve (heart) — *see* Endocarditis, pulmonary
  - racemose (peripheral) I72.9
    - congenital — *see* Aneurysm, congenital
  - radial I72.1
  - Rasmussen NEC A15.Ø
  - renal (artery) I72.2
  - retina — *see also* Disorder, retina, microaneurysms
    - congenital Q14.1
    - diabetic — *see* EØ8-E13 with .3-
  - sinus of Valsalva Q25.49
  - specified NEC I72.8
  - spinal (cord) I72.8
    - syphilitic (hemorrhage) A52.Ø9
  - splenic I72.8
  - subclavian (artery) (ruptured) I72.8
    - syphilitic A52.Ø9
  - superior mesenteric I72.8
  - syphilitic (aorta) A52.Ø1
    - central nervous system A52.Ø5
    - congenital (late) A5Ø.54 *[I79.Ø]*
    - spine, spinal A52.Ø9
  - thoracoabdominal (aorta) I71.6Ø
    - ruptured I71.5Ø
    - syphilitic A52.Ø1
  - thorax, thoracic (aorta) (arch) (nonsyphilitic) — *see* Aneurysm, aorta, thorax
    - ruptured — *see* Aneurysm, aorta, thorax, ruptured
    - syphilitic A52.Ø1
  - traumatic (complication) (early), specified site — *see* Injury, blood vessel
  - tricuspid (heart) (valve) IØ7.8
  - ulnar I72.1
  - upper limb (ruptured) I72.1
  - valve, valvular — *see* Endocarditis
  - venous — *see also* Varix I86.8
    - congenital Q27.8
      - digestive system Q27.8
      - lower limb Q27.8
      - specified site NEC Q27.8
      - upper limb Q27.8
  - ventricle — *see* Aneurysm, heart
  - vertebral artery I72.6
  - visceral NEC I72.8
- **Angelman syndrome** Q93.51
- **Anger** R45.4
- **Angiectasis, angiectopia** I99.8
- **Angiitis** I77.6
  - allergic granulomatous M3Ø.1
  - hypersensitivity M31.Ø
  - necrotizing M31.9
    - specified NEC M31.8
  - nervous system, granulomatous I67.7
- **Angina** (attack) (cardiac) (chest) (heart) (pectoris) (syndrome) (vasomotor) I2Ø.9
  - with
    - atherosclerotic heart disease — *see* Arteriosclerosis, coronary (artery),
    - documented spasm I2Ø.1
  - abdominal K55.1
  - accelerated — *see* Angina, unstable
  - agranulocytic — *see* Agranulocytosis
  - angiospastic — *see* Angina, with documented spasm
  - aphthous BØ8.5
  - crescendo — *see* Angina, unstable
  - croupous JØ5.Ø
  - cruris I73.9
  - de novo effort — *see* Angina, unstable
  - diphtheritic, membranous A36.Ø
  - equivalent I2Ø.8
  - exudative, chronic J37.Ø
  - following acute myocardial infarction I23.7
  - gangrenous diphtheritic A36.Ø
  - intestinal K55.1
  - Ludovici K12.2
  - Ludwig's K12.2
  - malignant diphtheritic A36.Ø
  - membranous JØ5.Ø
    - diphtheritic A36.Ø
    - Vincent's A69.1
  - mesenteric K55.1
  - monocytic — *see* Mononucleosis, infectious

- **Angina** — *continued*
  - of effort — *see* Angina, specified NEC
  - phlegmonous J36
    - diphtheritic A36.Ø
  - post-infarctional I23.7
  - pre-infarctional — *see* Angina, unstable
  - Prinzmetal — *see* Angina, with documented spasm
  - progressive — *see* Angina, unstable
  - pseudomembranous A69.1
  - pultaceous, diphtheritic A36.Ø
  - refractory I2Ø.2
  - spasm-induced — *see* Angina, with documented spasm
  - specified NEC I2Ø.8
  - stable I2Ø.8
  - stenocardia — *see* Angina, specified NEC
  - stridulous, diphtheritic A36.2
  - tonsil J36
  - trachealis JØ5.Ø
  - unstable I2Ø.Ø
  - variant — *see* Angina, with documented spasm
  - Vincent's A69.1
  - worsening effort — *see* Angina, unstable
- **Angioblastoma** — *see* Neoplasm, connective tissue, uncertain behavior
- **Angiocholecystitis** — *see* Cholecystitis, acute
- **Angiocholitis** — *see also* Cholecystitis, acute K83.Ø9
- **Angiodysgenesis spinalis** G95.19
- **Angiodysplasia** (cecum) (colon) K55.2Ø
  - with bleeding K55.21
  - duodenum (and stomach) K31.819
    - with bleeding K31.811
  - stomach (and duodenum) K31.819
    - with bleeding K31.811
- **Angioedema** (allergic) (any site) (with urticaria) T78.3 ☑
  - episodic, with eosinophilia D72.118
  - hereditary D84.1
- **Angioendothelioma** — *see* Neoplasm, uncertain behavior, by site
  - benign D18.ØØ
    - intra-abdominal D18.Ø3
    - intracranial D18.Ø2
    - skin D18.Ø1
    - specified site NEC D18.Ø9
  - bone — *see* Neoplasm, bone, malignant
  - Ewing's — *see* Neoplasm, bone, malignant
- **Angioendotheliomatosis** C85.8- ☑
- **Angiofibroma** — *see also* Neoplasm, benign, by site
  - juvenile
    - specified site — *see* Neoplasm, benign, by site
    - unspecified site D1Ø.6
- **Angiohemophilia** (A) (B) — *see* Disease, von Willebrand
- **Angioid streaks** (choroid) (macula) (retina) H35.33
- **Angiokeratoma** — *see* Neoplasm, skin, benign
  - corporis diffusum E75.21
- **Angioleiomyoma** — *see* Neoplasm, connective tissue, benign
- **Angiolipoma** — *see also* Lipoma
  - infiltrating — *see* Lipoma
- **Angioma** — *see also* Hemangioma, by site
  - capillary I78.1
  - hemorrhagicum hereditaria I78.Ø
  - intra-abdominal D18.Ø3
  - intracranial D18.Ø2
  - malignant — *see* Neoplasm, connective tissue, malignant
  - plexiform D18.ØØ
    - intra-abdominal D18.Ø3
    - intracranial D18.Ø2
    - skin D18.Ø1
    - specified site NEC D18.Ø9
  - senile I78.1
  - serpiginosum L81.7
  - skin D18.Ø1
  - specified site NEC D18.Ø9
  - spider I78.1
  - stellate I78.1
  - venous Q28.3
- **Angiomatosis** Q82.8
  - bacillary A79.89
  - encephalotrigeminal Q85.89
  - hemorrhagic familial I78.Ø
  - hereditary familial I78.Ø
  - liver K76.4
- **Angiomyolipoma** — *see* Lipoma
- **Angiomyoliposarcoma** — *see* Neoplasm, connective tissue, malignant
- **Angiomyoma** — *see* Neoplasm, connective tissue, benign

- **Anorchia, anorchism, anorchidism** Q55.Ø
- **Anorexia** R63.Ø
  - hysterical F44.89
  - nervosa F5Ø.ØØ
    - atypical F5Ø.9
    - binge-eating type F5Ø.2
      - with purging F5Ø.Ø2
    - restricting type F5Ø.Ø1
- **Anorgasmy, psychogenic** (female) F52.31
  - male F52.32
- **Anosmia** R43.Ø
  - hysterical F44.6
  - postinfectional J39.8
- **Anosognosia** R41.89
- **Anosteoplasia** Q78.9
- **Anovulatory cycle** N97.Ø
- **Anoxemia** RØ9.Ø2
  - newborn P84
- **Anoxia** (pathological) RØ9.Ø2
  - altitude T7Ø.29 ☑
  - cerebral G93.1
    - complicating
      - anesthesia (general) (local) or other sedation T88.59 ☑
        - in labor and delivery O74.3
        - in pregnancy O29.21- ☑
        - postpartum, puerperal O89.2
      - delivery (cesarean) (instrumental) O75.4
    - during a procedure G97.81
    - newborn P84
    - resulting from a procedure G97.82
  - due to
    - drowning T75.1 ☑
    - high altitude T7Ø.29 ☑
  - heart — *see* Insufficiency, coronary
  - intrauterine P84
  - myocardial — *see* Insufficiency, coronary
  - newborn P84
  - spinal cord G95.11
  - systemic (by suffocation) (low content in atmosphere) — *see* Asphyxia, traumatic
- **Anteflexion** — *see* Anteversion
- **Antenatal**
  - care (normal pregnancy) Z34.9Ø
  - screening (encounter for) of mother — *see also* Encounter, antenatal screening Z36.9
- **Antepartum** — *see* condition
- **Anterior** — *see* condition
- **Antero-occlusion** M26.22Ø
- **Anteversion**
  - cervix — *see* Anteversion, uterus
  - femur (neck), congenital Q65.89
  - uterus, uterine (cervix) (postinfectional) (postpartal, old) N85.4
    - congenital Q51.818
    - in pregnancy or childbirth — *see* Pregnancy, complicated by
- **Anthophobia** F4Ø.228
- **Anthracosilicosis** J6Ø
- **Anthracosis** (lung) (occupational) J6Ø
  - lingua K14.3
- **Anthrax** A22.9
  - with pneumonia A22.1
  - cerebral A22.8
  - colitis A22.2
  - cutaneous A22.Ø
  - gastrointestinal A22.2
  - inhalation A22.1
  - intestinal A22.2
  - meningitis A22.8
  - pulmonary A22.1
  - respiratory A22.1
  - sepsis A22.7
  - specified manifestation NEC A22.8
- **Anthropoid pelvis** Q74.2
  - with disproportion (fetopelvic) O33.Ø
- **Anthropophobia** F4Ø.1Ø
  - generalized F4Ø.11
- **Antibodies, maternal** (blood group) — *see* Isoimmunization, affecting management of pregnancy
  - anti-D — *see* Isoimmunization, affecting management of pregnancy, Rh
    - newborn P55.Ø
- **Antibody**
  - anticardiolipin R76.Ø
    - with
      - hemorrhagic disorder D68.312
      - hypercoagulable state D68.61
- **Antibody** — *continued*
  - antiphosphatidylglycerol R76.Ø
    - with
      - hemorrhagic disorder D68.312
      - hypercoagulable state D68.61
  - antiphosphatidylinositol R76.Ø
    - with
      - hemorrhagic disorder D68.312
      - hypercoagulable state D68.61
  - antiphosphatidylserine R76.Ø
    - with
      - hemorrhagic disorder D68.312
      - hypercoagulable state D68.61
  - antiphospholipid R76.Ø
    - with
      - hemorrhagic disorder D68.312
      - hypercoagulable state D68.61
- **Anticardiolipin syndrome** D68.61
- **Anticoagulant, circulating** (intrinsic) — *see also* Disorder, hemorrhagic D68.318
  - drug-induced (extrinsic) — *see also* Disorder, hemorrhagic D68.32
  - iatrogenic D68.32
- **Antidiuretic hormone syndrome** E22.2
- **Antimonial cholera** — *see* Poisoning, antimony
- **Antiphospholipid**
  - antibody
    - with hemorrhagic disorder D68.312
    - syndrome D68.61
- **Antisocial personality** F6Ø.2
- **Antithrombinemia** — *see* Circulating anticoagulants
- **Antithromboplastinemia** D68.318
- **Antithromboplastinogenemia** D68.318
- **Antitoxin complication or reaction** — *see* Complications, vaccination
- **Antlophobia** F4Ø.228
- **Antritis** J32.Ø
  - maxilla J32.Ø
    - acute JØ1.ØØ
      - recurrent JØ1.Ø1
  - stomach K29.5Ø
    - with bleeding K29.51
- **Antrum, antral** — *see* condition
- **Anuria** R34
  - calculous (impacted) (recurrent) — *see also* Calculus, urinary N2Ø.9
  - following
    - abortion — *see* Abortion by type complicated by, renal failure
    - ectopic or molar pregnancy OØ8.4
  - newborn P96.Ø
  - postprocedural N99.Ø
  - postrenal N13.8
  - traumatic (following crushing) T79.5 ☑
- **Anus, anal** — *see* condition
- **Anusitis** K62.89
- **Anxiety** F41.9
  - depression F41.8
  - episodic paroxysmal F41.Ø
  - generalized F41.1
  - hysteria F41.8
  - neurosis F41.1
  - panic type F41.Ø
  - reaction F41.1
  - separation, abnormal (of childhood) F93.Ø
  - specified NEC F41.8
  - state F41.1
- **Aorta, aortic** — *see* condition
- **Aortectasia** — *see* Ectasia, aorta
  - with aneurysm — *see* Aneurysm, aorta
- **Aortitis** (nonsyphilitic) (calcific) I77.6
  - arteriosclerotic I7Ø.Ø
  - Doehle-Heller A52.Ø2
  - luetic A52.Ø2
  - rheumatic — *see* Endocarditis, acute, rheumatic
  - specific (syphilitic) A52.Ø2
  - syphilitic A52.Ø2
    - congenital A5Ø.54 *[I79.1]*
- **Apathetic thyroid storm** — *see* Thyrotoxicosis
- **Apathy** R45.3
- **Apeirophobia** F4Ø.228
- **Apepsia** K3Ø
  - psychogenic F45.8
- **Aperistalsis, esophagus** K22.Ø
- **Apertognathia** M26.29
- **Apert's syndrome** Q87.Ø
- **Aphagia** R13.Ø
  - psychogenic F5Ø.9
- **Aphakia** (acquired) (postoperative) H27.Ø- ☑
  - congenital Q12.3
- **Aphasia** (amnestic) (global) (nominal) (semantic) (syntactic) R47.Ø1
  - acquired, with epilepsy (Landau-Kleffner syndrome) — *see* Epilepsy, specified NEC
  - auditory (developmental) F8Ø.2
  - developmental (receptive type) F8Ø.2
    - expressive type F8Ø.1
    - Wernicke's F8Ø.2
  - following
    - cerebrovascular disease I69.92Ø
      - cerebral infarction I69.32Ø
      - intracerebral hemorrhage I69.12Ø
      - nontraumatic intracranial hemorrhage NEC I69.22Ø
      - specified disease NEC I69.82Ø
      - subarachnoid hemorrhage I69.Ø2Ø
  - primary progressive — *see also* Dementia, in, diseases specified elsewhere G31.Ø1 *[FØ2.8Ø]*
    - with behavioral disturbance — *see also* Dementia, in, diseases specified elsewhere G31.Ø1 *[FØ2.81-]* ☑
  - progressive isolated — *see also* Dementia, in, diseases specified elsewhere G31.Ø1 *[FØ2.8Ø]*
    - with behavioral disturbance — *see also* Dementia, in, diseases specified elsewhere G31.Ø1 *[FØ2.81-]* ☑
  - sensory F8Ø.2
  - syphilis, tertiary A52.19
  - Wernicke's (developmental) F8Ø.2
- **Aphonia** (organic) R49.1
  - hysterical F44.4
  - psychogenic F44.4
- **Aphthae, aphthous** — *see also* condition
  - Bednar's K12.Ø
  - cachectic K14.Ø
  - epizootic BØ8.8
  - fever BØ8.8
  - oral (recurrent) K12.Ø
  - stomatitis (major) (minor) K12.Ø
  - thrush B37.Ø
  - ulcer (oral) (recurrent) K12.Ø
    - genital organ(s) NEC
      - female N76.6
      - male N5Ø.89
    - larynx J38.7
- **Apical** — *see* condition
- **Apiphobia** F4Ø.218
- **Aplasia** — *see also* Agenesis
  - abdominal muscle syndrome Q79.4
  - alveolar process (acquired) — *see* Anomaly, alveolar
    - congenital Q38.6
  - aorta (congenital) Q25.41
  - axialis extracorticalis (congenita) E75.29
  - bone marrow (myeloid) D61.9
    - congenital D61.Ø1
  - brain QØØ.Ø
    - part of QØ4.3
  - bronchus Q32.4
  - cementum KØØ.4
  - cerebellum QØ4.3
  - cervix (congenital) Q51.5
  - congenital pure red cell D61.Ø1
  - corpus callosum QØ4.Ø
  - cutis congenita Q84.8
  - erythrocyte congenital D61.Ø1
  - extracortical axial E75.29
  - eye Q11.1
  - fovea centralis (congenital) Q14.1
  - gallbladder, congenital Q44.Ø
  - iris Q13.1
  - labyrinth, membranous Q16.5
  - limb (congenital) Q73.8
    - lower — *see* Defect, reduction, lower limb
    - upper — *see* Agenesis, arm
  - lung, congenital (bilateral) (unilateral) Q33.3
  - pancreas Q45.Ø
  - parathyroid-thymic D82.1
  - Pelizaeus-Merzbacher E75.29
  - penis Q55.5
  - prostate Q55.4
  - red cell (with thymoma) D6Ø.9
    - acquired D6Ø.9
      - due to drugs D6Ø.9
    - adult D6Ø.9
    - chronic D6Ø.Ø
    - congenital D61.Ø1

- **Aplasia** — *continued*
  - red cell — *continued*
    - constitutional D61.01
    - due to drugs D60.9
    - hereditary D61.01
    - of infants D61.01
    - primary D61.01
    - pure D61.01
      - due to drugs D60.9
    - specified type NEC D60.8
    - transient D60.1
  - round ligament Q52.8
  - skin Q84.8
  - spermatic cord Q55.4
  - spleen Q89.01
  - testicle Q55.0
  - thymic, with immunodeficiency D82.1
  - thyroid (congenital) (with myxedema) E03.1
  - uterus Q51.0
  - ventral horn cell Q06.1
- **Apnea, apneic** (of) (spells) R06.81
  - newborn P28.40
    - central P28.41
    - mixed P28.43
    - obstructive P28.42
    - sleep
      - primary P28.30
        - central P28.31
        - mixed P28.33
        - obstructive P28.32
        - specified NEC P28.39
    - specified NEC P28.49
  - prematurity P28.49
  - sleep G47.30
    - central (primary) G47.31
      - idiopathic G47.31
      - in conditions classified elsewhere G47.37
    - obstructive (adult) (pediatric) G47.33
      - hypopnea G47.33
    - primary central G47.31
    - specified NEC G47.39
- **Apneumatosis, newborn** P28.0
- **Apocrine metaplasia** (breast) — *see* Dysplasia, mammary, specified type NEC
- **Apophysitis** (bone) — *see also* Osteochondropathy
  - calcaneus M92.8
  - juvenile M92.9
- **Apoplectiform convulsions** (cerebral ischemia) I67.82
- **Apoplexia, apoplexy, apoplectic**
  - adrenal A39.1
  - heart (auricle) (ventricle) — *see* Infarct, myocardium
  - heat T67.01 ☑
  - hemorrhagic (stroke) — *see* Hemorrhage, intracranial
  - meninges, hemorrhagic — *see* Hemorrhage, intracranial, subarachnoid
  - uremic N18.9 *[I68.8]*
- **Appearance**
  - bizarre R46.1
  - specified NEC R46.89
  - very low level of personal hygiene R46.0
- **Appendage**
  - epididymal (organ of Morgagni) Q55.4
  - intestine (epiploic) Q43.8
  - preauricular Q17.0
  - testicular (organ of Morgagni) Q55.29
- **Appendicitis** (pneumococcal) (retrocecal) K37
  - with
    - gangrene K35.891
      - with localized peritonitis K35.31
    - perforation NOS K35.32
    - peritoneal abscess K35.33
    - peritonitis NEC K35.33
      - generalized (with perforation or rupture) K35.20
        - with abscess K35.21
      - localized K35.30
        - with
          - gangrene K35.31
          - perforation K35.32
            - and abscess K35.33
    - rupture (with localized peritonitis) K35.32
  - acute (catarrhal) (fulminating) (obstructive) (retrocecal) (suppurative) K35.80
    - with
      - gangrene K35.891
      - peritoneal abscess K35.33
      - peritonitis NEC K35.33
        - generalized (with perforation or rupture) K35.20
- **Appendicitis** — *continued*
  - acute — *continued*
    - with — *continued*
      - peritonitis — *continued*
        - generalized — *continued*
          - with abscess K35.21
        - localized K35.30
          - with
            - gangrene K35.31
            - perforation K35.32
              - and abscess K35.33
    - specified NEC K35.890
      - with gangrene K35.891
        - with localized peritonitis K35.31
  - amebic A06.89
  - chronic (recurrent) K36
  - exacerbation — *see* Appendicitis, with, gangrene
  - gangrenous — *see* Appendicitis, acute
  - healed (obliterative) K36
  - interval K36
  - neurogenic K36
  - obstructive K36
  - recurrent K36
  - relapsing K36
  - ruptured NOS (with localized peritonitis) K35.32
  - subacute (adhesive) K36
  - subsiding K36
  - suppurative — *see* Appendicitis, acute
  - tuberculous A18.32
- **Appendicopathia oxyurica** B80
- **Appendix, appendicular** — *see also* condition
  - epididymis Q55.4
  - Morgagni
    - female Q50.5
    - male (epididymal) Q55.4
      - testicular Q55.29
  - testis Q55.29
- **Appetite**
  - depraved — *see* Pica
  - excessive R63.2
  - lack or loss — *see also* Anorexia R63.0
    - nonorganic origin F50.89
    - psychogenic F50.89
  - perverted (hysterical) — *see* Pica
- **Apple peel syndrome** Q41.1
- **Apprehension state** F41.1
- **Apprehensiveness, abnormal** F41.9
- **Approximal wear** K03.0
- **Apraxia** (classic) (ideational) (ideokinetic) (ideomotor) (motor) (verbal) R48.2
  - following
    - cerebrovascular disease I69.990
      - cerebral infarction I69.390
      - intracerebral hemorrhage I69.190
      - nontraumatic intracranial hemorrhage NEC I69.290
      - specified disease NEC I69.890
      - subarachnoid hemorrhage I69.090
  - oculomotor, congenital H51.8
- **Aptyalism** K11.7
- **Apudoma** — *see* Neoplasm, uncertain behavior, by site
- **Aqueous misdirection** H40.83- ☑
- **Arabicum elephantiasis** — *see* Infestation, filarial
- **Arachnitis** — *see* Meningitis
- **Arachnodactyly** — *see* Syndrome, Marfan's
- **Arachnoiditis** (acute) (adhesive) (basal) (brain) (cerebrospinal) — *see* Meningitis
- **Arachnophobia** F40.210
- **Arboencephalitis, Australian** A83.4
- **Arborization block** (heart) I45.5
- **ARC** (AIDS-related complex) B20
- **Arch**
  - aortic Q25.49
  - bovine Q25.49
- **Arches** — *see* condition
- **Arcuate uterus** Q51.810
- **Arcuatus uterus** Q51.810
- **Arcus** (cornea) senilis — *see* Degeneration, cornea, senile
- **Arc-welder's lung** J63.4
- **Areflexia** R29.2
- **Areola** — *see* condition
- **Argentaffinoma** — *see also* Neoplasm, uncertain behavior, by site
  - malignant — *see* Neoplasm, malignant, by site
  - syndrome E34.0
- **Argininemia** E72.21
- **Arginosuccinic aciduria** E72.22
- **Argyll Robertson phenomenon, pupil or syndrome** (syphilitic) A52.19
  - atypical H57.09
  - nonsyphilitic H57.09
- **Argyria, argyriasis**
  - conjunctival H11.13- ☑
  - from drug or medicament — *see* Table of Drugs and Chemicals, by substance
- **Argyrosis, conjunctival** H11.13- ☑
- **Arhinencephaly** Q04.1
- **Ariboflavinosis** E53.0
- **Arm** — *see* condition
- **Arnold-Chiari disease, obstruction or syndrome** (type II) Q07.00
  - with
    - hydrocephalus Q07.02
      - with spina bifida Q07.03
    - spina bifida Q07.01
      - with hydrocephalus Q07.03
  - type III — *see* Encephalocele
  - type IV Q04.8
- **Aromatic amino-acid metabolism disorder** E70.9
  - specified NEC E70.89
- **Arousals, confusional** G47.51
- **Arrest, arrested**
  - cardiac I46.9
    - complicating
      - abortion — *see* Abortion, by type, complicated by, cardiac arrest
      - anesthesia (general) (local) or other sedation — *see* Table of Drugs and Chemicals, by drug
        - in labor and delivery O74.2
        - in pregnancy O29.11- ☑
        - postpartum, puerperal O89.1
      - delivery (cesarean) (instrumental) O75.4
    - due to
      - cardiac condition I46.2
      - specified condition NEC I46.8
    - intraoperative I97.71- ☑
    - newborn P29.81
    - personal history, successfully resuscitated Z86.74
    - postprocedural I97.12- ☑
      - obstetric procedure O75.4
  - cardiorespiratory — *see* Arrest, cardiac
  - circulatory — *see* Arrest, cardiac
  - deep transverse O64.0 ☑
  - development or growth
    - bone — *see* Disorder, bone, development or growth
    - child R62.50
    - tracheal rings Q32.1
  - epiphyseal
    - complete
      - femur M89.15- ☑
      - humerus M89.12- ☑
      - tibia M89.16- ☑
      - ulna M89.13- ☑
    - forearm M89.13- ☑
      - specified NEC M89.13- ☑
      - ulna — *see* Arrest, epiphyseal, by type, ulna
    - lower leg M89.16- ☑
      - specified NEC M89.168
      - tibia — *see* Arrest, epiphyseal, by type, tibia
    - partial
      - femur M89.15- ☑
      - humerus M89.12- ☑
      - tibia M89.16- ☑
      - ulna M89.13- ☑
    - specified NEC M89.18
  - granulopoiesis — *see* Agranulocytosis
  - growth plate — *see* Arrest, epiphyseal
  - heart — *see* Arrest, cardiac
  - legal, anxiety concerning Z65.3
  - physeal — *see* Arrest, epiphyseal
  - respiratory R09.2
    - newborn P28.81
  - sinus I45.5
  - spermatogenesis (complete) — *see* Azoospermia
    - incomplete — *see* Oligospermia
  - transverse (deep) O64.0 ☑
- **Arrhenoblastoma**
  - benign
    - specified site — *see* Neoplasm, benign, by site
    - unspecified site
      - female D27.9
      - male D29.20
  - malignant
    - specified site — *see* Neoplasm, malignant, by site

- **Arrhenoblastoma** — *continued*
  - malignant — *continued*
    - unspecified site
      - female C56.9
      - male C62.9Ø
  - specified site — *see* Neoplasm, uncertain behavior, by site
  - unspecified site
    - female D39.1Ø
    - male D4Ø.1Ø
- **Arrhythmia** (auricle) (cardiac) (juvenile) (nodal) (reflex) (supraventricular) (transitory) (ventricle) I49.9
  - block I45.9
  - extrasystolic I49.49
  - newborn
    - bradycardia P29.12
    - occurring before birth PØ3.819
      - before onset of labor PØ3.81Ø
      - during labor PØ3.811
    - tachycardia P29.11
  - psychogenic F45.8
  - sinus I49.8
  - specified NEC I49.8
  - vagal R55
  - ventricular re-entry I47.Ø
- **Arrillaga-Ayerza syndrome** (pulmonary sclerosis with pulmonary hypertension) I27.Ø
- **Arsenical pigmentation** L81.8
  - from drug or medicament — *see* Table of Drugs and Chemicals
- **Arsenism** — *see* Poisoning, arsenic
- **Arterial** — *see* condition
- **Arteriofibrosis** — *see* Arteriosclerosis
- **Arteriolar sclerosis** — *see* Arteriosclerosis
- **Arteriolith** — *see* Arteriosclerosis
- **Arteriolitis** I77.6
  - necrotizing, kidney I77.5
  - renal — *see* Hypertension, kidney
- **Arteriolosclerosis** — *see* Arteriosclerosis
- **Arterionephrosclerosis** — *see* Hypertension, kidney
- **Arteriopathy** I77.9
  - cerebral autosomal dominant, with subcortical infarcts and leukoencephalopathy (CADASIL) I67.85Ø
- **Arteriosclerosis, arteriosclerotic** (diffuse) (obliterans) (of) (senile) (with calcification) I7Ø.9Ø
  - with
    - chronic limb-threatening ischemia — *see* Arteriosclerosis, with critical limb ischemia
    - critical limb ischemia
      - bypass graft I7Ø.329
        - autologous vein graft I7Ø.429
          - leg I7Ø.429
            - with
              - gangrene (and intermittent claudication, rest pain, and ulcer) I7Ø.469
              - rest pain (and intermittent claudication) I7Ø.429
            - bilateral I7Ø.423
              - with
                - gangrene (and intermittent claudication, rest pain, and ulcer) I7Ø.463
                - rest pain (and intermittent claudication) I7Ø.423
            - left I7Ø.422
              - with
                - gangrene (and intermittent claudication, rest pain, and ulcer) I7Ø.462
                - rest pain (and intermittent claudication) I7Ø.422
                - ulceration (and intermittent claudication and rest pain) I7Ø.449
                  - ankle I7Ø.443
                  - calf I7Ø.442
                  - foot site NEC I7Ø.445
                  - heel I7Ø.444
                  - lower leg NEC I7Ø.448
                  - mid foot I7Ø.444
                  - thigh I7Ø.441
            - right I7Ø.421
              - with
                - gangrene (and intermittent claudication, rest pain, and ulcer) I7Ø.461

- **Arteriosclerosis, arteriosclerotic** — *continued*
  - with — *continued*
    - critical limb ischemia — *continued*
      - bypass graft — *continued*
        - autologous vein graft — *continued*
          - leg — *continued*
            - right — *continued*
              - with — *continued*
                - rest pain (and intermittent claudication) I7Ø.421
                - ulceration (and intermittent claudication and rest pain) I7Ø.439
                  - ankle I7Ø.433
                  - calf I7Ø.432
                  - foot site NEC I7Ø.435
                  - heel I7Ø.434
                  - lower leg NEC I7Ø.438
                  - midfoot I7Ø.434
                  - thigh I7Ø.431
        - leg I7Ø.329
          - with
            - gangrene (and intermittent claudication, rest pain, and ulcer) I7Ø.369
            - rest pain (and intermittent claudication) I7Ø.329
          - bilateral I7Ø.323
            - with
              - gangrene (and intermittent claudication, rest pain, and ulcer) I7Ø.363
              - rest pain (and intermittent claudication) I7Ø.323
          - left I7Ø.322
            - with
              - gangrene (and intermittent claudication, rest pain, and ulcer) I7Ø.362
              - rest pain (and intermittent claudication) I7Ø.322
              - ulceration (and intermittent claudication and rest pain) I7Ø.349
                - ankle I7Ø.343
                - calf I7Ø.342
                - foot site NEC I7Ø.345
                - heel I7Ø.344
                - lower leg NEC I7Ø.348
                - midfoot I7Ø.344
                - thigh I7Ø.341
          - right I7Ø.321
            - with
              - gangrene (and intermittent claudication, rest pain, and ulcer) I7Ø.361
              - rest pain (and intermittent claudication) I7Ø.321
              - ulceration (and intermittent claudication and rest pain) I7Ø.339
                - ankle I7Ø.333
                - calf I7Ø.332
                - foot site NEC I7Ø.335
                - heel I7Ø.334
                - lower leg NEC I7Ø.338
                - midfoot I7Ø.334
                - thigh I7Ø.331
        - nonautologous biological graft I7Ø.529
          - leg I7Ø.529
            - with
              - gangrene (and intermittent claudication, rest pain, and ulcer) I7Ø.569
              - rest pain (and intermittent claudication) I7Ø.529
            - bilateral I7Ø.523
              - with
                - gangrene (and intermittent claudication, rest pain, and ulcer) I7Ø.563
                - rest pain (and intermittent claudication) I7Ø.523
            - left I7Ø.522
              - with
                - gangrene (and intermittent claudication, rest pain, and ulcer) I7Ø.562
                - rest pain (and intermittent claudication) I7Ø.522

- **Arteriosclerosis, arteriosclerotic** — *continued*
  - with — *continued*
    - critical limb ischemia — *continued*
      - bypass graft — *continued*
        - nonautologous biological graft — *continued*
          - leg — *continued*
            - left — *continued*
              - with — *continued*
                - ulceration (and intermittent claudication and rest pain) I7Ø.549
                  - ankle I7Ø.543
                  - calf I7Ø.542
                  - foot site NEC I7Ø.545
                  - heel I7Ø.544
                  - lower leg NEC I7Ø.548
                  - midfoot I7Ø.544
                  - thigh I7Ø.541
            - right I7Ø.521
              - with
                - gangrene (and intermittent claudication, rest pain, and ulcer) I7Ø.561
                - rest pain (and intermittent claudication) I7Ø.521
                - ulceration (and intermittent claudication and rest pain) I7Ø.539
                  - ankle I7Ø.533
                  - calf I7Ø.532
                  - foot site NEC I7Ø.535
                  - heel I7Ø.534
                  - lower leg NEC I7Ø.538
                  - midfoot I7Ø.534
                  - thigh I7Ø.531
        - nonbiological graft I7Ø.629
          - leg I7Ø.629
            - with
              - gangrene (and intermittent claudication, rest pain, and ulcer) I7Ø.669
              - rest pain (and intermittent claudication) I7Ø.629
            - bilateral I7Ø.623
              - with
                - gangrene (and intermittent claudication, rest pain, and ulcer) I7Ø.663
                - rest pain (intermittent claudication) I7Ø.623
            - left I7Ø.622
              - with
                - gangrene (and intermittent claudication, rest pain, and ulcer) I7Ø.662
                - rest pain (and intermittent claudication) I7Ø.622
                - ulceration (and intermittent claudication and rest pain) I7Ø.649
                  - ankle I7Ø.643
                  - calf I7Ø.642
                  - foot site NEC I7Ø.645
                  - heel I7Ø.644
                  - lower leg NEC I7Ø.648
                  - midfoot I7Ø.644
                  - thigh I7Ø.641
            - right I7Ø.621
              - with
                - gangrene (and intermittent claudication, rest pain, and ulcer) I7Ø.661
                - rest pain (and intermittent claudication) I7Ø.621
                - ulceration (and intermittent claudication and rest pain) I7Ø.639
                  - ankle I7Ø.633
                  - calf I7Ø.632
                  - foot site NEC I7Ø.635
                  - heel I7Ø.634
                  - lower leg NEC I7Ø.638
                  - midfoot I7Ø.634
                  - thigh I7Ø.631
        - specified graft NEC I7Ø.729
          - leg I7Ø.729

Arthritis, arthritic — *continued*
- in — *continued*
  - Mediterranean fever, familial — *see also* subcategory M14.8- MØ4.1
  - Meningococcus A39.83
  - metabolic disorder NEC — *see also* subcategory M14.8- E88.9
  - multiple myelomatosis C9Ø.Ø- ☑ *[M36.1]*
  - mumps B26.85
  - mycosis NEC — *see also* category MØ1 B49
  - myelomatosis (multiple) C9Ø.Ø- ☑ *[M36.1]*
  - neurological disorder NEC G98.Ø
  - ochronosis — *see also* subcategory M14.8- E7Ø.29
  - O'nyong-nyong — *see also* category MØ1 A92.1
  - parasitic disease NEC — *see also* category MØ1 B89
  - paratyphoid fever — *see also* category MØ1 AØ1.4
  - Pseudomonas — *see* Arthritis, pyogenic, bacterial NEC
  - psoriasis L4Ø.5Ø
  - pyogenic organism NEC — *see* Arthritis, pyogenic, bacterial NEC
  - Reiter's disease — *see* Reiter's disease
  - respiratory disorder NEC — *see also* subcategory M14.8- J98.9
  - reticulosis, malignant — *see also* subcategory M14.8- C86.Ø
  - rubella BØ6.82
  - Salmonella (arizonae) (cholerae-suis) (enteritidis) (typhimurium) AØ2.23
  - sarcoidosis D86.86
  - specified bacteria NEC — *see* Arthritis, pyogenic, bacterial NEC
  - sporotrichosis B42.82
  - syringomyelia G95.Ø
  - thalassemia NEC D56.9 *[M36.3]*
  - tuberculosis — *see* Tuberculosis, arthritis
  - typhoid fever AØ1.Ø4
  - urethritis, Reiter's — *see* Reiter's disease
  - viral disease NEC — *see also* category MØ1 B34.9
- infectious or infective — *see also* Arthritis, pyogenic or pyemic
  - spine — *see* Spondylopathy, infective
- juvenile MØ8.9Ø
  - with systemic onset — *see* Still's disease
  - ankle MØ8.97- ☑
  - elbow MØ8.92- ☑
  - foot joint MØ8.97- ☑
  - hand joint MØ8.94- ☑
  - hip MØ8.95- ☑
  - knee MØ8.96- ☑
  - multiple site MØ8.99
  - pauciarticular MØ8.4Ø
    - ankle MØ8.47- ☑
    - elbow MØ8.42- ☑
    - foot joint MØ8.47- ☑
    - hand joint MØ8.44- ☑
    - hip MØ8.45- ☑
    - knee MØ8.46- ☑
    - shoulder MØ8.41- ☑
    - specified site NEC MØ8.4A
    - vertebrae MØ8.48
    - wrist MØ8.43- ☑
  - psoriatic L4Ø.54
  - rheumatoid — *see* Arthritis, rheumatoid, juvenile
  - shoulder MØ8.91- ☑
  - specified site NEC MØ8.9A
  - specified type NEC MØ8.8Ø
    - ankle MØ8.87- ☑
    - elbow MØ8.82- ☑
    - foot joint MØ8.87- ☑
    - hand joint MØ8.84- ☑
    - hip MØ8.85- ☑
    - knee MØ8.86- ☑
    - multiple site MØ8.89
    - shoulder MØ8.81- ☑
    - specified joint NEC MØ8.88
    - vertebrae MØ8.88
    - wrist MØ8.83- ☑
  - wrist MØ8.93- ☑
- meaning osteoarthritis — *see* Osteoarthritis
- meningococcal A39.83
- menopausal (any site) NEC — *see* Arthritis, specified form NEC
- mutilans (psoriatic) L4Ø.52
- mycotic NEC — *see also* category MØ1 B49
- neuropathic (Charcot) — *see* Arthropathy, neuropathic
  - diabetic — *see* Diabetes, arthropathy, neuropathic

Arthritis, arthritic — *continued*
- neuropathic — *see* Arthropathy, neuropathic — *continued*
  - nonsyphilitic NEC G98.Ø
  - syringomyelic G95.Ø
- ochronotic — *see also* subcategory M14.8- E7Ø.29
- palindromic (any site) — *see* Rheumatism, palindromic
- pneumococcal MØØ.1Ø
  - ankle MØØ.17- ☑
  - elbow MØØ.12- ☑
  - foot joint — *see* Arthritis, pneumococcal, ankle
  - hand joint MØØ.14- ☑
  - hip MØØ.15- ☑
  - knee MØØ.16- ☑
  - multiple site MØØ.19
  - shoulder MØØ.11- ☑
  - vertebra MØØ.18
  - wrist MØØ.13- ☑
- postdysenteric — *see* Arthropathy, postdysenteric
- postmeningococcal A39.84
- postrheumatic, chronic — *see* Arthropathy, postrheumatic, chronic
- primary progressive — *see also* Arthritis, specified form NEC
  - spine — *see* Spondylitis, ankylosing
- psoriatic L4Ø.5Ø
- purulent (any site except spine) — *see* Arthritis, pyogenic or pyemic
  - spine — *see* Spondylopathy, infective
- pyogenic or pyemic (any site except spine) MØØ.9
  - bacterial NEC MØØ.8Ø
    - ankle MØØ.87- ☑
    - elbow MØØ.82- ☑
    - foot joint — *see* Arthritis, pyogenic, bacterial NEC, ankle
    - hand joint MØØ.84- ☑
    - hip MØØ.85- ☑
    - knee MØØ.86- ☑
    - multiple site MØØ.89
    - shoulder MØØ.81- ☑
    - vertebra MØØ.88
    - wrist MØØ.83- ☑
  - pneumococcal — *see* Arthritis, pneumococcal
  - spine — *see* Spondylopathy, infective
  - staphylococcal — *see* Arthritis, staphylococcal
  - streptococcal — *see* Arthritis, streptococcal NEC
    - pneumococcal — *see* Arthritis, pneumococcal
- reactive — *see* Reiter's disease
- rheumatic — *see also* Arthritis, rheumatoid
  - acute or subacute — *see* Fever, rheumatic
- rheumatoid MØ6.9
  - with
    - carditis — *see* Rheumatoid, carditis
    - endocarditis — *see* Rheumatoid, carditis
    - heart involvement NEC — *see* Rheumatoid, carditis
    - lung involvement — *see* Rheumatoid, lung
    - myocarditis — *see* Rheumatoid, carditis
    - myopathy — *see* Rheumatoid, myopathy
    - pericarditis — *see* Rheumatoid, carditis
    - polyneuropathy — *see* Rheumatoid, polyneuropathy
    - rheumatoid factor — *see* Arthritis, rheumatoid, seropositive
    - splenoadenomegaly and leukopenia — *see* Felty's syndrome
    - vasculitis — *see* Rheumatoid, vasculitis
    - visceral involvement NEC — *see* Rheumatoid, arthritis, with involvement of organs NEC
  - juvenile (with or without rheumatoid factor) MØ8.ØØ
    - with systemic onset — *see* Still's disease
    - ankle MØ8.Ø7- ☑
    - elbow MØ8.Ø2- ☑
    - foot joint MØ8.Ø7- ☑
    - hand joint MØ8.Ø4- ☑
    - hip MØ8.Ø5- ☑
    - knee MØ8.Ø6- ☑
    - multiple site MØ8.Ø9
    - shoulder MØ8.Ø1- ☑
    - specified site NEC MØ8.ØA
    - vertebra MØ8.Ø8
    - wrist MØ8.Ø3- ☑
  - seronegative MØ6.ØØ
    - ankle MØ6.Ø7- ☑
    - elbow MØ6.Ø2- ☑
    - foot joint MØ6.Ø7- ☑
    - hand joint MØ6.Ø4- ☑

Arthritis, arthritic — *continued*
- rheumatoid — *continued*
  - seronegative — *continued*
    - hip MØ6.Ø5- ☑
    - knee MØ6.Ø6- ☑
    - multiple site MØ6.Ø9
    - shoulder MØ6.Ø1- ☑
    - specified site NEC MØ6.ØA
    - vertebra MØ6.Ø8
    - wrist MØ6.Ø3- ☑
  - seropositive MØ5.9
    - specified NEC MØ5.8Ø
      - ankle MØ5.87- ☑
      - elbow MØ5.82- ☑
      - foot joint MØ5.87- ☑
      - hand joint MØ5.84- ☑
      - hip MØ5.85- ☑
      - knee MØ5.86- ☑
      - multiple sites MØ5.89
      - shoulder MØ5.81- ☑
      - specified site NEC MØ5.8A
      - vertebra — *see* Spondylitis, ankylosing
      - wrist MØ5.83- ☑
    - without organ involvement MØ5.7Ø
      - ankle MØ5.77- ☑
      - elbow MØ5.72- ☑
      - foot joint MØ5.77- ☑
      - hand joint MØ5.74- ☑
      - hip MØ5.75- ☑
      - knee MØ5.76- ☑
      - multiple sites MØ5.79
      - shoulder MØ5.71- ☑
      - specified site NEC MØ5.7A
      - vertebra — *see* Spondylitis, ankylosing
      - wrist MØ5.73- ☑
  - specified type NEC MØ6.8Ø
    - ankle MØ6.87- ☑
    - elbow MØ6.82- ☑
    - foot joint MØ6.87- ☑
    - hand joint MØ6.84- ☑
    - hip MØ6.85- ☑
    - knee MØ6.86- ☑
    - multiple site MØ6.89
    - shoulder MØ6.81- ☑
    - specified site NEC MØ6.8A
    - vertebra MØ6.88
    - wrist MØ6.83- ☑
  - spine — *see* Spondylitis, ankylosing
- rubella BØ6.82
- scorbutic — *see also* subcategory M14.8- E54
- senile or senescent — *see* Osteoarthritis
- septic (any site except spine) — *see* Arthritis, pyogenic or pyemic
  - spine — *see* Spondylopathy, infective
- serum (nontherapeutic) (therapeutic) — *see* Arthropathy, postimmunization
- specified form NEC M13.8Ø
  - ankle M13.87- ☑
  - elbow M13.82- ☑
  - foot joint M13.87- ☑
  - hand joint M13.84- ☑
  - hip M13.85- ☑
  - knee M13.86- ☑
  - multiple site M13.89
  - shoulder M13.81- ☑
  - specified joint NEC M13.88
  - wrist M13.83- ☑
- spine — *see also* Spondylosis
  - infectious or infective NEC — *see* Spondylopathy, infective
  - Marie-Strümpell — *see* Spondylitis, ankylosing
  - pyogenic — *see* Spondylopathy, infective
  - rheumatoid — *see* Spondylitis, ankylosing
  - traumatic (old) — *see* Spondylopathy, traumatic
  - tuberculous A18.Ø1
- staphylococcal MØØ.ØØ
  - ankle MØØ.Ø7- ☑
  - elbow MØØ.Ø2- ☑
  - foot joint — *see* Arthritis, staphylococcal, ankle
  - hand joint MØØ.Ø4- ☑
  - hip MØØ.Ø5- ☑
  - knee MØØ.Ø6- ☑
  - multiple site MØØ.Ø9
  - shoulder MØØ.Ø1- ☑
  - vertebra MØØ.Ø8
  - wrist MØØ.Ø3- ☑
- streptococcal NEC MØØ.2Ø

- **Arthritis, arthritic** — *continued*
  - streptococcal — *continued*
    - ankle MØØ.27- ☑
    - elbow MØØ.22- ☑
    - foot joint — *see* Arthritis, streptococcal, ankle
    - hand joint MØØ.24- ☑
    - hip MØØ.25- ☑
    - knee MØØ.26- ☑
    - multiple site MØØ.29
    - shoulder MØØ.21- ☑
    - vertebra MØØ.28
    - wrist MØØ.23- ☑
  - suppurative — *see* Arthritis, pyogenic or pyemic
  - syphilitic (late) A52.16
    - congenital A5Ø.55 *[M12.8Ø]*
  - syphilitica deformans (Charcot) A52.16
  - temporomandibular joint M26.64- ☑
  - toxic of menopause (any site) — *see* Arthritis, specified form NEC
  - transient — *see* Arthropathy, specified form NEC
  - traumatic (chronic) — *see* Arthropathy, traumatic
  - tuberculous A18.Ø2
    - spine A18.Ø1
  - uratic — *see* Gout
  - urethritica (Reiter's) — *see* Reiter's disease
  - vertebral — *see* Spondylopathy, inflammatory
  - villous (any site) — *see* Arthropathy, specified form NEC
- **Arthrocele** — *see* Effusion, joint
- **Arthrodesis status** Z98.1
- **Arthrodynia** — *see also* Pain, joint
- **Arthrodysplasia** Q74.9
- **Arthrofibrosis, joint** — *see* Ankylosis
- **Arthrogryposis** (congenital) Q68.8
  - multiplex congenita Q74.3
- **Arthrokatadysis** M24.7
- **Arthropathy** — *see also* Arthritis M12.9
  - Charcot's — *see* Arthropathy, neuropathic
    - diabetic — *see* Diabetes, arthropathy, neuropathic
    - syringomyelic G95.Ø
  - cricoarytenoid J38.7
  - crystal (-induced) — *see* Arthritis, in, crystals
  - diabetic NEC — *see* Diabetes, arthropathy
  - distal interphalangeal, psoriatic L4Ø.51
  - enteropathic MØ7.6Ø
    - ankle MØ7.67- ☑
    - elbow MØ7.62- ☑
    - foot joint MØ7.67- ☑
    - hand joint MØ7.64- ☑
    - hip MØ7.65- ☑
    - knee MØ7.66- ☑
    - multiple site MØ7.69
    - shoulder MØ7.61- ☑
    - vertebra MØ7.68
    - wrist MØ7.63- ☑
  - facet joint — *see also* Spondylosis M47.819
  - following intestinal bypass MØ2.ØØ
    - ankle MØ2.Ø7- ☑
    - elbow MØ2.Ø2- ☑
    - foot joint MØ2.Ø7- ☑
    - hand joint MØ2.Ø4- ☑
    - hip MØ2.Ø5- ☑
    - knee MØ2.Ø6- ☑
    - multiple site MØ2.Ø9
    - shoulder MØ2.Ø1- ☑
    - vertebra MØ2.Ø8
    - wrist MØ2.Ø3- ☑
  - gouty — *see also* Gout
    - in (due to)
      - Lesch-Nyhan syndrome E79.1 *[M14.8-]* ☑
      - sickle-cell disorders D57- ☑ *[M14.8-]* ☑
  - hemophilic NEC D66 *[M36.2]*
    - in (due to)
      - hyperparathyroidism NEC E21.3 *[M14.8-]* ☑
      - metabolic disease NOS E88.9 *[M14.8-]* ☑
  - in (due to)
    - acromegaly E22.Ø *[M14.8-]* ☑
    - amyloidosis E85.4 *[M14.8-]* ☑
    - blood disorder NOS D75.9 *[M36.3]*
    - diabetes — *see* Diabetes, arthropathy
    - endocrine disease NOS E34.9 *[M14.8-]* ☑
    - erythema
      - multiforme L51.9 *[M14.8-]* ☑
      - nodosum L52 *[M14.8-]* ☑
    - hemochromatosis E83.118 *[M14.8-]* ☑
    - hemoglobinopathy NEC D58.2 *[M36.3]*

- **Arthropathy** — *continued*
  - in — *continued*
    - hemophilia NEC D66 *[M36.2]*
    - Henoch-Schönlein purpura D69.Ø *[M36.4]*
    - hyperthyroidism EØ5.9Ø *[M14.8-]* ☑
    - hypothyroidism EØ3.9 *[M14.8-]* ☑
    - infective endocarditis I33.Ø *[M12.8Ø]*
    - leukemia NEC C95.9- ☑ *[M36.1]*
    - malignant histiocytosis C96.A *[M36.1]*
    - metabolic disease NOS E88.9 *[M14.8-]* ☑
    - multiple myeloma C9Ø.Ø- ☑ *[M36.1]*
    - neoplastic disease NOS (*see also* Neoplasm) D49.9 *[M36.1]*
    - nutritional deficiency — *see also* subcategory M14.8- E63.9
    - psoriasis NOS L4Ø.5Ø
    - sarcoidosis D86.86
    - syphilis (late) A52.77
      - congenital A5Ø.55 *[M12.8Ø]*
    - thyrotoxicosis — *see also* subcategory M14.8- EØ5.9Ø
    - ulcerative colitis K51.9Ø *[MØ7.6Ø]*
    - viral hepatitis (postinfectious) NEC B19.9 *[M12.8Ø]*
    - Whipple's disease — *see also* subcategory M14.8- K9Ø.81
  - Jaccoud — *see* Arthropathy, postrheumatic, chronic
  - juvenile — *see* Arthritis, juvenile
    - psoriatic L4Ø.54
  - mutilans (psoriatic) L4Ø.52
  - neuropathic (Charcot) M14.6Ø
    - ankle M14.67- ☑
    - diabetic — *see* Diabetes, arthropathy, neuropathic
    - elbow M14.62- ☑
    - foot joint M14.67- ☑
    - hand joint M14.64- ☑
    - hip M14.65- ☑
    - knee M14.66- ☑
    - multiple site M14.69
    - nonsyphilitic NEC G98.Ø
    - shoulder M14.61- ☑
    - syringomyelic G95.Ø
    - vertebra M14.68
    - wrist M14.63- ☑
  - osteopulmonary — *see* Osteoarthropathy, hypertrophic, specified NEC
  - postdysenteric MØ2.1Ø
    - ankle MØ2.17- ☑
    - elbow MØ2.12- ☑
    - foot joint MØ2.17- ☑
    - hand joint MØ2.14- ☑
    - hip MØ2.15- ☑
    - knee MØ2.16- ☑
    - multiple site MØ2.19
    - shoulder MØ2.11- ☑
    - vertebra MØ2.18
    - wrist MØ2.13- ☑
  - postimmunization MØ2.2Ø
    - ankle MØ2.27- ☑
    - elbow MØ2.22- ☑
    - foot joint MØ2.27- ☑
    - hand joint MØ2.24- ☑
    - hip MØ2.25- ☑
    - knee MØ2.26- ☑
    - multiple site MØ2.29
    - shoulder MØ2.21- ☑
    - vertebra MØ2.28
    - wrist MØ2.23- ☑
  - postinfectious NEC B99 ☑ *[M12.8Ø]*
    - in (due to)
      - enteritis due to Yersinia enterocolitica AØ4.6 *[M12.8Ø]*
      - syphilis A52.77
      - viral hepatitis NEC B19.9 *[M12.8Ø]*
  - postrheumatic, chronic (Jaccoud) M12.ØØ
    - ankle M12.Ø7- ☑
    - elbow M12.Ø2- ☑
    - foot joint M12.Ø7- ☑
    - hand joint M12.Ø4- ☑
    - hip M12.Ø5- ☑
    - knee M12.Ø6- ☑
    - multiple site M12.Ø9
    - shoulder M12.Ø1- ☑
    - specified joint NEC M12.Ø8
    - vertebrae M12.Ø8
    - wrist M12.Ø3- ☑
  - psoriatic NEC L4Ø.59
    - interphalangeal, distal L4Ø.51

- **Arthropathy** — *continued*
  - reactive MØ2.9
    - in (due to)
      - infective endocarditis I33.Ø *[MØ2.9]*
    - specified type NEC MØ2.8Ø
      - ankle MØ2.87- ☑
      - elbow MØ2.82- ☑
      - foot joint MØ2.87- ☑
      - hand joint MØ2.84- ☑
      - hip MØ2.85- ☑
      - knee MØ2.86- ☑
      - multiple site MØ2.89
      - shoulder MØ2.81- ☑
      - vertebra MØ2.88
      - wrist MØ2.83- ☑
  - specified form NEC M12.8Ø
    - ankle M12.87- ☑
    - elbow M12.82- ☑
    - foot joint M12.87- ☑
    - hand joint M12.84- ☑
    - hip M12.85- ☑
    - knee M12.86- ☑
    - multiple site M12.89
    - shoulder M12.81- ☑
    - specified joint NEC M12.88
    - vertebrae M12.88
    - wrist M12.83- ☑
  - syringomyelic G95.Ø
  - tabes dorsalis A52.16
  - tabetic A52.16
  - temporomandibular joint M26.65- ☑
  - transient — *see* Arthropathy, specified form NEC
  - traumatic M12.5Ø
    - ankle M12.57- ☑
    - elbow M12.52- ☑
    - foot joint M12.57- ☑
    - hand joint M12.54- ☑
    - hip M12.55- ☑
    - knee M12.56- ☑
    - multiple site M12.59
    - shoulder M12.51- ☑
    - specified joint NEC M12.58
    - vertebrae M12.58
    - wrist M12.53- ☑
- **Arthropyosis** — *see* Arthritis, pyogenic or pyemic
- **Arthrosis** (deformans) (degenerative) (localized) — *see also* Osteoarthritis M19.9Ø
  - spine — *see* Spondylosis
- **Arthus' phenomenon or reaction** T78.41 ☑
  - due to
    - drug — *see* Table of Drugs and Chemicals, by drug
- **Articular** — *see* condition
- **Articulation, reverse** (teeth) M26.24
- **Artificial**
  - insemination complication — *see* Complications, artificial, fertilization
  - opening status (functioning) (without complication) Z93.9
    - anus (colostomy) Z93.3
    - colostomy Z93.3
    - cystostomy Z93.5Ø
      - appendico-vesicostomy Z93.52
      - cutaneous Z93.51
      - specified NEC Z93.59
    - enterostomy Z93.4
    - gastrostomy Z93.1
    - ileostomy Z93.2
    - intestinal tract NEC Z93.4
    - jejunostomy Z93.4
    - nephrostomy Z93.6
    - specified site NEC Z93.8
    - tracheostomy Z93.Ø
    - ureterostomy Z93.6
    - urethrostomy Z93.6
    - urinary tract NEC Z93.6
    - vagina Z93.8
  - vagina status Z93.8
- **Arytenoid** — *see* condition
- **Asbestosis** (occupational) J61
- **Ascariasis** B77.9
  - with
    - complications NEC B77.89
    - intestinal complications B77.Ø
    - pneumonia, pneumonitis B77.81
- **Ascaridosis, ascaridiasis** — *see* Ascariasis
- **Ascaris** (infection) (infestation) (lumbricoides) — *see* Ascariasis

- **Asthma, asthmatic** — *continued*
  - allergic extrinsic — *continued*
    - with — *continued*
      - status asthmaticus J45.902
  - atopic — *see* Asthma, allergic extrinsic
  - cardiac — *see* Failure, ventricular, left
  - cardiobronchial I50.1
  - childhood J45.909
    - with
      - exacerbation (acute) J45.901
      - status asthmaticus J45.902
  - chronic obstructive J44.9
    - with
      - acute lower respiratory infection J44.0
      - exacerbation (acute) J44.1
  - collier's J60
  - cough variant J45.991
  - detergent J69.8
  - due to
    - detergent J69.8
    - inhalation of fumes J68.3
  - eosinophilic J82.83
  - extrinsic, allergic — *see* Asthma, allergic extrinsic
  - grinder's J62.8
  - hay — *see* Asthma, allergic extrinsic
  - heart I50.1
  - idiosyncratic — *see* Asthma, nonallergic
  - intermittent (mild) J45.20
    - with
      - exacerbation (acute) J45.21
      - status asthmaticus J45.22
  - intrinsic, nonallergic — *see* Asthma, nonallergic
  - Kopp's E32.8
  - late-onset J45.909
    - with
      - exacerbation (acute) J45.901
      - status asthmaticus J45.902
  - mild intermittent J45.20
    - with
      - exacerbation (acute) J45.21
      - status asthmaticus J45.22
  - mild persistent J45.30
    - with
      - exacerbation (acute) J45.31
      - status asthmaticus J45.32
  - Millar's (laryngismus stridulus) J38.5
  - miner's J60
  - mixed J45.909
    - with
      - exacerbation (acute) J45.901
      - status asthmaticus J45.902
  - moderate persistent J45.40
    - with
      - exacerbation (acute) J45.41
      - status asthmaticus J45.42
  - nervous — *see* Asthma, nonallergic
  - nonallergic (intrinsic) J45.909
    - with
      - exacerbation (acute) J45.901
      - status asthmaticus J45.902
  - persistent
    - mild J45.30
      - with
        - exacerbation (acute) J45.31
        - status asthmaticus J45.32
    - moderate J45.40
      - with
        - exacerbation (acute) J45.41
        - status asthmaticus J45.42
    - severe J45.50
      - with
        - exacerbation (acute) J45.51
        - status asthmaticus J45.52
  - platinum J45.998
  - pneumoconiotic NEC J64
  - potter's J62.8
  - predominantly allergic J45.909
  - psychogenic F54
  - pulmonary eosinophilic J82.83
  - red cedar J67.8
  - Rostan's I50.1
  - sandblaster's J62.8
  - sequoiosis J67.8
  - severe persistent J45.50
    - with
      - exacerbation (acute) J45.51
      - status asthmaticus J45.52
  - specified NEC J45.998
- **Asthma, asthmatic** — *continued*
  - stonemason's J62.8
  - thymic E32.8
  - tuberculous — *see* Tuberculosis, pulmonary
  - Wichmann's (laryngismus stridulus) J38.5
  - wood J67.8
- **Astigmatism** (compound) (congenital) H52.20- ☑
  - irregular H52.21- ☑
  - regular H52.22- ☑
- **Astraphobia** F40.220
- **Astroblastoma**
  - specified site — *see* Neoplasm, malignant, by site
  - unspecified site C71.9
- **Astrocytoma** (cystic)
  - anaplastic
    - specified site — *see* Neoplasm, malignant, by site
    - unspecified site C71.9
  - fibrillary
    - specified site — *see* Neoplasm, malignant, by site
    - unspecified site C71.9
  - fibrous
    - specified site — *see* Neoplasm, malignant, by site
    - unspecified site C71.9
  - gemistocytic
    - specified site — *see* Neoplasm, malignant, by site
    - unspecified site C71.9
  - juvenile
    - specified site — *see* Neoplasm, malignant, by site
    - unspecified site C71.9
  - pilocytic
    - specified site — *see* Neoplasm, malignant, by site
    - unspecified site C71.9
  - piloid
    - specified site — *see* Neoplasm, malignant, by site
    - unspecified site C71.9
  - protoplasmic
    - specified site — *see* Neoplasm, malignant, by site
    - unspecified site C71.9
  - specified site NEC — *see* Neoplasm, malignant, by site
  - subependymal D43.2
    - giant cell
      - specified site — *see* Neoplasm, uncertain behavior, by site
      - unspecified site D43.2
    - specified site — *see* Neoplasm, uncertain behavior, by site
    - unspecified site D43.2
  - unspecified site C71.9
- **Astroglioma**
  - specified site — *see* Neoplasm, malignant, by site
  - unspecified site C71.9
- **Asymbolia** R48.8
- **Asymmetry** — *see also* Distortion
  - between native and reconstructed breast N65.1
  - face Q67.0
  - jaw (lower) — *see* Anomaly, dentofacial, jaw-cranial base relationship, asymmetry
- **Asynergia, asynergy** R27.8
  - ventricular I51.89
- **Asystole** (heart) — *see* Arrest, cardiac
- **At risk**
  - for
    - dental caries Z91.849
      - high Z91.843
      - low Z91.841
      - moderate Z91.842
    - falling Z91.81
- **Ataxia, ataxy, ataxic** R27.0
  - acute R27.8
  - autosomal recessive Friedreich G11.11
  - brain (hereditary) G11.9
  - cerebellar (hereditary) G11.9
    - with defective DNA repair G11.3
    - alcoholic G31.2
    - early-onset G11.10
      - with
        - essential tremor G11.19
        - myoclonus [Hunt's ataxia] G11.19
        - retained tendon reflexes G11.19
    - in
      - alcoholism G31.2
      - myxedema E03.9 *[G13.2]*
      - neoplastic disease — *see also* Neoplasm D49.9 *[G32.81]*
      - specified disease NEC G32.81
    - late-onset (Marie's) G11.2
  - cerebral (hereditary) G11.9
  - congenital nonprogressive G11.0
- **Ataxia, ataxy, ataxic** — *continued*
  - family, familial — *see* Ataxia, hereditary
  - following
    - cerebrovascular disease I69.993
      - cerebral infarction I69.393
      - intracerebral hemorrhage I69.193
      - nontraumatic intracranial hemorrhage NEC I69.293
      - specified disease NEC I69.893
      - subarachnoid hemorrhage I69.093
  - Friedreich's (heredofamilial) (cerebellar) (spinal) (with retained reflexes) G11.11
  - gait R26.0
    - hysterical F44.4
  - general R27.8
  - gluten M35.9 *[G32.81]*
    - with celiac disease K90.0 *[G32.81]*
  - hereditary G11.9
    - with neuropathy G60.2
    - cerebellar — *see* Ataxia, cerebellar
    - spastic G11.4
    - specified NEC G11.8
    - spinal (Friedreich's) G11.11
  - heredofamilial — *see* Ataxia, hereditary
  - Hunt's G11.19
  - hysterical F44.4
  - locomotor (progressive) (syphilitic) (partial) (spastic) A52.11
    - diabetic — *see* Diabetes, ataxia
  - Marie's (cerebellar) (heredofamilial) (late- onset) G11.2
  - nonorganic origin F44.4
  - nonprogressive, congenital G11.0
  - psychogenic F44.4
  - Roussy-Lévy G60.0
  - Sanger-Brown's (hereditary) G11.2
  - spastic hereditary G11.4
  - spinal
    - hereditary (Friedreich's) G11.11
    - progressive (syphilitic) A52.11
  - spinocerebellar, X-linked recessive G11.19
  - telangiectasia (Louis-Bar) G11.3
- **Ataxia-telangiectasia** (Louis-Bar) G11.3
- **Atelectasis** (massive) (partial) (pressure) (pulmonary) J98.11
  - newborn P28.10
    - due to resorption P28.11
    - partial P28.19
    - primary P28.0
    - secondary P28.19
  - primary (newborn) P28.0
  - tuberculous — *see* Tuberculosis, pulmonary
- **Atelocardia** Q24.9
- **Atelomyelia** Q06.1
- **Atheroembolism**
  - of
    - extremities
      - lower I75.02- ☑
      - upper I75.01- ☑
    - kidney I75.81
    - specified NEC I75.89
- **Atheroma, atheromatous** — *see also* Arteriosclerosis I70.90
  - aorta, aortic I70.0
    - valve — *see also* Endocarditis, aortic I35.8
  - aorto-iliac I70.0
  - artery — *see* Arteriosclerosis
  - basilar (artery) I67.2
  - carotid (artery) (common) (internal) I67.2
  - cerebral (arteries) I67.2
  - coronary (artery) I25.10
    - with angina pectoris — *see* Arteriosclerosis, coronary (artery),
  - degeneration — *see* Arteriosclerosis
  - heart, cardiac — *see* Disease, heart, ischemic, atherosclerotic
  - mitral (valve) I34.89
  - myocardium, myocardial — *see* Disease, heart, ischemic, atherosclerotic
  - pulmonary valve (heart) — *see also* Endocarditis, pulmonary I37.8
  - tricuspid (heart) (valve) I36.8
  - valve, valvular — *see* Endocarditis
  - vertebral (artery) I67.2
- **Atheromatosis** — *see* Arteriosclerosis
- **Atherosclerosis** — *see also* Arteriosclerosis
  - coronary
    - artery I25.10

Atrophy, atrophic — *continued*
- Déjérine-Thomas G23.8
- disuse NEC — *see* Atrophy, muscle
- Duchenne-Aran G12.21
- ear H93.8- ☑
- edentulous alveolar ridge K08.2Ø
- endometrium (senile) N85.8
  - cervix N88.8
- enteric K63.89
- epididymis N5Ø.89
- eyeball — *see* Disorder, globe, degenerated condition, atrophy
- eyelid (senile) — *see* Disorder, eyelid, degenerative
- facial (skin) L9Ø.9
- fallopian tube (senile) N83.32- ☑
  - with ovary N83.33- ☑
- fascioscapulohumeral (Landouzy- Déjérine) G71.Ø2
- fatty, thymus (gland) E32.8
- gallbladder K82.8
- gastric K29.4Ø
  - with bleeding K29.41
- gastrointestinal K63.89
- glandular I89.8
- globe H44.52- ☑
- gum — *see* Recession, gingival
- hair L67.8
- heart (brown) — *see* Degeneration, myocardial
- hemifacial Q67.4
  - Romberg G51.8
- infantile E41
  - paralysis, acute — *see* Poliomyelitis, paralytic
- intestine K63.89
- iris (essential) (progressive) H21.26- ☑
  - specified NEC H21.29
- kidney (senile) (terminal) — *see also* Sclerosis, renal N26.1
  - congenital or infantile Q6Ø.5
    - bilateral Q6Ø.4
    - unilateral Q6Ø.3
  - hydronephrotic — *see* Hydronephrosis
- lacrimal gland (primary) HØ4.14- ☑
  - secondary HØ4.15- ☑
- Landouzy-Déjérine G71.Ø2
- laryngitis, infective J37.Ø
- larynx J38.7
- Leber's optic (hereditary) H47.22
- lip K13.Ø
- liver (yellow) K72.9Ø
  - with coma K72.91
  - acute, subacute K72.ØØ
    - with coma K72.Ø1
  - chronic K72.1Ø
    - with coma K72.11
- lung (senile) J98.4
- macular (dermatological) L9Ø.8
  - syphilitic, skin A51.39
    - striated A52.79
- mandible (edentulous) KØ8.2Ø
  - minimal KØ8.21
  - moderate KØ8.22
  - severe KØ8.23
- maxilla KØ8.2Ø
  - minimal KØ8.24
  - moderate KØ8.25
  - severe KØ8.26
- muscle, muscular (diffuse) (general) (idiopathic) (primary) M62.5Ø
  - ankle M62.57- ☑
  - back M62.5A9
    - cervical M62.5AØ
    - lumbosacral M62.5A2
    - thoracic M62.5A1
  - Duchenne-Aran G12.21
  - foot M62.57- ☑
  - forearm M62.53- ☑
  - hand M62.54- ☑
  - infantile spinal G12.Ø
  - lower leg M62.56- ☑
  - multiple sites M62.59
  - myelopathic — *see* Atrophy, muscle, spinal
  - myotonic G71.11
  - neuritic G58.9
  - neuropathic (peroneal) (progressive) G6Ø.Ø
  - pelvic (disuse) N81.84
  - peroneal G6Ø.Ø
  - progressive (bulbar) G12.21
    - adult G12.1
    - infantile (spinal) G12.Ø

Atrophy, atrophic — *continued*
- muscle, muscular — *continued*
  - progressive — *continued*
    - spinal G12.25
      - adult G12.1
      - infantile G12.Ø
  - pseudohypertrophic G71.Ø2
  - shoulder region M62.51- ☑
  - specified site NEC M62.58
  - spinal G12.9
    - adult form G12.1
    - Aran-Duchenne G12.21
    - childhood form, type II G12.1
    - distal G12.1
    - hereditary NEC G12.1
    - infantile, type I (Werdnig-Hoffmann) G12.Ø
    - juvenile form, type III (Kugelberg- Welander) G12.1
    - progressive G12.25
    - scapuloperoneal form G12.1
    - specified NEC G12.8
  - syphilitic A52.78
  - thigh M62.55- ☑
  - upper arm M62.52- ☑
- myocardium — *see* Degeneration, myocardial
- myometrium (senile) N85.8
  - cervix N88.8
- myopathic NEC — *see* Atrophy, muscle
- myotonia G71.11
- nail L6Ø.3
- nasopharynx J31.1
- nerve — *see also* Disorder, nerve
  - abducens — *see* Strabismus, paralytic, sixth nerve
  - accessory G52.8
  - acoustic or auditory H93.3 ☑
  - cranial G52.9
    - eighth (auditory) H93.3 ☑
    - eleventh (accessory) G52.8
    - fifth (trigeminal) G5Ø.8
    - first (olfactory) G52.Ø
    - fourth (trochlear) — *see* Strabismus, paralytic, fourth nerve
    - second (optic) H47.2Ø
    - sixth (abducens) — *see* Strabismus, paralytic, sixth nerve
    - tenth (pneumogastric) (vagus) G52.2
    - third (oculomotor) — *see* Strabismus, paralytic, third nerve
    - twelfth (hypoglossal) G52.3
  - hypoglossal G52.3
  - oculomotor — *see* Strabismus, paralytic, third nerve
  - olfactory G52.Ø
  - optic (papillomacular bundle)
    - syphilitic (late) A52.15
      - congenital A5Ø.44
  - pneumogastric G52.2
  - trigeminal G5Ø.8
  - trochlear — *see* Strabismus, paralytic, fourth nerve
  - vagus (pneumogastric) G52.2
- neurogenic, bone, tabetic A52.11
- nutritional E43
  - with marasmus E41
- old age R54
- olivopontocerebellar G23.8
- optic (nerve) H47.2Ø
  - glaucomatous H47.23- ☑
  - hereditary H47.22
  - primary H47.21- ☑
  - specified type NEC H47.29- ☑
  - syphilitic (late) A52.15
    - congenital A5Ø.44
- orbit HØ5.31- ☑
- ovary (senile) N83.31- ☑
  - with fallopian tube N83.33- ☑
- oviduct (senile) — *see* Atrophy, fallopian tube
- palsy, diffuse (progressive) G12.22
- pancreas (duct) (senile) K86.89
- parotid gland K11.Ø
- pelvic muscle N81.84
- penis N48.89
- pharynx J39.2
- pluriglandular E31.8
  - autoimmune E31.Ø
- polyarthritis M15.9
- prostate N42.89
- pseudohypertrophic (muscle) G71.Ø2
- renal — *see also* Sclerosis, renal N26.1
- retina, retinal (postinfectional) H35.89

Atrophy, atrophic — *continued*
- rhinitis J31.Ø
- salivary gland K11.Ø
- scar L9Ø.5
- sclerosis, lobar (of brain) — *see also* Dementia, in, diseases specified elsewhere G31.Ø9 *[FØ2.8Ø]*
  - with behavioral disturbance — *see also* Dementia, in, diseases specified elsewhere G31.Ø9 *[FØ2.81-]* ☑
- scrotum N5Ø.89
- seminal vesicle N5Ø.89
- senile R54
  - due to radiation (nonionizing) (solar) L57.8
- skin (patches) (spots) L9Ø.9
  - degenerative (senile) L9Ø.8
  - due to radiation (nonionizing) (solar) L57.8
  - senile L9Ø.8
- spermatic cord N5Ø.89
- spinal (acute) (cord) G95.89
  - muscular — *see* Atrophy, muscle, spinal
  - paralysis G12.2Ø
    - acute — *see* Poliomyelitis, paralytic
    - meaning progressive muscular atrophy G12.25
- spine (column) — *see* Spondylopathy, specified NEC
- spleen (senile) D73.Ø
- stomach K29.4Ø
  - with bleeding K29.41
- striate (skin) L9Ø.6
  - syphilitic A52.79
- subcutaneous L9Ø.9
- sublingual gland K11.Ø
- submandibular gland K11.Ø
- submaxillary gland K11.Ø
- Sudeck's — *see* Algoneurodystrophy
- suprarenal (capsule) (gland) E27.49
  - primary E27.1
- systemic affecting central nervous system
  - in
    - myxedema EØ3.9 *[G13.2]*
    - neoplastic disease — *see also* Neoplasm D49.9 *[G13.1]*
  - specified disease NEC G13.8
- tarso-orbital fascia, congenital Q1Ø.3
- testis N5Ø.Ø
- thenar, partial — *see* Syndrome, carpal tunnel
- thymus (fatty) E32.8
- thyroid (gland) (acquired) EØ3.4
  - with cretinism EØ3.1
  - congenital (with myxedema) EØ3.1
- tongue (senile) K14.8
  - papillae K14.4
- trachea J39.8
- tunica vaginalis N5Ø.89
- turbinate J34.89
- tympanic membrane (nonflaccid) H73.82- ☑
  - flaccid H73.81- ☑
- upper respiratory tract J39.8
- uterus, uterine (senile) N85.8
  - cervix N88.8
  - due to radiation (intended effect) N85.8
    - adverse effect or misadventure N99.89
- vagina (senile) N95.2
- vas deferens N5Ø.89
- vascular I99.8
- vertebra (senile) — *see* Spondylopathy, specified NEC
- vulva (senile) N9Ø.5
- Werdnig-Hoffmann G12.Ø
- yellow — *see* Failure, hepatic

Attack, attacks
- with alteration of consciousness (with automatisms) — *see* Epilepsy, localization-related, symptomatic, with complex partial seizures
- Adams-Stokes I45.9
- akinetic — *see* Epilepsy, generalized, specified NEC
- angina — *see* Angina
- atonic — *see* Epilepsy, generalized, specified NEC
- benign shuddering G25.83
- cataleptic — *see* Catalepsy
- coronary — *see* Infarct, myocardium
- cyanotic, newborn P28.2
- drop NEC R55
- epileptic — *see* Epilepsy
- heart — *see* infarct, myocardium
- hysterical F44.9
- jacksonian — *see* Epilepsy, localization-related, symptomatic, with simple partial seizures
- myocardium, myocardial — *see* Infarct, myocardium
- myoclonic — *see* Epilepsy, generalized, specified NEC

- **Attack, attacks** — *continued*
  - panic F41.Ø
  - psychomotor — *see* Epilepsy, localization-related, symptomatic, with complex partial seizures
  - salaam — *see* Epilepsy, spasms
  - schizophreniform, brief F23
  - shuddering, benign G25.83
  - Stokes-Adams I45.9
  - syncope R55
  - transient ischemic (TIA) G45.9
    - specified NEC G45.8
  - unconsciousness R55
    - hysterical F44.89
  - vasomotor R55
  - vasovagal (paroxysmal) (idiopathic) R55
  - without alteration of consciousness — *see* Epilepsy, localization-related, symptomatic, with simple partial seizures
- **Attention** (to)
  - artificial
    - opening (of) Z43.9
      - digestive tract NEC Z43.4
        - colon Z43.3
        - ilium Z43.2
        - stomach Z43.1
      - specified NEC Z43.8
      - trachea Z43.Ø
      - urinary tract NEC Z43.6
        - cystostomy Z43.5
        - nephrostomy Z43.6
        - ureterostomy Z43.6
        - urethrostomy Z43.6
      - vagina Z43.7
  - colostomy Z43.3
  - cystostomy Z43.5
  - deficit disorder or syndrome F98.8
    - with hyperactivity — *see* Disorder, attention-deficit hyperactivity
  - gastrostomy Z43.1
  - ileostomy Z43.2
  - jejunostomy Z43.4
  - nephrostomy Z43.6
  - surgical dressings Z48.Ø1
  - sutures Z48.Ø2
  - tracheostomy Z43.Ø
  - ureterostomy Z43.6
  - urethrostomy Z43.6
- **Attrition**
  - gum — *see* Recession, gingival
  - tooth, teeth (excessive) (hard tissues) KØ3.Ø
- **Atypical, atypism** — *see also* condition
  - cells (on cytolgocial smear) (endocervical) (endometrial) (glandular)
    - cervix R87.619
    - vagina R87.629
  - cervical N87.9
  - endometrium N85.9
    - hyperplasia N85.ØØ
  - parenting situation Z62.9
- **Auditory** — *see* condition
- **Aujeszky's disease** B33.8
- **Aurantiasis, cutis** E67.1
- **Auricle, auricular** — *see also* condition
  - cervical Q18.2
- **Auriculotemporal syndrome** G5Ø.8
- **Austin Flint murmur** (aortic insufficiency) I35.1
- **Australian**
  - Q fever A78
  - X disease A83.4
- **Autism, autistic** (childhood) (infantile) F84.Ø
  - atypical F84.9
  - spectrum disorder F84.Ø
- **Autodigestion** R68.89
- **Autoerythrocyte sensitization** (syndrome) D69.2
- **Autographism** L5Ø.3
- **Autoimmune**
  - disease (systemic) M35.9
  - inhibitors to clotting factors D68.311
  - lymphoproliferative syndrome [ALPS] D89.82
  - thyroiditis EØ6.3
- **Autointoxication** R68.89
- **Automatism** G93.89
  - with temporal sclerosis G93.81
  - epileptic — *see* Epilepsy, localization-related, symptomatic, with complex partial seizures
  - paroxysmal, idiopathic — *see* Epilepsy, localization-related, symptomatic, with complex partial seizures
- **Autonomic, autonomous**
  - bladder (neurogenic) N31.2
  - hysteria seizure F44.5
- **Autosensitivity, erythrocyte** D69.2
- **Autosensitization, cutaneous** L3Ø.2
- **Autosome** — *see* condition by chromosome involved
- **Autotopagnosia** R48.1
- **Autotoxemia** R68.89
- **Autumn** — *see* condition
- **Avellis' syndrome** G46.8
- **Aversion**
  - oral R63.39
    - newborn P92.- ☑
    - nonorganic origin F98.2 ☑
  - sexual F52.1
- **Aviator's**
  - disease or sickness — *see* Effect, adverse, high altitude
  - ear T7Ø.Ø ☑
- **Avitaminosis** (multiple) — *see also* Deficiency, vitamin E56.9
  - B E53.9
    - with
      - beriberi E51.11
      - pellagra E52
  - B2 E53.Ø
  - B6 E53.1
  - B12 E53.8
  - D E55.9
    - with rickets E55.Ø
  - G E53.Ø
  - K E56.1
  - nicotinic acid E52
- **AVNRT** (atrioventricular nodal re-entrant tachycardia) I47.1
- **AVRT** (atrioventricular nodal re-entrant tachycardia) I47.1
- **Avulsion** (traumatic)
  - blood vessel — *see* Injury, blood vessel
  - bone — *see* Fracture, by site
  - cartilage — *see also* Dislocation, by site
    - symphyseal (inner), complicating delivery O71.6
  - external site other than limb — *see* Wound, open, by site
  - eye SØ5.7- ☑
  - head (intracranial)
    - external site NEC SØ8.89 ☑
    - scalp SØ8.Ø ☑
  - internal organ or site — *see* Injury, by site
  - joint — *see also* Dislocation, by site
    - capsule — *see* Sprain, by site
  - kidney S37.Ø6- ☑
  - ligament — *see* Sprain, by site
  - limb — *see also* Amputation, traumatic, by site
    - skin and subcutaneous tissue — *see* Wound, open, by site
  - muscle — *see* Injury, muscle
  - nerve (root) — *see* Injury, nerve
  - scalp SØ8.Ø ☑
  - skin and subcutaneous tissue — *see* Wound, open, by site
  - spleen S36.Ø32 ☑
  - symphyseal cartilage (inner), complicating delivery O71.6
  - tendon — *see* Injury, muscle
  - tooth SØ3.2 ☑
- **Awareness of heart beat** RØØ.2
- **Axenfeld's**
  - anomaly or syndrome Q15.Ø
  - degeneration (calcareous) Q13.4
- **Axilla, axillary** — *see also* condition
  - breast Q83.1
- **Axonotmesis** — *see* Injury, nerve
- **Ayerza's disease or syndrome** (pulmonary artery sclerosis with pulmonary hypertension) I27.Ø
- **Azoospermia** (organic) N46.Ø1
  - due to
    - drug therapy N46.Ø21
    - efferent duct obstruction N46.Ø23
    - infection N46.Ø22
    - radiation N46.Ø24
    - specified cause NEC N46.Ø29
    - systemic disease N46.Ø25
- **Azotemia** R79.89
  - meaning uremia N19
- **Aztec ear** Q17.3
- **Azygos**
  - continuation inferior vena cava Q26.8
  - lobe (lung) Q33.1

B

- **Baastrup's disease** — *see* Kissing spine
- **Babesiosis** B6Ø.ØØ
  - due to
    - Babesia
      - divergens B6Ø.Ø3
      - duncani B6Ø.Ø2
      - KO-1 B6Ø.Ø9
      - microti B6Ø.Ø1
      - MO-1 B6Ø.Ø3
      - species
        - unspecified B6Ø.ØØ
      - venatorum B6Ø.Ø9
    - specified NEC B6Ø.Ø9
- **Babington's disease** (familial hemorrhagic telangiectasia) I78.Ø
- **Babinski's syndrome** A52.79
- **Baby**
  - crying constantly R68.11
  - floppy (syndrome) P94.2
- **Bacillary** — *see* condition
- **Bacilluria** R82.71
- **Bacillus** — *see also* Infection, bacillus
  - abortus infection A23.1
  - anthracis infection A22.9
  - coli infection — *see also* Escherichia coli B96.2Ø
  - Flexner's AØ3.1
  - mallei infection A24.Ø
  - Shiga's AØ3.Ø
  - suipestifer infection — *see* Infection, salmonella
- **Back** — *see* condition
- **Backache** (postural) M54.9
  - sacroiliac M53.3
  - specified NEC M54.89
- **Backflow** — *see* Reflux
- **Backward reading** (dyslexia) F81.Ø
- **Bacteremia** R78.81
  - with sepsis — *see* Sepsis
- **Bactericholia** — *see* Cholecystitis, acute
- **Bacterid, bacteride** (pustular) L4Ø.3
- **Bacterium, bacteria, bacterial**
  - agent NEC, as cause of disease classified elsewhere B96.89
  - in blood — *see* Bacteremia
  - in urine — *see* Bacteriuria
- **Bacteriuria, bacteruria** R82.71
  - asymptomatic R82.71
- **Bacteroides**
  - fragilis, as cause of disease classified elsewhere B96.6
- **Bad**
  - heart — *see* Disease, heart
  - trip
    - due to drug abuse — *see* Abuse, drug, hallucinogen
    - due to drug dependence — *see* Dependence, drug, hallucinogen
- **Baelz's disease** (cheilitis glandularis apostematosa) K13.Ø
- **Baerensprung's disease** (eczema marginatum) B35.6
- **Bagasse disease or pneumonitis** J67.1
- **Bagassosis** J67.1
- **Baker's cyst** — *see* Cyst, Baker's
- **Bakwin-Krida syndrome** (metaphyseal dysplasia) Q78.5
- **Balancing side interference** M26.56
- **Balanitis** (circinata) (erosiva) (gangrenosa) (phagedenic) (vulgaris) N48.1
  - amebic AØ6.82
  - candidal B37.42
  - due to Haemophilus ducreyi A57
  - gonococcal (acute) (chronic) A54.23
  - xerotica obliterans N48.Ø
- **Balanoposthitis** N47.6
  - gonococcal (acute) (chronic) A54.23
  - ulcerative (specific) A63.8
- **Balanorrhagia** — *see* Balanitis
- **Balantidiasis, balantidiosis** AØ7.Ø
- **Bald tongue** K14.4
- **Baldness** — *see also* Alopecia
  - male-pattern — *see* Alopecia, androgenic
- **Balkan grippe** A78
- **Balloon disease** — *see* Effect, adverse, high altitude
- **Balo's disease** (concentric sclerosis) G37.5
- **Bamberger-Marie disease** — *see* Osteoarthropathy, hypertrophic, specified type NEC
- **Bancroft's filariasis** B74.Ø
- **Band**(s)
  - adhesive — *see* Adhesions, peritoneum

- **Bite**(s) — *continued*
  - genital organs, external
    - female S31.552 ☑
      - superficial NEC S3Ø.876 ☑
        - insect S3Ø.866 ☑
      - vagina and vulva — *see* Bite, vulva
    - male S31.551 ☑
      - penis — *see* Bite, penis
      - scrotum — *see* Bite, scrotum
      - superficial NEC S3Ø.875 ☑
        - insect S3Ø.865 ☑
      - testes — *see* Bite, testis
  - groin — *see* Bite, abdomen, wall
  - gum — *see* Bite, oral cavity
  - hand S61.45- ☑
    - finger — *see* Bite, finger
    - superficial NEC S6Ø.57- ☑
      - insect S6Ø.56- ☑
    - thumb — *see* Bite, thumb
  - head SØ1.95 ☑
    - cheek — *see* Bite, cheek
    - ear — *see* Bite, ear
    - eyelid — *see* Bite, eyelid
    - lip — *see* Bite, lip
    - nose — *see* Bite, nose
    - oral cavity — *see* Bite, oral cavity
    - scalp — *see* Bite, scalp
    - specified site NEC SØ1.85 ☑
      - superficial NEC SØØ.87 ☑
        - insect SØØ.86 ☑
    - superficial NEC SØØ.97 ☑
      - insect SØØ.96 ☑
    - temporomandibular area — *see* Bite, cheek
  - heel — *see* Bite, foot
  - hip S71.Ø5- ☑
    - superficial NEC S7Ø.27- ☑
      - insect S7Ø.26- ☑
  - hymen S31.45 ☑
  - hypochondrium — *see* Bite, abdomen, wall
  - hypogastric region — *see* Bite, abdomen, wall
  - inguinal region — *see* Bite, abdomen, wall
  - insect — *see* Bite, by site, superficial, insect
  - instep — *see* Bite, foot
  - interscapular region — *see* Bite, thorax, back
  - jaw — *see* Bite, head, specified site NEC
  - knee S81.Ø5- ☑
    - superficial NEC S8Ø.27- ☑
      - insect S8Ø.26- ☑
  - labium (majus) (minus) — *see* Bite, vulva
  - lacrimal duct — *see* Bite, eyelid
  - larynx S11.Ø15 ☑
    - superficial NEC S1Ø.17 ☑
      - insect S1Ø.16 ☑
  - leg (lower) S81.85- ☑
    - ankle — *see* Bite, ankle
    - foot — *see* Bite, foot
    - knee — *see* Bite, knee
    - superficial NEC S8Ø.87- ☑
      - insect S8Ø.86- ☑
    - toe — *see* Bite, toe
    - upper — *see* Bite, thigh
  - lip SØ1.551 ☑
    - superficial NEC SØØ.571 ☑
      - insect SØØ.561 ☑
  - lizard (venomous) — *see* Venom, bite, reptile
  - loin — *see* Bite, abdomen, wall
  - lower back — *see* Bite, back, lower
  - lumbar region — *see* Bite, back, lower
  - malar region — *see* Bite, head, specified site NEC
  - mammary — *see* Bite, breast
  - marine animals (venomous) — *see* Toxicity, venom, marine animal
  - mastoid region — *see* Bite, head, specified site NEC
  - mouth — *see* Bite, oral cavity
  - nail
    - finger — *see* Bite, finger
    - toe — *see* Bite, toe
  - nape — *see* Bite, neck, specified site NEC
  - nasal (septum) (sinus) — *see* Bite, nose
  - nasopharynx — *see* Bite, head, specified site NEC
  - neck S11.95 ☑
    - involving
      - cervical esophagus — *see* Bite, esophagus, cervical
      - larynx — *see* Bite, larynx
      - pharynx — *see* Bite, pharynx

- **Bite**(s) — *continued*
  - neck — *continued*
    - involving — *continued*
      - thyroid gland S11.15 ☑
      - trachea — *see* Bite, trachea
    - specified site NEC S11.85 ☑
      - superficial NEC S1Ø.87 ☑
        - insect S1Ø.86 ☑
    - superficial NEC S1Ø.97 ☑
      - insect S1Ø.96 ☑
    - throat S11.85 ☑
      - superficial NEC S1Ø.17 ☑
        - insect S1Ø.16 ☑
  - nose (septum) (sinus) SØ1.25 ☑
    - superficial NEC SØØ.37 ☑
      - insect SØØ.36 ☑
  - occipital region — *see* Bite, scalp
  - oral cavity SØ1.552 ☑
    - superficial NEC SØØ.572 ☑
      - insect SØØ.562 ☑
  - orbital region — *see* Bite, eyelid
  - palate — *see* Bite, oral cavity
  - palm — *see* Bite, hand
  - parietal region — *see* Bite, scalp
  - pelvis S31.Ø5Ø ☑
    - with penetration into retroperitoneal space S31.Ø51 ☑
    - superficial NEC S3Ø.87Ø ☑
      - insect S3Ø.86Ø ☑
  - penis S31.25 ☑
    - superficial NEC S3Ø.872 ☑
      - insect S3Ø.862 ☑
  - perineum
    - female — *see* Bite, vulva
    - male — *see* Bite, pelvis
  - periocular area (with or without lacrimal passages) — *see* Bite, eyelid
  - phalanges
    - finger — *see* Bite, finger
    - toe — *see* Bite, toe
  - pharynx S11.25 ☑
    - superficial NEC S1Ø.17 ☑
      - insect S1Ø.16 ☑
  - pinna — *see* Bite, ear
  - poisonous — *see* Venom
  - popliteal space — *see* Bite, knee
  - prepuce — *see* Bite, penis
  - pubic region — *see* Bite, abdomen, wall
  - rectovaginal septum — *see* Bite, vulva
  - red bug B88.Ø
  - reptile NEC — *see also* Venom, bite, reptile
    - nonvenomous — *see* Bite, by site
    - snake — *see* Venom, bite, snake
  - sacral region — *see* Bite, back, lower
  - sacroiliac region — *see* Bite, back, lower
  - salivary gland — *see* Bite, oral cavity
  - scalp SØ1.Ø5 ☑
    - superficial NEC SØØ.Ø7 ☑
      - insect SØØ.Ø6 ☑
  - scapular region — *see* Bite, shoulder
  - scrotum S31.35 ☑
    - superficial NEC S3Ø.873 ☑
      - insect S3Ø.863 ☑
  - sea-snake (venomous) — *see* Toxicity, venom, snake, sea snake
  - shin — *see* Bite, leg
  - shoulder S41.Ø5- ☑
    - superficial NEC S4Ø.27- ☑
      - insect S4Ø.26- ☑
  - snake — *see also* Venom, bite, snake
    - nonvenomous — *see* Bite, by site
  - spermatic cord — *see* Bite, testis
  - spider (venomous) — *see* Toxicity, venom, spider
    - nonvenomous — *see* Bite, by site, superficial, insect
  - sternal region — *see* Bite, thorax, front
  - submaxillary region — *see* Bite, head, specified site NEC
  - submental region — *see* Bite, head, specified site NEC
  - subungual
    - finger(s) — *see* Bite, finger
    - toe — *see* Bite, toe
  - superficial — *see* Bite, by site, superficial
  - supraclavicular fossa S11.85 ☑
  - supraorbital — *see* Bite, head, specified site NEC
  - temple, temporal region — *see* Bite, head, specified site NEC

- **Bite**(s) — *continued*
  - temporomandibular area — *see* Bite, cheek
  - testis S31.35 ☑
    - superficial NEC S3Ø.873 ☑
      - insect S3Ø.863 ☑
  - thigh S71.15- ☑
    - superficial NEC S7Ø.37- ☑
      - insect S7Ø.36- ☑
  - thorax, thoracic (wall) S21.95 ☑
    - back S21.25- ☑
      - with penetration into thoracic cavity S21.45- ☑
    - breast — *see* Bite, breast
    - front S21.15- ☑
      - with penetration into thoracic cavity S21.35- ☑
    - superficial NEC S2Ø.97 ☑
      - back S2Ø.47- ☑
      - front S2Ø.37- ☑
      - insect S2Ø.96 ☑
        - back S2Ø.46- ☑
        - front S2Ø.36- ☑
  - throat — *see* Bite, neck, throat
  - thumb S61.Ø5- ☑
    - with
      - damage to nail S61.15- ☑
    - superficial NEC S6Ø.37- ☑
      - insect S6Ø.36- ☑
  - thyroid S11.15 ☑
    - superficial NEC S1Ø.87 ☑
      - insect S1Ø.86 ☑
  - toe(s) S91.15- ☑
    - with
      - damage to nail S91.25- ☑
    - great S91.15- ☑
      - with
        - damage to nail S91.25- ☑
    - lesser S91.15- ☑
      - with
        - damage to nail S91.25- ☑
    - superficial NEC S9Ø.47- ☑
      - great S9Ø.47- ☑
      - insect S9Ø.46- ☑
        - great S9Ø.46- ☑
  - tongue SØ1.552 ☑
  - trachea S11.Ø25 ☑
    - superficial NEC S1Ø.17 ☑
      - insect S1Ø.16 ☑
  - tunica vaginalis — *see* Bite, testis
  - tympanum, tympanic membrane — *see* Bite, ear
  - umbilical region S31.155 ☑
  - uvula — *see* Bite, oral cavity
  - vagina — *see* Bite, vulva
  - venomous — *see* Venom
  - vocal cords S11.Ø35 ☑
    - superficial NEC S1Ø.17 ☑
      - insect S1Ø.16 ☑
  - vulva S31.45 ☑
    - superficial NEC S3Ø.874 ☑
      - insect S3Ø.864 ☑
  - wrist S61.55- ☑
    - superficial NEC S6Ø.87- ☑
      - insect S6Ø.86- ☑
- **Biting, cheek or lip** K13.1
- **Biventricular failure** (heart) I5Ø.82
- **Björck** (-Thorson) **syndrome** (malignant carcinoid) E34.Ø
- **Black**
  - death A2Ø.9
  - eye SØØ.1- ☑
  - hairy tongue K14.3
  - heel (foot) S9Ø.3- ☑
  - lung (disease) J6Ø
  - palm (hand) S6Ø.22- ☑
- **Blackfan-Diamond anemia or syndrome** (congenital hypoplastic anemia) D61.Ø1
- **Blackhead** L7Ø.Ø
- **Blackout** R55
- **Bladder** — *see* condition
- **Blast** (air) (hydraulic) (immersion) (underwater)
  - blindness SØ5.8X- ☑
  - injury
    - abdomen or thorax — *see* Injury, by site
    - ear (acoustic nerve trauma) — *see* Injury, nerve, acoustic, specified type NEC
  - syndrome NEC T7Ø.8 ☑
- **Blastoma** — *see* Neoplasm, malignant, by site
  - pulmonary — *see* Neoplasm, lung, malignant
- **Blastomycosis, blastomycotic** B4Ø.9

Body, bodies — *continued*
- mass index — *continued*
  - adult — *continued*
    - 50.0-59.9 Z68.43
    - 60.0-69.9 Z68.44
    - 70 and over Z68.45
  - pediatric
    - 5th percentile to less than 85th percentile for age Z68.52
    - 85th percentile to less than 95th percentile for age Z68.53
    - greater than or equal to ninety-fifth percentile for age Z68.54
    - less than fifth percentile for age Z68.51
- Mooser's A75.2
- rice — *see also* Loose, body, joint
  - knee M23.4- ☑
- rocking F98.4

Boeck's
- disease or sarcoid — *see* Sarcoidosis
- lupoid (miliary) D86.3

Boerhaave's syndrome (spontaneous esophageal rupture) K22.3

Boggy
- cervix N88.8
- uterus N85.8

Boil — *see also* Furuncle, by site
- Aleppo B55.1
- Baghdad B55.1
- Delhi B55.1
- lacrimal
  - gland — *see* Dacryoadenitis
  - passages (duct) (sac) — *see* Inflammation, lacrimal, passages, acute
- Natal B55.1
- orbit, orbital — *see* Abscess, orbit
- tropical B55.1

Bold hives — *see* Urticaria

Bombé, iris — *see* Membrane, pupillary

Bone — *see* condition

Bonnevie-Ullrich syndrome — *see also* Turner's syndrome Q87.19

Bonnier's syndrome H81.8 ☑

Bonvale dam fever T73.3 ☑

Bony block of joint — *see* Ankylosis

BOOP (bronchiolitis obliterans organized pneumonia) J84.89

Borderline
- diabetes mellitus R73.03
- hypertension R03.0
- osteopenia M85.8- ☑
- pelvis, with obstruction during labor O65.1
- personality F60.3

Borna disease A83.9

Bornholm disease B33.0

Boston exanthem A88.0

Botalli, ductus (patent) (persistent) Q25.0

Bothriocephalus latus infestation B70.0

Botulism (foodborne intoxication) A05.1
- infant A48.51
- non-foodborne A48.52
- wound A48.52

Bouba — *see* Yaws

Bouchard's nodes (with arthropathy) M15.2

Bouffée délirante F23

Bouillaud's disease or syndrome (rheumatic heart disease) I01.9

Bourneville's disease Q85.1

Boutonniere deformity (finger) — *see* Deformity, finger, boutonniere

Bouveret (-Hoffmann) **syndrome** (paroxysmal tachycardia) I47.9

Bovine heart — *see* Hypertrophy, cardiac

Bowel — *see* condition

Bowen's
- dermatosis (precancerous) — *see* Neoplasm, skin, in situ
- disease — *see* Neoplasm, skin, in situ
- epithelioma — *see* Neoplasm, skin, in situ
- type
  - epidermoid carcinoma-in-situ — *see* Neoplasm, skin, in situ
  - intraepidermal squamous cell carcinoma — *see* Neoplasm, skin, in situ

Bowing
- femur — *see also* Deformity, limb, specified type NEC, thigh

Bowing — *continued*
- femur — *see also* Deformity, limb, specified type, thigh — *continued*
  - congenital Q68.3
- fibula — *see also* Deformity, limb, specified type NEC, lower leg
  - congenital Q68.4
- forearm — *see* Deformity, limb, specified type NEC, forearm
- leg(s), long bones, congenital Q68.5
- radius — *see* Deformity, limb, specified type NEC, forearm
- tibia — *see also* Deformity, limb, specified type NEC, lower leg
  - congenital Q68.4

Bowleg(s) (acquired) M21.16- ☑
- congenital Q68.5
- rachitic E64.3

Boyd's dysentery A03.2

Brachial — *see* condition

Brachycardia R00.1

Brachycephaly Q75.0

Bradley's disease A08.19

Bradyarrhythmia, cardiac I49.8

Bradycardia (sinoatrial) (sinus) (vagal) R00.1
- neonatal P29.12
- reflex G90.09
- tachycardia syndrome I49.5

Bradykinesia R25.8

Bradypnea R06.89

Bradytachycardia I49.5

Brailsford's disease or osteochondrosis — *see* Osteochondrosis, juvenile, radius

Brain — *see also* condition
- death G93.82
- syndrome — *see* Syndrome, brain

Branched-chain amino-acid disorder E71.2

Branchial — *see* condition
- cartilage, congenital Q18.2

Branchiogenic remnant (in neck) Q18.0

Brandt's syndrome (acrodermatitis enteropathica) E83.2

Brash (water) R12

Bravais-jacksonian epilepsy — *see* Epilepsy, localization-related, symptomatic, with simple partial seizures

Braxton Hicks contractions — *see* False, labor

Brazilian leishmaniasis B55.2

BRBPR K62.5

Break, retina (without detachment) H33.30- ☑
- with retinal detachment — *see* Detachment, retina
- horseshoe tear H33.31- ☑
- multiple H33.33- ☑
- round hole H33.32- ☑

Breakdown
- device, graft or implant — *see also* Complications, by site and type, mechanical T85.618 ☑
  - arterial graft NEC — *see* Complication, cardiovascular device, mechanical, vascular
  - breast (implant) T85.41 ☑
  - catheter NEC T85.618 ☑
    - cystostomy T83.010 ☑
    - dialysis (renal) T82.41 ☑
      - intraperitoneal T85.611 ☑
    - Hopkins T83.018 ☑
    - ileostomy T83.018 ☑
    - infusion NEC T82.514 ☑
      - cranial T85.610- ☑
      - epidural T85.610 ☑
      - intrathecal T85.610 ☑
      - spinal T85.610 ☑
      - subarachnoid T85.610 ☑
      - subdural T85.610 ☑
    - nephrostomy T83.012 ☑
    - urethral indwelling T83.011 ☑
    - urinary NEC T83.018 ☑
    - urostomy T83.018 ☑
  - electronic (electrode) (pulse generator) (stimulator)
    - bone T84.310 ☑
    - cardiac T82.119 ☑
      - electrode T82.110 ☑
      - pulse generator T82.111 ☑
      - specified type NEC T82.118 ☑
    - nervous system — *see* Complication, prosthetic device, mechanical, electronic nervous system stimulator
    - urinary — *see* Complication, genitourinary, device, urinary, mechanical

Breakdown — *continued*
- device, graft or implant — *see also* Complications, by site and type, mechanical — *continued*
  - fixation, internal (orthopedic) NEC — *see* Complication, fixation device, mechanical
  - gastrointestinal — *see* Complications, prosthetic device, mechanical, gastrointestinal device
  - genital NEC T83.418 ☑
    - intrauterine contraceptive device T83.31 ☑
    - penile prosthesis (cylinder) (implanted) (pump) (resevoir) T83.410 ☑
    - testicular prosthesis T83.411 ☑
  - heart NEC — *see* Complication, cardiovascular device, mechanical
  - intrathecal infusion pump T85.615 ☑
  - joint prosthesis — *see* Complications, joint prosthesis, internal, mechanical, by site
  - nervous system, specified device NEC T85.615 ☑
  - ocular NEC — *see* Complications, prosthetic device, mechanical, ocular device
  - orthopedic NEC — *see* Complication, orthopedic, device, mechanical
  - specified NEC T85.618 ☑
  - subcutaneous device pocket
    - nervous system prosthetic device, implant, or graft T85.890 ☑
    - other internal prosthetic device, implant, or graft T85.898 ☑
  - sutures, permanent T85.612 ☑
    - used in bone repair — *see* Complications, fixation device, internal (orthopedic), mechanical
  - urinary NEC T83.118 ☑
    - graft T83.21 ☑
    - sphincter, implanted T83.111 ☑
    - stent (ileal conduit) (nephroureteral) T83.113 ☑
      - ureteral indwelling T83.112 ☑
  - vascular NEC — *see* Complication, cardiovascular device, mechanical
  - ventricular intracranial shunt T85.01 ☑
- nervous F48.8
- perineum O90.1
- respirator J95.850
  - specified NEC J95.859
- ventilator J95.850
  - specified NEC J95.859

Breast — *see also* condition
- buds E30.1
  - in newborn P96.89
- dense R92.2
- nodule — *see also* Lump, breast N63.0

Breath
- foul R19.6
- holder, child R06.89
- holding spell R06.89
- shortness R06.02

Breathing
- labored — *see* Hyperventilation
- mouth R06.5
  - causing malocclusion M26.5 ☑
- periodic R06.3
  - high altitude G47.32

Breathlessness R06.81

Breda's disease — *see* Yaws

Breech presentation (mother) O32.1 ☑
- causing obstructed labor O64.1 ☑
- footling O32.8 ☑
  - causing obstructed labor O64.8 ☑
- incomplete O32.8 ☑
  - causing obstructed labor O64.8 ☑

Breisky's disease N90.4

Brennemann's syndrome I88.0

Brenner
- tumor (benign) D27.9
  - borderline malignancy D39.1- ☑
  - malignant C56 ☑
  - proliferating D39.1- ☑

Bretonneau's disease or angina A36.0

Breus' mole O02.0

Brevicollis Q76.49

Brickmakers' anemia B76.9 *[D63.8]*

Bridge, myocardial Q24.5

Bright red blood per rectum (BRBPR) K62.5

Bright's disease — *see also* Nephritis
- arteriosclerotic — *see* Hypertension, kidney

Brill (-Zinsser) **disease** (recrudescent typhus) A75.1

Brill-Symmers' disease C82.90

Brion-Kayser disease — *see* Fever, parathyroid

- **Bubo** — *continued*
  - scrofulous (tuberculous) A18.2
  - soft chancre A57
  - suppurating — *see* Lymphadenitis, acute
  - syphilitic (primary) A51.Ø
    - congenital A5Ø.Ø7
  - tropical A55
  - virulent (chancroidal) A57
- **Bubonic plague** A2Ø.Ø
- **Bubonocele** — *see* Hernia, inguinal
- **Buccal** — *see* condition
- **Buchanan's disease or osteochondrosis** M91.Ø
- **Buchem's syndrome** (hyperostosis corticalis) M85.2
- **Bucket-handle fracture or tear** (semilunar cartilage) — *see* Tear, meniscus
- **Budd-Chiari syndrome** (hepatic vein thrombosis) I82.Ø
- **Budgerigar fancier's disease or lung** J67.2
- **Buds**
  - breast E3Ø.1
    - in newborn P96.89
- **Buerger's disease** (thromboangiitis obliterans) I73.1
- **Bulbar** — *see* condition
- **Bulbus cordis** (left ventricle) (persistent) Q21.8
- **Bulimia** (nervosa) F5Ø.2
  - atypical F5Ø.9
  - normal weight F5Ø.9
- **Bulky**
  - stools R19.5
  - uterus N85.2
- **Bulla** (e) R23.8
  - lung (emphysematous) (solitary) J43.9
    - newborn P25.8
- **Bullet wound** — *see also* Puncture
  - fracture — *code as* Fracture, by site
  - internal organ — *see* Injury, by site
- **Bundle**
  - branch block (complete) (false) (incomplete) — *see* Block, bundle-branch
  - of His — *see* condition
- **Bunion** M21.61- ☑
  - tailor's M21.62- ☑
- **Bunionette** M21.62- ☑
- **Buphthalmia, buphthalmos** (congenital) Q15.Ø
- **Burdwan fever** B55.Ø
- **Bürger-Grütz disease or syndrome** E78.3
- **Buried**
  - penis (congenital) Q55.64
    - acquired N48.83
  - roots KØ8.3
- **Burke's syndrome** K86.89
- **Burkitt**
  - cell leukemia C91.Ø- ☑
  - lymphoma (malignant) C83.7- ☑
    - small noncleaved, diffuse C83.7- ☑
    - spleen C83.77
    - undifferentiated C83.7- ☑
  - tumor C83.7- ☑
  - type
    - acute lymphoblastic leukemia C91.Ø- ☑
    - undifferentiated C83.7- ☑
- **Burn** (electricity) (flame) (hot gas, liquid or hot object) (radiation) (steam) (thermal) T3Ø.Ø
  - abdomen, abdominal (muscle) (wall) T21.Ø2 ☑
    - first degree T21.12 ☑
    - second degree T21.22 ☑
    - third degree T21.32 ☑
  - above elbow T22.Ø39 ☑
    - first degree T22.139 ☑
    - left T22.Ø32 ☑
      - first degree T22.132 ☑
      - second degree T22.232 ☑
      - third degree T22.332 ☑
    - right T22.Ø31 ☑
      - first degree T22.131 ☑
      - second degree T22.231 ☑
      - third degree T22.331 ☑
    - second degree T22.239 ☑
    - third degree T22.339 ☑
  - acid (caustic) (external) (internal) — *see* Corrosion, by site
  - alimentary tract NEC T28.2 ☑
    - esophagus T28.1 ☑
    - mouth T28.Ø ☑
    - pharynx T28.Ø ☑
  - alkaline (caustic) (external) (internal) — *see* Corrosion, by site

- **Burn** — *continued*
  - ankle T25.Ø19 ☑
    - first degree T25.119 ☑
    - left T25.Ø12 ☑
      - first degree T25.112 ☑
      - second degree T25.212 ☑
      - third degree T25.312 ☑
    - multiple with foot — *see* Burn, lower, limb, multiple, ankle and foot
    - right T25.Ø11 ☑
      - first degree T25.111 ☑
      - second degree T25.211 ☑
      - third degree T25.311 ☑
    - second degree T25.219 ☑
    - third degree T25.319 ☑
  - anus — *see* Burn, buttock
  - arm (lower) (upper) — *see* Burn, upper, limb
  - axilla T22.Ø49 ☑
    - first degree T22.149 ☑
    - left T22.Ø42 ☑
      - first degree T22.142 ☑
      - second degree T22.242 ☑
      - third degree T22.342 ☑
    - right T22.Ø41 ☑
      - first degree T22.141 ☑
      - second degree T22.241 ☑
      - third degree T22.341 ☑
    - second degree T22.249 ☑
    - third degree T22.349 ☑
  - back (lower) T21.Ø4 ☑
    - first degree T21.14 ☑
    - second degree T21.24 ☑
    - third degree T21.34 ☑
    - upper T21.Ø3 ☑
      - first degree T21.13 ☑
      - second degree T21.23 ☑
      - third degree T21.33 ☑
  - blisters — *code as* Burn, second degree, by site
  - breast(s) — *see* Burn, chest wall
  - buttock(s) T21.Ø5 ☑
    - first degree T21.15 ☑
    - second degree T21.25 ☑
    - third degree T21.35 ☑
  - calf T24.Ø39 ☑
    - first degree T24.139 ☑
    - left T24.Ø32 ☑
      - first degree T24.132 ☑
      - second degree T24.232 ☑
      - third degree T24.332 ☑
    - right T24.Ø31 ☑
      - first degree T24.131 ☑
      - second degree T24.231 ☑
      - third degree T24.331 ☑
    - second degree T24.239 ☑
    - third degree T24.339 ☑
  - canthus (eye) — *see* Burn, eyelid
  - caustic acid or alkaline — *see* Corrosion, by site
  - cervix T28.3 ☑
  - cheek T2Ø.Ø6 ☑
    - first degree T2Ø.16 ☑
    - second degree T2Ø.26 ☑
    - third degree T2Ø.36 ☑
  - chemical (acids) (alkalines) (caustics) (external) (internal) — *see* Corrosion, by site
  - chest wall T21.Ø1 ☑
    - first degree T21.11 ☑
    - second degree T21.21 ☑
    - third degree T21.31 ☑
  - chin T2Ø.Ø3 ☑
    - first degree T2Ø.13 ☑
    - second degree T2Ø.23 ☑
    - third degree T2Ø.33 ☑
  - colon T28.2 ☑
  - conjunctiva (and cornea) — *see* Burn, cornea
  - cornea (and conjunctiva) T26.1- ☑
    - chemical — *see* Corrosion, cornea
  - corrosion (external) (internal) — *see* Corrosion, by site
  - deep necrosis of underlying tissue — *code as* Burn, third degree, by site
  - dorsum of hand T23.Ø69 ☑
    - first degree T23.169 ☑
    - left T23.Ø62 ☑
      - first degree T23.162 ☑
      - second degree T23.262 ☑
      - third degree T23.362 ☑
    - right T23.Ø61 ☑

- **Burn** — *continued*
  - dorsum of hand — *continued*
    - right — *continued*
      - first degree T23.161 ☑
      - second degree T23.261 ☑
      - third degree T23.361 ☑
    - second degree T23.269 ☑
    - third degree T23.369 ☑
  - due to ingested chemical agent — *see* Corrosion, by site
  - ear (auricle) (external) (canal) T2Ø.Ø1 ☑
    - first degree T2Ø.11 ☑
    - second degree T2Ø.21 ☑
    - third degree T2Ø.31 ☑
  - elbow T22.Ø29 ☑
    - first degree T22.129 ☑
    - left T22.Ø22 ☑
      - first degree T22.122 ☑
      - second degree T22.222 ☑
      - third degree T22.322 ☑
    - right T22.Ø21 ☑
      - first degree T22.121 ☑
      - second degree T22.221 ☑
      - third degree T22.321 ☑
    - second degree T22.229 ☑
    - third degree T22.329 ☑
  - epidermal loss — *code as* Burn, second degree, by site
  - erythema, erythematous — *code as* Burn, first degree, by site
  - esophagus T28.1 ☑
  - extent (percentage of body surface)
    - less than 1Ø percent T31.Ø
    - 1Ø-19 percent T31.1Ø
      - with Ø-9 percent third degree burns T31.1Ø
      - with 1Ø-19 percent third degree burns T31.11
    - 2Ø-29 percent T31.2Ø
      - with Ø-9 percent third degree burns T31.2Ø
      - with 1Ø-19 percent third degree burns T31.21
      - with 2Ø-29 percent third degree burns T31.22
    - 3Ø-39 percent T31.3Ø
      - with Ø-9 percent third degree burns T31.3Ø
      - with 1Ø-19 percent third degree burns T31.31
      - with 2Ø-29 percent third degree burns T31.32
      - with 3Ø-39 percent third degree burns T31.33
    - 4Ø-49 percent T31.4Ø
      - with Ø-9 percent third degree burns T31.4Ø
      - with 1Ø-19 percent third degree burns T31.41
      - with 2Ø-29 percent third degree burns T31.42
      - with 3Ø-39 percent third degree burns T31.43
      - with 4Ø-49 percent third degree burns T31.44
    - 5Ø-59 percent T31.5Ø
      - with Ø-9 percent third degree burns T31.5Ø
      - with 1Ø-19 percent third degree burns T31.51
      - with 2Ø-29 percent third degree burns T31.52
      - with 3Ø-39 percent third degree burns T31.53
      - with 4Ø-49 percent third degree burns T31.54
      - with 5Ø-59 percent third degree burns T31.55
    - 6Ø-69 percent T31.6Ø
      - with Ø-9 percent third degree burns T31.6Ø
      - with 1Ø-19 percent third degree burns T31.61
      - with 2Ø-29 percent third degree burns T31.62
      - with 3Ø-39 percent third degree burns T31.63
      - with 4Ø-49 percent third degree burns T31.64
      - with 5Ø-59 percent third degree burns T31.65
      - with 6Ø-69 percent third degree burns T31.66
    - 7Ø-79 percent T31.7Ø
      - with Ø-9 percent third degree burns T31.7Ø
      - with 1Ø-19 percent third degree burns T31.71
      - with 2Ø-29 percent third degree burns T31.72
      - with 3Ø-39 percent third degree burns T31.73
      - with 4Ø-49 percent third degree burns T31.74
      - with 5Ø-59 percent third degree burns T31.75
      - with 6Ø-69 percent third degree burns T31.76
      - with 7Ø-79 percent third degree burns T31.77
    - 8Ø-89 percent T31.8Ø
      - with Ø-9 percent third degree burns T31.8Ø
      - with 1Ø-19 percent third degree burns T31.81
      - with 2Ø-29 percent third degree burns T31.82
      - with 3Ø-39 percent third degree burns T31.83
      - with 4Ø-49 percent third degree burns T31.84
      - with 5Ø-59 percent third degree burns T31.85
      - with 6Ø-69 percent third degree burns T31.86
      - with 7Ø-79 percent third degree burns T31.87
      - with 8Ø-89 percent third degree burns T31.88
    - 9Ø percent or more T31.9Ø
      - with Ø-9 percent third degree burns T31.9Ø
      - with 1Ø-19 percent third degree burns T31.91
      - with 2Ø-29 percent third degree burns T31.92

Burn — *continued*
  extent — *continued*
    9Ø percent or more — *continued*
      with 3Ø-39 percent third degree burns T31.93
      with 4Ø-49 percent third degree burns T31.94
      with 5Ø-59 percent third degree burns T31.95
      with 6Ø-69 percent third degree burns T31.96
      with 7Ø-79 percent third degree burns T31.97
      with 8Ø-89 percent third degree burns T31.98
      with 9Ø percent or more third degree burns T31.99
  extremity — *see* Burn, limb
  eye(s) and adnexa T26.4- ☑
    with resulting rupture and destruction of eyeball T26.2- ☑
    conjunctival sac — *see* Burn, cornea
    cornea — *see* Burn, cornea
    lid — *see* Burn, eyelid
    periocular area — *see* Burn, eyelid
    specified site NEC T26.3- ☑
  eyeball — *see* Burn, eye
  eyelid(s) T26.Ø- ☑
    chemical — *see* Corrosion, eyelid
  face — *see* Burn, head
  finger T23.Ø29 ☑
    first degree T23.129 ☑
    left T23.Ø22 ☑
      first degree T23.122 ☑
      second degree T23.222 ☑
      third degree T23.322 ☑
    multiple sites (without thumb) T23.Ø39 ☑
      with thumb T23.Ø49 ☑
        first degree T23.149 ☑
        left T23.Ø42 ☑
          first degree T23.142 ☑
          second degree T23.242 ☑
          third degree T23.342 ☑
        right T23.Ø41 ☑
          first degree T23.141 ☑
          second degree T23.241 ☑
          third degree T23.341 ☑
        second degree T23.249 ☑
        third degree T23.349 ☑
      first degree T23.139 ☑
      left T23.Ø32 ☑
        first degree T23.132 ☑
        second degree T23.232 ☑
        third degree T23.332 ☑
      right T23.Ø31 ☑
        first degree T23.131 ☑
        second degree T23.231 ☑
        third degree T23.331 ☑
      second degree T23.239 ☑
      third degree T23.339 ☑
    right T23.Ø21 ☑
      first degree T23.121 ☑
      second degree T23.221 ☑
      third degree T23.321 ☑
    second degree T23.229 ☑
    third degree T23.329 ☑
  flank — *see* Burn, abdominal wall
  foot T25.Ø29 ☑
    first degree T25.129 ☑
    left T25.Ø22 ☑
      first degree T25.122 ☑
      second degree T25.222 ☑
      third degree T25.322 ☑
    multiple with ankle — *see* Burn, lower, limb, multiple, ankle and foot
    right T25.Ø21 ☑
      first degree T25.121 ☑
      second degree T25.221 ☑
      third degree T25.321 ☑
    second degree T25.229 ☑
    third degree T25.329 ☑
  forearm T22.Ø19 ☑
    first degree T22.119 ☑
    left T22.Ø12 ☑
      first degree T22.112 ☑
      second degree T22.212 ☑
      third degree T22.312 ☑
    right T22.Ø11 ☑
      first degree T22.111 ☑
      second degree T22.211 ☑
      third degree T22.311 ☑
    second degree T22.219 ☑

Burn — *continued*
  forearm — *continued*
    third degree T22.319 ☑
  forehead T2Ø.Ø6 ☑
    first degree T2Ø.16 ☑
    second degree T2Ø.26 ☑
    third degree T2Ø.36 ☑
  fourth degree — *code as* Burn, third degree, by site
  friction — *see* Burn, by site
  from swallowing caustic or corrosive substance NEC — *see* Corrosion, by site
  full thickness skin loss — *code as* Burn, third degree, by site
  gastrointestinal tract NEC T28.2 ☑
    from swallowing caustic or corrosive substance T28.7 ☑
  genital organs
    external
      female T21.Ø7 ☑
        first degree T21.17 ☑
        second degree T21.27 ☑
        third degree T21.37 ☑
      male T21.Ø6 ☑
        first degree T21.16 ☑
        second degree T21.26 ☑
        third degree T21.36 ☑
    internal T28.3 ☑
      from caustic or corrosive substance T28.8 ☑
  groin — *see* Burn, abdominal wall
  hand(s) T23.ØØ9 ☑
    back — *see* Burn, dorsum of hand
    finger — *see* Burn, finger
    first degree T23.1Ø9 ☑
    left T23.ØØ2 ☑
      first degree T23.1Ø2 ☑
      second degree T23.2Ø2 ☑
      third degree T23.3Ø2 ☑
    multiple sites with wrist T23.Ø99 ☑
      first degree T23.199 ☑
      left T23.Ø92 ☑
        first degree T23.192 ☑
        second degree T23.292 ☑
        third degree T23.392 ☑
      right T23.Ø91 ☑
        first degree T23.191 ☑
        second degree T23.291 ☑
        third degree T23.391 ☑
      second degree T23.299 ☑
      third degree T23.399 ☑
    palm — *see* Burn, palm
    right T23.ØØ1 ☑
      first degree T23.1Ø1 ☑
      second degree T23.2Ø1 ☑
      third degree T23.3Ø1 ☑
    second degree T23.2Ø9 ☑
    third degree T23.3Ø9 ☑
    thumb — *see* Burn, thumb
  head (and face) (and neck) T2Ø.ØØ ☑
    cheek — *see* Burn, cheek
    chin — *see* Burn, chin
    ear — *see* Burn, ear
    eye(s) only — *see* Burn, eye
    first degree T2Ø.1Ø ☑
    forehead — *see* Burn, forehead
    lip — *see* Burn, lip
    multiple sites T2Ø.Ø9 ☑
      first degree T2Ø.19 ☑
      second degree T2Ø.29 ☑
      third degree T2Ø.39 ☑
    neck — *see* Burn, neck
    nose — *see* Burn, nose
    scalp — *see* Burn, scalp
    second degree T2Ø.2Ø ☑
    third degree T2Ø.3Ø ☑
  hip(s) — *see* Burn, thigh
  inhalation — *see* Burn, respiratory tract
    caustic or corrosive substance (fumes) — *see* Corrosion, respiratory tract
  internal organ(s) T28.4Ø ☑
    alimentary tract T28.2 ☑
      esophagus T28.1 ☑
    eardrum T28.41 ☑
    esophagus T28.1 ☑
    from caustic or corrosive substance (swallowing) NEC — *see* Corrosion, by site
    genitourinary T28.3 ☑

Burn — *continued*
  internal organ(s) — *continued*
    mouth T28.Ø ☑
    pharynx T28.Ø ☑
    respiratory tract — *see* Burn, respiratory tract
    specified organ NEC T28.49 ☑
  interscapular region — *see* Burn, back, upper
  intestine (large) (small) T28.2 ☑
  knee T24.Ø29 ☑
    first degree T24.129 ☑
    left T24.Ø22 ☑
      first degree T24.122 ☑
      second degree T24.222 ☑
      third degree T24.322 ☑
    right T24.Ø21 ☑
      first degree T24.121 ☑
      second degree T24.221 ☑
      third degree T24.321 ☑
    second degree T24.229 ☑
    third degree T24.329 ☑
  labium (majus) (minus) — *see* Burn, genital organs, external, female
  lacrimal apparatus, duct, gland or sac — *see* Burn, eye, specified site NEC
  larynx T27.Ø ☑
    with lung T27.1 ☑
  leg(s) (lower) (upper) — *see* Burn, lower, limb
  lightning — *see* Burn, by site
  limb(s)
    lower (except ankle or foot alone) — *see* Burn, lower, limb
    upper — *see* Burn, upper limb
  lip(s) T2Ø.Ø2 ☑
    first degree T2Ø.12 ☑
    second degree T2Ø.22 ☑
    third degree T2Ø.32 ☑
  lower
    back — *see* Burn, back
    limb T24.ØØ9 ☑
      ankle — *see* Burn, ankle
      calf — *see* Burn, calf
      first degree T24.1Ø9 ☑
      foot — *see* Burn, foot
      hip — *see* Burn, thigh
      knee — *see* Burn, knee
      left T24.ØØ2 ☑
        first degree T24.1Ø2 ☑
        second degree T24.2Ø2 ☑
        third degree T24.3Ø2 ☑
      multiple sites, except ankle and foot T24.Ø99 ☑
        ankle and foot T25.Ø99 ☑
          first degree T25.199 ☑
          left T25.Ø92 ☑
            first degree T25.192 ☑
            second degree T25.292 ☑
            third degree T25.392 ☑
          right T25.Ø91 ☑
            first degree T25.191 ☑
            second degree T25.291 ☑
            third degree T25.391 ☑
          second degree T25.299 ☑
          third degree T25.399 ☑
        first degree T24.199 ☑
        left T24.Ø92 ☑
          first degree T24.192 ☑
          second degree T24.292 ☑
          third degree T24.392 ☑
        right T24.Ø91 ☑
          first degree T24.191 ☑
          second degree T24.291 ☑
          third degree T24.391 ☑
        second degree T24.299 ☑
        third degree T24.399 ☑
      right T24.ØØ1 ☑
        first degree T24.1Ø1 ☑
        second degree T24.2Ø1 ☑
        third degree T24.3Ø1 ☑
      second degree T24.2Ø9 ☑
      thigh — *see* Burn, thigh
      third degree T24.3Ø9 ☑
      toe — *see* Burn, toe
  lung (with larynx and trachea) T27.1 ☑
  mouth T28.Ø ☑
  neck T2Ø.Ø7 ☑
    first degree T2Ø.17 ☑
    second degree T2Ø.27 ☑

- **Burn** — *continued*
  - wrist — *continued*
    - left — *continued*
      - first degree T23.172 ☑
      - second degree T23.272 ☑
      - third degree T23.372 ☑
    - multiple sites with hand T23.Ø99 ☑
      - first degree T23.199 ☑
      - left T23.Ø92 ☑
        - first degree T23.192 ☑
        - second degree T23.292 ☑
        - third degree T23.392 ☑
      - right T23.Ø91 ☑
        - first degree T23.191 ☑
        - second degree T23.291 ☑
        - third degree T23.391 ☑
      - second degree T23.299 ☑
      - third degree T23.399 ☑
    - right T23.Ø71 ☑
      - first degree T23.171 ☑
      - second degree T23.271 ☑
      - third degree T23.371 ☑
    - second degree T23.279 ☑
    - third degree T23.379 ☑
- **Burnett's syndrome** E83.52
- **Burning**
  - feet syndrome E53.9
  - sensation R2Ø.8
  - tongue K14.6
- **Burn-out** (state) Z73.Ø
- **Burns' disease or osteochondrosis** — *see* Osteochondrosis, juvenile, ulna
- **Bursa** — *see* condition
- **Bursitis** M71.9
  - Achilles — *see* Tendinitis, Achilles
  - adhesive — *see* Bursitis, specified NEC
  - ankle — *see* Enthesopathy, lower limb, ankle, specified type NEC
  - calcaneal — *see* Enthesopathy, foot, specified type NEC
  - collateral ligament, tibial — *see* Bursitis, tibial collateral
  - due to use, overuse, pressure — *see also* Disorder, soft tissue, due to use, specified type NEC
    - specified NEC — *see* Disorder, soft tissue, due to use, specified NEC
  - Duplay's M75.Ø ☑
  - elbow NEC M7Ø.3- ☑
    - olecranon M7Ø.2- ☑
  - finger — *see* Disorder, soft tissue, due to use, specified type NEC, hand
  - foot — *see* Enthesopathy, foot, specified type NEC
  - gonococcal A54.49
  - gouty — *see* Gout
  - hand M7Ø.1- ☑
  - hip NEC M7Ø.7- ☑
    - trochanteric M7Ø.6- ☑
  - infective NEC M71.1Ø
    - abscess — *see* Abscess, bursa
    - ankle M71.17- ☑
    - elbow M71.12- ☑
    - foot M71.17- ☑
    - hand M71.14- ☑
    - hip M71.15- ☑
    - knee M71.16- ☑
    - multiple sites M71.19
    - shoulder M71.11- ☑
    - specified site NEC M71.18
    - wrist M71.13- ☑
  - ischial — *see* Bursitis, hip
  - knee NEC M7Ø.5- ☑
    - prepatellar M7Ø.4- ☑
  - occupational NEC — *see also* Disorder, soft tissue, due to, use
  - olecranon — *see* Bursitis, elbow, olecranon
  - pharyngeal J39.1
  - popliteal — *see* Bursitis, knee
  - prepatellar M7Ø.4- ☑
  - radiohumeral M7Ø.3- ☑
  - rheumatoid MØ6.2Ø
    - ankle MØ6.27- ☑
    - elbow MØ6.22- ☑
    - foot joint MØ6.27- ☑
    - hand joint MØ6.24- ☑
    - hip MØ6.25- ☑
    - knee MØ6.26- ☑
    - multiple site MØ6.29
    - shoulder MØ6.21- ☑
- **Bursitis** — *continued*
  - rheumatoid — *continued*
    - vertebra MØ6.28
    - wrist MØ6.23- ☑
  - scapulohumeral — *see* Bursitis, shoulder
  - semimembranous muscle (knee) — *see* Bursitis, knee
  - shoulder M75.5- ☑
    - adhesive — *see* Capsulitis, adhesive
  - specified NEC M71.5Ø
    - ankle M71.57- ☑
    - due to use, overuse or pressure — *see* Disorder, soft tissue, due to, use
    - elbow M71.52- ☑
    - foot M71.57- ☑
    - hand M71.54- ☑
    - hip M71.55- ☑
    - knee M71.56- ☑
    - shoulder — *see* Bursitis, shoulder
    - specified site NEC M71.58
    - tibial collateral M76.4- ☑
    - wrist M71.53- ☑
  - subacromial — *see* Bursitis, shoulder
  - subcoracoid — *see* Bursitis, shoulder
  - subdeltoid — *see* Bursitis, shoulder
  - syphilitic A52.78
  - Thornwaldt, Tornwaldt J39.2
  - tibial collateral M76.4- ☑
  - toe — *see* Enthesopathy, foot, specified type NEC
  - trochanteric (area) — *see* Bursitis, hip, trochanteric
  - wrist — *see* Bursitis, hand
- **Bursopathy** M71.9
  - specified type NEC M71.8Ø
    - ankle M71.87- ☑
    - elbow M71.82- ☑
    - foot M71.87- ☑
    - hand M71.84- ☑
    - hip M71.85- ☑
    - knee M71.86- ☑
    - multiple sites M71.89
    - shoulder M71.81- ☑
    - specified site NEC M71.88
    - wrist M71.83- ☑
- **Burst stitches or sutures** (complication of surgery) T81.31 ☑
  - external operation wound T81.31 ☑
  - internal operation wound T81.32 ☑
- **Buruli ulcer** A31.1
- **Bury's disease** L95.1
- **Buschke's**
  - disease — *see* Cryptococcosis by site
  - scleredema — *see* Sclerosis, systemic
- **Busse-Buschke disease** — *see* Cryptococcosis by site
- **Buttock** — *see* condition
- **Button**
  - Biskra B55.1
  - Delhi B55.1
  - oriental B55.1
- **Buttonhole deformity** (finger) — *see* Deformity, finger, boutonniere
- **Bwamba fever** A92.8
- **Byssinosis** J66.Ø
- **Bywaters' syndrome** T79.5 ☑

C

- **Cachexia** R64
  - cancerous R64
  - cardiac — *see* Disease, heart
  - dehydration E86.Ø
  - due to malnutrition R64
  - exophthalmic — *see* Hyperthyroidism
  - heart — *see* Disease, heart
  - hypophyseal E23.Ø
  - hypopituitary E23.Ø
  - lead — *see* Poisoning, lead
  - malignant R64
  - marsh — *see* Malaria
  - nervous F48.8
  - old age R54
  - paludal — *see* Malaria
  - pituitary E23.Ø
  - pulmonary R64
  - renal N28.9
  - saturnine — *see* Poisoning, lead
  - senile R54
  - Simmonds' E23.Ø
  - splenica D73.Ø
- **Cachexia** — *continued*
  - strumipriva EØ3.4
  - tuberculous NEC — *see* Tuberculosis
- **CADASIL** (cerebral autosomal dominant arteriopathy with subcortical infarcts and leukoencephalopathy) I67.85Ø
- **Café, au lait spots** L81.3
- **Caffeine-induced**
  - anxiety disorder F15.98Ø
  - sleep disorder F15.982
- **Caffey's syndrome** Q78.8
- **Caisson disease** T7Ø.3 ☑
- **Cake kidney** Q63.1
- **Caked breast** (puerperal, postpartum) O92.79
- **Calabar swelling** B74.3
- **Calcaneal spur** — *see* Spur, bone, calcaneal
- **Calcaneo-apophysitis** M92.8
- **Calcareous** — *see* condition
- **Calcicosis** J62.8
- **Calciferol** (vitamin D) deficiency E55.9
  - with rickets E55.Ø
- **Calcification**
  - adrenal (capsule) (gland) E27.49
    - tuberculous B9Ø.8 *[E35]*
  - aorta I7Ø.Ø
  - artery (annular) — *see* Arteriosclerosis
  - auricle (ear) — *see* Disorder, pinna, specified type NEC
  - basal ganglia G23.8
  - bladder N32.89
    - due to Schistosoma hematobium B65.Ø
  - brain (cortex) — *see* Calcification, cerebral
  - bronchus J98.Ø9
  - bursa M71.4Ø
    - ankle M71.47- ☑
    - elbow M71.42- ☑
    - foot M71.47- ☑
    - hand M71.44- ☑
    - hip M71.45- ☑
    - knee M71.46- ☑
    - multiple sites M71.49
    - shoulder M75.3- ☑
    - specified site NEC M71.48
    - wrist M71.43- ☑
  - cardiac — *see* Degeneration, myocardial
  - cerebral (cortex) G93.89
    - artery I67.2
  - cervix (uteri) N88.8
  - choroid plexus G93.89
  - conjunctiva — *see* Concretion, conjunctiva
  - corpora cavernosa (penis) N48.89
  - cortex (brain) — *see* Calcification, cerebral
  - dental pulp (nodular) KØ4.2
  - dentinal papilla KØØ.4
  - fallopian tube N83.8
  - falx cerebri G96.198
  - gallbladder K82.8
  - general E83.59
  - heart — *see also* Degeneration, myocardial
    - valve — *see also* Endocarditis
      - mitral — *see* Calcification, mitral
  - idiopathic infantile arterial (IIAC) Q28.8
  - intervertebral cartilage or disc (postinfective) — *see* Disorder, disc, specified NEC
  - intracranial — *see* Calcification, cerebral
  - joint — *see* Disorder, joint, specified type NEC
  - kidney N28.89
    - tuberculous N29 *[B9Ø.1]*
  - larynx (senile) J38.7
  - lens — *see* Cataract, specified NEC
  - lung (active) (postinfectional) J98.4
    - tuberculous B9Ø.9
  - lymph gland or node (postinfectional) I89.8
    - tuberculous — *see also* Tuberculosis, lymph gland B9Ø.8
  - mammographic R92.1
  - massive (paraplegic) — *see* Myositis, ossificans, in, quadriplegia
  - medial — *see* Arteriosclerosis, extremities
  - meninges (cerebral) (spinal) G96.198
  - metastatic E83.59
  - mitral (valve)
    - annular I34.81
      - nonrheumatic I34.81
      - rheumatic IØ5.8
    - annulus I34.81
      - nonrheumatic I34.81
      - rheumatic IØ5.8

- **Calcification** — *continued*
  - Mönckeberg's — *see* Arteriosclerosis, extremities
  - muscle M61.9
    - due to burns — *see* Myositis, ossificans, in, burns
    - paralytic — *see* Myositis, ossificans, in, quadriplegia
    - specified type NEC M61.40
      - ankle M61.47- ☑
      - foot M61.47- ☑
      - forearm M61.43- ☑
      - hand M61.44- ☑
      - lower leg M61.46- ☑
      - multiple sites M61.49
      - pelvic region M61.45- ☑
      - shoulder region M61.41- ☑
      - specified site NEC M61.48
      - thigh M61.45- ☑
      - upper arm M61.42- ☑
  - myocardium, myocardial — *see* Degeneration, myocardial
  - ovary N83.8
  - pancreas K86.89
  - penis N48.89
  - periarticular — *see* Disorder, joint, specified type NEC
  - pericardium — *see also* Pericarditis I31.1
  - pineal gland E34.8
  - pleura J94.8
    - postinfectional J94.8
    - tuberculous NEC B90.9
  - pulpal (dental) (nodular) K04.2
  - sclera H15.89
  - spleen D73.89
  - subcutaneous L94.2
  - suprarenal (capsule) (gland) E27.49
  - tendon (sheath) — *see also* Tenosynovitis, specified type NEC
    - with bursitis, synovitis or tenosynovitis — *see* Tendinitis, calcific
  - trachea J39.8
  - ureter N28.89
  - uterus N85.8
  - vitreous — *see* Deposit, crystalline
- **Calcified** — *see* Calcification
- **Calcinosis** (interstitial) (tumoral) (universalis) E83.59
  - with Raynaud's phenomenon, esophageal dysfunction, sclerodactyly, telangiectasia (CREST syndrome) M34.1
  - circumscripta (skin) L94.2
  - cutis L94.2
- **Calciphylaxis** — *see also* Calcification, by site E83.59
- **Calcium**
  - deposits — *see* Calcification, by site
  - metabolism disorder E83.50
  - salts or soaps in vitreous — *see* Deposit, crystalline
- **Calciuria** R82.994
- **Calculi** — *see* Calculus
- **Calculosis, intrahepatic** — *see* Calculus, bile duct
- **Calculus, calculi, calculous**
  - ampulla of Vater — *see* Calculus, bile duct
  - anuria (impacted) (recurrent) — *see also* Calculus, urinary N20.9
  - appendix K38.1
  - bile duct (common) (hepatic) K80.50
    - with
      - calculus of gallbladder — *see* Calculus, gallbladder and bile duct
      - cholangitis K80.30
        - with
          - cholecystitis — *see* Calculus, bile duct, with cholecystitis
          - obstruction K80.31
        - acute K80.32
          - with
            - chronic cholangitis K80.36
              - with obstruction K80.37
            - obstruction K80.33
        - chronic K80.34
          - with
            - acute cholangitis K80.36
              - with obstruction K80.37
            - obstruction K80.35
      - cholecystitis (with cholangitis) K80.40
        - with obstruction K80.41
        - acute K80.42
          - with
            - chronic cholecystitis K80.46
              - with obstruction K80.47
            - obstruction K80.43
        - chronic K80.44

- **Calculus, calculi, calculous** — *continued*
  - bile duct — *continued*
    - with — *continued*
      - cholecystitis — *continued*
        - chronic — *continued*
          - with
            - acute cholecystitis K80.46
              - with obstruction K80.47
            - obstruction K80.45
  - biliary — *see also* Calculus, gallbladder
    - specified NEC K80.80
      - with obstruction K80.81
  - bilirubin, multiple — *see* Calculus, gallbladder
  - bladder (encysted) (impacted) (urinary) (diverticulum) N21.0
  - bronchus J98.09
  - calyx (kidney) (renal) — *see* Calculus, kidney
  - cholesterol (pure) (solitary) — *see* Calculus, gallbladder
  - common duct (bile) — *see* Calculus, bile duct
  - conjunctiva — *see* Concretion, conjunctiva
  - cystic N21.0
    - duct — *see* Calculus, gallbladder
  - dental (subgingival) (supragingival) K03.6
  - diverticulum
    - bladder N21.0
    - kidney N20.0
  - epididymis N50.89
  - gallbladder K80.20
    - with
      - bile duct calculus — *see* Calculus, gallbladder and bile duct
      - cholecystitis K80.10
        - with obstruction K80.11
        - acute K80.00
          - with
            - chronic cholecystitis K80.12
              - with obstruction K80.13
            - obstruction K80.01
        - chronic K80.10
          - with
            - acute cholecystitis K80.12
              - with obstruction K80.13
            - obstruction K80.11
        - specified NEC K80.18
          - with obstruction K80.19
      - obstruction K80.21
  - gallbladder and bile duct K80.70
    - with
      - cholecystitis K80.60
        - with obstruction K80.61
        - acute K80.62
          - with
            - chronic cholecystitis K80.66
              - with obstruction K80.67
            - obstruction K80.63
        - chronic K80.64
          - with
            - acute cholecystitis K80.66
              - with obstruction K80.67
            - obstruction K80.65
      - obstruction K80.71
  - hepatic (duct) — *see* Calculus, bile duct
  - ileal conduit N21.8
  - intestinal (impaction) (obstruction) K56.49
  - kidney (impacted) (multiple) (pelvis) (recurrent) (staghorn) N20.0
    - with calculus, ureter N20.2
    - congenital Q63.8
  - lacrimal passages — *see* Dacryolith
  - liver (impacted) — *see* Calculus, bile duct
  - lung J98.4
  - mammographic R92.1
  - nephritic (impacted) (recurrent) — *see* Calculus, kidney
  - nose J34.89
  - pancreas (duct) K86.89
  - parotid duct or gland K11.5
  - pelvis, encysted — *see* Calculus, kidney
  - prostate N42.0
  - pulmonary J98.4
  - pyelitis (impacted) (recurrent) N20.0
    - with hydronephrosis N13.6
  - pyelonephritis (impacted) (recurrent) — *see* category N20 ☑
    - with hydronephrosis N13.6
  - renal (impacted) (recurrent) — *see* Calculus, kidney
  - salivary (duct) (gland) K11.5
  - seminal vesicle N50.89
  - staghorn — *see* Calculus, kidney

- **Calculus, calculi, calculous** — *continued*
  - Stensen's duct K11.5
  - stomach K31.89
  - sublingual duct or gland K11.5
    - congenital Q38.4
  - submandibular duct, gland or region K11.5
  - submaxillary duct, gland or region K11.5
  - suburethral N21.8
  - tonsil J35.8
  - tooth, teeth (subgingival) (supragingival) K03.6
  - tunica vaginalis N50.89
  - ureter (impacted) (recurrent) N20.1
    - with calculus, kidney N20.2
      - with hydronephrosis N13.2
        - with infection N13.6
  - ureteropelvic junction N20.1
  - urethra (impacted) N21.1
  - urinary (duct) (impacted) (passage) (tract) N20.9
    - with hydronephrosis N13.2
      - with infection N13.6
    - in (due to)
    - lower N21.9
      - specified NEC N21.8
  - vagina N89.8
  - vesical (impacted) N21.0
  - Wharton's duct K11.5
  - xanthine E79.8 *[N22]*
- **Calicectasis** N28.89
- **Caliectasis** N28.89
- **California**
  - disease B38.9
  - encephalitis A83.5
- **Caligo cornea** — *see* Opacity, cornea, central
- **Callositas, callosity** (infected) L84
- **Callus** (infected) L84
  - bone — *see* Osteophyte
    - excessive, following fracture — *code as* Sequelae of fracture
- **CALME** (childhood asymmetric labium majus enlargement) N90.61
- **Calorie deficiency or malnutrition** — *see also* Malnutrition E46
- **Calpainopathy** (primary) G71.032
  - autosomal dominant G71.031
  - autosomal recessive G71.032
- **Calvé-Perthes disease** — *see* Legg-Calvé-Perthes disease
- **Calvé's disease** — *see* Osteochondrosis, juvenile, spine
- **Calvities** — *see* Alopecia, androgenic
- **Cameroon fever** — *see* Malaria
- **Camptocormia** (hysterical) F44.4
- **Camurati-Engelmann syndrome** Q78.3
- **Canal** — *see also* condition
  - atrioventricular Q21.20
    - common Q21.23
    - incomplete Q21.21
    - intermediate Q21.22
    - partial Q21.21
    - transitional Q21.22
- **Canaliculitis** (lacrimal) (acute) (subacute) H04.33- ☑
  - Actinomyces A42.89
  - chronic H04.42- ☑
- **Canavan's disease** E75.29
- **Canceled procedure** (surgical) Z53.9
  - because of
    - contraindication Z53.09
      - smoking Z53.01
    - left against medical advice (AMA) Z53.29
    - patient's decision Z53.20
      - for reasons of belief or group pressure Z53.1
      - specified reason NEC Z53.29
    - specified reason NEC Z53.8
- **Cancer** — *see also* Neoplasm, by site, malignant
  - bile duct type liver C22.1
  - blood — *see* Leukemia
  - breast — *see also* Neoplasm, breast, malignant C50.91- ☑
  - hepatocellular C22.0
  - lung — *see also* Neoplasm, lung, malignant C34.90
  - ovarian — *see also* Neoplasm, ovary, malignant C56.9
  - unspecified site (primary) C80.1
- **Cancer (o) phobia** F45.29
- **Cancerous** — *see* Neoplasm, malignant, by site
- **Cancrum oris** A69.0
- **Candidiasis, candidal** B37.9
  - balanitis B37.42
  - bronchitis B37.1
  - cheilitis B37.83

- **Carcinoma** — *continued*
  - Hurthle cell C73
  - in
    - adenomatous
      - polyposis coli C18.9
    - pleomorphic adenoma — *see* Neoplasm, salivary glands, malignant
    - situ — *see* Carcinoma-in-situ
  - infiltrating
    - duct
      - with lobular
        - specified site — *see* Neoplasm, malignant, by site
        - unspecified site (female) C5Ø.91- ☑
          - male C5Ø.92- ☑
      - with Paget's disease — *see* Neoplasm, breast, malignant
      - specified site — *see* Neoplasm, malignant
      - unspecified site (female) C5Ø.91- ☑
        - male C5Ø.92- ☑
    - ductular
      - specified site — *see* Neoplasm, malignant
      - unspecified site (female) C5Ø.91- ☑
        - male C5Ø.92- ☑
    - lobular
      - specified site — *see* Neoplasm, malignant
      - unspecified site (female) C5Ø.91- ☑
        - male C5Ø.92- ☑
  - inflammatory
    - specified site — *see* Neoplasm, malignant
    - unspecified site (female) C5Ø.91- ☑
      - male C5Ø.92- ☑
  - intestinal type
    - specified site — *see* Neoplasm, malignant, by site
    - unspecified site C16.9
  - intracystic
    - noninfiltrating — *see* Neoplasm, in situ, by site
  - intraductal (noninfiltrating)
    - with Paget's disease — *see* Neoplasm, breast, malignant
    - breast DØ5.1- ☑
    - papillary
      - with invasion
        - specified site — *see* Neoplasm, malignant, by site
        - unspecified site (female) C5Ø.91- ☑
          - male C5Ø.92- ☑
      - breast DØ5.1- ☑
      - specified site NEC — *see* Neoplasm, in situ, by site
      - unspecified site (female) DØ5.1- ☑
    - specified site NEC — *see* Neoplasm, in situ, by site
    - unspecified site (female) DØ5.1- ☑
  - intraepidermal — *see* Neoplasm, in situ
    - squamous cell, Bowen's type — *see* Neoplasm, skin, in situ
  - intraepithelial — *see* Neoplasm, in situ, by site
    - squamous cell — *see* Neoplasm, in situ, by site
  - intraosseous C41.1
    - upper jaw (bone) C41.Ø
  - islet cell
    - with exocrine, mixed
      - specified site — *see* Neoplasm, malignant, by site
      - unspecified site C25.9
    - pancreas C25.4
    - specified site NEC — *see* Neoplasm, malignant, by site
    - unspecified site C25.4
  - juvenile, breast — *see* Neoplasm, breast, malignant
  - large cell
    - small cell
      - specified site — *see* Neoplasm, malignant, by site
      - unspecified site C34.9Ø
  - Leydig cell (testis)
    - specified site — *see* Neoplasm, malignant, by site
    - unspecified site
      - female C56.9
      - male C62.9Ø
  - lipid-rich (female) C5Ø.91- ☑
    - male C5Ø.92- ☑
  - liver cell C22.Ø
  - liver NEC C22.7

- **Carcinoma** — *continued*
  - lobular (infiltrating)
    - with intraductal
      - specified site — *see* Neoplasm, malignant, by site
      - unspecified site (female) C5Ø.91- ☑
        - male C5Ø.92- ☑
    - noninfiltrating
      - breast DØ5.Ø- ☑
      - specified site NEC — *see* Neoplasm, in situ, by site
      - unspecified site DØ5.Ø- ☑
    - specified site — *see* Neoplasm, malignant, by site
    - unspecified site (female) C5Ø.91- ☑
      - male C5Ø.92- ☑
  - medullary
    - with
      - amyloid stroma
        - specified site — *see* Neoplasm, malignant, by site
        - unspecified site C73
      - lymphoid stroma
        - specified site — *see* Neoplasm, malignant, by site
        - unspecified site (female) C5Ø.91- ☑
          - male C5Ø.92- ☑
  - Merkel cell C4A.9 (*following* C43)
    - anal margin C4A.51 (*following* C43)
    - anal skin C4A.51 (*following* C43)
    - canthus C4A.1- ☑ (*following* C43)
    - ear and external auricular canal C4A.2- ☑ (*following* C43)
    - external auricular canal C4A.2- ☑ (*following* C43)
    - eyelid, including canthus C4A.1- ☑ (*following* C43)
    - face C4A.3Ø (*following* C43)
      - specified NEC C4A.39 (*following* C43)
    - hip C4A.7- ☑ (*following* C43)
    - lip C4A.Ø (*following* C43)
    - lower limb, including hip C4A.7- ☑ (*following* C43)
    - neck C4A.4 (*following* C43)
    - nodal presentation C7B.1 (*following* C75)
    - nose C4A.31 (*following* C43)
    - overlapping sites C4A.8 (*following* C43)
    - perianal skin C4A.51 (*following* C43)
    - scalp C4A.4 (*following* C43)
    - secondary C7B.1 (*following* C75)
    - shoulder C4A.6- ☑ (*following* C43)
    - skin of breast C4A.52 (*following* C43)
    - trunk NEC C4A.59 (*following* C43)
    - upper limb, including shoulder C4A.6- ☑ (*following* C43)
    - visceral metastatic C7B.1 (*following* C75)
  - metastatic — *see* Neoplasm, secondary, by site
  - metatypical — *see* Neoplasm, skin, malignant
  - morphea, basal cell — *see* Neoplasm, skin, malignant
  - mucoid
    - cell
      - specified site — *see* Neoplasm, malignant, by site
      - unspecified site C75.1
  - neuroendocrine — *see also* Tumor, neuroendocrine
    - high grade, any site C7A.1 (*following* C75)
    - poorly differentiated, any site C7A.1 (*following* C75)
  - nonencapsulated sclerosing C73
  - noninfiltrating
    - intracystic — *see* Neoplasm, in situ, by site
    - intraductal
      - breast DØ5.1- ☑
      - papillary
        - breast DØ5.1- ☑
        - specified site NEC — *see* Neoplasm, in situ, by site
        - unspecified site DØ5.1- ☑
      - specified site — *see* Neoplasm, in situ, by site
      - unspecified site DØ5.1- ☑
    - lobular
      - breast DØ5.Ø- ☑
      - specified site NEC — *see* Neoplasm, in situ, by site
      - unspecified site (female) DØ5.Ø- ☑
  - oat cell
    - specified site — *see* Neoplasm, malignant, by site
    - unspecified site C34.9Ø
  - odontogenic C41.1
    - upper jaw (bone) C41.Ø
  - papillary
    - with follicular (mixed) C73

- **Carcinoma** — *continued*
  - papillary — *continued*
    - follicular variant C73
    - intraductal (noninfiltrating)
      - with invasion
        - specified site — *see* Neoplasm, malignant, by site
        - unspecified site (female) C5Ø.91- ☑
          - male C5Ø.92- ☑
      - breast DØ5.1- ☑
      - specified site NEC — *see* Neoplasm, in situ, by site
      - unspecified site DØ5.1- ☑
    - serous
      - specified site — *see* Neoplasm, malignant, by site
      - surface
        - specified site — *see* Neoplasm, malignant, by site
        - unspecified site C56.9
      - unspecified site C56.9
  - papillocystic
    - specified site — *see* Neoplasm, malignant, by site
    - unspecified site C56.9
  - parafollicular cell
    - specified site — *see* Neoplasm, malignant, by site
    - unspecified site C73
  - pilomatrix — *see* Neoplasm, skin, malignant
  - pseudomucinous
    - specified site — *see* Neoplasm, malignant, by site
    - unspecified site C56.9
  - renal cell C64- ☑
  - Schmincke — *see* Neoplasm, nasopharynx, malignant
  - Schneiderian
    - specified site — *see* Neoplasm, malignant, by site
    - unspecified site C3Ø.Ø
  - sebaceous — *see* Neoplasm, skin, malignant
  - secondary — *see also* Neoplasm, secondary, by site
    - Merkel cell C7B.1 (*following* C75)
  - secretory, breast — *see* Neoplasm, breast, malignant
  - serous
    - papillary
      - specified site — *see* Neoplasm, malignant, by site
      - unspecified site C56.9
    - surface, papillary
      - specified site — *see* Neoplasm, malignant, by site
      - unspecified site C56.9
  - Sertoli cell
    - specified site — *see* Neoplasm, malignant, by site
    - unspecified site C62.9Ø
      - female C56.9
      - male C62.9Ø
  - skin appendage — *see* Neoplasm, skin, malignant
  - small cell
    - fusiform cell
      - specified site — *see* Neoplasm, malignant, by site
      - unspecified site C34.9Ø
    - intermediate cell
      - specified site — *see* Neoplasm, malignant, by site
      - unspecified site C34.9Ø
    - large cell
      - specified site — *see* Neoplasm, malignant, by site
      - unspecified site C34.9Ø
  - solid
    - with amyloid stroma
      - specified site — *see* Neoplasm, malignant, by site
      - unspecified site C73
    - microinvasive
      - specified site — *see* Neoplasm, malignant, by site
      - unspecified site C53.9
  - sweat gland — *see* Neoplasm, skin, malignant
  - theca cell C56.- ☑
  - thymic C37
  - unspecified site (primary) C8Ø.1
  - water-clear cell C75.Ø
- **Carcinoma-in-situ** — *see also* Neoplasm, in situ, by site
  - breast NOS DØ5.9- ☑
    - specified type NEC DØ5.8- ☑
  - epidermoid — *see also* Neoplasm, in situ, by site
    - with questionable stromal invasion
      - cervix DØ6.9

Index

Carcinoma — Carcinoma-in-situ

- **Cholecystitis** — *continued*
  - gangrenous — *see* Cholecystitis, acute
  - paratyphoidal, current AØ1.4
  - suppurative — *see* Cholecystitis, acute
  - typhoidal AØ1.Ø9
- **Cholecystolithiasis** — *see* Calculus, gallbladder
- **Choledochitis** (suppurative) K83.Ø9
- **Choledocholith** — *see* Calculus, bile duct
- **Choledocholithiasis** (common duct) (hepatic duct) — *see* Calculus, bile duct
  - cystic — *see* Calculus, gallbladder
  - typhoidal AØ1.Ø9
- **Cholelithiasis** (cystic duct) (gallbladder) (impacted) (multiple) — *see* Calculus, gallbladder
  - bile duct (common) (hepatic) — *see* Calculus, bile duct
  - hepatic duct — *see* Calculus, bile duct
  - specified NEC K8Ø.8Ø
    - with obstruction K8Ø.81
- **Cholemia** — *see also* Jaundice
  - familial (simple) (congenital) E8Ø.4
  - Gilbert's E8Ø.4
- **Choleperitoneum, choleperitonitis** K65.3
- **Cholera** (Asiatic) (epidemic) (malignant) AØØ.9
  - antimonial — *see* Poisoning, antimony
  - classical AØØ.Ø
  - due to Vibrio cholerae Ø1 AØØ.9
    - biovar cholerae AØØ.Ø
    - biovar eltor AØØ.1
    - el tor AØØ.1
  - el tor AØØ.1
- **Cholerine** — *see* Cholera
- **Cholestasis NEC** K83.1
  - with hepatocyte injury K71.Ø
  - due to total parenteral nutrition (TPN) K76.89
  - pure K71.Ø
- **Cholesteatoma** (ear) (middle) (with reaction) H71.9- ☑
  - attic H71.Ø- ☑
  - external ear (canal) H6Ø.4- ☑
  - mastoid H71.2- ☑
  - postmastoidectomy cavity (recurrent) — *see* Complications, postmastoidectomy, recurrent cholesteatoma
  - recurrent (postmastoidectomy) — *see* Complications, postmastoidectomy, recurrent cholesteatoma
  - tympanum H71.1- ☑
- **Cholesteatosis, diffuse** H71.3- ☑
- **Cholesteremia** E78.ØØ
- **Cholesterin in vitreous** — *see* Deposit, crystalline
- **Cholesterol**
  - deposit
    - retina H35.89
    - vitreous — *see* Deposit, crystalline
  - elevated (high) E78.ØØ
    - with elevated (high) triglycerides E78.2
    - screening for Z13.22Ø
  - imbibition of gallbladder K82.4
- **Cholesterolemia** (essential) (pure) E78.ØØ
  - familial E78.Ø1
  - hereditary E78.Ø1
- **Cholesterolosis, cholesterosis** (gallbladder) K82.4
  - cerebrotendinous E75.5
- **Cholocolic fistula** K82.3
- **Choluria** R82.2
- **Chondritis** M94.8X9
  - aurical H61.Ø3- ☑
  - costal (Tietze's) M94.Ø
  - external ear H61.Ø3- ☑
  - patella, posttraumatic — *see* Chondromalacia, patella
  - pinna H61.Ø3- ☑
  - purulent M94.8X- ☑
  - tuberculous NEC A18.Ø2
    - intervertebral A18.Ø1
- **Chondroblastoma** — *see also* Neoplasm, bone, benign
  - malignant — *see* Neoplasm, bone, malignant
- **Chondrocalcinosis** M11.2Ø
  - ankle M11.27- ☑
  - elbow M11.22- ☑
  - familial M11.1Ø
    - ankle M11.17- ☑
    - elbow M11.12- ☑
    - foot joint M11.17- ☑
    - hand joint M11.14- ☑
    - hip M11.15- ☑
    - knee M11.16- ☑
    - multiple site M11.19
    - shoulder M11.11- ☑
    - vertebrae M11.18
- **Chondrocalcinosis** — *continued*
  - familial — *continued*
    - wrist M11.13- ☑
  - foot joint M11.27- ☑
  - hand joint M11.24- ☑
  - hip M11.25- ☑
  - knee M11.26- ☑
  - multiple site M11.29
  - shoulder M11.21- ☑
  - specified type NEC M11.2Ø
    - ankle M11.27- ☑
    - elbow M11.22- ☑
    - foot joint M11.27- ☑
    - hand joint M11.24- ☑
    - hip M11.25- ☑
    - knee M11.26- ☑
    - multiple site M11.29
    - shoulder M11.21- ☑
    - vertebrae M11.28
    - wrist M11.23- ☑
  - vertebrae M11.28
  - wrist M11.23- ☑
- **Chondrodermatitis nodularis helicis or anthelicis** — *see* Perichondritis, ear
- **Chondrodysplasia** Q78.9
  - with hemangioma Q78.4
  - calcificans congenita Q77.3
  - fetalis Q77.4
  - metaphyseal (Jansen's) (McKusick's) (Schmid's) Q78.8
  - punctata Q77.3
- **Chondrodystrophy, chondrodystrophia** (familial) (fetalis) (hypoplastic) Q78.9
  - calcificans congenita Q77.3
  - myotonic (congenital) G71.13
  - punctata Q77.3
- **Chondroectodermal dysplasia** Q77.6
- **Chondrogenesis imperfecta** Q77.4
- **Chondrolysis** M94.35- ☑
- **Chondroma** — *see also* Neoplasm, cartilage, benign
  - juxtacortical — *see* Neoplasm, bone, benign
  - periosteal — *see* Neoplasm, bone, benign
- **Chondromalacia** (systemic) M94.2Ø
  - acromioclavicular joint M94.21- ☑
  - ankle M94.27- ☑
  - elbow M94.22- ☑
  - foot joint M94.27- ☑
  - glenohumeral joint M94.21- ☑
  - hand joint M94.24- ☑
  - hip M94.25- ☑
  - knee M94.26- ☑
    - patella M22.4- ☑
  - multiple sites M94.29
  - patella M22.4- ☑
  - rib M94.28
  - sacroiliac joint M94.259
  - shoulder M94.21- ☑
  - sternoclavicular joint M94.21- ☑
  - vertebral joint M94.28
  - wrist M94.23- ☑
- **Chondromatosis** — *see also* Neoplasm, cartilage, uncertain behavior
  - internal Q78.4
- **Chondromyxosarcoma** — *see* Neoplasm, cartilage, malignant
- **Chondro-osteodysplasia** (Morquio-Brailsford type) E76.219
- **Chondro-osteodystrophy** E76.29
- **Chondro-osteoma** — *see* Neoplasm, bone, benign
- **Chondropathia tuberosa** M94.Ø
- **Chondrosarcoma** — *see* Neoplasm, cartilage, malignant
  - juxtacortical — *see* Neoplasm, bone, malignant
  - mesenchymal — *see* Neoplasm, connective tissue, malignant
  - myxoid — *see* Neoplasm, cartilage, malignant
- **Chordee** (nonvenereal) N48.89
  - congenital Q54.4
  - gonococcal A54.Ø9
- **Chorditis** (fibrinous) (nodosa) (tuberosa) J38.2
- **Chordoma** — *see* Neoplasm, vertebral (column), malignant
- **Chorea** (chronic) (gravis) (posthemiplegic) (senile) (spasmodic) G25.5
  - with
    - heart involvement IØ2.Ø
      - active or acute (conditions in IØ1-) IØ2.Ø
      - rheumatic IØ2.9
        - with valvular disorder IØ2.Ø
- **Chorea** — *continued*
  - with — *continued*
    - rheumatic heart disease (chronic) (inactive) (quiescent) — *code to* rheumatic heart condition involved
  - drug-induced G25.4
  - habit F95.8
  - hereditary G1Ø
  - Huntington's G1Ø
  - hysterical F44.4
  - minor IØ2.9
    - with heart involvement IØ2.Ø
  - progressive G25.5
    - hereditary G1Ø
  - rheumatic (chronic) IØ2.9
    - with heart involvement IØ2.Ø
  - Sydenham's IØ2.9
    - with heart involvement — *see* Chorea, with rheumatic heart disease
    - nonrheumatic G25.5
- **Choreoathetosis** (paroxysmal) G25.5
- **Chorioadenoma** (destruens) D39.2
- **Chorioamnionitis** O41.12- ☑
- **Chorioangioma** D26.7
- **Choriocarcinoma** — *see* Neoplasm, malignant, by site
  - combined with
    - embryonal carcinoma — *see* Neoplasm, malignant, by site
    - other germ cell elements — *see* Neoplasm, malignant, by site
    - teratoma — *see* Neoplasm, malignant, by site
  - specified site — *see* Neoplasm, malignant, by site
  - unspecified site
    - female C58
    - male C62.9Ø
- **Chorioencephalitis** (acute) (lymphocytic) (serous) A87.2
- **Chorioepithelioma** — *see* Choriocarcinoma
- **Choriomeningitis** (acute) (lymphocytic) (serous) A87.2
- **Chorionepithelioma** — *see* Choriocarcinoma
- **Chorioretinitis** — *see also* Inflammation, chorioretinal
  - disseminated — *see also* Inflammation, chorioretinal, disseminated
    - in neurosyphilis A52.19
  - Egyptian B76.9 *[D63.8]*
  - focal — *see also* Inflammation, chorioretinal, focal
  - histoplasmic B39.9 *[H32]*
  - in (due to)
    - histoplasmosis B39.9 *[H32]*
    - syphilis (secondary) A51.43
      - late A52.71
    - toxoplasmosis (acquired) B58.Ø1
      - congenital (active) P37.1 *[H32]*
    - tuberculosis A18.53
  - juxtapapillary, juxtapapillaris — *see* Inflammation, chorioretinal, focal, juxtapapillary
  - leprous A3Ø.9 *[H32]*
  - miner's B76.9 *[D63.8]*
  - progressive myopia (degeneration) — *see also* Myopia, degenerative H44.2- ☑
  - syphilitic (secondary) A51.43
    - congenital (early) A5Ø.Ø1 *[H32]*
      - late A5Ø.32
    - late A52.71
  - tuberculous A18.53
- **Chorioretinopathy, central serous** H35.71- ☑
- **Choroid** — *see* condition
- **Choroideremia** H31.21
- **Choroiditis** — *see* Chorioretinitis
- **Choroidopathy** — *see* Disorder, choroid
- **Choroidoretinitis** — *see* Chorioretinitis
- **Choroidoretinopathy, central serous** — *see* Chorioretinopathy, central serous
- **Christian-Weber disease** M35.6
- **Christmas disease** D67
- **Chromaffinoma** — *see also* Neoplasm, benign, by site
  - malignant — *see* Neoplasm, malignant, by site
- **Chromatopsia** — *see* Deficiency, color vision
- **Chromhidrosis, chromidrosis** L75.1
- **Chromoblastomycosis** — *see* Chromomycosis
- **Chromoconversion** R82.91
- **Chromomycosis** B43.9
  - brain abscess B43.1
  - cerebral B43.1
  - cutaneous B43.Ø
  - skin B43.Ø
  - specified NEC B43.8
  - subcutaneous abscess or cyst B43.2

Cleft — *continued*
- thyroid cartilage Q31.8
- uvula Q35.7

Cleidocranial dysostosis Q74.Ø
Cleptomania F63.2
Clicking hip (newborn) R29.4
Climacteric (female) — *see also* Menopause
- arthritis (any site) NEC — *see* Arthritis, specified form NEC
- depression (single episode) F32.89
  - recurrent episode F33.8
- male (symptoms) (syndrome) NEC N5Ø.89
- melancholia (single episode) F32.89
  - recurrent episode F33.8
- paranoid state F22
- polyarthritis NEC — *see* Arthritis, specified form NEC
- symptoms (female) N95.1

Clinical research investigation (clinical trial) (control subject) (normal comparison) (participant) ZØØ.6
Clitoris — *see* condition
Cloaca (persistent) Q43.7
Clonorchiasis, clonorchis infection (liver) B66.1
Clonus R25.8
Closed bite M26.29
Clostridium (C.) **perfringens, as cause of disease classified elsewhere** B96.7
Closure
- congenital, nose Q3Ø.Ø
- cranial sutures, premature Q75.Ø
- defective or imperfect NEC — *see* Imperfect, closure
- fistula, delayed — *see* Fistula
- foramen ovale, imperfect Q21.12
- hymen N89.6
- interauricular septum, defective Q21.19
- interventricular septum, defective Q21.Ø
- lacrimal duct — *see also* Stenosis, lacrimal, duct
  - congenital Q1Ø.5
- nose (congenital) Q3Ø.Ø
  - acquired M95.Ø
- of artificial opening — *see* Attention to, artificial, opening
- vagina N89.5
- valve — *see* Endocarditis
- vulva N9Ø.5

Clot (blood) — *see also* Embolism
- artery (obstruction) (occlusion) — *see* Embolism
- bladder N32.89
- brain (intradural or extradural) — *see* Occlusion, artery, cerebral
- circulation I74.9
- heart — *see also* Infarct, myocardium
  - not resulting in infarction I51.3
- vein — *see* Thrombosis

Clouded state R4Ø.1
- epileptic — *see* Epilepsy, specified NEC
- paroxysmal — *see* Epilepsy, specified NEC

Cloudy antrum, antra J32.Ø
Clouston's (hidrotic) **ectodermal dysplasia** Q82.4
Clubbed nail pachydermoperiostosis M89.4Ø *[L62]*
Clubbing of finger(s) (nails) R68.3
Clubfinger R68.3
- congenital Q68.1

Clubfoot (congenital) Q66.89
- acquired — *see* Deformity, limb, clubfoot
- equinovarus Q66.Ø- ☑
- paralytic — *see* Deformity, limb, clubfoot

Clubhand (congenital) (radial) Q71.4- ☑
- acquired — *see* Deformity, limb, clubhand

Clubnail R68.3
- congenital Q84.6

Clump, kidney Q63.1
Clumsiness, clumsy child syndrome F82
Cluttering F8Ø.81
Clutton's joints A5Ø.51 *[M12.8Ø]*
Coagulation, intravascular (diffuse) (disseminated) — *see also* Defibrination syndrome
- complicating abortion — *see* Abortion, by type, complicated by, intravascular coagulation
- following ectopic or molar pregnancy OØ8.1

Coagulopathy — *see also* Defect, coagulation
- consumption D65
- intravascular D65
  - newborn P6Ø

Coalition
- calcaneo-scaphoid Q66.89
- tarsal Q66.89

Coalminer's
- elbow — *see* Bursitis, elbow, olecranon
- lung or pneumoconiosis J6Ø

Coalworker's lung or pneumoconiosis J6Ø
Coarctation
- aorta (preductal) (postductal) Q25.1
- pulmonary artery Q25.71

Coated tongue K14.3
Coats' disease (exudative retinopathy) — *see* Retinopathy, exudative
Cocaine-induced
- anxiety disorder F14.98Ø
- bipolar and related disorder F14.94
- depressive disorder F14.94
- obsessive-compulsive and related disorder F14.988
- psychotic disorder F14.959
- sexual dysfunction F14.981
- sleep disorder F14.982

Cocainism — *see* Disorder, cocaine use
Coccidioidomycosis B38.9
- cutaneous B38.3
- disseminated B38.7
- generalized B38.7
- meninges B38.4
- prostate B38.81
- pulmonary B38.2
  - acute B38.Ø
  - chronic B38.1
- skin B38.3
- specified NEC B38.89

Coccidioidosis — *see* Coccidioidomycosis
Coccidiosis (intestinal) AØ7.3
Coccydynia, coccygodynia M53.3
Coccyx — *see* condition
Cochin-China diarrhea K9Ø.1
Cockayne's syndrome Q87.19
Cocked up toe — *see* Deformity, toe, specified NEC
Cock's peculiar tumor L72.3
Codman's tumor — *see* Neoplasm, bone, benign
Coenurosis B71.8
Coffee-worker's lung J67.8
Cogan's syndrome H16.32- ☑
- oculomotor apraxia H51.8

Coitus, painful (female) N94.1Ø
- male N53.12
- psychogenic F52.6

Cold JØØ
- with influenza, flu, or grippe — *see* Influenza, with, respiratory manifestations NEC
- agglutinin disease or hemoglobinuria (chronic) D59.12
- bronchial — *see* Bronchitis
- chest — *see* Bronchitis
- common (head) JØØ
- effects of T69.9 ☑
  - specified effect NEC T69.8 ☑
- excessive, effects of T69.9 ☑
  - specified effect NEC T69.8 ☑
- exhaustion from T69.8 ☑
- exposure to T69.9 ☑
  - specified effect NEC T69.8 ☑
- head JØØ
- injury syndrome (newborn) P8Ø.Ø
- on lung — *see* Bronchitis
- rose J3Ø.1
- sensitivity, auto-immune D59.12
- symptoms JØØ
- virus JØØ

Coldsore BØØ.1
Colibacillosis A49.8
- as the cause of other disease — *see also* Escherichia coli B96.2Ø
- generalized A41.5Ø

Colic (bilious) (infantile) (intestinal) (recurrent) (spasmodic) R1Ø.83
- abdomen R1Ø.83
  - psychogenic F45.8
- appendix, appendicular K38.8
- bile duct — *see* Calculus, bile duct
- biliary — *see* Calculus, bile duct
- common duct — *see* Calculus, bile duct
- cystic duct — *see* Calculus, gallbladder
- Devonshire NEC — *see* Poisoning, lead
- gallbladder — *see* Calculus, gallbladder
- gallstone — *see* Calculus, gallbladder
  - gallbladder or cystic duct — *see* Calculus, gallbladder
- hepatic (duct) — *see* Calculus, bile duct

Colic — *continued*
- hysterical F45.8
- kidney N23
- lead NEC — *see* Poisoning, lead
- mucous K58.9
  - with diarrhea K58.Ø
  - psychogenic F54
- nephritic N23
- painter's NEC — *see* Poisoning, lead
- pancreas K86.89
- psychogenic F45.8
- renal N23
- saturnine NEC — *see* Poisoning, lead
- ureter N23
- urethral N36.8
  - due to calculus N21.1
- uterus NEC N94.89
  - menstrual — *see* Dysmenorrhea
- worm NOS B83.9

Colicystitis — *see* Cystitis
Colitis (acute) (catarrhal) (chronic) (noninfective) (hemorrhagic) — *see also* Enteritis K52.9
- allergic K52.29
  - with
    - food protein-induced enterocolitis syndrome K52.21
    - proctocolitis K52.29
- amebic (acute) — *see also* Amebiasis AØ6.Ø
  - nondysenteric AØ6.2
- anthrax A22.2
- bacillary — *see* Infection, Shigella
- balantidial AØ7.Ø
- Clostridium difficile
  - not specified as recurrent AØ4.72
  - recurrent AØ4.71
- coccidial AØ7.3
- collagenous K52.831
- cystica superficialis K52.89
- dietary counseling and surveillance (for) Z71.3
- dietetic — *see also* Colitis, allergic K52.29
- drug-induced K52.1
- due to radiation K52.Ø
- eosinophilic K52.82
- food hypersensitivity — *see also* Colitis, allergic K52.29
- giardial AØ7.1
- granulomatous — *see* Enteritis, regional, large intestine
- indeterminate, so stated K52.3
- infectious — *see* Enteritis, infectious
- ischemic K55.9
  - acute (subacute) — *see also* Ischemia, intestine, acute K55.Ø39
  - chronic K55.1
  - due to mesenteric artery insufficiency K55.1
  - fulminant (acute) — *see also* Ischemia, intestine, acute K55.Ø39
- left sided K51.5Ø
  - with
    - abscess K51.514
    - complication K51.519
      - specified NEC K51.518
    - fistula K51.513
    - obstruction K51.512
    - rectal bleeding K51.511
- lymphocytic K52.832
- membranous
  - psychogenic F54
- microscopic K52.839
  - specified NEC K52.838
- mucous — *see* Syndrome, irritable, bowel
  - psychogenic F54
- noninfective K52.9
  - specified NEC K52.89
- polyposa — *see* Polyp, colon, inflammatory
- protozoal AØ7.9
- pseudomembranous
  - not specified as recurrent AØ4.72
  - recurrent AØ4.71
- pseudomucinous — *see* Syndrome, irritable, bowel
- regional — *see* Enteritis, regional, large intestine
  - infectious AØ9
- segmental — *see* Enteritis, regional, large intestine
- septic — *see* Enteritis, infectious
- spastic K58.9
  - with diarrhea K58.Ø
  - psychogenic F54
- staphylococcal AØ4.8
  - foodborne AØ5.Ø

- **Communication**
  - between
    - base of aorta and pulmonary artery Q21.4
    - left ventricle and right atrium Q2Ø.5
    - pericardial sac and pleural sac Q34.8
    - pulmonary artery and pulmonary vein, congenital Q25.72
  - congenital between uterus and digestive or urinary tract Q51.7
- **Compartment syndrome** (deep) (posterior) (traumatic) T79.AØ ☑ (*following* T79.7)
  - abdomen T79.A3 ☑ (*following* T79.7)
  - lower extremity (hip, buttock, thigh, leg, foot, toes) T79.A2 ☑ (*following* T79.7)
  - nontraumatic
    - abdomen M79.A3 (*following* M79.7)
    - lower extremity (hip, buttock, thigh, leg, foot, toes) M79.A2- ☑ (*following* M79.7)
    - specified site NEC M79.A9 (*following* M79.7)
    - upper extremity (shoulder, arm, forearm, wrist, hand, fingers) M79.A1- ☑ (*following* M79.7)
  - specified site NEC T79.A9 ☑ (*following* T79.7)
  - upper extremity (shoulder, arm, forearm, wrist, hand, fingers) T79.A1- ☑ (*following* T79.7)
- **Compensation**
  - failure — *see* Disease, heart
  - neurosis, psychoneurosis — *see* Disorder, factitious
- **Complaint** — *see also* Disease
  - bowel, functional K59.9
    - psychogenic F45.8
  - intestine, functional K59.9
    - psychogenic F45.8
  - kidney — *see* Disease, renal
  - miners' J6Ø
- **Complete** — *see* condition
- **Complex**
  - Addison-Schilder E71.528
  - cardiorenal — *see* Hypertension, cardiorenal
  - Costen's M26.69
  - disseminated mycobacterium avium- intracellulare (DMAC) A31.2
  - Eisenmenger's (ventricular septal defect) I27.83
  - hypersexual F52.8
  - jumped process, spine — *see* Dislocation, vertebra
  - primary, tuberculous A15.7
  - Schilder-Addison E71.528
  - subluxation (vertebral) M99.19
    - abdomen M99.19
    - acromioclavicular M99.17
    - cervical region M99.11
    - cervicothoracic M99.11
    - costochondral M99.18
    - costovertebral M99.18
    - head region M99.1Ø
    - hip M99.15
    - lower extremity M99.16
    - lumbar region M99.13
    - lumbosacral M99.13
    - occipitocervical M99.1Ø
    - pelvic region M99.15
    - pubic M99.15
    - rib cage M99.18
    - sacral region M99.14
    - sacrococcygeal M99.14
    - sacroiliac M99.14
    - specified NEC M99.19
    - sternochondral M99.18
    - sternoclavicular M99.17
    - thoracic region M99.12
    - thoracolumbar M99.12
    - upper extremity M99.17
  - Taussig-Bing (transposition, aorta and overriding pulmonary artery) Q2Ø.1
- **Complication**(s) (from) (of)
  - accidental puncture or laceration during a procedure (of) — *see* Complications, intraoperative (intraprocedural), puncture or laceration
  - amputation stump (surgical) (late) NEC T87.9
    - dehiscence T87.81
    - infection or inflammation T87.4Ø
      - lower limb T87.4- ☑
      - upper limb T87.4- ☑
    - necrosis T87.5Ø
      - lower limb T87.5- ☑
      - upper limb T87.5- ☑
    - neuroma T87.3Ø
      - lower limb T87.3- ☑
      - upper limb T87.3- ☑

- **Complication**(s) — *continued*
  - amputation stump — *continued*
    - specified type NEC T87.89
  - anastomosis (and bypass) — *see also* Complications, prosthetic device or implant
    - intestinal (internal) NEC K91.89
      - involving urinary tract N99.89
    - urinary tract (involving intestinal tract) N99.89
    - vascular — *see* Complications, cardiovascular device or implant
  - anesthesia, anesthetic — *see also* Anesthesia, complication T88.59 ☑
    - brain, postpartum, puerperal O89.2
    - cardiac
      - in
        - labor and delivery O74.2
        - pregnancy O29.19- ☑
      - postpartum, puerperal O89.1
    - central nervous system
      - in
        - labor and delivery O74.3
        - pregnancy O29.29- ☑
      - postpartum, puerperal O89.2
    - difficult or failed intubation T88.4 ☑
      - in pregnancy O29.6- ☑
    - failed sedation (conscious) (moderate) during procedure T88.52 ☑
    - general, unintended awareness during procedure T88.53 ☑
    - hyperthermia, malignant T88.3 ☑
    - hypothermia T88.51 ☑
    - intubation failure T88.4 ☑
    - malignant hyperthermia T88.3 ☑
    - pulmonary
      - in
        - labor and delivery O74.1
        - pregnancy NEC O29.Ø9- ☑
      - postpartum, puerperal O89.Ø9
    - shock T88.2 ☑
    - spinal and epidural
      - in
        - labor and delivery NEC O74.6
          - headache O74.5
        - pregnancy NEC O29.5X- ☑
      - postpartum, puerperal NEC O89.5
        - headache O89.4
    - unintended awareness under general anesthesia during procedure T88.53 ☑
  - anti-reflux device — *see* Complications, esophageal anti-reflux device
  - aortic (bifurcation) graft — *see* Complications, graft, vascular
  - aortocoronary (bypass) graft — *see* Complications, coronary artery (bypass) graft
  - aortofemoral (bypass) graft — *see* Complications, extremity artery (bypass) graft
  - arteriovenous
    - fistula, surgically created T82.9 ☑
      - embolism T82.818 ☑
      - fibrosis T82.828 ☑
      - hemorrhage T82.838 ☑
      - infection or inflammation T82.7 ☑
      - mechanical
        - breakdown T82.51Ø ☑
        - displacement T82.52Ø ☑
        - leakage T82.53Ø ☑
        - malposition T82.52Ø ☑
        - obstruction T82.59Ø ☑
        - perforation T82.59Ø ☑
        - protrusion T82.59Ø ☑
      - pain T82.848 ☑
      - specified type NEC T82.898 ☑
      - stenosis T82.858 ☑
      - thrombosis T82.868 ☑
    - shunt, surgically created T82.9 ☑
      - embolism T82.818 ☑
      - fibrosis T82.828 ☑
      - hemorrhage T82.838 ☑
      - infection or inflammation T82.7 ☑
      - mechanical
        - breakdown T82.511 ☑
        - displacement T82.521 ☑
        - leakage T82.531 ☑
        - malposition T82.521 ☑
        - obstruction T82.591 ☑
        - perforation T82.591 ☑
        - protrusion T82.591 ☑

- **Complication**(s) — *continued*
  - arteriovenous — *continued*
    - shunt, surgically created — *continued*
      - pain T82.848 ☑
      - specified type NEC T82.898 ☑
      - stenosis T82.858 ☑
      - thrombosis T82.868 ☑
  - arthroplasty — *see* Complications, joint prosthesis
  - artificial
    - fertilization or insemination N98.9
      - attempted introduction (of)
        - embryo in embryo transfer N98.3
        - ovum following in vitro fertilization N98.2
      - hyperstimulation of ovaries N98.1
      - infection N98.Ø
      - specified NEC N98.8
    - heart T82.9 ☑
      - embolism T82.817 ☑
      - fibrosis T82.827 ☑
      - hemorrhage T82.837 ☑
      - infection or inflammation T82.7 ☑
      - mechanical
        - breakdown T82.512 ☑
        - displacement T82.522 ☑
        - leakage T82.532 ☑
        - malposition T82.522 ☑
        - obstruction T82.592 ☑
        - perforation T82.592 ☑
        - protrusion T82.592 ☑
      - pain T82.847 ☑
      - specified type NEC T82.897 ☑
      - stenosis T82.857 ☑
      - thrombosis T82.867 ☑
    - opening
      - cecostomy — *see* Complications, colostomy
      - colostomy — *see* Complications, colostomy
      - cystostomy — *see* Complications, cystostomy
      - enterostomy — *see* Complications, enterostomy
      - gastrostomy — *see* Complications, gastrostomy
      - ileostomy — *see* Complications, enterostomy
      - jejunostomy — *see* Complications, enterostomy
      - nephrostomy — *see* Complications, stoma, urinary tract
      - tracheostomy — *see* Complications, tracheostomy
      - ureterostomy — *see* Complications, stoma, urinary tract
      - urethrostomy — *see* Complications, stoma, urinary tract
  - balloon implant or device
    - gastrointestinal T85.9 ☑
      - embolism T85.818 ☑
      - fibrosis T85.828 ☑
      - hemorrhage T85.838 ☑
      - infection and inflammation T85.79 ☑
      - pain T85.848 ☑
      - specified type NEC T85.898 ☑
      - stenosis T85.858 ☑
      - thrombosis T85.868 ☑
    - vascular (counterpulsation) T82.9 ☑
      - embolism T82.818 ☑
      - fibrosis T82.828 ☑
      - hemorrhage T82.838 ☑
      - infection or inflammation T82.7 ☑
      - mechanical
        - breakdown T82.513 ☑
        - displacement T82.523 ☑
        - leakage T82.533 ☑
        - malposition T82.523 ☑
        - obstruction T82.593 ☑
        - perforation T82.593 ☑
        - protrusion T82.593 ☑
      - pain T82.848 ☑
      - specified type NEC T82.898 ☑
      - stenosis T82.858 ☑
      - thrombosis T82.868 ☑
  - bariatric procedure
    - gastric band procedure K95.Ø9
      - infection K95.Ø1
    - specified procedure NEC K95.89
      - infection K95.81
  - bile duct implant (prosthetic) T85.9 ☑
    - embolism T85.818 ☑
    - fibrosis T85.828 ☑
    - hemorrhage T85.838 ☑
    - infection and inflammation T85.79 ☑

- **Complication**(s) — *continued*
  - bile duct implant — *continued*
    - mechanical
      - breakdown T85.51Ø ☑
      - displacement T85.52Ø ☑
      - malfunction T85.51Ø ☑
      - malposition T85.52Ø ☑
      - obstruction T85.59Ø ☑
      - perforation T85.59Ø ☑
      - protrusion T85.59Ø ☑
      - specified NEC T85.59Ø ☑
    - pain T85.848 ☑
    - specified type NEC T85.898 ☑
    - stenosis T85.858 ☑
    - thrombosis T85.868 ☑
  - bladder device (auxiliary) — *see* Complications, genitourinary, device or implant, urinary system
  - bleeding (postoperative) — *see* Complication, postoperative, hemorrhage
    - intraoperative — *see* Complication, intraoperative, hemorrhage
  - blood vessel graft — *see* Complications, graft, vascular
  - bone
    - device NEC T84.9 ☑
      - embolism T84.81 ☑
      - fibrosis T84.82 ☑
      - hemorrhage T84.83 ☑
      - infection or inflammation T84.7 ☑
      - mechanical
        - breakdown T84.318 ☑
        - displacement T84.328 ☑
        - malposition T84.328 ☑
        - obstruction T84.398 ☑
        - perforation T84.398 ☑
        - protrusion T84.398 ☑
      - pain T84.84 ☑
      - specified type NEC T84.89 ☑
      - stenosis T84.85 ☑
      - thrombosis T84.86 ☑
    - graft — *see* Complications, graft, bone
    - growth stimulator (electrode) — *see* Complications, electronic stimulator device, bone
    - marrow transplant — *see* Complications, transplant, bone, marrow
  - brain neurostimulator (electrode) — *see* Complications, electronic stimulator device, brain
  - breast implant (prosthetic) T85.9 ☑
    - capsular contracture T85.44 ☑
    - embolism T85.818 ☑
    - fibrosis T85.828 ☑
    - hemorrhage T85.838 ☑
    - infection and inflammation T85.79 ☑
    - mechanical
      - breakdown T85.41 ☑
      - displacement T85.42 ☑
      - leakage T85.43 ☑
      - malposition T85.42 ☑
      - obstruction T85.49 ☑
      - perforation T85.49 ☑
      - protrusion T85.49 ☑
      - specified NEC T85.49 ☑
    - pain T85.848 ☑
    - specified type NEC T85.898 ☑
    - stenosis T85.858 ☑
    - thrombosis T85.868 ☑
  - bypass — *see also* Complications, prosthetic device or implant
    - aortocoronary — *see* Complications, coronary artery (bypass) graft
    - arterial — *see also* Complications, graft, vascular
      - extremity — *see* Complications, extremity artery (bypass) graft
  - cardiac — *see also* Disease, heart
    - device, implant or graft T82.9 ☑
      - embolism T82.817 ☑
      - fibrosis T82.827 ☑
      - hemorrhage T82.837 ☑
      - infection or inflammation T82.7 ☑
        - valve prosthesis T82.6 ☑
      - mechanical
        - breakdown T82.519 ☑
          - specified device NEC T82.518 ☑
        - displacement T82.529 ☑
          - specified device NEC T82.528 ☑
        - leakage T82.539 ☑
          - specified device NEC T82.538 ☑

- **Complication**(s) — *continued*
  - cardiac — *see also* Disease, heart — *continued*
    - device, implant or graft — *continued*
      - mechanical — *continued*
        - malposition T82.529 ☑
          - specified device NEC T82.528 ☑
        - obstruction T82.599 ☑
          - specified device NEC T82.598 ☑
        - perforation T82.599 ☑
          - specified device NEC T82.598 ☑
        - protrusion T82.599 ☑
          - specified device NEC T82.598 ☑
      - pain T82.847 ☑
      - specified type NEC T82.897 ☑
      - stenosis T82.857 ☑
      - thrombosis T82.867 ☑
  - cardiovascular device, graft or implant T82.9 ☑
    - aortic graft — *see* Complications, graft, vascular
    - arteriovenous
      - fistula, artificial — *see* Complication, arteriovenous, fistula, surgically created
      - shunt — *see* Complication, arteriovenous, shunt, surgically created
    - artificial heart — *see* Complication, artificial, heart
    - balloon (counterpulsation) device — *see* Complication, balloon implant, vascular
    - carotid artery graft — *see* Complications, graft, vascular
    - coronary bypass graft — *see* Complication, coronary artery (bypass) graft
    - dialysis catheter (vascular) — *see* Complication, catheter, dialysis
    - electronic T82.9 ☑
      - electrode T82.9 ☑
        - embolism T82.817 ☑
        - fibrosis T82.827 ☑
        - hemorrhage T82.837 ☑
        - infection T82.7 ☑
        - mechanical
          - breakdown T82.11Ø ☑
          - displacement T82.12Ø ☑
          - leakage T82.19Ø ☑
          - obstruction T82.19Ø ☑
          - perforation T82.19Ø ☑
          - protrusion T82.19Ø ☑
          - specified type NEC T82.19Ø ☑
        - pain T82.847 ☑
        - specified NEC T82.897 ☑
        - stenosis T82.857 ☑
        - thrombosis T82.867 ☑
      - embolism T82.817 ☑
      - fibrosis T82.827 ☑
      - hemorrhage T82.837 ☑
      - infection T82.7 ☑
      - mechanical
        - breakdown T82.119 ☑
        - displacement T82.129 ☑
        - leakage T82.199 ☑
        - obstruction T82.199 ☑
        - perforation T82.199 ☑
        - protrusion T82.199 ☑
        - specified type NEC T82.199 ☑
      - pain T82.847 ☑
      - pulse generator T82.9 ☑
        - embolism T82.817 ☑
        - fibrosis T82.827 ☑
        - hemorrhage T82.837 ☑
        - infection T82.7 ☑
        - mechanical
          - breakdown T82.111 ☑
          - displacement T82.121 ☑
          - leakage T82.191 ☑
          - obstruction T82.191 ☑
          - perforation T82.191 ☑
          - protrusion T82.191 ☑
          - specified type NEC T82.191 ☑
        - pain T82.847 ☑
        - specified NEC T82.897 ☑
        - stenosis T82.857 ☑
        - thrombosis T82.867 ☑
      - specified condition NEC T82.897 ☑
      - specified device NEC T82.9 ☑
        - embolism T82.817 ☑
        - fibrosis T82.827 ☑
        - hemorrhage T82.837 ☑
        - infection T82.7 ☑

- **Complication**(s) — *continued*
  - cardiovascular device, graft or implant — *continued*
    - electronic — *continued*
      - specified device — *continued*
        - mechanical
          - breakdown T82.118 ☑
          - displacement T82.128 ☑
          - leakage T82.198 ☑
          - obstruction T82.198 ☑
          - perforation T82.198 ☑
          - protrusion T82.198 ☑
          - specified type NEC T82.198 ☑
        - pain T82.847 ☑
        - specified NEC T82.897 ☑
        - stenosis T82.857 ☑
        - thrombosis T82.867 ☑
      - stenosis T82.857 ☑
      - thrombosis T82.867 ☑
    - extremity artery graft — *see* Complication, extremity artery (bypass) graft
    - femoral artery graft — *see* Complication, extremity artery (bypass) graft
    - heart
      - transplant — *see* Complication, transplant, heart
      - valve — *see* Complication, prosthetic device, heart valve
        - graft — *see* Complication, heart, valve, graft
    - heart-lung transplant — *see* Complication, transplant, heart, with lung
    - infection or inflammation T82.7 ☑
    - umbrella device — *see* Complication, umbrella device, vascular
    - vascular graft (or anastomosis) — *see* Complication, graft, vascular
  - carotid artery (bypass) graft — *see* Complications, graft, vascular
  - catheter (device) NEC — *see also* Complications, prosthetic device or implant
    - cranial infusion
      - infection and inflammation T85.735 ☑
      - mechanical
        - breakdown T85.61Ø ☑
        - displacement T85.62Ø ☑
        - leakage T85.63Ø ☑
        - malfunction T85.69Ø ☑
        - malposition T85.62Ø ☑
        - obstruction T85.69Ø ☑
        - perforation T85.69Ø ☑
        - protrusion T85.69Ø ☑
        - specified NEC T85.69Ø ☑
    - cystostomy T83.9 ☑
      - embolism T83.81 ☑
      - fibrosis T83.82 ☑
      - hemorrhage T83.83 ☑
      - infection and inflammation T83.51Ø ☑
      - mechanical
        - breakdown T83.Ø1Ø ☑
        - displacement T83.Ø2Ø ☑
        - leakage T83.Ø3Ø ☑
        - malposition T83.Ø2Ø ☑
        - obstruction T83.Ø9Ø ☑
        - perforation T83.Ø9Ø ☑
        - protrusion T83.Ø9Ø ☑
        - specified NEC T83.Ø9Ø ☑
      - pain T83.84 ☑
      - specified type NEC T83.89 ☑
      - stenosis T83.85 ☑
      - thrombosis T83.86 ☑
    - dialysis (vascular) T82.9 ☑
      - embolism T82.818 ☑
      - fibrosis T82.828 ☑
      - hemorrhage T82.838 ☑
      - infection and inflammation T82.7 ☑
      - intraperitoneal — *see* Complications, catheter, intraperitoneal
      - mechanical
        - breakdown T82.41 ☑
        - displacement T82.42 ☑
        - leakage T82.43 ☑
        - malposition T82.42 ☑
        - obstruction T82.49 ☑
        - perforation T82.49 ☑
        - protrusion T82.49 ☑
      - pain T82.848 ☑
      - specified type NEC T82.898 ☑
      - stenosis T82.858 ☑

- **Complication**(s) — *continued*
  - electronic stimulator device — *continued*
    - bone — *continued*
      - hemorrhage T84.83 ☑
      - infection or inflammation T84.7 ☑
      - malfunction T84.310 ☑
      - malposition T84.320 ☑
      - mechanical NEC T84.390 ☑
      - obstruction T84.390 ☑
      - pain T84.84 ☑
      - perforation T84.390 ☑
      - protrusion T84.390 ☑
      - specified type NEC T84.89 ☑
      - stenosis T84.85 ☑
      - thrombosis T84.86 ☑
    - brain T85.9 ☑
      - embolism T85.810 ☑
      - fibrosis T85.820 ☑
      - hemorrhage T85.830 ☑
      - infection and inflammation T85.731 ☑
      - mechanical
        - breakdown T85.110 ☑
        - displacement T85.120 ☑
        - leakage T85.190 ☑
        - malposition T85.120 ☑
        - obstruction T85.190 ☑
        - perforation T85.190 ☑
        - protrusion T85.190 ☑
        - specified NEC T85.190 ☑
      - pain T85.840 ☑
      - specified type NEC T85.890 ☑
      - stenosis T85.850 ☑
      - thrombosis T85.860 ☑
    - cardiac (defibrillator) (pacemaker) — *see* Complications, cardiovascular device or implant, electronic
    - generator (brain) (gastric) (peripheral) (sacral) (spinal)
      - breakdown T85.113 ☑
      - displacement T85.123 ☑
      - leakage T85.193 ☑
      - malposition T85.123 ☑
      - obstruction T85.193 ☑
      - perforation T85.193 ☑
      - protrusion T85.193 ☑
      - specified type NEC T85.193 ☑
    - muscle T84.9 ☑
      - breakdown T84.418 ☑
      - displacement T84.428 ☑
      - embolism T84.81 ☑
      - fibrosis T84.82 ☑
      - hemorrhage T84.83 ☑
      - infection or inflammation T84.7 ☑
      - mechanical NEC T84.498 ☑
      - pain T84.84 ☑
      - specified type NEC T84.89 ☑
      - stenosis T84.85 ☑
      - thrombosis T84.86 ☑
    - nervous system T85.9 ☑
      - brain — *see* Complications, electronic stimulator device, brain
      - cranial nerve — *see* Complications, electronic stimulator device, peripheral nerve
      - embolism T85.810 ☑
      - fibrosis T85.820 ☑
      - gastric nerve — *see* Complications, electronic stimulator device, peripheral nerve
      - hemorrhage T85.830 ☑
      - infection and inflammation T85.738 ☑
      - mechanical
        - breakdown T85.118 ☑
        - displacement T85.128 ☑
        - leakage T85.199 ☑
        - malposition T85.128 ☑
        - obstruction T85.199 ☑
        - perforation T85.199 ☑
        - protrusion T85.199 ☑
        - specified NEC T85.199 ☑
      - pain T85.840 ☑
      - peripheral nerve — *see* Complications, electronic stimulator device, peripheral nerve
      - sacral nerve — *see* Complications, electronic stimulator device, peripheral nerve
      - specified type NEC T85.890 ☑
      - spinal cord — *see* Complications, electronic stimulator device, spinal cord

- **Complication**(s) — *continued*
  - electronic stimulator device — *continued*
    - nervous system — *continued*
      - stenosis T85.850 ☑
      - thrombosis T85.860 ☑
      - vagal nerve — *see* Complications, electronic stimulator device, peripheral nerve
    - peripheral nerve T85.9 ☑
      - embolism T85.810 ☑
      - fibrosis T85.820 ☑
      - hemorrhage T85.830 ☑
      - infection and inflammation T85.732 ☑
      - mechanical
        - breakdown T85.111 ☑
        - displacement T85.121 ☑
        - leakage T85.191 ☑
        - malposition T85.121 ☑
        - obstruction T85.191 ☑
        - perforation T85.191 ☑
        - protrusion T85.191 ☑
        - specified NEC T85.191 ☑
      - pain T85.840 ☑
      - specified type NEC T85.890 ☑
      - stenosis T85.850 ☑
      - thrombosis T85.860 ☑
    - spinal cord T85.9 ☑
      - embolism T85.810 ☑
      - fibrosis T85.820 ☑
      - hemorrhage T85.830 ☑
      - infection and inflammation T85.733 ☑
      - mechanical
        - breakdown T85.112 ☑
        - displacement T85.122 ☑
        - leakage T85.192 ☑
        - malposition T85.122 ☑
        - obstruction T85.192 ☑
        - perforation T85.192 ☑
        - protrusion T85.192 ☑
        - specified NEC T85.192 ☑
      - pain T85.840 ☑
      - specified type NEC T85.890 ☑
      - stenosis T85.850 ☑
      - thrombosis T85.860 ☑
    - urinary T83.9 ☑
      - embolism T83.81 ☑
      - fibrosis T83.82 ☑
      - hemorrhage T83.83 ☑
      - infection and inflammation T83.598 ☑
      - mechanical
        - breakdown T83.110 ☑
        - displacement T83.120 ☑
        - malposition T83.120 ☑
        - perforation T83.190 ☑
        - protrusion T83.190 ☑
        - specified NEC T83.190 ☑
      - pain T83.84 ☑
      - specified type NEC T83.89 ☑
      - stenosis T83.85 ☑
      - thrombosis T83.86 ☑
  - electroshock therapy T88.9 ☑
    - specified NEC T88.8 ☑
  - endocrine E34.9
    - postprocedural
      - adrenal hypofunction E89.6
      - hypoinsulinemia E89.1
      - hypoparathyroidism E89.2
      - hypopituitarism E89.3
      - hypothyroidism E89.0
      - ovarian failure E89.40
        - asymptomatic E89.40
        - symptomatic E89.41
      - specified NEC E89.89
      - testicular hypofunction E89.5
  - endodontic treatment NEC M27.59
  - enterostomy (stoma) K94.10
    - hemorrhage K94.11
    - infection K94.12
    - malfunction K94.13
    - mechanical K94.13
    - specified complication NEC K94.19
  - episiotomy, disruption O90.1
  - esophageal anti-reflux device T85.9 ☑
    - embolism T85.818 ☑
    - fibrosis T85.828 ☑
    - hemorrhage T85.838 ☑
    - infection and inflammation T85.79 ☑

- **Complication**(s) — *continued*
  - esophageal anti-reflux device — *continued*
    - mechanical
      - breakdown T85.511 ☑
      - displacement T85.521 ☑
      - malfunction T85.511 ☑
      - malposition T85.521 ☑
      - obstruction T85.591 ☑
      - perforation T85.591 ☑
      - protrusion T85.591 ☑
      - specified NEC T85.591 ☑
    - pain T85.848 ☑
    - specified type NEC T85.898 ☑
    - stenosis T85.858 ☑
    - thrombosis T85.868 ☑
  - esophagostomy K94.30
    - hemorrhage K94.31
    - infection K94.32
    - malfunction K94.33
    - mechanical K94.33
    - specified complication NEC K94.39
  - extracorporeal circulation T80.90 ☑
  - extremity artery (bypass) graft T82.9 ☑
    - arteriosclerosis — *see* Arteriosclerosis, extremities, bypass graft
    - embolism T82.818 ☑
    - fibrosis T82.828 ☑
    - hemorrhage T82.838 ☑
    - infection and inflammation T82.7 ☑
    - mechanical
      - breakdown T82.318 ☑
        - femoral artery T82.312 ☑
      - displacement T82.328 ☑
        - femoral artery T82.322 ☑
      - leakage T82.338 ☑
        - femoral artery T82.332 ☑
      - malposition T82.328 ☑
        - femoral artery T82.322 ☑
      - obstruction T82.398 ☑
        - femoral artery T82.392 ☑
      - perforation T82.398 ☑
        - femoral artery T82.392 ☑
      - protrusion T82.398 ☑
        - femoral artery T82.392 ☑
    - pain T82.848 ☑
    - specified type NEC T82.898 ☑
    - stenosis T82.858 ☑
    - thrombosis T82.868 ☑
  - eye H57.9
    - corneal graft — *see* Complications, graft, cornea
    - implant (prosthetic) T85.9 ☑
      - embolism T85.818 ☑
      - fibrosis T85.828 ☑
      - hemorrhage T85.838 ☑
      - infection and inflammation T85.79 ☑
      - mechanical
        - breakdown T85.318 ☑
        - displacement T85.328 ☑
        - leakage T85.398 ☑
        - malposition T85.328 ☑
        - obstruction T85.398 ☑
        - perforation T85.398 ☑
        - protrusion T85.398 ☑
        - specified NEC T85.398 ☑
      - pain T85.848 ☑
      - specified type NEC T85.898 ☑
      - stenosis T85.858 ☑
      - thrombosis T85.868 ☑
    - intraocular lens — *see* Complications, intraocular lens
    - orbital prosthesis — *see* Complications, orbital prosthesis
  - female genital N94.9
    - device, implant or graft NEC — *see* Complications, genitourinary, device or implant, genital tract
  - femoral artery (bypass) graft — *see* Complication, extremity artery (bypass) graft
  - fixation device, internal (orthopedic) T84.9 ☑
    - infection and inflammation T84.60 ☑
      - arm T84.61- ☑
        - humerus T84.61- ☑
        - radius T84.61- ☑
        - ulna T84.61- ☑
      - leg T84.629 ☑
        - femur T84.62- ☑
        - fibula T84.62- ☑

Complication(s) — *continued*
- postprocedural — *see also* Complications, surgical procedure — *continued*
  - hemorrhage — *continued*
    - musculoskeletal structure
      - following musculoskeletal surgery M96.830
      - following non-orthopedic surgery M96.831
      - following orthopedic surgery M96.830
    - nervous system
      - following nervous system procedure G97.51
      - following other procedure G97.52
    - respiratory system
      - following a respiratory system procedure J95.830
      - following other procedure J95.831
    - skin and subcutaneous tissue
      - following a procedure on other organ L76.22
      - following dermatologic procedure L76.21
    - spleen
      - following procedure on other organ D78.22
      - following procedure on the spleen D78.21
  - seroma (of)
    - circulatory system organ or structure
      - following cardiac bypass I97.641
      - following cardiac catheterization I97.640
      - following other circulatory system procedure I97.648
      - following other procedure I97.622
    - digestive system
      - following procedure on digestive system K91.872
      - following procedure on other organ K91.873
    - ear
      - following other procedure H95.54
      - following procedure on ear and mastoid process H95.53
    - endocrine system
      - following endocrine system procedure E89.822
      - following other procedure E89.823
    - eye and adnexa
      - following ophthalmic procedure H59.35- ☑
      - following other procedure H59.36- ☑
    - genitourinary organ or structure
      - following procedure on genitourinary organ or structure N99.842
      - following procedure on other organ N99.843
    - mastoid process
      - following other procedure H95.54
      - following procedure on ear and mastoid process H95.53
    - musculoskeletal structure
      - following musculoskeletal surgery M96.842
      - following non-orthopedic surgery M96.843
      - following orthopedic surgery M96.842
    - nervous system
      - following nervous system procedure G97.63
      - following other procedure G97.64
    - respiratory system
      - following other procedure J95.863
      - following procedure on respiratory system organ or structure J95.862
    - skin and subcutaneous tissue
      - following dermatologic procedure L76.33
      - following procedure on other organ L76.34
    - spleen
      - following procedure on other organ D78.34
      - following procedure on the spleen D78.33
  - specified NEC
    - circulatory system I97.89
    - digestive K91.89
    - ear H95.89
    - endocrine E89.89
    - eye and adnexa H59.89
    - genitourinary N99.89
    - mastoid process H95.89
    - metabolic E89.89
    - musculoskeletal structure M96.89
    - nervous system G97.82
    - respiratory system J95.89
    - skin and subcutaneous tissue L76.82
    - spleen D78.89
- pregnancy NEC — *see* Pregnancy, complicated by
- prosthetic device or implant T85.9 ☑
  - bile duct — *see* Complications, bile duct implant
  - breast — *see* Complications, breast implant

Complication(s) — *continued*
- prosthetic device or implant — *continued*
  - bulking agent
    - ureteral
      - erosion T83.714 ☑
      - exposure T83.724 ☑
    - urethral
      - erosion T83.713 ☑
      - exposure T83.723 ☑
  - cardiac and vascular NEC — *see* Complications, cardiovascular device or implant
  - corneal transplant — *see* Complications, graft, cornea
  - electronic nervous system stimulator — *see* Complications, electronic stimulator device
  - epidural infusion catheter — *see* Complications, catheter, epidural
  - esophageal anti-reflux device — *see* Complications, esophageal anti-reflux device
  - genital organ or tract — *see* Complications, genitourinary, device or implant, genital tract
    - specified NEC T83.79- ☑
  - heart valve — *see* Complications, heart, valve, prosthesis
  - infection or inflammation T85.79 ☑
    - intestine transplant T86.852
    - liver transplant T86.43
    - lung transplant T86.812
    - pancreas transplant T86.892
    - skin graft T86.822
  - intraocular lens — *see* Complications, intraocular lens
  - intraperitoneal (dialysis) catheter — *see* Complication(s), catheter, intraperitoneal dialysis
  - joint — *see* Complications, joint prosthesis, internal
  - mechanical NEC T85.698 ☑
    - dialysis catheter (vascular) — *see also* Complication, catheter, dialysis, mechanical
      - peritoneal — *see* Complication(s), catheter, intraperitoneal dialysis
    - gastrointestinal device T85.598 ☑
    - ocular device T85.398 ☑
    - subdural (infusion) catheter T85.690 ☑
    - suture, permanent T85.692 ☑
      - that for bone repair — *see* Complications, fixation device, internal (orthopedic), mechanical
    - ventricular shunt
      - breakdown T85.01 ☑
      - displacement T85.02 ☑
      - leakage T85.03 ☑
      - malposition T85.02 ☑
      - obstruction T85.09 ☑
      - perforation T85.09 ☑
      - protrusion T85.09 ☑
      - specified NEC T85.09 ☑
  - mesh
    - erosion (to surrounding organ or tissue) T83.718 ☑
      - urethral (into pelvic floor muscles) T83.712 ☑
      - vaginal (into pelvic floor muscles) T83.711 ☑
    - exposure (into surrounding organ or tissue) T83.728 ☑
      - urethral (through urethral wall) T83.722 ☑
      - vaginal (into vagina) (through vaginal wall) T83.721 ☑
  - orbital — *see* Complications, orbital prosthesis
  - penile T83.9 ☑
    - embolism T83.81 ☑
    - fibrosis T83.82 ☑
    - hemorrhage T83.83 ☑
    - infection and inflammation T83.61 ☑
    - mechanical
      - breakdown T83.410 ☑
      - displacement T83.420 ☑
      - leakage T83.490 ☑
      - malposition T83.420 ☑
      - obstruction T83.490 ☑
      - perforation T83.490 ☑
      - protrusion T83.490 ☑
      - specified NEC T83.490 ☑
    - pain T83.84 ☑
    - specified type NEC T83.89 ☑
    - stenosis T83.85 ☑
    - thrombosis T83.86 ☑

Complication(s) — *continued*
- prosthetic device or implant — *continued*
  - prosthetic materials NEC
    - erosion (to surrounding organ or tissue) T83.718 ☑
    - exposure (into surrounding organ or tissue) T83.728 ☑
  - skin graft T86.829
    - artificial skin or decellularized allodermis
      - embolism T85.818 ☑
      - fibrosis T85.828 ☑
      - hemorrhage T85.838 ☑
      - infection and inflammation T85.79 ☑
      - mechanical
        - breakdown T85.613 ☑
        - displacement T85.623 ☑
        - malfunction T85.613 ☑
        - malposition T85.623 ☑
        - obstruction T85.693 ☑
        - perforation T85.693 ☑
        - protrusion T85.693 ☑
        - specified NEC T85.693 ☑
      - pain T85.848 ☑
      - specified type NEC T85.898 ☑
      - stenosis T85.858 ☑
      - thrombosis T85.868 ☑
    - failure T86.821
    - infection T86.822
    - rejection T86.820
    - specified NEC T86.828
  - sling
    - urethral (female) (male)
      - erosion T83.712 ☑
      - exposure T83.722 ☑
  - specified NEC T85.9 ☑
    - embolism T85.818 ☑
    - fibrosis T85.828 ☑
    - hemorrhage T85.838 ☑
    - infection and inflammation T85.79 ☑
    - mechanical
      - breakdown T85.618 ☑
      - displacement T85.628 ☑
      - leakage T85.638 ☑
      - malfunction T85.618 ☑
      - malposition T85.628 ☑
      - obstruction T85.698 ☑
      - perforation T85.698 ☑
      - protrusion T85.698 ☑
      - specified NEC T85.698 ☑
    - pain T85.848 ☑
    - specified type NEC T85.898 ☑
    - stenosis T85.858 ☑
    - thrombosis T85.868 ☑
  - subdural infusion catheter — *see* Complications, catheter, subdural
  - sutures — *see* Complications, sutures
  - urinary organ or tract NEC — *see* Complications, genitourinary, device or implant, urinary system
  - vascular — *see* Complications, cardiovascular device or implant
  - ventricular shunt — *see* Complications, ventricular shunt (device)
- puerperium — *see* Puerperal
- puncture, spinal G97.1
  - cerebrospinal fluid leak G97.0
  - headache or reaction G97.1
- pyelogram N99.89
- radiation
  - kyphosis M96.2
  - scoliosis M96.5
- reattached
  - extremity (infection) (rejection)
    - lower T87.1X- ☑
    - upper T87.0X- ☑
  - specified body part NEC T87.2
- reconstructed breast
  - asymmetry between native and reconstructed breast N65.1
  - deformity N65.0
  - disproportion between native and reconstructed breast N65.1
  - excess tissue N65.0
  - misshappen N65.0
- reimplant NEC — *see also* Complications, prosthetic device or implant

Complication(s) — *continued*
- transfusion — *continued*
  - febrile nonhemolytic transfusion reaction R5Ø.84
  - hemochromatosis E83.111
  - hemolysis T8Ø.89 ☑
  - hemolytic reaction (antigen unspecified) T8Ø.919 ☑
  - incompatibility reaction (antigen unspecified) T8Ø.919 ☑
    - ABO T8Ø.3Ø ☑
      - delayed serologic (DSTR) T8Ø.39 ☑
      - hemolytic transfusion reaction (HTR) (unspecified time after transfusion) T8Ø.319 ☑
        - acute (AHTR) (less than 24 hours after transfusion) T8Ø.31Ø ☑
        - delayed (DHTR) (24 hours or more after transfusion) T8Ø.311 ☑
      - specified NEC T8Ø.39 ☑
    - acute (antigen unspecified) T8Ø.91Ø ☑
    - delayed (antigen unspecified) T8Ø.911 ☑
    - delayed serologic (DSTR) T8Ø.89 ☑
    - non-ABO (minor antigens (Duffy) (K) (Kell) (Kidd) (Lewis) (M) (N) (P) (S)) T8Ø.AØ ☑ *(following* T8Ø.4)
      - delayed serologic (DSTR) T8Ø.A9 ☑ *(following* T8Ø.4)
      - hemolytic transfusion reaction (HTR) (unspecified time after transfusion) T8Ø.A19 ☑ *(following* T8Ø.4)
        - acute (AHTR) (less than 24 hours after transfusion) T8Ø.A1Ø ☑ *(following* T8Ø.4)
        - delayed (DHTR) (24 hours or more after transfusion) T8Ø.A11 ☑ *(following* T8Ø.4)
      - specified NEC T8Ø.A9 ☑ *(following* T8Ø.4)
    - Rh (antigens (C) (c) (D) (E) (e)) (factor) T8Ø.4Ø ☑
      - delayed serologic (DSTR) T8Ø.49 ☑
      - hemolytic transfusion reaction (HTR) (unspecified time after transfusion) T8Ø.419 ☑
        - acute (AHTR) (less than 24 hours after transfusion) T8Ø.41Ø ☑
        - delayed (DHTR) (24 hours or more after transfusion) T8Ø.411 ☑
      - specified NEC T8Ø.49 ☑
  - infection T8Ø.29 ☑
    - acute T8Ø.22- ☑
  - reaction NEC T8Ø.89 ☑
  - sepsis T8Ø.29 ☑
  - shock T8Ø.89 ☑
- transplant T86.9Ø
  - bone T86.839
    - failure T86.831
    - infection T86.832
    - rejection T86.83Ø
    - specified type NEC T86.838
  - bone marrow T86.ØØ
    - failure T86.Ø2
    - infection T86.Ø3
    - rejection T86.Ø1
    - specified type NEC T86.Ø9
  - cornea T86.849- ☑
    - failure T86.841- ☑
    - infection T86.842- ☑
    - rejection T86.84Ø- ☑
    - specified type NEC T86.848- ☑
  - failure T86.92
  - heart T86.2Ø
    - with lung T86.3Ø
    - cardiac allograft vasculopathy T86.29Ø
      - failure T86.32
      - infection T86.33
      - rejection T86.31
      - specified type NEC T86.39
    - failure T86.22
    - infection T86.23
    - rejection T86.21
    - specified type NEC T86.298
  - infection T86.93
  - intestine T86.859
    - failure T86.851
    - infection T86.852
    - rejection T86.85Ø
    - specified type NEC T86.858
  - kidney T86.1Ø
    - failure T86.12
    - infection T86.13
    - rejection T86.11

Complication(s) — *continued*
- transplant — *continued*
  - kidney — *continued*
    - specified type NEC T86.19
  - liver T86.4Ø
    - failure T86.42
    - infection T86.43
    - rejection T86.41
    - specified type NEC T86.49
  - lung T86.819
    - with heart T86.3Ø
      - failure T86.32
      - infection T86.33
      - rejection T86.31
      - specified type NEC T86.39
    - failure T86.811
    - infection T86.812
    - rejection T86.81Ø
    - specified type NEC T86.818
  - malignant neoplasm C8Ø.2
  - pancreas T86.899
    - failure T86.891
    - infection T86.892
    - rejection T86.89Ø
    - specified type NEC T86.898
  - peripheral blood stem cells T86.5
  - post-transplant lymphoproliferative disorder (PTLD) D47.Z1 *(following* D47.4)
  - rejection T86.91
  - skin T86.829
    - failure T86.821
    - infection T86.822
    - rejection T86.82Ø
    - specified type NEC T86.828
  - specified
    - tissue T86.899
      - failure T86.891
      - infection T86.892
      - rejection T86.89Ø
      - specified type NEC T86.898
    - type NEC T86.99
  - stem cell (from peripheral blood) (from umbilical cord) T86.5
  - umbilical cord stem cells T86.5
- trauma (early) T79.9 ☑
  - specified NEC T79.8 ☑
- ultrasound therapy NEC T88.9 ☑
- umbilical cord NEC
  - complicating delivery O69.9 ☑
    - specified NEC O69.89 ☑
- umbrella device, vascular T82.9 ☑
  - embolism T82.818 ☑
  - fibrosis T82.828 ☑
  - hemorrhage T82.838 ☑
  - infection or inflammation T82.7 ☑
  - mechanical
    - breakdown T82.515 ☑
    - displacement T82.525 ☑
    - leakage T82.535 ☑
    - malposition T82.525 ☑
    - obstruction T82.595 ☑
    - perforation T82.595 ☑
    - protrusion T82.595 ☑
  - pain T82.848 ☑
  - specified type NEC T82.898 ☑
  - stenosis T82.858 ☑
  - thrombosis T82.868 ☑
- urethral catheter — *see* Complications, catheter, urethral, indwelling
- vaccination T88.1 ☑
  - anaphylaxis NEC T8Ø.52 ☑
  - arthropathy — *see* Arthropathy, postimmunization
  - cellulitis T88.Ø ☑
  - encephalitis or encephalomyelitis GØ4.Ø2
  - infection (general) (local) NEC T88.Ø ☑
  - meningitis GØ3.8
  - myelitis GØ4.Ø2
  - protein sickness T8Ø.62 ☑
  - rash T88.1 ☑
  - reaction (allergic) T88.1 ☑
    - serum T8Ø.62 ☑
  - sepsis T88.Ø ☑
  - serum intoxication, sickness, rash, or other serum reaction NEC T8Ø.62 ☑
    - anaphylactic shock T8Ø.52 ☑
  - shock (allergic) (anaphylactic) T8Ø.52 ☑
  - vaccinia (generalized) (localized) T88.1 ☑

Complication(s) — *continued*
- vas deferens device or implant — *see* Complications, genitourinary, device or implant, genital tract
- vascular I99.9
  - device or implant T82.9 ☑
    - embolism T82.818 ☑
    - fibrosis T82.828 ☑
    - hemorrhage T82.838 ☑
    - infection or inflammation T82.7 ☑
    - mechanical
      - breakdown T82.519 ☑
        - specified device NEC T82.518 ☑
      - displacement T82.529 ☑
        - specified device NEC T82.528 ☑
      - leakage T82.539 ☑
        - specified device NEC T82.538 ☑
      - malposition T82.529 ☑
        - specified device NEC T82.528 ☑
      - obstruction T82.599 ☑
        - specified device NEC T82.598 ☑
      - perforation T82.599 ☑
        - specified device NEC T82.598 ☑
      - protrusion T82.599 ☑
        - specified device NEC T82.598 ☑
    - pain T82.848 ☑
    - specified type NEC T82.898 ☑
    - stenosis T82.858 ☑
    - thrombosis T82.868 ☑
  - dialysis catheter — *see* Complication, catheter, dialysis
  - following infusion, therapeutic injection or transfusion T8Ø.1 ☑
  - graft T82.9 ☑
    - embolism T82.818 ☑
    - fibrosis T82.828 ☑
    - hemorrhage T82.838 ☑
    - mechanical
      - breakdown T82.319 ☑
        - aorta (bifurcation) T82.31Ø ☑
        - carotid artery T82.311 ☑
        - specified vessel NEC T82.318 ☑
      - displacement T82.329 ☑
        - aorta (bifurcation) T82.32Ø ☑
        - carotid artery T82.321 ☑
        - specified vessel NEC T82.328 ☑
      - leakage T82.339 ☑
        - aorta (bifurcation) T82.33Ø ☑
        - carotid artery T82.331 ☑
        - femoral artery T82.332 ☑
        - specified vessel NEC T82.338 ☑
      - malposition T82.329 ☑
        - aorta (bifurcation) T82.32Ø ☑
        - carotid artery T82.321 ☑
        - specified vessel NEC T82.328 ☑
      - obstruction T82.399 ☑
        - aorta (bifurcation) T82.39Ø ☑
        - carotid artery T82.391 ☑
        - specified vessel NEC T82.398 ☑
      - perforation T82.399 ☑
        - aorta (bifurcation) T82.39Ø ☑
        - carotid artery T82.391 ☑
        - specified vessel NEC T82.398 ☑
      - protrusion T82.399 ☑
        - aorta (bifurcation) T82.39Ø ☑
        - carotid artery T82.391 ☑
        - specified vessel NEC T82.398 ☑
    - pain T82.848 ☑
    - specified complication NEC T82.898 ☑
    - stenosis T82.858 ☑
    - thrombosis T82.868 ☑
  - postoperative — *see* Complications, postoperative, circulatory
- vena cava device (filter) (sieve) (umbrella) — *see* Complications, umbrella device, vascular
- ventilation therapy NEC T81.81 ☑
- ventilator
  - mechanical J95.85Ø
    - specified NEC J95.859
- ventricular (communicating) shunt (device) T85.9 ☑
  - embolism T85.81Ø ☑
  - fibrosis T85.82Ø ☑
  - hemorrhage T85.83Ø ☑
  - infection and inflammation T85.73Ø ☑
  - mechanical
    - breakdown T85.Ø1 ☑
    - displacement T85.Ø2 ☑

Complication(s) — *continued*
- ventricular shunt — *continued*
  - mechanical — *continued*
    - leakage T85.Ø3 ☑
    - malposition T85.Ø2 ☑
    - obstruction T85.Ø9 ☑
    - perforation T85.Ø9 ☑
    - protrusion T85.Ø9 ☑
    - specified NEC T85.Ø9 ☑
  - pain T85.84Ø ☑
  - specified type NEC T85.89Ø ☑
  - stenosis T85.85Ø ☑
  - thrombosis T85.86Ø ☑
- wire suture, permanent (implanted) — *see* Complications, suture, permanent

Compressed air disease T7Ø.3 ☑

Compression
- with injury — *code by* Nature of injury
- artery I77.1
  - celiac, syndrome I77.4
- brachial plexus G54.Ø
- brain (stem) G93.5
  - due to
    - contusion (diffuse) — *see also* Injury, intracranial, diffuse SØ6.AØ ☑
      - with herniation SØ6.A1 ☑
    - focal — *see also* Injury, intracranial, focal SØ6.AØ ☑
      - with herniation SØ6.A1 ☑
    - injury NEC — *see also* Injury, intracranial, diffuse SØ6.AØ ☑
  - nontraumatic G93.5
  - traumatic — *see also* Injury, intracranial, diffuse SØ6.AØ ☑
    - with herniation SØ6.A1 ☑
- bronchus J98.Ø9
- cauda equina G83.4
- celiac (artery) (axis) I77.4
- cerebral — *see* Compression, brain
- cervical plexus G54.2
- cord
  - spinal — *see* Compression, spinal
  - umbilical — *see* Compression, umbilical cord
- cranial nerve G52.9
  - eighth H93.3 ☑
  - eleventh G52.8
  - fifth G5Ø.8
  - first G52.Ø
  - fourth — *see* Strabismus, paralytic, fourth nerve
  - ninth G52.1
  - second — *see* Disorder, nerve, optic
  - seventh G51.8
  - sixth — *see* Strabismus, paralytic, sixth nerve
  - tenth G52.2
  - third — *see* Strabismus, paralytic, third nerve
  - twelfth G52.3
- diver's squeeze T7Ø.3 ☑
- during birth (newborn) P15.9
- esophagus K22.2
- eustachian tube — *see* Obstruction, eustachian tube, cartilaginous
- facies Q67.1
- fracture
  - nontraumatic NOS — *see* Collapse, vertebra
  - pathological — *see* Fracture, pathological
  - traumatic — *see* Fracture, traumatic
- heart — *see* Disease, heart
- intestine — *see* Obstruction, intestine
- laryngeal nerve, recurrent G52.2
  - with paralysis of vocal cords and larynx J38.ØØ
    - bilateral J38.Ø2
    - unilateral J38.Ø1
- lumbosacral plexus G54.1
- lung J98.4
- lymphatic vessel I89.Ø
- medulla — *see* Compression, brain
- nerve — *see also* Disorder, nerve G58.9
  - arm NEC — *see* Mononeuropathy, upper limb
  - axillary G54.Ø
  - cranial — *see* Compression, cranial nerve
  - leg NEC — *see* Mononeuropathy, lower limb
  - median (in carpal tunnel) — *see* Syndrome, carpal tunnel
  - optic — *see* Disorder, nerve, optic
  - plantar — *see* Lesion, nerve, plantar
  - posterior tibial (in tarsal tunnel) — *see* Syndrome, tarsal tunnel

Compression — *continued*
- nerve — *see also* Disorder, nerve — *continued*
  - root or plexus NOS (in) G54.9
    - intervertebral disc disorder NEC — *see* Disorder, disc, with, radiculopathy
      - with myelopathy — *see* Disorder, disc, with, myelopathy
    - neoplastic disease — *see also* Neoplasm D49.9 *[G55]*
    - spondylosis — *see* Spondylosis, with radiculopathy
  - sciatic (acute) — *see* Lesion, nerve, sciatic
  - sympathetic G9Ø.8
  - traumatic — *see* Injury, nerve
  - ulnar — *see* Lesion, nerve, ulnar
  - upper extremity NEC — *see* Mononeuropathy, upper limb
- spinal (cord) G95.2Ø
  - by displacement of intervertebral disc NEC — *see also* Disorder, disc, with, myelopathy
  - nerve root NOS G54.9
    - due to displacement of intervertebral disc NEC — *see* Disorder, disc, with, radiculopathy
      - with myelopathy — *see* Disorder, disc, with, myelopathy
  - specified NEC G95.29
  - spondylogenic (cervical) (lumbar, lumbosacral) (thoracic) — *see* Spondylosis, with myelopathy NEC
    - anterior — *see* Syndrome, anterior, spinal artery, compression
  - traumatic — *see* Injury, spinal cord, by region
- subcostal nerve (syndrome) — *see* Mononeuropathy, upper limb, specified NEC
- sympathetic nerve NEC G9Ø.8
- syndrome T79.5 ☑
- trachea J39.8
- ulnar nerve (by scar tissue) — *see* Lesion, nerve, ulnar
- umbilical cord
  - complicating delivery O69.2 ☑
    - cord around neck O69.1 ☑
    - prolapse O69.Ø ☑
    - specified NEC O69.2 ☑
- ureter N13.5
- vein I87.1
- vena cava (inferior) (superior) I87.1

Compulsion, compulsive
- gambling F63.Ø
- neurosis F42.8
- personality F6Ø.5
- states F42.8
- swearing F42.8
  - in Gilles de la Tourette's syndrome F95.2
- tics and spasms F95.9

Concato's disease (pericardial polyserositis) A19.9
- nontubercular I31.1
- pleural — *see* Pleurisy, with effusion

Concavity chest wall M95.4

Concealed penis Q55.64

Concern (normal) **about sick person in family** Z63.6

Concrescence (teeth) KØØ.2

Concretio cordis I31.1
- rheumatic IØ9.2

Concretion — *see also* Calculus
- appendicular K38.1
- canaliculus — *see* Dacryolith
- clitoris N9Ø.89
- conjunctiva H11.12- ☑
- eyelid — *see* Disorder, eyelid, specified type NEC
- lacrimal passages — *see* Dacryolith
- prepuce (male) N47.8
- salivary gland (any) K11.5
- seminal vesicle N5Ø.89
- tonsil J35.8

Concussion (brain) (cerebral) (current) SØ6.ØX9 ☑
- with
  - loss of consciousness
    - 3Ø minutes or less SØ6.ØX1 ☑
    - brief SØ6.ØX1 ☑
    - status unknown SØ6.ØXA ☑
    - unspecified duration SØ6.ØX9 ☑
  - no loss of consciousness SØ6.ØXØ ☑
- blast (air) (hydraulic) (immersion) (underwater)
  - abdomen or thorax — *see* Injury, blast, by site
  - ear with acoustic nerve injury — *see* Injury, nerve, acoustic, specified type NEC
- cauda equina S34.3 ☑

Concussion — *continued*
- conus medullaris S34.Ø2 ☑
- ocular SØ5.8X- ☑
- spinal (cord)
  - cervical S14.Ø ☑
  - lumbar S34.Ø1 ☑
  - sacral S34.Ø2 ☑
  - thoracic S24.Ø ☑
- syndrome FØ7.81
- without loss of consciousness SØ6.ØXØ ☑

Condition — *see also* Disease
- post COVID-19 UØ9.9

Conditions arising in the perinatal period — *see* Newborn, affected by

Conduct disorder — *see* Disorder, conduct

Condyloma A63.Ø
- acuminatum A63.Ø
- gonorrheal A54.Ø9
- latum A51.31
- syphilitic A51.31
  - congenital A5Ø.Ø7
- venereal, syphilitic A51.31

Conflagration — *see also* Burn
- asphyxia (by inhalation of gases, fumes or vapors) — *see also* Table of Drugs and Chemicals T59.9- ☑

Conflict (with) — *see also* Discord
- family Z73.9
- marital Z63.Ø
  - involving divorce or estrangement Z63.5
- parent-child Z62.82Ø
  - parent-adopted child Z62.821
  - parent-biological child Z62.82Ø
  - parent-foster child Z62.822
- social role NEC Z73.5

Confluent — *see* condition

Confusion, confused R41.Ø
- epileptic FØ5
- mental state (psychogenic) F44.89
- psychogenic F44.89
- reactive (from emotional stress, psychological trauma) F44.89

Confusional arousals G47.51

Congelation T69.9 ☑

Congenital — *see also* condition
- aortic septum Q25.49
- intrinsic factor deficiency D51.Ø
- malformation — *see* Anomaly

Congestion, congestive
- bladder N32.89
- bowel K63.89
- brain G93.89
- breast N64.59
- bronchial J98.Ø9
- catarrhal J31.Ø
- chest RØ9.89
- chill, malarial — *see* Malaria
- circulatory NEC I99.8
- duodenum K31.89
- eye — *see* Hyperemia, conjunctiva
- facial, due to birth injury P15.4
- general R68.89
- glottis J37.Ø
- heart — *see* Failure, heart, congestive
- hepatic K76.1
- hypostatic (lung) — *see* Edema, lung
- intestine K63.89
- kidney N28.89
- labyrinth H83.8 ☑
- larynx J37.Ø
- liver K76.1
- lung RØ9.89
  - active or acute — *see* Pneumonia
- malaria, malarial — *see* Malaria
- nasal RØ9.81
- nose RØ9.81
- orbit, orbital — *see also* Exophthalmos
  - inflammatory (chronic) — *see* Inflammation, orbit
- ovary N83.8
- pancreas K86.89
- pelvic, female N94.89
- pleural J94.8
- prostate (active) N42.1
- pulmonary — *see* Congestion, lung
- renal N28.89
- retina H35.81
- seminal vesicle N5Ø.1
- spinal cord G95.19
- spleen (chronic) D73.2

- **Constriction** — *continued*
  - external — *continued*
    - subungual
      - finger(s) — *see* Constriction, external, finger
      - toe(s) — *see* Constriction, external, toe
    - supraclavicular fossa S1Ø.84 ☑
    - supraorbital SØØ.84 ☑
    - temple SØØ.84 ☑
    - temporal region SØØ.84 ☑
    - testis S3Ø.843 ☑
    - thigh S7Ø.34- ☑
    - thorax, thoracic (wall) S2Ø.94 ☑
      - back S2Ø.44- ☑
      - front S2Ø.34- ☑
    - throat S1Ø.14 ☑
    - thumb S6Ø.34- ☑
    - toe(s) (lesser) S9Ø.44- ☑
      - great S9Ø.44- ☑
    - tongue SØØ.542 ☑
    - trachea S1Ø.14 ☑
    - tunica vaginalis S3Ø.843 ☑
    - uvula SØØ.542 ☑
    - vagina S3Ø.844 ☑
    - vulva S3Ø.844 ☑
    - wrist S6Ø.84- ☑
  - gallbladder — *see* Obstruction, gallbladder
  - intestine — *see* Obstruction, intestine
  - larynx J38.6
    - congenital Q31.8
      - specified NEC Q31.8
      - subglottic Q31.1
  - organ or site, congenital NEC — *see* Atresia, by site
  - prepuce (acquired) (congenital) N47.1
  - pylorus (adult hypertrophic) K31.1
    - congenital or infantile Q4Ø.Ø
    - newborn Q4Ø.Ø
  - ring dystocia (uterus) O62.4
  - spastic — *see also* Spasm
    - ureter N13.5
  - ureter N13.5
    - with infection N13.6
  - urethra — *see* Stricture, urethra
  - visual field (peripheral) (functional) — *see* Defect, visual field
- **Constrictive** — *see* condition
- **Consultation**
  - medical — *see* Counseling, medical
  - religious Z71.81
  - specified reason NEC Z71.89
  - spiritual Z71.81
  - without complaint or sickness Z71.9
    - feared complaint unfounded Z71.1
    - specified reason NEC Z71.89
- **Consumption** — *see* Tuberculosis
- **Contact** (with) — *see also* Exposure (to)
  - acariasis Z2Ø.7
  - AIDS virus Z2Ø.6
  - air pollution Z77.11Ø
  - algae and algae toxins Z77.121
  - algae bloom Z77.121
  - anthrax Z2Ø.81Ø
  - aromatic amines Z77.Ø2Ø
  - aromatic (hazardous) compounds NEC Z77.Ø28
  - aromatic dyes NOS Z77.Ø28
  - arsenic Z77.Ø1Ø
  - asbestos Z77.Ø9Ø
  - bacterial disease NEC Z2Ø.818
  - benzene Z77.Ø21
  - blue-green algae bloom Z77.121
  - body fluids (potentially hazardous) Z77.21
  - brown tide Z77.121
  - chemicals (chiefly nonmedicinal) (hazardous) NEC Z77.Ø98
  - cholera Z2Ø.Ø9
  - chromium compounds Z77.Ø18
  - communicable disease Z2Ø.9
    - bacterial NEC Z2Ø.818
    - specified NEC Z2Ø.89
    - viral NEC Z2Ø.828
    - Zika virus Z2Ø.821
  - coronavirus (disease) (novel) 2Ø19 Z2Ø.822
  - COVID-19 Z2Ø.822
  - cyanobacteria bloom Z77.121
  - dyes Z77.Ø98
  - Escherichia coli (E. coli) Z2Ø.Ø1
  - fiberglass — *see* Table of Drugs and Chemicals, fiberglass
  - German measles Z2Ø.4
- **Contact** — *continued*
  - gonorrhea Z2Ø.2
  - hazardous metals NEC Z77.Ø18
  - hazardous substances NEC Z77.29
  - hazards in the physical environment NEC Z77.128
  - hazards to health NEC Z77.9
  - HIV Z2Ø.6
  - HTLV-III/LAV Z2Ø.6
  - human immunodeficiency virus (HIV) Z2Ø.6
  - infection Z2Ø.9
    - specified NEC Z2Ø.89
  - infestation (parasitic) NEC Z2Ø.7
  - intestinal infectious disease NEC Z2Ø.Ø9
    - Escherichia coli (E. coli) Z2Ø.Ø1
  - lead Z77.Ø11
  - meningococcus Z2Ø.811
  - mold (toxic) Z77.12Ø
  - nickel dust Z77.Ø18
  - noise Z77.122
  - parasitic disease Z2Ø.7
  - pediculosis Z2Ø.7
  - pfiesteria piscicida Z77.121
  - poliomyelitis Z2Ø.89
  - pollution
    - air Z77.11Ø
    - environmental NEC Z77.118
    - soil Z77.112
    - water Z77.111
  - polycyclic aromatic hydrocarbons Z77.Ø28
  - positive maternal group B streptococcus PØØ.82
  - rabies Z2Ø.3
  - radiation, naturally occurring NEC Z77.123
  - radon Z77.123
  - red tide (Florida) Z77.121
  - rubella Z2Ø.4
  - SARS-CoV-2 Z2Ø.822
  - sexually-transmitted disease Z2Ø.2
  - smallpox (laboratory) Z2Ø.89
  - syphilis Z2Ø.2
  - tuberculosis Z2Ø.1
  - uranium Z77.Ø12
  - varicella Z2Ø.82Ø
  - venereal disease Z2Ø.2
  - viral disease NEC Z2Ø.828
  - viral hepatitis Z2Ø.5
  - water pollution Z77.111
  - Zika virus Z2Ø.821
- **Contamination, food** — *see* Intoxication, foodborne
- **Contraception, contraceptive**
  - advice Z3Ø.Ø9
  - counseling Z3Ø.Ø9
  - device (intrauterine) (in situ) Z97.5
    - causing menorrhagia T83.83 ☑
    - checking Z3Ø.431
    - complications — *see* Complications, intrauterine, contraceptive device
    - in place Z97.5
    - initial prescription Z3Ø.Ø14
    - reinsertion Z3Ø.433
    - removal Z3Ø.432
    - replacement Z3Ø.433
  - emergency (postcoital) Z3Ø.Ø12
  - initial prescription Z3Ø.Ø19
    - barrier Z3Ø.Ø18
    - diaphragm Z3Ø.Ø18
    - injectable Z3Ø.Ø13
    - intrauterine device Z3Ø.Ø14
    - pills Z3Ø.Ø11
    - postcoital (emergency) Z3Ø.Ø12
    - specified type NEC Z3Ø.Ø18
    - subdermal implantable Z3Ø.Ø17
    - transdermal patch hormonal Z3Ø.Ø16
    - vaginal ring hormonal Z3Ø.Ø15
  - maintenance Z3Ø.4Ø
    - barrier Z3Ø.49
    - diaphragm Z3Ø.49
    - examination Z3Ø.8
    - injectable Z3Ø.42
    - intrauterine device Z3Ø.431
    - pills Z3Ø.41
    - specified type NEC Z3Ø.49
    - subdermal implantable Z3Ø.46
    - transdermal patch hormonal Z3Ø.45
    - vaginal ring hormonal Z3Ø.44
  - management Z3Ø.9
    - specified NEC Z3Ø.8
  - postcoital (emergency) Z3Ø.Ø12
  - prescription Z3Ø.Ø19
    - repeat Z3Ø.4Ø
- **Contraception, contraceptive** — *continued*
  - sterilization Z3Ø.2
  - surveillance (drug) — *see* Contraception, maintenance
- **Contraction(s), contracture, contracted**
  - Achilles tendon — *see also* Short, tendon, Achilles
    - congenital Q66.89
  - amputation stump (surgical) (flexion) (late) (next proximal joint) T87.89
  - anus K59.89
  - bile duct (common) (hepatic) K83.8
  - bladder N32.89
    - neck or sphincter N32.Ø
  - bowel, cecum, colon or intestine, any part — *see* Obstruction, intestine
  - Braxton Hicks — *see* False, labor
  - breast implant, capsular T85.44 ☑
  - bronchial J98.Ø9
  - burn (old) — *see* Cicatrix
  - cervix — *see* Stricture, cervix
  - cicatricial — *see* Cicatrix
  - conjunctiva, trachomatous, active A71.1
    - sequelae (late effect) B94.Ø
  - Dupuytren's M72.Ø
  - eyelid — *see* Disorder, eyelid function
  - fascia (lata) (postural) M72.8
    - Dupuytren's M72.Ø
    - palmar M72.Ø
    - plantar M72.2
  - finger NEC — *see also* Deformity, finger
    - congenital Q68.1
    - joint — *see* Contraction, joint, hand
  - flaccid — *see* Contraction, paralytic
  - gallbladder K82.Ø
  - heart valve — *see* Endocarditis
  - hip — *see* Contraction, joint, hip
  - hourglass
    - bladder N32.89
      - congenital Q64.79
    - gallbladder K82.Ø
      - congenital Q44.1
    - stomach K31.89
      - congenital Q4Ø.2
      - psychogenic F45.8
    - uterus (complicating delivery) O62.4
  - hysterical F44.4
  - internal os — *see* Stricture, cervix
  - joint (abduction) (acquired) (adduction) (flexion) (rotation) M24.5Ø
    - ankle M24.57- ☑
    - congenital NEC Q68.8
      - hip Q65.89
    - elbow M24.52- ☑
    - foot joint M24.57- ☑
    - hand joint M24.54- ☑
    - hip M24.55- ☑
      - congenital Q65.89
    - hysterical F44.4
    - knee M24.56- ☑
    - shoulder M24.51- ☑
    - specified site NEC M24.59
    - wrist M24.53- ☑
  - kidney (granular) (secondary) N26.9
    - congenital Q63.8
    - hydronephritic — *see* Hydronephrosis
    - Page N26.2
    - pyelonephritic — *see* Pyelitis, chronic
    - tuberculous A18.11
  - ligament — *see also* Disorder, ligament
    - congenital Q79.8
  - muscle (postinfective) (postural) NEC M62.4Ø
    - with contracture of joint — *see* Contraction, joint
    - ankle M62.47- ☑
    - congenital Q79.8
      - sternocleidomastoid Q68.Ø
    - extraocular — *see* Strabismus
    - eye (extrinsic) — *see* Strabismus
    - foot M62.47- ☑
    - forearm M62.43- ☑
    - hand M62.44- ☑
    - hysterical F44.4
    - ischemic (Volkmann's) T79.6 ☑
    - lower leg M62.46- ☑
    - multiple sites M62.49
    - pelvic region M62.45- ☑
    - posttraumatic — *see* Strabismus, paralytic
    - psychogenic F45.8
      - conversion reaction F44.4

Contraction(s), contracture, contracted — *continued*
- muscle — *continued*
  - shoulder region M62.41- ☑
  - specified site NEC M62.48
  - thigh M62.45- ☑
  - upper arm M62.42- ☑
- neck — *see* Torticollis
- ocular muscle — *see* Strabismus
- organ or site, congenital NEC — *see* Atresia, by site
- outlet (pelvis) — *see* Contraction, pelvis
- palmar fascia M72.0
- paralytic
  - joint — *see* Contraction, joint
  - muscle — *see also* Contraction, muscle NEC
    - ocular — *see* Strabismus, paralytic
- pelvis (acquired) (general) M95.5
  - with disproportion (fetopelvic) O33.1
    - causing obstructed labor O65.1
    - inlet O33.2
    - mid-cavity O33.3 ☑
    - outlet O33.3 ☑
- plantar fascia M72.2
- premature
  - atrium I49.1
  - auriculoventricular I49.49
  - heart I49.49
  - junctional I49.2
  - supraventricular I49.1
  - ventricular I49.3
- prostate N42.89
- pylorus NEC — *see also* Pylorospasm
  - psychogenic F45.8
- rectum, rectal (sphincter) K59.89
- ring (Bandl's) (complicating delivery) O62.4
- scar — *see* Cicatrix
- spine — *see* Dorsopathy, deforming
- sternocleidomastoid (muscle), congenital Q68.0
- stomach K31.89
  - hourglass K31.89
    - congenital Q40.2
    - psychogenic F45.8
  - psychogenic F45.8
- tendon (sheath) M62.40
  - with contracture of joint — *see* Contraction, joint
  - Achilles — *see* Short, tendon, Achilles
  - ankle M62.47- ☑
    - Achilles — *see* Short, tendon, Achilles
  - foot M62.47- ☑
  - forearm M62.43- ☑
  - hand M62.44- ☑
  - lower leg M62.46- ☑
  - multiple sites M62.49
  - neck M62.48
  - pelvic region M62.45- ☑
  - shoulder region M62.41- ☑
  - specified site NEC M62.48
  - thigh M62.45- ☑
  - thorax M62.48
  - trunk M62.48
  - upper arm M62.42- ☑
- toe — *see* Deformity, toe, specified NEC
- ureterovesical orifice (postinfectional) N13.5
  - with infection N13.6
- urethra — *see also* Stricture, urethra
  - orifice N32.0
- uterus N85.8
  - abnormal NEC O62.9
  - clonic (complicating delivery) O62.4
  - dyscoordinate (complicating delivery) O62.4
  - hourglass (complicating delivery) O62.4
  - hypertonic O62.4
  - hypotonic NEC O62.2
  - inadequate
    - primary O62.0
    - secondary O62.1
  - incoordinate (complicating delivery) O62.4
  - poor O62.2
  - tetanic (complicating delivery) O62.4
- vagina (outlet) N89.5
- vesical N32.89
  - neck or urethral orifice N32.0
- visual field — *see* Defect, visual field, generalized
- Volkmann's (ischemic) T79.6 ☑

Contusion (skin surface intact) T14.8 ☑
- abdomen, abdominal (muscle) (wall) S30.1 ☑
- adnexa, eye NEC S05.8X- ☑
- adrenal gland S37.812 ☑
- alveolar process S00.532 ☑
- ankle S90.0- ☑
- antecubital space — *see* Contusion, forearm
- anus S30.3 ☑
- arm (upper) S40.02- ☑
  - lower (with elbow) — *see* Contusion, forearm
- auditory canal — *see* Contusion, ear
- auricle — *see* Contusion, ear
- axilla — *see* Contusion, arm, upper
- back — *see also* Contusion, thorax, back
  - lower S30.0 ☑
- bile duct S36.13 ☑
- bladder S37.22 ☑
- bone NEC T14.8 ☑
- brain (diffuse) — *see* Injury, intracranial, diffuse
  - focal — *see* Injury, intracranial, focal
- brainstem S06.38- ☑
- breast S20.0- ☑
- broad ligament S37.892 ☑
- brow S00.83 ☑
- buttock S30.0 ☑
- canthus, eye S00.1- ☑
- cauda equina S34.3 ☑
- cerebellar, traumatic S06.37- ☑
- cerebral S06.33- ☑
  - left side S06.32- ☑
  - right side S06.31- ☑
- cheek S00.83 ☑
  - internal S00.532 ☑
- chest (wall) — *see* Contusion, thorax
- chin S00.83 ☑
- clitoris S30.23 ☑
- colon — *see* Injury, intestine, large, contusion
- common bile duct S36.13 ☑
- conjunctiva S05.1- ☑
  - with foreign body (in conjunctival sac) — *see* Foreign body, conjunctival sac
- conus medullaris (spine) S34.139 ☑
- cornea — *see* Contusion, eyeball
  - with foreign body — *see* Foreign body, cornea
- corpus cavernosum S30.21 ☑
- cortex (brain) (cerebral) — *see* Injury, intracranial, diffuse
  - focal — *see* Injury, intracranial, focal
- costal region — *see* Contusion, thorax
- cystic duct S36.13 ☑
- diaphragm S27.802 ☑
- duodenum S36.420 ☑
- ear S00.43- ☑
- elbow S50.0- ☑
  - with forearm — *see* Contusion, forearm
- epididymis S30.22 ☑
- epigastric region S30.1 ☑
- epiglottis S10.0 ☑
- esophagus (thoracic) S27.812 ☑
  - cervical S10.0 ☑
- eyeball S05.1- ☑
- eyebrow S00.1- ☑
- eyelid (and periocular area) S00.1- ☑
- face NEC S00.83 ☑
- fallopian tube S37.529 ☑
  - bilateral S37.522 ☑
  - unilateral S37.521 ☑
- femoral triangle S30.1 ☑
- finger(s) S60.00 ☑
  - with damage to nail (matrix) S60.10 ☑
  - index S60.02- ☑
    - with damage to nail S60.12- ☑
  - little S60.05- ☑
    - with damage to nail S60.15- ☑
  - middle S60.03- ☑
    - with damage to nail S60.13- ☑
  - ring S60.04- ☑
    - with damage to nail S60.14- ☑
  - thumb — *see* Contusion, thumb
- flank S30.1 ☑
- foot (except toe(s) alone) S90.3- ☑
  - toe — *see* Contusion, toe
- forearm S50.1- ☑
  - elbow only — *see* Contusion, elbow
- forehead S00.83 ☑
- gallbladder S36.122 ☑
- genital organs, external
  - female S30.202 ☑
  - male S30.201 ☑
- globe (eye) — *see* Contusion, eyeball
- groin S30.1 ☑
- gum S00.532 ☑
- hand S60.22- ☑
  - finger(s) — *see* Contusion, finger
  - wrist — *see* Contusion, wrist
- head S00.93 ☑
  - ear — *see* Contusion, ear
  - eyelid — *see* Contusion, eyelid
  - lip S00.531 ☑
  - nose S00.33 ☑
  - oral cavity S00.532 ☑
  - scalp S00.03 ☑
  - specified part NEC S00.83 ☑
- heart — *see also* Injury, heart S26.91 ☑
- heel — *see* Contusion, foot
- hepatic duct S36.13 ☑
- hip S70.0- ☑
- ileum S36.428 ☑
- iliac region S30.1 ☑
- inguinal region S30.1 ☑
- interscapular region S20.229 ☑
- intra-abdominal organ S36.92 ☑
  - colon — *see* Injury, intestine, large, contusion
  - liver S36.112 ☑
  - pancreas — *see* Contusion, pancreas
  - rectum S36.62 ☑
  - small intestine — *see* Injury, intestine, small, contusion
  - specified organ NEC S36.892 ☑
  - spleen — *see* Contusion, spleen
  - stomach S36.32 ☑
- iris (eye) — *see* Contusion, eyeball
- jaw S00.83 ☑
- jejunum S36.428 ☑
- kidney S37.01- ☑
  - major (greater than 2 cm) S37.02- ☑
  - minor (less than 2 cm) S37.01- ☑
- knee S80.0- ☑
- labium (majus) (minus) S30.23 ☑
- lacrimal apparatus, gland or sac S05.8X- ☑
- larynx S10.0 ☑
- leg (lower) S80.1- ☑
  - knee — *see* Contusion, knee
- lens — *see* Contusion, eyeball
- lip S00.531 ☑
- liver S36.112 ☑
- lower back S30.0 ☑
- lumbar region S30.0 ☑
- lung S27.329 ☑
  - bilateral S27.322 ☑
  - unilateral S27.321 ☑
- malar region S00.83 ☑
- mastoid region S00.83 ☑
- membrane, brain — *see* Injury, intracranial, diffuse
  - focal — *see* Injury, intracranial, focal
- mesentery S36.892 ☑
- mesosalpinx S37.892 ☑
- mouth S00.532 ☑
- muscle — *see* Contusion, by site
- nail
  - finger — *see* Contusion, finger, with damage to nail
  - toe — *see* Contusion, toe, with damage to nail
- nasal S00.33 ☑
- neck S10.93 ☑
  - specified site NEC S10.83 ☑
  - throat S10.0 ☑
- nerve — *see* Injury, nerve
- newborn P54.5
- nose S00.33 ☑
- occipital
  - lobe (brain) — *see* Injury, intracranial, diffuse
    - focal — *see* Injury, intracranial, focal
  - region (scalp) S00.03 ☑
- orbit (region) (tissues) S05.1- ☑
- ovary S37.429 ☑
  - bilateral S37.422 ☑
  - unilateral S37.421 ☑
- palate S00.532 ☑
- pancreas S36.229 ☑
  - body S36.221 ☑
  - head S36.220 ☑
  - tail S36.222 ☑

- **Corrosion** — *continued*
  - trunk — *continued*
    - labia — *see* Corrosion, genital organs, external, female
    - lower back — *see* Corrosion, back
    - penis — *see* Corrosion, genital organs, external, male
    - perineum
      - female — *see* Corrosion, genital organs, external, female
      - male — *see* Corrosion, genital organs, external, male
    - scapular region — *see* Corrosion, upper limb
    - scrotum — *see* Corrosion, genital organs, external, male
    - second degree T21.6Ø ☑
    - shoulder — *see* Corrosion, upper limb
    - specified site NEC T21.49 ☑
      - first degree T21.59 ☑
      - second degree T21.69 ☑
      - third degree T21.79 ☑
    - testes — *see* Corrosion, genital organs, external, male
    - third degree T21.7Ø ☑
    - upper back — *see* Corrosion, back, upper
    - vagina T28.8 ☑
    - vulva — *see* Corrosion, genital organs, external, female
  - unspecified site with extent of body surface involved specified
    - less than 1Ø percent T32.Ø
    - 1Ø-19 percent (Ø-9 percent third degree) T32.1Ø
      - with 1Ø-19 percent third degree T32.11
    - 2Ø-29 percent (Ø-9 percent third degree) T32.2Ø
      - with
        - 1Ø-19 percent third degree T32.21
        - 2Ø-29 percent third degree T32.22
    - 3Ø-39 percent (Ø-9 percent third degree) T32.3Ø
      - with
        - 1Ø-19 percent third degree T32.31
        - 2Ø-29 percent third degree T32.32
        - 3Ø-39 percent third degree T32.33
    - 4Ø-49 percent (Ø-9 percent third degree) T32.4Ø
      - with
        - 1Ø-19 percent third degree T32.41
        - 2Ø-29 percent third degree T32.42
        - 3Ø-39 percent third degree T32.43
        - 4Ø-49 percent third degree T32.44
    - 5Ø-59 percent (Ø-9 percent third degree) T32.5Ø
      - with
        - 1Ø-19 percent third degree T32.51
        - 2Ø-29 percent third degree T32.52
        - 3Ø-39 percent third degree T32.53
        - 4Ø-49 percent third degree T32.54
        - 5Ø-59 percent third degree T32.55
    - 6Ø-69 percent (Ø-9 percent third degree) T32.6Ø
      - with
        - 1Ø-19 percent third degree T32.61
        - 2Ø-29 percent third degree T32.62
        - 3Ø-39 percent third degree T32.63
        - 4Ø-49 percent third degree T32.64
        - 5Ø-59 percent third degree T32.65
        - 6Ø-69 percent third degree T32.66
    - 7Ø-79 percent (Ø-9 percent third degree) T32.7Ø
      - with
        - 1Ø-19 percent third degree T32.71
        - 2Ø-29 percent third degree T32.72
        - 3Ø-39 percent third degree T32.73
        - 4Ø-49 percent third degree T32.74
        - 5Ø-59 percent third degree T32.75
        - 6Ø-69 percent third degree T32.76
        - 7Ø-79 percent third degree T32.77
    - 8Ø-89 percent (Ø-9 percent third degree) T32.8Ø
      - with
        - 1Ø-19 percent third degree T32.81
        - 2Ø-29 percent third degree T32.82
        - 3Ø-39 percent third degree T32.83
        - 4Ø-49 percent third degree T32.84
        - 5Ø-59 percent third degree T32.85
        - 6Ø-69 percent third degree T32.86
        - 7Ø-79 percent third degree T32.87
        - 8Ø-89 percent third degree T32.88
    - 9Ø percent or more (Ø-9 percent third degree) T32.9Ø
      - with
        - 1Ø-19 percent third degree T32.91
        - 2Ø-29 percent third degree T32.92
        - 3Ø-39 percent third degree T32.93
        - 4Ø-49 percent third degree T32.94

- **Corrosion** — *continued*
  - unspecified site with extent of body surface involved specified — *continued*
    - 9Ø percent or more — *continued*
      - with — *continued*
        - 5Ø-59 percent third degree T32.95
        - 6Ø-69 percent third degree T32.96
        - 7Ø-79 percent third degree T32.97
        - 8Ø-89 percent third degree T32.98
        - 9Ø-99 percent third degree T32.99
  - upper limb (axilla) (scapular region) T22.4Ø ☑
    - above elbow — *see* Corrosion, above elbow
    - axilla — *see* Corrosion, axilla
    - elbow — *see* Corrosion, elbow
    - first degree T22.5Ø ☑
    - forearm — *see* Corrosion, forearm
    - hand — *see* Corrosion, hand
    - interscapular region — *see* Corrosion, back, upper
    - multiple sites T22.499 ☑
      - first degree T22.599 ☑
      - left T22.492 ☑
        - first degree T22.592 ☑
        - second degree T22.692 ☑
        - third degree T22.792 ☑
      - right T22.491 ☑
        - first degree T22.591 ☑
        - second degree T22.691 ☑
        - third degree T22.791 ☑
      - second degree T22.699 ☑
      - third degree T22.799 ☑
    - scapular region — *see* Corrosion, scapular region
    - second degree T22.6Ø ☑
    - shoulder — *see* Corrosion, shoulder
    - third degree T22.7Ø ☑
    - wrist — *see* Corrosion, hand
  - uterus T28.8 ☑
  - vagina T28.8 ☑
  - vulva — *see* Corrosion, genital organs, external, female
  - wrist T23.479 ☑
    - first degree T23.579 ☑
    - left T23.472 ☑
      - first degree T23.572 ☑
      - second degree T23.672 ☑
      - third degree T23.772 ☑
    - multiple sites with hand T23.499 ☑
      - first degree T23.599 ☑
      - left T23.492 ☑
        - first degree T23.592 ☑
        - second degree T23.692 ☑
        - third degree T23.792 ☑
      - right T23.491 ☑
        - first degree T23.591 ☑
        - second degree T23.691 ☑
        - third degree T23.791 ☑
      - second degree T23.699 ☑
      - third degree T23.799 ☑
    - right T23.471 ☑
      - first degree T23.571 ☑
      - second degree T23.671 ☑
      - third degree T23.771 ☑
    - second degree T23.679 ☑
    - third degree T23.779 ☑
- **Corrosive burn** — *see* Corrosion
- **Corsican fever** — *see* Malaria
- **Cortical** — *see* condition
- **Cortico-adrenal** — *see* condition
- **Coryza** (acute) JØØ
  - with grippe or influenza — *see* Influenza, with, respiratory manifestations NEC
  - syphilitic
    - congenital (chronic) A5Ø.Ø5
- **Co-sleeping, child-caregiver** Z72.823
- **Costen's syndrome or complex** M26.69
- **Costiveness** — *see* Constipation
- **Costochondritis** M94.Ø
- **Cot death** R99
- **Cotard's syndrome** F22
- **Cotia virus** BØ8.8
- **Cotton wool spots** (retinal) H35.81
- **Cotungo's disease** — *see* Sciatica
- **Cough** (affected) (epidemic) (nervous) RØ5.9
  - with hemorrhage — *see* Hemoptysis
  - acute RØ5.1
  - bronchial RØ5.8
    - with grippe or influenza — *see* Influenza, with, respiratory manifestations NEC

- **Cough** — *continued*
  - chronic RØ5.3
  - functional F45.8
  - hysterical F45.8
  - laryngeal, spasmodic RØ5.8
  - paroxysmal, due to Bordetella pertussis (without pneumonia) A37.ØØ
    - with pneumonia A37.Ø1
  - persistent RØ5.3
  - psychogenic F45.8
  - refractory RØ5.3
  - smokers' J41.Ø
  - specified NEC RØ5.8
  - subacute RØ5.2
  - syncope RØ5.4
  - tea taster's B49
  - unexplained RØ5.3
- **Counseling** (for) Z71.9
  - abuse NEC
    - perpetrator Z69.82
    - victim Z69.81
  - alcohol abuser Z71.41
    - family Z71.42
  - child abuse
    - nonparental
      - perpetrator Z69.Ø21
      - victim Z69.Ø2Ø
    - parental
      - perpetrator Z69.Ø11
      - victim Z69.Ø1Ø
  - consanguinity Z71.89
  - contraceptive Z3Ø.Ø9
  - dietary Z71.3
  - drug abuser Z71.51
    - family member Z71.52
  - exercise Z71.82
  - family Z71.89
  - fertility preservation (prior to cancer therapy) (prior to removal of gonads) Z31.62
  - for non-attending third party Z71.Ø
    - related to sexual behavior or orientation Z7Ø.2
  - genetic
    - nonprocreative Z71.83
    - procreative NEC Z31.5
  - gestational carrier Z31.7
  - health (advice) (education) (instruction) — *see* Counseling, medical
    - risk for travel (international) Z71.84
  - human immunodeficiency virus (HIV) Z71.7
  - immunization safety Z71.85
  - impotence Z7Ø.1
  - insulin pump use Z46.81
  - medical (for) Z71.9
    - boarding school resident Z59.3
    - consanguinity Z71.89
    - feared complaint and no disease found Z71.1
    - human immunodeficiency virus (HIV) Z71.7
    - institutional resident Z59.3
    - on behalf of another Z71.Ø
      - related to sexual behavior or orientation Z7Ø.2
    - person living alone Z6Ø.2
    - specified reason NEC Z71.89
  - natural family planning
    - procreative Z31.61
    - to avoid pregnancy Z3Ø.Ø2
  - pediatric-to-adult transition Z71.87
  - perpetrator (of)
    - abuse NEC Z69.82
    - child abuse
      - non-parental Z69.Ø21
      - parental Z69.Ø11
    - rape NEC Z69.82
    - spousal abuse Z69.12
  - procreative NEC Z31.69
    - fertility preservation (prior to cancer therapy) (prior to removal of gonads) Z31.62
    - using natural family planning Z31.61
  - promiscuity Z7Ø.1
  - rape victim Z69.81
  - religious Z71.81
  - safety for travel (international) Z71.84
  - sex, sexual (related to) Z7Ø.9
    - attitude(s) Z7Ø.Ø
    - behavior or orientation Z7Ø.1
    - combined concerns Z7Ø.3
    - non-responsiveness Z7Ø.1
    - on behalf of third party Z7Ø.2
    - specified reason NEC Z7Ø.8
  - socioeconomic factors Z71.88

Cyst — *continued*
- bone — *continued*
  - solitary — *continued*
    - toe M85.47- ☑
    - ulna M85.43- ☑
    - vertebra M85.48
  - specified type NEC M85.6Ø
    - ankle M85.67- ☑
    - foot M85.67- ☑
    - forearm M85.63- ☑
    - hand M85.64- ☑
    - jaw M27.4Ø
      - developmental (nonodontogenic) KØ9.1
        - odontogenic KØ9.Ø
      - latent M27.Ø
    - lower leg M85.66- ☑
    - multiple site M85.69
    - neck M85.68
    - rib M85.68
    - shoulder M85.61- ☑
    - skull M85.68
    - specified site NEC M85.68
    - thigh M85.65- ☑
    - toe M85.67- ☑
    - upper arm M85.62- ☑
    - vertebra M85.68
- brain (acquired) G93.Ø
  - congenital QØ4.6
  - hydatid B67.99 *[G94]*
  - third ventricle (colloid), congenital QØ4.6
- branchial (cleft) Q18.Ø
- branchiogenic Q18.Ø
- breast (benign) (blue dome) (pedunculated) (solitary) N6Ø.Ø- ☑
  - involution — *see* Dysplasia, mammary, specified type NEC
  - sebaceous — *see* Dysplasia, mammary, specified type NEC
- broad ligament (benign) N83.8
- bronchogenic (mediastinal) (sequestration) J98.4
  - congenital Q33.Ø
- buccal KØ9.8
- bulbourethral gland N36.8
- bursa, bursal NEC M71.3Ø
  - with rupture — *see* Rupture, synovium
  - ankle M71.37- ☑
  - elbow M71.32- ☑
  - foot M71.37- ☑
  - hand M71.34- ☑
  - hip M71.35- ☑
  - multiple sites M71.39
  - pharyngeal J39.2
  - popliteal space — *see* Cyst, Baker's
  - shoulder M71.31- ☑
  - specified site NEC M71.38
  - wrist M71.33- ☑
- calcifying odontogenic D16.5
  - upper jaw (bone) (maxilla) D16.4
- canal of Nuck (female) N94.89
  - congenital Q52.4
- canthus — *see* Cyst, conjunctiva
- carcinomatous — *see* Neoplasm, malignant, by site
- cauda equina G95.89
- cavum septi pellucidi — *see* Cyst, brain
- celomic (pericardium) Q24.8
- cerebellopontine (angle) — *see* Cyst, brain
- cerebellum — *see* Cyst, brain
- cerebral — *see* Cyst, brain
- cervical lateral Q18.Ø
- cervix NEC N88.8
  - embryonic Q51.6
  - nabothian N88.8
- chiasmal optic NEC — *see* Disorder, optic, chiasm
- chocolate (ovary) N8Ø.1Ø- ☑
- choledochus, congenital Q44.4
- chorion O41.8X- ☑
- choroid plexus G93.Ø
  - congenital QØ4.6
- ciliary body — *see* Cyst, iris
- clitoris N9Ø.7
- colon K63.89
- common (bile) duct K83.5
- congenital NEC Q89.8
  - adrenal gland Q89.1
  - epiglottis Q31.8
  - esophagus Q39.8
  - fallopian tube Q5Ø.4

Cyst — *continued*
- congenital — *continued*
  - kidney Q61.ØØ
    - more than one (multiple) Q61.Ø2
      - specified as polycystic Q61.3
        - adult type Q61.2
        - infantile type NEC Q61.19
          - collecting duct dilation Q61.11
    - solitary Q61.Ø1
  - larynx Q31.8
  - liver Q44.6
  - lung Q33.Ø
  - mediastinum Q34.1
  - ovary Q5Ø.1
  - oviduct Q5Ø.4
  - periurethral (tissue) Q64.79
  - prepuce Q55.69
  - salivary gland (any) Q38.4
  - sublingual Q38.6
  - submaxillary gland Q38.6
  - thymus (gland) Q89.2
  - tongue Q38.3
  - ureterovesical orifice Q62.8
  - vulva Q52.79
- conjunctiva H11.44- ☑
- cornea H18.89- ☑
- corpora quadrigemina G93.Ø
- corpus
  - albicans N83.29- ☑
  - luteum (hemorrhagic) (ruptured) N83.1- ☑
- Cowper's gland (benign) (infected) N36.8
- cranial meninges G93.Ø
- craniobuccal pouch E23.6
- craniopharyngeal pouch E23.6
- cystic duct K82.8
- Cysticercus — *see* Cysticercosis
- Dandy-Walker QØ3.1
  - with spina bifida — *see* Spina bifida
- dental (root) KØ4.8
  - developmental KØ9.Ø
  - eruption KØ9.Ø
  - primordial KØ9.Ø
- dentigerous (mandible) (maxilla) KØ9.Ø
- dermoid — *see* Neoplasm, benign, by site
  - with malignant transformation C56.- ☑
  - implantation
    - external area or site (skin) NEC L72.Ø
    - iris — *see* Cyst, iris, implantation
    - vagina N89.8
    - vulva N9Ø.7
  - mouth KØ9.8
  - oral soft tissue KØ9.8
  - sacrococcygeal — *see* Cyst, pilonidal
- developmental KØ9.1
  - odontogenic KØ9.Ø
  - oral region (nonodontogenic) KØ9.1
  - ovary, ovarian Q5Ø.1
- dura (cerebral) G93.Ø
  - spinal G96.198
- ear (external) Q18.1
- echinococcal — *see* Echinococcus
- embryonic
  - cervix uteri Q51.6
  - fallopian tube Q5Ø.4
  - vagina Q52.4
- endometrium, endometrial (uterus) N85.8
  - ectopic — *see* Endometriosis
- enterogenous Q43.8
- epidermal, epidermoid (inclusion) (*see also* Cyst, skin) L72.Ø
  - mouth KØ9.8
  - oral soft tissue KØ9.8
- epididymis N5Ø.3
- epiglottis J38.7
- epiphysis cerebri E34.8
- epithelial (inclusion) L72.Ø
- epoophoron Q5Ø.5
- eruption KØ9.Ø
- esophagus K22.89
- ethmoid sinus J34.1
- external female genital organs NEC N9Ø.7
- eyelid (sebaceous) HØ2.829
  - infected — *see* Hordeolum
  - left HØ2.826
    - lower HØ2.825
    - upper HØ2.824
  - right HØ2.823
    - lower HØ2.822

Cyst — *continued*
- eyelid — *continued*
  - right — *continued*
    - upper HØ2.821
- eye NEC H57.89
  - congenital Q15.8
- fallopian tube N83.8
  - congenital Q5Ø.4
- fimbrial (twisted) Q5Ø.4
- fissural (oral region) KØ9.1
- follicle (graafian) (hemorrhagic) N83.Ø- ☑
  - nabothian N88.8
- follicular (atretic) (hemorrhagic) (ovarian) N83.Ø- ☑
  - dentigerous KØ9.Ø
  - odontogenic KØ9.Ø
  - skin L72.9
    - specified NEC L72.8
- frontal sinus J34.1
- gallbladder K82.8
- ganglion — *see* Ganglion
- Gartner's duct Q52.4
- gingiva KØ9.Ø
- gland of Moll — *see* Cyst, eyelid
- globulomaxillary KØ9.1
- graafian follicle (hemorrhagic) N83.Ø- ☑
- granulosal lutein (hemorrhagic) N83.1- ☑
- hemangiomatous D18.ØØ
  - intra-abdominal D18.Ø3
  - intracranial D18.Ø2
  - skin D18.Ø1
  - specified site NEC D18.Ø9
- hemorrhagic M27.49
- hydatid — *see also* Echinococcus B67.9Ø
  - brain B67.99 *[G94]*
  - liver — *see also* Cyst, liver, hydatid B67.8
  - lung NEC B67.99 *[J99]*
  - Morgagni
    - female Q5Ø.5
    - male (epididymal) Q55.4
      - testicular Q55.29
  - specified site NEC B67.99
- hymen N89.8
  - embryonic Q52.4
- hypopharynx J39.2
- hypophysis, hypophyseal (duct) (recurrent) E23.6
  - cerebri E23.6
- implantation (dermoid)
  - external area or site (skin) NEC L72.Ø
  - iris — *see* Cyst, iris, implantation
  - vagina N89.8
  - vulva N9Ø.7
- incisive canal KØ9.1
- inclusion (epidermal) (epithelial) (epidermoid) (squamous) L72.Ø
  - not of skin — *code under* Cyst, by site
- intestine (large) (small) K63.89
- intracranial — *see* Cyst, brain
- intraligamentous — *see also* Disorder, ligament
  - knee — *see* Derangement, knee
- intrasellar E23.6
- iris H21.3Ø9
  - exudative H21.31- ☑
  - idiopathic H21.3Ø- ☑
  - implantation H21.32- ☑
  - parasitic H21.33- ☑
  - pars plana (primary) H21.34- ☑
    - exudative H21.35- ☑
- jaw (bone) M27.4Ø
  - aneurysmal M27.49
  - developmental (odontogenic) KØ9.Ø
  - fissural KØ9.1
  - hemorrhagic M27.49
  - traumatic M27.49
- joint NEC — *see* Disorder, joint, specified type NEC
- kidney N28.1
  - acquired N28.1
  - calyceal — *see* Hydronephrosis
  - congenital Q61.ØØ
  - more than one (multiple) Q61.Ø2
    - specified as polycystic Q61.3
      - adult type (autosomal dominant) Q61.2
      - infantile type (autosomal recessive) NEC Q61.19
        - collecting duct dilation Q61.11
  - pyelogenic — *see* Hydronephrosis
  - simple N28.1
  - solitary (single) N28.1
    - acquired N28.1

- **Cyst** — *continued*
  - kidney — *continued*
    - solitary — *continued*
      - congenital Q61.Ø1
  - labium (majus) (minus) N9Ø.7
    - sebaceous N9Ø.7
  - lacrimal — *see also* Disorder, lacrimal system, specified NEC
    - gland HØ4.13- ☑
    - passages or sac — *see* Disorder, lacrimal system, specified NEC
  - larynx J38.7
  - lateral periodontal KØ9.Ø
  - lens H27.8
    - congenital Q12.8
  - lip (gland) K13.Ø
  - liver (idiopathic) (simple) K76.89
    - congenital Q44.6
    - hydatid B67.8
      - granulosus B67.Ø
      - multilocularis B67.5
  - lung J98.4
    - congenital Q33.Ø
    - giant bullous J43.9
  - lutein N83.1- ☑
  - lymphangiomatous D18.1
  - lymphoepithelial, oral soft tissue KØ9.8
  - macula — *see* Degeneration, macula, hole
  - malignant — *see* Neoplasm, malignant, by site
  - mammary gland — *see* Cyst, breast
  - mandible M27.4Ø
    - dentigerous KØ9.Ø
    - radicular KØ4.8
  - maxilla M27.4Ø
    - dentigerous KØ9.Ø
    - radicular KØ4.8
  - medial, face and neck Q18.8
  - median
    - anterior maxillary KØ9.1
    - palatal KØ9.1
  - mediastinum, congenital Q34.1
  - meibomian (gland) — *see* Chalazion
    - infected — *see* Hordeolum
  - membrane, brain G93.Ø
  - meninges (cerebral) G93.Ø
    - spinal G96.198
  - meniscus, knee — *see* Derangement, knee, meniscus, cystic
  - mesentery, mesenteric K66.8
    - chyle I89.8
  - mesonephric duct
    - female Q5Ø.5
    - male Q55.4
  - milk N64.89
  - Morgagni (hydatid)
    - female Q5Ø.5
    - male (epididymal) Q55.4
      - testicular Q55.29
  - mouth KØ9.8
  - Müllerian duct Q5Ø.4
    - appendix testis Q55.29
    - cervix Q51.6
    - fallopian tube Q5Ø.4
    - female Q5Ø.4
    - male Q55.29
    - prostatic utricle Q55.4
    - vagina (embryonal) Q52.4
  - multilocular (ovary) D39.1Ø
    - benign — *see* Neoplasm, benign, by site
  - myometrium N85.8
  - nabothian (follicle) (ruptured) N88.8
  - nasoalveolar KØ9.1
  - nasolabial KØ9.1
  - nasopalatine (anterior) (duct) KØ9.1
  - nasopharynx J39.2
  - neoplastic — *see* Neoplasm, uncertain behavior, by site
    - benign — *see* Neoplasm, benign, by site
  - nerve root
    - cervical G96.191
    - lumbar G96.191
    - sacral G96.191
    - thoracic G96.191
  - nervous system NEC G96.89
  - neuroenteric (congenital) QØ6.8
  - nipple — *see* Cyst, breast
  - nose (turbinates) J34.1
    - sinus J34.1

- **Cyst** — *continued*
  - odontogenic, developmental KØ9.Ø
  - omentum (lesser) K66.8
    - congenital Q45.8
  - ora serrata — *see* Cyst, retina, ora serrata
  - oral
    - region KØ9.9
      - developmental (nonodontogenic) KØ9.1
      - specified NEC KØ9.8
    - soft tissue KØ9.9
      - specified NEC KØ9.8
  - orbit HØ5.81- ☑
  - ovary, ovarian (twisted) N83.2Ø- ☑
    - adherent N83.2Ø- ☑
    - chocolate N8Ø.1Ø- ☑
    - corpus
      - albicans N83.29- ☑
      - luteum (hemorrhagic) N83.1- ☑
    - dermoid D27.9
    - developmental Q5Ø.1
    - due to failure of involution NEC N83.2Ø- ☑
    - endometrial N8Ø.1Ø- ☑
    - follicular (graafian) (hemorrhagic) N83.Ø- ☑
    - hemorrhagic N83.2Ø- ☑
    - in pregnancy or childbirth O34.8- ☑
      - with obstructed labor O65.5
    - multilocular D39.1Ø
    - pseudomucinous D27.9
    - retention N83.29- ☑
    - serous N83.2Ø- ☑
    - specified NEC N83.29- ☑
    - theca lutein (hemorrhagic) N83.1- ☑
    - tuberculous A18.18
  - oviduct N83.8
  - palate (median) (fissural) KØ9.1
  - palatine papilla (jaw) KØ9.1
  - pancreas, pancreatic (hemorrhagic) (true) K86.2
    - congenital Q45.2
    - false K86.3
  - paralabral
    - hip M24.85- ☑
    - shoulder S43.43- ☑
  - paramesonephric duct Q5Ø.4
    - female Q5Ø.4
    - male Q55.29
  - paranephric N28.1
  - paraphysis, cerebri, congenital QØ4.6
  - parasitic B89
  - parathyroid (gland) E21.4
  - paratubal N83.8
  - paraurethral duct N36.8
  - paroophoron Q5Ø.5
  - parotid gland K11.6
  - parovarian Q5Ø.5
  - pelvis, female N94.89
    - in pregnancy or childbirth O34.8- ☑
      - causing obstructed labor O65.5
  - penis (sebaceous) N48.89
  - periapical KØ4.8
  - pericardial (congenital) Q24.8
    - acquired (secondary) I31.8
  - pericoronal KØ9.Ø
  - perineural G96.191
  - periodontal KØ4.8
    - lateral KØ9.Ø
  - peripelvic (lymphatic) N28.1
  - peritoneum K66.8
    - chylous I89.8
  - periventricular, acquired, newborn P91.1
  - pharynx (wall) J39.2
  - pilar L72.11
  - pilonidal (infected) (rectum) LØ5.91
    - with abscess LØ5.Ø1
    - malignant C44.59- ☑
  - pituitary (duct) (gland) E23.6
  - placenta O43.19- ☑
  - pleura J94.8
  - popliteal — *see* Cyst, Baker's
  - porencephalic QØ4.6
    - acquired G93.Ø
  - postanal (infected) — *see* Cyst, pilonidal
  - postmastoidectomy cavity (mucosal) — *see* Complications, postmastoidectomy, cyst
  - preauricular Q18.1
  - prepuce N47.4
    - congenital Q55.69
  - primordial (jaw) KØ9.Ø
  - prostate N42.83

- **Cyst** — *continued*
  - pseudomucinous (ovary) D27.9
  - pupillary, miotic H21.27- ☑
  - radicular (residual) KØ4.8
  - radiculodental KØ4.8
  - ranular K11.8
  - Rathke's pouch E23.6
  - rectum (epithelium) (mucous) K62.89
  - renal — *see* Cyst, kidney
  - residual (radicular) KØ4.8
  - retention (ovary) N83.29- ☑
    - salivary gland K11.6
  - retina H33.19- ☑
    - ora serrata H33.11- ☑
    - parasitic H33.12- ☑
  - retroperitoneal K68.9
  - sacrococcygeal (dermoid) — *see* Cyst, pilonidal
  - salivary gland or duct (mucous extravasation or retention) K11.6
  - Sampson's N8Ø.1Ø- ☑
  - sclera H15.89
  - scrotum L72.9
    - sebaceous L72.3
  - sebaceous (duct) (gland) L72.3
    - breast — *see* Dysplasia, mammary, specified type NEC
    - eyelid — *see* Cyst, eyelid
    - genital organ NEC
      - female N94.89
      - male N5Ø.89
    - scrotum L72.3
  - semilunar cartilage (knee) (multiple) — *see* Derangement, knee, meniscus, cystic
  - seminal vesicle N5Ø.89
  - serous (ovary) N83.2Ø- ☑
  - sinus (accessory) (nasal) J34.1
  - Skene's gland N36.8
  - skin L72.9
    - breast — *see* Dysplasia, mammary, specified type NEC
    - epidermal, epidermoid L72.Ø
    - epithelial L72.Ø
    - eyelid — *see* Cyst, eyelid
    - genital organ NEC
      - female N9Ø.7
      - male N5Ø.89
    - inclusion L72.Ø
    - scrotum L72.9
    - sebaceous L72.3
    - sweat gland or duct L74.8
  - solitary
    - bone — *see* Cyst, bone, solitary
    - jaw M27.4Ø
    - kidney N28.1
  - spermatic cord N5Ø.89
  - sphenoid sinus J34.1
  - spinal meninges G96.198
  - spleen NEC D73.4
    - congenital Q89.Ø9
    - hydatid — *see also* Echinococcus B67.99 *[D77]*
  - Stafne's M27.Ø
  - subarachnoid intrasellar R93.Ø
  - subcutaneous, pheomycotic (chromomycotic) B43.2
  - subdural (cerebral) G93.Ø
    - spinal cord G96.198
  - sublingual gland K11.6
  - submandibular gland K11.6
  - submaxillary gland K11.6
  - suburethral N36.8
  - suprarenal gland E27.8
  - suprasellar — *see* Cyst, brain
  - sweat gland or duct L74.8
  - synovial — *see also* Cyst, bursa
    - ruptured — *see* Rupture, synovium
  - Tarlov G96.191
  - tarsal — *see* Chalazion
  - tendon (sheath) — *see* Disorder, tendon, specified type NEC
  - testis N44.2
    - tunica albuginea N44.1
  - theca lutein (ovary) N83.1- ☑
  - Thornwaldt's J39.2
  - thymus (gland) E32.8
  - thyroglossal duct (infected) (persistent) Q89.2
  - thyroid (gland) EØ4.1
  - thyrolingual duct (infected) (persistent) Q89.2
  - tongue K14.8
  - tonsil J35.8

- **Da Costa's syndrome** F45.8
- **Daae** (-Finsen) **disease** (epidemic pleurodynia) B33.Ø
- **Dabney's grip** B33.Ø
- **Dacryoadenitis, dacryadenitis** HØ4.ØØ- ☑
  - acute HØ4.Ø1- ☑
  - chronic HØ4.Ø2- ☑
- **Dacryocystitis** HØ4.3Ø- ☑
  - acute HØ4.32- ☑
  - chronic HØ4.41- ☑
  - neonatal P39.1
  - phlegmonous HØ4.31- ☑
  - syphilitic A52.71
    - congenital (early) A5Ø.Ø1
  - trachomatous, active A71.1
    - sequelae (late effect) B94.Ø
- **Dacryocystoblenorrhea** — *see* Inflammation, lacrimal, passages, chronic
- **Dacryocystocele** — *see* Disorder, lacrimal system, changes
- **Dacryolith, dacryolithiasis** HØ4.51- ☑
- **Dacryoma** — *see* Disorder, lacrimal system, changes
- **Dacryopericystitis** — *see* Dacryocystitis
- **Dacryops** HØ4.11- ☑
- **Dacryostenosis** — *see also* Stenosis, lacrimal
  - congenital Q1Ø.5
- **Dactylitis**
  - bone — *see* Osteomyelitis
  - sickle-cell D57.ØØ
    - Hb C D57.219
    - Hb SS D57.ØØ
    - specified NEC D57.819
  - skin LØ8.9
  - syphilitic A52.77
  - tuberculous A18.Ø3
- **Dactylolysis spontanea** (ainhum) L94.6
- **Dactylosymphysis** Q7Ø.9
  - fingers — *see* Syndactylism, complex, fingers
  - toes — *see* Syndactylism, complex, toes
- **Damage**
  - arteriosclerotic — *see* Arteriosclerosis
  - brain (nontraumatic) G93.9
    - anoxic, hypoxic G93.1
      - resulting from a procedure G97.82
    - child NEC G8Ø.9
    - due to birth injury P11.2
  - cardiorenal (vascular) — *see* Hypertension, cardiorenal
  - cerebral NEC — *see* Damage, brain
  - coccyx, complicating delivery O71.6
  - coronary — *see* Disease, heart, ischemic
  - deep tissue, pressure-induced — *see also* L89 with final character .6
  - eye, birth injury P15.3
  - liver (nontraumatic) K76.9
    - alcoholic K7Ø.9
    - due to drugs — *see* Disease, liver, toxic
    - toxic — *see* Disease, liver, toxic
  - lung
    - dabbing (related) UØ7.Ø
    - electronic cigarette (related) UØ7.Ø
    - vaping (associated) (device) (product) (use) UØ7.Ø
  - medication T88.7 ☑
  - organ
    - dabbing (related) UØ7.Ø
    - electronic cigarette (related) UØ7.Ø
    - vaping (associated) (device) (product) (use) UØ7.Ø
  - pelvic
    - joint or ligament, during delivery O71.6
    - organ NEC
      - during delivery O71.5
      - following ectopic or molar pregnancy OØ8.6
  - renal — *see* Disease, renal
  - subendocardium, subendocardial — *see* Degeneration, myocardial
  - vascular I99.9
- **Dana-Putnam syndrome** (subacute combined sclerosis with pernicious anemia) — *see* Degeneration, combined
- **Danbolt** (-Cross) **syndrome** (acrodermatitis enteropathica) E83.2
- **Dandruff** L21.Ø
- **Dandy-Walker syndrome** QØ3.1
  - with spina bifida — *see* Spina bifida
- **Danlos' syndrome** — *see also* Syndrome, Ehlers-Danlos Q79.6Ø
- **Darier** (-White) **disease** (congenital) Q82.8
  - meaning erythema annulare centrifugum L53.1
- **Darier-Roussy sarcoid** D86.3
- **Darling's disease or histoplasmosis** B39.4
- **Darwin's tubercle** Q17.8
- **Dawson's** (inclusion body) **encephalitis** A81.1
- **De Beurmann** (-Gougerot) **disease** B42.1
- **De la Tourette's syndrome** F95.2
- **De Lange's syndrome** Q87.19
- **De Morgan's spots** (senile angiomas) I78.1
- **De Quervain's**
  - disease (tendon sheath) M65.4
  - syndrome E34.51
  - thyroiditis (subacute granulomatous thyroiditis) EØ6.1
- **De Toni-Fanconi** (-Debré) **syndrome** E72.Ø9
  - with cystinosis E72.Ø4
- **Dead**
  - fetus, retained (mother) O36.4 ☑
    - early pregnancy OØ2.1
  - labyrinth H83.2 ☑
  - ovum, retained OØ2.Ø
- **Deaf nonspeaking NEC** H91.3
- **Deafmutism** (acquired) (congenital) NEC H91.3
  - hysterical F44.6
  - syphilitic, congenital — *see also* subcategory H94.8 A5Ø.Ø9
- **Deafness** (acquired) (complete) (hereditary) (partial) H91.9- ☑
  - with blue sclera and fragility of bone Q78.Ø
  - auditory fatigue — *see* Deafness, specified type NEC
  - aviation T7Ø.Ø ☑
    - nerve injury — *see* Injury, nerve, acoustic, specified type NEC
  - boilermaker's H83.3 ☑
  - central — *see* Deafness, sensorineural
  - conductive H9Ø.2
    - and sensorineural
      - mixed H9Ø.8
        - bilateral H9Ø.6
    - bilateral H9Ø.Ø
    - unilateral H9Ø.1- ☑
      - with restricted hearing on the contralateral side H9Ø.A- ☑
  - congenital H9Ø.5
    - with blue sclera and fragility of bone Q78.Ø
  - due to toxic agents — *see* Deafness, ototoxic
  - emotional (hysterical) F44.6
  - functional (hysterical) F44.6
  - high frequency H91.9- ☑
  - hysterical F44.6
  - low frequency H91.9- ☑
  - mental R48.8
  - mixed conductive and sensorineural H9Ø.8
    - bilateral H9Ø.6
    - unilateral H9Ø.7- ☑
  - nerve — *see* Deafness, sensorineural
  - neural — *see* Deafness, sensorineural
  - noise-induced — *see also* subcategory H83.3 ☑
    - nerve injury — *see* Injury, nerve, acoustic, specified type NEC
  - nonspeaking H91.3
  - ototoxic H91.Ø ☑
  - perceptive — *see* Deafness, sensorineural
  - psychogenic (hysterical) F44.6
  - sensorineural H9Ø.5
    - and conductive
      - bilateral H9Ø.6
      - mixed H9Ø.8
        - bilateral H9Ø.6
    - bilateral H9Ø.3
    - unilateral H9Ø.4- ☑
      - with restricted hearing on the contralateral side H9Ø.A- ☑
  - sensory — *see* Deafness, sensorineural
  - specified type NEC H91.8 ☑
  - sudden (idiopathic) H91.2- ☑
  - syphilitic A52.15
  - transient ischemic H93.Ø1- ☑
  - traumatic — *see* Injury, nerve, acoustic, specified type NEC
  - word (developmental) H93.25
- **Death** (cause unknown) (of) (unexplained) (unspecified cause) R99
  - brain G93.82
  - cardiac (sudden) (with successful resuscitation) — *see* Arrest, cardiac
    - family history of Z82.41
- **Death** — *continued*
  - cardiac — *see* Arrest, cardiac — *continued*
    - personal history of Z86.74
  - family member (assumed) Z63.4
- **Debility** (chronic) (general) (nervous) R53.81
  - congenital or neonatal NOS P96.9
  - nervous R53.81
  - old age R54
  - senile R54
- **Débove's disease** (splenomegaly) R16.1
- **Debt, burdensome** Z59.86
- **Decalcification**
  - bone — *see* Osteoporosis
  - teeth KØ3.89
- **Decapsulation, kidney** N28.89
- **Decay**
  - dental — *see* Caries, dental
  - senile R54
  - tooth, teeth — *see* Caries, dental
- **Deciduitis** (acute)
  - following ectopic or molar pregnancy OØ8.Ø
- **Decline** (general) — *see* Debility
  - cognitive, age-associated R41.81
- **Decompensation**
  - cardiac (acute) (chronic) — *see* Disease, heart
  - cardiovascular — *see* Disease, cardiovascular
  - heart — *see* Disease, heart
  - hepatic — *see* Failure, hepatic
  - myocardial (acute) (chronic) — *see* Disease, heart
  - respiratory J98.8
- **Decompression sickness** T7Ø.3 ☑
- **Decrease** (d)
  - absolute neutrophile count — *see* Neutropenia
  - blood
    - platelets — *see* Thrombocytopenia
    - pressure RØ3.1
      - due to shock following
        - injury T79.4 ☑
        - operation T81.19 ☑
  - estrogen E28.39
    - postablative E89.4Ø
      - asymptomatic E89.4Ø
      - symptomatic E89.41
  - fragility of erythrocytes D58.8
  - function
    - lipase (pancreatic) K9Ø.3
    - ovary in hypopituitarism E23.Ø
    - parenchyma of pancreas K86.89
    - pituitary (gland) (anterior) (lobe) E23.Ø
      - posterior (lobe) E23.Ø
  - functional activity R68.89
  - glucose R73.Ø9
  - hematocrit R71.Ø
  - hemoglobin R71.Ø
  - leukocytes D72.819
    - specified NEC D72.818
  - libido R68.82
  - lymphocytes D72.81Ø
  - platelets D69.6
  - respiration, due to shock following injury T79.4 ☑
  - sexual desire R68.82
  - tear secretion NEC — *see* Syndrome, dry eye
  - tolerance
    - fat K9Ø.49
    - glucose R73.Ø9
    - pancreatic K9Ø.3
    - salt and water E87.8
  - vision NEC H54.7
  - white blood cell count D72.819
    - specified NEC D72.818
- **Decubitus** (ulcer) — *see* Ulcer, pressure, by site
  - cervix N86
- **Deepening acetabulum** — *see* Derangement, joint, specified type NEC, hip
- **Defect, defective** Q89.9
  - 3-beta-hydroxysteroid dehydrogenase E25.Ø
  - 11-hydroxylase E25.Ø
  - 21-hydroxylase E25.Ø
  - abdominal wall, congenital Q79.59
  - antibody immunodeficiency D8Ø.9
  - aorticopulmonary septum Q21.4
  - atrial septal Q21.1Ø
    - coronary sinus Q21.13
    - following acute myocardial infarction (current complication) I23.1
    - ostium primum type (type I) Q21.2Ø

Deficiency, deficient — *continued*
- kappa-light chain D80.8
- labile factor (congenital) (hereditary) D68.2
  - acquired D68.4
- lacrimal fluid (acquired) — *see also* Syndrome, dry eye
  - congenital Q10.6
- lactase
  - congenital E73.0
  - secondary E73.1
- Laki-Lorand factor D68.2
- lecithin cholesterol acyltransferase E78.6
- lipocaic K86.89
- lipoprotein (familial) (high density) E78.6
- liver phosphorylase E74.09
- lysosomal alpha-1, 4 glucosidase E74.02
- magnesium E61.2
- major histocompatibility complex
  - class I D81.6
  - class II D81.7
- manganese E61.3
- menadione (vitamin K) E56.1
  - newborn P53
- mental (familial) (hereditary) — *see* Disability, intellectual
- methylenetetrahydrofolate reductase (MTHFR) E72.12
- mevalonate kinase M04.1
- mineralocorticoid E27.49
  - with glucocorticoid E27.49
- mineral NEC E61.8
- molybdenum (nutritional) E61.5
- moral F60.2
- multiple nutrient elements E61.7
- multiple sulfatase (MSD) E75.26
- muscle
  - carnitine (palmityltransferase) E71.314
  - phosphofructokinase E74.09
- myoadenylate deaminase E79.2
- myocardial — *see* Insufficiency, myocardial
- myophosphorylase E74.04
- NADH diaphorase or reductase (congenital) D74.0
- NADH-methemoglobin reductase (congenital) D74.0
- natrium E87.1
- niacin (amide) (-tryptophan) E52
- nicotinamide E52
- nicotinic acid E52
- number of teeth — *see* Anodontia
- nutrient element E61.9
  - multiple E61.7
  - specified NEC E61.8
- nutrition, nutritional — *see also* Nutrition deficient E63.9
  - sequelae — *see* Sequelae, nutritional deficiency
  - specified NEC E63.8
- of interleukin 1 receptor antagonist [DIRA] M04.8
- ornithine transcarbamylase E72.4
- ovarian E28.39
- oxygen — *see* Anoxia
- pantothenic acid E53.8
- parathyroid (gland) E20.9
- perineum (female) N81.89
- phenylalanine hydroxylase E70.1
- phosphoenolpyruvate carboxykinase E74.4
- phosphofructokinase E74.19
- phosphomannomutuse E74.818
- phosphomannose isomerase E74.818
- phosphomannosyl mutase E74.818
- phosphorylase kinase, liver E74.09
- pituitary hormone (isolated) E23.0
- plasma thromboplastin
  - antecedent (PTA) D68.1
  - component (PTC) D67
- plasminogen (type 1) (type 2) E88.02
- platelet NEC D69.1
  - constitutional — *see* Disease, von Willebrand
- polyglandular E31.8
  - autoimmune E31.0
- potassium (K) E87.6
- prepuce N47.3
- proaccelerin (congenital) (hereditary) D68.2
  - acquired D68.4
- proconvertin factor (congenital) (hereditary) D68.2
  - acquired D68.4
- protein — *see also* Malnutrition E46
  - anemia D53.0
  - C D68.59
  - S D68.59
- prothrombin (congenital) (hereditary) D68.2
  - acquired D68.4

Deficiency, deficient — *continued*
- Prower factor D68.2
- pseudocholinesterase E88.09
- PTA (plasma thromboplastin antecedent) D68.1
- PTC (plasma thromboplastin component) D67
- purine nucleoside phosphorylase (PNP) D81.5
- pyracin (alpha) (beta) E53.1
- pyridoxal E53.1
- pyridoxamine E53.1
- pyridoxine (derivatives) E53.1
- pyruvate
  - carboxylase E74.4
  - dehydrogenase E74.4
- riboflavin (vitamin B2) E53.0
- salt E87.1
- secretion
  - ovary E28.39
  - salivary gland (any) K11.7
  - urine R34
- selenium (dietary) E59
- serum antitrypsin, familial E88.01
- short stature homeobox gene (SHOX)
  - with
    - dyschondrosteosis Q78.8
    - short stature (idiopathic) E34.328
    - Turner's syndrome Q96.9
- sodium (Na) E87.1
- SPCA (factor VII) D68.2
- sphincter, intrinsic N36.42
  - with urethral hypermobility N36.43
- stable factor (congenital) (hereditary) D68.2
  - acquired D68.4
- Stuart-Prower (factor X) D68.2
- succinic semialdehyde dehydrogenase E72.81
- sucrase E74.39
- sulfatase E75.26
- sulfite oxidase E72.19
- thiamin, thiaminic (chloride) E51.9
  - beriberi (dry) E51.11
    - wet E51.12
- thrombokinase D68.2
  - newborn P53
- thyroid (gland) — *see* Hypothyroidism
- tocopherol E56.0
- tooth bud K00.0
- transcobalamine II (anemia) D51.2
- vanadium E61.6
- vascular I99.9
- vasopressin E23.2
- vertical ridge K06.8
- viosterol — *see* Deficiency, calciferol
- vitamin (multiple) NOS E56.9
  - A E50.9
    - with
      - Bitot's spot (corneal) E50.1
      - follicular keratosis E50.8
      - keratomalacia E50.4
      - manifestations NEC E50.8
      - night blindness E50.5
      - scar of cornea, xerophthalmic E50.6
      - xeroderma E50.8
      - xerophthalmia E50.7
      - xerosis
        - conjunctival E50.0
          - and Bitot's spot E50.1
        - cornea E50.2
          - and ulceration E50.3
    - sequelae E64.1
  - B (complex) NOS E53.9
    - with
      - beriberi (dry) E51.11
        - wet E51.12
      - pellagra E52
  - B1 NOS E51.9
    - beriberi (dry) E51.11
      - with circulatory system manifestations E51.11
      - wet E51.12
  - B12 E53.8
  - B2 (riboflavin) E53.0
  - B6 E53.1
  - C E54
    - sequelae E64.2
  - D E55.9
    - with
      - adult osteomalacia M83.8
      - rickets — *see* Rickets
    - 25-hydroxylase E83.32
  - E E56.0
  - folic acid E53.8

Deficiency, deficient — *continued*
- vitamin — *continued*
  - G E53.0
  - group B E53.9
    - specified NEC E53.8
  - H (biotin) E53.8
  - K E56.1
    - of newborn P53
  - nicotinic E52
  - P E56.8
  - PP (pellagra-preventing) E52
  - specified NEC E56.8
  - thiamin E51.9
    - beriberi — *see* Beriberi
- von Willebrand factor
  - partial quantitative — *see also* Disease, von Willebrand D68.01
  - total quantitative — *see also* Disease, von Willebrand D68.03
- zinc, dietary E60

Deficit — *see also* Deficiency
- attention and concentration R41.840
  - disorder — *see* Attention, deficit
  - following
    - cerebral infarction I69.310
    - cerebrovascular disease I69.910
      - specified disease NEC I69.810
    - nontraumatic
      - intracerebral hemorrhage I69.110
      - specified intracranial hemorrhage NEC I69.210
      - subarachnoid hemorrhage I69.010
- cognitive
  - communication R41.841
  - emotional
    - following
      - cerebral infarction I69.315
      - cerebrovascular disease I69.915
        - specified disease NEC I69.815
      - nontraumatic
        - intracerebral hemorrhage I69.115
        - specified intracranial hemorrhage NEC I69.215
        - subarachnoid hemorrhage I69.015
  - following
    - cerebral infarction I69.319
    - cerebrovascular disease I69.919
      - specified disease NEC I69.819
    - nontraumatic
      - intracerebral hemorrhage I69.119
      - specified intracranial hemorrhage NEC I69.219
      - subarachnoid hemorrhage I69.019
  - social
    - following
      - cerebral infarction I69.315
      - cerebrovascular disease I69.915
        - specified disease NEC I69.815
      - nontraumatic
        - intracerebral hemorrhage I69.115
        - specified intracranial hemorrhage NEC I69.215
        - subarachnoid hemorrhage I69.015
- cognitive NEC R41.89
  - following
    - cerebral infarction I69.318
    - cerebrovascular disease I69.918
      - specified disease NEC I69.818
    - nontraumatic
      - intracerebral hemorrhage I69.118
      - specified intracranial hemorrhage NEC I69.218
      - subarachnoid hemorrhage I69.018
- concentration R41.840
- executive function R41.844
  - following
    - cerebral infarction I69.314
    - cerebrovascular disease I69.914
      - specified disease NEC I69.814
    - nontraumatic
      - intracerebral hemorrhage I69.114
      - specified intracranial hemorrhage NEC I69.214
      - subarachnoid hemorrhage I69.014
- frontal lobe R41.844
  - following
    - cerebral infarction I69.314
    - cerebrovascular disease I69.914
      - specified disease NEC I69.814
    - nontraumatic
      - intracerebral hemorrhage I69.114
      - specified intracranial hemorrhage NEC I69.214
      - subarachnoid hemorrhage I69.014

Deficit — *continued*
- memory
  - following
    - cerebral infarction I69.311
    - cerebrovascular disease I69.911
      - specified disease NEC I69.811
    - nontraumatic
      - intracerebral hemorrhage I69.111
      - specified intracranial hemorrhage NEC I69.211
      - subarachnoid hemorrhage I69.Ø11
- neurologic NEC R29.818
  - ischemic
    - reversible (RIND) I63.9
      - prolonged (PRIND) I63.9
- oxygen RØ9.Ø2
- prolonged reversible ischemic neurologic (PRIND) I63.9
- psychomotor R41.843
  - following
    - cerebral infarction I69.313
    - cerebrovascular disease I69.913
      - specified disease NEC I69.813
    - nontraumatic
      - intracerebral hemorrhage I69.113
      - specified intracranial hemorrhage NEC I69.213
      - subarachnoid hemorrhage I69.Ø13
- visuospatial R41.842
  - following
    - cerebral infarction I69.312
    - cerebrovascular disease I69.912
      - specified disease NEC I69.812
    - nontraumatic
      - intracerebral hemorrhage I69.112
      - specified intracranial hemorrhage NEC I69.212
      - subarachnoid hemorrhage I69.Ø12

Deflection
- radius — *see* Deformity, limb, specified type NEC, forearm
- septum (acquired) (nasal) (nose) J34.2
- spine — *see* Curvature, spine
- turbinate (nose) J34.2

Defluvium
- capillorum — *see* Alopecia
- ciliorum — *see* Madarosis
- unguium L6Ø.8

Deformity Q89.9
- abdomen, congenital Q89.9
- abdominal wall
  - acquired M95.8
  - congenital Q79.59
- acquired (unspecified site) M95.9
- adrenal gland Q89.1
- alimentary tract, congenital Q45.9
  - upper Q4Ø.9
- ankle (joint) (acquired) — *see also* Deformity, limb, lower leg
  - abduction — *see* Contraction, joint, ankle
  - congenital Q68.8
  - contraction — *see* Contraction, joint, ankle
  - specified type NEC — *see* Deformity, limb, foot, specified NEC
- anus (acquired) K62.89
  - congenital Q43.9
- aorta (arch) (congenital) Q25.4Ø
  - acquired I77.89
- aortic
  - arch, acquired I77.89
  - cusp or valve (congenital) Q23.8
    - acquired — *see also* Endocarditis, aortic I35.8
- arm (acquired) (upper) — *see also* Deformity, limb, upper arm
  - congenital Q68.8
  - forearm — *see* Deformity, limb, forearm
- artery (congenital) (peripheral) NOS Q27.9
  - acquired I77.89
  - coronary (acquired) I25.9
    - congenital Q24.5
  - umbilical Q27.Ø
- atrial septal — *see also* Defect, atrial septal Q21.1Ø
- auditory canal (external) (congenital) — *see also* Malformation, ear, external
  - acquired — *see* Disorder, ear, external, specified type NEC
- auricle
  - ear (congenital) — *see also* Malformation, ear, external
    - acquired — *see* Disorder, pinna, deformity
- back — *see* Dorsopathy, deforming
- bile duct (common) (congenital) (hepatic) Q44.5

Deformity — *continued*
- bile duct — *continued*
  - acquired K83.8
- biliary duct or passage (congenital) Q44.5
  - acquired K83.8
- bladder (neck) (trigone) (sphincter) (acquired) N32.89
  - congenital Q64.79
- bone (acquired) NOS M95.9
  - congenital Q79.9
  - turbinate M95.Ø
- brain (congenital) QØ4.9
  - acquired G93.89
  - reduction QØ4.3
- breast (acquired) N64.89
  - congenital Q83.9
  - reconstructed N65.Ø
- bronchus (congenital) Q32.4
  - acquired NEC J98.Ø9
- bursa, congenital Q79.9
- canaliculi (lacrimalis) (acquired) — *see also* Disorder, lacrimal system, changes
  - congenital Q1Ø.6
- canthus, acquired — *see* Disorder, eyelid, specified type NEC
- capillary (acquired) I78.8
- cardiovascular system, congenital Q28.9
- caruncle, lacrimal (acquired) — *see also* Disorder, lacrimal system, changes
  - congenital Q1Ø.6
- cascade, stomach K31.2
- cecum (congenital) Q43.9
  - acquired K63.89
- cerebral, acquired G93.89
  - congenital QØ4.9
- cervix (uterus) (acquired) NEC N88.8
  - congenital Q51.9
- cheek (acquired) M95.2
  - congenital Q18.9
- chest (acquired) (wall) M95.4
  - congenital Q67.8
  - sequelae (late effect) of rickets E64.3
- chin (acquired) M95.2
  - congenital Q18.9
- choroid (congenital) Q14.3
  - acquired H31.8
  - plexus QØ7.8
    - acquired G96.198
- cicatricial — *see* Cicatrix
- cilia, acquired — *see* Disorder, eyelid, specified type NEC
- clavicle (acquired) M95.8
  - congenital Q68.8
- clitoris (congenital) Q52.6
  - acquired N9Ø.89
- clubfoot — *see* Clubfoot
- coccyx (acquired) — *see* subcategory M43.8 ☑
- colon (congenital) Q43.9
  - acquired K63.89
- concha (ear), congenital — *see also* Malformation, ear, external
  - acquired — *see* Disorder, pinna, deformity
- cornea (acquired) H18.7Ø
  - congenital Q13.4
  - descemetocele — *see* Descemetocele
  - ectasia — *see* Ectasia, cornea
  - specified NEC H18.79- ☑
  - staphyloma — *see* Staphyloma, cornea
- coronary artery (acquired) I25.9
  - congenital Q24.5
- cranium (acquired) — *see* Deformity, skull
- cricoid cartilage (congenital) Q31.8
  - acquired J38.7
- cystic duct (congenital) Q44.5
  - acquired K82.8
- Dandy-Walker QØ3.1
  - with spina bifida — *see* Spina bifida
- diaphragm (congenital) Q79.1
  - acquired J98.6
- digestive organ NOS Q45.9
- ductus arteriosus Q25.Ø
- duodenal bulb K31.89
- duodenum (congenital) Q43.9
  - acquired K31.89
- dura — *see* Deformity, meninges
- ear (acquired) — *see also* Disorder, pinna, deformity
  - congenital (external) Q17.9
    - internal Q16.5
    - middle Q16.4

Deformity — *continued*
- ear — *see also* Disorder, pinna, deformity — *continued*
  - congenital — *continued*
    - middle — *continued*
      - ossicles Q16.3
    - ossicles Q16.3
- ectodermal (congenital) NEC Q84.9
- ejaculatory duct (congenital) Q55.4
  - acquired N5Ø.89
- elbow (joint) (acquired) — *see also* Deformity, limb, upper arm
  - congenital Q68.8
  - contraction — *see* Contraction, joint, elbow
- endocrine gland NEC Q89.2
- epididymis (congenital) Q55.4
  - acquired N5Ø.89
- epiglottis (congenital) Q31.8
  - acquired J38.7
- esophagus (congenital) Q39.9
  - acquired K22.89
- eustachian tube (congenital) NEC Q17.8
- eye, congenital Q15.9
- eyebrow (congenital) Q18.8
- eyelid (acquired) — *see also* Disorder, eyelid, specified type NEC
  - congenital Q1Ø.3
- face (acquired) M95.2
  - congenital Q18.9
- fallopian tube, acquired N83.8
- femur (acquired) — *see* Deformity, limb, specified type NEC, thigh
- fetal
  - with fetopelvic disproportion O33.7 ☑
    - causing obstructed labor O66.3
- finger (acquired) M2Ø.ØØ- ☑
  - boutonniere M2Ø.Ø2- ☑
  - congenital Q68.1
  - flexion contracture — *see* Contraction, joint, hand
  - mallet finger M2Ø.Ø1- ☑
  - specified NEC M2Ø.Ø9- ☑
  - swan-neck M2Ø.Ø3- ☑
- flexion (joint) (acquired) — *see also* Deformity, limb, flexion M21.2Ø
  - congenital NOS Q74.9
    - hip Q65.89
- foot (acquired) — *see also* Deformity, limb, lower leg
  - cavovarus (congenital) Q66.1- ☑
  - congenital NOS Q66.9- ☑
    - specified type NEC Q66.89
  - specified type NEC — *see* Deformity, limb, foot, specified NEC
  - valgus (congenital) Q66.6
    - acquired — *see* Deformity, valgus, ankle
  - varus (congenital) NEC Q66.3- ☑
    - acquired — *see* Deformity, varus, ankle
- forearm (acquired) — *see also* Deformity, limb, forearm
  - congenital Q68.8
- forehead (acquired) M95.2
  - congenital Q75.8
- frontal bone (acquired) M95.2
  - congenital Q75.8
- gallbladder (congenital) Q44.1
  - acquired K82.8
- gastrointestinal tract (congenital) NOS Q45.9
  - acquired K63.89
- genitalia, genital organ(s) or system NEC
  - female (congenital) Q52.9
    - acquired N94.89
    - external Q52.7Ø
  - male (congenital) Q55.9
    - acquired N5Ø.89
- globe (eye) (congenital) Q15.8
  - acquired H44.89
- gum, acquired NEC KØ6.8
- hand (acquired) — *see* Deformity, limb, hand
  - congenital Q68.1
- head (acquired) M95.2
  - congenital Q75.8
- heart (congenital) Q24.9
  - septum Q21.9
    - auricular — *see also* Defect, atrial septal Q21.1Ø
    - ventricular Q21.Ø
  - valve (congenital) NEC Q24.8
    - acquired — *see* Endocarditis
- heel (acquired) — *see* Deformity, foot
- hepatic duct (congenital) Q44.5
  - acquired K83.8

Index — Deformity — Degeneration, degenerative

Degeneration, degenerative — *continued*
- intervertebral disc — *continued*
  - cervical, cervicothoracic — *see* Disorder, disc, cervical, degeneration — *continued*
    - with
      - myelopathy — *see* Disorder, disc, cervical, with myelopathy
      - neuritis, radiculitis or radiculopathy — *see* Disorder, disc, cervical, with neuritis
  - lumbar region M51.36
    - with
      - myelopathy M51.Ø6
      - neuritis, radiculitis, radiculopathy or sciatica M51.16
  - lumbosacral region M51.37
    - with
      - neuritis, radiculitis, radiculopathy or sciatica M51.17
  - sacrococcygeal region M53.3
  - thoracic region M51.34
    - with
      - myelopathy M51.Ø4
      - neuritis, radiculitis, radiculopathy M51.14
  - thoracolumbar region M51.35
    - with
      - myelopathy M51.Ø5
      - neuritis, radiculitis, radiculopathy M51.15
- intestine, amyloid E85.4
- iris (pigmentary) H21.23- ☑
- ischemic — *see* Ischemia
- joint disease — *see* Osteoarthritis
- kidney N28.89
  - amyloid E85.4 *[N29]*
  - cystic, congenital Q61.9
  - fatty N28.89
  - polycystic Q61.3
    - adult type (autosomal dominant) Q61.2
    - infantile type (autosomal recessive) NEC Q61.19
      - collecting duct dilatation Q61.11
- Kuhnt-Junius — *see also* Degeneration, macula H35.32- ☑
- lens — *see* Cataract
- lenticular (familial) (progressive) (Wilson's) (with cirrhosis of liver) E83.Ø1
- liver (diffuse) NEC K76.89
  - amyloid E85.4 *[K77]*
  - cystic K76.89
    - congenital Q44.6
  - fatty NEC K76.Ø
    - alcoholic K7Ø.Ø
  - hypertrophic K76.89
  - parenchymatous, acute or subacute K72.ØØ
    - with coma K72.Ø1
  - pigmentary K76.89
  - toxic (acute) K71.9
- lung J98.4
- lymph gland I89.8
  - hyaline I89.8
- macula, macular (acquired) (age-related) (senile) H35.3Ø
  - angioid streaks H35.33
  - atrophic age-related H35.31- ☑
  - congenital or hereditary — *see* Dystrophy, retina
  - cystoid H35.35- ☑
  - drusen H35.36- ☑
  - dry age-related H35.31- ☑
  - exudative H35.32- ☑
  - hole H35.34- ☑
  - nonexudative H35.31- ☑
  - puckering H35.37- ☑
  - toxic H35.38- ☑
  - wet age-related H35.32- ☑
- membranous labyrinth, congenital (causing impairment of hearing) Q16.5
- meniscus — *see* Derangement, meniscus
- mitral — *see* Insufficiency, mitral
- Mönckeberg's — *see* Arteriosclerosis, extremities
- motor centers, senile G31.1
- multi-system G9Ø.3
- mural — *see* Degeneration, myocardial
- muscle (fatty) (fibrous) (hyaline) (progressive) M62.89
  - heart — *see* Degeneration, myocardial
- myelin, central nervous system G37.9
- myocardial, myocardium (fatty) (hyaline) (senile) I51.5
  - with rheumatic fever (conditions in IØØ) IØ9.Ø
    - active, acute or subacute IØ1.2
      - with chorea IØ2.Ø
    - inactive or quiescent (with chorea) IØ9.Ø

Degeneration, degenerative — *continued*
- myocardial, myocardium — *continued*
  - hypertensive — *see* Hypertension, heart
  - rheumatic — *see* Degeneration, myocardial, with rheumatic fever
  - syphilitic A52.Ø6
- nasal sinus (mucosa) J32.9
  - frontal J32.1
  - maxillary J32.Ø
- nerve — *see* Disorder, nerve
- nervous system G31.9
  - alcoholic G31.2
  - amyloid E85.4 *[G99.8]*
  - autonomic G9Ø.9
  - fatty G31.89
  - specified NEC G31.89
- nipple N64.89
- olivopontocerebellar (hereditary) (familial) G23.8
- osseous labyrinth — *see* subcategory H83.8 ☑
- ovary N83.8
  - cystic N83.2Ø- ☑
  - microcystic N83.2Ø- ☑
- pallidal pigmentary (progressive) G23.Ø
- pancreas K86.89
  - tuberculous A18.83
- penis N48.89
- pigmentary (diffuse) (general)
  - localized — *see* Degeneration, by site
  - pallidal (progressive) G23.Ø
- pineal gland E34.8
- pituitary (gland) E23.6
- popliteal fat pad M79.4
- posterolateral (spinal cord) — *see* Degeneration, combined
- pulmonary valve (heart) I37.8
- pulp (tooth) KØ4.2
- pupillary margin H21.24- ☑
- renal — *see* Degeneration, kidney
- retina H35.9
  - hereditary (cerebroretinal) (congenital) (juvenile) (macula) (peripheral) (pigmentary) — *see* Dystrophy, retina
  - Kuhnt-Junius — *see also* Degeneration, macula H35.32- ☑
  - macula (cystic) (exudative) (hole) (nonexudative) (pseudohole) (senile) (toxic) — *see* Degeneration, macula
  - peripheral H35.4Ø
    - lattice H35.41- ☑
    - microcystoid H35.42- ☑
    - paving stone H35.43- ☑
    - secondary
      - pigmentary H35.45- ☑
      - vitreoretinal H35.46- ☑
    - senile reticular H35.44- ☑
  - pigmentary (primary) — *see also* Dystrophy, retina
    - secondary — *see* Degeneration, retina, peripheral, secondary
  - posterior pole — *see* Degeneration, macula
- saccule, congenital (causing impairment of hearing) Q16.5
- senile R54
  - brain G31.1
  - cardiac, heart or myocardium — *see* Degeneration, myocardial
  - motor centers G31.1
  - vascular — *see* Arteriosclerosis
- sinus (cystic) — *see also* Sinusitis
  - polypoid J33.1
- skin L98.8
  - amyloid E85.4 *[L99]*
  - colloid L98.8
- spinal (cord) G31.89
  - amyloid E85.4 *[G32.89]*
  - combined (subacute) — *see* Degeneration, combined
  - dorsolateral — *see* Degeneration, combined
  - familial NEC G31.89
  - fatty G31.89
  - funicular — *see* Degeneration, combined
  - posterolateral — *see* Degeneration, combined
  - subacute combined — *see* Degeneration, combined
  - tuberculous A17.81
- spleen D73.Ø
  - amyloid E85.4 *[D77]*
- stomach K31.89
- striatonigral G23.2
- suprarenal (capsule) (gland) E27.8

Degeneration, degenerative — *continued*
- synovial membrane (pulpy) — *see* Disorder, synovium, specified type NEC
- tapetoretinal — *see* Dystrophy, retina
- thymus (gland) E32.8
  - fatty E32.8
- thyroid (gland) EØ7.89
- tricuspid (heart) (valve) IØ7.9
- tuberculous NEC — *see* Tuberculosis
- turbinate J34.89
- uterus (cystic) N85.8
- vascular (senile) — *see* Arteriosclerosis
  - hypertensive — *see* Hypertension
- vitreoretinal, secondary — *see* Degeneration, retina, peripheral, secondary, vitreoretinal
- vitreous (body) H43.81- ☑
- Wallerian — *see* Disorder, nerve
- Wilson's hepatolenticular E83.Ø1

Deglutition
- paralysis R13.Ø
  - hysterical F44.4
- pneumonia J69.Ø

Degos' disease I77.89

Dehiscence (of)
- amputation stump T87.81
- cesarean wound O9Ø.Ø
- closure of
  - cornea T81.31 ☑
  - craniotomy T81.32 ☑
  - fascia (muscular) (superficial) T81.32 ☑
  - internal organ or tissue T81.32 ☑
  - laceration (external) (internal) T81.33 ☑
  - ligament T81.32 ☑
  - mucosa T81.31 ☑
  - muscle or muscle flap T81.32 ☑
  - ribs or rib cage T81.32 ☑
  - skin and subcutaneous tissue (full-thickness) (superficial) T81.31 ☑
  - skull T81.32 ☑
  - sternum (sternotomy) T81.32 ☑
  - tendon T81.32 ☑
  - traumatic laceration (external) (internal) T81.33 ☑
- episiotomy O9Ø.1
- operation wound NEC T81.31 ☑
  - external operation wound (superficial) T81.31 ☑
  - internal operation wound (deep) T81.32 ☑
- perineal wound (postpartum) O9Ø.1
- traumatic injury wound repair T81.33 ☑
- wound T81.3Ø ☑
  - traumatic repair T81.33 ☑

Dehydration E86.Ø
- newborn P74.1

Déjérine-Roussy syndrome G89.Ø

Déjérine-Sottas disease or neuropathy (hypertrophic) G6Ø.Ø

Déjérine-Thomas atrophy G23.8

Delay, delayed
- any plane in pelvis
  - complicating delivery O66.9
- birth or delivery NOS O63.9
- closure, ductus arteriosus (Botalli) P29.38
- coagulation — *see* Defect, coagulation
- conduction (cardiac) (ventricular) I45.9
- delivery, second twin, triplet, etc O63.2
- development R62.5Ø
  - global F88
  - intellectual (specific) F81.9
  - language F8Ø.9
    - due to hearing loss F8Ø.4
  - learning F81.9
  - milestone R62.Ø
  - pervasive F84.9
  - physiological R62.5Ø
    - specified stage NEC R62.Ø
  - reading F81.Ø
  - sexual E3Ø.Ø
  - speech F8Ø.9
    - due to hearing loss F8Ø.4
  - spelling F81.81
- ejaculation F52.32
- gastric emptying K3Ø
- menarche E3Ø.Ø
- menstruation (cause unknown) N91.Ø
- milestone R62.Ø
- passage of meconium (newborn) P76.Ø
- primary respiration P28.9
- puberty (constitutional) E3Ø.Ø

- **Dependence** — *continued*
  - drug — *continued*
    - inhalant F18.20
      - with
        - anxiety disorder F18.280
        - dementia, persisting F18.27
        - intoxication F18.229
          - with delirium F18.221
          - uncomplicated F18.220
        - mood disorder F18.24
        - other specified disorder F18.288
        - psychosis F18.259
          - delusions F18.250
          - hallucinations F18.251
        - unspecified disorder F18.29
      - in remission F18.21
    - nicotine F17.200
      - with disorder F17.209
        - in remission F17.201
        - specified disorder NEC F17.208
        - withdrawal F17.203
      - chewing tobacco F17.220
        - with disorder F17.229
          - in remission F17.221
          - specified disorder NEC F17.228
          - withdrawal F17.223
      - cigarettes F17.210
        - with disorder F17.219
          - in remission F17.211
          - specified disorder NEC F17.218
          - withdrawal F17.213
      - specified product NEC F17.290
        - with disorder F17.299
          - remission F17.291
          - specified disorder NEC F17.298
          - withdrawal F17.293
    - opioid F11.20
      - with
        - intoxication F11.229
          - with
            - delirium F11.221
            - perceptual disturbance F11.222
          - uncomplicated F11.220
        - mood disorder F11.24
        - other specified disorder F11.288
        - psychosis F11.259
          - delusions F11.250
          - hallucinations F11.251
        - sexual dysfunction F11.281
        - sleep disorder F11.282
        - unspecified disorder F11.29
        - withdrawal F11.23
      - in remission F11.21
    - psychoactive NEC F19.20
      - with
        - amnestic disorder F19.26
        - anxiety disorder F19.280
        - dementia F19.27
        - intoxication F19.229
          - with
            - delirium F19.221
            - perceptual disturbance F19.222
          - uncomplicated F19.220
        - mood disorder F19.24
        - other specified disorder F19.288
        - psychosis F19.259
          - delusions F19.250
          - hallucinations F19.251
        - sexual dysfunction F19.281
        - sleep disorder F19.282
        - unspecified disorder F19.29
        - withdrawal F19.239
          - with
            - delirium F19.231
            - perceptual disturbance F19.232
          - uncomplicated F19.230
    - sedative, hypnotic or anxiolytic F13.20
      - with
        - amnestic disorder F13.26
        - anxiety disorder F13.280
        - dementia, persisting F13.27
        - intoxication F13.229
          - with delirium F13.221
          - uncomplicated F13.220
        - mood disorder F13.24
        - other specified disorder F13.288
        - psychosis F13.259
          - delusions F13.250
          - hallucinations F13.251

- **Dependence** — *continued*
  - drug — *continued*
    - sedative, hypnotic or anxiolytic — *continued*
      - with — *continued*
        - sexual dysfunction F13.281
        - sleep disorder F13.282
        - unspecified disorder F13.29
        - withdrawal F13.239
          - with
            - delirium F13.231
            - perceptual disturbance F13.232
          - uncomplicated F13.230
      - in remission F13.21
    - stimulant NEC F15.20
      - with
        - anxiety disorder F15.280
        - intoxication F15.229
          - with
            - delirium F15.221
            - perceptual disturbance F15.222
          - uncomplicated F15.220
        - mood disorder F15.24
        - other specified disorder F15.288
        - psychosis F15.259
          - delusions F15.250
          - hallucinations F15.251
        - sexual dysfunction F15.281
        - sleep disorder F15.282
        - unspecified disorder F15.29
        - withdrawal F15.23
      - in remission F15.21
  - ethyl
    - alcohol (without remission) F10.20
      - with remission F10.21
    - bromide — *see* Dependence, drug, sedative
    - carbamate F19.20
    - chloride F19.20
    - morphine — *see* Dependence, drug, opioid
  - ganja — *see* Dependence, drug, cannabis
  - glue (airplane) (sniffing) — *see* Dependence, drug, inhalant
  - glutethimide — *see* Dependence, drug, sedative
  - hallucinogenics — *see* Dependence, drug, hallucinogen
  - hashish — *see* Dependence, drug, cannabis
  - hemp — *see* Dependence, drug, cannabis
  - heroin (salt) (any) — *see* Dependence, drug, opioid
  - hypnotic NEC — *see* Dependence, drug, sedative
  - Indian hemp — *see* Dependence, drug, cannabis
  - inhalants — *see* Dependence, drug, inhalant
  - khat — *see* Dependence, drug, stimulant NEC
  - laudanum — *see* Dependence, drug, opioid
  - LSD (-25) (derivatives) — *see* Dependence, drug, hallucinogen
  - luminal — *see* Dependence, drug, sedative
  - lysergic acid — *see* Dependence, drug, hallucinogen
  - maconha — *see* Dependence, drug, cannabis
  - marihuana — *see* Dependence, drug, cannabis
  - meprobamate — *see* Dependence, drug, sedative
  - mescaline — *see* Dependence, drug, hallucinogen
  - methadone — *see* Dependence, drug, opioid
  - methamphetamine(s) — *see* Dependence, drug, stimulant NEC
  - methaqualone — *see* Dependence, drug, sedative
  - methyl
    - alcohol (without remission) F10.20
      - with remission F10.21
    - bromide — *see* Dependence, drug, sedative
    - morphine — *see* Dependence, drug, opioid
    - phenidate — *see* Dependence, drug, stimulant NEC
    - sulfonal — *see* Dependence, drug, sedative
  - morphine (sulfate) (sulfite) (type) — *see* Dependence, drug, opioid
  - narcotic (drug) NEC — *see* Dependence, drug, opioid
  - nembutal — *see* Dependence, drug, sedative
  - neraval — *see* Dependence, drug, sedative
  - neravan — *see* Dependence, drug, sedative
  - neurobarb — *see* Dependence, drug, sedative
  - nicotine — *see* Dependence, drug, nicotine
  - nitrous oxide F19.20
  - nonbarbiturate sedatives and tranquilizers with similar effect — *see* Dependence, drug, sedative
  - on
    - artificial heart (fully implantable) (mechanical) Z95.812
    - aspirator Z99.0
    - care provider (because of) Z74.9
      - impaired mobility Z74.09

- **Dependence** — *continued*
  - on — *continued*
    - care provider — *continued*
      - need for
        - assistance with personal care Z74.1
        - continuous supervision Z74.3
      - no other household member able to render care Z74.2
      - specified reason NEC Z74.8
    - machine Z99.89
      - enabling NEC Z99.89
      - specified type NEC Z99.89
    - renal dialysis (hemodialysis) (peritoneal) Z99.2
    - respirator Z99.11
    - ventilator Z99.11
    - wheelchair Z99.3
  - opiate — *see* Dependence, drug, opioid
  - opioids — *see* Dependence, drug, opioid
  - opium (alkaloids) (derivatives) (tincture) — *see* Dependence, drug, opioid
  - oxygen (long-term) (supplemental) Z99.81
  - paraldehyde — *see* Dependence, drug, sedative
  - paregoric — *see* Dependence, drug, opioid
  - PCP (phencyclidine) (or related substance) — *see* Dependence, drug, hallucinogen
  - pentobarbital — *see* Dependence, drug, sedative
  - pentobarbitone (sodium) — *see* Dependence, drug, sedative
  - pentothal — *see* Dependence, drug, sedative
  - peyote — *see* Dependence, drug, hallucinogen
  - phencyclidine (PCP) (or related substance) — *see* Dependence, drug, hallucinogen
  - phenmetrazine — *see* Dependence, drug, stimulant NEC
  - phenobarbital — *see* Dependence, drug, sedative
  - polysubstance F19.20
  - psilocibin, psilocin, psilocyn, psilocyline — *see* Dependence, drug, hallucinogen
  - psychostimulant NEC — *see* Dependence, drug, stimulant NEC
  - secobarbital — *see* Dependence, drug, sedative
  - seconal — *see* Dependence, drug, sedative
  - sedative NEC — *see* Dependence, drug, sedative
  - specified drug NEC — *see* Dependence, drug
  - stimulant NEC — *see* Dependence, drug, stimulant NEC
  - substance NEC — *see* Dependence, drug
  - supplemental oxygen Z99.81
  - tobacco — *see* Dependence, drug, nicotine
    - counseling and surveillance Z71.6
  - tranquilizer NEC — *see* Dependence, drug, sedative
  - vitamin B6 E53.1
  - volatile solvents — *see* Dependence, drug, inhalant
- **Dependency**
  - care-provider Z74.9
  - passive F60.7
  - reactions (persistent) F60.7
- **Depersonalization** (in neurotic state) (neurotic) (syndrome) F48.1
- **Depletion**
  - extracellular fluid E86.9
  - plasma E86.1
  - potassium E87.6
    - nephropathy N25.89
  - salt or sodium E87.1
    - causing heat exhaustion or prostration T67.4 ☑
    - nephropathy N28.9
  - volume NOS E86.9
- **Deployment** (current) (military) status Z56.82
  - in theater or in support of military war, peacekeeping and humanitarian operations Z56.82
  - personal history of Z91.82
    - military war, peacekeeping and humanitarian deployment (current or past conflict) Z91.82
  - returned from Z91.82
- **Depolarization, premature** I49.40
  - atrial I49.1
  - junctional I49.2
  - specified NEC I49.49
  - ventricular I49.3
- **Deposit**
  - bone in Boeck's sarcoid D86.89
  - calcareous, calcium — *see* Calcification
  - cholesterol
    - retina H35.89
    - vitreous (body) (humor) — *see* Deposit, crystalline
  - conjunctiva H11.11- ☑
  - cornea H18.00- ☑
    - argentous H18.02- ☑

- **Deposit** — *continued*
  - cornea — *continued*
    - due to metabolic disorder H18.Ø3- ☑
    - Kayser-Fleischer ring H18.Ø4- ☑
    - pigmentation — *see* Pigmentation, cornea
  - crystalline, vitreous (body) (humor) H43.2- ☑
  - hemosiderin in old scars of cornea — *see* Pigmentation, cornea, stromal
  - metallic in lens — *see* Cataract, specified NEC
  - skin R23.8
  - tooth, teeth (betel) (black) (green) (materia alba) (orange) (tobacco) KØ3.6
  - urate, kidney — *see* Calculus, kidney
- **Depraved appetite** — *see* Pica
- **Depressed**
  - HDL cholesterol E78.6
- **Depression** (acute) (mental) F32.A
  - agitated (single episode) F32.2
  - anaclitic — *see* Disorder, adjustment
  - anxiety F41.8
    - persistent F34.1
  - arches — *see also* Deformity, limb, flat foot
  - atypical (single episode) F32.89
    - recurrent episode F33.8
  - basal metabolic rate R94.8
  - bone marrow D75.89
  - central nervous system RØ9.2
  - cerebral R29.818
    - newborn P91.4
  - cerebrovascular I67.9
  - chest wall M95.4
  - climacteric (single episode) F32.89
    - recurrent episode F33.8
  - endogenous (without psychotic symptoms) F33.2
    - with psychotic symptoms F33.3
  - functional activity R68.89
  - hysterical F44.89
  - involutional (single episode) F32.89
    - recurrent episode F33.8
  - major F32.9
    - with psychotic symptoms F32.3
    - recurrent — *see* Disorder, depressive, recurrent
  - manic-depressive — *see* Disorder, depressive, recurrent
  - masked (single episode) F32.89
  - medullary G93.89
  - menopausal (single episode) F32.89
    - recurrent episode F33.8
  - metatarsus — *see* Depression, arches
  - monopolar F33.9
  - nervous F34.1
  - neurotic F34.1
  - nose M95.Ø
  - postnatal (NOS) F53.Ø
  - postpartum (NOS) F53.Ø
  - post-psychotic of schizophrenia F32.89
  - post-schizophrenic F32.89
  - psychogenic (reactive) (single episode) F32.9
  - psychoneurotic F34.1
  - psychotic (single episode) F32.3
    - recurrent F33.3
  - reactive (psychogenic) (single episode) F32.9
    - psychotic (single episode) F32.3
  - recurrent — *see* Disorder, depressive, recurrent
  - respiratory center G93.89
  - seasonal — *see* Disorder, depressive, recurrent
  - senile FØ3 ☑
  - severe, single episode F32.2
  - situational F43.21
  - skull Q67.4
  - specified NEC (single episode) F32.89
  - sternum M95.4
  - visual field — *see* Defect, visual field
  - vital (recurrent) (without psychotic symptoms) F33.2
    - with psychotic symptoms F33.3
    - single episode F32.2
- **Deprivation**
  - cultural Z6Ø.3
  - effects NOS T73.9 ☑
    - specified NEC T73.8 ☑
  - emotional NEC Z65.8
    - affecting infant or child — *see* Maltreatment, child, psychological
  - food T73.Ø ☑
  - material Z59.87
  - protein — *see* Malnutrition
  - sleep Z72.82Ø
  - social Z6Ø.4
- **Deprivation** — *continued*
  - social — *continued*
    - affecting infant or child — *see* Maltreatment, child, psychological
  - specified NEC T73.8 ☑
  - vitamins — *see* Deficiency, vitamin
  - water T73.1 ☑
- **Derangement**
  - ankle (internal) — *see* Derangement, joint, articular cartilage, ankle
  - cartilage (articular) NEC — *see* Derangement, joint, articular cartilage, by site
    - recurrent — *see* Dislocation, recurrent
  - cruciate ligament, anterior, current injury — *see* Sprain, knee, cruciate, anterior
  - elbow (internal) — *see* Derangement, joint, articular cartilage, elbow
  - hip (joint) (internal) (old) — *see* Derangement, joint, articular cartilage, hip
  - joint (internal) M24.9
    - ankylosis — *see* Ankylosis
    - articular cartilage M24.1Ø
      - ankle M24.17- ☑
      - elbow M24.12- ☑
      - foot M24.17- ☑
      - hand M24.14- ☑
      - hip M24.15- ☑
      - knee NEC M23.9- ☑
      - loose body — *see* Loose, body
      - shoulder M24.11- ☑
      - specified site NEC M24.19
      - wrist M24.13- ☑
    - contracture — *see* Contraction, joint
    - current injury — *see also* Dislocation
      - knee, meniscus or cartilage — *see* Tear, meniscus
    - dislocation
      - pathological — *see* Dislocation, pathological
      - recurrent — *see* Dislocation, recurrent
    - knee — *see* Derangement, knee
    - ligament — *see* Disorder, ligament
    - loose body — *see* Loose, body
    - recurrent — *see* Dislocation, recurrent
    - specified type NEC M24.8Ø
      - ankle M24.87- ☑
      - elbow M24.82- ☑
      - foot joint M24.87- ☑
      - hand joint M24.84- ☑
      - hip M24.85- ☑
      - shoulder M24.81- ☑
      - specified site NEC M24.89
      - wrist M24.83- ☑
    - temporomandibular M26.69
  - knee (recurrent) M23.9- ☑
    - ligament disruption, spontaneous M23.6Ø- ☑
      - anterior cruciate M23.61- ☑
      - capsular M23.67- ☑
      - instability, chronic M23.5- ☑
      - lateral collateral M23.64- ☑
      - medial collateral M23.63- ☑
      - posterior cruciate M23.62- ☑
    - loose body M23.4- ☑
    - meniscus M23.3Ø- ☑
      - cystic M23.ØØ- ☑
        - lateral M23.ØØ2
          - anterior horn M23.Ø4- ☑
          - posterior horn M23.Ø5- ☑
          - specified NEC M23.Ø6- ☑
        - medial M23.ØØ5
          - anterior horn M23.Ø1- ☑
          - posterior horn M23.Ø2- ☑
          - specified NEC M23.Ø3- ☑
      - degenerate — *see* Derangement, knee, meniscus, specified NEC
      - detached — *see* Derangement, knee, meniscus, specified NEC
      - due to old tear or injury M23.2Ø- ☑
        - lateral M23.2Ø- ☑
          - anterior horn M23.24- ☑
          - posterior horn M23.25- ☑
          - specified NEC M23.26- ☑
        - medial M23.2Ø- ☑
          - anterior horn M23.21- ☑
          - posterior horn M23.22- ☑
          - specified NEC M23.23- ☑
      - retained — *see* Derangement, knee, meniscus, specified NEC
- **Derangement** — *continued*
  - knee — *continued*
    - meniscus — *continued*
      - specified NEC M23.3Ø- ☑
        - lateral M23.3Ø- ☑
          - anterior horn M23.34- ☑
          - posterior horn M23.35- ☑
          - specified NEC M23.36- ☑
        - medial M23.3Ø- ☑
          - anterior horn M23.31- ☑
          - posterior horn M23.32- ☑
          - specified NEC M23.33- ☑
    - old M23.8X- ☑
    - specified NEC — *see* subcategory M23.8 ☑
  - low back NEC — *see* Dorsopathy, specified NEC
  - meniscus — *see* Derangement, knee, meniscus
  - mental — *see* Psychosis
  - patella, specified NEC — *see* Disorder, patella, derangement NEC
  - semilunar cartilage (knee) — *see* Derangement, knee, meniscus, specified NEC
  - shoulder (internal) — *see* Derangement, joint, shoulder
- **Dercum's disease** E88.2
- **Derealization** (neurotic) F48.1
- **Dermal** — *see* condition
- **Dermaphytid** — *see* Dermatophytosis
- **Dermatitis** (eczematous) L3Ø.9
  - ab igne L59.Ø
  - acarine B88.Ø
  - actinic (due to sun) L57.8
    - other than from sun L59.8
  - allergic — *see* Dermatitis, contact, allergic
  - ambustionis, due to burn or scald — *see* Burn
  - amebic AØ6.7
  - ammonia L22
  - arsenical (ingested) L27.8
  - artefacta L98.1
    - psychogenic F54
  - atopic L2Ø.9
    - psychogenic F54
    - specified NEC L2Ø.89
  - autoimmune progesterone L3Ø.8
  - berlock, berloque L56.2
  - blastomycotic B4Ø.3
  - blister beetle L24.89
  - bullous, bullosa L13.9
    - mucosynechial, atrophic L12.1
    - seasonal L3Ø.8
    - specified NEC L13.8
  - calorica L59.Ø
    - due to burn or scald — *see* Burn
  - caterpillar L24.89
  - cercarial B65.3
  - combustionis L59.Ø
    - due to burn or scald — *see* Burn
  - congelationis T69.1 ☑
  - contact (occupational) L25.9
    - allergic L23.9
      - due to
        - adhesives L23.1
        - cement L23.5
        - chemical products NEC L23.5
        - chromium L23.Ø
        - cosmetics L23.2
        - dander (cat) (dog) L23.81
        - drugs in contact with skin L23.3
        - dyes L23.4
        - food in contact with skin L23.6
        - hair (cat) (dog) L23.81
        - insecticide L23.5
        - metals L23.Ø
        - nickel L23.Ø
        - plants, non-food L23.7
        - plastic L23.5
        - rubber L23.5
        - specified agent NEC L23.89
    - due to
      - cement L25.3
      - chemical products NEC L25.3
      - cosmetics L25.Ø
      - dander (cat) (dog) L23.81
      - drugs in contact with skin L25.1
      - dyes L25.2
      - food in contact with skin L25.4
      - hair (cat) (dog) L23.81
      - plants, non-food L25.5
      - specified agent NEC L25.8
    - irritant L24.9

Dermatitis — *continued*
- contact — *continued*
  - irritant — *continued*
    - due to
      - body fluids L24.AØ
        - incontinence (dual) (fecal) (urinary) L24.A2
        - saliva L24.A1
        - specified NEC L24.A9
      - cement L24.5
      - chemical products NEC L24.5
      - cosmetics L24.3
      - detergents L24.Ø
      - drugs in contact with skin L24.4
      - food in contact with skin L24.6
      - oils and greases L24.1
      - plants, non-food L24.7
      - solvents L24.2
      - specified agent NEC L24.89
    - related to
      - colostomy L24.B3
      - endotracheal tube L24.A9
      - enterocutaneous fistula L24.B3
      - gastrostomy L24.B1
      - ileostomy L24.B3
      - jejunostomy L24.B1
      - saliva or spit fistula L24.B1
      - stoma or fistula L24.BØ
        - digestive L24.B1
        - fecal or urinary L24.B3
        - respiratory L24.B2
      - tracheostomy L24.B2
- contusiformis L52
- desquamative L3Ø.8
- diabetic — *see* EØ8-E13 with .62Ø
- diaper L22
- diphtheritica A36.3
- dry skin L85.3
- due to
  - acetone (contact) (irritant) L24.2
  - acids (contact) (irritant) L24.5
  - adhesive(s) (allergic) (contact) (plaster) L23.1
    - irritant L24.5
  - alcohol (irritant) (skin contact) (substances in category T51) L24.2
    - taken internally L27.8
  - alkalis (contact) (irritant) L24.5
  - arsenic (ingested) L27.8
  - carbon disulfide (contact) (irritant) L24.2
  - caustics (contact) (irritant) L24.5
  - cement (contact) L25.3
  - cereal (ingested) L27.2
  - chemical(s) NEC L25.3
    - taken internally L27.8
  - chlorocompounds L24.2
  - chromium (contact) (irritant) L24.81
  - coffee (ingested) L27.2
  - cold weather L3Ø.8
  - cosmetics (contact) L25.Ø
    - allergic L23.2
    - irritant L24.3
  - cyclohexanes L24.2
  - dander (cat) (dog) L23.81
  - Demodex species B88.Ø
  - Dermanyssus gallinae B88.Ø
  - detergents (contact) (irritant) L24.Ø
  - dichromate L24.81
  - drugs and medicaments (generalized) (internal use) L27.Ø
    - external — *see* Dermatitis, due to, drugs, in contact with skin
    - in contact with skin L25.1
      - allergic L23.3
      - irritant L24.4
    - localized skin eruption L27.1
    - specified substance — *see* Table of Drugs and Chemicals
  - dyes (contact) L25.2
    - allergic L23.4
    - irritant L24.89
  - epidermophytosis — *see* Dermatophytosis
  - esters L24.2
  - external irritant NEC L24.9
  - fish (ingested) L27.2
  - flour (ingested) L27.2
  - food (ingested) L27.2
    - in contact with skin L25.4
  - fruit (ingested) L27.2
  - furs (allergic) (contact) L23.81

Dermatitis — *continued*
- due to — *continued*
  - glues — *see* Dermatitis, due to, adhesives
  - glycols L24.2
  - greases NEC (contact) (irritant) L24.1
  - hair (cat) (dog) L23.81
  - hot
    - objects and materials — *see* Burn
    - weather or places L59.Ø
  - hydrocarbons L24.2
  - infrared rays L59.8
  - ingestion, ingested substance L27.9
    - chemical NEC L27.8
    - drugs and medicaments — *see* Dermatitis, due to, drugs
    - food L27.2
    - specified NEC L27.8
  - insecticide in contact with skin L24.5
  - internal agent L27.9
    - drugs and medicaments (generalized) — *see* Dermatitis, due to, drugs
    - food L27.2
  - irradiation — *see* Dermatitis, due to, radioactive substance
  - ketones L24.2
  - lacquer tree (allergic) (contact) L23.7
  - light (sun) NEC L57.8
    - acute L56.8
    - other L59.8
  - Liponyssoides sanguineus B88.Ø
  - low temperature L3Ø.8
  - meat (ingested) L27.2
  - metals, metal salts (contact) (irritant) L24.81
  - milk (ingested) L27.2
  - nickel (contact) (irritant) L24.81
  - nylon (contact) (irritant) L24.5
  - oils NEC (contact) (irritant) L24.1
  - paint solvent (contact) (irritant) L24.2
  - petroleum products (contact) (irritant) (substances in T52.Ø) L24.2
  - plants NEC (contact) L25.5
    - allergic L23.7
    - irritant L24.7
  - plasters (adhesive) (any) (allergic) (contact) L23.1
    - irritant L24.5
  - plastic (contact) L25.3
  - preservatives (contact) — *see* Dermatitis, due to, chemical, in contact with skin
  - primrose (allergic) (contact) L23.7
  - primula (allergic) (contact) L23.7
  - radiation L59.8
    - nonionizing (chronic exposure) L57.8
    - sun NEC L57.8
      - acute L56.8
  - radioactive substance L58.9
    - acute L58.Ø
    - chronic L58.1
  - radium L58.9
    - acute L58.Ø
    - chronic L58.1
  - ragweed (allergic) (contact) L23.7
  - Rhus (allergic) (contact) (diversiloba) (radicans) (toxicodendron) (venenata) (verniciflua) L23.7
  - rubber (contact) L24.5
  - Senecio jacobaea (allergic) (contact) L23.7
  - solvents (contact) (irritant) (substances in category T52) L24.2
  - specified agent NEC (contact) L25.8
    - allergic L23.89
    - irritant L24.89
  - sunshine NEC L57.8
    - acute L56.8
  - tetrachlorethylene (contact) (irritant) L24.2
  - toluene (contact) (irritant) L24.2
  - turpentine (contact) L24.2
  - ultraviolet rays (sun NEC) (chronic exposure) L57.8
    - acute L56.8
  - vaccine or vaccination L27.Ø
    - specified substance — *see* Table of Drugs and Chemicals
  - varicose veins — *see* Varix, leg, with, inflammation
  - X-rays L58.9
    - acute L58.Ø
    - chronic L58.1
- dyshydrotic L3Ø.1
- dysmenorrheica N94.6
- escharotica — *see* Burn
- exfoliative, exfoliativa (generalized) L26

Dermatitis — *continued*
- exfoliative, exfoliativa — *continued*
  - neonatorum LØØ
- eyelid — *see also* Dermatosis, eyelid HØ1.9
  - allergic HØ1.119
    - left HØ1.116
      - lower HØ1.115
      - upper HØ1.114
    - right HØ1.113
      - lower HØ1.112
      - upper HØ1.111
  - contact — *see* Dermatitis, eyelid, allergic
  - due to
    - Demodex species B88.Ø
    - herpes (zoster) BØ2.39
      - simplex BØØ.59
  - eczematous HØ1.139
    - left HØ1.136
      - lower HØ1.135
      - upper HØ1.134
    - right HØ1.133
      - lower HØ1.132
      - upper HØ1.131
  - specified NEC HØ1.8
- facta, factitia, factitial L98.1
  - psychogenic F54
- flexural NEC L2Ø.82
- friction L3Ø.4
- fungus B36.9
  - specified type NEC B36.8
- gangrenosa, gangrenous infantum LØ8.Ø
- harvest mite B88.Ø
- heat L59.Ø
- herpesviral, vesicular (ear) (lip) BØØ.1
- herpetiformis (bullous) (erythematous) (pustular) (vesicular) L13.Ø
  - juvenile L12.2
  - senile L12.Ø
- hiemalis L3Ø.8
- hypostatic, hypostatica — *see* Varix, leg, with, inflammation
- infectious eczematoid L3Ø.3
- infective L3Ø.3
- irritant — *see* Dermatitis, contact, irritant
- Jacquet's (diaper dermatitis) L22
- Leptus B88.Ø
- lichenified NEC L28.Ø
- medicamentosa (generalized) (internal use) — *see* Dermatitis, due to drugs
- mite B88.Ø
- multiformis L13.Ø
  - juvenile L12.2
- napkin L22
- neurotica L13.Ø
- nummular L3Ø.Ø
- papillaris capillitii L73.Ø
- pellagrous E52
- perioral L71.Ø
- photocontact L56.2
- polymorpha dolorosa L13.Ø
- pruriginosa L13.Ø
- pruritic NEC L3Ø.8
- psychogenic F54
- purulent LØ8.Ø
- pustular
  - contagious BØ8.Ø2
  - subcorneal L13.1
- pyococcal LØ8.Ø
- pyogenica LØ8.Ø
- repens L4Ø.2
- Ritter's (exfoliativa) LØØ
- Schamberg's L81.7
- schistosome B65.3
- seasonal bullous L3Ø.8
- seborrheic L21.9
  - infantile L21.1
  - specified NEC L21.8
- sensitization NOS L23.9
- septic LØ8.Ø
- solare L57.8
- specified NEC L3Ø.8
- stasis I87.2
  - with
    - varicose ulcer — *see* Varix, leg, with ulcer, with inflammation
    - varicose veins — *see* Varix, leg, with, inflammation

☑ **Additional Character Required — Refer to the Tabular List for Character Selection**

Disease, diseased — *continued*
- glomerular — *see also* Glomerulonephritis — *continued*
  - acute — *see* Nephritis, acute
  - chronic — *see* Nephritis, chronic
  - minimal change N05.0
  - rapidly progressive N01.9
- glycogen storage E74.00
  - Andersen's E74.09
  - Cori's E74.03
  - Forbes' E74.03
  - generalized E74.00
  - glucose-6-phosphatase deficiency E74.01
  - heart E74.02 *[I43]*
  - hepatorenal E74.09
  - Hers' E74.09
  - liver and kidney E74.09
  - McArdle's E74.04
  - muscle phosphofructokinase E74.09
  - myocardium E74.02 *[I43]*
  - Pompe's E74.02
  - Tauri's E74.09
  - type 0 E74.09
  - type I E74.01
  - type II E74.02
  - type III E74.03
  - type IV E74.09
  - type V E74.04
  - type VI-XI E74.09
  - Von Gierke's E74.01
- Goldstein's (familial hemorrhagic telangiectasia) I78.0
- gonococcal NOS A54.9
- graft-versus-host (GVH) D89.813
  - acute D89.810
  - acute on chronic D89.812
  - chronic D89.811
- grainhandler's J67.8
- granulomatous (childhood) (chronic) D71
- Graves' (exophthalmic goiter) — *see* Hyperthyroidism, with, goiter (diffuse)
- Griesinger's — *see* Ancylostomiasis
- Grisel's M43.6
- Gruby's (tinea tonsurans) B35.0
- Guillain-Barré G61.0
- Guinon's (motor-verbal tic) F95.2
- gum K06.9
- gynecological N94.9
- H (Hartnup's) E72.02
- Haff — *see* Poisoning, mercury
- Hageman (congenital factor XII deficiency) D68.2
- hair (color) (shaft) L67.9
  - follicles L73.9
    - specified NEC L73.8
- Hamman's (spontaneous mediastinal emphysema) J98.2
- hand, foot and mouth B08.4
- Hansen's — *see* Leprosy
- Hantavirus, with pulmonary manifestations B33.4
  - with renal manifestations A98.5
- Harada's H30.81- ☑
- Hartnup (pellagra-cerebellar ataxia-renal aminoaciduria) E72.02
- Hart's (pellagra-cerebellar ataxia-renal aminoaciduria) E72.02
- Hashimoto's (struma lymphomatosa) E06.3
- Hb — *see* Disease, hemoglobin
- heart (organic) I51.9
  - with
    - pulmonary edema (acute) — *see also* Failure, ventricular, left I50.1
    - rheumatic fever (conditions in I00)
      - active I01.9
        - with chorea I02.0
        - specified NEC I01.8
      - inactive or quiescent (with chorea) I09.9
        - specified NEC I09.89
  - amyloid E85.4 *[I43]*
  - aortic (valve) I35.9
  - arteriosclerotic or sclerotic (senile) — *see* Disease, heart, ischemic, atherosclerotic
  - artery, arterial — *see* Disease, heart, ischemic, atherosclerotic
  - beer drinkers' I42.6
  - beriberi (wet) E51.12
  - black I27.0
  - congenital Q24.9
    - cyanotic Q24.9
    - specified NEC Q24.8

Disease, diseased — *continued*
- heart — *continued*
  - coronary — *see* Disease, heart, ischemic
  - cryptogenic I51.9
  - fibroid — *see* Myocarditis
  - functional I51.89
    - psychogenic F45.8
  - glycogen storage E74.02 *[I43]*
  - gonococcal A54.83
  - hypertensive — *see* Hypertension, heart
  - hyperthyroid — *see also* Hyperthyroidism E05.90 *[I43]*
    - with thyroid storm E05.91 *[I43]*
  - ischemic (chronic or with a stated duration of over 4 weeks) I25.9
    - atherosclerotic (of) I25.10
      - with angina pectoris — *see* Arteriosclerosis, coronary (artery)
      - coronary artery bypass graft — *see* Arteriosclerosis, coronary (artery),
    - cardiomyopathy I25.5
    - diagnosed on ECG or other special investigation, but currently presenting no symptoms I25.6
    - silent I25.6
    - specified form NEC I25.89
  - kyphoscoliotic I27.1
  - meningococcal A39.50
    - endocarditis A39.51
    - myocarditis A39.52
    - pericarditis A39.53
  - mitral I05.9
    - specified NEC I05.8
  - muscular — *see* Degeneration, myocardial
  - psychogenic (functional) F45.8
  - pulmonary (chronic) I27.9
    - in schistosomiasis B65.9 *[I52]*
    - specified NEC I27.89
  - rheumatic (chronic) (inactive) (old) (quiescent) (with chorea) I09.9
    - active or acute I01.9
      - with chorea (acute) (rheumatic) (Sydenham's) I02.0
    - specified NEC I09.89
  - senile — *see* Myocarditis
  - syphilitic A52.06
    - aortic A52.03
      - aneurysm A52.01
    - congenital A50.54 *[I52]*
  - thyrotoxic — *see also* Thyrotoxicosis E05.90 *[I43]*
    - with thyroid storm E05.91 *[I43]*
  - valve, valvular (obstructive) (regurgitant) — *see also* Endocarditis
    - congenital NEC Q24.8
      - pulmonary Q22.3
  - vascular — *see* Disease, cardiovascular
- heavy chain NEC C88.2
  - alpha C88.3
  - gamma C88.2
  - mu C88.2
- Hebra's
  - pityriasis
    - maculata et circinata L42
    - rubra pilaris L44.0
  - prurigo L28.2
- hematopoietic organs D75.9
- hemoglobin or Hb
  - abnormal (mixed) NEC D58.2
    - with thalassemia D56.9
  - AS genotype D57.3
  - Bart's D56.0
  - C (Hb-C) D58.2
    - with other abnormal hemoglobin NEC D58.2
    - elliptocytosis D58.1
    - Hb-S D57.2- ☑
    - sickle-cell D57.2- ☑
    - thalassemia D56.8
  - Constant Spring D58.2
  - D (Hb-D) D58.2
  - E (Hb-E) D58.2
  - E-beta thalassemia D56.5
  - elliptocytosis D58.1
  - H (Hb-H) (thalassemia) D56.0
    - with other abnormal hemoglobin NEC D56.9
    - Constant Spring D56.0
  - I thalassemia D56.9
  - M D74.0
  - S or SS D57.1

Disease, diseased — *continued*
- hemoglobin or Hb — *continued*
  - S or SS — *continued*
    - with
      - acute chest syndrome D57.01
      - cerebral vascular involvement D57.03
      - crisis (painful) D57.00
        - with complication specified NEC D57.09
      - splenic sequestration D57.02
      - vasoocclusive pain D57.00
    - beta plus D57.44
      - with
        - acute chest syndrome D57.451
        - cerebral vascular involvement D57.453
        - crisis D57.459
          - with specified complication NEC D57.458
        - splenic sequestration D57.452
        - vasoocclusive pain D57.459
      - without crisis D57.44
    - beta zero D57.42
      - with
        - acute chest syndrome D57.431
        - cerebral vascular involvement D57.433
        - crisis D57.439
          - with specified complication NEC D57.438
        - splenic sequestration D57.432
        - vasoocclusive pain
      - without crisis D57.42
  - SC D57.2- ☑
  - SD D57.8- ☑
  - SE D57.8- ☑
  - spherocytosis D58.0
  - unstable, hemolytic D58.2
- hemolytic (newborn) P55.9
  - autoimmune D59.10
    - cold type (primary) (secondary) (symptomatic) D59.12
    - mixed type (primary) (secondary) (symptomatic) D59.13
    - warm type (primary) (secondary) (symptomatic) D59.11
  - drug-induced D59.0
  - due to or with
    - incompatibility
      - ABO (blood group) P55.1
      - blood (group) (Duffy) (K) (Kell) (Kidd) (Lewis) (M) (S) NEC P55.8
      - Rh (blood group) (factor) P55.0
    - Rh negative mother P55.0
  - specified type NEC P55.8
  - unstable hemoglobin D58.2
- hemorrhagic D69.9
  - newborn P53
- Henoch (-Schönlein) (purpura nervosa) D69.0
- hepatic — *see* Disease, liver
- hepatolenticular E83.01
- heredodegenerative NEC
  - spinal cord G95.89
- herpesviral, disseminated B00.7
- Hers' (glycogenosis VI) E74.09
- Herter (-Gee) (-Heubner) (nontropical sprue) K90.0
- Heubner-Herter (nontropical sprue) K90.0
- high fetal gene or hemoglobin thalassemia D56.9
- Hildenbrand's — *see* Typhus
- hip (joint) M25.9
  - congenital Q65.89
  - suppurative M00.9
  - tuberculous A18.02
- His (-Werner) (trench fever) A79.0
- Hodgson's — *see also* Aneurysm, aorta, thorax I71.20
  - ruptured — *see also* Aneurysm, aorta, thorax, ruptured I71.10
- Holla — *see* Spherocytosis
- hookworm B76.9
  - specified NEC B76.8
- host-versus-graft D89.813
  - acute D89.810
  - acute on chronic D89.812
  - chronic D89.811
- human immunodeficiency virus (HIV) B20
- Huntington's G10
  - with dementia — *see also* Dementia, in, diseases specified elsewhere G10 *[F02.80]*
- Hutchinson's (cheiropompholyx) — *see* Hutchinson's disease
- hyaline (diffuse) (generalized)

Disease, diseased — *continued*
- lung — *continued*
  - interstitial — *continued*
    - with progressive fibrotic phenotype, in diseases classified elsewhere J84.17Ø
  - obstructive (chronic) J44.9
    - with
      - acute
        - bronchitis J44.Ø
        - exacerbation NEC J44.1
        - lower respiratory infection J44.Ø
      - alveolitis, allergic J67.9
      - asthma J44.9
      - bronchiectasis J47.9
        - with
          - exacerbation (acute) J47.1
          - lower respiratory infection J47.Ø
      - bronchitis J44.9
        - with
          - exacerbation (acute) J44.1
          - lower respiratory infection J44.Ø
      - emphysema J43.9
      - hypersensitivity pneumonitis J67.9
    - decompensated J44.1
      - with
        - exacerbation (acute) J44.1
  - polycystic J98.4
    - congenital Q33.Ø
  - rheumatoid (diffuse) (interstitial) — *see* Rheumatoid, lung
  - vaping (associated) (device) (product) (use) UØ7.Ø
- Lutembacher's (atrial septal defect with mitral stenosis) Q21.19
- Lyme A69.2Ø
- lymphatic (gland) (system) (channel) (vessel) I89.9
- lymphoproliferative D47.9
  - specified NEC D47.Z9 (*following* D47.4)
  - T-gamma D47.Z9 (*following* D47.4)
  - X-linked D82.3
- Magitot's M27.2
- malarial — *see* Malaria
- malignant — *see also* Neoplasm, malignant, by site
- Manson's B65.1
- maple bark J67.6
- maple-syrup-urine E71.Ø
- Marburg (virus) A98.3
- Marion's (bladder neck obstruction) N32.Ø
- Marsh's (exophthalmic goiter) — *see* Hyperthyroidism, with, goiter (diffuse)
- mastoid (process) — *see* Disorder, ear, middle
- Mathieu's (leptospiral jaundice) A27.Ø
- Maxcy's A75.2
- McArdle (-Schmid-Pearson) (glycogenosis V) E74.Ø4
- mediastinum J98.59
- medullary center (idiopathic) (respiratory) G93.89
- Meige's (chronic hereditary edema) Q82.Ø
- meningococcal — *see* Infection, meningococcal
- mental F99
  - organic FØ9
- mesenchymal M35.9
- mesenteric embolic — *see also* Ischemia, intestine, acute K55.Ø39
- metabolic, metabolism E88.9
  - bilirubin E8Ø.7
- metal-polisher's J62.8
- metastatic — *see also* Neoplasm, secondary, by site C79.9
- microvascular - code to condition
- microvillus
  - atrophy Q43.8
  - inclusion (MVD) Q43.8
- middle ear — *see* Disorder, ear, middle
- Mikulicz' (dryness of mouth, absent or decreased lacrimation) K11.8
- Milroy's (chronic hereditary edema) Q82.Ø
- Minamata — *see* Poisoning, mercury
- minicore G71.29
- Minor's G95.19
- Minot's (hemorrhagic disease, newborn) P53
- Minot-von Willebrand-Jürgens (angiohemophilia) — *see* Disease, von Willebrand
- Mitchell's (erythromelalgia) I73.81
- mitral (valve) IØ5.9
  - nonrheumatic I34.9
- mixed connective tissue M35.1
- moldy hay J67.Ø
- Monge's T7Ø.29 ☑

Disease, diseased — *continued*
- Morgagni-Adams-Stokes (syncope with heart block) I45.9
- Morgagni's (syndrome) (hyperostosis frontalis interna) M85.2
- Morton's (with metatarsalgia) — *see* Lesion, nerve, plantar
- Morvan's G6Ø.8
- motor neuron (bulbar) (mixed type) (spinal) G12.2Ø
  - amyotrophic lateral sclerosis G12.21
  - familial G12.24
  - progressive bulbar palsy G12.22
  - specified NEC G12.29
- moyamoya I67.5
- mu heavy chain disease C88.2
- multicore G71.29
- multiminicore G71.29
- muscle — *see also* Disorder, muscle
  - inflammatory — *see* Myositis
  - ocular (external) — *see* Strabismus
- musculoskeletal system, soft tissue — *see also* Disorder, soft tissue
  - specified NEC — *see* Disorder, soft tissue, specified type NEC
- mushroom workers' J67.5
- mycotic B49
- myelodysplastic — *see also* Syndrome, myelodysplasia C94.6
- myelodysplastic/myeloproliferative neoplasm, unclassifiable C94.6
- myeloproliferative D47.1
  - chronic D47.1
  - not classified C94.6
  - specified NEC C94.6
  - unclassifiable C94.6
- myocardium, myocardial — *see also* Degeneration, myocardial I51.5
  - primary (idiopathic) I42.9
- myoneural G7Ø.9
- Naegeli's D69.1
- nails L6Ø.9
  - specified NEC L6Ø.8
- Nairobi (sheep virus) A93.8
- nasal J34.9
- nemaline body G71.21
- nerve — *see* Disorder, nerve
- nervous system G98.8
  - autonomic G9Ø.9
  - central G96.9
    - specified NEC G96.89
  - congenital QØ7.9
  - parasympathetic G9Ø.9
  - specified NEC G98.8
  - sympathetic G9Ø.9
  - vegetative G9Ø.9
- neuromuscular system G7Ø.9
- Newcastle B3Ø.8
- Nicolas (-Durand)-Favre (climatic bubo) A55
- nipple N64.9
  - Paget's C5Ø.Ø1- ☑
    - female C5Ø.Ø1- ☑
    - male C5Ø.Ø2- ☑
- Nishimoto (-Takeuchi) I67.5
- nonarthropod-borne NOS (viral) B34.9
  - enterovirus NEC B34.1
- nonautoimmune hemolytic D59.4
  - drug-induced D59.2
- Nonne-Milroy-Meige (chronic hereditary edema) Q82.Ø
- nose J34.9
- nucleus pulposus — *see* Disorder, disc
- nutritional E63.9
- oast-house-urine E72.19
- ocular
  - herpesviral BØØ.5Ø
  - zoster BØ2.3Ø
- obliterative vascular I77.1
- Ohara's — *see* Tularemia
- Opitz's (congestive splenomegaly) D73.2
- Oppenheim-Urbach (necrobiosis lipoidica diabeticorum) — *see* EØ8-E13 with .62Ø
- optic nerve NEC — *see* Disorder, nerve, optic
- orbit — *see* Disorder, orbit
- organ
  - dabbing (related) UØ7.Ø
  - electronic cigarette (related) UØ7.Ø
  - vaping (associated) (device) (product) (use) UØ7.Ø
- Oriental liver fluke B66.1
- Oriental lung fluke B66.4

Disease, diseased — *continued*
- Ormond's N13.5
- Oropouche virus A93.Ø
- Osler-Rendu (familial hemorrhagic telangiectasia) I78.Ø
- osteofibrocystic E21.Ø
- Otto's M24.7
- outer ear — *see* Disorder, ear, external
- ovary (noninflammatory) N83.9
  - cystic N83.2Ø- ☑
  - inflammatory — *see* Salpingo-oophoritis
  - polycystic E28.2
  - specified NEC N83.8
- Owren's (congenital) — *see* Defect, coagulation
- p11Ød-activating mutation causing senescent T cells, lymphadenopathy, and immunodeficiency [PASLI] D81.82
- pancreas K86.9
  - cystic K86.2
  - fibrocystic E84.9
  - specified NEC K86.89
- panvalvular IØ8.9
  - specified NEC IØ8.8
- parametrium (noninflammatory) N83.9
- parasitic B89
  - cerebral NEC B71.9 *[G94]*
  - intestinal NOS B82.9
  - mouth B37.Ø
  - skin NOS B88.9
  - specified type — *see* Infestation
  - tongue B37.Ø
- parathyroid (gland) E21.5
  - specified NEC E21.4
- Parkinson's G2Ø
- parodontal KØ5.6
- Parrot's (syphilitic osteochondritis) A5Ø.Ø2
- Parry's (exophthalmic goiter) — *see* Hyperthyroidism, with, goiter (diffuse)
- Parson's (exophthalmic goiter) — *see* Hyperthyroidism, with, goiter (diffuse)
- Paxton's (white piedra) B36.2
- pearl-worker's — *see* Osteomyelitis, specified type NEC
- Pellegrini-Stieda (calcification, knee joint) — *see* Bursitis, tibial collateral
- pelvis, pelvic
  - female NOS N94.9
    - specified NEC N94.89
  - gonococcal (acute) (chronic) A54.24
  - inflammatory (female) N73.9
    - acute N73.Ø
    - chlamydial A56.11
    - chronic N73.1
    - specified NEC N73.8
    - syphilitic (secondary) A51.42
      - late A52.76
    - tuberculous A18.17
  - organ, female N94.9
  - peritoneum, female NEC N94.89
- penis N48.9
  - inflammatory N48.29
    - abscess N48.21
    - cellulitis N48.22
  - specified NEC N48.89
- periapical tissues NOS KØ4.9Ø
- periodontal KØ5.6
  - specified NEC KØ5.5
- periosteum — *see* Disorder, bone, specified type NEC
- peripheral
  - arterial I73.9
  - autonomic nervous system G9Ø.9
  - nerves — *see* Polyneuropathy
  - vascular NOS I73.9
- peritoneum K66.9
  - pelvic, female NEC N94.89
  - specified NEC K66.8
- persistent mucosal (middle ear) H66.2Ø
  - left H66.22
    - with right H66.23
  - right H66.21
    - with left H66.23
- Petit's — *see* Hernia, abdomen, specified site NEC
- pharynx J39.2
  - specified NEC J39.2
- Phocas' — *see* Mastopathy, cystic
- photochromogenic (acid-fast bacilli) (pulmonary) A31.Ø
  - nonpulmonary A31.9
- Pick's — *see also* Dementia, in, diseases specified elsewhere G31.Ø1 *[FØ2.8Ø]*

Disease, diseased — *continued*
  Pick's — *see also* Dementia, in, diseases specified elsewhere — *continued*
    with behavioral disturbance — *see also* Dementia, in, diseases specified elsewhere G31.Ø1 *[FØ2.81-]* ☑
    brain G31.Ø1 *[FØ2.8Ø]*
      with behavioral disturbance — *see also* Dementia, in, diseases specified elsewhere G31.Ø1 *[FØ2.81-]* ☑
    of pericardium (pericardial pseudocirrhosis of liver) I31.1
  pigeon fancier's J67.2
  pineal gland E34.8
  pink — *see* Poisoning, mercury
  Pinkus' (lichen nitidus) L44.1
  pinworm B8Ø
  Piry virus A93.8
  pituitary (gland) E23.7
  pituitary-snuff-taker's J67.8
  pleura (cavity) J94.9
    specified NEC J94.8
  pneumatic drill (hammer) T75.21 ☑
  Pollitzer's (hidradenitis suppurativa) L73.2
  polycystic
    kidney or renal Q61.3
      adult type Q61.2
      childhood type NEC Q61.19
        collecting duct dilatation Q61.11
    liver or hepatic Q44.6
    lung or pulmonary J98.4
      congenital Q33.Ø
    ovary, ovaries E28.2
    spleen Q89.Ø9
  polyethylene T84.Ø5- ☑
  Pompe's (glycogenosis II) E74.Ø2
  Posadas-Wernicke B38.9
  Potain's (pulmonary edema) — *see* Edema, lung
  prepuce N47.8
    inflammatory N47.7
      balanoposthitis N47.6
  Pringle's (tuberous sclerosis) Q85.1
  prion, central nervous system A81.9
    specified NEC A81.89
  prostate N42.9
    specified NEC N42.89
  protozoal B64
    acanthamebiasis — *see* Acanthamebiasis
    African trypanosomiasis — *see* African trypanosomiasis
    babesiosis — *see also* Babesiosis B6Ø.ØØ
    Chagas disease — *see* Chagas disease
    intestine, intestinal AØ7.9
    leishmaniasis — *see* Leishmaniasis
    malaria — *see* Malaria
    naegleriasis B6Ø.2
    pneumocystosis B59
    specified organism NEC B6Ø.8
    toxoplasmosis — *see* Toxoplasmosis
  pseudo-Hurler's E77.Ø
  psychiatric F99
  psychotic — *see* Psychosis
  Puente's (simple glandular cheilitis) K13.Ø
  puerperal — *see also* Puerperal O9Ø.89
  pulmonary — *see also* Disease, lung
    artery I28.9
    chronic obstructive J44.9
      with
        acute bronchitis J44.Ø
        exacerbation (acute) J44.1
        lower respiratory infection (acute) J44.Ø
      decompensated J44.1
        with
          exacerbation (acute) J44.1
    heart I27.9
      specified NEC I27.89
    hypertensive (vascular) — *see also* Hypertension, pulmonary I27.2Ø
      NEC I27.2 ☑
      primary (idiopathic) I27.Ø
    valve I37.9
      rheumatic IØ9.89
  pulp (dental) NOS KØ4.9Ø
  pulseless M31.4
  Putnam's (subacute combined sclerosis with pernicious anemia) D51.Ø
  Pyle (-Cohn) (metaphyseal dysplasia) Q78.5
  ragpicker's or ragsorter's A22.1

Disease, diseased — *continued*
  Raynaud's — *see* Raynaud's disease
  reactive airway — *see* Asthma
  Reclus' (cystic) — *see* Mastopathy, cystic
  rectum K62.9
    specified NEC K62.89
  Refsum's (heredopathia atactica polyneuritiformis) G6Ø.1
  renal (functional) (pelvis) — *see also* Disease, kidney N28.9
    with
      edema — *see* Nephrosis
      glomerular lesion — *see* Glomerulonephritis
        with edema — *see* Nephrosis
      interstitial nephritis N12
    acute N28.9
    chronic — *see also* Disease, kidney, chronic N18.9
    cystic, congenital Q61.9
    diabetic — *see* EØ8-E13 with .22
    end-stage (failure) N18.6
      due to hypertension I12.Ø
    fibrocystic (congenital) Q61.8
    hypertensive — *see* Hypertension, kidney
    lupus M32.14
    phosphate-losing (tubular) N25.Ø
    polycystic (congenital) Q61.3
      adult type Q61.2
      childhood type NEC Q61.19
        collecting duct dilatation Q61.11
    rapidly progressive NØ1.9
    subacute NØ1.9
  Rendu-Osler-Weber (familial hemorrhagic telangiectasia) I78.Ø
  renovascular (arteriosclerotic) — *see* Hypertension, kidney
  respiratory (tract) J98.9
    acute or subacute NOS JØ6.9
      due to
        chemicals, gases, fumes or vapors (inhalation) J68.3
        external agent J7Ø.9
          specified NEC J7Ø.8
        radiation J7Ø.Ø
        smoke inhalation J7Ø.5
      noninfectious J39.8
    chronic NOS J98.9
      due to
        chemicals, gases, fumes or vapors J68.4
        external agent J7Ø.9
          specified NEC J7Ø.8
        radiation J7Ø.1
      newborn P27.9
        specified NEC P27.8
    due to
      chemicals, gases, fumes or vapors J68.9
        acute or subacute NEC J68.3
        chronic J68.4
      external agent J7Ø.9
        specified NEC J7Ø.8
    newborn P28.9
      specified type NEC P28.89
    upper J39.9
      acute or subacute JØ6.9
      noninfectious NEC J39.8
      specified NEC J39.8
      streptococcal JØ6.9
  retina, retinal H35.9
    Batten's or Batten-Mayou E75.4 *[H36]*
    specified NEC H35.89
  rheumatoid — *see* Arthritis, rheumatoid
  rickettsial NOS A79.9
    specified type NEC A79.89
  Riga (-Fede) (cachectic aphthae) K14.Ø
  Riggs' (compound periodontitis) — *see* Periodontitis
  Ritter's LØØ
  Rivalta's (cervicofacial actinomycosis) A42.2
  Robles' (onchocerciasis) B73.Ø1
  rod body G71.21
  Roger's (congenital interventricular septal defect) Q21.Ø
  Rosenthal's (factor XI deficiency) D68.1
  Ross River B33.1
  Rossbach's (hyperchlorhydria) K31.89
    psychogenic F45.8
  Rotes Quérol — *see* Hyperostosis, ankylosing
  Roth (-Bernhardt) — *see* Mononeuropathy, lower limb, meralgia paresthetica
  Runeberg's (progressive pernicious anemia) D51.Ø
  sacroiliac NEC M53.3

Disease, diseased — *continued*
  salivary gland or duct K11.9
    inclusion B25.9
    specified NEC K11.8
    virus B25.9
  sandworm B76.9
  Schimmelbusch's — *see* Mastopathy, cystic
  Schmorl's — *see* Schmorl's disease or nodes
  Schönlein (-Henoch) (purpura rheumatica) D69.Ø
  Schottmüller's — *see* Fever, paratyphoid
  Schultz's (agranulocytosis) — *see* Agranulocytosis
  Schwalbe-Ziehen-Oppenheim G24.1
  Schwartz-Jampel G71.13
  sclera H15.9
    specified NEC H15.89
  scrofulous (tuberculous) A18.2
  scrotum N5Ø.9
  sebaceous glands L73.9
  semilunar cartilage, cystic — *see also* Derangement, knee, meniscus, cystic
  seminal vesicle N5Ø.9
  serum NEC — *see also* Reaction, serum T8Ø.69 ☑
  sexually transmitted A64
    anogenital
      herpesviral infection — *see* Herpes, anogenital warts A63.Ø
    chancroid A57
    chlamydial infection — *see* Chlamydia
    gonorrhea — *see* Gonorrhea
    granuloma inguinale A58
    specified organism NEC A63.8
    syphilis — *see* Syphilis
    trichomoniasis — *see* Trichomoniasis
  Sézary C84.1- ☑
  shimamushi (scrub typhus) A75.3
  shipyard B3Ø.Ø
  sickle-cell D57.1
    with
      acute chest syndrome D57.Ø1
      cerebral vascular involvement D57.Ø3
      crisis (painful) D57.ØØ
        with complication specified NEC D57.Ø9
      splenic sequestration D57.Ø2
      vasoocclusive pain D57.ØØ
    elliptocytosis D57.8- ☑
    Hb-C D57.2Ø
      with
        acute chest syndrome D57.211
        cerebral vascular involvement D57.213
        crisis D57.219
          with specified complication NEC D57.218
        splenic sequestration D57.212
        vasoocclusive pain D57.219
      without crisis D57.2Ø
    Hb-SD D57.8Ø
      with
        acute chest syndrome D57.811
        cerebral vascular involvement D57.813
        crisis D57.819
          with complication specified NEC D57.818
        splenic sequestration D57.812
        vasoocclusive pain D57.819
      without crisis D57.8Ø
    Hb-SE D57.8Ø
      with
        acute chest syndrome D57.811
        cerebral vascular involvement D57.813
        crisis D57.819
          with complication specified NEC D57.818
        splenic sequestration D57.812
        vasoocclusive pain D57.819
      without crisis D57.8Ø
    specified NEC D57.8Ø
      with
        acute chest syndrome D57.811
        cerebral vascular involvement D57.813
        crisis D57.819
          with complication specified NEC D57.818
        splenic sequestration D57.812
        vasoocclusive pain D57.819
      without crisis D57.8Ø
    spherocytosis D57.8Ø
      with
        acute chest syndrome D57.811
        cerebral vascular involvement D57.813
        crisis D57.819
          with complication specified NEC D57.818
        splenic sequestration D57.812

- **Disorder** — *continued*
  - bone — *continued*
    - density and structure — *continued*
      - specified type — *continued*
        - skull M85.88
        - thigh M85.85- ☑
        - upper arm M85.82- ☑
        - vertebra M85.88
    - development and growth NEC M89.2Ø
      - carpus M89.24- ☑
      - clavicle M89.21- ☑
      - femur M89.25- ☑
      - fibula M89.26- ☑
      - finger M89.24- ☑
      - humerus M89.22- ☑
      - ilium M89.259
      - ischium M89.259
      - metacarpus M89.24- ☑
      - metatarsus M89.27- ☑
      - multiple sites M89.29
      - neck M89.28
      - radius M89.23- ☑
      - rib M89.28
      - scapula M89.21- ☑
      - skull M89.28
      - tarsus M89.27- ☑
      - tibia M89.26- ☑
      - toe M89.27- ☑
      - ulna M89.23- ☑
      - vertebra M89.28
    - specified type NEC M89.8X- ☑
  - brachial plexus G54.Ø
  - branched-chain amino-acid metabolism E71.2
    - specified NEC E71.19
  - breast N64.9
    - agalactia — *see* Agalactia
    - associated with
      - lactation O92.7Ø
        - specified NEC O92.79
      - pregnancy O92.2Ø
        - specified NEC O92.29
      - puerperium O92.2Ø
        - specified NEC O92.29
    - cracked nipple — *see* Cracked nipple
    - galactorrhea — *see* Galactorrhea
    - hypogalactia O92.4
    - lactation disorder NEC O92.79
    - mastitis — *see* Mastitis
    - nipple infection — *see* Infection, nipple
    - retracted nipple — *see* Retraction, nipple
    - specified type NEC N64.89
  - Briquet's F45.Ø
  - bullous, in diseases classified elsewhere L14
  - caffeine use
    - mild
      - with
        - caffeine-induced
          - anxiety disorder F15.18Ø
          - sleep disorder F15.182
    - moderate or severe
      - with
        - caffeine-induced
          - anxiety disorder F15.28Ø
          - sleep disorder F15.282
  - cannabis use
    - mild F12.1Ø
      - with
        - cannabis intoxication delirium F12.121
          - with perceptual disturbances F12.122
          - without perceptual disturbances F12.129
        - cannabis-induced
          - anxiety disorder F12.18Ø
          - psychotic disorder F12.159
          - sleep disorder F12.188
      - in remission (early) (sustained) F12.11
    - moderate or severe F12.2Ø
      - with
        - cannabis intoxication
          - with perceptual disturbances F12.222
          - without perceptual disturbances F12.229
        - cannabis-induced
          - anxiety disorder F12.28Ø
          - psychotic disorder F12.259
          - sleep disorder F12.288
        - delirium F12.221
      - in remission (early) (sustained) F12.21
  - carbohydrate
    - absorption, intestinal NEC E74.39

- **Disorder** — *continued*
  - carbohydrate — *continued*
    - metabolism (congenital) E74.9
      - specified NEC E74.89
  - cardiac, functional I51.89
  - carnitine metabolism E71.4Ø
  - cartilage M94.9
    - articular NEC — *see* Derangement, joint, articular cartilage
    - chondrocalcinosis — *see* Chondrocalcinosis
    - specified type NEC M94.8X- ☑
      - articular — *see* Derangement, joint, articular cartilage
      - multiple sites M94.8XØ
  - catatonia (due to known physiological condition) (with another mental disorder) FØ6.1
  - catatonic
    - due to (secondary to) known physiological condition FØ6.1
    - organic FØ6.1
  - central auditory processing H93.25
  - cervical
    - region NEC M53.82
    - root (nerve) NEC G54.2
  - character NOS F6Ø.9
  - childhood disintegrative NEC F84.3
  - cholesterol and bile acid metabolism E78.7Ø
    - Barth syndrome E78.71
    - other specified E78.79
    - Smith-Lemli-Opitz syndrome E78.72
  - choroid H31.9
    - atrophy — *see* Atrophy, choroid
    - degeneration — *see* Degeneration, choroid
    - detachment — *see* Detachment, choroid
    - dystrophy — *see* Dystrophy, choroid
    - hemorrhage — *see* Hemorrhage, choroid
    - rupture — *see* Rupture, choroid
    - scar — *see* Scar, chorioretinal
    - solar retinopathy — *see* Retinopathy, solar
    - specified type NEC H31.8
  - ciliary body — *see* Disorder, iris
    - degeneration — *see* Degeneration, ciliary body
  - coagulation (factor) — *see also* Defect, coagulation D68.9
    - newborn, transient P61.6
  - cocaine use
    - mild F14.1Ø
      - with
        - amphetamine, cocaine, or other stimulant intoxication
          - with perceptual disturbances F14.122
          - without perceptual disturbances F14.129
        - cocaine intoxication delirium F14.121
        - cocaine-induced
          - anxiety disorder F14.18Ø
          - bipolar and related disorder F14.14
          - depressive disorder F14.14
          - obsessive-compulsive and related disorder F14.188
          - psychotic disorder F14.159
          - sexual dysfunction F14.181
          - sleep disorder F14.182
      - in remission (early) (sustained) F14.11
    - moderate or severe F14.2Ø
      - with
        - amphetamine, cocaine, or other stimulant intoxication
          - with perceptual disturbances F14.222
          - without perceptual disturbances F14.229
        - cocaine intoxication delirium F14.221
        - cocaine-induced
          - anxiety disorder F14.28Ø
          - bipolar and related disorder F14.24
          - depressive disorder F14.24
          - obsessive-compulsive and related disorder F14.288
          - psychotic disorder F14.259
          - sexual dysfunction F14.281
          - sleep disorder F14.282
      - in remission (early) (sustained) F14.21
  - coccyx NEC M53.3
  - cognitive FØ9
    - due to (secondary to) general medical condition FØ9
    - persisting R41.89
      - due to
        - alcohol F1Ø.97
          - with dependence F1Ø.27
        - anxiolytics F13.97

- **Disorder** — *continued*
  - cognitive — *continued*
    - persisting — *continued*
      - due to — *continued*
        - anxiolytics — *continued*
          - with dependence F13.27
        - hypnotics F13.97
          - with dependence F13.27
        - sedatives F13.97
          - with dependence F13.27
        - specified substance NEC F19.97
          - with
            - abuse F19.17
            - dependence F19.27
  - communication F8Ø.9
    - social pragmatic F8Ø.82
  - conduct (childhood) F91.9
    - adjustment reaction — *see* Disorder, adjustment
    - adolescent onset type F91.2
    - childhood onset type F91.1
    - compulsive F63.9
    - confined to family context F91.Ø
    - depressive F91.8
    - group type F91.2
    - hyperkinetic — *see* Disorder, attention-deficit hyperactivity
    - oppositional defiance F91.3
    - socialized F91.2
    - solitary aggressive type F91.1
    - specified NEC F91.8
    - unsocialized (aggressive) F91.1
  - conduction, heart I45.9
  - congenital glycosylation (CDG) E74.89
  - conjunctiva H11.9
    - infection — *see* Conjunctivitis
  - connective tissue, localized L94.9
    - specified NEC L94.8
  - conversion (functional neurological symptom disorder)
    - with
      - abnormal movement F44.4
      - anesthesia or sensory loss F44.6
      - attacks or seizures F44.5
      - mixed symptoms F44.7
      - special sensory symptoms F44.6
      - speech symptoms F44.4
      - swallowing symptoms F44.4
      - weakness or paralysis F44.4
  - convulsive (secondary) — *see* Convulsions
  - cornea H18.9
    - deformity — *see* Deformity, cornea
    - degeneration — *see* Degeneration, cornea
    - deposits — *see* Deposit, cornea
    - due to contact lens H18.82- ☑
      - specified as edema — *see* Edema, cornea
    - edema — *see* Edema, cornea
    - keratitis — *see* Keratitis
    - keratoconjunctivitis — *see* Keratoconjunctivitis
    - membrane change — *see* Change, corneal membrane
    - neovascularization — *see* Neovascularization, cornea
    - scar — *see* Opacity, cornea
    - specified type NEC H18.89- ☑
    - ulcer — *see* Ulcer, cornea
  - corpus cavernosum N48.9
  - cranial nerve — *see* Disorder, nerve, cranial
  - Cyclin-Dependent Kinase-Like 5 Deficiency (CDKL5) G4Ø.42
  - cyclothymic F34.Ø
  - defiant oppositional F91.3
  - delusional (persistent) (systematized) F22
    - induced F24
  - depersonalization F48.1
  - depressive F32.A
    - due to known physiological condition
      - with
        - depressive features FØ6.31
        - major depressive-like episode FØ6.32
        - mixed features FØ6.34
    - major F32.9
      - with psychotic symptoms F32.3
      - in remission (full) F32.5
        - partial F32.4
      - recurrent F33.9
        - with psychotic features F33.3
      - single episode F32.9
        - mild F32.Ø
        - moderate F32.1

Disorder — *continued*
- depressive — *continued*
  - major — *continued*
    - single episode — *continued*
      - severe (without psychotic symptoms) F32.2
        - with psychotic symptoms F32.3
  - organic FØ6.31
  - persistent F34.1
  - recurrent F33.9
    - current episode
      - mild F33.Ø
      - moderate F33.1
      - severe (without psychotic symptoms) F33.2
        - with psychotic symptoms F33.3
    - in remission F33.4Ø
      - full F33.42
      - partial F33.41
    - specified NEC F33.8
  - single episode — *see* Episode, depressive
  - specified NEC F32.89
- developmental F89
  - arithmetical skills F81.2
  - coordination (motor) F82
  - expressive writing F81.81
  - language F8Ø.9
    - expressive F8Ø.1
    - mixed receptive and expressive F8Ø.2
    - receptive type F8Ø.2
    - specified NEC F8Ø.89
  - learning F81.9
    - arithmetical F81.2
    - reading F81.Ø
  - mixed F88
  - motor coordination or function F82
  - pervasive F84.9
    - specified NEC F84.8
  - phonological F8Ø.Ø
  - reading F81.Ø
  - scholastic skills — *see also* Disorder, learning
    - mixed F81.89
  - specified NEC F88
  - speech F8Ø.9
    - articulation F8Ø.Ø
    - specified NEC F8Ø.89
  - written expression F81.81
- diaphragm J98.6
- digestive (system) K92.9
  - newborn P78.9
    - specified NEC P78.89
  - postprocedural — *see* Complication, gastrointestinal
  - psychogenic F45.8
- disc (intervertebral) M51.9
  - with
    - myelopathy
      - cervical region M5Ø.ØØ
      - cervicothoracic region M5Ø.Ø3
      - high cervical region M5Ø.Ø1
      - lumbar region M51.Ø6
      - mid-cervical region M5Ø.Ø2Ø
      - sacrococcygeal region M53.3
      - thoracic region M51.Ø4
      - thoracolumbar region M51.Ø5
    - radiculopathy
      - cervical region M5Ø.1Ø
      - cervicothoracic region M5Ø.13
      - high cervical region M5Ø.11
      - lumbar region M51.16
      - lumbosacral region M51.17
      - mid-cervical region M5Ø.12Ø
      - sacrococcygeal region M53.3
      - thoracic region M51.14
      - thoracolumbar region M51.15
  - cervical M5Ø.9Ø
    - with
      - myelopathy M5Ø.ØØ
        - C2-C3 M5Ø.Ø1
        - C3-C4 M5Ø.Ø1
        - C4-C5 M5Ø.Ø21
        - C5-C6 M5Ø.Ø22
        - C6-C7 M5Ø.Ø23
        - C7-T1 M5Ø.Ø3
        - cervicothoracic region M5Ø.Ø3
        - high cervical region M5Ø.Ø1
        - mid-cervical region M5Ø.Ø2Ø
      - neuritis, radiculitis or radiculopathy M5Ø.1Ø
        - C2-C3 M5Ø.11
        - C3-C4 M5Ø.11
        - C4-C5 M5Ø.121
        - C5-C6 M5Ø.122

Disorder — *continued*
- disc — *continued*
  - cervical — *continued*
    - with — *continued*
      - neuritis, radiculitis or radiculopathy — *continued*
        - C6-C7 M5Ø.123
        - C7-T1 M5Ø.13
        - cervicothoracic region M5Ø.13
        - high cervical region M5Ø.11
        - mid-cervical region M5Ø.12Ø
    - C2-C3 M5Ø.91
    - C3-C4 M5Ø.91
    - C4-C5 M5Ø.921
    - C5-C6 M5Ø.922
    - C6-C7 M5Ø.923
    - C7-T1 M5Ø.93
    - cervicothoracic region M5Ø.93
    - degeneration M5Ø.3Ø
      - C2-C3 M5Ø.31
      - C3-C4 M5Ø.31
      - C4-C5 M5Ø.321
      - C5-C6 M5Ø.322
      - C6-C7 M5Ø.323
      - C7-T1 M5Ø.33
      - cervicothoracic region M5Ø.33
      - high cervical region M5Ø.31
      - mid-cervical region M5Ø.32Ø
    - displacement M5Ø.2Ø
      - C2-C3 M5Ø.21
      - C3-C4 M5Ø.21
      - C4-C5 M5Ø.221
      - C5-C6 M5Ø.222
      - C6-C7 M5Ø.223
      - C7-T1 M5Ø.23
      - cervicothoracic region M5Ø.23
      - high cervical region M5Ø.21
      - mid-cervical region M5Ø.22Ø
    - high cervical region M5Ø.91
    - mid-cervical region M5Ø.92Ø
    - specified type NEC M5Ø.8Ø
      - C2-C3 M5Ø.81
      - C3-C4 M5Ø.81
      - C4-C5 M5Ø.821
      - C5-C6 M5Ø.822
      - C6-C7 M5Ø.823
      - C7-T1 M5Ø.83
      - cervicothoracic region M5Ø.83
      - high cervical region M5Ø.81
      - mid-cervical region M5Ø.82Ø
  - specified NEC
    - lumbar region M51.86
    - lumbosacral region M51.87
    - sacrococcygeal region M53.3
    - thoracic region M51.84
    - thoracolumbar region M51.85
- disinhibited attachment (childhood) F94.2
- disintegrative, childhood NEC F84.3
- disruptive F91.9
  - mood dysregulation F34.81
  - specified NEC F91.8
- disruptive behavior — *see* Disorder, conduct
- dissocial personality F6Ø.2
- dissociative F44.9
  - affecting
    - motor function F44.4
      - and sensation F44.7
    - sensation F44.6
      - and motor function F44.7
  - brief reactive F43.Ø
  - due to (secondary to) general medical condition FØ6.8
  - mixed F44.7
  - organic FØ6.8
  - other specified NEC F44.89
- double heterozygous sickling — *see* Disease, sickle-cell
- dream anxiety F51.5
- drug induced hemorrhagic D68.32
- drug related F19.99
  - abuse — *see* Abuse, drug
  - dependence — *see* Dependence, drug
- dysmorphic body F45.22
- dysthymic F34.1
- ear H93.9- ☑
  - bleeding — *see* Otorrhagia
  - deafness — *see* Deafness
  - degenerative H93.Ø9- ☑
  - discharge — *see* Otorrhea

Disorder — *continued*
- ear — *continued*
  - external H61.9- ☑
    - auditory canal stenosis — *see* Stenosis, external ear canal
    - exostosis — *see* Exostosis, external ear canal
    - impacted cerumen — *see* Impaction, cerumen
    - otitis — *see* Otitis, externa
    - perichondritis — *see* Perichondritis, ear
    - pinna — *see* Disorder, pinna
    - specified type NEC H61.89- ☑
  - inner H83.9- ☑
    - vestibular dysfunction — *see* Disorder, vestibular function
  - middle H74.9- ☑
    - adhesive H74.1- ☑
    - ossicle — *see* Abnormal, ear ossicles
    - polyp — *see* Polyp, ear (middle)
    - specified NEC, in diseases classified elsewhere H75.8- ☑
  - postprocedural — *see* Complications, ear, procedure
  - specified NEC, in diseases classified elsewhere H94.8- ☑
- eating (adult) (psychogenic) F5Ø.9
  - anorexia — *see* Anorexia
  - binge F5Ø.81
  - bulimia F5Ø.2
  - child F98.29
    - pica F98.3
    - rumination disorder F98.21
  - pica F5Ø.89
    - childhood F98.3
- electrolyte (balance) NEC E87.8
  - with
    - abortion — *see* Abortion by type complicated by specified condition NEC
    - ectopic pregnancy OØ8.5
    - molar pregnancy OØ8.5
  - acidosis (lactic) (metabolic) E87.2Ø
    - acute E87.21
    - chronic E87.22
    - respiratory E87.29
    - specified NEC E87.29
  - alkalosis (metabolic) (respiratory) E87.3
- elimination, transepidermal L87.9
  - specified NEC L87.8
- emotional (persistent) F34.9
  - of childhood F93.9
    - specified NEC F93.8
- endocrine E34.9
  - postprocedural E89.89
    - specified NEC E89.89
- erectile (male) (organic) — *see also* Dysfunction, sexual, male, erectile N52.9
  - nonorganic F52.21
- erythematous — *see* Erythema
- esophagus K22.9
  - functional K22.4
  - psychogenic F45.8
- eustachian tube H69.9- ☑
  - infection — *see* Salpingitis, eustachian
  - obstruction — *see* Obstruction, eustachian tube
  - patulous — *see* Patulous, eustachian tube
  - specified NEC H69.8- ☑
- exhibitionistic F65.2
- extrapyramidal G25.9
  - in deseases classified elsewhere — *see* category G26
  - specified type NEC G25.89
- eye H57.9
  - postprocedural — *see* Complication, postprocedural, eye
- eyelid HØ2.9
  - cyst — *see* Cyst, eyelid
  - degenerative HØ2.7Ø
    - chloasma — *see* Chloasma, eyelid
    - madarosis — *see* Madarosis
    - specified type NEC HØ2.79
    - vitiligo — *see* Vitiligo, eyelid
    - xanthelasma — *see* Xanthelasma
  - dermatochalasis — *see* Dermatochalasis
  - edema — *see* Edema, eyelid
  - elephantiasis — *see* Elephantiasis, eyelid
  - foreign body, retained — *see* Foreign body, retained, eyelid
  - function HØ2.59

- **Disorder** — *continued*
  - temperature regulation, newborn — *continued*
    - specified NEC P81.8
  - temporomandibular joint M26.6Ø- ☑
  - tendon M67.9Ø
    - acromioclavicular M67.91- ☑
    - ankle M67.97- ☑
    - contracture — *see* Contracture, tendon
    - elbow M67.92- ☑
    - foot M67.97- ☑
    - forearm M67.93- ☑
    - hand M67.94- ☑
    - hip M67.95- ☑
    - knee M67.96- ☑
    - multiple sites M67.99
    - rupture — *see* Rupture, tendon
    - shoulder M67.91- ☑
    - specified type NEC M67.8Ø
      - acromioclavicular M67.81- ☑
      - ankle M67.87- ☑
      - elbow M67.82- ☑
      - foot M67.87- ☑
      - hand M67.84- ☑
      - hip M67.85- ☑
      - knee M67.86- ☑
      - multiple sites M67.89
      - trunk M67.88
      - wrist M67.83- ☑
    - synovitis — *see* Synovitis
    - tendinitis — *see* Tendinitis
    - tenosynovitis — *see* Tenosynovitis
    - trunk M67.98
    - upper arm M67.92- ☑
    - wrist M67.93- ☑
  - thoracic root (nerve) NEC G54.3
  - thyrocalcitonin hypersecretion EØ7.Ø
  - thyroid (gland) EØ7.9
    - function NEC, neonatal, transitory P72.2
    - iodine-deficiency related EØ1.8
    - specified NEC EØ7.89
  - tic — *see* Tic
  - tobacco use
    - chewing tobacco (mild) (moderate) (severe)
      - in remission (early) (sustained) F17.221
    - cigarettes (mild) (moderate) (severe)
      - in remission (early) (sustained) F17.211
    - mild F17.2ØØ
      - in remission (early) (sustained) F17.2Ø1
    - moderate F17.2ØØ
      - in remission (early) (sustained) F17.2Ø1
    - severe F17.2ØØ
      - in remission (early) (sustained) F17.2Ø1
    - specified product NEC (mild) (moderate) (severe)
      - in remission (early) (sustained) F17.291
  - tooth KØ8.9
    - development KØØ.9
      - specified NEC KØØ.8
    - eruption KØØ.6
  - Tourette's F95.2
  - trance and possession F44.89
  - transvestic F65.1
  - trauma and stressor-related NOS F43.9
    - other specified F43.89
    - unspecified F43.9
  - tricuspid (valve) — *see* Endocarditis, tricuspid
  - tryptophan metabolism E7Ø.5
  - tubular, phosphate-losing N25.Ø
  - tubulo-interstitial (in)
    - brucellosis A23.9 *[N16]*
    - cystinosis E72.Ø4
    - diphtheria A36.84
    - glycogen storage disease E74.ØØ *[N16]*
    - leukemia NEC C95.9- ☑ *[N16]*
    - lymphoma NEC C85.9- ☑ *[N16]*
    - mixed cryoglobulinemia D89.1 *[N16]*
    - multiple myeloma C9Ø.Ø- ☑ *[N16]*
    - Salmonella infection AØ2.25
    - sarcoidosis D86.84
    - sepsis A41.9 *[N16]*
      - streptococcal A4Ø.9 *[N16]*
    - systemic lupus erythematosus M32.15
    - toxoplasmosis B58.83
    - transplant rejection T86.91 *[N16]*
    - Wilson's disease E83.Ø1 *[N16]*
  - tubulo-renal function, impaired N25.9
    - specified NEC N25.89
  - tympanic membrane H73.9- ☑

- **Disorder** — *continued*
  - tympanic membrane — *continued*
    - atrophy — *see* Atrophy, tympanic membrane
    - infection — *see* Myringitis
    - perforation — *see* Perforation, tympanum
    - specified NEC H73.89- ☑
  - unsocialized aggressive F91.1
  - urea cycle metabolism E72.2Ø
    - argininemia E72.21
    - arginosuccinic aciduria E72.22
    - citrullinemia E72.23
    - ornithine transcarbamylase deficiency E72.4
    - other specified E72.29
  - ureter (in) N28.9
    - schistosomiasis B65.Ø *[N29]*
    - tuberculosis A18.11
  - urethra N36.9
    - specified NEC N36.8
  - urinary system N39.9
    - specified NEC N39.8
  - valve, heart
    - aortic — *see* Endocarditis, aortic
    - mitral — *see* Endocarditis, mitral
    - pulmonary — *see* Endocarditis, pulmonary
    - rheumatic
      - aortic — *see* Endocarditis, aortic, rheumatic
      - mitral — *see* Endocarditis, mitral
      - pulmonary — *see* Endocarditis, pulmonary, rheumatic
      - tricuspid — *see* Endocarditis, tricuspid
    - tricuspid — *see* Endocarditis, tricuspid
  - vestibular function H81.9- ☑
    - specified NEC — *see* subcategory H81.8 ☑
      - in diseases classified elsewhere H82.- ☑
    - vertigo — *see* Vertigo
  - vision, binocular H53.3Ø
    - abnormal retinal correspondence H53.31
    - diplopia H53.2
    - fusion with defective stereopsis H53.32
    - simultaneous perception H53.33
    - suppression H53.34
  - visual
    - cortex
      - blindness H47.619
        - left brain H47.612
        - right brain H47.611
      - due to
        - inflammatory disorder H47.629
          - left brain H47.622
          - right brain H47.621
        - neoplasm H47.639
          - left brain H47.632
          - right brain H47.631
        - vascular disorder H47.649
          - left brain H47.642
          - right brain H47.641
    - pathway H47.9
      - due to
        - inflammatory disorder H47.51- ☑
        - neoplasm H47.52- ☑
        - vascular disorder H47.53- ☑
      - optic chiasm — *see* Disorder, optic, chiasm
  - vitreous body H43.9
    - crystalline deposits — *see* Deposit, crystalline
    - degeneration — *see* Degeneration, vitreous
    - hemorrhage — *see* Hemorrhage, vitreous
    - opacities — *see* Opacity, vitreous
    - prolapse — *see* Prolapse, vitreous
    - specified type NEC H43.89
  - voice R49.9
    - specified type NEC R49.8
  - volatile solvent use
    - due to drug abuse — *see* Abuse, drug, inhalant
    - due to drug dependence — *see* Dependence, drug, inhalant
  - voyeuristic F65.3
  - white blood cells D72.9
    - specified NEC D72.89
  - withdrawing, child or adolescent F4Ø.1Ø
- **Disorientation** R41.Ø
- **Displacement, displaced**
  - acquired traumatic of bone, cartilage, joint, tendon NEC — *see* Dislocation
  - adrenal gland (congenital) Q89.1
  - appendix, retrocecal (congenital) Q43.8
  - auricle (congenital) Q17.4
  - bladder (acquired) N32.89
    - congenital Q64.19

- **Displacement, displaced** — *continued*
  - brachial plexus (congenital) QØ7.8
  - brain stem, caudal (congenital) QØ4.8
  - canaliculus (lacrimalis), congenital Q1Ø.6
  - cardia through esophageal hiatus (congenital) Q4Ø.1
  - cerebellum, caudal (congenital) QØ4.8
  - cervix — *see* Malposition, uterus
  - colon (congenital) Q43.3
  - device, implant or graft — *see also* Complications, by site and type, mechanical T85.628 ☑
    - arterial graft NEC — *see* Complication, cardiovascular device, mechanical, vascular
    - breast (implant) T85.42 ☑
    - catheter NEC T85.628 ☑
      - dialysis (renal) T82.42 ☑
        - intraperitoneal T85.621 ☑
      - infusion NEC T82.524 ☑
        - spinal (epidural) (subdural) T85.62Ø ☑
      - urinary
        - cystostomy T83.Ø2Ø ☑
        - Hopkins T83.Ø28 ☑
        - ileostomy T83.Ø28 ☑
        - indwelling T83.Ø21 ☑
        - nephrostomy T83.Ø22 ☑
        - specified NEC T83.Ø28 ☑
        - urostomy T83.Ø28 ☑
    - electronic (electrode) (pulse generator) (stimulator) — *see* Complication, electronic stimulator
    - fixation, internal (orthopedic) NEC — *see* Complication, fixation device, mechanical
    - gastrointestinal — *see* Complications, prosthetic device, mechanical, gastrointestinal device
    - genital NEC T83.428 ☑
      - intrauterine contraceptive device (string) T83.32 ☑
      - penile prosthesis (cylinder) (implanted) (pump) (reservoir) T83.42Ø ☑
      - testicular prosthesis T83.421 ☑
    - heart NEC — *see* Complication, cardiovascular device, mechanical
    - joint prosthesis — *see* Complications, joint prosthesis, mechanical
    - ocular — *see* Complications, prosthetic device, mechanical, ocular device
    - orthopedic NEC — *see* Complication, orthopedic, device or graft, mechanical
    - specified NEC T85.628 ☑
    - urinary NEC T83.128 ☑
      - graft T83.22 ☑
      - sphincter, implanted T83.121 ☑
      - stent (ileal conduit) (nephroureteral) T83.123 ☑
        - ureteral indwelling T83.122 ☑
    - vascular NEC — *see* Complication, cardiovascular device, mechanical
    - ventricular intracranial shunt T85.Ø2 ☑
  - electronic stimulator
    - bone T84.32Ø ☑
    - cardiac — *see* Complications, cardiac device, electronic
    - nervous system — *see* Complication, prosthetic device, mechanical, electronic nervous system stimulator
    - urinary — *see* Complications, electronic stimulator, urinary
  - esophageal mucosa into cardia of stomach, congenital Q39.8
  - esophagus (acquired) K22.89
    - congenital Q39.8
  - eyeball (acquired) (lateral) (old) — *see* Displacement, globe
    - congenital Q15.8
    - current — *see* Avulsion, eye
  - fallopian tube (acquired) N83.4- ☑
    - congenital Q5Ø.6
    - opening (congenital) Q5Ø.6
  - gallbladder (congenital) Q44.1
  - gastric mucosa (congenital) Q4Ø.2
  - globe (acquired) (old) (lateral) HØ5.21- ☑
    - current — *see* Avulsion, eye
  - heart (congenital) Q24.8
    - acquired I51.89
  - hymen (upward) (congenital) Q52.4
  - intervertebral disc NEC
    - with myelopathy — *see* Disorder, disc, with, myelopathy
    - cervical, cervicothoracic (with) M5Ø.2Ø

- **Displacement, displaced** — *continued*
  - intervertebral disc — *continued*
    - cervical, cervicothoracic — *continued*
      - myelopathy — *see* Disorder, disc, cervical, with myelopathy
      - neuritis, radiculitis or radiculopathy — *see* Disorder, disc, cervical, with neuritis
    - due to trauma — *see* Dislocation, vertebra
    - lumbar region M51.26
      - with
        - myelopathy M51.Ø6
        - neuritis, radiculitis, radiculopathy or sciatica M51.16
    - lumbosacral region M51.27
      - with
        - neuritis, radiculitis, radiculopathy or sciatica M51.17
    - sacrococcygeal region M53.3
    - thoracic region M51.24
      - with
        - myelopathy M51.Ø4
        - neuritis, radiculitis, radiculopathy M51.14
    - thoracolumbar region M51.25
      - with
        - myelopathy M51.Ø5
        - neuritis, radiculitis, radiculopathy M51.15
  - intrauterine device (string) T83.32 ☑
  - kidney (acquired) N28.83
    - congenital Q63.2
  - lachrymal, lacrimal apparatus or duct (congenital) Q1Ø.6
  - lens, congenital Q12.1
  - macula (congenital) Q14.1
  - Meckel's diverticulum Q43.Ø
    - malignant — *see* Table of Neoplasms, small intestine, malignant
  - nail (congenital) Q84.6
    - acquired L6Ø.8
  - opening of Wharton's duct in mouth Q38.4
  - organ or site, congenital NEC — *see* Malposition, congenital
  - ovary (acquired) N83.4- ☑
    - congenital Q5Ø.39
    - free in peritoneal cavity (congenital) Q5Ø.39
    - into hernial sac N83.4- ☑
  - oviduct (acquired) N83.4- ☑
    - congenital Q5Ø.6
  - parathyroid (gland) E21.4
  - parotid gland (congenital) Q38.4
  - punctum lacrimale (congenital) Q1Ø.6
  - sacro-iliac (joint) (congenital) Q74.2
    - current injury S33.2 ☑
    - old — *see* subcategory M53.2 ☑
  - salivary gland (any) (congenital) Q38.4
  - spleen (congenital) Q89.Ø9
  - stomach, congenital Q4Ø.2
  - sublingual duct Q38.4
  - tongue (downward) (congenital) Q38.3
  - tooth, teeth, fully erupted M26.3Ø
    - horizontal M26.33
    - vertical M26.34
  - trachea (congenital) Q32.1
  - ureter or ureteric opening or orifice (congenital) Q62.62
  - uterine opening of oviducts or fallopian tubes Q5Ø.6
  - uterus, uterine — *see* Malposition, uterus
  - ventricular septum Q21.Ø
    - with rudimentary ventricle Q2Ø.4
- **Disproportion**
  - between native and reconstructed breast N65.1
  - fiber-type G71.2Ø
    - congenital G71.29
- **Disruptio uteri** — *see* Rupture, uterus
- **Disruption** (of)
  - ciliary body NEC H21.89
  - closure of
    - cornea T81.31 ☑
    - craniotomy T81.32 ☑
    - fascia (muscular) (superficial) T81.32 ☑
    - internal organ or tissue T81.32 ☑
    - laceration (external) (internal) T81.33 ☑
    - ligament T81.32 ☑
    - mucosa T81.31 ☑
    - muscle or muscle flap T81.32 ☑
    - ribs or rib cage T81.32 ☑
    - skin and subcutaneous tissue (full-thickness) (superficial) T81.31 ☑
    - skull T81.32 ☑
    - sternum (sternotomy) T81.32 ☑
    - tendon T81.32 ☑
- **Disruption** — *continued*
  - closure of — *continued*
    - traumatic laceration (external) (internal) T81.33 ☑
  - family Z63.8
    - due to
      - absence of family member due to military deployment Z63.31
      - absence of family member NEC Z63.32
      - alcoholism and drug addiction in family Z63.72
      - bereavement Z63.4
      - death (assumed) or disappearance of family member Z63.4
      - divorce or separation Z63.5
      - drug addiction in family Z63.72
      - return of family member from military deployment (current or past conflict) Z63.71
      - stressful life events NEC Z63.79
  - iris NEC H21.89
  - ligament(s) — *see also* Sprain
    - knee
      - current injury — *see* Dislocation, knee
      - old (chronic) — *see* Derangement, knee, instability
      - spontaneous NEC — *see* Derangement, knee, disruption ligament
  - ossicular chain — *see* Discontinuity, ossicles, ear
  - pelvic ring (stable) S32.81Ø ☑
    - unstable S32.811 ☑
  - traumatic injury wound repair T81.33 ☑
  - wound T81.3Ø ☑
    - episiotomy O9Ø.1
    - operation T81.31 ☑
      - cesarean O9Ø.Ø
      - external operation wound (superficial) T81.31 ☑
      - internal operation wound (deep) T81.32 ☑
    - perineal (obstetric) O9Ø.1
    - traumatic injury repair T81.33 ☑
- **Dissatisfaction with**
  - employment Z56.9
  - school environment Z55.4
- **Dissecting** — *see* condition
- **Dissection**
  - aorta I71.ØØ
    - abdominal I71.Ø2
    - thoracic I71.Ø19
      - aortic arch I71.Ø11
      - ascending aorta I71.Ø1Ø
      - descending thoracic aorta I71.Ø12
    - thoracoabdominal I71.Ø3
  - artery I77.7Ø
    - basilar (trunk) I77.75
    - carotid I77.71
    - cerebral (nonruptured) I67.Ø
      - ruptured — *see* Hemorrhage, intracranial, subarachnoid
    - coronary I25.42
    - extremity
      - lower I77.77
      - upper I77.76
    - iliac I77.72
    - precerebral
      - congenital (nonruptured) Q28.1
      - specified site NEC I77.75
    - renal I77.73
    - specified NEC I77.79
    - vertebral I77.74
  - precerebral artery, congenital (nonruptured) Q28.1
  - Heartland A93.8
  - traumatic — *see* Wound, open, by site
  - vascular I99.8
  - wound — *see* Wound, open
- **Disseminated** — *see* condition
- **Dissociation**
  - auriculoventricular or atrioventricular (AV) (any degree) (isorhythmic) I45.89
    - with heart block I44.2
  - interference I45.89
- **Dissociative reaction, state** F44.9
- **Dissolution, vertebra** — *see* Osteoporosis
- **Distension, distention**
  - abdomen R14.Ø
  - bladder N32.89
  - cecum K63.89
  - colon K63.89
  - gallbladder K82.8
  - intestine K63.89
  - kidney N28.89
  - liver K76.89
- **Distension, distention** — *continued*
  - seminal vesicle N5Ø.89
  - stomach K31.89
    - acute K31.Ø
    - psychogenic F45.8
  - ureter — *see* Dilatation, ureter
  - uterus N85.8
- **Distoma hepaticum infestation** B66.3
- **Distomiasis** B66.9
  - bile passages B66.3
  - hemic B65.9
  - hepatic B66.3
    - due to Clonorchis sinensis B66.1
  - intestinal B66.5
  - liver B66.3
    - due to Clonorchis sinensis B66.1
  - lung B66.4
  - pulmonary B66.4
- **Distomolar** (fourth molar) KØØ.1
- **Disto-occlusion** (Division I) (Division II) M26.212
- **Distortion**(s) (congenital)
  - adrenal (gland) Q89.1
  - arm NEC Q68.8
  - bile duct or passage Q44.5
  - bladder Q64.79
  - brain QØ4.9
  - cervix (uteri) Q51.9
  - chest (wall) Q67.8
    - bones Q76.8
  - clavicle Q74.Ø
  - clitoris Q52.6
  - coccyx Q76.49
  - common duct Q44.5
  - coronary Q24.5
  - cystic duct Q44.5
  - ear (auricle) (external) Q17.3
    - inner Q16.5
    - middle Q16.4
      - ossicles Q16.3
  - endocrine NEC Q89.2
  - eustachian tube Q17.8
  - eye (adnexa) Q15.8
  - face bone(s) NEC Q75.8
  - fallopian tube Q5Ø.6
  - femur NEC Q68.8
  - fibula NEC Q68.8
  - finger(s) Q68.1
  - foot Q66.9- ☑
  - genitalia, genital organ(s)
    - female Q52.8
      - external Q52.79
      - internal NEC Q52.8
  - gyri QØ4.8
  - hand bone(s) Q68.1
  - heart (auricle) (ventricle) Q24.8
    - valve (cusp) Q24.8
  - hepatic duct Q44.5
  - humerus NEC Q68.8
  - hymen Q52.4
  - intrafamilial communications Z63.8
  - jaw NEC M26.89
  - labium (majus) (minus) Q52.79
  - leg NEC Q68.8
  - lens Q12.8
  - liver Q44.7
  - lumbar spine Q76.49
    - with disproportion O33.8
      - causing obstructed labor O65.Ø
  - lumbosacral (joint) (region) Q76.49
    - kyphosis — *see* Kyphosis, congenital
    - lordosis — *see* Lordosis, congenital
  - nerve QØ7.8
  - nose Q3Ø.8
  - organ
    - of Corti Q16.5
    - or site not listed — *see* Anomaly, by site
  - ossicles, ear Q16.3
  - oviduct Q5Ø.6
  - pancreas Q45.3
  - parathyroid (gland) Q89.2
  - pituitary (gland) Q89.2
  - radius NEC Q68.8
  - sacroiliac joint Q74.2
  - sacrum Q76.49
  - scapula Q74.Ø
  - shoulder girdle Q74.Ø
  - skull bone(s) NEC Q75.8

- **Disturbance(s)** — *continued*
  - sensation — *continued*
    - smell — *continued*
      - parosmia R43.1
      - specified NEC R43.8
    - taste R43.9
      - and smell (mixed) R43.8
      - parageusia R43.2
      - specified NEC R43.8
  - sensory — *see* Disturbance, sensation
  - situational (transient) — *see also* Disorder, adjustment
    - acute F43.0
  - sleep G47.9
    - nonorganic origin F51.9
  - smell — *see* Disturbance, sensation, smell
  - sociopathic F60.2
  - sodium balance, newborn
    - hypernatremia P74.21
    - hyponatremia P74.22
  - speech R47.9
    - developmental F80.9
    - specified NEC R47.89
  - stomach (functional) K31.9
  - sympathetic (nerve) G90.9
  - taste — *see* Disturbance, sensation, taste
  - temperature
    - regulation, newborn P81.9
      - specified NEC P81.8
    - sense R20.8
      - hysterical F44.6
  - tooth
    - eruption K00.6
    - formation K00.4
    - structure, hereditary NEC K00.5
  - touch — *see* Disturbance, sensation
  - vascular I99.9
    - arteriosclerotic — *see* Arteriosclerosis
  - vasomotor I73.9
  - vasospastic I73.9
  - vision, visual H53.9
    - following
      - cerebral infarction I69.398
      - cerebrovascular disease I69.998
        - specified NEC I69.898
      - intracerebral hemorrhage I69.198
      - nontraumatic intracranial hemorrhage NEC I69.298
      - specified disease NEC I69.898
      - subarachnoid hemorrhage I69.098
    - psychophysical H53.16
    - specified NEC H53.8
    - subjective H53.10
      - day blindness H53.11
      - discomfort H53.14- ☑
      - distortions of shape and size H53.15
      - loss
        - sudden H53.13- ☑
        - transient H53.12- ☑
      - specified type NEC H53.19
  - voice R49.9
    - psychogenic F44.4
    - specified NEC R49.8
- **Diuresis** R35.89
- **Diver's palsy, paralysis or squeeze** T70.3 ☑
- **Diverticulitis** (acute) K57.92
  - bladder — *see* Cystitis
  - ileum — *see* Diverticulitis, intestine, small
  - intestine K57.92
    - with
      - abscess, perforation K57.80
        - with bleeding K57.81
      - bleeding K57.93
    - congenital Q43.8
    - large K57.32
      - with
        - abscess, perforation K57.20
          - with bleeding K57.21
        - bleeding K57.33
        - small intestine K57.52
          - with
            - abscess, perforation K57.40
              - with bleeding K57.41
            - bleeding K57.53
    - small K57.12
      - with
        - abscess, perforation K57.00
          - with bleeding K57.01
        - bleeding K57.13
- **Diverticulitis** — *continued*
  - intestine — *continued*
    - small — *continued*
      - with — *continued*
        - large intestine K57.52
          - with
            - abscess, perforation K57.40
              - with bleeding K57.41
            - bleeding K57.53
- **Diverticulosis** K57.90
  - with bleeding K57.91
  - large intestine K57.30
    - with
      - bleeding K57.31
      - small intestine K57.50
        - with bleeding K57.51
  - small intestine K57.10
    - with
      - bleeding K57.11
      - large intestine K57.50
        - with bleeding K57.51
- **Diverticulum, diverticula** (multiple) K57.90
  - appendix (noninflammatory) K38.2
  - bladder (sphincter) N32.3
    - congenital Q64.6
  - bronchus (congenital) Q32.4
    - acquired J98.09
  - calyx, calyceal (kidney) N28.89
  - cardia (stomach) K31.4
  - cecum — *see* Diverticulosis, intestine, large
    - congenital Q43.8
  - colon — *see* Diverticulosis, intestine, large
    - congenital Q43.8
  - duodenum — *see* Diverticulosis, intestine, small
    - congenital Q43.8
  - epiphrenic (esophagus) K22.5
  - esophagus (congenital) Q39.6
    - acquired (epiphrenic) (pulsion) (traction) K22.5
  - eustachian tube — *see* Disorder, eustachian tube, specified NEC
  - fallopian tube N83.8
  - gastric K31.4
  - heart (congenital) Q24.8
  - ileum — *see* Diverticulosis, intestine, small
  - jejunum — *see* Diverticulosis, intestine, small
  - kidney (pelvis) (calyces) N28.89
    - with calculus — *see* Calculus, kidney
  - Meckel's (displaced) (hypertrophic) Q43.0
    - malignant — *see* Table of Neoplasms, small intestine, malignant
  - midthoracic K22.5
  - organ or site, congenital NEC — *see* Distortion
  - pericardium (congenital) (cyst) Q24.8
    - acquired I31.8
  - pharyngoesophageal (congenital) Q39.6
    - acquired K22.5
  - pharynx (congenital) Q38.7
  - rectosigmoid — *see* Diverticulosis, intestine, large
    - congenital Q43.8
  - rectum — *see* Diverticulosis, intestine, large
  - Rokitansky's K22.5
  - seminal vesicle N50.89
  - sigmoid — *see* Diverticulosis, intestine, large
    - congenital Q43.8
  - stomach (acquired) K31.4
    - congenital Q40.2
  - trachea (acquired) J39.8
  - ureter (acquired) N28.89
    - congenital Q62.8
  - ureterovesical orifice N28.89
  - urethra (acquired) N36.1
    - congenital Q64.79
  - ventricle, left (congenital) Q24.8
  - vesical N32.3
    - congenital Q64.6
  - Zenker's (esophagus) K22.5
- **Division**
  - cervix uteri (acquired) N88.8
  - glans penis Q55.69
  - labia minora (congenital) Q52.79
  - ligament (partial or complete) (current) — *see also* Sprain
    - with open wound — *see* Wound, open
  - muscle (partial or complete) (current) — *see also* Injury, muscle
    - with open wound — *see* Wound, open
  - nerve (traumatic) — *see* Injury, nerve
  - spinal cord — *see* Injury, spinal cord, by region
- **Division** — *continued*
  - vein I87.8
- **Divorce, causing family disruption** Z63.5
- **Dix-Hallpike neurolabyrinthitis** — *see* Neuronitis, vestibular
- **Dizziness** R42
  - hysterical F44.89
  - psychogenic F45.8
- **DMAC** (disseminated mycobacterium avium- intracellulare complex) A31.2
- **DNR** (do not resuscitate) Z66
- **Doan-Wiseman syndrome** (primary splenic neutropenia) — *see* Agranulocytosis
- **Doehle-Heller aortitis** A52.02
- **Dog bite** — *see* Bite
- **Dohle body panmyelopathic syndrome** D72.0
- **Dolichocephaly** Q67.2
- **Dolichocolon** Q43.8
- **Dolichostenomelia** — *see* Syndrome, Marfan's
- **Donohue's syndrome** E34.8
- **Donor** (organ or tissue) Z52.9
  - blood (whole) Z52.000
    - autologous Z52.010
    - specified component (lymphocytes) (platelets) NEC Z52.008
      - autologous Z52.018
      - specified donor NEC Z52.098
    - specified donor NEC Z52.090
    - stem cells Z52.001
      - autologous Z52.011
      - specified donor NEC Z52.091
  - bone Z52.20
    - autologous Z52.21
    - marrow Z52.3
    - specified type NEC Z52.29
  - cornea Z52.5
  - egg (Oocyte) Z52.819
    - age 35 and over Z52.812
      - anonymous recipient Z52.812
      - designated recipient Z52.813
    - under age 35 Z52.810
      - anonymous recipient Z52.810
      - designated recipient Z52.811
  - kidney Z52.4
  - liver Z52.6
  - lung Z52.89
  - lymphocyte — *see* Donor, blood, specified components NEC
  - Oocyte — *see* Donor, egg
  - platelets Z52.008
  - potential, examination of Z00.5
  - semen Z52.89
  - skin Z52.10
    - autologous Z52.11
    - specified type NEC Z52.19
  - specified organ or tissue NEC Z52.89
  - sperm Z52.89
- **Donovanosis** A58
- **Dorsalgia** M54.9
  - psychogenic F45.41
  - specified NEC M54.89
- **Dorsopathy** M53.9
  - deforming M43.9
    - specified NEC — *see* subcategory M43.8 ☑
  - specified NEC M53.80
    - cervical region M53.82
    - cervicothoracic region M53.83
    - lumbar region M53.86
    - lumbosacral region M53.87
    - occipito-atlanto-axial region M53.81
    - sacrococcygeal region M53.88
    - thoracic region M53.84
    - thoracolumbar region M53.85
- **Double**
  - albumin E88.09
  - aortic arch Q25.45
  - auditory canal Q17.8
  - auricle (heart) Q20.8
  - bladder Q64.79
  - cervix Q51.820
    - with doubling of uterus (and vagina) Q51.10
      - with obstruction Q51.11
  - inlet ventricle Q20.4
  - kidney with double pelvis (renal) Q63.0
  - meatus urinarius Q64.75
  - monster Q89.4
  - outlet
    - left ventricle Q20.2

- **Double** — *continued*
  - outlet — *continued*
    - right ventricle Q2Ø.1
  - pelvis (renal) with double ureter Q62.5
  - tongue Q38.3
  - ureter (one or both sides) Q62.5
    - with double pelvis (renal) Q62.5
  - urethra Q64.74
  - urinary meatus Q64.75
  - uterus Q51.28
    - with
      - doubling of cervix (and vagina) Q51.1Ø
        - with obstruction Q51.11
    - complete Q51.21
    - in pregnancy or childbirth O34.Ø- ☑
      - causing obstructed labor O65.5
    - partial Q51.22
    - specified NEC Q51.28
  - vagina Q52.1Ø
    - with doubling of uterus (and cervix) Q51.1Ø
      - with obstruction Q51.11
  - vision H53.2
  - vulva Q52.79
- **Doubled up** Z59.Ø1
- **Douglas' pouch, cul-de-sac** — *see* condition
- **Down syndrome** Q9Ø.9
  - meiotic nondisjunction Q9Ø.Ø
  - mitotic nondisjunction Q9Ø.1
  - mosaicism Q9Ø.1
  - translocation Q9Ø.2
- **DPD** (dihydropyrimidine dehydrogenase deficiency) E88.89
- **Dracontiasis** B72
- **Dracunculiasis, dracunculosis** B72
- **Dream state, hysterical** F44.89
- **Drepanocytic anemia** — *see* Disease, sickle-cell
- **Dresbach's syndrome** (elliptocytosis) D58.1
- **Dreschlera** (hawaiiensis) (infection) B43.8
- **Dressler's syndrome** I24.1
- **Drift, ulnar** — *see* Deformity, limb, specified type NEC, forearm
- **Drinking** (alcohol)
  - excessive, to excess NEC (without dependence) F1Ø.1Ø
    - habitual (continual) (without remission) F1Ø.2Ø
      - with remission F1Ø.21
- **Drip, postnasal** (chronic) RØ9.82
  - due to
    - allergic rhinitis — *see* Rhinitis, allergic
    - common cold JØØ
    - gastroesophageal reflux — *see* Reflux, gastroesophageal
    - nasopharyngitis — *see* Nasopharyngitis
    - other known condition — *code to* condition
    - sinusitis — *see* Sinusitis
- **Droop**
  - facial R29.81Ø
    - cerebrovascular disease I69.992
      - cerebral infarction I69.392
      - intracerebral hemorrhage I69.192
      - nontraumatic intracranial hemorrhage NEC I69.292
      - specified disease NEC I69.892
      - subarachnoid hemorrhage I69.Ø92
- **Drop** (in)
  - attack NEC R55
  - finger — *see* Deformity, finger
  - foot — *see* Deformity, limb, foot, drop
  - hematocrit (precipitous) R71.Ø
  - hemoglobin R71.Ø
  - toe — *see* Deformity, toe, specified NEC
  - wrist — *see* Deformity, limb, wrist drop
- **Dropped heart beats** I45.9
- **Dropsy, dropsical** — *see also* Hydrops
  - abdomen R18.8
  - brain — *see* Hydrocephalus
  - cardiac, heart — *see* Failure, heart, congestive
  - gangrenous — *see* Gangrene
  - heart — *see* Failure, heart, congestive
  - kidney — *see* Nephrosis
  - lung — *see* Edema, lung
  - newborn due to isoimmunization P56.Ø
  - pericardium — *see* Pericarditis
- **Drowned, drowning** (near) T75.1 ☑
- **Drowsiness** R4Ø.Ø
- **Drug**
  - abuse counseling and surveillance Z71.51
  - addiction — *see* Dependence
- **Drug** — *continued*
  - dependence — *see* Dependence
  - habit — *see* Dependence
  - harmful use — *see* Abuse, drug
  - induced fever R5Ø.2
  - overdose — *see* Table of Drugs and Chemicals, by drug, poisoning
  - poisoning — *see* Table of Drugs and Chemicals, by drug, poisoning
  - resistant organism infection — *see also* Resistant, organism, to, drug Z16.3Ø
  - therapy
    - long term (current) (prophylactic) — *see* Therapy, drug long-term (current) (prophylactic)
    - short term — *omit code*
  - wrong substance given or taken in error — *see* Table of Drugs and Chemicals, by drug, poisoning
- **Drunkenness** (without dependence) F1Ø.129
  - acute in alcoholism F1Ø.229
  - chronic (without remission) F1Ø.2Ø
    - with remission F1Ø.21
  - pathological (without dependence) F1Ø.129
    - with dependence F1Ø.229
  - sleep F51.9
- **Drusen**
  - macula (degenerative) (retina) — *see* Degeneration, macula, drusen
  - optic disc H47.32- ☑
- **Dry, dryness** — *see also* condition
  - larynx J38.7
  - mouth R68.2
    - due to dehydration E86.Ø
  - nose J34.89
  - socket (teeth) M27.3
  - throat J39.2
- **DSAP** L56.5
- **Duane's syndrome** H5Ø.81- ☑
- **Dubin-Johnson disease or syndrome** E8Ø.6
- **Dubois' disease** (thymus gland) A5Ø.59 *[E35]*
- **Dubowitz' syndrome** Q87.19
- **Duchenne-Aran muscular atrophy** G12.21
- **Duchenne-Griesinger disease** G71.Ø1
- **Duchenne's**
  - disease or syndrome
    - motor neuron disease G12.22
    - muscular dystrophy G71.Ø1
  - locomotor ataxia (syphilitic) A52.11
  - paralysis
    - birth injury P14.Ø
    - due to or associated with
      - motor neuron disease G12.22
      - muscular dystrophy G71.Ø1
- **Ducrey's chancre** A57
- **Duct, ductus** — *see* condition
- **Duhring's disease** (dermatitis herpetiformis) L13.Ø
- **Dullness, cardiac** (decreased) (increased) RØ1.2
- **Dumb ague** — *see* Malaria
- **Dumbness** — *see* Aphasia
- **Dumdum fever** B55.Ø
- **Dumping syndrome** (postgastrectomy) K91.1
- **Duodenitis** (nonspecific) (peptic) K29.8Ø
  - with bleeding K29.81
- **Duodenocholangitis** — *see* Cholangitis
- **Duodenum, duodenal** — *see* condition
- **Duplay's bursitis or periarthritis** M75.Ø ☑
- **Duplication, duplex** — *see also* Accessory
  - alimentary tract Q45.8
  - anus Q43.4
  - appendix (and cecum) Q43.4
  - biliary duct (any) Q44.5
  - bladder Q64.79
  - cecum (and appendix) Q43.4
  - cervix Q51.82Ø
  - chromosome NEC
    - with complex rearrangements NEC Q92.5
    - seen only at prometaphase Q92.8
  - cystic duct Q44.5
  - digestive organs Q45.8
  - esophagus Q39.8
  - frontonasal process Q75.8
  - intestine (large) (small) Q43.4
  - kidney Q63.Ø
  - liver Q44.7
  - pancreas Q45.3
  - penis Q55.69
  - respiratory organs NEC Q34.8
  - salivary duct Q38.4
  - spinal cord (incomplete) QØ6.2
- **Duplication, duplex** — *continued*
  - stomach Q4Ø.2
- **Dupré's disease** (meningism) R29.1
- **Dupuytren's contraction or disease** M72.Ø
- **Durand-Nicolas-Favre disease** A55
- **Durotomy** (inadvertent) (incidental) G97.41
- **Duroziez's disease** (congenital mitral stenosis) Q23.2
- **Dutton's relapsing fever** (West African) A68.1
- **Dwarfism** — *see also* Stature, short E34.328
  - achondroplastic Q77.4
  - congenital — *see also* Stature, short E34.328
  - constitutional E34.31
  - hypochondroplastic Q77.4
  - hypophyseal E23.Ø
  - infantile — *see also* Stature, short E34.328
  - Laron-type — *see also* Stature, short E34.321
  - Lorain (-Levi) type E23.Ø
  - metatropic Q77.8
  - nephrotic-glycosuric (with hypophosphatemic rickets) E72.Ø9
  - nutritional E45
  - pancreatic K86.89
  - pituitary E23.Ø
  - renal N25.Ø
  - thanatophoric Q77.1
- **Dyke-Young anemia** (secondary) (symptomatic) D59.19
- **Dysacusis** — *see* Abnormal, auditory perception
- **Dysadrenocortism** E27.9
  - hyperfunction E27.Ø
- **Dysarthria** R47.1
  - following
    - cerebral infarction I69.322
    - cerebrovascular disease I69.922
      - specified disease NEC I69.822
    - intracerebral hemorrhage I69.122
    - nontraumatic intracranial hemorrhage NEC I69.222
    - subarachnoid hemorrhage I69.Ø22
- **Dysautonomia** (familial) G9Ø.1
- **Dysbarism** T7Ø.3 ☑
- **Dysbasia** R26.2
  - angiosclerotica intermittens I73.9
  - hysterical F44.4
  - lordotica (progressiva) G24.1
  - nonorganic origin F44.4
  - psychogenic F44.4
- **Dysbetalipoproteinemia** (familial) E78.2
- **Dyscalculia** R48.8
  - developmental F81.2
- **Dyschezia** K59.ØØ
- **Dyschondroplasia** (with hemangiomata) Q78.4
- **Dyschromia** (skin) L81.9
- **Dyscollagenosis** M35.9
- **Dyscranio-pygo-phalangy** Q87.Ø
- **Dyscrasia**
  - blood (with) D75.9
    - antepartum hemorrhage — *see* Hemorrhage, antepartum, with coagulation defect
    - intrapartum hemorrhage O67.Ø
    - newborn P61.9
      - specified type NEC P61.8
    - puerperal, postpartum O72.3
  - polyglandular, pluriglandular E31.9
- **Dysendocrinism** E34.9
- **Dysentery, dysenteric** (catarrhal) (diarrhea) (epidemic) (hemorrhagic) (infectious) (sporadic) (tropical) AØ9
  - abscess, liver AØ6.4
  - amebic — *see also* Amebiasis AØ6.Ø
    - with abscess — *see* Abscess, amebic
    - acute AØ6.Ø
    - chronic AØ6.1
  - arthritis — *see also* category MØ1 AØ9
    - bacillary (*see also* category MØ1) AØ3.9
  - bacillary AØ3.9
    - arthritis — *see also* category MØ1 AØ3.9
    - Boyd AØ3.2
    - Flexner AØ3.1
    - Schmitz (-Stutzer) AØ3.Ø
    - Shiga (-Kruse) AØ3.Ø
    - Shigella AØ3.9
      - boydii AØ3.2
      - dysenteriae AØ3.Ø
      - flexneri AØ3.1
      - group A AØ3.Ø
      - group B AØ3.1
      - group C AØ3.2
      - group D AØ3.3
      - sonnei AØ3.3
    - specified type NEC AØ3.8

Dysfunction — *continued*
- temporomandibular (joint) M26.69
  - joint-pain syndrome M26.62- ☑
- testicular (endocrine) E29.9
  - specified NEC E29.8
- thymus E32.9
- thyroid EØ7.9
- ureterostomy (stoma) — *see* Complications, stoma, urinary tract
- urethrostomy (stoma) — *see* Complications, stoma, urinary tract
- uterus, complicating delivery O62.9
  - hypertonic O62.4
  - hypotonic O62.2
    - primary O62.Ø
    - secondary O62.1
- ventricular I51.9
  - with congestive heart failure — *see also* Failure, heart I5Ø.9
  - left, reversible, following sudden emotional stress I51.81

Dysgenesis
- gonadal (due to chromosomal anomaly) Q96.9
  - pure Q99.1
- renal Q6Ø.5
  - bilateral Q6Ø.4
  - unilateral Q6Ø.3
- reticular D72.Ø
- tidal platelet D69.3

Dysgerminoma
- specified site — *see* Neoplasm, malignant, by site
- unspecified site
  - female C56.9
  - male C62.9Ø

Dysgeusia R43.2

Dysgraphia R27.8

Dyshidrosis, dysidrosis L3Ø.1

Dyskaryotic cervical smear R87.619

Dyskeratosis L85.8
- cervix — *see* Dysplasia, cervix
- congenital Q82.8
- uterus NEC N85.8

Dyskinesia G24.9
- biliary (cystic duct or gallbladder) K82.8
- drug induced
  - orofacial G24.Ø1
- esophagus K22.4
- hysterical F44.4
- intestinal K59.89
- nonorganic origin F44.4
- orofacial (idiopathic) G24.4
  - drug induced G24.Ø1
- psychogenic F44.4
- subacute, drug induced G24.Ø1
- tardive G24.Ø1
  - neuroleptic induced G24.Ø1
- trachea J39.8
- tracheobronchial J98.Ø9

Dyslalia (developmental) F8Ø.Ø

Dyslexia R48.Ø
- developmental F81.Ø

Dyslipidemia E78.5
- depressed HDL cholesterol E78.6
- elevated fasting triglycerides E78.1

Dysmaturity — *see also* Light for dates
- pulmonary (newborn) (Wilson-Mikity) P27.Ø

Dysmenorrhea (essential) (exfoliative) N94.6
- congestive (syndrome) N94.6
- primary N94.4
- psychogenic F45.8
- secondary N94.5

Dysmetabolic syndrome X E88.81

Dysmetria R27.8

Dysmorphism (due to)
- alcohol Q86.Ø
- exogenous cause NEC Q86.8
- hydantoin Q86.1
- warfarin Q86.2

Dysmorphophobia (nondelusional) F45.22
- delusional F22

Dysnomia R47.Ø1

Dysorexia R63.Ø
- psychogenic F5Ø.89

Dysostosis
- cleidocranial, cleidocranialis Q74.Ø
- craniofacial Q75.1
- Fairbank's (idiopathic familial generalized osteophytosis) Q78.9

Dysostosis — *continued*
- mandibulofacial (incomplete) Q75.4
- multiplex E76.Ø1
- oculomandibular Q75.5

Dyspareunia (female) N94.1Ø
- deep N94.12
- male N53.12
- nonorganic F52.6
- psychogenic F52.6
- secondary N94.19
- specified NEC N94.19
- superficial (introital) N94.11

Dyspepsia R1Ø.13
- atonic K3Ø
- functional (allergic) (congenital) (gastrointestinal) (occupational) (reflex) K3Ø
- intestinal K59.89
- nervous F45.8
- neurotic F45.8
- psychogenic F45.8

Dysphagia R13.1Ø
- cervical R13.19
- following
  - cerebral infarction I69.391
  - cerebrovascular disease I69.991
    - specified NEC I69.891
  - intracerebral hemorrhage I69.191
  - nontraumatic intracranial hemorrhage NEC I69.291
  - specified disease NEC I69.891
  - subarachnoid hemorrhage I69.Ø91
- functional (hysterical) F45.8
- hysterical F45.8
- nervous (hysterical) F45.8
- neurogenic R13.19
- oral phase R13.11
- oropharyngeal phase R13.12
- pharyngeal phase R13.13
- pharyngoesophageal phase R13.14
- psychogenic F45.8
- sideropenic D5Ø.1
- spastica K22.4
- specified NEC R13.19

Dysphagocytosis, congenital D71

Dysphasia R47.Ø2
- developmental
  - expressive type F8Ø.1
  - receptive type F8Ø.2
- following
  - cerebrovascular disease I69.921
    - cerebral infarction I69.321
    - intracerebral hemorrhage I69.121
    - nontraumatic intracranial hemorrhage NEC I69.221
    - specified disease NEC I69.821
    - subarachnoid hemorrhage I69.Ø21

Dysphonia R49.Ø
- functional F44.4
- hysterical F44.4
- psychogenic F44.4
- spastica J38.3

Dysphoria
- gender F64.9
  - in
    - adolescence and adulthood F64.Ø
    - children F64.2
  - specified NEC F64.8
- postpartal O9Ø.6

Dyspituitarism E23.3

Dysplasia — *see also* Anomaly
- acetabular, congenital Q65.89
- alveolar capillary, with vein misalignment J84.843
- anus (histologically confirmed) (mild) (moderate) K62.82
  - severe DØ1.3
- arrhythmogenic right ventricular I42.8
- arterial, fibromuscular I77.3
- asphyxiating thoracic (congenital) Q77.2
- brain QØ7.9
- bronchopulmonary, perinatal P27.1
- cervix (uteri) N87.9
  - mild N87.Ø
  - moderate N87.1
  - severe DØ6.9
- chondroectodermal Q77.6
- colon D12.6
- craniometaphyseal Q78.8
- dentinal KØØ.5
- diaphyseal, progressive Q78.3

Dysplasia — *continued*
- dystrophic Q77.5
- ectodermal (anhidrotic) (congenital) (hereditary) Q82.4
  - hydrotic Q82.8
- epithelial, uterine cervix — *see* Dysplasia, cervix
- eye (congenital) Q11.2
- fibrous
  - bone NEC (monostotic) M85.ØØ
    - ankle M85.Ø7- ☑
    - foot M85.Ø7- ☑
    - forearm M85.Ø3- ☑
    - hand M85.Ø4- ☑
    - lower leg M85.Ø6- ☑
    - multiple site M85.Ø9
    - neck M85.Ø8
    - rib M85.Ø8
    - shoulder M85.Ø1- ☑
    - skull M85.Ø8
    - specified site NEC M85.Ø8
    - thigh M85.Ø5- ☑
    - toe M85.Ø7- ☑
    - upper arm M85.Ø2- ☑
    - vertebra M85.Ø8
  - diaphyseal, progressive Q78.3
  - jaw M27.8
  - polyostotic Q78.1
- florid osseous — *see also* Cyst, calcifying odontogenic
- high grade, focal D12.6
- hip, congenital Q65.89
- joint, congenital Q74.8
- kidney Q61.4
  - multicystic Q61.4
- leg Q74.2
- lung, congenital (not associated with short gestation) Q33.6
- mammary (gland) (benign) N6Ø.9- ☑
  - cyst (solitary) — *see* Cyst, breast
  - cystic — *see* Mastopathy, cystic
  - duct ectasia — *see* Ectasia, mammary duct
  - fibroadenosis — *see* Fibroadenosis, breast
  - fibrosclerosis — *see* Fibrosclerosis, breast
  - specified type NEC N6Ø.8- ☑
- metaphyseal Q78.5
- muscle Q79.8
- oculodentodigital Q87.Ø
- periapical (cemental) (cemento-osseous) — *see* Cyst, calcifying odontogenic
- periosteum — *see* Disorder, bone, specified type NEC
- polyostotic fibrous Q78.1
- prostate — *see also* Neoplasia, intraepithelial, prostate N42.3Ø
  - severe DØ7.5
  - specified NEC N42.39
- renal Q61.4
  - multicystic Q61.4
- retinal, congenital Q14.1
- right ventricular, arrhythmogenic I42.8
- septo-optic QØ4.4
- skin L98.8
- spinal cord QØ6.1
- spondyloepiphyseal Q77.7
- thymic, with immunodeficiency D82.1
- vagina N89.3
  - mild N89.Ø
  - moderate N89.1
  - severe NEC DØ7.2
- vulva N9Ø.3
  - mild N9Ø.Ø
  - moderate N9Ø.1
  - severe NEC DØ7.1

Dysplasminogenemia E88.Ø2

Dyspnea (nocturnal) (paroxysmal) RØ6.ØØ
- asthmatic (bronchial) J45.9Ø9
  - with
    - bronchitis J45.9Ø9
      - with
        - exacerbation (acute) J45.9Ø1
        - status asthmaticus J45.9Ø2
      - chronic J44.9
    - exacerbation (acute) J45.9Ø1
    - status asthmaticus J45.9Ø2
  - cardiac — *see* Failure, ventricular, left
- cardiac — *see* Failure, ventricular, left
- functional F45.8
- hyperventilation RØ6.4
- hysterical F45.8
- newborn P28.89
- orthopnea RØ6.Ø1

Dyspnea — *continued*
- psychogenic F45.8
- shortness of breath R06.02
- specified type NEC R06.09
- transfusion-associated [TAD] J95.87

Dyspraxia R27.8
- developmental (syndrome) F82

Dysproteinemia E88.09

Dysreflexia, autonomic G90.4

Dysrhythmia
- cardiac I49.9
  - newborn
    - bradycardia P29.12
    - occurring before birth P03.819
      - before onset of labor P03.810
      - during labor P03.811
    - tachycardia P29.11
  - postoperative I97.89
- cerebral or cortical — *see* Epilepsy

Dyssomnia — *see* Disorder, sleep

Dyssynergia
- biliary K83.8
- bladder sphincter N36.44
- cerebellaris myoclonica (Hunt's ataxia) G11.19

Dysthymia F34.1

Dysthyroidism E07.9

Dystocia O66.9
- affecting newborn P03.1
- cervical (hypotonic) O62.2
  - affecting newborn P03.6
  - primary O62.0
  - secondary O62.1
- contraction ring O62.4
- fetal O66.9
  - abnormality NEC O66.3
  - conjoined twins O66.3
  - oversize O66.2
- maternal O66.9
- positional O64.9 ☑
- shoulder (girdle) O66.0
  - causing obstructed labor O66.0
- uterine NEC O62.4

Dystonia G24.9
- cervical G24.3
- deformans progressiva G24.1
- drug induced NEC G24.09
  - acute G24.02
  - specified NEC G24.09
- familial G24.1
- idiopathic G24.1
  - familial G24.1
  - nonfamilial G24.2
  - orofacial G24.4
- lenticularis G24.8
- musculorum deformans G24.1
- neuroleptic induced (acute) G24.02
- orofacial (idiopathic) G24.4
- oromandibular G24.4
  - due to drug G24.01
- specified NEC G24.8
- torsion (familial) (idiopathic) G24.1
  - acquired G24.8
  - genetic G24.1
  - symptomatic (nonfamilial) G24.2

Dystonic movements R25.8

Dystrophy, dystrophia
- adiposogenital E23.6
- autosomal recessive, childhood type, muscular dystrophy resembling Duchenne or Becker G71.01
- Becker's type G71.01
- cervical sympathetic G90.2
- choroid (hereditary) H31.20
  - central areolar H31.22
  - choroideremia H31.21
  - gyrate atrophy H31.23
  - specified type NEC H31.29
- cornea (hereditary) H18.50- ☑
  - endothelial H18.51- ☑
  - epithelial H18.52- ☑
  - granular H18.53- ☑
  - lattice H18.54- ☑
  - macular H18.55- ☑
  - specified type NEC H18.59- ☑
- Duchenne's type G71.01
- due to malnutrition E45
- Erb's G71.02
- Fuchs' H18.51- ☑
- Gower's muscular G71.01

Dystrophy, dystrophia — *continued*
- hair L67.8
- infantile neuraxonal G31.89
- Landouzy-Déjérine G71.02
- Leyden-Möbius — *see also* Dystrophy, muscular, limb-girdle, by type G71.039
  - meaning Limb girdle muscular dystrophy NOS G71.039
  - meaning Limb girdle muscular dystrophy, other specified type — *see* by type
  - meaning Limb girdle muscular dystrophy, specified type NEC G71.038
  - meaning Limb girdle muscular dystrophy type 2A (autosomal recessive) G71.032
- muscular G71.00
  - autosomal recessive, childhood type, muscular dystrophy resembling Duchenne or Becker G71.01
  - benign (Becker type) G71.01
    - scapuloperoneal with early contractures [Emery-Dreifuss] G71.09
  - congenital (hereditary) (progressive) (with specific morphological abnormalities of the muscle fiber) G71.09
    - myotonic G71.11
  - distal G71.09
  - Duchenne type G71.01
  - Emery-Dreifuss G71.09
  - Erb type G71.02
  - facioscapulohumeral G71.02
  - Gower's G71.01
  - hereditary (progressive) — *see also* Dystrophy, muscular, by type G71.09
  - Landouzy-Déjérine type G71.02
  - limb-girdle G71.039
    - alpha-sarcoglycan-relate G71.0341
    - anoctamin-5-related autosomal recessive (R12) G71.035
    - autosomal recessive NEC G71.038
    - beta-sarcoglycan-related G71.0342
    - calpain-3-related G71.032
      - autosomal dominant G71.031
      - autosomal recessive G71.032
    - collagen VI related
      - autosomal dominant G71.031
      - autosomal recessive G71.038
    - D1 (autosomal dominant) G71.031
    - D2 (autosomal dominant) G71.031
    - D3 (autosomal dominant) G71.031
    - D4 (autosomal dominant) G71.031
    - D5 (autosomal dominant) G71.031
    - delta-sarcoglycan-related G71.0349
    - due to
      - alpha sarcoglycan dysfunction G71.0341
      - anoctamin-5 dysfunction G71.035
      - beta sarcoglycan dysfunction G71.0342
      - fukutin related protein dysfunction G71.038
      - sarcoglycan dysfunction, specified NEC G71.0349
    - FKRP-related autosomal recessive G71.038
    - gamma-sarcoglycan-related G71.0349
    - R1 (autosomal recessive) G71.032
    - R2 (autosomal recessive) G71.033
    - R3 (autosomal recessive) G71.0341
    - R4 (autosomal recessive) G71.0342
    - R5 (autosomal recessive) G71.0349
    - R6 (autosomal recessive) G71.0349
    - R7 (autosomal recessive) G71.038
    - R8 (autosomal recessive) G71.038
    - R9 (autosomal recessive) G71.038
    - R10 (autosomal recessive) G71.038
    - R11 (autosomal recessive) G71.038
    - R12 (autosomal recessive) G71.035
    - R13 (autosomal recessive) G71.038
    - R14 (autosomal recessive) G71.038
    - R15 (autosomal recessive) G71.038
    - R16 (autosomal recessive) G71.038
    - R17 (autosomal recessive) G71.038
    - R18 (autosomal recessive) G71.038
    - R19 (autosomal recessive) G71.038
    - R20 (autosomal recessive) G71.038
    - R21 (autosomal recessive) G71.038
    - R22 (autosomal recessive) G71.038
    - R23 (autosomal recessive) G71.038
    - R24 (autosomal recessive) G71.038
    - type 1 (autosomal dominant) G71.031
    - type 1A (autosomal dominant) G71.031
    - type 1B (autosomal dominant) G71.031
    - type 1C (autosomal dominant) G71.031

Dystrophy, dystrophia — *continued*
- muscular — *continued*
  - limb-girdle — *continued*
    - type 1E (autosomal dominant) G71.031
    - type 1H (autosomal dominant) G71.031
    - type 1I (autosomal dominant) G71.031
    - type 2 (autosomal recessive) G71.038
      - specified NEC G71.038
    - type 2A (autosomal recessive) G71.032
    - type 2B (autosomal recessive) G71.033
    - type 2C (autosomal recessive) G71.0349
    - type 2D (autosomal recessive) G71.0341
    - type 2E (autosomal recessive) G71.0342
    - type 2F (autosomal recessive) G71.0349
    - type 2I (autosomal recessive) G71.038
    - type 2L (autosomal recessive) G71.035
  - myotonic G71.11
  - progressive (hereditary) — *see also* Dystrophy, muscular, by type G71.09
    - Charcot-Marie (-Tooth) type G60.0
  - pseudohypertrophic (infantile) G71.01
  - scapulohumeral G71.02
  - scapuloperoneal G71.09
  - severe (Duchenne type) G71.01
  - specified type NEC G71.09
- myocardium, myocardial — *see* Degeneration, myocardial
- nail L60.3
  - congenital Q84.6
- nutritional E45
- ocular G71.09
- oculocerebrorenal E72.03
- oculopharyngeal G71.09
- ovarian N83.8
- polyglandular E31.8
- reflex (neuromuscular) (sympathetic) — *see* Syndrome, pain, complex regional I
- retinal (hereditary) H35.50
  - in
    - lipid storage disorders E75.6 *[H36]*
    - systemic lipidoses E75.6 *[H36]*
  - involving
    - pigment epithelium H35.54
    - sensory area H35.53
  - pigmentary H35.52
  - vitreoretinal H35.51
- Salzmann's nodular — *see* Degeneration, cornea, nodular
- scapuloperoneal G71.09
- skin NEC L98.8
- sympathetic (reflex) — *see* Syndrome, pain, complex regional I
  - cervical G90.2
- tapetoretinal H35.54
- thoracic, asphyxiating Q77.2
- unguium L60.3
  - congenital Q84.6
- vitreoretinal H35.51
- vulva N90.4
- yellow (liver) — *see* Failure, hepatic

Dysuria R30.0
- psychogenic F45.8

E

Eales' disease H35.06- ☑

Ear — *see also* condition
- piercing Z41.3
- tropical NEC B36.9 *[H62.40]*
  - in
    - aspergillosis B44.89
    - candidiasis B37.84
    - moniliasis B37.84
- wax (impacted) H61.20
  - left H61.22
    - with right H61.23
  - right H61.21
    - with left H61.23

Earache — *see* subcategory H92.0 ☑

Early satiety R68.81

Eaton-Lambert syndrome — *see* Syndrome, Lambert-Eaton

Eberth's disease (typhoid fever) A01.00

Ebola virus disease A98.4

Ebstein's anomaly or syndrome (heart) Q22.5

Eccentro-osteochondrodysplasia E76.29

Ecchondroma — *see* Neoplasm, bone, benign

Ecchondrosis D48.0

Edema, edematous — *continued*
- lung — *continued*
  - chronic J81.1
    - due to
      - chemicals, gases, fumes or vapors (inhalation) J68.1
      - external agent J7Ø.9
        - specified NEC J7Ø.8
      - radiation J7Ø.1
  - due to
    - chemicals, fumes or vapors (inhalation) J68.1
    - external agent J7Ø.9
      - specified NEC J7Ø.8
    - high altitude T7Ø.29 ☑
    - near drowning T75.1 ☑
    - radiation J7Ø.Ø
  - meaning failure, left ventricle I5Ø.1
- lymphatic I89.Ø
  - due to mastectomy I97.2
- macula H35.81
  - cystoid, following cataract surgery — *see* Complications, postprocedural, following cataract surgery
  - diabetic — *see* Diabetes, by type, with, retinopathy, with macular edema
- malignant — *see* Gangrene, gas
- Milroy's Q82.Ø
- nasopharynx J39.2
- newborn P83.3Ø
  - hydrops fetalis — *see* Hydrops, fetalis
  - specified NEC P83.39
- nutritional — *see also* Malnutrition, severe
  - with dyspigmentation, skin and hair E4Ø
- optic disc or nerve — *see* Papilledema
- orbit HØ5.22- ☑
- pancreas K86.89
- papilla, optic — *see* Papilledema
- penis N48.89
- periodic T78.3 ☑
  - hereditary D84.1
- pharynx J39.2
- pulmonary — *see* Edema, lung
- Quincke's T78.3 ☑
  - hereditary D84.1
- renal — *see* Nephrosis
- retina H35.81
  - diabetic — *see* Diabetes, by type, with, retinopathy, with macular edema
- salt E87.Ø
- scrotum N5Ø.89
- seminal vesicle N5Ø.89
- spermatic cord N5Ø.89
- spinal (cord) (vascular) (nontraumatic) G95.19
- starvation — *see* Malnutrition, severe
- stasis — *see* Hypertension, venous, (chronic)
- subglottic — *see* Edema, glottis
- supraglottic — *see* Edema, glottis
- testis N44.8
- tunica vaginalis N5Ø.89
- vas deferens N5Ø.89
- vulva (acute) N9Ø.89

Edentulism — *see* Absence, teeth, acquired

Edsall's disease T67.2 ☑

Educational handicap Z55.9
- less than a high school diploma Z55.5
- no general equivalence degree (GED) Z55.5
- specified NEC Z55.8

Edward's syndrome — *see* Trisomy, 18

Effect(s) (of) (from) — *see* Effect, adverse NEC

Effect, adverse
- abnormal gravitational (G) forces or states T75.81 ☑
- abuse — *see* Maltreatment
- air pressure T7Ø.9 ☑
  - specified NEC T7Ø.8 ☑
- altitude (high) — *see* Effect, adverse, high altitude
- anesthesia — *see also* Anesthesia T88.59 ☑
  - in labor and delivery O74.9
  - local, toxic
    - in labor and delivery O74.4
    - in pregnancy NEC O29.3- ☑
    - postpartum, puerperal O89.3
  - postpartum, puerperal O89.9
  - specified NEC T88.59 ☑
    - in labor and delivery O74.8
    - postpartum, puerperal O89.8
  - spinal and epidural T88.59 ☑
    - headache T88.59 ☑

Effect, adverse — *continued*
- anesthesia — *see also* Anesthesia — *continued*
  - spinal and epidural — *continued*
    - headache — *continued*
      - in labor and delivery O74.5
      - postpartum, puerperal O89.4
    - specified NEC
      - in labor and delivery O74.6
      - postpartum, puerperal O89.5
- antitoxin — *see* Complications, vaccination
- atmospheric pressure T7Ø.9 ☑
  - due to explosion T7Ø.8 ☑
  - high T7Ø.3 ☑
  - low — *see* Effect, adverse, high altitude
  - specified effect NEC T7Ø.8 ☑
- biological, correct substance properly administered — *see* Effect, adverse, drug
- blood (derivatives) (serum) (transfusion) — *see* Complications, transfusion
- chemical substance — *see* Table of Drugs and Chemicals
- cold (temperature) (weather) T69.9 ☑
  - chilblains T69.1 ☑
  - frostbite — *see* Frostbite
  - specified effect NEC T69.8 ☑
- drugs and medicaments T88.7 ☑
  - specified drug — *see* Table of Drugs and Chemicals, by drug, adverse effect
  - specified effect — *code to* condition
- electric current, electricity (shock) T75.4 ☑
  - burn — *see* Burn
- exertion (excessive) T73.3 ☑
- exposure — *see* Exposure
- external cause NEC T75.89 ☑
- foodstuffs T78.1 ☑
  - allergic reaction — *see* Allergy, food
    - causing anaphylaxis — *see* Shock, anaphylactic, due to food
  - noxious — *see* Poisoning, food, noxious
- gases, fumes, or vapors T59.9- ☑
  - specified agent — *see* Table of Drugs and Chemicals
- glue (airplane) sniffing
  - due to drug abuse — *see* Abuse, drug, inhalant
  - due to drug dependence — *see* Dependence, drug, inhalant
- heat — *see* Heat
- high altitude NEC T7Ø.29 ☑
  - anoxia T7Ø.29 ☑
  - on
    - ears T7Ø.Ø ☑
    - sinuses T7Ø.1 ☑
  - polycythemia D75.1
- high pressure fluids T7Ø.4 ☑
- hot weather — *see* Heat
- hunger T73.Ø ☑
- immersion, foot — *see* Immersion
- immunization — *see* Complications, vaccination
- immunological agents — *see* Complications, vaccination
- infrared (radiation) (rays) NOS T66 ☑
  - dermatitis or eczema L59.8
- infusion — *see* Complications, infusion
- lack of care of infants — *see* Maltreatment, child
- lightning — *see* Lightning
- medical care T88.9 ☑
  - specified NEC T88.8 ☑
- medicinal substance, correct, properly administered — *see* Effect, adverse, drug
- motion T75.3 ☑
- noise, on inner ear — *see* subcategory H83.3 ☑
- overheated places — *see* Heat
- psychosocial, of work environment Z56.5
- radiation (diagnostic) (infrared) (natural source) (therapeutic) (ultraviolet) (X-ray) NOS T66 ☑
  - dermatitis or eczema — *see* Dermatitis, due to, radiation
  - fibrosis of lung J7Ø.1
  - pneumonitis J7Ø.Ø
  - pulmonary manifestations
    - acute J7Ø.Ø
    - chronic J7Ø.1
  - skin L59.9
- radioactive substance NOS
  - dermatitis or eczema — *see* Radiodermatitis
- reduced temperature T69.9 ☑
  - immersion foot or hand — *see* Immersion
  - specified effect NEC T69.8 ☑

Effect, adverse — *continued*
- serum NEC — *see also* Reaction, serum T8Ø.69 ☑
- specified NEC T78.8 ☑
  - external cause NEC T75.89 ☑
- strangulation — *see* Asphyxia, traumatic
- submersion T75.1 ☑
- thirst T73.1 ☑
- toxic — *see* Toxicity
- transfusion — *see* Complications, transfusion
- ultraviolet (radiation) (rays) NOS T66 ☑
  - burn — *see* Burn
  - dermatitis or eczema — *see* Dermatitis, due to, ultraviolet rays
    - acute L56.8
- vaccine (any) — *see* Complications, vaccination
- vibration — *see* Vibration, adverse effects
- water pressure NEC T7Ø.9 ☑
  - specified NEC T7Ø.8 ☑
- weightlessness T75.82 ☑
- whole blood — *see* Complications, transfusion
- work environment Z56.5

Effects, late — *see* Sequelae

Effluvium
- anagen L65.1
- telogen L65.Ø

Effort syndrome (psychogenic) F45.8

Effusion
- amniotic fluid — *see* Pregnancy, complicated by, premature rupture of membranes
- brain (serous) G93.6
- bronchial — *see* Bronchitis
- cerebral G93.6
- cerebrospinal — *see also* Meningitis
  - vessel G93.6
- chest — *see* Effusion, pleura
- chylous, chyliform (pleura) J94.Ø
- intracranial G93.6
- joint M25.4Ø
  - ankle M25.47- ☑
  - elbow M25.42- ☑
  - foot joint M25.47- ☑
  - hand joint M25.44- ☑
  - hip M25.45- ☑
  - knee M25.46- ☑
  - shoulder M25.41- ☑
  - specified joint NEC M25.48
  - wrist M25.43- ☑
- malignant pleural J91.Ø
- meninges — *see* Meningitis
- pericardium, pericardial (noninflammatory) I31.39
  - acute — *see* Pericarditis, acute
  - malignant, in disease classified elsewhere I31.31
  - specified type, NEC I31.39
- peritoneal (chronic) R18.8
- pleura, pleurisy, pleuritic, pleuropericardial J9Ø
  - chylous, chyliform J94.Ø
  - due to systemic lupus erythematosis M32.13
  - in conditions classified elsewhere J91.8
  - influenzal — *see* Influenza, with, respiratory manifestations NEC
  - malignant J91.Ø
  - newborn P28.89
  - tuberculous NEC A15.6
    - primary (progressive) A15.7
- spinal — *see* Meningitis
- thorax, thoracic — *see* Effusion, pleura

Egg shell nails L6Ø.3
- congenital Q84.6

EGPA (eosinophilic granulomatosis with polyangiitis) M3Ø.1

Egyptian splenomegaly B65.1

Ehlers-Danlos syndrome — *see also* Syndrome, Ehlers-Danlos Q79.6Ø

Ehrlichiosis A77.4Ø
- due to
  - E. chafeensis A77.41
  - E. ewingii A77.49
  - E. muris euclairensis A77.49
  - E. sennetsu A79.81
  - specified organism NEC A77.49

Eichstedt's disease B36.Ø

Eisenmenger's
- complex or syndrome I27.83
- defect Q21.8

Ejaculation
- delayed F52.32
- painful N53.12

- **Ejaculation** — *continued*
  - premature F52.4
  - retarded N53.11
  - retrograde N53.14
  - semen, painful N53.12
    - psychogenic F52.6
- **Ekbom's syndrome** (restless legs) G25.81
- **Ekman's syndrome** (brittle bones and blue sclera) Q78.Ø
- **Elastic skin** Q82.8
  - acquired L57.4
- **Elastofibroma** — *see* Neoplasm, connective tissue, benign
- **Elastoma** (juvenile) Q82.8
  - Miescher's L87.2
- **Elastomyofibrosis** I42.4
- **Elastosis**
  - actinic, solar L57.8
  - atrophicans (senile) L57.4
  - perforans serpiginosa L87.2
  - senilis L57.4
- **Elbow** — *see* condition
- **Electric current, electricity, effects** (concussion) (fatal) (nonfatal) (shock) T75.4 ☑
  - burn — *see* Burn
- **Electric feet syndrome** E53.8
- **Electrocution** T75.4 ☑
  - from electroshock gun (taser) T75.4 ☑
- **Electrolyte imbalance** E87.8
  - with
    - abortion — *see* Abortion by type, complicated by, electrolyte imbalance
    - ectopic pregnancy OØ8.5
    - molar pregnancy OØ8.5
- **Elephantiasis** (nonfilarial) I89.Ø
  - arabicum — *see* Infestation, filarial
  - bancroftian B74.Ø
  - congenital (any site) (hereditary) Q82.Ø
  - due to
    - Brugia (malayi) B74.1
      - timori B74.2
    - mastectomy I97.2
    - Wuchereria (bancrofti) B74.Ø
  - eyelid HØ2.859
    - left HØ2.856
      - lower HØ2.855
      - upper HØ2.854
    - right HØ2.853
      - lower HØ2.852
      - upper HØ2.851
  - filarial, filariensis — *see* Infestation, filarial
  - glandular I89.Ø
  - graecorum A3Ø.9
  - lymphangiectatic I89.Ø
  - lymphatic vessel I89.Ø
    - due to mastectomy I97.2
  - scrotum (nonfilarial) I89.Ø
  - streptococcal I89.Ø
  - surgical I97.89
    - postmastectomy I97.2
  - telangiectodes I89.Ø
  - vulva (nonfilarial) N9Ø.89
- **Elevated, elevation**
  - alanine transaminase (ALT) R74.Ø1
  - ALT (alanine transaminase) R74.Ø1
  - antibody titer R76.Ø
  - aspartate transaminase (AST) R74.Ø1
  - AST (aspartate transaminase) R74.Ø1
  - basal metabolic rate R94.8
  - blood pressure — *see also* Hypertension
    - reading (incidental) (isolated) (nonspecific), no diagnosis of hypertension RØ3.Ø
  - blood sugar R73.9
  - body temperature (of unknown origin) R5Ø.9
  - cancer antigen 125 [CA 125] R97.1
  - carcinoembryonic antigen [CEA] R97.Ø
  - cholesterol E78.ØØ
    - with high triglycerides E78.2
  - conjugate, eye H51.Ø
  - C-reactive protein (CRP) R79.82
  - diaphragm, congenital Q79.1
  - erythrocyte sedimentation rate R7Ø.Ø
  - fasting glucose R73.Ø1
  - fasting triglycerides E78.1
  - finding on laboratory examination — *see* Findings, abnormal, inconclusive, without diagnosis, by type of exam
- **Elevated, elevation** — *continued*
  - GFR (glomerular filtration rate) — *see* Findings, abnormal, inconclusive, without diagnosis, by type of exam
  - glucose tolerance (oral) R73.Ø2
  - immunoglobulin level R76.8
  - indoleacetic acid R82.5
  - lactic acid dehydrogenase (LDH) level R74.Ø2
  - leukocytes D72.829
  - lipoprotein a (Lp(a)) level E78.41
  - liver function
    - study R94.5
    - test R79.89
      - alkaline phosphatase R74.8
      - aminotransferase R74.Ø1
      - bilirubin R17
      - hepatic enzyme R74.8
      - lactate dehydrogenase R74.Ø2
  - Lp(a) (lipoprotein(a)) E78.41
  - lymphocytes D72.82Ø
  - prostate specific antigen [PSA] R97.2Ø
  - Rh titer — *see* Complication(s), transfusion, incompatibility reaction, Rh (factor)
  - scapula, congenital Q74.Ø
  - sedimentation rate R7Ø.Ø
  - SGOT R74.Ø1
  - SGPT R74.Ø1
  - transaminase level R74.Ø1
  - triglycerides E78.1
    - with high cholesterol E78.2
  - troponin R77.8
  - tumor associated antigens [TAA] NEC R97.8
  - tumor specific antigens [TSA] NEC R97.8
  - urine level of
    - 17-ketosteroids R82.5
    - catecholamine R82.5
    - indoleacetic acid R82.5
    - steroids R82.5
    - vanillylmandelic acid (VMA) R82.5
  - venous pressure I87.8
  - white blood cell count D72.829
    - specified NEC D72.828
- **Elliptocytosis** (congenital) (hereditary) D58.1
  - Hb C (disease) D58.1
  - hemoglobin disease D58.1
  - sickle-cell (disease) D57.8- ☑
    - trait D57.3
- **Ellison-Zollinger syndrome** E16.4
- **Ellis-van Creveld syndrome** (chondroectodermal dysplasia) Q77.6
- **Elongated, elongation** (congenital) — *see also* Distortion
  - bone Q79.9
  - cervix (uteri) Q51.828
    - acquired N88.4
    - hypertrophic N88.4
  - colon Q43.8
  - common bile duct Q44.5
  - cystic duct Q44.5
  - frenulum, penis Q55.69
  - labia minora (acquired) N9Ø.69
  - ligamentum patellae Q74.1
  - petiolus (epiglottidis) Q31.8
  - tooth, teeth KØØ.2
  - uvula Q38.6
- **Eltor cholera** AØØ.1
- **Emaciation** R64
  - due to malnutrition E43
- **Embadomoniasis** AØ7.8
- **Embedded tooth, teeth** KØ1.Ø
  - root only KØ8.3
- **Embolic** — *see* condition
- **Embolism** (multiple) (paradoxical) I74.9
  - air (any site) (traumatic) T79.Ø ☑
    - following
      - abortion — *see* Abortion by type complicated by embolism
      - ectopic pregnancy OØ8.2
      - infusion, therapeutic injection or transfusion T8Ø.Ø ☑
      - molar pregnancy OØ8.2
      - procedure NEC
        - artery T81.719 ☑
          - mesenteric T81.71Ø ☑
          - renal T81.711 ☑
          - specified NEC T81.718 ☑
        - vein T81.72 ☑
- **Embolism** — *continued*
  - air — *continued*
    - in pregnancy, childbirth or puerperium — *see* Embolism, obstetric
  - amniotic fluid (pulmonary) — *see also* Embolism, obstetric
    - following
      - abortion — *see* Abortion by type complicated by embolism
      - ectopic pregnancy OØ8.2
      - molar pregnancy OØ8.2
  - aorta, aortic I74.1Ø
    - abdominal I74.Ø9
      - saddle I74.Ø1
    - bifurcation I74.Ø9
      - saddle I74.Ø1
    - thoracic I74.11
  - artery I74.9
    - auditory, internal I65.8
    - basilar — *see* Occlusion, artery, basilar
    - carotid (common) (internal) — *see* Occlusion, artery, carotid
    - cerebellar (anterior inferior) (posterior inferior) (superior) I66.3
    - cerebral — *see* Occlusion, artery, cerebral
    - choroidal (anterior) I65.8
    - communicating posterior I65.8
    - coronary — *see also* Infarct, myocardium
      - not resulting in infarction I24.Ø
    - extremity I74.4
      - lower I74.3
      - upper I74.2
    - hypophyseal I65.8
    - iliac I74.5
    - limb I74.4
      - lower I74.3
      - upper I74.2
    - mesenteric (with gangrene) — *see also* Ischemia, intestine, acute K55.Ø59
    - ophthalmic — *see* Occlusion, artery, retina
    - peripheral I74.4
    - pontine I65.8
    - precerebral — *see* Occlusion, artery, precerebral
    - pulmonary — *see* Embolism, pulmonary
    - renal N28.Ø
    - retinal — *see* Occlusion, artery, retina
    - septic I76
    - specified NEC I74.8
    - vertebral — *see* Occlusion, artery, vertebral
  - basilar (artery) I65.1
  - blood clot
    - following
      - abortion — *see* Abortion by type complicated by embolism
      - ectopic or molar pregnancy OØ8.2
    - in pregnancy, childbirth or puerperium — *see* Embolism, obstetric
  - brain — *see also* Occlusion, artery, cerebral
    - following
      - abortion — *see* Abortion by type complicated by embolism
      - ectopic or molar pregnancy OØ8.2
    - puerperal, postpartum, childbirth — *see* Embolism, obstetric
  - capillary I78.8
  - cardiac — *see also* Infarct, myocardium
    - not resulting in infarction I51.3
  - carotid (artery) (common) (internal) — *see* Occlusion, artery, carotid
  - cavernous sinus (venous) — *see* Embolism, intracranial venous sinus
  - cerebral — *see* Occlusion, artery, cerebral
  - cholesterol — *see* Atheroembolism
  - coronary (artery or vein) (systemic) — *see* Occlusion, coronary
  - due to device, implant or graft — *see also* Complications, by site and type, specified NEC
    - arterial graft NEC T82.818 ☑
    - breast (implant) T85.818 ☑
    - catheter NEC T85.818 ☑
      - dialysis (renal) T82.818 ☑
        - intraperitoneal T85.818 ☑
      - infusion NEC T82.818 ☑
        - spinal (epidural) (subdural) T85.81Ø ☑
      - urinary (indwelling) T83.81 ☑
    - electronic (electrode) (pulse generator) (stimulator)
      - bone T84.81 ☑
      - cardiac T82.817 ☑

- **Emphysema** — *continued*
  - centrilobular J43.2
  - compensatory J98.3
  - congenital (interstitial) P25.Ø
  - conjunctiva H11.89
  - connective tissue (traumatic) T79.7 ☑
    - surgical T81.82 ☑
  - due to chemicals, gases, fumes or vapors J68.4
  - eyelid(s) — *see* Disorder, eyelid, specified type NEC
    - surgical T81.82 ☑
    - traumatic T79.7 ☑
  - interstitial J98.2
    - congenital P25.Ø
    - perinatal period P25.Ø
  - laminated tissue T79.7 ☑
    - surgical T81.82 ☑
  - mediastinal J98.2
    - newborn P25.2
  - orbit, orbital — *see* Disorder, orbit, specified type NEC
  - panacinar J43.1
  - panlobular J43.1
  - specified NEC J43.8
  - subcutaneous (traumatic) T79.7 ☑
    - nontraumatic J98.2
    - postprocedural T81.82 ☑
    - surgical T81.82 ☑
  - surgical T81.82 ☑
  - thymus (gland) (congenital) E32.8
  - traumatic (subcutaneous) T79.7 ☑
  - unilateral J43.Ø
- **Empty nest syndrome** Z6Ø.Ø
- **Empyema** (acute) (chest) (double) (pleura) (supradiaphragmatic) (thorax) J86.9
  - with fistula J86.Ø
  - accessory sinus (chronic) — *see* Sinusitis
  - antrum (chronic) — *see* Sinusitis, maxillary
  - brain (any part) — *see* Abscess, brain
  - ethmoidal (chronic) (sinus) — *see* Sinusitis, ethmoidal
  - extradural — *see* Abscess, extradural
  - frontal (chronic) (sinus) — *see* Sinusitis, frontal
  - gallbladder K81.Ø
  - mastoid (process) (acute) — *see* Mastoiditis, acute
  - maxilla, maxillary M27.2
    - sinus (chronic) — *see* Sinusitis, maxillary
  - nasal sinus (chronic) — *see* Sinusitis
  - sinus (accessory) (chronic) (nasal) — *see* Sinusitis
  - sphenoidal (sinus) (chronic) — *see* Sinusitis, sphenoidal
  - subarachnoid — *see* Abscess, extradural
  - subdural — *see* Abscess, subdural
  - tuberculous A15.6
  - ureter — *see* Ureteritis
  - ventricular — *see* Abscess, brain
- **En coup de sabre lesion** L94.1
- **Enamel pearls** KØØ.2
- **Enameloma** KØØ.2
- **Enanthema, viral** BØ9
- **Encephalitis** (chronic) (hemorrhagic) (idiopathic) (nonepidemic) (spurious) (subacute) GØ4.9Ø
  - acute — *see also* Encephalitis, viral A86
    - disseminated GØ4.ØØ
      - infectious GØ4.Ø1
      - noninfectious GØ4.81
      - postimmunization (postvaccination) GØ4.Ø2
      - postinfectious GØ4.Ø1
    - inclusion body A85.8
    - necrotizing hemorrhagic GØ4.3Ø
      - postimmunization GØ4.32
      - postinfectious GØ4.31
      - specified NEC GØ4.39
  - arboviral, arbovirus NEC A85.2
  - arthropod-borne NEC (viral) A85.2
  - Australian A83.4
  - California (virus) A83.5
  - Central European (tick-borne) A84.1
  - Czechoslovakian A84.1
  - Dawson's (inclusion body) A81.1
  - diffuse sclerosing A81.1
  - disseminated, acute GØ4.ØØ
  - due to
    - cat scratch disease A28.1
    - human immunodeficiency virus (HIV) disease B2Ø *[GØ5.3]*
    - malaria — *see* Malaria
    - rickettsiosis — *see* Rickettsiosis
    - smallpox inoculation GØ4.Ø2
    - typhus — *see* Typhus
  - Eastern equine A83.2
- **Encephalitis** — *continued*
  - endemic (viral) A86
  - epidemic NEC (viral) A86
  - equine (acute) (infectious) (viral) A83.9
    - Eastern A83.2
    - Venezuelan A92.2
    - Western A83.1
  - Far Eastern (tick-borne) A84.Ø
  - following vaccination or other immunization procedure GØ4.Ø2
  - herpes zoster BØ2.Ø
  - herpesviral BØØ.4
    - due to herpesvirus 6 B1Ø.Ø1
    - due to herpesvirus 7 B1Ø.Ø9
    - specified NEC B1Ø.Ø9
  - Ilheus (virus) A83.8
  - in (due to)
    - actinomycosis A42.82
    - adenovirus A85.1
    - African trypanosomiasis B56.9 *[GØ5.3]*
    - Chagas' disease (chronic) B57.42
    - cytomegalovirus B25.8
    - enterovirus A85.Ø
    - herpes (simplex) virus BØØ.4
      - due to herpesvirus 6 B1Ø.Ø1
      - due to herpesvirus 7 B1Ø.Ø9
      - specified NEC B1Ø.Ø9
    - infectious disease NEC B99 ☑ *[GØ5.3]*
    - influenza — *see* Influenza, with, encephalopathy
    - listeriosis A32.12
    - measles BØ5.Ø
    - mumps B26.2
    - naegleriasis B6Ø.2
    - parasitic disease NEC B89 *[GØ5.3]*
    - poliovirus A8Ø.9 *[GØ5.3]*
    - rubella BØ6.Ø1
    - syphilis
      - congenital A5Ø.42
      - late A52.14
    - systemic lupus erythematosus M32.19
    - toxoplasmosis (acquired) B58.2
      - congenital P37.1
    - tuberculosis A17.82
    - zoster BØ2.Ø
  - inclusion body A81.1
  - infectious (acute) (virus) NEC A86
  - Japanese (B type) A83.Ø
  - La Crosse A83.5
  - lead — *see* Poisoning, lead
  - lethargica (acute) (infectious) A85.8
  - louping ill A84.89
  - lupus erythematosus, systemic M32.19
  - lymphatica A87.2
  - Mengo A85.8
  - meningococcal A39.81
  - Murray Valley A83.4
  - otitic NEC H66.4Ø *[GØ5.3]*
  - parasitic NOS B71.9
  - periaxial G37.Ø
  - periaxialis (concentrica) (diffuse) G37.5
  - postchickenpox BØ1.11
  - postexanthematous NEC BØ9
  - postimmunization GØ4.Ø2
  - postinfectious NEC GØ4.Ø1
  - postmeasles BØ5.Ø
  - postvaccinal GØ4.Ø2
  - postvaricella BØ1.11
  - postviral NEC A86
  - Powassan A84.81
  - Rasmussen GØ4.81
  - Rio Bravo A85.8
  - Russian
    - autumnal A83.Ø
    - spring-summer (taiga) A84.Ø
  - saturnine — *see* Poisoning, lead
  - specified NEC GØ4.81
  - St. Louis A83.3
  - subacute sclerosing A81.1
  - summer A83.Ø
  - suppurative GØ4.81
  - tick-borne A84.9
  - Torula, torular (cryptococcal) B45.1
  - toxic NEC G92.8
  - trichinosis B75 *[GØ5.3]*
  - type
    - B A83.Ø
    - C A83.3
  - van Bogaert's A81.1
- **Encephalitis** — *continued*
  - Venezuelan equine A92.2
  - Vienna A85.8
  - viral, virus A86
    - arthropod-borne NEC A85.2
      - mosquito-borne A83.9
        - Australian X disease A83.4
        - California virus A83.5
        - Eastern equine A83.2
        - Japanese (B type) A83.Ø
        - Murray Valley A83.4
        - specified NEC A83.8
        - St. Louis A83.3
        - type B A83.Ø
        - type C A83.3
        - Western equine A83.1
      - tick-borne A84.9
        - biundulant A84.1
        - central European A84.1
        - Czechoslovakian A84.1
        - diphasic meningoencephalitis A84.1
        - Far Eastern A84.Ø
        - Russian spring-summer (taiga) A84.Ø
        - specified NEC A84.89
    - specified type NEC A85.8
    - tick-borne, specified NEC A84.89
  - Western equine A83.1
- **Encephalocele** QØ1.9
  - frontal QØ1.Ø
  - nasofrontal QØ1.1
  - occipital QØ1.2
  - specified NEC QØ1.8
- **Encephalocystocele** — *see* Encephalocele
- **Encephaloduroarteriomyosynangiosis** (EDAMS) I67.5
- **Encephalomalacia** (brain) (cerebellar) (cerebral) — *see* Softening, brain
- **Encephalomeningitis** — *see* Meningoencephalitis
- **Encephalomeningocele** — *see* Encephalocele
- **Encephalomeningomyelitis** — *see* Meningoencephalitis
- **Encephalomyelitis** — *see also* Encephalitis GØ4.9Ø
  - acute disseminated GØ4.ØØ
    - infectious GØ4.Ø1
    - noninfectious GØ4.81
    - postimmunization GØ4.Ø2
    - postinfectious GØ4.Ø1
  - acute necrotizing hemorrhagic GØ4.3Ø
    - postimmunization GØ4.32
    - postinfectious GØ4.31
    - specified NEC GØ4.39
  - equine A83.9
    - Eastern A83.2
    - Venezuelan A92.2
    - Western A83.1
  - in diseases classified elsewhere GØ5.3
  - myalgic G93.32
    - chronic fatigue syndrome [ME/CFS] G93.32
  - postchickenpox BØ1.11
  - postinfectious NEC GØ4.Ø1
  - postmeasles BØ5.Ø
  - postvaccinal GØ4.Ø2
  - postvaricella BØ1.11
  - rubella BØ6.Ø1
  - specified NEC GØ4.81
  - Venezuelan equine A92.2
- **Encephalomyelocele** — *see* Encephalocele
- **Encephalomyelomeningitis** — *see* Meningoencephalitis
- **Encephalomyelopathy** G96.9
- **Encephalomyeloradiculitis** (acute) G61.Ø
- **Encephalomyeloradiculoneuritis** (acute) (Guillain-Barré) G61.Ø
- **Encephalomyeloradiculopathy** G96.9
- **Encephalopathia hyperbilirubinemica, newborn** P57.9
  - due to isoimmunization (conditions in P55) P57.Ø
- **Encephalopathy** (acute) G93.4Ø
  - acute necrotizing hemorrhagic GØ4.3Ø
    - postimmunization GØ4.32
    - postinfectious GØ4.31
    - specified NEC GØ4.39
  - alcoholic G31.2
  - anoxic — *see* Damage, brain, anoxic
  - arteriosclerotic I67.2
  - centrolobar progressive (Schilder) G37.Ø
  - congenital QØ7.9
  - degenerative, in specified disease NEC G32.89
  - demyelinating callosal G37.1

☑ Additional Character Required — Refer to the Tabular List for Character Selection

Endometriosis — *continued*
- deep
  - involving muscular wall of fallopian tube N8Ø.22 ☑
  - retrocervical N8Ø.Ø2
- diaphragm N8Ø.B39
  - deep N8Ø.B32
  - superficial N8Ø.B31
  - unspecified depth N8Ø.B39
- exocervix N8Ø.Ø1
- extra-pelvic abdominal peritoneum N8Ø.C4
- fallopian tube (unspecified depth) N8Ø.2Ø- ☑
  - deep N8Ø.22- ☑
  - superficial N8Ø.21- ☑
- female genital organ NEC N8Ø.8
- gallbladder N8Ø.8
- in scar of skin N8Ø.6
- inguinal canal N8Ø.C3
- internal N8Ø.Ø2
- intestine N8Ø.5Ø
- lung N8Ø.B2
- mediastinal space N8Ø.B5
- myometrium N8Ø.Ø3
- nerve
  - femoral N8Ø.D6
  - obturator N8Ø.D3
  - pelvic N8Ø.DØ
    - splanchnic N8Ø.D1
  - pudendal N8Ø.D5
  - retroperitoneum, NEC N8Ø.D9
  - sacral splanchnic N8Ø.D1
  - sciatic N8Ø.D4
  - specified, NEC N8Ø.D9
- ovary (unspecified depth) N8Ø.1Ø- ☑
  - deep N8Ø.12- ☑
  - superficial N8Ø.11- ☑
- parametrium N8Ø.399
- pelvic
  - brim N8Ø.38- ☑
    - deep N8Ø.37- ☑
    - superficial N8Ø.36- ☑
  - peritoneum N8Ø.3Ø
    - specified sites, NEC N8Ø.399
      - deep N8Ø.392
      - superficial N8Ø.391
  - sidewall N8Ø.35- ☑
    - deep N8Ø.34- ☑
    - superficial N8Ø.33- ☑
- pericardial space N8Ø.B4
- peritoneal (pelvic) N8Ø.3Ø
- pleura N8Ø.B1
- rectovaginal septum N8Ø.4Ø
  - with involvement of vagina N8Ø.42
  - without involvement of vagina N8Ø.41
- rectum N8Ø.519
  - deep (multifocal) N8Ø.512
  - superficial N8Ø.511
- retroperitoneum N8Ø.3Ø
- round ligament N8Ø.3C9
- sacral nerve roots N8Ø.D2
- skin (scar) N8Ø.6
- small N8Ø.569
  - deep (multifocal) N8Ø.562
  - superficial N8Ø.561
- specified site NEC N8Ø.8
- stromal D39.Ø
- thorax N8Ø.B- ☑
- umbilicus N8Ø.C2
- ureter N8Ø.A69
  - deep N8Ø.A5- ☑
  - extrinsic N8Ø.A4- ☑
  - intrinsic N8Ø.A5- ☑
  - superficial N8Ø.A4- ☑
  - unspecified depth N8Ø.A6- ☑
- uterosacral ligament(s) N8Ø.3C- ☑
  - deep N8Ø.3B- ☑
  - superficial N8Ø.3A- ☑
- uterus N8Ø.ØØ
  - deep N8Ø.Ø2
  - internal N8Ø.Ø2
  - superficial N8Ø.Ø1
- vagina N8Ø.42
- vulva N8Ø.8

Endometritis (decidual) (nonspecific) (purulent) (senile) (atrophic) (suppurative) N71.9
- with ectopic pregnancy OØ8.Ø
- acute N71.Ø
- blenorrhagic (gonococcal) (acute) (chronic) A54.24
- cervix, cervical (with erosion or ectropion) — *see also* Cervicitis
  - hyperplastic N72
- chlamydial A56.11
- chronic N71.1
- following
  - abortion — *see* Abortion by type complicated by genital infection
  - ectopic or molar pregnancy OØ8.Ø
- gonococcal, gonorrheal (acute) (chronic) A54.24
- hyperplastic — *see also* Hyperplasia, endometrial N85.ØØ
  - cervix N72
- puerperal, postpartum, childbirth O86.12
- subacute N71.Ø
- tuberculous A18.17

Endometrium — *see* condition
Endomyocardiopathy, South African I42.3
Endomyocarditis — *see* Endocarditis
Endomyofibrosis I42.3
Endomyometritis — *see* Endometritis
Endopericarditis — *see* Endocarditis
Endoperineuritis — *see* Disorder, nerve
Endophlebitis — *see* Phlebitis
Endophthalmia — *see* Endophthalmitis, purulent
Endophthalmitis (acute) (infective) (metastatic) (subacute) H44.ØØ9
- bleb associated — *see also* Bleb, inflamed (infected), postprocedural H59.4 ☑
- gonorrheal A54.39
- in (due to)
  - cysticercosis B69.1
  - onchocerciasis B73.Ø1
  - toxocariasis B83.Ø
- panuveitis — *see* Panuveitis
- parasitic H44.12- ☑
- purulent H44.ØØ- ☑
  - panophthalmitis — *see* Panophthalmitis
  - vitreous abscess H44.Ø2- ☑
- specified NEC H44.19
- sympathetic — *see* Uveitis, sympathetic

Endosalpingioma D28.2
Endosalpingiosis N94.89
Endosteitis — *see* Osteomyelitis
Endothelioma, bone — *see* Neoplasm, bone, malignant
Endotheliosis (hemorrhagic infectional) D69.8
Endotoxemia — code to condition
Endotrachelitis — *see* Cervicitis
Engelmann (-Camurati) **syndrome** Q78.3
English disease — *see* Rickets
Engman's disease L3Ø.3
Engorgement
- breast N64.59
  - newborn P83.4
  - puerperal, postpartum O92.79
- lung (passive) — *see* Edema, lung
- pulmonary (passive) — *see* Edema, lung
- stomach K31.89
- venous, retina — *see* Occlusion, retina, vein, engorgement

Enlargement, enlarged — *see also* Hypertrophy
- adenoids J35.2
  - with tonsils J35.3
- alveolar ridge KØ8.89
  - congenital — *see* Anomaly, alveolar
- apertures of diaphragm (congenital) Q79.1
- gingival KØ6.1
- heart, cardiac — *see* Hypertrophy, cardiac
- labium majus, childhood asymmetric (CALME) N9Ø.61
- lacrimal gland, chronic HØ4.Ø3- ☑
- liver — *see* Hypertrophy, liver
- lymph gland or node R59.9
  - generalized R59.1
  - localized R59.Ø
- orbit HØ5.34- ☑
- organ or site, congenital NEC — *see* Anomaly, by site
- parathyroid (gland) E21.Ø
- pituitary fossa R93.Ø
- prostate N4Ø.Ø
  - with lower urinary tract symptoms (LUTS) N4Ø.1
  - without lower urinary tract symtpoms (LUTS) N4Ø.Ø
- sella turcica R93.Ø
- spleen — *see* Splenomegaly
- thymus (gland) (congenital) E32.Ø
- thyroid (gland) — *see* Goiter
- tongue K14.8
- tonsils J35.1
  - with adenoids J35.3
- uterus N85.2
- vestibular aqueduct Q16.5

Enophthalmos HØ5.4Ø- ☑
- due to
  - orbital tissue atrophy HØ5.41- ☑
  - trauma or surgery HØ5.42- ☑

Enostosis M27.8
Entamebic, entamebiasis — *see* Amebiasis
Entanglement
- umbilical cord(s) O69.82 ☑
  - with compression O69.2 ☑
  - around neck (with compression) O69.81 ☑
    - with compression O69.1 ☑
    - without compression O69.81 ☑
  - of twins in monoamniotic sac O69.2 ☑
  - without compression O69.82 ☑

Enteralgia — *see* Pain, abdominal
Enteric — *see* condition
Enteritis (acute) (diarrheal) (hemorrhagic) (noninfective) K52.9
- adenovirus AØ8.2
- aertrycke infection AØ2.Ø
- allergic K52.29
  - with
    - eosinophilic gastritis or gastroenteritis K52.81
    - food protein-induced enterocolitis syndrome K52.21
    - food protein-induced enteropathy K52.22
    - FPIES K52.21
- amebic (acute) AØ6.Ø
  - with abscess — *see* Abscess, amebic
  - chronic AØ6.1
    - with abscess — *see* Abscess, amebic
    - nondysenteric AØ6.2
  - nondysenteric AØ6.2
- astrovirus AØ8.32
- bacillary NOS AØ3.9
- bacterial AØ4.9
  - specified NEC AØ4.8
- calicivirus AØ8.31
- candidal B37.82
- Chilomastix AØ7.8
- choleriformis AØØ.1
- chronic (noninfectious) K52.9
  - ulcerative — *see* Colitis, ulcerative
- cicatrizing (chronic) — *see* Enteritis, regional, small intestine
- Clostridium
  - botulinum (food poisoning) AØ5.1
  - difficile
    - not specified as recurrent AØ4.72
    - recurrent AØ4.71
- coccidial AØ7.3
- coxsackie virus AØ8.39
- dietetic — *see also* Enteritis, allergic K52.29
- drug-induced K52.1
- due to
  - astrovirus AØ8.32
  - calicivirus AØ8.31
  - coxsackie virus AØ8.39
  - drugs K52.1
  - echovirus AØ8.39
  - enterovirus NEC AØ8.39
  - food hypersensitivity — *see also* Enteritis, allergic K52.29
  - infectious organism (bacterial) (viral) — *see* Enteritis, infectious
  - torovirus AØ8.39
  - Yersinia enterocolitica AØ4.6
- echovirus AØ8.39
- eltor AØØ.1
- enterovirus NEC AØ8.39
- eosinophilic K52.81
- epidemic (infectious) AØ9
- fulminant — *see also* Ischemia, intestine, acute K55.Ø19
- gangrenous — *see* Enteritis, infectious
- giardial AØ7.1
- infectious NOS AØ9
  - due to
    - adenovirus AØ8.2
    - Aerobacter aerogenes AØ4.8
    - Arizona (bacillus) AØ2.Ø
    - bacteria NOS AØ4.9
      - specified NEC AØ4.8
    - Campylobacter AØ4.5

Enthesopathy — *continued*
- spinal — *continued*
  - cervical region M46.Ø2
  - cervicothoracic region M46.Ø3
  - lumbar region M46.Ø6
  - lumbosacral region M46.Ø7
  - multiple sites M46.Ø9
  - occipito-atlanto-axial region M46.Ø1
  - sacrococcygeal region M46.Ø8
  - thoracic region M46.Ø4
  - thoracolumbar region M46.Ø5
- tibial collateral bursitis — *see* Bursitis, tibial collateral
- upper arm M77.8
- wrist and carpus NEC M77.8
  - calcaneal spur — *see* Spur, bone, calcaneal
  - periarthritis of wrist — *see* Periarthritis, wrist

Entomophobia F4Ø.218

Entomophthoromycosis B46.8

Entrance, air into vein — *see* Embolism, air

Entrapment, nerve — *see* Neuropathy, entrapment

Entropion (eyelid) (paralytic) HØ2.ØØ9
- cicatricial HØ2.Ø19
  - left HØ2.Ø16
    - lower HØ2.Ø15
    - upper HØ2.Ø14
  - right HØ2.Ø13
    - lower HØ2.Ø12
    - upper HØ2.Ø11
- congenital Q1Ø.2
- left HØ2.ØØ6
  - lower HØ2.ØØ5
  - upper HØ2.ØØ4
- mechanical HØ2.Ø29
  - left HØ2.Ø26
    - lower HØ2.Ø25
    - upper HØ2.Ø24
  - right HØ2.Ø23
    - lower HØ2.Ø22
    - upper HØ2.Ø21
- right HØ2.ØØ3
  - lower HØ2.ØØ2
  - upper HØ2.ØØ1
- senile HØ2.Ø39
  - left HØ2.Ø36
    - lower HØ2.Ø35
    - upper HØ2.Ø34
  - right HØ2.Ø33
    - lower HØ2.Ø32
    - upper HØ2.Ø31
- spastic HØ2.Ø49
  - left HØ2.Ø46
    - lower HØ2.Ø45
    - upper HØ2.Ø44
  - right HØ2.Ø43
    - lower HØ2.Ø42
    - upper HØ2.Ø41

Enucleated eye (traumatic, current) SØ5.7- ☑

Enuresis R32
- functional F98.Ø
- habit disturbance F98.Ø
- nocturnal N39.44
  - psychogenic F98.Ø
- nonorganic origin F98.Ø
- psychogenic F98.Ø

Eosinopenia — *see* Agranulocytosis

Eosinophilia (allergic) (idiopathic) (secondary) D72.1Ø
- with
  - angiolymphoid hyperplasia (ALHE) D18.Ø1
- familial D72.19
- hereditary D72.19
- in disease classified elsewhere D72.18
- infiltrative — *see* Eosinophilia, pulmonary
- Löffler's J82.89
- peritoneal — *see* Peritonitis, eosinophilic
- pulmonary NEC J82.89
  - acute J82.82
  - asthmatic J82.83
  - chronic J82.81
- specified NEC D72.19
- tropical (pulmonary) J82.89

Eosinophilia-myalgia syndrome M35.89

Ependymitis (acute) (cerebral) (chronic) (granular) — *see* Encephalomyelitis

Ependymoblastoma
- specified site — *see* Neoplasm, malignant, by site
- unspecified site C71.9

Ependymoma (epithelial) (malignant)
- anaplastic
  - specified site — *see* Neoplasm, malignant, by site
  - unspecified site C71.9
- benign
  - specified site — *see* Neoplasm, benign, by site
  - unspecified site D33.2
- myxopapillary D43.2
  - specified site — *see* Neoplasm, uncertain behavior, by site
  - unspecified site D43.2
- papillary D43.2
  - specified site — *see* Neoplasm, uncertain behavior, by site
  - unspecified site D43.2
- specified site — *see* Neoplasm, malignant, by site
- unspecified site C71.9

Ependymopathy G93.89

Ephelis, ephelides L81.2

Epiblepharon (congenital) Q1Ø.3

Epicanthus, epicanthic fold (eyelid) (congenital) Q1Ø.3

Epicondylitis (elbow)
- lateral M77.1- ☑
- medial M77.Ø- ☑

Epicystitis — *see* Cystitis

Epidemic — *see* condition

Epidermidalization, cervix — *see* Dysplasia, cervix

Epidermis, epidermal — *see* condition

Epidermodysplasia verruciformis BØ7.8

Epidermolysis
- bullosa (congenital) Q81.9
  - acquired L12.3Ø
    - drug-induced L12.31
    - specified cause NEC L12.35
  - dystrophica Q81.2
  - letalis Q81.1
  - simplex Q81.Ø
  - specified NEC Q81.8
- necroticans combustiformis L51.2
  - due to drug — *see* Table of Drugs and Chemicals, by drug

Epidermophytid — *see* Dermatophytosis

Epidermophytosis (infected) — *see* Dermatophytosis

Epididymis — *see* condition

Epididymitis (acute) (nonvenereal) (recurrent) (residual) N45.1
- with orchitis N45.3
- blennorrhagic (gonococcal) A54.23
- caseous (tuberculous) A18.15
- chlamydial A56.19
- filarial — *see also* Infestation, filarial B74.9 *[N51]*
- gonococcal A54.23
- syphilitic A52.76
- tuberculous A18.15

Epididymo-orchitis — *see also* Epididymitis N45.3

Epidural — *see* condition

Epigastrium, epigastric — *see* condition

Epigastrocele — *see* Hernia, ventral

Epiglottis — *see* condition

Epiglottitis, epiglottiditis (acute) JØ5.1Ø
- with obstruction JØ5.11
- chronic J37.Ø

Epignathus Q89.4

Epilepsia partialis continua — *see also* Kozhevnikof's epilepsy G4Ø.1- ☑

Epilepsy, epileptic, epilepsia (attack) (cerebral) (convulsion) (fit) (seizure) G4Ø.9Ø9

Note: the following terms are to be considered equivalent to intractable: pharmacoresistant (pharmacologically resistant), treatment resistant, refractory (medically) and poorly controlled

- with
  - complex partial seizures — *see* Epilepsy, localization-related, symptomatic, with complex partial seizures
  - grand mal seizures on awakening — *see* Epilepsy, generalized, specified NEC
  - myoclonic absences — *see* Epilepsy, generalized, specified NEC
  - myoclonic-astatic seizures — *see* Epilepsy, generalized, specified NEC
  - simple partial seizures — *see* Epilepsy, localization-related, symptomatic, with simple partial seizures
- akinetic — *see* Epilepsy, generalized, specified NEC

Epilepsy, epileptic, epilepsia — *continued*
- benign childhood with centrotemporal EEG spikes — *see* Epilepsy, localization-related, idiopathic
- benign myoclonic in infancy G4Ø.8Ø- ☑
- Bravais-jacksonian — *see* Epilepsy, localization-related, symptomatic, with simple partial seizures
- childhood
  - with occipital EEG paroxysms — *see* Epilepsy, localization-related, idiopathic
  - absence G4Ø.AØ9 (*following* G4Ø.3)
    - intractable G4Ø.A19 (*following* G4Ø.3)
      - with status epilepticus G4Ø.A11 (*following* G4Ø.3)
      - without status epilepticus G4Ø.A19 (*following* G4Ø.3)
    - not intractable G4Ø.AØ9 (*following* G4Ø.3)
      - with status epilepticus G4Ø.AØ1 (*following* G4Ø.3)
      - without status epilepticus G4Ø.AØ9 (*following* G4Ø.3)
- climacteric — *see* Epilepsy, specified NEC
- cysticercosis B69.Ø
- deterioration (mental) FØ6.8
- due to syphilis A52.19
- focal — *see* Epilepsy, localization-related, symptomatic, with simple partial seizures
- generalized
  - idiopathic G4Ø.3Ø9
    - intractable G4Ø.319
      - with status epilepticus G4Ø.311
      - without status epilepticus G4Ø.319
    - not intractable G4Ø.3Ø9
      - with status epilepticus G4Ø.3Ø1
      - without status epilepticus G4Ø.3Ø9
  - specified NEC G4Ø.4Ø9
    - intractable G4Ø.419
      - with status epilepticus G4Ø.411
      - without status epilepticus G4Ø.419
    - not intractable G4Ø.4Ø9
      - with status epilepticus G4Ø.4Ø1
      - without status epilepticus G4Ø.4Ø9
- impulsive petit mal — *see* Epilepsy, juvenile myoclonic
- intractable G4Ø.919
  - with status epilepticus G4Ø.911
  - without status epilepticus G4Ø.919
- juvenile absence G4Ø.AØ9 (*following* G4Ø.3)
  - intractable G4Ø.A19 (*following* G4Ø.3)
    - with status epilepticus G4Ø.A11 (*following* G4Ø.3)
    - without status epilepticus G4Ø.A19 (*following* G4Ø.3)
  - not intractable G4Ø.AØ9 (*following* G4Ø.3)
    - with status epilepticus G4Ø.AØ1 (*following* G4Ø.3)
    - without status epilepticus G4Ø.AØ9 (*following* G4Ø.3)
- juvenile myoclonic G4Ø.BØ9 (*following* G4Ø.3)
  - intractable G4Ø.B19 (*following* G4Ø.3)
    - with status epilepticus G4Ø.B11 (*following* G4Ø.3)
    - without status epilepticus G4Ø.B19 (*following* G4Ø.3)
  - not intractable G4Ø.BØ9 (*following* G4Ø.3)
    - with status epilepticus G4Ø.BØ1 (*following* G4Ø.3)
    - without status epilepticus G4Ø.BØ9 (*following* G4Ø.3)
- localization-related (focal) (partial)
  - idiopathic G4Ø.ØØ9
    - with seizures of localized onset G4Ø.ØØ9
      - intractable G4Ø.Ø19
        - with status epilepticus G4Ø.Ø11
        - without status epilepticus G4Ø.Ø19
      - not intractable G4Ø.ØØ9
        - with status epilepticus G4Ø.ØØ1
        - without status epilepticus G4Ø.ØØ9
  - symptomatic
    - with complex partial seizures G4Ø.2Ø9
      - intractable G4Ø.219
        - with status epilepticus G4Ø.211
        - without status epilepticus G4Ø.219
      - not intractable G4Ø.2Ø9
        - with status epilepticus G4Ø.2Ø1
        - without status epilepticus G4Ø.2Ø9
    - with simple partial seizures G4Ø.1Ø9
      - intractable G4Ø.119
        - with status epilepticus G4Ø.111
        - without status epilepticus G4Ø.119
      - not intractable G4Ø.1Ø9
        - with status epilepticus G4Ø.1Ø1
        - without status epilepticus G4Ø.1Ø9

Epilepsy, epileptic, epilepsia — *continued*
- myoclonus, myoclonic — *see also* Epilepsy, generalized, specified NEC
  - progressive — *see* Epilepsy, generalized, idiopathic
  - severe, in infancy (SMEI) G4Ø.83- ☑
- not intractable G4Ø.9Ø9
  - with status epilepticus G4Ø.9Ø1
  - without status epilepticus G4Ø.9Ø9
- on awakening — *see* Epilepsy, generalized, specified NEC
- parasitic NOS B71.9 *[G94]*
- partialis continua — *see also* Kozhevnikof's epilepsy G4Ø.1- ☑
- peripheral — *see* Epilepsy, specified NEC
- polymorphic, in infancy (PMEI) G4Ø.83- ☑
- procursiva — *see* Epilepsy, localization-related, symptomatic, with simple partial seizures
- progressive (familial) myoclonic — *see* Epilepsy, generalized, idiopathic
- reflex — *see* Epilepsy, specified NEC
- related to
  - alcohol G4Ø.5Ø9
    - not intractable G4Ø.5Ø9
      - with status epilepticus G4Ø.5Ø1
      - without status eplilepticus G4Ø.5Ø9
  - drugs G4Ø.5Ø9
    - not intractable G4Ø.5Ø9
      - with status epilepticus G4Ø.5Ø1
      - without status eplilepticus G4Ø.5Ø9
  - external causes G4Ø.5Ø9
    - not intractable G4Ø.5Ø9
      - with status epilepticus G4Ø.5Ø1
      - without status eplilepticus G4Ø.5Ø9
  - hormonal changes G4Ø.5Ø9
    - not intractable G4Ø.5Ø9
      - with status epilepticus G4Ø.5Ø1
      - without status eplilepticus G4Ø.5Ø9
  - sleep deprivation G4Ø.5Ø9
    - not intractable G4Ø.5Ø9
      - with status epilepticus G4Ø.5Ø1
      - without status eplilepticus G4Ø.5Ø9
  - stress G4Ø.5Ø9
    - not intractable G4Ø.5Ø9
      - with status epilepticus G4Ø.5Ø1
      - without status eplilepticus G4Ø.5Ø9
- somatomotor — *see* Epilepsy, localization-related, symptomatic, with simple partial seizures
- somatosensory — *see* Epilepsy, localization-related, symptomatic, with simple partial seizures
- spasms G4Ø.822
  - intractable G4Ø.824
    - with status epilepticus G4Ø.823
    - without status epilepticus G4Ø.824
  - not intractable G4Ø.822
    - with status epilepticus G4Ø.821
    - without status epilepticus G4Ø.822
- specified NEC G4Ø.8Ø2
  - intractable G4Ø.8Ø4
    - with status epilepticus G4Ø.8Ø3
    - without status epilepticus G4Ø.8Ø4
  - not intractable G4Ø.8Ø2
    - with status epilepticus G4Ø.8Ø1
    - without status epilepticus G4Ø.8Ø2
- syndromes
  - generalized
    - idiopathic G4Ø.3Ø9
      - intractable G4Ø.319
        - with status epilepticus G4Ø.311
        - without status epilepticus G4Ø.319
      - not intractable G4Ø.3Ø9
        - with status epilepticus G4Ø.3Ø1
        - without status epilepticus G4Ø.3Ø9
    - specified NEC G4Ø.4Ø9
      - intractable G4Ø.419
        - with status epilepticus G4Ø.411
        - without status epilepticus G4Ø.419
      - not intractable G4Ø.4Ø9
        - with status epilepticus G4Ø.4Ø1
        - without status epilepticus G4Ø.4Ø9
  - localization-related (focal) (partial)
    - idiopathic G4Ø.ØØ9
      - with seizures of localized onset G4Ø.ØØ9
        - intractable G4Ø.Ø19
          - with status epilepticus G4Ø.Ø11
          - without status epilepticus G4Ø.Ø19
        - not intractable G4Ø.ØØ9
          - with status epilepticus G4Ø.ØØ1
          - without status epilepticus G4Ø.ØØ9

Epilepsy, epileptic, epilepsia — *continued*
- syndromes — *continued*
  - localization-related — *continued*
    - symptomatic
      - with complex partial seizures G4Ø.2Ø9
        - intractable G4Ø.219
          - with status epilepticus G4Ø.211
          - without status epilepticus G4Ø.219
        - not intractable G4Ø.2Ø9
          - with status epilepticus G4Ø.2Ø1
          - without status epilepticus G4Ø.2Ø9
      - with simple partial seizures G4Ø.1Ø9
        - intractable G4Ø.119
          - with status epilepticus G4Ø.111
          - without status epilepticus G4Ø.119
        - not intractable G4Ø.1Ø9
          - with status epilepticus G4Ø.1Ø1
          - without status epilepticus G4Ø.1Ø9
  - specified NEC G4Ø.8Ø2
    - intractable G4Ø.8Ø4
      - with status epilepticus G4Ø.8Ø3
      - without status epilepticus G4Ø.8Ø4
    - not intractable G4Ø.8Ø2
      - with status epilepticus G4Ø.8Ø1
      - without status epilepticus G4Ø.8Ø2
- tonic (-clonic) — *see* Epilepsy, generalized, specified NEC
- twilight FØ5
- uncinate (gyrus) — *see* Epilepsy, localization-related, symptomatic, with complex partial seizures
- Unverricht (-Lundborg) (familial myoclonic) — *see* Epilepsy, generalized, idiopathic
- visceral — *see* Epilepsy, specified NEC
- visual — *see* Epilepsy, specified NEC

Epiloia Q85.1

Epimenorrhea N92.Ø

Epipharyngitis — *see* Nasopharyngitis

Epiphora HØ4.2Ø- ☑
- due to
  - excess lacrimation HØ4.21- ☑
  - insufficient drainage HØ4.22- ☑

Epiphyseal arrest — *see* Arrest, epiphyseal

Epiphyseolysis, epiphysiolysis — *see* Osteochondropathy

Epiphysitis — *see also* Osteochondropathy
- juvenile M92.9
- syphilitic (congenital) A5Ø.Ø2

Epiplocele — *see* Hernia, abdomen

Epiploitis — *see* Peritonitis

Epiplosarcomphalocele — *see* Hernia, umbilicus

Episcleritis (suppurative) H15.1Ø- ☑
- in (due to)
  - syphilis A52.71
  - tuberculosis A18.51
- nodular H15.12- ☑
- periodica fugax H15.11- ☑
  - angioneurotic — *see* Edema, angioneurotic
- syphilitic (late) A52.71
- tuberculous A18.51

Episode
- affective, mixed F39
- depersonalization (in neurotic state) F48.1
- depressive F32.A
  - major F32.9
    - mild F32.Ø
    - moderate F32.1
    - severe (without psychotic symptoms) F32.2
      - with psychotic symptoms F32.3
  - recurrent F33.9
    - brief F33.8
  - specified NEC F32.89
- hypomanic F3Ø.8
- manic F3Ø.9
  - with
    - psychotic symptoms F3Ø.2
    - remission (full) F3Ø.4
      - partial F3Ø.3
  - other specified F3Ø.8
  - recurrent F31.89
  - without psychotic symptoms F3Ø.1Ø
    - mild F3Ø.11
    - moderate F3Ø.12
    - severe (without psychotic symptoms) F3Ø.13
      - with psychotic symptoms F3Ø.2
- psychotic F23
  - organic FØ6.8
- schizophrenic (acute) NEC, brief F23

Epispadias (female) (male) Q64.Ø

Episplenitis D73.89

Epistaxis (multiple) RØ4.Ø
- hereditary I78.Ø
- vicarious menstruation N94.89

Epithelioma (malignant) — *see also* Neoplasm, malignant, by site
- adenoides cysticum — *see* Neoplasm, skin, benign
- basal cell — *see* Neoplasm, skin, malignant
- benign — *see* Neoplasm, benign, by site
- Bowen's — *see* Neoplasm, skin, in situ
- calcifying, of Malherbe — *see* Neoplasm, skin, benign
- external site — *see* Neoplasm, skin, malignant
- intraepidermal, Jadassohn — *see* Neoplasm, skin, benign
- squamous cell — *see* Neoplasm, malignant, by site

Epitheliomatosis pigmented Q82.1

Epitheliopathy, multifocal placoid pigment H3Ø.14- ☑

Epithelium, epithelial — *see* condition

Epituberculosis (with atelectasis) (allergic) A15.7

Eponychia Q84.6

Epstein's
- nephrosis or syndrome — *see* Nephrosis
- pearl KØ9.8

Epulis (gingiva) (fibrous) (giant cell) KØ6.8

Equinia A24.Ø

Equinovarus (congenital) (talipes) Q66.Ø- ☑
- acquired — *see* Deformity, limb, clubfoot

Equivalent
- convulsive (abdominal) — *see* Epilepsy, specified NEC
- epileptic (psychic) — *see* Epilepsy, localization-related, symptomatic, with complex partial seizures

Erb (-Duchenne) **paralysis** (birth injury) (newborn) P14.Ø

Erb-Goldflam disease or syndrome G7Ø.ØØ
- with exacerbation (acute) G7Ø.Ø1
- in crisis G7Ø.Ø1

Erb's
- disease G71.Ø2
- palsy, paralysis (brachial) (birth) (newborn) P14.Ø
  - spinal (spastic) syphilitic A52.17
- pseudohypertrophic muscular dystrophy G71.Ø2

Erdheim's syndrome (acromegalic macrospondylitis) E22.Ø

Erection, painful (persistent) — *see* Priapism

Ergosterol deficiency (vitamin D) E55.9
- with
  - adult osteomalacia M83.8
  - rickets — *see* Rickets

Ergotism — *see also* Poisoning, food, noxious, plant
- from ergot used as drug (migraine therapy) — *see* Table of Drugs and Chemicals

Erosio interdigitalis blastomycetica B37.2

Erosion
- artery I77.2
  - without rupture I77.89
- bone — *see* Disorder, bone, density and structure, specified NEC
- bronchus J98.Ø9
- cartilage (joint) — *see* Disorder, cartilage, specified type NEC
- cervix (uteri) (acquired) (chronic) (congenital) N86
  - with cervicitis N72
- cornea (nontraumatic) — *see* Ulcer, cornea
  - recurrent H18.83- ☑
  - traumatic — *see* Abrasion, cornea
- dental (idiopathic) (occupational) (due to diet, drugs or vomiting) KØ3.2
- duodenum, postpyloric — *see* Ulcer, duodenum
- esophagus K22.1Ø
  - with bleeding K22.11
- gastric — *see* Ulcer, stomach
- gastrojejunal — *see* Ulcer, gastrojejunal
- implanted mesh — *see* Complications, prosthetic device or implant, mesh
- intestine K63.3
- lymphatic vessel I89.8
- pylorus, pyloric (ulcer) — *see* Ulcer, stomach
- spine, aneurysmal A52.Ø9
- stomach — *see* Ulcer, stomach
- subcutaneous device pocket
  - nervous system prosthetic device, implant, or graft T85.89Ø ☑
  - other internal prosthetic device, implant, or graft T85.898 ☑
- teeth (idiopathic) (occupational) (due to diet, drugs or vomiting) KØ3.2
- urethra N36.8

Erosion — *continued*
uterus N85.8
Erotomania F52.8
Error
metabolism, inborn — *see* Disorder, metabolism
refractive — *see* Disorder, refraction
Eructation R14.2
nervous or psychogenic F45.8
Eruption
creeping B76.9
drug (generalized) (taken internally) L27.Ø
fixed L27.1
in contact with skin — *see* Dermatitis, due to drugs
localized L27.1
Hutchinson, summer L56.4
Kaposi's varicelliform BØØ.Ø
napkin L22
polymorphous light (sun) L56.4
recalcitrant pustular L13.8
ringed R23.8
skin (nonspecific) R21
creeping (meaning hookworm) B76.9
due to inoculation/vaccination (generalized) — *see also* Dermatitis, due to, vaccine L27.Ø
localized L27.1
erysipeloid A26.Ø
feigned L98.1
Kaposi's varicelliform BØØ.Ø
lichenoid L28.Ø
meaning dermatitis — *see* Dermatitis
toxic NEC L53.Ø
tooth, teeth, abnormal (incomplete) (late) (premature) (sequence) KØØ.6
vesicular R23.8
Erysipelas (gangrenous) (infantile) (newborn) (phlegmonous) (suppurative) A46
external ear A46 *[H62.4Ø]*
puerperal, postpartum O86.89
Erysipeloid A26.9
cutaneous (Rosenbach's) A26.Ø
disseminated A26.8
sepsis A26.7
specified NEC A26.8
Erythema, erythematous (infectional) (inflammation) L53.9
ab igne L59.Ø
annulare (centrifugum) (rheumaticum) L53.1
arthriticum epidemicum A25.1
brucellum — *see* Brucellosis
chronic figurate NEC L53.3
chronicum migrans (Borrelia burgdorferi) A69.2Ø
diaper L22
due to
chemical NEC L53.Ø
in contact with skin L24.5
drug (internal use) — *see* Dermatitis, due to, drugs
elevatum diutinum L95.1
endemic E52
epidemic, arthritic A25.1
figuratum perstans L53.3
gluteal L22
heat — *code by site under* Burn, first degree
ichthyosiforme congenitum bullous Q8Ø.3
in diseases classified elsewhere L54
induratum (nontuberculous) L52
tuberculous A18.4
infectiosum BØ8.3
intertrigo L3Ø.4
iris L51.9
marginatum L53.2
in (due to) acute rheumatic fever IØØ
medicamentosum — *see* Dermatitis, due to, drugs
migrans A26.Ø
chronicum A69.2Ø
tongue K14.1
multiforme (major) (minor) L51.9
bullous, bullosum L51.1
conjunctiva L51.1
nonbullous L51.Ø
pemphigoides L12.Ø
specified NEC L51.8
napkin L22
neonatorum P83.88
toxic P83.1
nodosum L52
tuberculous A18.4
palmar L53.8
pernio T69.1 ☑

Erythema, erythematous — *continued*
rash, newborn P83.88
scarlatiniform (recurrent) (exfoliative) L53.8
solare L55.Ø
specified NEC L53.8
toxic, toxicum NEC L53.Ø
newborn P83.1
tuberculous (primary) A18.4
Erythematous, erythematosus — *see* condition
Erythermalgia (primary) I73.81
Erythralgia I73.81
Erythrasma LØ8.1
Erythredema (polyneuropathy) — *see* Poisoning, mercury
Erythremia (acute) C94.Ø- ☑
chronic D45
secondary D75.1
Erythroblastopenia — *see also* Aplasia, red cell D6Ø.9
congenital D61.Ø1
Erythroblastophthisis D61.Ø9
Erythroblastosis (fetalis) (newborn) P55.9
due to
ABO (antibodies) (incompatibility) (isoimmunization) P55.1
Rh (antibodies) (incompatibility) (isoimmunization) P55.Ø
Erythrocyanosis (crurum) I73.89
Erythrocythemia — *see* Erythremia
Erythrocytosis (megalosplenic) (secondary) D75.1
familial D75.Ø
oval, hereditary — *see* Elliptocytosis
secondary D75.1
stress D75.1
Erythroderma (secondary) — *see also* Erythema L53.9
bullous ichthyosiform, congenital Q8Ø.3
desquamativum L21.1
ichthyosiform, congenital (bullous) Q8Ø.3
neonatorum P83.88
psoriaticum L4Ø.8
Erythrodysesthesia, palmar plantar (PPE) L27.1
Erythrogenesis imperfecta D61.Ø9
Erythroleukemia C94.Ø- ☑
Erythromelalgia I73.81
Erythrophagocytosis D75.89
Erythrophobia F4Ø.298
Erythroplakia, oral epithelium, and tongue K13.29
Erythroplasia (Queyrat) DØ7.4
specified site — *see* Neoplasm, skin, in situ
unspecified site DØ7.4
Escherichia coli (E. coli), **as cause of disease classified elsewhere** B96.2Ø
non-O157 Shiga toxin-producing (with known O group) B96.22
non-Shiga toxin-producing B96.29
O157 B96.21
O157 with confirmation of Shiga toxin when H antigen is unknown, or is not H7 B96.21
O157:H- (nonmotile) with confirmation of Shiga toxin B96.21
O157:H7 with or without confirmation of Shiga toxin-production B96.21
specified NEC B96.22
Shiga toxin-producing (with unspecified O group) (STEC) B96.23
specified NEC B96.29
Esophagismus K22.4
Esophagitis (acute) (alkaline) (chemical) (chronic) (infectional) (necrotic) (peptic) (postoperative) (without bleeding) K2Ø.9Ø
with bleeding K2Ø.91
candidal B37.81
due to gastrointestinal reflux disease (without bleeding) K21.ØØ
with bleeding K21.Ø1
eosinophilic K2Ø.Ø
reflux K21.ØØ
specified NEC (without bleeding) K2Ø.8Ø
with bleeding K2Ø.81
tuberculous A18.83
ulcerative K22.1Ø
with bleeding K22.11
Esophagocele K22.5
Esophagomalacia K22.89
Esophagospasm K22.4
Esophagostenosis K22.2
Esophagostomiasis B81.8
Esophagotracheal — *see* condition
Esophagus — *see* condition

Esophoria H5Ø.51
convergence, excess H51.12
divergence, insufficiency H51.8
Esotropia — *see* Strabismus, convergent concomitant
Espundia B55.2
Essential — *see* condition
Esthesioneuroblastoma C3Ø.Ø
Esthesioneurocytoma C3Ø.Ø
Esthesioneuroepithelioma C3Ø.Ø
Esthiomene A55
Estivo-autumnal malaria (fever) B5Ø.9
Estrangement (marital) Z63.5
parent-child NEC Z62.89Ø
Estriasis — *see* Myiasis
Ethanolism — *see* Alcoholism
Etherism — *see* Dependence, drug, inhalant
Ethmoid, ethmoidal — *see* condition
Ethmoiditis (chronic) (nonpurulent) (purulent) — *see also* Sinusitis, ethmoidal
influenzal — *see* Influenza, with, respiratory manifestations NEC
Woakes' J33.1
Ethylism — *see* Alcoholism
Eulenburg's disease (congenital paramyotonia) G71.19
Eumycetoma B47.Ø
Eunuchoidism E29.1
hypogonadotropic E23.Ø
European blastomycosis — *see* Cryptococcosis
Eustachian — *see* condition
Evaluation (for) (of)
development state
adolescent ZØØ.3
period of
delayed growth in childhood ZØØ.7Ø
with abnormal findings ZØØ.71
rapid growth in childhood ZØØ.2
puberty ZØØ.3
growth and developmental state (period of rapid growth) ZØØ.2
delayed growth ZØØ.7Ø
with abnormal findings ZØØ.71
mental health (status) ZØØ.8
requested by authority ZØ4.6
period of
delayed growth in childhood ZØØ.7Ø
with abnormal findings ZØØ.71
rapid growth in childhood ZØØ.2
suspected condition — *see* Observation
Evans syndrome D69.41
Event
apparent life threatening in newborn and infant (ALTE) R68.13
brief resolved unexplained event (BRUE) R68.13
Eventration — *see also* Hernia, ventral
colon into chest — *see* Hernia, diaphragm
diaphragm (congenital) Q79.1
Eversion
bladder N32.89
cervix (uteri) N86
with cervicitis N72
foot NEC — *see also* Deformity, valgus, ankle
congenital Q66.6
punctum lacrimale (postinfectional) (senile) HØ4.52- ☑
ureter (meatus) N28.89
urethra (meatus) N36.8
uterus N81.4
Evidence
cytologic
of malignancy on anal smear R85.614
of malignancy on cervical smear R87.614
of malignancy on vaginal smear R87.624
Evisceration
birth injury P15.8
traumatic NEC
eye — *see* Enucleated eye
Evulsion — *see* Avulsion
Ewing's sarcoma or tumor — *see* Neoplasm, bone, malignant
Examination (for) (following) (general) (of) (routine) ZØØ.ØØ
with abnormal findings ZØØ.Ø1
abuse, physical (alleged), ruled out
adult ZØ4.71
child ZØ4.72
adolescent (development state) ZØØ.3
alleged rape or sexual assault (victim), ruled out
adult ZØ4.41
child ZØ4.42

Examination — *continued*
- allergy ZØ1.82
- annual (adult) (periodic) (physical) ZØØ.ØØ
  - with abnormal findings ZØØ.Ø1
  - gynecological ZØ1.419
    - with abnormal findings ZØ1.411
- antibody response ZØ1.84
- blood — *see* Examination, laboratory
- blood pressure ZØ1.3Ø
  - with abnormal findings ZØ1.31
- cancer staging — *see* Neoplasm, malignant, by site
- cervical Papanicolaou smear Z12.4
  - as part of routine gynecological examination ZØ1.419
    - with abnormal findings ZØ1.411
- child (over 28 days old) ZØØ.129
  - with abnormal findings ZØØ.121
  - under 28 days old — *see* Newborn, examination
- clinical research control or normal comparison (control) (participant) ZØØ.6
- contraceptive (drug) maintenance (routine) Z3Ø.8
  - device (intrauterine) Z3Ø.431
- dental ZØ1.2Ø
  - with abnormal findings ZØ1.21
- developmental — *see* Examination, child
- donor (potential) ZØØ.5
- ear ZØ1.1Ø
  - with abnormal findings NEC ZØ1.118
- eye ZØ1.ØØ
  - with abnormal findings ZØ1.Ø1
  - following failed vision screening ZØ1.Ø2Ø
    - with abnormal findings ZØ1.Ø21
- follow-up (routine) (following) ZØ9
  - chemotherapy NEC ZØ9
    - malignant neoplasm ZØ8
  - fracture ZØ9
  - malignant neoplasm ZØ8
  - postpartum Z39.2
  - psychotherapy ZØ9
  - radiotherapy NEC ZØ9
    - malignant neoplasm ZØ8
  - surgery NEC ZØ9
    - malignant neoplasm ZØ8
- following
  - accident NEC ZØ4.3
    - transport ZØ4.1
    - work ZØ4.2
  - assault, alleged, ruled out
    - adult ZØ4.71
    - child ZØ4.72
  - motor vehicle accident ZØ4.1
  - treatment (for) ZØ9
    - combined NEC ZØ9
      - fracture ZØ9
      - malignant neoplasm ZØ8
    - malignant neoplasm ZØ8
    - mental disorder ZØ9
    - specified condition NEC ZØ9
- forced sexual exploitation ZØ4.81
- forced labor exploitation ZØ4.82
- gynecological ZØ1.419
  - with abnormal findings ZØ1.411
  - for contraceptive maintenance Z3Ø.8
- health — *see* Examination, medical
- hearing ZØ1.1Ø
  - with abnormal findings NEC ZØ1.118
  - following failed hearing screening ZØ1.11Ø
  - infant or child (over 28 days old) ZØØ.129
    - with abnormal findings ZØØ.121
- immunity status testing ZØ1.84
- laboratory (as part of a general medical examination) ZØØ.ØØ
  - with abnormal findings ZØØ.Ø1
  - preprocedural ZØ1.812
- lactating mother Z39.1
- medical (adult) (for) (of) ZØØ.ØØ
  - with abnormal findings ZØØ.Ø1
  - administrative purpose only ZØ2.9
    - specified NEC ZØ2.89
  - admission to
    - armed forces ZØ2.3
    - old age home ZØ2.2
    - prison ZØ2.89
    - residential institution ZØ2.2
    - school ZØ2.Ø
      - following illness or medical treatment ZØ2.Ø
    - summer camp ZØ2.89
  - adoption ZØ2.82
  - blood alcohol or drug level ZØ2.83

Examination — *continued*
- medical — *continued*
  - camp (summer) ZØ2.89
  - clinical research, normal subject (control) (participant) ZØØ.6
  - control subject in clinical research (normal comparison) (participant) ZØØ.6
  - donor (potential) ZØØ.5
  - driving license ZØ2.4
  - general (adult) ZØØ.ØØ
    - with abnormal findings ZØØ.Ø1
  - immigration ZØ2.89
  - insurance purposes ZØ2.6
  - marriage ZØ2.89
  - medicolegal reasons NEC ZØ4.89
  - naturalization ZØ2.89
  - participation in sport ZØ2.5
  - paternity testing ZØ2.81
  - population survey ZØØ.8
  - pre-employment ZØ2.1
  - pre-operative — *see* Examination, pre-procedural
  - pre-procedural
    - cardiovascular ZØ1.81Ø
    - respiratory ZØ1.811
    - specified NEC ZØ1.818
  - preschool children
    - for admission to school ZØ2.Ø
  - prisoners
    - for entrance into prison ZØ2.89
  - recruitment for armed forces ZØ2.3
  - specified NEC ZØØ.8
  - sport competition ZØ2.5
- medicolegal reason NEC ZØ4.89
- following
  - forced sexual exploitation ZØ4.81
  - forced labor exploitation ZØ4.82
- newborn — *see* Newborn, examination
- pelvic (annual) (periodic) ZØ1.419
  - with abnormal findings ZØ1.411
- period of rapid growth in childhood ZØØ.2
- periodic (adult) (annual) (routine) ZØØ.ØØ
  - with abnormal findings ZØØ.Ø1
- physical (adult) — *see also* Examination, medical ZØØ.ØØ
  - sports ZØ2.5
- postpartum
  - immediately after delivery Z39.Ø
  - routine follow-up Z39.2
- pre-chemotherapy (antineoplastic) ZØ1.818
- prenatal (normal pregnancy) — *see also* Pregnancy, normal Z34.9- ☑
- pre-procedural (pre-operative)
  - cardiovascular ZØ1.81Ø
  - laboratory ZØ1.812
  - respiratory ZØ1.811
  - specified NEC ZØ1.818
- prior to chemotherapy (antineoplastic) ZØ1.818
- psychiatric NEC ZØØ.8
  - follow-up not needing further care ZØ9
  - requested by authority ZØ4.6
- radiological (as part of a general medical examination) ZØØ.ØØ
  - with abnormal findings ZØØ.Ø1
- repeat cervical smear to confirm findings of recent normal smear following initial abnormal smear ZØ1.42
- skin (hypersensitivity) ZØ1.82
- special — *see also* Examination, by type ZØ1.89
  - specified type NEC ZØ1.89
- specified type or reason NEC ZØ4.89
- teeth ZØ1.2Ø
  - with abnormal findings ZØ1.21
- urine — *see* Examination, laboratory
- vision ZØ1.ØØ
  - with abnormal findings ZØ1.Ø1
  - following failed vision screening ZØ1.Ø2Ø
    - with abnormal findings ZØ1.Ø21
  - infant or child (over 28 days old) ZØØ.129
    - with abnormal findings ZØØ.121

Exanthem, exanthema — *see also* Rash
- with enteroviral vesicular stomatitis BØ8.4
- Boston A88.Ø
- epidemic with meningitis A88.Ø *[GØ2]*
- subitum BØ8.2Ø
  - due to human herpesvirus 6 BØ8.21
  - due to human herpesvirus 7 BØ8.22
- viral, virus BØ9
  - specified type NEC BØ8.8

Excess, excessive, excessively
- alcohol level in blood R78.Ø
- androgen (ovarian) E28.1
- attrition, tooth, teeth KØ3.Ø
- carotene, carotin (dietary) E67.1
- cold, effects of T69.9 ☑
  - specified effect NEC T69.8 ☑
- convergence H51.12
- crying
  - in child, adolescent, or adult R45.83
  - in infant R68.11
- development, breast N62
- divergence H51.8
- drinking (alcohol) NEC (without dependence) F1Ø.1Ø
  - habitual (continual) (without remission) F1Ø.2Ø
- eating R63.2
- estrogen E28.Ø
- fat — *see also* Obesity
  - in heart — *see* Degeneration, myocardial
  - localized E65
- foreskin N47.8
- gas R14.Ø
- glucagon E16.3
- heat — *see* Heat
- intermaxillary vertical dimension of fully erupted teeth M26.37
- interocclusal distance of fully erupted teeth M26.37
- kalium E87.5
- large
  - colon K59.39
    - congenital Q43.8
  - infant PØ8.Ø
  - organ or site, congenital NEC — *see* Anomaly, by site
- long
  - organ or site, congenital NEC — *see* Anomaly, by site
- menstruation (with regular cycle) N92.Ø
  - with irregular cycle N92.1
- napping Z72.821
- natrium E87.Ø
- number of teeth KØØ.1
- nutrient (dietary) NEC R63.2
- potassium (K) E87.5
- salivation K11.7
- secretion — *see also* Hypersecretion
  - milk O92.6
  - sputum RØ9.3
  - sweat R61
- sexual drive F52.8
- short
  - organ or site, congenital NEC — *see* Anomaly, by site
  - umbilical cord in labor or delivery O69.3 ☑
- skin L98.7
  - and subcutaneous tissue L98.7
  - eyelid (acquired) — *see* Blepharochalasis
    - congenital Q1Ø.3
- sodium (Na) E87.Ø
- spacing of fully erupted teeth M26.32
- sputum RØ9.3
- sweating R61
- thirst R63.1
  - due to deprivation of water T73.1 ☑
- transportation time Z59.82
- tuberosity of jaw M26.Ø7
- vitamin
  - A (dietary) E67.Ø
    - administered as drug (prolonged intake) — *see* Table of Drugs and Chemicals, vitamins, adverse effect
    - overdose or wrong substance given or taken — *see* Table of Drugs and Chemicals, vitamins, poisoning
  - D (dietary) E67.3
    - administered as drug (prolonged intake) — *see* Table of Drugs and Chemicals, vitamins, adverse effect
    - overdose or wrong substance given or taken — *see* Table of Drugs and Chemicals, vitamins, poisoning
- weight
  - gain R63.5
  - loss R63.4

Excitability, abnormal, under minor stress (personality disorder) F6Ø.3

Excitation
- anomalous atrioventricular I45.6

Exudate
- pleural — *see* Effusion, pleura
- retina H35.89
- wound fluids L24.A9

Exudative — *see* condition

Eye, eyeball, eyelid — *see* condition

Eyestrain — *see* Disturbance, vision, subjective

Eyeworm disease of Africa B74.3

F

Faber's syndrome (achlorhydric anemia) D5Ø.9

Fabry (-Anderson) **disease** E75.21

Facet syndrome M47.89- ☑

Faciocephalalgia, autonomic — *see also* Neuropathy, peripheral, autonomic G9Ø.Ø9

Factor(s)
- psychic, associated with diseases classified elsewhere F54
- psychological
  - affecting physical conditions F54
  - or behavioral
    - affecting general medical condition F54
    - associated with disorders or diseases classified elsewhere F54

Fahr disease (of brain) G23.8

Fahr Volhard disease (of kidney) I12.- ☑

Failure, failed
- abortion — *see* Abortion, attempted
- aortic (valve) I35.8
  - rheumatic IØ6.8
- attempted abortion — *see* Abortion, attempted
- biventricular I5Ø.82
  - due to left heart failure I5Ø.814
- bone marrow — *see* Anemia, aplastic
- cardiac — *see* Failure, heart
- cardiorenal (chronic) — *see also* Failure, renal, and Failure, heart I5Ø.9
  - hypertensive I13.2
- cardiorespiratory — *see also* Failure, heart RØ9.2
- cardiovascular (chronic) — *see* Failure, heart
- cerebrovascular I67.9
- cervical dilatation in labor O62.Ø
- circulation, circulatory (peripheral) R57.9
  - newborn P29.89
- compensation — *see* Disease, heart
- compliance with medical treatment or regimen — *see* Noncompliance
- congestive — *see* Failure, heart, congestive
- dental implant (endosseous) M27.69
  - due to
    - failure of dental prosthesis M27.63
    - lack of attached gingiva M27.62
    - occlusal trauma (poor prosthetic design) M27.62
    - parafunctional habits M27.62
    - periodontal infection (peri-implantitis) M27.62
    - poor oral hygiene M27.62
  - osseointegration M27.61
    - due to
      - complications of systemic disease M27.61
      - poor bone quality M27.61
    - iatrogenic M27.61
  - post-osseointegration
    - biological M27.62
    - due to complications of systemic disease M27.62
    - iatrogenic M27.62
    - mechanical M27.63
  - pre-integration M27.61
  - pre-osseointegration M27.61
  - specified NEC M27.69
- descent of head (at term) of pregnancy (mother) O32.4 ☑
- endosseous dental implant — *see* Failure, dental implant
- engagement of head (term of pregnancy) (mother) O32.4 ☑
- erection (penile) — *see also* Dysfunction, sexual, male, erectile N52.9
  - nonorganic F52.21
- examination(s), anxiety concerning Z55.2
- expansion terminal respiratory units (newborn) (primary) P28.Ø
- forceps NOS (with subsequent cesarean delivery) O66.5
- gain weight (child over 28 days old) R62.51
  - adult R62.7
  - newborn P92.6
- genital response (male) F52.21
  - female F52.22

Failure, failed — *continued*
- heart (acute) (senile) (sudden) I5Ø.9
  - with
    - acute pulmonary edema — *see* Failure, ventricular, left
    - decompensation I5Ø.9
      - with
        - normal ejection fraction I5Ø.33
        - preserved ejection fraction I5Ø.33
        - reduced ejection fraction I5Ø.23
          - with diastolic dysfunction I5Ø.43
      - combined systolic and diastolic I5Ø.43
      - diastolic I5Ø.33
      - right I5Ø.813
      - systolic I5Ø.23
    - dilatation — *see* Disease, heart
    - hypertension — *see* Hypertension, heart
    - normal ejection fraction — *see* Failure, heart, diastolic
    - preserved ejection fraction — *see* Failure, heart, diastolic
    - reduced ejection fraction — *see* Failure, heart, systolic
  - arteriosclerotic I7Ø.9Ø
  - biventricular I5Ø.82
    - due to left heart failure I5Ø.814
  - combined left-right sided I5Ø.82
    - due to left heart failure I5Ø.814
  - compensated — *see also* Failure, heart, by type as diastolic or systolic, chronic I5Ø.9
  - complicating
    - anesthesia (general) (local) or other sedation
      - in labor and delivery O74.2
      - in pregnancy O29.12- ☑
      - postpartum, puerperal O89.1
    - delivery (cesarean) (instrumental) O75.4
  - congestive I5Ø.9
    - with rheumatic fever (conditions in IØØ)
      - active IØ1.8
      - inactive or quiescent (with chorea) IØ9.81
    - newborn P29.Ø
    - rheumatic (chronic) (inactive) (with chorea) IØ9.81
      - active or acute IØ1.8
        - with chorea IØ2.Ø
  - decompensated — *see also* Failure, heart, by type as diastolic or systolic, acute and chronic I5Ø.9
  - degenerative — *see* Degeneration, myocardial
  - diastolic (congestive) (left ventricular) I5Ø.3Ø
    - acute (congestive) I5Ø.31
      - and (on) chronic (congestive) I5Ø.33
    - chronic (congestive) I5Ø.32
      - and (on) acute (congestive) I5Ø.33
    - combined with systolic (congestive) I5Ø.4Ø
      - acute (congestive) I5Ø.41
        - and (on) chronic (congestive) I5Ø.43
      - chronic (congestive) I5Ø.42
        - and (on) acute (congestive) I5Ø.43
  - due to presence of cardiac prosthesis I97.13- ☑
  - end stage — *see also* Failure, heart, by type as diastolic or systolic, chronic I5Ø.84
  - following cardiac surgery I97.13- ☑
  - high output NOS I5Ø.83
  - hypertensive — *see* Hypertension, heart
  - left (ventricular) — *see also* Failure, ventricular, left
    - combined diastolic and systolic — *see* Failure, heart, diastolic, combined with systolic
    - diastolic — *see* Failure, heart, diastolic
    - systolic — *see* Failure, heart, systolic
  - low output (syndrome) NOS I5Ø.9
  - newborn P29.Ø
  - organic — *see* Disease, heart
  - peripartum O9Ø.3
  - postprocedural I97.13- ☑
  - rheumatic (chronic) (inactive) IØ9.9
  - right (isolated) (ventricular) I5Ø.81Ø
    - acute I5Ø.811
      - and (on) chronic I5Ø.813
    - chronic I5Ø.812
      - and acute I5Ø.813
    - secondary to left heart failure I5Ø.814
  - specified NEC I5Ø.89

Note: heart failure stages A, B, C, and D are based on the American College of Cardiology and American Heart Association stages of heart failure, which complement and should not be confused with the New York Heart Association Classification of Heart Failure, into Class I, Class II, Class III, and Class IV

Failure, failed — *continued*
- heart — *continued*
  - stage A Z91.89
  - stage B — *see also* Failure, heart, by type as diastolic or systolic I5Ø.9
  - stage C — *see also* Failure, heart, by type as diastolic or systolic I5Ø.9
  - stage D — *see also* Failure, heart, by type as diastolic or systolic, chronic I5Ø.84
  - systolic (congestive) (left ventricular) I5Ø.2Ø
    - acute (congestive) I5Ø.21
      - and (on) chronic (congestive) I5Ø.23
    - chronic (congestive) I5Ø.22
      - and (on) acute (congestive) I5Ø.23
    - combined with diastolic (congestive) I5Ø.4Ø
      - acute (congestive) I5Ø.41
        - and (on) chronic (congestive) I5Ø.43
      - chronic (congestive) I5Ø.42
        - and (on) acute (congestive) I5Ø.43
  - thyrotoxic — *see also* Thyrotoxicosis EØ5.9Ø *[I43]*
    - with
      - high output — *see also* Thyrotoxicosis I5Ø.83
      - thyroid storm EØ5.91 *[I43]*
        - high output — *see also* Thyrotoxicosis I5Ø.83
  - valvular — *see* Endocarditis
- hepatic K72.9Ø
  - with coma K72.91
  - acute or subacute K72.ØØ
    - with coma K72.Ø1
    - due to drugs K71.1Ø
      - with coma K71.11
  - alcoholic (acute) (chronic) (subacute) K7Ø.4Ø
    - with coma K7Ø.41
  - chronic K72.1Ø
    - with coma K72.11
    - due to drugs (acute) (subacute) (chronic) K71.1Ø
      - with coma K71.11
  - due to drugs (acute) (subacute) (chronic) K71.1Ø
    - with coma K71.11
  - postprocedural K91.82
- hepatorenal K76.7
- induction (of labor) O61.9
  - abortion — *see* Abortion, attempted
  - by
    - oxytocic drugs O61.Ø
    - prostaglandins O61.Ø
  - instrumental O61.1
  - mechanical O61.1
  - medical O61.Ø
  - specified NEC O61.8
  - surgical O61.1
- intubation during anesthesia T88.4 ☑
  - in pregnancy O29.6- ☑
  - labor and delivery O74.7
  - postpartum, puerperal O89.6
- involution, thymus (gland) E32.Ø
- kidney — *see also* Disease, kidney, chronic N19
  - acute — *see also* Failure, renal, acute N17.9
- lactation (complete) O92.3
  - partial O92.4
- Leydig's cell, adult E29.1
- liver — *see* Failure, hepatic
- menstruation at puberty N91.Ø
- mitral IØ5.8
- myocardial, myocardium — *see also* Failure, heart I5Ø.9
  - chronic — *see also* Failure, heart, congestive I5Ø.9
  - congestive — *see also* Failure, heart, congestive I5Ø.9
- newborn screening — *see* Abnormal, neonatal screening
  - neonatal congenital heart disease PØ9.5
- orgasm (female) (psychogenic) F52.31
  - male F52.32
- ovarian (primary) E28.39
  - iatrogenic E89.4Ø
    - asymptomatic E89.4Ø
    - symptomatic E89.41
  - postprocedural (postablative) (postirradiation) (postsurgical) E89.4Ø
    - asymptomatic E89.4Ø
    - symptomatic E89.41
- ovulation causing infertility N97.Ø
- polyglandular, autoimmune E31.Ø
- prosthetic joint implant — *see* Complications, joint prosthesis, mechanical, breakdown, by site
- renal N19

- **Failure, failed** — *continued*
  - renal — *continued*
    - with
      - tubular necrosis (acute) N17.Ø
    - acute N17.9
      - with
        - cortical necrosis N17.1
        - medullary necrosis N17.2
        - tubular necrosis N17.Ø
      - specified NEC N17.8
    - chronic N18.9
      - hypertensive — *see* Hypertension, kidney
    - congenital P96.Ø
    - end stage (chronic) N18.6
      - due to hypertension I12.Ø
    - following
      - abortion — *see* Abortion by type complicated by specified condition NEC
      - crushing T79.5 ☑
      - ectopic or molar pregnancy OØ8.4
      - labor and delivery (acute) O9Ø.4
    - hypertensive — *see* Hypertension, kidney
    - postprocedural N99.Ø
  - respiration, respiratory J96.9Ø
    - with
      - hypercapnia J96.92
      - hypercarbia J96.92
      - hypoxia J96.91
    - acute J96.ØØ
      - with
        - hypercapnia J96.Ø2
        - hypercarbia J96.Ø2
        - hypoxia J96.Ø1
    - center G93.89
    - acute and (on) chronic J96.2Ø
      - with
        - hypercapnia J96.22
        - hypercarbia J96.22
        - hypoxia J96.21
    - chronic J96.1Ø
      - with
        - hypercapnia J96.12
        - hypercarbia J96.12
        - hypoxia J96.11
    - newborn P28.5
    - postprocedural (acute) J95.821
      - acute and chronic J95.822
  - rotation
    - cecum Q43.3
    - colon Q43.3
    - intestine Q43.3
    - kidney Q63.2
  - sedation (conscious) (moderate) during procedure T88.52 ☑
    - history of Z92.83
  - segmentation — *see also* Fusion
    - fingers — *see* Syndactylism, complex, fingers
    - vertebra Q76.49
      - with scoliosis Q76.3
  - seminiferous tubule, adult E29.1
  - senile (general) R54
  - sexual arousal (male) F52.21
    - female F52.22
  - testicular endocrine function E29.1
  - to thrive (child over 28 days old) R62.51
    - adult R62.7
    - newborn P92.6
  - transplant T86.92
    - bone T86.831
      - marrow T86.Ø2
    - cornea T86.841- ☑
    - heart T86.22
      - with lung(s) T86.32
    - intestine T86.851
    - kidney T86.12
    - liver T86.42
    - lung(s) T86.811
      - with heart T86.32
    - pancreas T86.891
    - skin (allograft) (autograft) T86.821
    - specified organ or tissue NEC T86.891
    - stem cell (peripheral blood) (umbilical cord) T86.5
  - trial of labor (with subsequent cesarean delivery) O66.4Ø
    - following previous cesarean delivery O66.41
  - tubal ligation N99.89
  - urinary — *see* Disease, kidney, chronic
- **Failure, failed** — *continued*
  - vacuum extraction NOS (with subsequent cesarean delivery) O66.5
  - vasectomy N99.89
  - ventouse NOS (with subsequent cesarean delivery) O66.5
  - ventricular — *see also* Failure, heart I5Ø.9
    - left — *see also* Failure, heart, left I5Ø.1
      - with rheumatic fever (conditions in IØØ)
        - active IØ1.8
          - with chorea IØ2.Ø
        - inactive or quiescent (with chorea) IØ9.81
      - rheumatic (chronic) (inactive) (with chorea) IØ9.81
        - active or acute IØ1.8
          - with chorea IØ2.Ø
    - right — *see* Failure, heart, right
  - vital centers, newborn P91.88
- **Fainting** (fit) R55
- **Fallen arches** — *see* Deformity, limb, flat foot
- **Falling, falls** (repeated) R29.6
  - any organ or part — *see* Prolapse
- **Fallopian**
  - insufflation Z31.41
  - tube — *see* condition
- **Fallot's**
  - pentalogy Q21.8
  - tetrad or tetralogy Q21.3
  - triad or trilogy Q22.3
- **False** — *see also* condition
  - croup J38.5
  - joint — *see* Nonunion, fracture
  - labor (pains) O47.9
    - at or after 37 completed weeks of gestation O47.1
    - before 37 completed weeks of gestation O47.Ø- ☑
  - passage, urethra (prostatic) N36.5
  - pregnancy F45.8
- **Family, familial** — *see also* condition
  - disruption Z63.8
    - involving divorce or separation Z63.5
  - Li-Fraumeni (syndrome) Z15.Ø1
  - planning advice Z3Ø.Ø9
  - problem Z63.9
    - specified NEC Z63.8
  - retinoblastoma C69.2- ☑
- **Famine** (effects of) T73.Ø ☑
  - edema — *see* Malnutrition, severe
- **Fanconi** (-de Toni)(-Debré) **syndrome** E72.Ø9
  - with cystinosis E72.Ø4
- **Fanconi's anemia** (congenital pancytopenia) D61.Ø9
- **Farber's disease or syndrome** E75.29
- **Farcy** A24.Ø
- **Farmer's**
  - lung J67.Ø
  - skin L57.8
- **Farsightedness** — *see* Hypermetropia
- **Fascia** — *see* condition
- **Fasciculation** R25.3
- **Fasciitis** M72.9
  - diffuse (eosinophilic) M35.4
  - infective M72.8
    - necrotizing M72.6
  - necrotizing M72.6
  - nodular M72.4
  - perirenal (with ureteral obstruction) N13.5
    - with infection N13.6
  - plantar M72.2
  - specified NEC M72.8
  - traumatic (old) M72.8
    - current — *code by* site under Sprain
- **Fascioliasis** B66.3
- **Fasciolopsis, fasciolopsiasis** (intestinal) B66.5
- **Fascioscapulohumeral myopathy** G71.Ø2
- **Fast pulse** RØØ.Ø
- **Fat**
  - embolism — *see* Embolism, fat
  - excessive — *see also* Obesity
    - in heart — *see* Degeneration, myocardial
  - in stool R19.5
  - localized (pad) E65
    - heart — *see* Degeneration, myocardial
    - knee M79.4
    - retropatellar M79.4
  - necrosis
    - breast N64.1
    - mesentery K65.4
    - omentum K65.4
  - pad E65
- **Fat** — *continued*
  - pad — *continued*
    - knee M79.4
- **Fatigue** R53.83
  - auditory deafness — *see* Deafness
  - chronic R53.82
  - combat F43.Ø
  - general R53.83
    - psychogenic F48.8
  - heat (transient) T67.6 ☑
  - muscle M62.89
  - myocardium — *see* Failure, heart
  - neoplasm-related R53.Ø
  - nervous, neurosis F48.8
  - operational F48.8
  - psychogenic (general) F48.8
  - senile R54
  - voice R49.8
- **Fatness** — *see* Obesity
- **Fatty** — *see also* condition
  - apron E65
  - degeneration — *see* Degeneration, fatty
  - heart (enlarged) — *see* Degeneration, myocardial
  - liver NEC K76.Ø
    - alcoholic K7Ø.Ø
    - nonalcoholic K76.Ø
  - necrosis — *see* Degeneration, fatty
- **Fauces** — *see* condition
- **Fauchard's disease** (periodontitis) — *see* Periodontitis
- **Faucitis** JØ2.9
- **Favism** (anemia) D55.Ø
- **Favus** — *see* Dermatophytosis
- **Fazio-Londe disease or syndrome** G12.1
- **Fear complex or reaction** F4Ø.9
- **Fear of** — *see* Phobia
- **Feared complaint unfounded** Z71.1
- **Febris, febrile** — *see also* Fever
  - flava — *see also* Fever, yellow A95.9
  - melitensis A23.Ø
  - pestis — *see* Plague
  - recurrens — *see* Fever, relapsing
  - rubra A38.9
- **Fecal**
  - incontinence R15.9
  - smearing R15.1
  - soiling R15.1
  - urgency R15.2
- **Fecalith** (impaction) K56.41
  - appendix K38.1
  - congenital P76.8
- **Fede's disease** K14.Ø
- **Feeble rapid pulse due to shock following injury** T79.4 ☑
- **Feeble-minded** F7Ø
- **Feeding**
  - difficulties R63.3Ø
  - problem (elderly) (infant) R63.39
    - newborn P92.9
      - specified NEC P92.8
    - nonorganic (adult) — *see* Disorder, eating
- **Feeling** (of)
  - foreign body in throat RØ9.89
- **Feer's disease** — *see* Poisoning, mercury
- **Feet** — *see* condition
- **Feigned illness** Z76.5
- **Feil-Klippel syndrome** (brevicollis) Q76.1
- **Feinmesser's** (hidrotic) **ectodermal dysplasia** Q82.4
- **Felinophobia** F4Ø.218
- **Felon** — *see also* Cellulitis, digit
  - with lymphangitis — *see* Lymphangitis, acute, digit
- **Felty's syndrome** MØ5.ØØ
  - ankle MØ5.Ø7- ☑
  - elbow MØ5.Ø2- ☑
  - foot joint MØ5.Ø7- ☑
  - hand joint MØ5.Ø4- ☑
  - hip MØ5.Ø5- ☑
  - knee MØ5.Ø6- ☑
  - multiple site MØ5.Ø9
  - shoulder MØ5.Ø1- ☑
  - vertebra — *see* Spondylitis, ankylosing
  - wrist MØ5.Ø3- ☑
- **Female genital cutting status** — *see* Female genital mutilation status (FGM)
- **Female genital mutilation status** (FGM) N9Ø.81Ø
  - specified NEC N9Ø.818
  - type I (clitorectomy status) N9Ø.811

- **Fibrosarcoma** — *continued*
  - infantile — *see* Neoplasm, connective tissue, malignant
  - odontogenic C41.1
    - upper jaw (bone) C41.Ø
  - periosteal — *see* Neoplasm, bone, malignant
- **Fibrosclerosis**
  - breast N6Ø.3- ☑
  - multifocal M35.5
  - penis (corpora cavernosa) N48.6
- **Fibrosis, fibrotic**
  - adrenal (gland) E27.8
  - amnion O41.8X- ☑
  - anal papillae K62.89
  - arteriocapillary — *see* Arteriosclerosis
  - bladder N32.89
    - interstitial — *see* Cystitis, chronic, interstitial
    - localized submucosal — *see* Cystitis, chronic, interstitial
    - panmural — *see* Cystitis, chronic, interstitial
  - breast — *see* Fibrosclerosis, breast
  - capillary — *see also* Arteriosclerosis I7Ø.9Ø
    - lung (chronic) — *see* Fibrosis, lung
  - cardiac — *see* Myocarditis
  - cervix N88.8
  - chorion O41.8X- ☑
  - corpus cavernosum (sclerosing) N48.6
  - cystic (of pancreas) E84.9
    - with
      - distal intestinal obstruction syndrome E84.19
      - fecal impaction E84.19
      - intestinal manifestations NEC E84.19
      - pulmonary manifestations E84.Ø
      - specified manifestations NEC E84.8
  - due to device, implant or graft — *see also* Complications, by site and type, specified NEC T85.828 ☑
    - arterial graft NEC T82.828 ☑
    - breast (implant) T85.828 ☑
    - catheter NEC T85.828 ☑
      - dialysis (renal) T82.828 ☑
        - intraperitoneal T85.828 ☑
      - infusion NEC T82.828 ☑
        - spinal (epidural) (subdural) T85.82Ø ☑
      - urinary (indwelling) T83.82 ☑
    - electronic (electrode) (pulse generator) (stimulator)
      - bone T84.82 ☑
      - cardiac T82.827 ☑
      - nervous system (brain) (peripheral nerve) (spinal) T85.82Ø ☑
      - urinary T83.82 ☑
    - fixation, internal (orthopedic) NEC T84.82 ☑
    - gastrointestinal (bile duct) (esophagus) T85.828 ☑
    - genital NEC T83.82 ☑
    - heart NEC T82.827 ☑
    - joint prosthesis T84.82 ☑
    - ocular (corneal graft) (orbital implant) NEC T85.828 ☑
    - orthopedic NEC T84.82 ☑
    - specified NEC T85.828 ☑
    - urinary NEC T83.82 ☑
    - vascular NEC T82.828 ☑
    - ventricular intracranial shunt T85.82Ø ☑
  - ejaculatory duct N5Ø.89
  - endocardium — *see* Endocarditis
  - endomyocardial (tropical) I42.3
  - epididymis N5Ø.89
  - eye muscle — *see* Strabismus, mechanical
  - heart — *see* Myocarditis
  - hepatic — *see* Fibrosis, liver
  - hepatolienal (portal hypertension) K76.6
  - hepatosplenic (portal hypertension) K76.6
  - infrapatellar fat pad M79.4
  - intrascrotal N5Ø.89
  - kidney N26.9
  - liver K74.ØØ
    - with sclerosis K74.2
    - advanced K74.Ø2
    - alcoholic K7Ø.2
    - early K74.Ø1
    - stage
      - F1 or F2 K74.Ø1
      - F3 K74.Ø2
  - lung (atrophic) (chronic) (confluent) (massive) (perialveolar) (peribronchial) J84.1Ø
    - with
      - anthracosilicosis J6Ø
      - anthracosis J6Ø
      - asbestosis J61

- **Fibrosis, fibrotic** — *continued*
  - lung — *continued*
    - with — *continued*
      - bagassosis J67.1
      - bauxite J63.1
      - berylliosis J63.2
      - byssinosis J66.Ø
      - calcicosis J62.8
      - chalicosis J62.8
      - dust reticulation J64
      - farmer's lung J67.Ø
      - ganister disease J62.8
      - graphite J63.3
      - pneumoconiosis NOS J64
      - siderosis J63.4
      - silicosis J62.8
    - capillary J84.1Ø
    - congenital P27.8
    - diffuse (idiopathic) J84.1Ø
      - chemicals, gases, fumes or vapors (inhalation) J68.4
      - interstitial J84.1Ø
        - acute J84.114
      - talc J62.Ø
    - following radiation J7Ø.1
    - idiopathic J84.112
    - postinflammatory J84.1Ø
    - silicotic J62.8
    - tuberculous — *see* Tuberculosis, pulmonary
  - lymphatic gland I89.8
  - median bar — *see* Hyperplasia, prostate
  - mediastinum (idiopathic) J98.59
  - meninges G96.198
  - myocardium, myocardial — *see* Myocarditis
  - ovary N83.8
  - oviduct N83.8
  - pancreas K86.89
  - penis NEC N48.6
  - pericardium I31.Ø
  - perineum, in pregnancy or childbirth O34.7- ☑
    - causing obstructed labor O65.5
  - pleura J94.1
  - popliteal fat pad M79.4
  - prostate (chronic) — *see* Hyperplasia, prostate
  - pulmonary — *see also* Fibrosis, lung J84.1Ø
    - congenital P27.8
    - idiopathic J84.112
  - rectal sphincter K62.89
  - retroperitoneal, idiopathic (with ureteral obstruction) N13.5
    - with infection N13.6
  - sclerosing mesenteric (idiopathic) K65.4
  - scrotum N5Ø.89
  - seminal vesicle N5Ø.89
  - senile R54
  - skin L9Ø.5
  - spermatic cord N5Ø.89
  - spleen D73.89
    - in schistosomiasis (bilharziasis) B65.9 *[D77]*
  - subepidermal nodular — *see* Neoplasm, skin, benign
  - submucous (oral) (tongue) K13.5
  - testis N44.8
    - chronic, due to syphilis A52.76
  - thymus (gland) E32.8
  - tongue, submucous K13.5
  - tunica vaginalis N5Ø.89
  - uterus (non-neoplastic) N85.8
  - vagina N89.8
  - valve, heart — *see* Endocarditis
  - vas deferens N5Ø.89
  - vein I87.8
- **Fibrositis** (periarticular) M79.7
  - nodular, chronic (Jaccoud's) (rheumatoid) — *see* Arthropathy, postrheumatic, chronic
- **Fibrothorax** J94.1
- **Fibrotic** — *see* Fibrosis
- **Fibrous** — *see* condition
- **Fibroxanthoma** — *see also* Neoplasm, connective tissue, benign
  - atypical — *see* Neoplasm, connective tissue, uncertain behavior
  - malignant — *see* Neoplasm, connective tissue, malignant
- **Fibroxanthosarcoma** — *see* Neoplasm, connective tissue, malignant
- **Fiedler's**
  - disease (icterohemorrhagic leptospirosis) A27.Ø
  - myocarditis (acute) I4Ø.1

- **Fifth disease** BØ8.3
  - venereal A55
- **Filaria, filarial, filariasis** — *see* Infestation, filarial
- **Filatov's disease** — *see* Mononucleosis, infectious
- **File-cutter's disease** — *see* Poisoning, lead
- **Filling defect**
  - biliary tract R93.2
  - bladder R93.41
  - duodenum R93.3
  - gallbladder R93.2
  - gastrointestinal tract R93.3
  - intestine R93.3
  - kidney R93.42- ☑
  - stomach R93.3
  - ureter R93.41
  - urinary organs, specified NEC R93.49
- **Fimbrial cyst** Q5Ø.4
- **Financial problem affecting care NOS** Z59.9
  - bankruptcy Z59.89
  - foreclosure on loan Z59.89
    - home loan Z59.81- ☑
  - strain Z59.86
- **Findings, abnormal, inconclusive, without diagnosis** — *see also* Abnormal
  - 17-ketosteroids, elevated R82.5
  - acetonuria R82.4
  - alcohol in blood R78.Ø
  - anisocytosis R71.8
  - antenatal screening of mother O28.9
    - biochemical O28.1
    - chromosomal O28.5
    - cytological O28.2
    - genetic O28.5
    - hematological O28.Ø
    - radiological O28.4
    - specified NEC O28.8
    - ultrasonic O28.3
  - antibody titer, elevated R76.Ø
  - anticardiolipin antibody R76.Ø
  - antiphosphatidylglycerol antibody R76.Ø
  - antiphosphatidylinositol antibody R76.Ø
  - antiphosphatidylserine antibody R76.Ø
  - antiphospholipid antibody R76.Ø
  - bacteriuria R82.71
  - bicarbonate E87.8
  - bile in urine R82.2
  - blood sugar R73.Ø9
    - high R73.9
    - low (transient) E16.2
  - body fluid or substance, specified NEC R88.8
  - casts, urine R82.998
  - catecholamines R82.5
  - cells, urine R82.998
  - chloride E87.8
  - cholesterol E78.9
    - high E78.ØØ
      - with high triglycerides E78.2
  - chyluria R82.Ø
  - cloudy
    - dialysis effluent R88.Ø
    - urine R82.9Ø
  - creatinine clearance R94.4
  - crystals, urine R82.998
  - culture
    - blood R78.81
    - positive — *see* Positive, culture
  - echocardiogram R93.1
  - electrolyte level, urinary R82.998
  - function study NEC R94.8
    - bladder R94.8
    - endocrine NEC R94.7
      - thyroid R94.6
    - kidney R94.4
    - liver R94.5
    - pancreas R94.8
    - placenta R94.8
    - pulmonary R94.2
    - spleen R94.8
  - gallbladder, nonvisualization R93.2
  - glucose (tolerance test) (non-fasting) R73.Ø9
  - glycosuria R81
  - heart
    - shadow R93.1
    - sounds RØ1.2
  - hematinuria R82.3
  - hematocrit drop (precipitous) R71.Ø
  - hemoglobinuria R82.3

- **Fit** — *continued*
  - fainting R55
  - hysterical F44.5
  - newborn P9Ø
- **Fitting** (and adjustment) (of)
  - artificial
    - arm — *see* Admission, adjustment, artificial, arm
    - breast Z44.3 ☑
    - eye Z44.2 ☑
    - leg — *see* Admission, adjustment, artificial, leg
  - automatic implantable cardiac defibrillator (with synchronous cardiac pacemaker) Z45.Ø2
  - brain neuropacemaker Z46.2
    - implanted Z45.42
  - cardiac defibrillator — *see* Fitting (and adjustment) (of), automatic implantable cardiac defibrillator
  - catheter, non-vascular Z46.82
  - colostomy belt Z46.89
  - contact lenses Z46.Ø
  - CRT-D (resynchronization therapy defibrillator) Z45.Ø2
  - CRT-P (cardiac resynchronization therapy pacemaker) Z45.Ø18
    - pulse generator Z45.Ø1Ø
  - cystostomy device Z46.6
  - defibrillator, cardiac — *see* Fitting (and adjustment) (of), automatic implantable cardiac defibrillator
  - dentures Z46.3
  - device NOS Z46.9
    - abdominal Z46.89
    - gastrointestinal NEC Z46.59
    - implanted NEC Z45.89
    - nervous system Z46.2
      - implanted — *see* Admission, adjustment, device, implanted, nervous system
    - orthodontic Z46.4
    - orthoptic Z46.Ø
    - orthotic Z46.89
    - prosthetic (external) Z44.9
      - breast Z44.3 ☑
      - dental Z46.3
      - eye Z44.2 ☑
      - specified NEC Z44.8
    - specified NEC Z46.89
    - substitution
      - auditory Z46.2
        - implanted — *see* Admission, adjustment, device, implanted, hearing device
      - nervous system Z46.2
        - implanted — *see* Admission, adjustment, device, implanted, nervous system
      - visual Z46.2
        - implanted Z45.31
    - urinary Z46.6
  - gastric lap band Z46.51
  - gastrointestinal appliance NEC Z46.59
  - glasses (reading) Z46.Ø
  - hearing aid Z46.1
  - ileostomy device Z46.89
  - insulin pump Z46.81
  - intestinal appliance NEC Z46.89
  - myringotomy device (stent) (tube) Z45.82
  - neuropacemaker Z46.2
    - implanted Z45.42
  - non-vascular catheter Z46.82
  - orthodontic device Z46.4
  - orthopedic device (brace) (cast) (corset) (shoes) Z46.89
  - pacemaker (cardiac) (cardiac resynchronization therapy (CRT-P)) Z45.Ø18
    - nervous system (brain) (peripheral nerve) (spinal cord) Z46.2
      - implanted Z45.42
    - pulse generator Z45.Ø1Ø
  - portacath (port-a-cath) Z45.2
  - prosthesis (external) Z44.9
    - arm — *see* Admission, adjustment, artificial, arm
    - breast Z44.3 ☑
    - dental Z46.3
    - eye Z44.2 ☑
    - leg — *see* Admission, adjustment, artificial, leg
    - specified NEC Z44.8
  - spectacles Z46.Ø
  - wheelchair Z46.89
- **Fitzhugh-Curtis syndrome**
  - due to
    - Chlamydia trachomatis A74.81
    - Neisseria gonorrhorea (gonococcal peritonitis) A54.85
- **Fitz's syndrome** (acute hemorrhagic pancreatitis) — *see also* Pancreatitis, acute K85.8Ø
- **Fixation**
  - joint — *see* Ankylosis
  - larynx J38.7
  - stapes — *see* Ankylosis, ear ossicles
    - deafness — *see* Deafness, conductive
  - uterus (acquired) — *see* Malposition, uterus
  - vocal cord J38.3
- **Flabby ridge** KØ6.8
- **Flaccid** — *see also* condition
  - palate, congenital Q38.5
- **Flail**
  - chest S22.5 ☑
    - associated with chest compression and cardiopulmonary resuscitation M96.A4
    - newborn (birth injury) P13.8
  - joint (paralytic) M25.2Ø
    - ankle M25.27- ☑
    - elbow M25.22- ☑
    - foot joint M25.27- ☑
    - hand joint M25.24- ☑
    - hip M25.25- ☑
    - knee M25.26- ☑
    - shoulder M25.21- ☑
    - specified joint NEC M25.28
    - wrist M25.23- ☑
- **Flajani's disease** — *see* Hyperthyroidism, with, goiter (diffuse)
- **Flap, liver** K71.3
- **Flashbacks** (residual to hallucinogen use) F16.283
- **Flat**
  - chamber (eye) — *see* Disorder, globe, hypotony, flat anterior chamber
  - chest, congenital Q67.8
  - foot (acquired) (fixed type) (painful) (postural) — *see also* Deformity, limb, flat foot
    - congenital (rigid) (spastic (everted)) Q66.5- ☑
    - rachitic sequelae (late effect) E64.3
  - organ or site, congenital NEC — *see* Anomaly, by site
  - pelvis M95.5
    - with disproportion (fetopelvic) O33.Ø
      - causing obstructed labor O65.Ø
    - congenital Q74.2
- **Flatau-Schilder disease** G37.Ø
- **Flatback syndrome** M4Ø.3Ø
  - lumbar region M4Ø.36
  - lumbosacral region M4Ø.37
  - thoracolumbar region M4Ø.35
- **Flattening**
  - head, femur M89.8X5
  - hip — *see* Coxa, plana
  - lip (congenital) Q18.8
  - nose (congenital) Q67.4
    - acquired M95.Ø
- **Flatulence** R14.3
  - psychogenic F45.8
- **Flatus** R14.3
  - vaginalis N89.8
- **Flax-dresser's disease** J66.1
- **Flea bite** — *see* Injury, bite, by site, superficial, insect
- **Flecks, glaucomatous** (subcapsular) — *see* Cataract, complicated
- **Fleischer** (-Kayser) **ring** (cornea) H18.Ø4- ☑
- **Fleshy mole** OØ2.Ø
- **Flexibilitas cerea** — *see* Catalepsy
- **Flexion**
  - amputation stump (surgical) T87.89
  - cervix — *see* Malposition, uterus
  - contracture, joint — *see* Contraction, joint
  - deformity, joint — *see also* Deformity, limb, flexion M21.2Ø
    - hip, congenital Q65.89
  - uterus — *see also* Malposition, uterus
    - lateral — *see* Lateroversion, uterus
- **Flexner-Boyd dysentery** AØ3.2
- **Flexner's dysentery** AØ3.1
- **Flexure** — *see* Flexion
- **Flint murmur** (aortic insufficiency) I35.1
- **Floater, vitreous** — *see* Opacity, vitreous
- **Floating**
  - cartilage (joint) — *see also* Loose, body, joint
    - knee — *see* Derangement, knee, loose body
  - gallbladder, congenital Q44.1
  - kidney N28.89
    - congenital Q63.8
  - spleen D73.89
- **Flooding** N92.Ø
- **Floor** — *see* condition
- **Floppy**
  - baby syndrome (nonspecific) P94.2
  - iris syndrome (intraoperative) (IFIS) H21.81
  - nonrheumatic mitral valve syndrome I34.1
- **Flu** — *see also* Influenza
  - avian — *see also* Influenza, due to, identified novel influenza A virus JØ9.X2
  - bird — *see also* Influenza, due to, identified novel influenza A virus JØ9.X2
  - intestinal NEC AØ8.4
  - swine (viruses that normally cause infections in pigs) — *see also* Influenza, due to, identified novel influenza A virus JØ9.X2
- **Fluctuating blood pressure** I99.8
- **Fluid**
  - abdomen R18.8
  - chest J94.8
  - heart — *see* Failure, heart, congestive
  - joint — *see* Effusion, joint
  - loss (acute) E86.9
  - lung — *see* Edema, lung
  - overload E87.7Ø
    - specified NEC E87.79
  - peritoneal cavity R18.8
  - pleural cavity J94.8
  - retention R6Ø.9
- **Flukes NEC** — *see also* Infestation, fluke
  - blood NEC — *see* Schistosomiasis
  - liver B66.3
- **Fluor** (vaginalis) N89.8
  - trichomonal or due to Trichomonas (vaginalis) A59.ØØ
- **Fluorosis**
  - dental KØØ.3
  - skeletal M85.1Ø
    - ankle M85.17- ☑
    - foot M85.17- ☑
    - forearm M85.13- ☑
    - hand M85.14- ☑
    - lower leg M85.16- ☑
    - multiple site M85.19
    - neck M85.18
    - rib M85.18
    - shoulder M85.11- ☑
    - skull M85.18
    - specified site NEC M85.18
    - thigh M85.15- ☑
    - toe M85.17- ☑
    - upper arm M85.12- ☑
    - vertebra M85.18
- **Flush syndrome** E34.Ø
- **Flushing** R23.2
  - menopausal N95.1
- **Flutter**
  - atrial or auricular I48.92
    - atypical I48.4
    - type I I48.3
    - type II I48.4
    - typical I48.3
  - heart I49.8
    - atrial or auricular I48.92
      - atypical I48.4
      - type I I48.3
      - type II I48.4
      - typical I48.3
    - ventricular I49.Ø2
  - ventricular I49.Ø2
- **FNHTR** (febrile nonhemolytic transfusion reaction) R5Ø.84
- **Fochier's abscess** — *code by* site under Abscess
- **Focus, Assmann's** — *see* Tuberculosis, pulmonary
- **Fogo selvagem** L1Ø.3
- **Foix-Alajouanine syndrome** G95.19
- **Fold, folds** (anomalous) — *see also* Anomaly, by site
  - Descemet's membrane — *see* Change, corneal membrane, Descemet's, fold
  - epicanthic Q1Ø.3
  - heart Q24.8
- **Folie à deux** F24
- **Follicle**
  - cervix (nabothian) (ruptured) N88.8
  - graafian, ruptured, with hemorrhage N83.Ø- ☑
  - nabothian N88.8
- **Follicular** — *see* condition
- **Folliculitis** (superficial) L73.9
  - abscedens et suffodiens L66.3
  - cyst N83.Ø- ☑

- **Folliculitis** — *continued*
  - decalvans L66.2
  - deep — *see* Furuncle, by site
  - gonococcal (acute) (chronic) A54.Ø1
  - keloid, keloidalis L73.Ø
  - pustular LØ1.Ø2
  - ulerythematosa reticulata L66.4
- **Folliculome lipidique**
  - specified site — *see* Neoplasm, benign, by site
  - unspecified site
    - female D27.9
    - male D29.2Ø
- **Følling's disease** E7Ø.Ø
- **Follow-up** — *see* Examination, follow-up
- **Fong's syndrome** (hereditary osteo-onychodysplasia) Q87.2
- **Food**
  - allergy L27.2
  - asphyxia (from aspiration or inhalation) — *see* Foreign body, by site
  - choked on — *see* Foreign body, by site
  - deprivation T73.Ø ☑
    - specified kind of food NEC E63.8
  - insecurity Z59.41
  - intoxication — *see* Poisoning, food
  - lack of T73.Ø ☑
  - poisoning — *see* Poisoning, food
  - rejection NEC — *see* Disorder, eating
  - strangulation or suffocation — *see* Foreign body, by site
  - toxemia — *see* Poisoning, food
- **Foot** — *see* condition
- **Foramen ovale** (nonclosure) (patent) (persistent) Q21.12
- **Forbes' glycogen storage disease** E74.Ø3
- **Fordyce-Fox disease** L75.2
- **Fordyce's disease** (mouth) Q38.6
- **Forearm** — *see* condition
- **Foreclosure on loan** Z59.89
- **Foreign body**
  - with
    - laceration — *see* Laceration, by site, with foreign body
    - puncture wound — *see* Puncture, by site, with foreign body
  - accidentally left following a procedure T81.5Ø9 ☑
    - aspiration T81.5Ø6 ☑
      - resulting in
        - adhesions T81.516 ☑
        - obstruction T81.526 ☑
        - perforation T81.536 ☑
        - specified complication NEC T81.596 ☑
    - cardiac catheterization T81.5Ø5 ☑
      - resulting in
        - acute reaction T81.6Ø ☑
          - aseptic peritonitis T81.61 ☑
          - specified NEC T81.69 ☑
        - adhesions T81.515 ☑
        - obstruction T81.525 ☑
        - perforation T81.535 ☑
        - specified complication NEC T81.595 ☑
    - causing
      - acute reaction T81.6Ø ☑
        - aseptic peritonitis T81.61 ☑
        - specified complication NEC T81.69 ☑
      - adhesions T81.519 ☑
      - aseptic peritonitis T81.61 ☑
      - obstruction T81.529 ☑
      - perforation T81.539 ☑
      - specified complication NEC T81.599 ☑
    - endoscopy T81.5Ø4 ☑
      - resulting in
        - adhesions T81.514 ☑
        - obstruction T81.524 ☑
        - perforation T81.534 ☑
        - specified complication NEC T81.594 ☑
    - immunization T81.5Ø3 ☑
      - resulting in
        - adhesions T81.513 ☑
        - obstruction T81.523 ☑
        - perforation T81.533 ☑
        - specified complication NEC T81.593 ☑
    - infusion T81.5Ø1 ☑
      - resulting in
        - adhesions T81.511 ☑
        - obstruction T81.521 ☑
        - perforation T81.531 ☑

- **Foreign body** — *continued*
  - accidentally left following a procedure — *continued*
    - infusion — *continued*
      - resulting in — *continued*
        - specified complication NEC T81.591 ☑
    - injection T81.5Ø3 ☑
      - resulting in
        - adhesions T81.513 ☑
        - obstruction T81.523 ☑
        - perforation T81.533 ☑
        - specified complication NEC T81.593 ☑
    - kidney dialysis T81.5Ø2 ☑
      - resulting in
        - adhesions T81.512 ☑
        - obstruction T81.522 ☑
        - perforation T81.532 ☑
        - specified complication NEC T81.592 ☑
    - packing removal T81.5Ø7 ☑
      - resulting in
        - acute reaction T81.6Ø ☑
          - aseptic peritonitis T81.61 ☑
          - specified NEC T81.69 ☑
        - adhesions T81.517 ☑
        - obstruction T81.527 ☑
        - perforation T81.537 ☑
        - specified complication NEC T81.597 ☑
    - puncture T81.5Ø6 ☑
      - resulting in
        - adhesions T81.516 ☑
        - obstruction T81.526 ☑
        - perforation T81.536 ☑
        - specified complication NEC T81.596 ☑
    - specified procedure NEC T81.5Ø8 ☑
      - resulting in
        - acute reaction T81.6Ø ☑
          - aseptic peritonitis T81.61 ☑
          - specified NEC T81.69 ☑
        - adhesions T81.518 ☑
        - obstruction T81.528 ☑
        - perforation T81.538 ☑
        - specified complication NEC T81.598 ☑
    - surgical operation T81.5ØØ ☑
      - resulting in
        - acute reaction T81.6Ø ☑
          - aseptic peritonitis T81.61 ☑
          - specified NEC T81.69 ☑
        - adhesions T81.51Ø ☑
        - obstruction T81.52Ø ☑
        - perforation T81.53Ø ☑
        - specified complication NEC T81.59Ø ☑
    - transfusion T81.5Ø1 ☑
      - resulting in
        - adhesions T81.511 ☑
        - obstruction T81.521 ☑
        - perforation T81.531 ☑
        - specified complication NEC T81.591 ☑
  - alimentary tract T18.9 ☑
    - anus T18.5 ☑
    - colon T18.4 ☑
    - esophagus — *see* Foreign body, esophagus
    - mouth T18.Ø ☑
    - multiple sites T18.8 ☑
    - rectosigmoid (junction) T18.5 ☑
    - rectum T18.5 ☑
    - small intestine T18.3 ☑
    - specified site NEC T18.8 ☑
    - stomach T18.2 ☑
  - anterior chamber (eye) SØ5.5- ☑
  - auditory canal — *see* Foreign body, entering through orifice, ear
  - bronchus T17.5Ø8 ☑
    - causing
      - asphyxiation T17.5ØØ ☑
        - food (bone) (seed) T17.52Ø ☑
        - gastric contents (vomitus) T17.51Ø ☑
        - specified type NEC T17.59Ø ☑
      - injury NEC T17.5Ø8 ☑
        - food (bone) (seed) T17.528 ☑
        - gastric contents (vomitus) T17.518 ☑
        - specified type NEC T17.598 ☑
  - canthus — *see* Foreign body, conjunctival sac
  - ciliary body (eye) SØ5.5- ☑
  - conjunctival sac T15.1- ☑
  - cornea T15.Ø- ☑
  - entering through orifice
    - accessory sinus T17.Ø ☑

- **Foreign body** — *continued*
  - entering through orifice — *continued*
    - alimentary canal T18.9 ☑
      - multiple parts T18.8 ☑
      - specified part NEC T18.8 ☑
    - alveolar process T18.Ø ☑
    - antrum (Highmore's) T17.Ø ☑
    - anus T18.5 ☑
    - appendix T18.4 ☑
    - auditory canal — *see* Foreign body, entering through orifice, ear
    - auricle — *see* Foreign body, entering through orifice, ear
    - bladder T19.1 ☑
    - bronchioles — *see* Foreign body, respiratory tract, specified site NEC
    - bronchus (main) — *see* Foreign body, bronchus
    - buccal cavity T18.Ø ☑
    - canthus (inner) — *see* Foreign body, conjunctival sac
    - cecum T18.4 ☑
    - cervix (canal) (uteri) T19.3 ☑
    - colon T18.4 ☑
    - conjunctival sac — *see* Foreign body, conjunctival sac
    - cornea — *see* Foreign body, cornea
    - digestive organ or tract NOS T18.9 ☑
      - multiple parts T18.8 ☑
      - specified part NEC T18.8 ☑
    - duodenum T18.3 ☑
    - ear (external) T16.- ☑
    - esophagus — *see* Foreign body, esophagus
    - eye (external) NOS T15.9- ☑
      - conjunctival sac — *see* Foreign body, conjunctival sac
      - cornea — *see* Foreign body, cornea
      - specified part NEC T15.8- ☑
    - eyeball — *see also* Foreign body, entering through orifice, eye, specified part NEC
      - with penetrating wound — *see* Puncture, eyeball
    - eyelid — *see also* Foreign body, conjunctival sac
      - with
        - laceration — *see* Laceration, eyelid, with foreign body
        - puncture — *see* Puncture, eyelid, with foreign body
        - superficial injury — *see* Foreign body, superficial, eyelid
    - gastrointestinal tract T18.9 ☑
      - multiple parts T18.8 ☑
      - specified part NEC T18.8 ☑
    - genitourinary tract T19.9 ☑
      - multiple parts T19.8 ☑
      - specified part NEC T19.8 ☑
    - globe — *see* Foreign body, entering through orifice, eyeball
    - gum T18.Ø ☑
    - Highmore's antrum T17.Ø ☑
    - hypopharynx — *see* Foreign body, pharynx
    - ileum T18.3 ☑
    - intestine (small) T18.3 ☑
      - large T18.4 ☑
    - lacrimal apparatus (punctum) — *see* Foreign body, entering through orifice, eye, specified part NEC
    - large intestine T18.4 ☑
    - larynx — *see* Foreign body, larynx
    - lung — *see* Foreign body, respiratory tract, specified site NEC
    - maxillary sinus T17.Ø ☑
    - mouth T18.Ø ☑
    - nasal sinus T17.Ø ☑
    - nasopharynx — *see* Foreign body, pharynx
    - nose (passage) T17.1 ☑
    - nostril T17.1 ☑
    - oral cavity T18.Ø ☑
    - palate T18.Ø ☑
    - penis T19.4 ☑
    - pharynx — *see* Foreign body, pharynx
    - piriform sinus — *see* Foreign body, pharynx
    - rectosigmoid (junction) T18.5 ☑
    - rectum T18.5 ☑
    - respiratory tract — *see* Foreign body, respiratory tract
    - sinus (accessory) (frontal) (maxillary) (nasal) T17.Ø ☑
      - piriform — *see* Foreign body, pharynx

- **Foreign body** — *continued*
  - entering through orifice — *continued*
    - small intestine T18.3 ☑
    - stomach T18.2 ☑
    - suffocation by — *see* Foreign body, by site
    - tear ducts or glands — *see* Foreign body, entering through orifice, eye, specified part NEC
    - throat — *see* Foreign body, pharynx
    - tongue T18.0 ☑
    - tonsil, tonsillar (fossa) — *see* Foreign body, pharynx
    - trachea — *see* Foreign body, trachea
    - ureter T19.8 ☑
    - urethra T19.0 ☑
    - uterus (any part) T19.3 ☑
    - vagina T19.2 ☑
    - vulva T19.2 ☑
  - esophagus T18.108 ☑
    - causing
      - injury NEC T18.108 ☑
        - food (bone) (seed) T18.128 ☑
        - gastric contents (vomitus) T18.118 ☑
        - specified type NEC T18.198 ☑
      - tracheal compression T18.100 ☑
        - food (bone) (seed) T18.120 ☑
        - gastric contents (vomitus) T18.110 ☑
        - specified type NEC T18.190 ☑
  - feeling of, in throat R09.89
  - fragment — *see* Retained, foreign body fragments (type of)
  - genitourinary tract T19.9 ☑
    - bladder T19.1 ☑
    - multiple parts T19.8 ☑
    - penis T19.4 ☑
    - specified site NEC T19.8 ☑
    - urethra T19.0 ☑
    - uterus T19.3 ☑
      - IUD Z97.5
    - vagina T19.2 ☑
      - contraceptive device Z97.5
    - vulva T19.2 ☑
  - granuloma (old) (soft tissue) — *see also* Granuloma, foreign body
    - skin L92.3
  - in
    - laceration — *see* Laceration, by site, with foreign body
    - puncture wound — *see* Puncture, by site, with foreign body
    - soft tissue (residual) M79.5
  - inadvertently left in operation wound — *see* Foreign body, accidentally left during a procedure
  - ingestion, ingested NOS T18.9 ☑
  - inhalation or inspiration — *see* Foreign body, by site
  - internal organ, not entering through a natural orifice — code as specific injury with foreign body
  - intraocular S05.5- ☑
    - old, retained (nonmagnetic) H44.70- ☑
      - anterior chamber H44.71- ☑
      - ciliary body H44.72- ☑
      - iris H44.72- ☑
      - lens H44.73- ☑
      - magnetic H44.60- ☑
        - anterior chamber H44.61- ☑
        - ciliary body H44.62- ☑
        - iris H44.62- ☑
        - lens H44.63- ☑
        - posterior wall H44.64- ☑
        - specified site NEC H44.69- ☑
        - vitreous body H44.65- ☑
      - posterior wall H44.74- ☑
      - specified site NEC H44.79- ☑
      - vitreous body H44.75- ☑
  - iris — *see* Foreign body, intraocular
  - lacrimal punctum — *see* Foreign body, entering through orifice, eye, specified part NEC
  - larynx T17.308 ☑
    - causing
      - asphyxiation T17.300 ☑
        - food (bone) (seed) T17.320 ☑
        - gastric contents (vomitus) T17.310 ☑
        - specified type NEC T17.390 ☑
      - injury NEC T17.308 ☑
        - food (bone) (seed) T17.328 ☑
        - gastric contents (vomitus) T17.318 ☑
        - specified type NEC T17.398 ☑
  - lens — *see* Foreign body, intraocular

- **Foreign body** — *continued*
  - ocular muscle S05.4- ☑
    - old, retained — *see* Foreign body, orbit, old
  - old or residual
    - soft tissue (residual) M79.5
  - operation wound, left accidentally — *see* Foreign body, accidentally left during a procedure
  - orbit S05.4- ☑
    - old, retained H05.5- ☑
  - pharynx T17.208 ☑
    - causing
      - asphyxiation T17.200 ☑
        - food (bone) (seed) T17.220 ☑
        - gastric contents (vomitus) T17.210 ☑
        - specified type NEC T17.290 ☑
      - injury NEC T17.208 ☑
        - food (bone) (seed) T17.228 ☑
        - gastric contents (vomitus) T17.218 ☑
        - specified type NEC T17.298 ☑
  - respiratory tract T17.908 ☑
    - bronchioles — *see* Foreign body, respiratory tract, specified site NEC
    - bronchus — *see* Foreign body, bronchus
    - causing
      - asphyxiation T17.900 ☑
        - food (bone) (seed) T17.920 ☑
        - gastric contents (vomitus) T17.910 ☑
        - specified type NEC T17.990 ☑
      - injury NEC T17.908 ☑
        - food (bone) (seed) T17.928 ☑
        - gastric contents (vomitus) T17.918 ☑
        - specified type NEC T17.998 ☑
    - larynx — *see* Foreign body, larynx
    - lung — *see* Foreign body, respiratory tract, specified site NEC
    - multiple parts — *see* Foreign body, respiratory tract, specified site NEC
    - nasal sinus T17.0 ☑
    - nasopharynx — *see* Foreign body, pharynx
    - nose T17.1 ☑
    - nostril T17.1 ☑
    - pharynx — *see* Foreign body, pharynx
    - specified site NEC T17.808 ☑
      - causing
        - asphyxiation T17.800 ☑
          - food (bone) (seed) T17.820 ☑
          - gastric contents (vomitus) T17.810 ☑
          - specified type NEC T17.890 ☑
        - injury NEC T17.808 ☑
          - food (bone) (seed) T17.828 ☑
          - gastric contents (vomitus) T17.818 ☑
          - specified type NEC T17.898 ☑
    - throat — *see* Foreign body, pharynx
    - trachea — *see* Foreign body, trachea
  - retained (old) (nonmagnetic) (in)
    - anterior chamber (eye) — *see* Foreign body, intraocular, old, retained, anterior chamber
      - magnetic — *see* Foreign body, intraocular, old, retained, magnetic, anterior chamber
    - ciliary body — *see* Foreign body, intraocular, old, retained, ciliary body
      - magnetic — *see* Foreign body, intraocular, old, retained, magnetic, ciliary body
    - eyelid H02.819
      - left H02.816
        - lower H02.815
        - upper H02.814
      - right H02.813
        - lower H02.812
        - upper H02.811
    - fragments — *see* Retained, foreign body fragments (type of)
    - globe — *see* Foreign body, intraocular, old, retained
      - magnetic — *see* Foreign body, intraocular, old, retained, magnetic
    - intraocular — *see* Foreign body, intraocular, old, retained
      - magnetic — *see* Foreign body, intraocular, old, retained, magnetic
    - iris — *see* Foreign body, intraocular, old, retained, iris
      - magnetic — *see* Foreign body, intraocular, old, retained, magnetic, iris
    - lens — *see* Foreign body, intraocular, old, retained, lens
      - magnetic — *see* Foreign body, intraocular, old, retained, magnetic, lens

- **Foreign body** — *continued*
  - retained — *continued*
    - muscle — *see* Foreign body, retained, soft tissue
    - orbit — *see* Foreign body, orbit, old
    - posterior wall of globe — *see* Foreign body, intraocular, old, retained, posterior wall
      - magnetic — *see* Foreign body, intraocular, old, retained, magnetic, posterior wall
    - retrobulbar — *see* Foreign body, orbit, old, retrobulbar
    - soft tissue M79.5
    - vitreous — *see* Foreign body, intraocular, old, retained, vitreous body
      - magnetic — *see* Foreign body, intraocular, old, retained, magnetic, vitreous body
  - retina S05.5- ☑
  - superficial, without open wound
    - abdomen, abdominal (wall) S30.851 ☑
    - alveolar process S00.552 ☑
    - ankle S90.55- ☑
    - antecubital space — *see* Foreign body, superficial, forearm
    - anus S30.857 ☑
    - arm (upper) S40.85- ☑
    - auditory canal — *see* Foreign body, superficial, ear
    - auricle — *see* Foreign body, superficial, ear
    - axilla — *see* Foreign body, superficial, arm
    - back, lower S30.850 ☑
    - breast S20.15- ☑
    - brow S00.85 ☑
    - buttock S30.850 ☑
    - calf — *see* Foreign body, superficial, leg
    - canthus — *see* Foreign body, superficial, eyelid
    - cheek S00.85 ☑
      - internal S00.552 ☑
    - chest wall — *see* Foreign body, superficial, thorax
    - chin S00.85 ☑
    - clitoris S30.854 ☑
    - costal region — *see* Foreign body, superficial, thorax
    - digit(s)
      - foot — *see* Foreign body, superficial, toe
      - hand — *see* Foreign body, superficial, finger
    - ear S00.45- ☑
    - elbow S50.35- ☑
    - epididymis S30.853 ☑
    - epigastric region S30.851 ☑
    - epiglottis S10.15 ☑
    - esophagus, cervical S10.15 ☑
    - eyebrow — *see* Foreign body, superficial, eyelid
    - eyelid S00.25- ☑
    - face S00.85 ☑
    - finger(s) S60.459 ☑
      - index S60.45- ☑
      - little S60.45- ☑
      - middle S60.45- ☑
      - ring S60.45- ☑
    - flank S30.851 ☑
    - foot (except toe(s) alone) S90.85- ☑
      - toe — *see* Foreign body, superficial, toe
    - forearm S50.85- ☑
      - elbow only — *see* Foreign body, superficial, elbow
    - forehead S00.85 ☑
    - genital organs, external
      - female S30.856 ☑
      - male S30.855 ☑
    - groin S30.851 ☑
    - gum S00.552 ☑
    - hand S60.55- ☑
    - head S00.95 ☑
      - ear — *see* Foreign body, superficial, ear
      - eyelid — *see* Foreign body, superficial, eyelid
      - lip S00.551 ☑
      - nose S00.35 ☑
      - oral cavity S00.552 ☑
      - scalp S00.05 ☑
      - specified site NEC S00.85 ☑
    - heel — *see* Foreign body, superficial, foot
    - hip S70.25- ☑
    - inguinal region S30.851 ☑
    - interscapular region S20.459 ☑
    - jaw S00.85 ☑
    - knee S80.25- ☑
    - labium (majus) (minus) S30.854 ☑
    - larynx S10.15 ☑
    - leg (lower) S80.85- ☑

Fracture, traumatic — *continued*
femur, femoral — *continued*
upper end — *continued*
intracapsular S72.Ø1- ☑
midcervical (displaced) S72.Ø3- ☑
nondisplaced S72.Ø3- ☑
neck S72.ØØ- ☑
base (displaced) S72.Ø4- ☑
nondisplaced S72.Ø4- ☑
specified NEC S72.Ø9- ☑
pertrochanteric — *see* Fracture, femur, upper end, trochanteric
physeal S79.ØØ- ☑
Salter-Harris type I S79.Ø1- ☑
specified NEC S79.Ø9- ☑
subcapital (displaced) S72.Ø1- ☑
subtrochanteric (displaced) S72.2- ☑
nondisplaced S72.2- ☑
transcervical — *see* Fracture, femur, upper end, midcervical
trochanteric S72.1Ø- ☑
greater (displaced) S72.11- ☑
nondisplaced S72.11- ☑
lesser (displaced) S72.12- ☑
nondisplaced S72.12- ☑
fibula (shaft) (styloid) S82.4Ø- ☑
comminuted (displaced) S82.45- ☑
nondisplaced S82.45- ☑
following insertion of implant, prosthesis or plate M96.67- ☑
involving ankle or malleolus — *see* Fracture, fibula, lateral malleolus
lateral malleolus (displaced) S82.6- ☑
nondisplaced S82.6- ☑
lower end
physeal S89.3Ø- ☑
Salter-Harris
Type I S89.31- ☑
Type II S89.32- ☑
specified NEC S89.39- ☑
specified NEC S82.83- ☑
torus S82.82- ☑
oblique (displaced) S82.43- ☑
nondisplaced S82.43- ☑
segmental (displaced) S82.46- ☑
nondisplaced S82.46- ☑
specified NEC S82.49- ☑
spiral (displaced) S82.44- ☑
nondisplaced S82.44- ☑
transverse (displaced) S82.42- ☑
nondisplaced S82.42- ☑
upper end
physeal S89.2Ø- ☑
Salter-Harris
Type I S89.21- ☑
Type II S89.22- ☑
specified NEC S89.29- ☑
specified NEC S82.83- ☑
torus S82.81- ☑
finger (except thumb) S62.6Ø- ☑
distal phalanx (displaced) S62.63- ☑
nondisplaced S62.66- ☑
index S62.6Ø- ☑
distal phalanx (displaced) S62.63- ☑
nondisplaced S62.66- ☑
middle phalanx (displaced) S62.62- ☑
nondisplaced S62.65- ☑
proximal phalanx (displaced) S62.61- ☑
nondisplaced S62.64- ☑
little S62.6Ø- ☑
distal phalanx (displaced) S62.63- ☑
nondisplaced S62.66- ☑
middle phalanx (displaced) S62.62- ☑
nondisplaced S62.65- ☑
proximal phalanx (displaced) S62.61- ☑
nondisplaced S62.64- ☑
middle S62.6Ø- ☑
distal phalanx (displaced) S62.63- ☑
nondisplaced S62.66- ☑
middle phalanx (displaced) S62.62- ☑
nondisplaced S62.65- ☑
proximal phalanx (displaced) S62.61- ☑
nondisplaced S62.64- ☑
middle phalanx (displaced) S62.62- ☑
nondisplaced S62.65- ☑
proximal phalanx (displaced) S62.61- ☑

Fracture, traumatic — *continued*
finger — *continued*
proximal phalanx — *continued*
nondisplaced S62.64- ☑
ring S62.6Ø- ☑
distal phalanx (displaced) S62.63- ☑
nondisplaced S62.66- ☑
middle phalanx (displaced) S62.62- ☑
nondisplaced S62.65- ☑
proximal phalanx (displaced) S62.61- ☑
nondisplaced S62.64- ☑
thumb — *see* Fracture, thumb
following insertion (intraoperative) (postoperative) of orthopedic implant, joint prosthesis or bone plate M96.69
femur M96.66- ☑
fibula M96.67- ☑
humerus M96.62- ☑
pelvis M96.65
radius M96.63- ☑
specified bone NEC M96.69
tibia M96.67- ☑
ulna M96.63- ☑
foot S92.9Ø- ☑
astragalus — *see* Fracture, tarsal, talus
calcaneus — *see* Fracture, tarsal, calcaneus
cuboid — *see* Fracture, tarsal, cuboid
cuneiform — *see* Fracture, tarsal, cuneiform
metatarsal — *see* Fracture, metatarsal
navicular — *see* Fracture, tarsal, navicular
sesamoid S92.81- ☑
specified NEC S92.81- ☑
talus — *see* Fracture, tarsal, talus
tarsal — *see* Fracture, tarsal
toe — *see* Fracture, toe
forearm S52.9- ☑
radius — *see* Fracture, radius
ulna — *see* Fracture, ulna
fossa (anterior) (middle) (posterior) SØ2.19 ☑
fragility — *see* Fracture, pathological, due to osteoporosis
frontal (bone) (skull) SØ2.Ø ☑
sinus SØ2.19 ☑
glenoid (cavity) (scapula) — *see* Fracture, scapula, glenoid cavity
greenstick — *see* Fracture, by site
hallux — *see* Fracture, toe, great
hand S62.9- ☑
carpal — *see* Fracture, carpal bone
finger (except thumb) — *see* Fracture, finger
metacarpal — *see* Fracture, metacarpal
navicular (scaphoid) (hand) — *see* Fracture, carpal bone, navicular
thumb — *see* Fracture, thumb
healed or old
with complications — *code by* Nature of the complication
heel bone — *see* Fracture, tarsal, calcaneus
Hill-Sachs S42.29- ☑
hip — *see* Fracture, femur, neck
humerus S42.3Ø- ☑
anatomical neck — *see* Fracture, humerus, upper end
articular process — *see* Fracture, humerus, lower end
capitellum — *see* Fracture, humerus, lower end, condyle, lateral
distal end — *see* Fracture, humerus, lower end
epiphysis
lower — *see* Fracture, humerus, lower end, physeal
upper — *see* Fracture, humerus, upper end, physeal
external condyle — *see* Fracture, humerus, lower end, condyle, lateral
following insertion of implant, prosthesis or plate M96.62- ☑
great tuberosity — *see* Fracture, humerus, upper end, greater tuberosity
intercondylar — *see* Fracture, humerus, lower end
internal epicondyle — *see* Fracture, humerus, lower end, epicondyle, medial
lesser tuberosity — *see* Fracture, humerus, upper end, lesser tuberosity
lower end S42.4Ø- ☑
condyle
lateral (displaced) S42.45- ☑

Fracture, traumatic — *continued*
humerus — *continued*
lower end — *continued*
condyle — *continued*
lateral — *continued*
nondisplaced S42.45- ☑
medial (displaced) S42.46- ☑
nondisplaced S42.46- ☑
epicondyle
lateral (displaced) S42.43- ☑
nondisplaced S42.43- ☑
medial (displaced) S42.44- ☑
incarcerated S42.44- ☑
nondisplaced S42.44- ☑
physeal S49.1Ø- ☑
Salter-Harris
Type I S49.11- ☑
Type II S49.12- ☑
Type III S49.13- ☑
Type IV S49.14- ☑
specified NEC S49.19- ☑
specified NEC (displaced) S42.49- ☑
nondisplaced S42.49- ☑
supracondylar (simple) (displaced) S42.41- ☑
with intercondylar fracture — *see* Fracture, humerus, lower end
comminuted (displaced) S42.42- ☑
nondisplaced S42.42- ☑
nondisplaced S42.41- ☑
torus S42.48- ☑
transcondylar (displaced) S42.47- ☑
nondisplaced S42.47- ☑
proximal end — *see* Fracture, humerus, upper end
shaft S42.3Ø- ☑
comminuted (displaced) S42.35- ☑
nondisplaced S42.35- ☑
greenstick S42.31- ☑
oblique (displaced) S42.33- ☑
nondisplaced S42.33- ☑
segmental (displaced) S42.36- ☑
nondisplaced S42.36- ☑
specified NEC S42.39- ☑
spiral (displaced) S42.34- ☑
nondisplaced S42.34- ☑
transverse (displaced) S42.32- ☑
nondisplaced S42.32- ☑
supracondylar — *see* Fracture, humerus, lower end
surgical neck — *see* Fracture, humerus, upper end, surgical neck
trochlea — *see* Fracture, humerus, lower end, condyle, medial
tuberosity — *see* Fracture, humerus, upper end
upper end S42.2Ø- ☑
anatomical neck — *see* Fracture, humerus, upper end, specified NEC
articular head — *see* Fracture, humerus, upper end, specified NEC
epiphysis — *see* Fracture, humerus, upper end, physeal
greater tuberosity (displaced) S42.25- ☑
nondisplaced S42.25- ☑
lesser tuberosity (displaced) S42.26- ☑
nondisplaced S42.26- ☑
physeal S49.ØØ- ☑
Salter-Harris
Type I S49.Ø1- ☑
Type II S49.Ø2- ☑
Type III S49.Ø3- ☑
Type IV S49.Ø4- ☑
specified NEC S49.Ø9- ☑
specified NEC (displaced) S42.29- ☑
nondisplaced S42.29- ☑
surgical neck (displaced) S42.21- ☑
four-part S42.24- ☑
nondisplaced S42.21- ☑
three-part S42.23- ☑
two-part (displaced) S42.22- ☑
nondisplaced S42.22- ☑
torus S42.27- ☑
transepiphyseal — *see* Fracture, humerus, upper end, physeal
hyoid bone S12.8 ☑
ilium S32.3Ø- ☑
with disruption of pelvic ring — *see* Disruption, pelvic ring
avulsion (displaced) S32.31- ☑

- **Fracture, traumatic** — *continued*
  - vertebra, vertebral — *continued*
    - lumbar — *continued*
      - first — *continued*
        - wedge compression S32.Ø1Ø ☑
      - fourth S32.Ø49 ☑
        - burst (stable) S32.Ø41 ☑
          - unstable S32.Ø42 ☑
        - specified type NEC S32.Ø48 ☑
        - wedge compression S32.Ø4Ø ☑
      - second S32.Ø29 ☑
        - burst (stable) S32.Ø21 ☑
          - unstable S32.Ø22 ☑
        - specified type NEC S32.Ø28 ☑
        - wedge compression S32.Ø2Ø ☑
      - specified type NEC S32.ØØ8 ☑
      - third S32.Ø39 ☑
        - burst (stable) S32.Ø31 ☑
          - unstable S32.Ø32 ☑
        - specified type NEC S32.Ø38 ☑
        - wedge compression S32.Ø3Ø ☑
      - wedge compression S32.ØØØ ☑
    - metastatic — *see* Collapse, vertebra, in, specified disease NEC — *see also* Neoplasm
    - newborn (birth injury) P11.5
    - sacrum S32.1Ø ☑
      - specified NEC S32.19 ☑
      - Type
        - 1 S32.14 ☑
        - 2 S32.15 ☑
        - 3 S32.16 ☑
        - 4 S32.17 ☑
      - Zone
        - I S32.119 ☑
          - displaced (minimally) S32.111 ☑
            - severely S32.112 ☑
          - nondisplaced S32.11Ø ☑
        - II S32.129 ☑
          - displaced (minimally) S32.121 ☑
            - severely S32.122 ☑
          - nondisplaced S32.12Ø ☑
        - III S32.139 ☑
          - displaced (minimally) S32.131 ☑
            - severely S32.132 ☑
          - nondisplaced S32.13Ø ☑
    - thoracic — *see* Fracture, thorax, vertebra
  - vertex SØ2.Ø ☑
  - vomer (bone) SØ2.2 ☑
  - wrist S62.1Ø- ☑
    - carpal — *see* Fracture, carpal bone
    - navicular (scaphoid) (hand) — *see* Fracture, carpal, navicular
  - xiphisternum, xiphoid (process) S22.24 ☑
    - associated with chest compression and cardiopulmonary resuscitation M96.A1
  - zygoma SØ2.4Ø2 ☑
    - left side SØ2.4ØF ☑
    - right side SØ2.4ØE ☑
- **Fragile, fragility**
  - autosomal site Q95.5
  - bone, congenital (with blue sclera) Q78.Ø
  - capillary (hereditary) D69.8
  - hair L67.8
  - nails L6Ø.3
  - non-sex chromosome site Q95.5
  - X chromosome Q99.2
- **Fragilitas**
  - crinium L67.8
  - ossium (with blue sclerae) (hereditary) Q78.Ø
  - unguium L6Ø.3
    - congenital Q84.6
- **Fragments, cataract** (lens), **following cataract surgery** H59.Ø2- ☑
  - retained foreign body — *see* Retained, foreign body fragments (type of)
- **Frailty** (frail) R54
  - mental R41.81
- **Frambesia, frambesial** (tropica) — *see also* Yaws
  - initial lesion or ulcer A66.Ø
  - primary A66.Ø
- **Frambeside**
  - gummatous A66.4
  - of early yaws A66.2
- **Frambesioma** A66.1
- **Franceschetti-Klein** (-Wildervanck) **disease or syndrome** Q75.4
- **Francis' disease** — *see* Tularemia
- **Franklin disease** C88.2
- **Frank's essential thrombocytopenia** D69.3
- **Fraser's syndrome** Q87.Ø
- **Freckle**(s) L81.2
  - malignant melanoma in — *see* Melanoma
  - melanotic (Hutchinson's) — *see* Melanoma, in situ
  - retinal D49.81
- **Frederickson's hyperlipoproteinemia, type**
  - I and V E78.3
  - IIA E78.ØØ
  - IIB and III E78.2
  - IV E78.1
- **Freeman Sheldon syndrome** Q87.Ø
- **Freezing** — *see also* Effect, adverse, cold T69.9 ☑
- **Freiberg's disease** (infraction of metatarsal head or osteochondrosis) — *see* Osteochondrosis, juvenile, metatarsus
- **Frei's disease** A55
- **Fremitus, friction, cardiac** RØ1.2
- **Frenum, frenulum**
  - external os Q51.828
  - tongue (shortening) (congenital) Q38.1
- **Frequency micturition** (nocturnal) R35.Ø
  - psychogenic F45.8
- **Frey's syndrome**
  - auriculotemporal G5Ø.8
  - hyperhidrosis L74.52
- **Friction**
  - burn — *see* Burn, by site
  - fremitus, cardiac RØ1.2
  - precordial RØ1.2
  - sounds, chest RØ9.89
- **Friderichsen-Waterhouse syndrome or disease** A39.1
- **Friedländer's B** (bacillus) **NEC** — *see also* condition A49.8
- **Friedreich's**
  - ataxia G11.11
  - combined systemic disease G11.11
  - facial hemihypertrophy Q67.4
  - sclerosis (cerebellum) (spinal cord) G11.11
- **Frigidity** F52.22
- **Fröhlich's syndrome** E23.6
- **Frontal** — *see also* condition
  - lobe syndrome FØ7.Ø
- **Frostbite** (superficial) T33.9Ø ☑
  - with
    - partial thickness skin loss — *see* Frostbite (superficial), by site
    - tissue necrosis T34.9Ø ☑
  - abdominal wall T33.3 ☑
    - with tissue necrosis T34.3 ☑
  - ankle T33.81- ☑
    - with tissue necrosis T34.81- ☑
  - arm T33.4- ☑
    - with tissue necrosis T34.4- ☑
    - finger(s) — *see* Frostbite, finger
    - hand — *see* Frostbite, hand
    - wrist — *see* Frostbite, wrist
  - ear T33.Ø1- ☑
    - with tissue necrosis T34.Ø1- ☑
  - face T33.Ø9 ☑
    - with tissue necrosis T34.Ø9 ☑
  - finger T33.53- ☑
    - with tissue necrosis T34.53- ☑
  - foot T33.82- ☑
    - with tissue necrosis T34.82- ☑
  - hand T33.52- ☑
    - with tissue necrosis T34.52- ☑
  - head T33.Ø9 ☑
    - with tissue necrosis T34.Ø9 ☑
    - ear — *see* Frostbite, ear
    - nose — *see* Frostbite, nose
  - hip (and thigh) T33.6- ☑
    - with tissue necrosis T34.6- ☑
  - knee T33.7- ☑
    - with tissue necrosis T34.7- ☑
  - leg T33.9- ☑
    - with tissue necrosis T34.9- ☑
    - ankle — *see* Frostbite, ankle
    - foot — *see* Frostbite, foot
    - knee — *see* Frostbite, knee
    - lower T33.7- ☑
      - with tissue necrosis T34.7- ☑
    - thigh — *see* Frostbite, hip
    - toe — *see* Frostbite, toe
  - limb
    - lower T33.99 ☑
- **Frostbite** — *continued*
  - limb — *continued*
    - lower — *continued*
      - with tissue necrosis T34.99 ☑
    - upper — *see* Frostbite, arm
  - neck T33.1 ☑
    - with tissue necrosis T34.1 ☑
  - nose T33.Ø2 ☑
    - with tissue necrosis T34.Ø2 ☑
  - pelvis T33.3 ☑
    - with tissue necrosis T34.3 ☑
  - specified site NEC T33.99 ☑
    - with tissue necrosis T34.99 ☑
  - thigh — *see* Frostbite, hip
  - thorax T33.2 ☑
    - with tissue necrosis T34.2 ☑
  - toes T33.83- ☑
    - with tissue necrosis T34.83- ☑
  - trunk T33.99 ☑
    - with tissue necrosis T34.99 ☑
  - wrist T33.51- ☑
    - with tissue necrosis T34.51- ☑
- **Frotteurism** F65.81
- **Frozen** — *see also* Effect, adverse, cold T69.9 ☑
  - pelvis (female) N94.89
    - male K66.8
  - shoulder — *see* Capsulitis, adhesive
- **Fructokinase deficiency** E74.11
- **Fructose 1,6 diphosphatase deficiency** E74.19
- **Fructosemia** (benign) (essential) E74.12
- **Fructosuria** (benign) (essential) E74.11
- **Fuchs'**
  - black spot (myopic) — *see also* Myopia, degenerative H44.2- ☑
  - dystrophy (corneal endothelium) H18.51- ☑
  - heterochromic cyclitis — *see* Cyclitis, Fuchs' heterochromic
- **Fucosidosis** E77.1
- **Fugue** R68.89
  - dissociative F44.1
  - hysterical (dissociative) F44.1
  - postictal in epilepsy — *see* Epilepsy
  - reaction to exceptional stress (transient) F43.Ø
- **Fulminant, fulminating** — *see* condition
- **Functional** — *see also* condition
  - bleeding (uterus) N93.8
- **Functioning, intellectual, borderline** R41.83
- **Fundus** — *see* condition
- **Fungemia NOS** B49
- **Fungus, fungous**
  - cerebral G93.89
  - disease NOS B49
  - infection — *see* Infection, fungus
- **Funiculitis** (acute) (chronic) (endemic) N49.1
  - gonococcal (acute) (chronic) A54.23
  - tuberculous A18.15
- **Funnel**
  - breast (acquired) M95.4
    - congenital Q67.6
    - sequelae (late effect) of rickets E64.3
  - chest (acquired) M95.4
    - congenital Q67.6
    - sequelae (late effect) of rickets E64.3
  - pelvis (acquired) M95.5
    - with disproportion (fetopelvic) O33.3 ☑
      - causing obstructed labor O65.3
    - congenital Q74.2
- **FUO** (fever of unknown origin) R5Ø.9
- **Furfur** L21.Ø
  - microsporon B36.Ø
- **Furrier's lung** J67.8
- **Furrowed** K14.5
  - nail(s) (transverse) L6Ø.4
    - congenital Q84.6
  - tongue K14.5
    - congenital Q38.3
- **Furuncle** LØ2.92
  - abdominal wall LØ2.221
  - ankle — *see* Furuncle, lower limb
  - antecubital space — *see* Furuncle, upper limb
  - anus K61.Ø
  - arm — *see* Furuncle, upper limb
  - auditory canal, external — *see* Abscess, ear, external
  - auricle (ear) — *see* Abscess, ear, external
  - axilla (region) LØ2.42- ☑
  - back (any part) LØ2.222
  - breast N61.1

G

- **Gain in weight** (abnormal) (excessive) — *see also* Weight, gain
- **Gaisböck's disease** (polycythemia hypertonica) D75.1
- **Gait abnormality** R26.9
  - ataxic R26.Ø
  - falling R29.6
  - hysterical (ataxic) (staggering) F44.4
  - paralytic R26.1
  - spastic R26.1
  - specified type NEC R26.89
  - staggering R26.Ø
  - unsteadiness R26.81
  - walking difficulty NEC R26.2
- **Galactocele** (breast) N64.89
  - puerperal, postpartum O92.79
- **Galactokinase deficiency** E74.29
- **Galactophoritis** N61.Ø
  - gestational, puerperal, postpartum O91.2- ☑
- **Galactorrhea** O92.6
  - not associated with childbirth N64.3
- **Galactosemia** (classic) (congenital) E74.21
- **Galactosuria** E74.29
- **Galacturia** R82.Ø
  - schistosomiasis (bilharziasis) B65.Ø
- **GALD** (gestational alloimmune liver disease) P78.84
- **Galeazzi's fracture** S52.37- ☑
- **Galen's vein** — *see* condition
- **Galeophobia** F4Ø.218
- **Gall duct** — *see* condition
- **Gallbladder** — *see also* condition
  - acute K81.Ø
- **Gallop rhythm** RØØ.8
- **Gallstone** (colic) (cystic duct) (gallbladder) (impacted) (multiple) — *see also* Calculus, gallbladder
  - with
    - cholecystitis — *see* Calculus, gallbladder, with cholecystitis
  - bile duct (common) (hepatic) — *see* Calculus, bile duct
  - causing intestinal obstruction K56.3
  - specified NEC K8Ø.8Ø
    - with obstruction K8Ø.81
- **Gambling** Z72.6
  - pathological (compulsive) F63.Ø
- **Gammopathy** (of undetermined significance [MGUS]) D47.2
  - associated with lymphoplasmacytic dyscrasia D47.2
  - monoclonal D47.2
  - polyclonal D89.Ø
- **Gamna's disease** (siderotic splenomegaly) D73.1
- **Gamophobia** F4Ø.298
- **Gampsodactylia** (congenital) Q66.7- ☑
- **Gamstorp's disease** (adynamia episodica hereditaria) G72.3
- **Gandy-Nanta disease** (siderotic splenomegaly) D73.1
- **Gang**
  - membership offenses Z72.81Ø
- **Gangliocytoma** D36.1Ø
- **Ganglioglioma** — *see* Neoplasm, uncertain behavior, by site
- **Ganglion** (compound) (diffuse) (joint) (tendon (sheath)) M67.4Ø
  - ankle M67.47- ☑
  - foot M67.47- ☑
  - forearm M67.43- ☑
  - hand M67.44- ☑
  - lower leg M67.46- ☑
  - multiple sites M67.49
  - of yaws (early) (late) A66.6
  - pelvic region M67.45- ☑
  - periosteal — *see* Periostitis
  - shoulder region M67.41- ☑
  - specified site NEC M67.48
  - thigh region M67.45- ☑
  - tuberculous A18.Ø9
  - upper arm M67.42- ☑
  - wrist M67.43- ☑
- **Ganglioneuroblastoma** — *see* Neoplasm, nerve, malignant
- **Ganglioneuroma** D36.1Ø
  - malignant — *see* Neoplasm, nerve, malignant
- **Ganglioneuromatosis** D36.1Ø
- **Ganglionitis**
  - fifth nerve — *see* Neuralgia, trigeminal
  - gasserian (postherpetic) (postzoster) BØ2.21
- **Ganglionitis** — *continued*
  - geniculate G51.1
    - newborn (birth injury) P11.3
    - postherpetic, postzoster BØ2.21
  - herpes zoster BØ2.21
  - postherpetic geniculate BØ2.21
- **Gangliosidosis** E75.1Ø
  - GM1 E75.19
  - GM2 E75.ØØ
    - other specified E75.Ø9
    - Sandhoff disease E75.Ø1
    - Tay-Sachs disease E75.Ø2
  - GM3 E75.19
  - mucolipidosis IV E75.11
- **Gangosa** A66.5
- **Gangrene, gangrenous** (connective tissue) (dropsical) (dry) (moist) (skin) (ulcer) — *see also* Necrosis I96
  - with diabetes (mellitus) — *see* Diabetes, with, gangrene
  - abdomen (wall) I96
  - alveolar M27.3
  - appendix K35.8Ø
    - with
      - peritonitis, localized — *see also* Appendicitis K35.31
  - arteriosclerotic (general) (senile) — *see* Arteriosclerosis, extremities, with, gangrene
  - auricle I96
  - Bacillus welchii A48.Ø
  - bladder (infectious) — *see* Cystitis, specified type NEC
  - bowel, cecum, or colon — *see* Gangrene, intestine
  - Clostridium perfringens or welchii A48.Ø
  - cornea H18.89- ☑
  - corpora cavernosa N48.29
    - noninfective N48.89
  - cutaneous, spreading I96
  - decubital — *see* Ulcer, pressure, by site
  - diabetic (any site) — *see* Diabetes, with, gangrene
  - emphysematous — *see* Gangrene, gas
  - epidemic — *see* Poisoning, food, noxious, plant
  - epididymis (infectional) N45.1
  - erysipelas — *see* Erysipelas
  - extremity (lower) (upper) I96
  - Fournier N49.3
    - female N76.82
      - vagina and vulva N76.82
  - fusospirochetal A69.Ø
  - gallbladder — *see* Cholecystitis, acute
  - gas (bacillus) A48.Ø
    - following
      - abortion — *see* Abortion by type complicated by infection
      - ectopic or molar pregnancy OØ8.Ø
  - glossitis K14.Ø
  - hernia — *see* Hernia, by site, with gangrene
  - intestine, intestinal (hemorrhagic) (massive) — *see also* Infarct, intestine K55.Ø69
    - with
      - mesenteric embolism — *see also* Infarct, intestine K55.Ø69
      - obstruction — *see* Obstruction, intestine
  - laryngitis JØ4.Ø
  - limb (lower) (upper) I96
  - lung J85.Ø
    - spirochetal A69.8
  - lymphangitis I89.1
  - Meleney's (synergistic) — *see* Ulcer, skin
  - mesentery — *see also* Infarct, intestine K55.Ø69
    - with
      - embolism — *see also* Infarct, intestine K55.Ø69
      - intestinal obstruction — *see* Obstruction, intestine
  - mouth A69.Ø
  - ovary — *see* Oophoritis
  - pancreas — *see* Pancreatitis, acute
  - penis N48.29
    - noninfective N48.89
  - perineum I96
  - pharynx — *see also* Pharyngitis
    - Vincent's A69.1
  - presenile I73.1
  - progressive synergistic — *see* Ulcer, skin
  - pulmonary J85.Ø
  - pulpal (dental) KØ4.1
  - quinsy J36
  - Raynaud's (symmetric gangrene) I73.Ø1
  - retropharyngeal J39.2
  - scrotum N49.3
    - noninfective N5Ø.89
- **Gangrene, gangrenous** — *continued*
  - senile (atherosclerotic) — *see* Arteriosclerosis, extremities, with, gangrene
  - spermatic cord N49.1
    - noninfective N5Ø.89
  - spine I96
  - spirochetal NEC A69.8
  - spreading cutaneous I96
  - stomatitis A69.Ø
  - symmetrical I73.Ø1
  - testis (infectional) N45.2
    - noninfective N44.8
  - throat — *see also* Pharyngitis
    - diphtheritic A36.Ø
    - Vincent's A69.1
  - thyroid (gland) EØ7.89
  - tooth (pulp) KØ4.1
  - tuberculous NEC — *see* Tuberculosis
  - tunica vaginalis N49.1
    - noninfective N5Ø.89
  - umbilicus I96
  - uterus — *see* Endometritis
  - uvulitis K12.2
  - vas deferens N49.1
    - noninfective N5Ø.89
  - vulva N76.82
- **Ganister disease** J62.8
- **Ganser's syndrome** (hysterical) F44.89
- **Gardner-Diamond syndrome** (autoerythrocyte sensitization) D69.2
- **Gargoylism** E76.Ø1
- **Garré's disease, osteitis** (sclerosing), osteomyelitis — *see* Osteomyelitis, specified type NEC
- **Garrod's pad, knuckle** M72.1
- **Gartner's duct**
  - cyst Q52.4
  - persistent Q5Ø.6
- **Gas** R14.3
  - asphyxiation, inhalation, poisoning, suffocation NEC — *see* Table of Drugs and Chemicals
  - excessive R14.Ø
  - gangrene A48.Ø
    - following
      - abortion — *see* Abortion by type complicated by infection
      - ectopic or molar pregnancy OØ8.Ø
  - on stomach R14.Ø
  - pains R14.1
- **Gastralgia** — *see also* Pain, abdominal
- **Gastrectasis** K31.Ø
  - psychogenic F45.8
- **Gastric** — *see* condition
- **Gastrinoma**
  - malignant
    - pancreas C25.4
    - specified site NEC — *see* Neoplasm, malignant, by site
    - unspecified site C25.4
  - specified site — *see* Neoplasm, uncertain behavior
  - unspecified site D37.9
- **Gastritis** (simple) K29.7Ø
  - with bleeding K29.71
  - acute (erosive) K29.ØØ
    - with bleeding K29.Ø1
  - alcoholic K29.2Ø
    - with bleeding K29.21
  - allergic K29.6Ø
    - with bleeding K29.61
  - atrophic (chronic) K29.4Ø
    - with bleeding K29.41
  - chronic (antral) (fundal) K29.5Ø
    - with bleeding K29.51
    - atrophic K29.4Ø
      - with bleeding K29.41
    - superficial K29.3Ø
      - with bleeding K29.31
  - dietary counseling and surveillance Z71.3
  - due to diet deficiency E63.9
  - eosinophilic K52.81
  - giant hypertrophic K29.6Ø
    - with bleeding K29.61
  - granulomatous K29.6Ø
    - with bleeding K29.61
  - hypertrophic (mucosa) K29.6Ø
    - with bleeding K29.61
  - nervous F54
  - spastic K29.6Ø
    - with bleeding K29.61

Glycogen
- infiltration — *see* Disease, glycogen storage
- storage disease — *see* Disease, glycogen storage

Glycogenosis (diffuse) (generalized) — *see also* Disease, glycogen storage
- cardiac E74.02 *[I43]*
- diabetic, secondary — *see* Diabetes, glycogenosis, secondary
- pulmonary interstitial J84.842

Glycopenia E16.2

Glycosuria R81
- renal E74.818

Gnathostoma spinigerum (infection) (infestation), **gnathostomiasis** (wandering swelling) B83.1

Goiter (plunging) (substernal) E04.9
- with
  - hyperthyroidism (recurrent) — *see* Hyperthyroidism, with, goiter
  - thyrotoxicosis — *see* Hyperthyroidism, with, goiter
- adenomatous — *see* Goiter, nodular
- cancerous C73
- congenital (nontoxic) E03.0
  - diffuse E03.0
  - parenchymatous E03.0
  - transitory, with normal functioning P72.0
- cystic E04.2
  - due to iodine-deficiency E01.1
- due to
  - enzyme defect in synthesis of thyroid hormone E07.1
  - iodine-deficiency (endemic) E01.2
- dyshormonogenetic (familial) E07.1
- endemic (iodine-deficiency) E01.2
  - diffuse E01.0
  - multinodular E01.1
- exophthalmic — *see* Hyperthyroidism, with, goiter
- iodine-deficiency (endemic) E01.2
  - diffuse E01.0
  - multinodular E01.1
  - nodular E01.1
- lingual Q89.2
- lymphadenoid E06.3
- malignant C73
- multinodular (cystic) (nontoxic) E04.2
  - toxic or with hyperthyroidism E05.20
    - with thyroid storm E05.21
- neonatal NEC P72.0
- nodular (nontoxic) (due to) E04.9
  - with
    - hyperthyroidism E05.20
      - with thyroid storm E05.21
    - thyrotoxicosis E05.20
      - with thyroid storm E05.21
  - endemic E01.1
  - iodine-deficiency E01.1
  - sporadic E04.9
  - toxic E05.20
    - with thyroid storm E05.21
- nontoxic E04.9
  - diffuse (colloid) E04.0
  - multinodular E04.2
  - simple E04.0
  - specified NEC E04.8
  - uninodular E04.1
- simple E04.0
- toxic — *see* Hyperthyroidism, with, goiter
- uninodular (nontoxic) E04.1
  - toxic or with hyperthyroidism E05.10
    - with thyroid storm E05.11

Goiter-deafness syndrome E07.1

Goldberg syndrome Q89.8

Goldberg-Maxwell syndrome E34.51

Goldblatt's hypertension or kidney I70.1

Goldenhar (-Gorlin) **syndrome** Q87.0

Goldflam-Erb disease or syndrome G70.00
- with exacerbation (acute) G70.01
- in crisis G70.01

Goldscheider's disease Q81.8

Goldstein's disease (familial hemorrhagic telangiectasia) I78.0

Golfer's elbow — *see* Epicondylitis, medial

Gonadoblastoma
- specified site — *see* Neoplasm, uncertain behavior, by site
- unspecified site
  - female D39.10
  - male D40.10

Gonecystitis — *see* Vesiculitis

Gongylonemiasis B83.8

Goniosynechiae — *see* Adhesions, iris, goniosynechiae

Gonococcemia A54.86

Gonococcus, gonococcal (disease) (infection) — *see also* condition A54.9
- anus A54.6
- bursa, bursitis A54.49
- conjunctiva, conjunctivitis (neonatorum) A54.31
- endocardium A54.83
- eye A54.30
  - conjunctivitis A54.31
  - iridocyclitis A54.32
  - keratitis A54.33
  - newborn A54.31
  - other specified A54.39
- fallopian tubes (acute) (chronic) A54.24
- genitourinary (organ) (system) (tract) (acute)
  - lower A54.00
    - with abscess (accessory gland) (periurethral) A54.1
  - upper — *see also* condition A54.29
- heart A54.83
- iridocyclitis A54.32
- joint A54.42
- lymphatic (gland) (node) A54.89
- meninges, meningitis A54.81
- musculoskeletal A54.40
  - arthritis A54.42
  - osteomyelitis A54.43
  - other specified A54.49
  - spondylopathy A54.41
- pelviperitonitis A54.24
- pelvis (acute) (chronic) A54.24
- pharynx A54.5
- proctitis A54.6
- pyosalpinx (acute) (chronic) A54.24
- rectum A54.6
- skin A54.89
- specified site NEC A54.89
- tendon sheath A54.49
- throat A54.5
- urethra (acute) (chronic) A54.01
  - with abscess (accessory gland) (periurethral) A54.1
- vulva (acute) (chronic) A54.02

Gonocytoma
- specified site — *see* Neoplasm, uncertain behavior, by site
- unspecified site
  - female D39.10
  - male D40.10

Gonorrhea (acute) (chronic) A54.9
- Bartholin's gland (acute) (chronic) (purulent) A54.02
  - with abscess (accessory gland) (periurethral) A54.1
- bladder A54.01
- cervix A54.03
- conjunctiva, conjunctivitis (neonatorum) A54.31
- contact Z20.2
- Cowper's gland (with abscess) A54.1
- exposure to Z20.2
- fallopian tube (acute) (chronic) A54.24
- kidney (acute) (chronic) A54.21
- lower genitourinary tract A54.00
  - with abscess (accessory gland) (periurethral) A54.1
- ovary (acute) (chronic) A54.24
- pelvis (acute) (chronic) A54.24
  - female pelvic inflammatory disease A54.24
- penis A54.09
- prostate (acute) (chronic) A54.22
- seminal vesicle (acute) (chronic) A54.23
- specified site not listed — *see also* Gonococcus A54.89
- spermatic cord (acute) (chronic) A54.23
- urethra A54.01
  - with abscess (accessory gland) (periurethral) A54.1
- vagina A54.02
- vas deferens (acute) (chronic) A54.23
- vulva A54.02

Goodall's disease A08.19

Goodpasture's syndrome M31.0

Gopalan's syndrome (burning feet) E53.0

Gorlin-Chaudry-Moss syndrome Q87.0

Gottron's papules L94.4

Gougerot-Blum syndrome (pigmented purpuric lichenoid dermatitis) L81.7

Gougerot-Carteaud disease or syndrome (confluent reticulate papillomatosis) L83

Gougerot's syndrome (trisymptomatic) L81.7

Gouley's syndrome (constrictive pericarditis) I31.1

Goundou A66.6

Gout, chronic — *see also* Gout, gouty M1A.9 ☑ *(following M08)*
- drug-induced M1A.20 ☑ *(following M08)*
  - ankle M1A.27- ☑ *(following M08)*
  - elbow M1A.22- ☑ *(following M08)*
  - foot joint M1A.27- ☑ *(following M08)*
  - hand joint M1A.24- ☑ *(following M08)*
  - hip M1A.25- ☑ *(following M08)*
  - knee M1A.26- ☑ *(following M08)*
  - multiple site M1A.29- ☑ *(following M08)*
  - shoulder M1A.21- ☑ *(following M08)*
  - vertebrae M1A.28 ☑ *(following M08)*
  - wrist M1A.23- ☑ *(following M08)*
- idiopathic M1A.00 ☑ *(following M08)*
  - ankle M1A.07- ☑ *(following M08)*
  - elbow M1A.02- ☑ *(following M08)*
  - foot joint M1A.07- ☑ *(following M08)*
  - hand joint M1A.04- ☑ *(following M08)*
  - hip M1A.05- ☑ *(following M08)*
  - knee M1A.06- ☑ *(following M08)*
  - multiple site M1A.09 ☑ *(following M08)*
  - shoulder M1A.01- ☑ *(following M08)*
  - vertebrae M1A.08 ☑ *(following M08)*
  - wrist M1A.03- ☑ *(following M08)*
- in (due to) renal impairment M1A.30 ☑ *(following M08)*
  - ankle M1A.37- ☑ *(following M08)*
  - elbow M1A.32- ☑ *(following M08)*
  - foot joint M1A.37- ☑ *(following M08)*
  - hand joint M1A.34- ☑ *(following M08)*
  - hip M1A.35- ☑ *(following M08)*
  - knee M1A.36- ☑ *(following M08)*
  - multiple site M1A.39 ☑ *(following M08)*
  - shoulder M1A.31- ☑ *(following M08)*
  - vertebrae M1A.38 ☑ *(following M08)*
  - wrist M1A.33- ☑ *(following M08)*
- lead-induced M1A.10 ☑ *(following M08)*
  - ankle M1A.17- ☑ *(following M08)*
  - elbow M1A.12- ☑ *(following M08)*
  - foot joint M1A.17- ☑ *(following M08)*
  - hand joint M1A.14- ☑ *(following M08)*
  - hip M1A.15- ☑ *(following M08)*
  - knee M1A.16- ☑ *(following M08)*
  - multiple site M1A.19 ☑ *(following M08)*
  - shoulder M1A.11- ☑ *(following M08)*
  - vertebrae M1A.18 ☑ *(following M08)*
  - wrist M1A.13- ☑ *(following M08)*
- primary — *see* Gout, chronic, idiopathic
- saturnine — *see* Gout, chronic, lead-induced
- secondary NEC M1A.40 ☑ *(following M08)*
  - ankle M1A.47- ☑ *(following M08)*
  - elbow M1A.42- ☑ *(following M08)*
  - foot joint M1A.47- ☑ *(following M08)*
  - hand joint M1A.44- ☑ *(following M08)*
  - hip M1A.45- ☑ *(following M08)*
  - knee M1A.46- ☑ *(following M08)*
  - multiple site M1A.49 ☑ *(following M08)*
  - shoulder M1A.41- ☑ *(following M08)*
  - vertebrae M1A.48 ☑ *(following M08)*
  - wrist M1A.43- ☑ *(following M08)*
- syphilitic — *see also* subcategory M14.8- A52.77
- tophi M1A.9 ☑ *(following M08)*

Gout, gouty (acute) (attack) (flare) — *see also* Gout, chronic M10.9
- drug-induced M10.20
  - ankle M10.27- ☑
  - elbow M10.22- ☑
  - foot joint M10.27- ☑
  - hand joint M10.24- ☑
  - hip M10.25- ☑
  - knee M10.26- ☑
  - multiple site M10.29
  - shoulder M10.21- ☑
  - vertebrae M10.28
  - wrist M10.23- ☑
- idiopathic M10.00
  - ankle M10.07- ☑
  - elbow M10.02- ☑
  - foot joint M10.07- ☑
  - hand joint M10.04- ☑
  - hip M10.05- ☑
  - knee M10.06- ☑
  - multiple site M10.09
  - shoulder M10.01- ☑
  - vertebrae M10.08
  - wrist M10.03- ☑
- in (due to) renal impairment M10.30

- **Gout, gouty** — *continued*
  - in renal impairment — *continued*
    - ankle M1Ø.37- ☑
    - elbow M1Ø.32- ☑
    - foot joint M1Ø.37- ☑
    - hand joint M1Ø.34- ☑
    - hip M1Ø.35- ☑
    - knee M1Ø.36- ☑
    - multiple site M1Ø.39
    - shoulder M1Ø.31- ☑
    - vertebrae M1Ø.38
    - wrist M1Ø.33- ☑
  - lead-induced M1Ø.1Ø
    - ankle M1Ø.17- ☑
    - elbow M1Ø.12- ☑
    - foot joint M1Ø.17- ☑
    - hand joint M1Ø.14- ☑
    - hip M1Ø.15- ☑
    - knee M1Ø.16- ☑
    - multiple site M1Ø.19
    - shoulder M1Ø.11- ☑
    - vertebrae M1Ø.18
    - wrist M1Ø.13- ☑
  - primary — *see* Gout, idiopathic
  - saturnine — *see* Gout, lead-induced
  - secondary NEC M1Ø.4Ø
    - ankle M1Ø.47- ☑
    - elbow M1Ø.42- ☑
    - foot joint M1Ø.47- ☑
    - hand joint M1Ø.44- ☑
    - hip M1Ø.45- ☑
    - knee M1Ø.46- ☑
    - multiple site M1Ø.49
    - shoulder M1Ø.41- ☑
    - vertebrae M1Ø.48
    - wrist M1Ø.43- ☑
  - syphilitic — *see also* subcategory M14.8- A52.77
  - tophi — *see* Gout, chronic
- **Gower's**
  - muscular dystrophy G71.Ø1
  - syndrome (vasovagal attack) R55
- **Gradenigo's syndrome** — *see* Otitis, media, suppurative, acute
- **Graefe's disease** — *see* Strabismus, paralytic, ophthalmoplegia, progressive
- **Graft-versus-host disease** D89.813
  - acute D89.81Ø
  - acute on chronic D89.812
  - chronic D89.811
- **Grain mite** (itch) B88.Ø
- **Grainhandler's disease or lung** J67.8
- **Grand mal** — *see* Epilepsy, generalized, specified NEC
- **Grand multipara status only** (not pregnant) Z64.1
  - pregnant — *see* Pregnancy, complicated by, grand multiparity
- **Granite worker's lung** J62.8
- **Granular** — *see also* condition
  - inflammation, pharynx J31.2
  - kidney (contracting) — *see* Sclerosis, renal
  - liver K74.69
- **Granulation tissue** (abnormal) (excessive) L92.9
  - postmastoidectomy cavity — *see* Complications, postmastoidectomy, granulation
- **Granulocytopenia** (primary) (malignant) — *see* Agranulocytosis
- **Granuloma** L92.9
  - abdomen K66.8
    - from residual foreign body L92.3
    - pyogenicum L98.Ø
  - actinic L57.5
  - annulare (perforating) L92.Ø
  - apical KØ4.5
  - aural — *see* Otitis, externa, specified NEC
  - beryllium (skin) L92.3
  - bone
    - eosinophilic C96.6
    - from residual foreign body — *see* Osteomyelitis, specified type NEC
    - lung C96.6
  - brain (any site) GØ6.Ø
    - schistosomiasis B65.9 *[GØ7]*
  - canaliculus lacrimalis — *see* Granuloma, lacrimal
  - candidal (cutaneous) B37.2
  - cerebral (any site) GØ6.Ø
  - coccidioidal (primary) (progressive) B38.7
    - lung B38.1
    - meninges B38.4
- **Granuloma** — *continued*
  - colon K63.89
  - conjunctiva H11.22- ☑
  - dental KØ4.5
  - ear, middle — *see* Cholesteatoma
  - eosinophilic C96.6
    - bone C96.6
    - lung C96.6
    - oral mucosa K13.4
    - skin L92.2
  - eyelid HØ1.8
  - facial (e) L92.2
  - foreign body (in soft tissue) NEC M6Ø.2Ø
    - ankle M6Ø.27- ☑
    - foot M6Ø.27- ☑
    - forearm M6Ø.23- ☑
    - hand M6Ø.24- ☑
    - in operation wound — *see* Foreign body, accidentally left during a procedure
    - lower leg M6Ø.26- ☑
    - pelvic region M6Ø.25- ☑
    - shoulder region M6Ø.21- ☑
    - skin L92.3
    - specified site NEC M6Ø.28
    - subcutaneous tissue L92.3
    - thigh M6Ø.25- ☑
    - upper arm M6Ø.22- ☑
  - gangraenescens M31.2
  - genito-inguinale A58
  - giant cell (central) (reparative) (jaw) M27.1
    - gingiva (peripheral) KØ6.8
  - gland (lymph) I88.8
  - hepatic NEC K75.3
    - in (due to)
      - berylliosis J63.2 *[K77]*
      - sarcoidosis D86.89
  - Hodgkin C81.9 ☑
  - ileum K63.89
  - infectious B99.9
    - specified NEC B99.8
  - inguinale (Donovan) (venereal) A58
  - intestine NEC K63.89
  - intracranial (any site) GØ6.Ø
  - intraspinal (any part) GØ6.1
  - iridocyclitis — *see* Iridocyclitis, chronic
  - jaw (bone) (central) M27.1
    - reparative giant cell M27.1
  - kidney — *see also* Infection, kidney N15.8
  - lacrimal HØ4.81- ☑
  - larynx J38.7
  - lethal midline (faciale(e)) M31.2
  - liver NEC — *see* Granuloma, hepatic
  - lung (infectious) — *see also* Fibrosis, lung
    - coccidioidal B38.1
    - eosinophilic C96.6
  - Majocchi's B35.8
  - malignant (facial(e)) M31.2
  - mandible (central) M27.1
  - midline (lethal) M31.2
  - monilial (cutaneous) B37.2
  - nasal sinus — *see* Sinusitis
  - operation wound T81.89 ☑
    - foreign body — *see* Foreign body, accidentally left during a procedure
    - stitch T81.89 ☑
    - talc — *see* Foreign body, accidentally left during a procedure
  - oral mucosa K13.4
  - orbit, orbital HØ5.11- ☑
  - paracoccidioidal B41.8
  - penis, venereal A58
  - periapical KØ4.5
  - peritoneum K66.8
    - due to ova of helminths NOS — *see also* Helminthiasis B83.9 *[K67]*
  - postmastoidectomy cavity — *see* Complications, postmastoidectomy, recurrent cholesteatoma
  - prostate N42.89
  - pudendi (ulcerating) A58
  - pulp, internal (tooth) KØ3.3
  - pyogenic, pyogenicum (of) (skin) L98.Ø
    - gingiva KØ6.8
    - maxillary alveolar ridge KØ4.5
    - oral mucosa K13.4
  - rectum K62.89
  - reticulohistiocytic D76.3
  - rubrum nasi L74.8
  - Schistosoma — *see* Schistosomiasis
- **Granuloma** — *continued*
  - septic (skin) L98.Ø
  - silica (skin) L92.3
  - sinus (accessory) (infective) (nasal) — *see* Sinusitis
  - skin L92.9
    - from residual foreign body L92.3
    - pyogenicum L98.Ø
  - spine
    - syphilitic (epidural) A52.19
    - tuberculous A18.Ø1
  - stitch (postoperative) T81.89 ☑
  - suppurative (skin) L98.Ø
  - swimming pool A31.1
  - talc — *see also* Granuloma, foreign body
    - in operation wound — *see* Foreign body, accidentally left during a procedure
  - telangiectaticum (skin) L98.Ø
  - tracheostomy J95.Ø9
  - trichophyticum B35.8
  - tropicum A66.4
  - umbilical P83.81
  - umbilicus P83.81
  - urethra N36.8
  - uveitis — *see* Iridocyclitis, chronic
  - vagina A58
  - venereum A58
  - vocal cord J38.3
- **Granulomatosis** L92.9
  - with polyangiitis M31.3- ☑
  - eosinophilic, with polyangiitis [EGPA] M3Ø.1
  - lymphoid C83.8- ☑
  - miliary (listerial) A32.89
  - necrotizing, respiratory M31.3Ø
  - progressive septic D71
  - specified NEC L92.8
  - Wegener's M31.3Ø
    - with renal involvement M31.31
- **Granulomatous tissue** (abnormal) (excessive) L92.9
- **Granulosis rubra nasi** L74.8
- **Graphite fibrosis** (of lung) J63.3
- **Graphospasm** F48.8
  - organic G25.89
- **Grating scapula** M89.8X1
- **Gravel** (urinary) — *see* Calculus, urinary
- **Graves' disease** — *see* Hyperthyroidism, with, goiter
- **Gravis** — *see* condition
- **Grawitz tumor** C64.- ☑
- **Gray syndrome** (newborn) P93.Ø
- **Grayness, hair** (premature) L67.1
  - congenital Q84.2
- **Green sickness** D5Ø.8
- **Greenfield's disease**
  - meaning
    - concentric sclerosis (encephalitis periaxialis concentrica) G37.5
    - metachromatic leukodystrophy E75.25
- **Greenstick fracture** — *code as* Fracture, by site
- **Grey syndrome** (newborn) P93.Ø
- **Grief** F43.21
  - complicated F34.81
  - prolonged F43.29
  - reaction — *see also* Disorder, adjustment F43.2Ø
- **Griesinger's disease** B76.Ø
- **Grinder's lung or pneumoconiosis** J62.8
- **Grinding, teeth**
  - psychogenic F45.8
  - sleep related G47.63
- **Grip**
  - Dabney's B33.Ø
  - devil's B33.Ø
- **Grippe, grippal** — *see also* Influenza
  - Balkan A78
  - summer, of Italy A93.1
- **Grisel's disease** M43.6
- **Groin** — *see* condition
- **Grooved tongue** K14.5
- **Ground itch** B76.9
- **Grover's disease or syndrome** L11.1
- **Growing pains, children** R29.898
- **Growth** (fungoid) (neoplastic) (new) — *see also* Neoplasm
  - adenoid (vegetative) J35.8
  - benign — *see* Neoplasm, benign, by site
  - malignant — *see* Neoplasm, malignant, by site
  - rapid, childhood ZØØ.2
  - secondary — *see* Neoplasm, secondary, by site
- **Gruby's disease** B35.Ø
- **Gubler-Millard paralysis or syndrome** G46.3

Hematocele
  female NEC N94.89
    with ectopic pregnancy OØØ.9Ø
      with intrauterine pregnancy OØØ.91
    ovary N83.8
  male N5Ø.1
Hematochezia — *see also* Melena K92.1
Hematochyluria — *see also* Infestation, filarial
  schistosomiasis (bilharziasis) B65.Ø
Hematocolpos (with hematometra or hematosalpinx) N89.7
Hematocornea — *see* Pigmentation, cornea, stromal
Hematogenous — *see* condition
Hematoma (traumatic) (skin surface intact) — *see also* Contusion
  with
    injury of internal organs — *see* Injury, by site
    open wound — *see* Wound, open
  amputation stump (surgical) (late) T87.89
  aorta, dissecting I71.ØØ
    abdominal I71.Ø2
    thoracic — *see also* Dissection, aorta, thoracic I71.Ø19
    thoracoabdominal I71.Ø3
  aortic intramural — *see* Dissection, aorta
  arterial (complicating trauma) — *see* Injury, blood vessel, by site
  auricle — *see* Contusion, ear
    nontraumatic — *see* Disorder, pinna, hematoma
  birth injury NEC P15.8
  brain (traumatic)
    with
      cerebral laceration or contusion (diffuse) — *see* Injury, intracranial, diffuse
        focal — *see* Injury, intracranial, focal
    cerebellar, traumatic SØ6.37- ☑
    intracerebral, traumatic — *see* Injury, intracranial, intracerebral hemorrhage
    newborn NEC P52.4
      birth injury P1Ø.1
    nontraumatic — *see* Hemorrhage, intracranial
    subarachnoid, arachnoid, traumatic — *see* Injury, intracranial, subarachnoid hemorrhage
    subdural, traumatic — *see* Injury, intracranial, subdural hemorrhage
  breast (nontraumatic) N64.89
  broad ligament (nontraumatic) N83.7
    traumatic S37.892 ☑
  cerebellar, traumatic SØ6.37- ☑
  cerebral — *see* Hematoma, brain
  cerebrum SØ6.36- ☑
    left SØ6.35- ☑
    right SØ6.34- ☑
  cesarean delivery wound O9Ø.2
  complicating delivery (perineal) (pelvic) (vagina) (vulva) O71.7
  corpus cavernosum (nontraumatic) N48.89
  epididymis (nontraumatic) N5Ø.1
  epidural (traumatic) — *see* Injury, intracranial, epidural hemorrhage
    spinal — *see* Injury, spinal cord, by region
  episiotomy O9Ø.2
  face, birth injury P15.4
  genital organ NEC (nontraumatic)
    female (nonobstetric) N94.89
      traumatic S3Ø.2Ø2 ☑
    male N5Ø.1
      traumatic S3Ø.2Ø1 ☑
  internal organs — *see* Injury, by site
  intracerebral, traumatic — *see* Injury, intracranial, intracerebral hemorrhage
  intraoperative — *see* Complications, intraoperative, hemorrhage
  labia (nontraumatic) (nonobstetric) N9Ø.89
  liver (subcapsular) (nontraumatic) K76.89
    birth injury P15.Ø
  mediastinum — *see* Injury, intrathoracic
  mesosalpinx (nontraumatic) N83.7
    traumatic S37.898 ☑
  muscle — code by site under Contusion
  nontraumatic
    muscle M79.81
    soft tissue M79.81
  obstetrical surgical wound O9Ø.2
  orbit, orbital (nontraumatic) — *see also* Hemorrhage, orbit
    traumatic — *see* Contusion, orbit

Hematoma — *continued*
  pelvis (female) (nontraumatic) (nonobstetric) N94.89
    obstetric O71.7
    traumatic — *see* Injury, by site
  penis (nontraumatic) N48.89
    birth injury P15.5
  perianal (nontraumatic) K64.5
  perineal S3Ø.23 ☑
    complicating delivery O71.7
  perirenal — *see* Injury, kidney
  pinna — *see* Contusion, ear
    nontraumatic — *see* Disorder, pinna, hematoma
  placenta O43.89- ☑
  postoperative (postprocedural) — *see* Complication, postprocedural, hematoma
  retroperitoneal (nontraumatic) K66.1
    traumatic S36.892 ☑
  scrotum, superficial S3Ø.22 ☑
    birth injury P15.5
  seminal vesicle (nontraumatic) N5Ø.1
    traumatic S37.892 ☑
  spermatic cord (traumatic) S37.892 ☑
    nontraumatic N5Ø.1
  spinal (cord) (meninges) — *see also* Injury, spinal cord, by region
    newborn (birth injury) P11.5
  spleen D73.5
    intraoperative — *see* Complications, intraoperative, hemorrhage, spleen
    postprocedural (postoperative) — *see* Complications, postprocedural, hemorrhage, spleen
  sternocleidomastoid, birth injury P15.2
  sternomastoid, birth injury P15.2
  subarachnoid (traumatic) — *see* Injury, intracranial, subarachnoid hemorrhage
    newborn (nontraumatic) P52.5
      due to birth injury P1Ø.3
    nontraumatic — *see* Hemorrhage, intracranial, subarachnoid
  subdural (traumatic) — *see* Injury, intracranial, subdural hemorrhage
    newborn (localized) P52.8
      birth injury P1Ø.Ø
    nontraumatic — *see* Hemorrhage, intracranial, subdural
  superficial, newborn P54.5
  testis (nontraumatic) N5Ø.1
    birth injury P15.5
  tunica vaginalis (nontraumatic) N5Ø.1
  umbilical cord, complicating delivery O69.5 ☑
  uterine ligament (broad) (nontraumatic) N83.7
    traumatic S37.892 ☑
  vagina (ruptured) (nontraumatic) N89.8
    complicating delivery O71.7
  vas deferens (nontraumatic) N5Ø.1
    traumatic S37.892 ☑
  vitreous — *see* Hemorrhage, vitreous
  vulva (nontraumatic) (nonobstetric) N9Ø.89
    complicating delivery O71.7
    newborn (birth injury) P15.5
Hematometra N85.7
  with hematocolpos N89.7
Hematomyelia (central) G95.19
  newborn (birth injury) P11.5
  traumatic T14.8 ☑
Hematomyelitis GØ4.9Ø
Hematoperitoneum — *see* Hemoperitoneum
Hematophobia F4Ø.23Ø
Hematopneumothorax (see Hemothorax)
Hematopoiesis, cyclic D7Ø.4
Hematoporphyria — *see* Porphyria
Hematorachis, hematorrhachis G95.19
  newborn (birth injury) P11.5
Hematosalpinx N83.6
  with
    hematocolpos N89.7
    hematometra N85.7
      with hematocolpos N89.7
  infectional — *see* Salpingitis
Hematospermia R36.1
Hematothorax (see Hemothorax)
Hematuria R31.9
  benign (familial) (of childhood) — *see also* Hematuria, idiopathic
    essential microscopic R31.1
  due to sulphonamide, sulfonamide — *see* Table of Drugs and Chemicals, by drug

Hematuria — *continued*
  endemic — *see also* Schistosomiasis B65.Ø
  gross R31.Ø
  idiopathic NØ2.9
    with glomerular lesion
      C3
        glomerulonephritis NØ2.A
        glomerulopathy NØ2.A
          with dense deposit disease NØ2.6
      crescentic (diffuse) glomerulonephritis NØ2.7
      dense deposit disease NØ2.6
      endocapillary proliferative glomerulonephritis NØ2.4
      focal and segmental hyalinosis or sclerosis NØ2.1
      membranoproliferative (diffuse) NØ2.5
      membranous (diffuse) NØ2.2
      mesangial proliferative (diffuse) NØ2.3
      mesangiocapillary (diffuse) NØ2.5
      minor abnormality NØ2.Ø
      proliferative NEC NØ2.8
      specified pathology NEC NØ2.8
  intermittent — *see* Hematuria, idiopathic
  malarial B5Ø.8
  microscopic NEC (with symptoms) R31.29
    asymptomatic R31.21
    benign essential R31.1
  paroxysmal — *see also* Hematuria, idiopathic
    nocturnal D59.5
  persistent — *see* Hematuria, idiopathic
  recurrent — *see* Hematuria, idiopathic
  tropical — *see also* Schistosomiasis B65.Ø
  tuberculous A18.13
Hemeralopia (day blindness) H53.11
  vitamin A deficiency E5Ø.5
Hemi-akinesia R41.4
Hemianalgesia R2Ø.Ø
Hemianencephaly QØØ.Ø
Hemianesthesia R2Ø.Ø
Hemianopia, hemianopsia (heteronymous) H53.47
  homonymous H53.46- ☑
  syphilitic A52.71
Hemiathetosis R25.8
Hemiatrophy R68.89
  cerebellar G31.9
  face, facial, progressive (Romberg) G51.8
  tongue K14.8
Hemiballism (us) G25.5
Hemicardia Q24.8
Hemicephalus, hemicephaly QØØ.Ø
Hemichorea G25.5
Hemicolitis, left — *see* Colitis, left sided
Hemicrania
  congenital malformation QØØ.Ø
  continua G44.51
  meaning migraine — *see also* Migraine G43.9Ø9
  paroxysmal G44.Ø39
    chronic G44.Ø49
      intractable G44.Ø41
      not intractable G44.Ø49
    episodic G44.Ø39
      intractable G44.Ø31
      not intractable G44.Ø39
    intractable G44.Ø31
    not intractable G44.Ø39
Hemidystrophy — *see* Hemiatrophy
Hemiectromelia Q73.8
Hemihypalgesia R2Ø.8
Hemihypesthesia R2Ø.1
Hemi-inattention R41.4
Hemimelia Q73.8
  lower limb — *see* Defect, reduction, lower limb, specified type NEC
  upper limb — *see* Defect, reduction, upper limb, specified type NEC
Hemiparalysis — *see* Hemiplegia
Hemiparesis — *see* Hemiplegia
Hemiparesthesia R2Ø.2
Hemiparkinsonism G2Ø
Hemiplegia G81.9- ☑
  alternans facialis G83.89
  ascending NEC G81.9Ø
    spinal G95.89
  congenital (cerebral) G8Ø.8
    spastic G8Ø.2
  embolic (current episode) I63.4- ☑
  flaccid G81.Ø- ☑
  following
    cerebrovascular disease I69.959

Hemorrhage, hemorrhagic — *continued*
- epicranial subaponeurotic (massive), birth injury P12.2
- epidural (traumatic) — *see also* Injury, intracranial, epidural hemorrhage
  - nontraumatic I62.1
- esophagus K22.89
  - varix I85.Ø1
    - secondary I85.11
- excessive, following ectopic gestation (subsequent episode) OØ8.1
- extradural (traumatic) — *see* Injury, intracranial, epidural hemorrhage
  - birth injury P1Ø.8
  - newborn (anoxic) (nontraumatic) P52.8
  - nontraumatic I62.1
- eye NEC H57.89
  - fundus — *see* Hemorrhage, retina
  - lid — *see* Disorder, eyelid, specified type NEC
- fallopian tube N83.6
- fibrinogenolysis — *see* Fibrinolysis
- fibrinolytic (acquired) — *see* Fibrinolysis
- from
  - ear (nontraumatic) — *see* Otorrhagia
  - tracheostomy stoma J95.Ø1
- fundus, eye — *see* Hemorrhage, retina
- funis — *see* Hemorrhage, umbilicus, cord
- gastric — *see* Hemorrhage, stomach
- gastroenteric K92.2
  - newborn P54.3
- gastrointestinal (tract) K92.2
  - newborn P54.3
- genital organ, male N5Ø.1
- genitourinary (tract) NOS R31.9
- gingiva KØ6.8
- globe (eye) — *see* Hemophthalmos
- graafian follicle cyst (ruptured) N83.Ø- ☑
- gum KØ6.8
- heart I51.89
- hypopharyngeal (throat) RØ4.1
- intermenstrual (regular) N92.3
  - irregular N92.1
- internal (organs) NEC R58
  - capsule I61.Ø
  - ear — *see* subcategory H83.8 ☑
  - newborn P54.8
- intestine K92.2
  - newborn P54.3
- intra-abdominal R58
- intra-alveolar (lung), newborn P26.8
- intracerebral (nontraumatic) — *see* Hemorrhage, intracranial, intracerebral
- intracranial (nontraumatic) I62.9
  - birth injury P1Ø.9
  - epidural, nontraumatic I62.1
  - extradural, nontraumatic I62.1
  - intracerebral (nontraumatic) (in) I61.9
    - brain stem I61.3
    - cerebellum I61.4
    - hemisphere I61.2
      - cortical (superficial) I61.1
      - subcortical (deep) I61.Ø
    - intraoperative
      - during a nervous system procedure G97.31
      - during other procedure G97.32
    - intraventricular I61.5
    - multiple localized I61.6
    - newborn P52.4
      - birth injury P1Ø.1
    - postprocedural
      - following a nervous system procedure G97.51
      - following other procedure G97.52
    - specified NEC I61.8
    - superficial I61.1
    - traumatic (diffuse) — *see* Injury, intracranial, diffuse
      - focal — *see* Injury, intracranial, focal
  - newborn P52.9
    - specified NEC P52.8
  - subarachnoid (nontraumatic) (from) I6Ø.9
    - intracranial (cerebral) artery I6Ø.7
      - anterior communicating I6Ø.2
      - basilar I6Ø.4
      - carotid siphon and bifurcation I6Ø.Ø- ☑
      - communicating I6Ø.7
        - anterior I6Ø.2
        - posterior I6Ø.3- ☑
      - middle cerebral I6Ø.1- ☑
      - posterior communicating I6Ø.3- ☑

Hemorrhage, hemorrhagic — *continued*
- intracranial — *continued*
  - subarachnoid — *continued*
    - intracranial artery — *continued*
      - specified artery NEC I6Ø.6
      - vertebral I6Ø.5- ☑
    - newborn P52.5
      - birth injury P1Ø.3
    - specified NEC I6Ø.8
    - traumatic SØ6.6X- ☑
  - subdural (nontraumatic) I62.ØØ
    - acute I62.Ø1
    - birth injury P1Ø.Ø
    - chronic I62.Ø3
    - newborn (anoxic) (hypoxic) P52.8
      - birth injury P1Ø.Ø
    - spinal G95.19
    - subacute I62.Ø2
    - traumatic — *see* Injury, intracranial, subdural hemorrhage
  - traumatic — *see* Injury, intracranial, focal brain injury
- intramedullary NEC G95.19
- intraocular — *see* Hemophthalmos
- intraoperative, intraprocedural — *see* Complication, hemorrhage (hematoma), intraoperative (intraprocedural), by site
- intrapartum — *see* Hemorrhage, complicating, delivery
- intrapelvic
  - female N94.89
  - male K66.1
- intraperitoneal K66.1
- intrapontine I61.3
- intraprocedural — *see* Complication, hemorrhage (hematoma), intraoperative (intraprocedural), by site
- intrauterine N85.7
  - complicating delivery — *see also* Hemorrhage, complicating, delivery O67.9
  - postpartum — *see* Hemorrhage, postpartum
- intraventricular I61.5
  - newborn (nontraumatic) — *see also* Newborn, affected by, hemorrhage P52.3
    - due to birth injury P1Ø.2
    - grade
      - 1 P52.Ø
      - 2 P52.1
      - 3 P52.21
      - 4 P52.22
- intravesical N32.89
- iris (postinfectional) (postinflammatory) (toxic) — *see* Hyphema
- joint (nontraumatic) — *see* Hemarthrosis
- kidney N28.89
- knee (joint) (nontraumatic) — *see* Hemarthrosis, knee
- labyrinth — *see* subcategory H83.8 ☑
- lenticular striate artery I61.Ø
- ligature, vessel — *see* Hemorrhage, postoperative
- liver K76.89
- lung RØ4.89
  - newborn P26.9
    - massive P26.1
    - specified NEC P26.8
  - tuberculous — *see* Tuberculosis, pulmonary
- massive umbilical, newborn P51.Ø
- mediastinum — *see* Hemorrhage, lung
- medulla I61.3
- membrane (brain) I6Ø.8
  - spinal cord — *see* Hemorrhage, spinal cord
- meninges, meningeal (brain) (middle) I6Ø.8
  - spinal cord — *see* Hemorrhage, spinal cord
- mesentery K66.1
- metritis — *see* Endometritis
- mouth K13.79
- mucous membrane NEC R58
  - newborn P54.8
- muscle M62.89
- nail (subungual) L6Ø.8
- nasal turbinate RØ4.Ø
  - newborn P54.8
- navel, newborn P51.9
- newborn P54.9
  - specified NEC P54.8
- nipple N64.59
- nose RØ4.Ø
  - newborn P54.8
- omentum K66.1
- optic nerve (sheath) H47.Ø2- ☑

Hemorrhage, hemorrhagic — *continued*
- orbit, orbital HØ5.23- ☑
- ovary NEC N83.8
- oviduct N83.6
- pancreas K86.89
- parathyroid (gland) (spontaneous) E21.4
- parturition — *see* Hemorrhage, complicating, delivery
- penis N48.89
- pericardium, pericarditis I31.2
- peritoneum, peritoneal K66.1
- peritonsillar tissue J35.8
  - due to infection J36
- petechial R23.3
  - due to autosensitivity, erythrocyte D69.2
- pituitary (gland) E23.6
- pleura — *see* Hemorrhage, lung
- polioencephalitis, superior E51.2
- polymyositis — *see* Polymyositis
- pons, pontine I61.3
- posterior fossa (nontraumatic) I61.8
  - newborn P52.6
- postmenopausal N95.Ø
- postnasal RØ4.Ø
- postoperative — *see* Complications, postprocedural, hemorrhage, by site
- postpartum NEC (following delivery of placenta) O72.1
  - delayed or secondary O72.2
  - retained placenta O72.Ø
  - third stage O72.Ø
- pregnancy — *see* Hemorrhage, antepartum
- preretinal — *see* Hemorrhage, retina
- prostate N42.1
- puerperal — *see* Hemorrhage, postpartum
  - delayed or secondary O72.2
- pulmonary RØ4.89
  - newborn P26.9
    - massive P26.1
    - specified NEC P26.8
  - tuberculous — *see* Tuberculosis, pulmonary
- purpura (primary) D69.3
- rectum (sphincter) K62.5
  - newborn P54.2
- recurring, following initial hemorrhage at time of injury T79.2 ☑
- renal N28.89
- respiratory passage or tract RØ4.9
  - specified NEC RØ4.89
- retina, retinal (vessels) H35.6- ☑
  - diabetic — *see* Microaneurysm, retinal, diabetic
- retroperitoneal R58
- scalp R58
- scrotum N5Ø.1
- secondary (nontraumatic) R58
  - following initial hemorrhage at time of injury T79.2 ☑
- seminal vesicle N5Ø.1
- skin R23.3
  - newborn P54.5
- slipped umbilical ligature P51.8
- spermatic cord N5Ø.1
- spinal (cord) G95.19
  - newborn (birth injury) P11.5
- spleen D73.5
  - intraoperative — *see* Complications, intraoperative, hemorrhage, spleen
  - postprocedural — *see* Complications, postprocedural, hemorrhage, spleen
- stomach K92.2
  - newborn P54.3
  - ulcer — *see* Ulcer, stomach, with hemorrhage
- subarachnoid (nontraumatic) — *see* Hemorrhage, intracranial, subarachnoid
- subconjunctival — *see also* Hemorrhage, conjunctiva
  - birth injury P15.3
- subcortical (brain) I61.Ø
- subcutaneous R23.3
- subdiaphragmatic R58
- subdural (acute) (nontraumatic) — *see* Hemorrhage, intracranial, subdural
- subependymal
  - newborn P52.Ø
    - with intraventricular extension P52.1
      - and intracerebral extension P52.22
- subgaleal P12.2
- subhyaloid — *see* Hemorrhage, retina
- subperiosteal — *see* Disorder, bone, specified type NEC
- subretinal — *see* Hemorrhage, retina
- subtentorial — *see* Hemorrhage, intracranial, subdural

- **Hemorrhage, hemorrhagic** — *continued*
  - subungual L6Ø.8
  - suprarenal (capsule) (gland) E27.49
    - newborn P54.4
  - tentorium (traumatic) NEC — *see* Hemorrhage, brain
    - newborn (birth injury) P1Ø.4
  - testis N5Ø.1
  - third stage (postpartum) O72.Ø
  - thorax — *see* Hemorrhage, lung
  - throat RØ4.1
  - thymus (gland) E32.8
  - thyroid (cyst) (gland) EØ7.89
  - tongue K14.8
  - tonsil J35.8
  - trachea — *see* Hemorrhage, lung
  - tracheobronchial RØ4.89
    - newborn P26.Ø
  - traumatic — *code to* specific injury
    - cerebellar — *see* Hemorrhage, brain
    - intracranial — *see* Hemorrhage, brain
    - recurring or secondary (following initial hemorrhage at time of injury) T79.2 ☑
  - tuberculous NEC — *see also* Tuberculosis, pulmonary A15.Ø
  - tunica vaginalis N5Ø.1
  - ulcer — *code by* site under Ulcer, with hemorrhage K27.4
  - umbilicus, umbilical
    - cord
      - after birth, newborn P51.9
      - complicating delivery O69.5 ☑
    - newborn P51.9
      - massive P51.Ø
      - slipped ligature P51.8
    - stump P51.9
  - urethra (idiopathic) N36.8
  - uterus, uterine (abnormal) N93.9
    - climacteric N92.4
    - complicating delivery — *see* Hemorrhage, complicating, delivery
    - dysfunctional or functional N93.8
    - intermenstrual (regular) N92.3
      - irregular N92.1
    - postmenopausal N95.Ø
    - postpartum — *see* Hemorrhage, postpartum
    - preclimacteric or premenopausal N92.4
    - prepubertal N93.8
    - pubertal N92.2
  - vagina (abnormal) N93.9
    - newborn P54.6
  - vas deferens N5Ø.1
  - vasa previa O69.4 ☑
  - ventricular I61.5
  - vesical N32.89
  - viscera NEC R58
    - newborn P54.8
  - vitreous (humor) (intraocular) H43.1- ☑
  - vulva N9Ø.89
- **Hemorrhoids** (bleeding) (without mention of degree) K64.9
  - 1st degree (grade/stage I) (without prolapse outside of anal canal) K64.Ø
  - 2nd degree (grade/stage II) (that prolapse with straining but retract spontaneously) K64.1
  - 3rd degree (grade/stage III) (that prolapse with straining and require manual replacement back inside anal canal) K64.2
  - 4th degree (grade/stage IV) (with prolapsed tissue that cannot be manually replaced) K64.3
  - complicating
    - pregnancy O22.4 ☑
    - puerperium O87.2
  - external K64.4
    - with
      - thrombosis K64.5
  - internal (without mention of degree) K64.8
  - prolapsed K64.8
  - skin tags
    - anus K64.4
    - residual K64.4
  - specified NEC K64.8
  - strangulated — *see also* Hemorrhoids, by degree K64.8
  - thrombosed — *see also* Hemorrhoids, by degree K64.5
  - ulcerated — *see also* Hemorrhoids, by degree K64.8
- **Hemosalpinx** N83.6
  - with
    - hematocolpos N89.7
    - hematometra N85.7
- **Hemosalpinx** — *continued*
  - with — *continued*
    - hematometra — *continued*
      - with hematocolpos N89.7
- **Hemosiderosis** (dietary) E83.19
  - pulmonary, idiopathic E83.1- ☑ *[J84.Ø3]*
  - transfusion T8Ø.89 ☑
- **Hemothorax** (bacterial) (nontuberculous) J94.2
  - newborn P54.8
  - traumatic S27.1 ☑
    - with pneumothorax S27.2 ☑
  - tuberculous NEC A15.6
- **Henoch** (-Schönlein) **disease or syndrome** (purpura) D69.Ø
- **Henpue, henpuye** A66.6
- **Hepar lobatum** (syphilitic) A52.74
- **Hepatalgia** K76.89
- **Hepatitis** K75.9
  - acute B17.9
    - with coma K72.Ø1
    - with hepatic failure — *see* Failure, hepatic
    - alcoholic — *see* Hepatitis, alcoholic
    - infectious B17.9
    - non-viral K72.Ø ☑
    - viral B17.9
  - alcoholic (acute) (chronic) K7Ø.1Ø
    - with ascites K7Ø.11
  - amebic — *see* Abscess, liver, amebic
  - anicteric, (viral) — *see* Hepatitis, viral
  - antigen-associated (HAA) — *see* Hepatitis, B
  - Australia-antigen (positive) — *see* Hepatitis, B
  - autoimmune K75.4
  - B B19.1Ø
    - with hepatic coma B19.11
    - acute B16.9
      - with
        - delta-agent (coinfection) (without hepatic coma) B16.1
          - with hepatic coma B16.Ø
        - hepatic coma (without delta-agent coinfection) B16.2
    - chronic B18.1
      - with delta-agent B18.Ø
  - bacterial NEC K75.89
  - C (viral) B19.2Ø
    - with hepatic coma B19.21
    - acute B17.1Ø
      - with hepatic coma B17.11
    - chronic B18.2
  - catarrhal (acute) B15.9
    - with hepatic coma B15.Ø
  - cholangiolitic K75.89
  - cholestatic K75.89
  - chronic K73.9
    - active NEC K73.2
    - lobular NEC K73.1
    - persistent NEC K73.Ø
    - specified NEC K73.8
  - cytomegaloviral B25.1
  - due to ethanol (acute) (chronic) — *see* Hepatitis, alcoholic
  - epidemic B15.9
    - with hepatic coma B15.Ø
  - fulminant NEC (viral) — *see* Hepatitis, viral
  - granulomatous NEC K75.3
  - herpesviral BØØ.81
  - history of
    - B Z86.19
    - C Z86.19
  - homologous serum — *see* Hepatitis, viral, type B
  - in (due to)
    - mumps B26.81
    - toxoplasmosis (acquired) B58.1
      - congenital (active) P37.1 *[K77]*
  - infectious, infective B15.9
    - acute (subacute) B17.9
    - chronic B18.9
  - inoculation — *see* Hepatitis, viral, type B
  - interstitial (chronic) K74.69
  - ischemia, ischemic K72.ØØ
  - lupoid NEC K75.4
  - malignant NEC (with hepatic failure) K72.9Ø
    - with coma K72.91
  - neonatal (idiopathic) (toxic) P59.29
  - neonatal giant cell P59.29
  - newborn P59.29
  - non-viral K72.Ø ☑
  - postimmunization — *see* Hepatitis, viral, type B
- **Hepatitis** — *continued*
  - post-transfusion — *see* Hepatitis, viral, type B
  - reactive, nonspecific K75.2
  - serum — *see* Hepatitis, viral, type B
  - shock K72.ØØ
  - specified type NEC
    - with hepatic failure — *see* Failure, hepatic
  - syphilitic (late) A52.74
    - congenital (early) A5Ø.Ø8 *[K77]*
      - late A5Ø.59 *[K77]*
    - secondary A51.45
  - toxic — *see also* Disease, liver, toxic K71.6
  - tuberculous A18.83
  - viral, virus B19.9
    - with hepatic coma B19.Ø
    - acute B17.9
    - chronic B18.9
      - specified NEC B18.8
      - type
        - B B18.1
          - with delta-agent B18.Ø
        - C B18.2
    - congenital P35.3
    - coxsackie B33.8 *[K77]*
    - cytomegalic inclusion B25.1
    - in remission, any type — *code to* Hepatitis, chronic, by type
    - non-A, non-B B17.8
    - specified type NEC (with or without coma) B17.8
    - type
      - A B15.9
        - with hepatic coma B15.Ø
      - B B19.1Ø
        - with hepatic coma B19.11
        - acute B16.9
          - with
            - delta-agent (coinfection) (without hepatic coma) B16.1
              - with hepatic coma B16.Ø
            - hepatic coma (without delta-agent coinfection) B16.2
        - chronic B18.1
          - with delta-agent B18.Ø
      - C B19.2Ø
        - with hepatic coma B19.21
        - acute B17.1Ø
          - with hepatic coma B17.11
        - chronic B18.2
      - E B17.2
      - non-A, non-B B17.8
- **Hepatization lung** (acute) — *see* Pneumonia, lobar
- **Hepatoblastoma** C22.2
- **Hepatocarcinoma** C22.Ø
- **Hepatocholangiocarcinoma** C22.Ø
- **Hepatocholangioma, benign** D13.4
- **Hepatocholangitis** K75.89
- **Hepatolenticular degeneration** E83.Ø1
- **Hepatoma** (malignant) C22.Ø
  - benign D13.4
  - embryonal C22.Ø
- **Hepatomegaly** — *see also* Hypertrophy, liver
  - with splenomegaly R16.2
  - congenital Q44.7
  - in mononucleosis
    - gammaherpesviral B27.Ø9
    - infectious specified NEC B27.89
- **Hepatoptosis** K76.89
- **Hepatorenal syndrome following labor and delivery** O9Ø.4
- **Hepatosis** K76.89
- **Hepatosplenomegaly** R16.2
  - hyperlipemic (Bürger-Grütz type) E78.3 *[K77]*
- **Hereditary** — *see* condition
- **Hereditary alpha tryptasemia** (syndrome) D89.44
- **Heredodegeneration, macular** — *see* Dystrophy, retina
- **Heredopathia atactica polyneuritiformis** G6Ø.1
- **Heredosyphilis** — *see* Syphilis, congenital
- **Herlitz' syndrome** Q81.1
- **Hermansky-Pudlak syndrome** E7Ø.331
- **Hermaphrodite, hermaphroditism** (true) Q56.Ø
  - 46,XX with streak gonads Q99.1
  - 46,XX/46,XY Q99.Ø
  - 46,XY with streak gonads Q99.1
  - chimera 46,XX/46,XY Q99.Ø
- **Hernia, hernial** (acquired) (recurrent) K46.9
  - with
    - gangrene — *see* Hernia, by site, with, gangrene
    - incarceration — *see* Hernia, by site, with, obstruction

Hernia, hernial — *continued*
with — *continued*
irreducible — *see* Hernia, by site, with, obstruction
obstruction — *see* Hernia, by site, with, obstruction
strangulation — *see* Hernia, by site, with, obstruction
abdomen, abdominal K46.9
with
gangrene (and obstruction) K46.1
obstruction K46.Ø
femoral — *see* Hernia, femoral
incisional — *see* Hernia, incisional
inguinal — *see* Hernia, inguinal
specified site NEC K45.8
with
gangrene (and obstruction) K45.1
obstruction K45.Ø
umbilical — *see* Hernia, umbilical
wall — *see* Hernia, ventral
appendix — *see* Hernia, abdomen
bladder (mucosa) (sphincter)
congenital (female) (male) Q79.51
female — *see* Cystocele
male N32.89
brain, congenital — *see* Encephalocele
cartilage, vertebra — *see* Displacement, intervertebral disc
cerebral, congenital — *see also* Encephalocele
endaural QØ1.8
ciliary body (traumatic) SØ5.2- ☑
colon — *see* Hernia, abdomen
Cooper's — *see* Hernia, abdomen, specified site NEC
crural — *see* Hernia, femoral
diaphragm, diaphragmatic K44.9
with
gangrene (and obstruction) K44.1
obstruction K44.Ø
congenital Q79.Ø
direct (inguinal) — *see* Hernia, inguinal
diverticulum, intestine — *see* Hernia, abdomen
double (inguinal) — *see* Hernia, inguinal, bilateral
due to adhesions (with obstruction) K56.5Ø
epigastric — *see also* Hernia, ventral K43.9
esophageal hiatus — *see* Hernia, hiatal
external (inguinal) — *see* Hernia, inguinal
fallopian tube N83.4- ☑
fascia M62.89
femoral K41.9Ø
with
gangrene (and obstruction) K41.4Ø
not specified as recurrent K41.4Ø
recurrent K41.41
obstruction K41.3Ø
not specified as recurrent K41.3Ø
recurrent K41.31
not specified as recurrent K41.9Ø
recurrent K41.91
bilateral K41.2Ø
with
gangrene (and obstruction) K41.1Ø
not specified as recurrent K41.1Ø
recurrent K41.11
obstruction K41.ØØ
not specified as recurrent K41.ØØ
recurrent K41.Ø1
not specified as recurrent K41.2Ø
recurrent K41.21
unilateral K41.9Ø
with
gangrene (and obstruction) K41.4Ø
not specified as recurrent K41.4Ø
recurrent K41.41
obstruction K41.3Ø
not specified as recurrent K41.3Ø
recurrent K41.31
not specified as recurrent K41.9Ø
recurrent K41.91
foramen magnum G93.5
congenital QØ1.8
funicular (umbilical) — *see also* Hernia, umbilicus
spermatic (cord) — *see* Hernia, inguinal
gastrointestinal tract — *see* Hernia, abdomen
Hesselbach's — *see* Hernia, femoral, specified site NEC
hiatal (esophageal) (sliding) K44.9
with
gangrene (and obstruction) K44.1
obstruction K44.Ø
congenital Q4Ø.1

Hernia, hernial — *continued*
hypogastric — *see* Hernia, ventral
incarcerated — *see also* Hernia, by site, with obstruction
with gangrene — *see* Hernia, by site, with gangrene
incisional K43.2
with
gangrene (and obstruction) K43.1
obstruction K43.Ø
indirect (inguinal) — *see* Hernia, inguinal
inguinal (direct) (external) (funicular) (indirect) (internal) (oblique) (scrotal) (sliding) K4Ø.9Ø
with
gangrene (and obstruction) K4Ø.4Ø
not specified as recurrent K4Ø.4Ø
recurrent K4Ø.41
obstruction K4Ø.3Ø
not specified as recurrent K4Ø.3Ø
recurrent K4Ø.31
not specified as recurrent K4Ø.9Ø
recurrent K4Ø.91
bilateral K4Ø.2Ø
with
gangrene (and obstruction) K4Ø.1Ø
not specified as recurrent K4Ø.1Ø
recurrent K4Ø.11
obstruction K4Ø.ØØ
not specified as recurrent K4Ø.ØØ
recurrent K4Ø.Ø1
not specified as recurrent K4Ø.2Ø
recurrent K4Ø.21
unilateral K4Ø.9Ø
with
gangrene (and obstruction) K4Ø.4Ø
not specified as recurrent K4Ø.4Ø
recurrent K4Ø.41
obstruction K4Ø.3Ø
not specified as recurrent K4Ø.3Ø
recurrent K4Ø.31
not specified as recurrent K4Ø.9Ø
recurrent K4Ø.91
internal — *see also* Hernia, abdomen
inguinal — *see* Hernia, inguinal
interstitial — *see* Hernia, abdomen
intervertebral cartilage or disc — *see* Displacement, intervertebral disc
intestine, intestinal — *see* Hernia, by site
intra-abdominal — *see* Hernia, abdomen
iris (traumatic) SØ5.2- ☑
irreducible — *see also* Hernia, by site, with obstruction
with gangrene — *see* Hernia, by site, with gangrene
ischiatic — *see* Hernia, abdomen, specified site NEC
ischiorectal — *see* Hernia, abdomen, specified site NEC
lens (traumatic) SØ5.2- ☑
linea (alba) (semilunaris) — *see* Hernia, ventral
Littre's — *see* Hernia, abdomen
lumbar — *see* Hernia, abdomen, specified site NEC
lung (subcutaneous) J98.4
mediastinum J98.59
mesenteric (internal) — *see* Hernia, abdomen
midline — *see* Hernia, ventral
muscle (sheath) M62.89
nucleus pulposus — *see* Displacement, intervertebral disc
oblique (inguinal) — *see* Hernia, inguinal
obstructive — *see also* Hernia, by site, with obstruction
with gangrene — *see* Hernia, by site, with gangrene
obturator — *see* Hernia, abdomen, specified site NEC
omental — *see* Hernia, abdomen
ovary N83.4- ☑
oviduct N83.4- ☑
paraesophageal — *see also* Hernia, diaphragm
congenital Q4Ø.1
parastomal K43.5
with
gangrene (and obstruction) K43.4
obstruction K43.3
paraumbilical — *see* Hernia, umbilicus
perineal — *see* Hernia, abdomen, specified site NEC
Petit's — *see* Hernia, abdomen, specified site NEC
postoperative — *see* Hernia, incisional
pregnant uterus — *see* Abnormal, uterus in pregnancy or childbirth
prevesical N32.89
properitoneal — *see* Hernia, abdomen, specified site NEC
pudendal — *see* Hernia, abdomen, specified site NEC
rectovaginal N81.6

Hernia, hernial — *continued*
retroperitoneal — *see* Hernia, abdomen, specified site NEC
Richter's — *see* Hernia, abdomen, with obstruction
Rieux's, Riex's — *see* Hernia, abdomen, specified site NEC
sac condition (adhesion) (dropsy) (inflammation) (laceration) (suppuration) — *code by site under* Hernia
sciatic — *see* Hernia, abdomen, specified site NEC
scrotum, scrotal — *see* Hernia, inguinal
sliding (inguinal) — *see also* Hernia, inguinal
hiatus — *see* Hernia, hiatal
spigelian — *see* Hernia, ventral
spinal — *see* Spina bifida
strangulated — *see also* Hernia, by site, with obstruction
with gangrene — *see* Hernia, by site, with gangrene
subxiphoid — *see* Hernia, ventral
supra-umbilicus — *see* Hernia, ventral
tendon — *see* Disorder, tendon, specified type NEC
Treitz's (fossa) — *see* Hernia, abdomen, specified site NEC
tunica vaginalis Q55.29
umbilicus, umbilical K42.9
with
gangrene (and obstruction) K42.1
obstruction K42.Ø
ureter N28.89
urethra, congenital Q64.79
urinary meatus, congenital Q64.79
uterus N81.4
pregnant — *see* Abnormal, uterus in pregnancy or childbirth
vaginal (anterior) (wall) — *see* Cystocele
Velpeau's — *see* Hernia, femoral
ventral K43.9
with
gangrene (and obstruction) K43.7
obstruction K43.6
incisional K43.2
with
gangrene (and obstruction) K43.1
obstruction K43.Ø
recurrent — *see* Hernia, incisional
specified NEC K43.9
with
gangrene (and obstruction) K43.7
obstruction K43.6
vesical
congenital (female) (male) Q79.51
female — *see* Cystocele
male N32.89
vitreous (into wound) SØ5.2- ☑
into anterior chamber — *see* Prolapse, vitreous
Herniation — *see also* Hernia
brain (stem) G93.5
nontraumatic G93.5
traumatic SØ6.A1 ☑
cerebellar SØ6.A1 ☑
subfalcine (cingulate) SØ6.A1 ☑
tonsillar SØ6.A1 ☑
transtentorial (central) (upward cerebellar) SØ6.A1 ☑
uncal SØ6.A1 ☑
cerebral G93.5
nontraumatic G93.5
traumatic SØ6.A1 ☑
mediastinum J98.59
nucleus pulposus — *see* Displacement, intervertebral disc
Herpangina BØ8.5
Herpes, herpesvirus, herpetic BØØ.9
anogenital A6Ø.9
perianal skin A6Ø.1
rectum A6Ø.1
urogenital tract A6Ø.ØØ
cervix A6Ø.Ø3
male genital organ NEC A6Ø.Ø2
penis A6Ø.Ø1
specified site NEC A6Ø.Ø9
vagina A6Ø.Ø4
vulva A6Ø.Ø4
blepharitis (zoster) BØ2.39
simplex BØØ.59
circinatus B35.4
bullosus L12.Ø
conjunctivitis (simplex) BØØ.53

- **Herpes, herpesvirus, herpetic** — *continued*
  - conjunctivitis — *continued*
    - zoster B02.31
  - cornea B02.33
  - encephalitis B00.4
    - due to herpesvirus 6 B10.01
    - due to herpesvirus 7 B10.09
    - specified NEC B10.09
  - eye (zoster) B02.30
    - simplex B00.50
  - eyelid (zoster) B02.39
    - simplex B00.59
  - facialis B00.1
  - febrilis B00.1
  - geniculate ganglionitis B02.21
  - genital, genitalis A60.00
    - female A60.09
    - male A60.02
  - gestational, gestationis O26.4- ☑
  - gingivostomatitis B00.2
  - human B00.9
    - 1 — *see* Herpes, simplex
    - 2 — *see* Herpes, simplex
    - 3 — *see* Varicella
    - 4 — *see* Mononucleosis, Epstein-Barr (virus)
    - 5 — *see* Disease, cytomegalic inclusion (generalized)
    - 6
      - encephalitis B10.01
      - specified NEC B10.81
    - 7
      - encephalitis B10.09
      - specified NEC B10.82
    - 8 B10.89
  - infection NEC B10.89
    - Kaposi's sarcoma associated B10.89
  - iridocyclitis (simplex) B00.51
    - zoster B02.32
  - iris (vesicular erythema multiforme) L51.9
  - iritis (simplex) B00.51
  - Kaposi's sarcoma associated B10.89
  - keratitis (simplex) (dendritic) (disciform) (interstitial) B00.52
    - zoster (interstitial) B02.33
  - keratoconjunctivitis (simplex) B00.52
    - zoster B02.33
  - labialis B00.1
  - lip B00.1
  - meningitis (simplex) B00.3
    - zoster B02.1
  - ophthalmicus (zoster) NEC B02.30
    - simplex B00.50
  - penis A60.01
  - perianal skin A60.1
  - pharyngitis, pharyngotonsillitis B00.2
  - rectum A60.1
  - scrotum A60.02
  - sepsis B00.7
  - simplex B00.9
    - complicated NEC B00.89
    - congenital P35.2
    - conjunctivitis B00.53
    - external ear B00.1
    - eyelid B00.59
    - hepatitis B00.81
    - keratitis (interstitial) B00.52
    - myleitis B00.82
    - specified complication NEC B00.89
    - visceral B00.89
  - stomatitis B00.2
  - tonsurans B35.0
  - visceral B00.89
  - vulva A60.04
  - whitlow B00.89
  - zoster — *see also* condition B02.9
    - auricularis B02.21
    - complicated NEC B02.8
    - conjunctivitis B02.31
    - disseminated B02.7
    - encephalitis B02.0
    - eye (lid) B02.39
    - geniculate ganglionitis B02.21
    - keratitis (interstitial) B02.33
    - meningitis B02.1
    - myelitis B02.24
    - neuritis, neuralgia B02.29
    - ophthalmicus NEC B02.30
    - oticus B02.21
    - polyneuropathy B02.23
- **Herpes, herpesvirus, herpetic** — *continued*
  - zoster — *see also* condition — *continued*
    - specified complication NEC B02.8
    - trigeminal neuralgia B02.22
- **Herpesvirus** (human) — *see* Herpes
- **Herpetophobia** F40.218
- **Herrick's anemia** — *see* Disease, sickle-cell
- **Hers' disease** E74.09
- **Herter-Gee syndrome** K90.0
- **Herxheimer's reaction** R68.89
- **Hesitancy**
  - of micturition R39.11
  - urinary R39.11
- **Hesselbach's hernia** — *see* Hernia, femoral, specified site NEC
- **Heterochromia** (congenital) Q13.2
  - cataract — *see* Cataract, complicated
  - cyclitis (Fuchs) — *see* Cyclitis, Fuchs' heterochromic
  - hair L67.1
  - iritis — *see* Cyclitis, Fuchs' heterochromic
  - retained metallic foreign body (nonmagnetic) — *see* Foreign body, intraocular, old, retained
    - magnetic — *see* Foreign body, intraocular, old, retained, magnetic
  - uveitis — *see* Cyclitis, Fuchs' heterochromic
- **Heterophoria** — *see* Strabismus, heterophoria
- **Heterophyes, heterophyiasis** (small intestine) B66.8
- **Heterotopia, heterotopic** — *see also* Malposition, congenital
  - cerebralis Q04.8
- **Heterotropia** — *see* Strabismus
- **Heubner-Herter disease** K90.0
- **Hexadactylism** Q69.9
- **HGSIL** (cytology finding) (high grade squamous intraepithelial lesion on cytologic smear) (Pap smear finding)
  - anus R85.613
  - cervix R87.613
    - biopsy (histology) finding — *see* Neoplasia, intraepithelial, cervix, grade II or grade III
  - vagina R87.623
    - biopsy (histology) finding — *see* Neoplasia, intraepithelial, cervix, grade II or grade III
- **Hibernoma** — *see* Lipoma
- **Hiccup, hiccough** R06.6
  - epidemic B33.0
  - psychogenic F45.8
- **Hidden penis** (congenital) Q55.64
  - acquired N48.83
- **Hidradenitis** (axillaris) (suppurative) L73.2
- **Hidradenoma** (nodular) — *see also* Neoplasm, skin, benign
  - clear cell — *see* Neoplasm, skin, benign
  - papillary — *see* Neoplasm, skin, benign
- **Hidrocystoma** — *see* Neoplasm, skin, benign
- **High**
  - altitude effects T70.20 ☑
    - anoxia T70.29 ☑
    - on
      - ears T70.0 ☑
      - sinuses T70.1 ☑
    - polycythemia D75.1
  - arch
    - foot Q66.7- ☑
    - palate, congenital Q38.5
  - arterial tension — *see* Hypertension
  - basal metabolic rate R94.8
  - blood pressure — *see also* Hypertension
    - borderline R03.0
    - reading (incidental) (isolated) (nonspecific), without diagnosis of hypertension R03.0
  - cholesterol E78.00
    - with high triglycerides E78.2
  - diaphragm (congenital) Q79.1
  - expressed emotional level within family Z63.8
  - head at term O32.4 ☑
  - palate, congenital Q38.5
  - risk
    - infant NEC Z76.2
    - sexual behavior (heterosexual) Z72.51
      - bisexual Z72.53
      - homosexual Z72.52
  - scrotal testis, testes
    - bilateral Q53.23
    - unilateral Q53.13
  - temperature (of unknown origin) R50.9
  - thoracic rib Q76.6
- **High** — *continued*
  - triglycerides E78.1
    - with high cholesterol E78.2
- **Hildenbrand's disease** A75.0
- **Hilum** — *see* condition
- **Hip** — *see* condition
- **Hippel's disease** Q85.83
- **Hippophobia** F40.218
- **Hippus** H57.09
- **Hirschsprung's disease or megacolon** Q43.1
- **Hirsutism, hirsuties** L68.0
- **Hirudiniasis**
  - external B88.3
  - internal B83.4
- **Hiss-Russell dysentery** A03.1
- **Histidinemia, histidinuria** E70.41
- **Histiocytoma** — *see also* Neoplasm, skin, benign
  - fibrous — *see also* Neoplasm, skin, benign
    - atypical — *see* Neoplasm, connective tissue, uncertain behavior
    - malignant — *see* Neoplasm, connective tissue, malignant
- **Histiocytosis** D76.3
  - acute differentiated progressive C96.0
  - Langerhans' cell NEC C96.6
    - multifocal X
      - multisystemic (disseminated) C96.0
      - unisystemic C96.5
    - pulmonary, adult (adult PLCH) J84.82
    - unifocal (X) C96.6
  - lipid, lipoid D76.3
    - essential E75.29
  - malignant C96.A (*following* C96.6)
  - mononuclear phagocytes NEC D76.1
    - Langerhans' cells C96.6
  - non-Langerhans cell D76.3
  - polyostotic sclerosing D76.3
  - sinus, with massive lymphadenopathy D76.3
  - syndrome NEC D76.3
  - X NEC C96.6
    - acute (progressive) C96.0
    - chronic C96.6
    - multifocal C96.5
    - multisystemic C96.0
    - unifocal C96.6
- **Histoplasmosis** B39.9
  - with pneumonia NEC B39.2
  - African B39.5
  - American — *see* Histoplasmosis, capsulati
  - capsulati B39.4
    - disseminated B39.3
    - generalized B39.3
    - pulmonary B39.2
      - acute B39.0
      - chronic B39.1
  - Darling's B39.4
  - duboisii B39.5
  - lung NEC B39.2
- **History**
  - family (of) — *see also* History, personal (of)
    - alcohol abuse Z81.1
    - allergy NEC Z84.89
    - anemia Z83.2
    - arthritis Z82.61
    - asthma Z82.5
    - blindness Z82.1
    - cardiac death (sudden) Z82.41
    - carrier of genetic disease Z84.81
    - chromosomal anomaly Z82.79
    - chronic
      - disabling disease NEC Z82.8
      - lower respiratory disease Z82.5
    - colonic polyps Z83.71
    - congenital malformations and deformations Z82.79
      - polycystic kidney Z82.71
    - consanguinity Z84.3
    - deafness Z82.2
    - diabetes mellitus Z83.3
    - disability NEC Z82.8
    - disease or disorder (of)
      - allergic NEC Z84.89
      - behavioral NEC Z81.8
      - blood and blood-forming organs Z83.2
      - cardiovascular NEC Z82.49
      - chronic disabling NEC Z82.8
      - digestive Z83.79
      - ear NEC Z83.52
      - elevated lipoprotein (a) (Lp(a)) Z83.430

History — *continued*
- personal — *see also* History, family — *continued*
  - dysplasia — *continued*
    - cervical — *continued*
      - severe (grade III) Z86.001
    - prostatic Z87.430
    - vaginal (mild) (moderate) Z87.411
      - severe (grade III) Z86.002
    - vulvar (mild) (moderate) Z87.412
      - severe (grade III) Z86.002
  - embolism (venous) Z86.718
    - pulmonary Z86.711
  - encephalitis Z86.61
  - estrogen therapy Z92.23
  - extracorporeal membrane oxygenation (ECMO) Z92.81
  - failed conscious sedation Z92.83
  - failed moderate sedation Z92.83
  - fall, falling Z91.81
  - forced labor or sexual exploitation Z91.42
    - in childhood Z62.813
  - fracture (healed)
    - fatigue Z87.312
    - fragility Z87.310
    - osteoporosis Z87.310
    - pathological NEC Z87.311
    - stress Z87.312
    - traumatic Z87.81
  - gene therapy Z92.86
  - gestational diabetes Z86.32
  - hepatitis
    - B Z86.19
    - C Z86.19
  - Hodgkin disease Z85.71
  - hyperthermia, malignant Z88.4
  - hypospadias (corrected) Z87.710
  - hysterectomy Z90.710
  - immunosuppression therapy Z92.25
  - in situ neoplasm
    - breast Z86.000
    - cervix uteri Z86.001
    - digestive organs, specified NEC Z86.004
    - esophagus Z86.003
    - genital organs, specified NEC Z86.002
    - melanoma Z86.006
    - middle ear Z86.005
    - oral cavity Z86.003
    - respiratory system Z86.005
    - skin Z86.007
    - specified NEC Z86.008
    - stomach Z86.003
  - in utero procedure during pregnancy Z98.870
  - in utero procedure while a fetus Z98.871
  - infection NEC Z86.19
    - central nervous system Z86.61
    - coronavirus (disease) (novel) 2019 Z86.16
    - COVID-19 Z86.16
    - latent tuberculosis Z86.15
    - Methicillin resistant Staphylococcus aureus (MRSA) Z86.14
    - SARS-CoV-2 Z86.16
    - urinary (recurrent) (tract) Z87.440
  - injury NEC Z87.828
  - irradiation Z92.3
  - kidney stones Z87.442
  - latent tuberculosis infection Z86.15
  - leukemia Z85.6
  - lymphoma (non-Hodgkin) Z85.72
  - malignant melanoma (skin) Z85.820
  - malignant neoplasm (of) Z85.9
    - accessory sinuses Z85.22
    - anus NEC Z85.048
      - carcinoid Z85.040
    - bladder Z85.51
    - bone Z85.830
    - brain Z85.841
    - breast Z85.3
    - bronchus NEC Z85.118
      - carcinoid Z85.110
    - carcinoid — *see* History, personal (of), malignant neoplasm, by site, carcinioid
    - cervix Z85.41
    - colon NEC Z85.038
      - carcinoid Z85.030
    - digestive organ Z85.00
      - specified NEC Z85.09
    - endocrine gland NEC Z85.858
    - epididymis Z85.48
    - esophagus Z85.01

History — *continued*
- personal — *see also* History, family — *continued*
  - malignant neoplasm — *continued*
    - eye Z85.840
    - gastrointestinal tract — *see* History, malignant neoplasm, digestive organ
    - genital organ
      - female Z85.40
        - specified NEC Z85.44
      - male Z85.45
        - specified NEC Z85.49
    - hematopoietic NEC Z85.79
    - intrathoracic organ Z85.20
    - kidney NEC Z85.528
      - carcinoid Z85.520
    - large intestine NEC Z85.038
      - carcinoid Z85.030
    - larynx Z85.21
    - liver Z85.05
    - lung NEC Z85.118
      - carcinoid Z85.110
    - mediastinum Z85.29
    - Merkel cell Z85.821
    - middle ear Z85.22
    - nasal cavities Z85.22
    - nervous system NEC Z85.848
    - oral cavity Z85.819
      - specified site NEC Z85.818
    - ovary Z85.43
    - pancreas Z85.07
    - pelvis Z85.53
    - pharynx Z85.819
      - specified site NEC Z85.818
    - pleura Z85.29
    - prostate Z85.46
    - rectosigmoid junction NEC Z85.048
      - carcinoid Z85.040
    - rectum NEC Z85.048
      - carcinoid Z85.040
    - respiratory organ Z85.20
    - sinuses, accessory Z85.22
    - skin NEC Z85.828
      - melanoma Z85.820
      - Merkel cell Z85.821
    - small intestine NEC Z85.068
      - carcinoid Z85.060
    - soft tissue Z85.831
    - specified site NEC Z85.89
    - stomach NEC Z85.028
      - carcinoid Z85.020
    - testis Z85.47
    - thymus NEC Z85.238
      - carcinoid Z85.230
    - thyroid Z85.850
    - tongue Z85.810
    - trachea Z85.12
    - urinary organ or tract Z85.50
      - specified NEC Z85.59
    - uterus Z85.42
  - maltreatment Z91.89
  - medical treatment NEC Z92.89
  - melanoma Z85.820
    - in situ Z86.006
    - malignant (skin) Z85.820
  - meningitis Z86.61
  - mental disorder Z86.59
  - Merkel cell carcinoma (skin) Z85.821
  - Methicillin resistant Staphylococcus aureus (MRSA) Z86.14
  - military deployment Z91.82
  - military war, peacekeeping and humanitarian deployment (current or past conflict) Z91.82
  - myocardial infarction (old) I25.2
  - necrotizing enterocolitis of newborn (corrected) Z87.61
  - neglect (in)
    - adult Z91.412
    - childhood Z62.812
  - neoplasia
    - anal intraepithelial, III [AIN III] Z86.004
    - high-grade prostatic intraepithelial, III [HGPIN III] Z86.002
    - vaginal intraepithelial, III [VAIN III] Z86.002
    - vulvar intraepithelial, III [VIN III] Z86.002
  - neoplasm
    - benign Z86.018
      - brain Z86.011
      - colon polyp Z86.010

History — *continued*
- personal — *see also* History, family — *continued*
  - neoplasm — *continued*
    - in situ
      - breast Z86.000
      - cervix uteri Z86.001
      - digestive organs, specified NEC Z86.004
      - esophagus Z86.003
      - genital organs, specified NEC Z86.002
      - melanoma Z86.006
      - middle ear Z86.005
      - oral cavity Z86.003
      - respiratory system Z86.005
      - skin Z86.007
      - specified NEC Z86.008
      - stomach Z86.003
    - malignant — *see* History of, malignant neoplasm
    - uncertain behavior Z86.03
  - nephrotic syndrome Z87.441
  - nicotine dependence Z87.891
  - noncompliance with medical treatment or regimen — *see* Noncompliance
  - nutritional deficiency Z86.39
  - obstetric complications Z87.59
    - childbirth Z87.59
    - pregnancy Z87.59
    - pre-term labor Z87.51
    - puerperium Z87.59
  - osteoporosis fractures Z87.31 ☑
  - parasuicide (attempt) Z91.51
  - physical trauma NEC Z87.828
    - self-harm or suicide attempt Z91.51
  - pneumonia (recurrent) Z87.01
  - poisoning NEC Z91.89
    - self-harm or suicide attempt Z91.51
  - poor personal hygiene Z91.89
  - preterm labor Z87.51
  - procedure during pregnancy Z98.870
  - procedure while a fetus Z98.871
  - prolonged reversible ischemic neurologic deficit (PRIND) Z86.73
  - prostatic dysplasia Z87.430
  - psychological
    - abuse
      - adult Z91.411
      - child Z62.811
    - trauma, specified NEC Z91.49
  - radiation therapy Z92.3
  - removal
    - implant
      - breast Z98.86
  - renal calculi Z87.442
  - respiratory condition NEC Z87.09
  - retained foreign body fully removed Z87.821
  - risk factors NEC Z91.89
  - SARS-CoV-2 infection Z86.16
  - self-harm
    - nonsuicidal Z91.52
    - suicidal Z91.51
  - self-inflicted injury without suicidal intent Z91.52
  - self-injury
    - nonsuicidal Z91.52
  - self-mutilation Z91.52
  - self-poisoning attempt Z91.51
  - sex reassignment Z87.890
  - sleep-wake cycle problem Z72.821
  - specified NEC Z87.898
  - steroid therapy (systemic) Z92.241
    - inhaled Z92.240
  - stroke without residual deficits Z86.73
  - substance abuse NEC F10-F19
  - sudden cardiac arrest Z86.74
  - sudden cardiac death successfully resuscitated Z86.74
  - suicidal behavior Z91.51
  - suicide attempt Z91.51
  - surgery NEC Z98.890
    - with uterine scar Z98.891
    - sex reassignment Z87.890
    - transplant — *see* Transplant
  - thrombophlebitis Z86.72
  - thrombosis (venous) Z86.718
    - pulmonary Z86.711
  - tobacco dependence Z87.891
  - tracheoesophageal
    - atresia Z87.731
    - fistula Z87.731
  - transient ischemic attack (TIA) without residual deficits Z86.73

- **History** — *continued*
  - personal — *see also* History, family — *continued*
    - trauma (physical) NEC Z87.828
      - psychological NEC Z91.49
      - self-harm Z91.51
    - traumatic brain injury Z87.82Ø
    - tuberculosis, latent infection Z86.15
    - unhealthy sleep-wake cycle Z72.821
    - unintended awareness under general anesthesia Z92.84
    - urinary calculi Z87.442
    - urinary (recurrent) (tract) infection(s) Z87.44Ø
    - uterine scar from previous surgery Z98.891
    - vaginal dysplasia Z87.411
    - venous thrombosis or embolism Z86.718
      - pulmonary Z86.711
    - vulvar dysplasia Z87.412
- **His-Werner disease** A79.Ø
- **HIV** — *see also* Human, immunodeficiency virus B2Ø
  - laboratory evidence (nonconclusive) R75
  - nonconclusive test (in infants) R75
  - positive, seropositive Z21
- **Hives** (bold) — *see* Urticaria
- **Hoarseness** R49.Ø
- **Hobo** Z59.ØØ
- **Hodgkin disease** — *see* Lymphoma, Hodgkin
- **Hodgson's** — *see also* Aneurysm, aorta, thorax I71.2Ø
  - ruptured — *see also* Aneurysm, aorta, thorax, ruptured I71.1Ø
- **Hoffa-Kastert disease** E88.89
- **Hoffa's disease** E88.89
- **Hoffmann-Bouveret syndrome** I47.9
- **Hoffmann's syndrome** EØ3.9 *[G73.7]*
- **Hole** (round)
  - macula H35.34- ☑
  - retina (without detachment) — *see* Break, retina, round hole
    - with detachment — *see* Detachment, retina, with retinal, break
- **Holiday relief care** Z75.5
- **Hollenhorst's plaque** — *see* Occlusion, artery, retina
- **Hollow foot** (congenital) Q66.7- ☑
  - acquired — *see* Deformity, limb, foot, specified NEC
- **Holoprosencephaly** QØ4.2
- **Holt-Oram syndrome** Q87.2
- **Homelessness** Z59.ØØ
  - sheltered Z59.Ø1
  - unsheltered Z59.Ø2
- **Homesickness** — *see* Disorder, adjustment
- **Homocysteinemia** R79.83
- **Homocystinemia, homocystinuria** E72.11
- **Homogentisate 1,2-dioxygenase deficiency** E7Ø.29
- **Homologous serum hepatitis** (prophylactic) (therapeutic) — *see* Hepatitis, viral, type B
- **Honeycomb lung** J98.4
  - congenital Q33.Ø
- **Hooded**
  - clitoris Q52.6
  - penis Q55.69
- **Hookworm** (disease) (infection) (infestation) B76.9
  - with anemia B76.9 *[D63.8]*
  - specified NEC B76.8
- **Hordeolum** (eyelid) (externum) (recurrent) HØØ.Ø19
  - internum HØØ.Ø29
    - left HØØ.Ø26
      - lower HØØ.Ø25
      - upper HØØ.Ø24
    - right HØØ.Ø23
      - lower HØØ.Ø22
      - upper HØØ.Ø21
  - left HØØ.Ø16
    - lower HØØ.Ø15
    - upper HØØ.Ø14
  - right HØØ.Ø13
    - lower HØØ.Ø12
    - upper HØØ.Ø11
- **Horn**
  - cutaneous L85.8
  - nail L6Ø.2
    - congenital Q84.6
- **Horner** (-Claude Bernard) **syndrome** G9Ø.2
  - traumatic — *see* Injury, nerve, cervical sympathetic
- **Horseshoe kidney** (congenital) Q63.1
- **Horton's headache or neuralgia** G44.Ø99
  - intractable G44.Ø91
  - not intractable G44.Ø99
- **Hospital hopper syndrome** — *see* Disorder, factitious
- **Hospitalism in children** — *see* Disorder, adjustment
- **Hostility** R45.5
  - towards child Z62.3
- **Hot flashes**
  - menopausal N95.1
- **Hourglass** (contracture) — *see also* Contraction, hourglass
  - stomach K31.89
    - congenital Q4Ø.2
    - stricture K31.2
- **Household, housing circumstance affecting care** Z59.9
  - specified NEC Z59.89
- **Housemaid's knee** — *see* Bursitis, prepatellar
- **HSCT-TMA** (hematopoietic stem cell transplantation-associated thrombotic microangiopathy) M31.11
- **Hudson** (-Stähli) **line** (cornea) — *see* Pigmentation, cornea, anterior
- **Human**
  - bite (open wound) — *see also* Bite
    - intact skin surface — *see* Bite, superficial
  - herpesvirus — *see* Herpes
  - immunodeficiency virus (HIV) disease (infection) B2Ø
    - asymptomatic status Z21
    - contact Z2Ø.6
    - counseling Z71.7
    - dementia — *see also* Dementia, in, diseases specified elsewhere B2Ø *[FØ2.8Ø]*
      - with behavioral disturbance — *see also* Dementia, in, diseases specified elsewhere B2Ø *[FØ2.81-]* ☑
    - exposure to Z2Ø.6
    - laboratory evidence R75
    - type-2 (HIV 2) as cause of disease classified elsewhere B97.35
  - papillomavirus (HPV)
    - DNA test positive
      - high risk
        - cervix R87.81Ø
        - vagina R87.811
      - low risk
        - cervix R87.82Ø
        - vagina R87.821
    - screening for Z11.51
  - T-cell lymphotropic virus
    - type-1 (HTLV-I) infection B33.3
      - as cause of disease classified elsewhere B97.33
      - carrier Z22.6
    - type-2 (HTLV-II) as cause of disease classified elsewhere B97.34
- **Humidifier lung or pneumonitis** J67.7
- **Humiliation** (experience) **in childhood** Z62.898
- **Humpback** (acquired) — *see* Kyphosis
- **Hunchback** (acquired) — *see* Kyphosis
- **Hunger** T73.Ø ☑
  - air, psychogenic F45.8
- **Hungry bone syndrome** E83.81
- **Hunner's ulcer** — *see* Cystitis, chronic, interstitial
- **Hunter's**
  - glossitis D51.Ø
  - syndrome E76.1
- **Huntington's disease or chorea** G1Ø
  - with dementia — *see also* Dementia, in, diseases specified elsewhere G1Ø *[FØ2.8Ø]*
    - with behavioral disturbance — *see also* Dementia, in, diseases specified elsewhere G1Ø *[FØ2.81-]* ☑
- **Hunt's**
  - disease or syndrome (herpetic geniculate ganglionitis) BØ2.21
    - dyssynergia cerebellaris myoclonica G11.19
  - neuralgia BØ2.21
- **Hurler** (-Scheie) **disease or syndrome** E76.Ø2
- **Hurst's disease** G36.1
- **Hurthle cell**
  - adenocarcinoma C73
  - adenoma D34
  - carcinoma C73
  - tumor D34
- **Hutchinson-Boeck disease or syndrome** — *see* Sarcoidosis
- **Hutchinson-Gilford disease or syndrome** E34.8
- **Hutchinson's**
  - disease, meaning
    - angioma serpiginosum L81.7
    - pompholyx (cheiropompholyx) L3Ø.1
    - prurigo estivalis L56.4
    - summer eruption or summer prurigo L56.4
- **Hutchinson's** — *continued*
  - melanotic freckle — *see* Melanoma, in situ
    - malignant melanoma in — *see* Melanoma
  - teeth or incisors (congenital syphilis) A5Ø.52
  - triad (congenital syphilis) A5Ø.53
- **Hyalin plaque, sclera, senile** H15.89
- **Hyaline membrane** (disease) (lung) (pulmonary) (newborn) P22.Ø
- **Hyalinosis**
  - cutis (et mucosae) E78.89
  - focal and segmental (glomerular) — *see also* NØØ-NØ7 with fourth character .1 NØ5.1
- **Hyalitis, hyalosis, asteroid** — *see also* Deposit, crystalline
  - syphilitic (late) A52.71
- **Hydatid**
  - cyst or tumor — *see* Echinococcus
  - mole — *see* Hydatidiform mole
  - Morgagni
    - female Q5Ø.5
    - male (epididymal) Q55.4
      - testicular Q55.29
- **Hydatidiform mole** (benign) (complicating pregnancy) (delivered) (undelivered) OØ1.9
  - classical OØ1.Ø
  - complete OØ1.Ø
  - incomplete OØ1.1
  - invasive D39.2
  - malignant D39.2
  - partial OØ1.1
- **Hydatidosis** — *see* Echinococcus
- **Hydradenitis** (axillaris) (suppurative) L73.2
- **Hydradenoma** — *see* Hidradenoma
- **Hydramnios** O4Ø.- ☑
- **Hydrancephaly, hydranencephaly** QØ4.3
  - with spina bifida — *see* Spina bifida, with hydrocephalus
- **Hydrargyrism NEC** — *see* Poisoning, mercury
- **Hydrarthrosis** — *see also* Effusion, joint
  - gonococcal A54.42
  - intermittent M12.4Ø
    - ankle M12.47- ☑
    - elbow M12.42- ☑
    - foot joint M12.47- ☑
    - hand joint M12.44- ☑
    - hip M12.45- ☑
    - knee M12.46- ☑
    - multiple site M12.49
    - shoulder M12.41- ☑
    - specified joint NEC M12.48
    - wrist M12.43- ☑
  - of yaws (early) (late) — *see also* subcategory M14.8- A66.6
  - syphilitic (late) A52.77
    - congenital A5Ø.55 *[M12.8Ø]*
- **Hydremia** D64.89
- **Hydrencephalocele** (congenital) — *see* Encephalocele
- **Hydrencephalomeningocele** (congenital) — *see* Encephalocele
- **Hydroa** R23.8
  - aestivale L56.4
  - vacciniforme L56.4
- **Hydroadenitis** (axillaris) (suppurative) L73.2
- **Hydrocalycosis** — *see* Hydronephrosis
- **Hydrocele** (spermatic cord) (testis) (tunica vaginalis) N43.3
  - canal of Nuck N94.89
  - communicating N43.2
    - congenital P83.5
  - congenital P83.5
  - encysted N43.Ø
  - female NEC N94.89
  - infected N43.1
  - newborn P83.5
  - round ligament N94.89
  - specified NEC N43.2
  - spinalis — *see* Spina bifida
  - vulva N9Ø.89
- **Hydrocephalus** (acquired) (external) (internal) (malignant) (recurrent) G91.9
  - aqueduct Sylvius stricture QØ3.Ø
  - causing disproportion O33.6 ☑
    - with obstructed labor O66.3
  - communicating G91.Ø
  - congenital (external) (internal) QØ3.9
    - with spina bifida QØ5.4
      - cervical QØ5.Ø

- **Hyperplasia, hyperplastic** — *continued*
  - mandible, mandibular — *continued*
    - alveolar M26.72
    - unilateral condylar M27.8
  - maxilla, maxillary M26.Ø1
    - alveolar M26.71
  - myometrium, myometrial N85.2
  - neuroendocrine cell, of infancy J84.841
  - nose
    - lymphoid J34.89
    - polypoid J33.9
  - oral mucosa (irritative) K13.6
  - organ or site, congenital NEC — *see* Anomaly, by site
  - ovary N83.8
  - palate, papillary (irritative) K13.6
  - pancreatic islet cells E16.9
    - alpha E16.8
      - with excess
        - gastrin E16.4
        - glucagon E16.3
    - beta E16.1
  - parathyroid (gland) E21.Ø
  - pharynx (lymphoid) J39.2
  - prostate (adenofibromatous) (nodular) N4Ø.Ø
    - with lower urinary tract symptoms (LUTS) N4Ø.1
    - without lower urinary tract symtpoms (LUTS) N4Ø.Ø
  - renal artery I77.89
  - reticulo-endothelial (cell) D75.89
  - salivary gland (any) K11.1
  - Schimmelbusch's — *see* Mastopathy, cystic
  - suprarenal capsule (gland) E27.8
  - thymus (gland) (persistent) E32.Ø
  - thyroid (gland) — *see* Goiter
  - tonsils (faucial) (infective) (lingual) (lymphoid) J35.1
    - with adenoids J35.3
  - unilateral condylar M27.8
  - uterus, uterine N85.2
    - endometrium (glandular) — *see also* Hyperplasia, endometrial N85.ØØ
  - vulva N9Ø.69
    - epithelial N9Ø.3
- **Hyperpnea** — *see* Hyperventilation
- **Hyperpotassemia** E87.5
- **Hyperprebetalipoproteinemia** (familial) E78.1
- **Hyperprolactinemia** E22.1
- **Hyperprolinemia** (type I) (type II) E72.59
- **Hyperproteinemia** E88.Ø9
- **Hyperprothrombinemia, causing coagulation factor deficiency** D68.4
- **Hyperpyrexia** R5Ø.9
  - heat (effects) T67.Ø1 ☑
  - malignant, due to anesthetic T88.3 ☑
  - rheumatic — *see* Fever, rheumatic
  - unknown origin R5Ø.9
- **Hyper-reflexia** R29.2
- **Hypersalivation** K11.7
- **Hypersecretion**
  - ACTH (not associated with Cushing's syndrome) E27.Ø
    - pituitary E24.Ø
  - adrenaline E27.5
  - adrenomedullary E27.5
  - androgen (testicular) E29.Ø
    - ovarian (drug-induced) (iatrogenic) E28.1
  - calcitonin EØ7.Ø
  - catecholamine E27.5
  - corticoadrenal E24.9
  - cortisol E24.9
  - epinephrine E27.5
  - estrogen E28.Ø
  - gastric K31.89
    - psychogenic F45.8
  - gastrin E16.4
  - glucagon E16.3
  - hormone(s)
    - ACTH (not associated with Cushing's syndrome) E27.Ø
      - pituitary E24.Ø
    - antidiuretic E22.2
    - growth E22.Ø
    - intestinal NEC E34.1
    - ovarian androgen E28.1
    - pituitary E22.9
    - testicular E29.Ø
    - thyroid stimulating EØ5.8Ø
      - with thyroid storm EØ5.81
  - insulin — *see* Hyperinsulinism
  - lacrimal glands — *see* Epiphora
  - medulloadrenal E27.5
- **Hypersecretion** — *continued*
  - milk O92.6
  - ovarian androgens E28.1
  - salivary gland (any) K11.7
  - thyrocalcitonin EØ7.Ø
  - upper respiratory J39.8
- **Hypersegmentation, leukocytic, hereditary** D72.Ø
- **Hypersensitive, hypersensitiveness, hypersensitivity** — *see also* Allergy
  - carotid sinus G9Ø.Ø1
  - colon — *see* Irritable, colon
  - drug T88.7 ☑
  - gastrointestinal K52.29
    - immediate K52.29
    - psychogenic F45.8
  - labyrinth — *see* subcategory H83.2 ☑
  - pain R2Ø.8
  - pneumonitis — *see* Pneumonitis, allergic
  - reaction T78.4Ø ☑
    - upper respiratory tract NEC J39.3
- **Hypersomnia** (organic) G47.1Ø
  - due to
    - alcohol
      - abuse F1Ø.182
      - dependence F1Ø.282
      - use F1Ø.982
    - amphetamines
      - abuse F15.182
      - dependence F15.282
      - use F15.982
    - caffeine
      - abuse F15.182
      - dependence F15.282
      - use F15.982
    - cocaine
      - abuse F14.182
      - dependence F14.282
      - use F14.982
    - drug NEC
      - abuse F19.182
      - dependence F19.282
      - use F19.982
    - medical condition G47.14
    - mental disorder F51.13
    - opioid
      - abuse F11.182
      - dependence F11.282
      - use F11.982
    - psychoactive substance NEC
      - abuse F19.182
      - dependence F19.282
      - use F19.982
    - sedative, hypnotic, or anxiolytic
      - abuse F13.182
      - dependence F13.282
      - use F13.982
    - stimulant NEC
      - abuse F15.182
      - dependence F15.282
      - use F15.982
  - idiopathic G47.11
    - with long sleep time G47.11
    - without long sleep time G47.12
  - menstrual related G47.13
  - nonorganic origin F51.11
    - specified NEC F51.19
  - not due to a substance or known physiological condition F51.11
    - specified NEC F51.19
  - primary F51.11
  - recurrent G47.13
  - specified NEC G47.19
- **Hypersplenia, hypersplenism** D73.1
- **Hyperstimulation, ovaries** (associated with induced ovulation) N98.1
- **Hypersusceptibility** — *see* Allergy
- **Hypertelorism** (ocular) (orbital) Q75.2
- **Hypertension, hypertensive** (accelerated) (benign) (essential) (idiopathic) (malignant) (systemic) I1Ø
  - with
    - heart failure (congestive) I11.Ø
    - heart involvement (conditions in I5Ø.- or I51.4-I51.7, I51.89, I51.9, due to hypertension) — *see* Hypertension, heart
    - kidney involvement — *see* Hypertension, kidney
  - benign, intracranial G93.2
  - borderline RØ3.Ø
  - cardiorenal (disease) I13.1Ø
- **Hypertension, hypertensive** — *continued*
  - cardiorenal — *continued*
    - with heart failure I13.Ø
      - with stage 1 through stage 4 chronic kidney disease I13.Ø
      - with stage 5 or end stage renal disease I13.2
    - without heart failure I13.1Ø
      - with stage 1 through stage 4 chronic kidney disease I13.1Ø
      - with stage 5 or end stage renal disease I13.11
  - cardiovascular
    - disease (arteriosclerotic) (sclerotic) — *see* Hypertension, heart
    - renal (disease) — *see* Hypertension, cardiorenal
  - chronic venous — *see* Hypertension, venous (chronic)
  - complicating
    - childbirth (labor) O16.4
      - pre-existing O1Ø.92
        - with
          - heart disease O1Ø.12
            - with renal disease O1Ø.32
          - pre-eclampsia O11.4
          - renal disease O1Ø.22
            - with heart disease O1Ø.32
        - essential O1Ø.Ø2
        - secondary O1Ø.42
    - pregnancy O16.- ☑
      - with edema — *see also* Pre-eclampsia O14.9- ☑
      - gestational (pregnancy induced) (without proteinuria) O13.- ☑
        - with proteinuria O14.9- ☑
          - mild pre-eclampsia O14.Ø- ☑
          - moderate pre-eclampsia O14.Ø- ☑
          - severe pre-eclampsia O14.1- ☑
            - with hemolysis, elevated liver enzymes and low platelet count (HELLP) O14.2- ☑
      - pre-existing O1Ø.91- ☑
        - with
          - heart disease O1Ø.11- ☑
            - with renal disease O1Ø.31- ☑
          - pre-eclampsia — *see* category O11
          - renal disease O1Ø.21- ☑
            - with heart disease O1Ø.31- ☑
        - essential O1Ø.Ø1- ☑
        - secondary O1Ø.41- ☑
      - transient O13- ☑
    - puerperium, pre-existing O16.5
      - pre-existing
        - with
          - heart disease O1Ø.13
            - with renal disease O1Ø.33
          - pre-eclampsia O11.5
          - renal disease O1Ø.23
            - with heart disease O1Ø.33
        - essential O1Ø.Ø3
      - pregnancy-induced O13.9
      - secondary O1Ø.43
  - crisis I16.9
  - due to
    - endocrine disorders I15.2
    - pheochromocytoma I15.2
    - renal disorders NEC I15.1
      - arterial I15.Ø
    - renovascular disorders I15.Ø
    - specified disease NEC I15.8
  - emergency I16.1
  - encephalopathy I67.4
  - gestational (without significant proteinuria) (pregnancy-induced) (transient) O13.- ☑
    - with significant proteinuria — *see* Pre-eclampsia
    - complicating
      - delivery O13.4
      - puerperium O13.5
  - Goldblatt's I7Ø.1
  - heart (disease) (conditions in I51.4-I51.9 due to hypertension) I11.9
    - with
      - heart failure (congestive) I11.Ø
      - kidney disease (chronic) — *see* Hypertension, cardiorenal
  - intracranial, benign G93.2
  - kidney I12.9
    - with
      - heart disease — *see* Hypertension, cardiorenal
      - stage 1 through stage 4 chronic kidney disease I12.9

Hypertrophy, hypertrophic — *continued*
  nasal — *continued*
    turbinate J34.3
  nasopharynx, lymphoid (infectional) (tissue) (wall) J35.2
  nipple N62
  organ or site, congenital NEC — *see* Anomaly, by site
  ovary N83.8
  palate (hard) M27.8
    soft K13.79
  pancreas, congenital Q45.3
  parathyroid (gland) E21.Ø
  parotid gland K11.1
  penis N48.89
  pharyngeal tonsil J35.2
  pharynx J39.2
    lymphoid (infectional) (tissue) (wall) J35.2
  pituitary (anterior) (fossa) (gland) E23.6
  prepuce (congenital) N47.8
    female N9Ø.89
  prostate — *see* Enlargement, enlarged, prostate
    congenital Q55.4
  pseudomuscular — *see also* Dystrophy, muscular, by type, if applicable G71.Ø9
  pylorus (adult) (muscle) (sphincter) K31.1
    congenital or infantile Q4Ø.Ø
  rectal, rectum (sphincter) K62.89
  rhinitis (turbinate) J31.Ø
  salivary gland (any) K11.1
    congenital Q38.4
  scaphoid (tarsal) — *see* Hypertrophy, bone, tarsus
  scar L91.Ø
  scrotum N5Ø.89
  seminal vesicle N5Ø.89
  sigmoid — *see* Megacolon
  skin L91.9
    specified NEC L91.8
  spermatic cord N5Ø.89
  spleen — *see* Splenomegaly
  spondylitis — *see* Spondylosis
  stomach K31.89
  sublingual gland K11.1
  submandibular gland K11.1
  suprarenal cortex (gland) E27.8
  synovial NEC M67.2Ø
    acromioclavicular M67.21- ☑
    ankle M67.27- ☑
    elbow M67.22- ☑
    foot M67.27- ☑
    hand M67.24- ☑
    hip M67.25- ☑
    knee M67.26- ☑
    multiple sites M67.29
    specified site NEC M67.28
    wrist M67.23- ☑
  tendon — *see* Disorder, tendon, specified type NEC
  testis N44.8
    congenital Q55.29
  thymic, thymus (gland) (congenital) E32.Ø
  thyroid (gland) — *see* Goiter
  toe (congenital) Q74.2
    acquired — *see also* Deformity, toe, specified NEC
  tongue K14.8
    congenital Q38.2
    papillae (foliate) K14.3
  tonsils (faucial) (infective) (lingual) (lymphoid) J35.1
    with adenoids J35.3
  tunica vaginalis N5Ø.89
  ureter N28.89
  urethra N36.8
  uterus N85.2
    neck (with elongation) N88.4
    puerperal O9Ø.89
  uvula K13.79
  vagina N89.8
  vas deferens N5Ø.89
  vein I87.8
  ventricle, ventricular (heart) — *see also* Hypertrophy, cardiac
    congenital Q24.8
    in tetralogy of Fallot Q21.3
  verumontanum N36.8
  vocal cord J38.3
  vulva N9Ø.6Ø
    stasis (nonfilarial) N9Ø.69
Hypertropia H5Ø.2- ☑
Hypertyrosinemia E7Ø.21
Hyperuricemia (asymptomatic) E79.Ø
Hyperuricosuria R82.993
Hypervalinemia E71.19
Hyperventilation (tetany) RØ6.4
  hysterical F45.8
  psychogenic F45.8
  syndrome F45.8
Hypervitaminosis (dietary) NEC E67.8
  A E67.Ø
    administered as drug (prolonged intake) — *see* Table of Drugs and Chemicals, vitamins, adverse effect
    overdose or wrong substance given or taken — *see* Table of Drugs and Chemicals, vitamins, poisoning
  B6 E67.2
  D E67.3
    administered as drug (prolonged intake) — *see* Table of Drugs and Chemicals, vitamins, adverse effect
    overdose or wrong substance given or taken — *see* Table of Drugs and Chemicals, vitamins, poisoning
  K E67.8
    administered as drug (prolonged intake) — *see* Table of Drugs and Chemicals, vitamins, adverse effect
    overdose or wrong substance given or taken — *see* Table of Drugs and Chemicals, vitamins, poisoning
Hypervolemia E87.7Ø
  specified NEC E87.79
Hypesthesia R2Ø.1
  cornea — *see* Anesthesia, cornea
Hyphema H21.Ø- ☑
  traumatic SØ5.1- ☑
Hypoacidity, gastric K31.89
  psychogenic F45.8
Hypoadrenalism, hypoadrenia E27.4Ø
  primary E27.1
  tuberculous A18.7
Hypoadrenocorticism E27.4Ø
  pituitary E23.Ø
  primary E27.1
Hypoalbuminemia E88.Ø9
Hypoaldosteronism E27.4Ø
Hypoalphalipoproteinemia E78.6
Hypobarism T7Ø.29 ☑
Hypobaropathy T7Ø.29 ☑
Hypobetalipoproteinemia (familial) E78.6
Hypocalcemia E83.51
  dietary E58
  neonatal P71.1
    due to cow's milk P71.Ø
  phosphate-loading (newborn) P71.1
Hypochloremia E87.8
Hypochlorhydria K31.89
  neurotic F45.8
  psychogenic F45.8
Hypochondria, hypochondriac, hypochondriasis (reaction) F45.21
  sleep F51.Ø3
Hypochondrogenesis Q77.Ø
Hypochondroplasia Q77.4
Hypochromasia, blood cells D5Ø.8
Hypocitraturia R82.991
Hypodontia — *see* Anodontia
Hypoeosinophilia D72.89
Hypoesthesia R2Ø.1
Hypofibrinogenemia D68.8
  acquired D65
  congenital (hereditary) D68.2
Hypofunction
  adrenocortical E27.4Ø
    drug-induced E27.3
    postprocedural E89.6
    primary E27.1
  adrenomedullary, postprocedural E89.6
  cerebral R29.818
  corticoadrenal NEC E27.4Ø
  intestinal K59.89
  labyrinth — *see* subcategory H83.2 ☑
  ovary E28.39
  pituitary (gland) (anterior) E23.Ø
  testicular E29.1
    postprocedural (postsurgical) (postirradiation) (iatrogenic) E89.5
Hypogalactia O92.4
Hypogammaglobulinemia — *see also* Agammaglobulinemia D8Ø.1
  hereditary D8Ø.Ø
  nonfamilial D8Ø.1
  transient, of infancy D8Ø.7
Hypogenitalism (congenital) — *see* Hypogonadism
Hypoglossia Q38.3
Hypoglycemia (spontaneous) E16.2
  coma E15
    diabetic — *see* Diabetes, by type, with hypoglycemia, with coma
  diabetic — *see* Diabetes, hypoglycemia
  dietary counseling and surveillance Z71.3
  drug-induced E16.Ø
    with coma (nondiabetic) E15
  due to insulin E16.Ø
    with coma (nondiabetic) E15
    therapeutic misadventure — *see* subcategory T38.3 ☑
  functional, nonhyperinsulinemic E16.1
  iatrogenic E16.Ø
    with coma (nondiabetic) E15
  in infant of diabetic mother P7Ø.1
    gestational diabetes P7Ø.Ø
  infantile E16.1
  leucine-induced E71.19
  neonatal (transitory) P7Ø.4
    iatrogenic P7Ø.3
  reactive (not drug-induced) E16.1
  transitory neonatal P7Ø.4
Hypogonadism
  female E28.39
  hypogonadotropic E23.Ø
  male E29.1
  ovarian (primary) E28.39
  pituitary E23.Ø
  testicular (primary) E29.1
Hypohidrosis, hypoidrosis L74.4
Hypoinsulinemia, postprocedural E89.1
Hypokalemia E87.6
Hypoleukocytosis — *see* Agranulocytosis
Hypolipoproteinemia (alpha) (beta) E78.6
Hypomagnesemia E83.42
  neonatal P71.2
Hypomania, hypomanic reaction F3Ø.8
Hypomenorrhea — *see* Oligomenorrhea
Hypometabolism R63.8
Hypomotility
  gastrointestinal (tract) K31.89
    psychogenic F45.8
  intestine K59.89
    psychogenic F45.8
  stomach K31.89
    psychogenic F45.8
Hyponasality R49.22
Hyponatremia E87.1
Hypo-osmolality E87.1
Hypo-ovarianism, hypo-ovarism E28.39
Hypoparathyroidism E2Ø.9
  familial E2Ø.8
  idiopathic E2Ø.Ø
  neonatal, transitory P71.4
  postprocedural E89.2
  specified NEC E2Ø.8
Hypoperfusion (in)
  newborn P96.89
Hypopharyngitis — *see* Laryngopharyngitis
Hypophoria H5Ø.53
Hypophosphatemia, hypophosphatasia (acquired) (congenital) (renal) E83.39
  familial E83.31
Hypophyseal, hypophysis — *see also* condition
  dwarfism E23.Ø
  gigantism E22.Ø
Hypopiesis — *see* Hypotension
Hypopinealism E34.8
Hypopituitarism (juvenile) E23.Ø
  drug-induced E23.1
  due to
    hypophysectomy E89.3
    radiotherapy E89.3
  iatrogenic NEC E23.1
  postirradiation E89.3
  postpartum O99.285
  postprocedural E89.3
Hypoplasia, hypoplastic
  adrenal (gland), congenital Q89.1
  alimentary tract, congenital Q45.8

☑ **Additional Character Required — Refer to the Tabular List for Character Selection**

Hypoplasia, hypoplastic — *continued*
- alimentary tract, congenital — *continued*
  - upper Q4Ø.8
- anus, anal (canal) Q42.3
  - with fistula Q42.2
- aorta, aortic Q25.42
  - ascending, in hypoplastic left heart syndrome Q23.4
  - valve Q23.1
    - in hypoplastic left heart syndrome Q23.4
- areola, congenital Q83.8
- arm (congenital) — *see* Defect, reduction, upper limb
- artery (peripheral) Q27.8
  - brain (congenital) Q28.3
  - coronary Q24.5
  - digestive system Q27.8
  - lower limb Q27.8
  - pulmonary Q25.79
    - functional, unilateral J43.Ø
  - retinal (congenital) Q14.1
  - specified site NEC Q27.8
  - umbilical Q27.Ø
  - upper limb Q27.8
- auditory canal Q17.8
  - causing impairment of hearing Q16.9
- biliary duct or passage Q44.5
- bone NOS Q79.9
  - face Q75.8
  - marrow D61.9
    - megakaryocytic D69.49
  - skull — *see* Hypoplasia, skull
- brain QØ2
  - gyri QØ4.3
  - part of QØ4.3
- breast (areola) N64.82
- bronchus Q32.4
- cardiac Q24.8
- carpus — *see* Defect, reduction, upper limb, specified type NEC
- cartilage hair Q78.8
- cecum Q42.8
- cementum KØØ.4
- cephalic QØ2
- cerebellum QØ4.3
- cervix (uteri), congenital Q51.821
- clavicle (congenital) Q74.Ø
- coccyx Q76.49
- colon Q42.9
  - specified NEC Q42.8
- corpus callosum QØ4.Ø
- cricoid cartilage Q31.2
- digestive organ(s) or tract NEC Q45.8
  - upper (congenital) Q4Ø.8
- ear (auricle) (lobe) Q17.2
  - middle Q16.4
- enamel of teeth (neonatal) (postnatal) (prenatal) KØØ.4
- endocrine (gland) NEC Q89.2
- endometrium N85.8
- epididymis (congenital) Q55.4
- epiglottis Q31.2
- erythroid, congenital D61.Ø1
- esophagus (congenital) Q39.8
- eustachian tube Q17.8
- eye Q11.2
- eyelid (congenital) Q1Ø.3
- face Q18.8
  - bone(s) Q75.8
- femur (congenital) — *see* Defect, reduction, lower limb, specified type NEC
- fibula (congenital) — *see* Defect, reduction, lower limb, specified type NEC
- finger (congenital) — *see* Defect, reduction, upper limb, specified type NEC
- focal dermal Q82.8
- foot — *see* Defect, reduction, lower limb, specified type NEC
- gallbladder Q44.Ø
- genitalia, genital organ(s)
  - female, congenital Q52.8
    - external Q52.79
    - internal NEC Q52.8
  - in adiposogenital dystrophy E23.6
- glottis Q31.2
- hair Q84.2
- hand (congenital) — *see* Defect, reduction, upper limb, specified type NEC
- heart Q24.8
- humerus (congenital) — *see* Defect, reduction, upper limb, specified type NEC

Hypoplasia, hypoplastic — *continued*
- intestine (small) Q41.9
  - large Q42.9
    - specified NEC Q42.8
- jaw M26.Ø9
  - alveolar M26.79
  - lower M26.Ø4
    - alveolar M26.74
  - upper M26.Ø2
    - alveolar M26.73
- kidney(s) Q6Ø.5
  - bilateral Q6Ø.4
  - unilateral Q6Ø.3
- labium (majus) (minus), congenital Q52.79
- larynx Q31.2
- left heart syndrome Q23.4
- leg (congenital) — *see* Defect, reduction, lower limb
- limb Q73.8
  - lower (congenital) — *see* Defect, reduction, lower limb
  - upper (congenital) — *see* Defect, reduction, upper limb
- liver Q44.7
- lung (lobe) (not associated with short gestation) Q33.6
  - associated with immaturity, low birth weight, prematurity, or short gestation P28.Ø
- mammary (areola), congenital Q83.8
- mandible, mandibular M26.Ø4
  - alveolar M26.74
  - unilateral condylar M27.8
- maxillary M26.Ø2
  - alveolar M26.73
- medullary D61.9
- megakaryocytic D69.49
- metacarpus — *see* Defect, reduction, upper limb, specified type NEC
- metatarsus — *see* Defect, reduction, lower limb, specified type NEC
- muscle Q79.8
- nail(s) Q84.6
- nose, nasal Q3Ø.1
- optic nerve H47.Ø3- ☑
- osseous meatus (ear) Q17.8
- ovary, congenital Q5Ø.39
- pancreas Q45.Ø
- parathyroid (gland) Q89.2
- parotid gland Q38.4
- patella Q74.1
- pelvis, pelvic girdle Q74.2
- penis (congenital) Q55.62
- peripheral vascular system Q27.8
  - digestive system Q27.8
  - lower limb Q27.8
  - specified site NEC Q27.8
  - upper limb Q27.8
- pituitary (gland) (congenital) Q89.2
- pulmonary (not associated with short gestation) Q33.6
  - artery, functional J43.Ø
  - associated with short gestation P28.Ø
- radioulnar — *see* Defect, reduction, upper limb, specified type NEC
- radius — *see* Defect, reduction, upper limb
- rectum Q42.1
  - with fistula Q42.Ø
- respiratory system NEC Q34.8
- rib Q76.6
- right heart syndrome Q22.6
- sacrum Q76.49
- scapula Q74.Ø
- scrotum Q55.1
- shoulder girdle Q74.Ø
- skin Q82.8
- skull (bone) Q75.8
  - with
    - anencephaly QØØ.Ø
    - encephalocele — *see* Encephalocele
    - hydrocephalus QØ3.9
      - with spina bifida — *see* Spina bifida, by site, with hydrocephalus
    - microcephaly QØ2
- spinal (cord) (ventral horn cell) QØ6.1
- spine Q76.49
- sternum Q76.7
- tarsus — *see* Defect, reduction, lower limb, specified type NEC
- testis Q55.1
- thymic, with immunodeficiency D82.1
- thymus (gland) Q89.2

Hypoplasia, hypoplastic — *continued*
- thymus — *continued*
  - with immunodeficiency D82.1
- thyroid (gland) EØ3.1
  - cartilage Q31.2
- tibiofibular (congenital) — *see* Defect, reduction, lower limb, specified type NEC
- toe — *see* Defect, reduction, lower limb, specified type NEC
- tongue Q38.3
- Turner's KØØ.4
- ulna (congenital) — *see* Defect, reduction, upper limb
- umbilical artery Q27.Ø
- unilateral condylar M27.8
- ureter Q62.8
- uterus, congenital Q51.811
- vagina Q52.4
- vascular NEC peripheral Q27.8
  - brain Q28.3
  - digestive system Q27.8
  - lower limb Q27.8
  - specified site NEC Q27.8
  - upper limb Q27.8
- vein(s) (peripheral) Q27.8
  - brain Q28.3
  - digestive system Q27.8
  - great Q26.8
  - lower limb Q27.8
  - specified site NEC Q27.8
  - upper limb Q27.8
- vena cava (inferior) (superior) Q26.8
- vertebra Q76.49
- vulva, congenital Q52.79
- zonule (ciliary) Q12.8

Hypoplasminogenemia E88.Ø2

Hypopnea, obstructive sleep apnea G47.33

Hypopotassemia E87.6

Hypoproconvertinemia, congenital (hereditary) D68.2

Hypoproteinemia E77.8

Hypoprothrombinemia (congenital) (hereditary) (idiopathic) D68.2
- acquired D68.4
- newborn, transient P61.6

Hypoptyalism K11.7

Hypopyon (eye) (anterior chamber) — *see* Iridocyclitis, acute, hypopyon

Hypopyrexia R68.Ø

Hyporeflexia R29.2

Hyposecretion
- ACTH E23.Ø
- antidiuretic hormone E23.2
- ovary E28.39
- salivary gland (any) K11.7
- vasopressin E23.2

Hyposegmentation, leukocytic, hereditary D72.Ø

Hyposiderinemia D5Ø.9

Hypospadias Q54.9
- balanic Q54.Ø
- coronal Q54.Ø
- glandular Q54.Ø
- penile Q54.1
- penoscrotal Q54.2
- perineal Q54.3
- specified NEC Q54.8

Hypospermatogenesis — *see* Oligospermia

Hyposplenism D73.Ø

Hypostasis pulmonary, passive — *see* Edema, lung

Hypostatic — *see* condition

Hyposthenuria N28.89

Hypotension (arterial) (constitutional) I95.9
- chronic I95.89
- due to (of) hemodialysis I95.3
- drug-induced I95.2
- iatrogenic I95.89
- idiopathic (permanent) I95.Ø
- intracranial G96.81Ø
  - following
    - lumbar cerebrospinal fluid shunting G97.83
    - specified procedure NEC G97.84
    - ventricular shunting (ventriculostomy) G97.2
  - specified NEC G96.819
  - spontaneous G96.811
- intra-dialytic I95.3
- maternal, syndrome (following labor and delivery) O26.5- ☑
- neurogenic, orthostatic G9Ø.3
- orthostatic (chronic) I95.1
  - due to drugs I95.2

- **Immunization** — *continued*
  - not done — *see also* Underimmunization status — *continued*
    - because (of)
      - acute illness of patient Z28.Ø1
      - allergy to vaccine (or component) Z28.Ø4
      - caregiver refusal Z28.82
      - chronic illness of patient Z28.Ø2
      - contraindication NEC Z28.Ø9
      - delay in delivery of vaccine Z28.83
      - group pressure Z28.1
      - guardian refusal Z28.82
      - immune compromised state of patient Z28.Ø3
      - lack of availability of vaccine Z28.83
      - manufacturer delay of vaccine Z28.83
      - parent refusal Z28.82
      - patient had disease being vaccinated against Z28.81
      - patient refusal Z28.21
      - patient's belief Z28.1
      - religious beliefs of patient Z28.1
      - specified reason NEC Z28.89
        - of patient Z28.29
      - unavailability of vaccine Z28.83
      - unspecified patient reason Z28.2Ø
  - partial — *see also* Underimmunization status
    - for COVID-19 Z28.311
  - Rh factor
    - affecting management of pregnancy NEC O36.Ø9- ☑
      - anti-D antibody O36.Ø1- ☑
    - from transfusion — *see* Complication(s), transfusion, incompatibility reaction, Rh (factor)
- **Immunocompromised NOS** D84.9
- **Immunocytoma** C83.Ø- ☑
- **Immunodeficiency** D84.9
  - with
    - adenosine-deaminase deficiency — *see also* Deficiency, adenosine deaminase D81.3Ø
    - antibody defects D8Ø.9
      - specified type NEC D8Ø.8
    - hyperimmunoglobulinemia D8Ø.6
    - increased immunoglobulin M (IgM) D8Ø.5
    - major defect D82.9
      - specified type NEC D82.8
    - partial albinism D82.8
    - short-limbed stature D82.2
    - thrombocytopenia and eczema D82.Ø
  - antibody with
    - hyperimmunoglobulinemia D8Ø.6
    - near-normal immunoglobulins D8Ø.6
  - autosomal recessive, Swiss type D8Ø.Ø
  - combined D81.9
    - biotin-dependent carboxylase D81.819
      - biotinidase D81.81Ø
      - holocarboxylase synthetase D81.818
      - specified type NEC D81.818
    - severe (SCID) D81.9
      - with
        - low or normal B-cell numbers D81.2
        - low T- and B-cell numbers D81.1
        - reticular dysgenesis D81.Ø
    - specified type NEC D81.89
  - common variable D83.9
    - with
      - abnormalities of B-cell numbers and function D83.Ø
      - autoantibodies to B- or T-cells D83.2
      - immunoregulatory T-cell disorders D83.1
    - specified type NEC D83.8
  - due to
    - conditions classified elsewhere D84.81
    - drugs D84.821
    - external causes D84.822
    - medication (current or past) D84.821
  - following hereditary defective response to Epstein-Barr virus (EBV) D82.3
  - selective, immunoglobulin
    - A (IgA) D8Ø.2
    - G (IgG) (subclasses) D8Ø.3
    - M (IgM) D8Ø.4
  - severe combined (SCID) D81.9
    - due to adenosine deaminase deficiency D81.31
  - specified type NEC D84.89
  - X-linked, with increased IgM D8Ø.5
- **Immunodeficient NOS** D84.9
- **Immunosuppressed NOS** D84.9
- **Immunotherapy** (encounter for)
  - antineoplastic Z51.12
- **Impaction, impacted**
  - bowel, colon, rectum — *see also* Impaction, fecal K56.49
    - by gallstone K56.3
  - calculus — *see* Calculus
  - cerumen (ear) (external) H61.2- ☑
  - cuspid — *see* Impaction, tooth
  - dental (same or adjacent tooth) KØ1.1
  - fecal, feces K56.41
  - fracture — *see* Fracture, by site
  - gallbladder — *see* Calculus, gallbladder
  - gallstone(s) — *see* Calculus, gallbladder
    - bile duct (common) (hepatic) — *see* Calculus, bile duct
    - cystic duct — *see* Calculus, gallbladder
    - in intestine, with obstruction (any part) K56.3
  - intestine (calculous) NEC — *see also* Impaction, fecal K56.49
    - gallstone, with ileus K56.3
  - intrauterine device (IUD) T83.39 ☑
  - molar — *see* Impaction, tooth
  - shoulder, causing obstructed labor O66.Ø
  - tooth, teeth KØ1.1
  - turbinate J34.89
- **Impaired, impairment** (function)
  - auditory discrimination — *see* Abnormal, auditory perception
  - cognitive, mild, of uncertain or unknown etiology G31.84
  - dual sensory Z73.82
  - fasting glucose R73.Ø1
  - glucose tolerance (oral) R73.Ø2
  - hearing — *see* Deafness
  - heart — *see* Disease, heart
  - kidney N28.9
    - disorder resulting from N25.9
      - specified NEC N25.89
  - liver K72.9Ø
    - with coma K72.91
  - mastication KØ8.89
  - mild cognitive G31.84
    - of uncertain or unknown etiology G31.84
  - mild neurocognitive
    - due to known physiological condition (without behavioral disturbance) FØ6.7Ø
      - with behavioral disturbance FØ6.71
  - mobility
    - ear ossicles — *see* Ankylosis, ear ossicles
    - requiring care provider Z74.Ø9
  - myocardium, myocardial — *see* Insufficiency, myocardial
  - rectal sphincter R19.8
  - renal (acute) (chronic) N28.9
    - disorder resulting from N25.9
      - specified NEC N25.89
  - vision NEC H54.7
    - both eyes H54.3
- **Impediment, speech** — *see also* Disorder, speech R47.9
  - psychogenic (childhood) F98.8
  - slurring R47.81
  - specified NEC R47.89
- **Impending**
  - coronary syndrome I2Ø.Ø
  - delirium tremens F1Ø.239
  - myocardial infarction I2Ø.Ø
- **Imperception auditory** (acquired) — *see also* Deafness
  - congenital H93.25
- **Imperfect**
  - aeration, lung (newborn) NEC — *see* Atelectasis
  - closure (congenital)
    - alimentary tract NEC Q45.8
      - lower Q43.8
      - upper Q4Ø.8
    - atrioventricular ostium Q21.2Ø
    - atrium (secundum) Q21.11
    - branchial cleft NOS Q18.2
      - cyst Q18.Ø
      - fistula Q18.Ø
      - sinus Q18.Ø
    - choroid Q14.3
    - cricoid cartilage Q31.8
    - cusps, heart valve NEC Q24.8
      - pulmonary Q22.3
    - ductus
      - arteriosus Q25.Ø
      - Botalli Q25.Ø
    - ear drum (causing impairment of hearing) Q16.4
- **Imperfect** — *continued*
  - closure — *continued*
    - esophagus with communication to bronchus or trachea Q39.1
    - eyelid Q1Ø.3
    - foramen
      - botalli Q21.12
      - ovale Q21.12
    - genitalia, genital organ(s) or system
      - female Q52.8
        - external Q52.79
        - internal NEC Q52.8
      - male Q55.8
    - glottis Q31.8
    - interatrial ostium or septum Q21.19
    - interauricular ostium or septum Q21.19
    - interventricular ostium or septum Q21.Ø
    - larynx Q31.8
    - lip — *see* Cleft, lip
    - nasal septum Q3Ø.3
    - nose Q3Ø.2
    - omphalomesenteric duct Q43.Ø
    - optic nerve entry Q14.2
    - organ or site not listed — *see* Anomaly, by site
    - ostium
      - interatrial Q21.19
      - interauricular Q21.19
      - interventricular Q21.Ø
    - palate — *see* Cleft, palate
    - preauricular sinus Q18.1
    - retina Q14.1
    - roof of orbit Q75.8
    - sclera Q13.5
    - septum
      - aorticopulmonary Q21.4
      - atrial (secundum) Q21.19
      - between aorta and pulmonary artery Q21.4
      - heart Q21.9
      - interatrial (secundum) Q21.19
      - interauricular (secundum) Q21.19
      - interventricular Q21.Ø
        - in tetralogy of Fallot Q21.3
      - nasal Q3Ø.3
      - ventricular Q21.Ø
        - with pulmonary stenosis or atresia, dextraposition of aorta, and hypertrophy of right ventricle Q21.3
        - in tetralogy of Fallot Q21.3
    - skull Q75.Ø
      - with
        - anencephaly QØØ.Ø
        - encephalocele — *see* Encephalocele
        - hydrocephalus QØ3.9
          - with spina bifida — *see* Spina bifida, by site, with hydrocephalus
        - microcephaly QØ2
    - spine (with meningocele) — *see* Spina bifida
    - trachea Q32.1
    - tympanic membrane (causing impairment of hearing) Q16.4
    - uterus Q51.818
    - vitelline duct Q43.Ø
  - erection — *see* Dysfunction, sexual, male, erectile
  - fusion — *see* Imperfect, closure
  - inflation, lung (newborn) — *see* Atelectasis
  - posture R29.3
  - rotation, intestine Q43.3
  - septum, ventricular Q21.Ø
- **Imperfectly descended testis** — *see* Cryptorchid
- **Imperforate** (congenital) — *see also* Atresia
  - anus Q42.3
    - with fistula Q42.2
  - cervix (uteri) Q51.828
  - esophagus Q39.Ø
    - with tracheoesophageal fistula Q39.1
  - hymen Q52.3
  - jejunum Q41.1
  - pharynx Q38.8
  - rectum Q42.1
    - with fistula Q42.Ø
  - urethra Q64.39
  - vagina Q52.4
- **Impervious** (congenital) — *see also* Atresia
  - anus Q42.3
    - with fistula Q42.2
  - bile duct Q44.2
  - esophagus Q39.Ø
    - with tracheoesophageal fistula Q39.1

- **Impervious** — *continued*
  - intestine (small) Q41.9
    - large Q42.9
      - specified NEC Q42.8
  - rectum Q42.1
    - with fistula Q42.Ø
  - ureter — *see* Atresia, ureter
  - urethra Q64.39
- **Impetiginization of dermatoses** LØ1.1
- **Impetigo** (any organism) (any site) (circinate) (contagiosa) (simplex) (vulgaris) LØ1.ØØ
  - Bockhart's LØ1.Ø2
  - bullous, bullosa LØ1.Ø3
  - external ear LØ1.ØØ *[H62.4Ø]*
  - follicularis LØ1.Ø2
  - furfuracea L3Ø.5
  - herpetiformis L4Ø.1
    - nonobstetrical L4Ø.1
  - neonatorum LØ1.Ø3
  - nonbullous LØ1.Ø1
  - specified type NEC LØ1.Ø9
  - ulcerative LØ1.Ø9
- **Impingement** (on teeth)
  - joint — *see* Disorder, joint, specified type NEC
  - soft tissue
    - anterior M26.81
    - posterior M26.82
- **Implant, endometrial** N8Ø.9
- **Implantation**
  - anomalous — *see* Anomaly, by site
    - ureter Q62.63
  - cyst
    - external area or site (skin) NEC L72.Ø
    - iris — *see* Cyst, iris, implantation
    - vagina N89.8
    - vulva N9Ø.7
  - dermoid (cyst) — *see* Implantation, cyst
- **Impotence** (sexual) N52.9
  - counseling Z7Ø.1
  - organic origin — *see also* Dysfunction, sexual, male, erectile N52.9
  - psychogenic F52.21
- **Impression, basilar** Q75.8
- **Imprisonment, anxiety concerning** Z65.1
- **Improper care** (child) (newborn) — *see* Maltreatment
- **Improperly tied umbilical cord** (causing hemorrhage) P51.8
- **Impulsiveness** (impulsive) R45.87
- **Inability to swallow** — *see* Aphagia
  - comply with dietary regimen Z91.118
  - swallow — *see* Aphagia
- **Inaccessible, inaccessibility**
  - health care NEC Z75.3
    - due to
      - waiting period Z75.2
        - for admission to facility elsewhere Z75.1
  - other helping agencies Z75.4
  - transportation Z59.82
- **Inactive** — *see* condition
- **Inadequate, inadequacy**
  - aesthetics of dental restoration KØ8.56
  - biologic, constitutional, functional, or social F6Ø.7
  - development
    - child R62.5Ø
    - genitalia
      - after puberty NEC E3Ø.Ø
      - congenital
        - female Q52.8
          - external Q52.79
          - internal Q52.8
        - male Q55.8
    - lungs Q33.6
      - associated with short gestation P28.Ø
    - organ or site not listed — *see* Anomaly, by site
  - diet (causing nutritional deficiency) E63.9
  - drinking-water supply Z58.6
  - eating habits Z72.4
  - environment, household Z59.1
  - family support Z63.8
  - food (supply) NEC Z59.48
    - hunger effects T73.Ø ☑
  - functional F6Ø.7
  - household care, due to
    - family member
      - handicapped or ill Z74.2
      - on vacation Z75.5
      - temporarily away from home Z74.2
    - technical defects in home Z59.1

- **Inadequate, inadequacy** — *continued*
  - household care, due to — *continued*
    - temporary absence from home of person rendering care Z74.2
  - housing (heating) (space) Z59.1
  - income (financial) Z59.6
  - intrafamilial communication Z63.8
  - material resources Z59.87
  - mental — *see* Disability, intellectual
  - parental supervision or control of child Z62.Ø
  - personality F6Ø.7
  - pulmonary
    - function RØ6.89
      - newborn P28.5
    - ventilation, newborn P28.5
  - sample of cytologic smear
    - anus R85.615
    - cervix R87.615
    - vagina R87.625
  - social F6Ø.7
    - insurance Z59.7
    - skills NEC Z73.4
  - supervision of child by parent Z62.Ø
  - teaching affecting education Z55.8
  - transportation Z59.82
  - welfare support Z59.7
- **Inanition** R64
  - with edema — *see* Malnutrition, severe
  - due to
    - deprivation of food T73.Ø ☑
    - malnutrition — *see* Malnutrition
  - fever R5Ø.9
- **Inappropriate**
  - change in quantitative human chorionic gonadotropin (hCG) in early pregnancy OØ2.81
  - diet or eating habits Z72.4
  - level of quantitative human chorionic gonadotropin (hCG) for gestational age in early pregnancy OØ2.81
  - secretion
    - antidiuretic hormone (ADH) (excessive) E22.2
      - deficiency E23.2
    - pituitary (posterior) E22.2
- **Inattention at or after birth** — *see* Neglect
- **Incarceration, incarcerated**
  - enterocele K46.Ø
    - gangrenous K46.1
  - epiplocele K46.Ø
    - gangrenous K46.1
  - exomphalos K42.Ø
    - gangrenous K42.1
  - hernia — *see also* Hernia, by site, with obstruction
    - with gangrene — *see* Hernia, by site, with gangrene
  - iris, in wound — *see* Injury, eye, laceration, with prolapse
  - lens, in wound — *see* Injury, eye, laceration, with prolapse
  - omphalocele K42.Ø
  - prison, anxiety concerning Z65.1
  - rupture — *see* Hernia, by site
  - sarcoepiplocele K46.Ø
    - gangrenous K46.1
  - sarcoepiplomphalocele K42.Ø
    - with gangrene K42.1
  - uterus N85.8
    - gravid O34.51- ☑
      - causing obstructed labor O65.5
- **Incised wound**
  - external — *see* Laceration
  - internal organs — *see* Injury, by site
- **Incision, incisional**
  - hernia K43.2
    - with
      - gangrene (and obstruction) K43.1
      - obstruction K43.Ø
  - surgical, complication — *see* Complications, surgical procedure
  - traumatic
    - external — *see* Laceration
    - internal organs — *see* Injury, by site
- **Inclusion**
  - azurophilic leukocytic D72.Ø
  - blennorrhea (neonatal) (newborn) P39.1
  - gallbladder in liver (congenital) Q44.1
- **Incompatibility**
  - ABO
    - affecting management of pregnancy O36.11- ☑
      - anti-A sensitization O36.11- ☑

- **Incompatibility** — *continued*
  - ABO — *continued*
    - affecting management of pregnancy — *continued*
      - anti-B sensitization O36.19- ☑
      - specified NEC O36.19- ☑
    - infusion or transfusion reaction — *see* Complication(s), transfusion, incompatibility reaction, ABO
    - newborn P55.1
  - blood (group) (Duffy) (K) (Kell) (Kidd) (Lewis) (M) (S) NEC
    - affecting management of pregnancy O36.11- ☑
      - anti-A sensitization O36.11- ☑
      - anti-B sensitization O36.19- ☑
    - infusion or transfusion reaction T8Ø.89 ☑
    - newborn P55.8
  - divorce or estrangement Z63.5
  - Rh (blood group) (factor) Z31.82
    - affecting management of pregnancy NEC O36.Ø9- ☑
      - anti-D antibody O36.Ø1- ☑
    - infusion or transfusion reaction — *see* Complication(s), transfusion, incompatibility reaction, Rh (factor)
    - newborn P55.Ø
  - rhesus — *see* Incompatibility, Rh
- **Incompetency, incompetent, incompetence**
  - annular
    - aortic (valve) — *see* Insufficiency, aortic
    - mitral (valve) I34.Ø
    - pulmonary valve (heart) I37.1
  - aortic (valve) — *see* Insufficiency, aortic
  - cardiac valve — *see* Endocarditis
  - cervix, cervical (os) N88.3
    - in pregnancy O34.3- ☑
  - chronotropic I45.89
    - with
      - autonomic dysfunction G9Ø.8
      - ischemic heart disease I25.89
      - left ventricular dysfunction I51.89
      - sinus node dysfunction I49.8
  - esophagogastric (junction) (sphincter) K22.Ø
  - mitral (valve) — *see* Insufficiency, mitral
  - pelvic fundus N81.89
  - pubocervical tissue N81.82
  - pulmonary valve (heart) I37.1
    - congenital Q22.3
  - rectovaginal tissue N81.83
  - tricuspid (annular) (valve) — *see* Insufficiency, tricuspid
  - valvular — *see* Endocarditis
    - congenital Q24.8
  - vein, venous (saphenous) (varicose) — *see* Varix, leg
- **Incomplete** — *see also* condition
  - atrioventricular
    - canal Q21.21
    - septal defect Q21.21
  - bladder, emptying R33.9
  - defecation R15.Ø
  - endocardial cushion defect Q21.21
  - expansion lungs (newborn) NEC — *see* Atelectasis
  - rotation, intestine Q43.3
- **Inconclusive**
  - diagnostic imaging due to excess body fat of patient R93.9
  - findings on diagnostic imaging of breast NEC R92.8
  - mammogram (due to dense breasts) R92.2
- **Incontinence** R32
  - anal sphincter R15.9
  - coital N39.491
  - feces R15.9
    - nonorganic origin F98.1
  - insensible (urinary) N39.42
  - overflow N39.49Ø
  - postural (urinary) N39.492
  - psychogenic F45.8
  - rectal R15.9
  - reflex N39.498
  - stress (female) (male) N39.3
    - and urge N39.46
  - urethral sphincter R32
  - urge N39.41
    - and stress (female) (male) N39.46
  - urine (urinary) R32
    - continuous N39.45
    - due to cognitive impairment, or severe physical disability or immobility R39.81
    - functional R39.81
    - insensible N39.42

Index

Incontinence — Infarct, infarction

Infection, infected, infective — *continued*
- candiru B88.8
- Capillaria (intestinal) B81.1
  - hepatica B83.8
  - philippinensis B81.1
- cartilage — *see* Disorder, cartilage, specified type NEC
- cat liver fluke B66.Ø
- catheter-related bloodstream (CRBSI) T8Ø.211 ☑
- cellulitis — *code by* site under Cellulitis
- central line-associated T8Ø.219 ☑
  - bloodstream (CLABSI) T8Ø.211 ☑
  - specified NEC T8Ø.218 ☑
- Cephalosporium falciforme B47.Ø
- cerebrospinal — *see* Meningitis
- cervical gland (lymph) LØ4.Ø
- cervix — *see* Cervicitis
- cesarean delivery wound (puerperal) O86.ØØ
- cestodes — *see* Infestation, cestodes
- chest J22
- Chilomastix (intestinal) AØ7.8
- Chlamydia, chlamydial A74.9
  - anus A56.3
  - genitourinary tract A56.2
    - lower A56.ØØ
    - specified NEC A56.19
  - lymphogranuloma A55
  - pharynx A56.4
  - psittaci A7Ø
  - rectum A56.3
  - sexually transmitted NEC A56.8
- cholera — *see* Cholera
- Cladosporium
  - bantianum (brain abscess) B43.1
  - carrionii B43.Ø
  - castellanii B36.1
  - trichoides (brain abscess) B43.1
  - werneckii B36.1
- Clonorchis (sinensis) (liver) B66.1
- Clostridium NEC
  - bifermentans A48.Ø
  - botulinum (food poisoning) AØ5.1
    - infant A48.51
    - wound A48.52
  - difficile
    - as cause of disease classified elsewhere B96.89
    - foodborne (disease)
      - not specified as recurrent AØ4.72
      - recurrent AØ4.71
    - gas gangrene A48.Ø
    - necrotizing enterocolitis
      - not specified as recurrent AØ4.72
      - recurrent AØ4.71
    - sepsis A41.4
  - gas-forming NEC A48.Ø
  - histolyticum A48.Ø
  - novyi, causing gas gangrene A48.Ø
  - oedematiens A48.Ø
  - perfringens
    - as cause of disease classified elsewhere B96.7
    - due to food AØ5.2
    - foodborne (disease) AØ5.2
    - gas gangrene A48.Ø
    - sepsis A41.4
  - septicum, causing gas gangrene A48.Ø
  - sordellii, causing gas gangrene A48.Ø
  - welchii
    - as cause of disease classified elsewhere B96.7
    - foodborne (disease) AØ5.2
    - gas gangrene A48.Ø
    - necrotizing enteritis AØ5.2
    - sepsis A41.4
- Coccidioides (immitis) — *see* Coccidioidomycosis
- colon — *see* Enteritis, infectious
- colostomy K94.Ø2
- common duct — *see* Cholangitis
- congenital P39.9
  - Candida (albicans) P37.5
  - cytomegalovirus P35.1
  - hepatitis, viral P35.3
  - herpes simplex P35.2
  - infectious or parasitic disease P37.9
    - specified NEC P37.8
  - listeriosis (disseminated) P37.2
  - malaria NEC P37.4
    - falciparum P37.3
  - Plasmodium falciparum P37.3
  - poliomyelitis P35.8
  - rubella P35.Ø

Infection, infected, infective — *continued*
- congenital — *continued*
  - skin P39.4
  - toxoplasmosis (acute) (subacute) (chronic) P37.1
  - tuberculosis P37.Ø
  - urinary (tract) P39.3
  - vaccinia P35.8
  - virus P35.9
    - specified type NEC P35.8
- Conidiobolus B46.8
- coronavirus-2Ø19 UØ7.1
- coronavirus NEC B34.2
  - as cause of disease classified elsewhere B97.29
  - severe acute respiratory syndrome (SARS associated) B97.21
- corpus luteum — *see* Salpingo-oophoritis
- Corynebacterium diphtheriae — *see* Diphtheria
- cotia virus BØ8.8
- COVID-19 — *see also* COVID-19 UØ7.1
- Coxiella burnetii A78
- coxsackie — *see* Coxsackie
- Cryptococcus neoformans — *see* Cryptococcosis
- Cryptosporidium AØ7.2
- Cunninghamella — *see* Mucormycosis
- cyst — *see* Cyst
- cystic duct — *see also* Cholecystitis K81.9
- Cysticercus cellulosae — *see* Cysticercosis
- cytomegalovirus, cytomegaloviral B25.9
  - congenital P35.1
  - maternal, maternal care for (suspected) damage to fetus O35.3 ☑
  - mononucleosis B27.1Ø
    - with
      - complication NEC B27.19
      - meningitis B27.12
      - polyneuropathy B27.11
- delta-agent (acute), in hepatitis B carrier B17.Ø
- dental (pulpal origin) KØ4.7
- Deuteromycetes B47.Ø
- Dicrocoelium dendriticum B66.2
- Dipetalonema (perstans) (streptocerca) B74.4
- diphtherial — *see* Diphtheria
- Diphyllobothrium (adult) (latum) (pacificum) B7Ø.Ø
  - larval B7Ø.1
- Diplogonoporus (grandis) B71.8
- Dipylidium caninum B67.4
- Dirofilaria B74.8
- Dracunculus medinensis B72
- Drechslera (hawaiiensis) B43.8
- Ducrey Haemophilus (any location) A57
- due to or resulting from
  - artificial insemination N98.Ø
  - Babesia
    - divergens (-like) strain B6Ø.Ø3
    - duncani (-type) species B6Ø.Ø2
    - microti B6Ø.Ø1
    - species
      - specified NEC B6Ø.Ø9
  - central venous catheter T8Ø.219 ☑
    - bloodstream T8Ø.211 ☑
    - exit or insertion site T8Ø.212 ☑
    - localized T8Ø.212 ☑
    - port or reservoir T8Ø.212 ☑
    - specified NEC T8Ø.218 ☑
    - tunnel T8Ø.212 ☑
  - device, implant or graft — *see also* Complications, by site and type, infection or inflammation T85.79 ☑
    - arterial graft NEC T82.7 ☑
    - breast (implant) T85.79 ☑
    - catheter NEC T85.79 ☑
      - dialysis (renal) T82.7 ☑
        - central line T8Ø.211 ☑
        - intraperitoneal T85.71 ☑
      - infusion NEC T82.7 ☑
        - cranial T85.735 ☑
        - intrathecal T85.735 ☑
        - spinal (epidural) (subdural) T85.735 ☑
        - subarachnoid T85.735 ☑
      - urinary T83.518 ☑
        - cystostomy T83.51Ø ☑
        - Hopkins T83.518 ☑
        - ileostomy T83.518 ☑
        - nephrostomy T83.512 ☑
        - specified NEC T83.518 ☑
        - urethral indwelling T83.511 ☑
        - urostomy T83.518 ☑

Infection, infected, infective — *continued*
- due to or resulting from — *continued*
  - device, implant or graft — *see also* Complications, by site and type, infection or inflammation — *continued*
    - electronic (electrode) (pulse generator) (stimulator)
      - bone T84.7 ☑
      - cardiac T82.7 ☑
      - nervous system T85.738 ☑
        - brain T85.731 ☑
        - cranial nerve T85.732 ☑
        - gastric nerve T85.732 ☑
        - generator pocket T85.734 ☑
        - neurostimulator generator T85.734 ☑
        - peripheral nerve T85.732 ☑
        - sacral nerve T85.732 ☑
        - spinal cord T85.733 ☑
        - vagal nerve T85.732 ☑
      - urinary (indwelling) T83.51 ☑
    - fixation, internal (orthopedic) NEC — *see* Complication, fixation device, infection
    - gastrointestinal (bile duct) (esophagus) T85.79 ☑
      - neurostimulator electrode (lead) T85.732 ☑
    - genital NEC T83.69 ☑
    - heart NEC T82.7 ☑
      - valve (prosthesis) T82.6 ☑
        - graft T82.7 ☑
    - joint prosthesis — *see* Complication, joint prosthesis, infection
    - ocular (corneal graft) (orbital implant) NEC T85.79 ☑
    - orthopedic NEC T84.7 ☑
    - penile (cylinder) (pump) (resevoir) T83.61 ☑
    - specified NEC T85.79 ☑
    - testicular T83.62 ☑
    - urinary NEC T83.598 ☑
      - ileal conduit stent T83.593 ☑
      - implanted neurostimulation T83.59Ø ☑
      - implanted sphincter T83.591 ☑
      - indwelling ureteral stent T83.592 ☑
      - nephroureteral stent T83.593 ☑
      - specified stent NEC T83.593 ☑
    - vascular NEC T82.7 ☑
    - ventricular intracranial (communicating) shunt T85.73Ø ☑
  - Hickman catheter T8Ø.219 ☑
    - bloodstream T8Ø.211 ☑
    - localized T8Ø.212 ☑
    - specified NEC T8Ø.218 ☑
  - immunization or vaccination T88.Ø ☑
  - infusion, injection or transfusion NEC T8Ø.29 ☑
  - injury NEC — *code by* site under Wound, open
  - peripherally inserted central catheter (PICC) T8Ø.219 ☑
    - bloodstream T8Ø.211 ☑
    - localized T8Ø.212 ☑
    - specified NEC T8Ø.218 ☑
  - portacath (port-a-cath) T8Ø.219 ☑
    - bloodstream T8Ø.211 ☑
    - localized T8Ø.212 ☑
    - specified NEC T8Ø.218 ☑
  - protozoa of the order Piroplasmida NEC B6Ø.Ø9
  - pulmonary artery catheter — *see* Infection, due to or resulting from, central venous catheter
  - surgery T81.4Ø ☑
  - Swan Ganz catheter — *see* Infection, due to or resulting from, central venous catheter
  - triple lumen catheter T8Ø.219 ☑
    - bloodstream T8Ø.211 ☑
    - localized T8Ø.212 ☑
    - specified NEC T8Ø.218 ☑
  - umbilical venous catheter T8Ø.219 ☑
    - bloodstream T8Ø.211 ☑
    - localized T8Ø.212 ☑
    - specified NEC T8Ø.218 ☑
- during labor NEC O75.3
- ear (middle) — *see also* Otitis media
  - external — *see* Otitis, externa, infective
  - inner — *see* subcategory H83.Ø ☑
- Eberthella typhosa AØ1.ØØ
- Echinococcus — *see* Echinococcus
- echovirus
  - as cause of disease classified elsewhere B97.12
  - unspecified nature or site B34.1
- endocardium I33.Ø

- **Infestation** — *continued*
  - Parastrongylus
    - cantonensis B83.2
    - costaricensis B81.3
  - Pediculus B85.2
    - body B85.1
    - capitis (humanus) (any site) B85.Ø
    - corporis (humanus) (any site) B85.1
    - head B85.Ø
    - mixed (classifiable to more than one of the titles B85.Ø - B85.3) B85.4
    - pubis (any site) B85.3
  - Pentastoma B88.8
  - Phthirus (pubis) (any site) B85.3
    - with any infestation classifiable to B85.Ø - B85.2 B85.4
  - pinworm B8Ø
  - pork tapeworm (adult) B68.Ø
  - protozoal NEC B64
    - intestinal AØ7.9
      - specified NEC AØ7.8
    - specified NEC B6Ø.8
  - pubic, louse B85.3
  - rat tapeworm B71.Ø
  - red bug B88.Ø
  - roundworm (large) NEC B82.Ø
    - Ascariasis — *see also* Ascariasis B77.9
  - sandflea B88.1
  - Sarcoptes scabiei B86
  - scabies B86
  - Schistosoma B65.9
    - bovis B65.8
    - cercariae B65.3
    - haematobium B65.Ø
    - intercalatum B65.8
    - japonicum B65.2
    - mansoni B65.1
    - mattheei B65.8
    - mekongi B65.8
    - specified type NEC B65.8
    - spindale B65.8
  - screw worms — *see* Myiasis
  - skin NOS B88.9
  - Sparganum (mansoni) (proliferum) (baxteri) B7Ø.1
    - larval B7Ø.1
  - specified type NEC B88.8
  - Spirometra larvae B7Ø.1
  - Stellantchasmus falcatus B66.8
  - Strongyloides stercoralis — *see* Strongyloidiasis
  - Taenia B68.9
    - diminuta B71.Ø
    - echinococcus — *see* Echinococcus
    - mediocanellata B68.1
    - nana B71.Ø
    - saginata B68.1
    - solium (intestinal form) B68.Ø
      - larval form — *see* Cysticercosis
  - Taeniarhynchus saginatus B68.1
  - tapeworm B71.9
    - beef B68.1
    - broad B7Ø.Ø
      - larval B7Ø.1
    - dog B67.4
    - dwarf B71.Ø
    - fish B7Ø.Ø
      - larval B7Ø.1
    - pork B68.Ø
    - rat B71.Ø
  - Ternidens diminutus B81.8
  - Tetranychus molestissimus B88.Ø
  - threadworm B8Ø
  - tongue B37.Ø
  - Toxocara (canis) (cati) (felis) B83.Ø
  - trematode(s) NEC — *see* Infestation, fluke
  - Trichinella (spiralis) B75
  - Trichocephalus B79
  - Trichomonas — *see* Trichomoniasis
  - Trichostrongylus B81.2
  - Trichuris (trichiura) B79
  - Trombicula (irritans) B88.Ø
  - Tunga penetrans B88.1
  - Uncinaria americana B76.1
  - Vandellia cirrhosa B88.8
  - whipworm B79
  - worms B83.9
    - intestinal B82.Ø
  - Wuchereria (bancrofti) B74.Ø
- **Infiltrate, infiltration**
  - amyloid (generalized) (localized) — *see* Amyloidosis
  - calcareous NEC R89.7
    - localized — *see* Degeneration, by site
  - calcium salt R89.7
  - cardiac
    - fatty — *see* Degeneration, myocardial
    - glycogenic E74.Ø2 *[I43]*
  - corneal — *see* Edema, cornea
  - eyelid — *see* Inflammation, eyelid
  - glycogen, glycogenic — *see* Disease, glycogen storage
  - heart, cardiac
    - fatty — *see* Degeneration, myocardial
    - glycogenic E74.Ø2 *[I43]*
  - inflammatory in vitreous H43.89
  - kidney N28.89
  - leukemic — *see* Leukemia
  - liver K76.89
    - fatty — *see* Fatty, liver NEC
    - glycogen — *see also* Disease, glycogen storage E74.Ø3 *[K77]*
  - lung R91.8
    - eosinophilic — *see* Eosinophilia, pulmonary
  - lymphatic — *see also* Leukemia, lymphatic C91.9- ☑
    - gland I88.9
  - muscle, fatty M62.89
  - myocardium, myocardial
    - fatty — *see* Degeneration, myocardial
    - glycogenic E74.Ø2 *[I43]*
  - on chest x-ray R91.8
  - pulmonary R91.8
    - with eosinophilia — *see* Eosinophilia, pulmonary
  - skin (lymphocytic) L98.6
  - thymus (gland) (fatty) E32.8
  - urine R39.Ø
  - vesicant agent
    - antineoplastic chemotherapy T8Ø.81Ø ☑
    - other agent NEC T8Ø.818 ☑
  - vitreous body H43.89
- **Infirmity** R68.89
  - senile R54
- **Inflammation, inflamed, inflammatory** (with exudation)
  - abducent (nerve) — *see* Strabismus, paralytic, sixth nerve
  - accessory sinus (chronic) — *see* Sinusitis
  - adrenal (gland) E27.8
  - alveoli, teeth M27.3
    - scorbutic E54
  - anal canal, anus K62.89
  - antrum (chronic) — *see* Sinusitis, maxillary
  - appendix — *see* Appendicitis
  - arachnoid — *see* Meningitis
  - areola N61.Ø
    - puerperal, postpartum or gestational — *see* Infection, nipple
  - areolar tissue NOS LØ8.9
  - artery — *see* Arteritis
  - auditory meatus (external) — *see* Otitis, externa
  - Bartholin's gland N75.8
  - bile duct (common) (hepatic) or passage — *see* Cholangitis
  - bladder — *see* Cystitis
  - bone — *see* Osteomyelitis
  - brain — *see also* Encephalitis
    - membrane — *see* Meningitis
  - breast N61.Ø
    - puerperal, postpartum, gestational — *see* Mastitis, obstetric
  - broad ligament — *see* Disease, pelvis, inflammatory
  - bronchi — *see* Bronchitis
  - catarrhal JØØ
  - cecum — *see* Appendicitis
  - cerebral — *see also* Encephalitis
    - membrane — *see* Meningitis
  - cerebrospinal
    - meningococcal A39.Ø
  - cervix (uteri) — *see* Cervicitis
  - chest J98.8
  - chorioretinal H3Ø.9- ☑
    - cyclitis — *see* Cyclitis
    - disseminated H3Ø.1Ø- ☑
      - generalized H3Ø.13- ☑
      - peripheral H3Ø.12- ☑
      - posterior pole H3Ø.11- ☑
    - epitheliopathy — *see* Epitheliopathy
    - focal H3Ø.ØØ- ☑

Inflammation, inflamed, inflammatory — *continued*

- chorioretinal — *continued*
  - focal — *continued*
    - juxtapapillary H3Ø.Ø1- ☑
    - macular H3Ø.Ø4- ☑
    - paramacular — *see* Inflammation, chorioretinal, focal, macular
    - peripheral H3Ø.Ø3- ☑
    - posterior pole H3Ø.Ø2- ☑
  - specified type NEC H3Ø.89- ☑
- choroid — *see* Inflammation, chorioretinal
- chronic, postmastoidectomy cavity — *see* Complications, postmastoidectomy, inflammation
- colon — *see* Enteritis
- connective tissue (diffuse) NEC — *see* Disorder, soft tissue, specified type NEC
- cornea — *see* Keratitis
- corpora cavernosa N48.29
- cranial nerve — *see* Disorder, nerve, cranial
- Douglas' cul-de-sac or pouch (chronic) N73.Ø
- due to device, implant or graft — *see also* Complications, by site and type, infection or inflammation
  - arterial graft T82.7 ☑
  - breast (implant) T85.79 ☑
  - catheter T85.79 ☑
    - dialysis (renal) T82.7 ☑
      - intraperitoneal T85.71 ☑
    - infusion T82.7 ☑
      - cranial T85.735 ☑
      - intrathecal T85.735 ☑
      - spinal (epidural) (subdural) T85.735 ☑
      - subarachnoid T85.735 ☑
    - urinary T83.518 ☑
      - cystostomy T83.51Ø ☑
      - Hopkins T83.518 ☑
      - ileostomy T83.518 ☑
      - nephrostomy T83.512 ☑
      - specified NEC T83.518 ☑
      - urethral indwelling T83.511 ☑
      - urostomy T83.518 ☑
  - electronic (electrode) (pulse generator) (stimulator)
    - bone T84.7 ☑
    - cardiac T82.7 ☑
    - nervous system T85.738 ☑
      - brain T85.731 ☑
      - cranial nerve T85.732 ☑
      - gastric nerve T85.732 ☑
      - neurostimulator generator T85.734 ☑
      - peripheral nerve T85.732 ☑
      - sacral nerve T85.732 ☑
      - spinal cord T85.733 ☑
      - vagal nerve T85.732 ☑
    - urinary T83.59Ø ☑
  - fixation, internal (orthopedic) NEC — *see* Complication, fixation device, infection
  - gastrointestinal (bile duct) (esophagus) T85.79 ☑
    - neurostimulator electrode (lead) T85.732 ☑
  - genital NEC T83.69 ☑
  - heart NEC T82.7 ☑
    - valve (prosthesis) T82.6 ☑
      - graft T82.7 ☑
  - joint prosthesis — *see* Complication, joint prosthesis, infection
  - ocular (corneal graft) (orbital implant) NEC T85.79 ☑
  - orthopedic NEC T84.7 ☑
  - penile (cylinder) (pump) (resevoir) T83.61 ☑
  - specified NEC T85.79 ☑
  - testicular T83.62 ☑
  - urinary NEC T83.598 ☑
    - ileal conduit stent T83.593 ☑
    - implanted neurostimulation T83.59Ø ☑
    - implanted sphincter T83.591 ☑
    - indwelling ureteral stent T83.592 ☑
    - nephroureteral stent T83.593 ☑
    - specified stent NEC T83.593 ☑
  - vascular NEC T82.7 ☑
  - ventricular intracranial (communicating) shunt T85.73Ø ☑
- duodenum K29.8Ø
  - with bleeding K29.81
- dura mater — *see* Meningitis
- ear (middle) — *see also* Otitis, media
  - external — *see* Otitis, externa
  - inner — *see* subcategory H83.Ø ☑
- epididymis — *see* Epididymitis

Inflammation, inflamed, inflammatory — *continued*
- esophagus — *see* Esophagitis
- ethmoidal (sinus) (chronic) — *see* Sinusitis, ethmoidal
- eustachian tube (catarrhal) — *see* Salpingitis, eustachian
- eyelid HØ1.9
  - abscess — *see* Abscess, eyelid
  - blepharitis — *see* Blepharitis
  - chalazion — *see* Chalazion
  - dermatosis (noninfectious) — *see* Dermatosis, eyelid
  - hordeolum — *see* Hordeolum
  - specified NEC HØ1.8
- fallopian tube — *see* Salpingo-oophoritis
- fascia — *see* Myositis
- follicular, pharynx J31.2
- frontal (sinus) (chronic) — *see* Sinusitis, frontal
- gallbladder — *see* Cholecystitis
- gastric — *see* Gastritis
- gastrointestinal — *see* Enteritis
- genital organ (internal) (diffuse)
  - female — *see* Disease, pelvis, inflammatory
  - male N49.9
    - multiple sites N49.8
    - specified NEC N49.8
- gland (lymph) — *see* Lymphadenitis
- glottis — *see* Laryngitis
- granular, pharynx J31.2
- gum KØ5.1Ø
  - nonplaque induced KØ5.11
  - plaque induced KØ5.1Ø
- heart — *see* Carditis
- hepatic duct — *see* Cholangitis
- ileoanal (internal) pouch K91.85Ø
- ileum — *see also* Enteritis
  - regional or terminal — *see* Enteritis, regional
- intestinal pouch K91.85Ø
- intestine (any part) — *see* Enteritis
- jaw (acute) (bone) (chronic) (lower) (suppurative) (upper) M27.2
- joint NEC — *see* Arthritis
  - sacroiliac M46.1
- kidney — *see* Nephritis
- knee (joint) M13.169
  - tuberculous A18.Ø2
- labium (majus) (minus) — *see* Vulvitis
- lacrimal
  - gland — *see* Dacryoadenitis
  - passages (duct) (sac) — *see also* Dacryocystitis
    - canaliculitis — *see* Canaliculitis, lacrimal
- larynx — *see* Laryngitis
- leg NOS LØ8.9
- lip K13.Ø
- liver (capsule) — *see also* Hepatitis
  - chronic K73.9
  - suppurative K75.Ø
- lung (acute) — *see also* Pneumonia
  - chronic J98.4
- lymph gland or node — *see* Lymphadenitis
- lymphatic vessel — *see* Lymphangitis
- maxilla, maxillary M27.2
  - sinus (chronic) — *see* Sinusitis, maxillary
- membranes of brain or spinal cord — *see* Meningitis
- meninges — *see* Meningitis
- mouth K12.1
- muscle — *see* Myositis
- myocardium — *see* Myocarditis
- nasal sinus (chronic) — *see* Sinusitis
- nasopharynx — *see* Nasopharyngitis
- navel LØ8.82
- nerve NEC — *see* Neuritis
- nipple N61.Ø
  - puerperal, postpartum or gestational — *see* Infection, nipple
- nose — *see* Rhinitis
- oculomotor (nerve) — *see* Strabismus, paralytic, third nerve
- optic nerve — *see* Neuritis, optic
- orbit (chronic) HØ5.1Ø
  - acute HØ5.ØØ
    - abscess — *see* Abscess, orbit
    - cellulitis — *see* Cellulitis, orbit
    - osteomyelitis — *see* Osteomyelitis, orbit
    - periostitis — *see* Periostitis, orbital
    - tenonitis — *see* Tenonitis, eye
  - granuloma — *see* Granuloma, orbit
  - myositis — *see* Myositis, orbital

Inflammation, inflamed, inflammatory — *continued*
- ovary — *see* Salpingo-oophoritis
- oviduct — *see* Salpingo-oophoritis
- pancreas (acute) — *see* Pancreatitis
- parametrium N73.Ø
- parotid region LØ8.9
- pelvis, female — *see* Disease, pelvis, inflammatory
- penis (corpora cavernosa) N48.29
- perianal K62.89
- pericardium — *see* Pericarditis
- perineum (female) (male) LØ8.9
- perirectal K62.89
- peritoneum — *see* Peritonitis
- periuterine — *see* Disease, pelvis, inflammatory
- perivesical — *see* Cystitis
- petrous bone (acute) (chronic) — *see* Petrositis
- pharynx (acute) — *see* Pharyngitis
- pia mater — *see* Meningitis
- pleura — *see* Pleurisy
- polyp, colon — *see also* Polyp, colon, inflammatory K51.4Ø
- prostate — *see also* Prostatitis
  - specified type NEC N41.8
- rectosigmoid — *see* Rectosigmoiditis
- rectum — *see also* Proctitis K62.89
- respiratory, upper — *see also* Infection, respiratory, upper JØ6.9
  - acute, due to radiation J7Ø.Ø
  - chronic, due to external agent — *see* condition, respiratory, chronic, due to
  - due to
    - chemicals, gases, fumes or vapors (inhalation) J68.2
    - radiation J7Ø.1
- retina — *see* Chorioretinitis
- retrocecal — *see* Appendicitis
- retroperitoneal — *see* Peritonitis
- salivary duct or gland (any) (suppurative) — *see* Sialoadenitis
- scorbutic, alveoli, teeth E54
- scrotum N49.2
- seminal vesicle — *see* Vesiculitis
- sigmoid — *see* Enteritis
- sinus — *see* Sinusitis
- Skene's duct or gland — *see* Urethritis
- skin LØ8.9
- spermatic cord N49.1
- sphenoidal (sinus) — *see* Sinusitis, sphenoidal
- spinal
  - cord — *see* Encephalitis
  - membrane — *see* Meningitis
  - nerve — *see* Disorder, nerve
- spine — *see* Spondylopathy, inflammatory
- spleen (capsule) D73.89
- stomach — *see* Gastritis
- subcutaneous tissue LØ8.9
- suprarenal (gland) E27.8
- synovial — *see* Tenosynovitis
- tendon (sheath) NEC — *see* Tenosynovitis
- testis — *see* Orchitis
- throat (acute) — *see* Pharyngitis
- thymus (gland) E32.8
- thyroid (gland) — *see* Thyroiditis
- tongue K14.Ø
- tonsil — *see* Tonsillitis
- trachea — *see* Tracheitis
- trochlear (nerve) — *see* Strabismus, paralytic, fourth nerve
- tubal — *see* Salpingo-oophoritis
- tuberculous NEC — *see* Tuberculosis
- tubo-ovarian — *see* Salpingo-oophoritis
- tunica vaginalis N49.1
- tympanic membrane — *see* Tympanitis
- umbilicus, umbilical LØ8.82
- uterine ligament — *see* Disease, pelvis, inflammatory
- uterus (catarrhal) — *see* Endometritis
- uveal tract (anterior) NOS — *see also* Iridocyclitis
  - posterior — *see* Chorioretinitis
- vagina — *see* Vaginitis
- vas deferens N49.1
- vein — *see also* Phlebitis
  - intracranial or intraspinal (septic) GØ8
  - thrombotic I8Ø.9
    - leg — *see* Phlebitis, leg
    - lower extremity — *see* Phlebitis, leg
- vocal cord J38.3

Inflammation, inflamed, inflammatory — *continued*
- vulva — *see* Vulvitis
- Wharton's duct (suppurative) — *see* Sialoadenitis

Inflation, lung, imperfect (newborn) — *see* Atelectasis

Influenza (bronchial) (epidemic) (respiratory (upper)) (unidentified influenza virus) J11.1
- with
  - digestive manifestations J11.2
  - encephalopathy J11.81
  - enteritis J11.2
  - gastroenteritis J11.2
  - gastrointestinal manifestations J11.2
  - laryngitis J11.1
  - myocarditis J11.82
  - otitis media J11.83
  - pharyngitis J11.1
  - pneumonia J11.ØØ
    - specified type J11.Ø8
  - respiratory manifestations NEC J11.1
  - specified manifestation NEC J11.89
- A (non-novel) J1Ø- ☑
- A/H5N1 — *see also* Influenza, due to, identified novel influenza A virus JØ9.X2
- avian — *see also* Influenza, due to, identified novel influenza A virus JØ9.X2
- B J1Ø- ☑
- bird — *see also* Influenza, due to, identified novel influenza A virus JØ9.X2
- C J1Ø- ☑
- due to
  - avian — *see also* Influenza, due to, identified novel influenza A virus JØ9.X2
  - identified influenza virus NEC J1Ø.1
    - with
      - digestive manifestations J1Ø.2
      - encephalopathy J1Ø.81
      - enteritis J1Ø.2
      - gastroenteritis J1Ø.2
      - gastrointestinal manifestations J1Ø.2
      - laryngitis J1Ø.1
      - myocarditis J1Ø.82
      - otitis media J1Ø.83
      - pharyngitis J1Ø.1
      - pneumonia (unspecified type) J1Ø.ØØ
        - with same identified influenza virus J1Ø.Ø1
        - specified type NEC J1Ø.Ø8
      - respiratory manifestations NEC J1Ø.1
      - specified manifestation NEC J1Ø.89
  - identified novel influenza A virus JØ9.X2
    - with
      - digestive manifestations JØ9.X3
      - encephalopathy JØ9.X9
      - enteritis JØ9.X3
      - gastroenteritis JØ9.X3
      - gastrointestinal manifestations JØ9.X3
      - laryngitis JØ9.X2
      - myocarditis JØ9.X9
      - otitis media JØ9.X9
      - pharyngitis JØ9.X2
      - pneumonia JØ9.X1
      - respiratory manifestations NEC JØ9.X2
      - specified manifestation NEC JØ9.X9
      - upper respiratory symptoms JØ9.X2
- novel (2ØØ9) H1N1 influenza — *see also* Influenza, due to, identified influenza virus NEC J1Ø.1
- novel influenza A/H1N1 — *see also* Influenza, due to, identified influenza virus NEC J1Ø.1
- of other animal origin, not bird or swine — *see also* Influenza, due to, identified novel influenza A virus JØ9.X2
- swine (viruses that normally cause infections in pigs) — *see also* Influenza, due to, identified novel influenza A virus JØ9.X2

Influenzal — *see* Influenza

Influenza-like disease — *see* Influenza

Infraction, Freiberg's (metatarsal head) — *see* Osteochondrosis, juvenile, metatarsus

Infraeruption of tooth (teeth) M26.34

Infusion complication, misadventure, or reaction — *see* Complications, infusion

Ingestion
- chemical — *see* Table of Drugs and Chemicals, by substance, poisoning

Ingestion — *continued*
- drug or medicament
  - correct substance properly administered — *see* Table of Drugs and Chemicals, by drug, adverse effect
  - overdose or wrong substance given or taken — *see* Table of Drugs and Chemicals, by drug, poisoning
- foreign body — *see* Foreign body, alimentary tract
- multiple drug — *see* Table of Drugs and Chemicals, multiple
- tularemia A21.3

Ingrowing
- hair (beard) L73.1
- nail (finger) (toe) L60.0

Inguinal — *see also* condition
- testicle Q53.9
  - bilateral Q53.212
  - unilateral Q53.112

Inhalant-induced
- anxiety disorder F18.980
- depressive disorder F18.94
- major neurocognitive disorder F18.97
- mild neurocognitive disorder F18.988
- psychotic disorder F18.959

Inhalation
- anthrax A22.1
- flame T27.3 ☑
- food or foreign body — *see* Foreign body, by site
- gases, fumes, or vapors T59.9- ☑
  - specified agent NEC — *see* Table of Drugs and Chemicals, by substance T59.89- ☑
- liquid or vomitus — *see* Asphyxia
- meconium (newborn) P24.00
  - with
    - with respiratory symptoms P24.01
    - pneumonia (pneumonitis) P24.01
- mucus — *see* Asphyxia, mucus
- oil or gasoline (causing suffocation) — *see* Foreign body, by site
- smoke T59.81- ☑
  - with respiratory conditions J70.5
    - due to chemicals, gases, fumes and vapors J68.9
- steam — *see also* Burn, respiratory tract T59.9- ☑
- stomach contents or secretions — *see* Foreign body, by site
  - due to anesthesia (general) (local) or other sedation T88.59 ☑
    - in labor and delivery O74.0
    - in pregnancy O29.01- ☑
    - postpartum, puerperal O89.01

Inhibition, orgasm
- female F52.31
- male F52.32

Inhibitor, systemic lupus erythematosus (presence of) D68.62

Iniencephalus, iniencephaly Q00.2

Injection, traumatic jet (air) (industrial) (water) (paint or dye) T70.4 ☑

Injury — *see also* specified injury type T14.90 ☑
- abdomen, abdominal S39.91 ☑
  - blood vessel — *see* Injury, blood vessel, abdomen
  - cavity — *see* Injury, intra-abdominal
  - contusion S30.1 ☑
  - internal — *see* Injury, intra-abdominal
  - intra-abdominal organ — *see* Injury, intra-abdominal
  - nerve — *see* Injury, nerve, abdomen
  - open — *see* Wound, open, abdomen
  - specified NEC S39.81 ☑
  - superficial — *see* Injury, superficial, abdomen
- Achilles tendon S86.00- ☑
  - laceration S86.02- ☑
  - specified type NEC S86.09- ☑
  - strain S86.01- ☑
- acoustic, resulting in deafness — *see* Injury, nerve, acoustic
- adrenal (gland) S37.819 ☑
  - contusion S37.812 ☑
  - laceration S37.813 ☑
  - specified type NEC S37.818 ☑
- alveolar (process) S09.93 ☑
- ankle S99.91- ☑
  - contusion — *see* Contusion, ankle
  - dislocation — *see* Dislocation, ankle
  - fracture — *see* Fracture, ankle
  - nerve — *see* Injury, nerve, ankle

Injury — *continued*
- ankle — *continued*
  - open — *see* Wound, open, ankle
  - specified type NEC S99.81- ☑
  - sprain — *see* Sprain, ankle
  - superficial — *see* Injury, superficial, ankle
- anterior chamber, eye — *see* Injury, eye, specified site NEC
- anus — *see* Injury, abdomen
- aorta (thoracic) S25.00 ☑
  - abdominal S35.00 ☑
    - laceration (minor) (superficial) S35.01 ☑
      - major S35.02 ☑
    - specified type NEC S35.09 ☑
  - laceration (minor) (superficial) S25.01 ☑
    - major S25.02 ☑
  - specified type NEC S25.09 ☑
- arm (upper) S49.9- ☑
  - blood vessel — *see* Injury, blood vessel, arm
  - contusion — *see* Contusion, arm, upper
  - fracture — *see* Fracture, humerus
  - lower — *see* Injury, forearm
  - muscle — *see* Injury, muscle, shoulder
  - nerve — *see* Injury, nerve, arm
  - open — *see* Wound, open, arm
  - specified type NEC S49.8- ☑
  - superficial — *see* Injury, superficial, arm
- artery (complicating trauma) — *see also* Injury, blood vessel, by site
  - cerebral or meningeal — *see* Injury, intracranial
- auditory canal (external) (meatus) S09.91 ☑
- auricle, auris, ear S09.91 ☑
- axilla — *see* Injury, shoulder
- back — *see* Injury, back, lower
- bile duct S36.13 ☑
- birth — *see also* Birth, injury P15.9
- bladder (sphincter) S37.20 ☑
  - at delivery O71.5
  - contusion S37.22 ☑
  - laceration S37.23 ☑
  - obstetrical trauma O71.5
  - specified type NEC S37.29 ☑
- blast (air) (hydraulic) (immersion) (underwater) NEC T14.8 ☑
  - acoustic nerve trauma — *see* Injury, nerve, acoustic
  - bladder — *see* Injury, bladder
  - brain — *see* Concussion
    - primary, specified NEC S06.8A- ☑
  - colon — *see* Injury, intestine, large
  - ear (primary) S09.31- ☑
    - secondary S09.39- ☑
  - generalized T70.8 ☑
  - lung — *see* Injury, intrathoracic, lung
  - multiple body organs T70.8 ☑
  - peritoneum S36.81 ☑
  - rectum S36.61 ☑
  - retroperitoneum S36.898 ☑
  - small intestine S36.419 ☑
    - duodenum S36.410 ☑
    - specified site NEC S36.418 ☑
  - specified
    - intra-abdominal organ NEC S36.898 ☑
    - pelvic organ NEC S37.899 ☑
- blood vessel NEC T14.8 ☑
  - abdomen S35.9 ☑
    - aorta — *see* Injury, aorta, abdominal
    - celiac artery — *see* Injury, blood vessel, celiac artery
    - iliac vessel — *see* Injury, blood vessel, iliac
    - laceration S35.91 ☑
    - mesenteric vessel — *see* Injury, mesenteric
    - portal vein — *see* Injury, blood vessel, portal vein
    - renal vessel — *see* Injury, blood vessel, renal
    - specified vessel NEC S35.8X- ☑
    - splenic vessel — *see* Injury, blood vessel, splenic
    - vena cava — *see* Injury, vena cava, inferior
  - ankle — *see* Injury, blood vessel, foot
  - aorta (abdominal) (thoracic) — *see* Injury, aorta
  - arm (upper) NEC S45.90- ☑
    - forearm — *see* Injury, blood vessel, forearm
    - laceration S45.91- ☑
    - specified
      - site NEC S45.80- ☑
        - laceration S45.81- ☑
        - specified type NEC S45.89- ☑
      - type NEC S45.99- ☑

Injury — *continued*
- blood vessel — *continued*
  - arm — *continued*
    - superficial vein S45.30- ☑
      - laceration S45.31- ☑
      - specified type NEC S45.39- ☑
  - axillary
    - artery S45.00- ☑
      - laceration S45.01- ☑
      - specified type NEC S45.09- ☑
    - vein S45.20- ☑
      - laceration S45.21- ☑
      - specified type NEC S45.29- ☑
  - azygos vein — *see* Injury, blood vessel, thoracic, specified site NEC
  - brachial
    - artery S45.10- ☑
      - laceration S45.11- ☑
      - specified type NEC S45.19- ☑
    - vein S45.20- ☑
      - laceration S45.219 ☑
      - specified type NEC S45.29- ☑
  - carotid artery (common) (external) (internal, extracranial) S15.00- ☑
    - internal, intracranial S06.8- ☑
    - laceration (minor) (superficial) S15.01- ☑
      - major S15.02- ☑
    - specified type NEC S15.09- ☑
  - celiac artery S35.219 ☑
    - branch S35.299 ☑
      - laceration (minor) (superficial) S35.291 ☑
        - major S35.292 ☑
      - specified NEC S35.298 ☑
    - laceration (minor) (superficial) S35.211 ☑
      - major S35.212 ☑
    - specified type NEC S35.218 ☑
  - cerebral — *see* Injury, intracranial
  - deep plantar — *see* Injury, blood vessel, plantar artery
  - digital (hand) — *see* Injury, blood vessel, finger
  - dorsal
    - artery (foot) S95.00- ☑
      - laceration S95.01- ☑
      - specified type NEC S95.09- ☑
    - vein (foot) S95.20- ☑
      - laceration S95.21- ☑
      - specified type NEC S95.29- ☑
  - due to accidental laceration during procedure — *see* Laceration, accidental complicating surgery
  - extremity — *see* Injury, blood vessel, limb
  - femoral
    - artery (common) (superficial) S75.00- ☑
      - laceration (minor) (superficial) S75.01- ☑
        - major S75.02- ☑
      - specified type NEC S75.09- ☑
    - vein (hip level) (thigh level) S75.10- ☑
      - laceration (minor) (superficial) S75.11- ☑
        - major S75.12- ☑
      - specified type NEC S75.19- ☑
  - finger S65.50- ☑
    - index S65.50- ☑
      - laceration S65.51- ☑
      - specified type NEC S65.59- ☑
    - laceration S65.51- ☑
    - little S65.50- ☑
      - laceration S65.51- ☑
      - specified type NEC S65.59- ☑
    - middle S65.50- ☑
      - laceration S65.51- ☑
      - specified type NEC S65.59- ☑
    - specified type NEC S65.59- ☑
    - thumb — *see* Injury, blood vessel, thumb
  - foot S95.90- ☑
    - dorsal
      - artery — *see* Injury, blood vessel, dorsal, artery
      - vein — *see* Injury, blood vessel, dorsal, vein
    - laceration S95.91- ☑
    - plantar artery — *see* Injury, blood vessel, plantar artery
    - specified
      - site NEC S95.80- ☑
        - laceration S95.81- ☑
        - specified type NEC S95.89- ☑
      - specified type NEC S95.99- ☑

Index

Injury — Injury

Injury — *continued*
- intrathoracic — *continued*
  - diaphragm S27.8Ø9 ☑
    - contusion S27.8Ø2 ☑
    - laceration S27.8Ø3 ☑
    - specified type NEC S27.8Ø8 ☑
  - esophagus (thoracic) S27.819 ☑
    - contusion S27.812 ☑
    - laceration S27.813 ☑
    - specified type NEC S27.818 ☑
  - heart — *see* Injury, heart
  - hemopneumothorax S27.2 ☑
  - hemothorax S27.1 ☑
  - lung S27.3Ø9 ☑
    - aspiration J69.Ø
    - bilateral S27.3Ø2 ☑
    - blast injury (primary) S27.319 ☑
      - bilateral S27.312 ☑
      - secondary — *see* Injury, intrathoracic, lung, specified type NEC
      - unilateral S27.311 ☑
    - contusion S27.329 ☑
      - bilateral S27.322 ☑
      - unilateral S27.321 ☑
    - laceration S27.339 ☑
      - bilateral S27.332 ☑
      - unilateral S27.331 ☑
    - specified type NEC S27.399 ☑
      - bilateral S27.392 ☑
      - unilateral S27.391 ☑
    - unilateral S27.3Ø1 ☑
  - pleura S27.6Ø ☑
    - laceration S27.63 ☑
    - specified type NEC S27.69 ☑
  - pneumothorax S27.Ø ☑
  - specified organ NEC S27.899 ☑
    - contusion S27.892 ☑
    - laceration S27.893 ☑
    - specified type NEC S27.898 ☑
  - thoracic duct — *see* Injury, intrathoracic, specified organ NEC
  - thymus gland — *see* Injury, intrathoracic, specified organ NEC
  - trachea, thoracic S27.5Ø ☑
    - blast (primary) S27.51 ☑
    - contusion S27.52 ☑
    - laceration S27.53 ☑
    - specified type NEC S27.59 ☑
- iris — *see* Injury, eye, specified site NEC
  - penetrating — *see* Injury, eyeball, penetrating
- jaw SØ9.93 ☑
- jejunum — *see* Injury, intestine, small
- joint NOS T14.8 ☑
  - old or residual — *see* Disorder, joint, specified type NEC
- kidney S37.ØØ- ☑
  - acute (nontraumatic) N17.9
  - contusion — *see* Contusion, kidney
  - laceration — *see* Laceration, kidney
  - specified NEC S37.Ø9- ☑
- knee S89.9- ☑
  - contusion — *see* Contusion, knee
  - dislocation — *see* Dislocation, knee
  - meniscus (lateral) (medial) — *see* Sprain, knee, specified site NEC
    - old injury or tear — *see* Derangement, knee, meniscus, due to old injury
  - open — *see* Wound, open, knee
  - specified NEC S89.8- ☑
  - sprain — *see* Sprain, knee
  - superficial — *see* Injury, superficial, knee
- labium (majus) (minus) S39.94 ☑
- labyrinth, ear SØ9.3Ø- ☑
- lacrimal apparatus, duct, gland, or sac — *see* Injury, eye, specified site NEC
- larynx NEC S19.81 ☑
- leg (lower) S89.9- ☑
  - blood vessel — *see* Injury, blood vessel, leg
  - contusion — *see* Contusion, leg
  - fracture — *see* Fracture, leg
  - muscle — *see* Injury, muscle, leg
  - nerve — *see* Injury, nerve, leg
  - open — *see* Wound, open, leg
  - specified NEC S89.8- ☑
  - superficial — *see* Injury, superficial, leg
- lens, eye — *see* Injury, eye, specified site NEC

Injury — *continued*
- lens, eye — *see* Injury, eye, specified site — *continued*
  - penetrating — *see* Injury, eyeball, penetrating
- limb NEC T14.8 ☑
- lip SØ9.93 ☑
- liver S36.119 ☑
  - contusion S36.112 ☑
  - laceration S36.113 ☑
    - major (stellate) S36.116 ☑
    - minor S36.114 ☑
    - moderate S36.115 ☑
  - specified NEC S36.118 ☑
- lower back S39.92 ☑
  - specified NEC S39.82 ☑
- lumbar, lumbosacral (region) S39.92 ☑
  - plexus — *see* Injury, lumbosacral plexus
- lumbosacral plexus S34.4 ☑
- lung — *see also* Injury, intrathoracic, lung
  - aspiration J69.Ø
  - dabbing (related) UØ7.Ø
  - electronic cigarette (related) UØ7.Ø
  - EVALI - [e-cigarette, or vaping, product use associated] UØ7.Ø
  - transfusion-related (TRALI) J95.84
  - vaping (associated) (device) (product) (use) UØ7.Ø
- lymphatic thoracic duct — *see* Injury, intrathoracic, specified organ NEC
- malar region SØ9.93 ☑
- mastoid region SØ9.9Ø ☑
- maxilla SØ9.93 ☑
- mediastinum — *see* Injury, intrathoracic, specified organ NEC
- membrane, brain — *see* Injury, intracranial
- meningeal artery — *see* Injury, intracranial, subdural hemorrhage
- meninges (cerebral) — *see* Injury, intracranial
- mesenteric
  - artery
    - branch S35.299 ☑
      - laceration (minor) (superficial) S35.291 ☑
        - major S35.292 ☑
      - specified NEC S35.298 ☑
    - inferior S35.239 ☑
      - laceration (minor) (superficial) S35.231 ☑
        - major S35.232 ☑
      - specified NEC S35.238 ☑
    - superior S35.229 ☑
      - laceration (minor) (superficial) S35.221 ☑
        - major S35.222 ☑
      - specified NEC S35.228 ☑
  - plexus (inferior) (superior) — *see* Injury, nerve, lumbosacral, sympathetic
  - vein
    - inferior S35.349 ☑
      - laceration S35.341 ☑
      - specified NEC S35.348 ☑
    - superior S35.339 ☑
      - laceration S35.331 ☑
      - specified NEC S35.338 ☑
- mesentery — *see* Injury, intra-abdominal, specified site NEC
- mesosalpinx — *see* Injury, pelvic organ, specified site NEC
- middle ear SØ9.3Ø- ☑
- midthoracic region NOS S29.9 ☑
- mouth SØ9.93 ☑
- multiple NOS TØ7 ☑
- muscle (and fascia) (and tendon)
  - abdomen S39.ØØ1 ☑
    - laceration S39.Ø21 ☑
    - specified type NEC S39.Ø91 ☑
    - strain S39.Ø11 ☑
  - abductor
    - thumb, forearm level — *see* Injury, muscle, thumb, abductor
  - adductor
    - thigh S76.2Ø- ☑
      - laceration S76.22- ☑
      - specified type NEC S76.29- ☑
      - strain S76.21- ☑
  - ankle — *see* Injury, muscle, foot
  - anterior muscle group, at leg level (lower) S86.2Ø- ☑
    - laceration S86.22- ☑
    - specified type NEC S86.29- ☑
    - strain S86.21- ☑

Injury — *continued*
- muscle — *continued*
  - arm (upper) — *see* Injury, muscle, shoulder
  - biceps (parts NEC) S46.2Ø- ☑
    - laceration S46.22- ☑
    - long head S46.1Ø- ☑
      - laceration S46.12- ☑
      - specified type NEC S46.19- ☑
      - strain S46.11- ☑
    - specified type NEC S46.29- ☑
    - strain S46.21- ☑
  - extensor
    - finger(s) (other than thumb) — *see* Injury, muscle, finger by site, extensor
    - forearm level, specified NEC — *see* Injury, muscle, forearm, extensor
    - thumb — *see* Injury, muscle, thumb, extensor
    - toe (large) (ankle level) (foot level) — *see* Injury, muscle, toe, extensor
  - finger
    - extensor (forearm level) S56.4Ø- ☑
      - hand level S66.3Ø9 ☑
        - laceration S66.329 ☑
        - specified type NEC S66.399 ☑
        - strain S66.319 ☑
      - laceration S56.429 ☑
      - specified type NEC S56.499 ☑
      - strain S56.419 ☑
    - flexor (forearm level) S56.1Ø- ☑
      - hand level S66.1Ø9 ☑
        - laceration S66.129 ☑
        - specified type NEC S66.199 ☑
        - strain S66.119 ☑
      - laceration S56.129 ☑
      - specified type NEC S56.199 ☑
      - strain S56.119 ☑
    - index
      - extensor (forearm level)
        - hand level S66.3Ø8 ☑
          - laceration S66.32- ☑
          - specified type NEC S66.39- ☑
          - strain S66.31- ☑
        - specified type NEC S56.492- ☑
      - flexor (forearm level)
        - hand level S66.1Ø8 ☑
          - laceration S66.12- ☑
          - specified type NEC S66.19- ☑
          - strain S66.11- ☑
        - specified type NEC S56.19- ☑
        - strain S56.11- ☑
      - intrinsic S66.5Ø- ☑
        - laceration S66.52- ☑
        - specified type NEC S66.59- ☑
        - strain S66.51- ☑
    - intrinsic S66.5Ø9 ☑
      - laceration S66.529 ☑
      - specified type NEC S66.599 ☑
      - strain S66.519 ☑
    - little
      - extensor (forearm level)
        - hand level S66.3Ø- ☑
          - laceration S66.32- ☑
          - specified type NEC S66.39- ☑
          - strain S66.31- ☑
        - laceration S56.42- ☑
        - specified type NEC S56.49- ☑
        - strain S56.41- ☑
      - flexor (forearm level)
        - hand level S66.1Ø- ☑
          - laceration S66.12- ☑
          - specified type NEC S66.19- ☑
          - strain S66.11- ☑
        - laceration S56.12- ☑
        - specified type NEC S56.19- ☑
        - strain S56.11- ☑
      - intrinsic S66.5Ø- ☑
        - laceration S66.52- ☑
        - specified type NEC S66.59- ☑
        - strain S66.51- ☑
    - middle
      - extensor (forearm level)
        - hand level S66.3Ø- ☑
          - laceration S66.32- ☑
          - specified type NEC S66.39- ☑
          - strain S66.31- ☑
        - laceration S56.42- ☑

- **Injury** — *continued*
  - muscle — *continued*
    - finger — *continued*
      - middle — *continued*
        - extensor — *continued*
          - specified type NEC S56.49- ☑
          - strain S56.41- ☑
        - flexor (forearm level)
          - hand level S66.10- ☑
            - laceration S66.12- ☑
            - specified type NEC S66.19- ☑
            - strain S66.11- ☑
          - laceration S56.12- ☑
          - specified type NEC S56.19- ☑
          - strain S56.11- ☑
        - intrinsic S66.50- ☑
          - laceration S66.52- ☑
          - specified type NEC S66.59- ☑
          - strain S66.51- ☑
      - ring
        - extensor (forearm level)
          - hand level S66.30- ☑
            - laceration S66.32- ☑
            - specified type NEC S66.39- ☑
            - strain S66.31- ☑
          - laceration S56.42- ☑
          - specified type NEC S56.49- ☑
          - strain S56.41- ☑
        - flexor (forearm level)
          - hand level S66.10- ☑
            - laceration S66.12- ☑
            - specified type NEC S66.19- ☑
            - strain S66.11- ☑
          - laceration S56.12- ☑
          - specified type NEC S56.19- ☑
          - strain S56.11- ☑
        - intrinsic S66.50- ☑
          - laceration S66.52- ☑
          - specified type NEC S66.59- ☑
          - strain S66.51- ☑
    - flexor
      - finger(s) (other than thumb) — *see* Injury, muscle, finger
      - forearm level, specified NEC — *see* Injury, muscle, forearm, flexor
      - thumb — *see* Injury, muscle, thumb, flexor
      - toe (long) (ankle level) (foot level) — *see* Injury, muscle, toe, flexor
    - foot S96.90- ☑
      - intrinsic S96.20- ☑
        - laceration S96.22- ☑
        - specified type NEC S96.29- ☑
        - strain S96.21- ☑
      - laceration S96.92- ☑
      - long extensor, toe — *see* Injury, muscle, toe, extensor
      - long flexor, toe — *see* Injury, muscle, toe, flexor
      - specified
        - site NEC S96.80- ☑
          - laceration S96.82- ☑
          - specified type NEC S96.89- ☑
          - strain S96.81- ☑
        - type S96.99- ☑
      - strain S96.91- ☑
    - forearm (level) S56.90- ☑
      - extensor S56.50- ☑
        - laceration S56.52- ☑
        - specified type NEC S56.59- ☑
        - strain S56.51- ☑
      - flexor S56.20- ☑
        - laceration S56.22- ☑
        - specified type NEC S56.29- ☑
        - strain S56.21- ☑
      - laceration S56.92- ☑
      - specified S56.99- ☑
        - site NEC S56.80- ☑
          - laceration S56.82- ☑
          - strain S56.81- ☑
          - type NEC S56.89- ☑
      - strain S56.91- ☑
    - hand (level) S66.90- ☑
      - laceration S66.92- ☑
      - specified
        - site NEC S66.80- ☑
          - laceration S66.82- ☑
          - specified type NEC S66.89- ☑

- **Injury** — *continued*
  - muscle — *continued*
    - hand — *continued*
      - specified — *continued*
        - site — *continued*
          - strain S66.81- ☑
        - type NEC S66.99- ☑
      - strain S66.91- ☑
    - head S09.10 ☑
      - laceration S09.12 ☑
      - specified type NEC S09.19 ☑
      - strain S09.11 ☑
    - hip NEC S76.00- ☑
      - laceration S76.02- ☑
      - specified type NEC S76.09- ☑
      - strain S76.01- ☑
    - intrinsic
      - ankle and foot level — *see* Injury, muscle, foot, intrinsic
      - finger (other than thumb) — *see* Injury, muscle, finger by site, intrinsic
      - foot (level) — *see* Injury, muscle, foot, intrinsic
      - thumb — *see* Injury, muscle, thumb, intrinsic
    - leg (level) (lower) S86.90- ☑
      - Achilles tendon — *see* Injury, Achilles tendon
      - anterior muscle group — *see* Injury, muscle, anterior muscle group
      - laceration S86.92- ☑
      - peroneal muscle group — *see* Injury, muscle, peroneal muscle group
      - posterior muscle group — *see* Injury, muscle, posterior muscle group, leg level
      - specified
        - site NEC S86.80- ☑
          - laceration S86.82- ☑
          - specified type NEC S86.89- ☑
          - strain S86.81- ☑
        - type NEC S86.99- ☑
      - strain S86.91- ☑
    - long
      - extensor toe, at ankle and foot level — *see* Injury, muscle, toe, extensor
      - flexor, toe, at ankle and foot level — *see* Injury, muscle, toe, flexor
      - head, biceps — *see* Injury, muscle, biceps, long head
    - lower back S39.002 ☑
      - laceration S39.022 ☑
      - specified type NEC S39.092 ☑
      - strain S39.012 ☑
    - neck (level) S16.9 ☑
      - laceration S16.2 ☑
      - specified type NEC S16.8 ☑
      - strain S16.1 ☑
    - pelvis S39.003 ☑
      - laceration S39.023 ☑
      - specified type NEC S39.093 ☑
      - strain S39.013 ☑
    - peroneal muscle group, at leg level (lower) S86.30- ☑
      - laceration S86.32- ☑
      - specified type NEC S86.39- ☑
      - strain S86.31- ☑
    - posterior muscle (group)
      - leg level (lower) S86.10- ☑
        - laceration S86.12- ☑
        - specified type NEC S86.19- ☑
        - strain S86.11- ☑
      - thigh level S76.30- ☑
        - laceration S76.32- ☑
        - specified type NEC S76.39- ☑
        - strain S76.31- ☑
    - quadriceps (thigh) S76.10- ☑
      - laceration S76.12- ☑
      - specified type NEC S76.19- ☑
      - strain S76.11- ☑
    - shoulder S46.90- ☑
      - laceration S46.92- ☑
      - rotator cuff — *see* Injury, rotator cuff
      - specified site NEC S46.80- ☑
        - laceration S46.82- ☑
        - specified type NEC S46.89- ☑
        - strain S46.81- ☑
      - specified type NEC S46.99- ☑
      - strain S46.91- ☑
    - thigh NEC (level) S76.90- ☑

- **Injury** — *continued*
  - muscle — *continued*
    - thigh — *continued*
      - adductor — *see* Injury, muscle, adductor, thigh
      - laceration S76.92- ☑
      - posterior muscle (group) — *see* Injury, muscle, posterior muscle, thigh level
      - quadriceps — *see* Injury, muscle, quadriceps
      - specified
        - site NEC S76.80- ☑
          - laceration S76.82- ☑
          - specified type NEC S76.89- ☑
          - strain S76.81- ☑
        - type NEC S76.99- ☑
      - strain S76.91- ☑
    - thorax (level) S29.009 ☑
      - back wall S29.002 ☑
      - front wall S29.001 ☑
      - laceration S29.029 ☑
        - back wall S29.022 ☑
        - front wall S29.021 ☑
      - specified type NEC S29.099 ☑
        - back wall S29.092 ☑
        - front wall S29.091 ☑
      - strain S29.019 ☑
        - back wall S29.012 ☑
        - front wall S29.011 ☑
    - thumb
      - abductor (forearm level) S56.30- ☑
        - laceration S56.32- ☑
        - specified type NEC S56.39- ☑
        - strain S56.31- ☑
      - extensor (forearm level) S56.30- ☑
        - hand level S66.20- ☑
          - laceration S66.22- ☑
          - specified type NEC S66.29- ☑
          - strain S66.21- ☑
        - laceration S56.32- ☑
        - specified type NEC S56.39- ☑
        - strain S56.31- ☑
      - flexor (forearm level) S56.00- ☑
        - hand level S66.00- ☑
          - laceration S66.02- ☑
          - specified type NEC S66.09- ☑
          - strain S66.01- ☑
        - laceration S56.02- ☑
        - specified type NEC S56.09- ☑
        - strain S56.01- ☑
        - wrist level — *see* Injury, muscle, thumb, flexor, hand level
      - intrinsic S66.40- ☑
        - laceration S66.42- ☑
        - specified type NEC S66.49- ☑
        - strain S66.41- ☑
    - toe — *see also* Injury, muscle, foot
      - extensor, long S96.10- ☑
        - laceration S96.12- ☑
        - specified type NEC S96.19- ☑
        - strain S96.11- ☑
      - flexor, long S96.00- ☑
        - laceration S96.02- ☑
        - specified type NEC S96.09- ☑
        - strain S96.01- ☑
    - triceps S46.30- ☑
      - laceration S46.32- ☑
      - specified type NEC S46.39- ☑
      - strain S46.31- ☑
    - wrist (and hand) level — *see* Injury, muscle, hand
  - musculocutaneous nerve — *see* Injury, nerve, musculocutaneous
  - myocardial (acute) (chronic) (non-ischemic) (non-traumatic) I5A
    - traumatic — *see* Injury, heart
  - myocardium — *see also* Injury, heart
    - non-traumatic — *see* Injury, myocardial
  - nape — *see* Injury, neck
  - nasal (septum) (sinus) S09.92 ☑
  - nasopharynx S09.92 ☑
  - neck S19.9 ☑
    - specified NEC S19.80 ☑
      - specified site NEC S19.89 ☑
  - nerve NEC T14.8 ☑
    - abdomen S34.9 ☑
      - peripheral S34.6 ☑
      - specified site NEC S34.8 ☑
    - abducens S04.4- ☑

- Injury — *continued*
  - nerve — *continued*
    - abducens — *continued*
      - contusion S04.4- ☑
      - laceration S04.4- ☑
      - specified type NEC S04.4- ☑
    - abducent — *see* Injury, nerve, abducens
    - accessory S04.7- ☑
      - contusion S04.7- ☑
      - laceration S04.7- ☑
      - specified type NEC S04.7- ☑
    - acoustic S04.6- ☑
      - contusion S04.6- ☑
      - laceration S04.6- ☑
      - specified type NEC S04.6- ☑
    - ankle S94.9- ☑
      - cutaneous sensory S94.3- ☑
      - specified site NEC — *see* subcategory S94.8 ☑
    - anterior crural, femoral — *see* Injury, nerve, femoral
    - arm (upper) S44.9- ☑
      - axillary — *see* Injury, nerve, axillary
      - cutaneous — *see* Injury, nerve, cutaneous, arm
      - median — *see* Injury, nerve, median, upper arm
      - musculocutaneous — *see* Injury, nerve, musculocutaneous
      - radial — *see* Injury, nerve, radial, upper arm
      - specified site NEC — *see* subcategory S44.8 ☑
      - ulnar — *see* Injury, nerve, ulnar, arm
    - auditory — *see* Injury, nerve, acoustic
    - axillary S44.3- ☑
    - brachial plexus — *see* Injury, brachial plexus
    - cervical sympathetic S14.5 ☑
    - cranial S04.9 ☑
      - contusion S04.9 ☑
      - eighth (acoustic or auditory) — *see* Injury, nerve, acoustic
      - eleventh (accessory) — *see* Injury, nerve, accessory
      - fifth (trigeminal) — *see* Injury, nerve, trigeminal
      - first (olfactory) — *see* Injury, nerve, olfactory
      - fourth (trochlear) — *see* Injury, nerve, trochlear
      - laceration S04.9 ☑
      - ninth (glossopharyngeal) — *see* Injury, nerve, glossopharyngeal
      - second (optic) — *see* Injury, nerve, optic
      - seventh (facial) — *see* Injury, nerve, facial
      - sixth (abducent) — *see* Injury, nerve, abducens
      - specified
        - nerve NEC S04.89- ☑
          - contusion S04.89- ☑
          - laceration S04.89- ☑
          - specified type NEC S04.89- ☑
        - type NEC S04.9 ☑
      - tenth (pneumogastric or vagus) — *see* Injury, nerve, vagus
      - third (oculomotor) — *see* Injury, nerve, oculomotor
      - twelfth (hypoglossal) — *see* Injury, nerve, hypoglossal
    - cutaneous sensory
      - ankle (level) S94.3- ☑
      - arm (upper) (level) S44.5- ☑
      - foot (level) — *see* Injury, nerve, cutaneous sensory, ankle
      - forearm (level) S54.3- ☑
      - hip (level) S74.2- ☑
      - leg (lower level) S84.2- ☑
      - shoulder (level) — *see* Injury, nerve, cutaneous sensory, arm
      - thigh (level) — *see* Injury, nerve, cutaneous sensory, hip
    - deep peroneal — *see* Injury, nerve, peroneal, foot
    - digital
      - finger S64.4- ☑
        - index S64.49- ☑
        - little S64.49- ☑
        - middle S64.49- ☑
        - ring S64.49- ☑
      - thumb S64.3- ☑
      - toe — *see* Injury, nerve, ankle, specified site NEC
    - eighth cranial (acoustic or auditory) — *see* Injury, nerve, acoustic
    - eleventh cranial (accessory) — *see* Injury, nerve, accessory
    - facial S04.5- ☑
      - contusion S04.5- ☑
      - laceration S04.5- ☑
      - newborn P11.3
      - specified type NEC S04.5- ☑
    - femoral (hip level) (thigh level) S74.1- ☑
    - fifth cranial (trigeminal) — *see* Injury, nerve, trigeminal
    - finger (digital) — *see* Injury, nerve, digital, finger
    - first cranial (olfactory) — *see* Injury, nerve, olfactory
    - foot S94.9- ☑
      - cutaneous sensory S94.3- ☑
      - deep peroneal S94.2- ☑
      - lateral plantar S94.0- ☑
      - medial plantar S94.1- ☑
      - specified site NEC — *see* subcategory S94.8 ☑
    - forearm (level) S54.9- ☑
      - cutaneous sensory — *see* Injury, nerve, cutaneous sensory, forearm
      - median — *see* Injury, nerve, median
      - radial — *see* Injury, nerve, radial
      - specified site NEC — *see* subcategory S54.8 ☑
      - ulnar — *see* Injury, nerve, ulnar
    - fourth cranial (trochlear) — *see* Injury, nerve, trochlear
    - glossopharyngeal S04.89- ☑
      - specified type NEC S04.89- ☑
    - hand S64.9- ☑
      - median — *see* Injury, nerve, median, hand
      - radial — *see* Injury, nerve, radial, hand
      - specified NEC — *see* subcategory S64.8 ☑
      - ulnar — *see* Injury, nerve, ulnar, hand
    - hip (level) S74.9- ☑
      - cutaneous sensory — *see* Injury, nerve, cutaneous sensory, hip
      - femoral — *see* Injury, nerve, femoral
      - sciatic — *see* Injury, nerve, sciatic
      - specified site NEC — *see* subcategory S74.8 ☑
    - hypoglossal S04.89- ☑
      - specified type NEC S04.89- ☑
    - lateral plantar S94.0- ☑
    - leg (lower) S84.9- ☑
      - cutaneous sensory — *see* Injury, nerve, cutaneous sensory, leg
      - peroneal — *see* Injury, nerve, peroneal
      - specified site NEC — *see* subcategory S84.8 ☑
      - tibial — *see* Injury, nerve, tibial
      - upper — *see* Injury, nerve, thigh
    - lower
      - back — *see* Injury, nerve, abdomen, specified site NEC
        - peripheral — *see* Injury, nerve, abdomen, peripheral
      - limb — *see* Injury, nerve, leg
    - lumbar plexus — *see* Injury, nerve, lumbosacral, sympathetic
    - lumbar spinal — *see* Injury, spinal, lumbar
      - peripheral S34.6 ☑
      - root S34.21 ☑
      - sympathetic S34.5 ☑
    - lumbosacral
      - plexus — *see* Injury, nerve, lumbosacral, sympathetic
      - sympathetic S34.5 ☑
    - medial plantar S94.1- ☑
    - median (forearm level) S54.1- ☑
      - hand (level) S64.1- ☑
      - upper arm (level) S44.1- ☑
      - wrist (level) — *see* Injury, nerve, median, hand
    - musculocutaneous S44.4- ☑
    - musculospiral (upper arm level) — *see* Injury, nerve, radial, upper arm
    - neck S14.9 ☑
      - peripheral S14.4 ☑
      - specified site NEC S14.8 ☑
      - sympathetic S14.5 ☑
    - ninth cranial (glossopharyngeal) — *see* Injury, nerve, glossopharyngeal
    - oculomotor S04.1- ☑
      - contusion S04.1- ☑
      - laceration S04.1- ☑
      - specified type NEC S04.1- ☑
    - olfactory S04.81- ☑
      - specified type NEC S04.81- ☑
    - optic S04.01- ☑
      - contusion S04.01- ☑
      - laceration S04.01- ☑
      - specified type NEC S04.01- ☑
    - pelvic girdle — *see* Injury, nerve, hip
    - pelvis — *see* Injury, nerve, abdomen, specified site NEC
      - peripheral — *see* Injury, nerve, abdomen, peripheral
    - peripheral NEC T14.8 ☑
      - abdomen — *see* Injury, nerve, abdomen, peripheral
      - lower back — *see* Injury, nerve, abdomen, peripheral
      - neck — *see* Injury, nerve, neck, peripheral
      - pelvis — *see* Injury, nerve, abdomen, peripheral
      - specified NEC T14.8 ☑
    - peroneal (lower leg level) S84.1- ☑
      - foot S94.2- ☑
    - plexus
      - brachial — *see* Injury, brachial plexus
      - celiac, coeliac — *see* Injury, nerve, lumbosacral, sympathetic
      - mesenteric, inferior — *see* Injury, nerve, lumbosacral, sympathetic
      - sacral — *see* Injury, lumbosacral plexus
      - spinal
        - brachial — *see* Injury, brachial plexus
        - lumbosacral — *see* Injury, lumbosacral plexus
    - pneumogastric — *see* Injury, nerve, vagus
    - radial (forearm level) S54.2- ☑
      - hand (level) S64.2- ☑
      - upper arm (level) S44.2- ☑
      - wrist (level) — *see* Injury, nerve, radial, hand
    - root — *see* Injury, nerve, spinal, root
    - sacral plexus — *see* Injury, lumbosacral plexus
    - sacral spinal — *see* Injury, spinal, sacral
      - peripheral S34.6 ☑
      - root S34.22 ☑
      - sympathetic S34.5 ☑
    - sciatic (hip level) (thigh level) S74.0- ☑
    - second cranial (optic) — *see* Injury, nerve, optic
    - seventh cranial (facial) — *see* Injury, nerve, facial
    - shoulder — *see* Injury, nerve, arm
    - sixth cranial (abducent) — *see* Injury, nerve, abducens
    - spinal
      - plexus — *see* Injury, nerve, plexus, spinal
      - root
        - cervical S14.2 ☑
        - dorsal S24.2 ☑
        - lumbar S34.21 ☑
        - sacral S34.22 ☑
        - thoracic — *see* Injury, nerve, spinal, root, dorsal
    - splanchnic — *see* Injury, nerve, lumbosacral, sympathetic
    - sympathetic NEC — *see* Injury, nerve, lumbosacral, sympathetic
      - cervical — *see* Injury, nerve, cervical sympathetic
    - tenth cranial (pneumogastric or vagus) — *see* Injury, nerve, vagus
    - thigh (level) — *see* Injury, nerve, hip
      - cutaneous sensory — *see* Injury, nerve, cutaneous sensory, hip
      - femoral — *see* Injury, nerve, femoral
      - sciatic — *see* Injury, nerve, sciatic
      - specified NEC — *see* Injury, nerve, hip
    - third cranial (oculomotor) — *see* Injury, nerve, oculomotor
    - thorax S24.9 ☑
      - peripheral S24.3 ☑
      - specified site NEC S24.8 ☑
      - sympathetic S24.4 ☑
    - thumb, digital — *see* Injury, nerve, digital, thumb
    - tibial (lower leg level) (posterior) S84.0- ☑
    - toe — *see* Injury, nerve, ankle
    - trigeminal S04.3- ☑
      - contusion S04.3- ☑
      - laceration S04.3- ☑
      - specified type NEC S04.3- ☑
    - trochlear S04.2- ☑
      - contusion S04.2- ☑
      - laceration S04.2- ☑

Injury — *continued*
  toe — *continued*
    specified type NEC S99.82- ☑
    sprain — *see* Sprain, toe
    superficial — *see* Injury, superficial, toe
  tongue S09.93 ☑
  tonsil S09.93 ☑
  tooth S09.93 ☑
  trachea (cervical) NEC S19.82 ☑
    thoracic — *see* Injury, intrathoracic, trachea, thoracic
  transfusion-related acute lung (TRALI) J95.84
  tunica vaginalis S39.94 ☑
  twelfth cranial nerve (hypoglossal) — *see* Injury, nerve, hypoglossal
  ureter S37.10 ☑
    contusion S37.12 ☑
    laceration S37.13 ☑
    specified type NEC S37.19 ☑
  urethra (sphincter) S37.30 ☑
    at delivery O71.5
    contusion S37.32 ☑
    laceration S37.33 ☑
    specified type NEC S37.39 ☑
  urinary organ S37.90 ☑
    contusion S37.92 ☑
    laceration S37.93 ☑
    specified
      site NEC S37.899 ☑
        contusion S37.892 ☑
        laceration S37.893 ☑
        specified type NEC S37.898 ☑
      type NEC S37.99 ☑
  uterus, uterine S37.60 ☑
    with ectopic or molar pregnancy O08.6
    blood vessel — *see* Injury, blood vessel, iliac
    contusion S37.62 ☑
    laceration S37.63 ☑
      cervix at delivery O71.3
    rupture associated with obstetrics — *see* Rupture, uterus
    specified type NEC S37.69 ☑
  uvula S09.93 ☑
  vagina S39.93 ☑
    abrasion S30.814 ☑
    bite S31.45 ☑
      insect S30.864 ☑
      superficial NEC S30.874 ☑
    contusion S30.23 ☑
    crush S38.03 ☑
    during delivery — *see* Laceration, vagina, during delivery
    external constriction S30.844 ☑
    insect bite S30.864 ☑
    laceration S31.41 ☑
      with foreign body S31.42 ☑
    open wound S31.40 ☑
    puncture S31.43 ☑
      with foreign body S31.44 ☑
    superficial S30.95 ☑
      foreign body S30.854 ☑
  vas deferens — *see* Injury, pelvic organ, specified site NEC
  vascular NEC T14.8 ☑
  vein — *see* Injury, blood vessel
  vena cava (superior) S25.20 ☑
    inferior S35.10 ☑
      laceration (minor) (superficial) S35.11 ☑
        major S35.12 ☑
      specified type NEC S35.19 ☑
    laceration (minor) (superficial) S25.21 ☑
      major S25.22 ☑
    specified type NEC S25.29 ☑
  vesical (sphincter) — *see* Injury, bladder
  visual cortex S04.04- ☑
  vitreous (humor) S05.90 ☑
    specified NEC S05.8X- ☑
  vocal cord NEC S19.83 ☑
  vulva S39.94 ☑
    abrasion S30.814 ☑
    bite S31.45 ☑
      insect S30.864 ☑
      superficial NEC S30.874 ☑
    contusion S30.23 ☑
    crush S38.03 ☑
    during delivery — *see* Laceration, perineum, female, during delivery

Injury — *continued*
  vulva — *continued*
    external constriction S30.844 ☑
    insect bite S30.864 ☑
    laceration S31.41 ☑
      with foreign body S31.42 ☑
    open wound S31.40 ☑
    puncture S31.43 ☑
      with foreign body S31.44 ☑
    superficial S30.95 ☑
      foreign body S30.854 ☑
  whiplash (cervical spine) S13.4 ☑
  wrist S69.9- ☑
    blood vessel — *see* Injury, blood vessel, hand
    contusion — *see* Contusion, wrist
    dislocation — *see* Dislocation, wrist
    fracture — *see* Fracture, wrist
    muscle — *see* Injury, muscle, hand
    nerve — *see* Injury, nerve, hand
    open — *see* Wound, open, wrist
    specified NEC S69.8- ☑
    sprain — *see* Sprain, wrist
    superficial — *see* Injury, superficial, wrist

Inoculation — *see also* Vaccination
  complication or reaction — *see* Complications, vaccination

Insanity, insane — *see also* Psychosis
  adolescent — *see* Schizophrenia
  confusional F28
    acute or subacute F05
  delusional F22
  senile F03 ☑

Insect
  bite — *see* Bite, by site, superficial, insect
  venomous, poisoning NEC (by) — *see* Venom, arthropod

Insecurity
  financial Z59.86
  food Z59.41
  transportation Z59.82

Insensitivity
  adrenocorticotropin hormone (ACTH) E27.49
  androgen E34.50
    complete E34.51
    partial E34.52

Insertion
  cord (umbilical) lateral or velamentous O43.12- ☑
  intrauterine contraceptive device (encounter for) — *see* Intrauterine contraceptive device

Insolation (sunstroke) T67.01 ☑

Insomnia (organic) G47.00
  adjustment F51.02
  adjustment disorder F51.02
  behavioral, of childhood Z73.819
    combined type Z73.812
    limit setting type Z73.811
    sleep-onset association type Z73.810
  childhood Z73.819
  chronic F51.04
    somatized tension F51.04
  conditioned F51.04
  due to
    alcohol
      abuse F10.182
      dependence F10.282
      use F10.982
    amphetamines
      abuse F15.182
      dependence F15.282
      use F15.982
    anxiety disorder F51.05
    caffeine
      abuse F15.182
      dependence F15.282
      use F15.982
    cocaine
      abuse F14.182
      dependence F14.282
      use F14.982
    depression F51.05
    drug NEC
      abuse F19.182
      dependence F19.282
      use F19.982
    medical condition G47.01
    mental disorder NEC F51.05

Insomnia — *continued*
  due to — *continued*
    opioid
      abuse F11.182
      dependence F11.282
      use F11.982
    psychoactive substance NEC
      abuse F19.182
      dependence F19.182
      use F19.982
    sedative, hypnotic, or anxiolytic
      abuse F13.182
      dependence F13.282
      use F13.982
    stimulant NEC
      abuse F15.182
      dependence F15.282
      use F15.982
  fatal familial (FFI) A81.83
  idiopathic F51.01
  learned F51.3
  nonorganic origin F51.01
  not due to a substance or known physiological condition F51.01
    specified NEC F51.09
  paradoxical F51.03
  primary F51.01
  psychiatric F51.05
  psychophysiologic F51.04
  related to psychopathology F51.05
  short-term F51.02
  specified NEC G47.09
  stress-related F51.02
  transient F51.02
  without objective findings F51.02

Inspiration
  food or foreign body — *see* Foreign body, by site
  mucus — *see* Asphyxia, mucus

Inspissated bile syndrome (newborn) P59.1

Instability
  emotional (excessive) F60.3
  housing
    housed Z59.819
      with risk of homelessness Z59.811
      homelessness in past 12 months Z59.812
  joint (post-traumatic) M25.30
    ankle M25.37- ☑
    due to old ligament injury — *see* Disorder, ligament
    elbow M25.32- ☑
    flail — *see* Flail, joint
    foot M25.37- ☑
    hand M25.34- ☑
    hip M25.35- ☑
    knee M25.36- ☑
    lumbosacral — *see* subcategory M53.2 ☑
    prosthesis — *see* Complications, joint prosthesis, mechanical, displacement, by site
    sacroiliac — *see* subcategory M53.2 ☑
    secondary to
      old ligament injury — *see* Disorder, ligament
      removal of joint prosthesis M96.89
    shoulder (region) M25.31- ☑
    specified site NEC M25.39
    spine — *see* subcategory M53.2 ☑
    wrist M25.33- ☑
  knee (chronic) M23.5- ☑
  lumbosacral — *see* subcategory M53.2 ☑
  nervous F48.8
  personality (emotional) F60.3
  spine — *see* Instability, joint, spine
  vasomotor R55

Institutional syndrome (childhood) F94.2

Institutionalization, affecting child Z62.22
  disinhibited attachment F94.2

Insufficiency, insufficient
  accommodation, old age H52.4
  adrenal (gland) E27.40
    primary E27.1
  adrenocortical E27.40
    drug-induced E27.3
    iatrogenic E27.3
    primary E27.1
  anatomic crown height K08.89
  anterior (occlusal) guidance M26.54
  anus K62.89
  aortic (valve) I35.1
    with
      mitral (valve) disease I08.0

Index

Insufficiency, insufficient — Intoxication

J

- **Jaundice** — *continued*
  - acholuric (familial) (splenomegalic) — *see also* Spherocytosis
    - acquired D59.8
  - breast-milk (inhibitor) P59.3
  - catarrhal (acute) B15.9
    - with hepatic coma B15.Ø
  - cholestatic (benign) R17
  - due to or associated with
    - delayed conjugation P59.8
      - associated with (due to) preterm delivery P59.Ø
    - preterm delivery P59.Ø
  - epidemic (catarrhal) B15.9
    - with hepatic coma B15.Ø
    - leptospiral A27.Ø
    - spirochetal A27.Ø
  - familial nonhemolytic (congenital) (Gilbert) E8Ø.4
    - Crigler-Najjar E8Ø.5
  - febrile (acute) B15.9
    - with hepatic coma B15.Ø
    - leptospiral A27.Ø
    - spirochetal A27.Ø
  - hematogenous D59.9
  - hemolytic (acquired) D59.9
    - congenital — *see* Spherocytosis
  - hemorrhagic (acute) (leptospiral) (spirochetal) A27.Ø
  - infectious (acute) (subacute) B15.9
    - with hepatic coma B15.Ø
    - leptospiral A27.Ø
    - spirochetal A27.Ø
  - leptospiral (hemorrhagic) A27.Ø
  - malignant (without coma) K72.9Ø
    - with coma K72.91
  - neonatal — *see* Jaundice, newborn
  - newborn P59.9
    - due to or associated with
      - ABO
        - antibodies P55.1
        - incompatibility, maternal/fetal P55.1
        - isoimmunization P55.1
      - absence or deficiency of enzyme system for bilirubin conjugation (congenital) P59.8
      - bleeding P58.1
      - breast milk inhibitors to conjugation P59.3
        - associated with preterm delivery P59.Ø
      - bruising P58.Ø
      - Crigler-Najjar syndrome E8Ø.5
      - delayed conjugation P59.8
        - associated with preterm delivery P59.Ø
      - drugs or toxins
        - given to newborn P58.42
        - transmitted from mother P58.41
      - excessive hemolysis P58.9
        - due to
          - bleeding P58.1
          - bruising P58.Ø
          - drugs or toxins
            - given to newborn P58.42
            - transmitted from mother P58.41
          - infection P58.2
          - polycythemia P58.3
          - swallowed maternal blood P58.5
        - specified type NEC P58.8
      - galactosemia E74.21
      - Gilbert syndrome E8Ø.4
      - hemolytic disease P55.9
        - ABO isoimmunization P55.1
        - Rh isoimmunization P55.Ø
        - specified NEC P55.8
      - hepatocellular damage P59.2Ø
        - specified NEC P59.29
      - hereditary hemolytic anemia P58.8
      - hypothyroidism, congenital EØ3.1
      - incompatibility, maternal/fetal NOS P55.9
      - infection P58.2
      - inspissated bile syndrome P59.1
      - isoimmunization NOS P55.9
      - mucoviscidosis E84.9
      - polycythemia P58.3
      - preterm delivery P59.Ø
      - Rh
        - antibodies P55.Ø
        - incompatibility, maternal/fetal P55.Ø
        - isoimmunization P55.Ø
      - specified cause NEC P59.8
      - swallowed maternal blood P58.5
    - spherocytosis (congenital) D58.Ø
  - nonhemolytic congenital familial (Gilbert) E8Ø.4
- **Jaundice** — *continued*
  - nuclear, newborn — *see also* Kernicterus of newborn P57.9
  - obstructive — *see also* Obstruction, bile duct K83.1
  - post-immunization — *see* Hepatitis, viral, type, B
  - post-transfusion — *see* Hepatitis, viral, type, B
  - regurgitation — *see also* Obstruction, bile duct K83.1
  - serum (homologous) (prophylactic) (therapeutic) — *see* Hepatitis, viral, type, B
  - spirochetal (hemorrhagic) A27.Ø
  - symptomatic R17
    - newborn P59.9
- **Jaw** — *see* condition
- **Jaw-winking phenomenon or syndrome** QØ7.8
- **Jealousy**
  - alcoholic F1Ø.988
  - childhood F93.8
  - sibling F93.8
- **Jejunitis** — *see* Enteritis
- **Jejunostomy status** Z93.4
- **Jejunum, jejunal** — *see* condition
- **Jensen's disease** — *see* Inflammation, chorioretinal, focal, juxtapapillary
- **Jerks, myoclonic** G25.3
- **Jervell-Lange-Nielsen syndrome** I45.81
- **Jeune's disease** Q77.2
- **Jigger disease** B88.1
- **Job's syndrome** (chronic granulomatous disease) D71
- **Joint** — *see also* condition
  - mice — *see* Loose, body, joint
    - knee M23.4- ☑
- **Jordan's anomaly or syndrome** D72.Ø
- **Joseph-Diamond-Blackfan anemia** (congenital hypoplastic) D61.Ø1
- **Jungle yellow fever** A95.Ø
- **Jüngling's disease** — *see* Sarcoidosis
- **Juvenile** — *see* condition

K

- **Kahler's disease** C9Ø.Ø- ☑
- **Kakke** E51.11
- **Kala-azar** B55.Ø
- **Kallmann's syndrome** E23.Ø
- **Kanner's syndrome** (autism) — *see* Psychosis, childhood
- **Kaposi's**
  - dermatosis (xeroderma pigmentosum) Q82.1
  - lichen ruber L44.Ø
    - acuminatus L44.Ø
  - sarcoma
    - colon C46.4
    - connective tissue C46.1
    - gastrointestinal organ C46.4
    - lung C46.5- ☑
    - lymph node (multiple) C46.3
    - palate (hard) (soft) C46.2
    - rectum C46.4
    - skin (multiple sites) C46.Ø
    - specified site NEC C46.7
    - stomach C46.4
    - unspecified site C46.9
  - varicelliform eruption BØØ.Ø
    - vaccinia T88.1 ☑
- **Kartagener's syndrome or triad** (sinusitis, bronchiectasis, situs inversus) Q89.3
- **Karyotype**
  - with abnormality except iso (Xq) Q96.2
  - 45,X Q96.Ø
  - 46,X
    - iso (Xq) Q96.1
  - 46,XX Q98.3
    - with streak gonads Q5Ø.32
    - hermaphrodite (true) Q99.1
    - male Q98.3
  - 46,XY
    - with streak gonads Q56.1
    - female Q97.3
    - hermaphrodite (true) Q99.1
  - 47,XXX Q97.Ø
  - 47,XXY Q98.Ø
  - 47,XYY Q98.5
- **Kaschin-Beck disease** — *see* Disease, Kaschin-Beck
- **Katayama's disease or fever** B65.2
- **Kawasaki's syndrome** M3Ø.3
- **Kayser-Fleischer ring** (cornea) (pseudosclerosis) H18.Ø4- ☑
- **Kaznelson's syndrome** (congenital hypoplastic anemia) D61.Ø1
- **Kearns-Sayre syndrome** H49.81- ☑
- **Kedani fever** A75.3
- **Kelis** L91.Ø
- **Kelly (-Patterson) syndrome** (sideropenic dysphagia) D5Ø.1
- **Keloid, cheloid** L91.Ø
  - acne L73.Ø
  - Addison's L94.Ø
  - cornea — *see* Opacity, cornea
  - Hawkin's L91.Ø
  - scar L91.Ø
- **Keloma** L91.Ø
- **Kenya fever** A77.1
- **Keratectasia** — *see also* Ectasia, cornea
  - congenital Q13.4
- **Keratinization of alveolar ridge mucosa**
  - excessive K13.23
  - minimal K13.22
- **Keratinized residual ridge mucosa**
  - excessive K13.23
  - minimal K13.22
- **Keratitis** (nodular) (nonulcerative) (simple) (zonular) H16.9
  - with ulceration (central) (marginal) (perforated) (ring) — *see* Ulcer, cornea
  - actinic — *see* Photokeratitis
  - arborescens (herpes simplex) BØØ.52
  - areolar H16.11- ☑
  - bullosa H16.8
  - deep H16.3Ø9
    - specified type NEC H16.399
  - dendritic (a) (herpes simplex) BØØ.52
  - disciform (is) (herpes simplex) BØØ.52
    - varicella BØ1.81
  - filamentary H16.12- ☑
  - gonococcal (congenital or prenatal) A54.33
  - herpes, herpetic (simplex) BØØ.52
    - zoster BØ2.33
  - in (due to)
    - acanthamebiasis B6Ø.13
    - adenovirus B3Ø.Ø
    - exanthema — *see also* Exanthem BØ9
    - herpes (simplex) virus BØØ.52
    - measles BØ5.81
    - syphilis A5Ø.31
    - tuberculosis A18.52
    - zoster BØ2.33
  - interstitial (nonsyphilitic) H16.3Ø- ☑
    - diffuse H16.32- ☑
    - herpes, herpetic (simplex) BØØ.52
      - zoster BØ2.33
    - sclerosing H16.33- ☑
    - specified type NEC H16.39- ☑
    - syphilitic (congenital) (late) A5Ø.31
    - tuberculous A18.52
  - macular H16.11- ☑
  - nummular H16.11- ☑
  - oyster shuckers' H16.8
  - parenchymatous — *see* Keratitis, interstitial
  - petrificans H16.8
  - postmeasles BØ5.81
  - punctata
    - leprosa A3Ø.9 *[H16.14-]* ☑
    - syphilitic (profunda) A5Ø.31
  - punctate H16.14- ☑
  - purulent H16.8
  - rosacea L71.8
  - sclerosing H16.33- ☑
  - specified type NEC H16.8
  - stellate H16.11- ☑
  - striate H16.11- ☑
  - superficial H16.1Ø- ☑
    - with conjunctivitis — *see* Keratoconjunctivitis
    - due to light — *see* Photokeratitis
  - suppurative H16.8
  - syphilitic (congenital) (prenatal) A5Ø.31
  - trachomatous A71.1
    - sequelae B94.Ø
  - tuberculous A18.52
  - vesicular H16.8
  - xerotic — *see also* Keratomalacia H16.8
    - vitamin A deficiency E5Ø.4
- **Keratoacanthoma** L85.8
- **Keratocele** — *see* Descemetocele
- **Keratoconjunctivitis** H16.2Ø- ☑

- **Keratoconjunctivitis** — *continued*
  - Acanthamoeba B6Ø.13
  - adenoviral B3Ø.Ø
  - epidemic B3Ø.Ø
  - exposure H16.21- ☑
  - herpes, herpetic (simplex) BØØ.52
    - zoster BØ2.33
  - in exanthema — *see also* Exanthem BØ9
  - infectious B3Ø.Ø
  - lagophthalmic — *see* Keratoconjunctivitis, specified type NEC
  - neurotrophic H16.23- ☑
  - phlyctenular H16.25- ☑
  - postmeasles BØ5.81
  - shipyard B3Ø.Ø
  - sicca (Sjogren's) M35.Ø- ☑
    - not Sjogren's H16.22- ☑
  - specified type NEC H16.29- ☑
  - tuberculous (phlyctenular) A18.52
  - vernal H16.26- ☑
- **Keratoconus** H18.6Ø- ☑
  - congenital Q13.4
  - stable H18.61- ☑
  - unstable H18.62- ☑
- **Keratocyst** (dental) (odontogenic) — *see* Cyst, calcifying odontogenic
- **Keratoderma, keratodermia** (congenital) (palmaris et plantaris) (symmetrical) Q82.8
  - acquired L85.1
    - in diseases classified elsewhere L86
  - climactericum L85.1
  - gonococcal A54.89
  - gonorrheal A54.89
  - punctata L85.2
  - Reiter's — *see* Reiter's disease
- **Keratodermatocele** — *see* Descemetocele
- **Keratoglobus** H18.79 ☑
  - congenital Q15.8
    - with glaucoma Q15.Ø
- **Keratohemia** — *see* Pigmentation, cornea, stromal
- **Keratoiritis** — *see also* Iridocyclitis
  - syphilitic A5Ø.39
  - tuberculous A18.54
- **Keratoma** L57.Ø
  - palmaris and plantaris hereditarium Q82.8
  - senile L57.Ø
- **Keratomalacia** H18.44- ☑
  - vitamin A deficiency E5Ø.4
- **Keratomegaly** Q13.4
- **Keratomycosis** B49
  - nigrans, nigricans (palmaris) B36.1
- **Keratopathy** H18.9
  - band H18.42- ☑
  - bullous (aphakic), following cataract surgery H59.Ø1- ☑
  - bullous H18.1- ☑
- **Keratoscleritis, tuberculous** A18.52
- **Keratosis** L57.Ø
  - actinic L57.Ø
  - arsenical L85.8
  - congenital, specified NEC Q8Ø.8
  - female genital NEC N94.89
  - follicularis Q82.8
    - acquired L11.Ø
    - congenita Q82.8
    - et parafollicularis in cutem penetrans L87.Ø
    - spinulosa (decalvans) Q82.8
    - vitamin A deficiency E5Ø.8
  - gonococcal A54.89
  - male genital (external) N5Ø.89
  - nigricans L83
  - obturans, external ear (canal) — *see* Cholesteatoma, external ear
  - palmaris et plantaris (inherited) (symmetrical) Q82.8
    - acquired L85.1
  - penile N48.89
  - pharynx J39.2
  - pilaris, acquired L85.8
  - punctata (palmaris et plantaris) L85.2
  - scrotal N5Ø.89
  - seborrheic L82.1
    - inflamed L82.Ø
  - senile L57.Ø
  - solar L57.Ø
  - tonsillaris J35.8
  - vagina N89.4
  - vegetans Q82.8
  - vitamin A deficiency E5Ø.8
  - vocal cord J38.3
- **Kerato-uveitis** — *see* Iridocyclitis
- **Kerion** (celsi) B35.Ø
- **Kernicterus of newborn** (not due to isoimmunization) P57.9
  - due to isoimmunization (conditions in P55.Ø-P55.9) P57.Ø
  - specified type NEC P57.8
- **Kerunoparalysis** T75.Ø9 ☑
- **Keshan disease** E59
- **Ketoacidosis** E87.29
  - diabetic — *see* Diabetes, by type, with ketoacidosis
- **Ketonuria** R82.4
- **Ketosis NEC** E88.89
  - diabetic — *see* Diabetes, by type, with ketoacidosis
- **Kew Garden fever** A79.1
- **Kidney** — *see* condition
- **Kienböck's disease** — *see also* Osteochondrosis, juvenile, hand, carpal lunate
  - adult M93.1
- **Kimmelstiel** (-Wilson) **disease** — *see* Diabetes, Kimmelstiel (-Wilson) disease
- **Kink, kinking**
  - artery I77.1
  - hair (acquired) L67.8
  - ileum or intestine — *see* Obstruction, intestine
  - Lane's — *see* Obstruction, intestine
  - organ or site, congenital NEC — *see* Anomaly, by site
  - ureter (pelvic junction) N13.5
    - with
      - hydronephrosis N13.1
        - with infection N13.6
      - pyelonephritis (chronic) N11.1
    - congenital Q62.39
  - vein(s) I87.8
    - caval I87.1
    - peripheral I87.1
- **Kinnier Wilson's disease** (hepatolenticular degeneration) E83.Ø1
- **Kissing spine** M48.2Ø
  - cervical region M48.22
  - cervicothoracic region M48.23
  - lumbar region M48.26
  - lumbosacral region M48.27
  - occipito-atlanto-axial region M48.21
  - thoracic region M48.24
  - thoracolumbar region M48.25
- **Klatskin's tumor** C22.1
- **Klauder's disease** A26.8
- **Klebs' disease** — *see also* Glomerulonephritis NØ5- ☑
- **Klebsiella** (K.) **pneumoniae, as cause of disease classified elsewhere** B96.1
- **Klein** (e)**-Levin syndrome** G47.13
- **Kleptomania** F63.2
- **Klinefelter's syndrome** Q98.4
  - karyotype 47,XXY Q98.Ø
  - male with more than two X chromosomes Q98.1
- **Klippel-Feil deficiency, disease, or syndrome** (brevicollis) Q76.1
- **Klippel's disease** I67.2
- **Klippel-Trenaunay** (-Weber) **syndrome** Q87.2
- **Klumpke** (-Déjerine) **palsy, paralysis** (birth) (newborn) P14.1
- **Knee** — *see* condition
- **Knock knee** (acquired) M21.Ø6- ☑
  - congenital Q74.1
- **Knot**(s)
  - intestinal, syndrome (volvulus) K56.2
  - surfer S89.8- ☑
  - umbilical cord (true) O69.2 ☑
- **Knotting** (of)
  - hair L67.8
  - intestine K56.2
- **Knuckle pad** (Garrod's) M72.1
- **Koch's**
  - infection — *see* Tuberculosis
  - relapsing fever A68.9
- **Koch-Weeks' conjunctivitis** — *see* Conjunctivitis, acute, mucopurulent
- **Köebner's syndrome** Q81.8
- **Köenig's disease** (osteochondritis dissecans) — *see* Osteochondritis, dissecans
- **Köhler-Pellegrini-Steida disease or syndrome** (calcification, knee joint) — *see* Bursitis, tibial collateral
- **Köhler's disease**
  - patellar — *see* Osteochondrosis, juvenile, patella
  - tarsal navicular — *see* Osteochondrosis, juvenile, tarsus
- **Koilonychia** L6Ø.3
- **Koilonychia** — *continued*
  - congenital Q84.6
- **Kojevnikov's, epilepsy** — *see* Kozhevnikof's epilepsy
- **Koplik's spots** BØ5.9
- **Kopp's asthma** E32.8
- **Korsakoff's** (Wernicke) **disease, psychosis or syndrome** (alcoholic) F1Ø.96
  - with dependence F1Ø.26
  - drug-induced
    - due to drug abuse — *see* Abuse, drug, by type, with amnestic disorder
    - due to drug dependence — *see* Dependence, drug, by type, with amnestic disorder
  - nonalcoholic FØ4
- **Korsakov's disease, psychosis or syndrome** — *see* Korsakoff's disease
- **Korsakow's disease, psychosis or syndrome** — *see* Korsakoff's disease
- **Kostmann's disease or syndrome** (infantile genetic agranulocytosis) — *see* Agranulocytosis
- **Kozhevnikof's epilepsy** G4Ø.1Ø9
  - intractable G4Ø.119
    - with status epilepticus G4Ø.111
    - without status epilepticus G4Ø.119
  - not intractable G4Ø.1Ø9
    - with status epilepticus G4Ø.1Ø1
    - without status epilepticus G4Ø.1Ø9
- **Krabbe's**
  - disease E75.23
  - syndrome, congenital muscle hypoplasia Q79.8
- **Kraepelin-Morel disease** — *see* Schizophrenia
- **Kraft-Weber-Dimitri disease** Q85.89
- **Kraurosis**
  - ani K62.89
  - penis N48.Ø
  - vagina N89.8
  - vulva N9Ø.4
- **Kreotoxism** AØ5.9
- **Krukenberg's**
  - spindle — *see* Pigmentation, cornea, posterior
  - tumor C79.6- ☑
- **Kufs' disease** E75.4
- **Kugelberg-Welander disease** G12.1
- **Kuhnt-Junius degeneration** — *see also* Degeneration, macula H35.32- ☑
- **Kümmell's disease or spondylitis** — *see* Spondylopathy, traumatic
- **Kupffer cell sarcoma** C22.3
- **Kuru** A81.81
- **Kussmaul's**
  - disease M3Ø.Ø
  - respiration E87.29
    - in diabetic acidosis — *see* Diabetes, by type, with ketoacidosis
- **Kwashiorkor** E4Ø
  - marasmic, marasmus type E42
- **Kyasanur Forest disease** A98.2
- **Kyphoscoliosis, kyphoscoliotic** (acquired) — *see also* Scoliosis M41.9
  - congenital Q67.5
  - heart (disease) I27.1
  - sequelae of rickets E64.3
  - tuberculous A18.Ø1
- **Kyphosis, kyphotic** (acquired) M4Ø.2Ø9
  - cervical region M4Ø.2Ø2
  - cervicothoracic region M4Ø.2Ø3
  - congenital Q76.419
    - cervical region Q76.412
    - cervicothoracic region Q76.413
    - occipito-atlanto-axial region Q76.411
    - thoracic region Q76.414
    - thoracolumbar region Q76.415
  - Morquio-Brailsford type (spinal) — *see also* subcategory M49.8 E76.219
  - postlaminectomy M96.3
  - postradiation therapy M96.2
  - postural (adolescent) M4Ø.ØØ
    - cervicothoracic region M4Ø.Ø3
    - thoracic region M4Ø.Ø4
    - thoracolumbar region M4Ø.Ø5
  - secondary NEC M4Ø.1Ø
    - cervical region M4Ø.12
    - cervicothoracic region M4Ø.13
    - thoracic region M4Ø.14
    - thoracolumbar region M4Ø.15
  - sequelae of rickets E64.3
  - specified type NEC M4Ø.299
    - cervical region M4Ø.292

- **Kyphosis, kyphotic** — *continued*
  - specified type — *continued*
    - cervicothoracic region M4Ø.293
    - thoracic region M4Ø.294
    - thoracolumbar region M4Ø.295
  - syphilitic, congenital A5Ø.56
  - thoracic region M4Ø.2Ø4
  - thoracolumbar region M4Ø.2Ø5
  - tuberculous A18.Ø1
- **Kyrle disease** L87.Ø

L

- **Labia, labium** — *see* condition
- **Labile**
  - blood pressure RØ9.89
  - vasomotor system I73.9
- **Labioglossal paralysis** G12.29
- **Labium leporinum** — *see* Cleft, lip
- **Labor** — *see* Delivery
- **Labored breathing** — *see* Hyperventilation
- **Labyrinthitis** (circumscribed) (destructive) (diffuse) (inner ear) (latent) (purulent) (suppurative) — *see also* subcategory H83.Ø ☑
  - syphilitic A52.79
- **Laceration**
  - with abortion — *see* Abortion, by type, complicated by laceration of pelvic organs
  - abdomen, abdominal
    - wall S31.119 ☑
      - with
        - foreign body S31.129 ☑
        - penetration into peritoneal cavity S31.619 ☑
          - with foreign body S31.629 ☑
      - epigastric region S31.112 ☑
        - with
          - foreign body S31.122 ☑
          - penetration into peritoneal cavity S31.612 ☑
            - with foreign body S31.622 ☑
      - left
        - lower quadrant S31.114 ☑
          - with
            - foreign body S31.124 ☑
            - penetration into peritoneal cavity S31.614 ☑
              - with foreign body S31.624 ☑
        - upper quadrant S31.111 ☑
          - with
            - foreign body S31.121 ☑
            - penetration into peritoneal cavity S31.611 ☑
              - with foreign body S31.621 ☑
      - periumbilic region S31.115 ☑
        - with
          - foreign body S31.125 ☑
          - penetration into peritoneal cavity S31.615 ☑
            - with foreign body S31.625 ☑
      - right
        - lower quadrant S31.113 ☑
          - with
            - foreign body S31.123 ☑
            - penetration into peritoneal cavity S31.613 ☑
              - with foreign body S31.623 ☑
        - upper quadrant S31.11Ø ☑
          - with
            - foreign body S31.12Ø ☑
            - penetration into peritoneal cavity S31.61Ø ☑
              - with foreign body S31.62Ø ☑
  - accidental, complicating surgery — *see* Complications, surgical, accidental puncture or laceration
  - Achilles tendon S86.Ø2- ☑
  - adrenal gland S37.813 ☑
  - alveolar (process) — *see* Laceration, oral cavity
  - ankle S91.Ø1- ☑
    - with
      - foreign body S91.Ø2- ☑
  - antecubital space — *see* Laceration, elbow
  - anus (sphincter) S31.831 ☑
    - with
      - ectopic or molar pregnancy OØ8.6
      - foreign body S31.832 ☑
    - complicating delivery — *see* Delivery, complicated, by, laceration, anus (sphincter)

Laceration — *continued*

- anus — *continued*
  - following ectopic or molar pregnancy OØ8.6
  - nontraumatic, nonpuerperal — *see* Fissure, anus
- arm (upper) S41.11- ☑
  - with foreign body S41.12- ☑
  - lower — *see* Laceration, forearm
- auditory canal (external) (meatus) — *see* Laceration, ear
- auricle, ear — *see* Laceration, ear
- axilla — *see* Laceration, arm
- back — *see also* Laceration, thorax, back
  - lower S31.Ø1Ø ☑
    - with
      - foreign body S31.Ø2Ø ☑
        - with penetration into retroperitoneal space S31.Ø21 ☑
      - penetration into retroperitoneal space S31.Ø11 ☑
- bile duct S36.13 ☑
- bladder S37.23 ☑
  - with ectopic or molar pregnancy OØ8.6
  - following ectopic or molar pregnancy OØ8.6
  - obstetrical trauma O71.5
- blood vessel — *see* Injury, blood vessel
- bowel — *see also* Laceration, intestine
  - with ectopic or molar pregnancy OØ8.6
  - complicating abortion — *see* Abortion, by type, complicated by, specified condition NEC
  - following ectopic or molar pregnancy OØ8.6
  - obstetrical trauma O71.5
- brain (any part) (cortex) (diffuse) (membrane) — *see also* Injury, intracranial, diffuse
  - during birth P1Ø.8
    - with hemorrhage P1Ø.1
  - focal — *see* Injury, intracranial, focal brain injury
- brainstem SØ6.38- ☑
- breast S21.Ø1- ☑
  - with foreign body S21.Ø2- ☑
- broad ligament S37.893 ☑
  - with ectopic or molar pregnancy OØ8.6
  - following ectopic or molar pregnancy OØ8.6
  - laceration syndrome N83.8
  - obstetrical trauma O71.6
  - syndrome (laceration) N83.8
- buttock S31.8Ø1 ☑
  - with foreign body S31.8Ø2 ☑
  - left S31.821 ☑
    - with foreign body S31.822 ☑
  - right S31.811 ☑
    - with foreign body S31.812 ☑
- calf — *see* Laceration, leg
- canaliculus lacrimalis — *see* Laceration, eyelid
- canthus, eye — *see* Laceration, eyelid
- capsule, joint — *see* Sprain
- causing eversion of cervix uteri (old) N86
- central (perineal), complicating delivery O7Ø.9
- cerebellum, traumatic SØ6.37- ☑
- cerebral SØ6.33- ☑
  - during birth P1Ø.8
    - with hemorrhage P1Ø.1
  - left side SØ6.32- ☑
  - right side SØ6.31- ☑
- cervix (uteri)
  - with ectopic or molar pregnancy OØ8.6
  - following ectopic or molar pregnancy OØ8.6
  - nonpuerperal, nontraumatic N88.1
  - obstetrical trauma (current) O71.3
  - old (postpartal) N88.1
  - traumatic S37.63 ☑
- cheek (external) SØ1.41- ☑
  - with foreign body SØ1.42- ☑
  - internal — *see* Laceration, oral cavity
- chest wall — *see* Laceration, thorax
- chin — *see* Laceration, head, specified site NEC
- chordae tendinae NEC I51.1
  - concurrent with acute myocardial infarction — *see* Infarct, myocardium
  - following acute myocardial infarction (current complication) I23.4
- clitoris — *see* Laceration, vulva
- colon — *see* Laceration, intestine, large, colon
- common bile duct S36.13 ☑
- cortex (cerebral) — *see* Injury, intracranial, diffuse
- costal region — *see* Laceration, thorax
- cystic duct S36.13 ☑
- diaphragm S27.8Ø3 ☑

Laceration — *continued*

- digit(s)
  - foot — *see* Laceration, toe
  - hand — *see* Laceration, finger
- duodenum S36.43Ø ☑
- ear (canal) (external) SØ1.31- ☑
  - with foreign body SØ1.32- ☑
  - drum SØ9.2- ☑
- elbow S51.Ø1- ☑
  - with
    - foreign body S51.Ø2- ☑
- epididymis — *see* Laceration, testis
- epigastric region — *see* Laceration, abdomen, wall, epigastric region
- esophagus K22.89
  - traumatic
    - cervical S11.21 ☑
      - with foreign body S11.22 ☑
    - thoracic S27.813 ☑
- eye (ball) SØ5.3- ☑
  - with prolapse or loss of intraocular tissue SØ5.2- ☑
  - penetrating SØ5.6- ☑
- eyebrow — *see* Laceration, eyelid
- eyelid SØ1.11- ☑
  - with foreign body SØ1.12- ☑
- face NEC — *see* Laceration, head, specified site NEC
- fallopian tube S37.539 ☑
  - bilateral S37.532 ☑
  - unilateral S37.531 ☑
- finger(s) S61.219 ☑
  - with
    - damage to nail S61.319 ☑
      - with
        - foreign body S61.329 ☑
    - foreign body S61.229 ☑
  - index S61.218 ☑
    - with
      - damage to nail S61.318 ☑
        - with
          - foreign body S61.328 ☑
      - foreign body S61.228 ☑
    - left S61.211 ☑
      - with
        - damage to nail S61.311 ☑
          - with
            - foreign body S61.321 ☑
        - foreign body S61.221 ☑
    - right S61.21Ø ☑
      - with
        - damage to nail S61.31Ø ☑
          - with
            - foreign body S61.32Ø ☑
        - foreign body S61.22Ø ☑
  - little S61.218 ☑
    - with
      - damage to nail S61.318 ☑
        - with
          - foreign body S61.328 ☑
      - foreign body S61.228 ☑
    - left S61.217 ☑
      - with
        - damage to nail S61.317 ☑
          - with
            - foreign body S61.327 ☑
        - foreign body S61.227 ☑
    - right S61.216 ☑
      - with
        - damage to nail S61.316 ☑
          - with
            - foreign body S61.326 ☑
        - foreign body S61.226 ☑
  - middle S61.218 ☑
    - with
      - damage to nail S61.318 ☑
        - with
          - foreign body S61.328 ☑
      - foreign body S61.228 ☑
    - left S61.213 ☑
      - with
        - damage to nail S61.313 ☑
          - with
            - foreign body S61.323 ☑
        - foreign body S61.223 ☑
    - right S61.212 ☑
      - with
        - damage to nail S61.312 ☑

- **Lithemia** E79.Ø
- **Lithiasis** — *see* Calculus
- **Lithosis** J62.8
- **Lithuria** R82.998
- **Litigation, anxiety concerning** Z65.3
- **Little leaguer's elbow** — *see* Epicondylitis, medial
- **Little's disease** G8Ø.9
- **Littre's**
  - gland — *see* condition
  - hernia — *see* Hernia, abdomen
- **Littritis** — *see* Urethritis
- **Livedo** (annularis) (racemosa) (reticularis) R23.1
- **Liver** — *see* condition
- **Living alone** (problems with) Z6Ø.2
  - with handicapped person Z74.2
- **Living in a shelter** (motel) (scattered site housing) (temporary or transitional living situation) Z59.Ø1
- **Lloyd's syndrome** — *see* Adenomatosis, endocrine
- **Loa loa, loaiasis, loasis** B74.3
- **Lobar** — *see* condition
- **Lobomycosis** B48.Ø
- **Lobo's disease** B48.Ø
- **Lobotomy syndrome** FØ7.Ø
- **Lobstein** (-Ekman) **disease or syndrome** Q78.Ø
- **Lobster-claw hand** Q71.6- ☑
- **Lobulation** (congenital) — *see also* Anomaly, by site
  - kidney, Q63.1
  - liver, abnormal Q44.7
  - spleen Q89.Ø9
- **Lobule, lobular** — *see* condition
- **Local, localized** — *see* condition
- **Locked twins causing obstructed labor** O66.1
- **Locked-in state** G83.5
- **Locking**
  - joint — *see* Derangement, joint, specified type NEC
    - knee — *see* Derangement, knee
- **Lockjaw** — *see* Tetanus
- **Löffler's**
  - endocarditis I42.3
  - eosinophilia J82.89
  - pneumonia J82.89
  - syndrome (eosinophilic pneumonitis) J82.89
- **Loiasis** (with conjunctival infestation) (eyelid) B74.3
- **Lone Star fever** A77.Ø
- **Long**
  - COVID (-19) — *see also* COVID-19 UØ9.9
  - labor O63.9
    - first stage O63.Ø
    - second stage O63.1
  - QT syndrome I45.81
- **Longitudinal stripes or grooves, nails** L6Ø.8
  - congenital Q84.6
- **Long-term** (current) (prophylactic) **drug therapy** (use of)
  - 5-fluorouracil Z79.631
  - 6-mercaptopurine Z79.631
  - adalimumab Z79.62Ø
  - agents affecting estrogen receptors and estrogen levels NEC Z79.818
  - alkylating agent Z79.63Ø
  - anastrozole (Arimidex) Z79.811
  - antibiotics Z79.2
    - short-term use — *omit code*
  - anticoagulants Z79.Ø1
  - antidiabetic drugs, injectable, non-insulin Z79.85
  - anti-inflammatory, non-steroidal (NSAID) Z79.1
  - antimetabolite agent Z79.631
  - antiplatelet Z79.Ø2
  - antithrombotics Z79.Ø2
  - antitumor antibiotic Z79.632
  - apremilast Z79.61
  - aromatase inhibitors Z79.811
  - aspirin Z79.82
  - azathioprine Z79.624
  - birth control pill or patch Z79.3
  - bisphosphonates Z79.83
  - bleomycin Z79.632
  - calcineurin inhibitor Z79.621
  - chlorambucil Z79.63Ø
  - cisplatin Z79.63Ø
  - contraceptive, oral Z79.3
  - cyclophosphamide Z79.63Ø
  - cyclosporine Z79.621
  - cytarabine Z79.631
  - doxorubicin Z79.632
  - drug, specified NEC Z79.899
  - estrogen receptor downregulators Z79.818

Long-term (current) (prophylactic) **drug therapy** — *continued*

  - etanercept Z79.62Ø
  - etoposide Z79.634
  - Evista Z79.81Ø
  - exemestane (Aromasin) Z79.811
  - Fareston Z79.81Ø
  - fulvestrant (Faslodex) Z79.818
  - gonadotropin-releasing hormone (GnRH) agonist Z79.818
  - goserelin acetate (Zoladex) Z79.818
  - hormone replacement Z79.89Ø
  - hydroxyurea Z79.64
  - immunomodulators, unspecified Z79.6Ø
    - specified NEC Z79.69
  - immunomodulatory imide drug Z79.61
  - immunosuppressants, unspecified Z79.6Ø
    - specified NEC Z79.69
  - immunosuppressive biologic Z79.62Ø
  - infliximab Z79.62Ø
  - inhibitors of nucleotide synthesis Z79.624
  - insulin Z79.4
  - irinotecan Z79.634
  - Janus kinase inhibitor Z79.622
  - lenalidomide Z79.61
  - letrozole (Femara) Z79.811
  - leuprolide acetate (leuprorelin) (Lupron) Z79.818
  - mammalian target of rapamycin (mTOR) inhibitor Z79.623
  - megestrol acetate (Megace) Z79.818
  - methadone for pain management Z79.891
  - mitomycin C Z79.632
  - mitotic inhibitor Z79.633
  - monoclonal antibodies Z79.62Ø
  - myelosuppressive agent Z79.64
  - Nolvadex Z79.81Ø
  - non-insulin antidiabetic drug, injectable Z79.899
  - non-steroidal anti-inflammatories (NSAID) Z79.1
  - omycophenolate Z79.624
  - opiate analgesic Z79.891
  - oral
    - antidiabetic Z79.84
    - contraceptive Z79.3
    - hypoglycemic Z79.84
  - paclitaxel Z79.633
  - plant alkaloids Z79.633
  - pomalidomide Z79.61
  - purine synthesis (IMDH) inhibitors Z79.624
  - raloxifene (Evista) Z79.81Ø
  - selective estrogen receptor modulators (SERMs) Z79.81Ø
  - sirolimus Z79.623
  - steroids
    - inhaled Z79.51
    - systemic Z79.52
  - tacrolimus Z79.621
  - tamoxifen (Nolvadex) Z79.81Ø
  - tofacitinib Z79.622
  - topoisomerase inhibitor Z79.634
  - topotecan Z79.634
  - toremifene (Fareston) Z79.81Ø
  - vinblastine Z79.633
  - vincristine Z79.633
- **Loop**
  - intestine — *see* Volvulus
  - vascular on papilla (optic) Q14.2
- **Loose** — *see also* condition
  - body
    - joint M24.ØØ
      - ankle M24.Ø7- ☑
      - elbow M24.Ø2- ☑
      - hand M24.Ø4- ☑
      - hip M24.Ø5- ☑
      - knee M23.4- ☑
      - shoulder (region) M24.Ø1- ☑
      - specified site NEC M24.Ø8
      - toe M24.Ø7- ☑
      - vertebra M24.Ø8
      - wrist M24.Ø3- ☑
    - knee M23.4- ☑
    - sheath, tendon — *see* Disorder, tendon, specified type NEC
  - cartilage — *see* Loose, body, joint
  - skin and subcutaneous tissue (following bariatric surgery weight loss) (following dietary weight loss) L98.7
  - tooth, teeth KØ8.89
- **Loosening**
  - aseptic
    - joint prosthesis — *see* Complications, joint prosthesis, mechanical, loosening, by site
  - epiphysis — *see* Osteochondropathy
  - mechanical
    - joint prosthesis — *see* Complications, joint prosthesis, mechanical, loosening, by site
- **Looser-Milkman** (-Debray) **syndrome** M83.8
- **Lop ear** (deformity) Q17.3
- **Lorain** (-Levi) **short stature syndrome** E23.Ø
- **Lordosis** M4Ø.5Ø
  - acquired — *see* Lordosis, specified type NEC
  - congenital Q76.429
    - lumbar region Q76.426
    - lumbosacral region Q76.427
    - sacral region Q76.428
    - sacrococcygeal region Q76.428
    - thoracolumbar region Q76.425
  - lumbar region M4Ø.56
  - lumbosacral region M4Ø.57
  - postsurgical M96.4
  - postural — *see* Lordosis, specified type NEC
  - rachitic (late effect) (sequelae) E64.3
  - sequelae of rickets E64.3
  - specified type NEC M4Ø.4Ø
    - lumbar region M4Ø.46
    - lumbosacral region M4Ø.47
    - thoracolumbar region M4Ø.45
  - thoracolumbar region M4Ø.55
  - tuberculous A18.Ø1
- **Loss** (of)
  - appetite — *see also* Anorexia R63.Ø
    - hysterical F5Ø.89
    - nonorganic origin F5Ø.89
    - psychogenic F5Ø.89
  - blood — *see* Hemorrhage
  - bone —*see* Loss, substance of, bone
  - consciousness, transient R55
    - traumatic — *see* Injury, intracranial
  - control, sphincter, rectum R15.9
    - nonorganic origin F98.1
  - elasticity, skin R23.4
  - family (member) in childhood Z62.898
  - fluid (acute) E86.9
  - function of labyrinth — *see* subcategory H83.2 ☑
  - hair, nonscarring — *see* Alopecia
  - hearing — *see also* Deafness
    - central NOS H9Ø.5
    - conductive H9Ø.2
      - bilateral H9Ø.Ø
      - unilateral
        - with
          - restricted hearing on the contralateral side H9Ø.A1- ☑
          - unrestricted hearing on the contralateral side H9Ø.1- ☑
    - mixed conductive and sensorineural hearing loss H9Ø.8
      - bilateral H9Ø.6
      - unilateral
        - with
          - restricted hearing on the contralateral side H9Ø.A3- ☑
          - unrestricted hearing on the contralateral side H9Ø.7- ☑
    - neural NOS H9Ø.5
    - perceptive NOS H9Ø.5
    - sensorineural NOS H9Ø.5
      - bilateral H9Ø.3
      - unilateral
        - with
          - restricted hearing onthe contralateral side H9Ø.A2- ☑
          - unrestricted hearing on the contralateral side H9Ø.4- ☑
    - sensory NOS H9Ø.5
  - height R29.89Ø
  - limb or member, traumatic, current — *see* Amputation, traumatic
  - love relationship in childhood Z62.898
  - memory — *see also* Amnesia
    - mild, following organic brain damage FØ6.8
  - mind — *see* Psychosis
  - occlusal vertical dimension of fully erupted teeth M26.37
  - organ or part — *see* Absence, by site, acquired
  - ossicles, ear (partial) H74.32- ☑

M

- **Malformation** — *continued*
  - auricle — *continued*
    - ear — *continued*
      - acquired H61.119
        - left H61.112
          - with right H61.113
        - right H61.111
          - with left H61.113
  - bile duct Q44.5
  - bladder Q64.79
    - aplasia Q64.5
    - diverticulum Q64.6
    - exstrophy — *see* Exstrophy, bladder
    - neck obstruction Q64.31
  - bone Q79.9
    - face Q75.9
      - specified type NEC Q75.8
    - skull Q75.9
      - specified type NEC Q75.8
  - brain (multiple) QØ4.9
    - arteriovenous Q28.2
    - specified type NEC QØ4.8
  - branchial cleft Q18.2
  - breast Q83.9
    - specified type NEC Q83.8
  - broad ligament Q5Ø.6
  - bronchus Q32.4
  - bursa Q79.9
  - cardiac
    - chambers Q2Ø.9
      - specified type NEC Q2Ø.8
    - septum Q21.9
      - specified type NEC Q21.8
  - cerebral QØ4.9
    - vessels Q28.3
  - cervix uteri Q51.9
    - specified type NEC Q51.828
  - Chiari
    - Type I G93.5
    - Type II QØ7.Ø1
  - choroid (congenital) Q14.3
    - plexus QØ7.8
  - circulatory system Q28.9
  - cochlea Q16.5
  - cornea Q13.4
  - coronary vessels Q24.5
  - corpus callosum (congenital) QØ4.Ø
  - diaphragm Q79.1
  - digestive system NEC, specified type NEC Q45.8
  - dura QØ7.9
    - brain QØ4.9
    - spinal QØ6.9
  - ear Q17.9
    - causing impairment of hearing Q16.9
    - external Q17.9
      - accessory auricle Q17.Ø
      - causing impairment of hearing Q16.9
        - absence of
          - auditory canal Q16.1
          - auricle Q16.Ø
      - macrotia Q17.1
      - microtia Q17.2
      - misplacement Q17.4
      - misshapen NEC Q17.3
      - prominence Q17.5
      - specified type NEC Q17.8
    - inner Q16.5
    - middle Q16.4
      - absence of eustachian tube Q16.2
      - ossicles (fusion) Q16.3
    - ossicles Q16.3
    - specified type NEC Q17.8
  - epididymis Q55.4
  - esophagus Q39.9
    - specified type NEC Q39.8
  - eye Q15.9
    - lid Q1Ø.3
    - specified NEC Q15.8
  - fallopian tube Q5Ø.6
  - genital organ — *see* Anomaly, genitalia
  - great
    - artery Q25.9
      - aorta — *see* Malformation, aorta
      - pulmonary artery — *see* Malformation, pulmonary, artery
      - specified type NEC Q25.8
    - vein Q26.9
      - anomalous
        - portal venous connection Q26.5
- **Malformation** — *continued*
  - great — *continued*
    - vein — *continued*
      - anomalous — *continued*
        - pulmonary venous connection Q26.4
          - partial Q26.3
          - total Q26.2
      - persistent left superior vena cava Q26.1
      - portal vein-hepatic artery fistula Q26.6
      - specified type NEC Q26.8
      - vena cava stenosis, congenital Q26.Ø
  - gum Q38.6
  - hair Q84.2
  - heart Q24.9
    - specified type NEC Q24.8
  - integument Q84.9
    - specified type NEC Q84.8
  - internal ear Q16.5
  - intestine Q43.9
    - specified type NEC Q43.8
  - iris Q13.2
  - joint Q74.9
    - ankle Q74.2
    - lumbosacral Q76.49
    - sacroiliac Q74.2
    - specified type NEC Q74.8
  - kidney Q63.9
    - accessory Q63.Ø
    - giant Q63.3
    - horseshoe Q63.1
    - hydronephrosis Q62.Ø
    - malposition Q63.2
    - specified type NEC Q63.8
  - lacrimal apparatus Q1Ø.6
  - lingual Q38.3
  - lip Q38.Ø
  - liver Q44.7
  - lung Q33.9
  - meninges or membrane (congenital) QØ7.9
    - cerebral QØ4.8
    - spinal (cord) QØ6.9
  - middle ear Q16.4
    - ossicles Q16.3
  - mitral valve Q23.9
    - specified NEC Q23.8
  - Mondini's (congenital) (malformation, cochlea) Q16.5
  - mouth (congenital) Q38.6
  - multiple types NEC Q89.7
  - musculoskeletal system Q79.9
  - myocardium Q24.8
  - nail Q84.6
  - nervous system (central) QØ7.9
  - nose Q3Ø.9
    - specified type NEC Q3Ø.8
  - optic disc Q14.2
  - orbit Q1Ø.7
  - ovary Q5Ø.39
  - palate Q38.5
  - parathyroid gland Q89.2
  - pelvic organs or tissues NEC
    - in pregnancy or childbirth O34.8- ☑
      - causing obstructed labor O65.5
  - penis Q55.69
    - aplasia Q55.5
    - curvature (lateral) Q55.61
    - hypoplasia Q55.62
  - pericardium Q24.8
  - peripheral vascular system Q27.9
    - specified type NEC Q27.8
  - pharynx Q38.8
  - precerebral vessels Q28.1
  - prostate Q55.4
  - pulmonary
    - arteriovenous Q25.72
    - artery Q25.9
      - atresia Q25.5
      - specified type NEC Q25.79
      - stenosis Q25.6
    - valve Q22.3
  - renal artery Q27.2
  - respiratory system Q34.9
  - retina Q14.1
  - scrotum — *see* Malformation, testis and scrotum
  - seminal vesicles Q55.4
  - sense organs NEC QØ7.9
  - skin Q82.9
  - specified NEC Q89.8
  - spinal
    - cord QØ6.9
- **Malformation** — *continued*
  - spinal — *continued*
    - nerve root QØ7.8
  - spine Q76.49
    - kyphosis — *see* Kyphosis, congenital
    - lordosis — *see* Lordosis, congenital
  - spleen Q89.Ø9
  - stomach Q4Ø.3
    - specified type NEC Q4Ø.2
  - teeth, tooth KØØ.9
  - tendon Q79.9
  - testis and scrotum Q55.2Ø
    - aplasia Q55.Ø
    - hypoplasia Q55.1
    - polyorchism Q55.21
    - retractile testis Q55.22
    - scrotal transposition Q55.23
    - specified NEC Q55.29
  - thorax, bony Q76.9
  - throat Q38.8
  - thyroid gland Q89.2
  - tongue (congenital) Q38.3
    - hypertrophy Q38.2
    - tie Q38.1
  - trachea Q32.1
  - tricuspid valve Q22.9
    - specified type NEC Q22.8
  - umbilical cord NEC (complicating delivery) O69.89 ☑
  - umbilicus Q89.9
  - ureter Q62.8
    - agenesis Q62.4
    - duplication Q62.5
    - malposition — *see* Malposition, congenital, ureter
    - obstructive defect — *see* Defect, obstructive, ureter
    - vesico-uretero-renal reflux Q62.7
  - urethra Q64.79
    - aplasia Q64.5
    - duplication Q64.74
    - posterior valves Q64.2
    - prolapse Q64.71
    - stricture Q64.32
  - urinary system Q64.9
  - uterus Q51.9
    - specified type NEC Q51.818
  - vagina Q52.4
  - vas deferens Q55.4
    - atresia Q55.3
  - vascular system, peripheral Q27.9
  - venous — *see* Anomaly, vein(s)
  - vulva Q52.7Ø
- **Malfunction** — *see also* Dysfunction
  - cardiac electronic device T82.119 ☑
    - electrode T82.11Ø ☑
    - pulse generator T82.111 ☑
    - specified type NEC T82.118 ☑
  - catheter device NEC T85.618 ☑
    - cystostomy T83.Ø1Ø ☑
    - dialysis (renal) (vascular) T82.41 ☑
      - intraperitoneal T85.611 ☑
    - infusion NEC T82.514 ☑
      - cranial T85.61Ø ☑
      - epidural T85.61Ø ☑
      - intrathecal T85.61Ø ☑
      - spinal T85.61Ø ☑
      - subarachnoid T85.61Ø ☑
      - subdural T85.61Ø ☑
    - urinary — *see also* Breakdown, device, catheter T83.Ø18 ☑
  - colostomy K94.Ø3
    - valve K94.Ø3
  - cystostomy (stoma) N99.512
    - catheter T83.Ø1Ø ☑
  - enteric stoma K94.13
  - enterostomy K94.13
  - esophagostomy K94.33
  - gastroenteric K31.89
  - gastrostomy K94.23
  - ileostomy K94.13
    - valve K94.13
  - intrathecal infusion pump T85.615 ☑
  - jejunostomy K94.13
  - nervous system device, implant or graft, specified NEC T85.615 ☑
  - pacemaker — *see* Malfunction, cardiac electronic device
  - prosthetic device, internal — *see* Complications, prosthetic device, by site, mechanical
  - tracheostomy J95.Ø3

- **Mastoiditis** — *continued*
  - in (due to)
    - infectious disease NEC B99 ☑ *[H75.Ø-]* ☑
    - parasitic disease NEC B89 *[H75.Ø-]* ☑
    - tuberculosis A18.Ø3
  - petrositis — *see* Petrositis
  - postauricular fistula — *see* Fistula, postauricular
  - specified NEC H7Ø.89- ☑
  - tuberculous A18.Ø3
- **Mastopathy, mastopathia** N64.9
  - chronica cystica — *see* Mastopathy, cystic
  - cystic (chronic) (diffuse) N6Ø.1- ☑
    - with epithelial proliferation N6Ø.3- ☑
  - diffuse cystic — *see* Mastopathy, cystic
  - estrogenic, oestrogenica N64.89
  - ovarian origin N64.89
- **Mastoplasia, mastoplastia** N62
- **Masturbation** (excessive) F98.8
- **Maternal care** (for) — *see* Pregnancy (complicated by) (management affected by)
- **Matheiu's disease** (leptospiral jaundice) A27.Ø
- **Mauclaire's disease or osteochondrosis** — *see* Osteochondrosis, juvenile, hand, metacarpal
- **Maxcy's disease** A75.2
- **Maxilla, maxillary** — *see* condition
- **May** (-Hegglin) **anomaly or syndrome** D72.Ø
- **McArdle** (-Schmid)(-Pearson) **disease** (glycogen storage) E74.Ø4
- **McCune-Albright syndrome** Q78.1
- **McQuarrie's syndrome** (idiopathic familial hypoglycemia) E16.2
- **Meadow's syndrome** Q86.1
- **Measles** (black) (hemorrhagic) (suppressed) BØ5.9
  - with
    - complications NEC BØ5.89
    - encephalitis BØ5.Ø
    - intestinal complications BØ5.4
    - keratitis (keratoconjunctivitis) BØ5.81
    - meningitis BØ5.1
    - otitis media BØ5.3
    - pneumonia BØ5.2
  - French — *see* Rubella
  - German — *see* Rubella
  - Liberty — *see* Rubella
- **Meatitis, urethral** — *see* Urethritis
- **Meatus, meatal** — *see* condition
- **Meat-wrappers' asthma** J68.9
- **ME/CFS** (myalgic encephalomyelitis/chronic fatigue syndrome) G93.32
- **Meckel-Gruber syndrome** Q61.9
- **Meckel's diverticulitis, diverticulum** (displaced) (hypertrophic) Q43.Ø
  - malignant — *see* Table of Neoplasms, small intestine, malignant
- **Meconium**
  - ileus, newborn P76.Ø
    - in cystic fibrosis E84.11
    - meaning meconium plug (without cystic fibrosis) P76.Ø
  - obstruction, newborn P76.Ø
    - due to fecaliths P76.Ø
    - in mucoviscidosis E84.11
  - peritonitis P78.Ø
  - plug syndrome (newborn) NEC P76.Ø
- **Median** — *see also* condition
  - arcuate ligament syndrome I77.4
  - bar (prostate) (vesical orifice) — *see* Hyperplasia, prostate
  - rhomboid glossitis K14.2
- **Mediastinal shift** R93.89
- **Mediastinitis** (acute) (chronic) J98.51
  - syphilitic A52.73
  - tuberculous A15.8
- **Mediastinopericarditis** — *see also* Pericarditis
  - acute I3Ø.9
  - adhesive I31.Ø
  - chronic I31.8
    - rheumatic IØ9.2
- **Mediastinum, mediastinal** — *see* condition
- **Medicine poisoning** — *see* Table of Drugs and Chemicals, by drug, poisoning
- **Mediterranean**
  - fever — *see* Brucellosis
    - familial MØ4.1
    - tick A77.1
  - kala-azar B55.Ø
  - leishmaniasis B55.Ø
- **Mediterranean** — *continued*
  - tick fever A77.1
- **Medulla** — *see* condition
- **Medullary cystic kidney** Q61.5
- **Medullated fibers**
  - optic (nerve) Q14.8
  - retina Q14.1
- **Medulloblastoma**
  - desmoplastic C71.6
  - specified site — *see* Neoplasm, malignant, by site
  - unspecified site C71.6
- **Medulloepithelioma** — *see also* Neoplasm, malignant, by site
  - teratoid — *see* Neoplasm, malignant, by site
- **Medullomyoblastoma**
  - specified site — *see* Neoplasm, malignant, by site
  - unspecified site C71.6
- **Meekeren-Ehlers-Danlos syndrome** — *see also* Syndrome, Ehlers-Danlos Q79.69
- **Megacolon** (acquired) (functional) (not Hirschsprung's disease) (in) K59.39
  - Chagas' disease B57.32
  - congenital, congenitum (aganglionic) Q43.1
  - Hirschsprung's (disease) Q43.1
  - toxic NEC K59.31
    - due to Clostridium difficile
      - not specified as recurrent AØ4.72
      - recurrent AØ4.71
- **Megaesophagus** (functional) K22.Ø
  - congenital Q39.5
  - in (due to) Chagas' disease B57.31
- **Megalencephaly** QØ4.5
- **Megalerythema** (epidemic) BØ8.3
- **Megaloappendix** Q43.8
- **Megalocephalus, megalocephaly NEC** Q75.3
- **Megalocornea** Q15.8
  - with glaucoma Q15.Ø
- **Megalocytic anemia** D53.1
- **Megalodactylia** (fingers) (thumbs) (congenital) Q74.Ø
  - toes Q74.2
- **Megaloduodenum** Q43.8
- **Megaloesophagus** (functional) K22.Ø
  - congenital Q39.5
- **Megalogastria** (acquired) K31.89
  - congenital Q4Ø.2
- **Megalophthalmos** Q11.3
- **Megalopsia** H53.15
- **Megalosplenia** — *see* Splenomegaly
- **Megaloureter** N28.82
  - congenital Q62.2
- **Megarectum** K62.89
- **Megasigmoid** K59.39
  - congenital Q43.2
- **Megaureter** N28.82
  - congenital Q62.2
- **Megavitamin-B6 syndrome** E67.2
- **Megrim** — *see* Migraine
- **Meibomian**
  - cyst, infected — *see* Hordeolum
  - gland — *see* condition
  - sty, stye — *see* Hordeolum
- **Meibomitis** — *see* Hordeolum
- **Meige-Milroy disease** (chronic hereditary edema) Q82.Ø
- **Meige's syndrome** Q82.Ø
- **Melalgia, nutritional** E53.8
- **Melancholia** F32.A
  - climacteric (single episode) F32.89
    - recurrent episode F33.8
  - hypochondriac F45.29
  - intermittent (single episode) F32.89
    - recurrent episode F33.8
  - involutional (single episode) F32.89
    - recurrent episode F33.8
  - menopausal (single episode) F32.89
    - recurrent episode F33.8
  - puerperal F32.89
  - reactive (emotional stress or trauma) F32.3
  - recurrent F33.9
  - senile FØ3 ☑
  - stuporous (single episode) F32.89
    - recurrent episode F33.8
- **Melanemia** R79.89
- **Melanoameloblastoma** — *see* Neoplasm, bone, benign
- **Melanoblastoma** — *see* Melanoma
- **Melanocarcinoma** — *see* Melanoma
- **Melanocytoma, eyeball** D31.9- ☑
- **Melanocytosis, neurocutaneous** Q82.8
- **Melanoderma, melanodermia** L81.4
- **Melanodontia, infantile** KØ3.89
- **Melanodontoclasia** KØ3.89
- **Melanoepithelioma** — *see* Melanoma
- **Melanoma** (malignant) C43.9
  - acral lentiginous, malignant — *see* Melanoma, skin, by site
  - amelanotic — *see* Melanoma, skin, by site
  - balloon cell — *see* Melanoma, skin, by site
  - benign — *see* Nevus
  - desmoplastic, malignant — *see* Melanoma, skin, by site
  - epithelioid cell — *see* Melanoma, skin, by site
    - with spindle cell, mixed — *see* Melanoma, skin, by site
  - in
    - giant pigmented nevus — *see* Melanoma, skin, by site
    - Hutchinson's melanotic freckle — *see* Melanoma, skin, by site
    - junctional nevus — *see* Melanoma, skin, by site
    - precancerous melanosis — *see* Melanoma, skin, by site
  - in situ DØ3.9
    - abdominal wall DØ3.59
    - ala nasi DØ3.39
    - ankle DØ3.7- ☑
    - anus, anal (margin) (skin) DØ3.51
    - arm DØ3.6- ☑
    - auditory canal DØ3.2- ☑
    - auricle (ear) DØ3.2- ☑
    - auricular canal (external) DØ3.2- ☑
    - axilla, axillary fold DØ3.59
    - back DØ3.59
    - breast DØ3.52
    - brow DØ3.39
    - buttock DØ3.59
    - canthus (eye) DØ3.1- ☑
    - cheek (external) DØ3.39
    - chest wall DØ3.59
    - chin DØ3.39
    - choroid DØ3.8
    - conjunctiva DØ3.8
    - ear (external) DØ3.2- ☑
    - external meatus (ear) DØ3.2- ☑
    - eye DØ3.8
    - eyebrow DØ3.39
    - eyelid (lower) (upper) DØ3.1- ☑
    - face DØ3.3Ø
      - specified NEC DØ3.39
    - female genital organ (external) NEC DØ3.8
    - finger DØ3.6- ☑
    - flank DØ3.59
    - foot DØ3.7- ☑
    - forearm DØ3.6- ☑
    - forehead DØ3.39
    - foreskin DØ3.8
    - gluteal region DØ3.59
    - groin DØ3.59
    - hand DØ3.6- ☑
    - heel DØ3.7- ☑
    - helix DØ3.2- ☑
    - hip DØ3.7- ☑
    - interscapular region DØ3.59
    - iris DØ3.8
    - jaw DØ3.39
    - knee DØ3.7- ☑
    - labium (majus) (minus) DØ3.8
    - lacrimal gland DØ3.8
    - leg DØ3.7- ☑
    - lip (lower) (upper) DØ3.Ø
    - lower limb NEC DØ3.7- ☑
    - male genital organ (external) NEC DØ3.8
    - nail DØ3.9
      - finger DØ3.6- ☑
      - toe DØ3.7- ☑
    - neck DØ3.4
    - nose (external) DØ3.39
    - orbit DØ3.8
    - penis DØ3.8
    - perianal skin DØ3.51
    - perineum DØ3.51
    - pinna DØ3.2- ☑
    - popliteal fossa or space DØ3.7- ☑
    - prepuce DØ3.8
    - pudendum DØ3.8
    - retina DØ3.8

- **Melanoma** — *continued*
  - in situ — *continued*
    - retrobulbar DØ3.8
    - scalp DØ3.4
    - scrotum DØ3.8
    - shoulder DØ3.6- ☑
    - specified site NEC DØ3.8
    - submammary fold DØ3.52
    - temple DØ3.39
    - thigh DØ3.7- ☑
    - toe DØ3.7- ☑
    - trunk NEC DØ3.59
    - umbilicus DØ3.59
    - upper limb NEC DØ3.6- ☑
    - vulva DØ3.8
  - juvenile — *see* Nevus
  - malignant, of soft parts except skin — *see* Neoplasm, connective tissue, malignant
  - metastatic
    - breast C79.81
    - genital organ C79.82
    - specified site NEC C79.89
  - neurotropic, malignant — *see* Melanoma, skin, by site
  - nodular — *see* Melanoma, skin, by site
  - regressing, malignant — *see* Melanoma, skin, by site
  - skin C43.9
    - abdominal wall C43.59
    - ala nasi C43.31
    - ankle C43.7- ☑
    - anus, anal (skin) C43.51
    - arm C43.6- ☑
    - auditory canal (external) C43.2- ☑
    - auricle (ear) C43.2- ☑
    - auricular canal (external) C43.2- ☑
    - axilla, axillary fold C43.59
    - back C43.59
    - breast (female) (male) C43.52
    - brow C43.39
    - buttock C43.59
    - canthus (eye) C43.1- ☑
    - cheek (external) C43.39
    - chest wall C43.59
    - chin C43.39
    - ear (external) C43.2- ☑
    - elbow C43.6- ☑
    - external meatus (ear) C43.2- ☑
    - eyebrow C43.39
    - eyelid (lower) (upper) C43.1- ☑
    - face C43.3Ø
      - specified NEC C43.39
    - female genital organ (external) NEC C51.9
    - finger C43.6- ☑
    - flank C43.59
    - foot C43.7- ☑
    - forearm C43.6- ☑
    - forehead C43.39
    - foreskin C6Ø.Ø
    - glabella C43.39
    - gluteal region C43.59
    - groin C43.59
    - hand C43.6- ☑
    - heel C43.7- ☑
    - helix C43.2- ☑
    - hip C43.7- ☑
    - interscapular region C43.59
    - jaw (external) C43.39
    - knee C43.7- ☑
    - labium C51.9
      - majus C51.Ø
      - minus C51.1
    - leg C43.7- ☑
    - lip (lower) (upper) C43.Ø
    - lower limb NEC C43.7- ☑
    - male genital organ (external) NEC C63.9
    - nail
      - finger C43.6- ☑
      - toe C43.7- ☑
    - nasolabial groove C43.39
    - nates C43.59
    - neck C43.4
    - nose (external) C43.31
    - overlapping site C43.8
    - palpebra C43.1- ☑
    - penis C6Ø.9
    - perianal skin C43.51
    - perineum C43.51
    - pinna C43.2- ☑
- **Melanoma** — *continued*
  - skin — *continued*
    - popliteal fossa or space C43.7- ☑
    - prepuce C6Ø.Ø
    - pudendum C51.9
    - scalp C43.4
    - scrotum C63.2
    - shoulder C43.6- ☑
    - skin NEC C43.9
    - submammary fold C43.52
    - temple C43.39
    - thigh C43.7- ☑
    - toe C43.7- ☑
    - trunk NEC C43.59
    - umbilicus C43.59
    - upper limb NEC C43.6- ☑
    - vulva C51.9
      - overlapping sites C51.8
  - spindle cell
    - with epithelioid, mixed — *see* Melanoma, skin, by site
    - type A C69.4- ☑
    - type B C69.4- ☑
  - superficial spreading — *see* Melanoma, skin, by site
- **Melanosarcoma** — *see also* Melanoma
  - epithelioid cell — *see* Melanoma
- **Melanosis** L81.4
  - addisonian E27.1
    - tuberculous A18.7
  - adrenal E27.1
  - colon K63.89
  - conjunctiva — *see* Pigmentation, conjunctiva
    - congenital Q13.89
  - cornea (presenile) (senile) — *see also* Pigmentation, cornea
    - congenital Q13.4
  - eye NEC H57.89
    - congenital Q15.8
  - lenticularis progressiva Q82.1
  - liver K76.89
  - precancerous — *see also* Melanoma, in situ
    - malignant melanoma in — *see* Melanoma
  - Riehl's L81.4
  - sclera H15.89
    - congenital Q13.89
  - suprarenal E27.1
  - tar L81.4
  - toxic L81.4
- **Melanuria** R82.998
- **MELAS syndrome** E88.41
- **Melasma** L81.1
  - adrenal (gland) E27.1
  - suprarenal (gland) E27.1
- **Melena** K92.1
  - with ulcer — *code by* site under Ulcer, with hemorrhage K27.4
  - due to swallowed maternal blood P78.2
  - newborn, neonatal P54.1
    - due to swallowed maternal blood P78.2
- **Meleney's**
  - gangrene (cutaneous) — *see* Ulcer, skin
  - ulcer (chronic undermining) — *see* Ulcer, skin
- **Melioidosis** A24.9
  - acute A24.1
  - chronic A24.2
  - fulminating A24.1
  - pneumonia A24.1
  - pulmonary (chronic) A24.2
    - acute A24.1
    - subacute A24.2
  - sepsis A24.1
  - specified NEC A24.3
  - subacute A24.2
- **Melitensis, febris** A23.Ø
- **Melkersson** (-Rosenthal) **syndrome** G51.2
- **Mellitus, diabetes** — *see* Diabetes
- **Melorheostosis** (bone) — *see* Disorder, bone, density and structure, specified NEC
- **Meloschisis** Q18.4
- **Melotia** Q17.4
- **Membrana**
  - capsularis lentis posterior Q13.89
  - epipapillaris Q14.2
- **Membranacea placenta** O43.19- ☑
- **Membranaceous uterus** N85.8
- **Membrane**(s), membranous — *see also* condition
  - cyclitic — *see* Membrane, pupillary
- **Membrane(s), membranous** — *continued*
  - folds, congenital — *see* Web
  - Jackson's Q43.3
  - over face of newborn P28.9
  - premature rupture — *see* Rupture, membranes, premature
  - pupillary H21.4- ☑
    - persistent Q13.89
  - retained (with hemorrhage) (complicating delivery) O72.2
    - without hemorrhage O73.1
  - secondary cataract — *see* Cataract, secondary
  - unruptured (causing asphyxia) — *see* Asphyxia, newborn
  - vitreous — *see* Opacity, vitreous, membranes and strands
- **Membranitis** — *see* Chorioamnionitis
- **Memory disturbance, lack or loss** — *see also* Amnesia
  - mild, following organic brain damage FØ6.8
- **Menadione deficiency** E56.1
- **Menarche**
  - delayed E3Ø.Ø
  - precocious E3Ø.1
- **Mendacity, pathologic** F6Ø.2
- **Mendelson's syndrome** (due to anesthesia) J95.4
  - in labor and delivery O74.Ø
  - in pregnancy O29.Ø1- ☑
  - obstetric O74.Ø
  - postpartum, puerperal O89.Ø1
- **Ménétrier's disease or syndrome** K29.6Ø
  - with bleeding K29.61
- **Ménière's disease, syndrome or vertigo** H81.Ø- ☑
- **Meninges, meningeal** — *see* condition
- **Meningioma** — *see also* Neoplasm, meninges, benign
  - angioblastic — *see* Neoplasm, meninges, benign
  - angiomatous — *see* Neoplasm, meninges, benign
  - atypical — *see* Neoplasm, meninges, uncertain behavior
  - endotheliomatous — *see* Neoplasm, meninges, benign
  - fibroblastic — *see* Neoplasm, meninges, benign
  - fibrous — *see* Neoplasm, meninges, benign
  - hemangioblastic — *see* Neoplasm, meninges, benign
  - hemangiopericytic — *see* Neoplasm, meninges, benign
  - malignant — *see* Neoplasm, meninges, malignant
  - meningiothelial — *see* Neoplasm, meninges, benign
  - meningotheliomatous — *see* Neoplasm, meninges, benign
  - mixed — *see* Neoplasm, meninges, benign
  - multiple — *see* Neoplasm, meninges, uncertain behavior
  - papillary — *see* Neoplasm, meninges, uncertain behavior
  - psammomatous — *see* Neoplasm, meninges, benign
  - syncytial — *see* Neoplasm, meninges, benign
  - transitional — *see* Neoplasm, meninges, benign
- **Meningiomatosis** (diffuse) — *see* Neoplasm, meninges, uncertain behavior
- **Meningism** — *see* Meningismus
- **Meningismus** (infectional) (pneumococcal) R29.1
  - due to serum or vaccine R29.1
  - influenzal — *see* Influenza, with, manifestations NEC
- **Meningitis** (basal) (basic) (brain) (cerebral) (cervical) (congestive) (diffuse) (hemorrhagic) (infantile) (membranous) (metastatic) (nonspecific) (pontine) (progressive) (simple) (spinal) (subacute) (sympathetic) (toxic) GØ3.9
  - abacterial GØ3.Ø
  - actinomycotic A42.81
  - adenoviral A87.1
  - arbovirus A87.8
  - aseptic (acute) GØ3.Ø
  - bacterial GØØ.9
    - Escherichia coli (E. coli) GØØ.8
    - Friedländer (bacillus) GØØ.8
    - gram-negative GØØ.9
    - H. influenzae GØØ.Ø
    - Klebsiella GØØ.8
    - pneumococcal GØØ.1
    - specified organism NEC GØØ.8
    - staphylococcal GØØ.3
    - streptococcal (acute) GØØ.2
  - benign recurrent (Mollaret) GØ3.2
  - candidal B37.5
  - caseous (tuberculous) A17.Ø
  - cerebrospinal A39.Ø
  - chronic NEC GØ3.1
  - clear cerebrospinal fluid NEC GØ3.Ø

- **Mental** — *continued*
  - retardation — *see* Disability, intellectual
  - subnormality — *see* Disability, intellectuall
  - upset — *see* Disorder, mental
- **Meralgia paresthetica** G57.1- ☑
- **Mercurial** — *see* condition
- **Mercurialism** — *see* subcategory T56.1 ☑
- **Merkel cell tumor** — *see* Carcinoma, Merkel cell
- **Merocele** — *see* Hernia, femoral
- **Meromelia**
  - lower limb — *see* Defect, reduction, lower limb
    - intercalary
      - femur — *see* Defect, reduction, lower limb, specified type NEC
        - tibiofibular (complete) (incomplete) — *see* Defect, reduction, lower limb
  - upper limb — *see* Defect, reduction, upper limb
    - intercalary, humeral, radioulnar — *see* Agenesis, arm, with hand present
- **MERRF syndrome** (myoclonic epilepsy associated with ragged-red fiber) E88.42
- **Merzbacher-Pelizaeus disease** E75.29
- **Mesaortitis** — *see* Aortitis
- **Mesarteritis** — *see* Arteritis
- **Mesencephalitis** — *see* Encephalitis
- **Mesenchymoma** — *see also* Neoplasm, connective tissue, uncertain behavior
  - benign — *see* Neoplasm, connective tissue, benign
  - malignant — *see* Neoplasm, connective tissue, malignant
- **Mesenteritis**
  - retractile K65.4
  - sclerosing K65.4
- **Mesentery, mesenteric** — *see* condition
- **Mesiodens, mesiodentes** KØØ.1
- **Mesio-occlusion** M26.213
- **Mesocolon** — *see* condition
- **Mesonephroma** (malignant) — *see* Neoplasm, malignant, by site
  - benign — *see* Neoplasm, benign, by site
- **Mesophlebitis** — *see* Phlebitis
- **Mesostromal dysgenesia** Q13.89
- **Mesothelioma** (malignant) C45.9
  - benign
    - mesentery D19.1
    - mesocolon D19.1
    - omentum D19.1
    - peritoneum D19.1
    - pleura D19.Ø
    - specified site NEC D19.7
    - unspecified site D19.9
  - biphasic C45.9
    - benign
      - mesentery D19.1
      - mesocolon D19.1
      - omentum D19.1
      - peritoneum D19.1
      - pleura D19.Ø
      - specified site NEC D19.7
      - unspecified site D19.9
  - cystic D48.4
  - epithelioid C45.9
    - benign
      - mesentery D19.1
      - mesocolon D19.1
      - omentum D19.1
      - peritoneum D19.1
      - pleura D19.Ø
      - specified site NEC D19.7
      - unspecified site D19.9
  - fibrous C45.9
    - benign
      - mesentery D19.1
      - mesocolon D19.1
      - omentum D19.1
      - peritoneum D19.1
      - pleura D19.Ø
      - specified site NEC D19.7
      - unspecified site D19.9
  - site classification
    - liver C45.7
    - lung C45.7
    - mediastinum C45.7
    - mesentery C45.1
    - mesocolon C45.1
    - omentum C45.1
    - pericardium C45.2
    - peritoneum C45.1
- **Mesothelioma** — *continued*
  - site classification — *continued*
    - pleura C45.Ø
      - parietal C45.Ø
    - retroperitoneum C45.7
    - specified site NEC C45.7
    - unspecified C45.9
- **Metabolic syndrome** E88.81
- **Metagonimiasis** B66.8
- **Metagonimus infestation** (intestine) B66.8
- **Metal**
  - pigmentation L81.8
  - polisher's disease J62.8
- **Metamorphopsia** H53.15
- **Metaplasia**
  - apocrine (breast) — *see* Dysplasia, mammary, specified type NEC
  - cervix (squamous) — *see* Dysplasia, cervix
  - endometrium (squamous) (uterus) N85.8
  - esophagus K22.7- ☑
  - gastric intestinal K31.AØ
    - with dysplasia K31.A29
      - high grade K31.A22
      - low grade K31.A21
    - indefinite for dysplasia K31.AØ
    - without dysplasia K31.A19
      - involving
        - antrum K31.A11
        - body (corpus) K31.A12
        - cardia K31.A14
        - fundus K31.A13
        - multiple sites K31.A15
  - kidney (pelvis) (squamous) N28.89
  - myelogenous D73.1
  - myeloid (agnogenic) (megakaryocytic) D73.1
  - spleen D73.1
  - squamous cell, bladder N32.89
- **Metastasis, metastatic**
  - abscess — *see* Abscess
  - calcification E83.59
  - cancer
    - from specified site — *see* Neoplasm, malignant, by site
    - to specified site — *see* Neoplasm, secondary, by site
  - deposits (in) — *see* Neoplasm, secondary, by site
  - disease — *see also* Neoplasm, secondary, by site C79.9
  - spread (to) — *see* Neoplasm, secondary, by site
- **Metastrongyliasis** B83.8
- **Metatarsalgia** M77.4- ☑
  - anterior G57.6- ☑
  - Morton's G57.6- ☑
- **Metatarsus, metatarsal** — *see also* condition
  - adductus, congenital Q66.22- ☑
  - valgus (abductus), congenital Q66.6
  - varus (congenital) Q66.22- ☑
    - primus Q66.21- ☑
- **Methadone use** — *see* Use, opioid
- **Methemoglobinemia** D74.9
  - acquired (with sulfhemoglobinemia) D74.8
  - congenital D74.Ø
  - enzymatic (congenital) D74.Ø
  - Hb M disease D74.Ø
  - hereditary D74.Ø
  - toxic D74.8
- **Methemoglobinuria** — *see* Hemoglobinuria
- **Methioninemia** E72.19
- **Methylmalonic acidemia** E71.12Ø
- **Metritis** (catarrhal) (hemorrhagic) (septic) (suppurative) — *see also* Endometritis
  - cervical — *see* Cervicitis
- **Metropathia hemorrhagica** N93.8
- **Metroperitonitis** — *see* Peritonitis, pelvic, female
- **Metrorrhagia** N92.1
  - climacteric N92.4
  - menopausal N92.4
  - perimenopausal N92.4
  - postpartum NEC (atonic) (following delivery of placenta) O72.1
    - delayed or secondary O72.2
  - preclimacteric or premenopausal N92.4
  - psychogenic F45.8
- **Metrorrhexis** — *see* Rupture, uterus
- **Metrosalpingitis** N7Ø.91
- **Metrostaxis** N93.8
- **Metrovaginitis** — *see* Endometritis
- **Meyer-Schwickerath and Weyers syndrome** Q87.Ø
- **Meynert's amentia** (nonalcoholic) FØ4
- **Meynert's amentia** — *continued*
  - alcoholic F1Ø.96
    - with dependence F1Ø.26
- **Mibelli's disease** (porokeratosis) Q82.8
- **Mice, joint** — *see* Loose, body, joint
  - knee M23.4- ☑
- **Micrencephalon, micrencephaly** QØ2
- **Microalbuminuria** R8Ø.9
- **Microaneurysm, retinal** — *see also* Disorder, retina, microaneurysms
  - diabetic — *see* EØ8-E13 with .31
- **Microangiopathy** (peripheral) I73.9
  - thrombotic M31.1Ø
    - hematopoietic stem cell transplantation-associated [HSCT-TMA] M31.1Ø
- **Microcalcifications, breast** R92.Ø
- **Microcephalus, microcephalic, microcephaly** QØ2
  - due to toxoplasmosis (congenital) P37.1
- **Microcheilia** Q18.7
- **Microcolon** (congenital) Q43.8
- **Microcornea** (congenital) Q13.4
- **Microcytic** — *see* condition
- **Microdeletions NEC** Q93.88
- **Microdontia** KØØ.2
- **Microdrepanocytosis** D57.4Ø
  - with
    - acute chest syndrome D57.411
    - cerebral vascular involvement D57.413
    - crisis (painful) D57.419
      - with specified complication NEC D57.418
    - splenic sequestration D57.412
    - vasoocclusive pain D57.419
- **Microembolism**
  - atherothrombotic — *see* Atheroembolism
  - retinal — *see* Occlusion, artery, retina
- **Microencephalon** QØ2
- **Microfilaria streptocerca infestation** — *see* Onchocerciasis
- **Microgastria** (congenital) Q4Ø.2
- **Microgenia** M26.Ø6
- **Microgenitalia, congenital**
  - female Q52.8
  - male Q55.8
- **Microglioma** — *see* Lymphoma, non-Hodgkin, specified NEC
- **Microglossia** (congenital) Q38.3
- **Micrognathia, micrognathism** (congenital) (mandibular) (maxillary) M26.Ø9
- **Microgyria** (congenital) QØ4.3
- **Microinfarct of heart** — *see* Insufficiency, coronary
- **Microlentia** (congenital) Q12.8
- **Microlithiasis, alveolar, pulmonary** J84.Ø2
- **Micromastia** N64.82
- **Micromyelia** (congenital) QØ6.8
- **Micropenis** Q55.62
- **Microphakia** (congenital) Q12.8
- **Microphthalmos, microphthalmia** (congenital) Q11.2
  - due to toxoplasmosis P37.1
- **Micropsia** H53.15
- **Microscopic polyangiitis** (polyarteritis) M31.7
- **Microsporidiosis** B6Ø.8
  - intestinal AØ7.8
- **Microsporon furfur infestation** B36.Ø
- **Microsporosis** — *see also* Dermatophytosis
  - nigra B36.1
- **Microstomia** (congenital) Q18.5
- **Microtia** (congenital) (external ear) Q17.2
- **Microtropia** H5Ø.4Ø
- **Microvillus inclusion disease** (MVD) (MVID) Q43.8
- **Micturition**
  - disorder NEC — *see also* Difficulty, micturition R39.198
    - psychogenic F45.8
  - frequency R35.Ø
    - psychogenic F45.8
  - hesitancy R39.11
  - incomplete emptying R39.14
  - nocturnal R35.1
  - painful R3Ø.9
    - dysuria R3Ø.Ø
    - psychogenic F45.8
    - tenesmus R3Ø.1
  - poor stream R39.12
  - position dependent R39.192
  - split stream R39.13
  - straining R39.16
  - urgency R39.15
- **Mid plane** — *see* condition

Middle
- ear — *see* condition
- lobe (right) syndrome J98.19

Miescher's elastoma L87.2

Mietens' syndrome Q87.2

Migraine (idiopathic) G43.9Ø9
- with refractory migraine G43.919
  - with status migrainosus G43.911
  - without status migrainosus G43.919
- with aura (acute-onset) (prolonged) (typical) (without headache) G43.1Ø9
  - with refractory migraine G43.119
    - with status migrainosus G43.111
    - without status migrainosus G43.119
  - intractable G43.119
    - with status migrainosus G43.111
    - without status migrainosus G43.119
  - not intractable G43.1Ø9
    - with status migrainosus G43.1Ø1
    - without status migrainosus G43.1Ø9
  - persistent G43.5Ø9
    - with cerebral infarction G43.6Ø9
      - with refractory migraine G43.619
        - with status migrainosus G43.611
        - without status migrainosus G43.619
      - intractable G43.619
        - with status migrainosus G43.611
        - without status migrainosus G43.619
      - not intractable G43.6Ø9
        - with status migrainosus G43.6Ø1
        - without status migrainosus G43.6Ø9
      - without refractory migraine G43.6Ø9
        - with status migrainosus G43.6Ø1
        - without status migrainosus G43.6Ø9
    - without cerebral infarction G43.5Ø9
      - with refractory migraine G43.519
        - with status migrainosus G43.511
        - without status migrainosus G43.519
      - intractable G43.519
        - with status migrainosus G43.511
        - without status migrainosus G43.519
      - not intractable G43.5Ø9
        - with status migrainosus G43.5Ø1
        - without status migrainosus G43.5Ø9
      - without refractory migraine G43.5Ø9
        - with status migrainosus G43.5Ø1
        - without status migrainosus G43.5Ø9
  - without mention of refractory migraine G43.1Ø9
    - with status migrainosus G43.1Ø1
    - without status migrainosus G43.1Ø9
- abdominal G43.DØ (*following* G43.7)
  - with refractory migraine G43.D1 (*following* G43.7)
  - intractable G43.D1 (*following* G43.7)
  - not intractable G43.DØ (*following* G43.7)
  - without refractory migraine G43.DØ (*following* G43.7)
- basilar — *see* Migraine, with aura
- classical — *see* Migraine, with aura
- common — *see* Migraine, without aura
- complicated G43.1Ø9
- equivalents — *see* Migraine, with aura
- familiar — *see* Migraine, hemiplegic
- hemiplegic G43.4Ø9
  - with refractory migraine G43.419
    - with status migrainosus G43.411
    - without status migrainosus G43.419
  - intractable G43.419
    - with status migrainosus G43.411
    - without status migrainosus G43.419
  - not intractable G43.4Ø9
    - with status migrainosus G43.4Ø1
    - without status migrainosus G43.4Ø9
  - without refractory migraine G43.4Ø9
    - with status migrainosus G43.4Ø1
    - without status migrainosus G43.4Ø9
- intractable G43.919
  - with status migrainosus G43.911
  - without status migrainosus G43.919
- menstrual G43.829
  - with refractory migraine G43.839
    - with status migrainosus G43.831
    - without status migrainosus G43.839
  - intractable G43.839
    - with status migrainosus G43.831
    - without status migrainosus G43.839
  - not intractable G43.829
    - with status migrainosus G43.821
    - without status migrainosus G43.829
  - without refractory migraine G43.829

Migraine — *continued*
- menstrual — *continued*
  - without refractory migraine — *continued*
    - with status migrainosus G43.821
    - without status migrainosus G43.829
- menstrually related — *see* Migraine, menstrual
- not intractable G43.9Ø9
  - with status migrainosus G43.9Ø1
  - without status migrainosus G43.919
- ophthalmoplegic G43.BØ (*following* G43.7)
  - with refractory migraine G43.B1 (*following* G43.7)
  - intractable G43.B1 (*following* G43.7)
  - not intractable G43.BØ (*following* G43.7)
  - without refractory migraine G43.BØ (*following* G43.7)
- persistent aura (with, without) cerebral infarction — *see* Migraine, with aura, persistent
- preceded or accompanied by transient focal neurological phenomena — *see* Migraine, with aura
- pre-menstrual — *see* Migraine, menstrual
- pure menstrual — *see* Migraine, menstrual
- retinal — *see* Migraine, with aura
- specified NEC G43.8Ø9
  - intractable G43.819
    - with status migrainosus G43.811
    - without status migrainosus G43.819
  - not intractable G43.8Ø9
    - with status migrainosus G43.8Ø1
    - without status migrainosus G43.8Ø9
- sporadic — *see* Migraine, hemiplegic
- transformed — *see* Migraine, without aura, chronic
- triggered seizures — *see* Migraine, with aura
- without aura G43.ØØ9
  - with refractory migraine G43.Ø19
    - with status migrainosus G43.Ø11
    - without status migrainosus G43.Ø19
  - chronic G43.7Ø9
    - with refractory migraine G43.719
      - with status migrainosus G43.711
      - without status migrainosus G43.719
    - intractable
      - with status migrainosus G43.711
      - without status migrainosus G43.719
    - not intractable
      - with status migrainosus G43.7Ø1
      - without status migrainosus G43.7Ø9
    - without refractory migraine G43.7Ø9
      - with status migrainosus G43.7Ø1
      - without status migrainosus G43.7Ø9
  - intractable
    - with status migrainosus G43.Ø11
    - without status migrainosus G43.Ø19
  - not intractable
    - with status migrainosus G43.ØØ1
    - without status migrainosus G43.ØØ9
  - without mention of refractory migraine G43.ØØ9
    - with status migrainosus G43.ØØ1
    - without status migrainosus G43.ØØ9
- without refractory migraine G43.9Ø9
  - with status migrainosus G43.9Ø1
  - without status migrainosus G43.9Ø9

Migrant, social Z59.ØØ

Migration, anxiety concerning Z6Ø.3

Migratory, migrating — *see also* condition
- person Z59.ØØ
- testis Q55.29

Mikity-Wilson disease or syndrome P27.Ø

Mikulicz' disease or syndrome K11.8

Miliaria L74.3
- alba L74.1
- apocrine L75.2
- crystallina L74.1
- profunda L74.2
- rubra L74.Ø
- tropicalis L74.2

Miliary — *see* condition

Milium L72.Ø
- colloid L57.8

Milk
- crust L21.Ø
- excessive secretion O92.6
- poisoning — *see* Poisoning, food, noxious
- retention O92.79
- sickness — *see* Poisoning, food, noxious
- spots I31.Ø

Milk-alkali disease or syndrome E83.52

Milk-leg (deep vessels) (nonpuerperal) — *see* Embolism, vein, lower extremity
- complicating pregnancy O22.3- ☑

Milk-leg — *continued*
- puerperal, postpartum, childbirth O87.1

Milkman's disease or syndrome M83.8

Milky urine — *see* Chyluria

Millard-Gubler (-Foville) **paralysis or syndrome** G46.3

Millar's asthma J38.5

Miller Fisher syndrome G61.Ø

Mills' disease — *see* Hemiplegia

Millstone maker's pneumoconiosis J62.8

Milroy's disease (chronic hereditary edema) Q82.Ø

Minamata disease T56.1 ☑

Miners' asthma or lung J6Ø

Minkowski-Chauffard syndrome — *see* Spherocytosis

Minor — *see* condition

Minor's disease (hematomyelia) G95.19

Minot's disease (hemorrhagic disease), newborn P53

Minot-von Willebrand-Jurgens disease or syndrome (angiohemophilia) — *see* Disease, von Willebrand

Minus (and plus) **hand** (intrinsic) — *see* Deformity, limb, specified type NEC, forearm

Miosis (pupil) H57.Ø3

Mirizzi's syndrome (hepatic duct stenosis) K83.1

Mirror writing F81.Ø

MIS-A M35.81

Misadventure (of) (prophylactic) (therapeutic) — *see also* Complications T88.9 ☑
- administration of insulin (by accident) — *see* subcategory T38.3 ☑
- infusion — *see* Complications, infusion
- local applications (of fomentations, plasters, etc.) T88.9 ☑
  - burn or scald — *see* Burn
  - specified NEC T88.8 ☑
- medical care (early) (late) T88.9 ☑
  - adverse effect of drugs or chemicals — *see* Table of Drugs and Chemicals
  - burn or scald — *see* Burn
  - specified NEC T88.8 ☑
- specified NEC T88.8 ☑
- surgical procedure (early) (late) — *see* Complications, surgical procedure
- transfusion — *see* Complications, transfusion
- vaccination or other immunological procedure — *see* Complications, vaccination

MIS-C M35.81

Miscarriage OØ3.9

Misdirection, aqueous H4Ø.83- ☑

Misperception, sleep state F51.Ø2

Misplaced, misplacement
- ear Q17.4
- kidney (acquired) N28.89
  - congenital Q63.2
- organ or site, congenital NEC — *see* Malposition, congenital

Missed
- abortion OØ2.1
- delivery O36.4 ☑

Missing — *see also* Absence
- string of intrauterine contraceptive device T83.32- ☑

Misuse of drugs F19.99

Mitchell's disease (erythromelalgia) I73.81

Mite(s) (infestation) B88.9
- diarrhea B88.Ø
- grain (itch) B88.Ø
- hair follicle (itch) B88.Ø
- in sputum B88.Ø

Mitral — *see* condition

Mittelschmerz N94.Ø

Mixed — *see* condition

MMN (multifocal motor neuropathy) G61.82

MNGIE (Mitochondrial Neurogastrointestinal Encephalopathy) **syndrome** E88.49

Mobile, mobility
- cecum Q43.3
- excessive — *see* Hypermobility
- gallbladder, congenital Q44.1
- kidney N28.89
- organ or site, congenital NEC — *see* Malposition, congenital

Mobitz heart block (atrioventricular) I44.1

Moebius, Möbius
- disease (ophthalmoplegic migraine) — *see* Migraine, ophthalmoplegic
- syndrome Q87.Ø
  - congenital oculofacial paralysis (with other anomalies) Q87.Ø

- **Moebius, Möbius** — *continued*
  - syndrome — *continued*
    - ophthalmoplegic migraine — *see* Migraine, ophthalmoplegic
- **Moeller's glossitis** K14.0
- **Mohr's syndrome** (Types I and II) Q87.0
- **Mola destruens** D39.2
- **Molar pregnancy** O02.0
- **Molarization of premolars** K00.2
- **Molding, head** (during birth) — *omit code*
- **Mole** (pigmented) — *see also* Nevus
  - blood O02.0
  - Breus' O02.0
  - cancerous — *see* Melanoma
  - carneous O02.0
  - destructive D39.2
  - fleshy O02.0
  - hydatid, hydatidiform (benign) (complicating pregnancy) (delivered) (undelivered) O01.9
    - classical O01.0
    - complete O01.0
    - incomplete O01.1
    - invasive D39.2
    - malignant D39.2
    - partial O01.1
  - intrauterine O02.0
  - invasive (hydatidiform) D39.2
  - malignant
    - meaning
      - malignant hydatidiform mole D39.2
      - melanoma — *see* Melanoma
  - nonhydatidiform O02.0
  - nonpigmented — *see* Nevus
  - pregnancy NEC O02.0
  - skin — *see* Nevus
  - tubal O00.10- ☑
    - with intrauterine pregnancy O00.11- ☑
  - vesicular — *see* Mole, hydatidiform
- **Molimen, molimina** (menstrual) N94.3
- **Molluscum contagiosum** (epitheliale) B08.1
- **Mönckeberg's arteriosclerosis, disease, or sclerosis** — *see* Arteriosclerosis, extremities
- **Mondini's malformation** (cochlea) Q16.5
- **Mondor's disease** I80.8
- **Monge's disease** T70.29 ☑
- **Monilethrix** (congenital) Q84.1
- **Moniliasis** — *see also* Candidiasis B37.9
  - neonatal P37.5
- **Monitoring** (encounter for)
  - therapeutic drug level Z51.81
- **Monkey malaria** B53.1
- **Monkeypox** B04
- **Monoarthritis** M13.10
  - ankle M13.17- ☑
  - elbow M13.12- ☑
  - foot joint M13.17- ☑
  - hand joint M13.14- ☑
  - hip M13.15- ☑
  - knee M13.16- ☑
  - shoulder M13.11- ☑
  - wrist M13.13- ☑
- **Monoblastic** — *see* condition
- **Monochromat** (ism), monochromatopsia (acquired) (congenital) H53.51
- **Monocytic** — *see* condition
- **Monocytopenia** D72.818
- **Monocytosis** (symptomatic) D72.821
- **Monomania** — *see* Psychosis
- **Mononeuritis** G58.9
  - cranial nerve — *see* Disorder, nerve, cranial
  - femoral nerve G57.2- ☑
  - lateral
    - cutaneous nerve of thigh G57.1- ☑
    - popliteal nerve G57.3- ☑
  - lower limb G57.9- ☑
    - specified nerve NEC G57.8- ☑
  - medial popliteal nerve G57.4- ☑
  - median nerve G56.1- ☑
  - multiplex G58.7
  - plantar nerve G57.6- ☑
  - posterior tibial nerve G57.5- ☑
  - radial nerve G56.3- ☑
  - sciatic nerve G57.0- ☑
  - specified NEC G58.8
  - tibial nerve G57.4- ☑
  - ulnar nerve G56.2- ☑
  - upper limb G56.9- ☑
- **Mononeuritis** — *continued*
  - upper limb — *continued*
    - specified nerve NEC G56.8- ☑
  - vestibular — *see* subcategory H93.3 ☑
- **Mononeuropathy** G58.9
  - carpal tunnel syndrome — *see* Syndrome, carpal tunnel
  - diabetic NEC — *see* E08-E13 with .41
  - femoral nerve — *see* Lesion, nerve, femoral
  - ilioinguinal nerve G57.8- ☑
  - in diseases classified elsewhere — *see* category G59
  - intercostal G58.0
  - lower limb G57.9- ☑
    - causalgia — *see* Causalgia, lower limb
    - femoral nerve — *see* Lesion, nerve, femoral
    - meralgia paresthetica G57.1- ☑
    - plantar nerve — *see* Lesion, nerve, plantar
    - popliteal nerve — *see* Lesion, nerve, popliteal
    - sciatic nerve — *see* Lesion, nerve, sciatic
    - specified NEC G57.8- ☑
    - tarsal tunnel syndrome — *see* Syndrome, tarsal tunnel
  - median nerve — *see* Lesion, nerve, median
  - multiplex G58.7
  - obturator nerve G57.8- ☑
  - popliteal nerve — *see* Lesion, nerve, popliteal
  - radial nerve — *see* Lesion, nerve, radial
  - saphenous nerve G57.8- ☑
  - specified NEC G58.8
  - tarsal tunnel syndrome — *see* Syndrome, tarsal tunnel
  - tuberculous A17.83
  - ulnar nerve — *see* Lesion, nerve, ulnar
  - upper limb G56.9- ☑
    - carpal tunnel syndrome — *see* Syndrome, carpal tunnel
    - causalgia — *see* Causalgia
    - median nerve — *see* Lesion, nerve, median
    - radial nerve — *see* Lesion, nerve, radial
    - specified site NEC G56.8- ☑
    - ulnar nerve — *see* Lesion, nerve, ulnar
- **Mononucleosis, infectious** B27.90
  - with
    - complication NEC B27.99
    - meningitis B27.92
    - polyneuropathy B27.91
  - cytomegaloviral B27.10
    - with
      - complication NEC B27.19
      - meningitis B27.12
      - polyneuropathy B27.11
  - Epstein-Barr (virus) B27.00
    - with
      - complication NEC B27.09
      - meningitis B27.02
      - polyneuropathy B27.01
  - gammaherpesviral B27.00
    - with
      - complication NEC B27.09
      - meningitis B27.02
      - polyneuropathy B27.01
  - specified NEC B27.80
    - with
      - complication NEC B27.89
      - meningitis B27.82
      - polyneuropathy B27.81
- **Monoplegia** G83.3- ☑
  - congenital (cerebral) G80.8
    - spastic G80.1
  - embolic (current episode) I63.4- ☑
  - following
    - cerebrovascular disease
      - cerebral infarction
        - lower limb I69.34- ☑
        - upper limb I69.33- ☑
      - intracerebral hemorrhage
        - lower limb I69.14- ☑
        - upper limb I69.13- ☑
      - lower limb I69.94- ☑
      - nontraumatic intracranial hemorrhage NEC
        - lower limb I69.24- ☑
        - upper limb I69.23- ☑
      - specified disease NEC
        - lower limb I69.84- ☑
        - upper limb I69.83- ☑
      - stroke NOS
        - lower limb I69.34- ☑
        - upper limb I69.33- ☑
- **Monoplegia** — *continued*
  - following — *continued*
    - cerebrovascular disease — *continued*
      - subarachnoid hemorrhage
        - lower limb I69.04- ☑
        - upper limb I69.03- ☑
      - upper limb I69.93- ☑
  - hysterical (transient) F44.4
  - lower limb G83.1- ☑
  - psychogenic (conversion reaction) F44.4
  - thrombotic (current episode) I63.3- ☑
  - transient R29.818
  - upper limb G83.2- ☑
- **Monorchism, monorchidism** Q55.0
- **Monosomy** — *see also* Deletion, chromosome Q93.9
  - specified NEC Q93.89
  - whole chromosome
    - meiotic nondisjunction Q93.0
    - mitotic nondisjunction Q93.1
    - mosaicism Q93.1
  - X Q96.9
- **Monster, monstrosity** (single) Q89.7
  - acephalic Q00.0
  - twin Q89.4
- **Monteggia's fracture** (-dislocation) S52.27- ☑
- **Mooren's ulcer** (cornea) — *see* Ulcer, cornea, Mooren's
- **Moore's syndrome** — *see* Epilepsy, specified NEC
- **Mooser-Neill reaction** A75.2
- **Mooser's bodies** A75.2
- **Morbidity not stated or unknown** R69
- **Morbilli** — *see* Measles
- **Morbus** — *see also* Disease
  - angelicus, anglorum E55.0
  - Beigel B36.2
  - caducus — *see* Epilepsy
  - celiacus K90.0
  - comitialis — *see* Epilepsy
  - cordis — *see also* Disease, heart I51.9
    - valvulorum — *see* Endocarditis
  - coxae senilis M16.9
    - tuberculous A18.02
  - hemorrhagicus neonatorum P53
  - maculosus neonatorum P54.5
- **Morel** (-Stewart)(-Morgagni) **syndrome** M85.2
- **Morel-Kraepelin disease** — *see* Schizophrenia
- **Morel-Moore syndrome** M85.2
- **Morgagni's**
  - cyst, organ, hydatid, or appendage
    - female Q50.5
    - male (epididymal) Q55.4
      - testicular Q55.29
  - syndrome M85.2
- **Morgagni-Stewart-Morel syndrome** M85.2
- **Morgagni-Stokes-Adams syndrome** I45.9
- **Morgagni-Turner** (-Albright) **syndrome** Q96.9
- **Moria** F07.0
- **Moron** (I.Q. 50-69) F70
- **Morphea** L94.0
- **Morphinism** (without remission) F11.20
  - with remission F11.21
- **Morphinomania** (without remission) F11.20
  - with remission F11.21
- **Morquio** (-Ullrich)(-Brailsford) **disease or syndrome** — *see* Mucopolysaccharidosis
- **Mortification** (dry) (moist) — *see* Gangrene
- **Morton's metatarsalgia** (neuralgia) (neuroma) (syndrome) G57.6- ☑
- **Morvan's disease or syndrome** G60.8
- **Mosaicism, mosaic** (autosomal) (chromosomal)
  - 45,X/46,XX Q96.3
  - 45,X/other cell lines NEC with abnormal sex chromosome Q96.4
  - sex chromosome
    - female Q97.8
    - lines with various numbers of X chromosomes Q97.2
    - male Q98.7
  - XY Q96.3
- **Moschowitz' disease** M31.19
- **Mother yaw** A66.0
- **Motion sickness** (from travel, any vehicle) (from roundabouts or swings) T75.3 ☑
- **Mottled, mottling, teeth** (enamel) (endemic) (nonendemic) K00.3
- **Mounier-Kuhn syndrome** Q32.4
  - with bronchiectasis J47.9
    - exacerbation (acute) J47.1
    - lower respiratory infection J47.0

Index

Mycosis, mycotic — Myofibrosis

N

Nematodiasis — *continued*
- Ancylostoma B76.Ø

Neonatal — *see also* Newborn
- acne L7Ø.4
- bradycardia P29.12
- screening, abnormal findings on — *see* Abnormal, neonatal screening
- tachycardia P29.11
- tooth, teeth KØØ.6

Neonatorum — *see* condition

Neoplasia
- endocrine, multiple (MEN) E31.2Ø
  - type I E31.21
  - type IIA E31.22
  - type IIB E31.23
- intraepithelial (histologically confirmed)
  - anal (AIN) (histologically confirmed) K62.82
    - grade I K62.82
    - grade II K62.82
    - severe DØ1.3
  - cervical glandular (histologically confirmed) DØ6.9
  - cervix (uteri) (CIN) (histologically confirmed) N87.9
    - glandular DØ6.9
    - grade I N87.Ø
    - grade II N87.1
    - grade III (severe dysplasia) — *see also* Carcinoma, cervix uteri, in situ DØ6.9
  - prostate (histologically confirmed) (PIN) N42.31
    - grade I N42.31
    - grade II N42.31
    - grade III (severe dysplasia) DØ7.5
  - vagina (histologically confirmed) (VAIN) N89.3
    - grade I N89.Ø
    - grade II N89.1
    - grade III (severe dysplasia) DØ7.2
  - vulva (histologically confirmed) (VIN) N9Ø.3
    - grade I N9Ø.Ø
    - grade II N9Ø.1
    - grade III (severe dysplasia) DØ7.1

Neoplasm, neoplastic — *see also* Table of Neoplasms
- lipomatous, benign — *see* Lipoma
- malignant mast cell C96.2Ø
  - specified type NEC C96.29
- mast cell, of uncertain behavior NEC D47.Ø9
- myelodysplastic/myeloproliferative, unclassifiable C94.6

Neovascularization
- ciliary body — *see* Disorder, iris, vascular
- cornea H16.4Ø- ☑
  - deep H16.44- ☑
  - ghost vessels — *see* Ghost, vessels
  - localized H16.43- ☑
  - pannus — *see* Pannus
- iris — *see* Disorder, iris, vascular
- retina H35.Ø5- ☑

Nephralgia N23

Nephritis, nephritic (albuminuric) (azotemic) (congenital) (disseminated) (epithelial) (familial) (focal) (granulomatous) (hemorrhagic) (infantile) (nonsuppurative, excretory) (uremic) NØ5.9
- with
  - C3
    - glomerulonephritis NØ5.A
    - glomerulopathy NØ5.A
      - with dense deposit disease NØ5.6
  - dense deposit disease NØ5.6
  - diffuse
    - crescentic glomerulonephritis NØ5.7
    - endocapillary proliferative glomerulonephritis NØ5.4
    - membranous glomerulonephritis NØ5.2
    - mesangial proliferative glomerulonephritis NØ5.3
    - mesangiocapillary glomerulonephritis NØ5.5
  - edema — *see* Nephrosis
  - focal and segmental glomerular lesions NØ5.1
  - foot process disease NØ4.9
  - glomerular lesion
    - diffuse sclerosing NØ5.8
    - hypocomplementemic — *see* Nephritis, membranoproliferative
    - IgA — *see* Nephropathy, IgA
    - lobular, lobulonodular — *see* Nephritis, membranoproliferative
    - nodular — *see* Nephritis, membranoproliferative
  - lesion of
    - glomerulonephritis, proliferative NØ5.8
    - renal necrosis NØ5.9
  - minor glomerular abnormality NØ5.Ø

Nephritis, nephritic — *continued*
- with — *continued*
  - specified morphological changes NEC NØ5.8
- acute NØØ.9
  - with
    - C3
      - glomerulonephritis NØØ.A
      - glomerulopathy NØØ.A
        - with dense deposit disease NØØ.6
    - dense deposit disease NØØ.6
    - diffuse
      - crescentic glomerulonephritis NØØ.7
      - endocapillary proliferative glomerulonephritis NØØ.4
      - membranous glomerulonephritis NØØ.2
      - mesangial proliferative glomerulonephritis NØØ.3
      - mesangiocapillary glomerulonephritis NØØ.5
    - focal and segmental glomerular lesions NØØ.1
    - minor glomerular abnormality NØØ.Ø
    - specified morphological changes NEC NØØ.8
- amyloid E85.4 *[NØ8]*
- antiglomerular basement membrane (anti-GBM) antibody NEC
  - in Goodpasture's syndrome M31.Ø
- antitubular basement membrane (tubulo-interstitial) NEC N12
  - toxic — *see* Nephropathy, toxic
- arteriolar — *see* Hypertension, kidney
- arteriosclerotic — *see* Hypertension, kidney
- ascending — *see* Nephritis, tubulo-interstitial
- atrophic NØ3.9
- Balkan (endemic) N15.Ø
- calculous, calculus — *see* Calculus, kidney
- cardiac — *see* Hypertension, kidney
- cardiovascular — *see* Hypertension, kidney
- chronic NØ3.9
  - with
    - C3
      - glomerulonephritis NØ3.A
      - glomerulopathy NØ3.A
        - with dense deposit disease NØ3.6
    - dense deposit disease NØ3.6
    - diffuse
      - crescentic glomerulonephritis NØ3.7
      - endocapillary proliferative glomerulonephritis NØ3.4
      - membranous glomerulonephritis NØ3.2
      - mesangial proliferative glomerulonephritis NØ3.3
      - mesangiocapillary glomerulonephritis NØ3.5
    - focal and segmental glomerular lesions NØ3.1
    - minor glomerular abnormality NØ3.Ø
    - specified morphological changes NEC NØ3.8
  - arteriosclerotic — *see* Hypertension, kidney
- cirrhotic N26.9
- complicating pregnancy O26.83- ☑
- croupous NØØ.9
- degenerative — *see* Nephrosis
- diffuse sclerosing NØ5.8
- due to
  - diabetes mellitus — *see* EØ8-E13 with .21
  - subacute bacterial endocarditis I33.Ø
  - systemic lupus erythematosus (chronic) M32.14
  - typhoid fever AØ1.Ø9
- gonococcal (acute) (chronic) A54.21
- hypocomplementemic — *see* Nephritis, membranoproliferative
- IgA — *see* Nephropathy, IgA
- immune complex (circulating) NEC NØ5.8
- infective — *see* Nephritis, tubulo-interstitial
- interstitial — *see* Nephritis, tubulo-interstitial
- lead N14.3
- membranoproliferative (diffuse) (type 1 or 3) — *see also* NØØ-NØ7 with fourth character .5 NØ5.5
  - type 2 — *see also* NØØ-NØ7 with fourth character .6 NØ5.6
- minimal change NØ5.Ø
- necrotic, necrotizing NEC — *see also* NØØ-NØ7 with fourth character .8 NØ5.8
- nephrotic — *see* Nephrosis
- nodular — *see* Nephritis, membranoproliferative
- polycystic Q61.3
  - adult type Q61.2
  - autosomal
    - dominant Q61.2
    - recessive NEC Q61.19
  - childhood type NEC Q61.19

Nephritis, nephritic — *continued*
- polycystic — *continued*
  - infantile type NEC Q61.19
- poststreptococcal NØ5.9
  - acute NØØ.9
  - chronic NØ3.9
  - rapidly progressive NØ1.9
- proliferative NEC — *see also* NØØ-NØ7 with fourth character .8 NØ5.8
- purulent — *see* Nephritis, tubulo-interstitial
- rapidly progressive NØ1.9
  - with
    - C3
      - glomerulonephritis NØ1.A
      - glomerulopathy NØ1.A
        - with dense deposit disease NØ1.6
    - dense deposit disease NØ1.6
    - diffuse
      - crescentic glomerulonephritis NØ1.7
      - endocapillary proliferative glomerulonephritis NØ1.4
      - membranous glomerulonephritis NØ1.2
      - mesangial proliferative glomerulonephritis NØ1.3
      - mesangiocapillary glomerulonephritis NØ1.5
    - focal and segmental glomerular lesions NØ1.1
    - minor glomerular abnormality NØ1.Ø
    - specified morphological changes NEC NØ1.8
- salt losing or wasting NEC N28.89
- saturnine N14.3
- sclerosing, diffuse NØ5.8
- septic — *see* Nephritis, tubulo-interstitial
- specified pathology NEC — *see also* NØØ-NØ7 with fourth character .8 NØ5.8
- subacute NØ1.9
- suppurative — *see* Nephritis, tubulo-interstitial
- syphilitic (late) A52.75
  - congenital A5Ø.59 *[NØ8]*
  - early (secondary) A51.44
- toxic — *see* Nephropathy, toxic
- tubal, tubular — *see* Nephritis, tubulo-interstitial
- tuberculous A18.11
- tubulo-interstitial (in) N12
  - acute (infectious) N1Ø
  - chronic (infectious) N11.9
    - nonobstructive N11.8
      - reflux-associated N11.Ø
    - obstructive N11.1
    - specified NEC N11.8
  - due to
    - brucellosis A23.9 *[N16]*
    - cryoglobulinemia D89.1 *[N16]*
    - glycogen storage disease E74.ØØ *[N16]*
  - Sjögren's syndrome M35.Ø4
- vascular — *see* Hypertension, kidney
- war NØØ.9

Nephroblastoma (epithelial) (mesenchymal) C64- ☑

Nephrocalcinosis E83.59 *[N29]*

Nephrocystitis, pustular — *see* Nephritis, tubulo-interstitial

Nephrolithiasis (congenital) (pelvis) (recurrent) — *see also* Calculus, kidney

Nephroma C64- ☑
- mesoblastic D41.Ø- ☑

Nephronephritis — *see* Nephrosis

Nephronophthisis Q61.5

Nephropathia epidemica A98.5

Nephropathy — *see also* Nephritis N28.9
- with
  - edema — *see* Nephrosis
  - glomerular lesion — *see* Glomerulonephritis
- amyloid, hereditary E85.Ø
- analgesic N14.Ø
  - with medullary necrosis, acute N17.2
- Balkan (endemic) N15.Ø
- chemical — *see* Nephropathy, toxic
- contrast medium, radiography N14.11
- contrast-induced N14.11
- diabetic — *see* EØ8-E13 with .21
- drug-induced N14.2
  - contrast-induced N14.11
  - specified NEC N14.19
- focal and segmental hyalinosis or sclerosis NØ2.1
- heavy metal-induced N14.3
- hereditary NEC NØ7.9
  - with
    - C3
      - glomerulonephritis NØ7.A

- **Newborn** — *continued*
  - affected by — *continued*
    - hemorrhage — *continued*
      - intracranial — *continued*
        - specified NEC P52.8
      - intraventricular (nontraumatic) P52.3
        - grade 1 P52.0
        - grade 2 P52.1
        - grade 3 P52.21
        - grade 4 P52.22
      - posterior fossa (nontraumatic) P52.6
      - subarachnoid (nontraumatic) P52.5
      - subependymal P52.0
        - with intracerebral extension P52.22
        - with intraventricular extension P52.1
          - with enlargment of ventricles P52.21
        - without intraventricular extension P52.0
    - hypoxic ischemic encephalopathy [HIE] P91.60
      - mild P91.61
      - moderate P91.62
      - severe P91.63
    - induction of labor P03.89
    - intestinal perforation P78.0
    - intrauterine (fetal) blood loss P50.9
      - due to (from)
        - cut end of co-twin cord P50.5
        - hemorrhage into
          - co-twin P50.3
          - maternal circulation P50.4
        - placenta P50.2
        - ruptured cord blood P50.1
        - vasa previa P50.0
      - specified NEC P50.8
    - intrauterine (fetal) hemorrhage P50.9
    - intrauterine (in utero) procedure P96.5
    - malpresentation (malposition) NEC P03.1
    - maternal (complication of) (use of)
      - alcohol P04.3
      - amphetamines P04.16
      - analgesia (maternal) P04.0
      - anesthesia (maternal) P04.0
      - anticonvulsants P04.13
      - antidepressants P04.15
      - antineoplastic chemotherapy P04.11
      - anxiolytics P04.1A
      - blood loss P02.1
      - cannabis P04.81
      - circulatory disease P00.3
      - condition P00.9
        - specified NEC P00.89
      - cytotoxic drugs P04.12
      - delivery P03.9
        - Cesarean P03.4
        - forceps P03.2
        - vacuum extractor P03.3
      - diabetes mellitus (pre-existing) P70.1
      - disorder P00.9
        - specified NEC P00.89
      - drugs (addictive) (illegal) NEC P04.49
      - ectopic pregnancy P01.4
      - gestational diabetes P70.0
      - group B streptococcus (GBS) colonization (positive) P00.82
      - hemorrhage P02.1
      - hypertensive disorder P00.0
      - incompetent cervix P01.0
      - infectious disease P00.2
      - injury P00.5
      - labor and delivery P03.9
      - malpresentation before labor P01.7
      - maternal death P01.6
      - medical procedure P00.7
      - medication P04.19
        - specified type NEC P04.18
      - multiple pregnancy P01.5
      - nutritional disorder P00.4
      - oligohydramnios P01.2
      - opiates P04.14
        - administered for procedures during pregnancy or labor and delivery P04.0
      - parasitic disease P00.2
      - periodontal disease P00.81
      - placenta previa P02.0
      - polyhydramnios P01.3
      - precipitate delivery P03.5
      - pregnancy P01.9
        - specified P01.8
      - premature rupture of membranes P01.1
      - renal disease P00.1
- **Newborn** — *continued*
  - affected by — *continued*
    - maternal — *continued*
      - respiratory disease P00.3
      - sedative-hypnotics P04.17
      - surgical procedure P00.6
      - tranquilizers administered for procedures during pregnancy or labor and delivery P04.0
      - urinary tract disease P00.1
      - uterine contraction (abnormal) P03.6
    - meconium peritonitis P78.0
    - medication (legal) (maternal use) (prescribed) P04.19
    - membrane abnormalities P02.9
      - specified NEC P02.8
    - membranitis P02.78
    - methamphetamine(s) P04.49
    - mixed metabolic and respiratory acidosis P84
    - neonatal abstinence syndrome P96.1
    - noxious substances transmitted via placenta or breast milk P04.9
      - cannabis P04.81
      - specified NEC P04.89
    - nutritional supplements P04.5
    - placenta previa P02.0
    - placental
      - abnormality (functional) (morphological) P02.20
        - specified NEC P02.29
      - dysfunction P02.29
      - infarction P02.29
      - insufficiency P02.29
      - separation NEC P02.1
      - transfusion syndromes P02.3
    - placentitis P02.78
    - precipitate delivery P03.5
    - prolapsed cord P02.4
    - respiratory arrest P28.81
    - slow intrauterine growth P05.9
    - tobacco P04.2
    - twin to twin transplacental transfusion P02.3
    - umbilical cord (tightly) around neck P02.5
    - umbilical cord condition P02.60
      - short cord P02.69
      - specified NEC P02.69
    - uterine contractions (abnormal) P03.6
    - vasa previa P02.69
      - from intrauterine blood loss P50.0
  - apnea — *see also* Apnea, newborn P28.40
    - obstructive P28.42
    - primary — *see also* Apnea, newborn, sleep, primary P28.30
    - sleep (central) (obstructive) (primary) — *see also* Apnea, newborn, sleep, primary P28.30
  - born in hospital Z38.00
    - by cesarean Z38.01
  - born outside hospital Z38.1
  - breast buds P96.89
  - breast engorgement P83.4
  - check-up — *see* Newborn, examination
  - convulsion P90
  - dehydration P74.1
  - examination
    - 8 to 28 days old Z00.111
    - under 8 days old Z00.110
  - fever P81.9
    - environmentally-induced P81.0
  - hyperbilirubinemia P59.9
    - of prematurity P59.0
  - hypernatremia P74.21
  - hyponatremia P74.22
  - infection P39.9
    - candidal P37.5
    - specified NEC P39.8
    - urinary tract P39.3
  - jaundice P59.9
    - due to
      - breast milk inhibitor P59.3
      - hepatocellular damage P59.20
        - specified NEC P59.29
      - preterm delivery P59.0
    - of prematurity P59.0
    - specified NEC P59.8
  - late metabolic acidosis P74.0
  - mastitis P39.0
    - infective P39.0
    - noninfective P83.4
  - multiple born NEC Z38.8
    - born in hospital Z38.68
      - by cesarean Z38.69
- **Newborn** — *continued*
  - multiple born — *continued*
    - born outside hospital Z38.7
  - omphalitis P38.9
    - with mild hemorrhage P38.1
    - without hemorrhage P38.9
  - post-term P08.21
  - prolonged gestation (over 42 completed weeks) P08.22
  - quadruplet Z38.8
    - born in hospital Z38.63
      - by cesarean Z38.64
    - born outside hospital Z38.7
  - quintuplet Z38.8
    - born in hospital Z38.65
      - by cesarean Z38.66
    - born outside hospital Z38.7
  - seizure P90
  - sepsis (congenital) P36.9
    - due to
      - anaerobes NEC P36.5
      - Escherichia coli P36.4
      - Staphylococcus P36.30
        - aureus P36.2
        - specified NEC P36.39
      - Streptococcus P36.10
        - group B P36.0
        - specified NEC P36.19
    - specified NEC P36.8
  - triplet Z38.8
    - born in hospital Z38.61
      - by cesarean Z38.62
    - born outside hospital Z38.7
  - twin Z38.5
    - born in hospital Z38.30
      - by cesarean Z38.31
    - born outside hospital Z38.4
  - vomiting P92.09
    - bilious P92.01
  - weight check Z00.111
- **Newcastle conjunctivitis or disease** B30.8
- **Nezelof's syndrome** (pure alymphocytosis) D81.4
- **Niacin** (amide) **deficiency** E52
- **Nicolas** (-Durand)-**Favre disease** A55
- **Nicotine** — *see* Tobacco
- **Nicotinic acid deficiency** E52
- **Niemann-Pick disease or syndrome** E75.249
  - specified NEC E75.248
  - type
    - A E75.240
    - A/B E75.244
    - B E75.241
    - C E75.242
    - D E75.243
- **Night**
  - blindness — *see* Blindness, night
  - sweats R61
  - terrors (child) F51.4
- **Nightmares** (REM sleep type) F51.5
- **NIHSS** (National Institutes of Health Stroke Scale) **score** R29.7- ☑
- **Nipple** — *see* condition
- **Nisbet's chancre** A57
- **Nishimoto** (-Takeuchi) **disease** I67.5
- **Nitritoid crisis or reaction** — *see* Crisis, nitritoid
- **Nitrosohemoglobinemia** D74.8
- **Njovera** A65
- **No general equivalence degree** (GED) Z55.5
- **Nocardiosis, nocardiasis** A43.9
  - cutaneous A43.1
  - lung A43.0
  - pneumonia A43.0
  - pulmonary A43.0
  - specified site NEC A43.8
- **Nocturia** R35.1
  - psychogenic F45.8
- **Nocturnal** — *see* condition
- **Nodal rhythm** I49.8
- **Node**(s) — *see also* Nodule
  - Bouchard's (with arthropathy) M15.2
  - Haygarth's M15.8
  - Heberden's (with arthropathy) M15.1
  - larynx J38.7
  - lymph — *see* condition
  - milker's B08.03
  - Osler's I33.0
  - Schmorl's — *see* Schmorl's disease
  - singer's J38.2
  - teacher's J38.2

O

Obliteration
- appendix (lumen) K38.8
- artery I77.1
- bile duct (noncalculous) K83.1
- common duct (noncalculous) K83.1
- cystic duct — *see* Obstruction, gallbladder
- disease, arteriolar I77.1
- endometrium N85.8
- eye, anterior chamber — *see* Disorder, globe, hypotony
- fallopian tube N97.1
- lymphatic vessel I89.Ø
  - due to mastectomy I97.2
- organ or site, congenital NEC — *see* Atresia, by site
- ureter N13.5
  - with infection N13.6
- urethra — *see* Stricture, urethra
- vein I87.8
- vestibule (oral) KØ8.89

Observation (following) (for) (without need for further medical care) ZØ4.9
- accident NEC ZØ4.3
  - at work ZØ4.2
  - transport ZØ4.1
- adverse effect of drug ZØ3.6
- alleged rape or sexual assault (victim), ruled out
  - adult ZØ4.41
  - child ZØ4.42
- criminal assault ZØ4.89
- development state
  - adolescent ZØØ.3
  - period of rapid growth in childhood ZØØ.2
  - puberty ZØØ.3
- disease, specified NEC ZØ3.89
- following work accident ZØ4.2
- forced sexual exploitation ZØ4.81
- forced labor exploitation ZØ4.82
- growth and development state — *see* Observation, development state
- injuries (accidental) NEC — *see also* Observation, accident
- newborn (for)
  - suspected condition, related to exposure from the mother or birth process — *see* Newborn, affected by, maternal
    - ruled out ZØ5.9
      - cardiac ZØ5.Ø
      - connective tissue ZØ5.73
      - gastrointestinal ZØ5.5
      - genetic ZØ5.41
      - genitourinary ZØ5.6
      - immunologic ZØ5.43
      - infectious ZØ5.1
      - metabolic ZØ5.42
      - musculoskeletal ZØ5.72
      - neurological ZØ5.2
      - respiratory ZØ5.3
      - skin and subcutaneous tissue ZØ5.71
      - specified condition NEC ZØ5.8
- postpartum
  - immediately after delivery Z39.Ø
  - routine follow-up Z39.2
- pregnancy (normal) (without complication) Z34.9- ☑
  - high risk OØ9.9- ☑
- suicide attempt, alleged NEC ZØ3.89
  - self-poisoning ZØ3.6
- suspected, ruled out — *see also* Suspected condition, ruled out
  - abuse, physical
    - adult ZØ4.71
    - child ZØ4.72
  - accident at work ZØ4.2
  - adult battering victim ZØ4.71
  - child battering victim ZØ4.72
  - condition NEC ZØ3.89
    - newborn — *see also* Observation, newborn (for), suspected condition, ruled out ZØ5.9
  - drug poisoning or adverse effect ZØ3.6
  - exposure (to)
    - anthrax ZØ3.81Ø
    - biological agent NEC ZØ3.818
  - foreign body
    - aspirated (inhaled) ZØ3.822
    - ingested ZØ3.821
    - inserted (injected), in (eye) (orifice) (skin) ZØ3.823
  - inflicted injury NEC ZØ4.89
  - suicide attempt, alleged ZØ3.89
    - self-poisoning ZØ3.6

Observation — *continued*
- suspected, ruled out — *see also* Suspected condition, ruled out — *continued*
  - toxic effects from ingested substance (drug) (poison) ZØ3.6
- toxic effects from ingested substance (drug) (poison) ZØ3.6

Obsession, obsessional state F42.8
- mixed thoughts and acts F42.2

Obsessive-compulsive neurosis or reaction F42.8

Obstetric embolism, septic — *see* Embolism, obstetric, septic

Obstetrical trauma (complicating delivery) O71.9
- with or following ectopic or molar pregnancy OØ8.6
- specified type NEC O71.89

Obstipation — *see* Constipation

Obstruction, obstructed, obstructive
- airway J98.8
  - with
    - allergic alveolitis J67.9
    - asthma J45.9Ø9
      - with
        - exacerbation (acute) J45.9Ø1
        - status asthmaticus J45.9Ø2
    - bronchiectasis J47.9
      - with
        - exacerbation (acute) J47.1
        - lower respiratory infection J47.Ø
    - bronchitis (chronic) J44.9
    - emphysema J43.9
  - chronic J44.9
    - with
      - allergic alveolitis — *see* Pneumonitis, hypersensitivity
      - bronchiectasis J47.9
        - with
          - exacerbation (acute) J47.1
          - lower respiratory infection J47.Ø
  - due to
    - foreign body — *see* Foreign body, by site, causing asphyxia
    - inhalation of fumes or vapors J68.9
    - laryngospasm J38.5
- ampulla of Vater K83.1
- aortic (heart) (valve) — *see* Stenosis, aortic
- aortoiliac I74.Ø9
- aqueduct of Sylvius G91.1
  - congenital QØ3.Ø
    - with spina bifida — *see* Spina bifida, by site, with hydrocephalus
- Arnold-Chiari — *see* Arnold-Chiari disease
- artery — *see also* Atherosclerosis, artery I7Ø.9 ☑
  - basilar (complete) (partial) — *see* Occlusion, artery, basilar
  - carotid (complete) (partial) — *see* Occlusion, artery, carotid
  - cerebellar — *see* Occlusion, artery, cerebellar
  - cerebral (anterior) (middle) (posterior) — *see* Occlusion, artery, cerebral
  - precerebral — *see* Occlusion, artery, precerebral
  - renal N28.Ø
  - retinal NEC — *see* Occlusion, artery, retina
  - stent — *see* Restenosis, stent
  - vertebral (complete) (partial) — *see* Occlusion, artery, vertebral
- band (intestinal) — *see also* Obstruction, intestine, specified NEC K56.699
- bile duct or passage (common) (hepatic) (noncalculous) K83.1
  - with calculus K8Ø.51
  - congenital (causing jaundice) Q44.3
- biliary (duct) (tract) K83.1
  - gallbladder K82.Ø
- bladder-neck (acquired) N32.Ø
  - congenital Q64.31
  - due to hyperplasia (hypertrophy) of prostate — *see* Hyperplasia, prostate
- bowel — *see* Obstruction, intestine
- bronchus J98.Ø9
- canal, ear — *see* Stenosis, external ear canal
- cardia K22.2
- caval veins (inferior) (superior) I87.1
- cecum — *see* Obstruction, intestine
- circulatory I99.8
- colon — *see* Obstruction, intestine
- common duct (noncalculous) K83.1
- coronary (artery) — *see* Occlusion, coronary
- cystic duct — *see also* Obstruction, gallbladder

Obstruction, obstructed, obstructive — *continued*
- cystic duct — *see also* Obstruction, gallbladder — *continued*
  - with calculus K8Ø.21
- device, implant or graft — *see also* Complications, by site and type, mechanical T85.698 ☑
  - arterial graft NEC — *see* Complication, cardiovascular device, mechanical, vascular
  - catheter NEC T85.628 ☑
    - cystostomy T83.Ø9Ø ☑
    - dialysis (renal) T82.49 ☑
      - intraperitoneal T85.691 ☑
    - Hopkins T83.Ø98 ☑
    - ileostomy T83.Ø98 ☑
    - infusion NEC T82.594 ☑
      - spinal (epidural) (subdural) T85.69Ø ☑
    - nephrostomy T83.Ø92 ☑
    - urethral indwelling T83.Ø91 ☑
    - urinary T83.Ø98 ☑
    - urostomy T83.Ø98 ☑
  - due to infection T85.79 ☑
  - gastrointestinal — *see* Complications, prosthetic device, mechanical, gastrointestinal device
  - genital NEC T83.498 ☑
    - intrauterine contraceptive device T83.39 ☑
    - penile prosthesis (cylinder) (implanted) (pump) (resevoir) T83.49Ø ☑
    - testicular prosthesis T83.491 ☑
  - heart NEC — *see* Complication, cardiovascular device, mechanical
  - joint prosthesis — *see* Complications, joint prosthesis, mechanical, specified NEC, by site
  - orthopedic NEC — *see* Complication, orthopedic, device, mechanical
  - specified NEC T85.628 ☑
  - urinary NEC — *see also* Complication, genitourinary, device, urinary, mechanical
    - graft T83.29 ☑
  - vascular NEC — *see* Complication, cardiovascular device, mechanical
  - ventricular intracranial shunt T85.Ø9 ☑
- due to foreign body accidentally left in operative wound T81.529 ☑
- duodenum K31.5
- ejaculatory duct N5Ø.89
- esophagus K22.2
- eustachian tube (complete) (partial) H68.1Ø- ☑
  - cartilagenous (extrinsic) H68.13- ☑
    - intrinsic H68.12- ☑
  - osseous H68.11- ☑
- fallopian tube (bilateral) N97.1
- fecal K56.41
  - with hernia — *see* Hernia, by site, with obstruction
- foramen of Monro (congenital) QØ3.8
  - with spina bifida — *see* Spina bifida, by site, with hydrocephalus
- foreign body — *see* Foreign body
- gallbladder K82.Ø
  - with calculus, stones K8Ø.21
  - congenital Q44.1
- gastric outlet K31.1
- gastrointestinal — *see* Obstruction, intestine
- hepatic K76.89
  - duct (noncalculous) K83.1
- ileum — *see* Obstruction, intestine
- iliofemoral (artery) I74.5
- intestine K56.6Ø9
  - with
    - adhesions (intestinal) (peritoneal) K56.5Ø
      - complete K56.52
      - incomplete K56.51
      - partial K56.51
  - adynamic K56.Ø
  - by gallstone K56.3
  - complete K56.6Ø1
  - congenital (small) Q41.9
    - large Q42.9
      - specified part NEC Q42.8
  - incomplete K56.6ØØ
  - neurogenic K56.Ø
    - Hirschsprung's disease or megacolon Q43.1
  - newborn P76.9
    - due to
      - fecaliths P76.8
      - inspissated milk P76.2
      - meconium (plug) P76.Ø
        - in mucoviscidosis E84.11

Obstruction, obstructed, obstructive — *continued*
- intestine — *continued*
  - newborn — *continued*
    - specified NEC P76.8
  - partial K56.600
  - postoperative K91.30
    - complete K91.32
    - incomplete K91.31
    - partial K91.31
  - reflex K56.0
  - specified NEC K56.699
    - complete K56.691
    - incomplete K56.690
    - partial K56.690
  - volvulus K56.2
- intracardiac ball valve prosthesis T82.09 ☑
- jejunum — *see* Obstruction, intestine
- joint prosthesis — *see* Complications, joint prosthesis, mechanical, specified NEC, by site
- kidney (calices) — *see also* Hydronephrosis N28.89
- labor — *see* Delivery
- lacrimal (passages) (duct)
  - by
    - dacryolith — *see* Dacryolith
    - stenosis — *see* Stenosis, lacrimal
  - congenital Q10.5
  - neonatal H04.53- ☑
- lacrimonasal duct — *see* Obstruction, lacrimal
- lacteal, with steatorrhea K90.2
- laryngitis — *see* Laryngitis
- larynx NEC J38.6
  - congenital Q31.8
- lung J98.4
  - disease, chronic J44.9
- lymphatic I89.0
- meconium (plug)
  - newborn P76.0
    - due to fecaliths P76.0
    - in mucoviscidosis E84.11
- mitral — *see* Stenosis, mitral
- nasal J34.89
- nasolacrimal duct — *see also* Obstruction, lacrimal
  - congenital Q10.5
- nasopharynx J39.2
- nose J34.89
- organ or site, congenital NEC — *see* Atresia, by site
- pancreatic duct K86.89
- parotid duct or gland K11.8
- pelviureteral junction N13.5
  - with hydronephrosis N13.0
  - congenital Q62.39
- pharynx J39.2
- portal (circulation) (vein) I81
- prostate — *see also* Hyperplasia, prostate
  - valve (urinary) N32.0
- pulmonary valve (heart) I37.0
- pyelonephritis (chronic) N11.1
- pylorus
  - adult K31.1
  - congenital or infantile Q40.0
- rectosigmoid — *see* Obstruction, intestine
- rectum K62.4
- renal — *see also* Hydronephrosis N28.89
  - outflow N13.8
  - pelvis, congenital Q62.39
- respiratory J98.8
  - chronic J44.9
- retinal (vessels) H34.9
- salivary duct (any) K11.8
  - with calculus K11.5
- sigmoid — *see* Obstruction, intestine
- sinus (accessory) (nasal) J34.89
- Stensen's duct K11.8
- stomach NEC K31.89
  - acute K31.0
  - congenital Q40.2
  - due to pylorospasm K31.3
- submandibular duct K11.8
- submaxillary gland K11.8
  - with calculus K11.5
- thoracic duct I89.0
- thrombotic — *see* Thrombosis
- trachea J39.8
- tracheostomy airway J95.03
- tricuspid (valve) — *see* Stenosis, tricuspid
- upper respiratory, congenital Q34.8
- ureter (functional) (pelvic junction) NEC N13.5

Obstruction, obstructed, obstructive — *continued*
- ureter — *continued*
  - with
    - hydronephrosis N13.1
      - with infection N13.6
      - congenital Q62.39
    - pyelonephritis (chronic) N11.1
  - congenital Q62.39
  - due to calculus — *see* Calculus, ureter
- urethra NEC N36.8
  - congenital Q64.39
- urinary (moderate) N13.9
  - due to hyperplasia (hypertrophy) of prostate — *see* Hyperplasia, prostate
  - organ or tract (lower) N13.9
  - prostatic valve N32.0
  - specified NEC N13.8
- uropathy N13.9
- uterus N85.8
- vagina N89.5
- valvular — *see* Endocarditis
- vein, venous I87.1
  - caval (inferior) (superior) I87.1
  - thrombotic — *see* Thrombosis
- vena cava (inferior) (superior) I87.1
- vesical NEC N32.0
- vesicourethral orifice N32.0
  - congenital Q64.31
- vessel NEC I99.8
  - stent — *see* Restenosis, stent

Obturator — *see* condition

Occlusal wear, teeth K03.0

Occlusio pupillae — *see* Membrane, pupillary

Occlusion, occluded
- anus K62.4
  - congenital Q42.3
    - with fistula Q42.2
- aortoiliac (chronic) I74.09
- aqueduct of Sylvius G91.1
  - congenital Q03.0
    - with spina bifida — *see* Spina bifida, by site, with hydrocephalus
- artery — *see also* Atherosclerosis, artery I70.9 ☑
  - auditory, internal I65.8
  - basilar I65.1
    - with
      - infarction I63.22
        - due to
          - embolism I63.12
          - thrombosis I63.02
  - brain or cerebral I66.9
    - with infarction (due to) I63.5- ☑
      - embolism I63.4- ☑
      - thrombosis I63.3- ☑
  - carotid I65.2- ☑
    - with
      - infarction I63.23- ☑
        - due to
          - embolism I63.13- ☑
          - thrombosis I63.03- ☑
  - cerebellar (anterior inferior) (posterior inferior) (superior) I66.3
    - with infarction I63.54- ☑
      - due to
        - embolism I63.44- ☑
        - thrombosis I63.34- ☑
  - cerebral I66.9
    - with infarction I63.50
      - due to
        - embolism I63.40
          - specified NEC I63.49
        - thrombosis I63.30
          - specified NEC I63.39
    - anterior I66.1- ☑
      - with infarction I63.52- ☑
        - due to
          - embolism I63.42- ☑
          - thrombosis I63.32- ☑
    - middle I66.0- ☑
      - with infarction I63.51- ☑
        - due to
          - embolism I63.41- ☑
          - thrombosis I63.31- ☑
    - posterior I66.2- ☑
      - with infarction I63.53- ☑
        - due to
          - embolism I63.43- ☑

Occlusion, occluded — *continued*
- artery — *see also* Atherosclerosis, artery — *continued*
  - cerebral — *continued*
    - posterior — *continued*
      - with infarction — *continued*
        - due to — *continued*
          - thrombosis I63.33- ☑
    - specified NEC I66.8
      - with infarction I63.59
        - due to
          - embolism I63.4- ☑
          - thrombosis I63.3- ☑
  - choroidal (anterior) — *see* Occlusion, artery, precerebral, specified NEC
  - communicating posterior — *see* Occlusion, artery, precerebral, specified NEC
  - complete
    - coronary I25.82
    - extremities I70.92
  - coronary (acute) (thrombotic) (without myocardial infarction) I24.0
    - with myocardial infarction — *see* Infarction, myocardium
    - chronic total I25.82
    - complete I25.82
    - healed or old I25.2
    - total (chronic) I25.82
  - hypophyseal — *see* Occlusion, artery, precerebral, specified NEC
  - iliac I74.5
  - lower extremities due to stenosis or stricture I77.1
  - mesenteric (embolic) (thrombotic) — *see also* Infarct, intestine K55.069
  - perforating — *see* Occlusion, artery, cerebral, specified NEC
  - peripheral I77.9
    - thrombotic or embolic I74.4
  - pontine — *see* Occlusion, artery, precerebral, specified NEC
  - precerebral I65.9
    - with infarction I63.20
      - specified NEC I63.29
      - due to
        - embolism I63.10
          - specified NEC I63.19
        - thrombosis I63.00
          - specified NEC I63.09
    - basilar — *see* Occlusion, artery, basilar
    - carotid — *see* Occlusion, artery, carotid
    - puerperal O88.23
    - specified NEC I65.8
      - with infarction I63.29
        - due to
          - embolism I63.19
          - thrombosis I63.09
    - vertebral — *see* Occlusion, artery, vertebral
  - renal N28.0
  - retinal
    - branch H34.23- ☑
    - central H34.1- ☑
    - partial H34.21- ☑
    - transient H34.0- ☑
  - spinal — *see* Occlusion, artery, precerebral, vertebral
  - total (chronic)
    - oronary I25.82
    - extremities I70.92
  - vertebral I65.0- ☑
    - with
      - infarction I63.21- ☑
        - due to
          - embolism I63.11- ☑
          - thrombosis I63.01- ☑
- basilar artery — *see* Occlusion, artery, basilar
- bile duct (common) (hepatic) (noncalculous) K83.1
- bowel — *see* Obstruction, intestine
- carotid (artery) (common) (internal) — *see* Occlusion, artery, carotid
- centric (of teeth) M26.59
  - maximum intercuspation discrepancy M26.55
- cerebellar (artery) — *see* Occlusion, artery, cerebellar
- cerebral (artery) — *see* Occlusion, artery, cerebral
- cerebrovascular — *see also* Occlusion, artery, cerebral
  - with infarction I63.5- ☑
- cervical canal — *see* Stricture, cervix
- cervix (uteri) — *see* Stricture, cervix
- choanal Q30.0

Osteoarthritis — *continued*
- hip — *continued*
  - secondary — *see* Osteoarthritis, secondary, hip
  - unilateral M16.1- ☑
    - due to hip dysplasia M16.3- ☑
    - post-traumatic M16.5- ☑
    - primary M16.1- ☑
    - secondary NEC M16.7
- interphalangeal
  - distal (Heberden) M15.1
  - proximal (Bouchard) M15.2
- knee M17.9
  - bilateral M17.Ø
    - post-traumatic M17.2
    - secondary M17.4
  - post-traumatic — *see* Osteoarthritis, post-traumatic, knee
  - primary M17.1- ☑
    - bilateral M17.Ø
  - secondary — *see* Osteoarthritis, secondary, knee
  - unilateral M17.1- ☑
    - post-traumatic M17.3- ☑
    - primary M17.1- ☑
    - secondary NEC M17.5
- post-traumatic NEC M19.92
  - ankle M19.17- ☑
  - elbow M19.12- ☑
  - foot joint M19.17- ☑
  - hand joint M19.14- ☑
    - first carpometacarpal joint M18.3- ☑
      - bilateral M18.2
  - hip M16.5- ☑
    - bilateral M16.4
  - knee M17.3- ☑
    - bilateral M17.2
  - shoulder M19.11- ☑
  - specified site NEC M19.19
  - wrist M19.13- ☑
- primary M19.91
  - ankle M19.Ø7- ☑
  - elbow M19.Ø2- ☑
  - foot joint M19.Ø7- ☑
  - hand joint M19.Ø4- ☑
    - first carpometacarpal joint M18.1- ☑
      - bilateral M18.Ø
  - hip M16.1- ☑
    - bilateral M16.Ø
  - knee M17.1- ☑
    - bilateral M17.Ø
  - multiple sites M15.9
  - shoulder M19.Ø1- ☑
  - specified site NEC M19.Ø9
  - spine — *see* Spondylosis
  - wrist M19.Ø3- ☑
- secondary M19.93
  - ankle M19.27- ☑
  - elbow M19.22- ☑
  - foot joint M19.27- ☑
  - hand joint M19.24- ☑
    - first carpometacarpal joint M18.5- ☑
      - bilateral M18.4
  - hip M16.7-
    - bilateral M16.6
  - knee M17.5-
    - bilateral M17.4
  - multiple M15.3
  - shoulder M19.21- ☑
  - specified site NEC M19.29
  - spine — *see* Spondylosis
  - wrist M19.23- ☑
- shoulder M19.Ø1- ☑
  - post-traumatic M19.11- ☑
  - primary M19.Ø1- ☑
  - secondary M19.21- ☑
- specified site NEC M19.Ø9
- spine — *see* Spondylosis
- wrist M19.Ø3- ☑
  - first carpometacarpal joint — *see* Osteoarthritis, hand joint, first carpometacarpal joint
  - post-traumatic M19.13- ☑
  - primary M19.Ø3- ☑
  - secondary M19.23 ☑

Osteoarthropathy (hypertrophic) M19.9Ø
- ankle — *see* Osteoarthritis, primary, ankle
- elbow — *see* Osteoarthritis, primary, elbow
- foot joint — *see* Osteoarthritis, primary, foot
- hand joint — *see* Osteoarthritis, primary, hand joint
- knee joint — *see* Osteoarthritis, primary, knee
- multiple site — *see* Osteoarthritis, primary, multiple joint
- pulmonary — *see also* Osteoarthropathy, specified type NEC
  - hypertrophic — *see* Osteoarthropathy, hypertrophic, specified type NEC
- secondary — *see* Osteoarthropathy, specified type NEC
- secondary hypertrophic — *see* Osteoarthropathy, specified type NEC
- shoulder — *see* Osteoarthritis, primary, shoulder
- specified joint NEC — *see* Osteoarthritis, primary, specified joint NEC
- specified type NEC M89.4Ø
  - carpus M89.44- ☑
  - clavicle M89.41- ☑
  - femur M89.45- ☑
  - fibula M89.46- ☑
  - finger M89.44- ☑
  - humerus M89.42- ☑
  - ilium M89.459
  - ischium M89.459
  - metacarpus M89.44- ☑
  - metatarsus M89.47- ☑
  - multiple sites M89.49
  - neck M89.48
  - radius M89.43- ☑
  - rib M89.48
  - scapula M89.41- ☑
  - skull M89.48
  - tarsus M89.47- ☑
  - tibia M89.46- ☑
  - toe M89.47- ☑
  - ulna M89.43- ☑
  - vertebra M89.48
- spine — *see* Spondylosis
- wrist — *see* Osteoarthritis, primary, wrist

Osteoarthrosis (degenerative) (hypertrophic) (joint) — *see also* Osteoarthritis
- deformans alkaptonurica E7Ø.29 *[M36.8]*
- erosive M15.4
- generalized M15.9
  - primary M15.Ø
- polyarticular M15.9
- spine — *see* Spondylosis

Osteoblastoma — *see* Neoplasm, bone, benign
- aggressive — *see* Neoplasm, bone, uncertain behavior

Osteochondritis — *see also* Osteochondropathy, by site
- Brailsford's — *see* Osteochondrosis, juvenile, radius
- dissecans M93.2Ø
  - ankle M93.27- ☑
  - elbow M93.22- ☑
  - foot M93.27- ☑
  - hand M93.24- ☑
  - hip M93.25- ☑
  - knee M93.26- ☑
  - multiple sites M93.29
  - shoulder joint M93.21- ☑
  - specified site NEC M93.28
  - wrist M93.23- ☑
- juvenile M92.9
  - patellar — *see* Osteochondrosis, juvenile, patella
- syphilitic (congenital) (early) A5Ø.Ø2 *[M9Ø.8Ø]*
  - ankle A5Ø.Ø2 *[M9Ø.87-]* ☑
  - elbow A5Ø.Ø2 *[M9Ø.82-]* ☑
  - foot A5Ø.Ø2 *[M9Ø.87-]* ☑
  - forearm A5Ø.Ø2 *[M9Ø.83-]* ☑
  - hand A5Ø.Ø2 *[M9Ø.84-]* ☑
  - hip A5Ø.Ø2 *[M9Ø.85-]* ☑
  - knee A5Ø.Ø2 *[M9Ø.86-]* ☑
  - multiple sites A5Ø.Ø2 *[M9Ø.89]*
  - shoulder joint A5Ø.Ø2 *[M9Ø.81-]* ☑
  - specified site NEC A5Ø.Ø2 *[M9Ø.88]*

Osteochondroarthrosis deformans endemica — *see* Disease, Kaschin-Beck

Osteochondrodysplasia Q78.9
- with defects of growth of tubular bones and spine Q77.9
  - specified NEC Q77.8
- specified NEC Q78.8

Osteochondrodystrophy E78.9

Osteochondrolysis — *see* Osteochondritis, dissecans

Osteochondroma — *see* Neoplasm, bone, benign

Osteochondromatosis D16.9
- syndrome Q78.4

Osteochondromyxosarcoma — *see* Neoplasm, bone, malignant

Osteochondropathy M93.9Ø
- ankle M93.97- ☑
- elbow M93.92- ☑
- foot M93.97- ☑
- hand M93.94- ☑
- hip M93.95- ☑
- Kienböck's disease of adults M93.1
- knee M93.96- ☑
- multiple joints M93.99
- osteochondritis dissecans — *see* Osteochondritis, dissecans
- osteochondrosis — *see* Osteochondrosis
- shoulder region M93.91- ☑
- slipped upper femoral epiphysis — *see* Slipped, epiphysis, upper femoral
- specified joint NEC M93.98
- specified type NEC M93.8Ø
  - ankle M93.87- ☑
  - elbow M93.82- ☑
  - foot M93.87- ☑
  - hand M93.84- ☑
  - hip M93.85- ☑
  - knee M93.86- ☑
  - multiple joints M93.89
  - shoulder region M93.81- ☑
  - specified joint NEC M93.88
  - wrist M93.83- ☑
- syphilitic, congenital
  - early A5Ø.Ø2 *[M9Ø.8Ø]*
  - late A5Ø.56 *[M9Ø.8Ø]*
- wrist M93.93- ☑

Osteochondrosarcoma — *see* Neoplasm, bone, malignant

Osteochondrosis — *see also* Osteochondropathy, by site
- acetabulum (juvenile) M91.Ø
- adult — *see* Osteochondropathy, specified type NEC, by site
- astragalus (juvenile) — *see* Osteochondrosis, juvenile, tarsus
- Blount M92.51- ☑
- Buchanan's M91.Ø
- Burns' — *see* Osteochondrosis, juvenile, ulna
- calcaneus (juvenile) — *see* Osteochondrosis, juvenile, tarsus
- capitular epiphysis (femur) (juvenile) — *see* Legg-Calvé-Perthes disease
- carpal (juvenile) (lunate) (scaphoid) — *see* Osteochondrosis, juvenile, hand, carpal lunate
  - adult M93.1
- coxae juvenilis — *see* Legg-Calvé-Perthes disease
- deformans juvenilis, coxae — *see* Legg-Calvé-Perthes disease
- Diaz's — *see* Osteochondrosis, juvenile, tarsus
- dissecans (knee) (shoulder) — *see* Osteochondritis, dissecans
- femoral capital epiphysis (juvenile) — *see* Legg-Calvé-Perthes disease
- femur (head), juvenile — *see* Legg-Calvé-Perthes disease
- fibula (juvenile) — *see* Osteochondrosis, juvenile, fibula
- foot NEC (juvenile) M92.8
- Freiberg's — *see* Osteochondrosis, juvenile, metatarsus
- Haas' (juvenile) — *see* Osteochondrosis, juvenile, humerus
- Haglund's — *see* Osteochondrosis, juvenile, tarsus
- hip (juvenile) — *see* Legg-Calvé-Perthes disease
- humerus (capitulum) (head) (juvenile) — *see* Osteochondrosis, juvenile, humerus
- ilium, iliac crest (juvenile) M91.Ø
- ischiopubic synchondrosis M91.Ø
- Iselin's — *see* Osteochondrosis, juvenile, metatarsus
- juvenile, juvenilis M92.9
  - after congenital dislocation of hip reduction — *see* Osteochondrosis, juvenile, hip, specified NEC
  - arm — *see* Osteochondrosis, juvenile, upper limb NEC
  - capitular epiphysis (femur) — *see* Legg-Calvé-Perthes disease
  - clavicle, sternal epiphysis — *see* Osteochondrosis, juvenile, upper limb NEC
  - coxae — *see* Legg-Calvé-Perthes disease
  - deformans M92.9
  - fibula M92.5Ø- ☑

- **Osteomyelitis** — *continued*
  - chronic — *continued*
    - with draining sinus — *continued*
      - multiple sites M86.49
      - neck M86.48
      - orbit HØ5.Ø2- ☑
      - petrous bone — *see* Petrositis
      - radius M86.43- ☑
      - rib M86.48
      - scapula M86.41- ☑
      - skull M86.48
      - tarsus M86.47- ☑
      - tibia M86.46- ☑
      - toe M86.47- ☑
      - ulna M86.43- ☑
      - vertebra — *see* Osteomyelitis, vertebra
    - carpus M86.64- ☑
    - clavicle M86.61- ☑
    - femur M86.65- ☑
    - fibula M86.66- ☑
    - finger M86.64- ☑
    - hematogenous NEC M86.5Ø
      - carpus M86.54- ☑
      - clavicle M86.51- ☑
      - femur M86.55- ☑
      - fibula M86.56- ☑
      - finger M86.54- ☑
      - humerus M86.52- ☑
      - ilium M86.559
      - ischium M86.559
      - mandible M27.2
      - metacarpus M86.54- ☑
      - metatarsus M86.57- ☑
      - multifocal M86.3Ø
        - carpus M86.34- ☑
        - clavicle M86.31- ☑
        - femur M86.35- ☑
        - fibula M86.36- ☑
        - finger M86.34- ☑
        - humerus M86.32- ☑
        - ilium M86.359
        - ischium M86.359
        - metacarpus M86.34- ☑
        - metatarsus M86.37- ☑
        - multiple sites M86.39
        - neck M86.38
        - radius M86.33- ☑
        - rib M86.38
        - scapula M86.31- ☑
        - skull M86.38
        - tarsus M86.37- ☑
        - tibia M86.36- ☑
        - toe M86.37- ☑
        - ulna M86.33- ☑
        - vertebra — *see* Osteomyelitis, vertebra
      - multiple sites M86.59
      - neck M86.58
      - orbit HØ5.Ø2- ☑
      - petrous bone — *see* Petrositis
      - radius M86.53- ☑
      - rib M86.58
      - scapula M86.51- ☑
      - skull M86.58
      - tarsus M86.57- ☑
      - tibia M86.56- ☑
      - toe M86.57- ☑
      - ulna M86.53- ☑
      - vertebra — *see* Osteomyelitis, vertebra
    - humerus M86.62- ☑
    - ilium M86.659
    - ischium M86.659
    - mandible M27.2
    - metacarpus M86.64- ☑
    - metatarsus M86.67- ☑
    - multifocal — *see* Osteomyelitis, chronic, hematogenous, multifocal
    - multiple sites M86.69
    - neck M86.68
    - orbit HØ5.Ø2- ☑
    - petrous bone — *see* Petrositis
    - radius M86.63- ☑
    - rib M86.68
    - scapula M86.61- ☑
    - skull M86.68
    - tarsus M86.67- ☑
    - tibia M86.66- ☑
    - toe M86.67- ☑

- **Osteomyelitis** — *continued*
  - chronic — *continued*
    - ulna M86.63- ☑
    - vertebra — *see* Osteomyelitis, vertebra
  - echinococcal B67.2
  - Garr's — *see* Osteomyelitis, specified type NEC
  - in diabetes mellitus — *see* EØ8-E13 with .69
  - jaw (acute) (chronic) (lower) (neonatal) (suppurative) (upper) M27.2
  - nonsuppurating — *see* Osteomyelitis, specified type NEC
  - orbit HØ5.Ø2- ☑
  - petrous bone — *see* Petrositis
  - Salmonella (arizonae) (cholerae-suis) (enteritidis) (typhimurium) AØ2.24
  - sclerosing, nonsuppurative — *see* Osteomyelitis, specified type NEC
  - specified type NEC — *see also* subcategory M86.8X- ☑
    - mandible M27.2
    - orbit HØ5.Ø2- ☑
    - petrous bone — *see* Petrositis
    - vertebra — *see* Osteomyelitis, vertebra
  - subacute M86.2Ø
    - carpus M86.24- ☑
    - clavicle M86.21- ☑
    - femur M86.25- ☑
    - fibula M86.26- ☑
    - finger M86.24- ☑
    - humerus M86.22- ☑
    - mandible M27.2
    - metacarpus M86.24- ☑
    - metatarsus M86.27- ☑
    - multiple sites M86.29
    - neck M86.28
    - orbit HØ5.Ø2- ☑
    - petrous bone — *see* Petrositis
    - radius M86.23- ☑
    - rib M86.28
    - scapula M86.21- ☑
    - skull M86.28
    - tarsus M86.27- ☑
    - tibia M86.26- ☑
    - toe M86.27- ☑
    - ulna M86.23- ☑
    - vertebra — *see* Osteomyelitis, vertebra
  - syphilitic A52.77
    - congenital (early) A5Ø.Ø2 *[M9Ø.8Ø]*
  - tuberculous — *see* Tuberculosis, bone
  - typhoid AØ1.Ø5
  - vertebra M46.2Ø
    - cervical region M46.22
    - cervicothoracic region M46.23
    - lumbar region M46.26
    - lumbosacral region M46.27
    - occipito-atlanto-axial region M46.21
    - sacrococcygeal region M46.28
    - thoracic region M46.24
    - thoracolumbar region M46.25
- **Osteomyelofibrosis** D47.4
- **Osteomyelosclerosis** D75.89
- **Osteonecrosis** M87.9
  - due to
    - drugs — *see* Osteonecrosis, secondary, due to, drugs
    - trauma — *see* Osteonecrosis, secondary, due to, trauma
  - idiopathic aseptic M87.ØØ
    - ankle M87.Ø7- ☑
    - carpus M87.Ø3- ☑
    - clavicle M87.Ø1- ☑
    - femur M87.Ø5- ☑
    - fibula M87.Ø6- ☑
    - finger M87.Ø4- ☑
    - humerus M87.Ø2- ☑
    - ilium M87.Ø5Ø
    - ischium M87.Ø5Ø
    - metacarpus M87.Ø4- ☑
    - metatarsus M87.Ø7- ☑
    - multiple sites M87.Ø9
    - neck M87.Ø8
    - pelvis M87.Ø5Ø
    - radius M87.Ø3- ☑
    - rib M87.Ø8
    - scapula M87.Ø1- ☑
    - skull M87.Ø8
    - tarsus M87.Ø7- ☑
    - tibia M87.Ø6- ☑
    - toe M87.Ø7- ☑

- **Osteonecrosis** — *continued*
  - idiopathic aseptic — *continued*
    - ulna M87.Ø3- ☑
    - vertebra M87.Ø8
  - secondary NEC M87.3Ø
    - carpus M87.33- ☑
    - clavicle M87.31- ☑
    - due to
      - drugs M87.1Ø
        - carpus M87.13- ☑
        - clavicle M87.11- ☑
        - femur M87.15- ☑
        - fibula M87.16- ☑
        - finger M87.14- ☑
        - humerus M87.12- ☑
        - ilium M87.159
        - ischium M87.159
        - jaw M87.18Ø
        - metacarpus M87.14- ☑
        - metatarsus M87.17- ☑
        - multiple sites M87.19
        - neck M87.18 ☑
        - radius M87.13- ☑
        - rib M87.18 ☑
        - scapula M87.11- ☑
        - skull M87.18 ☑
        - tarsus M87.17- ☑
        - tibia M87.16- ☑
        - toe M87.17- ☑
        - ulna M87.13- ☑
        - vertebra M87.18 ☑
      - hemoglobinopathy NEC D58.2 *[M9Ø.5Ø]*
        - carpus D58.2 *[M9Ø.54-]* ☑
        - clavicle D58.2 *[M9Ø.51-]* ☑
        - femur D58.2 *[M9Ø.55-]* ☑
        - fibula D58.2 *[M9Ø.56-]* ☑
        - finger D58.2 *[M9Ø.54-]* ☑
        - humerus D58.2 *[M9Ø.52-]* ☑
        - ilium D58.2 *[M9Ø.55-]* ☑
        - ischium D58.2 *[M9Ø.55-]* ☑
        - metacarpus D58.2 *[M9Ø.54-]* ☑
        - metatarsus D58.2 *[M9Ø.57-]* ☑
        - multiple sites D58.2 *[M9Ø.58]*
        - neck D58.2 *[M9Ø.58]*
        - radius D58.2 *[M9Ø.53-]* ☑
        - rib D58.2 *[M9Ø.58]*
        - scapula D58.2 *[M9Ø.51-]* ☑
        - skull D58.2 *[M9Ø.58]*
        - tarsus D58.2 *[M9Ø.57-]* ☑
        - tibia D58.2 *[M9Ø.56-]* ☑
        - toe D58.2 *[M9Ø.57-]* ☑
        - ulna D58.2 *[M9Ø.53-]* ☑
        - vertebra D58.2 *[M9Ø.58]*
      - trauma (previous) M87.2Ø
        - carpus M87.23- ☑
        - clavicle M87.21- ☑
        - femur M87.25- ☑
        - fibula M87.26- ☑
        - finger M87.24- ☑
        - humerus M87.22- ☑
        - ilium M87.25- ☑
        - ischium M87.25- ☑
        - metacarpus M87.24- ☑
        - metatarsus M87.27- ☑
        - multiple sites M87.29
        - neck M87.28
        - radius M87.23- ☑
        - rib M87.28
        - scapula M87.21- ☑
        - skull M87.28
        - tarsus M87.27- ☑
        - tibia M87.26- ☑
        - toe M87.27- ☑
        - ulna M87.23- ☑
        - vertebra M87.28
    - femur M87.35- ☑
    - fibula M87.36- ☑
    - finger M87.34- ☑
    - humerus M87.32- ☑
    - ilium M87.35Ø
    - in
      - caisson disease T7Ø.3 ☑ *[M9Ø.5Ø]*
        - carpus T7Ø.3 ☑ *[M9Ø.54-]* ☑
        - clavicle T7Ø.3 ☑ *[M9Ø.51-]* ☑
        - femur T7Ø.3 ☑ *[M9Ø.55-]* ☑
        - fibula T7Ø.3 ☑ *[M9Ø.56-]* ☑

Osteonecrosis — *continued*
- secondary — *continued*
  - in — *continued*
    - caisson disease — *continued*
      - finger T7Ø.3 ☑ *[M9Ø.54-]* ☑
      - humerus T7Ø.3 ☑ *[M9Ø.52-]* ☑
      - ilium T7Ø.3 ☑ *[M9Ø.55-]* ☑
      - ischium T7Ø.3 ☑ *[M9Ø.55-]* ☑
      - metacarpus T7Ø.3 ☑ *[M9Ø.54-]* ☑
      - metatarsus T7Ø.3 ☑ *[M9Ø.57-]* ☑
      - multiple sites T7Ø.3 ☑ *[M9Ø.59]*
      - neck T7Ø.3 ☑ *[M9Ø.58]*
      - radius T7Ø.3 ☑ *[M9Ø.53-]* ☑
      - rib T7Ø.3 ☑ *[M9Ø.58]*
      - scapula T7Ø.3 ☑ *[M9Ø.51-]* ☑
      - skull T7Ø.3 ☑ *[M9Ø.58]*
      - tarsus T7Ø.3 ☑ *[M9Ø.57-]* ☑
      - tibia T7Ø.3 ☑ *[M9Ø.56-]* ☑
      - toe T7Ø.3 ☑ *[M9Ø.57-]* ☑
      - ulna T7Ø.3 ☑ *[M9Ø.53-]* ☑
      - vertebra T7Ø.3 ☑ *[M9Ø.58]*
  - ischium M87.35Ø
  - metacarpus M87.34- ☑
  - metatarsus M87.37- ☑
  - multiple site M87.39
  - neck M87.38
  - radius M87.33- ☑
  - rib M87.38
  - scapula M87.319
  - skull M87.38
  - tarsus M87.379
  - tibia M87.366
  - toe M87.379
  - ulna M87.33- ☑
  - vertebra M87.38
- specified type NEC M87.8Ø
  - carpus M87.83- ☑
  - clavicle M87.81- ☑
  - femur M87.85- ☑
  - fibula M87.86- ☑
  - finger M87.84- ☑
  - humerus M87.82- ☑
  - ilium M87.85- ☑
  - ischium M87.85- ☑
  - metacarpus M87.84- ☑
  - metatarsus M87.87- ☑
  - multiple sites M87.89
  - neck M87.88
  - radius M87.83- ☑
  - rib M87.88
  - scapula M87.81- ☑
  - skull M87.88
  - tarsus M87.87- ☑
  - tibia M87.86- ☑
  - toe M87.87- ☑
  - ulna M87.83- ☑
  - vertebra M87.88

Osteo-onycho-arthro-dysplasia Q87.2

Osteo-onychodysplasia, hereditary Q87.2

Osteopathia condensans disseminata Q78.8

Osteopathy — *see also* Osteomyelitis, Osteonecrosis, Osteoporosis
- after poliomyelitis M89.6Ø
  - carpus M89.64- ☑
  - clavicle M89.61- ☑
  - femur M89.65- ☑
  - fibula M89.66- ☑
  - finger M89.64- ☑
  - humerus M89.62- ☑
  - ilium M89.659
  - ischium M89.659
  - metacarpus M89.64- ☑
  - metatarsus M89.67- ☑
  - multiple sites M89.69
  - neck M89.68
  - radius M89.63- ☑
  - rib M89.68
  - scapula M89.61- ☑
  - skull M89.68
  - tarsus M89.67- ☑
  - tibia M89.66- ☑
  - toe M89.67- ☑
  - ulna M89.63- ☑
  - vertebra M89.68
- in (due to)
  - renal osteodystrophy N25.Ø

Osteopathy — *continued*
- in — *continued*
  - specified diseases classified elsewhere — *see* subcategory M9Ø.8 ☑

Osteopenia M85.8- ☑
- borderline M85.8- ☑

Osteoperiostitis — *see* Osteomyelitis, specified type NEC

Osteopetrosis (familial) Q78.2

Osteophyte M25.7Ø
- ankle M25.77- ☑
- elbow M25.72- ☑
- foot joint M25.77- ☑
- hand joint M25.74- ☑
- hip M25.75- ☑
- knee M25.76- ☑
- shoulder M25.71- ☑
- spine M25.78
- vertebrae M25.78
- wrist M25.73- ☑

Osteopoikilosis Q78.8

Osteoporosis (female) (male) M81.Ø
- with current pathological fracture M8Ø.ØØ ☑
- age-related M81.Ø
  - with current pathologic fracture M8Ø.ØØ ☑
    - carpus M8Ø.Ø4- ☑
    - clavicle M8Ø.Ø1- ☑
    - fibula M8Ø.Ø6- ☑
    - finger M8Ø.Ø4- ☑
    - humerus M8Ø.Ø2- ☑
    - ilium M8Ø.Ø5- ☑
    - ischium M8Ø.Ø5- ☑
    - metacarpus M8Ø.Ø4- ☑
    - metatarsus M8Ø.Ø7- ☑
    - pelvis M8Ø.Ø5- ☑
    - radius M8Ø.Ø3- ☑
    - rib(s) — *see* Osteoporosis, specified site NEC
    - scapula M8Ø.Ø1- ☑
    - site specified NEC M8Ø.ØA ☑
    - specified site NEC M8Ø.ØA ☑
    - tarsus M8Ø.Ø7- ☑
    - tibia M8Ø.Ø6- ☑
    - toe M8Ø.Ø7- ☑
    - ulna M8Ø.Ø3- ☑
    - vertebra M8Ø.Ø8 ☑
- disuse M81.8
  - with current pathological fracture M8Ø.8Ø ☑
    - carpus M8Ø.84- ☑
    - clavicle M8Ø.81- ☑
    - fibula M8Ø.86- ☑
    - finger M8Ø.84- ☑
    - humerus M8Ø.82- ☑
    - ilium M8Ø.85- ☑
    - ischium M8Ø.85- ☑
    - metacarpus M8Ø.84- ☑
    - metatarsus M8Ø.87- ☑
    - pelvis M8Ø.85- ☑
    - radius M8Ø.83- ☑
    - scapula M8Ø.81- ☑
    - site specified NEC M8Ø.8A ☑
    - tarsus M8Ø.87- ☑
    - tibia M8Ø.86- ☑
    - toe M8Ø.87- ☑
    - ulna M8Ø.83- ☑
    - vertebra M8Ø.88 ☑
- drug-induced — *see* Osteoporosis, specified type NEC
- idiopathic — *see* Osteoporosis, specified type NEC
- involutional — *see* Osteoporosis, age-related
- Lequesne M81.6
- localized M81.6
- postmenopausal M81.Ø
  - with pathological fracture M8Ø.ØØ ☑
    - carpus M8Ø.Ø4- ☑
    - clavicle M8Ø.Ø1- ☑
    - fibula M8Ø.Ø6- ☑
    - finger M8Ø.Ø4- ☑
    - humerus M8Ø.Ø2- ☑
    - ilium M8Ø.Ø5- ☑
    - ischium M8Ø.Ø5- ☑
    - metacarpus M8Ø.Ø4- ☑
    - metatarsus M8Ø.Ø7- ☑
    - pelvis M8Ø.Ø5- ☑
    - radius M8Ø.Ø3- ☑
    - scapula M8Ø.Ø1- ☑
    - site specified NEC M8Ø.ØA ☑
    - tarsus M8Ø.Ø7- ☑

Osteoporosis — *continued*
- postmenopausal — *continued*
  - with pathological fracture — *continued*
    - tibia M8Ø.Ø6- ☑
    - toe M8Ø.Ø7- ☑
    - ulna M8Ø.Ø3- ☑
    - vertebra M8Ø.Ø8 ☑
- postoophorectomy — *see* Osteoporosis, specified type NEC
- postsurgical malabsorption — *see* Osteoporosis, specified type NEC
- post-traumatic — *see* Osteoporosis, specified type NEC
- senile — *see* Osteoporosis, age-related
- specified type NEC M81.8
  - with pathological fracture M8Ø.8Ø ☑
    - carpus M8Ø.84- ☑
    - clavicle M8Ø.81- ☑
    - fibula M8Ø.86- ☑
    - finger M8Ø.84- ☑
    - humerus M8Ø.82- ☑
    - ilium M8Ø.85- ☑
    - ischium M8Ø.85- ☑
    - metacarpus M8Ø.84- ☑
    - metatarsus M8Ø.87- ☑
    - pelvis M8Ø.85- ☑
    - radius M8Ø.83- ☑
    - scapula M8Ø.81- ☑
    - site specified NEC M8Ø.8A ☑
    - tarsus M8Ø.87- ☑
    - tibia M8Ø.86- ☑
    - toe M8Ø.87- ☑
    - ulna M8Ø.83- ☑
    - vertebra M8Ø.88 ☑

Osteopsathyrosis (idiopathica) Q78.Ø

Osteoradionecrosis, jaw (acute) (chronic) (lower) (suppurative) (upper) M27.2

Osteosarcoma (any form) — *see* Neoplasm, bone, malignant

Osteosclerosis Q78.2
- acquired M85.8- ☑
- congenita Q77.4
- fragilitas (generalisata) Q78.2
- myelofibrosis D75.81

Osteosclerotic anemia D64.89

Osteosis
- cutis L94.2
- renal fibrocystic N25.Ø

Österreicher-Turner syndrome Q87.2

Ostium
- atrioventriculare commune Q21.23
- primum (arteriosum) (defect) (persistent) Q21.2Ø
- secundum (arteriosum) (defect) (patent) (persistent) Q21.11

Ostrum-Furst syndrome Q75.8

Otalgia H92.Ø ☑

Otitis (acute) H66.9Ø
- with effusion — *see also* Otitis, media, nonsuppurative
  - purulent — *see* Otitis, media, suppurative
- adhesive — *see* subcategory H74.1 ☑
- chronic — *see also* Otitis, media, chronic
  - with effusion — *see also* Otitis, media, nonsuppurative, chronic
- externa H6Ø.9- ☑
  - abscess — *see* Abscess, ear, external
  - acute (noninfective) H6Ø.5Ø- ☑
    - actinic H6Ø.51- ☑
    - chemical H6Ø.52- ☑
    - contact H6Ø.53- ☑
    - eczematoid H6Ø.54- ☑
    - infective — *see* Otitis, externa, infective
    - reactive H6Ø.55- ☑
    - specified NEC H6Ø.59- ☑
  - cellulitis — *see* Cellulitis, ear
  - chronic H6Ø.6- ☑
  - diffuse — *see* Otitis, externa, infective, diffuse
  - hemorrhagic — *see* Otitis, externa, infective, hemorrhagic
  - in (due to)
    - aspergillosis B44.89
    - candidiasis B37.84
    - erysipelas A46 *[H62.4Ø]*
    - herpes (simplex) virus infection BØØ.1
      - zoster BØ2.8
    - impetigo LØ1.ØØ *[H62.4Ø]*
    - infectious disease NEC B99 ☑ *[H62.4-]* ☑
    - mycosis NEC B36.9 *[H62.4Ø]*

Index

Otitis — Ovulation

Paralysis, paralytic — *continued*
- digestive organs NEC K59.89
- diplegic — *see* Diplegia
- divergence (nuclear) H51.8
- diver's T7Ø.3 ☑
- Duchenne's
  - birth injury P14.Ø
  - due to or associated with
    - motor neuron disease G12.22
    - muscular dystrophy G71.Ø1
- due to intracranial or spinal birth injury — *see* Palsy, cerebral
- embolic (current episode) I63.4- ☑
- Erb (-Duchenne) (birth) (newborn) P14.Ø
- Erb's syphilitic spastic spinal A52.17
- esophagus K22.89
- eye muscle (extrinsic) H49.9
  - intrinsic — *see also* Paresis, of accommodation
- facial (nerve) G51.Ø
  - birth injury P11.3
  - congenital P11.3
  - following operation NEC — *see* Puncture, accidental complicating surgery
  - newborn (birth injury) P11.3
- familial (recurrent) (periodic) G72.3
  - spastic G11.4
- fauces J39.2
- finger G56.9- ☑
- gait R26.1
- gastric nerve (nondiabetic) G52.2
- gaze, conjugate H51.Ø
- general (progressive) (syphilitic) A52.17
  - juvenile A5Ø.45
- glottis J38.ØØ
  - bilateral J38.Ø2
  - unilateral J38.Ø1
- gluteal G54.1
- Gubler (-Millard) G46.3
- hand — *see* Monoplegia, upper limb
- heart — *see* Arrest, cardiac
- hemiplegic — *see* Hemiplegia
- hyperkalemic periodic (familial) G72.3
- hypoglossal (nerve) G52.3
- hypokalemic periodic G72.3
- hysterical F44.4
- ileus K56.Ø
- infantile — *see also* Poliomyelitis, paralytic A8Ø.3Ø
  - bulbar — *see* Poliomyelitis, paralytic
  - cerebral — *see* Palsy, cerebral
  - spastic — *see* Palsy, cerebral, spastic
- infective — *see* Poliomyelitis, paralytic
- inferior nuclear G83.9
- internuclear — *see* Ophthalmoplegia, internuclear
- intestine K56.Ø
- iris H57.Ø9
  - due to diphtheria (toxin) A36.89
- ischemic, Volkmann's (complicating trauma) T79.6 ☑
- Jackson's G83.89
- jake — *see* Poisoning, food, noxious, plant
- Jamaica ginger (jake) G62.2
- juvenile general A5Ø.45
- Klumpke (-Déjérine) (birth) (newborn) P14.1
- labioglossal (laryngeal) (pharyngeal) G12.29
- Landry's G61.Ø
- laryngeal nerve (recurrent) (superior) (unilateral) J38.ØØ
  - bilateral J38.Ø2
  - unilateral J38.Ø1
- larynx J38.ØØ
  - bilateral J38.Ø2
  - due to diphtheria (toxin) A36.2
  - unilateral J38.Ø1
- lateral G12.23
- lead T56.Ø ☑
- left side — *see* Hemiplegia
- leg G83.1- ☑
  - both — *see* Paraplegia
  - crossed G83.89
  - hysterical F44.4
  - psychogenic F44.4
  - transient or transitory R29.818
    - traumatic NEC — *see* Injury, nerve, leg
- levator palpebrae superioris — *see* Blepharoptosis, paralytic
- limb — *see* Monoplegia
- lip K13.Ø
- Lissauer's A52.17
- lower limb — *see* Monoplegia, lower limb
  - both — *see* Paraplegia

Paralysis, paralytic — *continued*
- lung J98.4
- median nerve G56.1- ☑
- medullary (tegmental) G83.89
- mesencephalic NEC G83.89
  - tegmental G83.89
- middle alternating G83.89
- Millard-Gubler-Foville G46.3
- monoplegic — *see* Monoplegia
- motor G83.9
- muscle, muscular NEC G72.89
  - due to nerve lesion G58.9
  - eye (extrinsic) H49.9
    - intrinsic — *see* Paresis, of accommodation
    - oblique — *see* Strabismus, paralytic, fourth nerve
  - iris sphincter H21.9
  - ischemic (Volkmann's) (complicating trauma) T79.6 ☑
  - progressive G12.21
  - progressive, spinal G12.25
  - pseudohypertrophic G71.Ø2
  - spinal progressive G12.25
- musculocutaneous nerve G56.9- ☑
- musculospiral G56.9- ☑
- nerve — *see also* Disorder, nerve
  - abducent — *see* Strabismus, paralytic, sixth nerve
  - accessory G52.8
  - auditory (except Deafness) H93.3 ☑
  - birth injury P14.9
  - cranial or cerebral G52.9
  - facial G51.Ø
    - birth injury P11.3
    - congenital P11.3
    - newborn (birth injury) P11.3
  - fourth or trochlear — *see* Strabismus, paralytic, fourth nerve
  - newborn (birth injury) P14.9
  - oculomotor — *see* Strabismus, paralytic, third nerve
  - phrenic (birth injury) P14.2
  - radial G56.3- ☑
  - seventh or facial G51.Ø
    - newborn (birth injury) P11.3
  - sixth or abducent — *see* Strabismus, paralytic, sixth nerve
  - syphilitic A52.15
  - third or oculomotor — *see* Strabismus, paralytic, third nerve
  - trigeminal G5Ø.9
  - trochlear — *see* Strabismus, paralytic, fourth nerve
  - ulnar G56.2- ☑
- normokalemic periodic G72.3
- ocular H49.9
  - alternating G83.89
- oculofacial, congenital (Moebius) Q87.Ø
- oculomotor (external bilateral) (nerve) — *see* Strabismus, paralytic, third nerve
- palate (soft) K13.79
- paratrigeminal G5Ø.9
- periodic (familial) (hyperkalemic) (hypokalemic) (myotonic) (normokalemic) (potassium sensitive) (secondary) G72.3
- peripheral autonomic nervous system — *see* Neuropathy, peripheral, autonomic
- peroneal (nerve) G57.3- ☑
- pharynx J39.2
- phrenic nerve G56.8- ☑
- plantar nerve(s) G57.6- ☑
- pneumogastric nerve G52.2
- poliomyelitis (current) — *see* Poliomyelitis, paralytic
- popliteal nerve G57.3- ☑
- postepileptic transitory G83.84
- progressive (atrophic) (bulbar) (spinal) G12.22
  - general A52.17
  - infantile acute — *see* Poliomyelitis, paralytic
  - supranuclear G23.1
- pseudobulbar G12.29
- pseudohypertrophic (muscle) — *see also* Dystrophy, muscular, by type, if applicable G71.Ø9
- psychogenic F44.4
- quadriceps G57.9- ☑
- quadriplegic — *see* Tetraplegia
- radial nerve G56.3- ☑
- rectus muscle (eye) H49.9
- recurrent isolated sleep G47.53
- respiratory (muscle) (system) (tract) RØ6.81
  - center NEC G93.89
  - congenital P28.89
  - newborn P28.89

Paralysis, paralytic — *continued*
- right side — *see* Hemiplegia
- saturnine T56.Ø ☑
- sciatic nerve G57.Ø- ☑
- senile G83.9
- shaking — *see* Parkinsonism
- shoulder G56.9- ☑
- sleep, recurrent isolated G47.53
- spastic G83.9
  - cerebral — *see* Palsy, cerebral, spastic
  - congenital (cerebral) — *see* Palsy, cerebral, spastic
  - familial G11.4
  - hereditary G11.4
  - quadriplegic G8Ø.Ø
  - syphilitic (spinal) A52.17
- sphincter, bladder — *see* Paralysis, bladder
- spinal (cord) G83.9
  - accessory nerve G52.8
  - acute — *see* Poliomyelitis, paralytic
  - ascending acute G61.Ø
  - atrophic (acute) — *see also* Poliomyelitis, paralytic
    - spastic, syphilitic A52.17
  - congenital NEC — *see* Palsy, cerebral
  - hereditary G95.89
  - infantile — *see* Poliomyelitis, paralytic
  - progressive G12.21
    - muscle G12.25
  - sequelae NEC G83.89
- sternomastoid G52.8
- stomach K31.84
  - diabetic — *see* Diabetes, by type, with gastroparesis
  - nerve G52.2
    - diabetic — *see* Diabetes, by type, with gastroparesis
- stroke — *see* Infarct, brain
- subcapsularis G56.8- ☑
- supranuclear (progressive) G23.1
- sympathetic G9Ø.8
  - cervical G9Ø.Ø9
  - nervous system — *see* Neuropathy, peripheral, autonomic
- syndrome G83.9
  - specified NEC G83.89
- syphilitic spastic spinal (Erb's) A52.17
- thigh G57.9- ☑
- throat J39.2
  - diphtheritic A36.Ø
  - muscle J39.2
- thrombotic (current episode) I63.3- ☑
- thumb G56.9- ☑
- tick — *see* Toxicity, venom, arthropod, specified NEC
- Todd's (postepileptic transitory paralysis) G83.84
- toe G57.6- ☑
- tongue K14.8
- transient R29.5
  - arm or leg NEC R29.818
  - traumatic NEC — *see* Injury, nerve
- trapezius G52.8
- traumatic, transient NEC — *see* Injury, nerve
- trembling — *see* Parkinsonism
- triceps brachii G56.9- ☑
- trigeminal nerve G5Ø.9
- trochlear (nerve) — *see* Strabismus, paralytic, fourth nerve
- ulnar nerve G56.2- ☑
- upper limb — *see* Monoplegia, upper limb
- uremic N18.9 *[G99.8]*
- uveoparotitic D86.89
- uvula K13.79
  - postdiphtheritic A36.Ø
- vagus nerve G52.2
- vasomotor NEC G9Ø.8
- velum palati K13.79
- vesical — *see* Paralysis, bladder
- vestibular nerve (except Vertigo) H93.3 ☑
- vocal cords J38.ØØ
  - bilateral J38.Ø2
  - unilateral J38.Ø1
- Volkmann's (complicating trauma) T79.6 ☑
- wasting G12.29
- Weber's G46.3
- wrist G56.9- ☑

Paramedial urethrovesical orifice Q64.79

Paramenia N92.6

Parametritis — *see also* Disease, pelvis, inflammatory N73.2
- acute N73.Ø

Parametritis — *continued*
- complicating abortion — *see* Abortion, by type, complicated by, parametritis

Parametrium, parametric — *see* condition
Paramnesia — *see* Amnesia
Paramolar KØØ.1
Paramyloidosis E85.89
Paramyoclonus multiplex G25.3
Paramyotonia (congenita) G71.19
Parangi — *see* Yaws
Paranoia (querulans) F22
- senile FØ3 ☑

Paranoid
- dementia (senile) FØ3 ☑
  - praecox — *see* Schizophrenia
- personality F6Ø.Ø
- psychosis (climacteric) (involutional) (menopausal) F22
  - psychogenic (acute) F23
  - senile FØ3 ☑
- reaction (acute) F23
  - chronic F22
- schizophrenia F2Ø.Ø
- state (climacteric) (involutional) (menopausal) (simple) F22
  - senile FØ3 ☑
- tendencies F6Ø.Ø
- traits F6Ø.Ø
- trends F6Ø.Ø
- type, psychopathic personality F6Ø.Ø

Paraparesis — *see* Paraplegia
Paraphasia R47.Ø2
Paraphilia F65.9
Paraphimosis (congenital) N47.2
- chancroidal A57

Paraphrenia, paraphrenic (late) F22
- schizophrenia F2Ø.Ø

Paraplegia (lower) G82.2Ø
- ataxic — *see* Degeneration, combined, spinal cord
- complete G82.21
- congenital (cerebral) G8Ø.8
  - spastic G8Ø.1
- familial spastic G11.4
- functional (hysterical) F44.4
- hereditary, spastic G11.4
- hysterical F44.4
- incomplete G82.22
- Pott's A18.Ø1
- psychogenic F44.4
- spastic
  - Erb's spinal, syphilitic A52.17
  - hereditary G11.4
  - tropical GØ4.1
- syphilitic (spastic) A52.17
- traumatic
  - current injury — code to injury with seventh character A
    - sequela of previous injury — code to injury with seventh character S
- tropical spastic GØ4.1

Parapoxvirus BØ8.6Ø
- specified NEC BØ8.69

Paraproteinemia D89.2
- benign (familial) D89.2
- monoclonal D47.2
- secondary to malignant disease D47.2

Parapsoriasis L41.9
- en plaques L41.4
- guttata L41.1
- large plaque L41.4
- retiform, retiformis L41.5
- small plaque L41.3
- specified NEC L41.8
- varioliformis (acuta) L41.Ø

Parasitic — *see also* condition
- disease NEC B89
- stomatitis B37.Ø
- sycosis (beard) (scalp) B35.Ø
- twin Q89.4

Parasitism B89
- intestinal B82.9
- skin B88.9
- specified — *see* Infestation

Parasitophobia F4Ø.218
Parasomnia G47.5Ø
- due to
  - alcohol
    - abuse F1Ø.182
    - dependence F1Ø.282
    - use F1Ø.982
  - amphetamines
    - abuse F15.182
    - dependence F15.282
    - use F15.982
  - caffeine
    - abuse F15.182
    - dependence F15.282
    - use F15.982
  - cocaine
    - abuse F14.182
    - dependence F14.282
    - use F14.982
  - drug NEC
    - abuse F19.182
    - dependence F19.282
    - use F19.982
  - opioid
    - abuse F11.182
    - dependence F11.282
    - use F11.982
  - psychoactive substance NEC
    - abuse F19.182
    - dependence F19.282
    - use F19.982
  - sedative, hypnotic, or anxiolytic
    - abuse F13.182
    - dependence F13.282
    - use F13.982
  - stimulant NEC
    - abuse F15.182
    - dependence F15.282
    - use F15.982
- in conditions classified elsewhere G47.54
- nonorganic origin F51.8
- organic G47.5Ø
- specified NEC G47.59

Paraspadias Q54.9
Paraspasmus facialis G51.8
Parasuicide (attempt)
- history of (personal) Z91.51
  - in family Z81.8

Parathyroid gland — *see* condition
Parathyroid tetany E2Ø.9
Paratrachoma A74.Ø
Paratyphilitis — *see* Appendicitis
Paratyphoid (fever) — *see* Fever, paratyphoid
Paratyphus — *see* Fever, paratyphoid
Paraurethral duct Q64.79
Paraurethritis — *see also* Urethritis
- gonococcal (acute) (chronic) (with abscess) A54.1

Paravaccinia NEC BØ8.Ø4
Paravaginitis — *see* Vaginitis
Parencephalitis — *see also* Encephalitis
- sequelae GØ9

Parent-child conflict — *see* Conflict, parent-child
- estrangement NEC Z62.89Ø

Paresis — *see also* Paralysis
- accommodation — *see* Paresis, of accommodation
- Bernhardt's G57.1- ☑
- bladder (sphincter) — *see also* Paralysis, bladder
  - tabetic A52.17
- bowel, colon or intestine K56.Ø
- extrinsic muscle, eye H49.9
- general (progressive) (syphilitic) A52.17
  - juvenile A5Ø.45
- heart — *see* Failure, heart
- insane (syphilitic) A52.17
- juvenile (general) A5Ø.45
- of accommodation H52.52- ☑
- peripheral progressive (idiopathic) G6Ø.3
- pseudohypertrophic — *see also* Dystrophy, muscular, by type, if applicable G71.Ø9
- senile G83.9
- syphilitic (general) A52.17
  - congenital A5Ø.45
- vesical NEC N31.2

Paresthesia — *see also* Disturbance, sensation, skin R2Ø.2
- Bernhardt G57.1- ☑

Paretic — *see* condition
Parinaud's
- conjunctivitis H1Ø.89
- oculoglandular syndrome H1Ø.89
- ophthalmoplegia H49.88- ☑

Parkinsonism (idiopathic) (primary) G2Ø
- with neurogenic orthostatic hypotension (symptomatic) G9Ø.3
- arteriosclerotic G21.4
- dementia — *see also* Dementia, in, diseases specified elsewhere G2Ø *[FØ2.8Ø]*
  - with behavioral disturbance — *see also* Dementia, in, diseases specified elsewhere G2Ø *[FØ2.81-]* ☑
- due to
  - drugs NEC G21.19
    - neuroleptic G21.11
- medication-induced NEC G21.19
- neuroleptic induced G21.11
- postencephalitic G21.3
- secondary G21.9
  - due to
    - arteriosclerosis G21.4
    - drugs NEC G21.19
      - neuroleptic G21.11
    - encephalitis G21.3
    - external agents NEC G21.2
    - syphilis A52.19
  - specified NEC G21.8
- syphilitic A52.19
- treatment-induced NEC G21.19
- vascular G21.4

Parkinson's disease, syndrome or tremor — *see* Parkinsonism
Parodontitis — *see* Periodontitis
Parodontosis KØ5.4
Paronychia — *see also* Cellulitis, digit
- with lymphangitis — *see* Lymphangitis, acute, digit
- candidal (chronic) B37.2
- tuberculous (primary) A18.4

Parorexia (psychogenic) F5Ø.89
Parosmia R43.1
- psychogenic F45.8

Parotid gland — *see* condition
Parotitis, parotiditis (allergic) (nonspecific toxic) (purulent) (septic) (suppurative) — *see also* Sialoadenitis
- epidemic — *see* Mumps
- infectious — *see* Mumps
- postoperative K91.89
- surgical K91.89

Parrot fever A7Ø
Parrot's disease (early congenital syphilitic pseudoparalysis) A5Ø.Ø2
Parry-Romberg syndrome G51.8
Parry's disease or syndrome EØ5.ØØ
- with thyroid storm EØ5.Ø1

Pars planitis — *see* Cyclitis
Parsonage (-Aldren)-**Turner syndrome** G54.5
Parson's disease (exophthalmic goiter) EØ5.ØØ
- with thyroid storm EØ5.Ø1

Particolored infant Q82.8
Parturition — *see* Delivery
Parulis KØ4.7
- with sinus KØ4.6

Parvovirus, as cause of disease classified elsewhere B97.6
Pasini and Pierini's atrophoderma L9Ø.3
Passage
- false, urethra N36.5
- meconium (newborn) during delivery PØ3.82
- of sounds or bougies — *see* Attention to, artificial, opening

Passive — *see* condition
- smoking Z77.22

Past due on rent or mortgage Z59.81- ☑
Pasteurella septica A28.Ø
Pasteurellosis — *see* Infection, Pasteurella
PAT (paroxysmal atrial tachycardia) I47.1
Patau's syndrome — *see* Trisomy, 13
Patches
- mucous (syphilitic) A51.39
  - congenital A5Ø.Ø7
- smokers' (mouth) K13.24

Patellar — *see* condition
Patent — *see also* Imperfect, closure
- canal of Nuck Q52.4
- cervix N88.3
- ductus arteriosus or Botallo's Q25.Ø
- foramen
  - botalli Q21.12
  - ovale Q21.12
- interauricular septum Q21.19

- **Patent** — *continued*
  - interventricular septum Q21.Ø
  - omphalomesenteric duct Q43.Ø
  - os (uteri) — *see* Patent, cervix
  - ostium secundum (type II) Q21.11
  - urachus Q64.4
  - vitelline duct Q43.Ø
- **Paterson** (-Brown) (-Kelly) **syndrome or web** D5Ø.1
- **Pathologic, pathological** — *see also* condition
  - asphyxia RØ9.Ø1
  - fire-setting F63.1
  - gambling F63.Ø
  - ovum OØ2.Ø
  - resorption, tooth KØ3.3
  - stealing F63.2
- **Pathology** (of) — *see* Disease
  - periradicular, associated with previous endodontic treatment NEC M27.59
- **Pattern, sleep-wake, irregular** G47.23
- **Patulous** — *see also* Imperfect, closure (congenital)
  - alimentary tract Q45.8
    - lower Q43.8
    - upper Q4Ø.8
  - eustachian tube H69.Ø- ☑
- **Pause, sinoatrial** I49.5
- **Paxton's disease** B36.2
- **Pearl(s)**
  - enamel KØØ.2
  - Epstein's KØ9.8
- **Pearl-worker's disease** — *see* Osteomyelitis, specified type NEC
- **Pectenosis** K62.4
- **Pectoral** — *see* condition
- **Pectus**
  - carinatum (congenital) Q67.7
    - acquired M95.4
    - rachitic sequelae (late effect) E64.3
  - excavatum (congenital) Q67.6
    - acquired M95.4
    - rachitic sequelae (late effect) E64.3
  - recurvatum (congenital) Q67.6
- **Pedatrophia** E41
- **Pederosis** F65.4
- **Pediatric inflammatory multisystem syndrome** M35.81
- **Pediculosis** (infestation) B85.2
  - capitis (head-louse) (any site) B85.Ø
  - corporis (body-louse) (any site) B85.1
  - eyelid B85.Ø
  - mixed (classifiable to more than one of the titles B85.Ø-B85.3) B85.4
  - pubis (pubic louse) (any site) B85.3
  - vestimenti B85.1
  - vulvae B85.3
- **Pediculus** (infestation) — *see* Pediculosis
- **Pedophilia** F65.4
- **Peg-shaped teeth** KØØ.2
- **Pelade** — *see* Alopecia, areata
- **Pelger-Huët anomaly or syndrome** D72.Ø
- **Peliosis** (rheumatica) D69.Ø
  - hepatis K76.4
    - with toxic liver disease K71.8
- **Pelizaeus-Merzbacher disease** E75.29
- **Pellagra** (alcoholic) (with polyneuropathy) E52
- **Pellagra-cerebellar-ataxia-renal aminoaciduria syndrome** E72.Ø2
- **Pellegrini** (-Stieda) **disease or syndrome** — *see* Bursitis, tibial collateral
- **Pellizzi's syndrome** E34.8
- **Pel's crisis** A52.11
- **Pelvic** — *see also* condition
  - examination (periodic) (routine) ZØ1.419
    - with abnormal findings ZØ1.411
  - kidney, congenital Q63.2
- **Pelviolithiasis** — *see* Calculus, kidney
- **Pelviperitonitis** — *see also* Peritonitis, pelvic
  - gonococcal A54.24
  - puerperal O85
- **Pelvis** — *see* condition or type
- **Pemphigoid** L12.9
  - benign, mucous membrane L12.1
  - bullous L12.Ø
  - cicatricial L12.1
  - juvenile L12.2
  - ocular L12.1
  - specified NEC L12.8
- **Pemphigus** L1Ø.9
  - benign familial (chronic) Q82.8
- **Pemphigus** — *continued*
  - Brazilian L1Ø.3
  - circinatus L13.Ø
  - conjunctiva L12.1
  - drug-induced L1Ø.5
  - erythematosus L1Ø.4
  - foliaceus L1Ø.2
  - gangrenous — *see* Gangrene
  - neonatorum LØ1.Ø3
  - ocular L12.1
  - paraneoplastic L1Ø.81
  - specified NEC L1Ø.89
  - syphilitic (congenital) A5Ø.Ø6
  - vegetans L1Ø.1
  - vulgaris L1Ø.Ø
  - wildfire L1Ø.3
- **Pendred's syndrome** EØ7.1
- **Pendulous**
  - abdomen, in pregnancy — *see* Pregnancy, complicated by, abnormal, pelvic organs or tissues NEC
  - breast N64.89
- **Penetrating wound** — *see also* Puncture
  - with internal injury — *see* Injury, by site
  - eyeball — *see* Puncture, eyeball
  - orbit (with or without foreign body) — *see* Puncture, orbit
  - uterus by instrument with or following ectopic or molar pregnancy OØ8.6
- **Penicillosis** B48.4
- **Penis** — *see* condition
- **Penitis** N48.29
- **Pentalogy of Fallot** Q21.8
- **Pentasomy X syndrome** Q97.1
- **Pentosuria** (essential) E74.89
- **Percreta placenta -** O43.23 ☑
- **Peregrinating patient** — *see* Disorder, factitious
- **Perforation, perforated** (nontraumatic) (of)
  - accidental during procedure (blood vessel) (nerve) (organ) — *see* Complication, accidental puncture or laceration
  - antrum — *see* Sinusitis, maxillary
  - appendix K35.32
    - with localized peritonitis K35.32
  - atrial septum, multiple Q21.19
  - attic, ear — *see* Perforation, tympanum, attic
  - bile duct (common) (hepatic) K83.2
    - cystic K82.2
  - bladder (urinary)
    - with or following ectopic or molar pregnancy OØ8.6
    - obstetrical trauma O71.5
    - traumatic S37.29 ☑
      - at delivery O71.5
  - bowel K63.1
    - with or following ectopic or molar pregnancy OØ8.6
    - newborn P78.Ø
    - obstetrical trauma O71.5
    - traumatic — *see* Laceration, intestine
  - broad ligament N83.8
    - with or following ectopic or molar pregnancy OØ8.6
    - obstetrical trauma O71.6
  - by
    - device, implant or graft — *see also* Complications, by site and type, mechanical T85.628 ☑
      - arterial graft NEC — *see* Complication, cardiovascular device, mechanical, vascular
      - breast (implant) T85.49 ☑
      - catheter NEC T85.698 ☑
        - cystostomy T83.Ø9Ø ☑
        - dialysis (renal) T82.49 ☑
          - intraperitoneal T85.691 ☑
        - infusion NEC T82.594 ☑
          - spinal (epidural) (subdural) T85.69Ø ☑
        - urinary — *see also* Complications, catheter, urinary T83.Ø98 ☑
      - electronic (electrode) (pulse generator) (stimulator)
        - bone T84.39Ø ☑
        - cardiac T82.199 ☑
          - electrode T82.19Ø ☑
          - pulse generator T82.191 ☑
          - specified type NEC T82.198 ☑
        - nervous system — *see* Complication, prosthetic device, mechanical, electronic nervous system stimulator
        - urinary — *see* Complication, genitourinary, device, urinary, mechanical
- **Perforation, perforated** — *continued*
  - by — *continued*
    - device, implant or graft — *see also* Complications, by site and type, mechanical — *continued*
      - fixation, internal (orthopedic) NEC — *see* Complication, fixation device, mechanical
      - gastrointestinal — *see* Complications, prosthetic device, mechanical, gastrointestinal device
      - genital NEC T83.498 ☑
        - intrauterine contraceptive device T83.39 ☑
        - penile prosthesis T83.49Ø ☑
      - heart NEC — *see* Complication, cardiovascular device, mechanical
      - joint prosthesis — *see* Complications, joint prosthesis, mechanical, specified NEC, by site
      - ocular NEC — *see* Complications, prosthetic device, mechanical, ocular device
      - orthopedic NEC — *see* Complication, orthopedic, device, mechanical
      - specified NEC T85.628 ☑
      - urinary NEC — *see also* Complication, genitourinary, device, urinary, mechanical
        - graft T83.29 ☑
      - vascular NEC — *see* Complication, cardiovascular device, mechanical
      - ventricular intracranial shunt T85.Ø9 ☑
    - foreign body left accidentally in operative wound T81.539 ☑
    - instrument (any) during a procedure, accidental — *see* Puncture, accidental complicating surgery
  - cecum K35.32
    - with localized peritonitis K35.32
  - cervix (uteri) N88.8
    - with or following ectopic or molar pregnancy OØ8.6
    - obstetrical trauma O71.3
  - colon K63.1
    - newborn P78.Ø
    - obstetrical trauma O71.5
    - traumatic — *see* Laceration, intestine, large
  - common duct (bile) K83.2
  - cornea (due to ulceration) — *see* Ulcer, cornea, perforated
  - cystic duct K82.2
  - diverticulum (intestine) K57.8Ø
    - with bleeding K57.81
    - large intestine K57.2Ø
      - with
        - bleeding K57.21
        - small intestine K57.4Ø
          - with bleeding K57.41
    - small intestine K57.ØØ
      - with
        - bleeding K57.Ø1
        - large intestine K57.4Ø
          - with bleeding K57.41
  - ear drum — *see* Perforation, tympanum
  - esophagus K22.3
  - ethmoidal sinus — *see* Sinusitis, ethmoidal
  - frontal sinus — *see* Sinusitis, frontal
  - gallbladder K82.2
  - heart valve — *see* Endocarditis
  - ileum K63.1
    - newborn P78.Ø
    - obstetrical trauma O71.5
    - traumatic — *see* Laceration, intestine, small
  - instrumental, surgical (accidental) (blood vessel) (nerve) (organ) — *see* Puncture, accidental complicating surgery
  - intestine NEC K63.1
    - with ectopic or molar pregnancy OØ8.6
    - newborn P78.Ø
    - obstetrical trauma O71.5
    - traumatic — *see* Laceration, intestine
    - ulcerative NEC K63.1
      - newborn P78.Ø
  - jejunum, jejunal K63.1
    - obstetrical trauma O71.5
    - traumatic — *see* Laceration, intestine, small
    - ulcer — *see* Ulcer, gastrojejunal, with perforation
  - joint prosthesis — *see* Complications, joint prosthesis, mechanical, specified NEC, by site
  - mastoid (antrum) (cell) — *see* Disorder, mastoid, specified NEC
  - maxillary sinus — *see* Sinusitis, maxillary
  - membrana tympani — *see* Perforation, tympanum
  - nasal
    - septum J34.89

- **Perforation, perforated** — *continued*
  - nasal — *continued*
    - septum — *continued*
      - congenital Q3Ø.3
      - syphilitic A52.73
    - sinus J34.89
      - congenital Q3Ø.8
      - due to sinusitis — *see* Sinusitis
  - palate — *see also* Cleft, palate Q35.9
    - syphilitic A52.79
  - palatine vault — *see also* Cleft, palate, hard Q35.1
    - syphilitic A52.79
      - congenital A5Ø.59
  - pars flaccida (ear drum) — *see* Perforation, tympanum, attic
  - pelvic
    - floor S31.Ø3Ø ☑
      - with
        - ectopic or molar pregnancy OØ8.6
        - penetration into retroperitoneal space S31.Ø31 ☑
        - retained foreign body S31.Ø4Ø ☑
          - with penetration into retroperitoneal space S31.Ø41 ☑
      - following ectopic or molar pregnancy OØ8.6
      - obstetrical trauma O7Ø.1
    - organ S37.99 ☑
      - adrenal gland S37.818 ☑
      - bladder — *see* Perforation, bladder
      - fallopian tube S37.599 ☑
        - bilateral S37.592 ☑
        - unilateral S37.591 ☑
      - kidney S37.Ø9- ☑
      - obstetrical trauma O71.5
      - ovary S37.499 ☑
        - bilateral S37.492 ☑
        - unilateral S37.491 ☑
      - prostate S37.828 ☑
      - specified organ NEC S37.898 ☑
      - ureter — *see* Perforation, ureter
      - urethra — *see* Perforation, urethra
      - uterus — *see* Perforation, uterus
  - perineum — *see* Laceration, perineum
  - pharynx J39.2
  - rectum K63.1
    - newborn P78.Ø
    - obstetrical trauma O71.5
    - traumatic S36.63 ☑
  - root canal space due to endodontic treatment M27.51
  - sigmoid K63.1
    - newborn P78.Ø
    - obstetrical trauma O71.5
    - traumatic S36.533 ☑
  - sinus (accessory) (chronic) (nasal) J34.89
  - sphenoidal sinus — *see* Sinusitis, sphenoidal
  - surgical (accidental) (by instrument) (blood vessel) (nerve) (organ) — *see* Puncture, accidental complicating surgery
  - traumatic
    - external — *see* Puncture
    - eye — *see* Puncture, eyeball
    - internal organ — *see* Injury, by site
  - tympanum, tympanic (membrane) (persistent post-traumatic) (postinflammatory) H72.9- ☑
    - attic H72.1- ☑
      - multiple — *see* Perforation, tympanum, multiple
      - total — *see* Perforation, tympanum, total
    - central H72.Ø- ☑
      - multiple — *see* Perforation, tympanum, multiple
      - total — *see* Perforation, tympanum, total
    - marginal NEC — *see* subcategory H72.2 ☑
    - multiple H72.81- ☑
    - pars flaccida — *see* Perforation, tympanum, attic
    - total H72.82- ☑
    - traumatic, current episode SØ9.2- ☑
  - typhoid, gastrointestinal — *see* Typhoid
  - ulcer — *see* Ulcer, by site, with perforation
  - ureter N28.89
    - traumatic S37.19 ☑
  - urethra N36.8
    - with ectopic or molar pregnancy OØ8.6
    - following ectopic or molar pregnancy OØ8.6
    - obstetrical trauma O71.5
    - traumatic S37.39 ☑
      - at delivery O71.5
  - uterus
    - with ectopic or molar pregnancy OØ8.6

- **Perforation, perforated** — *continued*
  - uterus — *continued*
    - by intrauterine contraceptive device T83.39 ☑
    - following ectopic or molar pregnancy OØ8.6
    - obstetrical trauma O71.1
    - traumatic S37.69 ☑
      - obstetric O71.1
  - uvula K13.79
    - syphilitic A52.79
  - vagina O71.4
    - obstetrical trauma O71.4
    - other trauma — *see* Puncture, vagina
- **Periadenitis mucosa necrotica recurrens** K12.Ø
- **Periappendicitis** (acute) — *see* Appendicitis
- **Periarteritis nodosa** (disseminated) (infectious) (necrotizing) M3Ø.Ø
- **Periarthritis** (joint) — *see also* Enthesopathy
  - Duplay's M75.Ø- ☑
  - gonococcal A54.42
  - humeroscapularis — *see* Capsulitis, adhesive
  - scapulohumeral — *see* Capsulitis, adhesive
  - shoulder — *see* Capsulitis, adhesive
  - wrist M77.2- ☑
- **Periarthrosis** (angioneural) — *see* Enthesopathy
- **Pericapsulitis, adhesive** (shoulder) — *see* Capsulitis, adhesive
- **Pericarditis** (with decompensation) (with effusion) I31.9
  - with rheumatic fever (conditions in IØØ)
    - active — *see* Pericarditis, rheumatic
    - inactive or quiescent IØ9.2
  - acute (hemorrhagic) (nonrheumatic) (Sicca) I3Ø.9
    - with chorea (acute) (rheumatic) (Sydenham's) IØ2.Ø
    - benign I3Ø.8
    - nonspecific I3Ø.Ø
    - rheumatic IØ1.Ø
      - with chorea (acute) (Sydenham's) IØ2.Ø
  - adhesive or adherent (chronic) (external) (internal) I31.Ø
    - acute — *see* Pericarditis, acute
    - rheumatic IØ9.2
  - bacterial (acute) (subacute) (with serous or seropurulent effusion) I3Ø.1
  - calcareous I31.1
  - cholesterol (chronic) I31.8
    - acute I3Ø.9
  - chronic (nonrheumatic) I31.9
    - rheumatic IØ9.2
  - constrictive (chronic) I31.1
  - coxsackie B33.23
  - fibrinocaseous (tuberculous) A18.84
  - fibrinopurulent I3Ø.1
  - fibrinous I3Ø.8
  - fibrous I31.Ø
  - gonococcal A54.83
  - idiopathic I3Ø.Ø
  - in systemic lupus erythematosus M32.12
  - infective I3Ø.1
  - meningococcal A39.53
  - neoplastic (chronic) I31.8
    - acute I3Ø.9
  - obliterans, obliterating I31.Ø
  - plastic I31.Ø
  - pneumococcal I3Ø.1
  - postinfarction I24.1
  - purulent I3Ø.1
  - rheumatic (active) (acute) (with effusion) (with pneumonia) IØ1.Ø
    - with chorea (acute) (rheumatic) (Sydenham's) IØ2.Ø
    - chronic or inactive (with chorea) IØ9.2
  - rheumatoid — *see* Rheumatoid, carditis
  - septic I3Ø.1
  - serofibrinous I3Ø.8
  - staphylococcal I3Ø.1
  - streptococcal I3Ø.1
  - suppurative I3Ø.1
  - syphilitic A52.Ø6
  - tuberculous A18.84
  - uremic N18.9 *[I32]*
  - viral I3Ø.1
- **Pericardium, pericardial** — *see* condition
- **Pericellulitis** — *see* Cellulitis
- **Pericementitis** (chronic) (suppurative) — *see also* Periodontitis
  - acute KØ5.2Ø
    - generalized — *see* Periodontitis, aggressive, generalized
    - localized — *see* Periodontitis, aggressive, localized
- **Perichondritis**
  - auricle — *see* Perichondritis, ear

- **Perichondritis** — *continued*
  - bronchus J98.Ø9
  - ear (external) H61.ØØ- ☑
    - acute H61.Ø1- ☑
    - chronic H61.Ø2- ☑
  - external auditory canal — *see* Perichondritis, ear
  - larynx J38.7
    - syphilitic A52.73
    - typhoid AØ1.Ø9
  - nose J34.89
  - pinna — *see* Perichondritis, ear
  - trachea J39.8
- **Periclasia** KØ5.4
- **Pericoronitis** — *see* Periodontitis
- **Pericystitis** N3Ø.9Ø
  - with hematuria N3Ø.91
- **Peridiverticulitis** (intestine) K57.92
  - cecum — *see* Diverticulitis, intestine, large
  - colon — *see* Diverticulitis, intestine, large
  - duodenum — *see* Diverticulitis, intestine, small
  - intestine — *see* Diverticulitis, intestine
  - jejunum — *see* Diverticulitis, intestine, small
  - rectosigmoid — *see* Diverticulitis, intestine, large
  - rectum — *see* Diverticulitis, intestine, large
  - sigmoid — *see* Diverticulitis, intestine, large
- **Periendocarditis** — *see* Endocarditis
- **Periepididymitis** N45.1
- **Perifolliculitis** LØ1.Ø2
  - abscedens, caput, scalp L66.3
  - capitis, abscedens (et suffodiens) L66.3
  - superficial pustular LØ1.Ø2
- **Perihepatitis** K65.8
- **Perilabyrinthitis** (acute) — *see* subcategory H83.Ø ☑
- **Perimeningitis** — *see* Meningitis
- **Perimetritis** — *see* Endometritis
- **Perimetrosalpingitis** — *see* Salpingo-oophoritis
- **Perineocele** N81.81
- **Perinephric, perinephritic** — *see* condition
- **Perinephritis** — *see also* Infection, kidney
  - purulent — *see* Abscess, kidney
- **Perineum, perineal** — *see* condition
- **Perineuritis NEC** — *see* Neuralgia
- **Periodic** — *see* condition
- **Periodontitis** (chronic) (complex) (compound) (local) (simplex) KØ5.3Ø
  - acute KØ5.2Ø
    - generalized KØ5.229
      - moderate KØ5.222
      - severe KØ5.223
      - slight KØ5.221
    - localized KØ5.219
      - moderate KØ5.212
      - severe KØ5.213
      - slight KØ5.211
  - aggressive KØ5.2Ø
    - generalized KØ5.229
      - moderate KØ5.222
      - severe KØ5.223
      - slight KØ5.221
    - localized KØ5.219
      - moderate KØ5.212
      - severe KØ5.213
      - slight KØ5.211
  - apical KØ4.5
    - acute (pulpal origin) KØ4.4
  - generalized KØ5.329
    - moderate KØ5.322
    - severe KØ5.323
    - slight KØ5.321
  - localized KØ5.319
    - moderate KØ5.312
    - severe KØ5.313
    - slight KØ5.311
- **Periodontoclasia** KØ5.4
- **Periodontosis** (juvenile) KØ5.4
- **Periods** — *see also* Menstruation
  - heavy N92.Ø
  - irregular N92.6
  - shortened intervals (irregular) N92.1
- **Perionychia** — *see also* Cellulitis, digit
  - with lymphangitis — *see* Lymphangitis, acute, digit
- **Perioophoritis** — *see* Salpingo-oophoritis
- **Periorchitis** N45.2
- **Periosteum, periosteal** — *see* condition
- **Periostitis** (albuminosa) (circumscribed) (diffuse) (infective) (monomelic) — *see also* Osteomyelitis
  - alveolar M27.3

Periostitis — *continued*
- alveolodental M27.3
- dental M27.3
- gonorrheal A54.43
- jaw (lower) (upper) M27.2
- orbit H05.03- ☑
- syphilitic A52.77
  - congenital (early) A50.02 *[M90.80]*
  - secondary A51.46
- tuberculous — *see* Tuberculosis, bone
- yaws (hypertrophic) (early) (late) A66.6 *[M90.80]*

Periostosis (hyperplastic) — *see also* Disorder, bone, specified type NEC
- with osteomyelitis — *see* Osteomyelitis, specified type NEC

Peripartum
- cardiomyopathy O90.3

Periphlebitis — *see* Phlebitis
Periproctitis K62.89
Periprostatitis — *see* Prostatitis
Perirectal — *see* condition
Perirenal — *see* condition
Perisalpingitis — *see* Salpingo-oophoritis
Perisplenitis (infectional) D73.89
Peristalsis, visible or reversed R19.2
Peritendinitis — *see* Enthesopathy
Peritoneum, peritoneal — *see* condition
Peritonitis (adhesive) (bacterial) (fibrinous) (hemorrhagic) (idiopathic) (localized) (perforative) (primary) (with adhesions) (with effusion) K65.9
- with or following
  - abscess K65.1
  - appendicitis
    - with perforation or rupture K35.32
    - generalized — *see also* Appendicitis K35.20
    - localized — *see also* Appendicitis K35.30
  - diverticular disease (intestine) K57.80
    - with bleeding K57.81
    - ectopic or molar pregnancy O08.0
    - large intestine K57.20
      - with
        - bleeding K57.21
        - small intestine K57.40
          - with bleeding K57.41
    - small intestine K57.00
      - with
        - bleeding K57.01
        - large intestine K57.40
          - with bleeding K57.41
- acute (generalized) K65.0
- aseptic T81.61 ☑
- bile, biliary K65.3
- chemical T81.61 ☑
- chlamydial A74.81
- chronic proliferative K65.8
- complicating abortion — *see* Abortion, by type, complicated by, pelvic peritonitis
- congenital P78.1
- diaphragmatic K65.0
- diffuse K65.0
- diphtheritic A36.89
- disseminated K65.0
- due to
  - bile K65.3
  - foreign
    - body or object accidentally left during a procedure (instrument) (sponge) (swab) T81.599 ☑
    - substance accidentally left during a procedure (chemical) (powder) (talc) T81.61 ☑
  - talc T81.61 ☑
  - urine K65.8
- eosinophilic K65.8
  - acute K65.0
- fibrocaseous (tuberculous) A18.31
- fibropurulent K65.0
- following ectopic or molar pregnancy O08.0
- general (ized) K65.0
- gonococcal A54.85
- meconium (newborn) P78.0
- neonatal P78.1
  - meconium P78.0
- pancreatic K65.0
- paroxysmal, familial E85.0
  - benign E85.0
- pelvic
  - female N73.5
    - acute N73.3

Peritonitis — *continued*
- pelvic — *continued*
  - female — *continued*
    - chronic N73.4
      - with adhesions N73.6
  - male K65.0
- periodic, familial E85.0
- proliferative, chronic K65.8
- puerperal, postpartum, childbirth O85
- purulent K65.0
- septic K65.0
- specified NEC K65.8
- spontaneous bacterial K65.2
- subdiaphragmatic K65.0
- subphrenic K65.0
- suppurative K65.0
- syphilitic A52.74
  - congenital (early) A50.08 *[K67]*
- talc T81.61 ☑
- tuberculous A18.31
- urine K65.8

Peritonsillar — *see* condition
Peritonsillitis J36
Perityphlitis — *see also* Cecitis K37
Periureteritis N28.89
Periurethral — *see* condition
Periurethritis (gangrenous) — *see* Urethritis
Periuterine — *see* condition
Perivaginitis — *see* Vaginitis
Perivasculitis, retinal H35.06- ☑
Perivasitis (chronic) N49.1
Perivesiculitis (seminal) — *see* Vesiculitis
Perlèche NEC K13.0
- due to
  - candidiasis B37.83
  - moniliasis B37.83
  - riboflavin deficiency E53.0
  - vitamin B2 (riboflavin) deficiency E53.0

Pernicious — *see* condition
Pernio, perniosis T69.1 ☑
Perpetrator (of abuse) — *see* Index to External Causes of Injury, Perpetrator
Persecution
- delusion F22
- social Z60.5

Perseveration (tonic) R48.8
Persistence, persistent (congenital)
- anal membrane Q42.3
  - with fistula Q42.2
- arteria stapedia Q16.3
- atrioventricular canal Q21.20
- branchial cleft NOS Q18.2
  - cyst Q18.0
  - fistula Q18.0
  - sinus Q18.0
- bulbus cordis in left ventricle Q21.8
- canal of Cloquet Q14.0
- capsule (opaque) Q12.8
- cilioretinal artery or vein Q14.8
- cloaca Q43.7
- communication — *see* Fistula, congenital
- convolutions
  - aortic arch Q25.46
  - fallopian tube Q50.6
  - oviduct Q50.6
  - uterine tube Q50.6
- double aortic arch Q25.45
- ductus arteriosus (Botalli) Q25.0
- fetal
  - circulation P29.38
  - form of cervix (uteri) Q51.828
  - hemoglobin, hereditary (HPFH) D56.4
- foramen
  - Botalli Q21.12
  - ovale Q21.12
- Gartner's duct Q52.4
- hemoglobin, fetal (hereditary) (HPFH) D56.4
- hyaloid
  - artery (generally incomplete) Q14.0
  - system Q14.8
- hymen, in pregnancy or childbirth — *see* Pregnancy, complicated by, abnormal, vulva
- lanugo Q84.2
- left
  - posterior cardinal vein Q26.8
  - root with right arch of aorta Q25.49
  - superior vena cava Q26.1
- Meckel's diverticulum Q43.0

Persistence, persistent — *continued*
- Meckel's diverticulum — *continued*
  - malignant — *see* Table of Neoplasms, small intestine, malignant
- mucosal disease (middle ear) — *see* Otitis, media, suppurative, chronic, tubotympanic
- nail(s), anomalous Q84.6
- omphalomesenteric duct Q43.0
- organ or site not listed — *see* Anomaly, by site
- ostium
  - atrioventriculare commune Q21.23
  - primum Q21.20
  - secundum Q21.11
- ovarian rests in fallopian tube Q50.6
- pancreatic tissue in intestinal tract Q43.8
- primary (deciduous)
  - teeth K00.6
  - vitreous hyperplasia Q14.0
- pupillary membrane Q13.89
- rhesus (Rh) titer — *see* Complication(s), transfusion, incompatibility reaction, Rh (factor)
- right aortic arch Q25.47
- sinus
  - urogenitalis
    - female Q52.8
    - male Q55.8
  - venosus with imperfect incorporation in right auricle Q26.8
- thymus (gland) (hyperplasia) E32.0
- thyroglossal duct Q89.2
- thyrolingual duct Q89.2
- truncus arteriosus or communis Q20.0
- tunica vasculosa lentis Q12.2
- umbilical sinus Q64.4
- urachus Q64.4
- vitelline duct Q43.0

Person (with)
- admitted for clinical research, as a control subject (normal comparison) (participant) Z00.6
- awaiting admission to adequate facility elsewhere Z75.1
- concern (normal) about sick person in family Z63.6
- consulting on behalf of another Z71.0
- feigning illness Z76.5
- living (in)
  - alone Z60.2
  - boarding school Z59.3
  - residential institution Z59.3
  - without
    - adequate housing (heating) (space) Z59.1
    - housing (permanent) (temporary) Z59.00
    - person able to render necessary care Z74.2
    - shelter Z59.02
- on waiting list Z75.1
- sick or handicapped in family Z63.6

Personality (disorder) F60.9
- accentuation of traits (type A pattern) Z73.1
- affective F34.0
- aggressive F60.3
- amoral F60.2
- anacastic, anankastic F60.5
- antisocial F60.2
- anxious F60.6
- asocial F60.2
- asthenic F60.7
- avoidant F60.6
- borderline F60.3
- change due to organic condition (enduring) F07.0
- compulsive F60.5
- cycloid F34.0
- cyclothymic F34.0
- dependent F60.7
- depressive F34.1
- dissocial F60.2
- dual F44.81
- eccentric F60.89
- emotionally unstable F60.3
- expansive paranoid F60.0
- explosive F60.3
- fanatic F60.0
- haltlose type F60.89
- histrionic F60.4
- hyperthymic F34.0
- hypothymic F34.1
- hysterical F60.4
- immature F60.89
- inadequate F60.7
- labile (emotional) F60.3
- mixed (nonspecific) F60.89

- **Personality** — *continued*
  - morally defective F6Ø.2
  - multiple F44.81
  - narcissistic F6Ø.81
  - obsessional F6Ø.5
  - obsessive (-compulsive) F6Ø.5
  - organic FØ7.Ø
  - overconscientious F6Ø.5
  - paranoid F6Ø.Ø
  - passive (-dependent) F6Ø.7
  - passive-aggressive F6Ø.89
  - pathologic F6Ø.9
  - pattern defect or disturbance F6Ø.9
  - pseudopsychopathic (organic) FØ7.Ø
  - pseudoretarded (organic) FØ7.Ø
  - psychoinfantile F6Ø.4
  - psychoneurotic NEC F6Ø.89
  - psychopathic F6Ø.2
  - querulant F6Ø.Ø
  - sadistic F6Ø.89
  - schizoid F6Ø.1
  - self-defeating F6Ø.89
  - sensitive paranoid F6Ø.Ø
  - sociopathic (amoral) (antisocial) (asocial) (dissocial) F6Ø.2
  - specified NEC F6Ø.89
  - type A Z73.1
  - unstable (emotional) F6Ø.3
- **Perthes' disease** — *see* Legg-Calvé-Perthes disease
- **Pertussis** — *see also* Whooping cough A37.9Ø
- **Perversion, perverted**
  - appetite F5Ø.89
    - psychogenic F5Ø.89
  - function
    - pituitary gland E23.2
      - posterior lobe E22.2
  - sense of smell and taste R43.8
    - psychogenic F45.8
  - sexual — *see* Deviation, sexual
- **Pervious, congenital** — *see also* Imperfect, closure
  - ductus arteriosus Q25.Ø
- **Pes** (congenital) — *see also* Talipes
  - acquired — *see also* Deformity, limb, foot, specified NEC
    - planus — *see* Deformity, limb, flat foot
  - adductus Q66.89
  - cavus Q66.7- ☑
  - deformity NEC, acquired — *see* Deformity, limb, foot, specified NEC
  - planus (acquired) (any degree) — *see also* Deformity, limb, flat foot
    - rachitic sequelae (late effect) E64.3
  - valgus Q66.6
- **Pest, pestis** — *see* Plague
- **Petechia, petechiae** R23.3
  - newborn P54.5
- **Petechial typhus** A75.9
- **Peter's anomaly** Q13.4
- **Petit mal seizure** — *see* Epilepsy, childhood, absence
- **Petit's hernia** — *see* Hernia, abdomen, specified site NEC
- **Petrellidosis** B48.2
- **Petrositis** H7Ø.2Ø- ☑
  - acute H7Ø.21- ☑
  - chronic H7Ø.22- ☑
- **Peutz-Jeghers disease or syndrome** Q85.89
- **Peyronie's disease** N48.6
- **PFAPA** (periodic fever, aphthous stomatitis, pharyngitis, and adenopathy syndrome) MØ4.8
- **Pfeiffer's disease** — *see* Mononucleosis, infectious
- **Phagedena** (dry) (moist) (sloughing) — *see also* Gangrene
  - geometric L88
  - penis N48.29
  - tropical — *see* Ulcer, skin
  - vulva N76.6
- **Phagedenic** — *see* condition
- **Phakoma** H35.89
- **Phakomatosis** — *see also* specific eponymous syndromes Q85.9
  - Bourneville's Q85.1
  - specified NEC Q85.89
- **Phantom limb syndrome** (without pain) G54.7
  - with pain G54.6
- **Pharyngeal pouch syndrome** D82.1
- **Pharyngitis** (acute) (catarrhal) (gangrenous) (infective) (malignant) (membranous) (phlegmonous) (pseudomembranous) (simple) (subacute) (suppurative) (ulcerative) (viral) JØ2.9
- **Pharyngitis** — *continued*
  - with influenza, flu, or grippe — *see* Influenza, with, pharyngitis
  - aphthous BØ8.5
  - atrophic J31.2
  - chlamydial A56.4
  - chronic (atrophic) (granular) (hypertrophic) J31.2
  - coxsackievirus BØ8.5
  - diphtheritic A36.Ø
  - enteroviral vesicular BØ8.5
  - follicular (chronic) J31.2
  - fusospirochetal A69.1
  - gonococcal A54.5
  - granular (chronic) J31.2
  - herpesviral BØØ.2
  - hypertrophic J31.2
  - infectional, chronic J31.2
  - influenzal — *see* Influenza, with, respiratory manifestations NEC
  - lymphonodular, acute (enteroviral) BØ8.8
  - pneumococcal JØ2.8
  - purulent JØ2.9
  - putrid JØ2.9
  - septic JØ2.Ø
  - sicca J31.2
  - specified organism NEC JØ2.8
  - staphylococcal JØ2.8
  - streptococcal JØ2.Ø
  - syphilitic, congenital (early) A5Ø.Ø3
  - tuberculous A15.8
  - vesicular, enteroviral BØ8.5
  - viral NEC JØ2.8
- **Pharyngoconjunctivitis, viral** B3Ø.2
- **Pharyngolaryngitis** (acute) JØ6.Ø
  - chronic J37.Ø
- **Pharyngoplegia** J39.2
- **Pharyngotonsillitis, herpesviral** BØØ.2
- **Pharyngotracheitis, chronic** J42
- **Pharynx, pharyngeal** — *see* condition
- **Phencyclidine-induced**
  - anxiety disorder F16.98Ø
  - bipolar and related disorder F16.94
  - depressive disorder F16.94
  - psychotic disorder F16.959
- **Phenomenon**
  - Arthus' — *see* Arthus' phenomenon
  - jaw-winking QØ7.8
  - lupus erythematosus (LE) cell M32.9
  - Raynaud's (secondary) I73.ØØ
    - with gangrene I73.Ø1
  - vasomotor R55
  - vasospastic I73.9
  - vasovagal R55
  - Wenckebach's I44.1
- **Phenylketonuria** E7Ø.1
  - classical E7Ø.Ø
  - maternal E7Ø.1
- **Pheochromoblastoma**
  - specified site — *see* Neoplasm, malignant, by site
  - unspecified site C74.1Ø
- **Pheochromocytoma**
  - malignant
    - specified site — *see* Neoplasm, malignant, by site
    - unspecified site C74.1Ø
  - specified site — *see* Neoplasm, benign, by site
  - unspecified site D35.ØØ
- **Pheohyphomycosis** — *see* Chromomycosis
- **Pheomycosis** — *see* Chromomycosis
- **Phimosis** (congenital) (due to infection) N47.1
  - chancroidal A57
- **Phlebectasia** — *see also* Varix
  - congenital Q27.4
- **Phlebitis** (infective) (pyemic) (septic) (suppurative) I8Ø.9
  - antepartum — *see* Thrombophlebitis, antepartum
  - blue — *see* Phlebitis, leg, deep
  - breast, superficial I8Ø.8
  - calf muscular vein (NOS) I8Ø.25- ☑
  - cavernous (venous) sinus — *see* Phlebitis, intracranial (venous) sinus
  - cerebral (venous) sinus — *see* Phlebitis, intracranial (venous) sinus
  - chest wall, superficial I8Ø.8
  - cranial (venous) sinus — *see* Phlebitis, intracranial (venous) sinus
  - deep (vessels) — *see* Phlebitis, leg, deep
  - due to implanted device — *see* Complications, by site and type, specified NEC
  - during or resulting from a procedure T81.72 ☑
- **Phlebitis** — *continued*
  - femoral vein (superficial) I8Ø.1- ☑
  - femoropopliteal vein I8Ø.Ø- ☑
  - gastrocnemial vein I8Ø.25- ☑
  - gestational — *see* Phlebopathy, gestational
  - hepatic veins I8Ø.8
  - iliac vein (common) (external) (internal) I8Ø.21- ☑
  - iliofemoral — *see* Phlebitis, femoral vein
  - intracranial (venous) sinus (any) GØ8
    - nonpyogenic I67.6
  - intraspinal venous sinuses and veins GØ8
    - nonpyogenic G95.19
  - lateral (venous) sinus — *see* Phlebitis, intracranial (venous) sinus
  - leg I8Ø.3
    - antepartum — *see* Thrombophlebitis, antepartum
    - deep (vessels) NEC I8Ø.2Ø- ☑
      - iliac I8Ø.21- ☑
      - popliteal vein I8Ø.22- ☑
      - specified vessel NEC I8Ø.29- ☑
      - tibial vein (anterior) (posterior) I8Ø.23- ☑
    - femoral vein (superficial) I8Ø.1- ☑
    - superficial (vessels) I8Ø.Ø- ☑
  - longitudinal sinus — *see* Phlebitis, intracranial (venous) sinus
  - lower limb — *see* Phlebitis, leg
  - migrans, migrating (superficial) I82.1
  - pelvic
    - with ectopic or molar pregnancy OØ8.Ø
    - following ectopic or molar pregnancy OØ8.Ø
    - puerperal, postpartum O87.1
  - peroneal vein I8Ø.24- ☑
  - popliteal vein — *see* Phlebitis, leg, deep, popliteal
  - portal (vein) K75.1
  - postoperative T81.72 ☑
  - pregnancy — *see* Thrombophlebitis, antepartum
  - puerperal, postpartum, childbirth O87.Ø
    - deep O87.1
    - pelvic O87.1
    - superficial O87.Ø
  - retina — *see* Vasculitis, retina
  - saphenous (accessory) (great) (long) (small) — *see* Phlebitis, leg, superficial
  - sinus (meninges) — *see* Phlebitis, intracranial (venous) sinus
  - soleal vein I8Ø.25- ☑
  - specified site NEC I8Ø.8
  - syphilitic A52.Ø9
  - tibial vein — *see* Phlebitis, leg, deep, tibial
  - ulcerative I8Ø.9
    - leg — *see* Phlebitis, leg
  - umbilicus I8Ø.8
  - uterus (septic) — *see* Endometritis
  - varicose (leg) (lower limb) — *see* Varix, leg, with, inflammation
- **Phlebofibrosis** I87.8
- **Phleboliths** I87.8
- **Phlebopathy,**
  - gestational O22.9- ☑
  - puerperal O87.9
- **Phlebosclerosis** I87.8
- **Phlebothrombosis** — *see also* Thrombosis
  - antepartum — *see* Thrombophlebitis, antepartum
  - pregnancy — *see* Thrombophlebitis, antepartum
  - puerperal — *see* Thrombophlebitis, puerperal
- **Phlebotomus fever** A93.1
- **Phlegmasia**
  - alba dolens O87.1
    - nonpuerperal — *see* Phlebitis, femoral vein
  - cerulea dolens — *see* Phlebitis, leg, deep
- **Phlegmon** — *see* Abscess
- **Phlegmonous** — *see* condition
- **Phlyctenulosis** (allergic) (keratoconjunctivitis) (nontuberculous) — *see also* Keratoconjunctivitis
  - cornea — *see* Keratoconjunctivitis
  - tuberculous A18.52
- **Phobia, phobic** F4Ø.9
  - animal F4Ø.218
    - spiders F4Ø.21Ø
  - examination F4Ø.298
  - reaction F4Ø.9
  - simple F4Ø.298
  - social F4Ø.1Ø
    - generalized F4Ø.11
  - specific (isolated) F4Ø.298
    - animal F4Ø.218
      - spiders F4Ø.21Ø

- **Pleuralgia** RØ7.81
- **Pleurisy** (acute) (adhesive) (chronic) (costal) (diaphragmatic) (double) (dry) (fibrinous) (fibrous) (interlobar) (latent) (plastic) (primary) (residual) (sicca) (sterile) (subacute) (unresolved) RØ9.1
  - with
    - adherent pleura J86.Ø
    - effusion J9Ø
      - chylous, chyliform J94.Ø
      - tuberculous (non primary) A15.6
        - primary (progressive) A15.7
    - tuberculosis — *see* Pleurisy, tuberculous (non primary)
  - encysted — *see* Pleurisy, with effusion
  - exudative — *see* Pleurisy, with effusion
  - fibrinopurulent, fibropurulent — *see* Pyothorax
  - hemorrhagic — *see* Hemothorax
  - pneumococcal J9Ø
  - purulent — *see* Pyothorax
  - septic — *see* Pyothorax
  - serofibrinous — *see* Pleurisy, with effusion
  - seropurulent — *see* Pyothorax
  - serous — *see* Pleurisy, with effusion
  - staphylococcal J86.9
  - streptococcal J9Ø
  - suppurative — *see* Pyothorax
  - traumatic (post) (current) — *see* Injury, intrathoracic, pleura
  - tuberculous (with effusion) (non primary) A15.6
    - primary (progressive) A15.7
- **Pleuritis sicca** — *see* Pleurisy
- **Pleurobronchopneumonia** — *see* Pneumonia, broncho-
- **Pleurodynia** RØ7.81
  - epidemic B33.Ø
  - viral B33.Ø
- **Pleuropericarditis** — *see also* Pericarditis
  - acute I3Ø.9
- **Pleuropneumonia** (acute) (bilateral) (double) (septic) — *see also* Pneumonia J18.8
  - chronic — *see* Fibrosis, lung
- **Pleuro-pneumonia-like-organism** (PPLO), as cause of disease classified elsewhere B96.Ø
- **Pleurorrhea** — *see* Pleurisy, with effusion
- **Plexitis, brachial** G54.Ø
- **Plica**
  - polonica B85.Ø
  - syndrome, knee M67.5- ☑
  - tonsil J35.8
- **Plicated tongue** K14.5
- **Plug**
  - bronchus NEC J98.Ø9
  - meconium (newborn) NEC syndrome P76.Ø
  - mucus — *see* Asphyxia, mucus
- **Plumbism** — *see* subcategory T56.Ø ☑
- **Plummer's disease** EØ5.2Ø
  - with thyroid storm EØ5.21
- **Plummer-Vinson syndrome** D5Ø.1
- **Pluricarential syndrome of infancy** E4Ø
- **Plus** (and minus) **hand** (intrinsic) — *see* Deformity, limb, specified type NEC, forearm
- **PMEI** (polymorphic epilepsy in infancy) G4Ø.83- ☑
- **Pneumathemia** — *see* Air, embolism
- **Pneumatic hammer** (drill) syndrome T75.21 ☑
- **Pneumatocele** (lung) J98.4
  - intracranial G93.89
  - tension J44.9
- **Pneumatosis**
  - cystoides intestinalis K63.89
  - intestinalis K63.89
  - peritonei K66.8
- **Pneumaturia** R39.89
- **Pneumoblastoma** — *see* Neoplasm, lung, malignant
- **Pneumocephalus** G93.89
- **Pneumococcemia** A4Ø.3
- **Pneumococcus, pneumococcal** — *see* condition
- **Pneumoconiosis** (due to) (inhalation of) J64
  - with tuberculosis (any type in A15) J65
  - aluminum J63.Ø
  - asbestos J61
  - bagasse, bagassosis J67.1
  - bauxite J63.1
  - beryllium J63.2
  - coal miners' (simple) J6Ø
  - coalworkers' (simple) J6Ø
  - collier's J6Ø
  - cotton dust J66.Ø
  - diatomite (diatomaceous earth) J62.8
- **Pneumoconiosis** — *continued*
  - dust
    - inorganic NEC J63.6
    - lime J62.8
    - marble J62.8
    - organic NEC J66.8
  - fumes or vapors (from silo) J68.9
  - graphite J63.3
  - grinder's J62.8
  - kaolin J62.8
  - mica J62.8
  - millstone maker's J62.8
  - mineral fibers NEC J61
  - miner's J6Ø
  - moldy hay J67.Ø
  - potter's J62.8
  - rheumatoid — *see* Rheumatoid, lung
  - sandblaster's J62.8
  - silica, silicate NEC J62.8
    - with carbon J6Ø
  - stonemason's J62.8
  - talc (dust) J62.Ø
- **Pneumocystis carinii pneumonia** B59
- **Pneumocystis jiroveci** (pneumonia) B59
- **Pneumocystosis** (with pneumonia) B59
- **Pneumohemopericardium** I31.2
- **Pneumohemothorax** J94.2
  - traumatic S27.2 ☑
- **Pneumohydropericardium** — *see* Pericarditis
- **Pneumohydrothorax** — *see* Hydrothorax
- **Pneumomediastinum** J98.2
  - congenital or perinatal P25.2
- **Pneumomycosis** B49 *[J99]*
- **Pneumonia** (acute) (double) (migratory) (purulent) (septic) (unresolved) J18.9
  - with
    - influenza — *see* Influenza, with, pneumonia
    - lung abscess J85.1
      - due to specified organism — *see* Pneumonia, in (due to)
  - 2Ø19 (novel) coronavirus J12.82
  - adenoviral J12.Ø
  - adynamic J18.2
  - alba A5Ø.Ø4
  - allergic — *see also* Pneumonitis, hypersensitivity J82.89
  - alveolar — *see* Pneumonia, lobar
  - anaerobes J15.8
  - anthrax A22.1
  - apex, apical — *see* Pneumonia, lobar
  - Ascaris B77.81
  - aspiration J69.Ø
    - due to
      - aspiration of microorganisms
        - bacterial J15.9
        - viral J12.9
      - food (regurgitated) J69.Ø
      - gastric secretions J69.Ø
      - milk (regurgitated) J69.Ø
      - oils, essences J69.1
      - solids, liquids NEC J69.8
      - vomitus J69.Ø
    - newborn P24.81
      - amniotic fluid (clear) P24.11
      - blood P24.21
      - food (regurgitated) P24.31
      - liquor (amnii) P24.11
      - meconium P24.Ø1
      - milk P24.31
      - mucus P24.11
      - specified NEC P24.81
      - stomach contents P24.31
    - postprocedural J95.4
  - atypical NEC J18.9
  - bacillus J15.9
    - specified NEC J15.8
  - bacterial J15.9
    - specified NEC J15.8
  - Bacteroides (fragilis) (oralis) (melaninogenicus) J15.8
  - basal, basic, basilar — *see* Pneumonia, by type
  - bronchiolitis obliterans organized (BOOP) J84.89
  - broncho-, bronchial (confluent) (croupous) (diffuse) (disseminated) (hemorrhagic) (involving lobes) (lobar) (terminal) J18.Ø
    - allergic — *see also* Pneumonitis, hypersensitivity J82.89
    - aspiration — *see* Pneumonia, aspiration
    - bacterial J15.9
      - specified NEC J15.8
- **Pneumonia** — *continued*
  - broncho-, bronchial — *continued*
    - chronic — *see* Fibrosis, lung
    - diplococcal J13
    - Eaton's agent J15.7
    - Escherichia coli (E. coli) J15.5
    - Friedländer's bacillus J15.Ø
    - Hemophilus influenzae J14
    - hypostatic J18.2
    - inhalation — *see also* Pneumonia, aspiration
      - due to fumes or vapors (chemical) J68.Ø
      - of oils or essences J69.1
    - Klebsiella (pneumoniae) J15.Ø
    - lipid, lipoid J69.1
      - endogenous J84.89
    - Mycoplasma (pneumoniae) J15.7
    - pleuro-pneumonia-like-organisms (PPLO) J15.7
    - pneumococcal J13
    - Proteus J15.6
    - Pseudomonas J15.1
    - Serratia marcescens J15.6
    - specified organism NEC J16.8
    - staphylococcal — *see* Pneumonia, staphylococcal
    - streptococcal NEC J15.4
      - group B J15.3
      - pneumoniae J13
    - viral, virus — *see* Pneumonia, viral
  - Butyrivibrio (fibriosolvens) J15.8
  - Candida B37.1
  - caseous — *see* Tuberculosis, pulmonary
  - catarrhal — *see* Pneumonia, broncho
  - chlamydial J16.Ø
    - congenital P23.1
  - cholesterol J84.89
  - cirrhotic (chronic) — *see* Fibrosis, lung
  - Clostridium (haemolyticum) (novyi) J15.8
  - confluent — *see* Pneumonia, broncho
  - congenital (infective) P23.9
    - due to
      - bacterium NEC P23.6
      - Chlamydia P23.1
      - Escherichia coli P23.4
      - Haemophilus influenzae P23.6
      - infective organism NEC P23.8
      - Klebsiella pneumoniae P23.6
      - Mycoplasma P23.6
      - Pseudomonas P23.5
      - Staphylococcus P23.2
      - Streptococcus (except group B) P23.6
        - group B P23.3
      - viral agent P23.Ø
    - specified NEC P23.8
  - coronavirus (novel) (disease) 2Ø19 J12.82
  - COVID-19 J12.82
  - croupous — *see* Pneumonia, lobar
  - cryptogenic organizing J84.116
  - cytomegalic inclusion B25.Ø
  - cytomegaloviral B25.Ø
  - deglutition — *see* Pneumonia, aspiration
  - desquamative interstitial J84.117
  - diffuse — *see* Pneumonia, broncho
  - diplococcal, diplococcus (broncho-) (lobar) J13
  - disseminated (focal) — *see* Pneumonia, broncho
  - Eaton's agent J15.7
  - embolic, embolism — *see* Embolism, pulmonary
  - Enterobacter J15.6
  - eosinophilic J82.81
    - acute J82.82
    - chronic J82.81
  - Escherichia coli (E. coli) J15.5
  - Eubacterium J15.8
  - fibrinous — *see* Pneumonia, lobar
  - fibroid, fibrous (chronic) — *see* Fibrosis, lung
  - Friedländer's bacillus J15.Ø
  - Fusobacterium (nucleatum) J15.8
  - gangrenous J85.Ø
  - giant cell (measles) BØ5.2
  - gonococcal A54.84
  - gram-negative bacteria NEC J15.6
    - anaerobic J15.8
  - Hemophilus influenzae (broncho) (lobar) J14
  - human metapneumovirus J12.3
  - hypostatic (broncho) (lobar) J18.2
  - in (due to)
    - actinomycosis A42.Ø
    - adenovirus J12.Ø
    - anthrax A22.1
    - ascariasis B77.81

- **Pneumonitis** — *continued*
  - interstitial — *continued*
    - acute J84.114
    - lymphoid J84.2
    - non-specific J84.89
      - idiopathic J84.113
  - lymphoid, interstitial J84.2
  - meconium P24.Ø1
  - postanesthetic J95.4
    - correct substance properly administered — *see* Table of Drugs and Chemicals, by drug, adverse effect
    - in labor and delivery O74.Ø
    - in pregnancy O29.Ø1- ☑
    - obstetric O74.Ø
    - overdose or wrong substance given or taken (by accident) — *see* Table of Drugs and Chemicals, by drug, poisoning
    - postpartum, puerperal O89.Ø1
  - postoperative J95.4
    - obstetric O74.Ø
  - radiation J7Ø.Ø
  - rubella, congenital P35.Ø
  - ventilation (air-conditioning) J67.7
  - ventilator associated J95.851
  - wood-dust J67.8
- **Pneumonoconiosis** — *see* Pneumoconiosis
- **Pneumoparotid** K11.8
- **Pneumopathy NEC** J98.4
  - alveolar J84.Ø9
  - due to organic dust NEC J66.8
  - parietoalveolar J84.Ø9
- **Pneumopericarditis** — *see also* Pericarditis
  - acute I3Ø.9
- **Pneumopericardium** — *see also* Pericarditis
  - congenital P25.3
  - newborn P25.3
  - traumatic (post) — *see* Injury, heart
- **Pneumophagia** (psychogenic) F45.8
- **Pneumopleurisy, pneumopleuritis** — *see also* Pneumonia J18.8
- **Pneumopyopericardium** I3Ø.1
- **Pneumopyothorax** — *see* Pyopneumothorax
  - with fistula J86.Ø
- **Pneumorrhagia** — *see also* Hemorrhage, lung
  - tuberculous — *see* Tuberculosis, pulmonary
- **Pneumothorax NOS** J93.9
  - acute J93.83
  - chronic J93.81
  - congenital P25.1
  - perinatal period P25.1
  - postprocedural J95.811
  - specified NEC J93.83
  - spontaneous NOS J93.83
    - newborn P25.1
    - primary J93.11
    - secondary J93.12
    - tension J93.Ø
  - tense valvular, infectional J93.Ø
  - tension (spontaneous) J93.Ø
  - traumatic S27.Ø ☑
    - with hemothorax S27.2 ☑
  - tuberculous — *see* Tuberculosis, pulmonary
- **Podagra** — *see also* Gout M1Ø.9
- **Podencephalus** QØ1.9
- **Poikilocytosis** R71.8
- **Poikiloderma** L81.6
  - Civatte's L57.3
  - congenital Q82.8
  - vasculare atrophicans L94.5
- **Poikilodermatomyositis** M33.1Ø
  - with
    - myopathy M33.12
    - respiratory involvement M33.11
    - specified organ involvement NEC M33.19
  - amyopathic M33.13
  - without myopathy M33.13
- **Pointed ear** (congenital) Q17.3
- **Poison ivy, oak, sumac or other plant dermatitis** (allergic) (contact) L23.7
- **Poisoning** (acute) — *see also* Table of Drugs and Chemicals
  - algae and toxins T65.82- ☑
  - Bacillus B (aertrycke) (cholerae (suis)) (paratyphosus) (suipestifer) AØ2.9
    - botulinus AØ5.1
  - bacterial toxins AØ5.9
  - berries, noxious — *see* Poisoning, food, noxious, berries
- **Poisoning** — *continued*
  - botulism AØ5.1
  - ciguatera fish T61.Ø- ☑
  - Clostridium botulinum AØ5.1
  - death-cap (Amanita phalloides) (Amanita verna) — *see* Poisoning, food, noxious, mushrooms
  - drug — *see* Table of Drugs and Chemicals, by drug, poisoning
  - epidemic, fish (noxious) — *see* Poisoning, seafood
    - bacterial AØ5.9
  - fava bean D55.Ø
  - fish (noxious) T61.9- ☑
    - bacterial — *see* Intoxication, foodborne, by agent
    - ciguatera fish — *see* Poisoning, ciguatera fish
    - scombroid fish — *see* Poisoning, scombroid fish
    - specified type NEC T61.77- ☑
  - food NEC AØ5.9
    - bacterial — *see* Intoxication, foodborne, by agent
    - due to
      - Bacillus (aertrycke) (choleraesuis) (paratyphosus) (suipestifer) AØ2.9
        - botulinus AØ5.1
      - Clostridium (perfringens) (Welchii) AØ5.2
      - salmonella (aertrycke) (callinarum) (choleraesuis) (enteritidis) (paratyphi) (suipestifer) AØ2.9
        - with
          - gastroenteritis AØ2.Ø
          - sepsis AØ2.1
      - staphylococcus AØ5.Ø
      - Vibrio
        - parahaemolyticus AØ5.3
        - vulnificus AØ5.5
    - noxious or naturally toxic T62.9- ☑
      - berries — *see* subcategory T62.1 ☑
      - fish — *see* Poisoning, seafood
      - mushrooms — *see* subcategory T62.ØX ☑
      - plants NEC — *see* subcategory T62.2X ☑
      - seafood — *see* Poisoning, seafood
      - specified NEC — *see* subcategory T62.8X ☑
  - ichthyotoxism — *see* Poisoning, seafood
  - kreotoxism, food AØ5.9
  - latex T65.81- ☑
  - lead T56.Ø- ☑
  - mushroom — *see* Poisoning, food, noxious, mushroom
  - mussels — *see also* Poisoning, shellfish
    - bacterial — *see* Intoxication, foodborne, by agent
  - nicotine (tobacco) T65.2- ☑
  - noxious foodstuffs — *see* Poisoning, food, noxious
  - plants, noxious — *see* Poisoning, food, noxious, plants NEC
  - ptomaine — *see* Poisoning, food
  - radiation J7Ø.Ø
  - Salmonella (arizonae) (cholerae-suis) (enteritidis) (typhimurium) AØ2.9
  - scombroid fish T61.1- ☑
  - seafood (noxious) T61.9- ☑
    - bacterial — *see* Intoxication, foodborne, by agent
    - fish — *see* Poisoning, fish
    - shellfish — *see* Poisoning, shellfish
    - specified NEC — *see* subcategory T61.8X ☑
  - shellfish (amnesic) (azaspiracid) (diarrheic) (neurotoxic) (noxious) (paralytic) T61.78- ☑
    - bacterial — *see* Intoxication, foodborne, by agent
    - ciguatera mollusk — *see* Poisoning, ciguatera fish
  - specified substance NEC T65.891 ☑
  - Staphylococcus, food AØ5.Ø
  - tobacco (nicotine) T65.2- ☑
  - water E87.79
- **Poker spine** — *see* Spondylitis, ankylosing
- **Poland syndrome** Q79.8
- **Polioencephalitis** (acute) (bulbar) A8Ø.9
  - inferior G12.22
  - influenzal — *see* Influenza, with, encephalopathy
  - superior hemorrhagic (acute) (Wernicke's) E51.2
  - Wernicke's E51.2
- **Polioencephalomyelitis** (acute) (anterior) A8Ø.9
  - with beriberi E51.2
- **Polioencephalopathy, superior hemorrhagic** E51.2
  - with
    - beriberi E51.11
    - pellagra E52
- **Poliomeningoencephalitis** — *see* Meningoencephalitis
- **Poliomyelitis** (acute) (anterior) (epidemic) A8Ø.9
  - with paralysis (bulbar) — *see* Poliomyelitis, paralytic
  - abortive A8Ø.4
  - ascending (progressive) — *see* Poliomyelitis, paralytic
  - bulbar (paralytic) — *see* Poliomyelitis, paralytic
- **Poliomyelitis** — *continued*
  - congenital P35.8
  - nonepidemic A8Ø.9
  - nonparalytic A8Ø.4
  - paralytic A8Ø.3Ø
    - specified NEC A8Ø.39
    - vaccine-associated A8Ø.Ø
    - wild virus
      - imported A8Ø.1
      - indigenous A8Ø.2
  - spinal, acute A8Ø.9
- **Poliosis** (eyebrow) (eyelashes) L67.1
  - circumscripta, acquired L67.1
- **Pollakiuria** R35.Ø
  - psychogenic F45.8
- **Pollinosis** J3Ø.1
- **Pollitzer's disease** L73.2
- **Polyadenitis** — *see also* Lymphadenitis
  - malignant A2Ø.Ø
- **Polyalgia** M79.89
- **Polyangiitis** M3Ø.Ø
  - microscopic M31.7
  - overlap syndrome M3Ø.8
- **Polyarteritis**
  - microscopic M31.7
  - nodosa M3Ø.Ø
    - with lung involvement M3Ø.1
    - juvenile M3Ø.2
    - related condition NEC M3Ø.8
- **Polyarthralgia** — *see* Pain, joint
- **Polyarthritis, polyarthropathy** — *see also* Arthritis M13.Ø
  - due to or associated with other specified conditions — *see* Arthritis
  - epidemic (Australian) (with exanthema) B33.1
  - infective — *see* Arthritis, pyogenic or pyemic
  - inflammatory MØ6.4
  - juvenile (chronic) (seronegative) MØ8.3
  - migratory M13.8- ☑
  - rheumatic, acute — *see* Fever, rheumatic
- **Polyarthrosis** M15.9
  - post-traumatic M15.3
  - primary M15.Ø
  - specified NEC M15.8
- **Polycarential syndrome of infancy** E4Ø
- **Polychondritis** (atrophic) (chronic) — *see also* Disorder, cartilage, specified type NEC
  - relapsing M94.1
- **Polycoria** Q13.2
- **Polycystic** (disease)
  - degeneration, kidney Q61.3
    - autosomal dominant (adult type) Q61.2
    - autosomal recessive (infantile type) NEC Q61.19
  - kidney Q61.3
    - autosomal
      - dominant Q61.2
      - recessive NEC Q61.19
    - autosomal dominant (adult type) Q61.2
    - autosomal recessive (childhood type) NEC Q61.19
    - infantile type NEC Q61.19
  - liver Q44.6
  - lung J98.4
    - congenital Q33.Ø
  - ovary, ovaries E28.2
  - spleen Q89.Ø9
- **Polycythemia** (secondary) D75.1
  - acquired D75.1
  - benign (familial) D75.Ø
  - due to
    - donor twin P61.1
    - erythropoietin D75.1
    - fall in plasma volume D75.1
    - high altitude D75.1
    - maternal-fetal transfusion P61.1
    - stress D75.1
  - emotional D75.1
  - erythropoietin D75.1
  - familial (benign) D75.Ø
  - Gaisböck's (hypertonica) D75.1
  - high altitude D75.1
  - hypertonica D75.1
  - hypoxemic D75.1
  - neonatorum P61.1
  - nephrogenous D75.1
  - relative D75.1
  - secondary D75.1
  - spurious D75.1
  - stress D75.1

☑ **Additional Character Required — Refer to the Tabular List for Character Selection**

Polycythemia *— continued*
  vera D45
Polycytosis cryptogenica D75.1
Polydactylism, polydactyly Q69.9
  toes Q69.2
Polydipsia R63.1
Polydystrophy, pseudo-Hurler E77.Ø
Polyembryoma *— see* Neoplasm, malignant, by site
Polyglandular
  deficiency E31.Ø
  dyscrasia E31.9
  dysfunction E31.9
  syndrome E31.8
Polyhydramnios O4Ø.- ☑
Polymastia Q83.1
Polymenorrhea N92.Ø
Polymyalgia M35.3
  arteritica, giant cell M31.5
  rheumatica M35.3
    with giant cell arteritis M31.5
Polymyositis (acute) (chronic) (hemorrhagic) M33.2Ø
  with
    myopathy M33.22
    respiratory involvement M33.21
    skin involvement *— see* Dermatopolymyositis
    specified organ involvement NEC M33.29
  ossificans (generalisata) (progressiva) *— see* Myositis, ossificans, progressiva
Polyneuritis, polyneuritic *— see also* Polyneuropathy
  acute (post-)infective G61.Ø
  alcoholic G62.1
  cranialis G52.7
  demyelinating, chronic inflammatory (CIDP) G61.81
  diabetic *— see* Diabetes, polyneuropathy
  diphtheritic A36.83
  due to lack of vitamin NEC E56.9 *[G63]*
  endemic E51.11
  erythredema *— see* subcategory T56.1 ☑
  febrile, acute G61.Ø
  hereditary ataxic G6Ø.1
  idiopathic, acute G61.Ø
  infective (acute) G61.Ø
  inflammatory, chronic demyelinating (CIDP) G61.81
  nutritional E63.9 *[G63]*
  postinfective (acute) G61.Ø
  specified NEC G62.89
Polyneuropathy (peripheral) G62.9
  alcoholic G62.1
  amyloid (Portuguese) E85.1 *[G63]*
    transthyretin-related (ATTR) familial E85.1 *[G63]*
  arsenical G62.2
  critical illness G62.81
  demyelinating, chronic inflammatory (CIDP) G61.81
  diabetic *— see* Diabetes, polyneuropathy
  drug-induced G62.Ø
  hereditary G6Ø.9
    specified NEC G6Ø.8
  idiopathic G6Ø.9
    progressive G6Ø.3
  in (due to)
    alcohol G62.1
      sequelae G65.2
    amyloidosis, familial (Portuguese) E85.1 *[G63]*
    antitetanus serum G61.1
    arsenic G62.2
      sequelae G65.2
    avitaminosis NEC E56.9 *[G63]*
    beriberi E51.11
    collagen vascular disease NEC M35.9 *[G63]*
    deficiency (of)
      B (-complex) vitamins E53.9 *[G63]*
      vitamin B6 E53.1 *[G63]*
    diabetes *— see* Diabetes, polyneuropathy
    diphtheria A36.83
    drug or medicament G62.Ø
      correct substance properly administered *— see* Table of Drugs and Chemicals, by drug, adverse effect
      overdose or wrong substance given or taken *— see* Table of Drugs and Chemicals, by drug, poisoning
    endocrine disease NEC E34.9 *[G63]*
    herpes zoster BØ2.23
    hypoglycemia E16.2 *[G63]*
    infectious
      disease NEC B99 ☑ *[G63]*
      mononucleosis B27.91
    lack of vitamin NEC E56.9 *[G63]*

Polyneuropathy *— continued*
  in *— continued*
    lead G62.2
      sequelae G65.2
    leprosy A3Ø.9 *[G63]*
    Lyme disease A69.22
    metabolic disease NEC E88.9 *[G63]*
    microscopic polyangiitis M31.7 *[G63]*
    mumps B26.84
    neoplastic disease *— see also* Neoplasm D49.9 *[G63]*
    nutritional deficiency NEC E63.9 *[G63]*
    organophosphate compounds G62.2
      sequelae G65.2
    parasitic disease NEC B89 *[G63]*
    pellagra E52 *[G63]*
    polyarteritis nodosa M3Ø.Ø
    porphyria E8Ø.2Ø *[G63]*
    radiation G62.82
    rheumatoid arthritis *— see* Rheumatoid, polyneuropathy
    sarcoidosis D86.89
    serum G61.1
    syphilis (late) A52.15
      congenital A5Ø.43
    systemic
      connective tissue disorder M35.9 *[G63]*
      lupus erythematosus M32.19
    toxic agent NEC G62.2
      sequelae G65.2
    transthyretin-related (ATTR) familial amyloid E85.1
    triorthocresyl phosphate G62.2
      sequelae G65.2
    tuberculosis A17.89
    uremia N18.9 *[G63]*
    vitamin B12 deficiency E53.8 *[G63]*
      with anemia (pernicious) D51.Ø *[G63]*
        due to dietary deficiency D51.3, G63
    zoster BØ2.23
  inflammatory G61.9
    chronic demyelinating (CIDP) G61.81
    sequelae G65.1
    specified NEC G61.89
  lead G62.2
    sequelae G65.2
  nutritional NEC E63.9 *[G63]*
  postherpetic (zoster) BØ2.23
  progressive G6Ø.3
  radiation-induced G62.82
  sensory (hereditary) (idiopathic) G6Ø.8
  specified NEC G62.89
  syphilitic (late) A52.15
    congenital A5Ø.43
Polyopia H53.8
Polyorchism, polyorchidism Q55.21
Polyosteoarthritis *— see also* Osteoarthritis, generalized M15.9
  post-traumatic M15.3
  specified NEC M15.8
Polyostotic fibrous dysplasia Q78.1
Polyotia Q17.Ø
Polyp, polypus
  accessory sinus J33.8
  adenocarcinoma in *— see* Neoplasm, malignant, by site
  adenocarcinoma in situ in *— see* Neoplasm, in situ, by site
  adenoid tissue J33.Ø
  adenomatous *— see also* Neoplasm, benign, by site
    adenocarcinoma in *— see* Neoplasm, malignant, by site
    adenocarcinoma in situ in *— see* Neoplasm, in situ, by site
    carcinoma in *— see* Neoplasm, malignant, by site
    carcinoma in situ in *— see* Neoplasm, in situ, by site
    multiple *— see* Neoplasm, benign
      adenocarcinoma in *— see* Neoplasm, malignant, by site
      adenocarcinoma in situ in *— see* Neoplasm, in situ, by site
  antrum J33.8
  anus, anal (canal) K62.Ø
  Bartholin's gland N84.3
  bladder D41.4
  carcinoma in *— see* Neoplasm, malignant, by site
  carcinoma in situ in *— see* Neoplasm, in situ, by site
  cecum D12.Ø
  cervix (uteri) N84.1

Polyp, polypus *— continued*
  cervix *— continued*
    in pregnancy or childbirth *— see* Pregnancy, complicated by, abnormal, cervix
    mucous N84.1
    nonneoplastic N84.1
  choanal J33.Ø
  cholesterol K82.4
  clitoris N84.3
  colon K63.5
    adenomatous D12.6
      ascending D12.2
      cecum D12.Ø
      descending D12.4
      sigmoid D12.5
      transverse D12.3
    ascending K63.5
    cecum K63.5
    descending K63.5
    hyperplastic, (any site) K63.5
    inflammatory K51.4Ø
      with
        abscess K51.414
        complication K51.419
          specified NEC K51.418
        fistula K51.413
        intestinal obstruction K51.412
        rectal bleeding K51.411
    sigmoid K63.5
    transverse K63.5
  corpus uteri N84.Ø
  dental KØ4.Ø1
    irreversible KØ4.Ø2
    reversible KØ4.Ø1
  duodenum K31.7
  ear (middle) H74.4- ☑
  endometrium N84.Ø
  esophageal K22.81
  esophagogastric junction K22.82
  ethmoidal (sinus) J33.8
  fallopian tube N84.8
  female genital tract N84.9
    specified NEC N84.8
  frontal (sinus) J33.8
  gallbladder K82.4
  gingiva, gum KØ6.8
  labia, labium (majus) (minus) N84.3
  larynx (mucous) J38.1
    adenomatous D14.1
  malignant *— see* Neoplasm, malignant, by site
  maxillary (sinus) J33.8
  middle ear *— see* Polyp, ear (middle)
  myometrium N84.Ø
  nares
    anterior J33.9
    posterior J33.Ø
  nasal (mucous) J33.9
    cavity J33.Ø
    septum J33.Ø
  nasopharyngeal J33.Ø
  nose (mucous) J33.9
  oviduct N84.8
  pharynx J39.2
  placenta O9Ø.89
  prostate *— see* Enlargement, enlarged, prostate
  pudenda, pudendum N84.3
  pulpal (dental) KØ4.Ø1
    irreversible KØ4.Ø2
    reversible KØ4.Ø1
  rectum (nonadenomatous) K62.1
    adenomatous *— see* Polyp, adenomatous
  septum (nasal) J33.Ø
  sinus (accessory) (ethmoidal) (frontal) (maxillary) (sphenoidal) J33.8
  sphenoidal (sinus) J33.8
  stomach K31.7
    adenomatous D13.1
  tube, fallopian N84.8
  turbinate, mucous membrane J33.8
  umbilical, newborn P83.6
  ureter N28.89
  urethra N36.2
  uterus (body) (corpus) (mucous) N84.Ø
    cervix N84.1
    in pregnancy or childbirth *— see* Pregnancy, complicated by, tumor, uterus
  vagina N84.2
  vocal cord (mucous) J38.1

- **Polyp, polypus** — *continued*
  - vulva N84.3
- **Polyphagia** R63.2
- **Polyploidy** Q92.7
- **Polypoid** — *see* condition
- **Polyposis** — *see also* Polyp
  - coli (adenomatous) D12.6
    - adenocarcinoma in C18.9
    - adenocarcinoma in situ in — *see* Neoplasm, in situ, by site
    - carcinoma in C18.9
  - colon (adenomatous) D12.6
  - familial D12.6
    - adenocarcinoma in situ in — *see* Neoplasm, in situ, by site
  - intestinal (adenomatous) D12.6
  - malignant lymphomatous C83.1- ☑
  - multiple, adenomatous — *see also* Neoplasm, benign D36.9
- **Polyradiculitis** — *see* Polyneuropathy
- **Polyradiculoneuropathy** (acute) (postinfective) (segmentally demyelinating) G61.Ø
- **Polyserositis**
  - due to pericarditis I31.1
  - pericardial I31.1
  - periodic, familial E85.Ø
  - tuberculous A19.9
    - acute A19.1
    - chronic A19.8
- **Polysplenia syndrome** Q89.Ø9
- **Polysyndactyly** — *see also* Syndactylism, syndactyly Q7Ø.4
- **Polytrichia** L68.3
- **Polyunguia** Q84.6
- **Polyuria** R35.89
  - nocturnal R35.81
  - psychogenic F45.8
  - specified NEC R35.89
- **Pompe's disease** (glycogen storage) E74.Ø2
- **Pompholyx** L3Ø.1
- **Poncet's disease** (tuberculous rheumatism) A18.Ø9
- **Pond fracture** — *see* Fracture, skull
- **Ponos** B55.Ø
- **Pons, pontine** — *see* condition
- **Poor**
  - aesthetic of existing restoration of tooth KØ8.56
  - contractions, labor O62.2
  - gingival margin to tooth restoration KØ8.51
  - personal hygiene R46.Ø
  - prenatal care, affecting management of pregnancy — *see* Pregnancy, complicated by, insufficient, prenatal care
  - sucking reflex (newborn) R29.2
  - urinary stream R39.12
  - vision NEC H54.7
- **Poradenitis, nostras inguinalis or venerea** A55
- **Porencephaly** (congenital) (developmental) (true) QØ4.6
  - acquired G93.Ø
  - nondevelopmental G93.Ø
  - traumatic (post) FØ7.89
- **Porocephaliasis** B88.8
- **Porokeratosis** Q82.8
- **Poroma, eccrine** — *see* Neoplasm, skin, benign
- **Porphyria** (South African) E8Ø.2Ø
  - acquired E8Ø.2Ø
  - acute intermittent (hepatic) (Swedish) E8Ø.21
  - cutanea tarda (hereditary) (symptomatic) E8Ø.1
  - due to drugs E8Ø.2Ø
    - correct substance properly administered — *see* Table of Drugs and Chemicals, by drug, adverse effect
    - overdose or wrong substance given or taken — *see* Table of Drugs and Chemicals, by drug, poisoning
  - erythropoietic (congenital) (hereditary) E8Ø.Ø
  - hepatocutaneous type E8Ø.1
  - secondary E8Ø.2Ø
  - toxic NEC E8Ø.2Ø
  - variegata E8Ø.2Ø
- **Porphyrinuria** — *see* Porphyria
- **Porphyruria** — *see* Porphyria
- **Port wine nevus, mark, or stain** Q82.5
- **Portal** — *see* condition
- **Posadas-Wernicke disease** B38.9
- **Positive**
  - culture (nonspecific)
    - blood R78.81
    - bronchial washings R84.5
- **Positive** — *continued*
  - culture — *continued*
    - cerebrospinal fluid R83.5
    - cervix uteri R87.5
    - nasal secretions R84.5
    - nipple discharge R89.5
    - nose R84.5
      - staphylococcus (Methicillin susceptible) Z22.321
        - Methicillin resistant Z22.322
    - peritoneal fluid R85.5
    - pleural fluid R84.5
    - prostatic secretions R86.5
    - saliva R85.5
    - seminal fluid R86.5
    - sputum R84.5
    - synovial fluid R89.5
    - throat scrapings R84.5
    - urine R82.79
    - vagina R87.5
    - vulva R87.5
    - wound secretions R89.5
  - PPD (skin test) R76.11
  - serology for syphilis A53.Ø
    - false R76.8
    - with signs or symptoms — *code as* Syphilis, by site and stage
  - skin test, tuberculin (without active tuberculosis) R76.11
  - test, human immunodeficiency virus (HIV) R75
  - VDRL A53.Ø
    - with signs or symptoms — *code by* site and stage under Syphilis A53.9
  - Wassermann reaction A53.Ø
- **Post COVID-19 condition, unspecified** UØ9.9
- **Postcardiotomy syndrome** I97.Ø
- **Postcaval ureter** Q62.62
- **Postcholecystectomy syndrome** K91.5
- **Postclimacteric bleeding** N95.Ø
- **Postcommissurotomy syndrome** I97.Ø
- **Postconcussional syndrome** FØ7.81
- **Postcontusional syndrome** FØ7.81
- **Postcricoid region** — *see* condition
- **Post-dates** (4Ø-42 weeks) (pregnancy) (mother) O48.Ø
  - more than 42 weeks gestation O48.1
- **Postencephalitic syndrome** FØ7.89
- **Posterior** — *see* condition
- **Posterolateral sclerosis** (spinal cord) — *see* Degeneration, combined
- **Postexanthematous** — *see* condition
- **Postfebrile** — *see* condition
- **Postgastrectomy dumping syndrome** K91.1
- **Posthemiplegic chorea** — *see* Monoplegia
- **Posthemorrhagic anemia** (chronic) D5Ø.Ø
  - acute D62
  - newborn P61.3
- **Postherpetic neuralgia** (zoster) BØ2.29
  - trigeminal BØ2.22
- **Posthitis** N47.7
- **Postimmunization complication or reaction** — *see* Complications, vaccination
- **Postinfectious** — *see* condition
- **Postlaminectomy syndrome NEC** M96.1
- **Postleukotomy syndrome** FØ7.Ø
- **Postmastectomy lymphedema** (syndrome) I97.2
- **Postmaturity, postmature** (over 42 weeks)
  - maternal (over 42 weeks gestation) O48.1
  - newborn PØ8.22
- **Postmeasles complication NEC** — *see also* condition BØ5.89
- **Postmenopausal**
  - endometrium (atrophic) N95.8
    - suppurative — *see also* Endometritis N71.9
  - osteoporosis — *see* Osteoporosis, postmenopausal
- **Postnasal drip** RØ9.82
  - due to
    - allergic rhinitis — *see* Rhinitis, allergic
    - common cold JØØ
    - gastroesophageal reflux — *see* Reflux, gastroesophageal
    - nasopharyngitis — *see* Nasopharyngitis
    - other known condition — *code to* condition
    - sinusitis — *see* Sinusitis
- **Postnatal** — *see* condition
- **Postoperative** (postprocedural) — *see* Complication, postoperative
  - pneumothorax, therapeutic Z98.3
  - state NEC Z98.89Ø
- **Postpancreatectomy hyperglycemia** E89.1
- **Postpartum** — *see* Puerperal
- **Postphlebitic syndrome** — *see* Syndrome, postthrombotic
- **Postpolio** (myelitic) **syndrome** G14
- **Postpoliomyelitic** — *see also* condition
  - osteopathy — *see* Osteopathy, after poliomyelitis
- **Postprocedural** — *see also* Postoperative
  - hypoinsulinemia E89.1
- **Postschizophrenic depression** F32.89
- **Postsurgery status** — *see also* Status (post)
  - pneumothorax, therapeutic Z98.3
- **Post-term** (4Ø-42 weeks) (pregnancy) (mother) O48.Ø
  - infant PØ8.21
  - more than 42 weeks gestation (mother) O48.1
- **Post-traumatic brain syndrome, nonpsychotic** FØ7.81
- **Post-typhoid abscess** AØ1.Ø9
- **Postures, hysterical** F44.2
- **Postvaccinal reaction or complication** — *see* Complications, vaccination
- **Postvalvulotomy syndrome** I97.Ø
- **Potain's**
  - disease (pulmonary edema) — *see* Edema, lung
  - syndrome (gastrectasis with dyspepsia) K31.Ø
- **POTS** (postural orthostatic tachycardia syndrome) G9Ø.A
- **Potter's**
  - asthma J62.8
  - facies Q6Ø.6
  - lung J62.8
  - syndrome (with renal agenesis) Q6Ø.6
- **Pott's**
  - curvature (spinal) A18.Ø1
  - disease or paraplegia A18.Ø1
  - spinal curvature A18.Ø1
  - tumor, puffy — *see* Osteomyelitis, specified type NEC
- **Pouch**
  - bronchus Q32.4
  - Douglas' — *see* condition
  - esophagus, esophageal, congenital Q39.6
    - acquired K22.5
  - gastric K31.4
  - Hartmann's K82.8
  - pharynx, pharyngeal (congenital) Q38.7
- **Pouchitis** K91.85Ø
- **Poultrymen's itch** B88.Ø
- **Poverty NEC** Z59.6
  - extreme Z59.5
- **Poxvirus NEC** BØ8.8
- **Prader-Willi syndrome** Q87.11
- **Prader-Willi-like syndrome** Q87.19
- **Preauricular appendage or tag** Q17.Ø
- **Prebetalipoproteinemia** (acquired) (essential) (familial) (hereditary) (primary) (secondary) E78.1
  - with chylomicronemia E78.3
- **Precipitate labor or delivery** O62.3
- **Preclimacteric bleeding** (menorrhagia) N92.4
- **Precocious**
  - adrenarche E3Ø.1
  - menarche E3Ø.1
  - menstruation E3Ø.1
  - pubarche E3Ø.1
  - puberty E3Ø.1
    - central E22.8
  - sexual development NEC E3Ø.1
  - thelarche E3Ø.8
- **Precocity, sexual** (constitutional) (cryptogenic) (female) (idiopathic) (male) E3Ø.1
  - with adrenal hyperplasia E25.9
    - congenital E25.Ø
- **Precordial pain** RØ7.2
- **Predeciduous teeth** KØØ.2
- **Prediabetes, prediabetic** R73.Ø3
  - complicating
    - pregnancy — *see* Pregnancy, complicated by, diseases of, specified type or system NEC
    - puerperium O99.893
- **Predislocation status of hip at birth** Q65.6
- **Pre-eclampsia** O14.9- ☑
  - with pre-existing hypertension — *see* Hypertension, complicating pregnancy, pre-existing, with, pre-eclampsia
  - complicating
    - childbirth O14.94
    - puerperium O14.95
  - mild O14.Ø- ☑
    - complicating
      - childbirth O14.Ø4
      - puerperium O14.Ø5

Pre-eclampsia — *continued*
- moderate O14.Ø- ☑
  - complicating
    - childbirth O14.Ø4
    - puerperium O14.Ø5
- severe O14.1- ☑
  - with hemolysis, elevated liver enzymes and low platelet count (HELLP) O14.2- ☑
    - complicating
      - childbirth O14.24
      - puerperium O14.25
  - complicating
    - childbirth O14.14
    - puerperium O14.15

Pre-eruptive color change, teeth, tooth KØØ.8
Pre-excitation atrioventricular conduction I45.6
Preglaucoma H4Ø.ØØ- ☑
Pregnancy (single) (uterine) — *see also* Delivery and Puerperal Z33.1

> *Note: The Tabular must be reviewed for assignment of appropriate seventh character for multiple gestation codes in Chapter 15*

> *Note: The Tabular must be reviewed for assignment of the appropriate character indicating the trimester of the pregnancy*

- abdominal (ectopic) OØØ.ØØ
  - with intrauterine pregnancy OØØ.Ø1
  - with viable fetus O36.7- ☑
- ampullar OØØ.1Ø- ☑
  - with intrauterine pregnancy OØØ.11- ☑
- biochemical OØ2.81
- broad ligament OØØ.8Ø
  - with intrauterine pregnancy OØØ.81
- cervical OØØ.8
  - with intrauterine pregnancy OØØ.81
- chemical OØ2.81
- complicated by (care of) (management affected by)
  - abnormal, abnormality
    - cervix O34.4- ☑
      - causing obstructed labor O65.5
    - cord (umbilical) O69.9 ☑
    - fetal heart rate or rhythm O36.83- ☑
    - findings on antenatal screening of mother O28.9
      - biochemical O28.1
      - chromosomal O28.5
      - cytological O28.2
      - genetic O28.5
      - hematological O28.Ø
      - radiological O28.4
      - specified NEC O28.8
      - ultrasonic O28.3
    - glucose (tolerance) NEC O99.81Ø
    - pelvic organs O34.9- ☑
      - specified NEC O34.8- ☑
        - causing obstructed labor O65.5
    - pelvis (bony) (major) NEC O33.Ø
    - perineum O34.7- ☑
    - position
      - placenta O44.Ø- ☑
        - with hemorrhage O44.1- ☑
      - uterus O34.59- ☑
    - uterus O34.59- ☑
      - causing obstructed labor O65.5
      - congenital O34.Ø- ☑
    - vagina O34.6- ☑
      - causing obstructed labor O65.5
    - vulva O34.7- ☑
      - causing obstructed labor O65.5
  - abruptio placentae — *see* Abruptio placentae
  - abscess or cellulitis
    - bladder O23.1- ☑
    - breast O91.11- ☑
    - genital organ or tract O23.9- ☑
  - abuse
    - physical O9A.31 ☑ (*following* O99)
    - psychological O9A.51 ☑ (*following* O99)
    - sexual O9A.41 ☑ (*following* O99)
  - adverse effect anesthesia O29.9- ☑
    - aspiration pneumonitis O29.Ø1- ☑
    - cardiac arrest O29.11- ☑
    - cardiac complication NEC O29.19- ☑
    - cardiac failure O29.12- ☑
    - central nervous system complication NEC O29.29- ☑
    - cerebral anoxia O29.21- ☑

Pregnancy — *continued*
- complicated by — *continued*
  - adverse effect anesthesia — *continued*
    - failed or difficult intubation O29.6- ☑
    - inhalation of stomach contents or secretions NOS O29.Ø1- ☑
    - local, toxic reaction O29.3X ☑
    - Mendelson's syndrome O29.Ø1- ☑
    - pressure collapse of lung O29.Ø2- ☑
    - pulmonary complications NEC O29.Ø9- ☑
    - specified NEC O29.8X- ☑
    - spinal and epidural type NEC O29.5X ☑
      - induced headache O29.4- ☑
  - albuminuria — *see also* Proteinuria, gestational O12.1- ☑
  - alcohol use O99.31- ☑
  - amnionitis O41.12- ☑
  - anaphylactoid syndrome of pregnancy O88.Ø1- ☑
  - anemia (conditions in D5Ø-D64) (pre-existing) O99.Ø1- ☑
    - complicating the puerperium O99.Ø3
  - antepartum hemorrhage O46.9- ☑
    - with coagulation defect — *see* Hemorrhage, antepartum, with coagulation defect
    - specified NEC O46.8X- ☑
  - appendicitis O99.61- ☑
  - atrophy (yellow) (acute) liver (subacute) O26.61- ☑
  - bariatric surgery status O99.84- ☑
  - bicornis or bicornuate uterus O34.Ø- ☑
  - biliary tract problems O26.61- ☑
  - breech presentation O32.1 ☑
  - cardiovascular diseases (conditions in IØØ-IØ9, I2Ø-I52, I7Ø-I99) O99.41- ☑
  - cerebrovascular disorders (conditions in I6Ø-I69) O99.41- ☑
  - cervical shortening O26.87- ☑
  - cervicitis O23.51- ☑
  - cesarean scar defect (isthmocele) O34.22
  - chloasma (gravidarum) O26.89- ☑
  - cholecystitis O99.61- ☑
  - cholestasis (intrahepatic) O26.61- ☑
  - chorioamnionitis O41.12- ☑
  - circulatory system disorder (conditions in IØØ-IØ9, I2Ø-I99, O99.41-)
  - compound presentation O32.6 ☑
  - conjoined twins O3Ø.Ø2- ☑
  - connective system disorders (conditions in MØØ-M99) O99.891
  - contracted pelvis (general) O33.1
    - inlet O33.2
    - outlet O33.3 ☑
  - convulsions (eclamptic) (uremic) — *see also* Eclampsia O15.9
  - cracked nipple O92.11- ☑
  - cystitis O23.1- ☑
  - cystocele O34.8- ☑
  - death of fetus (near term) O36.4 ☑
    - early pregnancy OØ2.1
    - of one fetus or more in multiple gestation O31.2- ☑
  - deciduitis O41.14- ☑
  - decreased fetal movement O36.81- ☑
  - dental problems O99.61- ☑
  - diabetes (mellitus) O24.91- ☑
    - gestational (pregnancy induced) — *see* Diabetes, gestational
    - pre-existing O24.31- ☑
      - specified NEC O24.81- ☑
      - type 1 O24.Ø1- ☑
      - type 2 O24.11- ☑
  - digestive system disorders (conditions in KØØ-K93) O99.61- ☑
  - diseases of — *see* Pregnancy, complicated by, specified body system disease
    - biliary tract O26.61- ☑
    - blood NEC (conditions in D65-D77) O99.11- ☑
    - liver O26.61- ☑
    - specified NEC O99.891
  - disorders of — *see* Pregnancy, complicated by, specified body system disorder
    - amniotic fluid and membranes O41.9- ☑
      - specified NEC O41.8X- ☑
    - biliary tract O26.61- ☑
    - ear and mastoid process (conditions in H6Ø-H95) O99.891
    - eye and adnexa (conditions in HØØ-H59) O99.891

Pregnancy — *continued*
- complicated by — *continued*
  - disorders of — *see* Pregnancy, complicated by, specified body system disorder — *continued*
    - liver O26.61- ☑
    - skin (conditions in LØØ-L99) O99.71- ☑
    - specified NEC O99.891
  - displacement, uterus NEC O34.59- ☑
    - causing obstructed labor O65.5
  - disproportion (due to) O33.9
    - fetal (ascites) (hydrops) (meningomyelocele) (sacral teratoma) (tumor) deformities NEC O33.7 ☑
    - generally contracted pelvis O33.1
    - hydrocephalic fetus O33.6 ☑
    - inlet contraction of pelvis O33.2
    - mixed maternal and fetal origin O33.4 ☑
    - specified NEC O33.8
  - double uterus O34.Ø- ☑
    - causing obstructed labor O65.5
  - drug use (conditions in F11-F19) O99.32- ☑
  - eclampsia, eclamptic (coma) (convulsions) (delirium) (nephritis) (uremia) — *see also* Eclampsia O15.- ☑
  - ectopic pregnancy — *see* Pregnancy, ectopic
  - edema O12.Ø- ☑
    - with
      - gestational hypertension, mild — *see also* Pre-eclampsia O14.Ø- ☑
      - proteinuria O12.2- ☑
  - effusion, amniotic fluid — *see* Pregnancy, complicated by, premature rupture of membranes
  - elderly
    - multigravida OØ9.52- ☑
    - primigravida OØ9.51- ☑
  - embolism — *see also* Embolism, obstetric, pregnancy O88.- ☑
  - endocrine diseases NEC O99.28- ☑
  - endometritis O86.12
  - excessive weight gain O26.Ø- ☑
  - exhaustion O26.81- ☑
    - during labor and delivery O75.81
  - face presentation O32.3 ☑
  - failed induction of labor O61.9
    - instrumental O61.1
    - mechanical O61.1
    - medical O61.Ø
    - specified NEC O61.8
    - surgical O61.1
  - failed or difficult intubation for anesthesia O29.6- ☑
  - false labor (pains) O47.9
    - at or after 37 completed weeks of pregnancy O47.1
    - before 37 completed weeks of pregnancy O47.Ø- ☑
  - fatigue O26.81- ☑
    - during labor and delivery O75.81
  - fatty metamorphosis of liver O26.61- ☑
  - female genital mutilation O34.8- ☑ *[N9Ø.81-]* ☑
  - fetal (maternal care for)
    - abnormality or damage O35.9 ☑
      - acid-base balance O68
      - specified type NEC O35.8 ☑
    - acidemia O68
    - acidosis O68
    - agenesis of corpus callosum O35.Ø1 ☑
    - alkalosis O68
    - anemia and thrombocytopenia O36.82- ☑
    - anencephaly O35.Ø2 ☑
    - bradycardia O36.83- ☑
    - cardiac anomalies O35.B ☑
    - central nervous system malformation or damage O35.ØØ ☑
      - specified type NEC O35.Ø9 ☑
    - choroid plexus cysts O35.Ø3 ☑
    - chromosomal abnormality (conditions in Q9Ø-Q99) O35.1Ø ☑
      - sex chromosome O35.15 ☑
      - specified NEC O35.19 ☑
      - Trisomy 13 O35.11 ☑
      - Trisomy 18 O35.12 ☑
      - Trisomy 21 O35.13 ☑
      - Turner Syndrome O35.14 ☑
    - conjoined twins O3Ø.Ø2- ☑
    - damage from
      - amniocentesis O35.7 ☑

Index Pre-eclampsia — Pregnancy

- **Pregnancy** — *continued*
  - complicated by — *continued*
    - fetal — *continued*
      - damage from — *continued*
        - biopsy procedures O35.7 ☑
        - drug addiction O35.5 ☑
        - hematological investigation O35.7 ☑
        - intrauterine contraceptive device O35.7 ☑
        - maternal
          - alcohol addiction O35.4 ☑
          - cytomegalovirus infection O35.3 ☑
          - disease NEC O35.8 ☑
          - drug addiction O35.5 ☑
          - listeriosis O35.8 ☑
          - rubella O35.3 ☑
          - toxoplasmosis O35.8 ☑
          - viral infection O35.3 ☑
        - medical procedure NEC O35.7 ☑
        - radiation O35.6 ☑
      - death (near term) O36.4 ☑
        - early pregnancy OØ2.1
      - decreased movement O36.81- ☑
      - depressed heart rate tones O36.83- ☑
      - disproportion due to deformity (fetal) O33.7 ☑
      - encephalocele O35.Ø4 ☑
      - excessive growth (large for dates) O36.6- ☑
      - facial anomalies O35.A ☑
      - gastrointestinal anomalies O35.D ☑
      - genitourinary anomalies O35.E ☑
      - growth retardation O36.59- ☑
        - light for dates O36.59- ☑
        - small for dates O36.59- ☑
      - heart rate irregularity (abnormal variability) (bradycardia) (decelerations) (tachycardia) O36.83- ☑
      - hereditary disease O35.2 ☑
      - holoprosencephaly O35.Ø5 ☑
      - hydrocephalus O35.Ø6 ☑
      - hydrocephaly O35.Ø6 ☑
      - intrauterine death O36.4 ☑
      - microcephaly O35.Ø7 ☑
      - musculoskeletal anomalies
        - lower extremities O35.H ☑
        - trunk O35.F ☑
        - upper extremities O35.G ☑
      - non-reassuring heart rate or rhythm O36.83- ☑
      - poor growth O36.59- ☑
        - light for dates O36.59- ☑
        - small for dates O36.59- ☑
      - problem O36.9- ☑
        - specified NEC O36.89- ☑
      - pulmonary anomalies O35.C ☑
      - reduction (elective) O31.3- ☑
      - selective termination O31.3- ☑
      - spina bifida O35.Ø8 ☑
      - thrombocytopenia O36.82- ☑
    - fibroid (tumor) (uterus) O34.1- ☑
    - fissure of nipple O92.11- ☑
    - gallstones O99.61- ☑
    - gastric banding status O99.84- ☑
    - gastric bypass status O99.84- ☑
    - genital herpes (asymptomatic) (history of) (inactive) O98.3- ☑
    - genital tract infection O23.9- ☑
    - glomerular diseases (conditions in NØØ-NØ7) O26.83- ☑
      - with hypertension, pre-existing — *see* Hypertension, complicating, pregnancy, pre-existing, with, renal disease
    - gonorrhea O98.21- ☑
    - grand multiparity OØ9.4 ☑
    - habitual aborter — *see* Pregnancy, complicated by, recurrent pregnancy loss
    - HELLP syndrome (hemolysis, elevated liver enzymes and low platelet count) O14.2- ☑
    - hemorrhage
      - antepartum — *see* Hemorrhage, antepartum
      - before 2Ø completed weeks gestation O2Ø.9
        - specified NEC O2Ø.8
      - due to premature separation, placenta — *see also* Abruptio placentae O45.9- ☑
      - early O2Ø.9
        - specified NEC O2Ø.8
      - threatened abortion O2Ø.Ø
    - hemorrhoids O22.4- ☑
    - hepatitis (viral) O98.41- ☑

- **Pregnancy** — *continued*
  - complicated by — *continued*
    - herniation of uterus O34.59- ☑
    - high
      - head at term O32.4 ☑
      - risk — *see* Supervision (of) (for), high-risk
    - history of in utero procedure during previous pregnancy OØ9.82- ☑
    - HIV O98.71- ☑
    - human immunodeficiency virus (HIV) disease O98.71- ☑
    - hydatidiform mole — *see also* Mole, hydatidiform OØ1.9
    - hydramnios O4Ø.- ☑
    - hydrocephalic fetus (disproportion) O33.6 ☑
    - hydrops
      - amnii O4Ø.- ☑
      - fetalis O36.2- ☑
        - associated with isoimmunization — *see also* Pregnancy, complicated by, isoimmunization O36.11- ☑
    - hydrorrhea O42.9Ø
    - hyperemesis (gravidarum) (mild) — *see also* Hyperemesis, gravidarum O21.Ø
    - hypertension — *see* Hypertension, complicating pregnancy
    - hypertensive
      - heart and renal disease, pre-existing — *see* Hypertension, complicating, pregnancy, pre-existing, with, heart disease, with renal disease
      - heart disease, pre-existing — *see* Hypertension, complicating, pregnancy, pre-existing, with, heart disease
      - renal disease, pre-existing — *see* Hypertension, complicating, pregnancy, pre-existing, with, renal disease
    - hypotension O26.5- ☑
    - immune disorders NEC (conditions in D8Ø-D89) O99.11- ☑
    - incarceration, uterus O34.51- ☑
    - incompetent cervix O34.3- ☑
    - inconclusive fetal viability O36.8Ø ☑
    - infection(s) O98.91- ☑
      - amniotic fluid or sac O41.1Ø- ☑
      - bladder O23.1- ☑
      - carrier state NEC O99.83Ø
        - streptococcus B O99.82Ø
      - genital organ or tract O23.9- ☑
        - specified NEC O23.59- ☑
      - genitourinary tract O23.9- ☑
      - gonorrhea O98.21- ☑
      - hepatitis (viral) O98.41- ☑
      - HIV O98.71- ☑
      - human immunodeficiency virus (HIV) O98.71- ☑
      - intrauterine O41.12 ☑
      - kidney O23.Ø- ☑
      - nipple O91.Ø1- ☑
      - parasitic disease O98.91- ☑
        - specified NEC O98.81- ☑
      - protozoal disease O98.61- ☑
      - sexually transmitted NEC O98.31- ☑
      - specified type NEC O98.81- ☑
      - syphilis O98.11- ☑
      - tuberculosis O98.Ø1- ☑
      - urethra O23.2- ☑
      - urinary (tract) O23.4- ☑
        - specified NEC O23.3- ☑
      - viral disease O98.51- ☑
    - inflammation
      - intrauterine O41.12 ☑
    - injury or poisoning (conditions in SØØ-T88) O9A.21- ☑ (*following* O99)
      - due to abuse
        - physical O9A.31- ☑ (*following* O99)
        - psychological O9A.51- ☑ (*following* O99)
        - sexual O9A.41- ☑ (*following* O99)
    - insufficient
      - prenatal care OØ9.3- ☑
      - weight gain O26.1- ☑
    - insulin resistance O26.89 ☑
    - intrauterine fetal death (near term) O36.4 ☑
      - early pregnancy OØ2.1
      - multiple gestation (one fetus or more) O31.2- ☑
    - isoimmunization O36.11- ☑
      - anti-A sensitization O36.11- ☑

- **Pregnancy** — *continued*
  - complicated by — *continued*
    - isoimmunization — *continued*
      - anti-B sensitization O36.19- ☑
      - Rh O36.Ø9- ☑
        - anti-D antibody O36.Ø1- ☑
      - specified NEC O36.19- ☑
    - laceration of uterus NEC O71.81
    - malformation
      - central nervous system O35.ØØ ☑
        - specified type NEC O35.Ø9 ☑
      - placenta, placental (vessel) O43.1Ø- ☑
        - specified NEC O43.19- ☑
      - uterus (congenital) O34.Ø- ☑
    - malnutrition (conditions in E4Ø-E46) O25.1- ☑
    - maternal hypotension syndrome O26.5- ☑
    - mental disorders (conditions in FØ1-FØ9, F2Ø-F52 and F54-F99) O99.34- ☑
      - alcohol use O99.31- ☑
      - drug use O99.32- ☑
      - smoking O99.33- ☑
    - mentum presentation O32.3 ☑
    - metabolic disorders O99.28- ☑
    - missed
      - abortion OØ2.1
      - delivery O36.4 ☑
    - multiple gestations O3Ø.9- ☑
      - conjoined twins O3Ø.Ø2- ☑
      - quadruplet — *see* Pregnancy, quadruplet
      - specified complication NEC O31.8X- ☑
      - specified number of multiples NEC — *see* Pregnancy, multiple (gestation), specified NEC
      - triplet — *see* Pregnancy, triplet
      - twin — *see* Pregnancy, twin
    - musculoskeletal condition (conditions is MØØ-M99) O99.891
    - necrosis, liver (conditions in K72) O26.61- ☑
    - neoplasm
      - benign
        - cervix O34.4- ☑
        - corpus uteri O34.1- ☑
        - uterus O34.1- ☑
      - malignant O9A.11- ☑ (*following* O99)
    - nephropathy NEC O26.83- ☑
    - nervous system condition (conditions in GØØ-G99) O99.35- ☑
    - nutritional diseases NEC O99.28- ☑
    - obesity (pre-existing) O99.21- ☑
    - obesity surgery status O99.84- ☑
    - oblique lie or presentation O32.2 ☑
    - older mother — *see* Pregnancy, complicated by, elderly
    - oligohydramnios O41.Ø- ☑
      - with premature rupture of membranes — *see also* Pregnancy, complicated by, premature rupture of membranes O42.- ☑
    - onset (spontaneous) of labor after 37 completed weeks of gestation but before 39 completed weeks gestation, with delivery by (planned) cesarean section O75.82
    - oophoritis O23.52- ☑
    - overdose, drug — *see also* Table of Drugs and Chemicals, by drug, poisoning O9A.21- ☑ (*following* O99)
    - oversize fetus O33.5 ☑
    - papyraceous fetus O31.Ø- ☑
    - pelvic inflammatory disease O99.891
    - periodontal disease O99.61- ☑
    - peripheral neuritis O26.82- ☑
    - peritoneal (pelvic) adhesions O99.891
    - phlebitis O22.9- ☑
    - phlebopathy O22.9- ☑
    - phlebothrombosis (superficial) O22.2- ☑
      - deep O22.3- ☑
    - placenta accreta O43.21- ☑
    - placenta increta O43.22- ☑
    - placenta percreta O43.23- ☑
    - placenta previa O44.Ø- ☑
      - complete O44.Ø- ☑
        - with hemorrhage O44.1- ☑
      - marginal O44.2- ☑
        - with hemorrhage O44.3- ☑
      - partial O44.2- ☑
        - with hemorrhage O44.3- ☑
    - placental disorder O43.9- ☑
      - specified NEC O43.89- ☑

Index

Presbycusis, presbyacusia — Primigravida

- **Primipara**
  - elderly, affecting management of pregnancy, labor and delivery (supervision only) — *see* Pregnancy, complicated by, elderly, primigravida
  - older, affecting management of pregnancy, labor and delivery (supervision only) — *see* Pregnancy, complicated by, elderly, primigravida
  - very young, affecting management of pregnancy, labor and delivery (supervision only) — *see* Pregnancy, complicated by, young mother, primigravida
- **Primus varus** Q66.21- ☑
- **PRIND** (Prolonged reversible ischemic neurologic deficit) I63.9
- **Pringle's disease** (tuberous sclerosis) Q85.1
- **Prinzmetal angina** I2Ø.1
- **Prizefighter ear** — *see* Cauliflower ear
- **Problem** (with) (related to)
  - academic Z55.8
  - acculturation Z6Ø.3
  - adjustment (to)
    - change of job Z56.1
    - life-cycle transition Z6Ø.Ø
    - pension Z6Ø.Ø
    - retirement Z6Ø.Ø
  - adopted child Z62.821
  - alcoholism in family Z63.72
  - atypical parenting situation Z62.9
  - bankruptcy Z59.89
  - behavioral (adult) F69
    - drug seeking Z76.5
  - birth of sibling affecting child Z62.898
  - care (of)
    - provider dependency Z74.9
      - specified NEC Z74.8
    - sick or handicapped person in family or household Z63.6
  - child
    - abuse (affecting the child) — *see* Maltreatment, child
    - custody or support proceedings Z65.3
    - in care of non-parental family member Z62.21
    - in foster care Z62.21
    - in welfare custody Z62.21
    - living in orphanage or group home Z62.22
  - child-rearing Z62.9
    - specified NEC Z62.898
  - communication (developmental) F8Ø.9
  - conflict or discord (with)
    - boss Z56.4
    - classmates Z55.4
    - counselor Z64.4
    - employer Z56.4
    - family Z63.9
      - specified NEC Z63.8
    - probation officer Z64.4
    - social worker Z64.4
    - teachers Z55.4
    - workmates Z56.4
  - conviction in legal proceedings Z65.Ø
    - with imprisonment Z65.1
  - counselor Z64.4
  - creditors Z59.89
  - digestive K92.9
  - drug addict in family Z63.72
  - ear — *see* Disorder, ear
  - economic Z59.9
    - affecting care Z59.9
    - specified NEC Z59.89
    - strain Z59.86
  - education Z55.9
    - specified NEC Z55.8
  - employment Z56.9
    - change of job Z56.1
    - discord Z56.4
    - environment Z56.5
    - sexual harassment Z56.81
    - specified NEC Z56.89
    - stressful schedule Z56.3
    - stress NEC Z56.6
    - threat of job loss Z56.2
    - unemployment Z56.Ø
  - enuresis, child F98.Ø
  - eye H57.9
  - failed examinations (school) Z55.2
  - falling Z91.81
  - family — *see also* Disruption, family Z63.9
    - specified NEC Z63.8
  - feeding (elderly) (infant) R63.39

- **Problem** — *continued*
  - feeding — *continued*
    - newborn P92.9
      - breast P92.5
      - overfeeding P92.4
      - slow P92.2
      - specified NEC P92.8
      - underfeeding P92.3
    - nonorganic F5Ø.89
  - finance Z59.9
    - specified NEC Z59.89
  - foreclosure on loan Z59.89
  - foster child Z62.822
  - frightening experience(s) in childhood Z62.898
  - genital NEC
    - female N94.9
    - male N5Ø.9
  - health care Z75.9
    - specified NEC Z75.8
  - hearing — *see* Deafness
  - homelessness Z59.ØØ
  - housing Z59.9
    - inadequate Z59.1
    - isolated Z59.89
    - specified NEC Z59.89
  - identity (of childhood) F93.8
  - illegitimate pregnancy (unwanted) Z64.Ø
  - illiteracy Z55.Ø
  - impaired mobility Z74.Ø9
  - imprisonment or incarceration Z65.1
  - inadequate teaching affecting education Z55.8
  - inappropriate (excessive) parental pressure Z62.6
  - influencing health status NEC Z78.9
  - in-law Z63.1
  - institutionalization, affecting child Z62.22
  - intrafamilial communication Z63.8
  - jealousy, child F93.8
  - landlord Z59.2
  - language (developmental) F8Ø.9
  - learning (developmental) F81.9
  - legal Z65.3
    - conviction without imprisonment Z65.Ø
    - imprisonment Z65.1
    - release from prison Z65.2
  - life-management Z73.9
    - specified NEC Z73.89
  - life-style Z72.9
    - gambling Z72.6
    - high-risk sexual behavior (heterosexual) Z72.51
      - bisexual Z72.53
      - homosexual Z72.52
    - inappropriate eating habits Z72.4
    - self-damaging behavior NEC Z72.89
    - specified NEC Z72.89
    - tobacco use Z72.Ø
  - literacy Z55.9
    - low level Z55.Ø
    - specified NEC Z55.8
  - living alone Z6Ø.2
  - lodgers Z59.2
  - loss of love relationship in childhood Z62.898
  - marital Z63.Ø
    - involving
      - divorce Z63.5
      - estrangement Z63.5
      - gender identity F66
  - mastication KØ8.89
  - medical
    - care, within family Z63.6
    - facilities Z75.9
      - specified NEC Z75.8
  - mental F48.9
  - money Z59.86
  - multiparity Z64.1
  - negative life events in childhood Z62.9
    - altered pattern of family relationships Z62.898
    - frightening experience Z62.898
    - loss of
      - love relationship Z62.898
      - self-esteem Z62.898
    - physical abuse (alleged) — *see* Maltreatment, child
    - removal from home Z62.29
    - specified event NEC Z62.898
  - neighbor Z59.2
  - neurological NEC R29.818
  - new step-parent affecting child Z62.898
  - none (feared complaint unfounded) Z71.1
  - occupational NEC Z56.89
  - parent-child — *see* Conflict, parent-child

- **Problem** — *continued*
  - personal hygiene Z91.89
  - personality F69
  - phase-of-life transition, adjustment Z6Ø.Ø
  - presence of sick or disabled person in family or household Z63.79
    - needing care Z63.6
  - primary support group (family) Z63.9
    - specified NEC Z63.8
  - probation officer Z64.4
  - psychiatric F99
  - psychosexual (development) F66
  - psychosocial Z65.9
    - religious or spiritual Z65.8
    - specified NEC Z65.8
  - relationship Z63.9
    - childhood F93.8
  - release from prison Z65.2
    - religious or spiritual Z65.8
  - removal from home affecting child Z62.29
  - seeking and accepting known hazardous and harmful
    - behavioral or psychological interventions Z65.8
    - chemical, nutritional or physical interventions Z65.8
  - sexual function (nonorganic) F52.9
  - sight H54.7
  - sleep disorder, child F51.9
  - smell — *see* Disturbance, sensation, smell
  - social
    - environment Z6Ø.9
      - specified NEC Z6Ø.8
    - exclusion and rejection Z6Ø.4
    - worker Z64.4
  - speech R47.9
    - developmental F8Ø.9
    - specified NEC R47.89
  - swallowing — *see* Dysphagia
  - taste — *see* Disturbance, sensation, taste
  - tic, child F95.Ø
  - underachievement in school Z55.3
  - unemployment Z56.Ø
    - threatened Z56.2
  - unwanted pregnancy Z64.Ø
  - upbringing Z62.9
    - specified NEC Z62.898
  - urinary N39.9
  - voice production R47.89
  - work schedule (stressful) Z56.3
- **Procedure** (surgical)
  - converted
    - arthroscopic to open Z53.33
    - laparoscopic to open Z53.31
    - specified procedure NEC to open Z53.39
    - thoracoscopic to open Z53.32
  - for purpose other than remedying health state Z41.9
    - specified NEC Z41.8
  - not done Z53.9
    - because of
      - administrative reasons Z53.8
      - contraindication Z53.Ø9
        - smoking Z53.Ø1
      - patient's decision Z53.2Ø
        - for reasons of belief or group pressure Z53.1
        - left against medical advice (AMA) Z53.29
        - left without being seen Z53.21
        - specified reason NEC Z53.29
      - specified reason NEC Z53.8
- **Procidentia** (uteri) N81.3
- **Proctalgia** K62.89
  - fugax K59.4
  - spasmodic K59.4
- **Proctitis** K62.89
  - amebic (acute) AØ6.Ø
  - chlamydial A56.3
  - gonococcal A54.6
  - granulomatous — *see* Enteritis, regional, large intestine
  - herpetic A6Ø.1
  - radiation K62.7
  - tuberculous A18.32
  - ulcerative (chronic) K51.2Ø
    - with
      - complication K51.219
        - abscess K51.214
        - fistula K51.213
        - obstruction K51.212
        - rectal bleeding K51.211
        - specified NEC K51.218
- **Proctocele**
  - female (without uterine prolapse) N81.6

- **Proctocele** — *continued*
  - female — *continued*
    - with uterine prolapse N81.2
      - complete N81.3
  - male K62.3
- **Proctocolitis**
  - allergic K52.29
  - food protein-induced K52.29
  - food-induced eosinophilic K52.29
  - milk protein-induced K52.29
  - mucosal — *see* Rectosigmoiditis, ulcerative
- **Proctoptosis** K62.3
- **Proctorrhagia** K62.5
- **Proctosigmoiditis** K63.89
  - ulcerative (chronic) — *see* Rectosigmoiditis, ulcerative
- **Proctospasm** K59.4
  - psychogenic F45.8
- **Profichet's disease** — *see* Disorder, soft tissue, specified type NEC
- **Progeria** E34.8
- **Prognathism** (mandibular) (maxillary) M26.19
- **Progonoma** (melanotic) — *see* Neoplasm, benign, by site
- **Progressive** — *see* condition
- **Prolactinoma**
  - specified site — *see* Neoplasm, benign, by site
  - unspecified site D35.2
- **Prolapse, prolapsed**
  - anus, anal (canal) (sphincter) K62.2
  - arm or hand O32.2 ☑
    - causing obstructed labor O64.4 ☑
  - bladder (mucosa) (sphincter) (acquired)
    - congenital Q79.4
    - female — *see* Cystocele
    - male N32.89
  - breast implant (prosthetic) T85.49 ☑
  - cecostomy K94.Ø9
  - cecum K63.4
  - cervix, cervical (hypertrophied) N81.2
    - anterior lip, obstructing labor O65.5
    - congenital Q51.828
    - postpartal, old N81.2
    - stump N81.85
  - ciliary body (traumatic) — *see* Laceration, eye(ball), with prolapse or loss of interocular tissue
  - colon (pedunculated) K63.4
  - colostomy K94.Ø9
  - disc (intervertebral) — *see* Displacement, intervertebral disc
  - eye implant (orbital) T85.398 ☑
    - lens (ocular) — *see* Complications, intraocular lens
  - fallopian tube N83.4- ☑
  - gastric (mucosa) K31.89
  - genital, female N81.9
    - specified NEC N81.89
  - globe, nontraumatic — *see* Luxation, globe
  - ileostomy bud K94.19
  - intervertebral disc — *see* Displacement, intervertebral disc
  - intestine (small) K63.4
  - iris (traumatic) — *see* Laceration, eye(ball), with prolapse or loss of interocular tissue
    - nontraumatic H21.89
  - kidney N28.83
    - congenital Q63.2
  - laryngeal muscles or ventricle J38.7
  - liver K76.89
  - meatus urinarius N36.8
  - mitral (valve) I34.1
  - ocular lens implant — *see* Complications, intraocular lens
  - organ or site, congenital NEC — *see* Malposition, congenital
  - ovary N83.4- ☑
  - pelvic floor, female N81.89
  - perineum, female N81.89
  - rectum (mucosa) (sphincter) K62.3
    - due to trichuris trichuria B79
  - spleen D73.89
  - stomach K31.89
  - umbilical cord
    - complicating delivery O69.Ø ☑
  - urachus, congenital Q64.4
  - ureter N28.89
    - with obstruction N13.5
      - with infection N13.6
  - ureterovesical orifice N28.89
  - urethra (acquired) (infected) (mucosa) N36.8
- **Prolapse, prolapsed** — *continued*
  - urethra — *continued*
    - congenital Q64.71
  - urinary meatus N36.8
    - congenital Q64.72
  - uterovaginal N81.4
    - complete N81.3
    - incomplete N81.2
  - uterus (with prolapse of vagina) N81.4
    - complete N81.3
    - congenital Q51.818
    - first degree N81.2
    - in pregnancy or childbirth — *see* Pregnancy, complicated by, abnormal, uterus
    - incomplete N81.2
    - postpartal (old) N81.4
    - second degree N81.2
    - third degree N81.3
  - uveal (traumatic) — *see* Laceration, eye(ball), with prolapse or loss of interocular tissue
  - vagina (anterior) (wall) — *see* Cystocele
    - with prolapse of uterus N81.4
      - complete N81.3
      - incomplete N81.2
    - posterior wall N81.6
    - posthysterectomy N99.3
  - vitreous (humor) H43.Ø- ☑
    - in wound — *see* Laceration, eye(ball), with prolapse or loss of interocular tissue
  - womb — *see* Prolapse, uterus
- **Prolapsus, female** N81.9
  - specified NEC N81.89
- **Proliferation(s)**
  - primary cutaneous CD3Ø-positive large T-cell C86.6
  - prostate, atypical small acinar N42.32
- **Proliferative** — *see* condition
- **Prolonged, prolongation** (of)
  - bleeding (time) (idiopathic) R79.1
  - coagulation (time) R79.1
  - gestation (over 42 completed weeks)
    - mother O48.1
    - newborn PØ8.22
  - interval I44.Ø
  - labor O63.9
    - first stage O63.Ø
    - second stage O63.1
  - partial thromboplastin time (PTT) R79.1
  - pregnancy (more than 42 weeks gestation) O48.1
  - prothrombin time R79.1
  - QT interval R94.31
  - uterine contractions in labor O62.4
- **Prominence, prominent**
  - auricle (congenital) (ear) Q17.5
  - ischial spine or sacral promontory with disproportion (fetopelvic) O33.Ø
    - causing obstructed labor O65.Ø
  - nose (congenital) acquired M95.Ø
- **Promiscuity** — *see* High, risk, sexual behavior
- **Pronation**
  - ankle — *see* Deformity, limb, foot, specified NEC
  - foot — *see also* Deformity, limb, foot, specified NEC
    - congenital Q74.2
- **Prophylactic**
  - administration of
    - antibiotics, long-term Z79.2
      - short-term use — *omit code*
    - drug — *see also* Long-term (current) drug therapy (use of) Z79.899
  - medication Z79.899
  - organ removal (for neoplasia management) Z4Ø.ØØ
    - breast Z4Ø.Ø1
    - fallopian tube(s) Z4Ø.Ø3
      - with ovary(s) Z4Ø.Ø2
    - ovary(s) Z4Ø.Ø2
    - specified site NEC Z4Ø.Ø9
  - surgery Z4Ø.9
    - for risk factors related to malignant neoplasm — *see* Prophylactic, organ removal
    - specified NEC Z4Ø.8
  - vaccination Z23
- **Propionic acidemia** E71.121
- **Proptosis** (ocular) — *see also* Exophthalmos
  - thyroid — *see* Hyperthyroidism, with goiter
- **Prosecution, anxiety concerning** Z65.3
- **Prosopagnosia** R48.3
- **Prostadynia** N42.81
- **Prostate, prostatic** — *see* condition
- **Prostatism** — *see* Hyperplasia, prostate
- **Prostatitis** (congestive) (suppurative) (with cystitis) N41.9
  - acute N41.Ø
  - cavitary N41.8
  - chronic N41.1
  - diverticular N41.8
  - due to Trichomonas (vaginalis) A59.Ø2
  - fibrous N41.1
  - gonococcal (acute) (chronic) A54.22
  - granulomatous N41.4
  - hypertrophic N41.1
  - subacute N41.1
  - trichomonal A59.Ø2
  - tuberculous A18.14
- **Prostatocystitis** N41.3
- **Prostatorrhea** N42.89
- **Prostatosis** N42.82
- **Prostration** R53.83
  - heat — *see also* Heat, exhaustion
    - anhydrotic T67.3 ☑
    - due to
      - salt (and water) depletion T67.4 ☑
      - water depletion T67.3 ☑
  - nervous F48.8
  - senile R54
- **Protanomaly** (anomalous trichromat) H53.54
- **Protanopia** (complete) (incomplete) H53.54
- **Protection** (against) (from) — *see* Prophylactic
- **Protein**
  - deficiency NEC — *see* Malnutrition
  - malnutrition — *see* Malnutrition
  - sickness — *see also* Reaction, serum T8Ø.69 ☑
- **Proteinemia** R77.9
- **Proteinosis**
  - alveolar (pulmonary) J84.Ø1
  - lipid or lipoid (of Urbach) E78.89
- **Proteinuria** R8Ø.9
  - Bence Jones R8Ø.3
  - complicating pregnancy — *see* Proteinuria, gestational
  - gestational
    - complicating
      - childbirth O12.14
      - pregnancy O12.1- ☑
        - with edema O12.2- ☑
      - puerperium O12.15
  - idiopathic R8Ø.Ø
  - isolated R8Ø.Ø
    - with glomerular lesion NØ6.9
      - C3
        - glomerulonephritis NØ6.A
        - glomerulopathy NØ6.A
          - with dense deposit disease NØ6.6
      - dense deposit disease NØ6.6
      - diffuse
        - crescentic glomerulonephritis NØ6.7
        - endocapillary proliferative glomerulonephritis NØ6.4
        - mesangiocapillary glomerulonephritis NØ6.5
      - focal and segmental hyalinosis or sclerosis NØ6.1
      - membranous (diffuse) NØ6.2
      - mesangial proliferative (diffuse) NØ6.3
      - minimal change NØ6.Ø
      - specified pathology NEC NØ6.8
  - orthostatic R8Ø.2
    - with glomerular lesion — *see* Proteinuria, isolated, with glomerular lesion
  - persistent R8Ø.1
    - with glomerular lesion — *see* Proteinuria, isolated, with glomerular lesion
  - postural R8Ø.2
    - with glomerular lesion — *see* Proteinuria, isolated, with glomerular lesion
  - pre-eclamptic — *see* Pre-eclampsia
  - puerperal O12.15
  - specified type NEC R8Ø.8
- **Proteolysis, pathologic** D65
- **Proteus** (mirabilis) (morganii), **as cause of disease classified elsewhere** B96.4
- **Prothrombin gene mutation** D68.52
- **Protoporphyria, erythropoietic** E8Ø.Ø
- **Protozoal** — *see also* condition
  - disease B64
    - specified NEC B6Ø.8
- **Protrusion, protrusio**
  - acetabuli M24.7
  - acetabulum (into pelvis) M24.7
  - device, implant or graft — *see also* Complications, by site and type, mechanical T85.698 ☑

Protrusion, protrusio — *continued*
- device, implant or graft — *see also* Complications, by site and type, mechanical — *continued*
  - arterial graft NEC — *see* Complication, cardiovascular device, mechanical, vascular
  - breast (implant) T85.49 ☑
  - catheter NEC T85.698 ☑
    - cystostomy T83.Ø9Ø ☑
    - dialysis (renal) T82.49 ☑
      - intraperitoneal T85.691 ☑
    - infusion NEC T82.594 ☑
      - spinal (epidural) (subdural) T85.69Ø ☑
    - urinary — *see also* Complications, catheter, urinary T83.Ø98 ☑
  - electronic (electrode) (pulse generator) (stimulator)
    - bone T84.39Ø ☑
    - nervous system — *see* Complication, prosthetic device, mechanical, electronic nervous system stimulator
  - fixation, internal (orthopedic) NEC — *see* Complication, fixation device, mechanical
  - gastrointestinal — *see* Complications, prosthetic device, mechanical, gastrointestinal device
  - genital NEC T83.498 ☑
    - intrauterine contraceptive device T83.39 ☑
    - penile prosthesis (cylinder) (implanted) (pump) (resevoir) T83.49Ø ☑
    - testicular prosthesis T83.491 ☑
  - heart NEC — *see* Complication, cardiovascular device, mechanical
  - joint prosthesis — *see* Complications, joint prosthesis, mechanical, specified NEC, by site
  - ocular NEC — *see* Complications, prosthetic device, mechanical, ocular device
  - orthopedic NEC — *see* Complication, orthopedic, device, mechanical
  - specified NEC T85.628 ☑
  - urinary NEC — *see also* Complication, genitourinary, device, urinary, mechanical
    - graft T83.29 ☑
  - vascular NEC — *see* Complication, cardiovascular device, mechanical
  - ventricular intracranial shunt T85.Ø9 ☑
- intervertebral disc — *see* Displacement, intervertebral disc
- joint prosthesis — *see* Complications, joint prosthesis, mechanical, specified NEC, by site
- nucleus pulposus — *see* Displacement, intervertebral disc

Prune belly (syndrome) Q79.4
Prurigo (ferox) (gravis) (Hebrae) (Hebra's) (mitis) (simplex) L28.2
- Besnier's L2Ø.Ø
- estivalis L56.4
- nodularis L28.1
- psychogenic F45.8

Pruritus, pruritic (essential) L29.9
- ani, anus L29.Ø
  - psychogenic F45.8
- anogenital L29.3
  - psychogenic F45.8
- due to onchocerca volvulus B73.1
- gravidarum — *see* Pregnancy, complicated by, specified pregnancy-related condition NEC
- hiemalis L29.8
- neurogenic (any site) F45.8
- perianal L29.Ø
- psychogenic (any site) F45.8
- scroti, scrotum L29.1
  - psychogenic F45.8
- senile, senilis L29.8
- specified NEC L29.8
  - psychogenic F45.8
- Trichomonas A59.9
- vulva, vulvae L29.2
  - psychogenic F45.8

Pseudarthrosis, pseudoarthrosis (bone) — *see* Nonunion, fracture
- clavicle, congenital Q74.Ø
- joint, following fusion or arthrodesis M96.Ø

Pseudoaneurysm — *see* Aneurysm
Pseudoangina (pectoris) — *see* Angina
Pseudoangioma I81
Pseudoarteriosus Q28.8
Pseudoarthrosis — *see* Pseudarthrosis
Pseudobulbar affect (PBA) F48.2
Pseudochromhidrosis L67.8
Pseudocirrhosis, liver, pericardial I31.1
Pseudocowpox BØ8.Ø3
Pseudocoxalgia M91.3- ☑
Pseudocroup J38.5
Pseudo-Cushing's syndrome, alcohol-induced E24.4
Pseudocyesis F45.8
Pseudocyst
- lung J98.4
- pancreas K86.3
- retina — *see* Cyst, retina

Pseudoelephantiasis neuroarthritica Q82.Ø
Pseudoexfoliation, capsule (lens) — *see* Cataract, specified NEC
Pseudofolliculitis barbae L73.1
Pseudoglioma H44.89
Pseudohemophilia (Bernuth's) (hereditary) (type B) — *see* Disease, von Willebrand
- Type A D69.8
- vascular D69.8

Pseudohermaphroditism Q56.3
- adrenal E25.8
- female — *see also* Disorder, adrenogenital Q56.2
  - with adrenocortical disorder E25.8
  - without adrenocortical disorder Q56.2
  - adrenal (congenital) E25.Ø
- male — *see also* Disorder, adrenogenital Q56.1
  - with
    - 5-alpha-reductase deficiency E29.1
    - adrenocortical disorder E25.8
    - androgen resistance E34.51
    - cleft scrotum Q56.1
    - feminizing testis E34.51
  - without gonadal disorder Q56.1
  - adrenal E25.8

Pseudo-Hurler's polydystrophy E77.Ø
Pseudohydrocephalus G93.2
Pseudohypertrophic muscular dystrophy (Erb's) G71.Ø2
Pseudohypertrophy, muscle — *see also* Dystrophy, muscular, by type, if applicable G71.Ø9
Pseudohypoparathyroidism E2Ø.1
Pseudoinsomnia F51.Ø3
Pseudoleukemia, infantile D64.89
Pseudomembranous — *see* condition
Pseudomeningocele (cerebral) (infective) (post-traumatic) G96.198
- postprocedural (spinal) G97.82

Pseudomenses (newborn) P54.6
Pseudomenstruation (newborn) P54.6
Pseudomonas
- aeruginosa, as cause of disease classified elsewhere B96.5
- mallei infection A24.Ø
  - as cause of disease classified elsewhere B96.5
- pseudomallei, as cause of disease classified elsewhere B96.5

Pseudomyotonia G71.19
Pseudomyxoma peritonei C78.6
Pseudoneuritis, optic (nerve) (disc) (papilla), **congenital** Q14.2
Pseudo-obstruction intestine (acute) (chronic) (idiopathic) (intermittent secondary) (primary) K59.89
- colonic K59.81

Pseudopapilledema H47.33- ☑
- congenital Q14.2

Pseudoparalysis
- arm or leg R29.818
- atonic, congenital P94.2

Pseudopelade L66.Ø
Pseudophakia Z96.1
Pseudopolyarthritis, rhizomelic M35.3
Pseudopolycythemia D75.1
Pseudopseudohypoparathyroidism E2Ø.1
Pseudopterygium H11.81- ☑
Pseudoptosis (eyelid) — *see* Blepharochalasis
Pseudopuberty, precocious
- female heterosexual E25.8
- male isosexual E25.8

Pseudorickets (renal) N25.Ø
Pseudorubella BØ8.2Ø
Pseudosclerema, newborn P83.88
Pseudosclerosis (brain)
- Jakob's — *see* Creutzfeldt-Jakob disease or syndrome
- of Westphal (Strümpell) E83.Ø1
- spastic — *see* Creutzfeldt-Jakob disease or syndrome

Pseudotetanus — *see* Convulsions
Pseudotetany R29.Ø
Pseudotetany — *continued*
- hysterical F44.5

Pseudotruncus arteriosus Q25.49
Pseudotuberculosis A28.2
- enterocolitis AØ4.8
- pasteurella (infection) A28.Ø

Pseudotumor G93.2
- cerebri G93.2
- orbital HØ5.11 ☑

Pseudoxanthoma elasticum Q82.8
Psilosis (sprue) (tropical) K9Ø.1
- nontropical K9Ø.Ø

Psittacosis A7Ø
Psoitis M6Ø.88
Psoriasis L4Ø.9
- arthropathic L4Ø.5Ø
  - arthritis mutilans L4Ø.52
  - distal interphalangeal L4Ø.51
  - juvenile L4Ø.54
  - other specified L4Ø.59
  - spondylitis L4Ø.53
- buccal K13.29
- flexural L4Ø.8
- guttate L4Ø.4
- mouth K13.29
- nummular L4Ø.Ø
- plaque L4Ø.Ø
- psychogenic F54
- pustular (generalized) L4Ø.1
  - palmaris et plantaris L4Ø.3
- specified NEC L4Ø.8
- vulgaris L4Ø.Ø

Psychasthenia F48.8
Psychiatric disorder or problem F99
Psychogenic — *see also* condition
- factors associated with physical conditions F54

Psychological and behavioral factors affecting medical condition F59
Psychoneurosis, psychoneurotic — *see also* Neurosis
- anxiety (state) F41.1
- depersonalization F48.1
- hypochondriacal F45.21
- hysteria F44.9
- neurasthenic F48.8
- personality NEC F6Ø.89

Psychopathy, psychopathic
- affectionless F94.2
- autistic F84.5
- constitution, post-traumatic FØ7.81
- personality — *see* Disorder, personality
- sexual — *see* Deviation, sexual
- state F6Ø.2

Psychosexual identity disorder of childhood F64.2
Psychosis, psychotic F29
- acute (transient) F23
  - hysterical F44.9
- affective — *see* Disorder, mood
- alcoholic F1Ø.959
  - with
    - abuse F1Ø.159
    - anxiety disorder F1Ø.98Ø
      - with
        - abuse F1Ø.18Ø
        - dependence F1Ø.28Ø
    - delirium tremens F1Ø.231
    - delusions F1Ø.95Ø
      - with
        - abuse F1Ø.15Ø
        - dependence F1Ø.25Ø
    - dementia F1Ø.97
      - with dependence F1Ø.27
    - dependence F1Ø.259
    - hallucinosis F1Ø.951
      - with
        - abuse F1Ø.151
        - dependence F1Ø.251
    - mood disorder F1Ø.94
      - with
        - abuse F1Ø.14
        - dependence F1Ø.24
    - paranoia F1Ø.95Ø
      - with
        - abuse F1Ø.15Ø
        - dependence F1Ø.25Ø
    - persisting amnesia F1Ø.96
      - with dependence F1Ø.26
  - amnestic confabulatory F1Ø.96
    - with dependence F1Ø.26

- **Psychosis, psychotic** — *continued*
  - alcoholic — *continued*
    - delirium tremens F1Ø.231
    - Korsakoff's, Korsakov's, Korsakow's F1Ø.26
    - paranoid type F1Ø.95Ø
      - with
        - abuse F1Ø.15Ø
        - dependence F1Ø.25Ø
  - anergastic — *see* Psychosis, organic
  - arteriosclerotic (simple type) (uncomplicated) — *see also* Dementia, vascular FØ1.5Ø
    - with behavioral disturbance — *see* Dementia, vascular
  - childhood F84.Ø
    - atypical F84.8
  - climacteric — *see* Psychosis, involutional
  - confusional F29
    - acute or subacute FØ5
    - reactive F23
  - cycloid F23
  - depressive — *see* Disorder, depressive
  - disintegrative (childhood) F84.3
  - drug-induced — *see* F11-F19 with .X59
    - paranoid and hallucinatory states — *see* F11-F19 with .X5Ø or .X51
  - due to or associated with
    - addiction, drug — *see* F11-F19 with .X59
    - dependence
      - alcohol F1Ø.259
      - drug — *see* F11-F19 with .X59
    - epilepsy FØ6.8
    - Huntington's chorea FØ6.8
    - ischemia, cerebrovascular (generalized) FØ6.8
    - multiple sclerosis FØ6.8
    - physical disease FØ6.8
    - presenile dementia FØ3 ☑
    - senile dementia FØ3 ☑
    - vascular disease (arteriosclerotic) (cerebral) — *see also* Dementia, vascular FØ1.5Ø
      - with behavioral disturbance — *see* Dementia, vascular
  - epileptic FØ6.8
  - episode F23
    - due to or associated with physical condition FØ6.8
  - exhaustive F43.Ø
  - hallucinatory, chronic F28
  - hypomanic F3Ø.8
  - hysterical (acute) F44.9
  - induced F24
  - infantile F84.Ø
    - atypical F84.8
  - infective (acute) (subacute) FØ5
  - involutional F28
    - depressive — *see* Disorder, depressive
    - melancholic — *see* Disorder, depressive
    - paranoid (state) F22
  - Korsakoff's, Korsakov's, Korsakow's (nonalcoholic) FØ4
    - alcoholic F1Ø.96
      - in dependence F1Ø.26
    - induced by other psychoactive substance — *see* categories F11-F19 with .X5X
  - mania, manic (single episode) F3Ø.2
    - recurrent type F31.89
  - manic-depressive — *see* Disorder, bipolar
  - menopausal — *see* Psychosis, involutional
  - mixed schizophrenic and affective F25.8
  - multi-infarct (cerebrovascular) — *see also* Dementia, vascular FØ1.5Ø
    - with behavioral disturbance — *see* Dementia, vascular
  - nonorganic F29
    - specified NEC F28
  - organic FØ9
    - due to or associated with
      - arteriosclerosis (cerebral) — *see* Psychosis, arteriosclerotic
      - cerebrovascular disease, arteriosclerotic — *see* Psychosis, arteriosclerotic
      - childbirth — *see* Psychosis, puerperal
      - Creutzfeldt-Jakob disease or syndrome — *see* Creutzfeldt-Jakob disease or syndrome
      - dependence, alcohol F1Ø.259
      - disease
        - alcoholic liver F1Ø.259
        - brain, arteriosclerotic — *see* Psychosis, arteriosclerotic
        - cerebrovascular — *see also* Dementia, vascular FØ1.5Ø

- **Psychosis, psychotic** — *continued*
  - organic — *continued*
    - due to or associated with — *continued*
      - disease — *continued*
        - cerebrovascular — *see also* Dementia, vascular — *continued*
          - with behavioral disturbance — *see* Dementia, vascular
        - Creutzfeldt-Jakob — *see* Creutzfeldt-Jakob disease or syndrome
        - endocrine or metabolic FØ6.8
          - acute or subacute FØ5
        - liver, alcoholic F1Ø.259
      - epilepsy transient (acute) FØ5
      - infection
        - brain (intracranial) FØ6.8
          - acute or subacute FØ5
      - intoxication
        - alcoholic (acute) F1Ø.259
        - drug F11-F19 with .x59
      - ischemia, cerebrovascular (generalized) — *see* Psychosis, arteriosclerotic
      - puerperium — *see* Psychosis, puerperal
      - trauma, brain (birth) (from electric current) (surgical) FØ6.8
        - acute or subacute FØ5
    - infective FØ6.8
      - acute or subacute FØ5
    - post-traumatic FØ6.8
      - acute or subacute FØ5
  - paranoiac F22
  - paranoid (climacteric) (involutional) (menopausal) F22
    - psychogenic (acute) F23
    - schizophrenic F2Ø.Ø
    - senile FØ3 ☑
  - postpartum (NOS) F53.1
  - presbyophrenic (type) FØ3 ☑
  - presenile FØ3 ☑
  - psychogenic (paranoid) F23
    - depressive F32.3
  - puerperal (NOS) F53.1
    - specified type — *see* Psychosis, by type
  - reactive (brief) (transient) (emotional stress) (psychological trauma) F23
    - depressive F32.3
      - recurrent F33.3
    - excitative type F3Ø.8
  - schizoaffective F25.9
    - depressive type F25.1
    - manic type F25.Ø
  - schizophrenia, schizophrenic — *see* Schizophrenia
  - schizophrenia-like, in epilepsy FØ6.2
  - schizophreniform F2Ø.81
    - affective type F25.9
    - brief F23
    - confusional type F23
    - mixed type F25.Ø
  - senile NEC FØ3 ☑
    - depressed or paranoid type FØ3 ☑
    - simple deterioration FØ3 ☑
    - specified type — *code to* condition
  - shared F24
  - situational (reactive) F23
  - symbiotic (childhood) F84.3
  - symptomatic FØ9
- **Psychosomatic** — *see* Disorder, psychosomatic
- **Psychosyndrome, organic** FØ7.9
- **Psychotic episode due to or associated with physical condition** FØ6.8
- **Pterygium** (eye) H11.ØØ- ☑
  - amyloid H11.Ø1- ☑
  - central H11.Ø2- ☑
  - colli Q18.3
  - double H11.Ø3- ☑
  - peripheral
    - progressive H11.Ø5- ☑
    - stationary H11.Ø4- ☑
  - recurrent H11.Ø6- ☑
- **Ptilosis** (eyelid) — *see* Madarosis
- **Ptomaine** (poisoning) — *see* Poisoning, food
- **Ptosis** — *see also* Blepharoptosis
  - adiposa (false) — *see* Blepharoptosis
  - breast N64.81-
  - brow H57.81- ☑
  - cecum K63.4
  - colon K63.4
  - congenital (eyelid) Q1Ø.Ø
    - specified site NEC — *see* Anomaly, by site

- **Ptosis** — *continued*
  - eyebrow H57.81- ☑
  - eyelid — *see* Blepharoptosis
    - congenital Q1Ø.Ø
  - gastric K31.89
  - intestine K63.4
  - kidney N28.83
  - liver K76.89
  - renal N28.83
  - splanchnic K63.4
  - spleen D73.89
  - stomach K31.89
  - viscera K63.4
- **PTP** D69.51
- **Ptyalism** (periodic) K11.7
  - hysterical F45.8
  - pregnancy — *see* Pregnancy, complicated by, specified pregnancy-related condition NEC
  - psychogenic F45.8
- **Ptyalolithiasis** K11.5
- **Pubarche, precocious** E3Ø.1
- **Pubertas praecox** E3Ø.1
- **Puberty** (development state) ZØØ.3
  - bleeding (excessive) N92.2
  - delayed E3Ø.Ø
  - precocious (constitutional) (cryptogenic) (idiopathic) E3Ø.1
    - central E22.8
    - due to
      - ovarian hyperfunction E28.1
        - estrogen E28.Ø
      - testicular hyperfunction E29.Ø
  - premature E3Ø.1
    - due to
      - adrenal cortical hyperfunction E25.8
      - pineal tumor E34.8
      - pituitary (anterior) hyperfunction E22.8
- **Puckering, macula** — *see* Degeneration, macula, puckering
- **Pudenda, pudendum** — *see* condition
- **Puente's disease** (simple glandular cheilitis) K13.Ø
- **Puerperal, puerperium** (complicated by, complications)
  - abnormal glucose (tolerance test) O99.815
  - abscess
    - areola O91.Ø2
      - associated with lactation O91.Ø3
    - Bartholin's gland O86.19
    - breast O91.12
      - associated with lactation O91.13
    - cervix (uteri) O86.11
    - genital organ NEC O86.19
    - kidney O86.21
    - mammary O91.12
      - associated with lactation O91.13
    - nipple O91.Ø2
      - associated with lactation O91.Ø3
    - peritoneum O85
    - subareolar O91.12
      - associated with lactation O91.13
    - urinary tract — *see* Puerperal, infection, urinary
    - uterus O86.12
    - vagina (wall) O86.13
    - vaginorectal O86.13
    - vulvovaginal gland O86.13
  - adnexitis O86.19
  - afibrinogenemia, or other coagulation defect O72.3
  - albuminuria (acute) (subacute) — *see* Proteinuria, gestational
  - alcohol use O99.315
  - anemia O9Ø.81
    - pre-existing (pre-pregnancy) O99.Ø3
  - anesthetic death O89.8
  - apoplexy O99.43
  - bariatric surgery status O99.845
  - blood disorder NEC O99.13
  - blood dyscrasia O72.3
  - cardiomyopathy O9Ø.3
  - cerebrovascular disorder (conditions in I6Ø-I69) O99.43
  - cervicitis O86.11
  - circulatory system disorder O99.43
  - coagulopathy (any) O99.13
    - with hemorrhage O72.3
  - complications O9Ø.9
    - specified NEC O9Ø.89
  - convulsions — *see* Eclampsia
  - cystitis O86.22
  - cystopyelitis O86.29
  - delirium NEC FØ5

Puncture — *continued*
- genital organs, external — *continued*
  - female — *continued*
    - vagina — *see* Puncture, vagina
    - vulva — *see* Puncture, vulva
  - male S31.531 ☑
    - with foreign body S31.541 ☑
    - penis — *see* Puncture, penis
    - scrotum — *see* Puncture, scrotum
    - testis — *see* Puncture, testis
- groin — *see* Puncture, abdomen, wall
- gum — *see* Puncture, oral cavity
- hand S61.439 ☑
  - with
    - foreign body S61.449 ☑
  - finger — *see* Puncture, finger
  - left S61.432 ☑
    - with
      - foreign body S61.442 ☑
  - right S61.431 ☑
    - with
      - foreign body S61.441 ☑
  - thumb — *see* Puncture, thumb
- head SØ1.93 ☑
  - with foreign body SØ1.94 ☑
  - cheek — *see* Puncture, cheek
  - ear — *see* Puncture, ear
  - eyelid — *see* Puncture, eyelid
  - lip — *see* Puncture, oral cavity
  - nose — *see* Puncture, nose
  - oral cavity — *see* Puncture, oral cavity
  - scalp SØ1.Ø3 ☑
    - with foreign body SØ1.Ø4 ☑
  - specified site NEC SØ1.83 ☑
    - with foreign body SØ1.84 ☑
  - temporomandibular area — *see* Puncture, cheek
- heart S26.99 ☑
  - with hemopericardium S26.Ø9 ☑
  - without hemopericardium S26.19 ☑
- heel — *see* Puncture, foot
- hip S71.Ø39 ☑
  - with foreign body S71.Ø49 ☑
  - left S71.Ø32 ☑
    - with foreign body S71.Ø42 ☑
  - right S71.Ø31 ☑
    - with foreign body S71.Ø41 ☑
- hymen — *see* Puncture, vagina
- hypochondrium — *see* Puncture, abdomen, wall
- hypogastric region — *see* Puncture, abdomen, wall
- inguinal region — *see* Puncture, abdomen, wall
- instep — *see* Puncture, foot
- internal organs — *see* Injury, by site
- interscapular region — *see* Puncture, thorax, back
- intestine
  - large
    - colon S36.599 ☑
      - ascending S36.59Ø ☑
      - descending S36.592 ☑
      - sigmoid S36.593 ☑
      - specified site NEC S36.598 ☑
      - transverse S36.591 ☑
    - rectum S36.69 ☑
  - small S36.499 ☑
    - duodenum S36.49Ø ☑
    - specified site NEC S36.498 ☑
- intra-abdominal organ S36.99 ☑
  - gallbladder S36.128 ☑
  - intestine — *see* Puncture, intestine
  - liver S36.118 ☑
  - pancreas — *see* Puncture, pancreas
  - peritoneum S36.81 ☑
  - specified site NEC S36.898 ☑
  - spleen S36.Ø9 ☑
  - stomach S36.39 ☑
- jaw — *see* Puncture, head, specified site NEC
- knee S81.Ø39 ☑
  - with foreign body S81.Ø49 ☑
  - left S81.Ø32 ☑
    - with foreign body S81.Ø42 ☑
  - right S81.Ø31 ☑
    - with foreign body S81.Ø41 ☑
- labium (majus) (minus) — *see* Puncture, vulva
- lacrimal duct — *see* Puncture, eyelid
- larynx S11.Ø13 ☑
  - with foreign body S11.Ø14 ☑
- leg (lower) S81.839 ☑

Puncture — *continued*
- leg — *continued*
  - with foreign body S81.849 ☑
  - foot — *see* Puncture, foot
  - knee — *see* Puncture, knee
  - left S81.832 ☑
    - with foreign body S81.842 ☑
  - right S81.831 ☑
    - with foreign body S81.841 ☑
  - upper — *see* Puncture, thigh
- lip SØ1.531 ☑
  - with foreign body SØ1.541 ☑
- loin — *see* Puncture, abdomen, wall
- lower back — *see* Puncture, back, lower
- lumbar region — *see* Puncture, back, lower
- malar region — *see* Puncture, head, specified site NEC
- mammary — *see* Puncture, breast
- mastoid region — *see* Puncture, head, specified site NEC
- mouth — *see* Puncture, oral cavity
- nail
  - finger — *see* Puncture, finger, with damage to nail
  - toe — *see* Puncture, toe, with damage to nail
- nasal (septum) (sinus) — *see* Puncture, nose
- nasopharynx — *see* Puncture, head, specified site NEC
- neck S11.93 ☑
  - with foreign body S11.94 ☑
  - involving
    - cervical esophagus — *see* Puncture, cervical esophagus
    - larynx — *see* Puncture, larynx
    - pharynx — *see* Puncture, pharynx
    - thyroid gland — *see* Puncture, thyroid gland
    - trachea — *see* Puncture, trachea
  - specified site NEC S11.83 ☑
    - with foreign body S11.84 ☑
- nose (septum) (sinus) SØ1.23 ☑
  - with foreign body SØ1.24 ☑
- ocular — *see* Puncture, eyeball
- oral cavity SØ1.532 ☑
  - with foreign body SØ1.542 ☑
- orbit SØ5.4- ☑
- palate — *see* Puncture, oral cavity
- palm — *see* Puncture, hand
- pancreas S36.299 ☑
  - body S36.291 ☑
  - head S36.29Ø ☑
  - tail S36.292 ☑
- pelvis — *see* Puncture, back, lower
- penis S31.23 ☑
  - with foreign body S31.24 ☑
- perineum
  - female S31.43 ☑
    - with foreign body S31.44 ☑
  - male S31.139 ☑
    - with foreign body S31.149 ☑
- periocular area (with or without lacrimal passages) — *see* Puncture, eyelid
- phalanges
  - finger — *see* Puncture, finger
  - toe — *see* Puncture, toe
- pharynx S11.23 ☑
  - with foreign body S11.24 ☑
- pinna — *see* Puncture, ear
- popliteal space — *see* Puncture, knee
- prepuce — *see* Puncture, penis
- pubic region S31.139 ☑
  - with foreign body S31.149 ☑
- pudendum — *see* Puncture, genital organs, external
- rectovaginal septum — *see* Puncture, vagina
- sacral region — *see* Puncture, back, lower
- sacroiliac region — *see* Puncture, back, lower
- salivary gland — *see* Puncture, oral cavity
- scalp SØ1.Ø3 ☑
  - with foreign body SØ1.Ø4 ☑
- scapular region — *see* Puncture, shoulder
- scrotum S31.33 ☑
  - with foreign body S31.34 ☑
- shin — *see* Puncture, leg
- shoulder S41.Ø39 ☑
  - with foreign body S41.Ø49 ☑
  - left S41.Ø32 ☑
    - with foreign body S41.Ø42 ☑
  - right S41.Ø31 ☑
    - with foreign body S41.Ø41 ☑
- spermatic cord — *see* Puncture, testis

Puncture — *continued*
- sternal region — *see* Puncture, thorax, front
- submaxillary region — *see* Puncture, head, specified site NEC
- submental region — *see* Puncture, head, specified site NEC
- subungual
  - finger(s) — *see* Puncture, finger, with damage to nail
  - toe — *see* Puncture, toe, with damage to nail
- supraclavicular fossa — *see* Puncture, neck, specified site NEC
- temple, temporal region — *see* Puncture, head, specified site NEC
- temporomandibular area — *see* Puncture, cheek
- testis S31.33 ☑
  - with foreign body S31.34 ☑
- thigh S71.139 ☑
  - with foreign body S71.149 ☑
  - left S71.132 ☑
    - with foreign body S71.142 ☑
  - right S71.131 ☑
    - with foreign body S71.141 ☑
- thorax, thoracic (wall) S21.93 ☑
  - with foreign body S21.94 ☑
  - back S21.23- ☑
    - with
      - foreign body S21.24- ☑
        - with penetration S21.44 ☑
      - penetration S21.43 ☑
  - breast — *see* Puncture, breast
  - front S21.13- ☑
    - with
      - foreign body S21.14- ☑
        - with penetration S21.34 ☑
      - penetration S21.33 ☑
- throat — *see* Puncture, neck
- thumb S61.Ø39 ☑
  - with
    - damage to nail S61.139 ☑
      - with
        - foreign body S61.149 ☑
    - foreign body S61.Ø49 ☑
  - left S61.Ø32 ☑
    - with
      - damage to nail S61.132 ☑
        - with
          - foreign body S61.142 ☑
      - foreign body S61.Ø42 ☑
  - right S61.Ø31 ☑
    - with
      - damage to nail S61.131 ☑
        - with
          - foreign body S61.141 ☑
      - foreign body S61.Ø41 ☑
- thyroid gland S11.13 ☑
  - with foreign body S11.14 ☑
- toe(s) S91.139 ☑
  - with
    - damage to nail S91.239 ☑
      - with
        - foreign body S91.249 ☑
    - foreign body S91.149 ☑
  - great S91.133 ☑
    - with
      - damage to nail S91.233 ☑
        - with
          - foreign body S91.243 ☑
      - foreign body S91.143 ☑
    - left S91.132 ☑
      - with
        - damage to nail S91.232 ☑
          - with
            - foreign body S91.242 ☑
        - foreign body S91.142 ☑
    - right S91.131 ☑
      - with
        - damage to nail S91.231 ☑
          - with
            - foreign body S91.241 ☑
        - foreign body S91.141 ☑
  - lesser S91.136 ☑
    - with
      - damage to nail S91.236 ☑
        - with
          - foreign body S91.246 ☑

- **Puncture** — *continued*
  - toe(s) — *continued*
    - lesser — *continued*
      - with — *continued*
        - foreign body S91.146 ☑
      - left S91.135 ☑
        - with
          - damage to nail S91.235 ☑
            - with
              - foreign body S91.245 ☑
          - foreign body S91.145 ☑
      - right S91.134 ☑
        - with
          - damage to nail S91.234 ☑
            - with
              - foreign body S91.244 ☑
          - foreign body S91.144 ☑
  - tongue — *see* Puncture, oral cavity
  - trachea S11.Ø23 ☑
    - with foreign body S11.Ø24 ☑
  - tunica vaginalis — *see* Puncture, testis
  - tympanum, tympanic membrane SØ9.2- ☑
  - umbilical region S31.135 ☑
    - with foreign body S31.145 ☑
  - uvula — *see* Puncture, oral cavity
  - vagina S31.43 ☑
    - with foreign body S31.44 ☑
  - vocal cords S11.Ø33 ☑
    - with foreign body S11.Ø34 ☑
  - vulva S31.43 ☑
    - with foreign body S31.44 ☑
  - wrist S61.539 ☑
    - with
      - foreign body S61.549 ☑
    - left S61.532 ☑
      - with
        - foreign body S61.542 ☑
    - right S61.531 ☑
      - with
        - foreign body S61.541 ☑
- **PUO** (pyrexia of unknown origin) R5Ø.9
- **Pupillary membrane** (persistent) Q13.89
- **Pupillotonia** — *see* Anomaly, pupil, function, tonic pupil
- **Purpura** D69.2
  - abdominal D69.Ø
  - allergic D69.Ø
  - anaphylactoid D69.Ø
  - annularis telangiectodes L81.7
  - arthritic D69.Ø
  - autoerythrocyte sensitization D69.2
  - autoimmune D69.Ø
  - bacterial D69.Ø
  - Bateman's (senile) D69.2
  - capillary fragility (hereditary) (idiopathic) D69.8
  - cryoglobulinemic D89.1
  - Devil's pinches D69.2
  - fibrinolytic — *see* Fibrinolysis
  - fulminans, fulminous D65
  - gangrenous D65
  - hemorrhagic, hemorrhagica D69.3
    - not due to thrombocytopenia D69.Ø
  - Henoch (-Schönlein) (allergic) D69.Ø
  - hypergammaglobulinemic (benign) (Waldenström) D89.Ø
  - idiopathic (thrombocytopenic) D69.3
    - nonthrombocytopenic D69.Ø
  - immune thrombocytopenic D69.3
  - infectious D69.Ø
  - malignant D69.Ø
  - neonatorum P54.5
  - nervosa D69.Ø
  - newborn P54.5
  - nonthrombocytopenic D69.2
    - hemorrhagic D69.Ø
    - idiopathic D69.Ø
  - nonthrombopenic D69.2
  - peliosis rheumatica D69.Ø
  - posttransfusion (post-transfusion) (from (fresh) whole blood or blood products) D69.51
  - primary D69.49
  - red cell membrane sensitivity D69.2
  - rheumatica D69.Ø
  - Schönlein (-Henoch) (allergic) D69.Ø
  - scorbutic E54 *[D77]*
  - senile D69.2
  - simplex D69.2
  - symptomatica D69.Ø

- **Purpura** — *continued*
  - telangiectasia annularis L81.7
  - thrombocytopenic D69.49
    - congenital D69.42
    - hemorrhagic D69.3
    - hereditary D69.42
    - idiopathic D69.3
    - immune D69.3
    - neonatal, transitory P61.Ø
    - thrombotic M31.19
  - thrombohemolytic — *see* Fibrinolysis
  - thrombolytic — *see* Fibrinolysis
  - thrombopenic D69.49
  - thrombotic, thrombocytopenic M31.19
  - toxic D69.Ø
  - vascular D69.Ø
  - visceral symptoms D69.Ø
- **Purpuric spots** R23.3
- **Purulent** — *see* condition
- **Pus**
  - in
    - stool R19.5
    - urine N39.Ø
  - tube (rupture) — *see* Salpingo-oophoritis
- **Pustular rash** LØ8.Ø
- **Pustule** (nonmalignant) LØ8.9
  - malignant A22.Ø
- **Pustulosis palmaris et plantaris** L4Ø.3
- **Putnam** (-Dana) **disease or syndrome** — *see* Degeneration, combined
- **Putrescent pulp** (dental) KØ4.1
- **Pyarthritis, pyarthrosis** — *see* Arthritis, pyogenic or pyemic
  - tuberculous — *see* Tuberculosis, joint
- **Pyelectasis** — *see* Hydronephrosis
- **Pyelitis** (congenital) (uremic) — *see also* Pyelonephritis
  - with
    - calculus — *see* category N2Ø ☑
      - with hydronephrosis N13.6
    - contracted kidney N11.9
  - acute N1Ø
  - chronic N11.9
    - with calculus — *see* category N2Ø ☑
      - with hydronephrosis N13.6
  - cystica N28.84
  - puerperal (postpartum) O86.21
  - tuberculous A18.11
- **Pyelocystitis** — *see* Pyelonephritis
- **Pyelonephritis** — *see also* Nephritis, tubulo-interstitial
  - with
    - calculus — *see* category N2Ø ☑
      - with hydronephrosis N13.6
    - contracted kidney N11.9
  - acute N1Ø
  - calculous — *see* category N2Ø ☑
    - with hydronephrosis N13.6
  - chronic N11.9
    - with calculus — *see* category N2Ø ☑
      - with hydronephrosis N13.6
    - associated with ureteral obstruction or stricture N11.1
    - nonobstructive N11.8
      - with reflux (vesicoureteral) N11.Ø
    - obstructive N11.1
    - specified NEC N11.8
  - in (due to)
    - brucellosis A23.9 *[N16]*
    - cryoglobulinemia (mixed) D89.1 *[N16]*
    - cystinosis E72.Ø4
    - diphtheria A36.84
    - glycogen storage disease E74.Ø9 *[N16]*
    - leukemia NEC C95.9- ☑ *[N16]*
    - lymphoma NEC C85.9Ø *[N16]*
    - multiple myeloma C9Ø.Ø- ☑ *[N16]*
    - obstruction N11.1
    - Salmonella infection AØ2.25
    - sarcoidosis D86.84
    - sepsis A41.9 *[N16]*
    - Sjögren's disease M35.Ø4
    - toxoplasmosis B58.83
    - transplant rejection T86.91 *[N16]*
    - Wilson's disease E83.Ø1 *[N16]*
  - nonobstructive N12
    - with reflux (vesicoureteral) N11.Ø
    - chronic N11.8
  - syphilitic A52.75
- **Pyelonephrosis** (obstructive) N11.1
  - chronic N11.9

- **Pyelophlebitis** I8Ø.8
- **Pyeloureteritis cystica** N28.85
- **Pyemia, pyemic** (fever) (infection) (purulent) — *see also* Sepsis
  - joint — *see* Arthritis, pyogenic or pyemic
  - liver K75.1
  - pneumococcal A4Ø.3
  - portal K75.1
  - postvaccinal T88.Ø ☑
  - puerperal, postpartum, childbirth O85
  - specified organism NEC A41.89
  - tuberculous — *see* Tuberculosis, miliary
- **Pygopagus** Q89.4
- **Pyknoepilepsy** (idiopathic) — *see* Pyknolepsy
- **Pyknolepsy** G4Ø.AØ9 (*following* G4Ø.3)
  - intractable G4Ø.A19 (*following* G4Ø.3)
    - with status epilepticus G4Ø.A11 (*following* G4Ø.3)
    - without status epilepticus G4Ø.A19 (*following* G4Ø.3)
  - not intractable G4Ø.AØ9 (*following* G4Ø.3)
    - with status epilepticus G4Ø.AØ1 (*following* G4Ø.3)
    - without status epilepticus G4Ø.AØ9 (*following* G4Ø.3)
- **Pylephlebitis** K75.1
- **Pyle's syndrome** Q78.5
- **Pylethrombophlebitis** K75.1
- **Pylethrombosis** K75.1
- **Pyloritis** K29.9Ø
  - with bleeding K29.91
- **Pylorospasm** (reflex) **NEC** K31.3
  - congenital or infantile Q4Ø.Ø
  - neurotic F45.8
  - newborn Q4Ø.Ø
  - psychogenic F45.8
- **Pylorus, pyloric** — *see* condition
- **Pyoarthrosis** — *see* Arthritis, pyogenic or pyemic
- **Pyocele**
  - mastoid — *see* Mastoiditis, acute
  - sinus (accessory) — *see* Sinusitis
  - turbinate (bone) J32.9
  - urethra — *see also* Urethritis N34.Ø
- **Pyocolpos** — *see* Vaginitis
- **Pyocystitis** N3Ø.8Ø
  - with hematuria N3Ø.81
- **Pyoderma, pyodermia** LØ8.Ø
  - gangrenosum L88
  - newborn P39.4
  - phagedenic L88
  - vegetans LØ8.81
- **Pyodermatitis** LØ8.Ø
  - vegetans LØ8.81
- **Pyogenic** — *see* condition
- **Pyohydronephrosis** N13.6
- **Pyometra, pyometrium, pyometritis** — *see* Endometritis
- **Pyomyositis** (tropical) — *see* Myositis, infective
- **Pyonephritis** N12
- **Pyonephrosis** N13.6
  - tuberculous A18.11
- **Pyo-oophoritis** — *see* Salpingo-oophoritis
- **Pyo-ovarium** — *see* Salpingo-oophoritis
- **Pyopericarditis, pyopericardium** I3Ø.1
- **Pyophlebitis** — *see* Phlebitis
- **Pyopneumopericardium** I3Ø.1
- **Pyopneumothorax** (infective) J86.9
  - with fistula J86.Ø
  - tuberculous NEC A15.6
- **Pyosalpinx, pyosalpingitis** — *see also* Salpingo-oophoritis
- **Pyothorax** J86.9
  - with fistula J86.Ø
  - tuberculous NEC A15.6
- **Pyoureter** N28.89
  - tuberculous A18.11
- **Pyramidopallidonigral syndrome** G2Ø
- **Pyrexia** (of unknown origin) R5Ø.9
  - atmospheric T67.Ø1 ☑
  - during labor NEC O75.2
  - heat T67.Ø1 ☑
  - newborn P81.9
    - environmentally-induced P81.Ø
  - persistent R5Ø.9
  - puerperal O86.4
- **Pyroglobulinemia NEC** E88.Ø9
- **Pyromania** F63.1
- **Pyrosis** R12
- **Pyuria** (bacterial) (sterile) R82.81

- **Retained** — *see also* Retention
  - cholelithiasis following cholecystectomy K91.86
  - foreign body fragments (type of) Z18.9
    - acrylics Z18.2
    - animal quill(s) or spines Z18.31
    - cement Z18.83
    - concrete Z18.83
    - crystalline Z18.83
    - depleted isotope Z18.Ø9
    - depleted uranium Z18.Ø1
    - diethylhexyl phthalates Z18.2
    - glass Z18.81
    - isocyanate Z18.2
    - magnetic metal Z18.11
    - metal Z18.1Ø
    - nonmagnectic metal Z18.12
    - nontherapeutic radioactive Z18.Ø9
    - organic NEC Z18.39
    - plastic Z18.2
    - quill(s) (animal) Z18.31
    - radioactive (nontherapeutic) NEC Z18.Ø9
    - specified NEC Z18.89
    - spine(s) (animal) Z18.31
    - stone Z18.83
    - tooth (teeth) Z18.32
    - wood Z18.33
  - fragments (type of) Z18.9
    - acrylics Z18.2
    - animal quill(s) or spines Z18.31
    - cement Z18.83
    - concrete Z18.83
    - crystalline Z18.83
    - depleted isotope Z18.Ø9
    - depleted uranium Z18.Ø1
    - diethylhexyl phthalates Z18.2
    - glass Z18.81
    - isocyanate Z18.2
    - magnetic metal Z18.11
    - metal Z18.1Ø
    - nonmagnectic metal Z18.12
    - nontherapeutic radioactive Z18.Ø9
    - organic NEC Z18.39
    - plastic Z18.2
    - quill(s) (animal) Z18.31
    - radioactive (nontherapeutic) NEC Z18.Ø9
    - specified NEC Z18.89
    - spine(s) (animal) Z18.31
    - stone Z18.83
    - tooth (teeth) Z18.32
    - wood Z18.33
  - gallstones, following cholecystectomy K91.86
- **Retardation**
  - development, developmental, specific — *see* Disorder, developmental
  - endochondral bone growth — *see* Disorder, bone, development or growth
  - growth R62.5Ø
    - due to malnutrition E45
  - mental — *see* Disability, intellectual
  - motor function, specific F82
  - physical (child) R62.52
    - due to malnutrition E45
  - reading (specific) F81.Ø
  - spelling (specific) (without reading disorder) F81.81
- **Retching** — *see* Vomiting
- **Retention** — *see also* Retained
  - bladder — *see* Retention, urine
  - carbon dioxide E87.29
  - cholelithiasis following cholecystectomy K91.86
  - cyst — *see* Cyst
  - dead
    - fetus (at or near term) (mother) O36.4 ☑
      - early fetal death OØ2.1
    - ovum OØ2.Ø
  - decidua (fragments) (following delivery) (with hemorrhage) O72.2
    - without hemorrhage O73.1
  - deciduous tooth KØØ.6
  - dental root KØ8.3
  - fecal — *see* Constipation
  - fetus
    - dead O36.4 ☑
      - early OØ2.1
  - fluid R6Ø.9
  - foreign body — *see also* Foreign body, retained
    - current trauma — *code as* Foreign body, by site or type
  - gallstones, following cholecystectomy K91.86

- **Retention** — *continued*
  - gastric K31.89
  - intrauterine contraceptive device, in pregnancy — *see* Pregnancy, complicated by, retention, intrauterine device
  - membranes (complicating delivery) (with hemorrhage) O72.2
    - with abortion — *see* Abortion, by type
    - without hemorrhage O73.1
  - meniscus — *see* Derangement, meniscus
  - menses N94.89
  - milk (puerperal, postpartum) O92.79
  - nitrogen, extrarenal R39.2
  - ovary syndrome N99.83
  - placenta (total) (with hemorrhage) O72.Ø
    - without hemorrhage O73.Ø
    - portions or fragments (with hemorrhage) O72.2
      - without hemorrhage O73.1
  - products of conception
    - early pregnancy (dead fetus) OØ2.1
    - following
      - delivery (with hemorrhage) O72.2
        - without hemorrhage O73.1
  - secundines (following delivery) (with hemorrhage) O72.Ø
    - without hemorrhage O73.Ø
    - complicating puerperium (delayed hemorrhage) O72.2
    - partial O72.2
      - without hemorrhage O73.1
  - smegma, clitoris N9Ø.89
  - urine R33.9
    - due to hyperplasia (hypertrophy) of prostate — *see* Hyperplasia, prostate
    - drug-induced R33.Ø
    - organic R33.8
      - drug-induced R33.Ø
    - psychogenic F45.8
    - specified NEC R33.8
  - water (in tissues) — *see* Edema
- **Reticulation, dust** — *see* Pneumoconiosis
- **Reticulocytosis** R7Ø.1
- **Reticuloendotheliosis**
  - acute infantile C96.Ø
  - leukemic C91.4- ☑
  - nonlipid C96.Ø
- **Reticulohistiocytoma** (giant-cell) D76.3
- **Reticuloid, actinic** L57.1
- **Reticulosis** (skin)
  - acute of infancy C96.Ø
  - hemophagocytic, familial D76.1
  - histiocytic medullary C96.A (*following* C96.6)
  - lipomelanotic I89.8
  - malignant (midline) C86.Ø
  - polymorphic C83.8- ☑
  - Sézary — *see* Sézary disease
- **Retina, retinal** — *see also* condition
  - dark area D49.81
- **Retinitis** — *see also* Inflammation, chorioretinal
  - albuminurica N18.9 *[H32]*
  - diabetic — *see* Diabetes, retinitis
  - disciformis — *see* Degeneration, macula
  - focal — *see* Inflammation, chorioretinal, focal
  - gravidarum — *see* Pregnancy, complicated by, specified pregnancy-related condition NEC
  - juxtapapillaris — *see* Inflammation, chorioretinal, focal, juxtapapillary
  - luetic — *see* Retinitis, syphilitic
  - pigmentosa H35.52
  - proliferans — *see* Disorder, globe, degenerative, specified type NEC
  - proliferating — *see* Disorder, globe, degenerative, specified type NEC
  - renal N18.9 *[H32]*
  - syphilitic (early) (secondary) A51.43
    - central, recurrent A52.71
    - congenital (early) A5Ø.Ø1 *[H32]*
    - late A52.71
  - tuberculous A18.53
- **Retinoblastoma** C69.2- ☑
  - differentiated C69.2- ☑
  - undifferentiated C69.2- ☑
- **Retinochoroiditis** — *see also* Inflammation, chorioretinal
  - disseminated — *see* Inflammation, chorioretinal, disseminated
    - syphilitic A52.71
  - focal — *see* Inflammation, chorioretinal

- **Retinochoroiditis** — *continued*
  - juxtapapillaris — *see* Inflammation, chorioretinal, focal, juxtapapillary
- **Retinopathy** (background) H35.ØØ
  - arteriosclerotic I7Ø.8 *[H35.Ø-]* ☑
  - atherosclerotic I7Ø.8 *[H35.Ø-]* ☑
  - central serous — *see* Chorioretinopathy, central serous
  - Coats H35.Ø2- ☑
  - diabetic — *see* Diabetes, retinopathy
  - exudative H35.Ø2- ☑
  - hypertensive H35.Ø3- ☑
  - in (due to)
    - diabetes — *see* Diabetes, retinopathy
    - sickle-cell disorders D57.- ☑ *[H36]*
  - of prematurity H35.1Ø- ☑
    - stage Ø H35.11- ☑
    - stage 1 H35.12- ☑
    - stage 2 H35.13- ☑
    - stage 3 H35.14- ☑
    - stage 4 H35.15- ☑
    - stage 5 H35.16- ☑
  - pigmentary, congenital — *see* Dystrophy, retina
  - proliferative NEC H35.2- ☑
    - diabetic — *see* Diabetes, retinopathy, proliferative
    - sickle-cell D57.- ☑ *[H36]*
  - solar H31.Ø2- ☑
- **Retinoschisis** H33.1Ø- ☑
  - congenital Q14.1
  - specified type NEC H33.19- ☑
- **Retortamoniasis** AØ7.8
- **Retractile testis** Q55.22
- **Retraction**
  - cervix — *see* Retroversion, uterus
  - drum (membrane) — *see* Disorder, tympanic membrane, specified NEC
  - finger — *see* Deformity, finger
  - lid HØ2.539
    - left HØ2.536
      - lower HØ2.535
      - upper HØ2.534
    - right HØ2.533
      - lower HØ2.532
      - upper HØ2.531
  - lung J98.4
  - mediastinum J98.59
  - nipple N64.53
    - associated with
      - lactation O92.Ø3
      - pregnancy O92.Ø1- ☑
      - puerperium O92.Ø2
    - congenital Q83.8
  - palmar fascia M72.Ø
  - pleura — *see* Pleurisy
  - ring, uterus (Bandl's) (pathological) O62.4
  - sternum (congenital) Q76.7
    - acquired M95.4
  - uterus — *see* Retroversion, uterus
  - valve (heart) — *see* Endocarditis
- **Retrobulbar** — *see* condition
- **Retrocecal** — *see* condition
- **Retrocession** — *see* Retroversion
- **Retrodisplacement** — *see* Retroversion
- **Retroflection, retroflexion** — *see* Retroversion
- **Retrognathia, retrognathism** (mandibular) (maxillary) M26.19
- **Retrograde menstruation** N92.5
- **Retroperineal** — *see* condition
- **Retroperitoneal** — *see* condition
- **Retroperitonitis** K68.9
- **Retropharyngeal** — *see* condition
- **Retroplacental** — *see* condition
- **Retroposition** — *see* Retroversion
- **Retroprosthetic membrane** T85.398 ☑
- **Retrosternal thyroid** (congenital) Q89.2
- **Retroversion, retroverted**
  - cervix — *see* Retroversion, uterus
  - female NEC — *see* Retroversion, uterus
  - iris H21.89
  - testis (congenital) Q55.29
  - uterus (acquired) (acute) (any degree) (asymptomatic) (cervix) (postinfectional) (postpartal, old) N85.4
    - congenital Q51.818
    - in pregnancy O34.53- ☑
- **Retrovirus, as cause of disease classified elsewhere** B97.3Ø
  - human
    - immunodeficiency, type 2 (HIV 2) B97.35

Rietti-Greppi-Micheli anemia D56.9
Rieux's hernia — *see* Hernia, abdomen, specified site NEC
Riga (-Fede) **disease** K14.Ø
Riggs' disease — *see* Periodontitis
Right aortic arch Q25.47
Right middle lobe syndrome J98.11
Rigid, rigidity — *see also* condition
- abdominal R19.3Ø
  - with severe abdominal pain R1Ø.Ø
  - epigastric R19.36
  - generalized R19.37
  - left lower quadrant R19.34
  - left upper quadrant R19.32
  - periumbilic R19.35
  - right lower quadrant R19.33
  - right upper quadrant R19.31
- articular, multiple, congenital Q68.8
- cervix (uteri) in pregnancy — *see* Pregnancy, complicated by, abnormal, cervix
- hymen (acquired) (congenital) N89.6
- nuchal R29.1
- pelvic floor in pregnancy — *see* Pregnancy, complicated by, abnormal, pelvic organs or tissues NEC
- perineum or vulva in pregnancy — *see* Pregnancy, complicated by, abnormal, vulva
- spine — *see* Dorsopathy, specified NEC
- vagina in pregnancy — *see* Pregnancy, complicated by, abnormal, vagina

Rigors R68.89
- with fever R5Ø.9

Riley-Day syndrome G9Ø.1
RIND (reversible ischemic neurologic deficit) I63.9
Ring(s)
- aorta (vascular) Q25.45
- Bandl's O62.4
- contraction, complicating delivery O62.4
- esophageal, lower (muscular) K22.2
- Fleischer's (cornea) H18.Ø4- ☑
- hymenal, tight (acquired) (congenital) N89.6
- Kayser-Fleischer (cornea) H18.Ø4- ☑
- retraction, uterus, pathological O62.4
- Schatzki's (esophagus) (lower) K22.2
  - congenital Q39.3
- Soemmerring's — *see* Cataract, secondary
- vascular (congenital) Q25.8
  - aorta Q25.45

Ringed hair (congenital) Q84.1
Ringworm B35.9
- beard B35.Ø
- black dot B35.Ø
- body B35.4
- Burmese B35.5
- corporeal B35.4
- foot B35.3
- groin B35.6
- hand B35.2
- honeycomb B35.Ø
- nails B35.1
- perianal (area) B35.6
- scalp B35.Ø
- specified NEC B35.8
- Tokelau B35.5

Rise, venous pressure I87.8
Rising, PSA following treatment for malignant neoplasm of prostate R97.21
Risk
- for
  - dental caries Z91.849
    - high Z91.843
    - low Z91.841
    - moderate Z91.842
  - homelessness, imminent Z59.811
  - suffocation (smothering) under another while sleeping Z72.823
- suicidal
  - meaning personal history of attempted suicide Z91.51
  - meaning suicidal ideation — *see* Ideation, suicidal

Ritter's disease LØØ
Rivalry, sibling Z62.891
Rivalta's disease A42.2
River blindness B73.Ø1
Robert's pelvis Q74.2
- with disproportion (fetopelvic) O33.Ø
  - causing obstructed labor O65.Ø

Robin (-Pierre) **syndrome** Q87.Ø
Robinow-Silvermann-Smith syndrome Q87.19
Robinson's (hidrotic) **ectodermal dysplasia or syndrome** Q82.4
Robles' disease B73.Ø1
Rocky Mountain (spotted) **fever** A77.Ø
Roetheln — *see* Rubella
Roger's disease Q21.Ø
Rokitansky-Aschoff sinuses (gallbladder) K82.8
Rolando's fracture (displaced) S62.22- ☑
- nondisplaced S62.22- ☑

Romano-Ward (prolonged QT interval) **syndrome** I45.81
Romberg's disease or syndrome G51.8
Roof, mouth — *see* condition
Rosacea L71.9
- acne L71.9
- keratitis L71.8
- specified NEC L71.8

Rosary, rachitic E55.Ø
Rose
- cold J3Ø.1
- fever J3Ø.1
- rash R21
  - epidemic BØ6.9

Rosenbach's erysipeloid A26.Ø
Rosenthal's disease or syndrome D68.1
Roseola BØ9
- infantum BØ8.2Ø
  - due to human herpesvirus 6 BØ8.21
  - due to human herpesvirus 7 BØ8.22

Ross River disease or fever B33.1
Rossbach's disease K31.89
- psychogenic F45.8

Rostan's asthma (cardiac) — *see* Failure, ventricular, left
Rotation
- anomalous, incomplete or insufficient, intestine Q43.3
- cecum (congenital) Q43.3
- colon (congenital) Q43.3
- spine, incomplete or insufficient — *see* Dorsopathy, deforming, specified NEC
- tooth, teeth, fully erupted M26.35
- vertebra, incomplete or insufficient — *see* Dorsopathy, deforming, specified NEC

Rotes Quérol disease or syndrome — *see* Hyperostosis, ankylosing
Roth (-Bernhardt) **disease or syndrome** — *see* Meralgia paraesthetica
Rothmund (-Thomson) **syndrome** Q82.8
Rotor's disease or syndrome E8Ø.6
Round
- back (with wedging of vertebrae) — *see* Kyphosis
  - sequelae (late effect) of rickets E64.3
- worms (large) (infestation) NEC B82.Ø
  - Ascariasis — *see also* Ascariasis B77.9

Roussy-Lévy syndrome G6Ø.Ø
Rubella (German measles) BØ6.9
- complication NEC BØ6.Ø9
  - neurological BØ6.ØØ
- congenital P35.Ø
- contact Z2Ø.4
- exposure to Z2Ø.4
- maternal
  - care for (suspected) damage to fetus O35.3 ☑
  - manifest rubella in infant P35.Ø
  - suspected damage to fetus affecting management of pregnancy O35.3 ☑
- specified complications NEC BØ6.89

Rubeola (meaning measles) — *see* Measles
- meaning rubella — *see* Rubella

Rubeosis, iris — *see* Disorder, iris, vascular
Rubinstein-Taybi syndrome Q87.2
Rudimentary (congenital) — *see also* Agenesis
- arm — *see* Defect, reduction, upper limb
- bone Q79.9
- cervix uteri Q51.828
- eye Q11.2
- lobule of ear Q17.3
- patella Q74.1
- respiratory organs in thoracopagus Q89.4
- tracheal bronchus Q32.4
- uterus Q51.818
  - in male Q56.1
- vagina Q52.Ø

Ruled out condition — *see* Observation, suspected
Rumination R11.1Ø
- with nausea R11.2
- disorder of infancy F98.21
- neurotic F42.8
- newborn P92.1
- obsessional F42.8
- psychogenic F42.8

Runeberg's disease D51.Ø
Running out of money Z59.86
Runny nose RØ9.89
Rupia (syphilitic) A51.39
- congenital A5Ø.Ø6
- tertiary A52.79

Rupture, ruptured
- abscess (spontaneous) — *code by* site under Abscess
- aneurysm — *see* Aneurysm
- anus (sphincter) — *see* Laceration, anus
- aorta, aortic I71.8
  - abdominal I71.3Ø
    - infrarenal I71.33
    - juxtarenal I71.32
    - pararenal I71.31
  - arch I71.12
  - ascending I71.11
  - descending I71.8
    - abdominal I71.3Ø
    - thoracic I71.13
  - syphilitic A52.Ø1
  - thoracoabdominal I71.5Ø
    - paravisceral I71.52
    - supraceliac I71.51
  - thorax, thoracic I71.1Ø
  - transverse I71.12
  - traumatic — *see* Injury, aorta, laceration, major
  - valve or cusp — *see also* Endocarditis, aortic I35.8
- appendix (with peritonitis) — *see also* Appendicitis K35.32
  - with localized peritonitis — *see also* Appendicitis K35.32
- arteriovenous fistula, brain — *see* Fistula, arteriovenous, brain, ruptured
- artery I77.2
  - brain — *see* Hemorrhage, intracranial, intracerebral
  - coronary — *see* Infarct, myocardium
  - heart — *see* Infarct, myocardium
  - pulmonary I28.8
  - traumatic (complication) — *see* Injury, blood vessel
- bile duct (common) (hepatic) K83.2
  - cystic K82.2
- bladder (sphincter) (nontraumatic) (spontaneous) N32.89
  - following ectopic or molar pregnancy OØ8.6
  - obstetrical trauma O71.5
  - traumatic S37.29 ☑
- blood vessel — *see also* Hemorrhage
  - brain — *see* Hemorrhage, intracranial, intracerebral
  - heart — *see* Infarct, myocardium
  - traumatic (complication) — *see* Injury, blood vessel, laceration, major, by site
- bone — *see* Fracture
- bowel (nontraumatic) K63.1
- brain
  - aneurysm (congenital) — *see also* Hemorrhage, intracranial, subarachnoid
    - syphilitic A52.Ø5
  - hemorrhagic — *see* Hemorrhage, intracranial, intracerebral
- capillaries I78.8
- cardiac (auricle) (ventricle) (wall) I23.3
  - with hemopericardium I23.Ø
  - infectional I4Ø.9
  - traumatic — *see* Injury, heart
- cartilage (articular) (current) — *see also* Sprain
  - knee S83.3- ☑
  - semilunar — *see* Tear, meniscus
- cecum (with peritonitis) K65.Ø
  - with peritoneal abscess K35.33
  - traumatic S36.598 ☑
- celiac artery, traumatic — *see* Injury, blood vessel, celiac artery, laceration, major
- cerebral aneurysm (congenital) (see Hemorrhage, intracranial, subarachnoid)
- cervix (uteri)
  - with ectopic or molar pregnancy OØ8.6
  - following ectopic or molar pregnancy OØ8.6
  - obstetrical trauma O71.3
  - traumatic S37.69 ☑
- chordae tendineae NEC I51.1
  - concurrent with acute myocardial infarction — *see* Infarct, myocardium
  - following acute myocardial infarction (current complication) I23.4

- **Rupture, ruptured** — *continued*
  - choroid (direct) (indirect) (traumatic) H31.32- ☑
  - circle of Willis I6Ø.6
  - colon (nontraumatic) K63.1
    - traumatic — *see* Injury, intestine, large
  - cornea (traumatic) — *see* Injury, eye, laceration
  - coronary (artery) (thrombotic) — *see* Infarct, myocardium
  - corpus luteum (infected) (ovary) N83.1- ☑
  - cyst — *see* Cyst
  - cystic duct K82.2
  - Descemet's membrane — *see* Change, corneal membrane, Descemet's, rupture
    - traumatic — *see* Injury, eye, laceration
  - diaphragm, traumatic — *see* Injury, intrathoracic, diaphragm
  - disc — *see* Rupture, intervertebral disc
  - diverticulum (intestine) K57.8Ø
    - with bleeding K57.81
    - bladder N32.3
    - large intestine K57.2Ø
      - with
        - bleeding K57.21
        - small intestine K57.4Ø
          - with bleeding K57.41
    - small intestine K57.ØØ
      - with
        - bleeding K57.Ø1
        - large intestine K57.4Ø
          - with bleeding K57.41
  - duodenal stump K31.89
  - ear drum (nontraumatic) — *see also* Perforation, tympanum
    - traumatic SØ9.2- ☑
      - due to blast injury — *see* Injury, blast, ear
  - esophagus K22.3
  - eye (without prolapse or loss of intraocular tissue) — *see* Injury, eye, laceration
  - fallopian tube NEC (nonobstetric) (nontraumatic) N83.8
    - due to pregnancy OØØ.1Ø- ☑
      - with intrauterine pregnancy OØØ.11- ☑
  - fontanel P13.1
  - gallbladder K82.2
    - traumatic S36.128 ☑
  - gastric — *see also* Rupture, stomach
    - vessel K92.2
  - globe (eye) (traumatic) — *see* Injury, eye, laceration
  - graafian follicle (hematoma) N83.Ø- ☑
  - heart — *see* Rupture, cardiac
  - hymen (nontraumatic) (nonintentional) N89.8
  - internal organ, traumatic — *see* Injury, by site
  - intervertebral disc — *see* Displacement, intervertebral disc
    - traumatic — *see* Rupture, traumatic, intervertebral disc
  - intestine NEC (nontraumatic) K63.1
    - traumatic — *see* Injury, intestine
  - iris — *see also* Abnormality, pupillary
    - traumatic — *see* Injury, eye, laceration
  - joint capsule, traumatic — *see* Sprain
  - kidney (traumatic) S37.Ø6- ☑
    - birth injury P15.8
    - nontraumatic N28.89
  - lacrimal duct (traumatic) — *see* Injury, eye, specified site NEC
  - lens (cataract) (traumatic) — *see* Cataract, traumatic
  - ligament, traumatic — *see* Rupture, traumatic, ligament, by site
  - liver S36.116 ☑
    - birth injury P15.Ø
  - lymphatic vessel I89.8
  - marginal sinus (placental) (with hemorrhage) — *see* Hemorrhage, antepartum, specified cause NEC
  - membrana tympani (nontraumatic) — *see* Perforation, tympanum
  - membranes (spontaneous)
    - artificial
      - delayed delivery following O75.5
    - delayed delivery following — *see* Pregnancy, complicated by, premature rupture of membranes
  - meningeal artery I6Ø.8
  - meniscus (knee) — *see also* Tear, meniscus
    - old — *see* Derangement, meniscus
    - site other than knee — *code as* Sprain
  - mesenteric artery, traumatic — *see* Injury, mesenteric, artery, laceration, major
  - mesentery (nontraumatic) K66.8
- **Rupture, ruptured** — *continued*
  - mesentery — *continued*
    - traumatic — *see* Injury, intra-abdominal, specified, site NEC
  - mitral (valve) I34.89
  - muscle (traumatic) — *see also* Strain
    - diastasis — *see* Diastasis, muscle
    - nontraumatic M62.1Ø
      - ankle M62.17- ☑
      - foot M62.17- ☑
      - forearm M62.13- ☑
      - hand M62.14- ☑
      - lower leg M62.16- ☑
      - pelvic region M62.15- ☑
      - shoulder region M62.11- ☑
      - specified site NEC M62.18
      - thigh M62.15- ☑
      - upper arm M62.12- ☑
    - traumatic — *see* Strain, by site
  - musculotendinous junction NEC, nontraumatic — *see* Rupture, tendon, spontaneous
  - mycotic aneurysm causing cerebral hemorrhage — *see* Hemorrhage, intracranial, subarachnoid
  - myocardium, myocardial — *see* Rupture, cardiac
    - traumatic — *see* Injury, heart
  - nontraumatic, meaning hernia — *see* Hernia
  - obstructed — *see* Hernia, by site, obstructed
  - operation wound — *see* Disruption, wound, operation
  - ovary, ovarian N83.8
    - corpus luteum cyst N83.1- ☑
    - follicle (graafian) N83.Ø- ☑
  - oviduct (nonobstetric) (nontraumatic) N83.8
    - due to pregnancy OØØ.1Ø- ☑
      - with intrauterine pregnancy OØØ.11- ☑
  - pancreas (nontraumatic) K86.89
    - traumatic S36.299 ☑
  - papillary muscle NEC I51.2
    - following acute myocardial infarction (current complication) I23.5
  - pelvic
    - floor, complicating delivery O7Ø.1
    - organ NEC, obstetrical trauma O71.5
  - perineum (nonobstetric) (nontraumatic) N9Ø.89
    - complicating delivery — *see* Delivery, complicated, by, laceration, anus (sphincter)
  - postoperative wound — *see* Disruption, wound, operation
  - prostate (traumatic) S37.828 ☑
  - pulmonary
    - artery I28.8
    - valve (heart) I37.8
    - vein I28.8
    - vessel I28.8
  - pus tube — *see* Salpingitis
  - pyosalpinx — *see* Salpingitis
  - rectum (nontraumatic) K63.1
    - traumatic S36.69 ☑
  - retina, retinal (traumatic) (without detachment) — *see also* Break, retina
    - with detachment — *see* Detachment, retina, with retinal, break
  - rotator cuff (nontraumatic) M75.1Ø- ☑
    - complete M75.12- ☑
    - incomplete M75.11- ☑
  - sclera — *see* Injury, eye, laceration
  - sigmoid (nontraumatic) K63.1
    - traumatic S36.593 ☑
  - spinal cord — *see also* Injury, spinal cord, by region
    - due to injury at birth P11.5
    - newborn (birth injury) P11.5
  - spleen (traumatic) S36.Ø9 ☑
    - birth injury P15.1
    - congenital (birth injury) P15.1
    - due to P. vivax malaria B51.Ø
    - nontraumatic D73.5
    - spontaneous D73.5
  - splenic vein R58
    - traumatic — *see* Injury, blood vessel, splenic vein
  - stomach (nontraumatic) (spontaneous) K31.89
    - traumatic S36.39 ☑
  - supraspinatus (complete) (incomplete) (nontraumatic) — *see* Tear, rotator cuff
  - symphysis pubis
    - obstetric O71.6
    - traumatic S33.4 ☑
  - synovium (cyst) M66.1Ø
    - ankle M66.17- ☑
- **Rupture, ruptured** — *continued*
  - synovium — *continued*
    - elbow M66.12- ☑
    - finger M66.14- ☑
    - foot M66.17- ☑
    - forearm M66.13- ☑
    - hand M66.14- ☑
    - pelvic region M66.15- ☑
    - shoulder region M66.11- ☑
    - specified site NEC M66.18
    - thigh M66.15- ☑
    - toe M66.17- ☑
    - upper arm M66.12- ☑
    - wrist M66.13- ☑
  - tendon (traumatic) — *see* Strain
    - nontraumatic (spontaneous) M66.9
      - ankle M66.87- ☑
      - extensor M66.2Ø
        - ankle M66.27- ☑
        - foot M66.27- ☑
        - forearm M66.23- ☑
        - hand M66.24- ☑
        - lower leg M66.26- ☑
        - multiple sites M66.29
        - pelvic region M66.25- ☑
        - shoulder region M66.21- ☑
        - specified site NEC M66.28
        - thigh M66.25- ☑
        - upper arm M66.22- ☑
      - flexor M66.3Ø
        - ankle M66.37- ☑
        - foot M66.37- ☑
        - forearm M66.33- ☑
        - hand M66.34- ☑
        - lower leg M66.36- ☑
        - multiple sites M66.39
        - pelvic region M66.35- ☑
        - shoulder region M66.31- ☑
        - specified site NEC M66.38
        - thigh M66.35- ☑
        - upper arm M66.32- ☑
      - foot M66.87- ☑
      - forearm M66.83- ☑
      - hand M66.84- ☑
      - lower leg M66.86- ☑
      - multiple sites M66.89
      - pelvic region M66.85- ☑
      - shoulder region M66.81- ☑
      - specified
        - site NEC M66.88
        - tendon M66.8Ø
      - thigh M66.85- ☑
      - upper arm M66.82- ☑
  - thoracic duct I89.8
  - tonsil J35.8
  - traumatic
    - aorta — *see* Injury, aorta, laceration, major
    - diaphragm — *see* Injury, intrathoracic, diaphragm
    - external site — *see* Wound, open, by site
    - eye — *see* Injury, eye, laceration
    - internal organ — *see* Injury, by site
    - intervertebral disc
      - cervical S13.Ø ☑
      - lumbar S33.Ø ☑
      - thoracic S23.Ø ☑
    - kidney S37.Ø6- ☑
    - ligament — *see also* Sprain
      - ankle — *see* Sprain, ankle
      - carpus — *see* Rupture, traumatic, ligament, wrist
      - collateral (hand) — *see* Rupture, traumatic, ligament, finger, collateral
      - finger (metacarpophalangeal) (interphalangeal) S63.4Ø- ☑
        - collateral S63.41- ☑
          - index S63.41- ☑
          - little S63.41- ☑
          - middle S63.41- ☑
          - ring S63.41- ☑
        - index S63.4Ø- ☑
        - little S63.4Ø- ☑
        - middle S63.4Ø- ☑
        - palmar S63.42- ☑
          - index S63.42- ☑
          - little S63.42- ☑
          - middle S63.42- ☑
          - ring S63.42- ☑

- **Rupture, ruptured** — *continued*
  - traumatic — *continued*
    - ligament — *see also* Sprain — *continued*
      - finger — *continued*
        - ring S63.40- ☑
        - specified site NEC S63.499 ☑
          - index S63.49- ☑
          - little S63.49- ☑
          - middle S63.49- ☑
          - ring S63.49- ☑
        - volar plate S63.43- ☑
          - index S63.43- ☑
          - little S63.43- ☑
          - middle S63.43- ☑
          - ring S63.43- ☑
      - foot — *see* Sprain, foot
      - radial collateral S53.2- ☑
      - radiocarpal — *see* Rupture, traumatic, ligament, wrist, radiocarpal
      - ulnar collateral S53.3- ☑
      - ulnocarpal — *see* Rupture, traumatic, ligament, wrist, ulnocarpal
      - wrist S63.30- ☑
        - collateral S63.31- ☑
        - radiocarpal S63.32- ☑
        - specified site NEC S63.39- ☑
        - ulnocarpal (palmar) S63.33- ☑
    - liver S36.116 ☑
    - membrana tympani — *see* Rupture, ear drum, traumatic
    - muscle or tendon — *see* Strain
    - myocardium — *see* Injury, heart
    - pancreas S36.299 ☑
    - rectum S36.69 ☑
    - sigmoid S36.593 ☑
    - spleen S36.09 ☑
    - stomach S36.39 ☑
    - symphysis pubis S33.4 ☑
    - tympanum, tympanic (membrane) — *see* Rupture, ear drum, traumatic
    - ureter S37.19 ☑
    - uterus S37.69 ☑
    - vagina — *see* Injury, vagina
    - vena cava — *see* Injury, vena cava, laceration, major
  - tricuspid (heart) (valve) I07.8
  - tube, tubal (nonobstetric) (nontraumatic) N83.8
    - abscess — *see* Salpingitis
    - due to pregnancy O00.10- ☑
      - with intrauterine pregnancy O00.11- ☑
  - tympanum, tympanic (membrane) (nontraumatic) — *see also* Perforation, tympanic membrane H72.9- ☑
    - traumatic — *see* Rupture, ear drum, traumatic
  - umbilical cord, complicating delivery O69.89 ☑
  - ureter (traumatic) S37.19 ☑
    - nontraumatic N28.89
  - urethra (nontraumatic) N36.8
    - with ectopic or molar pregnancy O08.6
    - following ectopic or molar pregnancy O08.6
    - obstetrical trauma O71.5
    - traumatic S37.39 ☑
  - uterosacral ligament (nonobstetric) (nontraumatic) N83.8
  - uterus (traumatic) S37.69 ☑
    - before labor O71.0- ☑
    - during or after labor O71.1
    - nonpuerperal, nontraumatic N85.8
    - pregnant (during labor) O71.1
      - before labor O71.0- ☑
  - vagina — *see* Injury, vagina
  - valve, valvular (heart) — *see* Endocarditis
  - varicose vein — *see* Varix
  - varix — *see* Varix
  - vena cava R58
    - traumatic — *see* Injury, vena cava, laceration, major
  - vesical (urinary) N32.89
  - vessel (blood) R58
    - pulmonary I28.8
    - traumatic — *see* Injury, blood vessel
  - viscus R19.8
  - vulva complicating delivery O70.0
- **Russell-Silver syndrome** Q87.19
- **Russian spring-summer type encephalitis** A84.0
- **Rust's disease** (tuberculous cervical spondylitis) A18.01
- **Ruvalcaba-Myhre-Smith syndrome** E71.440
- **Rytand-Lipsitch syndrome** I44.2

S

- **Saber, sabre shin or tibia** (syphilitic) A50.56 *[M90.8-]* ☑
- **Sac lacrimal** — *see* condition
- **Saccharomyces infection** B37.9
- **Saccharopinuria** E72.3
- **Saccular** — *see* condition
- **Sacculation**
  - aorta (nonsyphilitic) — *see* Aneurysm, aorta
  - bladder N32.3
  - intralaryngeal (congenital) (ventricular) Q31.3
  - larynx (congenital) (ventricular) Q31.3
  - organ or site, congenital — *see* Distortion
  - pregnant uterus — *see* Pregnancy, complicated by, abnormal, uterus
  - ureter N28.89
  - urethra N36.1
  - vesical N32.3
- **Sachs' amaurotic familial idiocy or disease** E75.02
- **Sachs-Tay disease** E75.02
- **Sacks-Libman disease** M32.11
- **Sacralgia** M53.3
- **Sacralization** Q76.49
- **Sacrodynia** M53.3
- **Sacroiliac joint** — *see* condition
- **Sacroiliitis NEC** M46.1
- **Sacrum** — *see* condition
- **Saddle**
  - back — *see* Lordosis
  - embolus
    - abdominal aorta I74.01
    - pulmonary artery I26.92
      - with acute cor pulmonale I26.02
  - injury — *code to* condition
  - nose M95.0
    - due to syphilis A50.57
- **Sadism** (sexual) F65.52
- **Sadness, postpartal** O90.6
- **Sadomasochism** F65.50
- **Saemisch's ulcer** (cornea) — *see* Ulcer, cornea, central
- **Sagging**
  - skin and subcutaneous tissue (following bariatric surgery weight loss) (following dietary weight loss) L98.7
- **Sahib disease** B55.0
- **Sailors' skin** L57.8
- **Saint**
  - Anthony's fire — *see* Erysipelas
  - triad — *see* Hernia, diaphragm
  - Vitus' dance — *see* Chorea, Sydenham's
- **Salaam**
  - attack(s) — *see* Epilepsy, spasms
  - tic R25.8
- **Salicylism**
  - abuse F55.8
  - overdose or wrong substance given — *see* Table of Drugs and Chemicals, by drug, poisoning
- **Salivary duct or gland** — *see* condition
- **Salivation, excessive** K11.7
- **Salmonella** — *see* Infection, Salmonella
- **Salmonellosis** A02.0
- **Salpingitis** (catarrhal) (fallopian tube) (nodular) (pseudofollicular) (purulent) (septic) N70.91
  - with oophoritis N70.93
  - acute N70.01
    - with oophoritis N70.03
  - chlamydial A56.11
  - chronic N70.11
    - with oophoritis N70.13
  - complicating abortion — *see* Abortion, by type, complicated by, salpingitis
  - ear — *see* Salpingitis, eustachian
  - eustachian (tube) H68.00- ☑
    - acute H68.01- ☑
    - chronic H68.02- ☑
  - follicularis N70.11
    - with oophoritis N70.13
  - gonococcal (acute) (chronic) A54.24
  - interstitial, chronic N70.11
    - with oophoritis N70.13
  - isthmica nodosa N70.11
    - with oophoritis N70.13
  - specific (gonococcal) (acute) (chronic) A54.24
  - tuberculous (acute) (chronic) A18.17
  - venereal (gonococcal) (acute) (chronic) A54.24
- **Salpingocele** N83.4- ☑
- **Salpingo-oophoritis** (catarrhal) (purulent) (ruptured) (septic) (suppurative) N70.93
  - acute N70.03
    - with ectopic or molar pregnancy O08.0
    - following ectopic or molar pregnancy O08.0
    - gonococcal A54.24
  - chronic N70.13
  - following ectopic or molar pregnancy O08.0
  - gonococcal (acute) (chronic) A54.24
  - puerperal O86.19
  - specific (gonococcal) (acute) (chronic) A54.24
  - subacute N70.03
  - tuberculous (acute) (chronic) A18.17
  - venereal (gonococcal) (acute) (chronic) A54.24
- **Salpingo-ovaritis** — *see* Salpingo-oophoritis
- **Salpingoperitonitis** — *see* Salpingo-oophoritis
- **Salzmann's nodular dystrophy** — *see* Degeneration, cornea, nodular
- **Sampson's cyst or tumor** N80.10- ☑
- **San Joaquin** (Valley) **fever** B38.0
- **Sandblaster's asthma, lung or pneumoconiosis** J62.8
- **Sander's disease** (paranoia) F22
- **Sandfly fever** A93.1
- **Sandhoff's disease** E75.01
- **Sanfilippo** (Type B) (Type C) (Type D) **syndrome** E76.22
- **Sanger-Brown ataxia** G11.2
- **Sao Paulo fever or typhus** A77.0
- **Saponification, mesenteric** K65.8
- **Sarcocele** (benign)
  - syphilitic A52.76
    - congenital A50.59
- **Sarcocystosis** A07.8
- **Sarcoepiplocele** — *see* Hernia
- **Sarcoepiplomphalocele** Q79.2
- **Sarcoglycanopathy** G71.0340
  - alpha G71.0341
  - beta G71.0342
  - delta G71.0349
  - gamma G71.0349
- **Sarcoid** — *see also* Sarcoidosis
  - arthropathy D86.86
  - Boeck's D86.9
  - Darier-Roussy D86.3
  - iridocyclitis D86.83
  - meningitis D86.81
  - myocarditis D86.85
  - myositis D86.87
  - pyelonephritis D86.84
  - Spiegler-Fendt L08.89
- **Sarcoidosis** D86.9
  - with
    - cranial nerve palsies D86.82
    - hepatic granuloma D86.89
    - polyarthritis D86.86
    - tubulo-interstitial nephropathy D86.84
  - combined sites NEC D86.89
  - lung D86.0
    - and lymph nodes D86.2
  - lymph nodes D86.1
    - and lung D86.2
  - meninges D86.81
  - skin D86.3
  - specified type NEC D86.89
- **Sarcoma** (of) — *see also* Neoplasm, connective tissue, malignant
  - alveolar soft part — *see* Neoplasm, connective tissue, malignant
  - ameloblastic C41.1
    - upper jaw (bone) C41.0
  - botryoid — *see* Neoplasm, connective tissue, malignant
  - botryoides — *see* Neoplasm, connective tissue, malignant
  - cerebellar C71.6
    - circumscribed (arachnoidal) C71.6
  - circumscribed (arachnoidal) cerebellar C71.6
  - clear cell — *see also* Neoplasm, connective tissue, malignant
    - kidney C64.- ☑
  - dendritic cells (accessory cells) C96.4
  - embryonal — *see* Neoplasm, connective tissue, malignant
  - endometrial (stromal) C54.1
    - isthmus C54.0
  - epithelioid (cell) — *see* Neoplasm, connective tissue, malignant
  - Ewing's — *see* Neoplasm, bone, malignant
  - follicular dendritic cell C96.4

- **Schmincke's carcinoma or tumor** — *see* Neoplasm, nasopharynx, malignant
- **Schmitz** (-Stutzer) **dysentery** AØ3.Ø
- **Schmorl's disease or nodes**
  - lumbar region M51.46
  - lumbosacral region M51.47
  - sacrococcygeal region M53.3
  - thoracic region M51.44
  - thoracolumbar region M51.45
- **Schneiderian**
  - papilloma — *see* Neoplasm, nasopharynx, benign
    - specified site — *see* Neoplasm, benign, by site
    - unspecified site D14.Ø
  - specified site — *see* Neoplasm, malignant, by site
    - unspecified site C3Ø.Ø
- **Scholte's syndrome** (malignant carcinoid) E34.Ø
- **Scholz** (-Bielchowsky-Henneberg) **disease or syndrome** E75.25
- **Schönlein** (-Henoch) disease or purpura (primary) (rheumatic) D69.Ø
- **Schottmuller's disease** AØ1.4
- **Schroeder's syndrome** (endocrine hypertensive) E27.Ø
- **Schüller-Christian disease or syndrome** C96.5
- **Schultze's type acroparesthesia, simple** I73.89
- **Schultz's disease or syndrome** — *see* Agranulocytosis
- **Schwalbe-Ziehen-Oppenheim disease** G24.1
- **Schwannoma** — *see also* Neoplasm, nerve, benign
  - malignant — *see also* Neoplasm, nerve, malignant
    - with rhabdomyoblastic differentiation — *see* Neoplasm, nerve, malignant
  - melanocytic — *see* Neoplasm, nerve, benign
  - pigmented — *see* Neoplasm, nerve, benign
- **Schwannomatosis** Q85.Ø3
- **Schwartz** (-Jampel) **syndrome** G71.13
- **Schwartz-Bartter syndrome** E22.2
- **Schweniger-Buzzi anetoderma** L9Ø.1
- **Sciatic** — *see* condition
- **Sciatica** (infective) M54.3 ☑
  - with lumbago M54.4- ☑
    - due to intervertebral disc disorder — *see* Disorder, disc, with, radiculopathy
  - due to displacement of intervertebral disc (with lumbago) — *see* Disorder, disc, with, radiculopathy
  - wallet M54.3- ☑
- **Scimitar syndrome** Q26.8
- **Sclera** — *see* condition
- **Sclerectasia** H15.84- ☑
- **Scleredema**
  - adultorum — *see* Sclerosis, systemic
  - Buschke's — *see* Sclerosis, systemic
  - newborn P83.Ø
- **Sclerema** (adiposum) (edematosum) (neonatorum) (newborn) P83.Ø
  - adultorum — *see* Sclerosis, systemic
- **Scleriasis** — *see* Scleroderma
- **Scleritis** H15.ØØ- ☑
  - with corneal involvement H15.Ø4- ☑
  - anterior H15.Ø1- ☑
  - brawny H15.Ø2- ☑
  - in (due to) zoster BØ2.34
  - posterior H15.Ø3- ☑
  - specified type NEC H15.Ø9- ☑
  - syphilitic A52.71
  - tuberculous (nodular) A18.51
- **Sclerochoroiditis** H31.8
- **Scleroconjunctivitis** — *see* Scleritis
- **Sclerocystic ovary syndrome** E28.2
- **Sclerodactyly, sclerodactylia** L94.3
- **Scleroderma, sclerodermia** (acrosclerotic) (diffuse) (generalized) (progressive) (pulmonary) — *see also* Sclerosis, systemic M34.9
  - circumscribed L94.Ø
  - linear L94.1
  - localized L94.Ø
  - newborn P83.88
  - systemic M34.9
- **Sclerokeratitis** H16.8
  - tuberculous A18.52
- **Scleroma nasi** A48.8
- **Scleromalacia** (perforans) H15.Ø5- ☑
- **Scleromyxedema** L98.5
- **Sclérose en plaques** G35
- **Sclerosis, sclerotic**
  - adrenal (gland) E27.8
  - Alzheimer's — *see* Disease, Alzheimer's
  - amyotrophic (lateral) G12.21
  - aorta, aortic I7Ø.Ø

Sclerosis, sclerotic — *continued*

- aorta, aortic — *continued*
  - valve — *see* Endocarditis, aortic
- artery, arterial, arteriolar, arteriovascular — *see* Arteriosclerosis
- ascending multiple G35
- brain (generalized) (lobular) G37.9
  - artery, arterial I67.2
  - diffuse G37.Ø
  - disseminated G35
  - insular G35
  - Krabbe's E75.23
  - miliary G35
  - multiple G35
  - presenile (Alzheimer's) — *see* Disease, Alzheimer's, early onset
  - senile (arteriosclerotic) I67.2
  - stem, multiple G35
  - tuberous Q85.1
- bulbar, multiple G35
- bundle of His I44.39
- cardiac — *see* Disease, heart, ischemic, atherosclerotic
- cardiorenal — *see* Hypertension, cardiorenal
- cardiovascular — *see also* Disease, cardiovascular
  - renal — *see* Hypertension, cardiorenal
- cerebellar — *see* Sclerosis, brain
- cerebral — *see* Sclerosis, brain
- cerebrospinal (disseminated) (multiple) G35
- cerebrovascular I67.2
- choroid — *see* Degeneration, choroid
- combined (spinal cord) — *see also* Degeneration, combined
  - multiple G35
- concentric (Balo) G37.5
- cornea — *see* Opacity, cornea
- coronary (artery) I25.1Ø
  - with angina pectoris — *see* Arteriosclerosis, coronary (artery),
- corpus cavernosum
  - female N9Ø.89
  - male N48.6
- diffuse (brain) (spinal cord) G37.Ø
- disseminated G35
- dorsal G35
- dorsolateral (spinal cord) — *see* Degeneration, combined
- endometrium N85.5
- extrapyramidal G25.9
- eye, nuclear (senile) — *see* Cataract, senile, nuclear
- focal and segmental (glomerular) — *see also* NØØ-NØ7 with fourth character .1 NØ5.1
- Friedreich's (spinal cord) G11.11
- funicular (spermatic cord) N5Ø.89
- general (vascular) — *see* Arteriosclerosis
- gland (lymphatic) I89.8
- hepatic K74.1
  - alcoholic K7Ø.2
- hereditary
  - cerebellar G11.9
  - spinal (Friedreich's ataxia) G11.11
- hippocampal G93.81
- insular G35
- kidney — *see* Sclerosis, renal
- larynx J38.7
- lateral (amyotrophic) (descending) (spinal) G12.21
  - primary G12.23
- lens, senile nuclear — *see* Cataract, senile, nuclear
- liver K74.1
  - with fibrosis K74.2
    - alcoholic K7Ø.2
  - alcoholic K7Ø.2
  - cardiac K76.1
- lung — *see* Fibrosis, lung
- mastoid — *see* Mastoiditis, chronic
- mesial temporal G93.81
- mitral IØ5.8
- Mönckeberg's (medial) — *see* Arteriosclerosis, extremities
- multiple (brain stem) (cerebral) (generalized) (spinal cord) G35
- myocardium, myocardial — *see* Disease, heart, ischemic, atherosclerotic
- nuclear (senile), eye — *see* Cataract, senile, nuclear
- ovary N83.8
- pancreas K86.89
- penis N48.6
- peripheral arteries — *see* Arteriosclerosis, extremities
- plaques G35

Sclerosis, sclerotic — *continued*

- pluriglandular E31.8
- polyglandular E31.8
- posterolateral (spinal cord) — *see* Degeneration, combined
- presenile (Alzheimer's) — *see* Disease, Alzheimer's, early onset
- primary, lateral G12.23
- progressive, systemic M34.Ø
- pulmonary — *see* Fibrosis, lung
  - artery I27.Ø
  - valve (heart) — *see* Endocarditis, pulmonary
- renal N26.9
  - with
    - cystine storage disease E72.Ø9
    - hypertensive heart disease (conditions in I11) — *see* Hypertension, cardiorenal
  - arteriolar (hyaline) (hyperplastic) — *see* Hypertension, kidney
- retina (senile) (vascular) H35.ØØ
- senile (vascular) — *see* Arteriosclerosis
- spinal (cord) (progressive) G95.89
  - ascending G61.Ø
  - combined — *see also* Degeneration, combined
    - multiple G35
    - syphilitic A52.11
  - disseminated G35
  - dorsolateral — *see* Degeneration, combined
  - hereditary (Friedreich's) (mixed form) G11.11
  - lateral (amyotrophic) G12.21
    - progressive G12.23
  - multiple G35
  - posterior (syphilitic) A52.11
- stomach K31.89
- subendocardial, congenital I42.4
- systemic M34.9
  - with
    - lung involvement M34.81
    - myopathy M34.82
    - polyneuropathy M34.83
  - drug-induced M34.2
  - due to chemicals NEC M34.2
  - progressive M34.Ø
  - specified NEC M34.89
- temporal (mesial) G93.81
- tricuspid (heart) (valve) IØ7.8
- tuberous (brain) Q85.1
- tympanic membrane — *see* Disorder, tympanic membrane, specified NEC
- valve, valvular (heart) — *see* Endocarditis
- vascular — *see* Arteriosclerosis
- vein I87.8

- **Scoliosis** (acquired) (postural) M41.9
  - adolescent (idiopathic) — *see* Scoliosis, idiopathic, adolescent
  - congenital Q67.5
    - due to bony malformation Q76.3
    - failure of segmentation (hemivertebra) Q76.3
    - hemivertebra fusion Q76.3
    - postural Q67.5
  - degenerative M41.5- ☑
  - idiopathic M41.2Ø
    - adolescent M41.129
      - cervical region M41.122
      - cervicothoracic region M41.123
      - lumbar region M41.126
      - lumbosacral region M41.127
      - thoracic region M41.124
      - thoracolumbar region M41.125
    - cervical region M41.22
    - cervicothoracic region M41.23
    - infantile M41.ØØ
      - cervical region M41.Ø2
      - cervicothoracic region M41.Ø3
      - lumbar region M41.Ø6
      - lumbosacral region M41.Ø7
      - sacrococcygeal region M41.Ø8
      - thoracic region M41.Ø4
      - thoracolumbar region M41.Ø5
    - juvenile M41.119
      - cervical region M41.112
      - cervicothoracic region M41.113
      - lumbar region M41.116
      - lumbosacral region M41.117
      - thoracic region M41.114
      - thoracolumbar region M41.115
    - lumbar region M41.26
    - lumbosacral region M41.27

- **Scoliosis** — *continued*
  - idiopathic — *continued*
    - thoracic region M41.24
    - thoracolumbar region M41.25
  - infantile — *see* Scoliosis, idiopathic, infantile
  - neuromuscular M41.4Ø
    - cervical region M41.42
    - cervicothoracic region M41.43
    - lumbar region M41.46
    - lumbosacral region M41.47
    - occipito-atlanto-axial region M41.41
    - thoracic region M41.44
    - thoracolumbar region M41.45
  - paralytic — *see* Scoliosis, neuromuscular
  - postradiation therapy M96.5
  - rachitic (late effect or sequelae) E64.3 *[M49.8Ø]*
    - cervical region E64.3 *[M49.82]*
    - cervicothoracic region E64.3 *[M49.83]*
    - lumbar region E64.3 *[M49.86]*
    - lumbosacral region E64.3 *[M49.87]*
    - multiple sites E64.3 *[M49.89]*
    - occipito-atlanto-axial region E64.3 *[M49.81]*
    - sacrococcygeal region E64.3 *[M49.88]*
    - thoracic region E64.3 *[M49.84]*
    - thoracolumbar region E64.3 *[M49.85]*
  - sciatic M54.4- ☑
  - secondary (to) NEC M41.5Ø
    - cerebral palsy, Friedreich's ataxia, poliomyelitis, neuromuscular disorders — *see* Scoliosis, neuromuscular
    - cervical region M41.52
    - cervicothoracic region M41.53
    - lumbar region M41.56
    - lumbosacral region M41.57
    - thoracic region M41.54
    - thoracolumbar region M41.55
  - specified form NEC M41.8Ø
    - cervical region M41.82
    - cervicothoracic region M41.83
    - lumbar region M41.86
    - lumbosacral region M41.87
    - thoracic region M41.84
    - thoracolumbar region M41.85
  - thoracogenic M41.3Ø
    - thoracic region M41.34
    - thoracolumbar region M41.35
  - tuberculous A18.Ø1
- **Scoliotic pelvis**
  - with disproportion (fetopelvic) O33.Ø
    - causing obstructed labor O65.Ø
- **Scorbutus, scorbutic** — *see also* Scurvy
  - anemia D53.2
- **Score, NIHSS** (National Institutes of Health Stroke Scale) R29.7- ☑
- **Scotoma** (arcuate) (Bjerrum) (central) (ring) — *see also* Defect, visual field, localized, scotoma
  - scintillating H53.12- ☑
- **Scratch** — *see* Abrasion
- **Scratchy throat** RØ9.89
- **Screening** (for) Z13.9
  - alcoholism Z13.39
  - anemia Z13.Ø
  - anomaly, congenital Z13.89
  - antenatal, of mother — *see also* Encounter, antenatal screening Z36.9
  - arterial hypertension Z13.6
  - arthropod-borne viral disease NEC Z11.59
  - autism Z13.41
  - bacteriuria, asymptomatic Z13.89
  - behavioral disorder Z13.3Ø
    - specified NEC Z13.39
  - brain injury, traumatic Z13.85Ø
  - bronchitis, chronic Z13.83
  - brucellosis Z11.2
  - cardiovascular disorder Z13.6
  - cataract Z13.5
  - chlamydial diseases Z11.8
  - cholera Z11.Ø
  - chromosomal abnormalities (nonprocreative) NEC Z13.79
  - colonoscopy Z12.11
  - congenital
    - dislocation of hip Z13.89
    - eye disorder Z13.5
    - malformation or deformation Z13.89
  - contamination NEC Z13.88
  - coronavirus (disease) (novel) 2Ø19 Z11.52
  - COVID-19 Z11.52
- **Screening** — *continued*
  - cystic fibrosis Z13.228
  - dengue fever Z11.59
  - dental disorder Z13.84
  - depression (adult) (adolescent) (child) Z13.31
    - maternal Z13.32
    - perinatal Z13.32
  - developmental
    - delays Z13.4Ø
      - global (milestones) Z13.42
      - specified NEC Z13.49
    - handicap Z13.42
      - in early childhood Z13.42
  - diabetes mellitus Z13.1
  - diphtheria Z11.2
  - disability, intellectual Z13.39
  - disease or disorder Z13.9
    - bacterial NEC Z11.2
      - intestinal infectious Z11.Ø
      - respiratory tuberculosis Z11.1
    - behavioral Z13.3Ø
      - specified NEC Z13.39
    - blood or blood-forming organ Z13.Ø
    - cardiovascular Z13.6
    - Chagas' Z11.6
    - chlamydial Z11.8
    - coronavirus (novel) 2Ø19 Z11.52
    - COVID-19 Z11.52
    - dental Z13.89
    - developmental delays Z13.4Ø
      - global (milestones) Z13.42
      - specified NEC Z13.49
    - digestive tract NEC Z13.818
      - lower GI Z13.811
      - upper GI Z13.81Ø
    - ear Z13.5
    - endocrine Z13.29
    - eye Z13.5
    - genitourinary Z13.89
    - heart Z13.6
    - human immunodeficiency virus (HIV) infection Z11.4
    - immunity Z13.Ø
    - infection
      - intestinal Z11.Ø
        - specified NEC Z11.6
    - infectious Z11.9
    - mental health and behavioral Z13.3Ø
      - specified NEC Z13.39
    - metabolic Z13.228
    - neurological Z13.89
    - nutritional Z13.21
      - metabolic Z13.228
        - lipoid disorders Z13.22Ø
    - protozoal Z11.6
      - intestinal Z11.Ø
    - respiratory Z13.83
    - rheumatic Z13.828
    - rickettsial Z11.8
    - sexually-transmitted NEC Z11.3
      - human immunodeficiency virus (HIV) Z11.4
    - sickle-cell (trait) Z13.Ø
    - skin Z13.89
    - specified NEC Z13.89
    - spirochetal Z11.8
    - thyroid Z13.29
    - vascular Z13.6
    - venereal Z11.3
    - viral NEC Z11.59
      - coronavirus (novel) 2Ø19 Z11.52
      - COVID-19 Z11.52
      - human immunodeficiency virus (HIV) Z11.4
      - intestinal Z11.Ø
      - SARS-CoV-2 Z11.52
  - elevated titer Z13.89
  - emphysema Z13.83
  - encephalitis, viral (mosquito- or tick-borne) Z11.59
  - exposure to contaminants (toxic) Z13.88
  - fever
    - dengue Z11.59
    - hemorrhagic Z11.59
    - yellow Z11.59
  - filariasis Z11.6
  - galactosemia Z13.228
  - gastrointestinal condition Z13.818
  - genetic (nonprocreative) - for procreative management — *see* Testing, genetic, for procreative management
    - disease carrier status (nonprocreative) Z13.71
    - specified NEC (nonprocreative) Z13.79
- **Screening** — *continued*
  - genitourinary condition Z13.89
  - glaucoma Z13.5
  - gonorrhea Z11.3
  - gout Z13.89
  - helminthiasis (intestinal) Z11.6
  - hematopoietic malignancy Z12.89
  - hemoglobinopathies NEC Z13.Ø
  - hemorrhagic fever Z11.59
  - Hodgkin disease Z12.89
  - human immunodeficiency virus (HIV) Z11.4
  - human papillomavirus Z11.51
  - hypertension Z13.6
  - immunity disorders Z13.Ø
  - infant or child (over 28 days old) ZØØ.129
    - with abnormal findings ZØØ.121
  - infection
    - mycotic Z11.8
    - parasitic Z11.8
  - ingestion of radioactive substance Z13.88
  - intellectual disability Z13.39
  - intestinal
    - helminthiasis Z11.6
    - infectious disease Z11.Ø
  - leishmaniasis Z11.6
  - leprosy Z11.2
  - leptospirosis Z11.8
  - leukemia Z12.89
  - lymphoma Z12.89
  - malaria Z11.6
  - malnutrition Z13.29
    - metabolic Z13.228
    - nutritional Z13.21
  - measles Z11.59
  - mental health disorder Z13.3Ø
    - specified NEC Z13.39
  - metabolic errors, inborn Z13.228
  - multiphasic Z13.89
  - musculoskeletal disorder Z13.828
    - osteoporosis Z13.82Ø
  - mycoses Z11.8
  - myocardial infarction (acute) Z13.6
  - neoplasm (malignant) (of) Z12.9
    - bladder Z12.6
    - blood Z12.89
    - breast Z12.39
      - routine mammogram Z12.31
    - cervix Z12.4
    - colon Z12.11
    - genitourinary organs NEC Z12.79
      - bladder Z12.6
      - cervix Z12.4
      - ovary Z12.73
      - prostate Z12.5
      - testis Z12.71
      - vagina Z12.72
    - hematopoietic system Z12.89
    - intestinal tract Z12.1Ø
      - colon Z12.11
      - rectum Z12.12
      - small intestine Z12.13
    - lung Z12.2
    - lymph (glands) Z12.89
    - nervous system Z12.82
    - oral cavity Z12.81
    - prostate Z12.5
    - rectum Z12.12
    - respiratory organs Z12.2
    - skin Z12.83
    - small intestine Z12.13
    - specified site NEC Z12.89
    - stomach Z12.Ø
  - nephropathy Z13.89
  - nervous system disorders NEC Z13.858
  - neurological condition Z13.89
  - osteoporosis Z13.82Ø
  - parasitic infestation Z11.9
    - specified NEC Z11.8
  - phenylketonuria Z13.228
  - plague Z11.2
  - poisoning (chemical) (heavy metal) Z13.88
  - poliomyelitis Z11.59
  - postnatal, chromosomal abnormalities Z13.89
  - prenatal, of mother — *see also* Encounter, antenatal screening Z36.9
  - protozoal disease Z11.6
    - intestinal Z11.Ø
  - pulmonary tuberculosis Z11.1
  - radiation exposure Z13.88

- **Sepsis** — *continued*
  - due to device, implant or graft — *continued*
    - catheter — *continued*
      - urinary T83.518 ☑
    - ectopic or molar pregnancy O08.82
    - electronic (electrode) (pulse generator) (stimulator)
      - bone T84.7 ☑
      - cardiac T82.7 ☑
      - nervous system T85.738 ☑
        - brain T85.731 ☑
        - neurostimulator generator T85.734 ☑
        - peripheral nerve T85.732 ☑
        - spinal cord T85.733 ☑
      - urinary T83.590 ☑
    - fixation, internal (orthopedic) — *see* Complication, fixation device, infection
    - gastrointestinal (bile duct) (esophagus) T85.79 ☑
      - neurostimulator electrode (lead) T85.732 ☑
    - genital T83.69 ☑
    - heart NEC T82.7 ☑
      - valve (prosthesis) T82.6 ☑
        - graft T82.7 ☑
    - joint prosthesis — *see* Complication, joint prosthesis, infection
    - ocular (corneal graft) (orbital implant) T85.79 ☑
    - orthopedic NEC T84.7 ☑
      - fixation device, internal — *see* Complication, fixation device, infection
    - specified NEC T85.79 ☑
    - vascular T82.7 ☑
    - ventricular intracranial (communicating) shunt T85.730 ☑
  - during labor O75.3
  - Enterococcus A41.81
  - Erysipelothrix (rhusiopathiae) (erysipeloid) A26.7
  - Escherichia coli (E. coli) A41.5 ☑
  - extraintestinal yersiniosis A28.2
  - following
    - abortion (subsequent episode) O08.0
      - current episode — *see* Abortion
    - ectopic or molar pregnancy O08.82
    - immunization T88.0 ☑
    - infusion, therapeutic injection or transfusion NEC T80.29 ☑
    - obstetrical procedure O86.04
  - gangrenous A41.9
  - gonococcal A54.86
  - Gram-negative (organism) A41.5 ☑
    - anaerobic A41.4
  - Haemophilus influenzae A41.3
  - herpesviral B00.7
  - intra-abdominal K65.1
  - intraocular — *see* Endophthalmitis, purulent
  - Listeria monocytogenes A32.7
  - localized — *code to* specific localized infection
    - in operation wound T81.49 ☑
    - skin — *see* Abscess
  - malleus A24.0
  - melioidosis A24.1
  - meningeal — *see* Meningitis
  - meningococcal A39.4
    - acute A39.2
    - chronic A39.3
  - MSSA (Methicillin susceptible Staphylococcus aureus) A41.01
  - newborn P36.9
    - due to
      - anaerobes NEC P36.5
      - Escherichia coli P36.4
      - Staphylococcus P36.30
        - aureus P36.2
        - specified NEC P36.39
      - Streptococcus P36.10
        - group B P36.0
        - specified NEC P36.19
    - specified NEC P36.8
  - Pasteurella multocida A28.0
  - pelvic, puerperal, postpartum, childbirth O85
  - pneumococcal A40.3
  - postprocedural T81.44 ☑
  - puerperal, postpartum, childbirth (pelvic) O85
  - Salmonella (arizonae) (cholerae-suis) (enteritidis) (typhimurium) A02.1
  - severe R65.20
    - with septic shock R65.21
  - Shigella — *see also* Dysentery, bacillary A03.9
  - skin, localized — *see* Abscess
- **Sepsis** — *continued*
  - specified organism NEC A41.89
  - Staphylococcus, staphylococcal A41.2
    - aureus (methicillin susceptible) (MSSA) A41.01
      - methicillin resistant (MRSA) A41.02
    - coagulase-negative A41.1
    - specified NEC A41.1
  - Streptococcus, streptococcal A40.9
    - agalactiae A40.1
    - group
      - A A40.0
      - B A40.1
      - D A41.81
    - neonatal P36.10
      - group B P36.0
      - specified NEC P36.19
    - pneumoniae A40.3
    - pyogenes A40.0
    - specified NEC A40.8
  - tracheostomy stoma J95.02
  - tularemic A21.7
  - umbilical, umbilical cord (newborn) — *see* Sepsis, newborn
  - Yersinia pestis A20.7
- **Septate** — *see* Septum
- **Septic** — *see* condition
  - arm — *see* Cellulitis, upper limb
    - with lymphangitis — *see* Lymphangitis, acute, upper limb
  - embolus — *see* Embolism
  - finger — *see* Cellulitis, digit
    - with lymphangitis — *see* Lymphangitis, acute, digit
  - foot — *see* Cellulitis, lower limb
    - with lymphangitis — *see* Lymphangitis, acute, lower limb
  - gallbladder (acute) K81.0
  - hand — *see* Cellulitis, upper limb
    - with lymphangitis — *see* Lymphangitis, acute, upper limb
  - joint — *see* Arthritis, pyogenic or pyemic
  - leg — *see* Cellulitis, lower limb
    - with lymphangitis — *see* Lymphangitis, acute, lower limb
  - nail — *see also* Cellulitis, digit
    - with lymphangitis — *see* Lymphangitis, acute, digit
  - sore — *see also* Abscess
    - throat J02.0
      - streptococcal J02.0
  - spleen (acute) D73.89
  - teeth, tooth (pulpal origin) K04.4
  - throat — *see* Pharyngitis
  - thrombus — *see* Thrombosis
  - toe — *see* Cellulitis, digit
    - with lymphangitis — *see* Lymphangitis, acute, digit
  - tonsils, chronic J35.01
    - with adenoiditis J35.03
  - uterus — *see* Endometritis
- **Septicemia** A41.9
  - meaning sepsis — *see* Sepsis
- **Septum, septate** (congenital) — *see also* Anomaly, by site
  - anal Q42.3
    - with fistula Q42.2
  - aqueduct of Sylvius Q03.0
    - with spina bifida — *see* Spina bifida, by site, with hydrocephalus
  - uterus Q51.28
    - complete Q51.21
    - partial Q51.22
    - specified NEC Q51.28
  - vagina Q52.10
    - in pregnancy — *see* Pregnancy, complicated by, abnormal vagina
      - causing obstructed labor O65.5
    - longitudinal Q52.129
      - microperforate
        - left side Q52.124
        - right side Q52.123
      - nonobstruction Q52.120
      - obstructing Q52.129
        - left side Q52.122
        - right side Q52.121
    - transverse Q52.11
- **Sequelae** (of) — *see also* condition
  - abscess, intracranial or intraspinal (conditions in G06) G09
- **Sequelae** — *continued*
  - amputation — *code to* injury with seventh character S
  - burn and corrosion — *code to* injury with seventh character S
  - calcium deficiency E64.8
  - cerebrovascular disease — *see* Sequelae, disease, cerebrovascular
  - childbirth O94
  - contusion — *code to* injury with seventh character S
  - corrosion — *see* Sequelae, burn and corrosion
  - COVID-19 (post acute) U09.9
  - crushing injury — *code to* injury with seventh character S
  - disease
    - cerebrovascular I69.90
      - alteration of sensation I69.998
      - aphasia I69.920
      - apraxia I69.990
      - ataxia I69.993
      - cognitive deficits I69.91 ☑
      - disturbance of vision I69.998
      - dysarthria I69.922
      - dysphagia I69.991
      - dysphasia I69.921
      - facial droop I69.992
      - facial weakness I69.992
      - fluency disorder I69.923
      - hemiplegia I69.95- ☑
      - hemorrhage
        - intracerebral — *see* Sequelae, hemorrhage, intracerebral
        - intracranial, nontraumatic NEC — *see* Sequelae, hemorrhage, intracranial, nontraumatic
        - subarachnoid — *see* Sequelae, hemorrhage, subarachnoid
      - language deficit I69.928
      - monoplegia
        - lower limb I69.94- ☑
        - upper limb I69.93- ☑
      - paralytic syndrome I69.96- ☑
      - specified effect NEC I69.998
      - specified type NEC I69.80
        - alteration of sensation I69.898
        - aphasia I69.820
        - apraxia I69.890
        - ataxia I69.893
        - cognitive deficits I69.81 ☑
        - disturbance of vision I69.898
        - dysarthria I69.822
        - dysphagia I69.891
        - dysphasia I69.821
        - facial droop I69.892
        - facial weakness I69.892
        - fluency disorder I69.823
        - hemiplegia I69.85- ☑
        - language deficit I69.828
        - monoplegia
          - lower limb I69.84- ☑
          - upper limb I69.83- ☑
        - paralytic syndrome I69.86- ☑
        - specified effect NEC I69.898
      - speech deficit I69.928
        - speech deficit I69.828
      - stroke NOS — *see* Sequelae, stroke NOS
  - dislocation — *code to* injury with seventh character S
  - encephalitis or encephalomyelitis (conditions in G04) G09
    - in infectious disease NEC B94.8
    - viral B94.1
  - external cause — *code to* injury with seventh character S
  - foreign body entering natural orifice — *code to* injury with seventh character S
  - fracture — *code to* injury with seventh character S
  - frostbite — *code to* injury with seventh character S
  - Hansen's disease B92
  - hemorrhage
    - intracerebral I69.10
      - alteration of sensation I69.198
      - aphasia I69.120
      - apraxia I69.190
      - ataxia I69.193
      - cognitive deficits I69.11 ☑
      - disturbance of vision I69.198
      - dysarthria I69.122
      - dysphagia I69.191

- **Shellshock** — *continued*
  - lasting state — *see* Disorder, post-traumatic stress
- **Shield kidney** Q63.1
- **Shift**
  - auditory threshold (temporary) H93.24- ☑
  - mediastinal R93.89
- **Shifting sleep-work schedule** (affecting sleep) G47.26
- **Shiga** (-Kruse) **dysentery** AØ3.Ø
- **Shiga's bacillus** AØ3.Ø
- **Shigella** (dysentery) — *see* Dysentery, bacillary
- **Shigellosis** AØ3.9
  - Group A AØ3.Ø
  - Group B AØ3.1
  - Group C AØ3.2
  - Group D AØ3.3
- **Shin splints** S86.89- ☑
- **Shingles** — *see* Herpes, zoster
- **Shipyard disease or eye** B3Ø.Ø
- **Shirodkar suture, in pregnancy** — *see* Pregnancy, complicated by, incompetent cervix
- **Shock** R57.9
  - with ectopic or molar pregnancy OØ8.3
  - adrenal (cortical) (Addisonian) E27.2
  - adverse food reaction (anaphylactic) — *see* Shock, anaphylactic, due to food
  - allergic — *see* Shock, anaphylactic
  - anaphylactic T78.2 ☑
    - chemical — *see* Table of Drugs and Chemicals
    - due to drug or medicinal substance
      - correct substance properly administered T88.6 ☑
      - overdose or wrong substance given or taken (by accident) — *see* Table of Drugs and Chemicals, by drug, poisoning
    - due to food (nonpoisonous) T78.ØØ ☑
      - additives T78.Ø6 ☑
      - dairy products T78.Ø7 ☑
      - eggs T78.Ø8 ☑
      - fish T78.Ø3 ☑
        - shellfish T78.Ø2 ☑
      - fruit T78.Ø4 ☑
      - milk T78.Ø7 ☑
      - nuts T78.Ø5 ☑
        - multiple types T78.Ø5 ☑
        - peanuts T78.Ø1 ☑
      - peanuts T78.Ø1 ☑
      - seeds T78.Ø5 ☑
      - specified type NEC T78.Ø9 ☑
      - vegetable T78.Ø4 ☑
    - following sting(s) — *see* Venom
    - immunization T8Ø.52 ☑
    - serum T8Ø.59 ☑
      - blood and blood products T8Ø.51 ☑
      - immunization T8Ø.52 ☑
      - specified NEC T8Ø.59 ☑
      - vaccination T8Ø.52 ☑
  - anaphylactoid — *see* Shock, anaphylactic
  - anesthetic
    - correct substance properly administered T88.2 ☑
    - overdose or wrong substance given or taken — *see* Table of Drugs and Chemicals, by drug, poisoning
    - specified anesthetic — *see* Table of Drugs and Chemicals, by drug, poisoning
  - cardiogenic R57.Ø
  - chemical substance — *see* Table of Drugs and Chemicals
  - complicating ectopic or molar pregnancy OØ8.3
  - culture — *see* Disorder, adjustment
  - drug
    - due to correct substance properly administered T88.6 ☑
    - overdose or wrong substance given or taken (by accident) — *see* Table of Drugs and Chemicals, by drug, poisoning
  - during or after labor and delivery O75.1
  - electric T75.4 ☑
    - (taser) T75.4 ☑
  - endotoxic R65.21
    - postprocedural (resulting from a procedure, not elsewhere classified) T81.12 ☑
  - following
    - ectopic or molar pregnancy OØ8.3
    - injury (immediate) (delayed) T79.4 ☑
    - labor and delivery O75.1
  - food (anaphylactic) — *see* Shock, anaphylactic, due to food
  - from electroshock gun (taser) T75.4 ☑
- **Shock** — *continued*
  - gram-negative R65.21
    - postprocedural (resulting from a procedure, not elsewhere classified) T81.12 ☑
  - hematologic R57.8
  - hemorrhagic R57.8
    - surgery (intraoperative) (postoperative) T81.19 ☑
    - trauma T79.4 ☑
  - hypovolemic R57.1
    - surgical T81.19 ☑
    - traumatic T79.4 ☑
  - insulin E15
    - therapeutic misadventure — *see* subcategory T38.3 ☑
  - kidney N17.Ø
    - traumatic (following crushing) T79.5 ☑
  - lightning T75.Ø1 ☑
  - liver K72.ØØ
  - lung J8Ø
  - obstetric O75.1
    - with ectopic or molar pregnancy OØ8.3
    - following ectopic or molar pregnancy OØ8.3
  - pleural (surgical) T81.19 ☑
    - due to trauma T79.4 ☑
  - postprocedural (postoperative) T81.1Ø ☑
    - with ectopic or molar pregnancy OØ8.3
    - cardiogenic T81.11 ☑
    - endotoxic T81.12 ☑
    - following ectopic or molar pregnancy OØ8.3
    - gram-negative T81.12 ☑
    - hypovolemic T81.19 ☑
    - septic T81.12 ☑
    - specified type NEC T81.19 ☑
  - psychic F43.Ø
  - septic (due to severe sepsis) R65.21
  - specified NEC R57.8
  - surgical T81.1Ø ☑
  - taser gun (taser) T75.4 ☑
  - therapeutic misadventure NEC T81.1Ø ☑
  - thyroxin
    - overdose or wrong substance given or taken — *see* Table of Drugs and Chemicals, by drug, poisoning
  - toxic, syndrome A48.3
  - transfusion — *see* Complications, transfusion
  - traumatic (immediate) (delayed) T79.4 ☑
- **Shoemaker's chest** M95.4
- **Short, shortening, shortness**
  - arm (acquired) — *see also* Deformity, limb, unequal length
    - congenital Q71.81- ☑
    - forearm — *see* Deformity, limb, unequal length
  - bowel syndrome K91.2
  - breath RØ6.Ø2
  - cervical (complicating pregnancy) O26.87- ☑
    - non-gravid uterus N88.3
  - common bile duct, congenital Q44.5
  - cord (umbilical), complicating delivery O69.3 ☑
  - cystic duct, congenital Q44.5
  - esophagus (congenital) Q39.8
  - femur (acquired) — *see* Deformity, limb, unequal length, femur
    - congenital — *see* Defect, reduction, lower limb, longitudinal, femur
  - frenum, frenulum, linguae (congenital) Q38.1
  - hip (acquired) — *see also* Deformity, limb, unequal length
    - congenital Q65.89
  - leg (acquired) — *see also* Deformity, limb, unequal length
    - congenital Q72.81- ☑
    - lower leg — *see also* Deformity, limb, unequal length
  - limbed stature, with immunodeficiency D82.2
  - lower limb (acquired) — *see also* Deformity, limb, unequal length
    - congenital Q72.81- ☑
  - organ or site, congenital NEC — *see* Distortion
  - palate, congenital Q38.5
  - radius (acquired) — *see also* Deformity, limb, unequal length
    - congenital — *see* Defect, reduction, upper limb, longitudinal, radius
  - rib syndrome Q77.2
  - stature (child) (hereditary) (idiopathic) NEC R62.52
    - constitutional E34.31
- **Short, shortening, shortness** — *continued*
  - stature — *continued*
    - due to
      - endocrine disorder E34.3Ø
        - specified type NEC, due to endocrine dosorder E34.39
      - genetic causes E34.329
        - ACAN gene variant E34.328
        - acid-labile subunit gene (IGFALS) defect E34.321
        - aggrecan deficiency E34.328
        - genetic syndrome with resistance to insulin-like growth factor-1 E34.322
        - growth hormone gene 1 (GH1) defect with growth hormone neutralizing antibodies E34.321
        - growth hormone insensitivity syndrome (GHIS) E34.321
        - insulin-like growth factor 1 gene (IGF1) defect E34.321
        - insulin-like growth factor-1 receptor (IGF-1R) defect E34.322
        - insulin-like growth factor-1 (IGF-1) resistance E34.322
        - NPR-2 gene variant E34.328
        - post-insulin-like growth factor-1 receptor signaling defect E34.322
        - primary insulin-like growth factor-1 (IGF-1) deficiency E34.321
        - severe primary insulin-like growth factor-1 deficiency (SPIGFD) E34.321
        - signal transducer and activator of transcription 5B gene (STAT5b) defect E34.321
        - specified genetic cause NEC E34.328
    - Laron-type E34.321
  - tendon — *see also* Contraction, tendon
    - with contracture of joint — *see* Contraction, joint
    - Achilles (acquired) M67.Ø- ☑
      - congenital Q66.89
    - congenital Q79.8
  - thigh (acquired) — *see also* Deformity, limb, unequal length, femur
    - congenital — *see* Defect, reduction, lower limb, longitudinal, femur
  - tibialis anterior (tendon) — *see* Contraction, tendon
  - umbilical cord
    - complicating delivery O69.3 ☑
  - upper limb, congenital — *see* Defect, reduction, upper limb, specified type NEC
  - urethra N36.8
  - uvula, congenital Q38.5
  - vagina (congenital) Q52.4
- **Shortsightedness** — *see* Myopia
- **Shoshin** (acute fulminating beriberi) E51.11
- **Shoulder** — *see* condition
- **Shovel-shaped incisors** KØØ.2
- **Shower, thromboembolic** — *see* Embolism
- **Shunt**
  - arterial-venous (dialysis) Z99.2
  - arteriovenous, pulmonary (acquired) I28.Ø
    - congenital Q25.72
  - cerebral ventricle (communicating) in situ Z98.2
  - surgical, prosthetic, with complications — *see* Complications, cardiovascular, device or implant
- **Shutdown, renal** N28.9
- **Shy-Drager syndrome** G9Ø.3
- **Sialadenitis, sialadenosis** (any gland) (chronic) (periodic) (suppurative) — *see* Sialoadenitis
- **Sialectasia** K11.8
- **Sialidosis** E77.1
- **Sialitis, silitis** (any gland) (chronic) (suppurative) — *see* Sialoadenitis
- **Sialoadenitis** (any gland) (periodic) (suppurative) K11.2Ø
  - acute K11.21
    - recurrent K11.22
  - chronic K11.23
- **Sialoadenopathy** K11.9
- **Sialoangitis** — *see* Sialoadenitis
- **Sialodochitis** (fibrinosa) — *see* Sialoadenitis
- **Sialodocholithiasis** K11.5
- **Sialolithiasis** K11.5
- **Sialometaplasia, necrotizing** K11.8
- **Sialorrhea** — *see also* Ptyalism
  - periodic — *see* Sialoadenitis
- **Sialosis** K11.7
- **Siamese twin** Q89.4
- **Sibling rivalry** Z62.891
- **Sicard's syndrome** G52.7

Sicca syndrome — *see* Syndrome, Sjögren
Sick R69
- or handicapped person in family Z63.79
  - needing care at home Z63.6
- sinus (syndrome) I49.5

Sick-euthyroid syndrome EØ7.81
Sickle-cell
- anemia — *see* Disease, sickle-cell
- beta plus — *see* Disease, sickle-cell, thalassemia, beta plus
- beta zero — *see* Disease, sickle-cell, thalassemia, beta zero
- trait D57.3

Sicklemia — *see also* Disease, sickle-cell
- trait D57.3

Sickness
- air (travel) T75.3 ☑
- airplane T75.3 ☑
- alpine T7Ø.29 ☑
- altitude T7Ø.2Ø ☑
- Andes T7Ø.29 ☑
- aviator's T7Ø.29 ☑
- balloon T7Ø.29 ☑
- car T75.3 ☑
- compressed air T7Ø.3 ☑
- decompression T7Ø.3 ☑
- green D5Ø.8
- milk — *see* Poisoning, food, noxious
- motion T75.3 ☑
- mountain T7Ø.29 ☑
  - acute D75.1
- protein — *see also* Reaction, serum T8Ø.69 ☑
- radiation T66 ☑
- roundabout (motion) T75.3 ☑
- sea T75.3 ☑
- serum NEC — *see also* Reaction, serum T8Ø.69 ☑
- sleeping (African) B56.9
  - by Trypanosoma B56.9
    - brucei
      - gambiense B56.Ø
      - rhodesiense B56.1
  - East African B56.1
  - Gambian B56.Ø
  - Rhodesian B56.1
  - West African B56.Ø
- swing (motion) T75.3 ☑
- train (railway) (travel) T75.3 ☑
- travel (any vehicle) T75.3 ☑

Sideropenia — *see* Anemia, iron deficiency
Siderosilicosis J62.8
Siderosis (lung) J63.4
- brain G93.89
- eye (globe) — *see* Disorder, globe, degenerative, siderosis

Siemens' syndrome (ectodermal dysplasia) Q82.8
Sighing RØ6.89
- psychogenic F45.8

Sigmoid — *see also* condition
- flexure — *see* condition
- kidney Q63.1

Sigmoiditis — *see also* Enteritis K52.9
- infectious AØ9
- noninfectious K52.9

Silfverskïöld's syndrome Q78.9
Silicosiderosis J62.8
Silicosis, silicotic (simple) (complicated) J62.8
- with tuberculosis J65

Silicotuberculosis J65
Silo-fillers' disease J68.8
- bronchitis J68.Ø
- pneumonitis J68.Ø
- pulmonary edema J68.1

Silver's syndrome Q87.19
Simian malaria B53.1
Simmonds' cachexia or disease E23.Ø
Simons' disease or syndrome (progressive lipodystrophy) E88.1
Simple, simplex — *see* condition
Simulation, conscious (of illness) Z76.5
Simultanagnosia (asimultagnosia) R48.3
Sin Nombre virus disease (Hantavirus) (cardio)-pulmonary syndrome) B33.4
Sinding-Larsen disease or osteochondrosis — *see* Osteochondrosis, juvenile, patella
Singapore hemorrhagic fever A91
Singer's node or nodule J38.2
Single
- atrium Q21.2Ø
- coronary artery Q24.5
- umbilical artery Q27.Ø
- ventricle Q2Ø.4

Singultus RØ6.6
- epidemicus B33.Ø

Sinus — *see also* Fistula
- abdominal K63.89
- arrest I45.5
- arrhythmia I49.8
- bradycardia RØØ.1
- branchial cleft (internal) (external) Q18.Ø
- coccygeal — *see* Sinus, pilonidal
- dental KØ4.6
- dermal (congenital) QØ6.8
  - with abscess QØ6.8
  - coccygeal, pilonidal — *see* Sinus, coccygeal
- infected, skin NEC LØ8.89
- marginal, ruptured or bleeding — *see* Hemorrhage, antepartum, specified cause NEC
- medial, face and neck Q18.8
- pause I45.5
- pericranii QØ1.9
- pilonidal (infected) (rectum) LØ5.92
  - with abscess LØ5.Ø2
- preauricular Q18.1
- rectovaginal N82.3
- Rokitansky-Aschoff (gallbladder) K82.8
- sacrococcygeal (dermoid) (infected) — *see* Sinus, pilonidal
- tachycardia RØØ.Ø
  - paroxysmal I47.1
- tarsi syndrome M25.57- ☑
- testis N5Ø.89
- tract (postinfective) — *see* Fistula
- urachus Q64.4

Sinusitis (accessory) (chronic) (hyperplastic) (nasal) (nonpurulent) (purulent) J32.9
- acute JØ1.9Ø
  - ethmoidal JØ1.2Ø
    - recurrent JØ1.21
  - frontal JØ1.1Ø
    - recurrent JØ1.11
  - involving more than one sinus, other than pansinusitis JØ1.8Ø
    - recurrent JØ1.81
  - maxillary JØ1.ØØ
    - recurrent JØ1.Ø1
  - pansinusitis JØ1.4Ø
    - recurrent JØ1.41
  - recurrent JØ1.91
  - specified NEC JØ1.8Ø
    - recurrent JØ1.81
  - sphenoidal JØ1.3Ø
    - recurrent JØ1.31
- allergic — *see* Rhinitis, allergic
- due to high altitude T7Ø.1 ☑
- ethmoidal J32.2
  - acute JØ1.2Ø
    - recurrent JØ1.21
- frontal J32.1
  - acute JØ1.1Ø
    - recurrent JØ1.11
- influenzal — *see* Influenza, with, respiratory manifestations NEC
- involving more than one sinus but not pansinusitis J32.8
  - acute JØ1.8Ø
    - recurrent JØ1.81
- maxillary J32.Ø
  - acute JØ1.ØØ
    - recurrent JØ1.Ø1
- sphenoidal J32.3
  - acute JØ1.3Ø
    - recurrent JØ1.31
- tuberculous, any sinus A15.8

Sinusitis-bronchiectasis-situs inversus (syndrome) (triad) Q89.3
Sipple's syndrome E31.22
Sirenomelia (syndrome) Q87.2
Siriasis T67.Ø1 ☑
Sirkari's disease B55.Ø
Siti A65
Situation, psychiatric F99
Situational
- disturbance (transient) — *see* Disorder, adjustment
  - acute F43.Ø

Situational — *continued*
- maladjustment — *see* Disorder, adjustment
- reaction — *see* Disorder, adjustment
  - acute F43.Ø

Situs inversus or transversus (abdominalis) (thoracis) Q89.3
Sixth disease BØ8.2Ø
- due to human herpesvirus 6 BØ8.21
- due to human herpesvirus 7 BØ8.22

Sjögren-Larsson syndrome Q87.19
Sjögren's syndrome or disease — *see* Syndrome, Sjögren
Skeletal — *see* condition
Skene's gland — *see* condition
Skenitis — *see* Urethritis
Skerljevo A65
Skevas-Zerfus disease — *see* Toxicity, venom, marine animal, sea anemone
Skin — *see also* condition
- clammy R23.1
- donor — *see* Donor, skin
- dry L85.3
- hidebound M35.9

Slate-dressers' or slate-miners' lung J62.8
Sleep
- apnea — *see* Apnea, sleep
- deprivation Z72.82Ø
- disorder or disturbance G47.9
  - child F51.9
  - nonorganic origin F51.9
  - specified NEC G47.8
- disturbance G47.9
  - nonorganic origin F51.9
- drunkenness F51.9
- rhythm inversion G47.2- ☑
- terrors F51.4
- walking F51.3
  - hysterical F44.89

Sleep hygiene
- abuse Z72.821
- inadequate Z72.821
- poor Z72.821

Sleeping sickness — *see* Sickness, sleeping
Sleeplessness — *see* Insomnia
- menopausal N95.1

Sleep-wake schedule disorder G47.2Ø
Slim disease (in HIV infection) B2Ø
Slipped, slipping
- epiphysis (traumatic) — *see also* Osteochondropathy, specified type NEC
  - capital femoral (traumatic) [SCFE]
    - acute (on chronic) S79.Ø1- ☑
    - nontraumatic M93.ØØ- ☑
  - current traumatic — *code as* Fracture, by site
  - upper femoral (nontraumatic) [SUFE] M93.ØØ- ☑
    - acute M93.Ø1- ☑
      - on chronic M93.Ø3- ☑
    - chronic M93.Ø2- ☑
- intervertebral disc — *see* Displacement, intervertebral disc
- ligature, umbilical P51.8
- patella — *see* Disorder, patella, derangement NEC
- rib M89.8X8
- sacroiliac joint — *see* subcategory M53.2 ☑
- tendon — *see* Disorder, tendon
- ulnar nerve, nontraumatic — *see* Lesion, nerve, ulnar
- vertebra NEC — *see* Spondylolisthesis

Slocumb's syndrome E27.Ø
Sloughing (multiple) (phagedena) (skin) — *see also* Gangrene
- abscess — *see* Abscess
- appendix K38.8
- fascia — *see* Disorder, soft tissue, specified type NEC
- scrotum N5Ø.89
- tendon — *see* Disorder, tendon
- transplanted organ — *see* Rejection, transplant
- ulcer — *see* Ulcer, skin

Slow
- feeding, newborn P92.2
- flow syndrome, coronary I2Ø.8
- heart (beat) RØØ.1

Slowing, urinary stream R39.198
Sluder's neuralgia (syndrome) G44.89
Slurred, slurring speech R47.81
Small (ness)
- for gestational age — *see* Small for dates
- introitus, vagina N89.6

Small — *continued*
- kidney (unknown cause) N27.9
  - bilateral N27.1
  - unilateral N27.Ø
- ovary (congenital) Q5Ø.39
- pelvis
  - with disproportion (fetopelvic) O33.1
    - causing obstructed labor O65.1
- uterus N85.8
- white kidney NØ3.9

Small-and-light-for-dates — *see* Small for dates

Small-for-dates (infant) PØ5.1Ø
- with weight of
  - 499 grams or less PØ5.11
  - 5ØØ-749 grams PØ5.12
  - 75Ø-999 grams PØ5.13
  - 1ØØØ-1249 grams PØ5.14
  - 125Ø-1499 grams PØ5.15
  - 15ØØ-1749 grams PØ5.16
  - 175Ø-1999 grams PØ5.17
  - 2ØØØ-2499 grams PØ5.18
  - 25ØØ grams and over PØ5.19
- specified NEC PØ5.19

Smallpox BØ3

Smearing, fecal R15.1

SMEI (severe myoclonic epilepsy in infancy) G4Ø.83- ☑

Smith-Lemli-Opitz syndrome E78.72

Smith's fracture S52.54- ☑

Smoker — *see* Dependence, drug, nicotine

Smoker's
- bronchitis J41.Ø
- cough J41.Ø
- palate K13.24
- throat J31.2
- tongue K13.24

Smoking
- passive Z77.22

Smothering spells RØ6.81

Snaggle teeth, tooth M26.39

Snapping
- finger — *see* Trigger finger
- hip — *see* Derangement, joint, specified type NEC, hip
  - involving the iliotiblial band M76.3- ☑
- knee — *see* Derangement, knee
  - involving the iliotiblial band M76.3- ☑

Sneddon-Wilkinson disease or syndrome (sub-corneal pustular dermatosis) L13.1

Sneezing (intractable) RØ6.7

Sniffing
- cocaine
  - abuse — *see* Abuse, drug, cocaine
  - dependence — *see* Dependence, drug, cocaine
- gasoline
  - abuse — *see* Abuse, drug, inhalant
  - dependence — *see* Dependence, drug, inhalant
- glue (airplane)
  - abuse — *see* Abuse, drug, inhalant
  - drug dependence — *see* Dependence, drug, inhalant

Sniffles
- newborn P28.89

Snoring RØ6.83

Snow blindness — *see* Photokeratitis

Snuffles (non-syphilitic) RØ6.5
- newborn P28.89
- syphilitic (infant) A5Ø.Ø5 *[J99]*

Social
- exclusion Z6Ø.4
  - due to discrimination or persecution (perceived) Z6Ø.5
- migrant Z59.ØØ
  - acculturation difficulty Z6Ø.3
- rejection Z6Ø.4
  - due to discrimination or persecution Z6Ø.5
- role conflict NEC Z73.5
- skills inadequacy NEC Z73.4
- transplantation Z6Ø.3

Sodoku A25.Ø

Soemmerring's ring — *see* Cataract, secondary

Soft — *see also* condition
- nails L6Ø.3

Softening
- bone — *see* Osteomalacia
- brain (necrotic) (progressive) G93.89
  - congenital QØ4.8
  - embolic I63.4- ☑

Softening — *continued*
- brain — *continued*
  - hemorrhagic — *see* Hemorrhage, intracranial, intracerebral
  - occlusive I63.5- ☑
  - thrombotic I63.3- ☑
- cartilage M94.2- ☑
  - patella M22.4- ☑
- cerebellar — *see* Softening, brain
- cerebral — *see* Softening, brain
- cerebrospinal — *see* Softening, brain
- myocardial, heart — *see* Degeneration, myocardial
- spinal cord G95.89
- stomach K31.89

Soldier's
- heart F45.8
- patches I31.Ø

Solitary
- cyst, kidney N28.1
- kidney, congenital Q6Ø.Ø

Solvent abuse — *see* Abuse, drug, inhalant
- dependence — *see* Dependence, drug, inhalant

Somatization reaction, somatic reaction — *see* Disorder, somatoform

Somnambulism F51.3
- hysterical F44.89

Somnolence R4Ø.Ø
- nonorganic origin F51.11

Sonne dysentery AØ3.3

Soor B37.Ø

Sore
- bed — *see* Ulcer, pressure, by site
- chiclero B55.1
- Delhi B55.1
- desert — *see* Ulcer, skin
- eye H57.1- ☑
- Lahore B55.1
- mouth K13.79
  - canker K12.Ø
- muscle M79.1Ø
- Naga — *see* Ulcer, skin
- of skin — *see* Ulcer, skin
- oriental B55.1
- pressure — *see* Ulcer, pressure, by site
- skin L98.9
- soft A57
- throat (acute) — *see also* Pharyngitis
  - with influenza, flu, or grippe — *see* Influenza, with, respiratory manifestations NEC
  - chronic J31.2
  - coxsackie (virus) BØ8.5
  - diphtheritic A36.Ø
  - herpesviral BØØ.2
  - influenzal — *see* Influenza, with, respiratory manifestations NEC
  - septic JØ2.Ø
  - streptococcal (ulcerative) JØ2.Ø
  - viral NEC JØ2.8
    - coxsackie BØ8.5
- tropical — *see* Ulcer, skin
- veldt — *see* Ulcer, skin

Soto's syndrome (cerebral gigantism) Q87.3

South African cardiomyopathy syndrome I42.8

Southeast Asian hemorrhagic fever A91

Spacing
- abnormal, tooth, teeth, fully erupted M26.3Ø
- excessive, tooth, fully erupted M26.32

Spade-like hand (congenital) Q68.1

Spading nail L6Ø.8
- congenital Q84.6

Spanish collar N47.1

Sparganosis B7Ø.1

Spasm(s), spastic, spasticity — *see also* condition R25.2
- accommodation — *see* Spasm, of accommodation
- ampulla of Vater K83.4
- anus, ani (sphincter) (reflex) K59.4
  - psychogenic F45.8
- artery I73.9
  - cerebral G45.9
- Bell's G51.3- ☑
- bladder (sphincter, external or internal) N32.89
  - psychogenic F45.8
- bronchus, bronchiole J98.Ø1
- cardia K22.Ø
- cardiac I2Ø.1
- carpopedal — *see* Tetany
- cerebral (arteries) (vascular) G45.9

Spasm(s), spastic, spasticity — *continued*
- cervix, complicating delivery O62.4
- ciliary body (of accommodation) — *see* Spasm, of accommodation
- colon — *see also* Irritable, bowel K58.9
  - with diarrhea K58.Ø
  - psychogenic F45.8
- common duct K83.8
- compulsive — *see* Tic
- conjugate H51.8
- coronary (artery) I2Ø.1
- diaphragm (reflex) RØ6.6
  - epidemic B33.Ø
  - psychogenic F45.8
- duodenum K59.89
- epidemic diaphragmatic (transient) B33.Ø
- esophagus (diffuse) K22.4
  - psychogenic F45.8
- facial G51.3- ☑
- fallopian tube N83.8
- gastrointestinal (tract) K31.89
  - psychogenic F45.8
- glottis J38.5
  - hysterical F44.4
  - psychogenic F45.8
    - conversion reaction F44.4
  - reflex through recurrent laryngeal nerve J38.5
- habit — *see* Tic
- heart I2Ø.1
- hemifacial (clonic) G51.3- ☑
- hourglass — *see* Contraction, hourglass
- hysterical F44.4
- infantile — *see* Epilepsy, spasms
- inferior oblique, eye H51.8
- intestinal — *see also* Syndrome, irritable bowel K58.9
  - psychogenic F45.8
- larynx, laryngeal J38.5
  - hysterical F44.4
  - psychogenic F45.8
    - conversion reaction F44.4
- levator palpebrae superioris — *see* Disorder, eyelid function
- muscle NEC M62.838
  - back M62.83Ø
- nerve, trigeminal G51.Ø
- nervous F45.8
- nodding F98.4
- occupational F48.8
- oculogyric H51.8
  - psychogenic F45.8
- of accommodation H52.53- ☑
- ophthalmic artery — *see* Occlusion, artery, retina
- perineal, female N94.89
- peroneo-extensor — *see also* Deformity, limb, flat foot
- pharynx (reflex) J39.2
  - hysterical F45.8
  - psychogenic F45.8
- psychogenic F45.8
- pylorus NEC K31.3
  - adult hypertrophic K31.89
  - congenital or infantile Q4Ø.Ø
  - psychogenic F45.8
- rectum (sphincter) K59.4
  - psychogenic F45.8
- retinal (artery) — *see* Occlusion, artery, retina
- sigmoid — *see also* Syndrome, irritable bowel K58.9
  - psychogenic F45.8
- sphincter of Oddi K83.4
- stomach K31.89
  - neurotic F45.8
- throat J39.2
  - hysterical F45.8
  - psychogenic F45.8
- tic F95.9
  - chronic F95.1
  - transient of childhood F95.Ø
- tongue K14.8
- torsion (progressive) G24.1
- trigeminal nerve — *see* Neuralgia, trigeminal
- ureter N13.5
- urethra (sphincter) N35.919
- uterus N85.8
  - complicating labor O62.4
- vagina N94.2
  - psychogenic F52.5
- vascular I73.9
- vasomotor I73.9
- vein NEC I87.8

☑ **Additional Character Required — Refer to the Tabular List for Character Selection**

- **Stenosis, stenotic** — *continued*
  - aortic — *continued*
    - rheumatic — *continued*
      - with — *continued*
        - mitral disease — *continued*
          - with tricuspid (valve) disease I08.3
        - tricuspid (valve) disease I08.2
          - with mitral (valve) disease I08.3
    - specified cause NEC I35.Ø
    - syphilitic A52.Ø3
  - aqueduct of Sylvius (congenital) QØ3.Ø
    - with spina bifida — *see* Spina bifida, by site, with hydrocephalus
    - acquired G91.1
  - artery NEC — *see also* Arteriosclerosis I77.1
    - celiac I77.4
    - cerebral — *see* Occlusion, artery, cerebral
    - extremities — *see* Arteriosclerosis, extremities
    - precerebral — *see* Occlusion, artery, precerebral
    - pulmonary (congenital) Q25.6
      - acquired I28.8
    - renal I7Ø.1
    - stent
      - coronary T82.855 ☑
      - peripheral T82.856 ☑
  - bile duct (common) (hepatic) K83.1
    - congenital Q44.3
  - bladder-neck (acquired) N32.Ø
    - congenital Q64.31
  - brain G93.89
  - bronchus J98.Ø9
    - congenital Q32.3
    - syphilitic A52.72
  - cardia (stomach) K22.2
    - congenital Q39.3
  - cardiovascular — *see* Disease, cardiovascular
  - caudal M48.Ø8
  - cervix, cervical (canal) N88.2
    - congenital Q51.828
    - in pregnancy or childbirth — *see* Pregnancy, complicated by, abnormal cervix
  - colon — *see also* Obstruction, intestine
    - congenital Q42.9
      - specified NEC Q42.8
  - colostomy K94.Ø3
  - common (bile) duct K83.1
    - congenital Q44.3
  - coronary (artery) — *see* Disease, heart, ischemic, atherosclerotic
  - cystic duct — *see* Obstruction, gallbladder
  - due to presence of device, implant or graft — *see also* Complications, by site and type, specified NEC T85.858 ☑
    - arterial graft NEC T82.858 ☑
    - breast (implant) T85.858 ☑
    - catheter T85.858 ☑
      - dialysis (renal) T82.858 ☑
        - intraperitoneal T85.858 ☑
      - infusion NEC T82.858 ☑
        - spinal (epidural) (subdural) T85.85Ø ☑
      - urinary (indwelling) T83.85 ☑
    - fixation, internal (orthopedic) NEC T84.85 ☑
    - gastrointestinal (bile duct) (esophagus) T85.858 ☑
    - genital NEC T83.85 ☑
    - heart NEC T82.857 ☑
    - joint prosthesis T84.85 ☑
    - ocular (corneal graft) (orbital implant) NEC T85.858 ☑
    - orthopedic NEC T84.85 ☑
    - specified NEC T85.858 ☑
    - urinary NEC T83.85 ☑
    - vascular NEC T82.858 ☑
    - ventricular intracranial shunt T85.85Ø ☑
  - duodenum K31.5
    - congenital Q41.Ø
  - ejaculatory duct NEC N5Ø.89
    - stent
      - vascular
        - end stent
          - adjacent to stent — *see* Arteriosclerosis
          - within the stent
            - coronary T82.855 ☑
            - peripheral T82.856 ☑
        - in stent
          - coronary vessel T82.855 ☑
          - peripheral vessel T82.856 ☑
  - endocervical os — *see* Stenosis, cervix

- **Stenosis, stenotic** — *continued*
  - enterostomy K94.13
  - esophagus K22.2
    - congenital Q39.3
    - syphilitic A52.79
      - congenital A5Ø.59 *[K23]*
  - eustachian tube — *see* Obstruction, eustachian tube
  - external ear canal (acquired) H61.3Ø- ☑
    - congenital Q16.1
    - due to
      - inflammation H61.32- ☑
      - trauma H61.31- ☑
    - postprocedural H95.81- ☑
    - specified cause NEC H61.39- ☑
  - gallbladder — *see* Obstruction, gallbladder
  - glottis J38.6
  - heart valve — *see also* Endocarditis I38
    - aortic — *see* Stenosis, aortic
    - congenital Q24.8
    - mitral — *see* Stenosis, mitral
    - pulmonary — *see* Stenosis, pulmonary valve
    - tricuspid — *see* Stenosis, tricuspid
  - hepatic duct K83.1
  - hymen N89.6
  - hypertrophic subaortic (idiopathic) I42.1
  - ileum — *see also* Obstruction, intestine, specified NEC K56.699
    - congenital Q41.2
  - infundibulum cardia Q24.3
  - intervertebral foramina — *see also* Lesion, biomechanical, specified NEC
    - connective tissue M99.79
      - abdomen M99.79
      - cervical region M99.71
      - cervicothoracic M99.71
      - head region M99.7Ø
      - lumbar region M99.73
      - lumbosacral M99.73
      - occipitocervical M99.7Ø
      - sacral region M99.74
      - sacrococcygeal M99.74
      - sacroiliac M99.74
      - specified NEC M99.79
      - thoracic region M99.72
      - thoracolumbar M99.72
    - disc M99.79
      - abdomen M99.79
      - cervical region M99.71
      - cervicothoracic M99.71
      - head region M99.7Ø
      - lower extremity M99.76
      - lumbar region M99.73
      - lumbosacral M99.73
      - occipitocervical M99.7Ø
      - pelvic M99.75
      - rib cage M99.78
      - sacral region M99.74
      - sacrococcygeal M99.74
      - sacroiliac M99.74
      - specified NEC M99.79
      - thoracic region M99.72
      - thoracolumbar M99.72
      - upper extremity M99.77
    - osseous M99.69
      - abdomen M99.69
      - cervical region M99.61
      - cervicothoracic M99.61
      - head region M99.6Ø
      - lower extremity M99.66
      - lumbar region M99.63
      - lumbosacral M99.63
      - occipitocervical M99.6Ø
      - pelvic M99.65
      - rib cage M99.68
      - sacral region M99.64
      - sacrococcygeal M99.64
      - sacroiliac M99.64
      - specified NEC M99.69
      - thoracic region M99.62
      - thoracolumbar M99.62
      - upper extremity M99.67
    - subluxation — *see* Stenosis, intervertebral foramina, osseous
  - intestine — *see also* Obstruction, intestine
    - congenital (small) Q41.9
      - large Q42.9
        - specified NEC Q42.8
      - specified NEC Q41.8

- **Stenosis, stenotic** — *continued*
  - jejunum — *see also* Obstruction, intestine, specified NEC K56.699
    - congenital Q41.1
  - lacrimal (passage)
    - canaliculi HØ4.54- ☑
    - congenital Q1Ø.5
    - duct HØ4.55- ☑
    - punctum HØ4.56- ☑
    - sac HØ4.57- ☑
  - lacrimonasal duct — *see* Stenosis, lacrimal, duct
    - congenital Q1Ø.5
  - larynx J38.6
    - congenital NEC Q31.8
      - subglottic Q31.1
    - syphilitic A52.73
      - congenital A5Ø.59 *[J99]*
  - mitral (chronic) (inactive) (valve) IØ5.Ø
    - with
      - aortic valve disease IØ8.Ø
      - incompetency, insufficiency or regurgitation IØ5.2
    - active or acute IØ1.1
      - with rheumatic or Sydenham's chorea IØ2.Ø
    - congenital Q23.2
    - specified cause, except rheumatic I34.2
    - syphilitic A52.Ø3
  - myocardium, myocardial — *see also* Degeneration, myocardial
    - hypertrophic subaortic (idiopathic) I42.1
  - nares (anterior) (posterior) J34.89
    - congenital Q3Ø.Ø
  - nasal duct — *see also* Stenosis, lacrimal, duct
    - congenital Q1Ø.5
  - nasolacrimal duct — *see also* Stenosis, lacrimal, duct
    - congenital Q1Ø.5
  - neural canal — *see also* Lesion, biomechanical, specified NEC
    - connective tissue M99.49
      - abdomen M99.49
      - cervical region M99.41
      - cervicothoracic M99.41
      - head region M99.4Ø
      - lower extremity M99.46
      - lumbar region M99.43
      - lumbosacral M99.43
      - occipitocervical M99.4Ø
      - pelvic M99.45
      - rib cage M99.48
      - sacral region M99.44
      - sacrococcygeal M99.44
      - sacroiliac M99.44
      - specified NEC M99.49
      - thoracic region M99.42
      - thoracolumbar M99.42
      - upper extremity M99.47
    - intervertebral disc M99.59
      - abdomen M99.59
      - cervical region M99.51
      - cervicothoracic M99.51
      - head region M99.5Ø
      - lower extremity M99.56
      - lumbar region M99.53
      - lumbosacral M99.53
      - occipitocervical M99.5Ø
      - pelvic M99.55
      - rib cage M99.58
      - sacral region M99.54
      - sacrococcygeal M99.54
      - sacroiliac M99.54
      - specified NEC M99.59
      - thoracic region M99.52
      - thoracolumbar M99.52
      - upper extremity M99.57
    - osseous M99.39
      - abdomen M99.39
      - cervical region M99.31
      - cervicothoracic M99.31
      - head region M99.3Ø
      - lower extremity M99.36
      - lumbar region M99.33
      - lumbosacral M99.33
      - occipitocervical M99.3Ø
      - pelvic M99.35
      - rib cage M99.38
      - sacral region M99.34
      - sacrococcygeal M99.34
      - sacroiliac M99.34

- **Storm, thyroid** — *see* Thyrotoxicosis
- **Strabismus** (congenital) (nonparalytic) H50.9
  - concomitant H50.40
    - convergent — *see* Strabismus, convergent concomitant
    - divergent — *see* Strabismus, divergent concomitant
  - convergent concomitant H50.00
    - accommodative component H50.43
    - alternating H50.05
      - with
        - A pattern H50.06
        - specified nonconcomitances NEC H50.08
        - V pattern H50.07
    - monocular H50.01- ☑
      - with
        - A pattern H50.02- ☑
        - specified nonconcomitances NEC H50.04- ☑
        - V pattern H50.03- ☑
      - intermittent H50.31- ☑
        - alternating H50.32
  - cyclotropia H50.41 ☑
  - divergent concomitant H50.10
    - alternating H50.15
      - with
        - A pattern H50.16
        - specified noncomitances NEC H50.18
        - V pattern H50.17
    - monocular H50.11- ☑
      - with
        - A pattern H50.12- ☑
        - specified noncomitances NEC H50.14- ☑
        - V pattern H50.13- ☑
      - intermittent H50.33 ☑
        - alternating H50.34
  - Duane's syndrome H50.81- ☑
  - due to adhesions, scars H50.69
  - heterophoria H50.50
    - alternating H50.55
    - cyclophoria H50.54
    - esophoria H50.51
    - exophoria H50.52
    - vertical H50.53
  - heterotropia H50.40
    - intermittent H50.30
  - hypertropia H50.2- ☑
  - hypotropia — *see* Hypertropia
  - latent H50.50
  - mechanical H50.60
    - Brown's sheath syndrome H50.61- ☑
    - specified type NEC H50.69
  - monofixation syndrome H50.42
  - paralytic H49.9
    - abducens nerve H49.2- ☑
    - fourth nerve H49.1- ☑
    - Kearns-Sayre syndrome H49.81- ☑
    - ophthalmoplegia (external)
      - progressive H49.4- ☑
        - with pigmentary retinopathy H49.81- ☑
      - total H49.3- ☑
    - sixth nerve H49.2- ☑
    - specified type NEC H49.88- ☑
    - third nerve H49.0- ☑
    - trochlear nerve H49.1- ☑
  - specified type NEC H50.89
  - vertical H50.2- ☑
- **Strain**
  - back S39.012 ☑
  - cervical S16.1 ☑
  - eye NEC — *see* Disturbance, vision, subjective
  - heart — *see* Disease, heart
  - low back S39.012 ☑
  - mental NOS Z73.3
    - work-related Z56.6
  - muscle (tendon) — *see* Injury, muscle, by site, strain
  - neck S16.1 ☑
  - physical NOS Z73.3
    - work-related Z56.6
  - postural — *see also* Disorder, soft tissue, due to use
  - psychological NEC Z73.3
  - tendon — *see* Injury, muscle, by site, strain
- **Straining, on urination** R39.16
- **Strand, vitreous** — *see* Opacity, vitreous, membranes and strands
- **Strangulation, strangulated** — *see also* Asphyxia, traumatic
  - appendix K38.8
  - bladder-neck N32.0
  - bowel or colon K56.2
  - food or foreign body — *see* Foreign body, by site
  - hemorrhoids — *see* Hemorrhoids, with complication
  - hernia — *see also* Hernia, by site, with obstruction
    - with gangrene — *see* Hernia, by site, with gangrene
  - intestine (large) (small) K56.2
    - with hernia — *see also* Hernia, by site, with obstruction
      - with gangrene — *see* Hernia, by site, with gangrene
  - mesentery K56.2
  - mucus — *see* Asphyxia, mucus
  - omentum K56.2
  - organ or site, congenital NEC — *see* Atresia, by site
  - ovary — *see* Torsion, ovary
  - penis N48.89
    - foreign body T19.4 ☑
  - rupture — *see* Hernia, by site, with obstruction
  - stomach due to hernia — *see also* Hernia, by site, with obstruction
    - with gangrene — *see* Hernia, by site, with gangrene
  - vesicourethral orifice N32.0
- **Strangury** R30.0
- **Straw itch** B88.0
- **Strawberry**
  - gallbladder K82.4
  - mark Q82.5
  - tongue (red) (white) K14.3
- **Streak**(s)
  - macula, angioid H35.33
  - ovarian Q50.32
- **Strephosymbolia** F81.0
  - secondary to organic lesion R48.8
- **Streptobacillary fever** A25.1
- **Streptobacillosis** A25.1
- **Streptobacillus moniliformis** A25.1
- **Streptococcus, streptococcal** — *see also* condition
  - as cause of disease classified elsewhere B95.5
  - group
    - A, as cause of disease classified elsewhere B95.0
    - B, as cause of disease classified elsewhere B95.1
    - D, as cause of disease classified elsewhere B95.2
  - pneumoniae, as cause of disease classified elsewhere B95.3
  - specified NEC, as cause of disease classified elsewhere B95.4
- **Streptomycosis** B47.1
- **Streptotrichosis** A48.8
- **Stress** F43.9
  - family — *see* Disruption, family
  - fetal P84
    - complicating pregnancy O77.9
      - due to drug administration O77.1
  - mental NEC Z73.3
    - work-related Z56.6
  - physical NEC Z73.3
    - work-related Z56.6
  - polycythemia D75.1
  - reaction — *see also* Reaction, stress F43.9
  - work schedule Z56.3
- **Stretching, nerve** — *see* Injury, nerve
- **Striae albicantes, atrophicae or distensae** (cutis) L90.6
- **Stricture** — *see also* Stenosis
  - ampulla of Vater K83.1
  - anus (sphincter) K62.4
    - congenital Q42.3
      - with fistula Q42.2
    - infantile Q42.3
      - with fistula Q42.2
  - aorta (ascending) (congenital) Q25.1
    - arteriosclerotic I70.0
    - calcified I70.0
    - supravalvular, congenital Q25.3
  - aortic (valve) — *see* Stenosis, aortic
  - aqueduct of Sylvius (congenital) Q03.0
    - with spina bifida — *see* Spina bifida, by site, with hydrocephalus
    - acquired G91.1
  - artery I77.1
    - basilar — *see* Occlusion, artery, basilar
    - carotid — *see* Occlusion, artery, carotid
    - celiac I77.4
    - congenital (peripheral) Q27.8
      - cerebral Q28.3
      - coronary Q24.5
      - digestive system Q27.8
      - lower limb Q27.8
      - retinal Q14.1
      - specified site NEC Q27.8
      - umbilical Q27.0
      - upper limb Q27.8
    - coronary — *see* Disease, heart, ischemic, atherosclerotic
      - congenital Q24.5
    - precerebral — *see* Occlusion, artery, precerebral
    - pulmonary (congenital) Q25.6
      - acquired I28.8
    - renal I70.1
    - vertebral — *see* Occlusion, artery, vertebral
  - auditory canal (external) (congenital)
    - acquired — *see* Stenosis, external ear canal
  - bile duct (common) (hepatic) K83.1
    - congenital Q44.3
    - postoperative K91.89
  - bladder N32.89
    - neck N32.0
  - bowel — *see* Obstruction, intestine
  - brain G93.89
  - bronchus J98.09
    - congenital Q32.3
    - syphilitic A52.72
  - cardia (stomach) K22.2
    - congenital Q39.3
  - cardiac — *see also* Disease, heart
    - orifice (stomach) K22.2
  - cecum — *see* Obstruction, intestine
  - cervix, cervical (canal) N88.2
    - congenital Q51.828
    - in pregnancy — *see* Pregnancy, complicated by, abnormal cervix
      - causing obstructed labor O65.5
  - colon — *see also* Obstruction, intestine
    - congenital Q42.9
      - specified NEC Q42.8
  - colostomy K94.03
  - common (bile) duct K83.1
  - coronary (artery) — *see* Disease, heart, ischemic, atherosclerotic
  - cystic duct — *see* Obstruction, gallbladder
  - digestive organs NEC, congenital Q45.8
  - duodenum K31.5
    - congenital Q41.0
  - ear canal (external) (congenital) Q16.1
    - acquired — *see* Stricture, auditory canal, acquired
  - ejaculatory duct N50.89
  - enterostomy K94.13
  - esophagus K22.2
    - congenital Q39.3
    - syphilitic A52.79
      - congenital A50.59 *[K23]*
  - eustachian tube — *see also* Obstruction, eustachian tube
    - congenital Q17.8
  - fallopian tube N97.1
    - gonococcal A54.24
    - tuberculous A18.17
  - gallbladder — *see* Obstruction, gallbladder
  - glottis J38.6
  - heart — *see also* Disease, heart
    - valve — *see also* Endocarditis I38
      - aortic Q23.0
      - mitral Q23.2
      - pulmonary Q22.1
      - tricuspid Q22.4
  - hepatic duct K83.1
  - hourglass, of stomach K31.2
  - hymen N89.6
  - hypopharynx J39.2
  - ileum — *see also* Obstruction, intestine, specified NEC K56.699
    - congenital Q41.2
  - intestine — *see also* Obstruction, intestine
    - congenital (small) Q41.9
      - large Q42.9
        - specified NEC Q42.8
      - specified NEC Q41.8
    - ischemic K55.1
  - jejunum — *see also* Obstruction, intestine, specified NEC K56.699
    - congenital Q41.1
  - lacrimal passages — *see also* Stenosis, lacrimal
    - congenital Q10.5

- **Stricture** — *continued*
  - larynx J38.6
    - congenital NEC Q31.8
      - subglottic Q31.1
    - syphilitic A52.73
      - congenital A5Ø.59 *[J99]*
  - meatus
    - ear (congenital) Q16.1
      - acquired — *see* Stricture, auditory canal, acquired
    - osseous (ear) (congenital) Q16.1
      - acquired — *see* Stricture, auditory canal, acquired
    - urinarius — *see also* Stricture, urethra
      - congenital Q64.33
  - mitral (valve) — *see* Stenosis, mitral
  - myocardium, myocardial I51.5
    - hypertrophic subaortic (idiopathic) I42.1
  - nares (anterior) (posterior) J34.89
    - congenital Q3Ø.Ø
  - nasal duct — *see also* Stenosis, lacrimal, duct
    - congenital Q1Ø.5
  - nasolacrimal duct — *see also* Stenosis, lacrimal, duct
    - congenital Q1Ø.5
  - nasopharynx J39.2
    - syphilitic A52.73
  - nose J34.89
    - congenital Q3Ø.Ø
  - nostril (anterior) (posterior) J34.89
    - congenital Q3Ø.Ø
    - syphilitic A52.73
      - congenital A5Ø.59 *[J99]*
  - organ or site, congenital NEC — *see* Atresia, by site
  - os uteri — *see* Stricture, cervix
  - osseous meatus (ear) (congenital) Q16.1
    - acquired — *see* Stricture, auditory canal, acquired
  - oviduct — *see* Stricture, fallopian tube
  - pelviureteric junction (congenital) Q62.11
    - acquired, with hydronephrosis N13.Ø
  - penis, by foreign body T19.4 ☑
  - pharynx J39.2
  - prostate N42.89
  - pulmonary, pulmonic
    - artery (congenital) Q25.6
      - acquired I28.8
      - noncongenital I28.8
    - infundibulum (congenital) Q24.3
    - valve I37.Ø
      - congenital Q22.1
    - vein, acquired I28.8
    - vessel NEC I28.8
  - punctum lacrimale — *see also* Stenosis, lacrimal, punctum
    - congenital Q1Ø.5
  - pylorus (hypertrophic) K31.1
    - adult K31.1
    - congenital Q4Ø.Ø
    - infantile Q4Ø.Ø
  - rectosigmoid — *see also* Obstruction, intestine, specified NEC K56.699
  - rectum (sphincter) K62.4
    - congenital Q42.1
      - with fistula Q42.Ø
    - due to
      - chlamydial lymphogranuloma A55
      - irradiation K91.89
      - lymphogranuloma venereum A55
    - gonococcal A54.6
    - inflammatory (chlamydial) A55
    - syphilitic A52.74
    - tuberculous A18.32
  - renal artery I7Ø.1
    - congenital Q27.1
  - salivary duct or gland (any) K11.8
  - sigmoid (flexure) — *see* Obstruction, intestine
  - spermatic cord N5Ø.89
  - stoma (following) (of)
    - colostomy K94.Ø3
    - enterostomy K94.13
    - gastrostomy K94.23
    - ileostomy K94.13
    - tracheostomy J95.Ø3
  - stomach K31.89
    - congenital Q4Ø.2
    - hourglass K31.2
  - subaortic Q24.4
    - hypertrophic (acquired) (idiopathic) I42.1
  - subglottic J38.6

- **Stricture** — *continued*
  - syphilitic NEC A52.79
  - trachea J39.8
    - congenital Q32.1
    - syphilitic A52.73
    - tuberculous NEC A15.5
  - tracheostomy J95.Ø3
  - tricuspid (valve) — *see* Stenosis, tricuspid
  - tunica vaginalis N5Ø.89
  - ureter (postoperative) N13.5
    - with
      - hydronephrosis N13.1
        - with infection N13.6
      - pyelonephritis (chronic) N11.1
    - congenital — *see* Atresia, ureter
    - tuberculous A18.11
  - ureteropelvic junction (congenital) Q62.11
    - acquired, with hydronephrosis N13.Ø
  - ureterovesical orifice N13.5
    - with infection N13.6
  - urethra (organic) (spasmodic) — *see also* Stricture, urethra, male N35.919
    - associated with schistosomiasis B65.Ø *[N37]*
    - congenital Q64.39
      - valvular (posterior) Q64.2
    - due to
      - infection — *see* Stricture, urethra, postinfective
      - trauma — *see* Stricture, urethra, post-traumatic
    - female N35.92
    - gonococcal, gonorrheal A54.Ø1
    - infective NEC — *see* Stricture, urethra, postinfective
    - late effect (sequelae) of injury — *see* Stricture, urethra, post-traumatic
    - male N35.919
      - anterior urethra N35.914
      - bulbous urethra N35.912
      - meatal N35.911
      - membranous urethra N35.913
      - overlapping sites N35.916
    - postcatheterization — *see* Stricture, urethra, postprocedural
    - postinfective NEC
      - female N35.12
      - male N35.119
        - anterior urethra N35.114
        - bulbous urethra N35.112
        - meatal N35.111
        - membranous urethra N35.113
        - overlapping sites N35.116
    - postobstetric N35.Ø21
    - postoperative — *see* Stricture, urethra, postprocedural
    - postprocedural
      - female N99.12
      - male N99.114
        - anterior bulbous urethra N99.113
        - bulbous urethra N99.111
        - fossa navicularis N99.115
        - meatal N99.11Ø
        - membranous urethra N99.112
        - overlapping sites N99.116
    - post-traumatic
      - female N35.Ø28
        - due to childbirth N35.Ø21
      - male N35.Ø14
        - anterior urethra N35.Ø13
        - bulbous urethra N35.Ø11
        - meatal N35.Ø1Ø
        - membranous urethra N35.Ø12
        - overlapping sites N35.Ø16
    - sequela (late effect) of
      - childbirth N35.Ø21
      - injury — *see* Stricture, urethra, post-traumatic
    - specified cause NEC
      - female N35.82
      - male N35.819
        - anterior urethra N35.814
        - bulbous urethra N35.812
        - meatal N35.811
        - membranous urethra N35.813
        - overlapping sites N35.816
    - syphilitic A52.76
    - traumatic — *see* Stricture, urethra, post-traumatic
    - valvular (posterior), congenital Q64.2
  - urinary meatus — *see* Stricture, urethra
  - uterus, uterine (synechiae) N85.6
    - os (external) (internal) — *see* Stricture, cervix
  - vagina (outlet) — *see* Stenosis, vagina

- **Stricture** — *continued*
  - valve (cardiac) (heart) — *see also* Endocarditis
    - congenital
      - aortic Q23.Ø
      - mitral Q23.2
      - pulmonary Q22.1
      - tricuspid Q22.4
  - vas deferens N5Ø.89
    - congenital Q55.4
  - vein I87.1
  - vena cava (inferior) (superior) NEC I87.1
    - congenital Q26.Ø
  - vesicourethral orifice N32.Ø
    - congenital Q64.31
  - vulva (acquired) N9Ø.5
- **Stridor** RØ6.1
  - congenital (larynx) P28.89
- **Stridulous** — *see* condition
- **Stroke** (apoplectic) (brain) (embolic) (ischemic) (paralytic) (thrombotic) I63.9
  - cerebral, perinatal P91.82- ☑
  - cryptogenic — *see also* infarction, cerebral I63.9
  - epileptic — *see* Epilepsy
  - heat T67.Ø1 ☑
    - exertional T67.Ø2 ☑
    - specified NEC T67.Ø9 ☑
  - in evolution I63.9
  - intraoperative
    - during cardiac surgery I97.81Ø
    - during other surgery I97.811
  - ischemic, perinatal arterial P91.82- ☑
  - lightning — *see* Lightning
  - meaning
    - cerebral hemorrhage — *code to* Hemorrhage, intracranial
    - cerebral infarction — *code to* Infarction, cerebral
  - neonatal P91.82- ☑
  - postprocedural
    - following cardiac surgery I97.82Ø
    - following other surgery I97.821
  - sun T67.Ø1 ☑
    - specified NEC T67.Ø9 ☑
  - unspecified (NOS) I63.9
- **Stromatosis, endometrial** D39.Ø
- **Strongyloidiasis, strongyloidosis** B78.9
  - cutaneous B78.1
  - disseminated B78.7
  - intestinal B78.Ø
- **Strophulus pruriginosus** L28.2
- **Struck by lightning** — *see* Lightning
- **Struma** — *see also* Goiter
  - Hashimoto EØ6.3
  - lymphomatosa EØ6.3
  - nodosa (simplex) EØ4.9
    - endemic EØ1.2
      - multinodular EØ1.1
    - multinodular EØ4.2
      - iodine-deficiency related EØ1.1
    - toxic or with hyperthyroidism EØ5.2Ø
      - with thyroid storm EØ5.21
      - multinodular EØ5.2Ø
        - with thyroid storm EØ5.21
      - uninodular EØ5.1Ø
        - with thyroid storm EØ5.11
    - toxicosa EØ5.2Ø
      - with thyroid storm EØ5.21
      - multinodular EØ5.2Ø
        - with thyroid storm EØ5.21
      - uninodular EØ5.1Ø
        - with thyroid storm EØ5.11
    - uninodular EØ4.1
  - ovarii D27.- ☑
  - Riedel's EØ6.5
- **Strumipriva cachexia** EØ3.4
- **Strümpell-Marie spine** — *see* Spondylitis, ankylosing
- **Strümpell-Westphal pseudosclerosis** E83.Ø1
- **Stuart deficiency disease** (factor X) D68.2
- **Stuart-Prower factor deficiency** (factor X) D68.2
- **Student's elbow** — *see* Bursitis, elbow, olecranon
- **Stump** — *see* Amputation
- **Stunting, nutritional** E45
- **Stupor** (catatonic) R4Ø.1
  - depressive (single episode) F32.89
    - recurrent episode F33.8
  - dissociative F44.2
  - manic F3Ø.2
  - manic-depressive F31.89
  - psychogenic (anergic) F44.2

- **Substance** (other psychoactive) **-induced** — *continued*
  - mild neurocognitive disorder F19.988
  - obsessive-compulsive and related disorder F19.988
  - psychotic disorder F19.959
  - sexual dysfunction F19.981
  - sleep disorder F19.982
- **Substernal thyroid** EØ4.9
  - congenital Q89.2
- **Substitution disorder** F44.9
- **Subtentorial** — *see* condition
- **Subthyroidism** (acquired) — *see also* Hypothyroidism
  - congenital EØ3.1
- **Succenturiate placenta** O43.19- ☑
- **Sucking thumb, child** (excessive) F98.8
- **Sudamen, sudamina** L74.1
- **Sudanese kala-azar** B55.Ø
- **Sudden**
  - hearing loss — *see* Deafness, sudden
  - heart failure — *see* Failure, heart
- **Sudeck's atrophy, disease, or syndrome** — *see* Algoneurodystrophy
- **Suffocation** — *see* Asphyxia, traumatic
- **Sugar**
  - blood
    - high (transient) R73.9
    - low (transient) E16.2
  - in urine R81
- **Suicide, suicidal** (attempted) T14.91 ☑
  - by poisoning — *see* Table of Drugs and Chemicals
  - history of (personal) Z91.51
    - in family Z81.8
  - ideation — *see* Ideation, suicidal
  - risk
    - meaning personal history of attempted suicide Z91.51
    - meaning suicidal ideation — *see* Ideation, suicidal
  - tendencies
    - meaning personal history of attempted suicide Z91.51
    - meaning suicidal ideation — *see* Ideation, suicidal
  - trauma — *see* nature of injury by site
- **Suipestifer infection** — *see* Infection, salmonella
- **Sulfhemoglobinemia, sulphemoglobinemia** (acquired) (with methemoglobinemia) D74.8
- **Sumatran mite fever** A75.3
- **Summer** — *see* condition
- **Sunburn** L55.9
  - due to
    - tanning bed (acute) L56.8
      - chronic L57.8
    - ultraviolet radiation (acute) L56.8
      - chronic L57.8
  - first degree L55.Ø
  - second degree L55.1
  - third degree L55.2
- **SUNCT** (short lasting unilateral neuralgiform headache with conjunctival injection and tearing) G44.Ø59
  - intractable G44.Ø51
  - not intractable G44.Ø59
- **Sundowning** FØ5
- **Sunken acetabulum** — *see* Derangement, joint, specified type NEC, hip
- **Sunstroke** T67.Ø1 ☑
  - specified NEC T67.Ø9 ☑
- **Superfecundation** — *see* Pregnancy, multiple
- **Superfetation** — *see* Pregnancy, multiple
- **Superinvolution** (uterus) N85.8
- **Supernumerary** (congenital)
  - aortic cusps Q23.8
  - auditory ossicles Q16.3
  - bone Q79.8
  - breast Q83.1
  - carpal bones Q74.Ø
  - cusps, heart valve NEC Q24.8
    - aortic Q23.8
    - mitral Q23.2
    - pulmonary Q22.3
  - digit(s) Q69.9
  - ear (lobule) Q17.Ø
  - fallopian tube Q5Ø.6
  - finger Q69.Ø
  - hymen Q52.4
  - kidney Q63.Ø
  - lacrimonasal duct Q1Ø.6
  - lobule (ear) Q17.Ø
  - mitral cusps Q23.2
  - muscle Q79.8
- **Supernumerary** — *continued*
  - nipple(s) Q83.3
  - organ or site not listed — *see* Accessory
  - ossicles, auditory Q16.3
  - ovary Q5Ø.31
  - oviduct Q5Ø.6
  - pulmonary, pulmonic cusps Q22.3
  - rib Q76.6
    - cervical or first (syndrome) Q76.5
  - roots (of teeth) KØØ.2
  - spleen Q89.Ø9
  - tarsal bones Q74.2
  - teeth KØØ.1
  - testis Q55.29
  - thumb Q69.1
  - toe Q69.2
  - uterus Q51.28
  - vagina Q52.1 ☑
  - vertebra Q76.49
- **Supervision** (of)
  - contraceptive — *see* Prescription, contraceptives
  - dietary (for) Z71.3
    - allergy (food) Z71.3
    - colitis Z71.3
    - diabetes mellitus Z71.3
    - food allergy or intolerance Z71.3
    - gastritis Z71.3
    - hypercholesterolemia Z71.3
    - hypoglycemia Z71.3
    - intolerance (food) Z71.3
    - obesity Z71.3
    - specified NEC Z71.3
  - healthy infant or child Z76.2
    - foundling Z76.1
  - high-risk pregnancy — *see* Pregnancy, supervision of, high-risk
  - lactation Z39.1
  - pregnancy — *see* Pregnancy, supervision of
- **Supplemental teeth** KØØ.1
- **Suppression**
  - binocular vision H53.34
  - lactation O92.5
  - menstruation N94.89
  - ovarian secretion E28.39
  - renal N28.9
  - urine, urinary secretion R34
- **Suppuration, suppurative** — *see also* condition
  - accessory sinus (chronic) — *see* Sinusitis
  - adrenal gland
  - antrum (chronic) — *see* Sinusitis, maxillary
  - bladder — *see* Cystitis
  - brain GØ6.Ø
    - sequelae GØ9
  - breast N61.1
    - puerperal, postpartum or gestational — *see* Mastitis, obstetric, purulent
  - dental periosteum M27.3
  - ear (middle) — *see also* Otitis, media
    - external NEC — *see* Otitis, externa, infective
    - internal — *see* subcategory H83.Ø ☑
  - ethmoidal (chronic) (sinus) — *see* Sinusitis, ethmoidal
  - fallopian tube — *see* Salpingo-oophoritis
  - frontal (chronic) (sinus) — *see* Sinusitis, frontal
  - gallbladder (acute) K81.Ø
  - gum KØ5.2Ø
    - generalized — *see* Periodontitis, aggressive, generalized
    - localized — *see* Periodontitis, aggressive, localized
  - intracranial GØ6.Ø
  - joint — *see* Arthritis, pyogenic or pyemic
  - labyrinthine — *see* subcategory H83.Ø ☑
  - lung — *see* Abscess, lung
  - mammary gland N61.1
    - puerperal, postpartum O91.12
      - associated with lactation O91.13
  - maxilla, maxillary M27.2
    - sinus (chronic) — *see* Sinusitis, maxillary
  - muscle — *see* Myositis, infective
  - nasal sinus (chronic) — *see* Sinusitis
  - pancreas, acute — *see also* Pancreatitis, acute K85.8Ø
  - parotid gland — *see* Sialoadenitis
  - pelvis, pelvic
    - female — *see* Disease, pelvis, inflammatory
    - male K65.Ø
  - pericranial — *see* Osteomyelitis
  - salivary duct or gland (any) — *see* Sialoadenitis
  - sinus (accessory) (chronic) (nasal) — *see* Sinusitis
  - sphenoidal sinus (chronic) — *see* Sinusitis, sphenoidal
- **Suppuration, suppurative** — *continued*
  - thymus (gland) E32.1
  - thyroid (gland) EØ6.Ø
  - tonsil — *see* Tonsillitis
  - uterus — *see* Endometritis
- **Supraeruption of tooth** (teeth) M26.34
- **Supraglottitis** JØ4.3Ø
  - with obstruction JØ4.31
- **Suprarenal** (gland) — *see* condition
- **Suprascapular nerve** — *see* condition
- **Suprasellar** — *see* condition
- **Surfer's knots or nodules** S89.8- ☑
- **Surgical**
  - emphysema T81.82 ☑
  - procedures, complication or misadventure — *see* Complications, surgical procedures
  - shock T81.1Ø ☑
- **Surveillance** (of) (for) — *see also* Observation
  - alcohol abuse Z71.41
  - contraceptive — *see* Prescription, contraceptives
  - dietary Z71.3
  - drug abuse Z71.51
- **Susceptibility to disease, genetic** Z15.89
  - malignant neoplasm Z15.Ø9
    - breast Z15.Ø1
    - endometrium Z15.Ø4
    - ovary Z15.Ø2
    - prostate Z15.Ø3
    - specified NEC Z15.Ø9
  - multiple endocrine neoplasia Z15.81
- **Suspected condition, ruled out** — *see also* Observation, suspected
  - amniotic cavity and membrane ZØ3.71
  - cervical shortening ZØ3.75
  - fetal anomaly ZØ3.73
  - fetal growth ZØ3.74
  - maternal and fetal conditions NEC ZØ3.79
  - newborn — *see also* Observation, newborn, suspected condition ruled out ZØ5.9
  - oligohydramnios ZØ3.71
  - placental problem ZØ3.72
  - polyhydramnios ZØ3.71
- **Suspended uterus**
  - in pregnancy or childbirth — *see* Pregnancy, complicated by, abnormal uterus
- **Sutton's nevus** D22.9
- **Suture**
  - burst (in operation wound) T81.31 ☑
    - external operation wound T81.31 ☑
    - internal operation wound T81.32 ☑
  - inadvertently left in operation wound — *see* Foreign body, accidentally left during a procedure
  - removal Z48.Ø2
- **Swab inadvertently left in operation wound** — *see* Foreign body, accidentally left during a procedure
- **Swallowed, swallowing**
  - difficulty — *see* Dysphagia
  - foreign body — *see* Foreign body, alimentary tract
- **Swan-neck deformity** (finger) — *see* Deformity, finger, swan-neck
- **Swearing, compulsive** F42.8
  - in Gilles de la Tourette's syndrome F95.2
- **Sweat, sweats**
  - fetid L75.Ø
  - night R61
- **Sweating, excessive** R61
- **Sweeley-Klionsky disease** E75.21
- **Sweet's disease or dermatosis** L98.2
- **Swelling** (of) R6Ø.9
  - abdomen, abdominal (not referable to any particular organ) — *see* Mass, abdominal
  - ankle — *see* Effusion, joint, ankle
  - arm M79.89
    - forearm M79.89
  - breast — *see also* Lump, breast N63.Ø
  - Calabar B74.3
  - cervical gland R59.Ø
  - chest, localized R22.2
  - ear H93.8- ☑
  - extremity (lower) (upper) — *see* Disorder, soft tissue, specified type NEC
  - finger M79.89
  - foot M79.89
  - glands R59.9
    - generalized R59.1
    - localized R59.Ø
  - hand M79.89

- **Syndrome** — *continued*
  - immune effector cell-associated neurotoxicity — *continued*
    - grade — *continued*
      - unspecified G92.ØØ
  - immune reconstitution D89.3
  - immune reconstitution inflammatory [IRIS] D89.3
  - immunity deficiency, combined D81.9
  - immunodeficiency
    - acquired — *see* Human, immunodeficiency virus (HIV) disease
    - combined D81.9
  - impending coronary I2Ø.Ø
  - impingement, shoulder M75.4- ☑
  - inappropriate secretion of antidiuretic hormone E22.2
  - infant
    - gestational diabetes P7Ø.Ø
    - of diabetic mother P7Ø.1
  - infantilism (pituitary) E23.Ø
  - inferior vena cava I87.1
  - inspissated bile (newborn) P59.1
  - institutional (childhood) F94.2
  - insufficient sleep F51.12
  - intermediate coronary (artery) I2Ø.Ø
  - interspinous ligament — *see* Spondylopathy, specified NEC
  - intestinal
    - carcinoid E34.Ø
    - knot K56.2
  - intravascular coagulation-fibrinolysis (ICF) D65
  - iodine-deficiency, congenital EØØ.9
    - type
      - mixed EØØ.2
      - myxedematous EØØ.1
      - neurological EØØ.Ø
  - IRDS (idiopathic respiratory distress, newborn) P22.Ø
  - irritable
    - bowel K58.9
      - with
        - constipation K58.1
        - diarrhea K58.Ø
      - mixed K58.2
      - psychogenic F45.8
      - specified NEC K58.8
    - heart (psychogenic) F45.8
    - weakness F48.8
  - ischemic
    - bowel (transient) K55.9
      - chronic K55.1
      - due to mesenteric artery insufficiency K55.1
    - steal T82.898 ☑
  - IVC (intravascular coagulopathy) D65
  - Ivemark's Q89.Ø1
  - Jaccoud's — *see* Arthropathy, postrheumatic, chronic
  - Jackson's G83.89
  - Jakob-Creutzfeldt — *see* Creutzfeldt-Jakob disease or syndrome
  - jaw-winking QØ7.8
  - Jervell-Lange-Nielsen I45.81
  - jet lag G47.25
  - Job's D71
  - Joseph-Diamond-Blackfan D61.Ø1
  - jugular foramen G52.7
  - Kabuki Q89.8
  - Kanner's (autism) F84.Ø
  - Kartagener's Q89.3
  - Kelly's D5Ø.1
  - Kimmelstiel-Wilson — *see* Diabetes, specified type, with Kimmelstiel-Wilson disease
  - Klein (e)-Levine G47.13
  - Klippel-Feil (brevicollis) Q76.1
  - Köhler-Pellegrini-Steida — *see* Bursitis, tibial collateral
  - König's K59.89
  - Korsakoff (-Wernicke) (nonalcoholic) FØ4
    - alcoholic F1Ø.26
  - Kostmann's D7Ø.Ø
  - Krabbe's congenital muscle hypoplasia Q79.8
  - labyrinthine — *see* subcategory H83.2 ☑
  - lacunar NEC G46.7
  - Lambert-Eaton G7Ø.8Ø
    - in
      - neoplastic disease G73.1
      - specified disease NEC G7Ø.81
  - Landau-Kleffner — *see* Epilepsy, specified NEC
  - Larsen's Q74.8
  - lateral
    - cutaneous nerve of thigh G57.1- ☑
    - medullary G46.4

- **Syndrome** — *continued*
  - Launois' E22.Ø
  - lazy
    - leukocyte D7Ø.8
    - posture M62.3
  - Lemiere I8Ø.8
  - Lennox-Gastaut G4Ø.812
    - intractable G4Ø.814
      - with status epilepticus G4Ø.813
      - without status epilepticus G4Ø.814
    - not intractable G4Ø.812
      - with status epilepticus G4Ø.811
      - without status epilepticus G4Ø.812
  - lenticular, progressive E83.Ø1
  - Leopold-Levi's EØ5.9Ø
  - Lev's I44.2
  - Lichtheim's D51.Ø
  - Li-Fraumeni Z15.Ø1
  - Lightwood's N25.89
  - Lignac (de Toni) (-Fanconi) (-Debré) E72.Ø9
    - with cystinosis E72.Ø4
  - Likoff's I2Ø.8
  - limbic epilepsy personality FØ7.Ø
  - liver-kidney K76.7
  - lobotomy FØ7.Ø
  - Löffler's J82.89
  - long arm 18 or 21 deletion Q93.89
  - long QT I45.81
  - Louis-Barré G11.3
  - low
    - atmospheric pressure T7Ø.29 ☑
    - back M54.5Ø
    - output (cardiac) I5Ø.9
  - lower radicular, newborn (birth injury) P14.8
  - Luetscher's (dehydration) E86.Ø
  - Lupus anticoagulant D68.62
  - Lutembacher's Q21.19
  - macrophage activation D76.1
    - due to infection D76.2
  - magnesium-deficiency R29.Ø
  - Majeed MØ4.8
  - Mal de Debarquement R42
  - malabsorption K9Ø.9
    - postsurgical K91.2
  - malformation, congenital, due to
    - alcohol Q86.Ø
    - exogenous cause NEC Q86.8
    - hydantoin Q86.1
    - warfarin Q86.2
  - malignant
    - carcinoid E34.Ø
    - neuroleptic G21.Ø
  - Mallory-Weiss K22.6
  - mandibulofacial dysostosis Q75.4
  - manic-depressive — *see* Disorder, bipolar
  - maple-syrup-urine E71.Ø
  - Marable's I77.4
  - Marfan's Q87.4Ø
    - with
      - cardiovascular manifestations Q87.418
        - aortic dilation Q87.41Ø
      - ocular manifestations Q87.42
      - skeletal manifestations Q87.43
  - Marie's (acromegaly) E22.Ø
  - mast cell activation — *see* Activation, mast cell
  - maternal hypotension — *see* Syndrome, hypotension, maternal
  - May (-Hegglin) D72.Ø
  - McArdle (-Schmidt) (-Pearson) E74.Ø4
  - McQuarrie's E16.2
  - meconium plug (newborn) P76.Ø
  - median arcuate ligament I77.4
  - Meekeren-Ehlers-Danlos Q79.6 ☑
  - megavitamin-B6 E67.2
  - Meige G24.4
  - MELAS E88.41
  - Mendelson's O74.Ø
  - MERRF (myoclonic epilepsy associated with ragged-red fibers) E88.42
  - mesenteric
    - artery (superior) K55.1
    - vascular insufficiency K55.1
  - metabolic E88.81
  - metastatic carcinoid E34.Ø
  - micrognathia-glossoptosis Q87.Ø
  - midbrain NEC G93.89
  - middle lobe (lung) J98.19
  - middle radicular G54.Ø
  - migraine — *see also* Migraine G43.9Ø9

- **Syndrome** — *continued*
  - Mikulicz' K11.8
  - milk-alkali E83.52
  - Millard-Gubler G46.3
  - Miller-Dieker Q93.88
  - Miller-Fisher G61.Ø
  - Minkowski-Chauffard D58.Ø
  - Mirizzi's K83.1
  - MNGIE (Mitochondrial Neurogastrointestinal Encephalopathy) E88.49
  - Möbius, ophthalmoplegic migraine — *see* Migraine, ophthalmoplegic
  - monofixation H5Ø.42
  - Morel-Moore M85.2
  - Morel-Morgagni M85.2
  - Morgagni (-Morel) (-Stewart) M85.2
  - Morgagni-Adams-Stokes I45.9
  - Mounier-Kuhn Q32.4
    - with bronchiectasis J47.9
      - with
        - exacerbation (acute) J47.1
        - lower respiratory infection J47.Ø
    - acquired J98.Ø9
      - with bronchiectasis J47.9
        - with
          - exacerbation (acute) J47.1
          - lower respiratory infection J47.Ø
  - Muckle-Wells MØ4.2
  - mucocutaneous lymph node (acute febrile) (MCLS) M3Ø.3
  - multiple endocrine neoplasia (MEN) — *see* Neoplasia, endocrine, multiple (MEN)
  - multiple operations — *see* Disorder, factitious
  - multisystem inflammatory (in adults) (in children) M35.81
  - myasthenic G7Ø.9
    - in
      - diabetes mellitus — *see* Diabetes, amyotrophy
      - endocrine disease NEC E34.9 *[G73.3]*
      - neoplastic disease — *see also* Neoplasm D49.9 *[G73.3]*
      - thyrotoxicosis (hyperthyroidism) EØ5.9Ø *[G73.3]*
        - with thyroid storm EØ5.91 *[G73.3]*
  - myelodysplastic D46.9
    - with
      - 5q deletion D46.C (*following* D46.2)
      - isolated del (5q) chromosomal abnormality D46.C (*following* D46.2)
      - multilineage dysplasia D46.A (*following* D46.2)
        - with ringed sideroblasts D46.B (*following* D46.2)
    - lesions, low grade D46.2Ø
    - specified NEC D46.Z (*following* D46.4)
  - myeloid hypereosinophilic D72.118
  - myelopathic pain G89.Ø
  - myeloproliferative (chronic) D47.1
  - myofascial pain M79.18
  - Naffziger's G54.Ø
  - nail patella Q87.2
  - NARP (Neuropathy, Ataxia and Retinitis pigmentosa) E88.49
  - neonatal abstinence P96.1
  - nephritic — *see also* Nephritis
    - with edema — *see* Nephrosis
    - acute NØØ.9
    - chronic NØ3.9
    - rapidly progressive NØ1.9
  - nephrotic (congenital) — *see also* Nephrosis NØ4.9
    - with
      - C3
        - glomerulonephritis NØ4.A
        - glomerulopathy NØ4.A
          - with dense deposit disease NØ4.6
      - dense deposit disease NØ4.6
      - diffuse
        - crescentic glomerulonephritis NØ4.7
        - endocapillary proliferative glomerulonephritis NØ4.4
        - membranous glomerulonephritis NØ4.2
        - mesangial proliferative glomerulonephritis NØ4.3
        - mesangiocapillary glomerulonephritis NØ4.5
      - focal and segmental glomerular lesions NØ4.1
      - minor glomerular abnormality NØ4.Ø
      - specified morphological changes NEC NØ4.8
    - diabetic — *see* Diabetes, nephrosis
  - neurologic neglect R41.4
  - Nezelof's D81.4

Syndrome — *continued*
- Nonne-Milroy-Meige Q82.0
- Nothnagel's vasomotor acroparesthesia I73.89
- obesity hypoventilation (OHS) E66.2
- oculomotor H51.9
- Ogilvie K59.81
- ophthalmoplegia-cerebellar ataxia — *see* Strabismus, paralytic, third nerve
- oral allergy T78.1 ☑
- oral-facial-digital Q87.0
- organic
  - affective F06.30
  - amnesic (not alcohol- or drug-induced) F04
  - brain F09
  - depressive F06.31
  - hallucinosis F06.0
  - personality F07.0
- Ormond's N13.5
- oro-facial-digital Q87.0
- os trigonum Q68.8
- Osler-Weber-Rendu I78.0
- osteoporosis-osteomalacia M83.8
- Osterreicher-Turner Q87.2
- otolith — *see* subcategory H81.8 ☑
- oto-palatal-digital Q87.0
- outlet (thoracic) G54.0
- ovary
  - polycystic E28.2
  - resistant E28.39
  - sclerocystic E28.2
- Owren's D68.2
- Paget-Schroetter I82.890
- pain — *see also* Pain
  - complex regional I G90.50
    - lower limb G90.52- ☑
    - specified site NEC G90.59
    - upper limb G90.51- ☑
  - complex regional II — *see* Causalgia
- painful
  - bruising D69.2
  - feet E53.8
  - prostate N42.81
- paralysis agitans — *see* Parkinsonism
- paralytic G83.9
  - specified NEC G83.89
- Parinaud's H51.0
- parkinsonian — *see* Parkinsonism
- Parkinson's — *see* Parkinsonism
- paroxysmal facial pain G50.0
- Parry's E05.00
  - with thyroid storm E05.01
- Parsonage (-Aldren)-Turner G54.5
- patella clunk M25.86- ☑
- Paterson (-Brown) (-Kelly) D50.1
- pectoral girdle I77.89
- pectoralis minor I77.89
- pediatric autoimmune neuropsychiatric disorders associated with streptococcal infections (PANDAS) D89.89
- pediatric inflammatory multisystem M35.81
- Pelger-Huet D72.0
- pellagra-cerebellar ataxia-renal aminoaciduria E72.02
- pellagroid E52
- Pellegrini-Stieda — *see* Bursitis, tibial collateral
- pelvic congestion-fibrosis, female N94.89
- penta X Q97.1
- peptic ulcer — *see* Ulcer, peptic
- perabduction I77.89
- periodic fever M04.1
- periodic fever, aphthous stomatitis, pharyngitis, and adenopathy [PFAPA] M04.8
- periodic headache, in adults and children — *see* Headache, periodic syndromes in adults and children
- periurethral fibrosis N13.5
- Peutz-Jeghers Q85.89
- phantom limb (without pain) G54.7
  - with pain G54.6
- pharyngeal pouch D82.1
- Pick's — *see* Disease, Pick's
- Pickwickian E66.2
- PIE (pulmonary infiltration with eosinophilia) — *see also* Eosinophilia, pulmonary J82.89
- pigmentary pallidal degeneration (progressive) G23.0
- pineal E34.8
- pituitary E22.0
- placental transfusion — *see* Pregnancy, complicated by, placental transfusion syndromes

Syndrome — *continued*
- plantar fascia M72.2
- plateau iris (post-iridectomy) (postprocedural) H21.82
- Plummer-Vinson D50.1
- pluricarential of infancy E40
- plurideficiency E40
- pluriglandular (compensatory) E31.8
  - autoimmune E31.0
- pneumatic hammer T75.21 ☑
- polyangiitis overlap M30.8
- polycarential of infancy E40
- polyglandular E31.8
  - autoimmune E31.0
- polysplenia Q89.09
- pontine NEC G93.89
- popliteal
  - artery entrapment I77.89
  - web Q87.89
- post chemoembolization — *code to* associated conditions
- post endometrial ablation N99.85
- postbacterial fatigue G93.39
- postcardiac injury
  - postcardiotomy I97.0
  - postmyocardial infarction I24.1
- postcardiotomy I97.0
- postcholecystectomy K91.5
- postcommissurotomy I97.0
- postconcussional F07.81
- postcontusional F07.81
- post-COVID (-19) U09.9
- postencephalitic F07.89
- posterior
  - cervical sympathetic M53.0
  - cord G83.83
  - fossa compression G93.5
  - reversible encephalopathy (PRES) I67.83
- postgastrectomy (dumping) K91.1
- postgastric surgery K91.1
- postinfarction I24.1
- postinfectious fatigue G93.39
- postlaminectomy NEC M96.1
- postleukotomy F07.0
- postmastectomy lymphedema I97.2
- postmyocardial infarction I24.1
- postoperative NEC T81.9 ☑
  - blind loop K90.2
- postpartum panhypopituitary (Sheehan) E23.0
- postpolio (myelitic) G14
- postthrombotic I87.009
  - with
    - inflammation I87.02- ☑
      - with ulcer I87.03- ☑
    - specified complication NEC I87.09- ☑
    - ulcer I87.01- ☑
      - with inflammation I87.03- ☑
  - asymptomatic I87.00- ☑
- postural
  - orthostatic tachycardia [POTS] G90.A
  - tachycardia G90.A
- postvagotomy K91.1
- postvalvulotomy I97.0
- postviral NEC G93.31
  - fatigue G93.31
- Potain's K31.0
- potassium intoxication E87.5
- Prader-Willi Q87.11
- Prader-Willi-like Q87.19
- precerebral artery (multiple) (bilateral) G45.2
- preinfarction I20.0
- preleukemic D46.9
- premature senility E34.8
- premenstrual dysphoric F32.81
- premenstrual tension N94.3
- Prinzmetal-Massumi R07.1
- prune belly Q79.4
- pseudo -Turner's Q87.19
- pseudocarpal tunnel (sublimis) — *see* Syndrome, carpal tunnel
- pseudoparalytica G70.00
  - with exacerbation (acute) G70.01
  - in crisis G70.01
- psycho-organic (nonpsychotic severity) F07.9
  - acute or subacute F05
  - depressive type F06.31
  - hallucinatory type F06.0
  - nonpsychotic severity F07.0
  - specified NEC F07.89

Syndrome — *continued*
- PTEN (hamartoma) tumor Q85.81
- pulmonary
  - arteriosclerosis I27.0
  - dysmaturity (Wilson-Mikity) P27.0
  - hypoperfusion (idiopathic) P22.0
  - renal (hemorrhagic) (Goodpasture's) M31.0
- pure
  - motor lacunar G46.5
  - sensory lacunar G46.6
- Putnam-Dana D51.0
- pyogenic arthritis, pyoderma gangrenosum, and acne [PAPA] M04.8
- pyramidopallidonigral G20
- pyriformis — *see* Lesion, nerve, sciatic
- QT interval prolongation I45.81
- radicular NEC — *see* Radiculopathy
  - upper limbs, newborn (birth injury) P14.3
- rapid time-zone change G47.25
- Rasmussen G04.81
- Raymond (-Céstan) I65.8
- Raynaud's I73.00
  - with gangrene I73.01
- RDS (respiratory distress syndrome, newborn) P22.0
- reactive airways dysfunction J68.3
- Refsum's G60.1
- Reifenstein E34.52
- renal glomerulohyalinosis-diabetic — *see* Diabetes, nephrosis
- Rendu-Osler-Weber I78.0
- residual ovary N99.83
- resistant ovary E28.39
- respiratory
  - distress
    - acute J80
      - adult J80
      - child J80
      - idiopathic J84.114
    - newborn (idiopathic) (type I) P22.0
      - type II P22.1
- restless legs G25.81
- retinoblastoma (familial) C69.2 ☑
- retroperitoneal fibrosis N13.5
- retroviral seroconversion (acute) Z21
- Reye's G93.7
- Richter — *see* Leukemia, chronic lymphocytic, B-cell type
- Ridley's I50.1
- right
  - heart, hypoplastic Q22.6
  - ventricular obstruction — *see* Failure, heart, right
- Romano-Ward (prolonged QT interval) I45.81
- rotator cuff, shoulder — *see also* Tear, rotator cuff M75.10- ☑
- Rotes Quérol — *see* Hyperostosis, ankylosing
- Roth — *see* Meralgia paresthetica
- rubella (congenital) P35.0
- Ruvalcaba-Myhre-Smith E71.440
- Rytand-Lipsitch I44.2
- salt
  - depletion E87.1
    - due to heat NEC T67.8 ☑
      - causing heat exhaustion or prostration T67.4 ☑
  - low E87.1
- salt-losing N28.89
- SATB2-associated Q87.89
- Scaglietti-Dagnini E22.0
- scalenus anticus (anterior) G54.0
- scapulocostal — *see* Mononeuropathy, upper limb, specified site NEC
- scapuloperoneal G71.09
- schizophrenic, of childhood NEC F84.5
- Schnitzler D47.2
- Scholte's E34.0
- Schroeder's E27.0
- Schüller-Christian C96.5
- Schwachman's — *see* Syndrome, Shwachman's
- Schwartz (-Jampel) G71.13
- Schwartz-Bartter E22.2
- scimitar Q26.8
- sclerocystic ovary E28.2
- Seitelberger's G31.89
- septicemic adrenal hemorrhage A39.1
- seroconversion, retroviral (acute) Z21
- serous meningitis G93.2
- severe acute respiratory (SARS) J12.81
  - coronavirus 2 (*see also* COVID-19) U07.1

- **Synostosis** — *continued*
  - radioulnar Q74.Ø
- **Synovial sarcoma** — *see* Neoplasm, connective tissue, malignant
- **Synovioma** (malignant) — *see also* Neoplasm, connective tissue, malignant
  - benign — *see* Neoplasm, connective tissue, benign
- **Synoviosarcoma** — *see* Neoplasm, connective tissue, malignant
- **Synovitis** — *see also* Tenosynovitis M65.9
  - crepitant
    - hand M7Ø.Ø- ☑
    - wrist M7Ø.Ø3- ☑
  - gonococcal A54.49
  - gouty — *see* Gout
  - in (due to)
    - crystals M65.8- ☑
    - gonorrhea A54.49
    - syphilis (late) A52.78
    - use, overuse, pressure — *see* Disorder, soft tissue, due to use
  - infective NEC — *see* Tenosynovitis, infective NEC
  - specified NEC — *see* Tenosynovitis, specified type NEC
  - syphilitic A52.78
    - congenital (early) A5Ø.Ø2
  - toxic — *see* Synovitis, transient
  - transient M67.3- ☑
    - ankle M67.37- ☑
    - elbow M67.32- ☑
    - foot joint M67.37- ☑
    - hand joint M67.34- ☑
    - hip M67.35- ☑
    - knee M67.36- ☑
    - multiple site M67.39
    - pelvic region M67.35- ☑
    - shoulder M67.31- ☑
    - specified joint NEC M67.38
    - wrist M67.33- ☑
  - traumatic, current — *see* Sprain
  - tuberculous — *see* Tuberculosis, synovitis
  - villonodular (pigmented) M12.2- ☑
    - ankle M12.27- ☑
    - elbow M12.22- ☑
    - foot joint M12.27- ☑
    - hand joint M12.24- ☑
    - hip M12.25- ☑
    - knee M12.26- ☑
    - multiple site M12.29
    - pelvic region M12.25- ☑
    - shoulder M12.21- ☑
    - specified joint NEC M12.28
    - vertebrae M12.28
    - wrist M12.23- ☑
- **Syphilid** A51.39
  - congenital A5Ø.Ø6
  - newborn A5Ø.Ø6
  - tubercular (late) A52.79
- **Syphilis, syphilitic** (acquired) A53.9
  - abdomen (late) A52.79
  - acoustic nerve A52.15
  - adenopathy (secondary) A51.49
  - adrenal (gland) (with cortical hypofunction) A52.79
  - age under 2 years NOS — *see also* Syphilis, congenital, early
    - acquired A51.9
  - alopecia (secondary) A51.32
  - anemia (late) A52.79 *[D63.8]*
  - aneurysm (aorta) (ruptured) A52.Ø1
    - central nervous system A52.Ø5
    - congenital A5Ø.54 *[I79.Ø]*
  - anus (late) A52.74
    - primary A51.1
    - secondary A51.39
  - aorta (arch) (abdominal) (thoracic) A52.Ø2
    - aneurysm A52.Ø1
  - aortic (insufficiency) (regurgitation) (stenosis) A52.Ø3
    - aneurysm A52.Ø1
  - arachnoid (adhesive) (cerebral) (spinal) A52.13
  - asymptomatic — *see* Syphilis, latent
  - ataxia (locomotor) A52.11
  - atrophoderma maculatum A51.39
  - auricular fibrillation A52.Ø6
  - bladder (late) A52.76
  - bone A52.77
    - secondary A51.46
  - brain A52.17
  - breast (late) A52.79

- **Syphilis, syphilitic** — *continued*
  - bronchus (late) A52.72
  - bubo (primary) A51.Ø
  - bulbar palsy A52.19
  - bursa (late) A52.78
  - cardiac decompensation A52.Ø6
  - cardiovascular A52.ØØ
  - central nervous system (late) (recurrent) (relapse) (tertiary) A52.3
    - with
      - ataxia A52.11
      - general paralysis A52.17
        - juvenile A5Ø.45
      - paresis (general) A52.17
        - juvenile A5Ø.45
      - tabes (dorsalis) A52.11
        - juvenile A5Ø.45
      - taboparesis A52.17
        - juvenile A5Ø.45
    - aneurysm A52.Ø5
    - congenital A5Ø.4Ø
    - juvenile A5Ø.4Ø
    - remission in (sustained) A52.3
    - serology doubtful, negative, or positive A52.3
    - specified nature or site NEC A52.19
    - vascular A52.Ø5
  - cerebral A52.17
    - meningovascular A52.13
    - nerves (multiple palsies) A52.15
    - sclerosis A52.17
    - thrombosis A52.Ø5
  - cerebrospinal (tabetic type) A52.12
  - cerebrovascular A52.Ø5
  - cervix (late) A52.76
  - chancre (multiple) A51.Ø
    - extragenital A51.2
    - Rollet's A51.Ø
  - Charcot's joint A52.16
  - chorioretinitis A51.43
    - congenital A5Ø.Ø1
    - late A52.71
    - prenatal A5Ø.Ø1
  - choroiditis — *see* Syphilitic chorioretinitis
  - choroidoretinitis — *see* Syphilitic chorioretinitis
  - ciliary body (secondary) A51.43
    - late A52.71
  - colon (late) A52.74
  - combined spinal sclerosis A52.11
  - condyloma (latum) A51.31
  - congenital A5Ø.9
    - with
      - paresis (general) A5Ø.45
      - tabes (dorsalis) A5Ø.45
      - taboparesis A5Ø.45
    - chorioretinitis, choroiditis A5Ø.Ø1 *[H32]*
    - early, or less than 2 years after birth NEC A5Ø.2
      - with manifestations — *see* Syphilis, congenital, early, symptomatic
      - latent (without manifestations) A5Ø.1
        - negative spinal fluid test A5Ø.1
        - serology positive A5Ø.1
      - symptomatic A5Ø.Ø9
        - cutaneous A5Ø.Ø6
        - mucocutaneous A5Ø.Ø7
        - oculopathy A5Ø.Ø1
        - osteochondropathy A5Ø.Ø2
        - pharyngitis A5Ø.Ø3
        - pneumonia A5Ø.Ø4
        - rhinitis A5Ø.Ø5
        - visceral A5Ø.Ø8
    - interstitial keratitis A5Ø.31
    - juvenile neurosyphilis A5Ø.45
    - late, or 2 years or more after birth NEC A5Ø.7
      - chorioretinitis, choroiditis A5Ø.32
      - interstitial keratitis A5Ø.31
      - juvenile neurosyphilis A5Ø.45
      - latent (without manifestations) A5Ø.6
        - negative spinal fluid test A5Ø.6
        - serology positive A5Ø.6
      - symptomatic or with manifestations NEC A5Ø.59
        - arthropathy A5Ø.55
        - cardiovascular A5Ø.54
        - Clutton's joints A5Ø.51
        - Hutchinson's teeth A5Ø.52
        - Hutchinson's triad A5Ø.53
        - osteochondropathy A5Ø.56
        - saddle nose A5Ø.57
  - conjugal A53.9
    - tabes A52.11

- **Syphilis, syphilitic** — *continued*
  - conjunctiva (late) A52.71
  - contact Z2Ø.2
  - cord bladder A52.19
  - cornea, late A52.71
  - coronary (artery) (sclerosis) A52.Ø6
  - coryza, congenital A5Ø.Ø5
  - cranial nerve A52.15
    - multiple palsies A52.15
  - cutaneous — *see* Syphilis, skin
  - dacryocystitis (late) A52.71
  - degeneration, spinal cord A52.12
  - dementia paralytica A52.17
    - juvenilis A5Ø.45
  - destruction of bone A52.77
  - dilatation, aorta A52.Ø1
  - due to blood transfusion A53.9
  - dura mater A52.13
  - ear A52.79
    - inner A52.79
      - nerve (eighth) A52.15
      - neurorecurrence A52.15
  - early A51.9
    - cardiovascular A52.ØØ
    - central nervous system A52.3
    - latent (without manifestations) (less than 2 years after infection) A51.5
      - negative spinal fluid test A51.5
      - serological relapse after treatment A51.5
      - serology positive A51.5
    - relapse (treated, untreated) A51.9
    - skin A51.39
    - symptomatic A51.9
      - extragenital chancre A51.2
      - primary, except extragenital chancre A51.Ø
      - secondary — *see also* Syphilis, secondary A51.39
        - relapse (treated, untreated) A51.49
    - ulcer A51.39
  - eighth nerve (neuritis) A52.15
  - endemic A65
  - endocarditis A52.Ø3
    - aortic A52.Ø3
    - pulmonary A52.Ø3
  - epididymis (late) A52.76
  - epiglottis (late) A52.73
  - epiphysitis (congenital) (early) A5Ø.Ø2
  - episcleritis (late) A52.71
  - esophagus A52.79
  - eustachian tube A52.73
  - exposure to Z2Ø.2
  - eye A52.71
  - eyelid (late) (with gumma) A52.71
  - fallopian tube (late) A52.76
  - fracture A52.77
  - gallbladder (late) A52.74
  - gastric (polyposis) (late) A52.74
  - general A53.9
    - paralysis A52.17
      - juvenile A5Ø.45
  - genital (primary) A51.Ø
  - glaucoma A52.71
  - gumma NEC A52.79
    - cardiovascular system A52.ØØ
    - central nervous system A52.3
    - congenital A5Ø.59
  - heart (block) (decompensation) (disease) (failure) A52.Ø6 *[I52]*
    - valve NEC A52.Ø3
  - hemianesthesia A52.19
  - hemianopsia A52.71
  - hemiparesis A52.17
  - hemiplegia A52.17
  - hepatic artery A52.Ø9
  - hepatis A52.74
  - hepatomegaly, congenital A5Ø.Ø8
  - hereditaria tarda — *see* Syphilis, congenital, late
  - hereditary — *see* Syphilis, congenital
  - Hutchinson's teeth A5Ø.52
  - hyalitis A52.71
  - inactive — *see* Syphilis, latent
  - infantum — *see* Syphilis, congenital
  - inherited — *see* Syphilis, congenital
  - internal ear A52.79
  - intestine (late) A52.74
  - iris, iritis (secondary) A51.43
    - late A52.71
  - joint (late) A52.77
  - keratitis (congenital) (interstitial) (late) A5Ø.31

T

- **Tabacism, tabacosis, tabagism** — *see also* Poisoning, tobacco
  - meaning dependence (without remission) F17.200
    - with
      - disorder F17.299
        - in remission F17.211
        - specified disorder NEC F17.298
        - withdrawal F17.203
- **Tabardillo** A75.9
  - flea-borne A75.2
  - louse-borne A75.0
- **Tabes, tabetic** A52.10
  - with
    - central nervous system syphilis A52.10
    - Charcot's joint A52.16
    - cord bladder A52.19
    - crisis, viscera (any) A52.19
    - paralysis, general A52.17
    - paresis (general) A52.17
    - perforating ulcer (foot) A52.19
  - arthropathy (Charcot) A52.16
  - bladder A52.19
  - bone A52.11
  - cerebrospinal A52.12
  - congenital A50.45
  - conjugal A52.10
  - dorsalis A52.11
    - juvenile A50.49
  - juvenile A50.49
  - latent A52.19
  - mesenterica A18.39
  - paralysis, insane, general A52.17
  - spasmodic A52.17
  - syphilis (cerebrospinal) A52.12
- **Taboparalysis** A52.17
- **Taboparesis** (remission) A52.17
  - juvenile A50.45
- **TAC** (trigeminal autonomic cephalgia) **NEC** G44.099
  - intractable G44.091
  - not intractable G44.099
- **Tache noir** S60.22- ☑
- **Tachyalimentation** K91.2
- **Tachyarrhythmia, tachyrhythmia** — *see* Tachycardia
- **Tachycardia** R00.0
  - atrial (paroxysmal) I47.1
  - auricular I47.1
  - AV nodal re-entry (re-entrant) I47.1
  - junctional (paroxysmal) I47.1
  - newborn P29.11
  - nodal (paroxysmal) I47.1
  - non-paroxysmal AV nodal I45.89
  - paroxysmal (sustained) (nonsustained) I47.9
    - with sinus bradycardia I49.5
    - atrial (PAT) I47.1
    - atrioventricular (AV) (re-entrant) I47.1
      - psychogenic F54
    - junctional I47.1
      - ectopic I47.1
    - nodal I47.1
    - psychogenic (atrial) (supraventricular) (ventricular) F54
    - supraventricular (sustained) I47.1
      - psychogenic F54
    - ventricular I47.20
      - psychogenic F54
      - specified type NEC I47.29
  - psychogenic F45.8
  - sick sinus I49.5
  - sinoauricular NOS R00.0
    - paroxysmal I47.1
  - sinus [sinusal] NOS R00.0
    - paroxysmal I47.1
  - supraventricular I47.1
  - ventricular (paroxysmal) (sustained) I47.20
    - psychogenic F54
    - specified NEC I47.29
- **Tachygastria** K31.89
- **Tachypnea** R06.82
  - hysterical F45.8
  - newborn (idiopathic) (transitory) P22.1
  - psychogenic F45.8
  - transitory, of newborn P22.1
- **TACO** (transfusion associated circulatory overload) E87.71
- **TAD** (transfusion-associated dyspnea) J95.87
- **Taenia** (infection) (infestation) B68.9
- **Taenia** — *continued*
  - diminuta B71.0
  - echinococcal infestation B67.90
  - mediocanellata B68.1
  - nana B71.0
  - saginata B68.1
  - solium (intestinal form) B68.0
    - larval form — *see* Cysticercosis
- **Taeniasis** (intestine) — *see* Taenia
- **Tag** (hypertrophied skin) (infected) L91.8
  - adenoid J35.8
  - anus K64.4
  - hemorrhoidal K64.4
  - hymen N89.8
  - perineal N90.89
  - preauricular Q17.0
  - sentinel K64.4
  - skin L91.8
    - accessory (congenital) Q82.8
    - anus K64.4
    - congenital Q82.8
    - preauricular Q17.0
  - tonsil J35.8
  - urethra, urethral N36.8
  - vulva N90.89
- **Tahyna fever** B33.8
- **Takahara's disease** E80.3
- **Takayasu's disease or syndrome** M31.4
- **Talaromycosis** B48.4
- **Talcosis** (pulmonary) J62.0
- **Talipes** (congenital) Q66.89
  - acquired, planus — *see* Deformity, limb, flat foot
  - asymmetric Q66.89
  - calcaneovalgus Q66.4- ☑
  - calcaneovarus Q66.1- ☑
  - calcaneus Q66.89
  - cavus Q66.7- ☑
  - equinovalgus Q66.6
  - equinovarus Q66.0- ☑
  - equinus Q66.89
  - percavus Q66.7- ☑
  - planovalgus Q66.6
  - planus (acquired) (any degree) — *see also* Deformity, limb, flat foot
    - congenital Q66.5- ☑
    - due to rickets (sequelae) E64.3
  - valgus Q66.6
  - varus Q66.3- ☑
- **Tall stature, constitutional** E34.4
- **Talma's disease** M62.89
- **Talon noir** S90.3- ☑
  - hand S60.22- ☑
  - heel S90.3- ☑
  - toe S90.1- ☑
- **Tamponade, heart** I31.4
- **Tanapox** (virus disease) B08.71
- **Tangier disease** E78.6
- **Tantrum, child problem** F91.8
- **Tapeworm** (infection) (infestation) — *see* Infestation, tapeworm
- **Tapia's syndrome** G52.7
- **TAR** (thrombocytopenia with absent radius) **syndrome** Q87.2
- **Tarral-Besnier disease** L44.0
- **Tarsal tunnel syndrome** — *see* Syndrome, tarsal tunnel
- **Tarsalgia** — *see* Pain, limb, lower
- **Tarsitis** (eyelid) H01.8
  - syphilitic A52.71
  - tuberculous A18.4
- **Tartar** (teeth) (dental calculus) K03.6
- **Tattoo** (mark) L81.8
- **Tauri's disease** E74.09
- **Taurodontism** K00.2
- **Taussig-Bing syndrome** Q20.1
- **Taybi's syndrome** Q87.2
- **Tay-Sachs amaurotic familial idiocy or disease** E75.02
- **TBI** (traumatic brain injury) S06.9 ☑
- **Teacher's node or nodule** J38.2
- **Tear, torn** (traumatic) — *see also* Laceration
  - with abortion — *see* Abortion
  - annular fibrosis M51.35
  - anus, anal (sphincter) S31.831 ☑
    - complicating delivery
      - with third degree perineal laceration — *see also* Delivery, complicated, by, laceration, perineum, third degree O70.20
        - with mucosa O70.3
- **Tear, torn** — *continued*
  - anus, anal — *continued*
    - complicating delivery — *continued*
      - without third degree perineal laceration O70.4
    - nontraumatic (healed) (old) K62.81
  - articular cartilage, old — *see* Derangement, joint, articular cartilage, by site
  - bladder
    - with ectopic or molar pregnancy O08.6
    - following ectopic or molar pregnancy O08.6
    - obstetrical O71.5
    - traumatic — *see* Injury, bladder
  - bowel
    - with ectopic or molar pregnancy O08.6
    - following ectopic or molar pregnancy O08.6
    - obstetrical trauma O71.5
  - broad ligament
    - with ectopic or molar pregnancy O08.6
    - following ectopic or molar pregnancy O08.6
    - obstetrical trauma O71.6
  - bucket handle (knee) (meniscus) — *see* Tear, meniscus
  - capsule, joint — *see* Sprain
  - cartilage — *see also* Sprain
    - articular, old — *see* Derangement, joint, articular cartilage, by site
  - cervix
    - with ectopic or molar pregnancy O08.6
    - following ectopic or molar pregnancy O08.6
    - obstetrical trauma (current) O71.3
    - old N88.1
    - traumatic — *see* Injury, uterus
  - dural G97.41
    - nontraumatic G96.11
  - internal organ — *see* Injury, by site
  - knee cartilage
    - articular (current) S83.3- ☑
    - old — *see* Derangement, knee, meniscus, due to old tear
  - ligament — *see* Sprain
  - meniscus (knee) (current injury) S83.209 ☑
    - bucket-handle S83.20- ☑
    - lateral
      - bucket-handle S83.25- ☑
      - complex S83.27- ☑
      - peripheral S83.26- ☑
      - specified type NEC S83.28- ☑
    - medial
      - bucket-handle S83.21- ☑
      - complex S83.23- ☑
      - peripheral S83.22- ☑
      - specified type NEC S83.24- ☑
    - old — *see* Derangement, knee, meniscus, due to old tear
    - site other than knee — *code as* Sprain
    - specified type NEC S83.20- ☑
  - muscle — *see* Strain
  - pelvic
    - floor, complicating delivery O70.1
    - organ NEC, obstetrical trauma O71.5
      - with ectopic or molar pregnancy O08.6
      - following ectopic or molar pregnancy O08.6
  - perineal, secondary O90.1
  - periurethral tissue, obstetrical trauma O71.82
    - with ectopic or molar pregnancy O08.6
    - following ectopic or molar pregnancy O08.6
  - rectovaginal septum — *see* Laceration, vagina
  - retina, retinal (without detachment) (horseshoe) — *see also* Break, retina, horseshoe
    - with detachment — *see* Detachment, retina, with retinal, break
  - rotator cuff (nontraumatic) M75.10- ☑
    - complete M75.12- ☑
    - incomplete M75.11- ☑
    - traumatic S46.01- ☑
      - capsule S43.42- ☑
  - semilunar cartilage, knee — *see* Tear, meniscus
  - supraspinatus (complete) (incomplete) (nontraumatic) — *see also* Tear, rotator cuff M75.10- ☑
  - tendon — *see* Strain
  - tentorial, at birth P10.4
  - umbilical cord
    - complicating delivery O69.89 ☑
  - urethra
    - with ectopic or molar pregnancy O08.6
    - following ectopic or molar pregnancy O08.6
    - obstetrical trauma O71.5
  - uterus — *see* Injury, uterus

Test, tests, testing — *continued*
- vision Z01.ØØ
  - with abnormal findings Z01.Ø1
  - following failed vision screening Z01.Ø2Ø
    - with abnormal findings Z01.Ø21
  - infant or child (over 28 days old) ZØØ.129
    - with abnormal findings ZØØ.121
- Wassermann Z11.3
  - positive — *see* Serology for syphilis, positive

Testicle, testicular, testis — *see also* condition
- feminization syndrome — *see also* Syndrome, androgen insensitivity E34.51
- migrans Q55.29

Tetanus, tetanic (cephalic) (convulsions) A35
- with
  - abortion A34
  - ectopic or molar pregnancy OØ8.Ø
- following ectopic or molar pregnancy OØ8.Ø
- inoculation reaction (due to serum) — *see* Complications, vaccination
- neonatorum A33
- obstetrical A34
- puerperal, postpartum, childbirth A34

Tetany (due to) R29.Ø
- alkalosis E87.3
- associated with rickets E55.Ø
- convulsions R29.Ø
  - hysterical F44.5
- functional (hysterical) F44.5
- hyperkinetic R29.Ø
  - hysterical F44.5
- hyperpnea RØ6.4
  - hysterical F44.5
  - psychogenic F45.8
- hyperventilation — *see also* Hyperventilation RØ6.4
  - hysterical F44.5
- neonatal (without calcium or magnesium deficiency) P71.3
- parathyroid (gland) E2Ø.9
- parathyroprival E89.2
- post- (para)thyroidectomy E89.2
- postoperative E89.2
- pseudotetany R29.Ø
- psychogenic (conversion reaction) F44.5

Tetralogy of Fallot Q21.3

Tetraplegia (chronic) — *see also* Quadriplegia G82.5Ø

Thailand hemorrhagic fever A91

Thalassanemia — *see* Thalassemia

Thalassemia (anemia) (disease) D56.9
- with other hemoglobinopathy D56.8
- alpha (major) (severe) (triple gene defect) D56.Ø
  - minor D56.3
  - silent carrier D56.3
  - trait D56.3
- beta (severe) D56.1
  - homozygous D56.1
  - major D56.1
  - minor D56.3
  - trait D56.3
- delta-beta (homozygous) D56.2
  - minor D56.3
  - trait D56.3
- dominant D56.8
- hemoglobin
  - C D56.8
  - E-beta D56.5
- intermedia D56.1
- major D56.1
- minor D56.3
- mixed D56.8
- sickle-cell — *see* Disease, sickle-cell, thalassemia
- specified type NEC D56.8
- trait D56.3
- variants D56.8

Thanatophoric dwarfism or short stature Q77.1

Thaysen-Gee disease (nontropical sprue) K9Ø.Ø

Thaysen's disease K9Ø.Ø

Thecoma D27- ☑
- luteinized D27- ☑
- malignant C56- ☑

Thelarche, premature E3Ø.8

Thelaziasis B83.8

Thelitis N61.Ø
- puerperal, postpartum or gestational — *see* Infection, nipple

Therapeutic — *see* condition

Therapy
- drug, long-term (current) (prophylactic)
  - agents affecting estrogen receptors and estrogen levels NEC Z79.818
  - anastrozole (Arimidex) Z79.811
  - antibiotics Z79.2
    - short-term use — *omit code*
  - anticoagulants Z79.Ø1
  - anti-inflammatory Z79.1
  - antiplatelet Z79.Ø2
  - antithrombotics Z79.Ø2
  - aromatase inhibitors Z79.811
  - aspirin Z79.82
  - birth control pill or patch Z79.3
  - bisphosphonates Z79.83
  - contraceptive, oral Z79.3
  - drug, specified NEC Z79.899
  - estrogen receptor downregulators Z79.818
  - Evista Z79.81Ø
  - exemestane (Aromasin) Z79.811
  - Fareston Z79.81Ø
  - fulvestrant (Faslodex) Z79.818
  - gonadotropin-releasing hormone (GnRH) agonist Z79.818
  - goserelin acetate (Zoladex) Z79.818
  - hormone replacement Z79.89Ø
  - insulin Z79.4
  - letrozole (Femara) Z79.811
  - leuprolide acetate (leuprorelin) (Lupron) Z79.818
  - megestrol acetate (Megace) Z79.818
  - methadone
    - for pain management Z79.891
    - maintenance therapy F11.2Ø
  - Nolvadex Z79.81Ø
  - opiate analgesic Z79.891
  - oral contraceptive Z79.3
  - raloxifene (Evista) Z79.81Ø
  - selective estrogen receptor modulators (SERMs) Z79.81Ø
  - short term — *omit code*
  - steroids
    - inhaled Z79.51
    - systemic Z79.52
  - tamoxifen (Nolvadex) Z79.81Ø
  - toremifene (Fareston) Z79.81Ø

Thermic — *see* condition

Thermography (abnormal) — *see also* Abnormal, diagnostic imaging R93.89
- breast R92.8

Thermoplegia T67.Ø1 ☑

Thesaurismosis, glycogen — *see* Disease, glycogen storage

Thiamin deficiency E51.9
- specified NEC E51.8

Thiaminic deficiency with beriberi E51.11

Thibierge-Weissenbach syndrome — *see* Sclerosis, systemic

Thickening
- bone — *see* Hypertrophy, bone
- breast N64.59
- endometrium R93.89
- epidermal L85.9
  - specified NEC L85.8
- hymen N89.6
- larynx J38.7
- nail L6Ø.2
  - congenital Q84.5
- periosteal — *see* Hypertrophy, bone
- pleura J92.9
  - with asbestos J92.Ø
- skin R23.4
- subepiglottic J38.7
- tongue K14.8
- valve, heart — *see* Endocarditis

Thigh — *see* condition

Thinning vertebra — *see* Spondylopathy, specified NEC

Thirst, excessive R63.1
- due to deprivation of water T73.1 ☑

Thomsen disease G71.12

Thoracic — *see also* condition
- kidney Q63.2
- outlet syndrome G54.Ø

Thoracogastroschisis (congenital) Q79.8

Thoracopagus Q89.4

Thorax — *see* condition

Thorn's syndrome N28.89

Thorson-Björck syndrome E34.Ø

Threadworm (infection) (infestation) B8Ø

Threatened
- abortion O2Ø.Ø
  - with subsequent abortion OØ3.9
- job loss, anxiety concerning Z56.2
- labor (without delivery) O47.9
  - at or after 37 completed weeks of gestation O47.1
  - before 37 completed weeks of gestation O47.Ø- ☑
- loss of job, anxiety concerning Z56.2
- miscarriage O2Ø.Ø
- unemployment, anxiety concerning Z56.2

Three-day fever A93.1

Threshers' lung J67.Ø

Thrix annulata (congenital) Q84.1

Throat — *see* condition

Thrombasthenia (Glanzmann) (hemorrhagic) (hereditary) D69.1

Thromboangiitis I73.1
- obliterans (general) I73.1
  - cerebral I67.89
  - vessels
    - brain I67.89
    - spinal cord I67.89

Thromboarteritis — *see* Arteritis

Thromboasthenia (Glanzmann) (hemorrhagic) (hereditary) D69.1

Thrombocytasthenia (Glanzmann) D69.1

Thrombocythemia (hemorrhagic) *see also* Thrombocytosis D75.839
- essential D47.3
- idiopathic D47.3
- primary D47.3

Thrombocytopathy (dystrophic) (granulopenic) D69.1

Thrombocytopenia, thrombocytopenic D69.6
- with absent radius (TAR) Q87.2
- congenital D69.42
- dilutional D69.59
- due to
  - (massive) blood transfusion D69.59
  - drugs D69.59
  - extracorporeal circulation of blood D69.59
  - platelet alloimmunization D69.59
- essential D69.3
- heparin induced (HIT) D75.829
  - delayed-onset D75.828
  - immune-mediated D75.822
  - non-immune D75.821
  - persisting D75.828
  - syndrome
    - autoimmune D75.828
    - specified NEC D75.828
    - spontaneous (without heparin exposure) D75.84
  - type 1 D75.821
  - type 2 D75.822
- heparin-associated D75.821
- hereditary D69.42
- idiopathic D69.3
- neonatal, transitory P61.Ø
  - due to
    - exchange transfusion P61.Ø
    - idiopathic maternal thrombocytopenia P61.Ø
    - isoimmunization P61.Ø
- primary NEC D69.49
  - idiopathic D69.3
- puerperal, postpartum O72.3
- secondary D69.59
- transient neonatal P61.Ø
- vaccine-induced thrombotic D75.84

Thrombocytosis D75.839
- essential D47.3
- idiopathic D47.3
- primary D47.3
- reactive D75.838
- secondary D75.838
- specified NEC D75.838

Thromboembolism — *see* Embolism

Thrombopathy (Bernard-Soulier) D69.1
- constitutional — *see* Disease, von Willebrand
- Willebrand-Jurgens — *see* Disease, von Willebrand

Thrombopenia — *see* Thrombocytopenia

Thrombophilia D68.59
- primary NEC D68.59
- secondary NEC D68.69
- specified NEC D68.69

Thrombophlebitis I8Ø.9
- antepartum O22.2- ☑
  - deep O22.3- ☑
  - superficial O22.2- ☑
- calf muscular vein (NOS) I8Ø.25- ☑

Thrombosis, thrombotic — *continued*
- vas deferens N5Ø.1
- vein (acute) I82.9Ø
  - antecubital I82.61- ☑
    - chronic I82.71- ☑
  - axillary I82.A1- ☑ (*following* I82.7)
    - chronic I82.A2- ☑ (*following* I82.7)
  - basilic I82.61- ☑
    - chronic I82.71- ☑
  - brachial I82.62- ☑
    - chronic I82.72- ☑
  - brachiocephalic (innominate) I82.29Ø
    - chronic I82.291
  - cephalic I82.61- ☑
    - chronic I82.71- ☑
  - cerebral, nonpyogenic I67.6
  - chronic I82.91
  - deep (DVT) I82.4Ø- ☑
    - calf I82.4Z- ☑
      - chronic I82.5Z- ☑
    - lower leg I82.4Z- ☑
      - chronic I82.5Z- ☑
    - thigh I82.4Y- ☑
      - chronic I82.5Y- ☑
    - upper leg I82.4Y- ☑
      - chronic I82.5Y- ☑
  - femoral I82.41- ☑
    - chronic I82.51- ☑
  - iliac (iliofemoral) I82.42- ☑
    - chronic I82.52- ☑
  - innominate I82.29Ø
    - chronic I82.291
  - internal jugular I82.C1- ☑ (*following* I82.7)
    - chronic I82.C2- ☑ (*following* I82.7)
  - lower extremity
    - deep I82.4Ø- ☑
      - chronic I82.5Ø- ☑
      - specified NEC I82.49- ☑
        - chronic NEC I82.59- ☑
    - distal
      - deep I82.4Z- ☑
    - proximal
      - deep I82.4Y- ☑
        - chronic I82.5Y- ☑
    - superficial I82.81- ☑
  - perianal K64.5
  - popliteal I82.43- ☑
    - chronic I82.53- ☑
  - radial I82.62- ☑
    - chronic I82.72- ☑
  - renal I82.3
  - saphenous (greater) (lesser) I82.81- ☑
  - specified NEC I82.89Ø
    - chronic NEC I82.891
  - subclavian I82.B1- ☑ (*following* I82.7)
    - chronic I82.B2- ☑ (*following* I82.7)
  - thoracic NEC I82.29Ø
    - chronic I82.291
  - tibial I82.44- ☑
    - chronic I82.54- ☑
  - ulnar I82.62- ☑
    - chronic I82.72- ☑
  - upper extremity I82.6Ø- ☑
    - chronic I82.7Ø- ☑
    - deep I82.62- ☑
      - chronic I82.72- ☑
    - superficial I82.61- ☑
      - chronic I82.71- ☑
  - vena cava
    - inferior I82.22Ø
      - chronic I82.221
    - superior I82.21Ø
      - chronic I82.211
- venous, perianal K64.5
- ventricle — *see also* Infarct, myocardium
  - following acute myocardial infarction (current complication) I23.6
  - not resulting in infarction I24.Ø
  - old I51.3

Thrombus — *see* Thrombosis

Thrush — *see also* Candidiasis
- newborn P37.5
- oral B37.Ø
- vaginal (acute) B37.31
  - chronic (recurrent) B37.32

Thumb — *see also* condition
- sucking (child problem) F98.8

Thymitis E32.8

Thymoma — *see also* Neoplasm, thymus, by type
- malignant C37
- metaplastic C37
- microscopic D15.Ø
- sclerosing C37
- type A C37
- type AB C37
- type B1 C37
- type B2 C37
- type B3 C37

Thymus, thymic (gland) — *see* condition

Thyrocele — *see* Goiter

Thyroglossal — *see also* condition
- cyst Q89.2
- duct, persistent Q89.2

Thyroid (gland) (body) — *see also* condition
- hormone resistance EØ7.89
- lingual Q89.2
- nodule (cystic) (nontoxic) (single) EØ4.1

Thyroiditis EØ6.9
- acute (nonsuppurative) (pyogenic) (suppurative) EØ6.Ø
- autoimmune EØ6.3
- chronic (nonspecific) (sclerosing) EØ6.5
  - with thyrotoxicosis, transient EØ6.2
  - fibrous EØ6.5
  - lymphadenoid EØ6.3
  - lymphocytic EØ6.3
  - lymphoid EØ6.3
- de Quervain's EØ6.1
- drug-induced EØ6.4
- fibrous (chronic) EØ6.5
- giant-cell (follicular) EØ6.1
- granulomatous (de Quervain) (subacute) EØ6.1
- Hashimoto's (struma lymphomatosa) EØ6.3
- iatrogenic EØ6.4
- ligneous EØ6.5
- lymphocytic (chronic) EØ6.3
- lymphoid EØ6.3
- lymphomatous EØ6.3
- nonsuppurative EØ6.1
- postpartum, puerperal O9Ø.5
- pseudotuberculous EØ6.1
- pyogenic EØ6.Ø
- radiation EØ6.4
- Riedel's EØ6.5
- subacute (granulomatous) EØ6.1
- suppurative EØ6.Ø
- tuberculous A18.81
- viral EØ6.1
- woody EØ6.5

Thyrolingual duct, persistent Q89.2

Thyromegaly EØ1.Ø

Thyrotoxic
- crisis — *see* Thyrotoxicosis
- heart disease or failure — *see also* Thyrotoxicosis EØ5.9Ø *[I43]*
  - with thyroid storm EØ5.91 *[I43]*
- storm — *see* Thyrotoxicosis

Thyrotoxicosis (recurrent) EØ5.9Ø
- with
  - goiter (diffuse) EØ5.ØØ
    - with thyroid storm EØ5.Ø1
    - adenomatous uninodular EØ5.1Ø
      - with thyroid storm EØ5.11
    - multinodular EØ5.2Ø
      - with thyroid storm EØ5.21
    - nodular EØ5.2Ø
      - with thyroid storm EØ5.21
    - uninodular EØ5.1Ø
      - with thyroid storm EØ5.11
  - infiltrative
    - dermopathy EØ5.ØØ
      - with thyroid storm EØ5.Ø1
    - ophthalmopathy EØ5.ØØ
      - with thyroid storm EØ5.Ø1
  - single thyroid nodule EØ5.1Ø
    - with thyroid storm EØ5.11
  - thyroid storm EØ5.91
- due to
  - ectopic thyroid nodule or tissue EØ5.3Ø
    - with thyroid storm EØ5.31
  - ingestion of (excessive) thyroid material EØ5.4Ø
    - with thyroid storm EØ5.41
  - overproduction of thyroid-stimulating hormone EØ5.8Ø
    - with thyroid storm EØ5.81
  - specified cause NEC EØ5.8Ø

Thyrotoxicosis — *continued*
- due to — *continued*
  - specified cause — *continued*
    - with thyroid storm EØ5.81
- factitia EØ5.4Ø
  - with thyroid storm EØ5.41
- heart — *see also* Failure, heart, high-output EØ5.9Ø *[I43]*
  - with thyroid storm — *see also* Failure, heart, high-output EØ5.91 *[I43]*
  - failure — *see also* Failure, heart, high-output EØ5.9Ø *[I43]*
- neonatal (transient) P72.1
- transient with chronic thyroiditis EØ6.2

Tibia vara M92.51- ☑

Tic (disorder) F95.9
- breathing F95.8
- child problem F95.Ø
- compulsive F95.1
- de la Tourette F95.2
- degenerative (generalized) (localized) G25.69
  - facial G25.69
- disorder
  - chronic
    - motor F95.1
    - vocal F95.1
  - combined vocal and multiple motor F95.2
  - transient F95.Ø
- douloureux G5Ø.Ø
  - atypical G5Ø.1
  - postherpetic, postzoster BØ2.22
- drug-induced G25.61
- eyelid F95.8
- habit F95.9
  - chronic F95.1
  - transient of childhood F95.Ø
- lid, transient of childhood F95.Ø
- motor-verbal F95.2
- occupational F48.8
- orbicularis F95.8
  - transient of childhood F95.Ø
- organic origin G25.69
- postchoreic G25.69
- provisional F95.Ø
- psychogenic, compulsive F95.1
- salaam R25.8
- spasm (motor or vocal) F95.9
  - chronic F95.1
  - transient of childhood F95.Ø
- specified NEC F95.8

Tick-borne — *see* condition

Tietze's disease or syndrome M94.Ø

Tight, tightness
- anus K62.89
- chest RØ7.89
- fascia (lata) M62.89
- foreskin (congenital) N47.1
- hymen, hymenal ring N89.6
- introitus (acquired) (congenital) N89.6
- rectal sphincter K62.89
- tendon — *see* Short, tendon
- urethral sphincter N35.919

Tilting vertebra — *see* Dorsopathy, deforming, specified NEC

Timidity, child F93.8

Tinea (intersecta) (tarsi) B35.9
- amiantacea L44.8
- asbestina B35.Ø
- barbae B35.Ø
- beard B35.Ø
- black dot B35.Ø
- blanca B36.2
- capitis B35.Ø
- corporis B35.4
- cruris B35.6
- flava B36.Ø
- foot B35.3
- furfuracea B36.Ø
- imbricata (Tokelau) B35.5
- kerion B35.Ø
- manuum B35.2
- microsporic — *see* Dermatophytosis
- nigra B36.1
- nodosa — *see* Piedra
- pedis B35.3
- scalp B35.Ø
- specified NEC B35.8
- sycosis B35.Ø
- tonsurans B35.Ø

- **Tracheomalacia** — *continued*
  - congenital Q32.Ø
- **Tracheopharyngitis** (acute) JØ6.9
  - chronic J42
  - due to external agent — *see* Inflammation, respiratory, upper, due to
- **Tracheostenosis** J39.8
- **Tracheostomy**
  - complication — *see* Complication, tracheostomy
  - status Z93.Ø
    - attention to Z43.Ø
    - malfunctioning J95.Ø3
- **Trachoma, trachomatous** A71.9
  - active (stage) A71.1
  - contraction of conjunctiva A71.1
  - dubium A71.Ø
  - healed or sequelae B94.Ø
  - initial (stage) A71.Ø
  - pannus A71.1
  - Türck's J37.Ø
- **Traction, vitreomacular** H43.82- ☑
- **Train sickness** T75.3 ☑
- **Trait**(s)
  - Hb-S D57.3
  - hemoglobin
    - abnormal NEC D58.2
      - with thalassemia D56.3
    - C — *see* Disease, hemoglobin C
    - S (Hb-S) D57.3
  - Lepore D56.3
  - personality, accentuated Z73.1
  - sickle-cell D57.3
    - with elliptocytosis or spherocytosis D57.3
  - type A personality Z73.1
- **Tramp** Z59.ØØ
- **Trance** R41.89
  - hysterical F44.89
- **Transaminasemia** R74.Ø1
- **Transection**
  - abdomen (partial) S38.3 ☑
  - aorta (incomplete) — *see also* Injury, aorta
    - complete — *see* Injury, aorta, laceration, major
  - carotid artery (incomplete) — *see also* Injury, blood vessel, carotid, laceration
    - complete — *see* Injury, blood vessel, carotid, laceration, major
  - celiac artery (incomplete) S35.211 ☑
    - branch (incomplete) S35.291 ☑
      - complete S35.292 ☑
    - complete S35.212 ☑
  - innominate
    - artery (incomplete) — *see also* Injury, blood vessel, thoracic, innominate, artery, laceration
      - complete — *see* Injury, blood vessel, thoracic, innominate, artery, laceration, major
    - vein (incomplete) — *see also* Injury, blood vessel, thoracic, innominate, vein, laceration
      - complete — *see* Injury, blood vessel, thoracic, innominate, vein, laceration, major
  - jugular vein (external) (incomplete) — *see also* Injury, blood vessel, jugular vein, laceration
    - complete — *see* Injury, blood vessel, jugular vein, laceration, major
    - internal (incomplete) — *see also* Injury, blood vessel, jugular vein, internal, laceration
      - complete — *see* Injury, blood vessel, jugular vein, internal, laceration, major
  - mesenteric artery (incomplete) — *see also* Injury, mesenteric, artery, laceration
    - complete — *see* Injury, mesenteric artery, laceration, major
  - pulmonary vessel (incomplete) — *see also* Injury, blood vessel, thoracic, pulmonary, laceration
    - complete — *see* Injury, blood vessel, thoracic, pulmonary, laceration, major
  - subclavian — *see* Transection, innominate
  - vena cava (incomplete) — *see also* Injury, vena cava
    - complete — *see* Injury, vena cava, laceration, major
  - vertebral artery (incomplete) — *see also* Injury, blood vessel, vertebral, laceration
    - complete — *see* Injury, blood vessel, vertebral, laceration, major
- **Transfusion**
  - associated (red blood cell) hemochromatosis E83.111
  - blood
    - ABO incompatible — *see* Complication(s), transfusion, incompatibility reaction, ABO
- **Transfusion** — *continued*
  - blood — *continued*
    - minor blood group (Duffy) (E) (K) (Kell) (Kidd) (Lewis) (M) (N) (P) (S) T8Ø.89 ☑
    - reaction or complication — *see* Complications, transfusion
  - fetomaternal (mother) — *see* Pregnancy, complicated by, placenta, transfusion syndrome
  - maternofetal (mother) — *see* Pregnancy, complicated by, placenta, transfusion syndrome
  - placental (syndrome) (mother) — *see* Pregnancy, complicated by, placenta, transfusion syndrome
  - reaction (adverse) — *see* Complications, transfusion
  - related acute lung injury (TRALI) J95.84
  - twin-to-twin — *see* Pregnancy, complicated by, placenta, transfusion syndrome, fetus to fetus
- **Transient** (meaning homeless) — *see also* condition Z59.ØØ
- **Translocation**
  - balanced autosomal Q95.9
    - in normal individual Q95.Ø
  - chromosomes NEC Q99.8
    - balanced and insertion in normal individual Q95.Ø
  - Down syndrome Q9Ø.2
  - trisomy
    - 13 Q91.6
    - 18 Q91.2
    - 21 Q9Ø.2
- **Translucency, iris** — *see* Degeneration, iris
- **Transmission of chemical substances through the placenta** — *see* Absorption, chemical, through placenta
- **Transparency, lung, unilateral** J43.Ø
- **Transplant** (ed) (status) Z94.9
  - awaiting organ Z76.82
  - bone Z94.6
    - marrow Z94.81
  - candidate Z76.82
  - complication — *see* Complication, transplant
  - cornea Z94.7
  - heart Z94.1
    - and lung(s) Z94.3
    - valve Z95.2
      - prosthetic Z95.2
      - specified NEC Z95.4
      - xenogenic Z95.3
  - intestine Z94.82
  - kidney Z94.Ø
  - liver Z94.4
  - lung(s) Z94.2
    - and heart Z94.3
  - organ (failure) (infection) (rejection) Z94.9
    - removal status Z98.85
  - pancreas Z94.83
  - skin Z94.5
  - social Z6Ø.3
  - specified organ or tissue NEC Z94.89
  - stem cells Z94.84
  - tissue Z94.9
- **Transplants, ovarian, endometrial** N8Ø.1Ø- ☑
- **Transposed** — *see* Transposition
- **Transposition** (congenital) — *see also* Malposition, congenital
  - abdominal viscera Q89.3
  - aorta (dextra) Q2Ø.3
  - appendix Q43.8
  - colon Q43.8
  - corrected Q2Ø.5
  - great vessels (complete) (partial) Q2Ø.3
  - heart Q24.Ø
    - with complete transposition of viscera Q89.3
  - intestine (large) (small) Q43.8
  - reversed jejunal (for bypass) (status) Z98.Ø
  - scrotum Q55.23
  - stomach Q4Ø.2
    - with general transposition of viscera Q89.3
  - tooth, teeth, fully erupted M26.3Ø
  - vessels, great (complete) (partial) Q2Ø.3
  - viscera (abdominal) (thoracic) Q89.3
- **Transsexualism** F64.Ø
- **Transverse** — *see also* condition
  - arrest (deep), in labor O64.Ø ☑
  - lie (mother) O32.2 ☑
    - causing obstructed labor O64.8 ☑
- **Transvestism, transvestitism** (dual-role) F64.1
  - fetishistic F65.1
- **Trapped placenta** (with hemorrhage) O72.Ø
  - without hemorrhage O73.Ø
- **TRAPS** (tumor necrosis factor receptor associated periodic syndrome) MØ4.1
- **Trauma, traumatism** — *see also* Injury
  - acoustic — *see* subcategory H83.3 ☑
  - birth — *see* Birth, injury
  - complicating ectopic or molar pregnancy OØ8.6
  - during delivery O71.9
  - following ectopic or molar pregnancy OØ8.6
  - obstetric O71.9
    - specified NEC O71.89
  - occusal
    - primary KØ8.81
    - secondary KØ8.82
- **Traumatic** — *see also* condition
  - brain injury SØ6.9 ☑
- **Treacher Collins syndrome** Q75.4
- **Treitz's hernia** — *see* Hernia, abdomen, specified site NEC
- **Trematode infestation** — *see* Infestation, fluke
- **Trematodiasis** — *see* Infestation, fluke
- **Trembling paralysis** — *see* Parkinsonism
- **Tremor(s)** R25.1
  - drug induced G25.1
  - essential (benign) G25.Ø
  - familial G25.Ø
  - hereditary G25.Ø
  - hysterical F44.4
  - intention G25.2
  - medication induced postural G25.1
  - mercurial — *see* subcategory T56.1 ☑
  - Parkinson's — *see* Parkinsonism
  - psychogenic (conversion reaction) F44.4
  - senilis R54
  - specified type NEC G25.2
- **Trench**
  - fever A79.Ø
  - foot — *see* Immersion, foot
  - mouth A69.1
- **Treponema pallidum infection** — *see* Syphilis
- **Treponematosis**
  - due to
    - T. pallidum — *see* Syphilis
    - T. pertenue — *see* Yaws
- **Triad**
  - Hutchinson's (congenital syphilis) A5Ø.53
  - Kartagener's Q89.3
  - Saint's — *see* Hernia, diaphragm
- **Trichiasis** (eyelid) HØ2.Ø59
  - with entropion — *see* Entropion
  - left HØ2.Ø56
    - lower HØ2.Ø55
    - upper HØ2.Ø54
  - right HØ2.Ø53
    - lower HØ2.Ø52
    - upper HØ2.Ø51
- **Trichinella spiralis** (infection) (infestation) B75
- **Trichinellosis, trichiniasis, trichinelliasis, trichinosis** B75
  - with muscle disorder B75 *[M63.8Ø]*
    - ankle B75 *[M63.87-]* ☑
    - foot B75 *[M63.87-]* ☑
    - forearm B75 *[M63.83-]* ☑
    - hand B75 *[M63.84-]* ☑
    - lower leg B75 *[M63.86-]* ☑
    - multiple sites B75 *[M63.89]*
    - pelvic region B75 *[M63.85-]* ☑
    - shoulder region B75 *[M63.81-]* ☑
    - specified site NEC B75 *[M63.88]*
    - thigh B75 *[M63.85-]* ☑
    - upper arm B75 *[M63.82-]* ☑
- **Trichobezoar** T18.9 ☑
  - intestine T18.3 ☑
  - stomach T18.2 ☑
- **Trichocephaliasis, trichocephalosis** B79
- **Trichocephalus infestation** B79
- **Trichoclasis** L67.8
- **Trichoepithelioma** — *see also* Neoplasm, skin, benign
  - malignant — *see* Neoplasm, skin, malignant
- **Trichofolliculoma** — *see* Neoplasm, skin, benign
- **Tricholemmoma** — *see* Neoplasm, skin, benign
- **Trichomoniasis** A59.9
  - bladder A59.Ø3
  - cervix A59.Ø9
  - intestinal AØ7.8
  - prostate A59.Ø2
  - seminal vesicles A59.Ø9
  - specified site NEC A59.8

U

- **Ulcer, ulcerated, ulcerating, ulceration, ulcerative** — *continued*
  - pressure — *continued*
    - elbow L89.Ø- ☑
    - face L89.81- ☑
    - head L89.81- ☑
    - heel L89.6- ☑
    - hip L89.2- ☑
    - sacral region (tailbone) L89.15- ☑
    - specified site NEC L89.89- ☑
    - stage 1 (healing) (pre-ulcer skin changes limited to persistent focal edema)
      - ankle L89.5- ☑
      - back L89.1- ☑
      - buttock L89.3- ☑
      - coccyx L89.15- ☑
      - contiguous site of back, buttock, hip L89.4- ☑
      - elbow L89.Ø- ☑
      - face L89.81- ☑
      - head L89.81- ☑
      - heel L89.6- ☑
      - hip L89.2- ☑
      - sacral region (tailbone) L89.15- ☑
      - specified site NEC L89.89- ☑
    - stage 2 (healing) (abrasion, blister, partial thickness skin loss involving epidermis and/or dermis)
      - ankle L89.5- ☑
      - back L89.1- ☑
      - buttock L89.3- ☑
      - coccyx L89.15- ☑
      - contiguous site of back, buttock, hip L89.4- ☑
      - elbow L89.Ø- ☑
      - face L89.81- ☑
      - head L89.81- ☑
      - heel L89.6- ☑
      - hip L89.2- ☑
      - sacral region (tailbone) L89.15- ☑
      - specified site NEC L89.89- ☑
    - stage 3 (healing) (full thickness skin loss involving damage or necrosis of subcutaneous tissue)
      - ankle L89.5- ☑
      - back L89.1- ☑
      - buttock L89.3- ☑
      - coccyx L89.15- ☑
      - contiguous site of back, buttock, hip L89.4- ☑
      - elbow L89.Ø- ☑
      - face L89.81- ☑
      - head L89.81- ☑
      - heel L89.6- ☑
      - hip L89.2- ☑
      - sacral region (tailbone) L89.15- ☑
      - specified site NEC L89.89- ☑
    - stage 4 (healing) (necrosis of soft tissues through to underlying muscle, tendon, or bone)
      - ankle L89.5- ☑
      - back L89.1- ☑
      - buttock L89.3- ☑
      - coccyx L89.15- ☑
      - contiguous site of back, buttock, hip L89.4- ☑
      - elbow L89.Ø- ☑
      - face L89.81- ☑
      - head L89.81- ☑
      - heel L89.6- ☑
      - hip L89.2- ☑
      - sacral region (tailbone) L89.15- ☑
      - specified site NEC L89.89- ☑
    - unspecified stage
      - ankle L89.5- ☑
      - back L89.1- ☑
      - buttock L89.3- ☑
      - coccyx L89.15- ☑
      - contiguous site of back, buttock, hip L89.4- ☑
      - elbow L89.Ø- ☑
      - face L89.81- ☑
      - head L89.81- ☑
      - heel L89.6- ☑
      - hip L89.2- ☑
      - sacral region (tailbone) L89.15- ☑
      - specified site NEC L89.89- ☑
    - unstageable
      - ankle L89.5- ☑
      - back L89.1- ☑
      - buttock L89.3- ☑
      - coccyx L89.15- ☑
      - contiguous site of back, buttock, hip L89.4- ☑
      - elbow L89.Ø- ☑

- **Ulcer, ulcerated, ulcerating, ulceration, ulcerative** — *continued*
  - pressure — *continued*
    - unstageable — *continued*
      - face L89.81- ☑
      - head L89.81- ☑
      - heel L89.6- ☑
      - hip L89.2- ☑
      - sacral region (tailbone) L89.15- ☑
      - specified site NEC L89.89- ☑
  - primary of intestine K63.3
    - with perforation K63.1
  - prostate N41.9
  - pyloric — *see* Ulcer, stomach
  - rectosigmoid K63.3
    - with perforation K63.1
  - rectum (sphincter) (solitary) K62.6
    - stercoraceous, stercoral K62.6
  - retina — *see* Inflammation, chorioretinal
  - rodent — *see also* Neoplasm, skin, malignant
  - sclera — *see* Scleritis
  - scrofulous (tuberculous) A18.2
  - scrotum N5Ø.89
    - tuberculous A18.15
    - varicose I86.1
  - seminal vesicle N5Ø.89
  - sigmoid — *see* Ulcer, intestine
  - skin (atrophic) (chronic) (neurogenic) (non-healing) (perforating) (pyogenic) (trophic) (tropical) L98.499
    - with gangrene — *see* Gangrene
    - amebic AØ6.7
    - back — *see* Ulcer, back
    - buttock — *see* Ulcer, buttock
    - decubitus — *see* Ulcer, pressure
    - lower limb — *see* Ulcer, lower limb
    - mycobacterial A31.1
    - specified site NEC L98.499
      - with
        - bone involvement without evidence of necrosis L98.496
        - bone necrosis L98.494
        - exposed fat layer L98.492
        - muscle involvement without evidence of necrosis L98.495
        - muscle necrosis L98.493
        - skin breakdown only L98.491
        - specified severity NEC L98.498
    - tuberculous (primary) A18.4
    - varicose — *see* Ulcer, varicose
  - sloughing — *see* Ulcer, skin
  - solitary, anus or rectum (sphincter) K62.6
  - sore throat JØ2.9
    - streptococcal JØ2.Ø
  - spermatic cord N5Ø.89
  - spine (tuberculous) A18.Ø1
  - stasis (venous) — *see* Varix, leg, with, ulcer
    - without varicose veins I87.2
  - stercoraceous, stercoral K63.3
    - with perforation K63.1
    - anus or rectum K62.6
  - stoma, stomal — *see* Ulcer, gastrojejunal
  - stomach (eroded) (peptic) (round) K25.9
    - with
      - hemorrhage K25.4
        - and perforation K25.6
      - perforation K25.5
    - acute K25.3
      - with
        - hemorrhage K25.Ø
          - and perforation K25.2
        - perforation K25.1
    - chronic K25.7
      - with
        - hemorrhage K25.4
          - and perforation K25.6
        - perforation K25.5
  - stomal — *see* Ulcer, gastrojejunal
  - stomatitis K12.1
  - stress — *see* Ulcer, peptic
  - strumous (tuberculous) A18.2
  - submucosal, bladder — *see* Cystitis, interstitial
  - syphilitic (any site) (early) (secondary) A51.39
    - late A52.79
    - perforating A52.79
      - foot A52.11
  - testis N5Ø.89
  - thigh — *see* Ulcer, lower limb

- **Ulcer, ulcerated, ulcerating, ulceration, ulcerative** — *continued*
  - throat J39.2
    - diphtheritic A36.Ø
  - toe — *see* Ulcer, lower limb
  - tongue (traumatic) K14.Ø
  - tonsil J35.8
    - diphtheritic A36.Ø
  - trachea J39.8
  - trophic — *see* Ulcer, skin
  - tropical — *see* Ulcer, skin
  - tuberculous — *see* Tuberculosis, ulcer
  - tunica vaginalis N5Ø.89
  - turbinate J34.89
  - typhoid (perforating) — *see* Typhoid
  - unspecified site — *see* Ulcer, skin
  - urethra (meatus) — *see* Urethritis
  - uterus N85.8
    - cervix N86
      - with cervicitis N72
    - neck N86
      - with cervicitis N72
  - vagina N76.5
    - in Behçet's disease M35.2 *[N77.Ø]*
    - pessary N89.8
  - valve, heart I33.Ø
  - varicose (lower limb, any part) — *see also* Varix, leg, with, ulcer
    - broad ligament I86.2
    - esophagus — *see* Varix, esophagus
    - inflamed or infected — *see* Varix, leg, with ulcer, with inflammation
    - nasal septum I86.8
    - perineum I86.3
    - scrotum I86.1
    - specified site NEC I86.8
    - sublingual I86.Ø
    - vulva I86.3
  - vas deferens N5Ø.89
  - vulva (acute) (infectional) N76.6
    - in (due to)
      - Behçet's disease M35.2 *[N77.Ø]*
      - herpesviral (herpes simplex) infection A6Ø.Ø4
      - tuberculosis A18.18
  - vulvobuccal, recurring N76.6
  - X-ray L58.1
  - yaws A66.4
- **Ulcerosa scarlatina** A38.8
- **Ulcus** — *see also* Ulcer
  - cutis tuberculosum A18.4
  - duodeni — *see* Ulcer, duodenum
  - durum (syphilitic) A51.Ø
    - extragenital A51.2
  - gastrojejunale — *see* Ulcer, gastrojejunal
  - hypostaticum — *see* Ulcer, varicose
  - molle (cutis) (skin) A57
  - serpens corneae — *see* Ulcer, cornea, central
  - ventriculi — *see* Ulcer, stomach
- **Ulegyria** QØ4.8
- **Ulerythema**
  - ophryogenes, congenital Q84.2
  - sycosiforme L73.8
- **Ullrich** (-Bonnevie) (-Turner) **syndrome** — *see also* Turner's syndrome Q87.19
- **Ullrich-Feichtiger syndrome** Q87.Ø
- **Ulnar** — *see* condition
- **Ulorrhagia, ulorrhea** KØ6.8
- **Umbilicus, umbilical** — *see* condition
- **Unable to**
  - make ends meet Z59.86
  - obtain
    - adequate
      - childcare Z59.87
      - clothing Z59.87
      - utilities Z59.87
    - basic needs Z59.87
- **Unacceptable**
  - contours of tooth KØ8.54
  - morphology of tooth KØ8.54
- **Unaffordable transportation** Z59.82
- **Unavailability** (of)
  - bed at medical facility Z75.1
  - health service-related agencies Z75.4
  - medical facilities (at) Z75.3
    - due to
      - investigation by social service agency Z75.2
      - lack of services at home Z75.Ø
      - remoteness from facility Z75.3

- **Vasculitis** — *continued*
  - disseminated I77.6
  - hypocomplementemic M31.8
  - kidney I77.89
  - leukocytoclastic M31.Ø
  - livedoid L95.Ø
  - nodular L95.8
  - retina H35.Ø6- ☑
  - rheumatic — *see* Fever, rheumatic
  - rheumatoid — *see* Rheumatoid, vasculitis
  - skin (limited to) L95.9
    - specified NEC L95.8
  - systemic M31.8
- **Vasculopathy, necrotizing** M31.9
  - cardiac allograft T86.29Ø
  - specified NEC M31.8
- **Vasitis** (nodosa) N49.1
  - tuberculous A18.15
- **Vasodilation** I73.9
- **Vasomotor** — *see* condition
- **Vasoplasty, after previous sterilization** Z31.Ø
  - aftercare Z31.42
- **Vasospasm** (vasoconstriction) I73.9
  - cerebral (cerebrovascular) (artery) I67.848
    - reversible I67.841
  - coronary I2Ø.1
  - nerve
    - arm — *see* Mononeuropathy, upper limb
    - brachial plexus G54.Ø
    - cervical plexus G54.2
    - leg — *see* Mononeuropathy, lower limb
  - peripheral NOS I73.9
  - retina (artery) — *see* Occlusion, artery, retina
- **Vasospastic** — *see* condition
- **Vasovagal attack** (paroxysmal) R55
  - psychogenic F45.8
- **VATER syndrome** Q87.2
- **Vater's ampulla** — *see* condition
- **Vegetation, vegetative**
  - adenoid (nasal fossa) J35.8
  - endocarditis (acute) (any valve) (subacute) I33.Ø
  - heart (mycotic) (valve) I33.Ø
- **Veil**
  - Jackson's Q43.3
- **Vein, venous** — *see* condition
- **Veldt sore** — *see* Ulcer, skin
- **Velpeau's hernia** — *see* Hernia, femoral
- **Venereal**
  - bubo A55
  - disease A64
  - granuloma inguinale A58
  - lymphogranuloma (Durand-Nicolas-Favre) A55
- **Venofibrosis** I87.8
- **Venom, venomous** — *see* Table of Drugs and Chemicals, by animal or substance, poisoning
- **Venous** — *see* condition
- **Ventilator lung, newborn** P27.8
- **Ventral** — *see* condition
- **Ventricle, ventricular** — *see also* condition
  - escape I49.3
  - inversion Q2Ø.5
- **Ventriculitis** (cerebral) — *see also* Encephalitis GØ4.9Ø
- **Ventriculostomy status** Z98.2
- **Vernet's syndrome** G52.7
- **Verneuil's disease** (syphilitic bursitis) A52.78
- **Verruca** (due to HPV) (filiformis) (simplex) (viral) (vulgaris) BØ7.9
  - acuminata A63.Ø
  - necrogenica (primary) (tuberculosa) A18.4
  - plana BØ7.8
  - plantaris BØ7.Ø
  - seborrheica L82.1
    - inflamed L82.Ø
  - senile (seborrheic) L82.1
    - inflamed L82.Ø
  - tuberculosa (primary) A18.4
  - venereal A63.Ø
- **Verrucosities** — *see* Verruca
- **Verruga peruana, peruviana** A44.1
- **Version**
  - cervix — *see* Malposition, uterus
  - uterus (postinfectional) (postpartal, old) — *see* Malposition, uterus
- **Vertebra, vertebral** — *see* condition
- **Vertical talus** (congenital) Q66.8Ø
  - left foot Q66.82
  - right foot Q66.81
- **Vertigo** R42
  - auditory — *see* Vertigo, aural
  - aural H81.31- ☑
  - benign paroxysmal (positional) H81.1- ☑
  - central (origin) H81.4
  - cerebral H81.4
  - Dix and Hallpike (epidemic) — *see* Neuronitis, vestibular
  - due to infrasound T75.23 ☑
  - epidemic A88.1
    - Dix and Hallpike — *see* Neuronitis, vestibular
    - Pedersen's — *see* Neuronitis, vestibular
    - vestibular neuronitis — *see* Neuronitis, vestibular
  - hysterical F44.89
  - infrasound T75.23 ☑
  - labyrinthine — *see* subcategory H81.Ø ☑
  - laryngeal RØ5.4
  - malignant positional H81.4
  - Ménière's — *see* subcategory H81.Ø ☑
  - menopausal N95.1
  - otogenic — *see* Vertigo, aural
  - paroxysmal positional, benign — *see* Vertigo, benign paroxysmal
  - Pedersen's (epidemic) — *see* Neuronitis, vestibular
  - peripheral NEC H81.39- ☑
  - positional
    - benign paroxysmal — *see* Vertigo, benign paroxysmal
    - malignant H81.4
- **Very-low-density-lipoprotein-type** (VLDL) **hyperlipoproteinemia** E78.1
- **Vesania** — *see* Psychosis
- **Vesical** — *see* condition
- **Vesicle**
  - cutaneous R23.8
  - seminal — *see* condition
  - skin R23.8
- **Vesicocolic** — *see* condition
- **Vesicoperineal** — *see* condition
- **Vesicorectal** — *see* condition
- **Vesicourethrorectal** — *see* condition
- **Vesicovaginal** — *see* condition
- **Vesicular** — *see* condition
- **Vesiculitis** (seminal) N49.Ø
  - amebic AØ6.82
  - gonorrheal (acute) (chronic) A54.23
  - trichomonal A59.Ø9
  - tuberculous A18.15
- **Vestibulitis** (ear) — *see also* subcategory H83.Ø ☑
  - nose (external) J34.89
  - vulvar N94.81Ø
- **Vestibulopathy , acute peripheral** (recurrent) — *see* Neuronitis, vestibular
- **Vestige, vestigial** — *see also* Persistence
  - branchial Q18.Ø
  - structures in vitreous Q14.Ø
- **Vibration**
  - adverse effects T75.2Ø ☑
    - pneumatic hammer syndrome T75.21 ☑
    - specified effect NEC T75.29 ☑
    - vasospastic syndrome T75.22 ☑
    - vertigo from infrasound T75.23 ☑
  - exposure (occupational) Z57.7
  - vertigo T75.23 ☑
- **Vibriosis** A28.9
- **Victim** (of)
  - crime Z65.4
  - disaster Z65.5
  - terrorism Z65.4
  - torture Z65.4
  - war Z65.5
- **Vidal's disease** L28.Ø
- **Villaret's syndrome** G52.7
- **Villous** — *see* condition
- **VIN** — *see* Neoplasia, intraepithelial, vulva
- **Vincent's infection** (angina) (gingivitis) A69.1
  - stomatitis NEC A69.1
- **Vinson-Plummer syndrome** D5Ø.1
- **Violence, physical** R45.6
- **Viosterol deficiency** — *see* Deficiency, calciferol
- **Vipoma** — *see* Neoplasm, malignant, by site
- **Viremia** B34.9
- **Virilism** (adrenal) E25.9
  - congenital E25.Ø
- **Virilization** (female) (suprarenal) E25.9
  - congenital E25.Ø
  - isosexual E28.2
- **Virulent bubo** A57
- **Virus, viral** — *see also* condition
  - as cause of disease classified elsewhere B97.89
    - respiratory syncytial virus (RSV) — *see* Virus, respiratory syncytial (RSV)
  - cytomegalovirus B25.9
  - human immunodeficiency (HIV) — *see* Human, immunodeficiency virus (HIV) disease
  - infection — *see* Infection, virus
  - respiratory syncytial (RSV)
    - as cause of disease classified elsewhere B97.4
    - bronchiolitis J21.Ø
    - bronchitis J2Ø.5
    - bronchopneumonia J12.1
    - otitis media H65.- ☑ *[B97.4]*
    - pneumonia J12.1
    - upper respiratory infection JØ6.9 *[B97.4]*
  - specified NEC B34.8
  - swine influenza (viruses that normally cause infections in pigs) — *see also* Influenza, due to, identified novel influenza A virus JØ9.X2
  - West Nile (fever) A92.3Ø
    - with
      - complications NEC A92.39
      - cranial nerve disorders A92.32
      - encephalitis A92.31
      - encephalomyelitis A92.31
      - neurologic manifestation NEC A92.32
      - optic neuritis A92.32
      - polyradiculitis A92.32
- **Viscera, visceral** — *see* condition
- **Visceroptosis** K63.4
- **Visible peristalsis** R19.2
- **Vision, visual**
  - binocular, suppression H53.34
  - blurred, blurring H53.8
    - hysterical F44.6
  - defect, defective NEC H54.7
  - disorientation (syndrome) H53.8
  - disturbance H53.9
    - hysterical F44.6
  - double H53.2
  - examination ZØ1.ØØ
    - with abnormal findings ZØ1.Ø1
    - following failed vision screening ZØ1.Ø2Ø
      - with abnormal findings ZØ1.Ø21
  - field, limitation (defect) — *see* Defect, visual field
  - hallucinations R44.1
  - halos H53.19
  - loss — *see* Loss, vision
    - sudden — *see* Disturbance, vision, subjective, loss, sudden
  - low (both eyes) — *see* Low, vision
  - perception, simultaneous without fusion H53.33
- **Vitality, lack or want of** R53.83
  - newborn P96.89
- **Vitamin deficiency** — *see* Deficiency, vitamin
- **Vitelline duct, persistent** Q43.Ø
- **Vitiligo** L8Ø
  - eyelid HØ2.739
    - left HØ2.736
      - lower HØ2.735
      - upper HØ2.734
    - right HØ2.733
      - lower HØ2.732
      - upper HØ2.731
  - pinta A67.2
  - vulva N9Ø.89
- **Vitreal corneal syndrome** H59.Ø1- ☑
- **Vitreoretinopathy, proliferative** — *see also* Retinopathy, proliferative
  - with retinal detachment — *see* Detachment, retina, traction
- **Vitreous** — *see also* condition
  - touch syndrome — *see* Complication, postprocedural, following cataract surgery
- **Vocal cord** — *see* condition
- **Vogt-Koyanagi syndrome** H2Ø.82- ☑
- **Vogt's disease or syndrome** G8Ø.3
- **Vogt-Spielmeyer amaurotic idiocy or disease** E75.4
- **Voice**
  - change R49.9
    - specified NEC R49.8
  - loss — *see* Aphonia
- **Volhynian fever** A79.Ø
- **Volkmann's ischemic contracture or paralysis** (complicating trauma) T79.6 ☑
- **Volvulus** (bowel) (colon) (intestine) K56.2

Volvulus — *continued*
- with perforation K56.2
- congenital Q43.8
- duodenum K31.5
- fallopian tube — *see* Torsion, fallopian tube
- oviduct — *see* Torsion, fallopian tube
- stomach (due to absence of gastrocolic ligament) K31.89

Vomiting R11.10
- with nausea R11.2
- asphyxia — *see* Foreign body, by site, causing asphyxia, gastric contents
- bilious (cause unknown) R11.14
  - following gastro-intestinal surgery K91.0
  - in newborn P92.01
- blood — *see* Hematemesis
- causing asphyxia, choking, or suffocation — *see* Foreign body, by site
- cyclical, in migraine G43.A0 (*following* G43.7)
  - with refractory migraine G43.A1 (*following* G43.7)
  - intractable G43.A1 (*following* G43.7)
  - not intractable G43.A0 (*following* G43.7)
  - psychogenic F50.89
  - without refractory migraine G43.A0 (*following* G43.7)
- cyclical syndrome NOS (unrelated to migraine) R11.15
- fecal mater R11.13
- following gastrointestinal surgery K91.0
  - psychogenic F50.89
- functional K31.89
- hysterical F50.89
- nervous F50.89
- neurotic F50.89
- newborn NEC P92.09
  - bilious P92.01
- periodic R11.10
  - psychogenic F50.89
- persistent R11.15
- projectile R11.12
- psychogenic F50.89
- uremic — *see* Uremia
- without nausea R11.11

Vomito negro — *see* Fever, yellow
Von Bezold's abscess — *see* Mastoiditis, acute
Von Economo-Cruchet disease A85.8
Von Eulenburg's disease G71.19
Von Gierke's disease E74.01
Von Hippel (-Lindau) **disease or syndrome** Q85.83
Von Jaksch's anemia or disease D64.89
Von Recklinghausen
- disease (neurofibromatosis) Q85.01
  - bones E21.0

Von Schroetter's syndrome I82.890
Von Willebrand (-Jurgens) (-Minot) **disease or syndrome** — *see* Disease, von Willebrand
Von Zumbusch's disease L40.1
Voyeurism F65.3
Vrolik's disease Q78.0
Vulva — *see* condition
Vulvismus N94.2
Vulvitis (acute) (allergic) (atrophic) (hypertrophic) (intertriginous) (senile) N76.2
- with ectopic or molar pregnancy O08.0
- adhesive, congenital Q52.79
- blennorrhagic (gonococcal) A54.02
- candidal (acute) B37.31
  - chronic (recurrent) B37.32
- chlamydial A56.02
- due to Haemophilus ducreyi A57
- following ectopic or molar pregnancy O08.0
- gonococcal A54.02
  - with abscess (accessory gland) (periurethral) A54.1
- herpesviral A60.04
- leukoplakic N90.4
- monilial (acute) B37.31
  - chronic (recurrent) B37.32
- puerperal (postpartum) O86.19
- subacute or chronic N76.3
- syphilitic (early) A51.0
  - late A52.76
- trichomonal A59.01
- tuberculous A18.18

Vulvodynia N94.819
- specified NEC N94.818

Vulvorectal — *see* condition
Vulvovaginitis (acute) — *see* Vaginitis

W

Waiting list, person on Z75.1
- for organ transplant Z76.82
- undergoing social agency investigation Z75.2

Waldenström
- hypergammaglobulinemia D89.0
- syndrome or macroglobulinemia C88.0

Waldenström-Kjellberg syndrome D50.1
Walking
- difficulty R26.2
  - psychogenic F44.4
- sleep F51.3
  - hysterical F44.89

Wall, abdominal — *see* condition
Wallenberg's disease or syndrome G46.3
Wallgren's disease I87.8
Wandering
- gallbladder, congenital Q44.1
- in diseases classified elsewhere Z91.83
- kidney, congenital Q63.8
- organ or site, congenital NEC — *see* Malposition, congenital, by site
- pacemaker (heart) I49.8
- spleen D73.89

War neurosis F48.8
Wart (due to HPV) (filiform) (infectious) (viral) B07.9
- anogenital region (venereal) A63.0
- common B07.8
- external genital organs (venereal) A63.0
- flat B07.8
- Hassal-Henle's (of cornea) H18.49
- Peruvian A44.1
- plantar B07.0
- prosector (tuberculous) A18.4
- seborrheic L82.1
  - inflamed L82.0
- senile (seborrheic) L82.1
  - inflamed L82.0
- tuberculous A18.4
- venereal A63.0

Warthin's tumor — *see* Neoplasm, salivary gland, benign
Wassilieff's disease A27.0
Wasting
- disease R64
  - due to malnutrition E43
    - with marasmus E41
- extreme (due to malnutrition) E43
  - with marasmus E41
- muscle NEC — *see* Atrophy, muscle

Water
- clefts (senile cataract) — *see* Cataract, senile, incipient
- deprivation of T73.1 ☑
- intoxication E87.79
- itch B76.9
- lack of T73.1 ☑
  - safe drinking Z58.6
- loading E87.70
- on
  - brain — *see* Hydrocephalus
  - chest J94.8
- poisoning E87.79

Waterbrash R12
Waterhouse (-Friderichsen) **syndrome or disease** (meningococcal) A39.1
Water-losing nephritis N25.89
Watermelon stomach K31.819
- with hemorrhage K31.811
- without hemorrhage K31.819

Watsoniasis B66.8
Wax in ear — *see* Impaction, cerumen
Weak, weakening, weakness (generalized) R53.1
- arches (acquired) — *see also* Deformity, limb, flat foot
- bladder (sphincter) R32
- facial R29.810
  - following
    - cerebrovascular disease I69.992
      - cerebral infarction I69.392
      - intracerebral hemorrhage I69.192
      - nontraumatic intracranial hemorrhage NEC I69.292
      - specified disease NEC I69.892
      - stroke I69.392
      - subarachnoid hemorrhage I69.092
- foot (double) — *see also* Weak, arches
- heart, cardiac — *see* Failure, heart
- mind F70

Weak, weakening, weakness — *continued*
- muscle M62.81
- myocardium — *see* Failure, heart
- newborn P96.89
- pelvic fundus N81.89
- pubocervical tissue N81.82
- rectovaginal tissue N81.83
- senile R54
- urinary stream R39.12
- valvular — *see* Endocarditis

Wear, worn (with normal or routine use)
- articular bearing surface of internal joint prosthesis — *see* Complications, joint prosthesis, mechanical, wear of articular bearing surfaces, by site
- device, implant or graft — *see* Complications, by site, mechanical complication
- tooth, teeth (approximal) (hard tissues) (interproximal) (occlusal) K03.0

Weather, weathered
- effects of
  - cold T69.9 ☑
    - specified effect NEC T69.8 ☑
  - hot — *see* Heat
- skin L57.8

Weaver's syndrome Q87.3
Web, webbed (congenital)
- duodenal Q43.8
- esophagus Q39.4
- fingers Q70.1- ☑
- larynx (glottic) (subglottic) Q31.0
- neck (pterygium colli) Q18.3
- Paterson-Kelly D50.1
- popliteal syndrome Q87.89
- toes Q70.3- ☑

Weber-Christian disease M35.6
Weber-Cockayne syndrome (epidermolysis bullosa) Q81.8
Weber-Gubler syndrome G46.3
Weber-Leyden syndrome G46.3
Weber-Osler syndrome I78.0
Weber's paralysis or syndrome G46.3
Wedge-shaped or wedging vertebra — *see* Collapse, vertebra NEC
Wegener's granulomatosis or syndrome M31.30
- with
  - kidney involvement M31.31
  - lung involvement M31.30
    - with kidney involvement M31.31

Wegner's disease A50.02
Weight
- 1000-2499 grams at birth (low) — *see* Low, birthweight
- 999 grams or less at birth (extremely low) — *see* Low, birthweight, extreme
- and length below 10th percentile for gestational age P05.1- ☑
- below but length above 10th percentile for gestational age P05.0- ☑
- gain (abnormal) (excessive) R63.5
  - in pregnancy — *see* Pregnancy, complicated by, excessive weight gain
    - low — *see* Pregnancy, complicated by, insufficient, weight gain
- loss (abnormal) (cause unknown) R63.4

Weightlessness (effect of) T75.82 ☑
Weil (l)-Marchesani syndrome Q87.19
Weil's disease A27.0
Weingarten's syndrome J82.89
Weir Mitchell's disease I73.81
Weiss-Baker syndrome G90.09
Wells' disease L98.3
Wen — *see* Cyst, sebaceous
Wenckebach's block or phenomenon I44.1
Werdnig-Hoffmann syndrome (muscular atrophy) G12.0
Werlhof's disease D69.3
Wermer's disease or syndrome E31.21
Werner-His disease A79.0
Werner's disease or syndrome E34.8
Wernicke-Korsakoff's syndrome or psychosis (alcoholic) F10.96
- with dependence F10.26
- drug-induced
  - due to drug abuse — *see* Abuse, drug, by type, with amnestic disorder
  - due to drug dependence — *see* Dependence, drug, by type, with amnestic disorder
- nonalcoholic F04

- **Wernicke-Posadas disease** B38.9
- **Wernicke's**
  - developmental aphasia F8Ø.2
  - disease or syndrome E51.2
  - encephalopathy E51.2
  - polioencephalitis, superior E51.2
- **West African fever** B5Ø.8
- **Westphal-Strümpell syndrome** E83.Ø1
- **West's syndrome** — *see* Epilepsy, spasms
- **Wet**
  - feet, tropical (maceration) (syndrome) — *see* Immersion, foot
  - lung (syndrome), newborn P22.1
- **Wharton's duct** — *see* condition
- **Wheal** — *see* Urticaria
- **Wheezing** RØ6.2
- **Whiplash injury** S13.4 ☑
- **Whipple's disease** — *see also* subcategory M14.8- K9Ø.81
- **Whipworm** (disease) (infection) (infestation) B79
- **Whistling face** Q87.Ø
- **White** — *see also* condition
  - kidney, small NØ3.9
  - leg, puerperal, postpartum, childbirth O87.1
  - mouth B37.Ø
  - patches of mouth K13.29
  - spot lesions, teeth
    - chewing surface KØ2.51
    - pit and fissure surface KØ2.51
    - smooth surface KØ2.61
- **Whitehead** L7Ø.Ø
- **Whitlow** — *see also* Cellulitis, digit
  - with lymphangitis — *see* Lymphangitis, acute, digit
  - herpesviral BØØ.89
- **Whitmore's disease or fever** — *see* Melioidosis
- **Whooping cough** A37.9Ø
  - with pneumonia A37.91
    - due to Bordetella
      - bronchiseptica A37.81
      - parapertussis A37.11
      - pertussis A37.Ø1
    - specified organism NEC A37.81
  - due to
    - Bordetella
      - bronchiseptica A37.8Ø
        - with pneumonia A37.81
      - parapertussis A37.1Ø
        - with pneumonia A37.11
      - pertussis A37.ØØ
        - with pneumonia A37.Ø1
    - specified NEC A37.8Ø
      - with pneumonia A37.81
- **Wichman's asthma** J38.5
- **Wide cranial sutures, newborn** P96.3
- **Widening aorta** — *see* Ectasia, aorta
  - with aneurysm — *see* Aneurysm, aorta
- **Wilkie's disease or syndrome** K55.1
- **Wilkinson-Sneddon disease or syndrome** L13.1
- **Willebrand** (-Jürgens) **thrombopathy** — *see* Disease, von Willebrand
- **Williams syndrome** Q93.82
- **Willige-Hunt disease or syndrome** G23.1
- **Wilms' tumor** C64- ☑
- **Wilson-Mikity syndrome** P27.Ø
- **Wilson's**
  - disease or syndrome E83.Ø1
  - hepatolenticular degeneration E83.Ø1
  - lichen ruber L43.9
- **Window** — *see also* Imperfect, closure
  - aorticopulmonary Q21.4
- **Winter** — *see* condition
- **Wiskott-Aldrich syndrome** D82.Ø
- **Withdrawal state** — *see also* Dependence, drug by type, with withdrawal
  - alcohol
    - with perceptual disturbances F1Ø.232
      - due to alcohol abuse F1Ø.132
      - due to alcohol use F1Ø.932
    - abuse — *see* Abuse, alcohol, with, withdrawal
    - dependence — *see* Dependence, alcohol, with, withdrawal
    - use — *see* Use, alcohol, with, withdrawal
    - without perceptual disturbances F1Ø.239
      - due to alcohol abuse F1Ø.139
      - due to alcohol use F1Ø.939
  - caffeine F15.93
  - cannabis F12.23
- **Withdrawal state** — *continued*
  - newborn
    - correct therapeutic substance properly administered P96.2
    - infant of dependent mother P96.1
  - therapeutic substance, neonatal P96.2
- **Witts' anemia** D5Ø.8
- **Witzelsucht** FØ7.Ø
- **Woakes' ethmoiditis or syndrome** J33.1
- **Wolff-Hirschorn syndrome** Q93.3
- **Wolff-Parkinson-White syndrome** I45.6
- **Wolhynian fever** A79.Ø
- **Wolman's disease** E75.5
- **Wood lung or pneumonitis** J67.8
- **Woolly, wooly hair** (congenital) (nevus) Q84.1
- **Woolsorter's disease** A22.1
- **Word**
  - blindness (congenital) (developmental) F81.Ø
  - deafness (congenital) (developmental) H93.25
- **Worm(s)** (infection) (infestation) — *see also* Infestation, helminth
  - guinea B72
  - in intestine NEC B82.Ø
- **Worm-eaten soles** A66.3
- **Worn out** — *see* Exhaustion
  - cardiac
    - defibrillator (with synchronous cardiac pacemaker) Z45.Ø2
    - pacemaker
      - battery Z45.Ø1Ø
      - lead Z45.Ø18
  - device, implant or graft — *see* Complications, by site, mechanical
- **Worried well** Z71.1
- **Worries** R45.82
- **Wound check** Z48.Ø- ☑
  - due to injury — *code to* Injury, by site, using appropriate seventh character for subsequent encounter
- **Wound, open** T14.8- ☑
  - abdomen, abdominal
    - wall S31.1Ø9 ☑
      - with penetration into peritoneal cavity S31.6Ø9 ☑
      - bite — *see* Bite, abdomen, wall
      - epigastric region S31.1Ø2 ☑
        - with penetration into peritoneal cavity S31.6Ø2 ☑
        - bite — *see* Bite, abdomen, wall, epigastric region
        - laceration — *see* Laceration, abdomen, wall, epigastric region
        - puncture — *see* Puncture, abdomen, wall, epigastric region
      - laceration — *see* Laceration, abdomen, wall
      - left
        - lower quadrant S31.1Ø4 ☑
          - with penetration into peritoneal cavity S31.6Ø4 ☑
          - bite — *see* Bite, abdomen, wall, left, lower quadrant
          - laceration — *see* Laceration, abdomen, wall, left, lower quadrant
          - puncture — *see* Puncture, abdomen, wall, left, lower quadrant
        - upper quadrant S31.1Ø1 ☑
          - with penetration into peritoneal cavity S31.6Ø1 ☑
          - bite — *see* Bite, abdomen, wall, left, upper quadrant
          - laceration — *see* Laceration, abdomen, wall, left, upper quadrant
          - puncture — *see* Puncture, abdomen, wall, left, upper quadrant
      - periumbilic region S31.1Ø5 ☑
        - with penetration into peritoneal cavity S31.6Ø5 ☑
        - bite — *see* Bite, abdomen, wall, periumbilic region
        - laceration — *see* Laceration, abdomen, wall, periumbilic region
        - puncture — *see* Puncture, abdomen, wall, periumbilic region
      - puncture — *see* Puncture, abdomen, wall
      - right
        - lower quadrant S31.1Ø3 ☑
          - with penetration into peritoneal cavity S31.6Ø3 ☑
- **Wound, open** — *continued*
  - abdomen, abdominal — *continued*
    - wall — *continued*
      - right — *continued*
        - lower quadrant — *continued*
          - bite — *see* Bite, abdomen, wall, right, lower quadrant
          - laceration — *see* Laceration, abdomen, wall, right, lower quadrant
          - puncture — *see* Puncture, abdomen, wall, right, lower quadrant
        - upper quadrant S31.1ØØ ☑
          - with penetration into peritoneal cavity S31.6ØØ ☑
          - bite — *see* Bite, abdomen, wall, right, upper quadrant
          - laceration — *see* Laceration, abdomen, wall, right, upper quadrant
          - puncture — *see* Puncture, abdomen, wall, right, upper quadrant
  - alveolar (process) — *see* Wound, open, oral cavity
  - ankle S91.ØØ- ☑
    - bite — *see* Bite, ankle
    - laceration — *see* Laceration, ankle
    - puncture — *see* Puncture, ankle
  - antecubital space — *see* Wound, open, elbow
  - anterior chamber, eye — *see* Wound, open, ocular
  - anus S31.839 ☑
    - bite S31.835 ☑
    - laceration — *see* Laceration, anus
    - puncture — *see* Puncture, anus
  - arm (upper) S41.1Ø- ☑
    - with amputation — *see* Amputation, traumatic, arm
    - bite — *see* Bite, arm
    - forearm — *see* Wound, open, forearm
    - laceration — *see* Laceration, arm
    - puncture — *see* Puncture, arm
  - auditory canal (external) (meatus) — *see* Wound, open, ear
  - auricle, ear — *see* Wound, open, ear
  - axilla — *see* Wound, open, arm
  - back — *see also* Wound, open, thorax, back
    - lower S31.ØØØ ☑
      - with penetration into retroperitoneal space S31.ØØ1 ☑
      - bite — *see* Bite, back, lower
      - laceration — *see* Laceration, back, lower
      - puncture — *see* Puncture, back, lower
  - bite — *see* Bite
  - blood vessel — *see* Injury, blood vessel
  - breast S21.ØØ- ☑
    - with amputation — *see* Amputation, traumatic, breast
    - bite — *see* Bite, breast
    - laceration — *see* Laceration, breast
    - puncture — *see* Puncture, breast
  - buttock S31.8Ø9 ☑
    - bite — *see* Bite, buttock
    - laceration — *see* Laceration, buttock
    - left S31.829 ☑
    - puncture — *see* Puncture, buttock
    - right S31.819 ☑
  - calf — *see* Wound, open, leg
  - canaliculus lacrimalis — *see* Wound, open, eyelid
  - canthus, eye — *see* Wound, open, eyelid
  - cervical esophagus S11.2Ø ☑
    - bite S11.25 ☑
    - laceration — *see* Laceration, esophagus, traumatic, cervical
    - puncture — *see* Puncture, cervical esophagus
  - cheek (external) SØ1.4Ø- ☑
    - bite — *see* Bite, cheek
    - internal — *see* Wound, open, oral cavity
    - laceration — *see* Laceration, cheek
    - puncture — *see* Puncture, cheek
  - chest wall — *see* Wound, open, thorax
  - chin — *see* Wound, open, head, specified site NEC
  - choroid — *see* Wound, open, ocular
  - ciliary body (eye) — *see* Wound, open, ocular
  - clitoris S31.4Ø ☑
    - with amputation — *see* Amputation, traumatic, clitoris
    - bite S31.45 ☑
    - laceration — *see* Laceration, vulva
    - puncture — *see* Puncture, vulva
  - conjunctiva — *see* Wound, open, ocular

- **Wound, open** — *continued*
  - ocular — *continued*
    - orbit (penetrating) (with or without foreign body) SØ5.4- ☑
    - periocular area — *see* Wound, open, eyelid
    - specified NEC SØ5.8X- ☑
  - oral cavity SØ1.5Ø2 ☑
    - bite SØ1.552 ☑
    - laceration — *see* Laceration, oral cavity
    - puncture — *see* Puncture, oral cavity
  - orbit — *see* Wound, open, ocular, orbit
  - palate — *see* Wound, open, oral cavity
  - palm — *see* Wound, open, hand
  - pelvis, pelvic — *see also* Wound, open, back, lower
    - girdle — *see* Wound, open, hip
  - penetrating — *see* Puncture, by site
  - penis S31.2Ø ☑
    - with amputation — *see* Amputation, traumatic, penis
    - bite S31.25 ☑
    - laceration — *see* Laceration, penis
    - puncture — *see* Puncture, penis
  - perineum
    - bite — *see* Bite, perineum
    - female S31.5Ø2 ☑
    - laceration — *see* Laceration, perineum
    - male S31.5Ø1 ☑
    - puncture — *see* Puncture, perineum
  - periocular area (with or without lacrimal passages) — *see* Wound, open, eyelid
  - periumbilic region S31.1Ø5 ☑
    - with penetration into peritoneal cavity S31.6Ø5 ☑
    - bite — *see* Bite, abdomen, wall, periumbilic region
    - laceration — *see* Laceration, abdomen, wall, periumbilic region
    - puncture — *see* Puncture, abdomen, wall, periumbilic region
  - phalanges
    - finger — *see* Wound, open, finger
    - toe — *see* Wound, open, toe
  - pharynx S11.2Ø ☑
  - pinna — *see* Wound, open, ear
  - popliteal space — *see* Wound, open, knee
  - prepuce — *see* Wound, open, penis
  - pubic region — *see* Wound, open, back, lower
  - pudendum — *see* Wound, open, genital organs, external
  - puncture wound — *see* Puncture
  - rectovaginal septum — *see* Wound, open, vagina
  - right
    - lower quadrant S31.1Ø3 ☑
      - with penetration into peritoneal cavity S31.6Ø3 ☑
      - bite — *see* Bite, abdomen, wall, right, lower quadrant
      - laceration — *see* Laceration, abdomen, wall, right, lower quadrant
      - puncture — *see* Puncture, abdomen, wall, right, lower quadrant
    - upper quadrant S31.1ØØ ☑
      - with penetration into peritoneal cavity S31.6ØØ ☑
      - bite — *see* Bite, abdomen, wall, right, upper quadrant
      - laceration — *see* Laceration, abdomen, wall, right, upper quadrant
      - puncture — *see* Puncture, abdomen, wall, right, upper quadrant
  - sacral region — *see* Wound, open, back, lower
  - sacroiliac region — *see* Wound, open, back, lower
  - salivary gland — *see* Wound, open, oral cavity
  - scalp SØ1.ØØ ☑
    - bite SØ1.Ø5 ☑
    - laceration — *see* Laceration, scalp
    - puncture — *see* Puncture, scalp
  - scalpel, newborn (birth injury) P15.8
  - scapular region — *see* Wound, open, shoulder
  - sclera — *see* Wound, open, ocular
  - scrotum S31.3Ø ☑
    - with amputation — *see* Amputation, traumatic, scrotum
    - bite S31.35 ☑
    - laceration — *see* Laceration, scrotum
    - puncture — *see* Puncture, scrotum
  - shin — *see* Wound, open, leg
  - shoulder S41.ØØ- ☑

- **Wound, open** — *continued*
  - shoulder — *continued*
    - with amputation — *see* Amputation, traumatic, arm
    - bite — *see* Bite, shoulder
    - laceration — *see* Laceration, shoulder
    - puncture — *see* Puncture, shoulder
  - skin NOS T14.8 ☑
  - spermatic cord — *see* Wound, open, testis
  - sternal region — *see* Wound, open, thorax, front wall
  - submaxillary region — *see* Wound, open, head, specified site NEC
  - submental region — *see* Wound, open, head, specified site NEC
  - subungual
    - finger(s) — *see* Wound, open, finger
    - toe(s) — *see* Wound, open, toe
  - supraclavicular region — *see* Wound, open, neck, specified site NEC
  - temple, temporal region — *see* Wound, open, head, specified site NEC
  - temporomandibular area — *see* Wound, open, cheek
  - testis S31.3Ø ☑
    - with amputation — *see* Amputation, traumatic, testes
    - bite S31.35 ☑
    - laceration — *see* Laceration, testis
    - puncture — *see* Puncture, testis
  - thigh S71.1Ø- ☑
    - with amputation — *see* Amputation, traumatic, hip
    - bite — *see* Bite, thigh
    - laceration — *see* Laceration, thigh
    - puncture — *see* Puncture, thigh
  - thorax, thoracic (wall) S21.9Ø ☑
    - back S21.2Ø- ☑
      - with penetration S21.4Ø ☑
    - bite — *see* Bite, thorax
    - breast — *see* Wound, open, breast
    - front S21.1Ø- ☑
      - with penetration S21.3Ø ☑
    - laceration — *see* Laceration, thorax
    - puncture — *see* Puncture, thorax
  - throat — *see* Wound, open, neck
  - thumb S61.ØØ9 ☑
    - with
      - amputation — *see* Amputation, traumatic, thumb
      - damage to nail S61.1Ø9 ☑
    - bite — *see* Bite, thumb
    - laceration — *see* Laceration, thumb
    - left S61.ØØ2 ☑
      - with
        - damage to nail S61.1Ø2 ☑
    - puncture — *see* Puncture, thumb
    - right S61.ØØ1 ☑
      - with
        - damage to nail S61.1Ø1 ☑
  - thyroid (gland) — *see* Wound, open, neck, thyroid
  - toe(s) S91.1Ø9 ☑
    - with
      - amputation — *see* Amputation, traumatic, toe
      - damage to nail S91.2Ø9 ☑
    - bite — *see* Bite, toe
    - great S91.1Ø3 ☑
      - with
        - damage to nail S91.2Ø3 ☑
      - left S91.1Ø2 ☑
        - with
          - damage to nail S91.2Ø2 ☑
      - right S91.1Ø1 ☑
        - with
          - damage to nail S91.2Ø1 ☑
    - laceration — *see* Laceration, toe
    - lesser S91.1Ø6 ☑
      - with
        - damage to nail S91.2Ø6 ☑
      - left S91.1Ø5 ☑
        - with
          - damage to nail S91.2Ø5 ☑
      - right S91.1Ø4 ☑
        - with
          - damage to nail S91.2Ø4 ☑
    - puncture — *see* Puncture, toe
  - tongue — *see* Wound, open, oral cavity
  - trachea (cervical region) — *see* Wound, open, neck, trachea
  - tunica vaginalis — *see* Wound, open, testis

- **Wound, open** — *continued*
  - tympanum, tympanic membrane SØ9.2- ☑
    - laceration — *see* Laceration, ear, drum
    - puncture — *see* Puncture, tympanum
  - umbilical region — *see* Wound, open, abdomen, wall, periumbilic region
  - uvula — *see* Wound, open, oral cavity
  - vagina S31.4Ø ☑
    - bite S31.45 ☑
    - laceration — *see* Laceration, vagina
    - puncture — *see* Puncture, vagina
  - vitreous (humor) — *see* Wound, open, ocular
  - vocal cord S11.Ø39 ☑
    - bite — *see* Bite, vocal cord
    - laceration S11.Ø31 ☑
      - with foreign body S11.Ø32 ☑
    - puncture S11.Ø33 ☑
      - with foreign body S11.Ø34 ☑
  - vulva S31.4Ø ☑
    - with amputation — *see* Amputation, traumatic, vulva
    - bite S31.45 ☑
    - laceration — *see* Laceration, vulva
    - puncture — *see* Puncture, vulva
  - wrist S61.5Ø- ☑
    - bite — *see* Bite, wrist
    - laceration — *see* Laceration, wrist
    - puncture — *see* Puncture, wrist
- **Wound, superficial** — *see* Injury — *see also* specified injury type
- **Wright's syndrome** G54.Ø
- **Wrist** — *see* condition
- **Wrong drug** (by accident) (given in error) — *see* Table of Drugs and Chemicals, by drug, poisoning
- **Wry neck** — *see* Torticollis
- **Wuchereria** (bancrofti) **infestation** B74.Ø
- **Wuchereriasis** B74.Ø
- **Wucherende Struma Langhans** C73

X

- **Xanthelasma** (eyelid) (palpebrarum) HØ2.6Ø
  - left HØ2.66
    - lower HØ2.65
    - upper HØ2.64
  - right HØ2.63
    - lower HØ2.62
    - upper HØ2.61
- **Xanthelasmatosis** (essential) E78.2
- **Xanthinuria, hereditary** E79.8
- **Xanthoastrocytoma**
  - specified site — *see* Neoplasm, malignant, by site
  - unspecified site C71.9
- **Xanthofibroma** — *see* Neoplasm, connective tissue, benign
- **Xanthogranuloma** D76.3
- **Xanthoma(s), xanthomatosis** (primary) (familial) (hereditary) E75.5
  - with
    - hyperlipoproteinemia
      - Type I E78.3
      - Type III E78.2
      - Type IV E78.1
      - Type V E78.3
  - bone (generalisata) C96.5
  - cerebrotendinous E75.5
  - cutaneotendinous E75.5
  - disseminatum (skin) E78.2
  - eruptive E78.2
  - hypercholesterinemic E78.ØØ
  - hypercholesterolemic E78.ØØ
  - hyperlipidemic E78.5
  - joint E75.5
  - multiple (skin) E78.2
  - tendon (sheath) E75.5
  - tuberosum E78.2
  - tuberous E78.2
  - tubo-eruptive E78.2
  - verrucous, oral mucosa K13.4
- **Xanthosis** R23.8
- **Xenophobia** F4Ø.1Ø
- **Xeroderma** — *see also* Ichthyosis
  - acquired L85.Ø
    - eyelid HØ1.149
      - left HØ1.146
        - lower HØ1.145
        - upper HØ1.144

Y

Z

Note: The list below gives the code number for neoplasms by anatomical site. For each site there are six possible code numbers according to whether the neoplasm in question is malignant, benign, in situ, of uncertain behavior, or of unspecified nature. The description of the neoplasm will often indicate which of the six columns is appropriate; e.g., malignant melanoma of skin, benign fibroadenoma of breast, carcinoma in situ of cervix uteri. Where such descriptors are not present, the remainder of the Index should be consulted where guidance is given to the appropriate column for each morphological (histological) variety listed; e.g., Mesonephroma – see Neoplasm, malignant; Embryoma — see also Neoplasm, uncertain behavior; Disease, Bowen's – see Neoplasm, skin, in situ. However, the guidance in the Index can be overridden if one of the descriptors mentioned above is present; e.g., malignant adenoma of colon is coded to C18.9 and not to D12.6 as the adjective "malignant" overrides the Index entry "Adenoma — *see also* Neoplasm, benign, by site." Codes listed with a dash -, following the code have a required additional character for laterality. The tabular list must be reviewed for the complete code.

	Malignant Primary	Malignant Secondary	Ca in situ	Benign	Uncertain Behavior	Unspecified Behavior
Neoplasm, neoplastic	C80.1	C79.9	D09.9	D36.9	D48.9	D49.9
abdomen, abdominal	C76.2	C79.8-☑	D09.8	D36.7	D48.7	D49.89
cavity	C76.2	C79.8-☑	D09.8	D36.7	D48.7	D49.89
organ	C76.2	C79.8-☑	D09.8	D36.7	D48.7	D49.89
viscera	C76.2	C79.8-☑	D09.8	D36.7	D48.7	D49.89
wall — *see also* Neoplasm, abdomen, wall, skin	C44.509	C79.2	D04.5	D23.5	D48.5	D49.2
connective tissue	C49.4	C79.8-☑	—	D21.4	D48.1	D49.2
skin	C44.509					
basal cell carcinoma	C44.519	—	—	—	—	—
specified type NEC	C44.599	—	—	—	—	—
squamous cell carcinoma	C44.529	—	—	—	—	—
abdominopelvic	C76.8	C79.8-☑	—	D36.7	D48.7	D49.89
accessory sinus — *see* Neoplasm, sinus						
acoustic nerve	C72.4-☑	C79.49	—	D33.3	D43.3	D49.7
adenoid (pharynx) (tissue)	C11.1	C79.89	D00.08	D10.6	D37.05	D49.0
adipose tissue — *see also* Neoplasm, connective tissue	C49.4	C79.89	—	D21.9	D48.1	D49.2
adnexa (uterine)	C57.4	C79.89	D07.39	D28.7	D39.8	D49.59
adrenal	C74.9-☑	C79.7-☑	D09.3	D35.0-☑	D44.1-☑	D49.7
capsule	C74.9-☑	C79.7-☑	D09.3	D35.0-☑	D44.1-☑	D49.7
cortex	C74.0-☑	C79.7-☑	D09.3	D35.0-☑	D44.1-☑	D49.7
gland	C74.9-☑	C79.7-☑	D09.3	D35.0-☑	D44.1-☑	D49.7
medulla	C74.1-☑	C79.7-☑	D09.3	D35.0-☑	D44.1-☑	D49.7
ala nasi (external) — *see also* Neoplasm, skin, nose	C44.301	C79.2	D04.39	D23.39	D48.5	D49.2
alimentary canal or tract NEC	C26.9	C78.80	D01.9	D13.9	D37.9	D49.0
alveolar	C03.9	C79.89	D00.03	D10.39	D37.09	D49.0
mucosa	C03.9	C79.89	D00.03	D10.39	D37.09	D49.0
lower	C03.1	C79.89	D00.03	D10.39	D37.09	D49.0
upper	C03.0	C79.89	D00.03	D10.39	D37.09	D49.0
ridge or process	C41.1	C79.51	—	D16.5	D48.0	D49.2
carcinoma	C03.9	C79.8-☑	—	—	—	—
lower	C03.1	C79.8-☑	—	—	—	—
upper	C03.0	C79.8-☑	—	—	—	—
lower	C41.1	C79.51	—	D16.5	D48.0	D49.2
mucosa	C03.9	C79.89	D00.03	D10.39	D37.09	D49.0
lower	C03.1	C79.89	D00.03	D10.39	D37.09	D49.0
upper	C03.0	C79.89	D00.03	D10.39	D37.09	D49.0
upper	C41.0	C79.51	—	D16.4	D48.0	D49.2
sulcus	C06.1	C79.89	D00.02	D10.39	D37.09	D49.0
alveolus	C03.9	C79.89	D00.03	D10.39	D37.09	D49.0
lower	C03.1	C79.89	D00.03	D10.39	D37.09	D49.0
upper	C03.0	C79.89	D00.03	D10.39	D37.09	D49.0
ampulla of Vater	C24.1	C78.89	D01.5	D13.5	D37.6	D49.0
ankle NEC	C76.5-☑	C79.89	D04.7-☑	D36.7	D48.7	D49.89
anorectum, anorectal (junction)	C21.8	C78.5	D01.3	D12.9	D37.8	D49.0
antecubital fossa or space	C76.4-☑	C79.89	D04.6-☑	D36.7	D48.7	D49.89
Neoplasm, neoplastic — *continued*						
antrum (Highmore) (maxillary)	C31.0	C78.39	D02.3	D14.0	D38.5	D49.1
pyloric	C16.3	C78.89	D00.2	D13.1	D37.1	D49.0
tympanicum	C30.1	C78.39	D02.3	D14.0	D38.5	D49.1
anus, anal	C21.0	C78.5	D01.3	D12.9	D37.8	D49.0
canal	C21.1	C78.5	D01.3	D12.9	D37.8	D49.0
cloacogenic zone	C21.2	C78.5	D01.3	D12.9	D37.8	D49.0
margin — *see also* Neoplasm, anus, skin	C44.500	C79.2	D04.5	D23.5	D48.5	D49.2
overlapping lesion with rectosigmoid junction or rectum	C21.8	—	—	—	—	—
skin	C44.500	C79.2	D04.5	D23.5	D48.5	D49.2
basal cell carcinoma	C44.510	—	—	—	—	—
specified type NEC	C44.590	—	—	—	—	—
squamous cell carcinoma	C44.520	—	—	—	—	—
sphincter	C21.1	C78.5	D01.3	D12.9	D37.8	D49.0
aorta (thoracic)	C49.3	C79.89	—	D21.3	D48.1	D49.2
abdominal	C49.4	C79.89	—	D21.4	D48.1	D49.2
aortic body	C75.5	C79.89	—	D35.6	D44.7	D49.7
aponeurosis	C49.9	C79.89	—	D21.9	D48.1	D49.2
palmar	C49.1-☑	C79.89	—	D21.1-☑	D48.1	D49.2
plantar	C49.2-☑	C79.89	—	D21.2-☑	D48.1	D49.2
appendix	C18.1	C78.5	D01.0	D12.1	D37.3	D49.0
arachnoid	C70.9	C79.49	—	D32.9	D42.9	D49.7
cerebral	C70.0	C79.32	—	D32.0	D42.0	D49.7
spinal	C70.1	C79.49	—	D32.1	D42.1	D49.7
areola	C50.0-☑	C79.81	D05-☑	D24-☑	D48.6-☑	D49.3
arm NEC	C76.4-☑	C79.89	D04.6-☑	D36.7	D48.7	D49.89
artery — *see* Neoplasm, connective tissue						
aryepiglottic fold	C13.1	C79.89	D00.08	D10.7	D37.05	D49.0
hypopharyngeal aspect	C13.1	C79.89	D00.08	D10.7	D37.05	D49.0
laryngeal aspect	C32.1	C78.39	D02.0	D14.1	D38.0	D49.1
marginal zone	C13.1	C79.89	D00.08	D10.7	D37.05	D49.0
arytenoid (cartilage)	C32.3	C78.39	D02.0	D14.1	D38.0	D49.1
fold — *see* Neoplasm, aryepiglottic						
associated with transplanted organ	C80.2	—	—	—	—	—
atlas	C41.2	C79.51	—	D16.6	D48.0	D49.2
atrium, cardiac	C38.0	C79.89	—	D15.1	D48.7	D49.89
auditory						
canal (external) (skin)	C44.20-☑	C79.2	D04.2-☑	D23.2-☑	D48.5	D49.2
internal	C30.1	C78.39	D02.3	D14.0	D38.5	D49.1
nerve	C72.4-☑	C79.49	—	D33.3	D43.3	D49.7
tube	C30.1	C78.39	D02.3	D14.0	D38.5	D49.1
opening	C11.2	C79.89	D00.08	D10.6	D37.05	D49.0
auricle, ear — *see also* Neoplasm, skin, ear	C44.20-☑	C79.2	D04.2-☑	D23.2-☑	D48.5	D49.2
auricular canal (external) — *see also* Neoplasm, skin, ear	C44.20-☑	C79.2	D04.2-☑	D23.2-☑	D48.5	D49.2
internal	C30.1	C78.39	D02.3	D14.0	D38.5	D49.2
autonomic nerve or nervous system NEC (see Neoplasm, nerve, peripheral)						
axilla, axillary	C76.1	C79.89	D09.8	D36.7	D48.7	D49.89
fold — *see also* Neoplasm, skin, trunk	C44.509	C79.2	D04.5	D23.5	D48.5	D49.2
back NEC	C76.8	C79.89	D04.5	D36.7	D48.7	D49.89
Bartholin's gland	C51.0	C79.82	D07.1	D28.0	D39.8	D49.59
basal ganglia	C71.0	C79.31	—	D33.0	D43.0	D49.6
basis pedunculi	C71.7	C79.31	—	D33.1	D43.1	D49.6
bile or biliary (tract)	C24.9	C78.89	D01.5	D13.5	D37.6	D49.0

☑ **Additional Character Required — Refer to the Tabular List for Character Selection**

	Malignant Primary	Malignant Secondary	Ca in situ	Benign	Uncertain Behavior	Unspecified Behavior
Neoplasm, neoplastic *— continued*						
bile or biliary — *continued*						
canaliculi (biliferi) (intrahepatic)	C22.1	C78.7	D01.5	D13.4	D37.6	D49.0
canals, interlobular	C22.1	C78.89	D01.5	D13.4	D37.6	D49.0
duct or passage (common) (cystic) (extrahepatic)	C24.0	C78.89	D01.5	D13.5	D37.6	D49.0
interlobular	C22.1	C78.89	D01.5	D13.4	D37.6	D49.0
intrahepatic	C22.1	C78.7	D01.5	D13.4	D37.6	D49.0
and extrahepatic	C24.8	C78.89	D01.5	D13.5	D37.6	D49.0
bladder (urinary)	C67.9	C79.11	D09.0	D30.3	D41.4	D49.4
dome	C67.1	C79.11	D09.0	D30.3	D41.4	D49.4
neck	C67.5	C79.11	D09.0	D30.3	D41.4	D49.4
orifice	C67.9	C79.11	D09.0	D30.3	D41.4	D49.4
ureteric	C67.6	C79.11	D09.0	D30.3	D41.4	D49.4
urethral	C67.5	C79.11	D09.0	D30.3	D41.4	D49.4
overlapping lesion	C67.8	—	—	—	—	—
sphincter	C67.8	C79.11	D09.0	D30.3	D41.4	D49.4
trigone	C67.0	C79.11	D09.0	D30.3	D41.4	D49.4
urachus	C67.7	C79.11	D09.0	D30.3	D41.4	D49.4
wall	C67.9	C79.11	D09.0	D30.3	D41.4	D49.4
anterior	C67.3	C79.11	D09.0	D30.3	D41.4	D49.4
lateral	C67.2	C79.11	D09.0	D30.3	D41.4	D49.4
posterior	C67.4	C79.11	D09.0	D30.3	D41.4	D49.4
blood vessel — *see* Neoplasm, connective tissue						
bone (periosteum)	C41.9	C79.51	—	D16.9-	D48.0	D49.2
acetabulum						
ankle	C40.3-☑	C79.51	—	D16.3-☑	—	—
arm NEC	C40.0-☑	C79.51	—	D16.0-☑	—	—
astragalus	C40.3-☑	C79.51	—	D16.3-☑	—	—
atlas	C41.2	C79.51	—	D16.6	D48.0	D49.2
axis	C41.2	C79.51	—	D16.6	D48.0	D49.2
back NEC	C41.2	C79.51	—	D16.6	D48.0	D49.2
calcaneus	C40.3-☑	C79.51	—	D16.3-☑	—	—
calvarium	C41.0	C79.51	—	D16.4	D48.0	D49.2
carpus (any)	C40.1-☑	C79.51	—	D16.1-☑	—	—
cartilage NEC	C41.9	C79.51	—	D16.9	D48.0	D49.2
clavicle	C41.3	C79.51	—	D16.7	D48.0	D49.2
clivus	C41.0	C79.51	—	D16.4	D48.0	D49.2
coccygeal vertebra	C41.4	C79.51	—	D16.8	D48.0	D49.2
coccyx	C41.4	C79.51	—	D16.8	D48.0	D49.2
costal cartilage	C41.3	C79.51	—	D16.7	D48.0	D49.2
costovertebral joint	C41.3	C79.51	—	D16.7	D48.0	D49.2
cranial	C41.0	C79.51	—	D16.4	D48.0	D49.2
cuboid	C40.3-☑	C79.51	—	D16.3-☑	—	—
cuneiform	C41.9	C79.51	—	D16.9	D48.0	D49.2
elbow	C40.0-☑	C79.51	—	D16.0-☑	—	—
ethmoid (labyrinth)	C41.0	C79.51	—	D16.4	D48.0	D49.2
face	C41.0	C79.51	—	D16.4	D48.0	D49.2
femur (any part)	C40.2-☑	C79.51	—	D16.2-☑	—	—
fibula (any part)	C40.2-☑	C79.51	—	D16.2-☑	—	—
finger (any)	C40.1-☑	C79.51	—	D16.1-☑	—	—
foot	C40.3-☑	C79.51	—	D16.3-☑	—	—
forearm	C40.0-☑	C79.51	—	D16.0-☑	—	—
frontal	C41.0	C79.51	—	D16.4	D48.0	D49.2
hand	C40.1-☑	C79.51	—	D16.1-☑	—	—
heel	C40.3-☑	C79.51	—	D16.3-☑	—	—
hip	C41.4	C79.51	—	D16.8	D48.0	D49.2
humerus (any part)	C40.0-☑	C79.51	—	D16.0-☑	—	—
hyoid	C41.0	C79.51	—	D16.4	D48.0	D49.2
ilium	C41.4	C79.51	—	D16.8	D48.0	D49.2
innominate	C41.4	C79.51	—	D16.8	D48.0	D49.2
intervertebral cartilage or disc	C41.2	C79.51	—	D16.6	D48.0	D49.2
ischium	C41.4	C79.51	—	D16.8	D48.0	D49.2
jaw (lower)	C41.1	C79.51	—	D16.5	D48.0	D49.2
knee	C40.2-☑	C79.51	—	D16.2-☑	—	—
leg NEC	C40.2-☑	C79.51	—	D16.2-☑	—	—
limb NEC	C40.9-☑	C79.51	—	D16.9	—	—
Neoplasm, neoplastic *— continued*						
bone — *continued*						
limb — *continued*						
lower (long bones)	C40.2-☑	C79.51	—	D16.2-☑	—	—
short bones	C40.3-☑	C79.51	—	D16.3-☑	—	—
upper (long bones)	C40.0-☑	C79.51	—	D16.0-☑	—	—
short bones	C40.1-☑	C79.51	—	D16.1-☑	—	—
malar	C41.0	C79.51	—	D16.4	D48.0	D49.2
mandible	C41.1	C79.51	—	D16.5	D48.0	D49.2
marrow NEC (any bone)	C96.9	C79.52	—	—	D47.9	D49.89
mastoid	C41.0	C79.51	—	D16.4	D48.0	D49.2
maxilla, maxillary (superior)	C41.0	C79.51	—	D16.4	D48.0	D49.2
inferior	C41.1	C79.51	—	D16.5	D48.0	D49.2
metacarpus (any)	C40.1-☑	C79.51	—	D16.1-☑	—	—
metatarsus (any)	C40.3-☑	C79.51	—	D16.3-☑	—	—
navicular						
ankle	C40.3-☑	C79.51	—	—	—	—
hand	C40.1-☑	C79.51	—	—	—	—
nose, nasal	C41.0	C79.51	—	D16.4	D48.0	D49.2
occipital	C41.0	C79.51	—	D16.4	D48.0	D49.2
orbit	C41.0	C79.51	—	D16.4	D48.0	D49.2
overlapping sites	C40.8-☑	—	—	—	—	—
parietal	C41.0	C79.51	—	D16.4	D48.0	D49.2
patella	C40.2-☑	C79.51	—	—	—	—
pelvic	C41.4	C79.51	—	D16.8	D48.0	D49.2
phalanges						
foot	C40.3-☑	C79.51	—	—	—	—
hand	C40.1-☑	C79.51	—	—	—	—
pubic	C41.4	C79.51	—	D16.8	D48.0	D49.2
radius (any part)	C40.0-☑	C79.51	—	D16.0-☑	—	—
rib	C41.3	C79.51	—	D16.7	D48.0	D49.2
sacral vertebra	C41.4	C79.51	—	D16.8	D48.0	D49.2
sacrum	C41.4	C79.51	—	D16.8	D48.0	D49.2
scaphoid						
of ankle	C40.3-☑	C79.51	—	—	—	—
of hand	C40.1-☑	C79.51	—	—	—	—
scapula (any part)	C40.0-☑	C79.51	—	D16.0-☑	—	—
sella turcica	C41.0	C79.51	—	D16.4	D48.0	D49.2
shoulder	C40.0-☑	C79.51	—	D16.0-☑	—	—
skull	C41.0	C79.51	—	D16.4	D48.0	D49.2
sphenoid	C41.0	C79.51	—	D16.4	D48.0	D49.2
spine, spinal (column)	C41.2	C79.51	—	D16.6	D48.0	D49.2
coccyx	C41.4	C79.51	—	D16.8	D48.0	D49.2
sacrum	C41.4	C79.51	—	D16.8	D48.0	D49.2
sternum	C41.3	C79.51	—	D16.7	D48.0	D49.2
tarsus (any)	C40.3-☑	C79.51	—	—	—	—
temporal	C41.0	C79.51	—	D16.4	D48.0	D49.2
thumb	C40.1-☑	C79.51	—	—	—	—
tibia (any part)	C40.2-☑	C79.51	—	—	—	—
toe (any)	C40.3-☑	C79.51	—	—	—	—
trapezium	C40.1-☑	C79.51	—	—	—	—
trapezoid	C40.1-☑	C79.51	—	—	—	—
turbinate	C41.0	C79.51	—	D16.4	D48.0	D49.2
ulna (any part)	C40.0-☑	C79.51	—	D16.0-☑	—	—
unciform	C40.1-☑	C79.51	—	—	—	—
vertebra (column)	C41.2	C79.51	—	D16.6	D48.0	D49.2
coccyx	C41.4	C79.51	—	D16.8	D48.0	D49.2
sacrum	C41.4	C79.51	—	D16.8	D48.0	D49.2
vomer	C41.0	C79.51	—	D16.4	D48.0	D49.2
wrist	C40.1-☑	C79.51	—	—	—	—
xiphoid process	C41.3	C79.51	—	D16.7	D48.0	D49.2
zygomatic	C41.0	C79.51	—	D16.4	D48.0	D49.2
book-leaf (mouth) — *ventral surface of tongue and floor of mouth*	C06.89	C79.89	D00.00	D10.39	D37.09	D49.0
bowel — *see* Neoplasm, intestine						
brachial plexus	C47.1-☑	C79.89	—	D36.12	D48.2	D49.2
brain NEC	C71.9	C79.31	—	D33.2	D43.2	D49.6

	Malignant Primary	Malignant Secondary	Ca in situ	Benign	Uncertain Behavior	Unspecified Behavior
Neoplasm, neoplastic — *continued*						
brain — *continued*						
basal ganglia	C71.Ø	C79.31	—	D33.Ø	D43.Ø	D49.6
cerebellopontine angle	C71.6	C79.31	—	D33.1	D43.1	D49.6
cerebellum NOS	C71.6	C79.31	—	D33.1	D43.1	D49.6
cerebrum	C71.Ø	C79.31	—	D33.Ø	D43.Ø	D49.6
choroid plexus	C71.7	C79.31	—	D33.1	D43.1	D49.6
corpus callosum	C71.8	C79.31	—	D33.2	D43.2	D49.6
corpus striatum	C71.Ø	C79.31	—	D33.Ø	D43.Ø	D49.6
cortex (cerebral)	C71.Ø	C79.31	—	D33.Ø	D43.Ø	D49.6
frontal lobe	C71.1	C79.31	—	D33.Ø	D43.Ø	D49.6
globus pallidus	C71.Ø	C79.31	—	D33.Ø	D43.Ø	D49.6
hippocampus	C71.2	C79.31	—	D33.Ø	D43.Ø	D49.6
hypothalamus	C71.Ø	C79.31	—	D33.Ø	D43.Ø	D49.6
internal capsule	C71.Ø	C79.31	—	D33.Ø	D43.Ø	D49.6
medulla oblongata	C71.7	C79.31	—	D33.1	D43.1	D49.6
meninges	C7Ø.Ø	C79.32	—	D32.Ø	D42.Ø	D49.7
midbrain	C71.7	C79.31	—	D33.1	D43.1	D49.6
occipital lobe	C71.4	C79.31	—	D33.Ø	D43.Ø	D49.6
overlapping lesion	C71.8	C79.31	—	—	—	—
parietal lobe	C71.3	C79.31	—	D33.Ø	D43.Ø	D49.6
peduncle	C71.7	C79.31	—	D33.1	D43.1	D49.6
pons	C71.7	C79.31	—	D33.1	D43.1	D49.6
stem	C71.7	C79.31	—	D33.1	D43.1	D49.6
tapetum	C71.8	C79.31	—	D33.2	D43.2	D49.6
temporal lobe	C71.2	C79.31	—	D33.Ø	D43.Ø	D49.6
thalamus	C71.Ø	C79.31	—	D33.Ø	D43.Ø	D49.6
uncus	C71.2	C79.31	—	D33.Ø	D43.Ø	D49.6
ventricle (floor)	C71.5	C79.31	—	D33.Ø	D43.Ø	D49.6
fourth	C71.7	C79.31	—	D33.1	D43.1	D49.6
branchial (cleft) (cyst) (vestiges)	C1Ø.4	C79.89	DØØ.Ø8	D1Ø.5	D37.Ø5	D49.Ø
breast (connective tissue) (glandular tissue) (soft parts)	C5Ø.9-☑	C79.81	DØ5.-☑	D24.-☑	D48.6-☑	D49.3
areola	C5Ø.Ø-☑	C79.81	DØ5.-☑	D24.-☑	D48.6-☑	D49.3
axillary tail	C5Ø.6-☑	C79.81	DØ5.-☑	D24.-☑	D48.6-☑	D49.3
central portion	C5Ø.1-☑	C79.81	DØ5.-☑	D24.-☑	D48.6-☑	D49.3
inner	C5Ø.8-☑	C79.81	DØ5.-☑	D24.-☑	D48.6-☑	D49.3
lower	C5Ø.8-☑	C79.81	DØ5.-☑	D24.-☑	D48.6-☑	D49.3
lower-inner quadrant	C5Ø.3-☑	C79.81	DØ5.-☑	D24.-☑	D48.6-☑	D49.3
lower-outer quadrant	C5Ø.5-☑	C79.81	DØ5.-☑	D24.-☑	D48.6-☑	D49.3
mastectomy site (skin) — *see also* Neoplasm, breast, skin	C44.5Ø1	C79.2	—	—	—	—
specified as breast tissue	C5Ø.8-☑	C79.81	—	—	—	—
midline	C5Ø.8-☑	C79.81	DØ5.-☑	D24.-☑	D48.6-☑	D49.3
nipple	C5Ø.Ø-☑	C79.81	DØ5.-☑	D24.-☑	D48.6-☑	D49.3
outer	C5Ø.8-☑	C79.81	DØ5.-☑	D24.-☑	D48.6-☑	D49.3
overlapping lesion	C5Ø.8-☑	—	—	—	—	—
skin	C44.5Ø1	C79.2	DØ4.5	D23.5	D48.5	D49.2
basal cell carcinoma	C44.511	—	—	—	—	—
specified type NEC	C44.591	—	—	—	—	—
squamous cell carcinoma	C44.521	—	—	—	—	—
tail (axillary)	C5Ø.6-☑	C79.81	DØ5.-☑	D24.-☑	D48.6-☑	D49.3
upper	C5Ø.8-☑	C79.81	DØ5.-☑	D24.-☑	D48.6-☑	D49.3
upper-inner quadrant	C5Ø.2-☑	C79.81	DØ5.-☑	D24.-☑	D48.6-☑	D49.3
upper-outer quadrant	C5Ø.4-☑	C79.81	DØ5.-☑	D24.-☑	D48.6-☑	D49.3
broad ligament	C57.1-☑	C79.82	DØ7.39	D28.2	D39.8	D49.59
bronchiogenic, bronchogenic (lung)	C34.9-☑	C78.Ø-☑	DØ2.2-☑	D14.3-☑	D38.1	D49.1
bronchiole	C34.9-☑	C78.Ø-☑	DØ2.2-☑	D14.3-☑	D38.1	D49.1
bronchus	C34.9-☑	C78.Ø-☑	DØ2.2-☑	D14.3-☑	D38.1	D49.1
carina	C34.Ø-☑	C78.Ø-☑	DØ2.2-☑	D14.3-☑	D38.1	D49.1
lower lobe of lung	C34.3-☑	C78.Ø-☑	DØ2.2-☑	D14.3-☑	D38.1	D49.1

	Malignant Primary	Malignant Secondary	Ca in situ	Benign	Uncertain Behavior	Unspecified Behavior
Neoplasm, neoplastic — *continued*						
bronchus — *continued*						
main	C34.Ø-☑	C78.Ø-☑	DØ2.2-☑	D14.3-☑	D38.1	D49.1
middle lobe of lung	C34.2	C78.Ø-☑	DØ2.21	D14.31	D38.1	D49.1
overlapping lesion	C34.8-☑	—	—	—	—	—
upper lobe of lung	C34.1-☑	C78.Ø-☑	DØ2.2-☑	D14.3-☑	D38.1	D49.1
brow	C44.3Ø9	C79.2	DØ4.39	D23.39	D48.5	D49.2
basal cell carcinoma	C44.319	—	—	—	—	—
specified type NEC	C44.399	—	—	—	—	—
squamous cell carcinoma	C44.329	—	—	—	—	—
buccal (cavity)	CØ6.9	C79.89	DØØ.ØØ	D1Ø.39	D37.Ø9	D49.Ø
commissure	CØ6.Ø	C79.89	DØØ.Ø2	D1Ø.39	D37.Ø9	D49.Ø
groove (lower) (upper)	CØ6.1	C79.89	DØØ.Ø2	D1Ø.39	D37.Ø9	D49.Ø
mucosa	CØ6.Ø	C79.89	DØØ.Ø2	D1Ø.39	D37.Ø9	D49.Ø
sulcus (lower) (upper)	CØ6.1	C79.89	DØØ.Ø2	D1Ø.39	D37.Ø9	D49.Ø
bulbourethral gland	C68.Ø	C79.19	DØ9.19	D3Ø.4	D41.3	D49.59
bursa — *see* Neoplasm, connective tissue						
buttock NEC	C76.3	C79.89	DØ4.5	D36.7	D48.7	D49.89
calf	C76.5-☑	C79.89	DØ4.7-☑	D36.7	D48.7	D49.89
calvarium	C41.Ø	C79.51	—	D16.4	D48.Ø	D49.2
calyx, renal	C65.-☑	C79.Ø-☑	DØ9.19	D3Ø.1-☑	D41.1-☑	D49.51-☑
canal						
anal	C21.1	C78.5	DØ1.3	D12.9	D37.8	D49.Ø
auditory (external) — *see also* Neoplasm, skin, ear	C44.2Ø-☑	C79.2	DØ4.2-☑	D23.2-☑	D48.5	D49.2
auricular (external) — *see also* Neoplasm, skin, ear	C44.2Ø-☑	C79.2	DØ4.2-☑	D23.2-☑	D48.5	D49.2
canaliculi, biliary (biliferi) (intrahepatic)	C22.1	C78.7	DØ1.5	D13.4	D37.6	D49.Ø
canthus (eye) (inner) (outer)	C44.1Ø-☑	C79.2	DØ4.1-☑	D23.1-☑	D48.5	D49.2
basal cell carcinoma	C44.11-☑	—	—	—	—	—
sebaceous cell	C44.13-☑	—	—	—	—	—
specified type NEC	C44.19-☑	—	—	—	—	—
squamous cell carcinoma	C44.12-☑	—	—	—	—	—
capillary — *see* Neoplasm, connective tissue						
caput coli	C18.Ø	C78.5	DØ1.Ø	D12.Ø	D37.4	D49.Ø
carcinoid — *see* Tumor, carcinoid						
cardia (gastric)	C16.Ø	C78.89	DØØ.2	D13.1	D37.1	D49.Ø
cardiac orifice (stomach)	C16.Ø	C78.89	DØØ.2	D13.1	D37.1	D49.Ø
cardio-esophageal junction	C16.Ø	C78.89	DØØ.2	D13.1	D37.1	D49.Ø
cardio-esophagus	C16.Ø	C78.89	DØØ.2	D13.1	D37.1	D49.Ø
carina (bronchus)	C34.Ø-☑	C78.Ø-☑	DØ2.2-☑	D14.3-☑	D38.1	D49.1
carotid (artery)	C49.Ø	C79.89	—	D21.Ø	D48.1	D49.2
body	C75.4	C79.89	—	D35.5	D44.6	D49.7
carpus (any bone)	C4Ø.1-☑	C79.51	—	D16.1-☑	—	—
cartilage (articular) (joint) NEC — *see also* Neoplasm, bone	C41.9	C79.51	—	D16.9	D48.Ø	D49.2
arytenoid	C32.3	C78.39	DØ2.Ø	D14.1	D38.Ø	D49.1
auricular	C49.Ø	C79.89	—	D21.Ø	D48.1	D49.2
bronchi	C34.Ø-☑	C78.39	—	D14.3-☑	D38.1	D49.1
costal	C41.3	C79.51	—	D16.7	D48.Ø	D49.2
cricoid	C32.3	C78.39	DØ2.Ø	D14.1	D38.Ø	D49.1
cuneiform	C32.3	C78.39	DØ2.Ø	D14.1	D38.Ø	D49.1
ear (external)	C49.Ø	C79.89	—	D21.Ø	D48.1	D49.2
ensiform	C41.3	C79.51	—	D16.7	D48.Ø	D49.2
epiglottis	C32.1	C78.39	DØ2.Ø	D14.1	D38.Ø	D49.1

☑ **Additional Character Required — Refer to the Tabular List for Character Selection**

	Malignant Primary	Malignant Secondary	Ca in situ	Benign	Uncertain Behavior	Unspecified Behavior
Neoplasm, neoplastic — *continued*						
cartilage — *see also* Neoplasm, bone — *continued*						
epiglottis — *continued*						
anterior surface	C10.1	C79.89	D00.08	D10.5	D37.05	D49.0
eyelid	C49.0	C79.89	—	D21.0	D48.1	D49.2
intervertebral	C41.2	C79.51	—	D16.6	D48.0	D49.2
larynx, laryngeal	C32.3	C78.39	D02.0	D14.1	D38.0	D49.1
nose, nasal	C30.0	C78.39	D02.3	D14.0	D38.5	D49.1
pinna	C49.0	C79.89	—	D21.0	D48.1	D49.2
rib	C41.3	C79.51	—	D16.7	D48.0	D49.2
semilunar (knee)	C40.2-☑	C79.51	—	D16.2-☑	D48.0	D49.2
thyroid	C32.3	C78.39	D02.0	D14.1	D38.0	D49.1
trachea	C33	C78.39	D02.1	D14.2	D38.1	D49.1
cauda equina	C72.1	C79.49	—	D33.4	D43.4	D49.7
cavity						
buccal	C06.9	C79.89	D00.00	D10.30	D37.09	D49.0
nasal	C30.0	C78.39	D02.3	D14.0	D38.5	D49.1
oral	C06.9	C79.89	D00.00	D10.30	D37.09	D49.0
peritoneal	C48.2	C78.6	—	D20.1	D48.4	D49.0
tympanic	C30.1	C78.39	D02.3	D14.0	D38.5	D49.1
cecum	C18.0	C78.5	D01.0	D12.0	D37.4	D49.0
central nervous system	C72.9	C79.40	—	—	—	—
cerebellopontine (angle)	C71.6	C79.31	—	D33.1	D43.1	D49.6
cerebellum, cerebellar	C71.6	C79.31	—	D33.1	D43.1	D49.6
cerebrum, cerebra (cortex) (hemisphere) (white matter)	C71.0	C79.31	—	D33.0	D43.0	D49.6
meninges	C70.0	C79.32	—	D32.0	D42.0	D49.7
peduncle	C71.7	C79.31	—	D33.1	D43.1	D49.6
ventricle	C71.5	C79.31	—	D33.0	D43.0	D49.6
fourth	C71.7	C79.31	—	D33.1	D43.1	D49.6
cervical region	C76.0	C79.89	D09.8	D36.7	D48.7	D49.89
cervix (cervical) (uteri) (uterus)	C53.9	C79.82	D06.9	D26.0	D39.0	D49.59
canal	C53.0	C79.82	D06.0	D26.0	D39.0	D49.59
endocervix (canal) (gland)	C53.0	C79.82	D06.0	D26.0	D39.0	D49.59
exocervix	C53.1	C79.82	D06.1	D26.0	D39.0	D49.59
external os	C53.1	C79.82	D06.1	D26.0	D39.0	D49.59
internal os	C53.0	C79.82	D06.0	D26.0	D39.0	D49.59
nabothian gland	C53.0	C79.82	D06.0	D26.0	D39.0	D49.59
overlapping lesion	C53.8	—	—	—	—	—
squamocolumnar junction	C53.8	C79.82	D06.7	D26.0	D39.0	D49.59
stump	C53.8	C79.82	D06.7	D26.0	D39.0	D49.59
cheek	C76.0	C79.89	D09.8	D36.7	D48.7	D49.89
external	C44.309	C79.2	D04.39	D23.39	D48.5	D49.2
basal cell carcinoma	C44.319	—	—	—	—	—
specified type NEC	C44.399	—	—	—	—	—
squamous cell carcinoma	C44.329	—	—	—	—	—
inner aspect	C06.0	C79.89	D00.02	D10.39	D37.09	D49.0
internal	C06.0	C79.89	D00.02	D10.39	D37.09	D49.0
mucosa	C06.0	C79.89	D00.02	D10.39	D37.09	D49.0
chest (wall) NEC	C76.1	C79.89	D09.8	D36.7	D48.7	D49.89
chiasma opticum	C72.3-☑	C79.49	—	D33.3	D43.3	D49.7
chin	C44.309	C79.2	D04.39	D23.39	D48.5	D49.2
basal cell carcinoma	C44.319	—	—	—	—	—
specified type NEC	C44.399	—	—	—	—	—
squamous cell carcinoma	C44.329	—	—	—	—	—
choana	C11.3	C79.89	D00.08	D10.6	D37.05	D49.0
cholangiole	C22.1	C78.89	D01.5	D13.4	D37.6	D49.0
choledochal duct	C24.0	C78.89	D01.5	D13.5	D37.6	D49.0
choroid	C69.3-☑	C79.49	D09.2-☑	D31.3-☑	D48.7	D49.81
plexus	C71.5	C79.31	—	D33.0	D43.0	D49.6
ciliary body	C69.4-☑	C79.49	D09.2-☑	D31.4-☑	D48.7	D49.89
clavicle	C41.3	C79.51	—	D16.7	D48.0	D49.2
Neoplasm, neoplastic — *continued*						
clitoris	C51.2	C79.82	D07.1	D28.0	D39.8	D49.59
clivus	C41.0	C79.51	—	D16.4	D48.0	D49.2
cloacogenic zone	C21.2	C78.5	D01.3	D12.9	D37.8	D49.0
coccygeal						
body or glomus	C49.5	C79.89	—	D21.5	D48.1	D49.2
vertebra	C41.4	C79.51	—	D16.8	D48.0	D49.2
coccyx	C41.4	C79.51	—	D16.8	D48.0	D49.2
colon — *see also* Neoplasm, intestine, large	C18.9	C78.5	—	—	—	—
with rectum	C19	C78.5	D01.1	D12.7	D37.5	D49.0
columnella — *see also* Neoplasm, skin, face	C44.390	C79.2	D04.39	D23.39	D48.5	D49.2
column, spinal — *see* Neoplasm, spine						
commissure						
labial, lip	C00.6	C79.89	D00.01	D10.39	D37.01	D49.0
laryngeal	C32.0	C78.39	D02.0	D14.1	D38.0	D49.1
common (bile) duct	C24.0	C78.89	D01.5	D13.5	D37.6	D49.0
concha — *see also* Neoplasm, skin, ear	C44.20-☑	C79.2	D04.2-☑	D23.2-☑	D48.5	D49.2
nose	C30.0	C78.39	D02.3	D14.0	D38.5	D49.1
conjunctiva	C69.0-☑	C79.49	D09.2-☑	D31.0-☑	D48.7	D49.89
connective tissue NEC	C49.9	C79.89	—	D21.9	D48.1	D49.2

Note: For neoplasms of connective tissue (blood vessel, bursa, fascia, ligament, muscle, peripheral nerves, sympathetic and parasympathetic nerves and ganglia, synovia, tendon, etc.) or of morphological types that indicate connective tissue, code according to the list under "Neoplasm, connective tissue". For sites that do not appear in this list, code to neoplasm of that site; e.g., fibrosarcoma, pancreas (C25.9)

Note: Morphological types that indicate connective tissue appear in their proper place in the alphabetic index with the instruction "see Neoplasm, connective tissue ...."

	Malignant Primary	Malignant Secondary	Ca in situ	Benign	Uncertain Behavior	Unspecified Behavior
abdomen	C49.4	C79.89	—	D21.4	D48.1	D49.2
abdominal wall	C49.4	C79.89	—	D21.4	D48.1	D49.2
ankle	C49.2-☑	C79.89	—	D21.2-☑	D48.1	D49.2
antecubital fossa or space	C49.1-☑	C79.89	—	D21.1-☑	D48.1	D49.2
arm	C49.1-☑	C79.89	—	D21.1-☑	D48.1	D49.2
auricle (ear)	C49.0	C79.89	—	D21.0	D48.1	D49.2
axilla	C49.3	C79.89	—	D21.3	D48.1	D49.2
back	C49.6	C79.89	—	D21.6	D48.1	D49.2
breast — *see* Neoplasm, breast						
buttock	C49.5	C79.89	—	D21.5	D48.1	D49.2
calf	C49.2-☑	C79.89	—	D21.2-☑	D48.1	D49.2
cervical region	C49.0	C79.89	—	D21.0	D48.1	D49.2
cheek	C49.0	C79.89	—	D21.0	D48.1	D49.2
chest (wall)	C49.3	C79.89	—	D21.3	D48.1	D49.2
chin	C49.0	C79.89	—	D21.0	D48.1	D49.2
diaphragm	C49.3	C79.89	—	D21.3	D48.1	D49.2
ear (external)	C49.0	C79.89	—	D21.0	D48.1	D49.2
elbow	C49.1-☑	C79.89	—	D21.1-☑	D48.1	D49.2
extrarectal	C49.5	C79.89	—	D21.5	D48.1	D49.2
extremity	C49.9	C79.89	—	D21.9	D48.1	D49.2
lower	C49.2-☑	C79.89	—	D21.2-☑	D48.1	D49.2
upper	C49.1-☑	C79.89	—	D21.1-☑	D48.1	D49.2
eyelid	C49.0	C79.89	—	D21.0	D48.1	D49.2
face	C49.0	C79.89	—	D21.0	D48.1	D49.2
finger	C49.1-☑	C79.89	—	D21.1-☑	D48.1	D49.2
flank	C49.6	C79.89	—	D21.6	D48.1	D49.2
foot	C49.2-☑	C79.89	—	D21.2-☑	D48.1	D49.2
forearm	C49.1-☑	C79.89	—	D21.1-☑	D48.1	D49.2
forehead	C49.0	C79.89	—	D21.0	D48.1	D49.2
gastric	C49.4	C79.89	—	D21.4	D48.1	D49.2
gastrointestinal	C49.4	C79.89	—	D21.4	D48.1	D49.2
gluteal region	C49.5	C79.89	—	D21.5	D48.1	D49.2
great vessels NEC	C49.3	C79.89	—	D21.3	D48.1	D49.2
groin	C49.5	C79.89	—	D21.5	D48.1	D49.2
hand	C49.1-☑	C79.89	—	D21.1-☑	D48.1	D49.2
head	C49.0	C79.89	—	D21.0	D48.1	D49.2

	Malignant Primary	Malignant Secondary	Ca in situ	Benign	Uncertain Behavior	Unspecified Behavior
Neoplasm, neoplastic — *continued*						
connective tissue — *continued*						
heel	C49.2-☑	C79.89	—	D21.2-☑	D48.1	D49.2
hip	C49.2-☑	C79.89	—	D21.2-☑	D48.1	D49.2
hypochondrium	C49.4	C79.89	—	D21.4	D48.1	D49.2
iliopsoas muscle	C49.5	C79.89	—	D21.5	D48.1	D49.2
infraclavicular region	C49.3	C79.89	—	D21.3	D48.1	D49.2
inguinal (canal) (region)	C49.5	C79.89	—	D21.5	D48.1	D49.2
intestinal	C49.4	C79.89	—	D21.4	D48.1	D49.2
intrathoracic	C49.3	C79.89	—	D21.3	D48.1	D49.2
ischiorectal fossa	C49.5	C79.89	—	D21.5	D48.1	D49.2
jaw	C03.9	C79.89	D00.03	D10.39	D48.1	D49.0
knee	C49.2-☑	C79.89	—	D21.2-☑	D48.1	D49.2
leg	C49.2-☑	C79.89	—	D21.2-☑	D48.1	D49.2
limb NEC	C49.9	C79.89	—	D21.9	D48.1	D49.2
lower	C49.2-☑	C79.89	—	D21.2-☑	D48.1	D49.2
upper	C49.1-☑	C79.89	—	D21.1-☑	D48.1	D49.2
nates	C49.5	C79.89	—	D21.5	D48.1	D49.2
neck	C49.0	C79.89	—	D21.0	D48.1	D49.2
orbit	C69.6-☑	C79.49	D09.2-☑	D31.6-☑	D48.1	D49.89
overlapping lesion	C49.8	—	—	—	—	—
pararectal	C49.5	C79.89	—	D21.5	D48.1	D49.2
para-urethral	C49.5	C79.89	—	D21.5	D48.1	D49.2
paravaginal	C49.5	C79.89	—	D21.5	D48.1	D49.2
pelvis (floor)	C49.5	C79.89	—	D21.5	D48.1	D49.2
pelvo-abdominal	C49.8	C79.89	—	D21.6	D48.1	D49.2
perineum	C49.5	C79.89	—	D21.5	D48.1	D49.2
perirectal (tissue)	C49.5	C79.89	—	D21.5	D48.1	D49.2
periurethral (tissue)	C49.5	C79.89	—	D21.5	D48.1	D49.2
popliteal fossa or space	C49.2-☑	C79.89	—	D21.2-☑	D48.1	D49.2
presacral	C49.5	C79.89	—	D21.5	D48.1	D49.2
psoas muscle	C49.4	C79.89	—	D21.4	D48.1	D49.2
pterygoid fossa	C49.0	C79.89	—	D21.0	D48.1	D49.2
rectovaginal septum or wall	C49.5	C79.89	—	D21.5	D48.1	D49.2
rectovesical	C49.5	C79.89	—	D21.5	D48.1	D49.2
retroperitoneum	C48.0	C78.6	—	D20.0	D48.3	D49.0
sacrococcygeal region	C49.5	C79.89	—	D21.5	D48.1	D49.2
scalp	C49.0	C79.89	—	D21.0	D48.1	D49.2
scapular region	C49.3	C79.89	—	D21.3	D48.1	D49.2
shoulder	C49.1-☑	C79.89	—	D21.1-☑	D48.1	D49.2
skin (dermis) NEC — *see also* Neoplasm, skin, by site	C44.90	C79.2	D04.9	D23.9	D48.5	D49.2
stomach	C49.4	C79.89	—	D21.4	D48.1	D49.2
submental	C49.0	C79.89	—	D21.0	D48.1	D49.2
supraclavicular region	C49.0	C79.89	—	D21.0	D48.1	D49.2
temple	C49.0	C79.89	—	D21.0	D48.1	D49.2
temporal region	C49.0	C79.89	—	D21.0	D48.1	D49.2
thigh	C49.2-☑	C79.89	—	D21.2-☑	D48.1	D49.2
thoracic (duct) (wall)	C49.3	C79.89	—	D21.3	D48.1	D49.2
thorax	C49.3	C79.89	—	D21.3	D48.1	D49.2
thumb	C49.1-☑	C79.89	—	D21.1-☑	D48.1	D49.2
toe	C49.2-☑	C79.89	—	D21.2-☑	D48.1	D49.2
trunk	C49.6	C79.89	—	D21.6	D48.1	D49.2
umbilicus	C49.4	C79.89	—	D21.4	D48.1	D49.2
vesicorectal	C49.5	C79.89	—	D21.5	D48.1	D49.2
wrist	C49.1-☑	C79.89	—	D21.1-☑	D48.1	D49.2
conus medullaris	C72.0	C79.49	—	D33.4	D43.4	D49.7
cord (true) (vocal)	C32.0	C78.39	D02.0	D14.1	D38.0	D49.1
false	C32.1	C78.39	D02.0	D14.1	D38.0	D49.1
spermatic	C63.1-☑	C79.82	D07.69	D29.8	D40.8	D49.59
spinal (cervical) (lumbar) (thoracic)	C72.0	C79.49	—	D33.4	D43.4	D49.7
cornea (limbus)	C69.1-☑	C79.49	D09.2-☑	D31.1-☑	D48.7	D49.89
corpus						
albicans	C56.-☑	C79.6-☑	D07.39	D27.-☑	D39.1-☑	D49.59
callosum, brain	C71.0	C79.31	—	D33.2	D43.2	D49.6
Neoplasm, neoplastic — *continued*						
corpus — *continued*						
cavernosum	C60.2	C79.82	D07.4	D29.0	D40.8	D49.59
gastric	C16.2	C78.89	D00.2	D13.1	D37.1	D49.0
overlapping sites	C54.8	—	—	—	—	—
penis	C60.2	C79.82	D07.4	D29.0	D40.8	D49.59
striatum, cerebrum	C71.0	C79.31	—	D33.0	D43.0	D49.6
uteri	C54.9	C79.82	D07.0	D26.1	D39.0	D49.59
isthmus	C54.0	C79.82	D07.0	D26.1	D39.0	D49.59
cortex						
adrenal	C74.0-☑	C79.7-☑	D09.3	D35.0-☑	D44.1-☑	D49.7
cerebral	C71.0	C79.31	—	D33.0	D43.0	D49.6
costal cartilage	C41.3	C79.51	—	D16.7	D48.0	D49.2
costovertebral joint	C41.3	C79.51	—	D16.7	D48.0	D49.2
Cowper's gland	C68.0	C79.19	D09.19	D30.4	D41.3	D49.59
cranial (fossa, any)	C71.9	C79.31	—	D33.2	D43.2	D49.6
meninges	C70.0	C79.32	—	D32.0	D42.0	D49.7
nerve	C72.50	C79.49	—	D33.3	D43.3	D49.7
specified NEC	C72.59	C79.49	—	D33.3	D43.3	D49.7
craniobuccal pouch	C75.2	C79.89	D09.3	D35.2	D44.3	D49.7
craniopharyngeal (duct) (pouch)	C75.2	C79.89	D09.3	D35.3	D44.4	D49.7
cricoid	C13.0	C79.89	D00.08	D10.7	D37.05	D49.0
cartilage	C32.3	C78.39	D02.0	D14.1	D38.0	D49.1
cricopharynx	C13.0	C79.89	D00.08	D10.7	D37.05	D49.0
crypt of Morgagni	C21.8	C78.5	D01.3	D12.9	D37.8	D49.0
crystalline lens	C69.4-☑	C79.49	D09.2-☑	D31.4-☑	D48.7	D49.89
cul-de-sac (Douglas')	C48.1	C78.6	—	D20.1	D48.4	D49.0
cuneiform cartilage	C32.3	C78.39	D02.0	D14.1	D38.0	D49.1
cutaneous — *see* Neoplasm, skin						
cutis — *see* Neoplasm, skin						
cystic (bile) duct (common)	C24.0	C78.89	D01.5	D13.5	D37.6	D49.0
dermis — *see* Neoplasm, skin						
diaphragm	C49.3	C79.89	—	D21.3	D48.1	D49.2
digestive organs, system, tube, or tract NEC	C26.9	C78.89	D01.9	D13.9	D37.9	D49.0
disc, intervertebral	C41.2	C79.51	—	D16.6	D48.0	D49.2
disease, generalized	C80.0	—	—	—	—	—
disseminated	C80.0	—	—	—	—	—
Douglas' cul-de-sac or pouch	C48.1	C78.6	—	D20.1	D48.4	D49.0
duodenojejunal junction	C17.8	C78.4	D01.49	D13.39	D37.2	D49.0
duodenum	C17.0	C78.4	D01.49	D13.2	D37.2	D49.0
dura (cranial) (mater)	C70.9	C79.49	—	D32.9	D42.9	D49.7
cerebral	C70.0	C79.32	—	D32.0	D42.0	D49.7
spinal	C70.1	C79.49	—	D32.1	D42.1	D49.7
ear (external) — *see also* Neoplasm, skin, ear	C44.20-☑	C79.2	D04.2-☑	D23.2-☑	D48.5	D49.2
auricle or auris — *see also* Neoplasm, skin, ear	C44.20-☑	C79.2	D04.2-☑	D23.2-☑	D48.5	D49.2
canal, external — *see also* Neoplasm, skin, ear	C44.20-☑	C79.2	D04.2-☑	D23.2-☑	D48.5	D49.2
cartilage	C49.0	C79.89	—	D21.0	D48.1	D49.2
external meatus — *see also* Neoplasm, skin, ear	C44.20-☑	C79.2	D04.2-☑	D23.2-☑	D48.5	D49.2
inner	C30.1	C78.39	D02.3	D14.0	D38.5	D49.1
lobule — *see also* Neoplasm, skin, ear	C44.20-☑	C79.2	D04.2-☑	D23.2-☑	D48.5	D49.2
middle	C30.1	C78.39	D02.3	D14.0	D38.5	D49.1
overlapping lesion with accessory sinuses	C31.8	—	—	—	—	—

☑ Additional Character Required — Refer to the Tabular List for Character Selection

	Malignant Primary	Malignant Secondary	Ca in situ	Benign	Uncertain Behavior	Unspecified Behavior
Neoplasm, neoplastic — *continued*						
ear — *see also* Neoplasm, skin, ear — *continued*						
skin	C44.20-☑	C79.2	D04.2-☑	D23.2-☑	D48.5	D49.2
basal cell carcinoma	C44.21-☑	—	—	—	—	—
specified type NEC	C44.29-☑	—	—	—	—	—
squamous cell carcinoma	C44.22-☑	—	—	—	—	—
earlobe	C44.20-☑	C79.2	D04.2-☑	D23.2-☑	D48.5	D49.2
basal cell carcinoma	C44.21-☑	—	—	—	—	—
specified type NEC	C44.29-☑	—	—	—	—	—
squamous cell carcinoma	C44.22-☑	—	—	—	—	—
ejaculatory duct	C63.7	C79.82	D07.69	D29.8	D40.8	D49.59
elbow NEC	C76.4-☑	C79.89	D04.6-☑	D36.7	D48.7	D49.89
endocardium	C38.0	C79.89	—	D15.1	D48.7	D49.89
endocervix (canal) (gland)	C53.0	C79.82	D06.0	D26.0	D39.0	D49.59
endocrine gland NEC	C75.9	C79.89	D09.3	D35.9	D44.9	D49.7
pluriglandular	C75.8	C79.89	D09.3	D35.7	D44.9	D49.7
endometrium (gland) (stroma)	C54.1	C79.82	D07.0	D26.1	D39.0	D49.59
ensiform cartilage	C41.3	C79.51	—	D16.7	D48.0	D49.2
enteric — *see* Neoplasm, intestine						
ependyma (brain)	C71.5	C79.31	—	D33.0	D43.0	D49.6
fourth ventricle	C71.7	C79.31	—	D33.1	D43.1	D49.6
epicardium	C38.0	C79.89	—	D15.1	D48.7	D49.89
epididymis	C63.0-☑	C79.82	D07.69	D29.3-☑	D40.8	D49.59
epidural	C72.9	C79.49	—	D33.9	D43.9	D49.7
epiglottis	C32.1	C78.39	D02.0	D14.1	D38.0	D49.1
anterior aspect or surface	C10.1	C79.89	D00.08	D10.5	D37.05	D49.0
cartilage	C32.3	C78.39	D02.0	D14.1	D38.0	D49.1
free border (margin)	C10.1	C79.89	D00.08	D10.5	D37.05	D49.0
junctional region	C10.8	C79.89	D00.08	D10.5	D37.05	D49.0
posterior (laryngeal) surface	C32.1	C78.39	D02.0	D14.1	D38.0	D49.1
suprahyoid portion	C32.1	C78.39	D02.0	D14.1	D38.0	D49.1
esophagogastric junction	C16.0	C78.89	D00.2	D13.1	D37.1	D49.0
esophagus	C15.9	C78.89	D00.1	D13.0	D37.8	D49.0
abdominal	C15.5	C78.89	D00.1	D13.0	D37.8	D49.0
cervical	C15.3	C78.89	D00.1	D13.0	D37.8	D49.0
distal (third)	C15.5	C78.89	D00.1	D13.0	D37.8	D49.0
lower (third)	C15.5	C78.89	D00.1	D13.0	D37.8	D49.0
middle (third)	C15.4	C78.89	D00.1	D13.0	D37.8	D49.0
overlapping lesion	C15.8	—	—	—	—	—
proximal (third)	C15.3	C78.89	D00.1	D13.0	D37.8	D49.0
thoracic	C15.4	C78.89	D00.1	D13.0	D37.8	D49.0
upper (third)	C15.3	C78.89	D00.1	D13.0	D37.8	D49.0
ethmoid (sinus)	C31.1	C78.39	D02.3	D14.0	D38.5	D49.1
bone or labyrinth	C41.0	C79.51	—	D16.4	D48.0	D49.2
eustachian tube	C30.1	C78.39	D02.3	D14.0	D38.5	D49.1
exocervix	C53.1	C79.82	D06.1	D26.0	D39.0	D49.59
external						
meatus (ear) — *see also* Neoplasm, skin, ear	C44.20-☑	C79.2	D04.2-☑	D23.2-☑	D48.5	D49.2
os, cervix uteri	C53.1	C79.82	D06.1	D26.0	D39.0	D49.59
extradural	C72.9	C79.49	—	D33.9	D43.9	D49.7
extrahepatic (bile) duct	C24.0	C78.89	D01.5	D13.5	D37.6	D49.0
overlapping lesion with gallbladder	C24.8	—	—	—	—	—
extraocular muscle	C69.6-☑	C79.49	D09.2-☑	D31.6-☑	D48.7	D49.89
extrarectal	C76.3	C79.89	D09.8	D36.7	D48.7	D49.89
extremity	C76.8	C79.89	D04.8	D36.7	D48.7	D49.89

	Malignant Primary	Malignant Secondary	Ca in situ	Benign	Uncertain Behavior	Unspecified Behavior
Neoplasm, neoplastic — *continued*						
extremity — *continued*						
lower	C76.5-☑	C79.89	D04.7-☑	D36.7	D48.7	D49.89
upper	C76.4-☑	C79.89	D04.6-☑	D36.7	D48.7	D49.89
eyeball	C69.9-☑	C79.49	D09.2-☑	D31.9-☑	D48.7	D49.89
eyebrow	C44.309	C79.2	D04.39	D23.39	D48.5	D49.2
basal cell carcinoma	C44.319	—	—	—	—	—
specified type NEC	C44.399	—	—	—	—	—
squamous cell carcinoma	C44.329	—	—	—	—	—
eyelid (lower) (skin) (upper)	C44.10-☑	—	—	—	—	—
basal cell carcinoma	C44.11-☑	—	—	—	—	—
cartilage	C49.0	C79.89	—	D21.0	D48.1	D49.2
sebaceous cell	C44.13-☑	—	—	—	—	—
specified type NEC	C44.19-☑	—	—	—	—	—
squamous cell carcinoma	C44.12-☑	—	—	—	—	—
eye NEC	C69.9-☑	C79.49	D09.2-☑	D31.9-☑	D48.7	D49.89
overlapping sites	C69.8-☑	—	—	—	—	—
face NEC	C76.0	C79.89	D04.39	D36.7	D48.7	D49.89
fallopian tube (accessory)	C57.0-☑	C79.82	D07.39	D28.2	D39.8	D49.59
falx (cerebella) (cerebri)	C70.0	C79.32	—	D32.0	D42.0	D49.7
fascia — *see also* Neoplasm, connective tissue						
palmar	C49.1-☑	C79.89	—	D21.1-☑	D48.1	D49.2
plantar	C49.2-☑	C79.89	—	D21.2-☑	D48.1	D49.2
fatty tissue — *see* Neoplasm, connective tissue						
fauces, faucial NEC	C10.9	C79.89	D00.08	D10.5	D37.05	D49.0
pillars	C09.1	C79.89	D00.08	D10.5	D37.05	D49.0
tonsil	C09.9	C79.89	D00.08	D10.4	D37.05	D49.0
femur (any part)	C40.2-☑	—	—	D16.2-☑	—	—
fetal membrane	C58	C79.82	D07.0	D26.7	D39.2	D49.59
fibrous tissue — *see* Neoplasm, connective tissue						
fibula (any part)	C40.2-☑	C79.51	—	D16.2-☑	—	—
filum terminale	C72.0	C79.49	—	D33.4	D43.4	D49.7
finger NEC	C76.4-☑	C79.89	D04.6-☑	D36.7	D48.7	D49.89
flank NEC	C76.8	C79.89	D04.5	D36.7	D48.7	D49.89
follicle, nabothian	C53.0	C79.82	D06.0	D26.0	D39.0	D49.59
foot NEC	C76.5-☑	C79.89	D04.7-☑	D36.7	D48.7	D49.89
forearm NEC	C76.4-☑	C79.89	D04.6-☑	D36.7	D48.7	D49.89
forehead (skin)	C44.309	C79.2	D04.39	D23.39	D48.5	D49.2
basal cell carcinoma	C44.319	—	—	—	—	—
specified type NEC	C44.399	—	—	—	—	—
squamous cell carcinoma	C44.329	—	—	—	—	—
foreskin	C60.0	C79.82	D07.4	D29.0	D40.8	D49.59
fornix						
pharyngeal	C11.3	C79.89	D00.08	D10.6	D37.05	D49.0
vagina	C52	C79.82	D07.2	D28.1	D39.8	D49.59
fossa (of)						
anterior (cranial)	C71.9	C79.31	—	D33.2	D43.2	D49.6
cranial	C71.9	C79.31	—	D33.2	D43.2	D49.6
ischiorectal	C76.3	C79.89	D09.8	D36.7	D48.7	D49.89
middle (cranial)	C71.9	C79.31	—	D33.2	D43.2	D49.6
piriform	C12	C79.89	D00.08	D10.7	D37.05	D49.0
pituitary	C75.1	C79.89	D09.3	D35.2	D44.3	D49.7
posterior (cranial)	C71.9	C79.31	—	D33.2	D43.2	D49.6
pterygoid	C49.0	C79.89	—	D21.0	D48.1	D49.2
pyriform	C12	C79.89	D00.08	D10.7	D37.05	D49.0
Rosenmuller	C11.2	C79.89	D00.08	D10.6	D37.05	D49.0
tonsillar	C09.0	C79.89	D00.08	D10.5	D37.05	D49.0
fourchette	C51.9	C79.82	D07.1	D28.0	D39.8	D49.59
frenulum						
labii — *see* Neoplasm, lip, internal						

☑ **Additional Character Required — Refer to the Tabular List for Character Selection**

	Malignant Primary	Malignant Secondary	Ca in situ	Benign	Uncertain Behavior	Unspecified Behavior
Neoplasm, neoplastic — *continued*						
frenulum — *continued*						
linguae	C02.2	C79.89	D00.07	D10.1	D37.02	D49.Ø
frontal						
bone	C41.Ø	C79.51	—	D16.4	D48.Ø	D49.2
lobe, brain	C71.1	C79.31	—	D33.Ø	D43.Ø	D49.6
pole	C71.1	C79.31	—	D33.Ø	D43.Ø	D49.6
sinus	C31.2	C78.39	D02.3	D14.Ø	D38.5	D49.1
fundus						
stomach	C16.1	C78.89	DØØ.2	D13.1	D37.1	D49.Ø
uterus	C54.3	C79.82	D07.Ø	D26.1	D39.Ø	D49.59
gallbladder	C23	C78.89	DØ1.5	D13.5	D37.6	D49.Ø
overlapping lesion with extrahepatic bile ducts	C24.8	—	—	—	—	—
gall duct (extrahepatic)	C24.Ø	C78.89	DØ1.5	D13.5	D37.6	D49.Ø
intrahepatic	C22.1	C78.7	DØ1.5	D13.4	D37.6	D49.Ø
ganglia — *see also* Neoplasm, nerve, peripheral	C47.9	C79.89	—	D36.1Ø	D48.2	D49.2
basal	C71.Ø	C79.31	—	D33.Ø	D43.Ø	D49.6
cranial nerve	C72.5Ø	C79.49	—	D33.3	D43.3	D49.7
Gartner's duct	C52	C79.82	D07.2	D28.1	D39.8	D49.59
gastric — *see* Neoplasm, stomach						
gastrocolic	C26.9	C78.89	DØ1.9	D13.9	D37.9	D49.Ø
gastroesophageal junction	C16.Ø	C78.89	DØØ.2	D13.1	D37.1	D49.Ø
gastrointestinal (tract) NEC	C26.9	C78.89	DØ1.9	D13.9	D37.9	D49.Ø
generalized	C8Ø.Ø	—	—	—	—	—
genital organ or tract						
female NEC	C57.9	C79.82	D07.3Ø	D28.9	D39.9	D49.59
overlapping lesion	C57.8	—	—	—	—	—
specified site NEC	C57.7	C79.82	D07.39	D28.7	D39.8	D49.59
male NEC	C63.9	C79.82	D07.6Ø	D29.9	D4Ø.9	D49.59
overlapping lesion	C63.8	—	—	—	—	—
specified site NEC	C63.7	C79.82	D07.69	D29.8	D4Ø.8	D49.59
genitourinary tract						
female	C57.9	C79.82	D07.3Ø	D28.9	D39.9	D49.59
male	C63.9	C79.82	D07.6Ø	D29.9	D4Ø.9	D49.59
gingiva (alveolar) (marginal)	CØ3.9	C79.89	DØØ.Ø3	D1Ø.39	D37.Ø9	D49.Ø
lower	CØ3.1	C79.89	DØØ.Ø3	D1Ø.39	D37.Ø9	D49.Ø
mandibular	CØ3.1	C79.89	DØØ.Ø3	D1Ø.39	D37.Ø9	D49.Ø
maxillary	CØ3.Ø	C79.89	DØØ.Ø3	D1Ø.39	D37.Ø9	D49.Ø
upper	CØ3.Ø	C79.89	DØØ.Ø3	D1Ø.39	D37.Ø9	D49.Ø
gland, glandular (lymphatic) (system) — *see also* Neoplasm, lymph gland						
endocrine NEC	C75.9	C79.89	DØ9.3	D35.9	D44.9	D49.7
salivary — *see* Neoplasm, salivary gland						
glans penis	C6Ø.1	C79.82	D07.4	D29.Ø	D4Ø.8	D49.59
globus pallidus	C71.Ø	C79.31	—	D33.Ø	D43.Ø	D49.6
glomus						
coccygeal	C49.5	C79.89	—	D21.5	D48.1	D49.2
jugularis	C75.5	C79.89	—	D35.6	D44.7	D49.7
glosso-epiglottic fold(s)	C1Ø.1	C79.89	DØØ.Ø8	D1Ø.5	D37.Ø5	D49.Ø
glossopalatine fold	CØ9.1	C79.89	DØØ.Ø8	D1Ø.5	D37.Ø5	D49.Ø
glossopharyngeal sulcus	CØ9.Ø	C79.89	DØØ.Ø8	D1Ø.5	D37.Ø5	D49.Ø
glottis	C32.Ø	C78.39	DØ2.Ø	D14.1	D38.Ø	D49.1
gluteal region	C76.3	C79.89	DØ4.5	D36.7	D48.7	D49.89
great vessels NEC	C49.3	C79.89	—	D21.3	D48.1	D49.2
groin NEC	C76.3	C79.89	DØ4.5	D36.7	D48.7	D49.89
gum	CØ3.9	C79.89	DØØ.Ø3	D1Ø.39	D37.Ø9	D49.Ø
lower	CØ3.1	C79.89	DØØ.Ø3	D1Ø.39	D37.Ø9	D49.Ø
upper	CØ3.Ø	C79.89	DØØ.Ø3	D1Ø.39	D37.Ø9	D49.Ø
hand NEC	C76.4-☑	C79.89	DØ4.6-☑	D36.7	D48.7	D49.89
head NEC	C76.Ø	C79.89	DØ4.4	D36.7	D48.7	D49.89
heart	C38.Ø	C79.89	—	D15.1	D48.7	D49.89

	Malignant Primary	Malignant Secondary	Ca in situ	Benign	Uncertain Behavior	Unspecified Behavior
Neoplasm, neoplastic — *continued*						
heel NEC	C76.5-☑	C79.89	DØ4.7-☑	D36.7	D48.7	D49.89
helix — *see also* Neoplasm, skin, ear	C44.2Ø-☑	C79.2	DØ4.2-☑	D23.2-☑	D48.5	D49.2
hematopoietic, hemopoietic tissue NEC	C96.9	—	—	—	—	—
specified NEC	C96.Z	—	—	—	—	—
hemisphere, cerebral	C71.Ø	C79.31	—	D33.Ø	D43.Ø	D49.6
hemorrhoidal zone	C21.1	C78.5	DØ1.3	D12.9	D37.8	D49.Ø
hepatic — *see also* Index to disease, by histology	C22.9	C78.7	DØ1.5	D13.4	D37.6	D49.Ø
duct (bile)	C24.Ø	C78.89	DØ1.5	D13.5	D37.6	D49.Ø
flexure (colon)	C18.3	C78.5	DØ1.Ø	D12.3	D37.4	D49.Ø
primary	C22.8	C78.7	DØ1.5	D13.4	D37.6	D49.Ø
hepatobiliary	C24.9	C78.89	DØ1.5	D13.5	D37.6	D49.Ø
hepatoblastoma	C22.2	C78.7	DØ1.5	D13.4	D37.6	D49.Ø
hepatoma	C22.Ø	C78.7	DØ1.5	D13.4	D37.6	D49.Ø
hilus of lung	C34.Ø-☑	C78.Ø-☑	DØ2.2-☑	D14.3-☑	D38.1	D49.1
hippocampus, brain	C71.2	C79.31	—	D33.Ø	D43.Ø	D49.6
hip NEC	C76.5-☑	C79.89	DØ4.7-☑	D36.7	D48.7	D49.89
humerus (any part)	C4Ø.Ø-☑	C79.51	—	D16.Ø-☑	—	—
hymen	C52	C79.82	D07.2	D28.1	D39.8	D49.59
hypopharynx, hypopharyngeal NEC	C13.9	C79.89	DØØ.Ø8	D1Ø.7	D37.Ø5	D49.Ø
overlapping lesion	C13.8	—	—	—	—	—
postcricoid region	C13.Ø	C79.89	DØØ.Ø8	D1Ø.7	D37.Ø5	D49.Ø
posterior wall	C13.2	C79.89	DØØ.Ø8	D1Ø.7	D37.Ø5	D49.Ø
pyriform fossa (sinus)	C12	C79.89	DØØ.Ø8	D1Ø.7	D37.Ø5	D49.Ø
hypophysis	C75.1	C79.89	DØ9.3	D35.2	D44.3	D49.7
hypothalamus	C71.Ø	C79.31	—	D33.Ø	D43.Ø	D49.6
ileocecum, ileocecal (coil) (junction) (valve)	C18.Ø	C78.5	DØ1.Ø	D12.Ø	D37.4	D49.Ø
ileum	C17.2	C78.4	DØ1.49	D13.39	D37.2	D49.Ø
ilium	C41.4	C79.51	—	D16.8	D48.Ø	D49.2
immunoproliferative NEC	C88.9	—	—	—	—	—
infraclavicular (region)	C76.1	C79.89	DØ4.5	D36.7	D48.7	D49.89
inguinal (region)	C76.3	C79.89	DØ4.5	D36.7	D48.7	D49.89
insula	C71.Ø	C79.31	—	D33.Ø	D43.Ø	D49.6
insular tissue (pancreas)	C25.4	C78.89	DØ1.7	D13.7	D37.8	D49.Ø
brain	C71.Ø	C79.31	—	D33.Ø	D43.Ø	D49.6
interarytenoid fold	C13.1	C78.39	DØØ.Ø8	D1Ø.7	D37.Ø5	D49.Ø
hypopharyngeal aspect	C13.1	C79.89	DØØ.Ø8	D1Ø.7	D37.Ø5	D49.Ø
laryngeal aspect	C32.1	C78.39	DØ2.Ø	D14.1	D38.Ø	D49.1
marginal zone	C13.1	C79.89	DØØ.Ø8	D1Ø.7	D37.Ø5	D49.Ø
interdental papillae	CØ3.9	C79.89	DØØ.Ø3	D1Ø.39	D37.Ø9	D49.Ø
lower	CØ3.1	C79.89	DØØ.Ø3	D1Ø.39	D37.Ø9	D49.Ø
upper	CØ3.Ø	C79.89	DØØ.Ø3	D1Ø.39	D37.Ø9	D49.Ø
internal						
capsule	C71.Ø	C79.31	—	D33.Ø	D43.Ø	D49.6
os (cervix)	C53.Ø	C79.82	DØ6.Ø	D26.Ø	D39.Ø	D49.59
intervertebral cartilage or disc	C41.2	C79.51	—	D16.6	D48.Ø	D49.2
intestine, intestinal	C26.Ø	C78.8Ø	DØ1.4Ø	D13.9	D37.8	D49.Ø
large	C18.9	C78.5	DØ1.Ø	D12.6	D37.4	D49.Ø
appendix	C18.1	C78.5	DØ1.Ø	D12.1	D37.3	D49.Ø
caput coli	C18.Ø	C78.5	DØ1.Ø	D12.Ø	D37.4	D49.Ø
cecum	C18.Ø	C78.5	DØ1.Ø	D12.Ø	D37.4	D49.Ø
colon	C18.9	C78.5	DØ1.Ø	D12.6	D37.4	D49.Ø
and rectum	C19	C78.5	DØ1.1	D12.7	D37.5	D49.Ø
ascending	C18.2	C78.5	DØ1.Ø	D12.2	D37.4	D49.Ø
caput	C18.Ø	C78.5	DØ1.Ø	D12.Ø	D37.4	D49.Ø
descending	C18.6	C78.5	DØ1.Ø	D12.4	D37.4	D49.Ø
distal	C18.6	C78.5	DØ1.Ø	D12.4	D37.4	D49.Ø

	Malignant Primary	Malignant Secondary	Ca in situ	Benign	Uncertain Behavior	Unspecified Behavior
Neoplasm, neoplastic — *continued*						
intestine, intestinal — *continued*						
large — *continued*						
colon — *continued*						
left	C18.6	C78.5	DØ1.Ø	D12.4	D37.4	D49.Ø
overlapping lesion	C18.8	—	—	—	—	—
pelvic	C18.7	C78.5	DØ1.Ø	D12.5	D37.4	D49.Ø
right	C18.2	C78.5	DØ1.Ø	D12.2	D37.4	D49.Ø
sigmoid (flexure)	C18.7	C78.5	DØ1.Ø	D12.5	D37.4	D49.Ø
transverse	C18.4	C78.5	DØ1.Ø	D12.3	D37.4	D49.Ø
hepatic flexure	C18.3	C78.5	DØ1.Ø	D12.3	D37.4	D49.Ø
ileocecum, ileocecal (coil) (valve)	C18.Ø	C78.5	DØ1.Ø	D12.Ø	D37.4	D49.Ø
overlapping lesion	C18.8	—	—	—	—	—
sigmoid flexure (lower) (upper)	C18.7	C78.5	DØ1.Ø	D12.5	D37.4	D49.Ø
splenic flexure	C18.5	C78.5	DØ1.Ø	D12.3	D37.4	D49.Ø
small	C17.9	C78.4	DØ1.4Ø	D13.3Ø	D37.2	D49.Ø
duodenum	C17.Ø	C78.4	DØ1.49	D13.2	D37.2	D49.Ø
ileum	C17.2	C78.4	DØ1.49	D13.39	D37.2	D49.Ø
jejunum	C17.1	C78.4	DØ1.49	D13.39	D37.2	D49.Ø
overlapping lesion	C17.8	—	—	—	—	—
tract NEC	C26.Ø	C78.89	DØ1.4Ø	D13.9	D37.8	D49.Ø
intra-abdominal	C76.2	C79.89	DØ9.8	D36.7	D48.7	D49.89
intracranial NEC	C71.9	C79.31	—	D33.2	D43.2	D49.6
intrahepatic (bile) duct	C22.1	C78.7	DØ1.5	D13.4	D37.6	D49.Ø
intraocular	C69.9-☑	C79.49	DØ9.2-☑	D31.9-☑	D48.7	D49.89
intraorbital	C69.6-☑	C79.49	DØ9.2-☑	D31.6-☑	D48.7	D49.89
intrasellar	C75.1	C79.89	DØ9.3	D35.2	D44.3	D49.7
intrathoracic (cavity) (organs)	C76.1	C79.89	DØ9.8	D15.9	D48.7	D49.89
specified NEC	C76.1	C79.89	DØ9.8	D15.7	—	—
iris	C69.4-☑	C79.49	DØ9.2-☑	D31.4-☑	D48.7	D49.89
ischiorectal (fossa)	C76.3	C79.89	DØ9.8	D36.7	D48.7	D49.89
ischium	C41.4	C79.51	—	D16.8	D48.Ø	D49.2
island of Reil	C71.Ø	C79.31	—	D33.Ø	D43.Ø	D49.6
islands or islets of Langerhans	C25.4	C78.89	DØ1.7	D13.7	D37.8	D49.Ø
isthmus uteri	C54.Ø	C79.82	DØ7.Ø	D26.1	D39.Ø	D49.59
jaw	C76.Ø	C79.89	DØ9.8	D36.7	D48.7	D49.89
bone	C41.1	C79.51	—	D16.5	D48.Ø	D49.2
lower	C41.1	C79.51	—	D16.5	—	—
upper	C41.Ø	C79.51	—	D16.4	—	—
carcinoma (any type) (lower) (upper)	C76.Ø	C79.89	—	—	—	—
skin — *see also* Neoplasm, skin, face	C44.3Ø9	C79.2	DØ4.39	D23.39	D48.5	D49.2
soft tissues	CØ3.9	C79.89	DØØ.Ø3	D1Ø.39	D37.Ø9	D49.Ø
lower	CØ3.1	C79.89	DØØ.Ø3	D1Ø.39	D37.Ø9	D49.Ø
upper	CØ3.Ø	C79.89	DØØ.Ø3	D1Ø.39	D37.Ø9	D49.Ø
jejunum	C17.1	C78.4	DØ1.49	D13.39	D37.2	D49.Ø
joint NEC — *see also* Neoplasm, bone	C41.9	C79.51	—	D16.9	D48.Ø	D49.2
acromioclavicular	C4Ø.Ø-☑	C79.51	—	D16.Ø-☑	—	—
bursa or synovial membrane — *see* Neoplasm, connective tissue						
costovertebral	C41.3	C79.51	—	D16.7	D48.Ø	D49.2
sternocostal	C41.3	C79.51	—	D16.7	D48.Ø	D49.2
temporomandibular	C41.1	C79.51	—	D16.5	D48.Ø	D49.2
junction						
anorectal	C21.8	C78.5	DØ1.3	D12.9	D37.8	D49.Ø
cardioesophageal	C16.Ø	C78.89	DØØ.2	D13.1	D37.1	D49.Ø
esophagogastric	C16.Ø	C78.89	DØØ.2	D13.1	D37.1	D49.Ø
gastroesophageal	C16.Ø	C78.89	DØØ.2	D13.1	D37.1	D49.Ø
hard and soft palate	CØ5.9	C79.89	DØØ.ØØ	D1Ø.39	D37.Ø9	D49.Ø
ileocecal	C18.Ø	C78.5	DØ1.Ø	D12.Ø	D37.4	D49.Ø

	Malignant Primary	Malignant Secondary	Ca in situ	Benign	Uncertain Behavior	Unspecified Behavior
Neoplasm, neoplastic — *continued*						
junction — *continued*						
pelvirectal	C19	C78.5	DØ1.1	D12.7	D37.5	D49.Ø
pelviureteric	C65.-☑	C79.Ø-☑	DØ9.19	D3Ø.1-☑	D41.1-☑	D49.59
rectosigmoid	C19	C78.5	DØ1.1	D12.7	D37.5	D49.Ø
squamocolumnar, of cervix	C53.8	C79.82	DØ6.7	D26.Ø	D39.Ø	D49.59
Kaposi's sarcoma — *see* Kaposi's, sarcoma						
kidney (parenchymal)	C64.-☑	C79.Ø-☑	DØ9.19	D3Ø.Ø-☑	D41.Ø-☑	D49.51-☑
calyx	C65.-☑	C79.Ø-☑	DØ9.19	D3Ø.1-☑	D41.1-☑	D49.51-☑
hilus	C65.-☑	C79.Ø-☑	DØ9.19	D3Ø.1-☑	D41.1-☑	D49.51-☑
pelvis	C65.-☑	C79.Ø-☑	DØ9.19	D3Ø.1-☑	D41.1-☑	D49.51-☑
knee NEC	C76.5-☑	C79.89	DØ4.7-☑	D36.7	D48.7	D49.89
labia (skin)	C51.9	C79.82	DØ7.1	D28.Ø	D39.8	D49.59
majora	C51.Ø	C79.82	DØ7.1	D28.Ø	D39.8	D49.59
minora	C51.1	C79.82	DØ7.1	D28.Ø	D39.8	D49.59
labial — *see also* Neoplasm, lip	CØØ.9	C79.89	DØØ.Ø1	D1Ø.Ø	D37.Ø1	D49.Ø
sulcus (lower) (upper)	CØ6.1	C79.89	DØØ.Ø2	D1Ø.39	D37.Ø9	D49.Ø
labium (skin)	C51.9	C79.82	DØ7.1	D28.Ø	D39.8	D49.59
majus	C51.Ø	C79.82	DØ7.1	D28.Ø	D39.8	D49.59
minus	C51.1	C79.82	DØ7.1	D28.Ø	D39.8	D49.59
lacrimal						
canaliculi	C69.5-☑	C79.49	DØ9.2-☑	D31.5-☑	D48.7	D49.89
duct (nasal)	C69.5-☑	C79.49	DØ9.2-☑	D31.5-☑	D48.7	D49.89
gland	C69.5-☑	C79.49	DØ9.2-☑	D31.5-☑	D48.7	D49.89
punctum	C69.5-☑	C79.49	DØ9.2-☑	D31.5-☑	D48.7	D49.89
sac	C69.5-☑	C79.49	DØ9.2-☑	D31.5-☑	D48.7	D49.89
Langerhans, islands or islets	C25.4	C78.89	DØ1.7	D13.7	D37.8	D49.Ø
laryngopharynx	C13.9	C79.89	DØØ.Ø8	D1Ø.7	D37.Ø5	D49.Ø
larynx, laryngeal NEC	C32.9	C78.39	DØ2.Ø	D14.1	D38.Ø	D49.1
aryepiglottic fold	C32.1	C78.39	DØ2.Ø	D14.1	D38.Ø	D49.1
cartilage (arytenoid) (cricoid) (cuneiform) (thyroid)	C32.3	C78.39	DØ2.Ø	D14.1	D38.Ø	D49.1
commissure (anterior) (posterior)	C32.Ø	C78.39	DØ2.Ø	D14.1	D38.Ø	D49.1
extrinsic NEC	C32.1	C78.39	DØ2.Ø	D14.1	D38.Ø	D49.1
meaning hypopharynx	C13.9	C79.89	DØØ.Ø8	D1Ø.7	D37.Ø5	D49.Ø
interarytenoid fold	C32.1	C78.39	DØ2.Ø	D14.1	D38.Ø	D49.1
intrinsic	C32.Ø	C78.39	DØ2.Ø	D14.1	D38.Ø	D49.1
overlapping lesion	C32.8	—	—	—	—	—
ventricular band	C32.1	C78.39	DØ2.Ø	D14.1	D38.Ø	D49.1
leg NEC	C76.5-☑	C79.89	DØ4.7-☑	D36.7	D48.7	D49.89
lens, crystalline	C69.4-☑	C79.49	DØ9.2-☑	D31.4-☑	D48.7	D49.89
lid (lower) (upper)	C44.1Ø-☑	C79.2	DØ4.1-☑	D23.1-☑	D48.5	D49.2
basal cell carcinoma	C44.11-☑	—	—	—	—	—
sebaceous cell	C44.13-☑	—	—	—	—	—
specified type NEC	C44.19-☑	—	—	—	—	—
squamous cell carcinoma	C44.12-☑	—	—	—	—	—
ligament — *see also* Neoplasm, connective tissue						
broad	C57.1-☑	C79.82	DØ7.39	D28.2	D39.8	D49.59
Mackenrodt's	C57.7	C79.82	DØ7.39	D28.7	D39.8	D49.59
non-uterine — *see* Neoplasm, connective tissue						
round	C57.2-☑	C79.82	—	D28.2	D39.8	D49.59
sacro-uterine	C57.3	C79.82	—	D28.2	D39.8	D49.59
uterine	C57.3	C79.82	—	D28.2	D39.8	D49.59
utero-ovarian	C57.7	C79.82	DØ7.39	D28.2	D39.8	D49.59
uterosacral	C57.3	C79.82	—	D28.2	D39.8	D49.59
limb	C76.8	C79.89	DØ4.8	D36.7	D48.7	D49.89
lower	C76.5-☑	C79.89	DØ4.7-☑	D36.7	D48.7	D49.89
upper	C76.4-☑	C79.89	DØ4.6-☑	D36.7	D48.7	D49.89
limbus of cornea	C69.1-☑	C79.49	DØ9.2-☑	D31.1-☑	D48.7	D49.89

	Malignant Primary	Malignant Secondary	Ca in situ	Benign	Uncertain Behavior	Unspecified Behavior
Neoplasm, neoplastic — *continued*						
lingual NEC — *see also* Neoplasm, tongue	C02.9	C79.89	D00.07	D10.1	D37.02	D49.0
lingula, lung	C34.1-☑	C78.0-☑	D02.2-☑	D14.3-☑	D38.1	D49.1
lip	C00.9	C79.89	D00.01	D10.0	D37.01	D49.0
buccal aspect — *see* Neoplasm, lip, internal						
commissure	C00.6	C79.89	D00.01	D10.0	D37.01	D49.0
external	C00.2	C79.89	D00.01	D10.0	D37.01	D49.0
lower	C00.1	C79.89	D00.01	D10.0	D37.01	D49.0
upper	C00.0	C79.89	D00.01	D10.0	D37.01	D49.0
frenulum — *see* Neoplasm, lip, internal						
inner aspect — *see* Neoplasm, lip, internal						
internal	C00.5	C79.89	D00.01	D10.0	D37.01	D49.0
lower	C00.4	C79.89	D00.01	D10.0	D37.01	D49.0
upper	C00.3	C79.89	D00.01	D10.0	D37.01	D49.0
lipstick area	C00.2	C79.89	D00.01	D10.0	D37.01	D49.0
lower	C00.1	C79.89	D00.01	D10.0	D37.01	D49.0
upper	C00.0	C79.89	D00.01	D10.0	D37.01	D49.0
lower	C00.1	C79.89	D00.01	D10.0	D37.01	D49.0
internal	C00.4	C79.89	D00.01	D10.0	D37.01	D49.0
mucosa — *see* Neoplasm, lip, internal						
oral aspect — *see* Neoplasm, lip, internal						
overlapping lesion	C00.8	—	—	—	—	—
with oral cavity or pharynx	C14.8	—	—	—	—	—
skin (commissure) (lower) (upper)	C44.00	C79.2	D04.0	D23.0	D48.5	D49.2
basal cell carcinoma	C44.01	—	—	—	—	—
specified type NEC	C44.09	—	—	—	—	—
squamous cell carcinoma	C44.02	—	—	—	—	—
upper	C00.0	C79.89	D00.01	D10.0	D37.01	D49.0
internal	C00.3	C79.89	D00.01	D10.0	D37.01	D49.0
vermilion border	C00.2	C79.89	D00.01	D10.0	D37.01	D49.0
lower	C00.1	C79.89	D00.01	D10.0	D37.01	D49.0
upper	C00.0	C79.89	D00.01	D10.0	D37.01	D49.0
lipomatous — *see* Lipoma, by site						
liver — *see also* Index to disease, by histology	C22.9	C78.7	D01.5	D13.4	D37.6	D49.0
primary	C22.8	C78.7	D01.5	D13.4	D37.6	D49.0
lumbosacral plexus	C47.5	C79.89	—	D36.16	D48.2	D49.2
lung	C34.9-☑	C78.0-☑	D02.2-☑	D14.3-☑	D38.1	D49.1
azygos lobe	C34.1-☑	C78.0-☑	D02.2-☑	D14.3-☑	D38.1	D49.1
carina	C34.0-☑	C78.0-☑	D02.2-☑	D14.3-☑	D38.1	D49.1
hilus	C34.0-☑	C78.0-☑	D02.2-☑	D14.3-☑	D38.1	D49.1
linqula	C34.1-☑	C78.0-☑	D02.2-☑	D14.3-☑	D38.1	D49.1
lobe NEC	C34.9-☑	C78.0-☑	D02.2-☑	D14.3-☑	D38.1	D49.1
lower lobe	C34.3-☑	C78.0-☑	D02.2-☑	D14.3-☑	D38.1	D49.1
main bronchus	C34.0-☑	C78.0-☑	D02.2-☑	D14.3-☑	D38.1	D49.1
mesothelioma — *see* Mesothelioma						
middle lobe	C34.2	C78.0-☑	D02.21	D14.31	D38.1	D49.1
overlapping lesion	C34.8-☑	—	—	—	—	—
upper lobe	C34.1-☑	C78.0-☑	D02.2-☑	D14.3-☑	D38.1	D49.1
lymph, lymphatic channel NEC	C49.9	C79.89	—	D21.9	D48.1	D49.2
gland (secondary)	—	C77.9	—	D36.0	D48.7	D49.89
abdominal	—	C77.2	—	D36.0	D48.7	D49.89
aortic	—	C77.2	—	D36.0	D48.7	D49.89
arm	—	C77.3	—	D36.0	D48.7	D49.89
Neoplasm, neoplastic — *continued*						
lymph, lymphatic channel — *continued*						
gland — *continued*						
auricular (anterior) (posterior)	—	C77.0	—	D36.0	D48.7	D49.89
axilla, axillary	—	C77.3	—	D36.0	D48.7	D49.89
brachial	—	C77.3	—	D36.0	D48.7	D49.89
bronchial	—	C77.1	—	D36.0	D48.7	D49.89
bronchopulmonary	—	C77.1	—	D36.0	D48.7	D49.89
celiac	—	C77.2	—	D36.0	D48.7	D49.89
cervical	—	C77.0	—	D36.0	D48.7	D49.89
cervicofacial	—	C77.0	—	D36.0	D48.7	D49.89
Cloquet	—	C77.4	—	D36.0	D48.7	D49.89
colic	—	C77.2	—	D36.0	D48.7	D49.89
common duct	—	C77.2	—	D36.0	D48.7	D49.89
cubital	—	C77.3	—	D36.0	D48.7	D49.89
diaphragmatic	—	C77.1	—	D36.0	D48.7	D49.89
epigastric, inferior	—	C77.1	—	D36.0	D48.7	D49.89
epitrochlear	—	C77.3	—	D36.0	D48.7	D49.89
esophageal	—	C77.1	—	D36.0	D48.7	D49.89
face	—	C77.0	—	D36.0	D48.7	D49.89
femoral	—	C77.4	—	D36.0	D48.7	D49.89
gastric	—	C77.2	—	D36.0	D48.7	D49.89
groin	—	C77.4	—	D36.0	D48.7	D49.89
head	—	C77.0	—	D36.0	D48.7	D49.89
hepatic	—	C77.2	—	D36.0	D48.7	D49.89
hilar (pulmonary)	—	C77.1	—	D36.0	D48.7	D49.89
splenic	—	C77.2	—	D36.0	D48.7	D49.89
hypogastric	—	C77.5	—	D36.0	D48.7	D49.89
ileocolic	—	C77.2	—	D36.0	D48.7	D49.89
iliac	—	C77.5	—	D36.0	D48.7	D49.89
infraclavicular	—	C77.3	—	D36.0	D48.7	D49.89
inguina, inguinal	—	C77.4	—	D36.0	D48.7	D49.89
innominate	—	C77.1	—	D36.0	D48.7	D49.89
intercostal	—	C77.1	—	D36.0	D48.7	D49.89
intestinal	—	C77.2	—	D36.0	D48.7	D49.89
intrabdominal	—	C77.2	—	D36.0	D48.7	D49.89
intrapelvic	—	C77.5	—	D36.0	D48.7	D49.89
intrathoracic	—	C77.1	—	D36.0	D48.7	D49.89
jugular	—	C77.0	—	D36.0	D48.7	D49.89
leg	—	C77.4	—	D36.0	D48.7	D49.89
limb						
lower	—	C77.4	—	D36.0	D48.7	D49.89
upper	—	C77.3	—	D36.0	D48.7	D49.89
lower limb	—	C77.4	—	D36.0	D48.7	D49.89
lumbar	—	C77.2	—	D36.0	D48.7	D49.89
mandibular	—	C77.0	—	D36.0	D48.7	D49.89
mediastinal	—	C77.1	—	D36.0	D48.7	D49.89
mesenteric (inferior) (superior)	—	C77.2	—	D36.0	D48.7	D49.89
midcolic	—	C77.2	—	D36.0	D48.7	D49.89
multiple sites in categories C77.0 - C77.5	—	C77.8	—	D36.0	D48.7	D49.89
neck	—	C77.0	—	D36.0	D48.7	D49.89
obturator	—	C77.5	—	D36.0	D48.7	D49.89
occipital	—	C77.0	—	D36.0	D48.7	D49.89
pancreatic	—	C77.2	—	D36.0	D48.7	D49.89
para-aortic	—	C77.2	—	D36.0	D48.7	D49.89
paracervical	—	C77.5	—	D36.0	D48.7	D49.89
parametrial	—	C77.5	—	D36.0	D48.7	D49.89
parasternal	—	C77.1	—	D36.0	D48.7	D49.89
parotid	—	C77.0	—	D36.0	D48.7	D49.89
pectoral	—	C77.3	—	D36.0	D48.7	D49.89
pelvic	—	C77.5	—	D36.0	D48.7	D49.89
peri-aortic	—	C77.2	—	D36.0	D48.7	D49.89
peripancreatic	—	C77.2	—	D36.0	D48.7	D49.89
popliteal	—	C77.4	—	D36.0	D48.7	D49.89
porta hepatis	—	C77.2	—	D36.0	D48.7	D49.89
portal	—	C77.2	—	D36.0	D48.7	D49.89
preauricular	—	C77.0	—	D36.0	D48.7	D49.89
prelaryngeal	—	C77.0	—	D36.0	D48.7	D49.89
presymphysial	—	C77.5	—	D36.0	D48.7	D49.89
pretracheal	—	C77.0	—	D36.0	D48.7	D49.89
primary (any site) NEC	C96.9	—	—	—	—	—

☑ **Additional Character Required — Refer to the Tabular List for Character Selection**

	Malignant Primary	Malignant Secondary	Ca in situ	Benign	Uncertain Behavior	Unspecified Behavior
Neoplasm, neoplastic — *continued*						
lymph, lymphatic channel — *continued*						
gland — *continued*						
pulmonary (hiler)	—	C77.1	—	D36.0	D48.7	D49.89
pyloric	—	C77.2	—	D36.0	D48.7	D49.89
retroperitoneal	—	C77.2	—	D36.0	D48.7	D49.89
retropharyngeal	—	C77.0	—	D36.0	D48.7	D49.89
Rosenmuller's	—	C77.4	—	D36.0	D48.7	D49.89
sacral	—	C77.5	—	D36.0	D48.7	D49.89
scalene	—	C77.0	—	D36.0	D48.7	D49.89
site NEC	—	C77.9	—	D36.0	D48.7	D49.89
splenic (hilar)	—	C77.2	—	D36.0	D48.7	D49.89
subclavicular	—	C77.3	—	D36.0	D48.7	D49.89
subinguinal	—	C77.4	—	D36.0	D48.7	D49.89
sublingual	—	C77.0	—	D36.0	D48.7	D49.89
submandibular	—	C77.0	—	D36.0	D48.7	D49.89
submaxillary	—	C77.0	—	D36.0	D48.7	D49.89
submental	—	C77.0	—	D36.0	D48.7	D49.89
subscapular	—	C77.3	—	D36.0	D48.7	D49.89
supraclavicular	—	C77.0	—	D36.0	D48.7	D49.89
thoracic	—	C77.1	—	D36.0	D48.7	D49.89
tibial	—	C77.4	—	D36.0	D48.7	D49.89
tracheal	—	C77.1	—	D36.0	D48.7	D49.89
tracheobronchial	—	C77.1	—	D36.0	D48.7	D49.89
upper limb	—	C77.3	—	D36.0	D48.7	D49.89
Virchow's	—	C77.0	—	D36.0	D48.7	D49.89
node — *see also* Neoplasm, lymph gland						
primary NEC	C96.9	—	—	—	—	—
vessel — *see also* Neoplasm, connective tissue	C49.9	C79.89	—	D21.9	D48.1	D49.2
Mackenrodt's ligament	C57.7	C79.82	D07.39	D28.7	D39.8	D49.59
malar	C41.0	C79.51	—	D16.4	D48.0	D49.2
region — *see* Neoplasm, cheek						
mammary gland — *see* Neoplasm, breast						
mandible	C41.1	C79.51	—	D16.5	D48.0	D49.2
alveolar						
mucosa (carcinoma)	C03.1	C79.89	D00.03	D10.39	D37.09	D49.0
ridge or process	C41.1	C79.51	—	D16.5	D48.0	D49.2
marrow (bone) NEC	C96.9	C79.52	—	—	D47.9	D49.89
mastectomy site (skin) — *see also* Neoplasm, breast, skin	C44.501	C79.2	—	—	—	—
specified as breast tissue	C50.8-☑	C79.81	—	—	—	—
mastoid (air cells) (antrum) (cavity)	C30.1	C78.39	D02.3	D14.0	D38.5	D49.1
bone or process	C41.0	C79.51	—	D16.4	D48.0	D49.2
maxilla, maxillary (superior)	C41.0	C79.51	—	D16.4	D48.0	D49.2
alveolar						
mucosa	C03.0	C79.89	D00.03	D10.39	D37.09	D49.0
ridge or process (carcinoma)	C41.0	C79.51	—	D16.4	D48.0	D49.2
antrum	C31.0	C78.39	D02.3	D14.0	D38.5	D49.1
carcinoma	C03.0	C79.51	—	—	—	—
inferior — *see* Neoplasm, mandible						
sinus	C31.0	C78.39	D02.3	D14.0	D38.5	D49.1
meatus external (ear) — *see also* Neoplasm, skin, ear	C44.20-☑	C79.2	D04.2-☑	D23.2-☑	D48.5	D49.2
Meckel diverticulum, malignant	C17.3	C78.4	D01.49	D13.39	D37.2	D49.0
mediastinum, mediastinal	C38.3	C78.1	—	D15.2	D38.3	D49.89
anterior	C38.1	C78.1	—	D15.2	D38.3	D49.89

	Malignant Primary	Malignant Secondary	Ca in situ	Benign	Uncertain Behavior	Unspecified Behavior
Neoplasm, neoplastic — *continued*						
mediastinum, mediastinal — *continued*						
posterior	C38.2	C78.1	—	D15.2	D38.3	D49.89
medulla						
adrenal	C74.1-☑	C79.7-☑	D09.3	D35.0-☑	D44.1-☑	D49.7
oblongata	C71.7	C79.31	—	D33.1	D43.1	D49.6
meibomian gland	C44.10-☑	C79.2	D04.1-☑	D23.1-☑	D48.5	D49.2
basal cell carcinoma	C44.11-☑	—	—	—	—	—
sebaceous cell	C44.13-☑	—	—	—	—	—
specified type NEC	C44.19-☑	—	—	—	—	—
squamous cell carcinoma	C44.12-☑	—	—	—	—	—
melanoma — *see* Melanoma						
meninges	C70.9	C79.49	—	D32.9	D42.9	D49.7
brain	C70.0	C79.32	—	D32.0	D42.0	D49.7
cerebral	C70.0	C79.32	—	D32.0	D42.0	D49.7
crainial	C70.0	C79.32	—	D32.0	D42.0	D49.7
intracranial	C70.0	C79.32	—	D32.0	D42.0	D49.7
spinal (cord)	C70.1	C79.49	—	D32.1	D42.1	D49.7
meniscus, knee joint (lateral) (medial)	C40.2-☑	C79.51	—	D16.2-☑	D48.0	D49.2
Merkel cell — *see* Carcinoma, Merkel cell						
mesentery, mesenteric	C48.1	C78.6	—	D20.1	D48.4	D49.0
mesoappendix	C48.1	C78.6	—	D20.1	D48.4	D49.0
mesocolon	C48.1	C78.6	—	D20.1	D48.4	D49.0
mesopharynx — *see* Neoplasm, oropharynx						
mesosalpinx	C57.1-☑	C79.82	D07.39	D28.2	D39.8	D49.59
mesothelial tissue — *see* Mesothelioma						
mesothelioma — *see* Mesothelioma						
mesovarium	C57.1-☑	C79.82	D07.39	D28.2	D39.8	D49.59
metacarpus (any bone)	C40.1-☑	C79.51	—	D16.1-☑	—	—
metastatic NEC — *see also* Neoplasm, by site, secondary	—	C79.9	—	—	—	—
metatarsus (any bone)	C40.3-☑	C79.51	—	D16.3-☑	—	—
midbrain	C71.7	C79.31	—	D33.1	D43.1	D49.6
milk duct — *see* Neoplasm, breast						
mons						
pubis	C51.9	C79.82	D07.1	D28.0	D39.8	D49.59
veneris	C51.9	C79.82	D07.1	D28.0	D39.8	D49.59
motor tract	C72.9	C79.49	—	D33.9	D43.9	D49.7
brain	C71.9	C79.31	—	D33.2	D43.2	D49.6
cauda equina	C72.1	C79.49	—	D33.4	D43.4	D49.7
spinal	C72.0	C79.49	—	D33.4	D43.4	D49.7
mouth	C06.9	C79.89	D00.00	D10.30	D37.09	D49.0
book-leaf	C06.89	C79.89	—	—	—	—
floor	C04.9	C79.89	D00.06	D10.2	D37.09	D49.0
anterior portion	C04.0	C79.89	D00.06	D10.2	D37.09	D49.0
lateral portion	C04.1	C79.89	D00.06	D10.2	D37.09	D49.0
overlapping lesion	C04.8	—	—	—	—	—
overlapping NEC	C06.80	—	—	—	—	—
roof	C05.9	C79.89	D00.00	D10.39	D37.09	D49.0
specified part NEC	C06.89	C79.89	D00.00	D10.39	D37.09	D49.0
vestibule	C06.1	C79.89	D00.00	D10.39	D37.09	D49.0
mucosa						
alveolar (ridge or process)	C03.9	C79.89	D00.03	D10.39	D37.09	D49.0
lower	C03.1	C79.89	D00.03	D10.39	D37.09	D49.0
upper	C03.0	C79.89	D00.03	D10.39	D37.09	D49.0
buccal	C06.0	C79.89	D00.02	D10.39	D37.09	D49.0
cheek	C06.0	C79.89	D00.02	D10.39	D37.09	D49.0

	Malignant Primary	Malignant Secondary	Ca in situ	Benign	Uncertain Behavior	Unspecified Behavior
Neoplasm, neoplastic *— continued*						
mucosa *— continued*						
lip *— see* Neoplasm, lip, internal						
nasal	C30.0	C78.39	D02.3	D14.0	D38.5	D49.1
oral	C06.0	C79.89	D00.02	D10.39	D37.09	D49.0
Mullerian duct						
female	C57.7	C79.82	D07.39	D28.7	D39.8	D49.59
male	C63.7	C79.82	D07.69	D29.8	D40.8	D49.59
muscle *— see also* Neoplasm, connective tissue						
extraocular	C69.6-☑	C79.49	D09.2-☑	D31.6-☑	D48.7	D49.89
myocardium	C38.0	C79.89	—	D15.1	D48.7	D49.89
myometrium	C54.2	C79.82	D07.0	D26.1	D39.0	D49.59
myopericardium	C38.0	C79.89	—	D15.1	D48.7	D49.89
nabothian gland (follicle)	C53.0	C79.82	D06.0	D26.0	D39.0	D49.59
nail *— see also* Neoplasm, skin, limb	C44.90	C79.2	D04.9	D23.9	D48.5	D49.2
finger *— see also* Neoplasm, skin, limb, upper	C44.60-☑	C79.2	D04.6-☑	D23.6-☑	D48.5	D49.2
toe *— see also* Neoplasm, skin, limb, lower	C44.70-☑	C79.2	D04.7-☑	D23.7-☑	D48.5	D49.2
nares, naris (anterior) (posterior)	C30.0	C78.39	D02.3	D14.0	D38.5	D49.1
nasal *— see* Neoplasm, nose						
nasolabial groove *— see also* Neoplasm, skin, face	C44.309	C79.2	D04.39	D23.39	D48.5	D49.2
nasolacrimal duct	C69.5-☑	C79.49	D09.2-☑	D31.5-☑	D48.7	D49.89
nasopharynx, nasopharyngeal	C11.9	C79.89	D00.08	D10.6	D37.05	D49.0
floor	C11.3	C79.89	D00.08	D10.6	D37.05	D49.0
overlapping lesion	C11.8	—	—	—	—	—
roof	C11.0	C79.89	D00.08	D10.6	D37.05	D49.0
wall	C11.9	C79.89	D00.08	D10.6	D37.05	D49.0
anterior	C11.3	C79.89	D00.08	D10.6	D37.05	D49.0
lateral	C11.2	C79.89	D00.08	D10.6	D37.05	D49.0
posterior	C11.1	C79.89	D00.08	D10.6	D37.05	D49.0
superior	C11.0	C79.89	D00.08	D10.6	D37.05	D49.0
nates *— see also* Neoplasm, skin, trunk	C44.509	C79.2	D04.5	D23.5	D48.5	D49.2
neck NEC	C76.0	C79.89	D09.8	D36.7	D48.7	D49.89
skin	C44.40	—	—	—	—	—
basal cell carcinoma	C44.41	—	—	—	—	—
specified type NEC	C44.49	—	—	—	—	—
squamous cell carcinoma	C44.42	—	—	—	—	—
nerve (ganglion)	C47.9	C79.89	—	D36.10	D48.2	D49.2
abducens	C72.59	C79.49	—	D33.3	D43.3	D49.7
accessory (spinal)	C72.59	C79.49	—	D33.3	D43.3	D49.7
acoustic	C72.4-☑	C79.49	—	D33.3	D43.3	D49.7
auditory	C72.4-☑	C79.49	—	D33.3	D43.3	D49.7
autonomic NEC *— see also* Neoplasm, nerve, peripheral	C47.9	C79.89	—	D36.10	D48.2	D49.2
brachial	C47.1-☑	C79.89	—	D36.12	D48.2	D49.2
cranial	C72.50	C79.49	—	D33.3	D43.3	D49.7
specified NEC	C72.59	C79.49	—	D33.3	D43.3	D49.7
facial	C72.59	C79.49	—	D33.3	D43.3	D49.7
femoral	C47.2-☑	C79.89	—	D36.13	D48.2	D49.2
ganglion NEC *— see also* Neoplasm, nerve, peripheral	C47.9	C79.89	—	D36.10	D48.2	D49.2
glossopharyngeal	C72.59	C79.49	—	D33.3	D43.3	D49.7
hypoglossal	C72.59	C79.49	—	D33.3	D43.3	D49.7
intercostal	C47.3	C79.89	—	D36.14	D48.2	D49.2
lumbar	C47.6	C79.89	—	D36.17	D48.2	D49.2
median	C47.1-☑	C79.89	—	D36.12	D48.2	D49.2
obturator	C47.2-☑	C79.89	—	D36.13	D48.2	D49.2

	Malignant Primary	Malignant Secondary	Ca in situ	Benign	Uncertain Behavior	Unspecified Behavior
Neoplasm, neoplastic *— continued*						
nerve *— continued*						
oculomotor	C72.59	C79.49	—	D33.3	D43.3	D49.7
olfactory	C47.2-☑	C79.49	—	D33.3	D43.3	D49.7
optic	C72.3-☑	C79.49	—	D33.3	D43.3	D49.7
parasympathetic NEC	C47.9	C79.89	—	D36.10	D48.2	D49.2
peripheral NEC	C47.9	C79.89	—	D36.10	D48.2	D49.2
abdomen	C47.4	C79.89	—	D36.15	D48.2	D49.2
abdominal wall	C47.4	C79.89	—	D36.15	D48.2	D49.2
ankle	C47.2-☑	C79.89	—	D36.13	D48.2	D49.2
antecubital fossa or space	C47.1-☑	C79.89	—	D36.12	D48.2	D49.2
arm	C47.1-☑	C79.89	—	D36.12	D48.2	D49.2
auricle (ear)	C47.0	C79.89	—	D36.11	D48.2	D49.2
axilla	C47.3	C79.89	—	D36.12	D48.2	D49.2
back	C47.6	C79.89	—	D36.17	D48.2	D49.2
buttock	C47.5	C79.89	—	D36.16	D48.2	D49.2
calf	C47.2-☑	C79.89	—	D36.13	D48.2	D49.2
cervical region	C47.0	C79.89	—	D36.11	D48.2	D49.2
cheek	C47.0	C79.89	—	D36.11	D48.2	D49.2
chest (wall)	C47.3	C79.89	—	D36.14	D48.2	D49.2
chin	C47.0	C79.89	—	D36.11	D48.2	D49.2
ear (external)	C47.0	C79.89	—	D36.11	D48.2	D49.2
elbow	C47.1-☑	C79.89	—	D36.12	D48.2	D49.2
extrarectal	C47.5	C79.89	—	D36.16	D48.2	D49.2
extremity	C47.9	C79.89	—	D36.10	D48.2	D49.2
lower	C47.2-☑	C79.89	—	D36.13	D48.2	D49.2
upper	C47.1-☑	C79.89	—	D36.12	D48.2	D49.2
eyelid	C47.0	C79.89	—	D36.11	D48.2	D49.2
face	C47.0	C79.89	—	D36.11	D48.2	D49.2
finger	C47.1-☑	C79.89	—	D36.12	D48.2	D49.2
flank	C47.6	C79.89	—	D36.17	D48.2	D49.2
foot	C47.2-☑	C79.89	—	D36.13	D48.2	D49.2
forearm	C47.1-☑	C79.89	—	D36.12	D48.2	D49.2
forehead	C47.0	C79.89	—	D36.11	D48.2	D49.2
gluteal region	C47.5	C79.89	—	D36.16	D48.2	D49.2
groin	C47.5	C79.89	—	D36.16	D48.2	D49.2
hand	C47.1-☑	C79.89	—	D36.12	D48.2	D49.2
head	C47.0	C79.89	—	D36.11	D48.2	D49.2
heel	C47.2-☑	C79.89	—	D36.13	D48.2	D49.2
hip	C47.2-☑	C79.89	—	D36.13	D48.2	D49.2
infraclavicular region	C47.3	C79.89	—	D36.14	D48.2	D49.2
inguinal (canal) (region)	C47.5	C79.89	—	D36.16	D48.2	D49.2
intrathoracic	C47.3	C79.89	—	D36.14	D48.2	D49.2
ischiorectal fossa	C47.5	C79.89	—	D36.16	D48.2	D49.2
knee	C47.2-☑	C79.89	—	D36.13	D48.2	D49.2
leg	C47.2-☑	C79.89	—	D36.13	D48.2	D49.2
limb NEC	C47.9	C79.89	—	D36.10	D48.2	D49.2
lower	C47.2-☑	C79.89	—	D36.13	D48.2	D49.2
upper	C47.1-☑	C79.89	—	D36.12	D48.2	D49.2
nates	C47.5	C79.89	—	D36.16	D48.2	D49.2
neck	C47.0	C79.89	—	D36.11	D48.2	D49.2
orbit	C69.6-☑	C79.49	—	D31.6-☑	D48.7	D49.2
pararectal	C47.5	C79.89	—	D36.16	D48.2	D49.2
paraurethral	C47.5	C79.89	—	D36.16	D48.2	D49.2
paravaginal	C47.5	C79.89	—	D36.16	D48.2	D49.2
pelvis (floor)	C47.5	C79.89	—	D36.16	D48.2	D49.2
pelvoabdominal	C47.8	C79.89	—	D36.17	D48.2	D49.2
perineum	C47.5	C79.89	—	D36.16	D48.2	D49.2
perirectal (tissue)	C47.5	C79.89	—	D36.16	D48.2	D49.2
periurethral (tissue)	C47.5	C79.89	—	D36.16	D48.2	D49.2
popliteal fossa or space	C47.2-☑	C79.89	—	D36.13	D48.2	D49.2
presacral	C47.5	C79.89	—	D36.16	D48.2	D49.2
pterygoid fossa	C47.0	C79.89	—	D36.11	D48.2	D49.2
rectovaginal septum or wall	C47.5	C79.89	—	D36.16	D48.2	D49.2
rectovesical	C47.5	C79.89	—	D36.16	D48.2	D49.2
sacrococcygeal region	C47.5	C79.89	—	D36.16	D48.2	D49.2
scalp	C47.0	C79.89	—	D36.11	D48.2	D49.2

 ☑ **Additional Character Required — Refer to the Tabular List for Character Selection**

	Malignant Primary	Malignant Secondary	Ca in situ	Benign	Uncertain Behavior	Unspecified Behavior
Neoplasm, neoplastic — *continued*						
nerve — *continued*						
peripheral — *continued*						
scapular region	C47.3	C79.89	—	D36.14	D48.2	D49.2
shoulder	C47.1-☑	C79.89	—	D36.12	D48.2	D49.2
submental	C47.Ø	C79.89	—	D36.11	D48.2	D49.2
supraclavicular region	C47.Ø	C79.89	—	D36.11	D48.2	D49.2
temple	C47.Ø	C79.89	—	D36.11	D48.2	D49.2
temporal region	C47.Ø	C79.89	—	D36.11	D48.2	D49.2
thigh	C47.2-☑	C79.89	—	D36.13	D48.2	D49.2
thoracic (duct) (wall)	C47.3	C79.89	—	D36.14	D48.2	D49.2
thorax	C47.3	C79.89	—	D36.14	D48.2	D49.2
thumb	C47.1-☑	C79.89	—	D36.12	D48.2	D49.2
toe	C47.2-☑	C79.89	—	D36.13	D48.2	D49.2
trunk	C47.6	C79.89	—	D36.17	D48.2	D49.2
umbilicus	C47.4	C79.89	—	D36.15	D48.2	D49.2
vesicorectal	C47.5	C79.89	—	D36.16	D48.2	D49.2
wrist	C47.1-☑	C79.89	—	D36.12	D48.2	D49.2
radial	C47.1-☑	C79.89	—	D36.12	D48.2	D49.2
sacral	C47.5	C79.89	—	D36.16	D48.2	D49.2
sciatic	C47.2-☑	C79.89	—	D36.13	D48.2	D49.2
spinal NEC	C47.9	C79.89	—	D36.1Ø	D48.2	D49.2
accessory	C72.59	C79.49	—	D33.3	D43.3	D49.7
sympathetic NEC — *see also* Neoplasm, nerve, peripheral	C47.9	C79.89	—	D36.1Ø	D48.2	D49.2
trigeminal	C72.59	C79.49	—	D33.3	D43.3	D49.7
trochlear	C72.59	C79.49	—	D33.3	D43.3	D49.7
ulnar	C47.1-☑	C79.89	—	D36.12	D48.2	D49.2
vagus	C72.59	C79.49	—	D33.3	D43.3	D49.7
nervous system (central)	C72.9	C79.4Ø	—	D33.9	D43.9	D49.7
autonomic — *see* Neoplasm, nerve, peripheral						
parasympathetic — *see* Neoplasm, nerve, peripheral						
specified site NEC	—	C79.49	—	D33.7	D43.8	—
sympathetic — *see* Neoplasm, nerve, peripheral						
nevus — *see* Nevus						
nipple	C5Ø.Ø-☑	C79.81	DØ5.-☑	D24.-☑	—	—
nose, nasal	C76.Ø	C79.89	DØ9.8	D36.7	D48.7	D49.89
ala (external) (nasi) — *see also* Neoplasm, nose, skin	C44.3Ø1	C79.2	DØ4.39	D23.39	D48.5	D49.2
bone	C41.Ø	C79.51	—	D16.4	D48.Ø	D49.2
cartilage	C3Ø.Ø	C78.39	DØ2.3	D14.Ø	D38.5	D49.1
cavity	C3Ø.Ø	C78.39	DØ2.3	D14.Ø	D38.5	D49.1
choana	C11.3	C79.89	DØØ.Ø8	D1Ø.6	D37.Ø5	D49.Ø
external (skin) — *see also* Neoplasm, nose, skin	C44.3Ø1	C79.2	DØ4.39	D23.39	D48.5	D49.2
fossa	C3Ø.Ø	C78.39	DØ2.3	D14.Ø	D38.5	D49.1
internal	C3Ø.Ø	C78.39	DØ2.3	D14.Ø	D38.5	D49.1
mucosa	C3Ø.Ø	C78.39	DØ2.3	D14.Ø	D38.5	D49.1
septum	C3Ø.Ø	C78.39	DØ2.3	D14.Ø	D38.5	D49.1
posterior margin	C11.3	C79.89	DØØ.Ø8	D1Ø.6	D37.Ø5	D49.Ø
sinus — *see* Neoplasm, sinus						
skin	C44.3Ø1	C79.2	DØ4.39	D23.39	D48.5	D49.2
basal cell carcinoma	C44.311	—	—	—	—	—
specified type NEC	C44.391	—	—	—	—	—
squamous cell carcinoma	C44.321	—	—	—	—	—
turbinate (mucosa)	C3Ø.Ø	C78.39	DØ2.3	D14.Ø	D38.5	D49.1
bone	C41.Ø	C79.51	—	D16.4	D48.Ø	D49.2
vestibule	C3Ø.Ø	C78.39	DØ2.3	D14.Ø	D38.5	D49.1

	Malignant Primary	Malignant Secondary	Ca in situ	Benign	Uncertain Behavior	Unspecified Behavior
Neoplasm, neoplastic — *continued*						
nostril	C3Ø.Ø	C78.39	DØ2.3	D14.Ø	D38.5	D49.1
nucleus pulposus	C41.2	C79.51	—	D16.6	D48.Ø	D49.2
occipital						
bone	C41.Ø	C79.51	—	D16.4	D48.Ø	D49.2
lobe or pole, brain	C71.4	C79.31	—	D33.Ø	D43.Ø	D49.6
odontogenic — *see* Neoplasm, jaw bone						
olfactory nerve or bulb	C72.2-☑	C79.49	—	D33.3	D43.3	D49.7
olive (brain)	C71.7	C79.31	—	D33.1	D43.1	D49.6
omentum	C48.1	C78.6	—	D2Ø.1	D48.4	D49.Ø
operculum (brain)	C71.Ø	C79.31	—	D33.Ø	D43.Ø	D49.6
optic nerve, chiasm, or tract	C72.3-☑	C79.49	—	D33.3	D43.3	D49.7
oral (cavity)	CØ6.9	C79.89	DØØ.ØØ	D1Ø.3Ø	D37.Ø9	D49.Ø
ill-defined	C14.8	C79.89	DØØ.ØØ	D1Ø.3Ø	D37.Ø9	D49.Ø
mucosa	CØ6.Ø	C79.89	DØØ.Ø2	D1Ø.39	D37.Ø9	D49.Ø
orbit	C69.6-☑	C79.49	DØ9.2-☑	D31.6-☑	D48.7	D49.89
autonomic nerve	C69.6-☑	C79.49	—	D31.6-☑	D48.7	D49.2
bone	C41.Ø	C79.51	—	D16.4	D48.Ø	D49.2
eye	C69.6-☑	C79.49	DØ9.2-☑	D31.6-☑	D48.7	D49.89
peripheral nerves	C69.6-☑	C79.49	—	D31.6-☑	D48.7	D49.2
soft parts	C69.6-☑	C79.49	DØ9.2-☑	D31.6-☑	D48.7	D49.89
organ of Zuckerkandl	C75.5	C79.89	—	D35.6	D44.7	D49.7
oropharynx	C1Ø.9	C79.89	DØØ.Ø8	D1Ø.5	D37.Ø5	D49.Ø
branchial cleft (vestige)	C1Ø.4	C79.89	DØØ.Ø8	D1Ø.5	D37.Ø5	D49.Ø
junctional region	C1Ø.8	C79.89	DØØ.Ø8	D1Ø.5	D37.Ø5	D49.Ø
lateral wall	C1Ø.2	C79.89	DØØ.Ø8	D1Ø.5	D37.Ø5	D49.Ø
overlapping lesion	C1Ø.8	—	—	—	—	—
pillars or fauces	CØ9.1	C79.89	DØØ.Ø8	D1Ø.5	D37.Ø5	D49.Ø
posterior wall	C1Ø.3	C79.89	DØØ.Ø8	D1Ø.5	D37.Ø5	D49.Ø
vallecula	C1Ø.Ø	C79.89	DØØ.Ø8	D1Ø.5	D37.Ø5	D49.Ø
os						
external	C53.1	C79.82	DØ6.1	D26.Ø	D39.Ø	D49.59
internal	C53.Ø	C79.82	DØ6.Ø	D26.Ø	D39.Ø	D49.59
ovary	C56.-☑	C79.6-☑	DØ7.39	D27.-☑	D39.1-☑	D49.59
oviduct	C57.Ø-☑	C79.82	DØ7.39	D28.2	D39.8	D49.59
palate	CØ5.9	C79.89	DØØ.ØØ	D1Ø.39	D37.Ø9	D49.Ø
hard	CØ5.Ø	C79.89	DØØ.Ø5	D1Ø.39	D37.Ø9	D49.Ø
junction of hard and soft palate	CØ5.9	C79.89	DØØ.ØØ	D1Ø.39	D37.Ø9	D49.Ø
overlapping lesions	CØ5.8	—	—	—	—	—
soft	CØ5.1	C79.89	DØØ.Ø4	D1Ø.39	D37.Ø9	D49.Ø
nasopharyngeal surface	C11.3	C79.89	DØØ.Ø8	D1Ø.6	D37.Ø5	D49.Ø
posterior surface	C11.3	C79.89	DØØ.Ø8	D1Ø.6	D37.Ø5	D49.Ø
superior surface	C11.3	C79.89	DØØ.Ø8	D1Ø.6	D37.Ø5	D49.Ø
palatoglossal arch	CØ9.1	C79.89	DØØ.ØØ	D1Ø.5	D37.Ø9	D49.Ø
palatopharyngeal arch	CØ9.1	C79.89	DØØ.ØØ	D1Ø.5	D37.Ø9	D49.Ø
pallium	C71.Ø	C79.31	—	D33.Ø	D43.Ø	D49.6
palpebra	C44.1Ø-☑	C79.2	DØ4.1-☑	D23.1-☑	D48.5	D49.2
basal cell carcinoma	C44.11-☑	—	—	—	—	—
sebaceous cell	C44.13-☑	—	—	—	—	—
specified type NEC	C44.19-☑	—	—	—	—	—
squamous cell carcinoma	C44.12-☑	—	—	—	—	—
pancreas	C25.9	C78.89	DØ1.7	D13.6	D37.8	D49.Ø
body	C25.1	C78.89	DØ1.7	D13.6	D37.8	D49.Ø
duct (of Santorini) (of Wirsung)	C25.3	C78.89	DØ1.7	D13.6	D37.8	D49.Ø
ectopic tissue	C25.7	C78.89	—	D13.6	D37.8	D49.Ø
head	C25.Ø	C78.89	DØ1.7	D13.6	D37.8	D49.Ø
islet cells	C25.4	C78.89	DØ1.7	D13.7	D37.8	D49.Ø
neck	C25.7	C78.89	DØ1.7	D13.6	D37.8	D49.Ø
overlapping lesion	C25.8	—	—	—	—	—
tail	C25.2	C78.89	DØ1.7	D13.6	D37.8	D49.Ø

	Malignant Primary	Malignant Secondary	Ca in situ	Benign	Uncertain Behavior	Unspecified Behavior
Neoplasm, neoplastic — *continued*						
para-aortic body	C75.5	C79.89	—	D35.6	D44.7	D49.7
paraganglion NEC	C75.5	C79.89	—	D35.6	D44.7	D49.7
parametrium	C57.3	C79.82	—	D28.2	D39.8	D49.59
paranephric	C48.0	C78.6	—	D20.0	D48.3	D49.0
pararectal	C76.3	C79.89	—	D36.7	D48.7	D49.89
parasagittal (region)	C76.0	C79.89	D09.8	D36.7	D48.7	D49.89
parasellar	C72.9	C79.49	—	D33.9	D43.8	D49.7
parathyroid (gland)	C75.0	C79.89	D09.3	D35.1	D44.2	D49.7
paraurethral	C76.3	C79.89	—	D36.7	D48.7	D49.89
gland	C68.1	C79.19	D09.19	D30.8	D41.8	D49.59
paravaginal	C76.3	C79.89	—	D36.7	D48.7	D49.89
parenchyma, kidney	C64.-☑	C79.0-☑	D09.19	D30.0-☑	D41.0-☑	D49.51-☑
parietal						
bone	C41.0	C79.51	—	D16.4	D48.0	D49.2
lobe, brain	C71.3	C79.31	—	D33.0	D43.0	D49.6
paroophoron	C57.1-☑	C79.82	D07.39	D28.2	D39.8	D49.59
parotid (duct) (gland)	C07	C79.89	D00.00	D11.0	D37.030	D49.0
parovarium	C57.1-☑	C79.82	D07.39	D28.2	D39.8	D49.59
patella	C40.20	C79.51	—	—	—	—
peduncle, cerebral	C71.7	C79.31	—	D33.1	D43.1	D49.6
pelvirectal junction	C19	C78.5	D01.1	D12.7	D37.5	D49.0
pelvis, pelvic	C76.3	C79.89	D09.8	D36.7	D48.7	D49.89
bone	C41.4	C79.51	—	D16.8	D48.0	D49.2
floor	C76.3	C79.89	D09.8	D36.7	D48.7	D49.89
renal	C65.-☑	C79.0-☑	D09.19	D30.1-☑	D41.1-☑	D49.51-☑
viscera	C76.3	C79.89	D09.8	D36.7	D48.7	D49.89
wall	C76.3	C79.89	D09.8	D36.7	D48.7	D49.89
pelvo-abdominal	C76.8	C79.89	D09.8	D36.7	D48.7	D49.89
penis	C60.9	C79.82	D07.4	D29.0	D40.8	D49.59
body	C60.2	C79.82	D07.4	D29.0	D40.8	D49.59
corpus (cavernosum)	C60.2	C79.82	D07.4	D29.0	D40.8	D49.59
glans	C60.1	C79.82	D07.4	D29.0	D40.8	D49.59
overlapping sites	C60.8	—	—	—	—	—
skin NEC	C60.9	C79.82	D07.4	D29.0	D40.8	D49.59
periadrenal (tissue)	C48.0	C78.6	—	D20.0	D48.3	D49.0
perianal (skin) — *see also* Neoplasm, anus, skin	C44.500	C79.2	D04.5	D23.5	D48.5	D49.2
pericardium	C38.0	C79.89	—	D15.1	D48.7	D49.89
perinephric	C48.0	C78.6	—	D20.0	D48.3	D49.0
perineum	C76.3	C79.89	D09.8	D36.7	D48.7	D49.89
periodontal tissue NEC	C03.9	C79.89	D00.03	D10.39	D37.09	D49.0
periosteum — *see* Neoplasm, bone						
peripancreatic	C48.0	C78.6	—	D20.0	D48.3	D49.0
peripheral nerve NEC	C47.9	C79.89	—	D36.10	D48.2	D49.2
perirectal (tissue)	C76.3	C79.89	—	D36.7	D48.7	D49.89
perirenal (tissue)	C48.0	C78.6	—	D20.0	D48.3	D49.0
peritoneum, peritoneal (cavity)	C48.2	C78.6	—	D20.1	D48.4	D49.0
benign mesothelial tissue — *see* Mesothelioma, benign						
overlapping lesion	C48.8	—	—	—	—	—
with digestive organs	C26.9	—	—	—	—	—
parietal	C48.1	C78.6	—	D20.1	D48.4	D49.0
pelvic	C48.1	C78.6	—	D20.1	D48.4	D49.0
specified part NEC	C48.1	C78.6	—	D20.1	D48.4	D49.0
peritonsillar (tissue)	C76.0	C79.89	D09.8	D36.7	D48.7	D49.89
periurethral tissue	C76.3	C79.89	—	D36.7	D48.7	D49.89
phalanges						
foot	C40.3-☑	C79.51	—	D16.3-☑	—	—
hand	C40.1-☑	C79.51	—	D16.1-☑	—	—
pharynx, pharyngeal	C14.0	C79.89	D00.08	D10.9	D37.05	D49.0
bursa	C11.1	C79.89	D00.08	D10.6	D37.05	D49.0

	Malignant Primary	Malignant Secondary	Ca in situ	Benign	Uncertain Behavior	Unspecified Behavior
Neoplasm, neoplastic — *continued*						
pharynx, pharyngeal — *continued*						
fornix	C11.3	C79.89	D00.08	D10.6	D37.05	D49.0
recess	C11.2	C79.89	D00.08	D10.6	D37.05	D49.0
region	C14.0	C79.89	D00.08	D10.9	D37.05	D49.0
tonsil	C11.1	C79.89	D00.08	D10.6	D37.05	D49.0
wall (lateral) (posterior)	C14.0	C79.89	D00.08	D10.9	D37.05	D49.0
pia mater	C70.9	C79.40	—	D32.9	D42.9	D49.7
cerebral	C70.0	C79.32	—	D32.0	D42.0	D49.7
cranial	C70.0	C79.32	—	D32.0	D42.0	D49.7
spinal	C70.1	C79.49	—	D32.1	D42.1	D49.7
pillars of fauces	C09.1	C79.89	D00.08	D10.5	D37.05	D49.0
pineal (body) (gland)	C75.3	C79.89	D09.3	D35.4	D44.5	D49.7
pinna (ear) NEC — *see also* Neoplasm, skin, ear	C44.20-☑	C79.2	D04.2-☑	D23.2-☑	D48.5	D49.2
piriform fossa or sinus	C12	C79.89	D00.08	D10.7	D37.05	D49.0
pituitary (body) (fossa) (gland) (lobe)	C75.1	C79.89	D09.3	D35.2	D44.3	D49.7
placenta	C58	C79.82	D07.0	D26.7	D39.2	D49.59
pleura, pleural (cavity)	C38.4	C78.2	—	D19.0	D38.2	D49.1
overlapping lesion with heart or mediastinum	C38.8	—	—	—	—	—
parietal	C38.4	C78.2	—	D19.0	D38.2	D49.1
visceral	C38.4	C78.2	—	D19.0	D38.2	D49.1
plexus						
brachial	C47.1-☑	C79.89	—	D36.12	D48.2	D49.2
cervical	C47.0	C79.89	—	D36.11	D48.2	D49.2
choroid	C71.5	C79.31	—	D33.0	D43.0	D49.6
lumbosacral	C47.5	C79.89	—	D36.16	D48.2	D49.2
sacral	C47.5	C79.89	—	D36.16	D48.2	D49.2
pluriendocrine	C75.8	C79.89	D09.3	D35.7	D44.9	D49.7
pole						
frontal	C71.1	C79.31	—	D33.0	D43.0	D49.6
occipital	C71.4	C79.31	—	D33.0	D43.0	D49.6
pons (varolii)	C71.7	C79.31	—	D33.1	D43.1	D49.6
popliteal fossa or space	C76.5-☑	C79.89	D04.7-☑	D36.7	D48.7	D49.89
postcricoid (region)	C13.0	C79.89	D00.08	D10.7	D37.05	D49.0
posterior fossa (cranial)	C71.9	C79.31	—	D33.2	D43.2	D49.6
postnasal space	C11.9	C79.89	D00.08	D10.6	D37.05	D49.0
prepuce	C60.0	C79.82	D07.4	D29.0	D40.8	D49.59
prepylorus	C16.4	C78.89	D00.2	D13.1	D37.1	D49.0
presacral (region)	C76.3	C79.89	—	D36.7	D48.7	D49.89
prostate (gland)	C61	C79.82	D07.5	D29.1	D40.0	D49.59
utricle	C68.0	C79.19	D09.19	D30.4	D41.3	D49.59
pterygoid fossa	C49.0	C79.89	—	D21.0	D48.1	D49.2
pubic bone	C41.4	C79.51	—	D16.8	D48.0	D49.2
pudenda, pudendum (femaie)	C51.9	C79.82	D07.1	D28.0	D39.8	D49.59
pulmonary — *see also* Neoplasm, lung	C34.9-☑	C78.0-☑	D02.2-☑	D14.3-☑	D38.1	D49.1
putamen	C71.0	C79.31	—	D33.0	D43.0	D49.6
pyloric						
antrum	C16.3	C78.89	D00.2	D13.1	D37.1	D49.0
canal	C16.4	C78.89	D00.2	D13.1	D37.1	D49.0
pylorus	C16.4	C78.89	D00.2	D13.1	D37.1	D49.0
pyramid (brain)	C71.7	C79.31	—	D33.1	D43.1	D49.6
pyriform fossa or sinus	C12	C79.89	D00.08	D10.7	D37.05	D49.0
radius (any part)	C40.0-☑	C79.51	—	D16.0-☑	—	—
Rathke's pouch	C75.1	C79.89	D09.3	D35.2	D44.3	D49.7
rectosigmoid (junction)	C19	C78.5	D01.1	D12.7	D37.5	D49.0
overlapping lesion with anus or rectum	C21.8	—	—	—	—	—
rectouterine pouch	C48.1	C78.6	—	D20.1	D48.4	D49.0
rectovaginal septum or wall	C76.3	C79.89	D09.8	D36.7	D48.7	D49.89
rectovesical septum	C76.3	C79.89	D09.8	D36.7	D48.7	D49.89
rectum (ampulla)	C20	C78.5	D01.2	D12.8	D37.5	D49.0

☑ **Additional Character Required — Refer to the Tabular List for Character Selection**

	Malignant Primary	Malignant Secondary	Ca in situ	Benign	Uncertain Behavior	Unspecified Behavior
Neoplasm, neoplastic — *continued*						
rectum — *continued*						
and colon	C19	C78.5	D01.1	D12.7	D37.5	D49.0
overlapping lesion						
with anus or rectosigmoid junction	C21.8	—	—	—	—	—
renal	C64.-☑	C79.0-☑	D09.19	D30.0-☑	D41.0-☑	D49.51-☑
calyx	C65.-☑	C79.0-☑	D09.19	D30.1-☑	D41.1-☑	D49.51-☑
hilus	C65.-☑	C79.0-☑	D09.19	D30.1-☑	D41.1-☑	D49.51-☑
parenchyma	C64.-☑	C79.0-☑	D09.19	D30.0-☑	D41.0-☑	D49.51-☑
pelvis	C65.-☑	C79.0-☑	D09.19	D30.1-☑	D41.1-☑	D49.51-☑
respiratory						
organs or system NEC	C39.9	C78.30	D02.4	D14.4	D38.6	D49.1
tract NEC	C39.9	C78.30	D02.4	D14.4	D38.5	D49.1
upper	C39.0	C78.30	D02.4	D14.4	D38.5	D49.1
retina	C69.2-☑	C79.49	D09.2-☑	D31.2-☑	D48.7	D49.81
retrobulbar	C69.6-☑	C79.49	—	D31.6-☑	D48.7	D49.89
retrocecal	C48.0	C78.6	—	D20.0	D48.3	D49.0
retromolar (area) (triangle) (trigone)	C06.2	C79.89	D00.00	D10.39	D37.09	D49.0
retro-orbital	C76.0	C79.89	D09.8	D36.7	D48.7	D49.89
retroperitoneal (space) (tissue)	C48.0	C78.6	—	D20.0	D48.3	D49.0
retroperitoneum	C48.0	C78.6	—	D20.0	D48.3	D49.0
retropharyngeal	C14.0	C79.89	D00.08	D10.9	D37.05	D49.0
retrovesical (septum)	C76.3	C79.89	D09.8	D36.7	D48.7	D49.89
rhinencephalon	C71.0	C79.31	—	D33.0	D43.0	D49.6
rib	C41.3	C79.51	—	D16.7	D48.0	D49.2
Rosenmuller's fossa	C11.2	C79.89	D00.08	D10.6	D37.05	D49.0
round ligament	C57.2-☑	C79.82	—	D28.2	D39.8	D49.59
sacrococcyx, sacrococcygeal	C41.4	C79.51	—	D16.8	D48.0	D49.2
region	C76.3	C79.89	D09.8	D36.7	D48.7	D49.89
sacrouterine ligament	C57.3	C79.82	—	D28.2	D39.8	D49.59
sacrum, sacral (vertebra)	C41.4	C79.51	—	D16.8	D48.0	D49.2
salivary gland or duct (major)	C08.9	C79.89	D00.00	D11.9	D37.039	D49.0
minor NEC	C06.9	C79.89	D00.00	D10.39	D37.04	D49.0
overlapping lesion	C08.9	—	—	—	—	—
parotid	C07	C79.89	D00.00	D11.0	D37.030	D49.0
pluriglandular	C08.9	C79.89	D00.00	D11.9	D37.039	D49.0
sublingual	C08.1	C79.89	D00.00	D11.7	D37.031	D49.0
submandibular	C08.0	C79.89	D00.00	D11.7	D37.032	D49.0
submaxillary	C08.0	C79.89	D00.00	D11.7	D37.032	D49.0
salpinx (uterine)	C57.0-☑	C79.82	D07.39	D28.2	D39.8	D49.59
Santorini's duct	C25.3	C78.89	D01.7	D13.6	D37.8	D49.0
scalp	C44.40	C79.2	D04.4	D23.4	D48.5	D49.2
basal cell carcinoma	C44.41	—	—	—	—	—
specified type NEC	C44.49	—	—	—	—	—
squamous cell carcinoma	C44.42	—	—	—	—	—
scapula (any part)	C40.0-☑	C79.51	—	D16.0-☑	—	—
scapular region	C76.1	C79.89	D09.8	D36.7	D48.7	D49.89
scar NEC — *see also* Neoplasm, skin, by site	C44.90	C79.2	D04.9	D23.9	D48.5	D49.2
sciatic nerve	C47.2-☑	C79.89	—	D36.13	D48.2	D49.2
sclera	C69.4-☑	C79.49	D09.2-☑	D31.4-☑	D48.7	D49.89
scrotum (skin)	C63.2	C79.82	D07.61	D29.4	D40.8	D49.59
sebaceous gland — *see* Neoplasm, skin						
sella turcica	C75.1	C79.89	D09.3	D35.2	D44.3	D49.7
bone	C41.0	C79.51	—	D16.4	D48.0	D49.2
semilunar cartilage (knee)	C40.2-☑	C79.51	—	D16.2-☑	D48.0	D49.2
seminal vesicle	C63.7	C79.82	D07.69	D29.8	D40.8	D49.59
septum						
nasal	C30.0	C78.39	D02.3	D14.0	D38.5	D49.1
posterior margin	C11.3	C79.89	D00.08	D10.6	D37.05	D49.0
rectovaginal	C76.3	C79.89	D09.8	D36.7	D48.7	D49.89
rectovesical	C76.3	C79.89	D09.8	D36.7	D48.7	D49.89

	Malignant Primary	Malignant Secondary	Ca in situ	Benign	Uncertain Behavior	Unspecified Behavior
Neoplasm, neoplastic — *continued*						
septum — *continued*						
urethrovaginal	C57.9	C79.82	D07.30	D28.9	D39.9	D49.59
vesicovaginal	C57.9	C79.82	D07.30	D28.9	D39.9	D49.59
shoulder NEC	C76.4-☑	C79.89	D04.6-☑	D36.7	D48.7	D49.89
sigmoid flexure (lower) (upper)	C18.7	C78.5	D01.0	D12.5	D37.4	D49.0
sinus (accessory)	C31.9	C78.39	D02.3	D14.0	D38.5	D49.1
bone (any)	C41.0	C79.51	—	D16.4	D48.0	D49.2
ethmoidal	C31.1	C78.39	D02.3	D14.0	D38.5	D49.1
frontal	C31.2	C78.39	D02.3	D14.0	D38.5	D49.1
maxillary	C31.0	C78.39	D02.3	D14.0	D38.5	D49.1
nasal, paranasal NEC	C31.9	C78.39	D02.3	D14.0	D38.5	D49.1
overlapping lesion	C31.8	—	—	—	—	—
pyriform	C12	C79.89	D00.08	D10.7	D37.05	D49.0
sphenoid	C31.3	C78.39	D02.3	D14.0	D38.5	D49.1
skeleton, skeletal NEC	C41.9	C79.51	—	D16.9	D48.0	D49.2
Skene's gland	C68.1	C79.19	D09.19	D30.8	D41.8	D49.59
skin NOS	C44.90	C79.2	D04.9	D23.9	D48.5	D49.2
abdominal wall	C44.509	C79.2	D04.5	D23.5	D48.5	D49.2
basal cell carcinoma	C44.519	—	—	—	—	—
specified type NEC	C44.599	—	—	—	—	—
squamous cell carcinoma	C44.529	—	—	—	—	—
ala nasi — *see also* Neoplasm, nose, skin	C44.301	C79.2	D04.39	D23.39	D48.5	D49.2
ankle — *see also* Neoplasm, skin, limb, lower	C44.70-☑	C79.2	D04.7-☑	D23.7-☑	D48.5	D49.2
antecubital space — *see also* Neoplasm, skin, limb, upper	C44.60-☑	C79.2	D04.6-☑	D23.6-☑	D48.5	D49.2
anus	C44.500	C79.2	D04.5	D23.5	D48.5	D49.2
basal cell carcinoma	C44.510	—	—	—	—	—
specified type NEC	C44.590	—	—	—	—	—
squamous cell carcinoma	C44.520	—	—	—	—	—
arm — *see also* Neoplasm, skin, limb, upper	C44.60-☑	C79.2	D04.6-☑	D23.6-☑	D48.5	D49.2
auditory canal (external) — *see also* Neoplasm, skin, ear	C44.20-☑	C79.2	D04.2-☑	D23.2-☑	D48.5	D49.2
auricle (ear) — *see also* Neoplasm, skin, ear	C44.20-☑	C79.2	D04.2-☑	D23.2-☑	D48.5	D49.2
auricular canal (external) — *see also* Neoplasm, skin, ear	C44.20-☑	C79.2	D04.2-☑	D23.2-☑	D48.5	D49.2
axilla, axillary fold — *see also* Neoplasm, skin, trunk	C44.509	C79.2	D04.5	D23.5	D48.5	D49.2
back — *see also* Neoplasm, skin, trunk	C44.509	C79.2	D04.5	D23.5	D48.5	D49.2
basal cell carcinoma	C44.91	—	—	—	—	—
breast	C44.501	C79.2	D04.5	D23.5	D48.5	D49.2
basal cell carcinoma	C44.511	—	—	—	—	—
specified type NEC	C44.591	—	—	—	—	—
squamous cell carcinoma	C44.521	—	—	—	—	—
brow — *see also* Neoplasm, skin, face	C44.309	C79.2	D04.39	D23.39	D48.5	D49.2
buttock — *see also* Neoplasm, skin, trunk	C44.509	C79.2	D04.5	D23.5	D48.5	D49.2

	Malignant Primary	Malignant Secondary	Ca in situ	Benign	Uncertain Behavior	Unspecified Behavior
Neoplasm, neoplastic *— continued*						
skin *— continued*						
calf *— see also* Neoplasm, skin, limb, lower	C44.70-☑	C79.2	D04.7-☑	D23.7-☑	D48.5	D49.2
canthus (eye) (inner) (outer)	C44.10-☑	C79.2	D04.1-☑	D23.1-☑	D48.5	D49.2
basal cell carcinoma	C44.11-☑	—	—	—	—	—
sebaceous cell	C44.13-☑	—	—	—	—	—
specified type NEC	C44.19-☑	—	—	—	—	—
squamous cell carcinoma	C44.12-☑	—	—	—	—	—
cervical region *— see also* Neoplasm, skin, neck	C44.40	C79.2	D04.4	D23.4	D48.5	D49.2
cheek (external) *— see also* Neoplasm, skin, face	C44.309	C79.2	D04.39	D23.39	D48.5	D49.2
chest (wall) *— see also* Neoplasm, skin, trunk	C44.509	C79.2	D04.5	D23.5	D48.5	D49.2
chin *— see also* Neoplasm, skin, face	C44.309	C79.2	D04.39	D23.39	D48.5	D49.2
clavicular area *— see also* Neoplasm, skin, trunk	C44.509	C79.2	D04.5	D23.5	D48.5	D49.2
clitoris	C51.2	C79.82	D07.1	D28.0	D39.8	D49.59
columnella *— see also* Neoplasm, skin, face	C44.309	C79.2	D04.39	D23.39	D48.5	D49.2
concha *— see also* Neoplasm, skin, ear	C44.20-☑	C79.2	D04.2-☑	D23.2-☑	D48.5	D49.2
ear (external)	C44.20-☑	C79.2	D04.2-☑	D23.2-☑	D48.5	D49.2
basal cell carcinoma	C44.21-☑	—	—	—	—	—
specified type NEC	C44.29-☑	—	—	—	—	—
squamous cell carcinoma	C44.22-☑	—	—	—	—	—
elbow *— see also* Neoplasm, skin, limb, upper	C44.60-☑	C79.2	D04.6-☑	D23.6-☑	D48.5	D49.2
eyebrow *— see also* Neoplasm, skin, face	C44.309	C79.2	D04.39	D23.39	D48.5	D49.2
eyelid	C44.10-☑	C79.2	D04.1-☑	D23.1-☑	D48.5	D49.2
basal cell carcinoma	C44.11-☑	—	—	—	—	—
sebaceous cell	C44.13-☑	—	—	—	—	—
specified type NEC	C44.19-☑	—	—	—	—	—
squamous cell carcinoma	C44.12-☑	—	—	—	—	—
face NOS	C44.300	C79.2	D04.30	D23.30	D48.5	D49.2
basal cell carcinoma	C44.310	—	—	—	—	—
specified type NEC	C44.390	—	—	—	—	—
squamous cell carcinoma	C44.320	—	—	—	—	—
female genital organs (external)	C51.9	C79.82	D07.1	D28.0	D39.8	D49.59
clitoris	C51.2	C79.82	D07.1	D28.0	D39.8	D49.59
labium NEC	C51.9	C79.82	D07.1	D28.0	D39.8	D49.59
majus	C51.0	C79.82	D07.1	D28.0	D39.8	D49.59
minus	C51.1	C79.82	D07.1	D28.0	D39.8	D49.59
pudendum	C51.9	C79.82	D07.1	D28.0	D39.8	D49.59
vulva	C51.9	C79.82	D07.1	D28.0	D39.8	D49.59
finger *— see also* Neoplasm, skin, limb, upper	C44.60-☑	C79.2	D04.6-☑	D23.6-☑	D48.5	D49.2
flank *— see also* Neoplasm, skin, trunk	C44.509	C79.2	D04.5	D23.5	D48.5	D49.2
foot *— see also* Neoplasm, skin, limb, lower	C44.70-☑	C79.2	D04.7-☑	D23.7-☑	D48.5	D49.2
Neoplasm, neoplastic *— continued*						
skin *— continued*						
forearm *— see also* Neoplasm, skin, limb, upper	C44.60-☑	C79.2	D04.6-☑	D23.6-☑	D48.5	D49.2
forehead *— see also* Neoplasm, skin, face	C44.309	C79.2	D04.39	D23.39	D48.5	D49.2
glabella *— see also* Neoplasm, skin, face	C44.309	C79.2	D04.39	D23.39	D48.5	D49.2
gluteal region *— see also* Neoplasm, skin, trunk	C44.509	C79.2	D04.5	D23.5	D48.5	D49.2
groin *— see also* Neoplasm, skin, trunk	C44.509	C79.2	D04.5	D23.5	D48.5	D49.2
hand *— see also* Neoplasm, skin, limb, upper	C44.60-☑	C79.2	D04.6-☑	D23.6-☑	D48.5	D49.2
head NEC *— see also* Neoplasm, skin, scalp	C44.40	C79.2	D04.4	D23.4	D48.5	D49.2
heel *— see also* Neoplasm, skin, limb, lower	C44.70-☑	C79.2	D04.7-☑	D23.7-☑	D48.5	D49.2
helix *— see also* Neoplasm, skin, ear	C44.20-☑	C79.2	D04.2-☑	D23.2-☑	D48.5	D49.2
hip *— see also* Neoplasm, skin, limb, lower	C44.70-☑	C79.2	D04.7-☑	D23.7-☑	D48.5	D49.2
infraclavicular region *— see also* Neoplasm, skin, trunk	C44.509	C79.2	D04.5	D23.5	D48.5	D49.2
inguinal region *— see also* Neoplasm, skin, trunk	C44.509	C79.2	D04.5	D23.5	D48.5	D49.2
jaw *— see also* Neoplasm, skin, face	C44.309	C79.2	D04.39	D23.39	D48.5	D49.2
Kaposi's sarcoma *— see* Kaposi's, sarcoma, skin						
knee *— see also* Neoplasm, skin, limb, lower	C44.70-☑	C79.2	D04.7-☑	D23.7-☑	D48.5	D49.2
labia						
majora	C51.0	C79.82	D07.1	D28.0	D39.8	D49.59
minora	C51.1	C79.82	D07.1	D28.0	D39.8	D49.59
leg *— see also* Neoplasm, skin, limb, lower	C44.70-☑	C79.2	D04.7-☑	D23.7-☑	D48.5	D49.2
lid (lower) (upper)	C44.10-☑	C79.2	D04.1-☑	D23.1-☑	D48.5	D49.2
basal cell carcinoma	C44.11-☑	—	—	—	—	—
sebaceous cell	C44.13-☑	—	—	—	—	—
specified type NEC	C44.19-☑	—	—	—	—	—
squamous cell carcinoma	C44.12-☑	—	—	—	—	—
limb NEC	C44.90	C79.2	D04.9	D23.9	D48.5	D49.2
basal cell carcinoma	C44.91	—	—	—	—	—
lower	C44.70-☑	C79.2	D04.7-☑	D23.7-☑	D48.5	D49.2
basal cell carcinoma	C44.71-☑	—	—	—	—	—
specified type NEC	C44.79-☑	—	—	—	—	—
squamous cell carcinoma	C44.72-☑	—	—	—	—	—
upper	C44.60-☑	C79.2	D04.6-☑	D23.6-☑	D48.5	D49.2
basal cell carcinoma	C44.61-☑	—	—	—	—	—
specified type NEC	C44.69-☑	—	—	—	—	—
squamous cell carcinoma	C44.62-☑	—	—	—	—	—
lip (lower) (upper)	C44.00	C79.2	D04.0	D23.0	D48.5	D49.2

	Malignant Primary	Malignant Secondary	Ca in situ	Benign	Uncertain Behavior	Unspecified Behavior
Neoplasm, neoplastic — *continued*						
skin — *continued*						
lip — *continued*						
basal cell carcinoma	C44.01	—	—	—	—	—
specified type NEC	C44.09	—	—	—	—	—
squamous cell carcinoma	C44.02	—	—	—	—	—
male genital organs	C63.9	C79.82	D07.60	D29.9	D40.8	D49.59
penis	C60.9	C79.82	D07.4	D29.0	D40.8	D49.59
prepuce	C60.0	C79.82	D07.4	D29.0	D40.8	D49.59
scrotum	C63.2	C79.82	D07.61	D29.4	D40.8	D49.59
mastectomy site (skin) — *see also* Neoplasm, skin, breast	C44.501	C79.2	—	—	—	—
specified as breast tissue	C50.8-☑	C79.81	—	—	—	—
meatus, acoustic (external) — *see also* Neoplasm, skin, ear	C44.20-☑	C79.2	D04.2-☑	D23.2-☑	D48.5	D49.2
melanotic — *see* Melanoma						
Merkel cell — *see* Carcinoma, Merkel cell						
nates — *see also* Neoplasm, skin, trunk	C44.509	C79.2	D04.5	D23.5	D48.5	D49.2
neck	C44.40	C79.2	D04.4	D23.4	D48.5	D49.2
basal cell carcinoma	C44.41	—	—	—	—	—
specified type NEC	C44.49	—	—	—	—	—
squamous cell carcinoma	C44.42	—	—	—	—	—
nevus — *see* Nevus, skin						
nose (external) — *see also* Neoplasm, nose, skin	C44.301	C79.2	D04.39	D23.39	D48.5	D49.2
overlapping lesion	C44.80	—	—	—	—	—
basal cell carcinoma	C44.81	—	—	—	—	—
specified type NEC	C44.89	—	—	—	—	—
squamous cell carcinoma	C44.82	—	—	—	—	—
palm — *see also* Neoplasm, skin, limb, upper	C44.60-☑	C79.2	D04.6-☑	D23.6-☑	D48.5	D49.2
palpebra	C44.10-☑	C79.2	D04.1-☑	D23.1-☑	D48.5	D49.2
basal cell carcinoma	C44.11-☑	—	—	—	—	—
sebaceous cell	C44.13-☑	—	—	—	—	—
specified type NEC	C44.19-☑	—	—	—	—	—
squamous cell carcinoma	C44.12-☑	—	—	—	—	—
penis NEC	C60.9	C79.82	D07.4	D29.0	D40.8	D49.59
perianal — *see also* Neoplasm, skin, anus	C44.500	C79.2	D04.5	D23.5	D48.5	D49.2
perineum — *see also* Neoplasm, skin, anus	C44.500	C79.2	D04.5	D23.5	D48.5	D49.2
pinna — *see also* Neoplasm, skin, ear	C44.20-☑	C79.2	D04.2-☑	D23.2-☑	D48.5	D49.2
plantar — *see also* Neoplasm, skin, limb, lower	C44.70-☑	C79.2	D04.7-☑	D23.7-☑	D48.5	D49.2
popliteal fossa or space — *see also* Neoplasm, skin, limb, lower	C44.70-☑	C79.2	D04.7-☑	D23.7-☑	D48.5	D49.2
prepuce	C60.0	C79.82	D07.4	D29.0	D40.8	D49.59
pubes — *see also* Neoplasm, skin, trunk	C44.509	C79.2	D04.5	D23.5	D48.5	D49.2
sacrococcygeal region — *see also* Neoplasm, skin, trunk	C44.509	C79.2	D04.5	D23.5	D48.5	D49.2
scalp	C44.40	C79.2	D04.4	D23.4	D48.5	D49.2
basal cell carcinoma	C44.41	—	—	—	—	—
specified type NEC	C44.49	—	—	—	—	—
squamous cell carcinoma	C44.42	—	—	—	—	—
scapular region — *see also* Neoplasm, skin, trunk	C44.509	C79.2	D04.5	D23.5	D48.5	D49.2
scrotum	C63.2	C79.82	D07.61	D29.4	D40.8	D49.59
shoulder — *see also* Neoplasm, skin, limb, upper	C44.60-☑	C79.2	D04.6-☑	D23.6-☑	D48.5	D49.2
sole (foot) — *see also* Neoplasm, skin, limb, lower	C44.70-☑	C79.2	D04.7-☑	D23.7-☑	D48.5	D49.2
specified sites NEC	C44.80	C79.2	D04.8	D23.9	D48.5	D49.2
basal cell carcinoma	C44.81	—	—	—	—	—
specified type NEC	C44.89	—	—	—	—	—
squamous cell carcinoma	C44.82	—	—	—	—	—
specified type NEC	C44.99	—	—	—	—	—
squamous cell carcinoma	C44.92	—	—	—	—	—
submammary fold — *see also* Neoplasm, skin, trunk	C44.509	C79.2	D04.5	D23.5	D48.5	D49.2
supraclavicular region — *see also* Neoplasm, skin, neck	C44.40	C79.2	D04.4	D23.4	D48.5	D49.2
temple — *see also* Neoplasm, skin, face	C44.309	C79.2	D04.39	D23.39	D48.5	D49.2
thigh — *see also* Neoplasm, skin, limb, lower	C44.70-☑	C79.2	D04.7-☑	D23.7-☑	D48.5	D49.2
thoracic wall — *see also* Neoplasm, skin, trunk	C44.509	C79.2	D04.5	D23.5	D48.5	D49.2
thumb — *see also* Neoplasm, skin, limb, upper	C44.60-☑	C79.2	D04.6-☑	D23.6-☑	D48.5	D49.2
toe — *see also* Neoplasm, skin, limb, lower	C44.70-☑	C79.2	D04.7-☑	D23.7-☑	D48.5	D49.2
tragus — *see also* Neoplasm, skin, ear	C44.20-☑	C79.2	D04.2-☑	D23.2-☑	D48.5	D49.2
trunk	C44.509	C79.2	D04.5	D23.5	D48.5	D49.2
basal cell carcinoma	C44.519	—	—	—	—	—
specified type NEC	C44.599	—	—	—	—	—
squamous cell carcinoma	C44.529	—	—	—	—	—
umbilicus — *see also* Neoplasm, skin, trunk	C44.509	C79.2	D04.5	D23.5	D48.5	D49.2
vulva	C51.9	C79.82	D07.1	D28.0	D39.8	D49.59
overlapping lesion	C51.8	—	—	—	—	—
wrist — *see also* Neoplasm, skin, limb, upper	C44.60-☑	C79.2	D04.6-☑	D23.6-☑	D48.5	D49.2
skull	C41.0	C79.51	—	D16.4	D48.0	D49.2

☑ Additional Character Required — Refer to the Tabular List for Character Selection

	Malignant Primary	Malignant Secondary	Ca in situ	Benign	Uncertain Behavior	Unspecified Behavior
Neoplasm, neoplastic *— continued*						
soft parts or tissues — *see* Neoplasm, connective tissue						
specified site NEC	C76.8	C79.89	D09.8	D36.7	D48.7	D49.89
spermatic cord	C63.1-☑	C79.82	D07.69	D29.8	D40.8	D49.59
sphenoid	C31.3	C78.39	D02.3	D14.0	D38.5	D49.1
bone	C41.0	C79.51	—	D16.4	D48.0	D49.2
sinus	C31.3	C78.39	D02.3	D14.0	D38.5	D49.1
sphincter						
anal	C21.1	C78.5	D01.3	D12.9	D37.8	D49.0
of Oddi	C24.0	C78.89	D01.5	D13.5	D37.6	D49.0
spine, spinal (column)	C41.2	C79.51	—	D16.6	D48.0	D49.2
bulb	C71.7	C79.31	—	D33.1	D43.1	D49.6
coccyx	C41.4	C79.51	—	D16.8	D48.0	D49.2
cord (cervical) (lumbar) (sacral) (thoracic)	C72.0	C79.49	—	D33.4	D43.4	D49.7
dura mater	C70.1	C79.49	—	D32.1	D42.1	D49.7
lumbosacral	C41.2	C79.51	—	D16.6	D48.0	D49.2
marrow NEC	C96.9	C79.52	—	—	D47.9	D49.89
membrane	C70.1	C79.49	—	D32.1	D42.1	D49.7
meninges	C70.1	C79.49	—	D32.1	D42.1	D49.7
nerve (root)	C47.9	C79.89	—	D36.10	D48.2	D49.2
pia mater	C70.1	C79.49	—	D32.1	D42.1	D49.7
root	C47.9	C79.89	—	D36.10	D48.2	D49.2
sacrum	C41.4	C79.51	—	D16.8	D48.0	D49.2
spleen, splenic NEC	C26.1	C78.89	D01.7	D13.9	D37.8	D49.0
flexure (colon)	C18.5	C78.5	D01.0	D12.3	D37.4	D49.0
stem, brain	C71.7	C79.31	—	D33.1	D43.1	D49.6
Stensen's duct	C07	C79.89	D00.00	D11.0	D37.030	D49.0
sternum	C41.3	C79.51	—	D16.7	D48.0	D49.2
stomach	C16.9	C78.89	D00.2	D13.1	D37.1	D49.0
antrum (pyloric)	C16.3	C78.89	D00.2	D13.1	D37.1	D49.0
body	C16.2	C78.89	D00.2	D13.1	D37.1	D49.0
cardia	C16.0	C78.89	D00.2	D13.1	D37.1	D49.0
cardiac orifice	C16.0	C78.89	D00.2	D13.1	D37.1	D49.0
corpus	C16.2	C78.89	D00.2	D13.1	D37.1	D49.0
fundus	C16.1	C78.89	D00.2	D13.1	D37.1	D49.0
greater curvature NEC	C16.6	C78.89	D00.2	D13.1	D37.1	D49.0
lesser curvature NEC	C16.5	C78.89	D00.2	D13.1	D37.1	D49.0
overlapping lesion	C16.8	—	—	—	—	—
prepylorus	C16.4	C78.89	D00.2	D13.1	D37.1	D49.0
pylorus	C16.4	C78.89	D00.2	D13.1	D37.1	D49.0
wall NEC	C16.9	C78.89	D00.2	D13.1	D37.1	D49.0
anterior NEC	C16.8	C78.89	D00.2	D13.1	D37.1	D49.0
posterior NEC	C16.8	C78.89	D00.2	D13.1	D37.1	D49.0
stroma, endometrial	C54.1	C79.82	D07.0	D26.1	D39.0	D49.59
stump, cervical	C53.8	C79.82	D06.7	D26.0	D39.0	D49.59
subcutaneous (nodule) (tissue) NEC — *see* Neoplasm, connective tissue						
subdural	C70.9	C79.32	—	D32.9	D42.9	D49.7
subglottis, subglottic	C32.2	C78.39	D02.0	D14.1	D38.0	D49.1
sublingual	C04.9	C79.89	D00.06	D10.2	D37.09	D49.0
gland or duct	C08.1	C79.89	D00.00	D11.7	D37.031	D49.0
submandibular gland	C08.0	C79.89	D00.00	D11.7	D37.032	D49.0
submaxillary gland or duct	C08.0	C79.89	D00.00	D11.7	D37.032	D49.0
submental	C76.0	C79.89	D09.8	D36.7	D48.7	D49.89
subpleural	C34.9-☑	C78.0-☑	D02.2-☑	D14.3-☑	D38.1	D49.1
substernal	C38.1	C78.1	—	D15.2	D38.3	D49.89
sudoriferous, sudoriparous gland, site						
unspecified	C44.90	C79.2	D04.9	D23.9	D48.5	D49.2
specified site — *see* Neoplasm, skin						
supraclavicular region	C76.0	C79.89	D09.8	D36.7	D48.7	D49.89
supraglottis	C32.1	C78.39	D02.0	D14.1	D38.0	D49.1
suprarenal	C74.9-☑	C79.7-☑	D09.3	D35.0-☑	D44.1-☑	D49.7
capsule	C74.9-☑	C79.7-☑	D09.3	D35.0-☑	D44.1-☑	D49.7

	Malignant Primary	Malignant Secondary	Ca in situ	Benign	Uncertain Behavior	Unspecified Behavior
Neoplasm, neoplastic *— continued*						
suprarenal *— continued*						
cortex	C74.0-☑	C79.7-☑	D09.3	D35.0-☑	D44.1-☑	D49.7
gland	C74.9-☑	C79.7-☑	D09.3	D35.0-☑	D44.1-☑	D49.7
medulla	C74.1-☑	C79.7-☑	D09.3	D35.0-☑	D44.1-☑	D49.7
suprasellar (region)	C71.9	C79.31	—	D33.2	D43.2	D49.6
supratentorial (brain) NEC	C71.0	C79.31	—	D33.0	D43.0	D49.6
sweat gland (apocrine) (eccrine), site unspecified	C44.90	C79.2	D04.9	D23.9	D48.5	D49.2
specified site — *see* Neoplasm, skin						
sympathetic nerve or nervous system NEC	C47.9	C79.89	—	D36.10	D48.2	D49.2
symphysis pubis	C41.4	C79.51	—	D16.8	D48.0	D49.2
synovial membrane — *see* Neoplasm, connective tissue						
tapetum, brain	C71.8	C79.31	—	D33.2	D43.2	D49.6
tarsus (any bone)	C40.3-☑	C79.51	—	D16.3-☑	—	—
temple (skin) — *see also* Neoplasm, skin, face	C44.309	C79.2	D04.39	D23.39	D48.5	D49.2
temporal						
bone	C41.0	C79.51	—	D16.4	D48.0	D49.2
lobe or pole	C71.2	C79.31	—	D33.0	D43.0	D49.6
region	C76.0	C79.89	D09.8	D36.7	D48.7	D49.89
skin — *see also* Neoplasm, skin, face	C44.309	C79.2	D04.39	D23.39	D48.5	D49.2
tendon (sheath) — *see* Neoplasm, connective tissue						
tentorium (cerebelli)	C70.0	C79.32	—	D32.0	D42.0	D49.7
testis, testes	C62.9-☑	C79.82	D07.69	D29.2-☑	D40.1-☑	D49.59
descended	C62.1-☑	C79.82	D07.69	D29.2-☑	D40.1-☑	D49.59
ectopic	C62.0-☑	C79.82	D07.69	D29.2-☑	D40.1-☑	D49.59
retained	C62.0-☑	C79.82	D07.69	D29.2-☑	D40.1-☑	D49.59
scrotal	C62.1-☑	C79.82	D07.69	D29.2-☑	D40.1-☑	D49.59
undescended	C62.0-☑	C79.82	D07.69	D29.2-☑	D40.1-☑	D49.59
unspecified whether descended or undescended	C62.9-☑	C79.82	D07.69	D29.2-☑	D40.1-☑	D49.59
thalamus	C71.0	C79.31	—	D33.0	D43.0	D49.6
thigh NEC	C76.5-☑	C79.89	D04.7-☑	D36.7	D48.7	D49.89
thorax, thoracic (cavity) (organs NEC)	C76.1	C79.89	D09.8	D36.7	D48.7	D49.89
duct	C49.3	C79.89	—	D21.3	D48.1	D49.2
wall NEC	C76.1	C79.89	D09.8	D36.7	D48.7	D49.89
throat	C14.0	C79.89	D00.08	D10.9	D37.05	D49.0
thumb NEC	C76.4-☑	C79.89	D04.6-☑	D36.7	D48.7	D49.89
thymus (gland)	C37	C79.89	D09.3	D15.0	D38.4	D49.89
thyroglossal duct	C73	C79.89	D09.3	D34	D44.0	D49.7
thyroid (gland)	C73	C79.89	D09.3	D34	D44.0	D49.7
cartilage	C32.3	C78.39	D02.0	D14.1	D38.0	D49.1
tibia (any part)	C40.2-☑	C79.51	—	D16.2-☑	—	—
toe NEC	C76.5-☑	C79.89	D04.7-☑	D36.7	D48.7	D49.89
tongue	C02.9	C79.89	D00.07	D10.1	D37.02	D49.0
anterior (two-thirds) NEC	C02.3	C79.89	D00.07	D10.1	D37.02	D49.0
dorsal surface	C02.0	C79.89	D00.07	D10.1	D37.02	D49.0
ventral surface	C02.2	C79.89	D00.07	D10.1	D37.02	D49.0
base (dorsal surface)	C01	C79.89	D00.07	D10.1	D37.02	D49.0
border (lateral)	C02.1	C79.89	D00.07	D10.1	D37.02	D49.0
dorsal surface NEC	C02.0	C79.89	D00.07	D10.1	D37.02	D49.0
fixed part NEC	C01	C79.89	D00.07	D10.1	D37.02	D49.0
foreamen cecum	C02.0	C79.89	D00.07	D10.1	D37.02	D49.0
frenulum linguae	C02.2	C79.89	D00.07	D10.1	D37.02	D49.0
junctional zone	C02.8	C79.89	D00.07	D10.1	D37.02	D49.0
margin (lateral)	C02.1	C79.89	D00.07	D10.1	D37.02	D49.0
midline NEC	C02.0	C79.89	D00.07	D10.1	D37.02	D49.0
mobile part NEC	C02.3	C79.89	D00.07	D10.1	D37.02	D49.0

	Malignant Primary	Malignant Secondary	Ca in situ	Benign	Uncertain Behavior	Unspecified Behavior
Neoplasm, neoplastic — *continued*						
tongue — *continued*						
overlapping lesion	CØ2.8	—	—	—	—	—
posterior (third)	CØ1	C79.89	DØØ.Ø7	D1Ø.1	D37.Ø2	D49.Ø
root	CØ1	C79.89	DØØ.Ø7	D1Ø.1	D37.Ø2	D49.Ø
surface (dorsal)	CØ2.Ø	C79.89	DØØ.Ø7	D1Ø.1	D37.Ø2	D49.Ø
base	CØ1	C79.89	DØØ.Ø7	D1Ø.1	D37.Ø2	D49.Ø
ventral	CØ2.2	C79.89	DØØ.Ø7	D1Ø.1	D37.Ø2	D49.Ø
tip	CØ2.1	C79.89	DØØ.Ø7	D1Ø.1	D37.Ø2	D49.Ø
tonsil	CØ2.4	C79.89	DØØ.Ø7	D1Ø.1	D37.Ø2	D49.Ø
tonsil	CØ9.9	C79.89	DØØ.Ø8	D1Ø.4	D37.Ø5	D49.Ø
fauces, faucial	CØ9.9	C79.89	DØØ.Ø8	D1Ø.4	D37.Ø5	D49.Ø
lingual	CØ2.4	C79.89	DØØ.Ø7	D1Ø.1	D37.Ø2	D49.Ø
overlapping sites	CØ9.8	—	—	—	—	—
palatine	CØ9.9	C79.89	DØØ.Ø8	D1Ø.4	D37.Ø5	D49.Ø
pharyngeal	C11.1	C79.89	DØØ.Ø8	D1Ø.6	D37.Ø5	D49.Ø
pillar (anterior) (posterior)	CØ9.1	C79.89	DØØ.Ø8	D1Ø.5	D37.Ø5	D49.Ø
tonsillar fossa	CØ9.Ø	C79.89	DØØ.Ø8	D1Ø.5	D37.Ø5	D49.Ø
tooth socket NEC	CØ3.9	C79.89	DØØ.Ø3	D1Ø.39	D37.Ø9	D49.Ø
trachea (cartilage) (mucosa)	C33	C78.39	DØ2.1	D14.2	D38.1	D49.1
overlapping lesion with bronchus or lung	C34.8-☑	—	—	—	—	—
tracheobronchial	C34.8-☑	C78.39	DØ2.1	D14.2	D38.1	D49.1
overlapping lesion with lung	C34.8-☑	—	—	—	—	—
tragus — *see also* Neoplasm, skin, ear	C44.2Ø-☑	C79.2	DØ4.2-☑	D23.2-☑	D48.5	D49.2
trunk NEC	C76.8	C79.89	DØ4.5	D36.7	D48.7	D49.89
tubo-ovarian	C57.8	C79.82	DØ7.39	D28.7	D39.8	D49.59
tunica vaginalis	C63.7	C79.82	DØ7.69	D29.8	D4Ø.8	D49.59
turbinate (bone)	C41.Ø	C79.51	—	D16.4	D48.Ø	D49.2
nasal	C3Ø.Ø	C78.39	DØ2.3	D14.Ø	D38.5	D49.1
tympanic cavity	C3Ø.1	C78.39	DØ2.3	D14.Ø	D38.5	D49.1
ulna (any part)	C4Ø.Ø-☑	C79.51	—	D16.Ø-☑	—	—
umbilicus, umbilical — *see also* Neoplasm, skin, trunk	C44.5Ø9	C79.2	DØ4.5	D23.5	D48.5	D49.2
uncus, brain	C71.2	C79.31	—	D33.Ø	D43.Ø	D49.6
unknown site or unspecified	C8Ø.1	C79.9	DØ9.9	D36.9	D48.9	D49.9
urachus	C67.7	C79.11	DØ9.Ø	D3Ø.3	D41.4	D49.4
ureter-bladder (junction)	C67.6	C79.11	DØ9.Ø	D3Ø.3	D41.4	D49.4
ureter, ureteral	C66.-☑	C79.19	DØ9.19	D3Ø.2-☑	D41.2-☑	D49.59
orifice (bladder)	C67.6	C79.11	DØ9.Ø	D3Ø.3	D41.4	D49.4
urethra, urethral (gland)	C68.Ø	C79.19	DØ9.19	D3Ø.4	D41.3	D49.59
orifice, internal	C67.5	C79.11	DØ9.Ø	D3Ø.3	D41.4	D49.4
urethrovaginal (septum)	C57.9	C79.82	DØ7.3Ø	D28.9	D39.8	D49.59
urinary organ or system	C68.9	C79.1Ø	DØ9.1Ø	D3Ø.9	D41.9	D49.59
bladder — *see* Neoplasm, bladder						
overlapping lesion	C68.8	—	—	—	—	—
specified sites NEC	C68.8	C79.19	DØ9.19	D3Ø.8	D41.8	D49.59
utero-ovarian	C57.8	C79.82	DØ7.39	D28.7	D39.8	D49.59
ligament	C57.1-☑	C79.82	DØ7.39	D28.2	D39.8	D49.59
uterosacral ligament	C57.3	C79.82	—	D28.2	D39.8	D49.59
uterus, uteri, uterine	C55	C79.82	DØ7.Ø	D26.9	D39.Ø	D49.59
adnexa NEC	C57.4	C79.82	DØ7.39	D28.7	D39.8	D49.59
body	C54.9	C79.82	DØ7.Ø	D26.1	D39.Ø	D49.59
cervix	C53.9	C79.82	DØ6.9	D26.Ø	D39.Ø	D49.59
cornu	C54.9	C79.82	DØ7.Ø	D26.1	D39.Ø	D49.59
corpus	C54.9	C79.82	DØ7.Ø	D26.1	D39.Ø	D49.59
endocervix (canal) (gland)	C53.Ø	C79.82	DØ6.Ø	D26.Ø	D39.Ø	D49.59
endometrium	C54.1	C79.82	DØ7.Ø	D26.1	D39.Ø	D49.59
exocervix	C53.1	C79.82	DØ6.1	D26.Ø	D39.Ø	D49.59
external os	C53.1	C79.82	DØ6.1	D26.Ø	D39.Ø	D49.59
fundus	C54.3	C79.82	DØ7.Ø	D26.1	D39.Ø	D49.59
Neoplasm, neoplastic — *continued*						
uterus, uteri, uterine — *continued*						
internal os	C53.Ø	C79.82	DØ6.Ø	D26.Ø	D39.Ø	D49.59
isthmus	C54.Ø	C79.82	DØ7.Ø	D26.1	D39.Ø	D49.59
ligament	C57.3	C79.82	—	D28.2	D39.8	D49.59
broad	C57.1-☑	C79.82	DØ7.39	D28.2	D39.8	D49.59
round	C57.2-☑	C79.82	—	D28.2	D39.8	D49.59
lower segment	C54.Ø	C79.82	DØ7.Ø	D26.1	D39.Ø	D49.59
myometrium	C54.2	C79.82	DØ7.Ø	D26.1	D39.Ø	D49.59
overlapping sites	C54.8	—	—	—	—	—
squamocolumnar junction	C53.8	C79.82	DØ6.7	D26.Ø	D39.Ø	D49.59
tube	C57.Ø-☑	C79.82	DØ7.39	D28.2	D39.8	D49.59
utricle, prostatic	C68.Ø	C79.19	DØ9.19	D3Ø.4	D41.3	D49.59
uveal tract	C69.4-☑	C79.49	DØ9.2-☑	D31.4-☑	D48.7	D49.89
uvula	CØ5.2	C79.89	DØØ.Ø4	D1Ø.39	D37.Ø9	D49.Ø
vagina, vaginal (fornix) (vault) (wall)	C52	C79.82	DØ7.2	D28.1	D39.8	D49.59
vaginovesical	C57.9	C79.82	DØ7.3Ø	D28.9	D39.9	D49.59
septum	C57.9	C79.82	DØ7.3Ø	D28.9	D39.9	D49.59
vallecula (epiglottis)	C1Ø.Ø	C79.89	DØØ.Ø8	D1Ø.5	D37.Ø5	D49.Ø
vascular — *see* Neoplasm, connective tissue						
vas deferens	C63.1-☑	C79.82	DØ7.69	D29.8	D4Ø.8	D49.59
Vater's ampulla	C24.1	C78.89	DØ1.5	D13.5	D37.6	D49.Ø
vein, venous — *see* Neoplasm, connective tissue						
vena cava (abdominal) (inferior)	C49.4	C79.89	—	D21.4	D48.1	D49.2
superior	C49.3	C79.89	—	D21.3	D48.1	D49.2
ventricle (cerebral) (floor) (lateral) (third)	C71.5	C79.31	—	D33.Ø	D43.Ø	D49.6
cardiac (left) (right)	C38.Ø	C79.89	—	D15.1	D48.7	D49.89
fourth	C71.7	C79.31	—	D33.1	D43.1	D49.6
ventricular band of larynx	C32.1	C78.39	DØ2.Ø	D14.1	D38.Ø	D49.1
ventriculus — *see* Neoplasm, stomach						
vermillion border — *see* Neoplasm, lip						
vermis, cerebellum	C71.6	C79.31	—	D33.1	D43.1	D49.6
vertebra (column)	C41.2	C79.51	—	D16.6	D48.Ø	D49.2
coccyx	C41.4	C79.51	—	D16.8	D48.Ø	D49.2
marrow NEC	C96.9	C79.52	—	—	D47.9	D49.89
sacrum	C41.4	C79.51	—	D16.8	D48.Ø	D49.2
vesical — *see* Neoplasm, bladder						
vesicle, seminal	C63.7	C79.82	DØ7.69	D29.8	D4Ø.8	D49.59
vesicocervical tissue	C57.9	C79.82	DØ7.3Ø	D28.9	D39.9	D49.59
vesicorectal	C76.3	C79.82	DØ9.8	D36.7	D48.7	D49.89
vesicovaginal	C57.9	C79.82	DØ7.3Ø	D28.9	D39.9	D49.59
septum	C57.9	C79.82	DØ7.3Ø	D28.9	D39.8	D49.59
vessel (blood) — *see* Neoplasm, connective tissue						
vestibular gland, greater	C51.Ø	C79.82	DØ7.1	D28.Ø	D39.8	D49.59
vestibule						
mouth	CØ6.1	C79.89	DØØ.ØØ	D1Ø.39	D37.Ø9	D49.Ø
nose	C3Ø.Ø	C78.39	DØ2.3	D14.Ø	D38.5	D49.1
Virchow's gland	C77.Ø	C77.Ø	—	D36.Ø	D48.7	D49.89
viscera NEC	C76.8	C79.89	DØ9.8	D36.7	D48.7	D49.89
vocal cords (true)	C32.Ø	C78.39	DØ2.Ø	D14.1	D38.Ø	D49.1
false	C32.1	C78.39	DØ2.Ø	D14.1	D38.Ø	D49.1
vomer	C41.Ø	C79.51	—	D16.4	D48.Ø	D49.2
vulva	C51.9	C79.82	DØ7.1	D28.Ø	D39.8	D49.59
vulvovaginal gland	C51.Ø	C79.82	DØ7.1	D28.Ø	D39.8	D49.59
Waldeyer's ring	C14.2	C79.89	DØØ.Ø8	D1Ø.9	D37.Ø5	D49.Ø
Wharton's duct	CØ8.Ø	C79.89	DØØ.ØØ	D11.7	D37.Ø32	D49.Ø
white matter (central) (cerebral)	C71.Ø	C79.31	—	D33.Ø	D43.Ø	D49.6

	Malignant Primary	Malignant Secondary	Ca in situ	Benign	Uncertain Behavior	Unspecified Behavior
Neoplasm, neoplastic						
— *continued*						
windpipe	C33	C78.39	D02.1	D14.2	D38.1	D49.1
Wirsung's duct	C25.3	C78.89	D01.7	D13.6	D37.8	D49.0
wolffian (body) (duct)						
female	C57.7	C79.82	D07.39	D28.7	D39.8	D49.59
male	C63.7	C79.82	D07.69	D29.8	D40.8	D49.59
womb — *see* Neoplasm, uterus						
wrist NEC	C76.4-☑	C79.89	D04.6-☑	D36.7	D48.7	D49.89
xiphoid process	C41.3	C79.51	—	D16.7	D48.0	D49.2
Zuckerkandl organ	C75.5	C79.89	—	D35.6	D44.7	D49.7

Substance	Poisoning, Accidental (unintentional)	Poisoning, Intentional Self-harm	Poisoning, Assault	Poisoning, Undetermined	Adverse Effect	Under-dosing
14-hydroxydihydro-morphinone	T4Ø.2X1	T4Ø.2X2	T4Ø.2X3	T4Ø.2X4	T4Ø.2X5	T4Ø.2X6
1-Propanol	T51.3X1	T51.3X2	T51.3X3	T51.3X4	—	—
2,3,7,8-Tetrachlorodibenzo-p-dioxin	T53.7X1	T53.7X2	T53.7X3	T53.7X4	—	—
2,4,5-T (trichloro-phenoxyacetic acid)	T6Ø.1X1	T6Ø.1X2	T6Ø.1X3	T6Ø.1X4	—	—
2,4,5-Trichlorophen-oxyacetic acid	T6Ø.3X1	T6Ø.3X2	T6Ø.3X3	T6Ø.3X4	—	—
2,4-D (dichlorophen-oxyacetic acid)	T6Ø.3X1	T6Ø.3X2	T6Ø.3X3	T6Ø.3X4	—	—
2,4-Toluene diisocyanate	T65.ØX1	T65.ØX2	T65.ØX3	T65.ØX4	—	—
2-Deoxy-5-fluorouridine	T45.1X1	T45.1X2	T45.1X3	T45.1X4	T45.1X5	T45.1X6
2-Ethoxyethanol	T52.3X1	T52.3X2	T52.3X3	T52.3X4	—	—
2-Methoxyethanol	T52.3X1	T52.3X2	T52.3X3	T52.3X4	—	—
2-Propanol	T51.2X1	T51.2X2	T51.2X3	T51.2X4	—	—
3,4-methylenedioxymeth-amphetamine	T43.641	T43.642	T43.643	T43.644	—	—
4-Aminobutyric acid	T43.8X1	T43.8X2	T43.8X3	T43.8X4	T43.8X5	T43.8X6
4-Aminophenol derivatives	T39.1X1	T39.1X2	T39.1X3	T39.1X4	T39.1X5	T39.1X6
5-Deoxy-5-fluorouridine	T45.1X1	T45.1X2	T45.1X3	T45.1X4	T45.1X5	T45.1X6
5-Methoxypsoralen (5-MOP)	T5Ø.991	T5Ø.992	T5Ø.993	T5Ø.994	T5Ø.995	T5Ø.996
8-Aminoquinoline drugs	T37.2X1	T37.2X2	T37.2X3	T37.2X4	T37.2X5	T37.2X6
8-Methoxypsoralen (8-MOP)	T5Ø.991	T5Ø.992	T5Ø.993	T5Ø.994	T5Ø.995	T5Ø.996
9-hydoxyrisperidone*	T43.591	T43.592	T43.593	T43.594	T43.595	T43.596
ABOB	T37.5X1	T37.5X2	T37.5X3	T37.5X4	T37.5X5	T37.5X6
Abrine	T62.2X1	T62.2X2	T62.2X3	T62.2X4	—	—
Abrus (seed)	T62.2X1	T62.2X2	T62.2X3	T62.2X4	—	—
Absinthe	T51.ØX1	T51.ØX2	T51.ØX3	T51.ØX4	—	—
beverage	T51.ØX1	T51.ØX2	T51.ØX3	T51.ØX4	—	—
Acaricide	T6Ø.8X1	T6Ø.8X2	T6Ø.8X3	T6Ø.8X4	—	—
Acebutolol	T44.7X1	T44.7X2	T44.7X3	T44.7X4	T44.7X5	T44.7X6
Acecarbromal	T42.6X1	T42.6X2	T42.6X3	T42.6X4	T42.6X5	T42.6X6
Aceclidine	T44.1X1	T44.1X2	T44.1X3	T44.1X4	T44.1X5	T44.1X6
Acedapsone	T37.ØX1	T37.ØX2	T37.ØX3	T37.ØX4	T37.ØX5	T37.ØX6
Acefylline piperazine	T48.6X1	T48.6X2	T48.6X3	T48.6X4	T48.6X5	T48.6X6
Acemorphan	T4Ø.2X1	T4Ø.2X2	T4Ø.2X3	T4Ø.2X4	T4Ø.2X5	T4Ø.2X6
Acenocoumarin	T45.511	T45.512	T45.513	T45.514	T45.515	T45.516
Acenocoumarol	T45.511	T45.512	T45.513	T45.514	T45.515	T45.516
Aceon*	T46.4X1	T46.4X2	T46.4X3	T46.4X4	T46.4X5	T46.4X6
Acepifylline	T48.6X1	T48.6X2	T48.6X3	T48.6X4	T48.6X5	T48.6X6
Acepromazine	T43.3X1	T43.3X2	T43.3X3	T43.3X4	T43.3X5	T43.3X6
Acesulfamethoxypyridazine	T37.ØX1	T37.ØX2	T37.ØX3	T37.ØX4	T37.ØX5	T37.ØX6
Acetal	T52.8X1	T52.8X2	T52.8X3	T52.8X4	—	—
Acetaldehyde (vapor)	T52.8X1	T52.8X2	T52.8X3	T52.8X4	—	—
liquid	T65.891	T65.892	T65.893	T65.894	—	—
Acetaminophen	T39.1X1	T39.1X2	T39.1X3	T39.1X4	T39.1X5	T39.1X6
Acetaminosalol	T39.1X1	T39.1X2	T39.1X3	T39.1X4	T39.1X5	T39.1X6
Acetanilide	T39.1X1	T39.1X2	T39.1X3	T39.1X4	T39.1X5	T39.1X6
Acetarsol	T37.3X1	T37.3X2	T37.3X3	T37.3X4	T37.3X5	T37.3X6
Acetazolamide	T5Ø.2X1	T5Ø.2X2	T5Ø.2X3	T5Ø.2X4	T5Ø.2X5	T5Ø.2X6
Acetiamine	T45.2X1	T45.2X2	T45.2X3	T45.2X4	T45.2X5	T45.2X6
Acetic						
acid	T54.2X1	T54.2X2	T54.2X3	T54.2X4	—	—
with sodium acetate (ointment)	T49.3X1	T49.3X2	T49.3X3	T49.3X4	T49.3X5	T49.3X6
ester (solvent)(vapor)	T52.8X1	T52.8X2	T52.8X3	T52.8X4	—	—
irrigating solution	T5Ø.3X1	T5Ø.3X2	T5Ø.3X3	T5Ø.3X4	T5Ø.3X5	T5Ø.3X6
medicinal (lotion)	T49.2X1	T49.2X2	T49.2X3	T49.2X4	T49.2X5	T49.2X6
anhydride	T65.891	T65.892	T65.893	T65.894	—	—
ether (vapor)	T52.8X1	T52.8X2	T52.8X3	T52.8X4	—	—
Acetohexamide	T38.3X1	T38.3X2	T38.3X3	T38.3X4	T38.3X5	T38.3X6
Acetohydroxamic acid	T5Ø.991	T5Ø.992	T5Ø.993	T5Ø.994	T5Ø.995	T5Ø.996
Acetomenaphthone	T45.7X1	T45.7X2	T45.7X3	T45.7X4	T45.7X5	T45.7X6
Acetomorphine	T4Ø.1X1	T4Ø.1X2	T4Ø.1X3	T4Ø.1X4	—	—
Acetone (oils)	T52.4X1	T52.4X2	T52.4X3	T52.4X4	—	—
chlorinated	T52.4X1	T52.4X2	T52.4X3	T52.4X4	—	—
vapor	T52.4X1	T52.4X2	T52.4X3	T52.4X4	—	—
Acetonitrile	T52.8X1	T52.8X2	T52.8X3	T52.8X4	—	—
Acetophenazine	T43.3X1	T43.3X2	T43.3X3	T43.3X4	T43.3X5	T43.3X6
Acetophenetedin	T39.1X1	T39.1X2	T39.1X3	T39.1X4	T39.1X5	T39.1X6
Acetophenone	T52.4X1	T52.4X2	T52.4X3	T52.4X4	—	—
Acetorphine	T4Ø.2X1	T4Ø.2X2	T4Ø.2X3	T4Ø.2X4	—	—
Acetosulfone (sodium)	T37.1X1	T37.1X2	T37.1X3	T37.1X4	T37.1X5	T37.1X6
Acetrizoate (sodium)	T5Ø.8X1	T5Ø.8X2	T5Ø.8X3	T5Ø.8X4	T5Ø.8X5	T5Ø.8X6
Acetrizoic acid	T5Ø.8X1	T5Ø.8X2	T5Ø.8X3	T5Ø.8X4	T5Ø.8X5	T5Ø.8X6
Acetyl						
bromide	T53.6X1	T53.6X2	T53.6X3	T53.6X4	—	—
chloride	T53.6X1	T53.6X2	T53.6X3	T53.6X4	—	—
Acetylcarbromal	T42.6X1	T42.6X2	T42.6X3	T42.6X4	T42.6X5	T42.6X6
Acetylcholine						

Substance	Poisoning, Accidental (unintentional)	Poisoning, Intentional Self-harm	Poisoning, Assault	Poisoning, Undetermined	Adverse Effect	Under-dosing
Acetylcholine — *continued*						
chloride	T44.1X1	T44.1X2	T44.1X3	T44.1X4	T44.1X5	T44.1X6
derivative	T44.1X1	T44.1X2	T44.1X3	T44.1X4	T44.1X5	T44.1X6
Acetylcysteine	T48.4X1	T48.4X2	T48.4X3	T48.4X4	T48.4X5	T48.4X6
Acetyldigitoxin	T46.ØX1	T46.ØX2	T46.ØX3	T46.ØX4	T46.ØX5	T46.ØX6
Acetyldigoxin	T46.ØX1	T46.ØX2	T46.ØX3	T46.ØX4	T46.ØX5	T46.ØX6
Acetyldihydrocodeine	T4Ø.2X1	T4Ø.2X2	T4Ø.2X3	T4Ø.2X4	—	—
Acetyldihydrocodeinone	T4Ø.2X1	T4Ø.2X2	T4Ø.2X3	T4Ø.2X4	—	—
Acetylene (gas)	T59.891	T59.892	T59.893	T59.894	—	—
dichloride	T53.6X1	T53.6X2	T53.6X3	T53.6X4	—	—
incomplete combustion of	T58.11	T58.12	T58.13	T58.14	—	—
industrial	T59.891	T59.892	T59.893	T59.894	—	—
tetrachloride	T53.6X1	T53.6X2	T53.6X3	T53.6X4	—	—
vapor	T53.6X1	T53.6X2	T53.6X3	T53.6X4	—	—
Acetylpheneturide	T42.6X1	T42.6X2	T42.6X3	T42.6X4	T42.6X5	T42.6X6
Acetylphenylhydrazine	T39.8X1	T39.8X2	T39.8X3	T39.8X4	T39.8X5	T39.8X6
Acetylsalicylic acid (salts)	T39.Ø11	T39.Ø12	T39.Ø13	T39.Ø14	T39.Ø15	T39.Ø16
enteric coated	T39.Ø11	T39.Ø12	T39.Ø13	T39.Ø14	T39.Ø15	T39.Ø16
Acetylsulfamethoxypyridazine	T37.ØX1	T37.ØX2	T37.ØX3	T37.ØX4	T37.ØX5	T37.ØX6
Achromycin	T36.4X1	T36.4X2	T36.4X3	T36.4X4	T36.4X5	T36.4X6
ophthalmic preparation	T49.5X1	T49.5X2	T49.5X3	T49.5X4	T49.5X5	T49.5X6
topical NEC	T49.ØX1	T49.ØX2	T49.ØX3	T49.ØX4	T49.ØX5	T49.ØX6
Aciclovir	T37.5X1	T37.5X2	T37.5X3	T37.5X4	T37.5X5	T37.5X6
Acidifying agent NEC	T5Ø.9Ø1	T5Ø.9Ø2	T5Ø.9Ø3	T5Ø.9Ø4	T5Ø.9Ø5	T5Ø.9Ø6
Acid (corrosive) **NEC**	T54.2X1	T54.2X2	T54.2X3	T54.2X4	—	—
AcipHex*	T47.1X1	T47.1X2	T47.1X3	T47.1X4	T47.1X5	T47.1X6
Acipimox	T46.6X1	T46.6X2	T46.6X3	T46.6X4	T46.6X5	T46.6X6
Acitretin	T5Ø.991	T5Ø.992	T5Ø.993	T5Ø.994	T5Ø.995	T5Ø.996
Aclarubicin	T45.1X1	T45.1X2	T45.1X3	T45.1X4	T45.1X5	T45.1X6
Aclatonium napadisilate	T48.1X1	T48.1X2	T48.1X3	T48.1X4	T48.1X5	T48.1X6
Aconite (wild)	T46.991	T46.992	T46.993	T46.994	T46.995	T46.996
Aconitine	T46.991	T46.992	T46.993	T46.994	T46.995	T46.996
Aconitum ferox	T46.991	T46.992	T46.993	T46.994	T46.995	T46.996
Acridine	T65.6X1	T65.6X2	T65.6X3	T65.6X4	—	—
vapor	T59.891	T59.892	T59.893	T59.894	—	—
Acriflavine	T37.91	T37.92	T37.93	T37.94	T37.95	T37.96
Acriflavinium chloride	T49.ØX1	T49.ØX2	T49.ØX3	T49.ØX4	T49.ØX5	T49.ØX6
Acrinol	T49.ØX1	T49.ØX2	T49.ØX3	T49.ØX4	T49.ØX5	T49.ØX6
Acrisorcin	T49.ØX1	T49.ØX2	T49.ØX3	T49.ØX4	T49.ØX5	T49.ØX6
Acrivastine	T45.ØX1	T45.ØX2	T45.ØX3	T45.ØX4	T45.ØX5	T45.ØX6
Acrolein (gas)	T59.891	T59.892	T59.893	T59.894	—	—
liquid	T54.1X1	T54.1X2	T54.1X3	T54.1X4	—	—
Acrylamide	T65.891	T65.892	T65.893	T65.894	—	—
Acrylic resin	T49.3X1	T49.3X2	T49.3X3	T49.3X4	T49.3X5	T49.3X6
Acrylonitrile	T65.891	T65.892	T65.893	T65.894	—	—
Actaea spicata	T62.2X1	T62.2X2	T62.2X3	T62.2X4	—	—
berry	T62.1X1	T62.1X2	T62.1X3	T62.1X4	—	—
Acterol	T37.3X1	T37.3X2	T37.3X3	T37.3X4	T37.3X5	T37.3X6
ACTH	T38.811	T38.812	T38.813	T38.814	T38.815	T38.816
Actinomycin C	T45.1X1	T45.1X2	T45.1X3	T45.1X4	T45.1X5	T45.1X6
Actinomycin D	T45.1X1	T45.1X2	T45.1X3	T45.1X4	T45.1X5	T45.1X6
Activated charcoal — *see also* Charcoal, medicinal	T47.6X1	T47.6X2	T47.6X3	T47.6X4	T47.6X5	T47.6X6
Activella*	T38.5X1	T38.5X2	T38.5X3	T38.5X4	T38.5X5	T38.5X6
Acyclovir	T37.5X1	T37.5X2	T37.5X3	T37.5X4	T37.5X5	T37.5X6
Adenine	T45.2X1	T45.2X2	T45.2X3	T45.2X4	T45.2X5	T45.2X6
arabinoside	T37.5X1	T37.5X2	T37.5X3	T37.5X4	T37.5X5	T37.5X6
Adenosine (phosphate)	T46.2X1	T46.2X2	T46.2X3	T46.2X4	T46.2X5	T46.2X6
ADH	T38.891	T38.892	T38.893	T38.894	T38.895	T38.896
Adhesive NEC	T65.891	T65.892	T65.893	T65.894	—	—
Adicillin	T36.ØX1	T36.ØX2	T36.ØX3	T36.ØX4	T36.ØX5	T36.ØX6
Adiphenine	T44.3X1	T44.3X2	T44.3X3	T44.3X4	T44.3X5	T44.3X6
Adipiodone	T5Ø.8X1	T5Ø.8X2	T5Ø.8X3	T5Ø.8X4	T5Ø.8X5	T5Ø.8X6
Adjunct, pharmaceutical	T5Ø.9Ø1	T5Ø.9Ø2	T5Ø.9Ø3	T5Ø.9Ø4	T5Ø.9Ø5	T5Ø.9Ø6
Adrenal (extract, cortex or medulla) (glucocorticoids) (hormones) (mineralocorticoids)	T38.ØX1	T38.ØX2	T38.ØX3	T38.ØX4	T38.ØX5	T38.ØX6
ENT agent	T49.6X1	T49.6X2	T49.6X3	T49.6X4	T49.6X5	T49.6X6
ophthalmic preparation	T49.5X1	T49.5X2	T49.5X3	T49.5X4	T49.5X5	T49.5X6
topical NEC	T49.ØX1	T49.ØX2	T49.ØX3	T49.ØX4	T49.ØX5	T49.ØX6
Adrenalin — *see* Adrenaline						
Adrenaline	T44.5X1	T44.5X2	T44.5X3	T44.5X4	T44.5X5	T44.5X6
Adrenergic NEC	T44.9Ø1	T44.9Ø2	T44.9Ø3	T44.9Ø4	T44.9Ø5	T44.9Ø6
blocking agent NEC	T44.8X1	T44.8X2	T44.8X3	T44.8X4	T44.8X5	T44.8X6
beta, heart	T44.7X1	T44.7X2	T44.7X3	T44.7X4	T44.7X5	T44.7X6
specified NEC	T44.991	T44.992	T44.993	T44.994	T44.995	T44.996
Adrenochrome						
derivative	T46.991	T46.992	T46.993	T46.994	T46.995	T46.996
(mono) semicarbazone	T46.991	T46.992	T46.993	T46.994	T46.995	T46.996
Adrenocorticotrophic hormone	T38.811	T38.812	T38.813	T38.814	T38.815	T38.816
Adrenocorticotrophin	T38.811	T38.812	T38.813	T38.814	T38.815	T38.816

*Optum Value-Add

☑ Additional Character May Be Required — Refer to the Tabular List for Character Selection

Substance	Poisoning, Accidental (unintentional)	Poisoning, Intentional Self-harm	Poisoning, Assault	Poisoning, Undetermined	Adverse Effect	Under-dosing
Adriamycin	T45.1X1	T45.1X2	T45.1X3	T45.1X4	T45.1X5	T45.1X6
Adrucil*	T45.1X1	T45.1X2	T45.1X3	T45.1X4	T45.1X5	T45.1X6
Aerosol spray NEC	T65.91	T65.92	T65.93	T65.94	—	—
Aerosporin	T36.8X1	T36.8X2	T36.8X3	T36.8X4	T36.8X5	T36.8X6
ENT agent	T49.6X1	T49.6X2	T49.6X3	T49.6X4	T49.6X5	T49.6X6
ophthalmic preparation	T49.5X1	T49.5X2	T49.5X3	T49.5X4	T49.5X5	T49.5X6
topical NEC	T49.0X1	T49.0X2	T49.0X3	T49.0X4	T49.0X5	T49.0X6
Aethusa cynapium	T62.2X1	T62.2X2	T62.2X3	T62.2X4	—	—
Afghanistan black	T40.711	T40.712	T40.713	T40.714	T40.715	T40.716
Aflatoxin	T64.01	T64.02	T64.03	T64.04	—	—
Afloqualone	T42.8X1	T42.8X2	T42.8X3	T42.8X4	T42.8X5	T42.8X6
African boxwood	T62.2X1	T62.2X2	T62.2X3	T62.2X4	—	—
Agar	T47.4X1	T47.4X2	T47.4X3	T47.4X4	T47.4X5	T47.4X6
Agonist						
predominantly						
alpha-adrenoreceptor	T44.4X1	T44.4X2	T44.4X3	T44.4X4	T44.4X5	T44.4X6
beta-adrenoreceptor	T44.5X1	T44.5X2	T44.5X3	T44.5X4	T44.5X5	T44.5X6
Agricultural agent NEC	T65.91	T65.92	T65.93	T65.94	—	—
Agrypnal	T42.3X1	T42.3X2	T42.3X3	T42.3X4	T42.3X5	T42.3X6
AHLG	T50.Z11	T50.Z12	T50.Z13	T50.Z14	T50.Z15	T50.Z16
Air contaminant(s), source/type NOS	T65.91	T65.92	T65.93	T65.94	—	—
Ajmaline	T46.2X1	T46.2X2	T46.2X3	T46.2X4	T46.2X5	T46.2X6
Akee	T62.1X1	T62.1X2	T62.1X3	T62.1X4	—	—
Akne-Mycin*	T49.0X1	T49.0X2	T49.0X3	T49.0X4	T49.0X5	T49.0X6
Akrinol	T49.0X1	T49.0X2	T49.0X3	T49.0X4	T49.0X5	T49.0X6
Akritoin	T37.8X1	T37.8X2	T37.8X3	T37.8X4	T37.8X5	T37.8X6
Alacepril	T46.4X1	T46.4X2	T46.4X3	T46.4X4	T46.4X5	T46.4X6
Alantolactone	T37.4X1	T37.4X2	T37.4X3	T37.4X4	T37.4X5	T37.4X6
Albamycin	T36.8X1	T36.8X2	T36.8X3	T36.8X4	T36.8X5	T36.8X6
Albendazole	T37.4X1	T37.4X2	T37.4X3	T37.4X4	T37.4X5	T37.4X6
Albigutide*	T38.3X1	T38.3X2	T38.3X3	T38.3X4	T38.3X5	T38.3X6
Albumin						
bovine	T45.8X1	T45.8X2	T45.8X3	T45.8X4	T45.8X5	T45.8X6
human serum	T45.8X1	T45.8X2	T45.8X3	T45.8X4	T45.8X5	T45.8X6
salt-poor	T45.8X1	T45.8X2	T45.8X3	T45.8X4	T45.8X5	T45.8X6
normal human serum	T45.8X1	T45.8X2	T45.8X3	T45.8X4	T45.8X5	T45.8X6
Albuterol	T48.6X1	T48.6X2	T48.6X3	T48.6X4	T48.6X5	T48.6X6
Albutoin	T42.0X1	T42.0X2	T42.0X3	T42.0X4	T42.0X5	T42.0X6
Alclometasone	T49.0X1	T49.0X2	T49.0X3	T49.0X4	T49.0X5	T49.0X6
Alcohol	T51.91	T51.92	T51.93	T51.94	—	—
absolute	T51.0X1	T51.0X2	T51.0X3	T51.0X4	—	—
beverage	T51.0X1	T51.0X2	T51.0X3	T51.0X4	—	—
allyl	T51.8X1	T51.8X2	T51.8X3	T51.8X4	—	—
amyl	T51.3X1	T51.3X2	T51.3X3	T51.3X4	—	—
antifreeze	T51.1X1	T51.1X2	T51.1X3	T51.1X4	—	—
beverage	T51.0X1	T51.0X2	T51.0X3	T51.0X4	—	—
butyl	T51.3X1	T51.3X2	T51.3X3	T51.3X4	—	—
dehydrated	T51.0X1	T51.0X2	T51.0X3	T51.0X4	—	—
beverage	T51.0X1	T51.0X2	T51.0X3	T51.0X4	—	—
denatured	T51.0X1	T51.0X2	T51.0X3	T51.0X4	—	—
deterrent NEC	T50.6X1	T50.6X2	T50.6X3	T50.6X4	T50.6X5	T50.6X6
diagnostic (gastric function)	T50.8X1	T50.8X2	T50.8X3	T50.8X4	T50.8X5	T50.8X6
ethyl	T51.0X1	T51.0X2	T51.0X3	T51.0X4	—	—
beverage	T51.0X1	T51.0X2	T51.0X3	T51.0X4	—	—
grain	T51.0X1	T51.0X2	T51.0X3	T51.0X4	—	—
beverage	T51.0X1	T51.0X2	T51.0X3	T51.0X4	—	—
industrial	T51.0X1	T51.0X2	T51.0X3	T51.0X4	—	—
isopropyl	T51.2X1	T51.2X2	T51.2X3	T51.2X4	—	—
methyl	T51.1X1	T51.1X2	T51.1X3	T51.1X4	—	—
preparation for consumption	T51.0X1	T51.0X2	T51.0X3	T51.0X4	—	—
propyl	T51.3X1	T51.3X2	T51.3X3	T51.3X4	—	—
secondary	T51.2X1	T51.2X2	T51.2X3	T51.2X4	—	—
radiator	T51.1X1	T51.1X2	T51.1X3	T51.1X4	—	—
rubbing	T51.2X1	T51.2X2	T51.2X3	T51.2X4	—	—
specified type NEC	T51.8X1	T51.8X2	T51.8X3	T51.8X4	—	—
surgical	T51.0X1	T51.0X2	T51.0X3	T51.0X4	—	—
vapor (from any type of Alcohol)	T59.891	T59.892	T59.893	T59.894	—	—
wood	T51.1X1	T51.1X2	T51.1X3	T51.1X4	—	—
Alcuronium (chloride)	T48.1X1	T48.1X2	T48.1X3	T48.1X4	T48.1X5	T48.1X6
Aldactone	T50.0X1	T50.0X2	T50.0X3	T50.0X4	T50.0X5	T50.0X6
Aldesulfone sodium	T37.1X1	T37.1X2	T37.1X3	T37.1X4	T37.1X5	T37.1X6
Aldicarb	T60.0X1	T60.0X2	T60.0X3	T60.0X4	—	—
Aldomet	T46.5X1	T46.5X2	T46.5X3	T46.5X4	T46.5X5	T46.5X6
Aldosterone	T50.0X1	T50.0X2	T50.0X3	T50.0X4	T50.0X5	T50.0X6
Aldrin (dust)	T60.1X1	T60.1X2	T60.1X3	T60.1X4	—	—
Aleve — *see* Naproxen						
Alexitol sodium	T47.1X1	T47.1X2	T47.1X3	T47.1X4	T47.1X5	T47.1X6
Alfacalcidol	T45.2X1	T45.2X2	T45.2X3	T45.2X4	T45.2X5	T45.2X6
Alfadolone	T41.1X1	T41.1X2	T41.1X3	T41.1X4	T41.1X5	T41.1X6
Alfaxalone	T41.1X1	T41.1X2	T41.1X3	T41.1X4	T41.1X5	T41.1X6
Alfentanil	T40.411	T40.412	T40.413	T40.414	T40.415	T40.416
Alfuzosin (hydrochloride)	T44.8X1	T44.8X2	T44.8X3	T44.8X4	T44.8X5	T44.8X6
Algae (harmful) (toxin)	T65.821	T65.822	T65.823	T65.824	—	—
Algeldrate	T47.1X1	T47.1X2	T47.1X3	T47.1X4	T47.1X5	T47.1X6
Algin	T47.8X1	T47.8X2	T47.8X3	T47.8X4	T47.8X5	T47.8X6
Alglucerase	T45.3X1	T45.3X2	T45.3X3	T45.3X4	T45.3X5	T45.3X6
Alidase	T45.3X1	T45.3X2	T45.3X3	T45.3X4	T45.3X5	T45.3X6
Alimemazine	T43.3X1	T43.3X2	T43.3X3	T43.3X4	T43.3X5	T43.3X6
Aliphatic thiocyanates	T65.0X1	T65.0X2	T65.0X3	T65.0X4	—	—
Alitretinoin*	T49.0X1	T49.0X2	T49.0X3	T49.0X4	T49.0X5	T49.0X6
Alizapride	T45.0X1	T45.0X2	T45.0X3	T45.0X4	T45.0X5	T45.0X6
Alkali (caustic)	T54.3X1	T54.3X2	T54.3X3	T54.3X4	—	—
Alkaline antiseptic solution (aromatic)	T49.6X1	T49.6X2	T49.6X3	T49.6X4	T49.6X5	T49.6X6
Alkalinizing agents (medicinal)	T50.901	T50.902	T50.903	T50.904	T50.905	T50.906
Alkalizing agent NEC	T50.901	T50.902	T50.903	T50.904	T50.905	T50.906
Alka-seltzer	T39.011	T39.012	T39.013	T39.014	T39.015	T39.016
Alkavervir	T46.5X1	T46.5X2	T46.5X3	T46.5X4	T46.5X5	T46.5X6
Alkeran*	T45.1X1	T45.1X2	T45.1X3	T45.1X4	T45.1X5	T45.1X6
Alkonium (bromide)	T49.0X1	T49.0X2	T49.0X3	T49.0X4	T49.0X5	T49.0X6
Alkylating drug NEC	T45.1X1	T45.1X2	T45.1X3	T45.1X4	T45.1X5	T45.1X6
antimyeloproliferative	T45.1X1	T45.1X2	T45.1X3	T45.1X4	T45.1X5	T45.1X6
lymphatic	T45.1X1	T45.1X2	T45.1X3	T45.1X4	T45.1X5	T45.1X6
Alkylisocyanate	T65.0X1	T65.0X2	T65.0X3	T65.0X4	—	—
Allantoin	T49.4X1	T49.4X2	T49.4X3	T49.4X4	T49.4X5	T49.4X6
Allegron	T43.011	T43.012	T43.013	T43.014	T43.015	T43.016
Allethrin	T49.0X1	T49.0X2	T49.0X3	T49.0X4	T49.0X5	T49.0X6
Allobarbital	T42.3X1	T42.3X2	T42.3X3	T42.3X4	T42.3X5	T42.3X6
Allopurinol	T50.4X1	T50.4X2	T50.4X3	T50.4X4	T50.4X5	T50.4X6
Allyl						
alcohol	T51.8X1	T51.8X2	T51.8X3	T51.8X4	—	—
disulfide	T46.6X1	T46.6X2	T46.6X3	T46.6X4	T46.6X5	T46.6X6
Allylestrenol	T38.5X1	T38.5X2	T38.5X3	T38.5X4	T38.5X5	T38.5X6
Allylisopropylacetylurea	T42.6X1	T42.6X2	T42.6X3	T42.6X4	T42.6X5	T42.6X6
Allylisopropylmalonylurea	T42.3X1	T42.3X2	T42.3X3	T42.3X4	T42.3X5	T42.3X6
Allylthiourea	T49.3X1	T49.3X2	T49.3X3	T49.3X4	T49.3X5	T49.3X6
Allyltribromide	T42.6X1	T42.6X2	T42.6X3	T42.6X4	T42.6X5	T42.6X6
Allypropymal	T42.3X1	T42.3X2	T42.3X3	T42.3X4	T42.3X5	T42.3X6
Almagate	T47.1X1	T47.1X2	T47.1X3	T47.1X4	T47.1X5	T47.1X6
Almasilate	T47.1X1	T47.1X2	T47.1X3	T47.1X4	T47.1X5	T47.1X6
Almitrine	T50.7X1	T50.7X2	T50.7X3	T50.7X4	T50.7X5	T50.7X6
Aloes	T47.2X1	T47.2X2	T47.2X3	T47.2X4	T47.2X5	T47.2X6
Aloglutamol	T47.1X1	T47.1X2	T47.1X3	T47.1X4	T47.1X5	T47.1X6
Aloin	T47.2X1	T47.2X2	T47.2X3	T47.2X4	T47.2X5	T47.2X6
Aloxidone	T42.2X1	T42.2X2	T42.2X3	T42.2X4	T42.2X5	T42.2X6
Alpha						
acetyldigoxin	T46.0X1	T46.0X2	T46.0X3	T46.0X4	T46.0X5	T46.0X6
adrenergic blocking drug	T44.6X1	T44.6X2	T44.6X3	T44.6X4	T44.6X5	T44.6X6
amylase	T45.3X1	T45.3X2	T45.3X3	T45.3X4	T45.3X5	T45.3X6
tocoferol (acetate)	T45.2X1	T45.2X2	T45.2X3	T45.2X4	T45.2X5	T45.2X6
tocopherol	T45.2X1	T45.2X2	T45.2X3	T45.2X4	T45.2X5	T45.2X6
Alphadolone	T41.1X1	T41.1X2	T41.1X3	T41.1X4	T41.1X5	T41.1X6
Alphaprodine	T40.491	T40.492	T40.493	T40.494	T40.495	T40.496
Alphaxalone	T41.1X1	T41.1X2	T41.1X3	T41.1X4	T41.1X5	T41.1X6
Alprazolam	T42.4X1	T42.4X2	T42.4X3	T42.4X4	T42.4X5	T42.4X6
Alprenolol	T44.7X1	T44.7X2	T44.7X3	T44.7X4	T44.7X5	T44.7X6
Alprostadil	T46.7X1	T46.7X2	T46.7X3	T46.7X4	T46.7X5	T46.7X6
Alsactide	T38.811	T38.812	T38.813	T38.814	T38.815	T38.816
Alseroxylon	T46.5X1	T46.5X2	T46.5X3	T46.5X4	T46.5X5	T46.5X6
Alteplase	T45.611	T45.612	T45.613	T45.614	T45.615	T45.616
Altizide	T50.2X1	T50.2X2	T50.2X3	T50.2X4	T50.2X5	T50.2X6
Altoprev*	T46.6X1	T46.6X2	T46.6X3	T46.6X4	T46.6X5	T46.6X6
Altretamine	T45.1X1	T45.1X2	T45.1X3	T45.1X4	T45.1X5	T45.1X6
Alum (medicinal)	T49.4X1	T49.4X2	T49.4X3	T49.4X4	T49.4X5	T49.4X6
nonmedicinal (ammonium) (potassium)	T56.891	T56.892	T56.893	T56.894	—	—
Aluminium, aluminum						
acetate	T49.2X1	T49.2X2	T49.2X3	T49.2X4	T49.2X5	T49.2X6
solution	T49.0X1	T49.0X2	T49.0X3	T49.0X4	T49.0X5	T49.0X6
aspirin	T39.011	T39.012	T39.013	T39.014	T39.015	T39.016
bis (acetylsalicylate)	T39.011	T39.012	T39.013	T39.014	T39.015	T39.016
carbonate (gel, basic)	T47.1X1	T47.1X2	T47.1X3	T47.1X4	T47.1X5	T47.1X6
chlorhydroxide-complex	T47.1X1	T47.1X2	T47.1X3	T47.1X4	T47.1X5	T47.1X6
chloride	T49.2X1	T49.2X2	T49.2X3	T49.2X4	T49.2X5	T49.2X6
clofibrate	T46.6X1	T46.6X2	T46.6X3	T46.6X4	T46.6X5	T46.6X6
diacetate	T49.2X1	T49.2X2	T49.2X3	T49.2X4	T49.2X5	T49.2X6
glycinate	T47.1X1	T47.1X2	T47.1X3	T47.1X4	T47.1X5	T47.1X6
hydroxide (gel)	T47.1X1	T47.1X2	T47.1X3	T47.1X4	T47.1X5	T47.1X6
hydroxide-magnesium carb. gel	T47.1X1	T47.1X2	T47.1X3	T47.1X4	T47.1X5	T47.1X6
magnesium silicate	T47.1X1	T47.1X2	T47.1X3	T47.1X4	T47.1X5	T47.1X6

Substance	Poisoning, Accidental (unintentional)	Poisoning, Intentional Self-harm	Poisoning, Assault	Poisoning, Undetermined	Adverse Effect	Under-dosing
Aluminium, aluminum — *continued*						
nicotinate	T46.7X1	T46.7X2	T46.7X3	T46.7X4	T46.7X5	T46.7X6
ointment (surgical) (topical)	T49.3X1	T49.3X2	T49.3X3	T49.3X4	T49.3X5	T49.3X6
phosphate	T47.1X1	T47.1X2	T47.1X3	T47.1X4	T47.1X5	T47.1X6
salicylate	T39.Ø91	T39.Ø92	T39.Ø93	T39.Ø94	T39.Ø95	T39.Ø96
silicate	T47.1X1	T47.1X2	T47.1X3	T47.1X4	T47.1X5	T47.1X6
sodium silicate	T47.1X1	T47.1X2	T47.1X3	T47.1X4	T47.1X5	T47.1X6
subacetate	T49.2X1	T49.2X2	T49.2X3	T49.2X4	T49.2X5	T49.2X6
sulfate	T49.ØX1	T49.ØX2	T49.ØX3	T49.ØX4	T49.ØX5	T49.ØX6
tannate	T47.6X1	T47.6X2	T47.6X3	T47.6X4	T47.6X5	T47.6X6
topical NEC	T49.3X1	T49.3X2	T49.3X3	T49.3X4	T49.3X5	T49.3X6
Alurate	T42.3X1	T42.3X2	T42.3X3	T42.3X4	T42.3X5	T42.3X6
Alverine	T44.3X1	T44.3X2	T44.3X3	T44.3X4	T44.3X5	T44.3X6
Alvodine	T4Ø.2X1	T4Ø.2X2	T4Ø.2X3	T4Ø.2X4	T4Ø.2X5	T4Ø.2X6
Amanita phalloides	T62.ØX1	T62.ØX2	T62.ØX3	T62.ØX4	—	—
Amanitine	T62.ØX1	T62.ØX2	T62.ØX3	T62.ØX4	—	—
Amantadine	T42.8X1	T42.8X2	T42.8X3	T42.8X4	T42.8X5	T42.8X6
Ambazone	T49.6X1	T49.6X2	T49.6X3	T49.6X4	T49.6X5	T49.6X6
Ambenonium (chloride)	T44.ØX1	T44.ØX2	T44.ØX3	T44.ØX4	T44.ØX5	T44.ØX6
Ambroxol	T48.4X1	T48.4X2	T48.4X3	T48.4X4	T48.4X5	T48.4X6
Ambuphylline	T48.6X1	T48.6X2	T48.6X3	T48.6X4	T48.6X5	T48.6X6
Ambutonium bromide	T44.3X1	T44.3X2	T44.3X3	T44.3X4	T44.3X5	T44.3X6
Amcinonide	T49.ØX1	T49.ØX2	T49.ØX3	T49.ØX4	T49.ØX5	T49.ØX6
Amdinocilline	T36.ØX1	T36.ØX2	T36.ØX3	T36.ØX4	T36.ØX5	T36.ØX6
Americaine*	T41.3X1	T41.3X2	T41.3X3	T41.3X4	T41.3X5	T41.3X6
Ametazole	T5Ø.8X1	T5Ø.8X2	T5Ø.8X3	T5Ø.8X4	T5Ø.8X5	T5Ø.8X6
Amethocaine	T41.3X1	T41.3X2	T41.3X3	T41.3X4	T41.3X5	T41.3X6
regional	T41.3X1	T41.3X2	T41.3X3	T41.3X4	T41.3X5	T41.3X6
spinal	T41.3X1	T41.3X2	T41.3X3	T41.3X4	T41.3X5	T41.3X6
Amethopterin	T45.1X1	T45.1X2	T45.1X3	T45.1X4	T45.1X5	T45.1X6
Amezinium metilsulfate	T44.991	T44.992	T44.993	T44.994	T44.995	T44.996
Amfebutamone	T43.291	T43.292	T43.293	T43.294	T43.295	T43.296
Amfepramone	T5Ø.5X1	T5Ø.5X2	T5Ø.5X3	T5Ø.5X4	T5Ø.5X5	T5Ø.5X6
Amfetamine	T43.621	T43.622	T43.623	T43.624	T43.625	T43.626
Amfetaminil	T43.621	T43.622	T43.623	T43.624	T43.625	T43.626
Amfomycin	T36.8X1	T36.8X2	T36.8X3	T36.8X4	T36.8X5	T36.8X6
Amidefrine mesilate	T48.5X1	T48.5X2	T48.5X3	T48.5X4	T48.5X5	T48.5X6
Amidone	T4Ø.3X1	T4Ø.3X2	T4Ø.3X3	T4Ø.3X4	T4Ø.3X5	T4Ø.3X6
Amidopyrine	T39.2X1	T39.2X2	T39.2X3	T39.2X4	T39.2X5	T39.2X6
Amidotrizoate	T5Ø.8X1	T5Ø.8X2	T5Ø.8X3	T5Ø.8X4	T5Ø.8X5	T5Ø.8X6
Amiflamine	T43.1X1	T43.1X2	T43.1X3	T43.1X4	T43.1X5	T43.1X6
Amikacin	T36.5X1	T36.5X2	T36.5X3	T36.5X4	T36.5X5	T36.5X6
Amikhelline	T46.3X1	T46.3X2	T46.3X3	T46.3X4	T46.3X5	T46.3X6
Amiloride	T5Ø.2X1	T5Ø.2X2	T5Ø.2X3	T5Ø.2X4	T5Ø.2X5	T5Ø.2X6
Aminacrine	T49.ØX1	T49.ØX2	T49.ØX3	T49.ØX4	T49.ØX5	T49.ØX6
Amineptine	T43.Ø11	T43.Ø12	T43.Ø13	T43.Ø14	T43.Ø15	T43.Ø16
Aminitrozole	T37.3X1	T37.3X2	T37.3X3	T37.3X4	T37.3X5	T37.3X6
Aminoacetic acid (derivatives)	T5Ø.3X1	T5Ø.3X2	T5Ø.3X3	T5Ø.3X4	T5Ø.3X5	T5Ø.3X6
Amino acids	T5Ø.3X1	T5Ø.3X2	T5Ø.3X3	T5Ø.3X4	T5Ø.3X5	T5Ø.3X6
Aminoacridine	T49.ØX1	T49.ØX2	T49.ØX3	T49.ØX4	T49.ØX5	T49.ØX6
Aminobenzoic acid (-p)	T49.3X1	T49.3X2	T49.3X3	T49.3X4	T49.3X5	T49.3X6
Aminocaproic acid	T45.621	T45.622	T45.623	T45.624	T45.625	T45.626
Aminoethylisothiourium	T45.8X1	T45.8X2	T45.8X3	T45.8X4	T45.8X5	T45.8X6
Aminofenazone	T39.2X1	T39.2X2	T39.2X3	T39.2X4	T39.2X5	T39.2X6
Aminoglutethimide	T45.1X1	T45.1X2	T45.1X3	T45.1X4	T45.1X5	T45.1X6
Aminoglycosides*	T36.5X1	T36.5X2	T36.5X3	T36.5X4	T36.5X5	T36.5X6
Aminohippuric acid	T5Ø.8X1	T5Ø.8X2	T5Ø.8X3	T5Ø.8X4	T5Ø.8X5	T5Ø.8X6
Aminomethylbenzoic acid	T45.691	T45.692	T45.693	T45.694	T45.695	T45.696
Aminometradine	T5Ø.2X1	T5Ø.2X2	T5Ø.2X3	T5Ø.2X4	T5Ø.2X5	T5Ø.2X6
Aminopentamide	T44.3X1	T44.3X2	T44.3X3	T44.3X4	T44.3X5	T44.3X6
Aminophenazone	T39.2X1	T39.2X2	T39.2X3	T39.2X4	T39.2X5	T39.2X6
Aminophenol	T54.ØX1	T54.ØX2	T54.ØX3	T54.ØX4	—	—
Aminophenylpyridone	T43.591	T43.592	T43.593	T43.594	T43.595	T43.596
Aminophylline	T48.6X1	T48.6X2	T48.6X3	T48.6X4	T48.6X5	T48.6X6
Aminopterin sodium	T45.1X1	T45.1X2	T45.1X3	T45.1X4	T45.1X5	T45.1X6
Aminopyrine	T39.2X1	T39.2X2	T39.2X3	T39.2X4	T39.2X5	T39.2X6
Aminorex	T5Ø.5X1	T5Ø.5X2	T5Ø.5X3	T5Ø.5X4	T5Ø.5X5	T5Ø.5X6
Aminosalicylic acid	T37.1X1	T37.1X2	T37.1X3	T37.1X4	T37.1X5	T37.1X6
Aminosalylum	T37.1X1	T37.1X2	T37.1X3	T37.1X4	T37.1X5	T37.1X6
Amiodarone	T46.2X1	T46.2X2	T46.2X3	T46.2X4	T46.2X5	T46.2X6
Amiphenazole	T5Ø.7X1	T5Ø.7X2	T5Ø.7X3	T5Ø.7X4	T5Ø.7X5	T5Ø.7X6
Amiquinsin	T46.5X1	T46.5X2	T46.5X3	T46.5X4	T46.5X5	T46.5X6
Amisometradine	T5Ø.2X1	T5Ø.2X2	T5Ø.2X3	T5Ø.2X4	T5Ø.2X5	T5Ø.2X6
Amisulpride	T43.591	T43.592	T43.593	T43.594	T43.595	T43.596
Amitriptyline	T43.Ø11	T43.Ø12	T43.Ø13	T43.Ø14	T43.Ø15	T43.Ø16
Amitriptylinoxide	T43.Ø11	T43.Ø12	T43.Ø13	T43.Ø14	T43.Ø15	T43.Ø16
Amlexanox	T48.6X1	T48.6X2	T48.6X3	T48.6X4	T48.6X5	T48.6X6
Ammonia (fumes) (gas) (vapor)	T59.891	T59.892	T59.893	T59.894	—	—
aromatic spirit	T48.991	T48.992	T48.993	T48.994	T48.995	T48.996

Substance	Poisoning, Accidental (unintentional)	Poisoning, Intentional Self-harm	Poisoning, Assault	Poisoning, Undetermined	Adverse Effect	Under-dosing
Ammonia — *continued*						
liquid (household)	T54.3X1	T54.3X2	T54.3X3	T54.3X4	—	—
Ammoniated mercury	T49.ØX1	T49.ØX2	T49.ØX3	T49.ØX4	T49.ØX5	T49.ØX6
Ammonium						
acid tartrate	T49.5X1	T49.5X2	T49.5X3	T49.5X4	T49.5X5	T49.5X6
bromide	T42.6X1	T42.6X2	T42.6X3	T42.6X4	T42.6X5	T42.6X6
carbonate	T54.3X1	T54.3X2	T54.3X3	T54.3X4	—	—
chloride	T5Ø.991	T5Ø.992	T5Ø.993	T5Ø.994	T5Ø.995	T5Ø.996
expectorant	T48.4X1	T48.4X2	T48.4X3	T48.4X4	T48.4X5	T48.4X6
compounds (household) NEC	T54.3X1	T54.3X2	T54.3X3	T54.3X4	—	—
fumes (any usage)	T59.891	T59.892	T59.893	T59.894	—	—
industrial	T54.3X1	T54.3X2	T54.3X3	T54.3X4	—	—
ichthyosulronate	T49.4X1	T49.4X2	T49.4X3	T49.4X4	T49.4X5	T49.4X6
mandelate	T37.91	T37.92	T37.93	T37.94	T37.95	T37.96
sulfamate	T6Ø.3X1	T6Ø.3X2	T6Ø.3X3	T6Ø.3X4	—	—
sulfonate resin	T47.8X1	T47.8X2	T47.8X3	T47.8X4	T47.8X5	T47.8X6
Amobarbital (sodium)	T42.3X1	T42.3X2	T42.3X3	T42.3X4	T42.3X5	T42.3X6
Amodiaquine	T37.2X1	T37.2X2	T37.2X3	T37.2X4	T37.2X5	T37.2X6
Amopyroquin (e)	T37.2X1	T37.2X2	T37.2X3	T37.2X4	T37.2X5	T37.2X6
Amoxapine	T43.Ø11	T43.Ø12	T43.Ø13	T43.Ø14	T43.Ø15	T43.Ø16
Amoxicillin	T36.ØX1	T36.ØX2	T36.ØX3	T36.ØX4	T36.ØX5	T36.ØX6
Amperozide	T43.591	T43.592	T43.593	T43.594	T43.595	T43.596
Amphenidone	T43.591	T43.592	T43.593	T43.594	T43.595	T43.596
Amphetamine NEC	T43.621	T43.622	T43.623	T43.624	T43.625	T43.626
Amphogel*	T47.1X1	T47.1X2	T47.1X3	T47.1X4	T47.1X5	T47.1X6
Amphomycin	T36.8X1	T36.8X2	T36.8X3	T36.8X4	T36.8X5	T36.8X6
Amphotalide	T37.4X1	T37.4X2	T37.4X3	T37.4X4	T37.4X5	T37.4X6
Amphotericin B	T36.7X1	T36.7X2	T36.7X3	T36.7X4	T36.7X5	T36.7X6
topical	T49.ØX1	T49.ØX2	T49.ØX3	T49.ØX4	T49.ØX5	T49.ØX6
Ampicillin	T36.ØX1	T36.ØX2	T36.ØX3	T36.ØX4	T36.ØX5	T36.ØX6
Amprotropine	T44.3X1	T44.3X2	T44.3X3	T44.3X4	T44.3X5	T44.3X6
Amsacrine	T45.1X1	T45.1X2	T45.1X3	T45.1X4	T45.1X5	T45.1X6
Amygdaline	T62.2X1	T62.2X2	T62.2X3	T62.2X4	—	—
Amyl						
acetate	T52.8X1	T52.8X2	T52.8X3	T52.8X4	—	—
vapor	T59.891	T59.892	T59.893	T59.894	—	—
alcohol	T51.3X1	T51.3X2	T51.3X3	T51.3X4	—	—
chloride	T53.6X1	T53.6X2	T53.6X3	T53.6X4	—	—
formate	T52.8X1	T52.8X2	T52.8X3	T52.8X4	—	—
nitrite	T46.3X1	T46.3X2	T46.3X3	T46.3X4	T46.3X5	T46.3X6
propionate	T65.891	T65.892	T65.893	T65.894	—	—
Amylase	T47.5X1	T47.5X2	T47.5X3	T47.5X4	T47.5X5	T47.5X6
Amyleine, regional	T41.3X1	T41.3X2	T41.3X3	T41.3X4	T41.3X5	T41.3X6
Amylene						
dichloride	T53.6X1	T53.6X2	T53.6X3	T53.6X4	—	—
hydrate	T51.3X1	T51.3X2	T51.3X3	T51.3X4	—	—
Amylmetacresol	T49.6X1	T49.6X2	T49.6X3	T49.6X4	T49.6X5	T49.6X6
Amylobarbitone	T42.3X1	T42.3X2	T42.3X3	T42.3X4	T42.3X5	T42.3X6
Amylocaine, regional	T41.3X1	T41.3X2	T41.3X3	T41.3X4	T41.3X5	T41.3X6
infiltration (subcutaneous)	T41.3X1	T41.3X2	T41.3X3	T41.3X4	T41.3X5	T41.3X6
nerve block (peripheral) (plexus)	T41.3X1	T41.3X2	T41.3X3	T41.3X4	T41.3X5	T41.3X6
spinal	T41.3X1	T41.3X2	T41.3X3	T41.3X4	T41.3X5	T41.3X6
topical (surface)	T41.3X1	T41.3X2	T41.3X3	T41.3X4	T41.3X5	T41.3X6
Amylopectin	T47.6X1	T47.6X2	T47.6X3	T47.6X4	T47.6X5	T47.6X6
Amytal (sodium)	T42.3X1	T42.3X2	T42.3X3	T42.3X4	T42.3X5	T42.3X6
Anabolic steroid	T38.7X1	T38.7X2	T38.7X3	T38.7X4	T38.7X5	T38.7X6
Anacaine*	T41.3X1	T41.3X2	T41.3X3	T41.3X4	T41.3X5	T41.3X6
Analeptic NEC	T5Ø.7X1	T5Ø.7X2	T5Ø.7X3	T5Ø.7X4	T5Ø.7X5	T5Ø.7X6
Analgesic	T39.91	T39.92	T39.93	T39.94	T39.95	T39.96
anti-inflammatory NEC	T39.91	T39.92	T39.93	T39.94	T39.95	T39.96
propionic acid derivative	T39.311	T39.312	T39.313	T39.314	T39.315	T39.316
antirheumatic NEC	T39.4X1	T39.4X2	T39.4X3	T39.4X4	T39.4X5	T39.4X6
aromatic NEC	T39.1X1	T39.1X2	T39.1X3	T39.1X4	T39.1X5	T39.1X6
narcotic NEC	T4Ø.6Ø1	T4Ø.6Ø2	T4Ø.6Ø3	T4Ø.6Ø4	T4Ø.6Ø5	T4Ø.6Ø6
combination	T4Ø.6Ø1	T4Ø.6Ø2	T4Ø.6Ø3	T4Ø.6Ø4	T4Ø.6Ø5	T4Ø.6Ø6
obstetric	T4Ø.6Ø1	T4Ø.6Ø2	T4Ø.6Ø3	T4Ø.6Ø4	T4Ø.6Ø5	T4Ø.6Ø6
non-narcotic NEC	T39.91	T39.92	T39.93	T39.94	T39.95	T39.96
combination	T39.91	T39.92	T39.93	T39.94	T39.95	T39.96
pyrazole	T39.2X1	T39.2X2	T39.2X3	T39.2X4	T39.2X5	T39.2X6
specified NEC	T39.8X1	T39.8X2	T39.8X3	T39.8X4	T39.8X5	T39.8X6
Analgin	T39.2X1	T39.2X2	T39.2X3	T39.2X4	T39.2X5	T39.2X6
Anamirta cocculus	T62.1X1	T62.1X2	T62.1X3	T62.1X4	—	—
Ancillin	T36.ØX1	T36.ØX2	T36.ØX3	T36.ØX4	T36.ØX5	T36.ØX6
Ancrod	T45.691	T45.692	T45.693	T45.694	T45.695	T45.696
Androgen	T38.7X1	T38.7X2	T38.7X3	T38.7X4	T38.7X5	T38.7X6
Androgen-estrogen mixture	T38.7X1	T38.7X2	T38.7X3	T38.7X4	T38.7X5	T38.7X6
Androstalone	T38.7X1	T38.7X2	T38.7X3	T38.7X4	T38.7X5	T38.7X6
Androstanolone	T38.7X1	T38.7X2	T38.7X3	T38.7X4	T38.7X5	T38.7X6
Androsterone	T38.7X1	T38.7X2	T38.7X3	T38.7X4	T38.7X5	T38.7X6
Anemone pulsatilla	T62.2X1	T62.2X2	T62.2X3	T62.2X4	—	—

Substance	Poisoning, Accidental (unintentional)	Poisoning, Intentional Self-harm	Poisoning, Assault	Poisoning, Undetermined	Adverse Effect	Under-dosing
Anesthesia						
caudal	T41.3X1	T41.3X2	T41.3X3	T41.3X4	T41.3X5	T41.3X6
endotracheal	T41.ØX1	T41.ØX2	T41.ØX3	T41.ØX4	T41.ØX5	T41.ØX6
epidural	T41.3X1	T41.3X2	T41.3X3	T41.3X4	T41.3X5	T41.3X6
inhalation	T41.ØX1	T41.ØX2	T41.ØX3	T41.ØX4	T41.ØX5	T41.ØX6
local	T41.3X1	T41.3X2	T41.3X3	T41.3X4	T41.3X5	T41.3X6
mucosal	T41.3X1	T41.3X2	T41.3X3	T41.3X4	T41.3X5	T41.3X6
muscle relaxation	T48.1X1	T48.1X2	T48.1X3	T48.1X4	T48.1X5	T48.1X6
nerve blocking	T41.3X1	T41.3X2	T41.3X3	T41.3X4	T41.3X5	T41.3X6
plexus blocking	T41.3X1	T41.3X2	T41.3X3	T41.3X4	T41.3X5	T41.3X6
potentiated	T41.2Ø1	T41.2Ø2	T41.2Ø3	T41.2Ø4	T41.2Ø5	T41.2Ø6
rectal	T41.2Ø1	T41.2Ø2	T41.2Ø3	T41.2Ø4	T41.2Ø5	T41.2Ø6
general	T41.2Ø1	T41.2Ø2	T41.2Ø3	T41.2Ø4	T41.2Ø5	T41.2Ø6
local	T41.3X1	T41.3X2	T41.3X3	T41.3X4	T41.3X5	T41.3X6
regional	T41.3X1	T41.3X2	T41.3X3	T41.3X4	T41.3X5	T41.3X6
surface	T41.3X1	T41.3X2	T41.3X3	T41.3X4	T41.3X5	T41.3X6
Anesthetic NEC — *see also* Anesthesia	T41.41	T41.42	T41.43	T41.44	T41.45	T41.46
with muscle relaxant	T41.2Ø1	T41.2Ø2	T41.2Ø3	T41.2Ø4	T41.2Ø5	T41.2Ø6
general	T41.2Ø1	T41.2Ø2	T41.2Ø3	T41.2Ø4	T41.2Ø5	T41.2Ø6
local	T41.3X1	T41.3X2	T41.3X3	T41.3X4	T41.3X5	T41.3X6
gaseous NEC	T41.ØX1	T41.ØX2	T41.ØX3	T41.ØX4	T41.ØX5	T41.ØX6
general NEC	T41.2Ø1	T41.2Ø2	T41.2Ø3	T41.2Ø4	T41.2Ø5	T41.2Ø6
halogenated hydrocarbon derivatives NEC	T41.ØX1	T41.ØX2	T41.ØX3	T41.ØX4	T41.ØX5	T41.ØX6
infiltration NEC	T41.3X1	T41.3X2	T41.3X3	T41.3X4	T41.3X5	T41.3X6
intravenous NEC	T41.1X1	T41.1X2	T41.1X3	T41.1X4	T41.1X5	T41.1X6
local NEC	T41.3X1	T41.3X2	T41.3X3	T41.3X4	T41.3X5	T41.3X6
rectal	T41.2Ø1	T41.2Ø2	T41.2Ø3	T41.2Ø4	T41.2Ø5	T41.2Ø6
general	T41.2Ø1	T41.2Ø2	T41.2Ø3	T41.2Ø4	T41.2Ø5	T41.2Ø6
local	T41.3X1	T41.3X2	T41.3X3	T41.3X4	T41.3X5	T41.3X6
regional NEC	T41.3X1	T41.3X2	T41.3X3	T41.3X4	T41.3X5	T41.3X6
spinal NEC	T41.3X1	T41.3X2	T41.3X3	T41.3X4	T41.3X5	T41.3X6
thiobarbiturate	T41.1X1	T41.1X2	T41.1X3	T41.1X4	T41.1X5	T41.1X6
topical	T41.3X1	T41.3X2	T41.3X3	T41.3X4	T41.3X5	T41.3X6
Aneurine	T45.2X1	T45.2X2	T45.2X3	T45.2X4	T45.2X5	T45.2X6
Angeliq*	T38.5X1	T38.5X2	T38.5X3	T38.5X4	T38.5X5	T38.5X6
Angio-Conray	T5Ø.8X1	T5Ø.8X2	T5Ø.8X3	T5Ø.8X4	T5Ø.8X5	T5Ø.8X6
Angiotensin	T44.5X1	T44.5X2	T44.5X3	T44.5X4	T44.5X5	T44.5X6
Angiotensinamide	T44.991	T44.992	T44.993	T44.994	T44.995	T44.996
Anhydrohydroxy-progesterone	T38.5X1	T38.5X2	T38.5X3	T38.5X4	T38.5X5	T38.5X6
Anhydron	T5Ø.2X1	T5Ø.2X2	T5Ø.2X3	T5Ø.2X4	T5Ø.2X5	T5Ø.2X6
Anileridine	T4Ø.491	T4Ø.492	T4Ø.493	T4Ø.494	T4Ø.495	T4Ø.496
Aniline (dye) (liquid)	T65.3X1	T65.3X2	T65.3X3	T65.3X4	—	—
analgesic	T39.1X1	T39.1X2	T39.1X3	T39.1X4	T39.1X5	T39.1X6
derivatives, therapeutic NEC	T39.1X1	T39.1X2	T39.1X3	T39.1X4	T39.1X5	T39.1X6
vapor	T65.3X1	T65.3X2	T65.3X3	T65.3X4	—	—
Aniscoropine	T44.3X1	T44.3X2	T44.3X3	T44.3X4	T44.3X5	T44.3X6
Anise oil	T47.5X1	T47.5X2	T47.5X3	T47.5X4	T47.5X5	T47.5X6
Anisidine	T65.3X1	T65.3X2	T65.3X3	T65.3X4	—	—
Anisindione	T45.511	T45.512	T45.513	T45.514	T45.515	T45.516
Anisotropine methyl-bromide	T44.3X1	T44.3X2	T44.3X3	T44.3X4	T44.3X5	T44.3X6
Anistreplase	T45.611	T45.612	T45.613	T45.614	T45.615	T45.616
Anorexiant (central)	T5Ø.5X1	T5Ø.5X2	T5Ø.5X3	T5Ø.5X4	T5Ø.5X5	T5Ø.5X6
Anorexic agents	T5Ø.5X1	T5Ø.5X2	T5Ø.5X3	T5Ø.5X4	T5Ø.5X5	T5Ø.5X6
Ansaid*	T39.311	T39.312	T39.313	T39.314	T39.315	T39.316
Ansamycin	T36.6X1	T36.6X2	T36.6X3	T36.6X4	T36.6X5	T36.6X6
Ant (bite) (sting)	T63.421	T63.422	T63.423	T63.424	—	—
Antabuse	T5Ø.6X1	T5Ø.6X2	T5Ø.6X3	T5Ø.6X4	T5Ø.6X5	T5Ø.6X6
Antacid NEC	T47.1X1	T47.1X2	T47.1X3	T47.1X4	T47.1X5	T47.1X6
Antagonist						
Aldosterone	T5Ø.ØX1	T5Ø.ØX2	T5Ø.ØX3	T5Ø.ØX4	T5Ø.ØX5	T5Ø.ØX6
alpha-adrenoreceptor	T44.6X1	T44.6X2	T44.6X3	T44.6X4	T44.6X5	T44.6X6
anticoagulant	T45.7X1	T45.7X2	T45.7X3	T45.7X4	T45.7X5	T45.7X6
beta-adrenoreceptor	T44.7X1	T44.7X2	T44.7X3	T44.7X4	T44.7X5	T44.7X6
extrapyramidal NEC	T44.3X1	T44.3X2	T44.3X3	T44.3X4	T44.3X5	T44.3X6
folic acid	T45.1X1	T45.1X2	T45.1X3	T45.1X4	T45.1X5	T45.1X6
H2 receptor	T47.ØX1	T47.ØX2	T47.ØX3	T47.ØX4	T47.ØX5	T47.ØX6
heavy metal	T45.8X1	T45.8X2	T45.8X3	T45.8X4	T45.8X5	T45.8X6
narcotic analgesic	T5Ø.7X1	T5Ø.7X2	T5Ø.7X3	T5Ø.7X4	T5Ø.7X5	T5Ø.7X6
opiate	T5Ø.7X1	T5Ø.7X2	T5Ø.7X3	T5Ø.7X4	T5Ø.7X5	T5Ø.7X6
pyrimidine	T45.1X1	T45.1X2	T45.1X3	T45.1X4	T45.1X5	T45.1X6
serotonin	T46.5X1	T46.5X2	T46.5X3	T46.5X4	T46.5X5	T46.5X6
Antazolin (e)	T45.ØX1	T45.ØX2	T45.ØX3	T45.ØX4	T45.ØX5	T45.ØX6
Anterior pituitary hormone NEC	T38.811	T38.812	T38.813	T38.814	T38.815	T38.816
Anthelmintic NEC	T37.4X1	T37.4X2	T37.4X3	T37.4X4	T37.4X5	T37.4X6
Anthiolimine	T37.4X1	T37.4X2	T37.4X3	T37.4X4	T37.4X5	T37.4X6
Anthralin	T49.4X1	T49.4X2	T49.4X3	T49.4X4	T49.4X5	T49.4X6
Anthramycin	T45.1X1	T45.1X2	T45.1X3	T45.1X4	T45.1X5	T45.1X6
Antiadrenergic NEC	T44.8X1	T44.8X2	T44.8X3	T44.8X4	T44.8X5	T44.8X6

Substance	Poisoning, Accidental (unintentional)	Poisoning, Intentional Self-harm	Poisoning, Assault	Poisoning, Undetermined	Adverse Effect	Under-dosing
Antiallergic NEC	T45.ØX1	T45.ØX2	T45.ØX3	T45.ØX4	T45.ØX5	T45.ØX6
Antiandrogen NEC	T38.6X1	T38.6X2	T38.6X3	T38.6X4	T38.6X5	T38.6X6
Anti-anemic (drug) (preparation)	T45.8X1	T45.8X2	T45.8X3	T45.8X4	T45.8X5	T45.8X6
Antianxiety drug NEC	T43.5Ø1	T43.5Ø2	T43.5Ø3	T43.5Ø4	T43.5Ø5	T43.5Ø6
Antiaris toxicaria	T65.891	T65.892	T65.893	T65.894	—	—
Antiarteriosclerotic drug	T46.6X1	T46.6X2	T46.6X3	T46.6X4	T46.6X5	T46.6X6
Antiasthmatic drug NEC	T48.6X1	T48.6X2	T48.6X3	T48.6X4	T48.6X5	T48.6X6
Antibiotic Otic Suspension (Solution)*	T49.6X1	T49.6X2	T49.6X3	T49.6X4	T49.6X5	T49.6X6
Antibiotic NEC	T36.91	T36.92	T36.93	T36.94	T36.95	T36.96
aminoglycoside	T36.5X1	T36.5X2	T36.5X3	T36.5X4	T36.5X5	T36.5X6
anticancer	T45.1X1	T45.1X2	T45.1X3	T45.1X4	T45.1X5	T45.1X6
antifungal	T36.7X1	T36.7X2	T36.7X3	T36.7X4	T36.7X5	T36.7X6
antimycobacterial	T36.5X1	T36.5X2	T36.5X3	T36.5X4	T36.5X5	T36.5X6
antineoplastic	T45.1X1	T45.1X2	T45.1X3	T45.1X4	T45.1X5	T45.1X6
b-lactam NEC	T36.1X1	T36.1X2	T36.1X3	T36.1X4	T36.1X5	T36.1X6
cephalosporin (group)	T36.1X1	T36.1X2	T36.1X3	T36.1X4	T36.1X5	T36.1X6
chloramphenicol (group)	T36.2X1	T36.2X2	T36.2X3	T36.2X4	T36.2X5	T36.2X6
ENT	T49.6X1	T49.6X2	T49.6X3	T49.6X4	T49.6X5	T49.6X6
eye	T49.5X1	T49.5X2	T49.5X3	T49.5X4	T49.5X5	T49.5X6
fungicidal (local)	T49.ØX1	T49.ØX2	T49.ØX3	T49.ØX4	T49.ØX5	T49.ØX6
intestinal	T36.8X1	T36.8X2	T36.8X3	T36.8X4	T36.8X5	T36.8X6
local	T49.ØX1	T49.ØX2	T49.ØX3	T49.ØX4	T49.ØX5	T49.ØX6
macrolides	T36.3X1	T36.3X2	T36.3X3	T36.3X4	T36.3X5	T36.3X6
polypeptide	T36.8X1	T36.8X2	T36.8X3	T36.8X4	T36.8X5	T36.8X6
specified NEC	T36.8X1	T36.8X2	T36.8X3	T36.8X4	T36.8X5	T36.8X6
tetracycline (group)	T36.4X1	T36.4X2	T36.4X3	T36.4X4	T36.4X5	T36.4X6
throat	T49.6X1	T49.6X2	T49.6X3	T49.6X4	T49.6X5	T49.6X6
Anticancer agents NEC	T45.1X1	T45.1X2	T45.1X3	T45.1X4	T45.1X5	T45.1X6
Anticholesterolemic drug NEC	T46.6X1	T46.6X2	T46.6X3	T46.6X4	T46.6X5	T46.6X6
Anticholinergic NEC	T44.3X1	T44.3X2	T44.3X3	T44.3X4	T44.3X5	T44.3X6
Anticholinesterase	T44.ØX1	T44.ØX2	T44.ØX3	T44.ØX4	T44.ØX5	T44.ØX6
organophosphorus	T44.ØX1	T44.ØX2	T44.ØX3	T44.ØX4	T44.ØX5	T44.ØX6
insecticide	T6Ø.ØX1	T6Ø.ØX2	T6Ø.ØX3	T6Ø.ØX4	—	—
nerve gas	T59.891	T59.892	T59.893	T59.894	—	—
reversible	T44.ØX1	T44.ØX2	T44.ØX3	T44.ØX4	T44.ØX5	T44.ØX6
ophthalmological	T49.5X1	T49.5X2	T49.5X3	T49.5X4	T49.5X5	T49.5X6
Anticoagulant NEC	T45.511	T45.512	T45.513	T45.514	T45.515	T45.516
Antagonist	T45.7X1	T45.7X2	T45.7X3	T45.7X4	T45.7X5	T45.7X6
Anti-common-cold drug NEC	T48.5X1	T48.5X2	T48.5X3	T48.5X4	T48.5X5	T48.5X6
Anticonvulsant	T42.71	T42.72	T42.73	T42.74	T42.75	T42.76
barbiturate	T42.3X1	T42.3X2	T42.3X3	T42.3X4	T42.3X5	T42.3X6
combination (with barbiturate)	T42.3X1	T42.3X2	T42.3X3	T42.3X4	T42.3X5	T42.3X6
hydantoin	T42.ØX1	T42.ØX2	T42.ØX3	T42.ØX4	T42.ØX5	T42.ØX6
hypnotic NEC	T42.6X1	T42.6X2	T42.6X3	T42.6X4	T42.6X5	T42.6X6
oxazolidinedione	T42.2X1	T42.2X2	T42.2X3	T42.2X4	T42.2X5	T42.2X6
pyrimidinedione	T42.6X1	T42.6X2	T42.6X3	T42.6X4	T42.6X5	T42.6X6
specified NEC	T42.6X1	T42.6X2	T42.6X3	T42.6X4	T42.6X5	T42.6X6
succinimide	T42.2X1	T42.2X2	T42.2X3	T42.2X4	T42.2X5	T42.2X6
Antidepressant	T43.2Ø1	T43.2Ø2	T43.2Ø3	T43.2Ø4	T43.2Ø5	T43.2Ø6
monoamine oxidase inhibitor	T43.1X1	T43.1X2	T43.1X3	T43.1X4	T43.1X5	T43.1X6
selective serotonin norepinephrine reuptake inhibitor	T43.211	T43.212	T43.213	T43.214	T43.215	T43.216
selective serotonin reuptake inhibitor	T43.221	T43.222	T43.223	T43.224	T43.225	T43.226
specified NEC	T43.291	T43.292	T43.293	T43.294	T43.295	T43.296
tetracyclic	T43.Ø21	T43.Ø22	T43.Ø23	T43.Ø24	T43.Ø25	T43.Ø26
triazolopyridine	T43.211	T43.212	T43.213	T43.214	T43.215	T43.216
tricyclic	T43.Ø11	T43.Ø12	T43.Ø13	T43.Ø14	T43.Ø15	T43.Ø16
Antidiabetic NEC	T38.3X1	T38.3X2	T38.3X3	T38.3X4	T38.3X5	T38.3X6
biguanide	T38.3X1	T38.3X2	T38.3X3	T38.3X4	T38.3X5	T38.3X6
and sulfonyl combined	T38.3X1	T38.3X2	T38.3X3	T38.3X4	T38.3X5	T38.3X6
combined	T38.3X1	T38.3X2	T38.3X3	T38.3X4	T38.3X5	T38.3X6
sulfonylurea	T38.3X1	T38.3X2	T38.3X3	T38.3X4	T38.3X5	T38.3X6
Antidiarrheal drug NEC	T47.6X1	T47.6X2	T47.6X3	T47.6X4	T47.6X5	T47.6X6
absorbent	T47.6X1	T47.6X2	T47.6X3	T47.6X4	T47.6X5	T47.6X6
Anti-D immunoglobulin (human)	T5Ø.Z11	T5Ø.Z12	T5Ø.Z13	T5Ø.Z14	T5Ø.Z15	T5Ø.Z16
Antidiphtheria serum	T5Ø.Z11	T5Ø.Z12	T5Ø.Z13	T5Ø.Z14	T5Ø.Z15	T5Ø.Z16
Antidiuretic hormone	T38.891	T38.892	T38.893	T38.894	T38.895	T38.896
Antidote NEC	T5Ø.6X1	T5Ø.6X2	T5Ø.6X3	T5Ø.6X4	T5Ø.6X5	T5Ø.6X6
heavy metal	T45.8X1	T45.8X2	T45.8X3	T45.8X4	T45.8X5	T45.8X6
Antidysrhythmic NEC	T46.2X1	T46.2X2	T46.2X3	T46.2X4	T46.2X5	T46.2X6
Antiemetic drug	T45.ØX1	T45.ØX2	T45.ØX3	T45.ØX4	T45.ØX5	T45.ØX6
Antiepilepsy agent	T42.71	T42.72	T42.73	T42.74	T42.75	T42.76
combination	T42.5X1	T42.5X2	T42.5X3	T42.5X4	T42.5X5	T42.5X6
mixed	T42.5X1	T42.5X2	T42.5X3	T42.5X4	T42.5X5	T42.5X6

Substance	Poisoning, Accidental (unintentional)	Poisoning, Intentional Self-harm	Poisoning, Assault	Poisoning, Undetermined	Adverse Effect	Under-dosing
Antiepilepsy agent — *continued*						
specified, NEC	T42.6X1	T42.6X2	T42.6X3	T42.6X4	T42.6X5	T42.6X6
Antiestrogen NEC	T38.6X1	T38.6X2	T38.6X3	T38.6X4	T38.6X5	T38.6X6
Antifertility pill	T38.4X1	T38.4X2	T38.4X3	T38.4X4	T38.4X5	T38.4X6
Antifibrinolytic drug	T45.621	T45.622	T45.623	T45.624	T45.625	T45.626
Antifilarial drug	T37.4X1	T37.4X2	T37.4X3	T37.4X4	T37.4X5	T37.4X6
Antiflatulent	T47.5X1	T47.5X2	T47.5X3	T47.5X4	T47.5X5	T47.5X6
Antifreeze	T65.91	T65.92	T65.93	T65.94	—	—
alcohol	T51.1X1	T51.1X2	T51.1X3	T51.1X4	—	—
ethylene glycol	T51.8X1	T51.8X2	T51.8X3	T51.8X4	—	—
Antifungal						
antibiotic (systemic)	T36.7X1	T36.7X2	T36.7X3	T36.7X4	T36.7X5	T36.7X6
anti-infective NEC	T37.91	T37.92	T37.93	T37.94	T37.95	T37.96
disinfectant, local	T49.0X1	T49.0X2	T49.0X3	T49.0X4	T49.0X5	T49.0X6
nonmedicinal (spray)	T60.3X1	T60.3X2	T60.3X3	T60.3X4	—	—
topical	T49.0X1	T49.0X2	T49.0X3	T49.0X4	T49.0X5	T49.0X6
Anti-gastric-secretion drug NEC	T47.1X1	T47.1X2	T47.1X3	T47.1X4	T47.1X5	T47.1X6
Antigonadotrophin NEC	T38.6X1	T38.6X2	T38.6X3	T38.6X4	T38.6X5	T38.6X6
Antihallucinogen	T43.501	T43.502	T43.503	T43.504	T43.505	T43.506
Antihelmintics	T37.4X1	T37.4X2	T37.4X3	T37.4X4	T37.4X5	T37.4X6
Antihemophilic						
factor	T45.8X1	T45.8X2	T45.8X3	T45.8X4	T45.8X5	T45.8X6
fraction	T45.8X1	T45.8X2	T45.8X3	T45.8X4	T45.8X5	T45.8X6
globulin concentrate	T45.7X1	T45.7X2	T45.7X3	T45.7X4	T45.7X5	T45.7X6
human plasma	T45.8X1	T45.8X2	T45.8X3	T45.8X4	T45.8X5	T45.8X6
plasma, dried	T45.7X1	T45.7X2	T45.7X3	T45.7X4	T45.7X5	T45.7X6
Antihemorrhoidal preparation	T49.2X1	T49.2X2	T49.2X3	T49.2X4	T49.2X5	T49.2X6
Antiheparin drug	T45.7X1	T45.7X2	T45.7X3	T45.7X4	T45.7X5	T45.7X6
Antihistamine	T45.0X1	T45.0X2	T45.0X3	T45.0X4	T45.0X5	T45.0X6
Antihookworm drug	T37.4X1	T37.4X2	T37.4X3	T37.4X4	T37.4X5	T37.4X6
Anti-human lymphocytic globulin	T50.Z11	T50.Z12	T50.Z13	T50.Z14	T50.Z15	T50.Z16
Antihyperlipidemic drug	T46.6X1	T46.6X2	T46.6X3	T46.6X4	T46.6X5	T46.6X6
Antihypertensive drug NEC	T46.5X1	T46.5X2	T46.5X3	T46.5X4	T46.5X5	T46.5X6
Anti-infective NEC	T37.91	T37.92	T37.93	T37.94	T37.95	T37.96
anthelmintic	T37.4X1	T37.4X2	T37.4X3	T37.4X4	T37.4X5	T37.4X6
antibiotics	T36.91	T36.92	T36.93	T36.94	T36.95	T36.96
specified NEC	T36.8X1	T36.8X2	T36.8X3	T36.8X4	T36.8X5	T36.8X6
antimalarial	T37.2X1	T37.2X2	T37.2X3	T37.2X4	T37.2X5	T37.2X6
antimycobacterial NEC	T37.1X1	T37.1X2	T37.1X3	T37.1X4	T37.1X5	T37.1X6
antibiotics	T36.5X1	T36.5X2	T36.5X3	T36.5X4	T36.5X5	T36.5X6
antiprotozoal NEC	T37.3X1	T37.3X2	T37.3X3	T37.3X4	T37.3X5	T37.3X6
blood	T37.2X1	T37.2X2	T37.2X3	T37.2X4	T37.2X5	T37.2X6
antiviral	T37.5X1	T37.5X2	T37.5X3	T37.5X4	T37.5X5	T37.5X6
arsenical	T37.8X1	T37.8X2	T37.8X3	T37.8X4	T37.8X5	T37.8X6
bismuth, local	T49.0X1	T49.0X2	T49.0X3	T49.0X4	T49.0X5	T49.0X6
ENT	T49.6X1	T49.6X2	T49.6X3	T49.6X4	T49.6X5	T49.6X6
eye NEC	T49.5X1	T49.5X2	T49.5X3	T49.5X4	T49.5X5	T49.5X6
heavy metals NEC	T37.8X1	T37.8X2	T37.8X3	T37.8X4	T37.8X5	T37.8X6
local NEC	T49.0X1	T49.0X2	T49.0X3	T49.0X4	T49.0X5	T49.0X6
specified NEC	T49.0X1	T49.0X2	T49.0X3	T49.0X4	T49.0X5	T49.0X6
mixed	T37.91	T37.92	T37.93	T37.94	T37.95	T37.96
ophthalmic preparation	T49.5X1	T49.5X2	T49.5X3	T49.5X4	T49.5X5	T49.5X6
topical NEC	T49.0X1	T49.0X2	T49.0X3	T49.0X4	T49.0X5	T49.0X6
Anti-inflammatory drug NEC	T39.391	T39.392	T39.393	T39.394	T39.395	T39.396
local	T49.0X1	T49.0X2	T49.0X3	T49.0X4	T49.0X5	T49.0X6
nonsteroidal NEC	T39.391	T39.392	T39.393	T39.394	T39.395	T39.396
propionic acid derivative	T39.311	T39.312	T39.313	T39.314	T39.315	T39.316
specified NEC	T39.391	T39.392	T39.393	T39.394	T39.395	T39.396
Antikaluretic	T50.3X1	T50.3X2	T50.3X3	T50.3X4	T50.3X5	T50.3X6
Antiknock (tetraethyl lead)	T56.0X1	T56.0X2	T56.0X3	T56.0X4	—	—
Antilipemic drug NEC	T46.6X1	T46.6X2	T46.6X3	T46.6X4	T46.6X5	T46.6X6
Antilysin*	T45.621	T45.622	T45.623	T45.624	T45.625	T45.626
Antimalarial	T37.2X1	T37.2X2	T37.2X3	T37.2X4	T37.2X5	T37.2X6
prophylactic NEC	T37.2X1	T37.2X2	T37.2X3	T37.2X4	T37.2X5	T37.2X6
pyrimidine derivative	T37.2X1	T37.2X2	T37.2X3	T37.2X4	T37.2X5	T37.2X6
Antimetabolite	T45.1X1	T45.1X2	T45.1X3	T45.1X4	T45.1X5	T45.1X6
Antimitotic agent	T45.1X1	T45.1X2	T45.1X3	T45.1X4	T45.1X5	T45.1X6
Antimony (compounds) (vapor) **NEC**	T56.891	T56.892	T56.893	T56.894	—	—
anti-infectives	T37.8X1	T37.8X2	T37.8X3	T37.8X4	T37.8X5	T37.8X6
dimercaptosuccinate	T37.3X1	T37.3X2	T37.3X3	T37.3X4	T37.3X5	T37.3X6
hydride	T56.891	T56.892	T56.893	T56.894	—	—
pesticide (vapor)	T60.8X1	T60.8X2	T60.8X3	T60.8X4	—	—
potassium (sodium) tartrate	T37.8X1	T37.8X2	T37.8X3	T37.8X4	T37.8X5	T37.8X6
sodium dimercaptosuccinate	T37.3X1	T37.3X2	T37.3X3	T37.3X4	T37.3X5	T37.3X6
tartrated	T37.8X1	T37.8X2	T37.8X3	T37.8X4	T37.8X5	T37.8X6

Substance	Poisoning, Accidental (unintentional)	Poisoning, Intentional Self-harm	Poisoning, Assault	Poisoning, Undetermined	Adverse Effect	Under-dosing
Antimuscarinic NEC	T44.3X1	T44.3X2	T44.3X3	T44.3X4	T44.3X5	T44.3X6
Antimycobacterial drug NEC	T37.1X1	T37.1X2	T37.1X3	T37.1X4	T37.1X5	T37.1X6
antibiotics	T36.5X1	T36.5X2	T36.5X3	T36.5X4	T36.5X5	T36.5X6
combination	T37.1X1	T37.1X2	T37.1X3	T37.1X4	T37.1X5	T37.1X6
Antinausea drug	T45.0X1	T45.0X2	T45.0X3	T45.0X4	T45.0X5	T45.0X6
Antinematode drug	T37.4X1	T37.4X2	T37.4X3	T37.4X4	T37.4X5	T37.4X6
Antineoplastic NEC	T45.1X1	T45.1X2	T45.1X3	T45.1X4	T45.1X5	T45.1X6
alkaloidal	T45.1X1	T45.1X2	T45.1X3	T45.1X4	T45.1X5	T45.1X6
antibiotics	T45.1X1	T45.1X2	T45.1X3	T45.1X4	T45.1X5	T45.1X6
combination	T45.1X1	T45.1X2	T45.1X3	T45.1X4	T45.1X5	T45.1X6
estrogen	T38.5X1	T38.5X2	T38.5X3	T38.5X4	T38.5X5	T38.5X6
steroid	T38.7X1	T38.7X2	T38.7X3	T38.7X4	T38.7X5	T38.7X6
Antiparasitic drug (systemic)	T37.91	T37.92	T37.93	T37.94	T37.95	T37.96
local	T49.0X1	T49.0X2	T49.0X3	T49.0X4	T49.0X5	T49.0X6
specified NEC	T37.8X1	T37.8X2	T37.8X3	T37.8X4	T37.8X5	T37.8X6
Antiparkinsonism drug NEC	T42.8X1	T42.8X2	T42.8X3	T42.8X4	T42.8X5	T42.8X6
Antiperspirant NEC	T49.2X1	T49.2X2	T49.2X3	T49.2X4	T49.2X5	T49.2X6
Antiphlogistic NEC	T39.4X1	T39.4X2	T39.4X3	T39.4X4	T39.4X5	T39.4X6
Antiplatyhelmintic drug	T37.4X1	T37.4X2	T37.4X3	T37.4X4	T37.4X5	T37.4X6
Antiprotozoal drug NEC	T37.3X1	T37.3X2	T37.3X3	T37.3X4	T37.3X5	T37.3X6
blood	T37.2X1	T37.2X2	T37.2X3	T37.2X4	T37.2X5	T37.2X6
local	T49.0X1	T49.0X2	T49.0X3	T49.0X4	T49.0X5	T49.0X6
Antipruritic drug NEC	T49.1X1	T49.1X2	T49.1X3	T49.1X4	T49.1X5	T49.1X6
Antipsychotic drug	T43.501	T43.502	T43.503	T43.504	T43.505	T43.506
specified NEC	T43.591	T43.592	T43.593	T43.594	T43.595	T43.596
Antipyretic	T39.91	T39.92	T39.93	T39.94	T39.95	T39.96
specified NEC	T39.8X1	T39.8X2	T39.8X3	T39.8X4	T39.8X5	T39.8X6
Antipyrine	T39.2X1	T39.2X2	T39.2X3	T39.2X4	T39.2X5	T39.2X6
Antirabies hyperimmune serum	T50.Z11	T50.Z12	T50.Z13	T50.Z14	T50.Z15	T50.Z16
Antirheumatic NEC	T39.4X1	T39.4X2	T39.4X3	T39.4X4	T39.4X5	T39.4X6
Antirigidity drug NEC	T42.8X1	T42.8X2	T42.8X3	T42.8X4	T42.8X5	T42.8X6
Antischistosomal drug	T37.4X1	T37.4X2	T37.4X3	T37.4X4	T37.4X5	T37.4X6
Antiscorpion sera	T50.Z11	T50.Z12	T50.Z13	T50.Z14	T50.Z15	T50.Z16
Antiseborrheics	T49.4X1	T49.4X2	T49.4X3	T49.4X4	T49.4X5	T49.4X6
Antiseptics (external) (medicinal)	T49.0X1	T49.0X2	T49.0X3	T49.0X4	T49.0X5	T49.0X6
Antistine	T45.0X1	T45.0X2	T45.0X3	T45.0X4	T45.0X5	T45.0X6
Antitapeworm drug	T37.4X1	T37.4X2	T37.4X3	T37.4X4	T37.4X5	T37.4X6
Antitetanus immunoglobulin	T50.Z11	T50.Z12	T50.Z13	T50.Z14	T50.Z15	T50.Z16
Antithrombin III*	T45.511	T45.512	T45.513	T45.514	T45.515	T45.516
Antithrombotic	T45.521	T45.522	T45.523	T45.524	T45.525	T45.526
Antithyroid drug NEC	T38.2X1	T38.2X2	T38.2X3	T38.2X4	T38.2X5	T38.2X6
Antitoxin	T50.Z11	T50.Z12	T50.Z13	T50.Z14	T50.Z15	T50.Z16
diphtheria	T50.Z11	T50.Z12	T50.Z13	T50.Z14	T50.Z15	T50.Z16
gas gangrene	T50.Z11	T50.Z12	T50.Z13	T50.Z14	T50.Z15	T50.Z16
tetanus	T50.Z11	T50.Z12	T50.Z13	T50.Z14	T50.Z15	T50.Z16
Antitrichomonal drug	T37.3X1	T37.3X2	T37.3X3	T37.3X4	T37.3X5	T37.3X6
Antituberculars	T37.1X1	T37.1X2	T37.1X3	T37.1X4	T37.1X5	T37.1X6
antibiotics	T36.5X1	T36.5X2	T36.5X3	T36.5X4	T36.5X5	T36.5X6
Antitussive NEC	T48.3X1	T48.3X2	T48.3X3	T48.3X4	T48.3X5	T48.3X6
codeine mixture	T40.2X1	T40.2X2	T40.2X3	T40.2X4	T40.2X5	T40.2X6
opiate	T40.2X1	T40.2X2	T40.2X3	T40.2X4	T40.2X5	T40.2X6
Antivaricose drug	T46.8X1	T46.8X2	T46.8X3	T46.8X4	T46.8X5	T46.8X6
Antivenin, antivenom (sera)	T50.Z11	T50.Z12	T50.Z13	T50.Z14	T50.Z15	T50.Z16
crotaline	T50.Z11	T50.Z12	T50.Z13	T50.Z14	T50.Z15	T50.Z16
spider bite	T50.Z11	T50.Z12	T50.Z13	T50.Z14	T50.Z15	T50.Z16
Antivert*	T45.0X1	T45.0X2	T45.0X3	T45.0X4	T45.0X5	T45.0X6
Antivertigo drug	T45.0X1	T45.0X2	T45.0X3	T45.0X4	T45.0X5	T45.0X6
Antiviral drug NEC	T37.5X1	T37.5X2	T37.5X3	T37.5X4	T37.5X5	T37.5X6
eye	T49.5X1	T49.5X2	T49.5X3	T49.5X4	T49.5X5	T49.5X6
Antiwhipworm drug	T37.4X1	T37.4X2	T37.4X3	T37.4X4	T37.4X5	T37.4X6
Ant poison — *see* Insecticide						
Antrol — *see also* by specific chemical substance	T60.91	T60.92	T60.93	T60.94	—	—
fungicide	T60.91	T60.92	T60.93	T60.94	—	—
ANTU (alpha naphthylthiourea)	T60.4X1	T60.4X2	T60.4X3	T60.4X4	—	—
Apalcillin	T36.0X1	T36.0X2	T36.0X3	T36.0X4	T36.0X5	T36.0X6
APC	T48.5X1	T48.5X2	T48.5X3	T48.5X4	T48.5X5	T48.5X6
Aplonidine	T44.4X1	T44.4X2	T44.4X3	T44.4X4	T44.4X5	T44.4X6
Apomorphine	T47.7X1	T47.7X2	T47.7X3	T47.7X4	T47.7X5	T47.7X6
Appetite depressants, central	T50.5X1	T50.5X2	T50.5X3	T50.5X4	T50.5X5	T50.5X6
Apraclonidine (hydrochloride)	T44.4X1	T44.4X2	T44.4X3	T44.4X4	T44.4X5	T44.4X6
Apresoline	T46.5X1	T46.5X2	T46.5X3	T46.5X4	T46.5X5	T46.5X6
Apri*	T38.4X1	T38.4X2	T38.4X3	T38.4X4	T38.4X5	T38.4X6

Substance	Poisoning, Accidental (unintentional)	Poisoning, Intentional Self-harm	Poisoning, Assault	Poisoning, Undetermined	Adverse Effect	Under-dosing
Aprindine	T46.2X1	T46.2X2	T46.2X3	T46.2X4	T46.2X5	T46.2X6
Aprobarbital	T42.3X1	T42.3X2	T42.3X3	T42.3X4	T42.3X5	T42.3X6
Apronalide	T42.6X1	T42.6X2	T42.6X3	T42.6X4	T42.6X5	T42.6X6
Aprotinin	T45.621	T45.622	T45.623	T45.624	T45.625	T45.626
Aptocaine	T41.3X1	T41.3X2	T41.3X3	T41.3X4	T41.3X5	T41.3X6
Aqua fortis	T54.2X1	T54.2X2	T54.2X3	T54.2X4	—	—
Ara-A	T37.5X1	T37.5X2	T37.5X3	T37.5X4	T37.5X5	T37.5X6
Ara-C	T45.1X1	T45.1X2	T45.1X3	T45.1X4	T45.1X5	T45.1X6
Arachis oil	T49.3X1	T49.3X2	T49.3X3	T49.3X4	T49.3X5	T49.3X6
cathartic	T47.4X1	T47.4X2	T47.4X3	T47.4X4	T47.4X5	T47.4X6
Aralen	T37.2X1	T37.2X2	T37.2X3	T37.2X4	T37.2X5	T37.2X6
Arecoline	T44.1X1	T44.1X2	T44.1X3	T44.1X4	T44.1X5	T44.1X6
Arginine	T50.991	T50.992	T50.993	T50.994	T50.995	T50.996
glutamate	T50.991	T50.992	T50.993	T50.994	T50.995	T50.996
Argyrol	T49.0X1	T49.0X2	T49.0X3	T49.0X4	T49.0X5	T49.0X6
ENT agent	T49.6X1	T49.6X2	T49.6X3	T49.6X4	T49.6X5	T49.6X6
ophthalmic preparation	T49.5X1	T49.5X2	T49.5X3	T49.5X4	T49.5X5	T49.5X6
Aristocort	T38.0X1	T38.0X2	T38.0X3	T38.0X4	T38.0X5	T38.0X6
ENT agent	T49.6X1	T49.6X2	T49.6X3	T49.6X4	T49.6X5	T49.6X6
ophthalmic preparation	T49.5X1	T49.5X2	T49.5X3	T49.5X4	T49.5X5	T49.5X6
topical NEC	T49.0X1	T49.0X2	T49.0X3	T49.0X4	T49.0X5	T49.0X6
Aromatics, corrosive	T54.1X1	T54.1X2	T54.1X3	T54.1X4	—	—
disinfectants	T54.1X1	T54.1X2	T54.1X3	T54.1X4	—	—
Arsenate of lead	T57.0X1	T57.0X2	T57.0X3	T57.0X4	—	—
herbicide	T57.0X1	T57.0X2	T57.0X3	T57.0X4	—	—
Arsenic, arsenicals (compounds) (dust) (vapor) **NEC**	T57.0X1	T57.0X2	T57.0X3	T57.0X4	—	—
anti-infectives	T37.8X1	T37.8X2	T37.8X3	T37.8X4	T37.8X5	T37.8X6
pesticide (dust) (fumes)	T57.0X1	T57.0X2	T57.0X3	T57.0X4	—	—
Arsine (gas)	T57.0X1	T57.0X2	T57.0X3	T57.0X4	—	—
Arsobal*	T37.3X1	T37.3X2	T37.3X3	T37.3X4	T37.3X5	T37.3X6
Arsphenamine (silver)	T37.8X1	T37.8X2	T37.8X3	T37.8X4	T37.8X5	T37.8X6
Arsthinol	T37.3X1	T37.3X2	T37.3X3	T37.3X4	T37.3X5	T37.3X6
Artane	T44.3X1	T44.3X2	T44.3X3	T44.3X4	T44.3X5	T44.3X6
Arthropod (venomous) **NEC**	T63.481	T63.482	T63.483	T63.484	—	—
Articaine	T41.3X1	T41.3X2	T41.3X3	T41.3X4	T41.3X5	T41.3X6
Asbestos	T57.8X1	T57.8X2	T57.8X3	T57.8X4	—	—
Ascaridole	T37.4X1	T37.4X2	T37.4X3	T37.4X4	T37.4X5	T37.4X6
Ascorbic acid	T45.2X1	T45.2X2	T45.2X3	T45.2X4	T45.2X5	T45.2X6
Asiaticoside	T49.0X1	T49.0X2	T49.0X3	T49.0X4	T49.0X5	T49.0X6
Asparaginase	T45.1X1	T45.1X2	T45.1X3	T45.1X4	T45.1X5	T45.1X6
Aspidium (oleoresin)	T37.4X1	T37.4X2	T37.4X3	T37.4X4	T37.4X5	T37.4X6
Aspirin (aluminum) (soluble)	T39.011	T39.012	T39.013	T39.014	T39.015	T39.016
Aspoxicillin	T36.0X1	T36.0X2	T36.0X3	T36.0X4	T36.0X5	T36.0X6
Astemizole	T45.0X1	T45.0X2	T45.0X3	T45.0X4	T45.0X5	T45.0X6
Astringent (local)	T49.2X1	T49.2X2	T49.2X3	T49.2X4	T49.2X5	T49.2X6
specified NEC	T49.2X1	T49.2X2	T49.2X3	T49.2X4	T49.2X5	T49.2X6
Astromicin	T36.5X1	T36.5X2	T36.5X3	T36.5X4	T36.5X5	T36.5X6
Ataractic drug NEC	T43.501	T43.502	T43.503	T43.504	T43.505	T43.506
Atenolol	T44.7X1	T44.7X2	T44.7X3	T44.7X4	T44.7X5	T44.7X6
Atonia drug, intestinal	T47.4X1	T47.4X2	T47.4X3	T47.4X4	T47.4X5	T47.4X6
Atophan	T50.4X1	T50.4X2	T50.4X3	T50.4X4	T50.4X5	T50.4X6
Atracurium besilate	T48.1X1	T48.1X2	T48.1X3	T48.1X4	T48.1X5	T48.1X6
Atropine	T44.3X1	T44.3X2	T44.3X3	T44.3X4	T44.3X5	T44.3X6
derivative	T44.3X1	T44.3X2	T44.3X3	T44.3X4	T44.3X5	T44.3X6
methonitrate	T44.3X1	T44.3X2	T44.3X3	T44.3X4	T44.3X5	T44.3X6
Atrovent*	T48.6X1	T48.6X2	T48.6X3	T48.6X4	T48.6X5	T48.6X6
Attapulgite	T47.6X1	T47.6X2	T47.6X3	T47.6X4	T47.6X5	T47.6X6
Auramine	T65.891	T65.892	T65.893	T65.894	—	—
dye	T65.6X1	T65.6X2	T65.6X3	T65.6X4	—	—
fungicide	T60.3X1	T60.3X2	T60.3X3	T60.3X4	—	—
Auranofin	T39.4X1	T39.4X2	T39.4X3	T39.4X4	T39.4X5	T39.4X6
Aurantiin	T46.991	T46.992	T46.993	T46.994	T46.995	T46.996
Aureomycin	T36.4X1	T36.4X2	T36.4X3	T36.4X4	T36.4X5	T36.4X6
ophthalmic preparation	T49.5X1	T49.5X2	T49.5X3	T49.5X4	T49.5X5	T49.5X6
topical NEC	T49.0X1	T49.0X2	T49.0X3	T49.0X4	T49.0X5	T49.0X6
Aurothioglucose	T39.4X1	T39.4X2	T39.4X3	T39.4X4	T39.4X5	T39.4X6
Aurothioglycanide	T39.4X1	T39.4X2	T39.4X3	T39.4X4	T39.4X5	T39.4X6
Aurothiomalate sodium	T39.4X1	T39.4X2	T39.4X3	T39.4X4	T39.4X5	T39.4X6
Aurotioprol	T39.4X1	T39.4X2	T39.4X3	T39.4X4	T39.4X5	T39.4X6
Automobile fuel	T52.0X1	T52.0X2	T52.0X3	T52.0X4	—	—
Autonomic nervous system agent NEC	T44.901	T44.902	T44.903	T44.904	T44.905	T44.906
Avelox*	T36.8X1	T36.8X2	T36.8X3	T36.8X4	T36.8X5	T36.8X6
Avlosulfon	T37.1X1	T37.1X2	T37.1X3	T37.1X4	T37.1X5	T37.1X6
Avomine	T42.6X1	T42.6X2	T42.6X3	T42.6X4	T42.6X5	T42.6X6
Axerophthol	T45.2X1	T45.2X2	T45.2X3	T45.2X4	T45.2X5	T45.2X6
Azacitidine	T45.1X1	T45.1X2	T45.1X3	T45.1X4	T45.1X5	T45.1X6
Azacyclonol	T43.591	T43.592	T43.593	T43.594	T43.595	T43.596
Azadirachta	T60.2X1	T60.2X2	T60.2X3	T60.2X4	—	—
Azanidazole	T37.3X1	T37.3X2	T37.3X3	T37.3X4	T37.3X5	T37.3X6
Azapetine	T46.7X1	T46.7X2	T46.7X3	T46.7X4	T46.7X5	T46.7X6
Azapropazone	T39.2X1	T39.2X2	T39.2X3	T39.2X4	T39.2X5	T39.2X6
Azaribine	T45.1X1	T45.1X2	T45.1X3	T45.1X4	T45.1X5	T45.1X6
Azaserine	T45.1X1	T45.1X2	T45.1X3	T45.1X4	T45.1X5	T45.1X6
Azatadine	T45.0X1	T45.0X2	T45.0X3	T45.0X4	T45.0X5	T45.0X6
Azatepa	T45.1X1	T45.1X2	T45.1X3	T45.1X4	T45.1X5	T45.1X6
Azathioprine	T45.1X1	T45.1X2	T45.1X3	T45.1X4	T45.1X5	T45.1X6
Azelaic acid	T49.0X1	T49.0X2	T49.0X3	T49.0X4	T49.0X5	T49.0X6
Azelastine	T45.0X1	T45.0X2	T45.0X3	T45.0X4	T45.0X5	T45.0X6
Azidocillin	T36.0X1	T36.0X2	T36.0X3	T36.0X4	T36.0X5	T36.0X6
Azidothymidine	T37.5X1	T37.5X2	T37.5X3	T37.5X4	T37.5X5	T37.5X6
Azinphos (ethyl) (methyl)	T60.0X1	T60.0X2	T60.0X3	T60.0X4	—	—
Aziridine (chelating)	T54.1X1	T54.1X2	T54.1X3	T54.1X4	—	—
Azithromycin	T36.3X1	T36.3X2	T36.3X3	T36.3X4	T36.3X5	T36.3X6
Azlocillin	T36.0X1	T36.0X2	T36.0X3	T36.0X4	T36.0X5	T36.0X6
Azobenzene smoke	T65.3X1	T65.3X2	T65.3X3	T65.3X4	—	—
acaricide	T60.8X1	T60.8X2	T60.8X3	T60.8X4	—	—
Azo-Standard*	T49.0X1	T49.0X2	T49.0X3	T49.0X4	T49.0X5	T49.0X6
Azosulfamide	T37.0X1	T37.0X2	T37.0X3	T37.0X4	T37.0X5	T37.0X6
AZT	T37.5X1	T37.5X2	T37.5X3	T37.5X4	T37.5X5	T37.5X6
Aztreonam	T36.1X1	T36.1X2	T36.1X3	T36.1X4	T36.1X5	T36.1X6
Azulfidine	T37.0X1	T37.0X2	T37.0X3	T37.0X4	T37.0X5	T37.0X6
Azuresin	T50.8X1	T50.8X2	T50.8X3	T50.8X4	T50.8X5	T50.8X6
b-acetyldigoxin	T46.0X1	T46.0X2	T46.0X3	T46.0X4	T46.0X5	T46.0X6
P-Acetamidophenol	T39.1X1	T39.1X2	T39.1X3	T39.1X4	T39.1X5	T39.1X6
Bacampicillin	T36.0X1	T36.0X2	T36.0X3	T36.0X4	T36.0X5	T36.0X6
Bacillus						
lactobacillus	T47.8X1	T47.8X2	T47.8X3	T47.8X4	T47.8X5	T47.8X6
subtilis	T47.6X1	T47.6X2	T47.6X3	T47.6X4	T47.6X5	T47.6X6
Bacimycin	T49.0X1	T49.0X2	T49.0X3	T49.0X4	T49.0X5	T49.0X6
ophthalmic preparation	T49.5X1	T49.5X2	T49.5X3	T49.5X4	T49.5X5	T49.5X6
Bacitracin zinc	T49.0X1	T49.0X2	T49.0X3	T49.0X4	T49.0X5	T49.0X6
with neomycin	T49.0X1	T49.0X2	T49.0X3	T49.0X4	T49.0X5	T49.0X6
ENT agent	T49.6X1	T49.6X2	T49.6X3	T49.6X4	T49.6X5	T49.6X6
ophthalmic preparation	T49.5X1	T49.5X2	T49.5X3	T49.5X4	T49.5X5	T49.5X6
topical NEC	T49.0X1	T49.0X2	T49.0X3	T49.0X4	T49.0X5	T49.0X6
Baclofen	T42.8X1	T42.8X2	T42.8X3	T42.8X4	T42.8X5	T42.8X6
Baking soda	T50.991	T50.992	T50.993	T50.994	T50.995	T50.996
BAL	T45.8X1	T45.8X2	T45.8X3	T45.8X4	T45.8X5	T45.8X6
Bambuterol	T48.6X1	T48.6X2	T48.6X3	T48.6X4	T48.6X5	T48.6X6
Bamethan (sulfate)	T46.7X1	T46.7X2	T46.7X3	T46.7X4	T46.7X5	T46.7X6
Bamifylline	T48.6X1	T48.6X2	T48.6X3	T48.6X4	T48.6X5	T48.6X6
Bamipine	T45.0X1	T45.0X2	T45.0X3	T45.0X4	T45.0X5	T45.0X6
Baneberry — *see* Actaea spicata						
Banewort — *see* Belladonna						
Barbenyl	T42.3X1	T42.3X2	T42.3X3	T42.3X4	T42.3X5	T42.3X6
Barbexaclone	T42.6X1	T42.6X2	T42.6X3	T42.6X4	T42.6X5	T42.6X6
Barbital	T42.3X1	T42.3X2	T42.3X3	T42.3X4	T42.3X5	T42.3X6
sodium	T42.3X1	T42.3X2	T42.3X3	T42.3X4	T42.3X5	T42.3X6
Barbitone	T42.3X1	T42.3X2	T42.3X3	T42.3X4	T42.3X5	T42.3X6
Barbiturate NEC	T42.3X1	T42.3X2	T42.3X3	T42.3X4	T42.3X5	T42.3X6
with tranquilizer	T42.3X1	T42.3X2	T42.3X3	T42.3X4	T42.3X5	T42.3X6
anesthetic (intravenous)	T41.1X1	T41.1X2	T41.1X3	T41.1X4	T41.1X5	T41.1X6
Barium (carbonate) (chloride) (sulfite)	T57.8X1	T57.8X2	T57.8X3	T57.8X4	—	—
diagnostic agent	T50.8X1	T50.8X2	T50.8X3	T50.8X4	T50.8X5	T50.8X6
pesticide	T60.4X1	T60.4X2	T60.4X3	T60.4X4	—	—
rodenticide	T60.4X1	T60.4X2	T60.4X3	T60.4X4	—	—
sulfate (medicinal)	T50.8X1	T50.8X2	T50.8X3	T50.8X4	T50.8X5	T50.8X6
Barrier cream	T49.3X1	T49.3X2	T49.3X3	T49.3X4	T49.3X5	T49.3X6
Basic fuchsin	T49.0X1	T49.0X2	T49.0X3	T49.0X4	T49.0X5	T49.0X6
Basiliximab*	T45.1X1	T45.1X2	T45.1X3	T45.1X4	T45.1X5	T45.1X6
Battery acid or fluid	T54.2X1	T54.2X2	T54.2X3	T54.2X4	—	—
Bay rum	T51.8X1	T51.8X2	T51.8X3	T51.8X4	—	—
b-benzalbutyramide	T46.6X1	T46.6X2	T46.6X3	T46.6X4	T46.6X5	T46.6X6
BCG (vaccine)	T50.A91	T50.A92	T50.A93	T50.A94	T50.A95	T50.A96
BCNU	T45.1X1	T45.1X2	T45.1X3	T45.1X4	T45.1X5	T45.1X6
Bearsfoot	T62.2X1	T62.2X2	T62.2X3	T62.2X4	—	—
Beclamide	T42.6X1	T42.6X2	T42.6X3	T42.6X4	T42.6X5	T42.6X6
Beclomethasone	T44.5X1	T44.5X2	T44.5X3	T44.5X4	T44.5X5	T44.5X6
Bee (sting) (venom)	T63.441	T63.442	T63.443	T63.444	—	—
Befunolol	T49.5X1	T49.5X2	T49.5X3	T49.5X4	T49.5X5	T49.5X6
Bekanamycin	T36.5X1	T36.5X2	T36.5X3	T36.5X4	T36.5X5	T36.5X6
Belladonna — *see also* Nightshade						
alkaloids	T44.3X1	T44.3X2	T44.3X3	T44.3X4	T44.3X5	T44.3X6
extract	T44.3X1	T44.3X2	T44.3X3	T44.3X4	T44.3X5	T44.3X6
herb	T44.3X1	T44.3X2	T44.3X3	T44.3X4	T44.3X5	T44.3X6
Belviq*	T50.5X1	T50.5X2	T50.5X3	T50.5X4	T50.5X5	T50.5X6
Bemegride	T50.7X1	T50.7X2	T50.7X3	T50.7X4	T50.7X5	T50.7X6
Benactyzine	T44.3X1	T44.3X2	T44.3X3	T44.3X4	T44.3X5	T44.3X6
Benadryl	T45.0X1	T45.0X2	T45.0X3	T45.0X4	T45.0X5	T45.0X6
Benaprizine	T44.3X1	T44.3X2	T44.3X3	T44.3X4	T44.3X5	T44.3X6
Benazepril	T46.4X1	T46.4X2	T46.4X3	T46.4X4	T46.4X5	T46.4X6

Substance	Poisoning, Accidental (unintentional)	Poisoning, Intentional Self-harm	Poisoning, Assault	Poisoning, Undetermined	Adverse Effect	Under-dosing
Bencyclane	T46.7X1	T46.7X2	T46.7X3	T46.7X4	T46.7X5	T46.7X6
Bendazol	T46.3X1	T46.3X2	T46.3X3	T46.3X4	T46.3X5	T46.3X6
Bendrofluazide	T5Ø.2X1	T5Ø.2X2	T5Ø.2X3	T5Ø.2X4	T5Ø.2X5	T5Ø.2X6
Bendroflumethiazide	T5Ø.2X1	T5Ø.2X2	T5Ø.2X3	T5Ø.2X4	T5Ø.2X5	T5Ø.2X6
Benemid	T5Ø.4X1	T5Ø.4X2	T5Ø.4X3	T5Ø.4X4	T5Ø.4X5	T5Ø.4X6
Benethamine penicillin	T36.ØX1	T36.ØX2	T36.ØX3	T36.ØX4	T36.ØX5	T36.ØX6
Benexate	T47.1X1	T47.1X2	T47.1X3	T47.1X4	T47.1X5	T47.1X6
Benfluorex	T46.6X1	T46.6X2	T46.6X3	T46.6X4	T46.6X5	T46.6X6
Benfotiamine	T45.2X1	T45.2X2	T45.2X3	T45.2X4	T45.2X5	T45.2X6
Benisone	T49.ØX1	T49.ØX2	T49.ØX3	T49.ØX4	T49.ØX5	T49.ØX6
Benomyl	T6Ø.ØX1	T6Ø.ØX2	T6Ø.ØX3	T6Ø.ØX4	—	—
Benoquin	T49.8X1	T49.8X2	T49.8X3	T49.8X4	T49.8X5	T49.8X6
Benoxinate	T41.3X1	T41.3X2	T41.3X3	T41.3X4	T41.3X5	T41.3X6
Benperidol	T43.4X1	T43.4X2	T43.4X3	T43.4X4	T43.4X5	T43.4X6
Benproperine	T48.3X1	T48.3X2	T48.3X3	T48.3X4	T48.3X5	T48.3X6
Benserazide	T42.8X1	T42.8X2	T42.8X3	T42.8X4	T42.8X5	T42.8X6
Bentazepam	T42.4X1	T42.4X2	T42.4X3	T42.4X4	T42.4X5	T42.4X6
Bentiromide	T5Ø.8X1	T5Ø.8X2	T5Ø.8X3	T5Ø.8X4	T5Ø.8X5	T5Ø.8X6
Bentonite	T49.3X1	T49.3X2	T49.3X3	T49.3X4	T49.3X5	T49.3X6
Benzalbutyramide	T46.6X1	T46.6X2	T46.6X3	T46.6X4	T46.6X5	T46.6X6
Benzalkonium (chloride)	T49.ØX1	T49.ØX2	T49.ØX3	T49.ØX4	T49.ØX5	T49.ØX6
ophthalmic preparation	T49.5X1	T49.5X2	T49.5X3	T49.5X4	T49.5X5	T49.5X6
Benzamidosalicylate (calcium)	T37.1X1	T37.1X2	T37.1X3	T37.1X4	T37.1X5	T37.1X6
Benzamine	T41.3X1	T41.3X2	T41.3X3	T41.3X4	T41.3X5	T41.3X6
lactate	T49.1X1	T49.1X2	T49.1X3	T49.1X4	T49.1X5	T49.1X6
Benzamphetamine	T5Ø.5X1	T5Ø.5X2	T5Ø.5X3	T5Ø.5X4	T5Ø.5X5	T5Ø.5X6
Benzapril hydrochloride	T46.5X1	T46.5X2	T46.5X3	T46.5X4	T46.5X5	T46.5X6
Benzathine benzylpenicillin	T36.ØX1	T36.ØX2	T36.ØX3	T36.ØX4	T36.ØX5	T36.ØX6
Benzathine penicillin	T36.ØX1	T36.ØX2	T36.ØX3	T36.ØX4	T36.ØX5	T36.ØX6
Benzatropine	T42.8X1	T42.8X2	T42.8X3	T42.8X4	T42.8X5	T42.8X6
Benzbromarone	T5Ø.4X1	T5Ø.4X2	T5Ø.4X3	T5Ø.4X4	T5Ø.4X5	T5Ø.4X6
Benzcarbimine	T45.1X1	T45.1X2	T45.1X3	T45.1X4	T45.1X5	T45.1X6
Benzedrex	T44.991	T44.992	T44.993	T44.994	T44.995	T44.996
Benzedrine (amphetamine)	T43.621	T43.622	T43.623	T43.624	T43.625	T43.626
Benzenamine	T65.3X1	T65.3X2	T65.3X3	T65.3X4	—	—
Benzene	T52.1X1	T52.1X2	T52.1X3	T52.1X4	—	—
homologues (acetyl) (dimethyl) (methyl) (solvent)	T52.2X1	T52.2X2	T52.2X3	T52.2X4	—	—
Benzethonium (chloride)	T49.ØX1	T49.ØX2	T49.ØX3	T49.ØX4	T49.ØX5	T49.ØX6
Benzfetamine	T5Ø.5X1	T5Ø.5X2	T5Ø.5X3	T5Ø.5X4	T5Ø.5X5	T5Ø.5X6
Benzhexol	T44.3X1	T44.3X2	T44.3X3	T44.3X4	T44.3X5	T44.3X6
Benzhydramine (chloride)	T45.ØX1	T45.ØX2	T45.ØX3	T45.ØX4	T45.ØX5	T45.ØX6
Benzidine	T65.891	T65.892	T65.893	T65.894	—	—
Benzilonium bromide	T44.3X1	T44.3X2	T44.3X3	T44.3X4	T44.3X5	T44.3X6
Benzimidazole	T6Ø.3X1	T6Ø.3X2	T6Ø.3X3	T6Ø.3X4	—	—
Benzin (e) — *see* Ligroin						
Benziodarone	T46.3X1	T46.3X2	T46.3X3	T46.3X4	T46.3X5	T46.3X6
Benznidazole	T37.3X1	T37.3X2	T37.3X3	T37.3X4	T37.3X5	T37.3X6
Benzocaine	T41.3X1	T41.3X2	T41.3X3	T41.3X4	T41.3X5	T41.3X6
Benzocol*	T41.3X1	T41.3X2	T41.3X3	T41.3X4	T41.3X5	T41.3X6
Benzodiapin	T42.4X1	T42.4X2	T42.4X3	T42.4X4	T42.4X5	T42.4X6
Benzodiazepine NEC	T42.4X1	T42.4X2	T42.4X3	T42.4X4	T42.4X5	T42.4X6
Benzoic acid	T49.ØX1	T49.ØX2	T49.ØX3	T49.ØX4	T49.ØX5	T49.ØX6
with salicylic acid	T49.ØX1	T49.ØX2	T49.ØX3	T49.ØX4	T49.ØX5	T49.ØX6
Benzoin (tincture)	T48.5X1	T48.5X2	T48.5X3	T48.5X4	T48.5X5	T48.5X6
Benzol (benzene)	T52.1X1	T52.1X2	T52.1X3	T52.1X4	—	—
vapor	T52.ØX1	T52.ØX2	T52.ØX3	T52.ØX4	—	—
Benzomorphan	T4Ø.2X1	T4Ø.2X2	T4Ø.2X3	T4Ø.2X4	T4Ø.2X5	T4Ø.2X6
Benzonatate	T48.3X1	T48.3X2	T48.3X3	T48.3X4	T48.3X5	T48.3X6
Benzophenones	T49.3X1	T49.3X2	T49.3X3	T49.3X4	T49.3X5	T49.3X6
Benzopyrone	T46.991	T46.992	T46.993	T46.994	T46.995	T46.996
Benzothiadiazides	T5Ø.2X1	T5Ø.2X2	T5Ø.2X3	T5Ø.2X4	T5Ø.2X5	T5Ø.2X6
Benzoxonium chloride	T49.ØX1	T49.ØX2	T49.ØX3	T49.ØX4	T49.ØX5	T49.ØX6
Benzoylpas calcium	T37.1X1	T37.1X2	T37.1X3	T37.1X4	T37.1X5	T37.1X6
Benzoyl peroxide	T49.ØX1	T49.ØX2	T49.ØX3	T49.ØX4	T49.ØX5	T49.ØX6
Benzperidin	T43.591	T43.592	T43.593	T43.594	T43.595	T43.596
Benzperidol	T43.591	T43.592	T43.593	T43.594	T43.595	T43.596
Benzphetamine	T5Ø.5X1	T5Ø.5X2	T5Ø.5X3	T5Ø.5X4	T5Ø.5X5	T5Ø.5X6
Benzpyrinium bromide	T44.1X1	T44.1X2	T44.1X3	T44.1X4	T44.1X5	T44.1X6
Benzquinamide	T45.ØX1	T45.ØX2	T45.ØX3	T45.ØX4	T45.ØX5	T45.ØX6
Benzthiazide	T5Ø.2X1	T5Ø.2X2	T5Ø.2X3	T5Ø.2X4	T5Ø.2X5	T5Ø.2X6
Benztropine						
anticholinergic	T44.3X1	T44.3X2	T44.3X3	T44.3X4	T44.3X5	T44.3X6
antiparkinson	T42.8X1	T42.8X2	T42.8X3	T42.8X4	T42.8X5	T42.8X6
Benzydamine	T49.ØX1	T49.ØX2	T49.ØX3	T49.ØX4	T49.ØX5	T49.ØX6
Benzyl						
acetate	T52.8X1	T52.8X2	T52.8X3	T52.8X4	—	—
alcohol	T49.ØX1	T49.ØX2	T49.ØX3	T49.ØX4	T49.ØX5	T49.ØX6
benzoate	T49.ØX1	T49.ØX2	T49.ØX3	T49.ØX4	T49.ØX5	T49.ØX6
Benzoic acid	T49.ØX1	T49.ØX2	T49.ØX3	T49.ØX4	T49.ØX5	T49.ØX6
hydroquinone*	T49.4X1	T49.4X2	T49.4X3	T49.4X4	T49.4X5	T49.4X6
Benzyl — *continued*						
morphine	T4Ø.2X1	T4Ø.2X2	T4Ø.2X3	T4Ø.2X4	—	—
nicotinate	T46.6X1	T46.6X2	T46.6X3	T46.6X4	T46.6X5	T46.6X6
penicillin	T36.ØX1	T36.ØX2	T36.ØX3	T36.ØX4	T36.ØX5	T36.ØX6
Benzylhydrochlorthiazide	T5Ø.2X1	T5Ø.2X2	T5Ø.2X3	T5Ø.2X4	T5Ø.2X5	T5Ø.2X6
Benzylpenicillin	T36.ØX1	T36.ØX2	T36.ØX3	T36.ØX4	T36.ØX5	T36.ØX6
Benzylthiouracil	T38.2X1	T38.2X2	T38.2X3	T38.2X4	T38.2X5	T38.2X6
Bephenium hydroxynaphthoate	T37.4X1	T37.4X2	T37.4X3	T37.4X4	T37.4X5	T37.4X6
Bepridil	T46.1X1	T46.1X2	T46.1X3	T46.1X4	T46.1X5	T46.1X6
Bergamot oil	T65.891	T65.892	T65.893	T65.894	—	—
Bergapten	T5Ø.991	T5Ø.992	T5Ø.993	T5Ø.994	T5Ø.995	T5Ø.996
Berries, poisonous	T62.1X1	T62.1X2	T62.1X3	T62.1X4	—	—
Beryllium (compounds)	T56.7X1	T56.7X2	T56.7X3	T56.7X4	—	—
beta adrenergic blocking agent, heart	T44.7X1	T44.7X2	T44.7X3	T44.7X4	T44.7X5	T44.7X6
Betacarotene	T45.2X1	T45.2X2	T45.2X3	T45.2X4	T45.2X5	T45.2X6
Beta-Chlor	T42.6X1	T42.6X2	T42.6X3	T42.6X4	T42.6X5	T42.6X6
Betahistine	T46.7X1	T46.7X2	T46.7X3	T46.7X4	T46.7X5	T46.7X6
Betaine	T47.5X1	T47.5X2	T47.5X3	T47.5X4	T47.5X5	T47.5X6
Betamethasone	T49.ØX1	T49.ØX2	T49.ØX3	T49.ØX4	T49.ØX5	T49.ØX6
topical	T49.ØX1	T49.ØX2	T49.ØX3	T49.ØX4	T49.ØX5	T49.ØX6
Betamicin	T36.8X1	T36.8X2	T36.8X3	T36.8X4	T36.8X5	T36.8X6
Betanidine	T46.5X1	T46.5X2	T46.5X3	T46.5X4	T46.5X5	T46.5X6
Betaxolol	T44.7X1	T44.7X2	T44.7X3	T44.7X4	T44.7X5	T44.7X6
Betazole	T5Ø.8X1	T5Ø.8X2	T5Ø.8X3	T5Ø.8X4	T5Ø.8X5	T5Ø.8X6
Bethanechol	T44.1X1	T44.1X2	T44.1X3	T44.1X4	T44.1X5	T44.1X6
chloride	T44.1X1	T44.1X2	T44.1X3	T44.1X4	T44.1X5	T44.1X6
Bethanidine	T46.5X1	T46.5X2	T46.5X3	T46.5X4	T46.5X5	T46.5X6
Betoxycaine	T41.3X1	T41.3X2	T41.3X3	T41.3X4	T41.3X5	T41.3X6
Betula oil	T49.3X1	T49.3X2	T49.3X3	T49.3X4	T49.3X5	T49.3X6
Bevantolol	T44.7X1	T44.7X2	T44.7X3	T44.7X4	T44.7X5	T44.7X6
Bevonium metilsulfate	T44.3X1	T44.3X2	T44.3X3	T44.3X4	T44.3X5	T44.3X6
Bezafibrate	T46.6X1	T46.6X2	T46.6X3	T46.6X4	T46.6X5	T46.6X6
Bezitramide	T4Ø.491	T4Ø.492	T4Ø.493	T4Ø.494	T4Ø.495	T4Ø.496
BHA	T5Ø.991	T5Ø.992	T5Ø.993	T5Ø.994	T5Ø.995	T5Ø.996
Bhang	T4Ø.711	T4Ø.712	T4Ø.713	T4Ø.714	T4Ø.715	T4Ø.716
BHC (medicinal)	T49.ØX1	T49.ØX2	T49.ØX3	T49.ØX4	T49.ØX5	T49.ØX6
nonmedicinal (vapor)	T53.6X1	T53.6X2	T53.6X3	T53.6X4	—	—
Bialamicol	T37.3X1	T37.3X2	T37.3X3	T37.3X4	T37.3X5	T37.3X6
Bibenzonium bromide	T48.3X1	T48.3X2	T48.3X3	T48.3X4	T48.3X5	T48.3X6
Bibrocathol	T49.5X1	T49.5X2	T49.5X3	T49.5X4	T49.5X5	T49.5X6
Bichloride of mercury — *see* Mercury, chloride						
Bichromates (calcium) (potassium)(sodium) (crystals)	T57.8X1	T57.8X2	T57.8X3	T57.8X4	—	—
fumes	T56.2X1	T56.2X2	T56.2X3	T56.2X4	—	—
Biclotymol	T49.6X1	T49.6X2	T49.6X3	T49.6X4	T49.6X5	T49.6X6
BiCNU*	T45.1X1	T45.1X2	T45.1X3	T45.1X4	T45.1X5	T45.1X6
Bicucculine	T5Ø.7X1	T5Ø.7X2	T5Ø.7X3	T5Ø.7X4	T5Ø.7X5	T5Ø.7X6
Bifemelane	T43.291	T43.292	T43.293	T43.294	T43.295	T43.296
Biguanide derivatives, oral	T38.3X1	T38.3X2	T38.3X3	T38.3X4	T38.3X5	T38.3X6
Bile salts	T47.5X1	T47.5X2	T47.5X3	T47.5X4	T47.5X5	T47.5X6
Biligrafin	T5Ø.8X1	T5Ø.8X2	T5Ø.8X3	T5Ø.8X4	T5Ø.8X5	T5Ø.8X6
Bilopaque	T5Ø.8X1	T5Ø.8X2	T5Ø.8X3	T5Ø.8X4	T5Ø.8X5	T5Ø.8X6
Binifibrate	T46.6X1	T46.6X2	T46.6X3	T46.6X4	T46.6X5	T46.6X6
Binitrobenzol	T65.3X1	T65.3X2	T65.3X3	T65.3X4	—	—
Bioflavonoid(s)	T46.991	T46.992	T46.993	T46.994	T46.995	T46.996
Biological substance NEC	T5Ø.9Ø1	T5Ø.9Ø2	T5Ø.9Ø3	T5Ø.9Ø4	T5Ø.9Ø5	T5Ø.9Ø6
Biotin	T45.2X1	T45.2X2	T45.2X3	T45.2X4	T45.2X5	T45.2X6
Biperiden	T44.3X1	T44.3X2	T44.3X3	T44.3X4	T44.3X5	T44.3X6
Bisacodyl	T47.2X1	T47.2X2	T47.2X3	T47.2X4	T47.2X5	T47.2X6
Bisbentiamine	T45.2X1	T45.2X2	T45.2X3	T45.2X4	T45.2X5	T45.2X6
Bisbutiamine	T45.2X1	T45.2X2	T45.2X3	T45.2X4	T45.2X5	T45.2X6
Bisdequalinium (salts) (diacetate)	T49.6X1	T49.6X2	T49.6X3	T49.6X4	T49.6X5	T49.6X6
Bishydroxycoumarin	T45.511	T45.512	T45.513	T45.514	T45.515	T45.516
Bismarsen	T37.8X1	T37.8X2	T37.8X3	T37.8X4	T37.8X5	T37.8X6
Bismuth salts	T47.6X1	T47.6X2	T47.6X3	T47.6X4	T47.6X5	T47.6X6
aluminate	T47.1X1	T47.1X2	T47.1X3	T47.1X4	T47.1X5	T47.1X6
anti-infectives	T37.8X1	T37.8X2	T37.8X3	T37.8X4	T37.8X5	T37.8X6
formic iodide	T49.ØX1	T49.ØX2	T49.ØX3	T49.ØX4	T49.ØX5	T49.ØX6
glycolylarsenate	T49.ØX1	T49.ØX2	T49.ØX3	T49.ØX4	T49.ØX5	T49.ØX6
nonmedicinal (compounds) NEC	T65.91	T65.92	T65.93	T65.94	—	—
subcarbonate	T47.6X1	T47.6X2	T47.6X3	T47.6X4	T47.6X5	T47.6X6
subsalicylate	T37.8X1	T37.8X2	T37.8X3	T37.8X4	T37.8X5	T37.8X6
sulfarsphenamine	T37.8X1	T37.8X2	T37.8X3	T37.8X4	T37.8X5	T37.8X6
Bisoprolol	T44.7X1	T44.7X2	T44.7X3	T44.7X4	T44.7X5	T44.7X6
Bisoxatin	T47.2X1	T47.2X2	T47.2X3	T47.2X4	T47.2X5	T47.2X6
Bisulepin (hydrochloride)	T45.ØX1	T45.ØX2	T45.ØX3	T45.ØX4	T45.ØX5	T45.ØX6

*Optum Value-Add

Substance	Poisoning, Accidental (unintentional)	Poisoning, Intentional Self-harm	Poisoning, Assault	Poisoning, Undetermined	Adverse Effect	Under-dosing
Bithionol	T37.8X1	T37.8X2	T37.8X3	T37.8X4	T37.8X5	T37.8X6
anthelminthic	T37.4X1	T37.4X2	T37.4X3	T37.4X4	T37.4X5	T37.4X6
Bitolterol	T48.6X1	T48.6X2	T48.6X3	T48.6X4	T48.6X5	T48.6X6
Bitoscanate	T37.4X1	T37.4X2	T37.4X3	T37.4X4	T37.4X5	T37.4X6
Bitter almond oil	T62.8X1	T62.8X2	T62.8X3	T62.8X4	—	—
Bittersweet	T62.2X1	T62.2X2	T62.2X3	T62.2X4	—	—
Bivalirudin*	T45.511	T45.512	T45.513	T45.514	T45.515	T45.516
Black						
flag	T6Ø.91	T6Ø.92	T6Ø.93	T6Ø.94	—	—
henbane	T62.2X1	T62.2X2	T62.2X3	T62.2X4	—	—
leaf (40)	T6Ø.91	T6Ø.92	T6Ø.93	T6Ø.94	—	—
widow spider (bite)	T63.311	T63.312	T63.313	T63.314	—	—
antivenin	T5Ø.Z11	T5Ø.Z12	T5Ø.Z13	T5Ø.Z14	T5Ø.Z15	T5Ø.Z16
Blast furnace gas (carbon monoxide from)	T58.8X1	T58.8X2	T58.8X3	T58.8X4	—	—
Bleach	T54.91	T54.92	T54.93	T54.94	—	—
Bleaching agent (medicinal)	T49.4X1	T49.4X2	T49.4X3	T49.4X4	T49.4X5	T49.4X6
Bleomycin	T45.1X1	T45.1X2	T45.1X3	T45.1X4	T45.1X5	T45.1X6
Blockain	T41.3X1	T41.3X2	T41.3X3	T41.3X4	T41.3X5	T41.3X6
infiltration (subcutaneous)	T41.3X1	T41.3X2	T41.3X3	T41.3X4	T41.3X5	T41.3X6
nerve block (peripheral) (plexus)	T41.3X1	T41.3X2	T41.3X3	T41.3X4	T41.3X5	T41.3X6
topical (surface)	T41.3X1	T41.3X2	T41.3X3	T41.3X4	T41.3X5	T41.3X6
Blockers, calcium channel	T46.1X1	T46.1X2	T46.1X3	T46.1X4	T46.1X5	T46.1X6
Blood (derivatives) (natural) (plasma) (whole)	T45.8X1	T45.8X2	T45.8X3	T45.8X4	T45.8X5	T45.8X6
dried	T45.8X1	T45.8X2	T45.8X3	T45.8X4	T45.8X5	T45.8X6
drug affecting NEC	T45.91	T45.92	T45.93	T45.94	T45.95	T45.96
expander NEC	T45.8X1	T45.8X2	T45.8X3	T45.8X4	T45.8X5	T45.8X6
fraction NEC	T45.8X1	T45.8X2	T45.8X3	T45.8X4	T45.8X5	T45.8X6
substitute (macromolecular)	T45.8X1	T45.8X2	T45.8X3	T45.8X4	T45.8X5	T45.8X6
Blue velvet	T4Ø.2X1	T4Ø.2X2	T4Ø.2X3	T4Ø.2X4	—	—
Bone meal	T62.8X1	T62.8X2	T62.8X3	T62.8X4	—	—
Bonine	T45.ØX1	T45.ØX2	T45.ØX3	T45.ØX4	T45.ØX5	T45.ØX6
Bontril*	T5Ø.5X1	T5Ø.5X2	T5Ø.5X3	T5Ø.5X4	T5Ø.5X5	T5Ø.5X6
Bopindolol	T44.7X1	T44.7X2	T44.7X3	T44.7X4	T44.7X5	T44.7X6
Boracic acid	T49.ØX1	T49.ØX2	T49.ØX3	T49.ØX4	T49.ØX5	T49.ØX6
ENT agent	T49.6X1	T49.6X2	T49.6X3	T49.6X4	T49.6X5	T49.6X6
ophthalmic preparation	T49.5X1	T49.5X2	T49.5X3	T49.5X4	T49.5X5	T49.5X6
Borane complex	T57.8X1	T57.8X2	T57.8X3	T57.8X4	—	—
Borate(s)	T57.8X1	T57.8X2	T57.8X3	T57.8X4	—	—
buffer	T5Ø.991	T5Ø.992	T5Ø.993	T5Ø.994	T5Ø.995	T5Ø.996
cleanser	T54.91	T54.92	T54.93	T54.94	—	—
sodium	T57.8X1	T57.8X2	T57.8X3	T57.8X4	—	—
Borax (cleanser)	T54.91	T54.92	T54.93	T54.94	—	—
Bordeaux mixture	T6Ø.3X1	T6Ø.3X2	T6Ø.3X3	T6Ø.3X4	—	—
Boric acid	T49.ØX1	T49.ØX2	T49.ØX3	T49.ØX4	T49.ØX5	T49.ØX6
ENT agent	T49.6X1	T49.6X2	T49.6X3	T49.6X4	T49.6X5	T49.6X6
ophthalmic preparation	T49.5X1	T49.5X2	T49.5X3	T49.5X4	T49.5X5	T49.5X6
Bornaprine	T44.3X1	T44.3X2	T44.3X3	T44.3X4	T44.3X5	T44.3X6
Boron	T57.8X1	T57.8X2	T57.8X3	T57.8X4	—	—
hydride NEC	T57.8X1	T57.8X2	T57.8X3	T57.8X4	—	—
fumes or gas	T57.8X1	T57.8X2	T57.8X3	T57.8X4	—	—
trifluoride	T59.891	T59.892	T59.893	T59.894	—	—
Botox	T48.291	T48.292	T48.293	T48.294	T48.295	T48.296
Botulinus anti-toxin (type A, B)	T5Ø.Z11	T5Ø.Z12	T5Ø.Z13	T5Ø.Z14	T5Ø.Z15	T5Ø.Z16
Brake fluid vapor	T59.891	T59.892	T59.893	T59.894	—	—
Brallobarbital	T42.3X1	T42.3X2	T42.3X3	T42.3X4	T42.3X5	T42.3X6
Bran (wheat)	T47.4X1	T47.4X2	T47.4X3	T47.4X4	T47.4X5	T47.4X6
Brass (fumes)	T56.891	T56.892	T56.893	T56.894	—	—
Brasso	T52.ØX1	T52.ØX2	T52.ØX3	T52.ØX4	—	—
Bretylium tosilate	T46.2X1	T46.2X2	T46.2X3	T46.2X4	T46.2X5	T46.2X6
Brevital (sodium)	T41.1X1	T41.1X2	T41.1X3	T41.1X4	T41.1X5	T41.1X6
Brinase	T45.3X1	T45.3X2	T45.3X3	T45.3X4	T45.3X5	T45.3X6
British antilewisite	T45.8X1	T45.8X2	T45.8X3	T45.8X4	T45.8X5	T45.8X6
Brodalumab*	T5Ø.991	T5Ø.992	T5Ø.993	T5Ø.994	T5Ø.995	T5Ø.996
Brodifacoum	T6Ø.4X1	T6Ø.4X2	T6Ø.4X3	T6Ø.4X4	—	—
Bromal (hydrate)	T42.6X1	T42.6X2	T42.6X3	T42.6X4	T42.6X5	T42.6X6
Bromazepam	T42.4X1	T42.4X2	T42.4X3	T42.4X4	T42.4X5	T42.4X6
Bromazine	T45.ØX1	T45.ØX2	T45.ØX3	T45.ØX4	T45.ØX5	T45.ØX6
Brombenzylcyanide	T59.3X1	T59.3X2	T59.3X3	T59.3X4	—	—
Bromelains	T45.3X1	T45.3X2	T45.3X3	T45.3X4	T45.3X5	T45.3X6
Bromethalin	T6Ø.4X1	T6Ø.4X2	T6Ø.4X3	T6Ø.4X4	—	—
Bromhexine	T48.4X1	T48.4X2	T48.4X3	T48.4X4	T48.4X5	T48.4X6
Bromide salts	T42.6X1	T42.6X2	T42.6X3	T42.6X4	T42.6X5	T42.6X6
Bromindione	T45.511	T45.512	T45.513	T45.514	T45.515	T45.516
Bromine						
compounds (medicinal)	T42.6X1	T42.6X2	T42.6X3	T42.6X4	T42.6X5	T42.6X6
sedative	T42.6X1	T42.6X2	T42.6X3	T42.6X4	T42.6X5	T42.6X6
vapor	T59.891	T59.892	T59.893	T59.894	—	—

Substance	Poisoning, Accidental (unintentional)	Poisoning, Intentional Self-harm	Poisoning, Assault	Poisoning, Undetermined	Adverse Effect	Under-dosing
Bromisoval	T42.6X1	T42.6X2	T42.6X3	T42.6X4	T42.6X5	T42.6X6
Bromisovalum	T42.6X1	T42.6X2	T42.6X3	T42.6X4	T42.6X5	T42.6X6
Bromobenzylcyanide	T59.3X1	T59.3X2	T59.3X3	T59.3X4	—	—
Bromochlorosalicylani-lide	T49.ØX1	T49.ØX2	T49.ØX3	T49.ØX4	T49.ØX5	T49.ØX6
Bromocriptine	T42.8X1	T42.8X2	T42.8X3	T42.8X4	T42.8X5	T42.8X6
Bromodiphenhydramine	T45.ØX1	T45.ØX2	T45.ØX3	T45.ØX4	T45.ØX5	T45.ØX6
Bromoform	T42.6X1	T42.6X2	T42.6X3	T42.6X4	T42.6X5	T42.6X6
Bromophenol blue reagent	T5Ø.991	T5Ø.992	T5Ø.993	T5Ø.994	T5Ø.995	T5Ø.996
Bromopride	T47.8X1	T47.8X2	T47.8X3	T47.8X4	T47.8X5	T47.8X6
Bromosalicylchloranitide	T49.ØX1	T49.ØX2	T49.ØX3	T49.ØX4	T49.ØX5	T49.ØX6
Bromosalicylhydroxamic acid	T37.1X1	T37.1X2	T37.1X3	T37.1X4	T37.1X5	T37.1X6
Bromo-seltzer	T39.1X1	T39.1X2	T39.1X3	T39.1X4	T39.1X5	T39.1X6
Bromoxynil	T6Ø.3X1	T6Ø.3X2	T6Ø.3X3	T6Ø.3X4	—	—
Bromperidol	T43.4X1	T43.4X2	T43.4X3	T43.4X4	T43.4X5	T43.4X6
Brompheniramine	T45.ØX1	T45.ØX2	T45.ØX3	T45.ØX4	T45.ØX5	T45.ØX6
Bromsulfophthalein	T5Ø.8X1	T5Ø.8X2	T5Ø.8X3	T5Ø.8X4	T5Ø.8X5	T5Ø.8X6
Bromural	T42.6X1	T42.6X2	T42.6X3	T42.6X4	T42.6X5	T42.6X6
Bromvaletone	T42.6X1	T42.6X2	T42.6X3	T42.6X4	T42.6X5	T42.6X6
Bronchodilator NEC	T48.6X1	T48.6X2	T48.6X3	T48.6X4	T48.6X5	T48.6X6
Brotizolam	T42.4X1	T42.4X2	T42.4X3	T42.4X4	T42.4X5	T42.4X6
Brovincamine	T46.7X1	T46.7X2	T46.7X3	T46.7X4	T46.7X5	T46.7X6
Brown recluse spider (bite) (venom)	T63.331	T63.332	T63.333	T63.334	—	—
Brown spider (bite) (venom)	T63.391	T63.392	T63.393	T63.394	—	—
Broxaterol	T48.6X1	T48.6X2	T48.6X3	T48.6X4	T48.6X5	T48.6X6
Broxuridine	T45.1X1	T45.1X2	T45.1X3	T45.1X4	T45.1X5	T45.1X6
Broxyquinoline	T37.8X1	T37.8X2	T37.8X3	T37.8X4	T37.8X5	T37.8X6
Bruceine	T48.291	T48.292	T48.293	T48.294	T48.295	T48.296
Brucia	T62.2X1	T62.2X2	T62.2X3	T62.2X4	—	—
Brucine	T65.1X1	T65.1X2	T65.1X3	T65.1X4	—	—
Brunswick green — *see* Copper						
Bruten — *see* Ibuprofen						
Bryonia	T47.2X1	T47.2X2	T47.2X3	T47.2X4	T47.2X5	T47.2X6
Buclizine	T45.ØX1	T45.ØX2	T45.ØX3	T45.ØX4	T45.ØX5	T45.ØX6
Buclosamide	T49.ØX1	T49.ØX2	T49.ØX3	T49.ØX4	T49.ØX5	T49.ØX6
Budesonide	T44.5X1	T44.5X2	T44.5X3	T44.5X4	T44.5X5	T44.5X6
Budralazine	T46.5X1	T46.5X2	T46.5X3	T46.5X4	T46.5X5	T46.5X6
Bufferin	T39.Ø11	T39.Ø12	T39.Ø13	T39.Ø14	T39.Ø15	T39.Ø16
Buflomedil	T46.7X1	T46.7X2	T46.7X3	T46.7X4	T46.7X5	T46.7X6
Buformin	T38.3X1	T38.3X2	T38.3X3	T38.3X4	T38.3X5	T38.3X6
Bufotenine	T4Ø.991	T4Ø.992	T4Ø.993	T4Ø.994	—	—
Bufrolin	T48.6X1	T48.6X2	T48.6X3	T48.6X4	T48.6X5	T48.6X6
Bufylline	T48.6X1	T48.6X2	T48.6X3	T48.6X4	T48.6X5	T48.6X6
Bulgaricum IB*	T47.6X1	T47.6X2	T47.6X3	T47.6X4	T47.6X5	T47.6X6
Bulk filler	T5Ø.5X1	T5Ø.5X2	T5Ø.5X3	T5Ø.5X4	T5Ø.5X5	T5Ø.5X6
cathartic	T47.4X1	T47.4X2	T47.4X3	T47.4X4	T47.4X5	T47.4X6
Bumetanide	T5Ø.1X1	T5Ø.1X2	T5Ø.1X3	T5Ø.1X4	T5Ø.1X5	T5Ø.1X6
Bunaftine	T46.2X1	T46.2X2	T46.2X3	T46.2X4	T46.2X5	T46.2X6
Bunamiodyl	T5Ø.8X1	T5Ø.8X2	T5Ø.8X3	T5Ø.8X4	T5Ø.8X5	T5Ø.8X6
Bunazosin	T44.6X1	T44.6X2	T44.6X3	T44.6X4	T44.6X5	T44.6X6
Bunitrolol	T44.7X1	T44.7X2	T44.7X3	T44.7X4	T44.7X5	T44.7X6
Buphenine	T46.7X1	T46.7X2	T46.7X3	T46.7X4	T46.7X5	T46.7X6
Bupivacaine	T41.3X1	T41.3X2	T41.3X3	T41.3X4	T41.3X5	T41.3X6
infiltration (subcutaneous)	T41.3X1	T41.3X2	T41.3X3	T41.3X4	T41.3X5	T41.3X6
nerve block (peripheral) (plexus)	T41.3X1	T41.3X2	T41.3X3	T41.3X4	T41.3X5	T41.3X6
spinal	T41.3X1	T41.3X2	T41.3X3	T41.3X4	T41.3X5	T41.3X6
Bupranolol	T44.7X1	T44.7X2	T44.7X3	T44.7X4	T44.7X5	T44.7X6
Buprenorphine	T4Ø.491	T4Ø.492	T4Ø.493	T4Ø.494	T4Ø.495	T4Ø.496
Bupropion	T43.291	T43.292	T43.293	T43.294	T43.295	T43.296
Burimamide	T47.1X1	T47.1X2	T47.1X3	T47.1X4	T47.1X5	T47.1X6
Buserelin	T38.891	T38.892	T38.893	T38.894	T38.895	T38.896
Buspirone	T43.591	T43.592	T43.593	T43.594	T43.595	T43.596
Busulfan, busulphan	T45.1X1	T45.1X2	T45.1X3	T45.1X4	T45.1X5	T45.1X6
Busulfex*	T45.1X1	T45.1X2	T45.1X3	T45.1X4	T45.1X5	T45.1X6
Butabarbital (sodium)	T42.3X1	T42.3X2	T42.3X3	T42.3X4	T42.3X5	T42.3X6
Butabarbitone	T42.3X1	T42.3X2	T42.3X3	T42.3X4	T42.3X5	T42.3X6
Butabarpal	T42.3X1	T42.3X2	T42.3X3	T42.3X4	T42.3X5	T42.3X6
Butacaine	T41.3X1	T41.3X2	T41.3X3	T41.3X4	T41.3X5	T41.3X6
Butalamine	T46.7X1	T46.7X2	T46.7X3	T46.7X4	T46.7X5	T46.7X6
Butalbital	T42.3X1	T42.3X2	T42.3X3	T42.3X4	T42.3X5	T42.3X6
Butallylonal	T42.3X1	T42.3X2	T42.3X3	T42.3X4	T42.3X5	T42.3X6
Butamben	T41.3X1	T41.3X2	T41.3X3	T41.3X4	T41.3X5	T41.3X6
Butamirate	T48.3X1	T48.3X2	T48.3X3	T48.3X4	T48.3X5	T48.3X6
Butane (distributed in mobile container)	T59.891	T59.892	T59.893	T59.894	—	—
distributed through pipes	T59.891	T59.892	T59.893	T59.894	—	—
incomplete combustion	T58.11	T58.12	T58.13	T58.14	—	—
Butanilicaine	T41.3X1	T41.3X2	T41.3X3	T41.3X4	T41.3X5	T41.3X6
Butanol	T51.3X1	T51.3X2	T51.3X3	T51.3X4	—	—

Substance	Poisoning, Accidental (unintentional)	Poisoning, Intentional Self-harm	Poisoning, Assault	Poisoning, Undetermined	Adverse Effect	Under-dosing
Butanone, 2-butanone	T52.4X1	T52.4X2	T52.4X3	T52.4X4	—	—
Butantrone	T49.4X1	T49.4X2	T49.4X3	T49.4X4	T49.4X5	T49.4X6
Butaperazine	T43.3X1	T43.3X2	T43.3X3	T43.3X4	T43.3X5	T43.3X6
Butazolidin	T39.2X1	T39.2X2	T39.2X3	T39.2X4	T39.2X5	T39.2X6
Butetamate	T48.6X1	T48.6X2	T48.6X3	T48.6X4	T48.6X5	T48.6X6
Butethal	T42.3X1	T42.3X2	T42.3X3	T42.3X4	T42.3X5	T42.3X6
Butethamate	T44.3X1	T44.3X2	T44.3X3	T44.3X4	T44.3X5	T44.3X6
Buthalitone (sodium)	T41.1X1	T41.1X2	T41.1X3	T41.1X4	T41.1X5	T41.1X6
Butisol (sodium)	T42.3X1	T42.3X2	T42.3X3	T42.3X4	T42.3X5	T42.3X6
Butizide	T50.2X1	T50.2X2	T50.2X3	T50.2X4	T50.2X5	T50.2X6
Butobarbital	T42.3X1	T42.3X2	T42.3X3	T42.3X4	T42.3X5	T42.3X6
sodium	T42.3X1	T42.3X2	T42.3X3	T42.3X4	T42.3X5	T42.3X6
Butobarbitone	T42.3X1	T42.3X2	T42.3X3	T42.3X4	T42.3X5	T42.3X6
Butoconazole (nitrate)	T49.0X1	T49.0X2	T49.0X3	T49.0X4	T49.0X5	T49.0X6
Butorphanol	T40.491	T40.492	T40.493	T40.494	T40.495	T40.496
Butriptyline	T43.011	T43.012	T43.013	T43.014	T43.015	T43.016
Butropium bromide	T44.3X1	T44.3X2	T44.3X3	T44.3X4	T44.3X5	T44.3X6
Buttercups	T62.2X1	T62.2X2	T62.2X3	T62.2X4	—	—
Butter of antimony — *see* Antimony						
Butyl						
acetate (secondary)	T52.8X1	T52.8X2	T52.8X3	T52.8X4	—	—
alcohol	T51.3X1	T51.3X2	T51.3X3	T51.3X4	—	—
aminobenzoate	T41.3X1	T41.3X2	T41.3X3	T41.3X4	T41.3X5	T41.3X6
butyrate	T52.8X1	T52.8X2	T52.8X3	T52.8X4	—	—
carbinol	T51.3X1	T51.3X2	T51.3X3	T51.3X4	—	—
carbitol	T52.3X1	T52.3X2	T52.3X3	T52.3X4	—	—
cellosolve	T52.3X1	T52.3X2	T52.3X3	T52.3X4	—	—
chloral (hydrate)	T42.6X1	T42.6X2	T42.6X3	T42.6X4	T42.6X5	T42.6X6
formate	T52.8X1	T52.8X2	T52.8X3	T52.8X4	—	—
lactate	T52.8X1	T52.8X2	T52.8X3	T52.8X4	—	—
propionate	T52.8X1	T52.8X2	T52.8X3	T52.8X4	—	—
scopolamine bromide	T44.3X1	T44.3X2	T44.3X3	T44.3X4	T44.3X5	T44.3X6
thiobarbital sodium	T41.1X1	T41.1X2	T41.1X3	T41.1X4	T41.1X5	T41.1X6
Butylated hydroxyanisole	T50.991	T50.992	T50.993	T50.994	T50.995	T50.996
Butylchloral hydrate	T42.6X1	T42.6X2	T42.6X3	T42.6X4	T42.6X5	T42.6X6
Butyltoluene	T52.2X1	T52.2X2	T52.2X3	T52.2X4	—	—
Butyn	T41.3X1	T41.3X2	T41.3X3	T41.3X4	T41.3X5	T41.3X6
Butyrophenone (-based tranquilizers)	T43.4X1	T43.4X2	T43.4X3	T43.4X4	T43.4X5	T43.4X6
Cabazitaxel*	T45.1X1	T45.1X2	T45.1X3	T45.1X4	T45.1X5	T45.1X6
Cabergoline	T42.8X1	T42.8X2	T42.8X3	T42.8X4	T42.8X5	T42.8X6
Cacodyl, cacodylic acid	T57.0X1	T57.0X2	T57.0X3	T57.0X4	—	—
Cactinomycin	T45.1X1	T45.1X2	T45.1X3	T45.1X4	T45.1X5	T45.1X6
Cade oil	T49.4X1	T49.4X2	T49.4X3	T49.4X4	T49.4X5	T49.4X6
Cadexomer iodine	T49.0X1	T49.0X2	T49.0X3	T49.0X4	T49.0X5	T49.0X6
Cadmium (chloride) (fumes) (oxide)	T56.3X1	T56.3X2	T56.3X3	T56.3X4	—	—
sulfide (medicinal) NEC	T49.4X1	T49.4X2	T49.4X3	T49.4X4	T49.4X5	T49.4X6
Cadralazine	T46.5X1	T46.5X2	T46.5X3	T46.5X4	T46.5X5	T46.5X6
Caffeine	T43.611	T43.612	T43.613	T43.614	T43.615	T43.616
Calabar bean	T62.2X1	T62.2X2	T62.2X3	T62.2X4	—	—
Caladium seguinum	T62.2X1	T62.2X2	T62.2X3	T62.2X4	—	—
Calamine (lotion)	T49.3X1	T49.3X2	T49.3X3	T49.3X4	T49.3X5	T49.3X6
Calcifediol	T45.2X1	T45.2X2	T45.2X3	T45.2X4	T45.2X5	T45.2X6
Calciferol	T45.2X1	T45.2X2	T45.2X3	T45.2X4	T45.2X5	T45.2X6
Calcijex*	T45.2X1	T45.2X2	T45.2X3	T45.2X4	T45.2X5	T45.2X6
Calcitonin	T50.991	T50.992	T50.993	T50.994	T50.995	T50.996
Calcitriol	T45.2X1	T45.2X2	T45.2X3	T45.2X4	T45.2X5	T45.2X6
Calcium	T50.3X1	T50.3X2	T50.3X3	T50.3X4	T50.3X5	T50.3X6
actylsalicylate	T39.011	T39.012	T39.013	T39.014	T39.015	T39.016
benzamidosalicylate	T37.1X1	T37.1X2	T37.1X3	T37.1X4	T37.1X5	T37.1X6
bromide	T42.6X1	T42.6X2	T42.6X3	T42.6X4	T42.6X5	T42.6X6
bromolactobionate	T42.6X1	T42.6X2	T42.6X3	T42.6X4	T42.6X5	T42.6X6
carbaspirin	T39.011	T39.012	T39.013	T39.014	T39.015	T39.016
carbimide	T50.6X1	T50.6X2	T50.6X3	T50.6X4	T50.6X5	T50.6X6
carbonate	T47.1X1	T47.1X2	T47.1X3	T47.1X4	T47.1X5	T47.1X6
chloride	T50.991	T50.992	T50.993	T50.994	T50.995	T50.996
anhydrous	T50.991	T50.992	T50.993	T50.994	T50.995	T50.996
cyanide	T57.8X1	T57.8X2	T57.8X3	T57.8X4	—	—
dioctyl sulfosuccinate	T47.4X1	T47.4X2	T47.4X3	T47.4X4	T47.4X5	T47.4X6
disodium edathamil	T45.8X1	T45.8X2	T45.8X3	T45.8X4	T45.8X5	T45.8X6
disodium edetate	T45.8X1	T45.8X2	T45.8X3	T45.8X4	T45.8X5	T45.8X6
dobesilate	T46.991	T46.992	T46.993	T46.994	T46.995	T46.996
EDTA	T45.8X1	T45.8X2	T45.8X3	T45.8X4	T45.8X5	T45.8X6
ferrous citrate	T45.4X1	T45.4X2	T45.4X3	T45.4X4	T45.4X5	T45.4X6
folinate	T45.8X1	T45.8X2	T45.8X3	T45.8X4	T45.8X5	T45.8X6
glubionate	T50.3X1	T50.3X2	T50.3X3	T50.3X4	T50.3X5	T50.3X6
gluconate	T50.3X1	T50.3X2	T50.3X3	T50.3X4	T50.3X5	T50.3X6
gluconogalactogluconate	T50.3X1	T50.3X2	T50.3X3	T50.3X4	T50.3X5	T50.3X6
hydrate, hydroxide	T54.3X1	T54.3X2	T54.3X3	T54.3X4	—	—
hypochlorite	T54.3X1	T54.3X2	T54.3X3	T54.3X4	—	—
iodide	T48.4X1	T48.4X2	T48.4X3	T48.4X4	T48.4X5	T48.4X6

Substance	Poisoning, Accidental (unintentional)	Poisoning, Intentional Self-harm	Poisoning, Assault	Poisoning, Undetermined	Adverse Effect	Under-dosing
Calcium — *continued*						
ipodate	T50.8X1	T50.8X2	T50.8X3	T50.8X4	T50.8X5	T50.8X6
lactate	T50.3X1	T50.3X2	T50.3X3	T50.3X4	T50.3X5	T50.3X6
leucovorin	T45.8X1	T45.8X2	T45.8X3	T45.8X4	T45.8X5	T45.8X6
mandelate	T37.91	T37.92	T37.93	T37.94	T37.95	T37.96
oxide	T54.3X1	T54.3X2	T54.3X3	T54.3X4	—	—
pantothenate	T45.2X1	T45.2X2	T45.2X3	T45.2X4	T45.2X5	T45.2X6
phosphate	T50.3X1	T50.3X2	T50.3X3	T50.3X4	T50.3X5	T50.3X6
salicylate	T39.091	T39.092	T39.093	T39.094	T39.095	T39.096
salts	T50.3X1	T50.3X2	T50.3X3	T50.3X4	T50.3X5	T50.3X6
Calculus-dissolving drug	T50.991	T50.992	T50.993	T50.994	T50.995	T50.996
Calomel	T49.0X1	T49.0X2	T49.0X3	T49.0X4	T49.0X5	T49.0X6
Caloric agent	T50.3X1	T50.3X2	T50.3X3	T50.3X4	T50.3X5	T50.3X6
Calusterone	T38.7X1	T38.7X2	T38.7X3	T38.7X4	T38.7X5	T38.7X6
Camazepam	T42.4X1	T42.4X2	T42.4X3	T42.4X4	T42.4X5	T42.4X6
Camomile	T49.0X1	T49.0X2	T49.0X3	T49.0X4	T49.0X5	T49.0X6
Camoquin	T37.2X1	T37.2X2	T37.2X3	T37.2X4	T37.2X5	T37.2X6
Camphor						
insecticide	T60.2X1	T60.2X2	T60.2X3	T60.2X4	—	—
medicinal	T49.8X1	T49.8X2	T49.8X3	T49.8X4	T49.8X5	T49.8X6
Camylofin	T44.3X1	T44.3X2	T44.3X3	T44.3X4	T44.3X5	T44.3X6
Cancer chemotherapy drug regimen	T45.1X1	T45.1X2	T45.1X3	T45.1X4	T45.1X5	T45.1X6
Candeptin	T49.0X1	T49.0X2	T49.0X3	T49.0X4	T49.0X5	T49.0X6
Candicidin	T49.0X1	T49.0X2	T49.0X3	T49.0X4	T49.0X5	T49.0X6
Cankaid*	T49.6X1	T49.6X2	T49.6X3	T49.6X4	T49.6X5	T49.6X6
Cannabinoids, synthetic	T40.721	T40.722	T40.723	T40.724	T40.725	T40.726
Cannabinol	T40.711	T40.712	T40.713	T40.714	T40.715	T40.716
Cannabis (derivatives)	T40.711	T40.712	T40.713	T40.714	T40.715	T40.716
Canned heat	T51.1X1	T51.1X2	T51.1X3	T51.1X4	—	—
Canrenoic acid	T50.0X1	T50.0X2	T50.0X3	T50.0X4	T50.0X5	T50.0X6
Canrenone	T50.0X1	T50.0X2	T50.0X3	T50.0X4	T50.0X5	T50.0X6
Cantharides, cantharidin, cantharis	T49.8X1	T49.8X2	T49.8X3	T49.8X4	T49.8X5	T49.8X6
Canthaxanthin	T50.991	T50.992	T50.993	T50.994	T50.995	T50.996
Capillary-active drug NEC	T46.901	T46.902	T46.903	T46.904	T46.905	T46.906
Capreomycin	T36.8X1	T36.8X2	T36.8X3	T36.8X4	T36.8X5	T36.8X6
Capresla*	T45.1X1	T45.1X2	T45.1X3	T45.1X4	T45.1X5	T45.1X6
Capsicum	T49.4X1	T49.4X2	T49.4X3	T49.4X4	T49.4X5	T49.4X6
Captafol	T60.3X1	T60.3X2	T60.3X3	T60.3X4	—	—
Captan	T60.3X1	T60.3X2	T60.3X3	T60.3X4	—	—
Captodiame, captodiamine	T43.591	T43.592	T43.593	T43.594	T43.595	T43.596
Captopril	T46.4X1	T46.4X2	T46.4X3	T46.4X4	T46.4X5	T46.4X6
Caramiphen	T44.3X1	T44.3X2	T44.3X3	T44.3X4	T44.3X5	T44.3X6
Carazolol	T44.7X1	T44.7X2	T44.7X3	T44.7X4	T44.7X5	T44.7X6
Carbachol	T44.1X1	T44.1X2	T44.1X3	T44.1X4	T44.1X5	T44.1X6
Carbacrylamine (resin)	T50.3X1	T50.3X2	T50.3X3	T50.3X4	T50.3X5	T50.3X6
Carbamate (insecticide)	T60.0X1	T60.0X2	T60.0X3	T60.0X4	—	—
Carbamate (sedative)	T42.6X1	T42.6X2	T42.6X3	T42.6X4	T42.6X5	T42.6X6
herbicide	T60.0X1	T60.0X2	T60.0X3	T60.0X4	—	—
insecticide	T60.0X1	T60.0X2	T60.0X3	T60.0X4	—	—
Carbamazepine	T42.1X1	T42.1X2	T42.1X3	T42.1X4	T42.1X5	T42.1X6
Carbamide	T47.3X1	T47.3X2	T47.3X3	T47.3X4	T47.3X5	T47.3X6
peroxide	T49.0X1	T49.0X2	T49.0X3	T49.0X4	T49.0X5	T49.0X6
topical	T49.8X1	T49.8X2	T49.8X3	T49.8X4	T49.8X5	T49.8X6
Carbamylcholine chloride	T44.1X1	T44.1X2	T44.1X3	T44.1X4	T44.1X5	T44.1X6
Carbaril	T60.0X1	T60.0X2	T60.0X3	T60.0X4	—	—
Carbarsone	T37.3X1	T37.3X2	T37.3X3	T37.3X4	T37.3X5	T37.3X6
Carbaryl	T60.0X1	T60.0X2	T60.0X3	T60.0X4	—	—
Carbaspirin	T39.011	T39.012	T39.013	T39.014	T39.015	T39.016
Carbastat*	T49.5X1	T49.5X2	T49.5X3	T49.5X4	T49.5X5	T49.5X6
Carbazochrome (salicylate) (sodium sulfonate)	T49.4X1	T49.4X2	T49.4X3	T49.4X4	T49.4X5	T49.4X6
Carbenicillin	T36.0X1	T36.0X2	T36.0X3	T36.0X4	T36.0X5	T36.0X6
Carbenoxolone	T47.1X1	T47.1X2	T47.1X3	T47.1X4	T47.1X5	T47.1X6
Carbetapentane	T48.3X1	T48.3X2	T48.3X3	T48.3X4	T48.3X5	T48.3X6
Carbethyl salicylate	T39.091	T39.092	T39.093	T39.094	T39.095	T39.096
Carbidopa (with levodopa)	T42.8X1	T42.8X2	T42.8X3	T42.8X4	T42.8X5	T42.8X6
Carbimazole	T38.2X1	T38.2X2	T38.2X3	T38.2X4	T38.2X5	T38.2X6
Carbinol	T51.1X1	T51.1X2	T51.1X3	T51.1X4	—	—
Carbinoxamine	T45.0X1	T45.0X2	T45.0X3	T45.0X4	T45.0X5	T45.0X6
Carbiphene	T39.8X1	T39.8X2	T39.8X3	T39.8X4	T39.8X5	T39.8X6
Carbitol	T52.3X1	T52.3X2	T52.3X3	T52.3X4	—	—
Carbocaine	T41.3X1	T41.3X2	T41.3X3	T41.3X4	T41.3X5	T41.3X6
infiltration (subcutaneous)	T41.3X1	T41.3X2	T41.3X3	T41.3X4	T41.3X5	T41.3X6
nerve block (peripheral) (plexus)	T41.3X1	T41.3X2	T41.3X3	T41.3X4	T41.3X5	T41.3X6
topical (surface)	T41.3X1	T41.3X2	T41.3X3	T41.3X4	T41.3X5	T41.3X6
Carbocisteine	T48.4X1	T48.4X2	T48.4X3	T48.4X4	T48.4X5	T48.4X6
Carbocromen	T46.3X1	T46.3X2	T46.3X3	T46.3X4	T46.3X5	T46.3X6
Carbol fuchsin	T49.0X1	T49.0X2	T49.0X3	T49.0X4	T49.0X5	T49.0X6

Substance	Poisoning, Accidental (unintentional)	Poisoning, Intentional Self-harm	Poisoning, Assault	Poisoning, Undetermined	Adverse Effect	Under-dosing
Carbolic acid — *see also* Phenol	T54.ØX1	T54.ØX2	T54.ØX3	T54.ØX4	—	—
Carbolonium (bromide)	T48.1X1	T48.1X2	T48.1X3	T48.1X4	T48.1X5	T48.1X6
Carbo medicinalis	T47.6X1	T47.6X2	T47.6X3	T47.6X4	T47.6X5	T47.6X6
Carbomycin	T36.8X1	T36.8X2	T36.8X3	T36.8X4	T36.8X5	T36.8X6
Carbon						
bisulfide (liquid)	T65.4X1	T65.4X2	T65.4X3	T65.4X4	—	—
vapor	T65.4X1	T65.4X2	T65.4X3	T65.4X4	—	—
dioxide (gas)	T59.7X1	T59.7X2	T59.7X3	T59.7X4	—	—
medicinal	T41.5X1	T41.5X2	T41.5X3	T41.5X4	T41.5X5	T41.5X6
nonmedicinal	T59.7X1	T59.7X2	T59.7X3	T59.7X4	—	—
snow	T49.4X1	T49.4X2	T49.4X3	T49.4X4	T49.4X5	T49.4X6
disulfide (liquid)	T65.4X1	T65.4X2	T65.4X3	T65.4X4	—	—
vapor	T65.4X1	T65.4X2	T65.4X3	T65.4X4	—	—
monoxide (from incomplete combustion)	T58.91	T58.92	T58.93	T58.94	—	—
blast furnace gas	T58.8X1	T58.8X2	T58.8X3	T58.8X4	—	—
butane (distributed in mobile container)	T58.11	T58.12	T58.13	T58.14	—	—
distributed through pipes	T58.11	T58.12	T58.13	T58.14	—	—
charcoal fumes	T58.2X1	T58.2X2	T58.2X3	T58.2X4	—	—
coal	T58.2X1	T58.2X2	T58.2X3	T58.2X4	—	—
coke (in domestic stoves, fireplaces)	T58.2X1	T58.2X2	T58.2X3	T58.2X4	—	—
exhaust gas (motor) not in transit	T58.Ø1	T58.Ø2	T58.Ø3	T58.Ø4	—	—
combustion engine, any not in watercraft	T58.Ø1	T58.Ø2	T58.Ø3	T58.Ø4	—	—
farm tractor, not in transit	T58.Ø1	T58.Ø2	T58.Ø3	T58.Ø4	—	—
gas engine	T58.Ø1	T58.Ø2	T58.Ø3	T58.Ø4	—	—
motor pump	T58.Ø1	T58.Ø2	T58.Ø3	T58.Ø4	—	—
motor vehicle, not in transit	T58.Ø1	T58.Ø2	T58.Ø3	T58.Ø4	—	—
fuel (in domestic use)	T58.2X1	T58.2X2	T58.2X3	T58.2X4	—	—
gas (piped)	T58.11	T58.12	T58.13	T58.14	—	—
in mobile container	T58.11	T58.12	T58.13	T58.14	—	—
piped (natural)	T58.11	T58.12	T58.13	T58.14	—	—
utility	T58.11	T58.12	T58.13	T58.14	—	—
in mobile container	T58.11	T58.12	T58.13	T58.14	—	—
gas (piped)	T58.11	T58.12	T58.13	T58.14	—	—
illuminating gas	T58.11	T58.12	T58.13	T58.14	—	—
industrial fuels or gases, any	T58.8X1	T58.8X2	T58.8X3	T58.8X4	—	—
kerosene (in domestic stoves, fireplaces)	T58.2X1	T58.2X2	T58.2X3	T58.2X4	—	—
kiln gas or vapor	T58.8X1	T58.8X2	T58.8X3	T58.8X4	—	—
motor exhaust gas, not in transit	T58.Ø1	T58.Ø2	T58.Ø3	T58.Ø4	—	—
piped gas (manufactured) (natural)	T58.11	T58.12	T58.13	T58.14	—	—
producer gas	T58.8X1	T58.8X2	T58.8X3	T58.8X4	—	—
propane (distributed in mobile container)	T58.11	T58.12	T58.13	T58.14	—	—
distributed through pipes	T58.11	T58.12	T58.13	T58.14	—	—
solid (in domestic stoves, fireplaces)	T58.2X1	T58.2X2	T58.2X3	T58.2X4	—	—
specified source NEC	T58.8X1	T58.8X2	T58.8X3	T58.8X4	—	—
stove gas	T58.11	T58.12	T58.13	T58.14	—	—
piped	T58.11	T58.12	T58.13	T58.14	—	—
utility gas	T58.11	T58.12	T58.13	T58.14	—	—
piped	T58.11	T58.12	T58.13	T58.14	—	—
water gas	T58.11	T58.12	T58.13	T58.14	—	—
wood (in domestic stoves, fireplaces)	T58.2X1	T58.2X2	T58.2X3	T58.2X4	—	—
tetrachloride (vapor) NEC	T53.ØX1	T53.ØX2	T53.ØX3	T53.ØX4	—	—
liquid (cleansing agent) NEC	T53.ØX1	T53.ØX2	T53.ØX3	T53.ØX4	—	—
solvent	T53.ØX1	T53.ØX2	T53.ØX3	T53.ØX4	—	—
Carbonic acid gas	T59.7X1	T59.7X2	T59.7X3	T59.7X4	—	—
anhydrase inhibitor NEC	T5Ø.2X1	T5Ø.2X2	T5Ø.2X3	T5Ø.2X4	T5Ø.2X5	T5Ø.2X6
Carbophenothion	T6Ø.ØX1	T6Ø.ØX2	T6Ø.ØX3	T6Ø.ØX4	—	—
Carboplatin	T45.1X1	T45.1X2	T45.1X3	T45.1X4	T45.1X5	T45.1X6
Carboprost	T48.ØX1	T48.ØX2	T48.ØX3	T48.ØX4	T48.ØX5	T48.ØX6
Carboquone	T45.1X1	T45.1X2	T45.1X3	T45.1X4	T45.1X5	T45.1X6
Carbowax	T49.3X1	T49.3X2	T49.3X3	T49.3X4	T49.3X5	T49.3X6
Carboxymethylcellulose	T47.4X1	T47.4X2	T47.4X3	T47.4X4	T47.4X5	T47.4X6
Carbrital	T42.3X1	T42.3X2	T42.3X3	T42.3X4	T42.3X5	T42.3X6
Carbromal	T42.6X1	T42.6X2	T42.6X3	T42.6X4	T42.6X5	T42.6X6
Carbutamide	T38.3X1	T38.3X2	T38.3X3	T38.3X4	T38.3X5	T38.3X6
Carbuterol	T48.6X1	T48.6X2	T48.6X3	T48.6X4	T48.6X5	T48.6X6

Substance	Poisoning, Accidental (unintentional)	Poisoning, Intentional Self-harm	Poisoning, Assault	Poisoning, Undetermined	Adverse Effect	Under-dosing
Cardiac						
depressants	T46.2X1	T46.2X2	T46.2X3	T46.2X4	T46.2X5	T46.2X6
rhythm regulator	T46.2X1	T46.2X2	T46.2X3	T46.2X4	T46.2X5	T46.2X6
specified NEC	T46.2X1	T46.2X2	T46.2X3	T46.2X4	T46.2X5	T46.2X6
Cardiografin	T5Ø.8X1	T5Ø.8X2	T5Ø.8X3	T5Ø.8X4	T5Ø.8X5	T5Ø.8X6
Cardiogreen	T5Ø.8X1	T5Ø.8X2	T5Ø.8X3	T5Ø.8X4	T5Ø.8X5	T5Ø.8X6
Cardiotonic (glycoside) **NEC**	T46.ØX1	T46.ØX2	T46.ØX3	T46.ØX4	T46.ØX5	T46.ØX6
Cardiovascular drug NEC	T46.9Ø1	T46.9Ø2	T46.9Ø3	T46.9Ø4	T46.9Ø5	T46.9Ø6
Cardizem*	T46.1X1	T46.1X2	T46.1X3	T46.1X4	T46.1X5	T46.1X6
Cardrase	T5Ø.2X1	T5Ø.2X2	T5Ø.2X3	T5Ø.2X4	T5Ø.2X5	T5Ø.2X6
Carfecillin	T36.ØX1	T36.ØX2	T36.ØX3	T36.ØX4	T36.ØX5	T36.ØX6
Carfenazine	T43.3X1	T43.3X2	T43.3X3	T43.3X4	T43.3X5	T43.3X6
Carfusin	T49.ØX1	T49.ØX2	T49.ØX3	T49.ØX4	T49.ØX5	T49.ØX6
Carindacillin	T36.ØX1	T36.ØX2	T36.ØX3	T36.ØX4	T36.ØX5	T36.ØX6
Carisoprodol	T42.8X1	T42.8X2	T42.8X3	T42.8X4	T42.8X5	T42.8X6
Carmellose	T47.4X1	T47.4X2	T47.4X3	T47.4X4	T47.4X5	T47.4X6
Carminative	T47.5X1	T47.5X2	T47.5X3	T47.5X4	T47.5X5	T47.5X6
Carmofur	T45.1X1	T45.1X2	T45.1X3	T45.1X4	T45.1X5	T45.1X6
Carmustine	T45.1X1	T45.1X2	T45.1X3	T45.1X4	T45.1X5	T45.1X6
Carotene	T45.2X1	T45.2X2	T45.2X3	T45.2X4	T45.2X5	T45.2X6
Carphenazine	T43.3X1	T43.3X2	T43.3X3	T43.3X4	T43.3X5	T43.3X6
Carpipramine	T42.4X1	T42.4X2	T42.4X3	T42.4X4	T42.4X5	T42.4X6
Carprofen	T39.311	T39.312	T39.313	T39.314	T39.315	T39.316
Carpronium chloride	T44.3X1	T44.3X2	T44.3X3	T44.3X4	T44.3X5	T44.3X6
Carrageenan	T47.8X1	T47.8X2	T47.8X3	T47.8X4	T47.8X5	T47.8X6
Carteolol	T44.7X1	T44.7X2	T44.7X3	T44.7X4	T44.7X5	T44.7X6
Carter's Little Pills	T47.2X1	T47.2X2	T47.2X3	T47.2X4	T47.2X5	T47.2X6
Cartia*	T46.1X1	T46.1X2	T46.1X3	T46.1X4	T46.1X5	T46.1X6
Cascara (sagrada)	T47.2X1	T47.2X2	T47.2X3	T47.2X4	T47.2X5	T47.2X6
Cassava	T62.2X1	T62.2X2	T62.2X3	T62.2X4	—	—
Castellani's paint	T49.ØX1	T49.ØX2	T49.ØX3	T49.ØX4	T49.ØX5	T49.ØX6
Castor						
bean	T62.2X1	T62.2X2	T62.2X3	T62.2X4	—	—
oil	T47.2X1	T47.2X2	T47.2X3	T47.2X4	T47.2X5	T47.2X6
Catalase	T45.3X1	T45.3X2	T45.3X3	T45.3X4	T45.3X5	T45.3X6
Caterpillar (sting)	T63.431	T63.432	T63.433	T63.434	—	—
Catha (edulis) (tea)	T43.691	T43.692	T43.693	T43.694	—	—
Cathartic NEC	T47.4X1	T47.4X2	T47.4X3	T47.4X4	T47.4X5	T47.4X6
anthacene derivative	T47.2X1	T47.2X2	T47.2X3	T47.2X4	T47.2X5	T47.2X6
bulk	T47.4X1	T47.4X2	T47.4X3	T47.4X4	T47.4X5	T47.4X6
contact	T47.2X1	T47.2X2	T47.2X3	T47.2X4	T47.2X5	T47.2X6
emollient NEC	T47.4X1	T47.4X2	T47.4X3	T47.4X4	T47.4X5	T47.4X6
irritant NEC	T47.2X1	T47.2X2	T47.2X3	T47.2X4	T47.2X5	T47.2X6
mucilage	T47.4X1	T47.4X2	T47.4X3	T47.4X4	T47.4X5	T47.4X6
saline	T47.3X1	T47.3X2	T47.3X3	T47.3X4	T47.3X5	T47.3X6
vegetable	T47.2X1	T47.2X2	T47.2X3	T47.2X4	T47.2X5	T47.2X6
Cathine	T5Ø.5X1	T5Ø.5X2	T5Ø.5X3	T5Ø.5X4	T5Ø.5X5	T5Ø.5X6
Cathomycin	T36.8X1	T36.8X2	T36.8X3	T36.8X4	T36.8X5	T36.8X6
Cation exchange resin	T5Ø.3X1	T5Ø.3X2	T5Ø.3X3	T5Ø.3X4	T5Ø.3X5	T5Ø.3X6
Caustic(s) **NEC**	T54.91	T54.92	T54.93	T54.94	—	—
alkali	T54.3X1	T54.3X2	T54.3X3	T54.3X4	—	—
hydroxide	T54.3X1	T54.3X2	T54.3X3	T54.3X4	—	—
potash	T54.3X1	T54.3X2	T54.3X3	T54.3X4	—	—
soda	T54.3X1	T54.3X2	T54.3X3	T54.3X4	—	—
specified NEC	T54.91	T54.92	T54.93	T54.94	—	—
Ceepryn	T49.ØX1	T49.ØX2	T49.ØX3	T49.ØX4	T49.ØX5	T49.ØX6
ENT agent	T49.6X1	T49.6X2	T49.6X3	T49.6X4	T49.6X5	T49.6X6
lozenges	T49.6X1	T49.6X2	T49.6X3	T49.6X4	T49.6X5	T49.6X6
Cefacetrile	T36.1X1	T36.1X2	T36.1X3	T36.1X4	T36.1X5	T36.1X6
Cefaclor	T36.1X1	T36.1X2	T36.1X3	T36.1X4	T36.1X5	T36.1X6
Cefadroxil	T36.1X1	T36.1X2	T36.1X3	T36.1X4	T36.1X5	T36.1X6
Cefalexin	T36.1X1	T36.1X2	T36.1X3	T36.1X4	T36.1X5	T36.1X6
Cefaloglycin	T36.1X1	T36.1X2	T36.1X3	T36.1X4	T36.1X5	T36.1X6
Cefaloridine	T36.1X1	T36.1X2	T36.1X3	T36.1X4	T36.1X5	T36.1X6
Cefalosporins	T36.1X1	T36.1X2	T36.1X3	T36.1X4	T36.1X5	T36.1X6
Cefalotin	T36.1X1	T36.1X2	T36.1X3	T36.1X4	T36.1X5	T36.1X6
Cefamandole	T36.1X1	T36.1X2	T36.1X3	T36.1X4	T36.1X5	T36.1X6
Cefamycin antibiotic	T36.1X1	T36.1X2	T36.1X3	T36.1X4	T36.1X5	T36.1X6
Cefapirin	T36.1X1	T36.1X2	T36.1X3	T36.1X4	T36.1X5	T36.1X6
Cefatrizine	T36.1X1	T36.1X2	T36.1X3	T36.1X4	T36.1X5	T36.1X6
Cefazedone	T36.1X1	T36.1X2	T36.1X3	T36.1X4	T36.1X5	T36.1X6
Cefazolin	T36.1X1	T36.1X2	T36.1X3	T36.1X4	T36.1X5	T36.1X6
Cefbuperazone	T36.1X1	T36.1X2	T36.1X3	T36.1X4	T36.1X5	T36.1X6
Cefetamet	T36.1X1	T36.1X2	T36.1X3	T36.1X4	T36.1X5	T36.1X6
Cefixime	T36.1X1	T36.1X2	T36.1X3	T36.1X4	T36.1X5	T36.1X6
Cefmenoxime	T36.1X1	T36.1X2	T36.1X3	T36.1X4	T36.1X5	T36.1X6
Cefmetazole	T36.1X1	T36.1X2	T36.1X3	T36.1X4	T36.1X5	T36.1X6
Cefminox	T36.1X1	T36.1X2	T36.1X3	T36.1X4	T36.1X5	T36.1X6
Cefonicid	T36.1X1	T36.1X2	T36.1X3	T36.1X4	T36.1X5	T36.1X6
Cefoperazone	T36.1X1	T36.1X2	T36.1X3	T36.1X4	T36.1X5	T36.1X6
Ceforanide	T36.1X1	T36.1X2	T36.1X3	T36.1X4	T36.1X5	T36.1X6
Cefotaxime	T36.1X1	T36.1X2	T36.1X3	T36.1X4	T36.1X5	T36.1X6
Cefotetan	T36.1X1	T36.1X2	T36.1X3	T36.1X4	T36.1X5	T36.1X6

Substance	Poisoning, Accidental (unintentional)	Poisoning, Intentional Self-harm	Poisoning, Assault	Poisoning, Undetermined	Adverse Effect	Under-dosing
Cefotiam	T36.1X1	T36.1X2	T36.1X3	T36.1X4	T36.1X5	T36.1X6
Cefoxitin	T36.1X1	T36.1X2	T36.1X3	T36.1X4	T36.1X5	T36.1X6
Cefpimizole	T36.1X1	T36.1X2	T36.1X3	T36.1X4	T36.1X5	T36.1X6
Cefpiramide	T36.1X1	T36.1X2	T36.1X3	T36.1X4	T36.1X5	T36.1X6
Cefradine	T36.1X1	T36.1X2	T36.1X3	T36.1X4	T36.1X5	T36.1X6
Cefroxadine	T36.1X1	T36.1X2	T36.1X3	T36.1X4	T36.1X5	T36.1X6
Cefsulodin	T36.1X1	T36.1X2	T36.1X3	T36.1X4	T36.1X5	T36.1X6
Ceftazidime	T36.1X1	T36.1X2	T36.1X3	T36.1X4	T36.1X5	T36.1X6
Cefteram	T36.1X1	T36.1X2	T36.1X3	T36.1X4	T36.1X5	T36.1X6
Ceftezole	T36.1X1	T36.1X2	T36.1X3	T36.1X4	T36.1X5	T36.1X6
Ceftin*	T36.1X1	T36.1X2	T36.1X3	T36.1X4	T36.1X5	T36.1X6
Ceftizoxime	T36.1X1	T36.1X2	T36.1X3	T36.1X4	T36.1X5	T36.1X6
Ceftriaxone	T36.1X1	T36.1X2	T36.1X3	T36.1X4	T36.1X5	T36.1X6
Cefuroxime	T36.1X1	T36.1X2	T36.1X3	T36.1X4	T36.1X5	T36.1X6
Cefuzonam	T36.1X1	T36.1X2	T36.1X3	T36.1X4	T36.1X5	T36.1X6
Celestone	T38.0X1	T38.0X2	T38.0X3	T38.0X4	T38.0X5	T38.0X6
topical	T49.0X1	T49.0X2	T49.0X3	T49.0X4	T49.0X5	T49.0X6
Celiprolol	T44.7X1	T44.7X2	T44.7X3	T44.7X4	T44.7X5	T44.7X6
Cellosolve	T52.91	T52.92	T52.93	T52.94	—	—
Cell stimulants and proliferants	T49.8X1	T49.8X2	T49.8X3	T49.8X4	T49.8X5	T49.8X6
Cellulose						
cathartic	T47.4X1	T47.4X2	T47.4X3	T47.4X4	T47.4X5	T47.4X6
hydroxyethyl	T47.4X1	T47.4X2	T47.4X3	T47.4X4	T47.4X5	T47.4X6
nitrates (topical)	T49.3X1	T49.3X2	T49.3X3	T49.3X4	T49.3X5	T49.3X6
oxidized	T49.4X1	T49.4X2	T49.4X3	T49.4X4	T49.4X5	T49.4X6
Centipede (bite)	T63.411	T63.412	T63.413	T63.414	—	—
Central nervous system						
depressants	T42.71	T42.72	T42.73	T42.74	T42.75	T42.76
anesthetic (general) NEC	T41.201	T41.202	T41.203	T41.204	T41.205	T41.206
gases NEC	T41.0X1	T41.0X2	T41.0X3	T41.0X4	T41.0X5	T41.0X6
intravenous	T41.1X1	T41.1X2	T41.1X3	T41.1X4	T41.1X5	T41.1X6
barbiturates	T42.3X1	T42.3X2	T42.3X3	T42.3X4	T42.3X5	T42.3X6
benzodiazepines	T42.4X1	T42.4X2	T42.4X3	T42.4X4	T42.4X5	T42.4X6
bromides	T42.6X1	T42.6X2	T42.6X3	T42.6X4	T42.6X5	T42.6X6
cannabis sativa	T40.711	T40.712	T40.713	T40.714	T40.715	T40.716
chloral hydrate	T42.6X1	T42.6X2	T42.6X3	T42.6X4	T42.6X5	T42.6X6
ethanol	T51.0X1	T51.0X2	T51.0X3	T51.0X4	—	—
hallucinogenics	T40.901	T40.902	T40.903	T40.904	T40.905	T40.906
hypnotics	T42.71	T42.72	T42.73	T42.74	T42.75	T42.76
specified NEC	T42.6X1	T42.6X2	T42.6X3	T42.6X4	T42.6X5	T42.6X6
muscle relaxants	T42.8X1	T42.8X2	T42.8X3	T42.8X4	T42.8X5	T42.8X6
paraldehyde	T42.6X1	T42.6X2	T42.6X3	T42.6X4	T42.6X5	T42.6X6
sedatives; sedative-hypnotics	T42.71	T42.72	T42.73	T42.74	T42.75	T42.76
mixed NEC	T42.6X1	T42.6X2	T42.6X3	T42.6X4	T42.6X5	T42.6X6
specified NEC	T42.6X1	T42.6X2	T42.6X3	T42.6X4	T42.6X5	T42.6X6
muscle-tone depressants	T42.8X1	T42.8X2	T42.8X3	T42.8X4	T42.8X5	T42.8X6
stimulants	T43.601	T43.602	T43.603	T43.604	T43.605	T43.606
amphetamines	T43.621	T43.622	T43.623	T43.624	T43.625	T43.626
analeptics	T50.7X1	T50.7X2	T50.7X3	T50.7X4	T50.7X5	T50.7X6
antidepressants	T43.201	T43.202	T43.203	T43.204	T43.205	T43.206
opiate antagonists	T50.7X1	T50.7X2	T50.7X3	T50.7X4	T50.7X5	T50.7X6
specified NEC	T43.691	T43.692	T43.693	T43.694	T43.695	T43.696
Cepacol*	T41.3X1	T41.3X2	T41.3X3	T41.3X4	T41.3X5	T41.3X6
Cephalexin	T36.1X1	T36.1X2	T36.1X3	T36.1X4	T36.1X5	T36.1X6
Cephaloglycin	T36.1X1	T36.1X2	T36.1X3	T36.1X4	T36.1X5	T36.1X6
Cephaloridine	T36.1X1	T36.1X2	T36.1X3	T36.1X4	T36.1X5	T36.1X6
Cephalosporins	T36.1X1	T36.1X2	T36.1X3	T36.1X4	T36.1X5	T36.1X6
N (adicillin)	T36.0X1	T36.0X2	T36.0X3	T36.0X4	T36.0X5	T36.0X6
Cephalothin	T36.1X1	T36.1X2	T36.1X3	T36.1X4	T36.1X5	T36.1X6
Cephalotin	T36.1X1	T36.1X2	T36.1X3	T36.1X4	T36.1X5	T36.1X6
Cephradine	T36.1X1	T36.1X2	T36.1X3	T36.1X4	T36.1X5	T36.1X6
Cerbera (odallam)	T62.2X1	T62.2X2	T62.2X3	T62.2X4	—	—
Cerberin	T46.0X1	T46.0X2	T46.0X3	T46.0X4	T46.0X5	T46.0X6
Cerebral stimulants	T43.601	T43.602	T43.603	T43.604	T43.605	T43.606
psychotherapeutic	T43.601	T43.602	T43.603	T43.604	T43.605	T43.606
specified NEC	T43.691	T43.692	T43.693	T43.694	T43.695	T43.696
Cerium oxalate	T45.0X1	T45.0X2	T45.0X3	T45.0X4	T45.0X5	T45.0X6
Cerous oxalate	T45.0X1	T45.0X2	T45.0X3	T45.0X4	T45.0X5	T45.0X6
Ceruletide	T50.8X1	T50.8X2	T50.8X3	T50.8X4	T50.8X5	T50.8X6
Cetacort*	T49.0X1	T49.0X2	T49.0X3	T49.0X4	T49.0X5	T49.0X6
Cetalkonium (chloride)	T49.0X1	T49.0X2	T49.0X3	T49.0X4	T49.0X5	T49.0X6
Cethexonium chloride	T49.0X1	T49.0X2	T49.0X3	T49.0X4	T49.0X5	T49.0X6
Cetiedil	T46.7X1	T46.7X2	T46.7X3	T46.7X4	T46.7X5	T46.7X6
Cetirizine	T45.0X1	T45.0X2	T45.0X3	T45.0X4	T45.0X5	T45.0X6
Cetomacrogol	T50.991	T50.992	T50.993	T50.994	T50.995	T50.996
Cetotiamine	T45.2X1	T45.2X2	T45.2X3	T45.2X4	T45.2X5	T45.2X6
Cetoxime	T45.0X1	T45.0X2	T45.0X3	T45.0X4	T45.0X5	T45.0X6
Cetraxate	T47.1X1	T47.1X2	T47.1X3	T47.1X4	T47.1X5	T47.1X6
Cetrimide	T49.0X1	T49.0X2	T49.0X3	T49.0X4	T49.0X5	T49.0X6
Cetrimonium (bromide)	T49.0X1	T49.0X2	T49.0X3	T49.0X4	T49.0X5	T49.0X6
Cetylpyridinium chloride	T49.0X1	T49.0X2	T49.0X3	T49.0X4	T49.0X5	T49.0X6
Cetylpyridinium chloride — *continued*						
ENT agent	T49.6X1	T49.6X2	T49.6X3	T49.6X4	T49.6X5	T49.6X6
lozenges	T49.6X1	T49.6X2	T49.6X3	T49.6X4	T49.6X5	T49.6X6
Cevadilla — *see* Sabadilla						
Cevitamic acid	T45.2X1	T45.2X2	T45.2X3	T45.2X4	T45.2X5	T45.2X6
Chalk, precipitated	T47.1X1	T47.1X2	T47.1X3	T47.1X4	T47.1X5	T47.1X6
Chamomile	T49.0X1	T49.0X2	T49.0X3	T49.0X4	T49.0X5	T49.0X6
Ch'an su	T46.0X1	T46.0X2	T46.0X3	T46.0X4	T46.0X5	T46.0X6
Charcoal	T47.6X1	T47.6X2	T47.6X3	T47.6X4	T47.6X5	T47.6X6
activated — *see also* Charcoal, medicinal	T47.6X1	T47.6X2	T47.6X3	T47.6X4	T47.6X5	T47.6X6
fumes (Carbon monoxide)	T58.2X1	T58.2X2	T58.2X3	T58.2X4	—	—
industrial	T58.8X1	T58.8X2	T58.8X3	T58.8X4	—	—
medicinal (activated)	T47.6X1	T47.6X2	T47.6X3	T47.6X4	T47.6X5	T47.6X6
antidiarrheal	T47.6X1	T47.6X2	T47.6X3	T47.6X4	T47.6X5	T47.6X6
poison control	T47.8X1	T47.8X2	T47.8X3	T47.8X4	T47.8X5	T47.8X6
specified use other than for diarrhea	T47.8X1	T47.8X2	T47.8X3	T47.8X4	T47.8X5	T47.8X6
topical	T49.8X1	T49.8X2	T49.8X3	T49.8X4	T49.8X5	T49.8X6
Chaulmosulfone	T37.1X1	T37.1X2	T37.1X3	T37.1X4	T37.1X5	T37.1X6
Chelating agent NEC	T50.6X1	T50.6X2	T50.6X3	T50.6X4	T50.6X5	T50.6X6
Chelidonium majus	T62.2X1	T62.2X2	T62.2X3	T62.2X4	—	—
Chemical substance NEC	T65.91	T65.92	T65.93	T65.94	—	—
Chenodeoxycholic acid	T47.5X1	T47.5X2	T47.5X3	T47.5X4	T47.5X5	T47.5X6
Chenodiol	T47.5X1	T47.5X2	T47.5X3	T47.5X4	T47.5X5	T47.5X6
Chenopodium	T37.4X1	T37.4X2	T37.4X3	T37.4X4	T37.4X5	T37.4X6
Cherry laurel	T62.2X1	T62.2X2	T62.2X3	T62.2X4	—	—
Chiggertox*	T41.3X1	T41.3X2	T41.3X3	T41.3X4	T41.3X5	T41.3X6
Chinidin (e)	T46.2X1	T46.2X2	T46.2X3	T46.2X4	T46.2X5	T46.2X6
Chiniofon	T37.8X1	T37.8X2	T37.8X3	T37.8X4	T37.8X5	T37.8X6
Chlophedianol	T48.3X1	T48.3X2	T48.3X3	T48.3X4	T48.3X5	T48.3X6
Chloral	T42.6X1	T42.6X2	T42.6X3	T42.6X4	T42.6X5	T42.6X6
derivative	T42.6X1	T42.6X2	T42.6X3	T42.6X4	T42.6X5	T42.6X6
hydrate	T42.6X1	T42.6X2	T42.6X3	T42.6X4	T42.6X5	T42.6X6
Chloralamide	T42.6X1	T42.6X2	T42.6X3	T42.6X4	T42.6X5	T42.6X6
Chloralodol	T42.6X1	T42.6X2	T42.6X3	T42.6X4	T42.6X5	T42.6X6
Chloralose	T60.4X1	T60.4X2	T60.4X3	T60.4X4	—	—
Chlorambucil	T45.1X1	T45.1X2	T45.1X3	T45.1X4	T45.1X5	T45.1X6
Chloramine	T57.8X1	T57.8X2	T57.8X3	T57.8X4	—	—
T	T49.0X1	T49.0X2	T49.0X3	T49.0X4	T49.0X5	T49.0X6
topical	T49.0X1	T49.0X2	T49.0X3	T49.0X4	T49.0X5	T49.0X6
Chloramphenicol	T36.2X1	T36.2X2	T36.2X3	T36.2X4	T36.2X5	T36.2X6
ENT agent	T49.6X1	T49.6X2	T49.6X3	T49.6X4	T49.6X5	T49.6X6
ophthalmic preparation	T49.5X1	T49.5X2	T49.5X3	T49.5X4	T49.5X5	T49.5X6
topical NEC	T49.0X1	T49.0X2	T49.0X3	T49.0X4	T49.0X5	T49.0X6
Chlorate (potassium) (sodium) **NEC**	T60.3X1	T60.3X2	T60.3X3	T60.3X4	—	—
herbicide	T60.3X1	T60.3X2	T60.3X3	T60.3X4	—	—
Chlorazanil	T50.2X1	T50.2X2	T50.2X3	T50.2X4	T50.2X5	T50.2X6
Chlorbenzene, chlorbenzol	T53.7X1	T53.7X2	T53.7X3	T53.7X4	—	—
Chlorbenzoxamine	T44.3X1	T44.3X2	T44.3X3	T44.3X4	T44.3X5	T44.3X6
Chlorbutol	T42.6X1	T42.6X2	T42.6X3	T42.6X4	T42.6X5	T42.6X6
Chlorcyclizine	T45.0X1	T45.0X2	T45.0X3	T45.0X4	T45.0X5	T45.0X6
Chlordan (e) (dust)	T60.1X1	T60.1X2	T60.1X3	T60.1X4	—	—
Chlordantoin	T49.0X1	T49.0X2	T49.0X3	T49.0X4	T49.0X5	T49.0X6
Chlordiazepoxide	T42.4X1	T42.4X2	T42.4X3	T42.4X4	T42.4X5	T42.4X6
Chlordiethyl benzamide	T49.3X1	T49.3X2	T49.3X3	T49.3X4	T49.3X5	T49.3X6
Chloresium	T49.8X1	T49.8X2	T49.8X3	T49.8X4	T49.8X5	T49.8X6
Chlorethiazol	T42.6X1	T42.6X2	T42.6X3	T42.6X4	T42.6X5	T42.6X6
Chlorethyl — *see* Ethyl, chloride						
Chloretone	T42.6X1	T42.6X2	T42.6X3	T42.6X4	T42.6X5	T42.6X6
Chlorex	T53.6X1	T53.6X2	T53.6X3	T53.6X4	—	—
insecticide	T60.1X1	T60.1X2	T60.1X3	T60.1X4	—	—
Chlorfenvinphos	T60.0X1	T60.0X2	T60.0X3	T60.0X4	—	—
Chlorhexadol	T42.6X1	T42.6X2	T42.6X3	T42.6X4	T42.6X5	T42.6X6
Chlorhexamide	T45.1X1	T45.1X2	T45.1X3	T45.1X4	T45.1X5	T45.1X6
Chlorhexidine	T49.0X1	T49.0X2	T49.0X3	T49.0X4	T49.0X5	T49.0X6
Chlorhexidine Gluconate Oral Rinse*	T49.6X1	T49.6X2	T49.6X3	T49.6X4	T49.6X5	T49.6X6
Chlorhydroxyquinolin	T49.0X1	T49.0X2	T49.0X3	T49.0X4	T49.0X5	T49.0X6
Chloride of lime (bleach)	T54.3X1	T54.3X2	T54.3X3	T54.3X4	—	—
Chlorimipramine	T43.011	T43.012	T43.013	T43.014	T43.015	T43.016
Chlorinated						
camphene	T53.6X1	T53.6X2	T53.6X3	T53.6X4	—	—
diphenyl	T53.7X1	T53.7X2	T53.7X3	T53.7X4	—	—
hydrocarbons NEC	T53.91	T53.92	T53.93	T53.94	—	—
solvents	T53.91	T53.92	T53.93	T53.94	—	—
lime (bleach)	T54.3X1	T54.3X2	T54.3X3	T54.3X4	—	—
and boric acid solution	T49.0X1	T49.0X2	T49.0X3	T49.0X4	T49.0X5	T49.0X6
naphthalene (insecticide)	T60.1X1	T60.1X2	T60.1X3	T60.1X4	—	—

Substance	Poisoning, Accidental (unintentional)	Poisoning, Intentional Self-harm	Poisoning, Assault	Poisoning, Undetermined	Adverse Effect	Under-dosing
Chlorinated — *continued*						
naphthalene — *continued*						
industrial (non-pesticide)	T53.7X1	T53.7X2	T53.7X3	T53.7X4	—	—
pesticide NEC	T6Ø.8X1	T6Ø.8X2	T6Ø.8X3	T6Ø.8X4	—	—
soda — *see also* sodium hypochlorite						
solution	T49.ØX1	T49.ØX2	T49.ØX3	T49.ØX4	T49.ØX5	T49.ØX6
Chlorine (fumes) (gas)	T59.4X1	T59.4X2	T59.4X3	T59.4X4	—	—
bleach	T54.3X1	T54.3X2	T54.3X3	T54.3X4	—	—
compound gas NEC	T59.4X1	T59.4X2	T59.4X3	T59.4X4	—	—
disinfectant	T59.4X1	T59.4X2	T59.4X3	T59.4X4	—	—
releasing agents NEC	T59.4X1	T59.4X2	T59.4X3	T59.4X4	—	—
Chlorisondamine chloride	T46.991	T46.992	T46.993	T46.994	T46.995	T46.996
Chlormadinone	T38.5X1	T38.5X2	T38.5X3	T38.5X4	T38.5X5	T38.5X6
Chlormephos	T6Ø.ØX1	T6Ø.ØX2	T6Ø.ØX3	T6Ø.ØX4	—	—
Chlormerodrin	T5Ø.2X1	T5Ø.2X2	T5Ø.2X3	T5Ø.2X4	T5Ø.2X5	T5Ø.2X6
Chlormethiazole	T42.6X1	T42.6X2	T42.6X3	T42.6X4	T42.6X5	T42.6X6
Chlormethine	T45.1X1	T45.1X2	T45.1X3	T45.1X4	T45.1X5	T45.1X6
Chlormethylenecycline	T36.4X1	T36.4X2	T36.4X3	T36.4X4	T36.4X5	T36.4X6
Chlormezanone	T42.6X1	T42.6X2	T42.6X3	T42.6X4	T42.6X5	T42.6X6
Chloroacetic acid	T6Ø.3X1	T6Ø.3X2	T6Ø.3X3	T6Ø.3X4	—	—
Chloroacetone	T59.3X1	T59.3X2	T59.3X3	T59.3X4	—	—
Chloroacetophenone	T59.3X1	T59.3X2	T59.3X3	T59.3X4	—	—
Chloroaniline	T53.7X1	T53.7X2	T53.7X3	T53.7X4	—	—
Chlorobenzene, chlorobenzol	T53.7X1	T53.7X2	T53.7X3	T53.7X4	—	—
Chlorobromomethane (fire extinguisher)	T53.6X1	T53.6X2	T53.6X3	T53.6X4	—	—
Chlorobutanol	T49.ØX1	T49.ØX2	T49.ØX3	T49.ØX4	T49.ØX5	T49.ØX6
Chlorocresol	T49.ØX1	T49.ØX2	T49.ØX3	T49.ØX4	T49.ØX5	T49.ØX6
Chlorodehydromethyltestosterone	T38.7X1	T38.7X2	T38.7X3	T38.7X4	T38.7X5	T38.7X6
Chlorodeoxyadenosine*	T45.1X1	T45.1X2	T45.1X3	T45.1X4	T45.1X5	T45.1X6
Chlorodinitrobenzene	T53.7X1	T53.7X2	T53.7X3	T53.7X4	—	—
dust or vapor	T53.7X1	T53.7X2	T53.7X3	T53.7X4	—	—
Chlorodiphenyl	T53.7X1	T53.7X2	T53.7X3	T53.7X4	—	—
Chloroethane — *see* Ethyl, chloride						
Chloroethylene	T53.6X1	T53.6X2	T53.6X3	T53.6X4	—	—
Chlorofluorocarbons	T53.5X1	T53.5X2	T53.5X3	T53.5X4	—	—
Chloroform (fumes) (vapor)	T53.1X1	T53.1X2	T53.1X3	T53.1X4	—	—
anesthetic	T41.ØX1	T41.ØX2	T41.ØX3	T41.ØX4	T41.ØX5	T41.ØX6
solvent	T53.1X1	T53.1X2	T53.1X3	T53.1X4	—	—
water, concentrated	T41.ØX1	T41.ØX2	T41.ØX3	T41.ØX4	T41.ØX5	T41.ØX6
Chloroguanide	T37.2X1	T37.2X2	T37.2X3	T37.2X4	T37.2X5	T37.2X6
Chloromycetin	T36.2X1	T36.2X2	T36.2X3	T36.2X4	T36.2X5	T36.2X6
ENT agent	T49.6X1	T49.6X2	T49.6X3	T49.6X4	T49.6X5	T49.6X6
ophthalmic preparation	T49.5X1	T49.5X2	T49.5X3	T49.5X4	T49.5X5	T49.5X6
otic solution	T49.6X1	T49.6X2	T49.6X3	T49.6X4	T49.6X5	T49.6X6
topical NEC	T49.ØX1	T49.ØX2	T49.ØX3	T49.ØX4	T49.ØX5	T49.ØX6
Chloronitrobenzene	T53.7X1	T53.7X2	T53.7X3	T53.7X4	—	—
dust or vapor	T53.7X1	T53.7X2	T53.7X3	T53.7X4	—	—
Chlorophacinone	T6Ø.4X1	T6Ø.4X2	T6Ø.4X3	T6Ø.4X4	—	—
Chlorophenol	T53.7X1	T53.7X2	T53.7X3	T53.7X4	—	—
Chlorophenothane	T6Ø.1X1	T6Ø.1X2	T6Ø.1X3	T6Ø.1X4	—	—
Chlorophyll	T5Ø.991	T5Ø.992	T5Ø.993	T5Ø.994	T5Ø.995	T5Ø.996
Chloropicrin (fumes)	T53.6X1	T53.6X2	T53.6X3	T53.6X4	—	—
fumigant	T6Ø.8X1	T6Ø.8X2	T6Ø.8X3	T6Ø.8X4	—	—
fungicide	T6Ø.3X1	T6Ø.3X2	T6Ø.3X3	T6Ø.3X4	—	—
pesticide	T6Ø.8X1	T6Ø.8X2	T6Ø.8X3	T6Ø.8X4	—	—
Chloroprocaine	T41.3X1	T41.3X2	T41.3X3	T41.3X4	T41.3X5	T41.3X6
infiltration (subcutaneous)	T41.3X1	T41.3X2	T41.3X3	T41.3X4	T41.3X5	T41.3X6
nerve block (peripheral) (plexus)	T41.3X1	T41.3X2	T41.3X3	T41.3X4	T41.3X5	T41.3X6
spinal	T41.3X1	T41.3X2	T41.3X3	T41.3X4	T41.3X5	T41.3X6
Chloroptic	T49.5X1	T49.5X2	T49.5X3	T49.5X4	T49.5X5	T49.5X6
Chloropurine	T45.1X1	T45.1X2	T45.1X3	T45.1X4	T45.1X5	T45.1X6
Chloropyramine	T45.ØX1	T45.ØX2	T45.ØX3	T45.ØX4	T45.ØX5	T45.ØX6
Chloropyrifos	T6Ø.ØX1	T6Ø.ØX2	T6Ø.ØX3	T6Ø.ØX4	—	—
Chloropyrilene	T45.ØX1	T45.ØX2	T45.ØX3	T45.ØX4	T45.ØX5	T45.ØX6
Chloroquine	T37.2X1	T37.2X2	T37.2X3	T37.2X4	T37.2X5	T37.2X6
Chlorostat*	T49.ØX1	T49.ØX2	T49.ØX3	T49.ØX4	T49.ØX5	T49.ØX6
Chlorothalonil	T6Ø.3X1	T6Ø.3X2	T6Ø.3X3	T6Ø.3X4	—	—
Chlorothen	T45.ØX1	T45.ØX2	T45.ØX3	T45.ØX4	T45.ØX5	T45.ØX6
Chlorothiazide	T5Ø.2X1	T5Ø.2X2	T5Ø.2X3	T5Ø.2X4	T5Ø.2X5	T5Ø.2X6
Chlorothymol	T49.4X1	T49.4X2	T49.4X3	T49.4X4	T49.4X5	T49.4X6
Chlorotrianisene	T38.5X1	T38.5X2	T38.5X3	T38.5X4	T38.5X5	T38.5X6
Chlorovinyldichloroarsine, not in war	T57.ØX1	T57.ØX2	T57.ØX3	T57.ØX4	—	—
Chloroxine	T49.4X1	T49.4X2	T49.4X3	T49.4X4	T49.4X5	T49.4X6
Chloroxylenol	T49.ØX1	T49.ØX2	T49.ØX3	T49.ØX4	T49.ØX5	T49.ØX6
Chlorphenamine	T45.ØX1	T45.ØX2	T45.ØX3	T45.ØX4	T45.ØX5	T45.ØX6

Substance	Poisoning, Accidental (unintentional)	Poisoning, Intentional Self-harm	Poisoning, Assault	Poisoning, Undetermined	Adverse Effect	Under-dosing
Chlorphenesin	T42.8X1	T42.8X2	T42.8X3	T42.8X4	T42.8X5	T42.8X6
topical (antifungal)	T49.ØX1	T49.ØX2	T49.ØX3	T49.ØX4	T49.ØX5	T49.ØX6
Chlorpheniramine	T45.ØX1	T45.ØX2	T45.ØX3	T45.ØX4	T45.ØX5	T45.ØX6
Chlorphenoxamine	T45.ØX1	T45.ØX2	T45.ØX3	T45.ØX4	T45.ØX5	T45.ØX6
Chlorphentermine	T5Ø.5X1	T5Ø.5X2	T5Ø.5X3	T5Ø.5X4	T5Ø.5X5	T5Ø.5X6
Chlorprocaine — *see* Chloroprocaine						
Chlorproguanil	T37.2X1	T37.2X2	T37.2X3	T37.2X4	T37.2X5	T37.2X6
Chlorpromazine	T43.3X1	T43.3X2	T43.3X3	T43.3X4	T43.3X5	T43.3X6
Chlorpropamide	T38.3X1	T38.3X2	T38.3X3	T38.3X4	T38.3X5	T38.3X6
Chlorprothixene	T43.4X1	T43.4X2	T43.4X3	T43.4X4	T43.4X5	T43.4X6
Chlorquinaldol	T49.ØX1	T49.ØX2	T49.ØX3	T49.ØX4	T49.ØX5	T49.ØX6
Chlorquinol	T49.ØX1	T49.ØX2	T49.ØX3	T49.ØX4	T49.ØX5	T49.ØX6
Chlortalidone	T5Ø.2X1	T5Ø.2X2	T5Ø.2X3	T5Ø.2X4	T5Ø.2X5	T5Ø.2X6
Chlortetracycline	T36.4X1	T36.4X2	T36.4X3	T36.4X4	T36.4X5	T36.4X6
Chlorthalidone	T5Ø.2X1	T5Ø.2X2	T5Ø.2X3	T5Ø.2X4	T5Ø.2X5	T5Ø.2X6
Chlorthion	T6Ø.ØX1	T6Ø.ØX2	T6Ø.ØX3	T6Ø.ØX4	—	—
Chlorthiophos	T6Ø.ØX1	T6Ø.ØX2	T6Ø.ØX3	T6Ø.ØX4	—	—
Chlortrianisene	T38.5X1	T38.5X2	T38.5X3	T38.5X4	T38.5X5	T38.5X6
Chlor-Trimeton	T45.ØX1	T45.ØX2	T45.ØX3	T45.ØX4	T45.ØX5	T45.ØX6
Chlorzoxazone	T42.8X1	T42.8X2	T42.8X3	T42.8X4	T42.8X5	T42.8X6
Choke damp	T59.7X1	T59.7X2	T59.7X3	T59.7X4	—	—
Cholagogues	T47.5X1	T47.5X2	T47.5X3	T47.5X4	T47.5X5	T47.5X6
Cholebrine	T5Ø.8X1	T5Ø.8X2	T5Ø.8X3	T5Ø.8X4	T5Ø.8X5	T5Ø.8X6
Cholecalciferol	T45.2X1	T45.2X2	T45.2X3	T45.2X4	T45.2X5	T45.2X6
Cholecystokinin	T5Ø.8X1	T5Ø.8X2	T5Ø.8X3	T5Ø.8X4	T5Ø.8X5	T5Ø.8X6
Cholera vaccine	T5Ø.A91	T5Ø.A92	T5Ø.A93	T5Ø.A94	T5Ø.A95	T5Ø.A96
Choleretic	T47.5X1	T47.5X2	T47.5X3	T47.5X4	T47.5X5	T47.5X6
Cholesterol-lowering agents	T46.6X1	T46.6X2	T46.6X3	T46.6X4	T46.6X5	T46.6X6
Cholestyramine (resin)	T46.6X1	T46.6X2	T46.6X3	T46.6X4	T46.6X5	T46.6X6
Cholic acid	T47.5X1	T47.5X2	T47.5X3	T47.5X4	T47.5X5	T47.5X6
Choline	T48.6X1	T48.6X2	T48.6X3	T48.6X4	T48.6X5	T48.6X6
chloride	T5Ø.991	T5Ø.992	T5Ø.993	T5Ø.994	T5Ø.995	T5Ø.996
dihydrogen citrate	T5Ø.991	T5Ø.992	T5Ø.993	T5Ø.994	T5Ø.995	T5Ø.996
salicylate	T39.Ø91	T39.Ø92	T39.Ø93	T39.Ø94	T39.Ø95	T39.Ø96
theophyllinate	T48.6X1	T48.6X2	T48.6X3	T48.6X4	T48.6X5	T48.6X6
Cholinergic (drug) **NEC**	T44.1X1	T44.1X2	T44.1X3	T44.1X4	T44.1X5	T44.1X6
muscle tone enhancer	T44.1X1	T44.1X2	T44.1X3	T44.1X4	T44.1X5	T44.1X6
organophosphorus	T44.ØX1	T44.ØX2	T44.ØX3	T44.ØX4	T44.ØX5	T44.ØX6
insecticide	T6Ø.ØX1	T6Ø.ØX2	T6Ø.ØX3	T6Ø.ØX4	—	—
nerve gas	T59.891	T59.892	T59.893	T59.894	—	—
trimethyl ammonium propanediol	T44.1X1	T44.1X2	T44.1X3	T44.1X4	T44.1X5	T44.1X6
Cholinesterase reactivator	T5Ø.6X1	T5Ø.6X2	T5Ø.6X3	T5Ø.6X4	T5Ø.6X5	T5Ø.6X6
Cholografin	T5Ø.8X1	T5Ø.8X2	T5Ø.8X3	T5Ø.8X4	T5Ø.8X5	T5Ø.8X6
Chorionic gonadotropin	T38.891	T38.892	T38.893	T38.894	T38.895	T38.896
Chromate	T56.2X1	T56.2X2	T56.2X3	T56.2X4	—	—
dust or mist	T56.2X1	T56.2X2	T56.2X3	T56.2X4	—	—
lead — *see also* lead paint	T56.ØX1	T56.ØX2	T56.ØX3	T56.ØX4	—	—
Chromelin*	T49.3X1	T49.3X2	T49.3X3	T49.3X4	T49.3X5	T49.3X6
Chromic						
acid	T56.2X1	T56.2X2	T56.2X3	T56.2X4	—	—
dust or mist	T56.2X1	T56.2X2	T56.2X3	T56.2X4	—	—
phosphate 32P	T45.1X1	T45.1X2	T45.1X3	T45.1X4	T45.1X5	T45.1X6
Chromium	T56.2X1	T56.2X2	T56.2X3	T56.2X4	—	—
compounds — *see* Chromate						
sesquioxide	T5Ø.8X1	T5Ø.8X2	T5Ø.8X3	T5Ø.8X4	T5Ø.8X5	T5Ø.8X6
Chromomycin A3	T45.1X1	T45.1X2	T45.1X3	T45.1X4	T45.1X5	T45.1X6
Chromonar	T46.3X1	T46.3X2	T46.3X3	T46.3X4	T46.3X5	T46.3X6
Chromyl chloride	T56.2X1	T56.2X2	T56.2X3	T56.2X4	—	—
Chrysarobin	T49.4X1	T49.4X2	T49.4X3	T49.4X4	T49.4X5	T49.4X6
Chrysazin	T47.2X1	T47.2X2	T47.2X3	T47.2X4	T47.2X5	T47.2X6
Chymar	T45.3X1	T45.3X2	T45.3X3	T45.3X4	T45.3X5	T45.3X6
ophthalmic preparation	T49.5X1	T49.5X2	T49.5X3	T49.5X4	T49.5X5	T49.5X6
Chymopapain	T45.3X1	T45.3X2	T45.3X3	T45.3X4	T45.3X5	T45.3X6
Chymotrypsin	T45.3X1	T45.3X2	T45.3X3	T45.3X4	T45.3X5	T45.3X6
ophthalmic preparation	T49.5X1	T49.5X2	T49.5X3	T49.5X4	T49.5X5	T49.5X6
Cianidanol	T5Ø.991	T5Ø.992	T5Ø.993	T5Ø.994	T5Ø.995	T5Ø.996
Cianopramine	T43.Ø11	T43.Ø12	T43.Ø13	T43.Ø14	T43.Ø15	T43.Ø16
Cibenzoline	T46.2X1	T46.2X2	T46.2X3	T46.2X4	T46.2X5	T46.2X6
Ciclacillin	T36.ØX1	T36.ØX2	T36.ØX3	T36.ØX4	T36.ØX5	T36.ØX6
Ciclobarbital — *see* Hexobarbital						
Ciclonicate	T46.7X1	T46.7X2	T46.7X3	T46.7X4	T46.7X5	T46.7X6
Ciclopirox (olamine)	T49.ØX1	T49.ØX2	T49.ØX3	T49.ØX4	T49.ØX5	T49.ØX6
Ciclosporin	T45.1X1	T45.1X2	T45.1X3	T45.1X4	T45.1X5	T45.1X6
Cicuta maculata or virosa	T62.2X1	T62.2X2	T62.2X3	T62.2X4	—	—
Cicutoxin	T62.2X1	T62.2X2	T62.2X3	T62.2X4	—	—
Cigarette lighter fluid	T52.ØX1	T52.ØX2	T52.ØX3	T52.ØX4	—	—
Cigarettes (tobacco)	T65.221	T65.222	T65.223	T65.224	—	—
Ciguatoxin	T61.Ø1	T61.Ø2	T61.Ø3	T61.Ø4	—	—

Substance	Poisoning, Accidental (unintentional)	Poisoning, Intentional Self-harm	Poisoning, Assault	Poisoning, Undetermined	Adverse Effect	Under-dosing
Cilazapril	T46.4X1	T46.4X2	T46.4X3	T46.4X4	T46.4X5	T46.4X6
Cimetidine	T47.0X1	T47.0X2	T47.0X3	T47.0X4	T47.0X5	T47.0X6
Cimetropium bromide	T44.3X1	T44.3X2	T44.3X3	T44.3X4	T44.3X5	T44.3X6
Cinchocaine	T41.3X1	T41.3X2	T41.3X3	T41.3X4	T41.3X5	T41.3X6
topical (surface)	T41.3X1	T41.3X2	T41.3X3	T41.3X4	T41.3X5	T41.3X6
Cinchona	T37.2X1	T37.2X2	T37.2X3	T37.2X4	T37.2X5	T37.2X6
Cinchonine alkaloids	T37.2X1	T37.2X2	T37.2X3	T37.2X4	T37.2X5	T37.2X6
Cinchophen	T50.4X1	T50.4X2	T50.4X3	T50.4X4	T50.4X5	T50.4X6
Cinepazide	T46.7X1	T46.7X2	T46.7X3	T46.7X4	T46.7X5	T46.7X6
Cinnamedrine	T48.5X1	T48.5X2	T48.5X3	T48.5X4	T48.5X5	T48.5X6
Cinnarizine	T45.0X1	T45.0X2	T45.0X3	T45.0X4	T45.0X5	T45.0X6
Cinoxacin	T37.8X1	T37.8X2	T37.8X3	T37.8X4	T37.8X5	T37.8X6
Ciprofibrate	T46.6X1	T46.6X2	T46.6X3	T46.6X4	T46.6X5	T46.6X6
Ciprofloxacin	T36.8X1	T36.8X2	T36.8X3	T36.8X4	T36.8X5	T36.8X6
Cisapride	T47.8X1	T47.8X2	T47.8X3	T47.8X4	T47.8X5	T47.8X6
Cisplatin	T45.1X1	T45.1X2	T45.1X3	T45.1X4	T45.1X5	T45.1X6
Citalopram	T43.221	T43.222	T43.223	T43.224	T43.225	T43.226
Citanest	T41.3X1	T41.3X2	T41.3X3	T41.3X4	T41.3X5	T41.3X6
infiltration (subcutaneous)	T41.3X1	T41.3X2	T41.3X3	T41.3X4	T41.3X5	T41.3X6
nerve block (peripheral) (plexus)	T41.3X1	T41.3X2	T41.3X3	T41.3X4	T41.3X5	T41.3X6
Citracel*	T50.3X1	T50.3X2	T50.3X3	T50.3X4	T50.3X5	T50.3X6
Citric acid	T47.5X1	T47.5X2	T47.5X3	T47.5X4	T47.5X5	T47.5X6
Citrovorum (factor)	T45.8X1	T45.8X2	T45.8X3	T45.8X4	T45.8X5	T45.8X6
Claviceps purpurea	T62.2X1	T62.2X2	T62.2X3	T62.2X4	—	—
Clavulanic acid	T36.1X1	T36.1X2	T36.1X3	T36.1X4	T36.1X5	T36.1X6
Cleaner, cleansing agent, type not specified	T65.891	T65.892	T65.893	T65.894	—	—
of paint or varnish	T52.91	T52.92	T52.93	T52.94	—	—
specified type NEC	T65.891	T65.892	T65.893	T65.894	—	—
Clebopride	T47.8X1	T47.8X2	T47.8X3	T47.8X4	T47.8X5	T47.8X6
Clefamide	T37.3X1	T37.3X2	T37.3X3	T37.3X4	T37.3X5	T37.3X6
Clemastine	T45.0X1	T45.0X2	T45.0X3	T45.0X4	T45.0X5	T45.0X6
Clematis vitalba	T62.2X1	T62.2X2	T62.2X3	T62.2X4	—	—
Clemizole	T45.0X1	T45.0X2	T45.0X3	T45.0X4	T45.0X5	T45.0X6
penicillin	T36.0X1	T36.0X2	T36.0X3	T36.0X4	T36.0X5	T36.0X6
Clenbuterol	T48.6X1	T48.6X2	T48.6X3	T48.6X4	T48.6X5	T48.6X6
Clidinium bromide	T44.3X1	T44.3X2	T44.3X3	T44.3X4	T44.3X5	T44.3X6
Clinda-Derm*	T49.0X1	T49.0X2	T49.0X3	T49.0X4	T49.0X5	T49.0X6
Clindamycin	T36.8X1	T36.8X2	T36.8X3	T36.8X4	T36.8X5	T36.8X6
Clinofibrate	T46.6X1	T46.6X2	T46.6X3	T46.6X4	T46.6X5	T46.6X6
Clioquinol	T37.8X1	T37.8X2	T37.8X3	T37.8X4	T37.8X5	T37.8X6
Cliradon	T40.2X1	T40.2X2	T40.2X3	T40.2X4	—	—
Clobazam	T42.4X1	T42.4X2	T42.4X3	T42.4X4	T42.4X5	T42.4X6
Clobenzorex	T50.5X1	T50.5X2	T50.5X3	T50.5X4	T50.5X5	T50.5X6
Clobetasol	T49.0X1	T49.0X2	T49.0X3	T49.0X4	T49.0X5	T49.0X6
Clobetasone	T49.0X1	T49.0X2	T49.0X3	T49.0X4	T49.0X5	T49.0X6
Clobutinol	T48.3X1	T48.3X2	T48.3X3	T48.3X4	T48.3X5	T48.3X6
Clocortolone	T38.0X1	T38.0X2	T38.0X3	T38.0X4	T38.0X5	T38.0X6
Clodantoin	T49.0X1	T49.0X2	T49.0X3	T49.0X4	T49.0X5	T49.0X6
Clodronic acid	T50.991	T50.992	T50.993	T50.994	T50.995	T50.996
Clofazimine	T37.1X1	T37.1X2	T37.1X3	T37.1X4	T37.1X5	T37.1X6
Clofedanol	T48.3X1	T48.3X2	T48.3X3	T48.3X4	T48.3X5	T48.3X6
Clofenamide	T50.2X1	T50.2X2	T50.2X3	T50.2X4	T50.2X5	T50.2X6
Clofenotane	T49.0X1	T49.0X2	T49.0X3	T49.0X4	T49.0X5	T49.0X6
Clofezone	T39.2X1	T39.2X2	T39.2X3	T39.2X4	T39.2X5	T39.2X6
Clofibrate	T46.6X1	T46.6X2	T46.6X3	T46.6X4	T46.6X5	T46.6X6
Clofibride	T46.6X1	T46.6X2	T46.6X3	T46.6X4	T46.6X5	T46.6X6
Cloforex	T50.5X1	T50.5X2	T50.5X3	T50.5X4	T50.5X5	T50.5X6
Clomethiazole	T42.6X1	T42.6X2	T42.6X3	T42.6X4	T42.6X5	T42.6X6
Clometocillin	T36.0X1	T36.0X2	T36.0X3	T36.0X4	T36.0X5	T36.0X6
Clomifene	T38.5X1	T38.5X2	T38.5X3	T38.5X4	T38.5X5	T38.5X6
Clomiphene	T38.5X1	T38.5X2	T38.5X3	T38.5X4	T38.5X5	T38.5X6
Clomipramine	T43.011	T43.012	T43.013	T43.014	T43.015	T43.016
Clomocycline	T36.4X1	T36.4X2	T36.4X3	T36.4X4	T36.4X5	T36.4X6
Clonazepam	T42.4X1	T42.4X2	T42.4X3	T42.4X4	T42.4X5	T42.4X6
Clonidine	T46.5X1	T46.5X2	T46.5X3	T46.5X4	T46.5X5	T46.5X6
Clonixin	T39.8X1	T39.8X2	T39.8X3	T39.8X4	T39.8X5	T39.8X6
Clopamide	T50.2X1	T50.2X2	T50.2X3	T50.2X4	T50.2X5	T50.2X6
Clopenthixol	T43.4X1	T43.4X2	T43.4X3	T43.4X4	T43.4X5	T43.4X6
Cloperastine	T48.3X1	T48.3X2	T48.3X3	T48.3X4	T48.3X5	T48.3X6
Clophedianol	T48.3X1	T48.3X2	T48.3X3	T48.3X4	T48.3X5	T48.3X6
Cloponone	T36.2X1	T36.2X2	T36.2X3	T36.2X4	T36.2X5	T36.2X6
Cloprednol	T38.0X1	T38.0X2	T38.0X3	T38.0X4	T38.0X5	T38.0X6
Cloral betaine	T42.6X1	T42.6X2	T42.6X3	T42.6X4	T42.6X5	T42.6X6
Cloramfenicol	T36.2X1	T36.2X2	T36.2X3	T36.2X4	T36.2X5	T36.2X6
Clorazepate (dipotassium)	T42.4X1	T42.4X2	T42.4X3	T42.4X4	T42.4X5	T42.4X6
Clorexolone	T50.2X1	T50.2X2	T50.2X3	T50.2X4	T50.2X5	T50.2X6
Clorfenamine	T45.0X1	T45.0X2	T45.0X3	T45.0X4	T45.0X5	T45.0X6
Clorgiline	T43.1X1	T43.1X2	T43.1X3	T43.1X4	T43.1X5	T43.1X6
Clorotepine	T44.3X1	T44.3X2	T44.3X3	T44.3X4	T44.3X5	T44.3X6
Clorox (bleach)	T54.91	T54.92	T54.93	T54.94	—	—
Clorprenaline	T48.6X1	T48.6X2	T48.6X3	T48.6X4	T48.6X5	T48.6X6

Substance	Poisoning, Accidental (unintentional)	Poisoning, Intentional Self-harm	Poisoning, Assault	Poisoning, Undetermined	Adverse Effect	Under-dosing
Clortermine	T50.5X1	T50.5X2	T50.5X3	T50.5X4	T50.5X5	T50.5X6
Clotiapine	T43.591	T43.592	T43.593	T43.594	T43.595	T43.596
Clotiazepam	T42.4X1	T42.4X2	T42.4X3	T42.4X4	T42.4X5	T42.4X6
Clotibric acid	T46.6X1	T46.6X2	T46.6X3	T46.6X4	T46.6X5	T46.6X6
Clotrimazole	T49.0X1	T49.0X2	T49.0X3	T49.0X4	T49.0X5	T49.0X6
Cloxacillin	T36.0X1	T36.0X2	T36.0X3	T36.0X4	T36.0X5	T36.0X6
Cloxazolam	T42.4X1	T42.4X2	T42.4X3	T42.4X4	T42.4X5	T42.4X6
Cloxiquine	T49.0X1	T49.0X2	T49.0X3	T49.0X4	T49.0X5	T49.0X6
Clozapine	T42.4X1	T42.4X2	T42.4X3	T42.4X4	T42.4X5	T42.4X6
Coagulant NEC	T45.7X1	T45.7X2	T45.7X3	T45.7X4	T45.7X5	T45.7X6
Coal (carbon monoxide from) — *see also* Carbon, monoxide, coal	T58.2X1	T58.2X2	T58.2X3	T58.2X4	—	—
oil — *see* Kerosene						
tar	T49.1X1	T49.1X2	T49.1X3	T49.1X4	T49.1X5	T49.1X6
fumes	T59.891	T59.892	T59.893	T59.894	—	—
medicinal (ointment)	T49.4X1	T49.4X2	T49.4X3	T49.4X4	T49.4X5	T49.4X6
analgesics NEC	T39.2X1	T39.2X2	T39.2X3	T39.2X4	T39.2X5	T39.2X6
naphtha (solvent)	T52.0X1	T52.0X2	T52.0X3	T52.0X4	—	—
Coartem*	T37.2X1	T37.2X2	T37.2X3	T37.2X4	T37.2X5	T37.2X6
Cobalamine	T45.2X1	T45.2X2	T45.2X3	T45.2X4	T45.2X5	T45.2X6
Cobalt (nonmedicinal) (fumes) (industrial)	T56.891	T56.892	T56.893	T56.894	—	—
medicinal (trace) (chloride)	T45.8X1	T45.8X2	T45.8X3	T45.8X4	T45.8X5	T45.8X6
Cobra (venom)	T63.041	T63.042	T63.043	T63.044	—	—
Coca (leaf)	T40.5X1	T40.5X2	T40.5X3	T40.5X4	T40.5X5	T40.5X6
Cocaine	T40.5X1	T40.5X2	T40.5X3	T40.5X4	T40.5X5	T40.5X6
topical anesthetic	T41.3X1	T41.3X2	T41.3X3	T41.3X4	T41.3X5	T41.3X6
Cocarboxylase	T45.3X1	T45.3X2	T45.3X3	T45.3X4	T45.3X5	T45.3X6
Coccidioidin	T50.8X1	T50.8X2	T50.8X3	T50.8X4	T50.8X5	T50.8X6
Cocculus indicus	T62.1X1	T62.1X2	T62.1X3	T62.1X4	—	—
Cochineal	T65.6X1	T65.6X2	T65.6X3	T65.6X4	—	—
medicinal products	T50.991	T50.992	T50.993	T50.994	T50.995	T50.996
Codeine	T40.2X1	T40.2X2	T40.2X3	T40.2X4	T40.2X5	T40.2X6
Cod-liver oil	T45.2X1	T45.2X2	T45.2X3	T45.2X4	T45.2X5	T45.2X6
Coenzyme A	T50.991	T50.992	T50.993	T50.994	T50.995	T50.996
Coffee	T62.8X1	T62.8X2	T62.8X3	T62.8X4	—	—
Cogalactoisomerase	T50.991	T50.992	T50.993	T50.994	T50.995	T50.996
Cogentin	T44.3X1	T44.3X2	T44.3X3	T44.3X4	T44.3X5	T44.3X6
Coke fumes or gas (carbon monoxide)	T58.2X1	T58.2X2	T58.2X3	T58.2X4	—	—
industrial use	T58.8X1	T58.8X2	T58.8X3	T58.8X4	—	—
Colace	T47.4X1	T47.4X2	T47.4X3	T47.4X4	T47.4X5	T47.4X6
Colaspase	T45.1X1	T45.1X2	T45.1X3	T45.1X4	T45.1X5	T45.1X6
Colazal*	T47.8X1	T47.8X2	T47.8X3	T47.8X4	T47.8X5	T47.8X6
Colchicine	T50.4X1	T50.4X2	T50.4X3	T50.4X4	T50.4X5	T50.4X6
Colchicum	T62.2X1	T62.2X2	T62.2X3	T62.2X4	—	—
Cold cream	T49.3X1	T49.3X2	T49.3X3	T49.3X4	T49.3X5	T49.3X6
Colecalciferol	T45.2X1	T45.2X2	T45.2X3	T45.2X4	T45.2X5	T45.2X6
Colestipol	T46.6X1	T46.6X2	T46.6X3	T46.6X4	T46.6X5	T46.6X6
Colestyramine	T46.6X1	T46.6X2	T46.6X3	T46.6X4	T46.6X5	T46.6X6
Colimycin	T36.8X1	T36.8X2	T36.8X3	T36.8X4	T36.8X5	T36.8X6
Colistimethate	T36.8X1	T36.8X2	T36.8X3	T36.8X4	T36.8X5	T36.8X6
Colistin	T36.8X1	T36.8X2	T36.8X3	T36.8X4	T36.8X5	T36.8X6
sulfate (eye preparation)	T49.5X1	T49.5X2	T49.5X3	T49.5X4	T49.5X5	T49.5X6
Collagen	T50.991	T50.992	T50.993	T50.994	T50.995	T50.996
Collagenase	T49.4X1	T49.4X2	T49.4X3	T49.4X4	T49.4X5	T49.4X6
Collodion	T49.3X1	T49.3X2	T49.3X3	T49.3X4	T49.3X5	T49.3X6
Colocynth	T47.2X1	T47.2X2	T47.2X3	T47.2X4	T47.2X5	T47.2X6
Colophony adhesive	T49.3X1	T49.3X2	T49.3X3	T49.3X4	T49.3X5	T49.3X6
Colorant — *see also* Dye	T50.991	T50.992	T50.993	T50.994	T50.995	T50.996
Coloring matter — *see* Dye(s)						
Combustion gas (after combustion) — *see* Carbon, monoxide						
prior to combustion	T59.891	T59.892	T59.893	T59.894	—	—
Cometriq*	T45.1X1	T45.1X2	T45.1X3	T45.1X4	T45.1X5	T45.1X6
Compazine	T43.3X1	T43.3X2	T43.3X3	T43.3X4	T43.3X5	T43.3X6
Compound						
1080 (sodium fluoroacetate)	T60.4X1	T60.4X2	T60.4X3	T60.4X4	—	—
269 (endrin)	T60.1X1	T60.1X2	T60.1X3	T60.1X4	—	—
3422 (parathion)	T60.0X1	T60.0X2	T60.0X3	T60.0X4	—	—
3911 (phorate)	T60.0X1	T60.0X2	T60.0X3	T60.0X4	—	—
3956 (toxaphene)	T60.1X1	T60.1X2	T60.1X3	T60.1X4	—	—
4049 (malathion)	T60.0X1	T60.0X2	T60.0X3	T60.0X4	—	—
4069 (malathion)	T60.0X1	T60.0X2	T60.0X3	T60.0X4	—	—
4124 (dicapthon)	T60.0X1	T60.0X2	T60.0X3	T60.0X4	—	—
42 (warfarin)	T60.4X1	T60.4X2	T60.4X3	T60.4X4	—	—
497 (dieldrin)	T60.1X1	T60.1X2	T60.1X3	T60.1X4	—	—
E (cortisone)	T38.0X1	T38.0X2	T38.0X3	T38.0X4	T38.0X5	T38.0X6
F (hydrocortisone)	T38.0X1	T38.0X2	T38.0X3	T38.0X4	T38.0X5	T38.0X6
Comvax*	T50.A21	T50.A22	T50.A23	T50.A24	T50.A25	T50.A26

Substance	Poisoning, Accidental (unintentional)	Poisoning, Intentional Self-harm	Poisoning, Assault	Poisoning, Undetermined	Adverse Effect	Under-dosing
Congener, anabolic	T38.7X1	T38.7X2	T38.7X3	T38.7X4	T38.7X5	T38.7X6
Congo red	T5Ø.8X1	T5Ø.8X2	T5Ø.8X3	T5Ø.8X4	T5Ø.8X5	T5Ø.8X6
Coniine, conine	T62.2X1	T62.2X2	T62.2X3	T62.2X4	—	—
Conium (maculatum)	T62.2X1	T62.2X2	T62.2X3	T62.2X4	—	—
Conjugated estrogenic substances	T38.5X1	T38.5X2	T38.5X3	T38.5X4	T38.5X5	T38.5X6
Contac	T48.5X1	T48.5X2	T48.5X3	T48.5X4	T48.5X5	T48.5X6
Contact lens solution	T49.5X1	T49.5X2	T49.5X3	T49.5X4	T49.5X5	T49.5X6
Contraceptive (oral)	T38.4X1	T38.4X2	T38.4X3	T38.4X4	T38.4X5	T38.4X6
vaginal	T49.8X1	T49.8X2	T49.8X3	T49.8X4	T49.8X5	T49.8X6
Contrast medium, radiography	T5Ø.8X1	T5Ø.8X2	T5Ø.8X3	T5Ø.8X4	T5Ø.8X5	T5Ø.8X6
Convallaria glycosides	T46.ØX1	T46.ØX2	T46.ØX3	T46.ØX4	T46.ØX5	T46.ØX6
Convallaria majalis	T62.2X1	T62.2X2	T62.2X3	T62.2X4	—	—
berry	T62.1X1	T62.1X2	T62.1X3	T62.1X4	—	—
Copperhead snake (bite) (venom)	T63.Ø61	T63.Ø62	T63.Ø63	T63.Ø64	—	—
Copper (dust) (fumes) (nonmedicinal) **NEC**	T56.4X1	T56.4X2	T56.4X3	T56.4X4	—	—
arsenate, arsenite	T57.ØX1	T57.ØX2	T57.ØX3	T57.ØX4	—	—
insecticide	T6Ø.2X1	T6Ø.2X2	T6Ø.2X3	T6Ø.2X4	—	—
emetic	T47.7X1	T47.7X2	T47.7X3	T47.7X4	T47.7X5	T47.7X6
fungicide	T6Ø.3X1	T6Ø.3X2	T6Ø.3X3	T6Ø.3X4	—	—
gluconate	T49.ØX1	T49.ØX2	T49.ØX3	T49.ØX4	T49.ØX5	T49.ØX6
insecticide	T6Ø.2X1	T6Ø.2X2	T6Ø.2X3	T6Ø.2X4	—	—
medicinal (trace)	T45.8X1	T45.8X2	T45.8X3	T45.8X4	T45.8X5	T45.8X6
oleate	T49.ØX1	T49.ØX2	T49.ØX3	T49.ØX4	T49.ØX5	T49.ØX6
sulfate	T56.4X1	T56.4X2	T56.4X3	T56.4X4	—	—
cupric	T56.4X1	T56.4X2	T56.4X3	T56.4X4	—	—
fungicide	T6Ø.3X1	T6Ø.3X2	T6Ø.3X3	T6Ø.3X4	—	—
medicinal						
ear	T49.6X1	T49.6X2	T49.6X3	T49.6X4	T49.6X5	T49.6X6
emetic	T47.7X1	T47.7X2	T47.7X3	T47.7X4	T47.7X5	T47.7X6
eye	T49.5X1	T49.5X2	T49.5X3	T49.5X4	T49.5X5	T49.5X6
cuprous	T56.4X1	T56.4X2	T56.4X3	T56.4X4	—	—
fungicide	T6Ø.3X1	T6Ø.3X2	T6Ø.3X3	T6Ø.3X4	—	—
medicinal						
ear	T49.6X1	T49.6X2	T49.6X3	T49.6X4	T49.6X5	T49.6X6
emetic	T47.7X1	T47.7X2	T47.7X3	T47.7X4	T47.7X5	T47.7X6
eye	T49.5X1	T49.5X2	T49.5X3	T49.5X4	T49.5X5	T49.5X6
Coral (sting)	T63.691	T63.692	T63.693	T63.694	—	—
snake (bite) (venom)	T63.Ø21	T63.Ø22	T63.Ø23	T63.Ø24	—	—
Corbadrine	T49.6X1	T49.6X2	T49.6X3	T49.6X4	T49.6X5	T49.6X6
Cordite	T65.891	T65.892	T65.893	T65.894	—	—
vapor	T59.891	T59.892	T59.893	T59.894	—	—
Cordran	T49.ØX1	T49.ØX2	T49.ØX3	T49.ØX4	T49.ØX5	T49.ØX6
Cormax*	T49.ØX1	T49.ØX2	T49.ØX3	T49.ØX4	T49.ØX5	T49.ØX6
Corn cures	T49.4X1	T49.4X2	T49.4X3	T49.4X4	T49.4X5	T49.4X6
Cornhusker's lotion	T49.3X1	T49.3X2	T49.3X3	T49.3X4	T49.3X5	T49.3X6
Corn starch	T49.3X1	T49.3X2	T49.3X3	T49.3X4	T49.3X5	T49.3X6
Coronary vasodilator NEC	T46.3X1	T46.3X2	T46.3X3	T46.3X4	T46.3X5	T46.3X6
Corrosive NEC	T54.91	T54.92	T54.93	T54.94	—	—
acid NEC	T54.2X1	T54.2X2	T54.2X3	T54.2X4	—	—
aromatics	T54.1X1	T54.1X2	T54.1X3	T54.1X4	—	—
disinfectant	T54.1X1	T54.1X2	T54.1X3	T54.1X4	—	—
fumes NEC	T54.91	T54.92	T54.93	T54.94	—	—
specified NEC	T54.91	T54.92	T54.93	T54.94	—	—
sublimate	T56.1X1	T56.1X2	T56.1X3	T56.1X4	—	—
Cortate	T38.ØX1	T38.ØX2	T38.ØX3	T38.ØX4	T38.ØX5	T38.ØX6
Cort-Dome	T38.ØX1	T38.ØX2	T38.ØX3	T38.ØX4	T38.ØX5	T38.ØX6
ENT agent	T49.6X1	T49.6X2	T49.6X3	T49.6X4	T49.6X5	T49.6X6
ophthalmic preparation	T49.5X1	T49.5X2	T49.5X3	T49.5X4	T49.5X5	T49.5X6
topical NEC	T49.ØX1	T49.ØX2	T49.ØX3	T49.ØX4	T49.ØX5	T49.ØX6
Cortef	T38.ØX1	T38.ØX2	T38.ØX3	T38.ØX4	T38.ØX5	T38.ØX6
ENT agent	T49.6X1	T49.6X2	T49.6X3	T49.6X4	T49.6X5	T49.6X6
ophthalmic preparation	T49.5X1	T49.5X2	T49.5X3	T49.5X4	T49.5X5	T49.5X6
topical NEC	T49.ØX1	T49.ØX2	T49.ØX3	T49.ØX4	T49.ØX5	T49.ØX6
Corticosteroid	T38.ØX1	T38.ØX2	T38.ØX3	T38.ØX4	T38.ØX5	T38.ØX6
ENT agent	T49.6X1	T49.6X2	T49.6X3	T49.6X4	T49.6X5	T49.6X6
mineral	T5Ø.ØX1	T5Ø.ØX2	T5Ø.ØX3	T5Ø.ØX4	T5Ø.ØX5	T5Ø.ØX6
ophthalmic	T49.5X1	T49.5X2	T49.5X3	T49.5X4	T49.5X5	T49.5X6
topical NEC	T49.ØX1	T49.ØX2	T49.ØX3	T49.ØX4	T49.ØX5	T49.ØX6
Corticotropin	T38.811	T38.812	T38.813	T38.814	T38.815	T38.816
Cortisol	T49.ØX1	T49.ØX2	T49.ØX3	T49.ØX4	T49.ØX5	T49.ØX6
ENT agent	T49.6X1	T49.6X2	T49.6X3	T49.6X4	T49.6X5	T49.6X6
ophthalmic preparation	T49.5X1	T49.5X2	T49.5X3	T49.5X4	T49.5X5	T49.5X6
topical NEC	T49.ØX1	T49.ØX2	T49.ØX3	T49.ØX4	T49.ØX5	T49.ØX6
Cortisone (acetate)	T38.ØX1	T38.ØX2	T38.ØX3	T38.ØX4	T38.ØX5	T38.ØX6
ENT agent	T49.6X1	T49.6X2	T49.6X3	T49.6X4	T49.6X5	T49.6X6
ophthalmic preparation	T49.5X1	T49.5X2	T49.5X3	T49.5X4	T49.5X5	T49.5X6
topical NEC	T49.ØX1	T49.ØX2	T49.ØX3	T49.ØX4	T49.ØX5	T49.ØX6
Cortisporin*	T49.ØX1	T49.ØX2	T49.ØX3	T49.ØX4	T49.ØX5	T49.ØX6
Cortivazol	T38.ØX1	T38.ØX2	T38.ØX3	T38.ØX4	T38.ØX5	T38.ØX6

Substance	Poisoning, Accidental (unintentional)	Poisoning, Intentional Self-harm	Poisoning, Assault	Poisoning, Undetermined	Adverse Effect	Under-dosing
Cortogen	T38.ØX1	T38.ØX2	T38.ØX3	T38.ØX4	T38.ØX5	T38.ØX6
ENT agent	T49.6X1	T49.6X2	T49.6X3	T49.6X4	T49.6X5	T49.6X6
ophthalmic preparation	T49.5X1	T49.5X2	T49.5X3	T49.5X4	T49.5X5	T49.5X6
Cortone	T38.ØX1	T38.ØX2	T38.ØX3	T38.ØX4	T38.ØX5	T38.ØX6
ENT agent	T49.6X1	T49.6X2	T49.6X3	T49.6X4	T49.6X5	T49.6X6
ophthalmic preparation	T49.5X1	T49.5X2	T49.5X3	T49.5X4	T49.5X5	T49.5X6
Cortril	T38.ØX1	T38.ØX2	T38.ØX3	T38.ØX4	T38.ØX5	T38.ØX6
ENT agent	T49.6X1	T49.6X2	T49.6X3	T49.6X4	T49.6X5	T49.6X6
ophthalmic preparation	T49.5X1	T49.5X2	T49.5X3	T49.5X4	T49.5X5	T49.5X6
topical NEC	T49.ØX1	T49.ØX2	T49.ØX3	T49.ØX4	T49.ØX5	T49.ØX6
Corynebacterium parvum	T45.1X1	T45.1X2	T45.1X3	T45.1X4	T45.1X5	T45.1X6
Cosmetic preparation	T49.8X1	T49.8X2	T49.8X3	T49.8X4	T49.8X5	T49.8X6
Cosmetics	T49.8X1	T49.8X2	T49.8X3	T49.8X4	T49.8X5	T49.8X6
Cosyntropin	T38.811	T38.812	T38.813	T38.814	T38.815	T38.816
Cotarnine	T45.7X1	T45.7X2	T45.7X3	T45.7X4	T45.7X5	T45.7X6
Co-trimoxazole	T36.8X1	T36.8X2	T36.8X3	T36.8X4	T36.8X5	T36.8X6
Cottonseed oil	T49.3X1	T49.3X2	T49.3X3	T49.3X4	T49.3X5	T49.3X6
Cough mixture (syrup)	T48.4X1	T48.4X2	T48.4X3	T48.4X4	T48.4X5	T48.4X6
containing opiates	T4Ø.2X1	T4Ø.2X2	T4Ø.2X3	T4Ø.2X4	T4Ø.2X5	T4Ø.2X6
expectorants	T48.4X1	T48.4X2	T48.4X3	T48.4X4	T48.4X5	T48.4X6
Coumadin	T45.511	T45.512	T45.513	T45.514	T45.515	T45.516
rodenticide	T6Ø.4X1	T6Ø.4X2	T6Ø.4X3	T6Ø.4X4	—	—
Coumaphos	T6Ø.ØX1	T6Ø.ØX2	T6Ø.ØX3	T6Ø.ØX4	—	—
Coumarin	T45.511	T45.512	T45.513	T45.514	T45.515	T45.516
Coumetarol	T45.511	T45.512	T45.513	T45.514	T45.515	T45.516
Cowbane	T62.2X1	T62.2X2	T62.2X3	T62.2X4	—	—
Cozyme	T45.2X1	T45.2X2	T45.2X3	T45.2X4	T45.2X5	T45.2X6
Crack	T4Ø.5X1	T4Ø.5X2	T4Ø.5X3	T4Ø.5X4	—	—
Crataegus extract	T46.ØX1	T46.ØX2	T46.ØX3	T46.ØX4	T46.ØX5	T46.ØX6
Creolin	T54.1X1	T54.1X2	T54.1X3	T54.1X4	—	—
disinfectant	T54.1X1	T54.1X2	T54.1X3	T54.1X4	—	—
Creosol (compound)	T49.ØX1	T49.ØX2	T49.ØX3	T49.ØX4	T49.ØX5	T49.ØX6
Creosote (coal tar) (beechwood)	T49.ØX1	T49.ØX2	T49.ØX3	T49.ØX4	T49.ØX5	T49.ØX6
medicinal (expectorant)	T48.4X1	T48.4X2	T48.4X3	T48.4X4	T48.4X5	T48.4X6
syrup	T48.4X1	T48.4X2	T48.4X3	T48.4X4	T48.4X5	T48.4X6
Cresol(s)	T49.ØX1	T49.ØX2	T49.ØX3	T49.ØX4	T49.ØX5	T49.ØX6
and soap solution	T49.ØX1	T49.ØX2	T49.ØX3	T49.ØX4	T49.ØX5	T49.ØX6
Crestor*	T46.6X1	T46.6X2	T46.6X3	T46.6X4	T46.6X5	T46.6X6
Cresyl acetate	T49.ØX1	T49.ØX2	T49.ØX3	T49.ØX4	T49.ØX5	T49.ØX6
Cresylic acid	T49.ØX1	T49.ØX2	T49.ØX3	T49.ØX4	T49.ØX5	T49.ØX6
Crimidine	T6Ø.4X1	T6Ø.4X2	T6Ø.4X3	T6Ø.4X4	—	—
Croconazole	T37.8X1	T37.8X2	T37.8X3	T37.8X4	T37.8X5	T37.8X6
Cromoglicic acid	T48.6X1	T48.6X2	T48.6X3	T48.6X4	T48.6X5	T48.6X6
Cromolyn	T48.6X1	T48.6X2	T48.6X3	T48.6X4	T48.6X5	T48.6X6
Cromonar	T46.3X1	T46.3X2	T46.3X3	T46.3X4	T46.3X5	T46.3X6
Cropropamide	T39.8X1	T39.8X2	T39.8X3	T39.8X4	T39.8X5	T39.8X6
with crotethamide	T5Ø.7X1	T5Ø.7X2	T5Ø.7X3	T5Ø.7X4	T5Ø.7X5	T5Ø.7X6
Crotamiton	T49.ØX1	T49.ØX2	T49.ØX3	T49.ØX4	T49.ØX5	T49.ØX6
Crotethamide	T39.8X1	T39.8X2	T39.8X3	T39.8X4	T39.8X5	T39.8X6
with cropropamide	T5Ø.7X1	T5Ø.7X2	T5Ø.7X3	T5Ø.7X4	T5Ø.7X5	T5Ø.7X6
Croton (oil)	T47.2X1	T47.2X2	T47.2X3	T47.2X4	T47.2X5	T47.2X6
chloral	T42.6X1	T42.6X2	T42.6X3	T42.6X4	T42.6X5	T42.6X6
Crude oil	T52.ØX1	T52.ØX2	T52.ØX3	T52.ØX4	—	—
Cryogenine	T39.8X1	T39.8X2	T39.8X3	T39.8X4	T39.8X5	T39.8X6
Cryolite (vapor)	T6Ø.1X1	T6Ø.1X2	T6Ø.1X3	T6Ø.1X4	—	—
insecticide	T6Ø.1X1	T6Ø.1X2	T6Ø.1X3	T6Ø.1X4	—	—
Cryptenamine (tannates)	T46.5X1	T46.5X2	T46.5X3	T46.5X4	T46.5X5	T46.5X6
Crystal violet	T49.ØX1	T49.ØX2	T49.ØX3	T49.ØX4	T49.ØX5	T49.ØX6
Cuckoopint	T62.2X1	T62.2X2	T62.2X3	T62.2X4	—	—
Cumetharol	T45.511	T45.512	T45.513	T45.514	T45.515	T45.516
Cupric						
acetate	T6Ø.3X1	T6Ø.3X2	T6Ø.3X3	T6Ø.3X4	—	—
acetoarsenite	T57.ØX1	T57.ØX2	T57.ØX3	T57.ØX4	—	—
arsenate	T57.ØX1	T57.ØX2	T57.ØX3	T57.ØX4	—	—
gluconate	T49.ØX1	T49.ØX2	T49.ØX3	T49.ØX4	T49.ØX5	T49.ØX6
oleate	T49.ØX1	T49.ØX2	T49.ØX3	T49.ØX4	T49.ØX5	T49.ØX6
sulfate	T56.4X1	T56.4X2	T56.4X3	T56.4X4	—	—
Cuprimine*	T5Ø.6X1	T5Ø.6X2	T5Ø.6X3	T5Ø.6X4	T5Ø.6X5	T5Ø.6X6
Cuprous sulfate — *see also* Copper, sulfate	T56.4X1	T56.4X2	T56.4X3	T56.4X4	—	—
Curare, curarine	T48.1X1	T48.1X2	T48.1X3	T48.1X4	T48.1X5	T48.1X6
Cyamemazine	T43.3X1	T43.3X2	T43.3X3	T43.3X4	T43.3X5	T43.3X6
Cyamopsis tetragonoloba	T46.6X1	T46.6X2	T46.6X3	T46.6X4	T46.6X5	T46.6X6
Cyanacetyl hydrazide	T37.1X1	T37.1X2	T37.1X3	T37.1X4	T37.1X5	T37.1X6
Cyanic acid (gas)	T59.891	T59.892	T59.893	T59.894	—	—
Cyanide(s) (compounds) (potassium) (sodium) **NEC**	T65.ØX1	T65.ØX2	T65.ØX3	T65.ØX4	—	—
dust or gas (inhalation) NEC	T57.3X1	T57.3X2	T57.3X3	T57.3X4	—	—
fumigant	T65.ØX1	T65.ØX2	T65.ØX3	T65.ØX4	—	—
hydrogen	T57.3X1	T57.3X2	T57.3X3	T57.3X4	—	—

Substance	Poisoning, Accidental (unintentional)	Poisoning, Intentional Self-harm	Poisoning, Assault	Poisoning, Undetermined	Adverse Effect	Under-dosing
Cyanide(s) (compounds) (potassium) (sodium) **NEC** — *continued*						
mercuric — *see* Mercury						
pesticide (dust) (fumes)	T65.ØX1	T65.ØX2	T65.ØX3	T65.ØX4	—	—
Cyanoacrylate adhesive	T49.3X1	T49.3X2	T49.3X3	T49.3X4	T49.3X5	T49.3X6
Cyanocobalamin	T45.8X1	T45.8X2	T45.8X3	T45.8X4	T45.8X5	T45.8X6
Cyanogen (chloride) (gas) **NEC**	T59.891	T59.892	T59.893	T59.894	—	—
Cyclacillin	T36.ØX1	T36.ØX2	T36.ØX3	T36.ØX4	T36.ØX5	T36.ØX6
Cyclaine	T41.3X1	T41.3X2	T41.3X3	T41.3X4	T41.3X5	T41.3X6
Cyclamate	T5Ø.991	T5Ø.992	T5Ø.993	T5Ø.994	T5Ø.995	T5Ø.996
Cyclamen europaeum	T62.2X1	T62.2X2	T62.2X3	T62.2X4	—	—
Cyclandelate	T46.7X1	T46.7X2	T46.7X3	T46.7X4	T46.7X5	T46.7X6
Cyclazocine	T5Ø.7X1	T5Ø.7X2	T5Ø.7X3	T5Ø.7X4	T5Ø.7X5	T5Ø.7X6
Cyclizine	T45.ØX1	T45.ØX2	T45.ØX3	T45.ØX4	T45.ØX5	T45.ØX6
Cyclobarbital	T42.3X1	T42.3X2	T42.3X3	T42.3X4	T42.3X5	T42.3X6
Cyclobarbitone	T42.3X1	T42.3X2	T42.3X3	T42.3X4	T42.3X5	T42.3X6
Cyclobenzaprine	T48.1X1	T48.1X2	T48.1X3	T48.1X4	T48.1X5	T48.1X6
Cyclodrine	T44.3X1	T44.3X2	T44.3X3	T44.3X4	T44.3X5	T44.3X6
Cycloguanil embonate	T37.2X1	T37.2X2	T37.2X3	T37.2X4	T37.2X5	T37.2X6
Cyclohexane	T52.8X1	T52.8X2	T52.8X3	T52.8X4	—	—
Cyclohexanol	T51.8X1	T51.8X2	T51.8X3	T51.8X4	—	—
Cyclohexanone	T52.4X1	T52.4X2	T52.4X3	T52.4X4	—	—
Cycloheximide	T6Ø.3X1	T6Ø.3X2	T6Ø.3X3	T6Ø.3X4	—	—
Cyclohexyl acetate	T52.8X1	T52.8X2	T52.8X3	T52.8X4	—	—
Cycloleucin	T45.1X1	T45.1X2	T45.1X3	T45.1X4	T45.1X5	T45.1X6
Cyclomethycaine	T41.3X1	T41.3X2	T41.3X3	T41.3X4	T41.3X5	T41.3X6
Cyclopentamine	T44.4X1	T44.4X2	T44.4X3	T44.4X4	T44.4X5	T44.4X6
Cyclopenthiazide	T5Ø.2X1	T5Ø.2X2	T5Ø.2X3	T5Ø.2X4	T5Ø.2X5	T5Ø.2X6
Cyclopentolate	T44.3X1	T44.3X2	T44.3X3	T44.3X4	T44.3X5	T44.3X6
Cyclophosphamide	T45.1X1	T45.1X2	T45.1X3	T45.1X4	T45.1X5	T45.1X6
Cycloplegic drug	T49.5X1	T49.5X2	T49.5X3	T49.5X4	T49.5X5	T49.5X6
Cyclopropane	T41.291	T41.292	T41.293	T41.294	T41.295	T41.296
Cyclopyrabital	T39.8X1	T39.8X2	T39.8X3	T39.8X4	T39.8X5	T39.8X6
Cycloserine	T37.1X1	T37.1X2	T37.1X3	T37.1X4	T37.1X5	T37.1X6
Cyclosporin	T45.1X1	T45.1X2	T45.1X3	T45.1X4	T45.1X5	T45.1X6
Cyclothiazide	T5Ø.2X1	T5Ø.2X2	T5Ø.2X3	T5Ø.2X4	T5Ø.2X5	T5Ø.2X6
Cycrimine	T44.3X1	T44.3X2	T44.3X3	T44.3X4	T44.3X5	T44.3X6
Cyhalothrin	T6Ø.1X1	T6Ø.1X2	T6Ø.1X3	T6Ø.1X4	—	—
Cymarin	T46.ØX1	T46.ØX2	T46.ØX3	T46.ØX4	T46.ØX5	T46.ØX6
Cypermethrin	T6Ø.1X1	T6Ø.1X2	T6Ø.1X3	T6Ø.1X4	—	—
Cyphenothrin	T6Ø.2X1	T6Ø.2X2	T6Ø.2X3	T6Ø.2X4	—	—
Cyproheptadine	T45.ØX1	T45.ØX2	T45.ØX3	T45.ØX4	T45.ØX5	T45.ØX6
Cyproterone	T38.6X1	T38.6X2	T38.6X3	T38.6X4	T38.6X5	T38.6X6
Cystaran*	T49.5X1	T49.5X2	T49.5X3	T49.5X4	T49.5X5	T49.5X6
Cysteamine	T5Ø.6X1	T5Ø.6X2	T5Ø.6X3	T5Ø.6X4	T5Ø.6X5	T5Ø.6X6
Cytarabine	T45.1X1	T45.1X2	T45.1X3	T45.1X4	T45.1X5	T45.1X6
Cytisus						
laburnum	T62.2X1	T62.2X2	T62.2X3	T62.2X4	—	—
scoparius	T62.2X1	T62.2X2	T62.2X3	T62.2X4	—	—
Cytochrome C	T47.5X1	T47.5X2	T47.5X3	T47.5X4	T47.5X5	T47.5X6
Cytomel	T38.1X1	T38.1X2	T38.1X3	T38.1X4	T38.1X5	T38.1X6
Cytosine arabinoside	T45.1X1	T45.1X2	T45.1X3	T45.1X4	T45.1X5	T45.1X6
Cytoxan	T45.1X1	T45.1X2	T45.1X3	T45.1X4	T45.1X5	T45.1X6
Cytozyme	T45.7X1	T45.7X2	T45.7X3	T45.7X4	T45.7X5	T45.7X6
S-Carboxymethylcysteine	T48.4X1	T48.4X2	T48.4X3	T48.4X4	T48.4X5	T48.4X6
Dabigatran*	T45.511	T45.512	T45.513	T45.514	T45.515	T45.516
Dacarbazine	T45.1X1	T45.1X2	T45.1X3	T45.1X4	T45.1X5	T45.1X6
Dactinomycin	T45.1X1	T45.1X2	T45.1X3	T45.1X4	T45.1X5	T45.1X6
DADPS	T37.1X1	T37.1X2	T37.1X3	T37.1X4	T37.1X5	T37.1X6
Dakin's solution	T49.ØX1	T49.ØX2	T49.ØX3	T49.ØX4	T49.ØX5	T49.ØX6
Dalapon (sodium)	T6Ø.3X1	T6Ø.3X2	T6Ø.3X3	T6Ø.3X4	—	—
Dalmane	T42.4X1	T42.4X2	T42.4X3	T42.4X4	T42.4X5	T42.4X6
Danazol	T38.6X1	T38.6X2	T38.6X3	T38.6X4	T38.6X5	T38.6X6
Danilone	T45.511	T45.512	T45.513	T45.514	T45.515	T45.516
Danthron	T47.2X1	T47.2X2	T47.2X3	T47.2X4	T47.2X5	T47.2X6
Dantrolene	T42.8X1	T42.8X2	T42.8X3	T42.8X4	T42.8X5	T42.8X6
Dantron	T47.2X1	T47.2X2	T47.2X3	T47.2X4	T47.2X5	T47.2X6
Daphne (gnidium) (mezereum)	T62.2X1	T62.2X2	T62.2X3	T62.2X4	—	—
berry	T62.1X1	T62.1X2	T62.1X3	T62.1X4	—	—
Dapsone	T37.1X1	T37.1X2	T37.1X3	T37.1X4	T37.1X5	T37.1X6
Daraprim	T37.2X1	T37.2X2	T37.2X3	T37.2X4	T37.2X5	T37.2X6
Darnel	T62.2X1	T62.2X2	T62.2X3	T62.2X4	—	—
Darvon	T39.8X1	T39.8X2	T39.8X3	T39.8X4	T39.8X5	T39.8X6
Daunomycin	T45.1X1	T45.1X2	T45.1X3	T45.1X4	T45.1X5	T45.1X6
Daunorubicin	T45.1X1	T45.1X2	T45.1X3	T45.1X4	T45.1X5	T45.1X6
DBI	T38.3X1	T38.3X2	T38.3X3	T38.3X4	T38.3X5	T38.3X6
D-Con	T6Ø.91	T6Ø.92	T6Ø.93	T6Ø.94	—	—
insecticide	T6Ø.2X1	T6Ø.2X2	T6Ø.2X3	T6Ø.2X4	—	—
rodenticide	T6Ø.4X1	T6Ø.4X2	T6Ø.4X3	T6Ø.4X4	—	—
DDAVP	T38.891	T38.892	T38.893	T38.894	T38.895	T38.896
DDE (bis(chlorophenyl)-dichloroethylene)	T6Ø.2X1	T6Ø.2X2	T6Ø.2X3	T6Ø.2X4	—	—
DDS	T37.1X1	T37.1X2	T37.1X3	T37.1X4	T37.1X5	T37.1X6
DDT (dust)	T6Ø.1X1	T6Ø.1X2	T6Ø.1X3	T6Ø.1X4	—	—
Deadly nightshade — *see also* Belladonna	T62.2X1	T62.2X2	T62.2X3	T62.2X4	—	—
berry	T62.1X1	T62.1X2	T62.1X3	T62.1X4	—	—
Deamino-D-arginine vasopressin	T38.891	T38.892	T38.893	T38.894	T38.895	T38.896
Deanol (aceglumate)	T5Ø.991	T5Ø.992	T5Ø.993	T5Ø.994	T5Ø.995	T5Ø.996
Debrisoquine	T46.5X1	T46.5X2	T46.5X3	T46.5X4	T46.5X5	T46.5X6
Decaborane	T57.8X1	T57.8X2	T57.8X3	T57.8X4	—	—
fumes	T59.891	T59.892	T59.893	T59.894	—	—
Decadron	T38.ØX1	T38.ØX2	T38.ØX3	T38.ØX4	T38.ØX5	T38.ØX6
ENT agent	T49.6X1	T49.6X2	T49.6X3	T49.6X4	T49.6X5	T49.6X6
ophthalmic preparation	T49.5X1	T49.5X2	T49.5X3	T49.5X4	T49.5X5	T49.5X6
topical NEC	T49.ØX1	T49.ØX2	T49.ØX3	T49.ØX4	T49.ØX5	T49.ØX6
Decahydronaphthalene	T52.8X1	T52.8X2	T52.8X3	T52.8X4	—	—
Decalin	T52.8X1	T52.8X2	T52.8X3	T52.8X4	—	—
Decamethonium (bromide)	T48.1X1	T48.1X2	T48.1X3	T48.1X4	T48.1X5	T48.1X6
Decholin	T47.5X1	T47.5X2	T47.5X3	T47.5X4	T47.5X5	T47.5X6
Declomycin	T36.4X1	T36.4X2	T36.4X3	T36.4X4	T36.4X5	T36.4X6
Decongestant, nasal (mucosa)	T48.5X1	T48.5X2	T48.5X3	T48.5X4	T48.5X5	T48.5X6
combination	T48.5X1	T48.5X2	T48.5X3	T48.5X4	T48.5X5	T48.5X6
Deet	T6Ø.8X1	T6Ø.8X2	T6Ø.8X3	T6Ø.8X4	—	—
Deferoxamine	T45.8X1	T45.8X2	T45.8X3	T45.8X4	T45.8X5	T45.8X6
Deflazacort	T38.ØX1	T38.ØX2	T38.ØX3	T38.ØX4	T38.ØX5	T38.ØX6
Deglycyrrhizinized extract of licorice	T48.4X1	T48.4X2	T48.4X3	T48.4X4	T48.4X5	T48.4X6
Dehydrocholic acid	T47.5X1	T47.5X2	T47.5X3	T47.5X4	T47.5X5	T47.5X6
Dehydroemetine	T37.3X1	T37.3X2	T37.3X3	T37.3X4	T37.3X5	T37.3X6
Dekalin	T52.8X1	T52.8X2	T52.8X3	T52.8X4	—	—
Delafloxacin*	T36.8X1	T36.8X2	T36.8X3	T36.8X4	T36.8X5	T36.8X6
Delalutin	T38.5X1	T38.5X2	T38.5X3	T38.5X4	T38.5X5	T38.5X6
Delorazepam	T42.4X1	T42.4X2	T42.4X3	T42.4X4	T42.4X5	T42.4X6
Delphinium	T62.2X1	T62.2X2	T62.2X3	T62.2X4	—	—
Deltacortisone*	T38.ØX1	T38.ØX2	T38.ØX3	T38.ØX4	T38.ØX5	T38.ØX6
Deltamethrin	T6Ø.1X1	T6Ø.1X2	T6Ø.1X3	T6Ø.1X4	—	—
Deltasone	T38.ØX1	T38.ØX2	T38.ØX3	T38.ØX4	T38.ØX5	T38.ØX6
Deltra	T38.ØX1	T38.ØX2	T38.ØX3	T38.ØX4	T38.ØX5	T38.ØX6
Delvinal	T42.3X1	T42.3X2	T42.3X3	T42.3X4	T42.3X5	T42.3X6
Demecarium (bromide)	T49.5X1	T49.5X2	T49.5X3	T49.5X4	T49.5X5	T49.5X6
Demeclocycline	T36.4X1	T36.4X2	T36.4X3	T36.4X4	T36.4X5	T36.4X6
Demecolcine	T45.1X1	T45.1X2	T45.1X3	T45.1X4	T45.1X5	T45.1X6
Demegestone	T38.5X1	T38.5X2	T38.5X3	T38.5X4	T38.5X5	T38.5X6
Demelanizing agents	T49.8X1	T49.8X2	T49.8X3	T49.8X4	T49.8X5	T49.8X6
Demephion -O and -S	T6Ø.ØX1	T6Ø.ØX2	T6Ø.ØX3	T6Ø.ØX4	—	—
Demerol	T4Ø.2X1	T4Ø.2X2	T4Ø.2X3	T4Ø.2X4	T4Ø.2X5	T4Ø.2X6
Demethylchlortetracycline	T36.4X1	T36.4X2	T36.4X3	T36.4X4	T36.4X5	T36.4X6
Demethyltetracycline	T36.4X1	T36.4X2	T36.4X3	T36.4X4	T36.4X5	T36.4X6
Demeton -O and -S	T6Ø.ØX1	T6Ø.ØX2	T6Ø.ØX3	T6Ø.ØX4	—	—
Demulcent (external)	T49.3X1	T49.3X2	T49.3X3	T49.3X4	T49.3X5	T49.3X6
specified NEC	T49.3X1	T49.3X2	T49.3X3	T49.3X4	T49.3X5	T49.3X6
Demulen	T38.4X1	T38.4X2	T38.4X3	T38.4X4	T38.4X5	T38.4X6
Denatured alcohol	T51.ØX1	T51.ØX2	T51.ØX3	T51.ØX4	—	—
Dendrid	T49.5X1	T49.5X2	T49.5X3	T49.5X4	T49.5X5	T49.5X6
Dental drug, topical application NEC	T49.7X1	T49.7X2	T49.7X3	T49.7X4	T49.7X5	T49.7X6
Dentifrice	T49.7X1	T49.7X2	T49.7X3	T49.7X4	T49.7X5	T49.7X6
Deodorant spray (feminine hygiene)	T49.8X1	T49.8X2	T49.8X3	T49.8X4	T49.8X5	T49.8X6
Deoxycortone	T5Ø.ØX1	T5Ø.ØX2	T5Ø.ØX3	T5Ø.ØX4	T5Ø.ØX5	T5Ø.ØX6
Deoxyribonuclease (pancreatic)	T45.3X1	T45.3X2	T45.3X3	T45.3X4	T45.3X5	T45.3X6
Depilatory	T49.4X1	T49.4X2	T49.4X3	T49.4X4	T49.4X5	T49.4X6
Deprenalin	T42.8X1	T42.8X2	T42.8X3	T42.8X4	T42.8X5	T42.8X6
Deprenyl	T42.8X1	T42.8X2	T42.8X3	T42.8X4	T42.8X5	T42.8X6
Depressant						
appetite (central)	T5Ø.5X1	T5Ø.5X2	T5Ø.5X3	T5Ø.5X4	T5Ø.5X5	T5Ø.5X6
cardiac	T46.2X1	T46.2X2	T46.2X3	T46.2X4	T46.2X5	T46.2X6
central nervous system (anesthetic) — *see also* Central nervous system, depressants	T42.71	T42.72	T42.73	T42.74	T42.75	T42.76
general anesthetic	T41.2Ø1	T41.2Ø2	T41.2Ø3	T41.2Ø4	T41.2Ø5	T41.2Ø6
muscle tone	T42.8X1	T42.8X2	T42.8X3	T42.8X4	T42.8X5	T42.8X6
muscle tone, central	T42.8X1	T42.8X2	T42.8X3	T42.8X4	T42.8X5	T42.8X6
psychotherapeutic	T43.5Ø1	T43.5Ø2	T43.5Ø3	T43.5Ø4	T43.5Ø5	T43.5Ø6
Depressant, appetite	T5Ø.5X1	T5Ø.5X2	T5Ø.5X3	T5Ø.5X4	T5Ø.5X5	T5Ø.5X6
Deptropine	T45.ØX1	T45.ØX2	T45.ØX3	T45.ØX4	T45.ØX5	T45.ØX6
Dequalinium (chloride)	T49.ØX1	T49.ØX2	T49.ØX3	T49.ØX4	T49.ØX5	T49.ØX6
Derris root	T6Ø.2X1	T6Ø.2X2	T6Ø.2X3	T6Ø.2X4	—	—

*Optum Value-Add

Substance	Poisoning, Accidental (unintentional)	Poisoning, Intentional Self-harm	Poisoning, Assault	Poisoning, Undetermined	Adverse Effect	Under-dosing
Deserpidine	T46.5X1	T46.5X2	T46.5X3	T46.5X4	T46.5X5	T46.5X6
Desferrioxamine	T45.8X1	T45.8X2	T45.8X3	T45.8X4	T45.8X5	T45.8X6
Desipramine	T43.Ø11	T43.Ø12	T43.Ø13	T43.Ø14	T43.Ø15	T43.Ø16
Deslanoside	T46.ØX1	T46.ØX2	T46.ØX3	T46.ØX4	T46.ØX5	T46.ØX6
Desloughing agent	T49.4X1	T49.4X2	T49.4X3	T49.4X4	T49.4X5	T49.4X6
Desmethylimipramine	T43.Ø11	T43.Ø12	T43.Ø13	T43.Ø14	T43.Ø15	T43.Ø16
Desmopressin	T38.891	T38.892	T38.893	T38.894	T38.895	T38.896
Desocodeine	T4Ø.2X1	T4Ø.2X2	T4Ø.2X3	T4Ø.2X4	T4Ø.2X5	T4Ø.2X6
Desogestrel	T38.5X1	T38.5X2	T38.5X3	T38.5X4	T38.5X5	T38.5X6
Desomorphine	T4Ø.2X1	T4Ø.2X2	T4Ø.2X3	T4Ø.2X4	—	—
Desonide	T49.ØX1	T49.ØX2	T49.ØX3	T49.ØX4	T49.ØX5	T49.ØX6
Desoximetasone	T49.ØX1	T49.ØX2	T49.ØX3	T49.ØX4	T49.ØX5	T49.ØX6
Desoxycorticosteroid	T5Ø.ØX1	T5Ø.ØX2	T5Ø.ØX3	T5Ø.ØX4	T5Ø.ØX5	T5Ø.ØX6
Desoxycortone	T5Ø.ØX1	T5Ø.ØX2	T5Ø.ØX3	T5Ø.ØX4	T5Ø.ØX5	T5Ø.ØX6
Desoxyephedrine	T43.651	T43.652	T43.652	T43.654	T43.655	T43.656
Detaxtran	T46.6X1	T46.6X2	T46.6X3	T46.6X4	T46.6X5	T46.6X6
Detergent	T49.2X1	T49.2X2	T49.2X3	T49.2X4	T49.2X5	T49.2X6
external medication	T49.2X1	T49.2X2	T49.2X3	T49.2X4	T49.2X5	T49.2X6
local	T49.2X1	T49.2X2	T49.2X3	T49.2X4	T49.2X5	T49.2X6
medicinal	T49.2X1	T49.2X2	T49.2X3	T49.2X4	T49.2X5	T49.2X6
nonmedicinal	T55.1X1	T55.1X2	T55.1X3	T55.1X4	—	—
specified NEC	T55.1X1	T55.1X2	T55.1X3	T55.1X4	—	—
Deterrent, alcohol	T5Ø.6X1	T5Ø.6X2	T5Ø.6X3	T5Ø.6X4	T5Ø.6X5	T5Ø.6X6
Detoxifying agent	T5Ø.6X1	T5Ø.6X2	T5Ø.6X3	T5Ø.6X4	T5Ø.6X5	T5Ø.6X6
Detrothyronine	T38.1X1	T38.1X2	T38.1X3	T38.1X4	T38.1X5	T38.1X6
Dettol (external medication)	T49.ØX1	T49.ØX2	T49.ØX3	T49.ØX4	T49.ØX5	T49.ØX6
Dexamethasone	T38.ØX1	T38.ØX2	T38.ØX3	T38.ØX4	T38.ØX5	T38.ØX6
ENT agent	T49.6X1	T49.6X2	T49.6X3	T49.6X4	T49.6X5	T49.6X6
ophthalmic preparation	T49.5X1	T49.5X2	T49.5X3	T49.5X4	T49.5X5	T49.5X6
topical NEC	T49.ØX1	T49.ØX2	T49.ØX3	T49.ØX4	T49.ØX5	T49.ØX6
Dexamfetamine	T43.621	T43.622	T43.623	T43.624	T43.625	T43.626
Dexamphetamine	T43.621	T43.622	T43.623	T43.624	T43.625	T43.626
Dexbrompheniramine	T45.ØX1	T45.ØX2	T45.ØX3	T45.ØX4	T45.ØX5	T45.ØX6
Dexchlorpheniramine	T45.ØX1	T45.ØX2	T45.ØX3	T45.ØX4	T45.ØX5	T45.ØX6
Dexedrine	T43.621	T43.622	T43.623	T43.624	T43.625	T43.626
Dexetimide	T44.3X1	T44.3X2	T44.3X3	T44.3X4	T44.3X5	T44.3X6
Dexfenfluramine	T5Ø.5X1	T5Ø.5X2	T5Ø.5X3	T5Ø.5X4	T5Ø.5X5	T5Ø.5X6
Dexpanthenol	T45.2X1	T45.2X2	T45.2X3	T45.2X4	T45.2X5	T45.2X6
Dextran (40) (70) (150)	T45.8X1	T45.8X2	T45.8X3	T45.8X4	T45.8X5	T45.8X6
Dextriferron	T45.4X1	T45.4X2	T45.4X3	T45.4X4	T45.4X5	T45.4X6
Dextroamphetamine	T43.621	T43.622	T43.623	T43.624	T43.625	T43.626
Dextro calcium pantothenate	T45.2X1	T45.2X2	T45.2X3	T45.2X4	T45.2X5	T45.2X6
Dextromethorphan	T48.3X1	T48.3X2	T48.3X3	T48.3X4	T48.3X5	T48.3X6
Dextromoramide	T4Ø.491	T4Ø.492	T4Ø.493	T4Ø.494	—	—
topical	T49.8X1	T49.8X2	T49.8X3	T49.8X4	T49.8X5	T49.8X6
Dextro pantothenyl alcohol	T45.2X1	T45.2X2	T45.2X3	T45.2X4	T45.2X5	T45.2X6
Dextropropoxyphene	T4Ø.491	T4Ø.492	T4Ø.493	T4Ø.494	T4Ø.495	T4Ø.496
Dextrorphan	T4Ø.2X1	T4Ø.2X2	T4Ø.2X3	T4Ø.2X4	T4Ø.2X5	T4Ø.2X6
Dextrose	T5Ø.3X1	T5Ø.3X2	T5Ø.3X3	T5Ø.3X4	T5Ø.3X5	T5Ø.3X6
concentrated solution, intravenous	T46.8X1	T46.8X2	T46.8X3	T46.8X4	T46.8X5	T46.8X6
Dextrothyroxin	T38.1X1	T38.1X2	T38.1X3	T38.1X4	T38.1X5	T38.1X6
Dextrothyroxine sodium	T38.1X1	T38.1X2	T38.1X3	T38.1X4	T38.1X5	T38.1X6
DFP	T44.ØX1	T44.ØX2	T44.ØX3	T44.ØX4	T44.ØX5	T44.ØX6
DHE	T37.3X1	T37.3X2	T37.3X3	T37.3X4	T37.3X5	T37.3X6
45	T46.5X1	T46.5X2	T46.5X3	T46.5X4	T46.5X5	T46.5X6
DiaBeta*	T38.3X1	T38.3X2	T38.3X3	T38.3X4	T38.3X5	T38.3X6
Diabinese	T38.3X1	T38.3X2	T38.3X3	T38.3X4	T38.3X5	T38.3X6
Diacetone alcohol	T52.4X1	T52.4X2	T52.4X3	T52.4X4	—	—
Diacetyl monoxime	T5Ø.991	T5Ø.992	T5Ø.993	T5Ø.994	—	—
Diacetylmorphine	T4Ø.1X1	T4Ø.1X2	T4Ø.1X3	T4Ø.1X4	—	—
Diachylon plaster	T49.4X1	T49.4X2	T49.4X3	T49.4X4	T49.4X5	T49.4X6
Diaethylstilboestrolum	T38.5X1	T38.5X2	T38.5X3	T38.5X4	T38.5X5	T38.5X6
Diagnostic agent NEC	T5Ø.8X1	T5Ø.8X2	T5Ø.8X3	T5Ø.8X4	T5Ø.8X5	T5Ø.8X6
Dial (soap)	T49.2X1	T49.2X2	T49.2X3	T49.2X4	T49.2X5	T49.2X6
sedative	T42.3X1	T42.3X2	T42.3X3	T42.3X4	T42.3X5	T42.3X6
Dialkyl carbonate	T52.91	T52.92	T52.93	T52.94	—	—
Diallylbarbituric acid	T42.3X1	T42.3X2	T42.3X3	T42.3X4	T42.3X5	T42.3X6
Diallymal	T42.3X1	T42.3X2	T42.3X3	T42.3X4	T42.3X5	T42.3X6
Dialysis solution (intraperitoneal)	T5Ø.3X1	T5Ø.3X2	T5Ø.3X3	T5Ø.3X4	T5Ø.3X5	T5Ø.3X6
Diaminodiphenylsulfone	T37.1X1	T37.1X2	T37.1X3	T37.1X4	T37.1X5	T37.1X6
Diamorphine	T4Ø.1X1	T4Ø.1X2	T4Ø.1X3	T4Ø.1X4	—	—
Diamox	T5Ø.2X1	T5Ø.2X2	T5Ø.2X3	T5Ø.2X4	T5Ø.2X5	T5Ø.2X6
Diamthazole	T49.ØX1	T49.ØX2	T49.ØX3	T49.ØX4	T49.ØX5	T49.ØX6
Dianthone	T47.2X1	T47.2X2	T47.2X3	T47.2X4	T47.2X5	T47.2X6
Diaphenylsulfone	T37.ØX1	T37.ØX2	T37.ØX3	T37.ØX4	T37.ØX5	T37.ØX6
Diasone (sodium)	T37.1X1	T37.1X2	T37.1X3	T37.1X4	T37.1X5	T37.1X6
Diastase	T47.5X1	T47.5X2	T47.5X3	T47.5X4	T47.5X5	T47.5X6
Diastat*	T42.4X1	T42.4X2	T42.4X3	T42.4X4	T42.4X5	T42.4X6
Diatrizoate	T5Ø.8X1	T5Ø.8X2	T5Ø.8X3	T5Ø.8X4	T5Ø.8X5	T5Ø.8X6
Diazepam	T42.4X1	T42.4X2	T42.4X3	T42.4X4	T42.4X5	T42.4X6
Diazinon	T6Ø.ØX1	T6Ø.ØX2	T6Ø.ØX3	T6Ø.ØX4	—	—
Diazomethane (gas)	T59.891	T59.892	T59.893	T59.894	—	—
Diazoxide	T46.5X1	T46.5X2	T46.5X3	T46.5X4	T46.5X5	T46.5X6
Dibekacin	T36.5X1	T36.5X2	T36.5X3	T36.5X4	T36.5X5	T36.5X6
Dibenamine	T44.6X1	T44.6X2	T44.6X3	T44.6X4	T44.6X5	T44.6X6
Dibenzepin	T43.Ø11	T43.Ø12	T43.Ø13	T43.Ø14	T43.Ø15	T43.Ø16
Dibenzheptropine	T45.ØX1	T45.ØX2	T45.ØX3	T45.ØX4	T45.ØX5	T45.ØX6
Dibenzyline	T44.6X1	T44.6X2	T44.6X3	T44.6X4	T44.6X5	T44.6X6
Diborane (gas)	T59.891	T59.892	T59.893	T59.894	—	—
Dibromochloropropane	T6Ø.8X1	T6Ø.8X2	T6Ø.8X3	T6Ø.8X4	—	—
Dibromodulcitol	T45.1X1	T45.1X2	T45.1X3	T45.1X4	T45.1X5	T45.1X6
Dibromoethane	T53.6X1	T53.6X2	T53.6X3	T53.6X4	—	—
Dibromomannitol	T45.1X1	T45.1X2	T45.1X3	T45.1X4	T45.1X5	T45.1X6
Dibromopropamidine isethionate	T49.ØX1	T49.ØX2	T49.ØX3	T49.ØX4	T49.ØX5	T49.ØX6
Dibrompropamidine	T49.ØX1	T49.ØX2	T49.ØX3	T49.ØX4	T49.ØX5	T49.ØX6
Dibucaine	T41.3X1	T41.3X2	T41.3X3	T41.3X4	T41.3X5	T41.3X6
topical (surface)	T41.3X1	T41.3X2	T41.3X3	T41.3X4	T41.3X5	T41.3X6
Dibunate sodium	T48.3X1	T48.3X2	T48.3X3	T48.3X4	T48.3X5	T48.3X6
Dibutoline sulfate	T44.3X1	T44.3X2	T44.3X3	T44.3X4	T44.3X5	T44.3X6
Dicamba	T6Ø.3X1	T6Ø.3X2	T6Ø.3X3	T6Ø.3X4	—	—
Dicapthon	T6Ø.ØX1	T6Ø.ØX2	T6Ø.ØX3	T6Ø.ØX4	—	—
Dichlobenil	T6Ø.3X1	T6Ø.3X2	T6Ø.3X3	T6Ø.3X4	—	—
Dichlone	T6Ø.3X1	T6Ø.3X2	T6Ø.3X3	T6Ø.3X4	—	—
Dichloralphenozone	T42.6X1	T42.6X2	T42.6X3	T42.6X4	T42.6X5	T42.6X6
Dichlorbenzidine	T65.3X1	T65.3X2	T65.3X3	T65.3X4	—	—
Dichlorhydrin	T52.8X1	T52.8X2	T52.8X3	T52.8X4	—	—
Dichlorhydroxyquinoline	T37.8X1	T37.8X2	T37.8X3	T37.8X4	T37.8X5	T37.8X6
Dichlorobenzene	T53.7X1	T53.7X2	T53.7X3	T53.7X4	—	—
Dichlorobenzyl alcohol	T49.6X1	T49.6X2	T49.6X3	T49.6X4	T49.6X5	T49.6X6
Dichlorodifluoromethane	T53.5X1	T53.5X2	T53.5X3	T53.5X4	—	—
Dichloroethane	T52.8X1	T52.8X2	T52.8X3	T52.8X4	—	—
Dichloroethylene	T53.6X1	T53.6X2	T53.6X3	T53.6X4	—	—
Dichloroethyl sulfide, not in war	T59.891	T59.892	T59.893	T59.894	—	—
Dichloroformoxine, not in war	T59.891	T59.892	T59.893	T59.894	—	—
Dichlorohydrin, alpha-dichlorohydrin	T52.8X1	T52.8X2	T52.8X3	T52.8X4	—	—
Dichloromethane (solvent)	T53.4X1	T53.4X2	T53.4X3	T53.4X4	—	—
vapor	T53.4X1	T53.4X2	T53.4X3	T53.4X4	—	—
Dichloronaphthoquinone	T6Ø.3X1	T6Ø.3X2	T6Ø.3X3	T6Ø.3X4	—	—
Dichlorophen	T37.4X1	T37.4X2	T37.4X3	T37.4X4	T37.4X5	T37.4X6
Dichloropropene	T6Ø.3X1	T6Ø.3X2	T6Ø.3X3	T6Ø.3X4	—	—
Dichloropropionic acid	T6Ø.3X1	T6Ø.3X2	T6Ø.3X3	T6Ø.3X4	—	—
Dichlorphenamide	T5Ø.2X1	T5Ø.2X2	T5Ø.2X3	T5Ø.2X4	T5Ø.2X5	T5Ø.2X6
Dichlorvos	T6Ø.ØX1	T6Ø.ØX2	T6Ø.ØX3	T6Ø.ØX4	—	—
Dichysterol*	T45.2X1	T45.2X2	T45.2X3	T45.2X4	T45.2X5	T45.2X6
Diclofenac	T39.391	T39.392	T39.393	T39.394	T39.395	T39.396
Diclofenamide	T5Ø.2X1	T5Ø.2X2	T5Ø.2X3	T5Ø.2X4	T5Ø.2X5	T5Ø.2X6
Diclofensine	T43.291	T43.292	T43.293	T43.294	T43.295	T43.296
Diclonixine	T39.8X1	T39.8X2	T39.8X3	T39.8X4	T39.8X5	T39.8X6
Dicloxacillin	T36.ØX1	T36.ØX2	T36.ØX3	T36.ØX4	T36.ØX5	T36.ØX6
Dicophane	T49.ØX1	T49.ØX2	T49.ØX3	T49.ØX4	T49.ØX5	T49.ØX6
Dicoumarol, dicoumarin, dicumarol	T45.511	T45.512	T45.513	T45.514	T45.515	T45.516
Dicrotophos	T6Ø.ØX1	T6Ø.ØX2	T6Ø.ØX3	T6Ø.ØX4	—	—
Dicyanogen (gas)	T65.ØX1	T65.ØX2	T65.ØX3	T65.ØX4	—	—
Dicyclomine	T44.3X1	T44.3X2	T44.3X3	T44.3X4	T44.3X5	T44.3X6
Dicycloverine	T44.3X1	T44.3X2	T44.3X3	T44.3X4	T44.3X5	T44.3X6
Didanosine*	T37.5X1	T37.5X2	T37.5X3	T37.5X4	T37.5X5	T37.5X6
Dideoxycytidine	T37.5X1	T37.5X2	T37.5X3	T37.5X4	T37.5X5	T37.5X6
Dideoxyinosine	T37.5X1	T37.5X2	T37.5X3	T37.5X4	T37.5X5	T37.5X6
Dieldrin (vapor)	T6Ø.1X1	T6Ø.1X2	T6Ø.1X3	T6Ø.1X4	—	—
Diemal	T42.3X1	T42.3X2	T42.3X3	T42.3X4	T42.3X5	T42.3X6
Dienestrol	T38.5X1	T38.5X2	T38.5X3	T38.5X4	T38.5X5	T38.5X6
Dienoestrol	T38.5X1	T38.5X2	T38.5X3	T38.5X4	T38.5X5	T38.5X6
Dietetic drug NEC	T5Ø.9Ø1	T5Ø.9Ø2	T5Ø.9Ø3	T5Ø.9Ø4	T5Ø.9Ø5	T5Ø.9Ø6
Diethazine	T42.8X1	T42.8X2	T42.8X3	T42.8X4	T42.8X5	T42.8X6
Diethyl						
barbituric acid	T42.3X1	T42.3X2	T42.3X3	T42.3X4	T42.3X5	T42.3X6
carbamazine	T37.4X1	T37.4X2	T37.4X3	T37.4X4	T37.4X5	T37.4X6
carbinol	T51.3X1	T51.3X2	T51.3X3	T51.3X4	—	—
carbonate	T52.8X1	T52.8X2	T52.8X3	T52.8X4	—	—
ether (vapor) — *see also* ether	T41.ØX1	T41.ØX2	T41.ØX3	T41.ØX4	T41.ØX5	T41.ØX6
oxide	T52.8X1	T52.8X2	T52.8X3	T52.8X4	—	—
propion	T5Ø.5X1	T5Ø.5X2	T5Ø.5X3	T5Ø.5X4	T5Ø.5X5	T5Ø.5X6
stilbestrol	T38.5X1	T38.5X2	T38.5X3	T38.5X4	T38.5X5	T38.5X6
toluamide (nonmedicinal)	T6Ø.8X1	T6Ø.8X2	T6Ø.8X3	T6Ø.8X4	—	—
medicinal	T49.3X1	T49.3X2	T49.3X3	T49.3X4	T49.3X5	T49.3X6
Diethylcarbamazine	T37.4X1	T37.4X2	T37.4X3	T37.4X4	T37.4X5	T37.4X6

Substance	Poisoning, Accidental (unintentional)	Poisoning, Intentional Self-harm	Poisoning, Assault	Poisoning, Undetermined	Adverse Effect	Under-dosing
Diethylene						
dioxide	T52.8X1	T52.8X2	T52.8X3	T52.8X4	—	—
glycol (monoacetate)	T52.3X1	T52.3X2	T52.3X3	T52.3X4	—	—
(monobutyl ether)						
(monoethyl ether)						
Diethylhexylphthalate	T65.891	T65.892	T65.893	T65.894	—	—
Diethylpropion	T5Ø.5X1	T5Ø.5X2	T5Ø.5X3	T5Ø.5X4	T5Ø.5X5	T5Ø.5X6
Diethylstilbestrol	T38.5X1	T38.5X2	T38.5X3	T38.5X4	T38.5X5	T38.5X6
Diethylstilboestrol	T38.5X1	T38.5X2	T38.5X3	T38.5X4	T38.5X5	T38.5X6
Diethylsulfone-diethylmethane	T42.6X1	T42.6X2	T42.6X3	T42.6X4	T42.6X5	T42.6X6
Diethyltoluamide	T49.ØX1	T49.ØX2	T49.ØX3	T49.ØX4	T49.ØX5	T49.ØX6
Diethyltryptamine (DET)	T4Ø.991	T4Ø.992	T4Ø.993	T4Ø.994	—	—
Difebarbamate	T42.3X1	T42.3X2	T42.3X3	T42.3X4	T42.3X5	T42.3X6
Difencloxazine	T4Ø.2X1	T4Ø.2X2	T4Ø.2X3	T4Ø.2X4	T4Ø.2X5	T4Ø.2X6
Difenidol	T45.ØX1	T45.ØX2	T45.ØX3	T45.ØX4	T45.ØX5	T45.ØX6
Difenoxin	T47.6X1	T47.6X2	T47.6X3	T47.6X4	T47.6X5	T47.6X6
Difetarsone	T37.3X1	T37.3X2	T37.3X3	T37.3X4	T37.3X5	T37.3X6
Diffusin	T45.3X1	T45.3X2	T45.3X3	T45.3X4	T45.3X5	T45.3X6
Diflorasone	T49.ØX1	T49.ØX2	T49.ØX3	T49.ØX4	T49.ØX5	T49.ØX6
Diflos	T44.ØX1	T44.ØX2	T44.ØX3	T44.ØX4	T44.ØX5	T44.ØX6
Diflubenzuron	T6Ø.1X1	T6Ø.1X2	T6Ø.1X3	T6Ø.1X4	—	—
Diflucortolone	T49.ØX1	T49.ØX2	T49.ØX3	T49.ØX4	T49.ØX5	T49.ØX6
Diflunisal	T39.Ø91	T39.Ø92	T39.Ø93	T39.Ø94	T39.Ø95	T39.Ø96
Difluoromethyldopa	T42.8X1	T42.8X2	T42.8X3	T42.8X4	T42.8X5	T42.8X6
Difluorophate	T44.ØX1	T44.ØX2	T44.ØX3	T44.ØX4	T44.ØX5	T44.ØX6
Digestant NEC	T47.5X1	T47.5X2	T47.5X3	T47.5X4	T47.5X5	T47.5X6
Digitalin (e)	T46.ØX1	T46.ØX2	T46.ØX3	T46.ØX4	T46.ØX5	T46.ØX6
Digitalis (leaf)(glycoside)	T46.ØX1	T46.ØX2	T46.ØX3	T46.ØX4	T46.ØX5	T46.ØX6
lanata	T46.ØX1	T46.ØX2	T46.ØX3	T46.ØX4	T46.ØX5	T46.ØX6
purpurea	T46.ØX1	T46.ØX2	T46.ØX3	T46.ØX4	T46.ØX5	T46.ØX6
Digitoxin	T46.ØX1	T46.ØX2	T46.ØX3	T46.ØX4	T46.ØX5	T46.ØX6
Digitoxose	T46.ØX1	T46.ØX2	T46.ØX3	T46.ØX4	T46.ØX5	T46.ØX6
Digoxin	T46.ØX1	T46.ØX2	T46.ØX3	T46.ØX4	T46.ØX5	T46.ØX6
Digoxine	T46.ØX1	T46.ØX2	T46.ØX3	T46.ØX4	T46.ØX5	T46.ØX6
Dihydralazine	T46.5X1	T46.5X2	T46.5X3	T46.5X4	T46.5X5	T46.5X6
Dihydrazine	T46.5X1	T46.5X2	T46.5X3	T46.5X4	T46.5X5	T46.5X6
Dihydrocodeine	T4Ø.2X1	T4Ø.2X2	T4Ø.2X3	T4Ø.2X4	T4Ø.2X5	T4Ø.2X6
Dihydrocodeinone	T4Ø.2X1	T4Ø.2X2	T4Ø.2X3	T4Ø.2X4	T4Ø.2X5	T4Ø.2X6
Dihydroergocornine	T46.7X1	T46.7X2	T46.7X3	T46.7X4	T46.7X5	T46.7X6
Dihydroergocristine (mesilate)	T46.7X1	T46.7X2	T46.7X3	T46.7X4	T46.7X5	T46.7X6
Dihydroergokryptine	T46.7X1	T46.7X2	T46.7X3	T46.7X4	T46.7X5	T46.7X6
Dihydroergotamine	T46.5X1	T46.5X2	T46.5X3	T46.5X4	T46.5X5	T46.5X6
Dihydroergotoxine	T46.7X1	T46.7X2	T46.7X3	T46.7X4	T46.7X5	T46.7X6
mesilate	T46.7X1	T46.7X2	T46.7X3	T46.7X4	T46.7X5	T46.7X6
Dihydrohydroxycodeinone	T4Ø.2X1	T4Ø.2X2	T4Ø.2X3	T4Ø.2X4	T4Ø.2X5	T4Ø.2X6
Dihydrohydroxymorphinone	T4Ø.2X1	T4Ø.2X2	T4Ø.2X3	T4Ø.2X4	T4Ø.2X5	T4Ø.2X6
Dihydroisocodeine	T4Ø.2X1	T4Ø.2X2	T4Ø.2X3	T4Ø.2X4	T4Ø.2X5	T4Ø.2X6
Dihydromorphine	T4Ø.2X1	T4Ø.2X2	T4Ø.2X3	T4Ø.2X4	—	—
Dihydromorphinone	T4Ø.2X1	T4Ø.2X2	T4Ø.2X3	T4Ø.2X4	T4Ø.2X5	T4Ø.2X6
Dihydrostreptomycin	T36.5X1	T36.5X2	T36.5X3	T36.5X4	T36.5X5	T36.5X6
Dihydrotachysterol	T45.2X1	T45.2X2	T45.2X3	T45.2X4	T45.2X5	T45.2X6
Dihydroxyacetone*	T49.3X1	T49.3X2	T49.3X3	T49.3X4	T49.3X5	T49.3X6
Dihydroxyaluminum aminoacetate	T47.1X1	T47.1X2	T47.1X3	T47.1X4	T47.1X5	T47.1X6
Dihydroxyaluminum sodium carbonate	T47.1X1	T47.1X2	T47.1X3	T47.1X4	T47.1X5	T47.1X6
Dihydroxyanthraquinone	T47.2X1	T47.2X2	T47.2X3	T47.2X4	T47.2X5	T47.2X6
Dihydroxycodeinone	T4Ø.2X1	T4Ø.2X2	T4Ø.2X3	T4Ø.2X4	T4Ø.2X5	T4Ø.2X6
Dihydroxypropyl theophylline	T5Ø.2X1	T5Ø.2X2	T5Ø.2X3	T5Ø.2X4	T5Ø.2X5	T5Ø.2X6
Diiodohydroxyquin	T37.8X1	T37.8X2	T37.8X3	T37.8X4	T37.8X5	T37.8X6
topical	T49.ØX1	T49.ØX2	T49.ØX3	T49.ØX4	T49.ØX5	T49.ØX6
Diiodohydroxyquinoline	T37.8X1	T37.8X2	T37.8X3	T37.8X4	T37.8X5	T37.8X6
Diiodotyrosine	T38.2X1	T38.2X2	T38.2X3	T38.2X4	T38.2X5	T38.2X6
Diisopromine	T44.3X1	T44.3X2	T44.3X3	T44.3X4	T44.3X5	T44.3X6
Diisopropylamine	T46.3X1	T46.3X2	T46.3X3	T46.3X4	T46.3X5	T46.3X6
Diisopropylfluorophosphonate	T44.ØX1	T44.ØX2	T44.ØX3	T44.ØX4	T44.ØX5	T44.ØX6
Dilantin	T42.ØX1	T42.ØX2	T42.ØX3	T42.ØX4	T42.ØX5	T42.ØX6
Dilatrate*	T46.3X1	T46.3X2	T46.3X3	T46.3X4	T46.3X5	T46.3X6
Dilaudid	T4Ø.2X1	T4Ø.2X2	T4Ø.2X3	T4Ø.2X4	T4Ø.2X5	T4Ø.2X6
Dilazep	T46.3X1	T46.3X2	T46.3X3	T46.3X4	T46.3X5	T46.3X6
Dill	T47.5X1	T47.5X2	T47.5X3	T47.5X4	T47.5X5	T47.5X6
Diloxanide	T37.3X1	T37.3X2	T37.3X3	T37.3X4	T37.3X5	T37.3X6
Diltiazem	T46.1X1	T46.1X2	T46.1X3	T46.1X4	T46.1X5	T46.1X6
Dimazole	T49.ØX1	T49.ØX2	T49.ØX3	T49.ØX4	T49.ØX5	T49.ØX6
Dimefline	T5Ø.7X1	T5Ø.7X2	T5Ø.7X3	T5Ø.7X4	T5Ø.7X5	T5Ø.7X6
Dimefox	T6Ø.ØX1	T6Ø.ØX2	T6Ø.ØX3	T6Ø.ØX4	—	—
Dimemorfan	T48.3X1	T48.3X2	T48.3X3	T48.3X4	T48.3X5	T48.3X6
Dimenhydrinate	T45.ØX1	T45.ØX2	T45.ØX3	T45.ØX4	T45.ØX5	T45.ØX6
Dimercaprol (British anti-lewisite)	T45.8X1	T45.8X2	T45.8X3	T45.8X4	T45.8X5	T45.8X6
Dimercaptopropanol	T45.8X1	T45.8X2	T45.8X3	T45.8X4	T45.8X5	T45.8X6
Dimestrol	T38.5X1	T38.5X2	T38.5X3	T38.5X4	T38.5X5	T38.5X6
Dimetane	T45.ØX1	T45.ØX2	T45.ØX3	T45.ØX4	T45.ØX5	T45.ØX6
Dimethicone	T47.1X1	T47.1X2	T47.1X3	T47.1X4	T47.1X5	T47.1X6
Dimethindene	T45.ØX1	T45.ØX2	T45.ØX3	T45.ØX4	T45.ØX5	T45.ØX6
Dimethisoquin	T49.1X1	T49.1X2	T49.1X3	T49.1X4	T49.1X5	T49.1X6
Dimethisterone	T38.5X1	T38.5X2	T38.5X3	T38.5X4	T38.5X5	T38.5X6
Dimethoate	T6Ø.ØX1	T6Ø.ØX2	T6Ø.ØX3	T6Ø.ØX4	—	—
Dimethocaine	T41.3X1	T41.3X2	T41.3X3	T41.3X4	T41.3X5	T41.3X6
Dimethoxanate	T48.3X1	T48.3X2	T48.3X3	T48.3X4	T48.3X5	T48.3X6
Dimethyl						
arsine, arsinic acid	T57.ØX1	T57.ØX2	T57.ØX3	T57.ØX4	—	—
carbinol	T51.2X1	T51.2X2	T51.2X3	T51.2X4	—	—
carbonate	T52.8X1	T52.8X2	T52.8X3	T52.8X4	—	—
diguanide	T38.3X1	T38.3X2	T38.3X3	T38.3X4	T38.3X5	T38.3X6
ketone	T52.4X1	T52.4X2	T52.4X3	T52.4X4	—	—
vapor	T52.4X1	T52.4X2	T52.4X3	T52.4X4	—	—
meperidine	T4Ø.2X1	T4Ø.2X2	T4Ø.2X3	T4Ø.2X4	T4Ø.2X5	T4Ø.2X6
parathion	T6Ø.ØX1	T6Ø.ØX2	T6Ø.ØX3	T6Ø.ØX4	—	—
phthlate	T49.3X1	T49.3X2	T49.3X3	T49.3X4	T49.3X5	T49.3X6
polysiloxane	T47.8X1	T47.8X2	T47.8X3	T47.8X4	T47.8X5	T47.8X6
sulfate (fumes)	T59.891	T59.892	T59.893	T59.894	—	—
liquid	T65.891	T65.892	T65.893	T65.894	—	—
sulfoxide (nonmedicinal)	T52.8X1	T52.8X2	T52.8X3	T52.8X4	—	—
medicinal	T49.4X1	T49.4X2	T49.4X3	T49.4X4	T49.4X5	T49.4X6
tryptamine	T4Ø.991	T4Ø.992	T4Ø.993	T4Ø.994	—	—
tubocurarine	T48.1X1	T48.1X2	T48.1X3	T48.1X4	T48.1X5	T48.1X6
Dimethylamine sulfate	T49.4X1	T49.4X2	T49.4X3	T49.4X4	T49.4X5	T49.4X6
Dimethylcysteine*	T5Ø.6X1	T5Ø.6X2	T5Ø.6X3	T5Ø.6X4	T5Ø.6X5	T5Ø.6X6
Dimethylformamide	T52.8X1	T52.8X2	T52.8X3	T52.8X4	—	—
Dimethyltubocurarinium chloride	T48.1X1	T48.1X2	T48.1X3	T48.1X4	T48.1X5	T48.1X6
Dimeticone	T47.1X1	T47.1X2	T47.1X3	T47.1X4	T47.1X5	T47.1X6
Dimetilan	T6Ø.ØX1	T6Ø.ØX2	T6Ø.ØX3	T6Ø.ØX4	—	—
Dimetindene	T45.ØX1	T45.ØX2	T45.ØX3	T45.ØX4	T45.ØX5	T45.ØX6
Dimetotiazine	T43.3X1	T43.3X2	T43.3X3	T43.3X4	T43.3X5	T43.3X6
Dimorpholamine	T5Ø.7X1	T5Ø.7X2	T5Ø.7X3	T5Ø.7X4	T5Ø.7X5	T5Ø.7X6
Dimoxyline	T46.3X1	T46.3X2	T46.3X3	T46.3X4	T46.3X5	T46.3X6
Dinitrobenzene	T65.3X1	T65.3X2	T65.3X3	T65.3X4	—	—
vapor	T59.891	T59.892	T59.893	T59.894	—	—
Dinitrobenzol	T65.3X1	T65.3X2	T65.3X3	T65.3X4	—	—
vapor	T59.891	T59.892	T59.893	T59.894	—	—
Dinitrobutylphenol	T65.3X1	T65.3X2	T65.3X3	T65.3X4	—	—
Dinitro (-ortho-)cresol (pesticide) (spray)	T65.3X1	T65.3X2	T65.3X3	T65.3X4	—	—
Dinitrocyclohexylphenol	T65.3X1	T65.3X2	T65.3X3	T65.3X4	—	—
Dinitrophenol	T65.3X1	T65.3X2	T65.3X3	T65.3X4	—	—
Dinoprost	T48.ØX1	T48.ØX2	T48.ØX3	T48.ØX4	T48.ØX5	T48.ØX6
Dinoprostone	T48.ØX1	T48.ØX2	T48.ØX3	T48.ØX4	T48.ØX5	T48.ØX6
Dinoseb	T6Ø.3X1	T6Ø.3X2	T6Ø.3X3	T6Ø.3X4	—	—
Dioctyl sulfosuccinate (calcium) (sodium)	T47.4X1	T47.4X2	T47.4X3	T47.4X4	T47.4X5	T47.4X6
Diodone	T5Ø.8X1	T5Ø.8X2	T5Ø.8X3	T5Ø.8X4	T5Ø.8X5	T5Ø.8X6
Diodoquin	T37.8X1	T37.8X2	T37.8X3	T37.8X4	T37.8X5	T37.8X6
Dionin	T4Ø.2X1	T4Ø.2X2	T4Ø.2X3	T4Ø.2X4	T4Ø.2X5	T4Ø.2X6
Diosmin	T46.991	T46.992	T46.993	T46.994	T46.995	T46.996
Diovan*	T46.5X1	T46.5X2	T46.5X3	T46.5X4	T46.5X5	T46.5X6
Dioxane	T52.8X1	T52.8X2	T52.8X3	T52.8X4	—	—
Dioxathion	T6Ø.ØX1	T6Ø.ØX2	T6Ø.ØX3	T6Ø.ØX4	—	—
Dioxin	T53.7X1	T53.7X2	T53.7X3	T53.7X4	—	—
Dioxopromethazine	T43.3X1	T43.3X2	T43.3X3	T43.3X4	T43.3X5	T43.3X6
Dioxyline	T46.3X1	T46.3X2	T46.3X3	T46.3X4	T46.3X5	T46.3X6
Dipentene	T52.8X1	T52.8X2	T52.8X3	T52.8X4	—	—
Diperodon	T41.3X1	T41.3X2	T41.3X3	T41.3X4	T41.3X5	T41.3X6
Diphacinone	T6Ø.4X1	T6Ø.4X2	T6Ø.4X3	T6Ø.4X4	—	—
Diphemanil	T44.3X1	T44.3X2	T44.3X3	T44.3X4	T44.3X5	T44.3X6
metilsulfate	T44.3X1	T44.3X2	T44.3X3	T44.3X4	T44.3X5	T44.3X6
Diphenadione	T45.511	T45.512	T45.513	T45.514	T45.515	T45.516
rodenticide	T6Ø.4X1	T6Ø.4X2	T6Ø.4X3	T6Ø.4X4	—	—
Diphenhydramine	T45.ØX1	T45.ØX2	T45.ØX3	T45.ØX4	T45.ØX5	T45.ØX6
Diphenidol	T45.ØX1	T45.ØX2	T45.ØX3	T45.ØX4	T45.ØX5	T45.ØX6
Diphenoxylate	T47.6X1	T47.6X2	T47.6X3	T47.6X4	T47.6X5	T47.6X6
Diphenylamine	T65.3X1	T65.3X2	T65.3X3	T65.3X4	—	—
Diphenylbutazone	T39.2X1	T39.2X2	T39.2X3	T39.2X4	T39.2X5	T39.2X6
Diphenylchloroarsine, not in war	T57.ØX1	T57.ØX2	T57.ØX3	T57.ØX4	—	—
Diphenylhydantoin	T42.ØX1	T42.ØX2	T42.ØX3	T42.ØX4	T42.ØX5	T42.ØX6
Diphenylmethane dye	T52.1X1	T52.1X2	T52.1X3	T52.1X4	—	—
Diphenylpyraline	T45.ØX1	T45.ØX2	T45.ØX3	T45.ØX4	T45.ØX5	T45.ØX6
Diphtheria						
antitoxin	T5Ø.Z11	T5Ø.Z12	T5Ø.Z13	T5Ø.Z14	T5Ø.Z15	T5Ø.Z16

Substance	Poisoning, Accidental (unintentional)	Poisoning, Intentional Self-harm	Poisoning, Assault	Poisoning, Undetermined	Adverse Effect	Under-dosing
Diphtheria — *continued*						
toxoid	T5Ø.A91	T5Ø.A92	T5Ø.A93	T5Ø.A94	T5Ø.A95	T5Ø.A96
with tetanus toxoid	T5Ø.A21	T5Ø.A22	T5Ø.A23	T5Ø.A24	T5Ø.A25	T5Ø.A26
with pertussis component	T5Ø.A11	T5Ø.A12	T5Ø.A13	T5Ø.A14	T5Ø.A15	T5Ø.A16
vaccine	T5Ø.A91	T5Ø.A92	T5Ø.A93	T5Ø.A94	T5Ø.A95	T5Ø.A96
combination						
without pertussis	T5Ø.A21	T5Ø.A22	T5Ø.A23	T5Ø.A24	T5Ø.A25	T5Ø.A26
including pertussis	T5Ø.A11	T5Ø.A12	T5Ø.A13	T5Ø.A14	T5Ø.A15	T5Ø.A16
Diphylline	T5Ø.2X1	T5Ø.2X2	T5Ø.2X3	T5Ø.2X4	T5Ø.2X5	T5Ø.2X6
Dipipanone	T4Ø.491	T4Ø.492	T4Ø.493	T4Ø.494	—	—
Dipivefrine	T49.5X1	T49.5X2	T49.5X3	T49.5X4	T49.5X5	T49.5X6
Diplovax	T5Ø.B91	T5Ø.B92	T5Ø.B93	T5Ø.B94	T5Ø.B95	T5Ø.B96
Diprophylline	T5Ø.2X1	T5Ø.2X2	T5Ø.2X3	T5Ø.2X4	T5Ø.2X5	T5Ø.2X6
Dipropyline	T48.291	T48.292	T48.293	T48.294	T48.295	T48.296
Dipyridamole	T46.3X1	T46.3X2	T46.3X3	T46.3X4	T46.3X5	T46.3X6
Dipyrone	T39.2X1	T39.2X2	T39.2X3	T39.2X4	T39.2X5	T39.2X6
Diquat (dibromide)	T6Ø.3X1	T6Ø.3X2	T6Ø.3X3	T6Ø.3X4	—	—
Disinfectant	T65.891	T65.892	T65.893	T65.894	—	—
alkaline	T54.3X1	T54.3X2	T54.3X3	T54.3X4	—	—
aromatic	T54.1X1	T54.1X2	T54.1X3	T54.1X4	—	—
intestinal	T37.8X1	T37.8X2	T37.8X3	T37.8X4	T37.8X5	T37.8X6
Disipal	T42.8X1	T42.8X2	T42.8X3	T42.8X4	T42.8X5	T42.8X6
Disodium edetate	T5Ø.6X1	T5Ø.6X2	T5Ø.6X3	T5Ø.6X4	T5Ø.6X5	T5Ø.6X6
Disoprofol	T41.291	T41.292	T41.293	T41.294	T41.295	T41.296
Disopyramide*	T46.2X1	T46.2X2	T46.2X3	T46.2X4	T46.2X5	T46.2X6
Distigmine (bromide)	T44.ØX1	T44.ØX2	T44.ØX3	T44.ØX4	T44.ØX5	T44.ØX6
Disulfamide	T5Ø.2X1	T5Ø.2X2	T5Ø.2X3	T5Ø.2X4	T5Ø.2X5	T5Ø.2X6
Disulfanilamide	T37.ØX1	T37.ØX2	T37.ØX3	T37.ØX4	T37.ØX5	T37.ØX6
Disulfiram	T5Ø.6X1	T5Ø.6X2	T5Ø.6X3	T5Ø.6X4	T5Ø.6X5	T5Ø.6X6
Disulfoton	T6Ø.ØX1	T6Ø.ØX2	T6Ø.ØX3	T6Ø.ØX4	—	—
Dithiazanine iodide	T37.4X1	T37.4X2	T37.4X3	T37.4X4	T37.4X5	T37.4X6
Dithiocarbamate	T6Ø.ØX1	T6Ø.ØX2	T6Ø.ØX3	T6Ø.ØX4	—	—
Dithranol	T49.4X1	T49.4X2	T49.4X3	T49.4X4	T49.4X5	T49.4X6
Diucardin	T5Ø.2X1	T5Ø.2X2	T5Ø.2X3	T5Ø.2X4	T5Ø.2X5	T5Ø.2X6
Diupres	T5Ø.2X1	T5Ø.2X2	T5Ø.2X3	T5Ø.2X4	T5Ø.2X5	T5Ø.2X6
Diuretic NEC	T5Ø.2X1	T5Ø.2X2	T5Ø.2X3	T5Ø.2X4	T5Ø.2X5	T5Ø.2X6
benzothiadiazine	T5Ø.2X1	T5Ø.2X2	T5Ø.2X3	T5Ø.2X4	T5Ø.2X5	T5Ø.2X6
carbonic acid anhydrase inhibitors	T5Ø.2X1	T5Ø.2X2	T5Ø.2X3	T5Ø.2X4	T5Ø.2X5	T5Ø.2X6
furfuryl NEC	T5Ø.2X1	T5Ø.2X2	T5Ø.2X3	T5Ø.2X4	T5Ø.2X5	T5Ø.2X6
loop (high-ceiling)	T5Ø.1X1	T5Ø.1X2	T5Ø.1X3	T5Ø.1X4	T5Ø.1X5	T5Ø.1X6
mercurial NEC	T5Ø.2X1	T5Ø.2X2	T5Ø.2X3	T5Ø.2X4	T5Ø.2X5	T5Ø.2X6
osmotic	T5Ø.2X1	T5Ø.2X2	T5Ø.2X3	T5Ø.2X4	T5Ø.2X5	T5Ø.2X6
purine NEC	T5Ø.2X1	T5Ø.2X2	T5Ø.2X3	T5Ø.2X4	T5Ø.2X5	T5Ø.2X6
saluretic NEC	T5Ø.2X1	T5Ø.2X2	T5Ø.2X3	T5Ø.2X4	T5Ø.2X5	T5Ø.2X6
sulfonamide	T5Ø.2X1	T5Ø.2X2	T5Ø.2X3	T5Ø.2X4	T5Ø.2X5	T5Ø.2X6
thiazide NEC	T5Ø.2X1	T5Ø.2X2	T5Ø.2X3	T5Ø.2X4	T5Ø.2X5	T5Ø.2X6
xanthine	T5Ø.2X1	T5Ø.2X2	T5Ø.2X3	T5Ø.2X4	T5Ø.2X5	T5Ø.2X6
Diurgin	T5Ø.2X1	T5Ø.2X2	T5Ø.2X3	T5Ø.2X4	T5Ø.2X5	T5Ø.2X6
Diuril	T5Ø.2X1	T5Ø.2X2	T5Ø.2X3	T5Ø.2X4	T5Ø.2X5	T5Ø.2X6
Diuron	T6Ø.3X1	T6Ø.3X2	T6Ø.3X3	T6Ø.3X4	—	—
Divalproex	T42.6X1	T42.6X2	T42.6X3	T42.6X4	T42.6X5	T42.6X6
Divinyl ether	T41.ØX1	T41.ØX2	T41.ØX3	T41.ØX4	T41.ØX5	T41.ØX6
Dixanthogen	T49.ØX1	T49.ØX2	T49.ØX3	T49.ØX4	T49.ØX5	T49.ØX6
Dixyrazine	T43.3X1	T43.3X2	T43.3X3	T43.3X4	T43.3X5	T43.3X6
D-lysergic acid diethylamide	T4Ø.8X1	T4Ø.8X2	T4Ø.8X3	T4Ø.8X4	—	—
DMCT	T36.4X1	T36.4X2	T36.4X3	T36.4X4	T36.4X5	T36.4X6
DMSO — *see* Dimethyl, sulfoxide						
DNBP	T6Ø.3X1	T6Ø.3X2	T6Ø.3X3	T6Ø.3X4	—	—
DNOC	T65.3X1	T65.3X2	T65.3X3	T65.3X4	—	—
Dobutamine	T44.5X1	T44.5X2	T44.5X3	T44.5X4	T44.5X5	T44.5X6
DOCA	T38.ØX1	T38.ØX2	T38.ØX3	T38.ØX4	T38.ØX5	T38.ØX6
Docusate sodium	T47.4X1	T47.4X2	T47.4X3	T47.4X4	T47.4X5	T47.4X6
Dodicin	T49.ØX1	T49.ØX2	T49.ØX3	T49.ØX4	T49.ØX5	T49.ØX6
Dofamium chloride	T49.ØX1	T49.ØX2	T49.ØX3	T49.ØX4	T49.ØX5	T49.ØX6
Dolophine	T4Ø.3X1	T4Ø.3X2	T4Ø.3X3	T4Ø.3X4	T4Ø.3X5	T4Ø.3X6
Doloxene	T39.8X1	T39.8X2	T39.8X3	T39.8X4	T39.8X5	T39.8X6
Domestic gas (after combustion) — *see* Gas, utility						
prior to combustion	T59.891	T59.892	T59.893	T59.894	—	—
Domiodol	T48.4X1	T48.4X2	T48.4X3	T48.4X4	T48.4X5	T48.4X6
Domiphen (bromide)	T49.ØX1	T49.ØX2	T49.ØX3	T49.ØX4	T49.ØX5	T49.ØX6
Domperidone	T45.ØX1	T45.ØX2	T45.ØX3	T45.ØX4	T45.ØX5	T45.ØX6
Donepezil*	T44.ØX1	T44.ØX2	T44.ØX3	T44.ØX4	T44.ØX5	T44.ØX6
Dopa	T42.8X1	T42.8X2	T42.8X3	T42.8X4	T42.8X5	T42.8X6
Dopamine	T44.991	T44.992	T44.993	T44.994	T44.995	T44.996
Doriden	T42.6X1	T42.6X2	T42.6X3	T42.6X4	T42.6X5	T42.6X6
Dormiral	T42.3X1	T42.3X2	T42.3X3	T42.3X4	T42.3X5	T42.3X6
Dormison	T42.6X1	T42.6X2	T42.6X3	T42.6X4	T42.6X5	T42.6X6
Dornase	T48.4X1	T48.4X2	T48.4X3	T48.4X4	T48.4X5	T48.4X6
Dorsacaine	T41.3X1	T41.3X2	T41.3X3	T41.3X4	T41.3X5	T41.3X6

Substance	Poisoning, Accidental (unintentional)	Poisoning, Intentional Self-harm	Poisoning, Assault	Poisoning, Undetermined	Adverse Effect	Under-dosing
Dosulepin	T43.Ø11	T43.Ø12	T43.Ø13	T43.Ø14	T43.Ø15	T43.Ø16
Dothiepin	T43.Ø11	T43.Ø12	T43.Ø13	T43.Ø14	T43.Ø15	T43.Ø16
Doxantrazole	T48.6X1	T48.6X2	T48.6X3	T48.6X4	T48.6X5	T48.6X6
Doxapram	T5Ø.7X1	T5Ø.7X2	T5Ø.7X3	T5Ø.7X4	T5Ø.7X5	T5Ø.7X6
Doxazosin	T44.6X1	T44.6X2	T44.6X3	T44.6X4	T44.6X5	T44.6X6
Doxepin	T43.Ø11	T43.Ø12	T43.Ø13	T43.Ø14	T43.Ø15	T43.Ø16
Doxifluridine	T45.1X1	T45.1X2	T45.1X3	T45.1X4	T45.1X5	T45.1X6
Doxil*	T45.1X1	T45.1X2	T45.1X3	T45.1X4	T45.1X5	T45.1X6
Doxorubicin	T45.1X1	T45.1X2	T45.1X3	T45.1X4	T45.1X5	T45.1X6
Doxycycline	T36.4X1	T36.4X2	T36.4X3	T36.4X4	T36.4X5	T36.4X6
Doxylamine	T45.ØX1	T45.ØX2	T45.ØX3	T45.ØX4	T45.ØX5	T45.ØX6
Dramamine	T45.ØX1	T45.ØX2	T45.ØX3	T45.ØX4	T45.ØX5	T45.ØX6
Drano (drain cleaner)	T54.3X1	T54.3X2	T54.3X3	T54.3X4	—	—
Dressing, live pulp	T49.7X1	T49.7X2	T49.7X3	T49.7X4	T49.7X5	T49.7X6
Drocode	T4Ø.2X1	T4Ø.2X2	T4Ø.2X3	T4Ø.2X4	T4Ø.2X5	T4Ø.2X6
Dromoran	T4Ø.2X1	T4Ø.2X2	T4Ø.2X3	T4Ø.2X4	T4Ø.2X5	T4Ø.2X6
Dromostanolone	T38.7X1	T38.7X2	T38.7X3	T38.7X4	T38.7X5	T38.7X6
Dronabinol	T4Ø.711	T4Ø.712	T4Ø.713	T4Ø.714	T4Ø.715	T4Ø.716
Droperidol	T43.591	T43.592	T43.593	T43.594	T43.595	T43.596
Dropropizine	T48.3X1	T48.3X2	T48.3X3	T48.3X4	T48.3X5	T48.3X6
Drostanolone	T38.7X1	T38.7X2	T38.7X3	T38.7X4	T38.7X5	T38.7X6
Drotaverine	T44.3X1	T44.3X2	T44.3X3	T44.3X4	T44.3X5	T44.3X6
Drotrecogin alfa	T45.511	T45.512	T45.513	T45.514	T45.515	T45.516
Drug NEC	T5Ø.9Ø1	T5Ø.9Ø2	T5Ø.9Ø3	T5Ø.9Ø4	T5Ø.9Ø5	T5Ø.9Ø6
specified NEC	T5Ø.991	T5Ø.992	T5Ø.993	T5Ø.994	T5Ø.995	T5Ø.996
DTIC	T45.1X1	T45.1X2	T45.1X3	T45.1X4	T45.1X5	T45.1X6
Duboisine	T44.3X1	T44.3X2	T44.3X3	T44.3X4	T44.3X5	T44.3X6
Dulcolax	T47.2X1	T47.2X2	T47.2X3	T47.2X4	T47.2X5	T47.2X6
Duponol (C) (EP)	T49.2X1	T49.2X2	T49.2X3	T49.2X4	T49.2X5	T49.2X6
Durabolin	T38.7X1	T38.7X2	T38.7X3	T38.7X4	T38.7X5	T38.7X6
Durezol*	T49.5X1	T49.5X2	T49.5X3	T49.5X4	T49.5X5	T49.5X6
Dyclone	T41.3X1	T41.3X2	T41.3X3	T41.3X4	T41.3X5	T41.3X6
Dyclonine	T41.3X1	T41.3X2	T41.3X3	T41.3X4	T41.3X5	T41.3X6
Dydrogesterone	T38.5X1	T38.5X2	T38.5X3	T38.5X4	T38.5X5	T38.5X6
Dye NEC	T65.6X1	T65.6X2	T65.6X3	T65.6X4	—	—
antiseptic	T49.ØX1	T49.ØX2	T49.ØX3	T49.ØX4	T49.ØX5	T49.ØX6
diagnostic agents	T5Ø.8X1	T5Ø.8X2	T5Ø.8X3	T5Ø.8X4	T5Ø.8X5	T5Ø.8X6
pharmaceutical NEC	T5Ø.9Ø1	T5Ø.9Ø2	T5Ø.9Ø3	T5Ø.9Ø4	T5Ø.9Ø5	T5Ø.9Ø6
Dyflos	T44.ØX1	T44.ØX2	T44.ØX3	T44.ØX4	T44.ØX5	T44.ØX6
Dymelor	T38.3X1	T38.3X2	T38.3X3	T38.3X4	T38.3X5	T38.3X6
Dynamite	T65.3X1	T65.3X2	T65.3X3	T65.3X4	—	—
fumes	T59.891	T59.892	T59.893	T59.894	—	—
Dyphylline	T44.3X1	T44.3X2	T44.3X3	T44.3X4	T44.3X5	T44.3X6
b-eucaine	T49.1X1	T49.1X2	T49.1X3	T49.1X4	T49.1X5	T49.1X6
Ear drug NEC	T49.6X1	T49.6X2	T49.6X3	T49.6X4	T49.6X5	T49.6X6
Ear preparations	T49.6X1	T49.6X2	T49.6X3	T49.6X4	T49.6X5	T49.6X6
Echothiophate, echothiopate, ecothiopate	T49.5X1	T49.5X2	T49.5X3	T49.5X4	T49.5X5	T49.5X6
Econazole	T49.ØX1	T49.ØX2	T49.ØX3	T49.ØX4	T49.ØX5	T49.ØX6
Ecothiopate iodide	T49.5X1	T49.5X2	T49.5X3	T49.5X4	T49.5X5	T49.5X6
Ecstasy	T43.641	T43.642	T43.643	T43.644	—	—
Ectylurea	T42.6X1	T42.6X2	T42.6X3	T42.6X4	T42.6X5	T42.6X6
Edathamil disodium	T45.8X1	T45.8X2	T45.8X3	T45.8X4	T45.8X5	T45.8X6
Edecrin	T5Ø.1X1	T5Ø.1X2	T5Ø.1X3	T5Ø.1X4	T5Ø.1X5	T5Ø.1X6
Edetate, disodium (calcium)	T45.8X1	T45.8X2	T45.8X3	T45.8X4	T45.8X5	T45.8X6
Edoxudine	T49.5X1	T49.5X2	T49.5X3	T49.5X4	T49.5X5	T49.5X6
Edrophonium	T44.ØX1	T44.ØX2	T44.ØX3	T44.ØX4	T44.ØX5	T44.ØX6
chloride	T44.ØX1	T44.ØX2	T44.ØX3	T44.ØX4	T44.ØX5	T44.ØX6
EDTA	T5Ø.6X1	T5Ø.6X2	T5Ø.6X3	T5Ø.6X4	T5Ø.6X5	T5Ø.6X6
Eflornithine	T37.2X1	T37.2X2	T37.2X3	T37.2X4	T37.2X5	T37.2X6
Efloxate	T46.3X1	T46.3X2	T46.3X3	T46.3X4	T46.3X5	T46.3X6
Elase	T49.8X1	T49.8X2	T49.8X3	T49.8X4	T49.8X5	T49.8X6
Elastase	T47.5X1	T47.5X2	T47.5X3	T47.5X4	T47.5X5	T47.5X6
Elaterium	T47.2X1	T47.2X2	T47.2X3	T47.2X4	T47.2X5	T47.2X6
Elcatonin	T5Ø.991	T5Ø.992	T5Ø.993	T5Ø.994	T5Ø.995	T5Ø.996
Elder	T62.2X1	T62.2X2	T62.2X3	T62.2X4	—	—
berry, (unripe)	T62.1X1	T62.1X2	T62.1X3	T62.1X4	—	—
Electrolyte balance drug	T5Ø.3X1	T5Ø.3X2	T5Ø.3X3	T5Ø.3X4	T5Ø.3X5	T5Ø.3X6
Electrolytes NEC	T5Ø.3X1	T5Ø.3X2	T5Ø.3X3	T5Ø.3X4	T5Ø.3X5	T5Ø.3X6
Electrolytic agent NEC	T5Ø.3X1	T5Ø.3X2	T5Ø.3X3	T5Ø.3X4	T5Ø.3X5	T5Ø.3X6
Elemental diet	T5Ø.9Ø1	T5Ø.9Ø2	T5Ø.9Ø3	T5Ø.9Ø4	T5Ø.9Ø5	T5Ø.9Ø6
Elliptinium acetate	T45.1X1	T45.1X2	T45.1X3	T45.1X4	T45.1X5	T45.1X6
Elocon*	T49.ØX1	T49.ØX2	T49.ØX3	T49.ØX4	T49.ØX5	T49.ØX6
Embramine	T45.ØX1	T45.ØX2	T45.ØX3	T45.ØX4	T45.ØX5	T45.ØX6
Emepronium (salts)	T44.3X1	T44.3X2	T44.3X3	T44.3X4	T44.3X5	T44.3X6
bromide	T44.3X1	T44.3X2	T44.3X3	T44.3X4	T44.3X5	T44.3X6
Emetic NEC	T47.7X1	T47.7X2	T47.7X3	T47.7X4	T47.7X5	T47.7X6
Emetine	T37.3X1	T37.3X2	T37.3X3	T37.3X4	T37.3X5	T37.3X6
Emollient NEC	T49.3X1	T49.3X2	T49.3X3	T49.3X4	T49.3X5	T49.3X6
Emorfazone	T39.8X1	T39.8X2	T39.8X3	T39.8X4	T39.8X5	T39.8X6
Emylcamate	T43.591	T43.592	T43.593	T43.594	T43.595	T43.596
Enalapril	T46.4X1	T46.4X2	T46.4X3	T46.4X4	T46.4X5	T46.4X6

Substance	Poisoning, Accidental (unintentional)	Poisoning, Intentional Self-harm	Poisoning, Assault	Poisoning, Undetermined	Adverse Effect	Under-dosing
Enalaprilat	T46.4X1	T46.4X2	T46.4X3	T46.4X4	T46.4X5	T46.4X6
Enbrel*	T39.4X1	T39.4X2	T39.4X3	T39.4X4	T39.4X5	T39.4X6
Encainide	T46.2X1	T46.2X2	T46.2X3	T46.2X4	T46.2X5	T46.2X6
Endocaine	T41.3X1	T41.3X2	T41.3X3	T41.3X4	T41.3X5	T41.3X6
Endosulfan	T6Ø.2X1	T6Ø.2X2	T6Ø.2X3	T6Ø.2X4	—	—
Endothall	T6Ø.3X1	T6Ø.3X2	T6Ø.3X3	T6Ø.3X4	—	—
Endralazine	T46.5X1	T46.5X2	T46.5X3	T46.5X4	T46.5X5	T46.5X6
Endrin	T6Ø.1X1	T6Ø.1X2	T6Ø.1X3	T6Ø.1X4	—	—
Enflurane	T41.ØX1	T41.ØX2	T41.ØX3	T41.ØX4	T41.ØX5	T41.ØX6
Enfuvirtide*	T37.5X1	T37.5X2	T37.5X3	T37.5X4	T37.5X5	T37.5X6
Enhexymal	T42.3X1	T42.3X2	T42.3X3	T42.3X4	T42.3X5	T42.3X6
Enocitabine	T45.1X1	T45.1X2	T45.1X3	T45.1X4	T45.1X5	T45.1X6
Enovid	T38.4X1	T38.4X2	T38.4X3	T38.4X4	T38.4X5	T38.4X6
Enoxacin	T36.8X1	T36.8X2	T36.8X3	T36.8X4	T36.8X5	T36.8X6
Enoxaparin (sodium)	T45.511	T45.512	T45.513	T45.514	T45.515	T45.516
Enpiprazole	T43.591	T43.592	T43.593	T43.594	T43.595	T43.596
Enprofylline	T48.6X1	T48.6X2	T48.6X3	T48.6X4	T48.6X5	T48.6X6
Enprostil	T47.1X1	T47.1X2	T47.1X3	T47.1X4	T47.1X5	T47.1X6
Enterogastrone	T38.891	T38.892	T38.893	T38.894	T38.895	T38.896
ENT preparations (anti-infectives)	T49.6X1	T49.6X2	T49.6X3	T49.6X4	T49.6X5	T49.6X6
Enviomycin	T36.8X1	T36.8X2	T36.8X3	T36.8X4	T36.8X5	T36.8X6
Enzodase	T45.3X1	T45.3X2	T45.3X3	T45.3X4	T45.3X5	T45.3X6
Enzyme NEC	T45.3X1	T45.3X2	T45.3X3	T45.3X4	T45.3X5	T45.3X6
depolymerizing	T49.8X1	T49.8X2	T49.8X3	T49.8X4	T49.8X5	T49.8X6
fibrolytic	T45.3X1	T45.3X2	T45.3X3	T45.3X4	T45.3X5	T45.3X6
gastric	T47.5X1	T47.5X2	T47.5X3	T47.5X4	T47.5X5	T47.5X6
intestinal	T47.5X1	T47.5X2	T47.5X3	T47.5X4	T47.5X5	T47.5X6
local action	T49.4X1	T49.4X2	T49.4X3	T49.4X4	T49.4X5	T49.4X6
proteolytic	T49.4X1	T49.4X2	T49.4X3	T49.4X4	T49.4X5	T49.4X6
thrombolytic	T45.3X1	T45.3X2	T45.3X3	T45.3X4	T45.3X5	T45.3X6
EPAB	T41.3X1	T41.3X2	T41.3X3	T41.3X4	T41.3X5	T41.3X6
Epanutin	T42.ØX1	T42.ØX2	T42.ØX3	T42.ØX4	T42.ØX5	T42.ØX6
Ephedra	T44.991	T44.992	T44.993	T44.994	T44.995	T44.996
Ephedrine	T44.991	T44.992	T44.993	T44.994	T44.995	T44.996
Epichlorhydrin, epichlorohydrin	T52.8X1	T52.8X2	T52.8X3	T52.8X4	—	—
Epicillin	T36.ØX1	T36.ØX2	T36.ØX3	T36.ØX4	T36.ØX5	T36.ØX6
Epiestriol	T38.5X1	T38.5X2	T38.5X3	T38.5X4	T38.5X5	T38.5X6
Epilim — *see* Sodium, valproate						
Epimestrol	T38.5X1	T38.5X2	T38.5X3	T38.5X4	T38.5X5	T38.5X6
Epinephrine	T44.5X1	T44.5X2	T44.5X3	T44.5X4	T44.5X5	T44.5X6
EpiPen*	T44.5X1	T44.5X2	T44.5X3	T44.5X4	T44.5X5	T44.5X6
Epirubicin	T45.1X1	T45.1X2	T45.1X3	T45.1X4	T45.1X5	T45.1X6
Epitiostanol	T38.7X1	T38.7X2	T38.7X3	T38.7X4	T38.7X5	T38.7X6
Epitizide	T5Ø.2X1	T5Ø.2X2	T5Ø.2X3	T5Ø.2X4	T5Ø.2X5	T5Ø.2X6
EPN	T6Ø.ØX1	T6Ø.ØX2	T6Ø.ØX3	T6Ø.ØX4	—	—
EPO	T45.8X1	T45.8X2	T45.8X3	T45.8X4	T45.8X5	T45.8X6
Epoetin alpha	T45.8X1	T45.8X2	T45.8X3	T45.8X4	T45.8X5	T45.8X6
Epomediol	T5Ø.991	T5Ø.992	T5Ø.993	T5Ø.994	T5Ø.995	T5Ø.996
Epoprostenol	T45.521	T45.522	T45.523	T45.524	T45.525	T45.526
Epoxy resin	T65.891	T65.892	T65.893	T65.894	—	—
Eprazinone	T48.4X1	T48.4X2	T48.4X3	T48.4X4	T48.4X5	T48.4X6
Epsilon aminocaproic acid	T45.621	T45.622	T45.623	T45.624	T45.625	T45.626
Epsom salt	T47.3X1	T47.3X2	T47.3X3	T47.3X4	T47.3X5	T47.3X6
Eptazocine	T4Ø.491	T4Ø.492	T4Ø.493	T4Ø.494	T4Ø.495	T4Ø.496
Equanil	T43.591	T43.592	T43.593	T43.594	T43.595	T43.596
Equisetum	T62.2X1	T62.2X2	T62.2X3	T62.2X4	—	—
diuretic	T5Ø.2X1	T5Ø.2X2	T5Ø.2X3	T5Ø.2X4	T5Ø.2X5	T5Ø.2X6
Ergobasine	T48.ØX1	T48.ØX2	T48.ØX3	T48.ØX4	T48.ØX5	T48.ØX6
Ergocalciferol	T45.2X1	T45.2X2	T45.2X3	T45.2X4	T45.2X5	T45.2X6
Ergoloid mesylates	T46.7X1	T46.7X2	T46.7X3	T46.7X4	T46.7X5	T46.7X6
Ergometrine	T48.ØX1	T48.ØX2	T48.ØX3	T48.ØX4	T48.ØX5	T48.ØX6
Ergonovine	T48.ØX1	T48.ØX2	T48.ØX3	T48.ØX4	T48.ØX5	T48.ØX6
Ergotamine	T46.5X1	T46.5X2	T46.5X3	T46.5X4	T46.5X5	T46.5X6
Ergotocine	T48.ØX1	T48.ØX2	T48.ØX3	T48.ØX4	T48.ØX5	T48.ØX6
Ergotrate	T48.ØX1	T48.ØX2	T48.ØX3	T48.ØX4	T48.ØX5	T48.ØX6
Ergot NEC	T64.81	T64.82	T64.83	T64.84	—	—
derivative	T48.ØX1	T48.ØX2	T48.ØX3	T48.ØX4	T48.ØX5	T48.ØX6
medicinal (alkaloids)	T48.ØX1	T48.ØX2	T48.ØX3	T48.ØX4	T48.ØX5	T48.ØX6
prepared	T48.ØX1	T48.ØX2	T48.ØX3	T48.ØX4	T48.ØX5	T48.ØX6
Eritrityl tetranitrate	T46.3X1	T46.3X2	T46.3X3	T46.3X4	T46.3X5	T46.3X6
Erythrityl tetranitrate	T46.3X1	T46.3X2	T46.3X3	T46.3X4	T46.3X5	T46.3X6
Erythrol tetranitrate	T46.3X1	T46.3X2	T46.3X3	T46.3X4	T46.3X5	T46.3X6
Erythromycin (salts)	T36.3X1	T36.3X2	T36.3X3	T36.3X4	T36.3X5	T36.3X6
ophthalmic preparation	T49.5X1	T49.5X2	T49.5X3	T49.5X4	T49.5X5	T49.5X6
topical NEC	T49.ØX1	T49.ØX2	T49.ØX3	T49.ØX4	T49.ØX5	T49.ØX6
Erythropoietin	T45.8X1	T45.8X2	T45.8X3	T45.8X4	T45.8X5	T45.8X6
human	T45.8X1	T45.8X2	T45.8X3	T45.8X4	T45.8X5	T45.8X6
Esbriet*	T48.991	T48.992	T48.993	T48.994	T48.995	T48.996
Escin	T46.991	T46.992	T46.993	T46.994	T46.995	T46.996
Esculin	T45.2X1	T45.2X2	T45.2X3	T45.2X4	T45.2X5	T45.2X6
Esculoside	T45.2X1	T45.2X2	T45.2X3	T45.2X4	T45.2X5	T45.2X6

Substance	Poisoning, Accidental (unintentional)	Poisoning, Intentional Self-harm	Poisoning, Assault	Poisoning, Undetermined	Adverse Effect	Under-dosing
ESDT (ether-soluble tar distillate)	T49.1X1	T49.1X2	T49.1X3	T49.1X4	T49.1X5	T49.1X6
Eserine	T49.5X1	T49.5X2	T49.5X3	T49.5X4	T49.5X5	T49.5X6
Esflurbiprofen	T39.311	T39.312	T39.313	T39.314	T39.315	T39.316
Eskabarb	T42.3X1	T42.3X2	T42.3X3	T42.3X4	T42.3X5	T42.3X6
Eskalith	T43.8X1	T43.8X2	T43.8X3	T43.8X4	T43.8X5	T43.8X6
Esmolol	T44.7X1	T44.7X2	T44.7X3	T44.7X4	T44.7X5	T44.7X6
Estanozolol	T38.7X1	T38.7X2	T38.7X3	T38.7X4	T38.7X5	T38.7X6
Estazolam	T42.4X1	T42.4X2	T42.4X3	T42.4X4	T42.4X5	T42.4X6
Estradiol	T38.5X1	T38.5X2	T38.5X3	T38.5X4	T38.5X5	T38.5X6
with testosterone	T38.7X1	T38.7X2	T38.7X3	T38.7X4	T38.7X5	T38.7X6
benzoate	T38.5X1	T38.5X2	T38.5X3	T38.5X4	T38.5X5	T38.5X6
Estramustine	T45.1X1	T45.1X2	T45.1X3	T45.1X4	T45.1X5	T45.1X6
Estriol	T38.5X1	T38.5X2	T38.5X3	T38.5X4	T38.5X5	T38.5X6
Estrogen	T38.5X1	T38.5X2	T38.5X3	T38.5X4	T38.5X5	T38.5X6
with progesterone	T38.5X1	T38.5X2	T38.5X3	T38.5X4	T38.5X5	T38.5X6
conjugated	T38.5X1	T38.5X2	T38.5X3	T38.5X4	T38.5X5	T38.5X6
Estrone	T38.5X1	T38.5X2	T38.5X3	T38.5X4	T38.5X5	T38.5X6
Estropipate	T38.5X1	T38.5X2	T38.5X3	T38.5X4	T38.5X5	T38.5X6
Etacrynate sodium	T5Ø.1X1	T5Ø.1X2	T5Ø.1X3	T5Ø.1X4	T5Ø.1X5	T5Ø.1X6
Etacrynic acid	T5Ø.1X1	T5Ø.1X2	T5Ø.1X3	T5Ø.1X4	T5Ø.1X5	T5Ø.1X6
Etafedrine	T48.6X1	T48.6X2	T48.6X3	T48.6X4	T48.6X5	T48.6X6
Etafenone	T46.3X1	T46.3X2	T46.3X3	T46.3X4	T46.3X5	T46.3X6
Etambutol	T37.1X1	T37.1X2	T37.1X3	T37.1X4	T37.1X5	T37.1X6
Etamiphyllin	T48.6X1	T48.6X2	T48.6X3	T48.6X4	T48.6X5	T48.6X6
Etamivan	T5Ø.7X1	T5Ø.7X2	T5Ø.7X3	T5Ø.7X4	T5Ø.7X5	T5Ø.7X6
Etamsylate	T45.7X1	T45.7X2	T45.7X3	T45.7X4	T45.7X5	T45.7X6
Etebenecid	T5Ø.4X1	T5Ø.4X2	T5Ø.4X3	T5Ø.4X4	T5Ø.4X5	T5Ø.4X6
Ethacridine	T49.ØX1	T49.ØX2	T49.ØX3	T49.ØX4	T49.ØX5	T49.ØX6
Ethacrynate*	T5Ø.1X1	T5Ø.1X2	T5Ø.1X3	T5Ø.1X4	T5Ø.1X5	T5Ø.1X6
Ethacrynic acid	T5Ø.1X1	T5Ø.1X2	T5Ø.1X3	T5Ø.1X4	T5Ø.1X5	T5Ø.1X6
Ethadione	T42.2X1	T42.2X2	T42.2X3	T42.2X4	T42.2X5	T42.2X6
Ethambutol	T37.1X1	T37.1X2	T37.1X3	T37.1X4	T37.1X5	T37.1X6
Ethamide	T5Ø.2X1	T5Ø.2X2	T5Ø.2X3	T5Ø.2X4	T5Ø.2X5	T5Ø.2X6
Ethamivan	T5Ø.7X1	T5Ø.7X2	T5Ø.7X3	T5Ø.7X4	T5Ø.7X5	T5Ø.7X6
Ethamsylate	T45.7X1	T45.7X2	T45.7X3	T45.7X4	T45.7X5	T45.7X6
Ethanol	T51.ØX1	T51.ØX2	T51.ØX3	T51.ØX4	—	—
beverage	T51.ØX1	T51.ØX2	T51.ØX3	T51.ØX4	—	—
Ethanolamine oleate	T46.8X1	T46.8X2	T46.8X3	T46.8X4	T46.8X5	T46.8X6
Ethaverine	T44.3X1	T44.3X2	T44.3X3	T44.3X4	T44.3X5	T44.3X6
Ethchlorvynol	T42.6X1	T42.6X2	T42.6X3	T42.6X4	T42.6X5	T42.6X6
Ethebenecid	T5Ø.4X1	T5Ø.4X2	T5Ø.4X3	T5Ø.4X4	T5Ø.4X5	T5Ø.4X6
Ether (vapor)	T41.ØX1	T41.ØX2	T41.ØX3	T41.ØX4	T41.ØX5	T41.ØX6
anesthetic	T41.ØX1	T41.ØX2	T41.ØX3	T41.ØX4	T41.ØX5	T41.ØX6
divinyl	T41.ØX1	T41.ØX2	T41.ØX3	T41.ØX4	T41.ØX5	T41.ØX6
ethyl (medicinal)	T41.ØX1	T41.ØX2	T41.ØX3	T41.ØX4	T41.ØX5	T41.ØX6
nonmedicinal	T52.8X1	T52.8X2	T52.8X3	T52.8X4	—	—
petroleum — *see* Ligroin						
solvent	T52.8X1	T52.8X2	T52.8X3	T52.8X4	—	—
Ethiazide	T5Ø.2X1	T5Ø.2X2	T5Ø.2X3	T5Ø.2X4	T5Ø.2X5	T5Ø.2X6
Ethidium chloride (vapor)	T59.891	T59.892	T59.893	T59.894	—	—
Ethinamate	T42.6X1	T42.6X2	T42.6X3	T42.6X4	T42.6X5	T42.6X6
Ethinylestradiol, ethinyloestradiol	T38.5X1	T38.5X2	T38.5X3	T38.5X4	T38.5X5	T38.5X6
with						
levonorgestrel	T38.4X1	T38.4X2	T38.4X3	T38.4X4	T38.4X5	T38.4X6
norethisterone	T38.4X1	T38.4X2	T38.4X3	T38.4X4	T38.4X5	T38.4X6
Ethiodized oil (131 I)	T5Ø.8X1	T5Ø.8X2	T5Ø.8X3	T5Ø.8X4	T5Ø.8X5	T5Ø.8X6
Ethiofos*	T5Ø.991	T5Ø.992	T5Ø.993	T5Ø.994	T5Ø.995	T5Ø.996
Ethion	T6Ø.ØX1	T6Ø.ØX2	T6Ø.ØX3	T6Ø.ØX4	—	—
Ethionamide	T37.1X1	T37.1X2	T37.1X3	T37.1X4	T37.1X5	T37.1X6
Ethioniamide	T37.1X1	T37.1X2	T37.1X3	T37.1X4	T37.1X5	T37.1X6
Ethisterone	T38.5X1	T38.5X2	T38.5X3	T38.5X4	T38.5X5	T38.5X6
Ethobral	T42.3X1	T42.3X2	T42.3X3	T42.3X4	T42.3X5	T42.3X6
Ethocaine (infiltration) (topical)	T41.3X1	T41.3X2	T41.3X3	T41.3X4	T41.3X5	T41.3X6
nerve block (peripheral) (plexus)	T41.3X1	T41.3X2	T41.3X3	T41.3X4	T41.3X5	T41.3X6
spinal	T41.3X1	T41.3X2	T41.3X3	T41.3X4	T41.3X5	T41.3X6
Ethoheptazine	T4Ø.491	T4Ø.492	T4Ø.493	T4Ø.494	T4Ø.495	T4Ø.496
Ethopropazine	T44.3X1	T44.3X2	T44.3X3	T44.3X4	T44.3X5	T44.3X6
Ethosuximide	T42.2X1	T42.2X2	T42.2X3	T42.2X4	T42.2X5	T42.2X6
Ethotoin	T42.ØX1	T42.ØX2	T42.ØX3	T42.ØX4	T42.ØX5	T42.ØX6
Ethoxazene	T37.91	T37.92	T37.93	T37.94	T37.95	T37.96
Ethoxazorutoside	T46.991	T46.992	T46.993	T46.994	T46.995	T46.996
Ethoxzolamide	T5Ø.2X1	T5Ø.2X2	T5Ø.2X3	T5Ø.2X4	T5Ø.2X5	T5Ø.2X6
Ethyl						
acetate	T52.8X1	T52.8X2	T52.8X3	T52.8X4	—	—
alcohol	T51.ØX1	T51.ØX2	T51.ØX3	T51.ØX4	—	—
beverage	T51.ØX1	T51.ØX2	T51.ØX3	T51.ØX4	—	—
aldehyde (vapor)	T59.891	T59.892	T59.893	T59.894	—	—
liquid	T52.8X1	T52.8X2	T52.8X3	T52.8X4	—	—
aminobenzoate	T41.3X1	T41.3X2	T41.3X3	T41.3X4	T41.3X5	T41.3X6

Substance	Poisoning, Accidental (unintentional)	Poisoning, Intentional Self-harm	Poisoning, Assault	Poisoning, Undetermined	Adverse Effect	Under-dosing
Ethyl — *continued*						
aminophenothiazine	T43.3X1	T43.3X2	T43.3X3	T43.3X4	T43.3X5	T43.3X6
benzoate	T52.8X1	T52.8X2	T52.8X3	T52.8X4	—	—
biscoumacetate	T45.511	T45.512	T45.513	T45.514	T45.515	T45.516
bromide (anesthetic)	T41.ØX1	T41.ØX2	T41.ØX3	T41.ØX4	T41.ØX5	T41.ØX6
carbamate	T45.1X1	T45.1X2	T45.1X3	T45.1X4	T45.1X5	T45.1X6
carbinol	T51.3X1	T51.3X2	T51.3X3	T51.3X4	—	—
carbonate	T52.8X1	T52.8X2	T52.8X3	T52.8X4	—	—
chaulmoograte	T37.1X1	T37.1X2	T37.1X3	T37.1X4	T37.1X5	T37.1X6
chloride (anesthetic)	T41.ØX1	T41.ØX2	T41.ØX3	T41.ØX4	T41.ØX5	T41.ØX6
anesthetic (local)	T41.3X1	T41.3X2	T41.3X3	T41.3X4	T41.3X5	T41.3X6
inhaled	T41.ØX1	T41.ØX2	T41.ØX3	T41.ØX4	T41.ØX5	T41.ØX6
local	T49.4X1	T49.4X2	T49.4X3	T49.4X4	T49.4X5	T49.4X6
solvent	T53.6X1	T53.6X2	T53.6X3	T53.6X4	—	—
dibunate	T48.3X1	T48.3X2	T48.3X3	T48.3X4	T48.3X5	T48.3X6
dichloroarsine (vapor)	T57.ØX1	T57.ØX2	T57.ØX3	T57.ØX4	—	—
estranol	T38.7X1	T38.7X2	T38.7X3	T38.7X4	T38.7X5	T38.7X6
ether — *see also* ether	T52.8X1	T52.8X2	T52.8X3	T52.8X4	—	—
formate NEC (solvent)	T52.ØX1	T52.ØX2	T52.ØX3	T52.ØX4	—	—
fumarate	T49.4X1	T49.4X2	T49.4X3	T49.4X4	T49.4X5	T49.4X6
hydroxyisobutyrate NEC (solvent)	T52.8X1	T52.8X2	T52.8X3	T52.8X4	—	—
iodoacetate	T59.3X1	T59.3X2	T59.3X3	T59.3X4	—	—
lactate NEC (solvent)	T52.8X1	T52.8X2	T52.8X3	T52.8X4	—	—
loflazepate	T42.4X1	T42.4X2	T42.4X3	T42.4X4	T42.4X5	T42.4X6
mercuric chloride	T56.1X1	T56.1X2	T56.1X3	T56.1X4	—	—
methylcarbinol	T51.8X1	T51.8X2	T51.8X3	T51.8X4	—	—
morphine	T40.2X1	T40.2X2	T40.2X3	T40.2X4	T40.2X5	T40.2X6
noradrenaline	T48.6X1	T48.6X2	T48.6X3	T48.6X4	T48.6X5	T48.6X6
oxybutyrate NEC (solvent)	T52.8X1	T52.8X2	T52.8X3	T52.8X4	—	—
Ethylene (gas)	T59.891	T59.892	T59.893	T59.894	—	—
anesthetic (general)	T41.ØX1	T41.ØX2	T41.ØX3	T41.ØX4	T41.ØX5	T41.ØX6
chlorohydrin	T52.8X1	T52.8X2	T52.8X3	T52.8X4	—	—
vapor	T53.6X1	T53.6X2	T53.6X3	T53.6X4	—	—
dichloride	T52.8X1	T52.8X2	T52.8X3	T52.8X4	—	—
vapor	T53.6X1	T53.6X2	T53.6X3	T53.6X4	—	—
dinitrate	T52.3X1	T52.3X2	T52.3X3	T52.3X4	—	—
glycol(s)	T52.8X1	T52.8X2	T52.8X3	T52.8X4	—	—
dinitrate	T52.3X1	T52.3X2	T52.3X3	T52.3X4	—	—
monobutyl ether	T52.3X1	T52.3X2	T52.3X3	T52.3X4	—	—
imine	T54.1X1	T54.1X2	T54.1X3	T54.1X4	—	—
oxide (fumigant) (nonmedicinal)	T59.891	T59.892	T59.893	T59.894	—	—
medicinal	T49.ØX1	T49.ØX2	T49.ØX3	T49.ØX4	T49.ØX5	T49.ØX6
Ethylenediaminetetra-acetic acid	T50.6X1	T50.6X2	T50.6X3	T50.6X4	T50.6X5	T50.6X6
Ethylenediamine theophylline	T48.6X1	T48.6X2	T48.6X3	T48.6X4	T48.6X5	T48.6X6
Ethylenedinitrilotetra-acetate	T50.6X1	T50.6X2	T50.6X3	T50.6X4	T50.6X5	T50.6X6
Ethylestrenol	T38.7X1	T38.7X2	T38.7X3	T38.7X4	T38.7X5	T38.7X6
Ethylhydroxycellulose	T47.4X1	T47.4X2	T47.4X3	T47.4X4	T47.4X5	T47.4X6
Ethylidene						
chloride NEC	T53.6X1	T53.6X2	T53.6X3	T53.6X4	—	—
diacetate	T60.3X1	T60.3X2	T60.3X3	T60.3X4	—	—
dicoumarin	T45.511	T45.512	T45.513	T45.514	T45.515	T45.516
dicoumarol	T45.511	T45.512	T45.513	T45.514	T45.515	T45.516
diethyl ether	T52.ØX1	T52.ØX2	T52.ØX3	T52.ØX4	—	—
Ethylmorphine	T40.2X1	T40.2X2	T40.2X3	T40.2X4	T40.2X5	T40.2X6
Ethylnorepinephrine	T48.6X1	T48.6X2	T48.6X3	T48.6X4	T48.6X5	T48.6X6
Ethylparachlorophen-oxyisobutyrate	T46.6X1	T46.6X2	T46.6X3	T46.6X4	T46.6X5	T46.6X6
Ethynodiol	T38.4X1	T38.4X2	T38.4X3	T38.4X4	T38.4X5	T38.4X6
with mestranol diacetate	T38.4X1	T38.4X2	T38.4X3	T38.4X4	T38.4X5	T38.4X6
Ethyol*	T50.991	T50.992	T50.993	T50.994	T50.995	T50.996
Etidocaine	T41.3X1	T41.3X2	T41.3X3	T41.3X4	T41.3X5	T41.3X6
infiltration (subcutaneous)	T41.3X1	T41.3X2	T41.3X3	T41.3X4	T41.3X5	T41.3X6
nerve (peripheral) (plexus)	T41.3X1	T41.3X2	T41.3X3	T41.3X4	T41.3X5	T41.3X6
Etidronate	T50.991	T50.992	T50.993	T50.994	T50.995	T50.996
Etidronic acid (disodium salt)	T50.991	T50.992	T50.993	T50.994	T50.995	T50.996
Etifoxine	T42.6X1	T42.6X2	T42.6X3	T42.6X4	T42.6X5	T42.6X6
Etilefrine	T44.4X1	T44.4X2	T44.4X3	T44.4X4	T44.4X5	T44.4X6
Etilfen	T42.3X1	T42.3X2	T42.3X3	T42.3X4	T42.3X5	T42.3X6
Etinodiol	T38.4X1	T38.4X2	T38.4X3	T38.4X4	T38.4X5	T38.4X6
Etiroxate	T46.6X1	T46.6X2	T46.6X3	T46.6X4	T46.6X5	T46.6X6
Etizolam	T42.4X1	T42.4X2	T42.4X3	T42.4X4	T42.4X5	T42.4X6
Etodolac	T39.391	T39.392	T39.393	T39.394	T39.395	T39.396
Etofamide	T37.3X1	T37.3X2	T37.3X3	T37.3X4	T37.3X5	T37.3X6
Etofibrate	T46.6X1	T46.6X2	T46.6X3	T46.6X4	T46.6X5	T46.6X6
Etofylline	T46.7X1	T46.7X2	T46.7X3	T46.7X4	T46.7X5	T46.7X6
clofibrate	T46.6X1	T46.6X2	T46.6X3	T46.6X4	T46.6X5	T46.6X6
Etoglucid	T45.1X1	T45.1X2	T45.1X3	T45.1X4	T45.1X5	T45.1X6
Etomidate	T41.1X1	T41.1X2	T41.1X3	T41.1X4	T41.1X5	T41.1X6

Substance	Poisoning, Accidental (unintentional)	Poisoning, Intentional Self-harm	Poisoning, Assault	Poisoning, Undetermined	Adverse Effect	Under-dosing
Etomide	T39.8X1	T39.8X2	T39.8X3	T39.8X4	T39.8X5	T39.8X6
Etomidoline	T44.3X1	T44.3X2	T44.3X3	T44.3X4	T44.3X5	T44.3X6
Etoposide	T45.1X1	T45.1X2	T45.1X3	T45.1X4	T45.1X5	T45.1X6
Etorphine	T40.2X1	T40.2X2	T40.2X3	T40.2X4	T40.2X5	T40.2X6
Etoval	T42.3X1	T42.3X2	T42.3X3	T42.3X4	T42.3X5	T42.3X6
Etozolin	T50.1X1	T50.1X2	T50.1X3	T50.1X4	T50.1X5	T50.1X6
Etravirine*	T37.5X1	T37.5X2	T37.5X3	T37.5X4	T37.5X5	T37.5X6
Etretinate	T50.991	T50.992	T50.993	T50.994	T50.995	T50.996
Etryptamine	T43.691	T43.692	T43.693	T43.694	T43.695	T43.696
Etybenzatropine	T44.3X1	T44.3X2	T44.3X3	T44.3X4	T44.3X5	T44.3X6
Etynodiol	T38.4X1	T38.4X2	T38.4X3	T38.4X4	T38.4X5	T38.4X6
Eucaine	T41.3X1	T41.3X2	T41.3X3	T41.3X4	T41.3X5	T41.3X6
Eucalyptus oil	T49.7X1	T49.7X2	T49.7X3	T49.7X4	T49.7X5	T49.7X6
Eucatropine	T49.5X1	T49.5X2	T49.5X3	T49.5X4	T49.5X5	T49.5X6
Eucodal	T40.2X1	T40.2X2	T40.2X3	T40.2X4	T40.2X5	T40.2X6
Euneryl	T42.3X1	T42.3X2	T42.3X3	T42.3X4	T42.3X5	T42.3X6
Euphthalmine	T44.3X1	T44.3X2	T44.3X3	T44.3X4	T44.3X5	T44.3X6
Eurax	T49.ØX1	T49.ØX2	T49.ØX3	T49.ØX4	T49.ØX5	T49.ØX6
Euresol	T49.4X1	T49.4X2	T49.4X3	T49.4X4	T49.4X5	T49.4X6
Euthroid	T38.1X1	T38.1X2	T38.1X3	T38.1X4	T38.1X5	T38.1X6
Evans blue	T50.8X1	T50.8X2	T50.8X3	T50.8X4	T50.8X5	T50.8X6
Evipal	T42.3X1	T42.3X2	T42.3X3	T42.3X4	T42.3X5	T42.3X6
sodium	T41.1X1	T41.1X2	T41.1X3	T41.1X4	T41.1X5	T41.1X6
Evipan	T42.3X1	T42.3X2	T42.3X3	T42.3X4	T42.3X5	T42.3X6
sodium	T41.1X1	T41.1X2	T41.1X3	T41.1X4	T41.1X5	T41.1X6
Exalamide	T49.ØX1	T49.ØX2	T49.ØX3	T49.ØX4	T49.ØX5	T49.ØX6
Exalgin	T39.1X1	T39.1X2	T39.1X3	T39.1X4	T39.1X5	T39.1X6
Excipients, pharmaceutical	T50.901	T50.902	T50.903	T50.904	T50.905	T50.906
Exhaust gas (engine) (motor vehicle)	T58.Ø1	T58.Ø2	T58.Ø3	T58.Ø4	—	—
Ex-Lax (phenolphthalein)	T47.2X1	T47.2X2	T47.2X3	T47.2X4	T47.2X5	T47.2X6
Expectorant NEC	T48.4X1	T48.4X2	T48.4X3	T48.4X4	T48.4X5	T48.4X6
Extended insulin zinc suspension	T38.3X1	T38.3X2	T38.3X3	T38.3X4	T38.3X5	T38.3X6
External medications (skin) (mucous membrane)	T49.91	T49.92	T49.93	T49.94	T49.95	T49.96
dental agent	T49.7X1	T49.7X2	T49.7X3	T49.7X4	T49.7X5	T49.7X6
ENT agent	T49.6X1	T49.6X2	T49.6X3	T49.6X4	T49.6X5	T49.6X6
ophthalmic preparation	T49.5X1	T49.5X2	T49.5X3	T49.5X4	T49.5X5	T49.5X6
specified NEC	T49.8X1	T49.8X2	T49.8X3	T49.8X4	T49.8X5	T49.8X6
Extina*	T49.ØX1	T49.ØX2	T49.ØX3	T49.ØX4	T49.ØX5	T49.ØX6
Extrapyramidal antagonist NEC	T44.3X1	T44.3X2	T44.3X3	T44.3X4	T44.3X5	T44.3X6
Eye agents (anti-infective)	T49.5X1	T49.5X2	T49.5X3	T49.5X4	T49.5X5	T49.5X6
Eye drug NEC	T49.5X1	T49.5X2	T49.5X3	T49.5X4	T49.5X5	T49.5X6
FAC (fluorouracil + doxorubicin + cyclophosphamide)	T45.1X1	T45.1X2	T45.1X3	T45.1X4	T45.1X5	T45.1X6
Factor						
I (fibrinogen)	T45.8X1	T45.8X2	T45.8X3	T45.8X4	T45.8X5	T45.8X6
III (thromboplastin)	T45.8X1	T45.8X2	T45.8X3	T45.8X4	T45.8X5	T45.8X6
IX complex	T45.7X1	T45.7X2	T45.7X3	T45.7X4	T45.7X5	T45.7X6
human	T45.8X1	T45.8X2	T45.8X3	T45.8X4	T45.8X5	T45.8X6
VIII (antihemophilic Factor) (concentrate)	T45.8X1	T45.8X2	T45.8X3	T45.8X4	T45.8X5	T45.8X6
Famotidine	T47.ØX1	T47.ØX2	T47.ØX3	T47.ØX4	T47.ØX5	T47.ØX6
Fat suspension, intravenous	T50.991	T50.992	T50.993	T50.994	T50.995	T50.996
Fazadinium bromide	T48.1X1	T48.1X2	T48.1X3	T48.1X4	T48.1X5	T48.1X6
Febarbamate	T42.3X1	T42.3X2	T42.3X3	T42.3X4	T42.3X5	T42.3X6
Fecal softener	T47.4X1	T47.4X2	T47.4X3	T47.4X4	T47.4X5	T47.4X6
Fedrilate	T48.3X1	T48.3X2	T48.3X3	T48.3X4	T48.3X5	T48.3X6
Felodipine	T46.1X1	T46.1X2	T46.1X3	T46.1X4	T46.1X5	T46.1X6
Felypressin	T38.891	T38.892	T38.893	T38.894	T38.895	T38.896
Femizol*	T49.ØX1	T49.ØX2	T49.ØX3	T49.ØX4	T49.ØX5	T49.ØX6
Femoxetine	T43.221	T43.222	T43.223	T43.224	T43.225	T43.226
Fenalcomine	T46.3X1	T46.3X2	T46.3X3	T46.3X4	T46.3X5	T46.3X6
Fenamisal	T37.1X1	T37.1X2	T37.1X3	T37.1X4	T37.1X5	T37.1X6
Fenazone	T39.2X1	T39.2X2	T39.2X3	T39.2X4	T39.2X5	T39.2X6
Fenbendazole	T37.4X1	T37.4X2	T37.4X3	T37.4X4	T37.4X5	T37.4X6
Fenbutrazate	T50.5X1	T50.5X2	T50.5X3	T50.5X4	T50.5X5	T50.5X6
Fencamfamine	T43.691	T43.692	T43.693	T43.694	T43.695	T43.696
Fendiline	T46.1X1	T46.1X2	T46.1X3	T46.1X4	T46.1X5	T46.1X6
Fenetylline	T43.691	T43.692	T43.693	T43.694	T43.695	T43.696
Fenflumizole	T39.391	T39.392	T39.393	T39.394	T39.395	T39.396
Fenfluramine	T50.5X1	T50.5X2	T50.5X3	T50.5X4	T50.5X5	T50.5X6
Fenobarbital	T42.3X1	T42.3X2	T42.3X3	T42.3X4	T42.3X5	T42.3X6
Fenofibrate	T46.6X1	T46.6X2	T46.6X3	T46.6X4	T46.6X5	T46.6X6
Fenoprofen	T39.311	T39.312	T39.313	T39.314	T39.315	T39.316
Fenoterol	T48.6X1	T48.6X2	T48.6X3	T48.6X4	T48.6X5	T48.6X6
Fenoverine	T44.3X1	T44.3X2	T44.3X3	T44.3X4	T44.3X5	T44.3X6
Fenoxazoline	T48.5X1	T48.5X2	T48.5X3	T48.5X4	T48.5X5	T48.5X6
Fenproporex	T50.5X1	T50.5X2	T50.5X3	T50.5X4	T50.5X5	T50.5X6

Substance	Poisoning, Accidental (unintentional)	Poisoning, Intentional Self-harm	Poisoning, Assault	Poisoning, Undetermined	Adverse Effect	Under-dosing
Fenquizone	T5Ø.2X1	T5Ø.2X2	T5Ø.2X3	T5Ø.2X4	T5Ø.2X5	T5Ø.2X6
Fentanyl (analogs)	T4Ø.411	T4Ø.412	T4Ø.413	T4Ø.414	T4Ø.415	T4Ø.416
Fentazin	T43.3X1	T43.3X2	T43.3X3	T43.3X4	T43.3X5	T43.3X6
Fenthion	T6Ø.ØX1	T6Ø.ØX2	T6Ø.ØX3	T6Ø.ØX4	—	—
Fenticlor	T49.ØX1	T49.ØX2	T49.ØX3	T49.ØX4	T49.ØX5	T49.ØX6
Fenylbutazone	T39.2X1	T39.2X2	T39.2X3	T39.2X4	T39.2X5	T39.2X6
Feprazone	T39.2X1	T39.2X2	T39.2X3	T39.2X4	T39.2X5	T39.2X6
Fer de lance (bite) (venom)	T63.Ø61	T63.Ø62	T63.Ø63	T63.Ø64	—	—
Ferrex*	T45.4X1	T45.4X2	T45.4X3	T45.4X4	T45.4X5	T45.4X6
Ferric — *see also* Iron						
chloride	T45.4X1	T45.4X2	T45.4X3	T45.4X4	T45.4X5	T45.4X6
citrate	T45.4X1	T45.4X2	T45.4X3	T45.4X4	T45.4X5	T45.4X6
hydroxide						
colloidal	T45.4X1	T45.4X2	T45.4X3	T45.4X4	T45.4X5	T45.4X6
polymaltose	T45.4X1	T45.4X2	T45.4X3	T45.4X4	T45.4X5	T45.4X6
pyrophosphate	T45.4X1	T45.4X2	T45.4X3	T45.4X4	T45.4X5	T45.4X6
Ferritin	T45.4X1	T45.4X2	T45.4X3	T45.4X4	T45.4X5	T45.4X6
Ferrocholinate	T45.4X1	T45.4X2	T45.4X3	T45.4X4	T45.4X5	T45.4X6
Ferrodextrane	T45.4X1	T45.4X2	T45.4X3	T45.4X4	T45.4X5	T45.4X6
Ferropolimaler	T45.4X1	T45.4X2	T45.4X3	T45.4X4	T45.4X5	T45.4X6
Ferrous — *see also* Iron						
phosphate	T45.4X1	T45.4X2	T45.4X3	T45.4X4	T45.4X5	T45.4X6
salt	T45.4X1	T45.4X2	T45.4X3	T45.4X4	T45.4X5	T45.4X6
with folic acid	T45.4X1	T45.4X2	T45.4X3	T45.4X4	T45.4X5	T45.4X6
Ferrous fumerate, gluconate, lactate, salt NEC, sulfate (medicinal)	T45.4X1	T45.4X2	T45.4X3	T45.4X4	T45.4X5	T45.4X6
Ferrovanadium (fumes)	T59.891	T59.892	T59.893	T59.894	—	—
Ferrum — *see* Iron						
Fertilizers NEC	T65.891	T65.892	T65.893	T65.894	—	—
with herbicide mixture	T6Ø.3X1	T6Ø.3X2	T6Ø.3X3	T6Ø.3X4	—	—
Fetoxilate	T47.6X1	T47.6X2	T47.6X3	T47.6X4	T47.6X5	T47.6X6
Fiber, dietary	T47.4X1	T47.4X2	T47.4X3	T47.4X4	T47.4X5	T47.4X6
Fiberglass	T65.831	T65.832	T65.833	T65.834	—	—
Fibrinogen (human)	T45.8X1	T45.8X2	T45.8X3	T45.8X4	T45.8X5	T45.8X6
Fibrinolysin (human)	T45.691	T45.692	T45.693	T45.694	T45.695	T45.696
Fibrinolysis						
affecting drug	T45.6Ø1	T45.6Ø2	T45.6Ø3	T45.6Ø4	T45.6Ø5	T45.6Ø6
inhibitor NEC	T45.621	T45.622	T45.623	T45.624	T45.625	T45.626
Fibrinolytic drug	T45.611	T45.612	T45.613	T45.614	T45.615	T45.616
Filix mas	T37.4X1	T37.4X2	T37.4X3	T37.4X4	T37.4X5	T37.4X6
Filtering cream	T49.3X1	T49.3X2	T49.3X3	T49.3X4	T49.3X5	T49.3X6
Finacea*	T49.ØX1	T49.ØX2	T49.ØX3	T49.ØX4	T49.ØX5	T49.ØX6
Fiorinal	T39.Ø11	T39.Ø12	T39.Ø13	T39.Ø14	T39.Ø15	T39.Ø16
Firedamp	T59.891	T59.892	T59.893	T59.894	—	—
Fish, noxious, nonbacterial	T61.91	T61.92	T61.93	T61.94	—	—
ciguatera	T61.Ø1	T61.Ø2	T61.Ø3	T61.Ø4	—	—
scombroid	T61.11	T61.12	T61.13	T61.14	—	—
shell	T61.781	T61.782	T61.783	T61.784	—	—
specified NEC	T61.771	T61.772	T61.773	T61.774	—	—
Flagyl	T37.3X1	T37.3X2	T37.3X3	T37.3X4	T37.3X5	T37.3X6
Flavine adenine dinucleotide	T45.2X1	T45.2X2	T45.2X3	T45.2X4	T45.2X5	T45.2X6
Flavodic acid	T46.991	T46.992	T46.993	T46.994	T46.995	T46.996
Flavoxate	T44.3X1	T44.3X2	T44.3X3	T44.3X4	T44.3X5	T44.3X6
Flaxedil	T48.1X1	T48.1X2	T48.1X3	T48.1X4	T48.1X5	T48.1X6
Flaxseed (medicinal)	T49.3X1	T49.3X2	T49.3X3	T49.3X4	T49.3X5	T49.3X6
Flecainide	T46.2X1	T46.2X2	T46.2X3	T46.2X4	T46.2X5	T46.2X6
Fleroxacin	T36.8X1	T36.8X2	T36.8X3	T36.8X4	T36.8X5	T36.8X6
Floctafenine	T39.8X1	T39.8X2	T39.8X3	T39.8X4	T39.8X5	T39.8X6
Flomax	T44.6X1	T44.6X2	T44.6X3	T44.6X4	T44.6X5	T44.6X6
Flomoxef	T36.1X1	T36.1X2	T36.1X3	T36.1X4	T36.1X5	T36.1X6
Flopropione	T44.3X1	T44.3X2	T44.3X3	T44.3X4	T44.3X5	T44.3X6
FLORAjen*	T47.6X1	T47.6X2	T47.6X3	T47.6X4	T47.6X5	T47.6X6
Florantyrone	T47.5X1	T47.5X2	T47.5X3	T47.5X4	T47.5X5	T47.5X6
Floraquin	T37.8X1	T37.8X2	T37.8X3	T37.8X4	T37.8X5	T37.8X6
Florinef	T38.ØX1	T38.ØX2	T38.ØX3	T38.ØX4	T38.ØX5	T38.ØX6
ENT agent	T49.6X1	T49.6X2	T49.6X3	T49.6X4	T49.6X5	T49.6X6
ophthalmic preparation	T49.5X1	T49.5X2	T49.5X3	T49.5X4	T49.5X5	T49.5X6
topical NEC	T49.ØX1	T49.ØX2	T49.ØX3	T49.ØX4	T49.ØX5	T49.ØX6
Flowers of sulfur	T49.4X1	T49.4X2	T49.4X3	T49.4X4	T49.4X5	T49.4X6
Floxuridine	T45.1X1	T45.1X2	T45.1X3	T45.1X4	T45.1X5	T45.1X6
Fluanisone	T43.4X1	T43.4X2	T43.4X3	T43.4X4	T43.4X5	T43.4X6
Flubendazole	T37.4X1	T37.4X2	T37.4X3	T37.4X4	T37.4X5	T37.4X6
Fluclorolone acetonide	T49.ØX1	T49.ØX2	T49.ØX3	T49.ØX4	T49.ØX5	T49.ØX6
Flucloxacillin	T36.ØX1	T36.ØX2	T36.ØX3	T36.ØX4	T36.ØX5	T36.ØX6
Fluconazole	T37.8X1	T37.8X2	T37.8X3	T37.8X4	T37.8X5	T37.8X6
Flucytosine	T37.8X1	T37.8X2	T37.8X3	T37.8X4	T37.8X5	T37.8X6
Fludeoxyglucose (18F)	T5Ø.8X1	T5Ø.8X2	T5Ø.8X3	T5Ø.8X4	T5Ø.8X5	T5Ø.8X6
Fludiazepam	T42.4X1	T42.4X2	T42.4X3	T42.4X4	T42.4X5	T42.4X6
Fludrocortisone	T5Ø.ØX1	T5Ø.ØX2	T5Ø.ØX3	T5Ø.ØX4	T5Ø.ØX5	T5Ø.ØX6
ENT agent	T49.6X1	T49.6X2	T49.6X3	T49.6X4	T49.6X5	T49.6X6
Fludrocortisone — *continued*						
ophthalmic preparation	T49.5X1	T49.5X2	T49.5X3	T49.5X4	T49.5X5	T49.5X6
topical NEC	T49.ØX1	T49.ØX2	T49.ØX3	T49.ØX4	T49.ØX5	T49.ØX6
Fludroxycortide	T49.ØX1	T49.ØX2	T49.ØX3	T49.ØX4	T49.ØX5	T49.ØX6
Flufenamic acid	T39.391	T39.392	T39.393	T39.394	T39.395	T39.396
Fluindione	T45.511	T45.512	T45.513	T45.514	T45.515	T45.516
Flumequine	T37.8X1	T37.8X2	T37.8X3	T37.8X4	T37.8X5	T37.8X6
Flumethasone	T49.ØX1	T49.ØX2	T49.ØX3	T49.ØX4	T49.ØX5	T49.ØX6
Flumethiazide	T5Ø.2X1	T5Ø.2X2	T5Ø.2X3	T5Ø.2X4	T5Ø.2X5	T5Ø.2X6
Flumidin	T37.5X1	T37.5X2	T37.5X3	T37.5X4	T37.5X5	T37.5X6
Flunarizine	T46.7X1	T46.7X2	T46.7X3	T46.7X4	T46.7X5	T46.7X6
Flunidazole	T37.8X1	T37.8X2	T37.8X3	T37.8X4	T37.8X5	T37.8X6
Flunisolide	T48.6X1	T48.6X2	T48.6X3	T48.6X4	T48.6X5	T48.6X6
Flunitrazepam	T42.4X1	T42.4X2	T42.4X3	T42.4X4	T42.4X5	T42.4X6
Fluocinolone (acetonide)	T49.ØX1	T49.ØX2	T49.ØX3	T49.ØX4	T49.ØX5	T49.ØX6
Fluocinonide	T49.ØX1	T49.ØX2	T49.ØX3	T49.ØX4	T49.ØX5	T49.ØX6
Fluocortin (butyl)	T49.ØX1	T49.ØX2	T49.ØX3	T49.ØX4	T49.ØX5	T49.ØX6
Fluocortolone	T49.ØX1	T49.ØX2	T49.ØX3	T49.ØX4	T49.ØX5	T49.ØX6
Fluohydrocortisone	T38.ØX1	T38.ØX2	T38.ØX3	T38.ØX4	T38.ØX5	T38.ØX6
ENT agent	T49.6X1	T49.6X2	T49.6X3	T49.6X4	T49.6X5	T49.6X6
ophthalmic preparation	T49.5X1	T49.5X2	T49.5X3	T49.5X4	T49.5X5	T49.5X6
topical NEC	T49.ØX1	T49.ØX2	T49.ØX3	T49.ØX4	T49.ØX5	T49.ØX6
Fluonid	T49.ØX1	T49.ØX2	T49.ØX3	T49.ØX4	T49.ØX5	T49.ØX6
Fluopromazine	T43.3X1	T43.3X2	T43.3X3	T43.3X4	T43.3X5	T43.3X6
Fluoracetate	T6Ø.8X1	T6Ø.8X2	T6Ø.8X3	T6Ø.8X4	—	—
Fluorescein	T5Ø.8X1	T5Ø.8X2	T5Ø.8X3	T5Ø.8X4	T5Ø.8X5	T5Ø.8X6
Fluorhydrocortisone	T5Ø.ØX1	T5Ø.ØX2	T5Ø.ØX3	T5Ø.ØX4	T5Ø.ØX5	T5Ø.ØX6
Fluoride (nonmedicinal) (pesticide) (sodium) **NEC**	T6Ø.8X1	T6Ø.8X2	T6Ø.8X3	T6Ø.8X4	—	—
hydrogen — *see* Hydrofluoric acid						
medicinal NEC	T5Ø.991	T5Ø.992	T5Ø.993	T5Ø.994	T5Ø.995	T5Ø.996
dental use	T49.7X1	T49.7X2	T49.7X3	T49.7X4	T49.7X5	T49.7X6
not pesticide NEC	T54.91	T54.92	T54.93	T54.94	—	—
stannous	T49.7X1	T49.7X2	T49.7X3	T49.7X4	T49.7X5	T49.7X6
Fluorigard*	T47.7X1	T47.7X2	T47.7X3	T47.7X4	T47.7X5	T47.7X6
Fluorinated corticosteroids	T38.ØX1	T38.ØX2	T38.ØX3	T38.ØX4	T38.ØX5	T38.ØX6
Fluorine (gas)	T59.5X1	T59.5X2	T59.5X3	T59.5X4	—	—
salt — *see* Fluoride(s)						
Fluoristan	T49.7X1	T49.7X2	T49.7X3	T49.7X4	T49.7X5	T49.7X6
Fluormetholone	T49.ØX1	T49.ØX2	T49.ØX3	T49.ØX4	T49.ØX5	T49.ØX6
Fluoroacetate	T6Ø.8X1	T6Ø.8X2	T6Ø.8X3	T6Ø.8X4	—	—
Fluorocarbon monomer	T53.6X1	T53.6X2	T53.6X3	T53.6X4	—	—
Fluorocytosine	T37.8X1	T37.8X2	T37.8X3	T37.8X4	T37.8X5	T37.8X6
Fluorodeoxyuridine	T45.1X1	T45.1X2	T45.1X3	T45.1X4	T45.1X5	T45.1X6
Fluorometholone	T49.ØX1	T49.ØX2	T49.ØX3	T49.ØX4	T49.ØX5	T49.ØX6
ophthalmic preparation	T49.5X1	T49.5X2	T49.5X3	T49.5X4	T49.5X5	T49.5X6
Fluorophosphate insecticide	T6Ø.ØX1	T6Ø.ØX2	T6Ø.ØX3	T6Ø.ØX4	—	—
Fluorosol	T46.3X1	T46.3X2	T46.3X3	T46.3X4	T46.3X5	T46.3X6
Fluorouracil	T45.1X1	T45.1X2	T45.1X3	T45.1X4	T45.1X5	T45.1X6
Fluorphenylalanine	T49.5X1	T49.5X2	T49.5X3	T49.5X4	T49.5X5	T49.5X6
Fluothane	T41.ØX1	T41.ØX2	T41.ØX3	T41.ØX4	T41.ØX5	T41.ØX6
Fluoxetine	T43.221	T43.222	T43.223	T43.224	T43.225	T43.226
Fluoxymesterone	T38.7X1	T38.7X2	T38.7X3	T38.7X4	T38.7X5	T38.7X6
Flupenthixol	T43.4X1	T43.4X2	T43.4X3	T43.4X4	T43.4X5	T43.4X6
Flupentixol	T43.4X1	T43.4X2	T43.4X3	T43.4X4	T43.4X5	T43.4X6
Fluphenazine	T43.3X1	T43.3X2	T43.3X3	T43.3X4	T43.3X5	T43.3X6
Fluprednidene	T49.ØX1	T49.ØX2	T49.ØX3	T49.ØX4	T49.ØX5	T49.ØX6
Fluprednisolone	T38.ØX1	T38.ØX2	T38.ØX3	T38.ØX4	T38.ØX5	T38.ØX6
Fluradoline	T39.8X1	T39.8X2	T39.8X3	T39.8X4	T39.8X5	T39.8X6
Flurandrenolide	T49.ØX1	T49.ØX2	T49.ØX3	T49.ØX4	T49.ØX5	T49.ØX6
Flurandrenolone	T49.ØX1	T49.ØX2	T49.ØX3	T49.ØX4	T49.ØX5	T49.ØX6
Flurazepam	T42.4X1	T42.4X2	T42.4X3	T42.4X4	T42.4X5	T42.4X6
Flurbiprofen	T39.311	T39.312	T39.313	T39.314	T39.315	T39.316
Flurobate	T49.ØX1	T49.ØX2	T49.ØX3	T49.ØX4	T49.ØX5	T49.ØX6
Fluroxene	T41.ØX1	T41.ØX2	T41.ØX3	T41.ØX4	T41.ØX5	T41.ØX6
Fluspirilene	T43.591	T43.592	T43.593	T43.594	T43.595	T43.596
Flutamide	T38.6X1	T38.6X2	T38.6X3	T38.6X4	T38.6X5	T38.6X6
Flutazolam	T38.ØX1	T38.ØX2	T38.ØX3	T38.ØX4	T38.ØX5	T38.ØX6
Fluticasone propionate	T38.ØX1	T38.ØX2	T38.ØX3	T38.ØX4	T38.ØX5	T38.ØX6
Flutoprazepam	T42.4X1	T42.4X2	T42.4X3	T42.4X4	T42.4X5	T42.4X6
Flutropium bromide	T48.6X1	T48.6X2	T48.6X3	T48.6X4	T48.6X5	T48.6X6
Fluvoxamine	T43.221	T43.222	T43.223	T43.224	T43.225	T43.226
Folacin	T45.8X1	T45.8X2	T45.8X3	T45.8X4	T45.8X5	T45.8X6
Folic acid	T45.8X1	T45.8X2	T45.8X3	T45.8X4	T45.8X5	T45.8X6
with ferrous salt	T45.2X1	T45.2X2	T45.2X3	T45.2X4	T45.2X5	T45.2X6
antagonist	T45.1X1	T45.1X2	T45.1X3	T45.1X4	T45.1X5	T45.1X6
Folinic acid	T45.8X1	T45.8X2	T45.8X3	T45.8X4	T45.8X5	T45.8X6
Folium stramoniae	T48.6X1	T48.6X2	T48.6X3	T48.6X4	T48.6X5	T48.6X6
Follicle-stimulating hormone, human	T38.811	T38.812	T38.813	T38.814	T38.815	T38.816

Substance	Poisoning, Accidental (unintentional)	Poisoning, Intentional Self-harm	Poisoning, Assault	Poisoning, Undetermined	Adverse Effect	Under-dosing
Folpet	T60.3X1	T60.3X2	T60.3X3	T60.3X4	—	—
Fomepizole*	T50.6X1	T50.6X2	T50.6X3	T50.6X4	T50.6X5	T50.6X6
Fominoben	T48.3X1	T48.3X2	T48.3X3	T48.3X4	T48.3X5	T48.3X6
Food, foodstuffs, noxious, nonbacterial, NEC	T62.91	T62.92	T62.93	T62.94	—	—
berries	T62.1X1	T62.1X2	T62.1X3	T62.1X4	—	—
fish — *see also* Fish	T61.91	T61.92	T61.93	T61.94	—	—
mushrooms	T62.0X1	T62.0X2	T62.0X3	T62.0X4	—	—
plants	T62.2X1	T62.2X2	T62.2X3	T62.2X4	—	—
seafood	T61.91	T61.92	T61.93	T61.94	—	—
specified NEC	T61.8X1	T61.8X2	T61.8X3	T61.8X4	—	—
seeds	T62.2X1	T62.2X2	T62.2X3	T62.2X4	—	—
shellfish	T61.781	T61.782	T61.783	T61.784	—	—
specified NEC	T62.8X1	T62.8X2	T62.8X3	T62.8X4	—	—
Fool's parsley	T62.2X1	T62.2X2	T62.2X3	T62.2X4	—	—
Formaldehyde (solution), gas or vapor	T59.2X1	T59.2X2	T59.2X3	T59.2X4	—	—
fungicide	T60.3X1	T60.3X2	T60.3X3	T60.3X4	—	—
Formalin	T59.2X1	T59.2X2	T59.2X3	T59.2X4	—	—
fungicide	T60.3X1	T60.3X2	T60.3X3	T60.3X4	—	—
vapor	T59.2X1	T59.2X2	T59.2X3	T59.2X4	—	—
Formic acid	T54.2X1	T54.2X2	T54.2X3	T54.2X4	—	—
vapor	T59.891	T59.892	T59.893	T59.894	—	—
Formoterol*	T48.6X1	T48.6X2	T48.6X3	T48.6X4	T48.6X5	T48.6X6
Fortaz*	T36.1X1	T36.1X2	T36.1X3	T36.1X4	T36.1X5	T36.1X6
Foscarnet sodium	T37.5X1	T37.5X2	T37.5X3	T37.5X4	T37.5X5	T37.5X6
Fosfestrol	T38.5X1	T38.5X2	T38.5X3	T38.5X4	T38.5X5	T38.5X6
Fosfomycin	T36.8X1	T36.8X2	T36.8X3	T36.8X4	T36.8X5	T36.8X6
Fosfonet sodium	T37.5X1	T37.5X2	T37.5X3	T37.5X4	T37.5X5	T37.5X6
Fosinopril	T46.4X1	T46.4X2	T46.4X3	T46.4X4	T46.4X5	T46.4X6
sodium	T46.4X1	T46.4X2	T46.4X3	T46.4X4	T46.4X5	T46.4X6
Fowler's solution	T57.0X1	T57.0X2	T57.0X3	T57.0X4	—	—
Foxglove	T62.2X1	T62.2X2	T62.2X3	T62.2X4	—	—
Framycetin	T36.5X1	T36.5X2	T36.5X3	T36.5X4	T36.5X5	T36.5X6
Frangula	T47.2X1	T47.2X2	T47.2X3	T47.2X4	T47.2X5	T47.2X6
extract	T47.2X1	T47.2X2	T47.2X3	T47.2X4	T47.2X5	T47.2X6
Frei antigen	T50.8X1	T50.8X2	T50.8X3	T50.8X4	T50.8X5	T50.8X6
Freon	T53.5X1	T53.5X2	T53.5X3	T53.5X4	—	—
Fructose	T50.3X1	T50.3X2	T50.3X3	T50.3X4	T50.3X5	T50.3X6
Frusemide	T50.1X1	T50.1X2	T50.1X3	T50.1X4	T50.1X5	T50.1X6
FSH	T38.811	T38.812	T38.813	T38.814	T38.815	T38.816
Ftorafur	T45.1X1	T45.1X2	T45.1X3	T45.1X4	T45.1X5	T45.1X6
Fuel						
automobile	T52.0X1	T52.0X2	T52.0X3	T52.0X4	—	—
exhaust gas, not in transit	T58.01	T58.02	T58.03	T58.04	—	—
vapor NEC	T52.0X1	T52.0X2	T52.0X3	T52.0X4	—	—
gas (domestic use) — *see also* Carbon, monoxide, fuel, utility	T59.891	T59.892	T59.893	T59.894	—	—
utility	T59.891	T59.892	T59.893	T59.894	—	—
incomplete combustion of — *see* Carbon, monoxide, fuel, utility						
in mobile container	T59.891	T59.892	T59.893	T59.894	—	—
piped (natural)	T59.891	T59.892	T59.893	T59.894	—	—
industrial, incomplete combustion	T58.8X1	T58.8X2	T58.8X3	T58.8X4	—	—
Fugillin	T36.8X1	T36.8X2	T36.8X3	T36.8X4	T36.8X5	T36.8X6
Fulminate of mercury	T56.1X1	T56.1X2	T56.1X3	T56.1X4	—	—
Fulvicin	T36.7X1	T36.7X2	T36.7X3	T36.7X4	T36.7X5	T36.7X6
Fumadil	T36.8X1	T36.8X2	T36.8X3	T36.8X4	T36.8X5	T36.8X6
Fumagillin	T36.8X1	T36.8X2	T36.8X3	T36.8X4	T36.8X5	T36.8X6
Fumaric acid	T49.4X1	T49.4X2	T49.4X3	T49.4X4	T49.4X5	T49.4X6
Fumes (from)	T59.91	T59.92	T59.93	T59.94		
carbon monoxide — *see* Carbon, monoxide						
charcoal (domestic use) — *see* Charcoal, fumes						
chloroform — *see* Chloroform						
coke (in domestic stoves, fireplaces) — *see* Coke fumes						
corrosive NEC	T54.91	T54.92	T54.93	T54.94		
ether — *see* ether						
freons	T53.5X1	T53.5X2	T53.5X3	T53.5X4	—	—
hydrocarbons	T59.891	T59.892	T59.893	T59.894	—	—
petroleum (liquefied)	T59.891	T59.892	T59.893	T59.894	—	—
distributed through pipes (pure or mixed with air)	T59.891	T59.892	T59.893	T59.894	—	—
lead — *see* lead						

Substance	Poisoning, Accidental (unintentional)	Poisoning, Intentional Self-harm	Poisoning, Assault	Poisoning, Undetermined	Adverse Effect	Under-dosing
Fumes — *continued*						
metal — *see* Metals, or the specified metal						
nitrogen dioxide	T59.0X1	T59.0X2	T59.0X3	T59.0X4	—	—
pesticides — *see* Pesticide						
petroleum (liquefied)	T59.891	T59.892	T59.893	T59.894	—	—
distributed through pipes (pure or mixed with air)	T59.891	T59.892	T59.893	T59.894	—	—
polyester	T59.891	T59.892	T59.893	T59.894	—	—
specified source NEC — *see also* substance specified	T59.891	T59.892	T59.893	T59.894	—	—
sulfur dioxide	T59.1X1	T59.1X2	T59.1X3	T59.1X4	—	—
Fumigant NEC	T60.91	T60.92	T60.93	T60.94	—	—
Fungicide NEC (nonmedicinal)	T60.3X1	T60.3X2	T60.3X3	T60.3X4	—	—
Fungi, noxious, used as food	T62.0X1	T62.0X2	T62.0X3	T62.0X4	—	—
Fungizone	T36.7X1	T36.7X2	T36.7X3	T36.7X4	T36.7X5	T36.7X6
topical	T49.0X1	T49.0X2	T49.0X3	T49.0X4	T49.0X5	T49.0X6
Fungoid*	T49.0X1	T49.0X2	T49.0X3	T49.0X4	T49.0X5	T49.0X6
Furacin	T49.0X1	T49.0X2	T49.0X3	T49.0X4	T49.0X5	T49.0X6
Furadantin	T37.91	T37.92	T37.93	T37.94	T37.95	T37.96
Furazolidone	T37.8X1	T37.8X2	T37.8X3	T37.8X4	T37.8X5	T37.8X6
Furazolium chloride	T49.0X1	T49.0X2	T49.0X3	T49.0X4	T49.0X5	T49.0X6
Furfural	T52.8X1	T52.8X2	T52.8X3	T52.8X4	—	—
Furnace (coal burning) (domestic), gas from	T58.2X1	T58.2X2	T58.2X3	T58.2X4	—	—
industrial	T58.8X1	T58.8X2	T58.8X3	T58.8X4	—	—
Furniture polish	T65.891	T65.892	T65.893	T65.894	—	—
Furosemide	T50.1X1	T50.1X2	T50.1X3	T50.1X4	T50.1X5	T50.1X6
Furoxone	T37.91	T37.92	T37.93	T37.94	T37.95	T37.96
Fursultiamine	T45.2X1	T45.2X2	T45.2X3	T45.2X4	T45.2X5	T45.2X6
Fusafungine	T36.8X1	T36.8X2	T36.8X3	T36.8X4	T36.8X5	T36.8X6
Fusel oil (any) (amyl) (butyl) (propyl), vapor	T51.3X1	T51.3X2	T51.3X3	T51.3X4	—	—
Fusidate (ethanolamine) (sodium)	T36.8X1	T36.8X2	T36.8X3	T36.8X4	T36.8X5	T36.8X6
Fusidic acid	T36.8X1	T36.8X2	T36.8X3	T36.8X4	T36.8X5	T36.8X6
Fytic acid, nonasodium	T50.6X1	T50.6X2	T50.6X3	T50.6X4	T50.6X5	T50.6X6
b-Galactosidase	T47.5X1	T47.5X2	T47.5X3	T47.5X4	T47.5X5	T47.5X6
GABA	T43.8X1	T43.8X2	T43.8X3	T43.8X4	T43.8X5	T43.8X6
Gabitril*	T42.6X1	T42.6X2	T42.6X3	T42.6X4	T42.6X5	T42.6X6
Gadopentetic acid	T50.8X1	T50.8X2	T50.8X3	T50.8X4	T50.8X5	T50.8X6
Galactose	T50.3X1	T50.3X2	T50.3X3	T50.3X4	T50.3X5	T50.3X6
Galantamine	T44.0X1	T44.0X2	T44.0X3	T44.0X4	T44.0X5	T44.0X6
Gallamine (triethiodide)	T48.1X1	T48.1X2	T48.1X3	T48.1X4	T48.1X5	T48.1X6
Gallium citrate	T50.991	T50.992	T50.993	T50.994	T50.995	T50.996
Gallopamil	T46.1X1	T46.1X2	T46.1X3	T46.1X4	T46.1X5	T46.1X6
Gamboge	T47.2X1	T47.2X2	T47.2X3	T47.2X4	T47.2X5	T47.2X6
Gamimune	T50.Z11	T50.Z12	T50.Z13	T50.Z14	T50.Z15	T50.Z16
Gamma-aminobutyric acid	T43.8X1	T43.8X2	T43.8X3	T43.8X4	T43.8X5	T43.8X6
Gamma-benzene hexachloride (medicinal)	T49.0X1	T49.0X2	T49.0X3	T49.0X4	T49.0X5	T49.0X6
nonmedicinal, vapor	T53.6X1	T53.6X2	T53.6X3	T53.6X4	—	—
Gamma-BHC (medicinal) — *see also* Gamma-benzene hexachloride	T49.0X1	T49.0X2	T49.0X3	T49.0X4	T49.0X5	T49.0X6
Gamma globulin	T50.Z11	T50.Z12	T50.Z13	T50.Z14	T50.Z15	T50.Z16
Gamulin	T50.Z11	T50.Z12	T50.Z13	T50.Z14	T50.Z15	T50.Z16
Ganciclovir (sodium)	T37.5X1	T37.5X2	T37.5X3	T37.5X4	T37.5X5	T37.5X6
Ganglionic blocking drug NEC	T44.2X1	T44.2X2	T44.2X3	T44.2X4	T44.2X5	T44.2X6
specified NEC	T44.2X1	T44.2X2	T44.2X3	T44.2X4	T44.2X5	T44.2X6
Ganja	T40.711	T40.712	T40.713	T40.714	T40.715	T40.716
Garamycin	T36.5X1	T36.5X2	T36.5X3	T36.5X4	T36.5X5	T36.5X6
ophthalmic preparation	T49.5X1	T49.5X2	T49.5X3	T49.5X4	T49.5X5	T49.5X6
topical NEC	T49.0X1	T49.0X2	T49.0X3	T49.0X4	T49.0X5	T49.0X6
Gardenal	T42.3X1	T42.3X2	T42.3X3	T42.3X4	T42.3X5	T42.3X6
Gardepanyl	T42.3X1	T42.3X2	T42.3X3	T42.3X4	T42.3X5	T42.3X6
Gaseous substance — *see* Gas						
Gasoline	T52.0X1	T52.0X2	T52.0X3	T52.0X4	—	—
vapor	T52.0X1	T52.0X2	T52.0X3	T52.0X4	—	—
Gastric enzymes	T47.5X1	T47.5X2	T47.5X3	T47.5X4	T47.5X5	T47.5X6
Gastrografin	T50.8X1	T50.8X2	T50.8X3	T50.8X4	T50.8X5	T50.8X6
Gastrointestinal drug	T47.91	T47.92	T47.93	T47.94	T47.95	T47.96
biological	T47.8X1	T47.8X2	T47.8X3	T47.8X4	T47.8X5	T47.8X6
specified NEC	T47.8X1	T47.8X2	T47.8X3	T47.8X4	T47.8X5	T47.8X6
Gas NEC	T59.91	T59.92	T59.93	T59.94	—	—
acetylene	T59.891	T59.892	T59.893	T59.894	—	—
incomplete combustion of	T58.11	T58.12	T58.13	T58.14	—	—

Substance	Poisoning, Accidental (unintentional)	Poisoning, Intentional Self-harm	Poisoning, Assault	Poisoning, Undetermined	Adverse Effect	Under-dosing
Gas — *continued*						
air contaminants, source or type not specified	T59.91	T59.92	T59.93	T59.94	—	—
anesthetic	T41.ØX1	T41.ØX2	T41.ØX3	T41.ØX4	T41.ØX5	T41.ØX6
blast furnace	T58.8X1	T58.8X2	T58.8X3	T58.8X4	—	—
butane — *see* butane						
carbon monoxide — *see* Carbon, monoxide						
chlorine	T59.4X1	T59.4X2	T59.4X3	T59.4X4	—	—
coal	T58.2X1	T58.2X2	T58.2X3	T58.2X4	—	—
cyanide	T57.3X1	T57.3X2	T57.3X3	T57.3X4	—	—
dicyanogen	T65.ØX1	T65.ØX2	T65.ØX3	T65.ØX4	—	—
domestic — *see* Domestic gas						
exhaust	T58.Ø1	T58.Ø2	T58.Ø3	T58.Ø4	—	—
from utility (for cooking, heating, or lighting) (after combustion) — *see* Carbon, monoxide, fuel, utility						
prior to combustion	T59.891	T59.892	T59.893	T59.894	—	—
from wood- or coal-burning stove or fireplace	T58.2X1	T58.2X2	T58.2X3	T58.2X4	—	—
fuel (domestic use) (after combustion) — *see also* Carbon, monoxide, fuel						
industrial use	T58.8X1	T58.8X2	T58.8X3	T58.8X4	—	—
prior to combustion	T59.891	T59.892	T59.893	T59.894	—	—
utility	T59.891	T59.892	T59.893	T59.894	—	—
incomplete combustion of — *see* Carbon, monoxide, fuel, utility						
in mobile container	T59.891	T59.892	T59.893	T59.894	—	—
piped (natural)	T59.891	T59.892	T59.893	T59.894	—	—
garage	T58.Ø1	T58.Ø2	T58.Ø3	T58.Ø4	—	—
hydrocarbon NEC	T59.891	T59.892	T59.893	T59.894	—	—
incomplete combustion of — *see* Carbon, monoxide, fuel, utility						
liquefied — *see* butane						
piped	T59.891	T59.892	T59.893	T59.894	—	—
hydrocyanic acid	T65.ØX1	T65.ØX2	T65.ØX3	T65.ØX4	—	—
illuminating (after combustion)	T58.11	T58.12	T58.13	T58.14	—	—
prior to combustion	T59.891	T59.892	T59.893	T59.894	—	—
incomplete combustion, any — *see* Carbon, monoxide						
kiln	T58.8X1	T58.8X2	T58.8X3	T58.8X4	—	—
lacrimogenic	T59.3X1	T59.3X2	T59.3X3	T59.3X4	—	—
liquefied petroleum — *see* butane						
marsh	T59.891	T59.892	T59.893	T59.894	—	—
motor exhaust, not in transit	T58.Ø1	T58.Ø2	T58.Ø3	T58.Ø4	—	—
mustard, not in war	T59.891	T59.892	T59.893	T59.894	—	—
natural	T59.891	T59.892	T59.893	T59.894	—	—
nerve, not in war	T59.91	T59.92	T59.93	T59.94	—	—
oil	T52.ØX1	T52.ØX2	T52.ØX3	T52.ØX4	—	—
petroleum (liquefied) (distributed in mobile containers)	T59.891	T59.892	T59.893	T59.894	—	—
piped (pure or mixed with air)	T59.891	T59.892	T59.893	T59.894	—	—
piped (manufactured) (natural) NEC	T59.891	T59.892	T59.893	T59.894	—	—
producer	T58.8X1	T58.8X2	T58.8X3	T58.8X4	—	—
propane — *see* propane						
refrigerant (chlorofluoro-carbon)	T53.5X1	T53.5X2	T53.5X3	T53.5X4	—	—
not chlorofluoro-carbon	T59.891	T59.892	T59.893	T59.894	—	—
sewer	T59.91	T59.92	T59.93	T59.94	—	—
specified source NEC	T59.91	T59.92	T59.93	T59.94	—	—
stove (after combustion)	T58.11	T58.12	T58.13	T58.14	—	—
prior to combustion	T59.891	T59.892	T59.893	T59.894	—	—
tear	T59.3X1	T59.3X2	T59.3X3	T59.3X4	—	—
therapeutic	T41.5X1	T41.5X2	T41.5X3	T41.5X4	T41.5X5	T41.5X6
utility (for cooking, heating, or lighting) (piped) NEC	T59.891	T59.892	T59.893	T59.894	—	—
incomplete combustion of — *see* Carbon, monoxide, fuel, utility						
in mobile container	T59.891	T59.892	T59.893	T59.894	—	—
piped (natural)	T59.891	T59.892	T59.893	T59.894	—	—
water	T58.11	T58.12	T58.13	T58.14	—	—

Substance	Poisoning, Accidental (unintentional)	Poisoning, Intentional Self-harm	Poisoning, Assault	Poisoning, Undetermined	Adverse Effect	Under-dosing
Gas — *continued*						
water — *continued*						
incomplete combustion of — *see* Carbon, monoxide, fuel, utility						
Gaultheria procumbens	T62.2X1	T62.2X2	T62.2X3	T62.2X4	—	—
Gaviscon*	T47.1X1	T47.1X2	T47.1X3	T47.1X4	T47.1X5	T47.1X6
Gefarnate	T44.3X1	T44.3X2	T44.3X3	T44.3X4	T44.3X5	T44.3X6
Gelatin (intravenous)	T45.8X1	T45.8X2	T45.8X3	T45.8X4	T45.8X5	T45.8X6
absorbable (sponge)	T45.7X1	T45.7X2	T45.7X3	T45.7X4	T45.7X5	T45.7X6
Gelfilm	T49.8X1	T49.8X2	T49.8X3	T49.8X4	T49.8X5	T49.8X6
Gelfoam	T45.7X1	T45.7X2	T45.7X3	T45.7X4	T45.7X5	T45.7X6
Gelsemine	T5Ø.991	T5Ø.992	T5Ø.993	T5Ø.994	T5Ø.995	T5Ø.996
Gelsemium (sempervirens)	T62.2X1	T62.2X2	T62.2X3	T62.2X4	—	—
Gemeprost	T48.ØX1	T48.ØX2	T48.ØX3	T48.ØX4	T48.ØX5	T48.ØX6
Gemfibrozil	T46.6X1	T46.6X2	T46.6X3	T46.6X4	T46.6X5	T46.6X6
Gemonil	T42.3X1	T42.3X2	T42.3X3	T42.3X4	T42.3X5	T42.3X6
Gentamicin	T36.5X1	T36.5X2	T36.5X3	T36.5X4	T36.5X5	T36.5X6
ophthalmic preparation	T49.5X1	T49.5X2	T49.5X3	T49.5X4	T49.5X5	T49.5X6
topical NEC	T49.ØX1	T49.ØX2	T49.ØX3	T49.ØX4	T49.ØX5	T49.ØX6
Gentasol*	T49.5X1	T49.5X2	T49.5X3	T49.5X4	T49.5X5	T49.5X6
Gentian	T47.5X1	T47.5X2	T47.5X3	T47.5X4	T47.5X5	T47.5X6
violet	T49.ØX1	T49.ØX2	T49.ØX3	T49.ØX4	T49.ØX5	T49.ØX6
Gepefrine	T44.4X1	T44.4X2	T44.4X3	T44.4X4	T44.4X5	T44.4X6
Gestonorone caproate	T38.5X1	T38.5X2	T38.5X3	T38.5X4	T38.5X5	T38.5X6
Gexane	T49.ØX1	T49.ØX2	T49.ØX3	T49.ØX4	T49.ØX5	T49.ØX6
Gila monster (venom)	T63.111	T63.112	T63.113	T63.114	—	—
Ginger	T47.5X1	T47.5X2	T47.5X3	T47.5X4	T47.5X5	T47.5X6
Jamaica — *see* Jamaica, ginger						
Gitalin	T46.ØX1	T46.ØX2	T46.ØX3	T46.ØX4	T46.ØX5	T46.ØX6
amorphous	T46.ØX1	T46.ØX2	T46.ØX3	T46.ØX4	T46.ØX5	T46.ØX6
Gitaloxin	T46.ØX1	T46.ØX2	T46.ØX3	T46.ØX4	T46.ØX5	T46.ØX6
Gitoxin	T46.ØX1	T46.ØX2	T46.ØX3	T46.ØX4	T46.ØX5	T46.ØX6
Glafenine	T39.8X1	T39.8X2	T39.8X3	T39.8X4	T39.8X5	T39.8X6
Glandular extract (medicinal) NEC	T5Ø.Z91	T5Ø.Z92	T5Ø.Z93	T5Ø.Z94	T5Ø.Z95	T5Ø.Z96
Glaucarubin	T37.3X1	T37.3X2	T37.3X3	T37.3X4	T37.3X5	T37.3X6
Glibenclamide	T38.3X1	T38.3X2	T38.3X3	T38.3X4	T38.3X5	T38.3X6
Glibornuride	T38.3X1	T38.3X2	T38.3X3	T38.3X4	T38.3X5	T38.3X6
Gliclazide	T38.3X1	T38.3X2	T38.3X3	T38.3X4	T38.3X5	T38.3X6
Glimidine	T38.3X1	T38.3X2	T38.3X3	T38.3X4	T38.3X5	T38.3X6
Glipizide	T38.3X1	T38.3X2	T38.3X3	T38.3X4	T38.3X5	T38.3X6
Gliquidone	T38.3X1	T38.3X2	T38.3X3	T38.3X4	T38.3X5	T38.3X6
Glisolamide	T38.3X1	T38.3X2	T38.3X3	T38.3X4	T38.3X5	T38.3X6
Glisoxepide	T38.3X1	T38.3X2	T38.3X3	T38.3X4	T38.3X5	T38.3X6
Globin zinc insulin	T38.3X1	T38.3X2	T38.3X3	T38.3X4	T38.3X5	T38.3X6
Globulin						
antilymphocytic	T5Ø.Z11	T5Ø.Z12	T5Ø.Z13	T5Ø.Z14	T5Ø.Z15	T5Ø.Z16
antirhesus	T5Ø.Z11	T5Ø.Z12	T5Ø.Z13	T5Ø.Z14	T5Ø.Z15	T5Ø.Z16
antivenin	T5Ø.Z11	T5Ø.Z12	T5Ø.Z13	T5Ø.Z14	T5Ø.Z15	T5Ø.Z16
antiviral	T5Ø.Z11	T5Ø.Z12	T5Ø.Z13	T5Ø.Z14	T5Ø.Z15	T5Ø.Z16
Glucagon	T38.3X1	T38.3X2	T38.3X3	T38.3X4	T38.3X5	T38.3X6
Glucocorticoids	T38.ØX1	T38.ØX2	T38.ØX3	T38.ØX4	T38.ØX5	T38.ØX6
Glucocorticosteroid	T38.ØX1	T38.ØX2	T38.ØX3	T38.ØX4	T38.ØX5	T38.ØX6
Gluconic acid	T5Ø.991	T5Ø.992	T5Ø.993	T5Ø.994	T5Ø.995	T5Ø.996
Glucosamine sulfate	T39.4X1	T39.4X2	T39.4X3	T39.4X4	T39.4X5	T39.4X6
Glucose	T5Ø.3X1	T5Ø.3X2	T5Ø.3X3	T5Ø.3X4	T5Ø.3X5	T5Ø.3X6
with sodium chloride	T5Ø.3X1	T5Ø.3X2	T5Ø.3X3	T5Ø.3X4	T5Ø.3X5	T5Ø.3X6
Glucosulfone sodium	T37.1X1	T37.1X2	T37.1X3	T37.1X4	T37.1X5	T37.1X6
Glucotrol*	T38.3X1	T38.3X2	T38.3X3	T38.3X4	T38.3X5	T38.3X6
Glucurolactone	T47.8X1	T47.8X2	T47.8X3	T47.8X4	T47.8X5	T47.8X6
Glue NEC	T52.8X1	T52.8X2	T52.8X3	T52.8X4	—	—
Glutamic acid	T47.5X1	T47.5X2	T47.5X3	T47.5X4	T47.5X5	T47.5X6
Glutaral (medicinal)	T49.ØX1	T49.ØX2	T49.ØX3	T49.ØX4	T49.ØX5	T49.ØX6
nonmedicinal	T65.891	T65.892	T65.893	T65.894	—	—
Glutaraldehyde (nonmedicinal)	T65.891	T65.892	T65.893	T65.894	—	—
medicinal	T49.ØX1	T49.ØX2	T49.ØX3	T49.ØX4	T49.ØX5	T49.ØX6
Glutathione	T5Ø.6X1	T5Ø.6X2	T5Ø.6X3	T5Ø.6X4	T5Ø.6X5	T5Ø.6X6
Glutethimide	T42.6X1	T42.6X2	T42.6X3	T42.6X4	T42.6X5	T42.6X6
Glyburide	T38.3X1	T38.3X2	T38.3X3	T38.3X4	T38.3X5	T38.3X6
Glycerin	T47.4X1	T47.4X2	T47.4X3	T47.4X4	T47.4X5	T47.4X6
Glycerol	T47.4X1	T47.4X2	T47.4X3	T47.4X4	T47.4X5	T47.4X6
borax	T49.6X1	T49.6X2	T49.6X3	T49.6X4	T49.6X5	T49.6X6
intravenous	T5Ø.3X1	T5Ø.3X2	T5Ø.3X3	T5Ø.3X4	T5Ø.3X5	T5Ø.3X6
iodinated	T48.4X1	T48.4X2	T48.4X3	T48.4X4	T48.4X5	T48.4X6
Glycerophosphate	T5Ø.991	T5Ø.992	T5Ø.993	T5Ø.994	T5Ø.995	T5Ø.996
Glyceryl						
gualacolate	T48.4X1	T48.4X2	T48.4X3	T48.4X4	T48.4X5	T48.4X6
nitrate	T46.3X1	T46.3X2	T46.3X3	T46.3X4	T46.3X5	T46.3X6
triacetate (topical)	T49.ØX1	T49.ØX2	T49.ØX3	T49.ØX4	T49.ØX5	T49.ØX6
trinitrate	T46.3X1	T46.3X2	T46.3X3	T46.3X4	T46.3X5	T46.3X6
Glycine	T5Ø.3X1	T5Ø.3X2	T5Ø.3X3	T5Ø.3X4	T5Ø.3X5	T5Ø.3X6

Substance	Poisoning, Accidental (unintentional)	Poisoning, Intentional Self-harm	Poisoning, Assault	Poisoning, Undetermined	Adverse Effect	Under-dosing
Glyclopyramide	T38.3X1	T38.3X2	T38.3X3	T38.3X4	T38.3X5	T38.3X6
Glycobiarsol	T37.3X1	T37.3X2	T37.3X3	T37.3X4	T37.3X5	T37.3X6
Glycols (ether)	T52.3X1	T52.3X2	T52.3X3	T52.3X4	—	—
Glyconiazide	T37.1X1	T37.1X2	T37.1X3	T37.1X4	T37.1X5	T37.1X6
Glycopyrrolate	T44.3X1	T44.3X2	T44.3X3	T44.3X4	T44.3X5	T44.3X6
Glycopyrronium	T44.3X1	T44.3X2	T44.3X3	T44.3X4	T44.3X5	T44.3X6
bromide	T44.3X1	T44.3X2	T44.3X3	T44.3X4	T44.3X5	T44.3X6
Glycoside, cardiac (stimulant)	T46.ØX1	T46.ØX2	T46.ØX3	T46.ØX4	T46.ØX5	T46.ØX6
Glycyclamide	T38.3X1	T38.3X2	T38.3X3	T38.3X4	T38.3X5	T38.3X6
Glycyrrhiza extract	T48.4X1	T48.4X2	T48.4X3	T48.4X4	T48.4X5	T48.4X6
Glycyrrhizic acid	T48.4X1	T48.4X2	T48.4X3	T48.4X4	T48.4X5	T48.4X6
Glycyrrhizinate potassium	T48.4X1	T48.4X2	T48.4X3	T48.4X4	T48.4X5	T48.4X6
Glymidine sodium	T38.3X1	T38.3X2	T38.3X3	T38.3X4	T38.3X5	T38.3X6
Glyphosate	T6Ø.3X1	T6Ø.3X2	T6Ø.3X3	T6Ø.3X4	—	—
Glyphylline	T48.6X1	T48.6X2	T48.6X3	T48.6X4	T48.6X5	T48.6X6
Gold						
colloidal (I98Au)	T45.1X1	T45.1X2	T45.1X3	T45.1X4	T45.1X5	T45.1X6
salts	T39.4X1	T39.4X2	T39.4X3	T39.4X4	T39.4X5	T39.4X6
Golden sulfide of antimony	T56.891	T56.892	T56.893	T56.894	—	—
Goldylocks	T62.2X1	T62.2X2	T62.2X3	T62.2X4	—	—
Gonadal tissue extract	T38.9Ø1	T38.9Ø2	T38.9Ø3	T38.9Ø4	T38.9Ø5	T38.9Ø6
female	T38.5X1	T38.5X2	T38.5X3	T38.5X4	T38.5X5	T38.5X6
male	T38.7X1	T38.7X2	T38.7X3	T38.7X4	T38.7X5	T38.7X6
Gonadorelin	T38.891	T38.892	T38.893	T38.894	T38.895	T38.896
Gonadotropin	T38.891	T38.892	T38.893	T38.894	T38.895	T38.896
chorionic	T38.891	T38.892	T38.893	T38.894	T38.895	T38.896
pituitary	T38.811	T38.812	T38.813	T38.814	T38.815	T38.816
Goserelin	T45.1X1	T45.1X2	T45.1X3	T45.1X4	T45.1X5	T45.1X6
Grain alcohol	T51.ØX1	T51.ØX2	T51.ØX3	T51.ØX4	—	—
Gralise*	T42.6X1	T42.6X2	T42.6X3	T42.6X4	T42.6X5	T42.6X6
Gramicidin	T49.ØX1	T49.ØX2	T49.ØX3	T49.ØX4	T49.ØX5	T49.ØX6
Granisetron	T45.ØX1	T45.ØX2	T45.ØX3	T45.ØX4	T45.ØX5	T45.ØX6
Gratiola officinalis	T62.2X1	T62.2X2	T62.2X3	T62.2X4	—	—
Grease	T65.891	T65.892	T65.893	T65.894	—	—
Green hellebore	T62.2X1	T62.2X2	T62.2X3	T62.2X4	—	—
Green soap	T49.2X1	T49.2X2	T49.2X3	T49.2X4	T49.2X5	T49.2X6
Grifulvin	T36.7X1	T36.7X2	T36.7X3	T36.7X4	T36.7X5	T36.7X6
Griseofulvin	T36.7X1	T36.7X2	T36.7X3	T36.7X4	T36.7X5	T36.7X6
Growth hormone	T38.811	T38.812	T38.813	T38.814	T38.815	T38.816
Guaiacol derivatives	T48.4X1	T48.4X2	T48.4X3	T48.4X4	T48.4X5	T48.4X6
Guaiac reagent	T5Ø.991	T5Ø.992	T5Ø.993	T5Ø.994	T5Ø.995	T5Ø.996
Guaifenesin	T48.4X1	T48.4X2	T48.4X3	T48.4X4	T48.4X5	T48.4X6
Guaimesal	T48.4X1	T48.4X2	T48.4X3	T48.4X4	T48.4X5	T48.4X6
Guaiphenesin	T48.4X1	T48.4X2	T48.4X3	T48.4X4	T48.4X5	T48.4X6
Guaituss*	T48.4X1	T48.4X2	T48.4X3	T48.4X4	T48.4X5	T48.4X6
Guamecycline	T36.4X1	T36.4X2	T36.4X3	T36.4X4	T36.4X5	T36.4X6
Guanabenz	T46.5X1	T46.5X2	T46.5X3	T46.5X4	T46.5X5	T46.5X6
Guanacline	T46.5X1	T46.5X2	T46.5X3	T46.5X4	T46.5X5	T46.5X6
Guanadrel	T46.5X1	T46.5X2	T46.5X3	T46.5X4	T46.5X5	T46.5X6
Guanatol	T37.2X1	T37.2X2	T37.2X3	T37.2X4	T37.2X5	T37.2X6
Guanethidine	T46.5X1	T46.5X2	T46.5X3	T46.5X4	T46.5X5	T46.5X6
Guanfacine	T46.5X1	T46.5X2	T46.5X3	T46.5X4	T46.5X5	T46.5X6
Guano	T65.891	T65.892	T65.893	T65.894	—	—
Guanochlor	T46.5X1	T46.5X2	T46.5X3	T46.5X4	T46.5X5	T46.5X6
Guanoclor	T46.5X1	T46.5X2	T46.5X3	T46.5X4	T46.5X5	T46.5X6
Guanoctine	T46.5X1	T46.5X2	T46.5X3	T46.5X4	T46.5X5	T46.5X6
Guanoxabenz	T46.5X1	T46.5X2	T46.5X3	T46.5X4	T46.5X5	T46.5X6
Guanoxan	T46.5X1	T46.5X2	T46.5X3	T46.5X4	T46.5X5	T46.5X6
Guar gum (medicinal)	T46.6X1	T46.6X2	T46.6X3	T46.6X4	T46.6X5	T46.6X6
Hachimycin	T36.7X1	T36.7X2	T36.7X3	T36.7X4	T36.7X5	T36.7X6
Hair						
dye	T49.4X1	T49.4X2	T49.4X3	T49.4X4	T49.4X5	T49.4X6
preparation NEC	T49.4X1	T49.4X2	T49.4X3	T49.4X4	T49.4X5	T49.4X6
Halazepam	T42.4X1	T42.4X2	T42.4X3	T42.4X4	T42.4X5	T42.4X6
Halcinolone	T49.ØX1	T49.ØX2	T49.ØX3	T49.ØX4	T49.ØX5	T49.ØX6
Halcinonide	T49.ØX1	T49.ØX2	T49.ØX3	T49.ØX4	T49.ØX5	T49.ØX6
Halethazole	T49.ØX1	T49.ØX2	T49.ØX3	T49.ØX4	T49.ØX5	T49.ØX6
Hallucinogen NOS	T4Ø.9Ø1	T4Ø.9Ø2	T4Ø.9Ø3	T4Ø.9Ø4	T4Ø.9Ø5	T4Ø.9Ø6
specified NEC	T4Ø.991	T4Ø.992	T4Ø.993	T4Ø.994	T4Ø.995	T4Ø.996
Halofantrine	T37.2X1	T37.2X2	T37.2X3	T37.2X4	T37.2X5	T37.2X6
Halofenate	T46.6X1	T46.6X2	T46.6X3	T46.6X4	T46.6X5	T46.6X6
Halometasone	T49.ØX1	T49.ØX2	T49.ØX3	T49.ØX4	T49.ØX5	T49.ØX6
Haloperidol	T43.4X1	T43.4X2	T43.4X3	T43.4X4	T43.4X5	T43.4X6
Haloprogin	T49.ØX1	T49.ØX2	T49.ØX3	T49.ØX4	T49.ØX5	T49.ØX6
Halotex	T49.ØX1	T49.ØX2	T49.ØX3	T49.ØX4	T49.ØX5	T49.ØX6
Halothane	T41.ØX1	T41.ØX2	T41.ØX3	T41.ØX4	T41.ØX5	T41.ØX6
Haloxazolam	T42.4X1	T42.4X2	T42.4X3	T42.4X4	T42.4X5	T42.4X6
Halquinols	T49.ØX1	T49.ØX2	T49.ØX3	T49.ØX4	T49.ØX5	T49.ØX6
Hamamelis	T49.2X1	T49.2X2	T49.2X3	T49.2X4	T49.2X5	T49.2X6
Haptendextran	T45.8X1	T45.8X2	T45.8X3	T45.8X4	T45.8X5	T45.8X6
Harmonyl	T46.5X1	T46.5X2	T46.5X3	T46.5X4	T46.5X5	T46.5X6
Hartmann's solution	T5Ø.3X1	T5Ø.3X2	T5Ø.3X3	T5Ø.3X4	T5Ø.3X5	T5Ø.3X6
Hashish	T4Ø.711	T4Ø.712	T4Ø.713	T4Ø.714	T4Ø.715	T4Ø.716
Havrix*	T5Ø.B91	T5Ø.B92	T5Ø.B93	T5Ø.B94	T5Ø.B95	T5Ø.B96
Hawaiian Woodrose seeds	T4Ø.991	T4Ø.992	T4Ø.993	T4Ø.994	—	—
HCB	T6Ø.3X1	T6Ø.3X2	T6Ø.3X3	T6Ø.3X4	—	—
HCH	T53.6X1	T53.6X2	T53.6X3	T53.6X4	—	—
medicinal	T49.ØX1	T49.ØX2	T49.ØX3	T49.ØX4	T49.ØX5	T49.ØX6
HCN	T57.3X1	T57.3X2	T57.3X3	T57.3X4	—	—
Headache cures, drugs, powders NEC	T5Ø.9Ø1	T5Ø.9Ø2	T5Ø.9Ø3	T5Ø.9Ø4	T5Ø.9Ø5	T5Ø.9Ø6
Heavenly Blue (morning glory)	T4Ø.991	T4Ø.992	T4Ø.993	T4Ø.994	—	—
Heavy metal antidote	T45.8X1	T45.8X2	T45.8X3	T45.8X4	T45.8X5	T45.8X6
Hedaquinium	T49.ØX1	T49.ØX2	T49.ØX3	T49.ØX4	T49.ØX5	T49.ØX6
Hedge hyssop	T62.2X1	T62.2X2	T62.2X3	T62.2X4	—	—
Heet	T49.8X1	T49.8X2	T49.8X3	T49.8X4	T49.8X5	T49.8X6
Helenin	T37.4X1	T37.4X2	T37.4X3	T37.4X4	T37.4X5	T37.4X6
Helium (nonmedicinal) **NEC**	T59.891	T59.892	T59.893	T59.894	—	—
medicinal	T48.991	T48.992	T48.993	T48.994	T48.995	T48.996
Hellebore (black) (green) (white)	T62.2X1	T62.2X2	T62.2X3	T62.2X4	—	—
Hematin	T45.8X1	T45.8X2	T45.8X3	T45.8X4	T45.8X5	T45.8X6
Hematinic preparation	T45.8X1	T45.8X2	T45.8X3	T45.8X4	T45.8X5	T45.8X6
Hematological agent	T45.91	T45.92	T45.93	T45.94	T45.95	T45.96
specified NEC	T45.8X1	T45.8X2	T45.8X3	T45.8X4	T45.8X5	T45.8X6
Hemlock	T62.2X1	T62.2X2	T62.2X3	T62.2X4	—	—
Hemostatic	T45.621	T45.622	T45.623	T45.624	T45.625	T45.626
drug, systemic	T45.621	T45.622	T45.623	T45.624	T45.625	T45.626
Hemostyptic	T49.4X1	T49.4X2	T49.4X3	T49.4X4	T49.4X5	T49.4X6
Henbane	T62.2X1	T62.2X2	T62.2X3	T62.2X4	—	—
Heparin (sodium)	T45.511	T45.512	T45.513	T45.514	T45.515	T45.516
action reverser	T45.7X1	T45.7X2	T45.7X3	T45.7X4	T45.7X5	T45.7X6
Heparin-fraction	T45.511	T45.512	T45.513	T45.514	T45.515	T45.516
Heparinoid (systemic)	T45.511	T45.512	T45.513	T45.514	T45.515	T45.516
Hepatic secretion stimulant	T47.8X1	T47.8X2	T47.8X3	T47.8X4	T47.8X5	T47.8X6
Hepatitis A vaccine*	T5Ø.B91	T5Ø.B92	T5Ø.B93	T5Ø.B94	T5Ø.B95	T5Ø.B96
Hepatitis B						
immune globulin	T5Ø.Z11	T5Ø.Z12	T5Ø.Z13	T5Ø.Z14	T5Ø.Z15	T5Ø.Z16
vaccine	T5Ø.B91	T5Ø.B92	T5Ø.B93	T5Ø.B94	T5Ø.B95	T5Ø.B96
Hepronicate	T46.7X1	T46.7X2	T46.7X3	T46.7X4	T46.7X5	T46.7X6
Heptabarb	T42.3X1	T42.3X2	T42.3X3	T42.3X4	T42.3X5	T42.3X6
Heptabarbital	T42.3X1	T42.3X2	T42.3X3	T42.3X4	T42.3X5	T42.3X6
Heptabarbitone	T42.3X1	T42.3X2	T42.3X3	T42.3X4	T42.3X5	T42.3X6
Heptachlor	T6Ø.1X1	T6Ø.1X2	T6Ø.1X3	T6Ø.1X4	—	—
Heptalgin	T4Ø.2X1	T4Ø.2X2	T4Ø.2X3	T4Ø.2X4	T4Ø.2X5	T4Ø.2X6
Heptaminol	T46.3X1	T46.3X2	T46.3X3	T46.3X4	T46.3X5	T46.3X6
Herbicide NEC	T6Ø.3X1	T6Ø.3X2	T6Ø.3X3	T6Ø.3X4	—	—
Heroin	T4Ø.1X1	T4Ø.1X2	T4Ø.1X3	T4Ø.1X4	—	—
Herplex	T49.5X1	T49.5X2	T49.5X3	T49.5X4	T49.5X5	T49.5X6
HES	T45.8X1	T45.8X2	T45.8X3	T45.8X4	T45.8X5	T45.8X6
Hesperidin	T46.991	T46.992	T46.993	T46.994	T46.995	T46.996
Hetacillin	T36.ØX1	T36.ØX2	T36.ØX3	T36.ØX4	T36.ØX5	T36.ØX6
Hetastarch	T45.8X1	T45.8X2	T45.8X3	T45.8X4	T45.8X5	T45.8X6
HETP	T6Ø.ØX1	T6Ø.ØX2	T6Ø.ØX3	T6Ø.ØX4	—	—
Hexachlorobenzene (vapor)	T6Ø.3X1	T6Ø.3X2	T6Ø.3X3	T6Ø.3X4	—	—
Hexachlorocyclohexane	T53.6X1	T53.6X2	T53.6X3	T53.6X4	—	—
Hexachlorophene	T49.ØX1	T49.ØX2	T49.ØX3	T49.ØX4	T49.ØX5	T49.ØX6
Hexadiline	T46.3X1	T46.3X2	T46.3X3	T46.3X4	T46.3X5	T46.3X6
Hexadimethrine (bromide)	T45.7X1	T45.7X2	T45.7X3	T45.7X4	T45.7X5	T45.7X6
Hexadylamine	T46.3X1	T46.3X2	T46.3X3	T46.3X4	T46.3X5	T46.3X6
Hexaethyl tetraphosphate	T6Ø.ØX1	T6Ø.ØX2	T6Ø.ØX3	T6Ø.ØX4	—	—
Hexafluorenium bromide	T48.1X1	T48.1X2	T48.1X3	T48.1X4	T48.1X5	T48.1X6
Hexafluronium (bromide)	T48.1X1	T48.1X2	T48.1X3	T48.1X4	T48.1X5	T48.1X6
Hexa-germ	T49.2X1	T49.2X2	T49.2X3	T49.2X4	T49.2X5	T49.2X6
Hexahydrobenzol	T52.8X1	T52.8X2	T52.8X3	T52.8X4	—	—
Hexahydrocresol(s)	T51.8X1	T51.8X2	T51.8X3	T51.8X4	—	—
arsenide	T57.ØX1	T57.ØX2	T57.ØX3	T57.ØX4	—	—
arseniurated	T57.ØX1	T57.ØX2	T57.ØX3	T57.ØX4	—	—
cyanide	T57.3X1	T57.3X2	T57.3X3	T57.3X4	—	—
gas	T59.891	T59.892	T59.893	T59.894	—	—
Fluoride (liquid)	T57.8X1	T57.8X2	T57.8X3	T57.8X4	—	—
vapor	T59.891	T59.892	T59.893	T59.894	—	—
phophorated	T6Ø.ØX1	T6Ø.ØX2	T6Ø.ØX3	T6Ø.ØX4	—	—
sulfate	T57.8X1	T57.8X2	T57.8X3	T57.8X4	—	—
sulfide (gas)	T59.6X1	T59.6X2	T59.6X3	T59.6X4	—	—
arseniurated	T57.ØX1	T57.ØX2	T57.ØX3	T57.ØX4	—	—
sulfurated	T57.8X1	T57.8X2	T57.8X3	T57.8X4	—	—
Hexahydrophenol	T51.8X1	T51.8X2	T51.8X3	T51.8X4	—	—
Hexalen	T51.8X1	T51.8X2	T51.8X3	T51.8X4	—	—
Hexamethonium bromide	T44.2X1	T44.2X2	T44.2X3	T44.2X4	T44.2X5	T44.2X6
Hexamethylene	T52.8X1	T52.8X2	T52.8X3	T52.8X4	—	—

Substance	Poisoning, Accidental (unintentional)	Poisoning, Intentional Self-harm	Poisoning, Assault	Poisoning, Undetermined	Adverse Effect	Under-dosing
Hexamethylmelamine	T45.1X1	T45.1X2	T45.1X3	T45.1X4	T45.1X5	T45.1X6
Hexamidine	T49.ØX1	T49.ØX2	T49.ØX3	T49.ØX4	T49.ØX5	T49.ØX6
Hexamine (mandelate)	T37.8X1	T37.8X2	T37.8X3	T37.8X4	T37.8X5	T37.8X6
Hexanone, 2-hexanone	T52.4X1	T52.4X2	T52.4X3	T52.4X4	—	—
Hexanuorenium	T48.1X1	T48.1X2	T48.1X3	T48.1X4	T48.1X5	T48.1X6
Hexapropymate	T42.6X1	T42.6X2	T42.6X3	T42.6X4	T42.6X5	T42.6X6
Hexasonium iodide	T44.3X1	T44.3X2	T44.3X3	T44.3X4	T44.3X5	T44.3X6
Hexcarbacholine bromide	T48.1X1	T48.1X2	T48.1X3	T48.1X4	T48.1X5	T48.1X6
Hexemal	T42.3X1	T42.3X2	T42.3X3	T42.3X4	T42.3X5	T42.3X6
Hexestrol	T38.5X1	T38.5X2	T38.5X3	T38.5X4	T38.5X5	T38.5X6
Hexethal (sodium)	T42.3X1	T42.3X2	T42.3X3	T42.3X4	T42.3X5	T42.3X6
Hexetidine	T37.8X1	T37.8X2	T37.8X3	T37.8X4	T37.8X5	T37.8X6
Hexobarbital	T42.3X1	T42.3X2	T42.3X3	T42.3X4	T42.3X5	T42.3X6
rectal	T41.291	T41.292	T41.293	T41.294	T41.295	T41.296
sodium	T41.1X1	T41.1X2	T41.1X3	T41.1X4	T41.1X5	T41.1X6
Hexobendine	T46.3X1	T46.3X2	T46.3X3	T46.3X4	T46.3X5	T46.3X6
Hexocyclium	T44.3X1	T44.3X2	T44.3X3	T44.3X4	T44.3X5	T44.3X6
metilsulfate	T44.3X1	T44.3X2	T44.3X3	T44.3X4	T44.3X5	T44.3X6
Hexoestrol	T38.5X1	T38.5X2	T38.5X3	T38.5X4	T38.5X5	T38.5X6
Hexone	T52.4X1	T52.4X2	T52.4X3	T52.4X4	—	—
Hexoprenaline	T48.6X1	T48.6X2	T48.6X3	T48.6X4	T48.6X5	T48.6X6
Hexylcaine	T41.3X1	T41.3X2	T41.3X3	T41.3X4	T41.3X5	T41.3X6
Hexylresorcinol	T52.2X1	T52.2X2	T52.2X3	T52.2X4	—	—
HGH (human growth hormone)	T38.811	T38.812	T38.813	T38.814	T38.815	T38.816
Hibistat*	T49.ØX1	T49.ØX2	T49.ØX3	T49.ØX4	T49.ØX5	T49.ØX6
Hinkle's pills	T47.2X1	T47.2X2	T47.2X3	T47.2X4	T47.2X5	T47.2X6
Histalog	T5Ø.8X1	T5Ø.8X2	T5Ø.8X3	T5Ø.8X4	T5Ø.8X5	T5Ø.8X6
Histamine (phosphate)	T5Ø.8X1	T5Ø.8X2	T5Ø.8X3	T5Ø.8X4	T5Ø.8X5	T5Ø.8X6
Histolyn*	T5Ø.8X1	T5Ø.8X2	T5Ø.8X3	T5Ø.8X4	T5Ø.8X5	T5Ø.8X6
Histoplasmin	T5Ø.8X1	T5Ø.8X2	T5Ø.8X3	T5Ø.8X4	T5Ø.8X5	T5Ø.8X6
Holly berries	T62.2X1	T62.2X2	T62.2X3	T62.2X4	—	—
Homatropine	T44.3X1	T44.3X2	T44.3X3	T44.3X4	T44.3X5	T44.3X6
methylbromide	T44.3X1	T44.3X2	T44.3X3	T44.3X4	T44.3X5	T44.3X6
Homochlorcyclizine	T45.ØX1	T45.ØX2	T45.ØX3	T45.ØX4	T45.ØX5	T45.ØX6
Homosalate	T49.3X1	T49.3X2	T49.3X3	T49.3X4	T49.3X5	T49.3X6
Homo-tet	T5Ø.Z11	T5Ø.Z12	T5Ø.Z13	T5Ø.Z14	T5Ø.Z15	T5Ø.Z16
Hormone	T38.8Ø1	T38.8Ø2	T38.8Ø3	T38.8Ø4	T38.8Ø5	T38.8Ø6
adrenal cortical steroids	T38.ØX1	T38.ØX2	T38.ØX3	T38.ØX4	T38.ØX5	T38.ØX6
androgenic	T38.7X1	T38.7X2	T38.7X3	T38.7X4	T38.7X5	T38.7X6
anterior pituitary NEC	T38.811	T38.812	T38.813	T38.814	T38.815	T38.816
antidiabetic agents	T38.3X1	T38.3X2	T38.3X3	T38.3X4	T38.3X5	T38.3X6
antidiuretic	T38.891	T38.892	T38.893	T38.894	T38.895	T38.896
cancer therapy	T45.1X1	T45.1X2	T45.1X3	T45.1X4	T45.1X5	T45.1X6
follicle stimulating	T38.811	T38.812	T38.813	T38.814	T38.815	T38.816
gonadotropic	T38.891	T38.892	T38.893	T38.894	T38.895	T38.896
pituitary	T38.811	T38.812	T38.813	T38.814	T38.815	T38.816
growth	T38.811	T38.812	T38.813	T38.814	T38.815	T38.816
luteinizing	T38.811	T38.812	T38.813	T38.814	T38.815	T38.816
ovarian	T38.5X1	T38.5X2	T38.5X3	T38.5X4	T38.5X5	T38.5X6
oxytocic	T48.ØX1	T48.ØX2	T48.ØX3	T48.ØX4	T48.ØX5	T48.ØX6
parathyroid (derivatives)	T5Ø.991	T5Ø.992	T5Ø.993	T5Ø.994	T5Ø.995	T5Ø.996
pituitary (posterior) NEC	T38.891	T38.892	T38.893	T38.894	T38.895	T38.896
anterior	T38.811	T38.812	T38.813	T38.814	T38.815	T38.816
specified, NEC	T38.891	T38.892	T38.893	T38.894	T38.895	T38.896
thyroid	T38.1X1	T38.1X2	T38.1X3	T38.1X4	T38.1X5	T38.1X6
Hornet (sting)	T63.451	T63.452	T63.453	T63.454	—	—
Horse anti-human lymphocytic serum	T5Ø.Z11	T5Ø.Z12	T5Ø.Z13	T5Ø.Z14	T5Ø.Z15	T5Ø.Z16
Horticulture agent NEC	T65.91	T65.92	T65.93	T65.94	—	—
with pesticide	T6Ø.91	T6Ø.92	T6Ø.93	T6Ø.94	—	—
Human						
albumin	T45.8X1	T45.8X2	T45.8X3	T45.8X4	T45.8X5	T45.8X6
growth hormone (HGH)	T38.811	T38.812	T38.813	T38.814	T38.815	T38.816
immune serum	T5Ø.Z11	T5Ø.Z12	T5Ø.Z13	T5Ø.Z14	T5Ø.Z15	T5Ø.Z16
Hyaluronidase	T45.3X1	T45.3X2	T45.3X3	T45.3X4	T45.3X5	T45.3X6
Hyazyme	T45.3X1	T45.3X2	T45.3X3	T45.3X4	T45.3X5	T45.3X6
Hycodan	T4Ø.2X1	T4Ø.2X2	T4Ø.2X3	T4Ø.2X4	T4Ø.2X5	T4Ø.2X6
Hydantoin derivative NEC	T42.ØX1	T42.ØX2	T42.ØX3	T42.ØX4	T42.ØX5	T42.ØX6
Hydeltra	T38.ØX1	T38.ØX2	T38.ØX3	T38.ØX4	T38.ØX5	T38.ØX6
Hydergine	T44.6X1	T44.6X2	T44.6X3	T44.6X4	T44.6X5	T44.6X6
Hydrabamine penicillin	T36.ØX1	T36.ØX2	T36.ØX3	T36.ØX4	T36.ØX5	T36.ØX6
Hydralazine	T46.5X1	T46.5X2	T46.5X3	T46.5X4	T46.5X5	T46.5X6
Hydrargaphen	T49.ØX1	T49.ØX2	T49.ØX3	T49.ØX4	T49.ØX5	T49.ØX6
Hydrargyri aminochloridum	T49.ØX1	T49.ØX2	T49.ØX3	T49.ØX4	T49.ØX5	T49.ØX6
Hydrastine	T48.291	T48.292	T48.293	T48.294	T48.295	T48.296
Hydrazine	T54.1X1	T54.1X2	T54.1X3	T54.1X4	—	—
monoamine oxidase inhibitors	T43.1X1	T43.1X2	T43.1X3	T43.1X4	T43.1X5	T43.1X6
Hydrazoic acid, azides	T54.2X1	T54.2X2	T54.2X3	T54.2X4	—	—
Hydriodic acid	T48.4X1	T48.4X2	T48.4X3	T48.4X4	T48.4X5	T48.4X6
Hydrisalic*	T49.4X1	T49.4X2	T49.4X3	T49.4X4	T49.4X5	T49.4X6

Substance	Poisoning, Accidental (unintentional)	Poisoning, Intentional Self-harm	Poisoning, Assault	Poisoning, Undetermined	Adverse Effect	Under-dosing
Hydrocarbon gas	T59.891	T59.892	T59.893	T59.894	—	—
incomplete combustion of — *see* Carbon, monoxide, fuel, utility						
liquefied (mobile container)	T59.891	T59.892	T59.893	T59.894	—	—
piped (natural)	T59.891	T59.892	T59.893	T59.894	—	—
Hydrochloric acid (liquid)	T54.2X1	T54.2X2	T54.2X3	T54.2X4	—	—
medicinal (digestant)	T47.5X1	T47.5X2	T47.5X3	T47.5X4	T47.5X5	T47.5X6
vapor	T59.891	T59.892	T59.893	T59.894	—	—
Hydrochlorothiazide	T5Ø.2X1	T5Ø.2X2	T5Ø.2X3	T5Ø.2X4	T5Ø.2X5	T5Ø.2X6
Hydrocodone	T4Ø.2X1	T4Ø.2X2	T4Ø.2X3	T4Ø.2X4	T4Ø.2X5	T4Ø.2X6
Hydrocortisone (derivatives)	T38.ØX1	T38.ØX2	T38.ØX3	T38.ØX4	T38.ØX5	T38.ØX6
aceponate	T49.ØX1	T49.ØX2	T49.ØX3	T49.ØX4	T49.ØX5	T49.ØX6
ENT agent	T49.6X1	T49.6X2	T49.6X3	T49.6X4	T49.6X5	T49.6X6
ophthalmic preparation	T49.5X1	T49.5X2	T49.5X3	T49.5X4	T49.5X5	T49.5X6
topical NEC	T49.ØX1	T49.ØX2	T49.ØX3	T49.ØX4	T49.ØX5	T49.ØX6
Hydrocortone	T38.ØX1	T38.ØX2	T38.ØX3	T38.ØX4	T38.ØX5	T38.ØX6
ENT agent	T49.6X1	T49.6X2	T49.6X3	T49.6X4	T49.6X5	T49.6X6
ophthalmic preparation	T49.5X1	T49.5X2	T49.5X3	T49.5X4	T49.5X5	T49.5X6
topical NEC	T49.ØX1	T49.ØX2	T49.ØX3	T49.ØX4	T49.ØX5	T49.ØX6
Hydrocyanic acid (liquid)	T57.3X1	T57.3X2	T57.3X3	T57.3X4	—	—
gas	T65.ØX1	T65.ØX2	T65.ØX3	T65.ØX4	—	—
Hydroflumethiazide	T5Ø.2X1	T5Ø.2X2	T5Ø.2X3	T5Ø.2X4	T5Ø.2X5	T5Ø.2X6
Hydrofluoric acid (liquid)	T54.2X1	T54.2X2	T54.2X3	T54.2X4	—	—
vapor	T59.891	T59.892	T59.893	T59.894	—	—
Hydrogen	T59.891	T59.892	T59.893	T59.894	—	—
arsenide	T57.ØX1	T57.ØX2	T57.ØX3	T57.ØX4	—	—
arseniureted	T57.ØX1	T57.ØX2	T57.ØX3	T57.ØX4	—	—
chloride	T57.8X1	T57.8X2	T57.8X3	T57.8X4	—	—
cyanide (salts)	T57.3X1	T57.3X2	T57.3X3	T57.3X4	—	—
gas	T57.3X1	T57.3X2	T57.3X3	T57.3X4	—	—
Fluoride	T59.5X1	T59.5X2	T59.5X3	T59.5X4	—	—
vapor	T59.5X1	T59.5X2	T59.5X3	T59.5X4	—	—
peroxide	T49.ØX1	T49.ØX2	T49.ØX3	T49.ØX4	T49.ØX5	T49.ØX6
phosphureted	T57.1X1	T57.1X2	T57.1X3	T57.1X4	—	—
sulfide	T59.6X1	T59.6X2	T59.6X3	T59.6X4	—	—
arseniureted	T57.ØX1	T57.ØX2	T57.ØX3	T57.ØX4	—	—
sulfureted	T59.6X1	T59.6X2	T59.6X3	T59.6X4	—	—
Hydromethylpyridine	T46.7X1	T46.7X2	T46.7X3	T46.7X4	T46.7X5	T46.7X6
Hydromorphinol	T4Ø.2X1	T4Ø.2X2	T4Ø.2X3	T4Ø.2X4	—	—
Hydromorphinone	T4Ø.2X1	T4Ø.2X2	T4Ø.2X3	T4Ø.2X4	T4Ø.2X5	T4Ø.2X6
Hydromorphone	T4Ø.2X1	T4Ø.2X2	T4Ø.2X3	T4Ø.2X4	T4Ø.2X5	T4Ø.2X6
Hydromox	T5Ø.2X1	T5Ø.2X2	T5Ø.2X3	T5Ø.2X4	T5Ø.2X5	T5Ø.2X6
Hydrophilic lotion	T49.3X1	T49.3X2	T49.3X3	T49.3X4	T49.3X5	T49.3X6
Hydroquinidine	T46.2X1	T46.2X2	T46.2X3	T46.2X4	T46.2X5	T46.2X6
Hydroquinone	T52.2X1	T52.2X2	T52.2X3	T52.2X4	—	—
vapor	T59.891	T59.892	T59.893	T59.894	—	—
Hydro-ride*	T5Ø.2X1	T5Ø.2X2	T5Ø.2X3	T5Ø.2X4	T5Ø.2X5	T5Ø.2X6
Hydrosulfuric acid (gas)	T59.6X1	T59.6X2	T59.6X3	T59.6X4	—	—
Hydrotalcite	T47.1X1	T47.1X2	T47.1X3	T47.1X4	T47.1X5	T47.1X6
Hydrous wool fat	T49.3X1	T49.3X2	T49.3X3	T49.3X4	T49.3X5	T49.3X6
Hydroxide, caustic	T54.3X1	T54.3X2	T54.3X3	T54.3X4	—	—
Hydroxocobalamin	T45.8X1	T45.8X2	T45.8X3	T45.8X4	T45.8X5	T45.8X6
Hydroxyamphetamine	T49.5X1	T49.5X2	T49.5X3	T49.5X4	T49.5X5	T49.5X6
Hydroxycarbamide	T45.1X1	T45.1X2	T45.1X3	T45.1X4	T45.1X5	T45.1X6
Hydroxychloroquine	T37.8X1	T37.8X2	T37.8X3	T37.8X4	T37.8X5	T37.8X6
Hydroxydaunorubicin*	T45.1X1	T45.1X2	T45.1X3	T45.1X4	T45.1X5	T45.1X6
Hydroxydihydrocodeinone	T4Ø.2X1	T4Ø.2X2	T4Ø.2X3	T4Ø.2X4	T4Ø.2X5	T4Ø.2X6
Hydroxyestrone	T38.5X1	T38.5X2	T38.5X3	T38.5X4	T38.5X5	T38.5X6
Hydroxyethyl starch	T45.8X1	T45.8X2	T45.8X3	T45.8X4	T45.8X5	T45.8X6
Hydroxymethylpentanone	T52.4X1	T52.4X2	T52.4X3	T52.4X4	—	—
Hydroxyphenamate	T43.591	T43.592	T43.593	T43.594	T43.595	T43.596
Hydroxyphenylbutazone	T39.2X1	T39.2X2	T39.2X3	T39.2X4	T39.2X5	T39.2X6
Hydroxyprogesterone	T38.5X1	T38.5X2	T38.5X3	T38.5X4	T38.5X5	T38.5X6
caproate	T38.5X1	T38.5X2	T38.5X3	T38.5X4	T38.5X5	T38.5X6
Hydroxyquinoline (derivatives) **NEC**	T37.8X1	T37.8X2	T37.8X3	T37.8X4	T37.8X5	T37.8X6
Hydroxystilbamidine	T37.3X1	T37.3X2	T37.3X3	T37.3X4	T37.3X5	T37.3X6
Hydroxytoluene (nonmedicinal)	T54.ØX1	T54.ØX2	T54.ØX3	T54.ØX4	—	—
medicinal	T49.ØX1	T49.ØX2	T49.ØX3	T49.ØX4	T49.ØX5	T49.ØX6
Hydroxyurea	T45.1X1	T45.1X2	T45.1X3	T45.1X4	T45.1X5	T45.1X6
Hydroxyzine	T43.591	T43.592	T43.593	T43.594	T43.595	T43.596
Hyoscine	T44.3X1	T44.3X2	T44.3X3	T44.3X4	T44.3X5	T44.3X6
Hyoscyamine	T44.3X1	T44.3X2	T44.3X3	T44.3X4	T44.3X5	T44.3X6
Hyoscyamus	T44.3X1	T44.3X2	T44.3X3	T44.3X4	T44.3X5	T44.3X6
dry extract	T44.3X1	T44.3X2	T44.3X3	T44.3X4	T44.3X5	T44.3X6
Hypaque	T5Ø.8X1	T5Ø.8X2	T5Ø.8X3	T5Ø.8X4	T5Ø.8X5	T5Ø.8X6
HyperRAB*	T5Ø.Z11	T5Ø.Z12	T5Ø.Z13	T5Ø.Z14	T5Ø.Z15	T5Ø.Z16
Hypertussis	T5Ø.Z11	T5Ø.Z12	T5Ø.Z13	T5Ø.Z14	T5Ø.Z15	T5Ø.Z16
Hypnotic	T42.71	T42.72	T42.73	T42.74	T42.75	T42.76

Substance	Poisoning, Accidental (unintentional)	Poisoning, Intentional Self-harm	Poisoning, Assault	Poisoning, Undetermined	Adverse Effect	Under-dosing
Hypnotic — *continued*						
anticonvulsant	T42.71	T42.72	T42.73	T42.74	T42.75	T42.76
specified NEC	T42.6X1	T42.6X2	T42.6X3	T42.6X4	T42.6X5	T42.6X6
Hypochlorite	T49.ØX1	T49.ØX2	T49.ØX3	T49.ØX4	T49.ØX5	T49.ØX6
Hypophysis, posterior	T38.891	T38.892	T38.893	T38.894	T38.895	T38.896
Hypotensive NEC	T46.5X1	T46.5X2	T46.5X3	T46.5X4	T46.5X5	T46.5X6
Hypromellose	T49.5X1	T49.5X2	T49.5X3	T49.5X4	T49.5X5	T49.5X6
Ibacitabine	T37.5X1	T37.5X2	T37.5X3	T37.5X4	T37.5X5	T37.5X6
Ibopamine	T44.991	T44.992	T44.993	T44.994	T44.995	T44.996
Ibufenac	T39.311	T39.312	T39.313	T39.314	T39.315	T39.316
Ibuprofen	T39.311	T39.312	T39.313	T39.314	T39.315	T39.316
Ibuproxam	T39.311	T39.312	T39.313	T39.314	T39.315	T39.316
Ibuterol	T48.6X1	T48.6X2	T48.6X3	T48.6X4	T48.6X5	T48.6X6
Ichthammol	T49.ØX1	T49.ØX2	T49.ØX3	T49.ØX4	T49.ØX5	T49.ØX6
Ichthyol	T49.4X1	T49.4X2	T49.4X3	T49.4X4	T49.4X5	T49.4X6
Idarubicin	T45.1X1	T45.1X2	T45.1X3	T45.1X4	T45.1X5	T45.1X6
Idrocilamide	T42.8X1	T42.8X2	T42.8X3	T42.8X4	T42.8X5	T42.8X6
Ifenprodil	T46.7X1	T46.7X2	T46.7X3	T46.7X4	T46.7X5	T46.7X6
Ifosfamide	T45.1X1	T45.1X2	T45.1X3	T45.1X4	T45.1X5	T45.1X6
Iletin	T38.3X1	T38.3X2	T38.3X3	T38.3X4	T38.3X5	T38.3X6
Ilex	T62.2X1	T62.2X2	T62.2X3	T62.2X4	—	—
Illuminating gas (after combustion)	T58.11	T58.12	T58.13	T58.14	—	—
prior to combustion	T59.891	T59.892	T59.893	T59.894	—	—
Ilopan	T45.2X1	T45.2X2	T45.2X3	T45.2X4	T45.2X5	T45.2X6
Iloprost	T46.7X1	T46.7X2	T46.7X3	T46.7X4	T46.7X5	T46.7X6
Ilotycin	T36.3X1	T36.3X2	T36.3X3	T36.3X4	T36.3X5	T36.3X6
ophthalmic preparation	T49.5X1	T49.5X2	T49.5X3	T49.5X4	T49.5X5	T49.5X6
topical NEC	T49.ØX1	T49.ØX2	T49.ØX3	T49.ØX4	T49.ØX5	T49.ØX6
Imdur*	T46.3X1	T46.3X2	T46.3X3	T46.3X4	T46.3X5	T46.3X6
Imidazole-4-carboxamide	T45.1X1	T45.1X2	T45.1X3	T45.1X4	T45.1X5	T45.1X6
Iminostilbene	T42.1X1	T42.1X2	T42.1X3	T42.1X4	T42.1X5	T42.1X6
Imipenem	T36.ØX1	T36.ØX2	T36.ØX3	T36.ØX4	T36.ØX5	T36.ØX6
Imipramine	T43.Ø11	T43.Ø12	T43.Ø13	T43.Ø14	T43.Ø15	T43.Ø16
Immu-G	T5Ø.Z11	T5Ø.Z12	T5Ø.Z13	T5Ø.Z14	T5Ø.Z15	T5Ø.Z16
Immuglobin	T5Ø.Z11	T5Ø.Z12	T5Ø.Z13	T5Ø.Z14	T5Ø.Z15	T5Ø.Z16
Immune						
globulin	T5Ø.Z11	T5Ø.Z12	T5Ø.Z13	T5Ø.Z14	T5Ø.Z15	T5Ø.Z16
serum globulin	T5Ø.Z11	T5Ø.Z12	T5Ø.Z13	T5Ø.Z14	T5Ø.Z15	T5Ø.Z16
Immunoglobin human (intravenous) (normal)	T5Ø.Z11	T5Ø.Z12	T5Ø.Z13	T5Ø.Z14	T5Ø.Z15	T5Ø.Z16
unmodified	T5Ø.Z11	T5Ø.Z12	T5Ø.Z13	T5Ø.Z14	T5Ø.Z15	T5Ø.Z16
Immunosuppressive drug	T45.1X1	T45.1X2	T45.1X3	T45.1X4	T45.1X5	T45.1X6
Immu-tetanus	T5Ø.Z11	T5Ø.Z12	T5Ø.Z13	T5Ø.Z14	T5Ø.Z15	T5Ø.Z16
Indalpine	T43.221	T43.222	T43.223	T43.224	T43.225	T43.226
Indanazoline	T48.5X1	T48.5X2	T48.5X3	T48.5X4	T48.5X5	T48.5X6
Indandione (derivatives)	T45.511	T45.512	T45.513	T45.514	T45.515	T45.516
Indapamide	T46.5X1	T46.5X2	T46.5X3	T46.5X4	T46.5X5	T46.5X6
Indendione (derivatives)	T45.511	T45.512	T45.513	T45.514	T45.515	T45.516
Indenolol	T44.7X1	T44.7X2	T44.7X3	T44.7X4	T44.7X5	T44.7X6
Inderal	T44.7X1	T44.7X2	T44.7X3	T44.7X4	T44.7X5	T44.7X6
Indian						
hemp	T4Ø.711	T4Ø.712	T4Ø.713	T4Ø.714	T4Ø.715	T4Ø.716
tobacco	T62.2X1	T62.2X2	T62.2X3	T62.2X4	—	—
Indigo carmine	T5Ø.8X1	T5Ø.8X2	T5Ø.8X3	T5Ø.8X4	T5Ø.8X5	T5Ø.8X6
Indobufen	T45.521	T45.522	T45.523	T45.524	T45.525	T45.526
Indocin	T39.2X1	T39.2X2	T39.2X3	T39.2X4	T39.2X5	T39.2X6
Indocyanine green	T5Ø.8X1	T5Ø.8X2	T5Ø.8X3	T5Ø.8X4	T5Ø.8X5	T5Ø.8X6
Indometacin	T39.391	T39.392	T39.393	T39.394	T39.395	T39.396
Indomethacin	T39.391	T39.392	T39.393	T39.394	T39.395	T39.396
farnesil	T39.4X1	T39.4X2	T39.4X3	T39.4X4	T39.4X5	T39.4X6
Indoramin	T44.6X1	T44.6X2	T44.6X3	T44.6X4	T44.6X5	T44.6X6
Industrial						
alcohol	T51.ØX1	T51.ØX2	T51.ØX3	T51.ØX4	—	—
fumes	T59.891	T59.892	T59.893	T59.894	—	—
solvents (fumes) (vapors)	T52.91	T52.92	T52.93	T52.94	—	—
Inflectra*	T39.4X1	T39.4X2	T39.4X3	T39.4X4	T39.4X5	T39.4X6
Influenza vaccine	T5Ø.B91	T5Ø.B92	T5Ø.B93	T5Ø.B94	T5Ø.B95	T5Ø.B96
Ingested substance NEC	T65.91	T65.92	T65.93	T65.94	—	—
INH	T37.1X1	T37.1X2	T37.1X3	T37.1X4	T37.1X5	T37.1X6
Inhalation, gas (noxious) — *see* Gas						
Inhibitor						
angiotensin-converting enzyme	T46.4X1	T46.4X2	T46.4X3	T46.4X4	T46.4X5	T46.4X6
carbonic anhydrase	T5Ø.2X1	T5Ø.2X2	T5Ø.2X3	T5Ø.2X4	T5Ø.2X5	T5Ø.2X6
fibrinolysis	T45.621	T45.622	T45.623	T45.624	T45.625	T45.626
monoamine oxidase NEC	T43.1X1	T43.1X2	T43.1X3	T43.1X4	T43.1X5	T43.1X6
hydrazine	T43.1X1	T43.1X2	T43.1X3	T43.1X4	T43.1X5	T43.1X6
postsynaptic	T43.8X1	T43.8X2	T43.8X3	T43.8X4	T43.8X5	T43.8X6
prothrombin synthesis	T45.511	T45.512	T45.513	T45.514	T45.515	T45.516
Ink	T65.891	T65.892	T65.893	T65.894	—	—
Innopran*	T44.7X1	T44.7X2	T44.7X3	T44.7X4	T44.7X5	T44.7X6

Substance	Poisoning, Accidental (unintentional)	Poisoning, Intentional Self-harm	Poisoning, Assault	Poisoning, Undetermined	Adverse Effect	Under-dosing
Inorganic substance NEC	T57.91	T57.92	T57.93	T57.94	—	—
Inosine pranobex	T37.5X1	T37.5X2	T37.5X3	T37.5X4	T37.5X5	T37.5X6
Inositol	T5Ø.991	T5Ø.992	T5Ø.993	T5Ø.994	T5Ø.995	T5Ø.996
nicotinate	T46.7X1	T46.7X2	T46.7X3	T46.7X4	T46.7X5	T46.7X6
Inproquone	T45.1X1	T45.1X2	T45.1X3	T45.1X4	T45.1X5	T45.1X6
Insecticide NEC	T6Ø.91	T6Ø.92	T6Ø.93	T6Ø.94	—	—
carbamate	T6Ø.ØX1	T6Ø.ØX2	T6Ø.ØX3	T6Ø.ØX4	—	—
chlorinated	T6Ø.1X1	T6Ø.1X2	T6Ø.1X3	T6Ø.1X4	—	—
mixed	T6Ø.91	T6Ø.92	T6Ø.93	T6Ø.94	—	—
organochlorine	T6Ø.1X1	T6Ø.1X2	T6Ø.1X3	T6Ø.1X4	—	—
organophosphorus	T6Ø.ØX1	T6Ø.ØX2	T6Ø.ØX3	T6Ø.ØX4	—	—
Insect (sting), venomous	T63.481	T63.482	T63.483	T63.484	—	—
ant	T63.421	T63.422	T63.423	T63.424	—	—
bee	T63.441	T63.442	T63.443	T63.444	—	—
caterpillar	T63.431	T63.432	T63.433	T63.434	—	—
hornet	T63.451	T63.452	T63.453	T63.454	—	—
wasp	T63.461	T63.462	T63.463	T63.464	—	—
Insular tissue extract	T38.3X1	T38.3X2	T38.3X3	T38.3X4	T38.3X5	T38.3X6
Insulin (amorphous) (globin) (isophane) (Lente) (NPH) (Semilente) (Ultralente)	T38.3X1	T38.3X2	T38.3X3	T38.3X4	T38.3X5	T38.3X6
defalan	T38.3X1	T38.3X2	T38.3X3	T38.3X4	T38.3X5	T38.3X6
human	T38.3X1	T38.3X2	T38.3X3	T38.3X4	T38.3X5	T38.3X6
injection, soluble	T38.3X1	T38.3X2	T38.3X3	T38.3X4	T38.3X5	T38.3X6
biphasic	T38.3X1	T38.3X2	T38.3X3	T38.3X4	T38.3X5	T38.3X6
intermediate acting	T38.3X1	T38.3X2	T38.3X3	T38.3X4	T38.3X5	T38.3X6
protamine zinc	T38.3X1	T38.3X2	T38.3X3	T38.3X4	T38.3X5	T38.3X6
slow acting	T38.3X1	T38.3X2	T38.3X3	T38.3X4	T38.3X5	T38.3X6
zinc						
protamine injection	T38.3X1	T38.3X2	T38.3X3	T38.3X4	T38.3X5	T38.3X6
suspension (amorphous) (crystalline)	T38.3X1	T38.3X2	T38.3X3	T38.3X4	T38.3X5	T38.3X6
Interferon (alpha) (beta) (gamma)	T37.5X1	T37.5X2	T37.5X3	T37.5X4	T37.5X5	T37.5X6
Intestinal motility control drug	T47.6X1	T47.6X2	T47.6X3	T47.6X4	T47.6X5	T47.6X6
biological	T47.8X1	T47.8X2	T47.8X3	T47.8X4	T47.8X5	T47.8X6
Intranarcon	T41.1X1	T41.1X2	T41.1X3	T41.1X4	T41.1X5	T41.1X6
Intravenous						
amino acids	T5Ø.991	T5Ø.992	T5Ø.993	T5Ø.994	T5Ø.995	T5Ø.996
fat suspension	T5Ø.991	T5Ø.992	T5Ø.993	T5Ø.994	T5Ø.995	T5Ø.996
Inulin	T5Ø.8X1	T5Ø.8X2	T5Ø.8X3	T5Ø.8X4	T5Ø.8X5	T5Ø.8X6
Invanz*	T36.1X1	T36.1X2	T36.1X3	T36.1X4	T36.1X5	T36.1X6
Invert sugar	T5Ø.3X1	T5Ø.3X2	T5Ø.3X3	T5Ø.3X4	T5Ø.3X5	T5Ø.3X6
Inza — *see* Naproxen						
Iobenzamic acid	T5Ø.8X1	T5Ø.8X2	T5Ø.8X3	T5Ø.8X4	T5Ø.8X5	T5Ø.8X6
Iocarmic acid	T5Ø.8X1	T5Ø.8X2	T5Ø.8X3	T5Ø.8X4	T5Ø.8X5	T5Ø.8X6
Iocetamic acid	T5Ø.8X1	T5Ø.8X2	T5Ø.8X3	T5Ø.8X4	T5Ø.8X5	T5Ø.8X6
Iodamide	T5Ø.8X1	T5Ø.8X2	T5Ø.8X3	T5Ø.8X4	T5Ø.8X5	T5Ø.8X6
Iodide NEC — *see also* Iodine	T49.ØX1	T49.ØX2	T49.ØX3	T49.ØX4	T49.ØX5	T49.ØX6
mercury (ointment)	T49.ØX1	T49.ØX2	T49.ØX3	T49.ØX4	T49.ØX5	T49.ØX6
methylate	T49.ØX1	T49.ØX2	T49.ØX3	T49.ØX4	T49.ØX5	T49.ØX6
potassium (expectorant) NEC	T48.4X1	T48.4X2	T48.4X3	T48.4X4	T48.4X5	T48.4X6
Iodinated						
contrast medium	T5Ø.8X1	T5Ø.8X2	T5Ø.8X3	T5Ø.8X4	T5Ø.8X5	T5Ø.8X6
glycerol	T48.4X1	T48.4X2	T48.4X3	T48.4X4	T48.4X5	T48.4X6
human serum albumin (131I)	T5Ø.8X1	T5Ø.8X2	T5Ø.8X3	T5Ø.8X4	T5Ø.8X5	T5Ø.8X6
Iodine (antiseptic, external) (tincture) **NEC**	T49.ØX1	T49.ØX2	T49.ØX3	T49.ØX4	T49.ØX5	T49.ØX6
125 — *see also* Radiation sickness, and Exposure to radioactive isotopes	T5Ø.8X1	T5Ø.8X2	T5Ø.8X3	T5Ø.8X4	T5Ø.8X5	T5Ø.8X6
therapeutic	T5Ø.991	T5Ø.992	T5Ø.993	T5Ø.994	T5Ø.995	T5Ø.996
131 — *see also* Radiation sickness, and Exposure to radioactive isotopes	T5Ø.8X1	T5Ø.8X2	T5Ø.8X3	T5Ø.8X4	T5Ø.8X5	T5Ø.8X6
therapeutic	T38.2X1	T38.2X2	T38.2X3	T38.2X4	T38.2X5	T38.2X6
diagnostic	T5Ø.8X1	T5Ø.8X2	T5Ø.8X3	T5Ø.8X4	T5Ø.8X5	T5Ø.8X6
for thyroid conditions (antithyroid)	T38.2X1	T38.2X2	T38.2X3	T38.2X4	T38.2X5	T38.2X6
solution	T49.ØX1	T49.ØX2	T49.ØX3	T49.ØX4	T49.ØX5	T49.ØX6
vapor	T59.891	T59.892	T59.893	T59.894	—	—
Iodipamide	T5Ø.8X1	T5Ø.8X2	T5Ø.8X3	T5Ø.8X4	T5Ø.8X5	T5Ø.8X6
Iodized (poppy seed) oil	T5Ø.8X1	T5Ø.8X2	T5Ø.8X3	T5Ø.8X4	T5Ø.8X5	T5Ø.8X6
Iodobismitol	T37.8X1	T37.8X2	T37.8X3	T37.8X4	T37.8X5	T37.8X6
Iodochlorhydroxyquin	T37.8X1	T37.8X2	T37.8X3	T37.8X4	T37.8X5	T37.8X6
topical	T49.ØX1	T49.ØX2	T49.ØX3	T49.ØX4	T49.ØX5	T49.ØX6
Iodochlorhydroxyquinoline	T37.8X1	T37.8X2	T37.8X3	T37.8X4	T37.8X5	T37.8X6
Iodocholesterol (131I)	T5Ø.8X1	T5Ø.8X2	T5Ø.8X3	T5Ø.8X4	T5Ø.8X5	T5Ø.8X6
Iodoform	T49.ØX1	T49.ØX2	T49.ØX3	T49.ØX4	T49.ØX5	T49.ØX6

Substance	Poisoning, Accidental (unintentional)	Poisoning, Intentional Self-harm	Poisoning, Assault	Poisoning, Undetermined	Adverse Effect	Under-dosing
Iodohippuric acid	T5Ø.8X1	T5Ø.8X2	T5Ø.8X3	T5Ø.8X4	T5Ø.8X5	T5Ø.8X6
Iodopanoic acid	T5Ø.8X1	T5Ø.8X2	T5Ø.8X3	T5Ø.8X4	T5Ø.8X5	T5Ø.8X6
Iodophthalein (sodium)	T5Ø.8X1	T5Ø.8X2	T5Ø.8X3	T5Ø.8X4	T5Ø.8X5	T5Ø.8X6
Iodopyracet	T5Ø.8X1	T5Ø.8X2	T5Ø.8X3	T5Ø.8X4	T5Ø.8X5	T5Ø.8X6
Iodoquinol	T37.8X1	T37.8X2	T37.8X3	T37.8X4	T37.8X5	T37.8X6
Iodoxamic acid	T5Ø.8X1	T5Ø.8X2	T5Ø.8X3	T5Ø.8X4	T5Ø.8X5	T5Ø.8X6
Iofendylate	T5Ø.8X1	T5Ø.8X2	T5Ø.8X3	T5Ø.8X4	T5Ø.8X5	T5Ø.8X6
Ioglycamic acid	T5Ø.8X1	T5Ø.8X2	T5Ø.8X3	T5Ø.8X4	T5Ø.8X5	T5Ø.8X6
Iohexol	T5Ø.8X1	T5Ø.8X2	T5Ø.8X3	T5Ø.8X4	T5Ø.8X5	T5Ø.8X6
Ion exchange resin						
anion	T47.8X1	T47.8X2	T47.8X3	T47.8X4	T47.8X5	T47.8X6
cation	T5Ø.3X1	T5Ø.3X2	T5Ø.3X3	T5Ø.3X4	T5Ø.3X5	T5Ø.3X6
cholestyramine	T46.6X1	T46.6X2	T46.6X3	T46.6X4	T46.6X5	T46.6X6
intestinal	T47.8X1	T47.8X2	T47.8X3	T47.8X4	T47.8X5	T47.8X6
Iopamidol	T5Ø.8X1	T5Ø.8X2	T5Ø.8X3	T5Ø.8X4	T5Ø.8X5	T5Ø.8X6
Iopanoic acid	T5Ø.8X1	T5Ø.8X2	T5Ø.8X3	T5Ø.8X4	T5Ø.8X5	T5Ø.8X6
Iophenoic acid	T5Ø.8X1	T5Ø.8X2	T5Ø.8X3	T5Ø.8X4	T5Ø.8X5	T5Ø.8X6
Iopodate, sodium	T5Ø.8X1	T5Ø.8X2	T5Ø.8X3	T5Ø.8X4	T5Ø.8X5	T5Ø.8X6
Iopodic acid	T5Ø.8X1	T5Ø.8X2	T5Ø.8X3	T5Ø.8X4	T5Ø.8X5	T5Ø.8X6
Iopromide	T5Ø.8X1	T5Ø.8X2	T5Ø.8X3	T5Ø.8X4	T5Ø.8X5	T5Ø.8X6
Iopydol	T5Ø.8X1	T5Ø.8X2	T5Ø.8X3	T5Ø.8X4	T5Ø.8X5	T5Ø.8X6
Iotalamic acid	T5Ø.8X1	T5Ø.8X2	T5Ø.8X3	T5Ø.8X4	T5Ø.8X5	T5Ø.8X6
Iothalamate	T5Ø.8X1	T5Ø.8X2	T5Ø.8X3	T5Ø.8X4	T5Ø.8X5	T5Ø.8X6
Iothiouracil	T38.2X1	T38.2X2	T38.2X3	T38.2X4	T38.2X5	T38.2X6
Iotrol	T5Ø.8X1	T5Ø.8X2	T5Ø.8X3	T5Ø.8X4	T5Ø.8X5	T5Ø.8X6
Iotrolan	T5Ø.8X1	T5Ø.8X2	T5Ø.8X3	T5Ø.8X4	T5Ø.8X5	T5Ø.8X6
Iotroxate	T5Ø.8X1	T5Ø.8X2	T5Ø.8X3	T5Ø.8X4	T5Ø.8X5	T5Ø.8X6
Iotroxic acid	T5Ø.8X1	T5Ø.8X2	T5Ø.8X3	T5Ø.8X4	T5Ø.8X5	T5Ø.8X6
Ioversol	T5Ø.8X1	T5Ø.8X2	T5Ø.8X3	T5Ø.8X4	T5Ø.8X5	T5Ø.8X6
Ioxaglate	T5Ø.8X1	T5Ø.8X2	T5Ø.8X3	T5Ø.8X4	T5Ø.8X5	T5Ø.8X6
Ioxaglic acid	T5Ø.8X1	T5Ø.8X2	T5Ø.8X3	T5Ø.8X4	T5Ø.8X5	T5Ø.8X6
Ioxitalamic acid	T5Ø.8X1	T5Ø.8X2	T5Ø.8X3	T5Ø.8X4	T5Ø.8X5	T5Ø.8X6
Ipecac	T47.7X1	T47.7X2	T47.7X3	T47.7X4	T47.7X5	T47.7X6
Ipecacuanha	T48.4X1	T48.4X2	T48.4X3	T48.4X4	T48.4X5	T48.4X6
Ipodate, calcium	T5Ø.8X1	T5Ø.8X2	T5Ø.8X3	T5Ø.8X4	T5Ø.8X5	T5Ø.8X6
IPOL*	T5Ø.B91	T5Ø.B92	T5Ø.B93	T5Ø.B94	T5Ø.B95	T5Ø.B96
Ipral	T42.3X1	T42.3X2	T42.3X3	T42.3X4	T42.3X5	T42.3X6
Ipratropium (bromide)	T48.6X1	T48.6X2	T48.6X3	T48.6X4	T48.6X5	T48.6X6
Ipriflavone	T46.3X1	T46.3X2	T46.3X3	T46.3X4	T46.3X5	T46.3X6
Iprindole	T43.Ø11	T43.Ø12	T43.Ø13	T43.Ø14	T43.Ø15	T43.Ø16
Iproclozide	T43.1X1	T43.1X2	T43.1X3	T43.1X4	T43.1X5	T43.1X6
Iprofenin	T5Ø.8X1	T5Ø.8X2	T5Ø.8X3	T5Ø.8X4	T5Ø.8X5	T5Ø.8X6
Iproheptine	T49.2X1	T49.2X2	T49.2X3	T49.2X4	T49.2X5	T49.2X6
Iproniazid	T43.1X1	T43.1X2	T43.1X3	T43.1X4	T43.1X5	T43.1X6
Iproplatin	T45.1X1	T45.1X2	T45.1X3	T45.1X4	T45.1X5	T45.1X6
Iproveratril	T46.1X1	T46.1X2	T46.1X3	T46.1X4	T46.1X5	T46.1X6
Irinotecan*	T45.1X1	T45.1X2	T45.1X3	T45.1X4	T45.1X5	T45.1X6
Iron (compounds) (medicinal) **NEC**	T45.4X1	T45.4X2	T45.4X3	T45.4X4	T45.4X5	T45.4X6
ammonium	T45.4X1	T45.4X2	T45.4X3	T45.4X4	T45.4X5	T45.4X6
dextran injection	T45.4X1	T45.4X2	T45.4X3	T45.4X4	T45.4X5	T45.4X6
nonmedicinal	T56.891	T56.892	T56.893	T56.894	—	—
salts	T45.4X1	T45.4X2	T45.4X3	T45.4X4	T45.4X5	T45.4X6
sorbitex	T45.4X1	T45.4X2	T45.4X3	T45.4X4	T45.4X5	T45.4X6
sorbitol citric acid complex	T45.4X1	T45.4X2	T45.4X3	T45.4X4	T45.4X5	T45.4X6
Irrigating fluid (vaginal)	T49.8X1	T49.8X2	T49.8X3	T49.8X4	T49.8X5	T49.8X6
eye	T49.5X1	T49.5X2	T49.5X3	T49.5X4	T49.5X5	T49.5X6
Isepamicin	T36.5X1	T36.5X2	T36.5X3	T36.5X4	T36.5X5	T36.5X6
Isoaminile (citrate)	T48.3X1	T48.3X2	T48.3X3	T48.3X4	T48.3X5	T48.3X6
Isoamyl nitrite	T46.3X1	T46.3X2	T46.3X3	T46.3X4	T46.3X5	T46.3X6
Isobenzan	T6Ø.1X1	T6Ø.1X2	T6Ø.1X3	T6Ø.1X4	—	—
Isobutyl acetate	T52.8X1	T52.8X2	T52.8X3	T52.8X4	—	—
Isocarboxazid	T43.1X1	T43.1X2	T43.1X3	T43.1X4	T43.1X5	T43.1X6
Isoconazole	T49.ØX1	T49.ØX2	T49.ØX3	T49.ØX4	T49.ØX5	T49.ØX6
Isocyanate	T65.ØX1	T65.ØX2	T65.ØX3	T65.ØX4	—	—
Isoephedrine	T44.991	T44.992	T44.993	T44.994	T44.995	T44.996
Isoetarine	T48.6X1	T48.6X2	T48.6X3	T48.6X4	T48.6X5	T48.6X6
Isoethadione	T42.2X1	T42.2X2	T42.2X3	T42.2X4	T42.2X5	T42.2X6
Isoetharine	T44.5X1	T44.5X2	T44.5X3	T44.5X4	T44.5X5	T44.5X6
Isoflurane	T41.ØX1	T41.ØX2	T41.ØX3	T41.ØX4	T41.ØX5	T41.ØX6
Isoflurophate	T44.ØX1	T44.ØX2	T44.ØX3	T44.ØX4	T44.ØX5	T44.ØX6
Isomaltose, ferric complex	T45.4X1	T45.4X2	T45.4X3	T45.4X4	T45.4X5	T45.4X6
Isometheptene	T44.3X1	T44.3X2	T44.3X3	T44.3X4	T44.3X5	T44.3X6
Isoniazid	T37.1X1	T37.1X2	T37.1X3	T37.1X4	T37.1X5	T37.1X6
with						
rifampicin	T36.6X1	T36.6X2	T36.6X3	T36.6X4	T36.6X5	T36.6X6
thioacetazone	T37.1X1	T37.1X2	T37.1X3	T37.1X4	T37.1X5	T37.1X6
Isonicotinic acid hydrazide	T37.1X1	T37.1X2	T37.1X3	T37.1X4	T37.1X5	T37.1X6
Isonipecaine	T4Ø.491	T4Ø.492	T4Ø.493	T4Ø.494	T4Ø.495	T4Ø.496
Isopentaquine	T37.2X1	T37.2X2	T37.2X3	T37.2X4	T37.2X5	T37.2X6
Isophane insulin	T38.3X1	T38.3X2	T38.3X3	T38.3X4	T38.3X5	T38.3X6
Isophorone	T65.891	T65.892	T65.893	T65.894	—	—
Isophosphamide	T45.1X1	T45.1X2	T45.1X3	T45.1X4	T45.1X5	T45.1X6

Substance	Poisoning, Accidental (unintentional)	Poisoning, Intentional Self-harm	Poisoning, Assault	Poisoning, Undetermined	Adverse Effect	Under-dosing
Isopregnenone	T38.5X1	T38.5X2	T38.5X3	T38.5X4	T38.5X5	T38.5X6
Isoprenaline	T48.6X1	T48.6X2	T48.6X3	T48.6X4	T48.6X5	T48.6X6
Isopromethazine	T43.3X1	T43.3X2	T43.3X3	T43.3X4	T43.3X5	T43.3X6
Isopropamide	T44.3X1	T44.3X2	T44.3X3	T44.3X4	T44.3X5	T44.3X6
iodide	T44.3X1	T44.3X2	T44.3X3	T44.3X4	T44.3X5	T44.3X6
Isopropanol	T51.2X1	T51.2X2	T51.2X3	T51.2X4	—	—
Isopropyl						
acetate	T52.8X1	T52.8X2	T52.8X3	T52.8X4	—	—
alcohol	T51.2X1	T51.2X2	T51.2X3	T51.2X4	—	—
medicinal	T49.4X1	T49.4X2	T49.4X3	T49.4X4	T49.4X5	T49.4X6
ether	T52.8X1	T52.8X2	T52.8X3	T52.8X4	—	—
Isopropylaminophenazone	T39.2X1	T39.2X2	T39.2X3	T39.2X4	T39.2X5	T39.2X6
Isoproterenol	T48.6X1	T48.6X2	T48.6X3	T48.6X4	T48.6X5	T48.6X6
Isosorbide dinitrate	T46.3X1	T46.3X2	T46.3X3	T46.3X4	T46.3X5	T46.3X6
Isothipendyl	T45.ØX1	T45.ØX2	T45.ØX3	T45.ØX4	T45.ØX5	T45.ØX6
Isotretinoin	T5Ø.991	T5Ø.992	T5Ø.993	T5Ø.994	T5Ø.995	T5Ø.996
Isoxazolyl penicillin	T36.ØX1	T36.ØX2	T36.ØX3	T36.ØX4	T36.ØX5	T36.ØX6
Isoxicam	T39.391	T39.392	T39.393	T39.394	T39.395	T39.396
Isoxsuprine	T46.7X1	T46.7X2	T46.7X3	T46.7X4	T46.7X5	T46.7X6
Ispagula	T47.4X1	T47.4X2	T47.4X3	T47.4X4	T47.4X5	T47.4X6
husk	T47.4X1	T47.4X2	T47.4X3	T47.4X4	T47.4X5	T47.4X6
Isradipine	T46.1X1	T46.1X2	T46.1X3	T46.1X4	T46.1X5	T46.1X6
I-thyroxine sodium	T38.1X1	T38.1X2	T38.1X3	T38.1X4	T38.1X5	T38.1X6
Itraconazole	T37.8X1	T37.8X2	T37.8X3	T37.8X4	T37.8X5	T37.8X6
Itramin tosilate	T46.3X1	T46.3X2	T46.3X3	T46.3X4	T46.3X5	T46.3X6
Ivarest*	T41.3X1	T41.3X2	T41.3X3	T41.3X4	T41.3X5	T41.3X6
Ivermectin	T37.4X1	T37.4X2	T37.4X3	T37.4X4	T37.4X5	T37.4X6
Izoniazid	T37.1X1	T37.1X2	T37.1X3	T37.1X4	T37.1X5	T37.1X6
with thioacetazone	T37.1X1	T37.1X2	T37.1X3	T37.1X4	T37.1X5	T37.1X6
Jalap	T47.2X1	T47.2X2	T47.2X3	T47.2X4	T47.2X5	T47.2X6
Jamaica						
dogwood (bark)	T39.8X1	T39.8X2	T39.8X3	T39.8X4	T39.8X5	T39.8X6
ginger	T65.891	T65.892	T65.893	T65.894	—	—
root	T62.2X1	T62.2X2	T62.2X3	T62.2X4	—	—
Jantoven*	T45.511	T45.512	T45.513	T45.514	T45.515	T45.516
Jatropha	T62.2X1	T62.2X2	T62.2X3	T62.2X4	—	—
curcas	T62.2X1	T62.2X2	T62.2X3	T62.2X4	—	—
Jectofer	T45.4X1	T45.4X2	T45.4X3	T45.4X4	T45.4X5	T45.4X6
Jellyfish (sting)	T63.621	T63.622	T63.623	T63.624	—	—
Jequirity (bean)	T62.2X1	T62.2X2	T62.2X3	T62.2X4	—	—
Jimson weed (stramonium)	T62.2X1	T62.2X2	T62.2X3	T62.2X4	—	—
seeds	T62.2X1	T62.2X2	T62.2X3	T62.2X4	—	—
Josamycin	T36.3X1	T36.3X2	T36.3X3	T36.3X4	T36.3X5	T36.3X6
Juniper tar	T49.1X1	T49.1X2	T49.1X3	T49.1X4	T49.1X5	T49.1X6
Kaletra*	T37.5X1	T37.5X2	T37.5X3	T37.5X4	T37.5X5	T37.5X6
Kallidinogenase	T46.7X1	T46.7X2	T46.7X3	T46.7X4	T46.7X5	T46.7X6
Kallikrein	T46.7X1	T46.7X2	T46.7X3	T46.7X4	T46.7X5	T46.7X6
Kanamycin	T36.5X1	T36.5X2	T36.5X3	T36.5X4	T36.5X5	T36.5X6
Kantrex	T36.5X1	T36.5X2	T36.5X3	T36.5X4	T36.5X5	T36.5X6
Kaolin	T47.6X1	T47.6X2	T47.6X3	T47.6X4	T47.6X5	T47.6X6
light	T47.6X1	T47.6X2	T47.6X3	T47.6X4	T47.6X5	T47.6X6
Karaya (gum)	T47.4X1	T47.4X2	T47.4X3	T47.4X4	T47.4X5	T47.4X6
Kebuzone	T39.2X1	T39.2X2	T39.2X3	T39.2X4	T39.2X5	T39.2X6
Kelevan	T6Ø.1X1	T6Ø.1X2	T6Ø.1X3	T6Ø.1X4	—	—
Kemithal	T41.1X1	T41.1X2	T41.1X3	T41.1X4	T41.1X5	T41.1X6
Kenacort	T38.ØX1	T38.ØX2	T38.ØX3	T38.ØX4	T38.ØX5	T38.ØX6
Keratolytic drug NEC	T49.4X1	T49.4X2	T49.4X3	T49.4X4	T49.4X5	T49.4X6
anthracene	T49.4X1	T49.4X2	T49.4X3	T49.4X4	T49.4X5	T49.4X6
Keratoplastic NEC	T49.4X1	T49.4X2	T49.4X3	T49.4X4	T49.4X5	T49.4X6
Kerosene, kerosine (fuel) (solvent) **NEC**	T52.ØX1	T52.ØX2	T52.ØX3	T52.ØX4	—	—
insecticide	T52.ØX1	T52.ØX2	T52.ØX3	T52.ØX4	—	—
vapor	T52.ØX1	T52.ØX2	T52.ØX3	T52.ØX4	—	—
Ketamine	T41.291	T41.292	T41.293	T41.294	T41.295	T41.296
Ketazolam	T42.4X1	T42.4X2	T42.4X3	T42.4X4	T42.4X5	T42.4X6
Ketazon	T39.2X1	T39.2X2	T39.2X3	T39.2X4	T39.2X5	T39.2X6
Ketobemidone	T4Ø.491	T4Ø.492	T4Ø.493	T4Ø.494	—	—
Ketoconazole	T49.ØX1	T49.ØX2	T49.ØX3	T49.ØX4	T49.ØX5	T49.ØX6
Ketols	T52.4X1	T52.4X2	T52.4X3	T52.4X4	—	—
Ketone oils	T52.4X1	T52.4X2	T52.4X3	T52.4X4	—	—
Ketoprofen	T39.311	T39.312	T39.313	T39.314	T39.315	T39.316
Ketorolac	T39.8X1	T39.8X2	T39.8X3	T39.8X4	T39.8X5	T39.8X6
Ketotifen	T45.ØX1	T45.ØX2	T45.ØX3	T45.ØX4	T45.ØX5	T45.ØX6
Keytruda*	T45.1X1	T45.1X2	T45.1X3	T45.1X4	T45.1X5	T45.1X6
Khat	T43.691	T43.692	T43.693	T43.694	—	—
Khellin	T46.3X1	T46.3X2	T46.3X3	T46.3X4	T46.3X5	T46.3X6
Khelloside	T46.3X1	T46.3X2	T46.3X3	T46.3X4	T46.3X5	T46.3X6
Kiln gas or vapor (carbon monoxide)	T58.8X1	T58.8X2	T58.8X3	T58.8X4	—	—
Kineret*	T39.4X1	T39.4X2	T39.4X3	T39.4X4	T39.4X5	T39.4X6
Kitasamycin	T36.3X1	T36.3X2	T36.3X3	T36.3X4	T36.3X5	T36.3X6
Komgiblyze*	T38.3X1	T38.3X2	T38.3X3	T38.3X4	T38.3X5	T38.3X6
Konsyl	T47.4X1	T47.4X2	T47.4X3	T47.4X4	T47.4X5	T47.4X6

Substance	Poisoning, Accidental (unintentional)	Poisoning, Intentional Self-harm	Poisoning, Assault	Poisoning, Undetermined	Adverse Effect	Under-dosing
Kosam seed	T62.2X1	T62.2X2	T62.2X3	T62.2X4	—	—
Krait (venom)	T63.091	T63.092	T63.093	T63.094	—	—
Kwell (insecticide)	T60.1X1	T60.1X2	T60.1X3	T60.1X4	—	—
anti-infective (topical)	T49.0X1	T49.0X2	T49.0X3	T49.0X4	T49.0X5	T49.0X6
Labetalol	T44.8X1	T44.8X2	T44.8X3	T44.8X4	T44.8X5	T44.8X6
Laburnum (seeds)	T62.2X1	T62.2X2	T62.2X3	T62.2X4	—	—
leaves	T62.2X1	T62.2X2	T62.2X3	T62.2X4	—	—
Lachesine	T49.5X1	T49.5X2	T49.5X3	T49.5X4	T49.5X5	T49.5X6
Lacidipine	T46.5X1	T46.5X2	T46.5X3	T46.5X4	T46.5X5	T46.5X6
Lacquer	T65.6X1	T65.6X2	T65.6X3	T65.6X4	—	—
Lacrimogenic gas	T59.3X1	T59.3X2	T59.3X3	T59.3X4	—	—
Lactated potassic saline	T50.3X1	T50.3X2	T50.3X3	T50.3X4	T50.3X5	T50.3X6
Lactic acid	T49.8X1	T49.8X2	T49.8X3	T49.8X4	T49.8X5	T49.8X6
Lactobacillus						
acidophilus	T47.6X1	T47.6X2	T47.6X3	T47.6X4	T47.6X5	T47.6X6
compound	T47.6X1	T47.6X2	T47.6X3	T47.6X4	T47.6X5	T47.6X6
bifidus, lyophilized	T47.6X1	T47.6X2	T47.6X3	T47.6X4	T47.6X5	T47.6X6
bulgaricus	T47.6X1	T47.6X2	T47.6X3	T47.6X4	T47.6X5	T47.6X6
sporogenes	T47.6X1	T47.6X2	T47.6X3	T47.6X4	T47.6X5	T47.6X6
Lactoflavin	T45.2X1	T45.2X2	T45.2X3	T45.2X4	T45.2X5	T45.2X6
Lactose (as excipient)	T50.901	T50.902	T50.903	T50.904	T50.905	T50.906
Lactuca (virosa) (extract)	T42.6X1	T42.6X2	T42.6X3	T42.6X4	T42.6X5	T42.6X6
Lactucarium	T42.6X1	T42.6X2	T42.6X3	T42.6X4	T42.6X5	T42.6X6
Lactulose	T47.3X1	T47.3X2	T47.3X3	T47.3X4	T47.3X5	T47.3X6
Laevo — *see* Levo-						
Lanatosides	T46.0X1	T46.0X2	T46.0X3	T46.0X4	T46.0X5	T46.0X6
Lanolin	T49.3X1	T49.3X2	T49.3X3	T49.3X4	T49.3X5	T49.3X6
Lanoxin*	T46.0X1	T46.0X2	T46.0X3	T46.0X4	T46.0X5	T46.0X6
Largactil	T43.3X1	T43.3X2	T43.3X3	T43.3X4	T43.3X5	T43.3X6
Larkspur	T62.2X1	T62.2X2	T62.2X3	T62.2X4	—	—
Laroxyl	T43.011	T43.012	T43.013	T43.014	T43.015	T43.016
Lasix	T50.1X1	T50.1X2	T50.1X3	T50.1X4	T50.1X5	T50.1X6
Lassar's paste	T49.4X1	T49.4X2	T49.4X3	T49.4X4	T49.4X5	T49.4X6
Latamoxef	T36.1X1	T36.1X2	T36.1X3	T36.1X4	T36.1X5	T36.1X6
Latex	T65.811	T65.812	T65.813	T65.814	—	—
Lathyrus (seed)	T62.2X1	T62.2X2	T62.2X3	T62.2X4	—	—
Laudanum	T40.0X1	T40.0X2	T40.0X3	T40.0X4	T40.0X5	T40.0X6
Laudexium	T48.1X1	T48.1X2	T48.1X3	T48.1X4	T48.1X5	T48.1X6
Laughing gas	T41.0X1	T41.0X2	T41.0X3	T41.0X4	T41.0X5	T41.0X6
Laurel, black or cherry	T62.2X1	T62.2X2	T62.2X3	T62.2X4	—	—
Laurolinium	T49.0X1	T49.0X2	T49.0X3	T49.0X4	T49.0X5	T49.0X6
Lauryl sulfoacetate	T49.2X1	T49.2X2	T49.2X3	T49.2X4	T49.2X5	T49.2X6
Laxative NEC	T47.4X1	T47.4X2	T47.4X3	T47.4X4	T47.4X5	T47.4X6
osmotic	T47.3X1	T47.3X2	T47.3X3	T47.3X4	T47.3X5	T47.3X6
saline	T47.3X1	T47.3X2	T47.3X3	T47.3X4	T47.3X5	T47.3X6
stimulant	T47.2X1	T47.2X2	T47.2X3	T47.2X4	T47.2X5	T47.2X6
L-dopa	T42.8X1	T42.8X2	T42.8X3	T42.8X4	T42.8X5	T42.8X6
Lead (dust) (fumes) (vapor) NEC	T56.0X1	T56.0X2	T56.0X3	T56.0X4	—	—
acetate	T49.2X1	T49.2X2	T49.2X3	T49.2X4	T49.2X5	T49.2X6
alkyl (fuel additive)	T56.0X1	T56.0X2	T56.0X3	T56.0X4	—	—
anti-infectives	T37.8X1	T37.8X2	T37.8X3	T37.8X4	T37.8X5	T37.8X6
antiknock compound (tetraethyl)	T56.0X1	T56.0X2	T56.0X3	T56.0X4	—	—
arsenate, arsenite (dust)(herbicide) (insecticide) (vapor)	T57.0X1	T57.0X2	T57.0X3	T57.0X4	—	—
carbonate	T56.0X1	T56.0X2	T56.0X3	T56.0X4	—	—
paint	T56.0X1	T56.0X2	T56.0X3	T56.0X4	—	—
chromate	T56.0X1	T56.0X2	T56.0X3	T56.0X4	—	—
paint	T56.0X1	T56.0X2	T56.0X3	T56.0X4	—	—
dioxide	T56.0X1	T56.0X2	T56.0X3	T56.0X4	—	—
inorganic	T56.0X1	T56.0X2	T56.0X3	T56.0X4	—	—
iodide	T56.0X1	T56.0X2	T56.0X3	T56.0X4	—	—
pigment (paint)	T56.0X1	T56.0X2	T56.0X3	T56.0X4	—	—
monoxide (dust)	T56.0X1	T56.0X2	T56.0X3	T56.0X4	—	—
paint	T56.0X1	T56.0X2	T56.0X3	T56.0X4	—	—
organic	T56.0X1	T56.0X2	T56.0X3	T56.0X4	—	—
oxide	T56.0X1	T56.0X2	T56.0X3	T56.0X4	—	—
paint	T56.0X1	T56.0X2	T56.0X3	T56.0X4	—	—
paint	T56.0X1	T56.0X2	T56.0X3	T56.0X4	—	—
salts	T56.0X1	T56.0X2	T56.0X3	T56.0X4	—	—
specified compound NEC	T56.0X1	T56.0X2	T56.0X3	T56.0X4	—	—
tetra-ethyl	T56.0X1	T56.0X2	T56.0X3	T56.0X4	—	—
Lebanese red	T40.711	T40.712	T40.713	T40.714	T40.715	T40.716
Lefetamine	T39.8X1	T39.8X2	T39.8X3	T39.8X4	T39.8X5	T39.8X6
Lenperone	T43.4X1	T43.4X2	T43.4X3	T43.4X4	T43.4X5	T43.4X6
Lente lietin (insulin)	T38.3X1	T38.3X2	T38.3X3	T38.3X4	T38.3X5	T38.3X6
Leptazol	T50.7X1	T50.7X2	T50.7X3	T50.7X4	T50.7X5	T50.7X6
Leptophos	T60.0X1	T60.0X2	T60.0X3	T60.0X4	—	—
Leritine	T40.2X1	T40.2X2	T40.2X3	T40.2X4	T40.2X5	T40.2X6
Lescol*	T46.6X1	T46.6X2	T46.6X3	T46.6X4	T46.6X5	T46.6X6
Letosteine	T48.4X1	T48.4X2	T48.4X3	T48.4X4	T48.4X5	T48.4X6

Substance	Poisoning, Accidental (unintentional)	Poisoning, Intentional Self-harm	Poisoning, Assault	Poisoning, Undetermined	Adverse Effect	Under-dosing
Letter	T38.1X1	T38.1X2	T38.1X3	T38.1X4	T38.1X5	T38.1X6
Lettuce opium	T42.6X1	T42.6X2	T42.6X3	T42.6X4	T42.6X5	T42.6X6
Leucinocaine	T41.3X1	T41.3X2	T41.3X3	T41.3X4	T41.3X5	T41.3X6
Leucocianidol	T46.991	T46.992	T46.993	T46.994	T46.995	T46.996
Leucovorin (factor)	T45.8X1	T45.8X2	T45.8X3	T45.8X4	T45.8X5	T45.8X6
Leukeran	T45.1X1	T45.1X2	T45.1X3	T45.1X4	T45.1X5	T45.1X6
Leuprolide	T38.891	T38.892	T38.893	T38.894	T38.895	T38.896
Levalbuterol	T48.6X1	T48.6X2	T48.6X3	T48.6X4	T48.6X5	T48.6X6
Levallorphan	T50.7X1	T50.7X2	T50.7X3	T50.7X4	T50.7X5	T50.7X6
Levamisole	T37.4X1	T37.4X2	T37.4X3	T37.4X4	T37.4X5	T37.4X6
Levanil	T42.6X1	T42.6X2	T42.6X3	T42.6X4	T42.6X5	T42.6X6
Levarterenol	T44.4X1	T44.4X2	T44.4X3	T44.4X4	T44.4X5	T44.4X6
Levdropropizine	T48.3X1	T48.3X2	T48.3X3	T48.3X4	T48.3X5	T48.3X6
Levobunolol	T49.5X1	T49.5X2	T49.5X3	T49.5X4	T49.5X5	T49.5X6
Levocabastine (hydrochloride)	T45.0X1	T45.0X2	T45.0X3	T45.0X4	T45.0X5	T45.0X6
Levocarnitine	T50.991	T50.992	T50.993	T50.994	T50.995	T50.996
Levodopa	T42.8X1	T42.8X2	T42.8X3	T42.8X4	T42.8X5	T42.8X6
with carbidopa	T42.8X1	T42.8X2	T42.8X3	T42.8X4	T42.8X5	T42.8X6
Levo-dromoran	T40.2X1	T40.2X2	T40.2X3	T40.2X4	T40.2X5	T40.2X6
Levoglutamide	T50.991	T50.992	T50.993	T50.994	T50.995	T50.996
Levoid	T38.1X1	T38.1X2	T38.1X3	T38.1X4	T38.1X5	T38.1X6
Levo-isomethadone	T40.3X1	T40.3X2	T40.3X3	T40.3X4	T40.3X5	T40.3X6
Levomepromazine	T43.3X1	T43.3X2	T43.3X3	T43.3X4	T43.3X5	T43.3X6
Levonordefrin	T49.6X1	T49.6X2	T49.6X3	T49.6X4	T49.6X5	T49.6X6
Levonorgestrel	T38.4X1	T38.4X2	T38.4X3	T38.4X4	T38.4X5	T38.4X6
with ethinylestradiol	T38.5X1	T38.5X2	T38.5X3	T38.5X4	T38.5X5	T38.5X6
Levopromazine	T43.3X1	T43.3X2	T43.3X3	T43.3X4	T43.3X5	T43.3X6
Levoprome	T42.6X1	T42.6X2	T42.6X3	T42.6X4	T42.6X5	T42.6X6
Levopropoxyphene	T40.491	T40.492	T40.493	T40.494	T40.495	T40.496
Levopropylhexedrine	T50.5X1	T50.5X2	T50.5X3	T50.5X4	T50.5X5	T50.5X6
Levoproxyphylline	T48.6X1	T48.6X2	T48.6X3	T48.6X4	T48.6X5	T48.6X6
Levorphanol	T40.491	T40.492	T40.493	T40.494	T40.495	T40.496
Levothroid*	T38.1X1	T38.1X2	T38.1X3	T38.1X4	T38.1X5	T38.1X6
Levothyroxine	T38.1X1	T38.1X2	T38.1X3	T38.1X4	T38.1X5	T38.1X6
sodium	T38.1X1	T38.1X2	T38.1X3	T38.1X4	T38.1X5	T38.1X6
Levsin	T44.3X1	T44.3X2	T44.3X3	T44.3X4	T44.3X5	T44.3X6
Levulose	T50.3X1	T50.3X2	T50.3X3	T50.3X4	T50.3X5	T50.3X6
Lewisite (gas), not in war	T57.0X1	T57.0X2	T57.0X3	T57.0X4	—	—
Librium	T42.4X1	T42.4X2	T42.4X3	T42.4X4	T42.4X5	T42.4X6
Lidex	T49.0X1	T49.0X2	T49.0X3	T49.0X4	T49.0X5	T49.0X6
Lidocaine	T41.3X1	T41.3X2	T41.3X3	T41.3X4	T41.3X5	T41.3X6
regional	T41.3X1	T41.3X2	T41.3X3	T41.3X4	T41.3X5	T41.3X6
spinal	T41.3X1	T41.3X2	T41.3X3	T41.3X4	T41.3X5	T41.3X6
Lidofenin	T50.8X1	T50.8X2	T50.8X3	T50.8X4	T50.8X5	T50.8X6
Lidoflazine	T46.1X1	T46.1X2	T46.1X3	T46.1X4	T46.1X5	T46.1X6
Lighter fluid	T52.0X1	T52.0X2	T52.0X3	T52.0X4	—	—
Lignin hemicellulose	T47.6X1	T47.6X2	T47.6X3	T47.6X4	T47.6X5	T47.6X6
Lignocaine	T41.3X1	T41.3X2	T41.3X3	T41.3X4	T41.3X5	T41.3X6
regional	T41.3X1	T41.3X2	T41.3X3	T41.3X4	T41.3X5	T41.3X6
spinal	T41.3X1	T41.3X2	T41.3X3	T41.3X4	T41.3X5	T41.3X6
Ligroin (e) (solvent)	T52.0X1	T52.0X2	T52.0X3	T52.0X4	—	—
vapor	T59.891	T59.892	T59.893	T59.894	—	—
Ligustrum vulgare	T62.2X1	T62.2X2	T62.2X3	T62.2X4	—	—
Lily of the valley	T62.2X1	T62.2X2	T62.2X3	T62.2X4	—	—
Lime (chloride)	T54.3X1	T54.3X2	T54.3X3	T54.3X4	—	—
Limonene	T52.8X1	T52.8X2	T52.8X3	T52.8X4	—	—
Lincomycin	T36.8X1	T36.8X2	T36.8X3	T36.8X4	T36.8X5	T36.8X6
Lindane (insecticide) (nonmedicinal) (vapor)	T53.6X1	T53.6X2	T53.6X3	T53.6X4	—	—
medicinal	T49.0X1	T49.0X2	T49.0X3	T49.0X4	T49.0X5	T49.0X6
Liniments NEC	T49.91	T49.92	T49.93	T49.94	T49.95	T49.96
Linoleic acid	T46.6X1	T46.6X2	T46.6X3	T46.6X4	T46.6X5	T46.6X6
Linolenic acid	T46.6X1	T46.6X2	T46.6X3	T46.6X4	T46.6X5	T46.6X6
Linseed	T47.4X1	T47.4X2	T47.4X3	T47.4X4	T47.4X5	T47.4X6
Liothyronine	T38.1X1	T38.1X2	T38.1X3	T38.1X4	T38.1X5	T38.1X6
Liotrix	T38.1X1	T38.1X2	T38.1X3	T38.1X4	T38.1X5	T38.1X6
Lipancreatin	T47.5X1	T47.5X2	T47.5X3	T47.5X4	T47.5X5	T47.5X6
Lipo-alprostadil	T46.7X1	T46.7X2	T46.7X3	T46.7X4	T46.7X5	T46.7X6
Lipo-Lutin	T38.5X1	T38.5X2	T38.5X3	T38.5X4	T38.5X5	T38.5X6
Lipotropic drug NEC	T50.901	T50.902	T50.903	T50.904	T50.905	T50.906
Liquefied petroleum gases	T59.891	T59.892	T59.893	T59.894	—	—
piped (pure or mixed with air)	T59.891	T59.892	T59.893	T59.894	—	—
Liquid						
paraffin	T47.4X1	T47.4X2	T47.4X3	T47.4X4	T47.4X5	T47.4X6
petrolatum	T47.4X1	T47.4X2	T47.4X3	T47.4X4	T47.4X5	T47.4X6
topical	T49.3X1	T49.3X2	T49.3X3	T49.3X4	T49.3X5	T49.3X6
specified NEC	T65.891	T65.892	T65.893	T65.894	—	—
substance	T65.91	T65.92	T65.93	T65.94	—	—
Liquor creosolis compositus	T65.891	T65.892	T65.893	T65.894	—	—
Liquorice	T48.4X1	T48.4X2	T48.4X3	T48.4X4	T48.4X5	T48.4X6

Substance	Poisoning, Accidental (unintentional)	Poisoning, Intentional Self-harm	Poisoning, Assault	Poisoning, Undetermined	Adverse Effect	Under-dosing
Liquorice — *continued*						
extract	T47.8X1	T47.8X2	T47.8X3	T47.8X4	T47.8X5	T47.8X6
Liraglutide*	T38.3X1	T38.3X2	T38.3X3	T38.3X4	T38.3X5	T38.3X6
Lisinopril	T46.4X1	T46.4X2	T46.4X3	T46.4X4	T46.4X5	T46.4X6
Lisuride	T42.8X1	T42.8X2	T42.8X3	T42.8X4	T42.8X5	T42.8X6
Lithane	T43.8X1	T43.8X2	T43.8X3	T43.8X4	T43.8X5	T43.8X6
Lithium	T56.891	T56.892	T56.893	T56.894	—	—
gluconate	T43.591	T43.592	T43.593	T43.594	T43.595	T43.596
salts (carbonate)	T43.591	T43.592	T43.593	T43.594	T43.595	T43.596
Lithonate	T43.8X1	T43.8X2	T43.8X3	T43.8X4	T43.8X5	T43.8X6
Liver						
extract	T45.8X1	T45.8X2	T45.8X3	T45.8X4	T45.8X5	T45.8X6
for parenteral use	T45.8X1	T45.8X2	T45.8X3	T45.8X4	T45.8X5	T45.8X6
fraction 1	T45.8X1	T45.8X2	T45.8X3	T45.8X4	T45.8X5	T45.8X6
hydrolysate	T45.8X1	T45.8X2	T45.8X3	T45.8X4	T45.8X5	T45.8X6
Lizard (bite) (venom)	T63.121	T63.122	T63.123	T63.124	—	—
LMD	T45.8X1	T45.8X2	T45.8X3	T45.8X4	T45.8X5	T45.8X6
Lobelia	T62.2X1	T62.2X2	T62.2X3	T62.2X4	—	—
Lobeline	T5Ø.7X1	T5Ø.7X2	T5Ø.7X3	T5Ø.7X4	T5Ø.7X5	T5Ø.7X6
Local action drug NEC	T49.8X1	T49.8X2	T49.8X3	T49.8X4	T49.8X5	T49.8X6
Locorten	T49.ØX1	T49.ØX2	T49.ØX3	T49.ØX4	T49.ØX5	T49.ØX6
Lofepramine	T43.Ø11	T43.Ø12	T43.Ø13	T43.Ø14	T43.Ø15	T43.Ø16
Lolium temulentum	T62.2X1	T62.2X2	T62.2X3	T62.2X4	—	—
Lomotil	T47.6X1	T47.6X2	T47.6X3	T47.6X4	T47.6X5	T47.6X6
Lomustine	T45.1X1	T45.1X2	T45.1X3	T45.1X4	T45.1X5	T45.1X6
Lonidamine	T45.1X1	T45.1X2	T45.1X3	T45.1X4	T45.1X5	T45.1X6
LoOvral*	T38.4X1	T38.4X2	T38.4X3	T38.4X4	T38.4X5	T38.4X6
Loperamide	T47.6X1	T47.6X2	T47.6X3	T47.6X4	T47.6X5	T47.6X6
Loprazolam	T42.4X1	T42.4X2	T42.4X3	T42.4X4	T42.4X5	T42.4X6
Lorajmine	T46.2X1	T46.2X2	T46.2X3	T46.2X4	T46.2X5	T46.2X6
Loratidine	T45.ØX1	T45.ØX2	T45.ØX3	T45.ØX4	T45.ØX5	T45.ØX6
Lorazepam	T42.4X1	T42.4X2	T42.4X3	T42.4X4	T42.4X5	T42.4X6
Lorcainide	T46.2X1	T46.2X2	T46.2X3	T46.2X4	T46.2X5	T46.2X6
Lormetazepam	T42.4X1	T42.4X2	T42.4X3	T42.4X4	T42.4X5	T42.4X6
Lotions NEC	T49.91	T49.92	T49.93	T49.94	T49.95	T49.96
Lotrimin*	T49.ØX1	T49.ØX2	T49.ØX3	T49.ØX4	T49.ØX5	T49.ØX6
Lotusate	T42.3X1	T42.3X2	T42.3X3	T42.3X4	T42.3X5	T42.3X6
Lovastatin	T46.6X1	T46.6X2	T46.6X3	T46.6X4	T46.6X5	T46.6X6
Lowila	T49.2X1	T49.2X2	T49.2X3	T49.2X4	T49.2X5	T49.2X6
Loxapine	T43.591	T43.592	T43.593	T43.594	T43.595	T43.596
Lozenges (throat)	T49.6X1	T49.6X2	T49.6X3	T49.6X4	T49.6X5	T49.6X6
LSD	T4Ø.8X1	T4Ø.8X2	T4Ø.8X3	T4Ø.8X4	—	—
L-Tryptophan — *see* amino acid						
Lubricant, eye	T49.5X1	T49.5X2	T49.5X3	T49.5X4	T49.5X5	T49.5X6
Lubricating oil NEC	T52.ØX1	T52.ØX2	T52.ØX3	T52.ØX4	—	—
Lucanthone	T37.4X1	T37.4X2	T37.4X3	T37.4X4	T37.4X5	T37.4X6
Luminal	T42.3X1	T42.3X2	T42.3X3	T42.3X4	T42.3X5	T42.3X6
Lung irritant (gas) NEC	T59.91	T59.92	T59.93	T59.94		
Luteinizing hormone	T38.811	T38.812	T38.813	T38.814	T38.815	T38.816
Lutocylol	T38.5X1	T38.5X2	T38.5X3	T38.5X4	T38.5X5	T38.5X6
Lutromone	T38.5X1	T38.5X2	T38.5X3	T38.5X4	T38.5X5	T38.5X6
Lututrin	T48.291	T48.292	T48.293	T48.294	T48.295	T48.296
Luveris*	T38.891	T38.892	T38.893	T38.894	T38.895	T38.896
Lye (concentrated)	T54.3X1	T54.3X2	T54.3X3	T54.3X4	—	—
Lygranum (skin test)	T5Ø.8X1	T5Ø.8X2	T5Ø.8X3	T5Ø.8X4	T5Ø.8X5	T5Ø.8X6
Lymecycline	T36.4X1	T36.4X2	T36.4X3	T36.4X4	T36.4X5	T36.4X6
Lymphogranuloma venereum antigen	T5Ø.8X1	T5Ø.8X2	T5Ø.8X3	T5Ø.8X4	T5Ø.8X5	T5Ø.8X6
Lynestrenol	T38.4X1	T38.4X2	T38.4X3	T38.4X4	T38.4X5	T38.4X6
Lyovac Sodium Edecrin	T5Ø.1X1	T5Ø.1X2	T5Ø.1X3	T5Ø.1X4	T5Ø.1X5	T5Ø.1X6
Lypressin	T38.891	T38.892	T38.893	T38.894	T38.895	T38.896
Lysergic acid diethylamide	T4Ø.8X1	T4Ø.8X2	T4Ø.8X3	T4Ø.8X4	—	—
Lysergide	T4Ø.8X1	T4Ø.8X2	T4Ø.8X3	T4Ø.8X4	—	—
Lysine vasopressin	T38.891	T38.892	T38.893	T38.894	T38.895	T38.896
Lysol	T54.1X1	T54.1X2	T54.1X3	T54.1X4	—	—
Lysozyme	T49.ØX1	T49.ØX2	T49.ØX3	T49.ØX4	T49.ØX5	T49.ØX6
Lytta (vitatta)	T49.8X1	T49.8X2	T49.8X3	T49.8X4	T49.8X5	T49.8X6
Mace	T59.3X1	T59.3X2	T59.3X3	T59.3X4	—	—
Macrogol	T5Ø.991	T5Ø.992	T5Ø.993	T5Ø.994	T5Ø.995	T5Ø.996
Macrolide						
anabolic drug	T38.7X1	T38.7X2	T38.7X3	T38.7X4	T38.7X5	T38.7X6
antibiotic	T36.3X1	T36.3X2	T36.3X3	T36.3X4	T36.3X5	T36.3X6
Mafenide	T49.ØX1	T49.ØX2	T49.ØX3	T49.ØX4	T49.ØX5	T49.ØX6
Magaldrate	T47.1X1	T47.1X2	T47.1X3	T47.1X4	T47.1X5	T47.1X6
Magic mushroom	T4Ø.991	T4Ø.992	T4Ø.993	T4Ø.994	—	—
Magnamycin	T36.8X1	T36.8X2	T36.8X3	T36.8X4	T36.8X5	T36.8X6
Magnesia magma	T47.1X1	T47.1X2	T47.1X3	T47.1X4	T47.1X5	T47.1X6
Magnesium NEC	T56.891	T56.892	T56.893	T56.894	—	—
carbonate	T47.1X1	T47.1X2	T47.1X3	T47.1X4	T47.1X5	T47.1X6
citrate	T47.4X1	T47.4X2	T47.4X3	T47.4X4	T47.4X5	T47.4X6
hydroxide	T47.1X1	T47.1X2	T47.1X3	T47.1X4	T47.1X5	T47.1X6
oxide	T47.1X1	T47.1X2	T47.1X3	T47.1X4	T47.1X5	T47.1X6
peroxide	T49.ØX1	T49.ØX2	T49.ØX3	T49.ØX4	T49.ØX5	T49.ØX6
Magnesium — *continued*						
salicylate	T39.Ø91	T39.Ø92	T39.Ø93	T39.Ø94	T39.Ø95	T39.Ø96
silicofluoride	T5Ø.3X1	T5Ø.3X2	T5Ø.3X3	T5Ø.3X4	T5Ø.3X5	T5Ø.3X6
sulfate	T47.4X1	T47.4X2	T47.4X3	T47.4X4	T47.4X5	T47.4X6
thiosulfate	T45.ØX1	T45.ØX2	T45.ØX3	T45.ØX4	T45.ØX5	T45.ØX6
trisilicate	T47.1X1	T47.1X2	T47.1X3	T47.1X4	T47.1X5	T47.1X6
Malathion (medicinal)	T49.ØX1	T49.ØX2	T49.ØX3	T49.ØX4	T49.ØX5	T49.ØX6
insecticide	T6Ø.ØX1	T6Ø.ØX2	T6Ø.ØX3	T6Ø.ØX4	—	—
Male fern extract	T37.4X1	T37.4X2	T37.4X3	T37.4X4	T37.4X5	T37.4X6
M-AMSA	T45.1X1	T45.1X2	T45.1X3	T45.1X4	T45.1X5	T45.1X6
Mandelic acid	T37.8X1	T37.8X2	T37.8X3	T37.8X4	T37.8X5	T37.8X6
Manganese (dioxide) (salts)	T57.2X1	T57.2X2	T57.2X3	T57.2X4	—	—
medicinal	T5Ø.991	T5Ø.992	T5Ø.993	T5Ø.994	T5Ø.995	T5Ø.996
Mannitol	T47.3X1	T47.3X2	T47.3X3	T47.3X4	T47.3X5	T47.3X6
hexanitrate	T46.3X1	T46.3X2	T46.3X3	T46.3X4	T46.3X5	T46.3X6
Mannomustine	T45.1X1	T45.1X2	T45.1X3	T45.1X4	T45.1X5	T45.1X6
MAO inhibitors	T43.1X1	T43.1X2	T43.1X3	T43.1X4	T43.1X5	T43.1X6
Mapharsen	T37.8X1	T37.8X2	T37.8X3	T37.8X4	T37.8X5	T37.8X6
Maphenide	T49.ØX1	T49.ØX2	T49.ØX3	T49.ØX4	T49.ØX5	T49.ØX6
Maprotiline	T43.Ø21	T43.Ø22	T43.Ø23	T43.Ø24	T43.Ø25	T43.Ø26
Marcaine	T41.3X1	T41.3X2	T41.3X3	T41.3X4	T41.3X5	T41.3X6
infiltration (subcutaneous)	T41.3X1	T41.3X2	T41.3X3	T41.3X4	T41.3X5	T41.3X6
nerve block (peripheral) (plexus)	T41.3X1	T41.3X2	T41.3X3	T41.3X4	T41.3X5	T41.3X6
Marezine	T45.ØX1	T45.ØX2	T45.ØX3	T45.ØX4	T45.ØX5	T45.ØX6
Marihuana	T4Ø.711	T4Ø.712	T4Ø.713	T4Ø.714	T4Ø.715	T4Ø.716
Marijuana	T4Ø.711	T4Ø.712	T4Ø.713	T4Ø.714	T4Ø.715	T4Ø.716
Marine (sting)	T63.691	T63.692	T63.693	T63.694	—	—
animals (sting)	T63.691	T63.692	T63.693	T63.694	—	—
plants (sting)	T63.711	T63.712	T63.713	T63.714	—	—
Marplan	T43.1X1	T43.1X2	T43.1X3	T43.1X4	T43.1X5	T43.1X6
Marsh gas	T59.891	T59.892	T59.893	T59.894	—	—
Marsilid	T43.1X1	T43.1X2	T43.1X3	T43.1X4	T43.1X5	T43.1X6
Massengill*	T49.ØX1	T49.ØX2	T49.ØX3	T49.ØX4	T49.ØX5	T49.ØX6
Matulane	T45.1X1	T45.1X2	T45.1X3	T45.1X4	T45.1X5	T45.1X6
Mazindol	T5Ø.5X1	T5Ø.5X2	T5Ø.5X3	T5Ø.5X4	T5Ø.5X5	T5Ø.5X6
MCPA	T6Ø.3X1	T6Ø.3X2	T6Ø.3X3	T6Ø.3X4	—	—
MDMA	T43.641	T43.642	T43.643	T43.644	—	—
Meadow saffron	T62.2X1	T62.2X2	T62.2X3	T62.2X4	—	—
Measles virus vaccine (attenuated)	T5Ø.B91	T5Ø.B92	T5Ø.B93	T5Ø.B94	T5Ø.B95	T5Ø.B96
Meat, noxious	T62.8X1	T62.8X2	T62.8X3	T62.8X4	—	—
Meballymal	T42.3X1	T42.3X2	T42.3X3	T42.3X4	T42.3X5	T42.3X6
Mebanazine	T43.1X1	T43.1X2	T43.1X3	T43.1X4	T43.1X5	T43.1X6
Mebaral	T42.3X1	T42.3X2	T42.3X3	T42.3X4	T42.3X5	T42.3X6
Mebendazole	T37.4X1	T37.4X2	T37.4X3	T37.4X4	T37.4X5	T37.4X6
Mebeverine	T44.3X1	T44.3X2	T44.3X3	T44.3X4	T44.3X5	T44.3X6
Mebhydrolin	T45.ØX1	T45.ØX2	T45.ØX3	T45.ØX4	T45.ØX5	T45.ØX6
Mebumal	T42.3X1	T42.3X2	T42.3X3	T42.3X4	T42.3X5	T42.3X6
Mebutamate	T43.591	T43.592	T43.593	T43.594	T43.595	T43.596
Mecamylamine	T44.2X1	T44.2X2	T44.2X3	T44.2X4	T44.2X5	T44.2X6
Mechlorethamine	T45.1X1	T45.1X2	T45.1X3	T45.1X4	T45.1X5	T45.1X6
Mecillinam	T36.ØX1	T36.ØX2	T36.ØX3	T36.ØX4	T36.ØX5	T36.ØX6
Meclizine (hydrochloride)	T45.ØX1	T45.ØX2	T45.ØX3	T45.ØX4	T45.ØX5	T45.ØX6
Meclocycline	T36.4X1	T36.4X2	T36.4X3	T36.4X4	T36.4X5	T36.4X6
Meclofenamate	T39.391	T39.392	T39.393	T39.394	T39.395	T39.396
Meclofenamic acid	T39.391	T39.392	T39.393	T39.394	T39.395	T39.396
Meclofenoxate	T43.691	T43.692	T43.693	T43.694	T43.695	T43.696
Meclozine	T45.ØX1	T45.ØX2	T45.ØX3	T45.ØX4	T45.ØX5	T45.ØX6
Mecobalamin	T45.8X1	T45.8X2	T45.8X3	T45.8X4	T45.8X5	T45.8X6
Mecoprop	T6Ø.3X1	T6Ø.3X2	T6Ø.3X3	T6Ø.3X4	—	—
Mecrilate	T49.3X1	T49.3X2	T49.3X3	T49.3X4	T49.3X5	T49.3X6
Mecysteine	T48.4X1	T48.4X2	T48.4X3	T48.4X4	T48.4X5	T48.4X6
Medazepam	T42.4X1	T42.4X2	T42.4X3	T42.4X4	T42.4X5	T42.4X6
Medicament NEC	T5Ø.9Ø1	T5Ø.9Ø2	T5Ø.9Ø3	T5Ø.9Ø4	T5Ø.9Ø5	T5Ø.9Ø6
Medinal	T42.3X1	T42.3X2	T42.3X3	T42.3X4	T42.3X5	T42.3X6
Medomin	T42.3X1	T42.3X2	T42.3X3	T42.3X4	T42.3X5	T42.3X6
Medrogestone	T38.5X1	T38.5X2	T38.5X3	T38.5X4	T38.5X5	T38.5X6
Medroxalol	T44.8X1	T44.8X2	T44.8X3	T44.8X4	T44.8X5	T44.8X6
Medroxyprogesterone acetate (depot)	T38.5X1	T38.5X2	T38.5X3	T38.5X4	T38.5X5	T38.5X6
Medrysone	T49.ØX1	T49.ØX2	T49.ØX3	T49.ØX4	T49.ØX5	T49.ØX6
Mefenamic acid	T39.391	T39.392	T39.393	T39.394	T39.395	T39.396
Mefenorex	T5Ø.5X1	T5Ø.5X2	T5Ø.5X3	T5Ø.5X4	T5Ø.5X5	T5Ø.5X6
Mefloquine	T37.2X1	T37.2X2	T37.2X3	T37.2X4	T37.2X5	T37.2X6
Mefoxin*	T36.1X1	T36.1X2	T36.1X3	T36.1X4	T36.1X5	T36.1X6
Mefruside	T5Ø.2X1	T5Ø.2X2	T5Ø.2X3	T5Ø.2X4	T5Ø.2X5	T5Ø.2X6
Megahallucinogen	T4Ø.9Ø1	T4Ø.9Ø2	T4Ø.9Ø3	T4Ø.9Ø4	T4Ø.9Ø5	T4Ø.9Ø6
Megestrol	T38.5X1	T38.5X2	T38.5X3	T38.5X4	T38.5X5	T38.5X6
Meglumine						
antimoniate	T37.8X1	T37.8X2	T37.8X3	T37.8X4	T37.8X5	T37.8X6
diatrizoate	T5Ø.8X1	T5Ø.8X2	T5Ø.8X3	T5Ø.8X4	T5Ø.8X5	T5Ø.8X6
iodipamide	T5Ø.8X1	T5Ø.8X2	T5Ø.8X3	T5Ø.8X4	T5Ø.8X5	T5Ø.8X6

Substance	Poisoning, Accidental (unintentional)	Poisoning, Intentional Self-harm	Poisoning, Assault	Poisoning, Undetermined	Adverse Effect	Under-dosing
Meglumine — *continued*						
iotroxate	T5Ø.8X1	T5Ø.8X2	T5Ø.8X3	T5Ø.8X4	T5Ø.8X5	T5Ø.8X6
MEK (methyl ethyl ketone)	T52.4X1	T52.4X2	T52.4X3	T52.4X4	—	—
Meladinin	T49.3X1	T49.3X2	T49.3X3	T49.3X4	T49.3X5	T49.3X6
Meladrazine	T44.3X1	T44.3X2	T44.3X3	T44.3X4	T44.3X5	T44.3X6
Melaleuca alternifolia oil	T49.ØX1	T49.ØX2	T49.ØX3	T49.ØX4	T49.ØX5	T49.ØX6
Melanizing agents	T49.3X1	T49.3X2	T49.3X3	T49.3X4	T49.3X5	T49.3X6
Melanocyte-stimulating hormone	T38.891	T38.892	T38.893	T38.894	T38.895	T38.896
Melarsonyl potassium	T37.3X1	T37.3X2	T37.3X3	T37.3X4	T37.3X5	T37.3X6
Melarsoprol	T37.3X1	T37.3X2	T37.3X3	T37.3X4	T37.3X5	T37.3X6
Melia azedarach	T62.2X1	T62.2X2	T62.2X3	T62.2X4	—	—
Melitracen	T43.Ø11	T43.Ø12	T43.Ø13	T43.Ø14	T43.Ø15	T43.Ø16
Mellaril	T43.3X1	T43.3X2	T43.3X3	T43.3X4	T43.3X5	T43.3X6
Meloxicam*	T39.391	T39.392	T39.393	T39.394	T39.395	T39.396
Meloxine	T49.3X1	T49.3X2	T49.3X3	T49.3X4	T49.3X5	T49.3X6
Melperone	T43.4X1	T43.4X2	T43.4X3	T43.4X4	T43.4X5	T43.4X6
Melphalan	T45.1X1	T45.1X2	T45.1X3	T45.1X4	T45.1X5	T45.1X6
Memantine	T43.8X1	T43.8X2	T43.8X3	T43.8X4	T43.8X5	T43.8X6
Menadiol	T45.7X1	T45.7X2	T45.7X3	T45.7X4	T45.7X5	T45.7X6
sodium sulfate	T45.7X1	T45.7X2	T45.7X3	T45.7X4	T45.7X5	T45.7X6
Menadione	T45.7X1	T45.7X2	T45.7X3	T45.7X4	T45.7X5	T45.7X6
sodium bisulfite	T45.7X1	T45.7X2	T45.7X3	T45.7X4	T45.7X5	T45.7X6
Menaphthone	T45.7X1	T45.7X2	T45.7X3	T45.7X4	T45.7X5	T45.7X6
Menaquinone	T45.7X1	T45.7X2	T45.7X3	T45.7X4	T45.7X5	T45.7X6
Menatetrenone	T45.7X1	T45.7X2	T45.7X3	T45.7X4	T45.7X5	T45.7X6
Meningococcal vaccine	T5Ø.A91	T5Ø.A92	T5Ø.A93	T5Ø.A94	T5Ø.A95	T5Ø.A96
Menningovax (-AC) (-C)	T5Ø.A91	T5Ø.A92	T5Ø.A93	T5Ø.A94	T5Ø.A95	T5Ø.A96
Menotropins	T38.811	T38.812	T38.813	T38.814	T38.815	T38.816
Menthol	T48.5X1	T48.5X2	T48.5X3	T48.5X4	T48.5X5	T48.5X6
Mepacrine	T37.2X1	T37.2X2	T37.2X3	T37.2X4	T37.2X5	T37.2X6
Meparfynol	T42.6X1	T42.6X2	T42.6X3	T42.6X4	T42.6X5	T42.6X6
Mepartricin	T36.7X1	T36.7X2	T36.7X3	T36.7X4	T36.7X5	T36.7X6
Mepazine	T43.3X1	T43.3X2	T43.3X3	T43.3X4	T43.3X5	T43.3X6
Mepenzolate	T44.3X1	T44.3X2	T44.3X3	T44.3X4	T44.3X5	T44.3X6
bromide	T44.3X1	T44.3X2	T44.3X3	T44.3X4	T44.3X5	T44.3X6
Meperidine	T4Ø.491	T4Ø.492	T4Ø.493	T4Ø.494	T4Ø.495	T4Ø.496
Mephebarbital	T42.3X1	T42.3X2	T42.3X3	T42.3X4	T42.3X5	T42.3X6
Mephenamin (e)	T42.8X1	T42.8X2	T42.8X3	T42.8X4	T42.8X5	T42.8X6
Mephenesin	T42.8X1	T42.8X2	T42.8X3	T42.8X4	T42.8X5	T42.8X6
Mephenhydramine	T45.ØX1	T45.ØX2	T45.ØX3	T45.ØX4	T45.ØX5	T45.ØX6
Mephenoxalone	T42.8X1	T42.8X2	T42.8X3	T42.8X4	T42.8X5	T42.8X6
Mephentermine	T44.991	T44.992	T44.993	T44.994	T44.995	T44.996
Mephenytoin	T42.ØX1	T42.ØX2	T42.ØX3	T42.ØX4	T42.ØX5	T42.ØX6
with phenobarbital	T42.3X1	T42.3X2	T42.3X3	T42.3X4	T42.3X5	T42.3X6
Mephobarbital	T42.3X1	T42.3X2	T42.3X3	T42.3X4	T42.3X5	T42.3X6
Mephosfolan	T6Ø.ØX1	T6Ø.ØX2	T6Ø.ØX3	T6Ø.ØX4	—	—
Mepindolol	T44.7X1	T44.7X2	T44.7X3	T44.7X4	T44.7X5	T44.7X6
Mepiperphenidol	T44.3X1	T44.3X2	T44.3X3	T44.3X4	T44.3X5	T44.3X6
Mepitiostane	T38.7X1	T38.7X2	T38.7X3	T38.7X4	T38.7X5	T38.7X6
Mepivacaine	T41.3X1	T41.3X2	T41.3X3	T41.3X4	T41.3X5	T41.3X6
epidural	T41.3X1	T41.3X2	T41.3X3	T41.3X4	T41.3X5	T41.3X6
Meprednisone	T38.ØX1	T38.ØX2	T38.ØX3	T38.ØX4	T38.ØX5	T38.ØX6
Meprobam	T43.591	T43.592	T43.593	T43.594	T43.595	T43.596
Meprobamate	T43.591	T43.592	T43.593	T43.594	T43.595	T43.596
Meproscillarin	T46.ØX1	T46.ØX2	T46.ØX3	T46.ØX4	T46.ØX5	T46.ØX6
Meprylcaine	T41.3X1	T41.3X2	T41.3X3	T41.3X4	T41.3X5	T41.3X6
Meptazinol	T39.8X1	T39.8X2	T39.8X3	T39.8X4	T39.8X5	T39.8X6
Mepyramine	T45.ØX1	T45.ØX2	T45.ØX3	T45.ØX4	T45.ØX5	T45.ØX6
Mequinol*	T49.8X1	T49.8X2	T49.8X3	T49.8X4	T49.8X5	T49.8X6
Mequitazine	T43.3X1	T43.3X2	T43.3X3	T43.3X4	T43.3X5	T43.3X6
Meralluride	T5Ø.2X1	T5Ø.2X2	T5Ø.2X3	T5Ø.2X4	T5Ø.2X5	T5Ø.2X6
Merbaphen	T5Ø.2X1	T5Ø.2X2	T5Ø.2X3	T5Ø.2X4	T5Ø.2X5	T5Ø.2X6
Merbromin	T49.ØX1	T49.ØX2	T49.ØX3	T49.ØX4	T49.ØX5	T49.ØX6
Mercaptobenzothiazole salts	T49.ØX1	T49.ØX2	T49.ØX3	T49.ØX4	T49.ØX5	T49.ØX6
Mercaptomerin	T5Ø.2X1	T5Ø.2X2	T5Ø.2X3	T5Ø.2X4	T5Ø.2X5	T5Ø.2X6
Mercaptopurine	T45.1X1	T45.1X2	T45.1X3	T45.1X4	T45.1X5	T45.1X6
Mercumatilin	T5Ø.2X1	T5Ø.2X2	T5Ø.2X3	T5Ø.2X4	T5Ø.2X5	T5Ø.2X6
Mercuramide	T5Ø.2X1	T5Ø.2X2	T5Ø.2X3	T5Ø.2X4	T5Ø.2X5	T5Ø.2X6
Mercurochrome	T49.ØX1	T49.ØX2	T49.ØX3	T49.ØX4	T49.ØX5	T49.ØX6
Mercurophylline	T5Ø.2X1	T5Ø.2X2	T5Ø.2X3	T5Ø.2X4	T5Ø.2X5	T5Ø.2X6
Mercury, mercurial, mercuric, mercurous (compounds) (cyanide) (fumes) (nonmedicinal) (vapor) **NEC**	T56.1X1	T56.1X2	T56.1X3	T56.1X4	—	—
ammoniated	T49.ØX1	T49.ØX2	T49.ØX3	T49.ØX4	T49.ØX5	T49.ØX6
anti-infective						
local	T49.ØX1	T49.ØX2	T49.ØX3	T49.ØX4	T49.ØX5	T49.ØX6
systemic	T37.8X1	T37.8X2	T37.8X3	T37.8X4	T37.8X5	T37.8X6
topical	T49.ØX1	T49.ØX2	T49.ØX3	T49.ØX4	T49.ØX5	T49.ØX6
chloride (ammoniated)	T49.ØX1	T49.ØX2	T49.ØX3	T49.ØX4	T49.ØX5	T49.ØX6

Substance	Poisoning, Accidental (unintentional)	Poisoning, Intentional Self-harm	Poisoning, Assault	Poisoning, Undetermined	Adverse Effect	Under-dosing
Mercury, mercurial, mercuric, mercurous (compounds) (cyanide) (fumes) (nonmedicinal) (vapor) **NEC** — *continued*						
chloride — *continued*						
fungicide	T56.1X1	T56.1X2	T56.1X3	T56.1X4		
diuretic NEC	T5Ø.2X1	T5Ø.2X2	T5Ø.2X3	T5Ø.2X4	T5Ø.2X5	T5Ø.2X6
fungicide	T56.1X1	T56.1X2	T56.1X3	T56.1X4	—	—
organic (fungicide)	T56.1X1	T56.1X2	T56.1X3	T56.1X4	—	—
oxide, yellow	T49.ØX1	T49.ØX2	T49.ØX3	T49.ØX4	T49.ØX5	T49.ØX6
Mersalyl	T5Ø.2X1	T5Ø.2X2	T5Ø.2X3	T5Ø.2X4	T5Ø.2X5	T5Ø.2X6
Merthiolate	T49.ØX1	T49.ØX2	T49.ØX3	T49.ØX4	T49.ØX5	T49.ØX6
ophthalmic preparation	T49.5X1	T49.5X2	T49.5X3	T49.5X4	T49.5X5	T49.5X6
Meruvax	T5Ø.B91	T5Ø.B92	T5Ø.B93	T5Ø.B94	T5Ø.B95	T5Ø.B96
Mesalazine	T47.8X1	T47.8X2	T47.8X3	T47.8X4	T47.8X5	T47.8X6
Mescal buttons	T4Ø.991	T4Ø.992	T4Ø.993	T4Ø.994	—	—
Mescaline	T4Ø.991	T4Ø.992	T4Ø.993	T4Ø.994	—	—
Mesna	T48.4X1	T48.4X2	T48.4X3	T48.4X4	T48.4X5	T48.4X6
Mesoglycan	T46.6X1	T46.6X2	T46.6X3	T46.6X4	T46.6X5	T46.6X6
Mesoridazine	T43.3X1	T43.3X2	T43.3X3	T43.3X4	T43.3X5	T43.3X6
Mestanolone	T38.7X1	T38.7X2	T38.7X3	T38.7X4	T38.7X5	T38.7X6
Mesterolone	T38.7X1	T38.7X2	T38.7X3	T38.7X4	T38.7X5	T38.7X6
Mestranol	T38.5X1	T38.5X2	T38.5X3	T38.5X4	T38.5X5	T38.5X6
Mesulergine	T42.8X1	T42.8X2	T42.8X3	T42.8X4	T42.8X5	T42.8X6
Mesulfen	T49.ØX1	T49.ØX2	T49.ØX3	T49.ØX4	T49.ØX5	T49.ØX6
Mesuximide	T42.2X1	T42.2X2	T42.2X3	T42.2X4	T42.2X5	T42.2X6
Metabutethamine	T41.3X1	T41.3X2	T41.3X3	T41.3X4	T41.3X5	T41.3X6
Metactesylacetate	T49.ØX1	T49.ØX2	T49.ØX3	T49.ØX4	T49.ØX5	T49.ØX6
Metacycline	T36.4X1	T36.4X2	T36.4X3	T36.4X4	T36.4X5	T36.4X6
Metaldehyde (snail killer) **NEC**	T6Ø.8X1	T6Ø.8X2	T6Ø.8X3	T6Ø.8X4	—	—
Metals (heavy) (nonmedicinal)	T56.91	T56.92	T56.93	T56.94	—	—
dust, fumes, or vapor NEC	T56.91	T56.92	T56.93	T56.94	—	—
light NEC	T56.91	T56.92	T56.93	T56.94	—	—
dust, fumes, or vapor NEC	T56.91	T56.92	T56.93	T56.94	—	—
specified NEC	T56.891	T56.892	T56.893	T56.894	—	—
thallium	T56.811	T56.812	T56.813	T56.814	—	—
Metamfetamine	T43.651	T43.652	T43.652	T43.654	T43.655	T43.656
Metamizole sodium	T39.2X1	T39.2X2	T39.2X3	T39.2X4	T39.2X5	T39.2X6
Metampicillin	T36.ØX1	T36.ØX2	T36.ØX3	T36.ØX4	T36.ØX5	T36.ØX6
Metamucil	T47.4X1	T47.4X2	T47.4X3	T47.4X4	T47.4X5	T47.4X6
Metandienone	T38.7X1	T38.7X2	T38.7X3	T38.7X4	T38.7X5	T38.7X6
Metandrostenolone	T38.7X1	T38.7X2	T38.7X3	T38.7X4	T38.7X5	T38.7X6
Metaphen	T49.ØX1	T49.ØX2	T49.ØX3	T49.ØX4	T49.ØX5	T49.ØX6
Metaphos	T6Ø.ØX1	T6Ø.ØX2	T6Ø.ØX3	T6Ø.ØX4	—	—
Metapramine	T43.Ø11	T43.Ø12	T43.Ø13	T43.Ø14	T43.Ø15	T43.Ø16
Metaproterenol	T48.291	T48.292	T48.293	T48.294	T48.295	T48.296
Metaraminol	T44.4X1	T44.4X2	T44.4X3	T44.4X4	T44.4X5	T44.4X6
Metaxalone	T42.8X1	T42.8X2	T42.8X3	T42.8X4	T42.8X5	T42.8X6
Meted*	T49.4X1	T49.4X2	T49.4X3	T49.4X4	T49.4X5	T49.4X6
Metenolone	T38.7X1	T38.7X2	T38.7X3	T38.7X4	T38.7X5	T38.7X6
Metergoline	T42.8X1	T42.8X2	T42.8X3	T42.8X4	T42.8X5	T42.8X6
Metescufylline	T46.991	T46.992	T46.993	T46.994	T46.995	T46.996
Metetoin	T42.ØX1	T42.ØX2	T42.ØX3	T42.ØX4	T42.ØX5	T42.ØX6
Metformin	T38.3X1	T38.3X2	T38.3X3	T38.3X4	T38.3X5	T38.3X6
Methacholine	T44.1X1	T44.1X2	T44.1X3	T44.1X4	T44.1X5	T44.1X6
Methacycline	T36.4X1	T36.4X2	T36.4X3	T36.4X4	T36.4X5	T36.4X6
Methadone	T4Ø.3X1	T4Ø.3X2	T4Ø.3X3	T4Ø.3X4	T4Ø.3X5	T4Ø.3X6
Methadose*	T4Ø.3X1	T4Ø.3X2	T4Ø.3X3	T4Ø.3X4	T4Ø.3X5	T4Ø.3X6
Methallenestril	T38.5X1	T38.5X2	T38.5X3	T38.5X4	T38.5X5	T38.5X6
Methallenoestril	T38.5X1	T38.5X2	T38.5X3	T38.5X4	T38.5X5	T38.5X6
Methamphetamine	T43.651	T43.652	T43.652	T43.654	T43.655	T43.656
Methampyrone	T39.2X1	T39.2X2	T39.2X3	T39.2X4	T39.2X5	T39.2X6
Methandienone	T38.7X1	T38.7X2	T38.7X3	T38.7X4	T38.7X5	T38.7X6
Methandriol	T38.7X1	T38.7X2	T38.7X3	T38.7X4	T38.7X5	T38.7X6
Methandrostenolone	T38.7X1	T38.7X2	T38.7X3	T38.7X4	T38.7X5	T38.7X6
Methane	T59.891	T59.892	T59.893	T59.894	—	—
Methanethiol	T59.891	T59.892	T59.893	T59.894	—	—
Methaniazide	T37.1X1	T37.1X2	T37.1X3	T37.1X4	T37.1X5	T37.1X6
Methanol (vapor)	T51.1X1	T51.1X2	T51.1X3	T51.1X4	—	—
Methantheline	T44.3X1	T44.3X2	T44.3X3	T44.3X4	T44.3X5	T44.3X6
Methanthelinium bromide	T44.3X1	T44.3X2	T44.3X3	T44.3X4	T44.3X5	T44.3X6
Methaphenilene	T45.ØX1	T45.ØX2	T45.ØX3	T45.ØX4	T45.ØX5	T45.ØX6
Methapyrilene	T45.ØX1	T45.ØX2	T45.ØX3	T45.ØX4	T45.ØX5	T45.ØX6
Methaqualone (compound)	T42.6X1	T42.6X2	T42.6X3	T42.6X4	T42.6X5	T42.6X6
Metharbital	T42.3X1	T42.3X2	T42.3X3	T42.3X4	T42.3X5	T42.3X6
Methazolamide	T5Ø.2X1	T5Ø.2X2	T5Ø.2X3	T5Ø.2X4	T5Ø.2X5	T5Ø.2X6
Methdilazine	T43.3X1	T43.3X2	T43.3X3	T43.3X4	T43.3X5	T43.3X6
Methedrine	T43.651	T43.652	T43.653	T43.654	T43.655	T43.656
Methenamine (mandelate)	T37.8X1	T37.8X2	T37.8X3	T37.8X4	T37.8X5	T37.8X6
Methenolone	T38.7X1	T38.7X2	T38.7X3	T38.7X4	T38.7X5	T38.7X6

Substance	Poisoning, Accidental (unintentional)	Poisoning, Intentional Self-harm	Poisoning, Assault	Poisoning, Undetermined	Adverse Effect	Under-dosing
Methergine	T48.ØX1	T48.ØX2	T48.ØX3	T48.ØX4	T48.ØX5	T48.ØX6
Methetoin	T42.ØX1	T42.ØX2	T42.ØX3	T42.ØX4	T42.ØX5	T42.ØX6
Methiacil	T38.2X1	T38.2X2	T38.2X3	T38.2X4	T38.2X5	T38.2X6
Methicillin	T36.ØX1	T36.ØX2	T36.ØX3	T36.ØX4	T36.ØX5	T36.ØX6
Methimazole	T38.2X1	T38.2X2	T38.2X3	T38.2X4	T38.2X5	T38.2X6
Methiodal sodium	T5Ø.8X1	T5Ø.8X2	T5Ø.8X3	T5Ø.8X4	T5Ø.8X5	T5Ø.8X6
Methionine	T5Ø.991	T5Ø.992	T5Ø.993	T5Ø.994	T5Ø.995	T5Ø.996
Methisazone	T37.5X1	T37.5X2	T37.5X3	T37.5X4	T37.5X5	T37.5X6
Methisoprinol	T37.5X1	T37.5X2	T37.5X3	T37.5X4	T37.5X5	T37.5X6
Methitural	T42.3X1	T42.3X2	T42.3X3	T42.3X4	T42.3X5	T42.3X6
Methixene	T44.3X1	T44.3X2	T44.3X3	T44.3X4	T44.3X5	T44.3X6
Methobarbital, methobarbitone	T42.3X1	T42.3X2	T42.3X3	T42.3X4	T42.3X5	T42.3X6
Methocarbamol	T42.8X1	T42.8X2	T42.8X3	T42.8X4	T42.8X5	T42.8X6
skeletal muscle relaxant	T48.1X1	T48.1X2	T48.1X3	T48.1X4	T48.1X5	T48.1X6
Methohexital	T41.1X1	T41.1X2	T41.1X3	T41.1X4	T41.1X5	T41.1X6
Methohexitone	T41.1X1	T41.1X2	T41.1X3	T41.1X4	T41.1X5	T41.1X6
Methoin	T42.ØX1	T42.ØX2	T42.ØX3	T42.ØX4	T42.ØX5	T42.ØX6
Methopholine	T39.8X1	T39.8X2	T39.8X3	T39.8X4	T39.8X5	T39.8X6
Methopromazine	T43.3X1	T43.3X2	T43.3X3	T43.3X4	T43.3X5	T43.3X6
Methorate	T48.3X1	T48.3X2	T48.3X3	T48.3X4	T48.3X5	T48.3X6
Methoserpidine	T46.5X1	T46.5X2	T46.5X3	T46.5X4	T46.5X5	T46.5X6
Methotrexate	T45.1X1	T45.1X2	T45.1X3	T45.1X4	T45.1X5	T45.1X6
Methotrimeprazine	T43.3X1	T43.3X2	T43.3X3	T43.3X4	T43.3X5	T43.3X6
Methoxa-Dome	T49.3X1	T49.3X2	T49.3X3	T49.3X4	T49.3X5	T49.3X6
Methoxamine	T44.4X1	T44.4X2	T44.4X3	T44.4X4	T44.4X5	T44.4X6
Methoxsalen	T5Ø.991	T5Ø.992	T5Ø.993	T5Ø.994	T5Ø.995	T5Ø.996
Methoxyaniline	T65.3X1	T65.3X2	T65.3X3	T65.3X4	—	—
Methoxybenzyl penicillin	T36.ØX1	T36.ØX2	T36.ØX3	T36.ØX4	T36.ØX5	T36.ØX6
Methoxychlor	T53.7X1	T53.7X2	T53.7X3	T53.7X4	—	—
Methoxy-DDT	T53.7X1	T53.7X2	T53.7X3	T53.7X4	—	—
Methoxyflurane	T41.ØX1	T41.ØX2	T41.ØX3	T41.ØX4	T41.ØX5	T41.ØX6
Methoxyphenamine	T48.6X1	T48.6X2	T48.6X3	T48.6X4	T48.6X5	T48.6X6
Methoxypromazine	T43.3X1	T43.3X2	T43.3X3	T43.3X4	T43.3X5	T43.3X6
Methscopolamine bromide	T44.3X1	T44.3X2	T44.3X3	T44.3X4	T44.3X5	T44.3X6
Methsuximide	T42.2X1	T42.2X2	T42.2X3	T42.2X4	T42.2X5	T42.2X6
Methyclothiazide	T5Ø.2X1	T5Ø.2X2	T5Ø.2X3	T5Ø.2X4	T5Ø.2X5	T5Ø.2X6
Methyl						
acetate	T52.4X1	T52.4X2	T52.4X3	T52.4X4	—	—
acetone	T52.4X1	T52.4X2	T52.4X3	T52.4X4	—	—
acrylate	T65.891	T65.892	T65.893	T65.894	—	—
alcohol	T51.1X1	T51.1X2	T51.1X3	T51.1X4	—	—
aminophenol	T65.3X1	T65.3X2	T65.3X3	T65.3X4	—	—
amphetamine	T43.651	T43.652	T43.652	T43.654	T43.655	T43.656
androstanolone	T38.7X1	T38.7X2	T38.7X3	T38.7X4	T38.7X5	T38.7X6
atropine	T44.3X1	T44.3X2	T44.3X3	T44.3X4	T44.3X5	T44.3X6
benzene	T52.2X1	T52.2X2	T52.2X3	T52.2X4	—	—
benzoate	T52.8X1	T52.8X2	T52.8X3	T52.8X4	—	—
benzol	T52.2X1	T52.2X2	T52.2X3	T52.2X4	—	—
bromide (gas)	T59.891	T59.892	T59.893	T59.894	—	—
fumigant	T6Ø.8X1	T6Ø.8X2	T6Ø.8X3	T6Ø.8X4	—	—
butanol	T51.3X1	T51.3X2	T51.3X3	T51.3X4	—	—
carbinol	T51.1X1	T51.1X2	T51.1X3	T51.1X4	—	—
carbonate	T52.8X1	T52.8X2	T52.8X3	T52.8X4	—	—
CCNU	T45.1X1	T45.1X2	T45.1X3	T45.1X4	T45.1X5	T45.1X6
cellosolve	T52.91	T52.92	T52.93	T52.94	—	—
cellulose	T47.4X1	T47.4X2	T47.4X3	T47.4X4	T47.4X5	T47.4X6
chloride (gas)	T59.891	T59.892	T59.893	T59.894	—	—
chloroformate	T59.3X1	T59.3X2	T59.3X3	T59.3X4	—	—
cyclohexane	T52.8X1	T52.8X2	T52.8X3	T52.8X4	—	—
cyclohexanol	T51.8X1	T51.8X2	T51.8X3	T51.8X4	—	—
cyclohexanone	T52.8X1	T52.8X2	T52.8X3	T52.8X4	—	—
cyclohexyl acetate	T52.8X1	T52.8X2	T52.8X3	T52.8X4	—	—
demeton	T6Ø.ØX1	T6Ø.ØX2	T6Ø.ØX3	T6Ø.ØX4	—	—
dihydromorphinone	T4Ø.2X1	T4Ø.2X2	T4Ø.2X3	T4Ø.2X4	T4Ø.2X5	T4Ø.2X6
ergometrine	T48.ØX1	T48.ØX2	T48.ØX3	T48.ØX4	T48.ØX5	T48.ØX6
ergonovine	T48.ØX1	T48.ØX2	T48.ØX3	T48.ØX4	T48.ØX5	T48.ØX6
ethyl ketone	T52.4X1	T52.4X2	T52.4X3	T52.4X4	—	—
glucamine antimonate	T37.8X1	T37.8X2	T37.8X3	T37.8X4	T37.8X5	T37.8X6
hydrazine	T65.891	T65.892	T65.893	T65.894	—	—
iodide	T65.891	T65.892	T65.893	T65.894	—	—
isobutyl ketone	T52.4X1	T52.4X2	T52.4X3	T52.4X4	—	—
isothiocyanate	T6Ø.3X1	T6Ø.3X2	T6Ø.3X3	T6Ø.3X4	—	—
mercaptan	T59.891	T59.892	T59.893	T59.894	—	—
morphine NEC	T4Ø.2X1	T4Ø.2X2	T4Ø.2X3	T4Ø.2X4	T4Ø.2X5	T4Ø.2X6
nicotinate	T49.4X1	T49.4X2	T49.4X3	T49.4X4	T49.4X5	T49.4X6
paraben	T49.ØX1	T49.ØX2	T49.ØX3	T49.ØX4	T49.ØX5	T49.ØX6
parafynol	T42.6X1	T42.6X2	T42.6X3	T42.6X4	T42.6X5	T42.6X6
parathion	T6Ø.ØX1	T6Ø.ØX2	T6Ø.ØX3	T6Ø.ØX4	—	—
peridol	T43.4X1	T43.4X2	T43.4X3	T43.4X4	T43.4X5	T43.4X6
phenidate	T43.631	T43.632	T43.633	T43.634	T43.635	T43.636
prednisolone	T38.ØX1	T38.ØX2	T38.ØX3	T38.ØX4	T38.ØX5	T38.ØX6
Methyl — *continued*						
prednisolone — *continued*						
ENT agent	T49.6X1	T49.6X2	T49.6X3	T49.6X4	T49.6X5	T49.6X6
ophthalmic preparation	T49.5X1	T49.5X2	T49.5X3	T49.5X4	T49.5X5	T49.5X6
topical NEC	T49.ØX1	T49.ØX2	T49.ØX3	T49.ØX4	T49.ØX5	T49.ØX6
propylcarbinol	T51.3X1	T51.3X2	T51.3X3	T51.3X4	—	—
rosaniline NEC	T49.ØX1	T49.ØX2	T49.ØX3	T49.ØX4	T49.ØX5	T49.ØX6
salicylate	T49.2X1	T49.2X2	T49.2X3	T49.2X4	T49.2X5	T49.2X6
sulfate (fumes)	T59.891	T59.892	T59.893	T59.894	—	—
liquid	T52.8X1	T52.8X2	T52.8X3	T52.8X4	—	—
sulfonal	T42.6X1	T42.6X2	T42.6X3	T42.6X4	T42.6X5	T42.6X6
testosterone	T38.7X1	T38.7X2	T38.7X3	T38.7X4	T38.7X5	T38.7X6
thiouracil	T38.2X1	T38.2X2	T38.2X3	T38.2X4	T38.2X5	T38.2X6
Methylacetoxyprogesterone*	T38.5X1	T38.5X2	T38.5X3	T38.5X4	T38.5X5	T38.5X6
Methylamphetamine	T43.651	T43.652	T43.652	T43.654	T43.655	T43.656
Methylated spirit	T51.1X1	T51.1X2	T51.1X3	T51.1X4	—	—
Methylatropine nitrate	T44.3X1	T44.3X2	T44.3X3	T44.3X4	T44.3X5	T44.3X6
Methylbenactyzium bromide	T44.3X1	T44.3X2	T44.3X3	T44.3X4	T44.3X5	T44.3X6
Methylbenzethonium chloride	T49.ØX1	T49.ØX2	T49.ØX3	T49.ØX4	T49.ØX5	T49.ØX6
Methylcellulose	T47.4X1	T47.4X2	T47.4X3	T47.4X4	T47.4X5	T47.4X6
laxative	T47.4X1	T47.4X2	T47.4X3	T47.4X4	T47.4X5	T47.4X6
Methylchlorophenoxyacetic acid	T6Ø.3X1	T6Ø.3X2	T6Ø.3X3	T6Ø.3X4	—	—
Methyldopa	T46.5X1	T46.5X2	T46.5X3	T46.5X4	T46.5X5	T46.5X6
Methyldopate	T46.5X1	T46.5X2	T46.5X3	T46.5X4	T46.5X5	T46.5X6
Methylene						
blue	T5Ø.6X1	T5Ø.6X2	T5Ø.6X3	T5Ø.6X4	T5Ø.6X5	T5Ø.6X6
chloride or dichloride (solvent) NEC	T53.4X1	T53.4X2	T53.4X3	T53.4X4	—	—
Methylenedioxyamphetamine	T43.621	T43.622	T43.623	T43.624	T43.625	T43.626
Methylenedioxymeth-amphetamine	T43.641	T43.642	T43.643	T43.644	—	—
Methylergometrine	T48.ØX1	T48.ØX2	T48.ØX3	T48.ØX4	T48.ØX5	T48.ØX6
Methylergonovine	T48.ØX1	T48.ØX2	T48.ØX3	T48.ØX4	T48.ØX5	T48.ØX6
Methylestrenolone	T38.5X1	T38.5X2	T38.5X3	T38.5X4	T38.5X5	T38.5X6
Methylethyl cellulose	T5Ø.991	T5Ø.992	T5Ø.993	T5Ø.994	T5Ø.995	T5Ø.996
Methylhexabital	T42.3X1	T42.3X2	T42.3X3	T42.3X4	T42.3X5	T42.3X6
Methylmorphine	T4Ø.2X1	T4Ø.2X2	T4Ø.2X3	T4Ø.2X4	T4Ø.2X5	T4Ø.2X6
Methylparaben (ophthalmic)	T49.5X1	T49.5X2	T49.5X3	T49.5X4	T49.5X5	T49.5X6
Methylparafynol	T42.6X1	T42.6X2	T42.6X3	T42.6X4	T42.6X5	T42.6X6
Methylpentynol, methylpenthynol	T42.6X1	T42.6X2	T42.6X3	T42.6X4	T42.6X5	T42.6X6
Methylphenidate	T43.631	T43.632	T43.633	T43.634	T43.635	T43.636
Methylphenobarbital	T42.3X1	T42.3X2	T42.3X3	T42.3X4	T42.3X5	T42.3X6
Methylpolysiloxane	T47.1X1	T47.1X2	T47.1X3	T47.1X4	T47.1X5	T47.1X6
Methylprednisolone — *see* Methyl, prednisolone						
Methylrosaniline	T49.ØX1	T49.ØX2	T49.ØX3	T49.ØX4	T49.ØX5	T49.ØX6
Methylrosanilinium chloride	T49.ØX1	T49.ØX2	T49.ØX3	T49.ØX4	T49.ØX5	T49.ØX6
Methyltestosterone	T38.7X1	T38.7X2	T38.7X3	T38.7X4	T38.7X5	T38.7X6
Methylthionine chloride	T5Ø.6X1	T5Ø.6X2	T5Ø.6X3	T5Ø.6X4	T5Ø.6X5	T5Ø.6X6
Methylthioninium chloride	T5Ø.6X1	T5Ø.6X2	T5Ø.6X3	T5Ø.6X4	T5Ø.6X5	T5Ø.6X6
Methylthiouracil	T38.2X1	T38.2X2	T38.2X3	T38.2X4	T38.2X5	T38.2X6
Methyprylon	T42.6X1	T42.6X2	T42.6X3	T42.6X4	T42.6X5	T42.6X6
Methysergide	T46.5X1	T46.5X2	T46.5X3	T46.5X4	T46.5X5	T46.5X6
Metiamide	T47.1X1	T47.1X2	T47.1X3	T47.1X4	T47.1X5	T47.1X6
Meticillin	T36.ØX1	T36.ØX2	T36.ØX3	T36.ØX4	T36.ØX5	T36.ØX6
Meticrane	T5Ø.2X1	T5Ø.2X2	T5Ø.2X3	T5Ø.2X4	T5Ø.2X5	T5Ø.2X6
Metildigoxin	T46.ØX1	T46.ØX2	T46.ØX3	T46.ØX4	T46.ØX5	T46.ØX6
Metipranolol	T49.5X1	T49.5X2	T49.5X3	T49.5X4	T49.5X5	T49.5X6
Metirosine	T46.5X1	T46.5X2	T46.5X3	T46.5X4	T46.5X5	T46.5X6
Metisazone	T37.5X1	T37.5X2	T37.5X3	T37.5X4	T37.5X5	T37.5X6
Metixene	T44.3X1	T44.3X2	T44.3X3	T44.3X4	T44.3X5	T44.3X6
Metizoline	T48.5X1	T48.5X2	T48.5X3	T48.5X4	T48.5X5	T48.5X6
Metoclopramide	T45.ØX1	T45.ØX2	T45.ØX3	T45.ØX4	T45.ØX5	T45.ØX6
Metofenazate	T43.3X1	T43.3X2	T43.3X3	T43.3X4	T43.3X5	T43.3X6
Metofoline	T39.8X1	T39.8X2	T39.8X3	T39.8X4	T39.8X5	T39.8X6
Metolazone	T5Ø.2X1	T5Ø.2X2	T5Ø.2X3	T5Ø.2X4	T5Ø.2X5	T5Ø.2X6
Metopon	T4Ø.2X1	T4Ø.2X2	T4Ø.2X3	T4Ø.2X4	T4Ø.2X5	T4Ø.2X6
Metoprine	T45.1X1	T45.1X2	T45.1X3	T45.1X4	T45.1X5	T45.1X6
Metoprolol	T44.7X1	T44.7X2	T44.7X3	T44.7X4	T44.7X5	T44.7X6
Metrifonate	T6Ø.ØX1	T6Ø.ØX2	T6Ø.ØX3	T6Ø.ØX4	—	—
Metrizamide	T5Ø.8X1	T5Ø.8X2	T5Ø.8X3	T5Ø.8X4	T5Ø.8X5	T5Ø.8X6
Metrizoic acid	T5Ø.8X1	T5Ø.8X2	T5Ø.8X3	T5Ø.8X4	T5Ø.8X5	T5Ø.8X6
Metronidazole	T37.8X1	T37.8X2	T37.8X3	T37.8X4	T37.8X5	T37.8X6
Metycaine	T41.3X1	T41.3X2	T41.3X3	T41.3X4	T41.3X5	T41.3X6
infiltration (subcutaneous)	T41.3X1	T41.3X2	T41.3X3	T41.3X4	T41.3X5	T41.3X6

*Optum Value-Add

Substance	Poisoning, Accidental (unintentional)	Poisoning, Intentional Self-harm	Poisoning, Assault	Poisoning, Undetermined	Adverse Effect	Under-dosing
Metycaine — *continued*						
nerve block (peripheral) (plexus)	T41.3X1	T41.3X2	T41.3X3	T41.3X4	T41.3X5	T41.3X6
topical (surface)	T41.3X1	T41.3X2	T41.3X3	T41.3X4	T41.3X5	T41.3X6
Metyrapone	T50.8X1	T50.8X2	T50.8X3	T50.8X4	T50.8X5	T50.8X6
Mevacor*	T46.6X1	T46.6X2	T46.6X3	T46.6X4	T46.6X5	T46.6X6
Mevinphos	T60.0X1	T60.0X2	T60.0X3	T60.0X4	—	—
Mexazolam	T42.4X1	T42.4X2	T42.4X3	T42.4X4	T42.4X5	T42.4X6
Mexenone	T49.3X1	T49.3X2	T49.3X3	T49.3X4	T49.3X5	T49.3X6
Mexiletine	T46.2X1	T46.2X2	T46.2X3	T46.2X4	T46.2X5	T46.2X6
Mezereon	T62.2X1	T62.2X2	T62.2X3	T62.2X4	—	—
berries	T62.1X1	T62.1X2	T62.1X3	T62.1X4	—	—
Mezlocillin	T36.0X1	T36.0X2	T36.0X3	T36.0X4	T36.0X5	T36.0X6
Mianserin	T43.021	T43.022	T43.023	T43.024	T43.025	T43.026
Micatin	T49.0X1	T49.0X2	T49.0X3	T49.0X4	T49.0X5	T49.0X6
Miconazole	T49.0X1	T49.0X2	T49.0X3	T49.0X4	T49.0X5	T49.0X6
Micronomicin	T36.5X1	T36.5X2	T36.5X3	T36.5X4	T36.5X5	T36.5X6
Microzide*	T50.2X1	T50.2X2	T50.2X3	T50.2X4	T50.2X5	T50.2X6
Midazolam	T42.4X1	T42.4X2	T42.4X3	T42.4X4	T42.4X5	T42.4X6
Midecamycin	T36.3X1	T36.3X2	T36.3X3	T36.3X4	T36.3X5	T36.3X6
Mifepristone	T38.6X1	T38.6X2	T38.6X3	T38.6X4	T38.6X5	T38.6X6
Milk of magnesia	T47.1X1	T47.1X2	T47.1X3	T47.1X4	T47.1X5	T47.1X6
Millipede (tropical) (venomous)	T63.411	T63.412	T63.413	T63.414	—	—
Miltown	T43.591	T43.592	T43.593	T43.594	T43.595	T43.596
Milverine	T44.3X1	T44.3X2	T44.3X3	T44.3X4	T44.3X5	T44.3X6
Minaprine	T43.291	T43.292	T43.293	T43.294	T43.295	T43.296
Minaxolone	T41.291	T41.292	T41.293	T41.294	T41.295	T41.296
Mineral						
acids	T54.2X1	T54.2X2	T54.2X3	T54.2X4	—	—
oil (laxative)(medicinal)	T47.4X1	T47.4X2	T47.4X3	T47.4X4	T47.4X5	T47.4X6
emulsion	T47.2X1	T47.2X2	T47.2X3	T47.2X4	T47.2X5	T47.2X6
nonmedicinal	T52.0X1	T52.0X2	T52.0X3	T52.0X4	—	—
topical	T49.3X1	T49.3X2	T49.3X3	T49.3X4	T49.3X5	T49.3X6
salt NEC	T50.3X1	T50.3X2	T50.3X3	T50.3X4	T50.3X5	T50.3X6
spirits	T52.0X1	T52.0X2	T52.0X3	T52.0X4	—	—
Mineralocorticosteroid	T50.0X1	T50.0X2	T50.0X3	T50.0X4	T50.0X5	T50.0X6
Minocycline	T36.4X1	T36.4X2	T36.4X3	T36.4X4	T36.4X5	T36.4X6
Minoxidil	T46.7X1	T46.7X2	T46.7X3	T46.7X4	T46.7X5	T46.7X6
Miokamycin	T36.3X1	T36.3X2	T36.3X3	T36.3X4	T36.3X5	T36.3X6
Miotic drug	T49.5X1	T49.5X2	T49.5X3	T49.5X4	T49.5X5	T49.5X6
Mipafox	T60.0X1	T60.0X2	T60.0X3	T60.0X4	—	—
Mipomerson*	T46.6X1	T46.6X2	T46.6X3	T46.6X4	T46.6X5	T46.6X6
Mirex	T60.1X1	T60.1X2	T60.1X3	T60.1X4	—	—
Mirtazapine	T43.021	T43.022	T43.023	T43.024	T43.025	T43.026
Misonidazole	T37.3X1	T37.3X2	T37.3X3	T37.3X4	T37.3X5	T37.3X6
Misoprostol	T47.1X1	T47.1X2	T47.1X3	T47.1X4	T47.1X5	T47.1X6
Mithramycin	T45.1X1	T45.1X2	T45.1X3	T45.1X4	T45.1X5	T45.1X6
Mitobronitol	T45.1X1	T45.1X2	T45.1X3	T45.1X4	T45.1X5	T45.1X6
Mitoguazone	T45.1X1	T45.1X2	T45.1X3	T45.1X4	T45.1X5	T45.1X6
Mitolactol	T45.1X1	T45.1X2	T45.1X3	T45.1X4	T45.1X5	T45.1X6
Mitomycin	T45.1X1	T45.1X2	T45.1X3	T45.1X4	T45.1X5	T45.1X6
Mitopodozide	T45.1X1	T45.1X2	T45.1X3	T45.1X4	T45.1X5	T45.1X6
Mitotane	T45.1X1	T45.1X2	T45.1X3	T45.1X4	T45.1X5	T45.1X6
Mitoxantrone	T45.1X1	T45.1X2	T45.1X3	T45.1X4	T45.1X5	T45.1X6
Mivacurium chloride	T48.1X1	T48.1X2	T48.1X3	T48.1X4	T48.1X5	T48.1X6
Miyari bacteria	T47.6X1	T47.6X2	T47.6X3	T47.6X4	T47.6X5	T47.6X6
Moclobemide	T43.1X1	T43.1X2	T43.1X3	T43.1X4	T43.1X5	T43.1X6
Moderil	T46.5X1	T46.5X2	T46.5X3	T46.5X4	T46.5X5	T46.5X6
Mofebutazone	T39.2X1	T39.2X2	T39.2X3	T39.2X4	T39.2X5	T39.2X6
Mogadon — *see* Nitrazepam						
Molindone	T43.591	T43.592	T43.593	T43.594	T43.595	T43.596
Molsidomine	T46.3X1	T46.3X2	T46.3X3	T46.3X4	T46.3X5	T46.3X6
Mometasone	T49.0X1	T49.0X2	T49.0X3	T49.0X4	T49.0X5	T49.0X6
Monistat	T49.0X1	T49.0X2	T49.0X3	T49.0X4	T49.0X5	T49.0X6
Monkshood	T62.2X1	T62.2X2	T62.2X3	T62.2X4	—	—
Monoamine oxidase inhibitor NEC	T43.1X1	T43.1X2	T43.1X3	T43.1X4	T43.1X5	T43.1X6
hydrazine	T43.1X1	T43.1X2	T43.1X3	T43.1X4	T43.1X5	T43.1X6
Monobenzone	T49.4X1	T49.4X2	T49.4X3	T49.4X4	T49.4X5	T49.4X6
Monochloroacetic acid	T60.3X1	T60.3X2	T60.3X3	T60.3X4	—	—
Monochlorobenzene	T53.7X1	T53.7X2	T53.7X3	T53.7X4	—	—
Monoethanolamine	T46.8X1	T46.8X2	T46.8X3	T46.8X4	T46.8X5	T46.8X6
oleate	T46.8X1	T46.8X2	T46.8X3	T46.8X4	T46.8X5	T46.8X6
Monooctanoin	T50.991	T50.992	T50.993	T50.994	T50.995	T50.996
Monophenylbutazone	T39.2X1	T39.2X2	T39.2X3	T39.2X4	T39.2X5	T39.2X6
Monopril*	T46.4X1	T46.4X2	T46.4X3	T46.4X4	T46.4X5	T46.4X6
Monosodium glutamate	T65.891	T65.892	T65.893	T65.894	—	—
Monosulfiram	T49.0X1	T49.0X2	T49.0X3	T49.0X4	T49.0X5	T49.0X6
Monoxide, carbon — *see* Carbon, monoxide						
Monoxidine hydrochloride	T46.1X1	T46.1X2	T46.1X3	T46.1X4	T46.1X5	T46.1X6
Monuron	T60.3X1	T60.3X2	T60.3X3	T60.3X4	—	—
Moperone	T43.4X1	T43.4X2	T43.4X3	T43.4X4	T43.4X5	T43.4X6
Mopidamol	T45.1X1	T45.1X2	T45.1X3	T45.1X4	T45.1X5	T45.1X6
MOPP (mechloreth-amine + vincristine + prednisone + procarba-zine)	T45.1X1	T45.1X2	T45.1X3	T45.1X4	T45.1X5	T45.1X6
Morfin	T40.2X1	T40.2X2	T40.2X3	T40.2X4	T40.2X5	T40.2X6
Morinamide	T37.1X1	T37.1X2	T37.1X3	T37.1X4	T37.1X5	T37.1X6
Morning glory seeds	T40.991	T40.992	T40.993	T40.994	—	—
Moroxydine	T37.5X1	T37.5X2	T37.5X3	T37.5X4	T37.5X5	T37.5X6
Morphazinamide	T37.1X1	T37.1X2	T37.1X3	T37.1X4	T37.1X5	T37.1X6
Morphine	T40.2X1	T40.2X2	T40.2X3	T40.2X4	T40.2X5	T40.2X6
antagonist	T50.7X1	T50.7X2	T50.7X3	T50.7X4	T50.7X5	T50.7X6
Morpholinylethylmorphine	T40.2X1	T40.2X2	T40.2X3	T40.2X4	—	—
Morsuximide	T42.2X1	T42.2X2	T42.2X3	T42.2X4	T42.2X5	T42.2X6
Mosapramine	T43.591	T43.592	T43.593	T43.594	T43.595	T43.596
Moth balls — *see also* Pesticide	T60.2X1	T60.2X2	T60.2X3	T60.2X4	—	—
naphthalene	T60.2X1	T60.2X2	T60.2X3	T60.2X4	—	—
paradichlorobenzene	T60.1X1	T60.1X2	T60.1X3	T60.1X4	—	—
Motor exhaust gas	T58.01	T58.02	T58.03	T58.04	—	—
Motrin*	T39.311	T39.312	T39.313	T39.314	T39.315	T39.316
Mouthwash (antiseptic) (zinc chloride)	T49.6X1	T49.6X2	T49.6X3	T49.6X4	T49.6X5	T49.6X6
Moxastine	T45.0X1	T45.0X2	T45.0X3	T45.0X4	T45.0X5	T45.0X6
Moxaverine	T44.3X1	T44.3X2	T44.3X3	T44.3X4	T44.3X5	T44.3X6
Moxisylyte	T46.7X1	T46.7X2	T46.7X3	T46.7X4	T46.7X5	T46.7X6
Mucilage, plant	T47.4X1	T47.4X2	T47.4X3	T47.4X4	T47.4X5	T47.4X6
Mucolytic drug	T48.4X1	T48.4X2	T48.4X3	T48.4X4	T48.4X5	T48.4X6
Mucomyst	T48.4X1	T48.4X2	T48.4X3	T48.4X4	T48.4X5	T48.4X6
Mucous membrane agents (external)	T49.91	T49.92	T49.93	T49.94	T49.95	T49.96
specified NEC	T49.8X1	T49.8X2	T49.8X3	T49.8X4	T49.8X5	T49.8X6
Multaq*	T46.2X1	T46.2X2	T46.2X3	T46.2X4	T46.2X5	T46.2X6
Multiple unspecified drugs, medicaments and biological substances	T50.911	T50.912	T50.913	T50.914	T50.915	T50.916
Mumps						
immune globulin (human)	T50.Z11	T50.Z12	T50.Z13	T50.Z14	T50.Z15	T50.Z16
skin test antigen	T50.8X1	T50.8X2	T50.8X3	T50.8X4	T50.8X5	T50.8X6
vaccine	T50.B91	T50.B92	T50.B93	T50.B94	T50.B95	T50.B96
Mumpsvax	T50.B91	T50.B92	T50.B93	T50.B94	T50.B95	T50.B96
Mupirocin	T49.0X1	T49.0X2	T49.0X3	T49.0X4	T49.0X5	T49.0X6
Muriatic acid — *see* Hydrochloric acid						
Muromonab-CD3	T45.1X1	T45.1X2	T45.1X3	T45.1X4	T45.1X5	T45.1X6
Muscle-action drug NEC	T48.201	T48.202	T48.203	T48.204	T48.205	T48.206
Muscle affecting agents NEC	T48.201	T48.202	T48.203	T48.204	T48.205	T48.206
oxytocic	T48.0X1	T48.0X2	T48.0X3	T48.0X4	T48.0X5	T48.0X6
relaxants	T48.201	T48.202	T48.203	T48.204	T48.205	T48.206
central nervous system	T42.8X1	T42.8X2	T42.8X3	T42.8X4	T42.8X5	T42.8X6
skeletal	T48.1X1	T48.1X2	T48.1X3	T48.1X4	T48.1X5	T48.1X6
smooth	T44.3X1	T44.3X2	T44.3X3	T44.3X4	T44.3X5	T44.3X6
Muscle relaxant — *see* Relaxant, muscle						
Muscle-tone depressant, central NEC	T42.8X1	T42.8X2	T42.8X3	T42.8X4	T42.8X5	T42.8X6
specified NEC	T42.8X1	T42.8X2	T42.8X3	T42.8X4	T42.8X5	T42.8X6
Mushroom, noxious	T62.0X1	T62.0X2	T62.0X3	T62.0X4	—	—
Mussel, noxious	T61.781	T61.782	T61.783	T61.784	—	—
Mustard (emetic)	T47.7X1	T47.7X2	T47.7X3	T47.7X4	T47.7X5	T47.7X6
black	T47.7X1	T47.7X2	T47.7X3	T47.7X4	T47.7X5	T47.7X6
gas, not in war	T59.91	T59.92	T59.93	T59.94	—	—
nitrogen	T45.1X1	T45.1X2	T45.1X3	T45.1X4	T45.1X5	T45.1X6
Mustine	T45.1X1	T45.1X2	T45.1X3	T45.1X4	T45.1X5	T45.1X6
M-vac	T45.1X1	T45.1X2	T45.1X3	T45.1X4	T45.1X5	T45.1X6
Mycifradin	T36.5X1	T36.5X2	T36.5X3	T36.5X4	T36.5X5	T36.5X6
topical	T49.0X1	T49.0X2	T49.0X3	T49.0X4	T49.0X5	T49.0X6
Mycitracin	T36.8X1	T36.8X2	T36.8X3	T36.8X4	T36.8X5	T36.8X6
ophthalmic preparation	T49.5X1	T49.5X2	T49.5X3	T49.5X4	T49.5X5	T49.5X6
Mycostatin	T36.7X1	T36.7X2	T36.7X3	T36.7X4	T36.7X5	T36.7X6
topical	T49.0X1	T49.0X2	T49.0X3	T49.0X4	T49.0X5	T49.0X6
Mycotoxins	T64.81	T64.82	T64.83	T64.84	—	—
aflatoxin	T64.01	T64.02	T64.03	T64.04	—	—
specified NEC	T64.81	T64.82	T64.83	T64.84	—	—
Mydriacyl	T44.3X1	T44.3X2	T44.3X3	T44.3X4	T44.3X5	T44.3X6
Mydriatic drug	T49.5X1	T49.5X2	T49.5X3	T49.5X4	T49.5X5	T49.5X6
Myelobromal	T45.1X1	T45.1X2	T45.1X3	T45.1X4	T45.1X5	T45.1X6
Myleran	T45.1X1	T45.1X2	T45.1X3	T45.1X4	T45.1X5	T45.1X6
Myochrysin (e)	T39.2X1	T39.2X2	T39.2X3	T39.2X4	T39.2X5	T39.2X6
Myoneural blocking agents	T48.1X1	T48.1X2	T48.1X3	T48.1X4	T48.1X5	T48.1X6
Myrac*	T36.4X1	T36.4X2	T36.4X3	T36.4X4	T36.4X5	T36.4X6

Substance	Poisoning, Accidental (unintentional)	Poisoning, Intentional Self-harm	Poisoning, Assault	Poisoning, Undetermined	Adverse Effect	Under-dosing
Myralact	T49.0X1	T49.0X2	T49.0X3	T49.0X4	T49.0X5	T49.0X6
Myristica fragrans	T62.2X1	T62.2X2	T62.2X3	T62.2X4	—	—
Myristicin	T65.891	T65.892	T65.893	T65.894	—	—
Mysoline	T42.3X1	T42.3X2	T42.3X3	T42.3X4	T42.3X5	T42.3X6
Nabilone	T40.711	T40.712	T40.713	T40.714	T40.715	T40.716
Nabumetone	T39.391	T39.392	T39.393	T39.394	T39.395	T39.396
Nadolol	T44.7X1	T44.7X2	T44.7X3	T44.7X4	T44.7X5	T44.7X6
Nafcillin	T36.0X1	T36.0X2	T36.0X3	T36.0X4	T36.0X5	T36.0X6
Nafoxidine	T38.6X1	T38.6X2	T38.6X3	T38.6X4	T38.6X5	T38.6X6
Naftazone	T46.991	T46.992	T46.993	T46.994	T46.995	T46.996
Naftidrofuryl (oxalate)	T46.7X1	T46.7X2	T46.7X3	T46.7X4	T46.7X5	T46.7X6
Naftifine	T49.0X1	T49.0X2	T49.0X3	T49.0X4	T49.0X5	T49.0X6
Nail polish remover	T52.91	T52.92	T52.93	T52.94	—	—
Nalbuphine	T40.491	T40.492	T40.493	T40.494	T40.495	T40.496
Naled	T60.0X1	T60.0X2	T60.0X3	T60.0X4	—	—
Nalidixic acid	T37.8X1	T37.8X2	T37.8X3	T37.8X4	T37.8X5	T37.8X6
Nalorphine	T50.7X1	T50.7X2	T50.7X3	T50.7X4	T50.7X5	T50.7X6
Naloxone	T50.7X1	T50.7X2	T50.7X3	T50.7X4	T50.7X5	T50.7X6
Naltrexone	T50.7X1	T50.7X2	T50.7X3	T50.7X4	T50.7X5	T50.7X6
Namenda	T43.8X1	T43.8X2	T43.8X3	T43.8X4	T43.8X5	T43.8X6
Nandrolone	T38.7X1	T38.7X2	T38.7X3	T38.7X4	T38.7X5	T38.7X6
Naphazoline	T48.5X1	T48.5X2	T48.5X3	T48.5X4	T48.5X5	T48.5X6
Naphtha (painters') (petroleum)	T52.0X1	T52.0X2	T52.0X3	T52.0X4	—	—
- solvent	T52.0X1	T52.0X2	T52.0X3	T52.0X4	—	—
- vapor	T52.0X1	T52.0X2	T52.0X3	T52.0X4	—	—
Naphthalene (non-chlorinated)	T60.2X1	T60.2X2	T60.2X3	T60.2X4	—	—
- chlorinated	T60.1X1	T60.1X2	T60.1X3	T60.1X4	—	—
- - vapor	T60.1X1	T60.1X2	T60.1X3	T60.1X4	—	—
- insecticide or moth repellent	T60.2X1	T60.2X2	T60.2X3	T60.2X4	—	—
- - chlorinated	T60.1X1	T60.1X2	T60.1X3	T60.1X4	—	—
- vapor	T60.2X1	T60.2X2	T60.2X3	T60.2X4	—	—
- - chlorinated	T60.1X1	T60.1X2	T60.1X3	T60.1X4	—	—
Naphthol	T65.891	T65.892	T65.893	T65.894	—	—
Naphthylamine	T65.891	T65.892	T65.893	T65.894	—	—
Naphthylthiourea (ANTU)	T60.4X1	T60.4X2	T60.4X3	T60.4X4	—	—
Naprosyn — *see* Naproxen						
Naproxen	T39.311	T39.312	T39.313	T39.314	T39.315	T39.316
Narcotic (drug)	T40.601	T40.602	T40.603	T40.604	T40.605	T40.606
- analgesic NEC	T40.601	T40.602	T40.603	T40.604	T40.605	T40.606
- antagonist	T50.7X1	T50.7X2	T50.7X3	T50.7X4	T50.7X5	T50.7X6
- specified NEC	T40.691	T40.692	T40.693	T40.694	T40.695	T40.696
- synthetic	T40.491	T40.492	T40.493	T40.494	T40.495	T40.496
Narcotine	T48.3X1	T48.3X2	T48.3X3	T48.3X4	T48.3X5	T48.3X6
Nardil	T43.1X1	T43.1X2	T43.1X3	T43.1X4	T43.1X5	T43.1X6
Nasacort*	T49.5X1	T49.5X2	T49.5X3	T49.5X4	T49.5X5	T49.5X6
Nasal drug NEC	T49.6X1	T49.6X2	T49.6X3	T49.6X4	T49.6X5	T49.6X6
Natamycin	T49.0X1	T49.0X2	T49.0X3	T49.0X4	T49.0X5	T49.0X6
Natrium cyanide — *see* Cyanide(s)						
Natural						
- blood (product)	T45.8X1	T45.8X2	T45.8X3	T45.8X4	T45.8X5	T45.8X6
- gas (piped)	T59.891	T59.892	T59.893	T59.894	—	—
- - incomplete combustion	T58.11	T58.12	T58.13	T58.14	—	—
Nealbarbital	T42.3X1	T42.3X2	T42.3X3	T42.3X4	T42.3X5	T42.3X6
Nectadon	T48.3X1	T48.3X2	T48.3X3	T48.3X4	T48.3X5	T48.3X6
Nedocromil	T48.6X1	T48.6X2	T48.6X3	T48.6X4	T48.6X5	T48.6X6
Nefopam	T39.8X1	T39.8X2	T39.8X3	T39.8X4	T39.8X5	T39.8X6
Nematocyst (sting)	T63.691	T63.692	T63.693	T63.694	—	—
Nembutal	T42.3X1	T42.3X2	T42.3X3	T42.3X4	T42.3X5	T42.3X6
Nemonapride	T43.591	T43.592	T43.593	T43.594	T43.595	T43.596
Neoarsphenamine	T37.8X1	T37.8X2	T37.8X3	T37.8X4	T37.8X5	T37.8X6
Neocinchophen	T50.4X1	T50.4X2	T50.4X3	T50.4X4	T50.4X5	T50.4X6
Neomycin (derivatives)	T36.5X1	T36.5X2	T36.5X3	T36.5X4	T36.5X5	T36.5X6
- with						
- - bacitracin	T49.0X1	T49.0X2	T49.0X3	T49.0X4	T49.0X5	T49.0X6
- - neostigmine	T44.0X1	T44.0X2	T44.0X3	T44.0X4	T44.0X5	T44.0X6
- ENT agent	T49.6X1	T49.6X2	T49.6X3	T49.6X4	T49.6X5	T49.6X6
- ophthalmic preparation	T49.5X1	T49.5X2	T49.5X3	T49.5X4	T49.5X5	T49.5X6
- topical NEC	T49.0X1	T49.0X2	T49.0X3	T49.0X4	T49.0X5	T49.0X6
Neonal	T42.3X1	T42.3X2	T42.3X3	T42.3X4	T42.3X5	T42.3X6
Neopham*	T50.3X1	T50.3X2	T50.3X3	T50.3X4	T50.3X5	T50.3X6
Neoprontosil	T37.0X1	T37.0X2	T37.0X3	T37.0X4	T37.0X5	T37.0X6
Neosalvarsan	T37.8X1	T37.8X2	T37.8X3	T37.8X4	T37.8X5	T37.8X6
Neosilversalvarsan	T37.8X1	T37.8X2	T37.8X3	T37.8X4	T37.8X5	T37.8X6
Neosporin	T36.8X1	T36.8X2	T36.8X3	T36.8X4	T36.8X5	T36.8X6
- ENT agent	T49.6X1	T49.6X2	T49.6X3	T49.6X4	T49.6X5	T49.6X6
- opthalmic preparation	T49.5X1	T49.5X2	T49.5X3	T49.5X4	T49.5X5	T49.5X6
- topical NEC	T49.0X1	T49.0X2	T49.0X3	T49.0X4	T49.0X5	T49.0X6
Neostigmine bromide	T44.0X1	T44.0X2	T44.0X3	T44.0X4	T44.0X5	T44.0X6
Neraval	T42.3X1	T42.3X2	T42.3X3	T42.3X4	T42.3X5	T42.3X6

Substance	Poisoning, Accidental (unintentional)	Poisoning, Intentional Self-harm	Poisoning, Assault	Poisoning, Undetermined	Adverse Effect	Under-dosing
Neravan	T42.3X1	T42.3X2	T42.3X3	T42.3X4	T42.3X5	T42.3X6
Nerium oleander	T62.2X1	T62.2X2	T62.2X3	T62.2X4	—	—
Nerlynx*	T45.1X1	T45.1X2	T45.1X3	T45.1X4	T45.1X5	T45.1X6
Nerve gas, not in war	T59.91	T59.92	T59.93	T59.94	—	—
Nesacaine	T41.3X1	T41.3X2	T41.3X3	T41.3X4	T41.3X5	T41.3X6
- infiltration (subcutaneous)	T41.3X1	T41.3X2	T41.3X3	T41.3X4	T41.3X5	T41.3X6
- nerve block (peripheral) (plexus)	T41.3X1	T41.3X2	T41.3X3	T41.3X4	T41.3X5	T41.3X6
Netilmicin	T36.5X1	T36.5X2	T36.5X3	T36.5X4	T36.5X5	T36.5X6
Neurobarb	T42.3X1	T42.3X2	T42.3X3	T42.3X4	T42.3X5	T42.3X6
Neuroleptic drug NEC	T43.501	T43.502	T43.503	T43.504	T43.505	T43.506
Neuromuscular blocking drug	T48.1X1	T48.1X2	T48.1X3	T48.1X4	T48.1X5	T48.1X6
Neutral insulin injection	T38.3X1	T38.3X2	T38.3X3	T38.3X4	T38.3X5	T38.3X6
Neutral spirits	T51.0X1	T51.0X2	T51.0X3	T51.0X4	—	—
- beverage	T51.0X1	T51.0X2	T51.0X3	T51.0X4	—	—
Niacin	T46.7X1	T46.7X2	T46.7X3	T46.7X4	T46.7X5	T46.7X6
Niacinamide	T45.2X1	T45.2X2	T45.2X3	T45.2X4	T45.2X5	T45.2X6
Nialamide	T43.1X1	T43.1X2	T43.1X3	T43.1X4	T43.1X5	T43.1X6
Niaprazine	T42.6X1	T42.6X2	T42.6X3	T42.6X4	T42.6X5	T42.6X6
Nicametate	T46.7X1	T46.7X2	T46.7X3	T46.7X4	T46.7X5	T46.7X6
Nicardipine	T46.1X1	T46.1X2	T46.1X3	T46.1X4	T46.1X5	T46.1X6
Nicergoline	T46.7X1	T46.7X2	T46.7X3	T46.7X4	T46.7X5	T46.7X6
Nickel (carbonyl) (tetra-carbonyl) (fumes) (vapor)	T56.891	T56.892	T56.893	T56.894	—	—
Nickelocene	T56.891	T56.892	T56.893	T56.894	—	—
Niclosamide	T37.4X1	T37.4X2	T37.4X3	T37.4X4	T37.4X5	T37.4X6
Nicofuranose	T46.7X1	T46.7X2	T46.7X3	T46.7X4	T46.7X5	T46.7X6
Nicomorphine	T40.2X1	T40.2X2	T40.2X3	T40.2X4	—	—
Nicorandil	T46.3X1	T46.3X2	T46.3X3	T46.3X4	T46.3X5	T46.3X6
Nicotiana (plant)	T62.2X1	T62.2X2	T62.2X3	T62.2X4	—	—
Nicotinamide	T45.2X1	T45.2X2	T45.2X3	T45.2X4	T45.2X5	T45.2X6
Nicotine (insecticide) (spray) (sulfate) **NEC**	T60.2X1	T60.2X2	T60.2X3	T60.2X4	—	—
- from tobacco	T65.291	T65.292	T65.293	T65.294	—	—
- - cigarettes	T65.221	T65.222	T65.223	T65.224	—	—
- not insecticide	T65.291	T65.292	T65.293	T65.294	—	—
Nicotinic acid	T46.7X1	T46.7X2	T46.7X3	T46.7X4	T46.7X5	T46.7X6
Nicotinyl alcohol	T46.7X1	T46.7X2	T46.7X3	T46.7X4	T46.7X5	T46.7X6
Nicoumalone	T45.511	T45.512	T45.513	T45.514	T45.515	T45.516
Nifedipine	T46.1X1	T46.1X2	T46.1X3	T46.1X4	T46.1X5	T46.1X6
Nifenazone	T39.2X1	T39.2X2	T39.2X3	T39.2X4	T39.2X5	T39.2X6
Nifuraldezone	T37.91	T37.92	T37.93	T37.94	T37.95	T37.96
Nifuratel	T37.8X1	T37.8X2	T37.8X3	T37.8X4	T37.8X5	T37.8X6
Nifurtimox	T37.3X1	T37.3X2	T37.3X3	T37.3X4	T37.3X5	T37.3X6
Nifurtoinol	T37.8X1	T37.8X2	T37.8X3	T37.8X4	T37.8X5	T37.8X6
Nightshade, deadly (solanum) — *see also* Belladonna	T62.2X1	T62.2X2	T62.2X3	T62.2X4	—	—
- berry	T62.1X1	T62.1X2	T62.1X3	T62.1X4	—	—
Nikethamide	T50.7X1	T50.7X2	T50.7X3	T50.7X4	T50.7X5	T50.7X6
Nilstat	T36.7X1	T36.7X2	T36.7X3	T36.7X4	T36.7X5	T36.7X6
- topical	T49.0X1	T49.0X2	T49.0X3	T49.0X4	T49.0X5	T49.0X6
Nilutamide	T38.6X1	T38.6X2	T38.6X3	T38.6X4	T38.6X5	T38.6X6
Nimesulide	T39.391	T39.392	T39.393	T39.394	T39.395	T39.396
Nimetazepam	T42.4X1	T42.4X2	T42.4X3	T42.4X4	T42.4X5	T42.4X6
Nimodipine	T46.1X1	T46.1X2	T46.1X3	T46.1X4	T46.1X5	T46.1X6
Nimorazole	T37.3X1	T37.3X2	T37.3X3	T37.3X4	T37.3X5	T37.3X6
Nimustine	T45.1X1	T45.1X2	T45.1X3	T45.1X4	T45.1X5	T45.1X6
Nipent*	T45.1X1	T45.1X2	T45.1X3	T45.1X4	T45.1X5	T45.1X6
Niridazole	T37.4X1	T37.4X2	T37.4X3	T37.4X4	T37.4X5	T37.4X6
Nisentil	T40.2X1	T40.2X2	T40.2X3	T40.2X4	T40.2X5	T40.2X6
Nisoldipine	T46.1X1	T46.1X2	T46.1X3	T46.1X4	T46.1X5	T46.1X6
Nitramine	T65.3X1	T65.3X2	T65.3X3	T65.3X4	—	—
Nitrate, organic	T46.3X1	T46.3X2	T46.3X3	T46.3X4	T46.3X5	T46.3X6
Nitrazepam	T42.4X1	T42.4X2	T42.4X3	T42.4X4	T42.4X5	T42.4X6
Nitrefazole	T50.6X1	T50.6X2	T50.6X3	T50.6X4	T50.6X5	T50.6X6
Nitrendipine	T46.1X1	T46.1X2	T46.1X3	T46.1X4	T46.1X5	T46.1X6
Nitric						
- acid (liquid)	T54.2X1	T54.2X2	T54.2X3	T54.2X4	—	—
- - vapor	T59.891	T59.892	T59.893	T59.894	—	—
- oxide (gas)	T59.0X1	T59.0X2	T59.0X3	T59.0X4	—	—
Nitrimidazine	T37.3X1	T37.3X2	T37.3X3	T37.3X4	T37.3X5	T37.3X6
Nitrite, amyl (medicinal) (vapor)	T46.3X1	T46.3X2	T46.3X3	T46.3X4	T46.3X5	T46.3X6
Nitroaniline	T65.3X1	T65.3X2	T65.3X3	T65.3X4	—	—
- vapor	T59.891	T59.892	T59.893	T59.894	—	—
Nitrobenzene, nitrobenzol	T65.3X1	T65.3X2	T65.3X3	T65.3X4	—	—
- vapor	T65.3X1	T65.3X2	T65.3X3	T65.3X4	—	—
Nitrocellulose	T65.891	T65.892	T65.893	T65.894	—	—
- lacquer	T65.891	T65.892	T65.893	T65.894	—	—
Nitrodiphenyl	T65.3X1	T65.3X2	T65.3X3	T65.3X4	—	—
Nitrofural	T49.0X1	T49.0X2	T49.0X3	T49.0X4	T49.0X5	T49.0X6
Nitrofurantoin	T37.8X1	T37.8X2	T37.8X3	T37.8X4	T37.8X5	T37.8X6

Substance	Poisoning, Accidental (unintentional)	Poisoning, Intentional Self-harm	Poisoning, Assault	Poisoning, Undetermined	Adverse Effect	Under-dosing
Nitrofurazone	T49.ØX1	T49.ØX2	T49.ØX3	T49.ØX4	T49.ØX5	T49.ØX6
Nitrogen	T59.ØX1	T59.ØX2	T59.ØX3	T59.ØX4	—	—
mustard	T45.1X1	T45.1X2	T45.1X3	T45.1X4	T45.1X5	T45.1X6
Nitroglycerin, nitroglycerol (medicinal)	T46.3X1	T46.3X2	T46.3X3	T46.3X4	T46.3X5	T46.3X6
nonmedicinal	T65.5X1	T65.5X2	T65.5X3	T65.5X4	—	—
fumes	T65.5X1	T65.5X2	T65.5X3	T65.5X4	—	—
Nitroglycol	T52.3X1	T52.3X2	T52.3X3	T52.3X4	—	—
Nitrohydrochloric acid	T54.2X1	T54.2X2	T54.2X3	T54.2X4	—	—
Nitromersol	T49.ØX1	T49.ØX2	T49.ØX3	T49.ØX4	T49.ØX5	T49.ØX6
Nitronaphthalene	T65.891	T65.892	T65.893	T65.894	—	—
Nitrophenol	T54.ØX1	T54.ØX2	T54.ØX3	T54.ØX4	—	—
Nitropropane	T52.8X1	T52.8X2	T52.8X3	T52.8X4	—	—
Nitroprusside	T46.5X1	T46.5X2	T46.5X3	T46.5X4	T46.5X5	T46.5X6
Nitrosodimethylamine	T65.3X1	T65.3X2	T65.3X3	T65.3X4	—	—
Nitrothiazol	T37.4X1	T37.4X2	T37.4X3	T37.4X4	T37.4X5	T37.4X6
Nitrotoluene, nitrotoluol	T65.3X1	T65.3X2	T65.3X3	T65.3X4	—	—
vapor	T65.3X1	T65.3X2	T65.3X3	T65.3X4	—	—
Nitrous						
acid (liquid)	T54.2X1	T54.2X2	T54.2X3	T54.2X4	—	—
fumes	T59.891	T59.892	T59.893	T59.894	—	—
ether spirit	T46.3X1	T46.3X2	T46.3X3	T46.3X4	T46.3X5	T46.3X6
oxide	T41.ØX1	T41.ØX2	T41.ØX3	T41.ØX4	T41.ØX5	T41.ØX6
Nitroxoline	T37.8X1	T37.8X2	T37.8X3	T37.8X4	T37.8X5	T37.8X6
Nitrozone	T49.ØX1	T49.ØX2	T49.ØX3	T49.ØX4	T49.ØX5	T49.ØX6
Nizatidine	T47.ØX1	T47.ØX2	T47.ØX3	T47.ØX4	T47.ØX5	T47.ØX6
Nizofenone	T43.8X1	T43.8X2	T43.8X3	T43.8X4	T43.8X5	T43.8X6
Noctec	T42.6X1	T42.6X2	T42.6X3	T42.6X4	T42.6X5	T42.6X6
No Doz*	T43.611	T43.612	T43.613	T43.614	T43.615	T43.616
Noludar	T42.6X1	T42.6X2	T42.6X3	T42.6X4	T42.6X5	T42.6X6
Nomegestrol	T38.5X1	T38.5X2	T38.5X3	T38.5X4	T38.5X5	T38.5X6
Nomifensine	T43.291	T43.292	T43.293	T43.294	T43.295	T43.296
Nonoxinol	T49.8X1	T49.8X2	T49.8X3	T49.8X4	T49.8X5	T49.8X6
Nonylphenoxy (polyethoxyethanol)	T49.8X1	T49.8X2	T49.8X3	T49.8X4	T49.8X5	T49.8X6
Noptil	T42.3X1	T42.3X2	T42.3X3	T42.3X4	T42.3X5	T42.3X6
Noradrenaline	T44.4X1	T44.4X2	T44.4X3	T44.4X4	T44.4X5	T44.4X6
Noramidopyrine	T39.2X1	T39.2X2	T39.2X3	T39.2X4	T39.2X5	T39.2X6
methanesulfonate sodium	T39.2X1	T39.2X2	T39.2X3	T39.2X4	T39.2X5	T39.2X6
Norbormide	T6Ø.4X1	T6Ø.4X2	T6Ø.4X3	T6Ø.4X4	—	—
Nordazepam	T42.4X1	T42.4X2	T42.4X3	T42.4X4	T42.4X5	T42.4X6
Norepinephrine	T44.4X1	T44.4X2	T44.4X3	T44.4X4	T44.4X5	T44.4X6
Norethandrolone	T38.7X1	T38.7X2	T38.7X3	T38.7X4	T38.7X5	T38.7X6
Norethindrone	T38.4X1	T38.4X2	T38.4X3	T38.4X4	T38.4X5	T38.4X6
Norethisterone (acetate) (enantate)	T38.4X1	T38.4X2	T38.4X3	T38.4X4	T38.4X5	T38.4X6
with ethinylestradiol	T38.5X1	T38.5X2	T38.5X3	T38.5X4	T38.5X5	T38.5X6
Noretynodrel	T38.5X1	T38.5X2	T38.5X3	T38.5X4	T38.5X5	T38.5X6
Norfenefrine	T44.4X1	T44.4X2	T44.4X3	T44.4X4	T44.4X5	T44.4X6
Norfloxacin	T36.8X1	T36.8X2	T36.8X3	T36.8X4	T36.8X5	T36.8X6
Norgestrel	T38.4X1	T38.4X2	T38.4X3	T38.4X4	T38.4X5	T38.4X6
Norgestrienone	T38.4X1	T38.4X2	T38.4X3	T38.4X4	T38.4X5	T38.4X6
Norlestrin	T38.4X1	T38.4X2	T38.4X3	T38.4X4	T38.4X5	T38.4X6
Norlutin	T38.4X1	T38.4X2	T38.4X3	T38.4X4	T38.4X5	T38.4X6
Normal serum albumin (human), salt-poor	T45.8X1	T45.8X2	T45.8X3	T45.8X4	T45.8X5	T45.8X6
Normethandrone	T38.5X1	T38.5X2	T38.5X3	T38.5X4	T38.5X5	T38.5X6
Normison — *see* Benzodiazepines						
Normorphine	T4Ø.2X1	T4Ø.2X2	T4Ø.2X3	T4Ø.2X4	—	—
Norpseudoephedrine	T5Ø.5X1	T5Ø.5X2	T5Ø.5X3	T5Ø.5X4	T5Ø.5X5	T5Ø.5X6
Nortestosterone (furanpropionate)	T38.7X1	T38.7X2	T38.7X3	T38.7X4	T38.7X5	T38.7X6
Nortriptyline	T43.Ø11	T43.Ø12	T43.Ø13	T43.Ø14	T43.Ø15	T43.Ø16
Norvasc*	T46.1X1	T46.1X2	T46.1X3	T46.1X4	T46.1X5	T46.1X6
Noscapine	T48.3X1	T48.3X2	T48.3X3	T48.3X4	T48.3X5	T48.3X6
Nose preparations	T49.6X1	T49.6X2	T49.6X3	T49.6X4	T49.6X5	T49.6X6
Novobiocin	T36.5X1	T36.5X2	T36.5X3	T36.5X4	T36.5X5	T36.5X6
Novocain (infiltration) (topical)	T41.3X1	T41.3X2	T41.3X3	T41.3X4	T41.3X5	T41.3X6
nerve block (peripheral) (plexus)	T41.3X1	T41.3X2	T41.3X3	T41.3X4	T41.3X5	T41.3X6
spinal	T41.3X1	T41.3X2	T41.3X3	T41.3X4	T41.3X5	T41.3X6
Noxious foodstuff	T62.91	T62.92	T62.93	T62.94	—	—
specified NEC	T62.8X1	T62.8X2	T62.8X3	T62.8X4	—	—
Noxiptiline	T43.Ø11	T43.Ø12	T43.Ø13	T43.Ø14	T43.Ø15	T43.Ø16
Noxytiolin	T49.ØX1	T49.ØX2	T49.ØX3	T49.ØX4	T49.ØX5	T49.ØX6
NPH Iletin (insulin)	T38.3X1	T38.3X2	T38.3X3	T38.3X4	T38.3X5	T38.3X6
Numorphan	T4Ø.2X1	T4Ø.2X2	T4Ø.2X3	T4Ø.2X4	T4Ø.2X5	T4Ø.2X6
Nunol	T42.3X1	T42.3X2	T42.3X3	T42.3X4	T42.3X5	T42.3X6
Nupercaine (spinal anesthetic)	T41.3X1	T41.3X2	T41.3X3	T41.3X4	T41.3X5	T41.3X6
topical (surface)	T41.3X1	T41.3X2	T41.3X3	T41.3X4	T41.3X5	T41.3X6
Nutmeg oil (liniment)	T49.3X1	T49.3X2	T49.3X3	T49.3X4	T49.3X5	T49.3X6
Nutrilipid*	T5Ø.991	T5Ø.992	T5Ø.993	T5Ø.994	T5Ø.995	T5Ø.996
Nutritional supplement	T5Ø.9Ø1	T5Ø.9Ø2	T5Ø.9Ø3	T5Ø.9Ø4	T5Ø.9Ø5	T5Ø.9Ø6
Nux vomica	T65.1X1	T65.1X2	T65.1X3	T65.1X4	—	—
Nydrazid	T37.1X1	T37.1X2	T37.1X3	T37.1X4	T37.1X5	T37.1X6
Nylidrin	T46.7X1	T46.7X2	T46.7X3	T46.7X4	T46.7X5	T46.7X6
Nystatin	T36.7X1	T36.7X2	T36.7X3	T36.7X4	T36.7X5	T36.7X6
topical	T49.ØX1	T49.ØX2	T49.ØX3	T49.ØX4	T49.ØX5	T49.ØX6
Nytol	T45.ØX1	T45.ØX2	T45.ØX3	T45.ØX4	T45.ØX5	T45.ØX6
Obidoxime chloride	T5Ø.6X1	T5Ø.6X2	T5Ø.6X3	T5Ø.6X4	T5Ø.6X5	T5Ø.6X6
Octafonium (chloride)	T49.3X1	T49.3X2	T49.3X3	T49.3X4	T49.3X5	T49.3X6
Octamethyl pyrophosphoramide	T6Ø.ØX1	T6Ø.ØX2	T6Ø.ØX3	T6Ø.ØX4	—	—
Octanoin	T5Ø.991	T5Ø.992	T5Ø.993	T5Ø.994	T5Ø.995	T5Ø.996
Octatropine methylbromide	T44.3X1	T44.3X2	T44.3X3	T44.3X4	T44.3X5	T44.3X6
Octotiamine	T45.2X1	T45.2X2	T45.2X3	T45.2X4	T45.2X5	T45.2X6
Octoxinol (9)	T49.8X1	T49.8X2	T49.8X3	T49.8X4	T49.8X5	T49.8X6
Octreotide	T38.991	T38.992	T38.993	T38.994	T38.995	T38.996
Octyl nitrite	T46.3X1	T46.3X2	T46.3X3	T46.3X4	T46.3X5	T46.3X6
Oestradiol	T38.5X1	T38.5X2	T38.5X3	T38.5X4	T38.5X5	T38.5X6
Oestriol	T38.5X1	T38.5X2	T38.5X3	T38.5X4	T38.5X5	T38.5X6
Oestrogen	T38.5X1	T38.5X2	T38.5X3	T38.5X4	T38.5X5	T38.5X6
Oestrone	T38.5X1	T38.5X2	T38.5X3	T38.5X4	T38.5X5	T38.5X6
Ofloxacin	T36.8X1	T36.8X2	T36.8X3	T36.8X4	T36.8X5	T36.8X6
Oil (of)	T65.891	T65.892	T65.893	T65.894	—	—
bitter almond	T62.8X1	T62.8X2	T62.8X3	T62.8X4	—	—
cloves	T49.7X1	T49.7X2	T49.7X3	T49.7X4	T49.7X5	T49.7X6
colors	T65.6X1	T65.6X2	T65.6X3	T65.6X4	—	—
fumes	T59.891	T59.892	T59.893	T59.894	—	—
lubricating	T52.ØX1	T52.ØX2	T52.ØX3	T52.ØX4	—	—
Niobe	T52.8X1	T52.8X2	T52.8X3	T52.8X4	—	—
vitriol (liquid)	T54.2X1	T54.2X2	T54.2X3	T54.2X4	—	—
fumes	T54.2X1	T54.2X2	T54.2X3	T54.2X4	—	—
wintergreen (bitter) NEC	T49.3X1	T49.3X2	T49.3X3	T49.3X4	T49.3X5	T49.3X6
Oily preparation (for skin)	T49.3X1	T49.3X2	T49.3X3	T49.3X4	T49.3X5	T49.3X6
Ointment NEC	T49.3X1	T49.3X2	T49.3X3	T49.3X4	T49.3X5	T49.3X6
Olanzapine	T43.591	T43.592	T43.593	T43.594	T43.595	T43.596
Oleander	T62.2X1	T62.2X2	T62.2X3	T62.2X4	—	—
Oleandomycin	T36.3X1	T36.3X2	T36.3X3	T36.3X4	T36.3X5	T36.3X6
Oleandrin	T46.ØX1	T46.ØX2	T46.ØX3	T46.ØX4	T46.ØX5	T46.ØX6
Oleic acid	T46.6X1	T46.6X2	T46.6X3	T46.6X4	T46.6X5	T46.6X6
Oleovitamin A	T45.2X1	T45.2X2	T45.2X3	T45.2X4	T45.2X5	T45.2X6
Oleum ricini	T47.2X1	T47.2X2	T47.2X3	T47.2X4	T47.2X5	T47.2X6
Olive oil (medicinal) **NEC**	T47.4X1	T47.4X2	T47.4X3	T47.4X4	T47.4X5	T47.4X6
Olivomycin	T45.1X1	T45.1X2	T45.1X3	T45.1X4	T45.1X5	T45.1X6
Olodaterol*	T48.6X1	T48.6X2	T48.6X3	T48.6X4	T48.6X5	T48.6X6
Olsalazine	T47.8X1	T47.8X2	T47.8X3	T47.8X4	T47.8X5	T47.8X6
Omeprazole	T47.1X1	T47.1X2	T47.1X3	T47.1X4	T47.1X5	T47.1X6
OMPA	T6Ø.ØX1	T6Ø.ØX2	T6Ø.ØX3	T6Ø.ØX4	—	—
Oncovin	T45.1X1	T45.1X2	T45.1X3	T45.1X4	T45.1X5	T45.1X6
Ondansetron	T45.ØX1	T45.ØX2	T45.ØX3	T45.ØX4	T45.ØX5	T45.ØX6
Ophthaine	T41.3X1	T41.3X2	T41.3X3	T41.3X4	T41.3X5	T41.3X6
Ophthetic	T41.3X1	T41.3X2	T41.3X3	T41.3X4	T41.3X5	T41.3X6
Opiate NEC	T4Ø.6Ø1	T4Ø.6Ø2	T4Ø.6Ø3	T4Ø.6Ø4	T4Ø.6Ø5	T4Ø.6Ø6
antagonists	T5Ø.7X1	T5Ø.7X2	T5Ø.7X3	T5Ø.7X4	T5Ø.7X5	T5Ø.7X6
Opioid NEC	T4Ø.2X1	T4Ø.2X2	T4Ø.2X3	T4Ø.2X4	T4Ø.2X5	T4Ø.2X6
Opipramol	T43.Ø11	T43.Ø12	T43.Ø13	T43.Ø14	T43.Ø15	T43.Ø16
Opium alkaloids (total)	T4Ø.ØX1	T4Ø.ØX2	T4Ø.ØX3	T4Ø.ØX4	T4Ø.ØX5	T4Ø.ØX6
standardized powdered	T4Ø.ØX1	T4Ø.ØX2	T4Ø.ØX3	T4Ø.ØX4	T4Ø.ØX5	T4Ø.ØX6
tincture (camphorated)	T4Ø.ØX1	T4Ø.ØX2	T4Ø.ØX3	T4Ø.ØX4	T4Ø.ØX5	T4Ø.ØX6
Optivar*	T49.5X1	T49.5X2	T49.5X3	T49.5X4	T49.5X5	T49.5X6
Oracon	T38.4X1	T38.4X2	T38.4X3	T38.4X4	T38.4X5	T38.4X6
Oragrafin	T5Ø.8X1	T5Ø.8X2	T5Ø.8X3	T5Ø.8X4	T5Ø.8X5	T5Ø.8X6
Oral contraceptives	T38.4X1	T38.4X2	T38.4X3	T38.4X4	T38.4X5	T38.4X6
Oral rehydration salts	T5Ø.3X1	T5Ø.3X2	T5Ø.3X3	T5Ø.3X4	T5Ø.3X5	T5Ø.3X6
Orazamide	T5Ø.991	T5Ø.992	T5Ø.993	T5Ø.994	T5Ø.995	T5Ø.996
Orciprenaline	T48.291	T48.292	T48.293	T48.294	T48.295	T48.296
Organidin	T48.4X1	T48.4X2	T48.4X3	T48.4X4	T48.4X5	T48.4X6
Organonitrate NEC	T46.3X1	T46.3X2	T46.3X3	T46.3X4	T46.3X5	T46.3X6
Organophosphates	T6Ø.ØX1	T6Ø.ØX2	T6Ø.ØX3	T6Ø.ØX4	—	—
Orimune	T5Ø.B91	T5Ø.B92	T5Ø.B93	T5Ø.B94	T5Ø.B95	T5Ø.B96
Orinase	T38.3X1	T38.3X2	T38.3X3	T38.3X4	T38.3X5	T38.3X6
Ormeloxifene	T38.6X1	T38.6X2	T38.6X3	T38.6X4	T38.6X5	T38.6X6
Ornidazole	T37.3X1	T37.3X2	T37.3X3	T37.3X4	T37.3X5	T37.3X6
Ornithine aspartate	T5Ø.991	T5Ø.992	T5Ø.993	T5Ø.994	T5Ø.995	T5Ø.996
Ornoprostil	T47.1X1	T47.1X2	T47.1X3	T47.1X4	T47.1X5	T47.1X6
Orphenadrine (hydrochloride)	T42.8X1	T42.8X2	T42.8X3	T42.8X4	T42.8X5	T42.8X6
Ortal (sodium)	T42.3X1	T42.3X2	T42.3X3	T42.3X4	T42.3X5	T42.3X6
Orthoboric acid	T49.ØX1	T49.ØX2	T49.ØX3	T49.ØX4	T49.ØX5	T49.ØX6
ENT agent	T49.6X1	T49.6X2	T49.6X3	T49.6X4	T49.6X5	T49.6X6
ophthalmic preparation	T49.5X1	T49.5X2	T49.5X3	T49.5X4	T49.5X5	T49.5X6

Substance	Poisoning, Accidental (unintentional)	Poisoning, Intentional Self-harm	Poisoning, Assault	Poisoning, Undetermined	Adverse Effect	Under-dosing
Orthocaine	T41.3X1	T41.3X2	T41.3X3	T41.3X4	T41.3X5	T41.3X6
Orthodichlorobenzene	T53.7X1	T53.7X2	T53.7X3	T53.7X4	—	—
Ortho-Novum	T38.4X1	T38.4X2	T38.4X3	T38.4X4	T38.4X5	T38.4X6
Orthotolidine (reagent)	T54.2X1	T54.2X2	T54.2X3	T54.2X4	—	—
Osmic acid (liquid)	T54.2X1	T54.2X2	T54.2X3	T54.2X4	—	—
fumes	T54.2X1	T54.2X2	T54.2X3	T54.2X4	—	—
Osmotic diuretics	T5Ø.2X1	T5Ø.2X2	T5Ø.2X3	T5Ø.2X4	T5Ø.2X5	T5Ø.2X6
Otilonium bromide	T44.3X1	T44.3X2	T44.3X3	T44.3X4	T44.3X5	T44.3X6
Otorhinolaryngological drug NEC	T49.6X1	T49.6X2	T49.6X3	T49.6X4	T49.6X5	T49.6X6
Ouabain (e)	T46.ØX1	T46.ØX2	T46.ØX3	T46.ØX4	T46.ØX5	T46.ØX6
Ovarian						
hormone	T38.5X1	T38.5X2	T38.5X3	T38.5X4	T38.5X5	T38.5X6
stimulant	T38.5X1	T38.5X2	T38.5X3	T38.5X4	T38.5X5	T38.5X6
Ovide*	T49.ØX1	T49.ØX2	T49.ØX3	T49.ØX4	T49.ØX5	T49.ØX6
Ovral	T38.4X1	T38.4X2	T38.4X3	T38.4X4	T38.4X5	T38.4X6
Ovulen	T38.4X1	T38.4X2	T38.4X3	T38.4X4	T38.4X5	T38.4X6
Oxacillin	T36.ØX1	T36.ØX2	T36.ØX3	T36.ØX4	T36.ØX5	T36.ØX6
Oxalic acid	T54.2X1	T54.2X2	T54.2X3	T54.2X4	—	—
ammonium salt	T5Ø.991	T5Ø.992	T5Ø.993	T5Ø.994	T5Ø.995	T5Ø.996
Oxamniquine	T37.4X1	T37.4X2	T37.4X3	T37.4X4	T37.4X5	T37.4X6
Oxanamide	T43.591	T43.592	T43.593	T43.594	T43.595	T43.596
Oxandrolone	T38.7X1	T38.7X2	T38.7X3	T38.7X4	T38.7X5	T38.7X6
Oxantel	T37.4X1	T37.4X2	T37.4X3	T37.4X4	T37.4X5	T37.4X6
Oxapium iodide	T44.3X1	T44.3X2	T44.3X3	T44.3X4	T44.3X5	T44.3X6
Oxaprotiline	T43.Ø21	T43.Ø22	T43.Ø23	T43.Ø24	T43.Ø25	T43.Ø26
Oxaprozin	T39.311	T39.312	T39.313	T39.314	T39.315	T39.316
Oxatomide	T45.ØX1	T45.ØX2	T45.ØX3	T45.ØX4	T45.ØX5	T45.ØX6
Oxazepam	T42.4X1	T42.4X2	T42.4X3	T42.4X4	T42.4X5	T42.4X6
Oxazimedrine	T5Ø.5X1	T5Ø.5X2	T5Ø.5X3	T5Ø.5X4	T5Ø.5X5	T5Ø.5X6
Oxazolam	T42.4X1	T42.4X2	T42.4X3	T42.4X4	T42.4X5	T42.4X6
Oxazolidine derivatives	T42.2X1	T42.2X2	T42.2X3	T42.2X4	T42.2X5	T42.2X6
Oxazolidinedione (derivative)	T42.2X1	T42.2X2	T42.2X3	T42.2X4	T42.2X5	T42.2X6
Ox bile extract	T47.5X1	T47.5X2	T47.5X3	T47.5X4	T47.5X5	T47.5X6
Oxcarbazepine	T42.1X1	T42.1X2	T42.1X3	T42.1X4	T42.1X5	T42.1X6
Oxedrine	T44.4X1	T44.4X2	T44.4X3	T44.4X4	T44.4X5	T44.4X6
Oxeladin (citrate)	T48.3X1	T48.3X2	T48.3X3	T48.3X4	T48.3X5	T48.3X6
Oxendolone	T38.5X1	T38.5X2	T38.5X3	T38.5X4	T38.5X5	T38.5X6
Oxetacaine	T41.3X1	T41.3X2	T41.3X3	T41.3X4	T41.3X5	T41.3X6
Oxethazine	T41.3X1	T41.3X2	T41.3X3	T41.3X4	T41.3X5	T41.3X6
Oxetorone	T39.8X1	T39.8X2	T39.8X3	T39.8X4	T39.8X5	T39.8X6
Oxiconazole	T49.ØX1	T49.ØX2	T49.ØX3	T49.ØX4	T49.ØX5	T49.ØX6
Oxidizing agent NEC	T54.91	T54.92	T54.93	T54.94	—	—
Oxipurinol	T5Ø.4X1	T5Ø.4X2	T5Ø.4X3	T5Ø.4X4	T5Ø.4X5	T5Ø.4X6
Oxitriptan	T43.291	T43.292	T43.293	T43.294	T43.295	T43.296
Oxitropium bromide	T48.6X1	T48.6X2	T48.6X3	T48.6X4	T48.6X5	T48.6X6
Oxodipine	T46.1X1	T46.1X2	T46.1X3	T46.1X4	T46.1X5	T46.1X6
Oxolamine	T48.3X1	T48.3X2	T48.3X3	T48.3X4	T48.3X5	T48.3X6
Oxolinic acid	T37.8X1	T37.8X2	T37.8X3	T37.8X4	T37.8X5	T37.8X6
Oxomemazine	T43.3X1	T43.3X2	T43.3X3	T43.3X4	T43.3X5	T43.3X6
Oxophenarsine	T37.3X1	T37.3X2	T37.3X3	T37.3X4	T37.3X5	T37.3X6
Oxprenolol	T44.7X1	T44.7X2	T44.7X3	T44.7X4	T44.7X5	T44.7X6
Oxsoralen	T49.3X1	T49.3X2	T49.3X3	T49.3X4	T49.3X5	T49.3X6
Oxtriphylline	T48.6X1	T48.6X2	T48.6X3	T48.6X4	T48.6X5	T48.6X6
Oxybate sodium	T41.291	T41.292	T41.293	T41.294	T41.295	T41.296
Oxybuprocaine	T41.3X1	T41.3X2	T41.3X3	T41.3X4	T41.3X5	T41.3X6
Oxybutynin	T44.3X1	T44.3X2	T44.3X3	T44.3X4	T44.3X5	T44.3X6
Oxychlorosene	T49.ØX1	T49.ØX2	T49.ØX3	T49.ØX4	T49.ØX5	T49.ØX6
Oxycodone	T4Ø.2X1	T4Ø.2X2	T4Ø.2X3	T4Ø.2X4	T4Ø.2X5	T4Ø.2X6
OxyContin*	T4Ø.2X1	T4Ø.2X2	T4Ø.2X3	T4Ø.2X4	T4Ø.2X5	T4Ø.2X6
Oxyfedrine	T46.3X1	T46.3X2	T46.3X3	T46.3X4	T46.3X5	T46.3X6
Oxygen	T41.5X1	T41.5X2	T41.5X3	T41.5X4	T41.5X5	T41.5X6
Oxylone	T49.ØX1	T49.ØX2	T49.ØX3	T49.ØX4	T49.ØX5	T49.ØX6
ophthalmic preparation	T49.5X1	T49.5X2	T49.5X3	T49.5X4	T49.5X5	T49.5X6
Oxymesterone	T38.7X1	T38.7X2	T38.7X3	T38.7X4	T38.7X5	T38.7X6
Oxymetazoline	T48.5X1	T48.5X2	T48.5X3	T48.5X4	T48.5X5	T48.5X6
Oxymetholone	T38.7X1	T38.7X2	T38.7X3	T38.7X4	T38.7X5	T38.7X6
Oxymorphone	T4Ø.2X1	T4Ø.2X2	T4Ø.2X3	T4Ø.2X4	T4Ø.2X5	T4Ø.2X6
Oxypertine	T43.591	T43.592	T43.593	T43.594	T43.595	T43.596
Oxyphenbutazone	T39.2X1	T39.2X2	T39.2X3	T39.2X4	T39.2X5	T39.2X6
Oxyphencyclimine	T44.3X1	T44.3X2	T44.3X3	T44.3X4	T44.3X5	T44.3X6
Oxyphenisatine	T47.2X1	T47.2X2	T47.2X3	T47.2X4	T47.2X5	T47.2X6
Oxyphenonium bromide	T44.3X1	T44.3X2	T44.3X3	T44.3X4	T44.3X5	T44.3X6
Oxypolygelatin	T45.8X1	T45.8X2	T45.8X3	T45.8X4	T45.8X5	T45.8X6
Oxyquinoline (derivatives)	T37.8X1	T37.8X2	T37.8X3	T37.8X4	T37.8X5	T37.8X6
Oxytetracycline	T36.4X1	T36.4X2	T36.4X3	T36.4X4	T36.4X5	T36.4X6
Oxytocic drug NEC	T48.ØX1	T48.ØX2	T48.ØX3	T48.ØX4	T48.ØX5	T48.ØX6
Oxytocin (synthetic)	T48.ØX1	T48.ØX2	T48.ØX3	T48.ØX4	T48.ØX5	T48.ØX6
Oxytrol*	T44.3X1	T44.3X2	T44.3X3	T44.3X4	T44.3X5	T44.3X6
Ozone	T59.891	T59.892	T59.893	T59.894	—	—
PABA	T49.3X1	T49.3X2	T49.3X3	T49.3X4	T49.3X5	T49.3X6
Packed red cells	T45.8X1	T45.8X2	T45.8X3	T45.8X4	T45.8X5	T45.8X6
Padimate	T49.3X1	T49.3X2	T49.3X3	T49.3X4	T49.3X5	T49.3X6
Paint NEC	T65.6X1	T65.6X2	T65.6X3	T65.6X4	—	—
cleaner	T52.91	T52.92	T52.93	T52.94	—	—
fumes NEC	T59.891	T59.892	T59.893	T59.894	—	—
lead (fumes)	T56.ØX1	T56.ØX2	T56.ØX3	T56.ØX4	—	—
solvent NEC	T52.8X1	T52.8X2	T52.8X3	T52.8X4	—	—
stripper	T52.8X1	T52.8X2	T52.8X3	T52.8X4	—	—
Palfium	T4Ø.2X1	T4Ø.2X2	T4Ø.2X3	T4Ø.2X4	—	—
Palm kernel oil	T5Ø.991	T5Ø.992	T5Ø.993	T5Ø.994	T5Ø.995	T5Ø.996
Paludrine	T37.2X1	T37.2X2	T37.2X3	T37.2X4	T37.2X5	T37.2X6
PAM (pralidoxime)	T5Ø.6X1	T5Ø.6X2	T5Ø.6X3	T5Ø.6X4	T5Ø.6X5	T5Ø.6X6
Pamaquine (naphthoute)	T37.2X1	T37.2X2	T37.2X3	T37.2X4	T37.2X5	T37.2X6
Panadol	T39.1X1	T39.1X2	T39.1X3	T39.1X4	T39.1X5	T39.1X6
Pancreatic						
digestive secretion stimulant	T47.8X1	T47.8X2	T47.8X3	T47.8X4	T47.8X5	T47.8X6
dornase	T45.3X1	T45.3X2	T45.3X3	T45.3X4	T45.3X5	T45.3X6
Pancreatin	T47.5X1	T47.5X2	T47.5X3	T47.5X4	T47.5X5	T47.5X6
Pancrelipase	T47.5X1	T47.5X2	T47.5X3	T47.5X4	T47.5X5	T47.5X6
Pancuronium (bromide)	T48.1X1	T48.1X2	T48.1X3	T48.1X4	T48.1X5	T48.1X6
Pangamic acid	T45.2X1	T45.2X2	T45.2X3	T45.2X4	T45.2X5	T45.2X6
Panthenol	T45.2X1	T45.2X2	T45.2X3	T45.2X4	T45.2X5	T45.2X6
topical	T49.8X1	T49.8X2	T49.8X3	T49.8X4	T49.8X5	T49.8X6
Pantopon	T4Ø.ØX1	T4Ø.ØX2	T4Ø.ØX3	T4Ø.ØX4	T4Ø.ØX5	T4Ø.ØX6
Pantoprazole*	T47.1X1	T47.1X2	T47.1X3	T47.1X4	T47.1X5	T47.1X6
Pantothenic acid	T45.2X1	T45.2X2	T45.2X3	T45.2X4	T45.2X5	T45.2X6
Panwarfin	T45.511	T45.512	T45.513	T45.514	T45.515	T45.516
Papain	T47.5X1	T47.5X2	T47.5X3	T47.5X4	T47.5X5	T47.5X6
digestant	T47.5X1	T47.5X2	T47.5X3	T47.5X4	T47.5X5	T47.5X6
Papaveretum	T4Ø.ØX1	T4Ø.ØX2	T4Ø.ØX3	T4Ø.ØX4	T4Ø.ØX5	T4Ø.ØX6
Papaverine	T44.3X1	T44.3X2	T44.3X3	T44.3X4	T44.3X5	T44.3X6
Para-acetamidophenol	T39.1X1	T39.1X2	T39.1X3	T39.1X4	T39.1X5	T39.1X6
Para-aminobenzoic acid	T49.3X1	T49.3X2	T49.3X3	T49.3X4	T49.3X5	T49.3X6
Para-aminophenol derivatives	T39.1X1	T39.1X2	T39.1X3	T39.1X4	T39.1X5	T39.1X6
Para-aminosalicylic acid	T37.1X1	T37.1X2	T37.1X3	T37.1X4	T37.1X5	T37.1X6
Paracetaldehyde	T42.6X1	T42.6X2	T42.6X3	T42.6X4	T42.6X5	T42.6X6
Paracetamol	T39.1X1	T39.1X2	T39.1X3	T39.1X4	T39.1X5	T39.1X6
Parachlorophenol (camphorated)	T49.ØX1	T49.ØX2	T49.ØX3	T49.ØX4	T49.ØX5	T49.ØX6
Paracodin	T4Ø.2X1	T4Ø.2X2	T4Ø.2X3	T4Ø.2X4	T4Ø.2X5	T4Ø.2X6
Paradione	T42.2X1	T42.2X2	T42.2X3	T42.2X4	T42.2X5	T42.2X6
Paraffin(s) (wax)	T52.ØX1	T52.ØX2	T52.ØX3	T52.ØX4	—	—
liquid (medicinal)	T47.4X1	T47.4X2	T47.4X3	T47.4X4	T47.4X5	T47.4X6
nonmedicinal	T52.ØX1	T52.ØX2	T52.ØX3	T52.ØX4	—	—
Paraformaldehyde	T6Ø.3X1	T6Ø.3X2	T6Ø.3X3	T6Ø.3X4	—	—
Paraldehyde	T42.6X1	T42.6X2	T42.6X3	T42.6X4	T42.6X5	T42.6X6
Paramethadione	T42.2X1	T42.2X2	T42.2X3	T42.2X4	T42.2X5	T42.2X6
Paramethasone	T38.ØX1	T38.ØX2	T38.ØX3	T38.ØX4	T38.ØX5	T38.ØX6
acetate	T49.ØX1	T49.ØX2	T49.ØX3	T49.ØX4	T49.ØX5	T49.ØX6
Paraoxon	T6Ø.ØX1	T6Ø.ØX2	T6Ø.ØX3	T6Ø.ØX4	—	—
Paraquat	T6Ø.3X1	T6Ø.3X2	T6Ø.3X3	T6Ø.3X4	—	—
Parasympatholytic NEC	T44.3X1	T44.3X2	T44.3X3	T44.3X4	T44.3X5	T44.3X6
Parasympathomimetic drug NEC	T44.1X1	T44.1X2	T44.1X3	T44.1X4	T44.1X5	T44.1X6
Parathion	T6Ø.ØX1	T6Ø.ØX2	T6Ø.ØX3	T6Ø.ØX4	—	—
Parathormone	T5Ø.991	T5Ø.992	T5Ø.993	T5Ø.994	T5Ø.995	T5Ø.996
Parathyroid extract	T5Ø.991	T5Ø.992	T5Ø.993	T5Ø.994	T5Ø.995	T5Ø.996
Paratyphoid vaccine	T5Ø.A91	T5Ø.A92	T5Ø.A93	T5Ø.A94	T5Ø.A95	T5Ø.A96
Paredrine	T44.4X1	T44.4X2	T44.4X3	T44.4X4	T44.4X5	T44.4X6
Paregoric	T4Ø.ØX1	T4Ø.ØX2	T4Ø.ØX3	T4Ø.ØX4	T4Ø.ØX5	T4Ø.ØX6
Pargyline	T46.5X1	T46.5X2	T46.5X3	T46.5X4	T46.5X5	T46.5X6
Paris green	T57.ØX1	T57.ØX2	T57.ØX3	T57.ØX4	—	—
insecticide	T57.ØX1	T57.ØX2	T57.ØX3	T57.ØX4	—	—
Parnate	T43.1X1	T43.1X2	T43.1X3	T43.1X4	T43.1X5	T43.1X6
Paromomycin	T36.5X1	T36.5X2	T36.5X3	T36.5X4	T36.5X5	T36.5X6
Paroxypropione	T45.1X1	T45.1X2	T45.1X3	T45.1X4	T45.1X5	T45.1X6
Parsabiv*	T5Ø.991	T5Ø.992	T5Ø.993	T5Ø.994	T5Ø.995	T5Ø.996
Parzone	T4Ø.2X1	T4Ø.2X2	T4Ø.2X3	T4Ø.2X4	T4Ø.2X5	T4Ø.2X6
PAS	T37.1X1	T37.1X2	T37.1X3	T37.1X4	T37.1X5	T37.1X6
Pasiniazid	T37.1X1	T37.1X2	T37.1X3	T37.1X4	T37.1X5	T37.1X6
PBB (polybrominated biphenyls)	T65.891	T65.892	T65.893	T65.894	—	—
PCB	T65.891	T65.892	T65.893	T65.894	—	—
PCP						
meaning pentachlorophenol	T6Ø.1X1	T6Ø.1X2	T6Ø.1X3	T6Ø.1X4	—	—
fungicide	T6Ø.3X1	T6Ø.3X2	T6Ø.3X3	T6Ø.3X4	—	—
herbicide	T6Ø.3X1	T6Ø.3X2	T6Ø.3X3	T6Ø.3X4	—	—
insecticide	T6Ø.1X1	T6Ø.1X2	T6Ø.1X3	T6Ø.1X4	—	—
meaning phencyclidine	T4Ø.991	T4Ø.992	T4Ø.993	T4Ø.994	—	—
Peach kernel oil (emulsion)	T47.4X1	T47.4X2	T47.4X3	T47.4X4	T47.4X5	T47.4X6
Peanut oil (emulsion) **NEC**	T47.4X1	T47.4X2	T47.4X3	T47.4X4	T47.4X5	T47.4X6

Substance	Poisoning, Accidental (unintentional)	Poisoning, Intentional Self-harm	Poisoning, Assault	Poisoning, Undetermined	Adverse Effect	Under-dosing
Peanut oil (emulsion) **NEC** — *continued*						
topical	T49.3X1	T49.3X2	T49.3X3	T49.3X4	T49.3X5	T49.3X6
Pearly Gates (morning glory seeds)	T4Ø.991	T4Ø.992	T4Ø.993	T4Ø.994	—	—
Pecazine	T43.3X1	T43.3X2	T43.3X3	T43.3X4	T43.3X5	T43.3X6
Pectin	T47.6X1	T47.6X2	T47.6X3	T47.6X4	T47.6X5	T47.6X6
Pediaflor*	T49.7X1	T49.7X2	T49.7X3	T49.7X4	T49.7X5	T49.7X6
Pefloxacin	T37.8X1	T37.8X2	T37.8X3	T37.8X4	T37.8X5	T37.8X6
Pegademase, bovine	T5Ø.Z91	T5Ø.Z92	T5Ø.Z93	T5Ø.Z94	T5Ø.Z95	T5Ø.Z96
Pelletierine tannate	T37.4X1	T37.4X2	T37.4X3	T37.4X4	T37.4X5	T37.4X6
Pemirolast (potassium)	T48.6X1	T48.6X2	T48.6X3	T48.6X4	T48.6X5	T48.6X6
Pemoline	T5Ø.7X1	T5Ø.7X2	T5Ø.7X3	T5Ø.7X4	T5Ø.7X5	T5Ø.7X6
Pempidine	T44.2X1	T44.2X2	T44.2X3	T44.2X4	T44.2X5	T44.2X6
Penamecillin	T36.ØX1	T36.ØX2	T36.ØX3	T36.ØX4	T36.ØX5	T36.ØX6
Penbutolol	T44.7X1	T44.7X2	T44.7X3	T44.7X4	T44.7X5	T44.7X6
Penethamate	T36.ØX1	T36.ØX2	T36.ØX3	T36.ØX4	T36.ØX5	T36.ØX6
Penfluridol	T43.591	T43.592	T43.593	T43.594	T43.595	T43.596
Penflutizide	T5Ø.2X1	T5Ø.2X2	T5Ø.2X3	T5Ø.2X4	T5Ø.2X5	T5Ø.2X6
Pengitoxin	T46.ØX1	T46.ØX2	T46.ØX3	T46.ØX4	T46.ØX5	T46.ØX6
Penicillamine	T5Ø.6X1	T5Ø.6X2	T5Ø.6X3	T5Ø.6X4	T5Ø.6X5	T5Ø.6X6
Penicillin (any)	T36.ØX1	T36.ØX2	T36.ØX3	T36.ØX4	T36.ØX5	T36.ØX6
Penicillinase	T45.3X1	T45.3X2	T45.3X3	T45.3X4	T45.3X5	T45.3X6
Penicilloyl polylysine	T5Ø.8X1	T5Ø.8X2	T5Ø.8X3	T5Ø.8X4	T5Ø.8X5	T5Ø.8X6
Penimepicycline	T36.4X1	T36.4X2	T36.4X3	T36.4X4	T36.4X5	T36.4X6
Pentacel*	T5Ø.A11	T5Ø.A12	T5Ø.A13	T5Ø.A14	T5Ø.A15	T5Ø.A16
Pentachloroethane	T53.6X1	T53.6X2	T53.6X3	T53.6X4	—	—
Pentachloronaphthalene	T53.7X1	T53.7X2	T53.7X3	T53.7X4	—	—
Pentachlorophenol (pesticide)	T6Ø.1X1	T6Ø.1X2	T6Ø.1X3	T6Ø.1X4	—	—
fungicide	T6Ø.3X1	T6Ø.3X2	T6Ø.3X3	T6Ø.3X4	—	—
herbicide	T6Ø.3X1	T6Ø.3X2	T6Ø.3X3	T6Ø.3X4	—	—
insecticide	T6Ø.1X1	T6Ø.1X2	T6Ø.1X3	T6Ø.1X4	—	—
Pentaerythritol	T46.3X1	T46.3X2	T46.3X3	T46.3X4	T46.3X5	T46.3X6
chloral	T42.6X1	T42.6X2	T42.6X3	T42.6X4	T42.6X5	T42.6X6
tetranitrate NEC	T46.3X1	T46.3X2	T46.3X3	T46.3X4	T46.3X5	T46.3X6
Pentaerythrityl tetranitrate	T46.3X1	T46.3X2	T46.3X3	T46.3X4	T46.3X5	T46.3X6
Pentagastrin	T5Ø.8X1	T5Ø.8X2	T5Ø.8X3	T5Ø.8X4	T5Ø.8X5	T5Ø.8X6
Pentalin	T53.6X1	T53.6X2	T53.6X3	T53.6X4	—	—
Pentamethonium bromide	T44.2X1	T44.2X2	T44.2X3	T44.2X4	T44.2X5	T44.2X6
Pentamidine	T37.3X1	T37.3X2	T37.3X3	T37.3X4	T37.3X5	T37.3X6
Pentanol	T51.3X1	T51.3X2	T51.3X3	T51.3X4	—	—
Pentapyrrolinium (bitartrate)	T44.2X1	T44.2X2	T44.2X3	T44.2X4	T44.2X5	T44.2X6
Pentaquine	T37.2X1	T37.2X2	T37.2X3	T37.2X4	T37.2X5	T37.2X6
Pentazocine	T4Ø.491	T4Ø.492	T4Ø.493	T4Ø.494	T4Ø.495	T4Ø.496
Pentetrazole	T5Ø.7X1	T5Ø.7X2	T5Ø.7X3	T5Ø.7X4	T5Ø.7X5	T5Ø.7X6
Penthienate bromide	T44.3X1	T44.3X2	T44.3X3	T44.3X4	T44.3X5	T44.3X6
Pentifylline	T46.7X1	T46.7X2	T46.7X3	T46.7X4	T46.7X5	T46.7X6
Pentobarbital	T42.3X1	T42.3X2	T42.3X3	T42.3X4	T42.3X5	T42.3X6
sodium	T42.3X1	T42.3X2	T42.3X3	T42.3X4	T42.3X5	T42.3X6
Pentobarbitone	T42.3X1	T42.3X2	T42.3X3	T42.3X4	T42.3X5	T42.3X6
Pentolonium tartrate	T44.2X1	T44.2X2	T44.2X3	T44.2X4	T44.2X5	T44.2X6
Pentosan polysulfate (sodium)	T39.8X1	T39.8X2	T39.8X3	T39.8X4	T39.8X5	T39.8X6
Pentostatin	T45.1X1	T45.1X2	T45.1X3	T45.1X4	T45.1X5	T45.1X6
Pentothal	T41.1X1	T41.1X2	T41.1X3	T41.1X4	T41.1X5	T41.1X6
Pentoxifylline	T46.7X1	T46.7X2	T46.7X3	T46.7X4	T46.7X5	T46.7X6
Pentoxyverine	T48.3X1	T48.3X2	T48.3X3	T48.3X4	T48.3X5	T48.3X6
Pentrinat	T46.3X1	T46.3X2	T46.3X3	T46.3X4	T46.3X5	T46.3X6
Pentylenetetrazole	T5Ø.7X1	T5Ø.7X2	T5Ø.7X3	T5Ø.7X4	T5Ø.7X5	T5Ø.7X6
Pentylsalicylamide	T37.1X1	T37.1X2	T37.1X3	T37.1X4	T37.1X5	T37.1X6
Pentymal	T42.3X1	T42.3X2	T42.3X3	T42.3X4	T42.3X5	T42.3X6
Pepcid*	T47.ØX1	T47.ØX2	T47.ØX3	T47.ØX4	T47.ØX5	T47.ØX6
Peplomycin	T45.1X1	T45.1X2	T45.1X3	T45.1X4	T45.1X5	T45.1X6
Peppermint (oil)	T47.5X1	T47.5X2	T47.5X3	T47.5X4	T47.5X5	T47.5X6
Pepsin	T47.5X1	T47.5X2	T47.5X3	T47.5X4	T47.5X5	T47.5X6
digestant	T47.5X1	T47.5X2	T47.5X3	T47.5X4	T47.5X5	T47.5X6
Pepstatin	T47.1X1	T47.1X2	T47.1X3	T47.1X4	T47.1X5	T47.1X6
Peptavlon	T5Ø.8X1	T5Ø.8X2	T5Ø.8X3	T5Ø.8X4	T5Ø.8X5	T5Ø.8X6
Perazine	T43.3X1	T43.3X2	T43.3X3	T43.3X4	T43.3X5	T43.3X6
Percaine (spinal)	T41.3X1	T41.3X2	T41.3X3	T41.3X4	T41.3X5	T41.3X6
topical (surface)	T41.3X1	T41.3X2	T41.3X3	T41.3X4	T41.3X5	T41.3X6
Perchloroethylene	T53.3X1	T53.3X2	T53.3X3	T53.3X4	—	—
medicinal	T37.4X1	T37.4X2	T37.4X3	T37.4X4	T37.4X5	T37.4X6
vapor	T53.3X1	T53.3X2	T53.3X3	T53.3X4	—	—
Percodan	T4Ø.2X1	T4Ø.2X2	T4Ø.2X3	T4Ø.2X4	T4Ø.2X5	T4Ø.2X6
Percogesic — *see also* acetaminophen	T45.ØX1	T45.ØX2	T45.ØX3	T45.ØX4	T45.ØX5	T45.ØX6
Percorten	T38.ØX1	T38.ØX2	T38.ØX3	T38.ØX4	T38.ØX5	T38.ØX6
Pergolide	T42.8X1	T42.8X2	T42.8X3	T42.8X4	T42.8X5	T42.8X6
Pergonal	T38.811	T38.812	T38.813	T38.814	T38.815	T38.816

Substance	Poisoning, Accidental (unintentional)	Poisoning, Intentional Self-harm	Poisoning, Assault	Poisoning, Undetermined	Adverse Effect	Under-dosing
Perhexilene	T46.3X1	T46.3X2	T46.3X3	T46.3X4	T46.3X5	T46.3X6
Perhexiline (maleate)	T46.3X1	T46.3X2	T46.3X3	T46.3X4	T46.3X5	T46.3X6
Periactin	T45.ØX1	T45.ØX2	T45.ØX3	T45.ØX4	T45.ØX5	T45.ØX6
Periciazine	T43.3X1	T43.3X2	T43.3X3	T43.3X4	T43.3X5	T43.3X6
Periclor	T42.6X1	T42.6X2	T42.6X3	T42.6X4	T42.6X5	T42.6X6
Perindopril	T46.4X1	T46.4X2	T46.4X3	T46.4X4	T46.4X5	T46.4X6
Perisoxal	T39.8X1	T39.8X2	T39.8X3	T39.8X4	T39.8X5	T39.8X6
Peritoneal dialysis solution	T5Ø.3X1	T5Ø.3X2	T5Ø.3X3	T5Ø.3X4	T5Ø.3X5	T5Ø.3X6
Peritrate	T46.3X1	T46.3X2	T46.3X3	T46.3X4	T46.3X5	T46.3X6
Perlapine	T42.4X1	T42.4X2	T42.4X3	T42.4X4	T42.4X5	T42.4X6
Permanganate	T65.891	T65.892	T65.893	T65.894	—	—
Permapen*	T36.ØX1	T36.ØX2	T36.ØX3	T36.ØX4	T36.ØX5	T36.ØX6
Permethrin	T6Ø.1X1	T6Ø.1X2	T6Ø.1X3	T6Ø.1X4	—	—
Pernocton	T42.3X1	T42.3X2	T42.3X3	T42.3X4	T42.3X5	T42.3X6
Pernoston	T42.3X1	T42.3X2	T42.3X3	T42.3X4	T42.3X5	T42.3X6
Peronine	T4Ø.2X1	T4Ø.2X2	T4Ø.2X3	T4Ø.2X4	—	—
Perphenazine	T43.3X1	T43.3X2	T43.3X3	T43.3X4	T43.3X5	T43.3X6
Pertofrane	T43.Ø11	T43.Ø12	T43.Ø13	T43.Ø14	T43.Ø15	T43.Ø16
Pertussis						
immune serum (human)	T5Ø.Z11	T5Ø.Z12	T5Ø.Z13	T5Ø.Z14	T5Ø.Z15	T5Ø.Z16
vaccine (with diphtheria toxoid) (with tetanus toxoid)	T5Ø.A11	T5Ø.A12	T5Ø.A13	T5Ø.A14	T5Ø.A15	T5Ø.A16
Peruvian balsam	T49.ØX1	T49.ØX2	T49.ØX3	T49.ØX4	T49.ØX5	T49.ØX6
Peruvoside	T46.ØX1	T46.ØX2	T46.ØX3	T46.ØX4	T46.ØX5	T46.ØX6
Pesticide (dust) (fumes) (vapor) **NEC**	T6Ø.91	T6Ø.92	T6Ø.93	T6Ø.94	—	—
arsenic	T57.ØX1	T57.ØX2	T57.ØX3	T57.ØX4	—	—
chlorinated	T6Ø.1X1	T6Ø.1X2	T6Ø.1X3	T6Ø.1X4	—	—
cyanide	T65.ØX1	T65.ØX2	T65.ØX3	T65.ØX4	—	—
kerosene	T52.ØX1	T52.ØX2	T52.ØX3	T52.ØX4	—	—
mixture (of compounds)	T6Ø.91	T6Ø.92	T6Ø.93	T6Ø.94	—	—
naphthalene	T6Ø.2X1	T6Ø.2X2	T6Ø.2X3	T6Ø.2X4	—	—
organochlorine (compounds)	T6Ø.1X1	T6Ø.1X2	T6Ø.1X3	T6Ø.1X4	—	—
petroleum (distillate) (products) NEC	T6Ø.8X1	T6Ø.8X2	T6Ø.8X3	T6Ø.8X4	—	—
specified ingredient NEC	T6Ø.8X1	T6Ø.8X2	T6Ø.8X3	T6Ø.8X4	—	—
strychnine	T65.1X1	T65.1X2	T65.1X3	T65.1X4	—	—
thallium	T6Ø.4X1	T6Ø.4X2	T6Ø.4X3	T6Ø.4X4	—	—
Pethidine	T4Ø.491	T4Ø.492	T4Ø.493	T4Ø.494	T4Ø.495	T4Ø.496
Petrichloral	T42.6X1	T42.6X2	T42.6X3	T42.6X4	T42.6X5	T42.6X6
Petrol	T52.ØX1	T52.ØX2	T52.ØX3	T52.ØX4	—	—
vapor	T52.ØX1	T52.ØX2	T52.ØX3	T52.ØX4	—	—
Petrolatum	T49.3X1	T49.3X2	T49.3X3	T49.3X4	T49.3X5	T49.3X6
hydrophilic	T49.3X1	T49.3X2	T49.3X3	T49.3X4	T49.3X5	T49.3X6
liquid	T47.4X1	T47.4X2	T47.4X3	T47.4X4	T47.4X5	T47.4X6
topical	T49.3X1	T49.3X2	T49.3X3	T49.3X4	T49.3X5	T49.3X6
nonmedicinal	T52.ØX1	T52.ØX2	T52.ØX3	T52.ØX4	—	—
red veterinary	T49.3X1	T49.3X2	T49.3X3	T49.3X4	T49.3X5	T49.3X6
white	T49.3X1	T49.3X2	T49.3X3	T49.3X4	T49.3X5	T49.3X6
Petroleum (products) **NEC**	T52.ØX1	T52.ØX2	T52.ØX3	T52.ØX4	—	—
benzine(s) — *see* Ligroin						
ether — *see* Ligroin						
jelly — *see* Petrolatum						
naphtha — *see* Ligroin						
pesticide	T6Ø.8X1	T6Ø.8X2	T6Ø.8X3	T6Ø.8X4	—	—
solids	T52.ØX1	T52.ØX2	T52.ØX3	T52.ØX4	—	—
solvents	T52.ØX1	T52.ØX2	T52.ØX3	T52.ØX4	—	—
vapor	T52.ØX1	T52.ØX2	T52.ØX3	T52.ØX4	—	—
Peyote	T4Ø.991	T4Ø.992	T4Ø.993	T4Ø.994	—	—
Phanodorm, phanodorn	T42.3X1	T42.3X2	T42.3X3	T42.3X4	T42.3X5	T42.3X6
Phanquinone	T37.3X1	T37.3X2	T37.3X3	T37.3X4	T37.3X5	T37.3X6
Phanquone	T37.3X1	T37.3X2	T37.3X3	T37.3X4	T37.3X5	T37.3X6
Pharmaceutical						
adjunct NEC	T5Ø.9Ø1	T5Ø.9Ø2	T5Ø.9Ø3	T5Ø.9Ø4	T5Ø.9Ø5	T5Ø.9Ø6
excipient NEC	T5Ø.9Ø1	T5Ø.9Ø2	T5Ø.9Ø3	T5Ø.9Ø4	T5Ø.9Ø5	T5Ø.9Ø6
sweetener	T5Ø.9Ø1	T5Ø.9Ø2	T5Ø.9Ø3	T5Ø.9Ø4	T5Ø.9Ø5	T5Ø.9Ø6
viscous agent	T5Ø.9Ø1	T5Ø.9Ø2	T5Ø.9Ø3	T5Ø.9Ø4	T5Ø.9Ø5	T5Ø.9Ø6
Phazyme*	T47.1X1	T47.1X2	T47.1X3	T47.1X4	T47.1X5	T47.1X6
Phemitone	T42.3X1	T42.3X2	T42.3X3	T42.3X4	T42.3X5	T42.3X6
Phenacaine	T41.3X1	T41.3X2	T41.3X3	T41.3X4	T41.3X5	T41.3X6
Phenacemide	T42.6X1	T42.6X2	T42.6X3	T42.6X4	T42.6X5	T42.6X6
Phenacetin	T39.1X1	T39.1X2	T39.1X3	T39.1X4	T39.1X5	T39.1X6
Phenadoxone	T4Ø.2X1	T4Ø.2X2	T4Ø.2X3	T4Ø.2X4	—	—
Phenaglycodol	T43.591	T43.592	T43.593	T43.594	T43.595	T43.596
Phenantoin	T42.ØX1	T42.ØX2	T42.ØX3	T42.ØX4	T42.ØX5	T42.ØX6
Phenaphthazine reagent	T5Ø.991	T5Ø.992	T5Ø.993	T5Ø.994	T5Ø.995	T5Ø.996
Phenazocine	T4Ø.491	T4Ø.492	T4Ø.493	T4Ø.494	T4Ø.495	T4Ø.496
Phenazone	T39.2X1	T39.2X2	T39.2X3	T39.2X4	T39.2X5	T39.2X6
Phenazopyridine	T39.8X1	T39.8X2	T39.8X3	T39.8X4	T39.8X5	T39.8X6
Phenbenicillin	T36.ØX1	T36.ØX2	T36.ØX3	T36.ØX4	T36.ØX5	T36.ØX6
Phenbutrazate	T5Ø.5X1	T5Ø.5X2	T5Ø.5X3	T5Ø.5X4	T5Ø.5X5	T5Ø.5X6

Substance	Poisoning, Accidental (unintentional)	Poisoning, Intentional Self-harm	Poisoning, Assault	Poisoning, Undetermined	Adverse Effect	Under-dosing
Phencyclidine	T4Ø.991	T4Ø.992	T4Ø.993	T4Ø.994	T4Ø.995	T4Ø.996
Phendimetrazine	T5Ø.5X1	T5Ø.5X2	T5Ø.5X3	T5Ø.5X4	T5Ø.5X5	T5Ø.5X6
Phenelzine	T43.1X1	T43.1X2	T43.1X3	T43.1X4	T43.1X5	T43.1X6
Phenemal	T42.3X1	T42.3X2	T42.3X3	T42.3X4	T42.3X5	T42.3X6
Phenergan	T42.6X1	T42.6X2	T42.6X3	T42.6X4	T42.6X5	T42.6X6
Pheneticillin	T36.ØX1	T36.ØX2	T36.ØX3	T36.ØX4	T36.ØX5	T36.ØX6
Pheneturide	T42.6X1	T42.6X2	T42.6X3	T42.6X4	T42.6X5	T42.6X6
Phenformin	T38.3X1	T38.3X2	T38.3X3	T38.3X4	T38.3X5	T38.3X6
Phenglutarimide	T44.3X1	T44.3X2	T44.3X3	T44.3X4	T44.3X5	T44.3X6
Phenicarbazide	T39.8X1	T39.8X2	T39.8X3	T39.8X4	T39.8X5	T39.8X6
Phenindamine	T45.ØX1	T45.ØX2	T45.ØX3	T45.ØX4	T45.ØX5	T45.ØX6
Phenindione	T45.511	T45.512	T45.513	T45.514	T45.515	T45.516
Pheniprazine	T43.1X1	T43.1X2	T43.1X3	T43.1X4	T43.1X5	T43.1X6
Pheniramine	T45.ØX1	T45.ØX2	T45.ØX3	T45.ØX4	T45.ØX5	T45.ØX6
Phenisatin	T47.2X1	T47.2X2	T47.2X3	T47.2X4	T47.2X5	T47.2X6
Phenmetrazine	T5Ø.5X1	T5Ø.5X2	T5Ø.5X3	T5Ø.5X4	T5Ø.5X5	T5Ø.5X6
Phenobal	T42.3X1	T42.3X2	T42.3X3	T42.3X4	T42.3X5	T42.3X6
Phenobarbital	T42.3X1	T42.3X2	T42.3X3	T42.3X4	T42.3X5	T42.3X6
with						
mephenytoin	T42.3X1	T42.3X2	T42.3X3	T42.3X4	T42.3X5	T42.3X6
phenytoin	T42.3X1	T42.3X2	T42.3X3	T42.3X4	T42.3X5	T42.3X6
sodium	T42.3X1	T42.3X2	T42.3X3	T42.3X4	T42.3X5	T42.3X6
Phenobarbitone	T42.3X1	T42.3X2	T42.3X3	T42.3X4	T42.3X5	T42.3X6
Phenobutiodil	T5Ø.8X1	T5Ø.8X2	T5Ø.8X3	T5Ø.8X4	T5Ø.8X5	T5Ø.8X6
Phenoctide	T49.ØX1	T49.ØX2	T49.ØX3	T49.ØX4	T49.ØX5	T49.ØX6
Phenol	T49.ØX1	T49.ØX2	T49.ØX3	T49.ØX4	T49.ØX5	T49.ØX6
disinfectant	T54.ØX1	T54.ØX2	T54.ØX3	T54.ØX4	—	—
in oil injection	T46.8X1	T46.8X2	T46.8X3	T46.8X4	T46.8X5	T46.8X6
medicinal	T49.1X1	T49.1X2	T49.1X3	T49.1X4	T49.1X5	T49.1X6
nonmedicinal NEC	T54.ØX1	T54.ØX2	T54.ØX3	T54.ØX4	—	—
pesticide	T6Ø.8X1	T6Ø.8X2	T6Ø.8X3	T6Ø.8X4	—	—
red	T5Ø.8X1	T5Ø.8X2	T5Ø.8X3	T5Ø.8X4	T5Ø.8X5	T5Ø.8X6
Phenolic preparation	T49.1X1	T49.1X2	T49.1X3	T49.1X4	T49.1X5	T49.1X6
Phenolphthalein	T47.2X1	T47.2X2	T47.2X3	T47.2X4	T47.2X5	T47.2X6
Phenolsulfonphthalein	T5Ø.8X1	T5Ø.8X2	T5Ø.8X3	T5Ø.8X4	T5Ø.8X5	T5Ø.8X6
Phenomorphan	T4Ø.2X1	T4Ø.2X2	T4Ø.2X3	T4Ø.2X4	—	—
Phenonyl	T42.3X1	T42.3X2	T42.3X3	T42.3X4	T42.3X5	T42.3X6
Phenoperidine	T4Ø.491	T4Ø.492	T4Ø.493	T4Ø.494	—	—
Phenopyrazone	T46.991	T46.992	T46.993	T46.994	T46.995	T46.996
Phenoquin	T5Ø.4X1	T5Ø.4X2	T5Ø.4X3	T5Ø.4X4	T5Ø.4X5	T5Ø.4X6
Phenothiazine (psychotropic) **NEC**	T43.3X1	T43.3X2	T43.3X3	T43.3X4	T43.3X5	T43.3X6
insecticide	T6Ø.2X1	T6Ø.2X2	T6Ø.2X3	T6Ø.2X4	—	—
Phenothrin	T49.ØX1	T49.ØX2	T49.ØX3	T49.ØX4	T49.ØX5	T49.ØX6
Phenoxybenzamine	T46.7X1	T46.7X2	T46.7X3	T46.7X4	T46.7X5	T46.7X6
Phenoxyethanol	T49.ØX1	T49.ØX2	T49.ØX3	T49.ØX4	T49.ØX5	T49.ØX6
Phenoxymethyl penicillin	T36.ØX1	T36.ØX2	T36.ØX3	T36.ØX4	T36.ØX5	T36.ØX6
Phenprobamate	T42.8X1	T42.8X2	T42.8X3	T42.8X4	T42.8X5	T42.8X6
Phenprocoumon	T45.511	T45.512	T45.513	T45.514	T45.515	T45.516
Phensuximide	T42.2X1	T42.2X2	T42.2X3	T42.2X4	T42.2X5	T42.2X6
Phentermine	T5Ø.5X1	T5Ø.5X2	T5Ø.5X3	T5Ø.5X4	T5Ø.5X5	T5Ø.5X6
Phenthicillin	T36.ØX1	T36.ØX2	T36.ØX3	T36.ØX4	T36.ØX5	T36.ØX6
Phentolamine	T46.7X1	T46.7X2	T46.7X3	T46.7X4	T46.7X5	T46.7X6
Phenyl						
butazone	T39.2X1	T39.2X2	T39.2X3	T39.2X4	T39.2X5	T39.2X6
enediamine	T65.3X1	T65.3X2	T65.3X3	T65.3X4	—	—
hydrazine	T65.3X1	T65.3X2	T65.3X3	T65.3X4	—	—
antineoplastic	T45.1X1	T45.1X2	T45.1X3	T45.1X4	T45.1X5	T45.1X6
mercuric compounds — *see* Mercury						
salicylate	T49.3X1	T49.3X2	T49.3X3	T49.3X4	T49.3X5	T49.3X6
Phenylalanine mustard	T45.1X1	T45.1X2	T45.1X3	T45.1X4	T45.1X5	T45.1X6
Phenylbutazone	T39.2X1	T39.2X2	T39.2X3	T39.2X4	T39.2X5	T39.2X6
Phenylenediamine	T65.3X1	T65.3X2	T65.3X3	T65.3X4	—	—
Phenylephrine	T44.4X1	T44.4X2	T44.4X3	T44.4X4	T44.4X5	T44.4X6
Phenylethylbiguanide	T38.3X1	T38.3X2	T38.3X3	T38.3X4	T38.3X5	T38.3X6
Phenylmercuric						
acetate	T49.ØX1	T49.ØX2	T49.ØX3	T49.ØX4	T49.ØX5	T49.ØX6
borate	T49.ØX1	T49.ØX2	T49.ØX3	T49.ØX4	T49.ØX5	T49.ØX6
nitrate	T49.ØX1	T49.ØX2	T49.ØX3	T49.ØX4	T49.ØX5	T49.ØX6
Phenylmethylbarbitone	T42.3X1	T42.3X2	T42.3X3	T42.3X4	T42.3X5	T42.3X6
Phenylpropanol	T47.5X1	T47.5X2	T47.5X3	T47.5X4	T47.5X5	T47.5X6
Phenylpropanolamine	T44.991	T44.992	T44.993	T44.994	T44.995	T44.996
Phenylsulfthion	T6Ø.ØX1	T6Ø.ØX2	T6Ø.ØX3	T6Ø.ØX4	—	—
Phenyltoloxamine	T45.ØX1	T45.ØX2	T45.ØX3	T45.ØX4	T45.ØX5	T45.ØX6
Phenyramidol, phenyramidon	T39.8X1	T39.8X2	T39.8X3	T39.8X4	T39.8X5	T39.8X6
Phenytek*	T42.ØX1	T42.ØX2	T42.ØX3	T42.ØX4	T42.ØX5	T42.ØX6
Phenytoin	T42.ØX1	T42.ØX2	T42.ØX3	T42.ØX4	T42.ØX5	T42.ØX6
with Phenobarbital	T42.3X1	T42.3X2	T42.3X3	T42.3X4	T42.3X5	T42.3X6
pHisoHex	T49.2X1	T49.2X2	T49.2X3	T49.2X4	T49.2X5	T49.2X6
Pholcodine	T48.3X1	T48.3X2	T48.3X3	T48.3X4	T48.3X5	T48.3X6
Pholedrine	T46.991	T46.992	T46.993	T46.994	T46.995	T46.996

Substance	Poisoning, Accidental (unintentional)	Poisoning, Intentional Self-harm	Poisoning, Assault	Poisoning, Undetermined	Adverse Effect	Under-dosing
Phorate	T6Ø.ØX1	T6Ø.ØX2	T6Ø.ØX3	T6Ø.ØX4	—	—
Phosdrin	T6Ø.ØX1	T6Ø.ØX2	T6Ø.ØX3	T6Ø.ØX4	—	—
Phosfolan	T6Ø.ØX1	T6Ø.ØX2	T6Ø.ØX3	T6Ø.ØX4	—	—
Phosgene (gas)	T59.891	T59.892	T59.893	T59.894	—	—
Phosphamidon	T6Ø.ØX1	T6Ø.ØX2	T6Ø.ØX3	T6Ø.ØX4	—	—
Phosphate	T65.891	T65.892	T65.893	T65.894	—	—
laxative	T47.4X1	T47.4X2	T47.4X3	T47.4X4	T47.4X5	T47.4X6
organic	T6Ø.ØX1	T6Ø.ØX2	T6Ø.ØX3	T6Ø.ØX4	—	—
solvent	T52.91	T52.92	T52.93	T52.94	—	—
tricresyl	T65.891	T65.892	T65.893	T65.894	—	—
Phosphine	T57.1X1	T57.1X2	T57.1X3	T57.1X4	—	—
fumigant	T57.1X1	T57.1X2	T57.1X3	T57.1X4	—	—
Phospholine	T49.5X1	T49.5X2	T49.5X3	T49.5X4	T49.5X5	T49.5X6
Phosphoric acid	T54.2X1	T54.2X2	T54.2X3	T54.2X4	—	—
Phosphorus (compound) **NEC**	T57.1X1	T57.1X2	T57.1X3	T57.1X4	—	—
pesticide	T6Ø.ØX1	T6Ø.ØX2	T6Ø.ØX3	T6Ø.ØX4	—	—
Photrexa*	T49.5X1	T49.5X2	T49.5X3	T49.5X4	T49.5X5	T49.5X6
Phthalates	T65.891	T65.892	T65.893	T65.894	—	—
Phthalic anhydride	T65.891	T65.892	T65.893	T65.894	—	—
Phthalimidoglutarimide	T42.6X1	T42.6X2	T42.6X3	T42.6X4	T42.6X5	T42.6X6
Phthalylsulfathiazole	T37.ØX1	T37.ØX2	T37.ØX3	T37.ØX4	T37.ØX5	T37.ØX6
Phylloquinone	T45.7X1	T45.7X2	T45.7X3	T45.7X4	T45.7X5	T45.7X6
Physeptone	T4Ø.3X1	T4Ø.3X2	T4Ø.3X3	T4Ø.3X4	T4Ø.3X5	T4Ø.3X6
Physostigma venenosum	T62.2X1	T62.2X2	T62.2X3	T62.2X4	—	—
Physostigmine	T49.5X1	T49.5X2	T49.5X3	T49.5X4	T49.5X5	T49.5X6
Phytolacca decandra	T62.2X1	T62.2X2	T62.2X3	T62.2X4	—	—
berries	T62.1X1	T62.1X2	T62.1X3	T62.1X4	—	—
Phytomenadione	T45.7X1	T45.7X2	T45.7X3	T45.7X4	T45.7X5	T45.7X6
Phytonadione	T45.7X1	T45.7X2	T45.7X3	T45.7X4	T45.7X5	T45.7X6
Picoperine	T48.3X1	T48.3X2	T48.3X3	T48.3X4	T48.3X5	T48.3X6
Picosulfate (sodium)	T47.2X1	T47.2X2	T47.2X3	T47.2X4	T47.2X5	T47.2X6
Picric (acid)	T54.2X1	T54.2X2	T54.2X3	T54.2X4	—	—
Picrotoxin	T5Ø.7X1	T5Ø.7X2	T5Ø.7X3	T5Ø.7X4	T5Ø.7X5	T5Ø.7X6
Piketoprofen	T49.ØX1	T49.ØX2	T49.ØX3	T49.ØX4	T49.ØX5	T49.ØX6
Pilocarpine	T44.1X1	T44.1X2	T44.1X3	T44.1X4	T44.1X5	T44.1X6
Pilocarpus (jaborandi) extract	T44.1X1	T44.1X2	T44.1X3	T44.1X4	T44.1X5	T44.1X6
Pilsicainide (hydrochloride)	T46.2X1	T46.2X2	T46.2X3	T46.2X4	T46.2X5	T46.2X6
Pimaricin	T36.7X1	T36.7X2	T36.7X3	T36.7X4	T36.7X5	T36.7X6
Pimeclone	T5Ø.7X1	T5Ø.7X2	T5Ø.7X3	T5Ø.7X4	T5Ø.7X5	T5Ø.7X6
Pimelic ketone	T52.8X1	T52.8X2	T52.8X3	T52.8X4	—	—
Pimethixene	T45.ØX1	T45.ØX2	T45.ØX3	T45.ØX4	T45.ØX5	T45.ØX6
Piminodine	T4Ø.2X1	T4Ø.2X2	T4Ø.2X3	T4Ø.2X4	T4Ø.2X5	T4Ø.2X6
Pimozide	T43.591	T43.592	T43.593	T43.594	T43.595	T43.596
Pinacidil	T46.5X1	T46.5X2	T46.5X3	T46.5X4	T46.5X5	T46.5X6
Pinaverium bromide	T44.3X1	T44.3X2	T44.3X3	T44.3X4	T44.3X5	T44.3X6
Pinazepam	T42.4X1	T42.4X2	T42.4X3	T42.4X4	T42.4X5	T42.4X6
Pindolol	T44.7X1	T44.7X2	T44.7X3	T44.7X4	T44.7X5	T44.7X6
Pindone	T6Ø.4X1	T6Ø.4X2	T6Ø.4X3	T6Ø.4X4	—	—
Pine oil (disinfectant)	T65.891	T65.892	T65.893	T65.894	—	—
Pinkroot	T37.4X1	T37.4X2	T37.4X3	T37.4X4	T37.4X5	T37.4X6
Pipadone	T4Ø.2X1	T4Ø.2X2	T4Ø.2X3	T4Ø.2X4	—	—
Pipamazine	T45.ØX1	T45.ØX2	T45.ØX3	T45.ØX4	T45.ØX5	T45.ØX6
Pipamperone	T43.4X1	T43.4X2	T43.4X3	T43.4X4	T43.4X5	T43.4X6
Pipazetate	T48.3X1	T48.3X2	T48.3X3	T48.3X4	T48.3X5	T48.3X6
Pipemidic acid	T37.8X1	T37.8X2	T37.8X3	T37.8X4	T37.8X5	T37.8X6
Pipenzolate bromide	T44.3X1	T44.3X2	T44.3X3	T44.3X4	T44.3X5	T44.3X6
Piperacetazine	T43.3X1	T43.3X2	T43.3X3	T43.3X4	T43.3X5	T43.3X6
Piperacillin	T36.ØX1	T36.ØX2	T36.ØX3	T36.ØX4	T36.ØX5	T36.ØX6
Piperazine	T37.4X1	T37.4X2	T37.4X3	T37.4X4	T37.4X5	T37.4X6
estrone sulfate	T38.5X1	T38.5X2	T38.5X3	T38.5X4	T38.5X5	T38.5X6
Piper cubeba	T62.2X1	T62.2X2	T62.2X3	T62.2X4	—	—
Piperidione	T48.3X1	T48.3X2	T48.3X3	T48.3X4	T48.3X5	T48.3X6
Piperidolate	T44.3X1	T44.3X2	T44.3X3	T44.3X4	T44.3X5	T44.3X6
Piperocaine	T41.3X1	T41.3X2	T41.3X3	T41.3X4	T41.3X5	T41.3X6
infiltration (subcutaneous)	T41.3X1	T41.3X2	T41.3X3	T41.3X4	T41.3X5	T41.3X6
nerve block (peripheral) (plexus)	T41.3X1	T41.3X2	T41.3X3	T41.3X4	T41.3X5	T41.3X6
topical (surface)	T41.3X1	T41.3X2	T41.3X3	T41.3X4	T41.3X5	T41.3X6
Piperonyl butoxide	T6Ø.8X1	T6Ø.8X2	T6Ø.8X3	T6Ø.8X4	—	—
Pipethanate	T44.3X1	T44.3X2	T44.3X3	T44.3X4	T44.3X5	T44.3X6
Pipobroman	T45.1X1	T45.1X2	T45.1X3	T45.1X4	T45.1X5	T45.1X6
Pipotiazine	T43.3X1	T43.3X2	T43.3X3	T43.3X4	T43.3X5	T43.3X6
Pipoxizine	T45.ØX1	T45.ØX2	T45.ØX3	T45.ØX4	T45.ØX5	T45.ØX6
Pipradrol	T43.691	T43.692	T43.693	T43.694	T43.695	T43.696
Piprinhydrinate	T45.ØX1	T45.ØX2	T45.ØX3	T45.ØX4	T45.ØX5	T45.ØX6
Pirarubicin	T45.1X1	T45.1X2	T45.1X3	T45.1X4	T45.1X5	T45.1X6
Pirazinamide	T37.1X1	T37.1X2	T37.1X3	T37.1X4	T37.1X5	T37.1X6
Pirbuterol	T48.6X1	T48.6X2	T48.6X3	T48.6X4	T48.6X5	T48.6X6
Pirenzepine	T47.1X1	T47.1X2	T47.1X3	T47.1X4	T47.1X5	T47.1X6
Piretanide	T5Ø.1X1	T5Ø.1X2	T5Ø.1X3	T5Ø.1X4	T5Ø.1X5	T5Ø.1X6
Pirfenidone*	T48.991	T48.992	T48.993	T48.994	T48.995	T48.996

Table of Drugs and Chemicals

Substance	Poisoning, Accidental (unintentional)	Poisoning, Intentional Self-harm	Poisoning, Assault	Poisoning, Undetermined	Adverse Effect	Under-dosing
Piribedil	T42.8X1	T42.8X2	T42.8X3	T42.8X4	T42.8X5	T42.8X6
Piridoxilate	T46.3X1	T46.3X2	T46.3X3	T46.3X4	T46.3X5	T46.3X6
Piritramide	T4Ø.491	T4Ø.492	T4Ø.493	T4Ø.494	—	—
Piromidic acid	T37.8X1	T37.8X2	T37.8X3	T37.8X4	T37.8X5	T37.8X6
Piroxicam	T39.391	T39.392	T39.393	T39.394	T39.395	T39.396
beta-cyclodextrin complex	T39.8X1	T39.8X2	T39.8X3	T39.8X4	T39.8X5	T39.8X6
Pirozadil	T46.6X1	T46.6X2	T46.6X3	T46.6X4	T46.6X5	T46.6X6
Piscidia (bark) (erythrina)	T39.8X1	T39.8X2	T39.8X3	T39.8X4	T39.8X5	T39.8X6
Pitch	T65.891	T65.892	T65.893	T65.894	—	—
Pitkin's solution	T41.3X1	T41.3X2	T41.3X3	T41.3X4	T41.3X5	T41.3X6
Pitocin	T48.ØX1	T48.ØX2	T48.ØX3	T48.ØX4	T48.ØX5	T48.ØX6
Pitressin (tannate)	T38.891	T38.892	T38.893	T38.894	T38.895	T38.896
Pituitary extracts	T38.891	T38.892	T38.893	T38.894	T38.895	T38.896
(posterior)						
anterior	T38.811	T38.812	T38.813	T38.814	T38.815	T38.816
Pituitrin	T38.891	T38.892	T38.893	T38.894	T38.895	T38.896
Pivampicillin	T36.ØX1	T36.ØX2	T36.ØX3	T36.ØX4	T36.ØX5	T36.ØX6
Pivmecillinam	T36.ØX1	T36.ØX2	T36.ØX3	T36.ØX4	T36.ØX5	T36.ØX6
Placental hormone	T38.891	T38.892	T38.893	T38.894	T38.895	T38.896
Placidyl	T42.6X1	T42.6X2	T42.6X3	T42.6X4	T42.6X5	T42.6X6
Plague vaccine	T5Ø.A91	T5Ø.A92	T5Ø.A93	T5Ø.A94	T5Ø.A95	T5Ø.A96
Plant						
food or fertilizer NEC	T65.891	T65.892	T65.893	T65.894	—	—
containing herbicide	T6Ø.3X1	T6Ø.3X2	T6Ø.3X3	T6Ø.3X4	—	—
noxious, used as food	T62.2X1	T62.2X2	T62.2X3	T62.2X4	—	—
berries	T62.1X1	T62.1X2	T62.1X3	T62.1X4	—	—
seeds	T62.2X1	T62.2X2	T62.2X3	T62.2X4	—	—
specified type NEC	T62.2X1	T62.2X2	T62.2X3	T62.2X4	—	—
Plasma	T45.8X1	T45.8X2	T45.8X3	T45.8X4	T45.8X5	T45.8X6
expander NEC	T45.8X1	T45.8X2	T45.8X3	T45.8X4	T45.8X5	T45.8X6
protein fraction (human)	T45.8X1	T45.8X2	T45.8X3	T45.8X4	T45.8X5	T45.8X6
Plasmanate	T45.8X1	T45.8X2	T45.8X3	T45.8X4	T45.8X5	T45.8X6
Plasminogen (tissue)	T45.611	T45.612	T45.613	T45.614	T45.615	T45.616
activator						
Plaster dressing	T49.3X1	T49.3X2	T49.3X3	T49.3X4	T49.3X5	T49.3X6
Plastic dressing	T49.3X1	T49.3X2	T49.3X3	T49.3X4	T49.3X5	T49.3X6
Plavix*	T45.521	T45.522	T45.523	T45.524	T45.525	T45.526
Plegicil	T43.3X1	T43.3X2	T43.3X3	T43.3X4	T43.3X5	T43.3X6
Plicamycin	T45.1X1	T45.1X2	T45.1X3	T45.1X4	T45.1X5	T45.1X6
Podophyllotoxin	T49.8X1	T49.8X2	T49.8X3	T49.8X4	T49.8X5	T49.8X6
Podophyllum (resin)	T49.4X1	T49.4X2	T49.4X3	T49.4X4	T49.4X5	T49.4X6
Poisonous berries	T62.1X1	T62.1X2	T62.1X3	T62.1X4	—	—
Poison NEC	T65.91	T65.92	T65.93	T65.94	—	—
Pokeweed (any part)	T62.2X1	T62.2X2	T62.2X3	T62.2X4	—	—
Poldine metilsulfate	T44.3X1	T44.3X2	T44.3X3	T44.3X4	T44.3X5	T44.3X6
Polidexide (sulfate)	T46.6X1	T46.6X2	T46.6X3	T46.6X4	T46.6X5	T46.6X6
Polidocanol	T46.8X1	T46.8X2	T46.8X3	T46.8X4	T46.8X5	T46.8X6
Poliomyelitis vaccine	T5Ø.B91	T5Ø.B92	T5Ø.B93	T5Ø.B94	T5Ø.B95	T5Ø.B96
Polish (car) (floor) (furniture)	T65.891	T65.892	T65.893	T65.894	—	—
(metal) (porcelain)						
(silver)						
abrasive	T65.891	T65.892	T65.893	T65.894	—	—
porcelain	T65.891	T65.892	T65.893	T65.894	—	—
Poloxalkol	T47.4X1	T47.4X2	T47.4X3	T47.4X4	T47.4X5	T47.4X6
Poloxamer	T47.4X1	T47.4X2	T47.4X3	T47.4X4	T47.4X5	T47.4X6
Polyaminostyrene resins	T5Ø.3X1	T5Ø.3X2	T5Ø.3X3	T5Ø.3X4	T5Ø.3X5	T5Ø.3X6
Polycarbophil	T47.4X1	T47.4X2	T47.4X3	T47.4X4	T47.4X5	T47.4X6
Polychlorinated biphenyl	T65.891	T65.892	T65.893	T65.894	—	—
Polycycline	T36.4X1	T36.4X2	T36.4X3	T36.4X4	T36.4X5	T36.4X6
Polyester fumes	T59.891	T59.892	T59.893	T59.894	—	—
Polyester resin hardener	T52.91	T52.92	T52.93	T52.94	—	—
fumes	T59.891	T59.892	T59.893	T59.894	—	—
Polyestradiol phosphate	T38.5X1	T38.5X2	T38.5X3	T38.5X4	T38.5X5	T38.5X6
Polyethanolamine alkyl	T49.2X1	T49.2X2	T49.2X3	T49.2X4	T49.2X5	T49.2X6
sulfate						
Polyethylene adhesive	T49.3X1	T49.3X2	T49.3X3	T49.3X4	T49.3X5	T49.3X6
Polyferose	T45.4X1	T45.4X2	T45.4X3	T45.4X4	T45.4X5	T45.4X6
Polygeline	T45.8X1	T45.8X2	T45.8X3	T45.8X4	T45.8X5	T45.8X6
Polymyxin	T36.8X1	T36.8X2	T36.8X3	T36.8X4	T36.8X5	T36.8X6
B	T36.8X1	T36.8X2	T36.8X3	T36.8X4	T36.8X5	T36.8X6
ENT agent	T49.6X1	T49.6X2	T49.6X3	T49.6X4	T49.6X5	T49.6X6
ophthalmic preparation	T49.5X1	T49.5X2	T49.5X3	T49.5X4	T49.5X5	T49.5X6
topical NEC	T49.ØX1	T49.ØX2	T49.ØX3	T49.ØX4	T49.ØX5	T49.ØX6
E sulfate (eye preparation)	T49.5X1	T49.5X2	T49.5X3	T49.5X4	T49.5X5	T49.5X6
Polynoxylin	T49.ØX1	T49.ØX2	T49.ØX3	T49.ØX4	T49.ØX5	T49.ØX6
Polyoestradiol phosphate	T38.5X1	T38.5X2	T38.5X3	T38.5X4	T38.5X5	T38.5X6
Polyoxymethyleneurea	T49.ØX1	T49.ØX2	T49.ØX3	T49.ØX4	T49.ØX5	T49.ØX6
Poly-Pred*	T49.5X1	T49.5X2	T49.5X3	T49.5X4	T49.5X5	T49.5X6
Polysilane	T47.8X1	T47.8X2	T47.8X3	T47.8X4	T47.8X5	T47.8X6
Polytetrafluoroethylene	T59.891	T59.892	T59.893	T59.894	—	—
(inhaled)						
Polythiazide	T5Ø.2X1	T5Ø.2X2	T5Ø.2X3	T5Ø.2X4	T5Ø.2X5	T5Ø.2X6
Polyvidone	T45.8X1	T45.8X2	T45.8X3	T45.8X4	T45.8X5	T45.8X6

Substance	Poisoning, Accidental (unintentional)	Poisoning, Intentional Self-harm	Poisoning, Assault	Poisoning, Undetermined	Adverse Effect	Under-dosing
Polyvinylpyrrolidone	T45.8X1	T45.8X2	T45.8X3	T45.8X4	T45.8X5	T45.8X6
Pontocaine (hydrochloride)	T41.3X1	T41.3X2	T41.3X3	T41.3X4	T41.3X5	T41.3X6
(infiltration) (topical)						
nerve block (peripheral)	T41.3X1	T41.3X2	T41.3X3	T41.3X4	T41.3X5	T41.3X6
(plexus)						
spinal	T41.3X1	T41.3X2	T41.3X3	T41.3X4	T41.3X5	T41.3X6
Porfiromycin	T45.1X1	T45.1X2	T45.1X3	T45.1X4	T45.1X5	T45.1X6
Portactant alfa*	T48.991	T48.992	T48.993	T48.994	T48.995	T48.996
Posterior pituitary hormone	T38.891	T38.892	T38.893	T38.894	T38.895	T38.896
NEC						
Pot	T4Ø.711	T4Ø.712	T4Ø.713	T4Ø.714	T4Ø.715	T4Ø.716
Potash (caustic)	T54.3X1	T54.3X2	T54.3X3	T54.3X4	—	—
Potassic saline injection	T5Ø.3X1	T5Ø.3X2	T5Ø.3X3	T5Ø.3X4	T5Ø.3X5	T5Ø.3X6
(lactated)						
Potassium (salts) **NEC**	T5Ø.3X1	T5Ø.3X2	T5Ø.3X3	T5Ø.3X4	T5Ø.3X5	T5Ø.3X6
aminobenzoate	T45.8X1	T45.8X2	T45.8X3	T45.8X4	T45.8X5	T45.8X6
aminosalicylate	T37.1X1	T37.1X2	T37.1X3	T37.1X4	T37.1X5	T37.1X6
antimony ' tartrate'	T37.8X1	T37.8X2	T37.8X3	T37.8X4	T37.8X5	T37.8X6
arsenite (solution)	T57.ØX1	T57.ØX2	T57.ØX3	T57.ØX4	—	—
bichromate	T56.2X1	T56.2X2	T56.2X3	T56.2X4	—	—
bisulfate	T47.3X1	T47.3X2	T47.3X3	T47.3X4	T47.3X5	T47.3X6
bromide	T42.6X1	T42.6X2	T42.6X3	T42.6X4	T42.6X5	T42.6X6
canrenoate	T5Ø.ØX1	T5Ø.ØX2	T5Ø.ØX3	T5Ø.ØX4	T5Ø.ØX5	T5Ø.ØX6
carbonate	T54.3X1	T54.3X2	T54.3X3	T54.3X4	—	—
chlorate NEC	T65.891	T65.892	T65.893	T65.894	—	—
chloride	T5Ø.3X1	T5Ø.3X2	T5Ø.3X3	T5Ø.3X4	T5Ø.3X5	T5Ø.3X6
citrate	T5Ø.991	T5Ø.992	T5Ø.993	T5Ø.994	T5Ø.995	T5Ø.996
cyanide	T65.ØX1	T65.ØX2	T65.ØX3	T65.ØX4	—	—
ferric hexacyanoferrate	T5Ø.6X1	T5Ø.6X2	T5Ø.6X3	T5Ø.6X4	T5Ø.6X5	T5Ø.6X6
(medicinal)						
nonmedicinal	T65.891	T65.892	T65.893	T65.894	—	—
Fluoride	T57.8X1	T57.8X2	T57.8X3	T57.8X4	—	—
glucaldrate	T47.1X1	T47.1X2	T47.1X3	T47.1X4	T47.1X5	T47.1X6
hydroxide	T54.3X1	T54.3X2	T54.3X3	T54.3X4	—	—
iodate	T49.ØX1	T49.ØX2	T49.ØX3	T49.ØX4	T49.ØX5	T49.ØX6
iodide	T48.4X1	T48.4X2	T48.4X3	T48.4X4	T48.4X5	T48.4X6
nitrate	T57.8X1	T57.8X2	T57.8X3	T57.8X4	—	—
oxalate	T65.891	T65.892	T65.893	T65.894	—	—
perchlorate (nonmedicinal)	T65.891	T65.892	T65.893	T65.894	—	—
NEC						
antithyroid	T38.2X1	T38.2X2	T38.2X3	T38.2X4	T38.2X5	T38.2X6
medicinal	T38.2X1	T38.2X2	T38.2X3	T38.2X4	T38.2X5	T38.2X6
Permanganate	T65.891	T65.892	T65.893	T65.894	—	—
(nonmedicinal)						
medicinal	T49.ØX1	T49.ØX2	T49.ØX3	T49.ØX4	T49.ØX5	T49.ØX6
sulfate	T47.2X1	T47.2X2	T47.2X3	T47.2X4	T47.2X5	T47.2X6
Potassium-removing resin	T5Ø.3X1	T5Ø.3X2	T5Ø.3X3	T5Ø.3X4	T5Ø.3X5	T5Ø.3X6
Potassium-retaining drug	T5Ø.3X1	T5Ø.3X2	T5Ø.3X3	T5Ø.3X4	T5Ø.3X5	T5Ø.3X6
Povidone	T45.8X1	T45.8X2	T45.8X3	T45.8X4	T45.8X5	T45.8X6
iodine	T49.ØX1	T49.ØX2	T49.ØX3	T49.ØX4	T49.ØX5	T49.ØX6
Practolol	T44.7X1	T44.7X2	T44.7X3	T44.7X4	T44.7X5	T44.7X6
Prajmalium bitartrate	T46.2X1	T46.2X2	T46.2X3	T46.2X4	T46.2X5	T46.2X6
Pralidoxime (iodide)	T5Ø.6X1	T5Ø.6X2	T5Ø.6X3	T5Ø.6X4	T5Ø.6X5	T5Ø.6X6
chloride	T5Ø.6X1	T5Ø.6X2	T5Ø.6X3	T5Ø.6X4	T5Ø.6X5	T5Ø.6X6
Pramiverine	T44.3X1	T44.3X2	T44.3X3	T44.3X4	T44.3X5	T44.3X6
Pramlintide*	T38.3X1	T38.3X2	T38.3X3	T38.3X4	T38.3X5	T38.3X6
Pramocaine	T49.1X1	T49.1X2	T49.1X3	T49.1X4	T49.1X5	T49.1X6
Pramoxine	T49.1X1	T49.1X2	T49.1X3	T49.1X4	T49.1X5	T49.1X6
Prasterone	T38.7X1	T38.7X2	T38.7X3	T38.7X4	T38.7X5	T38.7X6
Pravastatin	T46.6X1	T46.6X2	T46.6X3	T46.6X4	T46.6X5	T46.6X6
Prazepam	T42.4X1	T42.4X2	T42.4X3	T42.4X4	T42.4X5	T42.4X6
Praziquantel	T37.4X1	T37.4X2	T37.4X3	T37.4X4	T37.4X5	T37.4X6
Prazitone	T43.291	T43.292	T43.293	T43.294	T43.295	T43.296
Prazosin	T44.6X1	T44.6X2	T44.6X3	T44.6X4	T44.6X5	T44.6X6
Prednicarbate	T49.ØX1	T49.ØX2	T49.ØX3	T49.ØX4	T49.ØX5	T49.ØX6
Prednimustine	T45.1X1	T45.1X2	T45.1X3	T45.1X4	T45.1X5	T45.1X6
Prednisolone	T38.ØX1	T38.ØX2	T38.ØX3	T38.ØX4	T38.ØX5	T38.ØX6
ENT agent	T49.6X1	T49.6X2	T49.6X3	T49.6X4	T49.6X5	T49.6X6
ophthalmic preparation	T49.5X1	T49.5X2	T49.5X3	T49.5X4	T49.5X5	T49.5X6
steaglate	T49.ØX1	T49.ØX2	T49.ØX3	T49.ØX4	T49.ØX5	T49.ØX6
topical NEC	T49.ØX1	T49.ØX2	T49.ØX3	T49.ØX4	T49.ØX5	T49.ØX6
Prednisone	T38.ØX1	T38.ØX2	T38.ØX3	T38.ØX4	T38.ØX5	T38.ØX6
Prednylidene	T38.ØX1	T38.ØX2	T38.ØX3	T38.ØX4	T38.ØX5	T38.ØX6
Pregnandiol	T38.5X1	T38.5X2	T38.5X3	T38.5X4	T38.5X5	T38.5X6
Pregneninolone	T38.5X1	T38.5X2	T38.5X3	T38.5X4	T38.5X5	T38.5X6
Preludin	T43.691	T43.692	T43.693	T43.694	T43.695	T43.696
Premarin	T38.5X1	T38.5X2	T38.5X3	T38.5X4	T38.5X5	T38.5X6
Premedication anesthetic	T41.2Ø1	T41.2Ø2	T41.2Ø3	T41.2Ø4	T41.2Ø5	T41.2Ø6
Prenalterol	T44.5X1	T44.5X2	T44.5X3	T44.5X4	T44.5X5	T44.5X6
Prenoxdiazine	T48.3X1	T48.3X2	T48.3X3	T48.3X4	T48.3X5	T48.3X6
Prenylamine	T46.3X1	T46.3X2	T46.3X3	T46.3X4	T46.3X5	T46.3X6
Preparation H	T49.8X1	T49.8X2	T49.8X3	T49.8X4	T49.8X5	T49.8X6
Preparation, local	T49.4X1	T49.4X2	T49.4X3	T49.4X4	T49.4X5	T49.4X6

Piribedil — Preparation, local

Substance	Poisoning, Accidental (unintentional)	Poisoning, Intentional Self-harm	Poisoning, Assault	Poisoning, Undetermined	Adverse Effect	Under-dosing
Preservative (nonmedicinal)	T65.891	T65.892	T65.893	T65.894	—	—
medicinal	T5Ø.9Ø1	T5Ø.9Ø2	T5Ø.9Ø3	T5Ø.9Ø4	T5Ø.9Ø5	T5Ø.9Ø6
wood	T6Ø.91	T6Ø.92	T6Ø.93	T6Ø.94	—	—
Prethcamide	T5Ø.7X1	T5Ø.7X2	T5Ø.7X3	T5Ø.7X4	T5Ø.7X5	T5Ø.7X6
Prevacid*	T47.1X1	T47.1X2	T47.1X3	T47.1X4	T47.1X5	T47.1X6
Pride of China	T62.2X1	T62.2X2	T62.2X3	T62.2X4	—	—
Pridinol	T44.3X1	T44.3X2	T44.3X3	T44.3X4	T44.3X5	T44.3X6
Prifinium bromide	T44.3X1	T44.3X2	T44.3X3	T44.3X4	T44.3X5	T44.3X6
Prilocaine	T41.3X1	T41.3X2	T41.3X3	T41.3X4	T41.3X5	T41.3X6
infiltration (subcutaneous)	T41.3X1	T41.3X2	T41.3X3	T41.3X4	T41.3X5	T41.3X6
nerve block (peripheral) (plexus)	T41.3X1	T41.3X2	T41.3X3	T41.3X4	T41.3X5	T41.3X6
regional	T41.3X1	T41.3X2	T41.3X3	T41.3X4	T41.3X5	T41.3X6
Primaquine	T37.2X1	T37.2X2	T37.2X3	T37.2X4	T37.2X5	T37.2X6
Primidone	T42.6X1	T42.6X2	T42.6X3	T42.6X4	T42.6X5	T42.6X6
Primula (veris)	T62.2X1	T62.2X2	T62.2X3	T62.2X4	—	—
Prinadol	T4Ø.2X1	T4Ø.2X2	T4Ø.2X3	T4Ø.2X4	T4Ø.2X5	T4Ø.2X6
Priscol, Priscoline	T44.6X1	T44.6X2	T44.6X3	T44.6X4	T44.6X5	T44.6X6
Pristinamycin	T36.3X1	T36.3X2	T36.3X3	T36.3X4	T36.3X5	T36.3X6
Pristiq*	T43.211	T43.212	T43.213	T43.214	T43.215	T43.216
Privet	T62.2X1	T62.2X2	T62.2X3	T62.2X4	—	—
berries	T62.1X1	T62.1X2	T62.1X3	T62.1X4	—	—
Privine	T44.4X1	T44.4X2	T44.4X3	T44.4X4	T44.4X5	T44.4X6
Pro-Banthine	T44.3X1	T44.3X2	T44.3X3	T44.3X4	T44.3X5	T44.3X6
Probarbital	T42.3X1	T42.3X2	T42.3X3	T42.3X4	T42.3X5	T42.3X6
Probenecid	T5Ø.4X1	T5Ø.4X2	T5Ø.4X3	T5Ø.4X4	T5Ø.4X5	T5Ø.4X6
Probucol	T46.6X1	T46.6X2	T46.6X3	T46.6X4	T46.6X5	T46.6X6
Procainamide	T46.2X1	T46.2X2	T46.2X3	T46.2X4	T46.2X5	T46.2X6
Procaine	T41.3X1	T41.3X2	T41.3X3	T41.3X4	T41.3X5	T41.3X6
benzylpenicillin	T36.ØX1	T36.ØX2	T36.ØX3	T36.ØX4	T36.ØX5	T36.ØX6
nerve block (periphreal) (plexus)	T41.3X1	T41.3X2	T41.3X3	T41.3X4	T41.3X5	T41.3X6
penicillin G	T36.ØX1	T36.ØX2	T36.ØX3	T36.ØX4	T36.ØX5	T36.ØX6
regional	T41.3X1	T41.3X2	T41.3X3	T41.3X4	T41.3X5	T41.3X6
spinal	T41.3X1	T41.3X2	T41.3X3	T41.3X4	T41.3X5	T41.3X6
Procalmidol	T43.591	T43.592	T43.593	T43.594	T43.595	T43.596
Procarbazine	T45.1X1	T45.1X2	T45.1X3	T45.1X4	T45.1X5	T45.1X6
Procaterol	T44.5X1	T44.5X2	T44.5X3	T44.5X4	T44.5X5	T44.5X6
Prochlorperazine	T43.3X1	T43.3X2	T43.3X3	T43.3X4	T43.3X5	T43.3X6
Procyclidine	T44.3X1	T44.3X2	T44.3X3	T44.3X4	T44.3X5	T44.3X6
Producer gas	T58.8X1	T58.8X2	T58.8X3	T58.8X4	—	—
Profadol	T4Ø.491	T4Ø.492	T4Ø.493	T4Ø.494	T4Ø.495	T4Ø.496
Profenamine	T44.3X1	T44.3X2	T44.3X3	T44.3X4	T44.3X5	T44.3X6
Profenil	T44.3X1	T44.3X2	T44.3X3	T44.3X4	T44.3X5	T44.3X6
Proflavine	T49.ØX1	T49.ØX2	T49.ØX3	T49.ØX4	T49.ØX5	T49.ØX6
Progabide	T42.6X1	T42.6X2	T42.6X3	T42.6X4	T42.6X5	T42.6X6
Progesterone	T38.5X1	T38.5X2	T38.5X3	T38.5X4	T38.5X5	T38.5X6
Progestin	T38.5X1	T38.5X2	T38.5X3	T38.5X4	T38.5X5	T38.5X6
oral contraceptive	T38.4X1	T38.4X2	T38.4X3	T38.4X4	T38.4X5	T38.4X6
Progestogen NEC	T38.5X1	T38.5X2	T38.5X3	T38.5X4	T38.5X5	T38.5X6
Progestone	T38.5X1	T38.5X2	T38.5X3	T38.5X4	T38.5X5	T38.5X6
Proglumide	T47.1X1	T47.1X2	T47.1X3	T47.1X4	T47.1X5	T47.1X6
Prograf*	T45.1X1	T45.1X2	T45.1X3	T45.1X4	T45.1X5	T45.1X6
Proguanil	T37.2X1	T37.2X2	T37.2X3	T37.2X4	T37.2X5	T37.2X6
Prolactin	T38.811	T38.812	T38.813	T38.814	T38.815	T38.816
Prolintane	T43.691	T43.692	T43.693	T43.694	T43.695	T43.696
Proloid	T38.1X1	T38.1X2	T38.1X3	T38.1X4	T38.1X5	T38.1X6
Proluton	T38.5X1	T38.5X2	T38.5X3	T38.5X4	T38.5X5	T38.5X6
Promacetin	T37.1X1	T37.1X2	T37.1X3	T37.1X4	T37.1X5	T37.1X6
Promazine	T43.3X1	T43.3X2	T43.3X3	T43.3X4	T43.3X5	T43.3X6
Promedol	T4Ø.2X1	T4Ø.2X2	T4Ø.2X3	T4Ø.2X4	—	—
Promegestone	T38.5X1	T38.5X2	T38.5X3	T38.5X4	T38.5X5	T38.5X6
Promethazine (teoclate)	T43.3X1	T43.3X2	T43.3X3	T43.3X4	T43.3X5	T43.3X6
Promin	T37.1X1	T37.1X2	T37.1X3	T37.1X4	T37.1X5	T37.1X6
Pronase	T45.3X1	T45.3X2	T45.3X3	T45.3X4	T45.3X5	T45.3X6
Pronestyl (hydrochloride)	T46.2X1	T46.2X2	T46.2X3	T46.2X4	T46.2X5	T46.2X6
Pronetalol	T44.7X1	T44.7X2	T44.7X3	T44.7X4	T44.7X5	T44.7X6
Prontosil	T37.ØX1	T37.ØX2	T37.ØX3	T37.ØX4	T37.ØX5	T37.ØX6
Propachlor	T6Ø.3X1	T6Ø.3X2	T6Ø.3X3	T6Ø.3X4	—	—
Propafenone	T46.2X1	T46.2X2	T46.2X3	T46.2X4	T46.2X5	T46.2X6
Propallylonal	T42.3X1	T42.3X2	T42.3X3	T42.3X4	T42.3X5	T42.3X6
Propamidine	T49.ØX1	T49.ØX2	T49.ØX3	T49.ØX4	T49.ØX5	T49.ØX6
Propane (distributed in mobile container)	T59.891	T59.892	T59.893	T59.894	—	—
distributed through pipes	T59.891	T59.892	T59.893	T59.894	—	—
incomplete combustion	T58.11	T58.12	T58.13	T58.14	—	—
Propanidid	T41.291	T41.292	T41.293	T41.294	T41.295	T41.296
Propanil	T6Ø.3X1	T6Ø.3X2	T6Ø.3X3	T6Ø.3X4	—	—
Propantheline	T44.3X1	T44.3X2	T44.3X3	T44.3X4	T44.3X5	T44.3X6
bromide	T44.3X1	T44.3X2	T44.3X3	T44.3X4	T44.3X5	T44.3X6
Proparacaine	T41.3X1	T41.3X2	T41.3X3	T41.3X4	T41.3X5	T41.3X6
Propatylnitrate	T46.3X1	T46.3X2	T46.3X3	T46.3X4	T46.3X5	T46.3X6

Substance	Poisoning, Accidental (unintentional)	Poisoning, Intentional Self-harm	Poisoning, Assault	Poisoning, Undetermined	Adverse Effect	Under-dosing
Propicillin	T36.ØX1	T36.ØX2	T36.ØX3	T36.ØX4	T36.ØX5	T36.ØX6
Propine*	T49.5X1	T49.5X2	T49.5X3	T49.5X4	T49.5X5	T49.5X6
Propiolactone	T49.ØX1	T49.ØX2	T49.ØX3	T49.ØX4	T49.ØX5	T49.ØX6
Propiomazine	T45.ØX1	T45.ØX2	T45.ØX3	T45.ØX4	T45.ØX5	T45.ØX6
Propionaldehyde (medicinal)	T42.6X1	T42.6X2	T42.6X3	T42.6X4	T42.6X5	T42.6X6
Propionate (calcium) (sodium)	T49.ØX1	T49.ØX2	T49.ØX3	T49.ØX4	T49.ØX5	T49.ØX6
Propion gel	T49.ØX1	T49.ØX2	T49.ØX3	T49.ØX4	T49.ØX5	T49.ØX6
Propitocaine	T41.3X1	T41.3X2	T41.3X3	T41.3X4	T41.3X5	T41.3X6
infiltration (subcutaneous)	T41.3X1	T41.3X2	T41.3X3	T41.3X4	T41.3X5	T41.3X6
nerve block (peripheral) (plexus)	T41.3X1	T41.3X2	T41.3X3	T41.3X4	T41.3X5	T41.3X6
Propofol	T41.291	T41.292	T41.293	T41.294	T41.295	T41.296
Propoxur	T6Ø.ØX1	T6Ø.ØX2	T6Ø.ØX3	T6Ø.ØX4	—	—
Propoxycaine	T41.3X1	T41.3X2	T41.3X3	T41.3X4	T41.3X5	T41.3X6
infiltration (subcutaneous)	T41.3X1	T41.3X2	T41.3X3	T41.3X4	T41.3X5	T41.3X6
nerve block (peripheral) (plexus)	T41.3X1	T41.3X2	T41.3X3	T41.3X4	T41.3X5	T41.3X6
topical (surface)	T41.3X1	T41.3X2	T41.3X3	T41.3X4	T41.3X5	T41.3X6
Propoxyphene	T4Ø.491	T4Ø.492	T4Ø.493	T4Ø.494	T4Ø.495	T4Ø.496
Propranolol	T44.7X1	T44.7X2	T44.7X3	T44.7X4	T44.7X5	T44.7X6
Propyl						
alcohol	T51.3X1	T51.3X2	T51.3X3	T51.3X4	—	—
carbinol	T51.3X1	T51.3X2	T51.3X3	T51.3X4	—	—
hexadrine	T44.4X1	T44.4X2	T44.4X3	T44.4X4	T44.4X5	T44.4X6
iodone	T5Ø.8X1	T5Ø.8X2	T5Ø.8X3	T5Ø.8X4	T5Ø.8X5	T5Ø.8X6
thiouracil	T38.2X1	T38.2X2	T38.2X3	T38.2X4	T38.2X5	T38.2X6
Propylaminophenothiazine	T43.3X1	T43.3X2	T43.3X3	T43.3X4	T43.3X5	T43.3X6
Propylene	T59.891	T59.892	T59.893	T59.894	—	—
Propylhexedrine	T48.5X1	T48.5X2	T48.5X3	T48.5X4	T48.5X5	T48.5X6
Propyliodone	T5Ø.8X1	T5Ø.8X2	T5Ø.8X3	T5Ø.8X4	T5Ø.8X5	T5Ø.8X6
Propylparaben (ophthalmic)	T49.5X1	T49.5X2	T49.5X3	T49.5X4	T49.5X5	T49.5X6
Propylthiouracil	T38.2X1	T38.2X2	T38.2X3	T38.2X4	T38.2X5	T38.2X6
Propyphenazone	T39.2X1	T39.2X2	T39.2X3	T39.2X4	T39.2X5	T39.2X6
Proquazone	T39.391	T39.392	T39.393	T39.394	T39.395	T39.396
Proscar*	T38.6X1	T38.6X2	T38.6X3	T38.6X4	T38.6X5	T38.6X6
Proscillaridin	T46.ØX1	T46.ØX2	T46.ØX3	T46.ØX4	T46.ØX5	T46.ØX6
Prostacyclin	T45.521	T45.522	T45.523	T45.524	T45.525	T45.526
Prostaglandin (I2)	T45.521	T45.522	T45.523	T45.524	T45.525	T45.526
E1	T46.7X1	T46.7X2	T46.7X3	T46.7X4	T46.7X5	T46.7X6
E2	T48.ØX1	T48.ØX2	T48.ØX3	T48.ØX4	T48.ØX5	T48.ØX6
F2 alpha	T48.ØX1	T48.ØX2	T48.ØX3	T48.ØX4	T48.ØX5	T48.ØX6
Prostigmin	T44.ØX1	T44.ØX2	T44.ØX3	T44.ØX4	T44.ØX5	T44.ØX6
Prosultiamine	T45.2X1	T45.2X2	T45.2X3	T45.2X4	T45.2X5	T45.2X6
Protamine sulfate	T45.7X1	T45.7X2	T45.7X3	T45.7X4	T45.7X5	T45.7X6
zinc insulin	T38.3X1	T38.3X2	T38.3X3	T38.3X4	T38.3X5	T38.3X6
Protease	T47.5X1	T47.5X2	T47.5X3	T47.5X4	T47.5X5	T47.5X6
Protectant, skin NEC	T49.3X1	T49.3X2	T49.3X3	T49.3X4	T49.3X5	T49.3X6
Protein hydrolysate	T5Ø.991	T5Ø.992	T5Ø.993	T5Ø.994	T5Ø.995	T5Ø.996
Prothiaden — *see* Dothiepin hydrochloride						
Prothionamide	T37.1X1	T37.1X2	T37.1X3	T37.1X4	T37.1X5	T37.1X6
Prothipendyl	T43.591	T43.592	T43.593	T43.594	T43.595	T43.596
Prothoate	T6Ø.ØX1	T6Ø.ØX2	T6Ø.ØX3	T6Ø.ØX4	—	—
Prothrombin						
activator	T45.7X1	T45.7X2	T45.7X3	T45.7X4	T45.7X5	T45.7X6
synthesis inhibitor	T45.511	T45.512	T45.513	T45.514	T45.515	T45.516
Protionamide	T37.1X1	T37.1X2	T37.1X3	T37.1X4	T37.1X5	T37.1X6
Protirelin	T38.891	T38.892	T38.893	T38.894	T38.895	T38.896
Protokylol	T48.6X1	T48.6X2	T48.6X3	T48.6X4	T48.6X5	T48.6X6
Protopam	T5Ø.6X1	T5Ø.6X2	T5Ø.6X3	T5Ø.6X4	T5Ø.6X5	T5Ø.6X6
Protoveratrine(s) (A) (B)	T46.5X1	T46.5X2	T46.5X3	T46.5X4	T46.5X5	T46.5X6
Protriptyline	T43.Ø11	T43.Ø12	T43.Ø13	T43.Ø14	T43.Ø15	T43.Ø16
Proventil*	T48.6X1	T48.6X2	T48.6X3	T48.6X4	T48.6X5	T48.6X6
Provera	T38.5X1	T38.5X2	T38.5X3	T38.5X4	T38.5X5	T38.5X6
Provitamin A	T45.2X1	T45.2X2	T45.2X3	T45.2X4	T45.2X5	T45.2X6
Proxibarbal	T42.3X1	T42.3X2	T42.3X3	T42.3X4	T42.3X5	T42.3X6
Proxymetacaine	T41.3X1	T41.3X2	T41.3X3	T41.3X4	T41.3X5	T41.3X6
Proxyphylline	T48.6X1	T48.6X2	T48.6X3	T48.6X4	T48.6X5	T48.6X6
Prozac — *see* Fluoxetine hydrochloride						
Prunus						
laurocerasus	T62.2X1	T62.2X2	T62.2X3	T62.2X4	—	—
virginiana	T62.2X1	T62.2X2	T62.2X3	T62.2X4	—	—
Prussian blue						
commercial	T65.891	T65.892	T65.893	T65.894	—	—
therapeutic	T5Ø.6X1	T5Ø.6X2	T5Ø.6X3	T5Ø.6X4	T5Ø.6X5	T5Ø.6X6
Prussic acid	T65.ØX1	T65.ØX2	T65.ØX3	T65.ØX4	—	—
vapor	T57.3X1	T57.3X2	T57.3X3	T57.3X4	—	—
Pseudoephedrine	T44.991	T44.992	T44.993	T44.994	T44.995	T44.996
Psilocin	T4Ø.991	T4Ø.992	T4Ø.993	T4Ø.994	—	—

Substance	Poisoning, Accidental (unintentional)	Poisoning, Intentional Self-harm	Poisoning, Assault	Poisoning, Undetermined	Adverse Effect	Under-dosing
Psilocybin	T4Ø.991	T4Ø.992	T4Ø.993	T4Ø.994	—	—
Psilocybine	T4Ø.991	T4Ø.992	T4Ø.993	T4Ø.994	—	—
Psoralene (nonmedicinal)	T65.891	T65.892	T65.893	T65.894	—	—
Psoralens (medicinal)	T5Ø.991	T5Ø.992	T5Ø.993	T5Ø.994	T5Ø.995	T5Ø.996
PSP (phenolsulfonphthalein)	T5Ø.8X1	T5Ø.8X2	T5Ø.8X3	T5Ø.8X4	T5Ø.8X5	T5Ø.8X6
Psychodysleptic drug NOS	T4Ø.9Ø1	T4Ø.9Ø2	T4Ø.9Ø3	T4Ø.9Ø4	T4Ø.9Ø5	T4Ø.9Ø6
specified NEC	T4Ø.991	T4Ø.992	T4Ø.993	T4Ø.994	T4Ø.995	T4Ø.996
Psychostimulant	T43.6Ø1	T43.6Ø2	T43.6Ø3	T43.6Ø4	T43.6Ø5	T43.6Ø6
amphetamine	T43.621	T43.622	T43.623	T43.624	T43.625	T43.626
caffeine	T43.611	T43.612	T43.613	T43.614	T43.615	T43.616
methylphenidate	T43.631	T43.632	T43.633	T43.634	T43.635	T43.636
specified NEC	T43.691	T43.692	T43.693	T43.694	T43.695	T43.696
Psychotherapeutic drug NEC	T43.91	T43.92	T43.93	T43.94	T43.95	T43.96
antidepressants — *see also* Antidepressant	T43.2Ø1	T43.2Ø2	T43.2Ø3	T43.2Ø4	T43.2Ø5	T43.2Ø6
specified NEC	T43.8X1	T43.8X2	T43.8X3	T43.8X4	T43.8X5	T43.8X6
tranquilizers NEC	T43.5Ø1	T43.5Ø2	T43.5Ø3	T43.5Ø4	T43.5Ø5	T43.5Ø6
Psychotomimetic agents	T4Ø.9Ø1	T4Ø.9Ø2	T4Ø.9Ø3	T4Ø.9Ø4	T4Ø.9Ø5	T4Ø.9Ø6
Psychotropic drug NEC	T43.91	T43.92	T43.93	T43.94	T43.95	T43.96
specified NEC	T43.8X1	T43.8X2	T43.8X3	T43.8X4	T43.8X5	T43.8X6
Psyllium hydrophilic mucilloid	T47.4X1	T47.4X2	T47.4X3	T47.4X4	T47.4X5	T47.4X6
Pteroylglutamic acid	T45.8X1	T45.8X2	T45.8X3	T45.8X4	T45.8X5	T45.8X6
Pteroyltriglutamate	T45.1X1	T45.1X2	T45.1X3	T45.1X4	T45.1X5	T45.1X6
PTFE — *see* Polytetrafluoroethylene						
Pulmicort*	T44.5X1	T44.5X2	T44.5X3	T44.5X4	T44.5X5	T44.5X6
Pulp						
devitalizing paste	T49.7X1	T49.7X2	T49.7X3	T49.7X4	T49.7X5	T49.7X6
dressing	T49.7X1	T49.7X2	T49.7X3	T49.7X4	T49.7X5	T49.7X6
Pulsatilla	T62.2X1	T62.2X2	T62.2X3	T62.2X4	—	—
Pumpkin seed extract	T37.4X1	T37.4X2	T37.4X3	T37.4X4	T37.4X5	T37.4X6
Purex (bleach)	T54.91	T54.92	T54.93	T54.94	—	—
Purgative NEC — *see also* Cathartic	T47.4X1	T47.4X2	T47.4X3	T47.4X4	T47.4X5	T47.4X6
Purine analogue (antineoplastic)	T45.1X1	T45.1X2	T45.1X3	T45.1X4	T45.1X5	T45.1X6
Purine diuretics	T5Ø.2X1	T5Ø.2X2	T5Ø.2X3	T5Ø.2X4	T5Ø.2X5	T5Ø.2X6
Purinethol	T45.1X1	T45.1X2	T45.1X3	T45.1X4	T45.1X5	T45.1X6
PVP	T45.8X1	T45.8X2	T45.8X3	T45.8X4	T45.8X5	T45.8X6
Pyrabital	T39.8X1	T39.8X2	T39.8X3	T39.8X4	T39.8X5	T39.8X6
Pyramidon	T39.2X1	T39.2X2	T39.2X3	T39.2X4	T39.2X5	T39.2X6
Pyrantel	T37.4X1	T37.4X2	T37.4X3	T37.4X4	T37.4X5	T37.4X6
Pyrathiazine	T45.ØX1	T45.ØX2	T45.ØX3	T45.ØX4	T45.ØX5	T45.ØX6
Pyrazinamide	T37.1X1	T37.1X2	T37.1X3	T37.1X4	T37.1X5	T37.1X6
Pyrazinoic acid (amide)	T37.1X1	T37.1X2	T37.1X3	T37.1X4	T37.1X5	T37.1X6
Pyrazole (derivatives)	T39.2X1	T39.2X2	T39.2X3	T39.2X4	T39.2X5	T39.2X6
Pyrazolone analgesic NEC	T39.2X1	T39.2X2	T39.2X3	T39.2X4	T39.2X5	T39.2X6
Pyrethrin, pyrethrum (nonmedicinal)	T6Ø.2X1	T6Ø.2X2	T6Ø.2X3	T6Ø.2X4	—	—
Pyrethrum extract	T49.ØX1	T49.ØX2	T49.ØX3	T49.ØX4	T49.ØX5	T49.ØX6
Pyribenzamine	T45.ØX1	T45.ØX2	T45.ØX3	T45.ØX4	T45.ØX5	T45.ØX6
Pyridine	T52.8X1	T52.8X2	T52.8X3	T52.8X4	—	—
aldoxime methiodide	T5Ø.6X1	T5Ø.6X2	T5Ø.6X3	T5Ø.6X4	T5Ø.6X5	T5Ø.6X6
aldoxime methyl chloride	T5Ø.6X1	T5Ø.6X2	T5Ø.6X3	T5Ø.6X4	T5Ø.6X5	T5Ø.6X6
vapor	T59.891	T59.892	T59.893	T59.894	—	—
Pyridium	T39.8X1	T39.8X2	T39.8X3	T39.8X4	T39.8X5	T39.8X6
Pyridostigmine bromide	T44.ØX1	T44.ØX2	T44.ØX3	T44.ØX4	T44.ØX5	T44.ØX6
Pyridoxal phosphate	T45.2X1	T45.2X2	T45.2X3	T45.2X4	T45.2X5	T45.2X6
Pyridoxine	T45.2X1	T45.2X2	T45.2X3	T45.2X4	T45.2X5	T45.2X6
Pyrilamine	T45.ØX1	T45.ØX2	T45.ØX3	T45.ØX4	T45.ØX5	T45.ØX6
Pyrimethamine	T37.2X1	T37.2X2	T37.2X3	T37.2X4	T37.2X5	T37.2X6
with sulfadoxine	T37.2X1	T37.2X2	T37.2X3	T37.2X4	T37.2X5	T37.2X6
Pyrimidine antagonist	T45.1X1	T45.1X2	T45.1X3	T45.1X4	T45.1X5	T45.1X6
Pyriminil	T6Ø.4X1	T6Ø.4X2	T6Ø.4X3	T6Ø.4X4	—	—
Pyrithione zinc	T49.4X1	T49.4X2	T49.4X3	T49.4X4	T49.4X5	T49.4X6
Pyrithyldione	T42.6X1	T42.6X2	T42.6X3	T42.6X4	T42.6X5	T42.6X6
Pyrogallic acid	T49.ØX1	T49.ØX2	T49.ØX3	T49.ØX4	T49.ØX5	T49.ØX6
Pyrogallol	T49.ØX1	T49.ØX2	T49.ØX3	T49.ØX4	T49.ØX5	T49.ØX6
Pyroxylin	T49.3X1	T49.3X2	T49.3X3	T49.3X4	T49.3X5	T49.3X6
Pyrrobutamine	T45.ØX1	T45.ØX2	T45.ØX3	T45.ØX4	T45.ØX5	T45.ØX6
Pyrrolizidine alkaloids	T62.8X1	T62.8X2	T62.8X3	T62.8X4	—	—
Pyrvinium chloride	T37.4X1	T37.4X2	T37.4X3	T37.4X4	T37.4X5	T37.4X6
PZI	T38.3X1	T38.3X2	T38.3X3	T38.3X4	T38.3X5	T38.3X6
Qbrelis*	T46.4X1	T46.4X2	T46.4X3	T46.4X4	T46.4X5	T46.4X6
Quaalude	T42.6X1	T42.6X2	T42.6X3	T42.6X4	T42.6X5	T42.6X6
Quarternary ammonium						
anti-infective	T49.ØX1	T49.ØX2	T49.ØX3	T49.ØX4	T49.ØX5	T49.ØX6
ganglion blocking	T44.2X1	T44.2X2	T44.2X3	T44.2X4	T44.2X5	T44.2X6
parasympatholytic	T44.3X1	T44.3X2	T44.3X3	T44.3X4	T44.3X5	T44.3X6
Quazepam	T42.4X1	T42.4X2	T42.4X3	T42.4X4	T42.4X5	T42.4X6
Quicklime	T54.3X1	T54.3X2	T54.3X3	T54.3X4	—	—
Quilbron-T*	T48.6X1	T48.6X2	T48.6X3	T48.6X4	T48.6X5	T48.6X6
Quillaja extract	T48.4X1	T48.4X2	T48.4X3	T48.4X4	T48.4X5	T48.4X6
Quinacrine	T37.2X1	T37.2X2	T37.2X3	T37.2X4	T37.2X5	T37.2X6
Quinaglute	T46.2X1	T46.2X2	T46.2X3	T46.2X4	T46.2X5	T46.2X6
Quinalbarbital	T42.3X1	T42.3X2	T42.3X3	T42.3X4	T42.3X5	T42.3X6
Quinalbarbitone sodium	T42.3X1	T42.3X2	T42.3X3	T42.3X4	T42.3X5	T42.3X6
Quinalphos	T6Ø.ØX1	T6Ø.ØX2	T6Ø.ØX3	T6Ø.ØX4	—	—
Quinapril	T46.4X1	T46.4X2	T46.4X3	T46.4X4	T46.4X5	T46.4X6
Quinestradiol	T38.5X1	T38.5X2	T38.5X3	T38.5X4	T38.5X5	T38.5X6
Quinestradol	T38.5X1	T38.5X2	T38.5X3	T38.5X4	T38.5X5	T38.5X6
Quinestrol	T38.5X1	T38.5X2	T38.5X3	T38.5X4	T38.5X5	T38.5X6
Quinethazone	T5Ø.2X1	T5Ø.2X2	T5Ø.2X3	T5Ø.2X4	T5Ø.2X5	T5Ø.2X6
Quingestanol	T38.4X1	T38.4X2	T38.4X3	T38.4X4	T38.4X5	T38.4X6
Quinidine	T46.2X1	T46.2X2	T46.2X3	T46.2X4	T46.2X5	T46.2X6
Quinine	T37.2X1	T37.2X2	T37.2X3	T37.2X4	T37.2X5	T37.2X6
Quiniobine	T37.8X1	T37.8X2	T37.8X3	T37.8X4	T37.8X5	T37.8X6
Quinisocaine	T49.1X1	T49.1X2	T49.1X3	T49.1X4	T49.1X5	T49.1X6
Quinocide	T37.2X1	T37.2X2	T37.2X3	T37.2X4	T37.2X5	T37.2X6
Quinoline (derivatives) **NEC**	T37.8X1	T37.8X2	T37.8X3	T37.8X4	T37.8X5	T37.8X6
Quinupramine	T43.Ø11	T43.Ø12	T43.Ø13	T43.Ø14	T43.Ø15	T43.Ø16
Quixin*	T49.5X1	T49.5X2	T49.5X3	T49.5X4	T49.5X5	T49.5X6
Quotane	T41.3X1	T41.3X2	T41.3X3	T41.3X4	T41.3X5	T41.3X6
Rabies						
immune globulin (human)	T5Ø.Z11	T5Ø.Z12	T5Ø.Z13	T5Ø.Z14	T5Ø.Z15	T5Ø.Z16
vaccine	T5Ø.B91	T5Ø.B92	T5Ø.B93	T5Ø.B94	T5Ø.B95	T5Ø.B96
Racemoramide	T4Ø.2X1	T4Ø.2X2	T4Ø.2X3	T4Ø.2X4	—	—
Racemorphan	T4Ø.2X1	T4Ø.2X2	T4Ø.2X3	T4Ø.2X4	T4Ø.2X5	T4Ø.2X6
Racepinefrin	T44.5X1	T44.5X2	T44.5X3	T44.5X4	T44.5X5	T44.5X6
Raclopride	T43.591	T43.592	T43.593	T43.594	T43.595	T43.596
Radiator alcohol	T51.1X1	T51.1X2	T51.1X3	T51.1X4	—	—
Radioactive drug NEC	T5Ø.8X1	T5Ø.8X2	T5Ø.8X3	T5Ø.8X4	T5Ø.8X5	T5Ø.8X6
Radio-opaque (drugs) (materials)	T5Ø.8X1	T5Ø.8X2	T5Ø.8X3	T5Ø.8X4	T5Ø.8X5	T5Ø.8X6
Ramifenazone	T39.2X1	T39.2X2	T39.2X3	T39.2X4	T39.2X5	T39.2X6
Ramipril	T46.4X1	T46.4X2	T46.4X3	T46.4X4	T46.4X5	T46.4X6
Ranitidine	T47.ØX1	T47.ØX2	T47.ØX3	T47.ØX4	T47.ØX5	T47.ØX6
Ranunculus	T62.2X1	T62.2X2	T62.2X3	T62.2X4	—	—
Rat poison NEC	T6Ø.4X1	T6Ø.4X2	T6Ø.4X3	T6Ø.4X4	—	—
Rattlesnake (venom)	T63.Ø11	T63.Ø12	T63.Ø13	T63.Ø14	—	—
Raubasine	T46.7X1	T46.7X2	T46.7X3	T46.7X4	T46.7X5	T46.7X6
Raudixin	T46.5X1	T46.5X2	T46.5X3	T46.5X4	T46.5X5	T46.5X6
Rautensin	T46.5X1	T46.5X2	T46.5X3	T46.5X4	T46.5X5	T46.5X6
Rautina	T46.5X1	T46.5X2	T46.5X3	T46.5X4	T46.5X5	T46.5X6
Rautotal	T46.5X1	T46.5X2	T46.5X3	T46.5X4	T46.5X5	T46.5X6
Rauwiloid	T46.5X1	T46.5X2	T46.5X3	T46.5X4	T46.5X5	T46.5X6
Rauwoldin	T46.5X1	T46.5X2	T46.5X3	T46.5X4	T46.5X5	T46.5X6
Rauwolfia (alkaloids)	T46.5X1	T46.5X2	T46.5X3	T46.5X4	T46.5X5	T46.5X6
Razadyne*	T44.ØX1	T44.ØX2	T44.ØX3	T44.ØX4	T44.ØX5	T44.ØX6
Razoxane	T45.1X1	T45.1X2	T45.1X3	T45.1X4	T45.1X5	T45.1X6
Realgar	T57.ØX1	T57.ØX2	T57.ØX3	T57.ØX4	—	—
Recombinant (R) — *see* specific protein						
Red blood cells, packed	T45.8X1	T45.8X2	T45.8X3	T45.8X4	T45.8X5	T45.8X6
Red squill (scilliroside)	T6Ø.4X1	T6Ø.4X2	T6Ø.4X3	T6Ø.4X4	—	—
Reducing agent, industrial NEC	T65.891	T65.892	T65.893	T65.894	—	—
Refrigerant gas (chlorofluorocarbon)	T53.5X1	T53.5X2	T53.5X3	T53.5X4	—	—
not chlorofluorocarbon	T59.891	T59.892	T59.893	T59.894	—	—
Regroton	T5Ø.2X1	T5Ø.2X2	T5Ø.2X3	T5Ø.2X4	T5Ø.2X5	T5Ø.2X6
Rehydration salts (oral)	T5Ø.3X1	T5Ø.3X2	T5Ø.3X3	T5Ø.3X4	T5Ø.3X5	T5Ø.3X6
Rela	T42.8X1	T42.8X2	T42.8X3	T42.8X4	T42.8X5	T42.8X6
Relaxant, muscle						
anesthetic	T48.1X1	T48.1X2	T48.1X3	T48.1X4	T48.1X5	T48.1X6
central nervous system	T42.8X1	T42.8X2	T42.8X3	T42.8X4	T42.8X5	T42.8X6
skeletal NEC	T48.1X1	T48.1X2	T48.1X3	T48.1X4	T48.1X5	T48.1X6
smooth NEC	T44.3X1	T44.3X2	T44.3X3	T44.3X4	T44.3X5	T44.3X6
Remoxipride	T43.591	T43.592	T43.593	T43.594	T43.595	T43.596
Renese	T5Ø.2X1	T5Ø.2X2	T5Ø.2X3	T5Ø.2X4	T5Ø.2X5	T5Ø.2X6
Renografin	T5Ø.8X1	T5Ø.8X2	T5Ø.8X3	T5Ø.8X4	T5Ø.8X5	T5Ø.8X6
Replacement solution	T5Ø.3X1	T5Ø.3X2	T5Ø.3X3	T5Ø.3X4	T5Ø.3X5	T5Ø.3X6
Reproterol	T48.6X1	T48.6X2	T48.6X3	T48.6X4	T48.6X5	T48.6X6
Rescinnamine	T46.5X1	T46.5X2	T46.5X3	T46.5X4	T46.5X5	T46.5X6
Reserpin (e)	T46.5X1	T46.5X2	T46.5X3	T46.5X4	T46.5X5	T46.5X6
Resorcin, resorcinol (nonmedicinal)	T65.891	T65.892	T65.893	T65.894	—	—
medicinal	T49.4X1	T49.4X2	T49.4X3	T49.4X4	T49.4X5	T49.4X6
Respaire	T48.4X1	T48.4X2	T48.4X3	T48.4X4	T48.4X5	T48.4X6
Respiratory drug NEC	T48.9Ø1	T48.9Ø2	T48.9Ø3	T48.9Ø4	T48.9Ø5	T48.9Ø6
antiasthmatic NEC	T48.6X1	T48.6X2	T48.6X3	T48.6X4	T48.6X5	T48.6X6
anti-common-cold NEC	T48.5X1	T48.5X2	T48.5X3	T48.5X4	T48.5X5	T48.5X6
expectorant NEC	T48.4X1	T48.4X2	T48.4X3	T48.4X4	T48.4X5	T48.4X6

Substance	Poisoning, Accidental (unintentional)	Poisoning, Intentional Self-harm	Poisoning, Assault	Poisoning, Undetermined	Adverse Effect	Under-dosing
Respiratory drug — *continued*						
stimulant	T48.9Ø1	T48.9Ø2	T48.9Ø3	T48.9Ø4	T48.9Ø5	T48.9Ø6
Restoril*	T42.4X1	T42.4X2	T42.4X3	T42.4X4	T42.4X5	T42.4X6
Retinoic acid	T49.ØX1	T49.ØX2	T49.ØX3	T49.ØX4	T49.ØX5	T49.ØX6
Retinol	T45.2X1	T45.2X2	T45.2X3	T45.2X4	T45.2X5	T45.2X6
Rh (D) **immune globulin** (human)	T5Ø.Z11	T5Ø.Z12	T5Ø.Z13	T5Ø.Z14	T5Ø.Z15	T5Ø.Z16
Rhodine	T39.Ø11	T39.Ø12	T39.Ø13	T39.Ø14	T39.Ø15	T39.Ø16
RhoGAM	T5Ø.Z11	T5Ø.Z12	T5Ø.Z13	T5Ø.Z14	T5Ø.Z15	T5Ø.Z16
Rhubarb						
dry extract	T47.2X1	T47.2X2	T47.2X3	T47.2X4	T47.2X5	T47.2X6
tincture, compound	T47.2X1	T47.2X2	T47.2X3	T47.2X4	T47.2X5	T47.2X6
Ribavirin	T37.5X1	T37.5X2	T37.5X3	T37.5X4	T37.5X5	T37.5X6
Riboflavin	T45.2X1	T45.2X2	T45.2X3	T45.2X4	T45.2X5	T45.2X6
Ribostamycin	T36.5X1	T36.5X2	T36.5X3	T36.5X4	T36.5X5	T36.5X6
Ricin	T62.2X1	T62.2X2	T62.2X3	T62.2X4	—	—
Ricinus communis	T62.2X1	T62.2X2	T62.2X3	T62.2X4	—	—
Rickettsial vaccine NEC	T5Ø.A91	T5Ø.A92	T5Ø.A93	T5Ø.A94	T5Ø.A95	T5Ø.A96
Rifabutin	T36.6X1	T36.6X2	T36.6X3	T36.6X4	T36.6X5	T36.6X6
Rifamide	T36.6X1	T36.6X2	T36.6X3	T36.6X4	T36.6X5	T36.6X6
Rifampicin	T36.6X1	T36.6X2	T36.6X3	T36.6X4	T36.6X5	T36.6X6
with isoniazid	T37.1X1	T37.1X2	T37.1X3	T37.1X4	T37.1X5	T37.1X6
Rifampin	T36.6X1	T36.6X2	T36.6X3	T36.6X4	T36.6X5	T36.6X6
Rifamycin	T36.6X1	T36.6X2	T36.6X3	T36.6X4	T36.6X5	T36.6X6
Rifaximin	T36.6X1	T36.6X2	T36.6X3	T36.6X4	T36.6X5	T36.6X6
Rimantadine	T37.5X1	T37.5X2	T37.5X3	T37.5X4	T37.5X5	T37.5X6
Rimazolium metilsulfate	T39.8X1	T39.8X2	T39.8X3	T39.8X4	T39.8X5	T39.8X6
Rimifon	T37.1X1	T37.1X2	T37.1X3	T37.1X4	T37.1X5	T37.1X6
Rimiterol	T48.6X1	T48.6X2	T48.6X3	T48.6X4	T48.6X5	T48.6X6
Ringer (lactate) **solution**	T5Ø.3X1	T5Ø.3X2	T5Ø.3X3	T5Ø.3X4	T5Ø.3X5	T5Ø.3X6
Risperdal*	T43.591	T43.592	T43.593	T43.594	T43.595	T43.596
Ristocetin	T36.8X1	T36.8X2	T36.8X3	T36.8X4	T36.8X5	T36.8X6
Ritalin	T43.631	T43.632	T43.633	T43.634	T43.635	T43.636
Ritodrine	T44.5X1	T44.5X2	T44.5X3	T44.5X4	T44.5X5	T44.5X6
Roach killer — *see* Insecticide						
Robitussin*	T48.3X1	T48.3X2	T48.3X3	T48.3X4	T48.3X5	T48.3X6
Rociverine	T44.3X1	T44.3X2	T44.3X3	T44.3X4	T44.3X5	T44.3X6
Rocky Mountain spotted fever vaccine	T5Ø.A91	T5Ø.A92	T5Ø.A93	T5Ø.A94	T5Ø.A95	T5Ø.A96
Rodenticide NEC	T6Ø.4X1	T6Ø.4X2	T6Ø.4X3	T6Ø.4X4	—	—
Rohypnol	T42.4X1	T42.4X2	T42.4X3	T42.4X4	T42.4X5	T42.4X6
Rokitamycin	T36.3X1	T36.3X2	T36.3X3	T36.3X4	T36.3X5	T36.3X6
Rolaids	T47.1X1	T47.1X2	T47.1X3	T47.1X4	T47.1X5	T47.1X6
Rolitetracycline	T36.4X1	T36.4X2	T36.4X3	T36.4X4	T36.4X5	T36.4X6
Romilar	T48.3X1	T48.3X2	T48.3X3	T48.3X4	T48.3X5	T48.3X6
Ronifibrate	T46.6X1	T46.6X2	T46.6X3	T46.6X4	T46.6X5	T46.6X6
Rosaprostol	T47.1X1	T47.1X2	T47.1X3	T47.1X4	T47.1X5	T47.1X6
Rose bengal sodium (131I)	T5Ø.8X1	T5Ø.8X2	T5Ø.8X3	T5Ø.8X4	T5Ø.8X5	T5Ø.8X6
Rose water ointment	T49.3X1	T49.3X2	T49.3X3	T49.3X4	T49.3X5	T49.3X6
Rosoxacin	T37.8X1	T37.8X2	T37.8X3	T37.8X4	T37.8X5	T37.8X6
Rotenone	T6Ø.2X1	T6Ø.2X2	T6Ø.2X3	T6Ø.2X4	—	—
Rotoxamine	T45.ØX1	T45.ØX2	T45.ØX3	T45.ØX4	T45.ØX5	T45.ØX6
Rough-on-rats	T6Ø.4X1	T6Ø.4X2	T6Ø.4X3	T6Ø.4X4	—	—
Roxatidine	T47.ØX1	T47.ØX2	T47.ØX3	T47.ØX4	T47.ØX5	T47.ØX6
Roxithromycin	T36.3X1	T36.3X2	T36.3X3	T36.3X4	T36.3X5	T36.3X6
Rt-PA	T45.611	T45.612	T45.613	T45.614	T45.615	T45.616
Rubbing alcohol	T51.2X1	T51.2X2	T51.2X3	T51.2X4	—	—
Rubefacient	T49.4X1	T49.4X2	T49.4X3	T49.4X4	T49.4X5	T49.4X6
Rubella vaccine	T5Ø.B91	T5Ø.B92	T5Ø.B93	T5Ø.B94	T5Ø.B95	T5Ø.B96
Rubeola vaccine	T5Ø.B91	T5Ø.B92	T5Ø.B93	T5Ø.B94	T5Ø.B95	T5Ø.B96
Rubidium chloride Rb82	T5Ø.8X1	T5Ø.8X2	T5Ø.8X3	T5Ø.8X4	T5Ø.8X5	T5Ø.8X6
Rubidomycin	T45.1X1	T45.1X2	T45.1X3	T45.1X4	T45.1X5	T45.1X6
Rue	T62.2X1	T62.2X2	T62.2X3	T62.2X4	—	—
Rufocromomycin	T45.1X1	T45.1X2	T45.1X3	T45.1X4	T45.1X5	T45.1X6
Russel's viper venin	T45.7X1	T45.7X2	T45.7X3	T45.7X4	T45.7X5	T45.7X6
Ruta (graveolens)	T62.2X1	T62.2X2	T62.2X3	T62.2X4	—	—
Rutinum	T46.991	T46.992	T46.993	T46.994	T46.995	T46.996
Rutoside	T46.991	T46.992	T46.993	T46.994	T46.995	T46.996
b-sitosterol(s)	T46.6X1	T46.6X2	T46.6X3	T46.6X4	T46.6X5	T46.6X6
Sabadilla (plant)	T62.2X1	T62.2X2	T62.2X3	T62.2X4	—	—
pesticide	T6Ø.2X1	T6Ø.2X2	T6Ø.2X3	T6Ø.2X4	—	—
Sabril*	T42.6X1	T42.6X2	T42.6X3	T42.6X4	T42.6X5	T42.6X6
Saccharated iron oxide	T45.8X1	T45.8X2	T45.8X3	T45.8X4	T45.8X5	T45.8X6
Saccharin	T5Ø.9Ø1	T5Ø.9Ø2	T5Ø.9Ø3	T5Ø.9Ø4	T5Ø.9Ø5	T5Ø.9Ø6
Saccharomyces boulardii	T47.6X1	T47.6X2	T47.6X3	T47.6X4	T47.6X5	T47.6X6
Safflower oil	T46.6X1	T46.6X2	T46.6X3	T46.6X4	T46.6X5	T46.6X6
Safrazine	T43.1X1	T43.1X2	T43.1X3	T43.1X4	T43.1X5	T43.1X6
Salazosulfapyridine	T37.ØX1	T37.ØX2	T37.ØX3	T37.ØX4	T37.ØX5	T37.ØX6
Salbutamol	T48.6X1	T48.6X2	T48.6X3	T48.6X4	T48.6X5	T48.6X6
Salicylamide	T39.Ø91	T39.Ø92	T39.Ø93	T39.Ø94	T39.Ø95	T39.Ø96
Salicylate NEC	T39.Ø91	T39.Ø92	T39.Ø93	T39.Ø94	T39.Ø95	T39.Ø96
methyl	T49.3X1	T49.3X2	T49.3X3	T49.3X4	T49.3X5	T49.3X6
theobromine calcium	T5Ø.2X1	T5Ø.2X2	T5Ø.2X3	T5Ø.2X4	T5Ø.2X5	T5Ø.2X6

Substance	Poisoning, Accidental (unintentional)	Poisoning, Intentional Self-harm	Poisoning, Assault	Poisoning, Undetermined	Adverse Effect	Under-dosing
Salicylazosulfapyridine	T37.ØX1	T37.ØX2	T37.ØX3	T37.ØX4	T37.ØX5	T37.ØX6
Salicylhydroxamic acid	T49.ØX1	T49.ØX2	T49.ØX3	T49.ØX4	T49.ØX5	T49.ØX6
Salicylic acid	T49.4X1	T49.4X2	T49.4X3	T49.4X4	T49.4X5	T49.4X6
with benzoic acid	T49.4X1	T49.4X2	T49.4X3	T49.4X4	T49.4X5	T49.4X6
congeners	T39.Ø91	T39.Ø92	T39.Ø93	T39.Ø94	T39.Ø95	T39.Ø96
derivative	T39.Ø91	T39.Ø92	T39.Ø93	T39.Ø94	T39.Ø95	T39.Ø96
salts	T39.Ø91	T39.Ø92	T39.Ø93	T39.Ø94	T39.Ø95	T39.Ø96
Salinazid	T37.1X1	T37.1X2	T37.1X3	T37.1X4	T37.1X5	T37.1X6
Salmeterol	T48.6X1	T48.6X2	T48.6X3	T48.6X4	T48.6X5	T48.6X6
Salol	T49.3X1	T49.3X2	T49.3X3	T49.3X4	T49.3X5	T49.3X6
Salsalate	T39.Ø91	T39.Ø92	T39.Ø93	T39.Ø94	T39.Ø95	T39.Ø96
Salt-replacing drug	T5Ø.9Ø1	T5Ø.9Ø2	T5Ø.9Ø3	T5Ø.9Ø4	T5Ø.9Ø5	T5Ø.9Ø6
Salt-retaining mineralocorticoid	T5Ø.ØX1	T5Ø.ØX2	T5Ø.ØX3	T5Ø.ØX4	T5Ø.ØX5	T5Ø.ØX6
Salt substitute	T5Ø.9Ø1	T5Ø.9Ø2	T5Ø.9Ø3	T5Ø.9Ø4	T5Ø.9Ø5	T5Ø.9Ø6
Saluretic NEC	T5Ø.2X1	T5Ø.2X2	T5Ø.2X3	T5Ø.2X4	T5Ø.2X5	T5Ø.2X6
Saluron	T5Ø.2X1	T5Ø.2X2	T5Ø.2X3	T5Ø.2X4	T5Ø.2X5	T5Ø.2X6
Salvarsan 606 (neosilver) (silver)	T37.8X1	T37.8X2	T37.8X3	T37.8X4	T37.8X5	T37.8X6
Sambucus canadensis	T62.2X1	T62.2X2	T62.2X3	T62.2X4	—	—
berry	T62.1X1	T62.1X2	T62.1X3	T62.1X4	—	—
Sandril	T46.5X1	T46.5X2	T46.5X3	T46.5X4	T46.5X5	T46.5X6
Sanguinaria canadensis	T62.2X1	T62.2X2	T62.2X3	T62.2X4	—	—
Saniflush (cleaner)	T54.2X1	T54.2X2	T54.2X3	T54.2X4	—	—
Santonin	T37.4X1	T37.4X2	T37.4X3	T37.4X4	T37.4X5	T37.4X6
Santyl	T49.8X1	T49.8X2	T49.8X3	T49.8X4	T49.8X5	T49.8X6
Saralasin	T46.5X1	T46.5X2	T46.5X3	T46.5X4	T46.5X5	T46.5X6
Sarcolysin	T45.1X1	T45.1X2	T45.1X3	T45.1X4	T45.1X5	T45.1X6
Sarilumab*	T39.4X1	T39.4X2	T39.4X3	T39.4X4	T39.4X5	T39.4X6
Sarkomycin	T45.1X1	T45.1X2	T45.1X3	T45.1X4	T45.1X5	T45.1X6
Saroten	T43.Ø11	T43.Ø12	T43.Ø13	T43.Ø14	T43.Ø15	T43.Ø16
Saturnine — *see* Lead						
Savin (oil)	T49.4X1	T49.4X2	T49.4X3	T49.4X4	T49.4X5	T49.4X6
Scammony	T47.2X1	T47.2X2	T47.2X3	T47.2X4	T47.2X5	T47.2X6
Scarlet red	T49.8X1	T49.8X2	T49.8X3	T49.8X4	T49.8X5	T49.8X6
Scheele's green	T57.ØX1	T57.ØX2	T57.ØX3	T57.ØX4	—	—
insecticide	T57.ØX1	T57.ØX2	T57.ØX3	T57.ØX4	—	—
Schizontozide (blood) (tissue)	T37.2X1	T37.2X2	T37.2X3	T37.2X4	T37.2X5	T37.2X6
Schradan	T6Ø.ØX1	T6Ø.ØX2	T6Ø.ØX3	T6Ø.ØX4	—	—
Schweinfurth green	T57.ØX1	T57.ØX2	T57.ØX3	T57.ØX4	—	—
insecticide	T57.ØX1	T57.ØX2	T57.ØX3	T57.ØX4	—	—
Scilla, rat poison	T6Ø.4X1	T6Ø.4X2	T6Ø.4X3	T6Ø.4X4	—	—
Scillaren	T6Ø.4X1	T6Ø.4X2	T6Ø.4X3	T6Ø.4X4	—	—
Sclerosing agent	T46.8X1	T46.8X2	T46.8X3	T46.8X4	T46.8X5	T46.8X6
Scombrotoxin	T61.11	T61.12	T61.13	T61.14	—	—
Scopolamine	T44.3X1	T44.3X2	T44.3X3	T44.3X4	T44.3X5	T44.3X6
Scopolia extract	T44.3X1	T44.3X2	T44.3X3	T44.3X4	T44.3X5	T44.3X6
Scouring powder	T65.891	T65.892	T65.893	T65.894	—	—
Sea						
anemone (sting)	T63.631	T63.632	T63.633	T63.634	—	—
cucumber (sting)	T63.691	T63.692	T63.693	T63.694	—	—
snake (bite) (venom)	T63.Ø91	T63.Ø92	T63.Ø93	T63.Ø94	—	—
urchin spine (puncture)	T63.691	T63.692	T63.693	T63.694	—	—
Seafood	T61.91	T61.92	T61.93	T61.94	—	—
specified NEC	T61.8X1	T61.8X2	T61.8X3	T61.8X4	—	—
Secbutabarbital	T42.3X1	T42.3X2	T42.3X3	T42.3X4	T42.3X5	T42.3X6
Secbutabarbitone	T42.3X1	T42.3X2	T42.3X3	T42.3X4	T42.3X5	T42.3X6
Secnidazole	T37.3X1	T37.3X2	T37.3X3	T37.3X4	T37.3X5	T37.3X6
Secobarbital	T42.3X1	T42.3X2	T42.3X3	T42.3X4	T42.3X5	T42.3X6
Seconal	T42.3X1	T42.3X2	T42.3X3	T42.3X4	T42.3X5	T42.3X6
Secretin	T5Ø.8X1	T5Ø.8X2	T5Ø.8X3	T5Ø.8X4	T5Ø.8X5	T5Ø.8X6
Sectral*	T44.7X1	T44.7X2	T44.7X3	T44.7X4	T44.7X5	T44.7X6
Sedative NEC	T42.71	T42.72	T42.73	T42.74	T42.75	T42.76
mixed NEC	T42.6X1	T42.6X2	T42.6X3	T42.6X4	T42.6X5	T42.6X6
Sedormid	T42.6X1	T42.6X2	T42.6X3	T42.6X4	T42.6X5	T42.6X6
Seed disinfectant or dressing	T6Ø.8X1	T6Ø.8X2	T6Ø.8X3	T6Ø.8X4	—	—
Seeds (poisonous)	T62.2X1	T62.2X2	T62.2X3	T62.2X4	—	—
Selegiline	T42.8X1	T42.8X2	T42.8X3	T42.8X4	T42.8X5	T42.8X6
Selenium NEC	T56.891	T56.892	T56.893	T56.894	—	—
disulfide or sulfide	T49.4X1	T49.4X2	T49.4X3	T49.4X4	T49.4X5	T49.4X6
fumes	T59.891	T59.892	T59.893	T59.894	—	—
sulfide	T49.4X1	T49.4X2	T49.4X3	T49.4X4	T49.4X5	T49.4X6
Selenomethionine (75Se)	T5Ø.8X1	T5Ø.8X2	T5Ø.8X3	T5Ø.8X4	T5Ø.8X5	T5Ø.8X6
Selsun	T49.4X1	T49.4X2	T49.4X3	T49.4X4	T49.4X5	T49.4X6
Semustine	T45.1X1	T45.1X2	T45.1X3	T45.1X4	T45.1X5	T45.1X6
Senega syrup	T48.4X1	T48.4X2	T48.4X3	T48.4X4	T48.4X5	T48.4X6
Senna	T47.2X1	T47.2X2	T47.2X3	T47.2X4	T47.2X5	T47.2X6
Sennoside A+B	T47.2X1	T47.2X2	T47.2X3	T47.2X4	T47.2X5	T47.2X6
Septisol	T49.2X1	T49.2X2	T49.2X3	T49.2X4	T49.2X5	T49.2X6
Seractide	T38.811	T38.812	T38.813	T38.814	T38.815	T38.816
Serax	T42.4X1	T42.4X2	T42.4X3	T42.4X4	T42.4X5	T42.4X6

*Optum Value-Add

Substance	Poisoning, Accidental (unintentional)	Poisoning, Intentional Self-harm	Poisoning, Assault	Poisoning, Undetermined	Adverse Effect	Under-dosing
Serenesil	T42.6X1	T42.6X2	T42.6X3	T42.6X4	T42.6X5	T42.6X6
Serenium (hydrochloride)	T37.91	T37.92	T37.93	T37.94	T37.95	T37.96
Serepax — *see* Oxazepam						
Serevent*	T48.6X1	T48.6X2	T48.6X3	T48.6X4	T48.6X5	T48.6X6
Sermorelin	T38.891	T38.892	T38.893	T38.894	T38.895	T38.896
Sernyl	T41.1X1	T41.1X2	T41.1X3	T41.1X4	T41.1X5	T41.1X6
Serotonin	T50.991	T50.992	T50.993	T50.994	T50.995	T50.996
Serpasil	T46.5X1	T46.5X2	T46.5X3	T46.5X4	T46.5X5	T46.5X6
Serrapeptase	T45.3X1	T45.3X2	T45.3X3	T45.3X4	T45.3X5	T45.3X6
Serum						
antibotulinus	T50.Z11	T50.Z12	T50.Z13	T50.Z14	T50.Z15	T50.Z16
anticytotoxic	T50.Z11	T50.Z12	T50.Z13	T50.Z14	T50.Z15	T50.Z16
antidiphtheria	T50.Z11	T50.Z12	T50.Z13	T50.Z14	T50.Z15	T50.Z16
antimeningococcus	T50.Z11	T50.Z12	T50.Z13	T50.Z14	T50.Z15	T50.Z16
anti-Rh	T50.Z11	T50.Z12	T50.Z13	T50.Z14	T50.Z15	T50.Z16
anti-snake-bite	T50.Z11	T50.Z12	T50.Z13	T50.Z14	T50.Z15	T50.Z16
antitetanic	T50.Z11	T50.Z12	T50.Z13	T50.Z14	T50.Z15	T50.Z16
antitoxic	T50.Z11	T50.Z12	T50.Z13	T50.Z14	T50.Z15	T50.Z16
complement (inhibitor)	T45.8X1	T45.8X2	T45.8X3	T45.8X4	T45.8X5	T45.8X6
convalescent	T50.Z11	T50.Z12	T50.Z13	T50.Z14	T50.Z15	T50.Z16
hemolytic complement	T45.8X1	T45.8X2	T45.8X3	T45.8X4	T45.8X5	T45.8X6
immune (human)	T50.Z11	T50.Z12	T50.Z13	T50.Z14	T50.Z15	T50.Z16
protective NEC	T50.Z11	T50.Z12	T50.Z13	T50.Z14	T50.Z15	T50.Z16
Setastine	T45.ØX1	T45.ØX2	T45.ØX3	T45.ØX4	T45.ØX5	T45.ØX6
Setoperone	T43.591	T43.592	T43.593	T43.594	T43.595	T43.596
Sewer gas	T59.91	T59.92	T59.93	T59.94	—	—
Shampoo	T55.ØX1	T55.ØX2	T55.ØX3	T55.ØX4	—	—
Shellfish, noxious, nonbacterial	T61.781	T61.782	T61.783	T61.784	—	—
Sildenafil	T46.7X1	T46.7X2	T46.7X3	T46.7X4	T46.7X5	T46.7X6
Silibinin	T50.991	T50.992	T50.993	T50.994	T50.995	T50.996
Silicone NEC	T65.891	T65.892	T65.893	T65.894	—	—
medicinal	T49.3X1	T49.3X2	T49.3X3	T49.3X4	T49.3X5	T49.3X6
Silvadene	T49.ØX1	T49.ØX2	T49.ØX3	T49.ØX4	T49.ØX5	T49.ØX6
Silver	T49.ØX1	T49.ØX2	T49.ØX3	T49.ØX4	T49.ØX5	T49.ØX6
anti-infectives	T49.ØX1	T49.ØX2	T49.ØX3	T49.ØX4	T49.ØX5	T49.ØX6
arsphenamine	T37.8X1	T37.8X2	T37.8X3	T37.8X4	T37.8X5	T37.8X6
colloidal	T49.ØX1	T49.ØX2	T49.ØX3	T49.ØX4	T49.ØX5	T49.ØX6
nitrate	T49.ØX1	T49.ØX2	T49.ØX3	T49.ØX4	T49.ØX5	T49.ØX6
ophthalmic preparation	T49.5X1	T49.5X2	T49.5X3	T49.5X4	T49.5X5	T49.5X6
toughened (keratolytic)	T49.4X1	T49.4X2	T49.4X3	T49.4X4	T49.4X5	T49.4X6
nonmedicinal (dust)	T56.891	T56.892	T56.893	T56.894	—	—
protein	T49.5X1	T49.5X2	T49.5X3	T49.5X4	T49.5X5	T49.5X6
salvarsan	T37.8X1	T37.8X2	T37.8X3	T37.8X4	T37.8X5	T37.8X6
sulfadiazine	T49.4X1	T49.4X2	T49.4X3	T49.4X4	T49.4X5	T49.4X6
Silymarin	T50.991	T50.992	T50.993	T50.994	T50.995	T50.996
Simaldrate	T47.1X1	T47.1X2	T47.1X3	T47.1X4	T47.1X5	T47.1X6
Simazine	T60.3X1	T60.3X2	T60.3X3	T60.3X4	—	—
Simethicone	T47.1X1	T47.1X2	T47.1X3	T47.1X4	T47.1X5	T47.1X6
Simfibrate	T46.6X1	T46.6X2	T46.6X3	T46.6X4	T46.6X5	T46.6X6
Simvastatin	T46.6X1	T46.6X2	T46.6X3	T46.6X4	T46.6X5	T46.6X6
Sincalide	T50.8X1	T50.8X2	T50.8X3	T50.8X4	T50.8X5	T50.8X6
Sinequan	T43.Ø11	T43.Ø12	T43.Ø13	T43.Ø14	T43.Ø15	T43.Ø16
Singoserp	T46.5X1	T46.5X2	T46.5X3	T46.5X4	T46.5X5	T46.5X6
Singulair*	T48.6X1	T48.6X2	T48.6X3	T48.6X4	T48.6X5	T48.6X6
Sintrom	T45.511	T45.512	T45.513	T45.514	T45.515	T45.516
Sisomicin	T36.5X1	T36.5X2	T36.5X3	T36.5X4	T36.5X5	T36.5X6
Sitosterols	T46.6X1	T46.6X2	T46.6X3	T46.6X4	T46.6X5	T46.6X6
Skeletal muscle relaxants	T48.1X1	T48.1X2	T48.1X3	T48.1X4	T48.1X5	T48.1X6
Skin						
agents (external)	T49.91	T49.92	T49.93	T49.94	T49.95	T49.96
specified NEC	T49.8X1	T49.8X2	T49.8X3	T49.8X4	T49.8X5	T49.8X6
test antigen	T50.8X1	T50.8X2	T50.8X3	T50.8X4	T50.8X5	T50.8X6
Sleep-eze	T45.ØX1	T45.ØX2	T45.ØX3	T45.ØX4	T45.ØX5	T45.ØX6
Sleeping draught, pill	T42.71	T42.72	T42.73	T42.74	T42.75	T42.76
Smallpox vaccine	T50.B11	T50.B12	T50.B13	T50.B14	T50.B15	T50.B16
Smelter fumes NEC	T56.91	T56.92	T56.93	T56.94	—	—
Smog	T59.1X1	T59.1X2	T59.1X3	T59.1X4	—	—
Smoke NEC	T59.811	T59.812	T59.813	T59.814	—	—
Smooth muscle relaxant	T44.3X1	T44.3X2	T44.3X3	T44.3X4	T44.3X5	T44.3X6
Snail killer NEC	T60.8X1	T60.8X2	T60.8X3	T60.8X4	—	—
Snake venom or bite	T63.ØØ1	T63.ØØ2	T63.ØØ3	T63.ØØ4	—	—
hemocoagulase	T45.7X1	T45.7X2	T45.7X3	T45.7X4	T45.7X5	T45.7X6
Snuff	T65.211	T65.212	T65.213	T65.214	—	—
Soap (powder) (product)	T55.ØX1	T55.ØX2	T55.ØX3	T55.ØX4	—	—
enema	T47.4X1	T47.4X2	T47.4X3	T47.4X4	T47.4X5	T47.4X6
medicinal, soft	T49.2X1	T49.2X2	T49.2X3	T49.2X4	T49.2X5	T49.2X6
superfatted	T49.2X1	T49.2X2	T49.2X3	T49.2X4	T49.2X5	T49.2X6
Sobrerol	T48.4X1	T48.4X2	T48.4X3	T48.4X4	T48.4X5	T48.4X6
Soda (caustic)	T54.3X1	T54.3X2	T54.3X3	T54.3X4	—	—
bicarb	T47.1X1	T47.1X2	T47.1X3	T47.1X4	T47.1X5	T47.1X6
chlorinated — *see* Sodium, hypochlorite						

Substance	Poisoning, Accidental (unintentional)	Poisoning, Intentional Self-harm	Poisoning, Assault	Poisoning, Undetermined	Adverse Effect	Under-dosing
Sodium						
acetosulfone	T37.1X1	T37.1X2	T37.1X3	T37.1X4	T37.1X5	T37.1X6
acetrizoate	T50.8X1	T50.8X2	T50.8X3	T50.8X4	T50.8X5	T50.8X6
acid phosphate	T50.3X1	T50.3X2	T50.3X3	T50.3X4	T50.3X5	T50.3X6
alginate	T47.8X1	T47.8X2	T47.8X3	T47.8X4	T47.8X5	T47.8X6
amidotrizoate	T50.8X1	T50.8X2	T50.8X3	T50.8X4	T50.8X5	T50.8X6
aminohippurate*	T50.8X1	T50.8X2	T50.8X3	T50.8X4	T50.8X5	T50.8X6
aminopterin	T45.1X1	T45.1X2	T45.1X3	T45.1X4	T45.1X5	T45.1X6
amylosulfate	T47.8X1	T47.8X2	T47.8X3	T47.8X4	T47.8X5	T47.8X6
amytal	T42.3X1	T42.3X2	T42.3X3	T42.3X4	T42.3X5	T42.3X6
antimony gluconate	T37.3X1	T37.3X2	T37.3X3	T37.3X4	T37.3X5	T37.3X6
arsenate	T57.ØX1	T57.ØX2	T57.ØX3	T57.ØX4	—	—
aurothiomalate	T39.4X1	T39.4X2	T39.4X3	T39.4X4	T39.4X5	T39.4X6
aurothiosulfate	T39.4X1	T39.4X2	T39.4X3	T39.4X4	T39.4X5	T39.4X6
barbiturate	T42.3X1	T42.3X2	T42.3X3	T42.3X4	T42.3X5	T42.3X6
basic phosphate	T47.4X1	T47.4X2	T47.4X3	T47.4X4	T47.4X5	T47.4X6
bicarbonate	T47.1X1	T47.1X2	T47.1X3	T47.1X4	T47.1X5	T47.1X6
bichromate	T57.8X1	T57.8X2	T57.8X3	T57.8X4	—	—
biphosphate	T50.3X1	T50.3X2	T50.3X3	T50.3X4	T50.3X5	T50.3X6
bisulfate	T65.891	T65.892	T65.893	T65.894	—	—
borate						
cleanser	T57.8X1	T57.8X2	T57.8X3	T57.8X4	—	—
eye	T49.5X1	T49.5X2	T49.5X3	T49.5X4	T49.5X5	T49.5X6
therapeutic	T49.8X1	T49.8X2	T49.8X3	T49.8X4	T49.8X5	T49.8X6
bromide	T42.6X1	T42.6X2	T42.6X3	T42.6X4	T42.6X5	T42.6X6
cacodylate (nonmedicinal)	T50.8X1	T50.8X2	T50.8X3	T50.8X4	T50.8X5	T50.8X6
NEC						
anti-infective	T37.8X1	T37.8X2	T37.8X3	T37.8X4	T37.8X5	T37.8X6
herbicide	T60.3X1	T60.3X2	T60.3X3	T60.3X4	—	—
calcium edetate	T45.8X1	T45.8X2	T45.8X3	T45.8X4	T45.8X5	T45.8X6
carbonate NEC	T54.3X1	T54.3X2	T54.3X3	T54.3X4	—	—
chlorate NEC	T65.891	T65.892	T65.893	T65.894	—	—
herbicide	T54.91	T54.92	T54.93	T54.94	—	—
chloride	T50.3X1	T50.3X2	T50.3X3	T50.3X4	T50.3X5	T50.3X6
with glucose	T50.3X1	T50.3X2	T50.3X3	T50.3X4	T50.3X5	T50.3X6
chromate	T65.891	T65.892	T65.893	T65.894	—	—
citrate	T50.991	T50.992	T50.993	T50.994	T50.995	T50.996
cromoglicate	T48.6X1	T48.6X2	T48.6X3	T48.6X4	T48.6X5	T48.6X6
cyanide	T65.ØX1	T65.ØX2	T65.ØX3	T65.ØX4	—	—
cyclamate	T50.3X1	T50.3X2	T50.3X3	T50.3X4	T50.3X5	T50.3X6
dehydrocholate	T45.8X1	T45.8X2	T45.8X3	T45.8X4	T45.8X5	T45.8X6
diatrizoate	T50.8X1	T50.8X2	T50.8X3	T50.8X4	T50.8X5	T50.8X6
dibunate	T48.4X1	T48.4X2	T48.4X3	T48.4X4	T48.4X5	T48.4X6
dioctyl sulfosuccinate	T47.4X1	T47.4X2	T47.4X3	T47.4X4	T47.4X5	T47.4X6
dipantoyl ferrate	T45.8X1	T45.8X2	T45.8X3	T45.8X4	T45.8X5	T45.8X6
edetate	T45.8X1	T45.8X2	T45.8X3	T45.8X4	T45.8X5	T45.8X6
ethacrynate	T50.1X1	T50.1X2	T50.1X3	T50.1X4	T50.1X5	T50.1X6
etidronate*	T50.991	T50.992	T50.993	T50.994	T50.995	T50.996
feredetate	T45.8X1	T45.8X2	T45.8X3	T45.8X4	T45.8X5	T45.8X6
Fluoride — *see* Fluoride						
fluoroacetate (dust) (pesticide)	T60.4X1	T60.4X2	T60.4X3	T60.4X4	—	—
free salt	T50.3X1	T50.3X2	T50.3X3	T50.3X4	T50.3X5	T50.3X6
fusidate	T36.8X1	T36.8X2	T36.8X3	T36.8X4	T36.8X5	T36.8X6
glucaldrate	T47.1X1	T47.1X2	T47.1X3	T47.1X4	T47.1X5	T47.1X6
glucosulfone	T37.1X1	T37.1X2	T37.1X3	T37.1X4	T37.1X5	T37.1X6
glutamate	T45.8X1	T45.8X2	T45.8X3	T45.8X4	T45.8X5	T45.8X6
hydrogen carbonate	T50.3X1	T50.3X2	T50.3X3	T50.3X4	T50.3X5	T50.3X6
hydroxide	T54.3X1	T54.3X2	T54.3X3	T54.3X4	—	—
hypochlorite (bleach) NEC	T54.3X1	T54.3X2	T54.3X3	T54.3X4	—	—
disinfectant	T54.3X1	T54.3X2	T54.3X3	T54.3X4	—	—
medicinal (anti-infective) (external)	T49.ØX1	T49.ØX2	T49.ØX3	T49.ØX4	T49.ØX5	T49.ØX6
vapor	T54.3X1	T54.3X2	T54.3X3	T54.3X4	—	—
hyposulfite	T49.ØX1	T49.ØX2	T49.ØX3	T49.ØX4	T49.ØX5	T49.ØX6
indigotin disulfonate	T50.8X1	T50.8X2	T50.8X3	T50.8X4	T50.8X5	T50.8X6
iodide	T50.991	T50.992	T50.993	T50.994	T50.995	T50.996
I-131	T50.8X1	T50.8X2	T50.8X3	T50.8X4	T50.8X5	T50.8X6
therapeutic	T38.2X1	T38.2X2	T38.2X3	T38.2X4	T38.2X5	T38.2X6
iodohippurate (131I)	T50.8X1	T50.8X2	T50.8X3	T50.8X4	T50.8X5	T50.8X6
iopodate	T50.8X1	T50.8X2	T50.8X3	T50.8X4	T50.8X5	T50.8X6
iothalamate	T50.8X1	T50.8X2	T50.8X3	T50.8X4	T50.8X5	T50.8X6
iron edetate	T45.4X1	T45.4X2	T45.4X3	T45.4X4	T45.4X5	T45.4X6
lactate (compound solution)	T45.8X1	T45.8X2	T45.8X3	T45.8X4	T45.8X5	T45.8X6
lauryl (sulfate)	T49.2X1	T49.2X2	T49.2X3	T49.2X4	T49.2X5	T49.2X6
L-triiodothyronine	T38.1X1	T38.1X2	T38.1X3	T38.1X4	T38.1X5	T38.1X6
magnesium citrate	T50.991	T50.992	T50.993	T50.994	T50.995	T50.996
mersalate	T50.2X1	T50.2X2	T50.2X3	T50.2X4	T50.2X5	T50.2X6
metasilicate	T65.891	T65.892	T65.893	T65.894	—	—
metrizoate	T50.8X1	T50.8X2	T50.8X3	T50.8X4	T50.8X5	T50.8X6
monofluoroacetate (pesticide)	T60.1X1	T60.1X2	T60.1X3	T60.1X4	—	—

Substance	Poisoning, Accidental (unintentional)	Poisoning, Intentional Self-harm	Poisoning, Assault	Poisoning, Undetermined	Adverse Effect	Under-dosing
Sodium — *continued*						
morrhuate	T46.8X1	T46.8X2	T46.8X3	T46.8X4	T46.8X5	T46.8X6
nafcillin	T36.ØX1	T36.ØX2	T36.ØX3	T36.ØX4	T36.ØX5	T36.ØX6
nitrate (oxidizing agent)	T65.891	T65.892	T65.893	T65.894	—	—
nitrite	T5Ø.6X1	T5Ø.6X2	T5Ø.6X3	T5Ø.6X4	T5Ø.6X5	T5Ø.6X6
nitroferricyanide	T46.5X1	T46.5X2	T46.5X3	T46.5X4	T46.5X5	T46.5X6
nitroprusside	T46.5X1	T46.5X2	T46.5X3	T46.5X4	T46.5X5	T46.5X6
oxalate	T65.891	T65.892	T65.893	T65.894	—	—
oxide/peroxide	T65.891	T65.892	T65.893	T65.894	—	—
oxybate	T41.291	T41.292	T41.293	T41.294	T41.295	T41.296
para-aminohippurate	T5Ø.8X1	T5Ø.8X2	T5Ø.8X3	T5Ø.8X4	T5Ø.8X5	T5Ø.8X6
perborate (nonmedicinal) NEC	T65.891	T65.892	T65.893	T65.894	—	—
medicinal	T49.ØX1	T49.ØX2	T49.ØX3	T49.ØX4	T49.ØX5	T49.ØX6
soap	T55.ØX1	T55.ØX2	T55.ØX3	T55.ØX4	—	—
percarbonate — *see* Sodium, perborate						
pertechnetate Tc99m	T5Ø.8X1	T5Ø.8X2	T5Ø.8X3	T5Ø.8X4	T5Ø.8X5	T5Ø.8X6
phosphate						
cellulose	T45.8X1	T45.8X2	T45.8X3	T45.8X4	T45.8X5	T45.8X6
dibasic	T47.2X1	T47.2X2	T47.2X3	T47.2X4	T47.2X5	T47.2X6
monobasic	T47.2X1	T47.2X2	T47.2X3	T47.2X4	T47.2X5	T47.2X6
phytate	T5Ø.6X1	T5Ø.6X2	T5Ø.6X3	T5Ø.6X4	T5Ø.6X5	T5Ø.6X6
picosulfate	T47.2X1	T47.2X2	T47.2X3	T47.2X4	T47.2X5	T47.2X6
polyhydroxyaluminium monocarbonate	T47.1X1	T47.1X2	T47.1X3	T47.1X4	T47.1X5	T47.1X6
polystyrene sulfonate	T5Ø.3X1	T5Ø.3X2	T5Ø.3X3	T5Ø.3X4	T5Ø.3X5	T5Ø.3X6
propionate	T49.ØX1	T49.ØX2	T49.ØX3	T49.ØX4	T49.ØX5	T49.ØX6
propyl hydroxybenzoate	T5Ø.991	T5Ø.992	T5Ø.993	T5Ø.994	T5Ø.995	T5Ø.996
psylliate	T46.8X1	T46.8X2	T46.8X3	T46.8X4	T46.8X5	T46.8X6
removing resins	T5Ø.3X1	T5Ø.3X2	T5Ø.3X3	T5Ø.3X4	T5Ø.3X5	T5Ø.3X6
salicylate	T39.Ø91	T39.Ø92	T39.Ø93	T39.Ø94	T39.Ø95	T39.Ø96
salt NEC	T5Ø.3X1	T5Ø.3X2	T5Ø.3X3	T5Ø.3X4	T5Ø.3X5	T5Ø.3X6
selenate	T6Ø.2X1	T6Ø.2X2	T6Ø.2X3	T6Ø.2X4	—	—
stibogluconate	T37.3X1	T37.3X2	T37.3X3	T37.3X4	T37.3X5	T37.3X6
sulfate	T47.4X1	T47.4X2	T47.4X3	T47.4X4	T47.4X5	T47.4X6
sulfoxone	T37.1X1	T37.1X2	T37.1X3	T37.1X4	T37.1X5	T37.1X6
tetradecyl sulfate	T46.8X1	T46.8X2	T46.8X3	T46.8X4	T46.8X5	T46.8X6
thiopental	T41.1X1	T41.1X2	T41.1X3	T41.1X4	T41.1X5	T41.1X6
thiosalicylate	T39.Ø91	T39.Ø92	T39.Ø93	T39.Ø94	T39.Ø95	T39.Ø96
thiosulfate	T5Ø.6X1	T5Ø.6X2	T5Ø.6X3	T5Ø.6X4	T5Ø.6X5	T5Ø.6X6
tolbutamide	T38.3X1	T38.3X2	T38.3X3	T38.3X4	T38.3X5	T38.3X6
(L)-triiodothyronine	T38.1X1	T38.1X2	T38.1X3	T38.1X4	T38.1X5	T38.1X6
tyropanoate	T5Ø.8X1	T5Ø.8X2	T5Ø.8X3	T5Ø.8X4	T5Ø.8X5	T5Ø.8X6
valproate	T42.6X1	T42.6X2	T42.6X3	T42.6X4	T42.6X5	T42.6X6
versenate	T5Ø.6X1	T5Ø.6X2	T5Ø.6X3	T5Ø.6X4	T5Ø.6X5	T5Ø.6X6
Sodium-free salt	T5Ø.9Ø1	T5Ø.9Ø2	T5Ø.9Ø3	T5Ø.9Ø4	T5Ø.9Ø5	T5Ø.9Ø6
Sodium-removing resin	T5Ø.3X1	T5Ø.3X2	T5Ø.3X3	T5Ø.3X4	T5Ø.3X5	T5Ø.3X6
Soft soap	T55.ØX1	T55.ØX2	T55.ØX3	T55.ØX4	—	—
Solanine	T62.2X1	T62.2X2	T62.2X3	T62.2X4	—	—
berries	T62.1X1	T62.1X2	T62.1X3	T62.1X4	—	—
Solanum dulcamara	T62.2X1	T62.2X2	T62.2X3	T62.2X4	—	—
berries	T62.1X1	T62.1X2	T62.1X3	T62.1X4	—	—
Solapsone	T37.1X1	T37.1X2	T37.1X3	T37.1X4	T37.1X5	T37.1X6
Solaquin*	T49.8X1	T49.8X2	T49.8X3	T49.8X4	T49.8X5	T49.8X6
Solar lotion	T49.3X1	T49.3X2	T49.3X3	T49.3X4	T49.3X5	T49.3X6
Solasulfone	T37.1X1	T37.1X2	T37.1X3	T37.1X4	T37.1X5	T37.1X6
Soldering fluid	T65.891	T65.892	T65.893	T65.894	—	—
Solid substance	T65.91	T65.92	T65.93	T65.94	—	—
specified NEC	T65.891	T65.892	T65.893	T65.894	—	—
Solvent, industrial NEC	T52.91	T52.92	T52.93	T52.94	—	—
naphtha	T52.ØX1	T52.ØX2	T52.ØX3	T52.ØX4	—	—
petroleum	T52.ØX1	T52.ØX2	T52.ØX3	T52.ØX4	—	—
specified NEC	T52.8X1	T52.8X2	T52.8X3	T52.8X4	—	—
Soma	T42.8X1	T42.8X2	T42.8X3	T42.8X4	T42.8X5	T42.8X6
Somatorelin	T38.891	T38.892	T38.893	T38.894	T38.895	T38.896
Somatostatin	T38.991	T38.992	T38.993	T38.994	T38.995	T38.996
Somatotropin	T38.811	T38.812	T38.813	T38.814	T38.815	T38.816
Somatrem	T38.811	T38.812	T38.813	T38.814	T38.815	T38.816
Somatropin	T38.811	T38.812	T38.813	T38.814	T38.815	T38.816
Sominex	T45.ØX1	T45.ØX2	T45.ØX3	T45.ØX4	T45.ØX5	T45.ØX6
Somnos	T42.6X1	T42.6X2	T42.6X3	T42.6X4	T42.6X5	T42.6X6
Somonal	T42.3X1	T42.3X2	T42.3X3	T42.3X4	T42.3X5	T42.3X6
Soneryl	T42.3X1	T42.3X2	T42.3X3	T42.3X4	T42.3X5	T42.3X6
Soothing syrup	T5Ø.9Ø1	T5Ø.9Ø2	T5Ø.9Ø3	T5Ø.9Ø4	T5Ø.9Ø5	T5Ø.9Ø6
Sopor	T42.6X1	T42.6X2	T42.6X3	T42.6X4	T42.6X5	T42.6X6
Soporific	T42.71	T42.72	T42.73	T42.74	T42.75	T42.76
Soporific drug	T42.71	T42.72	T42.73	T42.74	T42.75	T42.76
specified type NEC	T42.6X1	T42.6X2	T42.6X3	T42.6X4	T42.6X5	T42.6X6
Sorbide nitrate	T46.3X1	T46.3X2	T46.3X3	T46.3X4	T46.3X5	T46.3X6
Sorbitol	T47.4X1	T47.4X2	T47.4X3	T47.4X4	T47.4X5	T47.4X6
Sotalol	T44.7X1	T44.7X2	T44.7X3	T44.7X4	T44.7X5	T44.7X6
Sotradecol	T46.8X1	T46.8X2	T46.8X3	T46.8X4	T46.8X5	T46.8X6
Soysterol	T46.6X1	T46.6X2	T46.6X3	T46.6X4	T46.6X5	T46.6X6
Spacoline	T44.3X1	T44.3X2	T44.3X3	T44.3X4	T44.3X5	T44.3X6
Spanish fly	T49.8X1	T49.8X2	T49.8X3	T49.8X4	T49.8X5	T49.8X6
Sparine	T43.3X1	T43.3X2	T43.3X3	T43.3X4	T43.3X5	T43.3X6
Sparteine	T48.ØX1	T48.ØX2	T48.ØX3	T48.ØX4	T48.ØX5	T48.ØX6
Spasmolytic						
anticholinergics	T44.3X1	T44.3X2	T44.3X3	T44.3X4	T44.3X5	T44.3X6
autonomic	T44.3X1	T44.3X2	T44.3X3	T44.3X4	T44.3X5	T44.3X6
bronchial NEC	T48.6X1	T48.6X2	T48.6X3	T48.6X4	T48.6X5	T48.6X6
quaternary ammonium	T44.3X1	T44.3X2	T44.3X3	T44.3X4	T44.3X5	T44.3X6
skeletal muscle NEC	T48.1X1	T48.1X2	T48.1X3	T48.1X4	T48.1X5	T48.1X6
Spectinomycin	T36.5X1	T36.5X2	T36.5X3	T36.5X4	T36.5X5	T36.5X6
Spectracef*	T36.1X1	T36.1X2	T36.1X3	T36.1X4	T36.1X5	T36.1X6
Speed	T43.651	T43.652	T43.652	T43.654	T43.655	T43.656
Spermicide	T49.8X1	T49.8X2	T49.8X3	T49.8X4	T49.8X5	T49.8X6
Spider (bite) (venom)	T63.391	T63.392	T63.393	T63.394	—	—
antivenin	T5Ø.Z11	T5Ø.Z12	T5Ø.Z13	T5Ø.Z14	T5Ø.Z15	T5Ø.Z16
Spigelia (root)	T37.4X1	T37.4X2	T37.4X3	T37.4X4	T37.4X5	T37.4X6
Spindle inactivator	T5Ø.4X1	T5Ø.4X2	T5Ø.4X3	T5Ø.4X4	T5Ø.4X5	T5Ø.4X6
Spiperone	T43.4X1	T43.4X2	T43.4X3	T43.4X4	T43.4X5	T43.4X6
Spiramycin	T36.3X1	T36.3X2	T36.3X3	T36.3X4	T36.3X5	T36.3X6
Spirapril	T46.4X1	T46.4X2	T46.4X3	T46.4X4	T46.4X5	T46.4X6
Spirilene	T43.591	T43.592	T43.593	T43.594	T43.595	T43.596
Spirit(s) (neutral) **NEC**	T51.ØX1	T51.ØX2	T51.ØX3	T51.ØX4	—	—
beverage	T51.ØX1	T51.ØX2	T51.ØX3	T51.ØX4	—	—
industrial	T51.ØX1	T51.ØX2	T51.ØX3	T51.ØX4	—	—
mineral	T52.ØX1	T52.ØX2	T52.ØX3	T52.ØX4	—	—
of salt — *see* Hydrochloric acid						
surgical	T51.ØX1	T51.ØX2	T51.ØX3	T51.ØX4	—	—
Spiriva*	T44.3X1	T44.3X2	T44.3X3	T44.3X4	T44.3X5	T44.3X6
Spironolactone	T5Ø.ØX1	T5Ø.ØX2	T5Ø.ØX3	T5Ø.ØX4	T5Ø.ØX5	T5Ø.ØX6
Spiroperidol	T43.4X1	T43.4X2	T43.4X3	T43.4X4	T43.4X5	T43.4X6
Sponge, absorbable (gelatin)	T45.7X1	T45.7X2	T45.7X3	T45.7X4	T45.7X5	T45.7X6
Sporostacin	T49.ØX1	T49.ØX2	T49.ØX3	T49.ØX4	T49.ØX5	T49.ØX6
Spray (aerosol)	T65.91	T65.92	T65.93	T65.94	—	—
cosmetic	T65.891	T65.892	T65.893	T65.894	—	—
medicinal NEC	T5Ø.9Ø1	T5Ø.9Ø2	T5Ø.9Ø3	T5Ø.9Ø4	T5Ø.9Ø5	T5Ø.9Ø6
pesticides — *see* Pesticide						
specified content — *see specific* substance						
Spurge flax	T62.2X1	T62.2X2	T62.2X3	T62.2X4	—	—
Spurges	T62.2X1	T62.2X2	T62.2X3	T62.2X4	—	—
Sputum viscosity-lowering drug	T48.4X1	T48.4X2	T48.4X3	T48.4X4	T48.4X5	T48.4X6
Squill	T46.ØX1	T46.ØX2	T46.ØX3	T46.ØX4	T46.ØX5	T46.ØX6
rat poison	T6Ø.4X1	T6Ø.4X2	T6Ø.4X3	T6Ø.4X4	—	—
Squirting cucumber (cathartic)	T47.2X1	T47.2X2	T47.2X3	T47.2X4	T47.2X5	T47.2X6
Stains	T65.6X1	T65.6X2	T65.6X3	T65.6X4	—	—
Stannous fluoride	T49.7X1	T49.7X2	T49.7X3	T49.7X4	T49.7X5	T49.7X6
Stanolone	T38.7X1	T38.7X2	T38.7X3	T38.7X4	T38.7X5	T38.7X6
Stanozolol	T38.7X1	T38.7X2	T38.7X3	T38.7X4	T38.7X5	T38.7X6
Staphisagria or stavesacre (pediculicide)	T49.ØX1	T49.ØX2	T49.ØX3	T49.ØX4	T49.ØX5	T49.ØX6
Starch	T5Ø.9Ø1	T5Ø.9Ø2	T5Ø.9Ø3	T5Ø.9Ø4	T5Ø.9Ø5	T5Ø.9Ø6
Stavzor*	T42.6X1	T42.6X2	T42.6X3	T42.6X4	T42.6X5	T42.6X6
Stelazine	T43.3X1	T43.3X2	T43.3X3	T43.3X4	T43.3X5	T43.3X6
Stemetil	T43.3X1	T43.3X2	T43.3X3	T43.3X4	T43.3X5	T43.3X6
Stepronin	T48.4X1	T48.4X2	T48.4X3	T48.4X4	T48.4X5	T48.4X6
Sterculia	T47.4X1	T47.4X2	T47.4X3	T47.4X4	T47.4X5	T47.4X6
Sternutator gas	T59.891	T59.892	T59.893	T59.894	—	—
Steroid	T38.ØX1	T38.ØX2	T38.ØX3	T38.ØX4	T38.ØX5	T38.ØX6
anabolic	T38.7X1	T38.7X2	T38.7X3	T38.7X4	T38.7X5	T38.7X6
androgenic	T38.7X1	T38.7X2	T38.7X3	T38.7X4	T38.7X5	T38.7X6
antineoplastic, hormone	T38.7X1	T38.7X2	T38.7X3	T38.7X4	T38.7X5	T38.7X6
estrogen	T38.5X1	T38.5X2	T38.5X3	T38.5X4	T38.5X5	T38.5X6
ENT agent	T49.6X1	T49.6X2	T49.6X3	T49.6X4	T49.6X5	T49.6X6
ophthalmic preparation	T49.5X1	T49.5X2	T49.5X3	T49.5X4	T49.5X5	T49.5X6
topical NEC	T49.ØX1	T49.ØX2	T49.ØX3	T49.ØX4	T49.ØX5	T49.ØX6
Stibine	T56.891	T56.892	T56.893	T56.894	—	—
Stibogluconate	T37.3X1	T37.3X2	T37.3X3	T37.3X4	T37.3X5	T37.3X6
Stibophen	T37.4X1	T37.4X2	T37.4X3	T37.4X4	T37.4X5	T37.4X6
Stilbamidine (isetionate)	T37.3X1	T37.3X2	T37.3X3	T37.3X4	T37.3X5	T37.3X6
Stilbestrol	T38.5X1	T38.5X2	T38.5X3	T38.5X4	T38.5X5	T38.5X6
Stilboestrol	T38.5X1	T38.5X2	T38.5X3	T38.5X4	T38.5X5	T38.5X6
Stimulant						
central nervous system — *see also* Psychostimulant	T43.6Ø1	T43.6Ø2	T43.6Ø3	T43.6Ø4	T43.6Ø5	T43.6Ø6
analeptics	T5Ø.7X1	T5Ø.7X2	T5Ø.7X3	T5Ø.7X4	T5Ø.7X5	T5Ø.7X6
opiate antagonist	T5Ø.7X1	T5Ø.7X2	T5Ø.7X3	T5Ø.7X4	T5Ø.7X5	T5Ø.7X6

*Optum Value-Add

☑ Additional Character May Be Required — Refer to the Tabular List for Character Selection

Substance	Poisoning, Accidental (unintentional)	Poisoning, Intentional Self-harm	Poisoning, Assault	Poisoning, Undetermined	Adverse Effect	Under-dosing
Stimulant — *continued*						
central nervous system — *see also* Psychostimulant — *continued*						
psychotherapeutic NEC — *see also* Psychotherapeutic drug	T43.6Ø1	T43.6Ø2	T43.6Ø3	T43.6Ø4	T43.6Ø5	T43.6Ø6
specified NEC	T43.691	T43.692	T43.693	T43.694	T43.695	T43.696
respiratory	T48.9Ø1	T48.9Ø2	T48.9Ø3	T48.9Ø4	T48.9Ø5	T48.9Ø6
Stone-dissolving drug	T5Ø.9Ø1	T5Ø.9Ø2	T5Ø.9Ø3	T5Ø.9Ø4	T5Ø.9Ø5	T5Ø.9Ø6
Storage battery (cells) (acid)	T54.2X1	T54.2X2	T54.2X3	T54.2X4	—	—
Stovaine	T41.3X1	T41.3X2	T41.3X3	T41.3X4	T41.3X5	T41.3X6
infiltration (subcutaneous)	T41.3X1	T41.3X2	T41.3X3	T41.3X4	T41.3X5	T41.3X6
nerve block (peripheral) (plexus)	T41.3X1	T41.3X2	T41.3X3	T41.3X4	T41.3X5	T41.3X6
spinal	T41.3X1	T41.3X2	T41.3X3	T41.3X4	T41.3X5	T41.3X6
topical (surface)	T41.3X1	T41.3X2	T41.3X3	T41.3X4	T41.3X5	T41.3X6
Stovarsal	T37.8X1	T37.8X2	T37.8X3	T37.8X4	T37.8X5	T37.8X6
Stove gas — *see* Gas, stove						
Stoxil	T49.5X1	T49.5X2	T49.5X3	T49.5X4	T49.5X5	T49.5X6
Stramonium	T48.6X1	T48.6X2	T48.6X3	T48.6X4	T48.6X5	T48.6X6
natural state	T62.2X1	T62.2X2	T62.2X3	T62.2X4	—	—
Streptodornase	T45.3X1	T45.3X2	T45.3X3	T45.3X4	T45.3X5	T45.3X6
Streptoduocin	T36.5X1	T36.5X2	T36.5X3	T36.5X4	T36.5X5	T36.5X6
Streptokinase	T45.611	T45.612	T45.613	T45.614	T45.615	T45.616
Streptomycin (derivative)	T36.5X1	T36.5X2	T36.5X3	T36.5X4	T36.5X5	T36.5X6
Streptonivicin	T36.5X1	T36.5X2	T36.5X3	T36.5X4	T36.5X5	T36.5X6
Streptovarycin	T36.5X1	T36.5X2	T36.5X3	T36.5X4	T36.5X5	T36.5X6
Streptozocin	T45.1X1	T45.1X2	T45.1X3	T45.1X4	T45.1X5	T45.1X6
Streptozotocin	T45.1X1	T45.1X2	T45.1X3	T45.1X4	T45.1X5	T45.1X6
Stripper (paint) (solvent)	T52.8X1	T52.8X2	T52.8X3	T52.8X4	—	—
Strobane	T6Ø.1X1	T6Ø.1X2	T6Ø.1X3	T6Ø.1X4	—	—
Strofantina	T46.ØX1	T46.ØX2	T46.ØX3	T46.ØX4	T46.ØX5	T46.ØX6
Stromectol*	T37.4X1	T37.4X2	T37.4X3	T37.4X4	T37.4X5	T37.4X6
Strophanthin (g) (k)	T46.ØX1	T46.ØX2	T46.ØX3	T46.ØX4	T46.ØX5	T46.ØX6
Strophanthus	T46.ØX1	T46.ØX2	T46.ØX3	T46.ØX4	T46.ØX5	T46.ØX6
Strophantin	T46.ØX1	T46.ØX2	T46.ØX3	T46.ØX4	T46.ØX5	T46.ØX6
Strophantin-g	T46.ØX1	T46.ØX2	T46.ØX3	T46.ØX4	T46.ØX5	T46.ØX6
Strychnine (nonmedicinal) (pesticide) (salts)	T65.1X1	T65.1X2	T65.1X3	T65.1X4	—	—
medicinal	T48.291	T48.292	T48.293	T48.294	T48.295	T48.296
Strychnos (ignatii) — *see* Strychnine						
Styramate	T42.8X1	T42.8X2	T42.8X3	T42.8X4	T42.8X5	T42.8X6
Styrene	T65.891	T65.892	T65.893	T65.894	—	—
Succinimide, antiepileptic or anticonvulsant	T42.2X1	T42.2X2	T42.2X3	T42.2X4	T42.2X5	T42.2X6
mercuric — *see* Mercury						
Succinylcholine	T48.1X1	T48.1X2	T48.1X3	T48.1X4	T48.1X5	T48.1X6
Succinylsulfathiazole	T37.ØX1	T37.ØX2	T37.ØX3	T37.ØX4	T37.ØX5	T37.ØX6
Sucralfate	T47.1X1	T47.1X2	T47.1X3	T47.1X4	T47.1X5	T47.1X6
Sucrose	T5Ø.3X1	T5Ø.3X2	T5Ø.3X3	T5Ø.3X4	T5Ø.3X5	T5Ø.3X6
Sufentanil	T4Ø.411	T4Ø.412	T4Ø.413	T4Ø.414	T4Ø.415	T4Ø.416
Sulbactam	T36.ØX1	T36.ØX2	T36.ØX3	T36.ØX4	T36.ØX5	T36.ØX6
Sulbenicillin	T36.ØX1	T36.ØX2	T36.ØX3	T36.ØX4	T36.ØX5	T36.ØX6
Sulbentine	T49.ØX1	T49.ØX2	T49.ØX3	T49.ØX4	T49.ØX5	T49.ØX6
Sulconazole*	T49.ØX1	T49.ØX2	T49.ØX3	T49.ØX4	T49.ØX5	T49.ØX6
Sulfacetamide	T49.ØX1	T49.ØX2	T49.ØX3	T49.ØX4	T49.ØX5	T49.ØX6
ophthalmic preparation	T49.5X1	T49.5X2	T49.5X3	T49.5X4	T49.5X5	T49.5X6
Sulfachlorpyridazine	T37.ØX1	T37.ØX2	T37.ØX3	T37.ØX4	T37.ØX5	T37.ØX6
Sulfacitine	T37.ØX1	T37.ØX2	T37.ØX3	T37.ØX4	T37.ØX5	T37.ØX6
Sulfadiasulfone sodium	T37.ØX1	T37.ØX2	T37.ØX3	T37.ØX4	T37.ØX5	T37.ØX6
Sulfadiazine	T37.ØX1	T37.ØX2	T37.ØX3	T37.ØX4	T37.ØX5	T37.ØX6
silver (topical)	T49.ØX1	T49.ØX2	T49.ØX3	T49.ØX4	T49.ØX5	T49.ØX6
Sulfadimethoxine	T37.ØX1	T37.ØX2	T37.ØX3	T37.ØX4	T37.ØX5	T37.ØX6
Sulfadimidine	T37.ØX1	T37.ØX2	T37.ØX3	T37.ØX4	T37.ØX5	T37.ØX6
Sulfadoxine	T37.ØX1	T37.ØX2	T37.ØX3	T37.ØX4	T37.ØX5	T37.ØX6
with pyrimethamine	T37.2X1	T37.2X2	T37.2X3	T37.2X4	T37.2X5	T37.2X6
Sulfaethidole	T37.ØX1	T37.ØX2	T37.ØX3	T37.ØX4	T37.ØX5	T37.ØX6
Sulfafurazole	T37.ØX1	T37.ØX2	T37.ØX3	T37.ØX4	T37.ØX5	T37.ØX6
Sulfaguanidine	T37.ØX1	T37.ØX2	T37.ØX3	T37.ØX4	T37.ØX5	T37.ØX6
Sulfalene	T37.ØX1	T37.ØX2	T37.ØX3	T37.ØX4	T37.ØX5	T37.ØX6
Sulfaloxate	T37.ØX1	T37.ØX2	T37.ØX3	T37.ØX4	T37.ØX5	T37.ØX6
Sulfaloxic acid	T37.ØX1	T37.ØX2	T37.ØX3	T37.ØX4	T37.ØX5	T37.ØX6
Sulfamazone	T39.2X1	T39.2X2	T39.2X3	T39.2X4	T39.2X5	T39.2X6
Sulfamerazine	T37.ØX1	T37.ØX2	T37.ØX3	T37.ØX4	T37.ØX5	T37.ØX6
Sulfameter	T37.ØX1	T37.ØX2	T37.ØX3	T37.ØX4	T37.ØX5	T37.ØX6
Sulfamethazine	T37.ØX1	T37.ØX2	T37.ØX3	T37.ØX4	T37.ØX5	T37.ØX6
Sulfamethizole	T37.ØX1	T37.ØX2	T37.ØX3	T37.ØX4	T37.ØX5	T37.ØX6
Sulfamethoxazole	T37.ØX1	T37.ØX2	T37.ØX3	T37.ØX4	T37.ØX5	T37.ØX6
with trimethoprim	T36.8X1	T36.8X2	T36.8X3	T36.8X4	T36.8X5	T36.8X6
Sulfamethoxydiazine	T37.ØX1	T37.ØX2	T37.ØX3	T37.ØX4	T37.ØX5	T37.ØX6
Sulfamethoxypyridazine	T37.ØX1	T37.ØX2	T37.ØX3	T37.ØX4	T37.ØX5	T37.ØX6
Sulfamethylthiazole	T37.ØX1	T37.ØX2	T37.ØX3	T37.ØX4	T37.ØX5	T37.ØX6
Sulfametoxydiazine	T37.ØX1	T37.ØX2	T37.ØX3	T37.ØX4	T37.ØX5	T37.ØX6
Sulfamidopyrine	T39.2X1	T39.2X2	T39.2X3	T39.2X4	T39.2X5	T39.2X6
Sulfamonomethoxine	T37.ØX1	T37.ØX2	T37.ØX3	T37.ØX4	T37.ØX5	T37.ØX6
Sulfamoxole	T37.ØX1	T37.ØX2	T37.ØX3	T37.ØX4	T37.ØX5	T37.ØX6
Sulfamylon	T49.ØX1	T49.ØX2	T49.ØX3	T49.ØX4	T49.ØX5	T49.ØX6
Sulfan blue (diagnostic dye)	T5Ø.8X1	T5Ø.8X2	T5Ø.8X3	T5Ø.8X4	T5Ø.8X5	T5Ø.8X6
Sulfanilamide	T37.ØX1	T37.ØX2	T37.ØX3	T37.ØX4	T37.ØX5	T37.ØX6
Sulfanilylguanidine	T37.ØX1	T37.ØX2	T37.ØX3	T37.ØX4	T37.ØX5	T37.ØX6
Sulfaperin	T37.ØX1	T37.ØX2	T37.ØX3	T37.ØX4	T37.ØX5	T37.ØX6
Sulfaphenazole	T37.ØX1	T37.ØX2	T37.ØX3	T37.ØX4	T37.ØX5	T37.ØX6
Sulfaphenylthiazole	T37.ØX1	T37.ØX2	T37.ØX3	T37.ØX4	T37.ØX5	T37.ØX6
Sulfaproxyline	T37.ØX1	T37.ØX2	T37.ØX3	T37.ØX4	T37.ØX5	T37.ØX6
Sulfapyridine	T37.ØX1	T37.ØX2	T37.ØX3	T37.ØX4	T37.ØX5	T37.ØX6
Sulfapyrimidine	T37.ØX1	T37.ØX2	T37.ØX3	T37.ØX4	T37.ØX5	T37.ØX6
Sulfarsphenamine	T37.8X1	T37.8X2	T37.8X3	T37.8X4	T37.8X5	T37.8X6
Sulfasalazine	T37.ØX1	T37.ØX2	T37.ØX3	T37.ØX4	T37.ØX5	T37.ØX6
Sulfasuxidine	T37.ØX1	T37.ØX2	T37.ØX3	T37.ØX4	T37.ØX5	T37.ØX6
Sulfasymazine	T37.ØX1	T37.ØX2	T37.ØX3	T37.ØX4	T37.ØX5	T37.ØX6
Sulfated amylopectin	T47.8X1	T47.8X2	T47.8X3	T47.8X4	T47.8X5	T47.8X6
Sulfathiazole	T37.ØX1	T37.ØX2	T37.ØX3	T37.ØX4	T37.ØX5	T37.ØX6
Sulfatostearate	T49.2X1	T49.2X2	T49.2X3	T49.2X4	T49.2X5	T49.2X6
Sulfatrim*	T36.8X1	T36.8X2	T36.8X3	T36.8X4	T36.8X5	T36.8X6
Sulfinpyrazone	T5Ø.4X1	T5Ø.4X2	T5Ø.4X3	T5Ø.4X4	T5Ø.4X5	T5Ø.4X6
Sulfiram	T49.ØX1	T49.ØX2	T49.ØX3	T49.ØX4	T49.ØX5	T49.ØX6
Sulfisomidine	T37.ØX1	T37.ØX2	T37.ØX3	T37.ØX4	T37.ØX5	T37.ØX6
Sulfisoxazole	T37.ØX1	T37.ØX2	T37.ØX3	T37.ØX4	T37.ØX5	T37.ØX6
ophthalmic preparation	T49.5X1	T49.5X2	T49.5X3	T49.5X4	T49.5X5	T49.5X6
Sulfobromophthalein (sodium)	T5Ø.8X1	T5Ø.8X2	T5Ø.8X3	T5Ø.8X4	T5Ø.8X5	T5Ø.8X6
Sulfobromphthalein	T5Ø.8X1	T5Ø.8X2	T5Ø.8X3	T5Ø.8X4	T5Ø.8X5	T5Ø.8X6
Sulfogaiacol	T48.4X1	T48.4X2	T48.4X3	T48.4X4	T48.4X5	T48.4X6
Sulfomyxin	T36.8X1	T36.8X2	T36.8X3	T36.8X4	T36.8X5	T36.8X6
Sulfonal	T42.6X1	T42.6X2	T42.6X3	T42.6X4	T42.6X5	T42.6X6
Sulfonamide NEC	T37.ØX1	T37.ØX2	T37.ØX3	T37.ØX4	T37.ØX5	T37.ØX6
eye	T49.5X1	T49.5X2	T49.5X3	T49.5X4	T49.5X5	T49.5X6
Sulfonazide	T37.1X1	T37.1X2	T37.1X3	T37.1X4	T37.1X5	T37.1X6
Sulfones	T37.1X1	T37.1X2	T37.1X3	T37.1X4	T37.1X5	T37.1X6
Sulfonethylmethane	T42.6X1	T42.6X2	T42.6X3	T42.6X4	T42.6X5	T42.6X6
Sulfonmethane	T42.6X1	T42.6X2	T42.6X3	T42.6X4	T42.6X5	T42.6X6
Sulfonphthal, sulfonphthol	T5Ø.8X1	T5Ø.8X2	T5Ø.8X3	T5Ø.8X4	T5Ø.8X5	T5Ø.8X6
Sulfonylurea derivatives, oral	T38.3X1	T38.3X2	T38.3X3	T38.3X4	T38.3X5	T38.3X6
Sulforidazine	T43.3X1	T43.3X2	T43.3X3	T43.3X4	T43.3X5	T43.3X6
Sulfoxone	T37.1X1	T37.1X2	T37.1X3	T37.1X4	T37.1X5	T37.1X6
Sulfuric acid	T54.2X1	T54.2X2	T54.2X3	T54.2X4	—	—
Sulfur, sulfurated, sulfuric, sulfurous, sulfuryl (compounds NEC) (medicinal)	T49.4X1	T49.4X2	T49.4X3	T49.4X4	T49.4X5	T49.4X6
acid	T54.2X1	T54.2X2	T54.2X3	T54.2X4	—	—
dioxide (gas)	T59.1X1	T59.1X2	T59.1X3	T59.1X4	—	—
ether — *see* Ether(s)						
hydrogen	T59.6X1	T59.6X2	T59.6X3	T59.6X4	—	—
medicinal (keratolytic) (ointment) NEC	T49.4X1	T49.4X2	T49.4X3	T49.4X4	T49.4X5	T49.4X6
ointment	T49.ØX1	T49.ØX2	T49.ØX3	T49.ØX4	T49.ØX5	T49.ØX6
pesticide (vapor)	T6Ø.91	T6Ø.92	T6Ø.93	T6Ø.94	—	—
vapor NEC	T59.891	T59.892	T59.893	T59.894	—	—
Sulglicotide	T47.1X1	T47.1X2	T47.1X3	T47.1X4	T47.1X5	T47.1X6
Sulindac	T39.391	T39.392	T39.393	T39.394	T39.395	T39.396
Sulisatin	T47.2X1	T47.2X2	T47.2X3	T47.2X4	T47.2X5	T47.2X6
Sulisobenzone	T49.3X1	T49.3X2	T49.3X3	T49.3X4	T49.3X5	T49.3X6
Sulkowitch's reagent	T5Ø.8X1	T5Ø.8X2	T5Ø.8X3	T5Ø.8X4	T5Ø.8X5	T5Ø.8X6
Sulmetozine	T44.3X1	T44.3X2	T44.3X3	T44.3X4	T44.3X5	T44.3X6
Suloctidil	T46.7X1	T46.7X2	T46.7X3	T46.7X4	T46.7X5	T46.7X6
Sulph- — *see also* Sulf-						
Sulphadiazine	T37.ØX1	T37.ØX2	T37.ØX3	T37.ØX4	T37.ØX5	T37.ØX6
Sulphadimethoxine	T37.ØX1	T37.ØX2	T37.ØX3	T37.ØX4	T37.ØX5	T37.ØX6
Sulphadimidine	T37.ØX1	T37.ØX2	T37.ØX3	T37.ØX4	T37.ØX5	T37.ØX6
Sulphadione	T37.1X1	T37.1X2	T37.1X3	T37.1X4	T37.1X5	T37.1X6
Sulphafurazole	T37.ØX1	T37.ØX2	T37.ØX3	T37.ØX4	T37.ØX5	T37.ØX6
Sulphamethizole	T37.ØX1	T37.ØX2	T37.ØX3	T37.ØX4	T37.ØX5	T37.ØX6
Sulphamethoxazole	T37.ØX1	T37.ØX2	T37.ØX3	T37.ØX4	T37.ØX5	T37.ØX6
Sulphan blue	T5Ø.8X1	T5Ø.8X2	T5Ø.8X3	T5Ø.8X4	T5Ø.8X5	T5Ø.8X6
Sulphaphenazole	T37.ØX1	T37.ØX2	T37.ØX3	T37.ØX4	T37.ØX5	T37.ØX6
Sulphapyridine	T37.ØX1	T37.ØX2	T37.ØX3	T37.ØX4	T37.ØX5	T37.ØX6
Sulphasalazine	T37.ØX1	T37.ØX2	T37.ØX3	T37.ØX4	T37.ØX5	T37.ØX6
Sulphinpyrazone	T5Ø.4X1	T5Ø.4X2	T5Ø.4X3	T5Ø.4X4	T5Ø.4X5	T5Ø.4X6
Sulpiride	T43.591	T43.592	T43.593	T43.594	T43.595	T43.596
Sulprostone	T48.ØX1	T48.ØX2	T48.ØX3	T48.ØX4	T48.ØX5	T48.ØX6

Substance	Poisoning, Accidental (unintentional)	Poisoning, Intentional Self-harm	Poisoning, Assault	Poisoning, Undetermined	Adverse Effect	Under-dosing
Sulpyrine	T39.2X1	T39.2X2	T39.2X3	T39.2X4	T39.2X5	T39.2X6
Sultamicillin	T36.ØX1	T36.ØX2	T36.ØX3	T36.ØX4	T36.ØX5	T36.ØX6
Sulthiame	T42.6X1	T42.6X2	T42.6X3	T42.6X4	T42.6X5	T42.6X6
Sultiame	T42.6X1	T42.6X2	T42.6X3	T42.6X4	T42.6X5	T42.6X6
Sultopride	T43.591	T43.592	T43.593	T43.594	T43.595	T43.596
Sumatriptan	T39.8X1	T39.8X2	T39.8X3	T39.8X4	T39.8X5	T39.8X6
Sumavel*	T39.8X1	T39.8X2	T39.8X3	T39.8X4	T39.8X5	T39.8X6
Sunflower seed oil	T46.6X1	T46.6X2	T46.6X3	T46.6X4	T46.6X5	T46.6X6
Superinone	T48.4X1	T48.4X2	T48.4X3	T48.4X4	T48.4X5	T48.4X6
Suprofen	T39.311	T39.312	T39.313	T39.314	T39.315	T39.316
Suramin (sodium)	T37.4X1	T37.4X2	T37.4X3	T37.4X4	T37.4X5	T37.4X6
Surfacaine	T41.3X1	T41.3X2	T41.3X3	T41.3X4	T41.3X5	T41.3X6
Surital	T41.1X1	T41.1X2	T41.1X3	T41.1X4	T41.1X5	T41.1X6
Sutilains	T45.3X1	T45.3X2	T45.3X3	T45.3X4	T45.3X5	T45.3X6
Suxamethonium (chloride)	T48.1X1	T48.1X2	T48.1X3	T48.1X4	T48.1X5	T48.1X6
Suxethonium (chloride)	T48.1X1	T48.1X2	T48.1X3	T48.1X4	T48.1X5	T48.1X6
Suxibuzone	T39.2X1	T39.2X2	T39.2X3	T39.2X4	T39.2X5	T39.2X6
Sweetener	T5Ø.901	T5Ø.902	T5Ø.903	T5Ø.904	T5Ø.905	T5Ø.906
Sweet niter spirit	T46.3X1	T46.3X2	T46.3X3	T46.3X4	T46.3X5	T46.3X6
Sweet oil (birch)	T49.3X1	T49.3X2	T49.3X3	T49.3X4	T49.3X5	T49.3X6
Sylvant*	T45.1X1	T45.1X2	T45.1X3	T45.1X4	T45.1X5	T45.1X6
Sym-dichloroethyl ether	T53.6X1	T53.6X2	T53.6X3	T53.6X4	—	—
Sympatholytic NEC	T44.8X1	T44.8X2	T44.8X3	T44.8X4	T44.8X5	T44.8X6
haloalkylamine	T44.8X1	T44.8X2	T44.8X3	T44.8X4	T44.8X5	T44.8X6
Sympathomimetic NEC	T44.901	T44.902	T44.903	T44.904	T44.905	T44.906
anti-common-cold	T48.5X1	T48.5X2	T48.5X3	T48.5X4	T48.5X5	T48.5X6
bronchodilator	T48.6X1	T48.6X2	T48.6X3	T48.6X4	T48.6X5	T48.6X6
specified NEC	T44.991	T44.992	T44.993	T44.994	T44.995	T44.996
Synagis	T5Ø.B91	T5Ø.B92	T5Ø.B93	T5Ø.B94	T5Ø.B95	T5Ø.B96
Synalar	T49.ØX1	T49.ØX2	T49.ØX3	T49.ØX4	T49.ØX5	T49.ØX6
Synthetic cannabinoids	T4Ø.721	T4Ø.722	T4Ø.723	T4Ø.724	T4Ø.725	T4Ø.726
Synthroid	T38.1X1	T38.1X2	T38.1X3	T38.1X4	T38.1X5	T38.1X6
Syntocinon	T48.ØX1	T48.ØX2	T48.ØX3	T48.ØX4	T48.ØX5	T48.ØX6
Syrosingopine	T46.5X1	T46.5X2	T46.5X3	T46.5X4	T46.5X5	T46.5X6
Systemic drug	T45.91	T45.92	T45.93	T45.94	T45.95	T45.96
specified NEC	T45.8X1	T45.8X2	T45.8X3	T45.8X4	T45.8X5	T45.8X6
Tablets — *see also* specified substance	T5Ø.901	T5Ø.902	T5Ø.903	T5Ø.904	T5Ø.905	T5Ø.906
Tace	T38.5X1	T38.5X2	T38.5X3	T38.5X4	T38.5X5	T38.5X6
Tacrine	T44.ØX1	T44.ØX2	T44.ØX3	T44.ØX4	T44.ØX5	T44.ØX6
Tadalafil	T46.7X1	T46.7X2	T46.7X3	T46.7X4	T46.7X5	T46.7X6
Talampicillin	T36.ØX1	T36.ØX2	T36.ØX3	T36.ØX4	T36.ØX5	T36.ØX6
Talbutal	T42.3X1	T42.3X2	T42.3X3	T42.3X4	T42.3X5	T42.3X6
Talc powder	T49.3X1	T49.3X2	T49.3X3	T49.3X4	T49.3X5	T49.3X6
Talcum	T49.3X1	T49.3X2	T49.3X3	T49.3X4	T49.3X5	T49.3X6
Taleranol	T38.6X1	T38.6X2	T38.6X3	T38.6X4	T38.6X5	T38.6X6
Taltz*	T39.391	T39.392	T39.393	T39.394	T39.395	T39.396
Tamoxifen	T38.6X1	T38.6X2	T38.6X3	T38.6X4	T38.6X5	T38.6X6
Tamsulosin	T44.6X1	T44.6X2	T44.6X3	T44.6X4	T44.6X5	T44.6X6
Tandearil, tanderil	T39.2X1	T39.2X2	T39.2X3	T39.2X4	T39.2X5	T39.2X6
Tannic acid	T49.2X1	T49.2X2	T49.2X3	T49.2X4	T49.2X5	T49.2X6
medicinal (astringent)	T49.2X1	T49.2X2	T49.2X3	T49.2X4	T49.2X5	T49.2X6
Tannin — *see* Tannic acid						
Tansy	T62.2X1	T62.2X2	T62.2X3	T62.2X4	—	—
TAO	T36.3X1	T36.3X2	T36.3X3	T36.3X4	T36.3X5	T36.3X6
Tapazole	T38.2X1	T38.2X2	T38.2X3	T38.2X4	T38.2X5	T38.2X6
Taractan	T43.591	T43.592	T43.593	T43.594	T43.595	T43.596
Tarantula (venomous)	T63.321	T63.322	T63.323	T63.324	—	—
Tartar emetic	T37.8X1	T37.8X2	T37.8X3	T37.8X4	T37.8X5	T37.8X6
Tartaric acid	T65.891	T65.892	T65.893	T65.894	—	—
Tartrated antimony (anti-infective)	T37.8X1	T37.8X2	T37.8X3	T37.8X4	T37.8X5	T37.8X6
Tartrate, laxative	T47.4X1	T47.4X2	T47.4X3	T47.4X4	T47.4X5	T47.4X6
Tar NEC	T52.ØX1	T52.ØX2	T52.ØX3	T52.ØX4	—	—
camphor	T6Ø.1X1	T6Ø.1X2	T6Ø.1X3	T6Ø.1X4	—	—
distillate	T49.1X1	T49.1X2	T49.1X3	T49.1X4	T49.1X5	T49.1X6
fumes	T59.891	T59.892	T59.893	T59.894	—	—
medicinal	T49.1X1	T49.1X2	T49.1X3	T49.1X4	T49.1X5	T49.1X6
ointment	T49.1X1	T49.1X2	T49.1X3	T49.1X4	T49.1X5	T49.1X6
Tauromustine	T45.1X1	T45.1X2	T45.1X3	T45.1X4	T45.1X5	T45.1X6
TCA — *see* Trichloroacetic acid						
TCDD	T53.7X1	T53.7X2	T53.7X3	T53.7X4	—	—
TDI (vapor)	T65.ØX1	T65.ØX2	T65.ØX3	T65.ØX4	—	—
Tear						
gas	T59.3X1	T59.3X2	T59.3X3	T59.3X4	—	—
solution	T49.5X1	T49.5X2	T49.5X3	T49.5X4	T49.5X5	T49.5X6
Tecentriq*	T45.1X1	T45.1X2	T45.1X3	T45.1X4	T45.1X5	T45.1X6
Teclothiazide	T5Ø.2X1	T5Ø.2X2	T5Ø.2X3	T5Ø.2X4	T5Ø.2X5	T5Ø.2X6
Teclozan	T37.3X1	T37.3X2	T37.3X3	T37.3X4	T37.3X5	T37.3X6
Tegafur	T45.1X1	T45.1X2	T45.1X3	T45.1X4	T45.1X5	T45.1X6
Tegretol	T42.1X1	T42.1X2	T42.1X3	T42.1X4	T42.1X5	T42.1X6
Teicoplanin	T36.8X1	T36.8X2	T36.8X3	T36.8X4	T36.8X5	T36.8X6
Telepaque	T5Ø.8X1	T5Ø.8X2	T5Ø.8X3	T5Ø.8X4	T5Ø.8X5	T5Ø.8X6

Substance	Poisoning, Accidental (unintentional)	Poisoning, Intentional Self-harm	Poisoning, Assault	Poisoning, Undetermined	Adverse Effect	Under-dosing
Tellurium	T56.891	T56.892	T56.893	T56.894	—	—
fumes	T56.891	T56.892	T56.893	T56.894	—	—
TEM	T45.1X1	T45.1X2	T45.1X3	T45.1X4	T45.1X5	T45.1X6
Temazepam	T42.4X1	T42.4X2	T42.4X3	T42.4X4	T42.4X5	T42.4X6
Temocillin	T36.ØX1	T36.ØX2	T36.ØX3	T36.ØX4	T36.ØX5	T36.ØX6
Tenamfetamine	T43.621	T43.622	T43.623	T43.624	T43.625	T43.626
Tenecteplase*	T45.611	T45.612	T45.613	T45.614	T45.615	T45.616
Teniposide	T45.1X1	T45.1X2	T45.1X3	T45.1X4	T45.1X5	T45.1X6
Tenitramine	T46.3X1	T46.3X2	T46.3X3	T46.3X4	T46.3X5	T46.3X6
Tenoglicin	T48.4X1	T48.4X2	T48.4X3	T48.4X4	T48.4X5	T48.4X6
Tenonitrozole	T37.3X1	T37.3X2	T37.3X3	T37.3X4	T37.3X5	T37.3X6
Tenoxicam	T39.391	T39.392	T39.393	T39.394	T39.395	T39.396
TEPA	T45.1X1	T45.1X2	T45.1X3	T45.1X4	T45.1X5	T45.1X6
TEPP	T6Ø.ØX1	T6Ø.ØX2	T6Ø.ØX3	T6Ø.ØX4	—	—
Teprotide	T46.5X1	T46.5X2	T46.5X3	T46.5X4	T46.5X5	T46.5X6
Terazosin	T44.6X1	T44.6X2	T44.6X3	T44.6X4	T44.6X5	T44.6X6
Terbufos	T6Ø.ØX1	T6Ø.ØX2	T6Ø.ØX3	T6Ø.ØX4	—	—
Terbutaline	T48.6X1	T48.6X2	T48.6X3	T48.6X4	T48.6X5	T48.6X6
Terconazole	T49.ØX1	T49.ØX2	T49.ØX3	T49.ØX4	T49.ØX5	T49.ØX6
Terfenadine	T45.ØX1	T45.ØX2	T45.ØX3	T45.ØX4	T45.ØX5	T45.ØX6
Teriparatide (acetate)	T5Ø.991	T5Ø.992	T5Ø.993	T5Ø.994	T5Ø.995	T5Ø.996
Terizidone	T37.1X1	T37.1X2	T37.1X3	T37.1X4	T37.1X5	T37.1X6
Terlipressin	T38.891	T38.892	T38.893	T38.894	T38.895	T38.896
Terodiline	T46.3X1	T46.3X2	T46.3X3	T46.3X4	T46.3X5	T46.3X6
Teroxalene	T37.4X1	T37.4X2	T37.4X3	T37.4X4	T37.4X5	T37.4X6
Terpin (cis) **hydrate**	T48.4X1	T48.4X2	T48.4X3	T48.4X4	T48.4X5	T48.4X6
Terramycin	T36.4X1	T36.4X2	T36.4X3	T36.4X4	T36.4X5	T36.4X6
Tertatolol	T44.7X1	T44.7X2	T44.7X3	T44.7X4	T44.7X5	T44.7X6
Tessalon	T48.3X1	T48.3X2	T48.3X3	T48.3X4	T48.3X5	T48.3X6
Testolactone	T38.7X1	T38.7X2	T38.7X3	T38.7X4	T38.7X5	T38.7X6
Testosterone	T38.7X1	T38.7X2	T38.7X3	T38.7X4	T38.7X5	T38.7X6
Tetanus toxoid or vaccine	T5Ø.A91	T5Ø.A92	T5Ø.A93	T5Ø.A94	T5Ø.A95	T5Ø.A96
antitoxin	T5Ø.Z11	T5Ø.Z12	T5Ø.Z13	T5Ø.Z14	T5Ø.Z15	T5Ø.Z16
immune globulin (human)	T5Ø.Z11	T5Ø.Z12	T5Ø.Z13	T5Ø.Z14	T5Ø.Z15	T5Ø.Z16
toxoid	T5Ø.A91	T5Ø.A92	T5Ø.A93	T5Ø.A94	T5Ø.A95	T5Ø.A96
with diphtheria toxoid	T5Ø.A21	T5Ø.A22	T5Ø.A23	T5Ø.A24	T5Ø.A25	T5Ø.A26
with pertussis	T5Ø.A11	T5Ø.A12	T5Ø.A13	T5Ø.A14	T5Ø.A15	T5Ø.A16
Tetrabenazine	T43.591	T43.592	T43.593	T43.594	T43.595	T43.596
Tetracaine	T41.3X1	T41.3X2	T41.3X3	T41.3X4	T41.3X5	T41.3X6
nerve block (peripheral) (plexus)	T41.3X1	T41.3X2	T41.3X3	T41.3X4	T41.3X5	T41.3X6
regional	T41.3X1	T41.3X2	T41.3X3	T41.3X4	T41.3X5	T41.3X6
spinal	T41.3X1	T41.3X2	T41.3X3	T41.3X4	T41.3X5	T41.3X6
Tetrachlorethylene — *see* Tetrachloroethylene						
Tetrachlormethiazide	T5Ø.2X1	T5Ø.2X2	T5Ø.2X3	T5Ø.2X4	T5Ø.2X5	T5Ø.2X6
Tetrachloroethane	T53.6X1	T53.6X2	T53.6X3	T53.6X4	—	—
vapor	T53.6X1	T53.6X2	T53.6X3	T53.6X4	—	—
paint or varnish	T53.6X1	T53.6X2	T53.6X3	T53.6X4	—	—
Tetrachloroethylene (liquid)	T53.3X1	T53.3X2	T53.3X3	T53.3X4	—	—
medicinal	T37.4X1	T37.4X2	T37.4X3	T37.4X4	T37.4X5	T37.4X6
vapor	T53.3X1	T53.3X2	T53.3X3	T53.3X4	—	—
Tetrachloromethane — *see* Carbon tetrachloride						
Tetracosactide	T38.811	T38.812	T38.813	T38.814	T38.815	T38.816
Tetracosactrin	T38.811	T38.812	T38.813	T38.814	T38.815	T38.816
Tetracycline	T36.4X1	T36.4X2	T36.4X3	T36.4X4	T36.4X5	T36.4X6
ophthalmic preparation	T49.5X1	T49.5X2	T49.5X3	T49.5X4	T49.5X5	T49.5X6
topical NEC	T49.ØX1	T49.ØX2	T49.ØX3	T49.ØX4	T49.ØX5	T49.ØX6
Tetradifon	T6Ø.8X1	T6Ø.8X2	T6Ø.8X3	T6Ø.8X4	—	—
Tetradotoxin	T61.771	T61.772	T61.773	T61.774	—	—
Tetraethyl						
lead	T56.ØX1	T56.ØX2	T56.ØX3	T56.ØX4	—	—
pyrophosphate	T6Ø.ØX1	T6Ø.ØX2	T6Ø.ØX3	T6Ø.ØX4	—	—
Tetraethylammonium chloride	T44.2X1	T44.2X2	T44.2X3	T44.2X4	T44.2X5	T44.2X6
Tetraethylthiuram disulfide	T5Ø.6X1	T5Ø.6X2	T5Ø.6X3	T5Ø.6X4	T5Ø.6X5	T5Ø.6X6
Tetrahydroaminoacridine	T44.ØX1	T44.ØX2	T44.ØX3	T44.ØX4	T44.ØX5	T44.ØX6
Tetrahydrocannabinol	T4Ø.711	T4Ø.712	T4Ø.713	T4Ø.714	T4Ø.715	T4Ø.716
Tetrahydrofuran	T52.8X1	T52.8X2	T52.8X3	T52.8X4	—	—
Tetrahydrolipstatin*	T47.8X1	T47.8X2	T47.8X3	T47.8X4	T47.8X5	T47.8X6
Tetrahydronaphthalene	T52.8X1	T52.8X2	T52.8X3	T52.8X4	—	—
Tetrahydrozoline	T49.5X1	T49.5X2	T49.5X3	T49.5X4	T49.5X5	T49.5X6
Tetralin	T52.8X1	T52.8X2	T52.8X3	T52.8X4	—	—
Tetramethrin	T6Ø.2X1	T6Ø.2X2	T6Ø.2X3	T6Ø.2X4	—	—
Tetramethylthiuram (disulfide) **NEC**	T6Ø.3X1	T6Ø.3X2	T6Ø.3X3	T6Ø.3X4	—	—
medicinal	T49.ØX1	T49.ØX2	T49.ØX3	T49.ØX4	T49.ØX5	T49.ØX6
Tetramisole	T37.4X1	T37.4X2	T37.4X3	T37.4X4	T37.4X5	T37.4X6
Tetranicotinoyl fructose	T46.7X1	T46.7X2	T46.7X3	T46.7X4	T46.7X5	T46.7X6
Tetrazepam	T42.4X1	T42.4X2	T42.4X3	T42.4X4	T42.4X5	T42.4X6

Substance	Poisoning, Accidental (unintentional)	Poisoning, Intentional Self-harm	Poisoning, Assault	Poisoning, Undetermined	Adverse Effect	Under-dosing
Tetronal	T42.6X1	T42.6X2	T42.6X3	T42.6X4	T42.6X5	T42.6X6
Tetryl	T65.3X1	T65.3X2	T65.3X3	T65.3X4	—	—
Tetrylammonium chloride	T44.2X1	T44.2X2	T44.2X3	T44.2X4	T44.2X5	T44.2X6
Tetryzoline	T49.5X1	T49.5X2	T49.5X3	T49.5X4	T49.5X5	T49.5X6
Thalidomide	T45.1X1	T45.1X2	T45.1X3	T45.1X4	T45.1X5	T45.1X6
Thallium (compounds) (dust) **NEC**	T56.811	T56.812	T56.813	T56.814	—	—
pesticide	T6Ø.4X1	T6Ø.4X2	T6Ø.4X3	T6Ø.4X4	—	—
THC	T4Ø.711	T4Ø.712	T4Ø.713	T4Ø.714	T4Ø.715	T4Ø.716
Thebacon	T48.3X1	T48.3X2	T48.3X3	T48.3X4	T48.3X5	T48.3X6
Thebaine	T4Ø.2X1	T4Ø.2X2	T4Ø.2X3	T4Ø.2X4	T4Ø.2X5	T4Ø.2X6
Thenoic acid	T49.6X1	T49.6X2	T49.6X3	T49.6X4	T49.6X5	T49.6X6
Thenyldiamine	T45.ØX1	T45.ØX2	T45.ØX3	T45.ØX4	T45.ØX5	T45.ØX6
Theobromine (calcium salicylate)	T48.6X1	T48.6X2	T48.6X3	T48.6X4	T48.6X5	T48.6X6
sodium salicylate	T48.6X1	T48.6X2	T48.6X3	T48.6X4	T48.6X5	T48.6X6
Theolair*	T48.6X1	T48.6X2	T48.6X3	T48.6X4	T48.6X5	T48.6X6
Theophyllamine	T48.6X1	T48.6X2	T48.6X3	T48.6X4	T48.6X5	T48.6X6
Theophylline	T48.6X1	T48.6X2	T48.6X3	T48.6X4	T48.6X5	T48.6X6
aminobenzoic acid	T48.6X1	T48.6X2	T48.6X3	T48.6X4	T48.6X5	T48.6X6
ethylenediamine	T48.6X1	T48.6X2	T48.6X3	T48.6X4	T48.6X5	T48.6X6
piperazine p-amino-benzoate	T48.6X1	T48.6X2	T48.6X3	T48.6X4	T48.6X5	T48.6X6
Therevac*	T47.4X1	T47.4X2	T47.4X3	T47.4X4	T47.4X5	T47.4X6
Thiabendazole	T37.4X1	T37.4X2	T37.4X3	T37.4X4	T37.4X5	T37.4X6
Thialbarbital	T41.1X1	T41.1X2	T41.1X3	T41.1X4	T41.1X5	T41.1X6
Thiamazole	T38.2X1	T38.2X2	T38.2X3	T38.2X4	T38.2X5	T38.2X6
Thiambutosine	T37.1X1	T37.1X2	T37.1X3	T37.1X4	T37.1X5	T37.1X6
Thiamine	T45.2X1	T45.2X2	T45.2X3	T45.2X4	T45.2X5	T45.2X6
Thiamphenicol	T36.2X1	T36.2X2	T36.2X3	T36.2X4	T36.2X5	T36.2X6
Thiamylal	T41.1X1	T41.1X2	T41.1X3	T41.1X4	T41.1X5	T41.1X6
sodium	T41.1X1	T41.1X2	T41.1X3	T41.1X4	T41.1X5	T41.1X6
Thiazesim	T43.291	T43.292	T43.293	T43.294	T43.295	T43.296
Thiazides (diuretics)	T5Ø.2X1	T5Ø.2X2	T5Ø.2X3	T5Ø.2X4	T5Ø.2X5	T5Ø.2X6
Thiazinamium metilsulfate	T43.3X1	T43.3X2	T43.3X3	T43.3X4	T43.3X5	T43.3X6
Thiethylperazine	T43.3X1	T43.3X2	T43.3X3	T43.3X4	T43.3X5	T43.3X6
Thimerosal	T49.ØX1	T49.ØX2	T49.ØX3	T49.ØX4	T49.ØX5	T49.ØX6
ophthalmic preparation	T49.5X1	T49.5X2	T49.5X3	T49.5X4	T49.5X5	T49.5X6
Thioacetazone	T37.1X1	T37.1X2	T37.1X3	T37.1X4	T37.1X5	T37.1X6
with isoniazid	T37.1X1	T37.1X2	T37.1X3	T37.1X4	T37.1X5	T37.1X6
Thiobarbital sodium	T41.1X1	T41.1X2	T41.1X3	T41.1X4	T41.1X5	T41.1X6
Thiobarbiturate anesthetic	T41.1X1	T41.1X2	T41.1X3	T41.1X4	T41.1X5	T41.1X6
Thiobismol	T37.8X1	T37.8X2	T37.8X3	T37.8X4	T37.8X5	T37.8X6
Thiobutabarbital sodium	T41.1X1	T41.1X2	T41.1X3	T41.1X4	T41.1X5	T41.1X6
Thiocarbamate (insecticide)	T6Ø.ØX1	T6Ø.ØX2	T6Ø.ØX3	T6Ø.ØX4	—	—
Thiocarbamide	T38.2X1	T38.2X2	T38.2X3	T38.2X4	T38.2X5	T38.2X6
Thiocarbarsone	T37.8X1	T37.8X2	T37.8X3	T37.8X4	T37.8X5	T37.8X6
Thiocarlide	T37.1X1	T37.1X2	T37.1X3	T37.1X4	T37.1X5	T37.1X6
Thioctamide	T5Ø.991	T5Ø.992	T5Ø.993	T5Ø.994	T5Ø.995	T5Ø.996
Thioctic acid	T5Ø.991	T5Ø.992	T5Ø.993	T5Ø.994	T5Ø.995	T5Ø.996
Thiofos	T6Ø.ØX1	T6Ø.ØX2	T6Ø.ØX3	T6Ø.ØX4	—	—
Thioglycolate	T49.4X1	T49.4X2	T49.4X3	T49.4X4	T49.4X5	T49.4X6
Thioglycolic acid	T65.891	T65.892	T65.893	T65.894	—	—
Thioguanine	T45.1X1	T45.1X2	T45.1X3	T45.1X4	T45.1X5	T45.1X6
Thiomercaptomerin	T5Ø.2X1	T5Ø.2X2	T5Ø.2X3	T5Ø.2X4	T5Ø.2X5	T5Ø.2X6
Thiomerin	T5Ø.2X1	T5Ø.2X2	T5Ø.2X3	T5Ø.2X4	T5Ø.2X5	T5Ø.2X6
Thiomersal	T49.ØX1	T49.ØX2	T49.ØX3	T49.ØX4	T49.ØX5	T49.ØX6
Thionazin	T6Ø.ØX1	T6Ø.ØX2	T6Ø.ØX3	T6Ø.ØX4	—	—
Thiopental (sodium)	T41.1X1	T41.1X2	T41.1X3	T41.1X4	T41.1X5	T41.1X6
Thiopentone (sodium)	T41.1X1	T41.1X2	T41.1X3	T41.1X4	T41.1X5	T41.1X6
Thiopropazate	T43.3X1	T43.3X2	T43.3X3	T43.3X4	T43.3X5	T43.3X6
Thioproperazine	T43.3X1	T43.3X2	T43.3X3	T43.3X4	T43.3X5	T43.3X6
Thioridazine	T43.3X1	T43.3X2	T43.3X3	T43.3X4	T43.3X5	T43.3X6
Thiosinamine	T49.3X1	T49.3X2	T49.3X3	T49.3X4	T49.3X5	T49.3X6
Thiotepa	T45.1X1	T45.1X2	T45.1X3	T45.1X4	T45.1X5	T45.1X6
Thiothixene	T43.4X1	T43.4X2	T43.4X3	T43.4X4	T43.4X5	T43.4X6
Thiouracil (benzyl) (methyl) (propyl)	T38.2X1	T38.2X2	T38.2X3	T38.2X4	T38.2X5	T38.2X6
Thiourea	T38.2X1	T38.2X2	T38.2X3	T38.2X4	T38.2X5	T38.2X6
Thiphenamil	T44.3X1	T44.3X2	T44.3X3	T44.3X4	T44.3X5	T44.3X6
Thiram	T6Ø.3X1	T6Ø.3X2	T6Ø.3X3	T6Ø.3X4	—	—
medicinal	T49.2X1	T49.2X2	T49.2X3	T49.2X4	T49.2X5	T49.2X6
Thonzylamine (systemic)	T45.ØX1	T45.ØX2	T45.ØX3	T45.ØX4	T45.ØX5	T45.ØX6
mucosal decongestant	T48.5X1	T48.5X2	T48.5X3	T48.5X4	T48.5X5	T48.5X6
Thorazine	T43.3X1	T43.3X2	T43.3X3	T43.3X4	T43.3X5	T43.3X6
Thorium dioxide suspension	T5Ø.8X1	T5Ø.8X2	T5Ø.8X3	T5Ø.8X4	T5Ø.8X5	T5Ø.8X6
Thornapple	T62.2X1	T62.2X2	T62.2X3	T62.2X4	—	—
Throat drug NEC	T49.6X1	T49.6X2	T49.6X3	T49.6X4	T49.6X5	T49.6X6
Thrombate 111*	T45.511	T45.512	T45.513	T45.514	T45.515	T45.516
Thrombin	T45.7X1	T45.7X2	T45.7X3	T45.7X4	T45.7X5	T45.7X6
Thrombolysin	T45.611	T45.612	T45.613	T45.614	T45.615	T45.616
Thromboplastin	T45.7X1	T45.7X2	T45.7X3	T45.7X4	T45.7X5	T45.7X6
Thurfyl nicotinate	T46.7X1	T46.7X2	T46.7X3	T46.7X4	T46.7X5	T46.7X6
Thymol	T49.ØX1	T49.ØX2	T49.ØX3	T49.ØX4	T49.ØX5	T49.ØX6
Thymopentin	T37.5X1	T37.5X2	T37.5X3	T37.5X4	T37.5X5	T37.5X6
Thymoxamine	T46.7X1	T46.7X2	T46.7X3	T46.7X4	T46.7X5	T46.7X6
Thymus extract	T38.891	T38.892	T38.893	T38.894	T38.895	T38.896
Thyreotrophic hormone	T38.811	T38.812	T38.813	T38.814	T38.815	T38.816
Thyroglobulin	T38.1X1	T38.1X2	T38.1X3	T38.1X4	T38.1X5	T38.1X6
Thyroid (hormone)	T38.1X1	T38.1X2	T38.1X3	T38.1X4	T38.1X5	T38.1X6
Thyrolar	T38.1X1	T38.1X2	T38.1X3	T38.1X4	T38.1X5	T38.1X6
Thyrotrophin	T38.811	T38.812	T38.813	T38.814	T38.815	T38.816
Thyrotropic hormone	T38.811	T38.812	T38.813	T38.814	T38.815	T38.816
Thyroxine	T38.1X1	T38.1X2	T38.1X3	T38.1X4	T38.1X5	T38.1X6
Tiabendazole	T37.4X1	T37.4X2	T37.4X3	T37.4X4	T37.4X5	T37.4X6
Tiamizide	T5Ø.2X1	T5Ø.2X2	T5Ø.2X3	T5Ø.2X4	T5Ø.2X5	T5Ø.2X6
Tianeptine	T43.291	T43.292	T43.293	T43.294	T43.295	T43.296
Tiapamil	T46.1X1	T46.1X2	T46.1X3	T46.1X4	T46.1X5	T46.1X6
Tiapride	T43.591	T43.592	T43.593	T43.594	T43.595	T43.596
Tiaprofenic acid	T39.311	T39.312	T39.313	T39.314	T39.315	T39.316
Tiaramide	T39.8X1	T39.8X2	T39.8X3	T39.8X4	T39.8X5	T39.8X6
Ticagrelor*	T45.521	T45.522	T45.523	T45.524	T45.525	T45.526
Ticarcillin	T36.ØX1	T36.ØX2	T36.ØX3	T36.ØX4	T36.ØX5	T36.ØX6
Ticlatone	T49.ØX1	T49.ØX2	T49.ØX3	T49.ØX4	T49.ØX5	T49.ØX6
Ticlopidine	T45.521	T45.522	T45.523	T45.524	T45.525	T45.526
Ticrynafen	T5Ø.1X1	T5Ø.1X2	T5Ø.1X3	T5Ø.1X4	T5Ø.1X5	T5Ø.1X6
Tidiacic	T5Ø.991	T5Ø.992	T5Ø.993	T5Ø.994	T5Ø.995	T5Ø.996
Tiemonium	T44.3X1	T44.3X2	T44.3X3	T44.3X4	T44.3X5	T44.3X6
iodide	T44.3X1	T44.3X2	T44.3X3	T44.3X4	T44.3X5	T44.3X6
Tienilic acid	T5Ø.1X1	T5Ø.1X2	T5Ø.1X3	T5Ø.1X4	T5Ø.1X5	T5Ø.1X6
Tifenamil	T44.3X1	T44.3X2	T44.3X3	T44.3X4	T44.3X5	T44.3X6
Tigan	T45.ØX1	T45.ØX2	T45.ØX3	T45.ØX4	T45.ØX5	T45.ØX6
Tigloidine	T44.3X1	T44.3X2	T44.3X3	T44.3X4	T44.3X5	T44.3X6
Tilactase	T47.5X1	T47.5X2	T47.5X3	T47.5X4	T47.5X5	T47.5X6
Tiletamine	T41.291	T41.292	T41.293	T41.294	T41.295	T41.296
Tilidine	T4Ø.491	T4Ø.492	T4Ø.493	T4Ø.494	—	—
Timepidium bromide	T44.3X1	T44.3X2	T44.3X3	T44.3X4	T44.3X5	T44.3X6
Timiperone	T43.4X1	T43.4X2	T43.4X3	T43.4X4	T43.4X5	T43.4X6
Timolol	T44.7X1	T44.7X2	T44.7X3	T44.7X4	T44.7X5	T44.7X6
Tincture, iodine — *see* Iodine						
Tindal	T43.3X1	T43.3X2	T43.3X3	T43.3X4	T43.3X5	T43.3X6
Tinidazole	T37.3X1	T37.3X2	T37.3X3	T37.3X4	T37.3X5	T37.3X6
Tin (chloride) (dust) (oxide) **NEC**	T56.6X1	T56.6X2	T56.6X3	T56.6X4	—	—
anti-infectives	T37.8X1	T37.8X2	T37.8X3	T37.8X4	T37.8X5	T37.8X6
Tinoridine	T39.8X1	T39.8X2	T39.8X3	T39.8X4	T39.8X5	T39.8X6
Tiocarlide	T37.1X1	T37.1X2	T37.1X3	T37.1X4	T37.1X5	T37.1X6
Tioclomarol	T45.511	T45.512	T45.513	T45.514	T45.515	T45.516
Tioconazole	T49.ØX1	T49.ØX2	T49.ØX3	T49.ØX4	T49.ØX5	T49.ØX6
Tioguanine	T45.1X1	T45.1X2	T45.1X3	T45.1X4	T45.1X5	T45.1X6
Tiopronin	T5Ø.991	T5Ø.992	T5Ø.993	T5Ø.994	T5Ø.995	T5Ø.996
Tiotixene	T43.4X1	T43.4X2	T43.4X3	T43.4X4	T43.4X5	T43.4X6
Tioxolone	T49.4X1	T49.4X2	T49.4X3	T49.4X4	T49.4X5	T49.4X6
Tipepidine	T48.3X1	T48.3X2	T48.3X3	T48.3X4	T48.3X5	T48.3X6
Tiquizium bromide	T44.3X1	T44.3X2	T44.3X3	T44.3X4	T44.3X5	T44.3X6
Tiratricol	T38.1X1	T38.1X2	T38.1X3	T38.1X4	T38.1X5	T38.1X6
Tisopurine	T5Ø.4X1	T5Ø.4X2	T5Ø.4X3	T5Ø.4X4	T5Ø.4X5	T5Ø.4X6
Titanium (compounds) (vapor)	T56.891	T56.892	T56.893	T56.894	—	—
dioxide	T49.3X1	T49.3X2	T49.3X3	T49.3X4	T49.3X5	T49.3X6
ointment	T49.3X1	T49.3X2	T49.3X3	T49.3X4	T49.3X5	T49.3X6
oxide	T49.3X1	T49.3X2	T49.3X3	T49.3X4	T49.3X5	T49.3X6
tetrachloride	T56.891	T56.892	T56.893	T56.894	—	—
Titanocene	T56.891	T56.892	T56.893	T56.894	—	—
Titroid	T38.1X1	T38.1X2	T38.1X3	T38.1X4	T38.1X5	T38.1X6
Tizanidine	T42.8X1	T42.8X2	T42.8X3	T42.8X4	T42.8X5	T42.8X6
TMTD	T6Ø.3X1	T6Ø.3X2	T6Ø.3X3	T6Ø.3X4	—	—
TNT (fumes)	T65.3X1	T65.3X2	T65.3X3	T65.3X4	—	—
Toadstool	T62.ØX1	T62.ØX2	T62.ØX3	T62.ØX4	—	—
Tobacco NEC	T65.291	T65.292	T65.293	T65.294	—	—
cigarettes	T65.221	T65.222	T65.223	T65.224	—	—
Indian	T62.2X1	T62.2X2	T62.2X3	T62.2X4	—	—
smoke, second-hand	T65.221	T65.222	T65.223	T65.224	—	—
Tobraflex*	T49.5X1	T49.5X2	T49.5X3	T49.5X4	T49.5X5	T49.5X6
Tobramycin	T36.5X1	T36.5X2	T36.5X3	T36.5X4	T36.5X5	T36.5X6
Tocainide	T46.2X1	T46.2X2	T46.2X3	T46.2X4	T46.2X5	T46.2X6
Tocoferol	T45.2X1	T45.2X2	T45.2X3	T45.2X4	T45.2X5	T45.2X6
Tocopherol	T45.2X1	T45.2X2	T45.2X3	T45.2X4	T45.2X5	T45.2X6
acetate	T45.2X1	T45.2X2	T45.2X3	T45.2X4	T45.2X5	T45.2X6
Tocosamine	T48.ØX1	T48.ØX2	T48.ØX3	T48.ØX4	T48.ØX5	T48.ØX6
Todralazine	T46.5X1	T46.5X2	T46.5X3	T46.5X4	T46.5X5	T46.5X6
Tofisopam	T42.4X1	T42.4X2	T42.4X3	T42.4X4	T42.4X5	T42.4X6

Substance	Poisoning, Accidental (unintentional)	Poisoning, Intentional Self-harm	Poisoning, Assault	Poisoning, Undetermined	Adverse Effect	Under-dosing
Tofranil	T43.011	T43.012	T43.013	T43.014	T43.015	T43.016
Toilet deodorizer	T65.891	T65.892	T65.893	T65.894	—	—
Tolamolol	T44.7X1	T44.7X2	T44.7X3	T44.7X4	T44.7X5	T44.7X6
Tolazamide	T38.3X1	T38.3X2	T38.3X3	T38.3X4	T38.3X5	T38.3X6
Tolazoline	T46.7X1	T46.7X2	T46.7X3	T46.7X4	T46.7X5	T46.7X6
Tolbutamide (sodium)	T38.3X1	T38.3X2	T38.3X3	T38.3X4	T38.3X5	T38.3X6
Tolciclate	T49.0X1	T49.0X2	T49.0X3	T49.0X4	T49.0X5	T49.0X6
Tolmetin	T39.391	T39.392	T39.393	T39.394	T39.395	T39.396
Tolnaftate	T49.0X1	T49.0X2	T49.0X3	T49.0X4	T49.0X5	T49.0X6
Tolonidine	T46.5X1	T46.5X2	T46.5X3	T46.5X4	T46.5X5	T46.5X6
Toloxatone	T42.6X1	T42.6X2	T42.6X3	T42.6X4	T42.6X5	T42.6X6
Tolperisone	T44.3X1	T44.3X2	T44.3X3	T44.3X4	T44.3X5	T44.3X6
Tolserol	T42.8X1	T42.8X2	T42.8X3	T42.8X4	T42.8X5	T42.8X6
Toluene (liquid)	T52.2X1	T52.2X2	T52.2X3	T52.2X4	—	—
diisocyanate	T65.0X1	T65.0X2	T65.0X3	T65.0X4	—	—
Toluidine	T65.891	T65.892	T65.893	T65.894	—	—
vapor	T59.891	T59.892	T59.893	T59.894	—	—
Toluol (liquid)	T52.2X1	T52.2X2	T52.2X3	T52.2X4	—	—
vapor	T52.2X1	T52.2X2	T52.2X3	T52.2X4	—	—
Toluylenediamine	T65.3X1	T65.3X2	T65.3X3	T65.3X4	—	—
Tolylene-2,4-diisocyanate	T65.0X1	T65.0X2	T65.0X3	T65.0X4	—	—
Tonic NEC	T50.901	T50.902	T50.903	T50.904	T50.905	T50.906
Topical action drug NEC	T49.91	T49.92	T49.93	T49.94	T49.95	T49.96
ear, nose or throat	T49.6X1	T49.6X2	T49.6X3	T49.6X4	T49.6X5	T49.6X6
eye	T49.5X1	T49.5X2	T49.5X3	T49.5X4	T49.5X5	T49.5X6
skin	T49.91	T49.92	T49.93	T49.94	T49.95	T49.96
specified NEC	T49.8X1	T49.8X2	T49.8X3	T49.8X4	T49.8X5	T49.8X6
Toprol*	T44.7X1	T44.7X2	T44.7X3	T44.7X4	T44.7X5	T44.7X6
Toquizine	T44.3X1	T44.3X2	T44.3X3	T44.3X4	T44.3X5	T44.3X6
Toremifene	T38.6X1	T38.6X2	T38.6X3	T38.6X4	T38.6X5	T38.6X6
Tosylchloramide sodium	T49.8X1	T49.8X2	T49.8X3	T49.8X4	T49.8X5	T49.8X6
Toxaphene (dust) (spray)	T60.1X1	T60.1X2	T60.1X3	T60.1X4	—	—
Toxin, diphtheria (Schick Test)	T50.8X1	T50.8X2	T50.8X3	T50.8X4	T50.8X5	T50.8X6
Toxoid						
combined	T50.A21	T50.A22	T50.A23	T50.A24	T50.A25	T50.A26
diphtheria	T50.A91	T50.A92	T50.A93	T50.A94	T50.A95	T50.A96
tetanus	T50.A91	T50.A92	T50.A93	T50.A94	T50.A95	T50.A96
Trace element NEC	T45.8X1	T45.8X2	T45.8X3	T45.8X4	T45.8X5	T45.8X6
Tractor fuel NEC	T52.0X1	T52.0X2	T52.0X3	T52.0X4	—	—
Tragacanth	T50.991	T50.992	T50.993	T50.994	T50.995	T50.996
Tramadol	T40.421	T40.422	T40.423	T40.424	T40.425	T40.426
Tramazoline	T48.5X1	T48.5X2	T48.5X3	T48.5X4	T48.5X5	T48.5X6
Tranexamic acid	T45.621	T45.622	T45.623	T45.624	T45.625	T45.626
Tranilast	T45.0X1	T45.0X2	T45.0X3	T45.0X4	T45.0X5	T45.0X6
Tranquilizer NEC	T43.501	T43.502	T43.503	T43.504	T43.505	T43.506
with hypnotic or sedative	T42.6X1	T42.6X2	T42.6X3	T42.6X4	T42.6X5	T42.6X6
benzodiazepine NEC	T42.4X1	T42.4X2	T42.4X3	T42.4X4	T42.4X5	T42.4X6
butyrophenone NEC	T43.4X1	T43.4X2	T43.4X3	T43.4X4	T43.4X5	T43.4X6
carbamate	T43.591	T43.592	T43.593	T43.594	T43.595	T43.596
dimethylamine	T43.3X1	T43.3X2	T43.3X3	T43.3X4	T43.3X5	T43.3X6
ethylamine	T43.3X1	T43.3X2	T43.3X3	T43.3X4	T43.3X5	T43.3X6
hydroxyzine	T43.591	T43.592	T43.593	T43.594	T43.595	T43.596
major NEC	T43.501	T43.502	T43.503	T43.504	T43.505	T43.506
penothiazine NEC	T43.3X1	T43.3X2	T43.3X3	T43.3X4	T43.3X5	T43.3X6
phenothiazine-based	T43.3X1	T43.3X2	T43.3X3	T43.3X4	T43.3X5	T43.3X6
piperazine NEC	T43.3X1	T43.3X2	T43.3X3	T43.3X4	T43.3X5	T43.3X6
piperidine	T43.3X1	T43.3X2	T43.3X3	T43.3X4	T43.3X5	T43.3X6
propylamine	T43.3X1	T43.3X2	T43.3X3	T43.3X4	T43.3X5	T43.3X6
specified NEC	T43.591	T43.592	T43.593	T43.594	T43.595	T43.596
thioxanthene NEC	T43.591	T43.592	T43.593	T43.594	T43.595	T43.596
Tranxene	T42.4X1	T42.4X2	T42.4X3	T42.4X4	T42.4X5	T42.4X6
Tranylcypromine	T43.1X1	T43.1X2	T43.1X3	T43.1X4	T43.1X5	T43.1X6
Trapidil	T46.3X1	T46.3X2	T46.3X3	T46.3X4	T46.3X5	T46.3X6
Trasentine	T44.3X1	T44.3X2	T44.3X3	T44.3X4	T44.3X5	T44.3X6
Travert	T50.3X1	T50.3X2	T50.3X3	T50.3X4	T50.3X5	T50.3X6
Trazodone	T43.211	T43.212	T43.213	T43.214	T43.215	T43.216
Treanda*	T45.1X1	T45.1X2	T45.1X3	T45.1X4	T45.1X5	T45.1X6
Trecator	T37.1X1	T37.1X2	T37.1X3	T37.1X4	T37.1X5	T37.1X6
Treosulfan	T45.1X1	T45.1X2	T45.1X3	T45.1X4	T45.1X5	T45.1X6
Tretamine	T45.1X1	T45.1X2	T45.1X3	T45.1X4	T45.1X5	T45.1X6
Tretinoin	T49.0X1	T49.0X2	T49.0X3	T49.0X4	T49.0X5	T49.0X6
Tretoquinol	T48.6X1	T48.6X2	T48.6X3	T48.6X4	T48.6X5	T48.6X6
Triacetin	T49.0X1	T49.0X2	T49.0X3	T49.0X4	T49.0X5	T49.0X6
Triacetoxyanthracene	T49.4X1	T49.4X2	T49.4X3	T49.4X4	T49.4X5	T49.4X6
Triacetyloleandomycin	T36.3X1	T36.3X2	T36.3X3	T36.3X4	T36.3X5	T36.3X6
Triamcinolone	T38.0X1	T38.0X2	T38.0X3	T38.0X4	T38.0X5	T38.0X6
ENT agent	T49.6X1	T49.6X2	T49.6X3	T49.6X4	T49.6X5	T49.6X6
hexacetonide	T49.0X1	T49.0X2	T49.0X3	T49.0X4	T49.0X5	T49.0X6
ophthalmic preparation	T49.5X1	T49.5X2	T49.5X3	T49.5X4	T49.5X5	T49.5X6
topical NEC	T49.0X1	T49.0X2	T49.0X3	T49.0X4	T49.0X5	T49.0X6
Triampyzine	T44.3X1	T44.3X2	T44.3X3	T44.3X4	T44.3X5	T44.3X6
Triamterene	T50.2X1	T50.2X2	T50.2X3	T50.2X4	T50.2X5	T50.2X6

Substance	Poisoning, Accidental (unintentional)	Poisoning, Intentional Self-harm	Poisoning, Assault	Poisoning, Undetermined	Adverse Effect	Under-dosing
Triazine (herbicide)	T60.3X1	T60.3X2	T60.3X3	T60.3X4	—	—
Triaziquone	T45.1X1	T45.1X2	T45.1X3	T45.1X4	T45.1X5	T45.1X6
Triazolam	T42.4X1	T42.4X2	T42.4X3	T42.4X4	T42.4X5	T42.4X6
Triazole (herbicide)	T60.3X1	T60.3X2	T60.3X3	T60.3X4	—	—
Tribavirin*	T37.5X1	T37.5X2	T37.5X3	T37.5X4	T37.5X5	T37.5X6
Tribenoside	T46.991	T46.992	T46.993	T46.994	T46.995	T46.996
Tribromacetaldehyde	T42.6X1	T42.6X2	T42.6X3	T42.6X4	T42.6X5	T42.6X6
Tribromoethanol, rectal	T41.291	T41.292	T41.293	T41.294	T41.295	T41.296
Tribromomethane	T42.6X1	T42.6X2	T42.6X3	T42.6X4	T42.6X5	T42.6X6
Trichlorethane	T53.2X1	T53.2X2	T53.2X3	T53.2X4	—	—
Trichlorethylene	T53.2X1	T53.2X2	T53.2X3	T53.2X4	—	—
Trichlorfon	T60.0X1	T60.0X2	T60.0X3	T60.0X4	—	—
Trichlormethiazide	T50.2X1	T50.2X2	T50.2X3	T50.2X4	T50.2X5	T50.2X6
Trichlormethine	T45.1X1	T45.1X2	T45.1X3	T45.1X4	T45.1X5	T45.1X6
Trichloroacetic acid, Trichloracetic acid	T54.2X1	T54.2X2	T54.2X3	T54.2X4	—	—
medicinal	T49.4X1	T49.4X2	T49.4X3	T49.4X4	T49.4X5	T49.4X6
Trichloroethane	T53.2X1	T53.2X2	T53.2X3	T53.2X4	—	—
Trichloroethanol	T42.6X1	T42.6X2	T42.6X3	T42.6X4	T42.6X5	T42.6X6
Trichloroethylene (liquid) (vapor)	T53.2X1	T53.2X2	T53.2X3	T53.2X4	—	—
anesthetic (gas)	T41.0X1	T41.0X2	T41.0X3	T41.0X4	T41.0X5	T41.0X6
vapor NEC	T53.2X1	T53.2X2	T53.2X3	T53.2X4	—	—
Trichloroethyl phosphate	T42.6X1	T42.6X2	T42.6X3	T42.6X4	T42.6X5	T42.6X6
Trichlorofluoromethane NEC	T53.5X1	T53.5X2	T53.5X3	T53.5X4	—	—
Trichloronate	T60.0X1	T60.0X2	T60.0X3	T60.0X4	—	—
Trichloropropane	T53.6X1	T53.6X2	T53.6X3	T53.6X4	—	—
Trichlorotriethylamine	T45.1X1	T45.1X2	T45.1X3	T45.1X4	T45.1X5	T45.1X6
Trichomonacides NEC	T37.3X1	T37.3X2	T37.3X3	T37.3X4	T37.3X5	T37.3X6
Trichomycin	T36.7X1	T36.7X2	T36.7X3	T36.7X4	T36.7X5	T36.7X6
Triclobisonium chloride	T49.0X1	T49.0X2	T49.0X3	T49.0X4	T49.0X5	T49.0X6
Triclocarban	T49.0X1	T49.0X2	T49.0X3	T49.0X4	T49.0X5	T49.0X6
Triclofos	T42.6X1	T42.6X2	T42.6X3	T42.6X4	T42.6X5	T42.6X6
Triclosan	T49.0X1	T49.0X2	T49.0X3	T49.0X4	T49.0X5	T49.0X6
Tricosal*	T39.091	T39.092	T39.093	T39.094	T39.095	T39.096
Tricresyl phosphate	T65.891	T65.892	T65.893	T65.894	—	—
solvent	T52.91	T52.92	T52.93	T52.94	—	—
Tricyclamol chloride	T44.3X1	T44.3X2	T44.3X3	T44.3X4	T44.3X5	T44.3X6
Tridesilon	T49.0X1	T49.0X2	T49.0X3	T49.0X4	T49.0X5	T49.0X6
Tridihexethyl iodide	T44.3X1	T44.3X2	T44.3X3	T44.3X4	T44.3X5	T44.3X6
Tridione	T42.2X1	T42.2X2	T42.2X3	T42.2X4	T42.2X5	T42.2X6
Trientine	T45.8X1	T45.8X2	T45.8X3	T45.8X4	T45.8X5	T45.8X6
Triethanolamine NEC	T54.3X1	T54.3X2	T54.3X3	T54.3X4	—	—
detergent	T54.3X1	T54.3X2	T54.3X3	T54.3X4	—	—
trinitrate (biphosphate)	T46.3X1	T46.3X2	T46.3X3	T46.3X4	T46.3X5	T46.3X6
Triethanomelamine	T45.1X1	T45.1X2	T45.1X3	T45.1X4	T45.1X5	T45.1X6
Triethylenemelamine	T45.1X1	T45.1X2	T45.1X3	T45.1X4	T45.1X5	T45.1X6
Triethylenephosphoramide	T45.1X1	T45.1X2	T45.1X3	T45.1X4	T45.1X5	T45.1X6
Triethylenethiophosphoramide	T45.1X1	T45.1X2	T45.1X3	T45.1X4	T45.1X5	T45.1X6
Trifluoperazine	T43.3X1	T43.3X2	T43.3X3	T43.3X4	T43.3X5	T43.3X6
Trifluoroethyl vinyl ether	T41.0X1	T41.0X2	T41.0X3	T41.0X4	T41.0X5	T41.0X6
Trifluperidol	T43.4X1	T43.4X2	T43.4X3	T43.4X4	T43.4X5	T43.4X6
Triflupromazine	T43.3X1	T43.3X2	T43.3X3	T43.3X4	T43.3X5	T43.3X6
Trifluridine	T37.5X1	T37.5X2	T37.5X3	T37.5X4	T37.5X5	T37.5X6
Triflusal	T45.521	T45.522	T45.523	T45.524	T45.525	T45.526
Trihexyphenidyl	T44.3X1	T44.3X2	T44.3X3	T44.3X4	T44.3X5	T44.3X6
Triiodothyronine	T38.1X1	T38.1X2	T38.1X3	T38.1X4	T38.1X5	T38.1X6
Trilene	T41.0X1	T41.0X2	T41.0X3	T41.0X4	T41.0X5	T41.0X6
Trilostane	T38.991	T38.992	T38.993	T38.994	T38.995	T38.996
Trimebutine	T44.3X1	T44.3X2	T44.3X3	T44.3X4	T44.3X5	T44.3X6
Trimecaine	T41.3X1	T41.3X2	T41.3X3	T41.3X4	T41.3X5	T41.3X6
Trimeprazine (tartrate)	T44.3X1	T44.3X2	T44.3X3	T44.3X4	T44.3X5	T44.3X6
Trimetaphan camsilate	T44.2X1	T44.2X2	T44.2X3	T44.2X4	T44.2X5	T44.2X6
Trimetazidine	T46.7X1	T46.7X2	T46.7X3	T46.7X4	T46.7X5	T46.7X6
Trimethadione	T42.2X1	T42.2X2	T42.2X3	T42.2X4	T42.2X5	T42.2X6
Trimethaphan	T44.2X1	T44.2X2	T44.2X3	T44.2X4	T44.2X5	T44.2X6
Trimethidinium	T44.2X1	T44.2X2	T44.2X3	T44.2X4	T44.2X5	T44.2X6
Trimethobenzamide	T45.0X1	T45.0X2	T45.0X3	T45.0X4	T45.0X5	T45.0X6
Trimethoprim	T37.8X1	T37.8X2	T37.8X3	T37.8X4	T37.8X5	T37.8X6
with sulfamethoxazole	T36.8X1	T36.8X2	T36.8X3	T36.8X4	T36.8X5	T36.8X6
Trimethylcarbinol	T51.3X1	T51.3X2	T51.3X3	T51.3X4	—	—
Trimethylpsoralen	T49.3X1	T49.3X2	T49.3X3	T49.3X4	T49.3X5	T49.3X6
Trimeton	T45.0X1	T45.0X2	T45.0X3	T45.0X4	T45.0X5	T45.0X6
Trimetrexate	T45.1X1	T45.1X2	T45.1X3	T45.1X4	T45.1X5	T45.1X6
Trimipramine	T43.011	T43.012	T43.013	T43.014	T43.015	T43.016
Trimox*	T36.0X1	T36.0X2	T36.0X3	T36.0X4	T36.0X5	T36.0X6
Trimustine	T45.1X1	T45.1X2	T45.1X3	T45.1X4	T45.1X5	T45.1X6
Trinitrine	T46.3X1	T46.3X2	T46.3X3	T46.3X4	T46.3X5	T46.3X6
Trinitrobenzol	T65.3X1	T65.3X2	T65.3X3	T65.3X4	—	—
Trinitrophenol	T65.3X1	T65.3X2	T65.3X3	T65.3X4	—	—
Trinitrotoluene (fumes)	T65.3X1	T65.3X2	T65.3X3	T65.3X4	—	—

Substance	Poisoning, Accidental (unintentional)	Poisoning, Intentional Self-harm	Poisoning, Assault	Poisoning, Undetermined	Adverse Effect	Under-dosing
Trional	T42.6X1	T42.6X2	T42.6X3	T42.6X4	T42.6X5	T42.6X6
Triorthocresyl phosphate	T65.891	T65.892	T65.893	T65.894	—	—
Trioxide of arsenic	T57.ØX1	T57.ØX2	T57.ØX3	T57.ØX4	—	—
Trioxysalen	T49.4X1	T49.4X2	T49.4X3	T49.4X4	T49.4X5	T49.4X6
Tripamide	T5Ø.2X1	T5Ø.2X2	T5Ø.2X3	T5Ø.2X4	T5Ø.2X5	T5Ø.2X6
Triparanol	T46.6X1	T46.6X2	T46.6X3	T46.6X4	T46.6X5	T46.6X6
Tripelennamine	T45.ØX1	T45.ØX2	T45.ØX3	T45.ØX4	T45.ØX5	T45.ØX6
Triperiden	T44.3X1	T44.3X2	T44.3X3	T44.3X4	T44.3X5	T44.3X6
Triperidol	T43.4X1	T43.4X2	T43.4X3	T43.4X4	T43.4X5	T43.4X6
Triphenylphosphate	T65.891	T65.892	T65.893	T65.894	—	—
Triple						
bromides	T42.6X1	T42.6X2	T42.6X3	T42.6X4	T42.6X5	T42.6X6
carbonate	T47.1X1	T47.1X2	T47.1X3	T47.1X4	T47.1X5	T47.1X6
vaccine						
DPT	T5Ø.A11	T5Ø.A12	T5Ø.A13	T5Ø.A14	T5Ø.A15	T5Ø.A16
including pertussis	T5Ø.A11	T5Ø.A12	T5Ø.A13	T5Ø.A14	T5Ø.A15	T5Ø.A16
MMR	T5Ø.B91	T5Ø.B92	T5Ø.B93	T5Ø.B94	T5Ø.B95	T5Ø.B96
Triprolidine	T45.ØX1	T45.ØX2	T45.ØX3	T45.ØX4	T45.ØX5	T45.ØX6
Trisodium hydrogen edetate	T5Ø.6X1	T5Ø.6X2	T5Ø.6X3	T5Ø.6X4	T5Ø.6X5	T5Ø.6X6
Trisoralen	T49.3X1	T49.3X2	T49.3X3	T49.3X4	T49.3X5	T49.3X6
Trisulfapyrimidines	T37.ØX1	T37.ØX2	T37.ØX3	T37.ØX4	T37.ØX5	T37.ØX6
Trithiozine	T44.3X1	T44.3X2	T44.3X3	T44.3X4	T44.3X5	T44.3X6
Tritiozine	T44.3X1	T44.3X2	T44.3X3	T44.3X4	T44.3X5	T44.3X6
Tritoqualine	T45.ØX1	T45.ØX2	T45.ØX3	T45.ØX4	T45.ØX5	T45.ØX6
Trizivir*	T37.5X1	T37.5X2	T37.5X3	T37.5X4	T37.5X5	T37.5X6
Trofosfamide	T45.1X1	T45.1X2	T45.1X3	T45.1X4	T45.1X5	T45.1X6
Troleandomycin	T36.3X1	T36.3X2	T36.3X3	T36.3X4	T36.3X5	T36.3X6
Trolnitrate (phosphate)	T46.3X1	T46.3X2	T46.3X3	T46.3X4	T46.3X5	T46.3X6
Tromantadine	T37.5X1	T37.5X2	T37.5X3	T37.5X4	T37.5X5	T37.5X6
Trometamol	T5Ø.2X1	T5Ø.2X2	T5Ø.2X3	T5Ø.2X4	T5Ø.2X5	T5Ø.2X6
Tromethamine	T5Ø.2X1	T5Ø.2X2	T5Ø.2X3	T5Ø.2X4	T5Ø.2X5	T5Ø.2X6
Tronothane	T41.3X1	T41.3X2	T41.3X3	T41.3X4	T41.3X5	T41.3X6
Tropacine	T44.3X1	T44.3X2	T44.3X3	T44.3X4	T44.3X5	T44.3X6
Tropatepine	T44.3X1	T44.3X2	T44.3X3	T44.3X4	T44.3X5	T44.3X6
Tropicamide	T44.3X1	T44.3X2	T44.3X3	T44.3X4	T44.3X5	T44.3X6
Trospium chloride	T44.3X1	T44.3X2	T44.3X3	T44.3X4	T44.3X5	T44.3X6
Troxerutin	T46.991	T46.992	T46.993	T46.994	T46.995	T46.996
Troxidone	T42.2X1	T42.2X2	T42.2X3	T42.2X4	T42.2X5	T42.2X6
Tryparsamide	T37.3X1	T37.3X2	T37.3X3	T37.3X4	T37.3X5	T37.3X6
Trypsin	T45.3X1	T45.3X2	T45.3X3	T45.3X4	T45.3X5	T45.3X6
Tryptizol	T43.Ø11	T43.Ø12	T43.Ø13	T43.Ø14	T43.Ø15	T43.Ø16
TSH	T38.811	T38.812	T38.813	T38.814	T38.815	T38.816
Tuaminoheptane	T48.5X1	T48.5X2	T48.5X3	T48.5X4	T48.5X5	T48.5X6
Tuberculin, purified protein derivative (PPD)	T5Ø.8X1	T5Ø.8X2	T5Ø.8X3	T5Ø.8X4	T5Ø.8X5	T5Ø.8X6
Tubocurare	T48.1X1	T48.1X2	T48.1X3	T48.1X4	T48.1X5	T48.1X6
Tubocurarine (chloride)	T48.1X1	T48.1X2	T48.1X3	T48.1X4	T48.1X5	T48.1X6
Tulobuterol	T48.6X1	T48.6X2	T48.6X3	T48.6X4	T48.6X5	T48.6X6
Turpentine (spirits of)	T52.8X1	T52.8X2	T52.8X3	T52.8X4	—	—
vapor	T52.8X1	T52.8X2	T52.8X3	T52.8X4	—	—
Twinrix*	T5Ø.B91	T5Ø.B92	T5Ø.B93	T5Ø.B94	T5Ø.B95	T5Ø.B96
Tybamate	T43.591	T43.592	T43.593	T43.594	T43.595	T43.596
Tygacil*	T36.4X1	T36.4X2	T36.4X3	T36.4X4	T36.4X5	T36.4X6
Tyloxapol	T48.4X1	T48.4X2	T48.4X3	T48.4X4	T48.4X5	T48.4X6
Tymazoline	T48.5X1	T48.5X2	T48.5X3	T48.5X4	T48.5X5	T48.5X6
Tymlos*	T5Ø.991	T5Ø.992	T5Ø.993	T5Ø.994	T5Ø.995	T5Ø.996
Typhoid-paratyphoid vaccine	T5Ø.A91	T5Ø.A92	T5Ø.A93	T5Ø.A94	T5Ø.A95	T5Ø.A96
Typhus vaccine	T5Ø.A91	T5Ø.A92	T5Ø.A93	T5Ø.A94	T5Ø.A95	T5Ø.A96
Tyropanoate	T5Ø.8X1	T5Ø.8X2	T5Ø.8X3	T5Ø.8X4	T5Ø.8X5	T5Ø.8X6
Tyrothricin	T49.6X1	T49.6X2	T49.6X3	T49.6X4	T49.6X5	T49.6X6
ENT agent	T49.6X1	T49.6X2	T49.6X3	T49.6X4	T49.6X5	T49.6X6
ophthalmic preparation	T49.5X1	T49.5X2	T49.5X3	T49.5X4	T49.5X5	T49.5X6
Ufenamate	T39.391	T39.392	T39.393	T39.394	T39.395	T39.396
Ultraviolet light protectant	T49.3X1	T49.3X2	T49.3X3	T49.3X4	T49.3X5	T49.3X6
Unasyn*	T36.ØX1	T36.ØX2	T36.ØX3	T36.ØX4	T36.ØX5	T36.ØX6
Undecenoic acid	T49.ØX1	T49.ØX2	T49.ØX3	T49.ØX4	T49.ØX5	T49.ØX6
Undecoylium	T49.ØX1	T49.ØX2	T49.ØX3	T49.ØX4	T49.ØX5	T49.ØX6
Undecylenic acid (derivatives)	T49.ØX1	T49.ØX2	T49.ØX3	T49.ØX4	T49.ØX5	T49.ØX6
Unna's boot	T49.3X1	T49.3X2	T49.3X3	T49.3X4	T49.3X5	T49.3X6
Unsaturated fatty acid	T46.6X1	T46.6X2	T46.6X3	T46.6X4	T46.6X5	T46.6X6
Uracil mustard	T45.1X1	T45.1X2	T45.1X3	T45.1X4	T45.1X5	T45.1X6
Uramustine	T45.1X1	T45.1X2	T45.1X3	T45.1X4	T45.1X5	T45.1X6
Urapidil	T46.5X1	T46.5X2	T46.5X3	T46.5X4	T46.5X5	T46.5X6
Urari	T48.1X1	T48.1X2	T48.1X3	T48.1X4	T48.1X5	T48.1X6
Urate oxidase	T5Ø.4X1	T5Ø.4X2	T5Ø.4X3	T5Ø.4X4	T5Ø.4X5	T5Ø.4X6
Urea	T47.3X1	T47.3X2	T47.3X3	T47.3X4	T47.3X5	T47.3X6
peroxide	T49.ØX1	T49.ØX2	T49.ØX3	T49.ØX4	T49.ØX5	T49.ØX6
stibamine	T37.4X1	T37.4X2	T37.4X3	T37.4X4	T37.4X5	T37.4X6
topical	T49.8X1	T49.8X2	T49.8X3	T49.8X4	T49.8X5	T49.8X6

Substance	Poisoning, Accidental (unintentional)	Poisoning, Intentional Self-harm	Poisoning, Assault	Poisoning, Undetermined	Adverse Effect	Under-dosing
Ureaphil*	T48.ØX1	T48.ØX2	T48.ØX3	T48.ØX4	T48.ØX5	T48.ØX6
Urethane	T45.1X1	T45.1X2	T45.1X3	T45.1X4	T45.1X5	T45.1X6
Urginea (maritima) (scilla) — *see* Squill						
Uric acid metabolism drug NEC	T5Ø.4X1	T5Ø.4X2	T5Ø.4X3	T5Ø.4X4	T5Ø.4X5	T5Ø.4X6
Uricosuric agent	T5Ø.4X1	T5Ø.4X2	T5Ø.4X3	T5Ø.4X4	T5Ø.4X5	T5Ø.4X6
Urinary anti-infective	T37.8X1	T37.8X2	T37.8X3	T37.8X4	T37.8X5	T37.8X6
Urofollitropin	T38.811	T38.812	T38.813	T38.814	T38.815	T38.816
Urokinase	T45.611	T45.612	T45.613	T45.614	T45.615	T45.616
Urokon	T5Ø.8X1	T5Ø.8X2	T5Ø.8X3	T5Ø.8X4	T5Ø.8X5	T5Ø.8X6
Ursodeoxycholic acid	T5Ø.991	T5Ø.992	T5Ø.993	T5Ø.994	T5Ø.995	T5Ø.996
Ursodiol	T5Ø.991	T5Ø.992	T5Ø.993	T5Ø.994	T5Ø.995	T5Ø.996
Urtica	T62.2X1	T62.2X2	T62.2X3	T62.2X4	—	—
Utility gas — *see* Gas, utility						
Vaccine NEC	T5Ø.Z91	T5Ø.Z92	T5Ø.Z93	T5Ø.Z94	T5Ø.Z95	T5Ø.Z96
antineoplastic	T5Ø.Z91	T5Ø.Z92	T5Ø.Z93	T5Ø.Z94	T5Ø.Z95	T5Ø.Z96
bacterial NEC	T5Ø.A91	T5Ø.A92	T5Ø.A93	T5Ø.A94	T5Ø.A95	T5Ø.A96
with						
other bacterial component	T5Ø.A21	T5Ø.A22	T5Ø.A23	T5Ø.A24	T5Ø.A25	T5Ø.A26
pertussis component	T5Ø.A11	T5Ø.A12	T5Ø.A13	T5Ø.A14	T5Ø.A15	T5Ø.A16
viral-rickettsial component	T5Ø.A21	T5Ø.A22	T5Ø.A23	T5Ø.A24	T5Ø.A25	T5Ø.A26
mixed NEC	T5Ø.A21	T5Ø.A22	T5Ø.A23	T5Ø.A24	T5Ø.A25	T5Ø.A26
BCG	T5Ø.A91	T5Ø.A92	T5Ø.A93	T5Ø.A94	T5Ø.A95	T5Ø.A96
cholera	T5Ø.A91	T5Ø.A92	T5Ø.A93	T5Ø.A94	T5Ø.A95	T5Ø.A96
diphtheria	T5Ø.A91	T5Ø.A92	T5Ø.A93	T5Ø.A94	T5Ø.A95	T5Ø.A96
with tetanus	T5Ø.A21	T5Ø.A22	T5Ø.A23	T5Ø.A24	T5Ø.A25	T5Ø.A26
and pertussis	T5Ø.A11	T5Ø.A12	T5Ø.A13	T5Ø.A14	T5Ø.A15	T5Ø.A16
influenza	T5Ø.B91	T5Ø.B92	T5Ø.B93	T5Ø.B94	T5Ø.B95	T5Ø.B96
measles	T5Ø.B91	T5Ø.B92	T5Ø.B93	T5Ø.B94	T5Ø.B95	T5Ø.B96
with mumps and rubella	T5Ø.B91	T5Ø.B92	T5Ø.B93	T5Ø.B94	T5Ø.B95	T5Ø.B96
meningococcal	T5Ø.A91	T5Ø.A92	T5Ø.A93	T5Ø.A94	T5Ø.A95	T5Ø.A96
mumps	T5Ø.B91	T5Ø.B92	T5Ø.B93	T5Ø.B94	T5Ø.B95	T5Ø.B96
paratyphoid	T5Ø.A91	T5Ø.A92	T5Ø.A93	T5Ø.A94	T5Ø.A95	T5Ø.A96
pertussis	T5Ø.A11	T5Ø.A12	T5Ø.A13	T5Ø.A14	T5Ø.A15	T5Ø.A16
with diphtheria	T5Ø.A11	T5Ø.A12	T5Ø.A13	T5Ø.A14	T5Ø.A15	T5Ø.A16
and tetanus	T5Ø.A11	T5Ø.A12	T5Ø.A13	T5Ø.A14	T5Ø.A15	T5Ø.A16
with other component	T5Ø.A11	T5Ø.A12	T5Ø.A13	T5Ø.A14	T5Ø.A15	T5Ø.A16
plague	T5Ø.A91	T5Ø.A92	T5Ø.A93	T5Ø.A94	T5Ø.A95	T5Ø.A96
poliomyelitis	T5Ø.B91	T5Ø.B92	T5Ø.B93	T5Ø.B94	T5Ø.B95	T5Ø.B96
poliovirus	T5Ø.B91	T5Ø.B92	T5Ø.B93	T5Ø.B94	T5Ø.B95	T5Ø.B96
rabies	T5Ø.B91	T5Ø.B92	T5Ø.B93	T5Ø.B94	T5Ø.B95	T5Ø.B96
respiratory syncytial virus	T5Ø.B91	T5Ø.B92	T5Ø.B93	T5Ø.B94	T5Ø.B95	T5Ø.B96
rickettsial NEC	T5Ø.A91	T5Ø.A92	T5Ø.A93	T5Ø.A94	T5Ø.A95	T5Ø.A96
with						
bacterial component	T5Ø.A21	T5Ø.A22	T5Ø.A23	T5Ø.A24	T5Ø.A25	T5Ø.A26
Rocky Mountain spotted fever	T5Ø.A91	T5Ø.A92	T5Ø.A93	T5Ø.A94	T5Ø.A95	T5Ø.A96
rubella	T5Ø.B91	T5Ø.B92	T5Ø.B93	T5Ø.B94	T5Ø.B95	T5Ø.B96
sabin oral	T5Ø.B91	T5Ø.B92	T5Ø.B93	T5Ø.B94	T5Ø.B95	T5Ø.B96
smallpox	T5Ø.B11	T5Ø.B12	T5Ø.B13	T5Ø.B14	T5Ø.B15	T5Ø.B16
TAB	T5Ø.A91	T5Ø.A92	T5Ø.A93	T5Ø.A94	T5Ø.A95	T5Ø.A96
tetanus	T5Ø.A91	T5Ø.A92	T5Ø.A93	T5Ø.A94	T5Ø.A95	T5Ø.A96
typhoid	T5Ø.A91	T5Ø.A92	T5Ø.A93	T5Ø.A94	T5Ø.A95	T5Ø.A96
typhus	T5Ø.A91	T5Ø.A92	T5Ø.A93	T5Ø.A94	T5Ø.A95	T5Ø.A96
viral NEC	T5Ø.B91	T5Ø.B92	T5Ø.B93	T5Ø.B94	T5Ø.B95	T5Ø.B96
yellow fever	T5Ø.B91	T5Ø.B92	T5Ø.B93	T5Ø.B94	T5Ø.B95	T5Ø.B96
Vaccinia immune globulin	T5Ø.Z11	T5Ø.Z12	T5Ø.Z13	T5Ø.Z14	T5Ø.Z15	T5Ø.Z16
Vaginal contraceptives	T49.8X1	T49.8X2	T49.8X3	T49.8X4	T49.8X5	T49.8X6
Valacyclovir*	T37.5X1	T37.5X2	T37.5X3	T37.5X4	T37.5X5	T37.5X6
Valerian						
root	T42.6X1	T42.6X2	T42.6X3	T42.6X4	T42.6X5	T42.6X6
tincture	T42.6X1	T42.6X2	T42.6X3	T42.6X4	T42.6X5	T42.6X6
Valethamate bromide	T44.3X1	T44.3X2	T44.3X3	T44.3X4	T44.3X5	T44.3X6
Valisone	T49.ØX1	T49.ØX2	T49.ØX3	T49.ØX4	T49.ØX5	T49.ØX6
Valium	T42.4X1	T42.4X2	T42.4X3	T42.4X4	T42.4X5	T42.4X6
Valmid	T42.6X1	T42.6X2	T42.6X3	T42.6X4	T42.6X5	T42.6X6
Valnoctamide	T42.6X1	T42.6X2	T42.6X3	T42.6X4	T42.6X5	T42.6X6
Valproate (sodium)	T42.6X1	T42.6X2	T42.6X3	T42.6X4	T42.6X5	T42.6X6
Valproic acid	T42.6X1	T42.6X2	T42.6X3	T42.6X4	T42.6X5	T42.6X6
Valpromide	T42.6X1	T42.6X2	T42.6X3	T42.6X4	T42.6X5	T42.6X6
Vanadium	T56.891	T56.892	T56.893	T56.894	—	—
Vancomycin	T36.8X1	T36.8X2	T36.8X3	T36.8X4	T36.8X5	T36.8X6
Vandazole*	T49.ØX1	T49.ØX2	T49.ØX3	T49.ØX4	T49.ØX5	T49.ØX6
Vapor — *see also* Gas	T59.91	T59.92	T59.93	T59.94	—	—
kiln (carbon monoxide)	T58.8X1	T58.8X2	T58.8X3	T58.8X4	—	—
lead — *see* lead						
specified source NEC	T59.891	T59.892	T59.893	T59.894	—	—
Vardenafil	T46.7X1	T46.7X2	T46.7X3	T46.7X4	T46.7X5	T46.7X6
Varicose reduction drug	T46.8X1	T46.8X2	T46.8X3	T46.8X4	T46.8X5	T46.8X6
Varnish	T65.4X1	T65.4X2	T65.4X3	T65.4X4	—	—

Substance	Poisoning, Accidental (unintentional)	Poisoning, Intentional Self-harm	Poisoning, Assault	Poisoning, Undetermined	Adverse Effect	Under-dosing
Varnish — *continued*						
cleaner	T52.91	T52.92	T52.93	T52.94	—	—
Vaseline	T49.3X1	T49.3X2	T49.3X3	T49.3X4	T49.3X5	T49.3X6
Vasodilan	T46.7X1	T46.7X2	T46.7X3	T46.7X4	T46.7X5	T46.7X6
Vasodilator						
coronary NEC	T46.3X1	T46.3X2	T46.3X3	T46.3X4	T46.3X5	T46.3X6
peripheral NEC	T46.7X1	T46.7X2	T46.7X3	T46.7X4	T46.7X5	T46.7X6
Vasopressin	T38.891	T38.892	T38.893	T38.894	T38.895	T38.896
Vasopressor drugs	T38.891	T38.892	T38.893	T38.894	T38.895	T38.896
Vecuronium bromide	T48.1X1	T48.1X2	T48.1X3	T48.1X4	T48.1X5	T48.1X6
Vegetable extract, astringent	T49.2X1	T49.2X2	T49.2X3	T49.2X4	T49.2X5	T49.2X6
Venlafaxine	T43.211	T43.212	T43.213	T43.214	T43.215	T43.216
Venom, venomous (bite) (sting)	T63.91	T63.92	T63.93	T63.94	—	—
amphibian NEC	T63.831	T63.832	T63.833	T63.834	—	—
animal NEC	T63.891	T63.892	T63.893	T63.894	—	—
ant	T63.421	T63.422	T63.423	T63.424	—	—
arthropod NEC	T63.481	T63.482	T63.483	T63.484	—	—
bee	T63.441	T63.442	T63.443	T63.444	—	—
centipede	T63.411	T63.412	T63.413	T63.414	—	—
fish	T63.591	T63.592	T63.593	T63.594	—	—
frog	T63.811	T63.812	T63.813	T63.814	—	—
hornet	T63.451	T63.452	T63.453	T63.454	—	—
insect NEC	T63.481	T63.482	T63.483	T63.484	—	—
lizard	T63.121	T63.122	T63.123	T63.124	—	—
marine						
animals	T63.691	T63.692	T63.693	T63.694	—	—
bluebottle	T63.611	T63.612	T63.613	T63.614	—	—
jellyfish NEC	T63.621	T63.622	T63.623	T63.624	—	—
Portuguese Man-o-war	T63.611	T63.612	T63.613	T63.614	—	—
sea anemone	T63.631	T63.632	T63.633	T63.634	—	—
specified NEC	T63.691	T63.692	T63.693	T63.694	—	—
fish	T63.591	T63.592	T63.593	T63.594	—	—
plants	T63.711	T63.712	T63.713	T63.714	—	—
sting ray	T63.511	T63.512	T63.513	T63.514	—	—
millipede (tropical)	T63.411	T63.412	T63.413	T63.414	—	—
plant NEC	T63.791	T63.792	T63.793	T63.794	—	—
marine	T63.711	T63.712	T63.713	T63.714	—	—
reptile	T63.191	T63.192	T63.193	T63.194	—	—
gila monster	T63.111	T63.112	T63.113	T63.114	—	—
lizard NEC	T63.121	T63.122	T63.123	T63.124	—	—
scorpion	T63.2X1	T63.2X2	T63.2X3	T63.2X4	—	—
snake	T63.ØØ1	T63.ØØ2	T63.ØØ3	T63.ØØ4	—	—
African NEC	T63.Ø81	T63.Ø82	T63.Ø83	T63.Ø84	—	—
American (North) (South) NEC	T63.Ø61	T63.Ø62	T63.Ø63	T63.Ø64	—	—
Asian	T63.Ø81	T63.Ø82	T63.Ø83	T63.Ø84	—	—
Australian	T63.Ø71	T63.Ø72	T63.Ø73	T63.Ø74	—	—
cobra	T63.Ø41	T63.Ø42	T63.Ø43	T63.Ø44	—	—
coral snake	T63.Ø21	T63.Ø22	T63.Ø23	T63.Ø24	—	—
rattlesnake	T63.Ø11	T63.Ø12	T63.Ø13	T63.Ø14	—	—
specified NEC	T63.Ø91	T63.Ø92	T63.Ø93	T63.Ø94	—	—
taipan	T63.Ø31	T63.Ø32	T63.Ø33	T63.Ø34	—	—
specified NEC	T63.891	T63.892	T63.893	T63.894	—	—
spider	T63.3Ø1	T63.3Ø2	T63.3Ø3	T63.3Ø4	—	—
black widow	T63.311	T63.312	T63.313	T63.314	—	—
brown recluse	T63.331	T63.332	T63.333	T63.334	—	—
specified NEC	T63.391	T63.392	T63.393	T63.394	—	—
tarantula	T63.321	T63.322	T63.323	T63.324	—	—
sting ray	T63.511	T63.512	T63.513	T63.514	—	—
toad	T63.821	T63.822	T63.823	T63.824	—	—
wasp	T63.461	T63.462	T63.463	T63.464	—	—
Venous sclerosing drug NEC	T46.8X1	T46.8X2	T46.8X3	T46.8X4	T46.8X5	T46.8X6
Ventavis*	T46.7X1	T46.7X2	T46.7X3	T46.7X4	T46.7X5	T46.7X6
Ventolin — *see* Albuterol						
Veramon	T42.3X1	T42.3X2	T42.3X3	T42.3X4	T42.3X5	T42.3X6
Verapamil	T46.1X1	T46.1X2	T46.1X3	T46.1X4	T46.1X5	T46.1X6
Veratrine	T46.5X1	T46.5X2	T46.5X3	T46.5X4	T46.5X5	T46.5X6
Veratrum						
album	T62.2X1	T62.2X2	T62.2X3	T62.2X4	—	—
alkaloids	T46.5X1	T46.5X2	T46.5X3	T46.5X4	T46.5X5	T46.5X6
viride	T62.2X1	T62.2X2	T62.2X3	T62.2X4	—	—
Verdigris	T6Ø.3X1	T6Ø.3X2	T6Ø.3X3	T6Ø.3X4	—	—
Veronal	T42.3X1	T42.3X2	T42.3X3	T42.3X4	T42.3X5	T42.3X6
Veroxil	T37.4X1	T37.4X2	T37.4X3	T37.4X4	T37.4X5	T37.4X6
Versenate	T5Ø.6X1	T5Ø.6X2	T5Ø.6X3	T5Ø.6X4	T5Ø.6X5	T5Ø.6X6
Versidyne	T39.8X1	T39.8X2	T39.8X3	T39.8X4	T39.8X5	T39.8X6
Vetrabutine	T48.ØX1	T48.ØX2	T48.ØX3	T48.ØX4	T48.ØX5	T48.ØX6
Vexol*	T49.5X1	T49.5X2	T49.5X3	T49.5X4	T49.5X5	T49.5X6
Victrelis*	T37.5X1	T37.5X2	T37.5X3	T37.5X4	T37.5X5	T37.5X6
Vidarabine	T37.5X1	T37.5X2	T37.5X3	T37.5X4	T37.5X5	T37.5X6

Substance	Poisoning, Accidental (unintentional)	Poisoning, Intentional Self-harm	Poisoning, Assault	Poisoning, Undetermined	Adverse Effect	Under-dosing
Vienna						
green	T57.ØX1	T57.ØX2	T57.ØX3	T57.ØX4	—	—
insecticide	T6Ø.2X1	T6Ø.2X2	T6Ø.2X3	T6Ø.2X4	—	—
red	T57.ØX1	T57.ØX2	T57.ØX3	T57.ØX4	—	—
pharmaceutical dye	T5Ø.991	T5Ø.992	T5Ø.993	T5Ø.994	T5Ø.995	T5Ø.996
Vigabatrin	T42.6X1	T42.6X2	T42.6X3	T42.6X4	T42.6X5	T42.6X6
Viloxazine	T43.291	T43.292	T43.293	T43.294	T43.295	T43.296
Viminol	T39.8X1	T39.8X2	T39.8X3	T39.8X4	T39.8X5	T39.8X6
Vinbarbital, vinbarbitone	T42.3X1	T42.3X2	T42.3X3	T42.3X4	T42.3X5	T42.3X6
Vinblastine	T45.1X1	T45.1X2	T45.1X3	T45.1X4	T45.1X5	T45.1X6
Vinburnine	T46.7X1	T46.7X2	T46.7X3	T46.7X4	T46.7X5	T46.7X6
Vincamine	T45.1X1	T45.1X2	T45.1X3	T45.1X4	T45.1X5	T45.1X6
Vincristine	T45.1X1	T45.1X2	T45.1X3	T45.1X4	T45.1X5	T45.1X6
Vindesine	T45.1X1	T45.1X2	T45.1X3	T45.1X4	T45.1X5	T45.1X6
Vinesthene, vinethene	T41.ØX1	T41.ØX2	T41.ØX3	T41.ØX4	T41.ØX5	T41.ØX6
Vinorelbine tartrate	T45.1X1	T45.1X2	T45.1X3	T45.1X4	T45.1X5	T45.1X6
Vinpocetine	T46.7X1	T46.7X2	T46.7X3	T46.7X4	T46.7X5	T46.7X6
Vinyl						
acetate	T65.891	T65.892	T65.893	T65.894	—	—
bital	T42.3X1	T42.3X2	T42.3X3	T42.3X4	T42.3X5	T42.3X6
bromide	T65.891	T65.892	T65.893	T65.894	—	—
chloride	T59.891	T59.892	T59.893	T59.894	—	—
ether	T41.ØX1	T41.ØX2	T41.ØX3	T41.ØX4	T41.ØX5	T41.ØX6
Vinylbital	T42.3X1	T42.3X2	T42.3X3	T42.3X4	T42.3X5	T42.3X6
Vinylidene chloride	T65.891	T65.892	T65.893	T65.894	—	—
Vioform	T37.8X1	T37.8X2	T37.8X3	T37.8X4	T37.8X5	T37.8X6
topical	T49.ØX1	T49.ØX2	T49.ØX3	T49.ØX4	T49.ØX5	T49.ØX6
Viokase*	T47.5X1	T47.5X2	T47.5X3	T47.5X4	T47.5X5	T47.5X6
Viomycin	T36.8X1	T36.8X2	T36.8X3	T36.8X4	T36.8X5	T36.8X6
Viosterol	T45.2X1	T45.2X2	T45.2X3	T45.2X4	T45.2X5	T45.2X6
Viper (venom)	T63.Ø91	T63.Ø92	T63.Ø93	T63.Ø94	—	—
Viprynium	T37.4X1	T37.4X2	T37.4X3	T37.4X4	T37.4X5	T37.4X6
Viquidil	T46.7X1	T46.7X2	T46.7X3	T46.7X4	T46.7X5	T46.7X6
Viral vaccine NEC	T5Ø.B91	T5Ø.B92	T5Ø.B93	T5Ø.B94	T5Ø.B95	T5Ø.B96
Virginiamycin	T36.8X1	T36.8X2	T36.8X3	T36.8X4	T36.8X5	T36.8X6
Virugon	T37.5X1	T37.5X2	T37.5X3	T37.5X4	T37.5X5	T37.5X6
Viscous agent	T5Ø.9Ø1	T5Ø.9Ø2	T5Ø.9Ø3	T5Ø.9Ø4	T5Ø.9Ø5	T5Ø.9Ø6
Visine	T49.5X1	T49.5X2	T49.5X3	T49.5X4	T49.5X5	T49.5X6
Visnadine	T46.3X1	T46.3X2	T46.3X3	T46.3X4	T46.3X5	T46.3X6
Vitamin NEC	T45.2X1	T45.2X2	T45.2X3	T45.2X4	T45.2X5	T45.2X6
A	T45.2X1	T45.2X2	T45.2X3	T45.2X4	T45.2X5	T45.2X6
B1	T45.2X1	T45.2X2	T45.2X3	T45.2X4	T45.2X5	T45.2X6
B2	T45.2X1	T45.2X2	T45.2X3	T45.2X4	T45.2X5	T45.2X6
B6	T45.2X1	T45.2X2	T45.2X3	T45.2X4	T45.2X5	T45.2X6
B12	T45.2X1	T45.2X2	T45.2X3	T45.2X4	T45.2X5	T45.2X6
B15	T45.2X1	T45.2X2	T45.2X3	T45.2X4	T45.2X5	T45.2X6
B NEC	T45.2X1	T45.2X2	T45.2X3	T45.2X4	T45.2X5	T45.2X6
nicotinic acid	T46.7X1	T46.7X2	T46.7X3	T46.7X4	T46.7X5	T46.7X6
C	T45.2X1	T45.2X2	T45.2X3	T45.2X4	T45.2X5	T45.2X6
D	T45.2X1	T45.2X2	T45.2X3	T45.2X4	T45.2X5	T45.2X6
D2	T45.2X1	T45.2X2	T45.2X3	T45.2X4	T45.2X5	T45.2X6
D3	T45.2X1	T45.2X2	T45.2X3	T45.2X4	T45.2X5	T45.2X6
E	T45.2X1	T45.2X2	T45.2X3	T45.2X4	T45.2X5	T45.2X6
E acetate	T45.2X1	T45.2X2	T45.2X3	T45.2X4	T45.2X5	T45.2X6
hematopoietic	T45.8X1	T45.8X2	T45.8X3	T45.8X4	T45.8X5	T45.8X6
K1	T45.7X1	T45.7X2	T45.7X3	T45.7X4	T45.7X5	T45.7X6
K2	T45.7X1	T45.7X2	T45.7X3	T45.7X4	T45.7X5	T45.7X6
K NEC	T45.7X1	T45.7X2	T45.7X3	T45.7X4	T45.7X5	T45.7X6
PP	T45.2X1	T45.2X2	T45.2X3	T45.2X4	T45.2X5	T45.2X6
ulceroprotectant	T47.1X1	T47.1X2	T47.1X3	T47.1X4	T47.1X5	T47.1X6
Vleminckx's solution	T49.4X1	T49.4X2	T49.4X3	T49.4X4	T49.4X5	T49.4X6
Voltaren — *see* Diclofenac sodium						
Voraxaze*	T5Ø.6X1	T5Ø.6X2	T5Ø.6X3	T5Ø.6X4	T5Ø.6X5	T5Ø.6X6
Warfarin	T45.511	T45.512	T45.513	T45.514	T45.515	T45.516
rodenticide	T6Ø.4X1-	T6Ø.4X2-	T6Ø.4X3-	T6Ø.4X4-	—	—
sodium	T45.511	T45.512	T45.513	T45.514	T45.515	T45.516
Wasp (sting)	T63.461	T63.462	T63.463	T63.464	—	—
Water						
balance drug	T5Ø.3X1	T5Ø.3X2	T5Ø.3X3	T5Ø.3X4	T5Ø.3X5	T5Ø.3X6
distilled	T5Ø.3X1	T5Ø.3X2	T5Ø.3X3	T5Ø.3X4	T5Ø.3X5	T5Ø.3X6
gas — *see* Gas, water						
incomplete combustion of — *see* Carbon, monoxide, fuel, utility						
hemlock	T62.2X1	T62.2X2	T62.2X3	T62.2X4	—	—
moccasin (venom)	T63.Ø61	T63.Ø62	T63.Ø63	T63.Ø64	—	—
purified	T5Ø.3X1	T5Ø.3X2	T5Ø.3X3	T5Ø.3X4	T5Ø.3X5	T5Ø.3X6
Wax (paraffin) (petroleum)	T52.ØX1	T52.ØX2	T52.ØX3	T52.ØX4	—	—
automobile	T65.891	T65.892	T65.893	T65.894	—	—
floor	T52.ØX1	T52.ØX2	T52.ØX3	T52.ØX4	—	—
Weed killers NEC	T6Ø.3X1	T6Ø.3X2	T6Ø.3X3	T6Ø.3X4	—	—
Wellbutrin*	T43.291	T43.292	T43.293	T43.294	T43.295	T43.296

Substance	Poisoning, Accidental (unintentional)	Poisoning, Intentional Self-harm	Poisoning, Assault	Poisoning, Undetermined	Adverse Effect	Under-dosing
Welldorm	T42.6X1	T42.6X2	T42.6X3	T42.6X4	T42.6X5	T42.6X6
Westcort*	T49.0X1	T49.0X2	T49.0X3	T49.0X4	T49.0X5	T49.0X6
White						
arsenic	T57.0X1	T57.0X2	T57.0X3	T57.0X4	—	—
hellebore	T62.2X1	T62.2X2	T62.2X3	T62.2X4	—	—
lotion (keratolytic)	T49.4X1	T49.4X2	T49.4X3	T49.4X4	T49.4X5	T49.4X6
spirit	T52.0X1	T52.0X2	T52.0X3	T52.0X4	—	—
Whitewash	T65.891	T65.892	T65.893	T65.894	—	—
Whole blood (human)	T45.8X1	T45.8X2	T45.8X3	T45.8X4	T45.8X5	T45.8X6
Wild						
black cherry	T62.2X1	T62.2X2	T62.2X3	T62.2X4	—	—
poisonous plants NEC	T62.2X1	T62.2X2	T62.2X3	T62.2X4	—	—
Window cleaning fluid	T65.891	T65.892	T65.893	T65.894	—	—
Wintergreen (oil)	T49.3X1	T49.3X2	T49.3X3	T49.3X4	T49.3X5	T49.3X6
Wisterine	T62.2X1	T62.2X2	T62.2X3	T62.2X4	—	—
Witch hazel	T49.2X1	T49.2X2	T49.2X3	T49.2X4	T49.2X5	T49.2X6
Wood alcohol or spirit	T51.1X1	T51.1X2	T51.1X3	T51.1X4	—	—
Wool fat (hydrous)	T49.3X1	T49.3X2	T49.3X3	T49.3X4	T49.3X5	T49.3X6
Woorali	T48.1X1	T48.1X2	T48.1X3	T48.1X4	T48.1X5	T48.1X6
Wormseed, American	T37.4X1	T37.4X2	T37.4X3	T37.4X4	T37.4X5	T37.4X6
Xamoterol	T44.5X1	T44.5X2	T44.5X3	T44.5X4	T44.5X5	T44.5X6
Xanax*	T42.4X1	T42.4X2	T42.4X3	T42.4X4	T42.4X5	T42.4X6
Xanthine diuretics	T50.2X1	T50.2X2	T50.2X3	T50.2X4	T50.2X5	T50.2X6
Xanthinol nicotinate	T46.7X1	T46.7X2	T46.7X3	T46.7X4	T46.7X5	T46.7X6
Xanthotoxin	T49.3X1	T49.3X2	T49.3X3	T49.3X4	T49.3X5	T49.3X6
Xantinol nicotinate	T46.7X1	T46.7X2	T46.7X3	T46.7X4	T46.7X5	T46.7X6
Xantocillin	T36.0X1	T36.0X2	T36.0X3	T36.0X4	T36.0X5	T36.0X6
Xenon (127Xe) (133Xe)	T50.8X1	T50.8X2	T50.8X3	T50.8X4	T50.8X5	T50.8X6
Xenysalate	T49.4X1	T49.4X2	T49.4X3	T49.4X4	T49.4X5	T49.4X6
Xibornol	T37.8X1	T37.8X2	T37.8X3	T37.8X4	T37.8X5	T37.8X6
Xigris	T45.511	T45.512	T45.513	T45.514	T45.515	T45.516
Xipamide	T50.2X1	T50.2X2	T50.2X3	T50.2X4	T50.2X5	T50.2X6
Xylene (vapor)	T52.2X1	T52.2X2	T52.2X3	T52.2X4	—	—
Xylocaine (infiltration) (topical)	T41.3X1	T41.3X2	T41.3X3	T41.3X4	T41.3X5	T41.3X6
nerve block (peripheral) (plexus)	T41.3X1	T41.3X2	T41.3X3	T41.3X4	T41.3X5	T41.3X6
spinal	T41.3X1	T41.3X2	T41.3X3	T41.3X4	T41.3X5	T41.3X6
Xylol (vapor)	T52.2X1	T52.2X2	T52.2X3	T52.2X4	—	—
Xylometazoline	T48.5X1	T48.5X2	T48.5X3	T48.5X4	T48.5X5	T48.5X6
Xylose*	T50.8X1	T50.8X2	T50.8X3	T50.8X4	T50.8X5	T50.8X6
Yaz*	T38.4X1	T38.4X2	T38.4X3	T38.4X4	T38.4X5	T38.4X6
Yeast	T45.2X1	T45.2X2	T45.2X3	T45.2X4	T45.2X5	T45.2X6
dried	T45.2X1	T45.2X2	T45.2X3	T45.2X4	T45.2X5	T45.2X6
Yellow						
fever vaccine	T50.B91	T50.B92	T50.B93	T50.B94	T50.B95	T50.B96
jasmine	T62.2X1	T62.2X2	T62.2X3	T62.2X4	—	—
phenolphthalein	T47.2X1	T47.2X2	T47.2X3	T47.2X4	T47.2X5	T47.2X6
Yervoy*	T45.1X1	T45.1X2	T45.1X3	T45.1X4	T45.1X5	T45.1X6
Yew	T62.2X1	T62.2X2	T62.2X3	T62.2X4	—	—
Yohimbic acid	T40.991	T40.992	T40.993	T40.994	T40.995	T40.996
Zactane	T39.8X1	T39.8X2	T39.8X3	T39.8X4	T39.8X5	T39.8X6
Zalcitabine	T37.5X1	T37.5X2	T37.5X3	T37.5X4	T37.5X5	T37.5X6
Zanaflex*	T48.1X1	T48.1X2	T48.1X3	T48.1X4	T48.1X5	T48.1X6
Zaroxolyn	T50.2X1	T50.2X2	T50.2X3	T50.2X4	T50.2X5	T50.2X6
Zephiran (topical)	T49.0X1	T49.0X2	T49.0X3	T49.0X4	T49.0X5	T49.0X6
ophthalmic preparation	T49.5X1	T49.5X2	T49.5X3	T49.5X4	T49.5X5	T49.5X6
Zeranol	T38.7X1	T38.7X2	T38.7X3	T38.7X4	T38.7X5	T38.7X6
Zerone	T51.1X1	T51.1X2	T51.1X3	T51.1X4	—	—
Zidovudine	T37.5X1	T37.5X2	T37.5X3	T37.5X4	T37.5X5	T37.5X6
Zilactin*	T41.3X1	T41.3X2	T41.3X3	T41.3X4	T41.3X5	T41.3X6
Zimeldine	T43.221	T43.222	T43.223	T43.224	T43.225	T43.226
Zinc (compounds) (fumes) (vapor) NEC	T56.5X1	T56.5X2	T56.5X3	T56.5X4	—	—
anti-infectives	T49.0X1	T49.0X2	T49.0X3	T49.0X4	T49.0X5	T49.0X6
antivaricose	T46.8X1	T46.8X2	T46.8X3	T46.8X4	T46.8X5	T46.8X6
bacitracin	T49.0X1	T49.0X2	T49.0X3	T49.0X4	T49.0X5	T49.0X6
chloride (mouthwash)	T49.6X1	T49.6X2	T49.6X3	T49.6X4	T49.6X5	T49.6X6
chromate	T56.5X1	T56.5X2	T56.5X3	T56.5X4	—	—
gelatin	T49.3X1	T49.3X2	T49.3X3	T49.3X4	T49.3X5	T49.3X6
oxide	T49.3X1	T49.3X2	T49.3X3	T49.3X4	T49.3X5	T49.3X6
plaster	T49.3X1	T49.3X2	T49.3X3	T49.3X4	T49.3X5	T49.3X6
peroxide	T49.0X1	T49.0X2	T49.0X3	T49.0X4	T49.0X5	T49.0X6
pesticides	T56.5X1	T56.5X2	T56.5X3	T56.5X4	—	—
phosphide	T60.4X1	T60.4X2	T60.4X3	T60.4X4	—	—
pyrithionate	T49.4X1	T49.4X2	T49.4X3	T49.4X4	T49.4X5	T49.4X6
stearate	T49.3X1	T49.3X2	T49.3X3	T49.3X4	T49.3X5	T49.3X6
sulfate	T49.5X1	T49.5X2	T49.5X3	T49.5X4	T49.5X5	T49.5X6
ENT agent	T49.6X1	T49.6X2	T49.6X3	T49.6X4	T49.6X5	T49.6X6
ophthalmic solution	T49.5X1	T49.5X2	T49.5X3	T49.5X4	T49.5X5	T49.5X6
topical NEC	T49.0X1	T49.0X2	T49.0X3	T49.0X4	T49.0X5	T49.0X6
undecylenate	T49.0X1	T49.0X2	T49.0X3	T49.0X4	T49.0X5	T49.0X6
Zineb	T60.0X1	T60.0X2	T60.0X3	T60.0X4	—	—
Zinostatin	T45.1X1	T45.1X2	T45.1X3	T45.1X4	T45.1X5	T45.1X6
Zipeprol	T48.3X1	T48.3X2	T48.3X3	T48.3X4	T48.3X5	T48.3X6
Zofenopril	T46.4X1	T46.4X2	T46.4X3	T46.4X4	T46.4X5	T46.4X6
Zolpidem	T42.6X1	T42.6X2	T42.6X3	T42.6X4	T42.6X5	T42.6X6
Zomepirac	T39.391	T39.392	T39.393	T39.394	T39.395	T39.396
Zopiclone	T42.6X1	T42.6X2	T42.6X3	T42.6X4	T42.6X5	T42.6X6
Zorubicin	T45.1X1	T45.1X2	T45.1X3	T45.1X4	T45.1X5	T45.1X6
Zotepine	T43.591	T43.592	T43.593	T43.594	T43.595	T43.596
Zovant	T45.511	T45.512	T45.513	T45.514	T45.515	T45.516
Zoxazolamine	T42.8X1	T42.8X2	T42.8X3	T42.8X4	T42.8X5	T42.8X6
Zuclopenthixol	T43.4X1	T43.4X2	T43.4X3	T43.4X4	T43.4X5	T43.4X6
Zyflo*	T48.6X1	T48.6X2	T48.6X3	T48.6X4	T48.6X5	T48.6X6
Zygadenus (venenosus)	T62.2X1	T62.2X2	T62.2X3	T62.2X4	—	—
Zyprexa	T43.591	T43.592	T43.593	T43.594	T43.595	T43.596
Zyzal*	T45.0X1	T45.0X2	T45.0X3	T45.0X4	T45.0X5	T45.0X6

A

- **Abandonment** (causing exposure to weather conditions) (with intent to injure or kill) NEC X58 ☑
- **Abuse** (adult) (child) (mental) (physical) (sexual) X58 ☑
- **Accident** (to) X58 ☑
  - aircraft (in transit) (powered) — *see also* Accident, transport, aircraft
    - due to, caused by cataclysm — *see* Forces of nature, by type
  - animal-drawn vehicle — *see* Accident, transport, animal-drawn vehicle occupant
  - animal-rider — *see* Accident, transport, animal-rider
  - automobile — *see* Accident, transport, car occupant
  - bare foot water skier V94.4 ☑
  - boat, boating — *see also* Accident, watercraft
    - striking swimmer
      - powered V94.11 ☑
      - unpowered V94.12 ☑
  - bus — *see* Accident, transport, bus occupant
  - cable car, not on rails V98.0 ☑
    - on rails — *see* Accident, transport, streetcar occupant
  - car — *see* Accident, transport, car occupant
  - caused by, due to
    - animal NEC W64 ☑
    - chain hoist W24.0 ☑
    - cold (excessive) — *see* Exposure, cold
    - corrosive liquid, substance — *see* Table of Drugs and Chemicals
    - cutting or piercing instrument — *see* Contact, with, by type of instrument
    - drive belt W24.0 ☑
    - electric
      - current — *see* Exposure, electric current
      - motor — *see also* Contact, with, by type of machine W31.3 ☑
        - current (of) W86.8 ☑
    - environmental factor NEC X58 ☑
    - explosive material — *see* Explosion
    - fire, flames — *see* Exposure, fire
    - firearm missile — *see* Discharge, firearm by type
    - heat (excessive) — *see* Heat
    - hot — *see* Contact, with, hot
    - ignition — *see* Ignition
    - lifting device W24.0 ☑
    - lightning — *see* subcategory T75.0 ☑
      - causing fire — *see* Exposure, fire
    - machine, machinery — *see* Contact, with, by type of machine
    - natural factor NEC X58 ☑
    - pulley (block) W24.0 ☑
    - radiation — *see* Radiation
    - steam X13.1 ☑
      - inhalation X13.0 ☑
      - pipe X16 ☑
    - thunderbolt — *see* subcategory T75.0 ☑
      - causing fire — *see* Exposure, fire
    - transmission device W24.1 ☑
  - coach — *see* Accident, transport, bus occupant
  - coal car — *see* Accident, transport, industrial vehicle occupant
  - diving — *see also* Fall, into, water
    - with
      - drowning or submersion — *see* Drowning
  - forklift — *see* Accident, transport, industrial vehicle occupant
  - heavy transport vehicle NOS — *see* Accident, transport, truck occupant
  - ice yacht V98.2 ☑
  - in
    - medical, surgical procedure
      - as, or due to misadventure — *see* Misadventure
      - causing an abnormal reaction or later complication without mention of misadventure — *see also* Complication of or following, by type of procedure Y84.9
  - land yacht V98.1 ☑
  - late effect of — *see* W00-X58 with 7th character S
  - logging car — *see* Accident, transport, industrial vehicle occupant
  - machine, machinery — *see also* Contact, with, by type of machine
    - on board watercraft V93.69 ☑
      - explosion — *see* Explosion, in, watercraft

Accident — *continued*

  - machine, machinery — *see also* Contact, with, by type of machine — *continued*
    - on board watercraft — *continued*
      - fire — *see* Burn, on board watercraft
      - powered craft V93.63 ☑
        - ferry boat V93.61 ☑
        - fishing boat V93.62 ☑
        - jetskis V93.63 ☑
        - liner V93.61 ☑
        - merchant ship V93.60 ☑
        - passenger ship V93.61 ☑
        - sailboat V93.64 ☑
  - mine tram — *see* Accident, transport, industrial vehicle occupant
  - mobility scooter (motorized) — *see* Accident, transport, pedestrian, conveyance, specified type NEC
  - motor scooter — *see* Accident, transport, motorcyclist
  - motor vehicle NOS (traffic) — *see also* Accident, transport V89.2 ☑
    - nontraffic V89.0 ☑
    - three-wheeled NOS — *see* Accident, transport, three-wheeled motor vehicle occupant
  - motorcycle NOS — *see* Accident, transport, motorcyclist
  - nonmotor vehicle NOS (nontraffic) — *see also* Accident, transport V89.1 ☑
    - traffic NOS V89.3 ☑
  - nontraffic (victim's mode of transport NOS) V88.9 ☑
    - collision (between) V88.7 ☑
      - bus and truck V88.5 ☑
      - car and:
        - bus V88.3 ☑
        - pickup V88.2 ☑
        - three-wheeled motor vehicle V88.0 ☑
        - train V88.6 ☑
        - truck V88.4 ☑
        - two-wheeled motor vehicle V88.0 ☑
        - van V88.2 ☑
      - specified vehicle NEC and:
        - three-wheeled motor vehicle V88.1 ☑
        - two-wheeled motor vehicle V88.1 ☑
    - known mode of transport — *see* Accident, transport, by type of vehicle
    - noncollision V88.8 ☑
  - on board watercraft V93.89 ☑
    - powered craft V93.83 ☑
      - ferry boat V93.81 ☑
      - fishing boat V93.82 ☑
      - jetskis V93.83 ☑
      - liner V93.81 ☑
      - merchant ship V93.80 ☑
      - passenger ship V93.81 ☑
    - unpowered craft V93.88 ☑
      - canoe V93.85 ☑
      - inflatable V93.86 ☑
        - in tow
          - recreational V94.31 ☑
          - specified NEC V94.32 ☑
      - kayak V93.85 ☑
      - sailboat V93.84 ☑
      - surf-board V93.88 ☑
      - water skis V93.87 ☑
      - windsurfer V93.88 ☑
  - parachutist V97.29 ☑
    - entangled in object V97.21 ☑
    - injured on landing V97.22 ☑
  - pedal cycle — *see* Accident, transport, pedal cyclist
  - pedestrian (on foot)
    - with
      - another pedestrian W51 ☑
        - on pedestrian conveyance NEC V00.09 ☑
        - with fall W03 ☑
          - due to ice or snow W00.0 ☑
      - rider of
        - hoverboard V00.038 ☑
        - Segway V00.038 ☑
        - standing
          - electric scooter V00.031 ☑
          - micro-mobility pedestrian conveyance NEC V00.038 ☑
      - roller skater (in-line) V00.01 ☑
      - skate boarder V00.02 ☑
      - transport vehicle — *see* Accident, transport
    - on pedestrian conveyance — *see* Accident, transport, pedestrian, conveyance

Accident — *continued*

  - pick-up truck or van — *see* Accident, transport, pickup truck occupant
  - quarry truck — *see* Accident, transport, industrial vehicle occupant
  - railway vehicle (any) (in motion) — *see* Accident, transport, railway vehicle occupant
    - due to cataclysm — *see* Forces of nature, by type
  - scooter (non-motorized) — *see* Accident, transport, pedestrian, conveyance, scooter
  - sequelae of — *see* categories W00-X58 with 7th character S
  - skateboard — *see* Accident, transport, pedestrian, conveyance, skateboard
  - ski(ing) — *see* Accident, transport, pedestrian, conveyance
    - lift V98.3 ☑
  - specified cause NEC X58 ☑
  - streetcar — *see* Accident, transport, streetcar occupant
  - traffic (victim's mode of transport NOS) V87.9 ☑
    - collision (between) V87.7 ☑
      - bus and truck V87.5 ☑
      - car and:
        - bus V87.3 ☑
        - pickup V87.2 ☑
        - three-wheeled motor vehicle V87.0 ☑
        - train V87.6 ☑
        - truck V87.4 ☑
        - two-wheeled motor vehicle V87.0 ☑
        - van V87.2 ☑
      - specified vehicle NEC V86.39 ☑
        - and
          - three-wheeled motor vehicle V87.1 ☑
          - two-wheeled motor vehicle V87.1 ☑
        - driver V86.09 ☑
        - passenger V86.19 ☑
        - person on outside V86.29 ☑
        - while boarding or alighting V86.49 ☑
    - known mode of transport — *see* Accident, transport, by type of vehicle
    - noncollision V87.8 ☑
  - transport (involving injury to) V99 ☑
    - 18 wheeler — *see* Accident, transport, truck occupant
    - agricultural vehicle occupant (nontraffic) V84.9 ☑
      - driver V84.5 ☑
      - hanger-on V84.7 ☑
      - passenger V84.6 ☑
      - traffic V84.3 ☑
        - driver V84.0 ☑
        - hanger-on V84.2 ☑
        - passenger V84.1 ☑
      - while boarding or alighting V84.4 ☑
    - aircraft NEC V97.89 ☑
      - military NEC V97.818 ☑
        - civilian injured by V97.811 ☑
        - with civilian aircraft V97.810 ☑
      - occupant injured (in)
        - nonpowered craft accident V96.9 ☑
          - balloon V96.00 ☑
            - collision V96.03 ☑
            - crash V96.01 ☑
            - explosion V96.05 ☑
            - fire V96.04 ☑
            - forced landing V96.02 ☑
            - specified type NEC V96.09 ☑
          - glider V96.20 ☑
            - collision V96.23 ☑
            - crash V96.21 ☑
            - explosion V96.25 ☑
            - fire V96.24 ☑
            - forced landing V96.22 ☑
            - specified type NEC V96.29 ☑
          - hang glider V96.10 ☑
            - collision V96.13 ☑
            - crash V96.11 ☑
            - explosion V96.15 ☑
            - fire V96.14 ☑
            - forced landing V96.12 ☑
            - specified type NEC V96.19 ☑
          - specified craft NEC V96.8 ☑
        - powered craft accident V95.9 ☑
          - fixed wing NEC
            - commercial V95.30 ☑
              - collision V95.33 ☑
              - crash V95.31 ☑

External Causes Index

Abandonment — Accident

- **Accident** — *continued*
  - transport — *continued*
    - bus occupant — *continued*
      - hanger-on — *continued*
        - collision — *continued*
          - three wheeled motor vehicle (traffic) V72.7 ☑
            - nontraffic V72.2 ☑
          - truck (traffic) V74.7 ☑
            - nontraffic V74.2 ☑
          - two wheeled motor vehicle (traffic) V72.7 ☑
            - nontraffic V72.2 ☑
          - van (traffic) V73.7 ☑
            - nontraffic V73.2 ☑
        - noncollision accident (traffic) V78.7 ☑
          - nontraffic V78.2 ☑
      - noncollision accident (traffic) V78.9 ☑
        - nontraffic V78.3 ☑
        - while boarding or alighting V78.4 ☑
      - nontraffic V79.3 ☑
      - passenger
        - collision (with)
          - animal (traffic) V70.6 ☑
            - being ridden (traffic) V76.6 ☑
              - nontraffic V76.1 ☑
            - nontraffic V70.1 ☑
          - animal-drawn vehicle (traffic) V76.6 ☑
            - nontraffic V76.1 ☑
          - bus (traffic) V74.6 ☑
            - nontraffic V74.1 ☑
          - car (traffic) V73.6 ☑
            - nontraffic V73.1 ☑
          - motor vehicle NOS (traffic) V79.50 ☑
            - nontraffic V79.10 ☑
            - specified type NEC (traffic) V79.59 ☑
              - nontraffic V79.19 ☑
          - pedal cycle (traffic) V71.6 ☑
            - nontraffic V71.1 ☑
          - pickup truck (traffic) V73.6 ☑
            - nontraffic V73.1 ☑
          - railway vehicle (traffic) V75.6 ☑
            - nontraffic V75.1 ☑
          - specified vehicle NEC (traffic) V76.6 ☑
            - nontraffic V76.1 ☑
          - stationary object (traffic) V77.6 ☑
            - nontraffic V77.1 ☑
          - streetcar (traffic) V76.6 ☑
            - nontraffic V76.1 ☑
          - three wheeled motor vehicle (traffic) V72.6 ☑
            - nontraffic V72.1 ☑
          - truck (traffic) V74.6 ☑
            - nontraffic V74.1 ☑
          - two wheeled motor vehicle (traffic) V72.6 ☑
            - nontraffic V72.1 ☑
          - van (traffic) V73.6 ☑
            - nontraffic V73.1 ☑
        - noncollision accident (traffic) V78.6 ☑
          - nontraffic V78.1 ☑
      - specified type NEC V79.88 ☑
        - military vehicle V79.81 ☑
    - cable car, not on rails V98.0 ☑
      - on rails — *see* Accident, transport, streetcar occupant
    - car occupant V49.9 ☑
      - ambulance occupant — *see* Accident, transport, ambulance occupant
      - collision (with)
        - animal (traffic) V40.9 ☑
          - being ridden (traffic) V46.9 ☑
            - nontraffic V46.3 ☑
            - while boarding or alighting V46.4 ☑
          - nontraffic V40.3 ☑
          - while boarding or alighting V40.4 ☑
        - animal-drawn vehicle (traffic) V46.9 ☑
          - nontraffic V46.3 ☑
          - while boarding or alighting V46.4 ☑
        - bus (traffic) V44.9 ☑
          - nontraffic V44.3 ☑
          - while boarding or alighting V44.4 ☑
        - car (traffic) V43.92 ☑
          - nontraffic V43.32 ☑
          - while boarding or alighting V43.42 ☑
        - motor vehicle NOS (traffic) V49.60 ☑

- **Accident** — *continued*
  - transport — *continued*
    - car occupant — *continued*
      - collision — *continued*
        - motor vehicle — *continued*
          - nontraffic V49.20 ☑
          - specified type NEC (traffic) V49.69 ☑
            - nontraffic V49.29 ☑
        - pedal cycle (traffic) V41.9 ☑
          - nontraffic V41.3 ☑
          - while boarding or alighting V41.4 ☑
        - pickup truck (traffic) V43.93 ☑
          - nontraffic V43.33 ☑
          - while boarding or alighting V43.43 ☑
        - railway vehicle (traffic) V45.9 ☑
          - nontraffic V45.3 ☑
          - while boarding or alighting V45.4 ☑
        - specified vehicle NEC (traffic) V46.9 ☑
          - nontraffic V46.3 ☑
          - while boarding or alighting V46.4 ☑
        - sport utility vehicle (traffic) V43.91 ☑
          - nontraffic V43.31 ☑
          - while boarding or alighting V43.41 ☑
        - stationary object (traffic) V47.9 ☑
          - nontraffic V47.3 ☑
          - while boarding or alighting V47.4 ☑
        - streetcar (traffic) V46.9 ☑
          - nontraffic V46.3 ☑
          - while boarding or alighting V46.4 ☑
        - three wheeled motor vehicle (traffic) V42.9 ☑
          - nontraffic V42.3 ☑
          - while boarding or alighting V42.4 ☑
        - truck (traffic) V44.9 ☑
          - nontraffic V44.3 ☑
          - while boarding or alighting V44.4 ☑
        - two wheeled motor vehicle (traffic) V42.9 ☑
          - nontraffic V42.3 ☑
          - while boarding or alighting V42.4 ☑
        - van (traffic) V43.94 ☑
          - nontraffic V43.34 ☑
          - while boarding or alighting V43.44 ☑
      - driver
        - collision (with)
          - animal (traffic) V40.5 ☑
            - being ridden (traffic) V46.5 ☑
              - nontraffic V46.0 ☑
            - nontraffic V40.0 ☑
          - animal-drawn vehicle (traffic) V46.5 ☑
            - nontraffic V46.0 ☑
          - bus (traffic) V44.5 ☑
            - nontraffic V44.0 ☑
          - car (traffic) V43.52 ☑
            - nontraffic V43.02 ☑
          - motor vehicle NOS (traffic) V49.40 ☑
            - nontraffic V49.00 ☑
            - specified type NEC (traffic) V49.49 ☑
              - nontraffic V49.09 ☑
          - pedal cycle (traffic) V41.5 ☑
            - nontraffic V41.0 ☑
          - pickup truck (traffic) V43.53 ☑
            - nontraffic V43.03 ☑
          - railway vehicle (traffic) V45.5 ☑
            - nontraffic V45.0 ☑
          - specified vehicle NEC (traffic) V46.5 ☑
            - nontraffic V46.0 ☑
          - sport utility vehicle (traffic) V43.51 ☑
            - nontraffic V43.01 ☑
          - stationary object (traffic) V47.5 ☑
            - nontraffic V47.0 ☑
          - streetcar (traffic) V46.5 ☑
            - nontraffic V46.0 ☑
          - three wheeled motor vehicle (traffic) V42.5 ☑
            - nontraffic V42.0 ☑
          - truck (traffic) V44.5 ☑
            - nontraffic V44.0 ☑
          - two wheeled motor vehicle (traffic) V42.5 ☑
            - nontraffic V42.0 ☑
          - van (traffic) V43.54 ☑
            - nontraffic V43.04 ☑
        - noncollision accident (traffic) V48.5 ☑
          - nontraffic V48.0 ☑
      - hanger-on
        - collision (with)
          - animal (traffic) V40.7 ☑

- **Accident** — *continued*
  - transport — *continued*
    - car occupant — *continued*
      - hanger-on — *continued*
        - collision — *continued*
          - animal — *continued*
            - being ridden (traffic) V46.7 ☑
              - nontraffic V46.2 ☑
            - nontraffic V40.2 ☑
          - animal-drawn vehicle (traffic) V46.7 ☑
            - nontraffic V46.2 ☑
          - bus (traffic) V44.7 ☑
            - nontraffic V44.2 ☑
          - car (traffic) V43.72 ☑
            - nontraffic V43.22 ☑
          - pedal cycle (traffic) V41.7 ☑
            - nontraffic V41.2 ☑
          - pickup truck (traffic) V43.73 ☑
            - nontraffic V43.23 ☑
          - railway vehicle (traffic) V45.7 ☑
            - nontraffic V45.2 ☑
          - specified vehicle NEC (traffic) V46.7 ☑
            - nontraffic V46.2 ☑
          - sport utility vehicle (traffic) V43.71 ☑
            - nontraffic V43.21 ☑
          - stationary object (traffic) V47.7 ☑
            - nontraffic V47.2 ☑
          - streetcar (traffic) V46.7 ☑
            - nontraffic V46.2 ☑
          - three wheeled motor vehicle (traffic) V42.7 ☑
            - nontraffic V42.2 ☑
          - truck (traffic) V44.7 ☑
            - nontraffic V44.2 ☑
          - two wheeled motor vehicle (traffic) V42.7 ☑
            - nontraffic V42.2 ☑
          - van (traffic) V43.74 ☑
            - nontraffic V43.24 ☑
        - noncollision accident (traffic) V48.7 ☑
          - nontraffic V48.2 ☑
      - noncollision accident (traffic) V48.9 ☑
        - nontraffic V48.3 ☑
        - while boarding or alighting V48.4 ☑
      - nontraffic V49.3 ☑
      - passenger
        - collision (with)
          - animal (traffic) V40.6 ☑
            - being ridden (traffic) V46.6 ☑
              - nontraffic V46.1 ☑
            - nontraffic V40.1 ☑
          - animal-drawn vehicle (traffic) V46.6 ☑
            - nontraffic V46.1 ☑
          - bus (traffic) V44.6 ☑
            - nontraffic V44.1 ☑
          - car (traffic) V43.62 ☑
            - nontraffic V43.12 ☑
          - motor vehicle NOS (traffic) V49.50 ☑
            - nontraffic V49.10 ☑
            - specified type NEC (traffic) V49.59 ☑
              - nontraffic V49.19 ☑
          - pedal cycle (traffic) V41.6 ☑
            - nontraffic V41.1 ☑
          - pickup truck (traffic) V43.63 ☑
            - nontraffic V43.13 ☑
          - railway vehicle (traffic) V45.6 ☑
            - nontraffic V45.1 ☑
          - specified vehicle NEC (traffic) V46.6 ☑
            - nontraffic V46.1 ☑
          - sport utility vehicle (traffic) V43.61 ☑
            - nontraffic V43.11 ☑
          - stationary object (traffic) V47.6 ☑
            - nontraffic V47.1 ☑
          - streetcar (traffic) V46.6 ☑
            - nontraffic V46.1 ☑
          - three wheeled motor vehicle (traffic) V42.6 ☑
            - nontraffic V42.1 ☑
          - truck (traffic) V44.6 ☑
            - nontraffic V44.1 ☑
          - two wheeled motor vehicle (traffic) V42.6 ☑
            - nontraffic V42.1 ☑
          - van (traffic) V43.64 ☑
            - nontraffic V43.14 ☑
        - noncollision accident (traffic) V48.6 ☑

- **Accident** — *continued*
  - transport — *continued*
    - pedestrian — *continued*
      - conveyance — *continued*
        - flat-bottomed — *continued*
          - collision — *continued*
            - vehicle — *continued*
              - motor — *continued*
                - traffic V09.20 ☑
          - fall V00.381 ☑
          - nontraffic V09.1 ☑
            - involving motor vehicle NEC V09.00 ☑
          - snow
            - board — *see* Accident, transport, pedestrian, conveyance, snow board
            - ski — *see* Accident, transport, pedestrian, conveyance, skis (snow)
          - traffic V09.3 ☑
            - involving motor vehicle NEC V09.20 ☑
        - gliding type NEC V00.288 ☑
          - collision (with) V09.9 ☑
            - animal being ridden or animal drawn vehicle V06.99 ☑
              - nontraffic V06.09 ☑
              - traffic V06.19 ☑
            - bus or heavy transport V04.99 ☑
              - nontraffic V04.09 ☑
              - traffic V04.19 ☑
            - car V03.99 ☑
              - nontraffic V03.09 ☑
              - traffic V03.19 ☑
            - pedal cycle V01.99 ☑
              - nontraffic V01.09 ☑
              - traffic V01.19 ☑
            - pick-up truck or van V03.99 ☑
              - nontraffic V03.09 ☑
              - traffic V03.19 ☑
            - railway (train) (vehicle) V05.99 ☑
              - nontraffic V05.09 ☑
              - traffic V05.19 ☑
            - stationary object V00.282 ☑
            - streetcar V06.99 ☑
              - nontraffic V06.09 ☑
              - traffic V02.19 ☑
            - two- or three-wheeled motor vehicle V02.99 ☑
              - nontraffic V02.09 ☑
              - traffic V02.19 ☑
            - vehicle V09.9 ☑
              - animal-drawn V06.99 ☑
                - nontraffic V06.09 ☑
                - traffic V06.19 ☑
              - motor
                - nontraffic V09.00 ☑
                - traffic V09.20 ☑
          - fall V00.281 ☑
          - heelies — *see* Accident, transport, pedestrian, conveyance, heelies
          - ice skate — *see* Accident, transport, pedestrian, conveyance, ice skate
          - nontraffic V09.1 ☑
            - involving motor vehicle NEC V09.00 ☑
          - sled — *see* Accident, transport, pedestrian, conveyance, sled
          - traffic V09.3 ☑
            - involving motor vehicle NEC V09.20 ☑
          - wheelies — *see* Accident, transport, pedestrian, conveyance, heelies
        - heelies V00.158 ☑
          - colliding with stationary object V00.152 ☑
          - fall V00.151 ☑
        - hoverboard
          - collision with
            - animal being ridden or animal drawn vehicle V06.938 ☑
              - nontraffic V06.038 ☑
              - traffic V06.138 ☑
            - bus or heavy transport V04.938 ☑
              - nontraffic V04.038 ☑
              - traffic V04.138 ☑
            - car V03.938 ☑
              - nontraffic V03.038 ☑
              - traffic V03.138 ☑
            - pedal cycle V01.938 ☑

- **Accident** — *continued*
  - transport — *continued*
    - pedestrian — *continued*
      - conveyance — *continued*
        - hoverboard — *continued*
          - collision with — *continued*
            - pedal cycle — *continued*
              - nontraffic V01.038 ☑
              - traffic V01.138 ☑
            - pick-up or van V03.938 ☑
              - nontraffic V03.038 ☑
              - traffic V03.138 ☑
            - railway (train) (vehicle) V05.938 ☑
              - nontraffic V05.038 ☑
              - traffic V05.138 ☑
            - streetcar V06.938 ☑
              - nontraffic V06.038 ☑
              - traffic V06.138 ☑
            - three-wheeled motor vehicle V02.938 ☑
              - nontraffic V02.038 ☑
              - traffic V02.138 ☑
            - two-wheeled motor vehicle V02.938 ☑
              - nontraffic V02.038 ☑
              - traffic V02.138 ☑
            - vehicle, nonmotor, specified NEC V06.938 ☑
              - nontraffic V06.038 ☑
              - traffic V06.138 ☑
          - fall V00.848 ☑
        - ice skates V00.218 ☑
          - collision (with) V09.9 ☑
            - animal being ridden or animal drawn vehicle V06.99 ☑
              - nontraffic V06.09 ☑
              - traffic V06.19 ☑
            - bus or heavy transport V04.99 ☑
              - nontraffic V04.09 ☑
              - traffic V04.19 ☑
            - car V03.99 ☑
              - nontraffic V03.09 ☑
              - traffic V03.19 ☑
            - pedal cycle V01.99 ☑
              - nontraffic V01.09 ☑
              - traffic V01.19 ☑
            - pick-up truck or van V03.99 ☑
              - nontraffic V03.09 ☑
              - traffic V03.19 ☑
            - railway (train) (vehicle) V05.99 ☑
              - nontraffic V05.09 ☑
              - traffic V05.19 ☑
            - stationary object V00.212 ☑
            - streetcar V06.99 ☑
              - nontraffic V06.09 ☑
              - traffic V06.19 ☑
            - two- or three-wheeled motor vehicle V02.99 ☑
              - nontraffic V02.09 ☑
              - traffic V02.19 ☑
            - vehicle V09.9 ☑
              - animal-drawn V06.99 ☑
                - nontraffic V06.09 ☑
                - traffic V06.19 ☑
              - motor
                - nontraffic V09.00 ☑
                - traffic V09.20 ☑
          - fall V00.211 ☑
          - nontraffic V09.1 ☑
            - involving motor vehicle NEC V09.00 ☑
          - traffic V09.3 ☑
            - involving motor vehicle NEC V09.20 ☑
        - motorized mobility scooter V00.838 ☑
          - collision with stationary object V00.832 ☑
          - fall from V00.831 ☑
        - nontraffic V09.1 ☑
          - involving motor vehicle V09.00 ☑
            - military V09.01 ☑
            - specified type NEC V09.09 ☑
        - roller skates (non in-line) V00.128 ☑
          - collision (with) V09.9 ☑
            - animal being ridden or animal drawn vehicle V06.91 ☑
              - nontraffic V06.01 ☑
              - traffic V06.11 ☑

- **Accident** — *continued*
  - transport — *continued*
    - pedestrian — *continued*
      - conveyance — *continued*
        - roller skates — *continued*
          - collision — *continued*
            - bus or heavy transport V04.91 ☑
              - nontraffic V04.01 ☑
              - traffic V04.11 ☑
            - car V03.91 ☑
              - nontraffic V03.01 ☑
              - traffic V03.11 ☑
            - pedal cycle V01.91 ☑
              - nontraffic V01.01 ☑
              - traffic V01.11 ☑
            - pick-up truck or van V03.91 ☑
              - nontraffic V03.01 ☑
              - traffic V03.11 ☑
            - railway (train) (vehicle) V05.91 ☑
              - nontraffic V05.01 ☑
              - traffic V05.11 ☑
            - stationary object V00.122 ☑
            - streetcar V06.91 ☑
              - nontraffic V06.01 ☑
              - traffic V06.11 ☑
            - two- or three-wheeled motor vehicle V02.91 ☑
              - nontraffic V02.01 ☑
              - traffic V02.11 ☑
            - vehicle V09.9 ☑
              - animal-drawn V06.91 ☑
                - nontraffic V06.01 ☑
                - traffic V06.11 ☑
              - motor
                - nontraffic V09.00 ☑
                - traffic V09.20 ☑
          - fall V00.121 ☑
          - in-line V00.118 ☑
            - collision — *see* also Accident, transport, pedestrian, conveyance occupant, roller skates, collision
              - with stationary object V00.112 ☑
            - fall V00.111 ☑
          - nontraffic V09.1 ☑
            - involving motor vehicle NEC V09.00 ☑
          - traffic V09.3 ☑
            - involving motor vehicle NEC V09.20 ☑
        - rolling shoes V00.158 ☑
          - colliding with stationary object V00.152 ☑
          - fall V00.151 ☑
        - rolling type NEC V00.188 ☑
          - collision (with) V09.9 ☑
            - animal being ridden or animal drawn vehicle V06.99 ☑
              - nontraffic V06.09 ☑
              - traffic V06.19 ☑
            - bus or heavy transport V04.99 ☑
              - nontraffic V04.09 ☑
              - traffic V04.19 ☑
            - car V03.99 ☑
              - nontraffic V03.09 ☑
              - traffic V03.19 ☑
            - pedal cycle V01.99 ☑
              - nontraffic V01.09 ☑
              - traffic V01.19 ☑
            - pick-up truck or van V03.99 ☑
              - nontraffic V03.09 ☑
              - traffic V03.19 ☑
            - railway (train) (vehicle) V05.99 ☑
              - nontraffic V05.09 ☑
              - traffic V05.19 ☑
            - stationary object V00.182 ☑
            - streetcar V06.99 ☑
              - nontraffic V06.09 ☑
              - traffic V06.19 ☑
            - two- or three-wheeled motor vehicle V02.99 ☑
              - nontraffic V02.09 ☑
              - traffic V02.19 ☑
            - vehicle V09.9 ☑
              - animal-drawn V06.99 ☑
                - nontraffic V06.09 ☑
                - traffic V06.19 ☑
              - motor
                - nontraffic V09.00 ☑

- **Accident** — *continued*
  - transport — *continued*
    - pedestrian — *continued*
      - conveyance — *continued*
        - snow board — *continued*
          - collision — *continued*
            - railway — *continued*
              - traffic V05.19 ☑
            - stationary object VØØ.312 ☑
            - streetcar VØ6.99 ☑
              - nontraffic VØ6.Ø9 ☑
              - traffic VØ6.19 ☑
            - two- or three-wheeled motor vehicle VØ2.99 ☑
              - nontraffic VØ2.Ø9 ☑
              - traffic VØ2.19 ☑
            - vehicle VØ9.9 ☑
              - animal-drawn VØ6.99 ☑
                - nontraffic VØ6.Ø9 ☑
                - traffic VØ6.19 ☑
              - motor
                - nontraffic VØ9.ØØ ☑
                - traffic VØ9.2Ø ☑
          - fall VØØ.311 ☑
          - nontraffic VØ9.1 ☑
            - involving motor vehicle NEC VØ9.ØØ ☑
          - traffic VØ9.3 ☑
            - involving motor vehicle NEC VØ9.2Ø ☑
        - specified type NEC VØØ.898 ☑
          - collision (with) VØ9.9 ☑
            - animal being ridden or animal drawn vehicle VØ6.99 ☑
              - nontraffic VØ6.Ø9 ☑
              - traffic VØ6.19 ☑
            - bus or heavy transport VØ4.99 ☑
              - nontraffic VØ4.Ø9 ☑
              - traffic VØ4.19 ☑
            - car VØ3.99 ☑
              - nontraffic VØ3.Ø9 ☑
              - traffic VØ3.19 ☑
            - pedal cycle VØ1.99 ☑
              - nontraffic VØ1.Ø9 ☑
              - traffic VØ1.19 ☑
            - pick-up truck or van VØ3.99 ☑
              - nontraffic VØ3.Ø9 ☑
              - traffic VØ3.19 ☑
            - railway (train) (vehicle) VØ5.99 ☑
              - nontraffic VØ5.Ø9 ☑
              - traffic VØ5.19 ☑
            - stationary object VØØ.892 ☑
            - streetcar VØ6.99 ☑
              - nontraffic VØ6.Ø9 ☑
              - traffic VØ6.19 ☑
            - two- or three-wheeled motor vehicle VØ2.99 ☑
              - nontraffic VØ2.Ø9 ☑
              - traffic VØ2.19 ☑
            - vehicle VØ9.9 ☑
              - animal-drawn VØ6.99 ☑
                - nontraffic VØ6.Ø9 ☑
                - traffic VØ6.19 ☑
              - motor
                - nontraffic VØ9.ØØ ☑
                - traffic VØ9.2Ø ☑
          - fall VØØ.891 ☑
          - nontraffic VØ9.1 ☑
            - involving motor vehicle NEC VØ9.ØØ ☑
          - traffic VØ9.3 ☑
            - involving motor vehicle NEC VØ9.2Ø ☑
        - standing
          - electric scooter
            - collision with
              - animal being ridden or animal drawn vehicle VØ6.931 ☑
                - nontraffic VØ6.Ø31 ☑
                - traffic VØ6.131 ☑
              - bus or heavy transport VØ4.931 ☑
                - nontraffic VØ4.Ø31 ☑
                - traffic VØ4.131 ☑
              - car VØ3.931 ☑
                - nontraffic VØ4.Ø31 ☑
                - traffic VØ4.131 ☑
              - pedal cycle VØ1.931 ☑
                - nontraffic VØ1.Ø31 ☑
                - traffic VØ1.131 ☑
              - pick-up or van VØ3.931 ☑

- **Accident** — *continued*
  - transport — *continued*
    - pedestrian — *continued*
      - conveyance — *continued*
        - standing — *continued*
          - electric scooter — *continued*
            - collision with — *continued*
              - pick-up or van — *continued*
                - nontraffic VØ3.Ø31 ☑
                - traffic VØ3.131 ☑
              - railway (train) (vehicle) VØ5.931 ☑
                - nontraffic VØ5.Ø31 ☑
                - traffic VØ5.131 ☑
              - streetcar VØ6.931 ☑
                - nontraffic VØ6.Ø31 ☑
                - traffic VØ6.131 ☑
              - three-wheeled motor vehicle VØ2.931 ☑
                - nontraffic VØ2.Ø31 ☑
                - traffic VØ2.131 ☑
              - two-wheeled motor vehicle VØ2.931 ☑
                - nontraffic VØ2.Ø31 ☑
                - traffic VØ2.131 ☑
              - vehicle, nonmotor, specified NEC VØ6.931 ☑
                - nontraffic VØ6.Ø31 ☑
                - traffic VØ6.131 ☑
            - fall VØØ.841 ☑
          - micro-mobility pedestrian conveyance
            - collision with
              - animal being ridden or animal drawn vehicle VØ6.938 ☑
                - nontraffic VØ6.Ø38 ☑
                - traffic VØ6.138 ☑
              - bus or heavy transport VØ4.938 ☑
                - nontraffic VØ4.Ø38 ☑
                - traffic VØ4.138 ☑
              - car VØ3.938 ☑
                - nontraffic VØ3.Ø38 ☑
                - traffic VØ3.138 ☑
              - pedal cycle VØ1.938 ☑
                - nontraffic VØ1.Ø38 ☑
                - traffic VØ1.138 ☑
              - pick-up or van VØ3.938 ☑
                - nontraffic VØ3.Ø38 ☑
                - traffic VØ3.138 ☑
              - railway (train) (vehicle) VØ5.938 ☑
                - nontraffic VØ5.Ø38 ☑
                - traffic VØ5.138 ☑
              - stationary object VØØ.842 ☑
              - streetcar VØ6.938 ☑
                - nontraffic VØ6.Ø38 ☑
                - traffic VØ6.138 ☑
              - three-wheeled motor vehicle VØ2.938 ☑
                - nontraffic VØ2.Ø38 ☑
                - traffic VØ2.138 ☑
              - two-wheeled motor vehicle VØ2.938 ☑
                - nontraffic VØ2.Ø38 ☑
                - traffic VØ2.138 ☑
              - vehicle, nonmotor, specified NEC VØ6.938 ☑
                - nontraffic VØ6.Ø38 ☑
                - traffic VØ6.138 ☑
            - fall VØØ.848 ☑
        - traffic VØ9.3 ☑
          - involving motor vehicle VØ9.2Ø ☑
            - military VØ9.21 ☑
            - specified type NEC VØ9.29 ☑
        - wheelchair (powered) VØØ.818 ☑
          - collision (with) VØ9.9 ☑
            - animal being ridden or animal drawn vehicle VØ6.99 ☑
              - nontraffic VØ6.Ø9 ☑
              - traffic VØ6.19 ☑
            - bus or heavy transport VØ4.99 ☑
              - nontraffic VØ4.Ø9 ☑
              - traffic VØ4.19 ☑
            - car VØ3.99 ☑
              - nontraffic VØ3.Ø9 ☑
              - traffic VØ3.19 ☑
            - pedal cycle VØ1.99 ☑
              - nontraffic VØ1.Ø9 ☑
              - traffic VØ1.19 ☑

- **Accident** — *continued*
  - transport — *continued*
    - pedestrian — *continued*
      - conveyance — *continued*
        - wheelchair — *continued*
          - collision — *continued*
            - pick-up truck or van VØ3.99 ☑
              - nontraffic VØ3.Ø9 ☑
              - traffic VØ3.19 ☑
            - railway (train) (vehicle) VØ5.99 ☑
              - nontraffic VØ5.Ø9 ☑
              - traffic VØ5.19 ☑
            - stationary object VØØ.812 ☑
            - streetcar VØ6.99 ☑
              - nontraffic VØ6.Ø9 ☑
              - traffic VØ6.19 ☑
            - two- or three-wheeled motor vehicle VØ2.99 ☑
              - nontraffic VØ2.Ø9 ☑
              - traffic VØ2.19 ☑
            - vehicle VØ9.9 ☑
              - animal-drawn VØ6.99 ☑
                - nontraffic VØ6.Ø9 ☑
                - traffic VØ6.19 ☑
              - motor
                - nontraffic VØ9.ØØ ☑
                - traffic VØ9.2Ø ☑
          - fall VØØ.811 ☑
          - nontraffic VØ9.1 ☑
            - involving motor vehicle NEC VØ9.ØØ ☑
          - traffic VØ9.3 ☑
            - involving motor vehicle NEC VØ9.2Ø ☑
        - wheeled shoe VØØ.158 ☑
          - colliding with stationary object VØØ.152 ☑
          - fall VØØ.151 ☑
      - on foot — *see also* Accident, pedestrian
        - collision (with)
          - animal being ridden or animal drawn vehicle VØ6.9Ø ☑
            - nontraffic VØ6.ØØ ☑
            - traffic VØ6.1Ø ☑
          - bus or heavy transport VØ4.9Ø ☑
            - nontraffic VØ4.ØØ ☑
            - traffic VØ4.1Ø ☑
          - car VØ3.9Ø ☑
            - nontraffic VØ3.ØØ ☑
            - traffic VØ3.1Ø ☑
          - pedal cycle VØ1.9Ø ☑
            - nontraffic VØ1.ØØ ☑
            - traffic VØ1.1Ø ☑
          - pick-up truck or van VØ3.9Ø ☑
            - nontraffic VØ3.ØØ ☑
            - traffic VØ3.1Ø ☑
          - railway (train) (vehicle) VØ5.9Ø ☑
            - nontraffic VØ5.ØØ ☑
            - traffic VØ5.1Ø ☑
          - streetcar VØ6.9Ø ☑
            - nontraffic VØ6.ØØ ☑
            - traffic VØ6.1Ø ☑
          - two- or three-wheeled motor vehicle VØ2.9Ø ☑
            - nontraffic VØ2.ØØ ☑
            - traffic VØ2.1Ø ☑
          - vehicle VØ9.9 ☑
            - animal-drawn VØ6.9Ø ☑
              - nontraffic VØ6.ØØ ☑
              - traffic VØ6.1Ø ☑
            - motor
        - nontraffic VØ9.1 ☑
          - involving motor vehicle VØ9.ØØ ☑
            - military VØ9.Ø1 ☑
            - specified type NEC VØ9.Ø9 ☑
        - traffic VØ9.3 ☑
          - involving motor vehicle VØ9.2Ø ☑
            - military VØ9.21 ☑
            - specified type NEC VØ9.29 ☑
    - person NEC (unknown way or transportation) V99 ☑
      - collision (between)
        - bus (with)
          - heavy transport vehicle (traffic) V87.5 ☑
            - nontraffic V88.5 ☑
        - car (with)
          - bus (traffic) V87.3 ☑
            - nontraffic V88.3 ☑
          - heavy transport vehicle (traffic) V87.4 ☑

- **Accident** — *continued*
  - transport — *continued*
    - person — *continued*
      - collision — *continued*
        - car — *continued*
          - heavy transport vehicle — *continued*
            - nontraffic V88.4 ☑
          - nontraffic V88.5 ☑
          - pick-up truck or van (traffic) V87.2 ☑
            - nontraffic V88.2 ☑
          - train or railway vehicle (traffic) V87.6 ☑
            - nontraffic V88.6 ☑
          - two-or three-wheeled motor vehicle (traffic) V87.Ø ☑
            - nontraffic V88.Ø ☑
        - motor vehicle (traffic) NEC V87.7 ☑
          - nontraffic V88.7 ☑
        - two-or three-wheeled vehicle (with) (traffic) motor vehicle NEC V87.1 ☑
          - nontraffic V88.1 ☑
      - nonmotor vehicle (collision) (noncollision) (traffic) V87.9 ☑
        - nontraffic V88.9 ☑
    - pickup truck occupant V59.9 ☑
      - collision (with)
        - animal (traffic) V5Ø.9 ☑
          - being ridden (traffic) V56.9 ☑
            - nontraffic V56.3 ☑
            - while boarding or alighting V56.4 ☑
          - nontraffic V5Ø.3 ☑
          - while boarding or alighting V5Ø.4 ☑
        - animal-drawn vehicle (traffic) V56.9 ☑
          - nontraffic V56.3 ☑
          - while boarding or alighting V56.4 ☑
        - bus (traffic) V54.9 ☑
          - nontraffic V54.3 ☑
          - while boarding or alighting V54.4 ☑
        - car (traffic) V53.9 ☑
          - nontraffic V53.3 ☑
          - while boarding or alighting V53.4 ☑
        - motor vehicle NOS (traffic) V59.6Ø ☑
          - nontraffic V59.2Ø ☑
          - specified type NEC (traffic) V59.69 ☑
            - nontraffic V59.29 ☑
        - pedal cycle (traffic) V51.9 ☑
          - nontraffic V51.3 ☑
          - while boarding or alighting V51.4 ☑
        - pickup truck (traffic) V53.9 ☑
          - nontraffic V53.3 ☑
          - while boarding or alighting V53.4 ☑
        - railway vehicle (traffic) V55.9 ☑
          - nontraffic V55.3 ☑
          - while boarding or alighting V55.4 ☑
        - specified vehicle NEC (traffic) V56.9 ☑
          - nontraffic V56.3 ☑
          - while boarding or alighting V56.4 ☑
        - stationary object (traffic) V57.9 ☑
          - nontraffic V57.3 ☑
          - while boarding or alighting V57.4 ☑
        - streetcar (traffic) V56.9 ☑
          - nontraffic V56.3 ☑
          - while boarding or alighting V56.4 ☑
        - three wheeled motor vehicle (traffic) V52.9 ☑
          - nontraffic V52.3 ☑
          - while boarding or alighting V52.4 ☑
        - truck (traffic) V54.9 ☑
          - nontraffic V54.3 ☑
          - while boarding or alighting V54.4 ☑
        - two wheeled motor vehicle (traffic) V52.9 ☑
          - nontraffic V52.3 ☑
          - while boarding or alighting V52.4 ☑
        - van (traffic) V53.9 ☑
          - nontraffic V53.3 ☑
          - while boarding or alighting V53.4 ☑
      - driver
        - collision (with)
          - animal (traffic) V5Ø.5 ☑
            - being ridden (traffic) V56.5 ☑
              - nontraffic V56.Ø ☑
            - nontraffic V5Ø.Ø ☑
          - animal-drawn vehicle (traffic) V56.5 ☑
            - nontraffic V56.Ø ☑
          - bus (traffic) V54.5 ☑
            - nontraffic V54.Ø ☑
          - car (traffic) V53.5 ☑
            - nontraffic V53.Ø ☑

- **Accident** — *continued*
  - transport — *continued*
    - pickup truck occupant — *continued*
      - driver — *continued*
        - collision — *continued*
          - motor vehicle NOS (traffic) V59.4Ø ☑
            - nontraffic V59.ØØ ☑
            - specified type NEC (traffic) V59.49 ☑
              - nontraffic V59.Ø9 ☑
          - pedal cycle (traffic) V51.5 ☑
            - nontraffic V51.Ø ☑
          - pickup truck (traffic) V53.5 ☑
            - nontraffic V53.Ø ☑
          - railway vehicle (traffic) V55.5 ☑
            - nontraffic V55.Ø ☑
          - specified vehicle NEC (traffic) V56.5 ☑
            - nontraffic V56.Ø ☑
          - stationary object (traffic) V57.5 ☑
            - nontraffic V57.Ø ☑
          - streetcar (traffic) V56.5 ☑
            - nontraffic V56.Ø ☑
          - three wheeled motor vehicle (traffic) V52.5 ☑
            - nontraffic V52.Ø ☑
          - truck (traffic) V54.5 ☑
            - nontraffic V54.Ø ☑
          - two wheeled motor vehicle (traffic) V52.5 ☑
            - nontraffic V52.Ø ☑
          - van (traffic) V53.5 ☑
            - nontraffic V53.Ø ☑
        - noncollision accident (traffic) V58.5 ☑
          - nontraffic V58.Ø ☑
      - hanger-on
        - collision (with)
          - animal (traffic) V5Ø.7 ☑
            - being ridden (traffic) V56.7 ☑
              - nontraffic V56.2 ☑
            - nontraffic V5Ø.2 ☑
          - animal-drawn vehicle (traffic) V56.7 ☑
            - nontraffic V56.2 ☑
          - bus (traffic) V54.7 ☑
            - nontraffic V54.2 ☑
          - car (traffic) V53.7 ☑
            - nontraffic V53.2 ☑
          - pedal cycle (traffic) V51.7 ☑
            - nontraffic V51.2 ☑
          - pickup truck (traffic) V53.7 ☑
            - nontraffic V53.2 ☑
          - railway vehicle (traffic) V55.7 ☑
            - nontraffic V55.2 ☑
          - specified vehicle NEC (traffic) V56.7 ☑
            - nontraffic V56.2 ☑
          - stationary object (traffic) V57.7 ☑
            - nontraffic V57.2 ☑
          - streetcar (traffic) V56.7 ☑
            - nontraffic V56.2 ☑
          - three wheeled motor vehicle (traffic) V52.7 ☑
            - nontraffic V52.2 ☑
          - truck (traffic) V54.7 ☑
            - nontraffic V54.2 ☑
          - two wheeled motor vehicle (traffic) V52.7 ☑
            - nontraffic V52.2 ☑
          - van (traffic) V53.7 ☑
            - nontraffic V53.2 ☑
        - noncollision accident (traffic) V58.7 ☑
          - nontraffic V58.2 ☑
      - noncollision accident (traffic) V58.9 ☑
        - nontraffic V58.3 ☑
        - while boarding or alighting V58.4 ☑
      - nontraffic V59.3 ☑
      - passenger
        - collision (with)
          - animal (traffic) V5Ø.6 ☑
            - being ridden (traffic) V56.6 ☑
              - nontraffic V56.1 ☑
            - nontraffic V5Ø.1 ☑
          - animal-drawn vehicle (traffic) V56.6 ☑
            - nontraffic V56.1 ☑
          - bus (traffic) V54.6 ☑
            - nontraffic V54.1 ☑
          - car (traffic) V53.6 ☑
            - nontraffic V53.1 ☑
          - motor vehicle NOS (traffic) V59.5Ø ☑

- **Accident** — *continued*
  - transport — *continued*
    - pickup truck occupant — *continued*
      - passenger — *continued*
        - collision — *continued*
          - motor vehicle — *continued*
            - nontraffic V59.1Ø ☑
            - specified type NEC (traffic) V59.59 ☑
              - nontraffic V59.19 ☑
          - pedal cycle (traffic) V51.6 ☑
            - nontraffic V51.1 ☑
          - pickup truck (traffic) V53.6 ☑
            - nontraffic V53.1 ☑
          - railway vehicle (traffic) V55.6 ☑
            - nontraffic V55.1 ☑
          - specified vehicle NEC (traffic) V56.6 ☑
            - nontraffic V56.1 ☑
          - stationary object (traffic) V57.6 ☑
            - nontraffic V57.1 ☑
          - streetcar (traffic) V56.6 ☑
            - nontraffic V56.1 ☑
          - three wheeled motor vehicle (traffic) V52.6 ☑
            - nontraffic V52.1 ☑
          - truck (traffic) V54.6 ☑
            - nontraffic V54.1 ☑
          - two wheeled motor vehicle (traffic) V52.6 ☑
            - nontraffic V52.1 ☑
          - van (traffic) V53.6 ☑
            - nontraffic V53.1 ☑
        - noncollision accident (traffic) V58.6 ☑
          - nontraffic V58.1 ☑
      - specified type NEC V59.88 ☑
        - military vehicle V59.81 ☑
    - quarry truck — *see* Accident, transport, industrial vehicle occupant
    - race car — *see* Accident, transport, motor vehicle NEC occupant
    - railway vehicle occupant V81.9 ☑
      - collision (with) V81.3 ☑
        - motor vehicle (non-military) (traffic) V81.1 ☑
          - military V81.83 ☑
          - nontraffic V81.Ø ☑
        - rolling stock V81.2 ☑
        - specified object NEC V81.3 ☑
      - during derailment V81.7 ☑
        - with antecedent collision — *see* Accident, transport, railway vehicle occupant, collision
      - explosion V81.81 ☑
      - fall (in railway vehicle) V81.5 ☑
        - during derailment V81.7 ☑
          - with antecedent collision — *see* Accident, transport, railway vehicle occupant, collision
        - from railway vehicle V81.6 ☑
          - during derailment V81.7 ☑
            - with antecedent collision — *see* Accident, transport, railway vehicle occupant, collision
        - while boarding or alighting V81.4 ☑
      - fire V81.81 ☑
      - object falling onto train V81.82 ☑
      - specified type NEC V81.89 ☑
      - while boarding or alighting V81.4 ☑
    - Segway VØØ.848 ☑
    - ski lift V98.3 ☑
    - snowmobile occupant (nontraffic) V86.92 ☑
      - driver V86.52 ☑
      - hanger-on V86.72 ☑
      - passenger V86.62 ☑
      - traffic V86.32 ☑
        - driver V86.Ø2 ☑
        - hanger-on V86.22 ☑
        - passenger V86.12 ☑
      - while boarding or alighting V86.42 ☑
    - specified NEC V98.8 ☑
    - sport utility vehicle occupant — *see also* Accident, transport, pickup truck occupant
    - streetcar occupant V82.9 ☑
      - collision (with) V82.3 ☑
        - motor vehicle (traffic) V82.1 ☑
          - nontraffic V82.Ø ☑
        - rolling stock V82.2 ☑
      - during derailment V82.7 ☑

Accident — *continued*
- transport — *continued*
  - truck occupant — *continued*
    - collision — *continued*
      - truck (traffic) V64.9 ☑
        - nontraffic V64.3 ☑
        - while boarding or alighting V64.4 ☑
      - two wheeled motor vehicle (traffic) V62.9 ☑
        - nontraffic V62.3 ☑
        - while boarding or alighting V62.4 ☑
      - van (traffic) V63.9 ☑
        - nontraffic V63.3 ☑
        - while boarding or alighting V63.4 ☑
    - driver
      - collision (with)
        - animal (traffic) V6Ø.5 ☑
          - being ridden (traffic) V66.5 ☑
            - nontraffic V66.Ø ☑
          - nontraffic V6Ø.Ø ☑
        - animal-drawn vehicle (traffic) V66.5 ☑
          - nontraffic V66.Ø ☑
        - bus (traffic) V64.5 ☑
          - nontraffic V64.Ø ☑
        - car (traffic) V63.5 ☑
          - nontraffic V63.Ø ☑
        - motor vehicle NOS (traffic) V69.4Ø ☑
          - nontraffic V69.ØØ ☑
          - specified type NEC (traffic) V69.49 ☑
            - nontraffic V69.Ø9 ☑
        - pedal cycle (traffic) V61.5 ☑
          - nontraffic V61.Ø ☑
        - pickup truck (traffic) V63.5 ☑
          - nontraffic V63.Ø ☑
        - railway vehicle (traffic) V65.5 ☑
          - nontraffic V65.Ø ☑
        - specified vehicle NEC (traffic) V66.5 ☑
          - nontraffic V66.Ø ☑
        - stationary object (traffic) V67.5 ☑
          - nontraffic V67.Ø ☑
        - streetcar (traffic) V66.5 ☑
          - nontraffic V66.Ø ☑
        - three wheeled motor vehicle (traffic) V62.5 ☑
          - nontraffic V62.Ø ☑
        - truck (traffic) V64.5 ☑
          - nontraffic V64.Ø ☑
        - two wheeled motor vehicle (traffic) V62.5 ☑
          - nontraffic V62.Ø ☑
        - van (traffic) V63.5 ☑
          - nontraffic V63.Ø ☑
      - noncollision accident (traffic) V68.5 ☑
        - nontraffic V68.Ø ☑
    - dump — *see* Accident, transport, construction vehicle occupant
    - hanger-on
      - collision (with)
        - animal (traffic) V6Ø.7 ☑
          - being ridden (traffic) V66.7 ☑
            - nontraffic V66.2 ☑
          - nontraffic V6Ø.2 ☑
        - animal-drawn vehicle (traffic) V66.7 ☑
          - nontraffic V66.2 ☑
        - bus (traffic) V64.7 ☑
          - nontraffic V64.2 ☑
        - car (traffic) V63.7 ☑
          - nontraffic V63.2 ☑
        - pedal cycle (traffic) V61.7 ☑
          - nontraffic V61.2 ☑
        - pickup truck (traffic) V63.7 ☑
          - nontraffic V63.2 ☑
        - railway vehicle (traffic) V65.7 ☑
          - nontraffic V65.2 ☑
        - specified vehicle NEC (traffic) V66.7 ☑
          - nontraffic V66.2 ☑
        - stationary object (traffic) V67.7 ☑
          - nontraffic V67.2 ☑
        - streetcar (traffic) V66.7 ☑
          - nontraffic V66.2 ☑
        - three wheeled motor vehicle (traffic) V62.7 ☑
          - nontraffic V62.2 ☑
        - truck (traffic) V64.7 ☑
          - nontraffic V64.2 ☑
        - two wheeled motor vehicle (traffic) V62.7 ☑

Accident — *continued*
- transport — *continued*
  - truck occupant — *continued*
    - hanger-on — *continued*
      - collision — *continued*
        - two wheeled motor vehicle — *continued*
          - nontraffic V62.2 ☑
        - van (traffic) V63.7 ☑
          - nontraffic V63.2 ☑
      - noncollision accident (traffic) V68.7 ☑
        - nontraffic V68.2 ☑
    - noncollision accident (traffic) V68.9 ☑
      - nontraffic V68.3 ☑
      - while boarding or alighting V68.4 ☑
    - nontraffic V69.3 ☑
    - passenger
      - collision (with)
        - animal (traffic) V6Ø.6 ☑
          - being ridden (traffic) V66.6 ☑
            - nontraffic V66.1- ☑
          - nontraffic V6Ø.1 ☑
        - animal-drawn vehicle (traffic) V66.6 ☑
          - nontraffic V66.1 ☑
        - bus (traffic) V64.6 ☑
          - nontraffic V64.1 ☑
        - car (traffic) V63.6 ☑
          - nontraffic V63.1 ☑
        - motor vehicle NOS (traffic) V69.5Ø ☑
          - nontraffic V69.1Ø ☑
          - specified type NEC (traffic) V69.59 ☑
            - nontraffic V69.19 ☑
        - pedal cycle (traffic) V61.6 ☑
          - nontraffic V61.1 ☑
        - pickup truck (traffic) V63.6 ☑
          - nontraffic V63.1 ☑
        - railway vehicle (traffic) V65.6 ☑
          - nontraffic V65.1 ☑
        - specified vehicle NEC (traffic) V66.6 ☑
          - nontraffic V66.1 ☑
        - stationary object (traffic) V67.6 ☑
          - nontraffic V67.1 ☑
        - streetcar (traffic) V66.6 ☑
          - nontraffic V66.1 ☑
        - three wheeled motor vehicle (traffic) V62.6 ☑
          - nontraffic V62.1 ☑
        - truck (traffic) V64.6 ☑
          - nontraffic V64.1 ☑
        - two wheeled motor vehicle (traffic) V62.6 ☑
          - nontraffic V62.1 ☑
        - van (traffic) V63.6 ☑
          - nontraffic V63.1 ☑
      - noncollision accident (traffic) V68.6 ☑
        - nontraffic V68.1 ☑
    - pickup — *see* Accident, transport, pickup truck occupant
    - specified type NEC V69.88 ☑
      - military vehicle V69.81 ☑
  - van occupant V59.9 ☑
    - collision (with)
      - animal (traffic) V5Ø.9 ☑
        - being ridden (traffic) V56.9 ☑
          - nontraffic V56.3 ☑
          - while boarding or alighting V56.4 ☑
        - nontraffic V5Ø.3 ☑
        - while boarding or alighting V5Ø.4 ☑
      - animal-drawn vehicle (traffic) V56.9 ☑
        - nontraffic V56.3 ☑
        - while boarding or alighting V56.4 ☑
      - bus (traffic) V54.9 ☑
        - nontraffic V54.3 ☑
        - while boarding or alighting V54.4 ☑
      - car (traffic) V53.9 ☑
        - nontraffic V53.3 ☑
        - while boarding or alighting V53.4 ☑
      - motor vehicle NOS (traffic) V59.6Ø ☑
        - nontraffic V59.2Ø ☑
        - specified type NEC (traffic) V59.69 ☑
          - nontraffic V59.29 ☑
      - pedal cycle (traffic) V51.9 ☑
        - nontraffic V51.3 ☑
        - while boarding or alighting V51.4 ☑
      - pickup truck (traffic) V53.9 ☑
        - nontraffic V53.3 ☑

Accident — *continued*
- transport — *continued*
  - van occupant — *continued*
    - collision — *continued*
      - pickup truck — *continued*
        - while boarding or alighting V53.4 ☑
      - railway vehicle (traffic) V55.9 ☑
        - nontraffic V55.3 ☑
        - while boarding or alighting V55.4 ☑
      - specified vehicle NEC (traffic) V56.9 ☑
        - nontraffic V56.3 ☑
        - while boarding or alighting V56.4 ☑
      - stationary object (traffic) V57.9 ☑
        - nontraffic V57.3 ☑
        - while boarding or alighting V57.4 ☑
      - streetcar (traffic) V56.9 ☑
        - nontraffic V56.3 ☑
        - while boarding or alighting V56.4 ☑
      - three wheeled motor vehicle (traffic) V52.9 ☑
        - nontraffic V52.3 ☑
        - while boarding or alighting V52.4 ☑
      - truck (traffic) V54.9 ☑
        - nontraffic V54.3 ☑
        - while boarding or alighting V54.4 ☑
      - two wheeled motor vehicle (traffic) V52.9 ☑
        - nontraffic V52.3 ☑
        - while boarding or alighting V52.4 ☑
      - van (traffic) V53.9 ☑
        - nontraffic V53.3 ☑
        - while boarding or alighting V53.4 ☑
    - driver
      - collision (with)
        - animal (traffic) V5Ø.5 ☑
          - being ridden (traffic) V56.5 ☑
            - nontraffic V56.Ø ☑
          - nontraffic V5Ø.Ø ☑
        - animal-drawn vehicle (traffic) V56.5 ☑
          - nontraffic V56.Ø ☑
        - bus (traffic) V54.5 ☑
          - nontraffic V54.Ø ☑
        - car (traffic) V53.5 ☑
          - nontraffic V53.Ø ☑
        - motor vehicle NOS (traffic) V59.4Ø ☑
          - nontraffic V59.ØØ ☑
          - specified type NEC (traffic) V59.49 ☑
            - nontraffic V59.Ø9 ☑
        - pedal cycle (traffic) V51.5 ☑
          - nontraffic V51.Ø ☑
        - pickup truck (traffic) V53.5 ☑
          - nontraffic V53.Ø ☑
        - railway vehicle (traffic) V55.5 ☑
          - nontraffic V55.Ø ☑
        - specified vehicle NEC (traffic) V56.5 ☑
          - nontraffic V56.Ø ☑
        - stationary object (traffic) V57.5 ☑
          - nontraffic V57.Ø ☑
        - streetcar (traffic) V56.5 ☑
          - nontraffic V56.Ø ☑
        - three wheeled motor vehicle (traffic) V52.5 ☑
          - nontraffic V52.Ø ☑
        - truck (traffic) V54.5 ☑
          - nontraffic V54.Ø ☑
        - two wheeled motor vehicle (traffic) V52.5 ☑
          - nontraffic V52.Ø ☑
        - van (traffic) V53.5 ☑
          - nontraffic V53.Ø ☑
      - noncollision accident (traffic) V58.5 ☑
        - nontraffic V58.Ø ☑
    - hanger-on
      - collision (with)
        - animal (traffic) V5Ø.7 ☑
          - being ridden (traffic) V56.7 ☑
            - nontraffic V56.2 ☑
          - nontraffic V5Ø.2 ☑
        - animal-drawn vehicle (traffic) V56.7 ☑
          - nontraffic V56.2 ☑
        - bus (traffic) V54.7 ☑
          - nontraffic V54.2 ☑
        - car (traffic) V53.7 ☑
          - nontraffic V53.2 ☑
        - pedal cycle (traffic) V51.7 ☑
          - nontraffic V51.2 ☑
        - pickup truck (traffic) V53.7 ☑
          - nontraffic V53.2 ☑

External Causes Index

Accident — Activity

Activity — *continued*
- elliptical machine Y93.A1 (*following* Y93.7)
- exercise(s)
  - machines ((primarily) for)
    - cardiorespiratory conditioning Y93.A1 (*following* Y93.7)
    - muscle strengthening Y93.B1 (*following* Y93.7)
  - muscle strengthening (non-machine) NEC Y93.B9 (*following* Y93.7)
- external motion NEC Y93.I9 (*following* Y93.7)
  - rollercoaster Y93.I1 (*following* Y93.7)
- fainting game Y93.85
- field hockey Y93.65
- figure skating (pairs) (singles) Y93.21
- flag football Y93.62
- floor mopping and cleaning Y93.E5 (*following* Y93.7)
- food preparation and clean up Y93.G1 (*following* Y93.7)
- football (American) NOS Y93.61
  - flag Y93.62
  - tackle Y93.61
  - touch Y93.62
- four square Y93.6A
- free weights Y93.B3 (*following* Y93.7)
- frisbee (ultimate) Y93.74
- furniture
  - building Y93.D3 (*following* Y93.7)
  - finishing Y93.D3 (*following* Y93.7)
  - repair Y93.D3 (*following* Y93.7)
- game playing (electronic)
  - using interactive device Y93.C2 (*following* Y93.7)
  - using keyboard or other stationary device Y93.C1 (*following* Y93.7)
- gardening Y93.H2 (*following* Y93.7)
- golf Y93.53
- grass drills Y93.A6 (*following* Y93.7)
- grilling and smoking food Y93.G2 (*following* Y93.7)
- grooming and shearing an animal Y93.K3 (*following* Y93.7)
- guerilla drills Y93.A6 (*following* Y93.7)
- gymnastics (rhythmic) Y93.43
- hand held interactive electronic device Y93.C2 (*following* Y93.7)
- handball Y93.73
- handcrafts NEC Y93.D9 (*following* Y93.7)
- hang gliding Y93.35
- hiking (on level or elevated terrain) Y93.Ø1
- hockey (ice) Y93.22
  - field Y93.65
- horseback riding Y93.52
- household (interior) maintenance NEC Y93.E9 (*following* Y93.7)
- ice NEC Y93.29
  - dancing Y93.21
  - hockey Y93.22
  - skating Y93.21
- inline roller skating Y93.51
- ironing Y93.E4 (*following* Y93.7)
- judo Y93.75
- jumping jacks Y93.A2 (*following* Y93.7)
- jumping rope Y93.56
- jumping (off) NEC Y93.39
  - BASE (Building, Antenna, Span, Earth) Y93.33
  - bungee Y93.34
  - jacks Y93.A2 (*following* Y93.7)
  - rope Y93.56
- karate Y93.75
- kayaking (in calm and turbulent water) Y93.16
- keyboarding (computer) Y93.C1 (*following* Y93.7)
- kickball Y93.6A
- knitting Y93.D1 (*following* Y93.7)
- lacrosse Y93.65
- land maintenance NEC Y93.H9 (*following* Y93.7)
- landscaping Y93.H2 (*following* Y93.7)
- laundry Y93.E2 (*following* Y93.7)
- machines (exercise)
  - primarily for cardiorespiratory conditioning Y93.A1 (*following* Y93.7)
  - primarily for muscle strengthening Y93.B1 (*following* Y93.7)
- maintenance
  - exterior building NEC Y93.H9 (*following* Y93.7)
  - household (interior) NEC Y93.E9 (*following* Y93.7)
  - land Y93.H9 (*following* Y93.7)
  - property Y93.H9 (*following* Y93.7)
- marching (on level or elevated terrain) Y93.Ø1
- martial arts Y93.75
- microwave oven Y93.G3 (*following* Y93.7)
- milking an animal Y93.K2 (*following* Y93.7)
- mopping (floor) Y93.E5 (*following* Y93.7)

Activity — *continued*
- mountain climbing Y93.31
- muscle strengthening
  - exercises (non-machine) NEC Y93.B9 (*following* Y93.7)
  - machines Y93.B1 (*following* Y93.7)
- musical keyboard (electronic) playing Y93.J1 (*following* Y93.7)
- nordic skiing Y93.24
- obstacle course Y93.A5 (*following* Y93.7)
- oven (microwave) Y93.G3 (*following* Y93.7)
- packing up and unpacking in moving to a new residence Y93.E6 (*following* Y93.7)
- parasailing Y93.19
- pass out game Y93.85
- percussion instrument playing NEC Y93.J2 (*following* Y93.7)
- personal
  - bathing and showering Y93.E1 (*following* Y93.7)
  - hygiene NEC Y93.E8 (*following* Y93.7)
  - showering Y93.E1 (*following* Y93.7)
- physical games generally associated with school recess, summer camp and children Y93.6A
- physical training NEC Y93.A9 (*following* Y93.7)
- piano playing Y93.J1 (*following* Y93.7)
- pilates Y93.B4 (*following* Y93.7)
- platform diving Y93.12
- playing musical instrument
  - brass instrument Y93.J4 (*following* Y93.7)
  - drum Y93.J2 (*following* Y93.7)
  - musical keyboard (electronic) Y93.J1 (*following* Y93.7)
  - percussion instrument NEC Y93.J2 (*following* Y93.7)
  - piano Y93.J1 (*following* Y93.7)
  - string instrument Y93.J3 (*following* Y93.7)
  - winds instrument Y93.J4 (*following* Y93.7)
- property maintenance
  - exterior NEC Y93.H9 (*following* Y93.7)
  - interior NEC Y93.E9 (*following* Y93.7)
- pruning (garden and lawn) Y93.H2 (*following* Y93.7)
- pull-ups Y93.B2 (*following* Y93.7)
- push-ups Y93.B2 (*following* Y93.7)
- racquetball Y93.73
- rafting (in calm and turbulent water) Y93.16
- raking (leaves) Y93.H1 (*following* Y93.7)
- rappelling Y93.32
- refereeing a sports activity Y93.81
- residential relocation Y93.E6 (*following* Y93.7)
- rhythmic gymnastics Y93.43
- rhythmic movement NEC Y93.49
- riding
  - horseback Y93.52
  - rollercoaster Y93.I1 (*following* Y93.7)
- rock climbing Y93.31
- roller skating (inline) Y93.51
- rollercoaster riding Y93.I1 (*following* Y93.7)
- rough housing and horseplay Y93.83
- rowing (in calm and turbulent water) Y93.16
- rugby Y93.63
- running Y93.Ø2
- SCUBA diving Y93.15
- sewing Y93.D2 (*following* Y93.7)
- shoveling Y93.H1 (*following* Y93.7)
  - dirt Y93.H1 (*following* Y93.7)
  - snow Y93.H1 (*following* Y93.7)
- showering (personal) Y93.E1 (*following* Y93.7)
- sit-ups Y93.B2 (*following* Y93.7)
- skateboarding Y93.51
- skating (ice) Y93.21
  - roller Y93.51
- skiing (alpine) (downhill) Y93.23
  - cross country Y93.24
  - nordic Y93.24
  - water Y93.17
- sledding (snow) Y93.23
- sleeping (sleep) Y93.84
- smoking and grilling food Y93.G2 (*following* Y93.7)
- snorkeling Y93.15
- snow NEC Y93.29
  - boarding Y93.23
  - shoveling Y93.H1 (*following* Y93.7)
  - sledding Y93.23
  - tubing Y93.23
- soccer Y93.66
- softball Y93.64
- specified NEC Y93.89
- spectator at an event Y93.82
- sports NEC Y93.79
  - sports played as a team or group NEC Y93.69

Activity — *continued*
- sports — *continued*
  - sports played individually NEC Y93.59
- springboard diving Y93.12
- squash Y93.73
- stationary bike Y93.A1 (*following* Y93.7)
- step (stepping) exercise (class) Y93.A3 (*following* Y93.7)
- stepper machine Y93.A1 (*following* Y93.7)
- stove Y93.G3 (*following* Y93.7)
- string instrument playing Y93.J3 (*following* Y93.7)
- surfing Y93.18
  - wind Y93.18
- swimming Y93.11
- tackle football Y93.61
- tap dancing Y93.41
- tennis Y93.73
- tobogganing Y93.23
- touch football Y93.62
- track and field events (non-running) Y93.57
  - running Y93.Ø2
- trampoline Y93.44
- treadmill Y93.A1 (*following* Y93.7)
- trimming shrubs Y93.H2 (*following* Y93.7)
- tubing (in calm and turbulent water) Y93.16
  - snow Y93.23
- ultimate frisbee Y93.74
- underwater diving Y93.15
- unpacking in moving to a new residence Y93.E6 (*following* Y93.7)
- use of stove, oven and microwave oven Y93.G3 (*following* Y93.7)
- vacuuming Y93.E3 (*following* Y93.7)
- volleyball (beach) (court) Y93.68
- wake boarding Y93.17
- walking (on level or elevated terrain) Y93.Ø1
  - an animal Y93.K1 (*following* Y93.7)
- walking an animal Y93.K1 (*following* Y93.7)
- wall climbing Y93.31
- warm up and cool down exercises Y93.A2 (*following* Y93.7)
- water NEC Y93.19
  - aerobics Y93.14
  - craft NEC Y93.19
  - exercise Y93.14
  - polo Y93.13
  - skiing Y93.17
  - sliding Y93.18
  - survival training and testing Y93.19
- weeding (garden and lawn) Y93.H2 (*following* Y93.7)
- wind instrument playing Y93.J4 (*following* Y93.7)
- windsurfing Y93.18
- wrestling Y93.72
- yoga Y93.42

Adverse effect of drugs — *see* Table of Drugs and Chemicals

Aerosinusitis — *see* Air, pressure

After-effect, late — *see* Sequelae

Air
- blast in war operations — *see* War operations, air blast
- pressure
  - change, rapid
    - during
      - ascent W94.29 ☑
        - while (in) (surfacing from)
          - aircraft W94.23 ☑
          - deep water diving W94.21 ☑
          - underground W94.22 ☑
      - descent W94.39 ☑
        - in
          - aircraft W94.31 ☑
          - water W94.32 ☑
  - high, prolonged W94.Ø ☑
  - low, prolonged W94.12 ☑
    - due to residence or long visit at high altitude W94.11 ☑

Alpine sickness W94.11 ☑

Altitude sickness W94.11 ☑

Anaphylactic shock, anaphylaxis — *see* Table of Drugs and Chemicals

Andes disease W94.11 ☑

Arachnidism, arachnoidism X58 ☑

Arson (with intent to injure or kill) X97 ☑

Asphyxia, asphyxiation
- by
  - food (bone) (seed) — *see* categories T17 and T18 ☑
  - gas — *see also* Table of Drugs and Chemicals
    - legal
      - execution — *see* Legal, intervention, gas

- **Asphyxia, asphyxiation** — *continued*
  - by — *continued*
    - gas — *see also* Table of Drugs and Chemicals — *continued*
      - legal — *continued*
        - intervention — *see* Legal, intervention, gas
  - from
    - fire — *see also* Exposure, fire
      - in war operations — *see* War operations, fire
    - ignition — *see* Ignition
    - vomitus T17.81 ☑
  - in war operations — *see* War operations, restriction of airway
- **Aspiration**
  - food (any type) (into respiratory tract) (with asphyxia, obstruction respiratory tract, suffocation) — *see* categories T17 and T18 ☑
  - foreign body — *see* Foreign body, aspiration
  - vomitus (with asphyxia, obstruction respiratory tract, suffocation) T17.81 ☑
- **Assassination** (attempt) — *see* Assault
- **Assault** (homicidal) (by) (in) YØ9
  - arson X97 ☑
  - bite (of human being) YØ4.1 ☑
  - bodily force YØ4.8 ☑
    - bite YØ4.1 ☑
    - bumping into YØ4.2 ☑
    - sexual — *see* subcategories T74.Ø, T76.Ø ☑
    - unarmed fight YØ4.Ø ☑
  - bomb X96.9 ☑
    - antipersonnel X96.Ø ☑
    - fertilizer X96.3 ☑
    - gasoline X96.1 ☑
    - letter X96.2 ☑
    - petrol X96.1 ☑
    - pipe X96.3 ☑
    - specified NEC X96.8 ☑
  - brawl (hand) (fists) (foot) (unarmed) YØ4.Ø ☑
  - burning, burns (by fire) NEC X97 ☑
    - acid YØ8.89 ☑
    - caustic, corrosive substance YØ8.89 ☑
    - chemical from swallowing caustic, corrosive substance — *see* Table of Drugs and Chemicals
    - cigarette(s) X97 ☑
    - hot object X98.9 ☑
      - fluid NEC X98.2 ☑
      - household appliance X98.3 ☑
      - specified NEC X98.8 ☑
      - steam X98.Ø ☑
      - tap water X98.1 ☑
      - vapors X98.Ø ☑
    - scalding — *see* Assault, burning
    - steam X98.Ø ☑
    - vitriol YØ8.89 ☑
  - caustic, corrosive substance (gas) YØ8.89 ☑
  - crashing of
    - aircraft YØ8.81 ☑
    - motor vehicle YØ3.8 ☑
      - pushed in front of YØ2.Ø ☑
      - run over YØ3.Ø ☑
      - specified NEC YØ3.8 ☑
  - cutting or piercing instrument X99.9 ☑
    - dagger X99.2 ☑
    - glass X99.Ø ☑
    - knife X99.1 ☑
    - specified NEC X99.8 ☑
    - sword X99.2 ☑
  - dagger X99.2 ☑
  - drowning (in) X92.9 ☑
    - bathtub X92.Ø ☑
    - natural water X92.3 ☑
    - specified NEC X92.8 ☑
    - swimming pool X92.1 ☑
      - following fall X92.2 ☑
  - dynamite X96.8 ☑
  - explosive(s) (material) X96.9 ☑
  - fight (hand) (fists) (foot) (unarmed) YØ4.Ø ☑
    - with weapon — *see* Assault, by type of weapon
  - fire X97 ☑
  - firearm X95.9 ☑
    - airgun X95.Ø1 ☑
    - handgun X93 ☑
    - hunting rifle X94.1 ☑
    - larger X94.9 ☑
      - specified NEC X94.8 ☑
    - machine gun X94.2 ☑

- **Assault** — *continued*
  - firearm — *continued*
    - shotgun X94.Ø ☑
    - specified NEC X95.8 ☑
  - from high place YØ1 ☑
  - gunshot (wound) NEC — *see* Assault, firearm, by type
  - incendiary device X97 ☑
  - injury YØ9
    - to child due to criminal abortion attempt NEC YØ8.89 ☑
  - knife X99.1 ☑
  - late effect of — *see* categories X92-YØ8 with 7th character S
  - placing before moving object NEC YØ2.8 ☑
    - motor vehicle YØ2.Ø ☑
  - poisoning — *see* categories T36-T65 with 7th character S
  - puncture, any part of body — *see* Assault, cutting or piercing instrument
  - pushing
    - before moving object NEC YØ2.8 ☑
      - motor vehicle YØ2.Ø ☑
      - subway train YØ2.1 ☑
      - train YØ2.1 ☑
    - from high place YØ1 ☑
  - rape T74.2- ☑
  - scalding — *see* Assault, burning
  - sequelae of — *see* categories X92-YØ8 with 7th character S
  - sexual (by bodily force) T74.2- ☑
  - shooting — *see* Assault, firearm
  - specified means NEC YØ8.89 ☑
  - stab, any part of body — *see* Assault, cutting or piercing instrument
  - steam X98.Ø ☑
  - striking against
    - other person YØ4.2 ☑
    - sports equipment YØ8.Ø9 ☑
      - baseball bat YØ8.Ø2 ☑
      - hockey stick YØ8.Ø1 ☑
  - struck by
    - sports equipment YØ8.Ø9 ☑
      - baseball bat YØ8.Ø2 ☑
      - hockey stick YØ8.Ø1 ☑
  - submersion — *see* Assault, drowning
  - violence YØ9
  - weapon YØ9
    - blunt YØØ ☑
    - cutting or piercing — *see* Assault, cutting or piercing instrument
    - firearm — *see* Assault, firearm
  - wound YØ9
    - cutting — *see* Assault, cutting or piercing instrument
    - gunshot — *see* Assault, firearm
    - knife X99.1 ☑
    - piercing — *see* Assault, cutting or piercing instrument
    - puncture — *see* Assault, cutting or piercing instrument
    - stab — *see* Assault, cutting or piercing instrument
- **Attack by mammals NEC** W55.89 ☑
- **Avalanche** — *see* Landslide
- **Aviator's disease** — *see* Air, pressure

B

- **Barotitis, barodontalgia, barosinusitis, barotrauma** (otitic) (sinus) — *see* Air, pressure
- **Battered** (baby) (child) (person) (syndrome) X58 ☑
- **Bayonet wound** W26.1 ☑
  - in
    - legal intervention — *see* Legal, intervention, sharp object, bayonet
    - war operations — *see* War operations, combat
  - stated as undetermined whether accidental or intentional Y28.8 ☑
  - suicide (attempt) X78.2 ☑
- **Bean in nose** — *see* categories T17 and T18 ☑
- **Bed set on fire NEC** — *see* Exposure, fire, uncontrolled, building, bed
- **Beheading** (by guillotine)
  - homicide X99.9 ☑
  - legal execution — *see* Legal, intervention
- **Bending, injury in** (prolonged) (static) X5Ø.1 ☑
- **Bends** — *see* Air, pressure, change

- **Bite, bitten by**
  - alligator W58.Ø1 ☑
  - arthropod (nonvenomous) NEC W57 ☑
  - bull W55.21 ☑
  - cat W55.Ø1 ☑
  - cow W55.21 ☑
  - crocodile W58.11 ☑
  - dog W54.Ø ☑
  - goat W55.31 ☑
  - hoof stock NEC W55.31 ☑
  - horse W55.11 ☑
  - human being (accidentally) W5Ø.3 ☑
    - with intent to injure or kill YØ4.1 ☑
    - as, or caused by, a crowd or human stampede (with fall) W52 ☑
    - assault YØ4.1 ☑
    - homicide (attempt) YØ4.1 ☑
    - in
      - fight YØ4.1 ☑
  - insect (nonvenomous) W57 ☑
  - lizard (nonvenomous) W59.Ø1 ☑
  - mammal NEC W55.81 ☑
    - marine W56.31 ☑
  - marine animal (nonvenomous) W56.81 ☑
  - millipede W57 ☑
  - moray eel W56.51 ☑
  - mouse W53.Ø1 ☑
  - person(s) (accidentally) W5Ø.3 ☑
    - with intent to injure or kill YØ4.1 ☑
    - as, or caused by, a crowd or human stampede (with fall) W52 ☑
    - assault YØ4.1 ☑
    - homicide (attempt) YØ4.1 ☑
    - in
      - fight YØ4.1 ☑
  - pig W55.41 ☑
  - raccoon W55.51 ☑
  - rat W53.11 ☑
  - reptile W59.81 ☑
    - lizard W59.Ø1 ☑
    - snake W59.11 ☑
    - turtle W59.21 ☑
      - terrestrial W59.81 ☑
  - rodent W53.81 ☑
    - mouse W53.Ø1 ☑
    - rat W53.11 ☑
    - specified NEC W53.81 ☑
    - squirrel W53.21 ☑
  - shark W56.41 ☑
  - sheep W55.31 ☑
  - snake (nonvenomous) W59.11 ☑
  - spider (nonvenomous) W57 ☑
  - squirrel W53.21 ☑
- **Blast** (air) in war operations — *see* War operations, blast
- **Blizzard** X37.2 ☑
- **Blood alcohol level** Y9Ø.9
  - less than 2Ømg/1ØØml Y9Ø.Ø
  - presence in blood, level not specified Y9Ø.9
  - 2Ø-39mg/1ØØml Y9Ø.1
  - 4Ø-59mg/1ØØml Y9Ø.2
  - 6Ø-79mg/1ØØml Y9Ø.3
  - 8Ø-99mg/1ØØml Y9Ø.4
  - 1ØØ-119mg/1ØØml Y9Ø.5
  - 12Ø-199mg/1ØØml Y9Ø.6
  - 2ØØ-239mg/1ØØml Y9Ø.7
- **Blow** X58 ☑
  - by law-enforcing agent, police (on duty) — *see* Legal, intervention, manhandling
    - blunt object — *see* Legal, intervention, blunt object
- **Blowing up** — *see* Explosion
- **Brawl** (hand) (fists) (foot) YØ4.Ø ☑
- **Breakage** (accidental) (part of)
  - ladder (causing fall) W11 ☑
  - scaffolding (causing fall) W12 ☑
- **Broken**
  - glass, contact with — *see* Contact, with, glass
  - power line (causing electric shock) W85 ☑
- **Bumping against, into** (accidentally)
  - object NEC W22.8 ☑
    - caused by crowd or human stampede (with fall) W52 ☑
    - sports equipment W21.9 ☑
    - with fall — *see* Fall, due to, bumping against, object
  - person(s) W51 ☑
    - with fall WØ3 ☑
      - due to ice or snow WØØ.Ø ☑

Bumping against, into — *continued*
- person(s) — *continued*
  - assault Y04.2 ☑
  - caused by, a crowd or human stampede (with fall) W52 ☑
  - homicide (attempt) Y04.2 ☑
- sports equipment W21.9 ☑

Burn, burned, burning (accidental) (by) (from) (on)
- acid NEC — *see* Table of Drugs and Chemicals
- bed linen — *see* Exposure, fire, uncontrolled, in building, bed
- blowtorch X08.8 ☑
  - with ignition of clothing NEC X06.2 ☑
    - nightwear X05 ☑
- bonfire, campfire (controlled) — *see also* Exposure, fire, controlled, not in building)
  - uncontrolled — *see* Exposure, fire, uncontrolled, not in building
- candle X08.8 ☑
  - with ignition of clothing NEC X06.2 ☑
    - nightwear X05 ☑
- caustic liquid, substance (external) (internal) NEC — *see* Table of Drugs and Chemicals
- chemical (external) (internal) — *see also* Table of Drugs and Chemicals
  - in war operations — *see* War operations. fire
- cigar(s) or cigarette(s) X08.8 ☑
  - with ignition of clothing NEC X06.2 ☑
    - nightwear X05 ☑
- clothes, clothing NEC (from controlled fire) X06.2 ☑
  - with conflagration — *see* Exposure, fire, uncontrolled, building
  - not in building or structure — *see* Exposure, fire, uncontrolled, not in building
- cooker (hot) X15.8 ☑
  - stated as undetermined whether accidental or intentional Y27.3 ☑
  - suicide (attempt) X77.3 ☑
- electric blanket X16 ☑
- engine (hot) X17 ☑
- fire, flames — *see* Exposure, fire
- flare, Very pistol — *see* Discharge, firearm NEC
- heat
  - from appliance (electrical) (household) X15.8 ☑
    - cooker X15.8 ☑
    - hotplate X15.2 ☑
    - kettle X15.8 ☑
    - light bulb X15.8 ☑
    - saucepan X15.3 ☑
    - skillet X15.3 ☑
    - stated as undetermined whether accidental or intentional Y27.3 ☑
    - stove X15.0 ☑
    - suicide (attempt) X77.3 ☑
    - toaster X15.1 ☑
  - in local application or packing during medical or surgical procedure Y63.5
- heating
  - appliance, radiator or pipe X16 ☑
- homicide (attempt) — *see* Assault, burning
- hot
  - air X14.1 ☑
  - cooker X15.8 ☑
  - drink X10.0 ☑
  - engine X17 ☑
  - fat X10.2 ☑
  - fluid NEC X12 ☑
  - food X10.1 ☑
  - gases X14.1 ☑
  - heating appliance X16 ☑
  - household appliance NEC X15.8 ☑
  - kettle X15.8 ☑
  - liquid NEC X12 ☑
  - machinery X17 ☑
  - metal (molten) (liquid) NEC X18 ☑
  - object (not producing fire or flames) NEC X19 ☑
  - oil (cooking) X10.2 ☑
  - pipe(s) X16 ☑
  - radiator X16 ☑
  - saucepan (glass) (metal) X15.3 ☑
  - stove (kitchen) X15.0 ☑
  - substance NEC X19 ☑
    - caustic or corrosive NEC — *see* Table of Drugs and Chemicals
  - toaster X15.1 ☑
  - tool X17 ☑

Burn, burned, burning — *continued*
- hot — *continued*
  - vapor X13.1 ☑
  - water (tap) — *see* Contact, with, hot, tap water
- hotplate X15.2 ☑
  - suicide (attempt) X77.3 ☑
- ignition — *see* Ignition
- in war operations — *see* War operations, fire
- inflicted by other person X97 ☑
  - by hot objects, hot vapor, and steam — *see* Assault, burning, hot object
- internal, from swallowed caustic, corrosive liquid, substance — *see* Table of Drugs and Chemicals
- iron (hot) X15.8 ☑
  - stated as undetermined whether accidental or intentional Y27.3 ☑
  - suicide (attempt) X77.3 ☑
- kettle (hot) X15.8 ☑
  - stated as undetermined whether accidental or intentional Y27.3 ☑
  - suicide (attempt) X77.3 ☑
- lamp (flame) X08.8 ☑
  - with ignition of clothing NEC X06.2 ☑
    - nightwear X05 ☑
- lighter (cigar) (cigarette) X08.8 ☑
  - with ignition of clothing NEC X06.2 ☑
    - nightwear X05 ☑
- lightning — *see* subcategory T75.0 ☑
  - causing fire — *see* Exposure, fire
- liquid (boiling) (hot) NEC X12 ☑
  - stated as undetermined whether accidental or intentional Y27.2 ☑
  - suicide (attempt) X77.2 ☑
- local application of externally applied substance in medical or surgical care Y63.5
- machinery (hot) X17 ☑
- matches X08.8 ☑
  - with ignition of clothing NEC X06.2 ☑
    - nightwear X05 ☑
- mattress — *see* Exposure, fire, uncontrolled, building, bed
- medicament, externally applied Y63.5
- metal (hot) (liquid) (molten) NEC X18 ☑
- nightwear (nightclothes, nightdress, gown, pajamas, robe) X05 ☑
- object (hot) NEC X19 ☑
- on board watercraft
  - due to
    - accident to watercraft V91.09 ☑
      - powered craft V91.03 ☑
        - ferry boat V91.01 ☑
        - fishing boat V91.02 ☑
        - jetskis V91.03 ☑
        - liner V91.01 ☑
        - merchant ship V91.00 ☑
        - passenger ship V91.01 ☑
      - unpowered craft V91.08 ☑
        - canoe V91.05 ☑
        - inflatable V91.06 ☑
        - kayak V91.05 ☑
        - sailboat V91.04 ☑
        - surf-board V91.08 ☑
        - water skis V91.07 ☑
        - windsurfer V91.08 ☑
    - fire on board V93.09 ☑
      - ferry boat V93.01 ☑
      - fishing boat V93.02 ☑
      - jetskis V93.03 ☑
      - liner V93.01 ☑
      - merchant ship V93.00 ☑
      - passenger ship V93.01 ☑
      - powered craft NEC V93.03 ☑
      - sailboat V93.04 ☑
    - specified heat source NEC on board V93.19 ☑
      - ferry boat V93.11 ☑
      - fishing boat V93.12 ☑
      - jetskis V93.13 ☑
      - liner V93.11 ☑
      - merchant ship V93.10 ☑
      - passenger ship V93.11 ☑
      - powered craft NEC V93.13 ☑
      - sailboat V93.14 ☑
- pipe (hot) X16 ☑
  - smoking X08.8 ☑
    - with ignition of clothing NEC X06.2 ☑
      - nightwear X05 ☑

Burn, burned, burning — *continued*
- powder — *see* Powder burn
- radiator (hot) X16 ☑
- saucepan (hot) (glass) (metal) X15.3 ☑
  - stated as undetermined whether accidental or intentional Y27.3 ☑
  - suicide (attempt) X77.3 ☑
- self-inflicted X76 ☑
  - stated as undetermined whether accidental or intentional Y26 ☑
- stated as undetermined whether accidental or intentional Y27.0 ☑
- steam X13.1 ☑
  - pipe X16 ☑
    - stated as undetermined whether accidental or intentional Y27.8 ☑
  - stated as undetermined whether accidental or intentional Y27.0 ☑
  - suicide (attempt) X77.0 ☑
- stove (hot) (kitchen) X15.0 ☑
  - stated as undetermined whether accidental or intentional Y27.3 ☑
  - suicide (attempt) X77.3 ☑
- substance (hot) NEC X19 ☑
  - boiling X12 ☑
    - stated as undetermined whether accidental or intentional Y27.2 ☑
    - suicide (attempt) X77.2 ☑
  - molten (metal) X18 ☑
- suicide (attempt) NEC X76 ☑
  - hot
    - household appliance X77.3 ☑
    - object X77.9 ☑
- therapeutic misadventure
  - heat in local application or packing during medical or surgical procedure Y63.5
  - overdose of radiation Y63.2
- toaster (hot) X15.1 ☑
  - stated as undetermined whether accidental or intentional Y27.3 ☑
  - suicide (attempt) X77.3 ☑
- tool (hot) X17 ☑
- torch, welding X08.8 ☑
  - with ignition of clothing NEC X06.2 ☑
    - nightwear X05 ☑
- trash fire (controlled) — *see* Exposure, fire, controlled, not in building
  - uncontrolled — *see* Exposure, fire, uncontrolled, not in building
- vapor (hot) X13.1 ☑
  - stated as undetermined whether accidental or intentional Y27.0 ☑
  - suicide (attempt) X77.0 ☑
- Very pistol — *see* Discharge, firearm NEC

Butted by animal W55.82 ☑
- bull W55.22 ☑
- cow W55.22 ☑
- goat W55.32 ☑
- horse W55.12 ☑
- pig W55.42 ☑
- sheep W55.32 ☑

C

Caisson disease — *see* Air, pressure, change

Campfire (exposure to) (controlled) — *see also* Exposure, fire, controlled, not in building
- uncontrolled — *see* Exposure, fire, uncontrolled, not in building

Capital punishment (any means) — *see* Legal, intervention

Car sickness T75.3 ☑

Casualty (not due to war) NEC X58 ☑
- war — *see* War operations

Cat
- bite W55.01 ☑
- scratch W55.03 ☑

Cataclysm, cataclysmic (any injury) NEC — *see* Forces of nature

Catching fire — *see* Exposure, fire

Caught
- between
  - folding object W23.0 ☑
  - objects (moving) W23.0 ☑

Caught — *continued*
- between — *continued*
  - objects — *continued*
    - and
      - machinery — *see* Contact, with, by type of machine
      - stationary
    - stationary W23.1 ☑
    - and moving
  - sliding door and door frame W23.Ø ☑
- by, in
  - machinery (moving parts of) — *see* Contact, with, by type of machine
  - washing-machine wringer W23.Ø ☑
- under packing crate (due to losing grip) W23.1 ☑

Cave-in caused by cataclysmic earth surface movement or eruption — *see* Landslide

Change(s) in air pressure — *see* Air, pressure, change

Choked, choking (on) (any object except food or vomitus)
- food (bone) (seed) — *see* categories T17 and T18 ☑
- vomitus T17.81- ☑

Civil insurrection — *see* War operations

Cloudburst (any injury) X37.8 ☑

Cold, exposure to (accidental) (excessive) (extreme) (natural) (place) NEC — *see* Exposure, cold

Collapse
- building W2Ø.1 ☑
  - burning (uncontrolled fire) XØØ.2 ☑
- dam or man-made structure (causing earth movement) X36.Ø ☑
- machinery — *see* Contact, with, by type of machine
- structure W2Ø.1 ☑
  - burning (uncontrolled fire) XØØ.2 ☑

Collision (accidental) NEC — *see also* Accident, transport V89.9 ☑
- pedestrian W51 ☑
  - with fall WØ3 ☑
    - due to ice or snow WØØ.Ø ☑
    - involving pedestrian conveyance — *see* Accident, transport, pedestrian, conveyance
  - and
    - crowd or human stampede (with fall) W52 ☑
    - object W22.8 ☑
      - with fall — *see* Fall, due to, bumping against, object
- person(s) — *see* Collision, pedestrian
- transport vehicle NEC V89.9 ☑
  - and
    - avalanche, fallen or not moving — *see* Accident, transport
      - falling or moving — *see* Landslide
    - landslide, fallen or not moving — *see* Accident, transport
      - falling or moving — *see* Landslide
  - due to cataclysm — *see* Forces of nature, by type
  - intentional, purposeful suicide (attempt) — *see* Suicide, collision

Combustion, spontaneous — *see* Ignition

Complication (delayed) **of or following** (medical or surgical procedure) Y84.9
- with misadventure — *see* Misadventure
- amputation of limb(s) Y83.5
- anastomosis (arteriovenous) (blood vessel) (gastrojejunal) (tendon) (natural or artificial material) Y83.2
- aspiration (of fluid) Y84.4
  - tissue Y84.8
- biopsy Y84.8
- blood
  - sampling Y84.7
  - transfusion
    - procedure Y84.8
- bypass Y83.2
- catheterization (urinary) Y84.6
  - cardiac Y84.Ø
- colostomy Y83.3
- cystostomy Y83.3
- dialysis (kidney) Y84.1
- drug — *see* Table of Drugs and Chemicals
- due to misadventure — *see* Misadventure
- duodenostomy Y83.3
- electroshock therapy Y84.3
- external stoma, creation of Y83.3
- formation of external stoma Y83.3
- gastrostomy Y83.3
- graft Y83.2
- hypothermia (medically-induced) Y84.8

Complication (delayed) **of or following** — *continued*
- implant, implantation (of)
  - artificial
    - internal device (cardiac pacemaker) (electrodes in brain) (heart valve prosthesis) (orthopedic) Y83.1
    - material or tissue (for anastomosis or bypass) Y83.2
      - with creation of external stoma Y83.3
  - natural tissues (for anastomosis or bypass) Y83.2
    - with creation of external stoma Y83.3
- infusion
  - procedure Y84.8
- injection — *see* Table of Drugs and Chemicals
  - procedure Y84.8
- insertion of gastric or duodenal sound Y84.5
- insulin-shock therapy Y84.3
- paracentesis (abdominal) (thoracic) (aspirative) Y84.4
- procedures other than surgical operation — *see* Complication of or following, by type of procedure
- radiological procedure or therapy Y84.2
- removal of organ (partial) (total) NEC Y83.6
- sampling
  - blood Y84.7
  - fluid NEC Y84.4
  - tissue Y84.8
- shock therapy Y84.3
- surgical operation NEC — *see also* Complication of or following, by type of operation Y83.9
  - reconstructive NEC Y83.4
    - with
      - anastomosis, bypass or graft Y83.2
      - formation of external stoma Y83.3
  - specified NEC Y83.8
- transfusion — *see also* Table of Drugs and Chemicals
  - procedure Y84.8
- transplant, transplantation (heart) (kidney) (liver) (whole organ, any) Y83.Ø
  - partial organ Y83.4
- ureterostomy Y83.3
- vaccination — *see also* Table of Drugs and Chemicals
  - procedure Y84.8

Compression
- divers' squeeze — *see* Air, pressure, change
- trachea by
  - food (lodged in esophagus) — *see* categories T17 and T18 ☑
  - vomitus (lodged in esophagus) T17.81- ☑

Conflagration — *see* Exposure, fire, uncontrolled

Constriction (external)
- hair W49.Ø1 ☑
- jewelry W49.Ø4 ☑
- ring W49.Ø4 ☑
- rubber band W49.Ø3 ☑
- specified item NEC W49.Ø9 ☑
- string W49.Ø2 ☑
- thread W49.Ø2 ☑

Contact (accidental)
- with
  - abrasive wheel (metalworking) W31.1 ☑
  - alligator W58.Ø9 ☑
    - bite W58.Ø1 ☑
    - crushing W58.Ø3 ☑
    - strike W58.Ø2 ☑
  - amphibian W62.9 ☑
    - frog W62.Ø ☑
    - toad W62.1 ☑
  - animal (nonvenomous) NEC W64 ☑
    - marine W56.89 ☑
      - bite W56.81 ☑
      - dolphin — *see* Contact, with, dolphin
      - fish NEC — *see* Contact, with, fish
      - mammal — *see* Contact, with, mammal, marine
      - orca — *see* Contact, with, orca
      - sea lion — *see* Contact, with, sea lion
      - shark — *see* Contact, with, shark
      - strike W56.82 ☑
  - animate mechanical force NEC W64 ☑
  - arrow W21.89 ☑
    - not thrown, projected or falling W45.8 ☑
  - arthropods (nonvenomous) W57 ☑
  - axe W27.Ø ☑
  - band-saw (industrial) W31.2 ☑
  - bayonet — *see* Bayonet wound
  - bee(s) X58 ☑

Contact — *continued*
- with — *continued*
  - bench-saw (industrial) W31.2 ☑
  - bird W61.99 ☑
    - bite W61.91 ☑
    - chicken — *see* Contact, with, chicken
    - duck — *see* Contact, with, duck
    - goose — *see* Contact, with, goose
    - macaw — *see* Contact, with, macaw
    - parrot — *see* Contact, with, parrot
    - psittacine — *see* Contact, with, psittacine
    - strike W61.92 ☑
    - turkey — *see* Contact, with, turkey
  - blender W29.Ø ☑
  - boiling water X12 ☑
    - stated as undetermined whether accidental or intentional Y27.2 ☑
    - suicide (attempt) X77.2 ☑
  - bore, earth-drilling or mining (land) (seabed) W31.Ø ☑
  - buffalo — *see* Contact, with, hoof stock NEC
  - bull W55.29 ☑
    - bite W55.21 ☑
    - gored W55.22 ☑
    - strike W55.22 ☑
  - bumper cars W31.81 ☑
  - camel — *see* Contact, with, hoof stock NEC
  - can
    - lid W26.8 ☑
    - opener W27.4 ☑
      - powered W29.Ø ☑
  - cat W55.Ø9 ☑
    - bite W55.Ø1 ☑
    - scratch W55.Ø3 ☑
  - caterpillar (venomous) X58 ☑
  - centipede (venomous) X58 ☑
  - chain
    - hoist W24.Ø ☑
      - agricultural operations W3Ø.89 ☑
    - saw W29.3 ☑
  - chicken W61.39 ☑
    - peck W61.33 ☑
    - strike W61.32 ☑
  - chisel W27.Ø ☑
  - circular saw W31.2 ☑
  - cobra X58 ☑
  - combine (harvester) W3Ø.Ø ☑
  - conveyer belt W24.1 ☑
  - cooker (hot) X15.8 ☑
    - stated as undetermined whether accidental or intentional Y27.3 ☑
    - suicide (attempt) X77.3 ☑
  - coral X58 ☑
  - cotton gin W31.82 ☑
  - cow W55.29 ☑
    - bite W55.21 ☑
    - strike W55.22 ☑
  - crane W24.Ø ☑
    - agricultural operations W3Ø.89 ☑
  - crocodile W58.19 ☑
    - bite W58.11 ☑
    - crushing W58.13 ☑
    - strike W58.12 ☑
  - dagger W26.1 ☑
    - stated as undetermined whether accidental or intentional Y28.2 ☑
    - suicide (attempt) X78.2 ☑
  - dairy equipment W31.82 ☑
  - dart W21.89 ☑
    - not thrown, projected or falling W45.8 ☑
  - deer — *see* Contact, with, hoof stock NEC
  - derrick W24.Ø ☑
    - agricultural operations W3Ø.89 ☑
      - hay W3Ø.2 ☑
  - dog W54.8 ☑
    - bite W54.Ø ☑
    - strike W54.1 ☑
  - dolphin W56.Ø9 ☑
    - bite W56.Ø1 ☑
    - strike W56.Ø2 ☑
  - donkey — *see* Contact, with, hoof stock NEC
  - drill (powered) W29.8 ☑
    - earth (land) (seabed) W31.Ø ☑
    - nonpowered W27.8 ☑
  - drive belt W24.Ø ☑
    - agricultural operations W3Ø.89 ☑

- **Contact** — *continued*
  - with — *continued*
    - transmission device (belt, cable, chain, gear, pinion, shaft) W24.1 ☑
      - agricultural operations W3Ø.89 ☑
    - turbine (gas) (water-driven) W31.3 ☑
    - turkey W61.49 ☑
      - peck W61.43 ☑
      - strike W61.42 ☑
    - turtle (nonvenomous) W59.29 ☑
      - bite W59.21 ☑
      - strike W59.22 ☑
      - terrestrial W59.89 ☑
        - bite W59.81 ☑
        - crushing W59.83 ☑
        - strike W59.82 ☑
    - under-cutter W31.Ø ☑
    - urine — *see* Contact, with, by type of animal
    - vehicle
      - agricultural use (transport) — *see* Accident, transport, agricultural vehicle
        - not on public highway W3Ø.81 ☑
      - industrial use (transport) — *see* Accident, transport, industrial vehicle
        - not on public highway W31.83 ☑
      - off-road use (transport) — *see* Accident, transport, all-terrain or off-road vehicle
        - not on public highway W31.83 ☑
      - special construction use (transport) — *see* Accident, transport, construction vehicle
        - not on public highway W31.83 ☑
    - venomous
      - animal X58 ☑
      - arthropods X58 ☑
      - lizard X58 ☑
      - marine animal NEC X58 ☑
      - marine plant NEC X58 ☑
      - millipedes (tropical) X58 ☑
      - plant(s) X58 ☑
      - snake X58 ☑
      - spider X58 ☑
    - viper X58 ☑
    - washing-machine (powered) W29.2 ☑
    - wasp X58 ☑
    - weaving-machine W31.89 ☑
    - winch W24.Ø ☑
      - agricultural operations W3Ø.89 ☑
    - wire NEC W24.Ø ☑
      - agricultural operations W3Ø.89 ☑
    - wood slivers W45.8 ☑
    - yellow jacket X58 ☑
    - zebra — *see* Contact, with, hoof stock NEC
  - pressure X5Ø.9 ☑
  - stress X5Ø.9 ☑
- **Coup de soleil** X32 ☑
- **Crash**
  - aircraft (in transit) (powered) V95.9 ☑
    - balloon V96.Ø1 ☑
    - fixed wing NEC (private) V95.21 ☑
      - commercial V95.31 ☑
    - glider V96.21 ☑
      - hang V96.11 ☑
      - powered V95.11 ☑
    - helicopter V95.Ø1 ☑
    - in war operations — *see* War operations, destruction of aircraft
    - microlight V95.11 ☑
    - nonpowered V96.9 ☑
      - specified NEC V96.8 ☑
    - powered NEC V95.8 ☑
    - stated as
      - homicide (attempt) YØ8.81 ☑
      - suicide (attempt) X83.Ø ☑
    - ultralight V95.11 ☑
  - spacecraft V95.41 ☑
  - transport vehicle NEC — *see also* Accident, transport V89.9 ☑
    - homicide (attempt) YØ3.8 ☑
    - motor NEC (traffic) V89.2 ☑
      - homicide (attempt) YØ3.8 ☑
      - suicide (attempt) — *see* Suicide, collision
- **Cruelty** (mental) (physical) (sexual) X58 ☑
- **Crushed** (accidentally) X58 ☑
  - between objects (moving) (stationary and moving) W23.Ø ☑
    - stationary W23.1 ☑
- **Crushed** — *continued*
  - by
    - alligator W58.Ø3 ☑
    - avalanche NEC — *see* Landslide
    - cave-in W2Ø.Ø ☑
      - caused by cataclysmic earth surface movement — *see* Landslide
    - crocodile W58.13 ☑
    - crowd or human stampede W52 ☑
    - falling
      - aircraft V97.39 ☑
        - in war operations — *see* War operations, destruction of aircraft
      - earth, material W2Ø.Ø ☑
        - caused by cataclysmic earth surface movement — *see* Landslide
      - object NEC W2Ø.8 ☑
    - landslide NEC — *see* Landslide
    - lizard (nonvenomous) W59.Ø9 ☑
    - machinery — *see* Contact, with, by type of machine
    - reptile NEC W59.89 ☑
    - snake (nonvenomous) W59.13 ☑
  - in
    - machinery — *see* Contact, with, by type of machine
- **Cut, cutting** (any part of body) (accidental) — *see also* Contact, with, by object or machine
  - during medical or surgical treatment as misadventure — *see* Index to Diseases and Injuries, Complications
  - homicide (attempt) — *see* Assault, cutting or piercing instrument
  - inflicted by other person — *see* Assault, cutting or piercing instrument
  - legal
    - execution — *see* Legal, intervention
    - intervention — *see* Legal, intervention, sharp object
  - machine NEC — *see also* Contact, with, by type of machine W31.9 ☑
  - self-inflicted — *see* Suicide, cutting or piercing instrument
  - suicide (attempt) — *see* Suicide, cutting or piercing instrument
- **Cyclone** (any injury) X37.1 ☑

D

- **Decapitation** (accidental circumstances) NEC X58 ☑
  - homicide X99.9 ☑
  - legal execution — *see* Legal, intervention
- **Dehydration from lack of water** X58 ☑
- **Deprivation** X58 ☑
- **Derailment** (accidental)
  - railway (rolling stock) (train) (vehicle) (without antecedent collision) V81.7 ☑
    - with antecedent collision — *see* Accident, transport, railway vehicle occupant
  - streetcar (without antecedent collision) V82.7 ☑
    - with antecedent collision — *see* Accident, transport, streetcar occupant
- **Descent**
  - parachute (voluntary) (without accident to aircraft) V97.29 ☑
    - due to accident to aircraft — *see* Accident, transport, aircraft
- **Desertion** X58 ☑
- **Destitution** X58 ☑
- **Disability, late effect or sequela of injury** — *see* Sequelae
- **Discharge** (accidental)
  - airgun W34.Ø1Ø ☑
    - assault X95.Ø1 ☑
    - homicide (attempt) X95.Ø1 ☑
    - stated as undetermined whether accidental or intentional Y24.Ø ☑
    - suicide (attempt) X74.Ø1 ☑
  - BB gun — *see* Discharge, airgun
  - firearm (accidental) W34.ØØ ☑
    - assault X95.9 ☑
    - handgun (pistol) (revolver) W32.Ø ☑
      - assault X93 ☑
      - homicide (attempt) X93 ☑
      - legal intervention — *see* Legal, intervention, firearm, handgun
      - stated as undetermined whether accidental or intentional Y22 ☑
      - suicide (attempt) X72 ☑
- **Discharge** — *continued*
  - firearm — *continued*
    - homicide (attempt) X95.9 ☑
    - hunting rifle W33.Ø2 ☑
      - assault X94.1 ☑
      - homicide (attempt) X94.1 ☑
      - legal intervention
        - injuring
          - bystander Y35.Ø32 ☑
          - law enforcement personnel Y35.Ø31 ☑
          - suspect Y35.Ø33 ☑
          - unspecified person Y35.Ø39 ☑
      - stated as undetermined whether accidental or intentional Y23.1 ☑
      - suicide (attempt) X73.1 ☑
    - larger W33.ØØ ☑
      - assault X94.9 ☑
      - homicide (attempt) X94.9 ☑
      - hunting rifle — *see* Discharge, firearm, hunting rifle
      - legal intervention — *see* Legal, intervention, firearm by type of firearm
      - machine gun — *see* Discharge, firearm, machine gun
      - shotgun — *see* Discharge, firearm, shotgun
      - specified NEC W33.Ø9 ☑
        - assault X94.8 ☑
        - homicide (attempt) X94.8 ☑
        - legal intervention
          - injuring
            - bystander Y35.Ø92 ☑
            - law enforcement personnel Y35.Ø91 ☑
            - suspect Y35.Ø93 ☑
            - unspecified person Y35.Ø99 ☑
        - stated as undetermined whether accidental or intentional Y23.8 ☑
        - suicide (attempt) X73.8 ☑
      - stated as undetermined whether accidental or intentional Y23.9 ☑
      - suicide (attempt) X73.9 ☑
    - legal intervention
      - injuring
        - bystander Y35.ØØ2 ☑
        - law enforcement personnel Y35.ØØ1 ☑
        - suspect Y35.Ø3 ☑
        - unspecified person Y35.ØØ9 ☑
      - using rubber bullet
        - injuring
          - bystander Y35.Ø42 ☑
          - law enforcement personnel Y35.Ø41 ☑
          - suspect Y35.Ø43 ☑
          - unspecified person Y35.Ø49 ☑
    - machine gun W33.Ø3 ☑
      - assault X94.2 ☑
      - homicide (attempt) X94.2 ☑
      - legal intervention — *see* Legal, intervention, firearm, machine gun
      - stated as undetermined whether accidental or intentional Y23.3 ☑
      - suicide (attempt) X73.2 ☑
    - pellet gun — *see* Discharge, airgun
    - shotgun W33.Ø1 ☑
      - assault X94.Ø ☑
      - homicide (attempt) X94.Ø ☑
      - legal intervention — *see* Legal, intervention, firearm, specified NEC
      - stated as undetermined whether accidental or intentional Y23.Ø ☑
      - suicide (attempt) X73.Ø ☑
    - specified NEC W34.Ø9 ☑
      - assault X95.8 ☑
      - homicide (attempt) X95.8 ☑
      - legal intervention — *see* Legal, intervention, firearm, specified NEC
      - stated as undetermined whether accidental or intentional Y24.8 ☑
      - suicide (attempt) X74.8 ☑
    - stated as undetermined whether accidental or intentional Y24.9 ☑
    - suicide (attempt) X74.9 ☑
    - Very pistol W34.Ø9 ☑
      - assault X95.8 ☑
      - homicide (attempt) X95.8 ☑
      - stated as undetermined whether accidental or intentional Y24.8 ☑

- **Drowning** — *continued*
  - in — *continued*
    - bathtub — *continued*
      - assault X92.Ø ☑
      - following fall W16.211 ☑
        - stated as undetermined whether accidental or intentional Y21.1 ☑
      - stated as undetermined whether accidental or intentional Y21.Ø ☑
      - suicide (attempt) X71.Ø ☑
    - lake — *see* Drowning, in, natural water
    - natural water (lake) (open sea) (river) (stream) (pond) W69 ☑
      - assault X92.3 ☑
      - following
        - dive or jump W16.611 ☑
          - striking bottom W16.621 ☑
        - fall W16.111 ☑
          - striking
            - bottom W16.121 ☑
            - side W16.131 ☑
      - stated as undetermined whether accidental or intentional Y21.4 ☑
      - suicide (attempt) X71.3 ☑
    - quarry — *see* Drowning, in, specified place NEC
    - quenching tank — *see* Drowning, in, specified place NEC
    - reservoir — *see* Drowning, in, specified place NEC
    - river — *see* Drowning, in, natural water
    - sea — *see* Drowning, in, natural water
    - specified place NEC W73 ☑
      - assault X92.8 ☑
      - following
        - dive or jump W16.811 ☑
          - striking
            - bottom W16.821 ☑
            - wall W16.831 ☑
        - fall W16.311 ☑
          - striking
            - bottom W16.321 ☑
            - wall W16.331 ☑
      - stated as undetermined whether accidental or intentional Y21.8 ☑
      - suicide (attempt) X71.8 ☑
    - stream — *see* Drowning, in, natural water
    - swimming-pool W67 ☑
      - assault X92.1 ☑
        - following fall X92.2 ☑
      - following
        - dive or jump W16.511 ☑
          - striking
            - bottom W16.521 ☑
            - wall W16.531 ☑
        - fall W16.Ø11 ☑
          - striking
            - bottom W16.Ø21 ☑
            - wall W16.Ø31 ☑
      - stated as undetermined whether accidental or intentional Y21.2 ☑
        - following fall Y21.3 ☑
      - suicide (attempt) X71.1 ☑
        - following fall X71.2 ☑
    - war operations — *see* War operations, restriction of airway
  - resulting from accident to watercraft — *see* Drowning, due to, accident, watercraft
  - self-inflicted X71.9 ☑
  - stated as undetermined whether accidental or intentional Y21.9 ☑
  - suicide (attempt) X71.9 ☑

E

- **Earth falling** (on) W2Ø.Ø ☑
  - caused by cataclysmic earth surface movement or eruption — *see* Landslide
- **Earth** (surface) **movement NEC** — *see* Forces of nature, earth movement
- **Earthquake** (any injury) X34 ☑
- **Effect**(s) (adverse) **of**
  - air pressure (any) — *see* Air, pressure
  - cold, excessive (exposure to) — *see* Exposure, cold
  - heat (excessive) — *see* Heat
  - hot place (weather) — *see* Heat
  - insolation X3Ø ☑
  - late — *see* Sequelae
- **Effect**(s) (adverse) **of** — *continued*
  - motion — *see* Motion
  - nuclear explosion or weapon in war operations — *see* War operations, nuclear weapon
  - radiation — *see* Radiation
  - travel — *see* Travel
- **Electric shock** (accidental) (by) (in) — *see* Exposure, electric current
- **Electrocution** (accidental) — *see* Exposure, electric current
- **Endotracheal tube wrongly placed during anesthetic procedure**
- **Entanglement**
  - in
    - bed linen, causing suffocation T71 ☑
    - wheel of pedal cycle V19.88 ☑
- **Entry of foreign body or material** — *see* Foreign body
- **Environmental pollution related condition** — *see* category Z57 ☑
- **Execution, legal** (any method) — *see* Legal, intervention
- **Exhaustion**
  - cold — *see* Exposure, cold
  - due to excessive exertion — *see also* Overexertion X5Ø.9 ☑
  - heat — *see* Heat
- **Explosion** (accidental) (of) (with secondary fire) W4Ø.9 ☑
  - acetylene W4Ø.1 ☑
  - aerosol can W36.1 ☑
  - air tank (compressed) (in machinery) W36.2 ☑
  - aircraft (in transit) (powered) NEC V95.9 ☑
    - balloon V96.Ø5 ☑
    - fixed wing NEC (private) V95.25 ☑
      - commercial V95.35 ☑
    - glider V96.25 ☑
      - hang V96.15 ☑
      - powered V95.15 ☑
    - helicopter V95.Ø5 ☑
    - in war operations — *see* War operations, destruction of aircraft
    - microlight V95.15 ☑
    - nonpowered V96.9 ☑
      - specified NEC V96.8 ☑
    - powered NEC V95.8 ☑
    - stated as
      - homicide (attempt) YØ3.8 ☑
      - suicide (attempt) X83.Ø ☑
    - ultralight V95.15 ☑
  - anesthetic gas in operating room W4Ø.1 ☑
  - antipersonnel bomb W4Ø.8 ☑
    - assault X96.Ø ☑
    - homicide (attempt) X96.Ø ☑
    - suicide (attempt) X75 ☑
  - assault X96.9 ☑
  - bicycle tire W37.Ø ☑
  - blasting (cap) (materials) W4Ø.Ø ☑
  - boiler (machinery), not on transport vehicle W35 ☑
    - on watercraft — *see* Explosion, in, watercraft
  - butane W4Ø.1 ☑
  - caused by other person X96.9 ☑
  - coal gas W4Ø.1 ☑
  - detonator W4Ø.Ø ☑
  - dump (munitions) W4Ø.8 ☑
  - dynamite W4Ø.Ø ☑
    - in
      - assault X96.8 ☑
      - homicide (attempt) X96.8 ☑
      - legal intervention
        - injuring
          - bystander Y35.112 ☑
          - law enforcement personnel Y35.111 ☑
          - suspect Y35.113 ☑
          - unspecified person Y35.119 ☑
      - suicide (attempt) X75 ☑
  - explosive (material) W4Ø.9 ☑
    - gas W4Ø.1 ☑
    - in blasting operation W4Ø.Ø ☑
    - specified NEC W4Ø.8 ☑
      - in
        - assault X96.8 ☑
        - homicide (attempt) X96.8 ☑
        - legal intervention
          - injuring
            - bystander Y35.192 ☑
            - law enforcement personnel Y35.191 ☑
            - suspect Y35.193 ☑
- **Explosion** — *continued*
  - explosive — *continued*
    - specified — *continued*
      - in — *continued*
        - legal intervention — *continued*
          - injuring — *continued*
            - unspecified person Y35.199 ☑
        - suicide (attempt) X75 ☑
  - factory (munitions) W4Ø.8 ☑
  - fertilizer bomb W4Ø.8 ☑
    - assault X96.3 ☑
    - homicide (attempt) X96.3 ☑
    - suicide (attempt) X75 ☑
  - firearm (parts) NEC W34.19 ☑
    - airgun W34.11Ø ☑
    - BB gun W34.11Ø ☑
    - gas, air or spring-operated gun NEC W34.118 ☑
    - hangun W32.1 ☑
    - hunting rifle W33.12 ☑
    - larger firearm W33.1Ø ☑
      - specified NEC W33.19 ☑
    - machine gun W33.13 ☑
    - paintball gun W34.111 ☑
    - pellet gun W34.11Ø ☑
    - shotgun W33.11 ☑
    - Very pistol [flare] W34.19 ☑
  - fire-damp W4Ø.1 ☑
  - fireworks W39 ☑
  - gas (coal) (explosive) W4Ø.1 ☑
    - cylinder W36.9 ☑
      - aerosol can W36.1 ☑
      - air tank W36.2 ☑
      - pressurized W36.3 ☑
      - specified NEC W36.8 ☑
  - gasoline (fumes) (tank) not in moving motor vehicle W4Ø.1 ☑
    - bomb W4Ø.8 ☑
      - assault X96.1 ☑
      - homicide (attempt) X96.1 ☑
      - suicide (attempt) X75 ☑
    - in motor vehicle — *see* Accident, transport, by type of vehicle
  - grain store W4Ø.8 ☑
  - grenade W4Ø.8 ☑
    - in
      - assault X96.8 ☑
      - homicide (attempt) X96.8 ☑
      - legal intervention
        - injuring
          - bystander Y35.192 ☑
          - law enforcement personnel Y35.191 ☑
          - suspect Y35.193 ☑
          - unspecified person Y35.199 ☑
      - suicide (attempt) X75 ☑
  - handgun (parts) — *see* Explosion, firearm, hangun (parts)
  - homicide (attempt) X96.9 ☑
    - antipersonnel bomb — *see* Explosion, antipersonnel bomb
    - fertilizer bomb — *see* Explosion, fertilizer bomb
    - gasoline bomb — *see* Explosion, gasoline bomb
    - letter bomb — *see* Explosion, letter bomb
    - pipe bomb — *see* Explosion, pipe bomb
    - specified NEC X96.8 ☑
  - hose, pressurized W37.8 ☑
  - hot water heater, tank (in machinery) W35 ☑
    - on watercraft — *see* Explosion, in, watercraft
  - in, on
    - dump W4Ø.8 ☑
    - factory W4Ø.8 ☑
    - mine (of explosive gases) NEC W4Ø.1 ☑
    - watercraft V93.59 ☑
      - powered craft V93.53 ☑
        - ferry boat V93.51 ☑
        - fishing boat V93.52 ☑
        - jetskis V93.53 ☑
        - liner V93.51 ☑
        - merchant ship V93.5Ø ☑
        - passenger ship V93.51 ☑
        - sailboat V93.54 ☑
  - letter bomb W4Ø.8 ☑
    - assault X96.2 ☑
    - homicide (attempt) X96.2 ☑
    - suicide (attempt) X75 ☑
  - machinery — *see also* Contact, with, by type of machine

Exposure — *continued*
- gravitational forces (abnormal) W49.9 ☑
- heat (natural) NEC — *see* Heat
- high-pressure jet (hydraulic) (pneumatic) W49.9 ☑
- hydraulic jet W49.9 ☑
- inanimate mechanical force W49.9 ☑
- jet, high-pressure (hydraulic) (pneumatic) W49.9 ☑
- lightning — *see* subcategory T75.Ø ☑
  - causing fire — *see* Exposure, fire
- mechanical forces NEC W49.9 ☑
  - animate NEC W64 ☑
  - inanimate NEC W49.9 ☑
- noise W42.9 ☑
  - supersonic W42.Ø ☑
- noxious substance — *see* Table of Drugs and Chemicals
- pneumatic jet W49.9 ☑
- prolonged in deep-freeze unit or refrigerator W93.2 ☑
- radiation — *see* Radiation
- smoke — *see also* Exposure, fire
  - tobacco, second hand Z77.22
- specified factors NEC X58 ☑
- sunlight X32 ☑
  - man-made (sun lamp) W89.8 ☑
    - tanning bed W89.1 ☑
- supersonic waves W42.Ø ☑
- transmission line(s), electric W85 ☑
- vibration W49.9 ☑
- waves
  - infrasound W49.9 ☑
  - sound W42.9 ☑
  - supersonic W42.Ø ☑
- weather NEC — *see* Forces of nature

External cause status Y99.9
- child assisting in compensated work for family Y99.8
- civilian activity done for financial or other compensation Y99.Ø
- civilian activity done for income or pay Y99.Ø
- family member assisting in compensated work for other family member Y99.8
- hobby not done for income Y99.8
- leisure activity Y99.8
- military activity Y99.1
- off-duty activity of military personnel Y99.8
- recreation or sport not for income or while a student Y99.8
- specified NEC Y99.8
- student activity Y99.8
- volunteer activity Y99.2

F

Factors, supplemental
- alcohol
  - blood level
    - less than 2Ømg/1ØØml Y9Ø.Ø
    - presence in blood, level not specified Y9Ø.9
    - 2Ø-39mg/1ØØml Y9Ø.1
    - 4Ø-59mg/1ØØml Y9Ø.2
    - 6Ø-79mg/1ØØml Y9Ø.3
    - 8Ø-99mg/1ØØml Y9Ø.4
    - 1ØØ-119mg/1ØØml Y9Ø.5
    - 12Ø-199mg/1ØØml Y9Ø.6
    - 2ØØ-239mg/1ØØml Y9Ø.7
    - 24Ømg/1ØØml or more Y9Ø.8
  - presence in blood, but level not specified Y9Ø.9
- environmental-pollution-related condition- see Z57 ☑
- nosocomial condition Y95
- work-related condition Y99.Ø

Failure
- in suture or ligature during surgical procedure Y65.2
- mechanical, of instrument or apparatus (any) (during any medical or surgical procedure) Y65.8
- sterile precautions (during medical and surgical care) — *see* Misadventure, failure, sterile precautions, by type of procedure
- to
  - introduce tube or instrument Y65.4
    - endotracheal tube during anesthesia Y65.3
  - make curve (transport vehicle) NEC — *see* Accident, transport
  - remove tube or instrument Y65.4

Fall, falling (accidental) W19 ☑
- building W2Ø.1 ☑
  - burning (uncontrolled fire) XØØ.3 ☑
- down
  - embankment W17.81 ☑
  - escalator W1Ø.Ø ☑
  - hill W17.81 ☑
  - ladder W11 ☑
  - ramp W1Ø.2 ☑
  - stairs, steps W1Ø.9 ☑
- due to
  - bumping against
    - object W18.ØØ ☑
      - sharp glass W18.Ø2 ☑
      - specified NEC W18.Ø9 ☑
      - sports equipment W18.Ø1 ☑
    - person WØ3 ☑
      - due to ice or snow WØØ.Ø ☑
      - on pedestrian conveyance — *see* Accident, transport, pedestrian, conveyance
  - collision with another person WØ3 ☑
    - due to ice or snow WØØ.Ø ☑
    - involving pedestrian conveyance — *see* Accident, transport, pedestrian, conveyance
  - grocery cart tipping over W17.82 ☑
  - ice or snow WØØ.9 ☑
    - from one level to another WØØ.2 ☑
      - on stairs or steps WØØ.1 ☑
    - involving pedestrian conveyance — *see* Accident, transport, pedestrian, conveyance
    - on same level WØØ.Ø ☑
  - slipping (on moving sidewalk) WØ1.Ø ☑
    - with subsequent striking against object WØ1.1Ø ☑
      - furniture WØ1.19Ø ☑
      - sharp object WØ1.119 ☑
        - glass WØ1.11Ø ☑
        - power tool or machine WØ1.111 ☑
        - specified NEC WØ1.118 ☑
      - specified NEC WØ1.198 ☑
  - striking against
    - object W18.ØØ ☑
      - sharp glass W18.Ø2 ☑
      - specified NEC W18.Ø9 ☑
      - sports equipment W18.Ø1 ☑
    - person WØ3 ☑
      - due to ice or snow WØØ.Ø ☑
      - on pedestrian conveyance — *see* Accident, transport, pedestrian, conveyance
- earth (with asphyxia or suffocation (by pressure)) — *see* Earth, falling
- from, off, out of
  - aircraft NEC (with accident to aircraft NEC) V97.Ø ☑
    - while boarding or alighting V97.1 ☑
  - balcony W13.Ø ☑
  - bed WØ6 ☑
  - boat, ship, watercraft NEC (with drowning or submersion) — *see* Drowning, due to, fall overboard
    - with hitting bottom or object V94.Ø ☑
  - bridge W13.1 ☑
  - building W13.9 ☑
    - burning (uncontrolled fire) XØØ.3 ☑
  - cavity W17.2 ☑
  - chair WØ7 ☑
  - cherry picker W17.89 ☑
  - cliff W15 ☑
  - dock W17.4 ☑
  - embankment W17.81 ☑
  - escalator W1Ø.Ø ☑
  - flagpole W13.8 ☑
  - furniture NEC WØ8 ☑
  - grocery cart W17.82 ☑
  - haystack W17.89 ☑
  - high place NEC W17.89 ☑
    - stated as undetermined whether accidental or intentional Y3Ø ☑
  - hole W17.2 ☑
  - incline W1Ø.2 ☑
  - ladder W11 ☑
  - lifting device W17.89 ☑
  - machine, machinery — *see also* Contact, with, by type of machine
    - not in operation W17.89 ☑
  - manhole W17.1 ☑
  - mobile elevated work platform [MEWP] W17.89 ☑
  - motorized mobility scooter WØ5.2 ☑
  - one level to another NEC W17.89 ☑
    - intentional, purposeful, suicide (attempt) X8Ø ☑
    - stated as undetermined whether accidental or intentional Y3Ø ☑
  - pit W17.2 ☑
  - playground equipment WØ9.8 ☑
    - jungle gym WØ9.2 ☑
    - slide WØ9.Ø ☑
    - swing WØ9.1 ☑
  - quarry W17.89 ☑
  - railing W13.9 ☑
  - ramp W1Ø.2 ☑
  - roof W13.2 ☑
  - scaffolding W12 ☑
  - scooter (nonmotorized) WØ5.1 ☑
    - motorized mobility WØ5.2 ☑
  - sky lift W17.89 ☑
  - stairs, steps W1Ø.9 ☑
    - curb W1Ø.1 ☑
    - due to ice or snow WØØ.1 ☑
    - escalator W1Ø.Ø ☑
    - incline W1Ø.2 ☑
    - ramp W1Ø.2 ☑
    - sidewalk curb W1Ø.1 ☑
    - specified NEC W1Ø.8 ☑
  - standing
    - electric scooter VØØ.841 ☑
    - micro-mobility pedestrian conveyance VØØ.848 ☑
  - stepladder W11 ☑
  - stool WØ8 ☑
  - storm drain W17.1 ☑
  - streetcar NEC V82.6 ☑
    - while boarding or alighting V82.4 ☑
    - with antecedent collision — *see* Accident, transport, streetcar occupant
  - structure NEC W13.8 ☑
    - burning (uncontrolled fire) XØØ.3 ☑
  - table WØ8 ☑
  - toilet W18.11 ☑
    - with subsequent striking against object W18.12 ☑
  - train NEC V81.6 ☑
    - during derailment (without antecedent collision) V81.7 ☑
      - with antecedent collision — *see* Accident, transport, railway vehicle occupant
    - while boarding or alighting V81.4 ☑
  - transport vehicle after collision — *see* Accident, transport, by type of vehicle, collision
  - tree W14 ☑
  - vehicle (in motion) NEC — *see also* Accident, transport V89.9 ☑
    - motor NEC — *see also* Accident, transport, occupant, by type of vehicle V87.8 ☑
    - stationary W17.89 ☑
      - while boarding or alighting — *see* Accident, transport, by type of vehicle, while boarding or alighting
  - viaduct W13.8 ☑
  - wall W13.8 ☑
  - watercraft — *see also* Drowning, due to, fall overboard
    - with hitting bottom or object V94.Ø ☑
  - well W17.Ø ☑
  - wheelchair, non-moving WØ5.Ø ☑
    - powered — *see* Accident, transport, pedestrian, conveyance occupant, specified type NEC
  - window W13.4 ☑
- in, on
  - aircraft NEC V97.Ø ☑
    - while boarding or alighting V97.1 ☑
    - with accident to aircraft V97.Ø ☑
  - bathtub (empty) W18.2 ☑
    - filled W16.212 ☑
      - causing drowning W16.211 ☑
  - escalator W1Ø.Ø ☑
  - incline W1Ø.2 ☑
  - ladder W11 ☑
  - machine, machinery — *see* Contact, with, by type of machine
  - object, edged, pointed or sharp (with cut) — *see* Fall, by type
  - playground equipment WØ9.8 ☑
    - jungle gym WØ9.2 ☑

- **Forces of nature** — *continued*
  - tidal wave — *continued*
    - due to
      - earthquake X37.41 ☑
      - landslide X37.43 ☑
      - storm X37.42 ☑
      - volcanic eruption X37.41 ☑
  - tornado X37.1 ☑
  - tsunami X37.41 ☑
  - twister X37.1 ☑
  - typhoon X37.Ø ☑
  - volcanic eruption X35 ☑
- **Foreign body**
  - aspiration — *see* Index to Diseases and Injuries, Foreign body, respiratory tract
  - embedded in skin W45 ☑
  - entering through skin W45.8 ☑
    - can lid W26.8 ☑
    - nail W45.Ø ☑
    - paper W26.2 ☑
    - specified NEC W45.8 ☑
    - splinter W45.8 ☑
- **Forest fire** (exposure to) — *see* Exposure, fire, uncontrolled, not in building
- **Found injured** X58 ☑
  - from exposure (to) — *see* Exposure
  - on
    - highway, road(way), street V89.9 ☑
    - railway right of way V81.9 ☑
- **Fracture** (circumstances unknown or unspecified) X58 ☑
  - due to specified cause NEC X58 ☑
- **Freezing** — *see* Exposure, cold
- **Frostbite** X31 ☑
  - due to man-made conditions — *see* Exposure, cold, man-made
- **Frozen** — *see* Exposure, cold

G

- **Gored by bull** W55.22 ☑
- **Gunshot wound** W34.ØØ ☑

H

- **Hailstones, injured by** X39.8 ☑
- **Hanged herself or himself** — *see* Hanging, self-inflicted
- **Hanging** (accidental) — *see also* category T71 ☑
  - legal execution — *see* Legal, intervention, specified means NEC
- **Heat** (effects of) (excessive) X3Ø ☑
  - due to
    - man-made conditions W92 ☑
      - on board watercraft V93.29 ☑
        - fishing boat V93.22 ☑
        - merchant ship V93.2Ø ☑
        - passenger ship V93.21 ☑
        - sailboat V93.24 ☑
        - specified powered craft NEC V93.23 ☑
    - weather (conditions) X3Ø ☑
  - from
    - electric heating apparatus causing burning X16 ☑
    - nuclear explosion in war operations — *see* War operations, nuclear weapons
  - inappropriate in local application or packing in medical or surgical procedure Y63.5
- **Hemorrhage**
  - delayed following medical or surgical treatment without mention of misadventure — *see* Index to Diseases and Injuries, Complication(s)
  - during medical or surgical treatment as misadventure — *see* Index to Diseases and Injuries, Complication(s)
- **High**
  - altitude (effects) — *see* Air, pressure, low
  - level of radioactivity, effects — *see* Radiation
  - pressure (effects) — *see* Air, pressure, high
  - temperature, effects — *see* Heat
- **Hit, hitting** (accidental) by — *see* Struck by
- **Hitting against** — *see* Striking against
- **Homicide** (attempt) (justifiable) — *see* Assault
- **Hot**
  - place, effects — *see also* Heat
  - weather, effects X3Ø ☑
- **House fire** (uncontrolled) — *see* Exposure, fire, uncontrolled, building
- **Humidity, causing problem** X39.8 ☑
- **Hunger** X58 ☑
- **Hurricane** (any injury) X37.Ø ☑
- **Hypobarism, hypobaropathy** — *see* Air, pressure, low

I

- **Ictus**
  - caloris — *see also* Heat
  - solaris X3Ø ☑
- **Ignition** (accidental) — *see also* Exposure, fire XØ8.8 ☑
  - anesthetic gas in operating room W4Ø.1 ☑
  - apparel XØ6.2 ☑
    - from highly flammable material XØ4 ☑
    - nightwear XØ5 ☑
  - bed linen (sheets) (spreads) (pillows) (mattress) — *see* Exposure, fire, uncontrolled, building, bed
  - benzine XØ4 ☑
  - clothes, clothing NEC (from controlled fire) XØ6.2 ☑
    - from
      - highly flammable material XØ4 ☑
  - ether XØ4 ☑
    - in operating room W4Ø.1 ☑
  - explosive material — *see* Explosion
  - gasoline XØ4 ☑
  - jewelry (plastic) (any) XØ6.Ø ☑
  - kerosene XØ4 ☑
  - material
    - explosive — *see* Explosion
    - highly flammable with secondary explosion XØ4 ☑
  - nightwear XØ5 ☑
  - paraffin XØ4 ☑
  - petrol XØ4 ☑
- **Immersion** (accidental) — *see also* Drowning
  - hand or foot due to cold (excessive) X31 ☑
- **Implantation of quills of porcupine** W55.89 ☑
- **Inanition** (from) (hunger) X58 ☑
  - thirst X58 ☑
- **Inappropriate operation performed**
  - correct operation on wrong side or body part (wrong side) (wrong site) Y65.53
  - operation intended for another patient done on wrong patient Y65.52
  - wrong operation performed on correct patient Y65.51
- **Inattention after, at birth** (homicidal intent) (infanticidal intent) X58 ☑
- **Incident, adverse**
  - device
    - anesthesiology Y7Ø.8
      - accessory Y7Ø.2
      - diagnostic Y7Ø.Ø
      - miscellaneous Y7Ø.8
      - monitoring Y7Ø.Ø
      - prosthetic Y7Ø.2
      - rehabilitative Y7Ø.1
      - surgical Y7Ø.3
      - therapeutic Y7Ø.1
    - cardiovascular Y71.8
      - accessory Y71.2
      - diagnostic Y71.Ø
      - miscellaneous Y71.8
      - monitoring Y71.Ø
      - prosthetic Y71.2
      - rehabilitative Y71.1
      - surgical Y71.3
      - therapeutic Y71.1
    - gastroenterology Y73.8
      - accessory Y73.2
      - diagnostic Y73.Ø
      - miscellaneous Y73.8
      - monitoring Y73.Ø
      - prosthetic Y73.2
      - rehabilitative Y73.1
      - surgical Y73.3
      - therapeutic Y73.1
    - general
      - hospital Y74.8
        - accessory Y74.2
        - diagnostic Y74.Ø
        - miscellaneous Y74.8
        - monitoring Y74.Ø
        - prosthetic Y74.2
        - rehabilitative Y74.1
        - surgical Y74.3
        - therapeutic Y74.1
      - surgical Y81.8
        - accessory Y81.2
        - diagnostic Y81.Ø

- **Incident, adverse** — *continued*
  - device — *continued*
    - general — *continued*
      - surgical — *continued*
        - miscellaneous Y81.8
        - monitoring Y81.Ø
        - prosthetic Y81.2
        - rehabilitative Y81.1
        - surgical Y81.3
        - therapeutic Y81.1
    - gynecological Y76.8
      - accessory Y76.2
      - diagnostic Y76.Ø
      - miscellaneous Y76.8
      - monitoring Y76.Ø
      - prosthetic Y76.2
      - rehabilitative Y76.1
      - surgical Y76.3
      - therapeutic Y76.1
    - medical Y82.9
      - specified type NEC Y82.8
    - neurological Y75.8
      - accessory Y75.2
      - diagnostic Y75.Ø
      - miscellaneous Y75.8
      - monitoring Y75.Ø
      - prosthetic Y75.2
      - rehabilitative Y75.1
      - surgical Y75.3
      - therapeutic Y75.1
    - obstetrical Y76.8
      - accessory Y76.2
      - diagnostic Y76.Ø
      - miscellaneous Y76.8
      - monitoring Y76.Ø
      - prosthetic Y76.2
      - rehabilitative Y76.1
      - surgical Y76.3
      - therapeutic Y76.1
    - ophthalmic Y77.8
      - accessory Y77.2
      - contact lens (rigid gas permeable) (soft (hydrophilic)) Y77.11
      - diagnostic Y77.Ø
      - miscellaneous Y77.8
      - monitoring Y77.Ø
      - prosthetic Y77.2
      - rehabilitative Y77.19
      - surgical Y77.3
      - therapeutic Y77.19
    - orthopedic Y79.8
      - accessory Y79.2
      - diagnostic Y79.Ø
      - miscellaneous Y79.8
      - monitoring Y79.Ø
      - prosthetic Y79.2
      - rehabilitative Y79.1
      - surgical Y79.3
      - therapeutic Y79.1
    - otorhinolaryngological Y72.8
      - accessory Y72.2
      - diagnostic Y72.Ø
      - miscellaneous Y72.8
      - monitoring Y72.Ø
      - prosthetic Y72.2
      - rehabilitative Y72.1
      - surgical Y72.3
      - therapeutic Y72.1
    - personal use Y74.8
      - accessory Y74.2
      - diagnostic Y74.Ø
      - miscellaneous Y74.8
      - monitoring Y74.Ø
      - prosthetic Y74.2
      - rehabilitative Y74.1
      - surgical Y74.3
      - therapeutic Y74.1
    - physical medicine Y8Ø.8
      - accessory Y8Ø.2
      - diagnostic Y8Ø.Ø
      - miscellaneous Y8Ø.8
      - monitoring Y8Ø.Ø
      - prosthetic Y8Ø.2
      - rehabilitative Y8Ø.1
      - surgical Y8Ø.3
      - therapeutic Y8Ø.1
    - plastic surgical Y81.8
      - accessory Y81.2
      - diagnostic Y81.Ø

- **Legal** — *continued*
  - intervention — *continued*
    - cutting or piercing instrument — *see* Legal, intervention, sharp object
    - dynamite — *see* Legal, intervention, explosive, dynamite
    - electroshock device (taser)
      - injuring
        - bystander Y35.832 ☑
        - law enforcement personnel Y35.831 ☑
        - suspect Y35.833 ☑
        - unspecified person Y35.839 ☑
    - explosive(s)
      - dynamite
        - injuring
          - bystander Y35.112 ☑
          - law enforcement personnel Y35.111 ☑
          - suspect Y35.113 ☑
          - unspecified person Y35.119 ☑
      - grenade
        - injuring
          - bystander Y35.192 ☑
          - law enforcement personnel Y35.191 ☑
          - suspect Y35.193 ☑
          - unspecified person Y35.199 ☑
      - injuring
        - bystander Y35.1Ø2 ☑
        - law enforcement personnel Y35.1Ø1 ☑
        - suspect Y35.1Ø3 ☑
        - unspecified person Y35.1Ø9 ☑
      - mortar bomb
        - injuring
          - bystander Y35.192 ☑
          - law enforcement personnel Y35.191 ☑
          - suspect Y35.193 ☑
          - unspecified person Y35.199 ☑
      - shell
        - injuring
          - bystander Y35.122 ☑
          - law enforcement personnel Y35.121 ☑
          - suspect Y35.123 ☑
          - unspecified person Y35.129 ☑
      - specified NEC
        - injuring
          - bystander Y35.192 ☑
          - law enforcement personnel Y35.191 ☑
          - suspect Y35.193 ☑
          - unspecified person Y35.199 ☑
    - firearm(s) (discharge)
      - handgun
        - injuring
          - bystander Y35.Ø22 ☑
          - law enforcement personnel Y35.Ø21 ☑
          - suspect Y35.Ø23 ☑
          - unspecified person Y35.Ø29 ☑
      - injuring
        - bystander Y35.ØØ2 ☑
        - law enforcement personnel Y35.ØØ1 ☑
        - suspect Y35.ØØ3 ☑
        - unspecified person Y35.ØØ9 ☑
      - machine gun
        - injuring
          - bystander Y35.Ø12 ☑
          - law enforcement personnel Y35.Ø11 ☑
          - suspect Y35.Ø13 ☑
          - unspecified person Y35.Ø19 ☑
      - rifle pellet
        - injuring
          - bystander Y35.Ø32 ☑
          - law enforcement personnel Y35.Ø31 ☑
          - suspect Y35.Ø33 ☑
          - unspecified person Y35.Ø39 ☑
      - rubber bullet
        - injuring
          - bystander Y35.Ø42 ☑
          - law enforcement personnel Y35.Ø41 ☑
          - suspect Y35.Ø43 ☑
          - unspecified person Y35.Ø49 ☑
      - shotgun — *see* Legal, intervention, firearm, specified NEC
      - specified NEC
        - injuring
          - bystander Y35.Ø92 ☑
          - law enforcement personnel Y35.Ø91 ☑
          - suspect Y35.Ø93 ☑
          - unspecified person Y35.Ø99 ☑

- **Legal** — *continued*
  - intervention — *continued*
    - gas (asphyxiation) (poisoning)
      - injuring
        - bystander Y35.2Ø2 ☑
        - law enforcement personnel Y35.2Ø1 ☑
        - suspect Y35.2Ø3 ☑
        - unspecified person Y35.2Ø9 ☑
      - specified NEC
        - injuring
          - bystander Y35.292 ☑
          - law enforcement personnel Y35.291 ☑
          - suspect Y35.293 ☑
          - unspecified person Y35.299 ☑
      - tear gas
        - injuring
          - bystander Y35.212 ☑
          - law enforcement personnel Y35.211 ☑
          - suspect Y35.213 ☑
          - unspecified person Y35.219 ☑
    - grenade — *see* Legal, intervention, explosive, grenade
    - injuring
      - bystander Y35.92 ☑
      - law enforcement personnel Y35.91 ☑
      - suspect Y35.93 ☑
      - unspecified person Y35.99 ☑
    - late effect (of) — *see* with 7th character S Y35 ☑
    - manhandling
      - injuring
        - bystander Y35.812 ☑
        - law enforcement personnel Y35.811 ☑
        - suspect Y35.813 ☑
        - unspecified person Y35.819 ☑
    - sequelae (of) — *see* with 7th character S Y35 ☑
    - sharp objects
      - bayonet
        - injuring
          - bystander Y35.412 ☑
          - law enforcement personnel Y35.411 ☑
          - suspect Y35.413 ☑
          - unspecified person Y35.419 ☑
      - injuring
        - bystander Y35.4Ø2 ☑
        - law enforcement personnel Y35.4Ø1 ☑
        - suspect Y35.4Ø3 ☑
        - unspecified person Y35.4Ø9 ☑
      - specified NEC
        - injuring
          - bystander Y35.492 ☑
          - law enforcement personnel Y35.491 ☑
          - suspect Y35.493 ☑
          - unspecified person Y35.499 ☑
    - specified means NEC
      - injuring
        - bystander Y35.892 ☑
        - law enforcement personnel Y35.891 ☑
        - suspect Y35.893 ☑
        - unspecified person Y35.899 ☑
    - stabbing — *see* Legal, intervention, sharp object
    - stave — *see* Legal, intervention, blunt object, stave
    - stun gun
      - injuring
        - bystander Y35.832 ☑
        - law enforcement personnel Y35.831 ☑
        - suspect Y35.833 ☑
        - unspecified person Y35.839 ☑
    - taser
      - injuring
        - bystander Y35.832 ☑
        - law enforcement personnel Y35.831 ☑
        - suspect Y35.833 ☑
        - unspecified person Y35.839 ☑
    - tear gas — *see* Legal, intervention, gas, tear gas
    - truncheon — *see* Legal, intervention, blunt object, stave
- **Lifting** — *see also* Overexertion
  - heavy objects X5Ø.Ø ☑
  - weights X5Ø.Ø ☑
- **Lightning** (shock) (stroke) (struck by) — *see* subcategory T75.Ø ☑
  - causing fire — *see* Exposure, fire
- **Loss of control** (transport vehicle) NEC — *see* Accident, transport
- **Lost at sea NOS** — *see* Drowning, due to, fall overboard
- **Low**
  - pressure (effects) — *see* Air, pressure, low
  - temperature (effects) — *see* Exposure, cold
- **Lying before train, vehicle or other moving object** X81.8 ☑
  - subway train X81.1 ☑
  - train X81.1 ☑
  - undetermined whether accidental or intentional Y31 ☑
- **Lynching** — *see* Assault

M

- **Malfunction** (mechanism or component) (of)
  - firearm W34.1Ø ☑
    - airgun W34.11Ø ☑
    - BB gun W34.11Ø ☑
    - gas, air or spring-operated gun NEC W34.118 ☑
    - handgun W32.1 ☑
    - hunting rifle W33.12 ☑
    - larger firearm W33.1Ø ☑
      - specified NEC W33.19 ☑
    - machine gun W33.13 ☑
    - paintball gun W34.111 ☑
    - pellet gun W34.11Ø ☑
    - shotgun W33.11 ☑
    - specified NEC W34.19 ☑
    - Very pistol [flare] W34.19 ☑
  - handgun — *see* Malfunction, firearm, handgun
- **Maltreatment** — *see* Perpetrator
- **Mangled** (accidentally) NOS X58 ☑
- **Manhandling** (in brawl, fight) YØ4.Ø ☑
  - legal intervention — *see* Legal, intervention, manhandling
- **Manslaughter** (nonaccidental) — *see* Assault
- **Mauled by animal NEC** W55.89 ☑
- **Medical procedure, complication of** (delayed or as an abnormal reaction without mention of misadventure) — *see* Complication of or following, by specified type of procedure
  - due to or as a result of misadventure — *see* Misadventure
- **Melting** (due to fire) — *see also* Exposure, fire
  - apparel NEC XØ6.3 ☑
  - clothes, clothing NEC XØ6.3 ☑
    - nightwear XØ5 ☑
  - fittings or furniture (burning building) (uncontrolled fire) XØØ.8 ☑
  - nightwear XØ5 ☑
  - plastic jewelry XØ6.1 ☑
- **Mental cruelty** X58 ☑
- **Military operations** (injuries to military and civilians occuring during peacetime on military property and during routine military exercises and operations) (by) (from) (involving) Y37.9Ø- ☑
  - air blast Y37.2Ø- ☑
  - aircraft
    - destruction — *see* Military operations, destruction of aircraft
  - airway restriction — *see* Military operations, restriction of airways
  - asphyxiation — *see* Military operations, restriction of airways
  - biological weapons Y37.6X- ☑
  - blast Y37.2Ø- ☑
  - blast fragments Y37.2Ø- ☑
  - blast wave Y37.2Ø- ☑
  - blast wind Y37.2Ø- ☑
  - bomb Y37.2Ø- ☑
    - dirty Y37.5Ø- ☑
    - gasoline Y37.31- ☑
    - incendiary Y37.31- ☑
    - petrol Y37.31- ☑
  - bullet Y37.43- ☑
    - incendiary Y37.32- ☑
    - rubber Y37.41- ☑
  - chemical weapons Y37.7X- ☑
  - combat
    - hand to hand (unarmed) combat Y37.44- ☑
    - using blunt or piercing object Y37.45- ☑
  - conflagration — *see* Military operations, fire
  - conventional warfare NEC Y37.49- ☑
  - depth-charge Y37.Ø1- ☑
  - destruction of aircraft Y37.1Ø- ☑
    - due to
      - air to air missile Y37.11- ☑
      - collision with other aircraft Y37.12- ☑

N

O

- **Overheated** — *see* Heat
- **Overturning** (accidental)
  - machinery — *see* Contact, with, by type of machine
  - transport vehicle NEC — *see also* Accident, transport V89.9 ☑
  - watercraft (causing drowning, submersion) — *see also* Drowning, due to, accident to, watercraft, overturning
    - causing injury except drowning or submersion — *see* Accident, watercraft, causing, injury NEC

P

- **Parachute descent** (voluntary) (without accident to aircraft) V97.29 ☑
  - due to accident to aircraft — *see* Accident, transport, aircraft
- **Pecked by bird** W61.99 ☑
- **Perforation during medical or surgical treatment as misadventure** — *see* Index to Diseases and Injuries, Complication(s)
- **Perpetrator, perpetration, of assault, maltreatment and neglect** (by) YØ7.9
  - boyfriend YØ7.Ø3
  - brother YØ7.41Ø
    - stepbrother YØ7.435
  - coach YØ7.53
  - cousin
    - female YØ7.491
    - male YØ7.49Ø
  - daycare provider YØ7.519
    - at-home
      - adult care YØ7.512
      - childcare YØ7.51Ø
    - care center
      - adult care YØ7.513
      - childcare YØ7.511
  - family member NEC YØ7.499
  - father YØ7.11
    - adoptive YØ7.13
    - foster YØ7.42Ø
    - stepfather YØ7.43Ø
  - foster father YØ7.42Ø
  - foster mother YØ7.421
  - girl friend YØ7.Ø4
  - healthcare provider YØ7.529
    - mental health YØ7.521
    - specified NEC YØ7.528
  - husband YØ7.Ø1
  - instructor YØ7.53
  - mother YØ7.12
    - adoptive YØ7.14
    - foster YØ7.421
    - stepmother YØ7.433
  - multiple perpetrators YØ7.6
  - nonfamily member YØ7.5Ø
    - specified NEC YØ7.59
  - nurse YØ7.528
  - occupational therapist YØ7.528
  - partner of parent
    - female YØ7.434
    - male YØ7.432
  - physical therapist YØ7.528
  - sister YØ7.411
  - speech therapist YØ7.528
  - stepbrother YØ7.435
  - stepfather YØ7.43Ø
  - stepmother YØ7.433
  - stepsister YØ7.436
  - teacher YØ7.53
  - wife YØ7.Ø2
- **Piercing** — *see* Contact, with, by type of object or machine
- **Pinched**
  - between objects (moving) (stationary and moving) W23.Ø ☑
    - stationary W23.1 ☑
- **Pinned under machine**(ry) — *see* Contact, with, by type of machine
- **Place of occurrence** Y92.9
  - abandoned house Y92.89
  - airplane Y92.813
  - airport Y92.52Ø
  - ambulatory health services establishment NEC Y92.538
  - ambulatory surgery center Y92.53Ø
  - amusement park Y92.831
  - apartment (co-op) — *see* Place of occurrence, residence, apartment

Place of occurrence — *continued*

  - assembly hall Y92.29
  - bank Y92.51Ø
  - barn Y92.71
  - baseball field Y92.32Ø
  - basketball court Y92.31Ø
  - beach Y92.832
  - boarding house — *see* Place of occurrence, residence, boarding house
  - boat Y92.814
  - bowling alley Y92.39
  - bridge Y92.89
  - building under construction Y92.61
  - bus Y92.811
    - station Y92.521
  - cafe Y92.511
  - campsite Y92.833
  - campus — *see* Place of occurrence, school
  - canal Y92.89
  - car Y92.81Ø
  - casino Y92.59
  - children's home — *see* Place of occurrence, residence, institutional, orphanage
  - church Y92.22
  - cinema Y92.26
  - clubhouse Y92.29
  - coal pit Y92.64
  - college (community) Y92.214
  - condominium — *see* Place of occurrence, residence, apartment
  - construction area — *see* Place of occurrence, industrial and construction area
  - convalescent home — *see* Place of occurrence, residence, institutional, nursing home
  - court-house Y92.24Ø
  - cricket ground Y92.328
  - cultural building Y92.258
    - art gallery Y92.25Ø
    - museum Y92.251
    - music hall Y92.252
    - opera house Y92.253
    - specified NEC Y92.258
    - theater Y92.254
  - dancehall Y92.252
  - day nursery Y92.21Ø
  - dentist office Y92.531
  - derelict house Y92.89
  - desert Y92.82Ø
  - dockyard Y92.62
  - dock NOS Y92.89
  - doctor's office Y92.531
  - dormitory — *see* Place of occurrence, residence, institutional, school dormitory
  - dry dock Y92.62
  - factory (building) (premises) Y92.63
  - farm (land under cultivation) (outbuildings) Y92.79
    - barn Y92.71
    - chicken coop Y92.72
    - field Y92.73
    - hen house Y92.72
    - house — *see* Place of occurrence, residence, house
    - orchard Y92.74
    - specified NEC Y92.79
  - football field Y92.321
  - forest Y92.821
  - freeway Y92.411
  - gallery Y92.25Ø
  - garage (commercial) Y92.59
    - boarding house Y92.Ø44
    - military base Y92.135
    - mobile home Y92.Ø25
    - nursing home Y92.124
    - orphanage Y92.114
    - private house Y92.Ø15
    - reform school Y92.155
  - gas station Y92.524
  - gasworks Y92.69
  - golf course Y92.39
  - gravel pit Y92.64
  - grocery Y92.512
  - gymnasium Y92.39
  - handball court Y92.318
  - harbor Y92.89
  - harness racing course Y92.39
  - healthcare provider office Y92.531
  - highway Y92.41Ø
    - interstate Y92.411
  - hill Y92.828

Place of occurrence — *continued*

  - hockey rink Y92.33Ø
  - home — *see* Place of occurrence, residence
  - hospice — *see* Place of occurrence, residence, institutional, nursing home
  - hospital Y92.239
    - cafeteria Y92.233
    - corridor Y92.232
    - operating room Y92.234
    - patient
      - bathroom Y92.231
      - room Y92.23Ø
    - specified NEC Y92.238
  - hotel Y92.59
  - house — *see also* Place of occurrence, residence
    - abandoned Y92.89
    - under construction Y92.61
  - industrial and construction area (yard) Y92.69
    - building under construction Y92.61
    - dock Y92.62
    - dry dock Y92.62
    - factory Y92.63
    - gasworks Y92.69
    - mine Y92.64
    - oil rig Y92.65
    - pit Y92.64
    - power station Y92.69
    - shipyard Y92.62
    - specified NEC Y92.69
    - tunnel under construction Y92.69
    - workshop Y92.69
  - interstate Y92.411
  - kindergarten Y92.211
  - lacrosse field Y92.328
  - lake Y92.838
    - wilderness Y92.828
  - library Y92.241
  - mall Y92.59
  - market Y92.512
  - marsh Y92.828
  - military
    - base — *see* Place of occurrence, residence, institutional, military base
    - training ground Y92.84
  - mine Y92.64
  - mosque Y92.22
  - motel Y92.59
  - motorway (interstate) Y92.411
  - mountain Y92.828
  - movie-house Y92.26
  - museum Y92.251
  - music-hall Y92.252
  - not applicable Y92.9
  - nuclear power station Y92.69
  - nursing home — *see* Place of occurrence, residence, institutional, nursing home
  - office building Y92.59
  - offshore installation Y92.65
  - oil rig Y92.65
  - old people's home — *see* Place of occurrence, residence, institutional, specified NEC
  - opera-house Y92.253
  - orphanage — *see* Place of occurrence, residence, institutional, orphanage
  - outpatient surgery center Y92.53Ø
  - park (public) Y92.83Ø
    - amusement Y92.831
  - parking garage Y92.89
    - lot Y92.481
  - pavement Y92.48Ø
  - physician office Y92.531
  - polo field Y92.328
  - pond Y92.828
  - post office Y92.242
  - power station Y92.69
  - prairie Y92.828
  - prison — *see* Place of occurrence, residence, institutional, prison
  - public
    - administration building Y92.248
      - city hall Y92.243
      - courthouse Y92.24Ø
      - library Y92.241
      - post office Y92.242
      - specified NEC Y92.248
    - building NEC Y92.29
    - hall Y92.29
    - place NOS Y92.89

Place of occurrence — *continued*
- vehicle — *continued*
  - train Y92.815
  - truck Y92.812
- warehouse Y92.59
- water reservoir Y92.89
- wilderness area Y92.828
  - desert Y92.820
  - forest Y92.821
  - marsh Y92.828
  - mountain Y92.828
  - prairie Y92.828
  - specified NEC Y92.828
  - swamp Y92.828
- workshop Y92.69
- yard, private Y92.096
  - boarding house Y92.046
  - mobile home Y92.027
  - single family house Y92.017
- youth center Y92.29
- zoo (zoological garden) Y92.834

Plumbism — *see* Table of Drugs and Chemicals, lead

Poisoning (accidental) (by) — *see also* Table of Drugs and Chemicals
- by plant, thorns, spines, sharp leaves or other mechanisms NEC X58 ☑
- carbon monoxide
  - generated by
    - motor vehicle — *see* Accident, transport
    - watercraft (in transit) (not in transit) V93.89 ☑
      - ferry boat V93.81 ☑
      - fishing boat V93.82 ☑
      - jet skis V93.83 ☑
      - liner V93.81 ☑
      - merchant ship V93.80 ☑
      - passenger ship V93.81 ☑
      - powered craft NEC V93.83 ☑
- caused by injection of poisons into skin by plant thorns, spines, sharp leaves X58 ☑
  - marine or sea plants (venomous) X58 ☑
- execution — *see* Legal, intervention, gas
- intervention
  - by gas — *see* Legal, intervention, gas
  - other specified means — *see* Legal, intervention, specified means NEC
- exhaust gas
  - generated by
    - motor vehicle — *see* Accident, transport
    - watercraft (in transit) (not in transit) V93.89 ☑
      - ferry boat V93.81 ☑
      - fishing boat V93.82 ☑
      - jet skis V93.83 ☑
      - liner V93.81 ☑
      - merchant ship V93.80 ☑
      - passenger ship V93.81 ☑
      - powered craft NEC V93.83 ☑
- fumes or smoke due to
  - explosion — *see also* Explosion W40.9 ☑
  - fire — *see* Exposure, fire
  - ignition — *see* Ignition
- gas
  - in legal intervention — *see* Legal, intervention, gas
  - legal execution — *see* Legal, intervention, gas
- in war operations — *see* War operations
- legal

Powder burn (by) (from)
- airgun W34.110 ☑
- BB gun W34.110 ☑
- firearn NEC W34.19 ☑
- gas, air or spring-operated gun NEC W34.118 ☑
- handgun W32.1 ☑
- hunting rifle W33.12 ☑
- larger firearm W33.10 ☑
  - specified NEC W33.19 ☑
- machine gun W33.13 ☑
- paintball gun W34.111 ☑
- pellet gun W34.110 ☑
- shotgun W33.11 ☑
- Very pistol [flare] W34.19 ☑

Premature cessation (of) **surgical and medical care** Y66

Privation (food) (water) X58 ☑

Procedure (operation)
- correct, on wrong side or body part (wrong side) (wrong site) Y65.53
- intended for another patient done on wrong patient Y65.52
- performed on patient not scheduled for surgery Y65.52
- performed on wrong patient Y65.52
- wrong, performed on correct patient Y65.51

Prolonged
- sitting in transport vehicle — *see* Travel, by type of vehicle
- stay in
  - high altitude as cause of anoxia, barodontalgia, barotitis or hypoxia W94.11 ☑
  - weightless environment X52 ☑

Pulling, excessive — *see also* Overexertion X50.9- ☑

Puncture, puncturing — *see also* Contact, with, by type of object or machine
- by
  - plant thorns, spines, sharp leaves or other mechanisms NEC W60 ☑
- during medical or surgical treatment as misadventure — *see* Index to Diseases and Injuries, Complication(s)

Pushed, pushing (accidental) (injury in)
- by other person(s) (accidental) W51 ☑
  - as, or caused by, a crowd or human stampede (with fall) W52 ☑
  - before moving object NEC Y02.8 ☑
    - motor vehicle Y02.0 ☑
    - subway train Y02.1 ☑
    - train Y02.1 ☑
  - from
    - high place NEC
      - in accidental circumstances W17.89 ☑
      - stated as
        - intentional, homicide (attempt) Y01 ☑
        - undetermined whether accidental or intentional Y30 ☑
    - transport vehicle NEC — *see also* Accident, transport V89.9 ☑
      - stated as
        - intentional, homicide (attempt) Y08.89 ☑
  - with fall W03 ☑
    - due to ice or snow W00.0 ☑
- overexertion X50.9 ☑

R

Radiation (exposure to)
- arc lamps W89.0 ☑
- atomic power plant (malfunction) NEC W88.1 ☑
- complication of or abnormal reaction to medical radiotherapy Y84.2
- electromagnetic, ionizing W88.0 ☑
- gamma rays W88.1 ☑
- in
  - war operations (from or following nuclear explosion) — *see* War operations
- inadvertent exposure of patient (receiving test or therapy) Y63.3
- infrared (heaters and lamps) W90.1 ☑
  - excessive heat from W92 ☑
- ionized, ionizing (particles, artificially accelerated)
  - radioisotopes W88.1 ☑
  - specified NEC W88.8 ☑
  - x-rays W88.0 ☑
- isotopes, radioactive — *see* Radiation, radioactive isotopes
- laser(s) W90.2 ☑
  - in war operations — *see* War operations
  - misadventure in medical care Y63.2
- light sources (man-made visible and ultraviolet) W89.9 ☑
  - natural X32 ☑
  - specified NEC W89.8 ☑
  - tanning bed W89.1 ☑
  - welding light W89.0 ☑
- man-made visible light W89.9 ☑
  - specified NEC W89.8 ☑
  - tanning bed W89.1 ☑
  - welding light W89.0 ☑
- microwave W90.8 ☑
- misadventure in medical or surgical procedure Y63.2
- natural NEC X39.08 ☑
  - radon X39.01 ☑
- overdose (in medical or surgical procedure) Y63.2
- radar W90.0 ☑
- radioactive isotopes (any) W88.1 ☑
  - atomic power plant malfunction W88.1 ☑
  - misadventure in medical or surgical treatment Y63.2
- radiofrequency W90.0 ☑
- radium NEC W88.1 ☑
- sun X32 ☑
- ultraviolet (light) (man-made) W89.9 ☑
  - natural X32 ☑
  - specified NEC W89.8 ☑
  - tanning bed W89.1 ☑
  - welding light W89.0 ☑
- welding arc, torch, or light W89.0 ☑
  - excessive heat from W92 ☑
- x-rays (hard) (soft) W88.0 ☑

Range disease W94.11 ☑

Rape (attempted) T74.2- ☑

Rat bite W53.11 ☑

Reaching (prolonged) (static) X50.1 ☑

Reaction, abnormal to medical procedure — *see also* Complication of or following, by type of procedure Y84.9
- biologicals — *see* Table of Drugs and Chemicals
- drugs — *see* Table of Drugs and Chemicals
- vaccine — *see* Table of Drugs and Chemicals
- with misadventure — *see* Misadventure

Recoil
- airgun W34.110 ☑
- BB gun W34.110 ☑
- firearn NEC W34.19 ☑
- gas, air or spring-operated gun NEC W34.118 ☑
- handgun W32.1 ☑
- hunting rifle W33.12 ☑
- larger firearm W33.10 ☑
  - specified NEC W33.19 ☑
- machine gun W33.13 ☑
- paintball gun W34.111 ☑
- pellet W34.110 ☑
- shotgun W33.11 ☑
- Very pistol [flare] W34.19 ☑

Reduction in
- atmospheric pressure — *see* Air, pressure, change

Rock falling on or hitting (accidentally) (person) W20.8 ☑
- in cave-in W20.0 ☑

Run over (accidentally) (by)
- animal (not being ridden) NEC W55.89 ☑
- machinery — *see* Contact, with, by specified type of machine
- transport vehicle NEC — *see also* Accident, transport V09.9 ☑
  - intentional homicide (attempt) Y03.0 ☑
  - motor NEC V09.20 ☑
    - intentional homicide (attempt) Y03.0 ☑

Running
- before moving object X81.8 ☑
  - motor vehicle X81.0 ☑

Running off, away
- animal (being ridden) — *see also* Accident, transport V80.918 ☑
  - not being ridden W55.89 ☑
- animal-drawn vehicle NEC — *see also* Accident, transport V80.928 ☑
- highway, road(way), street
  - transport vehicle NEC — *see also* Accident, transport V89.9 ☑

Rupture pressurized devices — *see* Explosion, by type of device

S

Saturnism — *see* Table of Drugs and Chemicals, lead

Scald, scalding (accidental) (by) (from) (in) X19 ☑
- air (hot) X14.1 ☑
- gases (hot) X14.1 ☑
- homicide (attempt) — *see* Assault, burning, hot object
- inflicted by other person
  - stated as intentional, homicide (attempt) — *see* Assault, burning, hot object
- liquid (boiling) (hot) NEC X12 ☑
  - stated as undetermined whether accidental or intentional Y27.2 ☑
  - suicide (attempt) X77.2 ☑
- local application of externally applied substance in medical or surgical care Y63.5
- metal (molten) (liquid) (hot) NEC X18 ☑
- self-inflicted X77.9 ☑
- stated as undetermined whether accidental or intentional Y27.8 ☑

Scald, scalding — *continued*
  steam X13.1 ☑
    assault X98.Ø ☑
    stated as undetermined whether accidental or intentional Y27.Ø ☑
    suicide (attempt) X77.Ø ☑
  suicide (attempt) X77.9 ☑
  vapor (hot) X13.1 ☑
    assault X98.Ø ☑
    stated as undetermined whether accidental or intentional Y27.Ø ☑
    suicide (attempt) X77.Ø ☑
Scratched by
  cat W55.Ø3 ☑
  person(s) (accidentally) W5Ø.4 ☑
    with intent to injure or kill YØ4.Ø ☑
    as, or caused by, a crowd or human stampede (with fall) W52 ☑
    assault YØ4.Ø ☑
    homicide (attempt) YØ4.Ø ☑
    in
      fight YØ4.Ø ☑
      legal intervention
        injuring
          bystander Y35.892 ☑
          law enforcement personnel Y35.891 ☑
          suspect Y35.893 ☑
          unspecified person Y35.899 ☑
Seasickness T75.3 ☑
Self-harm NEC — *see also* External cause by type, undetermined whether accidental or intentional
  intentional — *see* Suicide
  poisoning NEC — *see* Table of Drugs and Chemicals, poisoning, accidental
Self-inflicted (injury) **NEC** — *see also* External cause by type, undetermined whether accidental or intentional
  intentional — *see* Suicide
  poisoning NEC — *see* Table of Drugs and Chemicals, poisoning, accidental
Sequelae (of)
  accident NEC — *see* WØØ-X58 with 7th character S
  assault (homicidal) (any means) — *see* X92-YØ8 with 7th character S
  homicide, attempt (any means) — *see* X92-YØ8 with 7th character S
  injury undetermined whether accidentally or purposely inflicted — *see* Y21-Y33 with 7th character S
  intentional self-harm (classifiable to X71-X83) — *see* X71-X83 with 7th character S
  legal intervention — *see* with 7th character S Y35 ☑
  motor vehicle accident — *see* VØØ-V99 with 7th character S
  suicide, attempt (any means) — *see* X71-X83 with 7th character S
  transport accident — *see* VØØ-V99 with 7th character S
  war operations — *see* War operations
Shock
  electric — *see* Exposure, electric current
  from electric appliance (any) (faulty) W86.8 ☑
    domestic W86.Ø ☑
    suicide (attempt) X83.1 ☑
Shooting, shot (accidental(ly)) — *see also* Discharge, firearm, by type
  herself or himself — *see* Discharge, firearm by type, self-inflicted
  homicide (attempt) — *see* Discharge, firearm by type, homicide
  in war operations — *see* War operations
  inflicted by other person — *see* Discharge, firearm by type, homicide
    accidental — *see* Discharge, firearm, by type of firearm
  legal
    execution — *see* Legal, intervention, firearm
    intervention — *see* Legal, intervention, firearm
  self-inflicted — *see* Discharge, firearm by type, suicide
    accidental — *see* Discharge, firearm, by type of firearm
  suicide (attempt) — *see* Discharge, firearm by type, suicide
Shoving (accidentally) **by other person** — *see* Pushed, by other person
Sickness
  alpine W94.11 ☑
  motion — *see* Motion
Sickness — *continued*
  mountain W94.11 ☑
Sinking (accidental)
  watercraft (causing drowning, submersion) — *see also* Drowning, due to, accident to, watercraft, sinking
    causing injury except drowning or submersion — *see* Accident, watercraft, causing, injury NEC
Siriasis X32 ☑
Sitting (prolonged) (static) X5Ø.1 ☑
Slashed wrists — *see* Cut, self-inflicted
Slipping (accidental) (on same level) (with fall) WØ1.Ø ☑
  on
    ice WØØ.Ø ☑
      with skates — *see* Accident, transport, pedestrian, conveyance
    mud WØ1.Ø ☑
    oil WØ1.Ø ☑
    snow WØØ.Ø ☑
      with skis — *see* Accident, transport, pedestrian, conveyance
    surface (slippery) (wet) NEC WØ1.Ø ☑
  without fall W18.4Ø ☑
    due to
      specified NEC W18.49 ☑
      stepping from one level to another W18.43 ☑
      stepping into hole or opening W18.42 ☑
      stepping on object W18.41 ☑
Sliver, wood, contact with W45.8 ☑
Smoldering (due to fire) — *see* Exposure, fire
Sodomy (attempted) **by force** T74.2 ☑
Sound waves (causing injury) W42.9 ☑
  supersonic W42.Ø ☑
Splinter, contact with W45.8 ☑
Stab, stabbing — *see* Cut
Standing (prolonged) (static) X5Ø.1 ☑
Starvation X58 ☑
Status of external cause Y99.9
  child assisting in compensated work for family Y99.8
  civilian activity done for financial or other compensation Y99.Ø
  civilian activity done for income or pay Y99.Ø
  family member assisting in compensated work for other family member Y99.8
  hobby not done for income Y99.8
  leisure activity Y99.8
  military activity Y99.1
  off-duty activity of military personnel Y99.8
  recreation or sport not for income or while a student Y99.8
  specified NEC Y99.8
  student activity Y99.8
  volunteer activity Y99.2
Stepped on
  by
    animal (not being ridden) NEC W55.89 ☑
    crowd or human stampede W52 ☑
    person W5Ø.Ø ☑
Stepping on
  object W22.8 ☑
    sports equipment W21.9 ☑
    stationary W22.Ø9 ☑
      sports equipment W21.89 ☑
    with fall W18.31 ☑
  person W51 ☑
    by crowd or human stampede W52 ☑
  sports equipment W21.9 ☑
Sting
  arthropod, nonvenomous W57 ☑
  insect, nonvenomous W57 ☑
Storm (cataclysmic) — *see* Forces of nature, cataclysmic storm
Straining, excessive — *see also* Overexertion X5Ø.9 ☑
Strangling — *see* Strangulation
Strangulation (accidental) T71 ☑
Strenuous movements — *see also* Overexertion X5Ø.9 ☑
Striking against
  airbag (automobile) W22.1Ø ☑
    driver side W22.11 ☑
    front passenger side W22.12 ☑
    specified NEC W22.19 ☑
  bottom when
    diving or jumping into water (in) W16.822 ☑
      causing drowning W16.821 ☑
      from boat W16.722 ☑
        causing drowning W16.721 ☑
Striking against — *continued*
  bottom when — *continued*
    diving or jumping into water — *continued*
      natural body W16.622 ☑
        causing drowning W16.821 ☑
      swimming pool W16.522 ☑
        causing drowning W16.521 ☑
    falling into water (in) W16.322 ☑
      causing drowning W16.321 ☑
      fountain — *see* Striking against, bottom when, falling into water, specified NEC
      natural body W16.122 ☑
        causing drowning W16.121 ☑
      reservoir — *see* Striking against, bottom when, falling into water, specified NEC
      specified NEC W16.322 ☑
        causing drowning W16.321 ☑
      swimming pool W16.Ø22 ☑
        causing drowning W16.Ø21 ☑
  diving board (swimming-pool) W21.4 ☑
  object W22.8 ☑
    caused by crowd or human stampede (with fall) W52 ☑
    furniture W22.Ø3 ☑
    lamppost W22.Ø2 ☑
    sports equipment W21.9 ☑
    stationary W22.Ø9 ☑
      sports equipment W21.89 ☑
    wall W22.Ø1 ☑
    with
      drowning or submersion — *see* Drowning
      fall — *see* Fall, due to, bumping against, object
  person(s) W51 ☑
    as, or caused by, a crowd or human stampede (with fall) W52 ☑
    assault YØ4.2 ☑
    homicide (attempt) YØ4.2 ☑
    with fall WØ3 ☑
      due to ice or snow WØØ.Ø ☑
  sports equipment W21.9 ☑
  wall (when) W22.Ø1 ☑
    diving or jumping into water (in) W16.832 ☑
      causing drowning W16.831 ☑
      swimming pool W16.532 ☑
        causing drowning W16.531 ☑
    falling into water (in) W16.332 ☑
      causing drowning W16.331 ☑
      fountain — *see* Striking against, wall when, falling into water, specified NEC
      natural body W16.132 ☑
        causing drowning W16.131 ☑
      reservoir — *see* Striking against, wall when, falling into water, specified NEC
      specified NEC W16.332 ☑
        causing drowning W16.331 ☑
      swimming pool W16.Ø32 ☑
        causing drowning W16.Ø31 ☑
    swimming pool (when) W22.Ø42 ☑
      causing drowning W22.Ø41 ☑
      diving or jumping into water W16.532 ☑
        causing drowning W16.531 ☑
      falling into water W16.Ø32 ☑
        causing drowning W16.Ø31 ☑
Struck (accidentally) **by**
  airbag (automobile) W22.1Ø ☑
    driver side W22.11 ☑
    front passenger side W22.12 ☑
    specified NEC W22.19 ☑
  alligator W58.Ø2 ☑
  animal (not being ridden) NEC W55.89 ☑
  avalanche — *see* Landslide
  ball (hit) (thrown) W21.ØØ ☑
    assault YØ8.Ø9 ☑
    baseball W21.Ø3 ☑
    basketball W21.Ø5 ☑
    football W21.Ø1 ☑
    golf ball W21.Ø4 ☑
    soccer W21.Ø2 ☑
    softball W21.Ø7 ☑
    specified NEC W21.Ø9 ☑
    volleyball W21.Ø6 ☑
  bat or racquet
    baseball bat W21.11 ☑
      assault YØ8.Ø2 ☑
    golf club W21.13 ☑
      assault YØ8.Ø9 ☑

Struck (accidentally) **by** — *continued*
- bat or racquet — *continued*
  - specified NEC W21.19 ☑
    - assault Y08.09 ☑
  - tennis racquet W21.12 ☑
    - assault Y08.09 ☑
- bullet — *see also* Discharge, firearm by type
  - in war operations — *see* War operations
- crocodile W58.12 ☑
- dog W54.1 ☑
- flare, Very pistol — *see* Discharge, firearm NEC
- hailstones X39.8 ☑
- hockey (ice)
  - field
    - puck W21.221 ☑
    - stick W21.211 ☑
  - puck W21.220 ☑
  - stick W21.210 ☑
    - assault Y08.01 ☑
- landslide — *see* Landslide
- law-enforcement agent (on duty) — *see* Legal, intervention, manhandling
  - with blunt object — *see* Legal, intervention, blunt object
- lightning T75.0 ☑
  - causing fire — *see* Exposure, fire
- machine — *see* Contact, with, by type of machine
- mammal NEC W55.89 ☑
  - marine W56.32 ☑
- marine animal W56.82 ☑
- missile
  - firearm — *see* Discharge, firearm by type
    - in war operations — *see* War operations, missile
- object W22.8 ☑
  - blunt W22.8 ☑
    - assault Y00 ☑
    - suicide (attempt) X79 ☑
    - undetermined whether accidental or intentional Y29 ☑
  - falling W20.8 ☑
    - from, in, on
      - building W20.1 ☑
        - burning (uncontrolled fire) X00.4 ☑
      - cataclysmic
        - earth surface movement NEC — *see* Landslide
        - storm — *see* Forces of nature, cataclysmic storm
      - cave-in W20.0 ☑
      - earthquake X34 ☑
      - machine (in operation) — *see* Contact, with, by type of machine
      - structure W20.1 ☑
        - burning X00.4 ☑
      - transport vehicle (in motion) — *see* Accident, transport, by type of vehicle
      - watercraft V93.49 ☑
        - due to
          - accident to craft V91.39 ☑
            - powered craft V91.33 ☑
              - ferry boat V91.31 ☑
              - fishing boat V91.32 ☑
              - jetskis V91.33 ☑
              - liner V91.31 ☑
              - merchant ship V91.30 ☑
              - passenger ship V91.31 ☑
            - unpowered craft V91.38 ☑
              - canoe V91.35 ☑
              - inflatable V91.36 ☑
              - kayak V91.35 ☑
              - sailboat V91.34 ☑
              - surf-board V91.38 ☑
              - windsurfer V91.38 ☑
        - powered craft V93.43 ☑
          - ferry boat V93.41 ☑
          - fishing boat V93.42 ☑
          - jetskis V93.43 ☑
          - liner V93.41 ☑
          - merchant ship V93.40 ☑
          - passenger ship V93.41 ☑
        - unpowered craft V93.48 ☑
          - sailboat V93.44 ☑
          - surf-board V93.48 ☑
          - windsurfer V93.48 ☑
  - moving NEC W20.8 ☑
  - projected W20.8 ☑

Struck (accidentally) **by** — *continued*
- object — *continued*
  - projected — *continued*
    - assault Y00 ☑
    - in sports W21.9 ☑
      - assault Y08.09 ☑
      - ball W21.00 ☑
        - baseball W21.03 ☑
        - basketball W21.05 ☑
        - football W21.01 ☑
        - golf ball W21.04 ☑
        - soccer W21.02 ☑
        - softball W21.07 ☑
        - specified NEC W21.09 ☑
        - volleyball W21.06 ☑
      - bat or racquet
        - baseball bat W21.11 ☑
          - assault Y08.02 ☑
        - golf club W21.13 ☑
          - assault Y08.09 ☑
        - specified NEC W21.19 ☑
          - assault Y08.09 ☑
        - tennis racquet W21.12 ☑
          - assault Y08.09 ☑
      - hockey (ice)
        - field
          - puck W21.221 ☑
          - stick W21.211 ☑
        - puck W21.220 ☑
        - stick W21.210 ☑
          - assault Y08.01 ☑
      - specified NEC W21.89 ☑
  - set in motion by explosion — *see* Explosion
  - thrown W20.8 ☑
    - assault Y00 ☑
    - in sports W21.9 ☑
      - assault Y08.09 ☑
      - ball W21.00 ☑
        - baseball W21.03 ☑
        - basketball W21.05 ☑
        - football W21.01 ☑
        - golf ball W21.04 ☑
        - soccer W21.02 ☑
        - soft ball W21.07 ☑
        - specified NEC W21.09 ☑
        - volleyball W21.06 ☑
      - bat or racquet
        - baseball bat W21.11 ☑
          - assault Y08.02 ☑
        - golf club W21.13 ☑
          - assault Y08.09 ☑
        - specified NEC W21.19 ☑
          - assault Y08.09 ☑
        - tennis racquet W21.12 ☑
          - assault Y08.09 ☑
      - hockey (ice)
        - field
          - puck W21.221 ☑
          - stick W21.211 ☑
        - puck W21.220 ☑
        - stick W21.210 ☑
          - assault Y08.01 ☑
      - specified NEC W21.89 ☑
- other person(s) W50.0 ☑
  - with
    - blunt object W22.8 ☑
      - intentional, homicide (attempt) Y00 ☑
      - sports equipment W21.9 ☑
      - undetermined whether accidental or intentional Y29 ☑
  - fall W03 ☑
    - due to ice or snow W00.0 ☑
  - as, or caused by, a crowd or human stampede (with fall) W52 ☑
  - assault Y04.2 ☑
  - homicide (attempt) Y04.2 ☑
  - in legal intervention
    - injuring
      - bystander Y35.812 ☑
      - law enforcement personnel Y35.811 ☑
      - suspect Y35.813 ☑
      - unspecified person Y35.819 ☑
  - sports equipment W21.9 ☑
- police (on duty) — *see* Legal, intervention, manhandling

Struck (accidentally) **by** — *continued*
- police — *see* Legal, intervention, manhandling — *continued*
  - with blunt object — *see* Legal, intervention, blunt object
- sports equipment W21.9 ☑
  - assault Y08.09 ☑
  - ball W21.00 ☑
    - baseball W21.03 ☑
    - basketball W21.05 ☑
    - football W21.01 ☑
    - golf ball W21.04 ☑
    - soccer W21.02 ☑
    - soft ball W21.07 ☑
    - specified NEC W21.09 ☑
    - volleyball W21.06 ☑
  - bat or racquet
    - baseball bat W21.11 ☑
      - assault Y08.02 ☑
    - golf club W21.13 ☑
      - assault Y08.09 ☑
    - specified NEC W21.19 ☑
      - assault Y08.09 ☑
    - tennis racquet W21.12 ☑
      - assault Y08.09 ☑
  - cleats (shoe) W21.31 ☑
  - foot wear NEC W21.39 ☑
  - football helmet W21.81 ☑
  - hockey (ice)
    - field
      - puck W21.221 ☑
      - stick W21.211 ☑
    - puck W21.220 ☑
    - stick W21.210 ☑
      - assault Y08.01 ☑
  - skate blades W21.32 ☑
  - specified NEC W21.89 ☑
    - assault Y08.09 ☑
- thunderbolt — *see* subcategory T75.0 ☑
  - causing fire — *see* Exposure, fire
- transport vehicle NEC — *see also* Accident, transport V09.9 ☑
  - intentional, homicide (attempt) Y03.0 ☑
  - motor NEC — *see also* Accident, transport V09.20 ☑
    - homicide Y03.0 ☑
- vehicle (transport) NEC — *see* Accident, transport, by type of vehicle
  - stationary (falling from jack, hydraulic lift, ramp) W20.8 ☑

Stumbling
- over
  - animal NEC W01.0 ☑
    - with fall W18.09 ☑
  - carpet, rug or (small) object W22.8 ☑
    - with fall W18.09 ☑
  - person W51 ☑
    - with fall W03 ☑
      - due to ice or snow W00.0 ☑
- without fall W18.40 ☑
  - due to
    - specified NEC W18.49 ☑
    - stepping from one level to another W18.43 ☑
    - stepping into hole or opening W18.42 ☑
    - stepping on object W18.41 ☑

Submersion (accidental) — *see* Drowning

Suffocation (accidental) (by external means) (by pressure) (mechanical) — *see also* category T71 ☑
- due to, by
  - avalanche — *see* Landslide
  - explosion — *see* Explosion
  - fire — *see* Exposure, fire
  - food, any type (aspiration) (ingestion) (inhalation) — *see* categories T17 and T18 ☑
  - ignition — *see* Ignition
  - landslide — *see* Landslide
  - machine(ry) — *see* Contact, with, by type of machine
  - vomitus (aspiration) (inhalation) T17.81- ☑
- in
  - burning building X00.8 ☑

Suicide, suicidal (attempted) (by) X83.8 ☑
- blunt object X79 ☑
- burning, burns X76 ☑
  - hot object X77.9 ☑
    - fluid NEC X77.2 ☑
    - household appliance X77.3 ☑
    - specified NEC X77.8 ☑

- **War operations** — *continued*
  - aircraft
    - destruction — *see* War operations, destruction of aircraft
  - airway restriction — *see* War operations, restriction of airways
  - asphyxiation — *see* War operations, restriction of airways
  - biological weapons Y36.6X- ☑
  - blast Y36.20- ☑
  - blast fragments Y36.20- ☑
  - blast wave Y36.20- ☑
  - blast wind Y36.20- ☑
  - bomb Y36.20- ☑
    - dirty Y36.50- ☑
    - gasoline Y36.31- ☑
    - incendiary Y36.31- ☑
    - petrol Y36.31- ☑
  - bullet Y36.43- ☑
    - incendiary Y36.32- ☑
    - rubber Y36.41- ☑
  - chemical weapons Y36.7X- ☑
  - combat
    - hand to hand (unarmed) combat Y36.44- ☑
    - using blunt or piercing object Y36.45- ☑
  - conflagration — *see* War operations, fire
  - conventional warfare NEC Y36.49- ☑
  - depth-charge Y36.01- ☑
  - destruction of aircraft Y36.10- ☑
    - due to
      - air to air missile Y36.11- ☑
      - collision with other aircraft Y36.12- ☑
      - detonation (accidental) of onboard munitions and explosives Y36.14- ☑
      - enemy fire or explosives Y36.11- ☑
      - explosive placed on aircraft Y36.11- ☑
      - onboard fire Y36.13- ☑
      - rocket propelled grenade [RPG] Y36.11- ☑
      - small arms fire Y36.11- ☑
      - surface to air missile Y36.11- ☑
    - specified NEC Y36.19- ☑
  - detonation (accidental) of
    - onboard marine weapons Y36.05- ☑
    - own munitions or munitions launch device Y36.24- ☑
  - dirty bomb Y36.50- ☑
  - explosion (of) Y36.20- ☑
    - aerial bomb Y36.21- ☑
    - after cessation of hostilities
      - bomb placed during war operations Y36.82- ☑
      - mine placed during war operations Y36.81- ☑

- **War operations** — *continued*
  - explosion — *continued*
    - bomb NOS — *see also* War operations, bomb(s) Y36.20- ☑
    - fragments Y36.20- ☑
    - grenade Y36.29- ☑
    - guided missile Y36.22- ☑
    - improvised explosive device [IED] (person-borne) (roadside) (vehicle-borne) Y36.23- ☑
    - land mine Y36.29- ☑
    - marine mine (at sea) (in harbor) Y36.02- ☑
    - marine weapon Y36.00- ☑
      - specified NEC Y36.09- ☑
    - own munitions or munitions launch device (accidental) Y36.24- ☑
    - sea-based artillery shell Y36.03- ☑
    - specified NEC Y36.29- ☑
    - torpedo Y36.04- ☑
  - fire Y36.30- ☑
    - specified NEC Y36.39- ☑
  - firearms
    - discharge Y36.43- ☑
    - pellets Y36.42- ☑
  - flamethrower Y36.33- ☑
  - fragments (from) (of)
    - improvised explosive device [IED] (person-borne) (roadside) (vehicle-borne) Y36.26- ☑
    - munitions Y36.25- ☑
    - specified NEC Y36.29- ☑
    - weapons Y36.27- ☑
  - friendly fire Y36.92 ☑
  - hand to hand (unarmed) combat Y36.44- ☑
  - hot substances — *see* War operations, fire
  - incendiary bullet Y36.32- ☑
  - nuclear weapon (effects of) Y36.50- ☑
    - acute radiation exposure Y36.54- ☑
    - blast pressure Y36.51- ☑
    - direct blast Y36.51- ☑
    - direct heat Y36.53- ☑
    - fallout exposure Y36.54- ☑
    - fireball Y36.53- ☑
    - indirect blast (struck or crushed by blast debris) (being thrown by blast) Y36.52- ☑
    - ionizing radiation (immediate exposure) Y36.54- ☑
    - nuclear radiation Y36.54- ☑
    - radiation
      - ionizing (immediate exposure) Y36.54- ☑
      - nuclear Y36.54- ☑
      - thermal Y36.53- ☑
    - secondary effects Y36.54- ☑

- **War operations** — *continued*
  - nuclear weapon — *continued*
    - specified NEC Y36.59- ☑
    - thermal radiation Y36.53- ☑
  - restriction of air (airway)
    - intentional Y36.46- ☑
    - unintentional Y36.47- ☑
  - rubber bullets Y36.41- ☑
  - shrapnel NOS Y36.29- ☑
  - suffocation — *see* War operations, restriction of airways
  - unconventional warfare NEC Y36.7X- ☑
  - underwater blast NOS Y36.00- ☑
  - warfare
    - conventional NEC Y36.49- ☑
    - unconventional NEC Y36.7X- ☑
  - weapon of mass destruction [WMD] Y36.91 ☑
  - weapons
    - biological weapons Y36.6X- ☑
    - chemical Y36.7X- ☑
    - nuclear (effects of) Y36.50- ☑
      - acute radiation exposure Y36.54- ☑
      - blast pressure Y36.51- ☑
      - direct blast Y36.51- ☑
      - direct heat Y36.53- ☑
      - fallout exposure Y36.54- ☑
      - fireball Y36.53- ☑
      - radiation
        - ionizing (immediate exposure) Y36.54- ☑
        - nuclear Y36.54- ☑
        - thermal Y36.53- ☑
      - secondary effects Y36.54- ☑
      - specified NEC Y36.59- ☑
    - of mass destruction [WMD] Y36.91 ☑
- **Washed**
  - away by flood — *see* Flood
  - off road by storm (transport vehicle) — *see* Forces of nature, cataclysmic storm
- **Weather exposure NEC** — *see* Forces of nature
- **Weightlessness** (causing injury) (effects of) (in spacecraft, real or simulated) X52 ☑
- **Work related condition** Y99.0
- **Wound** (accidental) NEC — *see also* Injury X58 ☑
  - battle — *see also* War operations Y36.90 ☑
  - gunshot — *see* Discharge, firearm by type
- **Wreck transport vehicle NEC** — *see also* Accident, transport V89.9 ☑
- **Wrong**
  - device implanted into correct surgical site Y65.51
  - fluid in infusion Y65.1
  - patient, procedure performed on Y65.52
  - procedure (operation) on correct patient Y65.51

ICD-10-CM Tabular List of Diseases and Injuries

Chapter 1. Certain Infectious and Parasitic Diseases (AØØ–B99)

Chapter-specific Guidelines with Coding Examples

The chapter-specific guidelines from the ICD-10-CM Official Guidelines for Coding and Reporting have been provided below. Along with these guidelines are coding examples, contained in the shaded boxes, that have been developed to help illustrate the coding and/or sequencing guidance found in these guidelines.

a. Human immunodeficiency virus (HIV) infections

1) Code only confirmed cases

Code only confirmed cases of HIV infection/illness. This is an exception to the hospital inpatient guideline Section II, H.

In this context, "confirmation" does not require documentation of positive serology or culture for HIV; the provider's diagnostic statement that the patient is HIV positive or has an HIV-related illness is sufficient.

Patient admitted with anemia with possible HIV infection

D64.9	**Anemia, unspecified**

Explanation: Only the anemia is coded in this scenario because it has not been confirmed that an HIV infection is present. This is an exception to the guideline Section II, H for hospital inpatient coding.

2) Selection and sequencing of HIV codes

(a) Patient admitted for HIV-related condition

If a patient is admitted for an HIV-related condition, the principal diagnosis should be B2Ø, Human immunodeficiency virus [HIV] disease followed by additional diagnosis codes for all reported HIV-related conditions.

An exception to this guideline is if the reason for admission is hemolytic-uremic syndrome associated with HIV disease. Assign code D59.31, Infection-associated hemolytic-uremic syndrome, followed by code B2Ø, Human immunodeficiency virus [HIV] disease.

(b) Patient with HIV disease admitted for unrelated condition

If a patient with HIV disease is admitted for an unrelated condition (such as a traumatic injury), the code for the unrelated condition (e.g., the nature of injury code) should be the principal diagnosis. Other diagnoses would be B2Ø followed by additional diagnosis codes for all reported HIV-related conditions.

Unstable angina, native coronary artery atherosclerosis, HIV

I25.11Ø	**Atherosclerotic heart disease of native coronary artery with unstable angina pectoris**
B2Ø	**Human immunodeficiency virus [HIV] disease**

Explanation: The arteriosclerotic coronary artery disease and the unstable angina are not related to HIV, so those conditions are reported first using a combination code, and HIV is reported secondarily.

(c) Whether the patient is newly diagnosed

Whether the patient is newly diagnosed or has had previous admissions/encounters for HIV conditions is irrelevant to the sequencing decision.

(d) Asymptomatic human immunodeficiency virus

Z21, Asymptomatic human immunodeficiency virus [HIV] infection status, is to be applied when the patient without any documentation of symptoms is listed as being "HIV positive," "known HIV," "HIV test positive," or similar terminology. Do not use this code if the term "AIDS" or "HIV disease" is used or if the patient is treated for any HIV-related illness or is described as having any condition(s) resulting from his/her HIV positive status; use B2Ø in these cases.

(e) Patients with inconclusive HIV serology

Patients with inconclusive HIV serology, but no definitive diagnosis or manifestations of the illness, may be assigned code R75, Inconclusive laboratory evidence of human immunodeficiency virus [HIV].

(f) Previously diagnosed HIV-related illness

Patients with any known prior diagnosis of an HIV-related illness should be coded to B2Ø. Once a patient has developed an HIV-related illness, the patient should always be assigned code B2Ø on every subsequent admission/encounter. Patients previously diagnosed with any HIV illness (B2Ø) should never be assigned to R75 or Z21, Asymptomatic human immunodeficiency virus [HIV] infection status.

(g) HIV infection in pregnancy, childbirth and the puerperium

During pregnancy, childbirth or the puerperium, a patient admitted (or presenting for a health care encounter) because of an HIV-related illness should receive a principal diagnosis code of O98.7-, Human immunodeficiency [HIV] disease complicating pregnancy, childbirth and the puerperium, followed by B2Ø and the code(s) for the HIV-related illness(es). Codes from Chapter 15 always take sequencing priority.

Patients with asymptomatic HIV infection status admitted (or presenting for a health care encounter) during pregnancy, childbirth, or the puerperium should receive codes of O98.7- and Z21.

(h) Encounters for testing for HIV

If a patient is being seen to determine his/her HIV status, use code Z11.4, Encounter for screening for human immunodeficiency virus [HIV]. Use additional codes for any associated high-risk behavior, if applicable.

If a patient with signs or symptoms is being seen for HIV testing, code the signs and symptoms. An additional counseling code Z71.7, Human immunodeficiency virus [HIV] counseling, may be used if counseling is provided during the encounter for the test.

When a patient returns to be informed of his/her HIV test results and the test result is negative, use code Z71.7, Human immunodeficiency virus [HIV] counseling.

If the results are positive, see previous guidelines and assign codes as appropriate.

(i) HIV managed by antiretroviral medication

If a patient with documented HIV disease, **HIV-related illness or AIDS** is currently managed on antiretroviral medications, assign code B2Ø, Human immunodeficiency virus [HIV] disease. Code Z79.899, Other long term (current) drug therapy, may be assigned as an additional code to identify the long-term (current) use of antiretroviral medications.

b. Infectious agents as the cause of diseases classified to other chapters

Certain infections are classified in chapters other than Chapter 1 and no organism is identified as part of the infection code. In these instances, it is necessary to use an additional code from Chapter 1 to identify the organism. A code from category B95, Streptococcus, Staphylococcus, and Enterococcus as the cause of diseases classified to other chapters, B96, Other bacterial agents as the cause of diseases classified to other chapters, or B97, Viral agents as the cause of diseases classified to other chapters, is to be used as an additional code to identify the organism. An instructional note will be found at the infection code advising that an additional organism code is required.

c. Infections resistant to antibiotics

Many bacterial infections are resistant to current antibiotics. It is necessary to identify all infections documented as antibiotic resistant. Assign a code from category Z16, Resistance to antimicrobial drugs, following the infection code only if the infection code does not identify drug resistance.

d. Sepsis, severe sepsis, and septic shock

1) Coding of sepsis and severe sepsis

(a) Sepsis

For a diagnosis of sepsis, assign the appropriate code for the underlying systemic infection. If the type of infection or causal organism is not further specified, assign code A41.9, Sepsis, unspecified organism.

A code from subcategory R65.2, Severe sepsis, should not be assigned unless severe sepsis or an associated acute organ dysfunction is documented.

(i) Negative or inconclusive blood cultures and sepsis

Negative or inconclusive blood cultures do not preclude a diagnosis of sepsis in patients with clinical evidence of the condition; however, the provider should be queried.

(ii) Urosepsis

The term urosepsis is a nonspecific term. It is not to be considered synonymous with sepsis. It has no default code in the Alphabetic Index. Should a provider use this term, he/she must be queried for clarification.

(iii) Sepsis with organ dysfunction

If a patient has sepsis and associated acute organ dysfunction or multiple organ dysfunction (MOD), follow the instructions for coding severe sepsis.

(iv) Acute organ dysfunction that is not clearly associated with the sepsis

If a patient has sepsis and an acute organ dysfunction, but the medical record documentation indicates that the acute organ dysfunction is related to a medical condition other than the sepsis, do not assign a code from subcategory R65.2, Severe sepsis. An acute organ dysfunction must be associated with the sepsis in order to assign the severe sepsis code. If the documentation is not clear as to whether an acute organ dysfunction is related to the sepsis or another medical condition, query the provider.

Sepsis and acute respiratory failure due to COPD exacerbation

A41.9	**Sepsis, unspecified organism**
J44.1	**Chronic obstructive pulmonary disease with (acute) exacerbation**
J96.ØØ	**Acute respiratory failure, unspecified whether with hypoxia or hypercapnia**

Explanation: Although acute organ dysfunction is present in the form of acute respiratory failure, severe sepsis (R65.2) is not coded in this example, as the acute respiratory failure is attributed to the COPD exacerbation rather than the sepsis. Sequencing of these codes would be determined by the circumstances of the admission.

(b) Severe sepsis

The coding of severe sepsis requires a minimum of 2 codes: first a code for the underlying systemic infection, followed by a code from subcategory R65.2, Severe sepsis. If the causal organism is not documented, assign code A41.9, Sepsis, unspecified organism, for the infection. Additional code(s) for the associated acute organ dysfunction are also required.

Due to the complex nature of severe sepsis, some cases may require querying the provider prior to assignment of the codes.

2) Septic shock

Septic shock generally refers to circulatory failure associated with severe sepsis, and therefore, it represents a type of acute organ dysfunction.

For cases of septic shock, the code for the systemic infection should be sequenced first, followed by code R65.21, Severe sepsis with septic shock or code T81.12, Postprocedural septic shock. Any additional codes for the other acute organ dysfunctions should also be assigned. As noted in the sequencing instructions in the Tabular List, the code for septic shock cannot be assigned as a principal diagnosis.

Sepsis with septic shock

A41.9	**Sepsis, unspecified organism**
R65.21	**Severe sepsis with septic shock**

Explanation: Documentation of septic shock automatically implies severe sepsis as it is a form of acute organ dysfunction. Septic shock is not coded as the principal diagnosis; it is always preceded by the code for the systemic infection.

3) Sequencing of severe sepsis

If severe sepsis is present on admission, and meets the definition of principal diagnosis, the underlying systemic infection should be assigned as principal diagnosis followed by the appropriate code from subcategory R65.2 as required by the sequencing rules in the Tabular List. A code from subcategory R65.2 can never be assigned as a principal diagnosis.

When severe sepsis develops during an encounter (it was not present on admission), the underlying systemic infection and the appropriate code from subcategory R65.2 should be assigned as secondary diagnoses.

Severe sepsis may be present on admission, but the diagnosis may not be confirmed until sometime after admission. If the documentation is not clear whether severe sepsis was present on admission, the provider should be queried.

For infection-associated hemolytic-uremic syndrome with severe sepsis, see guideline I.C.1.d.9.

4) Sepsis or severe sepsis with a localized infection

If the reason for admission is sepsis or severe sepsis and a localized infection, such as pneumonia or cellulitis, a code(s) for the underlying systemic infection should be assigned first and the code for the localized infection should be assigned as a secondary diagnosis. If the patient has severe sepsis, a code from subcategory R65.2 should also be assigned as a secondary diagnosis. If the patient is admitted with a localized infection, such as pneumonia, and sepsis/severe sepsis doesn't develop until after admission, the localized infection should be assigned first, followed by the appropriate sepsis/severe sepsis codes.

For hemolytic-uremic syndrome associated with sepsis, see guideline I.C.1.d.9.

Patient presents with acute renal failure due to severe sepsis from *Pseudomonas* pneumonia

A41.52	**Sepsis due to Pseudomonas**
J15.1	**Pneumonia due to Pseudomonas**
R65.2Ø	**Severe sepsis without septic shock**
N17.9	**Acute kidney failure, unspecified**

Explanation: If all conditions are present on admission, the systemic infection (sepsis) is sequenced first followed by the codes for the localized infection (pneumonia), severe sepsis and any organ dysfunction. If only the pneumonia was present on admission with the sepsis and resulting renal failure developing later in the admission, then the pneumonia would be sequenced first.

5) Sepsis due to a postprocedural infection

(a) Documentation of causal relationship

As with all postprocedural complications, code assignment is based on the provider's documentation of the relationship between the infection and the procedure.

(b) Sepsis due to a postprocedural infection

For infections following a procedure, a code from T81.4Ø, to T81.43 Infection following a procedure, or a code from O86.ØØ to O86.Ø3, Infection of obstetric surgical wound, that identifies the site of the infection should be coded first, if known. Assign an additional code for sepsis following a procedure (T81.44) or sepsis following an obstetrical procedure (O86.Ø4). Use an additional code to identify the infectious agent. If the patient has severe sepsis, the appropriate code from subcategory R65.2 should also be assigned with the additional code(s) for any acute organ dysfunction.

For infections following infusion, transfusion, therapeutic injection, or immunization, a code from subcategory T8Ø.2, Infections following infusion, transfusion, and therapeutic injection, or code T88.Ø-, Infection following immunization, should be coded first, followed by the code for the specific infection. If the patient has severe sepsis, the appropriate code from subcategory R65.2 should also be assigned, with the additional codes(s) for any acute organ dysfunction.

(c) Postprocedural infection and postprocedural septic shock

If a postprocedural infection has resulted in postprocedural septic shock, assign the codes indicated above for sepsis due to a postprocedural infection, followed by code T81.12-, Postprocedural septic shock. Do not assign code R65.21, Severe sepsis with septic shock. Additional code(s) should be assigned for any acute organ dysfunction.

Septic shock following abdominal procedure with intramuscular abscess

T81.42XA	**Infection following a procedure, deep incisional surgical site, initial encounter**
T81.44XA	**Sepsis following a procedure, initial encounter**
A41.9	**Sepsis, unspecified organism**
T81.12XA	**Postprocedural septic shock, initial encounter**

Explanation: The first code reported identifies the site of the postprocedural infection with intramuscular abscess coded to "deep incisional surgical site." If sepsis occurred as a result of the postprocedural infection, code T81.44- should be coded as a secondary diagnosis, followed by a code for the specific type of sepsis. Postprocedural septic shock is captured by code T81.12- and not with code R65.21. If any other acute organ dysfunction was documented as associated with the postprocedural sepsis, additional codes could be assigned to represent those conditions.

6) Sepsis and severe sepsis associated with a noninfectious process (condition)

In some cases, a noninfectious process (condition) such as trauma, may lead to an infection which can result in sepsis or severe sepsis. If sepsis or severe sepsis is documented as associated with a noninfectious condition, such as a burn or serious injury, and this condition meets the definition for principal diagnosis, the code for the noninfectious condition should be sequenced first, followed by the code for the resulting infection. If severe sepsis is present, a code from subcategory R65.2 should also be assigned with any associated organ dysfunction(s) codes. It is not necessary to assign a code from subcategory R65.1, Systemic inflammatory response syndrome (SIRS) of non-infectious origin, for these cases.

If the infection meets the definition of principal diagnosis, it should be sequenced before the non-infectious condition. When both the associated non-infectious condition and the infection meet the definition of principal diagnosis, either may be assigned as principal diagnosis.

Only one code from category R65, Symptoms and signs specifically associated with systemic inflammation and infection, should be assigned. Therefore, when a non-infectious condition leads to an infection resulting in severe sepsis, assign the appropriate code from subcategory R65.2, Severe sepsis. Do not additionally assign a code from subcategory R65.1, Systemic inflammatory response syndrome (SIRS) of non-infectious origin.

See Section I.C.18. SIRS due to non-infectious process.

Patient admitted with multiple third-degree burns of right upper arm develops severe MSSA sepsis with septic shock, three days into admission

T22.391A Burn of third degree of multiple sites of right shoulder and upper arm limb, except wrist and hand, initial encounter

A41.Ø1 Sepsis due to Methicillin susceptible Staphylococcus aureus

R65.21 Severe sepsis with septic shock

Explanation: Severe sepsis is coded rather than SIRS from R65 because it is documented as a severe systemic infectious response with septic shock to a noninfectious condition. The code for the systemic infection is not used as the principal diagnosis because it was not present on admission. The patient was admitted for the burn injury.

7) Sepsis and septic shock complicating abortion, pregnancy, childbirth, and the puerperium

See Section I.C.15. Sepsis and septic shock complicating abortion, pregnancy, childbirth and the puerperium

8) Newborn sepsis

See Section I.C.16. f. Bacterial sepsis of Newborn

9) Hemolytic-uremic syndrome associated with sepsis

If the reason for admission is hemolytic-uremic syndrome that is associated with sepsis, assign code D59.31, Infection-associated hemolytic-uremic syndrome, as the principal diagnosis. Codes for the underlying systemic infection and any other conditions (such as severe sepsis) should be assigned as secondary diagnoses.

e. Methicillin resistant Staphylococcus aureus (MRSA) conditions

1) Selection and sequencing of MRSA codes

(a) Combination codes for MRSA infection

When a patient is diagnosed with an infection that is due to methicillin resistant *Staphylococcus aureus* (MRSA), and that infection has a combination code that includes the causal organism (e.g., sepsis, pneumonia) assign the appropriate combination code for the condition (e.g., code A41.Ø2, Sepsis due to Methicillin resistant Staphylococcus aureus or code J15.212, Pneumonia due to Methicillin resistant Staphylococcus aureus). Do not assign code B95.62, Methicillin resistant Staphylococcus aureus infection as the cause of diseases classified elsewhere, as an additional code, because the combination code includes the type of infection and the MRSA organism. Do not assign a code from subcategory Z16.11, Resistance to penicillins, as an additional diagnosis.

See Section C.1. for instructions on coding and sequencing of sepsis and severe sepsis.

(b) Other codes for MRSA infection

When there is documentation of a current infection (e.g., wound infection, stitch abscess, urinary tract infection) due to MRSA, and that infection does not have a combination code that includes the causal organism, assign the appropriate code to identify the condition along with code B95.62, Methicillin resistant Staphylococcus aureus infection as the cause of diseases classified elsewhere for the MRSA infection. Do not assign a code from subcategory Z16.11, Resistance to penicillins.

(c) Methicillin susceptible Staphylococcus aureus (MSSA) and MRSA colonization

The condition or state of being colonized or carrying MSSA or MRSA is called colonization or carriage, while an individual person is described as being colonized or being a carrier.

Colonization means that MSSA or MSRA is present on or in the body without necessarily causing illness. A positive MRSA colonization test might be documented by the provider as "MRSA screen positive" or "MRSA nasal swab positive".

Assign code Z22.322, Carrier or suspected carrier of Methicillin resistant Staphylococcus aureus, for patients documented as having MRSA colonization. Assign code Z22.321, Carrier or suspected carrier of Methicillin susceptible Staphylococcus aureus, for patients documented as having MSSA colonization. Colonization is not necessarily indicative of a disease process or as the cause of a specific condition the patient may have unless documented as such by the provider.

(d) MRSA colonization and infection

If a patient is documented as having both MRSA colonization and infection during a hospital admission, code Z22.322, Carrier or suspected carrier of Methicillin resistant Staphylococcus aureus, and a code for the MRSA infection may both be assigned.

f. Zika virus infections

1) Code only confirmed cases

Code only a confirmed diagnosis of Zika virus (A92.5, Zika virus disease) as documented by the provider. This is an exception to the hospital inpatient guideline Section II, H. In this context, "confirmation" does not require documentation of the type of test performed; the provider's diagnostic statement that the condition is confirmed is sufficient. This code should be assigned regardless of the stated mode of transmission.

If the provider documents "suspected", "possible" or "probable" Zika, do not assign code A92.5. Assign a code(s) explaining the reason for encounter (such as fever, rash, or joint pain) or Z2Ø.821, Contact with and (suspected) exposure to Zika virus.

g. Coronavirus infections

1) COVID-19 infection (infection due to SARS-CoV-2)

(a) Code only confirmed cases

Code only a confirmed diagnosis of the 2019 novel coronavirus disease (COVID-19) as documented by the provider, or documentation of a positive COVID-19 test result. For a confirmed diagnosis, assign code UØ7.1, COVID-19. This is an exception to the hospital inpatient guideline Section II, H. In this context, "confirmation" does not require documentation of a positive test result for COVID-19; the provider's documentation that the individual has COVID-19 is sufficient.

If the provider documents "suspected," "possible," "probable," or "inconclusive" COVID-19, do not assign code UØ7.1. Instead, code the signs and symptoms reported. See guideline I.C.1.g.1.g.

An elderly patient who is a former smoker is admitted with a productive cough, fatigue, and chest discomfort. CXR and PFTs indicate acute bronchitis. Treatment includes cough suppressants and anti-inflammatory medication, along with isolation precautions. The provider documents acute bronchitis likely due to COVID-19. Laboratory tests were inconclusive.

J2Ø.9 Acute bronchitis, unspecified

Z87.891 History of tobacco dependence

Explanation: Because the COVID-19 diagnosis was documented as likely by the provider, code UØ7.1 cannot be assigned. Instead a code explaining the reason for the encounter is used, in this case the acute bronchitis. Code J2Ø.9 Acute bronchitis, unspecified, is used because the causative organism, specifically that which causes COVID-19, is not confirmed. Without further documentation of COVID-19 or another causative organism being present, code J2Ø.8 Acute bronchitis due to other specified organisms, does not apply.

(b) Sequencing of codes

When COVID-19 meets the definition of principal diagnosis, code UØ7.1, COVID-19, should be sequenced first, followed by the appropriate codes for associated manifestations, except when another guideline requires that certain codes be sequenced first, such as obstetrics, sepsis, or transplant complications.

The patient presents with acute hypoxic respiratory failure due to sepsis from COVID-19 related pneumonia.

A41.89 Other specified sepsis

UØ7.1 COVID-19

J12.82 Pneumonia due to coronavirus disease 2019

J96.Ø1 Acute respiratory failure with hypoxia

R65.2Ø Severe sepsis without septic shock

Explanation: If all conditions are present on admission, the systemic infection (sepsis) is sequenced first, followed by the code(s) for the localized infection (COVID-19 and pneumonia). The acute respiratory failure (acute organ dysfunction) is clearly documented as being associated with the sepsis, and therefore a severe sepsis code from subcategory R65.2- can also be assigned. If the sepsis had developed later in the admission, with or without any associated respiratory failure, the COVID-19 code would be sequenced first.

For a COVID-19 infection that progresses to sepsis, see Section I.C.1.d. Sepsis, Severe Sepsis, and Septic Shock

See Section I.C.15.s. for COVID-19 infection in pregnancy, childbirth, and the puerperium

See Section I.C.16.h. for COVID-19 infection in newborn

For a COVID-19 infection in a lung transplant patient, see Section I.C.19.g.3.a. Transplant complications other than kidney.

(c) Acute respiratory manifestations of COVID-19

When the reason for the encounter/admission is a respiratory manifestation of COVID-19, assign code UØ7.1, COVID-19, as the principal/first-listed diagnosis and assign code(s) for the respiratory manifestation(s) as additional diagnoses.

The following conditions are examples of common respiratory manifestations of COVID-19.

(i) Pneumonia

For a patient with pneumonia confirmed as due to COVID-19, assign codes UØ7.1, COVID-19, and J12.82, Pneumonia due to coronavirus disease 2019.

(ii) Acute bronchitis

For a patient with acute bronchitis confirmed as due to COVID-19, assign codes UØ7.1, and J2Ø.8, Acute bronchitis due to other specified organisms.

Bronchitis not otherwise specified (NOS) due to COVID-19 should be coded using code UØ7.1 and J4Ø, Bronchitis, not specified as acute or chronic.

(iii) Lower respiratory infection

If the COVID-19 is documented as being associated with a lower respiratory infection, not otherwise specified (NOS), or an acute respiratory infection, NOS, codes UØ7.1 and J22, Unspecified acute lower respiratory infection, should be assigned.

If the COVID-19 is documented as being associated with a respiratory infection, NOS, codes UØ7.1 and J98.8, Other specified respiratory disorders, should be assigned.

(iv) Acute respiratory distress syndrome

For acute respiratory distress syndrome (ARDS) due to COVID-19, assign codes UØ7.1, and J8Ø, Acute respiratory distress syndrome.

(v) Acute respiratory failure

For acute respiratory failure due to COVID-19, assign code UØ7.1, and code J96.Ø-, Acute respiratory failure.

(d) Non-respiratory manifestations of COVID-19

When the reason for the encounter/admission is a non-respiratory manifestation (e.g., viral enteritis) of COVID-19, assign code UØ7.1, COVID-19, as the principal/first-listed diagnosis and assign code(s) for the manifestation(s) as additional diagnoses.

(e) Exposure to COVID-19

For asymptomatic individuals with actual or suspected exposure to COVID-19, assign code Z2Ø.822, Contact with and (suspected) exposure to COVID-19.

For symptomatic individuals with actual or suspected exposure to COVID-19 and the infection has been ruled out, or test results are inconclusive or unknown, assign code Z2Ø.822, Contact with and (suspected) exposure to COVID-19. See guideline I.C.21.c.1, Contact/Exposure, for additional guidance regarding the use of category Z2Ø codes.

If COVID-19 is confirmed, see guideline I.C.1.g.1.a.

(f) Screening for COVID-19

During the COVID-19 pandemic, a screening code is generally not appropriate. Do not assign code Z11.52, Encounter for screening for COVID-19. For encounters for COVID-19 testing, including preoperative testing, code as exposure to COVID-19 (guideline I.C.1.g.1.e).

Coding guidance will be updated as new information concerning any changes in the pandemic status becomes available.

(g) Signs and symptoms without definitive diagnosis of COVID-19

For patients presenting with any signs/symptoms associated with COVID-19 (such as fever, etc.) but a definitive diagnosis has not been established, assign the appropriate code(s) for each of the presenting signs and symptoms such as:

- RØ5.1, Acute cough, or RØ5.9, Cough, unspecified
- RØ6.Ø2 Shortness of breath
- R5Ø.9 Fever, unspecified

If a patient with signs/symptoms associated with COVID-19 also has an actual or suspected contact with or exposure to COVID-19, assign Z2Ø.822, Contact with and (suspected) exposure to COVID19, as an additional code.

(h) Asymptomatic individuals who test positive for COVID-19

For asymptomatic individuals who test positive for COVID-19, see guideline I.C.1.g.1.a. Although the individual is asymptomatic, the individual has tested positive and is considered to have the COVID-19 infection.

(i) Personal history of COVID-19

For patients with a history of COVID-19, assign code Z86.16, Personal history of COVID-19.

(j) Follow-up visits after COVID-19 infection has resolved

For individuals who previously had COVID-19, without residual symptom(s) or condition(s), and are being seen for follow-up evaluation, and COVID-19 test results are negative, assign codes ZØ9, Encounter for follow-up examination after completed treatment for conditions other than malignant neoplasm, and Z86.16, Personal history of COVID-19.

For follow-up visits for individuals with symptom(s) or condition(s) related to a previous COVID-19 infection, see guideline I.C.1.g.1.m.

See Section I.C.21.c.8, Factors influencing health states and contact with health services, Follow-up

(k) Encounter for antibody testing

For an encounter for antibody testing that is not being performed to confirm a current COVID-19 infection, nor is a follow-up test after resolution of COVID-19, assign ZØ1.84, Encounter for antibody response examination.

Follow the applicable guidelines above if the individual is being tested to confirm a current COVID-19 infection.

For follow-up testing after a COVID-19 infection, see guideline I.C.1.g.1.j.

(l) Multisystem inflammatory syndrome

For individuals with multisystem inflammatory syndrome (MIS) and COVID-19, assign code UØ7.1, COVID-19, as the principal/first-listed diagnosis and assign code M35.81, Multisystem inflammatory syndrome, as an additional diagnosis.

If an individual with a history of COVID-19 develops MIS, assign codes M35.81, Multisystem inflammatory syndrome, and UØ9.9, Post COVID-19 condition, unspecified.

If an individual with a known or suspected exposure to COVID- 19, and no current COVID-19 infection or history of COVID-19, develops MIS, assign codes M35.81, Multisystem inflammatory syndrome, and Z2Ø.822, Contact with and (suspected) exposure to COVID-19.

Additional codes should be assigned for any associated complications of MIS.

(m) Post COVID-19 condition

For sequela of COVID-19, or associated symptoms or conditions that develop following a previous COVID-19 infection, assign a code(s) for the specific symptom(s) or condition(s) related to the previous COVID-19 infection, if known, and code UØ9.9, Post COVID-19 condition, unspecified.

Code UØ9.9 should not be assigned for manifestations of an active (current) COVID-19 infection.

If a patient has a condition(s) associated with a previous COVID-19 infection and develops a new active (current) COVID-19 infection, code UØ9.9 may be assigned in conjunction with code UØ7.1, COVID-19, to identify that the patient also has a condition(s) associated with a previous COVID-19 infection. Code(s) for the specific condition(s) associated with the previous COVID-19 infection and code(s) for manifestation(s) of the new active (current) COVID-19 infection should also be assigned.

(n) Underimmunization for COVID-19 Status

Code Z28.31Ø, Unvaccinated for COVID-19, may be assigned when the patient has not received **a** COVID-19 vaccine **of any type.** Code Z28.311, Partially vaccinated for COVID-19, may be assigned when the patient has **been partially vaccinated for COVID-19 as per the recommendations of** the Centers for Disease Control and Prevention (CDC) in place at the time of the encounter. For information, visit the CDC's website https://www.cdc.gov/coronavirus/2Ø19-ncov/vaccines/.

See Section I.B.14. for underimmunization documentation by clinicians other than patient's provider.

Chapter 1. Certain Infectious and Parasitic Diseases (A00-B99)

INCLUDES diseases generally recognized as communicable or transmissible

Use additional code to identify resistance to antimicrobial drugs (Z16.-)

EXCLUDES 1 *certain localized infections - see body system-related chapters*

EXCLUDES 2 *carrier or suspected carrier of infectious disease (Z22.-)*
infectious and parasitic diseases complicating pregnancy, childbirth and the puerperium (O98.-)
infectious and parasitic diseases specific to the perinatal period (P35-P39)
influenza and other acute respiratory infections (J00-J22)

This chapter contains the following blocks:

A00-A09	Intestinal infectious diseases
A15-A19	Tuberculosis
A20-A28	Certain zoonotic bacterial diseases
A30-A49	Other bacterial diseases
A50-A64	Infections with a predominantly sexual mode of transmission
A65-A69	Other spirochetal diseases
A70-A74	Other diseases caused by chlamydiae
A75-A79	Rickettsioses
A80-A89	Viral and prion infections of the central nervous system
A90-A99	Arthropod-borne viral fevers and viral hemorrhagic fevers
B00-B09	Viral infections characterized by skin and mucous membrane lesions
B10	Other human herpesviruses
B15-B19	Viral hepatitis
B20	Human immunodeficiency virus [HIV] disease
B25-B34	Other viral diseases
B35-B49	Mycoses
B50-B64	Protozoal diseases
B65-B83	Helminthiases
B85-B89	Pediculosis, acariasis and other infestations
B90-B94	Sequelae of infectious and parasitic diseases
B95-B97	Bacterial and viral infectious agents
B99	Other infectious diseases

Intestinal infectious diseases (A00-A09)

A00 Cholera

DEF: Acute infection of the bowel due to *Vibrio cholerae* that presents with profuse diarrhea, cramps, and vomiting, resulting in severe dehydration, electrolyte imbalance, and death. It is spread through ingestion of food or water contaminated with feces of infected persons.

A00.0 Cholera due to Vibrio cholerae 01, biovar cholerae CC
Classical cholera

A00.1 Cholera due to Vibrio cholerae 01, biovar eltor CC
Cholera eltor

A00.9 Cholera, unspecified CC

A01 Typhoid and paratyphoid fevers

DEF: Typhoid fever: Acute generalized illness caused by *Salmonella typhi*. Clinical features include fever, headache, abdominal pain, cough, toxemia, leukopenia, abnormal pulse, rose spots on the skin, bacteremia, hyperplasia of intestinal lymph nodes, mesenteric lymphadenopathy, and Peyer's patches in the intestines.

DEF: Paratyphoid fever: Prolonged febrile illness, caused by *Salmonella* serotypes other than *S. typhi*, especially *S. enterica* serotypes paratyphi A, B, and C.

A01.0 Typhoid fever
Infection due to Salmonella typhi

A01.00 Typhoid fever, unspecified CC
A01.01 Typhoid meningitis CC
A01.02 Typhoid fever with heart involvement CC
Typhoid endocarditis
Typhoid myocarditis
A01.03 Typhoid pneumonia CC HCC
A01.04 Typhoid arthritis CC HCC
A01.05 Typhoid osteomyelitis CC HCC
A01.09 Typhoid fever with other complications CC

A01.1 Paratyphoid fever A CC
A01.2 Paratyphoid fever B CC
A01.3 Paratyphoid fever C CC
A01.4 Paratyphoid fever, unspecified CC
Infection due to Salmonella paratyphi NOS

A02 Other salmonella infections

INCLUDES infection or foodborne intoxication due to any Salmonella species other than S. typhi and S. paratyphi

A02.0 Salmonella enteritis CC
Salmonellosis
TIP: Dehydration (E86.0) is a complication of salmonella enteritis and may be reported separately.

A02.1 Salmonella sepsis HIV MCC HCC

A02.2 Localized salmonella infections

A02.20 Localized salmonella infection, unspecified HIV
A02.21 Salmonella meningitis HIV MCC
A02.22 Salmonella pneumonia HIV MCC HCC
A02.23 Salmonella arthritis HIV CC HCC
A02.24 Salmonella osteomyelitis HIV CC HCC
A02.25 Salmonella pyelonephritis HIV CC
Salmonella tubulo-interstitial nephropathy
A02.29 Salmonella with other localized infection HIV CC

A02.8 Other specified salmonella infections HIV CC
A02.9 Salmonella infection, unspecified HIV CC

A03 Shigellosis

DEF: Infection caused by the genus *Shigella*, of the family *Enterobacteriaceae* that is known to cause an acute dysenteric infection of the bowel with fever, drowsiness, anorexia, nausea, vomiting, bloody diarrhea, abdominal cramps, and distention.

A03.0 Shigellosis due to Shigella dysenteriae CC
Group A shigellosis [Shiga-Kruse dysentery]

A03.1 Shigellosis due to Shigella flexneri
Group B shigellosis

A03.2 Shigellosis due to Shigella boydii
Group C shigellosis

A03.3 Shigellosis due to Shigella sonnei
Group D shigellosis

A03.8 Other shigellosis

A03.9 Shigellosis, unspecified
Bacillary dysentery NOS

A04 Other bacterial intestinal infections

EXCLUDES 1 *bacterial foodborne intoxications, NEC (A05.-)*
tuberculous enteritis (A18.32)

DEF: *Escherichia coli*: Gram-negative, anaerobic bacteria of the family *Enterobacteriaceae* found in the large intestine of warm-blooded animals, generally as a nonpathologic entity aiding in digestion. They become pathogenic when an opportunity to grow somewhere outside this relationship presents itself, such as ingestion of fecal-contaminated food or water.

A04.0 Enteropathogenic Escherichia coli infection CC
A04.1 Enterotoxigenic Escherichia coli infection CC
A04.2 Enteroinvasive Escherichia coli infection CC
A04.3 Enterohemorrhagic Escherichia coli infection CC
DEF: *E. coli* infection penetrating the intestinal mucosa, producing microscopic ulceration and bleeding.

A04.4 Other intestinal Escherichia coli infections CC
Escherichia coli enteritis NOS

A04.5 Campylobacter enteritis CC
TIP: For Guillain-Barre syndrome occurring as a sequela of *Campylobacter enteritis*, assign code G61.0 as the first-listed diagnosis followed by B94.8 for the sequelae.

A04.6 Enteritis due to Yersinia enterocolitica CC
EXCLUDES 1 *extraintestinal yersiniosis (A28.2)*

A04.7 Enterocolitis due to Clostridium difficile
Foodborne intoxication by Clostridium difficile
Pseudomembraneous colitis
AHA: 2017,4Q,4

A04.71 Enterocolitis due to Clostridium difficile, recurrent CC
AHA: 2020,1Q,18

A04.72 Enterocolitis due to Clostridium difficile, not specified as recurrent CC

A04.8 Other specified bacterial intestinal infections CC

A04.9 Bacterial intestinal infection, unspecified CC
Bacterial enteritis NOS

A05 Other bacterial foodborne intoxications, not elsewhere classified

EXCLUDES 1 *Clostridium difficile foodborne intoxication and infection (A04.7-)*
Escherichia coli infection (A04.0-A04.4)
listeriosis (A32.-)
salmonella foodborne intoxication and infection (A02.-)
toxic effect of noxious foodstuffs (T61-T62)

A05.0 Foodborne staphylococcal intoxication CC

TIP: Assign code A04.8 to report a staphylococcal infection when it is caused by the ingestion of contaminated food but not caused by *S. aureus* toxins.

A05.1 Botulism food poisoning CC

Botulism NOS
Classical foodborne intoxication due to Clostridium botulinum
EXCLUDES 1 *infant botulism (A48.51)*
wound botulism (A48.52)

DEF: Muscle-paralyzing neurotoxic disease caused by ingesting pre-formed toxin from the bacterium *Clostridium botulinum*. It causes vomiting and diarrhea, vision problems, slurred speech, difficulty swallowing, paralysis, and death.

A05.2 Foodborne Clostridium perfringens [Clostridium welchii] intoxication CC

Enteritis necroticans
Pig-bel

A05.3 Foodborne Vibrio parahaemolyticus intoxication CC

A05.4 Foodborne Bacillus cereus intoxication CC

A05.5 Foodborne Vibrio vulnificus intoxication CC

A05.8 Other specified bacterial foodborne intoxications CC

A05.9 Bacterial foodborne intoxication, unspecified

A06 Amebiasis

INCLUDES infection due to Entamoeba histolytica
EXCLUDES 1 *other protozoal intestinal diseases (A07.-)*
EXCLUDES 2 *acanthamebiasis (B60.1-)*
Naegleriasis (B60.2)

DEF: Infection with a single cell protozoan known as the amoeba. Transmission occurs through ingestion of feces, contaminated food or water, use of human feces as fertilizer, or person-to-person contact.

A06.0 Acute amebic dysentery CC

Acute amebiasis
Intestinal amebiasis NOS

A06.1 Chronic intestinal amebiasis CC

A06.2 Amebic nondysenteric colitis CC

A06.3 Ameboma of intestine CC

Ameboma NOS

A06.4 Amebic liver abscess MCC

Hepatic amebiasis

A06.5 Amebic lung abscess MCC HCC

Amebic abscess of lung (and liver)

A06.6 Amebic brain abscess MCC

Amebic abscess of brain (and liver) (and lung)

A06.7 Cutaneous amebiasis CC

A06.8 Amebic infection of other sites

A06.81 Amebic cystitis CC

A06.82 Other amebic genitourinary infections CC

Amebic balanitis
Amebic vesiculitis
Amebic vulvovaginitis

A06.89 Other amebic infections CC

Amebic appendicitis
Amebic splenic abscess

A06.9 Amebiasis, unspecified

A07 Other protozoal intestinal diseases

DEF: Protozoa: Group comprised of the simplest, single celled organisms, ranging in size from micro to macroscopic. They can live alone or in colonies, and do not show any differentiation in tissues. Most are motile and can live free in nature, but some are parasitic, causing disease in the variety of hosts they inhabit.

A07.0 Balantidiasis

Balantidial dysentery

A07.1 Giardiasis [lambliasis] CC

DEF: Infection caused by the flagellate protozoan *Giardia lamblia* causing gastrointestinal problems such as vomiting, chronic diarrhea, and weight loss. The most common parasite in the U.S., this is usually transmitted by ingesting contaminated water while in the cyst state, after which it latches onto the wall of the small intestine.

A07.2 Cryptosporidiosis CC HCC

DEF: Microscopic parasite found in water and one of the most common causes of waterborne gastrointestinal infectious disease in the United States. It is usually transmitted by ingesting contaminated drinking water or recreational water and causes profuse watery diarrhea, flatulence, abdominal pain, and cramping.

A07.3 Isosporiasis HIV CC

Infection due to Isospora belli and Isospora hominis
Intestinal coccidiosis
Isosporosis

A07.4 Cyclosporiasis CC

A07.8 Other specified protozoal intestinal diseases CC

Intestinal microsporidiosis
Intestinal trichomoniasis
Sarcocystosis
Sarcosporidiosis

A07.9 Protozoal intestinal disease, unspecified CC

Flagellate diarrhea
Protozoal colitis
Protozoal diarrhea
Protozoal dysentery

A08 Viral and other specified intestinal infections

EXCLUDES 1 *influenza with involvement of gastrointestinal tract (J09.X3, J10.2, J11.2)*

A08.0 Rotaviral enteritis CC

A08.1 Acute gastroenteropathy due to Norwalk agent and other small round viruses

A08.11 Acute gastroenteropathy due to Norwalk agent CC

Acute gastroenteropathy due to Norovirus
Acute gastroenteropathy due to Norwalk-like agent

A08.19 Acute gastroenteropathy due to other small round viruses CC

Acute gastroenteropathy due to small round virus [SRV] NOS

A08.2 Adenoviral enteritis CC

A08.3 Other viral enteritis

A08.31 Calicivirus enteritis CC

A08.32 Astrovirus enteritis CC

A08.39 Other viral enteritis CC

Coxsackie virus enteritis
Echovirus enteritis
Enterovirus enteritis NEC
Torovirus enteritis

A08.4 Viral intestinal infection, unspecified

Viral enteritis NOS
Viral gastroenteritis NOS
Viral gastroenteropathy NOS
AHA: 2016,3Q,12

A08.8 Other specified intestinal infections

A09 Infectious gastroenteritis and colitis, unspecified CC

Infectious colitis NOS
Infectious enteritis NOS
Infectious gastroenteritis NOS
EXCLUDES 1 *colitis NOS (K52.9)*
diarrhea NOS (R19.7)
enteritis NOS (K52.9)
gastroenteritis NOS (K52.9)
noninfective gastroenteritis and colitis, unspecified (K52.9)

DEF: Colitis: Inflammation of mucous membranes of the colon.
DEF: Enteritis: Inflammation of mucous membranes of the small intestine.
DEF: Gastroenteritis: Inflammation of mucous membranes of the stomach and intestines.

Tuberculosis (A15-A19)

INCLUDES infections due to Mycobacterium tuberculosis and Mycobacterium bovis

EXCLUDES 1 *congenital tuberculosis (P37.Ø)*
nonspecific reaction to test for tuberculosis without active tuberculosis (R76.1-)
pneumoconiosis associated with tuberculosis, any type in A15 (J65)
positive PPD (R76.11)
positive tuberculin skin test without active tuberculosis (R76.11)
sequelae of tuberculosis (B9Ø.-)
silicotuberculosis (J65)

DEF: Bacterial infection that typically spreads by inhalation of an airborne agent that usually attacks the lungs, but may also affect other organs.

✓4th **A15 Respiratory tuberculosis**

A15.Ø Tuberculosis of lung HIV CC
Tuberculous bronchiectasis
Tuberculous fibrosis of lung
Tuberculous pneumonia
Tuberculous pneumothorax

Tuberculosis of Lung

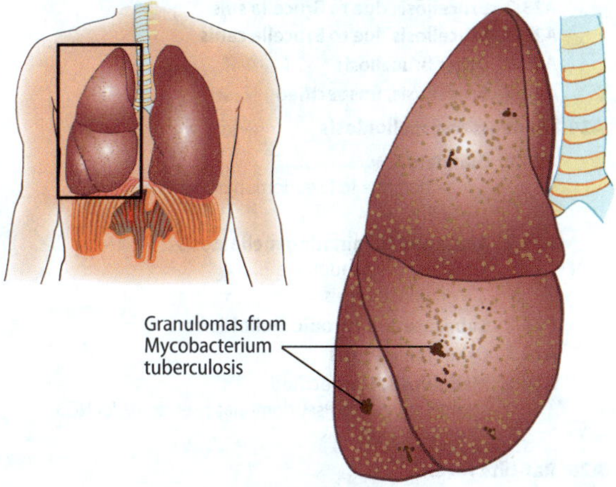

Granulomas from Mycobacterium tuberculosis

A15.4 Tuberculosis of intrathoracic lymph nodes HIV CC
Tuberculosis of hilar lymph nodes
Tuberculosis of mediastinal lymph nodes
Tuberculosis of tracheobronchial lymph nodes
EXCLUDES 1 *tuberculosis specified as primary (A15.7)*

A15.5 Tuberculosis of larynx, trachea and bronchus HIV CC
Tuberculosis of bronchus
Tuberculosis of glottis
Tuberculosis of larynx
Tuberculosis of trachea

A15.6 Tuberculous pleurisy HIV CC
Tuberculosis of pleura Tuberculous empyema
EXCLUDES 1 *primary respiratory tuberculosis (A15.7)*

A15.7 Primary respiratory tuberculosis HIV CC

A15.8 Other respiratory tuberculosis HIV CC
Mediastinal tuberculosis
Nasopharyngeal tuberculosis
Tuberculosis of nose
Tuberculosis of sinus [any nasal]

A15.9 Respiratory tuberculosis unspecified HIV CC

✓4th **A17 Tuberculosis of nervous system**

A17.Ø Tuberculous meningitis HIV MCC
Tuberculosis of meninges (cerebral)(spinal)
Tuberculous leptomeningitis
EXCLUDES 1 *tuberculous meningoencephalitis (A17.82)*

A17.1 Meningeal tuberculoma HIV MCC
Tuberculoma of meninges (cerebral) (spinal)
EXCLUDES 2 *tuberculoma of brain and spinal cord (A17.81)*

✓5th **A17.8 Other tuberculosis of nervous system**

A17.81 Tuberculoma of brain and spinal cord HIV MCC
Tuberculous abscess of brain and spinal cord

A17.82 Tuberculous meningoencephalitis HIV MCC
Tuberculous myelitis

A17.83 Tuberculous neuritis HIV MCC
Tuberculous mononeuropathy

A17.89 Other tuberculosis of nervous system HIV MCC
Tuberculous polyneuropathy

A17.9 Tuberculosis of nervous system, unspecified HIV CC

✓4th **A18 Tuberculosis of other organs**

✓5th **A18.Ø Tuberculosis of bones and joints**

A18.Ø1 Tuberculosis of spine HIV CC
Pott's disease or curvature of spine
Tuberculous arthritis
Tuberculous osteomyelitis of spine
Tuberculous spondylitis

A18.Ø2 Tuberculous arthritis of other joints HIV CC
Tuberculosis of hip (joint)
Tuberculosis of knee (joint)

A18.Ø3 Tuberculosis of other bones HIV CC
Tuberculous mastoiditis
Tuberculous osteomyelitis

A18.Ø9 Other musculoskeletal tuberculosis HIV CC
Tuberculous myositis
Tuberculous synovitis
Tuberculous tenosynovitis

✓5th **A18.1 Tuberculosis of genitourinary system**

A18.1Ø Tuberculosis of genitourinary system, unspecified HIV CC

A18.11 Tuberculosis of kidney and ureter HIV CC

A18.12 Tuberculosis of bladder HIV CC

A18.13 Tuberculosis of other urinary organs HIV CC
Tuberculous urethritis

A18.14 Tuberculosis of prostate HIV CC A ♂

A18.15 Tuberculosis of other male genital organs HIV CC ♂

A18.16 Tuberculosis of cervix HIV CC ♀

A18.17 Tuberculous female pelvic inflammatory disease HIV CC ♀
Tuberculous endometritis
Tuberculous oophoritis and salpingitis

A18.18 Tuberculosis of other female genital organs HIV CC ♀
Tuberculous ulceration of vulva

A18.2 Tuberculous peripheral lymphadenopathy HIV CC
Tuberculous adenitis
EXCLUDES 2 *tuberculosis of bronchial and mediastinal lymph nodes (A15.4)*
tuberculosis of mesenteric and retroperitoneal lymph nodes (A18.39)
tuberculous tracheobronchial adenopathy (A15.4)

✓5th **A18.3 Tuberculosis of intestines, peritoneum and mesenteric glands**

A18.31 Tuberculous peritonitis HIV MCC
Tuberculous ascites
DEF: Tuberculous inflammation of the membrane lining the abdomen.

A18.32 Tuberculous enteritis HIV CC
Tuberculosis of anus and rectum
Tuberculosis of intestine (large) (small)

A18.39 Retroperitoneal tuberculosis HIV CC
Tuberculosis of mesenteric glands
Tuberculosis of retroperitoneal (lymph glands)

A18.4 Tuberculosis of skin and subcutaneous tissue HIV CC
Erythema induratum, tuberculous
Lupus excedens
Lupus vulgaris NOS
Lupus vulgaris of eyelid
Scrofuloderma
Tuberculosis of external ear
EXCLUDES 2 *lupus erythematosus (L93.-)*
systemic lupus erythematosus (M32.-)

✓5th **A18.5 Tuberculosis of eye**
EXCLUDES 2 *lupus vulgaris of eyelid (A18.4)*

A18.5Ø Tuberculosis of eye, unspecified HIV CC

A18.51 Tuberculous episcleritis HIV CC

A18.52 Tuberculous keratitis HIV CC
Tuberculous interstitial keratitis
Tuberculous keratoconjunctivitis (interstitial) (phlyctenular)
A18.53 Tuberculous chorioretinitis HIV CC
A18.54 Tuberculous iridocyclitis HIV CC
A18.59 Other tuberculosis of eye HIV CC
Tuberculous conjunctivitis

A18.6 Tuberculosis of (inner) (middle) ear HIV CC
Tuberculous otitis media
EXCLUDES 2 *tuberculosis of external ear (A18.4)*
tuberculous mastoiditis (A18.Ø3)

A18.7 Tuberculosis of adrenal glands HIV CC
Tuberculous Addison's disease

5th **A18.8 Tuberculosis of other specified organs**
A18.81 Tuberculosis of thyroid gland HIV CC
A18.82 Tuberculosis of other endocrine glands HIV CC
Tuberculosis of pituitary gland
Tuberculosis of thymus gland
A18.83 Tuberculosis of digestive tract organs, not elsewhere classified HIV CC
EXCLUDES 1 *tuberculosis of intestine (A18.32)*
A18.84 Tuberculosis of heart HIV CC
Tuberculous cardiomyopathy
Tuberculous endocarditis
Tuberculous myocarditis
Tuberculous pericarditis
A18.85 Tuberculosis of spleen HIV CC
A18.89 Tuberculosis of other sites HIV CC
Tuberculosis of muscle
Tuberculous cerebral arteritis

4th **A19 Miliary tuberculosis**
INCLUDES disseminated tuberculosis
generalized tuberculosis
tuberculous polyserositis

A19.Ø Acute miliary tuberculosis of a single specified site HIV MCC
A19.1 Acute miliary tuberculosis of multiple sites HIV MCC
A19.2 Acute miliary tuberculosis, unspecified HIV MCC
A19.8 Other miliary tuberculosis HIV MCC
A19.9 Miliary tuberculosis, unspecified HIV MCC

Certain zoonotic bacterial diseases (A2Ø-A28)

4th **A2Ø Plague**
INCLUDES infection due to Yersinia pestis

A2Ø.Ø Bubonic plague MCC
A2Ø.1 Cellulocutaneous plague MCC
A2Ø.2 Pneumonic plague MCC HCC
A2Ø.3 Plague meningitis MCC
A2Ø.7 Septicemic plague MCC HCC
A2Ø.8 Other forms of plague MCC
Abortive plague
Asymptomatic plague
Pestis minor
A2Ø.9 Plague, unspecified MCC

4th **A21 Tularemia**
INCLUDES deer-fly fever
infection due to Francisella tularensis
rabbit fever

DEF: Febrile disease transmitted to humans by the bites of deer flies, fleas, and ticks, by inhaling aerosolized *F. tularensis*, or by ingesting contaminated food or water. Patients quickly develop fever, chills, weakness, headache, backache, and malaise.

A21.Ø Ulceroglandular tularemia CC
A21.1 Oculoglandular tularemia CC
Ophthalmic tularemia
A21.2 Pulmonary tularemia CC HCC
A21.3 Gastrointestinal tularemia CC
Abdominal tularemia
A21.7 Generalized tularemia CC
A21.8 Other forms of tularemia CC
A21.9 Tularemia, unspecified CC

4th **A22 Anthrax**
INCLUDES infection due to Bacillus anthracis

A22.Ø Cutaneous anthrax CC
Malignant carbuncle
Malignant pustule
A22.1 Pulmonary anthrax MCC HCC
Inhalation anthrax
Ragpicker's disease
Woolsorter's disease
A22.2 Gastrointestinal anthrax CC
A22.7 Anthrax sepsis MCC HCC
A22.8 Other forms of anthrax CC
Anthrax meningitis
A22.9 Anthrax, unspecified CC

4th **A23 Brucellosis**
INCLUDES Malta fever
Mediterranean fever
undulant fever

A23.Ø Brucellosis due to Brucella melitensis
A23.1 Brucellosis due to Brucella abortus
A23.2 Brucellosis due to Brucella suis
A23.3 Brucellosis due to Brucella canis
A23.8 Other brucellosis CC
A23.9 Brucellosis, unspecified CC

4th **A24 Glanders and melioidosis**

A24.Ø Glanders CC
Infection due to Pseudomonas mallei
Malleus
A24.1 Acute and fulminating melioidosis CC
Melioidosis pneumonia
Melioidosis sepsis
A24.2 Subacute and chronic melioidosis CC
A24.3 Other melioidosis CC
A24.9 Melioidosis, unspecified CC
Infection due to Pseudomonas pseudomallei NOS
Whitmore's disease

4th **A25 Rat-bite fevers**

A25.Ø Spirillosis CC
Sodoku
A25.1 Streptobacillosis CC
Epidemic arthritic erythema
Haverhill fever
Streptobacillary rat-bite fever
A25.9 Rat-bite fever, unspecified CC

4th **A26 Erysipeloid**
DEF: Acute cutaneous infection typically caused by trauma to the skin. Presenting as cellulitis, it may become systemic, affecting other organs. It is a gram-positive bacillus and mainly acquired by those who routinely handle meat.

A26.Ø Cutaneous erysipeloid
Erythema migrans
A26.7 Erysipelothrix sepsis MCC HCC
A26.8 Other forms of erysipeloid
A26.9 Erysipeloid, unspecified

4th **A27 Leptospirosis**

A27.Ø Leptospirosis icterohemorrhagica CC
Leptospiral or spirochetal jaundice (hemorrhagic)
Weil's disease
5th **A27.8 Other forms of leptospirosis**
A27.81 Aseptic meningitis in leptospirosis MCC
A27.89 Other forms of leptospirosis CC
A27.9 Leptospirosis, unspecified CC

4th **A28 Other zoonotic bacterial diseases, not elsewhere classified**

A28.Ø Pasteurellosis CC
A28.1 Cat-scratch disease CC
Cat-scratch fever
A28.2 Extraintestinal yersiniosis CC
EXCLUDES 1 *enteritis due to Yersinia enterocolitica (AØ4.6)*
plague (A2Ø.-)
A28.8 Other specified zoonotic bacterial diseases, not elsewhere classified CC
A28.9 Zoonotic bacterial disease, unspecified CC

Other bacterial diseases (A30-A49)

AHA: 2016,3Q,8-14

A30 Leprosy [Hansen's disease]
INCLUDES infection due to Mycobacterium leprae
EXCLUDES 1 *sequelae of leprosy (B92)*

A30.0 Indeterminate leprosy CC
I leprosy
A30.1 Tuberculoid leprosy CC
TT leprosy
A30.2 Borderline tuberculoid leprosy CC
BT leprosy
A30.3 Borderline leprosy CC
BB leprosy
A30.4 Borderline lepromatous leprosy CC
BL leprosy
A30.5 Lepromatous leprosy CC
LL leprosy
A30.8 Other forms of leprosy CC
A30.9 Leprosy, unspecified CC

A31 Infection due to other mycobacteria
EXCLUDES 2 *leprosy (A30.-)*
tuberculosis (A15-A19)

A31.0 Pulmonary mycobacterial infection CC HCC
Infection due to Mycobacterium avium
Infection due to Mycobacterium intracellulare [Battey bacillus]
Infection due to Mycobacterium kansasii
A31.1 Cutaneous mycobacterial infection CC
Buruli ulcer
Infection due to Mycobacterium marinum
Infection due to Mycobacterium ulcerans
A31.2 Disseminated mycobacterium avium-intracellulare complex (DMAC) HIV CC HCC
MAC sepsis
A31.8 Other mycobacterial infections HIV CC
A31.9 Mycobacterial infection, unspecified HIV CC
Atypical mycobacterial infection NOS
Mycobacteriosis NOS

A32 Listeriosis
INCLUDES listerial foodborne infection
EXCLUDES 1 *neonatal (disseminated) listeriosis (P37.2)*

A32.0 Cutaneous listeriosis CC
A32.1 Listerial meningitis and meningoencephalitis
A32.11 Listerial meningitis CC
A32.12 Listerial meningoencephalitis CC
A32.7 Listerial sepsis MCC HCC
A32.8 Other forms of listeriosis
A32.81 Oculoglandular listeriosis CC
A32.82 Listerial endocarditis CC
A32.89 Other forms of listeriosis CC
Listerial cerebral arteritis
A32.9 Listeriosis, unspecified CC

A33 Tetanus neonatorum MCC N
A34 Obstetrical tetanus CC M ♀
A35 Other tetanus MCC
Tetanus NOS
EXCLUDES 1 *obstetrical tetanus (A34)*
tetanus neonatorum (A33)

DEF: Tetanus: Acute, often fatal, infectious disease caused by the anaerobic, spore-forming bacillus *Clostridium tetani*. The bacillus enters the body through a contaminated wound, burns, surgical wounds, or cutaneous ulcers. Symptoms include lockjaw, spasms, seizures, and paralysis.

A36 Diphtheria
A36.0 Pharyngeal diphtheria CC
Diphtheritic membranous angina
Tonsillar diphtheria
A36.1 Nasopharyngeal diphtheria CC
A36.2 Laryngeal diphtheria CC
Diphtheritic laryngotracheitis
A36.3 Cutaneous diphtheria CC
EXCLUDES 2 *erythrasma (L08.1)*
A36.8 Other diphtheria
A36.81 Diphtheritic cardiomyopathy CC HCC
Diphtheritic myocarditis
A36.82 Diphtheritic radiculomyelitis CC
A36.83 Diphtheritic polyneuritis CC
A36.84 Diphtheritic tubulo-interstitial nephropathy CC
A36.85 Diphtheritic cystitis CC
A36.86 Diphtheritic conjunctivitis CC
A36.89 Other diphtheritic complications CC
Diphtheritic peritonitis
A36.9 Diphtheria, unspecified CC

A37 Whooping cough
DEF: Acute, highly contagious respiratory tract infection caused by *Bordetella pertussis* and *B. bronchiseptica*. Whooping cough is known by its characteristic paroxysmal cough.

A37.0 Whooping cough due to Bordetella pertussis
A37.00 Whooping cough due to Bordetella pertussis without pneumonia CC
Paroxysmal cough due to Bordetella pertussis without pneumonia
A37.01 Whooping cough due to Bordetella pertussis with pneumonia MCC
Paroxysmal cough due to Bordetella pertussis with pneumonia
A37.1 Whooping cough due to Bordetella parapertussis
A37.10 Whooping cough due to Bordetella parapertussis without pneumonia CC
A37.11 Whooping cough due to Bordetella parapertussis with pneumonia MCC
A37.8 Whooping cough due to other Bordetella species
A37.80 Whooping cough due to other Bordetella species without pneumonia CC
A37.81 Whooping cough due to other Bordetella species with pneumonia MCC
A37.9 Whooping cough, unspecified species
A37.90 Whooping cough, unspecified species without pneumonia CC
A37.91 Whooping cough, unspecified species with pneumonia MCC

A38 Scarlet fever
INCLUDES scarlatina
EXCLUDES 2 *streptococcal sore throat (J02.0)*
DEF: Acute contagious disease caused by Group A bacteria, the same bacterium that causes strep throat. Individuals with strep throat can develop scarlet fever particularly if the infection is not treated with antibiotics. It is characterized by a red blush to the skin of the chest and abdomen and swelling of the nose, throat, and mouth.

A38.0 Scarlet fever with otitis media CC
A38.1 Scarlet fever with myocarditis CC
A38.8 Scarlet fever with other complications CC
A38.9 Scarlet fever, uncomplicated CC
Scarlet fever, NOS

A39 Meningococcal infection
DEF: Condition caused by *Neisseria meningitidis*, a bacteria that may invade the spinal cord, brain, heart, joints, optic nerve, or bloodstream.

A39.0 Meningococcal meningitis MCC
A39.1 Waterhouse-Friderichsen syndrome MCC HCC
Meningococcal hemorrhagic adrenalitis
Meningococcic adrenal syndrome
A39.2 Acute meningococcemia MCC HCC
A39.3 Chronic meningococcemia MCC HCC
A39.4 Meningococcemia, unspecified MCC HCC
A39.5 Meningococcal heart disease
A39.50 Meningococcal carditis, unspecified MCC
A39.51 Meningococcal endocarditis MCC
A39.52 Meningococcal myocarditis MCC
A39.53 Meningococcal pericarditis MCC
A39.8 Other meningococcal infections
A39.81 Meningococcal encephalitis MCC
A39.82 Meningococcal retrobulbar neuritis CC
A39.83 Meningococcal arthritis CC HCC
A39.84 Postmeningococcal arthritis CC HCC

A39.89 Other meningococcal infections CC
Meningococcal conjunctivitis

A39.9 Meningococcal infection, unspecified CC
Meningococcal disease NOS

A40 Streptococcal sepsis
Code first:
postprocedural streptococcal sepsis (T81.4-)
streptococcal sepsis during labor (O75.3)
streptococcal sepsis following abortion or ectopic or molar pregnancy (O03-O07, O08.0)
streptococcal sepsis following immunization (T88.0)
streptococcal sepsis following infusion, transfusion or therapeutic injection (T80.2-)

EXCLUDES 1 *neonatal (P36.0-P36.1)*
puerperal sepsis (O85)
sepsis due to Streptococcus, group D (A41.81)

AHA: 2020,2Q,8,28; 2019,4Q,65; 2018,4Q,89; 2018,1Q,16; 2016,1Q,32

A40.0 Sepsis due to streptococcus, group A MCC HCC
A40.1 Sepsis due to streptococcus, group B MCC HCC
AHA: 2019,1Q,14
A40.3 Sepsis due to Streptococcus pneumoniae MCC HCC
Pneumococcal sepsis
A40.8 Other streptococcal sepsis MCC HCC
A40.9 Streptococcal sepsis, unspecified HIV MCC HCC

A41 Other sepsis
Code first:
postprocedural sepsis (T81.4-)
sepsis during labor (O75.3)
sepsis following abortion, ectopic or molar pregnancy (O03-O07, O08.0)
sepsis following immunization (T88.0)
sepsis following infusion, transfusion or therapeutic injection (T80.2-)

EXCLUDES 1 *bacteremia NOS (R78.81)*
neonatal (P36.-)
puerperal sepsis (O85)
streptococcal sepsis (A40.-)

EXCLUDES 2 *sepsis (due to) (in) actinomycotic (A42.7)*
sepsis (due to) (in) anthrax (A22.7)
sepsis (due to) (in) candidal (B37.7)
sepsis (due to) (in) Erysipelothrix (A26.7)
sepsis (due to) (in) extraintestinal yersiniosis (A28.2)
sepsis (due to) (in) gonococcal (A54.86)
sepsis (due to) (in) herpesviral (B00.7)
sepsis (due to) (in) listerial (A32.7)
sepsis (due to) (in) melioidosis (A24.1)
sepsis (due to) (in) meningococcal (A39.2-A39.4)
sepsis (due to) (in) plague (A20.7)
sepsis (due to) (in) tularemia (A21.7)
toxic shock syndrome (A48.3)

AHA: 2020,2Q,8,28; 2019,4Q,65; 2019,3Q,17; 2018,4Q,18; 2018,1Q,16; 2016,1Q,32; 2014,2Q,13

A41.0 Sepsis due to Staphylococcus aureus
A41.01 Sepsis due to Methicillin susceptible Staphylococcus aureus HIV MCC HCC
MSSA sepsis
Staphylococcus aureus sepsis NOS
AHA: 2020,2Q,17
A41.02 Sepsis due to Methicillin resistant Staphylococcus aureus HIV MCC HCC
A41.1 Sepsis due to other specified staphylococcus HIV MCC HCC
Coagulase negative staphylococcus sepsis
A41.2 Sepsis due to unspecified staphylococcus HIV MCC HCC
A41.3 Sepsis due to Hemophilus influenzae HIV MCC HCC
A41.4 Sepsis due to anaerobes HIV MCC HCC
EXCLUDES 1 *gas gangrene (A48.0)*
A41.5 Sepsis due to other Gram-negative organisms
A41.50 Gram-negative sepsis, unspecified HIV MCC HCC
Gram-negative sepsis NOS
AHA: 2020,2Q,28
A41.51 Sepsis due to Escherichia coli [E. coli] HIV MCC HCC
AHA: 2020,2Q,17
A41.52 Sepsis due to Pseudomonas HIV MCC HCC
Pseudomonas aeroginosa
A41.53 Sepsis due to Serratia HIV MCC HCC
A41.59 Other Gram-negative sepsis HIV MCC HCC
A41.8 Other specified sepsis
A41.81 Sepsis due to Enterococcus HIV MCC HCC
TIP: *E. faecium,* is a species of *Enterococcus* that is highly resistant to multiple antibiotics. Assign a code from category Z16 when resistance to antimicrobial drugs is documented.
A41.89 Other specified sepsis HIV MCC HCC
AHA: 2020,2Q,8; 2017,1Q,51; 2016,3Q,8-14
TIP: Viral sepsis is coded here; assign an additional code to identify the specific viral agent or illness.
A41.9 Sepsis, unspecified organism HIV MCC HCC
Septicemia NOS
AHA: 2022,2Q,5; 2022,1Q,35; 2020,2Q,28

A42 Actinomycosis
EXCLUDES 1 *actinomycetoma (B47.1)*
A42.0 Pulmonary actinomycosis HIV CC HCC
A42.1 Abdominal actinomycosis HIV CC
A42.2 Cervicofacial actinomycosis HIV CC
A42.7 Actinomycotic sepsis HIV MCC HCC
A42.8 Other forms of actinomycosis
A42.81 Actinomycotic meningitis HIV CC
A42.82 Actinomycotic encephalitis HIV CC
A42.89 Other forms of actinomycosis HIV CC
A42.9 Actinomycosis, unspecified HIV CC

A43 Nocardiosis
DEF: Rare bacterial infection occurring most often in those with weakened immune systems. Can be acquired in soil, decaying plants, or standing water. It typically begins in the lungs and has a tendency to spread to other body systems.
A43.0 Pulmonary nocardiosis HIV CC HCC
A43.1 Cutaneous nocardiosis HIV CC
A43.8 Other forms of nocardiosis HIV CC
A43.9 Nocardiosis, unspecified HIV CC

A44 Bartonellosis
A44.0 Systemic bartonellosis CC
Oroya fever
A44.1 Cutaneous and mucocutaneous bartonellosis CC
Verruga peruana
A44.8 Other forms of bartonellosis CC
A44.9 Bartonellosis, unspecified CC

A46 Erysipelas
EXCLUDES 1 *postpartum or puerperal erysipelas (O86.89)*
DEF: Skin infection affecting the upper dermis and superficial dermal lymphatics. Lesion edges are well-demarcated with distinct raised borders. It is often caused by group A *Streptococci.*

A48 Other bacterial diseases, not elsewhere classified
EXCLUDES 1 *actinomycetoma (B47.1)*
A48.0 Gas gangrene MCC HCC
Clostridial cellulitis
Clostridial myonecrosis
AHA: 2017,4Q,102
A48.1 Legionnaires' disease HIV MCC HCC
DEF: Severe and often fatal infection by *Legionella pneumophila.* Symptoms include high fever, gastrointestinal pain, headache, myalgia, dry cough, and pneumonia and it is usually transmitted through airborne water droplets via air conditioning systems or hot tubs.
A48.2 Nonpneumonic Legionnaires' disease [Pontiac fever]
A48.3 Toxic shock syndrome MCC HCC
Use additional code to identify the organism (B95, B96)
EXCLUDES 1 *endotoxic shock NOS (R57.8)*
sepsis NOS (A41.9)
AHA: 2022,1Q,35
DEF: Bacteria producing an endotoxin, such as *Staphylococci,* flood the body with the toxins producing a high fever, vomiting and diarrhea, decreasing blood pressure, a skin rash, and shock. *Synonym(s): TSS.*
A48.4 Brazilian purpuric fever
Systemic Hemophilus aegyptius infection

A48.5 Other specified botulism
Non-foodborne intoxication due to toxins of Clostridium botulinum [C. botulinum]
EXCLUDES 1 *food poisoning due to toxins of Clostridium botulinum (A05.1)*
A48.51 Infant botulism CC P
A48.52 Wound botulism CC
Non-foodborne botulism NOS
Use additional code for associated wound
A48.8 Other specified bacterial diseases

A49 Bacterial infection of unspecified site
EXCLUDES 1 *bacterial agents as the cause of diseases classified elsewhere (B95-B96)*
chlamydial infection NOS (A74.9)
meningococcal infection NOS (A39.9)
rickettsial infection NOS (A79.9)
spirochetal infection NOS (A69.9)
A49.0 Staphylococcal infection, unspecified site
A49.01 Methicillin susceptible Staphylococcus aureus infection, unspecified site
Methicillin susceptible Staphylococcus aureus (MSSA) infection
Staphylococcus aureus infection NOS
A49.02 Methicillin resistant Staphylococcus aureus infection, unspecified site
Methicillin resistant Staphylococcus aureus (MRSA) infection
A49.1 Streptococcal infection, unspecified site
A49.2 Hemophilus influenzae infection, unspecified site
A49.3 Mycoplasma infection, unspecified site
A49.8 Other bacterial infections of unspecified site
A49.9 Bacterial infection, unspecified
EXCLUDES 1 *bacteremia NOS (R78.81)*

Infections with a predominantly sexual mode of transmission (A50-A64)

EXCLUDES 1 *human immunodeficiency virus [HIV] disease (B20)*
nonspecific and nongonococcal urethritis (N34.1)
Reiter's disease (M02.3-)
AHA: 2021,2Q,6

A50 Congenital syphilis
A50.0 Early congenital syphilis, symptomatic
Any congenital syphilitic condition specified as early or manifest less than two years after birth.
A50.01 Early congenital syphilitic oculopathy CC
A50.02 Early congenital syphilitic osteochondropathy CC
A50.03 Early congenital syphilitic pharyngitis CC
Early congenital syphilitic laryngitis
A50.04 Early congenital syphilitic pneumonia CC
A50.05 Early congenital syphilitic rhinitis CC
A50.06 Early cutaneous congenital syphilis CC
A50.07 Early mucocutaneous congenital syphilis CC
A50.08 Early visceral congenital syphilis CC
A50.09 Other early congenital syphilis, symptomatic CC
A50.1 Early congenital syphilis, latent
Congenital syphilis without clinical manifestations, with positive serological reaction and negative spinal fluid test, less than two years after birth.
A50.2 Early congenital syphilis, unspecified CC
Congenital syphilis NOS less than two years after birth.
A50.3 Late congenital syphilitic oculopathy
EXCLUDES 1 *Hutchinson's triad (A50.53)*
A50.30 Late congenital syphilitic oculopathy, unspecified CC
A50.31 Late congenital syphilitic interstitial keratitis CC
A50.32 Late congenital syphilitic chorioretinitis CC
A50.39 Other late congenital syphilitic oculopathy CC
A50.4 Late congenital neurosyphilis [juvenile neurosyphilis]
Use additional code to identify any associated mental disorder
EXCLUDES 1 *Hutchinson's triad (A50.53)*
A50.40 Late congenital neurosyphilis, unspecified CC
Juvenile neurosyphilis NOS
A50.41 Late congenital syphilitic meningitis MCC
A50.42 Late congenital syphilitic encephalitis MCC
A50.43 Late congenital syphilitic polyneuropathy CC
A50.44 Late congenital syphilitic optic nerve atrophy CC
A50.45 Juvenile general paresis CC
Dementia paralytica juvenilis
Juvenile tabetoparetic neurosyphilis
A50.49 Other late congenital neurosyphilis CC
Juvenile tabes dorsalis
A50.5 Other late congenital syphilis, symptomatic
Any congenital syphilitic condition specified as late or manifest two years or more after birth.
A50.51 Clutton's joints CC
A50.52 Hutchinson's teeth CC
A50.53 Hutchinson's triad CC
A50.54 Late congenital cardiovascular syphilis CC
A50.55 Late congenital syphilitic arthropathy CC HCC
A50.56 Late congenital syphilitic osteochondropathy CC
A50.57 Syphilitic saddle nose CC
A50.59 Other late congenital syphilis, symptomatic CC
A50.6 Late congenital syphilis, latent
Congenital syphilis without clinical manifestations, with positive serological reaction and negative spinal fluid test, two years or more after birth.
A50.7 Late congenital syphilis, unspecified
Congenital syphilis NOS two years or more after birth.
A50.9 Congenital syphilis, unspecified

A51 Early syphilis
DEF: Syphilis: Sexually transmitted disease caused by the *Treponema pallidum* spirochete. Syphilis usually exhibits cutaneous manifestations and may exist for years without symptoms.
A51.0 Primary genital syphilis
Syphilitic chancre NOS
A51.1 Primary anal syphilis
A51.2 Primary syphilis of other sites
A51.3 Secondary syphilis of skin and mucous membranes
DEF: Transitory or chronic cutaneous eruptions that present within two to 10 weeks following an initial syphilis infection that may include nontender lymphadenopathy along with alopecia and condylomata lata.
A51.31 Condyloma latum CC
A51.32 Syphilitic alopecia CC
A51.39 Other secondary syphilis of skin CC
Syphilitic leukoderma
Syphilitic mucous patch
EXCLUDES 1 *late syphilitic leukoderma (A52.79)*
A51.4 Other secondary syphilis
A51.41 Secondary syphilitic meningitis MCC
A51.42 Secondary syphilitic female pelvic disease CC ♀
A51.43 Secondary syphilitic oculopathy CC
Secondary syphilitic chorioretinitis
Secondary syphilitic iridocyclitis, iritis
Secondary syphilitic uveitis
A51.44 Secondary syphilitic nephritis CC
A51.45 Secondary syphilitic hepatitis CC
A51.46 Secondary syphilitic osteopathy CC
A51.49 Other secondary syphilitic conditions CC
Secondary syphilitic lymphadenopathy
Secondary syphilitic myositis
A51.5 Early syphilis, latent
Syphilis (acquired) without clinical manifestations, with positive serological reaction and negative spinal fluid test, less than two years after infection.
A51.9 Early syphilis, unspecified

A52 Late syphilis
A52.0 Cardiovascular and cerebrovascular syphilis
A52.00 Cardiovascular syphilis, unspecified CC
A52.01 Syphilitic aneurysm of aorta CC
A52.02 Syphilitic aortitis CC
A52.03 Syphilitic endocarditis CC
Syphilitic aortic valve incompetence or stenosis
Syphilitic mitral valve stenosis
Syphilitic pulmonary valve regurgitation
A52.04 Syphilitic cerebral arteritis CC

A52.Ø5 Other cerebrovascular syphilis CC
Syphilitic cerebral aneurysm (ruptured) (non-ruptured)
Syphilitic cerebral thrombosis

A52.Ø6 Other syphilitic heart involvement CC
Syphilitic coronary artery disease
Syphilitic myocarditis
Syphilitic pericarditis

A52.Ø9 Other cardiovascular syphilis CC

✓5th **A52.1 Symptomatic neurosyphilis**

A52.1Ø Symptomatic neurosyphilis, unspecified CC

A52.11 Tabes dorsalis CC
Locomotor ataxia (progressive)
Tabetic neurosyphilis

A52.12 Other cerebrospinal syphilis CC

A52.13 Late syphilitic meningitis MCC

A52.14 Late syphilitic encephalitis MCC

A52.15 Late syphilitic neuropathy CC
Late syphilitic acoustic neuritis
Late syphilitic optic (nerve) atrophy
Late syphilitic polyneuropathy
Late syphilitic retrobulbar neuritis

A52.16 Charcôt's arthropathy (tabetic) CC
DEF: Progressive neurologic arthropathy in which chronic degeneration of joints in the weight-bearing areas with peripheral hypertrophy occurs as a complication of a neuropathy disorder. Supporting structures relax from a loss of sensation resulting in chronic joint instability.

A52.17 General paresis CC
Dementia paralytica

A52.19 Other symptomatic neurosyphilis CC
Syphilitic parkinsonism

A52.2 Asymptomatic neurosyphilis CC

A52.3 Neurosyphilis, unspecified CC
Gumma (syphilitic)
Syphilis (late)
Syphiloma
AHA: 2021,2Q,6

✓5th **A52.7 Other symptomatic late syphilis**

A52.71 Late syphilitic oculopathy CC
Late syphilitic chorioretinitis
Late syphilitic episcleritis

A52.72 Syphilis of lung and bronchus CC

A52.73 Symptomatic late syphilis of other respiratory organs CC

A52.74 Syphilis of liver and other viscera CC
Late syphilitic peritonitis

A52.75 Syphilis of kidney and ureter CC
Syphilitic glomerular disease

A52.76 Other genitourinary symptomatic late syphilis CC
Late syphilitic female pelvic inflammatory disease

A52.77 Syphilis of bone and joint CC

A52.78 Syphilis of other musculoskeletal tissue CC
Late syphilitic bursitis
Syphilis [stage unspecified] of bursa
Syphilis [stage unspecified] of muscle
Syphilis [stage unspecified] of synovium
Syphilis [stage unspecified] of tendon

A52.79 Other symptomatic late syphilis CC
Late syphilitic leukoderma
Syphilis of adrenal gland
Syphilis of pituitary gland
Syphilis of thyroid gland
Syphilitic splenomegaly
EXCLUDES 1 *syphilitic leukoderma (secondary) (A51.39)*

A52.8 Late syphilis, latent
Syphilis (acquired) without clinical manifestations, with positive serological reaction and negative spinal fluid test, two years or more after infection

A52.9 Late syphilis, unspecified

✓4th **A53 Other and unspecified syphilis**

A53.Ø Latent syphilis, unspecified as early or late
Latent syphilis NOS
Positive serological reaction for syphilis

A53.9 Syphilis, unspecified
Infection due to Treponema pallidum NOS
Syphilis (acquired) NOS
EXCLUDES 1 *syphilis NOS under two years of age (A5Ø.2)*

✓4th **A54 Gonococcal infection**
DEF: Sexually transmitted bacterial infection caused by *Neisseria gonorrhoeae.* Women are often asymptomatic, while men tend to develop urinary symptoms quickly.

✓5th **A54.Ø Gonococcal infection of lower genitourinary tract without periurethral or accessory gland abscess**
EXCLUDES 1 *gonococcal infection with genitourinary gland abscess (A54.1)*
gonococcal infection with periurethral abscess (A54.1)

A54.ØØ Gonococcal infection of lower genitourinary tract, unspecified CC

A54.Ø1 Gonococcal cystitis and urethritis, unspecified CC

A54.Ø2 Gonococcal vulvovaginitis, unspecified CC ♀

A54.Ø3 Gonococcal cervicitis, unspecified CC ♀

A54.Ø9 Other gonococcal infection of lower genitourinary tract CC

A54.1 Gonococcal infection of lower genitourinary tract with periurethral and accessory gland abscess CC
Gonococcal Bartholin's gland abscess

✓5th **A54.2 Gonococcal pelviperitonitis and other gonococcal genitourinary infection**

A54.21 Gonococcal infection of kidney and ureter CC

A54.22 Gonococcal prostatitis CC ♂

A54.23 Gonococcal infection of other male genital organs CC ♂
Gonococcal epididymitis
Gonococcal orchitis

A54.24 Gonococcal female pelvic inflammatory disease CC ♀
Gonococcal pelviperitonitis
EXCLUDES 1 *gonococcal peritonitis (A54.85)*

A54.29 Other gonococcal genitourinary infections CC

✓5th **A54.3 Gonococcal infection of eye**

A54.3Ø Gonococcal infection of eye, unspecified CC

A54.31 Gonococcal conjunctivitis CC
Ophthalmia neonatorum due to gonococcus

A54.32 Gonococcal iridocyclitis CC

A54.33 Gonococcal keratitis CC

A54.39 Other gonococcal eye infection CC
Gonococcal endophthalmia

✓5th **A54.4 Gonococcal infection of musculoskeletal system**

A54.4Ø Gonococcal infection of musculoskeletal system, unspecified CC HCC

A54.41 Gonococcal spondylopathy CC HCC

A54.42 Gonococcal arthritis CC HCC
EXCLUDES 2 *gonococcal infection of spine (A54.41)*

A54.43 Gonococcal osteomyelitis CC HCC
EXCLUDES 2 *gonococcal infection of spine (A54.41)*

A54.49 Gonococcal infection of other musculoskeletal tissue CC HCC
Gonococcal bursitis
Gonococcal myositis
Gonococcal synovitis
Gonococcal tenosynovitis

A54.5 Gonococcal pharyngitis

A54.6 Gonococcal infection of anus and rectum

✓5th **A54.8 Other gonococcal infections**

A54.81 Gonococcal meningitis MCC

A54.82 Gonococcal brain abscess CC

A54.83 Gonococcal heart infection CC
Gonococcal endocarditis
Gonococcal myocarditis
Gonococcal pericarditis

A54.84 Gonococcal pneumonia CC HCC

A54.85 Gonococcal peritonitis CC HCC

EXCLUDES 1 *gonococcal pelviperitonitis (A54.24)*

A54.86 Gonococcal sepsis MCC HCC

A54.89 Other gonococcal infections CC

Gonococcal keratoderma

Gonococcal lymphadenitis

A54.9 Gonococcal infection, unspecified CC

A55 Chlamydial lymphogranuloma (venereum)

Climatic or tropical bubo

Durand-Nicolas-Favre disease

Esthiomene

Lymphogranuloma inguinale

A56 Other sexually transmitted chlamydial diseases

INCLUDES sexually transmitted diseases due to Chlamydia trachomatis

EXCLUDES 1 *neonatal chlamydial conjunctivitis (P39.1)*

neonatal chlamydial pneumonia (P23.1)

EXCLUDES 2 *chlamydial lymphogranuloma (A55)*

conditions classified to A74.-

DEF: *Chlamydia trachomatis*: Bacterium that causes a common venereal disease. Symptoms of chlamydia are usually mild or absent, however, serious complications may cause irreversible damage, including cystitis, pelvic inflammatory disease, and infertility in women and discharge from the penis, prostatitis, and infertility in men. Genital chlamydial infection can cause arthritis, skin lesions, and inflammation of the eye and urethra. ***Synonym(s):*** *Reiter's syndrome.*

A56.Ø Chlamydial infection of lower genitourinary tract

A56.ØØ Chlamydial infection of lower genitourinary tract, unspecified

A56.Ø1 Chlamydial cystitis and urethritis

A56.Ø2 Chlamydial vulvovaginitis ♀

A56.Ø9 Other chlamydial infection of lower genitourinary tract

Chlamydial cervicitis

A56.1 Chlamydial infection of pelviperitoneum and other genitourinary organs

A56.11 Chlamydial female pelvic inflammatory disease ♀

A56.19 Other chlamydial genitourinary infection

Chlamydial epididymitis

Chlamydial orchitis

A56.2 Chlamydial infection of genitourinary tract, unspecified

A56.3 Chlamydial infection of anus and rectum

A56.4 Chlamydial infection of pharynx

A56.8 Sexually transmitted chlamydial infection of other sites

A57 Chancroid

Ulcus molle

DEF: Localized infection by *Haemophilus ducreyi*, causing genital ulcers and infecting the inguinal lymph nodes.

A58 Granuloma inguinale

Donovanosis

A59 Trichomoniasis

EXCLUDES 2 *intestinal trichomoniasis (AØ7.8)*

DEF: Infection with the parasitic, flagellated protozoa of the genus *Trichomonas*. This protozoon is found in the intestinal and genitourinary tracts of humans and in the mouth around tartar, cavities, and areas of periodontal disease.

A59.Ø Urogenital trichomoniasis

A59.ØØ Urogenital trichomoniasis, unspecified

Fluor (vaginalis) due to Trichomonas

Leukorrhea (vaginalis) due to Trichomonas

A59.Ø1 Trichomonal vulvovaginitis ♀

A59.Ø2 Trichomonal prostatitis ♂

A59.Ø3 Trichomonal cystitis and urethritis

A59.Ø9 Other urogenital trichomoniasis

Trichomonas cervicitis

A59.8 Trichomoniasis of other sites

A59.9 Trichomoniasis, unspecified

A6Ø Anogenital herpesviral [herpes simplex] infections

A6Ø.Ø Herpesviral infection of genitalia and urogenital tract

A6Ø.ØØ Herpesviral infection of urogenital system, unspecified HIV

A6Ø.Ø1 Herpesviral infection of penis HIV ♂

A6Ø.Ø2 Herpesviral infection of other male genital organs ♂

A6Ø.Ø3 Herpesviral cervicitis ♀

A6Ø.Ø4 Herpesviral vulvovaginitis HIV ♀

Herpesviral [herpes simplex] ulceration

Herpesviral [herpes simplex] vaginitis

Herpesviral [herpes simplex] vulvitis

A6Ø.Ø9 Herpesviral infection of other urogenital tract HIV

AHA: 2020,1Q,20

A6Ø.1 Herpesviral infection of perianal skin and rectum HIV

A6Ø.9 Anogenital herpesviral infection, unspecified HIV

A63 Other predominantly sexually transmitted diseases, not elsewhere classified

EXCLUDES 2 *molluscum contagiosum (BØ8.1)*

papilloma of cervix (D26.Ø)

A63.Ø Anogenital (venereal) warts

Anogenital warts due to (human) papillomavirus [HPV]

Condyloma acuminatum

A63.8 Other specified predominantly sexually transmitted diseases

A64 Unspecified sexually transmitted disease

Other spirochetal diseases (A65-A69)

EXCLUDES 2 *leptospirosis (A27.-)*

syphilis (A5Ø-A53)

A65 Nonvenereal syphilis

Bejel

Endemic syphilis

Njovera

A66 Yaws

INCLUDES bouba

frambesia (tropica)

pian

A66.Ø Initial lesions of yaws

Chancre of yaws

Frambesia, initial or primary

Initial frambesial ulcer

Mother yaw

A66.1 Multiple papillomata and wet crab yaws

Frambesioma

Pianoma

Plantar or palmar papilloma of yaws

A66.2 Other early skin lesions of yaws

Cutaneous yaws, less than five years after infection

Early yaws (cutaneous) (macular) (maculopapular) (micropapular) (papular)

Frambeside of early yaws

A66.3 Hyperkeratosis of yaws

Ghoul hand

Hyperkeratosis, palmar or plantar (early) (late) due to yaws

Worm-eaten soles

A66.4 Gummata and ulcers of yaws

Gummatous frambeside

Nodular late yaws (ulcerated)

A66.5 Gangosa

Rhinopharyngitis mutilans

A66.6 Bone and joint lesions of yaws HCC

Yaws ganglion

Yaws goundou

Yaws gumma, bone

Yaws gummatous osteitis or periostitis

Yaws hydrarthrosis

Yaws osteitis

Yaws periostitis (hypertrophic)

A66.7 Other manifestations of yaws

Juxta-articular nodules of yaws

Mucosal yaws

A66.8 Latent yaws

Yaws without clinical manifestations, with positive serology

A66.9 Yaws, unspecified

A67 Pinta [carate]

A67.Ø Primary lesions of pinta

Chancre (primary) of pinta

Papule (primary) of pinta

A67.1 Intermediate lesions of pinta
Erythematous plaques of pinta
Hyperchromic lesions of pinta
Hyperkeratosis of pinta
Pintids

A67.2 Late lesions of pinta
Achromic skin lesions of pinta
Cicatricial skin lesions of pinta
Dyschromic skin lesions of pinta

A67.3 Mixed lesions of pinta
Achromic with hyperchromic skin lesions of pinta [carate]

A67.9 Pinta, unspecified

A68 Relapsing fevers
INCLUDES recurrent fever
EXCLUDES 2 *Lyme disease (A69.2-)*

A68.Ø Louse-borne relapsing fever CC
Relapsing fever due to Borrelia recurrentis

A68.1 Tick-borne relapsing fever CC
Relapsing fever due to any Borrelia species other than Borrelia recurrentis

A68.9 Relapsing fever, unspecified CC

A69 Other spirochetal infections

A69.Ø Necrotizing ulcerative stomatitis
Cancrum oris
Fusospirochetal gangrene
Noma
Stomatitis gangrenosa

A69.1 Other Vincent's infections CC
Fusospirochetal pharyngitis
Necrotizing ulcerative (acute) gingivitis
Necrotizing ulcerative (acute) gingivostomatitis
Spirochetal stomatitis
Trench mouth
Vincent's angina
Vincent's gingivitis

A69.2 Lyme disease
Erythema chronicum migrans due to Borrelia burgdorferi
DEF: Recurrent multisystem disorder through tick bites that begins with lesions of erythema chronicum migrans and is followed by arthritis of the large joints, myalgia, malaise, and neurological and cardiac manifestations.

A69.2Ø Lyme disease, unspecified CC
AHA: 2021,4Q,5

A69.21 Meningitis due to Lyme disease CC

A69.22 Other neurologic disorders in Lyme disease CC
Cranial neuritis
Meningoencephalitis
Polyneuropathy

A69.23 Arthritis due to Lyme disease CC HCC

A69.29 Other conditions associated with Lyme disease CC
Myopericarditis due to Lyme disease
AHA: 2016,3Q,12

A69.8 Other specified spirochetal infections

A69.9 Spirochetal infection, unspecified

Other diseases caused by chlamydiae (A7Ø-A74)

EXCLUDES 1 *sexually transmitted chlamydial diseases (A55-A56)*

A7Ø Chlamydia psittaci infections CC
Ornithosis
Parrot fever
Psittacosis

A71 Trachoma
EXCLUDES 1 *sequelae of trachoma (B94.Ø)*

A71.Ø Initial stage of trachoma
Trachoma dubium

A71.1 Active stage of trachoma
Granular conjunctivitis (trachomatous)
Trachomatous follicular conjunctivitis
Trachomatous pannus

A71.9 Trachoma, unspecified

A74 Other diseases caused by chlamydiae
EXCLUDES 1 *neonatal chlamydial conjunctivitis (P39.1)*
neonatal chlamydial pneumonia (P23.1)
Reiter's disease (MØ2.3-)
sexually transmitted chlamydial diseases (A55-A56)
EXCLUDES 2 *chlamydial pneumonia (J16.Ø)*

A74.Ø Chlamydial conjunctivitis
Paratrachoma

A74.8 Other chlamydial diseases

A74.81 Chlamydial peritonitis

A74.89 Other chlamydial diseases

A74.9 Chlamydial infection, unspecified
Chlamydiosis NOS

Rickettsioses (A75-A79)

DEF: Rickettsia: Condition caused by bacteria that live in lice/ticks transmitted to humans through bites.

A75 Typhus fever
EXCLUDES 1 *rickettsiosis due to Ehrlichia sennetsu (A79.81)*

A75.Ø Epidemic louse-borne typhus fever due to Rickettsia prowazekii CC
Classical typhus (fever)
Epidemic (louse-borne) typhus

A75.1 Recrudescent typhus [Brill's disease] CC
Brill-Zinsser disease

A75.2 Typhus fever due to Rickettsia typhi CC
Murine (flea-borne) typhus

A75.3 Typhus fever due to Rickettsia tsutsugamushi CC
Scrub (mite-borne) typhus
Tsutsugamushi fever
Typhus fever due to Orientia Tsutsugamushi (scrub typhus)

A75.9 Typhus fever, unspecified CC
Typhus (fever) NOS

A77 Spotted fever [tick-borne rickettsioses]

A77.Ø Spotted fever due to Rickettsia rickettsii CC
Rocky Mountain spotted fever
Sao Paulo fever

A77.1 Spotted fever due to Rickettsia conorii CC
African tick typhus
Boutonneuse fever
India tick typhus
Kenya tick typhus
Marseilles fever
Mediterranean tick fever

A77.2 Spotted fever due to Rickettsia siberica CC
North Asian tick fever
Siberian tick typhus

A77.3 Spotted fever due to Rickettsia australis CC
Queensland tick typhus

A77.4 Ehrlichiosis
EXCLUDES 1 *anaplasmosis [A. phagocytophilum] (A79.82)*
rickettsiosis due to Ehrlichia sennetsu (A79.81)
AHA: 2021,4Q,5

A77.4Ø Ehrlichiosis, unspecified CC

A77.41 Ehrlichiosis chafeensis [E. chafeensis] CC

A77.49 Other ehrlichiosis CC
Ehrlichiosis due to E. ewingii
Ehrlichiosis due to E. muris euclairensis

A77.8 Other spotted fevers CC
Rickettsia 364D/R. philipii (Pacific Coast tick fever)
Spotted fever due to Rickettsia africae (African tick bite fever)
Spotted fever due to Rickettsia parkeri

A77.9 Spotted fever, unspecified CC
Tick-borne typhus NOS

A78 Q fever CC
Infection due to Coxiella burnetii
Nine Mile fever
Quadrilateral fever

A79 Other rickettsioses

A79.Ø Trench fever CC
Quintan fever
Wolhynian fever

A79.1 Rickettsialpox due to Rickettsia akari CC
Kew Garden fever
Vesicular rickettsiosis

A79.8 Other specified rickettsioses

A79.81 Rickettsiosis due to Ehrlichia sennetsu CC
Rickettsiosis due to Neorickettsia sennetsu

A79.82 Anaplasmosis [A. phagocytophilum] CC
Transfusion transmitted A. phagocytophilum
AHA: 2021,4Q,4-5

A79.89 Other specified rickettsioses CC

A79.9 Rickettsiosis, unspecified CC
Rickettsial infection NOS

Viral and prion infections of the central nervous system (A8Ø-A89)

EXCLUDES 1 *postpolio syndrome (G14)*
sequelae of poliomyelitis (B91)
sequelae of viral encephalitis (B94.1)

A8Ø Acute poliomyelitis

EXCLUDES 1 *acute flaccid myelitis (GØ4.82)*

A8Ø.Ø Acute paralytic poliomyelitis, vaccine-associated MCC
A8Ø.1 Acute paralytic poliomyelitis, wild virus, imported MCC
A8Ø.2 Acute paralytic poliomyelitis, wild virus, indigenous MCC
A8Ø.3 Acute paralytic poliomyelitis, other and unspecified
A8Ø.3Ø Acute paralytic poliomyelitis, unspecified MCC
A8Ø.39 Other acute paralytic poliomyelitis MCC
A8Ø.4 Acute nonparalytic poliomyelitis
A8Ø.9 Acute poliomyelitis, unspecified

A81 Atypical virus infections of central nervous system

INCLUDES diseases of the central nervous system caused by prions

▶Use additional code, if applicable, to identify:◀
▶dementia with anxiety (FØ2.84, FØ2.A4, FØ2.B4, FØ2.C4)◀
dementia with behavioral disturbance ▶(FØ2.81-, FØ2.A1-, FØ2.B1-, FØ2.C1-)◀
▶dementia with mood disturbance (FØ2.83, FØ2.A3, FØ2.B3, FØ2.C3)◀
▶dementia with psychotic disturbance (FØ2.82, FØ2.A2, FØ2.B2, FØ2.C2)◀
dementia without behavioral disturbance ▶(FØ2.8Ø, FØ2.AØ, FØ2.BØ, FØ2.CØ)◀
▶mild neurocognitive disorder due to known physiological condition (FØ6.7-)◀

A81.Ø Creutzfeldt-Jakob disease
DEF: Communicable, rare spongiform encephalopathy occurring later in life with progressive destruction of the pyramidal and extrapyramidal systems eventually leading to death. Progressive dementia, wasting of muscles, tremor, and other symptoms are present.

A81.ØØ Creutzfeldt-Jakob disease, unspecified CC HCC
Jakob-Creutzfeldt disease, unspecified

A81.Ø1 Variant Creutzfeldt-Jakob disease CC HCC
vCJD

A81.Ø9 Other Creutzfeldt-Jakob disease CC HCC
CJD
Familial Creutzfeldt-Jakob disease
Iatrogenic Creutzfeldt-Jakob disease
Sporadic Creutzfeldt-Jakob disease
Subacute spongiform encephalopathy (with dementia)

A81.1 Subacute sclerosing panencephalitis CC HCC
Dawson's inclusion body encephalitis
Van Bogaert's sclerosing leukoencephalopathy

A81.2 Progressive multifocal leukoencephalopathy HIV CC HCC
Multifocal leukoencephalopathy NOS

A81.8 Other atypical virus infections of central nervous system

A81.81 Kuru CC HCC

A81.82 Gerstmann-Sträussler-Scheinker syndrome HIV CC HCC
GSS syndrome

A81.83 Fatal familial insomnia HIV CC HCC
FFI

A81.89 Other atypical virus infections of central nervous system HIV CC HCC

A81.9 Atypical virus infection of central nervous system, unspecified HIV CC HCC
Prion diseases of the central nervous system NOS

A82 Rabies

A82.Ø Sylvatic rabies CC
A82.1 Urban rabies CC
A82.9 Rabies, unspecified CC

A83 Mosquito-borne viral encephalitis

INCLUDES mosquito-borne viral meningoencephalitis

EXCLUDES 2 *Venezuelan equine encephalitis (A92.2)*
West Nile fever (A92.3-)
West Nile virus (A92.3-)

A83.Ø Japanese encephalitis MCC
A83.1 Western equine encephalitis MCC
A83.2 Eastern equine encephalitis MCC
A83.3 St Louis encephalitis MCC
A83.4 Australian encephalitis MCC
Kunjin virus disease
A83.5 California encephalitis MCC
California meningoencephalitis
La Crosse encephalitis
A83.6 Rocio virus disease MCC
A83.8 Other mosquito-borne viral encephalitis MCC
A83.9 Mosquito-borne viral encephalitis, unspecified MCC

A84 Tick-borne viral encephalitis

INCLUDES tick-borne viral meningoencephalitis

A84.Ø Far Eastern tick-borne encephalitis [Russian spring-summer encephalitis] MCC
A84.1 Central European tick-borne encephalitis MCC
A84.8 Other tick-borne viral encephalitis
AHA: 2020,4Q,4-5

A84.81 Powassan virus disease MCC

A84.89 Other tick-borne viral encephalitis MCC
Louping ill
Code first, if applicable, transfusion related infection (T8Ø.22-)

A84.9 Tick-borne viral encephalitis, unspecified MCC

A85 Other viral encephalitis, not elsewhere classified

INCLUDES specified viral encephalomyelitis NEC
specified viral meningoencephalitis NEC

EXCLUDES 1 ~~*benign myalgic encephalomyelitis (G93.3)*~~
encephalitis due to cytomegalovirus (B25.8)
encephalitis due to herpesvirus NEC (B1Ø.Ø-)
encephalitis due to herpesvirus [herpes simplex] (BØØ.4)
encephalitis due to measles virus (BØ5.Ø)
encephalitis due to mumps virus (B26.2)
encephalitis due to poliomyelitis virus (A8Ø.-)
encephalitis due to zoster (BØ2.Ø)
lymphocytic choriomeningitis (A87.2)
▶*myalgic encephalomyelitis (G93.32)*◀

A85.Ø Enteroviral encephalitis HIV CC
Enteroviral encephalomyelitis

A85.1 Adenoviral encephalitis HIV CC
Adenoviral meningoencephalitis

A85.2 Arthropod-borne viral encephalitis, unspecified MCC
EXCLUDES 1 *West nile virus with encephalitis (A92.31)*

A85.8 Other specified viral encephalitis HIV CC
Encephalitis lethargica
Von Economo-Cruchet disease

A86 Unspecified viral encephalitis HIV CC
Viral encephalomyelitis NOS
Viral meningoencephalitis NOS

A87 Viral meningitis

EXCLUDES 1 *meningitis due to herpesvirus [herpes simplex] (B00.3)*
meningitis due to measles virus (B05.1)
meningitis due to mumps virus (B26.1)
meningitis due to poliomyelitis virus (A80.-)
meningitis due to zoster (B02.1)

DEF: Meningitis: Inflammation of the meningeal layers of the brain and spine.

A87.0 Enteroviral meningitis CC
Coxsackievirus meningitis
Echovirus meningitis

A87.1 Adenoviral meningitis CC

A87.2 Lymphocytic choriomeningitis CC
Lymphocytic meningoencephalitis

A87.8 Other viral meningitis CC

A87.9 Viral meningitis, unspecified CC

A88 Other viral infections of central nervous system, not elsewhere classified

EXCLUDES 1 *viral encephalitis NOS (A86)*
viral meningitis NOS (A87.9)

A88.0 Enteroviral exanthematous fever [Boston exanthem] CC

A88.1 Epidemic vertigo

A88.8 Other specified viral infections of central nervous system HIV CC

A89 Unspecified viral infection of central nervous system HIV CC

Arthropod-borne viral fevers and viral hemorrhagic fevers (A90-A99)

A90 Dengue fever [classical dengue] CC

EXCLUDES 1 *dengue hemorrhagic fever (A91)*

AHA: 2016,3Q,13

A91 Dengue hemorrhagic fever CC

A92 Other mosquito-borne viral fevers

EXCLUDES 1 *Ross River disease (B33.1)*

A92.0 Chikungunya virus disease CC
Chikungunya (hemorrhagic) fever

A92.1 O'nyong-nyong fever CC

A92.2 Venezuelan equine fever CC
Venezuelan equine encephalitis
Venezuelan equine encephalomyelitis virus disease

A92.3 West Nile virus infection
West Nile fever
AHA: 2016,3Q,12

A92.30 West Nile virus infection, unspecified MCC
West Nile fever NOS
West Nile fever without complications
West Nile virus NOS

A92.31 West Nile virus infection with encephalitis MCC
West Nile encephalitis
West Nile encephalomyelitis

A92.32 West Nile virus infection with other neurologic manifestation MCC
Use additional code to specify the neurologic manifestation

A92.39 West Nile virus infection with other complications MCC
Use additional code to specify the other conditions

A92.4 Rift Valley fever CC

A92.5 Zika virus disease CC
Zika virus fever
Zika virus infection
Zika NOS

EXCLUDES 1 *congenital Zika virus disease (P35.4)*

AHA: 2016,4Q,4-7

DEF: Virus transmitted via a bite from an infected Aedes species mosquito. Common symptoms of the virus include fever, rash, joint pain, and conjunctivitis; they are usually mild in nature and may last from several days to a week. Most people who have the Zika virus do not require medical attention; however, in pregnant women, the Zika virus can cause a serious birth defect called microcephaly, as well as other severe fetal brain defects.

TIP: Code only confirmed diagnoses of Zika virus; documentation by the physician that the disease is confirmed is sufficient.

A92.8 Other specified mosquito-borne viral fevers CC

A92.9 Mosquito-borne viral fever, unspecified CC

A93 Other arthropod-borne viral fevers, not elsewhere classified

A93.0 Oropouche virus disease CC
Oropouche fever

A93.1 Sandfly fever CC
Pappataci fever
Phlebotomus fever

A93.2 Colorado tick fever CC

A93.8 Other specified arthropod-borne viral fevers CC
Piry virus disease
Vesicular stomatitis virus disease [Indiana fever]

A94 Unspecified arthropod-borne viral fever CC
Arboviral fever NOS
Arbovirus infection NOS

A95 Yellow fever

A95.0 Sylvatic yellow fever CC
Jungle yellow fever

A95.1 Urban yellow fever CC

A95.9 Yellow fever, unspecified CC

A96 Arenaviral hemorrhagic fever

A96.0 Junin hemorrhagic fever CC
Argentinian hemorrhagic fever

A96.1 Machupo hemorrhagic fever CC
Bolivian hemorrhagic fever

A96.2 Lassa fever

A96.8 Other arenaviral hemorrhagic fevers CC

A96.9 Arenaviral hemorrhagic fever, unspecified CC

A98 Other viral hemorrhagic fevers, not elsewhere classified

EXCLUDES 1 *chikungunya hemorrhagic fever (A92.0)*
dengue hemorrhagic fever (A91)

A98.0 Crimean-Congo hemorrhagic fever CC
Central Asian hemorrhagic fever

A98.1 Omsk hemorrhagic fever CC

A98.2 Kyasanur Forest disease CC

A98.3 Marburg virus disease

A98.4 Ebola virus disease

A98.5 Hemorrhagic fever with renal syndrome CC
Epidemic hemorrhagic fever
Korean hemorrhagic fever
Russian hemorrhagic fever
Hantaan virus disease
Hantavirus disease with renal manifestations
Nephropathia epidemica
Songo fever

EXCLUDES 1 *hantavirus (cardio)-pulmonary syndrome (B33.4)*

A98.8 Other specified viral hemorrhagic fevers CC

A99 Unspecified viral hemorrhagic fever CC

Viral infections characterized by skin and mucous membrane lesions (B00-B09)

B00 Herpesviral [herpes simplex] infections

EXCLUDES 1 *congenital herpesviral infections (P35.2)*

EXCLUDES 2 *anogenital herpesviral infection (A60.-)*
gammaherpesviral mononucleosis (B27.0-)
herpangina (B08.5)

B00.0 Eczema herpeticum HIV
Kaposi's varicelliform eruption

B00.1 Herpesviral vesicular dermatitis HIV
Herpes simplex facialis
Herpes simplex labialis
Herpes simplex otitis externa
Vesicular dermatitis of ear
Vesicular dermatitis of lip

B00.2 Herpesviral gingivostomatitis and pharyngotonsillitis HIV CC
Herpesviral pharyngitis

B00.3 Herpesviral meningitis HIV MCC

B00.4 Herpesviral encephalitis HIV MCC
Herpesviral meningoencephalitis
Simian B disease

EXCLUDES 1 *herpesviral encephalitis due to herpesvirus 6 and 7 (B10.01, B10.09)*
non-simplex herpesviral encephalitis (B10.0-)

B00.5 Herpesviral ocular disease

B00.50 Herpesviral ocular disease, unspecified HIV CC

B00.51 Herpesviral iridocyclitis HIV CC
Herpesviral iritis
Herpesviral uveitis, anterior

B00.52 Herpesviral keratitis HIV CC
Herpesviral keratoconjunctivitis

B00.53 Herpesviral conjunctivitis HIV CC

B00.59 Other herpesviral disease of eye HIV CC
Herpesviral dermatitis of eyelid

B00.7 Disseminated herpesviral disease HIV MCC HCC
Herpesviral sepsis

B00.8 Other forms of herpesviral infections

B00.81 Herpesviral hepatitis HIV CC

B00.82 Herpes simplex myelitis MCC HCC

B00.89 Other herpesviral infection HIV CC
Herpesviral whitlow

B00.9 Herpesviral infection, unspecified HIV
Herpes simplex infection NOS

B01 Varicella [chickenpox]

B01.0 Varicella meningitis CC

B01.1 Varicella encephalitis, myelitis and encephalomyelitis
Postchickenpox encephalitis, myelitis and encephalomyelitis

B01.11 Varicella encephalitis and encephalomyelitis MCC
Postchickenpox encephalitis and encephalomyelitis

B01.12 Varicella myelitis MCC HCC
Postchickenpox myelitis

B01.2 Varicella pneumonia MCC

B01.8 Varicella with other complications

B01.81 Varicella keratitis CC

B01.89 Other varicella complications CC

B01.9 Varicella without complication CC
Varicella NOS

B02 Zoster [herpes zoster]
INCLUDES shingles
zona

B02.0 Zoster encephalitis HIV CC
Zoster meningoencephalitis

B02.1 Zoster meningitis HIV MCC
AHA: 2019,1Q,18

B02.2 Zoster with other nervous system involvement

B02.21 Postherpetic geniculate ganglionitis HIV CC

B02.22 Postherpetic trigeminal neuralgia HIV CC

B02.23 Postherpetic polyneuropathy HIV CC

B02.24 Postherpetic myelitis MCC HCC
Herpes zoster myelitis

B02.29 Other postherpetic nervous system involvement HIV CC
Postherpetic radiculopathy

B02.3 Zoster ocular disease

B02.30 Zoster ocular disease, unspecified HIV CC

B02.31 Zoster conjunctivitis HIV CC

B02.32 Zoster iridocyclitis HIV CC

B02.33 Zoster keratitis HIV CC
Herpes zoster keratoconjunctivitis

B02.34 Zoster scleritis HIV CC

B02.39 Other herpes zoster eye disease HIV CC
Zoster blepharitis

B02.7 Disseminated zoster HIV CC

B02.8 Zoster with other complications HIV CC
Herpes zoster otitis externa

B02.9 Zoster without complications HIV
Zoster NOS

B03 Smallpox CC

NOTE In 1980 the 33rd World Health Assembly declared that smallpox had been eradicated.
The classification is maintained for surveillance purposes.

B04 Monkeypox CC

B05 Measles
INCLUDES morbilli
EXCLUDES 1 *subacute sclerosing panencephalitis (A81.1)*

B05.0 Measles complicated by encephalitis MCC
Postmeasles encephalitis

B05.1 Measles complicated by meningitis CC
Postmeasles meningitis

B05.2 Measles complicated by pneumonia MCC
Postmeasles pneumonia

B05.3 Measles complicated by otitis media
Postmeasles otitis media

B05.4 Measles with intestinal complications CC

B05.8 Measles with other complications

B05.81 Measles keratitis and keratoconjunctivitis CC

B05.89 Other measles complications CC

B05.9 Measles without complication
Measles NOS

B06 Rubella [German measles]
EXCLUDES 1 *congenital rubella (P35.0)*
DEF: Highly contagious virus in which the symptoms are mild and short-lived in most people. Rubella during pregnancy, however, can result in abortion, stillbirth, or congenital defects.

B06.0 Rubella with neurological complications

B06.00 Rubella with neurological complication, unspecified CC

B06.01 Rubella encephalitis MCC
Rubella meningoencephalitis

B06.02 Rubella meningitis CC

B06.09 Other neurological complications of rubella CC

B06.8 Rubella with other complications

B06.81 Rubella pneumonia CC

B06.82 Rubella arthritis CC HCC

B06.89 Other rubella complications CC

B06.9 Rubella without complication
Rubella NOS

B07 Viral warts
INCLUDES verruca simplex
verruca vulgaris
viral warts due to human papillomavirus
EXCLUDES 2 *anogenital (venereal) warts (A63.0)*
papilloma of bladder (D41.4)
papilloma of cervix (D26.0)
papilloma larynx (D14.1)

B07.0 Plantar wart
Verruca plantaris

B07.8 Other viral warts
Common wart
Flat wart
Verruca plana

B07.9 Viral wart, unspecified

B08 Other viral infections characterized by skin and mucous membrane lesions, not elsewhere classified
EXCLUDES 1 *vesicular stomatitis virus disease (A93.8)*

B08.0 Other orthopoxvirus infections
EXCLUDES 2 *monkeypox (B04)*

B08.01 Cowpox and vaccinia not from vaccine

B08.010 Cowpox
DEF: Disease contracted by milking infected cows. The vesicles usually appear on the fingers, hands, and adjacent areas and usually disappear without scarring. Other symptoms include local edema, lymphangitis, and regional lymphadenitis with or without fever.

B08.011 Vaccinia not from vaccine
EXCLUDES 1 *vaccinia (from vaccination) (generalized) (T88.1)*

B08.02 Orf virus disease
Contagious pustular dermatitis
Ecthyma contagiosum

B08.03 Pseudocowpox [milker's node]

B08.04 Paravaccinia, unspecified

B08.09 Other orthopoxvirus infections
Orthopoxvirus infection NOS

B08.1 Molluscum contagiosum
DEF: Benign poxvirus infection causing small bumps on the skin or conjunctiva, transmitted by close contact.

B08.2 Exanthema subitum [sixth disease]
Roseola infantum

B08.20 Exanthema subitum [sixth disease], unspecified P
Roseola infantum, unspecified

B08.21 Exanthema subitum [sixth disease] due to human herpesvirus 6 P
Roseola infantum due to human herpesvirus 6

B08.22 Exanthema subitum [sixth disease] due to human herpesvirus 7 P
Roseola infantum due to human herpesvirus 7

B08.3 Erythema infectiosum [fifth disease] CC
DEF: Infection with human parvovirus B19, mainly occurring in children. Symptoms include a low-grade fever, malaise, or a "cold" a few days before the appearance of a mild rash illness that presents as a "slapped-cheek" rash on the face and a lacy red rash on the trunk and limbs.

B08.4 Enteroviral vesicular stomatitis with exanthem
Hand, foot and mouth disease

B08.5 Enteroviral vesicular pharyngitis
Herpangina
DEF: Acute infectious Coxsackie virus infection causing throat lesions, fever, and vomiting that generally affects children in the summer.

B08.6 Parapoxvirus infections

B08.60 Parapoxvirus infection, unspecified

B08.61 Bovine stomatitis

B08.62 Sealpox

B08.69 Other parapoxvirus infections

B08.7 Yatapoxvirus infections

B08.70 Yatapoxvirus infection, unspecified

B08.71 Tanapox virus disease CC

B08.72 Yaba pox virus disease
Yaba monkey tumor disease

B08.79 Other yatapoxvirus infections

B08.8 Other specified viral infections characterized by skin and mucous membrane lesions
Enteroviral lymphonodular pharyngitis
Foot-and-mouth disease
Poxvirus NEC

B09 Unspecified viral infection characterized by skin and mucous membrane lesions
Viral enanthema NOS
Viral exanthema NOS

Other human herpesviruses (B10)

B10 Other human herpesviruses
EXCLUDES 2 *cytomegalovirus (B25.9)*
Epstein-Barr virus (B27.0-)
herpes NOS (B00.9)
herpes simplex (B00.-)
herpes zoster (B02.-)
human herpesvirus NOS (B00.-)
human herpesvirus 1 and 2 (B00.-)
human herpesvirus 3 (B01.-, B02.-)
human herpesvirus 4 (B27.0-)
human herpesvirus 5 (B25.-)
varicella (B01.-)
zoster (B02.-)

B10.0 Other human herpesvirus encephalitis
EXCLUDES 2 *herpes encephalitis NOS (B00.4)*
herpes simplex encephalitis (B00.4)
human herpesvirus encephalitis (B00.4)
simian B herpes virus encephalitis (B00.4)

B10.01 Human herpesvirus 6 encephalitis HIV MCC

B10.09 Other human herpesvirus encephalitis HIV MCC
Human herpesvirus 7 encephalitis

B10.8 Other human herpesvirus infection

B10.81 Human herpesvirus 6 infection

B10.82 Human herpesvirus 7 infection

B10.89 Other human herpesvirus infection
Human herpesvirus 8 infection
Kaposi's sarcoma-associated herpesvirus infection

Viral hepatitis (B15-B19)

EXCLUDES 1 *sequelae of viral hepatitis (B94.2)*
EXCLUDES 2 *cytomegaloviral hepatitis (B25.1)*
herpesviral [herpes simplex] hepatitis (B00.81)

DEF: Hepatitis A: HAV infection that is self-limiting with flulike symptoms. Transmission is fecal-oral.
DEF: Hepatitis B: HBV infection that can be chronic and systemic. Transmission is bodily fluids.
DEF: Hepatitis C: HCV infection that can be chronic and systemic. Transmission is blood transfusion and unidentified agents.
DEF: Hepatitis D (delta): HDV that occurs only in the presence of hepatitis B virus. Transmission is contaminated blood in contact with mucous membranes.
DEF: Hepatitis E: HEV is an epidemic form. Transmission is fecal-oral, most often from contaminated water.

B15 Acute hepatitis A

B15.0 Hepatitis A with hepatic coma MCC

B15.9 Hepatitis A without hepatic coma CC
Hepatitis A (acute)(viral) NOS

B16 Acute hepatitis B
AHA: 2016,3Q,13

B16.0 Acute hepatitis B with delta-agent with hepatic coma MCC

B16.1 Acute hepatitis B with delta-agent without hepatic coma CC

B16.2 Acute hepatitis B without delta-agent with hepatic coma MCC

B16.9 Acute hepatitis B without delta-agent and without hepatic coma CC
Hepatitis B (acute) (viral) NOS

B17 Other acute viral hepatitis

B17.0 Acute delta-(super) infection of hepatitis B carrier CC

B17.1 Acute hepatitis C

B17.10 Acute hepatitis C without hepatic coma CC
Acute hepatitis C NOS

B17.11 Acute hepatitis C with hepatic coma MCC

B17.2 Acute hepatitis E CC

B17.8 Other specified acute viral hepatitis CC
Hepatitis non-A non-B (acute) (viral) NEC

B17.9 Acute viral hepatitis, unspecified CC
Acute hepatitis NOS
Acute infectious hepatitis NOS

B18 Chronic viral hepatitis
INCLUDES carrier of viral hepatitis
AHA: 2017,1Q,41

B18.0 Chronic viral hepatitis B with delta-agent CC HCC

B18.1 Chronic viral hepatitis B without delta-agent CC HCC
Carrier of viral hepatitis B
Chronic (viral) hepatitis B

B18.2 Chronic viral hepatitis C HCC
Carrier of viral hepatitis C
AHA: 2018,1Q,4

B18.8 Other chronic viral hepatitis CC HCC
Carrier of other viral hepatitis

B18.9 Chronic viral hepatitis, unspecified CC HCC
Carrier of unspecified viral hepatitis

B19 Unspecified viral hepatitis

B19.0 Unspecified viral hepatitis with hepatic coma MCC

B19.1 Unspecified viral hepatitis B

B19.10 Unspecified viral hepatitis B without hepatic coma CC
Unspecified viral hepatitis B NOS

B19.11 Unspecified viral hepatitis B with hepatic coma MCC

B19.2 Unspecified viral hepatitis C

B19.20 Unspecified viral hepatitis C without hepatic coma
Viral hepatitis C NOS

B19.21 Unspecified viral hepatitis C with hepatic coma MCC

B19.9 Unspecified viral hepatitis without hepatic coma CC
Viral hepatitis NOS

Human immunodeficiency virus [HIV] disease (B20)

B20 Human immunodeficiency virus [HIV] disease CC HCC

INCLUDES acquired immune deficiency syndrome [AIDS]
AIDS-related complex [ARC]
HIV infection, symptomatic

Code first Human immunodeficiency virus [HIV] disease complicating pregnancy, childbirth and the puerperium, if applicable (O98.7-)

Use additional code(s) to identify all manifestations of HIV infection

EXCLUDES 1 *asymptomatic human immunodeficiency virus [HIV] infection status (Z21)*
exposure to HIV virus (Z20.6)
inconclusive serologic evidence of HIV (R75)

AHA: 2022,1Q,36; 2021,2Q,6; 2021,1Q,52; 2020,4Q,97; 2020,2Q,12; 2019,1Q,8-11

Other viral diseases (B25-B34)

B25 Cytomegaloviral disease

EXCLUDES 1 *congenital cytomegalovirus infection (P35.1)*
cytomegaloviral mononucleosis (B27.1-)

B25.0 Cytomegaloviral pneumonitis MCC HCC
B25.1 Cytomegaloviral hepatitis CC HCC
B25.2 Cytomegaloviral pancreatitis MCC HCC
B25.8 Other cytomegaloviral diseases HIV CC HCC
Cytomegaloviral encephalitis
B25.9 Cytomegaloviral disease, unspecified HIV CC HCC

B26 Mumps

INCLUDES epidemic parotitis
infectious parotitis

B26.0 Mumps orchitis CC ♂
B26.1 Mumps meningitis MCC
B26.2 Mumps encephalitis MCC
B26.3 Mumps pancreatitis CC
B26.8 Mumps with other complications
B26.81 Mumps hepatitis CC
B26.82 Mumps myocarditis CC
B26.83 Mumps nephritis CC
B26.84 Mumps polyneuropathy CC
B26.85 Mumps arthritis CC HCC
B26.89 Other mumps complications CC
B26.9 Mumps without complication
Mumps NOS
Mumps parotitis NOS

B27 Infectious mononucleosis

INCLUDES glandular fever
monocytic angina
Pfeiffer's disease

B27.0 Gammaherpesviral mononucleosis
Mononucleosis due to Epstein-Barr virus
B27.00 Gammaherpesviral mononucleosis without complication
B27.01 Gammaherpesviral mononucleosis with polyneuropathy
B27.02 Gammaherpesviral mononucleosis with meningitis
B27.09 Gammaherpesviral mononucleosis with other complications
Hepatomegaly in gammaherpesviral mononucleosis
B27.1 Cytomegaloviral mononucleosis
B27.10 Cytomegaloviral mononucleosis without complications
B27.11 Cytomegaloviral mononucleosis with polyneuropathy
B27.12 Cytomegaloviral mononucleosis with meningitis
B27.19 Cytomegaloviral mononucleosis with other complication
Hepatomegaly in cytomegaloviral mononucleosis
B27.8 Other infectious mononucleosis
B27.80 Other infectious mononucleosis without complication
B27.81 Other infectious mononucleosis with polyneuropathy
B27.82 Other infectious mononucleosis with meningitis
B27.89 Other infectious mononucleosis with other complication
Hepatomegaly in other infectious mononucleosis
B27.9 Infectious mononucleosis, unspecified
B27.90 Infectious mononucleosis, unspecified without complication
B27.91 Infectious mononucleosis, unspecified with polyneuropathy
B27.92 Infectious mononucleosis, unspecified with meningitis
B27.99 Infectious mononucleosis, unspecified with other complication
Hepatomegaly in unspecified infectious mononucleosis

B30 Viral conjunctivitis

EXCLUDES 1 *herpesviral [herpes simplex] ocular disease (B00.5)*
ocular zoster (B02.3)

Viral Conjunctivitis

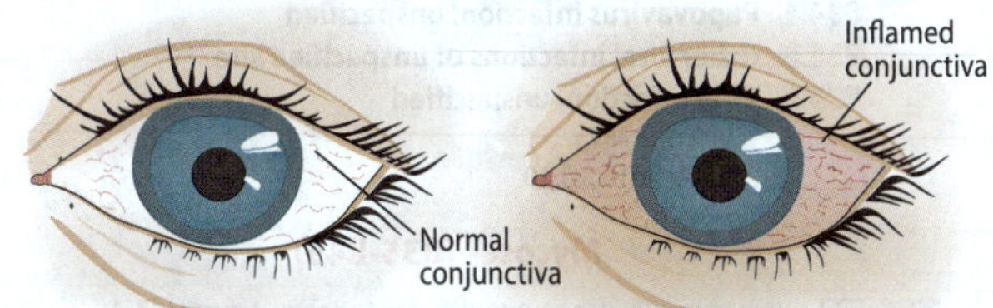

B30.0 Keratoconjunctivitis due to adenovirus
Epidemic keratoconjunctivitis
Shipyard eye
B30.1 Conjunctivitis due to adenovirus
Acute adenoviral follicular conjunctivitis
Swimming-pool conjunctivitis
B30.2 Viral pharyngoconjunctivitis
B30.3 Acute epidemic hemorrhagic conjunctivitis (enteroviral)
Conjunctivitis due to coxsackievirus 24
Conjunctivitis due to enterovirus 70
Hemorrhagic conjunctivitis (acute)(epidemic)
B30.8 Other viral conjunctivitis
Newcastle conjunctivitis
B30.9 Viral conjunctivitis, unspecified

B33 Other viral diseases, not elsewhere classified

B33.0 Epidemic myalgia
Bornholm disease
B33.1 Ross River disease CC
Epidemic polyarthritis and exanthema
Ross River fever
B33.2 Viral carditis
Coxsackie (virus) carditis
B33.20 Viral carditis, unspecified CC
B33.21 Viral endocarditis CC
B33.22 Viral myocarditis CC
B33.23 Viral pericarditis CC
B33.24 Viral cardiomyopathy HCC
B33.3 Retrovirus infections, not elsewhere classified
Retrovirus infection NOS
B33.4 Hantavirus (cardio)-pulmonary syndrome [HPS] [HCPS] CC
Hantavirus disease with pulmonary manifestations
Sin nombre virus disease
Use additional code to identify any associated acute kidney failure (N17.9)
EXCLUDES 1 *hantavirus disease with renal manifestations (A98.5)*
hemorrhagic fever with renal manifestations (A98.5)
B33.8 Other specified viral diseases
EXCLUDES 1 *anogenital human papillomavirus infection (A63.0)*
viral warts due to human papillomavirus infection (B07)

B34 Viral infection of unspecified site

EXCLUDES 1 *anogenital human papillomavirus infection (A63.0)*
cytomegaloviral disease NOS (B25.9)
herpesvirus [herpes simplex] infection NOS (B00.9)
retrovirus infection NOS (B33.3)
viral agents as the cause of diseases classified elsewhere (B97.-)
viral warts due to human papillomavirus infection (B07)

B34.0 Adenovirus infection, unspecified

B34.1 Enterovirus infection, unspecified
Coxsackievirus infection NOS
Echovirus infection NOS

B34.2 Coronavirus infection, unspecified
EXCLUDES 1 *COVID-19 (U07.1)*
pneumonia due to SARS-associated coronavirus (J12.81)
AHA: 2020,1Q,34-36

B34.3 Parvovirus infection, unspecified CC

B34.4 Papovavirus infection, unspecified

B34.8 Other viral infections of unspecified site

B34.9 Viral infection, unspecified
Viremia NOS
AHA: 2016,3Q,10

Mycoses (B35-B49)

EXCLUDES 2 *hypersensitivity pneumonitis due to organic dust (J67.-)*
mycosis fungoides (C84.0-)

B35 Dermatophytosis

INCLUDES favus
infections due to species of Epidermophyton, Micro-sporum and Trichophyton
tinea, any type except those in B36.-

DEF: Contagious superficial fungal infection of the skin that invades and grows in dead keratin.

B35.0 Tinea barbae and tinea capitis
Beard ringworm
Kerion
Scalp ringworm
Sycosis, mycotic

B35.1 Tinea unguium
Dermatophytic onychia
Dermatophytosis of nail
Onychomycosis
Ringworm of nails

B35.2 Tinea manuum
Dermatophytosis of hand
Hand ringworm

B35.3 Tinea pedis
Athlete's foot
Dermatophytosis of foot
Foot ringworm

B35.4 Tinea corporis
Ringworm of the body

B35.5 Tinea imbricata
Tokelau

B35.6 Tinea cruris
Dhobi itch
Groin ringworm
Jock itch

B35.8 Other dermatophytoses
Disseminated dermatophytosis
Granulomatous dermatophytosis

B35.9 Dermatophytosis, unspecified
Ringworm NOS

B36 Other superficial mycoses

B36.0 Pityriasis versicolor
Tinea flava
Tinea versicolor

B36.1 Tinea nigra
Keratomycosis nigricans palmaris
Microsporosis nigra
Pityriasis nigra

B36.2 White piedra
Tinea blanca

B36.3 Black piedra

B36.8 Other specified superficial mycoses

B36.9 Superficial mycosis, unspecified

B37 Candidiasis

INCLUDES candidosis
moniliasis

EXCLUDES 1 *neonatal candidiasis (P37.5)*

DEF: *Candida:* Genus of yeast-like fungi that are commonly found in the mouth, skin, intestinal tract, and vagina. It may cause a white, cheesy discharge.

B37.0 Candidal stomatitis HIV CC
Oral thrush

B37.1 Pulmonary candidiasis HIV MCC HCC
Candidal bronchitis
Candidal pneumonia

B37.2 Candidiasis of skin and nail HIV
Candidal onychia
Candidal paronychia
EXCLUDES 2 *diaper dermatitis (L22)*

▲ **B37.3 Candidiasis of vulva and vagina**
Candidal vulvovaginitis
Monilial vulvovaginitis
Vaginal thrush

● **B37.31 Acute candidiasis of vulva and vagina** ♀
Candidiasis of vulva and vagina NOS

● **B37.32 Chronic candidiasis of vulva and vagina** ♀
Recurrent candidiasis of vulva and vagina

B37.4 Candidiasis of other urogenital sites

B37.41 Candidal cystitis and urethritis CC H6

B37.42 Candidal balanitis ♂

B37.49 Other urogenital candidiasis CC H6
Candidal pyelonephritis

B37.5 Candidal meningitis HIV MCC

B37.6 Candidal endocarditis HIV MCC

B37.7 Candidal sepsis MCC HCC
Disseminated candidiasis
Systemic candidiasis
AHA: 2014,4Q,46
TIP: This code is assigned when sepsis is documented as due to any *Candida* type. If the nonspecific term "non-*Candida albicans*" is documented, code B48.8 Other specified mycoses, is assigned.

B37.8 Candidiasis of other sites

B37.81 Candidal esophagitis HIV CC HCC

B37.82 Candidal enteritis HIV CC
Candidal proctitis

B37.83 Candidal cheilitis HIV CC

B37.84 Candidal otitis externa HIV CC

B37.89 Other sites of candidiasis HIV CC
Candidal osteomyelitis

B37.9 Candidiasis, unspecified HIV
Thrush NOS

B38 Coccidioidomycosis

B38.0 Acute pulmonary coccidioidomycosis HIV CC HCC

B38.1 Chronic pulmonary coccidioidomycosis HIV CC HCC

B38.2 Pulmonary coccidioidomycosis, unspecified HIV CC HCC

B38.3 Cutaneous coccidioidomycosis HIV CC

B38.4 Coccidioidomycosis meningitis HIV MCC
DEF: *Coccidioides immitis* infection of the lining of the brain and/or spinal cord.

B38.7 Disseminated coccidioidomycosis HIV CC
Generalized coccidioidomycosis

B38.8 Other forms of coccidioidomycosis

B38.81 Prostatic coccidioidomycosis HIV CC ♂

B38.89 Other forms of coccidioidomycosis HIV CC

B38.9 Coccidioidomycosis, unspecified HIV CC

B39 Histoplasmosis

Code first associated AIDS (B2Ø)
Use additional code for any associated manifestations, such as:
- endocarditis (I39)
- meningitis (GØ2)
- pericarditis (I32)
- retinitis (H32)

DEF: Type of lung infection caused by breathing in fungal spores often found in the droppings of bats and birds or soil contaminated by their droppings.

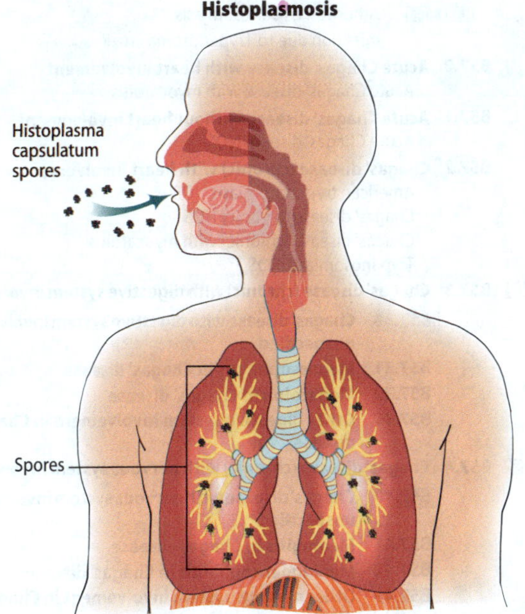

- **B39.Ø Acute pulmonary histoplasmosis capsulati** HIV MCC HCC
- **B39.1 Chronic pulmonary histoplasmosis capsulati** HIV MCC HCC
- **B39.2 Pulmonary histoplasmosis capsulati, unspecified** HIV MCC HCC
- **B39.3 Disseminated histoplasmosis capsulati** HIV CC
  Generalized histoplasmosis capsulati
- **B39.4 Histoplasmosis capsulati, unspecified** HIV
  American histoplasmosis
- **B39.5 Histoplasmosis duboisii** HIV
  African histoplasmosis
- **B39.9 Histoplasmosis, unspecified** HIV

B4Ø Blastomycosis

EXCLUDES 1 *Brazilian blastomycosis (B41.-)*
keloidal blastomycosis (B48.Ø)

- **B4Ø.Ø Acute pulmonary blastomycosis** CC HCC
- **B4Ø.1 Chronic pulmonary blastomycosis** CC HCC
- **B4Ø.2 Pulmonary blastomycosis, unspecified** CC HCC
- **B4Ø.3 Cutaneous blastomycosis** CC
- **B4Ø.7 Disseminated blastomycosis** CC
  Generalized blastomycosis
- **B4Ø.8 Other forms of blastomycosis**
  - **B4Ø.81 Blastomycotic meningoencephalitis** CC
    Meningomyelitis due to blastomycosis
  - **B4Ø.89 Other forms of blastomycosis** CC
- **B4Ø.9 Blastomycosis, unspecified** CC

B41 Paracoccidioidomycosis

INCLUDES Brazilian blastomycosis
Lutz' disease

- **B41.Ø Pulmonary paracoccidioidomycosis** CC HCC
- **B41.7 Disseminated paracoccidioidomycosis** CC
  Generalized paracoccidioidomycosis
- **B41.8 Other forms of paracoccidioidomycosis** CC
- **B41.9 Paracoccidioidomycosis, unspecified** CC

B42 Sporotrichosis

- **B42.Ø Pulmonary sporotrichosis**
- **B42.1 Lymphocutaneous sporotrichosis**
- **B42.7 Disseminated sporotrichosis**
  Generalized sporotrichosis
- **B42.8 Other forms of sporotrichosis**
  - **B42.81 Cerebral sporotrichosis**
    Meningitis due to sporotrichosis
  - **B42.82 Sporotrichosis arthritis** HCC
  - **B42.89 Other forms of sporotrichosis**
- **B42.9 Sporotrichosis, unspecified**

B43 Chromomycosis and pheomycotic abscess

- **B43.Ø Cutaneous chromomycosis**
  Dermatitis verrucosa
- **B43.1 Pheomycotic brain abscess**
  Cerebral chromomycosis
- **B43.2 Subcutaneous pheomycotic abscess and cyst**
- **B43.8 Other forms of chromomycosis**
- **B43.9 Chromomycosis, unspecified**

B44 Aspergillosis

INCLUDES aspergilloma

- **B44.Ø Invasive pulmonary aspergillosis** MCC HCC
- **B44.1 Other pulmonary aspergillosis** CC HCC
- **B44.2 Tonsillar aspergillosis** CC HCC
- **B44.7 Disseminated aspergillosis** CC HCC
  Generalized aspergillosis
- **B44.8 Other forms of aspergillosis**
  - **B44.81 Allergic bronchopulmonary aspergillosis** CC HCC
  - **B44.89 Other forms of aspergillosis** CC HCC
- **B44.9 Aspergillosis, unspecified** CC HCC

B45 Cryptococcosis

- **B45.Ø Pulmonary cryptococcosis** HIV CC HCC
- **B45.1 Cerebral cryptococcosis** MCC HCC
  Cryptococcal meningitis
  Cryptococcosis meningocerebralis
- **B45.2 Cutaneous cryptococcosis** HIV CC HCC
- **B45.3 Osseous cryptococcosis** HIV CC HCC
- **B45.7 Disseminated cryptococcosis** HIV CC HCC
  Generalized cryptococcosis
- **B45.8 Other forms of cryptococcosis** HIV CC HCC
- **B45.9 Cryptococcosis, unspecified** HIV CC HCC

B46 Zygomycosis

- **B46.Ø Pulmonary mucormycosis** MCC HCC
- **B46.1 Rhinocerebral mucormycosis** MCC HCC
- **B46.2 Gastrointestinal mucormycosis** MCC HCC
- **B46.3 Cutaneous mucormycosis** MCC HCC
  Subcutaneous mucormycosis
- **B46.4 Disseminated mucormycosis** MCC HCC
  Generalized mucormycosis
- **B46.5 Mucormycosis, unspecified** MCC HCC
- **B46.8 Other zygomycoses** MCC HCC
  Entomophthoromycosis
- **B46.9 Zygomycosis, unspecified** MCC HCC
  Phycomycosis NOS

B47 Mycetoma

- **B47.Ø Eumycetoma** CC
  Madura foot, mycotic
  Maduromycosis
- **B47.1 Actinomycetoma** HIV CC
- **B47.9 Mycetoma, unspecified** HIV CC
  Madura foot NOS

B48 Other mycoses, not elsewhere classified

- **B48.Ø Lobomycosis**
  Keloidal blastomycosis
  Lobo's disease
- **B48.1 Rhinosporidiosis**
- **B48.2 Allescheriasis** CC
  Infection due to Pseudallescheria boydii
  EXCLUDES 1 *eumycetoma (B47.Ø)*
- **B48.3 Geotrichosis** CC
  Geotrichum stomatitis
- **B48.4 Penicillosis** CC HCC
  Talaromycosis

B48.8 Other specified mycoses HIV CC HCC
Adiaspiromycosis
Infection of tissue and organs by Alternaria
Infection of tissue and organs by Drechslera
Infection of tissue and organs by Fusarium
Infection of tissue and organs by saprophytic fungi NEC
AHA: 2014,4Q,46; 2014,2Q,13
TIP: This code is assigned when the nonspecific term "non-*Candida albicans*" sepsis is documented. If sepsis is documented as due to any *Candida* type, code B37.7 Candidal sepsis, is assigned.

B49 Unspecified mycosis CC
Fungemia NOS

Protozoal diseases (B50-B64)

EXCLUDES 1 *amebiasis (A06.-)*
other protozoal intestinal diseases (A07.-)

B50 Plasmodium falciparum malaria
INCLUDES mixed infections of Plasmodium falciparum with any other Plasmodium species

B50.0 Plasmodium falciparum malaria with cerebral complications CC
Cerebral malaria NOS

B50.8 Other severe and complicated Plasmodium falciparum malaria CC
Severe or complicated Plasmodium falciparum malaria NOS

B50.9 Plasmodium falciparum malaria, unspecified MCC

B51 Plasmodium vivax malaria
INCLUDES mixed infections of Plasmodium vivax with other Plasmodium species, except Plasmodium falciparum
EXCLUDES 1 *Plasmodium vivax with Plasmodium falciparum (B50.-)*

B51.0 Plasmodium vivax malaria with rupture of spleen CC

B51.8 Plasmodium vivax malaria with other complications CC

B51.9 Plasmodium vivax malaria without complication CC
Plasmodium vivax malaria NOS

B52 Plasmodium malariae malaria
INCLUDES mixed infections of Plasmodium malariae with other Plasmodium species, except Plasmodium falciparum and Plasmodium vivax
EXCLUDES 1 *Plasmodium falciparum (B50.-)*
Plasmodium vivax (B51.-)

B52.0 Plasmodium malariae malaria with nephropathy CC

B52.8 Plasmodium malariae malaria with other complications CC

B52.9 Plasmodium malariae malaria without complication CC
Plasmodium malariae malaria NOS

B53 Other specified malaria

B53.0 Plasmodium ovale malaria CC
EXCLUDES 1 *Plasmodium ovale with Plasmodium falciparum (B50.-)*
Plasmodium ovale with Plasmodium malariae (B52.-)
Plasmodium ovale with Plasmodium vivax (B51.-)

B53.1 Malaria due to simian plasmodia CC
EXCLUDES 1 *malaria due to simian plasmodia with Plasmodium falciparum (B50.-)*
malaria due to simian plasmodia with Plasmodium malariae (B52.-)
malaria due to simian plasmodia with Plasmodium ovale (B53.0)
malaria due to simian plasmodia with Plasmodium vivax (B51.-)

B53.8 Other malaria, not elsewhere classified CC

B54 Unspecified malaria CC

B55 Leishmaniasis

B55.0 Visceral leishmaniasis CC
Kala-azar
Post-kala-azar dermal leishmaniasis

B55.1 Cutaneous leishmaniasis CC

B55.2 Mucocutaneous leishmaniasis CC

B55.9 Leishmaniasis, unspecified CC

B56 African trypanosomiasis

B56.0 Gambiense trypanosomiasis CC
Infection due to Trypanosoma brucei gambiense
West African sleeping sickness

B56.1 Rhodesiense trypanosomiasis CC
East African sleeping sickness
Infection due to Trypanosoma brucei rhodesiense

B56.9 African trypanosomiasis, unspecified CC
Sleeping sickness NOS

B57 Chagas' disease
INCLUDES American trypanosomiasis
infection due to Trypanosoma cruzi

B57.0 Acute Chagas' disease with heart involvement CC
Acute Chagas' disease with myocarditis

B57.1 Acute Chagas' disease without heart involvement CC
Acute Chagas' disease NOS

B57.2 Chagas' disease (chronic) with heart involvement CC
American trypanosomiasis NOS
Chagas' disease (chronic) NOS
Chagas' disease (chronic) with myocarditis
Trypanosomiasis NOS

B57.3 Chagas' disease (chronic) with digestive system involvement

B57.30 Chagas' disease with digestive system involvement, unspecified CC

B57.31 Megaesophagus in Chagas' disease CC

B57.32 Megacolon in Chagas' disease CC

B57.39 Other digestive system involvement in Chagas' disease CC

B57.4 Chagas' disease (chronic) with nervous system involvement

B57.40 Chagas' disease with nervous system involvement, unspecified CC

B57.41 Meningitis in Chagas' disease CC

B57.42 Meningoencephalitis in Chagas' disease CC

B57.49 Other nervous system involvement in Chagas' disease CC

B57.5 Chagas' disease (chronic) with other organ involvement CC

B58 Toxoplasmosis
INCLUDES infection due to Toxoplasma gondii
EXCLUDES 1 *congenital toxoplasmosis (P37.1)*

B58.0 Toxoplasma oculopathy

B58.00 Toxoplasma oculopathy, unspecified HIV CC

B58.01 Toxoplasma chorioretinitis HIV CC

B58.09 Other toxoplasma oculopathy HIV CC
Toxoplasma uveitis

B58.1 Toxoplasma hepatitis HIV CC

B58.2 Toxoplasma meningoencephalitis HIV MCC HCC

B58.3 Pulmonary toxoplasmosis HIV MCC HCC

B58.8 Toxoplasmosis with other organ involvement

B58.81 Toxoplasma myocarditis HIV MCC

B58.82 Toxoplasma myositis HIV CC

B58.83 Toxoplasma tubulo-interstitial nephropathy HIV CC
Toxoplasma pyelonephritis

B58.89 Toxoplasmosis with other organ involvement HIV CC

B58.9 Toxoplasmosis, unspecified HIV CC

B59 Pneumocystosis HIV MCC HCC
Pneumonia due to Pneumocystis carinii
Pneumonia due to Pneumocystis jiroveci

B60 Other protozoal diseases, not elsewhere classified
EXCLUDES 1 *cryptosporidiosis (A07.2)*
intestinal microsporidiosis (A07.8)
isosporiasis (A07.3)

B60.0 Babesiosis
AHA: 2020,4Q,5-6

B60.00 Babesiosis, unspecified CC
Babesiosis due to unspecified Babesia species
Piroplasmosis, unspecified

B60.01 Babesiosis due to Babesia microti CC
Infection due to B. microti

B60.02 Babesiosis due to Babesia duncani CC
Infection due to B. duncani and B. duncani-type species

B60.03 Babesiosis due to Babesia divergens CC
Babesiosis due to Babesia MO-1
Infection due to B. divergens and B. divergens-like strains

B60.09 Other babesiosis CC
Babesiosis due to Babesia KO-1
Babesiosis due to Babesia venatorum
Infection due to other Babesia species
Infection due to other protozoa of the order Piroplasmida
Other piroplasmosis

B60.1 Acanthamebiasis (5th)

B60.10 Acanthamebiasis, unspecified CC

B60.11 Meningoencephalitis due to Acanthamoeba (culbertsoni)

B60.12 Conjunctivitis due to Acanthamoeba

B60.13 Keratoconjunctivitis due to Acanthamoeba

B60.19 Other acanthamebic disease CC

B60.2 Naegleriasis CC
Primary amebic meningoencephalitis

B60.8 Other specified protozoal diseases HIV
Microsporidiosis

B64 Unspecified protozoal disease

Helminthiases (B65-B83)

B65 Schistosomiasis [bilharziasis] (4th)
INCLUDES snail fever

B65.0 Schistosomiasis due to Schistosoma haematobium [urinary schistosomiasis] CC

B65.1 Schistosomiasis due to Schistosoma mansoni [intestinal schistosomiasis] CC

B65.2 Schistosomiasis due to Schistosoma japonicum CC
Asiatic schistosomiasis

B65.3 Cercarial dermatitis CC
Swimmer's itch

B65.8 Other schistosomiasis CC
Infection due to Schistosoma intercalatum
Infection due to Schistosoma mattheei
Infection due to Schistosoma mekongi

B65.9 Schistosomiasis, unspecified CC

B66 Other fluke infections (4th)

B66.0 Opisthorchiasis CC
Infection due to cat liver fluke
Infection due to Opisthorchis (felineus)(viverrini)

B66.1 Clonorchiasis CC
Chinese liver fluke disease
Infection due to Clonorchis sinensis
Oriental liver fluke disease

B66.2 Dicroceliasis CC
Infection due to Dicrocoelium dendriticum
Lancet fluke infection

B66.3 Fascioliasis CC
Infection due to Fasciola gigantica
Infection due to Fasciola hepatica
Infection due to Fasciola indica
Sheep liver fluke disease

B66.4 Paragonimiasis CC HCC
Infection due to Paragonimus species
Lung fluke disease
Pulmonary distomiasis

B66.5 Fasciolopsiasis CC
Infection due to Fasciolopsis buski
Intestinal distomiasis

B66.8 Other specified fluke infections CC
Echinostomiasis
Heterophyiasis
Metagonimiasis
Nanophyetiasis
Watsoniasis

B66.9 Fluke infection, unspecified

B67 Echinococcosis (4th)
INCLUDES hydatidosis

B67.0 Echinococcus granulosus infection of liver CC

B67.1 Echinococcus granulosus infection of lung CC HCC

B67.2 Echinococcus granulosus infection of bone CC

B67.3 Echinococcus granulosus infection, other and multiple sites (5th)

B67.31 Echinococcus granulosus infection, thyroid gland CC

B67.32 Echinococcus granulosus infection, multiple sites CC

B67.39 Echinococcus granulosus infection, other sites CC

B67.4 Echinococcus granulosus infection, unspecified CC
Dog tapeworm (infection)

B67.5 Echinococcus multilocularis infection of liver CC

B67.6 Echinococcus multilocularis infection, other and multiple sites (5th)

B67.61 Echinococcus multilocularis infection, multiple sites CC

B67.69 Echinococcus multilocularis infection, other sites CC

B67.7 Echinococcus multilocularis infection, unspecified CC

B67.8 Echinococcosis, unspecified, of liver CC

B67.9 Echinococcosis, other and unspecified (5th)

B67.90 Echinococcosis, unspecified CC
Echinococcosis NOS

B67.99 Other echinococcosis CC

B68 Taeniasis (4th)
EXCLUDES 1 *cysticercosis (B69.-)*

B68.0 Taenia solium taeniasis CC
Pork tapeworm (infection)

B68.1 Taenia saginata taeniasis CC
Beef tapeworm (infection)
Infection due to adult tapeworm Taenia saginata

B68.9 Taeniasis, unspecified CC

B69 Cysticercosis (4th)
INCLUDES cysticerciasis infection due to larval form of Taenia solium
DEF: Condition that is developed when larvae or eggs of the tapeworm *Taenia solium* are ingested, most commonly in fecally contaminated water or undercooked pork.

B69.0 Cysticercosis of central nervous system CC

B69.1 Cysticercosis of eye CC

B69.8 Cysticercosis of other sites (5th)

B69.81 Myositis in cysticercosis CC

B69.89 Cysticercosis of other sites CC

B69.9 Cysticercosis, unspecified CC

B70 Diphyllobothriasis and sparganosis (4th)

B70.0 Diphyllobothriasis CC
Diphyllobothrium (adult) (latum) (pacificum) infection
Fish tapeworm (infection)
EXCLUDES 2 *larval diphyllobothriasis (B70.1)*

B70.1 Sparganosis CC
Infection due to Sparganum (mansoni) (proliferum)
Infection due to Spirometra larva
Larval diphyllobothriasis
Spirometrosis

B71 Other cestode infections (4th)

B71.0 Hymenolepiasis CC
Dwarf tapeworm infection
Rat tapeworm (infection)

B71.1 Dipylidiasis CC

B71.8 Other specified cestode infections CC
Coenurosis

B71.9 Cestode infection, unspecified
Tapeworm (infection) NOS

B72 Dracunculiasis CC
INCLUDES guinea worm infection
infection due to Dracunculus medinensis

4th B73 Onchocerciasis

INCLUDES onchocerca volvulus infection
onchocercosis
river blindness

5th B73.Ø Onchocerciasis with eye disease

B73.ØØ Onchocerciasis with eye involvement, unspecified CC

B73.Ø1 Onchocerciasis with endophthalmitis CC

B73.Ø2 Onchocerciasis with glaucoma CC

B73.Ø9 Onchocerciasis with other eye involvement CC
Infestation of eyelid due to onchocerciasis

B73.1 Onchocerciasis without eye disease CC

4th B74 Filariasis

EXCLUDES 2 *onchocerciasis (B73)*
tropical (pulmonary) eosinophilia NOS (J82.89)

B74.Ø Filariasis due to Wuchereria bancrofti CC
Bancroftian elephantiasis
Bancroftian filariasis

B74.1 Filariasis due to Brugia malayi CC

B74.2 Filariasis due to Brugia timori CC

B74.3 Loiasis CC
Calabar swelling
Eyeworm disease of Africa
Loa loa infection

B74.4 Mansonelliasis CC
Infection due to Mansonella ozzardi
Infection due to Mansonella perstans
Infection due to Mansonella streptocerca

B74.8 Other filariases CC
Dirofilariasis

B74.9 Filariasis, unspecified CC

B75 Trichinellosis CC

INCLUDES infection due to Trichinella species
trichiniasis

DEF: Infection by *Trichinella spiralis*, the smallest of the parasitic nematodes, that is transmitted by eating undercooked pork or bear meat. ***Synonym(s):*** *Trichinosis.*

4th B76 Hookworm diseases

INCLUDES uncinariasis

B76.Ø Ancylostomiasis CC
Infection due to Ancylostoma species

B76.1 Necatoriasis CC
Infection due to Necator americanus

B76.8 Other hookworm diseases CC

B76.9 Hookworm disease, unspecified CC
Cutaneous larva migrans NOS

4th B77 Ascariasis

INCLUDES ascaridiasis
roundworm infection

B77.Ø Ascariasis with intestinal complications CC

5th B77.8 Ascariasis with other complications

B77.81 Ascariasis pneumonia MCC

B77.89 Ascariasis with other complications CC

B77.9 Ascariasis, unspecified CC

4th B78 Strongyloidiasis

EXCLUDES 1 *trichostrongyliasis (B81.2)*

B78.Ø Intestinal strongyloidiasis HIV CC

B78.1 Cutaneous strongyloidiasis CC

B78.7 Disseminated strongyloidiasis HIV CC

B78.9 Strongyloidiasis, unspecified HIV CC

B79 Trichuriasis CC

INCLUDES trichocephaliasis
whipworm (disease)(infection)

B8Ø Enterobiasis CC

INCLUDES oxyuriasis
pinworm infection
threadworm infection

4th B81 Other intestinal helminthiases, not elsewhere classified

EXCLUDES 1 *angiostrongyliasis due to:*
angiostrongylus cantonensis (B83.2)
parastrongylus cantonensis (B83.2)

B81.Ø Anisakiasis CC
Infection due to Anisakis larva

B81.1 Intestinal capillariasis CC
Capillariasis NOS
Infection due to Capillaria philippinensis
EXCLUDES 2 *hepatic capillariasis (B83.8)*

B81.2 Trichostrongyliasis CC

B81.3 Intestinal angiostrongyliasis CC
Angiostrongyliasis due to:
Angiostrongylus costaricensis
Parastrongylus costaricensis

B81.4 Mixed intestinal helminthiases CC
Infection due to intestinal helminths classified to more than one of the categories B65.Ø-B81.3 and B81.8
Mixed helminthiasis NOS

B81.8 Other specified intestinal helminthiases CC
Infection due to Oesophagostomum species [esophagostomiasis]
Infection due to Ternidens diminutus [ternidensiasis]

4th B82 Unspecified intestinal parasitism

B82.Ø Intestinal helminthiasis, unspecified CC

B82.9 Intestinal parasitism, unspecified

4th B83 Other helminthiases

EXCLUDES 1 *capillariasis NOS (B81.1)*
EXCLUDES 2 *intestinal capillariasis (B81.1)*

B83.Ø Visceral larva migrans
Toxocariasis

B83.1 Gnathostomiasis
Wandering swelling

B83.2 Angiostrongyliasis due to Parastrongylus cantonensis
Eosinophilic meningoencephalitis due to Parastrongylus cantonensis
EXCLUDES 2 *intestinal angiostrongyliasis (B81.3)*

B83.3 Syngamiasis
Syngamosis

B83.4 Internal hirudiniasis
EXCLUDES 2 *external hirudiniasis (B88.3)*

B83.8 Other specified helminthiases
Acanthocephaliasis
Gongylonemiasis
Hepatic capillariasis
Metastrongyliasis
Thelaziasis

B83.9 Helminthiasis, unspecified
Worms NOS
EXCLUDES 1 *intestinal helminthiasis NOS (B82.Ø)*

Pediculosis, acariasis and other infestations (B85-B89)

4th B85 Pediculosis and phthiriasis

B85.Ø Pediculosis due to Pediculus humanus capitis
Head-louse infestation

B85.1 Pediculosis due to Pediculus humanus corporis
Body-louse infestation

B85.2 Pediculosis, unspecified

B85.3 Phthiriasis
Infestation by crab-louse
Infestation by Phthirus pubis

B85.4 Mixed pediculosis and phthiriasis
Infestation classifiable to more than one of the categories B85.Ø-B85.3

B86 Scabies
Sarcoptic itch
DEF: Mite infestation that is caused by *Sarcoptes scabiei*. Scabies causes intense itching and sometimes secondary infection.

4th B87 Myiasis

INCLUDES infestation by larva of flies

B87.Ø Cutaneous myiasis
Creeping myiasis

B87.1 Wound myiasis
Traumatic myiasis
B87.2 Ocular myiasis
B87.3 Nasopharyngeal myiasis
Laryngeal myiasis
B87.4 Aural myiasis
✓5th B87.8 Myiasis of other sites
B87.81 Genitourinary myiasis
B87.82 Intestinal myiasis
B87.89 Myiasis of other sites
B87.9 Myiasis, unspecified

✓4th **B88 Other infestations**
B88.Ø Other acariasis
Acarine dermatitis
Dermatitis due to Demodex species
Dermatitis due to Dermanyssus gallinae
Dermatitis due to Liponyssoides sanguineus
Trombiculosis
EXCLUDES 2 *scabies (B86)*
B88.1 Tungiasis [sandflea infestation]
B88.2 Other arthropod infestations
Scarabiasis
B88.3 External hirudiniasis
Leech infestation NOS
EXCLUDES 2 *internal hirudiniasis (B83.4)*
B88.8 Other specified infestations
Ichthyoparasitism due to Vandellia cirrhosa
Linguatulosis
Porocephaliasis
B88.9 Infestation, unspecified
Infestation (skin) NOS
Infestation by mites NOS
Skin parasites NOS

B89 Unspecified parasitic disease

Sequelae of infectious and parasitic diseases (B9Ø-B94)

NOTE Categories B9Ø-B94 are to be used to indicate conditions in categories AØØ-B89 as the cause of sequelae, which are themselves classified elsewhere. The "sequelae" include conditions specified as such; they also include residuals of diseases classifiable to the above categories if there is evidence that the disease itself is no longer present. Codes from these categories are not to be used for chronic infections. Code chronic current infections to active infectious disease as appropriate.

Code first condition resulting from (sequela) the infectious or parasitic disease

✓4th **B9Ø Sequelae of tuberculosis**
B9Ø.Ø Sequelae of central nervous system tuberculosis
B9Ø.1 Sequelae of genitourinary tuberculosis
B9Ø.2 Sequelae of tuberculosis of bones and joints
B9Ø.8 Sequelae of tuberculosis of other organs
EXCLUDES 2 *sequelae of respiratory tuberculosis (B9Ø.9)*
B9Ø.9 Sequelae of respiratory and unspecified tuberculosis
Sequelae of tuberculosis NOS

B91 Sequelae of poliomyelitis
EXCLUDES 1 *postpolio syndrome (G14)*

B92 Sequelae of leprosy

✓4th **B94 Sequelae of other and unspecified infectious and parasitic diseases**
B94.Ø Sequelae of trachoma
B94.1 Sequelae of viral encephalitis
B94.2 Sequelae of viral hepatitis
B94.8 Sequelae of other specified infectious and parasitic diseases
AHA: 2021,1Q,25-30,31-49; 2020,3Q,10-14; 2017,4Q,109
B94.9 Sequelae of unspecified infectious and parasitic disease
EXCLUDES 2 *post COVID-19 condition (UØ9.9)*

Bacterial and viral infectious agents (B95-B97)

NOTE These categories are provided for use as supplementary or additional codes to identify the infectious agent(s) in diseases classified elsewhere.

AHA: 2020,2Q,18; 2018,4Q,34; 2018,1Q,16

✓4th **B95 Streptococcus, Staphylococcus, and Enterococcus as the cause of diseases classified elsewhere**
B95.Ø Streptococcus, group A, as the cause of diseases classified elsewhere UPD
B95.1 Streptococcus, group B, as the cause of diseases classified elsewhere UPD
AHA: 2020,1Q,10; 2019,2Q,8-10
B95.2 Enterococcus as the cause of diseases classified elsewhere UPD
B95.3 Streptococcus pneumoniae as the cause of diseases classified elsewhere UPD
B95.4 Other streptococcus as the cause of diseases classified elsewhere UPD
B95.5 Unspecified streptococcus as the cause of diseases classified elsewhere UPD
✓5th B95.6 Staphylococcus aureus as the cause of diseases classified elsewhere
B95.61 Methicillin susceptible Staphylococcus aureus infection as the cause of diseases classified elsewhere UPD
Methicillin susceptible Staphylococcus aureus (MSSA) infection as the cause of diseases classified elsewhere
Staphylococcus aureus infection NOS as the cause of diseases classified elsewhere
B95.62 Methicillin resistant Staphylococcus aureus infection as the cause of diseases classified elsewhere UPD
Methicillin resistant staphylococcus aureus (MRSA) infection as the cause of diseases classified elsewhere
AHA: 2016,1Q,12
B95.7 Other staphylococcus as the cause of diseases classified elsewhere UPD
B95.8 Unspecified staphylococcus as the cause of diseases classified elsewhere UPD

✓4th **B96 Other bacterial agents as the cause of diseases classified elsewhere**
B96.Ø Mycoplasma pneumoniae [M. pneumoniae] as the cause of diseases classified elsewhere UPD
Pleuro-pneumonia-like-organism [PPLO]
B96.1 Klebsiella pneumoniae [K. pneumoniae] as the cause of diseases classified elsewhere UPD
✓5th B96.2 Escherichia coli [E. coli] as the cause of diseases classified elsewhere
AHA: 2022,1Q,31
B96.2Ø Unspecified Escherichia coli [E. coli] as the cause of diseases classified elsewhere UPD
Escherichia coli [E. coli] NOS
B96.21 Shiga toxin-producing Escherichia coli [E. coli] [STEC] O157 as the cause of diseases classified elsewhere UPD
E. coli O157:H- (nonmotile) with confirmation of Shiga toxin
E. coli O157 with confirmation of Shiga toxin when H antigen is unknown, or is not H7
O157:H7 Escherichia coli [E.coli] with or without confirmation of Shiga toxin-production
Shiga toxin-producing Escherichia coli [E.coli] O157:H7 with or without confirmation of Shiga toxin-production
STEC O157:H7 with or without confirmation of Shiga toxin-production
B96.22 Other specified Shiga toxin-producing Escherichia coli [E. coli] [STEC] as the cause of diseases classified elsewhere UPD
Non-O157 Shiga toxin-producing Escherichia coli [E.coli]
Non-O157 Shiga toxin-producing Escherichia coli [E.coli] with known O group
B96.23 Unspecified Shiga toxin-producing Escherichia coli [E. coli] [STEC] as the cause of diseases classified elsewhere UPD
Shiga toxin-producing Escherichia coli [E. coli] with unspecified O group
STEC NOS
B96.29 Other Escherichia coli [E. coli] as the cause of diseases classified elsewhere UPD
Non-Shiga toxin-producing E. coli
B96.3 Hemophilus influenzae [H. influenzae] as the cause of diseases classified elsewhere UPD
B96.4 Proteus (mirabilis) (morganii) as the cause of diseases classified elsewhere UPD

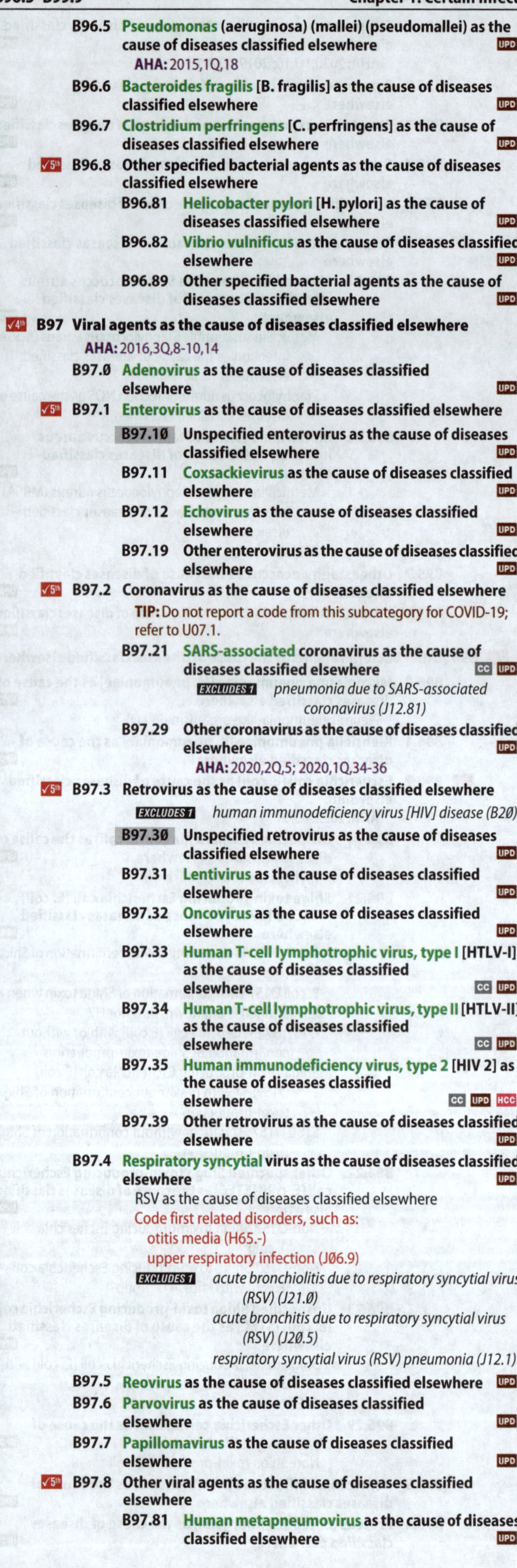

B96.5 **Pseudomonas** (aeruginosa) (mallei) (pseudomallei) as the cause of diseases classified elsewhere UPD
AHA: 2015,1Q,18

B96.6 **Bacteroides fragilis** [B. fragilis] as the cause of diseases classified elsewhere UPD

B96.7 **Clostridium perfringens** [C. perfringens] as the cause of diseases classified elsewhere UPD

✓5th **B96.8** Other specified bacterial agents as the cause of diseases classified elsewhere

B96.81 **Helicobacter pylori** [H. pylori] as the cause of diseases classified elsewhere UPD

B96.82 **Vibrio vulnificus** as the cause of diseases classified elsewhere UPD

B96.89 Other specified bacterial agents as the cause of diseases classified elsewhere UPD

✓4th **B97 Viral agents as the cause of diseases classified elsewhere**
AHA: 2016,3Q,8-10,14

B97.Ø **Adenovirus** as the cause of diseases classified elsewhere UPD

✓5th **B97.1** **Enterovirus** as the cause of diseases classified elsewhere

B97.1Ø Unspecified enterovirus as the cause of diseases classified elsewhere UPD

B97.11 **Coxsackievirus** as the cause of diseases classified elsewhere UPD

B97.12 **Echovirus** as the cause of diseases classified elsewhere UPD

B97.19 Other enterovirus as the cause of diseases classified elsewhere UPD

✓5th **B97.2** Coronavirus as the cause of diseases classified elsewhere
TIP: Do not report a code from this subcategory for COVID-19; refer to U07.1.

B97.21 **SARS-associated** coronavirus as the cause of diseases classified elsewhere CC UPD
EXCLUDES 1 *pneumonia due to SARS-associated coronavirus (J12.81)*

B97.29 Other coronavirus as the cause of diseases classified elsewhere UPD
AHA: 2020,2Q,5; 2020,1Q,34-36

✓5th **B97.3** Retrovirus as the cause of diseases classified elsewhere
EXCLUDES 1 *human immunodeficiency virus [HIV] disease (B2Ø)*

B97.3Ø Unspecified retrovirus as the cause of diseases classified elsewhere UPD

B97.31 **Lentivirus** as the cause of diseases classified elsewhere UPD

B97.32 **Oncovirus** as the cause of diseases classified elsewhere UPD

B97.33 **Human T-cell lymphotrophic virus, type I** [HTLV-I] as the cause of diseases classified elsewhere CC UPD

B97.34 **Human T-cell lymphotrophic virus, type II** [HTLV-II] as the cause of diseases classified elsewhere CC UPD

B97.35 **Human immunodeficiency virus, type 2** [HIV 2] as the cause of diseases classified elsewhere CC UPD HCC

B97.39 Other retrovirus as the cause of diseases classified elsewhere UPD

B97.4 **Respiratory syncytial** virus as the cause of diseases classified elsewhere UPD
RSV as the cause of diseases classified elsewhere
Code first related disorders, such as:
otitis media (H65.-)
upper respiratory infection (JØ6.9)
EXCLUDES 1 *acute bronchiolitis due to respiratory syncytial virus (RSV) (J21.Ø)*
acute bronchitis due to respiratory syncytial virus (RSV) (J2Ø.5)
respiratory syncytial virus (RSV) pneumonia (J12.1)

B97.5 **Reovirus** as the cause of diseases classified elsewhere UPD

B97.6 **Parvovirus** as the cause of diseases classified elsewhere UPD

B97.7 **Papillomavirus** as the cause of diseases classified elsewhere UPD

✓5th **B97.8** Other viral agents as the cause of diseases classified elsewhere

B97.81 **Human metapneumovirus** as the cause of diseases classified elsewhere UPD

B97.89 Other viral agents as the cause of diseases classified elsewhere UPD

Other infectious diseases (B99)

✓4th **B99 Other and unspecified infectious diseases**

B99.8 Other infectious disease HIV

B99.9 Unspecified infectious disease

Chapter 2. Neoplasms (CØØ–D49)

Chapter-specific Guidelines with Coding Examples

The chapter-specific guidelines from the ICD-10-CM Official Guidelines for Coding and Reporting have been provided below. Along with these guidelines are coding examples, contained in the shaded boxes, that have been developed to help illustrate the coding and/or sequencing guidance found in these guidelines.

General guidelines

Chapter 2 of the ICD-10-CM contains the codes for most benign and all malignant neoplasms. Certain benign neoplasms, such as prostatic adenomas, may be found in the specific body system chapters. To properly code a neoplasm, it is necessary to determine from the record if the neoplasm is benign, in-situ, malignant, or of uncertain histologic behavior. If malignant, any secondary (metastatic) sites should also be determined.

Primary malignant neoplasms overlapping site boundaries

A primary malignant neoplasm that overlaps two or more contiguous (next to each other) sites should be classified to the subcategory/code .8 ('overlapping lesion'), unless the combination is specifically indexed elsewhere. For multiple neoplasms of the same site that are not contiguous such as tumors in different quadrants of the same breast, codes for each site should be assigned.

A 73-year-old white female with a large rapidly growing malignant tumor in the left breast extending from the upper outer quadrant into the axillary tail

C5Ø.812	**Malignant neoplasm of overlapping sites of left female breast**

Explanation: Because this is a single large tumor that overlaps two contiguous sites, a single code for overlapping sites is assigned.

A 52-year old white female with two distinct lesions of the right breast, one (Ø.5 cm) in the upper outer quadrant and a second (1.5 cm) in the lower outer quadrant; path report indicates both lesions are malignant

C5Ø.411	**Malignant neoplasm of upper-outer quadrant of right female breast**
C5Ø.511	**Malignant neoplasm of lower-outer quadrant of right female breast**

Explanation: This patient has two distinct malignant lesions of right breast in adjacent quadrants. Because the lesions are not contiguous, two codes are reported.

Malignant neoplasm of ectopic tissue

Malignant neoplasms of ectopic tissue are to be coded to the site of origin mentioned, e.g., ectopic pancreatic malignant neoplasms involving the stomach are coded to malignant neoplasm of pancreas, unspecified (C25.9).

The neoplasm table in the Alphabetic Index should be referenced first. However, if the histological term is documented, that term should be referenced first, rather than going immediately to the Neoplasm Table, in order to determine which column in the Neoplasm Table is appropriate. For example, if the documentation indicates "adenoma," refer to the term in the Alphabetic Index to review the entries under this term and the instructional note to "see also neoplasm, by site, benign." The table provides the proper code based on the type of neoplasm and the site. It is important to select the proper column in the table that corresponds to the type of neoplasm. The Tabular List should then be referenced to verify that the correct code has been selected from the table and that a more specific site code does not exist.

See Section I.C.21. Factors influencing health status and contact with health services, Status, for information regarding Z15.Ø, codes for genetic susceptibility to cancer.

a. *Admission/Encounter for treatment of primary site*

If the malignancy **is chiefly responsible for occasioning the patient admission/encounter and treatment is directed at the primary site**, designate the **primary** malignancy as the principal/**first-listed** diagnosis.

The only exception to this guideline is if the administration of chemotherapy, immunotherapy or external beam radiation therapy **is chiefly responsible for occasioning the admission/encounter. In that case**, assign the appropriate Z51.-- code as the first-listed or principal diagnosis, and the **underlying** diagnosis or problem for which the service is being performed as a secondary diagnosis.

b. *Admission/Encounter for* treatment of secondary site

When a patient is admitted because of a primary neoplasm with metastasis and treatment is directed toward the secondary site only, the secondary neoplasm is designated as the principal diagnosis even though the primary malignancy is still present.

Patient with primary prostate cancer with metastasis to lungs admitted for wedge resection of mass in right lung

C78.Ø1	**Secondary malignant neoplasm of right lung**
C61	**Malignant neoplasm of prostate**

Explanation: Since the admission is for treatment of the lung metastasis, the secondary lung metastasis is sequenced before the primary prostate cancer.

c. Coding and sequencing of complications

Coding and sequencing of complications associated with the malignancies or with the therapy thereof are subject to the following guidelines:

1) Anemia associated with malignancy

When admission/encounter is for management of an anemia associated with the malignancy, and the treatment is only for anemia, the appropriate code for the malignancy is sequenced as the principal or first-listed diagnosis followed by the appropriate code for the anemia (such as code D63.Ø, Anemia in neoplastic disease).

Patient is admitted for treatment of anemia in advanced colon cancer

C18.9	**Malignant neoplasm of colon, unspecified**
D63.Ø	**Anemia in neoplastic disease**

Explanation: Even though the admission was solely to treat the anemia, this guideline indicates that the code for the malignancy is sequenced first.

2) Anemia associated with chemotherapy, immunotherapy and radiation therapy

When the admission/encounter is for management of an anemia associated with an adverse effect of the administration of chemotherapy or immunotherapy and the only treatment is for the anemia, the anemia code is sequenced first followed by the appropriate codes for the neoplasm and the adverse effect (T45.1X5, Adverse effect of antineoplastic and immunosuppressive drugs).

A 56-year-old Hispanic male with grade II follicular lymphoma involving multiple lymph node sites referred for blood transfusion to treat anemia due to chemotherapy

D64.81	**Anemia due to antineoplastic chemotherapy**
C82.18	**Follicular lymphoma grade II, lymph nodes of multiple sites**
T45.1X5A	**Adverse effect of antineoplastic and immunosuppressive drugs, initial encounter**

Explanation: The code for the anemia is sequenced first followed by the code for the malignant neoplasm and lastly the code for the adverse effect.

When the admission/encounter is for management of an anemia associated with an adverse effect of radiotherapy, the anemia code should be sequenced first, followed by the appropriate neoplasm code and code Y84.2, Radiological procedure and radiotherapy as the cause of abnormal reaction of the patient, or of later complication, without mention of misadventure at the time of the procedure.

A 55-year-old male with a large malignant rectal tumor has been receiving external radiation therapy to shrink the tumor prior to planned surgery. He is admitted today for a blood transfusion to treat anemia related to radiation therapy.

D64.89	**Other specified anemias**
C2Ø	**Malignant neoplasm of rectum**
Y84.2	**Radiological procedure and radiotherapy as the cause of abnormal reaction of the patient, or of later complication, without mention of misadventure at the time of the procedure**

Explanation: The code for the anemia is sequenced first, followed by the code for the malignancy, and lastly the code for the abnormal reaction due to radiotherapy.

3) Management of dehydration due to the malignancy

When the admission/encounter is for management of dehydration due to the malignancy and only the dehydration is being treated (intravenous rehydration), the dehydration is sequenced first, followed by the code(s) for the malignancy.

4) Treatment of a complication resulting from a surgical procedure

When the admission/encounter is for treatment of a complication resulting from a surgical procedure, designate the complication as the principal or first-listed diagnosis if treatment is directed at resolving the complication.

d. Primary malignancy previously excised

When a primary malignancy has been previously excised or eradicated from its site and there is no further treatment directed to that site and there is no evidence of any existing primary malignancy at that site, a code from category Z85, Personal history of malignant neoplasm, should be used to indicate the former site of the malignancy. Any mention of extension, invasion, or metastasis to another site is coded as a secondary malignant neoplasm to that site. The secondary site may be the principal or first-listed diagnosis with the Z85 code used as a secondary code.

See section I.C.2.t. Secondary malignant neoplasm of lymphoid tissue.

History of breast cancer, left radical mastectomy 18 months ago with no current treatment; bronchoscopy with lung biopsy shows metastatic disease in the right lung

C78.Ø1	**Secondary malignant neoplasm of right lung**
Z85.3	**Personal history of malignant neoplasm of breast**

Explanation: The patient has undergone a diagnostic procedure that revealed metastatic breast cancer in the right lung. The code for the secondary (metastatic) site is sequenced first followed by a personal history code to identify the former site of the primary malignancy.

e. Admissions/encounters involving chemotherapy, immunotherapy and radiation therapy

1) Episode of care involves surgical removal of neoplasm

When an episode of care involves the surgical removal of a neoplasm, primary or secondary site, followed by adjunct chemotherapy or radiation treatment during the same episode of care, the code for the neoplasm should be assigned as principal or first-listed diagnosis.

2) Patient admission/encounter solely for administration of chemotherapy, immunotherapy and radiation therapy

If a patient admission/encounter is solely for the administration of chemotherapy, immunotherapy or external beam radiation therapy assign code Z51.Ø, Encounter for antineoplastic radiation therapy, or Z51.11, Encounter for antineoplastic chemotherapy, or Z51.12, Encounter for antineoplastic immunotherapy as the first-listed or principal diagnosis. If a patient receives more than one of these therapies during the same admission more than one of these codes may be assigned, in any sequence.

The malignancy for which the therapy is being administered should be assigned as a secondary diagnosis.

If a patient admission/encounter is for the insertion or implantation of radioactive elements (e.g., brachytherapy) the appropriate code for the malignancy is sequenced as the principal or first-listed diagnosis. Code Z51.Ø should not be assigned.

3) Patient admitted for radiation therapy, chemotherapy or immunotherapy and develops complications

When a patient is admitted for the purpose of external beam radiotherapy, immunotherapy or chemotherapy and develops complications such as uncontrolled nausea and vomiting or dehydration, the principal or first-listed diagnosis is Z51.Ø, Encounter for antineoplastic radiation therapy, or Z51.11, Encounter for antineoplastic chemotherapy, or Z51.12, Encounter for antineoplastic immunotherapy followed by any codes for the complications.

When a patient is admitted for the purpose of insertion or implantation of radioactive elements (e.g., brachytherapy) and develops complications such as uncontrolled nausea and vomiting or dehydration, the principal or first-listed diagnosis is the appropriate code for the malignancy followed by any codes for the complications.

A patient with prostate cancer was admitted for brachytherapy seed implantation and consequently developed urinary retention.

C61	**Malignant neoplasm of prostate**
R33.9	**Retention of urine, unspecified**

Explanation: A code for the malignancy should be listed as the principal diagnosis when insertion of a radioactive element is the reason for admission, even when a complication related to that radioactive element occurs. Codes describing the complications should be listed as secondary codes.

f. Admission/encounter to determine extent of malignancy

When the reason for admission/encounter is to determine the extent of the malignancy, or for a procedure such as paracentesis or thoracentesis, the primary malignancy or appropriate metastatic site is designated as the principal or first-listed diagnosis, even though chemotherapy or radiotherapy is administered.

Patient with left lung cancer with malignant pleural effusion admitted for paracentesis and initiation/administration of chemotherapy

C34.92	**Malignant neoplasm of unspecified part of left bronchus or lung**
J91.Ø	**Malignant pleural effusion**
Z51.11	**Encounter for antineoplastic chemotherapy**

Explanation: The lung cancer is sequenced before the chemotherapy in this instance because the paracentesis for the malignant effusion is also being performed. An instructional note under the malignant effusion instructs that the lung cancer be sequenced first.

g. Symptoms, signs, and abnormal findings listed in Chapter 18 associated with neoplasms

Symptoms, signs, and ill-defined conditions listed in Chapter 18 characteristic of, or associated with, an existing primary or secondary site malignancy cannot be used to replace the malignancy as principal or first-listed diagnosis, regardless of the number of admissions or encounters for treatment and care of the neoplasm.

See Section I.C.21. Factors influencing health status and contact with health services, Encounter for prophylactic organ removal.

h. Admission/encounter for pain control/management

See Section I.C.6. for information on coding admission/encounter for pain control/management.

i. Malignancy in two or more noncontiguous sites

A patient may have more than one malignant tumor in the same organ. These tumors may represent different primaries or metastatic disease, depending on the site. Should the documentation be unclear, the provider should be queried as to the status of each tumor so that the correct codes can be assigned.

j. Disseminated malignant neoplasm, unspecified

Code C8Ø.Ø, Disseminated malignant neoplasm, unspecified, is for use only in those cases where the patient has advanced metastatic disease and no known primary or secondary sites are specified. It should not be used in place of assigning codes for the primary site and all known secondary sites.

Patient who has had no medical care for many years is seen today and diagnosed with carcinomatosis

C8Ø.Ø	**Disseminated malignant neoplasm, unspecified**

Explanation: Carcinomatosis NOS is an "includes" note under this code. Should seldom be used but is available for use in cases such as this.

k. Malignant neoplasm without specification of site

Code C80.1, Malignant (primary) neoplasm, unspecified, equates to Cancer, unspecified. This code should only be used when no determination can be made as to the primary site of a malignancy. This code should rarely be used in the inpatient setting.

l. Sequencing of neoplasm codes

1) Encounter for treatment of primary malignancy

If the reason for the encounter is for treatment of a primary malignancy, assign the malignancy as the principal/first-listed diagnosis. The primary site is to be sequenced first, followed by any metastatic sites.

2) Encounter for treatment of secondary malignancy

When an encounter is for a primary malignancy with metastasis and treatment is directed toward the metastatic (secondary) site(s) only, the metastatic site(s) is designated as the principal/first-listed diagnosis. The primary malignancy is coded as an additional code.

Patient has primary colon cancer with metastasis to rib and is evaluated for possible excision of portion of rib bone

C79.51	**Secondary malignant neoplasm of bone**
C18.9	**Malignant neoplasm of colon, unspecified**

Explanation: The treatment for this encounter is focused on the metastasis to the rib bone rather than the primary colon cancer, thus indicating that the bone metastasis is sequenced as the first-listed code.

3) Malignant neoplasm in a pregnant patient

When a pregnant patient has a malignant neoplasm, a code from subcategory O9A.1-, Malignant neoplasm complicating pregnancy, childbirth, and the puerperium, should be sequenced first, followed by the appropriate code from Chapter 2 to indicate the type of neoplasm.

A 30-year-old pregnant female in second trimester evaluated for thyroid malignancy

O9A.112	**Malignant neoplasm complicating pregnancy, second trimester**
C73	**Malignant neoplasm of thyroid gland**

Explanation: Codes from chapter 15 describing complications of pregnancy are sequenced as first-listed codes, further specified by codes from other chapters such as neoplastic, unless the pregnancy is documented as incidental to the condition. See also guideline 1.C.15.a.1.

4) Encounter for complication associated with a neoplasm

When an encounter is for management of a complication associated with a neoplasm, such as dehydration, and the treatment is only for the complication, the complication is coded first, followed by the appropriate code(s) for the neoplasm.

The exception to this guideline is anemia. When the admission/encounter is for management of an anemia associated with the malignancy, and the treatment is only for anemia, the appropriate code for the malignancy is sequenced as the principal or first-listed diagnosis followed by code D63.0, Anemia in neoplastic disease.

Patient with pancreatic cancer is seen for initiation of TPN for cancer-related moderate protein-calorie malnutrition

E44.0	**Moderate protein-calorie malnutrition**
C25.9	**Malignant neoplasm of pancreas, unspecified**

Explanation: The encounter is to initiate treatment for malnutrition, a common complication of many types of neoplasms, and is sequenced first.

5) Complication from surgical procedure for treatment of a neoplasm

When an encounter is for treatment of a complication resulting from a surgical procedure performed for the treatment of the neoplasm, designate the complication as the principal/first-listed diagnosis. See the guideline regarding the coding of a current malignancy versus personal history to determine if the code for the neoplasm should also be assigned.

6) Pathologic fracture due to a neoplasm

When an encounter is for a pathological fracture due to a neoplasm, and the focus of treatment is the fracture, a code from subcategory M84.5, Pathological fracture in neoplastic disease, should be sequenced first, followed by the code for the neoplasm.

If the focus of treatment is the neoplasm with an associated pathological fracture, the neoplasm code should be sequenced first, followed by a code from M84.5 for the pathological fracture.

m. Current malignancy versus personal history of malignancy

When a primary malignancy has been excised but further treatment, such as an additional surgery for the malignancy, radiation therapy or chemotherapy is directed to that site, the primary malignancy code should be used until treatment is completed.

Female patient with ongoing chemotherapy after right mastectomy for breast cancer

C50.911	**Malignant neoplasm of unspecified site of right female breast**
Z90.11	**Acquired absence of right breast and nipple**

Explanation: Even though the breast has been removed, the breast cancer is still being treated with chemotherapy and therefore is still coded as a current condition rather than personal history.

When a primary malignancy has been previously excised or eradicated from its site, there is no further treatment (of the malignancy) directed to that site, and there is no evidence of any existing primary malignancy at that site, a code from category Z85, Personal history of malignant neoplasm, should be used to indicate the former site of the malignancy.

Codes from subcategories Z85.0 – Z85.85 should only be assigned for the former site of a primary malignancy, not the site of a secondary malignancy. Code Z85.89 may be assigned for the former site(s) of either a primary or secondary malignancy.

See Section I.C.21. Factors influencing health status and contact with health services, History (of)

n. Leukemia, multiple myeloma, and malignant plasma cell neoplasms in remission versus personal history

The categories for leukemia, and category C90, Multiple myeloma and malignant plasma cell neoplasms, have codes indicating whether or not the leukemia has achieved remission. There are also codes Z85.6, Personal history of leukemia, and Z85.79, Personal history of other malignant neoplasms of lymphoid, hematopoietic and related tissues. If the documentation is unclear as to whether the leukemia has achieved remission, the provider should be queried.

See Section I.C.21. Factors influencing health status and contact with health services, History (of)

o. Aftercare following surgery for neoplasm

See Section I.C.21. Factors influencing health status and contact with health services, Aftercare

p. Follow-up care for completed treatment of a malignancy

See Section I.C.21. Factors influencing health status and contact with health services, Follow-up

q. Prophylactic organ removal for prevention of malignancy

See Section I.C. 21, Factors influencing health status and contact with health services, Prophylactic organ removal

r. Malignant neoplasm associated with transplanted organ

A malignant neoplasm of a transplanted organ should be coded as a transplant complication. Assign first the appropriate code from category T86.-, Complications of transplanted organs and tissue, followed by code C80.2, Malignant neoplasm associated with transplanted organ. Use an additional code for the specific malignancy.

s. Breast implant associated anaplastic large cell lymphoma

Breast implant associated anaplastic large cell lymphoma (BIA-ALCL) is a type of lymphoma that can develop around breast implants. Assign code C84.7A, Anaplastic large cell lymphoma, ALK-negative, breast, for BIA-ALCL. Do not assign a complication code from chapter 19.

t. Secondary malignant neoplasm of lymphoid tissue

When a malignant neoplasm of lymphoid tissue metastasizes beyond the lymph nodes, a code from categories C81-C85 with a final character "9" should be assigned identifying "extranodal and solid organ sites" rather than a code for the secondary neoplasm of the affected solid organ. For example, for metastasis of B-cell lymphoma to the lung, brain and left adrenal gland, assign code C83.39, Diffuse large B-cell lymphoma, extranodal and solid organ sites.

Chapter 2. Neoplasms (C00-D49)

NOTE

Functional activity

All neoplasms are classified in this chapter, whether they are functionally active or not. An additional code from Chapter 4 may be used, to identify functional activity associated with any neoplasm.

Morphology [Histology]

Chapter 2 classifies neoplasms primarily by site (topography), with broad groupings for behavior, malignant, in situ, benign, etc. The Table of Neoplasms should be used to identify the correct topography code. In a few cases, such as for malignant melanoma and certain neuroendocrine tumors, the morphology (histologic type) is included in the category and codes.

Primary malignant neoplasms overlapping site boundaries

A primary malignant neoplasm that overlaps two or more contiguous (next to each other) sites should be classified to the subcategory/code .8 ("overlapping lesion"), unless the combination is specifically indexed elsewhere. For multiple neoplasms of the same site that are not contiguous, such as tumors in different quadrants of the same breast, codes for each site should be assigned.

Malignant neoplasm of ectopic tissue

Malignant neoplasms of ectopic tissue are to be coded to the site mentioned, e.g., ectopic pancreatic malignant neoplasms are coded to pancreas, unspecified (C25.9).

AHA: 2017,4Q,103; 2017,1Q,4,5-6,8

This chapter contains the following blocks:

C00-C14	Malignant neoplasms of lip, oral cavity and pharynx
C15-C26	Malignant neoplasms of digestive organs
C30-C39	Malignant neoplasms of respiratory and intrathoracic organs
C40-C41	Malignant neoplasms of bone and articular cartilage
C43-C44	Melanoma and other malignant neoplasms of skin
C45-C49	Malignant neoplasms of mesothelial and soft tissue
C50	Malignant neoplasms of breast
C51-C58	Malignant neoplasms of female genital organs
C60-C63	Malignant neoplasms of male genital organs
C64-C68	Malignant neoplasms of urinary tract
C69-C72	Malignant neoplasms of eye, brain and other parts of central nervous system
C73-C75	Malignant neoplasms of thyroid and other endocrine glands
C7A	Malignant neuroendocrine tumors
C7B	Secondary neuroendocrine tumors
C76-C80	Malignant neoplasms of ill-defined, other secondary and unspecified sites
C81-C96	Malignant neoplasms of lymphoid, hematopoietic and related tissue
D00-D09	In situ neoplasms
D10-D36	Benign neoplasms, except benign neuroendocrine tumors
D3A	Benign neuroendocrine tumors
D37-D48	Neoplasms of uncertain behavior, polycythemia vera and myelodysplastic syndromes
D49	Neoplasms of unspecified behavior

MALIGNANT NEOPLASMS (C00-C96)

Malignant neoplasms, stated or presumed to be primary (of specified sites), and certain specified histologies, except neuroendocrine, and of lymphoid, hematopoietic and related tissue (C00-C75)

AHA: 2022,1Q,16

Malignant neoplasms of lip, oral cavity and pharynx (C00-C14)

4th C00 Malignant neoplasm of lip

Use additional code to identify:
- alcohol abuse and dependence (F10.-)
- history of tobacco dependence (Z87.891)
- tobacco dependence (F17.-)
- tobacco use (Z72.0)

EXCLUDES 1 *malignant melanoma of lip (C43.0)*
Merkel cell carcinoma of lip (C4A.0)
other and unspecified malignant neoplasm of skin of lip (C44.0-)

C00.0 Malignant neoplasm of external upper lip
- Malignant neoplasm of lipstick area of upper lip
- Malignant neoplasm of upper lip NOS
- Malignant neoplasm of vermilion border of upper lip

C00.1 Malignant neoplasm of external lower lip
- Malignant neoplasm of lower lip NOS
- Malignant neoplasm of lipstick area of lower lip
- Malignant neoplasm of vermilion border of lower lip

C00.2 Malignant neoplasm of external lip, unspecified
- Malignant neoplasm of vermilion border of lip NOS

C00.3 Malignant neoplasm of upper lip, inner aspect
- Malignant neoplasm of buccal aspect of upper lip
- Malignant neoplasm of frenulum of upper lip
- Malignant neoplasm of mucosa of upper lip
- Malignant neoplasm of oral aspect of upper lip

C00.4 Malignant neoplasm of lower lip, inner aspect
- Malignant neoplasm of buccal aspect of lower lip
- Malignant neoplasm of frenulum of lower lip
- Malignant neoplasm of mucosa of lower lip
- Malignant neoplasm of oral aspect of lower lip

C00.5 Malignant neoplasm of lip, unspecified, inner aspect
- Malignant neoplasm of buccal aspect of lip, unspecified
- Malignant neoplasm of frenulum of lip, unspecified
- Malignant neoplasm of mucosa of lip, unspecified
- Malignant neoplasm of oral aspect of lip, unspecified

C00.6 Malignant neoplasm of commissure of lip, unspecified

C00.8 Malignant neoplasm of overlapping sites of lip

C00.9 Malignant neoplasm of lip, unspecified

C01 Malignant neoplasm of base of tongue HCC
- Malignant neoplasm of dorsal surface of base of tongue
- Malignant neoplasm of fixed part of tongue NOS
- Malignant neoplasm of posterior third of tongue

Use additional code to identify:
- alcohol abuse and dependence (F10.-)
- history of tobacco dependence (Z87.891)
- tobacco dependence (F17.-)
- tobacco use (Z72.0)

Malignant Neoplasm of Tongue

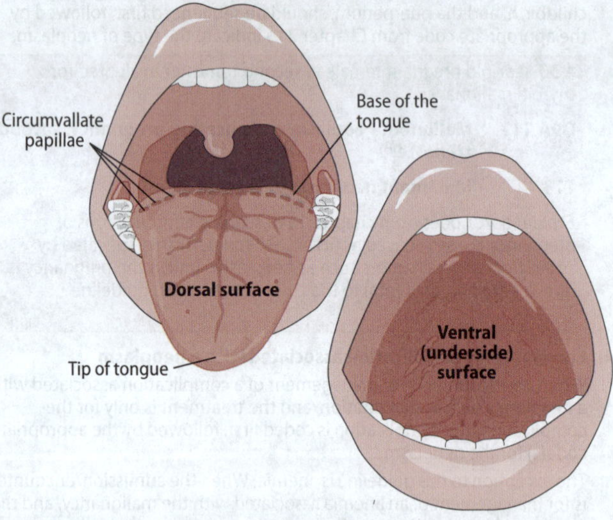

4th C02 Malignant neoplasm of other and unspecified parts of tongue

Use additional code to identify:
- alcohol abuse and dependence (F10.-)
- history of tobacco dependence (Z87.891)
- tobacco dependence (F17.-)
- tobacco use (Z72.0)

C02.0 Malignant neoplasm of dorsal surface of tongue HCC
- Malignant neoplasm of anterior two-thirds of tongue, dorsal surface

EXCLUDES 2 *malignant neoplasm of dorsal surface of base of tongue (C01)*

C02.1 Malignant neoplasm of border of tongue HCC
- Malignant neoplasm of tip of tongue

C02.2 Malignant neoplasm of ventral surface of tongue HCC
- Malignant neoplasm of anterior two-thirds of tongue, ventral surface
- Malignant neoplasm of frenulum linguae

C02.3 Malignant neoplasm of anterior two-thirds of tongue, part unspecified HCC
- Malignant neoplasm of middle third of tongue NOS
- Malignant neoplasm of mobile part of tongue NOS

C02.4 Malignant neoplasm of lingual tonsil HCC

EXCLUDES 2 *malignant neoplasm of tonsil NOS (C09.9)*

C02.8 Malignant neoplasm of overlapping sites of tongue HCC
Malignant neoplasm of two or more contiguous sites of tongue

C02.9 Malignant neoplasm of tongue, unspecified HCC

C03 Malignant neoplasm of gum
INCLUDES malignant neoplasm of alveolar (ridge) mucosa
malignant neoplasm of gingiva
Use additional code to identify:
alcohol abuse and dependence (F10.-)
history of tobacco dependence (Z87.891)
tobacco dependence (F17.-)
tobacco use (Z72.0)
EXCLUDES 2 *malignant odontogenic neoplasms (C41.0-C41.1)*

C03.0 Malignant neoplasm of upper gum HCC
C03.1 Malignant neoplasm of lower gum HCC
C03.9 Malignant neoplasm of gum, unspecified HCC

C04 Malignant neoplasm of floor of mouth
Use additional code to identify:
alcohol abuse and dependence (F10.-)
history of tobacco dependence (Z87.891)
tobacco dependence (F17.-)
tobacco use (Z72.0)

C04.0 Malignant neoplasm of anterior floor of mouth HCC
Malignant neoplasm of anterior to the premolar-canine junction
C04.1 Malignant neoplasm of lateral floor of mouth HCC
C04.8 Malignant neoplasm of overlapping sites of floor of mouth HCC
C04.9 Malignant neoplasm of floor of mouth, unspecified HCC

C05 Malignant neoplasm of palate
Use additional code to identify:
alcohol abuse and dependence (F10.-)
history of tobacco dependence (Z87.891)
tobacco dependence (F17.-)
tobacco use (Z72.0)
EXCLUDES 1 *Kaposi's sarcoma of palate (C46.2)*

C05.0 Malignant neoplasm of hard palate HCC
C05.1 Malignant neoplasm of soft palate HCC
EXCLUDES 2 *malignant neoplasm of nasopharyngeal surface of soft palate (C11.3)*
C05.2 Malignant neoplasm of uvula HCC
C05.8 Malignant neoplasm of overlapping sites of palate HCC
C05.9 Malignant neoplasm of palate, unspecified HCC
Malignant neoplasm of roof of mouth

C06 Malignant neoplasm of other and unspecified parts of mouth
Use additional code to identify:
alcohol abuse and dependence (F10.-)
history of tobacco dependence (Z87.891)
tobacco dependence (F17.-)
tobacco use (Z72.0)

C06.0 Malignant neoplasm of cheek mucosa HCC
Malignant neoplasm of buccal mucosa NOS
Malignant neoplasm of internal cheek
C06.1 Malignant neoplasm of vestibule of mouth HCC
Malignant neoplasm of buccal sulcus (upper) (lower)
Malignant neoplasm of labial sulcus (upper) (lower)
C06.2 Malignant neoplasm of retromolar area HCC
C06.8 Malignant neoplasm of overlapping sites of other and unspecified parts of mouth
C06.80 Malignant neoplasm of overlapping sites of unspecified parts of mouth HCC
C06.89 Malignant neoplasm of overlapping sites of other parts of mouth HCC
"book leaf" neoplasm [ventral surface of tongue and floor of mouth]
C06.9 Malignant neoplasm of mouth, unspecified HCC
Malignant neoplasm of minor salivary gland, unspecified site
Malignant neoplasm of oral cavity NOS

C07 Malignant neoplasm of parotid gland HCC
Use additional code to identify:
alcohol abuse and dependence (F10.-)
exposure to environmental tobacco smoke (Z77.22)
exposure to tobacco smoke in the perinatal period (P96.81)
history of tobacco dependence (Z87.891)
occupational exposure to environmental tobacco smoke (Z57.31)
tobacco dependence (F17.-)
tobacco use (Z72.0)

C08 Malignant neoplasm of other and unspecified major salivary glands
INCLUDES malignant neoplasm of salivary ducts
Use additional code to identify:
alcohol abuse and dependence (F10.-)
exposure to environmental tobacco smoke (Z77.22)
exposure to tobacco smoke in the perinatal period (P96.81)
history of tobacco dependence (Z87.891)
occupational exposure to environmental tobacco smoke (Z57.31)
tobacco dependence (F17.-)
tobacco use (Z72.0)
EXCLUDES 1 *malignant neoplasms of specified minor salivary glands which are classified according to their anatomical location*
EXCLUDES 2 *malignant neoplasms of minor salivary glands NOS (C06.9)*
malignant neoplasm of parotid gland (C07)

C08.0 Malignant neoplasm of submandibular gland HCC
Malignant neoplasm of submaxillary gland
C08.1 Malignant neoplasm of sublingual gland HCC
C08.9 Malignant neoplasm of major salivary gland, unspecified HCC
Malignant neoplasm of salivary gland (major) NOS

C09 Malignant neoplasm of tonsil
Use additional code to identify:
alcohol abuse and dependence (F10.-)
exposure to environmental tobacco smoke (Z77.22)
exposure to tobacco smoke in the perinatal period (P96.81)
history of tobacco dependence (Z87.891)
occupational exposure to environmental tobacco smoke (Z57.31)
tobacco dependence (F17.-)
tobacco use (Z72.0)
EXCLUDES 2 *malignant neoplasm of lingual tonsil (C02.4)*
malignant neoplasm of pharyngeal tonsil (C11.1)

C09.0 Malignant neoplasm of tonsillar fossa HCC
C09.1 Malignant neoplasm of tonsillar pillar (anterior) (posterior) HCC
C09.8 Malignant neoplasm of overlapping sites of tonsil HCC
C09.9 Malignant neoplasm of tonsil, unspecified HCC
Malignant neoplasm of tonsil NOS
Malignant neoplasm of faucial tonsils
Malignant neoplasm of palatine tonsils

C10 Malignant neoplasm of oropharynx
Use additional code to identify:
alcohol abuse and dependence (F10.-)
exposure to environmental tobacco smoke (Z77.22)
exposure to tobacco smoke in the perinatal period (P96.81)
history of tobacco dependence (Z87.891)
occupational exposure to environmental tobacco smoke (Z57.31)
tobacco dependence (F17.-)
tobacco use (Z72.0)
EXCLUDES 2 *malignant neoplasm of tonsil (C09.-)*
DEF: Oropharynx: Middle portion of pharynx (throat); communicates with the oral cavity, nasopharynx and laryngopharynx.

C10.0 Malignant neoplasm of vallecula HCC
C10.1 Malignant neoplasm of anterior surface of epiglottis HCC
Malignant neoplasm of epiglottis, free border [margin]
Malignant neoplasm of glossoepiglottic fold(s)
EXCLUDES 2 *malignant neoplasm of epiglottis (suprahyoid portion) NOS (C32.1)*
C10.2 Malignant neoplasm of lateral wall of oropharynx HCC
C10.3 Malignant neoplasm of posterior wall of oropharynx HCC
C10.4 Malignant neoplasm of branchial cleft HCC
Malignant neoplasm of branchial cyst [site of neoplasm]
C10.8 Malignant neoplasm of overlapping sites of oropharynx HCC
Malignant neoplasm of junctional region of oropharynx
C10.9 Malignant neoplasm of oropharynx, unspecified HCC

C11 Malignant neoplasm of nasopharynx
Use additional code to identify:
exposure to environmental tobacco smoke (Z77.22)
exposure to tobacco smoke in the perinatal period (P96.81)
history of tobacco dependence (Z87.891)
occupational exposure to environmental tobacco smoke (Z57.31)
tobacco dependence (F17.-)
tobacco use (Z72.Ø)
DEF: Nasopharynx: Upper portion of pharynx (throat); communicates with the nasal cavities, oropharynx and tympanic cavities.

C11.Ø Malignant neoplasm of superior wall of nasopharynx HCC
Malignant neoplasm of roof of nasopharynx

C11.1 Malignant neoplasm of posterior wall of nasopharynx HCC
Malignant neoplasm of adenoid
Malignant neoplasm of pharyngeal tonsil

C11.2 Malignant neoplasm of lateral wall of nasopharynx HCC
Malignant neoplasm of fossa of Rosenmüller
Malignant neoplasm of opening of auditory tube
Malignant neoplasm of pharyngeal recess

C11.3 Malignant neoplasm of anterior wall of nasopharynx HCC
Malignant neoplasm of floor of nasopharynx
Malignant neoplasm of nasopharyngeal (anterior) (posterior) surface of soft palate
Malignant neoplasm of posterior margin of nasal choana
Malignant neoplasm of posterior margin of nasal septum

C11.8 Malignant neoplasm of overlapping sites of nasopharynx HCC

C11.9 Malignant neoplasm of nasopharynx, unspecified HCC
Malignant neoplasm of nasopharyngeal wall NOS

C12 Malignant neoplasm of pyriform sinus HCC
Malignant neoplasm of pyriform fossa
Use additional code to identify:
exposure to environmental tobacco smoke (Z77.22)
exposure to tobacco smoke in the perinatal period (P96.81)
history of tobacco dependence (Z87.891)
occupational exposure to environmental tobacco smoke (Z57.31)
tobacco dependence (F17.-)
tobacco use (Z72.Ø)

C13 Malignant neoplasm of hypopharynx
Use additional code to identify:
exposure to environmental tobacco smoke (Z77.22)
exposure to tobacco smoke in the perinatal period (P96.81)
history of tobacco dependence (Z87.891)
occupational exposure to environmental tobacco smoke (Z57.31)
tobacco dependence (F17.-)
tobacco use (Z72.Ø)
EXCLUDES 2 *malignant neoplasm of pyriform sinus (C12)*
DEF: Hypopharynx: Lower portion of pharynx (throat); communicates with the oropharynx and the esophagus. ***Synonym(s):*** *laryngopharynx.*

C13.Ø Malignant neoplasm of postcricoid region HCC

C13.1 Malignant neoplasm of aryepiglottic fold, hypopharyngeal aspect HCC
Malignant neoplasm of aryepiglottic fold, marginal zone
Malignant neoplasm of aryepiglottic fold NOS
Malignant neoplasm of interarytenoid fold, marginal zone
Malignant neoplasm of interarytenoid fold NOS
EXCLUDES 2 *malignant neoplasm of aryepiglottic fold or interarytenoid fold, laryngeal aspect (C32.1)*

C13.2 Malignant neoplasm of posterior wall of hypopharynx HCC

C13.8 Malignant neoplasm of overlapping sites of hypopharynx HCC

C13.9 Malignant neoplasm of hypopharynx, unspecified HCC
Malignant neoplasm of hypopharyngeal wall NOS

C14 Malignant neoplasm of other and ill-defined sites in the lip, oral cavity and pharynx
Use additional code to identify:
alcohol abuse and dependence (F1Ø.-)
exposure to environmental tobacco smoke (Z77.22)
exposure to tobacco smoke in the perinatal period (P96.81)
history of tobacco dependence (Z87.891)
occupational exposure to environmental tobacco smoke (Z57.31)
tobacco dependence (F17.-)
tobacco use (Z72.Ø)
EXCLUDES 1 *malignant neoplasm of oral cavity NOS (CØ6.9)*

C14.Ø Malignant neoplasm of pharynx, unspecified HCC

C14.2 Malignant neoplasm of Waldeyer's ring HCC
DEF: Waldeyer's ring: Ring of lymphoid tissue that is made up of the two palatine tonsils, the pharyngeal tonsil (adenoid), and the lingual tonsil. It functions as the defense against infection and assists with the development of the immune system.

C14.8 Malignant neoplasm of overlapping sites of lip, oral cavity and pharynx HCC
Primary malignant neoplasm of two or more contiguous sites of lip, oral cavity and pharynx
EXCLUDES 1 *"book leaf" neoplasm [ventral surface of tongue and floor of mouth] (CØ6.89)*

Malignant neoplasms of digestive organs (C15-C26)

EXCLUDES 1 *Kaposi's sarcoma of gastrointestinal sites (C46.4)*
EXCLUDES 2 *gastrointestinal stromal tumors (C49.A-)*

C15 Malignant neoplasm of esophagus
Use additional code to identify:
alcohol abuse and dependence (F1Ø.-)

C15.3 Malignant neoplasm of upper third of esophagus CC HCC

C15.4 Malignant neoplasm of middle third of esophagus CC HCC

C15.5 Malignant neoplasm of lower third of esophagus CC HCC
EXCLUDES 1 *malignant neoplasm of cardio-esophageal junction (C16.Ø)*

C15.8 Malignant neoplasm of overlapping sites of esophagus CC HCC

C15.9 Malignant neoplasm of esophagus, unspecified CC HCC

C16 Malignant neoplasm of stomach
Use additional code to identify:
alcohol abuse and dependence (F1Ø.-)
EXCLUDES 2 *malignant carcinoid tumor of the stomach (C7A.Ø92)*

C16.Ø Malignant neoplasm of cardia CC HCC
Malignant neoplasm of cardiac orifice
Malignant neoplasm of cardio-esophageal junction
Malignant neoplasm of esophagus and stomach
Malignant neoplasm of gastro-esophageal junction

C16.1 Malignant neoplasm of fundus of stomach CC HCC

C16.2 Malignant neoplasm of body of stomach CC HCC

C16.3 Malignant neoplasm of pyloric antrum CC HCC
Malignant neoplasm of gastric antrum

C16.4 Malignant neoplasm of pylorus CC HCC
Malignant neoplasm of prepylorus
Malignant neoplasm of pyloric canal

C16.5 Malignant neoplasm of lesser curvature of stomach, unspecified CC HCC
Malignant neoplasm of lesser curvature of stomach, not classifiable to C16.1-C16.4

C16.6 Malignant neoplasm of greater curvature of stomach, unspecified CC HCC
Malignant neoplasm of greater curvature of stomach, not classifiable to C16.Ø-C16.4

C16.8 Malignant neoplasm of overlapping sites of stomach CC HCC

C16.9 Malignant neoplasm of stomach, unspecified CC HCC
Gastric cancer NOS

C17 Malignant neoplasm of small intestine
EXCLUDES 1 *malignant carcinoid tumors of the small intestine (C7A.Ø1)*
AHA: 2016,1Q,19

C17.Ø Malignant neoplasm of duodenum CC HCC

C17.1 Malignant neoplasm of jejunum CC HCC

C17.2 Malignant neoplasm of ileum CC HCC
EXCLUDES 1 *malignant neoplasm of ileocecal valve (C18.Ø)*

C17.3 Meckel's diverticulum, malignant CC HCC
EXCLUDES 1 *Meckel's diverticulum, congenital (Q43.Ø)*
DEF: Congenital, abnormal remnant of embryonic digestive system development that leaves a sacculation or outpouching from the wall of the small intestine near the terminal part of the ileum made of acid-secreting tissue as in the stomach.

C17.8 Malignant neoplasm of overlapping sites of small intestine CC HCC

C17.9 Malignant neoplasm of small intestine, unspecified CC HCC

C18 Malignant neoplasm of colon

EXCLUDES 1 *malignant carcinoid tumors of the colon (C7A.Ø2-)*

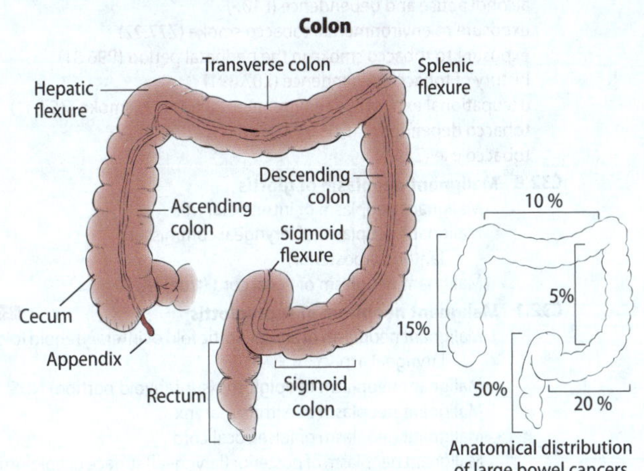

C18.Ø Malignant neoplasm of cecum CC HCC
Malignant neoplasm of ileocecal valve

C18.1 Malignant neoplasm of appendix CC HCC

C18.2 Malignant neoplasm of ascending colon CC HCC

C18.3 Malignant neoplasm of hepatic flexure CC HCC

C18.4 Malignant neoplasm of transverse colon CC HCC

C18.5 Malignant neoplasm of splenic flexure CC HCC

C18.6 Malignant neoplasm of descending colon CC HCC

C18.7 Malignant neoplasm of sigmoid colon CC HCC
Malignant neoplasm of sigmoid (flexure)
EXCLUDES 1 *malignant neoplasm of rectosigmoid junction (C19)*

C18.8 Malignant neoplasm of overlapping sites of colon CC HCC

C18.9 Malignant neoplasm of colon, unspecified CC HCC
Malignant neoplasm of large intestine NOS

C19 Malignant neoplasm of rectosigmoid junction CC HCC
Malignant neoplasm of colon with rectum
Malignant neoplasm of rectosigmoid (colon)
EXCLUDES 1 *malignant carcinoid tumors of the colon (C7A.Ø2-)*

C2Ø Malignant neoplasm of rectum CC HCC
Malignant neoplasm of rectal ampulla
EXCLUDES 1 *malignant carcinoid tumor of the rectum (C7A.Ø26)*

C21 Malignant neoplasm of anus and anal canal

EXCLUDES 2 *malignant carcinoid tumors of the colon (C7A.Ø2-)*
malignant melanoma of anal margin (C43.51)
malignant melanoma of anal skin (C43.51)
malignant melanoma of perianal skin (C43.51)
other and unspecified malignant neoplasm of anal margin (C44.5ØØ, C44.51Ø, C44.52Ø, C44.59Ø)
other and unspecified malignant neoplasm of anal skin (C44.5ØØ, C44.51Ø, C44.52Ø, C44.59Ø)
other and unspecified malignant neoplasm of perianal skin (C44.5ØØ, C44.51Ø, C44.52Ø, C44.59Ø)

C21.Ø Malignant neoplasm of anus, unspecified CC HCC

C21.1 Malignant neoplasm of anal canal CC HCC
Malignant neoplasm of anal sphincter

C21.2 Malignant neoplasm of cloacogenic zone CC HCC

C21.8 Malignant neoplasm of overlapping sites of rectum, anus and anal canal CC HCC
Malignant neoplasm of anorectal junction
Malignant neoplasm of anorectum
Primary malignant neoplasm of two or more contiguous sites of rectum, anus and anal canal

C22 Malignant neoplasm of liver and intrahepatic bile ducts

EXCLUDES 1 *malignant neoplasm of biliary tract NOS (C24.9)*
secondary malignant neoplasm of liver and intrahepatic bile duct (C78.7)

Use additional code to identify:
alcohol abuse and dependence (F1Ø.-)
hepatitis B (B16.-, B18.Ø-B18.1)
hepatitis C (B17.1-, B18.2)

C22.Ø Liver cell carcinoma CC HCC
Hepatocellular carcinoma
Hepatoma
AHA: 2016,1Q,18

C22.1 Intrahepatic bile duct carcinoma CC HCC
Cholangiocarcinoma
EXCLUDES 1 *malignant neoplasm of hepatic duct (C24.Ø)*

C22.2 Hepatoblastoma CC HCC

C22.3 Angiosarcoma of liver CC HCC
Kupffer cell sarcoma

C22.4 Other sarcomas of liver CC HCC

C22.7 Other specified carcinomas of liver CC HCC

C22.8 Malignant neoplasm of liver, primary, unspecified as to type CC HCC

C22.9 Malignant neoplasm of liver, not specified as primary or secondary CC HCC

C23 Malignant neoplasm of gallbladder CC HCC

C24 Malignant neoplasm of other and unspecified parts of biliary tract

EXCLUDES 1 *malignant neoplasm of intrahepatic bile duct (C22.1)*

C24.Ø Malignant neoplasm of extrahepatic bile duct CC HCC
Malignant neoplasm of biliary duct or passage NOS
Malignant neoplasm of common bile duct
Malignant neoplasm of cystic duct
Malignant neoplasm of hepatic duct

C24.1 Malignant neoplasm of ampulla of Vater CC HCC
DEF: Malignant neoplasm in the area of dilation at the juncture of the common bile and pancreatic ducts near the opening into the lumen of the duodenum.

C24.8 Malignant neoplasm of overlapping sites of biliary tract CC HCC
Malignant neoplasm involving both intrahepatic and extrahepatic bile ducts
Primary malignant neoplasm of two or more contiguous sites of biliary tract

C24.9 Malignant neoplasm of biliary tract, unspecified CC HCC

C25 Malignant neoplasm of pancreas

Code also if applicable exocrine pancreatic insufficiency (K86.81)
Use additional code to identify:
alcohol abuse and dependence (F1Ø.-)

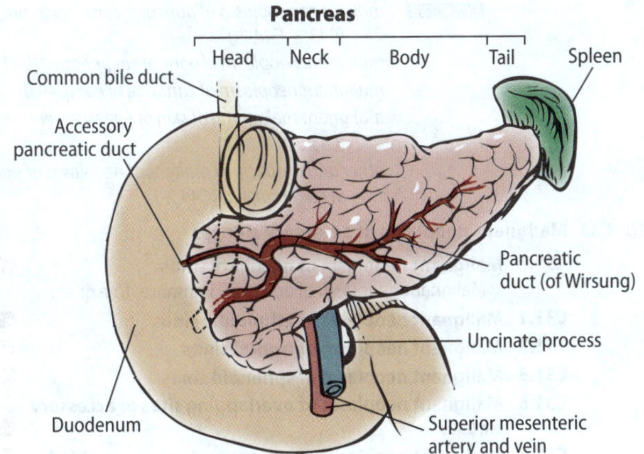

C25.Ø Malignant neoplasm of head of pancreas CC HCC

C25.1 Malignant neoplasm of body of pancreas CC HCC

C25.2 Malignant neoplasm of tail of pancreas CC HCC

C25.3 Malignant neoplasm of pancreatic duct CC HCC

C25.4 Malignant neoplasm of endocrine pancreas CC HCC
Malignant neoplasm of islets of Langerhans
Use additional code to identify any functional activity

C25.7 Malignant neoplasm of other parts of pancreas CC HCC
Malignant neoplasm of neck of pancreas

C25.8 Malignant neoplasm of overlapping sites of pancreas CC HCC

C25.9 Malignant neoplasm of pancreas, unspecified CC HCC

C26 Malignant neoplasm of other and ill-defined digestive organs
EXCLUDES 1 *malignant neoplasm of peritoneum and retroperitoneum (C48.-)*

C26.Ø Malignant neoplasm of intestinal tract, part unspecified HCC
Malignant neoplasm of intestine NOS

C26.1 Malignant neoplasm of spleen HCC
EXCLUDES 1 *Hodgkin lymphoma (C81.-)*
non-Hodgkin lymphoma (C82-C85)

C26.9 Malignant neoplasm of ill-defined sites within the digestive system HCC
Malignant neoplasm of alimentary canal or tract NOS
Malignant neoplasm of gastrointestinal tract NOS
EXCLUDES 1 *malignant neoplasm of abdominal NOS (C76.2)*
malignant neoplasm of intra-abdominal NOS (C76.2)

Malignant neoplasms of respiratory and intrathoracic organs (C3Ø-C39)

INCLUDES malignant neoplasm of middle ear
EXCLUDES 1 *mesothelioma (C45.-)*

C3Ø Malignant neoplasm of nasal cavity and middle ear

C3Ø.Ø Malignant neoplasm of nasal cavity HCC
Malignant neoplasm of cartilage of nose
Malignant neoplasm of nasal concha
Malignant neoplasm of internal nose
Malignant neoplasm of septum of nose
Malignant neoplasm of vestibule of nose
EXCLUDES 1 *malignant neoplasm of nasal bone (C41.Ø)*
malignant neoplasm of nose NOS (C76.Ø)
malignant neoplasm of olfactory bulb (C72.2-)
malignant neoplasm of posterior margin of nasal septum and choana (C11.3)
malignant melanoma of skin of nose (C43.31)
malignant neoplasm of turbinates (C41.Ø)
other and unspecified malignant neoplasm of skin of nose (C44.3Ø1, C44.311, C44.321, C44.391)

C3Ø.1 Malignant neoplasm of middle ear HCC
Malignant neoplasm of antrum tympanicum
Malignant neoplasm of auditory tube
Malignant neoplasm of eustachian tube
Malignant neoplasm of inner ear
Malignant neoplasm of mastoid air cells
Malignant neoplasm of tympanic cavity
EXCLUDES 1 *malignant neoplasm of auricular canal (external) (C43.2-, C44.2-)*
malignant neoplasm of bone of ear (meatus) (C41.Ø)
malignant neoplasm of cartilage of ear (C49.Ø)
malignant melanoma of skin of (external) ear (C43.2-)
other and unspecified malignant neoplasm of skin of (external) ear (C44.2-)

C31 Malignant neoplasm of accessory sinuses

C31.Ø Malignant neoplasm of maxillary sinus HCC
Malignant neoplasm of antrum (Highmore) (maxillary)

C31.1 Malignant neoplasm of ethmoidal sinus HCC

C31.2 Malignant neoplasm of frontal sinus HCC

C31.3 Malignant neoplasm of sphenoid sinus HCC

C31.8 Malignant neoplasm of overlapping sites of accessory sinuses HCC

C31.9 Malignant neoplasm of accessory sinus, unspecified HCC

C32 Malignant neoplasm of larynx
Use additional code to identify:
alcohol abuse and dependence (F1Ø.-)
exposure to environmental tobacco smoke (Z77.22)
exposure to tobacco smoke in the perinatal period (P96.81)
history of tobacco dependence (Z87.891)
occupational exposure to environmental tobacco smoke (Z57.31)
tobacco dependence (F17.-)
tobacco use (Z72.Ø)

C32.Ø Malignant neoplasm of glottis HCC
Malignant neoplasm of intrinsic larynx
Malignant neoplasm of laryngeal commissure (anterior)(posterior)
Malignant neoplasm of vocal cord (true) NOS

C32.1 Malignant neoplasm of supraglottis HCC
Malignant neoplasm of aryepiglottic fold or interarytenoid fold, laryngeal aspect
Malignant neoplasm of epiglottis (suprahyoid portion) NOS
Malignant neoplasm of extrinsic larynx
Malignant neoplasm of false vocal cord
Malignant neoplasm of posterior (laryngeal) surface of epiglottis
Malignant neoplasm of ventricular bands
EXCLUDES 2 *malignant neoplasm of anterior surface of epiglottis (C1Ø.1)*
malignant neoplasm of aryepiglottic fold or interarytenoid fold, hypopharyngeal aspect (C13.1)
malignant neoplasm of aryepiglottic fold or interarytenoid fold, marginal zone (C13.1)
malignant neoplasm of aryepiglottic fold or interarytenoid fold NOS (C13.1)

C32.2 Malignant neoplasm of subglottis HCC

C32.3 Malignant neoplasm of laryngeal cartilage HCC

C32.8 Malignant neoplasm of overlapping sites of larynx HCC

C32.9 Malignant neoplasm of larynx, unspecified HCC

C33 Malignant neoplasm of trachea CC HCC
Use additional code to identify:
exposure to environmental tobacco smoke (Z77.22)
exposure to tobacco smoke in the perinatal period (P96.81)
history of tobacco dependence (Z87.891)
occupational exposure to environmental tobacco smoke (Z57.31)
tobacco dependence (F17.-)
tobacco use (Z72.Ø)

C34 Malignant neoplasm of bronchus and lung
Use additional code to identify:
exposure to environmental tobacco smoke (Z77.22)
exposure to tobacco smoke in the perinatal period (P96.81)
history of tobacco dependence (Z87.891)
occupational exposure to environmental tobacco smoke (Z57.31)
tobacco dependence (F17.-)
tobacco use (Z72.Ø)
EXCLUDES 1 *Kaposi's sarcoma of lung (C46.5-)*
malignant carcinoid tumor of the bronchus and lung (C7A.Ø9Ø)

AHA: 2019,1Q,16

TIP: When documented, assign code I31.3 for associated malignant pericardial effusion. If the sole reason for admission is to treat the effusion with no treatment of the lung malignancy rendered, code I31.3 may be sequenced first.

C34.Ø Malignant neoplasm of main bronchus
Malignant neoplasm of carina
Malignant neoplasm of hilus (of lung)

C34.ØØ Malignant neoplasm of unspecified main bronchus CC HCC

C34.Ø1 Malignant neoplasm of right main bronchus CC HCC

C34.Ø2 Malignant neoplasm of left main bronchus CC HCC

C34.1 Malignant neoplasm of upper lobe, bronchus or lung

C34.1Ø Malignant neoplasm of upper lobe, unspecified bronchus or lung CC HCC

C34.11 Malignant neoplasm of upper lobe, right bronchus or lung CC HCC

C34.12 Malignant neoplasm of upper lobe, left bronchus or lung CC HCC

C34.2 Malignant neoplasm of middle lobe, bronchus or lung CC HCC

C34.3 Malignant neoplasm of lower lobe, bronchus or lung

C34.30 Malignant neoplasm of lower lobe, unspecified bronchus or lung CC HCC

C34.31 Malignant neoplasm of lower lobe, right bronchus or lung CC HCC

C34.32 Malignant neoplasm of lower lobe, left bronchus or lung CC HCC

C34.8 Malignant neoplasm of overlapping sites of bronchus and lung

C34.80 Malignant neoplasm of overlapping sites of unspecified bronchus and lung CC HCC

C34.81 Malignant neoplasm of overlapping sites of right bronchus and lung CC HCC

C34.82 Malignant neoplasm of overlapping sites of left bronchus and lung CC HCC

C34.9 Malignant neoplasm of unspecified part of bronchus or lung

C34.90 Malignant neoplasm of unspecified part of unspecified bronchus or lung CC HCC
Lung cancer NOS

C34.91 Malignant neoplasm of unspecified part of right bronchus or lung CC HCC

C34.92 Malignant neoplasm of unspecified part of left bronchus or lung CC HCC

C37 Malignant neoplasm of thymus CC HCC
EXCLUDES 1 *malignant carcinoid tumor of the thymus (C7A.Ø91)*

C38 Malignant neoplasm of heart, mediastinum and pleura
EXCLUDES 1 *mesothelioma (C45.-)*

C38.Ø Malignant neoplasm of heart CC HCC
Malignant neoplasm of pericardium
EXCLUDES 1 *malignant neoplasm of great vessels (C49.3)*

C38.1 Malignant neoplasm of anterior mediastinum CC HCC

C38.2 Malignant neoplasm of posterior mediastinum CC HCC

C38.3 Malignant neoplasm of mediastinum, part unspecified CC HCC

C38.4 Malignant neoplasm of pleura CC HCC

C38.8 Malignant neoplasm of overlapping sites of heart, mediastinum and pleura CC HCC

C39 Malignant neoplasm of other and ill-defined sites in the respiratory system and intrathoracic organs
Use additional code to identify:
exposure to environmental tobacco smoke (Z77.22)
exposure to tobacco smoke in the perinatal period (P96.81)
history of tobacco dependence (Z87.891)
occupational exposure to environmental tobacco smoke (Z57.31)
tobacco dependence (F17.-)
tobacco use (Z72.Ø)
EXCLUDES 1 *intrathoracic malignant neoplasm NOS (C76.1)*
thoracic malignant neoplasm NOS (C76.1)

C39.Ø Malignant neoplasm of upper respiratory tract, part unspecified HCC

C39.9 Malignant neoplasm of lower respiratory tract, part unspecified HCC
Malignant neoplasm of respiratory tract NOS

Malignant neoplasms of bone and articular cartilage (C4Ø-C41)

INCLUDES malignant neoplasm of cartilage (articular) (joint)
malignant neoplasm of periosteum
EXCLUDES 1 *malignant neoplasm of bone marrow NOS (C96.9)*
malignant neoplasm of synovia (C49.-)

C4Ø Malignant neoplasm of bone and articular cartilage of limbs
Use additional code to identify major osseous defect, if applicable (M89.7-)

C4Ø.Ø Malignant neoplasm of scapula and long bones of upper limb

C4Ø.ØØ Malignant neoplasm of scapula and long bones of unspecified upper limb CC HCC

C4Ø.Ø1 Malignant neoplasm of scapula and long bones of right upper limb CC HCC

C4Ø.Ø2 Malignant neoplasm of scapula and long bones of left upper limb CC HCC

C4Ø.1 Malignant neoplasm of short bones of upper limb

C4Ø.1Ø Malignant neoplasm of short bones of unspecified upper limb CC HCC

C4Ø.11 Malignant neoplasm of short bones of right upper limb CC HCC

C4Ø.12 Malignant neoplasm of short bones of left upper limb CC HCC

C4Ø.2 Malignant neoplasm of long bones of lower limb

C4Ø.2Ø Malignant neoplasm of long bones of unspecified lower limb CC HCC

C4Ø.21 Malignant neoplasm of long bones of right lower limb CC HCC

C4Ø.22 Malignant neoplasm of long bones of left lower limb CC HCC

C4Ø.3 Malignant neoplasm of short bones of lower limb

C4Ø.3Ø Malignant neoplasm of short bones of unspecified lower limb CC HCC

C4Ø.31 Malignant neoplasm of short bones of right lower limb CC HCC

C4Ø.32 Malignant neoplasm of short bones of left lower limb CC HCC

C4Ø.8 Malignant neoplasm of overlapping sites of bone and articular cartilage of limb

C4Ø.8Ø Malignant neoplasm of overlapping sites of bone and articular cartilage of unspecified limb CC HCC

C4Ø.81 Malignant neoplasm of overlapping sites of bone and articular cartilage of right limb CC HCC

C4Ø.82 Malignant neoplasm of overlapping sites of bone and articular cartilage of left limb CC HCC

C4Ø.9 Malignant neoplasm of unspecified bones and articular cartilage of limb

C4Ø.9Ø Malignant neoplasm of unspecified bones and articular cartilage of unspecified limb CC HCC

C4Ø.91 Malignant neoplasm of unspecified bones and articular cartilage of right limb CC HCC

C4Ø.92 Malignant neoplasm of unspecified bones and articular cartilage of left limb CC HCC

C41 Malignant neoplasm of bone and articular cartilage of other and unspecified sites
EXCLUDES 1 *malignant neoplasm of bones of limbs (C4Ø.-)*
malignant neoplasm of cartilage of ear (C49.Ø)
malignant neoplasm of cartilage of eyelid (C49.Ø)
malignant neoplasm of cartilage of larynx (C32.3)
malignant neoplasm of cartilage of limbs (C4Ø.-)
malignant neoplasm of cartilage of nose (C3Ø.Ø)

C41.Ø Malignant neoplasm of bones of skull and face CC HCC
Malignant neoplasm of maxilla (superior)
Malignant neoplasm of orbital bone
EXCLUDES 2 *carcinoma, any type except intraosseous or odontogenic of:*
maxillary sinus (C31.Ø)
upper jaw (CØ3.Ø)
malignant neoplasm of jaw bone (lower) (C41.1)

C41.1 Malignant neoplasm of mandible CC HCC
Malignant neoplasm of inferior maxilla
Malignant neoplasm of lower jaw bone
EXCLUDES 2 *carcinoma, any type except intraosseous or odontogenic of:*
jaw NOS (CØ3.9)
lower (CØ3.1)
malignant neoplasm of upper jaw bone (C41.Ø)

C41.2 Malignant neoplasm of vertebral column CC HCC
EXCLUDES 1 *malignant neoplasm of sacrum and coccyx (C41.4)*

C41.3 Malignant neoplasm of ribs, sternum and clavicle CC HCC

C41.4 Malignant neoplasm of pelvic bones, sacrum and coccyx CC HCC

C41.9 Malignant neoplasm of bone and articular cartilage, unspecified CC HCC

Melanoma and other malignant neoplasms of skin (C43-C44)

C43 Malignant melanoma of skin
EXCLUDES 1 *melanoma in situ (DØ3.-)*
EXCLUDES 2 *malignant melanoma of skin of genital organs (C51-C52, C6Ø.-, C63.-)*
Merkel cell carcinoma (C4A.-)
sites other than skin - code to malignant neoplasm of the site

C43.Ø Malignant melanoma of lip HCC
EXCLUDES 1 *malignant neoplasm of vermilion border of lip (CØØ.Ø-CØØ.2)*

✓5th **C43.1 Malignant melanoma of eyelid, including canthus**
AHA: 2018,4Q,4

C43.10 Malignant melanoma of unspecified eyelid, including canthus HCC

✓6th **C43.11 Malignant melanoma of right eyelid, including canthus**

C43.111 Malignant melanoma of right upper eyelid, including canthus HCC

C43.112 Malignant melanoma of right lower eyelid, including canthus HCC

✓6th **C43.12 Malignant melanoma of left eyelid, including canthus**

C43.121 Malignant melanoma of left upper eyelid, including canthus HCC

C43.122 Malignant melanoma of left lower eyelid, including canthus HCC

✓5th **C43.2 Malignant melanoma of ear and external auricular canal**

C43.20 Malignant melanoma of unspecified ear and external auricular canal HCC

C43.21 Malignant melanoma of right ear and external auricular canal HCC

C43.22 Malignant melanoma of left ear and external auricular canal HCC

✓5th **C43.3 Malignant melanoma of other and unspecified parts of face**

C43.30 Malignant melanoma of unspecified part of face HCC

C43.31 Malignant melanoma of nose HCC

C43.39 Malignant melanoma of other parts of face HCC

C43.4 Malignant melanoma of scalp and neck HCC

✓5th **C43.5 Malignant melanoma of trunk**

EXCLUDES 2 *malignant neoplasm of anus NOS (C21.0)*
malignant neoplasm of scrotum (C63.2)

C43.51 Malignant melanoma of anal skin HCC
Malignant melanoma of anal margin
Malignant melanoma of perianal skin

C43.52 Malignant melanoma of skin of breast HCC

C43.59 Malignant melanoma of other part of trunk HCC

✓5th **C43.6 Malignant melanoma of upper limb, including shoulder**

C43.60 Malignant melanoma of unspecified upper limb, including shoulder HCC

C43.61 Malignant melanoma of right upper limb, including shoulder HCC

C43.62 Malignant melanoma of left upper limb, including shoulder HCC

✓5th **C43.7 Malignant melanoma of lower limb, including hip**

C43.70 Malignant melanoma of unspecified lower limb, including hip HCC

C43.71 Malignant melanoma of right lower limb, including hip HCC

C43.72 Malignant melanoma of left lower limb, including hip HCC

C43.8 Malignant melanoma of overlapping sites of skin HCC

C43.9 Malignant melanoma of skin, unspecified HCC
Malignant melanoma of unspecified site of skin
Melanoma (malignant) NOS

✓4th **C4A Merkel cell carcinoma**

DEF: Malignant cutaneous cancer predominantly found in elderly patients with sun exposure that usually presents as a flesh-colored or bluish-red lump typically seen on the neck, head, and face.

C4A.0 Merkel cell carcinoma of lip HCC

EXCLUDES 1 *malignant neoplasm of vermilion border of lip (C00.0-C00.2)*

✓5th **C4A.1 Merkel cell carcinoma of eyelid, including canthus**
AHA: 2018,4Q,4

C4A.10 Merkel cell carcinoma of unspecified eyelid, including canthus HCC

✓6th **C4A.11 Merkel cell carcinoma of right eyelid, including canthus**

C4A.111 Merkel cell carcinoma of right upper eyelid, including canthus HCC

C4A.112 Merkel cell carcinoma of right lower eyelid, including canthus HCC

✓6th **C4A.12 Merkel cell carcinoma of left eyelid, including canthus**

C4A.121 Merkel cell carcinoma of left upper eyelid, including canthus HCC

C4A.122 Merkel cell carcinoma of left lower eyelid, including canthus HCC

✓5th **C4A.2 Merkel cell carcinoma of ear and external auricular canal**

C4A.20 Merkel cell carcinoma of unspecified ear and external auricular canal HCC

C4A.21 Merkel cell carcinoma of right ear and external auricular canal HCC

C4A.22 Merkel cell carcinoma of left ear and external auricular canal HCC

✓5th **C4A.3 Merkel cell carcinoma of other and unspecified parts of face**

C4A.30 Merkel cell carcinoma of unspecified part of face HCC

C4A.31 Merkel cell carcinoma of nose HCC

C4A.39 Merkel cell carcinoma of other parts of face HCC

C4A.4 Merkel cell carcinoma of scalp and neck HCC

✓5th **C4A.5 Merkel cell carcinoma of trunk**

EXCLUDES 2 *malignant neoplasm of anus NOS (C21.0)*
malignant neoplasm of scrotum (C63.2)

C4A.51 Merkel cell carcinoma of anal skin HCC
Merkel cell carcinoma of anal margin
Merkel cell carcinoma of perianal skin

C4A.52 Merkel cell carcinoma of skin of breast HCC

C4A.59 Merkel cell carcinoma of other part of trunk HCC

✓5th **C4A.6 Merkel cell carcinoma of upper limb, including shoulder**

C4A.60 Merkel cell carcinoma of unspecified upper limb, including shoulder HCC

C4A.61 Merkel cell carcinoma of right upper limb, including shoulder HCC

C4A.62 Merkel cell carcinoma of left upper limb, including shoulder HCC

✓5th **C4A.7 Merkel cell carcinoma of lower limb, including hip**

C4A.70 Merkel cell carcinoma of unspecified lower limb, including hip HCC

C4A.71 Merkel cell carcinoma of right lower limb, including hip HCC

C4A.72 Merkel cell carcinoma of left lower limb, including hip HCC

C4A.8 Merkel cell carcinoma of overlapping sites HCC

C4A.9 Merkel cell carcinoma, unspecified HCC
Merkel cell carcinoma of unspecified site
Merkel cell carcinoma NOS

✓4th **C44 Other and unspecified malignant neoplasm of skin**

INCLUDES malignant neoplasm of sebaceous glands
malignant neoplasm of sweat glands

EXCLUDES 1 *Kaposi's sarcoma of skin (C46.0)*
malignant melanoma of skin (C43.-)
malignant neoplasm of skin of genital organs (C51-C52, C60.-, C63.2)
Merkel cell carcinoma (C4A.-)

DEF: Basal cell carcinoma: Abnormal growth of skin cells that arises from the deepest layer of the epidermis and may present as an open sore, red patches, pink growth, or scar. Typically caused by sun exposure, it is one of the most common forms of skin cancer.

DEF: Squamous cell carcinoma: Uncontrolled growth of abnormal skin cells that arises from the outer layers of the skin (epidermis) and may present as an open sore. It is characterized by a firm, red nodule, elevated growth with a central depression, or a flat sore with a scaly crust.

✓5th **C44.0 Other and unspecified malignant neoplasm of skin of lip**

EXCLUDES 1 *malignant neoplasm of lip (C00.-)*

C44.00 Unspecified malignant neoplasm of skin of lip

C44.01 Basal cell carcinoma of skin of lip

C44.02 Squamous cell carcinoma of skin of lip

C44.09 Other specified malignant neoplasm of skin of lip

✓5th **C44.1 Other and unspecified malignant neoplasm of skin of eyelid, including canthus**

EXCLUDES 1 *connective tissue of eyelid (C49.0)*

AHA: 2018,4Q,4

✓6th **C44.10 Unspecified malignant neoplasm of skin of eyelid, including canthus**

C44.101 Unspecified malignant neoplasm of skin of unspecified eyelid, including canthus

✓7th **C44.102 Unspecified malignant neoplasm of skin of right eyelid, including canthus**

C44.1021 Unspecified malignant neoplasm of skin of right upper eyelid, including canthus

C44.1022 Unspecified malignant neoplasm of skin of right lower eyelid, including canthus
C44.109 Unspecified malignant neoplasm of skin of left eyelid, including canthus
C44.1091 Unspecified malignant neoplasm of skin of left upper eyelid, including canthus
C44.1092 Unspecified malignant neoplasm of skin of left lower eyelid, including canthus
C44.11 Basal cell carcinoma of skin of eyelid, including canthus
C44.111 Basal cell carcinoma of skin of unspecified eyelid, including canthus
C44.112 Basal cell carcinoma of skin of right eyelid, including canthus
C44.1121 Basal cell carcinoma of skin of right upper eyelid, including canthus
C44.1122 Basal cell carcinoma of skin of right lower eyelid, including canthus
C44.119 Basal cell carcinoma of skin of left eyelid, including canthus
C44.1191 Basal cell carcinoma of skin of left upper eyelid, including canthus
C44.1192 Basal cell carcinoma of skin of left lower eyelid, including canthus
C44.12 Squamous cell carcinoma of skin of eyelid, including canthus
C44.121 Squamous cell carcinoma of skin of unspecified eyelid, including canthus
C44.122 Squamous cell carcinoma of skin of right eyelid, including canthus
C44.1221 Squamous cell carcinoma of skin of right upper eyelid, including canthus
C44.1222 Squamous cell carcinoma of skin of right lower eyelid, including canthus
C44.129 Squamous cell carcinoma of skin of left eyelid, including canthus
C44.1291 Squamous cell carcinoma of skin of left upper eyelid, including canthus
C44.1292 Squamous cell carcinoma of skin of left lower eyelid, including canthus
C44.13 Sebaceous cell carcinoma of skin of eyelid, including canthus
C44.131 Sebaceous cell carcinoma of skin of unspecified eyelid, including canthus
C44.132 Sebaceous cell carcinoma of skin of right eyelid, including canthus
C44.1321 Sebaceous cell carcinoma of skin of right upper eyelid, including canthus
C44.1322 Sebaceous cell carcinoma of skin of right lower eyelid, including canthus
C44.139 Sebaceous cell carcinoma of skin of left eyelid, including canthus
C44.1391 Sebaceous cell carcinoma of skin of left upper eyelid, including canthus
C44.1392 Sebaceous cell carcinoma of skin of left lower eyelid, including canthus
C44.19 Other specified malignant neoplasm of skin of eyelid, including canthus
C44.191 Other specified malignant neoplasm of skin of unspecified eyelid, including canthus
C44.192 Other specified malignant neoplasm of skin of right eyelid, including canthus
C44.1921 Other specified malignant neoplasm of skin of right upper eyelid, including canthus
C44.1922 Other specified malignant neoplasm of skin of right lower eyelid, including canthus
C44.199 Other specified malignant neoplasm of skin of left eyelid, including canthus
C44.1991 Other specified malignant neoplasm of skin of left upper eyelid, including canthus
C44.1992 Other specified malignant neoplasm of skin of left lower eyelid, including canthus
C44.2 Other and unspecified malignant neoplasm of skin of ear and external auricular canal
EXCLUDES 1 *connective tissue of ear (C49.0)*
C44.20 Unspecified malignant neoplasm of skin of ear and external auricular canal
C44.201 Unspecified malignant neoplasm of skin of unspecified ear and external auricular canal
C44.202 Unspecified malignant neoplasm of skin of right ear and external auricular canal
C44.209 Unspecified malignant neoplasm of skin of left ear and external auricular canal
C44.21 Basal cell carcinoma of skin of ear and external auricular canal
C44.211 Basal cell carcinoma of skin of unspecified ear and external auricular canal
C44.212 Basal cell carcinoma of skin of right ear and external auricular canal
C44.219 Basal cell carcinoma of skin of left ear and external auricular canal
C44.22 Squamous cell carcinoma of skin of ear and external auricular canal
C44.221 Squamous cell carcinoma of skin of unspecified ear and external auricular canal
C44.222 Squamous cell carcinoma of skin of right ear and external auricular canal
C44.229 Squamous cell carcinoma of skin of left ear and external auricular canal
C44.29 Other specified malignant neoplasm of skin of ear and external auricular canal
C44.291 Other specified malignant neoplasm of skin of unspecified ear and external auricular canal
C44.292 Other specified malignant neoplasm of skin of right ear and external auricular canal
C44.299 Other specified malignant neoplasm of skin of left ear and external auricular canal
C44.3 Other and unspecified malignant neoplasm of skin of other and unspecified parts of face
C44.30 Unspecified malignant neoplasm of skin of other and unspecified parts of face
C44.300 Unspecified malignant neoplasm of skin of unspecified part of face
C44.301 Unspecified malignant neoplasm of skin of nose
C44.309 Unspecified malignant neoplasm of skin of other parts of face
C44.31 Basal cell carcinoma of skin of other and unspecified parts of face
C44.310 Basal cell carcinoma of skin of unspecified parts of face
C44.311 Basal cell carcinoma of skin of nose
C44.319 Basal cell carcinoma of skin of other parts of face
C44.32 Squamous cell carcinoma of skin of other and unspecified parts of face
C44.320 Squamous cell carcinoma of skin of unspecified parts of face
C44.321 Squamous cell carcinoma of skin of nose
C44.329 Squamous cell carcinoma of skin of other parts of face
C44.39 Other specified malignant neoplasm of skin of other and unspecified parts of face
C44.390 Other specified malignant neoplasm of skin of unspecified parts of face
C44.391 Other specified malignant neoplasm of skin of nose
C44.399 Other specified malignant neoplasm of skin of other parts of face

C44.4 Other and unspecified malignant neoplasm of skin of scalp and neck
- **C44.40 Unspecified malignant neoplasm of skin of scalp and neck**
- **C44.41 Basal cell carcinoma of skin of scalp and neck**
- **C44.42 Squamous cell carcinoma of skin of scalp and neck**
- **C44.49 Other specified malignant neoplasm of skin of scalp and neck**

C44.5 Other and unspecified malignant neoplasm of skin of trunk

EXCLUDES 1 *anus NOS (C21.0)*
scrotum (C63.2)

- **C44.50 Unspecified malignant neoplasm of skin of trunk**
  - **C44.500 Unspecified malignant neoplasm of anal skin**
    Unspecified malignant neoplasm of anal margin
    Unspecified malignant neoplasm of perianal skin
  - **C44.501 Unspecified malignant neoplasm of skin of breast**
  - **C44.509 Unspecified malignant neoplasm of skin of other part of trunk**
- **C44.51 Basal cell carcinoma of skin of trunk**
  - **C44.510 Basal cell carcinoma of anal skin**
    Basal cell carcinoma of anal margin
    Basal cell carcinoma of perianal skin
  - **C44.511 Basal cell carcinoma of skin of breast**
  - **C44.519 Basal cell carcinoma of skin of other part of trunk**
- **C44.52 Squamous cell carcinoma of skin of trunk**
  - **C44.520 Squamous cell carcinoma of anal skin**
    Squamous cell carcinoma of anal margin
    Squamous cell carcinoma of perianal skin
  - **C44.521 Squamous cell carcinoma of skin of breast**
  - **C44.529 Squamous cell carcinoma of skin of other part of trunk**
- **C44.59 Other specified malignant neoplasm of skin of trunk**
  - **C44.590 Other specified malignant neoplasm of anal skin**
    Other specified malignant neoplasm of anal margin
    Other specified malignant neoplasm of perianal skin
  - **C44.591 Other specified malignant neoplasm of skin of breast**
  - **C44.599 Other specified malignant neoplasm of skin of other part of trunk**

C44.6 Other and unspecified malignant neoplasm of skin of upper limb, including shoulder
- **C44.60 Unspecified malignant neoplasm of skin of upper limb, including shoulder**
  - **C44.601 Unspecified malignant neoplasm of skin of unspecified upper limb, including shoulder**
  - **C44.602 Unspecified malignant neoplasm of skin of right upper limb, including shoulder**
  - **C44.609 Unspecified malignant neoplasm of skin of left upper limb, including shoulder**
- **C44.61 Basal cell carcinoma of skin of upper limb, including shoulder**
  - **C44.611 Basal cell carcinoma of skin of unspecified upper limb, including shoulder**
  - **C44.612 Basal cell carcinoma of skin of right upper limb, including shoulder**
  - **C44.619 Basal cell carcinoma of skin of left upper limb, including shoulder**
- **C44.62 Squamous cell carcinoma of skin of upper limb, including shoulder**
  - **C44.621 Squamous cell carcinoma of skin of unspecified upper limb, including shoulder**
  - **C44.622 Squamous cell carcinoma of skin of right upper limb, including shoulder**
  - **C44.629 Squamous cell carcinoma of skin of left upper limb, including shoulder**
- **C44.69 Other specified malignant neoplasm of skin of upper limb, including shoulder**
  - **C44.691 Other specified malignant neoplasm of skin of unspecified upper limb, including shoulder**
  - **C44.692 Other specified malignant neoplasm of skin of right upper limb, including shoulder**
  - **C44.699 Other specified malignant neoplasm of skin of left upper limb, including shoulder**

C44.7 Other and unspecified malignant neoplasm of skin of lower limb, including hip
- **C44.70 Unspecified malignant neoplasm of skin of lower limb, including hip**
  - **C44.701 Unspecified malignant neoplasm of skin of unspecified lower limb, including hip**
  - **C44.702 Unspecified malignant neoplasm of skin of right lower limb, including hip**
  - **C44.709 Unspecified malignant neoplasm of skin of left lower limb, including hip**
- **C44.71 Basal cell carcinoma of skin of lower limb, including hip**
  - **C44.711 Basal cell carcinoma of skin of unspecified lower limb, including hip**
  - **C44.712 Basal cell carcinoma of skin of right lower limb, including hip**
  - **C44.719 Basal cell carcinoma of skin of left lower limb, including hip**
- **C44.72 Squamous cell carcinoma of skin of lower limb, including hip**
  - **C44.721 Squamous cell carcinoma of skin of unspecified lower limb, including hip**
  - **C44.722 Squamous cell carcinoma of skin of right lower limb, including hip**
  - **C44.729 Squamous cell carcinoma of skin of left lower limb, including hip**
- **C44.79 Other specified malignant neoplasm of skin of lower limb, including hip**
  - **C44.791 Other specified malignant neoplasm of skin of unspecified lower limb, including hip**
  - **C44.792 Other specified malignant neoplasm of skin of right lower limb, including hip**
  - **C44.799 Other specified malignant neoplasm of skin of left lower limb, including hip**

C44.8 Other and unspecified malignant neoplasm of overlapping sites of skin
- **C44.80 Unspecified malignant neoplasm of overlapping sites of skin**
- **C44.81 Basal cell carcinoma of overlapping sites of skin**
- **C44.82 Squamous cell carcinoma of overlapping sites of skin**
- **C44.89 Other specified malignant neoplasm of overlapping sites of skin**

C44.9 Other and unspecified malignant neoplasm of skin, unspecified
- **C44.90 Unspecified malignant neoplasm of skin, unspecified**
  Malignant neoplasm of unspecified site of skin
- **C44.91 Basal cell carcinoma of skin, unspecified**
- **C44.92 Squamous cell carcinoma of skin, unspecified**
- **C44.99 Other specified malignant neoplasm of skin, unspecified**

Malignant neoplasms of mesothelial and soft tissue (C45-C49)

C45 Mesothelioma

DEF: Rare type of cancer that forms in the thin layer of protective tissue that covers the majority of internal organs (mesothelium).

- **C45.0 Mesothelioma of pleura** CC HCC
  EXCLUDES 1 *other malignant neoplasm of pleura (C38.4)*
  AHA: 2017,2Q,11
  TIP: For pleural mesothelioma that has metastasized to the chest wall, assign this code for the primary site along with C79.89 for metastatic cancer in the chest wall.
- **C45.1 Mesothelioma of peritoneum** CC HCC
  Mesothelioma of cul-de-sac
  Mesothelioma of mesentery
  Mesothelioma of mesocolon
  Mesothelioma of omentum
  Mesothelioma of peritoneum (parietal) (pelvic)
  EXCLUDES 1 *other malignant neoplasm of soft tissue of peritoneum (C48.-)*
- **C45.2 Mesothelioma of pericardium** CC HCC
  EXCLUDES 1 *other malignant neoplasm of pericardium (C38.0)*
- **C45.7 Mesothelioma of other sites** HCC

C45.9 Mesothelioma, unspecified HCC

C46 Kaposi's sarcoma

Code first any human immunodeficiency virus [HIV] disease (B20)

DEF: Malignant neoplasm that causes patches of abnormal tissue to grow under the skin, in the lining of the mouth, nose, and throat, in lymph nodes, or in other visceral organs. Kaposi's sarcoma is caused by human herpesvirus8 (HHV8).

C46.0 Kaposi's sarcoma of skin HIV CC HCC

C46.1 Kaposi's sarcoma of soft tissue HIV CC HCC

Kaposi's sarcoma of blood vessel
Kaposi's sarcoma of connective tissue
Kaposi's sarcoma of fascia
Kaposi's sarcoma of ligament
Kaposi's sarcoma of lymphatic(s) NEC
Kaposi's sarcoma of muscle

EXCLUDES 2 *Kaposi's sarcoma of lymph glands and nodes (C46.3)*

C46.2 Kaposi's sarcoma of palate HIV CC HCC

C46.3 Kaposi's sarcoma of lymph nodes HIV CC HCC

C46.4 Kaposi's sarcoma of gastrointestinal sites HIV CC HCC

C46.5 Kaposi's sarcoma of lung

AHA: 2019,1Q,16

TIP: When associated malignant pericardial effusion is documented, assign code I31.3. If the sole reason for admission is to treat the effusion with no treatment of the lung malignancy rendered, code I31.3 may be sequenced first.

C46.50 Kaposi's sarcoma of unspecified lung HIV CC HCC

C46.51 Kaposi's sarcoma of right lung HIV CC HCC

C46.52 Kaposi's sarcoma of left lung HIV CC HCC

C46.7 Kaposi's sarcoma of other sites HIV CC HCC

C46.9 Kaposi's sarcoma, unspecified HIV CC HCC

Kaposi's sarcoma of unspecified site

C47 Malignant neoplasm of peripheral nerves and autonomic nervous system

INCLUDES malignant neoplasm of sympathetic and parasympathetic nerves and ganglia

EXCLUDES 1 *Kaposi's sarcoma of soft tissue (C46.1)*

C47.0 Malignant neoplasm of peripheral nerves of head, face and neck CC HCC

EXCLUDES 1 *malignant neoplasm of peripheral nerves of orbit (C69.6-)*

C47.1 Malignant neoplasm of peripheral nerves of upper limb, including shoulder

C47.10 Malignant neoplasm of peripheral nerves of unspecified upper limb, including shoulder CC HCC

C47.11 Malignant neoplasm of peripheral nerves of right upper limb, including shoulder CC HCC

C47.12 Malignant neoplasm of peripheral nerves of left upper limb, including shoulder CC HCC

C47.2 Malignant neoplasm of peripheral nerves of lower limb, including hip

C47.20 Malignant neoplasm of peripheral nerves of unspecified lower limb, including hip CC HCC

C47.21 Malignant neoplasm of peripheral nerves of right lower limb, including hip CC HCC

C47.22 Malignant neoplasm of peripheral nerves of left lower limb, including hip CC HCC

C47.3 Malignant neoplasm of peripheral nerves of thorax CC HCC

C47.4 Malignant neoplasm of peripheral nerves of abdomen CC HCC

C47.5 Malignant neoplasm of peripheral nerves of pelvis CC HCC

C47.6 Malignant neoplasm of peripheral nerves of trunk, unspecified CC HCC

Malignant neoplasm of peripheral nerves of unspecified part of trunk

C47.8 Malignant neoplasm of overlapping sites of peripheral nerves and autonomic nervous system CC HCC

C47.9 Malignant neoplasm of peripheral nerves and autonomic nervous system, unspecified CC HCC

Malignant neoplasm of unspecified site of peripheral nerves and autonomic nervous system

C48 Malignant neoplasm of retroperitoneum and peritoneum

EXCLUDES 1 *Kaposi's sarcoma of connective tissue (C46.1)*
mesothelioma (C45.-)

C48.0 Malignant neoplasm of retroperitoneum CC HCC

C48.1 Malignant neoplasm of specified parts of peritoneum CC HCC

Malignant neoplasm of cul-de-sac
Malignant neoplasm of mesentery
Malignant neoplasm of mesocolon
Malignant neoplasm of omentum
Malignant neoplasm of parietal peritoneum
Malignant neoplasm of pelvic peritoneum

C48.2 Malignant neoplasm of peritoneum, unspecified CC HCC

C48.8 Malignant neoplasm of overlapping sites of retroperitoneum and peritoneum CC HCC

C49 Malignant neoplasm of other connective and soft tissue

INCLUDES malignant neoplasm of blood vessel
malignant neoplasm of bursa
malignant neoplasm of cartilage
malignant neoplasm of fascia
malignant neoplasm of fat
malignant neoplasm of ligament, except uterine
malignant neoplasm of lymphatic vessel
malignant neoplasm of muscle
malignant neoplasm of synovia
malignant neoplasm of tendon (sheath)

EXCLUDES 1 *malignant neoplasm of cartilage (of):*
articular (C40-C41)
larynx (C32.3)
nose (C30.0)
malignant neoplasm of connective tissue of breast (C50.-)

EXCLUDES 2 *Kaposi's sarcoma of soft tissue (C46.1)*
malignant neoplasm of heart (C38.0)
malignant neoplasm of peripheral nerves and autonomic nervous system (C47.-)
malignant neoplasm of peritoneum (C48.2)
malignant neoplasm of retroperitoneum (C48.0)
malignant neoplasm of uterine ligament (C57.3)
mesothelioma (C45.-)

C49.0 Malignant neoplasm of connective and soft tissue of head, face and neck CC HCC

Malignant neoplasm of connective tissue of ear
Malignant neoplasm of connective tissue of eyelid

EXCLUDES 1 *connective tissue of orbit (C69.6-)*

C49.1 Malignant neoplasm of connective and soft tissue of upper limb, including shoulder

C49.10 Malignant neoplasm of connective and soft tissue of unspecified upper limb, including shoulder CC HCC

C49.11 Malignant neoplasm of connective and soft tissue of right upper limb, including shoulder CC HCC

C49.12 Malignant neoplasm of connective and soft tissue of left upper limb, including shoulder CC HCC

C49.2 Malignant neoplasm of connective and soft tissue of lower limb, including hip

C49.20 Malignant neoplasm of connective and soft tissue of unspecified lower limb, including hip CC HCC

C49.21 Malignant neoplasm of connective and soft tissue of right lower limb, including hip CC HCC

C49.22 Malignant neoplasm of connective and soft tissue of left lower limb, including hip CC HCC

C49.3 Malignant neoplasm of connective and soft tissue of thorax CC HCC

Malignant neoplasm of axilla
Malignant neoplasm of diaphragm
Malignant neoplasm of great vessels

EXCLUDES 1 *malignant neoplasm of breast (C50.-)*
malignant neoplasm of heart (C38.0)
malignant neoplasm of mediastinum (C38.1-C38.3)
malignant neoplasm of thymus (C37)

AHA: 2015,3Q,19

C49.4 Malignant neoplasm of connective and soft tissue of abdomen CC HCC

Malignant neoplasm of abdominal wall
Malignant neoplasm of hypochondrium

C49.5 Malignant neoplasm of connective and soft tissue of pelvis CC HCC

Malignant neoplasm of buttock
Malignant neoplasm of groin
Malignant neoplasm of perineum

C49.6 Malignant neoplasm of connective and soft tissue of trunk, unspecified CC HCC
Malignant neoplasm of back NOS

C49.8 Malignant neoplasm of overlapping sites of connective and soft tissue CC HCC
Primary malignant neoplasm of two or more contiguous sites of connective and soft tissue

C49.9 Malignant neoplasm of connective and soft tissue, unspecified CC HCC

√5th **C49.A Gastrointestinal stromal tumor**
AHA: 2016,4Q,8
DEF: Uncommon malignant tumor found in the GI tract that originates from interstitial cells of the autonomic nervous system. Most occur in the stomach or small intestine but can originate anywhere in the GI tract.

C49.AØ Gastrointestinal stromal tumor, unspecified site CC HCC
C49.A1 Gastrointestinal stromal tumor of esophagus CC HCC
C49.A2 Gastrointestinal stromal tumor of stomach CC HCC
C49.A3 Gastrointestinal stromal tumor of small intestine CC HCC
C49.A4 Gastrointestinal stromal tumor of large intestine CC HCC
C49.A5 Gastrointestinal stromal tumor of rectum CC HCC
C49.A9 Gastrointestinal stromal tumor of other sites CC HCC

Malignant neoplasms of breast (C5Ø)

√4th **C5Ø Malignant neoplasm of breast**
INCLUDES connective tissue of breast
Paget's disease of breast
Paget's disease of nipple
Use additional code to identify estrogen receptor status (Z17.Ø, Z17.1)
EXCLUDES 1 *skin of breast (C44.5Ø1, C44.511, C44.521, C44.591)*
AHA: 2017,4Q,19

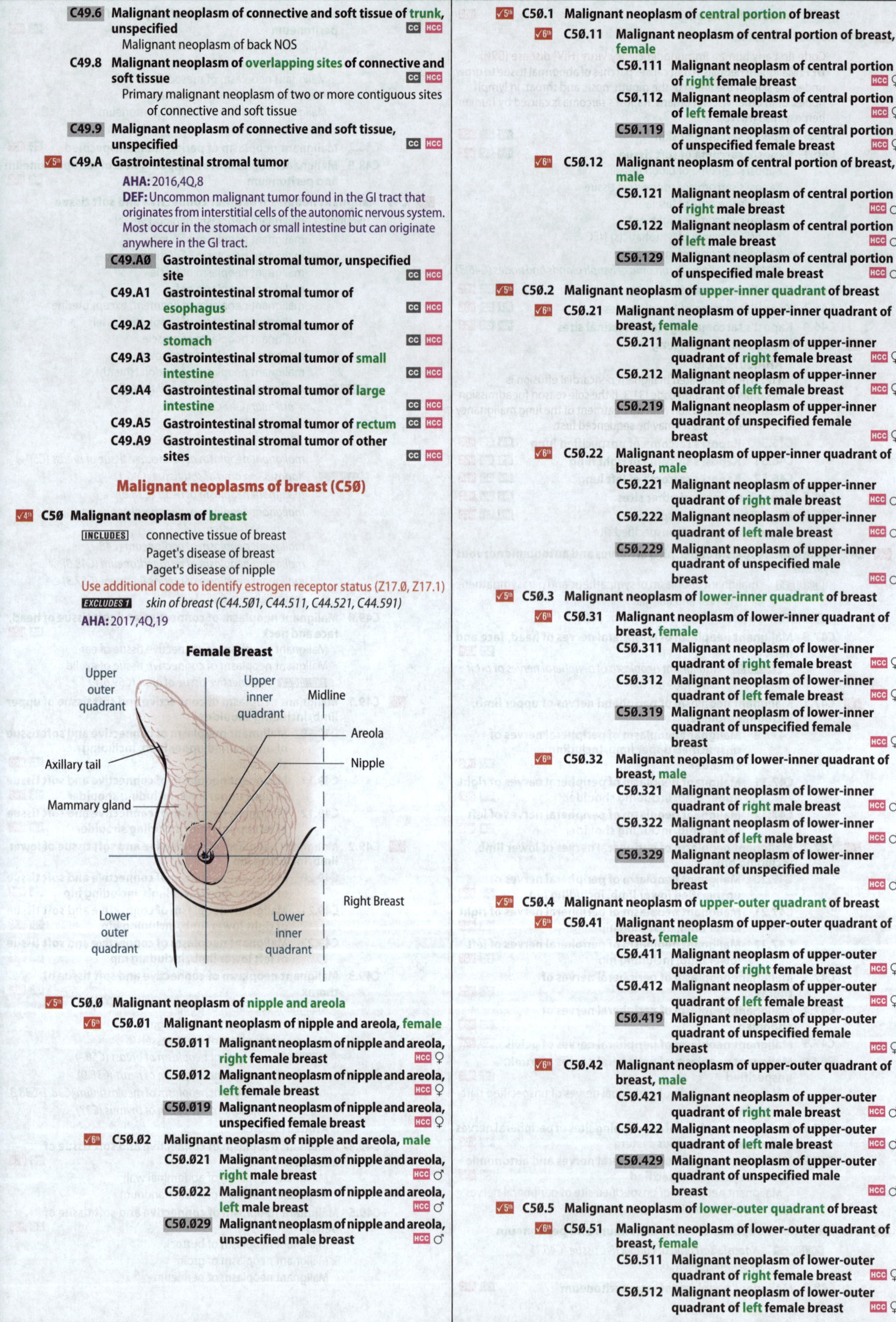

√5th **C5Ø.Ø Malignant neoplasm of nipple and areola**
√6th **C5Ø.Ø1 Malignant neoplasm of nipple and areola, female**
C5Ø.Ø11 Malignant neoplasm of nipple and areola, right female breast HCC ♀
C5Ø.Ø12 Malignant neoplasm of nipple and areola, left female breast HCC ♀
C5Ø.Ø19 Malignant neoplasm of nipple and areola, unspecified female breast HCC ♀
√6th **C5Ø.Ø2 Malignant neoplasm of nipple and areola, male**
C5Ø.Ø21 Malignant neoplasm of nipple and areola, right male breast HCC ♂
C5Ø.Ø22 Malignant neoplasm of nipple and areola, left male breast HCC ♂
C5Ø.Ø29 Malignant neoplasm of nipple and areola, unspecified male breast HCC ♂

√5th **C5Ø.1 Malignant neoplasm of central portion of breast**
√6th **C5Ø.11 Malignant neoplasm of central portion of breast, female**
C5Ø.111 Malignant neoplasm of central portion of right female breast HCC ♀
C5Ø.112 Malignant neoplasm of central portion of left female breast HCC ♀
C5Ø.119 Malignant neoplasm of central portion of unspecified female breast HCC ♀
√6th **C5Ø.12 Malignant neoplasm of central portion of breast, male**
C5Ø.121 Malignant neoplasm of central portion of right male breast HCC ♂
C5Ø.122 Malignant neoplasm of central portion of left male breast HCC ♂
C5Ø.129 Malignant neoplasm of central portion of unspecified male breast HCC ♂

√5th **C5Ø.2 Malignant neoplasm of upper-inner quadrant of breast**
√6th **C5Ø.21 Malignant neoplasm of upper-inner quadrant of breast, female**
C5Ø.211 Malignant neoplasm of upper-inner quadrant of right female breast HCC ♀
C5Ø.212 Malignant neoplasm of upper-inner quadrant of left female breast HCC ♀
C5Ø.219 Malignant neoplasm of upper-inner quadrant of unspecified female breast HCC ♀
√6th **C5Ø.22 Malignant neoplasm of upper-inner quadrant of breast, male**
C5Ø.221 Malignant neoplasm of upper-inner quadrant of right male breast HCC ♂
C5Ø.222 Malignant neoplasm of upper-inner quadrant of left male breast HCC ♂
C5Ø.229 Malignant neoplasm of upper-inner quadrant of unspecified male breast HCC ♂

√5th **C5Ø.3 Malignant neoplasm of lower-inner quadrant of breast**
√6th **C5Ø.31 Malignant neoplasm of lower-inner quadrant of breast, female**
C5Ø.311 Malignant neoplasm of lower-inner quadrant of right female breast HCC ♀
C5Ø.312 Malignant neoplasm of lower-inner quadrant of left female breast HCC ♀
C5Ø.319 Malignant neoplasm of lower-inner quadrant of unspecified female breast HCC ♀
√6th **C5Ø.32 Malignant neoplasm of lower-inner quadrant of breast, male**
C5Ø.321 Malignant neoplasm of lower-inner quadrant of right male breast HCC ♂
C5Ø.322 Malignant neoplasm of lower-inner quadrant of left male breast HCC ♂
C5Ø.329 Malignant neoplasm of lower-inner quadrant of unspecified male breast HCC ♂

√5th **C5Ø.4 Malignant neoplasm of upper-outer quadrant of breast**
√6th **C5Ø.41 Malignant neoplasm of upper-outer quadrant of breast, female**
C5Ø.411 Malignant neoplasm of upper-outer quadrant of right female breast HCC ♀
C5Ø.412 Malignant neoplasm of upper-outer quadrant of left female breast HCC ♀
C5Ø.419 Malignant neoplasm of upper-outer quadrant of unspecified female breast HCC ♀
√6th **C5Ø.42 Malignant neoplasm of upper-outer quadrant of breast, male**
C5Ø.421 Malignant neoplasm of upper-outer quadrant of right male breast HCC ♂
C5Ø.422 Malignant neoplasm of upper-outer quadrant of left male breast HCC ♂
C5Ø.429 Malignant neoplasm of upper-outer quadrant of unspecified male breast HCC ♂

√5th **C5Ø.5 Malignant neoplasm of lower-outer quadrant of breast**
√6th **C5Ø.51 Malignant neoplasm of lower-outer quadrant of breast, female**
C5Ø.511 Malignant neoplasm of lower-outer quadrant of right female breast HCC ♀
C5Ø.512 Malignant neoplasm of lower-outer quadrant of left female breast HCC ♀

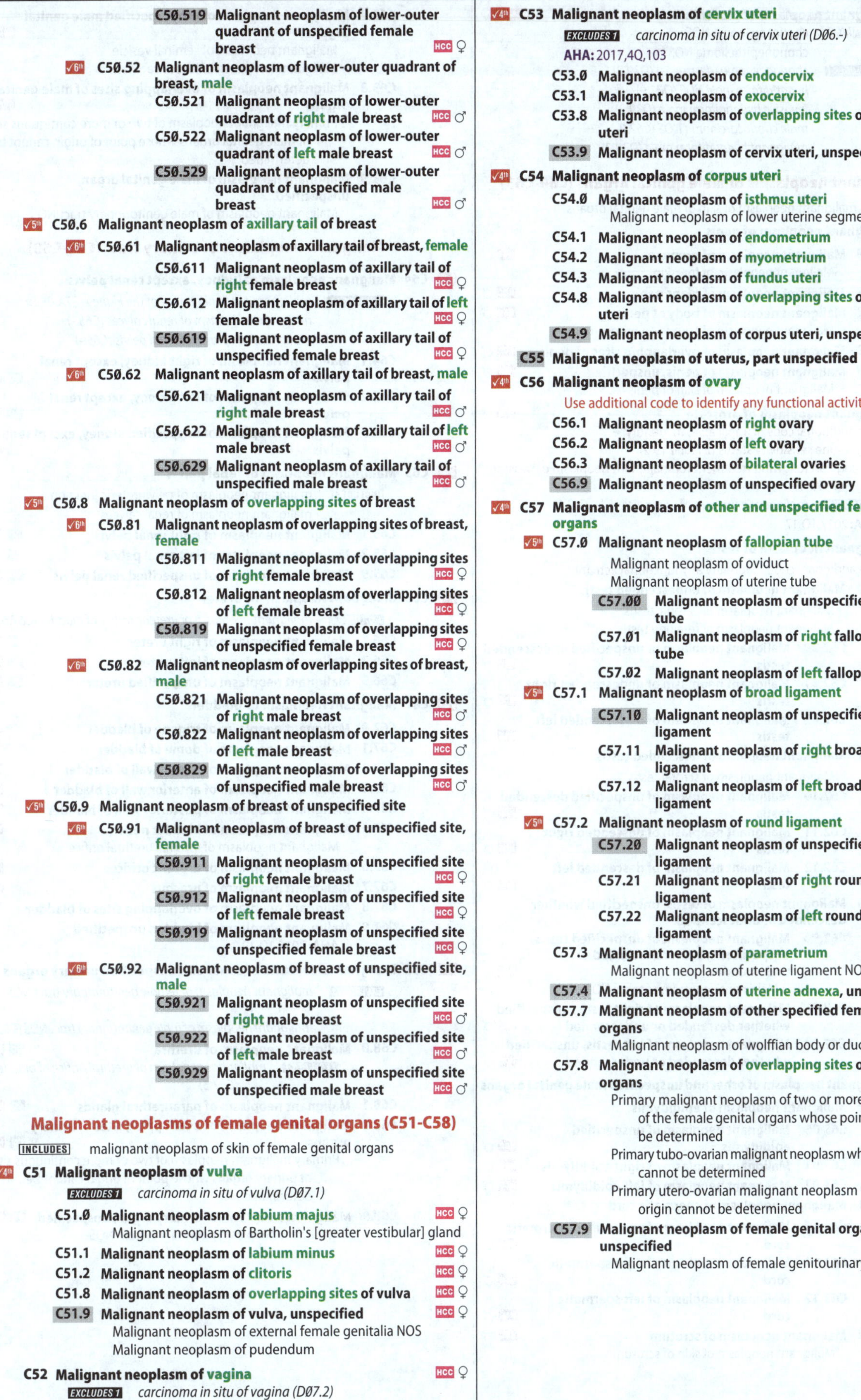

- **C5Ø.519 Malignant neoplasm of lower-outer quadrant of unspecified female breast** HCC ♀
- √6th **C5Ø.52 Malignant neoplasm of lower-outer quadrant of breast, male**
  - **C5Ø.521 Malignant neoplasm of lower-outer quadrant of right male breast** HCC ♂
  - **C5Ø.522 Malignant neoplasm of lower-outer quadrant of left male breast** HCC ♂
  - **C5Ø.529 Malignant neoplasm of lower-outer quadrant of unspecified male breast** HCC ♂
- √5th **C5Ø.6 Malignant neoplasm of axillary tail of breast**
  - √6th **C5Ø.61 Malignant neoplasm of axillary tail of breast, female**
    - **C5Ø.611 Malignant neoplasm of axillary tail of right female breast** HCC ♀
    - **C5Ø.612 Malignant neoplasm of axillary tail of left female breast** HCC ♀
    - **C5Ø.619 Malignant neoplasm of axillary tail of unspecified female breast** HCC ♀
  - √6th **C5Ø.62 Malignant neoplasm of axillary tail of breast, male**
    - **C5Ø.621 Malignant neoplasm of axillary tail of right male breast** HCC ♂
    - **C5Ø.622 Malignant neoplasm of axillary tail of left male breast** HCC ♂
    - **C5Ø.629 Malignant neoplasm of axillary tail of unspecified male breast** HCC ♂
- √5th **C5Ø.8 Malignant neoplasm of overlapping sites of breast**
  - √6th **C5Ø.81 Malignant neoplasm of overlapping sites of breast, female**
    - **C5Ø.811 Malignant neoplasm of overlapping sites of right female breast** HCC ♀
    - **C5Ø.812 Malignant neoplasm of overlapping sites of left female breast** HCC ♀
    - **C5Ø.819 Malignant neoplasm of overlapping sites of unspecified female breast** HCC ♀
  - √6th **C5Ø.82 Malignant neoplasm of overlapping sites of breast, male**
    - **C5Ø.821 Malignant neoplasm of overlapping sites of right male breast** HCC ♂
    - **C5Ø.822 Malignant neoplasm of overlapping sites of left male breast** HCC ♂
    - **C5Ø.829 Malignant neoplasm of overlapping sites of unspecified male breast** HCC ♂
- √5th **C5Ø.9 Malignant neoplasm of breast of unspecified site**
  - √6th **C5Ø.91 Malignant neoplasm of breast of unspecified site, female**
    - **C5Ø.911 Malignant neoplasm of unspecified site of right female breast** HCC ♀
    - **C5Ø.912 Malignant neoplasm of unspecified site of left female breast** HCC ♀
    - **C5Ø.919 Malignant neoplasm of unspecified site of unspecified female breast** HCC ♀
  - √6th **C5Ø.92 Malignant neoplasm of breast of unspecified site, male**
    - **C5Ø.921 Malignant neoplasm of unspecified site of right male breast** HCC ♂
    - **C5Ø.922 Malignant neoplasm of unspecified site of left male breast** HCC ♂
    - **C5Ø.929 Malignant neoplasm of unspecified site of unspecified male breast** HCC ♂

Malignant neoplasms of female genital organs (C51-C58)

INCLUDES malignant neoplasm of skin of female genital organs

√4th **C51 Malignant neoplasm of vulva**

EXCLUDES 1 *carcinoma in situ of vulva (DØ7.1)*

- **C51.Ø Malignant neoplasm of labium majus** HCC ♀
  Malignant neoplasm of Bartholin's [greater vestibular] gland
- **C51.1 Malignant neoplasm of labium minus** HCC ♀
- **C51.2 Malignant neoplasm of clitoris** HCC ♀
- **C51.8 Malignant neoplasm of overlapping sites of vulva** HCC ♀
- **C51.9 Malignant neoplasm of vulva, unspecified** HCC ♀
  Malignant neoplasm of external female genitalia NOS
  Malignant neoplasm of pudendum

C52 Malignant neoplasm of vagina HCC ♀

EXCLUDES 1 *carcinoma in situ of vagina (DØ7.2)*

√4th **C53 Malignant neoplasm of cervix uteri**

EXCLUDES 1 *carcinoma in situ of cervix uteri (DØ6.-)*

AHA: 2017,4Q,103

- **C53.Ø Malignant neoplasm of endocervix** HCC ♀
- **C53.1 Malignant neoplasm of exocervix** HCC ♀
- **C53.8 Malignant neoplasm of overlapping sites of cervix uteri** HCC ♀
- **C53.9 Malignant neoplasm of cervix uteri, unspecified** HCC ♀

√4th **C54 Malignant neoplasm of corpus uteri**

- **C54.Ø Malignant neoplasm of isthmus uteri** HCC ♀
  Malignant neoplasm of lower uterine segment
- **C54.1 Malignant neoplasm of endometrium** HCC ♀
- **C54.2 Malignant neoplasm of myometrium** HCC ♀
- **C54.3 Malignant neoplasm of fundus uteri** HCC ♀
- **C54.8 Malignant neoplasm of overlapping sites of corpus uteri** HCC ♀
- **C54.9 Malignant neoplasm of corpus uteri, unspecified** HCC ♀

C55 Malignant neoplasm of uterus, part unspecified HCC ♀

√4th **C56 Malignant neoplasm of ovary**

Use additional code to identify any functional activity

- **C56.1 Malignant neoplasm of right ovary** CC HCC ♀
- **C56.2 Malignant neoplasm of left ovary** CC HCC ♀
- **C56.3 Malignant neoplasm of bilateral ovaries** CC HCC ♀
- **C56.9 Malignant neoplasm of unspecified ovary** CC HCC ♀

√4th **C57 Malignant neoplasm of other and unspecified female genital organs**

- √5th **C57.Ø Malignant neoplasm of fallopian tube**
  Malignant neoplasm of oviduct
  Malignant neoplasm of uterine tube
  - **C57.ØØ Malignant neoplasm of unspecified fallopian tube** HCC ♀
  - **C57.Ø1 Malignant neoplasm of right fallopian tube** HCC ♀
  - **C57.Ø2 Malignant neoplasm of left fallopian tube** HCC ♀
- √5th **C57.1 Malignant neoplasm of broad ligament**
  - **C57.1Ø Malignant neoplasm of unspecified broad ligament** HCC ♀
  - **C57.11 Malignant neoplasm of right broad ligament** HCC ♀
  - **C57.12 Malignant neoplasm of left broad ligament** HCC ♀
- √5th **C57.2 Malignant neoplasm of round ligament**
  - **C57.2Ø Malignant neoplasm of unspecified round ligament** HCC ♀
  - **C57.21 Malignant neoplasm of right round ligament** HCC ♀
  - **C57.22 Malignant neoplasm of left round ligament** HCC ♀
- **C57.3 Malignant neoplasm of parametrium** HCC ♀
  Malignant neoplasm of uterine ligament NOS
- **C57.4 Malignant neoplasm of uterine adnexa, unspecified** HCC ♀
- **C57.7 Malignant neoplasm of other specified female genital organs** HCC ♀
  Malignant neoplasm of wolffian body or duct
- **C57.8 Malignant neoplasm of overlapping sites of female genital organs** HCC ♀
  Primary malignant neoplasm of two or more contiguous sites of the female genital organs whose point of origin cannot be determined
  Primary tubo-ovarian malignant neoplasm whose point of origin cannot be determined
  Primary utero-ovarian malignant neoplasm whose point of origin cannot be determined
- **C57.9 Malignant neoplasm of female genital organ, unspecified** HCC ♀
  Malignant neoplasm of female genitourinary tract NOS

C58 Malignant neoplasm of placenta HCC M ♀
INCLUDES choriocarcinoma NOS
chorionepithelioma NOS
EXCLUDES 1 *chorioadenoma (destruens) (D39.2)*
hydatidiform mole NOS (O01.9)
invasive hydatidiform mole (D39.2)
male choriocarcinoma NOS (C62.9-)
malignant hydatidiform mole (D39.2)

Malignant neoplasms of male genital organs (C60-C63)

INCLUDES malignant neoplasm of skin of male genital organs

C60 Malignant neoplasm of penis
- **C60.0 Malignant neoplasm of prepuce** HCC ♂
  Malignant neoplasm of foreskin
- **C60.1 Malignant neoplasm of glans penis** HCC ♂
- **C60.2 Malignant neoplasm of body of penis** HCC ♂
  Malignant neoplasm of corpus cavernosum
- **C60.8 Malignant neoplasm of overlapping sites of penis** HCC ♂
- **C60.9 Malignant neoplasm of penis, unspecified** HCC ♂
  Malignant neoplasm of skin of penis NOS

C61 Malignant neoplasm of prostate HCC ♂
▶Use additional code, if applicable, to identify:◀
hormone sensitivity status (Z19.1-Z19.2)
rising PSA following treatment for malignant neoplasm of prostate (R97.21)
EXCLUDES 1 *malignant neoplasm of seminal vesicle (C63.7)*
AHA: 2017,1Q,17

C62 Malignant neoplasm of testis
Use additional code to identify any functional activity
- **C62.0 Malignant neoplasm of undescended testis**
  Malignant neoplasm of ectopic testis
  Malignant neoplasm of retained testis
  - **C62.00 Malignant neoplasm of unspecified undescended testis** HCC ♂
  - **C62.01 Malignant neoplasm of undescended right testis** HCC ♂
  - **C62.02 Malignant neoplasm of undescended left testis** HCC ♂
- **C62.1 Malignant neoplasm of descended testis**
  Malignant neoplasm of scrotal testis
  - **C62.10 Malignant neoplasm of unspecified descended testis** HCC ♂
  - **C62.11 Malignant neoplasm of descended right testis** HCC ♂
  - **C62.12 Malignant neoplasm of descended left testis** HCC ♂
- **C62.9 Malignant neoplasm of testis, unspecified whether descended or undescended**
  - **C62.90 Malignant neoplasm of unspecified testis, unspecified whether descended or undescended** HCC ♂
    Malignant neoplasm of testis NOS
  - **C62.91 Malignant neoplasm of right testis, unspecified whether descended or undescended** HCC ♂
  - **C62.92 Malignant neoplasm of left testis, unspecified whether descended or undescended** HCC ♂

C63 Malignant neoplasm of other and unspecified male genital organs
- **C63.0 Malignant neoplasm of epididymis**
  - **C63.00 Malignant neoplasm of unspecified epididymis** HCC ♂
  - **C63.01 Malignant neoplasm of right epididymis** HCC ♂
  - **C63.02 Malignant neoplasm of left epididymis** HCC ♂
- **C63.1 Malignant neoplasm of spermatic cord**
  - **C63.10 Malignant neoplasm of unspecified spermatic cord** HCC ♂
  - **C63.11 Malignant neoplasm of right spermatic cord** HCC ♂
  - **C63.12 Malignant neoplasm of left spermatic cord** HCC ♂
- **C63.2 Malignant neoplasm of scrotum** HCC ♂
  Malignant neoplasm of skin of scrotum
- **C63.7 Malignant neoplasm of other specified male genital organs** HCC ♂
  Malignant neoplasm of seminal vesicle
  Malignant neoplasm of tunica vaginalis
- **C63.8 Malignant neoplasm of overlapping sites of male genital organs** HCC ♂
  Primary malignant neoplasm of two or more contiguous sites of male genital organs whose point of origin cannot be determined
- **C63.9 Malignant neoplasm of male genital organ, unspecified** HCC ♂
  Malignant neoplasm of male genitourinary tract NOS

Malignant neoplasms of urinary tract (C64-C68)

C64 Malignant neoplasm of kidney, except renal pelvis
EXCLUDES 1 *malignant carcinoid tumor of the kidney (C7A.093)*
malignant neoplasm of renal calyces (C65.-)
malignant neoplasm of renal pelvis (C65.-)
- **C64.1 Malignant neoplasm of right kidney, except renal pelvis** CC HCC
- **C64.2 Malignant neoplasm of left kidney, except renal pelvis** CC HCC
- **C64.9 Malignant neoplasm of unspecified kidney, except renal pelvis** CC HCC

C65 Malignant neoplasm of renal pelvis
INCLUDES malignant neoplasm of pelviureteric junction
malignant neoplasm of renal calyces
- **C65.1 Malignant neoplasm of right renal pelvis** CC HCC
- **C65.2 Malignant neoplasm of left renal pelvis** CC HCC
- **C65.9 Malignant neoplasm of unspecified renal pelvis** CC HCC

C66 Malignant neoplasm of ureter
EXCLUDES 1 *malignant neoplasm of ureteric orifice of bladder (C67.6)*
- **C66.1 Malignant neoplasm of right ureter** CC HCC
- **C66.2 Malignant neoplasm of left ureter** CC HCC
- **C66.9 Malignant neoplasm of unspecified ureter** CC HCC

C67 Malignant neoplasm of bladder
- **C67.0 Malignant neoplasm of trigone of bladder** HCC
- **C67.1 Malignant neoplasm of dome of bladder** HCC
- **C67.2 Malignant neoplasm of lateral wall of bladder** HCC
- **C67.3 Malignant neoplasm of anterior wall of bladder** HCC
- **C67.4 Malignant neoplasm of posterior wall of bladder** HCC
- **C67.5 Malignant neoplasm of bladder neck** HCC
  Malignant neoplasm of internal urethral orifice
- **C67.6 Malignant neoplasm of ureteric orifice** HCC
- **C67.7 Malignant neoplasm of urachus** HCC
- **C67.8 Malignant neoplasm of overlapping sites of bladder** HCC
- **C67.9 Malignant neoplasm of bladder, unspecified** HCC
  AHA: 2016,1Q,19

C68 Malignant neoplasm of other and unspecified urinary organs
EXCLUDES 1 *malignant neoplasm of female genitourinary tract NOS (C57.9)*
malignant neoplasm of male genitourinary tract NOS (C63.9)
- **C68.0 Malignant neoplasm of urethra** CC HCC
  EXCLUDES 1 *malignant neoplasm of urethral orifice of bladder (C67.5)*
- **C68.1 Malignant neoplasm of paraurethral glands** CC HCC
- **C68.8 Malignant neoplasm of overlapping sites of urinary organs** CC HCC
  Primary malignant neoplasm of two or more contiguous sites of urinary organs whose point of origin cannot be determined
- **C68.9 Malignant neoplasm of urinary organ, unspecified** CC HCC
  Malignant neoplasm of urinary system NOS

Malignant neoplasms of eye, brain and other parts of central nervous system (C69-C72)

C69 Malignant neoplasm of eye and adnexa

EXCLUDES 1 *malignant neoplasm of connective tissue of eyelid (C49.Ø)*
malignant neoplasm of eyelid (skin) (C43.1-, C44.1-)
malignant neoplasm of optic nerve (C72.3-)

C69.Ø Malignant neoplasm of conjunctiva
- **C69.ØØ Malignant neoplasm of unspecified conjunctiva** HCC
- **C69.Ø1 Malignant neoplasm of right conjunctiva** HCC
- **C69.Ø2 Malignant neoplasm of left conjunctiva** HCC

C69.1 Malignant neoplasm of cornea
- **C69.1Ø Malignant neoplasm of unspecified cornea** HCC
- **C69.11 Malignant neoplasm of right cornea** HCC
- **C69.12 Malignant neoplasm of left cornea** HCC

C69.2 Malignant neoplasm of retina

EXCLUDES 1 *dark area on retina (D49.81)*
neoplasm of unspecified behavior of retina and choroid (D49.81)
retinal freckle (D49.81)

- **C69.2Ø Malignant neoplasm of unspecified retina** HCC
- **C69.21 Malignant neoplasm of right retina** HCC
- **C69.22 Malignant neoplasm of left retina** HCC

C69.3 Malignant neoplasm of choroid
- **C69.3Ø Malignant neoplasm of unspecified choroid** HCC
- **C69.31 Malignant neoplasm of right choroid** HCC
- **C69.32 Malignant neoplasm of left choroid** HCC

C69.4 Malignant neoplasm of ciliary body
- **C69.4Ø Malignant neoplasm of unspecified ciliary body** HCC
- **C69.41 Malignant neoplasm of right ciliary body** HCC
- **C69.42 Malignant neoplasm of left ciliary body** HCC

C69.5 Malignant neoplasm of lacrimal gland and duct

Malignant neoplasm of lacrimal sac
Malignant neoplasm of nasolacrimal duct

- **C69.5Ø Malignant neoplasm of unspecified lacrimal gland and duct** HCC
- **C69.51 Malignant neoplasm of right lacrimal gland and duct** HCC
- **C69.52 Malignant neoplasm of left lacrimal gland and duct** HCC

C69.6 Malignant neoplasm of orbit

Malignant neoplasm of connective tissue of orbit
Malignant neoplasm of extraocular muscle
Malignant neoplasm of peripheral nerves of orbit
Malignant neoplasm of retrobulbar tissue
Malignant neoplasm of retro-ocular tissue

EXCLUDES 1 *malignant neoplasm of orbital bone (C41.Ø)*

- **C69.6Ø Malignant neoplasm of unspecified orbit** HCC
- **C69.61 Malignant neoplasm of right orbit** HCC
- **C69.62 Malignant neoplasm of left orbit** HCC

C69.8 Malignant neoplasm of overlapping sites of eye and adnexa
- **C69.8Ø Malignant neoplasm of overlapping sites of unspecified eye and adnexa** HCC
- **C69.81 Malignant neoplasm of overlapping sites of right eye and adnexa** HCC
- **C69.82 Malignant neoplasm of overlapping sites of left eye and adnexa** HCC

C69.9 Malignant neoplasm of unspecified site of eye

Malignant neoplasm of eyeball

- **C69.9Ø Malignant neoplasm of unspecified site of unspecified eye** HCC
- **C69.91 Malignant neoplasm of unspecified site of right eye** HCC
- **C69.92 Malignant neoplasm of unspecified site of left eye** HCC

C7Ø Malignant neoplasm of meninges
- **C7Ø.Ø Malignant neoplasm of cerebral meninges** CC HCC
- **C7Ø.1 Malignant neoplasm of spinal meninges** CC HCC
- **C7Ø.9 Malignant neoplasm of meninges, unspecified** CC HCC

C71 Malignant neoplasm of brain

EXCLUDES 1 *malignant neoplasm of cranial nerves (C72.2-C72.5)*
retrobulbar malignant neoplasm (C69.6-)

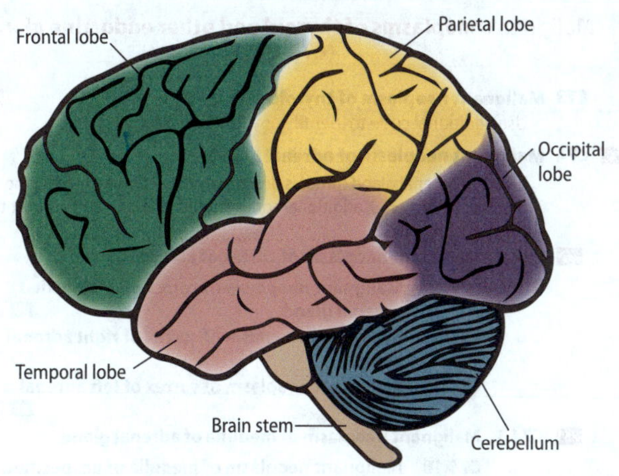

- **C71.Ø Malignant neoplasm of cerebrum, except lobes and ventricles** CC HCC
  Malignant neoplasm of supratentorial NOS
- **C71.1 Malignant neoplasm of frontal lobe** CC HCC
- **C71.2 Malignant neoplasm of temporal lobe** CC HCC
- **C71.3 Malignant neoplasm of parietal lobe** CC HCC
- **C71.4 Malignant neoplasm of occipital lobe** CC HCC
- **C71.5 Malignant neoplasm of cerebral ventricle** CC HCC
  EXCLUDES 1 *malignant neoplasm of fourth cerebral ventricle (C71.7)*
- **C71.6 Malignant neoplasm of cerebellum** CC HCC
- **C71.7 Malignant neoplasm of brain stem** CC HCC
  Malignant neoplasm of fourth cerebral ventricle
  Infratentorial malignant neoplasm NOS
- **C71.8 Malignant neoplasm of overlapping sites of brain** CC HCC
- **C71.9 Malignant neoplasm of brain, unspecified** CC HCC
  AHA: 2014,3Q,3

C72 Malignant neoplasm of spinal cord, cranial nerves and other parts of central nervous system

EXCLUDES 1 *malignant neoplasm of meninges (C7Ø.-)*
malignant neoplasm of peripheral nerves and autonomic nervous system (C47.-)

- **C72.Ø Malignant neoplasm of spinal cord** CC HCC
- **C72.1 Malignant neoplasm of cauda equina** CC HCC

C72.2 Malignant neoplasm of olfactory nerve

Malignant neoplasm of olfactory bulb

- **C72.2Ø Malignant neoplasm of unspecified olfactory nerve** CC HCC
- **C72.21 Malignant neoplasm of right olfactory nerve** CC HCC
- **C72.22 Malignant neoplasm of left olfactory nerve** CC HCC

C72.3 Malignant neoplasm of optic nerve
- **C72.3Ø Malignant neoplasm of unspecified optic nerve** CC HCC
- **C72.31 Malignant neoplasm of right optic nerve** CC HCC
- **C72.32 Malignant neoplasm of left optic nerve** CC HCC

C72.4 Malignant neoplasm of acoustic nerve
- **C72.4Ø Malignant neoplasm of unspecified acoustic nerve** CC HCC
- **C72.41 Malignant neoplasm of right acoustic nerve** CC HCC
- **C72.42 Malignant neoplasm of left acoustic nerve** CC HCC

C72.5 Malignant neoplasm of other and unspecified cranial nerves
- **C72.5Ø Malignant neoplasm of unspecified cranial nerve** CC HCC
  Malignant neoplasm of cranial nerve NOS
- **C72.59 Malignant neoplasm of other cranial nerves** CC HCC

C72.9 Malignant neoplasm of central nervous system, unspecified CC HCC
Malignant neoplasm of unspecified site of central nervous system
Malignant neoplasm of nervous system NOS

Malignant neoplasms of thyroid and other endocrine glands (C73-C75)

C73 Malignant neoplasm of thyroid gland HCC
Use additional code to identify any functional activity

C74 Malignant neoplasm of adrenal gland
TIP: If an adrenal gland tumor is described as functioning (producing too much of a hormone), additional codes should be assigned to report the functional activity.

C74.Ø Malignant neoplasm of cortex of adrenal gland
C74.ØØ Malignant neoplasm of cortex of unspecified adrenal gland CC HCC
C74.Ø1 Malignant neoplasm of cortex of right adrenal gland CC HCC
C74.Ø2 Malignant neoplasm of cortex of left adrenal gland CC HCC

C74.1 Malignant neoplasm of medulla of adrenal gland
C74.1Ø Malignant neoplasm of medulla of unspecified adrenal gland CC HCC
C74.11 Malignant neoplasm of medulla of right adrenal gland CC HCC
C74.12 Malignant neoplasm of medulla of left adrenal gland CC HCC

C74.9 Malignant neoplasm of unspecified part of adrenal gland
C74.9Ø Malignant neoplasm of unspecified part of unspecified adrenal gland CC HCC
C74.91 Malignant neoplasm of unspecified part of right adrenal gland CC HCC
C74.92 Malignant neoplasm of unspecified part of left adrenal gland CC HCC

C75 Malignant neoplasm of other endocrine glands and related structures
EXCLUDES 1 *malignant carcinoid tumors (C7A.Ø-)*
malignant neoplasm of adrenal gland (C74.-)
malignant neoplasm of endocrine pancreas (C25.4)
malignant neoplasm of islets of Langerhans (C25.4)
malignant neoplasm of ovary (C56.-)
malignant neoplasm of testis (C62.-)
malignant neoplasm of thymus (C37)
malignant neoplasm of thyroid gland (C73)
malignant neuroendocrine tumors (C7A.-)

C75.Ø Malignant neoplasm of parathyroid gland CC HCC
C75.1 Malignant neoplasm of pituitary gland CC HCC
C75.2 Malignant neoplasm of craniopharyngeal duct CC HCC
C75.3 Malignant neoplasm of pineal gland CC HCC
C75.4 Malignant neoplasm of carotid body CC HCC
C75.5 Malignant neoplasm of aortic body and other paraganglia CC HCC
C75.8 Malignant neoplasm with pluriglandular involvement, unspecified CC HCC
C75.9 Malignant neoplasm of endocrine gland, unspecified CC HCC

Malignant neuroendocrine tumors (C7A)

C7A Malignant neuroendocrine tumors
Code also any associated multiple endocrine neoplasia [MEN] syndromes (E31.2-)
Use additional code to identify any associated endocrine syndrome, such as:
carcinoid syndrome (E34.Ø)
EXCLUDES 2 *malignant pancreatic islet cell tumors (C25.4)*
Merkel cell carcinoma (C4A.-)
AHA: 2019,3Q,7
DEF: Tumors comprised of cells that are capable of producing hormonal syndromes in which the normal hormonal balance required to support body system function is adversely affected.

C7A.Ø Malignant carcinoid tumors
AHA: 2019,3Q,7
DEF: Specific type of slow-growing neuroendocrine tumors. Carcinoid tumors occur most commonly in the hormone producing cells of the gastrointestinal tracts and can also occur in the pancreas, testes, ovaries, or lungs.

C7A.ØØ Malignant carcinoid tumor of unspecified site CC HCC

C7A.Ø1 Malignant carcinoid tumors of the small intestine
C7A.Ø1Ø Malignant carcinoid tumor of the duodenum CC HCC
C7A.Ø11 Malignant carcinoid tumor of the jejunum CC HCC
C7A.Ø12 Malignant carcinoid tumor of the ileum CC HCC
C7A.Ø19 Malignant carcinoid tumor of the small intestine, unspecified portion CC HCC

C7A.Ø2 Malignant carcinoid tumors of the appendix, large intestine, and rectum
C7A.Ø2Ø Malignant carcinoid tumor of the appendix CC HCC
C7A.Ø21 Malignant carcinoid tumor of the cecum CC HCC
C7A.Ø22 Malignant carcinoid tumor of the ascending colon CC HCC
C7A.Ø23 Malignant carcinoid tumor of the transverse colon CC HCC
C7A.Ø24 Malignant carcinoid tumor of the descending colon CC HCC
C7A.Ø25 Malignant carcinoid tumor of the sigmoid colon CC HCC
C7A.Ø26 Malignant carcinoid tumor of the rectum CC HCC
C7A.Ø29 Malignant carcinoid tumor of the large intestine, unspecified portion CC HCC
Malignant carcinoid tumor of the colon NOS

C7A.Ø9 Malignant carcinoid tumors of other sites
C7A.Ø9Ø Malignant carcinoid tumor of the bronchus and lung CC HCC
AHA: 2019,1Q,16
TIP: When associated malignant pericardial effusion is documented, assign code I31.3. If the sole reason for admission is to treat the effusion with no treatment of the lung malignancy rendered, code I31.3 may be sequenced first.
C7A.Ø91 Malignant carcinoid tumor of the thymus CC HCC
C7A.Ø92 Malignant carcinoid tumor of the stomach CC HCC
C7A.Ø93 Malignant carcinoid tumor of the kidney CC HCC
C7A.Ø94 Malignant carcinoid tumor of the foregut, unspecified CC HCC
C7A.Ø95 Malignant carcinoid tumor of the midgut, unspecified CC HCC
C7A.Ø96 Malignant carcinoid tumor of the hindgut, unspecified CC HCC
C7A.Ø98 Malignant carcinoid tumors of other sites CC HCC

C7A.1 **Malignant poorly differentiated neuroendocrine tumors** CC HCC
Malignant poorly differentiated neuroendocrine tumor NOS
Malignant poorly differentiated neuroendocrine carcinoma, any site
High grade neuroendocrine carcinoma, any site

C7A.8 **Other malignant neuroendocrine tumors** CC HCC
AHA: 2019,3Q,7

Secondary neuroendocrine tumors (C7B)

√4th **C7B Secondary neuroendocrine tumors**
Use additional code to identify any functional activity

√5th C7B.Ø **Secondary carcinoid tumors**
AHA: 2019,3Q,7
DEF: Specific type of slow-growing neuroendocrine tumors. Carcinoid tumors occur most commonly in the hormone producing cells of the gastrointestinal tracts and can also occur in the pancreas, testes, ovaries, or lungs.

C7B.ØØ **Secondary carcinoid tumors, unspecified site** HCC
C7B.Ø1 **Secondary carcinoid tumors of distant lymph nodes** CC HCC
C7B.Ø2 **Secondary carcinoid tumors of liver** CC HCC
C7B.Ø3 **Secondary carcinoid tumors of bone** CC HCC
C7B.Ø4 **Secondary carcinoid tumors of peritoneum** CC HCC
Mesentary metastasis of carcinoid tumor
C7B.Ø9 **Secondary carcinoid tumors of other sites** CC HCC

C7B.1 **Secondary Merkel cell carcinoma** HCC
Merkel cell carcinoma nodal presentation
Merkel cell carcinoma visceral metastatic presentation

C7B.8 **Other secondary neuroendocrine tumors** CC HCC
AHA: 2019,3Q,7

Malignant neoplasms of ill-defined, other secondary and unspecified sites (C76-C8Ø)

√4th **C76 Malignant neoplasm of other and ill-defined sites**
EXCLUDES 1 *malignant neoplasm of female genitourinary tract NOS (C57.9)*
malignant neoplasm of male genitourinary tract NOS (C63.9)
malignant neoplasm of lymphoid, hematopoietic and related tissue (C81-C96)
malignant neoplasm of skin (C44.-)
malignant neoplasm of unspecified site NOS (C8Ø.1)

C76.Ø **Malignant neoplasm of head, face and neck** HCC
Malignant neoplasm of cheek NOS
Malignant neoplasm of nose NOS

C76.1 **Malignant neoplasm of thorax** HCC
Intrathoracic malignant neoplasm NOS
Malignant neoplasm of axilla NOS
Thoracic malignant neoplasm NOS

C76.2 **Malignant neoplasm of abdomen** HCC

C76.3 **Malignant neoplasm of pelvis** HCC
Malignant neoplasm of groin NOS
Malignant neoplasm of sites overlapping systems within the pelvis
Rectovaginal (septum) malignant neoplasm
Rectovesical (septum) malignant neoplasm

√5th C76.4 **Malignant neoplasm of upper limb**
C76.4Ø **Malignant neoplasm of unspecified upper limb** HCC
C76.41 **Malignant neoplasm of right upper limb** HCC
C76.42 **Malignant neoplasm of left upper limb** HCC

√5th C76.5 **Malignant neoplasm of lower limb**
C76.5Ø **Malignant neoplasm of unspecified lower limb** HCC
C76.51 **Malignant neoplasm of right lower limb** HCC
C76.52 **Malignant neoplasm of left lower limb** HCC

C76.8 **Malignant neoplasm of other specified ill-defined sites** HCC
Malignant neoplasm of overlapping ill-defined sites

√4th **C77 Secondary and unspecified malignant neoplasm of lymph nodes**
EXCLUDES 1 *malignant neoplasm of lymph nodes, specified as primary (C81-C86, C88, C96.-)*
mesentary metastasis of carcinoid tumor (C7B.Ø4)
secondary carcinoid tumors of distant lymph nodes (C7B.Ø1)

C77.Ø **Secondary and unspecified malignant neoplasm of lymph nodes of head, face and neck** CC HCC
Secondary and unspecified malignant neoplasm of supraclavicular lymph nodes

C77.1 **Secondary and unspecified malignant neoplasm of intrathoracic lymph nodes** CC HCC

C77.2 **Secondary and unspecified malignant neoplasm of intra-abdominal lymph nodes** CC HCC

C77.3 **Secondary and unspecified malignant neoplasm of axilla and upper limb lymph nodes** CC HCC
Secondary and unspecified malignant neoplasm of pectoral lymph nodes

C77.4 **Secondary and unspecified malignant neoplasm of inguinal and lower limb lymph nodes** CC HCC

C77.5 **Secondary and unspecified malignant neoplasm of intrapelvic lymph nodes** CC HCC

C77.8 **Secondary and unspecified malignant neoplasm of lymph nodes of multiple regions** CC HCC

C77.9 **Secondary and unspecified malignant neoplasm of lymph node, unspecified** CC HCC

√4th **C78 Secondary malignant neoplasm of respiratory and digestive organs**
EXCLUDES 1 *secondary carcinoid tumors of liver (C7B.Ø2)*
secondary carcinoid tumors of peritoneum (C7B.Ø4)
EXCLUDES 2 *lymph node metastases (C77.Ø)*

√5th C78.Ø **Secondary malignant neoplasm of lung**
AHA: 2019,1Q,16
C78.ØØ **Secondary malignant neoplasm of unspecified lung** CC HCC
C78.Ø1 **Secondary malignant neoplasm of right lung** CC HCC
C78.Ø2 **Secondary malignant neoplasm of left lung** CC HCC

C78.1 **Secondary malignant neoplasm of mediastinum** CC HCC
C78.2 **Secondary malignant neoplasm of pleura** CC HCC

√5th C78.3 **Secondary malignant neoplasm of other and unspecified respiratory organs**
C78.3Ø **Secondary malignant neoplasm of unspecified respiratory organ** CC HCC
C78.39 **Secondary malignant neoplasm of other respiratory organs** CC HCC

C78.4 **Secondary malignant neoplasm of small intestine** CC HCC
C78.5 **Secondary malignant neoplasm of large intestine and rectum** CC HCC
C78.6 **Secondary malignant neoplasm of retroperitoneum and peritoneum** CC HCC
AHA: 2017,2Q,12
C78.7 **Secondary malignant neoplasm of liver and intrahepatic bile duct** CC HCC

√5th C78.8 **Secondary malignant neoplasm of other and unspecified digestive organs**
C78.8Ø **Secondary malignant neoplasm of unspecified digestive organ** CC HCC
C78.89 **Secondary malignant neoplasm of other digestive organs** CC HCC
Code also exocrine pancreatic insufficiency (K86.81)

√4th **C79 Secondary malignant neoplasm of other and unspecified sites**
EXCLUDES 1 *secondary carcinoid tumors (C7B.-)*
secondary neuroendocrine tumors (C7B.-)

√5th C79.Ø **Secondary malignant neoplasm of kidney and renal pelvis**
C79.ØØ **Secondary malignant neoplasm of unspecified kidney and renal pelvis** CC HCC
C79.Ø1 **Secondary malignant neoplasm of right kidney and renal pelvis** CC HCC
C79.Ø2 **Secondary malignant neoplasm of left kidney and renal pelvis** CC HCC

√5th C79.1 **Secondary malignant neoplasm of bladder and other and unspecified urinary organs**
C79.1Ø **Secondary malignant neoplasm of unspecified urinary organs** CC HCC

C79.11 Secondary malignant neoplasm of bladder CC HCC

EXCLUDES 2 *lymph node metastases (C77.0)*

C79.19 Secondary malignant neoplasm of other urinary organs CC HCC

C79.2 Secondary malignant neoplasm of skin CC HCC

EXCLUDES 1 *secondary Merkel cell carcinoma (C7B.1)*

C79.3 Secondary malignant neoplasm of brain and cerebral meninges

C79.31 Secondary malignant neoplasm of brain CC HCC

C79.32 Secondary malignant neoplasm of cerebral meninges CC HCC

AHA: 2020,1Q,13

C79.4 Secondary malignant neoplasm of other and unspecified parts of nervous system

C79.40 Secondary malignant neoplasm of unspecified part of nervous system CC HCC

C79.49 Secondary malignant neoplasm of other parts of nervous system CC HCC

C79.5 Secondary malignant neoplasm of bone and bone marrow

EXCLUDES 1 *secondary carcinoid tumors of bone (C7B.03)*

C79.51 Secondary malignant neoplasm of bone CC HCC

TIP: Do not assign in addition to a code from subcategory C90.0 when multiple myeloma is described as metastatic to the bone; bone involvement is integral to multiple myeloma.

C79.52 Secondary malignant neoplasm of bone marrow CC HCC

C79.6 Secondary malignant neoplasm of ovary

C79.60 Secondary malignant neoplasm of unspecified ovary CC HCC ♀

C79.61 Secondary malignant neoplasm of right ovary CC HCC ♀

C79.62 Secondary malignant neoplasm of left ovary CC HCC ♀

C79.63 Secondary malignant neoplasm of bilateral ovaries CC HCC ♀

C79.7 Secondary malignant neoplasm of adrenal gland

C79.70 Secondary malignant neoplasm of unspecified adrenal gland CC HCC

C79.71 Secondary malignant neoplasm of right adrenal gland CC HCC

C79.72 Secondary malignant neoplasm of left adrenal gland CC HCC

C79.8 Secondary malignant neoplasm of other specified sites

C79.81 Secondary malignant neoplasm of breast CC HCC

C79.82 Secondary malignant neoplasm of genital organs CC HCC

C79.89 Secondary malignant neoplasm of other specified sites CC HCC

AHA: 2017,2Q,11

C79.9 Secondary malignant neoplasm of unspecified site CC HCC

Metastatic cancer NOS

Metastatic disease NOS

EXCLUDES 1 *carcinomatosis NOS (C80.0)*
generalized cancer NOS (C80.0)
malignant (primary) neoplasm of unspecified site (C80.1)

C80 Malignant neoplasm without specification of site

EXCLUDES 1 *malignant carcinoid tumor of unspecified site (C7A.00)*
malignant neoplasm of specified multiple sites - code to each site

C80.0 Disseminated malignant neoplasm, unspecified CC HCC

Carcinomatosis NOS

Generalized cancer, unspecified site (primary) (secondary)

Generalized malignancy, unspecified site (primary) (secondary)

C80.1 Malignant (primary) neoplasm, unspecified HCC

Cancer NOS

Cancer unspecified site (primary)

Carcinoma unspecified site (primary)

Malignancy unspecified site (primary)

EXCLUDES 1 *secondary malignant neoplasm of unspecified site (C79.9)*

C80.2 Malignant neoplasm associated with transplanted organ CC UPD HCC

Code first complication of transplanted organ (T86.-)

Use additional code to identify the specific malignancy

Malignant neoplasms of lymphoid, hematopoietic and related tissue (C81-C96)

EXCLUDES 2 *Kaposi's sarcoma of lymph nodes (C46.3)*
secondary and unspecified neoplasm of lymph nodes (C77.-)
secondary neoplasm of bone marrow (C79.52)
secondary neoplasm of spleen (C78.89)

C81 Hodgkin lymphoma

EXCLUDES 1 *personal history of Hodgkin lymphoma (Z85.71)*

DEF: Malignant disorder of lymphoid cells characterized by the presence of progressively swollen lymph nodes and spleen that may also involve the liver. A diagnosis of Hodgkin's lymphoma can be confirmed by the presence of Reed-Sternberg cells. ***Synonym(s):*** *Hodgkin disease.*

C81.0 Nodular lymphocyte predominant Hodgkin lymphoma

C81.00 Nodular lymphocyte predominant Hodgkin lymphoma, unspecified site CC HCC

C81.01 Nodular lymphocyte predominant Hodgkin lymphoma, lymph nodes of head, face, and neck CC HCC

C81.02 Nodular lymphocyte predominant Hodgkin lymphoma, intrathoracic lymph nodes CC HCC

C81.03 Nodular lymphocyte predominant Hodgkin lymphoma, intra-abdominal lymph nodes CC HCC

C81.04 Nodular lymphocyte predominant Hodgkin lymphoma, lymph nodes of axilla and upper limb CC HCC

C81.05 Nodular lymphocyte predominant Hodgkin lymphoma, lymph nodes of inguinal region and lower limb CC HCC

C81.06 Nodular lymphocyte predominant Hodgkin lymphoma, intrapelvic lymph nodes CC HCC

C81.07 Nodular lymphocyte predominant Hodgkin lymphoma, spleen CC HCC

C81.08 Nodular lymphocyte predominant Hodgkin lymphoma, lymph nodes of multiple sites CC HCC

C81.09 Nodular lymphocyte predominant Hodgkin lymphoma, extranodal and solid organ sites CC HCC

C81.1 Nodular sclerosis Hodgkin lymphoma

Nodular sclerosis classical Hodgkin lymphoma

C81.10 Nodular sclerosis Hodgkin lymphoma, unspecified site CC HCC

C81.11 Nodular sclerosis Hodgkin lymphoma, lymph nodes of head, face, and neck CC HCC

C81.12 Nodular sclerosis Hodgkin lymphoma, intrathoracic lymph nodes CC HCC

C81.13 Nodular sclerosis Hodgkin lymphoma, intra-abdominal lymph nodes CC HCC

C81.14 Nodular sclerosis Hodgkin lymphoma, lymph nodes of axilla and upper limb CC HCC

C81.15 Nodular sclerosis Hodgkin lymphoma, lymph nodes of inguinal region and lower limb CC HCC

C81.16 Nodular sclerosis Hodgkin lymphoma, intrapelvic lymph nodes CC HCC

C81.17 Nodular sclerosis Hodgkin lymphoma, spleen CC HCC

C81.18 Nodular sclerosis Hodgkin lymphoma, lymph nodes of multiple sites CC HCC

C81.19 Nodular sclerosis Hodgkin lymphoma, extranodal and solid organ sites CC HCC

C81.2 Mixed cellularity Hodgkin lymphoma

Mixed cellularity classical Hodgkin lymphoma

C81.20 Mixed cellularity Hodgkin lymphoma, unspecified site CC HCC

C81.21 Mixed cellularity Hodgkin lymphoma, lymph nodes of head, face, and neck CC HCC

C81.22 Mixed cellularity Hodgkin lymphoma, intrathoracic lymph nodes CC HCC

C81.23 Mixed cellularity Hodgkin lymphoma, intra-abdominal lymph nodes CC HCC

C81.24 Mixed cellularity Hodgkin lymphoma, lymph nodes of axilla and upper limb CC HCC

C81.25 Mixed cellularity Hodgkin lymphoma, lymph nodes of inguinal region and lower limb CC HCC

C81.26 Mixed cellularity Hodgkin lymphoma, intrapelvic lymph nodes CC HCC

C81.27 Mixed cellularity Hodgkin lymphoma, spleen CC HCC

C81.28 Mixed cellularity Hodgkin lymphoma, lymph nodes of multiple sites CC HCC

C81.29 Mixed cellularity Hodgkin lymphoma, extranodal and solid organ sites CC HCC

✓5th C81.3 Lymphocyte depleted Hodgkin lymphoma

Lymphocyte depleted classical Hodgkin lymphoma

C81.30 Lymphocyte depleted Hodgkin lymphoma, unspecified site CC HCC

C81.31 Lymphocyte depleted Hodgkin lymphoma, lymph nodes of head, face, and neck CC HCC

C81.32 Lymphocyte depleted Hodgkin lymphoma, intrathoracic lymph nodes CC HCC

C81.33 Lymphocyte depleted Hodgkin lymphoma, intra-abdominal lymph nodes CC HCC

C81.34 Lymphocyte depleted Hodgkin lymphoma, lymph nodes of axilla and upper limb CC HCC

C81.35 Lymphocyte depleted Hodgkin lymphoma, lymph nodes of inguinal region and lower limb CC HCC

C81.36 Lymphocyte depleted Hodgkin lymphoma, intrapelvic lymph nodes CC HCC

C81.37 Lymphocyte depleted Hodgkin lymphoma, spleen CC HCC

C81.38 Lymphocyte depleted Hodgkin lymphoma, lymph nodes of multiple sites CC HCC

C81.39 Lymphocyte depleted Hodgkin lymphoma, extranodal and solid organ sites CC HCC

✓5th C81.4 Lymphocyte-rich Hodgkin lymphoma

Lymphocyte-rich classical Hodgkin lymphoma

EXCLUDES 1 *nodular lymphocyte predominant Hodgkin lymphoma (C81.0-)*

C81.40 Lymphocyte-rich Hodgkin lymphoma, unspecified site CC HCC

C81.41 Lymphocyte-rich Hodgkin lymphoma, lymph nodes of head, face, and neck CC HCC

C81.42 Lymphocyte-rich Hodgkin lymphoma, intrathoracic lymph nodes CC HCC

C81.43 Lymphocyte-rich Hodgkin lymphoma, intra-abdominal lymph nodes CC HCC

C81.44 Lymphocyte-rich Hodgkin lymphoma, lymph nodes of axilla and upper limb CC HCC

C81.45 Lymphocyte-rich Hodgkin lymphoma, lymph nodes of inguinal region and lower limb CC HCC

C81.46 Lymphocyte-rich Hodgkin lymphoma, intrapelvic lymph nodes CC HCC

C81.47 Lymphocyte-rich Hodgkin lymphoma, spleen CC HCC

C81.48 Lymphocyte-rich Hodgkin lymphoma, lymph nodes of multiple sites CC HCC

C81.49 Lymphocyte-rich Hodgkin lymphoma, extranodal and solid organ sites CC HCC

✓5th C81.7 Other Hodgkin lymphoma

Classical Hodgkin lymphoma NOS

Other classical Hodgkin lymphoma

C81.70 Other Hodgkin lymphoma, unspecified site CC HCC

C81.71 Other Hodgkin lymphoma, lymph nodes of head, face, and neck CC HCC

C81.72 Other Hodgkin lymphoma, intrathoracic lymph nodes CC HCC

C81.73 Other Hodgkin lymphoma, intra-abdominal lymph nodes CC HCC

C81.74 Other Hodgkin lymphoma, lymph nodes of axilla and upper limb CC HCC

C81.75 Other Hodgkin lymphoma, lymph nodes of inguinal region and lower limb CC HCC

C81.76 Other Hodgkin lymphoma, intrapelvic lymph nodes CC HCC

C81.77 Other Hodgkin lymphoma, spleen CC HCC

C81.78 Other Hodgkin lymphoma, lymph nodes of multiple sites CC HCC

C81.79 Other Hodgkin lymphoma, extranodal and solid organ sites CC HCC

✓5th C81.9 Hodgkin lymphoma, unspecified

C81.90 Hodgkin lymphoma, unspecified, unspecified site CC HCC

C81.91 Hodgkin lymphoma, unspecified, lymph nodes of head, face, and neck CC HCC

C81.92 Hodgkin lymphoma, unspecified, intrathoracic lymph nodes CC HCC

C81.93 Hodgkin lymphoma, unspecified, intra-abdominal lymph nodes CC HCC

C81.94 Hodgkin lymphoma, unspecified, lymph nodes of axilla and upper limb CC HCC

C81.95 Hodgkin lymphoma, unspecified, lymph nodes of inguinal region and lower limb CC HCC

C81.96 Hodgkin lymphoma, unspecified, intrapelvic lymph nodes CC HCC

C81.97 Hodgkin lymphoma, unspecified, spleen CC HCC

C81.98 Hodgkin lymphoma, unspecified, lymph nodes of multiple sites CC HCC

C81.99 Hodgkin lymphoma, unspecified, extranodal and solid organ sites CC HCC

✓4th C82 Follicular lymphoma

INCLUDES follicular lymphoma with or without diffuse areas

EXCLUDES 1 *mature T/NK-cell lymphomas (C84.-)*

personal history of non-Hodgkin lymphoma (Z85.72)

DEF: Most common subgroup of non-Hodgkin lymphomas (NHL), accounting for 20 to 30 percent of all NHLs. NHL is a B-cell lymphoma that is slow growing and characterized by the circular pattern of malignant cell growth with the cells clustered into identifiable nodules or follicles.

✓5th C82.0 Follicular lymphoma grade I

C82.00 Follicular lymphoma grade I, unspecified site CC HCC

C82.01 Follicular lymphoma grade I, lymph nodes of head, face, and neck CC HCC

C82.02 Follicular lymphoma grade I, intrathoracic lymph nodes CC HCC

C82.03 Follicular lymphoma grade I, intra-abdominal lymph nodes CC HCC

C82.04 Follicular lymphoma grade I, lymph nodes of axilla and upper limb CC HCC

C82.05 Follicular lymphoma grade I, lymph nodes of inguinal region and lower limb CC HCC

C82.06 Follicular lymphoma grade I, intrapelvic lymph nodes CC HCC

C82.07 Follicular lymphoma grade I, spleen CC HCC

C82.08 Follicular lymphoma grade I, lymph nodes of multiple sites CC HCC

C82.09 Follicular lymphoma grade I, extranodal and solid organ sites CC HCC

✓5th C82.1 Follicular lymphoma grade II

C82.10 Follicular lymphoma grade II, unspecified site CC HCC

C82.11 Follicular lymphoma grade II, lymph nodes of head, face, and neck CC HCC

C82.12 Follicular lymphoma grade II, intrathoracic lymph nodes CC HCC

C82.13 Follicular lymphoma grade II, intra-abdominal lymph nodes CC HCC

C82.14 Follicular lymphoma grade II, lymph nodes of axilla and upper limb CC HCC

C82.15 Follicular lymphoma grade II, lymph nodes of inguinal region and lower limb CC HCC

C82.16 Follicular lymphoma grade II, intrapelvic lymph nodes CC HCC

C82.17 Follicular lymphoma grade II, spleen CC HCC

C82.18 Follicular lymphoma grade II, lymph nodes of multiple sites CC HCC

C82.19 Follicular lymphoma grade II, extranodal and solid organ sites CC HCC

✓5th C82.2 Follicular lymphoma grade III, unspecified

C82.20 Follicular lymphoma grade III, unspecified, unspecified site CC HCC

C82.21 Follicular lymphoma grade III, unspecified, lymph nodes of head, face, and neck CC HCC

C82.22 Follicular lymphoma grade III, unspecified, intrathoracic lymph nodes CC HCC

C82.23 Follicular lymphoma grade III, unspecified, intra-abdominal lymph nodes CC HCC

C82.24 Follicular lymphoma grade III, unspecified, lymph nodes of axilla and upper limb CC HCC

C82.25 Follicular lymphoma grade III, unspecified, lymph nodes of inguinal region and lower limb CC HCC

C82.26 Follicular lymphoma grade III, unspecified, intrapelvic lymph nodes CC HCC
C82.27 Follicular lymphoma grade III, unspecified, spleen CC HCC
C82.28 Follicular lymphoma grade III, unspecified, lymph nodes of multiple sites CC HCC
C82.29 Follicular lymphoma grade III, unspecified, extranodal and solid organ sites CC HCC

5th C82.3 Follicular lymphoma grade IIIa

C82.3Ø Follicular lymphoma grade IIIa, unspecified site CC HCC
C82.31 Follicular lymphoma grade IIIa, lymph nodes of head, face, and neck CC HCC
C82.32 Follicular lymphoma grade IIIa, intrathoracic lymph nodes CC HCC
C82.33 Follicular lymphoma grade IIIa, intra-abdominal lymph nodes CC HCC
C82.34 Follicular lymphoma grade IIIa, lymph nodes of axilla and upper limb CC HCC
C82.35 Follicular lymphoma grade IIIa, lymph nodes of inguinal region and lower limb CC HCC
C82.36 Follicular lymphoma grade IIIa, intrapelvic lymph nodes CC HCC
C82.37 Follicular lymphoma grade IIIa, spleen CC HCC
C82.38 Follicular lymphoma grade IIIa, lymph nodes of multiple sites CC HCC
C82.39 Follicular lymphoma grade IIIa, extranodal and solid organ sites CC HCC

5th C82.4 Follicular lymphoma grade IIIb

C82.4Ø Follicular lymphoma grade IIIb, unspecified site CC HCC
C82.41 Follicular lymphoma grade IIIb, lymph nodes of head, face, and neck CC HCC
C82.42 Follicular lymphoma grade IIIb, intrathoracic lymph nodes CC HCC
C82.43 Follicular lymphoma grade IIIb, intra-abdominal lymph nodes CC HCC
C82.44 Follicular lymphoma grade IIIb, lymph nodes of axilla and upper limb CC HCC
C82.45 Follicular lymphoma grade IIIb, lymph nodes of inguinal region and lower limb CC HCC
C82.46 Follicular lymphoma grade IIIb, intrapelvic lymph nodes CC HCC
C82.47 Follicular lymphoma grade IIIb, spleen CC HCC
C82.48 Follicular lymphoma grade IIIb, lymph nodes of multiple sites CC HCC
C82.49 Follicular lymphoma grade IIIb, extranodal and solid organ sites CC HCC

5th C82.5 Diffuse follicle center lymphoma

C82.5Ø Diffuse follicle center lymphoma, unspecified site HIV CC HCC
C82.51 Diffuse follicle center lymphoma, lymph nodes of head, face, and neck HIV CC HCC
C82.52 Diffuse follicle center lymphoma, intrathoracic lymph nodes HIV CC HCC
C82.53 Diffuse follicle center lymphoma, intra-abdominal lymph nodes HIV CC HCC
C82.54 Diffuse follicle center lymphoma, lymph nodes of axilla and upper limb HIV CC HCC
C82.55 Diffuse follicle center lymphoma, lymph nodes of inguinal region and lower limb HIV CC HCC
C82.56 Diffuse follicle center lymphoma, intrapelvic lymph nodes HIV CC HCC
C82.57 Diffuse follicle center lymphoma, spleen HIV CC HCC
C82.58 Diffuse follicle center lymphoma, lymph nodes of multiple sites HIV CC HCC
C82.59 Diffuse follicle center lymphoma, extranodal and solid organ sites HIV CC HCC

5th C82.6 Cutaneous follicle center lymphoma

C82.6Ø Cutaneous follicle center lymphoma, unspecified site CC HCC
C82.61 Cutaneous follicle center lymphoma, lymph nodes of head, face, and neck CC HCC
C82.62 Cutaneous follicle center lymphoma, intrathoracic lymph nodes CC HCC
C82.63 Cutaneous follicle center lymphoma, intra-abdominal lymph nodes CC HCC
C82.64 Cutaneous follicle center lymphoma, lymph nodes of axilla and upper limb CC HCC
C82.65 Cutaneous follicle center lymphoma, lymph nodes of inguinal region and lower limb CC HCC
C82.66 Cutaneous follicle center lymphoma, intrapelvic lymph nodes CC HCC
C82.67 Cutaneous follicle center lymphoma, spleen CC HCC
C82.68 Cutaneous follicle center lymphoma, lymph nodes of multiple sites CC HCC
C82.69 Cutaneous follicle center lymphoma, extranodal and solid organ sites CC HCC

5th C82.8 Other types of follicular lymphoma

C82.8Ø Other types of follicular lymphoma, unspecified site CC HCC
C82.81 Other types of follicular lymphoma, lymph nodes of head, face, and neck CC HCC
C82.82 Other types of follicular lymphoma, intrathoracic lymph nodes CC HCC
C82.83 Other types of follicular lymphoma, intra-abdominal lymph nodes CC HCC
C82.84 Other types of follicular lymphoma, lymph nodes of axilla and upper limb CC HCC
C82.85 Other types of follicular lymphoma, lymph nodes of inguinal region and lower limb CC HCC
C82.86 Other types of follicular lymphoma, intrapelvic lymph nodes CC HCC
C82.87 Other types of follicular lymphoma, spleen CC HCC
C82.88 Other types of follicular lymphoma, lymph nodes of multiple sites CC HCC
C82.89 Other types of follicular lymphoma, extranodal and solid organ sites CC HCC

5th C82.9 Follicular lymphoma, unspecified

C82.9Ø Follicular lymphoma, unspecified, unspecified site CC HCC
C82.91 Follicular lymphoma, unspecified, lymph nodes of head, face, and neck CC HCC
C82.92 Follicular lymphoma, unspecified, intrathoracic lymph nodes CC HCC
C82.93 Follicular lymphoma, unspecified, intra-abdominal lymph nodes CC HCC
C82.94 Follicular lymphoma, unspecified, lymph nodes of axilla and upper limb CC HCC
C82.95 Follicular lymphoma, unspecified, lymph nodes of inguinal region and lower limb CC HCC
C82.96 Follicular lymphoma, unspecified, intrapelvic lymph nodes CC HCC
C82.97 Follicular lymphoma, unspecified, spleen CC HCC
C82.98 Follicular lymphoma, unspecified, lymph nodes of multiple sites CC HCC
C82.99 Follicular lymphoma, unspecified, extranodal and solid organ sites CC HCC

4th C83 Non-follicular lymphoma

EXCLUDES 1 *personal history of non-Hodgkin lymphoma (Z85.72)*

5th C83.Ø Small cell B-cell lymphoma

Lymphoplasmacytic lymphoma
Nodal marginal zone lymphoma
Non-leukemic variant of B-CLL
Splenic marginal zone lymphoma

EXCLUDES 1 *chronic lymphocytic leukemia (C91.1)*
mature T/NK-cell lymphomas (C84.-)
Waldenström macroglobulinemia (C88.Ø)

DEF: Nonfollicular lymphoma that is rare, slow growing, and usually found in the older population.

C83.ØØ Small cell B-cell lymphoma, unspecified site HIV CC HCC
C83.Ø1 Small cell B-cell lymphoma, lymph nodes of head, face, and neck HIV CC HCC
C83.Ø2 Small cell B-cell lymphoma, intrathoracic lymph nodes HIV CC HCC
C83.Ø3 Small cell B-cell lymphoma, intra-abdominal lymph nodes HIV CC HCC
C83.Ø4 Small cell B-cell lymphoma, lymph nodes of axilla and upper limb HIV CC HCC
C83.Ø5 Small cell B-cell lymphoma, lymph nodes of inguinal region and lower limb HIV CC HCC

C83.Ø6 Small cell B-cell lymphoma, intrapelvic lymph nodes HIV CC HCC
C83.Ø7 Small cell B-cell lymphoma, spleen HIV CC HCC
C83.Ø8 Small cell B-cell lymphoma, lymph nodes of multiple sites HIV CC HCC
C83.Ø9 Small cell B-cell lymphoma, extranodal and solid organ sites HIV CC HCC

C83.1 Mantle cell lymphoma
Centrocytic lymphoma
Malignant lymphomatous polyposis
DEF: Rare form of B-cell non-Hodgkin lymphoma named for the location of the tumor cell production, the mantle zone of the lymph nodes.

C83.1Ø Mantle cell lymphoma, unspecified site HIV CC HCC
C83.11 Mantle cell lymphoma, lymph nodes of head, face, and neck HIV CC HCC
C83.12 Mantle cell lymphoma, intrathoracic lymph nodes HIV CC HCC
C83.13 Mantle cell lymphoma, intra-abdominal lymph nodes HIV CC HCC
C83.14 Mantle cell lymphoma, lymph nodes of axilla and upper limb HIV CC HCC
C83.15 Mantle cell lymphoma, lymph nodes of inguinal region and lower limb HIV CC HCC
C83.16 Mantle cell lymphoma, intrapelvic lymph nodes HIV CC HCC
C83.17 Mantle cell lymphoma, spleen HIV CC HCC
C83.18 Mantle cell lymphoma, lymph nodes of multiple sites HIV CC HCC
C83.19 Mantle cell lymphoma, extranodal and solid organ sites HIV CC HCC

C83.3 Diffuse large B-cell lymphoma
Anaplastic diffuse large B-cell lymphoma
CD3Ø-positive diffuse large B-cell lymphoma
Centroblastic diffuse large B-cell lymphoma
Diffuse large B-cell lymphoma, subtype not specified
Immunoblastic diffuse large B-cell lymphoma
Plasmablastic diffuse large B-cell lymphoma
T-cell rich diffuse large B-cell lymphoma
EXCLUDES 1 *mediastinal (thymic) large B-cell lymphoma (C85.2-)*
mature T/NK-cell lymphomas (C84.-)
DEF: Nonfollicular lymphoma that is one of the more common types of lymphoma. This cancer is fast growing and affects any age but is found mostly in the older population.

C83.3Ø Diffuse large B-cell lymphoma, unspecified site HIV CC HCC
C83.31 Diffuse large B-cell lymphoma, lymph nodes of head, face, and neck HIV CC HCC
C83.32 Diffuse large B-cell lymphoma, intrathoracic lymph nodes HIV CC HCC
C83.33 Diffuse large B-cell lymphoma, intra-abdominal lymph nodes HIV CC HCC
C83.34 Diffuse large B-cell lymphoma, lymph nodes of axilla and upper limb HIV CC HCC
C83.35 Diffuse large B-cell lymphoma, lymph nodes of inguinal region and lower limb HIV CC HCC
C83.36 Diffuse large B-cell lymphoma, intrapelvic lymph nodes HIV CC HCC
C83.37 Diffuse large B-cell lymphoma, spleen HIV CC HCC
C83.38 Diffuse large B-cell lymphoma, lymph nodes of multiple sites HIV CC HCC
C83.39 Diffuse large B-cell lymphoma, extranodal and solid organ sites HIV CC HCC

C83.5 Lymphoblastic (diffuse) lymphoma
B-precursor lymphoma
Lymphoblastic B-cell lymphoma
Lymphoblastic lymphoma NOS
Lymphoblastic T-cell lymphoma
T-precursor lymphoma
DEF: Type of non-Hodgkin lymphoma considered lymphoma or leukemia—the determination is made based on the amount of bone marrow involvement. The cells are small to medium immature T-cells that often originate in the thymus where many of the T-cells are made.

C83.5Ø Lymphoblastic (diffuse) lymphoma, unspecified site CC HCC
C83.51 Lymphoblastic (diffuse) lymphoma, lymph nodes of head, face, and neck CC HCC
C83.52 Lymphoblastic (diffuse) lymphoma, intrathoracic lymph nodes CC HCC
C83.53 Lymphoblastic (diffuse) lymphoma, intra-abdominal lymph nodes CC HCC
C83.54 Lymphoblastic (diffuse) lymphoma, lymph nodes of axilla and upper limb CC HCC
C83.55 Lymphoblastic (diffuse) lymphoma, lymph nodes of inguinal region and lower limb CC HCC
C83.56 Lymphoblastic (diffuse) lymphoma, intrapelvic lymph nodes CC HCC
C83.57 Lymphoblastic (diffuse) lymphoma, spleen CC HCC
C83.58 Lymphoblastic (diffuse) lymphoma, lymph nodes of multiple sites CC HCC
C83.59 Lymphoblastic (diffuse) lymphoma, extranodal and solid organ sites CC HCC

C83.7 Burkitt lymphoma
Atypical Burkitt lymphoma
Burkitt-like lymphoma
EXCLUDES 1 *mature B-cell leukemia Burkitt type (C91.A-)*
DEF: Malignancy of the lymphatic system, most often seen as a large bone-deteriorating lesion within the jaw or as an abdominal mass. It is a form of non-Hodgkin's lymphoma and is recognized as the fastest growing human tumor.

C83.7Ø Burkitt lymphoma, unspecified site HIV CC HCC
C83.71 Burkitt lymphoma, lymph nodes of head, face, and neck HIV CC HCC
C83.72 Burkitt lymphoma, intrathoracic lymph nodes HIV CC HCC
C83.73 Burkitt lymphoma, intra-abdominal lymph nodes HIV CC HCC
C83.74 Burkitt lymphoma, lymph nodes of axilla and upper limb HIV CC HCC
C83.75 Burkitt lymphoma, lymph nodes of inguinal region and lower limb HIV CC HCC
C83.76 Burkitt lymphoma, intrapelvic lymph nodes HIV CC HCC
C83.77 Burkitt lymphoma, spleen HIV CC HCC
C83.78 Burkitt lymphoma, lymph nodes of multiple sites HIV CC HCC
C83.79 Burkitt lymphoma, extranodal and solid organ sites HIV CC HCC

C83.8 Other non-follicular lymphoma
Intravascular large B-cell lymphoma
Lymphoid granulomatosis
Primary effusion B-cell lymphoma
EXCLUDES 1 *mediastinal (thymic) large B-cell lymphoma (C85.2-)*
T-cell rich B-cell lymphoma (C83.3-)

C83.8Ø Other non-follicular lymphoma, unspecified site HIV CC HCC
C83.81 Other non-follicular lymphoma, lymph nodes of head, face, and neck HIV CC HCC
C83.82 Other non-follicular lymphoma, intrathoracic lymph nodes HIV CC HCC
C83.83 Other non-follicular lymphoma, intra-abdominal lymph nodes HIV CC HCC
C83.84 Other non-follicular lymphoma, lymph nodes of axilla and upper limb HIV CC HCC
C83.85 Other non-follicular lymphoma, lymph nodes of inguinal region and lower limb HIV CC HCC
C83.86 Other non-follicular lymphoma, intrapelvic lymph nodes HIV CC HCC
C83.87 Other non-follicular lymphoma, spleen HIV CC HCC
C83.88 Other non-follicular lymphoma, lymph nodes of multiple sites HIV CC HCC
C83.89 Other non-follicular lymphoma, extranodal and solid organ sites HIV CC HCC

C83.9 Non-follicular (diffuse) lymphoma, unspecified

C83.9Ø Non-follicular (diffuse) lymphoma, unspecified, unspecified site HIV CC HCC
C83.91 Non-follicular (diffuse) lymphoma, unspecified, lymph nodes of head, face, and neck HIV CC HCC
C83.92 Non-follicular (diffuse) lymphoma, unspecified, intrathoracic lymph nodes HIV CC HCC
C83.93 Non-follicular (diffuse) lymphoma, unspecified, intra-abdominal lymph nodes HIV CC HCC
C83.94 Non-follicular (diffuse) lymphoma, unspecified, lymph nodes of axilla and upper limb HIV CC HCC

C83.95 Non-follicular (diffuse) lymphoma, unspecified, lymph nodes of inguinal region and lower limb HIV CC HCC

C83.96 Non-follicular (diffuse) lymphoma, unspecified, intrapelvic lymph nodes HIV CC HCC

C83.97 Non-follicular (diffuse) lymphoma, unspecified, spleen HIV CC HCC

C83.98 Non-follicular (diffuse) lymphoma, unspecified, lymph nodes of multiple sites HIV CC HCC

C83.99 Non-follicular (diffuse) lymphoma, unspecified, extranodal and solid organ sites HIV CC HCC

C84 Mature T/NK-cell lymphomas

EXCLUDES 1 *personal history of non-Hodgkin lymphoma (Z85.72)*

C84.0 Mycosis fungoides

EXCLUDES 1 *▶peripheral T-cell lymphoma, not elsewhere classified◀ (C84.4-)*

DEF: Most common form of cutaneous T-cell lymphoma. A type of non-Hodgkin lymphoma in which white blood cells become cancerous and affect the skin and sometimes internal organs.

Synonym(s): *Alibert-Bazin syndrome.*

C84.00 Mycosis fungoides, unspecified site CC HCC

C84.01 Mycosis fungoides, lymph nodes of head, face, and neck CC HCC

C84.02 Mycosis fungoides, intrathoracic lymph nodes CC HCC

C84.03 Mycosis fungoides, intra-abdominal lymph nodes CC HCC

C84.04 Mycosis fungoides, lymph nodes of axilla and upper limb CC HCC

C84.05 Mycosis fungoides, lymph nodes of inguinal region and lower limb CC HCC

C84.06 Mycosis fungoides, intrapelvic lymph nodes CC HCC

C84.07 Mycosis fungoides, spleen CC HCC

C84.08 Mycosis fungoides, lymph nodes of multiple sites CC HCC

C84.09 Mycosis fungoides, extranodal and solid organ sites CC HCC

C84.1 Sézary disease

DEF: Extension of mycosis fungoides that affects the blood and all of the skin, appearing as sunburn, rather than patches. It spreads to the lymph nodes and is often linked to a weakened immune system.

C84.10 Sézary disease, unspecified site CC HCC

C84.11 Sézary disease, lymph nodes of head, face, and neck CC HCC

C84.12 Sézary disease, intrathoracic lymph nodes CC HCC

C84.13 Sézary disease, intra-abdominal lymph nodes CC HCC

C84.14 Sézary disease, lymph nodes of axilla and upper limb CC HCC

C84.15 Sézary disease, lymph nodes of inguinal region and lower limb CC HCC

C84.16 Sézary disease, intrapelvic lymph nodes CC HCC

C84.17 Sézary disease, spleen CC HCC

C84.18 Sézary disease, lymph nodes of multiple sites CC HCC

C84.19 Sézary disease, extranodal and solid organ sites CC HCC

▲ **C84.4 Peripheral T-cell lymphoma, not elsewhere classified**

Lennert's lymphoma
Lymphoepithelioid lymphoma
Mature T-cell lymphoma, not elsewhere classified

▲ C84.40 Peripheral T-cell lymphoma, not elsewhere classified, unspecified site HIV CC HCC

▲ C84.41 Peripheral T-cell lymphoma, not elsewhere classified, lymph nodes of head, face, and neck HIV CC HCC

▲ C84.42 Peripheral T-cell lymphoma, not elsewhere classified, intrathoracic lymph nodes HIV CC HCC

▲ C84.43 Peripheral T-cell lymphoma, not elsewhere classified, intra-abdominal lymph nodes HIV CC HCC

▲ C84.44 Peripheral T-cell lymphoma, not elsewhere classified, lymph nodes of axilla and upper limb HIV CC HCC

▲ C84.45 Peripheral T-cell lymphoma, not elsewhere classified, lymph nodes of inguinal region and lower limb HIV CC HCC

▲ C84.46 Peripheral T-cell lymphoma, not elsewhere classified, intrapelvic lymph nodes HIV CC HCC

▲ C84.47 Peripheral T-cell lymphoma, not elsewhere classified, spleen HIV CC HCC

▲ C84.48 Peripheral T-cell lymphoma, not elsewhere classified, lymph nodes of multiple sites HIV CC HCC

▲ C84.49 Peripheral T-cell lymphoma, not elsewhere classified, extranodal and solid organ sites HIV CC HCC

C84.6 Anaplastic large cell lymphoma, ALK-positive

Anaplastic large cell lymphoma, CD30-positive

C84.60 Anaplastic large cell lymphoma, ALK-positive, unspecified site HIV CC HCC

C84.61 Anaplastic large cell lymphoma, ALK-positive, lymph nodes of head, face, and neck HIV CC HCC

C84.62 Anaplastic large cell lymphoma, ALK-positive, intrathoracic lymph nodes HIV CC HCC

C84.63 Anaplastic large cell lymphoma, ALK-positive, intra-abdominal lymph nodes HIV CC HCC

C84.64 Anaplastic large cell lymphoma, ALK-positive, lymph nodes of axilla and upper limb HIV CC HCC

C84.65 Anaplastic large cell lymphoma, ALK-positive, lymph nodes of inguinal region and lower limb HIV CC HCC

C84.66 Anaplastic large cell lymphoma, ALK-positive, intrapelvic lymph nodes HIV CC HCC

C84.67 Anaplastic large cell lymphoma, ALK-positive, spleen HIV CC HCC

C84.68 Anaplastic large cell lymphoma, ALK-positive, lymph nodes of multiple sites HIV CC HCC

C84.69 Anaplastic large cell lymphoma, ALK-positive, extranodal and solid organ sites HIV CC HCC

C84.7 Anaplastic large cell lymphoma, ALK-negative

EXCLUDES 1 *primary cutaneous CD30-positive T-cell proliferations (C86.6-)*

C84.70 Anaplastic large cell lymphoma, ALK-negative, unspecified site HIV CC HCC

C84.71 Anaplastic large cell lymphoma, ALK-negative, lymph nodes of head, face, and neck HIV CC HCC

C84.72 Anaplastic large cell lymphoma, ALK-negative, intrathoracic lymph nodes HIV CC HCC

C84.73 Anaplastic large cell lymphoma, ALK-negative, intra-abdominal lymph nodes HIV CC HCC

C84.74 Anaplastic large cell lymphoma, ALK-negative, lymph nodes of axilla and upper limb HIV CC HCC

C84.75 Anaplastic large cell lymphoma, ALK-negative, lymph nodes of inguinal region and lower limb HIV CC HCC

C84.76 Anaplastic large cell lymphoma, ALK-negative, intrapelvic lymph nodes HIV CC HCC

C84.77 Anaplastic large cell lymphoma, ALK-negative, spleen HIV CC HCC

C84.78 Anaplastic large cell lymphoma, ALK-negative, lymph nodes of multiple sites HIV CC HCC

C84.79 Anaplastic large cell lymphoma, ALK-negative, extranodal and solid organ sites HIV CC HCC

C84.7A Anaplastic large cell lymphoma, ALK-negative, breast HIV CC HCC

Breast implant associated anaplastic large cell lymphoma (BIA-ALCL)

Use additional code to identify:
breast implant status (Z98.82)
personal history of breast implant removal (Z98.86)

AHA: 2021,4Q,6

C84.A Cutaneous T-cell lymphoma, unspecified

AHA: 2021,2Q,6

C84.A0 Cutaneous T-cell lymphoma, unspecified, unspecified site HIV CC HCC

C84.A1 Cutaneous T-cell lymphoma, unspecified lymph nodes of head, face, and neck HIV CC HCC

C84.A2 Cutaneous T-cell lymphoma, unspecified, intrathoracic lymph nodes HIV CC HCC

C84.A3 Cutaneous T-cell lymphoma, unspecified, intra-abdominal lymph nodes HIV CC HCC

C84.A4 Cutaneous T-cell lymphoma, unspecified, lymph nodes of axilla and upper limb HIV CC HCC
C84.A5 Cutaneous T-cell lymphoma, unspecified, lymph nodes of inguinal region and lower limb HIV CC HCC
C84.A6 Cutaneous T-cell lymphoma, unspecified, intrapelvic lymph nodes HIV CC HCC
C84.A7 Cutaneous T-cell lymphoma, unspecified, spleen HIV CC HCC
C84.A8 Cutaneous T-cell lymphoma, unspecified, lymph nodes of multiple sites HIV CC HCC
C84.A9 Cutaneous T-cell lymphoma, unspecified, extranodal and solid organ sites HIV CC HCC

C84.Z Other mature T/NK-cell lymphomas

NOTE If T-cell lineage or involvement is mentioned in conjunction with a specific lymphoma, code to the more specific description.

EXCLUDES 1 *angioimmunoblastic T-cell lymphoma (C86.5)*
blastic NK-cell lymphoma (C86.4)
enteropathy-type T-cell lymphoma (C86.2)
extranodal NK-cell lymphoma, nasal type (C86.Ø)
hepatosplenic T-cell lymphoma (C86.1)
primary cutaneous CD3Ø-positive T-cell proliferations (C86.6)
subcutaneous panniculitis-like T-cell lymphoma (C86.3)
T-cell leukemia (C91.1-)

C84.ZØ Other mature T/NK-cell lymphomas, unspecified site HIV CC HCC
C84.Z1 Other mature T/NK-cell lymphomas, lymph nodes of head, face, and neck HIV CC HCC
C84.Z2 Other mature T/NK-cell lymphomas, intrathoracic lymph nodes HIV CC HCC
C84.Z3 Other mature T/NK-cell lymphomas, intra-abdominal lymph nodes HIV CC HCC
C84.Z4 Other mature T/NK-cell lymphomas, lymph nodes of axilla and upper limb HIV CC HCC
C84.Z5 Other mature T/NK-cell lymphomas, lymph nodes of inguinal region and lower limb HIV CC HCC
C84.Z6 Other mature T/NK-cell lymphomas, intrapelvic lymph nodes HIV CC HCC
C84.Z7 Other mature T/NK-cell lymphomas, spleen HIV CC HCC
C84.Z8 Other mature T/NK-cell lymphomas, lymph nodes of multiple sites HIV CC HCC
C84.Z9 Other mature T/NK-cell lymphomas, extranodal and solid organ sites HIV CC HCC

C84.9 Mature T/NK-cell lymphomas, unspecified

NK/T cell lymphoma NOS

EXCLUDES 1 *mature T-cell lymphoma, not elsewhere classified (C84.4-)*

C84.9Ø Mature T/NK-cell lymphomas, unspecified, unspecified site HIV CC HCC
C84.91 Mature T/NK-cell lymphomas, unspecified, lymph nodes of head, face, and neck HIV CC HCC
C84.92 Mature T/NK-cell lymphomas, unspecified, intrathoracic lymph nodes HIV CC HCC
C84.93 Mature T/NK-cell lymphomas, unspecified, intra-abdominal lymph nodes HIV CC HCC
C84.94 Mature T/NK-cell lymphomas, unspecified, lymph nodes of axilla and upper limb HIV CC HCC
C84.95 Mature T/NK-cell lymphomas, unspecified, lymph nodes of inguinal region and lower limb HIV CC HCC
C84.96 Mature T/NK-cell lymphomas, unspecified, intrapelvic lymph nodes HIV CC HCC
C84.97 Mature T/NK-cell lymphomas, unspecified, spleen HIV CC HCC
C84.98 Mature T/NK-cell lymphomas, unspecified, lymph nodes of multiple sites HIV CC HCC
C84.99 Mature T/NK-cell lymphomas, unspecified, extranodal and solid organ sites HIV CC HCC

C85 Other specified and unspecified types of non-Hodgkin lymphoma

EXCLUDES 1 *other specified types of T/NK-cell lymphoma (C86.-)*
personal history of non-Hodgkin lymphoma (Z85.72)

C85.1 Unspecified B-cell lymphoma

NOTE If B-cell lineage or involvement is mentioned in conjunction with a specific lymphoma, code to the more specific description.

C85.1Ø Unspecified B-cell lymphoma, unspecified site HIV CC HCC
C85.11 Unspecified B-cell lymphoma, lymph nodes of head, face, and neck HIV CC HCC
C85.12 Unspecified B-cell lymphoma, intrathoracic lymph nodes HIV CC HCC
C85.13 Unspecified B-cell lymphoma, intra-abdominal lymph nodes HIV CC HCC
C85.14 Unspecified B-cell lymphoma, lymph nodes of axilla and upper limb HIV CC HCC
C85.15 Unspecified B-cell lymphoma, lymph nodes of inguinal region and lower limb HIV CC HCC
C85.16 Unspecified B-cell lymphoma, intrapelvic lymph nodes HIV CC HCC
C85.17 Unspecified B-cell lymphoma, spleen HIV CC HCC
C85.18 Unspecified B-cell lymphoma, lymph nodes of multiple sites HIV CC HCC
C85.19 Unspecified B-cell lymphoma, extranodal and solid organ sites HIV CC HCC

C85.2 Mediastinal (thymic) large B-cell lymphoma

C85.2Ø Mediastinal (thymic) large B-cell lymphoma, unspecified site HIV CC HCC
C85.21 Mediastinal (thymic) large B-cell lymphoma, lymph nodes of head, face, and neck HIV CC HCC
C85.22 Mediastinal (thymic) large B-cell lymphoma, intrathoracic lymph nodes HIV CC HCC
C85.23 Mediastinal (thymic) large B-cell lymphoma, intra-abdominal lymph nodes HIV CC HCC
C85.24 Mediastinal (thymic) large B-cell lymphoma, lymph nodes of axilla and upper limb HIV CC HCC
C85.25 Mediastinal (thymic) large B-cell lymphoma, lymph nodes of inguinal region and lower limb HIV CC HCC
C85.26 Mediastinal (thymic) large B-cell lymphoma, intrapelvic lymph nodes HIV CC HCC
C85.27 Mediastinal (thymic) large B-cell lymphoma, spleen HIV CC HCC
C85.28 Mediastinal (thymic) large B-cell lymphoma, lymph nodes of multiple sites HIV CC HCC
C85.29 Mediastinal (thymic) large B-cell lymphoma, extranodal and solid organ sites HIV CC HCC

C85.8 Other specified types of non-Hodgkin lymphoma

C85.8Ø Other specified types of non-Hodgkin lymphoma, unspecified site HIV CC HCC
C85.81 Other specified types of non-Hodgkin lymphoma, lymph nodes of head, face, and neck HIV CC HCC
C85.82 Other specified types of non-Hodgkin lymphoma, intrathoracic lymph nodes HIV CC HCC
C85.83 Other specified types of non-Hodgkin lymphoma, intra-abdominal lymph nodes HIV CC HCC
C85.84 Other specified types of non-Hodgkin lymphoma, lymph nodes of axilla and upper limb HIV CC HCC
C85.85 Other specified types of non-Hodgkin lymphoma, lymph nodes of inguinal region and lower limb HIV CC HCC
C85.86 Other specified types of non-Hodgkin lymphoma, intrapelvic lymph nodes HIV CC HCC
C85.87 Other specified types of non-Hodgkin lymphoma, spleen HIV CC HCC
C85.88 Other specified types of non-Hodgkin lymphoma, lymph nodes of multiple sites HIV CC HCC
C85.89 Other specified types of non-Hodgkin lymphoma, extranodal and solid organ sites HIV CC HCC

C85.9 Non-Hodgkin lymphoma, unspecified

Lymphoma NOS
Malignant lymphoma NOS
Non-Hodgkin lymphoma NOS

C85.9Ø Non-Hodgkin lymphoma, unspecified, unspecified site HIV CC HCC
C85.91 Non-Hodgkin lymphoma, unspecified, lymph nodes of head, face, and neck HIV CC HCC

C85.92 Non-Hodgkin lymphoma, unspecified, intrathoracic lymph nodes HIV CC HCC

C85.93 Non-Hodgkin lymphoma, unspecified, intra-abdominal lymph nodes HIV CC HCC

C85.94 Non-Hodgkin lymphoma, unspecified, lymph nodes of axilla and upper limb HIV CC HCC

C85.95 Non-Hodgkin lymphoma, unspecified, lymph nodes of inguinal region and lower limb HIV CC HCC

C85.96 Non-Hodgkin lymphoma, unspecified, intrapelvic lymph nodes HIV CC HCC

C85.97 Non-Hodgkin lymphoma, unspecified, spleen HIV CC HCC

C85.98 Non-Hodgkin lymphoma, unspecified, lymph nodes of multiple sites HIV CC HCC

C85.99 Non-Hodgkin lymphoma, unspecified, extranodal and solid organ sites HIV CC HCC

✓4th C86 Other specified types of T/NK-cell lymphoma

EXCLUDES 1 *anaplastic large cell lymphoma, ALK negative (C84.7-)*
anaplastic large cell lymphoma, ALK positive (C84.6-)
mature T/NK-cell lymphomas (C84.-)
other specified types of non-Hodgkin lymphoma (C85.8-)

C86.Ø Extranodal NK/T-cell lymphoma, nasal type HIV CC HCC

C86.1 Hepatosplenic T-cell lymphoma HIV CC HCC
Alpha-beta and gamma delta types

C86.2 Enteropathy-type (intestinal) T-cell lymphoma HIV CC HCC
Enteropathy associated T-cell lymphoma

C86.3 Subcutaneous panniculitis-like T-cell lymphoma HIV CC HCC

C86.4 Blastic NK-cell lymphoma HIV CC HCC
Blastic plasmacytoid dendritic cell neoplasm (BPDCN)

C86.5 Angioimmunoblastic T-cell lymphoma HIV CC HCC
Angioimmunoblastic lymphadenopathy with dysproteinemia (AILD)

C86.6 Primary cutaneous CD3Ø-positive T-cell proliferations HIV CC HCC
Lymphomatoid papulosis
Primary cutaneous anaplastic large cell lymphoma
Primary cutaneous CD3Ø-positive large T-cell lymphoma

✓4th C88 Malignant immunoproliferative diseases and certain other B-cell lymphomas

EXCLUDES 1 *B-cell lymphoma, unspecified (C85.1-)*
personal history of other malignant neoplasms of lymphoid, hematopoietic and related tissues (Z85.79)

C88.Ø Waldenström macroglobulinemia HCC
Lymphoplasmacytic lymphoma with IgM-production
Macroglobulinemia (idiopathic) (primary)
EXCLUDES 1 *small cell B-cell lymphoma (C83.Ø)*

C88.2 Heavy chain disease CC HCC
Franklin disease
Gamma heavy chain disease
Mu heavy chain disease

C88.3 Immunoproliferative small intestinal disease CC HCC
Alpha heavy chain disease
Mediterranean lymphoma

C88.4 Extranodal marginal zone B-cell lymphoma of mucosa-associated lymphoid tissue [MALT-lymphoma] HIV CC HCC
Lymphoma of skin-associated lymphoid tissue [SALT-lymphoma]
Lymphoma of bronchial-associated lymphoid tissue [BALT-lymphoma]
EXCLUDES 1 *high malignant (diffuse large B-cell) lymphoma (C83.3-)*

C88.8 Other malignant immunoproliferative diseases CC HCC

C88.9 Malignant immunoproliferative disease, unspecified CC HCC
Immunoproliferative disease NOS

✓4th C9Ø Multiple myeloma and malignant plasma cell neoplasms

EXCLUDES 1 *personal history of other malignant neoplasms of lymphoid, hematopoietic and related tissues (Z85.79)*

AHA: 2019,2Q,30

✓5th C9Ø.Ø Multiple myeloma
Kahler's disease
Medullary plasmacytoma
Myelomatosis
Plasma cell myeloma
EXCLUDES 1 *solitary myeloma (C9Ø.3-)*
solitary plasmactyoma (C9Ø.3-)

AHA: 2021,3Q,5

TIP: Smoldering multiple myeloma (SMM) is a plasma cell disorder that has not yet progressed to active multiple myeloma. Code D47.2 should be used when only SMM is documented.

TIP: Do not assign an additional code for bone metastasis (C79.51) when multiple myeloma is described as metastatic to the bone; bone involvement is integral to this disease process.

C9Ø.ØØ Multiple myeloma not having achieved remission CC HCC
Multiple myeloma with failed remission
Multiple myeloma NOS

C9Ø.Ø1 Multiple myeloma in remission CC HCC

C9Ø.Ø2 Multiple myeloma in relapse CC HCC

✓5th C9Ø.1 Plasma cell leukemia
Plasmacytic leukemia

AHA: 2019,2Q,30

C9Ø.1Ø Plasma cell leukemia not having achieved remission CC HCC
Plasma cell leukemia with failed remission
Plasma cell leukemia NOS

C9Ø.11 Plasma cell leukemia in remission CC HCC

C9Ø.12 Plasma cell leukemia in relapse CC HCC

✓5th C9Ø.2 Extramedullary plasmacytoma

C9Ø.2Ø Extramedullary plasmacytoma not having achieved remission CC HCC
Extramedullary plasmacytoma with failed remission
Extramedullary plasmacytoma NOS

C9Ø.21 Extramedullary plasmacytoma in remission CC HCC

C9Ø.22 Extramedullary plasmacytoma in relapse CC HCC

✓5th C9Ø.3 Solitary plasmacytoma
Localized malignant plasma cell tumor NOS
Plasmacytoma NOS
Solitary myeloma

C9Ø.3Ø Solitary plasmacytoma not having achieved remission CC HCC
Solitary plasmacytoma with failed remission
Solitary plasmacytoma NOS

C9Ø.31 Solitary plasmacytoma in remission CC HCC

C9Ø.32 Solitary plasmacytoma in relapse CC HCC

✓4th C91 Lymphoid leukemia

EXCLUDES 1 *personal history of leukemia (Z85.6)*

AHA: 2020,1Q,13

DEF: Malignant proliferation of immature lymphocytes (white blood cells that make up lymphoid tissue), called lymphoblasts, that originate in the bone marrow. Can be acute (ALL) or chronic (CLL).

✓5th C91.Ø Acute lymphoblastic leukemia [ALL]

NOTE Codes in subcategory C91.Ø- should only be used for T-cell and B-cell precursor leukemia

C91.ØØ Acute lymphoblastic leukemia not having achieved remission CC HCC
Acute lymphoblastic leukemia with failed remission
Acute lymphoblastic leukemia NOS

C91.Ø1 Acute lymphoblastic leukemia, in remission CC HCC

C91.Ø2 Acute lymphoblastic leukemia, in relapse CC HCC

C91.1 Chronic lymphocytic leukemia of B-cell type
Lymphoplasmacytic leukemia
Richter syndrome
EXCLUDES 1 *lymphoplasmacytic lymphoma (C83.0-)*

C91.10 Chronic lymphocytic leukemia of B-cell type not having achieved remission CC HCC
Chronic lymphocytic leukemia of B-cell type with failed remission
Chronic lymphocytic leukemia of B-cell type NOS

C91.11 Chronic lymphocytic leukemia of B-cell type in remission CC HCC

C91.12 Chronic lymphocytic leukemia of B-cell type in relapse CC HCC

C91.3 Prolymphocytic leukemia of B-cell type

C91.30 Prolymphocytic leukemia of B-cell type not having achieved remission CC HCC
Prolymphocytic leukemia of B-cell type with failed remission
Prolymphocytic leukemia of B-cell type NOS

C91.31 Prolymphocytic leukemia of B-cell type, in remission CC HCC

C91.32 Prolymphocytic leukemia of B-cell type, in relapse CC HCC

C91.4 Hairy cell leukemia
Leukemic reticuloendotheliosis
DEF: Rare type of leukemia that is slow growing and often also considered a type of lymphoma. The small B-cell lymphocytes appear with "hairy" projections under a microscope and are found mostly in the bone marrow, spleen, and blood.

C91.40 Hairy cell leukemia not having achieved remission CC HCC
Hairy cell leukemia with failed remission
Hairy cell leukemia NOS

C91.41 Hairy cell leukemia, in remission CC HCC

C91.42 Hairy cell leukemia, in relapse CC HCC

C91.5 Adult T-cell lymphoma/leukemia (HTLV-1-associated)
Acute variant of adult T-cell lymphoma/leukemia (HTLV-1-associated)
Chronic variant of adult T-cell lymphoma/leukemia (HTLV-1-associated)
Lymphomatoid variant of adult T-cell lymphoma/leukemia (HTLV-1-associated)
Smouldering variant of adult T-cell lymphoma/leukemia (HTLV-1-associated)

C91.50 Adult T-cell lymphoma/leukemia (HTLV-1-associated) not having achieved remission CC HCC A
Adult T-cell lymphoma/leukemia (HTLV-1-associated) with failed remission
Adult T-cell lymphoma/leukemia (HTLV-1-associated) NOS

C91.51 Adult T-cell lymphoma/leukemia (HTLV-1-associated), in remission CC HCC A

C91.52 Adult T-cell lymphoma/leukemia (HTLV-1-associated), in relapse CC HCC A

C91.6 Prolymphocytic leukemia of T-cell type

C91.60 Prolymphocytic leukemia of T-cell type not having achieved remission CC HCC
Prolymphocytic leukemia of T-cell type with failed remission
Prolymphocytic leukemia of T-cell type NOS

C91.61 Prolymphocytic leukemia of T-cell type, in remission CC HCC

C91.62 Prolymphocytic leukemia of T-cell type, in relapse CC HCC

C91.A Mature B-cell leukemia Burkitt-type
EXCLUDES 1 *Burkitt lymphoma (C83.7-)*

C91.A0 Mature B-cell leukemia Burkitt-type not having achieved remission CC HCC
Mature B-cell leukemia Burkitt-type with failed remission
Mature B-cell leukemia Burkitt-type NOS

C91.A1 Mature B-cell leukemia Burkitt-type, in remission CC HCC

C91.A2 Mature B-cell leukemia Burkitt-type, in relapse CC HCC

C91.Z Other lymphoid leukemia
T-cell large granular lymphocytic leukemia (associated with rheumatoid arthritis)

C91.Z0 Other lymphoid leukemia not having achieved remission CC HCC
Other lymphoid leukemia with failed remission
Other lymphoid leukemia NOS

C91.Z1 Other lymphoid leukemia, in remission CC HCC

C91.Z2 Other lymphoid leukemia, in relapse CC HCC

C91.9 Lymphoid leukemia, unspecified

C91.90 Lymphoid leukemia, unspecified not having achieved remission CC HCC
Lymphoid leukemia with failed remission
Lymphoid leukemia NOS

C91.91 Lymphoid leukemia, unspecified, in remission CC HCC

C91.92 Lymphoid leukemia, unspecified, in relapse CC HCC

C92 Myeloid leukemia
INCLUDES granulocytic leukemia
myelogenous leukemia
EXCLUDES 1 *personal history of leukemia (Z85.6)*
AHA: 2020,1Q,13; 2019,1Q,16
DEF: Cancer that develops in immature myelocytes called myeloblasts. These are the cells that become white blood cells (except lymphocytes), red blood cells, or platelet-making cells. Can be acute (AML) or chronic (CML).
TIP: Pancytopenia, although common in some types of myeloid leukemias, is not always inherent. When it is documented, code D61.818 can be assigned in addition to a code from this category.

C92.0 Acute myeloblastic leukemia
Acute myeloblastic leukemia, minimal differentiation
Acute myeloblastic leukemia (with maturation)
Acute myeloblastic leukemia 1/ETO
Acute myeloblastic leukemia M0
Acute myeloblastic leukemia M1
Acute myeloblastic leukemia M2
Acute myeloblastic leukemia with t(8;21)
Acute myeloblastic leukemia (without a FAB classification) NOS
Refractory anemia with excess blasts in transformation [RAEBT]
EXCLUDES 1 *acute exacerbation of chronic myeloid leukemia (C92.10)*
refractory anemia with excess of blasts not in transformation (D46.2-)
AHA: 2018,4Q,87

C92.00 Acute myeloblastic leukemia, not having achieved remission CC HCC
Acute myeloblastic leukemia with failed remission
Acute myeloblastic leukemia NOS

C92.01 Acute myeloblastic leukemia, in remission CC HCC
AHA: 2021,3Q,4

C92.02 Acute myeloblastic leukemia, in relapse CC HCC

C92.1 Chronic myeloid leukemia, BCR/ABL-positive
Chronic myelogenous leukemia, Philadelphia chromosome (Ph1) positive
Chronic myelogenous leukemia, t(9;22) (q34;q11)
Chronic myelogenous leukemia with crisis of blast cells
EXCLUDES 1 *atypical chronic myeloid leukemia BCR/ABL-negative (C92.2-)*
chronic myelomonocytic leukemia (C93.1-)
chronic myeloproliferative disease (D47.1)

C92.10 Chronic myeloid leukemia, BCR/ABL-positive, not having achieved remission CC HCC
Chronic myeloid leukemia, BCR/ABL-positive with failed remission
Chronic myeloid leukemia, BCR/ABL-positive NOS

C92.11 Chronic myeloid leukemia, BCR/ABL-positive, in remission CC HCC

C92.12 Chronic myeloid leukemia, BCR/ABL-positive, in relapse CC HCC

✓5th **C92.2 Atypical chronic myeloid leukemia, BCR/ABL-negative**

C92.Ø0 Atypical chronic myeloid leukemia, BCR/ABL-negative, not having achieved remission CC HCC

Atypical chronic myeloid leukemia, BCR/ABL-negative with failed remission

Atypical chronic myeloid leukemia, BCR/ABL-negative NOS

C92.21 Atypical chronic myeloid leukemia, BCR/ABL-negative, in remission CC HCC

C92.22 Atypical chronic myeloid leukemia, BCR/ABL-negative, in relapse CC HCC

✓5th **C92.3 Myeloid sarcoma**

A malignant tumor of immature myeloid cells

Chloroma

Granulocytic sarcoma

C92.3Ø Myeloid sarcoma, not having achieved remission CC HCC

Myeloid sarcoma with failed remission

Myeloid sarcoma NOS

C92.31 Myeloid sarcoma, in remission CC HCC

C92.32 Myeloid sarcoma, in relapse CC HCC

✓5th **C92.4 Acute promyelocytic leukemia**

AML M3

AML Me with t(15;17) and variants

C92.4Ø Acute promyelocytic leukemia, not having achieved remission CC HCC

Acute promyelocytic leukemia with failed remission

Acute promyelocytic leukemia NOS

C92.41 Acute promyelocytic leukemia, in remission CC HCC

C92.42 Acute promyelocytic leukemia, in relapse CC HCC

✓5th **C92.5 Acute myelomonocytic leukemia**

AML M4

AML M4 Eo with inv(16) or t(16;16)

C92.5Ø Acute myelomonocytic leukemia, not having achieved remission CC HCC

Acute myelomonocytic leukemia with failed remission

Acute myelomonocytic leukemia NOS

C92.51 Acute myelomonocytic leukemia, in remission CC HCC

C92.52 Acute myelomonocytic leukemia, in relapse CC HCC

✓5th **C92.6 Acute myeloid leukemia with 11q23-abnormality**

Acute myeloid leukemia with variation of MLL-gene

C92.6Ø Acute myeloid leukemia with 11q23-abnormality not having achieved remission CC HCC

Acute myeloid leukemia with 11q23-abnormality with failed remission

Acute myeloid leukemia with 11q23-abnormality NOS

C92.61 Acute myeloid leukemia with 11q23-abnormality in remission CC HCC

C92.62 Acute myeloid leukemia with 11q23-abnormality in relapse CC HCC

✓5th **C92.A Acute myeloid leukemia with multilineage dysplasia**

Acute myeloid leukemia with dysplasia of remaining hematopoesis and/or myelodysplastic disease in its history

C92.AØ Acute myeloid leukemia with multilineage dysplasia, not having achieved remission CC HCC

Acute myeloid leukemia with multilineage dysplasia with failed remission

Acute myeloid leukemia with multilineage dysplasia NOS

C92.A1 Acute myeloid leukemia with multilineage dysplasia, in remission CC HCC

C92.A2 Acute myeloid leukemia with multilineage dysplasia, in relapse CC HCC

✓5th **C92.Z Other myeloid leukemia**

C92.ZØ Other myeloid leukemia not having achieved remission CC HCC

Myeloid leukemia NEC with failed remission

Myeloid leukemia NEC

C92.Z1 Other myeloid leukemia, in remission CC HCC

C92.Z2 Other myeloid leukemia, in relapse CC HCC

✓5th **C92.9 Myeloid leukemia, unspecified**

C92.9Ø Myeloid leukemia, unspecified, not having achieved remission CC HCC

Myeloid leukemia, unspecified with failed remission

Myeloid leukemia, unspecified NOS

C92.91 Myeloid leukemia, unspecified in remission CC HCC

C92.92 Myeloid leukemia, unspecified in relapse CC HCC

✓4th **C93 Monocytic leukemia**

INCLUDES monocytoid leukemia

EXCLUDES 1 *personal history of leukemia (Z85.6)*

AHA: 2020,1Q,13

✓5th **C93.Ø Acute monoblastic/monocytic leukemia**

AML M5

AML M5a

AML M5b

C93.ØØ Acute monoblastic/monocytic leukemia, not having achieved remission CC HCC

Acute monoblastic/monocytic leukemia with failed remission

Acute monoblastic/monocytic leukemia NOS

C93.Ø1 Acute monoblastic/monocytic leukemia, in remission CC HCC

C93.Ø2 Acute monoblastic/monocytic leukemia, in relapse CC HCC

✓5th **C93.1 Chronic myelomonocytic leukemia**

Chronic monocytic leukemia

CMML-1

CMML-2

CMML with eosinophilia

Code also, if applicable, eosinophilia (D72.18)

C93.1Ø Chronic myelomonocytic leukemia not having achieved remission CC HCC

Chronic myelomonocytic leukemia with failed remission

Chronic myelomonocytic leukemia NOS

C93.11 Chronic myelomonocytic leukemia, in remission CC HCC

C93.12 Chronic myelomonocytic leukemia, in relapse CC HCC

✓5th **C93.3 Juvenile myelomonocytic leukemia**

C93.3Ø Juvenile myelomonocytic leukemia, not having achieved remission CC HCC P

Juvenile myelomonocytic leukemia with failed remission

Juvenile myelomonocytic leukemia NOS

C93.31 Juvenile myelomonocytic leukemia, in remission CC HCC P

C93.32 Juvenile myelomonocytic leukemia, in relapse CC HCC P

✓5th **C93.Z Other monocytic leukemia**

C93.ZØ Other monocytic leukemia, not having achieved remission CC HCC

Other monocytic leukemia NOS

C93.Z1 Other monocytic leukemia, in remission CC HCC

C93.Z2 Other monocytic leukemia, in relapse CC HCC

✓5th **C93.9 Monocytic leukemia, unspecified**

C93.9Ø Monocytic leukemia, unspecified, not having achieved remission CC HCC

Monocytic leukemia, unspecified with failed remission

Monocytic leukemia, unspecified NOS

C93.91 Monocytic leukemia, unspecified in remission CC HCC

C93.92 Monocytic leukemia, unspecified in relapse CC HCC

C94 Other leukemias of specified cell type

EXCLUDES 1 *leukemic reticuloendotheliosis (C91.4-)*
myelodysplastic syndromes (D46.-)
personal history of leukemia (Z85.6)
plasma cell leukemia (C90.1-)

AHA: 2020,1Q,13

C94.0 Acute erythroid leukemia
Acute myeloid leukemia M6(a)(b)
Erythroleukemia
DEF: Erythroleukemia: Malignant blood dyscrasia (a myeloproliferative disorder).

C94.00 Acute erythroid leukemia, not having achieved remission CC HCC
Acute erythroid leukemia with failed remission
Acute erythroid leukemia NOS

C94.01 Acute erythroid leukemia, in remission CC HCC

C94.02 Acute erythroid leukemia, in relapse CC HCC

C94.2 Acute megakaryoblastic leukemia
Acute myeloid leukemia M7
Acute megakaryocytic leukemia

C94.20 Acute megakaryoblastic leukemia not having achieved remission CC HCC
Acute megakaryoblastic leukemia with failed remission
Acute megakaryoblastic leukemia NOS

C94.21 Acute megakaryoblastic leukemia, in remission CC HCC

C94.22 Acute megakaryoblastic leukemia, in relapse CC HCC

C94.3 Mast cell leukemia
AHA: 2017,4Q,5

C94.30 Mast cell leukemia not having achieved remission CC HCC
Mast cell leukemia with failed remission
Mast cell leukemia NOS

C94.31 Mast cell leukemia, in remission CC HCC

C94.32 Mast cell leukemia, in relapse CC HCC

C94.4 Acute panmyelosis with myelofibrosis
Acute myelofibrosis
EXCLUDES 1 *myelofibrosis NOS (D75.81)*
secondary myelofibrosis NOS (D75.81)

C94.40 Acute panmyelosis with myelofibrosis not having achieved remission CC HCC
Acute myelofibrosis NOS
Acute panmyelosis with myelofibrosis with failed remission
Acute panmyelosis NOS

C94.41 Acute panmyelosis with myelofibrosis, in remission CC HCC

C94.42 Acute panmyelosis with myelofibrosis, in relapse CC HCC

▲ **C94.6 Myelodysplastic disease, not elsewhere classified** CC HCC
▶Myelodysplastic/myeloproliferative neoplasm, unclassifiable◀
▶Myeloproliferative disease, not elsewhere classified◀

C94.8 Other specified leukemias
Aggressive NK-cell leukemia
Acute basophilic leukemia

C94.80 Other specified leukemias not having achieved remission CC HCC
Other specified leukemia with failed remission
Other specified leukemias NOS

C94.81 Other specified leukemias, in remission CC HCC

C94.82 Other specified leukemias, in relapse CC HCC

C95 Leukemia of unspecified cell type

EXCLUDES 1 *personal history of leukemia (Z85.6)*

AHA: 2020,1Q,13

C95.0 Acute leukemia of unspecified cell type
Acute bilineal leukemia
Acute mixed lineage leukemia
Biphenotypic acute leukemia
Stem cell leukemia of unclear lineage
EXCLUDES 1 *acute exacerbation of unspecified chronic leukemia (C95.10)*

C95.00 Acute leukemia of unspecified cell type not having achieved remission CC HCC
Acute leukemia of unspecified cell type with failed remission
Acute leukemia NOS

C95.01 Acute leukemia of unspecified cell type, in remission CC HCC

C95.02 Acute leukemia of unspecified cell type, in relapse CC HCC

C95.1 Chronic leukemia of unspecified cell type

C95.10 Chronic leukemia of unspecified cell type not having achieved remission CC HCC
Chronic leukemia of unspecified cell type with failed remission
Chronic leukemia NOS

C95.11 Chronic leukemia of unspecified cell type, in remission CC HCC

C95.12 Chronic leukemia of unspecified cell type, in relapse CC HCC

C95.9 Leukemia, unspecified

C95.90 Leukemia, unspecified not having achieved remission CC HCC
Leukemia, unspecified with failed remission
Leukemia NOS

C95.91 Leukemia, unspecified, in remission CC HCC

C95.92 Leukemia, unspecified, in relapse CC HCC

C96 Other and unspecified malignant neoplasms of lymphoid, hematopoietic and related tissue

EXCLUDES 1 *personal history of other malignant neoplasms of lymphoid, hematopoietic and related tissues (Z85.79)*

C96.0 Multifocal and multisystemic (disseminated) Langerhans-cell histiocytosis CC HCC
Histiocytosis X, multisystemic
Letterer-Siwe disease
EXCLUDES 1 *adult pulmonary Langerhans cell histiocytosis (J84.82)*
multifocal and unisystemic Langerhans-cell histiocytosis (C96.5)
unifocal Langerhans-cell histiocytosis (C96.6)

C96.2 Malignant mast cell neoplasm
EXCLUDES 1 *indolent mastocytosis (D47.02)*
mast cell leukemia (C94.30)
mastocytosis (congenital) (cutaneous) (Q82.2)

AHA: 2017,4Q,5

DEF: Mast cell: Type of white blood cell found in the loose connective tissue of blood vessels and bronchioles responsible for acute hypersensitivity reactions, including anaphylactic shock. The IgE receptors on these cells bind with allergens causing cell degranulation and diffuse, widespread histamine release that results in airway constriction and vasodilation with decreased systemic blood pressure.

C96.20 Malignant mast cell neoplasm, unspecified CC HCC

C96.21 Aggressive systemic mastocytosis CC HCC

C96.22 Mast cell sarcoma CC HCC

C96.29 Other malignant mast cell neoplasm CC HCC

C96.4 Sarcoma of dendritic cells (accessory cells) CC HCC
Follicular dendritic cell sarcoma
Interdigitating dendritic cell sarcoma
Langerhans cell sarcoma

C96.5 Multifocal and unisystemic Langerhans-cell histiocytosis CC HCC
Hand-Schüller-Christian disease
Histiocytosis X, multifocal
EXCLUDES 1 *multifocal and multisystemic (disseminated) Langerhans-cell histiocytosis (C96.0)*
unifocal Langerhans-cell histiocytosis (C96.6)

C96.6 Unifocal Langerhans-cell histiocytosis CC HCC
Eosinophilic granuloma
Histiocytosis X, unifocal
Histiocytosis X NOS
Langerhans-cell histiocytosis NOS
EXCLUDES 1 *multifocal and multisysemic (disseminated) Langerhans-cell histiocytosis (C96.0)*
multifocal and unisystemic Langerhans-cell histiocytosis (C96.5)

C96.A Histiocytic sarcoma CC HCC
Malignant histiocytosis

C96.Z Other specified malignant neoplasms of lymphoid, hematopoietic and related tissue CC HCC

C96.9 Malignant neoplasm of lymphoid, hematopoietic and related tissue, unspecified CC HCC

In situ neoplasms (D00-D09)

INCLUDES Bowen's disease
erythroplasia
grade III intraepithelial neoplasia
Queyrat's erythroplasia

4th D00 Carcinoma in situ of oral cavity, esophagus and stomach
EXCLUDES 1 *melanoma in situ (D03.-)*

5th D00.0 Carcinoma in situ of lip, oral cavity and pharynx
Use additional code to identify:
exposure to environmental tobacco smoke (Z77.22)
exposure to tobacco smoke in the perinatal period (P96.81)
history of tobacco dependence (Z87.891)
occupational exposure to environmental tobacco smoke (Z57.31)
tobacco dependence (F17.-)
tobacco use (Z72.0)
EXCLUDES 1 *carcinoma in situ of aryepiglottic fold or interarytenoid fold, laryngeal aspect (D02.0)*
carcinoma in situ of epiglottis NOS (D02.0)
carcinoma in situ of epiglottis suprahyoid portion (D02.0)
carcinoma in situ of skin of lip (D03.0, D04.0)

D00.00 Carcinoma in situ of oral cavity, unspecified site
D00.01 Carcinoma in situ of labial mucosa and vermilion border
D00.02 Carcinoma in situ of buccal mucosa
D00.03 Carcinoma in situ of gingiva and edentulous alveolar ridge
D00.04 Carcinoma in situ of soft palate
D00.05 Carcinoma in situ of hard palate
D00.06 Carcinoma in situ of floor of mouth
D00.07 Carcinoma in situ of tongue
D00.08 Carcinoma in situ of pharynx
Carcinoma in situ of aryepiglottic fold NOS
Carcinoma in situ of hypopharyngeal aspect of aryepiglottic fold
Carcinoma in situ of marginal zone of aryepiglottic fold

D00.1 Carcinoma in situ of esophagus
D00.2 Carcinoma in situ of stomach

4th D01 Carcinoma in situ of other and unspecified digestive organs
EXCLUDES 1 *melanoma in situ (D03.-)*

D01.0 Carcinoma in situ of colon
EXCLUDES 1 *carcinoma in situ of rectosigmoid junction (D01.1)*

D01.1 Carcinoma in situ of rectosigmoid junction
D01.2 Carcinoma in situ of rectum
D01.3 Carcinoma in situ of anus and anal canal
Anal intraepithelial neoplasia III [AIN III]
Severe dysplasia of anus
EXCLUDES 1 *anal intraepithelial neoplasia I and II [AIN I and AIN II] (K62.82)*
carcinoma in situ of anal margin (D04.5)
carcinoma in situ of anal skin (D04.5)
carcinoma in situ of perianal skin (D04.5)

5th D01.4 Carcinoma in situ of other and unspecified parts of intestine
EXCLUDES 1 *carcinoma in situ of ampulla of Vater (D01.5)*

D01.40 Carcinoma in situ of unspecified part of intestine
D01.49 Carcinoma in situ of other parts of intestine

D01.5 Carcinoma in situ of liver, gallbladder and bile ducts
Carcinoma in situ of ampulla of Vater

D01.7 Carcinoma in situ of other specified digestive organs
Carcinoma in situ of pancreas

D01.9 Carcinoma in situ of digestive organ, unspecified

4th D02 Carcinoma in situ of middle ear and respiratory system
Use additional code to identify:
exposure to environmental tobacco smoke (Z77.22)
exposure to tobacco smoke in the perinatal period (P96.81)
history of tobacco dependence (Z87.891)
occupational exposure to environmental tobacco smoke (Z57.31)
tobacco dependence (F17.-)
tobacco use (Z72.0)
EXCLUDES 1 *melanoma in situ (D03.-)*

D02.0 Carcinoma in situ of larynx
Carcinoma in situ of aryepiglottic fold or interarytenoid fold, laryngeal aspect
Carcinoma in situ of epiglottis (suprahyoid portion)
EXCLUDES 1 *carcinoma in situ of aryepiglottic fold or interarytenoid fold NOS (D00.08)*
carcinoma in situ of hypopharyngeal aspect (D00.08)
carcinoma in situ of marginal zone (D00.08)

D02.1 Carcinoma in situ of trachea

5th D02.2 Carcinoma in situ of bronchus and lung
D02.20 Carcinoma in situ of unspecified bronchus and lung
D02.21 Carcinoma in situ of right bronchus and lung
D02.22 Carcinoma in situ of left bronchus and lung

D02.3 Carcinoma in situ of other parts of respiratory system
Carcinoma in situ of accessory sinuses
Carcinoma in situ of middle ear
Carcinoma in situ of nasal cavities
EXCLUDES 1 *carcinoma in situ of ear (external) (skin) (D04.2-)*
carcinoma in situ of nose NOS (D09.8)
carcinoma in situ of skin of nose (D04.3)

D02.4 Carcinoma in situ of respiratory system, unspecified

4th D03 Melanoma in situ
D03.0 Melanoma in situ of lip HCC

5th D03.1 Melanoma in situ of eyelid, including canthus
AHA: 2018,4Q,4
D03.10 Melanoma in situ of unspecified eyelid, including canthus HCC
6th D03.11 Melanoma in situ of right eyelid, including canthus
D03.111 Melanoma in situ of right upper eyelid, including canthus HCC
D03.112 Melanoma in situ of right lower eyelid, including canthus HCC
6th D03.12 Melanoma in situ of left eyelid, including canthus
D03.121 Melanoma in situ of left upper eyelid, including canthus HCC
D03.122 Melanoma in situ of left lower eyelid, including canthus HCC

5th D03.2 Melanoma in situ of ear and external auricular canal
D03.20 Melanoma in situ of unspecified ear and external auricular canal HCC
D03.21 Melanoma in situ of right ear and external auricular canal HCC
D03.22 Melanoma in situ of left ear and external auricular canal HCC

5th D03.3 Melanoma in situ of other and unspecified parts of face
D03.30 Melanoma in situ of unspecified part of face HCC
D03.39 Melanoma in situ of other parts of face HCC

D03.4 Melanoma in situ of scalp and neck HCC

D03.5 Melanoma in situ of trunk

D03.51 Melanoma in situ of anal skin HCC
Melanoma in situ of anal margin
Melanoma in situ of perianal skin

D03.52 Melanoma in situ of breast (skin) (soft tissue) HCC

D03.59 Melanoma in situ of other part of trunk HCC

D03.6 Melanoma in situ of upper limb, including shoulder

D03.60 Melanoma in situ of unspecified upper limb, including shoulder HCC

D03.61 Melanoma in situ of right upper limb, including shoulder HCC

D03.62 Melanoma in situ of left upper limb, including shoulder HCC

D03.7 Melanoma in situ of lower limb, including hip

D03.70 Melanoma in situ of unspecified lower limb, including hip HCC

D03.71 Melanoma in situ of right lower limb, including hip HCC

D03.72 Melanoma in situ of left lower limb, including hip HCC

D03.8 Melanoma in situ of other sites HCC
Melanoma in situ of scrotum
EXCLUDES 1 *carcinoma in situ of scrotum (D07.61)*

D03.9 Melanoma in situ, unspecified HCC

D04 Carcinoma in situ of skin
EXCLUDES 1 *erythroplasia of Queyrat (penis) NOS (D07.4)*
melanoma in situ (D03.-)

D04.0 Carcinoma in situ of skin of lip
EXCLUDES 2 *carcinoma in situ of vermilion border of lip (D00.01)*

D04.1 Carcinoma in situ of skin of eyelid, including canthus
AHA: 2018,4Q,4

D04.10 Carcinoma in situ of skin of unspecified eyelid, including canthus

D04.11 Carcinoma in situ of skin of right eyelid, including canthus

D04.111 Carcinoma in situ of skin of right upper eyelid, including canthus

D04.112 Carcinoma in situ of skin of right lower eyelid, including canthus

D04.12 Carcinoma in situ of skin of left eyelid, including canthus

D04.121 Carcinoma in situ of skin of left upper eyelid, including canthus

D04.122 Carcinoma in situ of skin of left lower eyelid, including canthus

D04.2 Carcinoma in situ of skin of ear and external auricular canal

D04.20 Carcinoma in situ of skin of unspecified ear and external auricular canal

D04.21 Carcinoma in situ of skin of right ear and external auricular canal

D04.22 Carcinoma in situ of skin of left ear and external auricular canal

D04.3 Carcinoma in situ of skin of other and unspecified parts of face

D04.30 Carcinoma in situ of skin of unspecified part of face

D04.39 Carcinoma in situ of skin of other parts of face

D04.4 Carcinoma in situ of skin of scalp and neck

D04.5 Carcinoma in situ of skin of trunk
Carcinoma in situ of anal margin
Carcinoma in situ of anal skin
Carcinoma in situ of perianal skin
Carcinoma in situ of skin of breast
EXCLUDES 1 *carcinoma in situ of anus NOS (D01.3)*
carcinoma in situ of scrotum (D07.61)
carcinoma in situ of skin of genital organs (D07.-)

D04.6 Carcinoma in situ of skin of upper limb, including shoulder

D04.60 Carcinoma in situ of skin of unspecified upper limb, including shoulder

D04.61 Carcinoma in situ of skin of right upper limb, including shoulder

D04.62 Carcinoma in situ of skin of left upper limb, including shoulder

D04.7 Carcinoma in situ of skin of lower limb, including hip

D04.70 Carcinoma in situ of skin of unspecified lower limb, including hip

D04.71 Carcinoma in situ of skin of right lower limb, including hip

D04.72 Carcinoma in situ of skin of left lower limb, including hip

D04.8 Carcinoma in situ of skin of other sites

D04.9 Carcinoma in situ of skin, unspecified

D05 Carcinoma in situ of breast
EXCLUDES 1 *carcinoma in situ of skin of breast (D04.5)*
melanoma in situ of breast (skin) (D03.5)
Paget's disease of breast or nipple (C50.-)

D05.0 Lobular carcinoma in situ of breast

D05.00 Lobular carcinoma in situ of unspecified breast

D05.01 Lobular carcinoma in situ of right breast

D05.02 Lobular carcinoma in situ of left breast

D05.1 Intraductal carcinoma in situ of breast

D05.10 Intraductal carcinoma in situ of unspecified breast

D05.11 Intraductal carcinoma in situ of right breast

D05.12 Intraductal carcinoma in situ of left breast

D05.8 Other specified type of carcinoma in situ of breast

D05.80 Other specified type of carcinoma in situ of unspecified breast

D05.81 Other specified type of carcinoma in situ of right breast

D05.82 Other specified type of carcinoma in situ of left breast

D05.9 Unspecified type of carcinoma in situ of breast

D05.90 Unspecified type of carcinoma in situ of unspecified breast

D05.91 Unspecified type of carcinoma in situ of right breast

D05.92 Unspecified type of carcinoma in situ of left breast

D06 Carcinoma in situ of cervix uteri
INCLUDES cervical adenocarcinoma in situ
cervical intraepithelial glandular neoplasia
cervical intraepithelial neoplasia III [CIN III]
severe dysplasia of cervix uteri
EXCLUDES 1 *cervical intraepithelial neoplasia II [CIN II] (N87.1)*
cytologic evidence of malignancy of cervix without histologic confirmation (R87.614)
high grade squamous intraepithelial lesion (HGSIL) of cervix (R87.613)
melanoma in situ of cervix (D03.5)
moderate cervical dysplasia (N87.1)

D06.0 Carcinoma in situ of endocervix ♀

D06.1 Carcinoma in situ of exocervix ♀

D06.7 Carcinoma in situ of other parts of cervix ♀

D06.9 Carcinoma in situ of cervix, unspecified ♀

D07 Carcinoma in situ of other and unspecified genital organs
EXCLUDES 1 *melanoma in situ of trunk (D03.5)*

D07.0 Carcinoma in situ of endometrium ♀

D07.1 Carcinoma in situ of vulva ♀
Severe dysplasia of vulva
Vulvar intraepithelial neoplasia III [VIN III]
EXCLUDES 1 *moderate dysplasia of vulva (N90.1)*
vulvar intraepithelial neoplasia II [VIN II] (N90.1)

D07.2 Carcinoma in situ of vagina ♀
Severe dysplasia of vagina
Vaginal intraepithelial neoplasia III [VAIN III]
EXCLUDES 1 *moderate dysplasia of vagina (N89.1)*
vaginal intraepithelial neoplasia II [VIN II] (N89.1)

D07.3 Carcinoma in situ of other and unspecified female genital organs

D07.30 Carcinoma in situ of unspecified female genital organs ♀

D07.39 Carcinoma in situ of other female genital organs ♀

D07.4 Carcinoma in situ of penis ♂
Erythroplasia of Queyrat NOS

D07.5 Carcinoma in situ of prostate ♂
Prostatic intraepithelial neoplasia III (PIN III)
Severe dysplasia of prostate
EXCLUDES 1 *dysplasia (mild) (moderate) of prostate (N42.3-)*
prostatic intraepithelial neoplasia II [PIN II] (N42.3-)

D07.6 Carcinoma in situ of other and unspecified male genital organs

D07.60 Carcinoma in situ of unspecified male genital organs ♂

D07.61 Carcinoma in situ of scrotum ♂

D07.69 Carcinoma in situ of other male genital organs ♂

D09 Carcinoma in situ of other and unspecified sites

EXCLUDES 1 *melanoma in situ (D03.-)*

D09.0 Carcinoma in situ of bladder

D09.1 Carcinoma in situ of other and unspecified urinary organs

D09.10 Carcinoma in situ of unspecified urinary organ

D09.19 Carcinoma in situ of other urinary organs

D09.2 Carcinoma in situ of eye

EXCLUDES 1 *carcinoma in situ of skin of eyelid (D04.1-)*

D09.20 Carcinoma in situ of unspecified eye

D09.21 Carcinoma in situ of right eye

D09.22 Carcinoma in situ of left eye

D09.3 Carcinoma in situ of thyroid and other endocrine glands

EXCLUDES 1 *carcinoma in situ of endocrine pancreas (D01.7)*
carcinoma in situ of ovary (D07.39)
carcinoma in situ of testis (D07.69)

D09.8 Carcinoma in situ of other specified sites

D09.9 Carcinoma in situ, unspecified

Benign neoplasms, except benign neuroendocrine tumors (D10-D36)

D10 Benign neoplasm of mouth and pharynx

D10.0 Benign neoplasm of lip

Benign neoplasm of lip (frenulum) (inner aspect) (mucosa) (vermilion border)

EXCLUDES 1 *benign neoplasm of skin of lip (D22.0, D23.0)*

D10.1 Benign neoplasm of tongue

Benign neoplasm of lingual tonsil

D10.2 Benign neoplasm of floor of mouth

D10.3 Benign neoplasm of other and unspecified parts of mouth

D10.30 Benign neoplasm of unspecified part of mouth

D10.39 Benign neoplasm of other parts of mouth

Benign neoplasm of minor salivary gland NOS

EXCLUDES 1 *benign odontogenic neoplasms (D16.4-D16.5)*
benign neoplasm of mucosa of lip (D10.0)
benign neoplasm of nasopharyngeal surface of soft palate (D10.6)

D10.4 Benign neoplasm of tonsil

Benign neoplasm of tonsil (faucial) (palatine)

EXCLUDES 1 *benign neoplasm of lingual tonsil (D10.1)*
benign neoplasm of pharyngeal tonsil (D10.6)
benign neoplasm of tonsillar fossa (D10.5)
benign neoplasm of tonsillar pillars (D10.5)

D10.5 Benign neoplasm of other parts of oropharynx

Benign neoplasm of epiglottis, anterior aspect
Benign neoplasm of tonsillar fossa
Benign neoplasm of tonsillar pillars
Benign neoplasm of vallecula

EXCLUDES 1 *benign neoplasm of epiglottis NOS (D14.1)*
benign neoplasm of epiglottis, suprahyoid portion (D14.1)

DEF: Oropharynx: Middle portion of pharynx (throat); communicates with the oral cavity, nasopharynx and laryngopharynx.

D10.6 Benign neoplasm of nasopharynx

Benign neoplasm of pharyngeal tonsil
Benign neoplasm of posterior margin of septum and choanae

DEF: Nasopharynx: Upper portion of pharynx (throat); communicates with the nasal cavities, oropharynx and tympanic cavities.

D10.7 Benign neoplasm of hypopharynx

DEF: Hypopharynx: Lower portion of pharynx (throat); communicates with the oropharynx and the esophagus. ***Synonym(s):*** *laryngopharynx.*

D10.9 Benign neoplasm of pharynx, unspecified

D11 Benign neoplasm of major salivary glands

EXCLUDES 1 *benign neoplasms of specified minor salivary glands which are classified according to their anatomical location*
benign neoplasms of minor salivary glands NOS (D10.39)

D11.0 Benign neoplasm of parotid gland

D11.7 Benign neoplasm of other major salivary glands

Benign neoplasm of sublingual salivary gland
Benign neoplasm of submandibular salivary gland

D11.9 Benign neoplasm of major salivary gland, unspecified

D12 Benign neoplasm of colon, rectum, anus and anal canal

EXCLUDES 1 *benign carcinoid tumors of the large intestine, and rectum (D3A.02-)*
polyp of colon NOS (K63.5)

AHA: 2018,2Q,14; 2017,1Q,15; 2015,2Q,14

TIP: Code K63.5 Polyp of colon, is assigned when documentation states hyperplastic colon polyps, regardless of the site in the colon. Slow-growing, hyperplastic polyps are not precancerous and are classified differently from benign or adenomatous polyps.

D12.0 Benign neoplasm of cecum

Benign neoplasm of ileocecal valve

D12.1 Benign neoplasm of appendix

EXCLUDES 1 *benign carcinoid tumor of the appendix (D3A.020)*

D12.2 Benign neoplasm of ascending colon

D12.3 Benign neoplasm of transverse colon

Benign neoplasm of hepatic flexure
Benign neoplasm of splenic flexure

AHA: 2017,1Q,16

D12.4 Benign neoplasm of descending colon

D12.5 Benign neoplasm of sigmoid colon

D12.6 Benign neoplasm of colon, unspecified

Adenomatosis of colon
Benign neoplasm of large intestine NOS
Polyposis (hereditary) of colon

EXCLUDES 1 *inflammatory polyp of colon (K51.4-)*

D12.7 Benign neoplasm of rectosigmoid junction

D12.8 Benign neoplasm of rectum

EXCLUDES 1 *benign carcinoid tumor of the rectum (D3A.026)*

AHA: 2018,1Q,6

D12.9 Benign neoplasm of anus and anal canal

Benign neoplasm of anus NOS

EXCLUDES 1 *benign neoplasm of anal margin (D22.5, D23.5)*
benign neoplasm of anal skin (D22.5, D23.5)
benign neoplasm of perianal skin (D22.5, D23.5)

D13 Benign neoplasm of other and ill-defined parts of digestive system

EXCLUDES 1 *benign stromal tumors of digestive system (D21.4)*

D13.0 Benign neoplasm of esophagus

D13.1 Benign neoplasm of stomach

EXCLUDES 1 *benign carcinoid tumor of the stomach (D3A.092)*

D13.2 Benign neoplasm of duodenum

EXCLUDES 1 *benign carcinoid tumor of the duodenum (D3A.010)*

D13.3 Benign neoplasm of other and unspecified parts of small intestine

EXCLUDES 1 *benign carcinoid tumors of the small intestine (D3A.01-)*
benign neoplasm of ileocecal valve (D12.0)

D13.30 Benign neoplasm of unspecified part of small intestine

D13.39 Benign neoplasm of other parts of small intestine

D13.4 Benign neoplasm of liver

Benign neoplasm of intrahepatic bile ducts

D13.5 Benign neoplasm of extrahepatic bile ducts

D13.6 Benign neoplasm of pancreas

EXCLUDES 1 *benign neoplasm of endocrine pancreas (D13.7)*

D13.7 Benign neoplasm of endocrine pancreas

Benign neoplasm of islets of Langerhans
Islet cell tumor

Use additional code to identify any functional activity

D13.9 Benign neoplasm of ill-defined sites within the digestive system

Benign neoplasm of digestive system NOS
Benign neoplasm of intestine NOS
Benign neoplasm of spleen

D14 Benign neoplasm of middle ear and respiratory system

D14.0 Benign neoplasm of middle ear, nasal cavity and accessory sinuses
Benign neoplasm of cartilage of nose
EXCLUDES 1 *benign neoplasm of auricular canal (external) (D22.2-, D23.2-)*
benign neoplasm of bone of ear (D16.4)
benign neoplasm of bone of nose (D16.4)
benign neoplasm of cartilage of ear (D21.0)
benign neoplasm of ear (external)(skin) (D22.2-, D23.2-)
benign neoplasm of nose NOS (D36.7)
benign neoplasm of skin of nose (D22.39, D23.39)
benign neoplasm of olfactory bulb (D33.3)
benign neoplasm of posterior margin of septum and choanae (D10.6)
polyp of accessory sinus (J33.8)
polyp of ear (middle) (H74.4)
polyp of nasal (cavity) (J33.-)

D14.1 Benign neoplasm of larynx
Adenomatous polyp of larynx
Benign neoplasm of epiglottis (suprahyoid portion)
EXCLUDES 1 *benign neoplasm of epiglottis, anterior aspect (D10.5)*
polyp (nonadenomatous) of vocal cord or larynx (J38.1)

D14.2 Benign neoplasm of trachea

D14.3 Benign neoplasm of bronchus and lung
EXCLUDES 1 *benign carcinoid tumor of the bronchus and lung (D3A.090)*

D14.30 Benign neoplasm of unspecified bronchus and lung
D14.31 Benign neoplasm of right bronchus and lung
D14.32 Benign neoplasm of left bronchus and lung

D14.4 Benign neoplasm of respiratory system, unspecified

D15 Benign neoplasm of other and unspecified intrathoracic organs
EXCLUDES 1 *benign neoplasm of mesothelial tissue (D19.-)*

D15.0 Benign neoplasm of thymus
EXCLUDES 1 *benign carcinoid tumor of the thymus (D3A.091)*

D15.1 Benign neoplasm of heart
EXCLUDES 1 *benign neoplasm of great vessels (D21.3)*

D15.2 Benign neoplasm of mediastinum

D15.7 Benign neoplasm of other specified intrathoracic organs

D15.9 Benign neoplasm of intrathoracic organ, unspecified

D16 Benign neoplasm of bone and articular cartilage
EXCLUDES 1 *benign neoplasm of connective tissue of ear (D21.0)*
benign neoplasm of connective tissue of eyelid (D21.0)
benign neoplasm of connective tissue of larynx (D14.1)
benign neoplasm of connective tissue of nose (D14.0)
benign neoplasm of synovia (D21.-)

D16.0 Benign neoplasm of scapula and long bones of upper limb

D16.00 Benign neoplasm of scapula and long bones of unspecified upper limb
D16.01 Benign neoplasm of scapula and long bones of right upper limb
D16.02 Benign neoplasm of scapula and long bones of left upper limb

D16.1 Benign neoplasm of short bones of upper limb

D16.10 Benign neoplasm of short bones of unspecified upper limb
D16.11 Benign neoplasm of short bones of right upper limb
D16.12 Benign neoplasm of short bones of left upper limb

D16.2 Benign neoplasm of long bones of lower limb

D16.20 Benign neoplasm of long bones of unspecified lower limb
D16.21 Benign neoplasm of long bones of right lower limb
D16.22 Benign neoplasm of long bones of left lower limb

D16.3 Benign neoplasm of short bones of lower limb

D16.30 Benign neoplasm of short bones of unspecified lower limb
D16.31 Benign neoplasm of short bones of right lower limb
D16.32 Benign neoplasm of short bones of left lower limb

D16.4 Benign neoplasm of bones of skull and face
Benign neoplasm of maxilla (superior)
Benign neoplasm of orbital bone
Keratocyst of maxilla
Keratocystic odontogenic tumor of maxilla
EXCLUDES 2 *benign neoplasm of lower jaw bone (D16.5)*

D16.5 Benign neoplasm of lower jaw bone
Keratocyst of mandible
Keratocystic odontogenic tumor of mandible

D16.6 Benign neoplasm of vertebral column
EXCLUDES 1 *benign neoplasm of sacrum and coccyx (D16.8)*

D16.7 Benign neoplasm of ribs, sternum and clavicle

D16.8 Benign neoplasm of pelvic bones, sacrum and coccyx

D16.9 Benign neoplasm of bone and articular cartilage, unspecified

D17 Benign lipomatous neoplasm

D17.0 Benign lipomatous neoplasm of skin and subcutaneous tissue of head, face and neck

D17.1 Benign lipomatous neoplasm of skin and subcutaneous tissue of trunk

D17.2 Benign lipomatous neoplasm of skin and subcutaneous tissue of limb

D17.20 Benign lipomatous neoplasm of skin and subcutaneous tissue of unspecified limb
D17.21 Benign lipomatous neoplasm of skin and subcutaneous tissue of right arm
D17.22 Benign lipomatous neoplasm of skin and subcutaneous tissue of left arm
D17.23 Benign lipomatous neoplasm of skin and subcutaneous tissue of right leg
D17.24 Benign lipomatous neoplasm of skin and subcutaneous tissue of left leg

D17.3 Benign lipomatous neoplasm of skin and subcutaneous tissue of other and unspecified sites

D17.30 Benign lipomatous neoplasm of skin and subcutaneous tissue of unspecified sites
D17.39 Benign lipomatous neoplasm of skin and subcutaneous tissue of other sites

D17.4 Benign lipomatous neoplasm of intrathoracic organs

D17.5 Benign lipomatous neoplasm of intra-abdominal organs
EXCLUDES 1 *benign lipomatous neoplasm of peritoneum and retroperitoneum (D17.79)*

D17.6 Benign lipomatous neoplasm of spermatic cord ♂

D17.7 Benign lipomatous neoplasm of other sites

D17.71 Benign lipomatous neoplasm of kidney
D17.72 Benign lipomatous neoplasm of other genitourinary organ
D17.79 Benign lipomatous neoplasm of other sites
Benign lipomatous neoplasm of peritoneum
Benign lipomatous neoplasm of retroperitoneum

D17.9 Benign lipomatous neoplasm, unspecified
Lipoma NOS

D18 Hemangioma and lymphangioma, any site
EXCLUDES 1 *benign neoplasm of glomus jugulare (D35.6)*
blue or pigmented nevus (D22.-)
nevus NOS (D22.-)
vascular nevus (Q82.5)

D18.0 Hemangioma
Angioma NOS
Cavernous nevus
DEF: Common benign tumor usually occurring in infancy that is composed of newly formed blood vessels due to malformation of the angioblastic tissue.

D18.00 Hemangioma unspecified site
D18.01 Hemangioma of skin and subcutaneous tissue
D18.02 Hemangioma of intracranial structures HCC
D18.03 Hemangioma of intra-abdominal structures
D18.09 Hemangioma of other sites

D18.1 Lymphangioma, any site
AHA: 2018,3Q,31; 2018,2Q,13

D19 Benign neoplasm of mesothelial tissue

D19.0 Benign neoplasm of mesothelial tissue of pleura
D19.1 Benign neoplasm of mesothelial tissue of peritoneum
D19.7 Benign neoplasm of mesothelial tissue of other sites
D19.9 Benign neoplasm of mesothelial tissue, unspecified
Benign mesothelioma NOS

D20 Benign neoplasm of soft tissue of retroperitoneum and peritoneum

EXCLUDES 1 *benign lipomatous neoplasm of peritoneum and retroperitoneum (D17.79)*
benign neoplasm of mesothelial tissue (D19.-)

D20.0 Benign neoplasm of soft tissue of retroperitoneum

D20.1 Benign neoplasm of soft tissue of peritoneum

D21 Other benign neoplasms of connective and other soft tissue

INCLUDES benign neoplasm of blood vessel
benign neoplasm of bursa
benign neoplasm of cartilage
benign neoplasm of fascia
benign neoplasm of fat
benign neoplasm of ligament, except uterine
benign neoplasm of lymphatic channel
benign neoplasm of muscle
benign neoplasm of synovia
benign neoplasm of tendon (sheath)
benign stromal tumors

EXCLUDES 1 *benign neoplasm of articular cartilage (D16.-)*
benign neoplasm of cartilage of larynx (D14.1)
benign neoplasm of cartilage of nose (D14.0)
benign neoplasm of connective tissue of breast (D24.-)
benign neoplasm of peripheral nerves and autonomic nervous system (D36.1-)
benign neoplasm of peritoneum (D20.1)
benign neoplasm of retroperitoneum (D20.0)
benign neoplasm of uterine ligament, any (D28.2)
benign neoplasm of vascular tissue (D18.-)
hemangioma (D18.0-)
lipomatous neoplasm (D17.-)
lymphangioma (D18.1)
uterine leiomyoma (D25.-)

D21.0 Benign neoplasm of connective and other soft tissue of head, face and neck

Benign neoplasm of connective tissue of ear
Benign neoplasm of connective tissue of eyelid

EXCLUDES 1 *benign neoplasm of connective tissue of orbit (D31.6-)*

D21.1 Benign neoplasm of connective and other soft tissue of upper limb, including shoulder

D21.10 Benign neoplasm of connective and other soft tissue of unspecified upper limb, including shoulder

D21.11 Benign neoplasm of connective and other soft tissue of right upper limb, including shoulder

D21.12 Benign neoplasm of connective and other soft tissue of left upper limb, including shoulder

D21.2 Benign neoplasm of connective and other soft tissue of lower limb, including hip

D21.20 Benign neoplasm of connective and other soft tissue of unspecified lower limb, including hip

D21.21 Benign neoplasm of connective and other soft tissue of right lower limb, including hip

D21.22 Benign neoplasm of connective and other soft tissue of left lower limb, including hip

D21.3 Benign neoplasm of connective and other soft tissue of thorax

Benign neoplasm of axilla
Benign neoplasm of diaphragm
Benign neoplasm of great vessels

EXCLUDES 1 *benign neoplasm of heart (D15.1)*
benign neoplasm of mediastinum (D15.2)
benign neoplasm of thymus (D15.0)

D21.4 Benign neoplasm of connective and other soft tissue of abdomen

Benign stromal tumors of abdomen

D21.5 Benign neoplasm of connective and other soft tissue of pelvis

EXCLUDES 1 *benign neoplasm of any uterine ligament (D28.2)*
uterine leiomyoma (D25.-)

D21.6 Benign neoplasm of connective and other soft tissue of trunk, unspecified

Benign neoplasm of connective and other soft tissue of back NOS

D21.9 Benign neoplasm of connective and other soft tissue, unspecified

D22 Melanocytic nevi

INCLUDES atypical nevus
blue hairy pigmented nevus
nevus NOS

D22.0 Melanocytic nevi of lip

D22.1 Melanocytic nevi of eyelid, including canthus

AHA: 2018,4Q,4

D22.10 Melanocytic nevi of unspecified eyelid, including canthus

D22.11 Melanocytic nevi of right eyelid, including canthus

D22.111 Melanocytic nevi of right upper eyelid, including canthus

D22.112 Melanocytic nevi of right lower eyelid, including canthus

D22.12 Melanocytic nevi of left eyelid, including canthus

D22.121 Melanocytic nevi of left upper eyelid, including canthus

D22.122 Melanocytic nevi of left lower eyelid, including canthus

D22.2 Melanocytic nevi of ear and external auricular canal

D22.20 Melanocytic nevi of unspecified ear and external auricular canal

D22.21 Melanocytic nevi of right ear and external auricular canal

D22.22 Melanocytic nevi of left ear and external auricular canal

D22.3 Melanocytic nevi of other and unspecified parts of face

D22.30 Melanocytic nevi of unspecified part of face

D22.39 Melanocytic nevi of other parts of face

D22.4 Melanocytic nevi of scalp and neck

D22.5 Melanocytic nevi of trunk

Melanocytic nevi of anal margin
Melanocytic nevi of anal skin
Melanocytic nevi of perianal skin
Melanocytic nevi of skin of breast

D22.6 Melanocytic nevi of upper limb, including shoulder

D22.60 Melanocytic nevi of unspecified upper limb, including shoulder

D22.61 Melanocytic nevi of right upper limb, including shoulder

D22.62 Melanocytic nevi of left upper limb, including shoulder

D22.7 Melanocytic nevi of lower limb, including hip

D22.70 Melanocytic nevi of unspecified lower limb, including hip

D22.71 Melanocytic nevi of right lower limb, including hip

D22.72 Melanocytic nevi of left lower limb, including hip

D22.9 Melanocytic nevi, unspecified

D23 Other benign neoplasms of skin

INCLUDES benign neoplasm of hair follicles
benign neoplasm of sebaceous glands
benign neoplasm of sweat glands

EXCLUDES 1 *benign lipomatous neoplasms of skin (D17.0-D17.3)*

EXCLUDES 2 *melanocytic nevi (D22.-)*

D23.0 Other benign neoplasm of skin of lip

EXCLUDES 1 *benign neoplasm of vermilion border of lip (D10.0)*

D23.1 Other benign neoplasm of skin of eyelid, including canthus

AHA: 2018,4Q,4

D23.10 Other benign neoplasm of skin of unspecified eyelid, including canthus

D23.11 Other benign neoplasm of skin of right eyelid, including canthus

D23.111 Other benign neoplasm of skin of right upper eyelid, including canthus

D23.112 Other benign neoplasm of skin of right lower eyelid, including canthus

D23.12 Other benign neoplasm of skin of left eyelid, including canthus

D23.121 Other benign neoplasm of skin of left upper eyelid, including canthus

D23.122 Other benign neoplasm of skin of left lower eyelid, including canthus

D23.2 Other benign neoplasm of skin of ear and external auricular canal

D23.20 Other benign neoplasm of skin of unspecified ear and external auricular canal

D23.21 **Other benign neoplasm of skin of right ear and external auricular canal**

D23.22 **Other benign neoplasm of skin of left ear and external auricular canal**

5th D23.3 **Other benign neoplasm of skin of other and unspecified parts of face**

D23.30 **Other benign neoplasm of skin of unspecified part of face**

D23.39 **Other benign neoplasm of skin of other parts of face**

D23.4 **Other benign neoplasm of skin of scalp and neck**

D23.5 **Other benign neoplasm of skin of trunk**

Other benign neoplasm of anal margin
Other benign neoplasm of anal skin
Other benign neoplasm of perianal skin
Other benign neoplasm of skin of breast

EXCLUDES 1 *benign neoplasm of anus NOS (D12.9)*

5th D23.6 **Other benign neoplasm of skin of upper limb, including shoulder**

D23.60 **Other benign neoplasm of skin of unspecified upper limb, including shoulder**

D23.61 **Other benign neoplasm of skin of right upper limb, including shoulder**

D23.62 **Other benign neoplasm of skin of left upper limb, including shoulder**

5th D23.7 **Other benign neoplasm of skin of lower limb, including hip**

D23.70 **Other benign neoplasm of skin of unspecified lower limb, including hip**

D23.71 **Other benign neoplasm of skin of right lower limb, including hip**

D23.72 **Other benign neoplasm of skin of left lower limb, including hip**

D23.9 **Other benign neoplasm of skin, unspecified**

4th D24 **Benign neoplasm of breast**

INCLUDES benign neoplasm of connective tissue of breast
benign neoplasm of soft parts of breast
fibroadenoma of breast

EXCLUDES 2 *adenofibrosis of breast (N6Ø.2)*
benign cyst of breast (N6Ø.-)
benign mammary dysplasia (N6Ø.-)
benign neoplasm of skin of breast (D22.5, D23.5)
fibrocystic disease of breast (N6Ø.-)

D24.1 **Benign neoplasm of right breast**

D24.2 **Benign neoplasm of left breast**

D24.9 **Benign neoplasm of unspecified breast**

4th D25 **Leiomyoma of uterus**

INCLUDES uterine fibroid
uterine fibromyoma
uterine myoma

Uterine Leiomyomas (Fibroids)

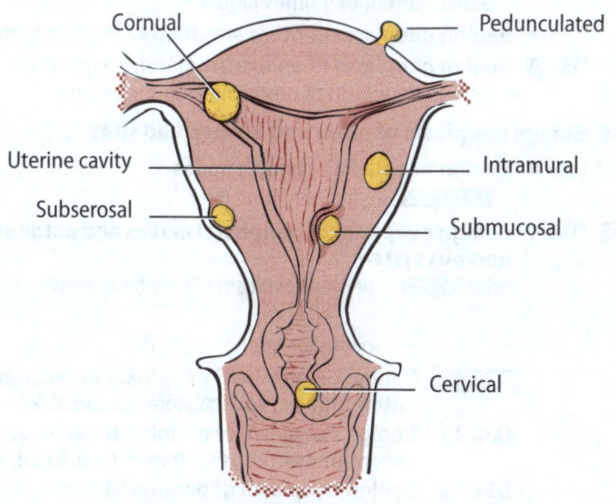

D25.Ø **Submucous leiomyoma of uterus** ♀

D25.1 **Intramural leiomyoma of uterus** ♀
Interstitial leiomyoma of uterus

D25.2 **Subserosal leiomyoma of uterus** ♀
Subperitoneal leiomyoma of uterus

D25.9 **Leiomyoma of uterus, unspecified** ♀

4th D26 **Other benign neoplasms of uterus**

D26.Ø **Other benign neoplasm of cervix uteri** ♀

D26.1 **Other benign neoplasm of corpus uteri** ♀

D26.7 **Other benign neoplasm of other parts of uterus** ♀

D26.9 **Other benign neoplasm of uterus, unspecified** ♀

4th D27 **Benign neoplasm of ovary**

Use additional code to identify any functional activity

EXCLUDES 2 *corpus albicans cyst (N83.2-)*
corpus luteum cyst (N83.1-)
endometrial cyst ▶(N8Ø.1-)◀
follicular (atretic) cyst (N83.Ø-)
graafian follicle cyst (N83.Ø-)
ovarian cyst NEC (N83.2-)
ovarian retention cyst (N83.2-)

D27.Ø **Benign neoplasm of right ovary** ♀

D27.1 **Benign neoplasm of left ovary** ♀

D27.9 **Benign neoplasm of unspecified ovary** ♀

4th D28 **Benign neoplasm of other and unspecified female genital organs**

INCLUDES adenomatous polyp
benign neoplasm of skin of female genital organs
benign teratoma

EXCLUDES 1 *epoophoron cyst (Q5Ø.5)*
fimbrial cyst (Q5Ø.4)
Gartner's duct cyst (Q52.4)
parovarian cyst (Q5Ø.5)

D28.Ø **Benign neoplasm of vulva** ♀

D28.1 **Benign neoplasm of vagina** ♀

D28.2 **Benign neoplasm of uterine tubes and ligaments** ♀
Benign neoplasm of fallopian tube
Benign neoplasm of uterine ligament (broad) (round)

D28.7 **Benign neoplasm of other specified female genital organs** ♀

D28.9 **Benign neoplasm of female genital organ, unspecified** ♀

4th D29 **Benign neoplasm of male genital organs**

INCLUDES benign neoplasm of skin of male genital organs

D29.Ø **Benign neoplasm of penis** ♂

D29.1 **Benign neoplasm of prostate** ♂

EXCLUDES 1 *enlarged prostate (N4Ø.-)*

5th D29.2 **Benign neoplasm of testis**

Use additional code to identify any functional activity

D29.20 **Benign neoplasm of unspecified testis** ♂

D29.21 **Benign neoplasm of right testis** ♂

D29.22 **Benign neoplasm of left testis** ♂

5th D29.3 **Benign neoplasm of epididymis**

D29.30 **Benign neoplasm of unspecified epididymis** ♂

D29.31 **Benign neoplasm of right epididymis** ♂

D29.32 **Benign neoplasm of left epididymis** ♂

D29.4 **Benign neoplasm of scrotum** ♂
Benign neoplasm of skin of scrotum

D29.8 **Benign neoplasm of other specified male genital organs** ♂
Benign neoplasm of seminal vesicle
Benign neoplasm of spermatic cord
Benign neoplasm of tunica vaginalis

D29.9 **Benign neoplasm of male genital organ, unspecified** ♂

4th D3Ø **Benign neoplasm of urinary organs**

5th D3Ø.Ø **Benign neoplasm of kidney**

EXCLUDES 1 *benign carcinoid tumor of the kidney (D3A.Ø93)*
benign neoplasm of renal calyces (D3Ø.1-)
benign neoplasm of renal pelvis (D3Ø.1-)

D3Ø.ØØ **Benign neoplasm of unspecified kidney**

D3Ø.Ø1 **Benign neoplasm of right kidney**

D3Ø.Ø2 **Benign neoplasm of left kidney**

5th D3Ø.1 **Benign neoplasm of renal pelvis**

D3Ø.10 **Benign neoplasm of unspecified renal pelvis**

D3Ø.11 **Benign neoplasm of right renal pelvis**

D3Ø.12 **Benign neoplasm of left renal pelvis**

5th D3Ø.2 **Benign neoplasm of ureter**

EXCLUDES 1 *benign neoplasm of ureteric orifice of bladder (D3Ø.3)*

D3Ø.20 **Benign neoplasm of unspecified ureter**

D3Ø.21 **Benign neoplasm of right ureter**

D3Ø.22 **Benign neoplasm of left ureter**

D30.3 Benign neoplasm of bladder
Benign neoplasm of ureteric orifice of bladder
Benign neoplasm of urethral orifice of bladder

D30.4 Benign neoplasm of urethra
EXCLUDES 1 *benign neoplasm of urethral orifice of bladder (D30.3)*

D30.8 Benign neoplasm of other specified urinary organs
Benign neoplasm of paraurethral glands

D30.9 Benign neoplasm of urinary organ, unspecified
Benign neoplasm of urinary system NOS

D31 Benign neoplasm of eye and adnexa
EXCLUDES 1 *benign neoplasm of connective tissue of eyelid (D21.0)*
benign neoplasm of optic nerve (D33.3)
benign neoplasm of skin of eyelid (D22.1-, D23.1-)

D31.0 Benign neoplasm of conjunctiva
D31.00 Benign neoplasm of unspecified conjunctiva
D31.01 Benign neoplasm of right conjunctiva
D31.02 Benign neoplasm of left conjunctiva

D31.1 Benign neoplasm of cornea
D31.10 Benign neoplasm of unspecified cornea
D31.11 Benign neoplasm of right cornea
D31.12 Benign neoplasm of left cornea

D31.2 Benign neoplasm of retina
EXCLUDES 1 *dark area on retina (D49.81)*
hemangioma of retina (D49.81)
neoplasm of unspecified behavior of retina and choroid (D49.81)
retinal freckle (D49.81)
D31.20 Benign neoplasm of unspecified retina
D31.21 Benign neoplasm of right retina
D31.22 Benign neoplasm of left retina

D31.3 Benign neoplasm of choroid
D31.30 Benign neoplasm of unspecified choroid
D31.31 Benign neoplasm of right choroid
D31.32 Benign neoplasm of left choroid

D31.4 Benign neoplasm of ciliary body
D31.40 Benign neoplasm of unspecified ciliary body
D31.41 Benign neoplasm of right ciliary body
D31.42 Benign neoplasm of left ciliary body

D31.5 Benign neoplasm of lacrimal gland and duct
Benign neoplasm of lacrimal sac
Benign neoplasm of nasolacrimal duct
D31.50 Benign neoplasm of unspecified lacrimal gland and duct
D31.51 Benign neoplasm of right lacrimal gland and duct
D31.52 Benign neoplasm of left lacrimal gland and duct

D31.6 Benign neoplasm of unspecified site of orbit
Benign neoplasm of connective tissue of orbit
Benign neoplasm of extraocular muscle
Benign neoplasm of peripheral nerves of orbit
Benign neoplasm of retrobulbar tissue
Benign neoplasm of retro-ocular tissue
EXCLUDES 1 *benign neoplasm of orbital bone (D16.4)*
D31.60 Benign neoplasm of unspecified site of unspecified orbit
D31.61 Benign neoplasm of unspecified site of right orbit
D31.62 Benign neoplasm of unspecified site of left orbit

D31.9 Benign neoplasm of unspecified part of eye
Benign neoplasm of eyeball
D31.90 Benign neoplasm of unspecified part of unspecified eye
D31.91 Benign neoplasm of unspecified part of right eye
D31.92 Benign neoplasm of unspecified part of left eye

D32 Benign neoplasm of meninges
D32.0 Benign neoplasm of cerebral meninges HCC
D32.1 Benign neoplasm of spinal meninges HCC
D32.9 Benign neoplasm of meninges, unspecified HCC
Meningioma NOS

D33 Benign neoplasm of brain and other parts of central nervous system
EXCLUDES 1 *angioma (D18.0-)*
benign neoplasm of meninges (D32.-)
benign neoplasm of peripheral nerves and autonomic nervous system (D36.1-)
hemangioma (D18.0-)
neurofibromatosis (Q85.0-)
retro-ocular benign neoplasm (D31.6-)

D33.0 Benign neoplasm of brain, supratentorial HCC
Benign neoplasm of cerebral ventricle
Benign neoplasm of cerebrum
Benign neoplasm of frontal lobe
Benign neoplasm of occipital lobe
Benign neoplasm of parietal lobe
Benign neoplasm of temporal lobe
EXCLUDES 1 *benign neoplasm of fourth ventricle (D33.1)*

D33.1 Benign neoplasm of brain, infratentorial HCC
Benign neoplasm of brain stem
Benign neoplasm of cerebellum
Benign neoplasm of fourth ventricle

D33.2 Benign neoplasm of brain, unspecified HCC

D33.3 Benign neoplasm of cranial nerves HCC
Benign neoplasm of olfactory bulb

D33.4 Benign neoplasm of spinal cord HCC

D33.7 Benign neoplasm of other specified parts of central nervous system HCC

D33.9 Benign neoplasm of central nervous system, unspecified HCC
Benign neoplasm of nervous system (central) NOS

D34 Benign neoplasm of thyroid gland
Use additional code to identify any functional activity

D35 Benign neoplasm of other and unspecified endocrine glands
Use additional code to identify any functional activity
EXCLUDES 1 *benign neoplasm of endocrine pancreas (D13.7)*
benign neoplasm of ovary (D27.-)
benign neoplasm of testis (D29.2.-)
benign neoplasm of thymus (D15.0)

D35.0 Benign neoplasm of adrenal gland
D35.00 Benign neoplasm of unspecified adrenal gland
D35.01 Benign neoplasm of right adrenal gland
D35.02 Benign neoplasm of left adrenal gland

D35.1 Benign neoplasm of parathyroid gland

D35.2 Benign neoplasm of pituitary gland HCC
AHA: 2014,3Q,22

D35.3 Benign neoplasm of craniopharyngeal duct HCC

D35.4 Benign neoplasm of pineal gland HCC

D35.5 Benign neoplasm of carotid body

D35.6 Benign neoplasm of aortic body and other paraganglia
Benign tumor of glomus jugulare

D35.7 Benign neoplasm of other specified endocrine glands

D35.9 Benign neoplasm of endocrine gland, unspecified
Benign neoplasm of unspecified endocrine gland

D36 Benign neoplasm of other and unspecified sites

D36.0 Benign neoplasm of lymph nodes
EXCLUDES 1 *lymphangioma (D18.1)*

D36.1 Benign neoplasm of peripheral nerves and autonomic nervous system
EXCLUDES 1 *benign neoplasm of peripheral nerves of orbit (D31.6-)*
neurofibromatosis (Q85.0-)
D36.10 Benign neoplasm of peripheral nerves and autonomic nervous system, unspecified
D36.11 Benign neoplasm of peripheral nerves and autonomic nervous system of face, head, and neck
D36.12 Benign neoplasm of peripheral nerves and autonomic nervous system, upper limb, including shoulder
D36.13 Benign neoplasm of peripheral nerves and autonomic nervous system of lower limb, including hip
D36.14 Benign neoplasm of peripheral nerves and autonomic nervous system of thorax
D36.15 Benign neoplasm of peripheral nerves and autonomic nervous system of abdomen

N Newborn: 0 · P Pediatric: 0-17 · M Maternity: 9-64 · A Adult: 15-124 · UNS Unspecified Site · MCC Major Complication/Comorbidity · CC Complication/Comorbidity

D36.16 Benign neoplasm of peripheral nerves and autonomic nervous system of pelvis

D36.17 Benign neoplasm of peripheral nerves and autonomic nervous system of trunk, unspecified

D36.7 Benign neoplasm of other specified sites
Benign neoplasm of back NOS
Benign neoplasm of nose NOS

D36.9 Benign neoplasm, unspecified site

Benign neuroendocrine tumors (D3A)

D3A Benign neuroendocrine tumors
Code also any associated multiple endocrine neoplasia [MEN] syndromes (E31.2-)
Use additional code to identify any associated endocrine syndrome, such as:
carcinoid syndrome (E34.Ø)
EXCLUDES 2 *benign pancreatic islet cell tumors (D13.7)*

D3A.Ø Benign carcinoid tumors
DEF: Specific type of slow-growing neuroendocrine tumors. Carcinoid tumors occur most commonly in the hormone producing cells of the gastrointestinal tracts and can also occur in the pancreas, testes, ovaries, or lungs.

D3A.ØØ Benign carcinoid tumor of unspecified site
Carcinoid tumor NOS

D3A.Ø1 Benign carcinoid tumors of the small intestine
D3A.Ø1Ø Benign carcinoid tumor of the duodenum
D3A.Ø11 Benign carcinoid tumor of the jejunum
D3A.Ø12 Benign carcinoid tumor of the ileum
D3A.Ø19 Benign carcinoid tumor of the small intestine, unspecified portion

D3A.Ø2 Benign carcinoid tumors of the appendix, large intestine, and rectum
D3A.Ø2Ø Benign carcinoid tumor of the appendix
D3A.Ø21 Benign carcinoid tumor of the cecum
D3A.Ø22 Benign carcinoid tumor of the ascending colon
D3A.Ø23 Benign carcinoid tumor of the transverse colon
D3A.Ø24 Benign carcinoid tumor of the descending colon
D3A.Ø25 Benign carcinoid tumor of the sigmoid colon
D3A.Ø26 Benign carcinoid tumor of the rectum
D3A.Ø29 Benign carcinoid tumor of the large intestine, unspecified portion
Benign carcinoid tumor of the colon NOS

D3A.Ø9 Benign carcinoid tumors of other sites
D3A.Ø9Ø Benign carcinoid tumor of the bronchus and lung
D3A.Ø91 Benign carcinoid tumor of the thymus
D3A.Ø92 Benign carcinoid tumor of the stomach
D3A.Ø93 Benign carcinoid tumor of the kidney
D3A.Ø94 Benign carcinoid tumor of the foregut, unspecified
D3A.Ø95 Benign carcinoid tumor of the midgut, unspecified
D3A.Ø96 Benign carcinoid tumor of the hindgut, unspecified
D3A.Ø98 Benign carcinoid tumors of other sites

D3A.8 Other benign neuroendocrine tumors
Neuroendocrine tumor NOS

Neoplasms of uncertain behavior, polycythemia vera and myelodysplastic syndromes (D37-D48)

NOTE Categories D37-D44, and D48 classify by site neoplasms of uncertain behavior, i.e., histologic confirmation whether the neoplasm is malignant or benign cannot be made.
EXCLUDES 1 *neoplasms of unspecified behavior (D49.-)*

D37 Neoplasm of uncertain behavior of oral cavity and digestive organs
EXCLUDES 1 *stromal tumors of uncertain behavior of digestive system (D48.1)*

D37.Ø Neoplasm of uncertain behavior of lip, oral cavity and pharynx
EXCLUDES 1 *neoplasm of uncertain behavior of aryepiglottic fold or interarytenoid fold, laryngeal aspect (D38.Ø)*
neoplasm of uncertain behavior of epiglottis NOS (D38.Ø)
neoplasm of uncertain behavior of skin of lip (D48.5)
neoplasm of uncertain behavior of suprahyoid portion of epiglottis (D38.Ø)

D37.Ø1 Neoplasm of uncertain behavior of lip
Neoplasm of uncertain behavior of vermilion border of lip

D37.Ø2 Neoplasm of uncertain behavior of tongue

D37.Ø3 Neoplasm of uncertain behavior of the major salivary glands
D37.Ø3Ø Neoplasm of uncertain behavior of the parotid salivary glands
D37.Ø31 Neoplasm of uncertain behavior of the sublingual salivary glands
D37.Ø32 Neoplasm of uncertain behavior of the submandibular salivary glands
D37.Ø39 Neoplasm of uncertain behavior of the major salivary glands, unspecified

D37.Ø4 Neoplasm of uncertain behavior of the minor salivary glands
Neoplasm of uncertain behavior of submucosal salivary glands of lip
Neoplasm of uncertain behavior of submucosal salivary glands of cheek
Neoplasm of uncertain behavior of submucosal salivary glands of hard palate
Neoplasm of uncertain behavior of submucosal salivary glands of soft palate

D37.Ø5 Neoplasm of uncertain behavior of pharynx
Neoplasm of uncertain behavior of aryepiglottic fold of pharynx NOS
Neoplasm of uncertain behavior of hypopharyngeal aspect of aryepiglottic fold of pharynx
Neoplasm of uncertain behavior of marginal zone of aryepiglottic fold of pharynx

D37.Ø9 Neoplasm of uncertain behavior of other specified sites of the oral cavity

D37.1 Neoplasm of uncertain behavior of stomach

D37.2 Neoplasm of uncertain behavior of small intestine

D37.3 Neoplasm of uncertain behavior of appendix

D37.4 Neoplasm of uncertain behavior of colon

D37.5 Neoplasm of uncertain behavior of rectum
Neoplasm of uncertain behavior of rectosigmoid junction

D37.6 Neoplasm of uncertain behavior of liver, gallbladder and bile ducts
Neoplasm of uncertain behavior of ampulla of Vater

D37.8 Neoplasm of uncertain behavior of other specified digestive organs
Neoplasm of uncertain behavior of anal canal
Neoplasm of uncertain behavior of anal sphincter
Neoplasm of uncertain behavior of anus NOS
Neoplasm of uncertain behavior of esophagus
Neoplasm of uncertain behavior of intestine NOS
Neoplasm of uncertain behavior of pancreas
EXCLUDES 1 *neoplasm of uncertain behavior of anal margin (D48.5)*
neoplasm of uncertain behavior of anal skin (D48.5)
neoplasm of uncertain behavior of perianal skin (D48.5)

D37.9 Neoplasm of uncertain behavior of digestive organ, unspecified

Chapter 2. Neoplasms

4th D38 Neoplasm of uncertain behavior of middle ear and respiratory and intrathoracic organs

EXCLUDES 1 *neoplasm of uncertain behavior of heart (D48.7)*

D38.Ø Neoplasm of uncertain behavior of larynx

Neoplasm of uncertain behavior of aryepiglottic fold or interarytenoid fold, laryngeal aspect

Neoplasm of uncertain behavior of epiglottis (suprahyoid portion)

EXCLUDES 1 *neoplasm of uncertain behavior of aryepiglottic fold or interarytenoid fold NOS (D37.Ø5)*

neoplasm of uncertain behavior of hypopharyngeal aspect of aryepiglottic fold (D37.Ø5)

neoplasm of uncertain behavior of marginal zone of aryepiglottic fold (D37.Ø5)

D38.1 Neoplasm of uncertain behavior of trachea, bronchus and lung

D38.2 Neoplasm of uncertain behavior of pleura

D38.3 Neoplasm of uncertain behavior of mediastinum

D38.4 Neoplasm of uncertain behavior of thymus

D38.5 Neoplasm of uncertain behavior of other respiratory organs

Neoplasm of uncertain behavior of accessory sinuses

Neoplasm of uncertain behavior of cartilage of nose

Neoplasm of uncertain behavior of middle ear

Neoplasm of uncertain behavior of nasal cavities

EXCLUDES 1 *neoplasm of uncertain behavior of ear (external) (skin) (D48.5)*

neoplasm of uncertain behavior of nose NOS (D48.7)

neoplasm of uncertain behavior of skin of nose (D48.5)

D38.6 Neoplasm of uncertain behavior of respiratory organ, unspecified UNS

4th D39 Neoplasm of uncertain behavior of female genital organs

D39.Ø Neoplasm of uncertain behavior of uterus ♀

5th D39.1 Neoplasm of uncertain behavior of ovary

Use additional code to identify any functional activity

D39.1Ø Neoplasm of uncertain behavior of unspecified ovary ♀

D39.11 Neoplasm of uncertain behavior of right ovary ♀

D39.12 Neoplasm of uncertain behavior of left ovary ♀

D39.2 Neoplasm of uncertain behavior of placenta M ♀

Chorioadenoma destruens

Invasive hydatidiform mole

Malignant hydatidiform mole

EXCLUDES 1 *hydatidiform mole NOS (OØ1.9)*

D39.8 Neoplasm of uncertain behavior of other specified female genital organs ♀

Neoplasm of uncertain behavior of skin of female genital organs

D39.9 Neoplasm of uncertain behavior of female genital organ, unspecified ♀

4th D4Ø Neoplasm of uncertain behavior of male genital organs

D4Ø.Ø Neoplasm of uncertain behavior of prostate ♂

5th D4Ø.1 Neoplasm of uncertain behavior of testis

D4Ø.1Ø Neoplasm of uncertain behavior of unspecified testis ♂

D4Ø.11 Neoplasm of uncertain behavior of right testis ♂

D4Ø.12 Neoplasm of uncertain behavior of left testis ♂

D4Ø.8 Neoplasm of uncertain behavior of other specified male genital organs ♂

Neoplasm of uncertain behavior of skin of male genital organs

D4Ø.9 Neoplasm of uncertain behavior of male genital organ, unspecified ♂

4th D41 Neoplasm of uncertain behavior of urinary organs

5th D41.Ø Neoplasm of uncertain behavior of kidney

EXCLUDES 1 *neoplasm of uncertain behavior of renal pelvis (D41.1-)*

D41.ØØ Neoplasm of uncertain behavior of unspecified kidney

D41.Ø1 Neoplasm of uncertain behavior of right kidney

D41.Ø2 Neoplasm of uncertain behavior of left kidney

5th D41.1 Neoplasm of uncertain behavior of renal pelvis

D41.1Ø Neoplasm of uncertain behavior of unspecified renal pelvis

D41.11 Neoplasm of uncertain behavior of right renal pelvis

D41.12 Neoplasm of uncertain behavior of left renal pelvis

5th D41.2 Neoplasm of uncertain behavior of ureter

D41.2Ø Neoplasm of uncertain behavior of unspecified ureter

D41.21 Neoplasm of uncertain behavior of right ureter

D41.22 Neoplasm of uncertain behavior of left ureter

D41.3 Neoplasm of uncertain behavior of urethra

D41.4 Neoplasm of uncertain behavior of bladder

D41.8 Neoplasm of uncertain behavior of other specified urinary organs

D41.9 Neoplasm of uncertain behavior of unspecified urinary organ

4th D42 Neoplasm of uncertain behavior of meninges

D42.Ø Neoplasm of uncertain behavior of cerebral meninges HCC

D42.1 Neoplasm of uncertain behavior of spinal meninges HCC

D42.9 Neoplasm of uncertain behavior of meninges, unspecified HCC

4th D43 Neoplasm of uncertain behavior of brain and central nervous system

EXCLUDES 1 *neoplasm of uncertain behavior of peripheral nerves and autonomic nervous system (D48.2)*

D43.Ø Neoplasm of uncertain behavior of brain, supratentorial HCC

Neoplasm of uncertain behavior of cerebral ventricle

Neoplasm of uncertain behavior of cerebrum

Neoplasm of uncertain behavior of frontal lobe

Neoplasm of uncertain behavior of occipital lobe

Neoplasm of uncertain behavior of parietal lobe

Neoplasm of uncertain behavior of temporal lobe

EXCLUDES 1 *neoplasm of uncertain behavior of fourth ventricle (D43.1)*

D43.1 Neoplasm of uncertain behavior of brain, infratentorial HCC

Neoplasm of uncertain behavior of brain stem

Neoplasm of uncertain behavior of cerebellum

Neoplasm of uncertain behavior of fourth ventricle

D43.2 Neoplasm of uncertain behavior of brain, unspecified HCC

D43.3 Neoplasm of uncertain behavior of cranial nerves HCC

D43.4 Neoplasm of uncertain behavior of spinal cord HCC

D43.8 Neoplasm of uncertain behavior of other specified parts of central nervous system HCC

D43.9 Neoplasm of uncertain behavior of central nervous system, unspecified HCC

Neoplasm of uncertain behavior of nervous system (central) NOS

4th D44 Neoplasm of uncertain behavior of endocrine glands

EXCLUDES 1 *multiple endocrine adenomatosis (E31.2-)*

multiple endocrine neoplasia (E31.2-)

neoplasm of uncertain behavior of endocrine pancreas (D37.8)

neoplasm of uncertain behavior of ovary (D39.1-)

neoplasm of uncertain behavior of testis (D4Ø.1-)

neoplasm of uncertain behavior of thymus (D38.4)

D44.Ø Neoplasm of uncertain behavior of thyroid gland

5th D44.1 Neoplasm of uncertain behavior of adrenal gland

Use additional code to identify any functional activity

D44.1Ø Neoplasm of uncertain behavior of unspecified adrenal gland

D44.11 Neoplasm of uncertain behavior of right adrenal gland

D44.12 Neoplasm of uncertain behavior of left adrenal gland

D44.2 Neoplasm of uncertain behavior of parathyroid gland

D44.3 Neoplasm of uncertain behavior of pituitary gland HCC

Use additional code to identify any functional activity

D44.4 Neoplasm of uncertain behavior of craniopharyngeal duct HCC

D44.5 Neoplasm of uncertain behavior of pineal gland HCC

D44.6 Neoplasm of uncertain behavior of carotid body HCC

D44.7 Neoplasm of uncertain behavior of aortic body and other paraganglia HCC

AHA: 2021,2Q,7; 2016,4Q,26

D44.9 Neoplasm of uncertain behavior of unspecified endocrine gland UNS

D45 Polycythemia vera HCC

EXCLUDES 1 *familial polycythemia (D75.Ø)*
secondary polycythemia (D75.1)

DEF: Abnormal proliferation of all bone marrow elements, increased red cell mass, and total blood volume. The etiology is unknown, but it is frequently associated with splenomegaly, leukocytosis, and thrombocythemia.

4th **D46 Myelodysplastic syndromes**

Use additional code for adverse effect, if applicable, to identify drug (T36-T5Ø with fifth or sixth character 5)

EXCLUDES 2 *drug-induced aplastic anemia (D61.1)*

D46.Ø Refractory anemia without ring sideroblasts, so stated HCC
Refractory anemia without sideroblasts, without excess of blasts

D46.1 Refractory anemia with ring sideroblasts HCC
RARS

5th **D46.2 Refractory anemia with excess of blasts [RAEB]**

D46.2Ø Refractory anemia with excess of blasts, unspecified HCC
RAEB NOS

D46.21 Refractory anemia with excess of blasts 1 HCC
RAEB 1

D46.22 Refractory anemia with excess of blasts 2 CC HCC
RAEB 2

D46.A Refractory cytopenia with multilineage dysplasia HCC

D46.B Refractory cytopenia with multilineage dysplasia and ring sideroblasts HCC
RCMD RS

D46.C Myelodysplastic syndrome with isolated del(5q) chromosomal abnormality CC HCC
Myelodysplastic syndrome with 5q deletion
5q minus syndrome NOS

D46.4 Refractory anemia, unspecified HCC

D46.Z Other myelodysplastic syndromes HCC

EXCLUDES 1 *chronic myelomonocytic leukemia (C93.1-)*

D46.9 Myelodysplastic syndrome, unspecified HCC
Myelodysplasia NOS

4th **D47 Other neoplasms of uncertain behavior of lymphoid, hematopoietic and related tissue**

5th **D47.Ø Mast cell neoplasms of uncertain behavior**

EXCLUDES 1 *congenital cutaneous mastocytosis (Q82.2)*
histiocytic neoplasms of uncertain behavior (D47.Z9)
malignant mast cell neoplasm (C96.2-)

AHA: 2017,4Q,5

D47.Ø1 Cutaneous mastocytosis CC
Diffuse cutaneous mastocytosis
Maculopapular cutaneous mastocytosis
Solitary mastocytoma
Telangiectasia macularis eruptiva perstans
Urticaria pigmentosa

EXCLUDES 1 *congenital (diffuse) (maculopapular) cutaneous mastocytosis (Q82.2)*
congenital urticaria pigmentosa (Q82.2)
extracutaneous mastocytoma (D47.Ø9)

D47.Ø2 Systemic mastocytosis CC
Indolent systemic mastocytosis
Isolated bone marrow mastocytosis
Smoldering systemic mastocytosis
Systemic mastocytosis, with an associated hematological non-mast cell lineage disease (SM-AHNMD)

Code also, if applicable, any associated hematological non-mast cell lineage disease, such as:
acute myeloid leukemia (C92.6-, C92.A-)
chronic myelomonocytic leukemia (C93.1-)
essential thrombocytosis (D47.3)
hypereosinophilic syndrome (D72.1)
myelodysplastic syndrome (D46.9)
myeloproliferative syndrome (D47.1)
non-Hodgkin lymphoma (C82-C85)
plasma cell myeloma (C9Ø.Ø-)
polycythemia vera (D45)

EXCLUDES 1 *aggressive systemic mastocytosis (C96.21)*
mast cell leukemia (C94.3-)

D47.Ø9 Other mast cell neoplasms of uncertain behavior CC
Extracutaneous mastocytoma
Mast cell tumor NOS
Mastocytoma NOS
Mastocytosis NOS

D47.1 Chronic myeloproliferative disease CC HCC
Chronic neutrophilic leukemia
Myeloproliferative disease, unspecified

EXCLUDES 1 *atypical chronic myeloid leukemia BCR/ABL-negative (C92.2-)*
chronic myeloid leukemia BCR/ABL-positive (C92.1-)
myelofibrosis NOS (D75.81)
myelophthisic anemia (D61.82)
myelophthisis (D61.82)
secondary myelofibrosis NOS (D75.81)

D47.2 Monoclonal gammopathy
Monoclonal gammopathy of undetermined significance [MGUS]

AHA: 2021,3Q,5

TIP: Smoldering multiple myeloma (SMM) is coded here.

D47.3 Essential (hemorrhagic) thrombocythemia HCC
Essential thrombocytosis
Idiopathic hemorrhagic thrombocythemia
Primary thrombocytosis

EXCLUDES 2 *reactive thrombocytosis (D75.838)*
secondary thrombocytosis (D75.838)
thrombocythemia NOS (D75.839)
thrombocytosis NOS (D75.839)

DEF: Chronic myeloproliferative neoplasm involving production of excess blood platelets that may result in abnormal clotting or hemorrhaging.

D47.4 Osteomyelofibrosis HCC
Chronic idiopathic myelofibrosis
Myelofibrosis (idiopathic) (with myeloid metaplasia)
Myelosclerosis (megakaryocytic) with myeloid metaplasia
Secondary myelofibrosis in myeloproliferative disease

EXCLUDES 1 *acute myelofibrosis (C94.4-)*

5th **D47.Z Other specified neoplasms of uncertain behavior of lymphoid, hematopoietic and related tissue**

AHA: 2016,4Q,8

D47.Z1 Post-transplant lymphoproliferative disorder (PTLD) CC UPD HCC

Code first complications of transplanted organs and tissue (T86.-)

DEF: Excessive proliferation of B-cell lymphocytes following Epstein-Barr virus infection in organ transplant patients. It may progress to non-Hodgkin lymphoma.

D47.Z2 Castleman disease CC HCC

Code also, if applicable, human herpesvirus 8 infection (B1Ø.89)

EXCLUDES 2 *Kaposi's sarcoma (C46.-)*

DEF: Rare disease of the lymph nodes and lymphoid tissues that closely mimics lymphoma.

D47.Z9 Other specified neoplasms of uncertain behavior of lymphoid, hematopoietic and related tissue CC HCC
Histiocytic tumors of uncertain behavior

D47.9 Neoplasm of uncertain behavior of lymphoid, hematopoietic and related tissue, unspecified CC HCC
Lymphoproliferative disease NOS

4th **D48 Neoplasm of uncertain behavior of other and unspecified sites**

EXCLUDES 1 *neurofibromatosis (nonmalignant) (Q85.Ø-)*

D48.Ø Neoplasm of uncertain behavior of bone and articular cartilage

EXCLUDES 1 *neoplasm of uncertain behavior of cartilage of ear (D48.1)*
neoplasm of uncertain behavior of cartilage of larynx (D38.Ø)
neoplasm of uncertain behavior of cartilage of nose (D38.5)
neoplasm of uncertain behavior of connective tissue of eyelid (D48.1)
neoplasm of uncertain behavior of synovia (D48.1)

D48.1 Neoplasm of uncertain behavior of connective and other soft tissue

Neoplasm of uncertain behavior of connective tissue of ear
Neoplasm of uncertain behavior of connective tissue of eyelid
Stromal tumors of uncertain behavior of digestive system

EXCLUDES 1 *neoplasm of uncertain behavior of articular cartilage (D48.Ø)*
neoplasm of uncertain behavior of cartilage of larynx (D38.Ø)
neoplasm of uncertain behavior of cartilage of nose (D38.5)
neoplasm of uncertain behavior of connective tissue of breast (D48.6-)

D48.2 Neoplasm of uncertain behavior of peripheral nerves and autonomic nervous system

EXCLUDES 1 *neoplasm of uncertain behavior of peripheral nerves of orbit (D48.7)*

D48.3 Neoplasm of uncertain behavior of retroperitoneum

D48.4 Neoplasm of uncertain behavior of peritoneum

D48.5 Neoplasm of uncertain behavior of skin

Neoplasm of uncertain behavior of anal margin
Neoplasm of uncertain behavior of anal skin
Neoplasm of uncertain behavior of perianal skin
Neoplasm of uncertain behavior of skin of breast

EXCLUDES 1 *neoplasm of uncertain behavior of anus NOS (D37.8)*
neoplasm of uncertain behavior of skin of genital organs (D39.8, D4Ø.8)
neoplasm of uncertain behavior of vermilion border of lip (D37.Ø)

√5th **D48.6 Neoplasm of uncertain behavior of breast**

Neoplasm of uncertain behavior of connective tissue of breast
Cystosarcoma phyllodes

EXCLUDES 1 *neoplasm of uncertain behavior of skin of breast (D48.5)*

D48.6Ø Neoplasm of uncertain behavior of unspecified breast

D48.61 Neoplasm of uncertain behavior of right breast

D48.62 Neoplasm of uncertain behavior of left breast

D48.7 Neoplasm of uncertain behavior of other specified sites

Neoplasm of uncertain behavior of eye
Neoplasm of uncertain behavior of heart
Neoplasm of uncertain behavior of peripheral nerves of orbit

EXCLUDES 1 *neoplasm of uncertain behavior of connective tissue (D48.1)*
neoplasm of uncertain behavior of skin of eyelid (D48.5)

D48.9 Neoplasm of uncertain behavior, unspecified

Neoplasms of unspecified behavior (D49)

√4th **D49 Neoplasms of unspecified behavior**

NOTE Category D49 classifies by site neoplasms of unspecified morphology and behavior. The term "mass", unless otherwise stated, is not to be regarded as a neoplastic growth.

INCLUDES "growth" NOS
neoplasm NOS
new growth NOS
tumor NOS

EXCLUDES 1 *neoplasms of uncertain behavior (D37-D44, D48)*

D49.Ø Neoplasm of unspecified behavior of digestive system

EXCLUDES 1 *neoplasm of unspecified behavior of margin of anus (D49.2)*
neoplasm of unspecified behavior of perianal skin (D49.2)
neoplasm of unspecified behavior of skin of anus (D49.2)

D49.1 Neoplasm of unspecified behavior of respiratory system

D49.2 Neoplasm of unspecified behavior of bone, soft tissue, and skin

EXCLUDES 1 *neoplasm of unspecified behavior of anal canal (D49.Ø)*
neoplasm of unspecified behavior of anus NOS (D49.Ø)
neoplasm of unspecified behavior of bone marrow (D49.89)
neoplasm of unspecified behavior of cartilage of larynx (D49.1)
neoplasm of unspecified behavior of cartilage of nose (D49.1)
neoplasm of unspecified behavior of connective tissue of breast (D49.3)
neoplasm of unspecified behavior of skin of genital organs (D49.59)
neoplasm of unspecified behavior of vermilion border of lip (D49.Ø)

D49.3 Neoplasm of unspecified behavior of breast

EXCLUDES 1 *neoplasm of unspecified behavior of skin of breast (D49.2)*

D49.4 Neoplasm of unspecified behavior of bladder

√5th **D49.5 Neoplasm of unspecified behavior of other genitourinary organs**

AHA: 2016,4Q,9

√6th **D49.51 Neoplasm of unspecified behavior of kidney**

D49.511 Neoplasm of unspecified behavior of right kidney

D49.512 Neoplasm of unspecified behavior of left kidney

D49.519 Neoplasm of unspecified behavior of unspecified kidney

D49.59 Neoplasm of unspecified behavior of other genitourinary organ

D49.6 Neoplasm of unspecified behavior of brain HCC

EXCLUDES 1 *neoplasm of unspecified behavior of cerebral meninges (D49.7)*
neoplasm of unspecified behavior of cranial nerves (D49.7)

D49.7 Neoplasm of unspecified behavior of endocrine glands and other parts of nervous system

EXCLUDES 1 *neoplasm of unspecified behavior of peripheral, sympathetic, and parasympathetic nerves and ganglia (D49.2)*

√5th **D49.8 Neoplasm of unspecified behavior of other specified sites**

EXCLUDES 1 *neoplasm of unspecified behavior of eyelid (skin) (D49.2)*
neoplasm of unspecified behavior of eyelid cartilage (D49.2)
neoplasm of unspecified behavior of great vessels (D49.2)
neoplasm of unspecified behavior of optic nerve (D49.7)

D49.81 Neoplasm of unspecified behavior of retina and choroid

Dark area on retina
Retinal freckle

D49.89 Neoplasm of unspecified behavior of other specified sites

D49.9 Neoplasm of unspecified behavior of unspecified site

N Newborn: 0 P Pediatric: 0-17 M Maternity: 9-64 A Adult: 15-124 UNS Unspecified Site MCC Major Complication/Comorbidity CC Complication/Comorbidity

Chapter 3. Diseases of the Blood and Blood-forming Organs and Certain Disorders Involving the Immune Mechanism (D5Ø–D89)

Chapter-specific Guidelines with Coding Examples

Reserved for future guideline expansion

Chapter 3. Diseases of the Blood and Blood-forming Organs and Certain Disorders Involving the Immune Mechanism (D5Ø-D89)

EXCLUDES 2 *autoimmune disease (systemic) NOS (M35.9)*
certain conditions originating in the perinatal period (PØØ-P96)
complications of pregnancy, childbirth and the puerperium (OØØ-O9A)
congenital malformations, deformations and chromosomal abnormalities (QØØ-Q99)
endocrine, nutritional and metabolic diseases (EØØ-E88)
human immunodeficiency virus [HIV] disease (B2Ø)
injury, poisoning and certain other consequences of external causes (SØØ-T88)
neoplasms (CØØ-D49)
symptoms, signs and abnormal clinical and laboratory findings, not elsewhere classified (RØØ-R94)

This chapter contains the following blocks:

D5Ø-D53 Nutritional anemias
D55-D59 Hemolytic anemias
D6Ø-D64 Aplastic and other anemias and other bone marrow failure syndromes
D65-D69 Coagulation defects, purpura and other hemorrhagic conditions
D7Ø-D77 Other disorders of blood and blood-forming organs
D78 Intraoperative and postprocedural complications of the spleen
D8Ø-D89 Certain disorders involving the immune mechanism

Nutritional anemias (D5Ø-D53)

DEF: Nutritional anemia: The result of inadequate intake or absorption of a vitamin or mineral that impacts the production of red blood cells or causes them to develop abnormally affecting the size and shape.
TIP: Documentation must identify a link between anemia and the nutritional deficiency; low levels of a particular nutrient may occur concurrently with anemia but not cause the anemia.

✓4th **D5Ø Iron deficiency anemia**
INCLUDES asiderotic anemia
hypochromic anemia

D5Ø.Ø Iron deficiency anemia secondary to blood loss (chronic)
Posthemorrhagic anemia (chronic)
EXCLUDES 1 *acute posthemorrhagic anemia (D62)*
congenital anemia from fetal blood loss (P61.3)
AHA: 2019,3Q,17

D5Ø.1 Sideropenic dysphagia
Kelly-Paterson syndrome
Plummer-Vinson syndrome

D5Ø.8 Other iron deficiency anemias
Iron deficiency anemia due to inadequate dietary iron intake

D5Ø.9 Iron deficiency anemia, unspecified

✓4th **D51 Vitamin B12 deficiency anemia**
EXCLUDES 1 *vitamin B12 deficiency (E53.8)*

D51.Ø Vitamin B12 deficiency anemia due to intrinsic factor deficiency
Addison anemia
Biermer anemia
Pernicious (congenital) anemia
Congenital intrinsic factor deficiency
DEF: Chronic progressive anemia due to vitamin B12 malabsorption, caused by lack of secretion of intrinsic factor, which is produced by the gastric mucosa of the stomach.

D51.1 Vitamin B12 deficiency anemia due to selective vitamin B12 malabsorption with proteinuria
Imerslund (Gräsbeck) syndrome
Megaloblastic hereditary anemia

D51.2 Transcobalamin II deficiency

D51.3 Other dietary vitamin B12 deficiency anemia
Vegan anemia

D51.8 Other vitamin B12 deficiency anemias

D51.9 Vitamin B12 deficiency anemia, unspecified

✓4th **D52 Folate deficiency anemia**
EXCLUDES 1 *folate deficiency without anemia (E53.8)*
DEF: Deficiency in a B complex vitamin needed for the production of healthy red blood cells. Lack of folate, or folic acid, and other absorption conditions can cause anemia resulting in large, misshapen red blood cells called megaloblasts.

D52.Ø Dietary folate deficiency anemia
Nutritional megaloblastic anemia
DEF: Result of a poor diet with inadequate intake of folate, which is needed to produce healthy red blood cells.

D52.1 Drug-induced folate deficiency anemia
Use additional code for adverse effect, if applicable, to identify drug (T36-T5Ø with fifth or sixth character 5)

D52.8 Other folate deficiency anemias

D52.9 Folate deficiency anemia, unspecified
Folic acid deficiency anemia NOS

✓4th **D53 Other nutritional anemias**
INCLUDES megaloblastic anemia unresponsive to vitamin B12 or folate therapy

D53.Ø Protein deficiency anemia
Amino-acid deficiency anemia
Orotaciduric anemia
EXCLUDES 1 *Lesch-Nyhan syndrome (E79.1)*

D53.1 Other megaloblastic anemias, not elsewhere classified
Megaloblastic anemia NOS
EXCLUDES 1 *Di Guglielmo's disease (C94.Ø)*

D53.2 Scorbutic anemia
EXCLUDES 1 *scurvy (E54)*

D53.8 Other specified nutritional anemias
Anemia associated with deficiency of copper
Anemia associated with deficiency of molybdenum
Anemia associated with deficiency of zinc
EXCLUDES 1 *nutritional deficiencies without anemia, such as:*
copper deficiency NOS (E61.Ø)
molybdenum deficiency NOS (E61.5)
zinc deficiency NOS (E6Ø)

D53.9 Nutritional anemia, unspecified
Simple chronic anemia
EXCLUDES 1 *anemia NOS (D64.9)*
AHA: 2018,4Q,88

Hemolytic anemias (D55-D59)

✓4th **D55 Anemia due to enzyme disorders**
EXCLUDES 1 *drug-induced enzyme deficiency anemia (D59.2)*

D55.Ø Anemia due to glucose-6-phosphate dehydrogenase [G6PD] deficiency HCC
Favism
G6PD deficiency anemia
EXCLUDES 1 *glucose-6-phosphate dehydrogenase (G6PD) deficiency without anemia (D75.A)*

D55.1 Anemia due to other disorders of glutathione metabolism HCC
Anemia (due to) enzyme deficiencies, except G6PD, related to the hexose monophosphate [HMP] shunt pathway
Anemia (due to) hemolytic nonspherocytic (hereditary), type I

✓5th **D55.2 Anemia due to disorders of glycolytic enzymes**
EXCLUDES 1 *disorders of glycolysis not associated with anemia (E74.81-)*
AHA: 2021,4Q,6-7

D55.21 Anemia due to pyruvate kinase deficiency HCC
PK deficiency anemia
Pyruvate kinase deficiency anemia

D55.29 Anemia due to other disorders of glycolytic enzymes HCC
Hexokinase deficiency anemia
Triose-phosphate isomerase deficiency anemia

D55.3 Anemia due to disorders of nucleotide metabolism HCC

D55.8 Other anemias due to enzyme disorders HCC

D55.9 Anemia due to enzyme disorder, unspecified HCC

D56 Thalassemia

EXCLUDES 1 *sickle-cell thalassemia (D57.4-)*

DEF: Group of inherited disorders of hemoglobin metabolism causing mild to severe anemia. It is usually found in people of Mediterranean, African, Chinese, or Asian descent.

Thalassemia

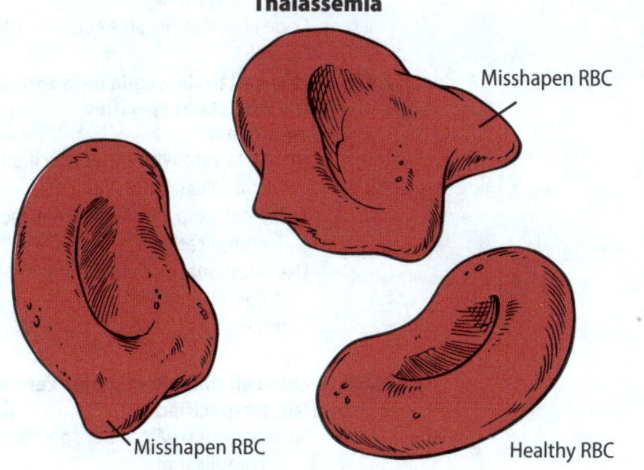

D56.Ø Alpha thalassemia HCC

Alpha thalassemia major
Hemoglobin H Constant Spring
Hemoglobin H disease
Hydrops fetalis due to alpha thalassemia
Severe alpha thalassemia
Triple gene defect alpha thalassemia

Use additional code, if applicable, for hydrops fetalis due to alpha thalassemia (P56.99)

EXCLUDES 1 *alpha thalassemia trait or minor (D56.3)*
asymptomatic alpha thalassemia (D56.3)
hydrops fetalis due to isoimmunization (P56.Ø)
hydrops fetalis not due to immune hemolysis (P83.2)

DEF: HBA1 and HBA2 genetic variant of chromosome 16 prevalent among those of African and Southeast Asian descent. Alpha thalassemia is associated with a wide spectrum of anemic presentation and includes hemoglobin H disease subtypes.

D56.1 Beta thalassemia HCC

Beta thalassemia major
Cooley's anemia
Homozygous beta thalassemia
Severe beta thalassemia
Thalassemia intermedia
Thalassemia major

EXCLUDES 1 *beta thalassemia minor (D56.3)*
beta thalassemia trait (D56.3)
delta-beta thalassemia (D56.2)
hemoglobin E-beta thalassemia (D56.5)
sickle-cell beta thalassemia (D57.4-)

D56.2 Delta-beta thalassemia HCC

Homozygous delta-beta thalassemia

EXCLUDES 1 *delta-beta thalassemia minor (D56.3)*
delta-beta thalassemia trait (D56.3)

D56.3 Thalassemia minor

Alpha thalassemia minor
Alpha thalassemia silent carrier
Alpha thalassemia trait
Beta thalassemia minor
Beta thalassemia trait
Delta-beta thalassemia minor
Delta-beta thalassemia trait
Thalassemia trait NOS

EXCLUDES 1 *alpha thalassemia (D56.Ø)*
beta thalassemia (D56.1)
delta-beta thalassemia (D56.2)
hemoglobin E-beta thalassemia (D56.5)
sickle-cell trait (D57.3)

DEF: Solitary abnormal gene that identifies a carrier of the disease, yet with an absence of symptoms or a clinically mild anemic presentation.

D56.4 Hereditary persistence of fetal hemoglobin [HPFH] HCC

D56.5 Hemoglobin E-beta thalassemia HCC

EXCLUDES 1 *beta thalassemia (D56.1)*
beta thalassemia minor (D56.3)
beta thalassemia trait (D56.3)
delta-beta thalassemia (D56.2)
delta-beta thalassemia trait (D56.3)
hemoglobin E disease (D58.2)
other hemoglobinopathies (D58.2)
sickle-cell beta thalassemia (D57.4-)

D56.8 Other thalassemias HCC

Dominant thalassemia
Hemoglobin C thalassemia
Mixed thalassemia
Thalassemia with other hemoglobinopathy

EXCLUDES 1 *hemoglobin C disease (D58.2)*
hemoglobin E disease (D58.2)
other hemoglobinopathies (D58.2)
sickle-cell anemia (D57.-)
sickle-cell thalassemia (D57.4)

D56.9 Thalassemia, unspecified

Mediterranean anemia (with other hemoglobinopathy)

D57 Sickle-cell disorders

Use additional code for any associated fever (R5Ø.81)

EXCLUDES 1 *other hemoglobinopathies (D58.-)*

AHA: 2022,2Q,28

DEF: Severe, chronic inherited diseases caused by a genetic variation in hemoglobin protein of the red blood cell. The gene mutation causes the red blood cell to become hard, sticky, and crescent or sickle shaped, making it harder for red blood cells to travel through the bloodstream, disrupting blood flow and decreasing oxygen transport to tissues.

Sickle cell

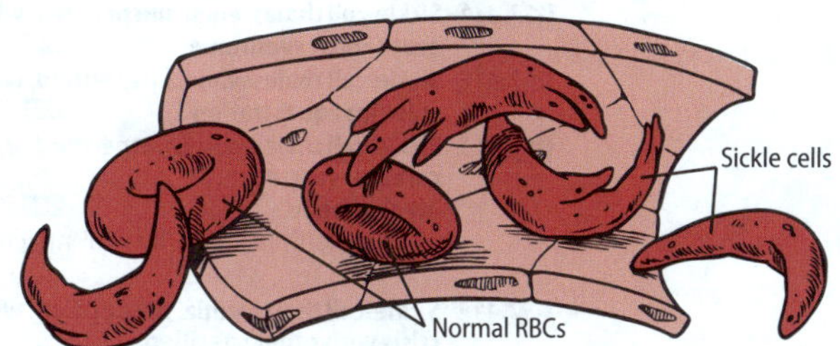

D57.Ø Hb-SS disease with crisis

Sickle-cell disease with crisis
Hb-SS disease with vasoocclusive pain

AHA: 2020,4Q,6-7

D57.ØØ Hb-SS disease with crisis, unspecified MCC HCC

Hb-SS disease with (painful) crisis NOS
Hb-SS disease with vasoocclusive pain NOS

D57.Ø1 Hb-SS disease with acute chest syndrome MCC HCC

D57.Ø2 Hb-SS disease with splenic sequestration MCC HCC

D57.Ø3 Hb-SS disease with cerebral vascular involvement MCC HCC

Code also, if applicable, cerebral infarction (I63.-)

D57.Ø9 Hb-SS disease with crisis with other specified complication MCC HCC

Use additional code to identify complications, such as:
cholelithiasis (K8Ø.-)
priapism (N48.32)

D57.1 Sickle-cell disease without crisis HCC

Hb-SS disease without crisis
Sickle-cell anemia NOS
Sickle-cell disease NOS
Sickle-cell disorder NOS

D57.2 Sickle-cell/Hb-C disease

Hb-SC disease
Hb-S/Hb-C disease

AHA: 2020,4Q,6-7

D57.2Ø Sickle-cell/Hb-C disease without crisis HCC

D57.21 Sickle-cell/Hb-C disease with crisis

D57.211 Sickle-cell/Hb-C disease with acute chest syndrome MCC HCC

D57.212 Sickle-cell/Hb-C disease with splenic sequestration MCC HCC

D57.213 Sickle-cell/Hb-C disease with cerebral vascular involvement MCC HCC

Code also, if applicable, cerebral infarction (I63.-)

D57.218 Sickle-cell/Hb-C disease with crisis with other specified complication MCC HCC

Use additional code to identify complications, such as:
cholelithiasis (K8Ø.-)
priapism (N48.32)

D57.219 Sickle-cell/Hb-C disease with crisis, unspecified MCC HCC

Sickle-cell/Hb-C disease with crisis NOS
Sickle-cell/Hb-C disease with vasoocclusive pain NOS

D57.3 Sickle-cell trait HCC

Hb-S trait
Heterozygous hemoglobin S

DEF: Heterozygous genetic makeup characterized by one gene for normal hemoglobin and one for sickle-cell hemoglobin. The clinical disease is rarely present.

√5th **D57.4 Sickle-cell thalassemia**

Sickle-cell beta thalassemia
Thalassemia Hb-S disease

AHA: 2020,4Q,6-7

D57.4Ø Sickle-cell thalassemia without crisis HCC

Microdrepanocytosis
Sickle-cell thalassemia NOS

√6th **D57.41 Sickle-cell thalassemia, unspecified, with crisis**

Sickle-cell thalassemia with (painful) crisis NOS
Sickle-cell thalassemia with vasoocclusive pain NOS

D57.411 Sickle-cell thalassemia, unspecified, with acute chest syndrome MCC HCC

D57.412 Sickle-cell thalassemia, unspecified, with splenic sequestration MCC HCC

D57.413 Sickle-cell thalassemia, unspecified, with cerebral vascular involvement MCC HCC

Code also, if applicable cerebral infarction (I63.-)

D57.418 Sickle-cell thalassemia, unspecified, with crisis with other specified complication MCC HCC

Use additional code to identify complications, such as:
cholelithiasis (K8Ø.-)
priapism (N48.32)

D57.419 Sickle-cell thalassemia, unspecified, with crisis MCC HCC

Sickle-cell thalassemia with (painful) crisis NOS
Sickle-cell thalassemia with vasoocclusive pain NOS

D57.42 Sickle-cell thalassemia beta zero without crisis HCC

HbS-beta zero without crisis
Sickle-cell beta zero without crisis

√6th **D57.43 Sickle-cell thalassemia beta zero with crisis**

HbS-beta zero with crisis
Sickle-cell beta zero with crisis

D57.431 Sickle-cell thalassemia beta zero with acute chest syndrome MCC HCC

HbS-beta zero with acute chest syndrome
Sickle-cell beta zero with acute chest syndrome

D57.432 Sickle-cell thalassemia beta zero with splenic sequestration MCC HCC

HbS-beta zero with splenic sequestration
Sickle-cell beta zero with splenic sequestration

D57.433 Sickle-cell thalassemia beta zero with cerebral vascular involvement MCC HCC

HbS-beta zero with cerebral vascular involvement
Sickle-cell beta zero with cerebral vascular involvement

Code also, if applicable cerebral infarction (I63.-)

D57.438 Sickle-cell thalassemia beta zero with crisis with other specified complication MCC HCC

HbS-beta zero with other specified complication
Sickle-cell beta zero with other specified complication

Use additional code to identify complications, such as:
cholelithiasis (K8Ø.-)
priapism (N48.32)

D57.439 Sickle-cell thalassemia beta zero with crisis, unspecified MCC HCC

HbS-beta zero with other specified complication
Sickle-cell beta zero with crisis unspecified
Sickle-cell thalassemia beta zero with (painful) crisis NOS
Sickle-cell thalassemia beta zero with vasoocclusive pain NOS

D57.44 Sickle-cell thalassemia beta plus without crisis HCC

HbS-beta plus without crisis
Sickle-cell beta plus without crisis

√6th **D57.45 Sickle-cell thalassemia beta plus with crisis**

HbS-beta plus with crisis
Sickle-cell beta plus with crisis

D57.451 Sickle-cell thalassemia beta plus with acute chest syndrome MCC HCC

HbS-beta plus with acute chest syndrome
Sickle-cell beta plus with acute chest syndrome

D57.452 Sickle-cell thalassemia beta plus with splenic sequestration MCC HCC

HbS-beta plus with splenic sequestration
Sickle-cell beta plus with splenic sequestration

D57.453 Sickle-cell thalassemia beta plus with cerebral vascular involvement MCC HCC

HbS-beta plus with cerebral vascular involvement
Sickle-cell beta plus with cerebral vascular involvement

Code also, if applicable cerebral infarction (I63.-)

D57.458 Sickle-cell thalassemia beta plus with crisis with other specified complication MCC HCC

HbS-beta plus with crisis with other specified complication
Sickle-cell beta plus with crisis with other specified complication

Use additional code to identify complications, such as:
cholelithiasis (K8Ø.-)
priapism (N48.32)

D57.459 Sickle-cell thalassemia beta plus with crisis, unspecified MCC HCC

HbS-beta plus with crisis with unspecified complication
Sickle-cell beta plus with crisis with unspecified complication
Sickle-cell thalassemia beta plus with (painful) crisis NOS
Sickle-cell thalassemia beta plus with vasoocclusive pain NOS

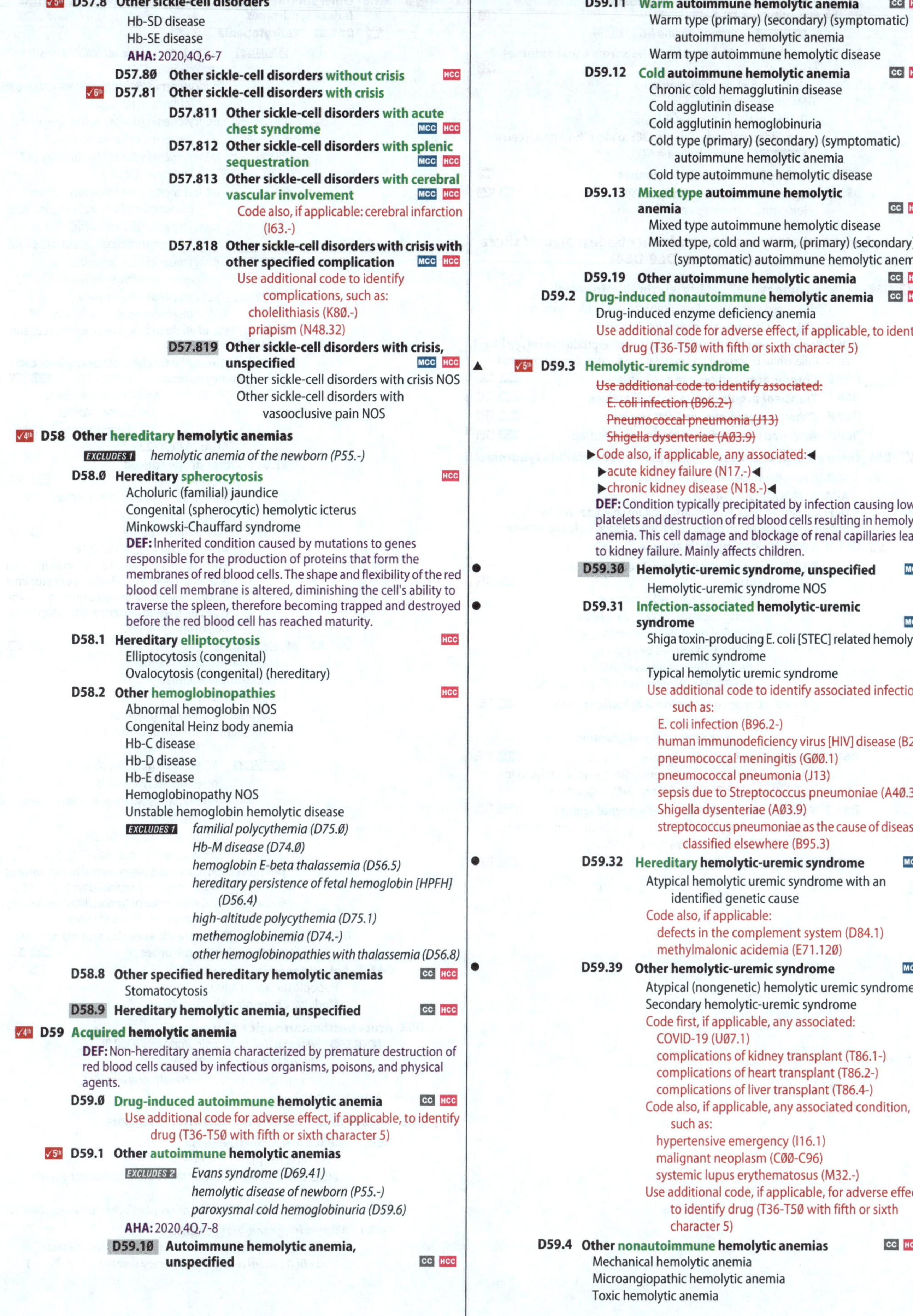

✓5th **D57.8 Other sickle-cell disorders**
Hb-SD disease
Hb-SE disease
AHA: 2020,4Q,6-7

D57.8Ø Other sickle-cell disorders without crisis HCC

✓6th **D57.81 Other sickle-cell disorders with crisis**

D57.811 Other sickle-cell disorders with acute chest syndrome MCC HCC

D57.812 Other sickle-cell disorders with splenic sequestration MCC HCC

D57.813 Other sickle-cell disorders with cerebral vascular involvement MCC HCC
Code also, if applicable: cerebral infarction (I63.-)

D57.818 Other sickle-cell disorders with crisis with other specified complication MCC HCC
Use additional code to identify complications, such as:
cholelithiasis (K8Ø.-)
priapism (N48.32)

D57.819 Other sickle-cell disorders with crisis, unspecified MCC HCC
Other sickle-cell disorders with crisis NOS
Other sickle-cell disorders with vasoocclusive pain NOS

✓4th **D58 Other hereditary hemolytic anemias**
EXCLUDES 1 *hemolytic anemia of the newborn (P55.-)*

D58.Ø Hereditary spherocytosis HCC
Acholuric (familial) jaundice
Congenital (spherocytic) hemolytic icterus
Minkowski-Chauffard syndrome
DEF: Inherited condition caused by mutations to genes responsible for the production of proteins that form the membranes of red blood cells. The shape and flexibility of the red blood cell membrane is altered, diminishing the cell's ability to traverse the spleen, therefore becoming trapped and destroyed before the red blood cell has reached maturity.

D58.1 Hereditary elliptocytosis HCC
Elliptocytosis (congenital)
Ovalocytosis (congenital) (hereditary)

D58.2 Other hemoglobinopathies HCC
Abnormal hemoglobin NOS
Congenital Heinz body anemia
Hb-C disease
Hb-D disease
Hb-E disease
Hemoglobinopathy NOS
Unstable hemoglobin hemolytic disease
EXCLUDES 1 *familial polycythemia (D75.Ø)*
Hb-M disease (D74.Ø)
hemoglobin E-beta thalassemia (D56.5)
hereditary persistence of fetal hemoglobin [HPFH] (D56.4)
high-altitude polycythemia (D75.1)
methemoglobinemia (D74.-)
other hemoglobinopathies with thalassemia (D56.8)

D58.8 Other specified hereditary hemolytic anemias CC HCC
Stomatocytosis

D58.9 Hereditary hemolytic anemia, unspecified CC HCC

✓4th **D59 Acquired hemolytic anemia**
DEF: Non-hereditary anemia characterized by premature destruction of red blood cells caused by infectious organisms, poisons, and physical agents.

D59.Ø Drug-induced autoimmune hemolytic anemia CC HCC
Use additional code for adverse effect, if applicable, to identify drug (T36-T5Ø with fifth or sixth character 5)

✓5th **D59.1 Other autoimmune hemolytic anemias**
EXCLUDES 2 *Evans syndrome (D69.41)*
hemolytic disease of newborn (P55.-)
paroxysmal cold hemoglobinuria (D59.6)
AHA: 2020,4Q,7-8

D59.1Ø Autoimmune hemolytic anemia, unspecified CC HCC

D59.11 Warm autoimmune hemolytic anemia CC HCC
Warm type (primary) (secondary) (symptomatic) autoimmune hemolytic anemia
Warm type autoimmune hemolytic disease

D59.12 Cold autoimmune hemolytic anemia CC HCC
Chronic cold hemagglutinin disease
Cold agglutinin disease
Cold agglutinin hemoglobinuria
Cold type (primary) (secondary) (symptomatic) autoimmune hemolytic anemia
Cold type autoimmune hemolytic disease

D59.13 Mixed type autoimmune hemolytic anemia CC HCC
Mixed type autoimmune hemolytic disease
Mixed type, cold and warm, (primary) (secondary) (symptomatic) autoimmune hemolytic anemia

D59.19 Other autoimmune hemolytic anemia CC HCC

D59.2 Drug-induced nonautoimmune hemolytic anemia CC HCC
Drug-induced enzyme deficiency anemia
Use additional code for adverse effect, if applicable, to identify drug (T36-T5Ø with fifth or sixth character 5)

▲ ✓5th **D59.3 Hemolytic-uremic syndrome**
~~Use additional code to identify associated:~~
~~E. coli infection (B96.2-)~~
~~Pneumococcal pneumonia (J13)~~
~~Shigella dysenteriae (AØ3.9)~~
►Code also, if applicable, any associated:◄
►acute kidney failure (N17.-)◄
►chronic kidney disease (N18.-)◄
DEF: Condition typically precipitated by infection causing low platelets and destruction of red blood cells resulting in hemolytic anemia. This cell damage and blockage of renal capillaries lead to kidney failure. Mainly affects children.

● **D59.3Ø Hemolytic-uremic syndrome, unspecified** MCC
Hemolytic-uremic syndrome NOS

● **D59.31 Infection-associated hemolytic-uremic syndrome** MCC
Shiga toxin-producing E. coli [STEC] related hemolytic uremic syndrome
Typical hemolytic uremic syndrome
Use additional code to identify associated infection, such as:
E. coli infection (B96.2-)
human immunodeficiency virus [HIV] disease (B2Ø)
pneumococcal meningitis (GØØ.1)
pneumococcal pneumonia (J13)
sepsis due to Streptococcus pneumoniae (A4Ø.3)
Shigella dysenteriae (AØ3.9)
streptococcus pneumoniae as the cause of diseases classified elsewhere (B95.3)

● **D59.32 Hereditary hemolytic-uremic syndrome** MCC
Atypical hemolytic uremic syndrome with an identified genetic cause
Code also, if applicable:
defects in the complement system (D84.1)
methylmalonic acidemia (E71.12Ø)

● **D59.39 Other hemolytic-uremic syndrome** MCC
Atypical (nongenetic) hemolytic uremic syndrome
Secondary hemolytic-uremic syndrome
Code first, if applicable, any associated:
COVID-19 (UØ7.1)
complications of kidney transplant (T86.1-)
complications of heart transplant (T86.2-)
complications of liver transplant (T86.4-)
Code also, if applicable, any associated condition, such as:
hypertensive emergency (I16.1)
malignant neoplasm (CØØ-C96)
systemic lupus erythematosus (M32.-)
Use additional code, if applicable, for adverse effect to identify drug (T36-T5Ø with fifth or sixth character 5)

D59.4 Other nonautoimmune hemolytic anemias CC HCC
Mechanical hemolytic anemia
Microangiopathic hemolytic anemia
Toxic hemolytic anemia

D59.5 Paroxysmal nocturnal hemoglobinuria [Marchiafava-Micheli] HCC

EXCLUDES 1 *hemoglobinuria NOS (R82.3)*

D59.6 Hemoglobinuria due to hemolysis from other external causes HCC

Hemoglobinuria from exertion

March hemoglobinuria

Paroxysmal cold hemoglobinuria

Use additional code (Chapter 2Ø) to identify external cause

EXCLUDES 1 *hemoglobinuria NOS (R82.3)*

D59.8 Other acquired hemolytic anemias HCC

D59.9 Acquired hemolytic anemia, unspecified CC HCC

Idiopathic hemolytic anemia, chronic

Aplastic and other anemias and other bone marrow failure syndromes (D6Ø-D64)

D6Ø Acquired pure red cell aplasia [erythroblastopenia] 4th

INCLUDES red cell aplasia (acquired) (adult) (with thymoma)

EXCLUDES 1 *congenital red cell aplasia (D61.Ø1)*

DEF: Bone marrow failure characterized by underproduction of red blood cells while white blood cell and platelet production remains normal.

D6Ø.Ø Chronic acquired pure red cell aplasia MCC HCC

D6Ø.1 Transient acquired pure red cell aplasia MCC HCC

D6Ø.8 Other acquired pure red cell aplasias MCC HCC

D6Ø.9 Acquired pure red cell aplasia, unspecified MCC HCC

D61 Other aplastic anemias and other bone marrow failure syndromes 4th

EXCLUDES 2 *neutropenia (D7Ø.-)*

AHA: 2020,3Q,22; 2014,4Q,22

DEF: Aplastic anemia: Bone marrow failure characterized by underproduction of red bloods cells, white blood cells and platelets.

D61.Ø Constitutional aplastic anemia 5th

D61.Ø1 Constitutional (pure) red blood cell aplasia CC HCC

Blackfan-Diamond syndrome

Congenital (pure) red cell aplasia

Familial hypoplastic anemia

Primary (pure) red cell aplasia

Red cell (pure) aplasia of infants

EXCLUDES 1 *acquired red cell aplasia (D6Ø.9)*

D61.Ø9 Other constitutional aplastic anemia CC HCC

Fanconi's anemia

Pancytopenia with malformations

D61.1 Drug-induced aplastic anemia MCC HCC

Use additional code for adverse effect, if applicable, to identify drug (T36-T5Ø with fifth or sixth character 5)

D61.2 Aplastic anemia due to other external agents MCC HCC

Code first, if applicable, toxic effects of substances chiefly nonmedicinal as to source (T51-T65)

D61.3 Idiopathic aplastic anemia MCC HCC

D61.8 Other specified aplastic anemias and other bone marrow failure syndromes 5th

D61.81 Pancytopenia 6th

EXCLUDES 1 *pancytopenia (due to) (with) aplastic anemia (D61.9)*

pancytopenia (due to) (with) bone marrow infiltration (D61.82)

pancytopenia (due to) (with) congenital (pure) red cell aplasia (D61.Ø1)

pancytopenia (due to) (with) hairy cell leukemia (C91.4-)

pancytopenia (due to) (with) human immunodeficiency virus disease (B2Ø)

pancytopenia (due to) (with) leukoerythroblastic anemia (D61.82)

pancytopenia (due to) (with) myeloproliferative disease (D47.1)

EXCLUDES 2 *pancytopenia (due to) (with) myelodysplastic syndromes (D46.-)*

DEF: Shortage of all three blood cells: white, red, and platelets.

D61.81Ø Antineoplastic chemotherapy induced pancytopenia MCC HCC

EXCLUDES 2 *aplastic anemia due to antineoplastic chemotherapy (D61.1)*

AHA: 2020,3Q,22

D61.811 Other drug-induced pancytopenia MCC HCC

EXCLUDES 2 *aplastic anemia due to drugs (D61.1)*

D61.818 Other pancytopenia CC HCC

AHA: 2020,3Q,24; 2019,1Q,16

TIP: Assign this code in addition to myeloid leukemia codes (C92.-) when pancytopenia is documented. Although common in some types of myeloid leukemia, pancytopenia is not always inherent.

D61.82 Myelophthisis CC HCC

Leukoerythroblastic anemia

Myelophthisic anemia

Panmyelophthisis

Code also the underlying disorder, such as:

malignant neoplasm of breast (C5Ø.-)

tuberculosis (A15.-)

EXCLUDES 1 *idiopathic myelofibrosis (D47.1)*

myelofibrosis NOS (D75.81)

myelofibrosis with myeloid metaplasia (D47.4)

primary myelofibrosis (D47.1)

secondary myelofibrosis (D75.81)

DEF: Condition that occurs when normal hematopoietic tissue in the bone marrow is replaced with abnormal tissue, such as fibrous tissue or tumors. Most commonly seen during the advanced stages of cancer.

D61.89 Other specified aplastic anemias and other bone marrow failure syndromes MCC HCC

D61.9 Aplastic anemia, unspecified CC HCC

Hypoplastic anemia NOS

Medullary hypoplasia

D62 Acute posthemorrhagic anemia CC

EXCLUDES 1 *anemia due to chronic blood loss (D5Ø.Ø)*

blood loss anemia NOS (D5Ø.Ø)

congenital anemia from fetal blood loss (P61.3)

AHA: 2019,3Q,11,17

D63 Anemia in chronic diseases classified elsewhere 4th

D63.Ø Anemia in neoplastic disease

Code first neoplasm (CØØ-D49)

EXCLUDES 1 *aplastic anemia due to antineoplastic chemotherapy (D61.1)*

EXCLUDES 2 *anemia due to antineoplastic chemotherapy (D64.81)*

D63.1 Anemia in chronic kidney disease

Erythropoietin resistant anemia (EPO resistant anemia)

Code first underlying chronic kidney disease (CKD) (N18.-)

D63.8 *Anemia in other chronic diseases classified elsewhere*
Code first underlying disease, such as:
diphyllobothriasis (B7Ø.Ø)
hookworm disease (B76.Ø-B76.9)
hypothyroidism (EØØ.Ø-EØ3.9)
malaria (B5Ø.Ø-B54)
symptomatic late syphilis (A52.79)
tuberculosis (A18.89)

✓4th **D64 Other anemias**
EXCLUDES 1 *refractory anemia (D46.-)*
refractory anemia with excess blasts in transformation [RAEB T] (C92.Ø-)
DEF: Sideroblastic anemia: Hereditary or secondary disorder in which the red blood cells cannot effectively use iron, a nutrient needed to make hemoglobin. Although the iron can enter the red blood cell it is not assimilated into the hemoglobin molecule and builds up ringed sideroblasts around the cell nucleus.

D64.Ø Hereditary sideroblastic anemia HCC
Sex-linked hypochromic sideroblastic anemia

D64.1 *Secondary sideroblastic anemia due to disease* HCC
Code first underlying disease

D64.2 Secondary sideroblastic anemia due to drugs and toxins HCC
Code first poisoning due to drug or toxin, if applicable (T36-T65 with fifth or sixth character 1-4 or 6)
Use additional code for adverse effect, if applicable, to identify drug (T36-T5Ø with fifth or sixth character 5)

D64.3 Other sideroblastic anemias HCC
Sideroblastic anemia NOS
Pyridoxine-responsive sideroblastic anemia NEC

D64.4 Congenital dyserythropoietic anemia
Dyshematopoietic anemia (congenital)
EXCLUDES 1 *Blackfan-Diamond syndrome (D61.Ø1)*
Di Guglielmo's disease (C94.Ø)

✓5th **D64.8 Other specified anemias**

D64.81 Anemia due to antineoplastic chemotherapy
Antineoplastic chemotherapy induced anemia
EXCLUDES 2 *anemia in neoplastic disease (D63.Ø)*
aplastic anemia due to antineoplastic chemotherapy (D61.1)
AHA: 2021,3Q,4; 2014,4Q,22

D64.89 Other specified anemias
Infantile pseudoleukemia

D64.9 Anemia, unspecified
AHA: 2020,3Q,24; 2018,4Q,88; 2017,1Q,7

Coagulation defects, purpura and other hemorrhagic conditions (D65-D69)

D65 Disseminated intravascular coagulation [defibrination syndrome] MCC HCC
Afibrinogenemia, acquired
Consumption coagulopathy
Diffuse or disseminated intravascular coagulation [DIC]
Fibrinolytic hemorrhage, acquired
Fibrinolytic purpura
Purpura fulminans
EXCLUDES 1 *disseminated intravascular coagulation (complicating):*
abortion or ectopic or molar pregnancy (OØØ-OØ7, OØ8.1)
in newborn (P6Ø)
pregnancy, childbirth and the puerperium (O45.Ø, O46.Ø, O67.Ø, O72.3)
AHA: 2021,1Q,39

Coagulation

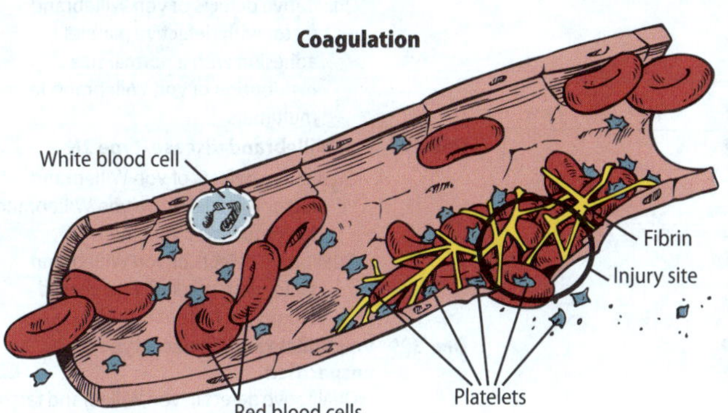

D66 Hereditary factor VIII deficiency MCC HCC
Classical hemophilia
Deficiency factor VIII (with functional defect)
Hemophilia NOS
Hemophilia A
EXCLUDES 1 *factor VIII deficiency with vascular defect* ▶*(D68.Ø-)*◀
DEF: Hereditary, sex-linked lack of antihemophilic globulin (AHG) (factor VIII) that causes abnormal coagulation characterized by increased bleeding; large bruises of skin; bleeding in the mouth, nose, and gastrointestinal tract; and hemorrhages into joints, resulting in swelling and impaired function.

D67 Hereditary factor IX deficiency MCC HCC
Christmas disease
Factor IX deficiency (with functional defect)
Hemophilia B
Plasma thromboplastin component [PTC] deficiency

✓4th **D68 Other coagulation defects**
EXCLUDES 1 ▶*abnormal coagulation profile NOS*◀ *(R79.1)*
~~*coagulation defects complicating abortion or ectopic or molar pregnancy (OØØ-OØ7, OØ8.1)*~~
~~*coagulation defects complicating pregnancy, childbirth and the puerperium (O45.Ø, O46.Ø, O67.Ø, O72.3)*~~
EXCLUDES 2 ▶*coagulation defects complicating abortion or ectopic or molar pregnancy (OØØ-OØ7, OØ8.1)*◀
▶*coagulation defects complicating pregnancy, childbirth and the puerperium (O45.Ø, O46.Ø, O67.Ø, O72.3)*◀
AHA: 2016,1Q,14

▲ ✓5th **D68.Ø Von Willebrand disease**
~~Angiohemophilia~~
~~Factor VIII deficiency with vascular defect~~
~~Vascular hemophilia~~
EXCLUDES 1 *capillary fragility (hereditary) (D69.8)*
factor VIII deficiency NOS (D66)
factor VIII deficiency with functional defect (D66)
DEF: Congenital, abnormal blood coagulation caused by deficient blood factor VII. Symptoms include excess or prolonged bleeding.

● **D68.ØØ Von Willebrand disease, unspecified** CC

● **D68.Ø1 Von Willebrand disease, type 1** CC
Partial quantitative deficiency of von Willebrand factor
Type 1C von Willebrand disease

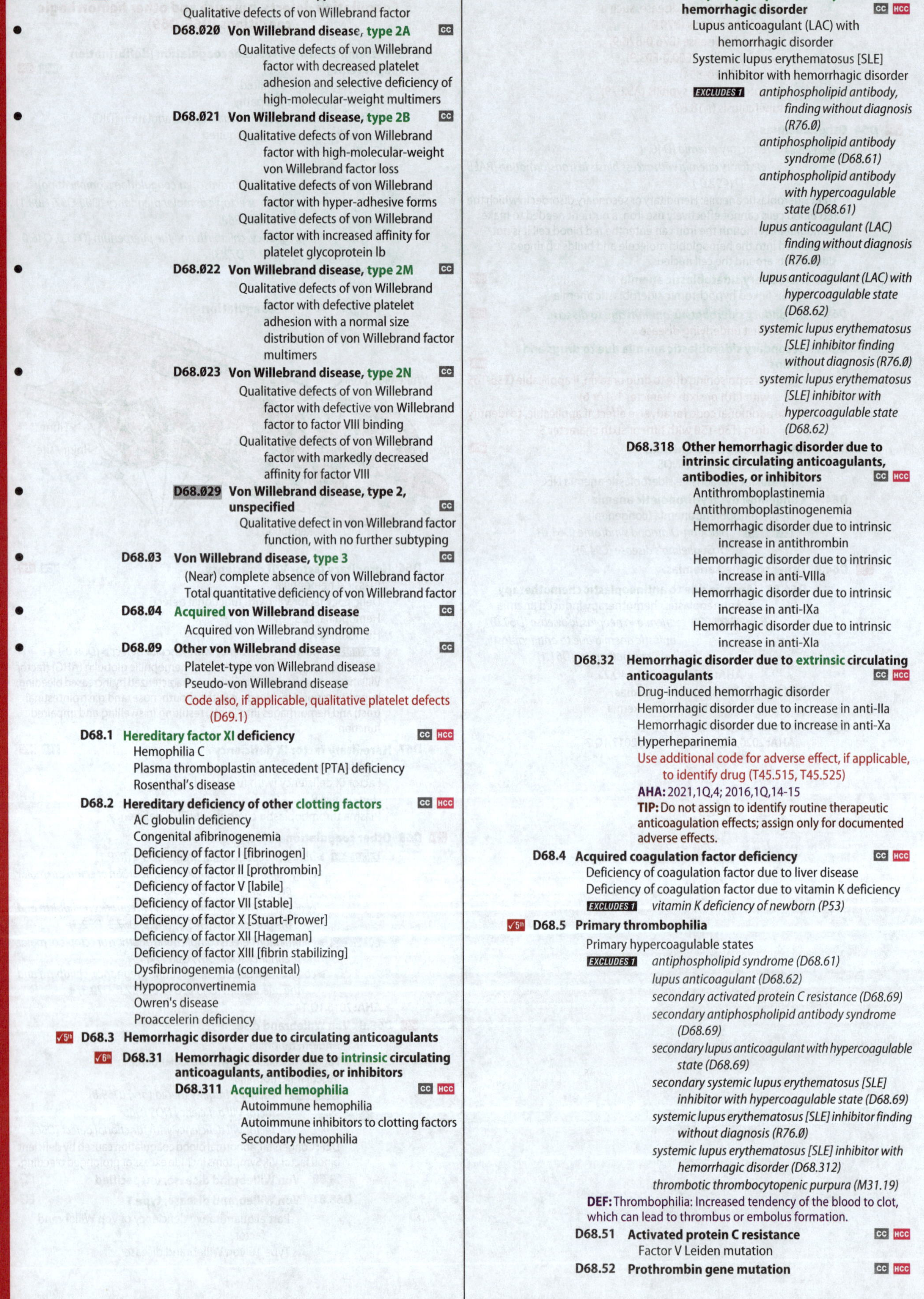

- **D68.02 Von Willebrand disease, type 2**
  Qualitative defects of von Willebrand factor
  - **D68.020 Von Willebrand disease, type 2A** CC
    Qualitative defects of von Willebrand factor with decreased platelet adhesion and selective deficiency of high-molecular-weight multimers
  - **D68.021 Von Willebrand disease, type 2B** CC
    Qualitative defects of von Willebrand factor with high-molecular-weight von Willebrand factor loss
    Qualitative defects of von Willebrand factor with hyper-adhesive forms
    Qualitative defects of von Willebrand factor with increased affinity for platelet glycoprotein Ib
  - **D68.022 Von Willebrand disease, type 2M** CC
    Qualitative defects of von Willebrand factor with defective platelet adhesion with a normal size distribution of von Willebrand factor multimers
  - **D68.023 Von Willebrand disease, type 2N** CC
    Qualitative defects of von Willebrand factor with defective von Willebrand factor to factor VIII binding
    Qualitative defects of von Willebrand factor with markedly decreased affinity for factor VIII
  - **D68.029 Von Willebrand disease, type 2, unspecified** CC
    Qualitative defect in von Willebrand factor function, with no further subtyping
- **D68.03 Von Willebrand disease, type 3** CC
  (Near) complete absence of von Willebrand factor
  Total quantitative deficiency of von Willebrand factor
- **D68.04 Acquired von Willebrand disease** CC
  Acquired von Willebrand syndrome
- **D68.09 Other von Willebrand disease** CC
  Platelet-type von Willebrand disease
  Pseudo-von Willebrand disease
  Code also, if applicable, qualitative platelet defects (D69.1)

D68.1 Hereditary factor XI deficiency CC HCC
Hemophilia C
Plasma thromboplastin antecedent [PTA] deficiency
Rosenthal's disease

D68.2 Hereditary deficiency of other clotting factors CC HCC
AC globulin deficiency
Congenital afibrinogenemia
Deficiency of factor I [fibrinogen]
Deficiency of factor II [prothrombin]
Deficiency of factor V [labile]
Deficiency of factor VII [stable]
Deficiency of factor X [Stuart-Prower]
Deficiency of factor XII [Hageman]
Deficiency of factor XIII [fibrin stabilizing]
Dysfibrinogenemia (congenital)
Hypoproconvertinemia
Owren's disease
Proaccelerin deficiency

D68.3 Hemorrhagic disorder due to circulating anticoagulants

D68.31 Hemorrhagic disorder due to intrinsic circulating anticoagulants, antibodies, or inhibitors

D68.311 Acquired hemophilia CC HCC
Autoimmune hemophilia
Autoimmune inhibitors to clotting factors
Secondary hemophilia

D68.312 Antiphospholipid antibody with hemorrhagic disorder CC HCC
Lupus anticoagulant (LAC) with hemorrhagic disorder
Systemic lupus erythematosus [SLE] inhibitor with hemorrhagic disorder
EXCLUDES 1 *antiphospholipid antibody, finding without diagnosis (R76.0)*
antiphospholipid antibody syndrome (D68.61)
antiphospholipid antibody with hypercoagulable state (D68.61)
lupus anticoagulant (LAC) finding without diagnosis (R76.0)
lupus anticoagulant (LAC) with hypercoagulable state (D68.62)
systemic lupus erythematosus [SLE] inhibitor finding without diagnosis (R76.0)
systemic lupus erythematosus [SLE] inhibitor with hypercoagulable state (D68.62)

D68.318 Other hemorrhagic disorder due to intrinsic circulating anticoagulants, antibodies, or inhibitors CC HCC
Antithromboplastinemia
Antithromboplastinogenemia
Hemorrhagic disorder due to intrinsic increase in antithrombin
Hemorrhagic disorder due to intrinsic increase in anti-VIIIa
Hemorrhagic disorder due to intrinsic increase in anti-IXa
Hemorrhagic disorder due to intrinsic increase in anti-XIa

D68.32 Hemorrhagic disorder due to extrinsic circulating anticoagulants CC HCC
Drug-induced hemorrhagic disorder
Hemorrhagic disorder due to increase in anti-IIa
Hemorrhagic disorder due to increase in anti-Xa
Hyperheparinemia
Use additional code for adverse effect, if applicable, to identify drug (T45.515, T45.525)
AHA: 2021,1Q,4; 2016,1Q,14-15
TIP: Do not assign to identify routine therapeutic anticoagulation effects; assign only for documented adverse effects.

D68.4 Acquired coagulation factor deficiency CC HCC
Deficiency of coagulation factor due to liver disease
Deficiency of coagulation factor due to vitamin K deficiency
EXCLUDES 1 *vitamin K deficiency of newborn (P53)*

D68.5 Primary thrombophilia
Primary hypercoagulable states
EXCLUDES 1 *antiphospholipid syndrome (D68.61)*
lupus anticoagulant (D68.62)
secondary activated protein C resistance (D68.69)
secondary antiphospholipid antibody syndrome (D68.69)
secondary lupus anticoagulant with hypercoagulable state (D68.69)
secondary systemic lupus erythematosus [SLE] inhibitor with hypercoagulable state (D68.69)
systemic lupus erythematosus [SLE] inhibitor finding without diagnosis (R76.0)
systemic lupus erythematosus [SLE] inhibitor with hemorrhagic disorder (D68.312)
thrombotic thrombocytopenic purpura (M31.19)
DEF: Thrombophilia: Increased tendency of the blood to clot, which can lead to thrombus or embolus formation.

D68.51 Activated protein C resistance CC HCC
Factor V Leiden mutation

D68.52 Prothrombin gene mutation CC HCC

D68.59 Other primary thrombophilia CC HCC
Antithrombin III deficiency
Hypercoagulable state NOS
Primary hypercoagulable state NEC
Primary thrombophilia NEC
Protein C deficiency
Protein S deficiency
Thrombophilia NOS
AHA: 2021,2Q,8

✓5th **D68.6 Other thrombophilia**
Other hypercoagulable states
EXCLUDES 1 *diffuse or disseminated intravascular coagulation [DIC] (D65)*
heparin induced thrombocytopenia (HIT) ▶(D75.82-)◀
hyperhomocysteinemia (E72.11)

D68.61 Antiphospholipid syndrome CC HCC
Anticardiolipin syndrome
Antiphospholipid antibody syndrome
EXCLUDES 1 *anti-phospholipid antibody, finding without diagnosis (R76.0)*
anti-phospholipid antibody with hemorrhagic disorder (D68.312)
lupus anticoagulant syndrome (D68.62)

D68.62 Lupus anticoagulant syndrome CC HCC
Lupus anticoagulant
Presence of systemic lupus erythematosus [SLE] inhibitor
EXCLUDES 1 *anticardiolipin syndrome (D68.61)*
antiphospholipid syndrome (D68.61)
lupus anticoagulant (LAC) finding without diagnosis (R76.0)
lupus anticoagulant (LAC) with hemorrhagic disorder (D68.312)

D68.69 Other thrombophilia CC HCC
Hypercoagulable states NEC
Secondary hypercoagulable state NOS
AHA: 2021,2Q,8

D68.8 Other specified coagulation defects CC HCC
EXCLUDES 1 *hemorrhagic disease of newborn (P53)*
AHA: 2021,1Q,39

D68.9 Coagulation defect, unspecified CC HCC

✓4th **D69 Purpura and other hemorrhagic conditions**
EXCLUDES 1 *benign hypergammaglobulinemic purpura (D89.0)*
cryoglobulinemic purpura (D89.1)
essential (hemorrhagic) thrombocythemia (D47.3)
hemorrhagic thrombocythemia (D47.3)
purpura fulminans (D65)
thrombotic thrombocytopenic purpura (M31.19)
Waldenström hypergammaglobulinemic purpura (D89.0)

D69.0 Allergic purpura CC HCC
Allergic vasculitis
Nonthrombocytopenic hemorrhagic purpura
Nonthrombocytopenic idiopathic purpura
Purpura anaphylactoid
Purpura Henoch(-Schönlein)
Purpura rheumatica
Vascular purpura
EXCLUDES 1 *thrombocytopenic hemorrhagic purpura (D69.3)*
AHA: 2020,3Q,26
DEF: Any hemorrhagic condition, thrombocytic or nonthrombocytopenic in origin, caused by a presumed allergic reaction.

D69.1 Qualitative platelet defects HCC
Bernard-Soulier [giant platelet] syndrome
Glanzmann's disease
Grey platelet syndrome
Thromboasthenia (hemorrhagic) (hereditary)
Thrombocytopathy
EXCLUDES 1 *▶hemolytic-uremic syndrome (D59.3-)◀*
~~*von Willebrand's disease (D68.0)*~~
EXCLUDES 2 *▶von Willebrand disease (D68.0-)◀*

D69.2 Other nonthrombocytopenic purpura HCC
Purpura NOS
Purpura simplex
Senile purpura

D69.3 Immune thrombocytopenic purpura CC HCC
Hemorrhagic (thrombocytopenic) purpura
Idiopathic thrombocytopenic purpura
Tidal platelet dysgenesis
DEF: Tidal platelet dysgenesis: Fluctuation of platelet counts from normal to very low within periods of 20 to 40 days and may involve autoimmune platelet destruction.

✓5th **D69.4 Other primary thrombocytopenia**
EXCLUDES 1 *transient neonatal thrombocytopenia (P61.0)*
Wiskott-Aldrich syndrome (D82.0)

D69.41 Evans syndrome CC HCC

D69.42 Congenital and hereditary thrombocytopenia purpura CC HCC
Congenital thrombocytopenia
Hereditary thrombocytopenia
Code first congenital or hereditary disorder, such as:
thrombocytopenia with absent radius (TAR syndrome) (Q87.2)

D69.49 Other primary thrombocytopenia HCC
Megakaryocytic hypoplasia
Primary thrombocytopenia NOS

✓5th **D69.5 Secondary thrombocytopenia**
EXCLUDES 1 *heparin induced thrombocytopenia (HIT) ▶(D75.82-)◀*
transient thrombocytopenia of newborn (P61.0)

D69.51 Posttransfusion purpura
Posttransfusion purpura from whole blood (fresh) or blood products
PTP

D69.59 Other secondary thrombocytopenia
AHA: 2014,4Q,22

D69.6 Thrombocytopenia, unspecified HCC
AHA: 2020,3Q,24

D69.8 Other specified hemorrhagic conditions HCC
Capillary fragility (hereditary)
Vascular pseudohemophilia

D69.9 Hemorrhagic condition, unspecified HCC

Other disorders of blood and blood-forming organs (D70-D77)

✓4th **D70 Neutropenia**
INCLUDES agranulocytosis
decreased absolute neurophile count (ANC)
Use additional code for any associated:
fever (R50.81)
mucositis (J34.81, K12.3-, K92.81, N76.81)
EXCLUDES 1 *neutropenic splenomegaly (D73.81)*
transient neonatal neutropenia (P61.5)
DEF: Abnormally low number of neutrophils. Neutrophils are phagocytic, meaning they surround and consume harmful pathogens, primarily bacteria. When neutrophil counts decrease the risk of infection increases.

D70.0 Congenital agranulocytosis HCC
Congenital neutropenia
Infantile genetic agranulocytosis
Kostmann's disease

D70.1 Agranulocytosis secondary to cancer chemotherapy HCC
Code also underlying neoplasm
Use additional code for adverse effect, if applicable, to identify drug (T45.1X5)
AHA: 2020,3Q,22; 2014,4Q,22

D70.2 Other drug-induced agranulocytosis HCC
Use additional code for adverse effect, if applicable, to identify drug (T36-T50 with fifth or sixth character 5)

D70.3 Neutropenia due to infection HCC

D70.4 Cyclic neutropenia HCC
Cyclic hematopoiesis
Periodic neutropenia

D70.8 Other neutropenia HCC

D70.9 Neutropenia, unspecified HCC
AHA: 2020,3Q,24

D71 Functional disorders of polymorphonuclear neutrophils HCC
Cell membrane receptor complex [CR3] defect
Chronic (childhood) granulomatous disease
Congenital dysphagocytosis
Progressive septic granulomatosis

✓4th **D72 Other disorders of white blood cells**
EXCLUDES 1 *basophilia (D72.824)*
immunity disorders (D8Ø-D89)
neutropenia (D7Ø)
preleukemia (syndrome) (D46.9)

D72.Ø Genetic anomalies of leukocytes HCC
Alder (granulation) (granulocyte) anomaly
Alder syndrome
Hereditary leukocytic hypersegmentation
Hereditary leukocytic hyposegmentation
Hereditary leukomelanopathy
May-Hegglin (granulation) (granulocyte) anomaly
May-Hegglin syndrome
Pelger-Huët (granulation) (granulocyte) anomaly
Pelger-Huët syndrome
EXCLUDES 1 *Chédiak (-Steinbrinck)-Higashi syndrome (E7Ø.33Ø)*

✓5th **D72.1 Eosinophilia**
EXCLUDES 2 *Löffler's syndrome (J82.89)*
pulmonary eosinophilia (J82.-)
AHA: 2020,4Q,8-10
DEF: Abnormally large accumulation or formation of eosinophils (nucleated, granular leukocytes) in the blood, characteristic of allergic states and infection.

D72.1Ø Eosinophilia, unspecified

✓6th **D72.11 Hypereosinophilic syndrome [HES]**

D72.11Ø Idiopathic hypereosinophilic syndrome [IHES]

D72.111 Lymphocytic Variant Hypereosinophilic Syndrome [LHES]
Lymphocyte variant hypereosinophilia
Code also, if applicable, any associated lymphocytic neoplastic disorder

D72.118 Other hypereosinophilic syndrome
Episodic angioedema with eosinophilia
Gleich's syndrome

D72.119 Hypereosinophilic syndrome [HES], unspecified

D72.12 Drug rash with eosinophilia and systemic symptoms syndrome
DRESS syndrome
Use additional code for adverse effect, if applicable, to identify drug (T36-T5Ø with fifth or sixth character 5)

D72.18 Eosinophilia in diseases classified elsewhere
Code first underlying disease, such as:
chronic myelomonocytic leukemia (C93.1-)

D72.19 Other eosinophilia
Familial eosinophilia
Hereditary eosinophilia

✓5th **D72.8 Other specified disorders of white blood cells**
EXCLUDES 1 *leukemia (C91-C95)*

✓6th **D72.81 Decreased white blood cell count**
EXCLUDES 1 *neutropenia (D7Ø.-)*

D72.81Ø Lymphocytopenia
Decreased lymphocytes

D72.818 Other decreased white blood cell count
Basophilic leukopenia
Eosinophilic leukopenia
Monocytopenia
Other decreased leukocytes
Plasmacytopenia

D72.819 Decreased white blood cell count, unspecified
Decreased leukocytes, unspecified
Leukocytopenia, unspecified
Leukopenia
EXCLUDES 1 *malignant leukopenia (D7Ø.9)*

✓6th **D72.82 Elevated white blood cell count**
EXCLUDES 1 *eosinophilia (D72.1)*

D72.82Ø Lymphocytosis (symptomatic)
Elevated lymphocytes

D72.821 Monocytosis (symptomatic)
EXCLUDES 1 *infectious mononucleosis (B27.-)*

D72.822 Plasmacytosis

D72.823 Leukemoid reaction
Basophilic leukemoid reaction
Leukemoid reaction NOS
Lymphocytic leukemoid reaction
Monocytic leukemoid reaction
Myelocytic leukemoid reaction
Neutrophilic leukemoid reaction

D72.824 Basophilia
DEF: Increase in the basophils of the blood, a type of white blood cell, often seen in conjunction with neoplastic disorders.

D72.825 Bandemia
Bandemia without diagnosis of specific infection
EXCLUDES 1 *confirmed infection - code to infection*
leukemia (C91.-, C92.-, C93.-, C94.-, C95.-)
DEF: Increase in early neutrophil cells, called band cells, that may indicate infection.

D72.828 Other elevated white blood cell count

D72.829 Elevated white blood cell count, unspecified
Elevated leukocytes, unspecified
Leukocytosis, unspecified

D72.89 Other specified disorders of white blood cells
Abnormality of white blood cells NEC

D72.9 Disorder of white blood cells, unspecified
Abnormal leukocyte differential NOS

✓4th **D73 Diseases of spleen**

D73.Ø Hyposplenism
Atrophy of spleen
EXCLUDES 1 *asplenia (congenital) (Q89.Ø1)*
postsurgical absence of spleen (Z9Ø.81)

D73.1 Hypersplenism
EXCLUDES 1 *neutropenic splenomegaly (D73.81)*
primary splenic neutropenia (D73.81)
splenitis, splenomegaly in late syphilis (A52.79)
splenitis, splenomegaly in tuberculosis (A18.85)
splenomegaly NOS (R16.1)
splenomegaly congenital (Q89.Ø)

D73.2 Chronic congestive splenomegaly

D73.3 Abscess of spleen

D73.4 Cyst of spleen

D73.5 Infarction of spleen
Splenic rupture, nontraumatic
Torsion of spleen
EXCLUDES 1 *rupture of spleen due to Plasmodium vivax malaria (B51.Ø)*
traumatic rupture of spleen (S36.Ø3-)

✓5th **D73.8 Other diseases of spleen**

D73.81 Neutropenic splenomegaly
Werner-Schultz disease

D73.89 Other diseases of spleen
Fibrosis of spleen NOS
Perisplenitis
Splenitis NOS

D73.9 Disease of spleen, unspecified

✓4th **D74 Methemoglobinemia**

D74.Ø Congenital methemoglobinemia CC
Congenital NADH-methemoglobin reductase deficiency
Hemoglobin-M [Hb-M] disease
Methemoglobinemia, hereditary

D74.8 Other methemoglobinemias CC
Acquired methemoglobinemia (with sulfhemoglobinemia)
Toxic methemoglobinemia

D74.9 Methemoglobinemia, unspecified CC

D75 Other and unspecified diseases of blood and blood-forming organs

EXCLUDES 2 *acute lymphadenitis (L04.-)*
chronic lymphadenitis (I88.1)
enlarged lymph nodes (R59.-)
hypergammaglobulinemia NOS (D89.2)
lymphadenitis NOS (I88.9)
mesenteric lymphadenitis (acute) (chronic) (I88.0)

D75.0 Familial erythrocytosis
Benign polycythemia
Familial polycythemia
EXCLUDES 1 *hereditary ovalocytosis (D58.1)*

D75.1 Secondary polycythemia
Acquired polycythemia
Emotional polycythemia
Erythrocytosis NOS
Hypoxemic polycythemia
Nephrogenous polycythemia
Polycythemia due to erythropoietin
Polycythemia due to fall in plasma volume
Polycythemia due to high altitude
Polycythemia due to stress
Polycythemia NOS
Relative polycythemia
EXCLUDES 1 *polycythemia neonatorum (P61.1)*
polycythemia vera (D45)
DEF: Elevated number of red blood cells in circulating blood as a result of reduced oxygen supply to the tissues.

D75.8 Other specified diseases of blood and blood-forming organs

D75.81 Myelofibrosis CC HCC
Myelofibrosis NOS
Secondary myelofibrosis NOS
Code first the underlying disorder, such as:
malignant neoplasm of breast (C50.-)
Use additional code, if applicable, for associated therapy-related myelodysplastic syndrome (D46.-)
Use additional code for adverse effect, if applicable, to identify drug (T45.1X5)
EXCLUDES 1 *acute myelofibrosis (C94.4-)*
idiopathic myelofibrosis (D47.1)
leukoerythroblastic anemia (D61.82)
myelofibrosis with myeloid metaplasia (D47.4)
myelophthisic anemia (D61.82)
myelophthisis (D61.82)
primary myelofibrosis (D47.1)

▲ **D75.82 Heparin induced thrombocytopenia (HIT)**
▶Use additional code, if applicable, for adverse effect of heparin (T45.515-)◀
DEF: Immune-mediated reaction to heparin therapy causing an abrupt fall in platelet count and serious complications such as pulmonary embolism, stroke, AMI, or DVT.

● **D75.821 Non-immune heparin-induced thrombocytopenia**
Non-immune HIT
Type 1 heparin-induced thrombocytopenia

● **D75.822 Immune-mediated heparin-induced thrombocytopenia**
Immune-mediated HIT
Type 2 heparin-induced thrombocytopenia

● **D75.828 Other heparin-induced thrombocytopenia syndrome**
Autoimmune heparin-induced thrombocytopenia syndrome
Delayed-onset heparin-induced thrombocytopenia
Persisting heparin-induced thrombocytopenia

● **D75.829 Heparin-induced thrombocytopenia, unspecified**

D75.83 Thrombocytosis
EXCLUDES 2 *essential thrombocythemia (D47.3)*
AHA: 2021,4Q,7-8

D75.838 Other thrombocytosis
Reactive thrombocytosis
Secondary thrombocytosis
Code also underlying condition, if known and applicable

D75.839 Thrombocytosis, unspecified
Thrombocythemia NOS
Thrombocytosis NOS

● **D75.84 Other platelet-activating anti-PF4 disorders**
Spontaneous heparin-induced thrombocytopenia syndrome (without heparin exposure)
Thrombosis with thrombocytopenia syndrome
Vaccine-induced thrombotic thrombocytopenia
Use additional code, if applicable, for adverse effect of other viral vaccine (T50.B95-)

D75.89 Other specified diseases of blood and blood-forming organs

D75.9 Disease of blood and blood-forming organs, unspecified

D75.A Glucose-6-phosphate dehydrogenase (G6PD) deficiency without anemia
EXCLUDES 1 *glucose-6-phosphate dehydrogenase (G6PD) deficiency with anemia (D55.0)*
AHA: 2019,4Q,4-5

D76 Other specified diseases with participation of lymphoreticular and reticulohistiocytic tissue

EXCLUDES 1 *(Abt-) Letterer-Siwe disease (C96.0)*
eosinophilic granuloma (C96.6)
Hand-Schüller-Christian disease (C96.5)
histiocytic medullary reticulosis (C96.9)
histiocytic sarcoma (C96.A)
histiocytosis X, multifocal (C96.5)
histiocytosis X, unifocal (C96.6)
Langerhans-cell histiocytosis, multifocal (C96.5)
Langerhans-cell histiocytosis NOS (C96.6)
Langerhans-cell histiocytosis, unifocal (C96.6)
leukemic reticuloendotheliosis (C91.4-)
lipomelanotic reticulosis (I89.8)
malignant histiocytosis (C96.A)
malignant reticulosis (C86.0)
nonlipid reticuloendotheliosis (C96.0)

D76.1 Hemophagocytic lymphohistiocytosis CC HCC
Familial hemophagocytic reticulosis
Histiocytoses of mononuclear phagocytes

D76.2 Hemophagocytic syndrome, infection-associated CC HCC
Use additional code to identify infectious agent or disease

D76.3 Other histiocytosis syndromes CC HCC
Reticulohistiocytoma (giant-cell)
Sinus histiocytosis with massive lymphadenopathy
Xanthogranuloma

D77 Other disorders of blood and blood-forming organs in diseases classified elsewhere
Code first underlying disease, such as:
amyloidosis (E85.-)
congenital early syphilis (A50.0)
echinococcosis (B67.0-B67.9)
malaria (B50.0-B54)
schistosomiasis [bilharziasis] (B65.0-B65.9)
vitamin C deficiency (E54)
EXCLUDES 1 *rupture of spleen due to Plasmodium vivax malaria (B51.0)*
splenitis, splenomegaly in late syphilis (A52.79)
splenitis, splenomegaly in tuberculosis (A18.85)

Intraoperative and postprocedural complications of the spleen (D78)

D78 Intraoperative and postprocedural complications of the spleen
AHA: 2016,4Q,9-10

D78.Ø Intraoperative hemorrhage and hematoma of the spleen complicating a procedure
EXCLUDES 1 *intraoperative hemorrhage and hematoma of the spleen due to accidental puncture or laceration during a procedure (D78.1-)*

D78.Ø1 Intraoperative hemorrhage and hematoma of the spleen complicating a procedure on the spleen CC

D78.Ø2 Intraoperative hemorrhage and hematoma of the spleen complicating other procedure CC

D78.1 Accidental puncture and laceration of the spleen during a procedure

D78.11 Accidental puncture and laceration of the spleen during a procedure on the spleen CC

D78.12 Accidental puncture and laceration of the spleen during other procedure CC
AHA: 2022,1Q,22

D78.2 Postprocedural hemorrhage of the spleen following a procedure

D78.21 Postprocedural hemorrhage of the spleen following a procedure on the spleen CC

D78.22 Postprocedural hemorrhage of the spleen following other procedure CC

D78.3 Postprocedural hematoma and seroma of the spleen following a procedure

D78.31 Postprocedural hematoma of the spleen following a procedure on the spleen CC

D78.32 Postprocedural hematoma of the spleen following other procedure CC

D78.33 Postprocedural seroma of the spleen following a procedure on the spleen CC

D78.34 Postprocedural seroma of the spleen following other procedure CC

D78.8 Other intraoperative and postprocedural complications of the spleen
Use additional code, if applicable, to further specify disorder

D78.81 Other intraoperative complications of the spleen CC

D78.89 Other postprocedural complications of the spleen CC

Certain disorders involving the immune mechanism (D8Ø-D89)

INCLUDES defects in the complement system
immunodeficiency disorders, except human immunodeficiency virus [HIV] disease
sarcoidosis

EXCLUDES 1 *autoimmune disease (systemic) NOS (M35.9)*
functional disorders of polymorphonuclear neutrophils (D71)
human immunodeficiency virus [HIV] disease (B2Ø)

D8Ø Immunodeficiency with predominantly antibody defects

D8Ø.Ø Hereditary hypogammaglobulinemia CC HCC
Autosomal recessive agammaglobulinemia (Swiss type)
X-linked agammaglobulinemia [Bruton] (with growth hormone deficiency)

D8Ø.1 Nonfamilial hypogammaglobulinemia CC HCC
Agammaglobulinemia with immunoglobulin-bearing B-lymphocytes
Common variable agammaglobulinemia [CVAgamma]
Hypogammaglobulinemia NOS

D8Ø.2 Selective deficiency of immunoglobulin A [IgA] CC HCC

D8Ø.3 Selective deficiency of immunoglobulin G [IgG] subclasses CC HCC

D8Ø.4 Selective deficiency of immunoglobulin M [IgM] CC HCC

D8Ø.5 Immunodeficiency with increased immunoglobulin M [IgM] CC HCC

D8Ø.6 Antibody deficiency with near-normal immunoglobulins or with hyperimmunoglobulinemia CC HCC

D8Ø.7 Transient hypogammaglobulinemia of infancy CC HCC

D8Ø.8 Other immunodeficiencies with predominantly antibody defects CC HCC
Kappa light chain deficiency

D8Ø.9 Immunodeficiency with predominantly antibody defects, unspecified CC HCC

D81 Combined immunodeficiencies
EXCLUDES 1 *autosomal recessive agammaglobulinemia (Swiss type) (D8Ø.Ø)*

D81.Ø Severe combined immunodeficiency [SCID] with reticular dysgenesis CC HCC

D81.1 Severe combined immunodeficiency [SCID] with low T- and B-cell numbers CC HCC

D81.2 Severe combined immunodeficiency [SCID] with low or normal B-cell numbers CC HCC

D81.3 Adenosine deaminase [ADA] deficiency
AHA: 2019,4Q,5-6

D81.3Ø Adenosine deaminase deficiency, unspecified CC HCC
ADA deficiency NOS

D81.31 Severe combined immunodeficiency due to adenosine deaminase deficiency CC HCC
ADA deficiency with SCID
Adenosine deaminase [ADA] deficiency with severe combined immunodeficiency

D81.32 Adenosine deaminase 2 deficiency CC HCC
ADA2 deficiency
Adenosine deaminase deficiency type 2
Code also, if applicable, any associated manifestations, such as:
polyarteritis nodosa (M3Ø.Ø)
stroke (I63.-)

D81.39 Other adenosine deaminase deficiency CC HCC
Adenosine deaminase [ADA] deficiency type 1, NOS
Adenosine deaminase [ADA] deficiency type 1, without SCID
Adenosine deaminase [ADA] deficiency type 1, without severe combined immunodeficiency
Partial ADA deficiency (type 1)
Partial adenosine deaminase deficiency (type 1)

D81.4 Nezelof's syndrome CC HCC

D81.5 Purine nucleoside phosphorylase [PNP] deficiency CC HCC

D81.6 Major histocompatibility complex class I deficiency CC HCC
Bare lymphocyte syndrome

D81.7 Major histocompatibility complex class II deficiency CC HCC

D81.8 Other combined immunodeficiencies

D81.81 Biotin-dependent carboxylase deficiency
Multiple carboxylase deficiency
EXCLUDES 1 *biotin-dependent carboxylase deficiency due to dietary deficiency of biotin (E53.8)*

D81.81Ø Biotinidase deficiency

D81.818 Other biotin-dependent carboxylase deficiency
Holocarboxylase synthetase deficiency
Other multiple carboxylase deficiency

D81.819 Biotin-dependent carboxylase deficiency, unspecified
Multiple carboxylase deficiency, unspecified

● **D81.82 Activated Phosphoinositide 3-kinase Delta Syndrome [APDS]** CC
p11Ød-activating mutation causing senescent T cells, lymphadenopathy, and immunodeficiency [PASLI] disease
Code also, if applicable, any associated manifestations, such as:
bronchiectasis (J47.-)
herpes virus infections (BØØ.-)
other acute respiratory tract infections (JØØ-JØ6; J2Ø-J22)
other infections (AØØ-B99)
pneumonia (J12-J18)

D81.89 Other combined immunodeficiencies CC HCC

D81.9 Combined immunodeficiency, unspecified CC HCC
Severe combined immunodeficiency disorder [SCID] NOS

D82 Immunodeficiency associated with other major defects
EXCLUDES 1 *ataxia telangiectasia [Louis-Bar] (G11.3)*

D82.Ø Wiskott-Aldrich syndrome CC HCC
Immunodeficiency with thrombocytopenia and eczema

D82.1 **Di George's syndrome** CC HCC
Pharyngeal pouch syndrome
Thymic alymphoplasia
Thymic aplasia or hypoplasia with immunodeficiency
AHA: 2019,3Q,14

D82.2 **Immunodeficiency with short-limbed stature** HCC

D82.3 **Immunodeficiency following hereditary defective response to Epstein-Barr virus** HCC
X-linked lymphoproliferative disease

D82.4 **Hyperimmunoglobulin E [IgE] syndrome** HCC

D82.8 **Immunodeficiency associated with other specified major defects** HCC

D82.9 **Immunodeficiency associated with major defect, unspecified** HCC

✓4th **D83 Common variable immunodeficiency**

D83.0 **Common variable immunodeficiency with predominant abnormalities of B-cell numbers and function** CC HCC

D83.1 **Common variable immunodeficiency with predominant immunoregulatory T-cell disorders** CC HCC

D83.2 **Common variable immunodeficiency with autoantibodies to B- or T-cells** CC HCC

D83.8 **Other common variable immunodeficiencies** CC HCC

D83.9 **Common variable immunodeficiency, unspecified** CC HCC

✓4th **D84 Other immunodeficiencies**

D84.0 **Lymphocyte function antigen-1 [LFA-1] defect** HCC

D84.1 **Defects in the complement system** HCC
C1 esterase inhibitor [C1-INH] deficiency

✓5th D84.8 **Other specified immunodeficiencies**
AHA: 2020,4Q,10-12

D84.81 ***Immunodeficiency due to conditions classified elsewhere*** CC HCC
Code first underlying condition, such as:
chromosomal abnormalities (Q90-Q99)
diabetes mellitus (E08-E13)
malignant neoplasms (C00-C96)
EXCLUDES 1 *certain disorders involving the immune mechanism (D80-D83, D84.0, D84.1, D84.9)*
human immunodeficiency virus [HIV] disease (B20)
AHA: 2021,1Q,52

✓6th D84.82 **Immunodeficiency due to drugs and external causes**

D84.821 **Immunodeficiency due to drugs** CC HCC
Immunodeficiency due to (current or past) medication
Use additional code for adverse effect if applicable, to identify adverse effect of drug (T36-T50 with fifth or six character 5)
Use additional code, if applicable, for associated long term (current) drug therapy drug or medication such as:
long term (current) drug therapy systemic steroids (Z79.52)
other long term (current) drug therapy (Z79.899)

D84.822 **Immunodeficiency due to external causes** CC HCC
Code also, if applicable, radiological procedure and radiotherapy (Y84.2)
Use additional code for external cause such as:
exposure to ionizing radiation (W88)

D84.89 **Other immunodeficiencies** CC HCC

D84.9 **Immunodeficiency, unspecified** CC HCC
Immunocompromised NOS
Immunodeficient NOS
Immunosuppressed NOS
AHA: 2020,4Q,10

✓4th **D86 Sarcoidosis**
DEF: Clustering of immune cells resulting in granuloma formation. Often affects the lungs and lymphatic system but can occur in other body sites.

D86.0 **Sarcoidosis of lung** HCC

D86.1 **Sarcoidosis of lymph nodes**

D86.2 **Sarcoidosis of lung with sarcoidosis of lymph nodes** HCC

D86.3 **Sarcoidosis of skin**

✓5th D86.8 **Sarcoidosis of other sites**

D86.81 **Sarcoid meningitis**

D86.82 **Multiple cranial nerve palsies in sarcoidosis** HCC

D86.83 **Sarcoid iridocyclitis**

D86.84 **Sarcoid pyelonephritis**
Tubulo-interstitial nephropathy in sarcoidosis

D86.85 **Sarcoid myocarditis**

D86.86 **Sarcoid arthropathy**
Polyarthritis in sarcoidosis

D86.87 **Sarcoid myositis**

D86.89 **Sarcoidosis of other sites**
Hepatic granuloma
Uveoparotid fever [Heerfordt]

D86.9 **Sarcoidosis, unspecified**

✓4th **D89 Other disorders involving the immune mechanism, not elsewhere classified**
EXCLUDES 1 *hyperglobulinemia NOS (R77.1)*
monoclonal gammopathy (of undetermined significance) (D47.2)
EXCLUDES 2 *transplant failure and rejection (T86.-)*

D89.0 **Polyclonal hypergammaglobulinemia**
Benign hypergammaglobulinemic purpura
Polyclonal gammopathy NOS

D89.1 **Cryoglobulinemia** HCC
Cryoglobulinemic purpura
Cryoglobulinemic vasculitis
Essential cryoglobulinemia
Idiopathic cryoglobulinemia
Mixed cryoglobulinemia
Primary cryoglobulinemia
Secondary cryoglobulinemia

D89.2 **Hypergammaglobulinemia, unspecified**

D89.3 **Immune reconstitution syndrome** HCC
Immune reconstitution inflammatory syndrome [IRIS]
Use additional code for adverse effect, if applicable, to identify drug (T36-T50 with fifth or sixth character 5)

✓5th D89.4 **Mast cell activation syndrome and related disorders**
EXCLUDES 1 *aggressive systemic mastocytosis (C96.21)*
congenital cutaneous mastocytosis (Q82.2)
(non-congenital) cutaneous mastocytosis (D47.01)
(indolent) systemic mastocytosis (D47.02)
malignant mast cell neoplasm (C96.2-)
malignant mastocytoma (C96.29)
mast cell leukemia (C94.3-)
mast cell sarcoma (C96.22)
mastocytoma NOS (D47.09)
other mast cell neoplasms of uncertain behavior (D47.09)
systemic mastocytosis associated with a clonal hematologic non-mast cell lineage disease (SM-AHNMD) (D47.02)
AHA: 2016,4Q,11

D89.40 **Mast cell activation, unspecified** HCC
Mast cell activation disorder, unspecified
Mast cell activation syndrome, NOS

D89.41 **Monoclonal mast cell activation syndrome** HCC

D89.42 **Idiopathic mast cell activation syndrome** HCC

D89.43 **Secondary mast cell activation** HCC
Secondary mast cell activation syndrome
Code also underlying etiology, if known

D89.44 **Hereditary alpha tryptasemia** HCC
Use additional code, if applicable, for:
allergy status, other than to drugs and biological substances (Z91.0-)
personal history of anaphylaxis (Z87.892)
AHA: 2021,4Q,8

D89.49 **Other mast cell activation disorder** HCC
Other mast cell activation syndrome

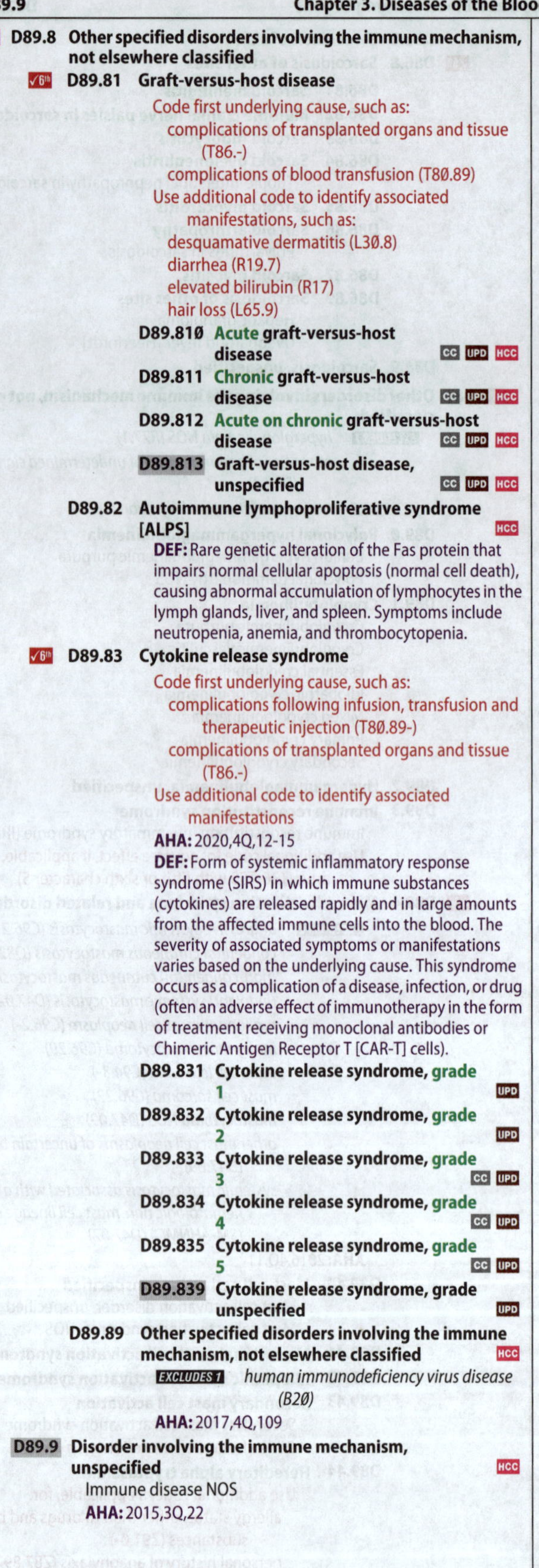

✓5th **D89.8 Other specified disorders involving the immune mechanism, not elsewhere classified**

✓6th **D89.81 Graft-versus-host disease**

Code first underlying cause, such as:
- complications of transplanted organs and tissue (T86.-)
- complications of blood transfusion (T8Ø.89)

Use additional code to identify associated manifestations, such as:
- desquamative dermatitis (L3Ø.8)
- diarrhea (R19.7)
- elevated bilirubin (R17)
- hair loss (L65.9)

D89.81Ø Acute graft-versus-host disease CC UPD HCC

D89.811 Chronic graft-versus-host disease CC UPD HCC

D89.812 Acute on chronic graft-versus-host disease CC UPD HCC

D89.813 Graft-versus-host disease, unspecified CC UPD HCC

D89.82 Autoimmune lymphoproliferative syndrome [ALPS] HCC

DEF: Rare genetic alteration of the Fas protein that impairs normal cellular apoptosis (normal cell death), causing abnormal accumulation of lymphocytes in the lymph glands, liver, and spleen. Symptoms include neutropenia, anemia, and thrombocytopenia.

✓6th **D89.83 Cytokine release syndrome**

Code first underlying cause, such as:
- complications following infusion, transfusion and therapeutic injection (T8Ø.89-)
- complications of transplanted organs and tissue (T86.-)

Use additional code to identify associated manifestations

AHA: 2020,4Q,12-15

DEF: Form of systemic inflammatory response syndrome (SIRS) in which immune substances (cytokines) are released rapidly and in large amounts from the affected immune cells into the blood. The severity of associated symptoms or manifestations varies based on the underlying cause. This syndrome occurs as a complication of a disease, infection, or drug (often an adverse effect of immunotherapy in the form of treatment receiving monoclonal antibodies or Chimeric Antigen Receptor T [CAR-T] cells).

D89.831 Cytokine release syndrome, grade 1 UPD

D89.832 Cytokine release syndrome, grade 2 UPD

D89.833 Cytokine release syndrome, grade 3 CC UPD

D89.834 Cytokine release syndrome, grade 4 CC UPD

D89.835 Cytokine release syndrome, grade 5 CC UPD

D89.839 Cytokine release syndrome, grade unspecified UPD

D89.89 Other specified disorders involving the immune mechanism, not elsewhere classified HCC

EXCLUDES 1 *human immunodeficiency virus disease (B2Ø)*

AHA: 2017,4Q,109

D89.9 Disorder involving the immune mechanism, unspecified HCC

Immune disease NOS

AHA: 2015,3Q,22

Chapter 4. Endocrine, Nutritional and Metabolic Diseases (E00–E89)

Chapter-specific Guidelines with Coding Examples

The chapter-specific guidelines from the ICD-10-CM Official Guidelines for Coding and Reporting have been provided below. Along with these guidelines are coding examples, contained in the shaded boxes, that have been developed to help illustrate the coding and/or sequencing guidance found in these guidelines.

a. Diabetes mellitus

The diabetes mellitus codes are combination codes that include the type of diabetes mellitus, the body system affected, and the complications affecting that body system. As many codes within a particular category as are necessary to describe all of the complications of the disease may be used. They should be sequenced based on the reason for a particular encounter. Assign as many codes from categories E08–E13 as needed to identify all of the associated conditions that the patient has.

Patient is seen for poorly controlled diabetes, type 2, with diabetic polyneuropathy and diabetic retinopathy with macular edema

E11.65 **Type 2 diabetes mellitus with hyperglycemia**

E11.311 **Type 2 diabetes mellitus with unspecified diabetic retinopathy with macular edema**

E11.42 **Type 2 diabetes mellitus with diabetic polyneuropathy**

Explanation: Use as many codes to describe the diabetic complications as needed. Many are combination codes that describe more than one condition. Code first the reason for the encounter. "Poorly controlled" is described as "with hyperglycemia." Diabetes documented as "uncontrolled" is not assumed to be hyperglycemic but can be classified to either hyperglycemia or hypoglycemia. If documentation is not clear, the provider must be queried so that the appropriate code can be reported.

1) Type of diabetes

The age of a patient is not the sole determining factor, though most type 1 diabetics develop the condition before reaching puberty. For this reason, type 1 diabetes mellitus is also referred to as juvenile diabetes.

A 45-year-old patient is diagnosed with type 1 diabetes

E10.9 **Type 1 diabetes mellitus without complications**

Explanation: Although most type 1 diabetics are diagnosed in childhood or adolescence, it can also begin in adults.

2) Type of diabetes mellitus not documented

If the type of diabetes mellitus is not documented in the medical record the default is E11.-, Type 2 diabetes mellitus.

H & P lists diabetes and hypertension on patient problem list

E11.9 **Type 2 diabetes mellitus without complications**

I10 **Essential (primary) hypertension**

Explanation: Since the type of diabetes was not documented and no complications were noted, the default code is E11.9.

3) Diabetes mellitus and the use of insulin, oral hypoglycemics, and injectable non-insulin drugs

If the documentation in a medical record does not indicate the type of diabetes but does indicate that the patient uses insulin, code E11-, Type 2 diabetes mellitus, should be assigned. Additional code(s) should be assigned from category Z79 to identify the long-term (current) use of insulin, oral hypoglycemic drugs, or injectable non-insulin antidiabetic, as follows:

If the patient is treated with both oral **hypoglycemic drugs** and insulin, both code Z79.4, Long term (current) use of insulin, and code Z79.84, Long term (current) use of oral hypoglycemic drugs, should be assigned.

If the patient is treated with both insulin and an injectable non-insulin antidiabetic drug, assign codes Z79.4, Long term (current) use of insulin, and **Z79.85, Long-term (current) use of injectable non-insulin antidiabetic drugs.**

If the patient is treated with both oral hypoglycemic drugs and an injectable non-insulin antidiabetic drug, assign codes Z79.84, Long term (current) use of oral hypoglycemic drugs, and **Z79.85, Long-term (current) use of injectable non-insulin antidiabetic drugs.**

Code Z79.4 should not be assigned if insulin is given temporarily to bring a type 2 patient's blood sugar under control during an encounter.

Type 2 diabetic patient on daily metformin and Victoza is admitted in ketoacidosis, insulin given to stabilize blood sugars and discontinued at discharge

E11.10 **Type 2 diabetes mellitus with ketoacidosis without coma**

Z79.84 **Long term (current) use of oral hypoglycemic drugs**

Z79.85 **Long term (current) use of injectable non-insulin anti-diabetic drugs**

Explanation: Documentation indicates the patient is on an oral antidiabetic medication (metformin) and an injectable noninsulin antidiabetic medication (Victoza). Although insulin was given to the patient during the encounter, it was discontinued at discharge, indicating that the patient does not regularly use insulin. A Z code representing long-term use of the oral drug and long-term use of the injectable medication can be applied. Applying code Z79.4 to represent long-term use of insulin would be inappropriate.

4) Diabetes mellitus in pregnancy and gestational diabetes

See Section I.C.15. Diabetes mellitus in pregnancy.

See Section I.C.15. Gestational (pregnancy induced) diabetes

5) Complications due to insulin pump malfunction

(a) Underdose of insulin due to insulin pump failure

An underdose of insulin due to an insulin pump failure should be assigned to a code from subcategory T85.6, Mechanical complication of other specified internal and external prosthetic devices, implants and grafts, that specifies the type of pump malfunction, as the principal or first-listed code, followed by code T38.3X6-, Underdosing of insulin and oral hypoglycemic [antidiabetic] drugs. Additional codes for the type of diabetes mellitus and any associated complications due to the underdosing should also be assigned.

A 24-year-old type 1 diabetic male treated in ED for hyperglycemia; insulin pump found to be malfunctioning and underdosing

T85.614A **Breakdown (mechanical) of insulin pump, initial encounter**

T38.3X6A **Underdosing of insulin and oral hypoglycemic [antidiabetic] drugs, initial encounter**

E10.65 **Type 1 diabetes mellitus with hyperglycemia**

Explanation: The complication code for the mechanical breakdown of the pump is sequenced first, followed by the underdosing code and type of diabetes with complication. Code all other diabetic complication codes necessary to describe the patient's condition.

(b) Overdose of insulin due to insulin pump failure

The principal or first-listed code for an encounter due to an insulin pump malfunction resulting in an overdose of insulin, should also be T85.6-, Mechanical complication of other specified internal and external prosthetic devices, implants and grafts, followed by code T38.3X1-, Poisoning by insulin and oral hypoglycemic [antidiabetic] drugs, accidental (unintentional).

A 24-year-old type 1 diabetic male found down with diabetic coma, brought into ED and treated for hypoglycemia; insulin pump found to be malfunctioning and overdosing

T85.614A **Breakdown (mechanical) of insulin pump, initial encounter**

T38.3X1A **Poisoning by insulin and oral hypoglycemic [antidiabetic] drugs, accidental (unintentional), initial encounter**

E10.641 **Type 1 diabetes mellitus with hypoglycemia with coma**

Explanation: The complication code for the mechanical breakdown of the pump is sequenced first, followed by the poisoning code and type of diabetes with complication. All the characters in the combination code must be used to form a valid code and to fully describe the type of diabetes, the hypoglycemia, and the coma.

6) **Secondary diabetes mellitus**

Codes under categories EØ8, Diabetes mellitus due to underlying condition, EØ9, Drug or chemical induced diabetes mellitus, and E13, Other specified diabetes mellitus, identify complications/manifestations associated with secondary diabetes mellitus. Secondary diabetes is always caused by another condition or event (e.g., cystic fibrosis, malignant neoplasm of pancreas, pancreatectomy, adverse effect of drug, or poisoning).

(a) **Secondary diabetes mellitus and the use of insulin or oral hypoglycemic drugs**

For patients with secondary diabetes mellitus who routinely use insulin, oral hypoglycemic drugs, or injectable non-insulin drugs, additional code(s) from category Z79 should be assigned to identify the long-term (current) use of insulin, oral hypoglycemic drugs, or non-injectable non-insulin drugs as follows:

If the patient is treated with both oral **hypoglycemic drugs** and insulin, both code Z79.4, Long term (current) use of insulin, and code Z79.84, Long term (current) use of oral hypoglycemic drugs, should be assigned.

If the patient is treated with both insulin and an injectable non-insulin antidiabetic drug, assign codes Z79.4, Long-term (current) use of insulin, and **Z79.85, Long-term (current) use of injectable non-insulin antidiabetic drugs**.

If the patient is treated with both oral hypoglycemic drugs and an injectable non-insulin antidiabetic drug, assign codes Z79.84, Long-term (current) use of oral hypoglycemic drugs, and **Z79.85, Long-term (current) use of injectable non-insulin antidiabetic drugs.**

Code Z79.4 should not be assigned if insulin is given temporarily to bring a secondary diabetic patient's blood sugar under control during an encounter

The patient, maintained on metformin and insulin, was admitted for treatment of diabetic gangrene. The patient developed diabetes secondary to Nelson's syndrome.

E24.1	**Nelson's syndrome**
EØ8.52	**Diabetes mellitus due to underlying condition with diabetic peripheral angiopathy with gangrene**
Z79.4	**Long term (current) use of insulin**
Z79.84	**Long term (current) use of oral hypoglycemic drugs**

Explanation: When diabetes is caused by an underlying condition, the underlying condition should always be sequenced before any codes representing the diabetes. Patients with secondary diabetes may be maintained on both insulin and an oral hypoglycemic. When maintained on both, report a code for the long term use of insulin and a code for the long term use of oral hypoglycemic.

(b) **Assigning and sequencing secondary diabetes codes and its causes**

The sequencing of the secondary diabetes codes in relationship to codes for the cause of the diabetes is based on the Tabular List instructions for categories EØ8, EØ9 and E13.

(i) **Secondary diabetes mellitus due to pancreatectomy**

For postpancreatectomy diabetes mellitus (lack of insulin due to the surgical removal of all or part of the pancreas), assign code E89.1, Postprocedural hypoinsulinemia. Assign a code from category E13 and a code from subcategory Z90.41, Acquired absence of pancreas, as additional codes.

Patient with newly diagnosed diabetes after surgical removal of part of pancreas is discharged with referral for consult to initiate insulin.

E89.1	**Postprocedural hypoinsulinemia**
E13.9	**Other specified diabetes mellitus without complications**
Z9Ø.411	**Acquired partial absence of pancreas**

Explanation: Sequence the postprocedural complication of the hypoinsulinemia due to the partial removal of the pancreas as the first-listed code, followed by codes for other specified diabetes (NEC) without complications and partial acquired absence of the pancreas. Code Z79.4 Long term (current) use of insulin, is not added because the insulin has not yet been started.

(ii) **Secondary diabetes due to drugs**

Secondary diabetes may be caused by an adverse effect of correctly administered medications, poisoning or sequela of poisoning.

See section I.C.19.e. for coding of adverse effects and poisoning, and section I.C.20 for external cause code reporting.

Initial encounter for corticosteroid-induced diabetes mellitus

EØ9.9	**Drug or chemical induced diabetes mellitus without complications**
T38.ØX5A	**Adverse effect of glucocorticoids and synthetic analogues, initial encounter**

Explanation: If the diabetes is caused by an adverse effect of a drug, the diabetic condition is coded first. If it occurs from a poisoning or overdose, the poisoning code causing the diabetes is sequenced first.

Chapter 4. Endocrine, Nutritional and Metabolic Diseases (E00-E89)

NOTE All neoplasms, whether functionally active or not, are classified in Chapter 2. Appropriate codes in this chapter (i.e. E05.8, E07.0, E16-E31, E34.-) may be used as additional codes to indicate either functional activity by neoplasms and ectopic endocrine tissue or hyperfunction and hypofunction of endocrine glands associated with neoplasms and other conditions classified elsewhere.

EXCLUDES 1 *transitory endocrine and metabolic disorders specific to newborn (P70-P74)*

AHA: 2018,2Q,6

This chapter contains the following blocks:

E00-E07 Disorders of thyroid gland
E08-E13 Diabetes mellitus
E15-E16 Other disorders of glucose regulation and pancreatic internal secretion
E20-E35 Disorders of other endocrine glands
E36 Intraoperative complications of endocrine system
E40-E46 Malnutrition
E50-E64 Other nutritional deficiencies
E65-E68 Overweight, obesity and other hyperalimentation
E70-E88 Metabolic disorders
E89 Postprocedural endocrine and metabolic complications and disorders, not elsewhere classified

Disorders of thyroid gland (E00-E07)

√4th **E00 Congenital iodine-deficiency syndrome**
Use additional code (F70-F79) to identify associated intellectual disabilities
EXCLUDES 1 *subclinical iodine-deficiency hypothyroidism (E02)*

E00.0 Congenital iodine-deficiency syndrome, neurological type
Endemic cretinism, neurological type

E00.1 Congenital iodine-deficiency syndrome, myxedematous type
Endemic hypothyroid cretinism
Endemic cretinism, myxedematous type

E00.2 Congenital iodine-deficiency syndrome, mixed type
Endemic cretinism, mixed type

E00.9 Congenital iodine-deficiency syndrome, unspecified
Congenital iodine-deficiency hypothyroidism NOS
Endemic cretinism NOS

√4th **E01 Iodine-deficiency related thyroid disorders and allied conditions**
EXCLUDES 1 *congenital iodine-deficiency syndrome (E00.-)*
subclinical iodine-deficiency hypothyroidism (E02)

E01.0 Iodine-deficiency related diffuse (endemic) goiter

E01.1 Iodine-deficiency related multinodular (endemic) goiter
Iodine-deficiency related nodular goiter

E01.2 Iodine-deficiency related (endemic) goiter, unspecified
Endemic goiter NOS

E01.8 Other iodine-deficiency related thyroid disorders and allied conditions
Acquired iodine-deficiency hypothyroidism NOS

E02 Subclinical iodine-deficiency hypothyroidism
AHA: 2021,1Q,8

√4th **E03 Other hypothyroidism**
EXCLUDES 1 *iodine-deficiency related hypothyroidism (E00-E02)*
postprocedural hypothyroidism (E89.0)
DEF: Hypothyroidism: Underproduction of thyroid hormone.

E03.0 Congenital hypothyroidism with diffuse goiter
Congenital parenchymatous goiter (nontoxic)
Congenital goiter (nontoxic) NOS
EXCLUDES 1 *transitory congenital goiter with normal function (P72.0)*

E03.1 Congenital hypothyroidism without goiter
Aplasia of thyroid (with myxedema)
Congenital atrophy of thyroid
Congenital hypothyroidism NOS

E03.2 Hypothyroidism due to medicaments and other exogenous substances
Code first poisoning due to drug or toxin, if applicable (T36-T65 with fifth or sixth character 1-4 or 6)
Use additional code for adverse effect, if applicable, to identify drug (T36-T50 with fifth or sixth character 5)

E03.3 Postinfectious hypothyroidism

E03.4 Atrophy of thyroid (acquired)
EXCLUDES 1 *congenital atrophy of thyroid (E03.1)*

E03.5 Myxedema coma MCC HCC

E03.8 Other specified hypothyroidism
AHA: 2021,1Q,8

E03.9 Hypothyroidism, unspecified
Myxedema NOS

√4th **E04 Other nontoxic goiter**
EXCLUDES 1 *congenital goiter (NOS) (diffuse) (parenchymatous) (E03.0)*
iodine-deficiency related goiter (E00-E02)

E04.0 Nontoxic diffuse goiter
Diffuse (colloid) nontoxic goiter
Simple nontoxic goiter

E04.1 Nontoxic single thyroid nodule
Colloid nodule (cystic) (thyroid)
Nontoxic uninodular goiter
Thyroid (cystic) nodule NOS
DEF: Enlarged thyroid, commonly due to decreased thyroid production, with a single nodule. No clinical hypothyroidism.

E04.2 Nontoxic multinodular goiter
Cystic goiter NOS
Multinodular (cystic) goiter NOS
DEF: Enlarged thyroid, commonly due to decreased thyroid production with multiple nodules. No clinical hypothyroidism.

E04.8 Other specified nontoxic goiter

E04.9 Nontoxic goiter, unspecified
Goiter NOS
Nodular goiter (nontoxic) NOS

√4th **E05 Thyrotoxicosis [hyperthyroidism]**
EXCLUDES 1 *chronic thyroiditis with transient thyrotoxicosis (E06.2)*
neonatal thyrotoxicosis (P72.1)
DEF: Excessive quantities of hormones from the thyroid gland caused by overproduction or loss of storage ability.

√5th **E05.0 Thyrotoxicosis with diffuse goiter**
Exophthalmic or toxic goiter NOS
Graves' disease
Toxic diffuse goiter
DEF: Diffuse thyroid enlargement accompanied by hyperthyroidism, bulging eyes, and dermopathy.

E05.00 Thyrotoxicosis with diffuse goiter without thyrotoxic crisis or storm

E05.01 Thyrotoxicosis with diffuse goiter with thyrotoxic crisis or storm MCC

Goiter

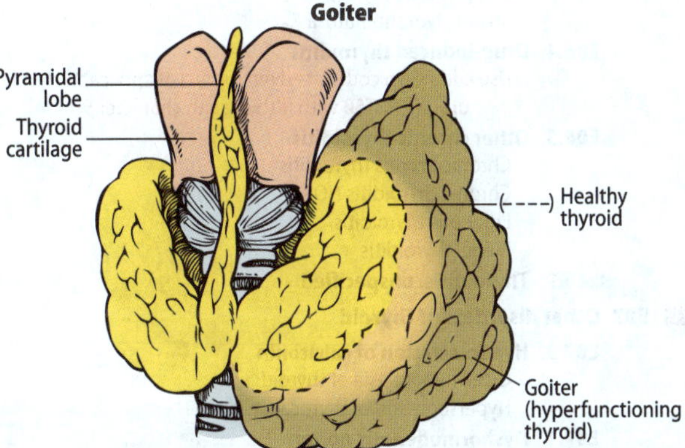

√5th **E05.1 Thyrotoxicosis with toxic single thyroid nodule**
Thyrotoxicosis with toxic uninodular goiter
DEF: Symptomatic hyperthyroidism with a single nodule on the enlarged thyroid gland. Onset of symptoms can be abrupt and include extreme nervousness, insomnia, weight loss, tremors, and psychosis or coma.

E05.10 Thyrotoxicosis with toxic single thyroid nodule without thyrotoxic crisis or storm

E05.11 Thyrotoxicosis with toxic single thyroid nodule with thyrotoxic crisis or storm MCC

√5th **E05.2 Thyrotoxicosis with toxic multinodular goiter**
Toxic nodular goiter NOS

E05.20 Thyrotoxicosis with toxic multinodular goiter without thyrotoxic crisis or storm

E05.21 Thyrotoxicosis with toxic multinodular goiter with thyrotoxic crisis or storm MCC

√5th **E05.3 Thyrotoxicosis from ectopic thyroid tissue**

E05.30 Thyrotoxicosis from ectopic thyroid tissue without thyrotoxic crisis or storm

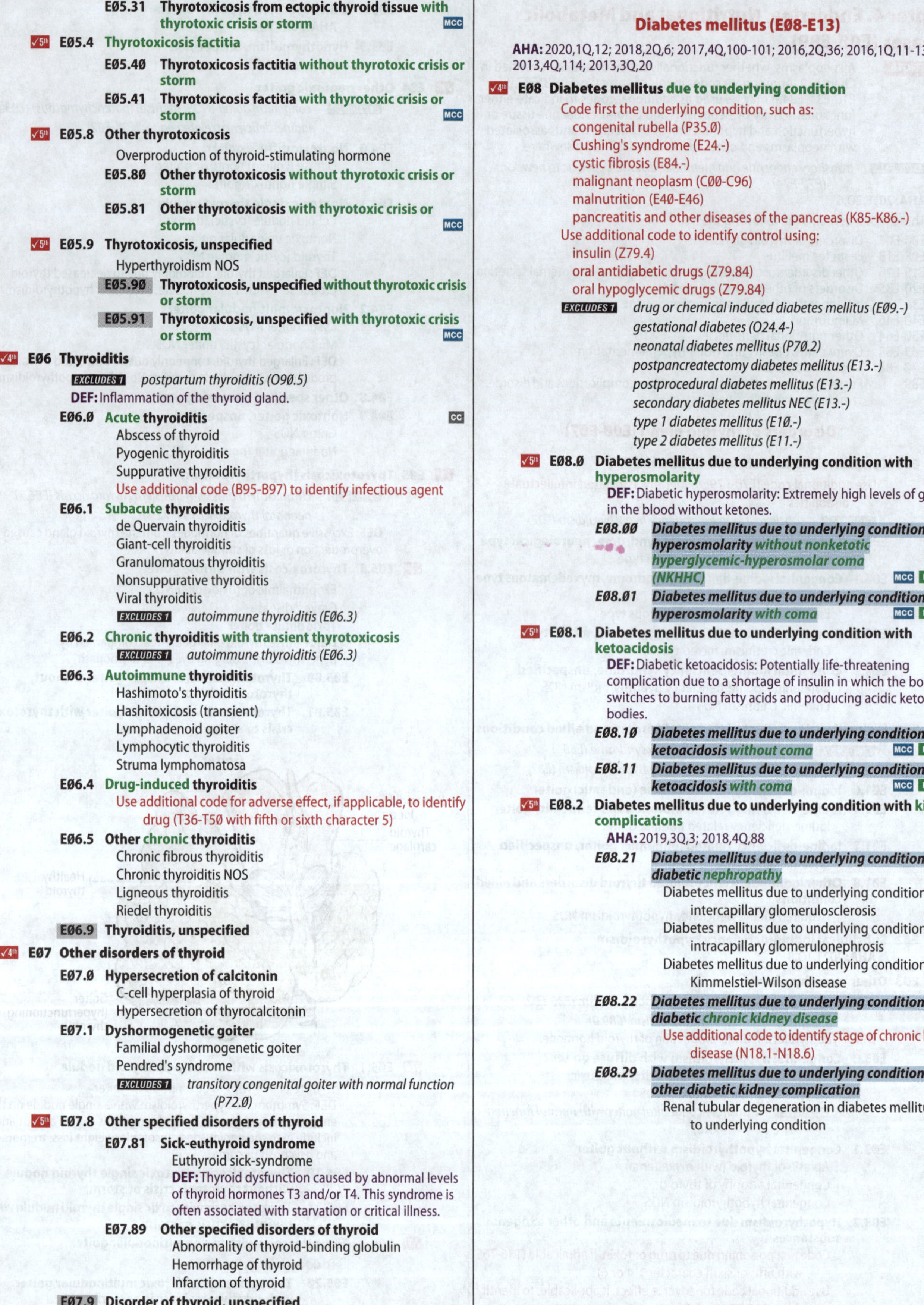

EØ5.31 Thyrotoxicosis from ectopic thyroid tissue with thyrotoxic crisis or storm MCC

✓5th **EØ5.4 Thyrotoxicosis factitia**

EØ5.4Ø Thyrotoxicosis factitia without thyrotoxic crisis or storm

EØ5.41 Thyrotoxicosis factitia with thyrotoxic crisis or storm MCC

✓5th **EØ5.8 Other thyrotoxicosis**

Overproduction of thyroid-stimulating hormone

EØ5.8Ø Other thyrotoxicosis without thyrotoxic crisis or storm

EØ5.81 Other thyrotoxicosis with thyrotoxic crisis or storm MCC

✓5th **EØ5.9 Thyrotoxicosis, unspecified**

Hyperthyroidism NOS

EØ5.9Ø Thyrotoxicosis, unspecified without thyrotoxic crisis or storm

EØ5.91 Thyrotoxicosis, unspecified with thyrotoxic crisis or storm MCC

✓4th **EØ6 Thyroiditis**

EXCLUDES 1 *postpartum thyroiditis (O9Ø.5)*

DEF: Inflammation of the thyroid gland.

EØ6.Ø Acute thyroiditis CC

Abscess of thyroid

Pyogenic thyroiditis

Suppurative thyroiditis

Use additional code (B95-B97) to identify infectious agent

EØ6.1 Subacute thyroiditis

de Quervain thyroiditis

Giant-cell thyroiditis

Granulomatous thyroiditis

Nonsuppurative thyroiditis

Viral thyroiditis

EXCLUDES 1 *autoimmune thyroiditis (EØ6.3)*

EØ6.2 Chronic thyroiditis with transient thyrotoxicosis

EXCLUDES 1 *autoimmune thyroiditis (EØ6.3)*

EØ6.3 Autoimmune thyroiditis

Hashimoto's thyroiditis

Hashitoxicosis (transient)

Lymphadenoid goiter

Lymphocytic thyroiditis

Struma lymphomatosa

EØ6.4 Drug-induced thyroiditis

Use additional code for adverse effect, if applicable, to identify drug (T36-T5Ø with fifth or sixth character 5)

EØ6.5 Other chronic thyroiditis

Chronic fibrous thyroiditis

Chronic thyroiditis NOS

Ligneous thyroiditis

Riedel thyroiditis

EØ6.9 Thyroiditis, unspecified

✓4th **EØ7 Other disorders of thyroid**

EØ7.Ø Hypersecretion of calcitonin

C-cell hyperplasia of thyroid

Hypersecretion of thyrocalcitonin

EØ7.1 Dyshormogenetic goiter

Familial dyshormogenetic goiter

Pendred's syndrome

EXCLUDES 1 *transitory congenital goiter with normal function (P72.Ø)*

✓5th **EØ7.8 Other specified disorders of thyroid**

EØ7.81 Sick-euthyroid syndrome

Euthyroid sick-syndrome

DEF: Thyroid dysfunction caused by abnormal levels of thyroid hormones T3 and/or T4. This syndrome is often associated with starvation or critical illness.

EØ7.89 Other specified disorders of thyroid

Abnormality of thyroid-binding globulin

Hemorrhage of thyroid

Infarction of thyroid

EØ7.9 Disorder of thyroid, unspecified

Diabetes mellitus (EØ8-E13)

AHA: 2020,1Q,12; 2018,2Q,6; 2017,4Q,100-101; 2016,2Q,36; 2016,1Q,11-13; 2013,4Q,114; 2013,3Q,20

✓4th **EØ8 Diabetes mellitus due to underlying condition**

Code first the underlying condition, such as:

- congenital rubella (P35.Ø)
- Cushing's syndrome (E24.-)
- cystic fibrosis (E84.-)
- malignant neoplasm (CØØ-C96)
- malnutrition (E4Ø-E46)
- pancreatitis and other diseases of the pancreas (K85-K86.-)

Use additional code to identify control using:

- insulin (Z79.4)
- oral antidiabetic drugs (Z79.84)
- oral hypoglycemic drugs (Z79.84)

EXCLUDES 1 *drug or chemical induced diabetes mellitus (EØ9.-)*
gestational diabetes (O24.4-)
neonatal diabetes mellitus (P7Ø.2)
postpancreatectomy diabetes mellitus (E13.-)
postprocedural diabetes mellitus (E13.-)
secondary diabetes mellitus NEC (E13.-)
type 1 diabetes mellitus (E1Ø.-)
type 2 diabetes mellitus (E11.-)

✓5th **EØ8.Ø Diabetes mellitus due to underlying condition with hyperosmolarity**

DEF: Diabetic hyperosmolarity: Extremely high levels of glucose in the blood without ketones.

EØ8.ØØ Diabetes mellitus due to underlying condition with hyperosmolarity without nonketotic hyperglycemic-hyperosmolar coma (NKHHC) MCC H9 HCC

EØ8.Ø1 Diabetes mellitus due to underlying condition with hyperosmolarity with coma MCC H9 HCC

✓5th **EØ8.1 Diabetes mellitus due to underlying condition with ketoacidosis**

DEF: Diabetic ketoacidosis: Potentially life-threatening complication due to a shortage of insulin in which the body switches to burning fatty acids and producing acidic ketone bodies.

EØ8.1Ø Diabetes mellitus due to underlying condition with ketoacidosis without coma MCC H9 HCC

EØ8.11 Diabetes mellitus due to underlying condition with ketoacidosis with coma MCC H9 HCC

✓5th **EØ8.2 Diabetes mellitus due to underlying condition with kidney complications**

AHA: 2019,3Q,3; 2018,4Q,88

EØ8.21 Diabetes mellitus due to underlying condition with diabetic nephropathy HCC

Diabetes mellitus due to underlying condition with intercapillary glomerulosclerosis

Diabetes mellitus due to underlying condition with intracapillary glomerulonephrosis

Diabetes mellitus due to underlying condition with Kimmelstiel-Wilson disease

EØ8.22 Diabetes mellitus due to underlying condition with diabetic chronic kidney disease HCC

Use additional code to identify stage of chronic kidney disease (N18.1-N18.6)

EØ8.29 Diabetes mellitus due to underlying condition with other diabetic kidney complication HCC

Renal tubular degeneration in diabetes mellitus due to underlying condition

E08.3 Diabetes mellitus due to underlying condition with ophthalmic complications

AHA: 2016,4Q,11-13

One of the following 7th characters is to be assigned to codes in subcategories E08.32, E08.33, E08.34, E08.35, and E08.37 to designate laterality of the disease:
1 right eye
2 left eye
3 bilateral
9 unspecified eye

E08.31 Diabetes mellitus due to underlying condition with unspecified diabetic retinopathy

DEF: Diabetic retinopathy: Diabetic complication from damage to the retinal vessels resulting in vision problems that can progress to blindness.

E08.311 *Diabetes mellitus due to underlying condition with unspecified diabetic retinopathy with macular edema* HCC

E08.319 *Diabetes mellitus due to underlying condition with unspecified diabetic retinopathy without macular edema* HCC

E08.32 Diabetes mellitus due to underlying condition with mild nonproliferative diabetic retinopathy

Diabetes mellitus due to underlying condition with nonproliferative diabetic retinopathy NOS

E08.321 *Diabetes mellitus due to underlying condition with mild nonproliferative diabetic retinopathy with macular edema* HCC

E08.329 *Diabetes mellitus due to underlying condition with mild nonproliferative diabetic retinopathy without macular edema* HCC

E08.33 Diabetes mellitus due to underlying condition with moderate nonproliferative diabetic retinopathy

E08.331 *Diabetes mellitus due to underlying condition with moderate nonproliferative diabetic retinopathy with macular edema* HCC

E08.339 *Diabetes mellitus due to underlying condition with moderate nonproliferative diabetic retinopathy without macular edema* HCC

E08.34 Diabetes mellitus due to underlying condition with severe nonproliferative diabetic retinopathy

E08.341 *Diabetes mellitus due to underlying condition with severe nonproliferative diabetic retinopathy with macular edema* HCC

E08.349 *Diabetes mellitus due to underlying condition with severe nonproliferative diabetic retinopathy without macular edema* HCC

E08.35 Diabetes mellitus due to underlying condition with proliferative diabetic retinopathy

E08.351 *Diabetes mellitus due to underlying condition with proliferative diabetic retinopathy with macular edema* HCC

E08.352 *Diabetes mellitus due to underlying condition with proliferative diabetic retinopathy with traction retinal detachment involving the macula* HCC

E08.353 *Diabetes mellitus due to underlying condition with proliferative diabetic retinopathy with traction retinal detachment not involving the macula* HCC

E08.354 *Diabetes mellitus due to underlying condition with proliferative diabetic retinopathy with combined traction retinal detachment and rhegmatogenous retinal detachment* HCC

E08.355 *Diabetes mellitus due to underlying condition with stable proliferative diabetic retinopathy* HCC

E08.359 *Diabetes mellitus due to underlying condition with proliferative diabetic retinopathy without macular edema* HCC

E08.36 *Diabetes mellitus due to underlying condition with diabetic cataract* HCC

AHA: 2019,2Q,30-31; 2016,4Q,142

E08.37 *Diabetes mellitus due to underlying condition with diabetic macular edema, resolved following treatment* HCC

E08.39 *Diabetes mellitus due to underlying condition with other diabetic ophthalmic complication* HCC

Use additional code to identify manifestation, such as:
diabetic glaucoma (H40-H42)

E08.4 Diabetes mellitus due to underlying condition with neurological complications

E08.40 *Diabetes mellitus due to underlying condition with diabetic neuropathy, unspecified* HCC

E08.41 *Diabetes mellitus due to underlying condition with diabetic mononeuropathy* HCC

E08.42 *Diabetes mellitus due to underlying condition with diabetic polyneuropathy* HCC

Diabetes mellitus due to underlying condition with diabetic neuralgia

E08.43 *Diabetes mellitus due to underlying condition with diabetic autonomic (poly)neuropathy* HCC

Diabetes mellitus due to underlying condition with diabetic gastroparesis

AHA: 2013,4Q,114

E08.44 *Diabetes mellitus due to underlying condition with diabetic amyotrophy* HCC

E08.49 *Diabetes mellitus due to underlying condition with other diabetic neurological complication* HCC

E08.5 Diabetes mellitus due to underlying condition with circulatory complications

E08.51 *Diabetes mellitus due to underlying condition with diabetic peripheral angiopathy without gangrene* HCC

AHA: 2018,3Q,3-4; 2018,2Q,7

E08.52 *Diabetes mellitus due to underlying condition with diabetic peripheral angiopathy with gangrene* CC HCC

Diabetes mellitus due to underlying condition with diabetic gangrene

AHA: 2020,2Q,18; 2018,3Q,3; 2018,2Q,7; 2017,4Q,102

E08.59 *Diabetes mellitus due to underlying condition with other circulatory complications* HCC

E08.6 Diabetes mellitus due to underlying condition with other specified complications

E08.61 Diabetes mellitus due to underlying condition with diabetic arthropathy

E08.610 *Diabetes mellitus due to underlying condition with diabetic neuropathic arthropathy* HCC

Diabetes mellitus due to underlying condition with Charcôt's joints

DEF: Charcot's joint: Progressive neurologic arthropathy in which chronic degeneration of joints in the weight-bearing areas with peripheral hypertrophy occurs as a complication of a neuropathy disorder. Supporting structures relax from a loss of sensation resulting in chronic joint instability.

E08.618 *Diabetes mellitus due to underlying condition with other diabetic arthropathy* HCC

AHA: 2018,2Q,6

E08.62 Diabetes mellitus due to underlying condition with skin complications

E08.620 *Diabetes mellitus due to underlying condition with diabetic dermatitis* HCC

Diabetes mellitus due to underlying condition with diabetic necrobiosis lipoidica

E08.621 *Diabetes mellitus due to underlying condition with foot ulcer* HCC

Use additional code to identify site of ulcer (L97.4-, L97.5-)

AHA: 2020,2Q,19

EØ8.622 ***Diabetes mellitus due to underlying condition with other skin ulcer*** HCC
Use additional code to identify site of ulcer (L97.1-L97.9, L98.41-L98.49)
AHA: 2021,1Q,7; 2017,4Q,17

EØ8.628 ***Diabetes mellitus due to underlying condition with other skin complications*** HCC

✓6th **EØ8.63 Diabetes mellitus due to underlying condition with oral complications**

EØ8.63Ø ***Diabetes mellitus due to underlying condition with periodontal disease*** HCC

EØ8.638 ***Diabetes mellitus due to underlying condition with other oral complications*** HCC

✓6th **EØ8.64 Diabetes mellitus due to underlying condition with hypoglycemia**
AHA: 2017,1Q,42

EØ8.641 ***Diabetes mellitus due to underlying condition with hypoglycemia with coma*** MCC HCC

EØ8.649 ***Diabetes mellitus due to underlying condition with hypoglycemia without coma*** HCC
AHA: 2016,3Q,42; 2015,3Q,21

EØ8.65 ***Diabetes mellitus due to underlying condition with hyperglycemia*** HCC
AHA: 2017,1Q,42; 2013,3Q,20

EØ8.69 ***Diabetes mellitus due to underlying condition with other specified complication*** HCC
Use additional code to identify complication
AHA: 2016,4Q,141; 2016,1Q,13

EØ8.8 ***Diabetes mellitus due to underlying condition with unspecified complications*** HCC

EØ8.9 ***Diabetes mellitus due to underlying condition without complications*** HCC
AHA: 2020,2Q,18

✓4th **EØ9 Drug or chemical induced diabetes mellitus**
Code first poisoning due to drug or toxin, if applicable (T36-T65 with fifth or sixth character 1-4 or 6)
Use additional code for adverse effect, if applicable, to identify drug (T36-T5Ø with fifth or sixth character 5)
Use additional code to identify control using:
insulin (Z79.4)
oral antidiabetic drugs (Z79.84)
oral hypoglycemic drugs (Z79.84)

EXCLUDES 1 *diabetes mellitus due to underlying condition (EØ8.-)*
gestational diabetes (O24.4-)
neonatal diabetes mellitus (P7Ø.2)
postpancreatectomy diabetes mellitus (E13.-)
postprocedural diabetes mellitus (E13.-)
secondary diabetes mellitus NEC (E13.-)
type 1 diabetes mellitus (E1Ø.-)
type 2 diabetes mellitus (E11.-)

✓5th **EØ9.Ø Drug or chemical induced diabetes mellitus with hyperosmolarity**
DEF: Diabetic hyperosmolarity: Extremely high levels of glucose in the blood without ketones.

EØ9.ØØ Drug or chemical induced diabetes mellitus with hyperosmolarity without nonketotic hyperglycemic-hyperosmolar coma (NKHHC) MCC H9 HCC

EØ9.Ø1 Drug or chemical induced diabetes mellitus with hyperosmolarity with coma MCC H9 HCC

✓5th **EØ9.1 Drug or chemical induced diabetes mellitus with ketoacidosis**
DEF: Diabetic ketoacidosis: Potentially life-threatening complication due to a shortage of insulin in which the body switches to burning fatty acids and producing acidic ketone bodies.

EØ9.1Ø Drug or chemical induced diabetes mellitus with ketoacidosis without coma MCC H9 HCC

EØ9.11 Drug or chemical induced diabetes mellitus with ketoacidosis with coma MCC H9 HCC

✓5th **EØ9.2 Drug or chemical induced diabetes mellitus with kidney complications**
AHA: 2019,3Q,3; 2018,4Q,88

EØ9.21 Drug or chemical induced diabetes mellitus with diabetic nephropathy HCC
Drug or chemical induced diabetes mellitus with intercapillary glomerulosclerosis
Drug or chemical induced diabetes mellitus with intracapillary glomerulonephrosis
Drug or chemical induced diabetes mellitus with Kimmelstiel-Wilson disease

EØ9.22 Drug or chemical induced diabetes mellitus with diabetic chronic kidney disease HCC
Use additional code to identify stage of chronic kidney disease (N18.1-N18.6)

EØ9.29 Drug or chemical induced diabetes mellitus with other diabetic kidney complication HCC
Drug or chemical induced diabetes mellitus with renal tubular degeneration

✓5th **EØ9.3 Drug or chemical induced diabetes mellitus with ophthalmic complications**
AHA: 2016,4Q,11-13

One of the following 7th characters is to be assigned to codes in subcategories EØ9.32, EØ9.33, EØ9.34, EØ9.35, and EØ9.37 to designate laterality of the disease:
1 right eye
2 left eye
3 bilateral
9 unspecified eye

✓6th **EØ9.31 Drug or chemical induced diabetes mellitus with unspecified diabetic retinopathy**
DEF: Diabetic retinopathy: Diabetic complication from damage to the retinal vessels resulting in vision problems that can progress to blindness.

EØ9.311 Drug or chemical induced diabetes mellitus with unspecified diabetic retinopathy with macular edema HCC

EØ9.319 Drug or chemical induced diabetes mellitus with unspecified diabetic retinopathy without macular edema HCC

✓6th **EØ9.32 Drug or chemical induced diabetes mellitus with mild nonproliferative diabetic retinopathy**
Drug or chemical induced diabetes mellitus with nonproliferative diabetic retinopathy NOS

✓7th **EØ9.321 Drug or chemical induced diabetes mellitus with mild nonproliferative diabetic retinopathy with macular edema** HCC

✓7th **EØ9.329 Drug or chemical induced diabetes mellitus with mild nonproliferative diabetic retinopathy without macular edema** HCC

✓6th **EØ9.33 Drug or chemical induced diabetes mellitus with moderate nonproliferative diabetic retinopathy**

✓7th **EØ9.331 Drug or chemical induced diabetes mellitus with moderate nonproliferative diabetic retinopathy with macular edema** HCC

✓7th **EØ9.339 Drug or chemical induced diabetes mellitus with moderate nonproliferative diabetic retinopathy without macular edema** HCC

✓6th **EØ9.34 Drug or chemical induced diabetes mellitus with severe nonproliferative diabetic retinopathy**

✓7th **EØ9.341 Drug or chemical induced diabetes mellitus with severe nonproliferative diabetic retinopathy with macular edema** HCC

✓7th **EØ9.349 Drug or chemical induced diabetes mellitus with severe nonproliferative diabetic retinopathy without macular edema** HCC

✓6th **EØ9.35 Drug or chemical induced diabetes mellitus with proliferative diabetic retinopathy**

✓7th **EØ9.351 Drug or chemical induced diabetes mellitus with proliferative diabetic retinopathy with macular edema** HCC

✓7th **EØ9.352 Drug or chemical induced diabetes mellitus with proliferative diabetic retinopathy with traction retinal detachment involving the macula** HCC

E09.353 Drug or chemical induced diabetes mellitus with proliferative diabetic retinopathy with traction retinal detachment not involving the macula HCC

E09.354 Drug or chemical induced diabetes mellitus with proliferative diabetic retinopathy with combined traction retinal detachment and rhegmatogenous retinal detachment HCC

E09.355 Drug or chemical induced diabetes mellitus with stable proliferative diabetic retinopathy HCC

E09.359 Drug or chemical induced diabetes mellitus with proliferative diabetic retinopathy without macular edema HCC

E09.36 Drug or chemical induced diabetes mellitus with diabetic cataract HCC
AHA: 2019,2Q,30-31; 2016,4Q,142

E09.37 Drug or chemical induced diabetes mellitus with diabetic macular edema, resolved following treatment HCC

E09.39 Drug or chemical induced diabetes mellitus with other diabetic ophthalmic complication HCC
Use additional code to identify manifestation, such as:
diabetic glaucoma (H40-H42)

E09.4 Drug or chemical induced diabetes mellitus with neurological complications

E09.40 Drug or chemical induced diabetes mellitus with neurological complications with diabetic neuropathy, unspecified HCC

E09.41 Drug or chemical induced diabetes mellitus with neurological complications with diabetic mononeuropathy HCC

E09.42 Drug or chemical induced diabetes mellitus with neurological complications with diabetic polyneuropathy HCC
Drug or chemical induced diabetes mellitus with diabetic neuralgia

E09.43 Drug or chemical induced diabetes mellitus with neurological complications with diabetic autonomic (poly)neuropathy HCC
Drug or chemical induced diabetes mellitus with diabetic gastroparesis
AHA: 2013,4Q,114

E09.44 Drug or chemical induced diabetes mellitus with neurological complications with diabetic amyotrophy HCC

E09.49 Drug or chemical induced diabetes mellitus with neurological complications with other diabetic neurological complication HCC

E09.5 Drug or chemical induced diabetes mellitus with circulatory complications

E09.51 Drug or chemical induced diabetes mellitus with diabetic peripheral angiopathy without gangrene HCC
AHA: 2018,3Q,3-4; 2018,2Q,7

E09.52 Drug or chemical induced diabetes mellitus with diabetic peripheral angiopathy with gangrene CC HCC
Drug or chemical induced diabetes mellitus with diabetic gangrene
AHA: 2020,2Q,18; 2018,3Q,3; 2018,2Q,7; 2017,4Q,102

E09.59 Drug or chemical induced diabetes mellitus with other circulatory complications HCC

E09.6 Drug or chemical induced diabetes mellitus with other specified complications

E09.61 Drug or chemical induced diabetes mellitus with diabetic arthropathy

E09.610 Drug or chemical induced diabetes mellitus with diabetic neuropathic arthropathy HCC
Drug or chemical induced diabetes mellitus with Charcôt's joints
DEF: Charcot's joint: Progressive neurologic arthropathy in which chronic degeneration of joints in the weight-bearing areas with peripheral hypertrophy occurs as a complication of a neuropathy disorder. Supporting structures relax from a loss of sensation resulting in chronic joint instability.

E09.618 Drug or chemical induced diabetes mellitus with other diabetic arthropathy HCC
AHA: 2018,2Q,6

E09.62 Drug or chemical induced diabetes mellitus with skin complications

E09.620 Drug or chemical induced diabetes mellitus with diabetic dermatitis HCC
Drug or chemical induced diabetes mellitus with diabetic necrobiosis lipoidica

E09.621 Drug or chemical induced diabetes mellitus with foot ulcer HCC
Use additional code to identify site of ulcer (L97.4-, L97.5-)
AHA: 2020,2Q,19

E09.622 Drug or chemical induced diabetes mellitus with other skin ulcer HCC
Use additional code to identify site of ulcer (L97.1-L97.9, L98.41-L98.49)
AHA: 2021,1Q,7; 2017,4Q,17

E09.628 Drug or chemical induced diabetes mellitus with other skin complications HCC

E09.63 Drug or chemical induced diabetes mellitus with oral complications

E09.630 Drug or chemical induced diabetes mellitus with periodontal disease HCC

E09.638 Drug or chemical induced diabetes mellitus with other oral complications HCC

E09.64 Drug or chemical induced diabetes mellitus with hypoglycemia
AHA: 2017,1Q,42

E09.641 Drug or chemical induced diabetes mellitus with hypoglycemia with coma MCC HCC

E09.649 Drug or chemical induced diabetes mellitus with hypoglycemia without coma HCC
AHA: 2016,3Q,42; 2015,3Q,21

E09.65 Drug or chemical induced diabetes mellitus with hyperglycemia HCC
AHA: 2017,1Q,42; 2013,3Q,20

E09.69 Drug or chemical induced diabetes mellitus with other specified complication HCC
Use additional code to identify complication
AHA: 2016,4Q,141; 2016,1Q,13

E09.8 Drug or chemical induced diabetes mellitus with unspecified complications HCC

E09.9 Drug or chemical induced diabetes mellitus without complications HCC
AHA: 2020,2Q,18

E10 Type 1 diabetes mellitus

INCLUDES brittle diabetes (mellitus)
diabetes (mellitus) due to autoimmune process
diabetes (mellitus) due to immune mediated pancreatic islet beta-cell destruction
idiopathic diabetes (mellitus)
juvenile onset diabetes (mellitus)
ketosis-prone diabetes (mellitus)

EXCLUDES 1 *diabetes mellitus due to underlying condition (E08.-)*
drug or chemical induced diabetes mellitus (E09.-)
gestational diabetes (O24.4-)
hyperglycemia NOS (R73.9)
neonatal diabetes mellitus (P70.2)
postpancreatectomy diabetes mellitus (E13.-)
postprocedural diabetes mellitus (E13.-)
secondary diabetes mellitus NEC (E13.-)
type 2 diabetes mellitus (E11.-)

AHA: 2020,3Q,30

E10.1 Type 1 diabetes mellitus with ketoacidosis
AHA: 2013,3Q,20
DEF: Diabetic ketoacidosis: Potentially life-threatening complication due to a shortage of insulin in which the body switches to burning fatty acids and producing acidic ketone bodies.

E10.10 Type 1 diabetes mellitus with ketoacidosis without coma MCC H9 HCC

E10.11 Type 1 diabetes mellitus with ketoacidosis with coma MCC H9 HCC

E10.2 Type 1 diabetes mellitus with kidney complications
AHA: 2019,3Q,3; 2018,4Q,88

E10.21 Type 1 diabetes mellitus with diabetic nephropathy HCC
Type 1 diabetes mellitus with intercapillary glomerulosclerosis
Type 1 diabetes mellitus with intracapillary glomerulonephrosis
Type 1 diabetes mellitus with Kimmelstiel-Wilson disease

E10.22 Type 1 diabetes mellitus with diabetic chronic kidney disease HCC
Use additional code to identify stage of chronic kidney disease (N18.1-N18.6)

E10.29 Type 1 diabetes mellitus with other diabetic kidney complication HCC
Type 1 diabetes mellitus with renal tubular degeneration
AHA: 2016,1Q,13

E10.3 Type 1 diabetes mellitus with ophthalmic complications
AHA: 2016,4Q,11-13

One of the following 7th characters is to be assigned to codes in subcategories E10.32, E10.33, E10.34, E10.35, and E10.37 to designate laterality of the disease:
1 right eye
2 left eye
3 bilateral
9 unspecified eye

E10.31 Type 1 diabetes mellitus with unspecified diabetic retinopathy
DEF: Diabetic retinopathy: Diabetic complication from damage to the retinal vessels resulting in vision problems that can progress to blindness.

E10.311 Type 1 diabetes mellitus with unspecified diabetic retinopathy with macular edema HCC

E10.319 Type 1 diabetes mellitus with unspecified diabetic retinopathy without macular edema HCC

E10.32 Type 1 diabetes mellitus with mild nonproliferative diabetic retinopathy
Type 1 diabetes mellitus with nonproliferative diabetic retinopathy NOS

E10.321 Type 1 diabetes mellitus with mild nonproliferative diabetic retinopathy with macular edema HCC

E10.329 Type 1 diabetes mellitus with mild nonproliferative diabetic retinopathy without macular edema HCC

E10.33 Type 1 diabetes mellitus with moderate nonproliferative diabetic retinopathy

E10.331 Type 1 diabetes mellitus with moderate nonproliferative diabetic retinopathy with macular edema HCC

E10.339 Type 1 diabetes mellitus with moderate nonproliferative diabetic retinopathy without macular edema HCC

E10.34 Type 1 diabetes mellitus with severe nonproliferative diabetic retinopathy

E10.341 Type 1 diabetes mellitus with severe nonproliferative diabetic retinopathy with macular edema HCC

E10.349 Type 1 diabetes mellitus with severe nonproliferative diabetic retinopathy without macular edema HCC

E10.35 Type 1 diabetes mellitus with proliferative diabetic retinopathy

E10.351 Type 1 diabetes mellitus with proliferative diabetic retinopathy with macular edema HCC

E10.352 Type 1 diabetes mellitus with proliferative diabetic retinopathy with traction retinal detachment involving the macula HCC

E10.353 Type 1 diabetes mellitus with proliferative diabetic retinopathy with traction retinal detachment not involving the macula HCC

E10.354 Type 1 diabetes mellitus with proliferative diabetic retinopathy with combined traction retinal detachment and rhegmatogenous retinal detachment HCC

E10.355 Type 1 diabetes mellitus with stable proliferative diabetic retinopathy HCC

E10.359 Type 1 diabetes mellitus with proliferative diabetic retinopathy without macular edema HCC

E10.36 Type 1 diabetes mellitus with diabetic cataract HCC
AHA: 2019,2Q,30-31; 2016,4Q,142

E10.37 Type 1 diabetes mellitus with diabetic macular edema, resolved following treatment HCC

E10.39 Type 1 diabetes mellitus with other diabetic ophthalmic complication HCC
Use additional code to identify manifestation, such as:
diabetic glaucoma (H40-H42)

E10.4 Type 1 diabetes mellitus with neurological complications

E10.40 Type 1 diabetes mellitus with diabetic neuropathy, unspecified HCC

E10.41 Type 1 diabetes mellitus with diabetic mononeuropathy HCC

E10.42 Type 1 diabetes mellitus with diabetic polyneuropathy HCC
Type 1 diabetes mellitus with diabetic neuralgia

E10.43 Type 1 diabetes mellitus with diabetic autonomic (poly)neuropathy HCC
Type 1 diabetes mellitus with diabetic gastroparesis
AHA: 2013,4Q,114

E10.44 Type 1 diabetes mellitus with diabetic amyotrophy HCC

E10.49 Type 1 diabetes mellitus with other diabetic neurological complication HCC

E10.5 Type 1 diabetes mellitus with circulatory complications

E10.51 Type 1 diabetes mellitus with diabetic peripheral angiopathy without gangrene HCC
AHA: 2018,3Q,3-4; 2018,2Q,7

E10.52 Type 1 diabetes mellitus with diabetic peripheral angiopathy with gangrene CC HCC
Type 1 diabetes mellitus with diabetic gangrene
AHA: 2020,2Q,18; 2018,3Q,3; 2018,2Q,7; 2017,4Q,102

E10.59 Type 1 diabetes mellitus with other circulatory complications HCC

E10.6 Type 1 diabetes mellitus with other specified complications

E10.61 Type 1 diabetes mellitus with diabetic arthropathy

E10.610 Type 1 diabetes mellitus with diabetic neuropathic arthropathy HCC

Type 1 diabetes mellitus with Charcôt's joints

DEF: Charcot's joint: Progressive neurologic arthropathy in which chronic degeneration of joints in the weight-bearing areas with peripheral hypertrophy occurs as a complication of a neuropathy disorder. Supporting structures relax from a loss of sensation resulting in chronic joint instability.

E10.618 Type 1 diabetes mellitus with other diabetic arthropathy HCC

AHA: 2018,2Q,6

E10.62 Type 1 diabetes mellitus with skin complications

E10.620 Type 1 diabetes mellitus with diabetic dermatitis HCC

Type 1 diabetes mellitus with diabetic necrobiosis lipoidica

E10.621 Type 1 diabetes mellitus with foot ulcer HCC

Use additional code to identify site of ulcer (L97.4-, L97.5-)

AHA: 2020,2Q,19

E10.622 Type 1 diabetes mellitus with other skin ulcer HCC

Use additional code to identify site of ulcer (L97.1-L97.9, L98.41-L98.49)

AHA: 2021,1Q,7; 2017,4Q,17

E10.628 Type 1 diabetes mellitus with other skin complications HCC

E10.63 Type 1 diabetes mellitus with oral complications

E10.630 Type 1 diabetes mellitus with periodontal disease HCC

E10.638 Type 1 diabetes mellitus with other oral complications HCC

E10.64 Type 1 diabetes mellitus with hypoglycemia

AHA: 2017,1Q,42

E10.641 Type 1 diabetes mellitus with hypoglycemia with coma MCC HCC

E10.649 Type 1 diabetes mellitus with hypoglycemia without coma HCC

AHA: 2016,3Q,42; 2016,1Q,13; 2015,3Q,21

E10.65 Type 1 diabetes mellitus with hyperglycemia HCC

AHA: 2022,1Q,28; 2017,1Q,42; 2013,3Q,20

E10.69 Type 1 diabetes mellitus with other specified complication HCC

Use additional code to identify complication

AHA: 2022,1Q,28; 2016,4Q,141; 2016,1Q,13

E10.8 Type 1 diabetes mellitus with unspecified complications HCC

E10.9 Type 1 diabetes mellitus without complications HCC

AHA: 2020,2Q,18

E11 Type 2 diabetes mellitus

INCLUDES diabetes (mellitus) due to insulin secretory defect
diabetes NOS
insulin resistant diabetes (mellitus)

Use additional code to identify control using:
insulin (Z79.4)
oral antidiabetic drugs (Z79.84)
oral hypoglycemic drugs (Z79.84)

EXCLUDES 1 *diabetes mellitus due to underlying condition (E08.-)*
drug or chemical induced diabetes mellitus (E09.-)
gestational diabetes (O24.4-)
neonatal diabetes mellitus (P70.2)
postpancreatectomy diabetes mellitus (E13.-)
postprocedural diabetes mellitus (E13.-)
secondary diabetes mellitus NEC (E13.-)
type 1 diabetes mellitus (E10.-)

AHA: 2020,3Q,30; 2020,1Q,12; 2016,2Q,10; 2013,1Q,26

E11.0 Type 2 diabetes mellitus with hyperosmolarity

DEF: Diabetic hyperosmolarity: Extremely high levels of glucose in the blood without ketones.

E11.00 Type 2 diabetes mellitus with hyperosmolarity without nonketotic hyperglycemic-hyperosmolar coma (NKHHC) MCC H9 HCC

AHA: 2022,1Q,28

E11.01 Type 2 diabetes mellitus with hyperosmolarity with coma MCC H9 HCC

E11.1 Type 2 diabetes mellitus with ketoacidosis

AHA: 2017,4Q,6

DEF: Diabetic ketoacidosis: Potentially life-threatening complication due to a shortage of insulin in which the body switches to burning fatty acids and producing acidic ketone bodies.

E11.10 Type 2 diabetes mellitus with ketoacidosis without coma MCC H9 HCC

E11.11 Type 2 diabetes mellitus with ketoacidosis with coma MCC H9 HCC

E11.2 Type 2 diabetes mellitus with kidney complications

AHA: 2019,3Q,3; 2018,4Q,88

E11.21 Type 2 diabetes mellitus with diabetic nephropathy HCC

Type 2 diabetes mellitus with intercapillary glomerulosclerosis

Type 2 diabetes mellitus with intracapillary glomerulonephrosis

Type 2 diabetes mellitus with Kimmelstiel-Wilson disease

E11.22 Type 2 diabetes mellitus with diabetic chronic kidney disease HCC

Use additional code to identify stage of chronic kidney disease (N18.1-N18.6)

E11.29 Type 2 diabetes mellitus with other diabetic kidney complication HCC

Type 2 diabetes mellitus with renal tubular degeneration

E11.3 Type 2 diabetes mellitus with ophthalmic complications

AHA: 2016,4Q,11-13

One of the following 7th characters is to be assigned to codes in subcategories E11.32, E11.33, E11.34, E11.35, and E11.37 to designate laterality of the disease:
1 right eye
2 left eye
3 bilateral
9 unspecified eye

E11.31 Type 2 diabetes mellitus with unspecified diabetic retinopathy

DEF: Diabetic retinopathy: Diabetic complication from damage to the retinal vessels resulting in vision problems that can progress to blindness.

E11.311 Type 2 diabetes mellitus with unspecified diabetic retinopathy with macular edema HCC

E11.319 Type 2 diabetes mellitus with unspecified diabetic retinopathy without macular edema HCC

√6th **E11.32 Type 2 diabetes mellitus with mild nonproliferative diabetic retinopathy**
Type 2 diabetes mellitus with nonproliferative diabetic retinopathy NOS

√7th **E11.321 Type 2 diabetes mellitus with mild nonproliferative diabetic retinopathy with macular edema** HCC

√7th **E11.329 Type 2 diabetes mellitus with mild nonproliferative diabetic retinopathy without macular edema** HCC

√6th **E11.33 Type 2 diabetes mellitus with moderate nonproliferative diabetic retinopathy**

√7th **E11.331 Type 2 diabetes mellitus with moderate nonproliferative diabetic retinopathy with macular edema** HCC

√7th **E11.339 Type 2 diabetes mellitus with moderate nonproliferative diabetic retinopathy without macular edema** HCC

√6th **E11.34 Type 2 diabetes mellitus with severe nonproliferative diabetic retinopathy**

√7th **E11.341 Type 2 diabetes mellitus with severe nonproliferative diabetic retinopathy with macular edema** HCC

√7th **E11.349 Type 2 diabetes mellitus with severe nonproliferative diabetic retinopathy without macular edema** HCC

√6th **E11.35 Type 2 diabetes mellitus with proliferative diabetic retinopathy**

√7th **E11.351 Type 2 diabetes mellitus with proliferative diabetic retinopathy with macular edema** HCC

√7th **E11.352 Type 2 diabetes mellitus with proliferative diabetic retinopathy with traction retinal detachment involving the macula** HCC

√7th **E11.353 Type 2 diabetes mellitus with proliferative diabetic retinopathy with traction retinal detachment not involving the macula** HCC

√7th **E11.354 Type 2 diabetes mellitus with proliferative diabetic retinopathy with combined traction retinal detachment and rhegmatogenous retinal detachment** HCC

√7th **E11.355 Type 2 diabetes mellitus with stable proliferative diabetic retinopathy** HCC

√7th **E11.359 Type 2 diabetes mellitus with proliferative diabetic retinopathy without macular edema** HCC

E11.36 Type 2 diabetes mellitus with diabetic cataract HCC
AHA: 2019,2Q,30-31; 2016,4Q,142

√x 7th **E11.37 Type 2 diabetes mellitus with diabetic macular edema, resolved following treatment** HCC

E11.39 Type 2 diabetes mellitus with other diabetic ophthalmic complication HCC
Use additional code to identify manifestation, such as:
diabetic glaucoma (H40-H42)

√5th **E11.4 Type 2 diabetes mellitus with neurological complications**

E11.40 Type 2 diabetes mellitus with diabetic neuropathy, unspecified HCC
AHA: 2013,4Q,129

E11.41 Type 2 diabetes mellitus with diabetic mononeuropathy HCC

E11.42 Type 2 diabetes mellitus with diabetic polyneuropathy HCC
Type 2 diabetes mellitus with diabetic neuralgia
AHA: 2020,1Q,12

E11.43 Type 2 diabetes mellitus with diabetic autonomic (poly)neuropathy HCC
Type 2 diabetes mellitus with diabetic gastroparesis
AHA: 2013,4Q,114

E11.44 Type 2 diabetes mellitus with diabetic amyotrophy HCC

E11.49 Type 2 diabetes mellitus with other diabetic neurological complication HCC

√5th **E11.5 Type 2 diabetes mellitus with circulatory complications**

E11.51 Type 2 diabetes mellitus with diabetic peripheral angiopathy without gangrene HCC
AHA: 2018,3Q,3-4; 2018,2Q,7

E11.52 Type 2 diabetes mellitus with diabetic peripheral angiopathy with gangrene CC HCC
Type 2 diabetes mellitus with diabetic gangrene
AHA: 2020,2Q,18; 2018,3Q,3; 2018,2Q,7; 2017,4Q,102

E11.59 Type 2 diabetes mellitus with other circulatory complications HCC

√5th **E11.6 Type 2 diabetes mellitus with other specified complications**

√6th **E11.61 Type 2 diabetes mellitus with diabetic arthropathy**

E11.610 Type 2 diabetes mellitus with diabetic neuropathic arthropathy HCC
Type 2 diabetes mellitus with Charcôt's joints
DEF: Charcot's joint: Progressive neurologic arthropathy in which chronic degeneration of joints in the weight-bearing areas with peripheral hypertrophy occurs as a complication of a neuropathy disorder. Supporting structures relax from a loss of sensation resulting in chronic joint instability.

E11.618 Type 2 diabetes mellitus with other diabetic arthropathy HCC
AHA: 2018,2Q,6

√6th **E11.62 Type 2 diabetes mellitus with skin complications**

E11.620 Type 2 diabetes mellitus with diabetic dermatitis HCC
Type 2 diabetes mellitus with diabetic necrobiosis lipoidica

E11.621 Type 2 diabetes mellitus with foot ulcer HCC
Use additional code to identify site of ulcer (L97.4-, L97.5-)
AHA: 2020,2Q,19; 2020,1Q,12

E11.622 Type 2 diabetes mellitus with other skin ulcer HCC
Use additional code to identify site of ulcer (L97.1-L97.9, L98.41-L98.49)
AHA: 2021,1Q,7; 2017,4Q,17

E11.628 Type 2 diabetes mellitus with other skin complications HCC

√6th **E11.63 Type 2 diabetes mellitus with oral complications**

E11.630 Type 2 diabetes mellitus with periodontal disease HCC

E11.638 Type 2 diabetes mellitus with other oral complications HCC

√6th **E11.64 Type 2 diabetes mellitus with hypoglycemia**
AHA: 2017,1Q,42

E11.641 Type 2 diabetes mellitus with hypoglycemia with coma MCC HCC

E11.649 Type 2 diabetes mellitus with hypoglycemia without coma HCC
AHA: 2016,3Q,42; 2015,3Q,21

E11.65 Type 2 diabetes mellitus with hyperglycemia HCC
AHA: 2022,1Q,28; 2017,1Q,42; 2013,3Q,20

E11.69 Type 2 diabetes mellitus with other specified complication HCC
Use additional code to identify complication
AHA: 2020,1Q,12; 2016,4Q,141; 2016,1Q,13

E11.8 Type 2 diabetes mellitus with unspecified complications HCC

E11.9 Type 2 diabetes mellitus without complications HCC
AHA: 2020,2Q,18

E13 Other specified diabetes mellitus

INCLUDES diabetes mellitus due to genetic defects of beta-cell function
diabetes mellitus due to genetic defects in insulin action
postpancreatectomy diabetes mellitus
postprocedural diabetes mellitus
secondary diabetes mellitus NEC

Use additional code to identify control using:
insulin (Z79.4)
oral antidiabetic drugs (Z79.84)
oral hypoglycemic drugs (Z79.84)

EXCLUDES 1 *diabetes (mellitus) due to autoimmune process (E1Ø.-)*
diabetes (mellitus) due to immune mediated pancreatic islet beta-cell destruction (E1Ø.-)
diabetes mellitus due to underlying condition (EØ8.-)
drug or chemical induced diabetes mellitus (EØ9.-)
gestational diabetes (O24.4-)
neonatal diabetes mellitus (P7Ø.2)
type 1 diabetes mellitus (E1Ø.-)

AHA: 2018,3Q,4; 2016,1Q,11-13

TIP: Use this category when the diabetes is documented as diabetes type 1.5. Synonymous terms used in the documentation may also include combined diabetes type 1 and type 2, latent autoimmune diabetes of adults (LADA), slow-progressing type 1 diabetes, or double diabetes.

TIP: When postprocedural or postpancreatectomy hypoinsulinemia (E89.1) is documented with postprocedural or postpancreatectomy diabetes mellitus (E13.-), code E89.1 should be sequenced first.

E13.Ø Other specified diabetes mellitus with hyperosmolarity

DEF: Diabetic hyperosmolarity: Extremely high levels of glucose in the blood without ketones.

E13.ØØ Other specified diabetes mellitus with hyperosmolarity without nonketotic hyperglycemic-hyperosmolar coma (NKHHC) MCC H9 HCC

EXCLUDES 2 *type 2 diabetes mellitus (E11.-)*

E13.Ø1 Other specified diabetes mellitus with hyperosmolarity with coma MCC H9 HCC

E13.1 Other specified diabetes mellitus with ketoacidosis

AHA: 2016,2Q,10; 2013,1Q,26

DEF: Diabetic ketoacidosis: Potentially life-threatening complication due to a shortage of insulin in which the body switches to burning fatty acids and producing acidic ketone bodies.

E13.1Ø Other specified diabetes mellitus with ketoacidosis without coma MCC H9 HCC

E13.11 Other specified diabetes mellitus with ketoacidosis with coma MCC H9 HCC

E13.2 Other specified diabetes mellitus with kidney complications

AHA: 2019,3Q,3; 2018,4Q,88

E13.21 Other specified diabetes mellitus with diabetic nephropathy HCC

Other specified diabetes mellitus with intercapillary glomerulosclerosis
Other specified diabetes mellitus with intracapillary glomerulonephrosis
Other specified diabetes mellitus with Kimmelstiel-Wilson disease

E13.22 Other specified diabetes mellitus with diabetic chronic kidney disease HCC

Use additional code to identify stage of chronic kidney disease (N18.1-N18.6)

E13.29 Other specified diabetes mellitus with other diabetic kidney complication HCC

Other specified diabetes mellitus with renal tubular degeneration

E13.3 Other specified diabetes mellitus with ophthalmic complications

AHA: 2016,4Q,11-13

One of the following 7th characters is to be assigned to codes in subcategories E13.32, E13.33, E13.34, E13.35, and E13.37 to designate laterality of the disease:
1 right eye
2 left eye
3 bilateral
9 unspecified eye

E13.31 Other specified diabetes mellitus with unspecified diabetic retinopathy

DEF: Diabetic retinopathy: Diabetic complication from damage to the retinal vessels resulting in vision problems that can progress to blindness.

E13.311 Other specified diabetes mellitus with unspecified diabetic retinopathy with macular edema HCC

E13.319 Other specified diabetes mellitus with unspecified diabetic retinopathy without macular edema HCC

E13.32 Other specified diabetes mellitus with mild nonproliferative diabetic retinopathy

Other specified diabetes mellitus with nonproliferative diabetic retinopathy NOS

E13.321 Other specified diabetes mellitus with mild nonproliferative diabetic retinopathy with macular edema HCC

E13.329 Other specified diabetes mellitus with mild nonproliferative diabetic retinopathy without macular edema HCC

E13.33 Other specified diabetes mellitus with moderate nonproliferative diabetic retinopathy

E13.331 Other specified diabetes mellitus with moderate nonproliferative diabetic retinopathy with macular edema HCC

E13.339 Other specified diabetes mellitus with moderate nonproliferative diabetic retinopathy without macular edema HCC

E13.34 Other specified diabetes mellitus with severe nonproliferative diabetic retinopathy

E13.341 Other specified diabetes mellitus with severe nonproliferative diabetic retinopathy with macular edema HCC

E13.349 Other specified diabetes mellitus with severe nonproliferative diabetic retinopathy without macular edema HCC

E13.35 Other specified diabetes mellitus with proliferative diabetic retinopathy

E13.351 Other specified diabetes mellitus with proliferative diabetic retinopathy with macular edema HCC

E13.352 Other specified diabetes mellitus with proliferative diabetic retinopathy with traction retinal detachment involving the macula HCC

E13.353 Other specified diabetes mellitus with proliferative diabetic retinopathy with traction retinal detachment not involving the macula HCC

E13.354 Other specified diabetes mellitus with proliferative diabetic retinopathy with combined traction retinal detachment and rhegmatogenous retinal detachment HCC

E13.355 Other specified diabetes mellitus with stable proliferative diabetic retinopathy HCC

E13.359 Other specified diabetes mellitus with proliferative diabetic retinopathy without macular edema HCC

E13.36 Other specified diabetes mellitus with diabetic cataract HCC

AHA: 2019,2Q,30-31; 2016,4Q,142

E13.37 Other specified diabetes mellitus with diabetic macular edema, resolved following treatment HCC

E13.39 Other specified diabetes mellitus with other diabetic ophthalmic complication HCC
Use additional code to identify manifestation, such as:
diabetic glaucoma (H40-H42)

✓5th **E13.4 Other specified diabetes mellitus with neurological complications**

E13.40 Other specified diabetes mellitus with diabetic neuropathy, unspecified HCC

E13.41 Other specified diabetes mellitus with diabetic mononeuropathy HCC

E13.42 Other specified diabetes mellitus with diabetic polyneuropathy HCC
Other specified diabetes mellitus with diabetic neuralgia

E13.43 Other specified diabetes mellitus with diabetic autonomic (poly)neuropathy HCC
Other specified diabetes mellitus with diabetic gastroparesis
AHA: 2013,4Q,114

E13.44 Other specified diabetes mellitus with diabetic amyotrophy HCC

E13.49 Other specified diabetes mellitus with other diabetic neurological complication HCC

✓5th **E13.5 Other specified diabetes mellitus with circulatory complications**

E13.51 Other specified diabetes mellitus with diabetic peripheral angiopathy without gangrene HCC
AHA: 2018,3Q,3-4; 2018,2Q,7

E13.52 Other specified diabetes mellitus with diabetic peripheral angiopathy with gangrene CC HCC
Other specified diabetes mellitus with diabetic gangrene
AHA: 2020,2Q,18; 2018,3Q,3; 2018,2Q,7; 2017,4Q,102

E13.59 Other specified diabetes mellitus with other circulatory complications HCC

✓5th **E13.6 Other specified diabetes mellitus with other specified complications**

✓6th **E13.61 Other specified diabetes mellitus with diabetic arthropathy**

E13.610 Other specified diabetes mellitus with diabetic neuropathic arthropathy HCC
Other specified diabetes mellitus with Charcôt's joints
DEF: Charcot's joint: Progressive neurologic arthropathy in which chronic degeneration of joints in the weight-bearing areas with peripheral hypertrophy occurs as a complication of a neuropathy disorder. Supporting structures relax from a loss of sensation resulting in chronic joint instability.

E13.618 Other specified diabetes mellitus with other diabetic arthropathy HCC
AHA: 2018,2Q,6

✓6th **E13.62 Other specified diabetes mellitus with skin complications**

E13.620 Other specified diabetes mellitus with diabetic dermatitis HCC
Other specified diabetes mellitus with diabetic necrobiosis lipoidica

E13.621 Other specified diabetes mellitus with foot ulcer HCC
Use additional code to identify site of ulcer (L97.4-, L97.5-)
AHA: 2020,2Q,19

E13.622 Other specified diabetes mellitus with other skin ulcer HCC
Use additional code to identify site of ulcer (L97.1-L97.9, L98.41-L98.49)
AHA: 2021,1Q,7; 2017,4Q,17

E13.628 Other specified diabetes mellitus with other skin complications HCC

✓6th **E13.63 Other specified diabetes mellitus with oral complications**

E13.630 Other specified diabetes mellitus with periodontal disease HCC

E13.638 Other specified diabetes mellitus with other oral complications HCC

✓6th **E13.64 Other specified diabetes mellitus with hypoglycemia**
AHA: 2017,1Q,42

E13.641 Other specified diabetes mellitus with hypoglycemia with coma MCC HCC

E13.649 Other specified diabetes mellitus with hypoglycemia without coma HCC
AHA: 2016,3Q,42; 2015,3Q,21

E13.65 Other specified diabetes mellitus with hyperglycemia HCC
AHA: 2017,1Q,42; 2013,3Q,20

E13.69 Other specified diabetes mellitus with other specified complication HCC
Use additional code to identify complication
AHA: 2016,4Q,141; 2016,1Q,13

E13.8 Other specified diabetes mellitus with unspecified complications HCC

E13.9 Other specified diabetes mellitus without complications HCC
AHA: 2020,2Q,18

Other disorders of glucose regulation and pancreatic internal secretion (E15-E16)

E15 Nondiabetic hypoglycemic coma CC H9 HCC
INCLUDES drug-induced insulin coma in nondiabetic
hyperinsulinism with hypoglycemic coma
hypoglycemic coma NOS

✓4th **E16 Other disorders of pancreatic internal secretion**

E16.0 Drug-induced hypoglycemia without coma
EXCLUDES 1 *diabetes with hypoglycemia without coma (E09.649)*
Use additional code for adverse effect, if applicable, to identify drug (T36-T50 with fifth or sixth character 5)

E16.1 Other hypoglycemia
Functional hyperinsulinism
Functional nonhyperinsulinemic hypoglycemia
Hyperinsulinism NOS
Hyperplasia of pancreatic islet beta cells NOS
EXCLUDES 1 *diabetes with hypoglycemia (E08.649, E10.649, E11.649, E13.649)*
hypoglycemia in infant of diabetic mother (P70.1)
neonatal hypoglycemia (P70.4)

E16.2 Hypoglycemia, unspecified
EXCLUDES 1 *diabetes with hypoglycemia (E08.649, E10.649, E11.649, E13.649)*
AHA: 2016,3Q,42
TIP: Assign for nondiabetic hypoglycemic encephalopathy not further clarified in the documentation.

E16.3 Increased secretion of glucagon
Hyperplasia of pancreatic endocrine cells with glucagon excess

E16.4 Increased secretion of gastrin
Hypergastrinemia
Hyperplasia of pancreatic endocrine cells with gastrin excess
Zollinger-Ellison syndrome

E16.8 Other specified disorders of pancreatic internal secretion
Increased secretion from endocrine pancreas of growth hormone-releasing hormone
Increased secretion from endocrine pancreas of pancreatic polypeptide
Increased secretion from endocrine pancreas of somatostatin
Increased secretion from endocrine pancreas of vasoactive-intestinal polypeptide

E16.9 Disorder of pancreatic internal secretion, unspecified
Islet-cell hyperplasia NOS
Pancreatic endocrine cell hyperplasia NOS

Disorders of other endocrine glands (E2Ø-E35)

EXCLUDES 1 *galactorrhea (N64.3)*
gynecomastia (N62)

E2Ø Hypoparathyroidism
EXCLUDES 1 *Di George's syndrome (D82.1)*
postprocedural hypoparathyroidism (E89.2)
tetany NOS (R29.Ø)
transitory neonatal hypoparathyroidism (P71.4)

E2Ø.Ø Idiopathic hypoparathyroidism HCC
DEF: Abnormally low secretion of parathyroid hormones, with unknown cause, which triggers decreased calcium and increased phosphorus in the blood that can result in cataracts, muscle cramps, tetany, tingling, or burning in the lips, fingers, and toes.

E2Ø.1 Pseudohypoparathyroidism

E2Ø.8 Other hypoparathyroidism HCC

E2Ø.9 Hypoparathyroidism, unspecified HCC
Parathyroid tetany

E21 Hyperparathyroidism and other disorders of parathyroid gland
EXCLUDES 1 *adult osteomalacia (M83.-)*
ectopic hyperparathyroidism (E34.2)
hungry bone syndrome (E83.81)
infantile and juvenile osteomalacia (E55.Ø)
EXCLUDES 2 *familial hypocalciuric hypercalcemia (E83.52)*

E21.Ø Primary hyperparathyroidism HCC
Hyperplasia of parathyroid
Osteitis fibrosa cystica generalisata [von Recklinghausen's disease of bone]
DEF: Parathyroid dysfunction commonly caused by hyperplasia of two or more glands. Symptoms include hypercalcemia and increased parathyroid hormone levels.

E21.1 Secondary hyperparathyroidism, not elsewhere classified HCC
EXCLUDES 1 *secondary hyperparathyroidism of renal origin (N25.81)*

E21.2 Other hyperparathyroidism HCC
Tertiary hyperparathyroidism
EXCLUDES 1 *familial hypocalciuric hypercalcemia (E83.52)*

E21.3 Hyperparathyroidism, unspecified HCC

E21.4 Other specified disorders of parathyroid gland HCC

E21.5 Disorder of parathyroid gland, unspecified HCC

E22 Hyperfunction of pituitary gland
EXCLUDES 1 *Cushing's syndrome (E24.-)*
Nelson's syndrome (E24.1)
overproduction of ACTH not associated with Cushing's disease (E27.Ø)
overproduction of pituitary ACTH (E24.Ø)
overproduction of thyroid-stimulating hormone (EØ5.8-)

E22.Ø Acromegaly and pituitary gigantism HCC
Overproduction of growth hormone
EXCLUDES 1 *constitutional gigantism (E34.4)*
constitutional tall stature (E34.4)
increased secretion from endocrine pancreas of growth hormone-releasing hormone (E16.8)
DEF: Acromegaly: Chronic condition caused by overproduction of the pituitary growth hormone resulting in enlarged skeletal parts and facial features.

E22.1 Hyperprolactinemia CC HCC
Use additional code for adverse effect, if applicable, to identify drug (T36-T5Ø with fifth or sixth character 5)

E22.2 Syndrome of inappropriate secretion of antidiuretic hormone CC HCC

E22.8 Other hyperfunction of pituitary gland CC HCC
Central precocious puberty

E22.9 Hyperfunction of pituitary gland, unspecified CC HCC

E23 Hypofunction and other disorders of the pituitary gland
INCLUDES the listed conditions whether the disorder is in the pituitary or the hypothalamus
EXCLUDES 1 *postprocedural hypopituitarism (E89.3)*
▶*short stature due to endocrine disorder (E34.3-)*◀

E23.Ø Hypopituitarism CC HCC
Fertile eunuch syndrome
Hypogonadotropic hypogonadism
Idiopathic growth hormone deficiency
Isolated deficiency of gonadotropin
Isolated deficiency of growth hormone
Isolated deficiency of pituitary hormone
Kallmann's syndrome
Lorain-Levi short stature
Necrosis of pituitary gland (postpartum)
Panhypopituitarism
Pituitary cachexia
Pituitary insufficiency NOS
Pituitary short stature
Sheehan's syndrome
Simmonds' disease

E23.1 Drug-induced hypopituitarism HCC
Use additional code for adverse effect, if applicable, to identify drug (T36-T5Ø with fifth or sixth character 5)

E23.2 Diabetes insipidus CC HCC
EXCLUDES 1 *nephrogenic diabetes insipidus (N25.1)*

E23.3 Hypothalamic dysfunction, not elsewhere classified HCC
EXCLUDES 1 *Prader-Willi syndrome (Q87.11)*
Russell-Silver syndrome (Q87.19)

E23.6 Other disorders of pituitary gland HCC
Abscess of pituitary
Adiposogenital dystrophy

E23.7 Disorder of pituitary gland, unspecified HCC

E24 Cushing's syndrome
EXCLUDES 1 *congenital adrenal hyperplasia (E25.Ø)*
DEF: Abdominal striae, acne, hypertension, decreased carbohydrate tolerance, moon face, obesity, protein catabolism, and psychiatric disturbances resulting from increased adrenocortical secretion of cortisol caused by ACTH-dependent adrenocortical hyperplasia or tumor, or by steroid effects.

E24.Ø Pituitary-dependent Cushing's disease CC HCC
Overproduction of pituitary ACTH
Pituitary-dependent hypercorticalism

E24.1 Nelson's syndrome HCC

E24.2 Drug-induced Cushing's syndrome CC HCC
Use additional code for adverse effect, if applicable, to identify drug (T36-T5Ø with fifth or sixth character 5)

E24.3 Ectopic ACTH syndrome CC HCC

E24.4 Alcohol-induced pseudo-Cushing's syndrome CC HCC

E24.8 Other Cushing's syndrome CC HCC

E24.9 Cushing's syndrome, unspecified CC HCC

E25 Adrenogenital disorders
INCLUDES adrenogenital syndromes, virilizing or feminizing, whether acquired or due to adrenal hyperplasia
consequent on inborn enzyme defects in hormone synthesis
female adrenal pseudohermaphroditism
female heterosexual precocious pseudopuberty
male isosexual precocious pseudopuberty
male macrogenitosomia praecox
male sexual precocity with adrenal hyperplasia
male virilization (female)
EXCLUDES 1 *indeterminate sex and pseudohermaphroditism (Q56)*
chromosomal abnormalities (Q9Ø-Q99)

E25.Ø Congenital adrenogenital disorders associated with enzyme deficiency HCC
Congenital adrenal hyperplasia
21-Hydroxylase deficiency
Salt-losing congenital adrenal hyperplasia

E25.8 Other adrenogenital disorders HCC
Idiopathic adrenogenital disorder
Use additional code for adverse effect, if applicable, to identify drug (T36-T5Ø with fifth or sixth character 5)

E25.9 Adrenogenital disorder, unspecified HCC
Adrenogenital syndrome NOS

E26 Hyperaldosteronism

E26.Ø Primary hyperaldosteronism

E26.Ø1 Conn's syndrome HCC
Code also adrenal adenoma (D35.Ø-)

E26.Ø2 Glucocorticoid-remediable aldosteronism HCC
Familial aldosteronism type I
DEF: Rare autosomal dominant familial form of primary aldosteronism in which the secretion of aldosterone is under the influence of adrenocorticotrophic hormone (ACTH) rather than the renin-angiotensin mechanism. Moderate hypersecretion of aldosterone and suppressed plasma renin activity that are rapidly reversed by administration of glucosteroids. Symptoms include hypertension and mild hypokalemia.

E26.Ø9 Other primary hyperaldosteronism HCC
Primary aldosteronism due to adrenal hyperplasia (bilateral)

E26.1 Secondary hyperaldosteronism HCC

E26.8 Other hyperaldosteronism

E26.81 Bartter's syndrome HCC

E26.89 Other hyperaldosteronism HCC

E26.9 Hyperaldosteronism, unspecified HCC
Aldosteronism NOS
Hyperaldosteronism NOS

E27 Other disorders of adrenal gland

E27.Ø Other adrenocortical overactivity CC HCC
Overproduction of ACTH, not associated with Cushing's disease
Premature adrenarche
EXCLUDES 1 *Cushing's syndrome (E24.-)*

E27.1 Primary adrenocortical insufficiency CC HCC
Addison's disease
Autoimmune adrenalitis
EXCLUDES 1 *Addison only phenotype adrenoleukodystrophy (E71.528)*
amyloidosis (E85.-)
tuberculous Addison's disease (A18.7)
Waterhouse-Friderichsen syndrome (A39.1)

E27.2 Addisonian crisis CC HCC
Adrenal crisis
Adrenocortical crisis
DEF: Life-threatening condition that occurs when there is not enough cortisol excreted from the adrenal glands. This condition may be due to injury to the adrenal glands or to the pituitary gland, which controls adrenal hormone secretion, or when a patient stops hydrocortisone treatment too quickly or too early.

E27.3 Drug-induced adrenocortical insufficiency CC HCC
Use additional code for adverse effect, if applicable, to identify drug (T36-T5Ø with fifth or sixth character 5)

E27.4 Other and unspecified adrenocortical insufficiency
EXCLUDES 1 *adrenoleukodystrophy [Addison-Schilder] (E71.528)*
Waterhouse-Friderichsen syndrome (A39.1)

E27.4Ø Unspecified adrenocortical insufficiency CC HCC
Adrenocortical insufficiency NOS
Hypoaldosteronism

E27.49 Other adrenocortical insufficiency CC HCC
Adrenal hemorrhage
Adrenal infarction

E27.5 Adrenomedullary hyperfunction CC HCC
Adrenomedullary hyperplasia
Catecholamine hypersecretion

E27.8 Other specified disorders of adrenal gland HCC
Abnormality of cortisol-binding globulin

E27.9 Disorder of adrenal gland, unspecified HCC

E28 Ovarian dysfunction
EXCLUDES 1 *isolated gonadotropin deficiency (E23.Ø)*
postprocedural ovarian failure (E89.4-)

E28.Ø Estrogen excess ♀
Use additional code for adverse effect, if applicable, to identify drug (T36-T5Ø with fifth or sixth character 5)

E28.1 Androgen excess ♀
Hypersecretion of ovarian androgens
Use additional code for adverse effect, if applicable, to identify drug (T36-T5Ø with fifth or sixth character 5)

E28.2 Polycystic ovarian syndrome ♀
Sclerocystic ovary syndrome
Stein-Leventhal syndrome
AHA: 2022,2Q,16
DEF: Common hormonal disorder among women of reproductive age that involves enlarged ovaries with numerous small cysts located along the outer ovarian edge.

E28.3 Primary ovarian failure
EXCLUDES 1 *pure gonadal dysgenesis (Q99.1)*
Turner's syndrome (Q96.-)

E28.31 Premature menopause

E28.31Ø Symptomatic premature menopause A ♀
Symptoms such as flushing, sleeplessness, headache, lack of concentration, associated with premature menopause

E28.319 Asymptomatic premature menopause A ♀
Premature menopause NOS

E28.39 Other primary ovarian failure ♀
Decreased estrogen
Resistant ovary syndrome

E28.8 Other ovarian dysfunction ♀
Ovarian hyperfunction NOS
EXCLUDES 1 *postprocedural ovarian failure (E89.4-)*

E28.9 Ovarian dysfunction, unspecified ♀

E29 Testicular dysfunction
EXCLUDES 1 *androgen insensitivity syndrome (E34.5-)*
azoospermia or oligospermia NOS (N46.Ø-N46.1)
isolated gonadotropin deficiency (E23.Ø)
Klinefelter's syndrome (Q98.Ø-Q98.1, Q98.4)

E29.Ø Testicular hyperfunction ♂
Hypersecretion of testicular hormones

E29.1 Testicular hypofunction ♂
Defective biosynthesis of testicular androgen NOS
5-delta-Reductase deficiency (with male pseudohermaphroditism)
Testicular hypogonadism NOS
Use additional code for adverse effect, if applicable, to identify drug (T36-T5Ø with fifth or sixth character 5)
EXCLUDES 1 *postprocedural testicular hypofunction (E89.5)*

E29.8 Other testicular dysfunction ♂

E29.9 Testicular dysfunction, unspecified ♂

E3Ø Disorders of puberty, not elsewhere classified

E3Ø.Ø Delayed puberty
Constitutional delay of puberty
Delayed sexual development

E3Ø.1 Precocious puberty P
Precocious menstruation
EXCLUDES 1 *Albright (-McCune) (-Sternberg) syndrome (Q78.1)*
central precocious puberty (E22.8)
congenital adrenal hyperplasia (E25.Ø)
female heterosexual precocious pseudopuberty (E25.-)
male isosexual precocious pseudopuberty (E25.-)

E3Ø.8 Other disorders of puberty P
Premature thelarche

E3Ø.9 Disorder of puberty, unspecified

E31 Polyglandular dysfunction
EXCLUDES 1 *ataxia telangiectasia [Louis-Bar] (G11.3)*
dystrophia myotonica [Steinert] (G71.11)
pseudohypoparathyroidism (E2Ø.1)

E31.Ø Autoimmune polyglandular failure HCC
Schmidt's syndrome

E31.1 Polyglandular hyperfunction HCC
EXCLUDES 1 *multiple endocrine adenomatosis (E31.2-)*
multiple endocrine neoplasia (E31.2-)

E31.2 **Multiple endocrine neoplasia [MEN] syndromes**
Multiple endocrine adenomatosis
Code also any associated malignancies and other conditions associated with the syndromes
DEF: Group of conditions in which several endocrine glands grow excessively (such as in adenomatous hyperplasia) and/or develop benign or malignant tumors. Tumors and hyperplasia associated with MEN often produce excess hormones, which impede normal physiology. There is no comprehensive cure known for MEN syndrome. Treatment is directed at the hyperplasia or tumors in each individual gland. Tumors are usually surgically removed and oral medications or hormonal injections are used to correct hormone imbalances.

E31.20 **Multiple endocrine neoplasia [MEN] syndrome, unspecified** HCC
Multiple endocrine adenomatosis NOS
Multiple endocrine neoplasia [MEN] syndrome NOS

E31.21 **Multiple endocrine neoplasia [MEN] type I** HCC
Wermer's syndrome

E31.22 **Multiple endocrine neoplasia [MEN] type IIA** HCC
Sipple's syndrome

E31.23 **Multiple endocrine neoplasia [MEN] type IIB** HCC

E31.8 **Other polyglandular dysfunction** HCC

E31.9 **Polyglandular dysfunction, unspecified** HCC

E32 **Diseases of thymus**
EXCLUDES 1 *aplasia or hypoplasia of thymus with immunodeficiency (D82.1)*
myasthenia gravis (G70.0)

E32.0 **Persistent hyperplasia of thymus** HCC
Hypertrophy of thymus

E32.1 **Abscess of thymus** CC HCC

E32.8 **Other diseases of thymus** HCC
EXCLUDES 1 *aplasia or hypoplasia with immunodeficiency (D82.1)*
thymoma (D15.0)

E32.9 **Disease of thymus, unspecified** HCC

E34 **Other endocrine disorders**
EXCLUDES 1 *pseudohypoparathyroidism (E20.1)*

E34.0 **Carcinoid syndrome** CC HCC
NOTE May be used as an additional code to identify functional activity associated with a carcinoid tumor.

E34.1 **Other hypersecretion of intestinal hormones**

E34.2 **Ectopic hormone secretion, not elsewhere classified**
EXCLUDES 1 *ectopic ACTH syndrome (E24.3)*

▲ E34.3 **Short stature due to endocrine disorder**
~~Constitutional short stature~~
~~Laron-type short stature~~
EXCLUDES 1 *achondroplastic short stature (Q77.4)*
hypochondroplastic short stature (Q77.4)
nutritional short stature (E45)
pituitary short stature (E23.0)
progeria (E34.8)
renal short stature (N25.0)
Russell-Silver syndrome (Q87.19)
short-limbed stature with immunodeficiency (D82.2)
▶short stature (child) (R62.52)◀
short stature in specific dysmorphic syndromes - code to syndrome - see Alphabetical Index
short stature NOS (R62.52)

● E34.30 **Short stature due to endocrine disorder, unspecified**

● E34.31 **Constitutional short stature**
Constitutional delay of growth, puberty, or maturation

● E34.32 **Genetic causes of short stature**

● E34.321 **Primary insulin-like growth factor-1 (IGF-1) deficiency**
Acid-labile subunit gene (IGFALS) defect
Growth hormone gene 1 (GH1) defect with growth hormone neutralizing antibodies
Growth hormone insensitivity syndrome (GHIS)
Insulin-like growth factor 1 gene (IGF1) defect
Laron type short stature
Severe primary insulin-like growth factor-1 deficiency (SPIGFD)
Signal transducer and activator of transcription 5B gene (STAT5b) defect

● E34.322 **Insulin-like growth factor-1 (IGF-1) resistance**
Genetic syndrome with resistance to insulin-like growth factor-1
Insulin-like growth factor-1 receptor (IGF-1R) defect
Post-insulin-like growth factor-1 receptor signaling defect

● E34.328 **Other genetic causes of short stature**
Short stature due to ACAN gene variant
Short stature due to aggrecan deficiency
Short stature due to NPR-2 gene variant

● E34.329 **Unspecified genetic causes of short stature**

● E34.39 **Other short stature due to endocrine disorder**

E34.4 **Constitutional tall stature** HCC
Constitutional gigantism

E34.5 **Androgen insensitivity syndrome**
DEF: X-linked recessive condition in which individuals that are chromosomally male fail to develop normal male external genitalia due to an abnormality on the X chromosome that prohibits the body, completely or in part, from recognizing the androgens produced. ***Synonym(s):*** *AIS*

E34.50 **Androgen insensitivity syndrome, unspecified**
Androgen insensitivity NOS

E34.51 **Complete androgen insensitivity syndrome**
Complete androgen insensitivity
de Quervain syndrome
Goldberg-Maxwell syndrome

E34.52 **Partial androgen insensitivity syndrome**
Partial androgen insensitivity
Reifenstein syndrome

E34.8 **Other specified endocrine disorders**
Pineal gland dysfunction
Progeria
EXCLUDES 2 *pseudohypoparathyroidism (E20.1)*

E34.9 **Endocrine disorder, unspecified**
Endocrine disturbance NOS
Hormone disturbance NOS

E35 Disorders of endocrine glands in diseases classified elsewhere
Code first underlying disease, such as:
late congenital syphilis of thymus gland [Dubois disease] (A50.5)
Use additional code, if applicable, to identify:
sequelae of tuberculosis of other organs (B90.8)
EXCLUDES 1 *Echinococcus granulosus infection of thyroid gland (B67.3)*
meningococcal hemorrhagic adrenalitis (A39.1)
syphilis of endocrine gland (A52.79)
tuberculosis of adrenal gland, except calcification (A18.7)
tuberculosis of endocrine gland NEC (A18.82)
tuberculosis of thyroid gland (A18.81)
Waterhouse-Friderichsen syndrome (A39.1)

Intraoperative complications of endocrine system (E36)

4th E36 Intraoperative complications of endocrine system
EXCLUDES 2 *postprocedural endocrine and metabolic complications and disorders, not elsewhere classified (E89.-)*

5th E36.Ø Intraoperative hemorrhage and hematoma of an endocrine system organ or structure complicating a procedure
EXCLUDES 1 *intraoperative hemorrhage and hematoma of an endocrine system organ or structure due to accidental puncture or laceration during a procedure (E36.1-)*

E36.Ø1 Intraoperative hemorrhage and hematoma of an endocrine system organ or structure complicating an endocrine system procedure CC
AHA: 2020,1Q,19

E36.Ø2 Intraoperative hemorrhage and hematoma of an endocrine system organ or structure complicating other procedure CC

5th E36.1 Accidental puncture and laceration of an endocrine system organ or structure during a procedure

E36.11 Accidental puncture and laceration of an endocrine system organ or structure during an endocrine system procedure CC

E36.12 Accidental puncture and laceration of an endocrine system organ or structure during other procedure CC

E36.8 Other intraoperative complications of endocrine system
Use additional code, if applicable, to further specify disorder

Malnutrition (E4Ø-E46)

EXCLUDES 1 *intestinal malabsorption (K9Ø.-)*
sequelae of protein-calorie malnutrition (E64.Ø)
EXCLUDES 2 *nutritional anemias (D5Ø-D53)*
starvation (T73.Ø)
AHA: 2020,1Q,4-7; 2017,4Q,108; 2017,3Q,25
TIP: Assign additional code for BMI from category Z68, when documented. BMI can be based on documentation from clinicians who are not the patient's provider.
TIP: Malnutrition is not considered integral to cancer; assign the appropriate code in addition to the code for the specific type of cancer.

E4Ø Kwashiorkor MCC HCC
Severe malnutrition with nutritional edema with dyspigmentation of skin and hair
EXCLUDES 1 *marasmic kwashiorkor (E42)*

E41 Nutritional marasmus MCC HCC
Severe malnutrition with marasmus
EXCLUDES 1 *marasmic kwashiorkor (E42)*
AHA: 2017,3Q,24
DEF: Protein-calorie malabsorption or malnutrition in children characterized by tissue wasting, dehydration, and subcutaneous fat depletion. It may occur with infectious disease.

E42 Marasmic kwashiorkor MCC HCC
Intermediate form severe protein-calorie malnutrition
Severe protein-calorie malnutrition with signs of both kwashiorkor and marasmus

E43 Unspecified severe protein-calorie malnutrition MCC HCC
Starvation edema
AHA: 2022,1Q,13; 2020,1Q,5,6; 2017,4Q,108
TIP: Assign code R64 when emaciation is documented without documentation of malnutrition.

4th E44 Protein-calorie malnutrition of moderate and mild degree
AHA: 2020,1Q,5

E44.Ø Moderate protein-calorie malnutrition CC HCC

E44.1 Mild protein-calorie malnutrition CC HCC

E45 Retarded development following protein-calorie malnutrition CC HCC
Nutritional short stature
Nutritional stunting
Physical retardation due to malnutrition

E46 Unspecified protein-calorie malnutrition CC HCC
Malnutrition NOS
Protein-calorie imbalance NOS
EXCLUDES 1 *nutritional deficiency NOS (E63.9)*
AHA: 2018,4Q,82

Other nutritional deficiencies (E5Ø-E64)

EXCLUDES 2 *nutritional anemias (D5Ø-D53)*

4th E5Ø Vitamin A deficiency
EXCLUDES 1 *sequelae of vitamin A deficiency (E64.1)*

E5Ø.Ø Vitamin A deficiency with conjunctival xerosis

E5Ø.1 Vitamin A deficiency with Bitot's spot and conjunctival xerosis
Bitot's spot in the young child
DEF: Vitamin A deficiency with conjunctival dryness and superficial spots of keratinized epithelium.

E5Ø.2 Vitamin A deficiency with corneal xerosis

E5Ø.3 Vitamin A deficiency with corneal ulceration and xerosis

E5Ø.4 Vitamin A deficiency with keratomalacia
DEF: Vitamin A deficiency creating corneal dryness that progresses to corneal insensitivity, softness, and necrosis. It is usually bilateral.

E5Ø.5 Vitamin A deficiency with night blindness

E5Ø.6 Vitamin A deficiency with xerophthalmic scars of cornea

E5Ø.7 Other ocular manifestations of vitamin A deficiency
Xerophthalmia NOS

E5Ø.8 Other manifestations of vitamin A deficiency
Follicular keratosis
Xeroderma

E5Ø.9 Vitamin A deficiency, unspecified
Hypovitaminosis A NOS

4th E51 Thiamine deficiency
EXCLUDES 1 *sequelae of thiamine deficiency (E64.8)*

5th E51.1 Beriberi

E51.11 Dry beriberi CC
Beriberi NOS
Beriberi with polyneuropathy

E51.12 Wet beriberi CC
Beriberi with cardiovascular manifestations
Cardiovascular beriberi
Shoshin disease

E51.2 Wernicke's encephalopathy CC
DEF: Deficiency of vitamin B1 resulting in a triad of acute mental confusion, ataxia, and ophthalmoplegia. The vast majority of affected patients are alcoholics.

E51.8 Other manifestations of thiamine deficiency CC

E51.9 Thiamine deficiency, unspecified CC

E52 Niacin deficiency [pellagra]
Niacin (-tryptophan) deficiency
Nicotinamide deficiency
Pellagra (alcoholic)
EXCLUDES 1 *sequelae of niacin deficiency (E64.8)*

4th E53 Deficiency of other B group vitamins
EXCLUDES 1 *sequelae of vitamin B deficiency (E64.8)*

E53.Ø Riboflavin deficiency CC
Ariboflavinosis
Vitamin B2 deficiency

E53.1 Pyridoxine deficiency
Vitamin B6 deficiency
EXCLUDES 1 *pyridoxine-responsive sideroblastic anemia (D64.3)*

E53.8 Deficiency of other specified B group vitamins
Biotin deficiency
Cyanocobalamin deficiency
Folate deficiency
Folic acid deficiency
Pantothenic acid deficiency
Vitamin B12 deficiency
EXCLUDES 1 *folate deficiency anemia (D52.-)*
vitamin B12 deficiency anemia (D51.-)

E53.9 Vitamin B deficiency, unspecified

E54 Ascorbic acid deficiency
Deficiency of vitamin C
Scurvy
EXCLUDES 1 *scorbutic anemia (D53.2)*
sequelae of vitamin C deficiency (E64.2)
DEF: Vitamin C deficiency causing swollen gums, myalgia, weight loss, and weakness.

E55 Vitamin D deficiency

EXCLUDES 1 *adult osteomalacia (M83.-)*
osteoporosis (M8Ø.-)
sequelae of rickets (E64.3)

E55.Ø Rickets, active CC
Infantile osteomalacia
Juvenile osteomalacia
EXCLUDES 1 *celiac rickets (K9Ø.Ø)*
Crohn's rickets (K5Ø.-)
hereditary vitamin D-dependent rickets (E83.32)
inactive rickets (E64.3)
renal rickets (N25.Ø)
sequelae of rickets (E64.3)
vitamin D-resistant rickets (E83.31)
DEF: Rickets: Softening or weakening of the bones due to a lack of vitamin D, calcium, and phosphate.

E55.9 Vitamin D deficiency, unspecified
Avitaminosis D

E56 Other vitamin deficiencies

EXCLUDES 1 *sequelae of other vitamin deficiencies (E64.8)*

E56.Ø Deficiency of vitamin E

E56.1 Deficiency of vitamin K
EXCLUDES 1 *deficiency of coagulation factor due to vitamin K deficiency (D68.4)*
vitamin K deficiency of newborn (P53)

E56.8 Deficiency of other vitamins

E56.9 Vitamin deficiency, unspecified

E58 Dietary calcium deficiency

EXCLUDES 1 *disorders of calcium metabolism (E83.5-)*
sequelae of calcium deficiency (E64.8)

E59 Dietary selenium deficiency

Keshan disease
EXCLUDES 1 *sequelae of selenium deficiency (E64.8)*

E6Ø Dietary zinc deficiency

E61 Deficiency of other nutrient elements

Use additional code for adverse effect, if applicable, to identify drug (T36-T5Ø with fifth or sixth character 5)
EXCLUDES 1 *disorders of mineral metabolism (E83.-)*
iodine deficiency related thyroid disorders (EØØ-EØ2)
sequelae of malnutrition and other nutritional deficiencies (E64.-)

E61.Ø Copper deficiency

E61.1 Iron deficiency
EXCLUDES 1 *iron deficiency anemia (D5Ø.-)*

E61.2 Magnesium deficiency

E61.3 Manganese deficiency

E61.4 Chromium deficiency

E61.5 Molybdenum deficiency

E61.6 Vanadium deficiency

E61.7 Deficiency of multiple nutrient elements

E61.8 Deficiency of other specified nutrient elements

E61.9 Deficiency of nutrient element, unspecified

E63 Other nutritional deficiencies

EXCLUDES 2 *dehydration (E86.Ø)*
failure to thrive, adult (R62.7)
failure to thrive, child (R62.51)
feeding problems in newborn (P92.-)
sequelae of malnutrition and other nutritional deficiencies (E64.-)

E63.Ø Essential fatty acid [EFA] deficiency

E63.1 Imbalance of constituents of food intake

E63.8 Other specified nutritional deficiencies

E63.9 Nutritional deficiency, unspecified

E64 Sequelae of malnutrition and other nutritional deficiencies

NOTE This category is to be used to indicate conditions in categories E43, E44, E46, E5Ø-E63 as the cause of sequelae, which are themselves classified elsewhere. The 'sequelae' include conditions specified as such; they also include the late effects of diseases classifiable to the above categories if the disease itself is no longer present

Code first condition resulting from (sequela) of malnutrition and other nutritional deficiencies

E64.Ø Sequelae of protein-calorie malnutrition CC HCC
EXCLUDES 2 *retarded development following protein-calorie malnutrition (E45)*

E64.1 Sequelae of vitamin A deficiency

E64.2 Sequelae of vitamin C deficiency

E64.3 Sequelae of rickets

E64.8 Sequelae of other nutritional deficiencies

E64.9 Sequelae of unspecified nutritional deficiency

Overweight, obesity and other hyperalimentation (E65-E68)

E65 Localized adiposity

Fat pad

E66 Overweight and obesity

Code first obesity complicating pregnancy, childbirth and the puerperium, if applicable (O99.21-)
Use additional code to identify body mass index (BMI), if known (Z68.-)
EXCLUDES 1 *adiposogenital dystrophy (E23.6)*
lipomatosis NOS (E88.2)
lipomatosis dolorosa [Dercum] (E88.2)
Prader-Willi syndrome (Q87.11)
AHA: 2018,4Q,77,79-80
TIP: Do not assign a BMI code (Z68.-) when a pregnant patient is documented as being overweight or obese. Only a code from subcategory O99.21- and a code from this category should be assigned.

E66.Ø Obesity due to excess calories

E66.Ø1 Morbid (severe) obesity due to excess calories H11 HCC
EXCLUDES 1 *morbid (severe) obesity with alveolar hypoventilation (E66.2)*
AHA: 2022,2Q,9

E66.Ø9 Other obesity due to excess calories

E66.1 Drug-induced obesity
Use additional code for adverse effect, if applicable, to identify drug (T36-T5Ø with fifth or sixth character 5)

E66.2 Morbid (severe) obesity with alveolar hypoventilation CC HCC
Obesity hypoventilation syndrome (OHS)
Pickwickian syndrome

E66.3 Overweight
AHA: 2018,4Q,78

E66.8 Other obesity

E66.9 Obesity, unspecified
Obesity NOS
AHA: 2021,2Q,10

E67 Other hyperalimentation

EXCLUDES 1 *hyperalimentation NOS (R63.2)*
sequelae of hyperalimentation (E68)

E67.Ø Hypervitaminosis A

E67.1 Hypercarotenemia
DEF: Elevated blood carotene level as a result of excessive carotenoid ingestion or an inability to convert carotenoids to vitamin A. Characteristics often include yellow discoloration of the skin, which may follow overeating of carotenoid-rich foods such as carrots, sweet potatoes, or squash.

E67.2 Megavitamin-B6 syndrome

E67.3 Hypervitaminosis D

E67.8 Other specified hyperalimentation

E68 Sequelae of hyperalimentation

Code first condition resulting from (sequela) of hyperalimentation

Metabolic disorders (E70-E88)

EXCLUDES 1 *androgen insensitivity syndrome (E34.5-)*
congenital adrenal hyperplasia (E25.0)
hemolytic anemias attributable to enzyme disorders (D55.-)
Marfan's syndrome (Q87.4)
5-alpha-reductase deficiency (E29.1)

EXCLUDES 2 *Ehlers-Danlos syndromes (Q79.6-)*

AHA: 2018,2Q,6

E70 Disorders of aromatic amino-acid metabolism

E70.0 Classical phenylketonuria CC HCC

E70.1 Other hyperphenylalaninemias CC HCC

E70.2 Disorders of tyrosine metabolism

EXCLUDES 1 *transitory tyrosinemia of newborn (P74.5)*

E70.20 Disorder of tyrosine metabolism, unspecified CC HCC

E70.21 Tyrosinemia CC HCC
Hypertyrosinemia

E70.29 Other disorders of tyrosine metabolism CC HCC
Alkaptonuria
Ochronosis

E70.3 Albinism

DEF: Absence of pigment in skin, hair, and eyes. This genetic condition is often accompanied by astigmatism, photophobia, and nystagmus.

E70.30 Albinism, unspecified CC HCC

E70.31 Ocular albinism

E70.310 X-linked ocular albinism CC HCC

E70.311 Autosomal recessive ocular albinism CC HCC

E70.318 Other ocular albinism CC HCC

E70.319 Ocular albinism, unspecified CC HCC

E70.32 Oculocutaneous albinism

EXCLUDES 1 *Chediak-Higashi syndrome (E70.330)*
Hermansky-Pudlak syndrome (E70.331)

E70.320 Tyrosinase negative oculocutaneous albinism CC HCC
Albinism I
Oculocutaneous albinism ty-neg

E70.321 Tyrosinase positive oculocutaneous albinism CC HCC
Albinism II
Oculocutaneous albinism ty-pos

E70.328 Other oculocutaneous albinism CC HCC
Cross syndrome

E70.329 Oculocutaneous albinism, unspecified CC HCC

E70.33 Albinism with hematologic abnormality

E70.330 Chediak-Higashi syndrome CC HCC

E70.331 Hermansky-Pudlak syndrome CC HCC

E70.338 Other albinism with hematologic abnormality CC HCC

E70.339 Albinism with hematologic abnormality, unspecified CC HCC

E70.39 Other specified albinism CC HCC
Piebaldism

E70.4 Disorders of histidine metabolism

E70.40 Disorders of histidine metabolism, unspecified CC HCC

E70.41 Histidinemia CC HCC

E70.49 Other disorders of histidine metabolism CC HCC

E70.5 Disorders of tryptophan metabolism CC HCC

E70.8 Other disorders of aromatic amino-acid metabolism

AHA: 2020,4Q,15-16

E70.81 Aromatic L-amino acid decarboxylase deficiency CC HCC
AADC deficiency

E70.89 Other disorders of aromatic amino-acid metabolism CC HCC

E70.9 Disorder of aromatic amino-acid metabolism, unspecified CC HCC

E71 Disorders of branched-chain amino-acid metabolism and fatty-acid metabolism

E71.0 Maple-syrup-urine disease CC HCC

E71.1 Other disorders of branched-chain amino-acid metabolism

E71.11 Branched-chain organic acidurias

E71.110 Isovaleric acidemia CC HCC

E71.111 3-methylglutaconic aciduria CC HCC

E71.118 Other branched-chain organic acidurias CC HCC

E71.12 Disorders of propionate metabolism

E71.120 Methylmalonic acidemia CC HCC

E71.121 Propionic acidemia CC HCC

E71.128 Other disorders of propionate metabolism CC HCC

E71.19 Other disorders of branched-chain amino-acid metabolism CC HCC
Hyperleucine-isoleucinemia
Hypervalinemia

E71.2 Disorder of branched-chain amino-acid metabolism, unspecified CC HCC

E71.3 Disorders of fatty-acid metabolism

EXCLUDES 1 *peroxisomal disorders (E71.5)*
Refsum's disease (G60.1)
Schilder's disease (G37.0)

EXCLUDES 2 *carnitine deficiency due to inborn error of metabolism (E71.42)*

E71.30 Disorder of fatty-acid metabolism, unspecified

E71.31 Disorders of fatty-acid oxidation

E71.310 Long chain/very long chain acyl CoA dehydrogenase deficiency CC HCC
LCAD
VLCAD

E71.311 Medium chain acyl CoA dehydrogenase deficiency CC HCC
MCAD

E71.312 Short chain acyl CoA dehydrogenase deficiency CC HCC
SCAD

E71.313 Glutaric aciduria type II CC HCC
Glutaric aciduria type II A
Glutaric aciduria type II B
Glutaric aciduria type II C

EXCLUDES 1 *glutaric aciduria (type 1) NOS (E72.3)*

E71.314 Muscle carnitine palmitoyltransferase deficiency CC HCC

E71.318 Other disorders of fatty-acid oxidation CC HCC

E71.32 Disorders of ketone metabolism CC HCC

E71.39 Other disorders of fatty-acid metabolism CC HCC

E71.4 Disorders of carnitine metabolism

EXCLUDES 1 *muscle carnitine palmitoyltransferase deficiency (E71.314)*

E71.40 Disorder of carnitine metabolism, unspecified HCC

E71.41 Primary carnitine deficiency HCC

E71.42 Carnitine deficiency due to inborn errors of metabolism HCC
Code also associated inborn error or metabolism

E71.43 Iatrogenic carnitine deficiency HCC
Carnitine deficiency due to hemodialysis
Carnitine deficiency due to Valproic acid therapy

E71.44 Other secondary carnitine deficiency

E71.440 Ruvalcaba-Myhre-Smith syndrome HCC

E71.448 Other secondary carnitine deficiency HCC

E71.5 Peroxisomal disorders

EXCLUDES 1 *Schilder's disease (G37.0)*

E71.50 Peroxisomal disorder, unspecified CC HCC

E71.51 Disorders of peroxisome biogenesis
Group 1 peroxisomal disorders

EXCLUDES 1 *Refsum's disease (G60.1)*

E71.510 Zellweger syndrome CC HCC

E71.511 Neonatal adrenoleukodystrophy CC HCC

EXCLUDES 1 *X-linked adrenoleukodystrophy (E71.42-)*

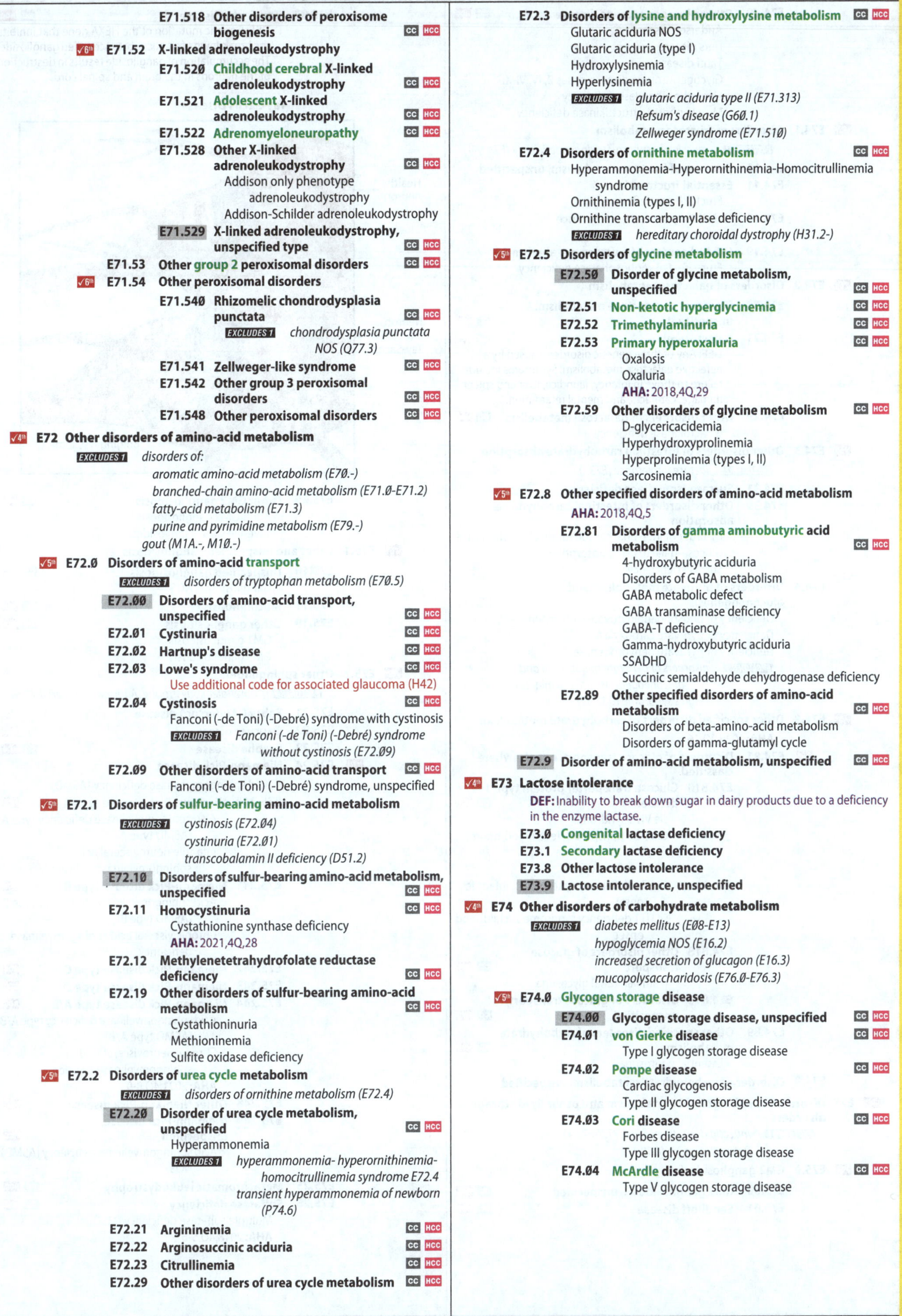

E71.518 Other disorders of peroxisome biogenesis CC HCC

✓6th **E71.52 X-linked adrenoleukodystrophy**

E71.520 Childhood cerebral X-linked adrenoleukodystrophy CC HCC

E71.521 Adolescent X-linked adrenoleukodystrophy CC HCC

E71.522 Adrenomyeloneuropathy CC HCC

E71.528 Other X-linked adrenoleukodystrophy CC HCC
- Addison only phenotype adrenoleukodystrophy
- Addison-Schilder adrenoleukodystrophy

E71.529 X-linked adrenoleukodystrophy, unspecified type CC HCC

E71.53 Other group 2 peroxisomal disorders CC HCC

✓6th **E71.54 Other peroxisomal disorders**

E71.540 Rhizomelic chondrodysplasia punctata CC HCC
- EXCLUDES 1 *chondrodysplasia punctata NOS (Q77.3)*

E71.541 Zellweger-like syndrome CC HCC

E71.542 Other group 3 peroxisomal disorders CC HCC

E71.548 Other peroxisomal disorders CC HCC

✓4th **E72 Other disorders of amino-acid metabolism**

EXCLUDES 1 *disorders of:*
- *aromatic amino-acid metabolism (E70.-)*
- *branched-chain amino-acid metabolism (E71.0-E71.2)*
- *fatty-acid metabolism (E71.3)*
- *purine and pyrimidine metabolism (E79.-)*

gout (M1A.-, M10.-)

✓5th **E72.0 Disorders of amino-acid transport**

EXCLUDES 1 *disorders of tryptophan metabolism (E70.5)*

E72.00 Disorders of amino-acid transport, unspecified CC HCC

E72.01 Cystinuria CC HCC

E72.02 Hartnup's disease CC HCC

E72.03 Lowe's syndrome CC HCC
- Use additional code for associated glaucoma (H42)

E72.04 Cystinosis CC HCC
- Fanconi (-de Toni) (-Debré) syndrome with cystinosis
- EXCLUDES 1 *Fanconi (-de Toni) (-Debré) syndrome without cystinosis (E72.09)*

E72.09 Other disorders of amino-acid transport CC HCC
- Fanconi (-de Toni) (-Debré) syndrome, unspecified

✓5th **E72.1 Disorders of sulfur-bearing amino-acid metabolism**

EXCLUDES 1 *cystinosis (E72.04)*
cystinuria (E72.01)
transcobalamin II deficiency (D51.2)

E72.10 Disorders of sulfur-bearing amino-acid metabolism, unspecified CC HCC

E72.11 Homocystinuria CC HCC
- Cystathionine synthase deficiency
- AHA: 2021,4Q,28

E72.12 Methylenetetrahydrofolate reductase deficiency CC HCC

E72.19 Other disorders of sulfur-bearing amino-acid metabolism CC HCC
- Cystathioninuria
- Methioninemia
- Sulfite oxidase deficiency

✓5th **E72.2 Disorders of urea cycle metabolism**

EXCLUDES 1 *disorders of ornithine metabolism (E72.4)*

E72.20 Disorder of urea cycle metabolism, unspecified CC HCC
- Hyperammonemia
- EXCLUDES 1 *hyperammonemia- hyperornithinemia-homocitrullinemia syndrome E72.4*
  transient hyperammonemia of newborn (P74.6)

E72.21 Argininemia CC HCC

E72.22 Arginosuccinic aciduria CC HCC

E72.23 Citrullinemia CC HCC

E72.29 Other disorders of urea cycle metabolism CC HCC

E72.3 Disorders of lysine and hydroxylysine metabolism CC HCC
- Glutaric aciduria NOS
- Glutaric aciduria (type I)
- Hydroxylysinemia
- Hyperlysinemia
- EXCLUDES 1 *glutaric aciduria type II (E71.313)*
  Refsum's disease (G60.1)
  Zellweger syndrome (E71.510)

E72.4 Disorders of ornithine metabolism CC HCC
- Hyperammonemia-Hyperornithinemia-Homocitrullinemia syndrome
- Ornithinemia (types I, II)
- Ornithine transcarbamylase deficiency
- EXCLUDES 1 *hereditary choroidal dystrophy (H31.2-)*

✓5th **E72.5 Disorders of glycine metabolism**

E72.50 Disorder of glycine metabolism, unspecified CC HCC

E72.51 Non-ketotic hyperglycinemia CC HCC

E72.52 Trimethylaminuria CC HCC

E72.53 Primary hyperoxaluria CC HCC
- Oxalosis
- Oxaluria
- AHA: 2018,4Q,29

E72.59 Other disorders of glycine metabolism CC HCC
- D-glycericacidemia
- Hyperhydroxyprolinemia
- Hyperprolinemia (types I, II)
- Sarcosinemia

✓5th **E72.8 Other specified disorders of amino-acid metabolism**

AHA: 2018,4Q,5

E72.81 Disorders of gamma aminobutyric acid metabolism CC HCC
- 4-hydroxybutyric aciduria
- Disorders of GABA metabolism
- GABA metabolic defect
- GABA transaminase deficiency
- GABA-T deficiency
- Gamma-hydroxybutyric aciduria
- SSADHD
- Succinic semialdehyde dehydrogenase deficiency

E72.89 Other specified disorders of amino-acid metabolism CC HCC
- Disorders of beta-amino-acid metabolism
- Disorders of gamma-glutamyl cycle

E72.9 Disorder of amino-acid metabolism, unspecified CC HCC

✓4th **E73 Lactose intolerance**

DEF: Inability to break down sugar in dairy products due to a deficiency in the enzyme lactase.

E73.0 Congenital lactase deficiency

E73.1 Secondary lactase deficiency

E73.8 Other lactose intolerance

E73.9 Lactose intolerance, unspecified

✓4th **E74 Other disorders of carbohydrate metabolism**

EXCLUDES 1 *diabetes mellitus (E08-E13)*
hypoglycemia NOS (E16.2)
increased secretion of glucagon (E16.3)
mucopolysaccharidosis (E76.0-E76.3)

✓5th **E74.0 Glycogen storage disease**

E74.00 Glycogen storage disease, unspecified CC HCC

E74.01 von Gierke disease CC HCC
- Type I glycogen storage disease

E74.02 Pompe disease CC HCC
- Cardiac glycogenosis
- Type II glycogen storage disease

E74.03 Cori disease CC HCC
- Forbes disease
- Type III glycogen storage disease

E74.04 McArdle disease CC HCC
- Type V glycogen storage disease

E74.Ø9 Other glycogen storage disease CC HCC
- Andersen disease
- Hers disease
- Tauri disease
- Glycogen storage disease, types Ø, IV, VI-XI
- Liver phosphorylase deficiency
- Muscle phosphofructokinase deficiency

✓5th **E74.1 Disorders of fructose metabolism**

EXCLUDES 1 *muscle phosphofructokinase deficiency (E74.Ø9)*

E74.1Ø Disorder of fructose metabolism, unspecified

E74.11 Essential fructosuria
- Fructokinase deficiency

E74.12 Hereditary fructose intolerance
- Fructosemia

E74.19 Other disorders of fructose metabolism
- Fructose-1, 6-diphosphatase deficiency

✓5th **E74.2 Disorders of galactose metabolism**

E74.2Ø Disorders of galactose metabolism, unspecified CC HCC

E74.21 Galactosemia CC HCC

DEF: Any of three genetic disorders caused by a defective galactose metabolism. Symptoms include failure to thrive in infancy, jaundice, liver and spleen damage, cataracts, and mental retardation.

E74.29 Other disorders of galactose metabolism CC HCC
- Galactokinase deficiency

✓5th **E74.3 Other disorders of intestinal carbohydrate absorption**

EXCLUDES 2 *lactose intolerance (E73.-)*

E74.31 Sucrase-isomaltase deficiency

E74.39 Other disorders of intestinal carbohydrate absorption
- Disorder of intestinal carbohydrate absorption NOS
- Glucose-galactose malabsorption
- Sucrase deficiency

E74.4 Disorders of pyruvate metabolism and gluconeogenesis CC HCC
- Deficiency of phosphoenolpyruvate carboxykinase
- Deficiency of pyruvate carboxylase
- Deficiency of pyruvate dehydrogenase

EXCLUDES 1 *disorders of pyruvate metabolism and gluconeogenesis with anemia (D55.-)*
Leigh's syndrome (G31.82)

✓5th **E74.8 Other specified disorders of carbohydrate metabolism**

AHA: 2020,4Q,16

✓6th **E74.81 Disorders of glucose transport, not elsewhere classified**

E74.81Ø Glucose transporter protein type 1 deficiency CC HCC
- De Vivo syndrome
- Glucose transport defect, blood-brain barrier
- Glut1 deficiency
- GLUT1 deficiency syndrome 1, infantile onset
- GLUT1 deficiency syndrome 2, childhood onset

E74.818 Other disorders of glucose transport CC HCC
- (Familial) renal glycosuria

E74.819 Disorders of glucose transport, unspecified CC HCC

E74.89 Other specified disorders of carbohydrate metabolism CC HCC
- Essential pentosuria

E74.9 Disorder of carbohydrate metabolism, unspecified HCC

✓4th **E75 Disorders of sphingolipid metabolism and other lipid storage disorders**

EXCLUDES 1 *mucolipidosis, types I-III (E77.Ø-E77.1)*
Refsum's disease (G6Ø.1)

✓5th **E75.Ø GM2 gangliosidosis**

E75.ØØ GM2 gangliosidosis, unspecified CC HCC

E75.Ø1 Sandhoff disease CC HCC

E75.Ø2 Tay-Sachs disease CC HCC

DEF: Genetic mutation of the HEXA gene that inhibits the breakdown of a toxic substance called ganglioside. The accumulation of ganglioside results in destruction of the neurons in the brain and spinal cord.

Tay-Sachs Disease

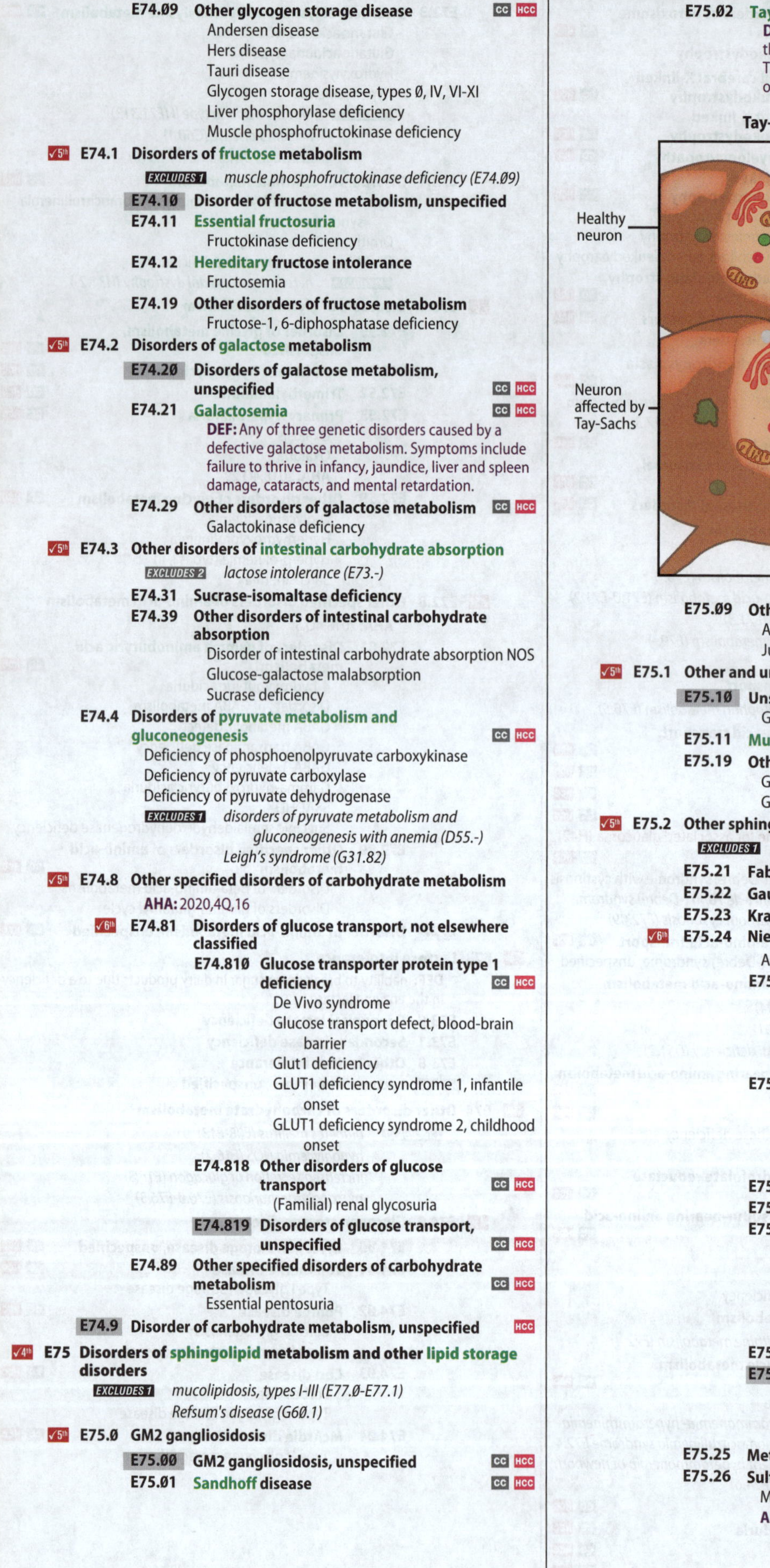

E75.Ø9 Other GM2 gangliosidosis CC HCC
- Adult GM2 gangliosidosis
- Juvenile GM2 gangliosidosis

✓5th **E75.1 Other and unspecified gangliosidosis**

E75.1Ø Unspecified gangliosidosis CC HCC
- Gangliosidosis NOS

E75.11 Mucolipidosis IV CC HCC

E75.19 Other gangliosidosis CC HCC
- GM1 gangliosidosis
- GM3 gangliosidosis

✓5th **E75.2 Other sphingolipidosis**

EXCLUDES 1 *adrenoleukodystrophy [Addison-Schilder] (E71.528)*

E75.21 Fabry (-Anderson) disease HCC

E75.22 Gaucher disease HCC

E75.23 Krabbe disease CC HCC

✓6th **E75.24 Niemann-Pick disease**
- Acid sphingomyelinase deficiency (ASMD)

E75.24Ø Niemann-Pick disease type A HCC
- Acid sphingomyelinase deficiency type A (ASMD type A)
- Infantile neurovisceral acid sphingomyelinase deficiency

E75.241 Niemann-Pick disease type B HCC
- Acid sphingomyelinase deficiency type B (ASMD type B)
- Chronic visceral acid sphingomyelinase deficiency

E75.242 Niemann-Pick disease type C HCC

E75.243 Niemann-Pick disease type D HCC

E75.244 Niemann-Pick disease type A/B HCC
- Acid sphingomyelinase deficiency type A/B (ASMD type A/B)
- Chronic neurovisceral acid sphingomyelinase deficiency

AHA: 2021,4Q,8-9

E75.248 Other Niemann-Pick disease HCC

E75.249 Niemann-Pick disease, unspecified HCC
- Acid sphingomyelinase deficiency (ASMD) NOS

E75.25 Metachromatic leukodystrophy CC HCC

E75.26 Sulfatase deficiency CC HCC
- Multiple sulfatase deficiency (MSD)

AHA: 2018,4Q,5-6

N Newborn: 0 P Pediatric: 0-17 M Maternity: 9-64 A Adult: 15-124 UNS Unspecified Site MCC Major Complication/Comorbidity CC Complication/Comorbidity

E75.29 Other sphingolipidosis CC HCC
Farber's syndrome
Sulfatide lipidosis

E75.3 Sphingolipidosis, unspecified HCC

E75.4 Neuronal ceroid lipofuscinosis CC HCC
Batten disease
Bielschowsky-Jansky disease
Kufs disease
Spielmeyer-Vogt disease

E75.5 Other lipid storage disorders
Cerebrotendinous cholesterosis [van Bogaert-Scherer-Epstein]
Wolman's disease

E75.6 Lipid storage disorder, unspecified

✓4th **E76 Disorders of glycosaminoglycan metabolism**

✓5th **E76.0 Mucopolysaccharidosis, type I**

E76.01 Hurler's syndrome CC HCC

E76.02 Hurler-Scheie syndrome CC HCC

E76.03 Scheie's syndrome CC HCC

E76.1 Mucopolysaccharidosis, type II CC HCC
Hunter's syndrome

✓5th **E76.2 Other mucopolysaccharidoses**

✓6th **E76.21 Morquio mucopolysaccharidoses**

E76.210 Morquio A mucopolysaccharidoses CC HCC
Classic Morquio syndrome
Morquio syndrome A
Mucopolysaccharidosis, type IVA

E76.211 Morquio B mucopolysaccharidoses CC HCC
Morquio-like mucopolysaccharidoses
Morquio-like syndrome
Morquio syndrome B
Mucopolysaccharidosis, type IVB

E76.219 Morquio mucopolysaccharidoses, unspecified CC HCC
Morquio syndrome
Mucopolysaccharidosis, type IV

E76.22 Sanfilippo mucopolysaccharidoses CC HCC
Mucopolysaccharidosis, type III (A) (B) (C) (D)
Sanfilippo A syndrome
Sanfilippo B syndrome
Sanfilippo C syndrome
Sanfilippo D syndrome

E76.29 Other mucopolysaccharidoses CC HCC
beta-Glucuronidase deficiency
Maroteaux-Lamy (mild) (severe) syndrome
Mucopolysaccharidosis, types VI, VII

E76.3 Mucopolysaccharidosis, unspecified CC HCC

E76.8 Other disorders of glucosaminoglycan metabolism CC HCC

E76.9 Glucosaminoglycan metabolism disorder, unspecified CC HCC

✓4th **E77 Disorders of glycoprotein metabolism**

E77.0 Defects in post-translational modification of lysosomal enzymes HCC
Mucolipidosis II [I-cell disease]
Mucolipidosis III [pseudo-Hurler polydystrophy]

E77.1 Defects in glycoprotein degradation HCC
Aspartylglucosaminuria
Fucosidosis
Mannosidosis
Sialidosis [mucolipidosis I]

E77.8 Other disorders of glycoprotein metabolism HCC

E77.9 Disorder of glycoprotein metabolism, unspecified HCC

✓4th **E78 Disorders of lipoprotein metabolism and other lipidemias**

EXCLUDES 1 *sphingolipidosis (E75.0-E75.3)*

✓5th **E78.0 Pure hypercholesterolemia**
AHA: 2016,4Q,13-14

E78.00 Pure hypercholesterolemia, unspecified
Fredrickson's hyperlipoproteinemia, type IIa
Hyperbetalipoproteinemia
Low-density-lipoprotein-type [LDL] hyperlipoproteinemia
(Pure) hypercholesterolemia NOS
AHA: 2022,2Q,5-6

E78.01 Familial hypercholesterolemia

E78.1 Pure hyperglyceridemia
Elevated fasting triglycerides
Endogenous hyperglyceridemia
Fredrickson's hyperlipoproteinemia, type IV
Hyperlipidemia, group B
Hyperprebetalipoproteinemia
Very-low-density-lipoprotein-type [VLDL] hyperlipoproteinemia

E78.2 Mixed hyperlipidemia
Broad- or floating-betalipoproteinemia
Combined hyperlipidemia NOS
Elevated cholesterol with elevated triglycerides NEC
Fredrickson's hyperlipoproteinemia, type IIb or III
Hyperbetalipoproteinemia with prebetalipoproteinemia
Hypercholesteremia with endogenous hyperglyceridemia
Hyperlipidemia, group C
Tubo-eruptive xanthoma
Xanthoma tuberosum

EXCLUDES 1 *cerebrotendinous cholesterosis [van Bogaert-Scherer-Epstein] (E75.5)*
familial combined hyperlipidemia (E78.49)

AHA: 2022,2Q,6

E78.3 Hyperchylomicronemia
Chylomicron retention disease
Fredrickson's hyperlipoproteinemia, type I or V
Hyperlipidemia, group D
Mixed hyperglyceridemia

✓5th **E78.4 Other hyperlipidemia**
AHA: 2018,4Q,6

E78.41 Elevated Lipoprotein(a)
Elevated Lp(a)

E78.49 Other hyperlipidemia
Familial combined hyperlipidemia

E78.5 Hyperlipidemia, unspecified
AHA: 2022,2Q,5

E78.6 Lipoprotein deficiency
Abetalipoproteinemia
Depressed HDL cholesterol
High-density lipoprotein deficiency
Hypoalphalipoproteinemia
Hypobetalipoproteinemia (familial)
Lecithin cholesterol acyltransferase deficiency
Tangier disease

✓5th **E78.7 Disorders of bile acid and cholesterol metabolism**

EXCLUDES 1 *Niemann-Pick disease type C (E75.242)*

E78.70 Disorder of bile acid and cholesterol metabolism, unspecified

E78.71 Barth syndrome CC

E78.72 Smith-Lemli-Opitz syndrome CC

E78.79 Other disorders of bile acid and cholesterol metabolism

✓5th **E78.8 Other disorders of lipoprotein metabolism**

E78.81 Lipoid dermatoarthritis

E78.89 Other lipoprotein metabolism disorders

E78.9 Disorder of lipoprotein metabolism, unspecified

✓4th **E79 Disorders of purine and pyrimidine metabolism**

EXCLUDES 1 *Ataxia-telangiectasia (Q87.19)*
Bloom's syndrome (Q82.8)
Cockayne's syndrome (Q87.19)
calculus of kidney (N20.0)
combined immunodeficiency disorders (D81.-)
Fanconi's anemia (D61.09)
gout (M1A.-, M10.-)
orotaciduric anemia (D53.0)
progeria (E34.8)
Werner's syndrome (E34.8)
xeroderma pigmentosum (Q82.1)

E79.0 Hyperuricemia without signs of inflammatory arthritis and tophaceous disease
Asymptomatic hyperuricemia

E79.1 Lesch-Nyhan syndrome CC HCC
HGPRT deficiency

E79.2 Myoadenylate deaminase deficiency CC HCC

E79.8 Other disorders of purine and pyrimidine metabolism CC HCC
Hereditary xanthinuria

Additional Character Required | x7th Placeholder | Questionable PDx | Manifestation | Unspecified | UPD Unacceptable PDx | H1-H14 HAC | HCC CMS-HCC Dx | 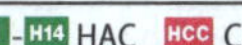 HIV Dx

E79.9 Disorder of purine and pyrimidine metabolism, unspecified CC HCC

E80 Disorders of porphyrin and bilirubin metabolism
INCLUDES defects of catalase and peroxidase

E80.0 Hereditary erythropoietic porphyria CC HCC
Congenital erythropoietic porphyria
Erythropoietic protoporphyria

E80.1 Porphyria cutanea tarda CC HCC

E80.2 Other and unspecified porphyria

E80.20 Unspecified porphyria CC HCC
Porphyria NOS

E80.21 Acute intermittent (hepatic) porphyria CC HCC

E80.29 Other porphyria CC HCC
Hereditary coproporphyria

E80.3 Defects of catalase and peroxidase CC HCC
Acatalasia [Takahara]

E80.4 Gilbert syndrome

E80.5 Crigler-Najjar syndrome

E80.6 Other disorders of bilirubin metabolism
Dubin-Johnson syndrome
Rotor's syndrome

E80.7 Disorder of bilirubin metabolism, unspecified

E83 Disorders of mineral metabolism
EXCLUDES 1 *dietary mineral deficiency (E58-E61)*
parathyroid disorders (E20-E21)
vitamin D deficiency (E55.-)

E83.0 Disorders of copper metabolism

E83.00 Disorder of copper metabolism, unspecified

E83.01 Wilson's disease
Code also associated Kayser Fleischer ring (H18.04-)

E83.09 Other disorders of copper metabolism
Menkes' (kinky hair) (steely hair) disease

E83.1 Disorders of iron metabolism
EXCLUDES 1 *iron deficiency anemia (D50.-)*
sideroblastic anemia (D64.0-D64.3)

E83.10 Disorder of iron metabolism, unspecified

E83.11 Hemochromatosis
EXCLUDES 1 *GALD (P78.84)*
gestational alloimmune liver disease (P78.84)
neonatal hemochromatosis (P78.84)

E83.110 Hereditary hemochromatosis HCC
Bronzed diabetes
Pigmentary cirrhosis (of liver)
Primary (hereditary) hemochromatosis

E83.111 Hemochromatosis due to repeated red blood cell transfusions
Iron overload due to repeated red blood cell transfusions
Transfusion (red blood cell) associated hemochromatosis

E83.118 Other hemochromatosis

E83.119 Hemochromatosis, unspecified

E83.19 Other disorders of iron metabolism
Use additional code, if applicable, for idiopathic pulmonary hemosiderosis (J84.03)

E83.2 Disorders of zinc metabolism
Acrodermatitis enteropathica

E83.3 Disorders of phosphorus metabolism and phosphatases
EXCLUDES 1 *adult osteomalacia (M83.-)*
osteoporosis (M80.-)

E83.30 Disorder of phosphorus metabolism, unspecified

E83.31 Familial hypophosphatemia
Vitamin D-resistant osteomalacia
Vitamin D-resistant rickets
EXCLUDES 1 *vitamin D-deficiency rickets (E55.0)*

E83.32 Hereditary vitamin D-dependent rickets (type 1) (type 2)
25-hydroxyvitamin D 1-alpha-hydroxylase deficiency
Pseudovitamin D deficiency
Vitamin D receptor defect

E83.39 Other disorders of phosphorus metabolism
Acid phosphatase deficiency
Hypophosphatasia

E83.4 Disorders of magnesium metabolism

E83.40 Disorders of magnesium metabolism, unspecified

E83.41 Hypermagnesemia
AHA: 2016,4Q,54

E83.42 Hypomagnesemia

E83.49 Other disorders of magnesium metabolism

E83.5 Disorders of calcium metabolism
EXCLUDES 1 *chondrocalcinosis (M11.1-M11.2)*
hungry bone syndrome (E83.81)
hyperparathyroidism (E21.0-E21.3)

E83.50 Unspecified disorder of calcium metabolism

E83.51 Hypocalcemia

E83.52 Hypercalcemia
Familial hypocalciuric hypercalcemia

E83.59 Other disorders of calcium metabolism

E83.8 Other disorders of mineral metabolism

E83.81 Hungry bone syndrome

E83.89 Other disorders of mineral metabolism

E83.9 Disorder of mineral metabolism, unspecified

E84 Cystic fibrosis
INCLUDES mucoviscidosis
Code also exocrine pancreatic insufficiency (K86.81)
DEF: Genetic disorder affecting the respiratory, digestive, and reproductive systems in infants to young adults by disturbing exocrine gland function and causing chronic pulmonary disease with excess mucus production and pancreatic deficiency.

E84.0 Cystic fibrosis with pulmonary manifestations MCC HCC
Use additional code to identify any infectious organism present, such as:
Pseudomonas (B96.5)
AHA: 2021,1Q,23

E84.1 Cystic fibrosis with intestinal manifestations

E84.11 Meconium ileus in cystic fibrosis MCC HCC N
EXCLUDES 1 *meconium ileus not due to cystic fibrosis (P76.0)*

E84.19 Cystic fibrosis with other intestinal manifestations CC HCC
Distal intestinal obstruction syndrome

E84.8 Cystic fibrosis with other manifestations CC HCC

E84.9 Cystic fibrosis, unspecified CC HCC

E85 Amyloidosis
EXCLUDES 2 *Alzheimer's disease (G30.0-)*
DEF: Conditions of diverse etiologies characterized by the accumulation of insoluble fibrillar proteins (amyloid) in various organs and tissues of the body, compromising vital functions.

E85.0 Non-neuropathic heredofamilial amyloidosis CC HCC
Hereditary amyloid nephropathy
Code also associated disorders, such as:
autoinflammatory syndromes (M04.-)
EXCLUDES 2 *transthyretin-related (ATTR) familial amyloid cardiomyopathy (E85.4)*

E85.1 Neuropathic heredofamilial amyloidosis CC HCC
Amyloid polyneuropathy (Portuguese)
Transthyretin-related (ATTR) familial amyloid polyneuropathy
AHA: 2012,4Q,99

E85.2 Heredofamilial amyloidosis, unspecified CC HCC

E85.3 Secondary systemic amyloidosis CC HCC
Hemodialysis-associated amyloidosis

E85.4 Organ-limited amyloidosis CC HCC
Localized amyloidosis
Transthyretin-related (ATTR) familial amyloid cardiomyopathy

E85.8 Other amyloidosis
AHA: 2017,4Q,7

E85.81 Light chain (AL) amyloidosis CC HCC

E85.82 Wild-type transthyretin-related (ATTR) amyloidosis CC HCC
Senile systemic amyloidosis (SSA)

E85.89 Other amyloidosis CC HCC

E85.9 Amyloidosis, unspecified CC HCC

E86 Volume depletion

Use additional code(s) for any associated disorders of electrolyte and acid-base balance (E87.-)

EXCLUDES 1 *dehydration of newborn (P74.1)*
postprocedural hypovolemic shock (T81.19)
traumatic hypovolemic shock (T79.4)

EXCLUDES 2 *hypovolemic shock NOS (R57.1)*

AHA: 2019,2Q,7; 2018,2Q,6

E86.Ø Dehydration
AHA: 2019,2Q,7; 2019,1Q,12; 2014,1Q,7
TIP: Can be assigned in addition to hypernatremia (E87.0) or hyponatremia (E87.1), when documented.

E86.1 Hypovolemia
Depletion of volume of plasma

E86.9 Volume depletion, unspecified
DEF: Depletion of total body water (dehydration) and/or contraction of total intravascular plasma (hypovolemia).

E87 Other disorders of fluid, electrolyte and acid-base balance

EXCLUDES 1 *diabetes insipidus (E23.2)*
electrolyte imbalance associated with hyperemesis gravidarum (O21.1)
electrolyte imbalance following ectopic or molar pregnancy (OØ8.5)
familial periodic paralysis (G72.3)

AHA: 2018,2Q,6

E87.Ø Hyperosmolality and hypernatremia CC
Sodium [Na] excess
Sodium [Na] overload
AHA: 2022,1Q,28; 2014,1Q,7
TIP: Assign an additional code for dehydration (E86.0), when documented.

E87.1 Hypo-osmolality and hyponatremia CC
Sodium [Na] deficiency
EXCLUDES 1 *syndrome of inappropriate secretion of antidiuretic hormone (E22.2)*
AHA: 2014,1Q,7
TIP: Assign an additional code for dehydration (E86.0), when documented.

▲ **E87.2 Acidosis**
~~Acidosis NOS~~
~~Lactic acidosis~~
~~Metabolic acidosis~~
~~Respiratory acidosis~~
EXCLUDES 1 *diabetic acidosis - see categories EØ8-E1Ø, E11, E13 with ketoacidosis*
AHA: 2020,3Q,30
DEF: Reduction of alkaline in the blood and tissues caused by an increase in acid and decrease in bicarbonate.

● **E87.2Ø Acidosis, unspecified** CC
Lactic acidosis NOS
Metabolic acidosis NOS
Code also, if applicable, respiratory failure with hypercapnia (J96. with 5th character 2)

● **E87.21 Acute metabolic acidosis** CC
Acute lactic acidosis

● **E87.22 Chronic metabolic acidosis** CC
Chronic lactic acidosis
Code first underlying etiology, if applicable

● **E87.29 Other acidosis** CC
Respiratory acidosis NOS
EXCLUDES 2 *acute respiratory acidosis (J96.Ø2)*
chronic respiratory acidosis (J96.12)

E87.3 Alkalosis CC
Alkalosis NOS
Metabolic alkalosis
Respiratory alkalosis

E87.4 Mixed disorder of acid-base balance CC

E87.5 Hyperkalemia
Potassium [K] excess
Potassium [K] overload

E87.6 Hypokalemia
Potassium [K] deficiency

E87.7 Fluid overload
EXCLUDES 1 *edema NOS (R6Ø.9)*
fluid retention (R6Ø.9)

E87.7Ø Fluid overload, unspecified

E87.71 Transfusion associated circulatory overload
Fluid overload due to transfusion (blood) (blood components)
TACO

E87.79 Other fluid overload

E87.8 Other disorders of electrolyte and fluid balance, not elsewhere classified
Electrolyte imbalance NOS
Hyperchloremia
Hypochloremia

E88 Other and unspecified metabolic disorders

Use additional codes for associated conditions

EXCLUDES 1 *histiocytosis X (chronic) (C96.6)*

E88.Ø Disorders of plasma-protein metabolism, not elsewhere classified
EXCLUDES 1 *monoclonal gammopathy (of undetermined significance) (D47.2)*
polyclonal hypergammaglobulinemia (D89.Ø)
Waldenström macroglobulinemia (C88.Ø)
EXCLUDES 2 *disorder of lipoprotein metabolism (E78.-)*

E88.Ø1 Alpha-1-antitrypsin deficiency HCC
AAT deficiency

E88.Ø2 Plasminogen deficiency CC
Dysplasminogenemia
Hypoplasminogenemia
Type 1 plasminogen deficiency
Type 2 plasminogen deficiency
Code also, if applicable, ligneous conjunctivitis (H1Ø.51)
Use additional code for associated findings, such as:
hydrocephalus (G91.4)
otitis media (H67.-)
respiratory disorder related to plasminogen deficiency (J99)
AHA: 2018,4Q,6-7

E88.Ø9 Other disorders of plasma-protein metabolism, not elsewhere classified
Bisalbuminemia

E88.1 Lipodystrophy, not elsewhere classified
Lipodystrophy NOS
EXCLUDES 1 *Whipple's disease (K9Ø.81)*

E88.2 Lipomatosis, not elsewhere classified
Lipomatosis NOS
Lipomatosis (Check) dolorosa [Dercum]

E88.3 Tumor lysis syndrome MCC
Tumor lysis syndrome (spontaneous)
Tumor lysis syndrome following antineoplastic drug chemotherapy
Use additional code for adverse effect, if applicable, to identify drug (T45.1X5)
AHA: 2020,1Q,37; 2019,2Q,24
DEF: Potentially fatal metabolic complication of tumor necrosis caused by spontaneous or treatment-related accumulation of byproducts from dying cancer cells. Symptoms include hyperkalemia, hyperphosphatemia, hypocalcemia, hyperuricemia, and hyperuricosuria.

E88.4 Mitochondrial metabolism disorders
EXCLUDES 1 *disorders of pyruvate metabolism (E74.4)*
Kearns-Sayre syndrome (H49.81)
Leber's disease (H47.22)
Leigh's encephalopathy (G31.82)
mitochondrial myopathy, NEC (G71.3)
Reye's syndrome (G93.7)

E88.4Ø Mitochondrial metabolism disorder, unspecified CC HCC

E88.41 MELAS syndrome CC HCC
Mitochondrial myopathy, encephalopathy, lactic acidosis and stroke-like episodes

E88.42 MERRF syndrome CC HCC
Myoclonic epilepsy associated with ragged-red fibers
Code also progressive myoclonic epilepsy (G4Ø.3-)

E88.49 Other mitochondrial metabolism disorders CC HCC

Chapter 4. Endocrine, Nutritional and Metabolic Diseases

✓5th **E88.8 Other specified metabolic disorders**

E88.81 Metabolic syndrome
Dysmetabolic syndrome X
Use additional codes for associated manifestations, such as:
obesity (E66.-)
DEF: Group of health risks that increase the likelihood of developing heart disease, stroke, and diabetes. These risks include certain parameters for blood pressure, cholesterol, and glucose levels.

E88.89 Other specified metabolic disorders HCC
Launois-Bensaude adenolipomatosis
EXCLUDES 1 *adult pulmonary Langerhans cell histiocytosis (J84.82)*

E88.9 Metabolic disorder, unspecified

Postprocedural endocrine and metabolic complications and disorders, not elsewhere classified (E89)

✓4th **E89 Postprocedural endocrine and metabolic complications and disorders, not elsewhere classified**
EXCLUDES 2 *intraoperative complications of endocrine system organ or structure (E36.Ø-, E36.1-, E36.8)*

E89.Ø Postprocedural hypothyroidism
Postirradiation hypothyroidism
Postsurgical hypothyroidism

E89.1 Postprocedural hypoinsulinemia CC
Postpancreatectomy hyperglycemia
Postsurgical hypoinsulinemia
Use additional code, if applicable, to identify:
acquired absence of pancreas (Z9Ø.41-)
diabetes mellitus (postpancreatectomy) (postprocedural) (E13.-)
insulin use (Z79.4)
EXCLUDES 1 *transient postprocedural hyperglycemia (R73.9)*
transient postprocedural hypoglycemia (E16.2)

E89.2 Postprocedural hypoparathyroidism HCC
Parathyroprival tetany

E89.3 Postprocedural hypopituitarism HCC
Postirradiation hypopituitarism

✓5th **E89.4 Postprocedural ovarian failure**

E89.4Ø Asymptomatic postprocedural ovarian failure ♀
Postprocedural ovarian failure NOS

E89.41 Symptomatic postprocedural ovarian failure ♀
Symptoms such as flushing, sleeplessness, headache, lack of concentration, associated with postprocedural menopause

E89.5 Postprocedural testicular hypofunction ♂

E89.6 Postprocedural adrenocortical (-medullary) hypofunction CC HCC

✓5th **E89.8 Other postprocedural endocrine and metabolic complications and disorders**
AHA: 2016,4Q,9-10

✓6th **E89.81 Postprocedural hemorrhage of an endocrine system organ or structure following a procedure**

E89.81Ø Postprocedural hemorrhage of an endocrine system organ or structure following an endocrine system procedure CC

E89.811 Postprocedural hemorrhage of an endocrine system organ or structure following other procedure CC

✓6th **E89.82 Postprocedural hematoma and seroma of an endocrine system organ or structure**

E89.82Ø Postprocedural hematoma of an endocrine system organ or structure following an endocrine system procedure CC

E89.821 Postprocedural hematoma of an endocrine system organ or structure following other procedure CC

E89.822 Postprocedural seroma of an endocrine system organ or structure following an endocrine system procedure CC

E89.823 Postprocedural seroma of an endocrine system organ or structure following other procedure CC

E89.89 Other postprocedural endocrine and metabolic complications and disorders CC
Use additional code, if applicable, to further specify disorder

Chapter 5. Mental, Behavioral and Neurodevelopmental Disorders (FØ1–F99)

Chapter-specific Guidelines with Coding Examples

The chapter-specific guidelines from the ICD-10-CM Official Guidelines for Coding and Reporting have been provided below. Along with these guidelines are coding examples, contained in the shaded boxes, that have been developed to help illustrate the coding and/or sequencing guidance found in these guidelines.

a. Pain disorders related to psychological factors

Assign code F45.41, for pain that is exclusively related to psychological disorders. As indicated by the Excludes 1 note under category G89, a code from category G89 should not be assigned with code F45.41.

> Perceived abdominal pain determined to be persistent somatoform pain disorder
>
> **F45.41 Pain disorder exclusively related to psychological factors**
>
> *Explanation*: This pain was diagnosed as being exclusively psychological; therefore, no code from category G89 is added.

Code F45.42, Pain disorders with related psychological factors, should be used with a code from category G89, Pain, not elsewhere classified, if there is documentation of a psychological component for a patient with acute or chronic pain.

See Section I.C.6. Pain

b. Mental and behavioral disorders due to psychoactive substance use

1) In remission

Selection of codes **describing** "in remission" for categories F1Ø-F19, Mental and behavioral disorders due to psychoactive substance use (categories F1Ø-F19 with -.11, -.21, **-.91**) requires the provider's clinical judgment **and** are assigned only on the basis of provider documentation (as defined in the Official Guidelines for Coding and Reporting), unless otherwise instructed by the classification.

Mild substance use disorders in early or sustained remission are classified to the appropriate codes for substance abuse in remission, and moderate or severe substance use disorders in early or sustained remission are classified to the appropriate codes for substance dependence in remission.

> Insomnia in patient with history of methamphetamine abuse; lab results indicate no current drug use
>
> **G47.ØØ Insomnia, unspecified**
>
> **F15.1Ø Other stimulant abuse, uncomplicated**
>
> *Explanation*: Insomnia is a common side-effect of stimulant use, such as methamphetamines. Although lab tests do not indicate that the patient is currently using methamphetamines, there is no specific documentation stating that the stimulant abuse is in remission. "History of" abuse does not equate to "in remission" in this instance.

2) Psychoactive substance use, abuse and dependence

When the provider documentation refers to use, abuse and dependence of the same substance (e.g. alcohol, opioid, cannabis, etc.), only one code should be assigned to identify the pattern of use based on the following hierarchy:

- If both use and abuse are documented, assign only the code for abuse
- If both abuse and dependence are documented, assign only the code for dependence
- If use, abuse and dependence are all documented, assign only the code for dependence
- If both use and dependence are documented, assign only the code for dependence.

> History and physical notes cannabis dependence; progress note says cannabis abuse
>
> **F12.2Ø Cannabis dependence, uncomplicated**
>
> *Explanation*: In the hierarchy, the dependence code is used if both abuse and dependence are documented.

> Discharge summary says cocaine abuse; progress notes list cocaine use
>
> **F14.1Ø Cocaine abuse, uncomplicated**
>
> *Explanation*: In the hierarchy, the abuse code is used if both abuse and use are documented.

3) Psychoactive substance use, unspecified

As with all other unspecified diagnoses, the codes for unspecified psychoactive substance use (F1Ø.9-, F11.9-, F12.9-, F13.9-, F14.9-, F15.9-, F16.9-, F18.9-, F19.9-) should only be assigned based on provider documentation and when they meet the definition of a reportable diagnosis (see Section III, Reporting Additional Diagnoses). These codes are to be used only when the psychoactive substance use is associated with a substance related disorder (chapter 5 disorders such as sexual dysfunction, sleep disorder, or a mental or behavioral disorder) or medical condition, and such a relationship is documented by the provider.

4) Medical conditions due to psychoactive substance use, abuse and dependence

Medical conditions due to substance use, abuse, and dependence are not classified as substance-induced disorders. Assign the diagnosis code for the medical condition as directed by the Alphabetical Index along with the appropriate psychoactive substance use, abuse or dependence code. For example, for alcoholic pancreatitis due to alcohol dependence, assign the appropriate code from subcategory K85.2, Alcohol induced acute pancreatitis, and the appropriate code from subcategory F1Ø.2, such as code F1Ø.2Ø, Alcohol dependence, uncomplicated. It would not be appropriate to assign code F1Ø.288, Alcohol dependence with other alcohol-induced disorder.

5) Blood alcohol level

A code from category Y9Ø, Evidence of alcohol involvement determined by blood alcohol level, may be assigned when this information is documented and the patient's provider has documented a condition classifiable to category F1Ø, Alcohol related disorders. The blood alcohol level does not need to be documented by the patient's provider in order for it to be coded.

See Section I.B.14. for blood alcohol level documentation by clinicians other than patient's provider.

c. Factitious disorder

Factitious disorder imposed on self or Munchausen's syndrome is a disorder in which a person falsely reports or causes his or her own physical or psychological signs or symptoms. For patients with documented factitious disorder on self or Munchausen's syndrome, assign the appropriate code from subcategory F68.1-, Factitious disorder imposed on self.

Munchausen's syndrome by proxy (MSBP) is a disorder in which a caregiver (perpetrator) falsely reports or causes an illness or injury in another person (victim) under his or her care, such as a child, an elderly adult, or a person who has a disability. The condition is also referred to as "factitious disorder imposed on another" or "factitious disorder by proxy." The perpetrator, not the victim, receives this diagnosis. Assign code F68.A, Factitious disorder imposed on another, to the perpetrator's record. For the victim of a patient suffering from MSBP, assign the appropriate code from categories T74, Adult and child abuse, neglect and other maltreatment, confirmed, or T76, Adult and child abuse, neglect and other maltreatment, suspected.

See Section I.C.19.f. Adult and child abuse, neglect and other maltreatment

d. Dementia

The ICD-10-CM classifies dementia (categories FØ1, FØ2, and FØ3) on the basis of the etiology and severity (unspecified, mild, moderate or severe). Selection of the appropriate severity level requires the provider's clinical judgment and codes should be assigned only on the basis of provider documentation (as defined in the *Official Guidelines for Coding and Reporting*), unless otherwise instructed by the classification. If the documentation does not provide information about the severity of the dementia, assign the appropriate code for unspecified severity.

If a patient is admitted to an inpatient acute care hospital or other inpatient facility setting with dementia at one severity level and it progresses to a higher severity level, assign one code for the highest severity level reported during the stay.

Chapter 5. Mental, Behavioral and Neurodevelopmental Disorders (F01-F99)

INCLUDES disorders of psychological development

EXCLUDES 2 *symptoms, signs and abnormal clinical laboratory findings, not elsewhere classified (R00-R99)*

This chapter contains the following blocks:

F01-F09 Mental disorders due to known physiological conditions
F10-F19 Mental and behavioral disorders due to psychoactive substance use
F20-F29 Schizophrenia, schizotypal, delusional, and other non-mood psychotic disorders
F30-F39 Mood [affective] disorders
F40-F48 Anxiety, dissociative, stress-related, somatoform and other nonpsychotic mental disorders
F50-F59 Behavioral syndromes associated with physiological disturbances and physical factors
F60-F69 Disorders of adult personality and behavior
F70-F79 Intellectual disabilities
F80-F89 Pervasive and specific developmental disorders
F90-F98 Behavioral and emotional disorders with onset usually occurring in childhood and adolescence
F99 Unspecified mental disorder

Mental disorders due to known physiological conditions (F01-F09)

NOTE This block comprises a range of mental disorders grouped together on the basis of their having in common a demonstrable etiology in cerebral disease, brain injury, or other insult leading to cerebral dysfunction. The dysfunction may be primary, as in diseases, injuries, and insults that affect the brain directly and selectively; or secondary, as in systemic diseases and disorders that attack the brain only as one of the multiple organs or systems of the body that are involved.

✓4th **F01 Vascular dementia**

Vascular dementia as a result of infarction of the brain due to vascular disease, including hypertensive cerebrovascular disease.

INCLUDES arteriosclerotic dementia
▶major neurocognitive disorder due to vascular disease◀
▶multi-infarct dementia◀

Code first the underlying physiological condition or sequelae of cerebrovascular disease.

▲ ✓5th **F01.5 Vascular dementia, unspecified severity**

▲ **F01.50 Vascular dementia, unspecified severity, without behavioral disturbance, psychotic disturbance, mood disturbance, and anxiety** HCC A

▶Major neurocognitive disorder due to vascular disease NOS◀
▶Vascular dementia NOS◀
AHA: 2021,2Q,4

▲ ✓6th **F01.51 Vascular dementia, unspecified severity, with behavioral disturbance**

Major neurocognitive disorder due to vascular disease, with behavioral disturbance
Major neurocognitive disorder with aggressive behavior
Major neurocognitive disorder with combative behavior
Major neurocognitive disorder with violent behavior
Vascular dementia with aggressive behavior
Vascular dementia with combative behavior
Vascular dementia with violent behavior

Use additional code, if applicable, to identify wandering in vascular dementia (Z91.83)

● **F01.511 Vascular dementia, unspecified severity, with agitation** CC UPD A

Major neurocognitive disorder due to vascular disease, unspecified severity, with aberrant motor behavior such as restlessness, rocking, pacing, or exit-seeking
Major neurocognitive disorder due to vascular disease, unspecified severity, with verbal or physical behaviors such as profanity, shouting, threatening, anger, aggression, combativeness, or violence
Vascular dementia, unspecified severity, with aberrant motor behavior such as restlessness, rocking, pacing, or exit-seeking
Vascular dementia, unspecified severity, with verbal or physical behaviors such as profanity, shouting, threatening, anger, aggression, combativeness, or violence

● **F01.518 Vascular dementia, unspecified severity, with other behavioral disturbance** CC UPD A

Major neurocognitive disorder due to vascular disease, unspecified severity, with behavioral disturbances such as sleep disturbance, social disinhibition, or sexual disinhibition
Vascular dementia, unspecified severity, with behavioral disturbances such as sleep disturbance, social disinhibition, or sexual disinhibition

Use additional code, if applicable, to identify wandering in vascular dementia (Z91.83)

● **F01.52 Vascular dementia, unspecified severity, with psychotic disturbance** CC UPD A

Major neurocognitive disorder due to vascular disease, unspecified severity, with psychotic disturbance such as hallucinations, paranoia, suspiciousness, or delusional state
Vascular dementia, unspecified severity, with psychotic disturbance such as hallucinations, paranoia, suspiciousness, or delusional state

● **F01.53 Vascular dementia, unspecified severity, with mood disturbance** CC UPD A

Major neurocognitive disorder due to vascular disease, unspecified severity, with mood disturbance such as depression, apathy, or anhedonia
Vascular dementia, unspecified severity, with mood disturbance such as depression, apathy, or anhedonia

● **F01.54 Vascular dementia, unspecified severity, with anxiety** CC UPD A

Major neurocognitive disorder due to vascular disease, unspecified severity, with anxiety

● √5th **FØ1.A Vascular dementia, mild**

EXCLUDES 1 *mild neurocognitive disorder due to known physiological condition with or without behavioral disturbance (FØ6.7-)*

● **FØ1.AØ Vascular dementia, mild, without behavioral disturbance, psychotic disturbance, mood disturbance, and anxiety** UPD A

Major neurocognitive disorder due to vascular disease, mild, NOS

Vascular dementia, mild, NOS

● √6th **FØ1.A1 Vascular dementia, mild, with behavioral disturbance**

● **FØ1.A11 Vascular dementia, mild, with agitation** CC UPD A

Major neurocognitive disorder due to vascular disease, mild, with aberrant motor behavior such as restlessness, rocking, pacing, or exit-seeking

Major neurocognitive disorder due to vascular disease, mild, with verbal or physical behaviors such as profanity, shouting, threatening, anger, aggression, combativeness, or violence

Vascular dementia, mild, with aberrant motor behavior such as restlessness, rocking, pacing, or exit-seeking

Vascular dementia, mild, with verbal or physical behaviors such as profanity, shouting, threatening, anger, aggression, combativeness, or violence

● **FØ1.A18 Vascular dementia, mild, with other behavioral disturbance** CC UPD A

Major neurocognitive disorder due to vascular disease, mild, with behavioral disturbances such as sleep disturbance, social disinhibition, or sexual disinhibition

Vascular dementia, mild, with behavioral disturbances such as sleep disturbance, social disinhibition, or sexual disinhibition

Use additional code, if applicable, to identify wandering in vascular dementia (Z91.83)

● **FØ1.A2 Vascular dementia, mild, with psychotic disturbance** CC UPD A

Major neurocognitive disorder due to vascular disease, mild, with psychotic disturbance such as hallucinations, paranoia, suspiciousness, or delusional state

Vascular dementia, mild, with psychotic disturbance such as hallucinations, paranoia, suspiciousness, or delusional state

● **FØ1.A3 Vascular dementia, mild, with mood disturbance** CC UPD A

Major neurocognitive disorder due to vascular disease, mild, with mood disturbance such as depression, apathy, or anhedonia

Vascular dementia, mild, with mood disturbance such as depression, apathy, or anhedonia

● **FØ1.A4 Vascular dementia, mild, with anxiety** CC UPD A

Major neurocognitive disorder due to vascular disease, mild, with anxiety

● √5th **FØ1.B Vascular dementia, moderate**

● **FØ1.BØ Vascular dementia, moderate, without behavioral disturbance, psychotic disturbance, mood disturbance, and anxiety** UPD A

Major neurocognitive disorder due to vascular disease, moderate, NOS

Vascular dementia, moderate, NOS

● √6th **FØ1.B1 Vascular dementia, moderate, with behavioral disturbance**

● **FØ1.B11 Vascular dementia, moderate, with agitation** CC UPD A

Major neurocognitive disorder due to vascular disease, moderate, with aberrant motor behavior such as restlessness, rocking, pacing, or exit-seeking

Major neurocognitive disorder due to vascular disease, moderate, with verbal or physical behaviors such as profanity, shouting, threatening, anger, aggression, combativeness, or violence

Vascular dementia, moderate, with aberrant motor behavior such as restlessness, rocking, pacing, or exit-seeking

Vascular dementia, moderate, with verbal or physical behaviors such as profanity, shouting, threatening, anger, aggression, combativeness, or violence

● **FØ1.B18 Vascular dementia, moderate, with other behavioral disturbance** CC UPD A

Major neurocognitive disorder due to vascular disease, moderate, with behavioral disturbances such as sleep disturbance, social disinhibition, or sexual disinhibition

Vascular dementia, moderate, with behavioral disturbances such as sleep disturbance, social disinhibition, or sexual disinhibition

Use additional code, if applicable, to identify wandering in vascular dementia (Z91.83)

● **FØ1.B2 Vascular dementia, moderate, with psychotic disturbance** CC UPD A

Major neurocognitive disorder due to vascular disease, moderate, with psychotic disturbance such as hallucinations, paranoia, suspiciousness, or delusional state

Vascular dementia, moderate, with psychotic disturbance such as hallucinations, paranoia, suspiciousness, or delusional state

● **FØ1.B3 Vascular dementia, moderate, with mood disturbance** CC UPD A

Major neurocognitive disorder due to vascular disease, moderate, with mood disturbance such as depression, apathy, or anhedonia

Vascular dementia, moderate, with mood disturbance such as depression, apathy, or anhedonia

● **FØ1.B4 Vascular dementia, moderate, with anxiety** CC UPD A

Major neurocognitive disorder due to vascular disease, moderate, with anxiety

● √5th **FØ1.C Vascular dementia, severe**

● **FØ1.CØ Vascular dementia, severe, without behavioral disturbance, psychotic disturbance, mood disturbance, and anxiety** UPD A

Major neurocognitive disorder due to vascular disease, severe, NOS

Vascular dementia, severe, NOS

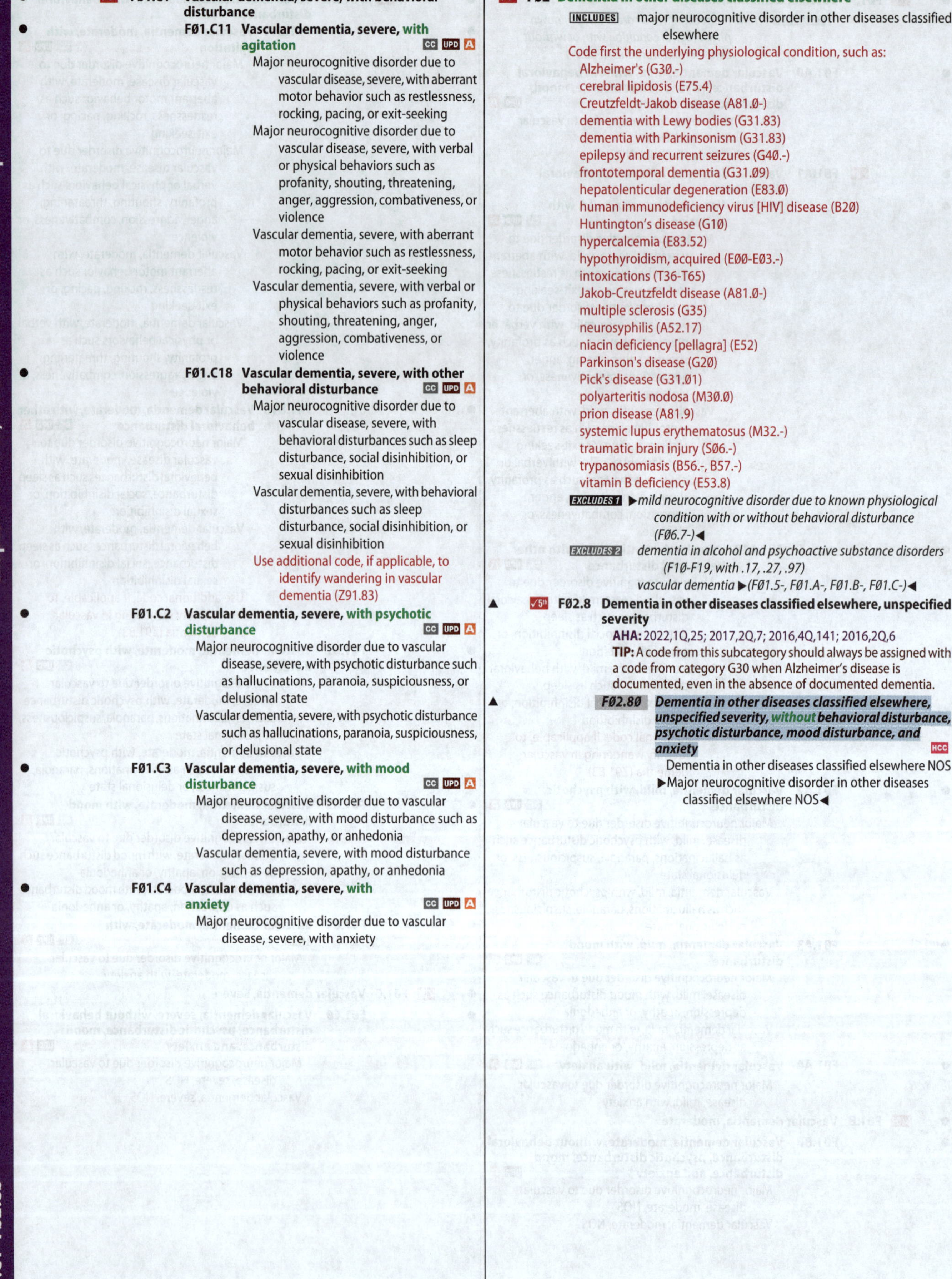

● F01.C1 **Vascular dementia, severe, with behavioral disturbance**

● F01.C11 **Vascular dementia, severe, with agitation** CC UPD A

Major neurocognitive disorder due to vascular disease, severe, with aberrant motor behavior such as restlessness, rocking, pacing, or exit-seeking

Major neurocognitive disorder due to vascular disease, severe, with verbal or physical behaviors such as profanity, shouting, threatening, anger, aggression, combativeness, or violence

Vascular dementia, severe, with aberrant motor behavior such as restlessness, rocking, pacing, or exit-seeking

Vascular dementia, severe, with verbal or physical behaviors such as profanity, shouting, threatening, anger, aggression, combativeness, or violence

● F01.C18 **Vascular dementia, severe, with other behavioral disturbance** CC UPD A

Major neurocognitive disorder due to vascular disease, severe, with behavioral disturbances such as sleep disturbance, social disinhibition, or sexual disinhibition

Vascular dementia, severe, with behavioral disturbances such as sleep disturbance, social disinhibition, or sexual disinhibition

Use additional code, if applicable, to identify wandering in vascular dementia (Z91.83)

● F01.C2 **Vascular dementia, severe, with psychotic disturbance** CC UPD A

Major neurocognitive disorder due to vascular disease, severe, with psychotic disturbance such as hallucinations, paranoia, suspiciousness, or delusional state

Vascular dementia, severe, with psychotic disturbance such as hallucinations, paranoia, suspiciousness, or delusional state

● F01.C3 **Vascular dementia, severe, with mood disturbance** CC UPD A

Major neurocognitive disorder due to vascular disease, severe, with mood disturbance such as depression, apathy, or anhedonia

Vascular dementia, severe, with mood disturbance such as depression, apathy, or anhedonia

● F01.C4 **Vascular dementia, severe, with anxiety** CC UPD A

Major neurocognitive disorder due to vascular disease, severe, with anxiety

√4th F02 **Dementia in other diseases classified elsewhere**

INCLUDES major neurocognitive disorder in other diseases classified elsewhere

Code first the underlying physiological condition, such as:
- Alzheimer's (G30.-)
- cerebral lipidosis (E75.4)
- Creutzfeldt-Jakob disease (A81.0-)
- dementia with Lewy bodies (G31.83)
- dementia with Parkinsonism (G31.83)
- epilepsy and recurrent seizures (G40.-)
- frontotemporal dementia (G31.09)
- hepatolenticular degeneration (E83.0)
- human immunodeficiency virus [HIV] disease (B20)
- Huntington's disease (G10)
- hypercalcemia (E83.52)
- hypothyroidism, acquired (E00-E03.-)
- intoxications (T36-T65)
- Jakob-Creutzfeldt disease (A81.0-)
- multiple sclerosis (G35)
- neurosyphilis (A52.17)
- niacin deficiency [pellagra] (E52)
- Parkinson's disease (G20)
- Pick's disease (G31.01)
- polyarteritis nodosa (M30.0)
- prion disease (A81.9)
- systemic lupus erythematosus (M32.-)
- traumatic brain injury (S06.-)
- trypanosomiasis (B56.-, B57.-)
- vitamin B deficiency (E53.8)

EXCLUDES 1 ►*mild neurocognitive disorder due to known physiological condition with or without behavioral disturbance (F06.7-)*◄

EXCLUDES 2 *dementia in alcohol and psychoactive substance disorders (F10-F19, with .17, .27, .97)*

vascular dementia ►*(F01.5-, F01.A-, F01.B-, F01.C-)*◄

▲ √5th F02.8 **Dementia in other diseases classified elsewhere, unspecified severity**

AHA: 2022,1Q,25; 2017,2Q,7; 2016,4Q,141; 2016,2Q,6

TIP: A code from this subcategory should always be assigned with a code from category G30 when Alzheimer's disease is documented, even in the absence of documented dementia.

▲ F02.80 ***Dementia in other diseases classified elsewhere, unspecified severity, without behavioral disturbance, psychotic disturbance, mood disturbance, and anxiety*** HCC

Dementia in other diseases classified elsewhere NOS

►Major neurocognitive disorder in other diseases classified elsewhere NOS◄

▲ ✓6th **F02.81 Dementia in other diseases classified elsewhere, unspecified severity, with behavioral disturbance**

~~Dementia in other diseases classified elsewhere with aggressive behavior~~

~~Dementia in other diseases classified elsewhere with combative behavior~~

~~Dementia in other diseases classified elsewhere with violent behavior~~

~~Major neurocognitive disorder in other diseases classified elsewhere with aggressive behavior~~

~~Major neurocognitive disorder in other diseases classified elsewhere with combative behavior~~

~~Major neurocognitive disorder in other diseases classified elsewhere with violent behavior~~

~~Use additional code, if applicable, to identify wandering in dementia in conditions classified elsewhere (Z91.83)~~

● ***F02.811 Dementia in other diseases classified elsewhere, unspecified severity, with agitation*** CC

Dementia in other diseases classified elsewhere, unspecified severity, with aberrant motor behavior such as restlessness, rocking, pacing, or exit-seeking

Dementia in other diseases classified elsewhere, unspecified severity, with verbal or physical behaviors such as profanity, shouting, threatening, anger, aggression, combativeness, or violence

Major neurocognitive disorder in other diseases classified elsewhere, unspecified severity, with aberrant motor behavior such as restlessness, rocking, pacing, or exit-seeking

Major neurocognitive disorder in other diseases classified elsewhere, unspecified severity, with verbal or physical behaviors such as profanity, shouting, threatening, anger, aggression, combativeness, or violence

● ***F02.818 Dementia in other diseases classified elsewhere, unspecified severity, with other behavioral disturbance*** CC

Dementia in other diseases classified elsewhere with sleep disturbance, social disinhibition, or sexual disinhibition

Major neurocognitive disorder in other diseases classified elsewhere with sleep disturbance, social disinhibition, or sexual disinhibition

Use additional code, if applicable, to identify wandering in dementia in conditions classified elsewhere (Z91.83)

● ***F02.82 Dementia in other diseases classified elsewhere, unspecified severity, with psychotic disturbance*** CC

Dementia in other diseases classified elsewhere, unspecified severity, with psychotic disturbance such as hallucinations, paranoia, suspiciousness, or delusional state

Major neurocognitive disorder in other diseases classified elsewhere, unspecified, with psychotic disturbance such as hallucinations, paranoia, suspiciousness, or delusional state

● ***F02.83 Dementia in other diseases classified elsewhere, unspecified severity, with mood disturbance*** CC

Dementia in other diseases classified elsewhere, unspecified severity, with mood disturbance such as depression, apathy, or anhedonia

Major neurocognitive disorder in other diseases classified elsewhere unspecified severity,with mood disturbance such as with depression, apathy, or anhedonia

● ***F02.84 Dementia in other diseases classified elsewhere, unspecified severity, with anxiety*** CC

Major neurocognitive disorder in other diseases classified elsewhere unspecified severity, with anxiety

● ✓5th **F02.A Dementia in other diseases classified elsewhere, mild**

EXCLUDES 1 *mild neurocognitive disorder due to known physiological condition with or without behavioral disturbance (F06.7-)*

● ***F02.A0 Dementia in other diseases classified elsewhere, mild, without behavioral disturbance, psychotic disturbance, mood disturbance, and anxiety***

Dementia in other diseases classified elsewhere, mild, NOS

Major neurocognitive disorder in other diseases classified elsewhere, mild, NOS

● ✓6th **F02.A1 Dementia in other diseases classified elsewhere, mild, with behavioral disturbance**

● ***F02.A11 Dementia in other diseases classified elsewhere, mild, with agitation*** CC

Dementia in other diseases classified elsewhere, mild, with aberrant motor behavior such as restlessness, rocking, pacing, or exit-seeking

Dementia in other diseases classified elsewhere, mild, with verbal or physical behaviors such as profanity, shouting, threatening, anger, aggression, combativeness, or violence

Major neurocognitive disorder in other diseases classified elsewhere, mild, with aberrant motor behavior such as restlessness, rocking, pacing, or exit-seeking

Major neurocognitive disorder in other diseases classified elsewhere, mild, with verbal or physical behaviors such as profanity, shouting, threatening, anger, aggression, combativeness, or violence

● ***F02.A18 Dementia in other diseases classified elsewhere, mild, with other behavioral disturbance*** CC

Dementia in other diseases classified elsewhere, mild, with behavioral disturbances such as sleep disturbance, social disinhibition, or sexual disinhibition

Major neurocognitive disorder in other diseases classified elsewhere, mild, with behavioral disturbances such as sleep disturbance, social disinhibition, or sexual disinhibition

Use additional code, if applicable, to identify wandering in dementia in conditions classified elsewhere (Z91.83)

● ***F02.A2 Dementia in other diseases classified elsewhere, mild, with psychotic disturbance*** CC

Dementia in other diseases classified elsewhere, mild, with psychotic disturbance such as hallucinations, paranoia, suspiciousness, or delusional state

Major neurocognitive disorder in other diseases classified elsewhere, mild, with psychotic disturbance such as hallucinations, paranoia, suspiciousness, or delusional state

● ***F02.A3 Dementia in other diseases classified elsewhere, mild, with mood disturbance*** CC

Dementia in other diseases classified elsewhere, mild, with mood disturbance such as depression, apathy, or anhedonia

Major neurocognitive disorder in other diseases classified elsewhere, mild, with mood disturbance such as depression, apathy, or anhedonia

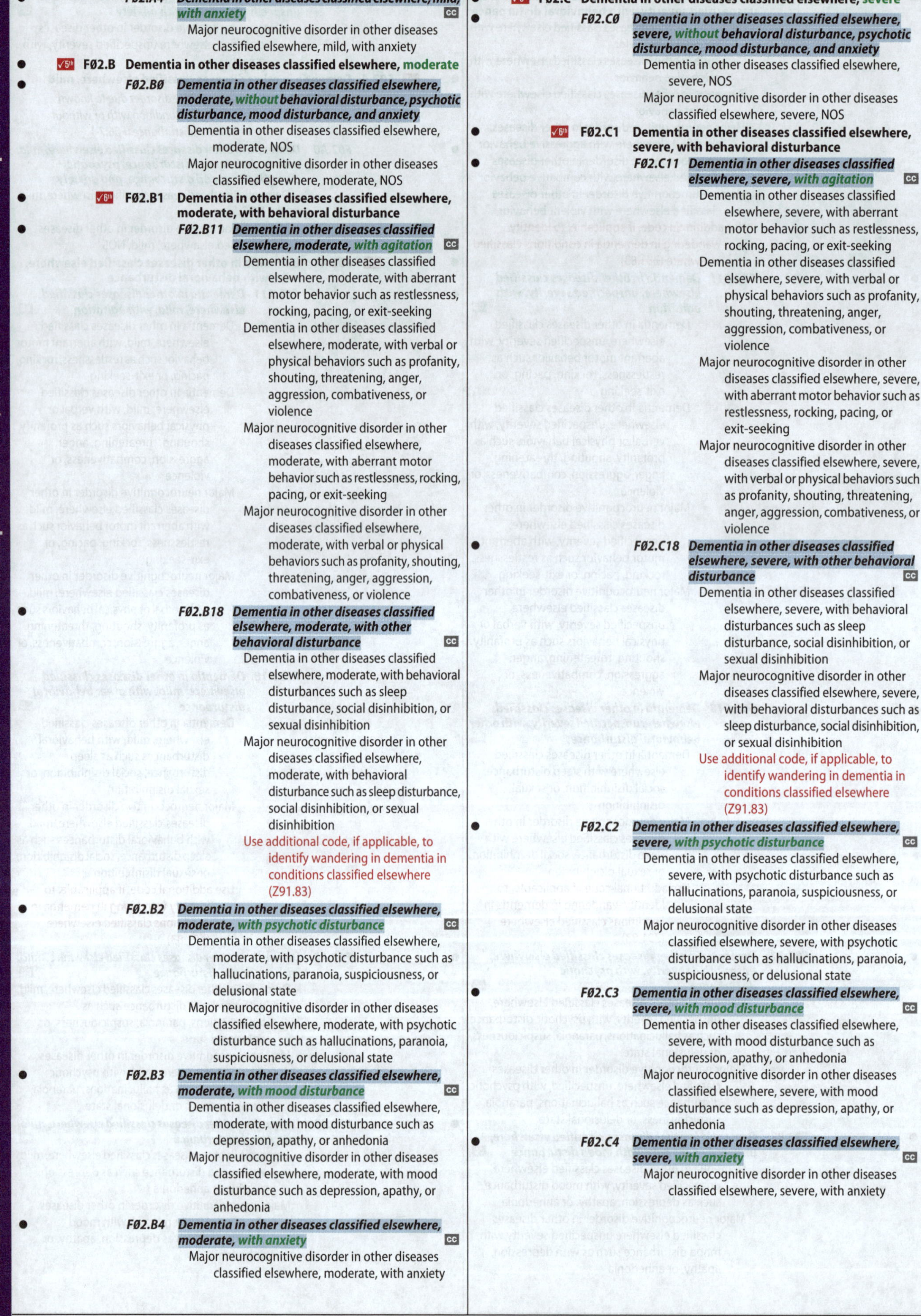

● **FØ2.A4** ***Dementia in other diseases classified elsewhere, mild, with anxiety*** CC
Major neurocognitive disorder in other diseases classified elsewhere, mild, with anxiety

● ✓5th **FØ2.B Dementia in other diseases classified elsewhere, moderate**

● **FØ2.BØ** ***Dementia in other diseases classified elsewhere, moderate, without behavioral disturbance, psychotic disturbance, mood disturbance, and anxiety***
Dementia in other diseases classified elsewhere, moderate, NOS
Major neurocognitive disorder in other diseases classified elsewhere, moderate, NOS

● ✓6th **FØ2.B1 Dementia in other diseases classified elsewhere, moderate, with behavioral disturbance**

● **FØ2.B11** ***Dementia in other diseases classified elsewhere, moderate, with agitation*** CC
Dementia in other diseases classified elsewhere, moderate, with aberrant motor behavior such as restlessness, rocking, pacing, or exit-seeking
Dementia in other diseases classified elsewhere, moderate, with verbal or physical behaviors such as profanity, shouting, threatening, anger, aggression, combativeness, or violence
Major neurocognitive disorder in other diseases classified elsewhere, moderate, with aberrant motor behavior such as restlessness, rocking, pacing, or exit-seeking
Major neurocognitive disorder in other diseases classified elsewhere, moderate, with verbal or physical behaviors such as profanity, shouting, threatening, anger, aggression, combativeness, or violence

● **FØ2.B18** ***Dementia in other diseases classified elsewhere, moderate, with other behavioral disturbance*** CC
Dementia in other diseases classified elsewhere, moderate, with behavioral disturbances such as sleep disturbance, social disinhibition, or sexual disinhibition
Major neurocognitive disorder in other diseases classified elsewhere, moderate, with behavioral disturbance such as sleep disturbance, social disinhibition, or sexual disinhibition
Use additional code, if applicable, to identify wandering in dementia in conditions classified elsewhere (Z91.83)

● **FØ2.B2** ***Dementia in other diseases classified elsewhere, moderate, with psychotic disturbance*** CC
Dementia in other diseases classified elsewhere, moderate, with psychotic disturbance such as hallucinations, paranoia, suspiciousness, or delusional state
Major neurocognitive disorder in other diseases classified elsewhere, moderate, with psychotic disturbance such as hallucinations, paranoia, suspiciousness, or delusional state

● **FØ2.B3** ***Dementia in other diseases classified elsewhere, moderate, with mood disturbance*** CC
Dementia in other diseases classified elsewhere, moderate, with mood disturbance such as depression, apathy, or anhedonia
Major neurocognitive disorder in other diseases classified elsewhere, moderate, with mood disturbance such as depression, apathy, or anhedonia

● **FØ2.B4** ***Dementia in other diseases classified elsewhere, moderate, with anxiety*** CC
Major neurocognitive disorder in other diseases classified elsewhere, moderate, with anxiety

● ✓5th **FØ2.C Dementia in other diseases classified elsewhere, severe**

● **FØ2.CØ** ***Dementia in other diseases classified elsewhere, severe, without behavioral disturbance, psychotic disturbance, mood disturbance, and anxiety***
Dementia in other diseases classified elsewhere, severe, NOS
Major neurocognitive disorder in other diseases classified elsewhere, severe, NOS

● ✓6th **FØ2.C1 Dementia in other diseases classified elsewhere, severe, with behavioral disturbance**

● **FØ2.C11** ***Dementia in other diseases classified elsewhere, severe, with agitation*** CC
Dementia in other diseases classified elsewhere, severe, with aberrant motor behavior such as restlessness, rocking, pacing, or exit-seeking
Dementia in other diseases classified elsewhere, severe, with verbal or physical behaviors such as profanity, shouting, threatening, anger, aggression, combativeness, or violence
Major neurocognitive disorder in other diseases classified elsewhere, severe, with aberrant motor behavior such as restlessness, rocking, pacing, or exit-seeking
Major neurocognitive disorder in other diseases classified elsewhere, severe, with verbal or physical behaviors such as profanity, shouting, threatening, anger, aggression, combativeness, or violence

● **FØ2.C18** ***Dementia in other diseases classified elsewhere, severe, with other behavioral disturbance*** CC
Dementia in other diseases classified elsewhere, severe, with behavioral disturbances such as sleep disturbance, social disinhibition, or sexual disinhibition
Major neurocognitive disorder in other diseases classified elsewhere, severe, with behavioral disturbances such as sleep disturbance, social disinhibition, or sexual disinhibition
Use additional code, if applicable, to identify wandering in dementia in conditions classified elsewhere (Z91.83)

● **FØ2.C2** ***Dementia in other diseases classified elsewhere, severe, with psychotic disturbance*** CC
Dementia in other diseases classified elsewhere, severe, with psychotic disturbance such as hallucinations, paranoia, suspiciousness, or delusional state
Major neurocognitive disorder in other diseases classified elsewhere, severe, with psychotic disturbance such as hallucinations, paranoia, suspiciousness, or delusional state

● **FØ2.C3** ***Dementia in other diseases classified elsewhere, severe, with mood disturbance*** CC
Dementia in other diseases classified elsewhere, severe, with mood disturbance such as depression, apathy, or anhedonia
Major neurocognitive disorder in other diseases classified elsewhere, severe, with mood disturbance such as depression, apathy, or anhedonia

● **FØ2.C4** ***Dementia in other diseases classified elsewhere, severe, with anxiety*** CC
Major neurocognitive disorder in other diseases classified elsewhere, severe, with anxiety

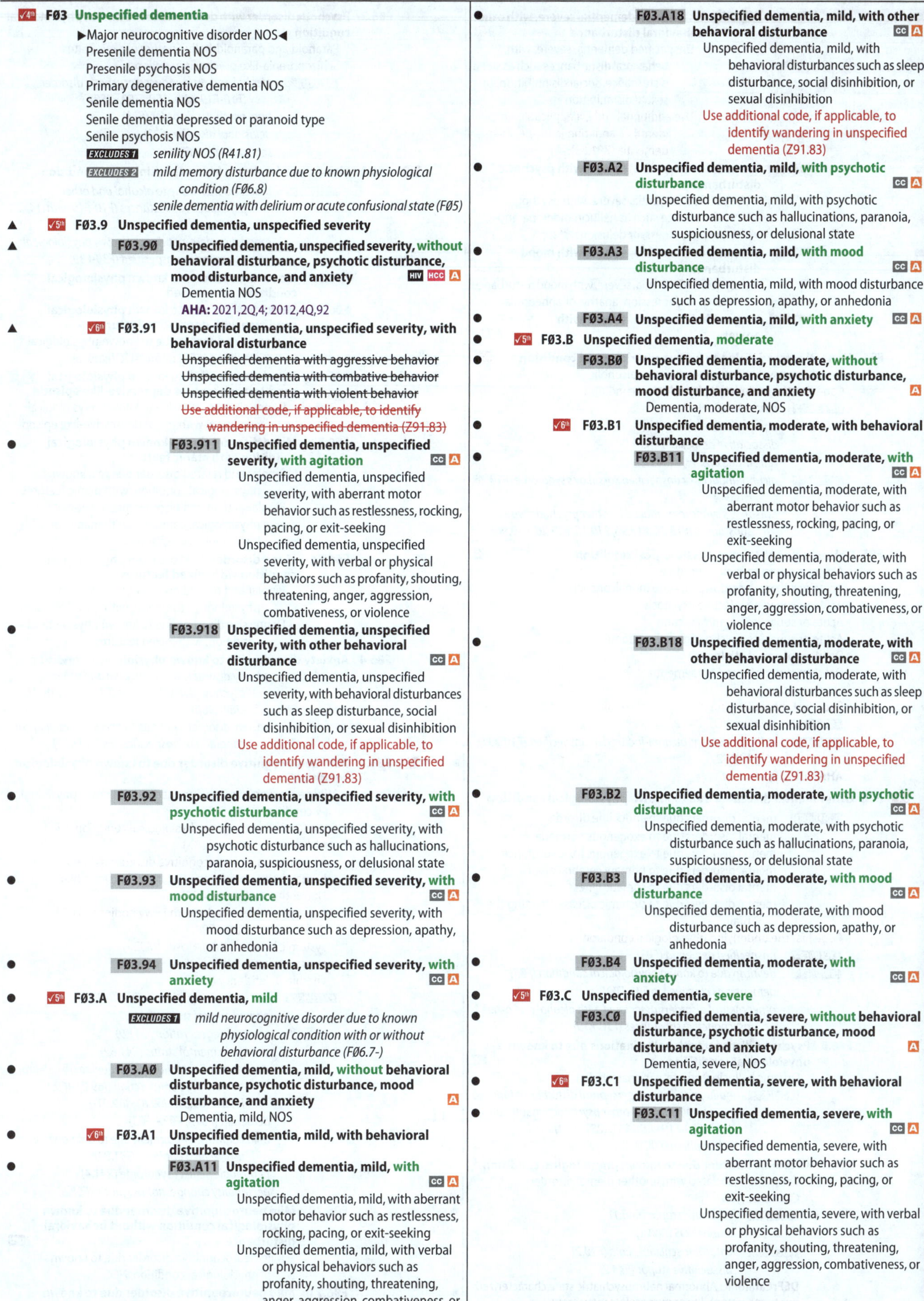

F03 Unspecified dementia

▶Major neurocognitive disorder NOS◀
Presenile dementia NOS
Presenile psychosis NOS
Primary degenerative dementia NOS
Senile dementia NOS
Senile dementia depressed or paranoid type
Senile psychosis NOS

EXCLUDES 1 *senility NOS (R41.81)*

EXCLUDES 2 *mild memory disturbance due to known physiological condition (F06.8)*
senile dementia with delirium or acute confusional state (F05)

▲ **F03.9 Unspecified dementia, unspecified severity**

▲ **F03.90 Unspecified dementia, unspecified severity, without behavioral disturbance, psychotic disturbance, mood disturbance, and anxiety** HIV HCC A
Dementia NOS
AHA: 2021,2Q,4; 2012,4Q,92

▲ **F03.91 Unspecified dementia, unspecified severity, with behavioral disturbance**
~~Unspecified dementia with aggressive behavior~~
~~Unspecified dementia with combative behavior~~
~~Unspecified dementia with violent behavior~~
~~Use additional code, if applicable, to identify wandering in unspecified dementia (Z91.83)~~

● **F03.911 Unspecified dementia, unspecified severity, with agitation** CC A
Unspecified dementia, unspecified severity, with aberrant motor behavior such as restlessness, rocking, pacing, or exit-seeking
Unspecified dementia, unspecified severity, with verbal or physical behaviors such as profanity, shouting, threatening, anger, aggression, combativeness, or violence

● **F03.918 Unspecified dementia, unspecified severity, with other behavioral disturbance** CC A
Unspecified dementia, unspecified severity, with behavioral disturbances such as sleep disturbance, social disinhibition, or sexual disinhibition
Use additional code, if applicable, to identify wandering in unspecified dementia (Z91.83)

● **F03.92 Unspecified dementia, unspecified severity, with psychotic disturbance** CC A
Unspecified dementia, unspecified severity, with psychotic disturbance such as hallucinations, paranoia, suspiciousness, or delusional state

● **F03.93 Unspecified dementia, unspecified severity, with mood disturbance** CC A
Unspecified dementia, unspecified severity, with mood disturbance such as depression, apathy, or anhedonia

● **F03.94 Unspecified dementia, unspecified severity, with anxiety** CC A

● **F03.A Unspecified dementia, mild**

EXCLUDES 1 *mild neurocognitive disorder due to known physiological condition with or without behavioral disturbance (F06.7-)*

● **F03.A0 Unspecified dementia, mild, without behavioral disturbance, psychotic disturbance, mood disturbance, and anxiety** A
Dementia, mild, NOS

● **F03.A1 Unspecified dementia, mild, with behavioral disturbance**

● **F03.A11 Unspecified dementia, mild, with agitation** CC A
Unspecified dementia, mild, with aberrant motor behavior such as restlessness, rocking, pacing, or exit-seeking
Unspecified dementia, mild, with verbal or physical behaviors such as profanity, shouting, threatening, anger, aggression, combativeness, or violence

● **F03.A18 Unspecified dementia, mild, with other behavioral disturbance** CC A
Unspecified dementia, mild, with behavioral disturbances such as sleep disturbance, social disinhibition, or sexual disinhibition
Use additional code, if applicable, to identify wandering in unspecified dementia (Z91.83)

● **F03.A2 Unspecified dementia, mild, with psychotic disturbance** CC A
Unspecified dementia, mild, with psychotic disturbance such as hallucinations, paranoia, suspiciousness, or delusional state

● **F03.A3 Unspecified dementia, mild, with mood disturbance** CC A
Unspecified dementia, mild, with mood disturbance such as depression, apathy, or anhedonia

● **F03.A4 Unspecified dementia, mild, with anxiety** CC A

● **F03.B Unspecified dementia, moderate**

● **F03.B0 Unspecified dementia, moderate, without behavioral disturbance, psychotic disturbance, mood disturbance, and anxiety** A
Dementia, moderate, NOS

● **F03.B1 Unspecified dementia, moderate, with behavioral disturbance**

● **F03.B11 Unspecified dementia, moderate, with agitation** CC A
Unspecified dementia, moderate, with aberrant motor behavior such as restlessness, rocking, pacing, or exit-seeking
Unspecified dementia, moderate, with verbal or physical behaviors such as profanity, shouting, threatening, anger, aggression, combativeness, or violence

● **F03.B18 Unspecified dementia, moderate, with other behavioral disturbance** CC A
Unspecified dementia, moderate, with behavioral disturbances such as sleep disturbance, social disinhibition, or sexual disinhibition
Use additional code, if applicable, to identify wandering in unspecified dementia (Z91.83)

● **F03.B2 Unspecified dementia, moderate, with psychotic disturbance** CC A
Unspecified dementia, moderate, with psychotic disturbance such as hallucinations, paranoia, suspiciousness, or delusional state

● **F03.B3 Unspecified dementia, moderate, with mood disturbance** CC A
Unspecified dementia, moderate, with mood disturbance such as depression, apathy, or anhedonia

● **F03.B4 Unspecified dementia, moderate, with anxiety** CC A

● **F03.C Unspecified dementia, severe**

● **F03.C0 Unspecified dementia, severe, without behavioral disturbance, psychotic disturbance, mood disturbance, and anxiety** A
Dementia, severe, NOS

● **F03.C1 Unspecified dementia, severe, with behavioral disturbance**

● **F03.C11 Unspecified dementia, severe, with agitation** CC A
Unspecified dementia, severe, with aberrant motor behavior such as restlessness, rocking, pacing, or exit-seeking
Unspecified dementia, severe, with verbal or physical behaviors such as profanity, shouting, threatening, anger, aggression, combativeness, or violence

● **FØ3.C18 Unspecified dementia, severe, with other behavioral disturbance** CC A

Unspecified dementia, severe, with behavioral disturbances such as sleep disturbance, social disinhibition, or sexual disinhibition

Use additional code, if applicable, to identify wandering in unspecified dementia (Z91.83)

● **FØ3.C2 Unspecified dementia, severe, with psychotic disturbance** CC A

Unspecified dementia, severe, with psychotic disturbance such as hallucinations, paranoia, suspiciousness, or delusional state

● **FØ3.C3 Unspecified dementia, severe, with mood disturbance** CC A

Unspecified dementia, severe, with mood disturbance such as depression, apathy, or anhedonia

● **FØ3.C4 Unspecified dementia, severe, with anxiety** CC A

FØ4 Amnestic disorder due to known physiological condition HCC

Korsakov's psychosis or syndrome, nonalcoholic

Code first the underlying physiological condition

EXCLUDES 1 *amnesia NOS (R41.3)*
anterograde amnesia (R41.1)
dissociative amnesia (F44.Ø)
retrograde amnesia (R41.2)

EXCLUDES 2 *alcohol-induced or unspecified Korsakov's syndrome (F1Ø.26, F1Ø.96)*
Korsakov's syndrome induced by other psychoactive substances (F13.26, F13.96, F19.16, F19.26, F19.96)

FØ5 Delirium due to known physiological condition CC

Acute or subacute brain syndrome
Acute or subacute confusional state (nonalcoholic)
Acute or subacute infective psychosis
Acute or subacute organic reaction
Acute or subacute psycho-organic syndrome
Delirium of mixed etiology
Delirium superimposed on dementia
Sundowning

Code first the underlying physiological condition

EXCLUDES 1 *delirium NOS (R41.Ø)*

EXCLUDES 2 *delirium tremens alcohol-induced or unspecified (F1Ø.231, F1Ø.921)*

AHA: 2019,2Q,34

√4th **FØ6 Other mental disorders due to known physiological condition**

INCLUDES mental disorders due to endocrine disorder
mental disorders due to exogenous hormone
mental disorders due to exogenous toxic substance
mental disorders due to primary cerebral disease
mental disorders due to somatic illness
mental disorders due to systemic disease affecting the brain

Code first the underlying physiological condition

EXCLUDES 1 *unspecified dementia (FØ3)*

EXCLUDES 2 *delirium due to known physiological condition (FØ5)*
dementia as classified in FØ1-FØ2
other mental disorders associated with alcohol and other psychoactive substances (F1Ø-F19)

FØ6.Ø Psychotic disorder with hallucinations due to known physiological condition CC

Organic hallucinatory state (nonalcoholic)

EXCLUDES 2 *hallucinations and perceptual disturbance induced by alcohol and other psychoactive substances (F1Ø-F19 with .151, .251, .951)*
schizophrenia (F2Ø.-)

FØ6.1 Catatonic disorder due to known physiological condition

Catatonia associated with another mental disorder
Catatonia NOS

EXCLUDES 1 *catatonic stupor (R4Ø.1)*
stupor NOS (R4Ø.1)

EXCLUDES 2 *catatonic schizophrenia (F2Ø.2)*
dissociative stupor (F44.2)

DEF: Catatonic: Abnormal neuropsychiatric state characterized by stupor, immobility or purposeless movements, or unresponsiveness in a person who otherwise appears awake.

FØ6.2 Psychotic disorder with delusions due to known physiological condition CC

Paranoid and paranoid-hallucinatory organic states
Schizophrenia-like psychosis in epilepsy

EXCLUDES 2 *alcohol and drug-induced psychotic disorder (F1Ø-F19 with .15Ø, .25Ø, .95Ø)*
brief psychotic disorder (F23)
delusional disorder (F22)
schizophrenia (F2Ø.-)

√5th **FØ6.3 Mood disorder due to known physiological condition**

EXCLUDES 2 *mood disorders due to alcohol and other psychoactive substances (F1Ø-F19 with .14, .24, .94)*
mood disorders, not due to known physiological condition or unspecified (F3Ø-F39)

FØ6.3Ø Mood disorder due to known physiological condition, unspecified

FØ6.31 Mood disorder due to known physiological condition with depressive features

Depressive disorder due to known physiological condition, with depressive features

FØ6.32 Mood disorder due to known physiological condition with major depressive-like episode

Depressive disorder due to known physiological condition, with major depressive-like episode

FØ6.33 Mood disorder due to known physiological condition with manic features

Bipolar and related disorder due to a known physiological condition, with manic features
Bipolar and related disorder due to known physiological condition, with manic- or hypomanic-like episodes

FØ6.34 Mood disorder due to known physiological condition with mixed features

Bipolar and related disorder due to known physiological condition, with mixed features
Depressive disorder due to known physiological condition, with mixed features

FØ6.4 Anxiety disorder due to known physiological condition

EXCLUDES 2 *anxiety disorders due to alcohol and other psychoactive substances (F1Ø-F19 with .18Ø, .28Ø, .98Ø)*
anxiety disorders, not due to known physiological condition or unspecified (F4Ø.-, F41.-)

● √5th **FØ6.7 Mild neurocognitive disorder due to known physiological condition**

Mild neurocognitive impairment due to a known physiological condition

Code first the underlying physiological condition, such as:
Alzheimer's disease (G3Ø.-)
frontotemporal neurocognitive disorder (G31.Ø9)
human immunodeficiency virus [HIV] disease (B2Ø)
Huntington's disease (G1Ø)
neurocognitive disorder with Lewy bodies (G31.83)
Parkinson's disease (G2Ø)
systemic lupus erythematosus (M32.-)
traumatic brain injury (SØ6.-)
vitamin B deficiency (E53.-)

EXCLUDES 1 *age related cognitive decline (R41.81)*
altered mental status (R41.82)
cerebral degeneration (G31.9)
change in mental status (R41.82)
cognitive deficits following (sequelae of) cerebral hemorrhage or infarction (I69.Ø1-I69.11-, I69.21-I69.31-, I69.81-I69.91-)
dementia (FØ1.-, FØ2.-, FØ3)
mild cognitive impairment due to unknown or unspecified etiology (G31.84)
neurologic neglect syndrome (R41.4)
personality change, nonpsychotic (F68.8)

● **FØ6.7Ø Mild neurocognitive disorder due to known physiological condition without behavioral disturbance** UPD

Mild neurocognitive disorder due to known physiological condition, NOS

● **FØ6.71 Mild neurocognitive disorder due to known physiological condition with behavioral disturbance** CC UPD

F06.8 Other specified mental disorders due to known physiological condition HIV
Epileptic psychosis NOS
Obsessive-compulsive and related disorder due to a known physiological condition
Organic dissociative disorder
Organic emotionally labile [asthenic] disorder

F07 Personality and behavioral disorders due to known physiological condition
Code first the underlying physiological condition

F07.0 Personality change due to known physiological condition
Frontal lobe syndrome
Limbic epilepsy personality syndrome
Lobotomy syndrome
Organic personality disorder
Organic pseudopsychopathic personality
Organic pseudoretarded personality
Postleucotomy syndrome
~~Code first underlying physiological condition~~
EXCLUDES 1 *mild cognitive impairment (G31.84)*
postconcussional syndrome (F07.81)
postencephalitic syndrome (F07.89)
signs and symptoms involving emotional state (R45.-)
EXCLUDES 2 *specific personality disorder (F60.-)*

F07.8 Other personality and behavioral disorders due to known physiological condition

F07.81 Postconcussional syndrome
Postcontusional syndrome (encephalopathy)
Post-traumatic brain syndrome, nonpsychotic
Use additional code to identify associated post-traumatic headache, if applicable (G44.3-)
EXCLUDES 1 *current concussion (brain) (S06.0-)*
postencephalitic syndrome (F07.89)
DEF: Concussion symptoms that persist for weeks or months after a head injury. These symptoms may include headache, giddiness, fatigue, insomnia, mood fluctuation, and a subjective feeling of impaired intellectual function with extreme reaction to normal stressors.

F07.89 Other personality and behavioral disorders due to known physiological condition UPD
Postencephalitic syndrome
Right hemispheric organic affective disorder

F07.9 Unspecified personality and behavioral disorder due to known physiological condition HIV
Organic psychosyndrome

F09 Unspecified mental disorder due to known physiological condition HIV
Mental disorder NOS due to known physiological condition
Organic brain syndrome NOS
Organic mental disorder NOS
Organic psychosis NOS
Symptomatic psychosis NOS
Code first the underlying physiological condition
EXCLUDES 1 ▶*mild neurocognitive disorder due to known physiological condition (F06.7-)*◀
psychosis NOS (F29)

Mental and behavioral disorders due to psychoactive substance use (F10-F19)

AHA: 2022,1Q,34; 2020,1Q,9; 2018,4Q,69-70; 2017,4Q,8; 2017,2Q,27
TIP: Psychoactive substance withdrawal can occur in individuals who do not have a diagnosis of dependence but who use the substance regularly (i.e., use or abuse) and then reduce or cease the use.

F10 Alcohol related disorders
Use additional code for blood alcohol level, if applicable (Y90.-)
AHA: 2019,3Q,8

F10.1 Alcohol abuse
EXCLUDES 1 *alcohol dependence (F10.2-)*
alcohol use, unspecified (F10.9-)
AHA: 2018,1Q,16; 2015,2Q,15

F10.10 Alcohol abuse, uncomplicated
Alcohol use disorder, mild

F10.11 Alcohol abuse, in remission
Alcohol use disorder, mild, in early remission
Alcohol use disorder, mild, in sustained remission
AHA: 2022,1Q,25

F10.12 Alcohol abuse with intoxication

F10.120 Alcohol abuse with intoxication, uncomplicated HCC

F10.121 Alcohol abuse with intoxication delirium CC HCC

F10.129 Alcohol abuse with intoxication, unspecified HCC

F10.13 Alcohol abuse, with withdrawal
AHA: 2020,4Q,16-17

F10.130 Alcohol abuse with withdrawal, uncomplicated CC HCC

F10.131 Alcohol abuse with withdrawal delirium CC HCC

F10.132 Alcohol abuse with withdrawal with perceptual disturbance CC HCC

F10.139 Alcohol abuse with withdrawal, unspecified CC HCC

F10.14 Alcohol abuse with alcohol-induced mood disorder CC HCC
Alcohol use disorder, mild, with alcohol-induced bipolar or related disorder
Alcohol use disorder, mild, with alcohol-induced depressive disorder

F10.15 Alcohol abuse with alcohol-induced psychotic disorder

F10.150 Alcohol abuse with alcohol-induced psychotic disorder with delusions HCC

F10.151 Alcohol abuse with alcohol-induced psychotic disorder with hallucinations CC HCC
DEF: Psychosis lasting less than six months with slight or no clouding of consciousness in which auditory hallucinations predominate.

F10.159 Alcohol abuse with alcohol-induced psychotic disorder, unspecified CC HCC

F10.18 Alcohol abuse with other alcohol-induced disorders
AHA: 2022,1Q,33

F10.180 Alcohol abuse with alcohol-induced anxiety disorder CC HCC
AHA: 2022,1Q,25,33

F10.181 Alcohol abuse with alcohol-induced sexual dysfunction CC HCC

F10.182 Alcohol abuse with alcohol-induced sleep disorder HCC

F10.188 Alcohol abuse with other alcohol-induced disorder CC HCC
AHA: 2022,1Q,25

F10.19 Alcohol abuse with unspecified alcohol-induced disorder CC HCC

F10.2 Alcohol dependence
EXCLUDES 1 *alcohol abuse (F10.1-)*
alcohol use, unspecified (F10.9-)
EXCLUDES 2 *toxic effect of alcohol (T51.0-)*

F10.20 Alcohol dependence, uncomplicated HCC
Alcohol use disorder, moderate
Alcohol use disorder, severe
AHA: 2020,1Q,9

F10.21 Alcohol dependence, in remission HCC
Alcohol use disorder, moderate, in early remission
Alcohol use disorder, moderate, in sustained remission
Alcohol use disorder, severe, in early remission
Alcohol use disorder, severe, in sustained remission

F10.22 Alcohol dependence with intoxication
Acute drunkenness (in alcoholism)
EXCLUDES 2 *alcohol dependence with withdrawal (F10.23-)*

F10.220 Alcohol dependence with intoxication, uncomplicated HCC

F10.221 Alcohol dependence with intoxication delirium CC HCC

F10.229 Alcohol dependence with intoxication, unspecified HCC

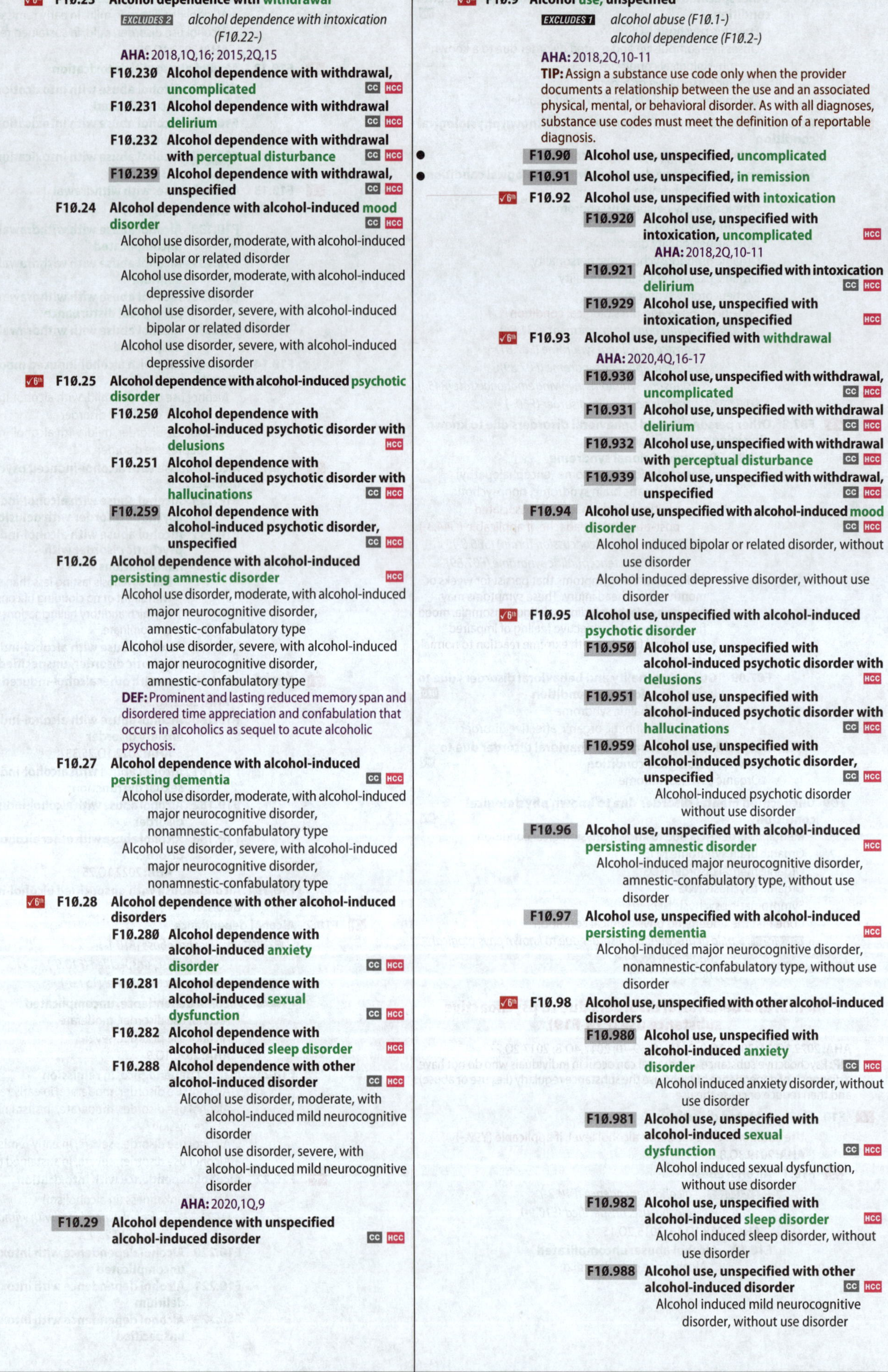

√6th **F1Ø.23 Alcohol dependence with withdrawal**

EXCLUDES 2 *alcohol dependence with intoxication (F1Ø.22-)*

AHA: 2018,1Q,16; 2015,2Q,15

F1Ø.23Ø Alcohol dependence with withdrawal, uncomplicated CC HCC

F1Ø.231 Alcohol dependence with withdrawal delirium CC HCC

F1Ø.232 Alcohol dependence with withdrawal with perceptual disturbance CC HCC

F1Ø.239 Alcohol dependence with withdrawal, unspecified CC HCC

F1Ø.24 Alcohol dependence with alcohol-induced mood disorder CC HCC

Alcohol use disorder, moderate, with alcohol-induced bipolar or related disorder

Alcohol use disorder, moderate, with alcohol-induced depressive disorder

Alcohol use disorder, severe, with alcohol-induced bipolar or related disorder

Alcohol use disorder, severe, with alcohol-induced depressive disorder

√6th **F1Ø.25 Alcohol dependence with alcohol-induced psychotic disorder**

F1Ø.25Ø Alcohol dependence with alcohol-induced psychotic disorder with delusions HCC

F1Ø.251 Alcohol dependence with alcohol-induced psychotic disorder with hallucinations CC HCC

F1Ø.259 Alcohol dependence with alcohol-induced psychotic disorder, unspecified CC HCC

F1Ø.26 Alcohol dependence with alcohol-induced persisting amnestic disorder HCC

Alcohol use disorder, moderate, with alcohol-induced major neurocognitive disorder, amnestic-confabulatory type

Alcohol use disorder, severe, with alcohol-induced major neurocognitive disorder, amnestic-confabulatory type

DEF: Prominent and lasting reduced memory span and disordered time appreciation and confabulation that occurs in alcoholics as sequel to acute alcoholic psychosis.

F1Ø.27 Alcohol dependence with alcohol-induced persisting dementia CC HCC

Alcohol use disorder, moderate, with alcohol-induced major neurocognitive disorder, nonamnestic-confabulatory type

Alcohol use disorder, severe, with alcohol-induced major neurocognitive disorder, nonamnestic-confabulatory type

√6th **F1Ø.28 Alcohol dependence with other alcohol-induced disorders**

F1Ø.28Ø Alcohol dependence with alcohol-induced anxiety disorder CC HCC

F1Ø.281 Alcohol dependence with alcohol-induced sexual dysfunction CC HCC

F1Ø.282 Alcohol dependence with alcohol-induced sleep disorder HCC

F1Ø.288 Alcohol dependence with other alcohol-induced disorder CC HCC

Alcohol use disorder, moderate, with alcohol-induced mild neurocognitive disorder

Alcohol use disorder, severe, with alcohol-induced mild neurocognitive disorder

AHA: 2020,1Q,9

F1Ø.29 Alcohol dependence with unspecified alcohol-induced disorder CC HCC

√5th **F1Ø.9 Alcohol use, unspecified**

EXCLUDES 1 *alcohol abuse (F1Ø.1-)*
alcohol dependence (F1Ø.2-)

AHA: 2018,2Q,10-11

TIP: Assign a substance use code only when the provider documents a relationship between the use and an associated physical, mental, or behavioral disorder. As with all diagnoses, substance use codes must meet the definition of a reportable diagnosis.

● **F1Ø.9Ø Alcohol use, unspecified, uncomplicated**

● **F1Ø.91 Alcohol use, unspecified, in remission**

√6th **F1Ø.92 Alcohol use, unspecified with intoxication**

F1Ø.92Ø Alcohol use, unspecified with intoxication, uncomplicated HCC

AHA: 2018,2Q,10-11

F1Ø.921 Alcohol use, unspecified with intoxication delirium CC HCC

F1Ø.929 Alcohol use, unspecified with intoxication, unspecified HCC

√6th **F1Ø.93 Alcohol use, unspecified with withdrawal**

AHA: 2020,4Q,16-17

F1Ø.93Ø Alcohol use, unspecified with withdrawal, uncomplicated CC HCC

F1Ø.931 Alcohol use, unspecified with withdrawal delirium CC HCC

F1Ø.932 Alcohol use, unspecified with withdrawal with perceptual disturbance CC HCC

F1Ø.939 Alcohol use, unspecified with withdrawal, unspecified CC HCC

F1Ø.94 Alcohol use, unspecified with alcohol-induced mood disorder CC HCC

Alcohol induced bipolar or related disorder, without use disorder

Alcohol induced depressive disorder, without use disorder

√6th **F1Ø.95 Alcohol use, unspecified with alcohol-induced psychotic disorder**

F1Ø.95Ø Alcohol use, unspecified with alcohol-induced psychotic disorder with delusions HCC

F1Ø.951 Alcohol use, unspecified with alcohol-induced psychotic disorder with hallucinations CC HCC

F1Ø.959 Alcohol use, unspecified with alcohol-induced psychotic disorder, unspecified CC HCC

Alcohol-induced psychotic disorder without use disorder

F1Ø.96 Alcohol use, unspecified with alcohol-induced persisting amnestic disorder HCC

Alcohol-induced major neurocognitive disorder, amnestic-confabulatory type, without use disorder

F1Ø.97 Alcohol use, unspecified with alcohol-induced persisting dementia HCC

Alcohol-induced major neurocognitive disorder, nonamnestic-confabulatory type, without use disorder

√6th **F1Ø.98 Alcohol use, unspecified with other alcohol-induced disorders**

F1Ø.98Ø Alcohol use, unspecified with alcohol-induced anxiety disorder CC HCC

Alcohol induced anxiety disorder, without use disorder

F1Ø.981 Alcohol use, unspecified with alcohol-induced sexual dysfunction CC HCC

Alcohol induced sexual dysfunction, without use disorder

F1Ø.982 Alcohol use, unspecified with alcohol-induced sleep disorder HCC

Alcohol induced sleep disorder, without use disorder

F1Ø.988 Alcohol use, unspecified with other alcohol-induced disorder CC HCC

Alcohol induced mild neurocognitive disorder, without use disorder

Chapter 5. Mental, Behavioral and Neurodevelopmental Disorders
F1Ø.23–F1Ø.988

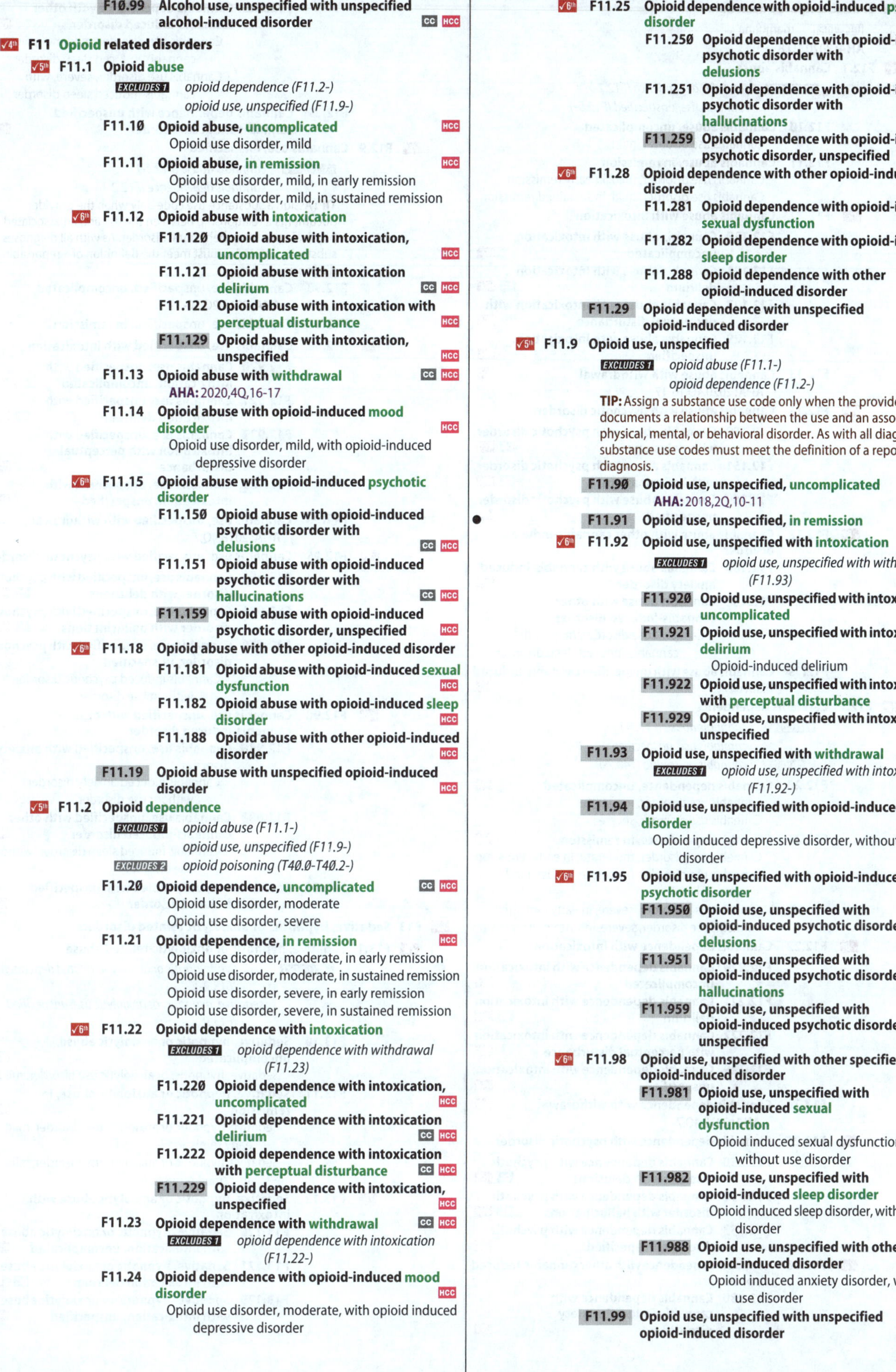

F10.99 Alcohol use, unspecified with unspecified alcohol-induced disorder CC HCC

F11 Opioid related disorders

F11.1 Opioid abuse

EXCLUDES 1 *opioid dependence (F11.2-)*
opioid use, unspecified (F11.9-)

F11.10 Opioid abuse, uncomplicated HCC
Opioid use disorder, mild

F11.11 Opioid abuse, in remission HCC
Opioid use disorder, mild, in early remission
Opioid use disorder, mild, in sustained remission

F11.12 Opioid abuse with intoxication

F11.120 Opioid abuse with intoxication, uncomplicated HCC

F11.121 Opioid abuse with intoxication delirium CC HCC

F11.122 Opioid abuse with intoxication with perceptual disturbance HCC

F11.129 Opioid abuse with intoxication, unspecified HCC

F11.13 Opioid abuse with withdrawal CC HCC
AHA: 2020,4Q,16-17

F11.14 Opioid abuse with opioid-induced mood disorder HCC
Opioid use disorder, mild, with opioid-induced depressive disorder

F11.15 Opioid abuse with opioid-induced psychotic disorder

F11.150 Opioid abuse with opioid-induced psychotic disorder with delusions CC HCC

F11.151 Opioid abuse with opioid-induced psychotic disorder with hallucinations CC HCC

F11.159 Opioid abuse with opioid-induced psychotic disorder, unspecified HCC

F11.18 Opioid abuse with other opioid-induced disorder

F11.181 Opioid abuse with opioid-induced sexual dysfunction HCC

F11.182 Opioid abuse with opioid-induced sleep disorder HCC

F11.188 Opioid abuse with other opioid-induced disorder HCC

F11.19 Opioid abuse with unspecified opioid-induced disorder HCC

F11.2 Opioid dependence

EXCLUDES 1 *opioid abuse (F11.1-)*
opioid use, unspecified (F11.9-)

EXCLUDES 2 *opioid poisoning (T40.0-T40.2-)*

F11.20 Opioid dependence, uncomplicated CC HCC
Opioid use disorder, moderate
Opioid use disorder, severe

F11.21 Opioid dependence, in remission HCC
Opioid use disorder, moderate, in early remission
Opioid use disorder, moderate, in sustained remission
Opioid use disorder, severe, in early remission
Opioid use disorder, severe, in sustained remission

F11.22 Opioid dependence with intoxication

EXCLUDES 1 *opioid dependence with withdrawal (F11.23)*

F11.220 Opioid dependence with intoxication, uncomplicated HCC

F11.221 Opioid dependence with intoxication delirium CC HCC

F11.222 Opioid dependence with intoxication with perceptual disturbance CC HCC

F11.229 Opioid dependence with intoxication, unspecified HCC

F11.23 Opioid dependence with withdrawal CC HCC

EXCLUDES 1 *opioid dependence with intoxication (F11.22-)*

F11.24 Opioid dependence with opioid-induced mood disorder HCC
Opioid use disorder, moderate, with opioid induced depressive disorder

F11.25 Opioid dependence with opioid-induced psychotic disorder

F11.250 Opioid dependence with opioid-induced psychotic disorder with delusions CC HCC

F11.251 Opioid dependence with opioid-induced psychotic disorder with hallucinations CC HCC

F11.259 Opioid dependence with opioid-induced psychotic disorder, unspecified CC HCC

F11.28 Opioid dependence with other opioid-induced disorder

F11.281 Opioid dependence with opioid-induced sexual dysfunction CC HCC

F11.282 Opioid dependence with opioid-induced sleep disorder CC HCC

F11.288 Opioid dependence with other opioid-induced disorder CC HCC

F11.29 Opioid dependence with unspecified opioid-induced disorder HCC

F11.9 Opioid use, unspecified

EXCLUDES 1 *opioid abuse (F11.1-)*
opioid dependence (F11.2-)

TIP: Assign a substance use code only when the provider documents a relationship between the use and an associated physical, mental, or behavioral disorder. As with all diagnoses, substance use codes must meet the definition of a reportable diagnosis.

F11.90 Opioid use, unspecified, uncomplicated
AHA: 2018,2Q,10-11

F11.91 Opioid use, unspecified, in remission

F11.92 Opioid use, unspecified with intoxication

EXCLUDES 1 *opioid use, unspecified with withdrawal (F11.93)*

F11.920 Opioid use, unspecified with intoxication, uncomplicated HCC

F11.921 Opioid use, unspecified with intoxication delirium CC HCC
Opioid-induced delirium

F11.922 Opioid use, unspecified with intoxication with perceptual disturbance HCC

F11.929 Opioid use, unspecified with intoxication, unspecified HCC

F11.93 Opioid use, unspecified with withdrawal CC HCC

EXCLUDES 1 *opioid use, unspecified with intoxication (F11.92-)*

F11.94 Opioid use, unspecified with opioid-induced mood disorder HCC
Opioid induced depressive disorder, without use disorder

F11.95 Opioid use, unspecified with opioid-induced psychotic disorder

F11.950 Opioid use, unspecified with opioid-induced psychotic disorder with delusions CC HCC

F11.951 Opioid use, unspecified with opioid-induced psychotic disorder with hallucinations CC HCC

F11.959 Opioid use, unspecified with opioid-induced psychotic disorder, unspecified HCC

F11.98 Opioid use, unspecified with other specified opioid-induced disorder

F11.981 Opioid use, unspecified with opioid-induced sexual dysfunction HCC
Opioid induced sexual dysfunction, without use disorder

F11.982 Opioid use, unspecified with opioid-induced sleep disorder HCC
Opioid induced sleep disorder, without use disorder

F11.988 Opioid use, unspecified with other opioid-induced disorder HCC
Opioid induced anxiety disorder, without use disorder

F11.99 Opioid use, unspecified with unspecified opioid-induced disorder HCC

Chapter 5. Mental, Behavioral and Neurodevelopmental Disorders

F10.99–F11.99

F12 Cannabis related disorders
INCLUDES marijuana
AHA: 2020,1Q,8

F12.1 Cannabis abuse
EXCLUDES 1 *cannabis dependence (F12.2-)*
cannabis use, unspecified (F12.9-)

F12.10 Cannabis abuse, uncomplicated
Cannabis use disorder, mild

F12.11 Cannabis abuse, in remission
Cannabis use disorder, mild, in early remission
Cannabis use disorder, mild, in sustained remission

F12.12 Cannabis abuse with intoxication

F12.120 Cannabis abuse with intoxication, uncomplicated HCC

F12.121 Cannabis abuse with intoxication delirium CC HCC

F12.122 Cannabis abuse with intoxication with perceptual disturbance HCC

F12.129 Cannabis abuse with intoxication, unspecified HCC

F12.13 Cannabis abuse with withdrawal HCC
AHA: 2020,4Q,16-17

F12.15 Cannabis abuse with psychotic disorder

F12.150 Cannabis abuse with psychotic disorder with delusions CC HCC

F12.151 Cannabis abuse with psychotic disorder with hallucinations CC HCC

F12.159 Cannabis abuse with psychotic disorder, unspecified HCC

F12.18 Cannabis abuse with other cannabis-induced disorder

F12.180 Cannabis abuse with cannabis-induced anxiety disorder HCC

F12.188 Cannabis abuse with other cannabis-induced disorder HCC
Cannabis use disorder, mild, with cannabis-induced sleep disorder

F12.19 Cannabis abuse with unspecified cannabis-induced disorder HCC

F12.2 Cannabis dependence
EXCLUDES 1 *cannabis abuse (F12.1-)*
cannabis use, unspecified (F12.9-)
EXCLUDES 2 *cannabis poisoning (T40.7-)*

F12.20 Cannabis dependence, uncomplicated HCC
Cannabis use disorder, moderate
Cannabis use disorder, severe

F12.21 Cannabis dependence, in remission HCC
Cannabis use disorder, moderate, in early remission
Cannabis use disorder, moderate, in sustained remission
Cannabis use disorder, severe, in early remission
Cannabis use disorder, severe, in sustained remission

F12.22 Cannabis dependence with intoxication

F12.220 Cannabis dependence with intoxication, uncomplicated HCC

F12.221 Cannabis dependence with intoxication delirium CC HCC

F12.222 Cannabis dependence with intoxication with perceptual disturbance HCC

F12.229 Cannabis dependence with intoxication, unspecified HCC

F12.23 Cannabis dependence with withdrawal HCC
AHA: 2018,4Q,7

F12.25 Cannabis dependence with psychotic disorder

F12.250 Cannabis dependence with psychotic disorder with delusions CC HCC

F12.251 Cannabis dependence with psychotic disorder with hallucinations CC HCC

F12.259 Cannabis dependence with psychotic disorder, unspecified HCC

F12.28 Cannabis dependence with other cannabis-induced disorder

F12.280 Cannabis dependence with cannabis-induced anxiety disorder HCC

F12.288 Cannabis dependence with other cannabis-induced disorder HCC
Cannabis use disorder, moderate, with cannabis-induced sleep disorder
Cannabis use disorder, severe, with cannabis-induced sleep disorder

F12.29 Cannabis dependence with unspecified cannabis-induced disorder HCC

F12.9 Cannabis use, unspecified
EXCLUDES 1 *cannabis abuse (F12.1-)*
cannabis dependence (F12.2-)
TIP: Assign a substance use code only when the provider documents a relationship between the use and an associated physical, mental, or behavioral disorder. As with all diagnoses, substance use codes must meet the definition of a reportable diagnosis.

F12.90 Cannabis use, unspecified, uncomplicated
AHA: 2018,2Q,10-11

● **F12.91 Cannabis use, unspecified, in remission**

F12.92 Cannabis use, unspecified with intoxication

F12.920 Cannabis use, unspecified with intoxication, uncomplicated HCC

F12.921 Cannabis use, unspecified with intoxication delirium CC HCC

F12.922 Cannabis use, unspecified with intoxication with perceptual disturbance HCC

F12.929 Cannabis use, unspecified with intoxication, unspecified HCC

F12.93 Cannabis use, unspecified with withdrawal HCC
AHA: 2018,4Q,7

F12.95 Cannabis use, unspecified with psychotic disorder

F12.950 Cannabis use, unspecified with psychotic disorder with delusions CC HCC

F12.951 Cannabis use, unspecified with psychotic disorder with hallucinations CC HCC

F12.959 Cannabis use, unspecified with psychotic disorder, unspecified HCC
Cannabis induced psychotic disorder, without use disorder

F12.98 Cannabis use, unspecified with other cannabis-induced disorder

F12.980 Cannabis use, unspecified with anxiety disorder HCC
Cannabis induced anxiety disorder, without use disorder

F12.988 Cannabis use, unspecified with other cannabis-induced disorder HCC
Cannabis induced sleep disorder, without use disorder

F12.99 Cannabis use, unspecified with unspecified cannabis-induced disorder HCC

F13 Sedative, hypnotic, or anxiolytic related disorders

F13.1 Sedative, hypnotic or anxiolytic-related abuse
EXCLUDES 1 *sedative, hypnotic or anxiolytic-related dependence (F13.2-)*
sedative, hypnotic, or anxiolytic use, unspecified (F13.9-)

F13.10 Sedative, hypnotic or anxiolytic abuse, uncomplicated HCC
Sedative, hypnotic, or anxiolytic use disorder, mild

F13.11 Sedative, hypnotic or anxiolytic abuse, in remission HCC
Sedative, hypnotic or anxiolytic use disorder, mild, in early remission
Sedative, hypnotic or anxiolytic use disorder, mild, in sustained remission

F13.12 Sedative, hypnotic or anxiolytic abuse with intoxication

F13.120 Sedative, hypnotic or anxiolytic abuse with intoxication, uncomplicated HCC

F13.121 Sedative, hypnotic or anxiolytic abuse with intoxication delirium CC HCC

F13.129 Sedative, hypnotic or anxiolytic abuse with intoxication, unspecified HCC

✓6th **F13.13 Sedative, hypnotic or anxiolytic abuse with withdrawal**
AHA: 2020,4Q,16-17
F13.13Ø Sedative, hypnotic or anxiolytic abuse with withdrawal, uncomplicated CC HCC
F13.131 Sedative, hypnotic or anxiolytic abuse with withdrawal delirium CC HCC
F13.132 Sedative, hypnotic or anxiolytic abuse with withdrawal with perceptual disturbance CC HCC
F13.139 Sedative, hypnotic or anxiolytic abuse with withdrawal, unspecified CC HCC
F13.14 Sedative, hypnotic or anxiolytic abuse with sedative, hypnotic or anxiolytic-induced mood disorder HCC
Sedative, hypnotic, or anxiolytic use disorder, mild, with sedative, hypnotic, or anxiolytic-induced bipolar or related disorder
Sedative, hypnotic, or anxiolytic use disorder, mild, with sedative, hypnotic, or anxiolytic-induced depressive disorder
✓6th **F13.15 Sedative, hypnotic or anxiolytic abuse with sedative, hypnotic or anxiolytic-induced psychotic disorder**
F13.15Ø Sedative, hypnotic or anxiolytic abuse with sedative, hypnotic or anxiolytic-induced psychotic disorder with delusions CC HCC
F13.151 Sedative, hypnotic or anxiolytic abuse with sedative, hypnotic or anxiolytic-induced psychotic disorder with hallucinations CC HCC
F13.159 Sedative, hypnotic or anxiolytic abuse with sedative, hypnotic or anxiolytic-induced psychotic disorder, unspecified HCC
✓6th **F13.18 Sedative, hypnotic or anxiolytic abuse with other sedative, hypnotic or anxiolytic-induced disorders**
F13.18Ø Sedative, hypnotic or anxiolytic abuse with sedative, hypnotic or anxiolytic-induced anxiety disorder HCC
F13.181 Sedative, hypnotic or anxiolytic abuse with sedative, hypnotic or anxiolytic-induced sexual dysfunction HCC
F13.182 Sedative, hypnotic or anxiolytic abuse with sedative, hypnotic or anxiolytic-induced sleep disorder HCC
F13.188 Sedative, hypnotic or anxiolytic abuse with other sedative, hypnotic or anxiolytic-induced disorder HCC
F13.19 Sedative, hypnotic or anxiolytic abuse with unspecified sedative, hypnotic or anxiolytic-induced disorder HCC
✓5th **F13.2 Sedative, hypnotic or anxiolytic-related dependence**
EXCLUDES 1 *sedative, hypnotic or anxiolytic-related abuse (F13.1-)*
sedative, hypnotic, or anxiolytic use, unspecified (F13.9-)
EXCLUDES 2 *sedative, hypnotic, or anxiolytic poisoning (T42.-)*
F13.2Ø Sedative, hypnotic or anxiolytic dependence, uncomplicated CC HCC
F13.21 Sedative, hypnotic or anxiolytic dependence, in remission HCC
Sedative, hypnotic or anxiolytic use disorder, moderate, in early remission
Sedative, hypnotic or anxiolytic use disorder, moderate, in sustained remission
Sedative, hypnotic or anxiolytic use disorder, severe, in early remission
Sedative, hypnotic or anxiolytic use disorder, severe, in sustained remission
✓6th **F13.22 Sedative, hypnotic or anxiolytic dependence with intoxication**
EXCLUDES 1 *sedative, hypnotic or anxiolytic dependence with withdrawal (F13.23-)*
F13.22Ø Sedative, hypnotic or anxiolytic dependence with intoxication, uncomplicated HCC
F13.221 Sedative, hypnotic or anxiolytic dependence with intoxication delirium CC HCC
F13.229 Sedative, hypnotic or anxiolytic dependence with intoxication, unspecified HCC
✓6th **F13.23 Sedative, hypnotic or anxiolytic dependence with withdrawal**
Sedative, hypnotic, or anxiolytic use disorder, moderate
Sedative, hypnotic, or anxiolytic use disorder, severe
EXCLUDES 1 *sedative, hypnotic or anxiolytic dependence with intoxication (F13.22-)*
F13.23Ø Sedative, hypnotic or anxiolytic dependence with withdrawal, uncomplicated CC HCC
F13.231 Sedative, hypnotic or anxiolytic dependence with withdrawal delirium CC HCC
F13.232 Sedative, hypnotic or anxiolytic dependence with withdrawal with perceptual disturbance CC HCC
Sedative, hypnotic, or anxiolytic withdrawal with perceptual disturbances
F13.239 Sedative, hypnotic or anxiolytic dependence with withdrawal, unspecified CC HCC
Sedative, hypnotic, or anxiolytic withdrawal without perceptual disturbances
F13.24 Sedative, hypnotic or anxiolytic dependence with sedative, hypnotic or anxiolytic-induced mood disorder HCC
Sedative, hypnotic, or anxiolytic use disorder, moderate, with sedative, hypnotic, or anxiolytic-induced bipolar or related disorder
Sedative, hypnotic, or anxiolytic use disorder, moderate, with sedative, hypnotic, or anxiolytic-induced depressive disorder
Sedative, hypnotic, or anxiolytic use disorder, severe, with sedative, hypnotic, or anxiolytic-induced bipolar or related disorder
Sedative, hypnotic, or anxiolytic use disorder, severe, with sedative, hypnotic, or anxiolytic-induced depressive disorder
✓6th **F13.25 Sedative, hypnotic or anxiolytic dependence with sedative, hypnotic or anxiolytic-induced psychotic disorder**
F13.25Ø Sedative, hypnotic or anxiolytic dependence with sedative, hypnotic or anxiolytic-induced psychotic disorder with delusions CC HCC
F13.251 Sedative, hypnotic or anxiolytic dependence with sedative, hypnotic or anxiolytic-induced psychotic disorder with hallucinations CC HCC
F13.259 Sedative, hypnotic or anxiolytic dependence with sedative, hypnotic or anxiolytic-induced psychotic disorder, unspecified CC HCC
F13.26 Sedative, hypnotic or anxiolytic dependence with sedative, hypnotic or anxiolytic-induced persisting amnestic disorder CC HCC
F13.27 Sedative, hypnotic or anxiolytic dependence with sedative, hypnotic or anxiolytic-induced persisting dementia CC HCC
Sedative, hypnotic, or anxiolytic use disorder, moderate, with sedative, hypnotic, or anxiolytic induced major neurocognitive disorder
Sedative, hypnotic, or anxiolytic use disorder, severe, with sedative, hypnotic, or anxiolytic-induced major neurocognitive disorder
✓6th **F13.28 Sedative, hypnotic or anxiolytic dependence with other sedative, hypnotic or anxiolytic-induced disorders**
F13.28Ø Sedative, hypnotic or anxiolytic dependence with sedative, hypnotic or anxiolytic-induced anxiety disorder CC HCC

F13.281 Sedative, hypnotic or anxiolytic dependence with sedative, hypnotic or anxiolytic-induced sexual dysfunction CC HCC

F13.282 Sedative, hypnotic or anxiolytic dependence with sedative, hypnotic or anxiolytic-induced sleep disorder CC HCC

F13.288 Sedative, hypnotic or anxiolytic dependence with other sedative, hypnotic or anxiolytic-induced disorder CC HCC

Sedative, hypnotic, or anxiolytic use disorder, moderate, with sedative, hypnotic, or anxiolytic-induced mild neurocognitive disorder

Sedative, hypnotic, or anxiolytic use disorder, severe, with sedative, hypnotic, or anxiolytic-induced mild neurocognitive disorder

F13.29 Sedative, hypnotic or anxiolytic dependence with unspecified sedative, hypnotic or anxiolytic-induced disorder HCC

5th **F13.9 Sedative, hypnotic or anxiolytic-related use, unspecified**

EXCLUDES 1 *sedative, hypnotic or anxiolytic-related abuse (F13.1-)*
sedative, hypnotic or anxiolytic-related dependence (F13.2-)

TIP: Assign a substance use code only when the provider documents a relationship between the use and an associated physical, mental, or behavioral disorder. As with all diagnoses, substance use codes must meet the definition of a reportable diagnosis.

F13.90 Sedative, hypnotic or anxiolytic use, unspecified, uncomplicated

AHA: 2018,2Q,10-11

● **F13.91 Sedative, hypnotic or anxiolytic use, unspecified, in remission**

6th **F13.92 Sedative, hypnotic or anxiolytic use, unspecified with intoxication**

EXCLUDES 1 *sedative, hypnotic or anxiolytic use, unspecified with withdrawal (F13.93-)*

F13.920 Sedative, hypnotic or anxiolytic use, unspecified with intoxication, uncomplicated HCC

F13.921 Sedative, hypnotic or anxiolytic use, unspecified with intoxication delirium CC HCC

Sedative, hypnotic, or anxiolytic-induced delirium

F13.929 Sedative, hypnotic or anxiolytic use, unspecified with intoxication, unspecified HCC

6th **F13.93 Sedative, hypnotic or anxiolytic use, unspecified with withdrawal**

EXCLUDES 1 *sedative, hypnotic or anxiolytic use, unspecified with intoxication (F13.92-)*

F13.930 Sedative, hypnotic or anxiolytic use, unspecified with withdrawal, uncomplicated CC HCC

F13.931 Sedative, hypnotic or anxiolytic use, unspecified with withdrawal delirium CC HCC

F13.932 Sedative, hypnotic or anxiolytic use, unspecified with withdrawal with perceptual disturbances CC HCC

F13.939 Sedative, hypnotic or anxiolytic use, unspecified with withdrawal, unspecified CC HCC

F13.94 Sedative, hypnotic or anxiolytic use, unspecified with sedative, hypnotic or anxiolytic-induced mood disorder HCC

Sedative, hypnotic, or anxiolytic-induced bipolar or related disorder, without use disorder

Sedative, hypnotic, or anxiolytic-induced depressive disorder, without use disorder

6th **F13.95 Sedative, hypnotic or anxiolytic use, unspecified with sedative, hypnotic or anxiolytic-induced psychotic disorder**

F13.950 Sedative, hypnotic or anxiolytic use, unspecified with sedative, hypnotic or anxiolytic-induced psychotic disorder with delusions CC HCC

F13.951 Sedative, hypnotic or anxiolytic use, unspecified with sedative, hypnotic or anxiolytic-induced psychotic disorder with hallucinations CC HCC

F13.959 Sedative, hypnotic or anxiolytic use, unspecified with sedative, hypnotic or anxiolytic-induced psychotic disorder, unspecified HCC

Sedative, hypnotic, or anxiolytic-induced psychotic disorder, without use disorder

F13.96 Sedative, hypnotic or anxiolytic use, unspecified with sedative, hypnotic or anxiolytic-induced persisting amnestic disorder HCC

F13.97 Sedative, hypnotic or anxiolytic use, unspecified with sedative, hypnotic or anxiolytic-induced persisting dementia CC HCC

Sedative, hypnotic, or anxiolytic-induced major neurocognitive disorder, without use disorder

6th **F13.98 Sedative, hypnotic or anxiolytic use, unspecified with other sedative, hypnotic or anxiolytic-induced disorders**

F13.980 Sedative, hypnotic or anxiolytic use, unspecified with sedative, hypnotic or anxiolytic-induced anxiety disorder HCC

Sedative, hypnotic, or anxiolytic-induced anxiety disorder, without use disorder

F13.981 Sedative, hypnotic or anxiolytic use, unspecified with sedative, hypnotic or anxiolytic-induced sexual dysfunction HCC

Sedative, hypnotic, or anxiolytic-induced sexual dysfunction disorder, without use disorder

F13.982 Sedative, hypnotic or anxiolytic use, unspecified with sedative, hypnotic or anxiolytic-induced sleep disorder HCC

Sedative, hypnotic, or anxiolytic-induced sleep disorder, without use disorder

F13.988 Sedative, hypnotic or anxiolytic use, unspecified with other sedative, hypnotic or anxiolytic-induced disorder HCC

Sedative, hypnotic, or anxiolytic-induced mild neurocognitive disorder

F13.99 Sedative, hypnotic or anxiolytic use, unspecified with unspecified sedative, hypnotic or anxiolytic-induced disorder HCC

4th **F14 Cocaine related disorders**

EXCLUDES 2 *other stimulant-related disorders (F15.-)*

5th **F14.1 Cocaine abuse**

EXCLUDES 1 *cocaine dependence (F14.2-)*
cocaine use, unspecified (F14.9-)

F14.10 Cocaine abuse, uncomplicated HCC

Cocaine use disorder, mild

F14.11 Cocaine abuse, in remission HCC

Cocaine use disorder, mild, in early remission

Cocaine use disorder, mild, in sustained remission

6th **F14.12 Cocaine abuse with intoxication**

F14.120 Cocaine abuse with intoxication, uncomplicated HCC

F14.121 Cocaine abuse with intoxication with delirium CC HCC

F14.122 Cocaine abuse with intoxication with perceptual disturbance HCC

F14.129 Cocaine abuse with intoxication, unspecified HCC

F14.13 Cocaine abuse, unspecified with withdrawal CC HCC

AHA: 2020,4Q,16-17

F14.14 Cocaine abuse with cocaine-induced mood disorder HCC
Cocaine use disorder, mild, with cocaine-induced bipolar or related disorder
Cocaine use disorder, mild, with cocaine-induced depressive disorder

✓6th **F14.15 Cocaine abuse with cocaine-induced psychotic disorder**

F14.150 Cocaine abuse with cocaine-induced psychotic disorder with delusions CC HCC

F14.151 Cocaine abuse with cocaine-induced psychotic disorder with hallucinations CC HCC

F14.159 Cocaine abuse with cocaine-induced psychotic disorder, unspecified HCC

✓6th **F14.18 Cocaine abuse with other cocaine-induced disorder**

F14.180 Cocaine abuse with cocaine-induced anxiety disorder HCC

F14.181 Cocaine abuse with cocaine-induced sexual dysfunction HCC

F14.182 Cocaine abuse with cocaine-induced sleep disorder HCC

F14.188 Cocaine abuse with other cocaine-induced disorder HCC
Cocaine use disorder, mild, with cocaine-induced obsessive compulsive or related disorder

F14.19 Cocaine abuse with unspecified cocaine-induced disorder HCC

✓5th **F14.2 Cocaine dependence**

EXCLUDES 1 *cocaine abuse (F14.1-)*
cocaine use, unspecified (F14.9-)

EXCLUDES 2 *cocaine poisoning (T40.5-)*

F14.20 Cocaine dependence, uncomplicated CC HCC
Cocaine use disorder, moderate
Cocaine use disorder, severe

F14.21 Cocaine dependence, in remission HCC
Cocaine use disorder, moderate, in early remission
Cocaine use disorder, moderate, in sustained remission
Cocaine use disorder, severe, in early remission
Cocaine use disorder, severe, in sustained remission

✓6th **F14.22 Cocaine dependence with intoxication**

EXCLUDES 1 *cocaine dependence with withdrawal (F14.23)*

F14.220 Cocaine dependence with intoxication, uncomplicated HCC

F14.221 Cocaine dependence with intoxication delirium CC HCC

F14.222 Cocaine dependence with intoxication with perceptual disturbance CC HCC

F14.229 Cocaine dependence with intoxication, unspecified CC HCC

F14.23 Cocaine dependence with withdrawal CC HCC

EXCLUDES 1 *cocaine dependence with intoxication (F14.22-)*

F14.24 Cocaine dependence with cocaine-induced mood disorder HCC
Cocaine use disorder, moderate, with cocaine-induced bipolar or related disorder
Cocaine use disorder, moderate, with cocaine-induced depressive disorder
Cocaine use disorder, severe, with cocaine-induced bipolar or related disorder
Cocaine use disorder, severe, with cocaine-induced depressive disorder

✓6th **F14.25 Cocaine dependence with cocaine-induced psychotic disorder**

F14.250 Cocaine dependence with cocaine-induced psychotic disorder with delusions CC HCC

F14.251 Cocaine dependence with cocaine-induced psychotic disorder with hallucinations CC HCC

F14.259 Cocaine dependence with cocaine-induced psychotic disorder, unspecified CC HCC

✓6th **F14.28 Cocaine dependence with other cocaine-induced disorder**

F14.280 Cocaine dependence with cocaine-induced anxiety disorder CC HCC

F14.281 Cocaine dependence with cocaine-induced sexual dysfunction CC HCC

F14.282 Cocaine dependence with cocaine-induced sleep disorder CC HCC

F14.288 Cocaine dependence with other cocaine-induced disorder CC HCC
Cocaine use disorder, moderate, with cocaine-induced obsessive compulsive or related disorder
Cocaine use disorder, severe, with cocaine-induced obsessive compulsive or related disorder

F14.29 Cocaine dependence with unspecified cocaine-induced disorder HCC

✓5th **F14.9 Cocaine use, unspecified**

EXCLUDES 1 *cocaine abuse (F14.1-)*
cocaine dependence (F14.2-)

TIP: Assign a substance use code only when the provider documents a relationship between the use and an associated physical, mental, or behavioral disorder. As with all diagnoses, substance use codes must meet the definition of a reportable diagnosis.

F14.90 Cocaine use, unspecified, uncomplicated
AHA: 2018,2Q,10-11

● **F14.91 Cocaine use, unspecified, in remission**

✓6th **F14.92 Cocaine use, unspecified with intoxication**

F14.920 Cocaine use, unspecified with intoxication, uncomplicated HCC

F14.921 Cocaine use, unspecified with intoxication delirium CC HCC

F14.922 Cocaine use, unspecified with intoxication with perceptual disturbance HCC

F14.929 Cocaine use, unspecified with intoxication, unspecified HCC

F14.93 Cocaine use, unspecified with withdrawal CC HCC
AHA: 2020,4Q,16-17

F14.94 Cocaine use, unspecified with cocaine-induced mood disorder HCC
Cocaine induced bipolar or related disorder, without use disorder
Cocaine induced depressive disorder, without use disorder

✓6th **F14.95 Cocaine use, unspecified with cocaine-induced psychotic disorder**

F14.950 Cocaine use, unspecified with cocaine-induced psychotic disorder with delusions CC HCC

F14.951 Cocaine use, unspecified with cocaine-induced psychotic disorder with hallucinations CC HCC

F14.959 Cocaine use, unspecified with cocaine-induced psychotic disorder, unspecified HCC
Cocaine induced psychotic disorder, without use disorder

✓6th **F14.98 Cocaine use, unspecified with other specified cocaine-induced disorder**

F14.980 Cocaine use, unspecified with cocaine-induced anxiety disorder HCC
Cocaine induced anxiety disorder, without use disorder

F14.981 Cocaine use, unspecified with cocaine-induced sexual dysfunction HCC
Cocaine induced sexual dysfunction, without use disorder

F14.982 Cocaine use, unspecified with cocaine-induced sleep disorder HCC
Cocaine induced sleep disorder, without use disorder

F14.988 Cocaine use, unspecified with other cocaine-induced disorder HCC
Cocaine induced obsessive compulsive or related disorder

F14.99 Cocaine use, unspecified with unspecified cocaine-induced disorder HCC

F15 Other stimulant related disorders
INCLUDES amphetamine-related disorders
caffeine
EXCLUDES 2 *cocaine-related disorders (F14.-)*

F15.1 Other stimulant abuse
EXCLUDES 1 *other stimulant dependence (F15.2-)*
other stimulant use, unspecified (F15.9-)

F15.10 Other stimulant abuse, uncomplicated HCC
Amphetamine type substance use disorder, mild
Other or unspecified stimulant use disorder, mild

F15.11 Other stimulant abuse, in remission HCC
Amphetamine type substance use disorder, mild, in early remission
Amphetamine type substance use disorder, mild, in sustained remission
Other or unspecified stimulant use disorder, mild, in early remission
Other or unspecified stimulant use disorder, mild, in sustained remission
AHA: 2021,3Q,8

F15.12 Other stimulant abuse with intoxication

F15.120 Other stimulant abuse with intoxication, uncomplicated HCC

F15.121 Other stimulant abuse with intoxication delirium CC HCC

F15.122 Other stimulant abuse with intoxication with perceptual disturbance HCC
Amphetamine or other stimulant use disorder, mild, with amphetamine or other stimulant intoxication, with perceptual disturbances

F15.129 Other stimulant abuse with intoxication, unspecified HCC
Amphetamine or other stimulant use disorder, mild, with amphetamine or other stimulant intoxication, without perceptual disturbances

F15.13 Other stimulant abuse with withdrawal CC HCC
AHA: 2020,4Q,16-17

F15.14 Other stimulant abuse with stimulant-induced mood disorder HCC
Amphetamine or other stimulant use disorder, mild, with amphetamine or other stimulant induced bipolar or related disorder
Amphetamine or other stimulant use disorder, mild, with amphetamine or other stimulant induced depressive disorder

F15.15 Other stimulant abuse with stimulant-induced psychotic disorder

F15.150 Other stimulant abuse with stimulant-induced psychotic disorder with delusions CC HCC

F15.151 Other stimulant abuse with stimulant-induced psychotic disorder with hallucinations CC HCC

F15.159 Other stimulant abuse with stimulant-induced psychotic disorder, unspecified HCC

F15.18 Other stimulant abuse with other stimulant-induced disorder

F15.180 Other stimulant abuse with stimulant-induced anxiety disorder HCC

F15.181 Other stimulant abuse with stimulant-induced sexual dysfunction HCC

F15.182 Other stimulant abuse with stimulant-induced sleep disorder HCC

F15.188 Other stimulant abuse with other stimulant-induced disorder HCC
Amphetamine or other stimulant use disorder, mild, with amphetamine or other stimulant induced obsessive-compulsive or related disorder

F15.19 Other stimulant abuse with unspecified stimulant-induced disorder HCC

F15.2 Other stimulant dependence
EXCLUDES 1 *other stimulant abuse (F15.1-)*
other stimulant use, unspecified (F15.9-)

F15.20 Other stimulant dependence, uncomplicated CC HCC
Amphetamine type substance use disorder, moderate
Amphetamine type substance use disorder, severe
Other or unspecified stimulant use disorder, moderate
Other or unspecified stimulant use disorder, severe

F15.21 Other stimulant dependence, in remission HCC
Amphetamine type substance use disorder, moderate, in early remission
Amphetamine type substance use disorder, moderate, in sustained remission
Amphetamine type substance use disorder, severe, in early remission
Amphetamine type substance use disorder, severe, in sustained remission
Other or unspecified stimulant use disorder, moderate, in early remission
Other or unspecified stimulant use disorder, moderate, in sustained remission
Other or unspecified stimulant use disorder, severe, in early remission
Other or unspecified stimulant use disorder, severe, in sustained remission

F15.22 Other stimulant dependence with intoxication
EXCLUDES 1 *other stimulant dependence with withdrawal (F15.23)*

F15.220 Other stimulant dependence with intoxication, uncomplicated HCC

F15.221 Other stimulant dependence with intoxication delirium CC HCC

F15.222 Other stimulant dependence with intoxication with perceptual disturbance CC HCC
Amphetamine or other stimulant use disorder, moderate, with amphetamine or other stimulant intoxication, with perceptual disturbances
Amphetamine or other stimulant use disorder, severe, with amphetamine or other stimulant intoxication, with perceptual disturbances

F15.229 Other stimulant dependence with intoxication, unspecified HCC
Amphetamine or other stimulant use disorder, moderate, with amphetamine or other stimulant intoxication, without perceptual disturbances
Amphetamine or other stimulant use disorder, severe, with amphetamine or other stimulant intoxication, without perceptual disturbances

F15.23 Other stimulant dependence with withdrawal CC HCC
Amphetamine or other stimulant withdrawal
EXCLUDES 1 *other stimulant dependence with intoxication (F15.22-)*

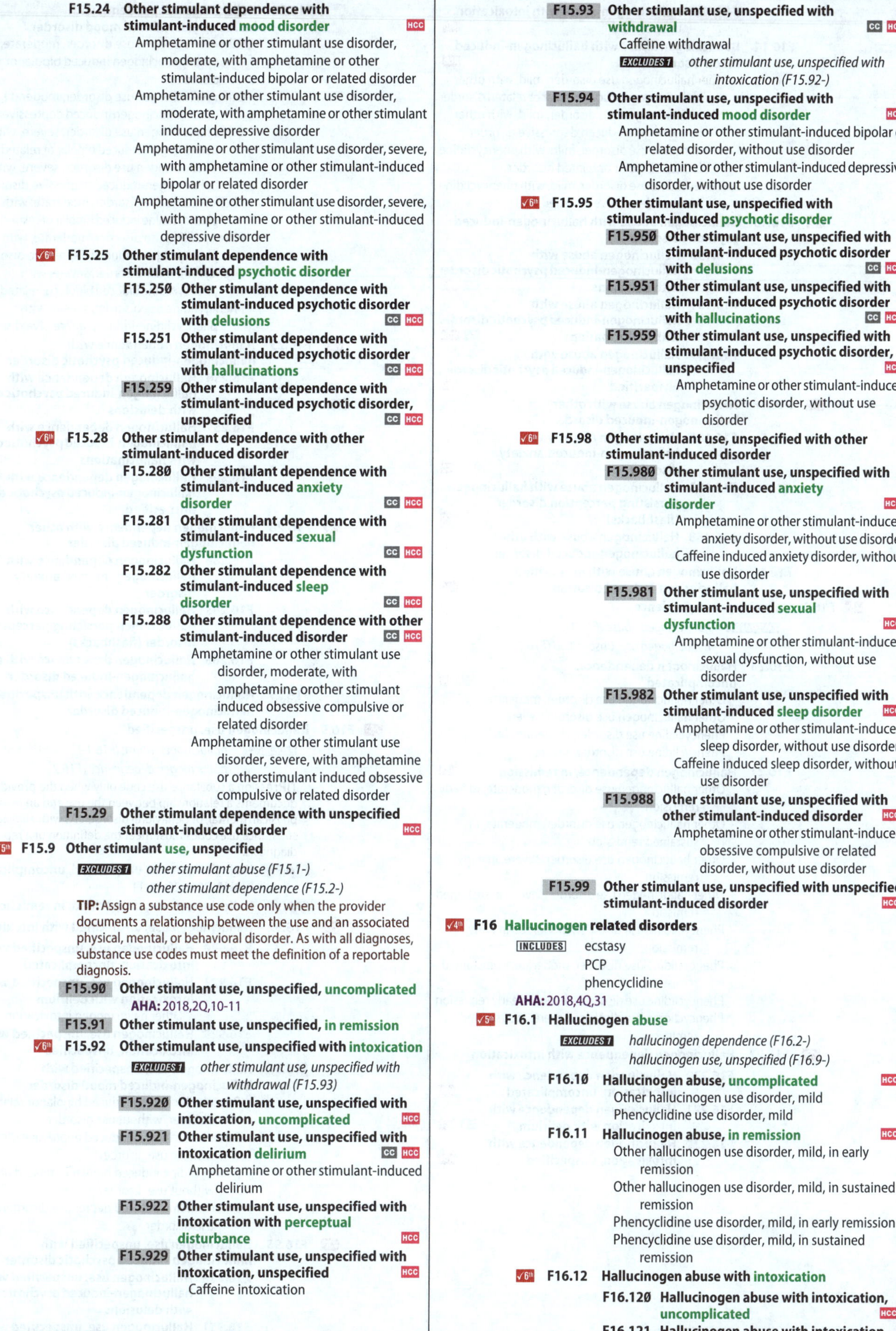

F15.24 Other stimulant dependence with stimulant-induced mood disorder HCC
Amphetamine or other stimulant use disorder, moderate, with amphetamine or other stimulant-induced bipolar or related disorder
Amphetamine or other stimulant use disorder, moderate, with amphetamine or other stimulant induced depressive disorder
Amphetamine or other stimulant use disorder, severe, with amphetamine or other stimulant-induced bipolar or related disorder
Amphetamine or other stimulant use disorder, severe, with amphetamine or other stimulant-induced depressive disorder

F15.25 Other stimulant dependence with stimulant-induced psychotic disorder

F15.250 Other stimulant dependence with stimulant-induced psychotic disorder with delusions CC HCC

F15.251 Other stimulant dependence with stimulant-induced psychotic disorder with hallucinations CC HCC

F15.259 Other stimulant dependence with stimulant-induced psychotic disorder, unspecified CC HCC

F15.28 Other stimulant dependence with other stimulant-induced disorder

F15.280 Other stimulant dependence with stimulant-induced anxiety disorder CC HCC

F15.281 Other stimulant dependence with stimulant-induced sexual dysfunction CC HCC

F15.282 Other stimulant dependence with stimulant-induced sleep disorder CC HCC

F15.288 Other stimulant dependence with other stimulant-induced disorder CC HCC
Amphetamine or other stimulant use disorder, moderate, with amphetamine orother stimulant induced obsessive compulsive or related disorder
Amphetamine or other stimulant use disorder, severe, with amphetamine or otherstimulant induced obsessive compulsive or related disorder

F15.29 Other stimulant dependence with unspecified stimulant-induced disorder HCC

F15.9 Other stimulant use, unspecified

EXCLUDES 1 *other stimulant abuse (F15.1-)*
other stimulant dependence (F15.2-)

TIP: Assign a substance use code only when the provider documents a relationship between the use and an associated physical, mental, or behavioral disorder. As with all diagnoses, substance use codes must meet the definition of a reportable diagnosis.

F15.90 Other stimulant use, unspecified, uncomplicated
AHA: 2018,2Q,10-11

• **F15.91 Other stimulant use, unspecified, in remission**

F15.92 Other stimulant use, unspecified with intoxication

EXCLUDES 1 *other stimulant use, unspecified with withdrawal (F15.93)*

F15.920 Other stimulant use, unspecified with intoxication, uncomplicated HCC

F15.921 Other stimulant use, unspecified with intoxication delirium CC HCC
Amphetamine or other stimulant-induced delirium

F15.922 Other stimulant use, unspecified with intoxication with perceptual disturbance HCC

F15.929 Other stimulant use, unspecified with intoxication, unspecified HCC
Caffeine intoxication

F15.93 Other stimulant use, unspecified with withdrawal CC HCC
Caffeine withdrawal

EXCLUDES 1 *other stimulant use, unspecified with intoxication (F15.92-)*

F15.94 Other stimulant use, unspecified with stimulant-induced mood disorder HCC
Amphetamine or other stimulant-induced bipolar or related disorder, without use disorder
Amphetamine or other stimulant-induced depressive disorder, without use disorder

F15.95 Other stimulant use, unspecified with stimulant-induced psychotic disorder

F15.950 Other stimulant use, unspecified with stimulant-induced psychotic disorder with delusions CC HCC

F15.951 Other stimulant use, unspecified with stimulant-induced psychotic disorder with hallucinations CC HCC

F15.959 Other stimulant use, unspecified with stimulant-induced psychotic disorder, unspecified HCC
Amphetamine or other stimulant-induced psychotic disorder, without use disorder

F15.98 Other stimulant use, unspecified with other stimulant-induced disorder

F15.980 Other stimulant use, unspecified with stimulant-induced anxiety disorder HCC
Amphetamine or other stimulant-induced anxiety disorder, without use disorder
Caffeine induced anxiety disorder, without use disorder

F15.981 Other stimulant use, unspecified with stimulant-induced sexual dysfunction HCC
Amphetamine or other stimulant-induced sexual dysfunction, without use disorder

F15.982 Other stimulant use, unspecified with stimulant-induced sleep disorder HCC
Amphetamine or other stimulant-induced sleep disorder, without use disorder
Caffeine induced sleep disorder, without use disorder

F15.988 Other stimulant use, unspecified with other stimulant-induced disorder HCC
Amphetamine or other stimulant-induced obsessive compulsive or related disorder, without use disorder

F15.99 Other stimulant use, unspecified with unspecified stimulant-induced disorder HCC

F16 Hallucinogen related disorders

INCLUDES ecstasy
PCP
phencyclidine

AHA: 2018,4Q,31

F16.1 Hallucinogen abuse

EXCLUDES 1 *hallucinogen dependence (F16.2-)*
hallucinogen use, unspecified (F16.9-)

F16.10 Hallucinogen abuse, uncomplicated HCC
Other hallucinogen use disorder, mild
Phencyclidine use disorder, mild

F16.11 Hallucinogen abuse, in remission HCC
Other hallucinogen use disorder, mild, in early remission
Other hallucinogen use disorder, mild, in sustained remission
Phencyclidine use disorder, mild, in early remission
Phencyclidine use disorder, mild, in sustained remission

F16.12 Hallucinogen abuse with intoxication

F16.120 Hallucinogen abuse with intoxication, uncomplicated HCC

F16.121 Hallucinogen abuse with intoxication with delirium CC HCC

F16.122 Hallucinogen abuse with intoxication with perceptual disturbance HCC

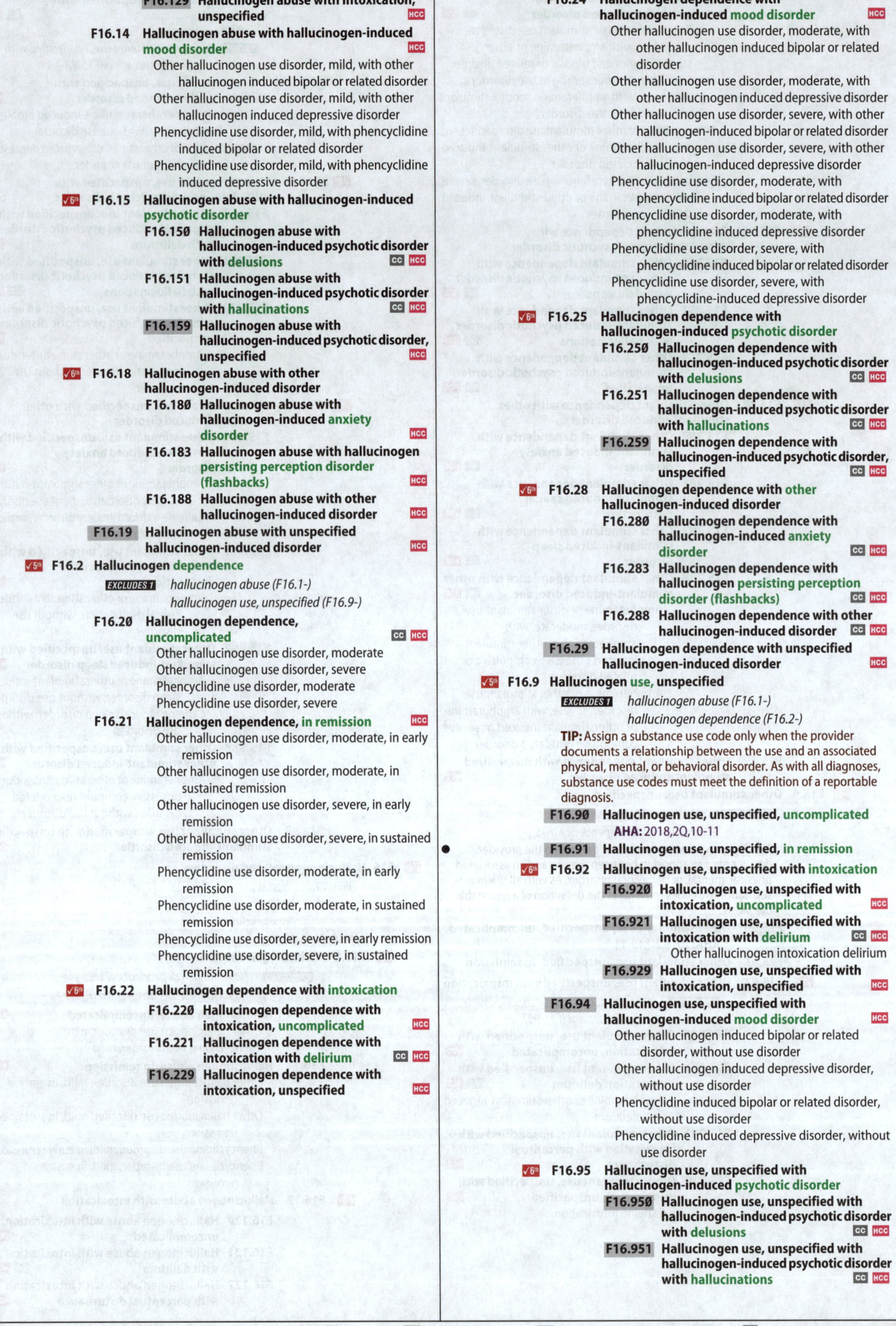

F16.129 Hallucinogen abuse with intoxication, unspecified HCC

F16.14 Hallucinogen abuse with hallucinogen-induced mood disorder HCC
- Other hallucinogen use disorder, mild, with other hallucinogen induced bipolar or related disorder
- Other hallucinogen use disorder, mild, with other hallucinogen induced depressive disorder
- Phencyclidine use disorder, mild, with phencyclidine induced bipolar or related disorder
- Phencyclidine use disorder, mild, with phencyclidine induced depressive disorder

√6th **F16.15 Hallucinogen abuse with hallucinogen-induced psychotic disorder**

F16.15Ø Hallucinogen abuse with hallucinogen-induced psychotic disorder with delusions CC HCC

F16.151 Hallucinogen abuse with hallucinogen-induced psychotic disorder with hallucinations CC HCC

F16.159 Hallucinogen abuse with hallucinogen-induced psychotic disorder, unspecified HCC

√6th **F16.18 Hallucinogen abuse with other hallucinogen-induced disorder**

F16.18Ø Hallucinogen abuse with hallucinogen-induced anxiety disorder HCC

F16.183 Hallucinogen abuse with hallucinogen persisting perception disorder (flashbacks) HCC

F16.188 Hallucinogen abuse with other hallucinogen-induced disorder HCC

F16.19 Hallucinogen abuse with unspecified hallucinogen-induced disorder HCC

√5th **F16.2 Hallucinogen dependence**

EXCLUDES 1 *hallucinogen abuse (F16.1-)*
hallucinogen use, unspecified (F16.9-)

F16.2Ø Hallucinogen dependence, uncomplicated CC HCC
- Other hallucinogen use disorder, moderate
- Other hallucinogen use disorder, severe
- Phencyclidine use disorder, moderate
- Phencyclidine use disorder, severe

F16.21 Hallucinogen dependence, in remission HCC
- Other hallucinogen use disorder, moderate, in early remission
- Other hallucinogen use disorder, moderate, in sustained remission
- Other hallucinogen use disorder, severe, in early remission
- Other hallucinogen use disorder, severe, in sustained remission
- Phencyclidine use disorder, moderate, in early remission
- Phencyclidine use disorder, moderate, in sustained remission
- Phencyclidine use disorder, severe, in early remission
- Phencyclidine use disorder, severe, in sustained remission

√6th **F16.22 Hallucinogen dependence with intoxication**

F16.22Ø Hallucinogen dependence with intoxication, uncomplicated HCC

F16.221 Hallucinogen dependence with intoxication with delirium CC HCC

F16.229 Hallucinogen dependence with intoxication, unspecified HCC

F16.24 Hallucinogen dependence with hallucinogen-induced mood disorder HCC
- Other hallucinogen use disorder, moderate, with other hallucinogen induced bipolar or related disorder
- Other hallucinogen use disorder, moderate, with other hallucinogen induced depressive disorder
- Other hallucinogen use disorder, severe, with other hallucinogen-induced bipolar or related disorder
- Other hallucinogen use disorder, severe, with other hallucinogen-induced depressive disorder
- Phencyclidine use disorder, moderate, with phencyclidine induced bipolar or related disorder
- Phencyclidine use disorder, moderate, with phencyclidine induced depressive disorder
- Phencyclidine use disorder, severe, with phencyclidine induced bipolar or related disorder
- Phencyclidine use disorder, severe, with phencyclidine-induced depressive disorder

√6th **F16.25 Hallucinogen dependence with hallucinogen-induced psychotic disorder**

F16.25Ø Hallucinogen dependence with hallucinogen-induced psychotic disorder with delusions CC HCC

F16.251 Hallucinogen dependence with hallucinogen-induced psychotic disorder with hallucinations CC HCC

F16.259 Hallucinogen dependence with hallucinogen-induced psychotic disorder, unspecified CC HCC

√6th **F16.28 Hallucinogen dependence with other hallucinogen-induced disorder**

F16.28Ø Hallucinogen dependence with hallucinogen-induced anxiety disorder CC HCC

F16.283 Hallucinogen dependence with hallucinogen persisting perception disorder (flashbacks) CC HCC

F16.288 Hallucinogen dependence with other hallucinogen-induced disorder CC HCC

F16.29 Hallucinogen dependence with unspecified hallucinogen-induced disorder HCC

√5th **F16.9 Hallucinogen use, unspecified**

EXCLUDES 1 *hallucinogen abuse (F16.1-)*
hallucinogen dependence (F16.2-)

TIP: Assign a substance use code only when the provider documents a relationship between the use and an associated physical, mental, or behavioral disorder. As with all diagnoses, substance use codes must meet the definition of a reportable diagnosis.

F16.9Ø Hallucinogen use, unspecified, uncomplicated
AHA: 2018,2Q,10-11

● **F16.91 Hallucinogen use, unspecified, in remission**

√6th **F16.92 Hallucinogen use, unspecified with intoxication**

F16.92Ø Hallucinogen use, unspecified with intoxication, uncomplicated HCC

F16.921 Hallucinogen use, unspecified with intoxication with delirium CC HCC
- Other hallucinogen intoxication delirium

F16.929 Hallucinogen use, unspecified with intoxication, unspecified HCC

F16.94 Hallucinogen use, unspecified with hallucinogen-induced mood disorder HCC
- Other hallucinogen induced bipolar or related disorder, without use disorder
- Other hallucinogen induced depressive disorder, without use disorder
- Phencyclidine induced bipolar or related disorder, without use disorder
- Phencyclidine induced depressive disorder, without use disorder

√6th **F16.95 Hallucinogen use, unspecified with hallucinogen-induced psychotic disorder**

F16.95Ø Hallucinogen use, unspecified with hallucinogen-induced psychotic disorder with delusions CC HCC

F16.951 Hallucinogen use, unspecified with hallucinogen-induced psychotic disorder with hallucinations CC HCC

F16.959 Hallucinogen use, unspecified with hallucinogen-induced psychotic disorder, unspecified HCC

Other hallucinogen induced psychotic disorder, without use disorder

Phencyclidine induced psychotic disorder, without use disorder

✓6th **F16.98 Hallucinogen use, unspecified with other specified hallucinogen-induced disorder**

F16.980 Hallucinogen use, unspecified with hallucinogen-induced anxiety disorder HCC

Other hallucinogen-induced anxiety disorder, without use disorder

Phencyclidine induced anxiety disorder, without use disorder

F16.983 Hallucinogen use, unspecified with hallucinogen persisting perception disorder (flashbacks) HCC

F16.988 Hallucinogen use, unspecified with other hallucinogen-induced disorder HCC

F16.99 Hallucinogen use, unspecified with unspecified hallucinogen-induced disorder HCC

✓4th **F17 Nicotine dependence**

EXCLUDES 1 *history of tobacco dependence (Z87.891)*

tobacco use NOS (Z72.0)

EXCLUDES 2 *tobacco use (smoking) during pregnancy, childbirth and the puerperium (O99.33-)*

toxic effect of nicotine (T65.2-)

AHA: 2013,4Q,108-109

✓5th **F17.2 Nicotine dependence**

✓6th **F17.20 Nicotine dependence, unspecified**

F17.200 Nicotine dependence, unspecified, uncomplicated UPD

Tobacco use disorder, mild

Tobacco use disorder, moderate

Tobacco use disorder, severe

AHA: 2016,1Q,36

TIP: Assign when provider documentation indicates "smoker" without further specification.

F17.201 Nicotine dependence, unspecified, in remission UPD

Tobacco use disorder, mild, in early remission

Tobacco use disorder, mild, in sustained remission

Tobacco use disorder, moderate, in early remission

Tobacco use disorder, moderate, in sustained remission

Tobacco use disorder, severe, in early remission

Tobacco use disorder, severe, in sustained remission

F17.203 Nicotine dependence unspecified, with withdrawal CC

Tobacco withdrawal

F17.208 Nicotine dependence, unspecified, with other nicotine-induced disorders

F17.209 Nicotine dependence, unspecified, with unspecified nicotine-induced disorders

✓6th **F17.21 Nicotine dependence, cigarettes**

F17.210 Nicotine dependence, cigarettes, uncomplicated UPD

AHA: 2017,2Q,28-29

F17.211 Nicotine dependence, cigarettes, in remission UPD

Tobacco use disorder, cigarettes, mild, in early remission

Tobacco use disorder, cigarettes, mild, in sustained remission

Tobacco use disorder, cigarettes, moderate, in early remission

Tobacco use disorder, cigarettes, moderate, in sustained remission

Tobacco use disorder, cigarettes, severe, in early remission

Tobacco use disorder, cigarettes, severe, in sustained remission

F17.213 Nicotine dependence, cigarettes, with withdrawal CC

F17.218 Nicotine dependence, cigarettes, with other nicotine-induced disorders

F17.219 Nicotine dependence, cigarettes, with unspecified nicotine-induced disorders

✓6th **F17.22 Nicotine dependence, chewing tobacco**

F17.220 Nicotine dependence, chewing tobacco, uncomplicated UPD

F17.221 Nicotine dependence, chewing tobacco, in remission UPD

Tobacco use disorder, chewing tobacco, mild, in early remission

Tobacco use disorder, chewing tobacco, mild, in sustained remission

Tobacco use disorder, chewing tobacco, moderate, in early remission

Tobacco use disorder, chewing tobacco, moderate, in sustained remission

Tobacco use disorder, chewing tobacco, severe, in early remission

Tobacco use disorder, chewing tobacco, severe, in sustained remission

F17.223 Nicotine dependence, chewing tobacco, with withdrawal CC

F17.228 Nicotine dependence, chewing tobacco, with other nicotine-induced disorders

F17.229 Nicotine dependence, chewing tobacco, with unspecified nicotine-induced disorders

✓6th **F17.29 Nicotine dependence, other tobacco product**

F17.290 Nicotine dependence, other tobacco product, uncomplicated UPD

AHA: 2017,2Q,28-29

F17.291 Nicotine dependence, other tobacco product, in remission UPD

Tobacco use disorder, other tobacco product, mild, in early remission

Tobacco use disorder, other tobacco product, mild, in sustained remission

Tobacco use disorder, other tobacco product, moderate, in early remission

Tobacco use disorder, other tobacco product, moderate, in sustained remission

Tobacco use disorder, other tobacco product, severe, in early remission

Tobacco use disorder, other tobacco product, severe, in sustained remission

F17.293 Nicotine dependence, other tobacco product, with withdrawal CC

F17.298 Nicotine dependence, other tobacco product, with other nicotine-induced disorders

F17.299 Nicotine dependence, other tobacco product, with unspecified nicotine-induced disorders

F18 Inhalant related disorders

INCLUDES volatile solvents

F18.1 Inhalant abuse

EXCLUDES 1 *inhalant dependence (F18.2-)*
inhalant use, unspecified (F18.9-)

F18.10 Inhalant abuse, uncomplicated HCC
Inhalant use disorder, mild

F18.11 Inhalant abuse, in remission HCC
Inhalant use disorder, mild, in early remission
Inhalant use disorder, mild, in sustained remission

F18.12 Inhalant abuse with intoxication

F18.120 Inhalant abuse with intoxication, uncomplicated HCC

F18.121 Inhalant abuse with intoxication delirium CC HCC

F18.129 Inhalant abuse with intoxication, unspecified HCC

F18.14 Inhalant abuse with inhalant-induced mood disorder HCC
Inhalant use disorder, mild, with inhalant induced depressive disorder

F18.15 Inhalant abuse with inhalant-induced psychotic disorder

F18.150 Inhalant abuse with inhalant-induced psychotic disorder with delusions CC HCC

F18.151 Inhalant abuse with inhalant-induced psychotic disorder with hallucinations CC HCC

F18.159 Inhalant abuse with inhalant-induced psychotic disorder, unspecified HCC

F18.17 Inhalant abuse with inhalant-induced dementia CC HCC
Inhalant use disorder, mild, with inhalant induced major neurocognitive disorder

F18.18 Inhalant abuse with other inhalant-induced disorders

F18.180 Inhalant abuse with inhalant-induced anxiety disorder HCC

F18.188 Inhalant abuse with other inhalant-induced disorder HCC
Inhalant use disorder, mild, with inhalant induced mild neurocognitive disorder

F18.19 Inhalant abuse with unspecified inhalant-induced disorder HCC

F18.2 Inhalant dependence

EXCLUDES 1 *inhalant abuse (F18.1-)*
inhalant use, unspecified (F18.9-)

F18.20 Inhalant dependence, uncomplicated CC HCC
Inhalant use disorder, moderate
Inhalant use disorder, severe

F18.21 Inhalant dependence, in remission HCC
Inhalant use disorder, moderate, in early remission
Inhalant use disorder, moderate, in sustained remission
Inhalant use disorder, severe, in early remission
Inhalant use disorder, severe, in sustained remission

F18.22 Inhalant dependence with intoxication

F18.220 Inhalant dependence with intoxication, uncomplicated HCC

F18.221 Inhalant dependence with intoxication delirium CC HCC

F18.229 Inhalant dependence with intoxication, unspecified HCC

F18.24 Inhalant dependence with inhalant-induced mood disorder HCC
Inhalant use disorder, moderate, with inhalant induced depressive disorder
Inhalant use disorder, severe, with inhalant induced depressive disorder

F18.25 Inhalant dependence with inhalant-induced psychotic disorder

F18.250 Inhalant dependence with inhalant-induced psychotic disorder with delusions CC HCC

F18.251 Inhalant dependence with inhalant-induced psychotic disorder with hallucinations CC HCC

F18.259 Inhalant dependence with inhalant-induced psychotic disorder, unspecified CC HCC

F18.27 Inhalant dependence with inhalant-induced dementia CC HCC
Inhalant use disorder, moderate, with inhalant induced major neurocognitive disorder
Inhalant use disorder, severe, with inhalant induced major neurocognitive disorder

F18.28 Inhalant dependence with other inhalant-induced disorders

F18.280 Inhalant dependence with inhalant-induced anxiety disorder CC HCC

F18.288 Inhalant dependence with other inhalant-induced disorder CC HCC
Inhalant use disorder, moderate, with inhalant-induced mild neurocognitive disorder
Inhalant use disorder, severe, with inhalant-induced mild neurocognitive disorder

F18.29 Inhalant dependence with unspecified inhalant-induced disorder HCC

F18.9 Inhalant use, unspecified

EXCLUDES 1 *inhalant abuse (F18.1-)*
inhalant dependence (F18.2-)

TIP: Assign a substance use code only when the provider documents a relationship between the use and an associated physical, mental, or behavioral disorder. As with all diagnoses, substance use codes must meet the definition of a reportable diagnosis.

F18.90 Inhalant use, unspecified, uncomplicated
AHA: 2018,2Q,10-11

● **F18.91 Inhalant use, unspecified, in remission**

F18.92 Inhalant use, unspecified with intoxication

F18.920 Inhalant use, unspecified with intoxication, uncomplicated HCC

F18.921 Inhalant use, unspecified with intoxication with delirium CC HCC

F18.929 Inhalant use, unspecified with intoxication, unspecified HCC

F18.94 Inhalant use, unspecified with inhalant-induced mood disorder HCC
Inhalant induced depressive disorder

F18.95 Inhalant use, unspecified with inhalant-induced psychotic disorder

F18.950 Inhalant use, unspecified with inhalant-induced psychotic disorder with delusions CC HCC

F18.951 Inhalant use, unspecified with inhalant-induced psychotic disorder with hallucinations CC HCC

F18.959 Inhalant use, unspecified with inhalant-induced psychotic disorder, unspecified HCC

F18.97 Inhalant use, unspecified with inhalant-induced persisting dementia CC HCC
Inhalant-induced major neurocognitive disorder

F18.98 Inhalant use, unspecified with other inhalant-induced disorders

F18.980 Inhalant use, unspecified with inhalant-induced anxiety disorder HCC

F18.988 Inhalant use, unspecified with other inhalant-induced disorder HCC
Inhalant-induced mild neurocognitive disorder

F18.99 Inhalant use, unspecified with unspecified inhalant-induced disorder HCC

F19 Other psychoactive substance related disorders

INCLUDES polysubstance drug use (indiscriminate drug use)

F19.1 Other psychoactive substance abuse

EXCLUDES 1 *other psychoactive substance dependence (F19.2-)*
other psychoactive substance use, unspecified (F19.9-)

F19.10 Other psychoactive substance abuse, uncomplicated HCC
Other (or unknown) substance use disorder, mild

F19.11 Other psychoactive substance abuse, in remission HCC
Other (or unknown) substance use disorder, mild, in early remission
Other (or unknown) substance use disorder, mild, in sustained remission

✓6th **F19.12 Other psychoactive substance abuse with intoxication**

F19.120 Other psychoactive substance abuse with intoxication, uncomplicated HCC

F19.121 Other psychoactive substance abuse with intoxication delirium CC HCC

F19.122 Other psychoactive substance abuse with intoxication with perceptual disturbances HCC

F19.129 Other psychoactive substance abuse with intoxication, unspecified HCC

✓6th **F19.13 Other psychoactive substance abuse with withdrawal**
AHA: 2020,4Q,16-17

F19.130 Other psychoactive substance abuse with withdrawal, uncomplicated CC HCC

F19.131 Other psychoactive substance abuse with withdrawal delirium CC HCC

F19.132 Other psychoactive substance abuse with withdrawal with perceptual disturbance CC HCC

F19.139 Other psychoactive substance abuse with withdrawal, unspecified CC HCC

F19.14 Other psychoactive substance abuse with psychoactive substance-induced mood disorder HCC
Other (or unknown) substance use disorder, mild, with other (or unknown) substance-induced bipolar or related disorder
Other (or unknown) substance use disorder, mild, with other (or unknown) substance-induced depressive disorder

✓6th **F19.15 Other psychoactive substance abuse with psychoactive substance-induced psychotic disorder**

F19.150 Other psychoactive substance abuse with psychoactive substance-induced psychotic disorder with delusions CC HCC

F19.151 Other psychoactive substance abuse with psychoactive substance-induced psychotic disorder with hallucinations CC HCC

F19.159 Other psychoactive substance abuse with psychoactive substance-induced psychotic disorder, unspecified HCC

F19.16 Other psychoactive substance abuse with psychoactive substance-induced persisting amnestic disorder HCC

F19.17 Other psychoactive substance abuse with psychoactive substance-induced persisting dementia CC HCC
Other (or unknown) substance use disorder, mild, with other (or unknown) substance-induced major neurocognitive disorder

✓6th **F19.18 Other psychoactive substance abuse with other psychoactive substance-induced disorders**

F19.180 Other psychoactive substance abuse with psychoactive substance-induced anxiety disorder HCC

F19.181 Other psychoactive substance abuse with psychoactive substance-induced sexual dysfunction HCC

F19.182 Other psychoactive substance abuse with psychoactive substance-induced sleep disorder HCC

F19.188 Other psychoactive substance abuse with other psychoactive substance-induced disorder HCC
Other (or unknown) substance use disorder, mild, with other (or unknown) substance induced mild neurocognitive disorder
Other (or unknown) substance use disorder, mild, with other (or unknown) substance induced obsessive-compulsive or related disorder

F19.19 Other psychoactive substance abuse with unspecified psychoactive substance-induced disorder HCC

✓5th **F19.2 Other psychoactive substance dependence**
EXCLUDES 1 *other psychoactive substance abuse (F19.1-)*
other psychoactive substance use, unspecified (F19.9-)

F19.20 Other psychoactive substance dependence, uncomplicated CC HCC
Other (or unknown) substance use disorder, moderate
Other (or unknown) substance use disorder, severe

F19.21 Other psychoactive substance dependence, in remission HCC
Other (or unknown) substance use disorder, moderate, in early remission
Other (or unknown) substance use disorder, moderate, in sustained remission
Other (or unknown) substance use disorder, severe, in early remission
Other (or unknown) substance use disorder, severe, in sustained remission

✓6th **F19.22 Other psychoactive substance dependence with intoxication**
EXCLUDES 1 *other psychoactive substance dependence with withdrawal (F19.23-)*

F19.220 Other psychoactive substance dependence with intoxication, uncomplicated HCC

F19.221 Other psychoactive substance dependence with intoxication delirium CC HCC

F19.222 Other psychoactive substance dependence with intoxication with perceptual disturbance CC HCC

F19.229 Other psychoactive substance dependence with intoxication, unspecified HCC

✓6th **F19.23 Other psychoactive substance dependence with withdrawal**
EXCLUDES 1 *other psychoactive substance dependence with intoxication (F19.22-)*

F19.230 Other psychoactive substance dependence with withdrawal, uncomplicated CC HCC

F19.231 Other psychoactive substance dependence with withdrawal delirium CC HCC

F19.232 Other psychoactive substance dependence with withdrawal with perceptual disturbance CC HCC

F19.239 Other psychoactive substance dependence with withdrawal, unspecified CC HCC

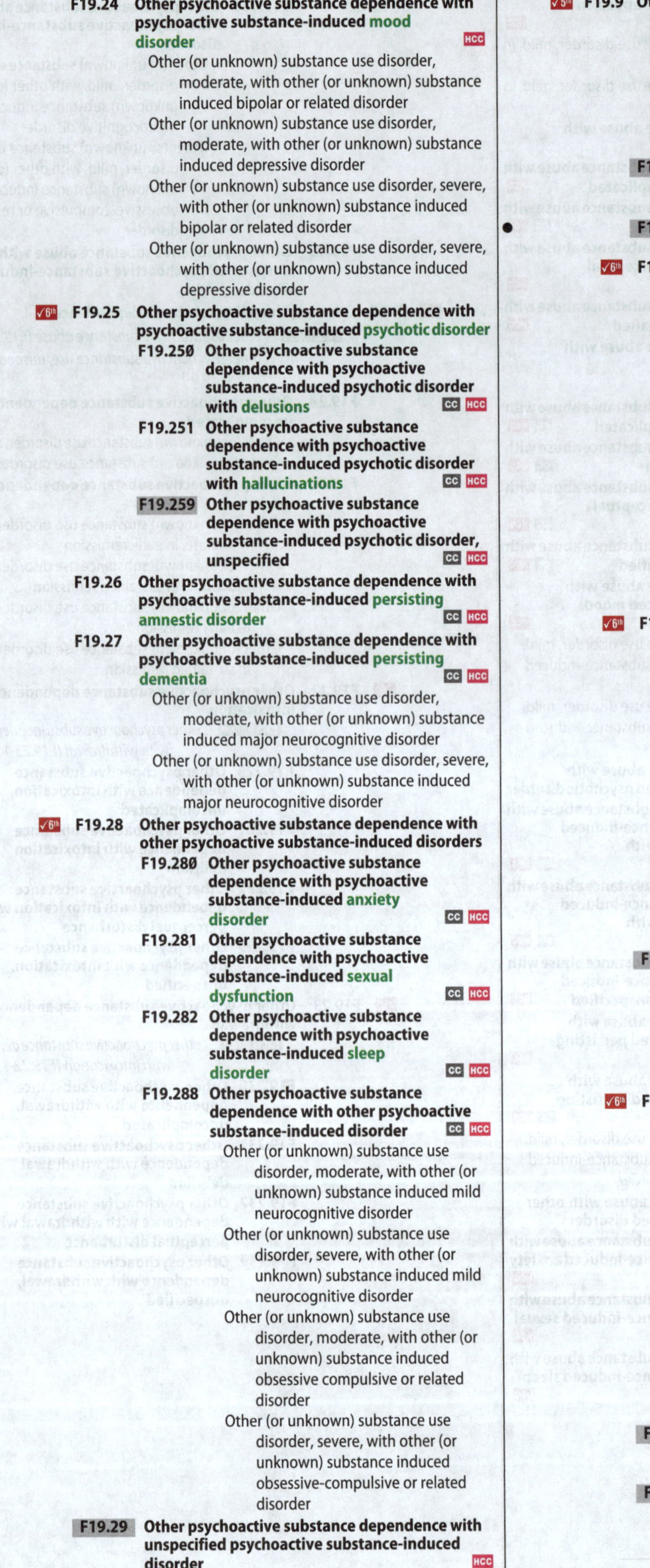

F19.24 Other psychoactive substance dependence with psychoactive substance-induced mood disorder HCC
- Other (or unknown) substance use disorder, moderate, with other (or unknown) substance induced bipolar or related disorder
- Other (or unknown) substance use disorder, moderate, with other (or unknown) substance induced depressive disorder
- Other (or unknown) substance use disorder, severe, with other (or unknown) substance induced bipolar or related disorder
- Other (or unknown) substance use disorder, severe, with other (or unknown) substance induced depressive disorder

✓6th **F19.25 Other psychoactive substance dependence with psychoactive substance-induced psychotic disorder**

F19.250 Other psychoactive substance dependence with psychoactive substance-induced psychotic disorder with delusions CC HCC

F19.251 Other psychoactive substance dependence with psychoactive substance-induced psychotic disorder with hallucinations CC HCC

F19.259 Other psychoactive substance dependence with psychoactive substance-induced psychotic disorder, unspecified CC HCC

F19.26 Other psychoactive substance dependence with psychoactive substance-induced persisting amnestic disorder CC HCC

F19.27 Other psychoactive substance dependence with psychoactive substance-induced persisting dementia CC HCC
- Other (or unknown) substance use disorder, moderate, with other (or unknown) substance induced major neurocognitive disorder
- Other (or unknown) substance use disorder, severe, with other (or unknown) substance induced major neurocognitive disorder

✓6th **F19.28 Other psychoactive substance dependence with other psychoactive substance-induced disorders**

F19.280 Other psychoactive substance dependence with psychoactive substance-induced anxiety disorder CC HCC

F19.281 Other psychoactive substance dependence with psychoactive substance-induced sexual dysfunction CC HCC

F19.282 Other psychoactive substance dependence with psychoactive substance-induced sleep disorder CC HCC

F19.288 Other psychoactive substance dependence with other psychoactive substance-induced disorder CC HCC
- Other (or unknown) substance use disorder, moderate, with other (or unknown) substance induced mild neurocognitive disorder
- Other (or unknown) substance use disorder, severe, with other (or unknown) substance induced mild neurocognitive disorder
- Other (or unknown) substance use disorder, moderate, with other (or unknown) substance induced obsessive compulsive or related disorder
- Other (or unknown) substance use disorder, severe, with other (or unknown) substance induced obsessive-compulsive or related disorder

F19.29 Other psychoactive substance dependence with unspecified psychoactive substance-induced disorder HCC

✓5th **F19.9 Other psychoactive substance use, unspecified**

EXCLUDES 1 *other psychoactive substance abuse (F19.1-)*
other psychoactive substance dependence (F19.2-)

TIP: Assign a substance use code only when the provider documents a relationship between the use and an associated physical, mental, or behavioral disorder. As with all diagnoses, substance use codes must meet the definition of a reportable diagnosis.

F19.90 Other psychoactive substance use, unspecified, uncomplicated
AHA: 2018,2Q,10-11

● **F19.91 Other psychoactive substance use, unspecified, in remission**

✓6th **F19.92 Other psychoactive substance use, unspecified with intoxication**

EXCLUDES 1 *other psychoactive substance use, unspecified with withdrawal (F19.93)*

F19.920 Other psychoactive substance use, unspecified with intoxication, uncomplicated HCC

F19.921 Other psychoactive substance use, unspecified with intoxication with delirium CC HCC
- Other (or unknown) substance-induced delirium

F19.922 Other psychoactive substance use, unspecified with intoxication with perceptual disturbance HCC

F19.929 Other psychoactive substance use, unspecified with intoxication, unspecified HCC

✓6th **F19.93 Other psychoactive substance use, unspecified with withdrawal**

EXCLUDES 1 *other psychoactive substance use, unspecified with intoxication (F19.92-)*

F19.930 Other psychoactive substance use, unspecified with withdrawal, uncomplicated CC HCC

F19.931 Other psychoactive substance use, unspecified with withdrawal delirium CC HCC

F19.932 Other psychoactive substance use, unspecified with withdrawal with perceptual disturbance CC HCC

F19.939 Other psychoactive substance use, unspecified with withdrawal, unspecified CC HCC

F19.94 Other psychoactive substance use, unspecified with psychoactive substance-induced mood disorder HCC
- Other (or unknown) substance-induced bipolar or related disorder, without use disorder
- Other (or unknown) substance-induced depressive disorder, without use disorder

✓6th **F19.95 Other psychoactive substance use, unspecified with psychoactive substance-induced psychotic disorder**

F19.950 Other psychoactive substance use, unspecified with psychoactive substance-induced psychotic disorder with delusions CC HCC

F19.951 Other psychoactive substance use, unspecified with psychoactive substance-induced psychotic disorder with hallucinations CC HCC

F19.959 Other psychoactive substance use, unspecified with psychoactive substance-induced psychotic disorder, unspecified HCC
- Other or unknown substance-induced psychotic disorder, without use disorder

F19.96 Other psychoactive substance use, unspecified with psychoactive substance-induced persisting amnestic disorder HCC

F19.97 Other psychoactive substance use, unspecified with psychoactive substance-induced persisting dementia CC HCC
- Other (or unknown) substance-induced major neurocognitive disorder, without use disorder

✓6th **F19.98 Other psychoactive substance use, unspecified with other psychoactive substance-induced disorders**

F19.980 Other psychoactive substance use, unspecified with psychoactive substance-induced anxiety disorder HCC
Other (or unknown) substance-induced anxiety disorder, without use disorder

F19.981 Other psychoactive substance use, unspecified with psychoactive substance-induced sexual dysfunction HCC
Other (or unknown) substance-induced sexual dysfunction, without use disorder

F19.982 Other psychoactive substance use, unspecified with psychoactive substance-induced sleep disorder HCC
Other (or unknown) substance-induced sleep disorder, without use disorder

F19.988 Other psychoactive substance use, unspecified with other psychoactive substance-induced disorder HCC
Other (or unknown) substance-induced mild neurocognitive disorder, without use disorder
Other (or unknown) substance-induced obsessive-compulsive or related disorder, without use disorder

F19.99 Other psychoactive substance use, unspecified with unspecified psychoactive substance-induced disorder HCC

Schizophrenia, schizotypal, delusional, and other non-mood psychotic disorders (F2Ø-F29)

✓4th **F2Ø Schizophrenia**

EXCLUDES 1 *brief psychotic disorder (F23)*
cyclic schizophrenia (F25.Ø)
mood [affective] disorders with psychotic symptoms (F3Ø.2, F31.2, F31.5, F31.64, F32.3, F33.3)
schizoaffective disorder (F25.-)
schizophrenic reaction NOS (F23)

EXCLUDES 2 *schizophrenic reaction in:*
alcoholism (F1Ø.15-, F1Ø.25-, F1Ø.95-)
brain disease (FØ6.2)
epilepsy (FØ6.2)
psychoactive drug use (F11-F19 with .15, .25, .95)
schizotypal disorder (F21)

DEF: Group of disorders with disturbances in thought (delusions, hallucinations), mood (blunted, flattened, inappropriate affect), and sense of self. Schizophrenia also includes bizarre, purposeless behavior, repetitious activity, or inactivity.

F2Ø.Ø Paranoid schizophrenia CC HCC
Paraphrenic schizophrenia
EXCLUDES 1 *involutional paranoid state (F22)*
paranoia (F22)
DEF: Preoccupied with delusional suspicions and auditory hallucinations related to a single theme. This type of schizophrenia is usually hostile, grandiose, threatening, persecutory, and occasionally hypochondriacal.

F2Ø.1 Disorganized schizophrenia CC HCC
Hebephrenic schizophrenia
Hebephrenia

F2Ø.2 Catatonic schizophrenia CC HCC
Schizophrenic catalepsy
Schizophrenic catatonia
Schizophrenic flexibilitas cerea
EXCLUDES 1 *catatonic stupor (R4Ø.1)*
DEF: Extreme changes in motor activity. One extreme is a decreased response or reaction to the environment and the other is spontaneous activity.

F2Ø.3 Undifferentiated schizophrenia HCC
Atypical schizophrenia
EXCLUDES 1 *acute schizophrenia-like psychotic disorder (F23)*
EXCLUDES 2 *post-schizophrenic depression (F32.89)*

F2Ø.5 Residual schizophrenia CC HCC
Restzustand (schizophrenic)
Schizophrenic residual state

✓5th **F2Ø.8 Other schizophrenia**

F2Ø.81 Schizophreniform disorder CC HCC
Schizophreniform psychosis NOS

F2Ø.89 Other schizophrenia CC HCC
Cenesthopathic schizophrenia
Simple schizophrenia

F2Ø.9 Schizophrenia, unspecified HCC
AHA: 2019,2Q,32

F21 Schizotypal disorder HCC
Borderline schizophrenia
Latent schizophrenia
Latent schizophrenic reaction
Prepsychotic schizophrenia
Prodromal schizophrenia
Pseudoneurotic schizophrenia
Pseudopsychopathic schizophrenia
Schizotypal personality disorder
EXCLUDES 2 *Asperger's syndrome (F84.5)*
schizoid personality disorder (F6Ø.1)
DEF: Disorder characterized by various oddities of thinking, perception, communication, and behavior that may be manifested as magical thinking, ideas of reference, paranoid ideation, recurrent illusions and derealization (depersonalization), or social isolation.

F22 Delusional disorders HCC
Delusional dysmorphophobia
Involutional paranoid state
Paranoia
Paranoia querulans
Paranoid psychosis
Paranoid state
Paraphrenia (late)
Sensitiver Beziehungswahn
EXCLUDES 1 *mood [affective] disorders with psychotic symptoms (F3Ø.2, F31.2, F31.5, F31.64, F32.3, F33.3)*
paranoid schizophrenia (F2Ø.Ø)
EXCLUDES 2 *paranoid personality disorder (F6Ø.Ø)*
paranoid psychosis, psychogenic (F23)
paranoid reaction (F23)

F23 Brief psychotic disorder CC HCC
Paranoid reaction
Psychogenic paranoid psychosis
EXCLUDES 2 *mood [affective] disorders with psychotic symptoms (F3Ø.2, F31.2, F31.5, F31.64, F32.3, F33.3)*
AHA: 2019,2Q,32

F24 Shared psychotic disorder HCC
Folie à deux
Induced paranoid disorder
Induced psychotic disorder

✓4th **F25 Schizoaffective disorders**
EXCLUDES 1 *mood [affective] disorders with psychotic symptoms (F3Ø.2, F31.2, F31.5, F31.64, F32.3, F33.3)*
schizophrenia (F2Ø.-)

F25.Ø Schizoaffective disorder, bipolar type HCC
Cyclic schizophrenia
Schizoaffective disorder, manic type
Schizoaffective disorder, mixed type
Schizoaffective psychosis, bipolar type

F25.1 Schizoaffective disorder, depressive type HCC
Schizoaffective psychosis, depressive type

F25.8 Other schizoaffective disorders HCC

F25.9 Schizoaffective disorder, unspecified HCC
Schizoaffective psychosis NOS

F28 Other psychotic disorder not due to a substance or known physiological condition HIV HCC
Chronic hallucinatory psychosis
Other specified schizophrenia spectrum and other psychotic disorder

F29 Unspecified psychosis not due to a substance or known physiological condition HIV HCC
Psychosis NOS
Unspecified schizophrenia spectrum and other psychotic disorder
EXCLUDES 1 *mental disorder NOS (F99)*
unspecified mental disorder due to known physiological condition (F09)

Mood [affective] disorders (F30-F39)

F30 Manic episode
INCLUDES bipolar disorder, single manic episode
mixed affective episode
EXCLUDES 1 *bipolar disorder (F31.-)*
major depressive disorder, recurrent (F33.-)
major depressive disorder, single episode (F32.-)
DEF: Mania: Characterized by abnormal states of elation or excitement out of keeping with the individual's circumstances and varying from enhanced liveliness (hypomania) to violent, almost uncontrollable, excitement. Aggression and anger, flight of ideas, distractibility, impaired judgment, and grandiose ideas are common.

F30.1 Manic episode without psychotic symptoms
F30.10 Manic episode without psychotic symptoms, unspecified CC HCC
F30.11 Manic episode without psychotic symptoms, mild CC HCC
F30.12 Manic episode without psychotic symptoms, moderate CC HCC
F30.13 Manic episode, severe, without psychotic symptoms CC HCC
F30.2 Manic episode, severe with psychotic symptoms CC HCC
Manic stupor
Mania with mood-congruent psychotic symptoms
Mania with mood-incongruent psychotic symptoms
F30.3 Manic episode in partial remission HCC
F30.4 Manic episode in full remission HCC
F30.8 Other manic episodes HCC
Hypomania
F30.9 Manic episode, unspecified CC HCC
Mania NOS

F31 Bipolar disorder
INCLUDES bipolar I disorder
bipolar type I disorder
manic-depressive illness
manic-depressive psychosis
manic-depressive reaction
▶seasonal bipolar disorder◀
EXCLUDES 1 *bipolar disorder, single manic episode (F30.-)*
major depressive disorder, recurrent (F33.-)
major depressive disorder, single episode (F32.-)
EXCLUDES 2 *cyclothymia (F34.0)*
AHA: 2020,1Q,23

F31.0 Bipolar disorder, current episode hypomanic CC HCC
F31.1 Bipolar disorder, current episode manic without psychotic features
F31.10 Bipolar disorder, current episode manic without psychotic features, unspecified CC HCC
F31.11 Bipolar disorder, current episode manic without psychotic features, mild CC HCC
F31.12 Bipolar disorder, current episode manic without psychotic features, moderate CC HCC
F31.13 Bipolar disorder, current episode manic without psychotic features, severe CC HCC
F31.2 Bipolar disorder, current episode manic severe with psychotic features CC HCC
Bipolar disorder, current episode manic with mood-congruent psychotic symptoms
Bipolar disorder, current episode manic with mood-incongruent psychotic symptoms
Bipolar I disorder, current or most recent episode manic with psychotic features
F31.3 Bipolar disorder, current episode depressed, mild or moderate severity
F31.30 Bipolar disorder, current episode depressed, mild or moderate severity, unspecified CC HCC
F31.31 Bipolar disorder, current episode depressed, mild CC HCC
F31.32 Bipolar disorder, current episode depressed, moderate CC HCC
F31.4 Bipolar disorder, current episode depressed, severe, without psychotic features CC HCC
F31.5 Bipolar disorder, current episode depressed, severe, with psychotic features CC HCC
Bipolar disorder, current episode depressed with mood-congruent psychotic symptoms
Bipolar disorder, current episode depressed with mood-incongruent psychotic symptoms
Bipolar I disorder, current or most recent episode depressed, with psychotic features
F31.6 Bipolar disorder, current episode mixed
F31.60 Bipolar disorder, current episode mixed, unspecified CC HCC
F31.61 Bipolar disorder, current episode mixed, mild CC HCC
F31.62 Bipolar disorder, current episode mixed, moderate CC HCC
F31.63 Bipolar disorder, current episode mixed, severe, without psychotic features CC HCC
F31.64 Bipolar disorder, current episode mixed, severe, with psychotic features CC HCC
Bipolar disorder, current episode mixed with mood-congruent psychotic symptoms
Bipolar disorder, current episode mixed with mood-incongruent psychotic symptoms
F31.7 Bipolar disorder, currently in remission
F31.70 Bipolar disorder, currently in remission, most recent episode unspecified HCC
F31.71 Bipolar disorder, in partial remission, most recent episode hypomanic HCC
F31.72 Bipolar disorder, in full remission, most recent episode hypomanic HCC
F31.73 Bipolar disorder, in partial remission, most recent episode manic HCC
F31.74 Bipolar disorder, in full remission, most recent episode manic HCC
F31.75 Bipolar disorder, in partial remission, most recent episode depressed HCC
F31.76 Bipolar disorder, in full remission, most recent episode depressed HCC
F31.77 Bipolar disorder, in partial remission, most recent episode mixed HCC
F31.78 Bipolar disorder, in full remission, most recent episode mixed HCC
F31.8 Other bipolar disorders
F31.81 Bipolar II disorder CC HCC
Bipolar disorder, type 2
F31.89 Other bipolar disorder CC HCC
Recurrent manic episodes NOS
F31.9 Bipolar disorder, unspecified HCC
Manic depression
AHA: 2020,1Q,23

F32 Depressive episode
INCLUDES single episode of agitated depression
single episode of depressive reaction
single episode of major depression
single episode of psychogenic depression
single episode of reactive depression
single episode of vital depression
EXCLUDES 1 *bipolar disorder (F31.-)*
manic episode (F30.-)
recurrent depressive disorder (F33.-)
EXCLUDES 2 *adjustment disorder (F43.2)*
AHA: 2020,1Q,23
DEF: Mood disorder that produces depression that may exhibit as sadness, low self-esteem, or guilt feelings. Other manifestations may be withdrawal from friends and family and interrupted sleep.
F32.0 Major depressive disorder, single episode, mild CC HCC
F32.1 Major depressive disorder, single episode, moderate CC HCC
F32.2 Major depressive disorder, single episode, severe without psychotic features CC HCC

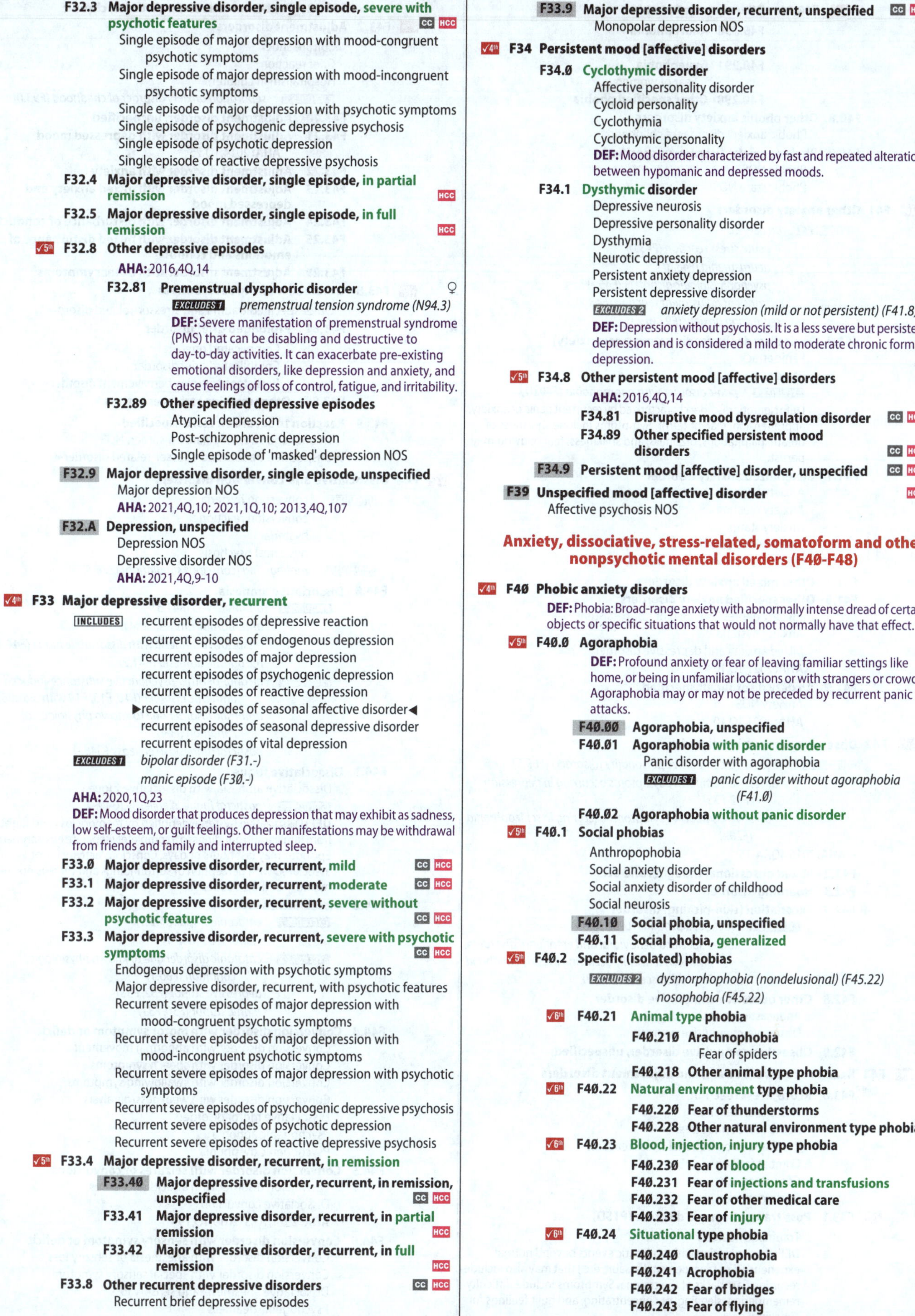

F32.3 Major depressive disorder, single episode, severe with psychotic features CC HCC
Single episode of major depression with mood-congruent psychotic symptoms
Single episode of major depression with mood-incongruent psychotic symptoms
Single episode of major depression with psychotic symptoms
Single episode of psychogenic depressive psychosis
Single episode of psychotic depression
Single episode of reactive depressive psychosis

F32.4 Major depressive disorder, single episode, in partial remission HCC

F32.5 Major depressive disorder, single episode, in full remission HCC

✓5th **F32.8 Other depressive episodes**
AHA: 2016,4Q,14

F32.81 Premenstrual dysphoric disorder ♀
EXCLUDES 1 *premenstrual tension syndrome (N94.3)*
DEF: Severe manifestation of premenstrual syndrome (PMS) that can be disabling and destructive to day-to-day activities. It can exacerbate pre-existing emotional disorders, like depression and anxiety, and cause feelings of loss of control, fatigue, and irritability.

F32.89 Other specified depressive episodes
Atypical depression
Post-schizophrenic depression
Single episode of 'masked' depression NOS

F32.9 Major depressive disorder, single episode, unspecified
Major depression NOS
AHA: 2021,4Q,10; 2021,1Q,10; 2013,4Q,107

F32.A Depression, unspecified
Depression NOS
Depressive disorder NOS
AHA: 2021,4Q,9-10

✓4th **F33 Major depressive disorder, recurrent**
INCLUDES recurrent episodes of depressive reaction
recurrent episodes of endogenous depression
recurrent episodes of major depression
recurrent episodes of psychogenic depression
recurrent episodes of reactive depression
►recurrent episodes of seasonal affective disorder◄
recurrent episodes of seasonal depressive disorder
recurrent episodes of vital depression
EXCLUDES 1 *bipolar disorder (F31.-)*
manic episode (F30.-)
AHA: 2020,1Q,23
DEF: Mood disorder that produces depression that may exhibit as sadness, low self-esteem, or guilt feelings. Other manifestations may be withdrawal from friends and family and interrupted sleep.

F33.0 Major depressive disorder, recurrent, mild CC HCC

F33.1 Major depressive disorder, recurrent, moderate CC HCC

F33.2 Major depressive disorder, recurrent, severe without psychotic features CC HCC

F33.3 Major depressive disorder, recurrent, severe with psychotic symptoms CC HCC
Endogenous depression with psychotic symptoms
Major depressive disorder, recurrent, with psychotic features
Recurrent severe episodes of major depression with mood-congruent psychotic symptoms
Recurrent severe episodes of major depression with mood-incongruent psychotic symptoms
Recurrent severe episodes of major depression with psychotic symptoms
Recurrent severe episodes of psychogenic depressive psychosis
Recurrent severe episodes of psychotic depression
Recurrent severe episodes of reactive depressive psychosis

✓5th **F33.4 Major depressive disorder, recurrent, in remission**

F33.40 Major depressive disorder, recurrent, in remission, unspecified CC HCC

F33.41 Major depressive disorder, recurrent, in partial remission HCC

F33.42 Major depressive disorder, recurrent, in full remission HCC

F33.8 Other recurrent depressive disorders CC HCC
Recurrent brief depressive episodes

F33.9 Major depressive disorder, recurrent, unspecified CC HCC
Monopolar depression NOS

✓4th **F34 Persistent mood [affective] disorders**

F34.0 Cyclothymic disorder
Affective personality disorder
Cycloid personality
Cyclothymia
Cyclothymic personality
DEF: Mood disorder characterized by fast and repeated alterations between hypomanic and depressed moods.

F34.1 Dysthymic disorder
Depressive neurosis
Depressive personality disorder
Dysthymia
Neurotic depression
Persistent anxiety depression
Persistent depressive disorder
EXCLUDES 2 *anxiety depression (mild or not persistent) (F41.8)*
DEF: Depression without psychosis. It is a less severe but persistent depression and is considered a mild to moderate chronic form of depression.

✓5th **F34.8 Other persistent mood [affective] disorders**
AHA: 2016,4Q,14

F34.81 Disruptive mood dysregulation disorder CC HCC

F34.89 Other specified persistent mood disorders CC HCC

F34.9 Persistent mood [affective] disorder, unspecified CC HCC

F39 Unspecified mood [affective] disorder HCC
Affective psychosis NOS

Anxiety, dissociative, stress-related, somatoform and other nonpsychotic mental disorders (F40-F48)

✓4th **F40 Phobic anxiety disorders**
DEF: Phobia: Broad-range anxiety with abnormally intense dread of certain objects or specific situations that would not normally have that effect.

✓5th **F40.0 Agoraphobia**
DEF: Profound anxiety or fear of leaving familiar settings like home, or being in unfamiliar locations or with strangers or crowds. Agoraphobia may or may not be preceded by recurrent panic attacks.

F40.00 Agoraphobia, unspecified

F40.01 Agoraphobia with panic disorder
Panic disorder with agoraphobia
EXCLUDES 1 *panic disorder without agoraphobia (F41.0)*

F40.02 Agoraphobia without panic disorder

✓5th **F40.1 Social phobias**
Anthropophobia
Social anxiety disorder
Social anxiety disorder of childhood
Social neurosis

F40.10 Social phobia, unspecified

F40.11 Social phobia, generalized

✓5th **F40.2 Specific (isolated) phobias**
EXCLUDES 2 *dysmorphophobia (nondelusional) (F45.22)*
nosophobia (F45.22)

✓6th **F40.21 Animal type phobia**
F40.210 Arachnophobia
Fear of spiders
F40.218 Other animal type phobia

✓6th **F40.22 Natural environment type phobia**
F40.220 Fear of thunderstorms
F40.228 Other natural environment type phobia

✓6th **F40.23 Blood, injection, injury type phobia**
F40.230 Fear of blood
F40.231 Fear of injections and transfusions
F40.232 Fear of other medical care
F40.233 Fear of injury

✓6th **F40.24 Situational type phobia**
F40.240 Claustrophobia
F40.241 Acrophobia
F40.242 Fear of bridges
F40.243 Fear of flying
F40.248 Other situational type phobia

Chapter 5. Mental, Behavioral and Neurodevelopmental Disorders

F32.3–F40.248

F40.29 Other specified phobia

F40.290 Androphobia
Fear of men

F40.291 Gynephobia
Fear of women

F40.298 Other specified phobia

F40.8 Other phobic anxiety disorders
Phobic anxiety disorder of childhood

F40.9 Phobic anxiety disorder, unspecified
Phobia NOS
Phobic state NOS

F41 Other anxiety disorders

EXCLUDES 2 *anxiety in:*
acute stress reaction (F43.0)
neurasthenia (F48.8)
psychophysiologic disorders (F45.-)
transient adjustment reaction (F43.2)
separation anxiety (F93.0)

F41.0 Panic disorder [episodic paroxysmal anxiety]
Panic attack
Panic state
EXCLUDES 1 *panic disorder with agoraphobia (F40.01)*
DEF: Neurotic disorder characterized by recurrent panic or anxiety, apprehension, fear, or terror. Symptoms include shortness of breath, palpitations, dizziness, and shakiness; fear of dying may persist.

F41.1 Generalized anxiety disorder
Anxiety neurosis
Anxiety reaction
Anxiety state
Overanxious disorder
EXCLUDES 2 *neurasthenia (F48.8)*

F41.3 Other mixed anxiety disorders

F41.8 Other specified anxiety disorders
Anxiety depression (mild or not persistent)
Anxiety hysteria
Mixed anxiety and depressive disorder
AHA: 2021,1Q,10

F41.9 Anxiety disorder, unspecified
Anxiety NOS
AHA: 2021,1Q,10

F42 Obsessive-compulsive disorder

EXCLUDES 2 *obsessive-compulsive personality (disorder) (F60.5)*
obsessive-compulsive symptoms occurring in depression (F32-F33)
obsessive-compulsive symptoms occurring in schizophrenia (F20.-)

AHA: 2016,4Q,14-15

F42.2 Mixed obsessional thoughts and acts

F42.3 Hoarding disorder

F42.4 Excoriation (skin-picking) disorder
EXCLUDES 1 *factitial dermatitis (L98.1)*
other specified behavioral and emotional disorders with onset usually occurring in early childhood and adolescence (F98.8)

F42.8 Other obsessive-compulsive disorder
Anancastic neurosis
Obsessive-compulsive neurosis

F42.9 Obsessive-compulsive disorder, unspecified

F43 Reaction to severe stress, and adjustment disorders

F43.0 Acute stress reaction
Acute crisis reaction
Acute reaction to stress
Combat and operational stress reaction
Combat fatigue
Crisis state
Psychic shock

F43.1 Post-traumatic stress disorder (PTSD)
Traumatic neurosis
DEF: Preoccupation with traumatic events beyond normal experience (i.e., rape, personal assault, etc.) that may also include recurring flashbacks of the trauma. Symptoms include difficulty remembering, sleeping, or concentrating, and guilt feelings for surviving.

F43.10 Post-traumatic stress disorder, unspecified

F43.11 Post-traumatic stress disorder, acute

F43.12 Post-traumatic stress disorder, chronic

F43.2 Adjustment disorders
Culture shock
Grief reaction
Hospitalism in children
EXCLUDES 2 *separation anxiety disorder of childhood (F93.0)*

F43.20 Adjustment disorder, unspecified

F43.21 Adjustment disorder with depressed mood
AHA: 2014,1Q,25

F43.22 Adjustment disorder with anxiety

F43.23 Adjustment disorder with mixed anxiety and depressed mood

F43.24 Adjustment disorder with disturbance of conduct

F43.25 Adjustment disorder with mixed disturbance of emotions and conduct

F43.29 Adjustment disorder with other symptoms

▲ **F43.8 Other reactions to severe stress**
Other specified trauma and stressor-related disorder

● **F43.81 Prolonged grief disorder**
Complicated grief
Complicated grief disorder
Persistent complex bereavement disorder

● **F43.89 Other reactions to severe stress**

F43.9 Reaction to severe stress, unspecified
Trauma and stressor-related disorder, NOS
▶Unspecified trauma and stressor-related disorder◀

F44 Dissociative and conversion disorders

INCLUDES conversion hysteria
conversion reaction
hysteria
hysterical psychosis

EXCLUDES 2 *malingering [conscious simulation] (Z76.5)*

F44.0 Dissociative amnesia HCC
EXCLUDES 1 *amnesia NOS (R41.3)*
anterograde amnesia (R41.1)
dissociative amnesia with dissociative fugue (F44.1)
retrograde amnesia (R41.2)
EXCLUDES 2 *alcohol-or other psychoactive substance-induced amnestic disorder (F10, F13, F19 with .26, .96)*
amnestic disorder due to known physiological condition (F04)
postictal amnesia in epilepsy (G40.-)

F44.1 Dissociative fugue HCC
Dissociative amnesia with dissociative fugue
EXCLUDES 2 *postictal fugue in epilepsy (G40.-)*
DEF: Dissociative hysteria identified by memory loss and flight from familiar surroundings to a completely separate environment. Episodes may last hours or days. Conscious activity is not associated with perception of surroundings and there is no later memory of the episode.

F44.2 Dissociative stupor
EXCLUDES 1 *catatonic stupor (R40.1)*
stupor NOS (R40.1)
EXCLUDES 2 *catatonic disorder due to known physiological condition (F06.1)*
depressive stupor (F32, F33)
manic stupor (F30, F31)

F44.4 Conversion disorder with motor symptom or deficit
Conversion disorder with abnormal movement
Conversion disorder with speech symptoms
Conversion disorder with swallowing symptoms
Conversion disorder with weakness/paralysis
Dissociative motor disorders
Psychogenic aphonia
Psychogenic dysphonia

F44.5 Conversion disorder with seizures or convulsions
Conversion disorder with attacks or seizures
Dissociative convulsions
AHA: 2021,1Q,3; 2019,1Q,19

F44.6 Conversion disorder with sensory symptom or deficit
Conversion disorder with anesthesia or sensory loss
Conversion disorder with special sensory symptoms
Dissociative anesthesia and sensory loss
Psychogenic deafness

F44.7 Conversion disorder with mixed symptom presentation

F44.8 Other dissociative and conversion disorders

F44.81 Dissociative identity disorder HCC
Multiple personality disorder

F44.89 Other dissociative and conversion disorders
Ganser's syndrome
Psychogenic confusion
Psychogenic twilight state
Trance and possession disorders

F44.9 Dissociative and conversion disorder, unspecified
Dissociative disorder NOS

F45 Somatoform disorders
EXCLUDES 2 *dissociative and conversion disorders (F44.-)*
factitious disorders (F68.1-, F68.A)
hair-plucking (F63.3)
lalling (F80.0)
lisping (F80.0)
malingering [conscious simulation] (Z76.5)
nail-biting (F98.8)
psychological or behavioral factors associated with disorders or diseases classified elsewhere (F54)
sexual dysfunction, not due to a substance or known physiological condition (F52.-)
thumb-sucking (F98.8)
tic disorders (in childhood and adolescence) (F95.-)
Tourette's syndrome (F95.2)
trichotillomania (F63.3)

DEF: Types of disorders causing inconsistent physical symptoms that cannot be explained.

F45.0 Somatization disorder
Briquet's disorder
Multiple psychosomatic disorder

F45.1 Undifferentiated somatoform disorder
Somatic symptom disorder
Undifferentiated psychosomatic disorder

F45.2 Hypochondriacal disorders
EXCLUDES 2 *delusional dysmorphophobia (F22)*
fixed delusions about bodily functions or shape (F22)

F45.20 Hypochondriacal disorder, unspecified

F45.21 Hypochondriasis
Hypochondriacal neurosis
Illness anxiety disorder

F45.22 Body dysmorphic disorder
Dysmorphophobia (nondelusional)
Nosophobia

F45.29 Other hypochondriacal disorders

F45.4 Pain disorders related to psychological factors
EXCLUDES 1 *pain NOS (R52)*

F45.41 Pain disorder exclusively related to psychological factors
Somatoform pain disorder (persistent)

F45.42 Pain disorder with related psychological factors
Code also associated acute or chronic pain (G89.-)

F45.8 Other somatoform disorders
Psychogenic dysmenorrhea
Psychogenic dysphagia, including 'globus hystericus'
Psychogenic pruritus
Psychogenic torticollis
Somatoform autonomic dysfunction
Teeth grinding
EXCLUDES 1 *sleep related teeth grinding (G47.63)*

F45.9 Somatoform disorder, unspecified
Psychosomatic disorder NOS

F48 Other nonpsychotic mental disorders

F48.1 Depersonalization-derealization syndrome HCC

F48.2 Pseudobulbar affect
Involuntary emotional expression disorder
Code first underlying cause, if known, such as:
amyotrophic lateral sclerosis (G12.21)
multiple sclerosis (G35)
sequelae of cerebrovascular disease (I69.-)
sequelae of traumatic intracranial injury (S06.-)

F48.8 Other specified nonpsychotic mental disorders
Dhat syndrome
Neurasthenia
Occupational neurosis, including writer's cramp
Psychasthenia
Psychasthenic neurosis
Psychogenic syncope

F48.9 Nonpsychotic mental disorder, unspecified
Neurosis NOS

Behavioral syndromes associated with physiological disturbances and physical factors (F50-F59)

F50 Eating disorders
EXCLUDES 1 *anorexia NOS (R63.0)*
feeding problems of newborn (P92.-)
polyphagia (R63.2)
EXCLUDES 2 *feeding difficulties (R63.3)*
feeding disorder in infancy or childhood (F98.2-)

AHA: 2022,1Q,13; 2018,4Q,82

TIP: Assign additional code for BMI from category Z68, when documented. BMI can be based on documentation from clinicians who are not the patient's provider.

F50.0 Anorexia nervosa
EXCLUDES 1 *loss of appetite (R63.0)*
psychogenic loss of appetite (F50.89)

DEF: Psychological eating disorder characterized by an intense fear of gaining weight and an unrealistic perception of body image that perpetuates the feeling of being fat or having too much fat. Avoidance of food and restrictive or unhealthy eating are common.

F50.00 Anorexia nervosa, unspecified CC

F50.01 Anorexia nervosa, restricting type CC

F50.02 Anorexia nervosa, binge eating/purging type CC
EXCLUDES 1 *bulimia nervosa (F50.2)*

F50.2 Bulimia nervosa CC
Bulimia NOS
Hyperorexia nervosa
EXCLUDES 1 *anorexia nervosa, binge eating/purging type (F50.02)*

DEF: Episodic pattern of overeating (binge eating) followed by purging or extreme exercise accompanied by an awareness of the abnormal eating pattern with a fear of not being able to stop eating.

F50.8 Other eating disorders
EXCLUDES 2 *pica of infancy and childhood (F98.3)*

AHA: 2017,4Q,9; 2016,4Q,15-16

F50.81 Binge eating disorder

F50.82 Avoidant/restrictive food intake disorder

F50.89 Other specified eating disorder
Pica in adults
Psychogenic loss of appetite

F50.9 Eating disorder, unspecified
Atypical anorexia nervosa
Atypical bulimia nervosa
Feeding or eating disorder, unspecified
Other specified feeding disorder

F51 Sleep disorders not due to a substance or known physiological condition
EXCLUDES 2 *organic sleep disorders (G47.-)*

F51.0 Insomnia not due to a substance or known physiological condition
EXCLUDES 2 *alcohol related insomnia (F10.182, F10.282, F10.982)*
drug-related insomnia (F11.182, F11.282, F11.982, F13.182, F13.282, F13.982, F14.182, F14.282, F14.982, F15.182, F15.282, F15.982, F19.182, F19.282, F19.982)
insomnia NOS (G47.0-)
insomnia due to known physiological condition (G47.0-)
organic insomnia (G47.0-)
sleep deprivation (Z72.820)

F51.01 Primary insomnia
Idiopathic insomnia

F51.02 Adjustment insomnia

F51.03 Paradoxical insomnia

F51.04 Psychophysiologic insomnia

F51.Ø5 Insomnia due to other mental disorder
Code also associated mental disorder

F51.Ø9 Other insomnia not due to a substance or known physiological condition

✓5th **F51.1 Hypersomnia not due to a substance or known physiological condition**
EXCLUDES 2 *alcohol related hypersomnia (F1Ø.182, F1Ø.282, F1Ø.982)*
drug-related hypersomnia (F11.182, F11.282, F11.982, F13.182, F13.282, F13.982, F14.182, F14.282, F14.982, F15.182, F15.282, F15.982, F19.182, F19.282, F19.982)
hypersomnia NOS (G47.1Ø)
hypersomnia due to known physiological condition (G47.1Ø)
idiopathic hypersomnia (G47.11, G47.12)
narcolepsy (G47.4-)

F51.11 Primary hypersomnia

F51.12 Insufficient sleep syndrome
EXCLUDES 1 *sleep deprivation (Z72.82Ø)*

F51.13 Hypersomnia due to other mental disorder
Code also associated mental disorder

F51.19 Other hypersomnia not due to a substance or known physiological condition

F51.3 Sleepwalking [somnambulism]
Non-rapid eye movement sleep arousal disorders, sleepwalking type

F51.4 Sleep terrors [night terrors]
Non-rapid eye movement sleep arousal disorders, sleep terror type

F51.5 Nightmare disorder
Dream anxiety disorder

F51.8 Other sleep disorders not due to a substance or known physiological condition

F51.9 Sleep disorder not due to a substance or known physiological condition, unspecified
Emotional sleep disorder NOS

✓4th **F52 Sexual dysfunction not due to a substance or known physiological condition**
EXCLUDES 2 *Dhat syndrome (F48.8)*

F52.Ø Hypoactive sexual desire disorder
Lack or loss of sexual desire
Male hypoactive sexual desire disorder
Sexual anhedonia
EXCLUDES 1 *decreased libido (R68.82)*

F52.1 Sexual aversion disorder
Sexual aversion and lack of sexual enjoyment

✓5th **F52.2 Sexual arousal disorders**
Failure of genital response

F52.21 Male erectile disorder ♂
Erectile disorder
Psychogenic impotence
EXCLUDES 1 *impotence of organic origin (N52.-)*
impotence NOS (N52.-)

F52.22 Female sexual arousal disorder ♀
Female sexual interest/arousal disorder

✓5th **F52.3 Orgasmic disorder**
Inhibited orgasm
Psychogenic anorgasmy

F52.31 Female orgasmic disorder ♀

F52.32 Male orgasmic disorder ♂
Delayed ejaculation

F52.4 Premature ejaculation ♂

F52.5 Vaginismus not due to a substance or known physiological condition ♀
Psychogenic vaginismus
EXCLUDES 2 *vaginismus (due to a known physiological condition) (N94.2)*
DEF: Psychogenic response resulting in painful contractions of the vaginal canal muscles. This condition can be severe enough to prevent sexual intercourse.

F52.6 Dyspareunia not due to a substance or known physiological condition
Genito-pelvic pain penetration disorder
Psychogenic dyspareunia
EXCLUDES 2 *dyspareunia (due to a known physiological condition) (N94.1-)*

F52.8 Other sexual dysfunction not due to a substance or known physiological condition
Excessive sexual drive
Nymphomania
Satyriasis

F52.9 Unspecified sexual dysfunction not due to a substance or known physiological condition UPD
Sexual dysfunction NOS

✓4th **F53 Mental and behavioral disorders associated with the puerperium, not elsewhere classified**
EXCLUDES 1 *mood disorders with psychotic features (F3Ø.2, F31.2, F31.5, F31.64, F32.3, F33.3)*
postpartum dysphoria (O9Ø.6)
psychosis in schizophrenia, schizotypal, delusional, and other psychotic disorders (F2Ø-F29)
AHA: 2018,4Q,8

F53.Ø Postpartum depression M ♀
Postnatal depression, NOS
Postpartum depression, NOS

F53.1 Puerperal psychosis HCC M ♀
Postpartum psychosis
Puerperal psychosis, NOS

F54 Psychological and behavioral factors associated with disorders or diseases classified elsewhere
Psychological factors affecting physical conditions
Code first the associated physical disorder, such as:
asthma (J45.-)
dermatitis (L23-L25)
gastric ulcer (K25.-)
mucous colitis (K58.-)
ulcerative colitis (K51.-)
urticaria (L5Ø.-)
EXCLUDES 2 *tension-type headache (G44.2)*

✓4th **F55 Abuse of non-psychoactive substances**
EXCLUDES 2 *abuse of psychoactive substances (F1Ø-F19)*

F55.Ø Abuse of antacids
F55.1 Abuse of herbal or folk remedies
F55.2 Abuse of laxatives
F55.3 Abuse of steroids or hormones
F55.4 Abuse of vitamins
F55.8 Abuse of other non-psychoactive substances

F59 Unspecified behavioral syndromes associated with physiological disturbances and physical factors
Psychogenic physiological dysfunction NOS

Disorders of adult personality and behavior (F6Ø-F69)

✓4th **F6Ø Specific personality disorders**

F6Ø.Ø Paranoid personality disorder HCC
Expansive paranoid personality (disorder)
Fanatic personality (disorder)
Paranoid personality (disorder)
Querulant personality (disorder)
Sensitive paranoid personality (disorder)
EXCLUDES 2 *paranoia (F22)*
paranoia querulans (F22)
paranoid psychosis (F22)
paranoid schizophrenia (F2Ø.Ø)
paranoid state (F22)

F6Ø.1 Schizoid personality disorder HCC
EXCLUDES 2 *Asperger's syndrome (F84.5)*
delusional disorder (F22)
schizoid disorder of childhood (F84.5)
schizophrenia (F2Ø.-)
schizotypal disorder (F21)

F6Ø.2 Antisocial personality disorder HCC
Amoral personality (disorder)
Asocial personality (disorder)
Dissocial personality disorder
Psychopathic personality (disorder)
Sociopathic personality (disorder)
EXCLUDES 1 *conduct disorders (F91.-)*
EXCLUDES 2 *borderline personality disorder (F6Ø.3)*

F6Ø.3 Borderline personality disorder HCC
Aggressive personality (disorder)
Emotionally unstable personality disorder
Explosive personality (disorder)
EXCLUDES 2 *antisocial personality disorder (F6Ø.2)*

F6Ø.4 Histrionic personality disorder HCC
Hysterical personality (disorder)
Psychoinfantile personality (disorder)

F6Ø.5 Obsessive-compulsive personality disorder HCC
Anankastic personality (disorder)
Compulsive personality (disorder)
Obsessional personality (disorder)
EXCLUDES 2 *obsessive-compulsive disorder (F42.-)*

F6Ø.6 Avoidant personality disorder HCC
Anxious personality disorder

F6Ø.7 Dependent personality disorder HCC
Asthenic personality (disorder)
Inadequate personality (disorder)
Passive personality (disorder)
DEF: Lack of self-confidence, fear of abandonment, and an obsessive need to be taken care of.

✓5th **F6Ø.8 Other specific personality disorders**

F6Ø.81 Narcissistic personality disorder HCC

F6Ø.89 Other specific personality disorders HCC
Eccentric personality disorder
"Haltlose" type personality disorder
Immature personality disorder
Passive-aggressive personality disorder
Psychoneurotic personality disorder
Self-defeating personality disorder

F6Ø.9 Personality disorder, unspecified HCC
Character disorder NOS
Character neurosis NOS
Pathological personality NOS

✓4th **F63 Impulse disorders**
EXCLUDES 2 *habitual excessive use of alcohol or psychoactive substances (F1Ø-F19)*
impulse disorders involving sexual behavior (F65.-)

F63.Ø Pathological gambling
Compulsive gambling
Gambling disorder
EXCLUDES 1 *gambling and betting NOS (Z72.6)*
EXCLUDES 2 *excessive gambling by manic patients (F3Ø, F31)*
gambling in antisocial personality disorder (F6Ø.2)

F63.1 Pyromania
Pathological fire-setting
EXCLUDES 2 *fire-setting (by) (in):*
adult with antisocial personality disorder (F6Ø.2)
alcohol or psychoactive substance intoxication (F1Ø-F19)
conduct disorders (F91.-)
mental disorders due to known physiological condition (FØ1-FØ9)
schizophrenia (F2Ø.-)

F63.2 Kleptomania
Pathological stealing
EXCLUDES 1 *shoplifting as the reason for observation for suspected mental disorder (ZØ3.8)*
EXCLUDES 2 *depressive disorder with stealing (F31-F33)*
stealing due to underlying mental condition - code to mental condition
stealing in mental disorders due to known physiological condition (FØ1-FØ9)

F63.3 Trichotillomania
Hair plucking
EXCLUDES 2 *other stereotyped movement disorder (F98.4)*

✓5th **F63.8 Other impulse disorders**

F63.81 Intermittent explosive disorder

F63.89 Other impulse disorders

F63.9 Impulse disorder, unspecified
Impulse control disorder NOS

✓4th **F64 Gender identity disorders**
AHA: 2016,4Q,16

F64.Ø Transsexualism
Gender identity disorder in adolescence and adulthood
Gender dysphoria in adolescents and adults

F64.1 Dual role transvestism
Use additional code to identify sex reassignment status (Z87.89Ø)
EXCLUDES 1 *gender identity disorder in childhood (F64.2)*
EXCLUDES 2 *fetishistic transvestism (F65.1)*

F64.2 Gender identity disorder of childhood P
Gender dysphoria in children
EXCLUDES 1 *gender identity disorder in adolescence and adulthood (F64.Ø)*
EXCLUDES 2 *sexual maturation disorder (F66)*

F64.8 Other gender identity disorders
Other specified gender dysphoria

F64.9 Gender identity disorder, unspecified
Gender dysphoria, unspecified
Gender-role disorder NOS

✓4th **F65 Paraphilias**

F65.Ø Fetishism
Fetishistic disorder

F65.1 Transvestic fetishism
Fetishistic transvestism
Transvestic disorder

F65.2 Exhibitionism
Exhibitionistic disorder

F65.3 Voyeurism
Voyeuristic disorder

F65.4 Pedophilia
Pedophilic disorder

✓5th **F65.5 Sadomasochism**

F65.5Ø Sadomasochism, unspecified

F65.51 Sexual masochism
Sexual masochism disorder

F65.52 Sexual sadism
Sexual sadism disorder

✓5th **F65.8 Other paraphilias**

F65.81 Frotteurism
Frotteuristic disorder

F65.89 Other paraphilias
Necrophilia
Other specified paraphilic disorder

F65.9 Paraphilia, unspecified
Paraphilic disorder, unspecified
Sexual deviation NOS

F66 Other sexual disorders
Sexual maturation disorder
Sexual relationship disorder

✓4th **F68 Other disorders of adult personality and behavior**
AHA: 2018,4Q,9,65

✓5th **F68.1 Factitious disorder imposed on self**
Compensation neurosis
Elaboration of physical symptoms for psychological reasons
Hospital hopper syndrome
Münchausen's syndrome
Peregrinating patient
EXCLUDES 2 *factitial dermatitis (L98.1)*
person feigning illness (with obvious motivation) (Z76.5)

F68.10 Factitious disorder imposed on self, unspecified CC

F68.11 Factitious disorder imposed on self, with predominantly psychological signs and symptoms

F68.12 Factitious disorder imposed on self, with predominantly physical signs and symptoms CC

F68.13 Factitious disorder imposed on self, with combined psychological and physical signs and symptoms

F68.A Factitious disorder imposed on another CC
Factitious disorder by proxy
Münchausen's by proxy

F68.8 Other specified disorders of adult personality and behavior

F69 Unspecified disorder of adult personality and behavior A

Intellectual disabilities (F70-F79)

Code first any associated physical or developmental disorders
EXCLUDES 1 *borderline intellectual functioning, IQ above 70 to 84 (R41.83)*

F70 Mild intellectual disabilities
IQ level 50-55 to approximately 70
Mild mental subnormality

F71 Moderate intellectual disabilities
IQ level 35-40 to 50-55
Moderate mental subnormality

F72 Severe intellectual disabilities CC
IQ 20-25 to 35-40
Severe mental subnormality

F73 Profound intellectual disabilities CC
IQ level below 20-25
Profound mental subnormality

✓4th **F78 Other intellectual disabilities**

✓5th **F78.A Other genetic related intellectual disabilities**
AHA: 2021,4Q,10-11

F78.A1 SYNGAP1-related intellectual disability
Code also, if applicable, any associated:
autism spectrum disorder (F84.0)
autistic disorder (F84.0)
encephalopathy (G93.4-)
epilepsy and recurrent seizures (G40.-)
other pervasive developmental disorders (F84.8)
pervasive developmental disorder, NOS (F84.9)

F78.A9 Other genetic related intellectual disability
Code also, if applicable, any associated disorders

F79 Unspecified intellectual disabilities
Mental deficiency NOS
Mental subnormality NOS

Pervasive and specific developmental disorders (F80-F89)

✓4th **F80 Specific developmental disorders of speech and language**

F80.0 Phonological disorder
Dyslalia
Functional speech articulation disorder
Lalling
Lisping
Phonological developmental disorder
Speech articulation developmental disorder
Speech-sound disorder
EXCLUDES 1 *speech articulation impairment due to aphasia NOS (R47.01)*
speech articulation impairment due to apraxia (R48.2)
EXCLUDES 2 *speech articulation impairment due to hearing loss (F80.4)*
speech articulation impairment due to intellectual disabilities (F70-F79)
speech articulation impairment with expressive language developmental disorder (F80.1)
speech articulation impairment with mixed receptive expressive language developmental disorder (F80.2)

F80.1 Expressive language disorder
Developmental dysphasia or aphasia, expressive type
EXCLUDES 1 *mixed receptive-expressive language disorder (F80.2)*
dysphasia and aphasia NOS (R47.-)
EXCLUDES 2 *acquired aphasia with epilepsy [Landau-Kleffner] (G40.80-)*
selective mutism (F94.0)
intellectual disabilities (F70-F79)
pervasive developmental disorders (F84.-)

F80.2 Mixed receptive-expressive language disorder
Developmental dysphasia or aphasia, receptive type
Developmental Wernicke's aphasia
EXCLUDES 1 *central auditory processing disorder (H93.25)*
dysphasia or aphasia NOS (R47.-)
expressive language disorder (F80.1)
expressive type dysphasia or aphasia (F80.1)
word deafness (H93.25)
EXCLUDES 2 *acquired aphasia with epilepsy [Landau-Kleffner] (G40.80-)*
pervasive developmental disorders (F84.-)
selective mutism (F94.0)
intellectual disabilities (F70-F79)

F80.4 Speech and language development delay due to hearing loss
Code also type of hearing loss (H90.-, H91.-)

✓5th **F80.8 Other developmental disorders of speech and language**
AHA: 2017,1Q,27

F80.81 Childhood onset fluency disorder
Cluttering NOS
Stuttering NOS
EXCLUDES 1 *adult onset fluency disorder (F98.5)*
fluency disorder in conditions classified elsewhere (R47.82)
fluency disorder (stuttering) following cerebrovascular disease (I69. with final characters -23)

F80.82 Social pragmatic communication disorder
EXCLUDES 1 *Asperger's syndrome (F84.5)*
autistic disorder (F84.0)
AHA: 2016,4Q,16

F80.89 Other developmental disorders of speech and language

F80.9 Developmental disorder of speech and language, unspecified
Communication disorder NOS
Language disorder NOS

✓4th **F81 Specific developmental disorders of scholastic skills**

F81.0 Specific reading disorder
"Backward reading"
Developmental dyslexia
Specific learning disorder, with impairment in reading
Specific reading retardation
EXCLUDES 1 *alexia NOS (R48.0)*
dyslexia NOS (R48.0)
DEF: Serious impairment of reading skills unexplained in relation to general intelligence and teaching processes.

F81.2 Mathematics disorder
Developmental acalculia
Developmental arithmetical disorder
Developmental Gerstmann's syndrome
Specific learning disorder, with impairment in mathematics
EXCLUDES 1 *acalculia NOS (R48.8)*
EXCLUDES 2 *arithmetical difficulties associated with a reading disorder (F81.0)*
arithmetical difficulties associated with a spelling disorder (F81.81)
arithmetical difficulties due to inadequate teaching (Z55.8)

✓5th **F81.8 Other developmental disorders of scholastic skills**

F81.81 Disorder of written expression
Specific learning disorder, with impairment in written expression
Specific spelling disorder

F81.89 Other developmental disorders of scholastic skills

F81.9 Developmental disorder of scholastic skills, unspecified UPD
Knowledge acquisition disability NOS
Learning disability NOS
Learning disorder NOS

F82 Specific developmental disorder of motor function
Clumsy child syndrome
Developmental coordination disorder
Developmental dyspraxia
EXCLUDES 1 *abnormalities of gait and mobility (R26.-)*
lack of coordination (R27.-)
EXCLUDES 2 *lack of coordination secondary to intellectual disabilities (F7Ø-F79)*

✓4th **F84 Pervasive developmental disorders**
Code also any associated medical condition and intellectual disabilities

F84.Ø Autistic disorder CC
Autism spectrum disorder
Infantile autism
Infantile psychosis
Kanner's syndrome
EXCLUDES 1 *Asperger's syndrome (F84.5)*
AHA: 2017,1Q,27

F84.2 Rett's syndrome CC
EXCLUDES 1 *Asperger's syndrome (F84.5)*
autistic disorder (F84.Ø)
other childhood disintegrative disorder (F84.3)

F84.3 Other childhood disintegrative disorder CC P
Dementia infantilis
Disintegrative psychosis
Heller's syndrome
Symbiotic psychosis
Use additional code to identify any associated neurological condition
EXCLUDES 1 *Asperger's syndrome (F84.5)*
autistic disorder (F84.Ø)
Rett's syndrome (F84.2)

F84.5 Asperger's syndrome CC
Asperger's disorder
Autistic psychopathy
Schizoid disorder of childhood
DEF: High-functioning form of autism. Children with this syndrome usually develop speech on schedule, are generally very intelligent, and communicate well, but have considerable social shortcomings. ***Synonym(s):*** *AS.*

F84.8 Other pervasive developmental disorders CC
Overactive disorder associated with intellectual disabilities and stereotyped movements

F84.9 Pervasive developmental disorder, unspecified CC
Atypical autism

F88 Other disorders of psychological development
Developmental agnosia
Global developmental delay
Other specified neurodevelopmental disorder

F89 Unspecified disorder of psychological development
Developmental disorder NOS
Neurodevelopmental disorder NOS

Behavioral and emotional disorders with onset usually occurring in childhood and adolescence (F9Ø-F98)

NOTE Codes within categories F9Ø-F98 may be used regardless of the age of a patient. These disorders generally have onset within the childhood or adolescent years, but may continue throughout life or not be diagnosed until adulthood

✓4th **F9Ø Attention-deficit hyperactivity disorders**
INCLUDES attention deficit disorder with hyperactivity
attention deficit syndrome with hyperactivity
EXCLUDES 2 *anxiety disorders (F4Ø.-, F41.-)*
mood [affective] disorders (F3Ø-F39)
pervasive developmental disorders (F84.-)
schizophrenia (F2Ø.-)

F9Ø.Ø Attention-deficit hyperactivity disorder, predominantly inattentive type
Attention-deficit/hyperactivity disorder, predominantly inattentive presentation

F9Ø.1 Attention-deficit hyperactivity disorder, predominantly hyperactive type
Attention-deficit/hyperactivity disorder, predominantly hyperactive impulsive presentation

F9Ø.2 Attention-deficit hyperactivity disorder, combined type
Attention-deficit/hyperactivity disorder, combined presentation

F9Ø.8 Attention-deficit hyperactivity disorder, other type

F9Ø.9 Attention-deficit hyperactivity disorder, unspecified type
Attention-deficit hyperactivity disorder of childhood or adolescence NOS
Attention-deficit hyperactivity disorder NOS

✓4th **F91 Conduct disorders**
EXCLUDES 1 *antisocial behavior (Z72.81-)*
antisocial personality disorder (F6Ø.2)
EXCLUDES 2 *conduct problems associated with attention-deficit hyperactivity disorder (F9Ø.-)*
mood [affective] disorders (F3Ø-F39)
pervasive developmental disorders (F84.-)
schizophrenia (F2Ø.-)

F91.Ø Conduct disorder confined to family context

F91.1 Conduct disorder, childhood-onset type
Unsocialized conduct disorder
Conduct disorder, solitary aggressive type
Unsocialized aggressive disorder

F91.2 Conduct disorder, adolescent-onset type
Socialized conduct disorder
Conduct disorder, group type

F91.3 Oppositional defiant disorder

F91.8 Other conduct disorders
Other specified conduct disorder
Other specified disruptive disorder

F91.9 Conduct disorder, unspecified
Behavioral disorder NOS
Conduct disorder NOS
Disruptive behavior disorder NOS
Disruptive disorder NOS

✓4th **F93 Emotional disorders with onset specific to childhood**

F93.Ø Separation anxiety disorder of childhood
EXCLUDES 2 *mood [affective] disorders (F3Ø-F39)*
nonpsychotic mental disorders (F4Ø-F48)
phobic anxiety disorder of childhood (F4Ø.8)
social phobia (F4Ø.1)

F93.8 Other childhood emotional disorders
Identity disorder
EXCLUDES 2 *gender identity disorder of childhood (F64.2)*

F93.9 Childhood emotional disorder, unspecified

✓4th **F94 Disorders of social functioning with onset specific to childhood and adolescence**

F94.Ø Selective mutism
Elective mutism
EXCLUDES 2 *pervasive developmental disorders (F84.-)*
schizophrenia (F2Ø.-)
specific developmental disorders of speech and language (F8Ø.-)
transient mutism as part of separation anxiety in young children (F93.Ø)

F94.1 Reactive attachment disorder of childhood
Use additional code to identify any associated failure to thrive or growth retardation
EXCLUDES 1 *disinhibited attachment disorder of childhood (F94.2)*
normal variation in pattern of selective attachment
EXCLUDES 2 *Asperger's syndrome (F84.5)*
maltreatment syndromes (T74.-)
sexual or physical abuse in childhood, resulting in psychosocial problems (Z62.81-)

F94.2 Disinhibited attachment disorder of childhood
Affectionless psychopathy
Institutional syndrome
EXCLUDES 1 *reactive attachment disorder of childhood (F94.1)*
EXCLUDES 2 *Asperger's syndrome (F84.5)*
attention-deficit hyperactivity disorders (F9Ø.-)
hospitalism in children (F43.2-)

F94.8 Other childhood disorders of social functioning

F94.9 Childhood disorder of social functioning, unspecified

✓4th **F95 Tic disorder**

F95.Ø Transient tic disorder
Provisional tic disorder

F95.1 Chronic motor or vocal tic disorder

F95.2 Tourette's disorder
Combined vocal and multiple motor tic disorder [de la Tourette]
Tourette's syndrome

F95.8 Other tic disorders

F95.9 Tic disorder, unspecified
Tic NOS

F98 Other behavioral and emotional disorders with onset usually occurring in childhood and adolescence
EXCLUDES 2 *breath-holding spells (R06.89)*
gender identity disorder of childhood (F64.2)
Kleine-Levin syndrome (G47.13)
obsessive-compulsive disorder (F42.-)
sleep disorders not due to a substance or known physiological condition (F51.-)

F98.0 Enuresis not due to a substance or known physiological condition
Enuresis (primary) (secondary) of nonorganic origin
Functional enuresis
Psychogenic enuresis
Urinary incontinence of nonorganic origin
EXCLUDES 1 *enuresis NOS (R32)*

F98.1 Encopresis not due to a substance or known physiological condition
Functional encopresis
Incontinence of feces of nonorganic origin
Psychogenic encopresis
Use additional code to identify the cause of any coexisting constipation
EXCLUDES 1 *encopresis NOS (R15.-)*

F98.2 Other feeding disorders of infancy and childhood
EXCLUDES 2 *anorexia nervosa and other eating disorders (F50.-)*
feeding difficulties (R63.3)
feeding problems of newborn (P92.-)
pica of infancy or childhood (F98.3)

F98.21 Rumination disorder of infancy

F98.29 Other feeding disorders of infancy and early childhood

F98.3 Pica of infancy and childhood

F98.4 Stereotyped movement disorders
Stereotype/habit disorder
EXCLUDES 1 *abnormal involuntary movements (R25.-)*
EXCLUDES 2 *compulsions in obsessive-compulsive disorder (F42.-)*
hair plucking (F63.3)
movement disorders of organic origin (G20-G25)
nail-biting (F98.8)
nose-picking (F98.8)
stereotypies that are part of a broader psychiatric condition (F01-F95)
thumb-sucking (F98.8)
tic disorders (F95.-)
trichotillomania (F63.3)

F98.5 Adult onset fluency disorder
EXCLUDES 1 *childhood onset fluency disorder (F80.81)*
dysphasia (R47.02)
fluency disorder in conditions classified elsewhere (R47.82)
fluency disorder (stuttering) following cerebrovascular disease (I69. with final characters -23)
tic disorders (F95.-)

F98.8 Other specified behavioral and emotional disorders with onset usually occurring in childhood and adolescence
Excessive masturbation
Nail-biting
Nose-picking
Thumb-sucking

F98.9 Unspecified behavioral and emotional disorders with onset usually occurring in childhood and adolescence

Unspecified mental disorder (F99)

F99 Mental disorder, not otherwise specified
Mental illness NOS
EXCLUDES 1 *unspecified mental disorder due to known physiological condition (F09)*

Chapter 6. Diseases of the Nervous System (GØØ-G99)

Chapter-specific Guidelines with Coding Examples

The chapter-specific guidelines from the ICD-10-CM Official Guidelines for Coding and Reporting have been provided below. Along with these guidelines are coding examples, contained in the shaded boxes, that have been developed to help illustrate the coding and/or sequencing guidance found in these guidelines.

a. Dominant/nondominant side

Codes from category G81, Hemiplegia and hemiparesis, and subcategories G83.1, Monoplegia of lower limb, G83.2, Monoplegia of upper limb, and G83.3, Monoplegia, unspecified, identify whether the dominant or nondominant side is affected. Should the affected side be documented, but not specified as dominant or nondominant, and the classification system does not indicate a default, code selection is as follows:

- For ambidextrous patients, the default should be dominant.
- If the left side is affected, the default is non-dominant.
- If the right side is affected, the default is dominant.

Hemiplegia affecting left side of ambidextrous patient

G81.92 Hemiplegia, unspecified affecting left dominant side

Explanation: Documentation states that the left side is affected and dominant is used for ambidextrous persons.

Right spastic hemiplegia, unknown whether patient is right- or left-handed

G81.11 Spastic hemiplegia affecting right dominant side

Explanation: Since it is unknown whether the patient is right- or left-handed, if the right side is affected, the default is dominant.

b. Pain—category G89

1) General coding information

Codes in category G89, Pain, not elsewhere classified, may be used in conjunction with codes from other categories and chapters to provide more detail about acute or chronic pain and neoplasm-related pain, unless otherwise indicated below.

If the pain is not specified as acute or chronic, post-thoracotomy, postprocedural, or neoplasm-related, do not assign codes from category G89.

A code from category G89 should not be assigned if the underlying (definitive) diagnosis is known, unless the reason for the encounter is pain control/ management and not management of the underlying condition.

When an admission or encounter is for a procedure aimed at treating the underlying condition (e.g., spinal fusion, kyphoplasty), a code for the underlying condition (e.g., vertebral fracture, spinal stenosis) should be assigned as the principal diagnosis. No code from category G89 should be assigned.

Elderly patient with back pain is admitted for kyphoplasty for age-related osteopathic compression fracture at vertebra T3

M8Ø.Ø8XA Age-related osteoporosis with current pathological fracture, vertebra(e), initial encounter for fracture

Explanation: No code is assigned for the pain as it is inherent in the underlying condition being treated.

(a) Category G89 codes as principal or first-listed diagnosis

Category G89 codes are acceptable as principal diagnosis or the first-listed code:

- When pain control or pain management is the reason for the admission/encounter (e.g., a patient with displaced intervertebral disc, nerve impingement and severe back pain presents for injection of steroid into the spinal canal). The underlying cause of the pain should be reported as an additional diagnosis, if known.
- When a patient is admitted for the insertion of a neurostimulator for pain control, assign the appropriate pain code as the principal or first-listed diagnosis. When an admission or encounter is for a procedure aimed at treating the underlying condition and a neurostimulator is inserted for pain control during the same admission/encounter, a code for the underlying condition should be assigned as the principal diagnosis and the appropriate pain code should be assigned as a secondary diagnosis.

Patient with chronic pain from lumbar spondylosis with radiculopathy not relieved by surgery is admitted for insertion of neurostimulator.

G89.29 Other chronic pain

M47.26 Other spondylosis with radiculopathy, lumbar region

Explanation: Since the patient is admitted specifically for a neurostimulator implantation for pain management and not to treat the underlying spondylosis, the chronic pain code is sequenced first, followed by the underlying condition. Neither code M54.16 nor M54.5 is necessary because M47.26 describes the radiculopathy and the site.

(b) Use of category G89 codes in conjunction with site specific pain codes

(i) Assigning category G89 and site-specific pain codes

Codes from category G89 may be used in conjunction with codes that identify the site of pain (including codes from chapter 18) if the category G89 code provides additional information. For example, if the code describes the site of the pain, but does not fully describe whether the pain is acute or chronic, then both codes should be assigned.

During hospital stay, patient is seen by orthopaedics to evaluate chronic left shoulder pain.

M25.512 Pain in left shoulder

G89.29 Other chronic pain

Explanation: No underlying condition has been determined yet so the pain would be the reason for the visit. The M25 pain code in this instance does not fully describe the condition as it does not represent that the pain is chronic. The G89 chronic pain code is assigned to provide specificity.

(ii) Sequencing of category G89 codes with site-specific pain codes

The sequencing of category G89 codes with site-specific pain codes (including chapter 18 codes), is dependent on the circumstances of the encounter/admission as follows:

- If the encounter is for pain control or pain management, assign the code from category G89 followed by the code identifying the specific site of pain (e.g., encounter for pain management for acute neck pain from trauma is assigned code G89.11, Acute pain due to trauma, followed by code M54.2, Cervicalgia, to identify the site of pain).

Management of acute, traumatic right knee pain

G89.11 Acute pain due to trauma

M25.561 Pain in right knee

Explanation: The reason for the encounter is to manage or control the pain, not to treat or evaluate an underlying condition. The G89 pain code is assigned as the principal diagnosis but in this instance does not fully describe the condition as it does not include the site and laterality. The M25 pain code is added to provide this information.

- If the encounter is for any other reason except pain control or pain management, and a related definitive diagnosis has not been established (confirmed) by the provider, assign the code for the specific site of pain first, followed by the appropriate code from category G89.

Tests are performed to investigate the source of the patient's chronic epigastric abdominal pain

R1Ø.13 Epigastric pain

G89.29 Other chronic pain

Explanation: In this instance the patient's epigastric pain is not being treated; rather the source of the pain is being investigated. A code from chapter 18 for epigastric pain is sequenced before the additional specificity of the G89 code for the chronic pain.

2) Pain due to devices, implants and grafts

See Section I.C.19. Pain due to medical devices

3) Postoperative pain

The provider's documentation should be used to guide the coding of postoperative pain, as well as *Section III. Reporting Additional Diagnoses* and *Section IV. Diagnostic Coding and Reporting in the Outpatient Setting.*

The default for post-thoracotomy and other postoperative pain not specified as acute or chronic is the code for the acute form.

Routine or expected postoperative pain immediately after surgery should not be coded.

Pain pump dose is increased for the patient's unexpected, extreme pain post-thoracotomy

G89.12 Acute post-thoracotomy pain

Explanation: When acute or chronic is not documented, default to acute. The use of "unexpected, extreme" and the increase of medication dosage indicate that the pain was more than routine or expected.

(a) Postoperative pain not associated with specific postoperative complication

Postoperative pain not associated with a specific postoperative complication is assigned to the appropriate postoperative pain code in category G89.

(b) Postoperative pain associated with specific postoperative complication

Postoperative pain associated with a specific postoperative complication (such as painful wire sutures) is assigned to the appropriate code(s) found in Chapter 19, Injury, poisoning, and certain other consequences of external causes. If appropriate, use additional code(s) from category G89 to identify acute or chronic pain (G89.18 or G89.28).

4) Chronic pain

Chronic pain is classified to subcategory G89.2. There is no time frame defining when pain becomes chronic pain. The provider's documentation should be used to guide use of these codes.

5) Neoplasm related pain

Code G89.3 is assigned to pain documented as being related, associated or due to cancer, primary or secondary malignancy, or tumor. This code is assigned regardless of whether the pain is acute or chronic.

This code may be assigned as the principal or first-listed code when the stated reason for the admission/encounter is documented as pain control/pain management. The underlying neoplasm should be reported as an additional diagnosis.

Pain medication adjustment for chronic pain from bone metastasis

G89.3 Neoplasm related pain (acute)(chronic)

C79.51 Secondary malignant neoplasm of bone

Explanation: Since the encounter was for pain medication management, the pain, rather than the neoplasm, was the reason for the encounter and is sequenced first. This "neoplasm-related pain" code includes both acute and chronic pain.

When the reason for the admission/encounter is management of the neoplasm and the pain associated with the neoplasm is also documented, code G89.3 may be assigned as an additional diagnosis. It is not necessary to assign an additional code for the site of the pain.

See Section I.C.2. for instructions on the sequencing of neoplasms for all other stated reasons for the admission/encounter (except for pain control/pain management).

Patient with lung cancer presents with acute hip pain and is evaluated and found to have iliac bone metastasis

C79.51 Secondary malignant neoplasm of bone

C34.9Ø Malignant neoplasm of unspecified part of unspecified bronchus or lung

G89.3 Neoplasm related pain (acute)(chronic)

Explanation: The reason for the encounter was the evaluation and diagnosis of the bone metastasis, whose code would be assigned as first-listed, followed by codes for the primary neoplasm and the pain due to the iliac bone metastasis.

6) Chronic pain syndrome

Central pain syndrome (G89.Ø) and chronic pain syndrome (G89.4) are different than the term "chronic pain," and therefore codes should only be used when the provider has specifically documented this condition.

See Section I.C.5. Pain disorders related to psychological factors

Chapter 6. Diseases of the Nervous System (G00-G99)

EXCLUDES 2 *certain conditions originating in the perinatal period (P04-P96)*
certain infectious and parasitic diseases (A00-B99)
complications of pregnancy, childbirth and the puerperium (O00-O9A)
congenital malformations, deformations, and chromosomal abnormalities (Q00-Q99)
endocrine, nutritional and metabolic diseases (E00-E88)
injury, poisoning and certain other consequences of external causes (S00-T88)
neoplasms (C00-D49)
symptoms, signs and abnormal clinical and laboratory findings, not elsewhere classified (R00-R94)

This chapter contains the following blocks:

G00-G09 Inflammatory diseases of the central nervous system
G10-G14 Systemic atrophies primarily affecting the central nervous system
G20-G26 Extrapyramidal and movement disorders
G30-G32 Other degenerative diseases of the nervous system
G35-G37 Demyelinating diseases of the central nervous system
G40-G47 Episodic and paroxysmal disorders
G50-G59 Nerve, nerve root and plexus disorders
G60-G65 Polyneuropathies and other disorders of the peripheral nervous system
G70-G73 Diseases of myoneural junction and muscle
G80-G83 Cerebral palsy and other paralytic syndromes
G89-G99 Other disorders of the nervous system

Inflammatory diseases of the central nervous system (G00-G09)

G00 Bacterial meningitis, not elsewhere classified (4th)
INCLUDES bacterial arachnoiditis
bacterial leptomeningitis
bacterial meningitis
bacterial pachymeningitis
EXCLUDES 1 *bacterial meningoencephalitis (G04.2)*
bacterial meningomyelitis (G04.2)

DEF: Inflammation of meningeal layers of the brain and spinal cord due to a bacterial infection.

G00.0 Hemophilus meningitis MCC
Meningitis due to Hemophilus influenzae

G00.1 Pneumococcal meningitis MCC
Meningtitis due to Streptococcal pneumoniae

G00.2 Streptococcal meningitis MCC
Use additional code to further identify organism (B95.0-B95.5)

G00.3 Staphylococcal meningitis MCC
Use additional code to further identify organism (B95.61-B95.8)

G00.8 Other bacterial meningitis MCC
Meningitis due to Escherichia coli
Meningitis due to Friedländer's bacillus
Meningitis due to Klebsiella
Use additional code to further identify organism (B96.-)

G00.9 Bacterial meningitis, unspecified MCC
Meningitis due to gram-negative bacteria, unspecified
Purulent meningitis NOS
Pyogenic meningitis NOS
Suppurative meningitis NOS

G01 Meningitis in bacterial diseases classified elsewhere MCC
Code first underlying disease
EXCLUDES 1 *meningitis (in):*
gonococcal (A54.81)
leptospirosis (A27.81)
listeriosis (A32.11)
Lyme disease (A69.21)
meningococcal (A39.0)
neurosyphilis (A52.13)
tuberculosis (A17.0)
meningoencephalitis and meningomyelitis in bacterial diseases classified elsewhere (G05)

G02 Meningitis in other infectious and parasitic diseases classified elsewhere MCC
Code first underlying disease, such as:
African trypanosomiasis (B56.-)
poliovirus infection (A80.-)
EXCLUDES 1 *candidal meningitis (B37.5)*
coccidioidomycosis meningitis (B38.4)
cryptococcal meningitis (B45.1)
herpesviral [herpes simplex] meningitis (B00.3)
infectious mononucleosis complicated by meningitis (B27.- with fifth character 2)
measles complicated by meningitis (B05.1)
meningoencephalitis and meningomyelitis in other infectious and parasitic diseases classified elsewhere (G05)
mumps meningitis (B26.1)
rubella meningitis (B06.02)
varicella [chickenpox] meningitis (B01.0)
zoster meningitis (B02.1)

G03 Meningitis due to other and unspecified causes (4th)
INCLUDES arachnoiditis NOS
leptomeningitis NOS
meningitis NOS
pachymeningitis NOS
EXCLUDES 1 *meningoencephalitis (G04.-)*
meningomyelitis (G04.-)

G03.0 Nonpyogenic meningitis MCC
Aseptic meningitis
Nonbacterial meningitis
DEF: Type of meningitis where no bacterial, viral, or other infectious source exists that explains the meningitis symptomology.

G03.1 Chronic meningitis CC

G03.2 Benign recurrent meningitis [Mollaret] CC
DEF: Aseptic or noninfectious inflammation of the meninges with the presence of Mollaret cells in the spinal fluid. The patient experiences recurrent bouts of inflammation, lasting anywhere from two to five days.

G03.8 Meningitis due to other specified causes MCC

G03.9 Meningitis, unspecified MCC
Arachnoiditis (spinal) NOS

G04 Encephalitis, myelitis and encephalomyelitis (4th)
INCLUDES acute ascending myelitis
meningoencephalitis
meningomyelitis
EXCLUDES 1 *encephalopathy NOS (G93.40)*
EXCLUDES 2 *acute transverse myelitis (G37.3-)*
alcoholic encephalopathy (G31.2)
~~*benign myalgic encephalomyelitis (G93.3)*~~
multiple sclerosis (G35)
►*myalgic encephalomyelitis (G93.32)*◄
subacute necrotizing myelitis (G37.4)
toxic encephalitis (G92.8)
toxic encephalopathy (G92.8)

DEF: Encephalitis: Inflammation of the brain, often caused by viral or bacterial infection.
DEF: Encephalomyelitis: Inflammatory disease, often viral in nature, that affects the brain and spinal cord.
DEF: Myelitis: Inflammation of the spinal cord.

G04.0 Acute disseminated encephalitis and encephalomyelitis (ADEM) (5th)
EXCLUDES 1 *acute necrotizing hemorrhagic encephalopathy (G04.3-)*
other noninfectious acute disseminated encephalomyelitis (noninfectious ADEM) (G04.81)

G04.00 Acute disseminated encephalitis and encephalomyelitis, unspecified MCC

G04.01 Postinfectious acute disseminated encephalitis and encephalomyelitis (postinfectious ADEM) MCC
EXCLUDES 1 *post chickenpox encephalitis (B01.1)*
post measles encephalitis (B05.0)
post measles myelitis (B05.1)

G04.02 Postimmunization acute disseminated encephalitis, myelitis and encephalomyelitis MCC
Encephalitis, post immunization
Encephalomyelitis, post immunization
Use additional code to identify the vaccine (T50.A-, T50.B-, T50.Z-)

G04.1 Tropical spastic paraplegia CC HCC

G04.2 Bacterial meningoencephalitis and meningomyelitis, not elsewhere classified MCC

G04.3 Acute necrotizing hemorrhagic encephalopathy (5th)
EXCLUDES 1 *acute disseminated encephalitis and encephalomyelitis (G04.0-)*

G04.30 Acute necrotizing hemorrhagic encephalopathy, unspecified MCC

G04.31 Postinfectious acute necrotizing hemorrhagic encephalopathy MCC

G04.32 Postimmunization acute necrotizing hemorrhagic encephalopathy MCC
Use additional code to identify the vaccine (T50.A-, T50.B-, T50.Z-)

G04.39 Other acute necrotizing hemorrhagic encephalopathy MCC
Code also underlying etiology, if applicable

G04.8 Other encephalitis, myelitis and encephalomyelitis (5th)
Code also any associated seizure (G40.-, R56.9)

G04.81 Other encephalitis and encephalomyelitis HIV MCC
Noninfectious acute disseminated encephalomyelitis (noninfectious ADEM)

G04.82 Acute flaccid myelitis MCC HCC
EXCLUDES 1 *transverse myelitis (G37.3)*
AHA: 2021,4Q,11

G04.89 Other myelitis HIV MCC HCC
AHA: 2020,1Q,14

G04.9 Encephalitis, myelitis and encephalomyelitis, unspecified (5th)

G04.90 Encephalitis and encephalomyelitis, unspecified HIV MCC
Ventriculitis (cerebral) NOS

G04.91 Myelitis, unspecified HIV MCC HCC

G05 Encephalitis, myelitis and encephalomyelitis in diseases classified elsewhere (4th)
Code first underlying disease, such as:
congenital toxoplasmosis encephalitis, myelitis and encephalomyelitis (P37.1)
cytomegaloviral encephalitis, myelitis and encephalomyelitis (B25.8)
encephalitis, myelitis and encephalomyelitis (in) systemic lupus erythematosus (M32.19)
eosinophilic meningoencephalitis (B83.2)
human immunodeficiency virus [HIV] disease (B20)
poliovirus (A80.-)
suppurative otitis media (H66.01-H66.4)
trichinellosis (B75)
EXCLUDES 1 *adenoviral encephalitis, myelitis and encephalomyelitis (A85.1)*
encephalitis, myelitis and encephalomyelitis (in) measles (B05.0)
enteroviral encephalitis, myelitis and encephalomyelitis (A85.0)
herpesviral [herpes simplex] encephalitis, myelitis and encephalomyelitis (B00.4)
listerial encephalitis, myelitis and encephalomyelitis (A32.12)
meningococcal encephalitis, myelitis and encephalomyelitis (A39.81)
mumps encephalitis, myelitis and encephalomyelitis (B26.2)
postchickenpox encephalitis, myelitis and encephalomyelitis (B01.1-)
rubella encephalitis, myelitis and encephalomyelitis (B06.01)
toxoplasmosis encephalitis, myelitis and encephalomyelitis (B58.2)
zoster encephalitis, myelitis and encephalomyelitis (B02.0)

G05.3 Encephalitis and encephalomyelitis in diseases classified elsewhere MCC
Meningoencephalitis in diseases classified elsewhere

G05.4 Myelitis in diseases classified elsewhere MCC HCC
Meningomyelitis in diseases classified elsewhere

G06 Intracranial and intraspinal abscess and granuloma (4th)
Use additional code (B95-B97) to identify infectious agent
DEF: Abscess: Circumscribed collection of pus resulting from bacteria, frequently associated with swelling and other signs of inflammation.
DEF: Granuloma: Abnormal, dense collections of cells forming a mass or nodule of chronically inflamed tissue with granulations that is usually associated with an infective process.

G06.0 Intracranial abscess and granuloma MCC
Brain [any part] abscess (embolic)
Cerebellar abscess (embolic)
Cerebral abscess (embolic)
Intracranial epidural abscess or granuloma
Intracranial extradural abscess or granuloma
Intracranial subdural abscess or granuloma
Otogenic abscess (embolic)
EXCLUDES 1 *tuberculous intracranial abscess and granuloma (A17.81)*

G06.1 Intraspinal abscess and granuloma MCC
Abscess (embolic) of spinal cord [any part]
Intraspinal epidural abscess or granuloma
Intraspinal extradural abscess or granuloma
Intraspinal subdural abscess or granuloma
EXCLUDES 1 *tuberculous intraspinal abscess and granuloma (A17.81)*

G06.2 Extradural and subdural abscess, unspecified MCC

G07 Intracranial and intraspinal abscess and granuloma in diseases classified elsewhere MCC
Code first underlying disease, such as:
schistosomiasis granuloma of brain (B65.-)
EXCLUDES 1 *abscess of brain:*
amebic (A06.6)
chromomycotic (B43.1)
gonococcal (A54.82)
tuberculous (A17.81)
tuberculoma of meninges (A17.1)

G08 Intracranial and intraspinal phlebitis and thrombophlebitis MCC
Septic embolism of intracranial or intraspinal venous sinuses and veins
Septic endophlebitis of intracranial or intraspinal venous sinuses and veins
Septic phlebitis of intracranial or intraspinal venous sinuses and veins
Septic thrombophlebitis of intracranial or intraspinal venous sinuses and veins
Septic thrombosis of intracranial or intraspinal venous sinuses and veins
EXCLUDES 1 *intracranial phlebitis and thrombophlebitis complicating:*
abortion, ectopic or molar pregnancy (O00-O07, O08.7)
pregnancy, childbirth and the puerperium (O22.5, O87.3)
nonpyogenic intracranial phlebitis and thrombophlebitis (I67.6)
EXCLUDES 2 *intracranial phlebitis and thrombophlebitis complicating nonpyogenic intraspinal phlebitis and thrombophlebitis (G95.1)*
DEF: Inflammation and formation of a blood clot in a vein within the brain or spine, or their linings.

G09 Sequelae of inflammatory diseases of central nervous system
NOTE Category G09 is to be used to indicate conditions whose primary classification is to G00-G08 as the cause of sequelae, themselves classifiable elsewhere. The "sequelae" include conditions specified as residuals.
Code first condition resulting from (sequela) of inflammatory diseases of central nervous system

Systemic atrophies primarily affecting the central nervous system (G10-G14)

G10 Huntington's disease CC HCC
Huntington's chorea
Huntington's dementia
▶Use additional code, if applicable, to identify:◀
▶dementia with anxiety (F02.84, F02.A4, F02.B4, F02.C4)◀
▶dementia with behavioral disturbance (F02.81-, F02.A1-, F02.B1-, F02.C1-)◀
▶dementia with mood disturbance (F02.83, F02.A3, F02.B3, F02.C3)◀
▶dementia with psychotic disturbance (F02.82, F02.A2, F02.B2, F02.C2)◀
▶dementia without behavioral disturbance (F02.80, F02.A0, F02.B0, F02.C0)◀
▶mild neurocognitive disorder due to known physiological condition (F06.7-)◀
~~Code also dementia in other diseases classified elsewhere without behavioral disturbance (F02.80)~~
DEF: Genetic disease caused by degeneration of nerve cells in the brain, characterized by chronic progressive mental deterioration. Dementia and death occur within 15 to 20 years of onset.

✓4th **G11 Hereditary ataxia**
EXCLUDES 2 *cerebral palsy (G80.-)*
hereditary and idiopathic neuropathy (G60.-)
metabolic disorders (E70-E88)
DEF: Ataxia: Defect in muscular control or coordination due to a central nervous system disorder, particularly when voluntary muscular movements are attempted.

G11.0 Congenital nonprogressive ataxia CC HCC

✓5th **G11.1 Early-onset cerebellar ataxia**
AHA: 2020,4Q,17-18

G11.10 Early-onset cerebellar ataxia, unspecified CC HCC
G11.11 Friedreich ataxia CC HCC
Autosomal recessive Friedreich ataxia
Friedreich ataxia with retained reflexes
G11.19 Other early-onset cerebellar ataxia CC HCC
Early-onset cerebellar ataxia with essential tremor
Early-onset cerebellar ataxia with myoclonus [Hunt's ataxia]
Early-onset cerebellar ataxia with retained tendon reflexes
X-linked recessive spinocerebellar ataxia

G11.2 Late-onset cerebellar ataxia CC HCC A
G11.3 Cerebellar ataxia with defective DNA repair CC HCC
Ataxia telangiectasia [Louis-Bar]
EXCLUDES 2 *Cockayne's syndrome (Q87.19)*
other disorders of purine and pyrimidine metabolism (E79.-)
xeroderma pigmentosum (Q82.1)
G11.4 Hereditary spastic paraplegia CC HCC
G11.8 Other hereditary ataxias CC HCC
G11.9 Hereditary ataxia, unspecified CC HCC
Hereditary cerebellar ataxia NOS
Hereditary cerebellar degeneration
Hereditary cerebellar disease
Hereditary cerebellar syndrome

✓4th **G12 Spinal muscular atrophy and related syndromes**

G12.0 Infantile spinal muscular atrophy, type I [Werdnig-Hoffman] CC HCC
G12.1 Other inherited spinal muscular atrophy CC HCC
Adult form spinal muscular atrophy
Childhood form, type II spinal muscular atrophy
Distal spinal muscular atrophy
Juvenile form, type III spinal muscular atrophy [Kugelberg-Welander]
Progressive bulbar palsy of childhood [Fazio-Londe]
Scapuloperoneal form spinal muscular atrophy

✓5th **G12.2 Motor neuron disease**
AHA: 2017,4Q,9-10

G12.20 Motor neuron disease, unspecified CC HCC
G12.21 Amyotrophic lateral sclerosis CC HCC A
G12.22 Progressive bulbar palsy CC HCC
G12.23 Primary lateral sclerosis CC HCC
G12.24 Familial motor neuron disease CC HCC
G12.25 Progressive spinal muscle atrophy CC HCC
G12.29 Other motor neuron disease CC HCC

G12.8 Other spinal muscular atrophies and related syndromes CC HCC
G12.9 Spinal muscular atrophy, unspecified CC HCC

✓4th **G13 Systemic atrophies primarily affecting central nervous system in diseases classified elsewhere**

G13.0 Paraneoplastic neuromyopathy and neuropathy HCC
Carcinomatous neuromyopathy
Sensorial paraneoplastic neuropathy [Denny Brown]
Code first underlying neoplasm (C00-D49)
G13.1 Other systemic atrophy primarily affecting central nervous system in neoplastic disease HCC
Paraneoplastic limbic encephalopathy
Code first underlying neoplasm (C00-D49)
G13.2 Systemic atrophy primarily affecting the central nervous system in myxedema HCC
Code first underlying disease, such as:
hypothyroidism (E03.-)
myxedematous congenital iodine deficiency (E00.1)
G13.8 Systemic atrophy primarily affecting central nervous system in other diseases classified elsewhere HCC
Code first underlying disease

G14 Postpolio syndrome
INCLUDES postpolio myelitic syndrome
EXCLUDES 1 *sequelae of poliomyelitis (B91)*

Extrapyramidal and movement disorders (G20-G26)

G20 Parkinson's disease HCC
Hemiparkinsonism
Idiopathic Parkinsonism or Parkinson's disease
Paralysis agitans
Parkinsonism or Parkinson's disease NOS
Primary Parkinsonism or Parkinson's disease
▶Use additional code, if applicable, to identify:◀
▶dementia with anxiety (F02.84, F02.A4, F02.B4, F02.C4)◀
dementia with behavioral disturbance ▶(F02.81-, F02.A1-, F02.B1-, F02.C1-)◀
▶dementia with mood disturbance (F02.83, F02.A3, F02.B3, F02.C3)◀
▶dementia with psychotic disturbance (F02.82, F02.A2, F02.B2, F02.C2)◀
dementia without behavioral disturbance ▶(F02.80, F02.A0, F02.B0, F02.C0)◀
▶mild neurocognitive disorder due to known physiological condition (F06.7-)◀
EXCLUDES 1 ~~*dementia with Parkinsonism (G31.83)*~~
AHA: 2017,2Q,7; 2016,2Q,6
TIP: Repeated falls (R29.6) are not integral to Parkinson's disease and can be separately coded.

✓4th **G21 Secondary parkinsonism**
EXCLUDES 1 *dementia with Parkinsonism (G31.83)*
Huntington's disease (G10)
Shy-Drager syndrome (G90.3)
syphilitic Parkinsonism (A52.19)

G21.0 Malignant neuroleptic syndrome MCC
Use additional code for adverse effect, if applicable, to identify drug (T43.3X5, T43.4X5, T43.505, T43.595)
EXCLUDES 1 *neuroleptic induced parkinsonism (G21.11)*

✓5th **G21.1 Other drug-induced secondary parkinsonism**

G21.11 Neuroleptic induced parkinsonism CC HCC
Use additional code for adverse effect, if applicable, to identify drug (T43.3X5, T43.4X5, T43.505, T43.595)
EXCLUDES 1 *malignant neuroleptic syndrome (G21.0)*
G21.19 Other drug induced secondary parkinsonism CC HCC
Other medication-induced parkinsonism
Use additional code for adverse effect, if applicable, to identify drug (T36-T50 with fifth or sixth character 5)

G21.2 Secondary parkinsonism due to other external agents CC HCC
Code first (T51-T65) to identify external agent
G21.3 Postencephalitic parkinsonism CC HCC
G21.4 Vascular parkinsonism HCC

G21.8 Other secondary parkinsonism CC HCC

G21.9 Secondary parkinsonism, unspecified CC HCC

✓4th **G23 Other degenerative diseases of basal ganglia**

EXCLUDES 2 *multi-system degeneration of the autonomic nervous system (G90.3)*

G23.0 Hallervorden-Spatz disease CC HCC
Pigmentary pallidal degeneration

G23.1 Progressive supranuclear ophthalmoplegia [Steele-Richardson-Olszewski] CC HCC
Progressive supranuclear palsy

G23.2 Striatonigral degeneration CC HCC

G23.8 Other specified degenerative diseases of basal ganglia CC HCC
Calcification of basal ganglia

G23.9 Degenerative disease of basal ganglia, unspecified CC HCC

✓4th **G24 Dystonia**

INCLUDES dyskinesia

EXCLUDES 2 *athetoid cerebral palsy (G80.3)*

DEF: Disorder of abnormal muscle tone, excessive or inadequate. Involuntary movements and prolonged muscle contractions result in tremors, abnormalities in posture, and twisting body motions that affect an isolated area or the whole body.

✓5th **G24.0 Drug induced dystonia**
Use additional code for adverse effect, if applicable, to identify drug (T36-T50 with fifth or sixth character 5)

G24.01 Drug induced subacute dyskinesia
Drug induced blepharospasm
Drug induced orofacial dyskinesia
Neuroleptic induced tardive dyskinesia
Tardive dyskinesia

G24.02 Drug induced acute dystonia CC
Acute dystonic reaction to drugs
Neuroleptic induced acute dystonia

G24.09 Other drug induced dystonia CC

G24.1 Genetic torsion dystonia
Dystonia deformans progressiva
Dystonia musculorum deformans
Familial torsion dystonia
Idiopathic familial dystonia
Idiopathic (torsion) dystonia NOS
(Schwalbe-) Ziehen-Oppenheim disease

G24.2 Idiopathic nonfamilial dystonia CC

G24.3 Spasmodic torticollis

EXCLUDES 1 *congenital torticollis (Q68.0)*
hysterical torticollis (F44.4)
ocular torticollis (R29.891)
psychogenic torticollis (F45.8)
torticollis NOS (M43.6)
traumatic recurrent torticollis (S13.4)

DEF: Twisted, unnatural position of the neck due to contracted cervical muscles that pull the head to one side or cause involuntary shaking of the head.

G24.4 Idiopathic orofacial dystonia
Orofacial dyskinesia

EXCLUDES 1 *drug induced orofacial dyskinesia (G24.01)*

G24.5 Blepharospasm

EXCLUDES 1 *drug induced blepharospasm (G24.01)*

DEF: Involuntary contraction of the orbicularis oculi muscle, resulting in the eyelids being completely closed.

G24.8 Other dystonia CC
Acquired torsion dystonia NOS

G24.9 Dystonia, unspecified
Dyskinesia NOS

✓4th **G25 Other extrapyramidal and movement disorders**

EXCLUDES 2 *sleep related movement disorders (G47.6-)*

G25.0 Essential tremor
Familial tremor

EXCLUDES 1 *tremor NOS (R25.1)*

G25.1 Drug-induced tremor
Use additional code for adverse effect, if applicable, to identify drug (T36-T50 with fifth or sixth character 5)

G25.2 Other specified forms of tremor
Intention tremor

G25.3 Myoclonus
Drug-induced myoclonus
Palatal myoclonus
Use additional code for adverse effect, if applicable, to identify drug (T36-T50 with fifth or sixth character 5)

EXCLUDES 1 *facial myokymia (G51.4)*
myoclonic epilepsy (G40.-)

DEF: Spasmodic, brief, involuntary muscle contractions that can be due to an undetermined etiology, drug-induced, or caused by a disease process.

G25.4 Drug-induced chorea
Use additional code for adverse effect, if applicable, to identify drug (T36-T50 with fifth or sixth character 5)

G25.5 Other chorea
Chorea NOS

EXCLUDES 1 *chorea NOS with heart involvement (I02.0)*
Huntington's chorea (G10)
rheumatic chorea (I02.-)
Sydenham's chorea (I02.-)

✓5th **G25.6 Drug induced tics and other tics of organic origin**

G25.61 Drug induced tics
Use additional code for adverse effect, if applicable, to identify drug (T36-T50 with fifth or sixth character 5)

G25.69 Other tics of organic origin

EXCLUDES 1 *habit spasm (F95.9)*
tic NOS (F95.9)
Tourette's syndrome (F95.2)

✓5th **G25.7 Other and unspecified drug induced movement disorders**
Use additional code for adverse effect, if applicable, to identify drug (T36-T50 with fifth or sixth character 5)

G25.70 Drug induced movement disorder, unspecified

G25.71 Drug induced akathisia
Drug induced acathisia
Neuroleptic induced acute akathisia
Tardive akathisia

G25.79 Other drug induced movement disorders

✓5th **G25.8 Other specified extrapyramidal and movement disorders**

G25.81 Restless legs syndrome
DEF: Neurological disorder of unknown etiology creating an irresistible urge to move the legs, which may temporarily relieve the symptoms. This syndrome is accompanied by motor restlessness and sensations of pain, burning, prickling, or tingling.

G25.82 Stiff-man syndrome CC

G25.83 Benign shuddering attacks

G25.89 Other specified extrapyramidal and movement disorders

G25.9 Extrapyramidal and movement disorder, unspecified CC

G26 Extrapyramidal and movement disorders in diseases classified elsewhere
Code first underlying disease

Other degenerative diseases of the nervous system (G30-G32)

G30 Alzheimer's disease

INCLUDES Alzheimer's dementia senile and presenile forms

▶Use additional code, if applicable, to identify:◀
- delirium, if applicable (F05)
- ▶dementia with anxiety (F02.84, F02.A4, F02.B4, F02.C4)◀
- dementia with behavioral disturbance ▶(F02.81-, F02.A1-, F02.B1-, F02.C1-)◀
- ▶dementia with mood disturbance (F02.83, F02.A3, F02.B3, F02.C3)◀
- ▶dementia with psychotic disturbance (F02.82, F02.A2, F02.B2, F02.C2)◀
- dementia without behavioral disturbance ▶(F02.80, F02.A0, F02.B0, F02.C0)◀
- ▶mild neurocognitive disorder due to known physiological condition (F06.7-)◀

EXCLUDES 1 *senile degeneration of brain NEC (G31.1)*
senile dementia NOS (F03)
senility NOS (R41.81)

AHA: 2017,1Q,43

TIP: A code from subcategory F02.8 should always be assigned with a code from this category, even in the absence of documented dementia.

TIP: Functional quadriplegia (R53.2) is not integral to Alzheimer's disease and can be coded in addition to codes from category G30.

G30.0 Alzheimer's disease with early onset HCC

G30.1 Alzheimer's disease with late onset HCC A

G30.8 Other Alzheimer's disease HCC

G30.9 Alzheimer's disease, unspecified HCC

AHA: 2016,2Q,6; 2012,4Q,95

G31 Other degenerative diseases of nervous system, not elsewhere classified

For codes G31.0 - G31.83, G31.85 - G31.9, use additional code, if applicable, to identify:
- ▶dementia with anxiety (F02.84, F02.A4, F02.B4, F02.C4)◀
- dementia with behavioral disturbance ▶(F02.81-, F02.A1-, F02.B1-, F02.C1-)◀
- ▶dementia with mood disturbance (F02.83, F02.A3, F02.B3, F02.C3)◀
- ▶dementia with psychotic disturbance (F02.82, F02.A2, F02.B2, F02.C2)◀
- dementia without behavioral disturbance ▶(F02.80, F02.A0, F02.B0, F02.C0)◀
- ▶mild neurocognitive disorder due to known physiological condition (F06.7-)◀

EXCLUDES 2 *Reye's syndrome (G93.7)*

G31.0 Frontotemporal dementia

G31.01 Pick's disease HCC

Primary progressive aphasia
Progressive isolated aphasia

DEF: Progressive frontotemporal dementia with asymmetrical atrophy of the frontal and temporal regions of the cerebral cortex and abnormal rounded brain cells called Pick cells with the presence of abnormal staining of protein (called tau). Symptoms include prominent apathy, behavioral changes such as disinhibition and restlessness, echolalia, impairment of language, memory, and intellect, increased carelessness, poor personal hygiene, and decreased attention span.

▲ **G31.09 Other frontotemporal neurocognitive disorder** HCC

Frontal dementia

▶Use additional code, if applicable, to identify mild neurocognitive disorders due to known physiological condition (F06.7-)◀

G31.1 Senile degeneration of brain, not elsewhere classified HCC

EXCLUDES 1 *Alzheimer's disease (G30.-)*
senility NOS (R41.81)

G31.2 Degeneration of nervous system due to alcohol HCC

Alcoholic cerebellar ataxia
Alcoholic cerebellar degeneration
Alcoholic cerebral degeneration
Alcoholic encephalopathy
Dysfunction of the autonomic nervous system due to alcohol
Code also associated alcoholism (F10.-)

G31.8 Other specified degenerative diseases of nervous system

G31.81 Alpers disease CC HCC

Grey-matter degeneration

G31.82 Leigh's disease CC HCC

Subacute necrotizing encephalopathy

▲ **G31.83 Neurocognitive disorder with Lewy bodies** HCC

~~Dementia with Parkinsonism~~
Lewy body dementia
Lewy body disease

▶Use additional code, if applicable, to identify mild neurocognitive disorders due to known physiological condition (F06.7-)◀

AHA: 2017,2Q,7; 2016,4Q,141

DEF: Cerebral dementia with neurophysiologic changes, increased hippocampal volume, hypoperfusion in the occipital lobes, beta amyloid deposits with neurofibrillary tangles, and atrophy of the cortex and brainstem. Hallmark neuropsychological characteristics include fluctuating cognition with pronounced variation in attention and alertness, recurrent hallucinations, and Parkinsonism.

▲ **G31.84 Mild cognitive impairment of uncertain or unknown etiology**

▶Mild cognitive disorder NOS◀
~~Mild neurocognitive disorder~~
▶Mild neurocognitive disorder of uncertain or unknown etiology◀

▶Use additional code to identify presence of:◀
- ▶alcohol abuse and dependence (F10.-)◀
- ▶exposure to environmental tobacco smoke (Z77.22)◀
- ▶history of tobacco dependence (Z87.891)◀
- ▶hypertension (I10-I16)◀
- ▶occupational exposure to environmental tobacco smoke (Z57.31)◀
- ▶tobacco dependence (F17.-)◀
- ▶tobacco use (Z72.0)◀

EXCLUDES 1 *age related cognitive decline (R41.81)*
altered mental status (R41.82)
cerebral degeneration (G31.9)
▶cerebrovascular diseases (I60-I69)◀
change in mental status (R41.82)
cognitive deficits following (sequelae of) cerebral hemorrhage or infarction (I69.01-, I69.11-, I69.21-, I69.31-, I69.81-, I69.91-)
cognitive impairment due to intracranial or head injury (S06.-)
dementia (F01.-, F02.-, F03)
~~mild memory disturbance (F06.8)~~
▶mild neurocognitive disorder due to a known physiological condition (F06.7-)◀
neurologic neglect syndrome (R41.4)
personality change, nonpsychotic (F68.8)

AHA: 2021,3Q,3

G31.85 Corticobasal degeneration HCC

G31.89 Other specified degenerative diseases of nervous system HCC

G31.9 Degenerative disease of nervous system, unspecified HCC

AHA: 2021,3Q,3

G32 Other degenerative disorders of nervous system in diseases classified elsewhere

G32.0 Subacute combined degeneration of spinal cord in diseases classified elsewhere CC HCC

Dana-Putnam syndrome
Sclerosis of spinal cord (combined) (dorsolateral) (posterolateral)

Code first underlying disease, such as:
- anemia (D51.9)
- dietary (D51.3)
- pernicious (D51.0)
- vitamin B12 deficiency (E53.8)

EXCLUDES 1 *syphilitic combined degeneration of spinal cord (A52.11)*

✓5th **G32.8 Other specified degenerative disorders of nervous system in diseases classified elsewhere**
Code first underlying disease, such as:
amyloidosis cerebral degeneration (E85.-)
cerebral degeneration (due to) hypothyroidism (E00.0-E03.9)
cerebral degeneration (due to) neoplasm (C00-D49)
cerebral degeneration (due to) vitamin B deficiency, except thiamine (E52-E53.-)
EXCLUDES 1 *superior hemorrhagic polioencephalitis [Wernicke's encephalopathy] (E51.2)*

G32.81 Cerebellar ataxia in diseases classified elsewhere CC HCC
Code first underlying disease, such as:
celiac disease (with gluten ataxia) (K90.0)
cerebellar ataxia (in) neoplastic disease (paraneoplastic cerebellar degeneration) (C00-D49)
non-celiac gluten ataxia (M35.9)
EXCLUDES 1 *systemic atrophy primarily affecting the central nervous system in alcoholic cerebellar ataxia (G31.2)*
systemic atrophy primarily affecting the central nervous system in myxedema (G13.2)

G32.89 Other specified degenerative disorders of nervous system in diseases classified elsewhere
Degenerative encephalopathy in diseases classified elsewhere

Demyelinating diseases of the central nervous system (G35-G37)

G35 Multiple sclerosis HCC
Disseminated multiple sclerosis
Generalized multiple sclerosis
Multiple sclerosis NOS
Multiple sclerosis of brain stem
Multiple sclerosis of cord
AHA: 2021,1Q,7

✓4th **G36 Other acute disseminated demyelination**
EXCLUDES 1 *postinfectious encephalitis and encephalomyelitis NOS (G04.01)*
DEF: Demyelination: Abnormal loss of myelin, the protective white matter that insulates nerve endings and facilitates neuroreception and neurotransmission. When this substance is damaged, the nerve is short-circuited, resulting in impaired or loss of function.

G36.0 Neuromyelitis optica [Devic] CC HCC
Demyelination in optic neuritis
EXCLUDES 1 *optic neuritis NOS (H46)*

G36.1 Acute and subacute hemorrhagic leukoencephalitis [Hurst] CC HCC

G36.8 Other specified acute disseminated demyelination CC HCC

G36.9 Acute disseminated demyelination, unspecified HIV CC HCC

✓4th **G37 Other demyelinating diseases of central nervous system**

G37.0 Diffuse sclerosis of central nervous system CC HCC
Periaxial encephalitis
Schilder's disease
EXCLUDES 1 *X linked adrenoleukodystrophy (E71.52-)*

G37.1 Central demyelination of corpus callosum CC HCC

G37.2 Central pontine myelinolysis CC HCC
AHA: 2022,2Q,10

G37.3 Acute transverse myelitis in demyelinating disease of central nervous system CC HCC
Acute transverse myelitis NOS
Acute transverse myelopathy
EXCLUDES 1 *acute flaccid myelitis (G04.82)*
multiple sclerosis (G35)
neuromyelitis optica [Devic] (G36.0)

G37.4 Subacute necrotizing myelitis of central nervous system HIV MCC HCC

G37.5 Concentric sclerosis [Balo] of central nervous system CC HCC

G37.8 Other specified demyelinating diseases of central nervous system CC HCC

G37.9 Demyelinating disease of central nervous system, unspecified HIV CC HCC

Episodic and paroxysmal disorders (G40-G47)

✓4th **G40 Epilepsy and recurrent seizures**
NOTE The following terms are to be considered equivalent to intractable: pharmacoresistant (pharmacologically resistant), treatment resistant, refractory (medically) and poorly controlled
EXCLUDES 1 *conversion disorder with seizures (F44.5)*
convulsions NOS (R56.9)
post traumatic seizures (R56.1)
seizure (convulsive) NOS (R56.9)
seizure of newborn (P90)
EXCLUDES 2 *hippocampal sclerosis (G93.81)*
mesial temporal sclerosis (G93.81)
temporal sclerosis (G93.81)
Todd's paralysis (G83.84)

✓5th **G40.0 Localization-related (focal) (partial) idiopathic epilepsy and epileptic syndromes with seizures of localized onset**
Benign childhood epilepsy with centrotemporal EEG spikes
Childhood epilepsy with occipital EEG paroxysms
EXCLUDES 1 *adult onset localization-related epilepsy (G40.1-, G40.2-)*

✓6th **G40.00 Localization-related (focal) (partial) idiopathic epilepsy and epileptic syndromes with seizures of localized onset, not intractable**
Localization-related (focal) (partial) idiopathic epilepsy and epileptic syndromes with seizures of localized onset without intractability

G40.001 Localization-related (focal) (partial) idiopathic epilepsy and epileptic syndromes with seizures of localized onset, not intractable, with status epilepticus CC HCC

G40.009 Localization-related (focal) (partial) idiopathic epilepsy and epileptic syndromes with seizures of localized onset, not intractable, without status epilepticus CC HCC
Localization-related (focal) (partial) idiopathic epilepsy and epileptic syndromes with seizures of localized onset NOS

✓6th **G40.01 Localization-related (focal) (partial) idiopathic epilepsy and epileptic syndromes with seizures of localized onset, intractable**

G40.011 Localization-related (focal) (partial) idiopathic epilepsy and epileptic syndromes with seizures of localized onset, intractable, with status epilepticus CC HCC

G40.019 Localization-related (focal) (partial) idiopathic epilepsy and epileptic syndromes with seizures of localized onset, intractable, without status epilepticus CC HCC

✓5th **G40.1 Localization-related (focal) (partial) symptomatic epilepsy and epileptic syndromes with simple partial seizures**
Attacks without alteration of consciousness
Epilepsia partialis continua [Kozhevnikof]
Simple partial seizures developing into secondarily generalized seizures

✓6th **G40.10 Localization-related (focal) (partial) symptomatic epilepsy and epileptic syndromes with simple partial seizures, not intractable**
Localization-related (focal) (partial) symptomatic epilepsy and epileptic syndromes with simple partial seizures without intractability

G40.101 Localization-related (focal) (partial) symptomatic epilepsy and epileptic syndromes with simple partial seizures, not intractable, with status epilepticus CC HCC

G40.109 Localization-related (focal) (partial) symptomatic epilepsy and epileptic syndromes with simple partial seizures, not intractable, without status epilepticus CC HCC

Localization-related (focal) (partial) symptomatic epilepsy and epileptic syndromes with simple partial seizures NOS

G40.11 Localization-related (focal) (partial) symptomatic epilepsy and epileptic syndromes with simple partial seizures, intractable

G40.111 Localization-related (focal) (partial) symptomatic epilepsy and epileptic syndromes with simple partial seizures, intractable, with status epilepticus CC HCC

G40.119 Localization-related (focal) (partial) symptomatic epilepsy and epileptic syndromes with simple partial seizures, intractable, without status epilepticus CC HCC

G40.2 Localization-related (focal) (partial) symptomatic epilepsy and epileptic syndromes with complex partial seizures

Attacks with alteration of consciousness, often with automatisms

Complex partial seizures developing into secondarily generalized seizures

G40.20 Localization-related (focal) (partial) symptomatic epilepsy and epileptic syndromes with complex partial seizures, not intractable

Localization-related (focal) (partial) symptomatic epilepsy and epileptic syndromes with complex partial seizures without intractability

G40.201 Localization-related (focal) (partial) symptomatic epilepsy and epileptic syndromes with complex partial seizures, not intractable, with status epilepticus CC HCC

G40.209 Localization-related (focal) (partial) symptomatic epilepsy and epileptic syndromes with complex partial seizures, not intractable, without status epilepticus CC HCC

Localization-related (focal) (partial) symptomatic epilepsy and epileptic syndromes with complex partial seizures NOS

G40.21 Localization-related (focal) (partial) symptomatic epilepsy and epileptic syndromes with complex partial seizures, intractable

G40.211 Localization-related (focal) (partial) symptomatic epilepsy and epileptic syndromes with complex partial seizures, intractable, with status epilepticus CC HCC

G40.219 Localization-related (focal) (partial) symptomatic epilepsy and epileptic syndromes with complex partial seizures, intractable, without status epilepticus CC HCC

G40.3 Generalized idiopathic epilepsy and epileptic syndromes

Code also MERRF syndrome, if applicable (E88.42)

G40.30 Generalized idiopathic epilepsy and epileptic syndromes, not intractable

Generalized idiopathic epilepsy and epileptic syndromes without intractability

G40.301 Generalized idiopathic epilepsy and epileptic syndromes, not intractable, with status epilepticus MCC HCC

G40.309 Generalized idiopathic epilepsy and epileptic syndromes, not intractable, without status epilepticus HCC

Generalized idiopathic epilepsy and epileptic syndromes NOS

G40.31 Generalized idiopathic epilepsy and epileptic syndromes, intractable

G40.311 Generalized idiopathic epilepsy and epileptic syndromes, intractable, with status epilepticus MCC HCC

G40.319 Generalized idiopathic epilepsy and epileptic syndromes, intractable, without status epilepticus MCC HCC

G40.A Absence epileptic syndrome

Childhood absence epilepsy [pyknolepsy]

Juvenile absence epilepsy

Absence epileptic syndrome, NOS

G40.A0 Absence epileptic syndrome, not intractable

G40.A01 Absence epileptic syndrome, not intractable, with status epilepticus HCC

G40.A09 Absence epileptic syndrome, not intractable, without status epilepticus HCC

G40.A1 Absence epileptic syndrome, intractable

G40.A11 Absence epileptic syndrome, intractable, with status epilepticus CC HCC

G40.A19 Absence epileptic syndrome, intractable, without status epilepticus CC HCC

G40.B Juvenile myoclonic epilepsy [impulsive petit mal]

G40.B0 Juvenile myoclonic epilepsy, not intractable

G40.B01 Juvenile myoclonic epilepsy, not intractable, with status epilepticus CC HCC

G40.B09 Juvenile myoclonic epilepsy, not intractable, without status epilepticus CC HCC

G40.B1 Juvenile myoclonic epilepsy, intractable

G40.B11 Juvenile myoclonic epilepsy, intractable, with status epilepticus CC HCC

G40.B19 Juvenile myoclonic epilepsy, intractable, without status epilepticus CC HCC

G40.4 Other generalized epilepsy and epileptic syndromes

Epilepsy with grand mal seizures on awakening

Epilepsy with myoclonic absences

Epilepsy with myoclonic-astatic seizures

Grand mal seizure NOS

Nonspecific atonic epileptic seizures

Nonspecific clonic epileptic seizures

Nonspecific myoclonic epileptic seizures

Nonspecific tonic epileptic seizures

Nonspecific tonic-clonic epileptic seizures

Symptomatic early myoclonic encephalopathy

G40.40 Other generalized epilepsy and epileptic syndromes, not intractable

Other generalized epilepsy and epileptic syndromes without intractability

Other generalized epilepsy and epileptic syndromes NOS

G40.401 Other generalized epilepsy and epileptic syndromes, not intractable, with status epilepticus HCC

G40.409 Other generalized epilepsy and epileptic syndromes, not intractable, without status epilepticus HCC

G40.41 Other generalized epilepsy and epileptic syndromes, intractable

G40.411 Other generalized epilepsy and epileptic syndromes, intractable, with status epilepticus CC HCC

G40.419 Other generalized epilepsy and epileptic syndromes, intractable, without status epilepticus CC HCC

G40.42 Cyclin-Dependent Kinase-Like 5 Deficiency Disorder HCC

CDKL5

Use additional code, if known, to identify associated manifestations, such as:

cortical blindness (H47.61-)

global development delay (F88)

AHA: 2020,4Q,18-19

G4Ø.5 Epileptic seizures related to external causes

Epileptic seizures related to alcohol
Epileptic seizures related to drugs
Epileptic seizures related to hormonal changes
Epileptic seizures related to sleep deprivation
Epileptic seizures related to stress

Code also, if applicable, associated epilepsy and recurrent seizures (G4Ø.-)

Use additional code for adverse effect, if applicable, to identify drug (T36-T5Ø with fifth or sixth character 5)

G4Ø.5Ø Epileptic seizures related to external causes, not intractable

G4Ø.5Ø1 Epileptic seizures related to external causes, not intractable, with status epilepticus CC HCC

G4Ø.5Ø9 Epileptic seizures related to external causes, not intractable, without status epilepticus CC HCC

Epileptic seizures related to external causes, NOS

G4Ø.8 Other epilepsy and recurrent seizures

Epilepsies and epileptic syndromes undetermined as to whether they are focal or generalized
Landau-Kleffner syndrome

G4Ø.8Ø Other epilepsy

G4Ø.8Ø1 Other epilepsy, not intractable, with status epilepticus CC HCC

Other epilepsy without intractability with status epilepticus

G4Ø.8Ø2 Other epilepsy, not intractable, without status epilepticus CC HCC

Other epilepsy NOS
Other epilepsy without intractability without status epilepticus

G4Ø.8Ø3 Other epilepsy, intractable, with status epilepticus CC HCC

G4Ø.8Ø4 Other epilepsy, intractable, without status epilepticus CC HCC

G4Ø.81 Lennox-Gastaut syndrome

DEF: Severe form of epilepsy with usual onset in early childhood. Seizures are frequent and difficult to treat, causing falls and intellectual impairment.

G4Ø.811 Lennox-Gastaut syndrome, not intractable, with status epilepticus CC HCC

G4Ø.812 Lennox-Gastaut syndrome, not intractable, without status epilepticus CC HCC

G4Ø.813 Lennox-Gastaut syndrome, intractable, with status epilepticus CC HCC

G4Ø.814 Lennox-Gastaut syndrome, intractable, without status epilepticus CC HCC

G4Ø.82 Epileptic spasms

Infantile spasms
Salaam attacks
West's syndrome

G4Ø.821 Epileptic spasms, not intractable, with status epilepticus CC HCC

G4Ø.822 Epileptic spasms, not intractable, without status epilepticus CC HCC

G4Ø.823 Epileptic spasms, intractable, with status epilepticus CC HCC

G4Ø.824 Epileptic spasms, intractable, without status epilepticus CC HCC

G4Ø.83 Dravet syndrome

Polymorphic epilepsy in infancy (PMEI)
Severe myoclonic epilepsy in infancy (SMEI)

AHA: 2020,4Q,19

G4Ø.833 Dravet syndrome, intractable, with status epilepticus CC HCC

G4Ø.834 Dravet syndrome, intractable, without status epilepticus CC HCC

Dravet syndrome NOS

G4Ø.89 Other seizures CC HCC

EXCLUDES 1 *post traumatic seizures (R56.1)*
recurrent seizures NOS (G4Ø.9Ø9)
seizure NOS (R56.9)

G4Ø.9 Epilepsy, unspecified

AHA: 2019,1Q,19

G4Ø.9Ø Epilepsy, unspecified, not intractable

Epilepsy, unspecified, without intractability

G4Ø.9Ø1 Epilepsy, unspecified, not intractable, with status epilepticus HCC

G4Ø.9Ø9 Epilepsy, unspecified, not intractable, without status epilepticus HCC

Epilepsy NOS
Epileptic convulsions NOS
Epileptic fits NOS
Epileptic seizures NOS
Recurrent seizures NOS
Seizure disorder NOS

AHA: 2021,2Q,3; 2021,1Q,3

G4Ø.91 Epilepsy, unspecified, intractable

Intractable seizure disorder NOS

G4Ø.911 Epilepsy, unspecified, intractable, with status epilepticus CC HCC

G4Ø.919 Epilepsy, unspecified, intractable, without status epilepticus CC HCC

G43 Migraine

NOTE The following terms are to be considered equivalent to intractable: pharmacoresistant (pharmacologically resistant), treatment resistant, refractory (medically) and poorly controlled

Use additional code for adverse effect, if applicable, to identify drug (T36-T5Ø with fifth or sixth character 5)

EXCLUDES 1 *headache NOS (R51.9)*
lower half migraine (G44.ØØ)

EXCLUDES 2 *headache syndromes (G44.-)*

DEF: Headaches that occur periodically on one or both sides of the head that may be associated with nausea and vomiting, sensitivity to light and sound, dizziness, distorted vision, and cognitive disturbances.

G43.Ø Migraine without aura

Common migraine

EXCLUDES 1 *chronic migraine without aura (G43.7-)*

G43.ØØ Migraine without aura, not intractable

Migraine without aura without mention of refractory migraine

G43.ØØ1 Migraine without aura, not intractable, with status migrainosus

G43.ØØ9 Migraine without aura, not intractable, without status migrainosus

Migraine without aura NOS

G43.Ø1 Migraine without aura, intractable

Migraine without aura with refractory migraine

G43.Ø11 Migraine without aura, intractable, with status migrainosus

G43.Ø19 Migraine without aura, intractable, without status migrainosus

G43.1 Migraine with aura

Basilar migraine
Classical migraine
Migraine equivalents
Migraine preceded or accompanied by transient focal neurological phenomena
Migraine triggered seizures
Migraine with acute-onset aura
Migraine with aura without headache (migraine equivalents)
Migraine with prolonged aura
Migraine with typical aura
Retinal migraine

Code also any associated seizure (G4Ø.-, R56.9)

EXCLUDES 1 *persistent migraine aura (G43.5-, G43.6-)*

G43.1Ø Migraine with aura, not intractable

Migraine with aura without mention of refractory migraine

G43.1Ø1 Migraine with aura, not intractable, with status migrainosus

G43.1Ø9 Migraine with aura, not intractable, without status migrainosus

Migraine with aura NOS

✓6th **G43.11 Migraine with aura, intractable**
Migraine with aura with refractory migraine
G43.111 Migraine with aura, intractable, with status migrainosus
G43.119 Migraine with aura, intractable, without status migrainosus

✓5th **G43.4 Hemiplegic migraine**
Familial migraine
Sporadic migraine

✓6th **G43.40 Hemiplegic migraine, not intractable**
Hemiplegic migraine without refractory migraine
G43.401 Hemiplegic migraine, not intractable, with status migrainosus
G43.409 Hemiplegic migraine, not intractable, without status migrainosus
Hemiplegic migraine NOS

✓6th **G43.41 Hemiplegic migraine, intractable**
Hemiplegic migraine with refractory migraine
G43.411 Hemiplegic migraine, intractable, with status migrainosus
G43.419 Hemiplegic migraine, intractable, without status migrainosus

✓5th **G43.5 Persistent migraine aura without cerebral infarction**

✓6th **G43.50 Persistent migraine aura without cerebral infarction, not intractable**
Persistent migraine aura without cerebral infarction, without refractory migraine
G43.501 Persistent migraine aura without cerebral infarction, not intractable, with status migrainosus
G43.509 Persistent migraine aura without cerebral infarction, not intractable, without status migrainosus
Persistent migraine aura NOS

✓6th **G43.51 Persistent migraine aura without cerebral infarction, intractable**
Persistent migraine aura without cerebral infarction, with refractory migraine
G43.511 Persistent migraine aura without cerebral infarction, intractable, with status migrainosus
G43.519 Persistent migraine aura without cerebral infarction, intractable, without status migrainosus

✓5th **G43.6 Persistent migraine aura with cerebral infarction**
Code also the type of cerebral infarction (I63.-)

✓6th **G43.60 Persistent migraine aura with cerebral infarction, not intractable**
Persistent migraine aura with cerebral infarction, without refractory migraine
G43.601 Persistent migraine aura with cerebral infarction, not intractable, with status migrainosus CC
G43.609 Persistent migraine aura with cerebral infarction, not intractable, without status migrainosus CC

✓6th **G43.61 Persistent migraine aura with cerebral infarction, intractable**
Persistent migraine aura with cerebral infarction, with refractory migraine
G43.611 Persistent migraine aura with cerebral infarction, intractable, with status migrainosus CC
G43.619 Persistent migraine aura with cerebral infarction, intractable, without status migrainosus CC

✓5th **G43.7 Chronic migraine without aura**
Transformed migraine
EXCLUDES 1 *migraine without aura (G43.0-)*

✓6th **G43.70 Chronic migraine without aura, not intractable**
Chronic migraine without aura, without refractory migraine
G43.701 Chronic migraine without aura, not intractable, with status migrainosus
G43.709 Chronic migraine without aura, not intractable, without status migrainosus
Chronic migraine without aura NOS

✓6th **G43.71 Chronic migraine without aura, intractable**
Chronic migraine without aura, with refractory migraine
G43.711 Chronic migraine without aura, intractable, with status migrainosus
G43.719 Chronic migraine without aura, intractable, without status migrainosus

✓5th **G43.A Cyclical vomiting**
EXCLUDES 1 *cyclical vomiting syndrome unrelated to migraine (R11.15)*
AHA: 2019,4Q,15
G43.A0 Cyclical vomiting, in migraine, not intractable
Cyclical vomiting, without refractory migraine
G43.A1 Cyclical vomiting, in migraine, intractable
Cyclical vomiting, with refractory migraine

✓5th **G43.B Ophthalmoplegic migraine**
G43.B0 Ophthalmoplegic migraine, not intractable
Ophthalmoplegic migraine, without refractory migraine
G43.B1 Ophthalmoplegic migraine, intractable
Ophthalmoplegic migraine, with refractory migraine

✓5th **G43.C Periodic headache syndromes in child or adult**
G43.C0 Periodic headache syndromes in child or adult, not intractable
Periodic headache syndromes in child or adult, without refractory migraine
G43.C1 Periodic headache syndromes in child or adult, intractable
Periodic headache syndromes in child or adult, with refractory migraine

✓5th **G43.D Abdominal migraine**
G43.D0 Abdominal migraine, not intractable
Abdominal migraine, without refractory migraine
G43.D1 Abdominal migraine, intractable
Abdominal migraine, with refractory migraine

✓5th **G43.8 Other migraine**

✓6th **G43.80 Other migraine, not intractable**
Other migraine, without refractory migraine
G43.801 Other migraine, not intractable, with status migrainosus
G43.809 Other migraine, not intractable, without status migrainosus

✓6th **G43.81 Other migraine, intractable**
Other migraine, with refractory migraine
G43.811 Other migraine, intractable, with status migrainosus
G43.819 Other migraine, intractable, without status migrainosus

✓6th **G43.82 Menstrual migraine, not intractable**
Menstrual headache, not intractable
Menstrual migraine, without refractory migraine
Menstrually related migraine, not intractable
Pre-menstrual headache, not intractable
Pre-menstrual migraine, not intractable
Pure menstrual migraine, not intractable
Code also associated premenstrual tension syndrome (N94.3)
G43.821 Menstrual migraine, not intractable, with status migrainosus ♀
G43.829 Menstrual migraine, not intractable, without status migrainosus ♀
Menstrual migraine NOS

✓6th **G43.83 Menstrual migraine, intractable**
Menstrual headache, intractable
Menstrual migraine, with refractory migraine
Menstrually related migraine, intractable
Pre-menstrual headache, intractable
Pre-menstrual migraine, intractable
Pure menstrual migraine, intractable
Code also associated premenstrual tension syndrome (N94.3)
G43.831 Menstrual migraine, intractable, with status migrainosus ♀
G43.839 Menstrual migraine, intractable, without status migrainosus ♀

G43.9 Migraine, unspecified

G43.90 Migraine, unspecified, not intractable
Migraine, unspecified, without refractory migraine

G43.901 Migraine, unspecified, not intractable, with status migrainosus
Status migrainosus NOS

G43.909 Migraine, unspecified, not intractable, without status migrainosus
Migraine NOS

G43.91 Migraine, unspecified, intractable
Migraine, unspecified, with refractory migraine

G43.911 Migraine, unspecified, intractable, with status migrainosus

G43.919 Migraine, unspecified, intractable, without status migrainosus

G44 Other headache syndromes

EXCLUDES 1 *headache NOS (R51.9)*

EXCLUDES 2 *atypical facial pain (G50.1)*
headache due to lumbar puncture (G97.1)
migraines (G43.-)
trigeminal neuralgia (G50.0)

G44.0 Cluster headaches and other trigeminal autonomic cephalgias (TAC)

DEF: Cluster headache: Characteristic grouping or clustering of headaches that can last for a number of weeks or months and then completely disappear for months or years. They are typically not associated with gastrointestinal upset or light sensitivity as experienced in migraines.

G44.00 Cluster headache syndrome, unspecified
Ciliary neuralgia
Cluster headache NOS
Histamine cephalgia
Lower half migraine
Migrainous neuralgia

G44.001 Cluster headache syndrome, unspecified, intractable

G44.009 Cluster headache syndrome, unspecified, not intractable
Cluster headache syndrome NOS

G44.01 Episodic cluster headache

G44.011 Episodic cluster headache, intractable

G44.019 Episodic cluster headache, not intractable
Episodic cluster headache NOS

G44.02 Chronic cluster headache

G44.021 Chronic cluster headache, intractable

G44.029 Chronic cluster headache, not intractable
Chronic cluster headache NOS

G44.03 Episodic paroxysmal hemicrania
Paroxysmal hemicrania NOS

G44.031 Episodic paroxysmal hemicrania, intractable

G44.039 Episodic paroxysmal hemicrania, not intractable
Episodic paroxysmal hemicrania NOS

G44.04 Chronic paroxysmal hemicrania

G44.041 Chronic paroxysmal hemicrania, intractable

G44.049 Chronic paroxysmal hemicrania, not intractable
Chronic paroxysmal hemicrania NOS

G44.05 Short lasting unilateral neuralgiform headache with conjunctival injection and tearing (SUNCT)

G44.051 Short lasting unilateral neuralgiform headache with conjunctival injection and tearing (SUNCT), intractable

G44.059 Short lasting unilateral neuralgiform headache with conjunctival injection and tearing (SUNCT), not intractable
Short lasting unilateral neuralgiform headache with conjunctival injection and tearing (SUNCT) NOS

G44.09 Other trigeminal autonomic cephalgias (TAC)

G44.091 Other trigeminal autonomic cephalgias (TAC), intractable

G44.099 Other trigeminal autonomic cephalgias (TAC), not intractable

G44.1 Vascular headache, not elsewhere classified

EXCLUDES 2 *cluster headache (G44.0)*
complicated headache syndromes (G44.5-)
drug-induced headache (G44.4-)
migraine (G43.-)
other specified headache syndromes (G44.8-)
post-traumatic headache (G44.3-)
tension-type headache (G44.2-)

G44.2 Tension-type headache

G44.20 Tension-type headache, unspecified

G44.201 Tension-type headache, unspecified, intractable

G44.209 Tension-type headache, unspecified, not intractable
Tension headache NOS

G44.21 Episodic tension-type headache

G44.211 Episodic tension-type headache, intractable

G44.219 Episodic tension-type headache, not intractable
Episodic tension-type headache NOS

G44.22 Chronic tension-type headache

G44.221 Chronic tension-type headache, intractable

G44.229 Chronic tension-type headache, not intractable
Chronic tension-type headache NOS

G44.3 Post-traumatic headache

G44.30 Post-traumatic headache, unspecified

G44.301 Post-traumatic headache, unspecified, intractable

G44.309 Post-traumatic headache, unspecified, not intractable
Post-traumatic headache NOS

G44.31 Acute post-traumatic headache

G44.311 Acute post-traumatic headache, intractable

G44.319 Acute post-traumatic headache, not intractable
Acute post-traumatic headache NOS

G44.32 Chronic post-traumatic headache

G44.321 Chronic post-traumatic headache, intractable

G44.329 Chronic post-traumatic headache, not intractable
Chronic post-traumatic headache NOS

G44.4 Drug-induced headache, not elsewhere classified
Medication overuse headache
Use additional code for adverse effect, if applicable, to identify drug (T36-T50 with fifth or sixth character 5)

G44.40 Drug-induced headache, not elsewhere classified, not intractable

G44.41 Drug-induced headache, not elsewhere classified, intractable

G44.5 Complicated headache syndromes

G44.51 Hemicrania continua

DEF: Persistent primary headache of unknown causation occurring on one side of the face and head. May last for more than three months, with daily and continuous pain of moderate intensity with severe exacerbations.

G44.52 New daily persistent headache (NDPH)

G44.53 Primary thunderclap headache

G44.59 Other complicated headache syndrome

G44.8 Other specified headache syndromes

EXCLUDES 2 *headache with orthostatic or positional component, not elsewhere classifed (R51.0)*

G44.81 Hypnic headache

G44.82 Headache associated with sexual activity
Orgasmic headache
Preorgasmic headache

G44.83 Primary cough headache

G44.84 Primary exertional headache

G44.85 Primary stabbing headache

G44.86 Cervicogenic headache
Code also associated cervical spinal condition, if known
AHA: 2021,4Q,11-12

G44.89 Other headache syndrome

G45 Transient cerebral ischemic attacks and related syndromes

EXCLUDES 1 *neonatal cerebral ischemia (P91.Ø)*
transient retinal artery occlusion (H34.Ø-)

AHA: 2018,2Q,9

DEF: Transient cerebral ischemic attack: Intermittent or brief cerebral dysfunction from lack of oxygenation with no persistent neurological deficits associated with occlusive vascular disease. TIA may denote an impending cerebrovascular accident.

G45.Ø Vertebro-basilar artery syndrome CC
G45.1 Carotid artery syndrome (hemispheric) CC
G45.2 Multiple and bilateral precerebral artery syndromes CC
G45.3 Amaurosis fugax CC
G45.4 Transient global amnesia
EXCLUDES 1 *amnesia NOS (R41.3)*
G45.8 Other transient cerebral ischemic attacks and related syndromes CC
G45.9 Transient cerebral ischemic attack, unspecified CC
Spasm of cerebral artery
TIA
Transient cerebral ischemia NOS

G46 Vascular syndromes of brain in cerebrovascular diseases
Code first underlying cerebrovascular disease (I6Ø-I69)

G46.Ø Middle cerebral artery syndrome CC
G46.1 Anterior cerebral artery syndrome CC
G46.2 Posterior cerebral artery syndrome CC
G46.3 Brain stem stroke syndrome
Benedikt syndrome
Claude syndrome
Foville syndrome
Millard-Gubler syndrome
Wallenberg syndrome
Weber syndrome
G46.4 Cerebellar stroke syndrome
G46.5 Pure motor lacunar syndrome
G46.6 Pure sensory lacunar syndrome
G46.7 Other lacunar syndromes
G46.8 Other vascular syndromes of brain in cerebrovascular diseases

G47 Sleep disorders

EXCLUDES 2 *nightmares (F51.5)*
nonorganic sleep disorders (F51.-)
sleep terrors (F51.4)
sleepwalking (F51.3)

G47.Ø Insomnia

EXCLUDES 2 *alcohol related insomnia (F1Ø.182, F1Ø.282, F1Ø.982)*
drug-related insomnia (F11.182, F11.282, F11.982, F13.182, F13.282, F13.982, F14.182, F14.282, F14.982, F15.182, F15.282, F15.982, F19.182, F19.282, F19.982)
idiopathic insomnia (F51.Ø1)
insomnia due to a mental disorder (F51.Ø5)
insomnia not due to a substance or known physiological condition (F51.Ø-)
nonorganic insomnia (F51.Ø-)
primary insomnia (F51.Ø1)
sleep apnea (G47.3-)

G47.ØØ Insomnia, unspecified
Insomnia NOS
G47.Ø1 Insomnia due to medical condition
Code also associated medical condition
G47.Ø9 Other insomnia

G47.1 Hypersomnia

EXCLUDES 2 *alcohol-related hypersomnia (F1Ø.182, F1Ø.282, F1Ø.982)*
drug-related hypersomnia (F11.182, F11.282, F11.982, F13.182, F13.282, F13.982, F14.182, F14.282, F14.982, F15.182, F15.282, F15.982, F19.182, F19.282, F19.982)
hypersomnia due to a mental disorder (F51.13)
hypersomnia not due to a substance or known physiological condition (F51.1-)
primary hypersomnia (F51.11)
sleep apnea (G47.3-)

G47.1Ø Hypersomnia, unspecified
Hypersomnia NOS
G47.11 Idiopathic hypersomnia with long sleep time
Idiopathic hypersomnia NOS
G47.12 Idiopathic hypersomnia without long sleep time
G47.13 Recurrent hypersomnia
Kleine-Levin syndrome
Menstrual related hypersomnia
G47.14 Hypersomnia due to medical condition
Code also associated medical condition
G47.19 Other hypersomnia

G47.2 Circadian rhythm sleep disorders
Disorders of the sleep wake schedule
Inversion of nyctohemeral rhythm
Inversion of sleep rhythm

DEF: Circadian rhythm: Daily cycle (24-hour period) of physical, mental, and behavioral changes. It is largely influenced by environmental cues, such as changes in light or temperature. *Synonym(s): sleep/wake cycle.*

G47.2Ø Circadian rhythm sleep disorder, unspecified type
Sleep wake schedule disorder NOS
G47.21 Circadian rhythm sleep disorder, delayed sleep phase type
Delayed sleep phase syndrome
G47.22 Circadian rhythm sleep disorder, advanced sleep phase type
G47.23 Circadian rhythm sleep disorder, irregular sleep wake type
Irregular sleep-wake pattern
G47.24 Circadian rhythm sleep disorder, free running type
Circadian rhythm sleep disorder, non-24-hour sleep-wake type
G47.25 Circadian rhythm sleep disorder, jet lag type
G47.26 Circadian rhythm sleep disorder, shift work type
G47.27 Circadian rhythm sleep disorder in conditions classified elsewhere
Code first underlying condition
G47.29 Other circadian rhythm sleep disorder

G47.3 Sleep apnea
Code also any associated underlying condition

EXCLUDES 1 *apnea NOS (RØ6.81)*
Cheyne-Stokes breathing (RØ6.3)
pickwickian syndrome (E66.2)
sleep apnea of newborn ►(P28.3-)◄

G47.3Ø Sleep apnea, unspecified
Sleep apnea NOS
G47.31 Primary central sleep apnea
Idiopathic central sleep apnea
G47.32 High altitude periodic breathing
G47.33 Obstructive sleep apnea (adult) (pediatric)
Obstructive sleep apnea hypopnea
EXCLUDES 1 *obstructive sleep apnea of newborn ►(P28.3-)◄*
G47.34 Idiopathic sleep related nonobstructive alveolar hypoventilation
Sleep related hypoxia
G47.35 Congenital central alveolar hypoventilation syndrome
G47.36 Sleep related hypoventilation in conditions classified elsewhere
Sleep related hypoxemia in conditions classified elsewhere
Code first underlying condition
G47.37 Central sleep apnea in conditions classified elsewhere
Code first underlying condition
G47.39 Other sleep apnea

G47.4 Narcolepsy and cataplexy

G47.41 Narcolepsy

G47.411 Narcolepsy with cataplexy

G47.419 Narcolepsy without cataplexy

Narcolepsy NOS

G47.42 Narcolepsy in conditions classified elsewhere

Code first underlying condition

G47.421 Narcolepsy in conditions classified elsewhere with cataplexy

G47.429 Narcolepsy in conditions classified elsewhere without cataplexy

G47.5 Parasomnia

EXCLUDES 1 *alcohol induced parasomnia (F1Ø.182, F1Ø.282, F1Ø.982)*

drug induced parasomnia (F11.182, F11.282, F11.982, F13.182, F13.282, F13.982, F14.182, F14.282, F14.982, F15.182, F15.282, F15.982, F19.182, F19.282, F19.982)

parasomnia not due to a substance or known physiological condition (F51.8)

G47.5Ø Parasomnia, unspecified

Parasomnia NOS

G47.51 Confusional arousals

G47.52 REM sleep behavior disorder

G47.53 Recurrent isolated sleep paralysis

G47.54 Parasomnia in conditions classified elsewhere

Code first underlying condition

G47.59 Other parasomnia

G47.6 Sleep related movement disorders

EXCLUDES 2 *restless legs syndrome (G25.81)*

G47.61 Periodic limb movement disorder

G47.62 Sleep related leg cramps

G47.63 Sleep related bruxism

EXCLUDES 1 *psychogenic bruxism (F45.8)*

G47.69 Other sleep related movement disorders

G47.8 Other sleep disorders

Other specified sleep-wake disorder

G47.9 Sleep disorder, unspecified

Sleep disorder NOS

Unspecified sleep-wake disorder

Nerve, nerve root and plexus disorders (G5Ø-G59)

EXCLUDES 1 *current traumatic nerve, nerve root and plexus disorders - see Injury, nerve by body region*

neuralgia NOS (M79.2)

neuritis NOS (M79.2)

peripheral neuritis in pregnancy (O26.82-)

radiculitis NOS (M54.1-)

G5Ø Disorders of trigeminal nerve

INCLUDES disorders of 5th cranial nerve

G5Ø.Ø Trigeminal neuralgia

Syndrome of paroxysmal facial pain

Tic douloureux

G5Ø.1 Atypical facial pain

G5Ø.8 Other disorders of trigeminal nerve

G5Ø.9 Disorder of trigeminal nerve, unspecified

G51 Facial nerve disorders

INCLUDES disorders of 7th cranial nerve

G51.Ø Bell's palsy

Facial palsy

G51.1 Geniculate ganglionitis

EXCLUDES 1 *postherpetic geniculate ganglionitis (BØ2.21)*

G51.2 Melkersson's syndrome

Melkersson-Rosenthal syndrome

G51.3 Clonic hemifacial spasm

AHA: 2018,4Q,10

G51.31 Clonic hemifacial spasm, right

G51.32 Clonic hemifacial spasm, left

G51.33 Clonic hemifacial spasm, bilateral

G51.39 Clonic hemifacial spasm, unspecified

G51.4 Facial myokymia

G51.8 Other disorders of facial nerve

G51.9 Disorder of facial nerve, unspecified

G52 Disorders of other cranial nerves

EXCLUDES 2 *disorders of acoustic [8th] nerve (H93.3)*

disorders of optic [2nd] nerve (H46, H47.Ø)

paralytic strabismus due to nerve palsy (H49.Ø-H49.2)

G52.Ø Disorders of olfactory nerve

Disorders of 1st cranial nerve

G52.1 Disorders of glossopharyngeal nerve

Disorder of 9th cranial nerve

Glossopharyngeal neuralgia

G52.2 Disorders of vagus nerve

Disorders of pneumogastric [1Øth] nerve

G52.3 Disorders of hypoglossal nerve

Disorders of 12th cranial nerve

G52.7 Disorders of multiple cranial nerves

Polyneuritis cranialis

G52.8 Disorders of other specified cranial nerves

G52.9 Cranial nerve disorder, unspecified

G53 Cranial nerve disorders in diseases classified elsewhere

Code first underlying disease, such as:

neoplasm (CØØ-D49)

EXCLUDES 1 *multiple cranial nerve palsy in sarcoidosis (D86.82)*

multiple cranial nerve palsy in syphilis (A52.15)

postherpetic geniculate ganglionitis (BØ2.21)

postherpetic trigeminal neuralgia (BØ2.22)

G54 Nerve root and plexus disorders

EXCLUDES 1 *current traumatic nerve root and plexus disorders - see nerve injury by body region*

intervertebral disc disorders (M5Ø-M51)

neuralgia or neuritis NOS (M79.2)

neuritis or radiculitis brachial NOS (M54.13)

neuritis or radiculitis lumbar NOS (M54.16)

neuritis or radiculitis lumbosacral NOS (M54.17)

neuritis or radiculitis thoracic NOS (M54.14)

radiculitis NOS (M54.1Ø)

radiculopathy NOS (M54.1Ø)

spondylosis (M47.-)

G54.Ø Brachial plexus disorders

Thoracic outlet syndrome

DEF: Acquired disorder affecting the spinal nerves that send signals to the shoulder, arm, and hand, causing corresponding motor and sensory dysfunction. This disorder is characterized by regional paresthesia, pain, muscle weakness, and in severe cases paralysis.

G54.1 Lumbosacral plexus disorders

G54.2 Cervical root disorders, not elsewhere classified

G54.3 Thoracic root disorders, not elsewhere classified

G54.4 Lumbosacral root disorders, not elsewhere classified

G54.5 Neuralgic amyotrophy

Parsonage-Aldren-Turner syndrome

Shoulder-girdle neuritis

EXCLUDES 1 *neuralgic amyotrophy in diabetes mellitus (EØ8-E13 with .44)*

G54.6 Phantom limb syndrome with pain HCC

G54.7 Phantom limb syndrome without pain HCC

Phantom limb syndrome NOS

G54.8 Other nerve root and plexus disorders

G54.9 Nerve root and plexus disorder, unspecified

G55 Nerve root and plexus compressions in diseases classified elsewhere

Code first underlying disease, such as:

neoplasm (CØØ-D49)

EXCLUDES 1 *nerve root compression (due to) (in) ankylosing spondylitis (M45.-)*

nerve root compression (due to) (in) dorsopathies (M53.-, M54.-)

nerve root compression (due to) (in) intervertebral disc disorders (M5Ø.1.-, M51.1.-)

nerve root compression (due to) (in) spondylopathies (M46.-, M48.-)

nerve root compression (due to) (in) spondylosis (M47.Ø-, M47.2-)

G56 Mononeuropathies of upper limb

EXCLUDES 1 *current traumatic nerve disorder - see nerve injury by body region*

AHA: 2016,4Q,17-18

G56.0 Carpal tunnel syndrome

DEF: Swelling and inflammation in the tendons or bursa surrounding the median nerve caused by repetitive activity. The resulting compression on the nerve causes pain, numbness, and tingling especially to the palm, index, middle finger, and thumb.

G56.00 Carpal tunnel syndrome, unspecified upper limb
G56.01 Carpal tunnel syndrome, right upper limb
G56.02 Carpal tunnel syndrome, left upper limb
G56.03 Carpal tunnel syndrome, bilateral upper limbs

G56.1 Other lesions of median nerve

G56.10 Other lesions of median nerve, unspecified upper limb
G56.11 Other lesions of median nerve, right upper limb
G56.12 Other lesions of median nerve, left upper limb
G56.13 Other lesions of median nerve, bilateral upper limbs

G56.2 Lesion of ulnar nerve

Tardy ulnar nerve palsy

G56.20 Lesion of ulnar nerve, unspecified upper limb
G56.21 Lesion of ulnar nerve, right upper limb
G56.22 Lesion of ulnar nerve, left upper limb
G56.23 Lesion of ulnar nerve, bilateral upper limbs

G56.3 Lesion of radial nerve

G56.30 Lesion of radial nerve, unspecified upper limb
G56.31 Lesion of radial nerve, right upper limb
G56.32 Lesion of radial nerve, left upper limb
G56.33 Lesion of radial nerve, bilateral upper limbs

G56.4 Causalgia of upper limb

Complex regional pain syndrome II of upper limb

EXCLUDES 1 *complex regional pain syndrome I of lower limb (G90.52-)*
complex regional pain syndrome I of upper limb (G90.51-)
complex regional pain syndrome II of lower limb (G57.7-)
reflex sympathetic dystrophy of lower limb (G90.52-)
reflex sympathetic dystrophy of upper limb (G90.51-)

G56.40 Causalgia of unspecified upper limb
G56.41 Causalgia of right upper limb
G56.42 Causalgia of left upper limb
G56.43 Causalgia of bilateral upper limbs

G56.8 Other specified mononeuropathies of upper limb

Interdigital neuroma of upper limb

G56.80 Other specified mononeuropathies of unspecified upper limb
G56.81 Other specified mononeuropathies of right upper limb
G56.82 Other specified mononeuropathies of left upper limb
G56.83 Other specified mononeuropathies of bilateral upper limbs

G56.9 Unspecified mononeuropathy of upper limb

G56.90 Unspecified mononeuropathy of unspecified upper limb
G56.91 Unspecified mononeuropathy of right upper limb
G56.92 Unspecified mononeuropathy of left upper limb
G56.93 Unspecified mononeuropathy of bilateral upper limbs

G57 Mononeuropathies of lower limb

EXCLUDES 1 *current traumatic nerve disorder - see nerve injury by body region*

AHA: 2016,4Q,17-18

G57.0 Lesion of sciatic nerve

EXCLUDES 1 *sciatica NOS (M54.3-)*
EXCLUDES 2 *sciatica attributed to intervertebral disc disorder (M51.1.-)*

G57.00 Lesion of sciatic nerve, unspecified lower limb
G57.01 Lesion of sciatic nerve, right lower limb
G57.02 Lesion of sciatic nerve, left lower limb
G57.03 Lesion of sciatic nerve, bilateral lower limbs

G57.1 Meralgia paresthetica

Lateral cutaneous nerve of thigh syndrome

G57.10 Meralgia paresthetica, unspecified lower limb
G57.11 Meralgia paresthetica, right lower limb
G57.12 Meralgia paresthetica, left lower limb
G57.13 Meralgia paresthetica, bilateral lower limbs

G57.2 Lesion of femoral nerve

G57.20 Lesion of femoral nerve, unspecified lower limb
G57.21 Lesion of femoral nerve, right lower limb
G57.22 Lesion of femoral nerve, left lower limb
G57.23 Lesion of femoral nerve, bilateral lower limbs

G57.3 Lesion of lateral popliteal nerve

Peroneal nerve palsy

AHA: 2020,3Q,12

G57.30 Lesion of lateral popliteal nerve, unspecified lower limb
G57.31 Lesion of lateral popliteal nerve, right lower limb
G57.32 Lesion of lateral popliteal nerve, left lower limb
G57.33 Lesion of lateral popliteal nerve, bilateral lower limbs

G57.4 Lesion of medial popliteal nerve

G57.40 Lesion of medial popliteal nerve, unspecified lower limb
G57.41 Lesion of medial popliteal nerve, right lower limb
G57.42 Lesion of medial popliteal nerve, left lower limb
G57.43 Lesion of medial popliteal nerve, bilateral lower limbs

G57.5 Tarsal tunnel syndrome

G57.50 Tarsal tunnel syndrome, unspecified lower limb
G57.51 Tarsal tunnel syndrome, right lower limb
G57.52 Tarsal tunnel syndrome, left lower limb
G57.53 Tarsal tunnel syndrome, bilateral lower limbs

G57.6 Lesion of plantar nerve

Morton's metatarsalgia

G57.60 Lesion of plantar nerve, unspecified lower limb
G57.61 Lesion of plantar nerve, right lower limb
G57.62 Lesion of plantar nerve, left lower limb
G57.63 Lesion of plantar nerve, bilateral lower limbs

G57.7 Causalgia of lower limb

Complex regional pain syndrome II of lower limb

EXCLUDES 1 *complex regional pain syndrome I of lower limb (G90.52-)*
complex regional pain syndrome I of upper limb (G90.51-)
complex regional pain syndrome II of upper limb (G56.4-)
reflex sympathetic dystrophy of lower limb (G90.52-)
reflex sympathetic dystrophy of upper limb (G90.51-)

G57.70 Causalgia of unspecified lower limb
G57.71 Causalgia of right lower limb
G57.72 Causalgia of left lower limb
G57.73 Causalgia of bilateral lower limbs

G57.8 Other specified mononeuropathies of lower limb

Interdigital neuroma of lower limb

G57.80 Other specified mononeuropathies of unspecified lower limb
G57.81 Other specified mononeuropathies of right lower limb
G57.82 Other specified mononeuropathies of left lower limb
G57.83 Other specified mononeuropathies of bilateral lower limbs

G57.9 Unspecified mononeuropathy of lower limb

G57.90 Unspecified mononeuropathy of unspecified lower limb
G57.91 Unspecified mononeuropathy of right lower limb
G57.92 Unspecified mononeuropathy of left lower limb
G57.93 Unspecified mononeuropathy of bilateral lower limbs

G58 Other mononeuropathies

G58.0 Intercostal neuropathy
G58.7 Mononeuritis multiplex
G58.8 Other specified mononeuropathies
G58.9 Mononeuropathy, unspecified

G59 *Mononeuropathy in diseases classified elsewhere*
Code first underlying disease
EXCLUDES 1 *diabetic mononeuropathy (E08-E13 with .41)*
syphilitic nerve paralysis (A52.19)
syphilitic neuritis (A52.15)
tuberculous mononeuropathy (A17.83)

Polyneuropathies and other disorders of the peripheral nervous system (G60-G65)

EXCLUDES 1 *neuralgia NOS (M79.2)*
neuritis NOS (M79.2)
peripheral neuritis in pregnancy (O26.82-)
radiculitis NOS (M54.10)

G60 Hereditary and idiopathic neuropathy

G60.0 Hereditary motor and sensory neuropathy
Charcôt-Marie-Tooth disease
Déjérine-Sottas disease
Hereditary motor and sensory neuropathy, types I-IV
Hypertrophic neuropathy of infancy
Peroneal muscular atrophy (axonal type) (hypertrophic type)
Roussy-Levy syndrome

G60.1 Refsum's disease CC
Infantile Refsum disease
DEF: Genetic disorder of the lipid metabolism characterized by retinitis pigmentosa, degenerative nerve disease, ataxia, and dry, rough, scaly skin.

G60.2 Neuropathy in association with hereditary ataxia

G60.3 Idiopathic progressive neuropathy

G60.8 Other hereditary and idiopathic neuropathies
Dominantly inherited sensory neuropathy
Morvan's disease
Nelaton's syndrome
Recessively inherited sensory neuropathy

G60.9 Hereditary and idiopathic neuropathy, unspecified

G61 Inflammatory polyneuropathy

G61.0 Guillain-Barre syndrome CC HCC
Acute (post-)infective polyneuritis
Miller Fisher syndrome
AHA: 2020,3Q,12; 2014,2Q,4
DEF: Autoimmune disorder due to an immune response to foreign antigens with paraplegia of limbs, flaccid paralysis, ophthalmoplegia, ataxia, and areflexia. In most cases, this disorder is triggered by a mild viral infection, surgery, or following an immunization.
TIP: Guillain-Barre syndrome can occur as a sequela of *Campylobacter* enteritis. Assign code B94.8 for the sequelae as an additional diagnosis.

G61.1 Serum neuropathy HCC
Use additional code for adverse effect, if applicable, to identify serum (T50.-)

G61.8 Other inflammatory polyneuropathies

G61.81 Chronic inflammatory demyelinating polyneuritis CC HCC

G61.82 Multifocal motor neuropathy HCC
MMN
AHA: 2016,4Q,18

G61.89 Other inflammatory polyneuropathies HCC

G61.9 Inflammatory polyneuropathy, unspecified HCC

G62 Other and unspecified polyneuropathies

G62.0 Drug-induced polyneuropathy HCC
Use additional code for adverse effect, if applicable, to identify drug (T36-T50 with fifth or sixth character 5)

G62.1 Alcoholic polyneuropathy HCC
AHA: 2019,3Q,8

G62.2 Polyneuropathy due to other toxic agents HCC
Code first (T51-T65) to identify toxic agent

G62.8 Other specified polyneuropathies

G62.81 Critical illness polyneuropathy CC HCC
Acute motor neuropathy

G62.82 Radiation-induced polyneuropathy HCC
Use additional external cause code (W88-W90, X39.0-) to identify cause

G62.89 Other specified polyneuropathies
AHA: 2016,2Q,11

G62.9 Polyneuropathy, unspecified
Neuropathy NOS

G63 *Polyneuropathy in diseases classified elsewhere* HCC
Code first underlying disease, such as:
amyloidosis (E85.-)
endocrine disease, except diabetes (E00-E07, E15-E16, E20-E34)
metabolic diseases (E70-E88)
neoplasm (C00-D49)
nutritional deficiency (E40-E64)
EXCLUDES 1 *polyneuropathy (in):*
diabetes mellitus (E08-E13 with .42)
diphtheria (A36.83)
infectious mononucleosis complicated by polyneuropathy (B27.0-B27.9 with fifth character 1)
Lyme disease (A69.22)
mumps (B26.84)
postherpetic (B02.23)
rheumatoid arthritis (M05.5-)
scleroderma (M34.83)
systemic lupus erythematosus (M32.19)
AHA: 2021,1Q,7; 2012,4Q,99

G64 Other disorders of peripheral nervous system
Disorder of peripheral nervous system NOS

G65 Sequelae of inflammatory and toxic polyneuropathies
Code first condition resulting from (sequela) of inflammatory and toxic polyneuropathies

G65.0 Sequelae of Guillain-Barré syndrome HCC

G65.1 Sequelae of other inflammatory polyneuropathy HCC

G65.2 Sequelae of toxic polyneuropathy HCC

Diseases of myoneural junction and muscle (G70-G73)

G70 Myasthenia gravis and other myoneural disorders
EXCLUDES 1 *botulism (A05.1, A48.51-A48.52)*
transient neonatal myasthenia gravis (P94.0)

G70.0 Myasthenia gravis
DEF: Autoimmune neuromuscular disorder caused by antibodies to the acetylcholine receptors at the neuromuscular junction, interfering with proper binding of the neurotransmitter from the neuron to the target muscle, causing muscle weakness, fatigue, and exhaustion, without pain or atrophy.

G70.00 Myasthenia gravis without (acute) exacerbation HCC
Myasthenia gravis NOS

G70.01 Myasthenia gravis with (acute) exacerbation MCC HCC
Myasthenia gravis in crisis

G70.1 Toxic myoneural disorders HCC
Code first (T51-T65) to identify toxic agent

G70.2 Congenital and developmental myasthenia HCC

G70.8 Other specified myoneural disorders

G70.80 Lambert-Eaton syndrome, unspecified CC HCC
Lambert-Eaton syndrome NOS

G70.81 *Lambert-Eaton syndrome in disease classified elsewhere* CC HCC
Code first underlying disease
EXCLUDES 1 *Lambert-Eaton syndrome in neoplastic disease (G73.1)*

G70.89 Other specified myoneural disorders HCC

G70.9 Myoneural disorder, unspecified HCC

G71 Primary disorders of muscles
EXCLUDES 2 *arthrogryposis multiplex congenita (Q74.3)*
metabolic disorders (E70-E88)
myositis (M60.-)

G71.0 Muscular dystrophy
AHA: 2018,4Q,11-12

G71.00 Muscular dystrophy, unspecified HCC

G71.01 Duchenne or Becker muscular dystrophy HCC
Autosomal recessive, childhood type, muscular dystrophy resembling Duchenne or Becker muscular dystrophy
Benign [Becker] muscular dystrophy
Severe [Duchenne] muscular dystrophy

G71.02 Facioscapulohumeral muscular dystrophy HCC
Scapulohumeral muscular dystrophy

● ✓6th G71.03 Limb girdle muscular dystrophies

● G71.031 Autosomal dominant limb girdle muscular dystrophy
LGMD D4 calpain-3-related
LGMD D5 collagen 6-related
Limb girdle muscular dystrophy type 1

● G71.032 Autosomal recessive limb girdle muscular dystrophy due to calpain-3 dysfunction
Limb girdle muscular dystrophy type 2A
LGMD R1 calpain-3-related
Primary calpainopathy

● G71.033 Limb girdle muscular dystrophy due to dysferlin dysfunction
Dysferlinopathy
LGMD R2 dysferlin-related
Limb girdle muscular dystrophy type 2B
Miyoshi Myopathy type 1

● ✓7th G71.034 Limb girdle muscular dystrophy due to sarcoglycan dysfunction

● G71.0340 Limb girdle muscular dystrophy due to sarcoglycan dysfunction, unspecified
Sarcoglycanopathy, NOS

● G71.0341 Limb girdle muscular dystrophy due to alpha sarcoglycan dysfunction
Alpha sarcoglycanopathy
Limb-girdle muscular dystrophy due to alpha-sarcoglycan deficiency
Limb girdle muscular dystrophy type 2D

● G71.0342 Limb girdle muscular dystrophy due to beta sarcoglycan dysfunction
Beta sarcoglycanopathy
Limb girdle muscular dystrophy due to beta-sarcoglycan deficiency
Limb girdle muscular dystrophy type 2E

● G71.0349 Limb girdle muscular dystrophy due to other sarcoglycan dysfunction
Delta sarcoglycanopathy
Delta-sarcoglycan-related LGMD R6
Gamma sarcoglycanopathy
Gamma-sarcoglycan-related LGMD R5
Limb girdle muscular dystrophy type 2C
Limb girdle muscular dystrophy type 2F

● G71.035 Limb girdle muscular dystrophy due to anoctamin-5 dysfunction
Anoctamin-5-related LGMD R12
Anoctaminopathy
Autosomal recessive limb girdle muscular dystrophy type 2L
Miyoshi myopathy type 3

● G71.038 Other limb girdle muscular dystrophy
LGMD R9 FKRP-related
LGMD R22 collagen 6-related
Limb girdle muscular dystrophy due to fukutin related protein dysfunction
Limb girdle muscular dystrophy type 2I
Other autosomal recessive limb girdle muscular dystrophy

● G71.039 Limb girdle muscular dystrophy, unspecified

G71.09 Other specified muscular dystrophies HCC
Benign scapuloperoneal muscular dystrophy with early contractures [Emery-Dreifuss]
Congenital muscular dystrophy NOS
Congenital muscular dystrophy with specific morphological abnormalities of the muscle fiber
Distal muscular dystrophy
~~Limb-girdle muscular dystrophy~~
Ocular muscular dystrophy
Oculopharyngeal muscular dystrophy
Scapuloperoneal muscular dystrophy

✓5th G71.1 Myotonic disorders

G71.11 Myotonic muscular dystrophy HCC
Dystrophia myotonica [Steinert]
Myotonia atrophica
Myotonic dystrophy
Proximal myotonic myopathy (PROMM)
Steinert disease

G71.12 Myotonia congenita
Acetazolamide responsive myotonia congenita
Dominant myotonia congenita [Thomsen disease]
Myotonia levior
Recessive myotonia congenita [Becker disease]

G71.13 Myotonic chondrodystrophy
Chondrodystrophic myotonia
Congenital myotonic chondrodystrophy
Schwartz-Jampel disease

G71.14 Drug induced myotonia
Use additional code for adverse effect, if applicable, to identify drug (T36-T50 with fifth or sixth character 5)

G71.19 Other specified myotonic disorders
Myotonia fluctuans
Myotonia permanens
Neuromyotonia [Isaacs]
Paramyotonia congenita (of von Eulenburg)
Pseudomyotonia
Symptomatic myotonia

✓5th G71.2 Congenital myopathies
EXCLUDES 2 *arthrogryposis multiplex congenita (Q74.3)*
AHA: 2020,4Q,19-21

G71.20 Congenital myopathy, unspecified CC HCC

G71.21 Nemaline myopathy CC HCC

✓6th G71.22 Centronuclear myopathy

G71.220 X-linked myotubular myopathy CC HCC
Myotubular (centronuclear) myopathy

G71.228 Other centronuclear myopathy CC HCC
Autosomal centronuclear myopathy
Autosomal dominant centronuclear myopathy
Autosomal recessive centronuclear myopathy
Centronuclear myopathy, NOS

G71.29 Other congenital myopathy CC HCC
Central core disease
Minicore disease
Multicore disease
Multiminicore disease

G71.3 Mitochondrial myopathy, not elsewhere classified
EXCLUDES 1 *Kearns-Sayre syndrome (H49.81)*
Leber's disease (H47.21)
Leigh's encephalopathy (G31.82)
mitochondrial metabolism disorders (E88.4.-)
Reye's syndrome (G93.7)

G71.8 Other primary disorders of muscles

G71.9 Primary disorder of muscle, unspecified
Hereditary myopathy NOS

4th G72 Other and unspecified myopathies

EXCLUDES 1 *arthrogryposis multiplex congenita (Q74.3)*
dermatopolymyositis (M33.-)
ischemic infarction of muscle (M62.2-)
myositis (M6Ø.-)
polymyositis (M33.2.-)

G72.Ø Drug-induced myopathy CC
Use additional code for adverse effect, if applicable, to identify drug (T36-T5Ø with fifth or sixth character 5)

G72.1 Alcoholic myopathy CC
Use additional code to identify alcoholism (F1Ø.-)

G72.2 Myopathy due to other toxic agents CC
Code first (T51-T65) to identify toxic agent

G72.3 Periodic paralysis
Familial periodic paralysis
Hyperkalemic periodic paralysis (familial)
Hypokalemic periodic paralysis (familial)
Myotonic periodic paralysis (familial)
Normokalemic paralysis (familial)
Potassium sensitive periodic paralysis
EXCLUDES 1 *paramyotonia congenita (of von Eulenburg) (G71.19)*

5th G72.4 Inflammatory and immune myopathies, not elsewhere classified

G72.41 Inclusion body myositis [IBM]

G72.49 Other inflammatory and immune myopathies, not elsewhere classified
Inflammatory myopathy NOS

5th G72.8 Other specified myopathies

G72.81 Critical illness myopathy CC
Acute necrotizing myopathy
Acute quadriplegic myopathy
Intensive care (ICU) myopathy
Myopathy of critical illness
AHA: 2020,3Q,12

G72.89 Other specified myopathies

G72.9 Myopathy, unspecified

4th G73 Disorders of myoneural junction and muscle in diseases classified elsewhere

G73.1 Lambert-Eaton syndrome in neoplastic disease CC UPD HCC
Code first underlying neoplasm (CØØ-D49)
EXCLUDES 1 *Lambert-Eaton syndrome not associated with neoplasm (G7Ø.8Ø-G7Ø.81)*

G73.3 Myasthenic syndromes in other diseases classified elsewhere CC HCC
Code first underlying disease, such as:
neoplasm (CØØ-D49)
thyrotoxicosis (EØ5.-)

G73.7 Myopathy in diseases classified elsewhere
Code first underlying disease, such as:
hyperparathyroidism (E21.Ø, E21.3)
hypoparathyroidism (E2Ø.-)
glycogen storage disease (E74.Ø)
lipid storage disorders (E75.-)
EXCLUDES 1 *myopathy in:*
rheumatoid arthritis (MØ5.32)
sarcoidosis (D86.87)
scleroderma (M34.82)
Sjögren syndrome (M35.Ø3)
systemic lupus erythematosus (M32.19)

Cerebral palsy and other paralytic syndromes (G8Ø-G83)

4th G8Ø Cerebral palsy
EXCLUDES 1 *hereditary spastic paraplegia (G11.4)*

G8Ø.Ø Spastic quadriplegic cerebral palsy MCC HCC
Congenital spastic paralysis (cerebral)

G8Ø.1 Spastic diplegic cerebral palsy CC HCC
Spastic cerebral palsy NOS

G8Ø.2 Spastic hemiplegic cerebral palsy CC HCC

G8Ø.3 Athetoid cerebral palsy CC HCC
Double athetosis (syndrome)
Dyskinetic cerebral palsy
Dystonic cerebral palsy
Vogt disease

G8Ø.4 Ataxic cerebral palsy HCC

G8Ø.8 Other cerebral palsy HCC
Mixed cerebral palsy syndromes

G8Ø.9 Cerebral palsy, unspecified HCC
Cerebral palsy NOS

4th G81 Hemiplegia and hemiparesis

NOTE This category is to be used only when hemiplegia (complete)(incomplete) is reported without further specification, or is stated to be old or longstanding but of unspecified cause. The category is also for use in multiple coding to identify these types of hemiplegia resulting from any cause.

EXCLUDES 1 *congenital cerebral palsy (G8Ø.-)*
hemiplegia and hemiparesis due to sequela of cerebrovascular disease (I69.Ø5-, I69.15-, I69.25-, I69.35-, I69.85-, I69.95-)

AHA: 2015,1Q,25

TIP: If the documentation specifies the affected side but not whether it is the dominant or nondominant side, the default is as follows: for ambidextrous patients, the default is dominant; when the left side is affected, the default is nondominant; and when the right side is affected, the default is dominant.

5th G81.Ø Flaccid hemiplegia

G81.ØØ Flaccid hemiplegia affecting unspecified side CC UNS HCC

G81.Ø1 Flaccid hemiplegia affecting right dominant side CC HCC

G81.Ø2 Flaccid hemiplegia affecting left dominant side CC HCC

G81.Ø3 Flaccid hemiplegia affecting right nondominant side CC HCC

G81.Ø4 Flaccid hemiplegia affecting left nondominant side CC HCC

5th G81.1 Spastic hemiplegia

G81.1Ø Spastic hemiplegia affecting unspecified side CC UNS HCC

G81.11 Spastic hemiplegia affecting right dominant side CC HCC

G81.12 Spastic hemiplegia affecting left dominant side CC HCC

G81.13 Spastic hemiplegia affecting right nondominant side CC HCC

G81.14 Spastic hemiplegia affecting left nondominant side CC HCC

5th G81.9 Hemiplegia, unspecified
AHA: 2014,1Q,23

G81.9Ø Hemiplegia, unspecified affecting unspecified side CC UNS HCC

G81.91 Hemiplegia, unspecified affecting right dominant side CC HCC

G81.92 Hemiplegia, unspecified affecting left dominant side CC HCC

G81.93 Hemiplegia, unspecified affecting right nondominant side CC HCC

G81.94 Hemiplegia, unspecified affecting left nondominant side CC HCC

4th G82 Paraplegia (paraparesis) and quadriplegia (quadriparesis)

NOTE This category is to be used only when the listed conditions are reported without further specification, or are stated to be old or longstanding but of unspecified cause. The category is also for use in multiple coding to identify these conditions resulting from any cause

EXCLUDES 1 *congenital cerebral palsy (G8Ø.-)*
functional quadriplegia (R53.2)
hysterical paralysis (F44.4)

5th G82.2 Paraplegia
Paralysis of both lower limbs NOS
Paraparesis (lower) NOS
Paraplegia (lower) NOS
AHA: 2017,3Q,3

G82.2Ø Paraplegia, unspecified CC HCC

G82.21 Paraplegia, complete CC HCC

G82.22 Paraplegia, incomplete CC HCC

5th G82.5 Quadriplegia

G82.5Ø Quadriplegia, unspecified MCC HCC

G82.51 Quadriplegia, C1-C4 complete MCC HCC

G82.52 Quadriplegia, C1-C4 incomplete MCC HCC

G82.53 **Quadriplegia, C5-C7 complete** MCC HCC

G82.54 **Quadriplegia, C5-C7 incomplete** MCC HCC

G83 Other paralytic syndromes

NOTE This category is to be used only when the listed conditions are reported without further specification, or are stated to be old or longstanding but of unspecified cause. The category is also for use in multiple coding to identify these conditions resulting from any cause.

INCLUDES paralysis (complete) (incomplete), except as in G8Ø-G82

G83.Ø Diplegia of upper limbs CC HCC

Diplegia (upper)

Paralysis of both upper limbs

G83.1 Monoplegia of lower limb

Paralysis of lower limb

EXCLUDES 1 *monoplegia of lower limbs due to sequela of cerebrovascular disease (I69.Ø4-, I69.14-, I69.24-, I69.34-, I69.84-, I69.94-)*

TIP: If the documentation specifies the affected side but not whether it is the dominant or nondominant side, the default is as follows: for ambidextrous patients, the default is dominant; when the left side is affected, the default is nondominant; and when the right side is affected, the default is dominant.

G83.1Ø **Monoplegia of lower limb affecting unspecified side** HCC

G83.11 **Monoplegia of lower limb affecting right dominant side** HCC

G83.12 **Monoplegia of lower limb affecting left dominant side** HCC

G83.13 **Monoplegia of lower limb affecting right nondominant side** HCC

G83.14 **Monoplegia of lower limb affecting left nondominant side** HCC

G83.2 Monoplegia of upper limb

Paralysis of upper limb

EXCLUDES 1 *monoplegia of upper limbs due to sequela of cerebrovascular disease (I69.Ø3-, I69.13-, I69.23-, I69.33-, I69.83-, I69.93-)*

TIP: If the documentation specifies the affected side but not whether it is the dominant or nondominant side, the default is as follows: for ambidextrous patients, the default is dominant; when the left side is affected, the default is nondominant; and when the right side is affected, the default is dominant.

G83.2Ø **Monoplegia of upper limb affecting unspecified side** HCC

G83.21 **Monoplegia of upper limb affecting right dominant side** HCC

G83.22 **Monoplegia of upper limb affecting left dominant side** HCC

G83.23 **Monoplegia of upper limb affecting right nondominant side** HCC

G83.24 **Monoplegia of upper limb affecting left nondominant side** HCC

G83.3 Monoplegia, unspecified

TIP: If the documentation specifies the affected side but not whether it is the dominant or nondominant side, the default is as follows: for ambidextrous patients, the default is dominant; when the left side is affected, the default is nondominant; and when the right side is affected, the default is dominant.

G83.3Ø **Monoplegia, unspecified affecting unspecified side** HCC

G83.31 **Monoplegia, unspecified affecting right dominant side** HCC

G83.32 **Monoplegia, unspecified affecting left dominant side** HCC

G83.33 **Monoplegia, unspecified affecting right nondominant side** HCC

G83.34 **Monoplegia, unspecified affecting left nondominant side** HCC

G83.4 Cauda equina syndrome CC HCC

Neurogenic bladder due to cauda equina syndrome

EXCLUDES 1 *cord bladder NOS (G95.89)*

neurogenic bladder NOS (N31.9)

AHA: 2020,3Q,24

DEF: Compression of the spinal nerve roots presenting with pain and tingling radiating down the buttocks, back of the thigh and calf, and into the foot in a sciatic manner with aching in the bladder, perineum, and sacrum. Loss of bowel and bladder control may also occur.

G83.5 Locked-in state MCC HCC

AHA: 2022,2Q,10

G83.8 Other specified paralytic syndromes

EXCLUDES 1 *paralytic syndromes due to current spinal cord injury - code to spinal cord injury (S14, S24, S34)*

G83.81 **Brown-Séquard syndrome** HCC

G83.82 **Anterior cord syndrome** HCC

G83.83 **Posterior cord syndrome** HCC

G83.84 **Todd's paralysis (postepileptic)** HCC

G83.89 **Other specified paralytic syndromes** HCC

G83.9 Paralytic syndrome, unspecified HCC

Other disorders of the nervous system (G89-G99)

G89 Pain, not elsewhere classified

Code also related psychological factors associated with pain (F45.42)

EXCLUDES 1 *generalized pain NOS (R52)*

pain disorders exclusively related to psychological factors (F45.41)

pain NOS (R52)

EXCLUDES 2 *atypical face pain (G5Ø.1)*

headache syndromes (G44.-)

localized pain, unspecified type - code to pain by site, such as:

abdomen pain (R1Ø.-)

back pain (M54.9)

breast pain (N64.4)

chest pain (RØ7.1-RØ7.9)

ear pain (H92.Ø-)

eye pain (H57.1)

headache (R51.9)

joint pain (M25.5-)

limb pain (M79.6-)

lumbar region pain (M54.5-)

painful urination (R3Ø.9)

pelvic and perineal pain (R1Ø.2)

renal colic (N23)

shoulder pain (M25.51-)

spine pain (M54.-)

throat pain (RØ7.Ø)

tongue pain (K14.6)

tooth pain (KØ8.8)

migraines (G43.-)

myalgia (M79.1-)

pain from prosthetic devices, implants, and grafts (T82.84, T83.84, T84.84, T85.84-)

phantom limb syndrome with pain (G54.6)

vulvar vestibulitis (N94.81Ø)

vulvodynia (N94.81-)

G89.Ø Central pain syndrome

Déjérine-Roussy syndrome

Myelopathic pain syndrome

Thalamic pain syndrome (hyperesthetic)

G89.1 Acute pain, not elsewhere classified

G89.11 **Acute pain due to trauma**

G89.12 **Acute post-thoracotomy pain**

Post-thoracotomy pain NOS

G89.18 **Other acute postprocedural pain**

Postoperative pain NOS

Postprocedural pain NOS

✓5th G89.2 Chronic pain, not elsewhere classified

EXCLUDES 1 *causalgia, lower limb (G57.7-)*
causalgia, upper limb (G56.4-)
central pain syndrome (G89.Ø)
chronic pain syndrome (G89.4)
complex regional pain syndrome II, lower limb (G57.7-)
complex regional pain syndrome II, upper limb (G56.4-)
neoplasm related chronic pain (G89.3)
reflex sympathetic dystrophy (G9Ø.5-)

G89.21 Chronic pain due to trauma

G89.22 Chronic post-thoracotomy pain

G89.28 Other chronic postprocedural pain
Other chronic postoperative pain

G89.29 Other chronic pain

G89.3 Neoplasm related pain (acute) (chronic)
Cancer associated pain
Pain due to malignancy (primary) (secondary)
Tumor associated pain

G89.4 Chronic pain syndrome
Chronic pain associated with significant psychosocial dysfunction

✓4th G9Ø Disorders of autonomic nervous system

EXCLUDES 1 *dysfunction of the autonomic nervous system due to alcohol (G31.2)*

✓5th G9Ø.Ø Idiopathic peripheral autonomic neuropathy

G9Ø.Ø1 Carotid sinus syncope
Carotid sinus syndrome
DEF: Vagal activation caused by pressure on the carotid sinus baroreceptors. Sympathetic nerve impulses may cause sinus arrest or AV block.

G9Ø.Ø9 Other idiopathic peripheral autonomic neuropathy
Idiopathic peripheral autonomic neuropathy NOS

G9Ø.1 Familial dysautonomia [Riley-Day] HCC

G9Ø.2 Horner's syndrome
Bernard(-Horner) syndrome
Cervical sympathetic dystrophy or paralysis

G9Ø.3 Multi-system degeneration of the autonomic nervous system CC HCC
Neurogenic orthostatic hypotension [Shy-Drager]
EXCLUDES 1 *orthostatic hypotension NOS (I95.1)*

G9Ø.4 Autonomic dysreflexia
Use additional code to identify the cause, such as:
fecal impaction (K56.41)
pressure ulcer (pressure area) (L89.-)
urinary tract infection (N39.Ø)

✓5th G9Ø.5 Complex regional pain syndrome I (CRPS I)
Reflex sympathetic dystrophy
EXCLUDES 1 *causalgia of lower limb (G57.7-)*
causalgia of upper limb (G56.4-)
complex regional pain syndrome II of lower limb (G57.7-)
complex regional pain syndrome II of upper limb (G56.4-)

G9Ø.5Ø Complex regional pain syndrome I, unspecified CC UNS

✓6th G9Ø.51 Complex regional pain syndrome I of upper limb

G9Ø.511 Complex regional pain syndrome I of right upper limb CC

G9Ø.512 Complex regional pain syndrome I of left upper limb CC

G9Ø.513 Complex regional pain syndrome I of upper limb, bilateral CC

G9Ø.519 Complex regional pain syndrome I of unspecified upper limb CC UNS

✓6th G9Ø.52 Complex regional pain syndrome I of lower limb

G9Ø.521 Complex regional pain syndrome I of right lower limb CC

G9Ø.522 Complex regional pain syndrome I of left lower limb CC

G9Ø.523 Complex regional pain syndrome I of lower limb, bilateral CC

G9Ø.529 Complex regional pain syndrome I of unspecified lower limb CC UNS

G9Ø.59 Complex regional pain syndrome I of other specified site CC

G9Ø.8 Other disorders of autonomic nervous system

G9Ø.9 Disorder of the autonomic nervous system, unspecified

● **G9Ø.A Postural orthostatic tachycardia syndrome [POTS]**
Chronic orthostatic intolerance
Postural tachycardia syndrome

✓4th G91 Hydrocephalus

INCLUDES acquired hydrocephalus
EXCLUDES 1 *Arnold-Chiari syndrome with hydrocephalus (QØ7.-)*
congenital hydrocephalus (QØ3.-)
spina bifida with hydrocephalus (QØ5.-)

DEF: Abnormal buildup of cerebrospinal fluid in the brain causing dilation of the ventricles.

Hydrocephalus (Acquired)

Normal ventricles — Hydrocephalic ventricles

G91.Ø Communicating hydrocephalus CC HCC
Secondary normal pressure hydrocephalus

G91.1 Obstructive hydrocephalus CC HCC
DEF: Obstruction of the cerebrospinal fluid passage from the brain into the spinal canal characterized by headaches, drowsiness, poor coordination, urinary incontinence, nausea, vomiting, and papilledema.

G91.2 (Idiopathic) normal pressure hydrocephalus CC HCC
Normal pressure hydrocephalus NOS

G91.3 Post-traumatic hydrocephalus, unspecified CC HCC

G91.4 Hydrocephalus in diseases classified elsewhere HCC
Code first underlying condition, such as:
congenital syphilis (A5Ø.4-)
neoplasm (CØØ-D49)
plasminogen deficiency (E88.Ø2)
EXCLUDES 1 *hydrocephalus due to congenital toxoplasmosis (P37.1)*
AHA: 2014,3Q,3

G91.8 Other hydrocephalus CC HCC

G91.9 Hydrocephalus, unspecified CC HCC

✓4th G92 Toxic encephalopathy

AHA: 2022,1Q,52; 2021,4Q,12-14; 2021,1Q,13; 2017,1Q,39-40
DEF: Brain tissue degeneration due to a toxic substance.

✓5th G92.Ø Immune effector cell-associated neurotoxicity syndrome
Code first underlying cause such as:
complications of immune effector cellular therapy (T8Ø.82)
Code also associated signs and symptoms, such as seizures and cerebral edema
Code also, if applicable:
cerebral edema (G93.6)
unspecified convulsions (R56.9)

G92.ØØ Immune effector cell-associated neurotoxicity syndrome, grade unspecified UPD
ICANS, grade unspecified

G92.Ø1 Immune effector cell-associated neurotoxicity syndrome, grade 1 UPD
ICANS, grade 1

G92.Ø2 Immune effector cell-associated neurotoxicity syndrome, grade 2 UPD
ICANS, grade 2

G92.Ø3 Immune effector cell-associated neurotoxicity syndrome, grade 3 CC UPD
ICANS, grade 3

G92.Ø4 Immune effector cell-associated neurotoxicity syndrome, grade 4 CC UPD
ICANS, grade 4

G92.Ø5 Immune effector cell-associated neurotoxicity syndrome, grade 5 CC UPD
ICANS, grade 5

G92.8 Other toxic encephalopathy MCC
Toxic encephalitis
Toxic metabolic encephalopathy
Code first poisoning due to drug or toxin, if applicable, (T36-T65 with fifth or sixth character 1-4 or 6)
Use additional code for adverse effect, if applicable, to identify drug (T36-T5Ø with fifth or sixth character 5)
AHA: 2022,1Q,52

G92.9 Unspecified toxic encephalopathy MCC
Code first poisoning due to drug or toxin, if applicable, (T36-T65 with fifth or sixth character 1-4 or 6)
Use additional code for adverse effect, if applicable, to identify drug (T36-T5Ø with fifth or sixth character 5)

✓4th **G93 Other disorders of brain**

G93.Ø Cerebral cysts
Arachnoid cyst
Porencephalic cyst, acquired
EXCLUDES 1 *acquired periventricular cysts of newborn (P91.1)*
congenital cerebral cysts (QØ4.6)

G93.1 Anoxic brain damage, not elsewhere classified CC HCC
EXCLUDES 1 *cerebral anoxia due to anesthesia during labor and delivery (O74.3)*
cerebral anoxia due to anesthesia during the puerperium (O89.2)
neonatal anoxia (P84)
DEF: Brain injury not resulting from birth trauma that is due to lack of oxygen. Brain cells, when deprived of oxygen, begin to expire after four minutes.

G93.2 Benign intracranial hypertension
Pseudotumor
EXCLUDES 1 *hypertensive encephalopathy (I67.4)*
obstructive hydrocephalus (G91.1)

▲ ✓5th **G93.3 Postviral and related fatigue syndromes**
~~Benign myalgic encephalomyelitis~~
▶Use additional code, if applicable, for post COVID-19 condition, unspecified (UØ9.9)◀
EXCLUDES 1 *chronic fatigue syndrome NOS (R53.82)*
▶neurasthenia (F48.8)◀

● **G93.31 Postviral fatigue syndrome**

● **G93.32 Myalgic encephalomyelitis/chronic fatigue syndrome**
Chronic fatigue syndrome
ME/CFS
Myalgic encephalomyelitis

● **G93.39 Other post infection and related fatigue syndromes**

✓5th **G93.4 Other and unspecified encephalopathy**
EXCLUDES 1 *alcoholic encephalopathy (G31.2)*
encephalopathy in diseases classified elsewhere (G94)
hypertensive encephalopathy (I67.4)
EXCLUDES 2 *toxic (metabolic) encephalopathy (G92.8)*

G93.4Ø Encephalopathy, unspecified HIV CC
AHA: 2017,2Q,8

G93.41 Metabolic encephalopathy HIV MCC
Septic encephalopathy
AHA: 2017,2Q,8; 2016,3Q,42; 2015,3Q,21
TIP: Assign separately when documented with diabetic hypoglycemia (EØ8.649, EØ9.649, E1Ø.649, E11.649, E13.649).

G93.49 Other encephalopathy HIV CC
Encephalopathy NEC
AHA: 2021,2Q,3; 2018,4Q,16; 2018,2Q,22,24; 2017,2Q,9

G93.5 Compression of brain MCC HCC
Arnold-Chiari type 1 compression of brain
Compression of brain (stem)
Herniation of brain (stem)
EXCLUDES 1 *traumatic compression of brain (SØ6.A-)*
AHA: 2020,2Q,31

G93.6 Cerebral edema MCC HCC
EXCLUDES 1 *cerebral edema due to birth injury (P11.Ø)*
traumatic cerebral edema (SØ6.1-)

G93.7 Reye's syndrome MCC HCC P
Code first poisoning due to salicylates, if applicable (T39.Ø-, with sixth character 1-4)
Use additional code for adverse effect due to salicylates, if applicable (T39.Ø-, with sixth character 5)
DEF: Rare childhood illness often developed after a viral upper respiratory infection. Symptoms include vomiting, elevated serum transaminase, brain swelling, disturbances of consciousness, seizures, and changes in liver and other viscera; it can be fatal.

✓5th **G93.8 Other specified disorders of brain**

G93.81 Temporal sclerosis
Hippocampal sclerosis
Mesial temporal sclerosis

G93.82 Brain death MCC

G93.89 Other specified disorders of brain
Postradiation encephalopathy
AHA: 2020,2Q,24; 2019,3Q,8

G93.9 Disorder of brain, unspecified HIV

G94 Other disorders of brain in diseases classified elsewhere
Code first underlying disease
EXCLUDES 1 *encephalopathy in congenital syphilis (A5Ø.49)*
encephalopathy in influenza (JØ9.X9, J1Ø.81, J11.81)
encephalopathy in syphilis (A52.19)
hydrocephalus in diseases classified elsewhere (G91.4)
AHA: 2018,2Q,22; 2017,2Q,8-9

✓4th **G95 Other and unspecified diseases of spinal cord**
EXCLUDES 2 *myelitis (GØ4.-)*

G95.Ø Syringomyelia and syringobulbia CC HCC

✓5th **G95.1 Vascular myelopathies**
EXCLUDES 2 *intraspinal phlebitis and thrombophlebitis, except non-pyogenic (GØ8)*

G95.11 Acute infarction of spinal cord (embolic) (nonembolic) MCC HCC
Anoxia of spinal cord
Arterial thrombosis of spinal cord

G95.19 Other vascular myelopathies MCC HCC
Edema of spinal cord
Hematomyelia
Nonpyogenic intraspinal phlebitis and thrombophlebitis
Subacute necrotic myelopathy

✓5th **G95.2 Other and unspecified cord compression**

G95.2Ø Unspecified cord compression HIV CC HCC

G95.29 Other cord compression HIV CC HCC

✓5th **G95.8 Other specified diseases of spinal cord**
EXCLUDES 1 *neurogenic bladder NOS (N31.9)*
neurogenic bladder due to cauda equina syndrome (G83.4)
neuromuscular dysfunction of bladder without spinal cord lesion (N31.-)

G95.81 Conus medullaris syndrome CC HCC

G95.89 Other specified diseases of spinal cord CC HCC
Cord bladder NOS
Drug-induced myelopathy
Radiation-induced myelopathy
EXCLUDES 1 *myelopathy NOS (G95.9)*

G95.9 Disease of spinal cord, unspecified HIV CC HCC
Myelopathy NOS

G96 Other disorders of central nervous system

G96.Ø Cerebrospinal fluid leak
Code also if applicable:
intracranial hypotension (G96.81-)
EXCLUDES 1 *cerebrospinal fluid leak from spinal puncture (G97.Ø)*
AHA: 2020,4Q,21-22; 2018,2Q,13

G96.ØØ Cerebrospinal fluid leak, unspecified CC
Code also if applicable:
head injury ►(SØØ-SØ9)◄

G96.Ø1 Cranial cerebrospinal fluid leak, spontaneous CC
Otorrhea due to spontaneous cerebrospinal fluid CSF leak
Rhinorrhea due to spontaneous cerebrospinal fluid CSF leak
Spontaneous cerebrospinal fluid leak from skull base

G96.Ø2 Spinal cerebrospinal fluid leak, spontaneous CC
Spontaneous cerebrospinal fluid leak from spine

G96.Ø8 Other cranial cerebrospinal fluid leak CC
Postoperative cranial cerebrospinal fluid leak
Traumatic cranial cerebrospinal fluid leak
Code also if applicable:
head injury (SØØ.- to SØ9.-)

G96.Ø9 Other spinal cerebrospinal fluid leak CC
Other spinal CSF leak
Postoperative spinal cerebrospinal fluid leak
Traumatic spinal cerebrospinal fluid leak
Code also if applicable:
head injury (SØØ.- to SØ9.-)

G96.1 Disorders of meninges, not elsewhere classified

G96.11 Dural tear CC
Code also intracranial hypotension, if applicable (G96.81-)
EXCLUDES 1 *accidental puncture or laceration of dura during a procedure (G97.41)*
AHA: 2014,4Q,24

G96.12 Meningeal adhesions (cerebral) (spinal)

G96.19 Other disorders of meninges, not elsewhere classified
AHA: 2020,4Q,22

G96.191 Perineural cyst
Cervical nerve root cyst
Lumbar nerve root cyst
Sacral nerve root cyst
Tarlov cyst
Thoracic nerve root cyst

G96.198 Other disorders of meninges, not elsewhere classified

G96.8 Other specified disorders of central nervous system
AHA: 2020,4Q,21,23-24

G96.81 Intracranial hypotension
Code also any associated diagnoses, such as:
brachial amyotrophy (G54.5)
cerebrospinal fluid leak from spine (G96.Ø2)
cranial nerve disorders in diseases classified elsewhere (G53)
nerve root and compressions in diseases classified elsewhere (G55)
nonpyogenic thrombosis of intracranial venous system (I67.6)
nontraumatic intracerebral hemorrhage (I61.-)
nontraumatic subdural hemorrhage (I62.Ø-)
other and unspecified cord compression (G95.2-)
other secondary parkinsonism (G21.8)
reversible cerebrovascular vasoconstriction syndrome (I67.841)
spinal cord herniation (G95.89)
stroke (I63.-)
syringomyelia (G95.Ø)

DEF: Central nervous system disorder resulting from a loss of cerebrospinal fluid (CSF) volume. More often associated with CSF leak at the level of the spine rather than the skull base, causes can be spontaneous, iatrogenic or traumatic spinal dura defects or holes, or overdrainage of CSF shunt devices. The most common symptom is headache.

G96.81Ø Intracranial hypotension, unspecified

G96.811 Intracranial hypotension, spontaneous

G96.819 Other intracranial hypotension

G96.89 Other specified disorders of central nervous system

G96.9 Disorder of central nervous system, unspecified HIV

G97 Intraoperative and postprocedural complications and disorders of nervous system, not elsewhere classified
EXCLUDES 2 *intraoperative and postprocedural cerebrovascular infarction (I97.81-, I97.82-)*
AHA: 2016,4Q,9-10

G97.Ø Cerebrospinal fluid leak from spinal puncture CC
Code also any associated diagnoses or complications, such as:
intracranial hypotension following a procedure (G97.83-G97.84)

Spinal Puncture

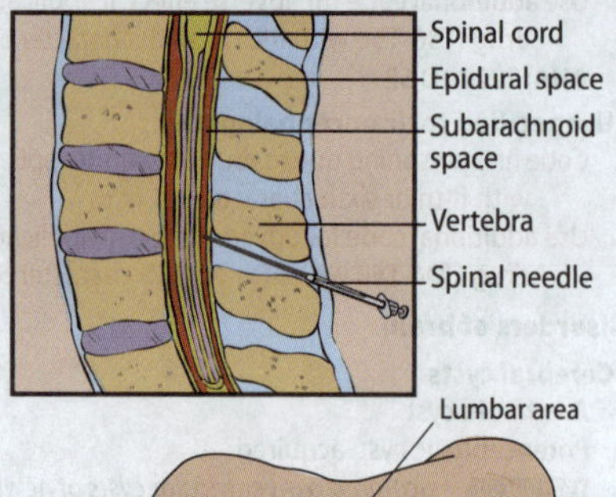

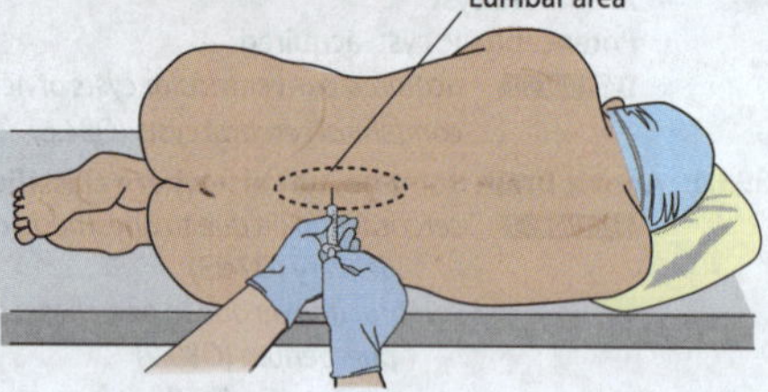

G97.1 Other reaction to spinal and lumbar puncture
Headache due to lumbar puncture
Other reaction to spinal dural puncture
Code also, if applicable, any associated headache with orthostatic component (R51.Ø)

G97.2 Intracranial hypotension following ventricular shunting CC
Code also any associated diagnoses or complications

G97.3 Intraoperative hemorrhage and hematoma of a nervous system organ or structure complicating a procedure
EXCLUDES 1 *intraoperative hemorrhage and hematoma of a nervous system organ or structure due to accidental puncture and laceration during a procedure (G97.4-)*

G97.31 Intraoperative hemorrhage and hematoma of a nervous system organ or structure complicating a nervous system procedure CC

G97.32 Intraoperative hemorrhage and hematoma of a nervous system organ or structure complicating other procedure CC

G97.4 Accidental puncture and laceration of a nervous system organ or structure during a procedure

G97.41 Accidental puncture or laceration of dura during a procedure CC
Incidental (inadvertent) durotomy
Code also any associated diagnoses or complications
AHA: 2014,4Q,24

G97.48 Accidental puncture and laceration of other nervous system organ or structure during a nervous system procedure CC

G97.49 Accidental puncture and laceration of other nervous system organ or structure during other procedure CC

G97.5 Postprocedural hemorrhage of a nervous system organ or structure following a procedure

G97.51 Postprocedural hemorrhage of a nervous system organ or structure following a nervous system procedure CC

G97.52 Postprocedural hemorrhage of a nervous system organ or structure following other procedure CC

G97.6 Postprocedural hematoma and seroma of a nervous system organ or structure following a procedure

G97.61 Postprocedural hematoma of a nervous system organ or structure following a nervous system procedure CC
AHA: 2020,3Q,24

G97.62 Postprocedural hematoma of a nervous system organ or structure following other procedure CC

G97.63 Postprocedural seroma of a nervous system organ or structure following a nervous system procedure CC

G97.64 Postprocedural seroma of a nervous system organ or structure following other procedure CC

G97.8 Other intraoperative and postprocedural complications and disorders of nervous system
Use additional code to further specify disorder
AHA: 2020,4Q,23

G97.81 Other intraoperative complications of nervous system CC

G97.82 Other postprocedural complications and disorders of nervous system CC
AHA: 2022,1Q,34

G97.83 Intracranial hypotension following lumbar cerebrospinal fluid shunting CC
Code also any associated diagnoses or complications

G97.84 Intracranial hypotension following other procedure CC
Code also, if applicable:
accidental puncture or laceration of dura during a procedure (G97.41)
cerebrospinal fluid leak from spinal puncture (G97.Ø)

G98 Other disorders of nervous system not elsewhere classified
INCLUDES nervous system disorder NOS

G98.Ø Neurogenic arthritis, not elsewhere classified
Nonsyphilitic neurogenic arthropathy NEC
Nonsyphilitic neurogenic spondylopathy NEC
EXCLUDES 1 *spondylopathy (in):*
syringomyelia and syringobulbia (G95.Ø)
tabes dorsalis (A52.11)

G98.8 Other disorders of nervous system HIV
Nervous system disorder NOS

G99 Other disorders of nervous system in diseases classified elsewhere

G99.Ø Autonomic neuropathy in diseases classified elsewhere CC
Code first underlying disease, such as:
amyloidosis (E85.-)
gout (M1A.-, M1Ø.-)
hyperthyroidism (EØ5.-)
EXCLUDES 1 *diabetic autonomic neuropathy (EØ8-E13 with .43)*

G99.2 Myelopathy in diseases classified elsewhere CC HCC
Code first underlying disease, such as:
neoplasm (CØØ-D49)
EXCLUDES 1 *myelopathy in:*
intervertebral disease (M5Ø.Ø-, M51.Ø-)
spondylosis (M47.Ø-, M47.1-)
AHA: 2018,3Q,18-19
TIP: Use this code in addition to a spondylolisthesis code (M43.1-) or a spinal stenosis code (M48.0-) when either of these disorders is documented as the cause of the myelopathy.

G99.8 Other specified disorders of nervous system in diseases classified elsewhere
Code first underlying disorder, such as:
amyloidosis (E85.-)
avitaminosis (E56.9)
EXCLUDES 1 *nervous system involvement in:*
cysticercosis (B69.Ø)
rubella (BØ6.Ø-)
syphilis (A52.1-)

Chapter 7. Diseases of the Eye and Adnexa (H00–H59)

Chapter-specific Guidelines with Coding Examples

The chapter-specific guidelines from the ICD-10-CM Official Guidelines for Coding and Reporting have been provided below. Along with these guidelines are coding examples, contained in the shaded boxes, that have been developed to help illustrate the coding and/or sequencing guidance found in these guidelines.

a. Glaucoma

1) Assigning glaucoma codes

Assign as many codes from category H40, Glaucoma, as needed to identify the type of glaucoma, the affected eye, and the glaucoma stage.

2) Bilateral glaucoma with same type and stage

When a patient has bilateral glaucoma and both eyes are documented as being the same type and stage, and there is a code for bilateral glaucoma, report only the code for the type of glaucoma, bilateral, with the seventh character for the stage.

> Bilateral severe stage pigmentary glaucoma
>
> **H40.1333 Pigmentary glaucoma, bilateral, severe stage**
>
> *Explanation*: In this scenario, the patient has the same type and stage of glaucoma in both eyes. As this type of glaucoma has a code for bilateral, assign only the code for the bilateral glaucoma with the seventh character for the stage.

When a patient has bilateral glaucoma and both eyes are documented as being the same type and stage, and the classification does not provide a code for bilateral glaucoma (i.e. subcategories H40.10 and H40.20) report only one code for the type of glaucoma with the appropriate seventh character for the stage.

> Bilateral open-angle glaucoma; not specified as to type and stage indeterminate in both eyes
>
> **H40.10X4 Unspecified open-angle glaucoma, indeterminate stage**
>
> *Explanation*: In this scenario, the patient has glaucoma of the same type and stage of both eyes, but there is no code specifically for bilateral glaucoma. Only one code is assigned with the appropriate seventh character for the stage.

3) Bilateral glaucoma stage with different types or stages

When a patient has bilateral glaucoma and each eye is documented as having a different type or stage, and the classification distinguishes laterality, assign the appropriate code for each eye rather than the code for bilateral glaucoma.

When a patient has bilateral glaucoma and each eye is documented as having a different type, and the classification does not distinguish laterality (i.e. subcategories H40.10 and H40.20), assign one code for each type of glaucoma with the appropriate seventh character for the stage.

> Documentation relates mild, unspecified primary angle-closure glaucoma of the left eye with mild unspecified open-angle glaucoma of the right eye
>
> **H40.20X1 Unspecified primary angle-closure glaucoma, mild stage**
>
> **H40.10X1 Unspecified open-angle glaucoma, mild stage**
>
> *Explanation*: In this scenario the patient has a different type of glaucoma in each eye and the classification does not distinguish laterality. A code for each type of glaucoma is assigned, each with the appropriate seventh character for the stage.

When a patient has bilateral glaucoma and each eye is documented as having the same type, but different stage, and the classification does not distinguish laterality (i.e. subcategories H40.10 and H40.20), assign a code for the type of glaucoma for each eye with the seventh character for the specific glaucoma stage documented for each eye.

> Bilateral open-angle glaucoma, not specified as to type; the right eye is documented to be in mild stage and the left eye as being in moderate stage
>
> **H40.10X1 Unspecified open-angle glaucoma, mild stage**
>
> **H40.10X2 Unspecified open-angle glaucoma, moderate stage**
>
> *Explanation*: In this scenario the patient has the same type of glaucoma in each eye but each eye is at a different stage, and the classification does not distinguish laterality at this subcategory level. Two codes are assigned; both codes represent the same type of glaucoma but each has a different seventh character identifying the appropriate stage for each eye.

4) Patient admitted with glaucoma and stage evolves during the admission

If a patient is admitted with glaucoma and the stage progresses during the admission, assign the code for highest stage documented.

> Patient admitted with mild low-tension glaucoma of the right eye, which progresses to moderate stage during the patient's stay
>
> **H40.1212 Low-tension glaucoma, right eye, moderate stage**
>
> *Explanation*: When the glaucoma stage progresses during an admission, assign only the code for the highest stage documented.

5) Indeterminate stage glaucoma

Assignment of the seventh character "4" for "indeterminate stage" should be based on the clinical documentation. The seventh character "4" is used for glaucomas whose stage cannot be clinically determined. This seventh character should not be confused with the seventh character "0", unspecified, which should be assigned when there is no documentation regarding the stage of the glaucoma.

b. Blindness

If "blindness" or "low vision" of both eyes is documented but the visual impairment category is not documented, assign code H54.3, Unqualified visual loss, both eyes. If "blindness" or "low vision" in one eye is documented but the visual impairment category is not documented, assign a code from H54.6-, Unqualified visual loss, one eye. If "blindness" or "visual loss" is documented without any information about whether one or both eyes are affected, assign code H54.7, Unspecified visual loss.

> Blindness in 89-year-old male
>
> **H54.7 Unspecified visual loss**
>
> *Explanation*: Blindness is stated, but there is no mention of whether one or both eyes are affected or the severity of this visual impairment.

Chapter 7. Diseases of the Eye and Adnexa (H00-H59)

NOTE Use an external cause code following the code for the eye condition, if applicable, to identify the cause of the eye condition

EXCLUDES 2 *certain conditions originating in the perinatal period (P04-P96)*
certain infectious and parasitic diseases (A00-B99)
complications of pregnancy, childbirth and the puerperium (O00-O9A)
congenital malformations, deformations, and chromosomal abnormalities (Q00-Q99)
diabetes mellitus related eye conditions (E09.3-, E10.3-, E11.3-, E13.3-)
endocrine, nutritional and metabolic diseases (E00-E88)
injury (trauma) of eye and orbit (S05.-)
injury, poisoning and certain other consequences of external causes (S00-T88)
neoplasms (C00-D49)
symptoms, signs and abnormal clinical and laboratory findings, not elsewhere classified (R00-R94)
syphilis related eye disorders (A50.01, A50.3-, A51.43, A52.71)

This chapter contains the following blocks:

H00-H05 Disorders of eyelid, lacrimal system and orbit
H10-H11 Disorders of conjunctiva
H15-H22 Disorders of sclera, cornea, iris and ciliary body
H25-H28 Disorders of lens
H30-H36 Disorders of choroid and retina
H40-H42 Glaucoma
H43-H44 Disorders of vitreous body and globe
H46-H47 Disorders of optic nerve and visual pathways
H49-H52 Disorders of ocular muscles, binocular movement, accommodation and refraction
H53-H54 Visual disturbances and blindness
H55-H57 Other disorders of eye and adnexa
H59 Intraoperative and postprocedural complications and disorders of eye and adnexa, not elsewhere classified

Disorders of eyelid, lacrimal system and orbit (H00-H05)

EXCLUDES 2 *open wound of eyelid (S01.1-)*
superficial injury of eyelid (S00.1-, S00.2-)

4th H00 Hordeolum and chalazion

5th H00.0 Hordeolum (externum) (internum) of eyelid

DEF: Acute localized infection of the gland of Zeis (external hordeolum) or Molt or of the meibomian glands (internal hordeolum) of the orbit.

6th H00.01 Hordeolum externum

Hordeolum NOS
Stye

H00.011 Hordeolum externum right upper eyelid
H00.012 Hordeolum externum right lower eyelid
H00.013 Hordeolum externum right eye, unspecified eyelid
H00.014 Hordeolum externum left upper eyelid
H00.015 Hordeolum externum left lower eyelid
H00.016 Hordeolum externum left eye, unspecified eyelid
H00.019 Hordeolum externum unspecified eye, unspecified eyelid

6th H00.02 Hordeolum internum

Infection of meibomian gland

H00.021 Hordeolum internum right upper eyelid
H00.022 Hordeolum internum right lower eyelid
H00.023 Hordeolum internum right eye, unspecified eyelid
H00.024 Hordeolum internum left upper eyelid
H00.025 Hordeolum internum left lower eyelid
H00.026 Hordeolum internum left eye, unspecified eyelid
H00.029 Hordeolum internum unspecified eye, unspecified eyelid

6th H00.03 Abscess of eyelid

Furuncle of eyelid

H00.031 Abscess of right upper eyelid
H00.032 Abscess of right lower eyelid
H00.033 Abscess of eyelid right eye, unspecified eyelid
H00.034 Abscess of left upper eyelid
H00.035 Abscess of left lower eyelid
H00.036 Abscess of eyelid left eye, unspecified eyelid
H00.039 Abscess of eyelid unspecified eye, unspecified eyelid

5th H00.1 Chalazion

Meibomian (gland) cyst

EXCLUDES 2 *infected meibomian gland (H00.02-)*

DEF: Noninfectious, obstructive mass in the oil gland of the eyelid that results in a small chronic lump or inflammation.

H00.11 Chalazion right upper eyelid
H00.12 Chalazion right lower eyelid
H00.13 Chalazion right eye, unspecified eyelid
H00.14 Chalazion left upper eyelid
H00.15 Chalazion left lower eyelid
H00.16 Chalazion left eye, unspecified eyelid
H00.19 Chalazion unspecified eye, unspecified eyelid

4th H01 Other inflammation of eyelid

5th H01.0 Blepharitis

EXCLUDES 1 *blepharoconjunctivitis (H10.5-)*

6th H01.00 Unspecified blepharitis

AHA: 2018,4Q,13

H01.001 Unspecified blepharitis right upper eyelid
H01.002 Unspecified blepharitis right lower eyelid
H01.003 Unspecified blepharitis right eye, unspecified eyelid
H01.004 Unspecified blepharitis left upper eyelid
H01.005 Unspecified blepharitis left lower eyelid
H01.006 Unspecified blepharitis left eye, unspecified eyelid
H01.009 Unspecified blepharitis unspecified eye, unspecified eyelid
H01.00A Unspecified blepharitis right eye, upper and lower eyelids
H01.00B Unspecified blepharitis left eye, upper and lower eyelids

6th H01.01 Ulcerative blepharitis

AHA: 2018,4Q,13

H01.011 Ulcerative blepharitis right upper eyelid
H01.012 Ulcerative blepharitis right lower eyelid
H01.013 Ulcerative blepharitis right eye, unspecified eyelid
H01.014 Ulcerative blepharitis left upper eyelid
H01.015 Ulcerative blepharitis left lower eyelid
H01.016 Ulcerative blepharitis left eye, unspecified eyelid
H01.019 Ulcerative blepharitis unspecified eye, unspecified eyelid
H01.01A Ulcerative blepharitis right eye, upper and lower eyelids
H01.01B Ulcerative blepharitis left eye, upper and lower eyelids

6th H01.02 Squamous blepharitis

AHA: 2018,4Q,13

H01.021 Squamous blepharitis right upper eyelid
H01.022 Squamous blepharitis right lower eyelid
H01.023 Squamous blepharitis right eye, unspecified eyelid
H01.024 Squamous blepharitis left upper eyelid
H01.025 Squamous blepharitis left lower eyelid
H01.026 Squamous blepharitis left eye, unspecified eyelid
H01.029 Squamous blepharitis unspecified eye, unspecified eyelid
H01.02A Squamous blepharitis right eye, upper and lower eyelids
H01.02B Squamous blepharitis left eye, upper and lower eyelids

5th H01.1 Noninfectious dermatoses of eyelid

6th H01.11 Allergic dermatitis of eyelid

Contact dermatitis of eyelid

H01.111 Allergic dermatitis of right upper eyelid
H01.112 Allergic dermatitis of right lower eyelid
H01.113 Allergic dermatitis of right eye, unspecified eyelid
H01.114 Allergic dermatitis of left upper eyelid
H01.115 Allergic dermatitis of left lower eyelid
H01.116 Allergic dermatitis of left eye, unspecified eyelid
H01.119 Allergic dermatitis of unspecified eye, unspecified eyelid

H01.12 Discoid lupus erythematosus of eyelid
- H01.121 Discoid lupus erythematosus of right upper eyelid
- H01.122 Discoid lupus erythematosus of right lower eyelid
- H01.123 Discoid lupus erythematosus of right eye, unspecified eyelid
- H01.124 Discoid lupus erythematosus of left upper eyelid
- H01.125 Discoid lupus erythematosus of left lower eyelid
- H01.126 Discoid lupus erythematosus of left eye, unspecified eyelid
- H01.129 Discoid lupus erythematosus of unspecified eye, unspecified eyelid

H01.13 Eczematous dermatitis of eyelid
- H01.131 Eczematous dermatitis of right upper eyelid
- H01.132 Eczematous dermatitis of right lower eyelid
- H01.133 Eczematous dermatitis of right eye, unspecified eyelid
- H01.134 Eczematous dermatitis of left upper eyelid
- H01.135 Eczematous dermatitis of left lower eyelid
- H01.136 Eczematous dermatitis of left eye, unspecified eyelid
- H01.139 Eczematous dermatitis of unspecified eye, unspecified eyelid

H01.14 Xeroderma of eyelid
- H01.141 Xeroderma of right upper eyelid
- H01.142 Xeroderma of right lower eyelid
- H01.143 Xeroderma of right eye, unspecified eyelid
- H01.144 Xeroderma of left upper eyelid
- H01.145 Xeroderma of left lower eyelid
- H01.146 Xeroderma of left eye, unspecified eyelid
- H01.149 Xeroderma of unspecified eye, unspecified eyelid

H01.8 Other specified inflammations of eyelid

H01.9 Unspecified inflammation of eyelid
Inflammation of eyelid NOS

H02 Other disorders of eyelid

EXCLUDES 1 *congenital malformations of eyelid (Q10.0-Q10.3)*

Entropion and Ectropion

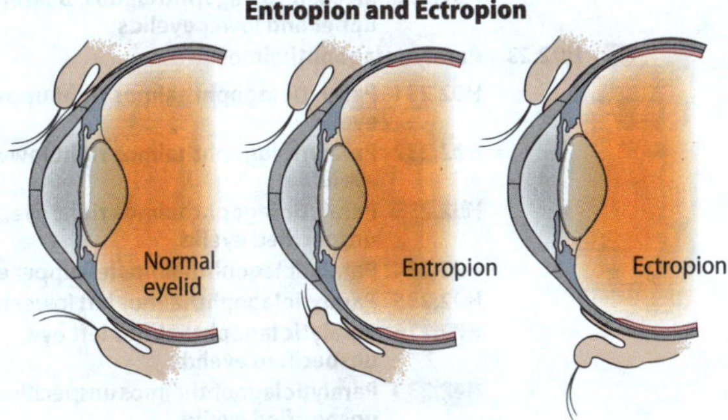

H02.0 Entropion and trichiasis of eyelid

DEF: Entropion: Inversion of the eyelid, turning the edge in toward the eyeball and causing irritation from contact of the lashes with the surface of the eye.
DEF: Trichiasis: Condition wherein the eyelid is in a normal position but lashes are ingrown or misdirected in their growth so that they irritate the tissues of the eye.

H02.00 Unspecified entropion of eyelid
- H02.001 Unspecified entropion of right upper eyelid
- H02.002 Unspecified entropion of right lower eyelid
- H02.003 Unspecified entropion of right eye, unspecified eyelid
- H02.004 Unspecified entropion of left upper eyelid
- H02.005 Unspecified entropion of left lower eyelid
- H02.006 Unspecified entropion of left eye, unspecified eyelid
- H02.009 Unspecified entropion of unspecified eye, unspecified eyelid

H02.01 Cicatricial entropion of eyelid
- H02.011 Cicatricial entropion of right upper eyelid
- H02.012 Cicatricial entropion of right lower eyelid
- H02.013 Cicatricial entropion of right eye, unspecified eyelid
- H02.014 Cicatricial entropion of left upper eyelid
- H02.015 Cicatricial entropion of left lower eyelid
- H02.016 Cicatricial entropion of left eye, unspecified eyelid
- H02.019 Cicatricial entropion of unspecified eye, unspecified eyelid

H02.02 Mechanical entropion of eyelid
- H02.021 Mechanical entropion of right upper eyelid
- H02.022 Mechanical entropion of right lower eyelid
- H02.023 Mechanical entropion of right eye, unspecified eyelid
- H02.024 Mechanical entropion of left upper eyelid
- H02.025 Mechanical entropion of left lower eyelid
- H02.026 Mechanical entropion of left eye, unspecified eyelid
- H02.029 Mechanical entropion of unspecified eye, unspecified eyelid

H02.03 Senile entropion of eyelid
- H02.031 Senile entropion of right upper eyelid A
- H02.032 Senile entropion of right lower eyelid A
- H02.033 Senile entropion of right eye, unspecified eyelid A
- H02.034 Senile entropion of left upper eyelid A
- H02.035 Senile entropion of left lower eyelid A
- H02.036 Senile entropion of left eye, unspecified eyelid A
- H02.039 Senile entropion of unspecified eye, unspecified eyelid A

H02.04 Spastic entropion of eyelid
- H02.041 Spastic entropion of right upper eyelid
- H02.042 Spastic entropion of right lower eyelid
- H02.043 Spastic entropion of right eye, unspecified eyelid
- H02.044 Spastic entropion of left upper eyelid
- H02.045 Spastic entropion of left lower eyelid
- H02.046 Spastic entropion of left eye, unspecified eyelid
- H02.049 Spastic entropion of unspecified eye, unspecified eyelid

H02.05 Trichiasis without entropion
- H02.051 Trichiasis without entropion right upper eyelid
- H02.052 Trichiasis without entropion right lower eyelid
- H02.053 Trichiasis without entropion right eye, unspecified eyelid
- H02.054 Trichiasis without entropion left upper eyelid
- H02.055 Trichiasis without entropion left lower eyelid
- H02.056 Trichiasis without entropion left eye, unspecified eyelid
- H02.059 Trichiasis without entropion unspecified eye, unspecified eyelid

H02.1 Ectropion of eyelid

DEF: Drooping of the lower eyelid away from the eye or outward turning or eversion of the edge of the eyelid, exposing the palpebral conjunctiva and causing irritation.

H02.10 Unspecified ectropion of eyelid
- H02.101 Unspecified ectropion of right upper eyelid
- H02.102 Unspecified ectropion of right lower eyelid
- H02.103 Unspecified ectropion of right eye, unspecified eyelid
- H02.104 Unspecified ectropion of left upper eyelid
- H02.105 Unspecified ectropion of left lower eyelid
- H02.106 Unspecified ectropion of left eye, unspecified eyelid

H02.109 Unspecified ectropion of unspecified eye, unspecified eyelid

H02.11 Cicatricial ectropion of eyelid
- H02.111 Cicatricial ectropion of right upper eyelid
- H02.112 Cicatricial ectropion of right lower eyelid
- H02.113 Cicatricial ectropion of right eye, unspecified eyelid
- H02.114 Cicatricial ectropion of left upper eyelid
- H02.115 Cicatricial ectropion of left lower eyelid
- H02.116 Cicatricial ectropion of left eye, unspecified eyelid
- H02.119 Cicatricial ectropion of unspecified eye, unspecified eyelid

H02.12 Mechanical ectropion of eyelid
- H02.121 Mechanical ectropion of right upper eyelid
- H02.122 Mechanical ectropion of right lower eyelid
- H02.123 Mechanical ectropion of right eye, unspecified eyelid
- H02.124 Mechanical ectropion of left upper eyelid
- H02.125 Mechanical ectropion of left lower eyelid
- H02.126 Mechanical ectropion of left eye, unspecified eyelid
- H02.129 Mechanical ectropion of unspecified eye, unspecified eyelid

H02.13 Senile ectropion of eyelid
- H02.131 Senile ectropion of right upper eyelid A
- H02.132 Senile ectropion of right lower eyelid A
- H02.133 Senile ectropion of right eye, unspecified eyelid A
- H02.134 Senile ectropion of left upper eyelid A
- H02.135 Senile ectropion of left lower eyelid A
- H02.136 Senile ectropion of left eye, unspecified eyelid A
- H02.139 Senile ectropion of unspecified eye, unspecified eyelid A

H02.14 Spastic ectropion of eyelid
- H02.141 Spastic ectropion of right upper eyelid
- H02.142 Spastic ectropion of right lower eyelid
- H02.143 Spastic ectropion of right eye, unspecified eyelid
- H02.144 Spastic ectropion of left upper eyelid
- H02.145 Spastic ectropion of left lower eyelid
- H02.146 Spastic ectropion of left eye, unspecified eyelid
- H02.149 Spastic ectropion of unspecified eye, unspecified eyelid

H02.15 Paralytic ectropion of eyelid

AHA: 2018,4Q,13
- H02.151 Paralytic ectropion of right upper eyelid
- H02.152 Paralytic ectropion of right lower eyelid
- H02.153 Paralytic ectropion of right eye, unspecified eyelid
- H02.154 Paralytic ectropion of left upper eyelid
- H02.155 Paralytic ectropion of left lower eyelid
- H02.156 Paralytic ectropion of left eye, unspecified eyelid
- H02.159 Paralytic ectropion of unspecified eye, unspecified eyelid

H02.2 Lagophthalmos

AHA: 2018,4Q,14

DEF: Condition of the eye that prevents it from closing completely.

H02.20 Unspecified lagophthalmos
- H02.201 Unspecified lagophthalmos right upper eyelid
- H02.202 Unspecified lagophthalmos right lower eyelid
- H02.203 Unspecified lagophthalmos right eye, unspecified eyelid
- H02.204 Unspecified lagophthalmos left upper eyelid
- H02.205 Unspecified lagophthalmos left lower eyelid
- H02.206 Unspecified lagophthalmos left eye, unspecified eyelid
- H02.209 Unspecified lagophthalmos unspecified eye, unspecified eyelid
- H02.20A Unspecified lagophthalmos right eye, upper and lower eyelids
- H02.20B Unspecified lagophthalmos left eye, upper and lower eyelids
- H02.20C Unspecified lagophthalmos, bilateral, upper and lower eyelids

H02.21 Cicatricial lagophthalmos
- H02.211 Cicatricial lagophthalmos right upper eyelid
- H02.212 Cicatricial lagophthalmos right lower eyelid
- H02.213 Cicatricial lagophthalmos right eye, unspecified eyelid
- H02.214 Cicatricial lagophthalmos left upper eyelid
- H02.215 Cicatricial lagophthalmos left lower eyelid
- H02.216 Cicatricial lagophthalmos left eye, unspecified eyelid
- H02.219 Cicatricial lagophthalmos unspecified eye, unspecified eyelid
- H02.21A Cicatricial lagophthalmos right eye, upper and lower eyelids
- H02.21B Cicatricial lagophthalmos left eye, upper and lower eyelids
- H02.21C Cicatricial lagophthalmos, bilateral, upper and lower eyelids

H02.22 Mechanical lagophthalmos
- H02.221 Mechanical lagophthalmos right upper eyelid
- H02.222 Mechanical lagophthalmos right lower eyelid
- H02.223 Mechanical lagophthalmos right eye, unspecified eyelid
- H02.224 Mechanical lagophthalmos left upper eyelid
- H02.225 Mechanical lagophthalmos left lower eyelid
- H02.226 Mechanical lagophthalmos left eye, unspecified eyelid
- H02.229 Mechanical lagophthalmos unspecified eye, unspecified eyelid
- H02.22A Mechanical lagophthalmos right eye, upper and lower eyelids
- H02.22B Mechanical lagophthalmos left eye, upper and lower eyelids
- H02.22C Mechanical lagophthalmos, bilateral, upper and lower eyelids

H02.23 Paralytic lagophthalmos
- H02.231 Paralytic lagophthalmos right upper eyelid
- H02.232 Paralytic lagophthalmos right lower eyelid
- H02.233 Paralytic lagophthalmos right eye, unspecified eyelid
- H02.234 Paralytic lagophthalmos left upper eyelid
- H02.235 Paralytic lagophthalmos left lower eyelid
- H02.236 Paralytic lagophthalmos left eye, unspecified eyelid
- H02.239 Paralytic lagophthalmos unspecified eye, unspecified eyelid
- H02.23A Paralytic lagophthalmos right eye, upper and lower eyelids
- H02.23B Paralytic lagophthalmos left eye, upper and lower eyelids
- H02.23C Paralytic lagophthalmos, bilateral, upper and lower eyelids

H02.3 Blepharochalasis

Pseudoptosis

DEF: Loss of elasticity and relaxation of skin of the eyelid, thickened or indurated skin on the eyelid associated with recurrent episodes of edema, and intracellular atrophy.
- H02.30 Blepharochalasis unspecified eye, unspecified eyelid
- H02.31 Blepharochalasis right upper eyelid
- H02.32 Blepharochalasis right lower eyelid
- H02.33 Blepharochalasis right eye, unspecified eyelid
- H02.34 Blepharochalasis left upper eyelid
- H02.35 Blepharochalasis left lower eyelid
- H02.36 Blepharochalasis left eye, unspecified eyelid

H02.4 Ptosis of eyelid

H02.40 Unspecified ptosis of eyelid

H02.401 Unspecified ptosis of right eyelid

H02.402 Unspecified ptosis of left eyelid

H02.403 Unspecified ptosis of bilateral eyelids

H02.409 Unspecified ptosis of unspecified eyelid

H02.41 Mechanical ptosis of eyelid

H02.411 Mechanical ptosis of right eyelid

H02.412 Mechanical ptosis of left eyelid

H02.413 Mechanical ptosis of bilateral eyelids

H02.419 Mechanical ptosis of unspecified eyelid

H02.42 Myogenic ptosis of eyelid

H02.421 Myogenic ptosis of right eyelid

H02.422 Myogenic ptosis of left eyelid

H02.423 Myogenic ptosis of bilateral eyelids

H02.429 Myogenic ptosis of unspecified eyelid

H02.43 Paralytic ptosis of eyelid

Neurogenic ptosis of eyelid

H02.431 Paralytic ptosis of right eyelid

H02.432 Paralytic ptosis of left eyelid

H02.433 Paralytic ptosis of bilateral eyelids

H02.439 Paralytic ptosis unspecified eyelid

H02.5 Other disorders affecting eyelid function

EXCLUDES 2 *blepharospasm (G24.5)*
organic tic (G25.69)
psychogenic tic (F95.-)

H02.51 Abnormal innervation syndrome

H02.511 Abnormal innervation syndrome right upper eyelid

H02.512 Abnormal innervation syndrome right lower eyelid

H02.513 Abnormal innervation syndrome right eye, unspecified eyelid

H02.514 Abnormal innervation syndrome left upper eyelid

H02.515 Abnormal innervation syndrome left lower eyelid

H02.516 Abnormal innervation syndrome left eye, unspecified eyelid

H02.519 Abnormal innervation syndrome unspecified eye, unspecified eyelid

H02.52 Blepharophimosis

Ankyloblepharon

H02.521 Blepharophimosis right upper eyelid

H02.522 Blepharophimosis right lower eyelid

H02.523 Blepharophimosis right eye, unspecified eyelid

H02.524 Blepharophimosis left upper eyelid

H02.525 Blepharophimosis left lower eyelid

H02.526 Blepharophimosis left eye, unspecified eyelid

H02.529 Blepharophimosis unspecified eye, unspecified lid

H02.53 Eyelid retraction

Eyelid lag

H02.531 Eyelid retraction right upper eyelid

H02.532 Eyelid retraction right lower eyelid

H02.533 Eyelid retraction right eye, unspecified eyelid

H02.534 Eyelid retraction left upper eyelid

H02.535 Eyelid retraction left lower eyelid

H02.536 Eyelid retraction left eye, unspecified eyelid

H02.539 Eyelid retraction unspecified eye, unspecified lid

H02.59 Other disorders affecting eyelid function

Deficient blink reflex
Sensory disorders

H02.6 Xanthelasma of eyelid

DEF: Condition in which there are small yellow tumors that occur on the eyelid, usually appearing near the nose.

H02.60 Xanthelasma of unspecified eye, unspecified eyelid

H02.61 Xanthelasma of right upper eyelid

H02.62 Xanthelasma of right lower eyelid

H02.63 Xanthelasma of right eye, unspecified eyelid

H02.64 Xanthelasma of left upper eyelid

H02.65 Xanthelasma of left lower eyelid

H02.66 Xanthelasma of left eye, unspecified eyelid

H02.7 Other and unspecified degenerative disorders of eyelid and periocular area

H02.70 Unspecified degenerative disorders of eyelid and periocular area

H02.71 Chloasma of eyelid and periocular area

Dyspigmentation of eyelid
Hyperpigmentation of eyelid

H02.711 Chloasma of right upper eyelid and periocular area

H02.712 Chloasma of right lower eyelid and periocular area

H02.713 Chloasma of right eye, unspecified eyelid and periocular area

H02.714 Chloasma of left upper eyelid and periocular area

H02.715 Chloasma of left lower eyelid and periocular area

H02.716 Chloasma of left eye, unspecified eyelid and periocular area

H02.719 Chloasma of unspecified eye, unspecified eyelid and periocular area

H02.72 Madarosis of eyelid and periocular area

Hypotrichosis of eyelid

H02.721 Madarosis of right upper eyelid and periocular area

H02.722 Madarosis of right lower eyelid and periocular area

H02.723 Madarosis of right eye, unspecified eyelid and periocular area

H02.724 Madarosis of left upper eyelid and periocular area

H02.725 Madarosis of left lower eyelid and periocular area

H02.726 Madarosis of left eye, unspecified eyelid and periocular area

H02.729 Madarosis of unspecified eye, unspecified eyelid and periocular area

H02.73 Vitiligo of eyelid and periocular area

Hypopigmentation of eyelid

H02.731 Vitiligo of right upper eyelid and periocular area

H02.732 Vitiligo of right lower eyelid and periocular area

H02.733 Vitiligo of right eye, unspecified eyelid and periocular area

H02.734 Vitiligo of left upper eyelid and periocular area

H02.735 Vitiligo of left lower eyelid and periocular area

H02.736 Vitiligo of left eye, unspecified eyelid and periocular area

H02.739 Vitiligo of unspecified eye, unspecified eyelid and periocular area

H02.79 Other degenerative disorders of eyelid and periocular area

H02.8 Other specified disorders of eyelid

H02.81 Retained foreign body in eyelid

Use additional code to identify the type of retained foreign body (Z18.-)

EXCLUDES 1 *laceration of eyelid with foreign body (S01.12-)*
retained intraocular foreign body (H44.6-, H44.7-)
superficial foreign body of eyelid and periocular area (S00.25-)

H02.811 Retained foreign body in right upper eyelid

H02.812 Retained foreign body in right lower eyelid

H02.813 Retained foreign body in right eye, unspecified eyelid

H02.814 Retained foreign body in left upper eyelid

H02.815 Retained foreign body in left lower eyelid

H02.816 Retained foreign body in left eye, unspecified eyelid

H02.819 Retained foreign body in unspecified eye, unspecified eyelid

H02.82 Cysts of eyelid

Sebaceous cyst of eyelid

H02.821 Cysts of right upper eyelid

H02.822 Cysts of right lower eyelid

Chapter 7. Diseases of the Eye and Adnexa

H02.4–H02.822

H02.823 Cysts of right eye, unspecified eyelid
H02.824 Cysts of left upper eyelid
H02.825 Cysts of left lower eyelid
H02.826 Cysts of left eye, unspecified eyelid
H02.829 Cysts of unspecified eye, unspecified eyelid

H02.83 Dermatochalasis of eyelid
DEF: Acquired form of connective tissue disorder associated with decreased elastic tissue and abnormal elastin formation, resulting in loss of elasticity of the skin of the eyelid. It is generally associated with aging.
H02.831 Dermatochalasis of right upper eyelid
H02.832 Dermatochalasis of right lower eyelid
H02.833 Dermatochalasis of right eye, unspecified eyelid
H02.834 Dermatochalasis of left upper eyelid
H02.835 Dermatochalasis of left lower eyelid
H02.836 Dermatochalasis of left eye, unspecified eyelid
H02.839 Dermatochalasis of unspecified eye, unspecified eyelid

H02.84 Edema of eyelid
Hyperemia of eyelid
H02.841 Edema of right upper eyelid
H02.842 Edema of right lower eyelid
H02.843 Edema of right eye, unspecified eyelid
H02.844 Edema of left upper eyelid
H02.845 Edema of left lower eyelid
H02.846 Edema of left eye, unspecified eyelid
H02.849 Edema of unspecified eye, unspecified eyelid

H02.85 Elephantiasis of eyelid
H02.851 Elephantiasis of right upper eyelid
H02.852 Elephantiasis of right lower eyelid
H02.853 Elephantiasis of right eye, unspecified eyelid
H02.854 Elephantiasis of left upper eyelid
H02.855 Elephantiasis of left lower eyelid
H02.856 Elephantiasis of left eye, unspecified eyelid
H02.859 Elephantiasis of unspecified eye, unspecified eyelid

H02.86 Hypertrichosis of eyelid
H02.861 Hypertrichosis of right upper eyelid
H02.862 Hypertrichosis of right lower eyelid
H02.863 Hypertrichosis of right eye, unspecified eyelid
H02.864 Hypertrichosis of left upper eyelid
H02.865 Hypertrichosis of left lower eyelid
H02.866 Hypertrichosis of left eye, unspecified eyelid
H02.869 Hypertrichosis of unspecified eye, unspecified eyelid

H02.87 Vascular anomalies of eyelid
H02.871 Vascular anomalies of right upper eyelid
H02.872 Vascular anomalies of right lower eyelid
H02.873 Vascular anomalies of right eye, unspecified eyelid
H02.874 Vascular anomalies of left upper eyelid
H02.875 Vascular anomalies of left lower eyelid
H02.876 Vascular anomalies of left eye, unspecified eyelid
H02.879 Vascular anomalies of unspecified eye, unspecified eyelid

H02.88 Meibomian gland dysfunction of eyelid
AHA: 2018,4Q,14-15
H02.881 Meibomian gland dysfunction right upper eyelid
H02.882 Meibomian gland dysfunction right lower eyelid
H02.883 Meibomian gland dysfunction of right eye, unspecified eyelid
H02.884 Meibomian gland dysfunction left upper eyelid
H02.885 Meibomian gland dysfunction left lower eyelid
H02.886 Meibomian gland dysfunction of left eye, unspecified eyelid
H02.889 Meibomian gland dysfunction of unspecified eye, unspecified eyelid
H02.88A Meibomian gland dysfunction right eye, upper and lower eyelids
H02.88B Meibomian gland dysfunction left eye, upper and lower eyelids

H02.89 Other specified disorders of eyelid
Hemorrhage of eyelid

H02.9 Unspecified disorder of eyelid
Disorder of eyelid NOS

H04 Disorders of lacrimal system

EXCLUDES 1 congenital malformations of lacrimal system (Q10.4-Q10.6)

H04.0 Dacryoadenitis
DEF: Inflammation of the lacrimal gland.

H04.00 Unspecified dacryoadenitis
H04.001 Unspecified dacryoadenitis, right lacrimal gland
H04.002 Unspecified dacryoadenitis, left lacrimal gland
H04.003 Unspecified dacryoadenitis, bilateral lacrimal glands
H04.009 Unspecified dacryoadenitis, unspecified lacrimal gland

H04.01 Acute dacryoadenitis
H04.011 Acute dacryoadenitis, right lacrimal gland
H04.012 Acute dacryoadenitis, left lacrimal gland
H04.013 Acute dacryoadenitis, bilateral lacrimal glands
H04.019 Acute dacryoadenitis, unspecified lacrimal gland

H04.02 Chronic dacryoadenitis
H04.021 Chronic dacryoadenitis, right lacrimal gland
H04.022 Chronic dacryoadenitis, left lacrimal gland
H04.023 Chronic dacryoadenitis, bilateral lacrimal gland
H04.029 Chronic dacryoadenitis, unspecified lacrimal gland

H04.03 Chronic enlargement of lacrimal gland
H04.031 Chronic enlargement of right lacrimal gland
H04.032 Chronic enlargement of left lacrimal gland
H04.033 Chronic enlargement of bilateral lacrimal glands
H04.039 Chronic enlargement of unspecified lacrimal gland

H04.1 Other disorders of lacrimal gland

H04.11 Dacryops
H04.111 Dacryops of right lacrimal gland
H04.112 Dacryops of left lacrimal gland
H04.113 Dacryops of bilateral lacrimal glands
H04.119 Dacryops of unspecified lacrimal gland

H04.12 Dry eye syndrome
Tear film insufficiency, NOS
H04.121 Dry eye syndrome of right lacrimal gland
H04.122 Dry eye syndrome of left lacrimal gland
H04.123 Dry eye syndrome of bilateral lacrimal glands
H04.129 Dry eye syndrome of unspecified lacrimal gland

H04.13 Lacrimal cyst
Lacrimal cystic degeneration
H04.131 Lacrimal cyst, right lacrimal gland
H04.132 Lacrimal cyst, left lacrimal gland
H04.133 Lacrimal cyst, bilateral lacrimal glands
H04.139 Lacrimal cyst, unspecified lacrimal gland

H04.14 Primary lacrimal gland atrophy
H04.141 Primary lacrimal gland atrophy, right lacrimal gland
H04.142 Primary lacrimal gland atrophy, left lacrimal gland
H04.143 Primary lacrimal gland atrophy, bilateral lacrimal glands
H04.149 Primary lacrimal gland atrophy, unspecified lacrimal gland

H04.15 Secondary lacrimal gland atrophy
H04.151 Secondary lacrimal gland atrophy, right lacrimal gland

H04.152 Secondary lacrimal gland atrophy, left lacrimal gland
H04.153 Secondary lacrimal gland atrophy, bilateral lacrimal glands
H04.159 Secondary lacrimal gland atrophy, unspecified lacrimal gland

√6th H04.16 Lacrimal gland dislocation
H04.161 Lacrimal gland dislocation, right lacrimal gland
H04.162 Lacrimal gland dislocation, left lacrimal gland
H04.163 Lacrimal gland dislocation, bilateral lacrimal glands
H04.169 Lacrimal gland dislocation, unspecified lacrimal gland

H04.19 Other specified disorders of lacrimal gland

√5th H04.2 Epiphora

DEF: Excessive tearing or overflow of tears down the cheeks often due to a stricture in the lacrimal passages but can be caused by other conditions.

√6th H04.20 Unspecified epiphora
H04.201 Unspecified epiphora, right side
H04.202 Unspecified epiphora, left side
H04.203 Unspecified epiphora, bilateral
H04.209 Unspecified epiphora, unspecified side

√6th H04.21 Epiphora due to excess lacrimation
H04.211 Epiphora due to excess lacrimation, right lacrimal gland
H04.212 Epiphora due to excess lacrimation, left lacrimal gland
H04.213 Epiphora due to excess lacrimation, bilateral lacrimal glands
H04.219 Epiphora due to excess lacrimation, unspecified lacrimal gland

√6th H04.22 Epiphora due to insufficient drainage
H04.221 Epiphora due to insufficient drainage, right side
H04.222 Epiphora due to insufficient drainage, left side
H04.223 Epiphora due to insufficient drainage, bilateral
H04.229 Epiphora due to insufficient drainage, unspecified side

√5th H04.3 Acute and unspecified inflammation of lacrimal passages

EXCLUDES 1 *neonatal dacryocystitis (P39.1)*

√6th H04.30 Unspecified dacryocystitis
H04.301 Unspecified dacryocystitis of right lacrimal passage
H04.302 Unspecified dacryocystitis of left lacrimal passage
H04.303 Unspecified dacryocystitis of bilateral lacrimal passages
H04.309 Unspecified dacryocystitis of unspecified lacrimal passage

√6th H04.31 Phlegmonous dacryocystitis
H04.311 Phlegmonous dacryocystitis of right lacrimal passage
H04.312 Phlegmonous dacryocystitis of left lacrimal passage
H04.313 Phlegmonous dacryocystitis of bilateral lacrimal passages
H04.319 Phlegmonous dacryocystitis of unspecified lacrimal passage

√6th H04.32 Acute dacryocystitis

Acute dacryopericystitis

H04.321 Acute dacryocystitis of right lacrimal passage
H04.322 Acute dacryocystitis of left lacrimal passage
H04.323 Acute dacryocystitis of bilateral lacrimal passages
H04.329 Acute dacryocystitis of unspecified lacrimal passage

√6th H04.33 Acute lacrimal canaliculitis
H04.331 Acute lacrimal canaliculitis of right lacrimal passage
H04.332 Acute lacrimal canaliculitis of left lacrimal passage
H04.333 Acute lacrimal canaliculitis of bilateral lacrimal passages
H04.339 Acute lacrimal canaliculitis of unspecified lacrimal passage

√5th H04.4 Chronic inflammation of lacrimal passages

√6th H04.41 Chronic dacryocystitis
H04.411 Chronic dacryocystitis of right lacrimal passage
H04.412 Chronic dacryocystitis of left lacrimal passage
H04.413 Chronic dacryocystitis of bilateral lacrimal passages
H04.419 Chronic dacryocystitis of unspecified lacrimal passage

√6th H04.42 Chronic lacrimal canaliculitis
H04.421 Chronic lacrimal canaliculitis of right lacrimal passage
H04.422 Chronic lacrimal canaliculitis of left lacrimal passage
H04.423 Chronic lacrimal canaliculitis of bilateral lacrimal passages
H04.429 Chronic lacrimal canaliculitis of unspecified lacrimal passage

√6th H04.43 Chronic lacrimal mucocele
H04.431 Chronic lacrimal mucocele of right lacrimal passage
H04.432 Chronic lacrimal mucocele of left lacrimal passage
H04.433 Chronic lacrimal mucocele of bilateral lacrimal passages
H04.439 Chronic lacrimal mucocele of unspecified lacrimal passage

√5th H04.5 Stenosis and insufficiency of lacrimal passages

√6th H04.51 Dacryolith
H04.511 Dacryolith of right lacrimal passage
H04.512 Dacryolith of left lacrimal passage
H04.513 Dacryolith of bilateral lacrimal passages
H04.519 Dacryolith of unspecified lacrimal passage

√6th H04.52 Eversion of lacrimal punctum
H04.521 Eversion of right lacrimal punctum
H04.522 Eversion of left lacrimal punctum
H04.523 Eversion of bilateral lacrimal punctum
H04.529 Eversion of unspecified lacrimal punctum

√6th H04.53 Neonatal obstruction of nasolacrimal duct

EXCLUDES 1 *congenital stenosis and stricture of lacrimal duct (Q10.5)*

H04.531 Neonatal obstruction of right nasolacrimal duct N
H04.532 Neonatal obstruction of left nasolacrimal duct N
H04.533 Neonatal obstruction of bilateral nasolacrimal duct N
H04.539 Neonatal obstruction of unspecified nasolacrimal duct N

√6th H04.54 Stenosis of lacrimal canaliculi
H04.541 Stenosis of right lacrimal canaliculi
H04.542 Stenosis of left lacrimal canaliculi
H04.543 Stenosis of bilateral lacrimal canaliculi
H04.549 Stenosis of unspecified lacrimal canaliculi

√6th H04.55 Acquired stenosis of nasolacrimal duct
H04.551 Acquired stenosis of right nasolacrimal duct
H04.552 Acquired stenosis of left nasolacrimal duct
H04.553 Acquired stenosis of bilateral nasolacrimal duct
H04.559 Acquired stenosis of unspecified nasolacrimal duct

√6th H04.56 Stenosis of lacrimal punctum
H04.561 Stenosis of right lacrimal punctum
H04.562 Stenosis of left lacrimal punctum
H04.563 Stenosis of bilateral lacrimal punctum
H04.569 Stenosis of unspecified lacrimal punctum

√6th H04.57 Stenosis of lacrimal sac
H04.571 Stenosis of right lacrimal sac
H04.572 Stenosis of left lacrimal sac
H04.573 Stenosis of bilateral lacrimal sac
H04.579 Stenosis of unspecified lacrimal sac

√5th **HØ4.6 Other changes of lacrimal passages**

√6th **HØ4.61 Lacrimal fistula**

HØ4.611 Lacrimal fistula right lacrimal passage

HØ4.612 Lacrimal fistula left lacrimal passage

HØ4.613 Lacrimal fistula bilateral lacrimal passages

HØ4.619 Lacrimal fistula unspecified lacrimal passage

HØ4.69 Other changes of lacrimal passages

√5th **HØ4.8 Other disorders of lacrimal system**

√6th **HØ4.81 Granuloma of lacrimal passages**

HØ4.811 Granuloma of right lacrimal passage

HØ4.812 Granuloma of left lacrimal passage

HØ4.813 Granuloma of bilateral lacrimal passages

HØ4.819 Granuloma of unspecified lacrimal passage

HØ4.89 Other disorders of lacrimal system

HØ4.9 Disorder of lacrimal system, unspecified

√4th **HØ5 Disorders of orbit**

EXCLUDES 1 *congenital malformation of orbit (Q1Ø.7)*

√5th **HØ5.Ø Acute inflammation of orbit**

HØ5.ØØ Unspecified acute inflammation of orbit

√6th **HØ5.Ø1 Cellulitis of orbit**

Abscess of orbit

HØ5.Ø11 Cellulitis of right orbit CC

HØ5.Ø12 Cellulitis of left orbit CC

HØ5.Ø13 Cellulitis of bilateral orbits CC

HØ5.Ø19 Cellulitis of unspecified orbit CC UNS

√6th **HØ5.Ø2 Osteomyelitis of orbit**

HØ5.Ø21 Osteomyelitis of right orbit CC

HØ5.Ø22 Osteomyelitis of left orbit CC

HØ5.Ø23 Osteomyelitis of bilateral orbits CC

HØ5.Ø29 Osteomyelitis of unspecified orbit CC UNS

√6th **HØ5.Ø3 Periostitis of orbit**

HØ5.Ø31 Periostitis of right orbit CC

HØ5.Ø32 Periostitis of left orbit CC

HØ5.Ø33 Periostitis of bilateral orbits CC

HØ5.Ø39 Periostitis of unspecified orbit CC UNS

√6th **HØ5.Ø4 Tenonitis of orbit**

HØ5.Ø41 Tenonitis of right orbit

HØ5.Ø42 Tenonitis of left orbit

HØ5.Ø43 Tenonitis of bilateral orbits

HØ5.Ø49 Tenonitis of unspecified orbit

√5th **HØ5.1 Chronic inflammatory disorders of orbit**

HØ5.1Ø Unspecified chronic inflammatory disorders of orbit

√6th **HØ5.11 Granuloma of orbit**

Pseudotumor (inflammatory) of orbit

HØ5.111 Granuloma of right orbit

HØ5.112 Granuloma of left orbit

HØ5.113 Granuloma of bilateral orbits

HØ5.119 Granuloma of unspecified orbit

√6th **HØ5.12 Orbital myositis**

HØ5.121 Orbital myositis, right orbit

HØ5.122 Orbital myositis, left orbit

HØ5.123 Orbital myositis, bilateral

HØ5.129 Orbital myositis, unspecified orbit

√5th **HØ5.2 Exophthalmic conditions**

HØ5.2Ø Unspecified exophthalmos

√6th **HØ5.21 Displacement (lateral) of globe**

HØ5.211 Displacement (lateral) of globe, right eye

HØ5.212 Displacement (lateral) of globe, left eye

HØ5.213 Displacement (lateral) of globe, bilateral

HØ5.219 Displacement (lateral) of globe, unspecified eye

√6th **HØ5.22 Edema of orbit**

Orbital congestion

HØ5.221 Edema of right orbit

HØ5.222 Edema of left orbit

HØ5.223 Edema of bilateral orbit

HØ5.229 Edema of unspecified orbit

√6th **HØ5.23 Hemorrhage of orbit**

HØ5.231 Hemorrhage of right orbit

HØ5.232 Hemorrhage of left orbit

HØ5.233 Hemorrhage of bilateral orbit

HØ5.239 Hemorrhage of unspecified orbit

√6th **HØ5.24 Constant exophthalmos**

HØ5.241 Constant exophthalmos, right eye

HØ5.242 Constant exophthalmos, left eye

HØ5.243 Constant exophthalmos, bilateral

HØ5.249 Constant exophthalmos, unspecified eye

√6th **HØ5.25 Intermittent exophthalmos**

HØ5.251 Intermittent exophthalmos, right eye

HØ5.252 Intermittent exophthalmos, left eye

HØ5.253 Intermittent exophthalmos, bilateral

HØ5.259 Intermittent exophthalmos, unspecified eye

√6th **HØ5.26 Pulsating exophthalmos**

HØ5.261 Pulsating exophthalmos, right eye

HØ5.262 Pulsating exophthalmos, left eye

HØ5.263 Pulsating exophthalmos, bilateral

HØ5.269 Pulsating exophthalmos, unspecified eye

√5th **HØ5.3 Deformity of orbit**

EXCLUDES 1 *congenital deformity of orbit (Q1Ø.7)*
hypertelorism (Q75.2)

HØ5.3Ø Unspecified deformity of orbit

√6th **HØ5.31 Atrophy of orbit**

HØ5.311 Atrophy of right orbit

HØ5.312 Atrophy of left orbit

HØ5.313 Atrophy of bilateral orbit

HØ5.319 Atrophy of unspecified orbit

√6th **HØ5.32 Deformity of orbit due to bone disease**

Code also associated bone disease

HØ5.321 Deformity of right orbit due to bone disease

HØ5.322 Deformity of left orbit due to bone disease

HØ5.323 Deformity of bilateral orbits due to bone disease

HØ5.329 Deformity of unspecified orbit due to bone disease

√6th **HØ5.33 Deformity of orbit due to trauma or surgery**

HØ5.331 Deformity of right orbit due to trauma or surgery

HØ5.332 Deformity of left orbit due to trauma or surgery

HØ5.333 Deformity of bilateral orbits due to trauma or surgery

HØ5.339 Deformity of unspecified orbit due to trauma or surgery

√6th **HØ5.34 Enlargement of orbit**

HØ5.341 Enlargement of right orbit

HØ5.342 Enlargement of left orbit

HØ5.343 Enlargement of bilateral orbits

HØ5.349 Enlargement of unspecified orbit

√6th **HØ5.35 Exostosis of orbit**

HØ5.351 Exostosis of right orbit

HØ5.352 Exostosis of left orbit

HØ5.353 Exostosis of bilateral orbits

HØ5.359 Exostosis of unspecified orbit

√5th **HØ5.4 Enophthalmos**

√6th **HØ5.4Ø Unspecified enophthalmos**

HØ5.4Ø1 Unspecified enophthalmos, right eye

HØ5.4Ø2 Unspecified enophthalmos, left eye

HØ5.4Ø3 Unspecified enophthalmos, bilateral

HØ5.4Ø9 Unspecified enophthalmos, unspecified eye

√6th **HØ5.41 Enophthalmos due to atrophy of orbital tissue**

HØ5.411 Enophthalmos due to atrophy of orbital tissue, right eye

HØ5.412 Enophthalmos due to atrophy of orbital tissue, left eye

HØ5.413 Enophthalmos due to atrophy of orbital tissue, bilateral

HØ5.419 Enophthalmos due to atrophy of orbital tissue, unspecified eye

√6th **HØ5.42 Enophthalmos due to trauma or surgery**

HØ5.421 Enophthalmos due to trauma or surgery, right eye

HØ5.422 Enophthalmos due to trauma or surgery, left eye

H05.423 Enophthalmos due to trauma or surgery, bilateral
H05.429 Enophthalmos due to trauma or surgery, unspecified eye

H05.5 Retained (old) foreign body following penetrating wound of orbit
Retrobulbar foreign body
Use additional code to identify the type of retained foreign body (Z18.-)
EXCLUDES 1 *current penetrating wound of orbit (S05.4-)*
EXCLUDES 2 *retained foreign body of eyelid (H02.81-)*
retained intraocular foreign body (H44.6-, H44.7-)
H05.50 Retained (old) foreign body following penetrating wound of unspecified orbit
H05.51 Retained (old) foreign body following penetrating wound of right orbit
H05.52 Retained (old) foreign body following penetrating wound of left orbit
H05.53 Retained (old) foreign body following penetrating wound of bilateral orbits

H05.8 Other disorders of orbit
H05.81 Cyst of orbit
Encephalocele of orbit
H05.811 Cyst of right orbit
H05.812 Cyst of left orbit
H05.813 Cyst of bilateral orbits
H05.819 Cyst of unspecified orbit
H05.82 Myopathy of extraocular muscles
H05.821 Myopathy of extraocular muscles, right orbit
H05.822 Myopathy of extraocular muscles, left orbit
H05.823 Myopathy of extraocular muscles, bilateral
H05.829 Myopathy of extraocular muscles, unspecified orbit
H05.89 Other disorders of orbit
H05.9 Unspecified disorder of orbit

Disorders of conjunctiva (H10-H11)

H10 Conjunctivitis
EXCLUDES 1 *keratoconjunctivitis (H16.2-)*

H10.0 Mucopurulent conjunctivitis
H10.01 Acute follicular conjunctivitis
H10.011 Acute follicular conjunctivitis, right eye
H10.012 Acute follicular conjunctivitis, left eye
H10.013 Acute follicular conjunctivitis, bilateral
H10.019 Acute follicular conjunctivitis, unspecified eye
H10.02 Other mucopurulent conjunctivitis
H10.021 Other mucopurulent conjunctivitis, right eye
H10.022 Other mucopurulent conjunctivitis, left eye
H10.023 Other mucopurulent conjunctivitis, bilateral
H10.029 Other mucopurulent conjunctivitis, unspecified eye

H10.1 Acute atopic conjunctivitis
Acute papillary conjunctivitis
H10.10 Acute atopic conjunctivitis, unspecified eye
H10.11 Acute atopic conjunctivitis, right eye
H10.12 Acute atopic conjunctivitis, left eye
H10.13 Acute atopic conjunctivitis, bilateral

H10.2 Other acute conjunctivitis
H10.21 Acute toxic conjunctivitis
Acute chemical conjunctivitis
Code first (T51-T65) to identify chemical and intent
EXCLUDES 1 *burn and corrosion of eye and adnexa (T26.-)*
H10.211 Acute toxic conjunctivitis, right eye
H10.212 Acute toxic conjunctivitis, left eye
H10.213 Acute toxic conjunctivitis, bilateral
H10.219 Acute toxic conjunctivitis, unspecified eye
H10.22 Pseudomembranous conjunctivitis
H10.221 Pseudomembranous conjunctivitis, right eye
H10.222 Pseudomembranous conjunctivitis, left eye
H10.223 Pseudomembranous conjunctivitis, bilateral
H10.229 Pseudomembranous conjunctivitis, unspecified eye
H10.23 Serous conjunctivitis, except viral
EXCLUDES 1 *viral conjunctivitis (B30.-)*
H10.231 Serous conjunctivitis, except viral, right eye
H10.232 Serous conjunctivitis, except viral, left eye
H10.233 Serous conjunctivitis, except viral, bilateral
H10.239 Serous conjunctivitis, except viral, unspecified eye

H10.3 Unspecified acute conjunctivitis
EXCLUDES 1 *ophthalmia neonatorum NOS (P39.1)*
H10.30 Unspecified acute conjunctivitis, unspecified eye
H10.31 Unspecified acute conjunctivitis, right eye
H10.32 Unspecified acute conjunctivitis, left eye
H10.33 Unspecified acute conjunctivitis, bilateral

H10.4 Chronic conjunctivitis
H10.40 Unspecified chronic conjunctivitis
H10.401 Unspecified chronic conjunctivitis, right eye
H10.402 Unspecified chronic conjunctivitis, left eye
H10.403 Unspecified chronic conjunctivitis, bilateral
H10.409 Unspecified chronic conjunctivitis, unspecified eye
H10.41 Chronic giant papillary conjunctivitis
H10.411 Chronic giant papillary conjunctivitis, right eye
H10.412 Chronic giant papillary conjunctivitis, left eye
H10.413 Chronic giant papillary conjunctivitis, bilateral
H10.419 Chronic giant papillary conjunctivitis, unspecified eye
H10.42 Simple chronic conjunctivitis
H10.421 Simple chronic conjunctivitis, right eye
H10.422 Simple chronic conjunctivitis, left eye
both–OU H10.423 Simple chronic conjunctivitis, bilateral
H10.429 Simple chronic conjunctivitis, unspecified eye
H10.43 Chronic follicular conjunctivitis
H10.431 Chronic follicular conjunctivitis, right eye
H10.432 Chronic follicular conjunctivitis, left eye
H10.433 Chronic follicular conjunctivitis, bilateral
H10.439 Chronic follicular conjunctivitis, unspecified eye
H10.44 Vernal conjunctivitis
EXCLUDES 1 *vernal keratoconjunctivitis with limbar and corneal involvement (H16.26-)*
H10.45 Other chronic allergic conjunctivitis

H10.5 Blepharoconjunctivitis
H10.50 Unspecified blepharoconjunctivitis
H10.501 Unspecified blepharoconjunctivitis, right eye
H10.502 Unspecified blepharoconjunctivitis, left eye
H10.503 Unspecified blepharoconjunctivitis, bilateral
H10.509 Unspecified blepharoconjunctivitis, unspecified eye
H10.51 Ligneous conjunctivitis
Code also underlying condition if known, such as: plasminogen deficiency (E88.02)
H10.511 Ligneous conjunctivitis, right eye
H10.512 Ligneous conjunctivitis, left eye
H10.513 Ligneous conjunctivitis, bilateral
H10.519 Ligneous conjunctivitis, unspecified eye

- ✓6th **H10.52 Angular blepharoconjunctivitis**
  - **H10.521 Angular blepharoconjunctivitis, right eye**
  - **H10.522 Angular blepharoconjunctivitis, left eye**
  - **H10.523 Angular blepharoconjunctivitis, bilateral**
  - **H10.529 Angular blepharoconjunctivitis, unspecified eye**
- ✓6th **H10.53 Contact blepharoconjunctivitis**
  - **H10.531 Contact blepharoconjunctivitis, right eye**
  - **H10.532 Contact blepharoconjunctivitis, left eye**
  - **H10.533 Contact blepharoconjunctivitis, bilateral**
  - **H10.539 Contact blepharoconjunctivitis, unspecified eye**

✓5th **H10.8 Other conjunctivitis**

- ✓6th **H10.81 Pingueculitis**

  EXCLUDES 1 *pinguecula (H11.15-)*
  - **H10.811 Pingueculitis, right eye**
  - **H10.812 Pingueculitis, left eye**
  - **H10.813 Pingueculitis, bilateral**
  - **H10.819 Pingueculitis, unspecified eye**
- ✓6th **H10.82 Rosacea conjunctivitis**

  Code first underlying rosacea dermatitis (L71.-)

  AHA: 2018,4Q,15
  - **H10.821 Rosacea conjunctivitis, right eye**
  - **H10.822 Rosacea conjunctivitis, left eye**
  - **H10.823 Rosacea conjunctivitis, bilateral**
  - **H10.829 Rosacea conjunctivitis, unspecified eye**
- **H10.89 Other conjunctivitis**

H10.9 Unspecified conjunctivitis

✓4th **H11 Other disorders of conjunctiva**

EXCLUDES 1 *keratoconjunctivitis (H16.2-)*

✓5th **H11.0 Pterygium of eye**

EXCLUDES 1 *pseudopterygium (H11.81-)*

DEF: Benign, wedge-shaped, conjunctival thickening that advances from the inner corner of the eye toward the cornea.

Pterygium

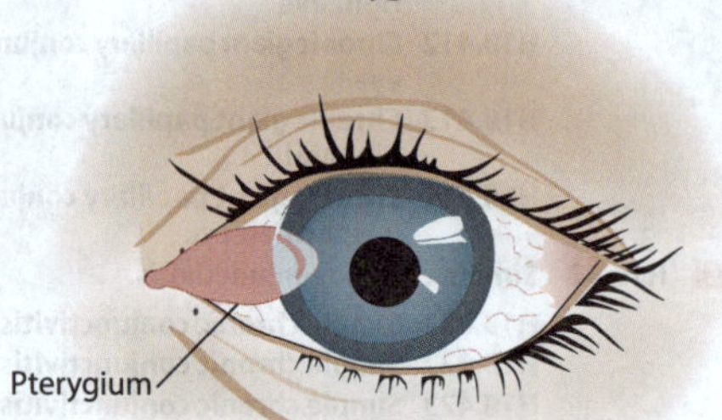

Pterygium

- ✓6th **H11.00 Unspecified pterygium of eye**
  - **H11.001 Unspecified pterygium of right eye**
  - **H11.002 Unspecified pterygium of left eye**
  - **H11.003 Unspecified pterygium of eye, bilateral**
  - **H11.009 Unspecified pterygium of unspecified eye**
- ✓6th **H11.01 Amyloid pterygium**
  - **H11.011 Amyloid pterygium of right eye**
  - **H11.012 Amyloid pterygium of left eye**
  - **H11.013 Amyloid pterygium of eye, bilateral**
  - **H11.019 Amyloid pterygium of unspecified eye**
- ✓6th **H11.02 Central pterygium of eye**
  - **H11.021 Central pterygium of right eye**
  - **H11.022 Central pterygium of left eye**
  - **H11.023 Central pterygium of eye, bilateral**
  - **H11.029 Central pterygium of unspecified eye**
- ✓6th **H11.03 Double pterygium of eye**
  - **H11.031 Double pterygium of right eye**
  - **H11.032 Double pterygium of left eye**
  - **H11.033 Double pterygium of eye, bilateral**
  - **H11.039 Double pterygium of unspecified eye**
- ✓6th **H11.04 Peripheral pterygium of eye, stationary**
  - **H11.041 Peripheral pterygium, stationary, right eye**
  - **H11.042 Peripheral pterygium, stationary, left eye**
  - **H11.043 Peripheral pterygium, stationary, bilateral**
  - **H11.049 Peripheral pterygium, stationary, unspecified eye**
- ✓6th **H11.05 Peripheral pterygium of eye, progressive**
  - **H11.051 Peripheral pterygium, progressive, right eye**
  - **H11.052 Peripheral pterygium, progressive, left eye**
  - **H11.053 Peripheral pterygium, progressive, bilateral**
  - **H11.059 Peripheral pterygium, progressive, unspecified eye**
- ✓6th **H11.06 Recurrent pterygium of eye**
  - **H11.061 Recurrent pterygium of right eye**
  - **H11.062 Recurrent pterygium of left eye**
  - **H11.063 Recurrent pterygium of eye, bilateral**
  - **H11.069 Recurrent pterygium of unspecified eye**

✓5th **H11.1 Conjunctival degenerations and deposits**

EXCLUDES 2 *pseudopterygium (H11.81)*

- **H11.10 Unspecified conjunctival degenerations**
- ✓6th **H11.11 Conjunctival deposits**
  - **H11.111 Conjunctival deposits, right eye**
  - **H11.112 Conjunctival deposits, left eye**
  - **H11.113 Conjunctival deposits, bilateral**
  - **H11.119 Conjunctival deposits, unspecified eye**
- ✓6th **H11.12 Conjunctival concretions**
  - **H11.121 Conjunctival concretions, right eye**
  - **H11.122 Conjunctival concretions, left eye**
  - **H11.123 Conjunctival concretions, bilateral**
  - **H11.129 Conjunctival concretions, unspecified eye**
- ✓6th **H11.13 Conjunctival pigmentations**

  Conjunctival argyrosis [argyria]
  - **H11.131 Conjunctival pigmentations, right eye**
  - **H11.132 Conjunctival pigmentations, left eye**
  - **H11.133 Conjunctival pigmentations, bilateral**
  - **H11.139 Conjunctival pigmentations, unspecified eye**
- ✓6th **H11.14 Conjunctival xerosis, unspecified**

  EXCLUDES 1 *xerosis of conjunctiva due to vitamin A deficiency (E50.0, E50.1)*

  DEF: Abnormal dryness of the conjunctiva due to lack of sufficient tears or conjunctival secretions.
  - **H11.141 Conjunctival xerosis, unspecified, right eye**
  - **H11.142 Conjunctival xerosis, unspecified, left eye**
  - **H11.143 Conjunctival xerosis, unspecified, bilateral**
  - **H11.149 Conjunctival xerosis, unspecified, unspecified eye**
- ✓6th **H11.15 Pinguecula**

  EXCLUDES 1 *pingueculitis (H10.81-)*

  DEF: Proliferation on the conjunctiva near the sclerocorneal junction, usually of the side of the nose and usually in older patients.

  Pinguecula

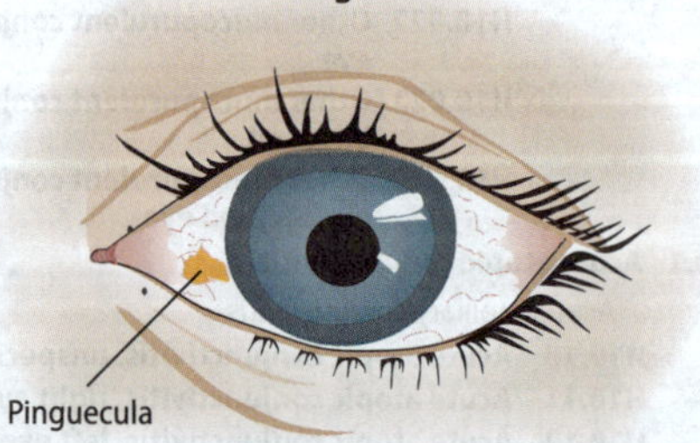

  Pinguecula
  - **H11.151 Pinguecula, right eye**
  - **H11.152 Pinguecula, left eye**
  - **H11.153 Pinguecula, bilateral**
  - **H11.159 Pinguecula, unspecified eye**

✓5th **H11.2 Conjunctival scars**

- ✓6th **H11.21 Conjunctival adhesions and strands (localized)**
  - **H11.211 Conjunctival adhesions and strands (localized), right eye**
  - **H11.212 Conjunctival adhesions and strands (localized), left eye**
  - **H11.213 Conjunctival adhesions and strands (localized), bilateral**
  - **H11.219 Conjunctival adhesions and strands (localized), unspecified eye**

H11.22 Conjunctival granuloma
H11.221 Conjunctival granuloma, right eye
H11.222 Conjunctival granuloma, left eye
H11.223 Conjunctival granuloma, bilateral
H11.229 Conjunctival granuloma, unspecified
H11.23 Symblepharon
H11.231 Symblepharon, right eye
H11.232 Symblepharon, left eye
H11.233 Symblepharon, bilateral
H11.239 Symblepharon, unspecified eye
H11.24 Scarring of conjunctiva
H11.241 Scarring of conjunctiva, right eye
H11.242 Scarring of conjunctiva, left eye
H11.243 Scarring of conjunctiva, bilateral
H11.249 Scarring of conjunctiva, unspecified eye
H11.3 Conjunctival hemorrhage
Subconjunctival hemorrhage
H11.30 Conjunctival hemorrhage, unspecified eye
H11.31 Conjunctival hemorrhage, right eye
H11.32 Conjunctival hemorrhage, left eye
H11.33 Conjunctival hemorrhage, bilateral
H11.4 Other conjunctival vascular disorders and cysts
H11.41 Vascular abnormalities of conjunctiva
Conjunctival aneurysm
H11.411 Vascular abnormalities of conjunctiva, right eye
H11.412 Vascular abnormalities of conjunctiva, left eye
H11.413 Vascular abnormalities of conjunctiva, bilateral
H11.419 Vascular abnormalities of conjunctiva, unspecified eye
H11.42 Conjunctival edema
H11.421 Conjunctival edema, right eye
H11.422 Conjunctival edema, left eye
H11.423 Conjunctival edema, bilateral
H11.429 Conjunctival edema, unspecified eye
H11.43 Conjunctival hyperemia
H11.431 Conjunctival hyperemia, right eye
H11.432 Conjunctival hyperemia, left eye
H11.433 Conjunctival hyperemia, bilateral
H11.439 Conjunctival hyperemia, unspecified eye
H11.44 Conjunctival cysts
H11.441 Conjunctival cysts, right eye
H11.442 Conjunctival cysts, left eye
H11.443 Conjunctival cysts, bilateral
H11.449 Conjunctival cysts, unspecified eye
H11.8 Other specified disorders of conjunctiva
H11.81 Pseudopterygium of conjunctiva
H11.811 Pseudopterygium of conjunctiva, right eye
H11.812 Pseudopterygium of conjunctiva, left eye
H11.813 Pseudopterygium of conjunctiva, bilateral
H11.819 Pseudopterygium of conjunctiva, unspecified eye
H11.82 Conjunctivochalasis
H11.821 Conjunctivochalasis, right eye
H11.822 Conjunctivochalasis, left eye
H11.823 Conjunctivochalasis, bilateral
H11.829 Conjunctivochalasis, unspecified eye
H11.89 Other specified disorders of conjunctiva
H11.9 Unspecified disorder of conjunctiva

Disorders of sclera, cornea, iris and ciliary body (H15-H22)

H15 Disorders of sclera
H15.0 Scleritis
H15.00 Unspecified scleritis
H15.001 Unspecified scleritis, right eye
H15.002 Unspecified scleritis, left eye
H15.003 Unspecified scleritis, bilateral
H15.009 Unspecified scleritis, unspecified eye
H15.01 Anterior scleritis
H15.011 Anterior scleritis, right eye
H15.012 Anterior scleritis, left eye
H15.013 Anterior scleritis, bilateral
H15.019 Anterior scleritis, unspecified eye
H15.02 Brawny scleritis
H15.021 Brawny scleritis, right eye
H15.022 Brawny scleritis, left eye
H15.023 Brawny scleritis, bilateral
H15.029 Brawny scleritis, unspecified eye
H15.03 Posterior scleritis
Sclerotenonitis
H15.031 Posterior scleritis, right eye
H15.032 Posterior scleritis, left eye
H15.033 Posterior scleritis, bilateral
H15.039 Posterior scleritis, unspecified eye
H15.04 Scleritis with corneal involvement
H15.041 Scleritis with corneal involvement, right eye
H15.042 Scleritis with corneal involvement, left eye
H15.043 Scleritis with corneal involvement, bilateral
H15.049 Scleritis with corneal involvement, unspecified eye
H15.05 Scleromalacia perforans
H15.051 Scleromalacia perforans, right eye
H15.052 Scleromalacia perforans, left eye
H15.053 Scleromalacia perforans, bilateral
H15.059 Scleromalacia perforans, unspecified eye
H15.09 Other scleritis
Scleral abscess
H15.091 Other scleritis, right eye
H15.092 Other scleritis, left eye
H15.093 Other scleritis, bilateral
H15.099 Other scleritis, unspecified eye
H15.1 Episcleritis
H15.10 Unspecified episcleritis
H15.101 Unspecified episcleritis, right eye
H15.102 Unspecified episcleritis, left eye
H15.103 Unspecified episcleritis, bilateral
H15.109 Unspecified episcleritis, unspecified eye
H15.11 Episcleritis periodica fugax
H15.111 Episcleritis periodica fugax, right eye
H15.112 Episcleritis periodica fugax, left eye
H15.113 Episcleritis periodica fugax, bilateral
H15.119 Episcleritis periodica fugax, unspecified eye
H15.12 Nodular episcleritis
H15.121 Nodular episcleritis, right eye
H15.122 Nodular episcleritis, left eye
H15.123 Nodular episcleritis, bilateral
H15.129 Nodular episcleritis, unspecified eye
H15.8 Other disorders of sclera
EXCLUDES 2 *blue sclera (Q13.5)*
degenerative myopia (H44.2-)
H15.81 Equatorial staphyloma
H15.811 Equatorial staphyloma, right eye
H15.812 Equatorial staphyloma, left eye
H15.813 Equatorial staphyloma, bilateral
H15.819 Equatorial staphyloma, unspecified eye
H15.82 Localized anterior staphyloma
H15.821 Localized anterior staphyloma, right eye
H15.822 Localized anterior staphyloma, left eye
H15.823 Localized anterior staphyloma, bilateral
H15.829 Localized anterior staphyloma, unspecified eye
H15.83 Staphyloma posticum
H15.831 Staphyloma posticum, right eye
H15.832 Staphyloma posticum, left eye
H15.833 Staphyloma posticum, bilateral
H15.839 Staphyloma posticum, unspecified eye
H15.84 Scleral ectasia
H15.841 Scleral ectasia, right eye
H15.842 Scleral ectasia, left eye
H15.843 Scleral ectasia, bilateral
H15.849 Scleral ectasia, unspecified eye
H15.85 Ring staphyloma
H15.851 Ring staphyloma, right eye

H15.852 Ring staphyloma, left eye
H15.853 Ring staphyloma, bilateral
H15.859 Ring staphyloma, unspecified eye
H15.89 Other disorders of sclera
H15.9 Unspecified disorder of sclera

H16 Keratitis
DEF: Condition in which the cornea becomes inflamed and irritated.

H16.0 Corneal ulcer
H16.00 Unspecified corneal ulcer
H16.001 Unspecified corneal ulcer, right eye
H16.002 Unspecified corneal ulcer, left eye
H16.003 Unspecified corneal ulcer, bilateral
H16.009 Unspecified corneal ulcer, unspecified eye
H16.01 Central corneal ulcer
H16.011 Central corneal ulcer, right eye
H16.012 Central corneal ulcer, left eye
H16.013 Central corneal ulcer, bilateral
H16.019 Central corneal ulcer, unspecified eye
H16.02 Ring corneal ulcer
H16.021 Ring corneal ulcer, right eye
H16.022 Ring corneal ulcer, left eye
H16.023 Ring corneal ulcer, bilateral
H16.029 Ring corneal ulcer, unspecified eye
H16.03 Corneal ulcer with hypopyon
H16.031 Corneal ulcer with hypopyon, right eye
H16.032 Corneal ulcer with hypopyon, left eye
H16.033 Corneal ulcer with hypopyon, bilateral
H16.039 Corneal ulcer with hypopyon, unspecified eye
H16.04 Marginal corneal ulcer
H16.041 Marginal corneal ulcer, right eye
H16.042 Marginal corneal ulcer, left eye
H16.043 Marginal corneal ulcer, bilateral
H16.049 Marginal corneal ulcer, unspecified eye
H16.05 Mooren's corneal ulcer
H16.051 Mooren's corneal ulcer, right eye
H16.052 Mooren's corneal ulcer, left eye
H16.053 Mooren's corneal ulcer, bilateral
H16.059 Mooren's corneal ulcer, unspecified eye
H16.06 Mycotic corneal ulcer
H16.061 Mycotic corneal ulcer, right eye
H16.062 Mycotic corneal ulcer, left eye
H16.063 Mycotic corneal ulcer, bilateral
H16.069 Mycotic corneal ulcer, unspecified eye
H16.07 Perforated corneal ulcer
H16.071 Perforated corneal ulcer, right eye
H16.072 Perforated corneal ulcer, left eye
H16.073 Perforated corneal ulcer, bilateral
H16.079 Perforated corneal ulcer, unspecified eye

H16.1 Other and unspecified superficial keratitis without conjunctivitis
H16.10 Unspecified superficial keratitis
H16.101 Unspecified superficial keratitis, right eye
H16.102 Unspecified superficial keratitis, left eye
H16.103 Unspecified superficial keratitis, bilateral
H16.109 Unspecified superficial keratitis, unspecified eye
H16.11 Macular keratitis
Areolar keratitis
Nummular keratitis
Stellate keratitis
Striate keratitis
H16.111 Macular keratitis, right eye
H16.112 Macular keratitis, left eye
H16.113 Macular keratitis, bilateral
H16.119 Macular keratitis, unspecified eye
H16.12 Filamentary keratitis
H16.121 Filamentary keratitis, right eye
H16.122 Filamentary keratitis, left eye
H16.123 Filamentary keratitis, bilateral
H16.129 Filamentary keratitis, unspecified eye
H16.13 Photokeratitis
Snow blindness
Welders keratitis
H16.131 Photokeratitis, right eye
H16.132 Photokeratitis, left eye
H16.133 Photokeratitis, bilateral
H16.139 Photokeratitis, unspecified eye
H16.14 Punctate keratitis
H16.141 Punctate keratitis, right eye
H16.142 Punctate keratitis, left eye
H16.143 Punctate keratitis, bilateral
H16.149 Punctate keratitis, unspecified eye

H16.2 Keratoconjunctivitis
H16.20 Unspecified keratoconjunctivitis
Superficial keratitis with conjunctivitis NOS
H16.201 Unspecified keratoconjunctivitis, right eye
H16.202 Unspecified keratoconjunctivitis, left eye
H16.203 Unspecified keratoconjunctivitis, bilateral
H16.209 Unspecified keratoconjunctivitis, unspecified eye
H16.21 Exposure keratoconjunctivitis
H16.211 Exposure keratoconjunctivitis, right eye
H16.212 Exposure keratoconjunctivitis, left eye
H16.213 Exposure keratoconjunctivitis, bilateral
H16.219 Exposure keratoconjunctivitis, unspecified eye
H16.22 Keratoconjunctivitis sicca, not specified as Sjögren's
EXCLUDES 1 *Sjögren's syndrome (M35.01)*
H16.221 Keratoconjunctivitis sicca, not specified as Sjögren's, right eye
H16.222 Keratoconjunctivitis sicca, not specified as Sjögren's, left eye
H16.223 Keratoconjunctivitis sicca, not specified as Sjögren's, bilateral
H16.229 Keratoconjunctivitis sicca, not specified as Sjögren's, unspecified eye
H16.23 Neurotrophic keratoconjunctivitis
H16.231 Neurotrophic keratoconjunctivitis, right eye
H16.232 Neurotrophic keratoconjunctivitis, left eye
H16.233 Neurotrophic keratoconjunctivitis, bilateral
H16.239 Neurotrophic keratoconjunctivitis, unspecified eye
H16.24 Ophthalmia nodosa
H16.241 Ophthalmia nodosa, right eye
H16.242 Ophthalmia nodosa, left eye
H16.243 Ophthalmia nodosa, bilateral
H16.249 Ophthalmia nodosa, unspecified eye
H16.25 Phlyctenular keratoconjunctivitis
H16.251 Phlyctenular keratoconjunctivitis, right eye
H16.252 Phlyctenular keratoconjunctivitis, left eye
H16.253 Phlyctenular keratoconjunctivitis, bilateral
H16.259 Phlyctenular keratoconjunctivitis, unspecified eye
H16.26 Vernal keratoconjunctivitis, with limbar and corneal involvement
EXCLUDES 1 *vernal conjunctivitis without limbar and corneal involvement (H10.44)*
H16.261 Vernal keratoconjunctivitis, with limbar and corneal involvement, right eye
H16.262 Vernal keratoconjunctivitis, with limbar and corneal involvement, left eye
H16.263 Vernal keratoconjunctivitis, with limbar and corneal involvement, bilateral
H16.269 Vernal keratoconjunctivitis, with limbar and corneal involvement, unspecified eye
H16.29 Other keratoconjunctivitis
H16.291 Other keratoconjunctivitis, right eye
H16.292 Other keratoconjunctivitis, left eye
H16.293 Other keratoconjunctivitis, bilateral
H16.299 Other keratoconjunctivitis, unspecified eye

H16.3 Interstitial and deep keratitis
H16.30 Unspecified interstitial keratitis
H16.301 Unspecified interstitial keratitis, right eye
H16.302 Unspecified interstitial keratitis, left eye

H16.303 Unspecified interstitial keratitis, bilateral
H16.309 Unspecified interstitial keratitis, unspecified eye

H16.31 Corneal abscess
- H16.311 Corneal abscess, right eye
- H16.312 Corneal abscess, left eye
- H16.313 Corneal abscess, bilateral
- H16.319 Corneal abscess, unspecified eye

H16.32 Diffuse interstitial keratitis
Cogan's syndrome
- H16.321 Diffuse interstitial keratitis, right eye
- H16.322 Diffuse interstitial keratitis, left eye
- H16.323 Diffuse interstitial keratitis, bilateral
- H16.329 Diffuse interstitial keratitis, unspecified eye

H16.33 Sclerosing keratitis
- H16.331 Sclerosing keratitis, right eye
- H16.332 Sclerosing keratitis, left eye
- H16.333 Sclerosing keratitis, bilateral
- H16.339 Sclerosing keratitis, unspecified eye

H16.39 Other interstitial and deep keratitis
- H16.391 Other interstitial and deep keratitis, right eye
- H16.392 Other interstitial and deep keratitis, left eye
- H16.393 Other interstitial and deep keratitis, bilateral
- H16.399 Other interstitial and deep keratitis, unspecified eye

H16.4 Corneal neovascularization

H16.40 Unspecified corneal neovascularization
- H16.401 Unspecified corneal neovascularization, right eye
- H16.402 Unspecified corneal neovascularization, left eye
- H16.403 Unspecified corneal neovascularization, bilateral
- H16.409 Unspecified corneal neovascularization, unspecified eye

H16.41 Ghost vessels (corneal)
- H16.411 Ghost vessels (corneal), right eye
- H16.412 Ghost vessels (corneal), left eye
- H16.413 Ghost vessels (corneal), bilateral
- H16.419 Ghost vessels (corneal), unspecified eye

H16.42 Pannus (corneal)
- H16.421 Pannus (corneal), right eye
- H16.422 Pannus (corneal), left eye
- H16.423 Pannus (corneal), bilateral
- H16.429 Pannus (corneal), unspecified eye

H16.43 Localized vascularization of cornea
- H16.431 Localized vascularization of cornea, right eye
- H16.432 Localized vascularization of cornea, left eye
- H16.433 Localized vascularization of cornea, bilateral
- H16.439 Localized vascularization of cornea, unspecified eye

H16.44 Deep vascularization of cornea
- H16.441 Deep vascularization of cornea, right eye
- H16.442 Deep vascularization of cornea, left eye
- H16.443 Deep vascularization of cornea, bilateral
- H16.449 Deep vascularization of cornea, unspecified eye

H16.8 Other keratitis UPD

H16.9 Unspecified keratitis

H17 Corneal scars and opacities

H17.0 Adherent leukoma
- H17.00 Adherent leukoma, unspecified eye
- H17.01 Adherent leukoma, right eye
- H17.02 Adherent leukoma, left eye
- H17.03 Adherent leukoma, bilateral

H17.1 Central corneal opacity
- H17.10 Central corneal opacity, unspecified eye
- H17.11 Central corneal opacity, right eye
- H17.12 Central corneal opacity, left eye
- H17.13 Central corneal opacity, bilateral

H17.8 Other corneal scars and opacities

H17.81 Minor opacity of cornea
Corneal nebula
- H17.811 Minor opacity of cornea, right eye
- H17.812 Minor opacity of cornea, left eye
- H17.813 Minor opacity of cornea, bilateral
- H17.819 Minor opacity of cornea, unspecified eye

H17.82 Peripheral opacity of cornea
- H17.821 Peripheral opacity of cornea, right eye
- H17.822 Peripheral opacity of cornea, left eye
- H17.823 Peripheral opacity of cornea, bilateral
- H17.829 Peripheral opacity of cornea, unspecified eye

H17.89 Other corneal scars and opacities

H17.9 Unspecified corneal scar and opacity

H18 Other disorders of cornea

H18.0 Corneal pigmentations and deposits

H18.00 Unspecified corneal deposit
- H18.001 Unspecified corneal deposit, right eye
- H18.002 Unspecified corneal deposit, left eye
- H18.003 Unspecified corneal deposit, bilateral
- H18.009 Unspecified corneal deposit, unspecified eye

H18.01 Anterior corneal pigmentations
Staehli's line
- H18.011 Anterior corneal pigmentations, right eye
- H18.012 Anterior corneal pigmentations, left eye
- H18.013 Anterior corneal pigmentations, bilateral
- H18.019 Anterior corneal pigmentations, unspecified eye

H18.02 Argentous corneal deposits
- H18.021 Argentous corneal deposits, right eye
- H18.022 Argentous corneal deposits, left eye
- H18.023 Argentous corneal deposits, bilateral
- H18.029 Argentous corneal deposits, unspecified eye

H18.03 Corneal deposits in metabolic disorders
Code also associated metabolic disorder
- H18.031 Corneal deposits in metabolic disorders, right eye
- H18.032 Corneal deposits in metabolic disorders, left eye
- H18.033 Corneal deposits in metabolic disorders, bilateral
- H18.039 Corneal deposits in metabolic disorders, unspecified eye

H18.04 Kayser-Fleischer ring
Code also associated Wilson's disease (E83.01)
- H18.041 Kayser-Fleischer ring, right eye
- H18.042 Kayser-Fleischer ring, left eye
- H18.043 Kayser-Fleischer ring, bilateral
- H18.049 Kayser-Fleischer ring, unspecified eye

H18.05 Posterior corneal pigmentations
Krukenberg's spindle
- H18.051 Posterior corneal pigmentations, right eye
- H18.052 Posterior corneal pigmentations, left eye
- H18.053 Posterior corneal pigmentations, bilateral
- H18.059 Posterior corneal pigmentations, unspecified eye

H18.06 Stromal corneal pigmentations
Hematocornea
- H18.061 Stromal corneal pigmentations, right eye
- H18.062 Stromal corneal pigmentations, left eye
- H18.063 Stromal corneal pigmentations, bilateral
- H18.069 Stromal corneal pigmentations, unspecified eye

H18.1 Bullous keratopathy

DEF: Corneal swelling due to a damaged corneal endothelium. Bullous keratopathy is characterized by recurring, rupturing epithelial blisters causing glaucoma, iridocyclitis, and Fuchs' dystrophy.

- H18.10 Bullous keratopathy, unspecified eye
- H18.11 Bullous keratopathy, right eye
- H18.12 Bullous keratopathy, left eye
- H18.13 Bullous keratopathy, bilateral

H18.2 Other and unspecified corneal edema

H18.20 Unspecified corneal edema

H18.21 Corneal edema secondary to contact lens

EXCLUDES 2 *other corneal disorders due to contact lens (H18.82-)*

H18.211 Corneal edema secondary to contact lens, right eye
H18.212 Corneal edema secondary to contact lens, left eye
H18.213 Corneal edema secondary to contact lens, bilateral
H18.219 Corneal edema secondary to contact lens, unspecified eye

H18.22 Idiopathic corneal edema

H18.221 Idiopathic corneal edema, right eye
H18.222 Idiopathic corneal edema, left eye
H18.223 Idiopathic corneal edema, bilateral
H18.229 Idiopathic corneal edema, unspecified eye

H18.23 Secondary corneal edema

H18.231 Secondary corneal edema, right eye
H18.232 Secondary corneal edema, left eye
H18.233 Secondary corneal edema, bilateral
H18.239 Secondary corneal edema, unspecified eye

H18.3 Changes of corneal membranes

H18.30 Unspecified corneal membrane change

H18.31 Folds and rupture in Bowman's membrane

H18.311 Folds and rupture in Bowman's membrane, right eye
H18.312 Folds and rupture in Bowman's membrane, left eye
H18.313 Folds and rupture in Bowman's membrane, bilateral
H18.319 Folds and rupture in Bowman's membrane, unspecified eye

H18.32 Folds in Descemet's membrane

H18.321 Folds in Descemet's membrane, right eye
H18.322 Folds in Descemet's membrane, left eye
H18.323 Folds in Descemet's membrane, bilateral
H18.329 Folds in Descemet's membrane, unspecified eye

H18.33 Rupture in Descemet's membrane

H18.331 Rupture in Descemet's membrane, right eye
H18.332 Rupture in Descemet's membrane, left eye
H18.333 Rupture in Descemet's membrane, bilateral
H18.339 Rupture in Descemet's membrane, unspecified eye

H18.4 Corneal degeneration

EXCLUDES 1 *Mooren's ulcer (H16.0-)*
recurrent erosion of cornea (H18.83-)

H18.40 Unspecified corneal degeneration

H18.41 Arcus senilis

Senile corneal changes

H18.411 Arcus senilis, right eye
H18.412 Arcus senilis, left eye
H18.413 Arcus senilis, bilateral
H18.419 Arcus senilis, unspecified eye

H18.42 Band keratopathy

H18.421 Band keratopathy, right eye
H18.422 Band keratopathy, left eye
H18.423 Band keratopathy, bilateral
H18.429 Band keratopathy, unspecified eye

H18.43 Other calcerous corneal degeneration

H18.44 Keratomalacia

EXCLUDES 1 *keratomalacia due to vitamin A deficiency (E50.4)*

H18.441 Keratomalacia, right eye
H18.442 Keratomalacia, left eye
H18.443 Keratomalacia, bilateral
H18.449 Keratomalacia, unspecified eye

H18.45 Nodular corneal degeneration

H18.451 Nodular corneal degeneration, right eye
H18.452 Nodular corneal degeneration, left eye
H18.453 Nodular corneal degeneration, bilateral
H18.459 Nodular corneal degeneration, unspecified eye

H18.46 Peripheral corneal degeneration

H18.461 Peripheral corneal degeneration, right eye
H18.462 Peripheral corneal degeneration, left eye
H18.463 Peripheral corneal degeneration, bilateral
H18.469 Peripheral corneal degeneration, unspecified eye

H18.49 Other corneal degeneration

H18.5 Hereditary corneal dystrophies

AHA: 2020,4Q,24

H18.50 Unspecified hereditary corneal dystrophies

H18.501 Unspecified hereditary corneal dystrophies, right eye
H18.502 Unspecified hereditary corneal dystrophies, left eye
H18.503 Unspecified hereditary corneal dystrophies, bilateral
H18.509 Unspecified hereditary corneal dystrophies, unspecified eye

H18.51 Endothelial corneal dystrophy

Fuchs' dystrophy

H18.511 Endothelial corneal dystrophy, right eye
H18.512 Endothelial corneal dystrophy, left eye
H18.513 Endothelial corneal dystrophy, bilateral
H18.519 Endothelial corneal dystrophy, unspecified eye

H18.52 Epithelial (juvenile) corneal dystrophy

H18.521 Epithelial (juvenile) corneal dystrophy, right eye
H18.522 Epithelial (juvenile) corneal dystrophy, left eye
H18.523 Epithelial (juvenile) corneal dystrophy, bilateral
H18.529 Epithelial (juvenile) corneal dystrophy, unspecified eye

H18.53 Granular corneal dystrophy

H18.531 Granular corneal dystrophy, right eye
H18.532 Granular corneal dystrophy, left eye
H18.533 Granular corneal dystrophy, bilateral
H18.539 Granular corneal dystrophy, unspecified eye

H18.54 Lattice corneal dystrophy

H18.541 Lattice corneal dystrophy, right eye
H18.542 Lattice corneal dystrophy, left eye
H18.543 Lattice corneal dystrophy, bilateral
H18.549 Lattice corneal dystrophy, unspecified eye

H18.55 Macular corneal dystrophy

H18.551 Macular corneal dystrophy, right eye
H18.552 Macular corneal dystrophy, left eye
H18.553 Macular corneal dystrophy, bilateral
H18.559 Macular corneal dystrophy, unspecified eye

H18.59 Other hereditary corneal dystrophies

H18.591 Other hereditary corneal dystrophies, right eye
H18.592 Other hereditary corneal dystrophies, left eye
H18.593 Other hereditary corneal dystrophies, bilateral
H18.599 Other hereditary corneal dystrophies, unspecified eye

H18.6 Keratoconus

H18.60 Keratoconus, unspecified

H18.601 Keratoconus, unspecified, right eye
H18.602 Keratoconus, unspecified, left eye
H18.603 Keratoconus, unspecified, bilateral
H18.609 Keratoconus, unspecified, unspecified eye

H18.61 Keratoconus, stable

H18.611 Keratoconus, stable, right eye
H18.612 Keratoconus, stable, left eye
H18.613 Keratoconus, stable, bilateral
H18.619 Keratoconus, stable, unspecified eye

N Newborn: 0 P Pediatric: 0-17 M Maternity: 9-64 A Adult: 15-124 UNS Unspecified Site MCC Major Complication/Comorbidity CC Complication/Comorbidity

H18.62 Keratoconus, unstable
Acute hydrops
H18.621 Keratoconus, unstable, right eye
H18.622 Keratoconus, unstable, left eye
H18.623 Keratoconus, unstable, bilateral
H18.629 Keratoconus, unstable, unspecified eye

H18.7 Other and unspecified corneal deformities
EXCLUDES 1 *congenital malformations of cornea (Q13.3-Q13.4)*
H18.70 Unspecified corneal deformity
H18.71 Corneal ectasia
H18.711 Corneal ectasia, right eye
H18.712 Corneal ectasia, left eye
H18.713 Corneal ectasia, bilateral
H18.719 Corneal ectasia, unspecified eye
H18.72 Corneal staphyloma
H18.721 Corneal staphyloma, right eye
H18.722 Corneal staphyloma, left eye
H18.723 Corneal staphyloma, bilateral
H18.729 Corneal staphyloma, unspecified eye
H18.73 Descemetocele
H18.731 Descemetocele, right eye
H18.732 Descemetocele, left eye
H18.733 Descemetocele, bilateral
H18.739 Descemetocele, unspecified eye
H18.79 Other corneal deformities
H18.791 Other corneal deformities, right eye
H18.792 Other corneal deformities, left eye
H18.793 Other corneal deformities, bilateral
H18.799 Other corneal deformities, unspecified eye

H18.8 Other specified disorders of cornea
H18.81 Anesthesia and hypoesthesia of cornea
H18.811 Anesthesia and hypoesthesia of cornea, right eye
H18.812 Anesthesia and hypoesthesia of cornea, left eye
H18.813 Anesthesia and hypoesthesia of cornea, bilateral
H18.819 Anesthesia and hypoesthesia of cornea, unspecified eye
H18.82 Corneal disorder due to contact lens
EXCLUDES 2 *corneal edema due to contact lens (H18.21-)*
H18.821 Corneal disorder due to contact lens, right eye
H18.822 Corneal disorder due to contact lens, left eye
H18.823 Corneal disorder due to contact lens, bilateral
H18.829 Corneal disorder due to contact lens, unspecified eye
H18.83 Recurrent erosion of cornea
H18.831 Recurrent erosion of cornea, right eye
H18.832 Recurrent erosion of cornea, left eye
H18.833 Recurrent erosion of cornea, bilateral
H18.839 Recurrent erosion of cornea, unspecified eye
H18.89 Other specified disorders of cornea
H18.891 Other specified disorders of cornea, right eye
H18.892 Other specified disorders of cornea, left eye
H18.893 Other specified disorders of cornea, bilateral
H18.899 Other specified disorders of cornea, unspecified eye

H18.9 Unspecified disorder of cornea

H20 Iridocyclitis

H20.0 Acute and subacute iridocyclitis
Acute anterior uveitis
Acute cyclitis
Acute iritis
Subacute anterior uveitis
Subacute cyclitis
Subacute iritis
EXCLUDES 1 *iridocyclitis, iritis, uveitis (due to) (in) diabetes mellitus (E08-E13 with .39)*
iridocyclitis, iritis, uveitis (due to) (in) diphtheria (A36.89)
iridocyclitis, iritis, uveitis (due to) (in) gonococcal (A54.32)
iridocyclitis, iritis, uveitis (due to) (in) herpes (simplex) (B00.51)
iridocyclitis, iritis, uveitis (due to) (in) herpes zoster (B02.32)
iridocyclitis, iritis, uveitis (due to) (in) late congenital syphilis (A50.39)
iridocyclitis, iritis, uveitis (due to) (in) late syphilis (A52.71)
iridocyclitis, iritis, uveitis (due to) (in) sarcoidosis (D86.83)
iridocyclitis, iritis, uveitis (due to) (in) syphilis (A51.43)
iridocyclitis, iritis, uveitis (due to) (in) toxoplasmosis (B58.09)
iridocyclitis, iritis, uveitis (due to) (in) tuberculosis (A18.54)
H20.00 Unspecified acute and subacute iridocyclitis CC
H20.01 Primary iridocyclitis
H20.011 Primary iridocyclitis, right eye CC
H20.012 Primary iridocyclitis, left eye CC
H20.013 Primary iridocyclitis, bilateral CC
H20.019 Primary iridocyclitis, unspecified eye CC UNS
H20.02 Recurrent acute iridocyclitis
H20.021 Recurrent acute iridocyclitis, right eye CC
H20.022 Recurrent acute iridocyclitis, left eye CC
H20.023 Recurrent acute iridocyclitis, bilateral CC
H20.029 Recurrent acute iridocyclitis, unspecified eye CC UNS
H20.03 Secondary infectious iridocyclitis
H20.031 Secondary infectious iridocyclitis, right eye CC
H20.032 Secondary infectious iridocyclitis, left eye CC
H20.033 Secondary infectious iridocyclitis, bilateral CC
H20.039 Secondary infectious iridocyclitis, unspecified eye CC UNS
H20.04 Secondary noninfectious iridocyclitis
H20.041 Secondary noninfectious iridocyclitis, right eye
H20.042 Secondary noninfectious iridocyclitis, left eye
H20.043 Secondary noninfectious iridocyclitis, bilateral
H20.049 Secondary noninfectious iridocyclitis, unspecified eye
H20.05 Hypopyon
H20.051 Hypopyon, right eye
H20.052 Hypopyon, left eye
H20.053 Hypopyon, bilateral
H20.059 Hypopyon, unspecified eye

H20.1 Chronic iridocyclitis
Use additional code for any associated cataract (H26.21-)
EXCLUDES 2 *posterior cyclitis (H30.2-)*
H20.10 Chronic iridocyclitis, unspecified eye
H20.11 Chronic iridocyclitis, right eye
H20.12 Chronic iridocyclitis, left eye
H20.13 Chronic iridocyclitis, bilateral

H2Ø.2 Lens-induced iridocyclitis
- **H2Ø.2Ø Lens-induced iridocyclitis, unspecified eye**
- **H2Ø.21 Lens-induced iridocyclitis, right eye**
- **H2Ø.22 Lens-induced iridocyclitis, left eye**
- **H2Ø.23 Lens-induced iridocyclitis, bilateral**

H2Ø.8 Other iridocyclitis

EXCLUDES 2 *glaucomatocyclitis crises (H4Ø.4-)*
posterior cyclitis (H3Ø.2-)
sympathetic uveitis (H44.13-)

H2Ø.81 Fuchs' heterochromic cyclitis
- **H2Ø.811 Fuchs' heterochromic cyclitis, right eye**
- **H2Ø.812 Fuchs' heterochromic cyclitis, left eye**
- **H2Ø.813 Fuchs' heterochromic cyclitis, bilateral**
- **H2Ø.819 Fuchs' heterochromic cyclitis, unspecified eye**

H2Ø.82 Vogt-Koyanagi syndrome
- **H2Ø.821 Vogt-Koyanagi syndrome, right eye**
- **H2Ø.822 Vogt-Koyanagi syndrome, left eye**
- **H2Ø.823 Vogt-Koyanagi syndrome, bilateral**
- **H2Ø.829 Vogt-Koyanagi syndrome, unspecified eye**

H2Ø.9 Unspecified iridocyclitis CC
Uveitis NOS

H21 Other disorders of iris and ciliary body

EXCLUDES 2 *sympathetic uveitis (H44.1-)*

H21.Ø Hyphema

EXCLUDES 1 *traumatic hyphema (SØ5.1-)*

Hyphema

Iris
Cornea
Hyphema

- **H21.ØØ Hyphema, unspecified eye**
- **H21.Ø1 Hyphema, right eye**
- **H21.Ø2 Hyphema, left eye**
- **H21.Ø3 Hyphema, bilateral**

H21.1 Other vascular disorders of iris and ciliary body
Neovascularization of iris or ciliary body
Rubeosis iridis
Rubeosis of iris

H21.1X Other vascular disorders of iris and ciliary body
- **H21.1X1 Other vascular disorders of iris and ciliary body, right eye**
- **H21.1X2 Other vascular disorders of iris and ciliary body, left eye**
- **H21.1X3 Other vascular disorders of iris and ciliary body, bilateral**
- **H21.1X9 Other vascular disorders of iris and ciliary body, unspecified eye**

H21.2 Degeneration of iris and ciliary body

H21.21 Degeneration of chamber angle
- **H21.211 Degeneration of chamber angle, right eye**
- **H21.212 Degeneration of chamber angle, left eye**
- **H21.213 Degeneration of chamber angle, bilateral**
- **H21.219 Degeneration of chamber angle, unspecified eye**

H21.22 Degeneration of ciliary body
- **H21.221 Degeneration of ciliary body, right eye**
- **H21.222 Degeneration of ciliary body, left eye**
- **H21.223 Degeneration of ciliary body, bilateral**
- **H21.229 Degeneration of ciliary body, unspecified eye**

H21.23 Degeneration of iris (pigmentary)
Translucency of iris
- **H21.231 Degeneration of iris (pigmentary), right eye**
- **H21.232 Degeneration of iris (pigmentary), left eye**
- **H21.233 Degeneration of iris (pigmentary), bilateral**
- **H21.239 Degeneration of iris (pigmentary), unspecified eye**

H21.24 Degeneration of pupillary margin
- **H21.241 Degeneration of pupillary margin, right eye**
- **H21.242 Degeneration of pupillary margin, left eye**
- **H21.243 Degeneration of pupillary margin, bilateral**
- **H21.249 Degeneration of pupillary margin, unspecified eye**

H21.25 Iridoschisis
- **H21.251 Iridoschisis, right eye**
- **H21.252 Iridoschisis, left eye**
- **H21.253 Iridoschisis, bilateral**
- **H21.259 Iridoschisis, unspecified eye**

H21.26 Iris atrophy (essential) (progressive)
- **H21.261 Iris atrophy (essential) (progressive), right eye**
- **H21.262 Iris atrophy (essential) (progressive), left eye**
- **H21.263 Iris atrophy (essential) (progressive), bilateral**
- **H21.269 Iris atrophy (essential) (progressive), unspecified eye**

H21.27 Miotic pupillary cyst
- **H21.271 Miotic pupillary cyst, right eye**
- **H21.272 Miotic pupillary cyst, left eye**
- **H21.273 Miotic pupillary cyst, bilateral**
- **H21.279 Miotic pupillary cyst, unspecified eye**

H21.29 Other iris atrophy

H21.3 Cyst of iris, ciliary body and anterior chamber

EXCLUDES 2 *miotic pupillary cyst (H21.27-)*

H21.3Ø Idiopathic cysts of iris, ciliary body or anterior chamber
Cyst of iris, ciliary body or anterior chamber NOS
- **H21.3Ø1 Idiopathic cysts of iris, ciliary body or anterior chamber, right eye**
- **H21.3Ø2 Idiopathic cysts of iris, ciliary body or anterior chamber, left eye**
- **H21.3Ø3 Idiopathic cysts of iris, ciliary body or anterior chamber, bilateral**
- **H21.3Ø9 Idiopathic cysts of iris, ciliary body or anterior chamber, unspecified eye**

H21.31 Exudative cysts of iris or anterior chamber
- **H21.311 Exudative cysts of iris or anterior chamber, right eye**
- **H21.312 Exudative cysts of iris or anterior chamber, left eye**
- **H21.313 Exudative cysts of iris or anterior chamber, bilateral**
- **H21.319 Exudative cysts of iris or anterior chamber, unspecified eye**

H21.32 Implantation cysts of iris, ciliary body or anterior chamber
- **H21.321 Implantation cysts of iris, ciliary body or anterior chamber, right eye**
- **H21.322 Implantation cysts of iris, ciliary body or anterior chamber, left eye**
- **H21.323 Implantation cysts of iris, ciliary body or anterior chamber, bilateral**
- **H21.329 Implantation cysts of iris, ciliary body or anterior chamber, unspecified eye**

H21.33 Parasitic cyst of iris, ciliary body or anterior chamber
- **H21.331 Parasitic cyst of iris, ciliary body or anterior chamber, right eye** CC
- **H21.332 Parasitic cyst of iris, ciliary body or anterior chamber, left eye** CC
- **H21.333 Parasitic cyst of iris, ciliary body or anterior chamber, bilateral** CC

H21.339 **Parasitic cyst of iris, ciliary body or anterior chamber, unspecified eye** CC UNS

√6th **H21.34** **Primary cyst of pars plana**
- **H21.341** **Primary cyst of pars plana, right eye**
- **H21.342** **Primary cyst of pars plana, left eye**
- **H21.343** **Primary cyst of pars plana, bilateral**
- **H21.349** **Primary cyst of pars plana, unspecified eye**

√6th **H21.35** **Exudative cyst of pars plana**

DEF: Protein, fatty-filled bullous elevation of the nonpigmented outermost ciliary epithelium of pars plana, due to fluid leak from blood vessels.
- **H21.351** **Exudative cyst of pars plana, right eye**
- **H21.352** **Exudative cyst of pars plana, left eye**
- **H21.353** **Exudative cyst of pars plana, bilateral**
- **H21.359** **Exudative cyst of pars plana, unspecified eye**

√5th **H21.4** **Pupillary membranes**

Iris bombé
Pupillary occlusion
Pupillary seclusion

EXCLUDES 1 *congenital pupillary membranes (Q13.8)*
- **H21.40** **Pupillary membranes, unspecified eye**
- **H21.41** **Pupillary membranes, right eye**
- **H21.42** **Pupillary membranes, left eye**
- **H21.43** **Pupillary membranes, bilateral**

√5th **H21.5** **Other and unspecified adhesions and disruptions of iris and ciliary body**

EXCLUDES 1 *corectopia (Q13.2)*

√6th **H21.50** **Unspecified adhesions of iris**

Synechia (iris) NOS
- **H21.501** **Unspecified adhesions of iris, right eye**
- **H21.502** **Unspecified adhesions of iris, left eye**
- **H21.503** **Unspecified adhesions of iris, bilateral**
- **H21.509** **Unspecified adhesions of iris and ciliary body, unspecified eye**

√6th **H21.51** **Anterior synechiae (iris)**
- **H21.511** **Anterior synechiae (iris), right eye**
- **H21.512** **Anterior synechiae (iris), left eye**
- **H21.513** **Anterior synechiae (iris), bilateral**
- **H21.519** **Anterior synechiae (iris), unspecified eye**

√6th **H21.52** **Goniosynechiae**
- **H21.521** **Goniosynechiae, right eye**
- **H21.522** **Goniosynechiae, left eye**
- **H21.523** **Goniosynechiae, bilateral**
- **H21.529** **Goniosynechiae, unspecified eye**

√6th **H21.53** **Iridodialysis**
- **H21.531** **Iridodialysis, right eye**
- **H21.532** **Iridodialysis, left eye**
- **H21.533** **Iridodialysis, bilateral**
- **H21.539** **Iridodialysis, unspecified eye**

√6th **H21.54** **Posterior synechiae (iris)**
- **H21.541** **Posterior synechiae (iris), right eye**
- **H21.542** **Posterior synechiae (iris), left eye**
- **H21.543** **Posterior synechiae (iris), bilateral**
- **H21.549** **Posterior synechiae (iris), unspecified eye**

√6th **H21.55** **Recession of chamber angle**
- **H21.551** **Recession of chamber angle, right eye**
- **H21.552** **Recession of chamber angle, left eye**
- **H21.553** **Recession of chamber angle, bilateral**
- **H21.559** **Recession of chamber angle, unspecified eye**

√6th **H21.56** **Pupillary abnormalities**

Deformed pupil
Ectopic pupil
Rupture of sphincter, pupil

EXCLUDES 1 *congenital deformity of pupil (Q13.2-)*
- **H21.561** **Pupillary abnormality, right eye**
- **H21.562** **Pupillary abnormality, left eye**
- **H21.563** **Pupillary abnormality, bilateral**
- **H21.569** **Pupillary abnormality, unspecified eye**

√5th **H21.8** **Other specified disorders of iris and ciliary body**

H21.81 **Floppy iris syndrome**

Intraoperative floppy iris syndrome (IFIS)

Use additional code for adverse effect, if applicable, to identify drug (T36-T50 with fifth or sixth character 5)

H21.82 **Plateau iris syndrome (post-iridectomy) (postprocedural)**

H21.89 **Other specified disorders of iris and ciliary body**

H21.9 **Unspecified disorder of iris and ciliary body**

H22 ***Disorders of iris and ciliary body in diseases classified elsewhere***

Code first underlying disease, such as:
- gout (M1A.-, M10.-)
- leprosy (A30.-)
- parasitic disease (B89)

Disorders of lens (H25-H28)

√4th **H25** **Age-related cataract**

Senile cataract

EXCLUDES 2 *capsular glaucoma with pseudoexfoliation of lens (H40.1-)*

Cataracts

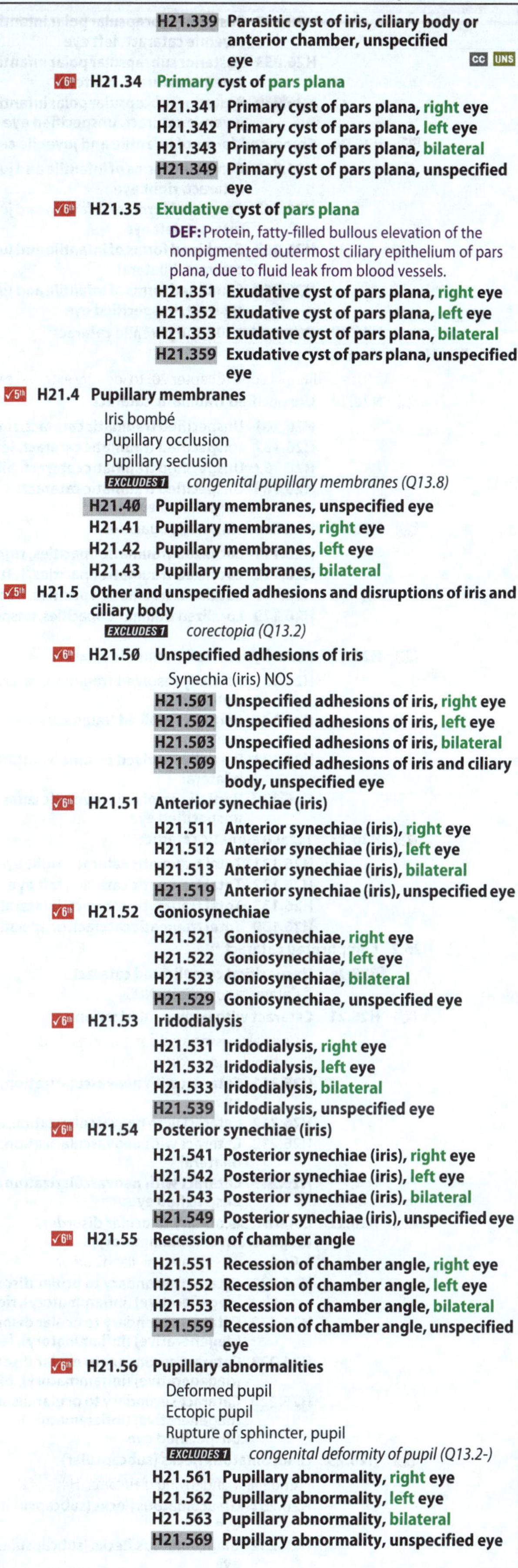

√5th **H25.0** **Age-related incipient cataract**

√6th **H25.01** **Cortical age-related cataract**
- **H25.011** **Cortical age-related cataract, right eye** A
- **H25.012** **Cortical age-related cataract, left eye** A
- **H25.013** **Cortical age-related cataract, bilateral** A
- **H25.019** **Cortical age-related cataract, unspecified eye** A

√6th **H25.03** **Anterior subcapsular polar age-related cataract**
- **H25.031** **Anterior subcapsular polar age-related cataract, right eye** A
- **H25.032** **Anterior subcapsular polar age-related cataract, left eye** A
- **H25.033** **Anterior subcapsular polar age-related cataract, bilateral** A
- **H25.039** **Anterior subcapsular polar age-related cataract, unspecified eye** A

√6th **H25.04** **Posterior subcapsular polar age-related cataract**
- **H25.041** **Posterior subcapsular polar age-related cataract, right eye** A
- **H25.042** **Posterior subcapsular polar age-related cataract, left eye** A
- **H25.043** **Posterior subcapsular polar age-related cataract, bilateral** A
- **H25.049** **Posterior subcapsular polar age-related cataract, unspecified eye** A

√6th **H25.09** **Other age-related incipient cataract**

Coronary age-related cataract
Punctate age-related cataract
Water clefts
- **H25.091** **Other age-related incipient cataract, right eye** A
- **H25.092** **Other age-related incipient cataract, left eye** A
- **H25.093** **Other age-related incipient cataract, bilateral** A

H25.Ø99 Other age-related incipient cataract, unspecified eye A

H25.1 Age-related nuclear cataract
- Cataracta brunescens
- Nuclear sclerosis cataract
- **AHA:** 2019,2Q,31; 2016,1Q,32

H25.1Ø Age-related nuclear cataract, unspecified eye A
H25.11 Age-related nuclear cataract, right eye A
H25.12 Age-related nuclear cataract, left eye A
H25.13 Age-related nuclear cataract, bilateral A

H25.2 Age-related cataract, morgagnian type
- Age-related hypermature cataract

H25.2Ø Age-related cataract, morgagnian type, unspecified eye A
H25.21 Age-related cataract, morgagnian type, right eye A
H25.22 Age-related cataract, morgagnian type, left eye A
H25.23 Age-related cataract, morgagnian type, bilateral A

H25.8 Other age-related cataract

H25.81 Combined forms of age-related cataract
- **AHA:** 2019,2Q,30

H25.811 Combined forms of age-related cataract, right eye A
H25.812 Combined forms of age-related cataract, left eye A
H25.813 Combined forms of age-related cataract, bilateral A
H25.819 Combined forms of age-related cataract, unspecified eye A
H25.89 Other age-related cataract A
H25.9 Unspecified age-related cataract A

H26 Other cataract

EXCLUDES 1 *congenital cataract (Q12.Ø)*

H26.Ø Infantile and juvenile cataract

H26.ØØ Unspecified infantile and juvenile cataract
H26.ØØ1 Unspecified infantile and juvenile cataract, right eye P
H26.ØØ2 Unspecified infantile and juvenile cataract, left eye P
H26.ØØ3 Unspecified infantile and juvenile cataract, bilateral P
H26.ØØ9 Unspecified infantile and juvenile cataract, unspecified eye P

H26.Ø1 Infantile and juvenile cortical, lamellar, or zonular cataract
H26.Ø11 Infantile and juvenile cortical, lamellar, or zonular cataract, right eye P
H26.Ø12 Infantile and juvenile cortical, lamellar, or zonular cataract, left eye P
H26.Ø13 Infantile and juvenile cortical, lamellar, or zonular cataract, bilateral P
H26.Ø19 Infantile and juvenile cortical, lamellar, or zonular cataract, unspecified eye P

H26.Ø3 Infantile and juvenile nuclear cataract
H26.Ø31 Infantile and juvenile nuclear cataract, right eye P
H26.Ø32 Infantile and juvenile nuclear cataract, left eye P
H26.Ø33 Infantile and juvenile nuclear cataract, bilateral P
H26.Ø39 Infantile and juvenile nuclear cataract, unspecified eye P

H26.Ø4 Anterior subcapsular polar infantile and juvenile cataract
H26.Ø41 Anterior subcapsular polar infantile and juvenile cataract, right eye P
H26.Ø42 Anterior subcapsular polar infantile and juvenile cataract, left eye P
H26.Ø43 Anterior subcapsular polar infantile and juvenile cataract, bilateral P
H26.Ø49 Anterior subcapsular polar infantile and juvenile cataract, unspecified eye P

H26.Ø5 Posterior subcapsular polar infantile and juvenile cataract
H26.Ø51 Posterior subcapsular polar infantile and juvenile cataract, right eye P
H26.Ø52 Posterior subcapsular polar infantile and juvenile cataract, left eye P
H26.Ø53 Posterior subcapsular polar infantile and juvenile cataract, bilateral P
H26.Ø59 Posterior subcapsular polar infantile and juvenile cataract, unspecified eye P

H26.Ø6 Combined forms of infantile and juvenile cataract
H26.Ø61 Combined forms of infantile and juvenile cataract, right eye P
H26.Ø62 Combined forms of infantile and juvenile cataract, left eye P
H26.Ø63 Combined forms of infantile and juvenile cataract, bilateral P
H26.Ø69 Combined forms of infantile and juvenile cataract, unspecified eye P
H26.Ø9 Other infantile and juvenile cataract P

H26.1 Traumatic cataract
- Use additional code (Chapter 2Ø) to identify external cause

H26.1Ø Unspecified traumatic cataract
H26.1Ø1 Unspecified traumatic cataract, right eye
H26.1Ø2 Unspecified traumatic cataract, left eye
H26.1Ø3 Unspecified traumatic cataract, bilateral
H26.1Ø9 Unspecified traumatic cataract, unspecified eye

H26.11 Localized traumatic opacities
H26.111 Localized traumatic opacities, right eye
H26.112 Localized traumatic opacities, left eye
H26.113 Localized traumatic opacities, bilateral
H26.119 Localized traumatic opacities, unspecified eye

H26.12 Partially resolved traumatic cataract
H26.121 Partially resolved traumatic cataract, right eye
H26.122 Partially resolved traumatic cataract, left eye
H26.123 Partially resolved traumatic cataract, bilateral
H26.129 Partially resolved traumatic cataract, unspecified eye

H26.13 Total traumatic cataract
H26.131 Total traumatic cataract, right eye
H26.132 Total traumatic cataract, left eye
H26.133 Total traumatic cataract, bilateral
H26.139 Total traumatic cataract, unspecified eye

H26.2 Complicated cataract
H26.2Ø Unspecified complicated cataract
- Cataracta complicata NOS

H26.21 Cataract with neovascularization
- Code also associated condition, such as: chronic iridocyclitis (H2Ø.1-)

H26.211 Cataract with neovascularization, right eye
H26.212 Cataract with neovascularization, left eye
H26.213 Cataract with neovascularization, bilateral
H26.219 Cataract with neovascularization, unspecified eye

H26.22 Cataract secondary to ocular disorders (degenerative) (inflammatory)
- Code also associated ocular disorder

H26.221 Cataract secondary to ocular disorders (degenerative) (inflammatory), right eye
H26.222 Cataract secondary to ocular disorders (degenerative) (inflammatory), left eye
H26.223 Cataract secondary to ocular disorders (degenerative) (inflammatory), bilateral
H26.229 Cataract secondary to ocular disorders (degenerative) (inflammatory), unspecified eye

H26.23 Glaucomatous flecks (subcapsular)
- Code first underlying glaucoma (H4Ø-H42)

H26.231 Glaucomatous flecks (subcapsular), right eye
H26.232 Glaucomatous flecks (subcapsular), left eye
H26.233 Glaucomatous flecks (subcapsular), bilateral
H26.239 Glaucomatous flecks (subcapsular), unspecified eye

H26.3 Drug-induced cataract
Toxic cataract
Use additional code for adverse effect, if applicable, to identify drug (T36-T50 with fifth or sixth character 5)
- **H26.30** Drug-induced cataract, unspecified eye
- **H26.31** Drug-induced cataract, right eye
- **H26.32** Drug-induced cataract, left eye
- **H26.33** Drug-induced cataract, bilateral

H26.4 Secondary cataract
- **H26.40** Unspecified secondary cataract
- **H26.41** Soemmering's ring
  - **H26.411** Soemmering's ring, right eye
  - **H26.412** Soemmering's ring, left eye
  - **H26.413** Soemmering's ring, bilateral
  - **H26.419** Soemmering's ring, unspecified eye
- **H26.49** Other secondary cataract
  AHA: 2018,2Q,14
  - **H26.491** Other secondary cataract, right eye
  - **H26.492** Other secondary cataract, left eye
  - **H26.493** Other secondary cataract, bilateral
  - **H26.499** Other secondary cataract, unspecified eye

H26.8 Other specified cataract
H26.9 Unspecified cataract

H27 Other disorders of lens
EXCLUDES 1 *congenital lens malformations (Q12.-)*
mechanical complications of intraocular lens implant (T85.2)
pseudophakia (Z96.1)

H27.0 Aphakia
Acquired absence of lens
Acquired aphakia
Aphakia due to trauma
EXCLUDES 1 *cataract extraction status (Z98.4-)*
congenital absence of lens (Q12.3)
congenital aphakia (Q12.3)
- **H27.00** Aphakia, unspecified eye
- **H27.01** Aphakia, right eye
- **H27.02** Aphakia, left eye
- **H27.03** Aphakia, bilateral

H27.1 Dislocation of lens
- **H27.10** Unspecified dislocation of lens
- **H27.11** Subluxation of lens
  - **H27.111** Subluxation of lens, right eye
  - **H27.112** Subluxation of lens, left eye
  - **H27.113** Subluxation of lens, bilateral
  - **H27.119** Subluxation of lens, unspecified eye
- **H27.12** Anterior dislocation of lens
  - **H27.121** Anterior dislocation of lens, right eye
  - **H27.122** Anterior dislocation of lens, left eye
  - **H27.123** Anterior dislocation of lens, bilateral
  - **H27.129** Anterior dislocation of lens, unspecified eye
- **H27.13** Posterior dislocation of lens
  - **H27.131** Posterior dislocation of lens, right eye
  - **H27.132** Posterior dislocation of lens, left eye
  - **H27.133** Posterior dislocation of lens, bilateral
  - **H27.139** Posterior dislocation of lens, unspecified eye

H27.8 Other specified disorders of lens
H27.9 Unspecified disorder of lens

H28 Cataract in diseases classified elsewhere
Code first underlying disease, such as:
hypoparathyroidism (E20.-)
myotonia (G71.1-)
myxedema (E03.-)
protein-calorie malnutrition (E40-E46)
EXCLUDES 1 *cataract in diabetes mellitus (E08.36, E09.36, E10.36, E11.36, E13.36)*

Disorders of choroid and retina (H30-H36)

H30 Chorioretinal inflammation

H30.0 Focal chorioretinal inflammation
Focal chorioretinitis
Focal choroiditis
Focal retinitis
Focal retinochoroiditis
- **H30.00** Unspecified focal chorioretinal inflammation
  Focal chorioretinitis NOS
  Focal choroiditis NOS
  Focal retinitis NOS
  Focal retinochoroiditis NOS
  - **H30.001** Unspecified focal chorioretinal inflammation, right eye
  - **H30.002** Unspecified focal chorioretinal inflammation, left eye
  - **H30.003** Unspecified focal chorioretinal inflammation, bilateral
  - **H30.009** Unspecified focal chorioretinal inflammation, unspecified eye
- **H30.01** Focal chorioretinal inflammation, juxtapapillary
  - **H30.011** Focal chorioretinal inflammation, juxtapapillary, right eye
  - **H30.012** Focal chorioretinal inflammation, juxtapapillary, left eye
  - **H30.013** Focal chorioretinal inflammation, juxtapapillary, bilateral
  - **H30.019** Focal chorioretinal inflammation, juxtapapillary, unspecified eye
- **H30.02** Focal chorioretinal inflammation of posterior pole
  - **H30.021** Focal chorioretinal inflammation of posterior pole, right eye
  - **H30.022** Focal chorioretinal inflammation of posterior pole, left eye
  - **H30.023** Focal chorioretinal inflammation of posterior pole, bilateral
  - **H30.029** Focal chorioretinal inflammation of posterior pole, unspecified eye
- **H30.03** Focal chorioretinal inflammation, peripheral
  - **H30.031** Focal chorioretinal inflammation, peripheral, right eye
  - **H30.032** Focal chorioretinal inflammation, peripheral, left eye
  - **H30.033** Focal chorioretinal inflammation, peripheral, bilateral
  - **H30.039** Focal chorioretinal inflammation, peripheral, unspecified eye
- **H30.04** Focal chorioretinal inflammation, macular or paramacular
  - **H30.041** Focal chorioretinal inflammation, macular or paramacular, right eye
  - **H30.042** Focal chorioretinal inflammation, macular or paramacular, left eye
  - **H30.043** Focal chorioretinal inflammation, macular or paramacular, bilateral
  - **H30.049** Focal chorioretinal inflammation, macular or paramacular, unspecified eye

H30.1 Disseminated chorioretinal inflammation
Disseminated chorioretinitis
Disseminated choroiditis
Disseminated retinitis
Disseminated retinochoroiditis
EXCLUDES 2 *exudative retinopathy (H35.02-)*
- **H30.10** Unspecified disseminated chorioretinal inflammation
  Disseminated chorioretinitis NOS
  Disseminated choroiditis NOS
  Disseminated retinitis NOS
  Disseminated retinochoroiditis NOS
  - **H30.101** Unspecified disseminated chorioretinal inflammation, right eye CC
  - **H30.102** Unspecified disseminated chorioretinal inflammation, left eye CC
  - **H30.103** Unspecified disseminated chorioretinal inflammation, bilateral CC
  - **H30.109** Unspecified disseminated chorioretinal inflammation, unspecified eye CC UNS

H30.11 Disseminated chorioretinal inflammation of posterior pole
- **H30.111 Disseminated chorioretinal inflammation of posterior pole, right eye** CC
- **H30.112 Disseminated chorioretinal inflammation of posterior pole, left eye** CC
- **H30.113 Disseminated chorioretinal inflammation of posterior pole, bilateral** CC
- **H30.119 Disseminated chorioretinal inflammation of posterior pole, unspecified eye** CC UNS

H30.12 Disseminated chorioretinal inflammation, peripheral
- **H30.121 Disseminated chorioretinal inflammation, peripheral right eye** CC
- **H30.122 Disseminated chorioretinal inflammation, peripheral, left eye** CC
- **H30.123 Disseminated chorioretinal inflammation, peripheral, bilateral** CC
- **H30.129 Disseminated chorioretinal inflammation, peripheral, unspecified eye** CC UNS

H30.13 Disseminated chorioretinal inflammation, generalized
- **H30.131 Disseminated chorioretinal inflammation, generalized, right eye** CC
- **H30.132 Disseminated chorioretinal inflammation, generalized, left eye** CC
- **H30.133 Disseminated chorioretinal inflammation, generalized, bilateral** CC
- **H30.139 Disseminated chorioretinal inflammation, generalized, unspecified eye** CC UNS

H30.14 Acute posterior multifocal placoid pigment epitheliopathy
- **H30.141 Acute posterior multifocal placoid pigment epitheliopathy, right eye** CC
- **H30.142 Acute posterior multifocal placoid pigment epitheliopathy, left eye** CC
- **H30.143 Acute posterior multifocal placoid pigment epitheliopathy, bilateral** CC
- **H30.149 Acute posterior multifocal placoid pigment epitheliopathy, unspecified eye** CC UNS

H30.2 Posterior cyclitis

Pars planitis
- **H30.20 Posterior cyclitis, unspecified eye**
- **H30.21 Posterior cyclitis, right eye**
- **H30.22 Posterior cyclitis, left eye**
- **H30.23 Posterior cyclitis, bilateral**

H30.8 Other chorioretinal inflammations

H30.81 Harada's disease
- **H30.811 Harada's disease, right eye**
- **H30.812 Harada's disease, left eye**
- **H30.813 Harada's disease, bilateral**
- **H30.819 Harada's disease, unspecified eye**

H30.89 Other chorioretinal inflammations
- **H30.891 Other chorioretinal inflammations, right eye** CC
- **H30.892 Other chorioretinal inflammations, left eye** CC
- **H30.893 Other chorioretinal inflammations, bilateral** CC
- **H30.899 Other chorioretinal inflammations, unspecified eye** CC UNS

H30.9 Unspecified chorioretinal inflammation

Chorioretinitis NOS
Choroiditis NOS
Neuroretinitis NOS
Retinitis NOS
Retinochoroiditis NOS
- **H30.90 Unspecified chorioretinal inflammation, unspecified eye** CC UNS
- **H30.91 Unspecified chorioretinal inflammation, right eye** CC
- **H30.92 Unspecified chorioretinal inflammation, left eye** CC
- **H30.93 Unspecified chorioretinal inflammation, bilateral** CC

H31 Other disorders of choroid

H31.0 Chorioretinal scars

EXCLUDES 2 *postsurgical chorioretinal scars (H59.81-)*

H31.00 Unspecified chorioretinal scars
- **H31.001 Unspecified chorioretinal scars, right eye**
- **H31.002 Unspecified chorioretinal scars, left eye**
- **H31.003 Unspecified chorioretinal scars, bilateral**
- **H31.009 Unspecified chorioretinal scars, unspecified eye**

H31.01 Macula scars of posterior pole (postinflammatory) (post-traumatic)

EXCLUDES 1 *postprocedural choriorentinal scar (H59.81-)*
- **H31.011 Macula scars of posterior pole (postinflammatory) (post-traumatic), right eye**
- **H31.012 Macula scars of posterior pole (postinflammatory) (post-traumatic), left eye**
- **H31.013 Macula scars of posterior pole (postinflammatory) (post-traumatic), bilateral**
- **H31.019 Macula scars of posterior pole (postinflammatory) (post-traumatic), unspecified eye**

H31.02 Solar retinopathy
- **H31.021 Solar retinopathy, right eye**
- **H31.022 Solar retinopathy, left eye**
- **H31.023 Solar retinopathy, bilateral**
- **H31.029 Solar retinopathy, unspecified eye**

H31.09 Other chorioretinal scars
- **H31.091 Other chorioretinal scars, right eye**
- **H31.092 Other chorioretinal scars, left eye**
- **H31.093 Other chorioretinal scars, bilateral**
- **H31.099 Other chorioretinal scars, unspecified eye**

H31.1 Choroidal degeneration

EXCLUDES 2 *angioid streaks of macula (H35.33)*

H31.10 Unspecified choroidal degeneration

Choroidal sclerosis NOS
- **H31.101 Choroidal degeneration, unspecified, right eye**
- **H31.102 Choroidal degeneration, unspecified, left eye**
- **H31.103 Choroidal degeneration, unspecified, bilateral**
- **H31.109 Choroidal degeneration, unspecified, unspecified eye**

H31.11 Age-related choroidal atrophy
- **H31.111 Age-related choroidal atrophy, right eye** A
- **H31.112 Age-related choroidal atrophy, left eye** A
- **H31.113 Age-related choroidal atrophy, bilateral** A
- **H31.119 Age-related choroidal atrophy, unspecified eye** A

H31.12 Diffuse secondary atrophy of choroid
- **H31.121 Diffuse secondary atrophy of choroid, right eye**
- **H31.122 Diffuse secondary atrophy of choroid, left eye**
- **H31.123 Diffuse secondary atrophy of choroid, bilateral**
- **H31.129 Diffuse secondary atrophy of choroid, unspecified eye**

H31.2 Hereditary choroidal dystrophy

EXCLUDES 2 *hyperornithinemia (E72.4)*
ornithinemia (E72.4)
- **H31.20 Hereditary choroidal dystrophy, unspecified**
- **H31.21 Choroideremia**
- **H31.22 Choroidal dystrophy (central areolar) (generalized) (peripapillary)**
- **H31.23 Gyrate atrophy, choroid**
- **H31.29 Other hereditary choroidal dystrophy**

H31.3 Choroidal hemorrhage and rupture

H31.30 Unspecified choroidal hemorrhage
- **H31.301 Unspecified choroidal hemorrhage, right eye**

H31.302 Unspecified choroidal hemorrhage, left eye
H31.303 Unspecified choroidal hemorrhage, bilateral
H31.309 Unspecified choroidal hemorrhage, unspecified eye

✓6th **H31.31 Expulsive choroidal hemorrhage**
H31.311 Expulsive choroidal hemorrhage, right eye
H31.312 Expulsive choroidal hemorrhage, left eye
H31.313 Expulsive choroidal hemorrhage, bilateral
H31.319 Expulsive choroidal hemorrhage, unspecified eye

✓6th **H31.32 Choroidal rupture**
H31.321 Choroidal rupture, right eye CC
H31.322 Choroidal rupture, left eye CC
H31.323 Choroidal rupture, bilateral CC
H31.329 Choroidal rupture, unspecified eye CC UNS

✓5th **H31.4 Choroidal detachment**

✓6th **H31.40 Unspecified choroidal detachment**
H31.401 Unspecified choroidal detachment, right eye CC
H31.402 Unspecified choroidal detachment, left eye CC
H31.403 Unspecified choroidal detachment, bilateral CC
H31.409 Unspecified choroidal detachment, unspecified eye CC UNS

✓6th **H31.41 Hemorrhagic choroidal detachment**
H31.411 Hemorrhagic choroidal detachment, right eye CC
H31.412 Hemorrhagic choroidal detachment, left eye CC
H31.413 Hemorrhagic choroidal detachment, bilateral CC
H31.419 Hemorrhagic choroidal detachment, unspecified eye CC UNS

✓6th **H31.42 Serous choroidal detachment**
H31.421 Serous choroidal detachment, right eye CC
H31.422 Serous choroidal detachment, left eye CC
H31.423 Serous choroidal detachment, bilateral CC
H31.429 Serous choroidal detachment, unspecified eye CC UNS

H31.8 Other specified disorders of choroid
H31.9 Unspecified disorder of choroid

H32 Chorioretinal disorders in diseases classified elsewhere
Code first underlying disease, such as:
congenital toxoplasmosis (P37.1)
histoplasmosis (B39.-)
leprosy (A30.-)

EXCLUDES 1 *chorioretinitis (in):*
toxoplasmosis (acquired) (B58.01)
tuberculosis (A18.53)

✓4th **H33 Retinal detachments and breaks**
EXCLUDES 1 *detachment of retinal pigment epithelium (H35.72-, H35.73-)*

Retinal Detachment

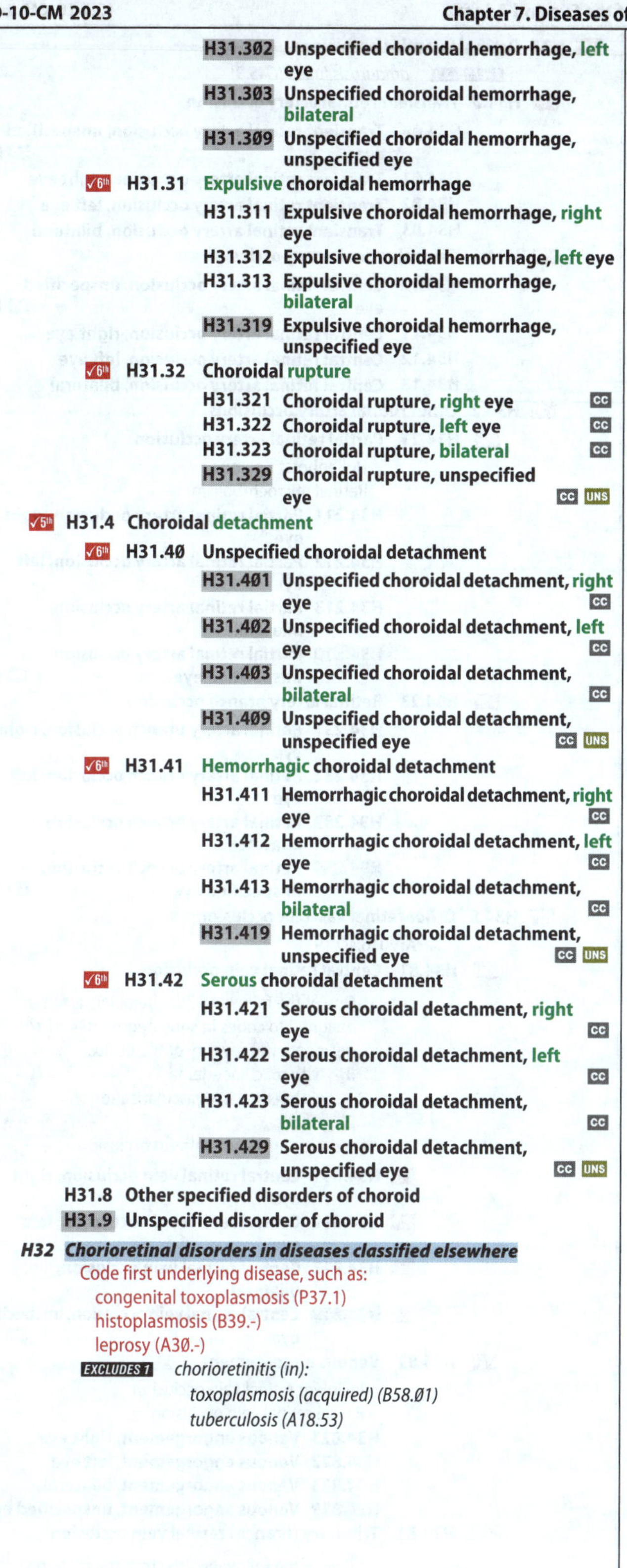

✓5th **H33.0 Retinal detachment with retinal break**
Rhegmatogenous retinal detachment
EXCLUDES 1 *serous retinal detachment (without retinal break) (H33.2-)*

✓6th **H33.00 Unspecified retinal detachment with retinal break**
H33.001 Unspecified retinal detachment with retinal break, right eye
H33.002 Unspecified retinal detachment with retinal break, left eye
H33.003 Unspecified retinal detachment with retinal break, bilateral
H33.009 Unspecified retinal detachment with retinal break, unspecified eye

✓6th **H33.01 Retinal detachment with single break**
H33.011 Retinal detachment with single break, right eye
H33.012 Retinal detachment with single break, left eye
H33.013 Retinal detachment with single break, bilateral
H33.019 Retinal detachment with single break, unspecified eye

✓6th **H33.02 Retinal detachment with multiple breaks**
H33.021 Retinal detachment with multiple breaks, right eye
H33.022 Retinal detachment with multiple breaks, left eye
H33.023 Retinal detachment with multiple breaks, bilateral
H33.029 Retinal detachment with multiple breaks, unspecified eye

✓6th **H33.03 Retinal detachment with giant retinal tear**
H33.031 Retinal detachment with giant retinal tear, right eye
H33.032 Retinal detachment with giant retinal tear, left eye
H33.033 Retinal detachment with giant retinal tear, bilateral
H33.039 Retinal detachment with giant retinal tear, unspecified eye

✓6th **H33.04 Retinal detachment with retinal dialysis**
H33.041 Retinal detachment with retinal dialysis, right eye
H33.042 Retinal detachment with retinal dialysis, left eye
H33.043 Retinal detachment with retinal dialysis, bilateral
H33.049 Retinal detachment with retinal dialysis, unspecified eye

✓6th **H33.05 Total retinal detachment**
H33.051 Total retinal detachment, right eye
H33.052 Total retinal detachment, left eye
H33.053 Total retinal detachment, bilateral
H33.059 Total retinal detachment, unspecified eye

✓5th **H33.1 Retinoschisis and retinal cysts**
EXCLUDES 1 *congenital retinoschisis (Q14.1)*
microcystoid degeneration of retina (H35.42-)

✓6th **H33.10 Unspecified retinoschisis**
H33.101 Unspecified retinoschisis, right eye
H33.102 Unspecified retinoschisis, left eye

H33.103 Unspecified retinoschisis, bilateral
H33.109 Unspecified retinoschisis, unspecified eye

H33.11 Cyst of ora serrata
- **H33.111** Cyst of ora serrata, right eye
- **H33.112** Cyst of ora serrata, left eye
- **H33.113** Cyst of ora serrata, bilateral
- **H33.119** Cyst of ora serrata, unspecified eye

H33.12 Parasitic cyst of retina
- **H33.121** Parasitic cyst of retina, right eye CC
- **H33.122** Parasitic cyst of retina, left eye CC
- **H33.123** Parasitic cyst of retina, bilateral CC
- **H33.129** Parasitic cyst of retina, unspecified eye CC UNS

H33.19 Other retinoschisis and retinal cysts

Pseudocyst of retina
- **H33.191** Other retinoschisis and retinal cysts, right eye
- **H33.192** Other retinoschisis and retinal cysts, left eye
- **H33.193** Other retinoschisis and retinal cysts, bilateral
- **H33.199** Other retinoschisis and retinal cysts, unspecified eye

H33.2 Serous retinal detachment

Retinal detachment NOS
Retinal detachment without retinal break

EXCLUDES 1 *central serous chorioretinopathy (H35.71-)*

- **H33.20** Serous retinal detachment, unspecified eye CC UNS
- **H33.21** Serous retinal detachment, right eye CC
- **H33.22** Serous retinal detachment, left eye CC
- **H33.23** Serous retinal detachment, bilateral CC

H33.3 Retinal breaks without detachment

EXCLUDES 1 *chorioretinal scars after surgery for detachment (H59.81-)*
peripheral retinal degeneration without break (H35.4-)

H33.30 Unspecified retinal break
- **H33.301** Unspecified retinal break, right eye
- **H33.302** Unspecified retinal break, left eye
- **H33.303** Unspecified retinal break, bilateral
- **H33.309** Unspecified retinal break, unspecified eye

H33.31 Horseshoe tear of retina without detachment

Operculum of retina without detachment
- **H33.311** Horseshoe tear of retina without detachment, right eye
- **H33.312** Horseshoe tear of retina without detachment, left eye
- **H33.313** Horseshoe tear of retina without detachment, bilateral
- **H33.319** Horseshoe tear of retina without detachment, unspecified eye

H33.32 Round hole of retina without detachment
- **H33.321** Round hole, right eye
- **H33.322** Round hole, left eye
- **H33.323** Round hole, bilateral
- **H33.329** Round hole, unspecified eye

H33.33 Multiple defects of retina without detachment
- **H33.331** Multiple defects of retina without detachment, right eye
- **H33.332** Multiple defects of retina without detachment, left eye
- **H33.333** Multiple defects of retina without detachment, bilateral
- **H33.339** Multiple defects of retina without detachment, unspecified eye

H33.4 Traction detachment of retina

Proliferative vitreo-retinopathy with retinal detachment
- **H33.40** Traction detachment of retina, unspecified eye CC UNS
- **H33.41** Traction detachment of retina, right eye CC
- **H33.42** Traction detachment of retina, left eye CC
- **H33.43** Traction detachment of retina, bilateral CC

H33.8 Other retinal detachments CC

H34 Retinal vascular occlusions

EXCLUDES 1 *amaurosis fugax (G45.3)*

H34.0 Transient retinal artery occlusion
- **H34.00** Transient retinal artery occlusion, unspecified eye CC UNS
- **H34.01** Transient retinal artery occlusion, right eye CC
- **H34.02** Transient retinal artery occlusion, left eye CC
- **H34.03** Transient retinal artery occlusion, bilateral CC

H34.1 Central retinal artery occlusion
- **H34.10** Central retinal artery occlusion, unspecified eye CC UNS
- **H34.11** Central retinal artery occlusion, right eye CC
- **H34.12** Central retinal artery occlusion, left eye CC
- **H34.13** Central retinal artery occlusion, bilateral CC

H34.2 Other retinal artery occlusions

H34.21 Partial retinal artery occlusion

Hollenhorst's plaque
Retinal microembolism
- **H34.211** Partial retinal artery occlusion, right eye CC
- **H34.212** Partial retinal artery occlusion, left eye CC
- **H34.213** Partial retinal artery occlusion, bilateral CC
- **H34.219** Partial retinal artery occlusion, unspecified eye CC UNS

H34.23 Retinal artery branch occlusion
- **H34.231** Retinal artery branch occlusion, right eye CC
- **H34.232** Retinal artery branch occlusion, left eye CC
- **H34.233** Retinal artery branch occlusion, bilateral CC
- **H34.239** Retinal artery branch occlusion, unspecified eye CC UNS

H34.8 Other retinal vascular occlusions

AHA: 2016,4Q,19

H34.81 Central retinal vein occlusion

One of the following 7th characters is to be assigned to codes in subcategory H34.81 to designate the severity of the occlusion:
- 0 with macular edema
- 1 with retinal neovascularization
- 2 stable
  old central retinal vein occlusion

- **H34.811** Central retinal vein occlusion, right eye CC
- **H34.812** Central retinal vein occlusion, left eye CC
- **H34.813** Central retinal vein occlusion, bilateral CC
- **H34.819** Central retinal vein occlusion, unspecified eye CC UNS

H34.82 Venous engorgement

Incipient retinal vein occlusion
Partial retinal vein occlusion
- **H34.821** Venous engorgement, right eye
- **H34.822** Venous engorgement, left eye
- **H34.823** Venous engorgement, bilateral
- **H34.829** Venous engorgement, unspecified eye

H34.83 Tributary (branch) retinal vein occlusion

One of the following 7th characters is to be assigned to codes in subcategory H34.83 to designate the severity of the occlusion:
- 0 with macular edema
- 1 with retinal neovascularization
- 2 stable
  old tributary (branch) retinal vein occlusion

- **H34.831** Tributary (branch) retinal vein occlusion, right eye
- **H34.832** Tributary (branch) retinal vein occlusion, left eye
- **H34.833** Tributary (branch) retinal vein occlusion, bilateral
- **H34.839** Tributary (branch) retinal vein occlusion, unspecified eye

H34.9 Unspecified retinal vascular occlusion CC

H35 Other retinal disorders

EXCLUDES 2 *diabetic retinal disorders (E08.311-E08.359, E09.311-E09.359, E10.311-E10.359, E11.311-E11.359, E13.311-E13.359)*

H35.0 Background retinopathy and retinal vascular changes

Code also any associated hypertension (I10)

- H35.00 Unspecified background retinopathy
- **H35.01 Changes in retinal vascular appearance**
  - Retinal vascular sheathing
  - H35.011 Changes in retinal vascular appearance, right eye
  - H35.012 Changes in retinal vascular appearance, left eye
  - H35.013 Changes in retinal vascular appearance, bilateral
  - H35.019 Changes in retinal vascular appearance, unspecified eye
- **H35.02 Exudative retinopathy**
  - Coats retinopathy
  - H35.021 Exudative retinopathy, right eye
  - H35.022 Exudative retinopathy, left eye
  - H35.023 Exudative retinopathy, bilateral
  - H35.029 Exudative retinopathy, unspecified eye
- **H35.03 Hypertensive retinopathy**
  - H35.031 Hypertensive retinopathy, right eye
  - H35.032 Hypertensive retinopathy, left eye
  - H35.033 Hypertensive retinopathy, bilateral
  - H35.039 Hypertensive retinopathy, unspecified eye
- **H35.04 Retinal micro-aneurysms, unspecified**
  - H35.041 Retinal micro-aneurysms, unspecified, right eye
  - H35.042 Retinal micro-aneurysms, unspecified, left eye
  - H35.043 Retinal micro-aneurysms, unspecified, bilateral
  - H35.049 Retinal micro-aneurysms, unspecified, unspecified eye
- **H35.05 Retinal neovascularization, unspecified**
  - H35.051 Retinal neovascularization, unspecified, right eye
  - H35.052 Retinal neovascularization, unspecified, left eye
  - H35.053 Retinal neovascularization, unspecified, bilateral
  - H35.059 Retinal neovascularization, unspecified, unspecified eye
- **H35.06 Retinal vasculitis**
  - Eales disease
  - Retinal perivasculitis
  - **DEF:** Sight-threatening intraocular inflammation of the retinal blood vessels that causes minimal, partial, or even complete blindness.
  - H35.061 Retinal vasculitis, right eye
  - H35.062 Retinal vasculitis, left eye
  - H35.063 Retinal vasculitis, bilateral
  - H35.069 Retinal vasculitis, unspecified eye
- **H35.07 Retinal telangiectasis**
  - H35.071 Retinal telangiectasis, right eye
  - H35.072 Retinal telangiectasis, left eye
  - H35.073 Retinal telangiectasis, bilateral
  - H35.079 Retinal telangiectasis, unspecified eye
- H35.09 Other intraretinal microvascular abnormalities
  - Retinal varices

H35.1 Retinopathy of prematurity

- **H35.10 Retinopathy of prematurity, unspecified**
  - Retinopathy of prematurity NOS
  - H35.101 Retinopathy of prematurity, unspecified, right eye
  - H35.102 Retinopathy of prematurity, unspecified, left eye
  - H35.103 Retinopathy of prematurity, unspecified, bilateral
  - H35.109 Retinopathy of prematurity, unspecified, unspecified eye
- **H35.11 Retinopathy of prematurity, stage 0**
  - H35.111 Retinopathy of prematurity, stage 0, right eye
  - H35.112 Retinopathy of prematurity, stage 0, left eye
  - H35.113 Retinopathy of prematurity, stage 0, bilateral
  - H35.119 Retinopathy of prematurity, stage 0, unspecified eye
- **H35.12 Retinopathy of prematurity, stage 1**
  - H35.121 Retinopathy of prematurity, stage 1, right eye
  - H35.122 Retinopathy of prematurity, stage 1, left eye
  - H35.123 Retinopathy of prematurity, stage 1, bilateral
  - H35.129 Retinopathy of prematurity, stage 1, unspecified eye
- **H35.13 Retinopathy of prematurity, stage 2**
  - H35.131 Retinopathy of prematurity, stage 2, right eye
  - H35.132 Retinopathy of prematurity, stage 2, left eye
  - H35.133 Retinopathy of prematurity, stage 2, bilateral
  - H35.139 Retinopathy of prematurity, stage 2, unspecified eye
- **H35.14 Retinopathy of prematurity, stage 3**
  - H35.141 Retinopathy of prematurity, stage 3, right eye
  - H35.142 Retinopathy of prematurity, stage 3, left eye
  - H35.143 Retinopathy of prematurity, stage 3, bilateral
  - H35.149 Retinopathy of prematurity, stage 3, unspecified eye
- **H35.15 Retinopathy of prematurity, stage 4**
  - H35.151 Retinopathy of prematurity, stage 4, right eye
  - H35.152 Retinopathy of prematurity, stage 4, left eye
  - H35.153 Retinopathy of prematurity, stage 4, bilateral
  - H35.159 Retinopathy of prematurity, stage 4, unspecified eye
- **H35.16 Retinopathy of prematurity, stage 5**
  - H35.161 Retinopathy of prematurity, stage 5, right eye
  - H35.162 Retinopathy of prematurity, stage 5, left eye
  - H35.163 Retinopathy of prematurity, stage 5, bilateral
  - H35.169 Retinopathy of prematurity, stage 5, unspecified eye
- **H35.17 Retrolental fibroplasia**
  - H35.171 Retrolental fibroplasia, right eye
  - H35.172 Retrolental fibroplasia, left eye
  - H35.173 Retrolental fibroplasia, bilateral
  - H35.179 Retrolental fibroplasia, unspecified eye

H35.2 Other non-diabetic proliferative retinopathy

Proliferative vitreo-retinopathy

EXCLUDES 1 *proliferative vitreo-retinopathy with retinal detachment (H33.4-)*

- H35.20 Other non-diabetic proliferative retinopathy, unspecified eye
- H35.21 Other non-diabetic proliferative retinopathy, right eye
- H35.22 Other non-diabetic proliferative retinopathy, left eye
- H35.23 Other non-diabetic proliferative retinopathy, bilateral

H35.3 Degeneration of macula and posterior pole

- H35.30 Unspecified macular degeneration A
  - Age-related macular degeneration

√6th **H35.31 Nonexudative age-related macular degeneration**
Atrophic age-related macular degeneration
Dry age-related macular degeneration
AHA: 2016,4Q,20-21

One of the following 7th characters is to be assigned to each code in subcategory H35.31 to designate the stage of the disease:
- 0 stage unspecified
- 1 early dry stage
- 2 intermediate dry stage
- 3 advanced atrophic without subfoveal involvement
  advanced dry stage
- 4 advanced atrophic with subfoveal involvement

√7th **H35.311 Nonexudative age-related macular degeneration, right eye** A
√7th **H35.312 Nonexudative age-related macular degeneration, left eye** A
√7th **H35.313 Nonexudative age-related macular degeneration, bilateral** A
√7th **H35.319 Nonexudative age-related macular degeneration, unspecified eye** A

√6th **H35.32 Exudative age-related macular degeneration**
Wet age-related macular degeneration
AHA: 2016,4Q,20-21

One of the following 7th characters is to be assigned to each code in subcategory H35.32 to designate the stage of the disease:
- 0 stage unspecified
- 1 with active choroidal neovascularization
- 2 with inactive choroidal neovascularization
  with involuted or regressed neovascularization
- 3 with inactive scar

√7th **H35.321 Exudative age-related macular degeneration, right eye** HCC A
√7th **H35.322 Exudative age-related macular degeneration, left eye** HCC A
√7th **H35.323 Exudative age-related macular degeneration, bilateral** HCC A
√7th **H35.329 Exudative age-related macular degeneration, unspecified eye** HCC A

H35.33 Angioid streaks of macula
DEF: Degeneration of the choroid, characterized by broad, irregular, dark brown streaks radiating from the optic disc; occurs with pseudoxanthoma elasticum or Paget's disease.

√6th **H35.34 Macular cyst, hole, or pseudohole**
H35.341 Macular cyst, hole, or pseudohole, right eye
H35.342 Macular cyst, hole, or pseudohole, left eye
H35.343 Macular cyst, hole, or pseudohole, bilateral
H35.349 Macular cyst, hole, or pseudohole, unspecified eye

√6th **H35.35 Cystoid macular degeneration**
EXCLUDES 1 *cystoid macular edema following cataract surgery (H59.03-)*
H35.351 Cystoid macular degeneration, right eye
H35.352 Cystoid macular degeneration, left eye
H35.353 Cystoid macular degeneration, bilateral
H35.359 Cystoid macular degeneration, unspecified eye

√6th **H35.36 Drusen (degenerative) of macula**
AHA: 2017,1Q,51; 2016,4Q,21
H35.361 Drusen (degenerative) of macula, right eye
H35.362 Drusen (degenerative) of macula, left eye
H35.363 Drusen (degenerative) of macula, bilateral
H35.369 Drusen (degenerative) of macula, unspecified eye

√6th **H35.37 Puckering of macula**
H35.371 Puckering of macula, right eye
H35.372 Puckering of macula, left eye
H35.373 Puckering of macula, bilateral
H35.379 Puckering of macula, unspecified eye

√6th **H35.38 Toxic maculopathy**
Code first poisoning due to drug or toxin, if applicable (T36-T65 with fifth or sixth character 1-4 or 6)
Use additional code for adverse effect, if applicable, to identify drug (T36-T50 with fifth or sixth character 5)
H35.381 Toxic maculopathy, right eye
H35.382 Toxic maculopathy, left eye
H35.383 Toxic maculopathy, bilateral
H35.389 Toxic maculopathy, unspecified eye

√5th **H35.4 Peripheral retinal degeneration**
EXCLUDES 1 *hereditary retinal degeneration (dystrophy) (H35.5-)*
peripheral retinal degeneration with retinal break (H33.3-)

H35.40 Unspecified peripheral retinal degeneration

√6th **H35.41 Lattice degeneration of retina**
Palisade degeneration of retina
DEF: Degeneration of the retina, often bilateral, that is usually benign. It is characterized by lines intersecting at irregular intervals in the peripheral retina. Retinal thinning and retinal holes may occur.
H35.411 Lattice degeneration of retina, right eye
H35.412 Lattice degeneration of retina, left eye
H35.413 Lattice degeneration of retina, bilateral
H35.419 Lattice degeneration of retina, unspecified eye

√6th **H35.42 Microcystoid degeneration of retina**
H35.421 Microcystoid degeneration of retina, right eye
H35.422 Microcystoid degeneration of retina, left eye
H35.423 Microcystoid degeneration of retina, bilateral
H35.429 Microcystoid degeneration of retina, unspecified eye

√6th **H35.43 Paving stone degeneration of retina**
H35.431 Paving stone degeneration of retina, right eye
H35.432 Paving stone degeneration of retina, left eye
H35.433 Paving stone degeneration of retina, bilateral
H35.439 Paving stone degeneration of retina, unspecified eye

√6th **H35.44 Age-related reticular degeneration of retina**
H35.441 Age-related reticular degeneration of retina, right eye A
H35.442 Age-related reticular degeneration of retina, left eye A
H35.443 Age-related reticular degeneration of retina, bilateral A
H35.449 Age-related reticular degeneration of retina, unspecified eye A

√6th **H35.45 Secondary pigmentary degeneration**
H35.451 Secondary pigmentary degeneration, right eye
H35.452 Secondary pigmentary degeneration, left eye
H35.453 Secondary pigmentary degeneration, bilateral
H35.459 Secondary pigmentary degeneration, unspecified eye

√6th **H35.46 Secondary vitreoretinal degeneration**
H35.461 Secondary vitreoretinal degeneration, right eye
H35.462 Secondary vitreoretinal degeneration, left eye
H35.463 Secondary vitreoretinal degeneration, bilateral
H35.469 Secondary vitreoretinal degeneration, unspecified eye

√5th **H35.5 Hereditary retinal dystrophy**
EXCLUDES 1 *dystrophies primarily involving Bruch's membrane (H31.1-)*

H35.50 Unspecified hereditary retinal dystrophy
H35.51 Vitreoretinal dystrophy

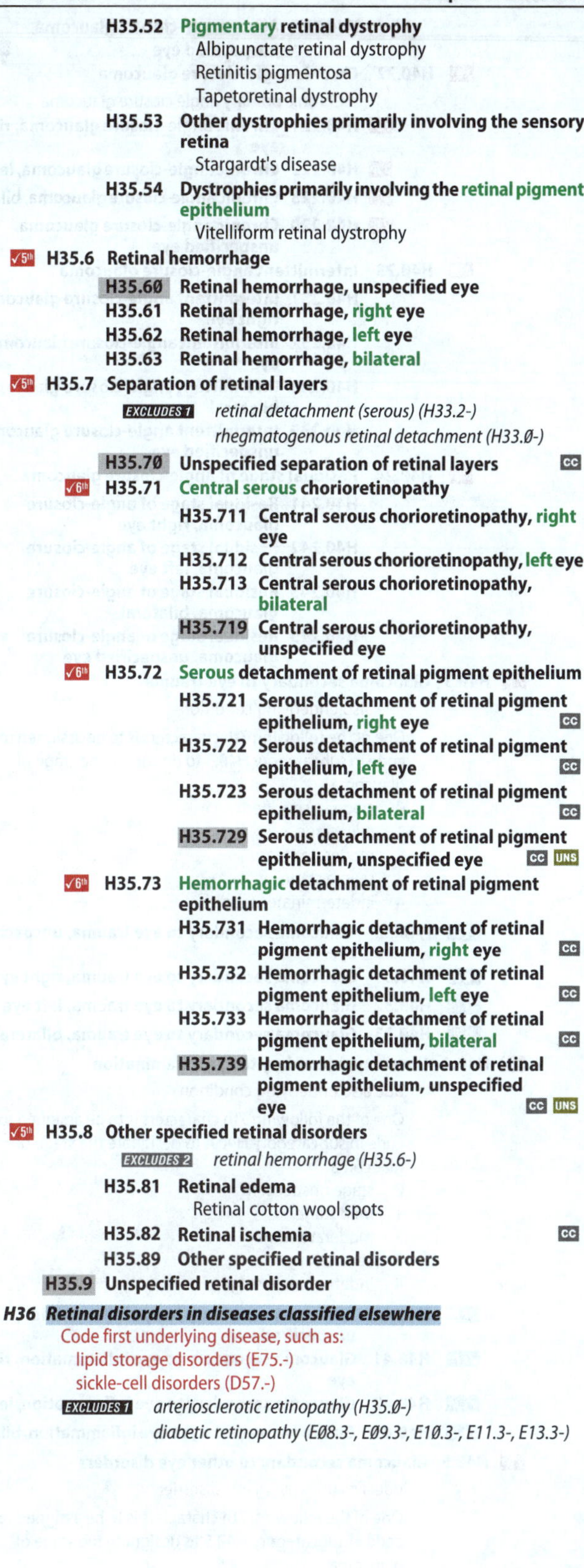

H35.52 Pigmentary retinal dystrophy
Albipunctate retinal dystrophy
Retinitis pigmentosa
Tapetoretinal dystrophy

H35.53 Other dystrophies primarily involving the sensory retina
Stargardt's disease

H35.54 Dystrophies primarily involving the retinal pigment epithelium
Vitelliform retinal dystrophy

H35.6 Retinal hemorrhage
- **H35.60 Retinal hemorrhage, unspecified eye**
- **H35.61 Retinal hemorrhage, right eye**
- **H35.62 Retinal hemorrhage, left eye**
- **H35.63 Retinal hemorrhage, bilateral**

H35.7 Separation of retinal layers
EXCLUDES 1 *retinal detachment (serous) (H33.2-)*
rhegmatogenous retinal detachment (H33.Ø-)

H35.70 Unspecified separation of retinal layers CC

H35.71 Central serous chorioretinopathy
- **H35.711 Central serous chorioretinopathy, right eye**
- **H35.712 Central serous chorioretinopathy, left eye**
- **H35.713 Central serous chorioretinopathy, bilateral**
- **H35.719 Central serous chorioretinopathy, unspecified eye**

H35.72 Serous detachment of retinal pigment epithelium
- **H35.721 Serous detachment of retinal pigment epithelium, right eye** CC
- **H35.722 Serous detachment of retinal pigment epithelium, left eye** CC
- **H35.723 Serous detachment of retinal pigment epithelium, bilateral** CC
- **H35.729 Serous detachment of retinal pigment epithelium, unspecified eye** CC UNS

H35.73 Hemorrhagic detachment of retinal pigment epithelium
- **H35.731 Hemorrhagic detachment of retinal pigment epithelium, right eye** CC
- **H35.732 Hemorrhagic detachment of retinal pigment epithelium, left eye** CC
- **H35.733 Hemorrhagic detachment of retinal pigment epithelium, bilateral** CC
- **H35.739 Hemorrhagic detachment of retinal pigment epithelium, unspecified eye** CC UNS

H35.8 Other specified retinal disorders
EXCLUDES 2 *retinal hemorrhage (H35.6-)*

H35.81 Retinal edema
Retinal cotton wool spots

H35.82 Retinal ischemia CC

H35.89 Other specified retinal disorders

H35.9 Unspecified retinal disorder

H36 Retinal disorders in diseases classified elsewhere
Code first underlying disease, such as:
lipid storage disorders (E75.-)
sickle-cell disorders (D57.-)
EXCLUDES 1 *arteriosclerotic retinopathy (H35.Ø-)*
diabetic retinopathy (EØ8.3-, EØ9.3-, E1Ø.3-, E11.3-, E13.3-)

Glaucoma (H4Ø-H42)

H4Ø Glaucoma
EXCLUDES 1 *absolute glaucoma (H44.51-)*
congenital glaucoma (Q15.Ø)
traumatic glaucoma due to birth injury (P15.3)

Open Angle/Angle Closure Glaucoma

Open angle
Closed angle
Fluid flow
Lens
Lens
Iris
Fluid flow
Cornea
Drainage canal

H4Ø.Ø Glaucoma suspect

H4Ø.ØØ Preglaucoma, unspecified
- **H4Ø.ØØ1 Preglaucoma, unspecified, right eye**
- **H4Ø.ØØ2 Preglaucoma, unspecified, left eye**
- **H4Ø.ØØ3 Preglaucoma, unspecified, bilateral**
- **H4Ø.ØØ9 Preglaucoma, unspecified, unspecified eye**

H4Ø.Ø1 Open angle with borderline findings, low risk
Open angle, low risk
- **H4Ø.Ø11 Open angle with borderline findings, low risk, right eye**
- **H4Ø.Ø12 Open angle with borderline findings, low risk, left eye**
- **H4Ø.Ø13 Open angle with borderline findings, low risk, bilateral**
- **H4Ø.Ø19 Open angle with borderline findings, low risk, unspecified eye**

H4Ø.Ø2 Open angle with borderline findings, high risk
Open angle, high risk
- **H4Ø.Ø21 Open angle with borderline findings, high risk, right eye**
- **H4Ø.Ø22 Open angle with borderline findings, high risk, left eye**
- **H4Ø.Ø23 Open angle with borderline findings, high risk, bilateral**
- **H4Ø.Ø29 Open angle with borderline findings, high risk, unspecified eye**

H4Ø.Ø3 Anatomical narrow angle
Primary angle closure suspect
- **H4Ø.Ø31 Anatomical narrow angle, right eye**
- **H4Ø.Ø32 Anatomical narrow angle, left eye**
- **H4Ø.Ø33 Anatomical narrow angle, bilateral**
- **H4Ø.Ø39 Anatomical narrow angle, unspecified eye**

H4Ø.Ø4 Steroid responder
- **H4Ø.Ø41 Steroid responder, right eye**
- **H4Ø.Ø42 Steroid responder, left eye**
- **H4Ø.Ø43 Steroid responder, bilateral**
- **H4Ø.Ø49 Steroid responder, unspecified eye**

H4Ø.Ø5 Ocular hypertension
- **H4Ø.Ø51 Ocular hypertension, right eye**
- **H4Ø.Ø52 Ocular hypertension, left eye**
- **H4Ø.Ø53 Ocular hypertension, bilateral**
- **H4Ø.Ø59 Ocular hypertension, unspecified eye**

H4Ø.Ø6 Primary angle closure without glaucoma damage
- **H4Ø.Ø61 Primary angle closure without glaucoma damage, right eye**
- **H4Ø.Ø62 Primary angle closure without glaucoma damage, left eye**
- **H4Ø.Ø63 Primary angle closure without glaucoma damage, bilateral**
- **H4Ø.Ø69 Primary angle closure without glaucoma damage, unspecified eye**

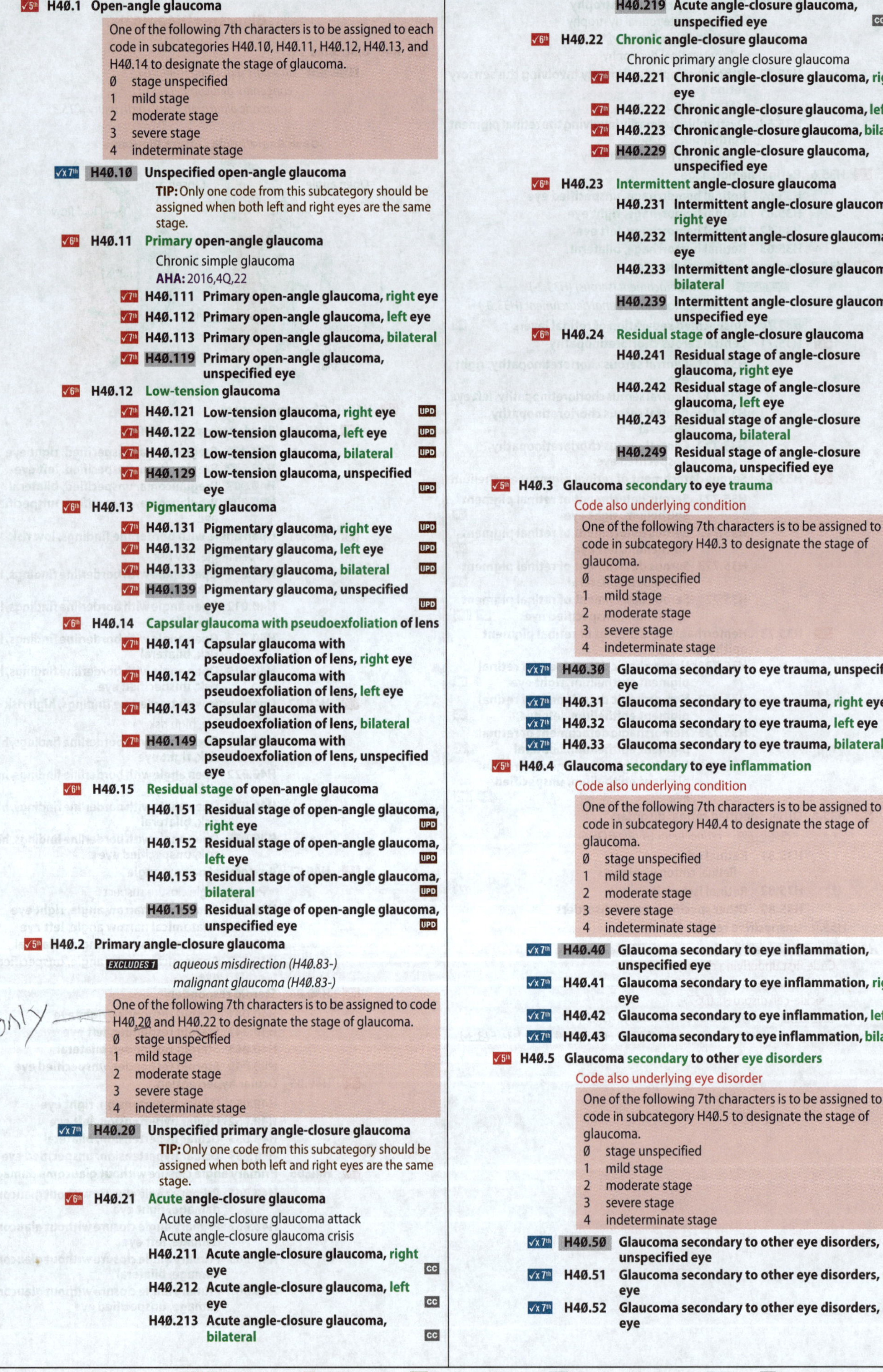

✓5th H4Ø.1 Open-angle glaucoma

One of the following 7th characters is to be assigned to each code in subcategories H4Ø.1Ø, H4Ø.11, H4Ø.12, H4Ø.13, and H4Ø.14 to designate the stage of glaucoma.
- Ø stage unspecified
- 1 mild stage
- 2 moderate stage
- 3 severe stage
- 4 indeterminate stage

✓x7th H4Ø.1Ø Unspecified open-angle glaucoma

TIP: Only one code from this subcategory should be assigned when both left and right eyes are the same stage.

✓6th H4Ø.11 Primary open-angle glaucoma

Chronic simple glaucoma

AHA: 2016,4Q,22

- **✓7th H4Ø.111 Primary open-angle glaucoma, right eye**
- **✓7th H4Ø.112 Primary open-angle glaucoma, left eye**
- **✓7th H4Ø.113 Primary open-angle glaucoma, bilateral**
- **✓7th H4Ø.119 Primary open-angle glaucoma, unspecified eye**

✓6th H4Ø.12 Low-tension glaucoma

- **✓7th H4Ø.121 Low-tension glaucoma, right eye** UPD
- **✓7th H4Ø.122 Low-tension glaucoma, left eye** UPD
- **✓7th H4Ø.123 Low-tension glaucoma, bilateral** UPD
- **✓7th H4Ø.129 Low-tension glaucoma, unspecified eye** UPD

✓6th H4Ø.13 Pigmentary glaucoma

- **✓7th H4Ø.131 Pigmentary glaucoma, right eye** UPD
- **✓7th H4Ø.132 Pigmentary glaucoma, left eye** UPD
- **✓7th H4Ø.133 Pigmentary glaucoma, bilateral** UPD
- **✓7th H4Ø.139 Pigmentary glaucoma, unspecified eye** UPD

✓6th H4Ø.14 Capsular glaucoma with pseudoexfoliation of lens

- **✓7th H4Ø.141 Capsular glaucoma with pseudoexfoliation of lens, right eye**
- **✓7th H4Ø.142 Capsular glaucoma with pseudoexfoliation of lens, left eye**
- **✓7th H4Ø.143 Capsular glaucoma with pseudoexfoliation of lens, bilateral**
- **✓7th H4Ø.149 Capsular glaucoma with pseudoexfoliation of lens, unspecified eye**

✓6th H4Ø.15 Residual stage of open-angle glaucoma

- **H4Ø.151 Residual stage of open-angle glaucoma, right eye** UPD
- **H4Ø.152 Residual stage of open-angle glaucoma, left eye** UPD
- **H4Ø.153 Residual stage of open-angle glaucoma, bilateral** UPD
- **H4Ø.159 Residual stage of open-angle glaucoma, unspecified eye** UPD

✓5th H4Ø.2 Primary angle-closure glaucoma

EXCLUDES 1 *aqueous misdirection (H4Ø.83-)*
malignant glaucoma (H4Ø.83-)

One of the following 7th characters is to be assigned to code H4Ø.2Ø and H4Ø.22 to designate the stage of glaucoma.
- Ø stage unspecified
- 1 mild stage
- 2 moderate stage
- 3 severe stage
- 4 indeterminate stage

✓x7th H4Ø.2Ø Unspecified primary angle-closure glaucoma

TIP: Only one code from this subcategory should be assigned when both left and right eyes are the same stage.

✓6th H4Ø.21 Acute angle-closure glaucoma

Acute angle-closure glaucoma attack
Acute angle-closure glaucoma crisis

- **H4Ø.211 Acute angle-closure glaucoma, right eye** CC
- **H4Ø.212 Acute angle-closure glaucoma, left eye** CC
- **H4Ø.213 Acute angle-closure glaucoma, bilateral** CC
- **H4Ø.219 Acute angle-closure glaucoma, unspecified eye** CC UNS

✓6th H4Ø.22 Chronic angle-closure glaucoma

Chronic primary angle closure glaucoma

- **✓7th H4Ø.221 Chronic angle-closure glaucoma, right eye**
- **✓7th H4Ø.222 Chronic angle-closure glaucoma, left eye**
- **✓7th H4Ø.223 Chronic angle-closure glaucoma, bilateral**
- **✓7th H4Ø.229 Chronic angle-closure glaucoma, unspecified eye**

✓6th H4Ø.23 Intermittent angle-closure glaucoma

- **H4Ø.231 Intermittent angle-closure glaucoma, right eye**
- **H4Ø.232 Intermittent angle-closure glaucoma, left eye**
- **H4Ø.233 Intermittent angle-closure glaucoma, bilateral**
- **H4Ø.239 Intermittent angle-closure glaucoma, unspecified eye**

✓6th H4Ø.24 Residual stage of angle-closure glaucoma

- **H4Ø.241 Residual stage of angle-closure glaucoma, right eye**
- **H4Ø.242 Residual stage of angle-closure glaucoma, left eye**
- **H4Ø.243 Residual stage of angle-closure glaucoma, bilateral**
- **H4Ø.249 Residual stage of angle-closure glaucoma, unspecified eye**

✓5th H4Ø.3 Glaucoma secondary to eye trauma

Code also underlying condition

One of the following 7th characters is to be assigned to each code in subcategory H4Ø.3 to designate the stage of glaucoma.
- Ø stage unspecified
- 1 mild stage
- 2 moderate stage
- 3 severe stage
- 4 indeterminate stage

- **✓x7th H4Ø.3Ø Glaucoma secondary to eye trauma, unspecified eye**
- **✓x7th H4Ø.31 Glaucoma secondary to eye trauma, right eye**
- **✓x7th H4Ø.32 Glaucoma secondary to eye trauma, left eye**
- **✓x7th H4Ø.33 Glaucoma secondary to eye trauma, bilateral**

✓5th H4Ø.4 Glaucoma secondary to eye inflammation

Code also underlying condition

One of the following 7th characters is to be assigned to each code in subcategory H4Ø.4 to designate the stage of glaucoma.
- Ø stage unspecified
- 1 mild stage
- 2 moderate stage
- 3 severe stage
- 4 indeterminate stage

- **✓x7th H4Ø.4Ø Glaucoma secondary to eye inflammation, unspecified eye**
- **✓x7th H4Ø.41 Glaucoma secondary to eye inflammation, right eye**
- **✓x7th H4Ø.42 Glaucoma secondary to eye inflammation, left eye**
- **✓x7th H4Ø.43 Glaucoma secondary to eye inflammation, bilateral**

✓5th H4Ø.5 Glaucoma secondary to other eye disorders

Code also underlying eye disorder

One of the following 7th characters is to be assigned to each code in subcategory H4Ø.5 to designate the stage of glaucoma.
- Ø stage unspecified
- 1 mild stage
- 2 moderate stage
- 3 severe stage
- 4 indeterminate stage

- **✓x7th H4Ø.5Ø Glaucoma secondary to other eye disorders, unspecified eye**
- **✓x7th H4Ø.51 Glaucoma secondary to other eye disorders, right eye**
- **✓x7th H4Ø.52 Glaucoma secondary to other eye disorders, left eye**

H40.53 Glaucoma secondary to other eye disorders, bilateral

H40.6 Glaucoma secondary to drugs

Use additional code for adverse effect, if applicable, to identify drug (T36-T50 with fifth or sixth character 5)

One of the following 7th characters is to be assigned to each code in subcategory H40.6 to designate the stage of glaucoma
- 0 stage unspecified
- 1 mild stage
- 2 moderate stage
- 3 severe stage
- 4 indeterminate stage

H40.60 Glaucoma secondary to drugs, unspecified eye
H40.61 Glaucoma secondary to drugs, right eye
H40.62 Glaucoma secondary to drugs, left eye
H40.63 Glaucoma secondary to drugs, bilateral

H40.8 Other glaucoma

H40.81 Glaucoma with increased episcleral venous pressure
H40.811 Glaucoma with increased episcleral venous pressure, right eye
H40.812 Glaucoma with increased episcleral venous pressure, left eye
H40.813 Glaucoma with increased episcleral venous pressure, bilateral
H40.819 Glaucoma with increased episcleral venous pressure, unspecified eye

H40.82 Hypersecretion glaucoma
H40.821 Hypersecretion glaucoma, right eye
H40.822 Hypersecretion glaucoma, left eye
H40.823 Hypersecretion glaucoma, bilateral
H40.829 Hypersecretion glaucoma, unspecified eye

H40.83 Aqueous misdirection
Malignant glaucoma
H40.831 Aqueous misdirection, right eye
H40.832 Aqueous misdirection, left eye
H40.833 Aqueous misdirection, bilateral
H40.839 Aqueous misdirection, unspecified eye

H40.89 Other specified glaucoma

H40.9 Unspecified glaucoma

H42 Glaucoma in diseases classified elsewhere

Code first underlying condition, such as:
- amyloidosis (E85.-)
- aniridia (Q13.1)
- glaucoma (in) diabetes mellitus (E08.39, E09.39, E10.39, E11.39, E13.39)
- Lowe's syndrome (E72.03)
- Reiger's anomaly (Q13.81)
- specified metabolic disorder (E70-E88)

EXCLUDES 1 *glaucoma (in) onchocerciasis (B73.02)*
glaucoma (in) syphilis (A52.71)
glaucoma (in) tuberculous (A18.59)

Disorders of vitreous body and globe (H43-H44)

H43 Disorders of vitreous body

H43.0 Vitreous prolapse

EXCLUDES 1 *traumatic vitreous prolapse (S05.2-)*
vitreous syndrome following cataract surgery (H59.0-)

H43.00 Vitreous prolapse, unspecified eye
H43.01 Vitreous prolapse, right eye
H43.02 Vitreous prolapse, left eye
H43.03 Vitreous prolapse, bilateral

H43.1 Vitreous hemorrhage
H43.10 Vitreous hemorrhage, unspecified eye HCC
H43.11 Vitreous hemorrhage, right eye HCC
H43.12 Vitreous hemorrhage, left eye HCC
H43.13 Vitreous hemorrhage, bilateral HCC

H43.2 Crystalline deposits in vitreous body
H43.20 Crystalline deposits in vitreous body, unspecified eye
H43.21 Crystalline deposits in vitreous body, right eye
H43.22 Crystalline deposits in vitreous body, left eye
H43.23 Crystalline deposits in vitreous body, bilateral

H43.3 Other vitreous opacities

H43.31 Vitreous membranes and strands
H43.311 Vitreous membranes and strands, right eye
H43.312 Vitreous membranes and strands, left eye
H43.313 Vitreous membranes and strands, bilateral
H43.319 Vitreous membranes and strands, unspecified eye

H43.39 Other vitreous opacities
Vitreous floaters
H43.391 Other vitreous opacities, right eye
H43.392 Other vitreous opacities, left eye
H43.393 Other vitreous opacities, bilateral
H43.399 Other vitreous opacities, unspecified eye

H43.8 Other disorders of vitreous body

EXCLUDES 1 *proliferative vitreo-retinopathy with retinal detachment (H33.4-)*
EXCLUDES 2 *vitreous abscess (H44.02-)*

H43.81 Vitreous degeneration
Vitreous detachment
H43.811 Vitreous degeneration, right eye
H43.812 Vitreous degeneration, left eye
H43.813 Vitreous degeneration, bilateral
H43.819 Vitreous degeneration, unspecified eye

H43.82 Vitreomacular adhesion
Vitreomacular traction
H43.821 Vitreomacular adhesion, right eye A
H43.822 Vitreomacular adhesion, left eye A
H43.823 Vitreomacular adhesion, bilateral A
H43.829 Vitreomacular adhesion, unspecified eye A

H43.89 Other disorders of vitreous body

H43.9 Unspecified disorder of vitreous body

H44 Disorders of globe

INCLUDES disorders affecting multiple structures of eye

H44.0 Purulent endophthalmitis

Use additional code to identify organism

EXCLUDES 1 *bleb associated endophthalmitis (H59.4-)*

H44.00 Unspecified purulent endophthalmitis
H44.001 Unspecified purulent endophthalmitis, right eye CC
H44.002 Unspecified purulent endophthalmitis, left eye CC
H44.003 Unspecified purulent endophthalmitis, bilateral CC
H44.009 Unspecified purulent endophthalmitis, unspecified eye CC UNS

H44.01 Panophthalmitis (acute)
H44.011 Panophthalmitis (acute), right eye CC
H44.012 Panophthalmitis (acute), left eye CC
H44.013 Panophthalmitis (acute), bilateral CC
H44.019 Panophthalmitis (acute), unspecified eye CC UNS

H44.02 Vitreous abscess (chronic)
H44.021 Vitreous abscess (chronic), right eye CC
H44.022 Vitreous abscess (chronic), left eye CC
H44.023 Vitreous abscess (chronic), bilateral CC
H44.029 Vitreous abscess (chronic), unspecified eye CC UNS

H44.1 Other endophthalmitis

EXCLUDES 1 *bleb associated endophthalmitis (H59.4-)*
EXCLUDES 2 *ophthalmia nodosa (H16.2-)*

H44.11 Panuveitis

DEF: Inflammation of all layers of the uvea of the eye, including the choroid, iris, and ciliary body. It also typically involves the lens, retina, optic nerve, and vitreous and causes reduced vision or blindness.

H44.111 Panuveitis, right eye CC
H44.112 Panuveitis, left eye CC
H44.113 Panuveitis, bilateral CC
H44.119 Panuveitis, unspecified eye CC UNS

- H44.12 Parasitic endophthalmitis, unspecified
  - H44.121 Parasitic endophthalmitis, unspecified, right eye CC
  - H44.122 Parasitic endophthalmitis, unspecified, left eye CC
  - H44.123 Parasitic endophthalmitis, unspecified, bilateral CC
  - H44.129 Parasitic endophthalmitis, unspecified, unspecified eye CC UNS
- H44.13 Sympathetic uveitis
  - H44.131 Sympathetic uveitis, right eye CC
  - H44.132 Sympathetic uveitis, left eye CC
  - H44.133 Sympathetic uveitis, bilateral CC
  - H44.139 Sympathetic uveitis, unspecified eye CC UNS
- H44.19 Other endophthalmitis CC

H44.2 Degenerative myopia

Malignant myopia

AHA: 2017,4Q,10-11

- H44.20 Degenerative myopia, unspecified eye
- H44.21 Degenerative myopia, right eye
- H44.22 Degenerative myopia, left eye
- H44.23 Degenerative myopia, bilateral
- H44.2A Degenerative myopia with choroidal neovascularization
  Use additional code for any associated choroid disorders (H31.-)
  - H44.2A1 Degenerative myopia with choroidal neovascularization, right eye
  - H44.2A2 Degenerative myopia with choroidal neovascularization, left eye
  - H44.2A3 Degenerative myopia with choroidal neovascularization, bilateral eye
  - H44.2A9 Degenerative myopia with choroidal neovascularization, unspecified eye
- H44.2B Degenerative myopia with macular hole
  - H44.2B1 Degenerative myopia with macular hole, right eye
  - H44.2B2 Degenerative myopia with macular hole, left eye
  - H44.2B3 Degenerative myopia with macular hole, bilateral eye
  - H44.2B9 Degenerative myopia with macular hole, unspecified eye
- H44.2C Degenerative myopia with retinal detachment
  Use additional code to identify the retinal detachment (H33.-)
  - H44.2C1 Degenerative myopia with retinal detachment, right eye
  - H44.2C2 Degenerative myopia with retinal detachment, left eye
  - H44.2C3 Degenerative myopia with retinal detachment, bilateral eye
  - H44.2C9 Degenerative myopia with retinal detachment, unspecified eye
- H44.2D Degenerative myopia with foveoschisis
  - H44.2D1 Degenerative myopia with foveoschisis, right eye
  - H44.2D2 Degenerative myopia with foveoschisis, left eye
  - H44.2D3 Degenerative myopia with foveoschisis, bilateral eye
  - H44.2D9 Degenerative myopia with foveoschisis, unspecified eye
- H44.2E Degenerative myopia with other maculopathy
  - H44.2E1 Degenerative myopia with other maculopathy, right eye
  - H44.2E2 Degenerative myopia with other maculopathy, left eye
  - H44.2E3 Degenerative myopia with other maculopathy, bilateral eye
  - H44.2E9 Degenerative myopia with other maculopathy, unspecified eye

H44.3 Other and unspecified degenerative disorders of globe

- H44.30 Unspecified degenerative disorder of globe
- H44.31 Chalcosis
  - H44.311 Chalcosis, right eye
  - H44.312 Chalcosis, left eye
  - H44.313 Chalcosis, bilateral
  - H44.319 Chalcosis, unspecified eye
- H44.32 Siderosis of eye
  DEF: Iron pigment deposits within tissue of the eyeball caused by high iron content of the blood. Symptoms include cataracts, rust-colored anterior subcapsular deposits, iris heterochromia, pupillary mydriasis, and depressed electroretinogram amplitudes.
  - H44.321 Siderosis of eye, right eye
  - H44.322 Siderosis of eye, left eye
  - H44.323 Siderosis of eye, bilateral
  - H44.329 Siderosis of eye, unspecified eye
- H44.39 Other degenerative disorders of globe
  - H44.391 Other degenerative disorders of globe, right eye
  - H44.392 Other degenerative disorders of globe, left eye
  - H44.393 Other degenerative disorders of globe, bilateral
  - H44.399 Other degenerative disorders of globe, unspecified eye

H44.4 Hypotony of eye

- H44.40 Unspecified hypotony of eye
- H44.41 Flat anterior chamber hypotony of eye
  - H44.411 Flat anterior chamber hypotony of right eye
  - H44.412 Flat anterior chamber hypotony of left eye
  - H44.413 Flat anterior chamber hypotony of eye, bilateral
  - H44.419 Flat anterior chamber hypotony of unspecified eye
- H44.42 Hypotony of eye due to ocular fistula
  - H44.421 Hypotony of right eye due to ocular fistula
  - H44.422 Hypotony of left eye due to ocular fistula
  - H44.423 Hypotony of eye due to ocular fistula, bilateral
  - H44.429 Hypotony of unspecified eye due to ocular fistula
- H44.43 Hypotony of eye due to other ocular disorders
  - H44.431 Hypotony of eye due to other ocular disorders, right eye
  - H44.432 Hypotony of eye due to other ocular disorders, left eye
  - H44.433 Hypotony of eye due to other ocular disorders, bilateral
  - H44.439 Hypotony of eye due to other ocular disorders, unspecified eye
- H44.44 Primary hypotony of eye
  - H44.441 Primary hypotony of right eye
  - H44.442 Primary hypotony of left eye
  - H44.443 Primary hypotony of eye, bilateral
  - H44.449 Primary hypotony of unspecified eye

H44.5 Degenerated conditions of globe

- H44.50 Unspecified degenerated conditions of globe
- H44.51 Absolute glaucoma
  - H44.511 Absolute glaucoma, right eye
  - H44.512 Absolute glaucoma, left eye
  - H44.513 Absolute glaucoma, bilateral
  - H44.519 Absolute glaucoma, unspecified eye
- H44.52 Atrophy of globe
  Phthisis bulbi
  - H44.521 Atrophy of globe, right eye
  - H44.522 Atrophy of globe, left eye
  - H44.523 Atrophy of globe, bilateral
  - H44.529 Atrophy of globe, unspecified eye
- H44.53 Leucocoria
  - H44.531 Leucocoria, right eye
  - H44.532 Leucocoria, left eye
  - H44.533 Leucocoria, bilateral
  - H44.539 Leucocoria, unspecified eye

H44.6 Retained (old) intraocular foreign body, magnetic

Use additional code to identify magnetic foreign body (Z18.11)

EXCLUDES 1 *current intraocular foreign body (S05.-)*

EXCLUDES 2 *retained foreign body in eyelid (H02.81-)*

retained (old) foreign body following penetrating wound of orbit (H05.5-)

retained (old) intraocular foreign body, nonmagnetic (H44.7-)

H44.60 Unspecified retained (old) intraocular foreign body, magnetic

H44.601 Unspecified retained (old) intraocular foreign body, magnetic, right eye

H44.602 Unspecified retained (old) intraocular foreign body, magnetic, left eye

H44.603 Unspecified retained (old) intraocular foreign body, magnetic, bilateral

H44.609 Unspecified retained (old) intraocular foreign body, magnetic, unspecified eye

H44.61 Retained (old) magnetic foreign body in anterior chamber

H44.611 Retained (old) magnetic foreign body in anterior chamber, right eye

H44.612 Retained (old) magnetic foreign body in anterior chamber, left eye

H44.613 Retained (old) magnetic foreign body in anterior chamber, bilateral

H44.619 Retained (old) magnetic foreign body in anterior chamber, unspecified eye

H44.62 Retained (old) magnetic foreign body in iris or ciliary body

H44.621 Retained (old) magnetic foreign body in iris or ciliary body, right eye

H44.622 Retained (old) magnetic foreign body in iris or ciliary body, left eye

H44.623 Retained (old) magnetic foreign body in iris or ciliary body, bilateral

H44.629 Retained (old) magnetic foreign body in iris or ciliary body, unspecified eye

H44.63 Retained (old) magnetic foreign body in lens

H44.631 Retained (old) magnetic foreign body in lens, right eye

H44.632 Retained (old) magnetic foreign body in lens, left eye

H44.633 Retained (old) magnetic foreign body in lens, bilateral

H44.639 Retained (old) magnetic foreign body in lens, unspecified eye

H44.64 Retained (old) magnetic foreign body in posterior wall of globe

H44.641 Retained (old) magnetic foreign body in posterior wall of globe, right eye

H44.642 Retained (old) magnetic foreign body in posterior wall of globe, left eye

H44.643 Retained (old) magnetic foreign body in posterior wall of globe, bilateral

H44.649 Retained (old) magnetic foreign body in posterior wall of globe, unspecified eye

H44.65 Retained (old) magnetic foreign body in vitreous body

H44.651 Retained (old) magnetic foreign body in vitreous body, right eye

H44.652 Retained (old) magnetic foreign body in vitreous body, left eye

H44.653 Retained (old) magnetic foreign body in vitreous body, bilateral

H44.659 Retained (old) magnetic foreign body in vitreous body, unspecified eye

H44.69 Retained (old) intraocular foreign body, magnetic, in other or multiple sites

H44.691 Retained (old) intraocular foreign body, magnetic, in other or multiple sites, right eye

H44.692 Retained (old) intraocular foreign body, magnetic, in other or multiple sites, left eye

H44.693 Retained (old) intraocular foreign body, magnetic, in other or multiple sites, bilateral

H44.699 Retained (old) intraocular foreign body, magnetic, in other or multiple sites, unspecified eye

H44.7 Retained (old) intraocular foreign body, nonmagnetic

Use additional code to identify nonmagnetic foreign body (Z18.01-Z18.10, Z18.12, Z18.2-Z18.9)

EXCLUDES 1 *current intraocular foreign body (S05.-)*

EXCLUDES 2 *retained foreign body in eyelid (H02.81-)*

retained (old) foreign body following penetrating wound of orbit (H05.5-)

retained (old) intraocular foreign body, magnetic (H44.6-)

H44.70 Unspecified retained (old) intraocular foreign body, nonmagnetic

H44.701 Unspecified retained (old) intraocular foreign body, nonmagnetic, right eye

H44.702 Unspecified retained (old) intraocular foreign body, nonmagnetic, left eye

H44.703 Unspecified retained (old) intraocular foreign body, nonmagnetic, bilateral

H44.709 Unspecified retained (old) intraocular foreign body, nonmagnetic, unspecified eye

Retained (old) intraocular foreign body NOS

H44.71 Retained (nonmagnetic) (old) foreign body in anterior chamber

H44.711 Retained (nonmagnetic) (old) foreign body in anterior chamber, right eye

H44.712 Retained (nonmagnetic) (old) foreign body in anterior chamber, left eye

H44.713 Retained (nonmagnetic) (old) foreign body in anterior chamber, bilateral

H44.719 Retained (nonmagnetic) (old) foreign body in anterior chamber, unspecified eye

H44.72 Retained (nonmagnetic) (old) foreign body in iris or ciliary body

H44.721 Retained (nonmagnetic) (old) foreign body in iris or ciliary body, right eye

H44.722 Retained (nonmagnetic) (old) foreign body in iris or ciliary body, left eye

H44.723 Retained (nonmagnetic) (old) foreign body in iris or ciliary body, bilateral

H44.729 Retained (nonmagnetic) (old) foreign body in iris or ciliary body, unspecified eye

H44.73 Retained (nonmagnetic) (old) foreign body in lens

H44.731 Retained (nonmagnetic) (old) foreign body in lens, right eye

H44.732 Retained (nonmagnetic) (old) foreign body in lens, left eye

H44.733 Retained (nonmagnetic) (old) foreign body in lens, bilateral

H44.739 Retained (nonmagnetic) (old) foreign body in lens, unspecified eye

H44.74 Retained (nonmagnetic) (old) foreign body in posterior wall of globe

H44.741 Retained (nonmagnetic) (old) foreign body in posterior wall of globe, right eye

H44.742 Retained (nonmagnetic) (old) foreign body in posterior wall of globe, left eye

H44.743 Retained (nonmagnetic) (old) foreign body in posterior wall of globe, bilateral

H44.749 Retained (nonmagnetic) (old) foreign body in posterior wall of globe, unspecified eye

H44.75 Retained (nonmagnetic) (old) foreign body in vitreous body

H44.751 Retained (nonmagnetic) (old) foreign body in vitreous body, right eye

H44.752 Retained (nonmagnetic) (old) foreign body in vitreous body, left eye

H44.753 Retained (nonmagnetic) (old) foreign body in vitreous body, bilateral

H44.759 Retained (nonmagnetic) (old) foreign body in vitreous body, unspecified eye

H44.79 Retained (old) intraocular foreign body, nonmagnetic, in other or multiple sites

H44.791 Retained (old) intraocular foreign body, nonmagnetic, in other or multiple sites, right eye

H44.792 Retained (old) intraocular foreign body, nonmagnetic, in other or multiple sites, left eye

H44.793 Retained (old) intraocular foreign body, nonmagnetic, in other or multiple sites, bilateral

H44.799 Retained (old) intraocular foreign body, nonmagnetic, in other or multiple sites, unspecified eye

H44.8 Other disorders of globe

H44.81 Hemophthalmos

DEF: Pool of blood within the eyeball, not from a current injury.

H44.811 Hemophthalmos, right eye
H44.812 Hemophthalmos, left eye
H44.813 Hemophthalmos, bilateral
H44.819 Hemophthalmos, unspecified eye

H44.82 Luxation of globe

H44.821 Luxation of globe, right eye
H44.822 Luxation of globe, left eye
H44.823 Luxation of globe, bilateral
H44.829 Luxation of globe, unspecified eye

H44.89 Other disorders of globe

AHA: 2022,1Q,33

H44.9 Unspecified disorder of globe

Disorders of optic nerve and visual pathways (H46-H47)

H46 Optic neuritis

EXCLUDES 2 *ischemic optic neuropathy (H47.01-)*
neuromyelitis optica [Devic] (G36.0)

H46.0 Optic papillitis

H46.00 Optic papillitis, unspecified eye CC UNS
H46.01 Optic papillitis, right eye CC
H46.02 Optic papillitis, left eye CC
H46.03 Optic papillitis, bilateral CC

H46.1 Retrobulbar neuritis

Retrobulbar neuritis NOS

EXCLUDES 1 *syphilitic retrobulbar neuritis (A52.15)*

H46.10 Retrobulbar neuritis, unspecified eye CC UNS
H46.11 Retrobulbar neuritis, right eye CC
H46.12 Retrobulbar neuritis, left eye CC
H46.13 Retrobulbar neuritis, bilateral CC

H46.2 Nutritional optic neuropathy

H46.3 Toxic optic neuropathy

Code first (T51-T65) to identify cause

H46.8 Other optic neuritis CC

H46.9 Unspecified optic neuritis CC

H47 Other disorders of optic [2nd] nerve and visual pathways

H47.0 Disorders of optic nerve, not elsewhere classified

H47.01 Ischemic optic neuropathy

H47.011 Ischemic optic neuropathy, right eye
H47.012 Ischemic optic neuropathy, left eye
H47.013 Ischemic optic neuropathy, bilateral
H47.019 Ischemic optic neuropathy, unspecified eye

H47.02 Hemorrhage in optic nerve sheath

H47.021 Hemorrhage in optic nerve sheath, right eye
H47.022 Hemorrhage in optic nerve sheath, left eye
H47.023 Hemorrhage in optic nerve sheath, bilateral
H47.029 Hemorrhage in optic nerve sheath, unspecified eye

H47.03 Optic nerve hypoplasia

H47.031 Optic nerve hypoplasia, right eye
H47.032 Optic nerve hypoplasia, left eye
H47.033 Optic nerve hypoplasia, bilateral
H47.039 Optic nerve hypoplasia, unspecified eye

H47.09 Other disorders of optic nerve, not elsewhere classified

Compression of optic nerve

H47.091 Other disorders of optic nerve, not elsewhere classified, right eye
H47.092 Other disorders of optic nerve, not elsewhere classified, left eye
H47.093 Other disorders of optic nerve, not elsewhere classified, bilateral
H47.099 Other disorders of optic nerve, not elsewhere classified, unspecified eye

H47.1 Papilledema

DEF: Swelling of the optic papilla, the raised area connected to the optic disk made up of nerves that enter the eyeball. It may be caused by increased intracranial pressure, decreased ocular pressure, or a retinal disorder.

H47.10 Unspecified papilledema CC
H47.11 Papilledema associated with increased intracranial pressure CC
H47.12 Papilledema associated with decreased ocular pressure
H47.13 Papilledema associated with retinal disorder

H47.14 Foster-Kennedy syndrome

H47.141 Foster-Kennedy syndrome, right eye
H47.142 Foster-Kennedy syndrome, left eye
H47.143 Foster-Kennedy syndrome, bilateral
H47.149 Foster-Kennedy syndrome, unspecified eye

H47.2 Optic atrophy

H47.20 Unspecified optic atrophy

H47.21 Primary optic atrophy

H47.211 Primary optic atrophy, right eye
H47.212 Primary optic atrophy, left eye
H47.213 Primary optic atrophy, bilateral
H47.219 Primary optic atrophy, unspecified eye

H47.22 Hereditary optic atrophy

Leber's optic atrophy

H47.23 Glaucomatous optic atrophy

H47.231 Glaucomatous optic atrophy, right eye
H47.232 Glaucomatous optic atrophy, left eye
H47.233 Glaucomatous optic atrophy, bilateral
H47.239 Glaucomatous optic atrophy, unspecified eye

H47.29 Other optic atrophy

Temporal pallor of optic disc

H47.291 Other optic atrophy, right eye
H47.292 Other optic atrophy, left eye
H47.293 Other optic atrophy, bilateral
H47.299 Other optic atrophy, unspecified eye

H47.3 Other disorders of optic disc

H47.31 Coloboma of optic disc

H47.311 Coloboma of optic disc, right eye
H47.312 Coloboma of optic disc, left eye
H47.313 Coloboma of optic disc, bilateral
H47.319 Coloboma of optic disc, unspecified eye

H47.32 Drusen of optic disc

H47.321 Drusen of optic disc, right eye
H47.322 Drusen of optic disc, left eye
H47.323 Drusen of optic disc, bilateral
H47.329 Drusen of optic disc, unspecified eye

H47.33 Pseudopapilledema of optic disc

H47.331 Pseudopapilledema of optic disc, right eye
H47.332 Pseudopapilledema of optic disc, left eye
H47.333 Pseudopapilledema of optic disc, bilateral
H47.339 Pseudopapilledema of optic disc, unspecified eye

H47.39 Other disorders of optic disc

H47.391 Other disorders of optic disc, right eye
H47.392 Other disorders of optic disc, left eye
H47.393 Other disorders of optic disc, bilateral
H47.399 Other disorders of optic disc, unspecified eye

H47.4 Disorders of optic chiasm

Code also underlying condition

H47.41 Disorders of optic chiasm in (due to) inflammatory disorders CC
H47.42 Disorders of optic chiasm in (due to) neoplasm CC
H47.43 Disorders of optic chiasm in (due to) vascular disorders CC
H47.49 Disorders of optic chiasm in (due to) other disorders CC

H47.5 Disorders of other visual pathways
Disorders of optic tracts, geniculate nuclei and optic radiations
Code also underlying condition

H47.51 Disorders of visual pathways in (due to) inflammatory disorders
H47.511 Disorders of visual pathways in (due to) inflammatory disorders, right side CC
H47.512 Disorders of visual pathways in (due to) inflammatory disorders, left side CC
H47.519 Disorders of visual pathways in (due to) inflammatory disorders, unspecified side CC UNS

H47.52 Disorders of visual pathways in (due to) neoplasm
H47.521 Disorders of visual pathways in (due to) neoplasm, right side CC
H47.522 Disorders of visual pathways in (due to) neoplasm, left side CC
H47.529 Disorders of visual pathways in (due to) neoplasm, unspecified side CC UNS

H47.53 Disorders of visual pathways in (due to) vascular disorders
H47.531 Disorders of visual pathways in (due to) vascular disorders, right side CC
H47.532 Disorders of visual pathways in (due to) vascular disorders, left side CC
H47.539 Disorders of visual pathways in (due to) vascular disorders, unspecified side CC UNS

H47.6 Disorders of visual cortex
Code also underlying condition
EXCLUDES 1 *injury to visual cortex SØ4.Ø4-*

H47.61 Cortical blindness
H47.611 Cortical blindness, right side of brain
H47.612 Cortical blindness, left side of brain
H47.619 Cortical blindness, unspecified side of brain

H47.62 Disorders of visual cortex in (due to) inflammatory disorders
H47.621 Disorders of visual cortex in (due to) inflammatory disorders, right side of brain CC
H47.622 Disorders of visual cortex in (due to) inflammatory disorders, left side of brain CC
H47.629 Disorders of visual cortex in (due to) inflammatory disorders, unspecified side of brain CC UNS

H47.63 Disorders of visual cortex in (due to) neoplasm
H47.631 Disorders of visual cortex in (due to) neoplasm, right side of brain CC
H47.632 Disorders of visual cortex in (due to) neoplasm, left side of brain CC
H47.639 Disorders of visual cortex in (due to) neoplasm, unspecified side of brain CC UNS

H47.64 Disorders of visual cortex in (due to) vascular disorders
H47.641 Disorders of visual cortex in (due to) vascular disorders, right side of brain CC
H47.642 Disorders of visual cortex in (due to) vascular disorders, left side of brain CC
H47.649 Disorders of visual cortex in (due to) vascular disorders, unspecified side of brain CC UNS

H47.9 Unspecified disorder of visual pathways

Disorders of ocular muscles, binocular movement, accommodation and refraction (H49-H52)

EXCLUDES 2 *nystagmus and other irregular eye movements (H55)*

H49 Paralytic strabismus
EXCLUDES 2 *internal ophthalmoplegia (H52.51-)*
internuclear ophthalmoplegia (H51.2-)
progressive supranuclear ophthalmoplegia (G23.1)
DEF: Strabismus: Misalignment of the eyes with the inability to move and focus in the same direction due to conditions affecting the muscles controlling them.

H49.Ø Third [oculomotor] nerve palsy
H49.ØØ Third [oculomotor] nerve palsy, unspecified eye
H49.Ø1 Third [oculomotor] nerve palsy, right eye
H49.Ø2 Third [oculomotor] nerve palsy, left eye
H49.Ø3 Third [oculomotor] nerve palsy, bilateral

H49.1 Fourth [trochlear] nerve palsy
H49.1Ø Fourth [trochlear] nerve palsy, unspecified eye
H49.11 Fourth [trochlear] nerve palsy, right eye
H49.12 Fourth [trochlear] nerve palsy, left eye
H49.13 Fourth [trochlear] nerve palsy, bilateral

H49.2 Sixth [abducent] nerve palsy
H49.2Ø Sixth [abducent] nerve palsy, unspecified eye
H49.21 Sixth [abducent] nerve palsy, right eye
H49.22 Sixth [abducent] nerve palsy, left eye
H49.23 Sixth [abducent] nerve palsy, bilateral

H49.3 Total (external) ophthalmoplegia
H49.3Ø Total (external) ophthalmoplegia, unspecified eye
H49.31 Total (external) ophthalmoplegia, right eye
H49.32 Total (external) ophthalmoplegia, left eye
H49.33 Total (external) ophthalmoplegia, bilateral

H49.4 Progressive external ophthalmoplegia
EXCLUDES 1 *Kearns-Sayre syndrome (H49.81-)*
H49.4Ø Progressive external ophthalmoplegia, unspecified eye
H49.41 Progressive external ophthalmoplegia, right eye
H49.42 Progressive external ophthalmoplegia, left eye
H49.43 Progressive external ophthalmoplegia, bilateral

H49.8 Other paralytic strabismus
H49.81 Kearns-Sayre syndrome
Progressive external ophthalmoplegia with pigmentary retinopathy
Use additional code for other manifestation, such as: heart block (I45.9)
H49.811 Kearns-Sayre syndrome, right eye CC HCC
H49.812 Kearns-Sayre syndrome, left eye CC HCC
H49.813 Kearns-Sayre syndrome, bilateral CC HCC
H49.819 Kearns-Sayre syndrome, unspecified eye CC UNS HCC

H49.88 Other paralytic strabismus
External ophthalmoplegia NOS
H49.881 Other paralytic strabismus, right eye
H49.882 Other paralytic strabismus, left eye
H49.883 Other paralytic strabismus, bilateral
H49.889 Other paralytic strabismus, unspecified eye

H49.9 Unspecified paralytic strabismus

H5Ø Other strabismus
DEF: Strabismus: Misalignment of the eyes with the inability to move and focus in the same direction due to conditions affecting the muscles controlling them.

H5Ø.Ø Esotropia
Convergent concomitant strabismus
EXCLUDES 1 *intermittent esotropia (H5Ø.31-, H5Ø.32)*
H5Ø.ØØ Unspecified esotropia
H5Ø.Ø1 Monocular esotropia
H5Ø.Ø11 Monocular esotropia, right eye
H5Ø.Ø12 Monocular esotropia, left eye
H5Ø.Ø2 Monocular esotropia with A pattern
H5Ø.Ø21 Monocular esotropia with A pattern, right eye

H50.022 Monocular esotropia with A pattern, left eye

✓6th **H50.03 Monocular esotropia with V pattern**

H50.031 Monocular esotropia with V pattern, right eye

H50.032 Monocular esotropia with V pattern, left eye

✓6th **H50.04 Monocular esotropia with other noncomitancies**

H50.041 Monocular esotropia with other noncomitancies, right eye

H50.042 Monocular esotropia with other noncomitancies, left eye

H50.05 Alternating esotropia

H50.06 Alternating esotropia with A pattern

H50.07 Alternating esotropia with V pattern

H50.08 Alternating esotropia with other noncomitancies

Eye Muscle Diseases

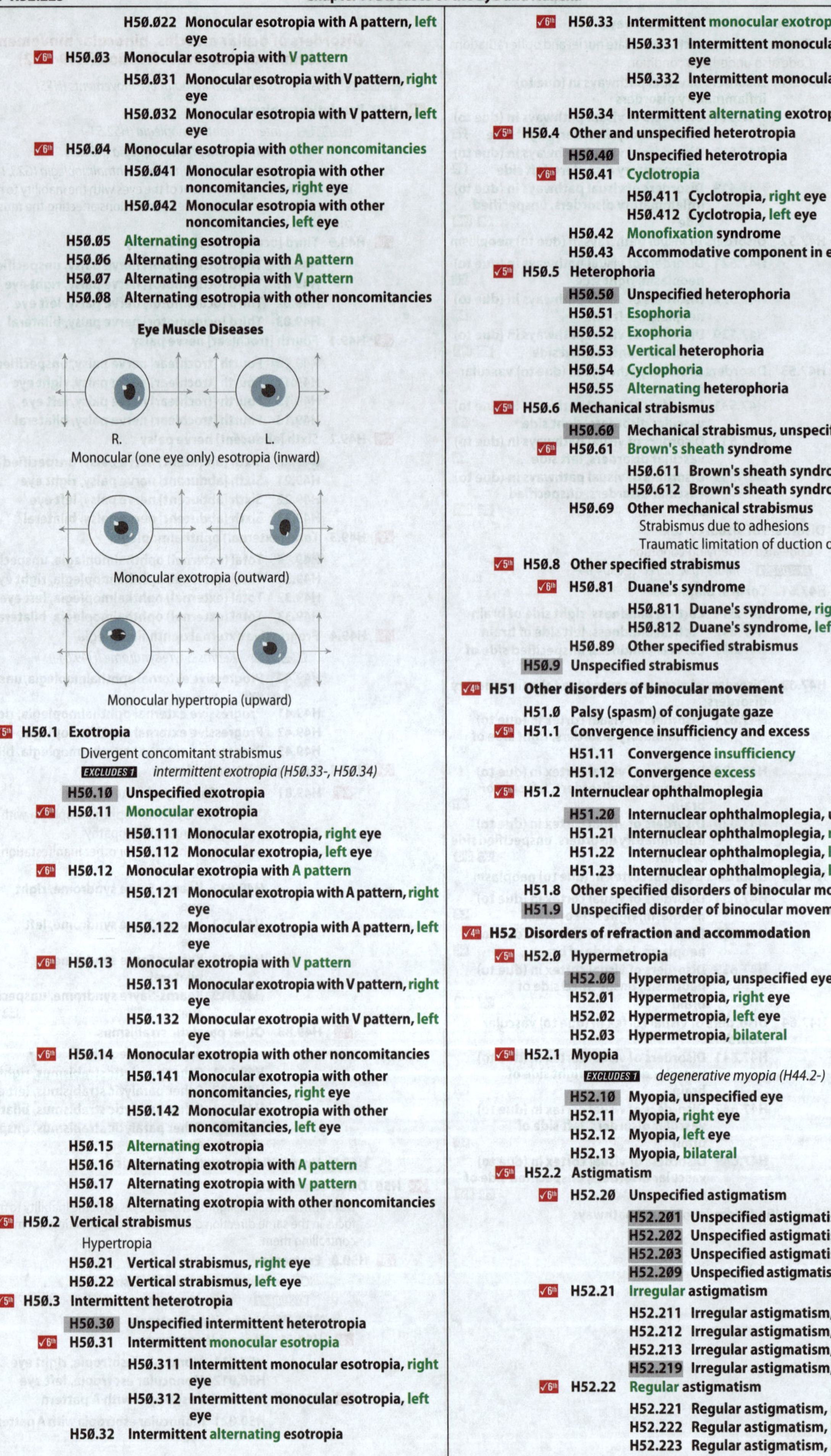

✓5th **H50.1 Exotropia**

Divergent concomitant strabismus

EXCLUDES 1 *intermittent exotropia (H50.33-, H50.34)*

H50.10 Unspecified exotropia

✓6th **H50.11 Monocular exotropia**

H50.111 Monocular exotropia, right eye

H50.112 Monocular exotropia, left eye

✓6th **H50.12 Monocular exotropia with A pattern**

H50.121 Monocular exotropia with A pattern, right eye

H50.122 Monocular exotropia with A pattern, left eye

✓6th **H50.13 Monocular exotropia with V pattern**

H50.131 Monocular exotropia with V pattern, right eye

H50.132 Monocular exotropia with V pattern, left eye

✓6th **H50.14 Monocular exotropia with other noncomitancies**

H50.141 Monocular exotropia with other noncomitancies, right eye

H50.142 Monocular exotropia with other noncomitancies, left eye

H50.15 Alternating exotropia

H50.16 Alternating exotropia with A pattern

H50.17 Alternating exotropia with V pattern

H50.18 Alternating exotropia with other noncomitancies

✓5th **H50.2 Vertical strabismus**

Hypertropia

H50.21 Vertical strabismus, right eye

H50.22 Vertical strabismus, left eye

✓5th **H50.3 Intermittent heterotropia**

H50.30 Unspecified intermittent heterotropia

✓6th **H50.31 Intermittent monocular esotropia**

H50.311 Intermittent monocular esotropia, right eye

H50.312 Intermittent monocular esotropia, left eye

H50.32 Intermittent alternating esotropia

✓6th **H50.33 Intermittent monocular exotropia**

H50.331 Intermittent monocular exotropia, right eye

H50.332 Intermittent monocular exotropia, left eye

H50.34 Intermittent alternating exotropia

✓5th **H50.4 Other and unspecified heterotropia**

H50.40 Unspecified heterotropia

✓6th **H50.41 Cyclotropia**

H50.411 Cyclotropia, right eye

H50.412 Cyclotropia, left eye

H50.42 Monofixation syndrome

H50.43 Accommodative component in esotropia

✓5th **H50.5 Heterophoria**

H50.50 Unspecified heterophoria

H50.51 Esophoria

H50.52 Exophoria

H50.53 Vertical heterophoria

H50.54 Cyclophoria

H50.55 Alternating heterophoria

✓5th **H50.6 Mechanical strabismus**

H50.60 Mechanical strabismus, unspecified

✓6th **H50.61 Brown's sheath syndrome**

H50.611 Brown's sheath syndrome, right eye

H50.612 Brown's sheath syndrome, left eye

H50.69 Other mechanical strabismus

Strabismus due to adhesions

Traumatic limitation of duction of eye muscle

✓5th **H50.8 Other specified strabismus**

✓6th **H50.81 Duane's syndrome**

H50.811 Duane's syndrome, right eye

H50.812 Duane's syndrome, left eye

H50.89 Other specified strabismus

H50.9 Unspecified strabismus

✓4th **H51 Other disorders of binocular movement**

H51.0 Palsy (spasm) of conjugate gaze

✓5th **H51.1 Convergence insufficiency and excess**

H51.11 Convergence insufficiency

H51.12 Convergence excess

✓5th **H51.2 Internuclear ophthalmoplegia**

H51.20 Internuclear ophthalmoplegia, unspecified eye

H51.21 Internuclear ophthalmoplegia, right eye

H51.22 Internuclear ophthalmoplegia, left eye

H51.23 Internuclear ophthalmoplegia, bilateral

H51.8 Other specified disorders of binocular movement

H51.9 Unspecified disorder of binocular movement

✓4th **H52 Disorders of refraction and accommodation**

✓5th **H52.0 Hypermetropia**

H52.00 Hypermetropia, unspecified eye

H52.01 Hypermetropia, right eye

H52.02 Hypermetropia, left eye

H52.03 Hypermetropia, bilateral

✓5th **H52.1 Myopia**

EXCLUDES 1 *degenerative myopia (H44.2-)*

H52.10 Myopia, unspecified eye

H52.11 Myopia, right eye

H52.12 Myopia, left eye

H52.13 Myopia, bilateral

✓5th **H52.2 Astigmatism**

✓6th **H52.20 Unspecified astigmatism**

H52.201 Unspecified astigmatism, right eye

H52.202 Unspecified astigmatism, left eye

H52.203 Unspecified astigmatism, bilateral

H52.209 Unspecified astigmatism, unspecified eye

✓6th **H52.21 Irregular astigmatism**

H52.211 Irregular astigmatism, right eye

H52.212 Irregular astigmatism, left eye

H52.213 Irregular astigmatism, bilateral

H52.219 Irregular astigmatism, unspecified eye

✓6th **H52.22 Regular astigmatism**

H52.221 Regular astigmatism, right eye

H52.222 Regular astigmatism, left eye

H52.223 Regular astigmatism, bilateral

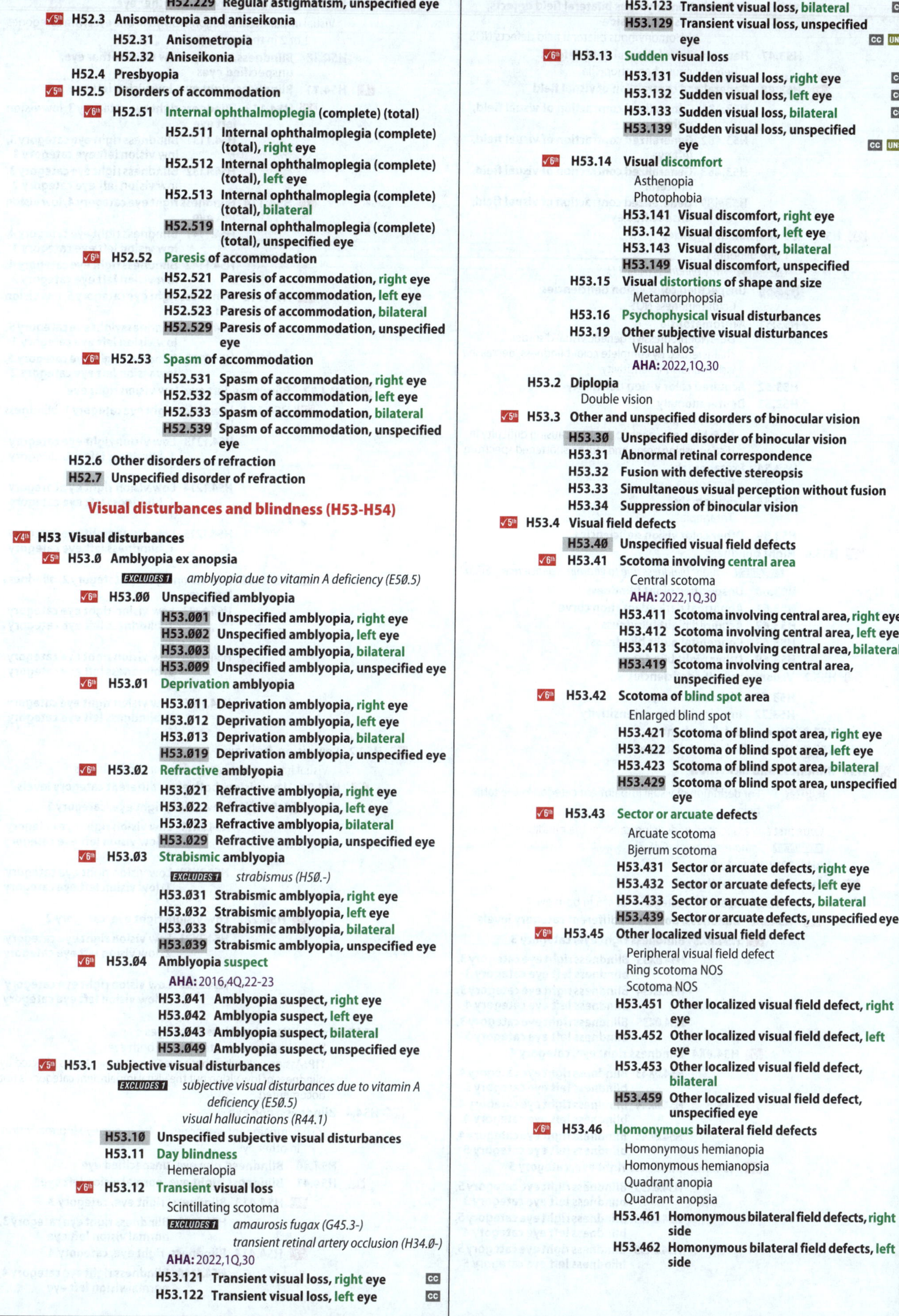

H52.229 Regular astigmatism, unspecified eye

H52.3 Anisometropia and aniseikonia
- H52.31 Anisometropia
- H52.32 Aniseikonia

H52.4 Presbyopia

H52.5 Disorders of accommodation
- H52.51 Internal ophthalmoplegia (complete) (total)
  - H52.511 Internal ophthalmoplegia (complete) (total), right eye
  - H52.512 Internal ophthalmoplegia (complete) (total), left eye
  - H52.513 Internal ophthalmoplegia (complete) (total), bilateral
  - H52.519 Internal ophthalmoplegia (complete) (total), unspecified eye
- H52.52 Paresis of accommodation
  - H52.521 Paresis of accommodation, right eye
  - H52.522 Paresis of accommodation, left eye
  - H52.523 Paresis of accommodation, bilateral
  - H52.529 Paresis of accommodation, unspecified eye
- H52.53 Spasm of accommodation
  - H52.531 Spasm of accommodation, right eye
  - H52.532 Spasm of accommodation, left eye
  - H52.533 Spasm of accommodation, bilateral
  - H52.539 Spasm of accommodation, unspecified eye

H52.6 Other disorders of refraction

H52.7 Unspecified disorder of refraction

Visual disturbances and blindness (H53-H54)

H53 Visual disturbances

H53.Ø Amblyopia ex anopsia

EXCLUDES 1 *amblyopia due to vitamin A deficiency (E5Ø.5)*

- H53.ØØ Unspecified amblyopia
  - H53.ØØ1 Unspecified amblyopia, right eye
  - H53.ØØ2 Unspecified amblyopia, left eye
  - H53.ØØ3 Unspecified amblyopia, bilateral
  - H53.ØØ9 Unspecified amblyopia, unspecified eye
- H53.Ø1 Deprivation amblyopia
  - H53.Ø11 Deprivation amblyopia, right eye
  - H53.Ø12 Deprivation amblyopia, left eye
  - H53.Ø13 Deprivation amblyopia, bilateral
  - H53.Ø19 Deprivation amblyopia, unspecified eye
- H53.Ø2 Refractive amblyopia
  - H53.Ø21 Refractive amblyopia, right eye
  - H53.Ø22 Refractive amblyopia, left eye
  - H53.Ø23 Refractive amblyopia, bilateral
  - H53.Ø29 Refractive amblyopia, unspecified eye
- H53.Ø3 Strabismic amblyopia

  EXCLUDES 1 *strabismus (H5Ø.-)*
  - H53.Ø31 Strabismic amblyopia, right eye
  - H53.Ø32 Strabismic amblyopia, left eye
  - H53.Ø33 Strabismic amblyopia, bilateral
  - H53.Ø39 Strabismic amblyopia, unspecified eye
- H53.Ø4 Amblyopia suspect

  AHA: 2016,4Q,22-23
  - H53.Ø41 Amblyopia suspect, right eye
  - H53.Ø42 Amblyopia suspect, left eye
  - H53.Ø43 Amblyopia suspect, bilateral
  - H53.Ø49 Amblyopia suspect, unspecified eye

H53.1 Subjective visual disturbances

EXCLUDES 1 *subjective visual disturbances due to vitamin A deficiency (E5Ø.5)*
visual hallucinations (R44.1)

- H53.1Ø Unspecified subjective visual disturbances
- H53.11 Day blindness
  Hemeralopia
- H53.12 Transient visual loss
  Scintillating scotoma

  EXCLUDES 1 *amaurosis fugax (G45.3-)*
  transient retinal artery occlusion (H34.Ø-)

  AHA: 2022,1Q,30
  - H53.121 Transient visual loss, right eye CC
  - H53.122 Transient visual loss, left eye CC
  - H53.123 Transient visual loss, bilateral CC
  - H53.129 Transient visual loss, unspecified eye CC UNS
- H53.13 Sudden visual loss
  - H53.131 Sudden visual loss, right eye CC
  - H53.132 Sudden visual loss, left eye CC
  - H53.133 Sudden visual loss, bilateral CC
  - H53.139 Sudden visual loss, unspecified eye CC UNS
- H53.14 Visual discomfort
  Asthenopia
  Photophobia
  - H53.141 Visual discomfort, right eye
  - H53.142 Visual discomfort, left eye
  - H53.143 Visual discomfort, bilateral
  - H53.149 Visual discomfort, unspecified
- H53.15 Visual distortions of shape and size
  Metamorphopsia
- H53.16 Psychophysical visual disturbances
- H53.19 Other subjective visual disturbances
  Visual halos
  AHA: 2022,1Q,30

H53.2 Diplopia
Double vision

H53.3 Other and unspecified disorders of binocular vision
- H53.3Ø Unspecified disorder of binocular vision
- H53.31 Abnormal retinal correspondence
- H53.32 Fusion with defective stereopsis
- H53.33 Simultaneous visual perception without fusion
- H53.34 Suppression of binocular vision

H53.4 Visual field defects
- H53.4Ø Unspecified visual field defects
- H53.41 Scotoma involving central area
  Central scotoma
  AHA: 2022,1Q,30
  - H53.411 Scotoma involving central area, right eye
  - H53.412 Scotoma involving central area, left eye
  - H53.413 Scotoma involving central area, bilateral
  - H53.419 Scotoma involving central area, unspecified eye
- H53.42 Scotoma of blind spot area
  Enlarged blind spot
  - H53.421 Scotoma of blind spot area, right eye
  - H53.422 Scotoma of blind spot area, left eye
  - H53.423 Scotoma of blind spot area, bilateral
  - H53.429 Scotoma of blind spot area, unspecified eye
- H53.43 Sector or arcuate defects
  Arcuate scotoma
  Bjerrum scotoma
  - H53.431 Sector or arcuate defects, right eye
  - H53.432 Sector or arcuate defects, left eye
  - H53.433 Sector or arcuate defects, bilateral
  - H53.439 Sector or arcuate defects, unspecified eye
- H53.45 Other localized visual field defect
  Peripheral visual field defect
  Ring scotoma NOS
  Scotoma NOS
  - H53.451 Other localized visual field defect, right eye
  - H53.452 Other localized visual field defect, left eye
  - H53.453 Other localized visual field defect, bilateral
  - H53.459 Other localized visual field defect, unspecified eye
- H53.46 Homonymous bilateral field defects
  Homonymous hemianopia
  Homonymous hemianopsia
  Quadrant anopia
  Quadrant anopsia
  - H53.461 Homonymous bilateral field defects, right side
  - H53.462 Homonymous bilateral field defects, left side

Additional Character Required · Placeholder · Questionable PDx · Manifestation · Unspecified · UPD Unacceptable PDx · H1-H14 HAC · HCC CMS-HCC Dx · HIV HIV Dx

H53.469 Homonymous bilateral field defects, unspecified side
Homonymous bilateral field defects NOS

H53.47 Heteronymous bilateral field defects
Heteronymous hemianop(s)ia

H53.48 Generalized contraction of visual field
- **H53.481 Generalized contraction of visual field, right eye**
- **H53.482 Generalized contraction of visual field, left eye**
- **H53.483 Generalized contraction of visual field, bilateral**
- **H53.489 Generalized contraction of visual field, unspecified eye**

H53.5 Color vision deficiencies
Color blindness
EXCLUDES 2 *day blindness (H53.11)*
- **H53.50 Unspecified color vision deficiencies**
  Color blindness NOS
- **H53.51 Achromatopsia**
  DEF: Nonprogressive genetic visual disorder characterized by complete color blindness, decreased vision, and light sensitivity.
- **H53.52 Acquired color vision deficiency**
- **H53.53 Deuteranomaly**
  Deuteranopia
  DEF: Male-only genetic disorder causing difficulty in distinguishing green and red; no shortened spectrum.
- **H53.54 Protanomaly**
  Protanopia
- **H53.55 Tritanomaly**
  Tritanopia
- **H53.59 Other color vision deficiencies**

H53.6 Night blindness
EXCLUDES 1 *night blindness due to vitamin A deficiency (E50.5)*
- **H53.60 Unspecified night blindness**
- **H53.61 Abnormal dark adaptation curve**
- **H53.62 Acquired night blindness**
- **H53.63 Congenital night blindness**
- **H53.69 Other night blindness**

H53.7 Vision sensitivity deficiencies
- **H53.71 Glare sensitivity**
- **H53.72 Impaired contrast sensitivity**

H53.8 Other visual disturbances

H53.9 Unspecified visual disturbance

H54 Blindness and low vision
NOTE For definition of visual impairment categories see table below
Code first any associated underlying cause of the blindness
EXCLUDES 1 *amaurosis fugax (G45.3)*
AHA: 2017,4Q,11-12

H54.0 Blindness, both eyes
Visual impairment categories 3, 4, 5 in both eyes.
- **H54.0X Blindness, both eyes, different category levels**
  - **H54.0X3 Blindness right eye, category 3**
    - **H54.0X33 Blindness right eye category 3, blindness left eye category 3**
    - **H54.0X34 Blindness right eye category 3, blindness left eye category 4**
    - **H54.0X35 Blindness right eye category 3, blindness left eye category 5**
  - **H54.0X4 Blindness right eye, category 4**
    - **H54.0X43 Blindness right eye category 4, blindness left eye category 3**
    - **H54.0X44 Blindness right eye category 4, blindness left eye category 4**
    - **H54.0X45 Blindness right eye category 4, blindness left eye category 5**
  - **H54.0X5 Blindness right eye, category 5**
    - **H54.0X53 Blindness right eye category 5, blindness left eye category 3**
    - **H54.0X54 Blindness right eye category 5, blindness left eye category 4**
    - **H54.0X55 Blindness right eye category 5, blindness left eye category 5**

H54.1 Blindness, one eye, low vision other eye
Visual impairment categories 3, 4, 5 in one eye, with categories 1 or 2 in the other eye.
- **H54.10 Blindness, one eye, low vision other eye, unspecified eyes**
- **H54.11 Blindness, right eye, low vision left eye**
  - **H54.113 Blindness right eye category 3, low vision left eye**
    - **H54.1131 Blindness right eye category 3, low vision left eye category 1**
    - **H54.1132 Blindness right eye category 3, low vision left eye category 2**
  - **H54.114 Blindness right eye category 4, low vision left eye**
    - **H54.1141 Blindness right eye category 4, low vision left eye category 1**
    - **H54.1142 Blindness right eye category 4, low vision left eye category 2**
  - **H54.115 Blindness right eye category 5, low vision left eye**
    - **H54.1151 Blindness right eye category 5, low vision left eye category 1**
    - **H54.1152 Blindness right eye category 5, low vision left eye category 2**
- **H54.12 Blindness, left eye, low vision right eye**
  - **H54.121 Low vision right eye category 1, blindness left eye**
    - **H54.1213 Low vision right eye category 1, blindness left eye category 3**
    - **H54.1214 Low vision right eye category 1, blindness left eye category 4**
    - **H54.1215 Low vision right eye category 1, blindness left eye category 5**
  - **H54.122 Low vision right eye category 2, blindness left eye**
    - **H54.1223 Low vision right eye category 2, blindness left eye category 3**
    - **H54.1224 Low vision right eye category 2, blindness left eye category 4**
    - **H54.1225 Low vision right eye category 2, blindness left eye category 5**

H54.2 Low vision, both eyes
Visual impairment categories 1 or 2 in both eyes.
- **H54.2X Low vision, both eyes, different category levels**
  - **H54.2X1 Low vision, right eye, category 1**
    - **H54.2X11 Low vision right eye category 1, low vision left eye category 1**
    - **H54.2X12 Low vision right eye category 1, low vision left eye category 2**
  - **H54.2X2 Low vision, right eye, category 2**
    - **H54.2X21 Low vision right eye category 2, low vision left eye category 1**
    - **H54.2X22 Low vision right eye category 2, low vision left eye category 2**

H54.3 Unqualified visual loss, both eyes
Visual impairment category 9 in both eyes.
TIP: Assign only when both eyes are documented as affected by blindness or low vision but the visual impairment category is not documented.

H54.4 Blindness, one eye
Visual impairment categories 3, 4, 5 in one eye [normal vision in other eye]
- **H54.40 Blindness, one eye, unspecified eye**
- **H54.41 Blindness, right eye, normal vision left eye**
  - **H54.413 Blindness, right eye, category 3**
    - **H54.413A Blindness right eye category 3, normal vision left eye**
  - **H54.414 Blindness, right eye, category 4**
    - **H54.414A Blindness right eye category 4, normal vision left eye**

√7th **H54.415 Blindness, right eye, category 5**
H54.415A Blindness right eye category 5, normal vision left eye

√6th **H54.42 Blindness, left eye, normal vision right eye**

√7th **H54.42A Blindness, left eye, category 3-5**
H54.42A3 Blindness left eye category 3, normal vision right eye
H54.42A4 Blindness left eye category 4, normal vision right eye
H54.42A5 Blindness left eye category 5, normal vision right eye

√5th **H54.5 Low vision, one eye**
Visual impairment categories 1 or 2 in one eye [normal vision in other eye].

H54.50 Low vision, one eye, unspecified eye

√6th **H54.51 Low vision, right eye, normal vision left eye**

√7th **H54.511 Low vision, right eye, category 1-2**
H54.511A Low vision right eye category 1, normal vision left eye
H54.512A Low vision right eye category 2, normal vision left eye

√7th **H54.52 Low vision, left eye, normal vision right eye**

√7th **H54.52A Low vision, left eye, category 1-2**
H54.52A1 Low vision left eye category 1, normal vision right eye
H54.52A2 Low vision left eye category 2, normal vision right eye

√5th **H54.6 Unqualified visual loss, one eye**
Visual impairment category 9 in one eye [normal vision in other eye].
TIP: Assign a code from this category only when one eye is documented as affected by blindness or low vision but the visual impairment category is not documented.

H54.60 Unqualified visual loss, one eye, unspecified
H54.61 Unqualified visual loss, right eye, normal vision left eye
H54.62 Unqualified visual loss, left eye, normal vision right eye

H54.7 Unspecified visual loss UPD
Visual impairment category 9 NOS
TIP: Assign only when documentation specifies blindness, visual loss, or low vision but not whether one or both eyes are affected or the visual impairment category.

H54.8 Legal blindness, as defined in USA
Blindness NOS according to USA definition
EXCLUDES 1 *legal blindness with specification of impairment level (H54.0-H54.7)*

NOTE The table below gives a classification of severity of visual impairment recommended by a WHO Study Group on the Prevention of Blindness, Geneva, 6-10 November 1972.

The term "low vision" in category H54 comprises categories 1 and 2 of the table, the term "blindness" categories 3, 4 and 5, and the term "unqualified visual loss" category 9.

If the extent of the visual field is taken into account, patients with a field no greater than 10 but greater than 5 around central fixation should be placed in category 3 and patients with a field no greater than 5 around central fixation should be placed in category 4, even if the central acuity is not impaired.

Category of visual impairment	Visual acuity with best possible correction	
	Maximum less than:	Minimum equal to or better than:
1	6/18 3/10 (0.3) 20/70	6/60 1/10 (0.1) 20/200
2	6/60 1/10 (0.1) 20/200	3/60 1/20 (0.05) 20/400
3	3/60 1/20 (0.05) 20/400	1/60 (finger counting at one meter) 1/50 (0.02) 5/300 (20/1200)
4	1/60 (finger counting at one meter) 1/50 (0.02) 5/300	Light perception
5	No light perception	
9	Undetermined or unspecified	

Other disorders of eye and adnexa (H55-H57)

√4th **H55 Nystagmus and other irregular eye movements**

√5th **H55.0 Nystagmus**
DEF: Rapid, rhythmic, involuntary movements of the eyeball in vertical, horizontal, rotational, or mixed directions.

H55.00 Unspecified nystagmus
H55.01 Congenital nystagmus
H55.02 Latent nystagmus
H55.03 Visual deprivation nystagmus
H55.04 Dissociated nystagmus
H55.09 Other forms of nystagmus

√5th **H55.8 Other irregular eye movements**
AHA: 2020,4Q,25
H55.81 Deficient saccadic eye movements
H55.82 Deficient smooth pursuit eye movements
H55.89 Other irregular eye movements

√4th **H57 Other disorders of eye and adnexa**

√5th **H57.0 Anomalies of pupillary function**
H57.00 Unspecified anomaly of pupillary function
H57.01 Argyll Robertson pupil, atypical
EXCLUDES 1 *syphilitic Argyll Robertson pupil (A52.19)*
H57.02 Anisocoria
H57.03 Miosis
H57.04 Mydriasis

√6th **H57.05 Tonic pupil**
H57.051 Tonic pupil, right eye
H57.052 Tonic pupil, left eye
H57.053 Tonic pupil, bilateral
H57.059 Tonic pupil, unspecified eye

H57.09 Other anomalies of pupillary function

H57.1 Ocular pain
- **H57.10 Ocular pain, unspecified eye**
- **H57.11 Ocular pain, right eye**
- **H57.12 Ocular pain, left eye**
- **H57.13 Ocular pain, bilateral**

H57.8 Other specified disorders of eye and adnexa
AHA: 2018,4Q,15-16
- **H57.81 Brow ptosis**
  - **H57.811 Brow ptosis, right**
  - **H57.812 Brow ptosis, left**
  - **H57.813 Brow ptosis, bilateral**
  - **H57.819 Brow ptosis, unspecified**
- **H57.89 Other specified disorders of eye and adnexa**

H57.9 Unspecified disorder of eye and adnexa UPD

Intraoperative and postprocedural complications and disorders of eye and adnexa, not elsewhere classified (H59)

H59 Intraoperative and postprocedural complications and disorders of eye and adnexa, not elsewhere classified
EXCLUDES 1 *mechanical complication of intraocular lens (T85.2)*
mechanical complication of other ocular prosthetic devices, implants and grafts (T85.3)
pseudophakia (Z96.1)
secondary cataracts (H26.4-)

H59.0 Disorders of the eye following cataract surgery
- **H59.01 Keratopathy (bullous aphakic) following cataract surgery**
  Vitreal corneal syndrome
  Vitreous (touch) syndrome
  - **H59.011 Keratopathy (bullous aphakic) following cataract surgery, right eye** CC
  - **H59.012 Keratopathy (bullous aphakic) following cataract surgery, left eye** CC
  - **H59.013 Keratopathy (bullous aphakic) following cataract surgery, bilateral** CC
  - **H59.019 Keratopathy (bullous aphakic) following cataract surgery, unspecified eye** CC UNS
- **H59.02 Cataract (lens) fragments in eye following cataract surgery**
  - **H59.021 Cataract (lens) fragments in eye following cataract surgery, right eye**
  - **H59.022 Cataract (lens) fragments in eye following cataract surgery, left eye**
  - **H59.023 Cataract (lens) fragments in eye following cataract surgery, bilateral**
  - **H59.029 Cataract (lens) fragments in eye following cataract surgery, unspecified eye**
- **H59.03 Cystoid macular edema following cataract surgery**
  - **H59.031 Cystoid macular edema following cataract surgery, right eye** CC
  - **H59.032 Cystoid macular edema following cataract surgery, left eye** CC
  - **H59.033 Cystoid macular edema following cataract surgery, bilateral** CC
  - **H59.039 Cystoid macular edema following cataract surgery, unspecified eye** CC UNS
- **H59.09 Other disorders of the eye following cataract surgery**
  - **H59.091 Other disorders of the right eye following cataract surgery** CC
  - **H59.092 Other disorders of the left eye following cataract surgery** CC
  - **H59.093 Other disorders of the eye following cataract surgery, bilateral** CC
  - **H59.099 Other disorders of unspecified eye following cataract surgery** CC UNS

H59.1 Intraoperative hemorrhage and hematoma of eye and adnexa complicating a procedure
EXCLUDES 1 *intraoperative hemorrhage and hematoma of eye and adnexa due to accidental puncture or laceration during a procedure (H59.2-)*
- **H59.11 Intraoperative hemorrhage and hematoma of eye and adnexa complicating an ophthalmic procedure**
  - **H59.111 Intraoperative hemorrhage and hematoma of right eye and adnexa complicating an ophthalmic procedure** CC
  - **H59.112 Intraoperative hemorrhage and hematoma of left eye and adnexa complicating an ophthalmic procedure** CC
  - **H59.113 Intraoperative hemorrhage and hematoma of eye and adnexa complicating an ophthalmic procedure, bilateral** CC
  - **H59.119 Intraoperative hemorrhage and hematoma of unspecified eye and adnexa complicating an ophthalmic procedure** CC UNS
- **H59.12 Intraoperative hemorrhage and hematoma of eye and adnexa complicating other procedure**
  - **H59.121 Intraoperative hemorrhage and hematoma of right eye and adnexa complicating other procedure** CC
  - **H59.122 Intraoperative hemorrhage and hematoma of left eye and adnexa complicating other procedure** CC
  - **H59.123 Intraoperative hemorrhage and hematoma of eye and adnexa complicating other procedure, bilateral** CC
  - **H59.129 Intraoperative hemorrhage and hematoma of unspecified eye and adnexa complicating other procedure** CC UNS

H59.2 Accidental puncture and laceration of eye and adnexa during a procedure
- **H59.21 Accidental puncture and laceration of eye and adnexa during an ophthalmic procedure**
  - **H59.211 Accidental puncture and laceration of right eye and adnexa during an ophthalmic procedure** CC
  - **H59.212 Accidental puncture and laceration of left eye and adnexa during an ophthalmic procedure** CC
  - **H59.213 Accidental puncture and laceration of eye and adnexa during an ophthalmic procedure, bilateral** CC
  - **H59.219 Accidental puncture and laceration of unspecified eye and adnexa during an ophthalmic procedure** CC UNS
- **H59.22 Accidental puncture and laceration of eye and adnexa during other procedure**
  - **H59.221 Accidental puncture and laceration of right eye and adnexa during other procedure** CC
  - **H59.222 Accidental puncture and laceration of left eye and adnexa during other procedure** CC
  - **H59.223 Accidental puncture and laceration of eye and adnexa during other procedure, bilateral** CC
  - **H59.229 Accidental puncture and laceration of unspecified eye and adnexa during other procedure** CC UNS

H59.3 Postprocedural hemorrhage, hematoma, and seroma of eye and adnexa following a procedure
AHA: 2016,4Q,9-10
- **H59.31 Postprocedural hemorrhage of eye and adnexa following an ophthalmic procedure**
  - **H59.311 Postprocedural hemorrhage of right eye and adnexa following an ophthalmic procedure** CC
  - **H59.312 Postprocedural hemorrhage of left eye and adnexa following an ophthalmic procedure** CC
  - **H59.313 Postprocedural hemorrhage of eye and adnexa following an ophthalmic procedure, bilateral** CC
  - **H59.319 Postprocedural hemorrhage of unspecified eye and adnexa following an ophthalmic procedure** CC UNS
- **H59.32 Postprocedural hemorrhage of eye and adnexa following other procedure**
  - **H59.321 Postprocedural hemorrhage of right eye and adnexa following other procedure** CC
  - **H59.322 Postprocedural hemorrhage of left eye and adnexa following other procedure** CC

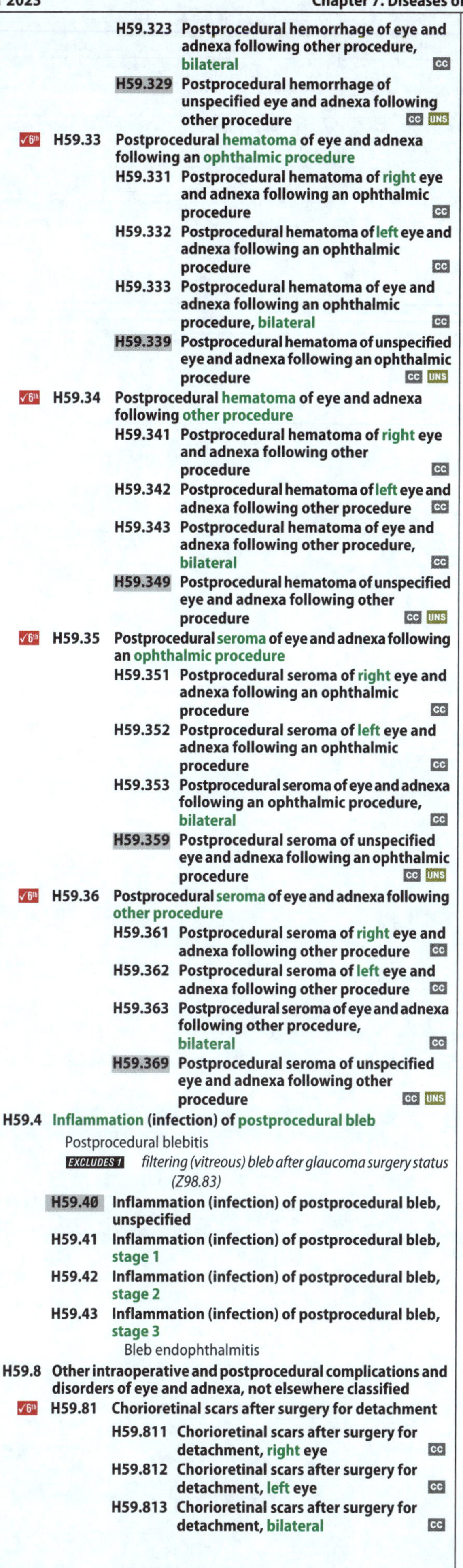

H59.323 Postprocedural hemorrhage of eye and adnexa following other procedure, bilateral CC

H59.329 Postprocedural hemorrhage of unspecified eye and adnexa following other procedure CC UNS

✓6th H59.33 Postprocedural hematoma of eye and adnexa following an ophthalmic procedure

H59.331 Postprocedural hematoma of right eye and adnexa following an ophthalmic procedure CC

H59.332 Postprocedural hematoma of left eye and adnexa following an ophthalmic procedure CC

H59.333 Postprocedural hematoma of eye and adnexa following an ophthalmic procedure, bilateral CC

H59.339 Postprocedural hematoma of unspecified eye and adnexa following an ophthalmic procedure CC UNS

✓6th H59.34 Postprocedural hematoma of eye and adnexa following other procedure

H59.341 Postprocedural hematoma of right eye and adnexa following other procedure CC

H59.342 Postprocedural hematoma of left eye and adnexa following other procedure CC

H59.343 Postprocedural hematoma of eye and adnexa following other procedure, bilateral CC

H59.349 Postprocedural hematoma of unspecified eye and adnexa following other procedure CC UNS

✓6th H59.35 Postprocedural seroma of eye and adnexa following an ophthalmic procedure

H59.351 Postprocedural seroma of right eye and adnexa following an ophthalmic procedure CC

H59.352 Postprocedural seroma of left eye and adnexa following an ophthalmic procedure CC

H59.353 Postprocedural seroma of eye and adnexa following an ophthalmic procedure, bilateral CC

H59.359 Postprocedural seroma of unspecified eye and adnexa following an ophthalmic procedure CC UNS

✓6th H59.36 Postprocedural seroma of eye and adnexa following other procedure

H59.361 Postprocedural seroma of right eye and adnexa following other procedure CC

H59.362 Postprocedural seroma of left eye and adnexa following other procedure CC

H59.363 Postprocedural seroma of eye and adnexa following other procedure, bilateral CC

H59.369 Postprocedural seroma of unspecified eye and adnexa following other procedure CC UNS

✓5th H59.4 Inflammation (infection) of postprocedural bleb

Postprocedural blebitis

EXCLUDES 1 *filtering (vitreous) bleb after glaucoma surgery status (Z98.83)*

H59.40 Inflammation (infection) of postprocedural bleb, unspecified

H59.41 Inflammation (infection) of postprocedural bleb, stage 1

H59.42 Inflammation (infection) of postprocedural bleb, stage 2

H59.43 Inflammation (infection) of postprocedural bleb, stage 3

Bleb endophthalmitis

✓5th H59.8 Other intraoperative and postprocedural complications and disorders of eye and adnexa, not elsewhere classified

✓6th H59.81 Chorioretinal scars after surgery for detachment

H59.811 Chorioretinal scars after surgery for detachment, right eye CC

H59.812 Chorioretinal scars after surgery for detachment, left eye CC

H59.813 Chorioretinal scars after surgery for detachment, bilateral CC

H59.819 Chorioretinal scars after surgery for detachment, unspecified eye CC UNS

H59.88 Other intraoperative complications of eye and adnexa, not elsewhere classified CC

H59.89 Other postprocedural complications and disorders of eye and adnexa, not elsewhere classified CC

AHA: 2020,3Q,29

Chapter 8. Diseases of the Ear and Mastoid Process (H60–H95)

Chapter-specific Guidelines with Coding Examples
Reserved for future guideline expansion.

Chapter 8. Diseases of the Ear and Mastoid Process (H60-H95)

NOTE Use an external cause code following the code for the ear condition, if applicable, to identify the cause of the ear condition

EXCLUDES 2 *certain conditions originating in the perinatal period (P04-P96)*
certain infectious and parasitic diseases (A00-B99)
complications of pregnancy, childbirth and the puerperium (O00-O9A)
congenital malformations, deformations and chromosomal abnormalities (Q00-Q99)
endocrine, nutritional and metabolic diseases (E00-E88)
injury, poisoning and certain other consequences of external causes (S00-T88)
neoplasms (C00-D49)
symptoms, signs and abnormal clinical and laboratory findings, not elsewhere classified (R00-R94)

This chapter contains the following blocks:

H60-H62 Diseases of external ear
H65-H75 Diseases of middle ear and mastoid
H80-H83 Diseases of inner ear
H90-H94 Other disorders of ear
H95 Intraoperative and postprocedural complications and disorders of ear and mastoid process, not elsewhere classified

Diseases of external ear (H60-H62)

H60 Otitis externa
TIP: When the specific infectious agent is identified, a code from Chapter 1 is assigned instead of a code from this category.

H60.0 Abscess of external ear
Boil of external ear
Carbuncle of auricle or external auditory canal
Furuncle of external ear
H60.00 Abscess of external ear, unspecified ear
H60.01 Abscess of right external ear
H60.02 Abscess of left external ear
H60.03 Abscess of external ear, bilateral

H60.1 Cellulitis of external ear
Cellulitis of auricle
Cellulitis of external auditory canal
H60.10 Cellulitis of external ear, unspecified ear
H60.11 Cellulitis of right external ear
H60.12 Cellulitis of left external ear
H60.13 Cellulitis of external ear, bilateral

H60.2 Malignant otitis externa
H60.20 Malignant otitis externa, unspecified ear CC UNS
H60.21 Malignant otitis externa, right ear CC
H60.22 Malignant otitis externa, left ear CC
H60.23 Malignant otitis externa, bilateral CC

H60.3 Other infective otitis externa
H60.31 Diffuse otitis externa
H60.311 Diffuse otitis externa, right ear
H60.312 Diffuse otitis externa, left ear
H60.313 Diffuse otitis externa, bilateral
H60.319 Diffuse otitis externa, unspecified ear
H60.32 Hemorrhagic otitis externa
H60.321 Hemorrhagic otitis externa, right ear
H60.322 Hemorrhagic otitis externa, left ear
H60.323 Hemorrhagic otitis externa, bilateral
H60.329 Hemorrhagic otitis externa, unspecified ear
H60.33 Swimmer's ear
DEF: Commonly occurs when water gets trapped in the ear after swimming.
H60.331 Swimmer's ear, right ear
H60.332 Swimmer's ear, left ear
H60.333 Swimmer's ear, bilateral
H60.339 Swimmer's ear, unspecified ear
H60.39 Other infective otitis externa
H60.391 Other infective otitis externa, right ear
H60.392 Other infective otitis externa, left ear
H60.393 Other infective otitis externa, bilateral
H60.399 Other infective otitis externa, unspecified ear

H60.4 Cholesteatoma of external ear
Keratosis obturans of external ear (canal)
EXCLUDES 2 *cholesteatoma of middle ear (H71.-)*
recurrent cholesteatoma of postmastoidectomy cavity (H95.0-)
DEF: Cholesteatoma: Noncancerous cyst-like mass of cell debris, including cholesterol and epithelial cells resulting from trauma, repeated or improperly healed infections, and congenital enclosure of epidermal cells.
H60.40 Cholesteatoma of external ear, unspecified ear
H60.41 Cholesteatoma of right external ear
H60.42 Cholesteatoma of left external ear
H60.43 Cholesteatoma of external ear, bilateral

H60.5 Acute noninfective otitis externa
H60.50 Unspecified acute noninfective otitis externa
Acute otitis externa NOS
H60.501 Unspecified acute noninfective otitis externa, right ear
H60.502 Unspecified acute noninfective otitis externa, left ear
H60.503 Unspecified acute noninfective otitis externa, bilateral
H60.509 Unspecified acute noninfective otitis externa, unspecified ear
H60.51 Acute actinic otitis externa
H60.511 Acute actinic otitis externa, right ear
H60.512 Acute actinic otitis externa, left ear
H60.513 Acute actinic otitis externa, bilateral
H60.519 Acute actinic otitis externa, unspecified ear
H60.52 Acute chemical otitis externa
H60.521 Acute chemical otitis externa, right ear
H60.522 Acute chemical otitis externa, left ear
H60.523 Acute chemical otitis externa, bilateral
H60.529 Acute chemical otitis externa, unspecified ear
H60.53 Acute contact otitis externa
H60.531 Acute contact otitis externa, right ear
H60.532 Acute contact otitis externa, left ear
H60.533 Acute contact otitis externa, bilateral
H60.539 Acute contact otitis externa, unspecified ear
H60.54 Acute eczematoid otitis externa
H60.541 Acute eczematoid otitis externa, right ear
H60.542 Acute eczematoid otitis externa, left ear
H60.543 Acute eczematoid otitis externa, bilateral
H60.549 Acute eczematoid otitis externa, unspecified ear
H60.55 Acute reactive otitis externa
H60.551 Acute reactive otitis externa, right ear
H60.552 Acute reactive otitis externa, left ear
H60.553 Acute reactive otitis externa, bilateral
H60.559 Acute reactive otitis externa, unspecified ear
H60.59 Other noninfective acute otitis externa
H60.591 Other noninfective acute otitis externa, right ear
H60.592 Other noninfective acute otitis externa, left ear
H60.593 Other noninfective acute otitis externa, bilateral
H60.599 Other noninfective acute otitis externa, unspecified ear

H60.6 Unspecified chronic otitis externa
H60.60 Unspecified chronic otitis externa, unspecified ear
H60.61 Unspecified chronic otitis externa, right ear
H60.62 Unspecified chronic otitis externa, left ear
H60.63 Unspecified chronic otitis externa, bilateral

H60.8 Other otitis externa
H60.8X Other otitis externa
H60.8X1 Other otitis externa, right ear
H60.8X2 Other otitis externa, left ear
H60.8X3 Other otitis externa, bilateral
H60.8X9 Other otitis externa, unspecified ear

H60.9 Unspecified otitis externa
H60.90 Unspecified otitis externa, unspecified ear
H60.91 Unspecified otitis externa, right ear

H60.92 Unspecified otitis externa, left ear

H60.93 Unspecified otitis externa, bilateral

H61 Other disorders of external ear

H61.0 Chondritis and perichondritis of external ear

Chondrodermatitis nodularis chronica helicis
Perichondritis of auricle
Perichondritis of pinna

H61.00 Unspecified perichondritis of external ear

- **H61.001** Unspecified perichondritis of right external ear
- **H61.002** Unspecified perichondritis of left external ear
- **H61.003** Unspecified perichondritis of external ear, bilateral
- **H61.009** Unspecified perichondritis of external ear, unspecified ear

H61.01 Acute perichondritis of external ear

- **H61.011** Acute perichondritis of right external ear
- **H61.012** Acute perichondritis of left external ear
- **H61.013** Acute perichondritis of external ear, bilateral
- **H61.019** Acute perichondritis of external ear, unspecified ear

H61.02 Chronic perichondritis of external ear

- **H61.021** Chronic perichondritis of right external ear
- **H61.022** Chronic perichondritis of left external ear
- **H61.023** Chronic perichondritis of external ear, bilateral
- **H61.029** Chronic perichondritis of external ear, unspecified ear

H61.03 Chondritis of external ear

Chondritis of auricle
Chondritis of pinna

AHA: 2015,1Q,18

DEF: Infection that has progressed into the cartilage and presents as indurated and edematous skin over the pinna. Vascular compromise occurs with tissue necrosis and deformity.

- **H61.031** Chondritis of right external ear
- **H61.032** Chondritis of left external ear
- **H61.033** Chondritis of external ear, bilateral
- **H61.039** Chondritis of external ear, unspecified ear

H61.1 Noninfective disorders of pinna

EXCLUDES 2 *cauliflower ear (M95.1-)*
gouty tophi of ear (M1A.-)

H61.10 Unspecified noninfective disorders of pinna

Disorder of pinna NOS

- **H61.101** Unspecified noninfective disorders of pinna, right ear
- **H61.102** Unspecified noninfective disorders of pinna, left ear
- **H61.103** Unspecified noninfective disorders of pinna, bilateral
- **H61.109** Unspecified noninfective disorders of pinna, unspecified ear

H61.11 Acquired deformity of pinna

Acquired deformity of auricle

EXCLUDES 2 *cauliflower ear (M95.1-)*

- **H61.111** Acquired deformity of pinna, right ear
- **H61.112** Acquired deformity of pinna, left ear
- **H61.113** Acquired deformity of pinna, bilateral
- **H61.119** Acquired deformity of pinna, unspecified ear

H61.12 Hematoma of pinna

Hematoma of auricle

- **H61.121** Hematoma of pinna, right ear
- **H61.122** Hematoma of pinna, left ear
- **H61.123** Hematoma of pinna, bilateral
- **H61.129** Hematoma of pinna, unspecified ear

H61.19 Other noninfective disorders of pinna

- **H61.191** Noninfective disorders of pinna, right ear
- **H61.192** Noninfective disorders of pinna, left ear
- **H61.193** Noninfective disorders of pinna, bilateral
- **H61.199** Noninfective disorders of pinna, unspecified ear

H61.2 Impacted cerumen

Wax in ear

- **H61.20** Impacted cerumen, unspecified ear
- **H61.21** Impacted cerumen, right ear
- **H61.22** Impacted cerumen, left ear
- **H61.23** Impacted cerumen, bilateral

H61.3 Acquired stenosis of external ear canal

Collapse of external ear canal

EXCLUDES 1 *postprocedural stenosis of external ear canal (H95.81-)*

H61.30 Acquired stenosis of external ear canal, unspecified

- **H61.301** Acquired stenosis of right external ear canal, unspecified
- **H61.302** Acquired stenosis of left external ear canal, unspecified
- **H61.303** Acquired stenosis of external ear canal, unspecified, bilateral
- **H61.309** Acquired stenosis of external ear canal, unspecified, unspecified ear

H61.31 Acquired stenosis of external ear canal secondary to trauma

- **H61.311** Acquired stenosis of right external ear canal secondary to trauma
- **H61.312** Acquired stenosis of left external ear canal secondary to trauma
- **H61.313** Acquired stenosis of external ear canal secondary to trauma, bilateral
- **H61.319** Acquired stenosis of external ear canal secondary to trauma, unspecified ear

H61.32 Acquired stenosis of external ear canal secondary to inflammation and infection

DEF: Narrowing of the external ear canal due to chronic inflammation or infection.

- **H61.321** Acquired stenosis of right external ear canal secondary to inflammation and infection
- **H61.322** Acquired stenosis of left external ear canal secondary to inflammation and infection
- **H61.323** Acquired stenosis of external ear canal secondary to inflammation and infection, bilateral
- **H61.329** Acquired stenosis of external ear canal secondary to inflammation and infection, unspecified ear

H61.39 Other acquired stenosis of external ear canal

- **H61.391** Other acquired stenosis of right external ear canal
- **H61.392** Other acquired stenosis of left external ear canal
- **H61.393** Other acquired stenosis of external ear canal, bilateral
- **H61.399** Other acquired stenosis of external ear canal, unspecified ear

H61.8 Other specified disorders of external ear

H61.81 Exostosis of external canal

- **H61.811** Exostosis of right external canal
- **H61.812** Exostosis of left external canal
- **H61.813** Exostosis of external canal, bilateral
- **H61.819** Exostosis of external canal, unspecified ear

H61.89 Other specified disorders of external ear

- **H61.891** Other specified disorders of right external ear
- **H61.892** Other specified disorders of left external ear
- **H61.893** Other specified disorders of external ear, bilateral
- **H61.899** Other specified disorders of external ear, unspecified ear

H61.9 Disorder of external ear, unspecified

- **H61.90** Disorder of external ear, unspecified, unspecified ear
- **H61.91** Disorder of right external ear, unspecified
- **H61.92** Disorder of left external ear, unspecified
- **H61.93** Disorder of external ear, unspecified, bilateral

H62 Disorders of external ear in diseases classified elsewhere

H62.4 Otitis externa in other diseases classified elsewhere

Code first underlying disease, such as:
erysipelas (A46)
impetigo (LØ1.Ø)

EXCLUDES 1 *otitis externa (in):*
candidiasis (B37.84)
herpes viral [herpes simplex] (BØØ.1)
herpes zoster (BØ2.8)

H62.4Ø Otitis externa in other diseases classified elsewhere, unspecified ear
H62.41 Otitis externa in other diseases classified elsewhere, right ear
H62.42 Otitis externa in other diseases classified elsewhere, left ear
H62.43 Otitis externa in other diseases classified elsewhere, bilateral

H62.8 Other disorders of external ear in diseases classified elsewhere

Code first underlying disease, such as:
gout (M1A.-, M1Ø.-)

H62.8X Other disorders of external ear in diseases classified elsewhere

H62.8X1 Other disorders of right external ear in diseases classified elsewhere
H62.8X2 Other disorders of left external ear in diseases classified elsewhere
H62.8X3 Other disorders of external ear in diseases classified elsewhere, bilateral
H62.8X9 Other disorders of external ear in diseases classified elsewhere, unspecified ear

Diseases of middle ear and mastoid (H65-H75)

H65 Nonsuppurative otitis media

INCLUDES nonsuppurative otitis media with myringitis

Use additional code for any associated perforated tympanic membrane (H72.-)

Use additional code, if applicable, to identify:
exposure to environmental tobacco smoke (Z77.22)
exposure to tobacco smoke in the perinatal period (P96.81)
history of tobacco dependence (Z87.891)
infectious agent (B95-B97)
occupational exposure to environmental tobacco smoke (Z57.31)
tobacco dependence (F17.-)
tobacco use (Z72.Ø)

H65.Ø Acute serous otitis media

Acute and subacute secretory otitis

H65.ØØ Acute serous otitis media, unspecified ear
H65.Ø1 Acute serous otitis media, right ear
H65.Ø2 Acute serous otitis media, left ear
H65.Ø3 Acute serous otitis media, bilateral
H65.Ø4 Acute serous otitis media, recurrent, right ear
H65.Ø5 Acute serous otitis media, recurrent, left ear
H65.Ø6 Acute serous otitis media, recurrent, bilateral
H65.Ø7 Acute serous otitis media, recurrent, unspecified ear

H65.1 Other acute nonsuppurative otitis media

EXCLUDES 1 *otitic barotrauma (T7Ø.Ø)*
otitis media (acute) NOS (H66.9)

H65.11 Acute and subacute allergic otitis media (mucoid) (sanguinous) (serous)

H65.111 Acute and subacute allergic otitis media (mucoid) (sanguinous) (serous), right ear
H65.112 Acute and subacute allergic otitis media (mucoid) (sanguinous) (serous), left ear
H65.113 Acute and subacute allergic otitis media (mucoid) (sanguinous) (serous), bilateral
H65.114 Acute and subacute allergic otitis media (mucoid) (sanguinous) (serous), recurrent, right ear
H65.115 Acute and subacute allergic otitis media (mucoid) (sanguinous) (serous), recurrent, left ear
H65.116 Acute and subacute allergic otitis media (mucoid) (sanguinous) (serous), recurrent, bilateral
H65.117 Acute and subacute allergic otitis media (mucoid) (sanguinous) (serous), recurrent, unspecified ear
H65.119 Acute and subacute allergic otitis media (mucoid) (sanguinous) (serous), unspecified ear

H65.19 Other acute nonsuppurative otitis media

Acute and subacute mucoid otitis media
Acute and subacute nonsuppurative otitis media NOS
Acute and subacute sanguinous otitis media
Acute and subacute seromucinous otitis media

H65.191 Other acute nonsuppurative otitis media, right ear
H65.192 Other acute nonsuppurative otitis media, left ear
H65.193 Other acute nonsuppurative otitis media, bilateral
H65.194 Other acute nonsuppurative otitis media, recurrent, right ear
H65.195 Other acute nonsuppurative otitis media, recurrent, left ear
H65.196 Other acute nonsuppurative otitis media, recurrent, bilateral
H65.197 Other acute nonsuppurative otitis media recurrent, unspecified ear
H65.199 Other acute nonsuppurative otitis media, unspecified ear

H65.2 Chronic serous otitis media

Chronic tubotympanal catarrh

H65.2Ø Chronic serous otitis media, unspecified ear
H65.21 Chronic serous otitis media, right ear
H65.22 Chronic serous otitis media, left ear
H65.23 Chronic serous otitis media, bilateral

H65.3 Chronic mucoid otitis media

Chronic mucinous otitis media
Chronic secretory otitis media
Chronic transudative otitis media
Glue ear

EXCLUDES 1 *adhesive middle ear disease (H74.1)*

H65.3Ø Chronic mucoid otitis media, unspecified ear
H65.31 Chronic mucoid otitis media, right ear
H65.32 Chronic mucoid otitis media, left ear
H65.33 Chronic mucoid otitis media, bilateral

H65.4 Other chronic nonsuppurative otitis media

H65.41 Chronic allergic otitis media

H65.411 Chronic allergic otitis media, right ear
H65.412 Chronic allergic otitis media, left ear
H65.413 Chronic allergic otitis media, bilateral
H65.419 Chronic allergic otitis media, unspecified ear

H65.49 Other chronic nonsuppurative otitis media

Chronic exudative otitis media
Chronic nonsuppurative otitis media NOS
Chronic otitis media with effusion (nonpurulent)
Chronic seromucinous otitis media

H65.491 Other chronic nonsuppurative otitis media, right ear
H65.492 Other chronic nonsuppurative otitis media, left ear
H65.493 Other chronic nonsuppurative otitis media, bilateral
H65.499 Other chronic nonsuppurative otitis media, unspecified ear

H65.9 Unspecified nonsuppurative otitis media

Allergic otitis media NOS
Catarrhal otitis media NOS
Exudative otitis media NOS
Mucoid otitis media NOS
Otitis media with effusion (nonpurulent) NOS
Secretory otitis media NOS
Seromucinous otitis media NOS
Serous otitis media NOS
Transudative otitis media NOS

H65.9Ø Unspecified nonsuppurative otitis media, unspecified ear
H65.91 Unspecified nonsuppurative otitis media, right ear
H65.92 Unspecified nonsuppurative otitis media, left ear
H65.93 Unspecified nonsuppurative otitis media, bilateral

H66 Suppurative and unspecified otitis media

INCLUDES suppurative and unspecified otitis media with myringitis

Use additional code to identify:
- exposure to environmental tobacco smoke (Z77.22)
- exposure to tobacco smoke in the perinatal period (P96.81)
- history of tobacco dependence (Z87.891)
- occupational exposure to environmental tobacco smoke (Z57.31)
- tobacco dependence (F17.-)
- tobacco use (Z72.Ø)

AHA: 2016,1Q,34

H66.Ø Acute suppurative otitis media

H66.ØØ Acute suppurative otitis media without spontaneous rupture of ear drum

H66.ØØ1 Acute suppurative otitis media without spontaneous rupture of ear drum, right ear

H66.ØØ2 Acute suppurative otitis media without spontaneous rupture of ear drum, left ear

H66.ØØ3 Acute suppurative otitis media without spontaneous rupture of ear drum, bilateral

H66.ØØ4 Acute suppurative otitis media without spontaneous rupture of ear drum, recurrent, right ear

H66.ØØ5 Acute suppurative otitis media without spontaneous rupture of ear drum, recurrent, left ear

H66.ØØ6 Acute suppurative otitis media without spontaneous rupture of ear drum, recurrent, bilateral

H66.ØØ7 Acute suppurative otitis media without spontaneous rupture of ear drum, recurrent, unspecified ear

H66.ØØ9 Acute suppurative otitis media without spontaneous rupture of ear drum, unspecified ear

H66.Ø1 Acute suppurative otitis media with spontaneous rupture of ear drum

DEF: Sudden, severe inflammation of the middle ear, causing pressure that perforates the ear drum tissue.

H66.Ø11 Acute suppurative otitis media with spontaneous rupture of ear drum, right ear

H66.Ø12 Acute suppurative otitis media with spontaneous rupture of ear drum, left ear

H66.Ø13 Acute suppurative otitis media with spontaneous rupture of ear drum, bilateral

H66.Ø14 Acute suppurative otitis media with spontaneous rupture of ear drum, recurrent, right ear

H66.Ø15 Acute suppurative otitis media with spontaneous rupture of ear drum, recurrent, left ear

H66.Ø16 Acute suppurative otitis media with spontaneous rupture of ear drum, recurrent, bilateral

H66.Ø17 Acute suppurative otitis media with spontaneous rupture of ear drum, recurrent, unspecified ear

H66.Ø19 Acute suppurative otitis media with spontaneous rupture of ear drum, unspecified ear

H66.1 Chronic tubotympanic suppurative otitis media

Benign chronic suppurative otitis media
Chronic tubotympanic disease

Use additional code for any associated perforated tympanic membrane (H72.-)

H66.1Ø Chronic tubotympanic suppurative otitis media, unspecified

H66.11 Chronic tubotympanic suppurative otitis media, right ear

H66.12 Chronic tubotympanic suppurative otitis media, left ear

H66.13 Chronic tubotympanic suppurative otitis media, bilateral

H66.2 Chronic atticoantral suppurative otitis media

Chronic atticoantral disease

Use additional code for any associated perforated tympanic membrane (H72.-)

H66.2Ø Chronic atticoantral suppurative otitis media, unspecified ear

H66.21 Chronic atticoantral suppurative otitis media, right ear

H66.22 Chronic atticoantral suppurative otitis media, left ear

H66.23 Chronic atticoantral suppurative otitis media, bilateral

H66.3 Other chronic suppurative otitis media

Chronic suppurative otitis media NOS

Use additional code for any associated perforated tympanic membrane (H72.-)

EXCLUDES 1 *tuberculous otitis media (A18.6)*

H66.3X Other chronic suppurative otitis media

H66.3X1 Other chronic suppurative otitis media, right ear

H66.3X2 Other chronic suppurative otitis media, left ear

H66.3X3 Other chronic suppurative otitis media, bilateral

H66.3X9 Other chronic suppurative otitis media, unspecified ear

H66.4 Suppurative otitis media, unspecified

Purulent otitis media NOS

Use additional code for any associated perforated tympanic membrane (H72.-)

H66.4Ø Suppurative otitis media, unspecified, unspecified ear

H66.41 Suppurative otitis media, unspecified, right ear

H66.42 Suppurative otitis media, unspecified, left ear

H66.43 Suppurative otitis media, unspecified, bilateral

H66.9 Otitis media, unspecified

Otitis media NOS
Acute otitis media NOS
Chronic otitis media NOS

Use additional code for any associated perforated tympanic membrane (H72.-)

H66.9Ø Otitis media, unspecified, unspecified ear

H66.91 Otitis media, unspecified, right ear

H66.92 Otitis media, unspecified, left ear

H66.93 Otitis media, unspecified, bilateral

H67 Otitis media in diseases classified elsewhere

Code first underlying disease, such as:
- plasminogen deficiency (E88.Ø2)
- viral disease NEC (BØØ-B34)

Use additional code for any associated perforated tympanic membrane (H72.-)

EXCLUDES 1 *otitis media in:*
- *influenza (JØ9.X9, J1Ø.83, J11.83)*
- *measles (BØ5.3)*
- *scarlet fever (A38.Ø)*
- *tuberculosis (A18.6)*

H67.1 *Otitis media in diseases classified elsewhere, right ear*

H67.2 *Otitis media in diseases classified elsewhere, left ear*

H67.3 *Otitis media in diseases classified elsewhere, bilateral*

H67.9 *Otitis media in diseases classified elsewhere, unspecified ear*

H68 Eustachian salpingitis and obstruction

DEF: Eustachian tube: Internal channel between the tympanic cavity and the nasopharynx that equalizes internal pressure to the outside pressure and drains mucous production from the middle ear.

H68.Ø Eustachian salpingitis

H68.ØØ Unspecified Eustachian salpingitis

H68.ØØ1 Unspecified Eustachian salpingitis, right ear

H68.ØØ2 Unspecified Eustachian salpingitis, left ear

H68.ØØ3 Unspecified Eustachian salpingitis, bilateral

H68.ØØ9 Unspecified Eustachian salpingitis, unspecified ear

H68.Ø1 Acute Eustachian salpingitis

H68.Ø11 Acute Eustachian salpingitis, right ear

H68.Ø12 Acute Eustachian salpingitis, left ear

H68.Ø13 Acute Eustachian salpingitis, bilateral

H68.Ø19 Acute Eustachian salpingitis, unspecified ear

H68.Ø2 Chronic Eustachian salpingitis

H68.Ø21 Chronic Eustachian salpingitis, right ear

H68.Ø22 Chronic Eustachian salpingitis, left ear

H68.023 Chronic Eustachian salpingitis, bilateral
H68.029 Chronic Eustachian salpingitis, unspecified ear

5th H68.1 Obstruction of Eustachian tube
Stenosis of Eustachian tube
Stricture of Eustachian tube

6th H68.10 Unspecified obstruction of Eustachian tube
H68.101 Unspecified obstruction of Eustachian tube, right ear
H68.102 Unspecified obstruction of Eustachian tube, left ear
H68.103 Unspecified obstruction of Eustachian tube, bilateral
H68.109 Unspecified obstruction of Eustachian tube, unspecified ear

6th H68.11 Osseous obstruction of Eustachian tube
H68.111 Osseous obstruction of Eustachian tube, right ear
H68.112 Osseous obstruction of Eustachian tube, left ear
H68.113 Osseous obstruction of Eustachian tube, bilateral
H68.119 Osseous obstruction of Eustachian tube, unspecified ear

6th H68.12 Intrinsic cartilagenous obstruction of Eustachian tube
H68.121 Intrinsic cartilagenous obstruction of Eustachian tube, right ear
H68.122 Intrinsic cartilagenous obstruction of Eustachian tube, left ear
H68.123 Intrinsic cartilagenous obstruction of Eustachian tube, bilateral
H68.129 Intrinsic cartilagenous obstruction of Eustachian tube, unspecified ear

6th H68.13 Extrinsic cartilagenous obstruction of Eustachian tube
Compression of Eustachian tube
H68.131 Extrinsic cartilagenous obstruction of Eustachian tube, right ear
H68.132 Extrinsic cartilagenous obstruction of Eustachian tube, left ear
H68.133 Extrinsic cartilagenous obstruction of Eustachian tube, bilateral
H68.139 Extrinsic cartilagenous obstruction of Eustachian tube, unspecified ear

4th H69 Other and unspecified disorders of Eustachian tube
DEF: Eustachian tube: Internal channel between the tympanic cavity and the nasopharynx that equalizes internal pressure to the outside pressure and drains mucous production from the middle ear.

5th H69.0 Patulous Eustachian tube
H69.00 Patulous Eustachian tube, unspecified ear
H69.01 Patulous Eustachian tube, right ear
H69.02 Patulous Eustachian tube, left ear
H69.03 Patulous Eustachian tube, bilateral

5th H69.8 Other specified disorders of Eustachian tube
H69.80 Other specified disorders of Eustachian tube, unspecified ear
H69.81 Other specified disorders of Eustachian tube, right ear
H69.82 Other specified disorders of Eustachian tube, left ear
H69.83 Other specified disorders of Eustachian tube, bilateral

5th H69.9 Unspecified Eustachian tube disorder
H69.90 Unspecified Eustachian tube disorder, unspecified ear
H69.91 Unspecified Eustachian tube disorder, right ear
H69.92 Unspecified Eustachian tube disorder, left ear
H69.93 Unspecified Eustachian tube disorder, bilateral

4th H70 Mastoiditis and related conditions

5th H70.0 Acute mastoiditis
Abscess of mastoid
Empyema of mastoid

6th H70.00 Acute mastoiditis without complications
H70.001 Acute mastoiditis without complications, right ear CC
H70.002 Acute mastoiditis without complications, left ear CC
H70.003 Acute mastoiditis without complications, bilateral CC
H70.009 Acute mastoiditis without complications, unspecified ear CC UNS

6th H70.01 Subperiosteal abscess of mastoid
H70.011 Subperiosteal abscess of mastoid, right ear CC
H70.012 Subperiosteal abscess of mastoid, left ear CC
H70.013 Subperiosteal abscess of mastoid, bilateral CC
H70.019 Subperiosteal abscess of mastoid, unspecified ear CC UNS

6th H70.09 Acute mastoiditis with other complications
H70.091 Acute mastoiditis with other complications, right ear CC
H70.092 Acute mastoiditis with other complications, left ear CC
H70.093 Acute mastoiditis with other complications, bilateral CC
H70.099 Acute mastoiditis with other complications, unspecified ear CC UNS

5th H70.1 Chronic mastoiditis
Caries of mastoid
Fistula of mastoid
EXCLUDES 1 *tuberculous mastoiditis (A18.03)*
H70.10 Chronic mastoiditis, unspecified ear
H70.11 Chronic mastoiditis, right ear
H70.12 Chronic mastoiditis, left ear
H70.13 Chronic mastoiditis, bilateral

5th H70.2 Petrositis
Inflammation of petrous bone

6th H70.20 Unspecified petrositis
H70.201 Unspecified petrositis, right ear
H70.202 Unspecified petrositis, left ear
H70.203 Unspecified petrositis, bilateral
H70.209 Unspecified petrositis, unspecified ear

6th H70.21 Acute petrositis
DEF: Sudden, severe inflammation of the petrous temporal bone behind the ear, associated with a middle ear infection.
H70.211 Acute petrositis, right ear
H70.212 Acute petrositis, left ear
H70.213 Acute petrositis, bilateral
H70.219 Acute petrositis, unspecified ear

6th H70.22 Chronic petrositis
H70.221 Chronic petrositis, right ear
H70.222 Chronic petrositis, left ear
H70.223 Chronic petrositis, bilateral
H70.229 Chronic petrositis, unspecified ear

5th H70.8 Other mastoiditis and related conditions
EXCLUDES 1 *preauricular sinus and cyst (Q18.1)*
sinus, fistula, and cyst of branchial cleft (Q18.0)

6th H70.81 Postauricular fistula
H70.811 Postauricular fistula, right ear
H70.812 Postauricular fistula, left ear
H70.813 Postauricular fistula, bilateral
H70.819 Postauricular fistula, unspecified ear

6th H70.89 Other mastoiditis and related conditions
H70.891 Other mastoiditis and related conditions, right ear
H70.892 Other mastoiditis and related conditions, left ear
H70.893 Other mastoiditis and related conditions, bilateral
H70.899 Other mastoiditis and related conditions, unspecified ear

5th H70.9 Unspecified mastoiditis
H70.90 Unspecified mastoiditis, unspecified ear
H70.91 Unspecified mastoiditis, right ear
H70.92 Unspecified mastoiditis, left ear
H70.93 Unspecified mastoiditis, bilateral

H71 Cholesteatoma of middle ear

EXCLUDES 2 *cholesteatoma of external ear (H60.4-)*
recurrent cholesteatoma of postmastoidectomy cavity (H95.0-)

AHA: 2021,3Q,8

DEF: Cholesteatoma: Noncancerous cyst-like mass of cell debris, including cholesterol and epithelial cells resulting from trauma, repeated or improperly healed infections, and congenital enclosure of epidermal cells.

Cholesteatoma of Middle Ear

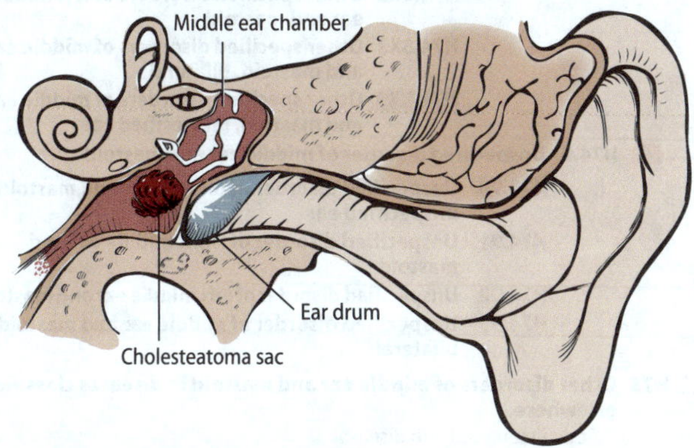

H71.0 Cholesteatoma of attic
- **H71.00** Cholesteatoma of attic, unspecified ear
- **H71.01** Cholesteatoma of attic, right ear
- **H71.02** Cholesteatoma of attic, left ear
- **H71.03** Cholesteatoma of attic, bilateral

H71.1 Cholesteatoma of tympanum
- **H71.10** Cholesteatoma of tympanum, unspecified ear
- **H71.11** Cholesteatoma of tympanum, right ear
- **H71.12** Cholesteatoma of tympanum, left ear
- **H71.13** Cholesteatoma of tympanum, bilateral

H71.2 Cholesteatoma of mastoid
- **H71.20** Cholesteatoma of mastoid, unspecified ear
- **H71.21** Cholesteatoma of mastoid, right ear
- **H71.22** Cholesteatoma of mastoid, left ear
- **H71.23** Cholesteatoma of mastoid, bilateral

H71.3 Diffuse cholesteatosis

AHA: 2021,3Q,8
- **H71.30** Diffuse cholesteatosis, unspecified ear
- **H71.31** Diffuse cholesteatosis, right ear
- **H71.32** Diffuse cholesteatosis, left ear
- **H71.33** Diffuse cholesteatosis, bilateral

H71.9 Unspecified cholesteatoma
- **H71.90** Unspecified cholesteatoma, unspecified ear
- **H71.91** Unspecified cholesteatoma, right ear
- **H71.92** Unspecified cholesteatoma, left ear
- **H71.93** Unspecified cholesteatoma, bilateral

H72 Perforation of tympanic membrane

INCLUDES persistent post-traumatic perforation of ear drum
postinflammatory perforation of ear drum

Code first any associated otitis media (H65.-, H66.1-, H66.2-, H66.3-, H66.4-, H66.9-, H67.-)

EXCLUDES 1 *acute suppurative otitis media with rupture of the tympanic membrane (H66.01-)*
traumatic rupture of ear drum (S09.2-)

H72.0 Central perforation of tympanic membrane
- **H72.00** Central perforation of tympanic membrane, unspecified ear
- **H72.01** Central perforation of tympanic membrane, right ear
- **H72.02** Central perforation of tympanic membrane, left ear
- **H72.03** Central perforation of tympanic membrane, bilateral

H72.1 Attic perforation of tympanic membrane

Perforation of pars flaccida
- **H72.10** Attic perforation of tympanic membrane, unspecified ear
- **H72.11** Attic perforation of tympanic membrane, right ear
- **H72.12** Attic perforation of tympanic membrane, left ear
- **H72.13** Attic perforation of tympanic membrane, bilateral

H72.2 Other marginal perforations of tympanic membrane

H72.2X Other marginal perforations of tympanic membrane
- **H72.2X1** Other marginal perforations of tympanic membrane, right ear
- **H72.2X2** Other marginal perforations of tympanic membrane, left ear
- **H72.2X3** Other marginal perforations of tympanic membrane, bilateral
- **H72.2X9** Other marginal perforations of tympanic membrane, unspecified ear

H72.8 Other perforations of tympanic membrane

H72.81 Multiple perforations of tympanic membrane
- **H72.811** Multiple perforations of tympanic membrane, right ear
- **H72.812** Multiple perforations of tympanic membrane, left ear
- **H72.813** Multiple perforations of tympanic membrane, bilateral
- **H72.819** Multiple perforations of tympanic membrane, unspecified ear

H72.82 Total perforations of tympanic membrane
- **H72.821** Total perforations of tympanic membrane, right ear
- **H72.822** Total perforations of tympanic membrane, left ear
- **H72.823** Total perforations of tympanic membrane, bilateral
- **H72.829** Total perforations of tympanic membrane, unspecified ear

H72.9 Unspecified perforation of tympanic membrane
- **H72.90** Unspecified perforation of tympanic membrane, unspecified ear
- **H72.91** Unspecified perforation of tympanic membrane, right ear
- **H72.92** Unspecified perforation of tympanic membrane, left ear
- **H72.93** Unspecified perforation of tympanic membrane, bilateral

H73 Other disorders of tympanic membrane

H73.0 Acute myringitis

EXCLUDES 1 *acute myringitis with otitis media (H65, H66)*

H73.00 Unspecified acute myringitis

Acute tympanitis NOS
- **H73.001** Acute myringitis, right ear
- **H73.002** Acute myringitis, left ear
- **H73.003** Acute myringitis, bilateral
- **H73.009** Acute myringitis, unspecified ear

H73.01 Bullous myringitis

DEF: Bacterial or viral otitis media that is characterized by the appearance of serous or hemorrhagic blebs on the ear drum and sudden onset of severe pain in ear.
- **H73.011** Bullous myringitis, right ear
- **H73.012** Bullous myringitis, left ear
- **H73.013** Bullous myringitis, bilateral
- **H73.019** Bullous myringitis, unspecified ear

H73.09 Other acute myringitis
- **H73.091** Other acute myringitis, right ear
- **H73.092** Other acute myringitis, left ear
- **H73.093** Other acute myringitis, bilateral
- **H73.099** Other acute myringitis, unspecified ear

H73.1 Chronic myringitis

Chronic tympanitis

EXCLUDES 1 *chronic myringitis with otitis media (H65, H66)*
- **H73.10** Chronic myringitis, unspecified ear
- **H73.11** Chronic myringitis, right ear
- **H73.12** Chronic myringitis, left ear
- **H73.13** Chronic myringitis, bilateral

H73.2 Unspecified myringitis
- **H73.20** Unspecified myringitis, unspecified ear
- **H73.21** Unspecified myringitis, right ear
- **H73.22** Unspecified myringitis, left ear
- **H73.23** Unspecified myringitis, bilateral

H73.8 Other specified disorders of tympanic membrane

H73.81 Atrophic flaccid tympanic membrane
- **H73.811** Atrophic flaccid tympanic membrane, right ear

H73.812 Atrophic flaccid tympanic membrane, left ear
H73.813 Atrophic flaccid tympanic membrane, bilateral
H73.819 Atrophic flaccid tympanic membrane, unspecified ear
H73.82 Atrophic nonflaccid tympanic membrane
H73.821 Atrophic nonflaccid tympanic membrane, right ear
H73.822 Atrophic nonflaccid tympanic membrane, left ear
H73.823 Atrophic nonflaccid tympanic membrane, bilateral
H73.829 Atrophic nonflaccid tympanic membrane, unspecified ear
H73.89 Other specified disorders of tympanic membrane
H73.891 Other specified disorders of tympanic membrane, right ear
H73.892 Other specified disorders of tympanic membrane, left ear
H73.893 Other specified disorders of tympanic membrane, bilateral
H73.899 Other specified disorders of tympanic membrane, unspecified ear
H73.9 Unspecified disorder of tympanic membrane
H73.90 Unspecified disorder of tympanic membrane, unspecified ear
H73.91 Unspecified disorder of tympanic membrane, right ear
H73.92 Unspecified disorder of tympanic membrane, left ear
H73.93 Unspecified disorder of tympanic membrane, bilateral

H74 Other disorders of middle ear mastoid
EXCLUDES 2 *mastoiditis (H70.-)*

H74.0 Tympanosclerosis
DEF: Calcification of tissue in the ear drum, middle ear bones, and middle ear canal.
H74.01 Tympanosclerosis, right ear
H74.02 Tympanosclerosis, left ear
H74.03 Tympanosclerosis, bilateral
H74.09 Tympanosclerosis, unspecified ear
H74.1 Adhesive middle ear disease
Adhesive otitis
EXCLUDES 1 *glue ear (H65.3-)*
H74.11 Adhesive right middle ear disease
H74.12 Adhesive left middle ear disease
H74.13 Adhesive middle ear disease, bilateral
H74.19 Adhesive middle ear disease, unspecified ear
H74.2 Discontinuity and dislocation of ear ossicles
H74.20 Discontinuity and dislocation of ear ossicles, unspecified ear
H74.21 Discontinuity and dislocation of right ear ossicles
H74.22 Discontinuity and dislocation of left ear ossicles
H74.23 Discontinuity and dislocation of ear ossicles, bilateral
H74.3 Other acquired abnormalities of ear ossicles
H74.31 Ankylosis of ear ossicles
H74.311 Ankylosis of ear ossicles, right ear
H74.312 Ankylosis of ear ossicles, left ear
H74.313 Ankylosis of ear ossicles, bilateral
H74.319 Ankylosis of ear ossicles, unspecified ear
H74.32 Partial loss of ear ossicles
H74.321 Partial loss of ear ossicles, right ear
H74.322 Partial loss of ear ossicles, left ear
H74.323 Partial loss of ear ossicles, bilateral
H74.329 Partial loss of ear ossicles, unspecified ear
H74.39 Other acquired abnormalities of ear ossicles
H74.391 Other acquired abnormalities of right ear ossicles
H74.392 Other acquired abnormalities of left ear ossicles
H74.393 Other acquired abnormalities of ear ossicles, bilateral
H74.399 Other acquired abnormalities of ear ossicles, unspecified ear
H74.4 Polyp of middle ear
H74.40 Polyp of middle ear, unspecified ear
H74.41 Polyp of right middle ear
H74.42 Polyp of left middle ear
H74.43 Polyp of middle ear, bilateral
H74.8 Other specified disorders of middle ear and mastoid
H74.8X Other specified disorders of middle ear and mastoid
H74.8X1 Other specified disorders of right middle ear and mastoid
H74.8X2 Other specified disorders of left middle ear and mastoid
H74.8X3 Other specified disorders of middle ear and mastoid, bilateral
H74.8X9 Other specified disorders of middle ear and mastoid, unspecified ear
H74.9 Unspecified disorder of middle ear and mastoid
H74.90 Unspecified disorder of middle ear and mastoid, unspecified ear
H74.91 Unspecified disorder of right middle ear and mastoid
H74.92 Unspecified disorder of left middle ear and mastoid
H74.93 Unspecified disorder of middle ear and mastoid, bilateral

H75 Other disorders of middle ear and mastoid in diseases classified elsewhere
Code first underlying disease

H75.0 Mastoiditis in infectious and parasitic diseases classified elsewhere
EXCLUDES 1 *mastoiditis (in):*
syphilis (A52.77)
tuberculosis (A18.03)
H75.00 Mastoiditis in infectious and parasitic diseases classified elsewhere, unspecified ear
H75.01 Mastoiditis in infectious and parasitic diseases classified elsewhere, right ear
H75.02 Mastoiditis in infectious and parasitic diseases classified elsewhere, left ear
H75.03 Mastoiditis in infectious and parasitic diseases classified elsewhere, bilateral
H75.8 Other specified disorders of middle ear and mastoid in diseases classified elsewhere
H75.80 Other specified disorders of middle ear and mastoid in diseases classified elsewhere, unspecified ear
H75.81 Other specified disorders of right middle ear and mastoid in diseases classified elsewhere
H75.82 Other specified disorders of left middle ear and mastoid in diseases classified elsewhere
H75.83 Other specified disorders of middle ear and mastoid in diseases classified elsewhere, bilateral

Diseases of inner ear (H80-H83)

H80 Otosclerosis
INCLUDES otospongiosis

H80.0 Otosclerosis involving oval window, nonobliterative
H80.00 Otosclerosis involving oval window, nonobliterative, unspecified ear
H80.01 Otosclerosis involving oval window, nonobliterative, right ear
H80.02 Otosclerosis involving oval window, nonobliterative, left ear
H80.03 Otosclerosis involving oval window, nonobliterative, bilateral
H80.1 Otosclerosis involving oval window, obliterative
H80.10 Otosclerosis involving oval window, obliterative, unspecified ear
H80.11 Otosclerosis involving oval window, obliterative, right ear
H80.12 Otosclerosis involving oval window, obliterative, left ear
H80.13 Otosclerosis involving oval window, obliterative, bilateral
H80.2 Cochlear otosclerosis
Otosclerosis involving otic capsule
Otosclerosis involving round window
H80.20 Cochlear otosclerosis, unspecified ear
H80.21 Cochlear otosclerosis, right ear
H80.22 Cochlear otosclerosis, left ear
H80.23 Cochlear otosclerosis, bilateral

H80.8 Other otosclerosis

H80.80 Other otosclerosis, unspecified ear
H80.81 Other otosclerosis, right ear
H80.82 Other otosclerosis, left ear
H80.83 Other otosclerosis, bilateral

H80.9 Unspecified otosclerosis

H80.90 Unspecified otosclerosis, unspecified ear
H80.91 Unspecified otosclerosis, right ear
H80.92 Unspecified otosclerosis, left ear
H80.93 Unspecified otosclerosis, bilateral

H81 Disorders of vestibular function

EXCLUDES 1 *epidemic vertigo (A88.1)*
vertigo NOS (R42)

H81.0 Ménière's disease

Labyrinthine hydrops
Ménière's syndrome or vertigo
DEF: Distended membranous labyrinth of the middle ear from fluctuating pressure of fluid (hydrops) that causes vertigo, tinnitus, pressure, and hearing loss that may last on and off for several hours. Episodes may occur in clusters or may subside for weeks, months, or even years.

H81.01 Ménière's disease, right ear
H81.02 Ménière's disease, left ear
H81.03 Ménière's disease, bilateral
H81.09 Ménière's disease, unspecified ear

H81.1 Benign paroxysmal vertigo

H81.10 Benign paroxysmal vertigo, unspecified ear
H81.11 Benign paroxysmal vertigo, right ear
H81.12 Benign paroxysmal vertigo, left ear
H81.13 Benign paroxysmal vertigo, bilateral

H81.2 Vestibular neuronitis

DEF: Transient benign vertigo caused by inflammation of the vestibular nerve. It is characterized by response to caloric stimulation on one side and nystagmus with rhythmic movement of the eyes. Normal auditory function is present.

H81.20 Vestibular neuronitis, unspecified ear
H81.21 Vestibular neuronitis, right ear
H81.22 Vestibular neuronitis, left ear
H81.23 Vestibular neuronitis, bilateral

H81.3 Other peripheral vertigo

H81.31 Aural vertigo

H81.311 Aural vertigo, right ear
H81.312 Aural vertigo, left ear
H81.313 Aural vertigo, bilateral
H81.319 Aural vertigo, unspecified ear

H81.39 Other peripheral vertigo

Lermoyez' syndrome
Otogenic vertigo
Peripheral vertigo NOS

H81.391 Other peripheral vertigo, right ear
H81.392 Other peripheral vertigo, left ear
H81.393 Other peripheral vertigo, bilateral
H81.399 Other peripheral vertigo, unspecified ear

H81.4 Vertigo of central origin

Central positional nystagmus

H81.8 Other disorders of vestibular function

H81.8X Other disorders of vestibular function

H81.8X1 Other disorders of vestibular function, right ear
H81.8X2 Other disorders of vestibular function, left ear
H81.8X3 Other disorders of vestibular function, bilateral
H81.8X9 Other disorders of vestibular function, unspecified ear
AHA: 2022,2Q,12

H81.9 Unspecified disorder of vestibular function

Vertiginous syndrome NOS

H81.90 Unspecified disorder of vestibular function, unspecified ear
H81.91 Unspecified disorder of vestibular function, right ear
H81.92 Unspecified disorder of vestibular function, left ear
H81.93 Unspecified disorder of vestibular function, bilateral

H82 Vertiginous syndromes in diseases classified elsewhere

Code first underlying disease

EXCLUDES 1 *epidemic vertigo (A88.1)*

H82.1 Vertiginous syndromes in diseases classified elsewhere, right ear
H82.2 Vertiginous syndromes in diseases classified elsewhere, left ear
H82.3 Vertiginous syndromes in diseases classified elsewhere, bilateral
H82.9 Vertiginous syndromes in diseases classified elsewhere, unspecified ear

H83 Other diseases of inner ear

H83.0 Labyrinthitis

DEF: Inflammation of the inner ear, or labyrinth, characterized by pus, vertigo, dizziness, nausea, and hearing loss.

H83.01 Labyrinthitis, right ear
H83.02 Labyrinthitis, left ear
H83.03 Labyrinthitis, bilateral
H83.09 Labyrinthitis, unspecified ear

H83.1 Labyrinthine fistula

H83.11 Labyrinthine fistula, right ear
H83.12 Labyrinthine fistula, left ear
H83.13 Labyrinthine fistula, bilateral
H83.19 Labyrinthine fistula, unspecified ear

H83.2 Labyrinthine dysfunction

Labyrinthine hypersensitivity
Labyrinthine hypofunction
Labyrinthine loss of function
DEF: Decreased function of the labyrinth sensors.

H83.2X Labyrinthine dysfunction

H83.2X1 Labyrinthine dysfunction, right ear
H83.2X2 Labyrinthine dysfunction, left ear
H83.2X3 Labyrinthine dysfunction, bilateral
H83.2X9 Labyrinthine dysfunction, unspecified ear

H83.3 Noise effects on inner ear

Acoustic trauma of inner ear
Noise-induced hearing loss of inner ear

H83.3X Noise effects on inner ear

H83.3X1 Noise effects on right inner ear
H83.3X2 Noise effects on left inner ear
H83.3X3 Noise effects on inner ear, bilateral
H83.3X9 Noise effects on inner ear, unspecified ear

H83.8 Other specified diseases of inner ear

H83.8X Other specified diseases of inner ear

H83.8X1 Other specified diseases of right inner ear
H83.8X2 Other specified diseases of left inner ear
H83.8X3 Other specified diseases of inner ear, bilateral
H83.8X9 Other specified diseases of inner ear, unspecified ear

H83.9 Unspecified disease of inner ear

H83.90 Unspecified disease of inner ear, unspecified ear
H83.91 Unspecified disease of right inner ear
H83.92 Unspecified disease of left inner ear
H83.93 Unspecified disease of inner ear, bilateral

Other disorders of ear (H90-H94)

H90 Conductive and sensorineural hearing loss

EXCLUDES 1 *deaf nonspeaking NEC (H91.3)*
deafness NOS (H91.9-)
hearing loss NOS (H91.9-)
noise-induced hearing loss (H83.3-)
ototoxic hearing loss (H91.0-)
sudden (idiopathic) hearing loss (H91.2-)

AHA: 2015,2Q,7
DEF: Conductive hearing loss: Hearing loss due to the inability of soundwaves to move from the outer (external) ear to the inner ear.
DEF: Sensorineural hearing loss: Hearing loss that occurs from damage to the hair cells of the inner ear or problems with the nerve pathways from the inner ear to the brain.

H90.0 Conductive hearing loss, bilateral

H90.1 **Conductive hearing loss, unilateral with unrestricted hearing on the contralateral side**
- H90.11 **Conductive hearing loss, unilateral, right ear, with unrestricted hearing on the contralateral side**
- H90.12 **Conductive hearing loss, unilateral, left ear, with unrestricted hearing on the contralateral side**

H90.2 **Conductive hearing loss, unspecified**
Conductive deafness NOS

H90.3 **Sensorineural hearing loss, bilateral**

H90.4 **Sensorineural hearing loss, unilateral with unrestricted hearing on the contralateral side**
- H90.41 **Sensorineural hearing loss, unilateral, right ear, with unrestricted hearing on the contralateral side**
- H90.42 **Sensorineural hearing loss, unilateral, left ear, with unrestricted hearing on the contralateral side**

H90.5 **Unspecified sensorineural hearing loss**
Central hearing loss NOS
Congenital deafness NOS
Neural hearing loss NOS
Perceptive hearing loss NOS
Sensorineural deafness NOS
Sensory hearing loss NOS
EXCLUDES 1 *abnormal auditory perception (H93.2-)*
psychogenic deafness (F44.6)

H90.6 **Mixed conductive and sensorineural hearing loss, bilateral**
AHA: 2015,2Q,7

H90.7 **Mixed conductive and sensorineural hearing loss, unilateral with unrestricted hearing on the contralateral side**
- H90.71 **Mixed conductive and sensorineural hearing loss, unilateral, right ear, with unrestricted hearing on the contralateral side**
- H90.72 **Mixed conductive and sensorineural hearing loss, unilateral, left ear, with unrestricted hearing on the contralateral side**

H90.8 **Mixed conductive and sensorineural hearing loss, unspecified**

H90.A **Conductive and sensorineural hearing loss with restricted hearing on the contralateral side**
AHA: 2016,4Q,23-25
- H90.A1 **Conductive hearing loss, unilateral, with restricted hearing on the contralateral side**
  - H90.A11 **Conductive hearing loss, unilateral, right ear with restricted hearing on the contralateral side**
  - H90.A12 **Conductive hearing loss, unilateral, left ear with restricted hearing on the contralateral side**
- H90.A2 **Sensorineural hearing loss, unilateral, with restricted hearing on the contralateral side**
  - H90.A21 **Sensorineural hearing loss, unilateral, right ear, with restricted hearing on the contralateral side**
  - H90.A22 **Sensorineural hearing loss, unilateral, left ear, with restricted hearing on the contralateral side**
- H90.A3 **Mixed conductive and sensorineural hearing loss, unilateral with restricted hearing on the contralateral side**
  - H90.A31 **Mixed conductive and sensorineural hearing loss, unilateral, right ear with restricted hearing on the contralateral side**
  - H90.A32 **Mixed conductive and sensorineural hearing, unilateral, left ear with restricted hearing on the contralateral side**

H91 Other and unspecified hearing loss
EXCLUDES 1 *abnormal auditory perception (H93.2-)*
hearing loss as classified in H90.-
impacted cerumen (H61.2-)
noise-induced hearing loss (H83.3-)
psychogenic deafness (F44.6)
transient ischemic deafness (H93.01-)

H91.0 **Ototoxic hearing loss**
Code first poisoning due to drug or toxin, if applicable (T36-T65 with fifth or sixth character 1-4 or 6)
Use additional code for adverse effect, if applicable, to identify drug (T36-T50 with fifth or sixth character 5)
- H91.01 **Ototoxic hearing loss, right ear**
- H91.02 **Ototoxic hearing loss, left ear**
- H91.03 **Ototoxic hearing loss, bilateral**
- H91.09 **Ototoxic hearing loss, unspecified ear**

H91.1 **Presbycusis**
Presbyacusia
- H91.10 **Presbycusis, unspecified ear**
- H91.11 **Presbycusis, right ear**
- H91.12 **Presbycusis, left ear**
- H91.13 **Presbycusis, bilateral**

H91.2 **Sudden idiopathic hearing loss**
Sudden hearing loss NOS
- H91.20 **Sudden idiopathic hearing loss, unspecified ear**
- H91.21 **Sudden idiopathic hearing loss, right ear**
- H91.22 **Sudden idiopathic hearing loss, left ear**
- H91.23 **Sudden idiopathic hearing loss, bilateral**

H91.3 **Deaf nonspeaking, not elsewhere classified**

H91.8 **Other specified hearing loss**
- H91.8X **Other specified hearing loss**
  - H91.8X1 **Other specified hearing loss, right ear**
  - H91.8X2 **Other specified hearing loss, left ear**
  - H91.8X3 **Other specified hearing loss, bilateral**
  - H91.8X9 **Other specified hearing loss, unspecified ear**

H91.9 **Unspecified hearing loss**
Deafness NOS
High frequency deafness
Low frequency deafness
- H91.90 **Unspecified hearing loss, unspecified ear**
- H91.91 **Unspecified hearing loss, right ear**
- H91.92 **Unspecified hearing loss, left ear**
- H91.93 **Unspecified hearing loss, bilateral**

H92 Otalgia and effusion of ear

H92.0 **Otalgia**
- H92.01 **Otalgia, right ear**
- H92.02 **Otalgia, left ear**
- H92.03 **Otalgia, bilateral**
- H92.09 **Otalgia, unspecified ear**

H92.1 **Otorrhea**
EXCLUDES 1 *leakage of cerebrospinal fluid through ear (G96.0)*
- H92.10 **Otorrhea, unspecified ear**
- H92.11 **Otorrhea, right ear**
- H92.12 **Otorrhea, left ear**
- H92.13 **Otorrhea, bilateral**

H92.2 **Otorrhagia**
EXCLUDES 1 *traumatic otorrhagia - code to injury*
- H92.20 **Otorrhagia, unspecified ear**
- H92.21 **Otorrhagia, right ear**
- H92.22 **Otorrhagia, left ear**
- H92.23 **Otorrhagia, bilateral**

H93 Other disorders of ear, not elsewhere classified

H93.0 **Degenerative and vascular disorders of ear**
EXCLUDES 1 *presbycusis (H91.1)*
- H93.01 **Transient ischemic deafness**
  - H93.011 **Transient ischemic deafness, right ear**
  - H93.012 **Transient ischemic deafness, left ear**
  - H93.013 **Transient ischemic deafness, bilateral**
  - H93.019 **Transient ischemic deafness, unspecified ear**
- H93.09 **Unspecified degenerative and vascular disorders of ear**
  - H93.091 **Unspecified degenerative and vascular disorders of right ear**
  - H93.092 **Unspecified degenerative and vascular disorders of left ear**
  - H93.093 **Unspecified degenerative and vascular disorders of ear, bilateral**
  - H93.099 **Unspecified degenerative and vascular disorders of unspecified ear**

H93.1 **Tinnitus**
- H93.11 **Tinnitus, right ear**
- H93.12 **Tinnitus, left ear**
- H93.13 **Tinnitus, bilateral**
- H93.19 **Tinnitus, unspecified ear**

H93.A **Pulsatile tinnitus**
AHA: 2016,4Q,25-26
- H93.A1 **Pulsatile tinnitus, right ear**
- H93.A2 **Pulsatile tinnitus, left ear**
- H93.A3 **Pulsatile tinnitus, bilateral**

H93.A9 Pulsatile tinnitus, unspecified ear

H93.2 Other abnormal auditory perceptions
EXCLUDES 2 *auditory hallucinations (R44.Ø)*

H93.21 Auditory recruitment
H93.211 Auditory recruitment, right ear
H93.212 Auditory recruitment, left ear
H93.213 Auditory recruitment, bilateral
H93.219 Auditory recruitment, unspecified ear

H93.22 Diplacusis
H93.221 Diplacusis, right ear
H93.222 Diplacusis, left ear
H93.223 Diplacusis, bilateral
H93.229 Diplacusis, unspecified ear

H93.23 Hyperacusis
DEF: Exceptionally acute sense of hearing caused by such conditions as Bell's palsy. This term may also refer to painful sensitivity to sounds.
H93.231 Hyperacusis, right ear
H93.232 Hyperacusis, left ear
H93.233 Hyperacusis, bilateral
H93.239 Hyperacusis, unspecified ear

H93.24 Temporary auditory threshold shift
H93.241 Temporary auditory threshold shift, right ear
H93.242 Temporary auditory threshold shift, left ear
H93.243 Temporary auditory threshold shift, bilateral
H93.249 Temporary auditory threshold shift, unspecified ear

H93.25 Central auditory processing disorder
Congenital auditory imperception
Word deafness
EXCLUDES 1 *mixed receptive-expressive language disorder (F8Ø.2)*

H93.29 Other abnormal auditory perceptions
H93.291 Other abnormal auditory perceptions, right ear
H93.292 Other abnormal auditory perceptions, left ear
H93.293 Other abnormal auditory perceptions, bilateral
H93.299 Other abnormal auditory perceptions, unspecified ear

H93.3 Disorders of acoustic nerve
Disorder of 8th cranial nerve
EXCLUDES 1 *acoustic neuroma (D33.3)*
syphilitic acoustic neuritis (A52.15)

H93.3X Disorders of acoustic nerve
H93.3X1 Disorders of right acoustic nerve
H93.3X2 Disorders of left acoustic nerve
H93.3X3 Disorders of bilateral acoustic nerves
H93.3X9 Disorders of unspecified acoustic nerve

H93.8 Other specified disorders of ear

H93.8X Other specified disorders of ear
H93.8X1 Other specified disorders of right ear
H93.8X2 Other specified disorders of left ear
H93.8X3 Other specified disorders of ear, bilateral
H93.8X9 Other specified disorders of ear, unspecified ear

H93.9 Unspecified disorder of ear
H93.90 Unspecified disorder of ear, unspecified ear UPD
H93.91 Unspecified disorder of right ear UPD
H93.92 Unspecified disorder of left ear UPD
H93.93 Unspecified disorder of ear, bilateral UPD

H94 Other disorders of ear in diseases classified elsewhere

H94.Ø Acoustic neuritis in infectious and parasitic diseases classified elsewhere
Code first underlying disease, such as:
parasitic disease (B65-B89)
EXCLUDES 1 *acoustic neuritis (in):*
herpes zoster (BØ2.29)
syphilis (A52.15)
H94.ØØ Acoustic neuritis in infectious and parasitic diseases classified elsewhere, unspecified ear
H94.Ø1 Acoustic neuritis in infectious and parasitic diseases classified elsewhere, right ear
H94.Ø2 Acoustic neuritis in infectious and parasitic diseases classified elsewhere, left ear
H94.Ø3 Acoustic neuritis in infectious and parasitic diseases classified elsewhere, bilateral

H94.8 Other specified disorders of ear in diseases classified elsewhere
Code first underlying disease, such as:
congenital syphilis (A5Ø.Ø)
EXCLUDES 1 *aural myiasis (B87.4)*
syphilitic labyrinthitis (A52.79)
H94.8Ø Other specified disorders of ear in diseases classified elsewhere, unspecified ear
H94.81 Other specified disorders of right ear in diseases classified elsewhere
H94.82 Other specified disorders of left ear in diseases classified elsewhere
H94.83 Other specified disorders of ear in diseases classified elsewhere, bilateral

Intraoperative and postprocedural complications and disorders of ear and mastoid process, not elsewhere classified (H95)

H95 Intraoperative and postprocedural complications and disorders of ear and mastoid process, not elsewhere classified
AHA: 2016,4Q,9-10

H95.Ø Recurrent cholesteatoma of postmastoidectomy cavity
H95.ØØ Recurrent cholesteatoma of postmastoidectomy cavity, unspecified ear
H95.Ø1 Recurrent cholesteatoma of postmastoidectomy cavity, right ear
H95.Ø2 Recurrent cholesteatoma of postmastoidectomy cavity, left ear
H95.Ø3 Recurrent cholesteatoma of postmastoidectomy cavity, bilateral ears

H95.1 Other disorders of ear and mastoid process following mastoidectomy

H95.11 Chronic inflammation of postmastoidectomy cavity
H95.111 Chronic inflammation of postmastoidectomy cavity, right ear
H95.112 Chronic inflammation of postmastoidectomy cavity, left ear
H95.113 Chronic inflammation of postmastoidectomy cavity, bilateral ears
H95.119 Chronic inflammation of postmastoidectomy cavity, unspecified ear

H95.12 Granulation of postmastoidectomy cavity
H95.121 Granulation of postmastoidectomy cavity, right ear
H95.122 Granulation of postmastoidectomy cavity, left ear
H95.123 Granulation of postmastoidectomy cavity, bilateral ears
H95.129 Granulation of postmastoidectomy cavity, unspecified ear

H95.13 Mucosal cyst of postmastoidectomy cavity
H95.131 Mucosal cyst of postmastoidectomy cavity, right ear
H95.132 Mucosal cyst of postmastoidectomy cavity, left ear
H95.133 Mucosal cyst of postmastoidectomy cavity, bilateral ears
H95.139 Mucosal cyst of postmastoidectomy cavity, unspecified ear

H95.19 Other disorders following mastoidectomy
H95.191 Other disorders following mastoidectomy, right ear
H95.192 Other disorders following mastoidectomy, left ear
H95.193 Other disorders following mastoidectomy, bilateral ears
H95.199 Other disorders following mastoidectomy, unspecified ear

H95.2 Intraoperative hemorrhage and hematoma of ear and mastoid process complicating a procedure

EXCLUDES 1 *intraoperative hemorrhage and hematoma of ear and mastoid process due to accidental puncture or laceration during a procedure (H95.3-)*

H95.21 Intraoperative hemorrhage and hematoma of ear and mastoid process complicating a procedure on the ear and mastoid process CC

H95.22 Intraoperative hemorrhage and hematoma of ear and mastoid process complicating other procedure CC

H95.3 Accidental puncture and laceration of ear and mastoid process during a procedure

H95.31 Accidental puncture and laceration of the ear and mastoid process during a procedure on the ear and mastoid process CC

H95.32 Accidental puncture and laceration of the ear and mastoid process during other procedure CC

H95.4 Postprocedural hemorrhage of ear and mastoid process following a procedure

H95.41 Postprocedural hemorrhage of ear and mastoid process following a procedure on the ear and mastoid process CC

H95.42 Postprocedural hemorrhage of ear and mastoid process following other procedure CC

H95.5 Postprocedural hematoma and seroma of ear and mastoid process following a procedure

H95.51 Postprocedural hematoma of ear and mastoid process following a procedure on the ear and mastoid process CC

H95.52 Postprocedural hematoma of ear and mastoid process following other procedure CC

H95.53 Postprocedural seroma of ear and mastoid process following a procedure on the ear and mastoid process CC

H95.54 Postprocedural seroma of ear and mastoid process following other procedure CC

H95.8 Other intraoperative and postprocedural complications and disorders of the ear and mastoid process, not elsewhere classified

EXCLUDES 2 *postprocedural complications and disorders following mastoidectomy (H95.Ø-, H95.1-)*

H95.81 Postprocedural stenosis of external ear canal

H95.811 Postprocedural stenosis of right external ear canal CC

H95.812 Postprocedural stenosis of left external ear canal CC

H95.813 Postprocedural stenosis of external ear canal, bilateral CC

H95.819 Postprocedural stenosis of unspecified external ear canal CC UNS

H95.88 Other intraoperative complications and disorders of the ear and mastoid process, not elsewhere classified CC

Use additional code, if applicable, to further specify disorder

H95.89 Other postprocedural complications and disorders of the ear and mastoid process, not elsewhere classified CC

Use additional code, if applicable, to further specify disorder

Chapter 9. Diseases of the Circulatory System (I00–I99)

Chapter-specific Guidelines with Coding Examples

The chapter-specific guidelines from the ICD-10-CM Official Guidelines for Coding and Reporting have been provided below. Along with these guidelines are coding examples, contained in the shaded boxes, that have been developed to help illustrate the coding and/or sequencing guidance found in these guidelines.

a. Hypertension

The classification presumes a causal relationship between hypertension and heart involvement and between hypertension and kidney involvement, as the two conditions are linked by the term "with" in the Alphabetic Index. These conditions should be coded as related even in the absence of provider documentation explicitly linking them, unless the documentation clearly states the conditions are unrelated.

For hypertension and conditions not specifically linked by relational terms such as "with," "associated with" or "due to" in the classification, provider documentation must link the conditions in order to code them as related.

1) Hypertension with heart disease

Hypertension with heart conditions classified to I50.- or I51.4-I51.7, I51.89, I51.9, are assigned to a code from category I11, Hypertensive heart disease. Use additional code(s) from category I50, Heart failure, to identify the type(s) of heart failure in those patients with heart failure.

The same heart conditions (I50.-, I51.4-I51.7, I51.89, I51.9) with hypertension are coded separately if the provider has documented they are unrelated to the hypertension. Sequence according to the circumstances of the admission/encounter.

Patient is admitted in left heart failure. Patient also has a history of hypertension managed by medication.

I11.0	**Hypertensive heart disease with heart failure**
I50.1	**Left ventricular failure, unspecified**

Explanation: Without a diagnostic statement to the contrary, hypertension and heart failure have an assumed causal relationship, and a combination code should be used. An additional code to identify the type of heart failure (I50.-) should also be provided.

2) Hypertensive chronic kidney disease

Assign codes from category I12, Hypertensive chronic kidney disease, when both hypertension and a condition classifiable to category N18, Chronic kidney disease (CKD), are present. CKD should not be coded as hypertensive if the provider indicates the CKD is not related to the hypertension.

The appropriate code from category N18 should be used as a secondary code with a code from category I12 to identify the stage of chronic kidney disease.

See Section I.C.14. Chronic kidney disease.

If a patient has hypertensive chronic kidney disease and acute renal failure, the acute renal failure should also be coded. Sequence according to the circumstances of the admission/encounter.

Patient is admitted with stage IV chronic kidney disease (CKD) due to polycystic kidney disease. Patient also is on lisinopril for hypertension.

N18.4	**Chronic kidney disease, stage 4 (severe)**
Q61.3	**Polycystic kidney, unspecified**
I10	**Essential (primary) hypertension**

Explanation: A combination code describing a relationship between hypertension and CKD is not used because the physician documentation identifies the polycystic kidney disease as the cause for the CKD.

3) Hypertensive heart and chronic kidney disease

Assign codes from combination category I13, Hypertensive heart and chronic kidney disease, when there is hypertension with both heart and kidney involvement. If heart failure is present, assign an additional code from category I50 to identify the type of heart failure.

The appropriate code from category N18, Chronic kidney disease, should be used as a secondary code with a code from category I13 to identify the stage of chronic kidney disease.

See Section I.C.14. Chronic kidney disease.

The codes in category I13, Hypertensive heart and chronic kidney disease, are combination codes that include hypertension, heart disease and chronic kidney disease. The Includes note at I13 specifies that the conditions included at I11 and I12 are included together in I13. If a patient has hypertension, heart disease and chronic kidney disease, then a code from I13 should be used, not individual codes for hypertension, heart disease and chronic kidney disease, or codes from I11 or I12.

For patients with both acute renal failure and chronic kidney disease, the acute renal failure should also be coded. Sequence according to the circumstances of the admission/encounter.

Patient admitted with acute tubular necrosis, history of hypertensive heart and kidney disease with congestive heart failure and stage 3a chronic kidney disease

N17.0	**Acute kidney failure with tubular necrosis**
I13.0	**Hypertensive heart and chronic kidney disease with heart failure and stage 1 through stage 4 chronic kidney disease, or unspecified chronic kidney disease**
I50.9	**Heart failure, unspecified**
N18.31	**Chronic kidney disease, stage 3a**

Explanation: It is appropriate to report an acute kidney failure code and a chronic kidney failure code when both conditions are treated during an encounter. In this instance, the acute renal failure was the focus of treatment and therefore sequenced as principal diagnosis. Combination codes in category I13 are used to report conditions classifiable to *both* categories I11 and I12. Do not report conditions classifiable to I11 and I12 separately. Use additional codes to report the type of heart failure and stage of CKD.

4) Hypertensive cerebrovascular disease

For hypertensive cerebrovascular disease, first assign the appropriate code from categories I60-I69, followed by the appropriate hypertension code.

Rupture of cerebral aneurysm caused by malignant hypertension

I60.7	**Nontraumatic subarachnoid hemorrhage from unspecified intracranial artery**
I10	**Essential (primary) hypertension**

Explanation: Hypertensive cerebrovascular disease requires two codes: the appropriate I60–I69 code followed by the appropriate hypertension code.

5) Hypertensive retinopathy

Subcategory H35.0, Background retinopathy and retinal vascular changes, should be used along with a code from categories I10-I15, in the Hypertensive diseases section, to include the systemic hypertension. The sequencing is based on the reason for the encounter.

6) Hypertension, secondary

Secondary hypertension is due to an underlying condition. Two codes are required: one to identify the underlying etiology and one from category I15 to identify the hypertension. Sequencing of codes is determined by the reason for admission/encounter.

Renovascular hypertension due to renal artery atherosclerosis

I15.0	**Renovascular hypertension**
I70.1	**Atherosclerosis of renal artery**

Explanation: Secondary hypertension requires two codes: a code to identify the etiology and the appropriate I15 code.

7) Hypertension, transient

Assign code R03.0, Elevated blood pressure reading without diagnosis of hypertension, unless patient has an established diagnosis of hypertension. Assign code O13.-, Gestational [pregnancy-induced] hypertension without significant proteinuria, or O14.-, Pre-eclampsia, for transient hypertension of pregnancy.

8) Hypertension, controlled

This diagnostic statement usually refers to an existing state of hypertension under control by therapy. Assign the appropriate code from categories I10-I15, Hypertensive diseases.

9) Hypertension, uncontrolled

Uncontrolled hypertension may refer to untreated hypertension or hypertension not responding to current therapeutic regimen. In either case, assign the appropriate code from categories I10-I15, Hypertensive diseases.

10) Hypertensive crisis

Assign a code from category I16, Hypertensive crisis, for documented hypertensive urgency, hypertensive emergency or unspecified hypertensive crisis. Code also any identified hypertensive disease (I10-I15). The sequencing is based on the reason for the encounter.

11) Pulmonary hypertension

Pulmonary hypertension is classified to category I27, Other pulmonary heart diseases. For secondary pulmonary hypertension (I27.1, I27.2-), code also any associated conditions or adverse effects of drugs or toxins. The sequencing is based on the reason for the encounter, except for adverse effects of drugs (See Section I.C.19.e.).

b. Atherosclerotic coronary artery disease and angina

ICD-10-CM has combination codes for atherosclerotic heart disease with angina pectoris. The subcategories for these codes are I25.11, Atherosclerotic heart disease of native coronary artery with angina pectoris and I25.7, Atherosclerosis of coronary artery bypass graft(s) and coronary artery of transplanted heart with angina pectoris.

When using one of these combination codes it is not necessary to use an additional code for angina pectoris. A causal relationship can be assumed in a patient with both atherosclerosis and angina pectoris, unless the documentation indicates the angina is due to something other than the atherosclerosis.

If a patient with coronary artery disease is admitted due to an acute myocardial infarction (AMI), the AMI should be sequenced before the coronary artery disease.

See Section I.C.9. Acute myocardial infarction (AMI)

c. Intraoperative and postprocedural cerebrovascular accident

Medical record documentation should clearly specify the cause- and- effect relationship between the medical intervention and the cerebrovascular accident in order to assign a code for intraoperative or postprocedural cerebrovascular accident.

Proper code assignment depends on whether it was an infarction or hemorrhage and whether it occurred intraoperatively or postoperatively. If it was a cerebral hemorrhage, code assignment depends on the type of procedure performed.

Embolic cerebral infarction of the right middle cerebral artery that occurred during hip replacement surgery. The surgeon documented as due to the surgery.

I97.811 **Intraoperative cerebrovascular infarction during other surgery**

I63.411 **Cerebral infarction due to embolism of right middle cerebral artery**

Explanation: Code assignment for intraoperative or postprocedural cerebrovascular accident is based on the provider's documentation of a cause-and-effect relationship between the condition and the procedure. Proper code assignment also depends on whether the cerebrovascular accident was an infarction or hemorrhage, occurred intraoperatively or postoperatively, and the type of procedure performed.

d. Sequelae of cerebrovascular disease

1) Category I69, Sequelae of cerebrovascular disease

Category I69 is used to indicate conditions classifiable to categories I60-I67 as the causes of sequela (neurologic deficits), themselves classified elsewhere. These "late effects" include neurologic deficits that persist after initial onset of conditions classifiable to categories I60-I67. The neurologic deficits caused by cerebrovascular disease may be present from the onset or may arise at any time after the onset of the condition classifiable to categories I60-I67.

Codes from category I69, Sequelae of cerebrovascular disease, that specify hemiplegia, hemiparesis and monoplegia identify whether the dominant or nondominant side is affected. Should the affected side be documented, but not specified as dominant or nondominant, and the classification system does not indicate a default, code selection is as follows:

- For ambidextrous patients, the default should be dominant.
- If the left side is affected, the default is non-dominant.
- If the right side is affected, the default is dominant.

2) Codes from category I69 with codes from I60-I67

Codes from category I69 may be assigned on a health care record with codes from I60-I67, if the patient has a current cerebrovascular disease and deficits from an old cerebrovascular disease.

3) Codes from category I69 and personal history of transient ischemic attack (TIA) and cerebral infarction (Z86.73)

Codes from category I69 should not be assigned if the patient does not have neurologic deficits.

See Section I.C.21.4. History (of) for use of personal history codes

e. Acute myocardial infarction (AMI)

1) Type 1 ST elevation myocardial infarction (STEMI) and non ST elevation myocardial infarction (NSTEMI)

The ICD-10-CM codes for type 1 acute myocardial infarction (AMI) identify the site, such as anterolateral wall or true posterior wall. Subcategories I21.0-I21.2 and code I21.3 are used for type 1 ST elevation myocardial infarction (STEMI). Code I21.4, Non-ST elevation (NSTEMI) myocardial infarction, is used for type 1 non-ST elevation myocardial infarction (NSTEMI) and nontransmural MIs.

If a type 1 NSTEMI evolves to STEMI, assign the STEMI code. If a type 1 STEMI converts to NSTEMI due to thrombolytic therapy, it is still coded as STEMI.

For encounters occurring while the myocardial infarction is equal to, or less than, four weeks old, including transfers to another acute setting or a postacute setting, and the myocardial infarction meets the definition for "other diagnoses" (see Section III, Reporting Additional Diagnoses), codes from category I21 may continue to be reported. For encounters after the 4-week time frame and the patient is still receiving care related to the myocardial infarction, the appropriate aftercare code should be assigned, rather than a code from category I21. For old or healed myocardial infarctions not requiring further care, code I25.2, Old myocardial infarction, may be assigned.

2) Acute myocardial infarction, unspecified

Code I21.9, Acute myocardial infarction, unspecified, is the default for unspecified acute myocardial infarction or unspecified type. If only type 1 STEMI or transmural MI without the site is documented, assign code I21.3, ST elevation (STEMI) myocardial infarction of unspecified site.

3) AMI documented as nontransmural or subendocardial but site provided

If an AMI is documented as nontransmural or subendocardial, but the site is provided, it is still coded as a subendocardial AMI.

See Section I.C.21.3. for information on coding status post administration of tPA in a different facility within the last 24 hours.

4) Subsequent acute myocardial infarction

A code from category I22, Subsequent ST elevation (STEMI) and non-ST elevation (NSTEMI) myocardial infarction, is to be used when a patient who has suffered a type 1 or unspecified AMI has a new AMI within the 4-week time frame of the initial AMI. A code from category I22 must be used in conjunction with a code from category I21. The sequencing of the I22 and I21 codes depends on the circumstances of the encounter.

Do not assign code I22 for subsequent myocardial infarctions other than type 1 or unspecified. For subsequent type 2 AMI assign only code I21.A1. For subsequent type 4 or type 5 AMI, assign only code I21.A9.

If a subsequent myocardial infarction of one type occurs within 4 weeks of a myocardial infarction of a different type, assign the appropriate codes from category I21 to identify each type. Do not assign a code from I22. Codes from category I22 should only be assigned if both the initial and subsequent myocardial infarctions are type 1 or unspecified.

5) Other types of myocardial infarction

The ICD-10-CM provides codes for different types of myocardial infarction. Type 1 myocardial infarctions are assigned to codes I21.0-I21.4.

Type 2 myocardial infarction (myocardial infarction due to demand ischemia or secondary to ischemic imbalance) is assigned to code I21.A1, Myocardial infarction type 2 with the underlying cause coded first. Do not assign code I24.8, Other forms of acute ischemic heart disease, for the demand ischemia. If a type 2 AMI is described as NSTEMI or STEMI, only assign code I21.A1. Codes I21.01-I21.4 should only be assigned for type 1 AMIs.

Acute myocardial infarctions type 3, 4a, 4b, 4c and 5 are assigned to code I21.A9, Other myocardial infarction type.

The "Code also" and "Code first" notes should be followed related to complications, and for coding of postprocedural myocardial infarctions during or following cardiac surgery.

Myocardial infarction involving the left circumflex artery occurring during PTCA with stent insertion to treat coronary artery disease

I25.10 **Atherosclerotic heart disease of native coronary artery without angina pectoris**

I97.790 **Other intraoperative cardiac functional disturbances during cardiac surgery**

I21.A9 **Other myocardial infarction type**

Explanation: A myocardial infarction occurring during a revascularization procedure is not considered a type 1 myocardial infarction (MI) and should not be coded to a type 1 MI code (I21.0-, I21.1-, I21.2-, I21.3) even when the specific site of the MI is documented. According to the code first instruction at I21.A9, the complication code (I97.790) should be sequenced before code I21.A9.

Chapter 9. Diseases of the Circulatory System (I00-I99)

EXCLUDES 2 *certain conditions originating in the perinatal period (P04-P96)*
certain infectious and parasitic diseases (A00-B99)
complications of pregnancy, childbirth and the puerperium (O00-O9A)
congenital malformations, deformations, and chromosomal abnormalities (Q00-Q99)
endocrine, nutritional and metabolic diseases (E00-E88)
injury, poisoning and certain other consequences of external causes (S00-T88)
neoplasms (C00-D49)
symptoms, signs and abnormal clinical and laboratory findings, not elsewhere classified (R00-R94)
systemic connective tissue disorders (M30-M36)
transient cerebral ischemic attacks and related syndromes (G45.-)

This chapter contains the following blocks:

I00-I02 Acute rheumatic fever
I05-I09 Chronic rheumatic heart diseases
I10-I16 Hypertensive diseases
I20-I25 Ischemic heart diseases
I26-I28 Pulmonary heart disease and diseases of pulmonary circulation
I30-I5A Other forms of heart disease
I60-I69 Cerebrovascular diseases
I70-I79 Diseases of arteries, arterioles and capillaries
I80-I89 Diseases of veins, lymphatic vessels and lymph nodes, not elsewhere classified
I95-I99 Other and unspecified disorders of the circulatory system

Acute rheumatic fever (I00-I02)

DEF: Rheumatic fever: Inflammatory disease that can follow a throat infection by group A *streptococci*. Complications can involve the joints (arthritis), subcutaneous tissue (nodules), skin (erythema marginatum), heart (carditis), or brain (chorea).

I00 Rheumatic fever without heart involvement
INCLUDES arthritis, rheumatic, acute or subacute
EXCLUDES 1 *rheumatic fever with heart involvement (I01.0-I01.9)*

✓4th **I01 Rheumatic fever with heart involvement**
EXCLUDES 1 *chronic diseases of rheumatic origin (I05-I09) unless rheumatic fever is also present or there is evidence of reactivation or activity of the rheumatic process*

I01.0 Acute rheumatic pericarditis CC
Any condition in I00 with pericarditis
Rheumatic pericarditis (acute)
EXCLUDES 1 *acute pericarditis not specified as rheumatic (I30.-)*

I01.1 Acute rheumatic endocarditis CC
Any condition in I00 with endocarditis or valvulitis
Acute rheumatic valvulitis

I01.2 Acute rheumatic myocarditis CC
Any condition in I00 with myocarditis

I01.8 Other acute rheumatic heart disease CC
Any condition in I00 with other or multiple types of heart involvement
Acute rheumatic pancarditis

I01.9 Acute rheumatic heart disease, unspecified CC
Any condition in I00 with unspecified type of heart involvement
Rheumatic carditis, acute
Rheumatic heart disease, active or acute

✓4th **I02 Rheumatic chorea**
INCLUDES Sydenham's chorea
EXCLUDES 1 *chorea NOS (G25.5)*
Huntington's chorea (G10)

I02.0 Rheumatic chorea with heart involvement CC
Chorea NOS with heart involvement
Rheumatic chorea with heart involvement of any type classifiable under I01.-

I02.9 Rheumatic chorea without heart involvement CC
Rheumatic chorea NOS

Chronic rheumatic heart diseases (I05-I09)

✓4th **I05 Rheumatic mitral valve diseases**
INCLUDES conditions classifiable to both I05.0 and I05.2-I05.9, whether specified as rheumatic or not
EXCLUDES 1 *mitral valve disease specified as nonrheumatic (I34.-)*
mitral valve disease with aortic and/or tricuspid valve involvement (I08.-)

I05.0 Rheumatic mitral stenosis
Mitral (valve) obstruction (rheumatic)

I05.1 Rheumatic mitral insufficiency
Rheumatic mitral incompetence
Rheumatic mitral regurgitation
EXCLUDES 1 *mitral insufficiency not specified as rheumatic (I34.0)*

I05.2 Rheumatic mitral stenosis with insufficiency
Rheumatic mitral stenosis with incompetence or regurgitation

I05.8 Other rheumatic mitral valve diseases
Rheumatic mitral (valve) failure

I05.9 Rheumatic mitral valve disease, unspecified
Rheumatic mitral (valve) disorder (chronic) NOS

✓4th **I06 Rheumatic aortic valve diseases**
EXCLUDES 1 *aortic valve disease not specified as rheumatic (I35.-)*
aortic valve disease with mitral and/or tricuspid valve involvement (I08.-)

I06.0 Rheumatic aortic stenosis
Rheumatic aortic (valve) obstruction

I06.1 Rheumatic aortic insufficiency
Rheumatic aortic incompetence
Rheumatic aortic regurgitation

I06.2 Rheumatic aortic stenosis with insufficiency
Rheumatic aortic stenosis with incompetence or regurgitation

I06.8 Other rheumatic aortic valve diseases

I06.9 Rheumatic aortic valve disease, unspecified
Rheumatic aortic (valve) disease NOS

✓4th **I07 Rheumatic tricuspid valve diseases**
INCLUDES rheumatic tricuspid valve diseases specified as rheumatic or unspecified
EXCLUDES 1 *tricuspid valve disease specified as nonrheumatic (I36.-)*
tricuspid valve disease with aortic and/or mitral valve involvement (I08.-)

I07.0 Rheumatic tricuspid stenosis
Tricuspid (valve) stenosis (rheumatic)

I07.1 Rheumatic tricuspid insufficiency
Tricuspid (valve) insufficiency (rheumatic)

I07.2 Rheumatic tricuspid stenosis and insufficiency

I07.8 Other rheumatic tricuspid valve diseases

I07.9 Rheumatic tricuspid valve disease, unspecified
Rheumatic tricuspid valve disorder NOS

✓4th **I08 Multiple valve diseases**
INCLUDES multiple valve diseases specified as rheumatic or unspecified
EXCLUDES 1 *endocarditis, valve unspecified (I38)*
multiple valve disease specified a nonrheumatic (I34.-, I35.-, I36.-, I37.-, I38.-, Q22.-, Q23.-, Q24.8-)
rheumatic valve disease NOS (I09.1)

I08.0 Rheumatic disorders of both mitral and aortic valves
Involvement of both mitral and aortic valves specified as rheumatic or unspecified
AHA: 2019,2Q,5

I08.1 Rheumatic disorders of both mitral and tricuspid valves

I08.2 Rheumatic disorders of both aortic and tricuspid valves

I08.3 Combined rheumatic disorders of mitral, aortic and tricuspid valves

I08.8 Other rheumatic multiple valve diseases

I08.9 Rheumatic multiple valve disease, unspecified

✓4th **I09 Other rheumatic heart diseases**

I09.0 Rheumatic myocarditis CC
EXCLUDES 1 *myocarditis not specified as rheumatic (I51.4)*

I09.1 Rheumatic diseases of endocardium, valve unspecified
Rheumatic endocarditis (chronic)
Rheumatic valvulitis (chronic)
EXCLUDES 1 *endocarditis, valve unspecified (I38)*

I09.2 Chronic rheumatic pericarditis CC
Adherent pericardium, rheumatic
Chronic rheumatic mediastinopericarditis
Chronic rheumatic myopericarditis
EXCLUDES 1 *chronic pericarditis not specified as rheumatic (I31.-)*

✓5th **I09.8 Other specified rheumatic heart diseases**

I09.81 Rheumatic heart failure CC HCC
Use additional code to identify type of heart failure (I50.-)

I09.89 Other specified rheumatic heart diseases
Rheumatic disease of pulmonary valve

I09.9 Rheumatic heart disease, unspecified
Rheumatic carditis
EXCLUDES 1 *rheumatoid carditis (M05.31)*

Hypertensive diseases (I10-I16)

Use additional code to identify:
exposure to environmental tobacco smoke (Z77.22)
history of tobacco dependence (Z87.891)
occupational exposure to environmental tobacco smoke (Z57.31)
tobacco dependence (F17.-)
tobacco use (Z72.0)

EXCLUDES 1 *neonatal hypertension (P29.2)*
primary pulmonary hypertension (I27.0)
EXCLUDES 2 *hypertensive disease complicating pregnancy, childbirth and the puerperium (O10-O11, O13-O16)*

I10 Essential (primary) hypertension
INCLUDES high blood pressure
hypertension (arterial) (benign) (essential) (malignant) (primary) (systemic)
EXCLUDES 1 *hypertensive disease complicating pregnancy, childbirth and the puerperium (O10-O11, O13-O16)*
EXCLUDES 2 *essential (primary) hypertension involving vessels of brain (I60-I69)*
essential (primary) hypertension involving vessels of eye (H35.0-)
AHA: 2022,1Q,36; 2020,1Q,12; 2018,2Q,9; 2016,4Q,27

✓4th **I11 Hypertensive heart disease**
INCLUDES any condition in I50.- or I51.4-I51.7, I51.89, I51.9 due to hypertension
AHA: 2018,2Q,9
TIP: Do not assign a code from this category when provider documentation indicates the heart disease is attributable to another cause.

I11.0 Hypertensive heart disease with heart failure HCC
Hypertensive heart failure
Use additional code to identify type of heart failure (I50.-)
AHA: 2017,1Q,47

I11.9 Hypertensive heart disease without heart failure
Hypertensive heart disease NOS

✓4th **I12 Hypertensive chronic kidney disease**
INCLUDES any condition in N18 and N26 — due to hypertension
arteriosclerosis of kidney
arteriosclerotic nephritis (chronic) (interstitial)
hypertensive nephropathy
nephrosclerosis
EXCLUDES 1 *hypertension due to kidney disease (I15.0, I15.1)*
renovascular hypertension (I15.0)
secondary hypertension (I15.-)
EXCLUDES 2 *acute kidney failure (N17.-)*
AHA: 2019,3Q,3; 2018,4Q,88; 2016,3Q,22
TIP: Do not assign a code from this category when provider documentation indicates the chronic kidney disease (CKD) is attributable to another cause.

I12.0 Hypertensive chronic kidney disease with stage 5 chronic kidney disease or end stage renal disease CC HCC
Use additional code to identify the stage of chronic kidney disease (N18.5, N18.6)

I12.9 Hypertensive chronic kidney disease with stage 1 through stage 4 chronic kidney disease, or unspecified chronic kidney disease
Hypertensive chronic kidney disease NOS
Hypertensive renal disease NOS
Use additional code to identify the stage of chronic kidney disease (N18.1-N18.4, N18.9)

✓4th **I13 Hypertensive heart and chronic kidney disease**
INCLUDES any condition in I11.- with any condition in I12.-
cardiorenal disease
cardiovascular renal disease
TIP: Do not assign a code from this category when provider documentation indicates the heart and/or chronic kidney disease is attributable to another cause.

I13.0 Hypertensive heart and chronic kidney disease with heart failure and stage 1 through stage 4 chronic kidney disease, or unspecified chronic kidney disease CC HCC
Use additional code to identify type of heart failure (I50.-)
Use additional code to identify stage of chronic kidney disease (N18.1-N18.4, N18.9)

✓5th **I13.1 Hypertensive heart and chronic kidney disease without heart failure**

I13.10 Hypertensive heart and chronic kidney disease without heart failure, with stage 1 through stage 4 chronic kidney disease, or unspecified chronic kidney disease
Hypertensive heart disease and hypertensive chronic kidney disease NOS
Use additional code to identify the stage of chronic kidney disease (N18.1-N18.4, N18.9)

I13.11 Hypertensive heart and chronic kidney disease without heart failure, with stage 5 chronic kidney disease, or end stage renal disease CC HCC
Use additional code to identify the stage of chronic kidney disease (N18.5, N18.6)

I13.2 Hypertensive heart and chronic kidney disease with heart failure and with stage 5 chronic kidney disease, or end stage renal disease CC HCC
Use additional code to identify type of heart failure (I50.-)
Use additional code to identify the stage of chronic kidney disease (N18.5, N18.6)

✓4th **I15 Secondary hypertension**
Code also underlying condition
EXCLUDES 1 *postprocedural hypertension (I97.3)*
EXCLUDES 2 *secondary hypertension involving vessels of brain (I60-I69)*
secondary hypertension involving vessels of eye (H35.0-)

I15.0 Renovascular hypertension
I15.1 Hypertension secondary to other renal disorders
AHA: 2016,3Q,22
I15.2 Hypertension secondary to endocrine disorders
I15.8 Other secondary hypertension
I15.9 Secondary hypertension, unspecified

✓4th **I16 Hypertensive crisis**
Code also any identified hypertensive disease (I10-I15)
AHA: 2016,4Q,26-28
I16.0 Hypertensive urgency
I16.1 Hypertensive emergency CC
I16.9 Hypertensive crisis, unspecified CC

Ischemic heart diseases (I20-I25)

Code also the presence of hypertension (I10-I16)

✓4th **I20 Angina pectoris**
Use additional code to identify:
exposure to environmental tobacco smoke (Z77.22)
history of tobacco dependence (Z87.891)
occupational exposure to environmental tobacco smoke (Z57.31)
tobacco dependence (F17.-)
tobacco use (Z72.0)
EXCLUDES 1 *angina pectoris with atherosclerotic heart disease of native coronary arteries (I25.1-)*
atherosclerosis of coronary artery bypass graft(s) and coronary artery of transplanted heart with angina pectoris (I25.7-)
postinfarction angina (I23.7)
DEF: Chest pain due to reduced blood flow resulting in a lack of oxygen to the heart muscles.

I20.0 Unstable angina CC HCC
Accelerated angina
Crescendo angina
De novo effort angina
Intermediate coronary syndrome
Preinfarction syndrome
Worsening effort angina

I20.1 Angina pectoris with documented spasm CC HCC
Angiospastic angina
Prinzmetal angina
Spasm-induced angina
Variant angina

● **I20.2 Refractory angina pectoris** CC

I2Ø.8 Other forms of angina pectoris HCC
Angina equivalent
Angina of effort
Coronary slow flow syndrome
Stable angina
Stenocardia
Use additional code(s) for symptoms associated with angina equivalent

I2Ø.9 Angina pectoris, unspecified HCC
Angina NOS
Anginal syndrome
Cardiac angina
Ischemic chest pain

✓4th I21 Acute myocardial infarction
INCLUDES cardiac infarction
coronary (artery) embolism
coronary (artery) occlusion
coronary (artery) rupture
coronary (artery) thrombosis
infarction of heart, myocardium, or ventricle
myocardial infarction specified as acute or with a stated duration of 4 weeks (28 days) or less from onset

Use additional code, if applicable, to identify:
exposure to environmental tobacco smoke (Z77.22)
history of tobacco dependence (Z87.891)
occupational exposure to environmental tobacco smoke (Z57.31)
status post administration of tPA (rtPA) in a different facility within the last 24 hours prior to admission to current facility (Z92.82)
tobacco dependence (F17.-)
tobacco use (Z72.Ø)

EXCLUDES 2 *old myocardial infarction (I25.2)*
postmyocardial infarction syndrome (I24.1)
subsequent type 1 myocardial infarction (I22.-)

AHA: 2019,2Q,5; 2018,4Q,68; 2018,3Q,5; 2017,4Q,12-14; 2017,1Q,44-45; 2016,4Q,140; 2015,2Q,16; 2013,1Q,25; 2012,4Q,96,102-103

TIP: When chronic total occlusion and myocardial infarction are documented as being in different vessels, assign code I25.82 Chronic total occlusion of coronary artery, in addition to the myocardial infarction code.

✓5th I21.Ø ST elevation (STEMI) myocardial infarction of anterior wall
Type 1 ST elevation myocardial infarction of anterior wall
DEF: ST elevation myocardial infarction: Complete obstruction of one or more coronary arteries causing decreased blood flow (ischemia) and necrosis of myocardial muscle cells.

I21.Ø1 ST elevation (STEMI) myocardial infarction involving left main coronary artery MCC HCC

I21.Ø2 ST elevation (STEMI) myocardial infarction involving left anterior descending coronary artery MCC HCC
ST elevation (STEMI) myocardial infarction involving diagonal coronary artery
AHA: 2013,1Q,25

I21.Ø9 ST elevation (STEMI) myocardial infarction involving other coronary artery of anterior wall MCC HCC
Acute transmural myocardial infarction of anterior wall
Anteroapical transmural (Q wave) infarction (acute)
Anterolateral transmural (Q wave) infarction (acute)
Anteroseptal transmural (Q wave) infarction (acute)
Transmural (Q wave) infarction (acute) (of) anterior (wall) NOS
AHA: 2012,4Q,102-103

✓5th I21.1 ST elevation (STEMI) myocardial infarction of inferior wall
Type 1 ST elevation myocardial infarction of inferior wall
DEF: ST elevation myocardial infarction: Complete obstruction of one or more coronary arteries causing decreased blood flow (ischemia) and necrosis of myocardial muscle cells.

I21.11 ST elevation (STEMI) myocardial infarction involving right coronary artery MCC HCC
Inferoposterior transmural (Q wave) infarction (acute)

I21.19 ST elevation (STEMI) myocardial infarction involving other coronary artery of inferior wall MCC HCC
Acute transmural myocardial infarction of inferior wall
Inferolateral transmural (Q wave) infarction (acute)
Transmural (Q wave) infarction (acute) (of) diaphragmatic wall
Transmural (Q wave) infarction (acute) (of) inferior (wall) NOS
EXCLUDES 2 *ST elevation (STEMI) myocardial infarction involving left circumflex coronary artery (I21.21)*
AHA: 2012,4Q,96

✓5th I21.2 ST elevation (STEMI) myocardial infarction of other sites
Type 1 ST elevation myocardial infarction of other sites
DEF: ST elevation myocardial infarction: Complete obstruction of one or more coronary arteries causing decreased blood flow (ischemia) and necrosis of myocardial muscle cells.

I21.21 ST elevation (STEMI) myocardial infarction involving left circumflex coronary artery MCC HCC
ST elevation (STEMI) myocardial infarction involving oblique marginal coronary artery

I21.29 ST elevation (STEMI) myocardial infarction involving other sites MCC HCC
Acute transmural myocardial infarction of other sites
Apical-lateral transmural (Q wave) infarction (acute)
Basal-lateral transmural (Q wave) infarction (acute)
High lateral transmural (Q wave) infarction (acute)
Lateral (wall) NOS transmural (Q wave) infarction (acute)
Posterior (true) transmural (Q wave) infarction (acute)
Posterobasal transmural (Q wave) infarction (acute)
Posterolateral transmural (Q wave) infarction (acute)
Posteroseptal transmural (Q wave) infarction (acute)
Septal transmural (Q wave) infarction (acute) NOS

I21.3 ST elevation (STEMI) myocardial infarction of unspecified site MCC HCC
Acute transmural myocardial infarction of unspecified site
Transmural (Q wave) myocardial infarction NOS
Type 1 ST elevation myocardial infarction of unspecified site
DEF: ST elevation myocardial infarction: Complete obstruction of one or more coronary arteries causing decreased blood flow (ischemia) and necrosis of myocardial muscle cells.

I21.4 Non-ST elevation (NSTEMI) myocardial infarction MCC HCC
Acute subendocardial myocardial infarction
Non-Q wave myocardial infarction NOS
Nontransmural myocardial infarction NOS
Type 1 non-ST elevation myocardial infarction
AHA: 2021,3Q,6; 2019,2Q,33; 2017,1Q,44-45
DEF: Partial obstruction of one or more coronary arteries that causes decreased blood flow (ischemia) and may cause partial thickness necrosis of myocardial muscle cells.

I21.9 Acute myocardial infarction, unspecified MCC HCC
Myocardial infarction (acute) NOS

✓5th I21.A Other type of myocardial infarction
AHA: 2019,2Q,5

I21.A1 Myocardial infarction type 2 MCC HCC
Myocardial infarction due to demand ischemia
Myocardial infarction secondary to ischemic imbalance
Code first the underlying cause, such as:
anemia (D5Ø.Ø-D64.9)
chronic obstructive pulmonary disease (J44.-)
paroxysmal tachycardia (I47.Ø-I47.9)
shock (R57.Ø-R57.9)
AHA: 2019,4Q,53; 2017,4Q,13-14
DEF: Often referred to as due to demand ischemia, myocardial infarction (MI) type 2 refers to an MI due to ischemia and necrosis resulting from an oxygen imbalance to the heart. This mismatch between oxygen decreased supply and increased demand is caused by conditions other than coronary artery disease such as vasospasm, embolism, anemia, hypertension, hypotension, or arrhythmias.

I21.A9 Other myocardial infarction type MCC HCC

Myocardial infarction associated with revascularization procedure
Myocardial infarction type 3
Myocardial infarction type 4a
Myocardial infarction type 4b
Myocardial infarction type 4c
Myocardial infarction type 5

Code first, if applicable, postprocedural myocardial infarction following cardiac surgery (I97.190), or postprocedural myocardial infarction during cardiac surgery (I97.790)

Code also complication, if known and applicable, such as:
(acute) stent occlusion (T82.897-)
(acute) stent stenosis (T82.855-)
(acute) stent thrombosis (T82.867-)
cardiac arrest due to underlying cardiac condition (I46.2)
complication of percutaneous coronary intervention (PCI) (I97.89)
occlusion of coronary artery bypass graft (T82.218-)

AHA: 2021,3Q,6; 2019,2Q,33

I22 Subsequent ST elevation (STEMI) and non-ST elevation (NSTEMI) myocardial infarction

INCLUDES acute myocardial infarction occurring within four weeks (28 days) of a previous acute myocardial infarction, regardless of site
cardiac infarction
coronary (artery) embolism
coronary (artery) occlusion
coronary (artery) rupture
coronary (artery) thrombosis
infarction of heart, myocardium, or ventricle
recurrent myocardial infarction
reinfarction of myocardium
rupture of heart, myocardium, or ventricle
subsequent type 1 myocardial infarction

Use additional code, if applicable, to identify:
exposure to environmental tobacco smoke (Z77.22)
history of tobacco dependence (Z87.891)
occupational exposure to environmental tobacco smoke (Z57.31)
status post administration of tPA (rtPA) in a different facility within the last 24 hours prior to admission to current facility (Z92.82)
tobacco dependence (F17.-)
tobacco use (Z72.0)

EXCLUDES 1 *subsequent myocardial infarction, type 2 (I21.A1)*
subsequent myocardial infarction of other type (type 3) (type 4) (type 5) (I21.A9)

AHA: 2018,4Q,68; 2018,3Q,5; 2017,4Q,12-13; 2017,2Q,11; 2013,1Q,25; 2012,4Q,97,102-103

DEF: Non-ST elevation myocardial infarction: Partial obstruction of one or more coronary arteries that causes decreased blood flow (ischemia) and may cause partial thickness necrosis of myocardial muscle cells.

DEF: ST elevation myocardial infarction: Complete obstruction of one or more coronary arteries causing decreased blood flow (ischemia) and necrosis of myocardial muscle cells.

TIP: When chronic total occlusion and myocardial infarction are documented as being in different vessels, assign code I25.82 Chronic total occlusion of coronary artery, in addition to the myocardial infarction code.

I22.0 Subsequent ST elevation (STEMI) myocardial infarction of anterior wall MCC HCC

Subsequent acute transmural myocardial infarction of anterior wall
Subsequent transmural (Q wave) infarction (acute)(of) anterior (wall) NOS
Subsequent anteroapical transmural (Q wave) infarction (acute)
Subsequent anterolateral transmural (Q wave) infarction (acute)
Subsequent anteroseptal transmural (Q wave) infarction (acute)

I22.1 Subsequent ST elevation (STEMI) myocardial infarction of inferior wall MCC HCC

Subsequent acute transmural myocardial infarction of inferior wall
Subsequent transmural (Q wave) infarction (acute)(of) diaphragmatic wall
Subsequent transmural (Q wave) infarction (acute)(of) inferior (wall) NOS
Subsequent inferolateral transmural (Q wave) infarction (acute)
Subsequent inferoposterior transmural (Q wave) infarction (acute)

AHA: 2012,4Q,102

I22.2 Subsequent non-ST elevation (NSTEMI) myocardial infarction MCC HCC

Subsequent acute subendocardial myocardial infarction
Subsequent non-Q wave myocardial infarction NOS
Subsequent nontransmural myocardial infarction NOS

I22.8 Subsequent ST elevation (STEMI) myocardial infarction of other sites MCC HCC

Subsequent acute transmural myocardial infarction of other sites
Subsequent apical-lateral transmural (Q wave) myocardial infarction (acute)
Subsequent basal-lateral transmural (Q wave) myocardial infarction (acute)
Subsequent high lateral transmural (Q wave) myocardial infarction (acute)
Subsequent transmural (Q wave) myocardial infarction (acute)(of) lateral (wall) NOS
Subsequent posterior (true) transmural (Q wave) myocardial infarction (acute)
Subsequent posterobasal transmural (Q wave) myocardial infarction (acute)
Subsequent posterolateral transmural (Q wave) myocardial infarction (acute)
Subsequent posteroseptal transmural (Q wave) myocardial infarction (acute)
Subsequent septal NOS transmural (Q wave) myocardial infarction (acute)

I22.9 Subsequent ST elevation (STEMI) myocardial infarction of unspecified site MCC HCC

Subsequent acute myocardial infarction of unspecified site
Subsequent myocardial infarction (acute) NOS

I23 Certain current complications following ST elevation (STEMI) and non-ST elevation (NSTEMI) myocardial infarction (within the 28 day period)

AHA: 2017,2Q,11

DEF: ST elevation myocardial infarction: Complete obstruction of one or more coronary arteries causing decreased blood flow (ischemia) and necrosis of myocardial muscle cells.

DEF: Non-ST elevation myocardial infarction: Partial obstruction of one or more coronary arteries that causes decreased blood flow (ischemia) and may cause partial thickness necrosis of myocardial muscle cells.

I23.0 Hemopericardium as current complication following acute myocardial infarction CC HCC A

EXCLUDES 1 *hemopericardium not specified as current complication following acute myocardial infarction (I31.2)*

I23.1 Atrial septal defect as current complication following acute myocardial infarction CC HCC A

EXCLUDES 1 *acquired atrial septal defect not specified as current complication following acute myocardial infarction (I51.0)*

I23.2 Ventricular septal defect as current complication following acute myocardial infarction CC HCC A

EXCLUDES 1 *acquired ventricular septal defect not specified as current complication following acute myocardial infarction (I51.0)*

I23.3 Rupture of cardiac wall without hemopericardium as current complication following acute myocardial infarction CC HCC A

I23.4 Rupture of chordae tendineae as current complication following acute myocardial infarction MCC HCC

EXCLUDES 1 *rupture of chordae tendineae not specified as current complication following acute myocardial infarction (I51.1)*

I23.5 Rupture of papillary muscle as current complication following acute myocardial infarction MCC HCC

EXCLUDES 1 *rupture of papillary muscle not specified as current complication following acute myocardial infarction (I51.2)*

I23.6 Thrombosis of atrium, auricular appendage, and ventricle as current complications following acute myocardial infarction CC HCC A

EXCLUDES 1 *thrombosis of atrium, auricular appendage, and ventricle not specified as current complication following acute myocardial infarction (I51.3)*

I23.7 Postinfarction angina CC HCC A

AHA: 2015,2Q,16

TIP: When postinfarction angina occurs with atherosclerotic coronary artery disease, code both I23.7 and I25.118 for atherosclerotic disease with other forms of angina pectoris.

I23.8 Other current complications following acute myocardial infarction CC HCC A

✓4th I24 Other acute ischemic heart diseases

EXCLUDES 1 *angina pectoris (I2Ø.-)*
transient myocardial ischemia in newborn (P29.4)

EXCLUDES 2 *non-ischemic myocardial injury (I5A)*

I24.Ø Acute coronary thrombosis not resulting in myocardial infarction CC HCC

Acute coronary (artery) (vein) embolism not resulting in myocardial infarction

Acute coronary (artery) (vein) occlusion not resulting in myocardial infarction

Acute coronary (artery) (vein) thromboembolism not resulting in myocardial infarction

EXCLUDES 1 *atherosclerotic heart disease (I25.1-)*

AHA: 2013,1Q,24

I24.1 Dressler's syndrome CC HCC

Postmyocardial infarction syndrome

EXCLUDES 1 *postinfarction angina (I23.7)*

DEF: Fever, leukocytosis, chest pain, evidence of pericarditis, pleurisy, and pneumonia occurring days or weeks after a myocardial infarction.

I24.8 Other forms of acute ischemic heart disease CC HCC

EXCLUDES 1 *myocardial infarction due to demand ischemia (I21.A1)*

AHA: 2019,4Q,53; 2017,4Q,13

I24.9 Acute ischemic heart disease, unspecified CC HCC

EXCLUDES 1 *ischemic heart disease (chronic) NOS (I25.9)*

✓4th I25 Chronic ischemic heart disease

Use additional code to identify:
- chronic total occlusion of coronary artery (I25.82)
- exposure to environmental tobacco smoke (Z77.22)
- history of tobacco dependence (Z87.891)
- occupational exposure to environmental tobacco smoke (Z57.31)
- tobacco dependence (F17.-)
- tobacco use (Z72.Ø)

EXCLUDES 2 *non-ischemic myocardial injury (I5A)*

✓5th I25.1 Atherosclerotic heart disease of native coronary artery

Atherosclerotic cardiovascular disease
Coronary (artery) atheroma
Coronary (artery) atherosclerosis
Coronary (artery) disease
Coronary (artery) sclerosis

Use additional code, if applicable, to identify:
- coronary atherosclerosis due to calcified coronary lesion (I25.84)
- coronary atherosclerosis due to lipid rich plaque (I25.83)

EXCLUDES 2 *atheroembolism (I75.-)*
atherosclerosis of coronary artery bypass graft(s) and transplanted heart (I25.7-)

Atheromas

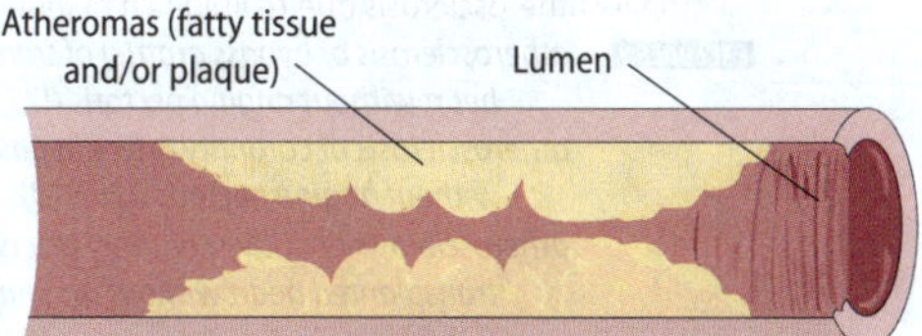

I25.1Ø Atherosclerotic heart disease of native coronary artery without angina pectoris A

Atherosclerotic heart disease NOS

AHA: 2021,3Q,6-7; 2015,2Q,16; 2012,4Q,92

✓6th I25.11 Atherosclerotic heart disease of native coronary artery with angina pectoris

I25.11Ø Atherosclerotic heart disease of native coronary artery with unstable angina pectoris CC HCC A

EXCLUDES 1 *unstable angina without atherosclerotic heart disease (I2Ø.Ø)*

I25.111 Atherosclerotic heart disease of native coronary artery with angina pectoris with documented spasm HCC A

EXCLUDES 1 *angina pectoris with documented spasm without atherosclerotic heart disease (I2Ø.1)*

● **I25.112 Atherosclerosic heart disease of native coronary artery with refractory angina pectoris** CC A

I25.118 Atherosclerotic heart disease of native coronary artery with other forms of angina pectoris HCC A

EXCLUDES 1 *other forms of angina pectoris without atherosclerotic heart disease (I2Ø.8)*

AHA: 2015,2Q,16

TIP: When postinfarction angina occurs with atherosclerotic coronary artery disease, code both I23.7 and I25.118 for atherosclerotic disease with other forms of angina pectoris.

I25.119 Atherosclerotic heart disease of native coronary artery with unspecified angina pectoris HCC A

Atherosclerotic heart disease with angina NOS

Atherosclerotic heart disease with ischemic chest pain

EXCLUDES 1 *unspecified angina pectoris without atherosclerotic heart disease (I2Ø.9)*

I25.2 Old myocardial infarction
Healed myocardial infarction
Past myocardial infarction diagnosed by ECG or other investigation, but currently presenting no symptoms

I25.3 Aneurysm of heart CC
Mural aneurysm
Ventricular aneurysm

✓5th **I25.4 Coronary artery aneurysm and dissection**

I25.41 Coronary artery aneurysm
Coronary arteriovenous fistula, acquired
EXCLUDES 1 *congenital coronary (artery) aneurysm (Q24.5)*

I25.42 Coronary artery dissection MCC
DEF: Tear in the intimal arterial wall of a coronary artery resulting in the sudden intrusion of blood within the layers of the wall.

I25.5 Ischemic cardiomyopathy
EXCLUDES 2 *coronary atherosclerosis (I25.1-, I25.7-)*

I25.6 Silent myocardial ischemia

✓5th **I25.7 Atherosclerosis of coronary artery bypass graft(s) and coronary artery of transplanted heart with angina pectoris**
Use additional code, if applicable, to identify:
coronary atherosclerosis due to calcified coronary lesion (I25.84)
coronary atherosclerosis due to lipid rich plaque (I25.83)
EXCLUDES 1 *atherosclerosis of bypass graft(s) of transplanted heart without angina pectoris (I25.812)*
atherosclerosis of coronary artery bypass graft(s) without angina pectoris (I25.810)
atherosclerosis of native coronary artery of transplanted heart without angina pectoris (I25.811)

✓6th **I25.70 Atherosclerosis of coronary artery bypass graft(s), unspecified, with angina pectoris**

I25.700 Atherosclerosis of coronary artery bypass graft(s), unspecified, with unstable angina pectoris CC HCC A
EXCLUDES 1 *unstable angina pectoris without atherosclerosis of coronary artery bypass graft (I20.0)*

I25.701 Atherosclerosis of coronary artery bypass graft(s), unspecified, with angina pectoris with documented spasm HCC A
EXCLUDES 1 *angina pectoris with documented spasm without atherosclerosis of coronary artery bypass graft (I20.1)*

● **I25.702 Atherosclerosis of coronary artery bypass graft(s), unspecified, with refractory angina pectoris** CC A

I25.708 Atherosclerosis of coronary artery bypass graft(s), unspecified, with other forms of angina pectoris HCC A
EXCLUDES 1 *other forms of angina pectoris without atherosclerosis of coronary artery bypass graft (I20.8)*

I25.709 Atherosclerosis of coronary artery bypass graft(s), unspecified, with unspecified angina pectoris HCC A
EXCLUDES 1 *unspecified angina pectoris without atherosclerosis of coronary artery bypass graft (I20.9)*

✓6th **I25.71 Atherosclerosis of autologous vein coronary artery bypass graft(s) with angina pectoris**

I25.710 Atherosclerosis of autologous vein coronary artery bypass graft(s) with unstable angina pectoris CC HCC A
EXCLUDES 1 *unstable angina without atherosclerosis of autologous vein coronary artery bypass graft(s) (I20.0)*
EXCLUDES 2 *embolism or thrombus of coronary artery bypass graft(s) (T82.8-)*

I25.711 Atherosclerosis of autologous vein coronary artery bypass graft(s) with angina pectoris with documented spasm CC HCC A
EXCLUDES 1 *angina pectoris with documented spasm without atherosclerosis of autologous vein coronary artery bypass graft(s) (I20.1)*

● **I25.712 Atherosclerosis of autologous vein coronary artery bypass graft(s) with refractory angina pectoris** CC A

I25.718 Atherosclerosis of autologous vein coronary artery bypass graft(s) with other forms of angina pectoris CC HCC A
EXCLUDES 1 *other forms of angina pectoris without atherosclerosis of autologous vein coronary artery bypass graft(s) (I20.8)*

I25.719 Atherosclerosis of autologous vein coronary artery bypass graft(s) with unspecified angina pectoris CC HCC A
EXCLUDES 1 *unspecified angina pectoris without atherosclerosis of autologous vein coronary artery bypass graft(s) (I20.9)*

✓6th **I25.72 Atherosclerosis of autologous artery coronary artery bypass graft(s) with angina pectoris**
Atherosclerosis of internal mammary artery graft with angina pectoris

I25.720 Atherosclerosis of autologous artery coronary artery bypass graft(s) with unstable angina pectoris CC HCC A
EXCLUDES 1 *unstable angina without atherosclerosis of autologous artery coronary artery bypass graft(s) (I20.0)*

I25.721 Atherosclerosis of autologous artery coronary artery bypass graft(s) with angina pectoris with documented spasm CC HCC A
EXCLUDES 1 *angina pectoris with documented spasm without atherosclerosis of autologous artery coronary artery bypass graft(s) (I20.1)*

● **I25.722 Atherosclerosis of autologous artery coronary artery bypass graft(s) with refractory angina pectoris** CC A

I25.728 Atherosclerosis of autologous artery coronary artery bypass graft(s) with other forms of angina pectoris CC HCC A
EXCLUDES 1 *other forms of angina pectoris without atherosclerosis of autologous artery coronary artery bypass graft(s) (I20.8)*

I25.729 Atherosclerosis of autologous artery coronary artery bypass graft(s) with unspecified angina pectoris CC HCC A

EXCLUDES 1 *unspecified angina pectoris without atherosclerosis of autologous artery coronary artery bypass graft(s) (I20.9)*

✓6th **I25.73 Atherosclerosis of nonautologous biological coronary artery bypass graft(s) with angina pectoris**

I25.730 Atherosclerosis of nonautologous biological coronary artery bypass graft(s) with unstable angina pectoris CC HCC A

EXCLUDES 1 *unstable angina without atherosclerosis of nonautologous biological coronary artery bypass graft(s) (I20.0)*

I25.731 Atherosclerosis of nonautologous biological coronary artery bypass graft(s) with angina pectoris with documented spasm CC HCC A

EXCLUDES 1 *angina pectoris with documented spasm without atherosclerosis of nonautologous biological coronary artery bypass graft(s) (I20.1)*

● **I25.732 Atherosclerosis of nonautologous biological coronary artery bypass graft(s) with refractory angina pectoris** CC A

I25.738 Atherosclerosis of nonautologous biological coronary artery bypass graft(s) with other forms of angina pectoris CC HCC A

EXCLUDES 1 *other forms of angina pectoris without atherosclerosis of nonautologous biological coronary artery bypass graft(s) (I20.8)*

I25.739 Atherosclerosis of nonautologous biological coronary artery bypass graft(s) with unspecified angina pectoris CC HCC A

EXCLUDES 1 *unspecified angina pectoris without atherosclerosis of nonautologous biological coronary artery bypass graft(s) (I20.9)*

✓6th **I25.75 Atherosclerosis of native coronary artery of transplanted heart with angina pectoris**

EXCLUDES 1 *atherosclerosis of native coronary artery of transplanted heart without angina pectoris (I25.811)*

I25.750 Atherosclerosis of native coronary artery of transplanted heart with unstable angina CC HCC

I25.751 Atherosclerosis of native coronary artery of transplanted heart with angina pectoris with documented spasm CC HCC

● **I25.752 Atherosclerosis of native coronary artery of transplanted heart with refractory angina pectoris** CC A

I25.758 Atherosclerosis of native coronary artery of transplanted heart with other forms of angina pectoris CC HCC

I25.759 Atherosclerosis of native coronary artery of transplanted heart with unspecified angina pectoris CC HCC

✓6th **I25.76 Atherosclerosis of bypass graft of coronary artery of transplanted heart with angina pectoris**

EXCLUDES 1 *atherosclerosis of bypass graft of coronary artery of transplanted heart without angina pectoris (I25.812)*

I25.760 Atherosclerosis of bypass graft of coronary artery of transplanted heart with unstable angina CC HCC A

I25.761 Atherosclerosis of bypass graft of coronary artery of transplanted heart with angina pectoris with documented spasm CC HCC A

● **I25.762 Atherosclerosis of bypass graft of coronary artery of transplanted heart with refractory angina pectoris** CC A

I25.768 Atherosclerosis of bypass graft of coronary artery of transplanted heart with other forms of angina pectoris CC HCC A

I25.769 Atherosclerosis of bypass graft of coronary artery of transplanted heart with unspecified angina pectoris CC HCC A

✓6th **I25.79 Atherosclerosis of other coronary artery bypass graft(s) with angina pectoris**

I25.790 Atherosclerosis of other coronary artery bypass graft(s) with unstable angina pectoris CC HCC A

EXCLUDES 1 *unstable angina without atherosclerosis of other coronary artery bypass graft(s) (I20.0)*

I25.791 Atherosclerosis of other coronary artery bypass graft(s) with angina pectoris with documented spasm CC HCC A

EXCLUDES 1 *angina pectoris with documented spasm without atherosclerosis of other coronary artery bypass graft(s) (I20.1)*

● **I25.792 Atherosclerosis of other coronary artery bypass graft(s) with refractory angina pectoris** CC A

I25.798 Atherosclerosis of other coronary artery bypass graft(s) with other forms of angina pectoris CC HCC A

EXCLUDES 1 *other forms of angina pectoris without atherosclerosis of other coronary artery bypass graft(s) (I20.8)*

I25.799 Atherosclerosis of other coronary artery bypass graft(s) with unspecified angina pectoris CC HCC A

EXCLUDES 1 *unspecified angina pectoris without atherosclerosis of other coronary artery bypass graft(s) (I20.9)*

✓5th **I25.8 Other forms of chronic ischemic heart disease**

✓6th **I25.81 Atherosclerosis of other coronary vessels without angina pectoris**

Use additional code, if applicable, to identify:

coronary atherosclerosis due to calcified coronary lesion (I25.84)

coronary atherosclerosis due to lipid rich plaque (I25.83)

EXCLUDES 2 *atherosclerotic heart disease of native coronary artery without angina pectoris (I25.10)*

I25.810 Atherosclerosis of coronary artery bypass graft(s) without angina pectoris CC A

Atherosclerosis of coronary artery bypass graft NOS

EXCLUDES 1 *atherosclerosis of coronary bypass graft(s) with angina pectoris (I25.70-I25.73-, I25.79-)*

I25.811 Atherosclerosis of native coronary artery of transplanted heart without angina pectoris CC

Atherosclerosis of native coronary artery of transplanted heart NOS

EXCLUDES 1 *atherosclerosis of native coronary artery of transplanted heart with angina pectoris (I25.75-)*

I25.812 Atherosclerosis of bypass graft of coronary artery of transplanted heart without angina pectoris CC A

Atherosclerosis of bypass graft of transplanted heart NOS

EXCLUDES 1 *atherosclerosis of bypass graft of transplanted heart with angina pectoris (I25.76)*

I25.82 Chronic total occlusion of coronary artery UPD

Complete occlusion of coronary artery

Total occlusion of coronary artery

Code first coronary atherosclerosis (I25.1-, I25.7-, I25.81-)

EXCLUDES 1 *acute coronary occulsion with myocardial infarction (I21.Ø-I21.9, I22.-)*

acute coronary occlusion without myocardial infarction (I24.Ø)

AHA: 2018,3Q,5

DEF: Complete blockage of the coronary artery due to plaque accumulation over an extended period of time, resulting in substantial reduction of blood flow. Symptoms include angina or chest pain.

TIP: Report this code in addition to a code from category I21 or I22 when the chronic total occlusion and the myocardial infarction are documented as being in different vessels.

I25.83 Coronary atherosclerosis due to lipid rich plaque UPD A

Code first coronary atherosclerosis (I25.1-, I25.7-, I25.81-)

I25.84 Coronary atherosclerosis due to calcified coronary lesion UPD

Coronary atherosclerosis due to severely calcified coronary lesion

Code first coronary atherosclerosis (I25.1-, I25.7-, I25.81-)

I25.89 Other forms of chronic ischemic heart disease

I25.9 Chronic ischemic heart disease, unspecified

Ischemic heart disease (chronic) NOS

Pulmonary heart disease and diseases of pulmonary circulation (I26-I28)

I26 Pulmonary embolism (4th)

INCLUDES pulmonary (acute)(artery)(vein) infarction

pulmonary (acute) (artery)(vein) thromboembolism

pulmonary (acute)(artery)(vein) thrombosis

EXCLUDES 2 *chronic pulmonary embolism (I27.82)*

personal history of pulmonary embolism (Z86.711)

pulmonary embolism complicating abortion, ectopic or molar pregnancy (OØØ-OØ7, OØ8.2)

pulmonary embolism complicating pregnancy, childbirth and the puerperium (O88.-)

pulmonary embolism due to trauma (T79.Ø, T79.1)

pulmonary embolism due to complications of surgical and medical care (T8Ø.Ø, T81.7-, T82.8-)

septic (non-pulmonary) arterial embolism (I76)

I26.Ø Pulmonary embolism with acute cor pulmonale (5th)

DEF: Cor pulmonale: Heart-lung disease appearing in identifiable forms as chronic or acute. The chronic form of this heart-lung disease is marked by dilation, hypertrophy and failure of the right ventricle due to a disease that has affected the function of the lungs, excluding congenital or left heart diseases and is also called chronic cardiopulmonary disease. The acute form is an overload of the right ventricle from a rapid onset of pulmonary hypertension, usually arising from a pulmonary embolism.

I26.Ø1 Septic pulmonary embolism with acute cor pulmonale MCC UPD HCC

Code first underlying infection

I26.Ø2 Saddle embolus of pulmonary artery with acute cor pulmonale MCC H10 HCC

I26.Ø9 Other pulmonary embolism with acute cor pulmonale MCC H10 HCC

Acute cor pulmonale NOS

AHA: 2014,4Q,21

I26.9 Pulmonary embolism without acute cor pulmonale (5th)

I26.9Ø Septic pulmonary embolism without acute cor pulmonale MCC UPD HCC

Code first underlying infection

I26.92 Saddle embolus of pulmonary artery without acute cor pulmonale MCC H10 HCC

I26.93 Single subsegmental pulmonary embolism without acute cor pulmonale MCC H10 HCC

Subsegmental pulmonary embolism NOS

AHA: 2021,2Q,9; 2019,4Q,6-7

I26.94 Multiple subsegmental pulmonary emboli without acute cor pulmonale MCC H10 HCC

AHA: 2022,2Q,13; 2021,2Q,9; 2019,4Q,6-7

I26.99 Other pulmonary embolism without acute cor pulmonale MCC H10 HCC

Acute pulmonary embolism NOS

Pulmonary embolism NOS

AHA: 2022,2Q,13; 2020,3Q,10-11; 2019,2Q,22

I27 Other pulmonary heart diseases (4th)

I27.Ø Primary pulmonary hypertension CC HCC

Heritable pulmonary arterial hypertension

Idiopathic pulmonary arterial hypertension

Primary group 1 pulmonary hypertension

Primary pulmonary arterial hypertension

EXCLUDES 1 *persistent pulmonary hypertension of newborn (P29.3Ø)*

pulmonary hypertension NOS (I27.2Ø)

secondary pulmonary arterial hypertension (I27.21)

secondary pulmonary hypertension (I27.29)

DEF: Condition that occurs when pressure within the pulmonary artery is elevated and vascular resistance is observed in the lungs.

I27.1 Kyphoscoliotic heart disease CC HCC

I27.2 Other secondary pulmonary hypertension (5th)

Code also associated underlying condition

EXCLUDES 1 *Eisenmenger's syndrome (I27.83)*

AHA: 2017,4Q,14-15; 2014,4Q,21

DEF: Condition that occurs when pressure within the pulmonary artery is elevated and vascular resistance is observed in the lungs.

I27.2Ø Pulmonary hypertension, unspecified HCC

Pulmonary hypertension NOS

I27.21 Secondary pulmonary arterial hypertension HCC

(Associated) (drug-induced) (toxin-induced) pulmonary arterial hypertension NOS

(Associated) (drug-induced) (toxin-induced) (secondary) group 1 pulmonary hypertension

Code also associated conditions if applicable, or adverse effects of drugs or toxins, such as:

adverse effect of appetite depressants (T5Ø.5X5)

congenital heart disease (Q2Ø-Q28)

human immunodeficiency virus [HIV] disease (B2Ø)

polymyositis (M33.2-)

portal hypertension (K76.6)

rheumatoid arthritis (MØ5.-)

schistosomiasis (B65.-)

Sjögren syndrome (M35.Ø-)

systemic sclerosis (M34.-)

I27.22 Pulmonary hypertension due to left heart disease HCC

Group 2 pulmonary hypertension

Code also associated left heart disease, if known, such as:

multiple valve disease (IØ8.-)

rheumatic aortic valve diseases (IØ6.-)

rheumatic mitral valve diseases (IØ5.-)

I27.23 Pulmonary hypertension due to lung diseases and hypoxia HCC

Group 3 pulmonary hypertension

Code also associated lung disease, if known, such as:

bronchiectasis (J47.-)

cystic fibrosis with pulmonary manifestations (E84.Ø)

interstitial lung disease (J84.-)

pleural effusion (J9Ø)

sleep apnea (G47.3-)

I27.24 Chronic thromboembolic pulmonary hypertension HCC
Group 4 pulmonary hypertension
Code also associated pulmonary embolism, if applicable (I26.-, I27.82)

I27.29 Other secondary pulmonary hypertension HCC
Group 5 pulmonary hypertension
Pulmonary hypertension with unclear multifactorial mechanisms
Pulmonary hypertension due to hematologic disorders
Pulmonary hypertension due to metabolic disorders
Pulmonary hypertension due to other systemic disorders
Code also other associated disorders, if known, such as:
chronic myeloid leukemia (C92.1Ø-C92.22)
essential thrombocythemia (D47.3)
Gaucher disease (E75.22)
hypertensive chronic kidney disease with end stage renal disease (I12.Ø, I13.11, I13.2)
hyperthyroidism (EØ5.-)
hypothyroidism (EØØ-EØ3)
polycythemia vera (D45)
sarcoidosis (D86.-)
AHA: 2016,2Q,8

✓5th **I27.8 Other specified pulmonary heart diseases**

I27.81 Cor pulmonale (chronic) HCC
Cor pulmonale NOS
EXCLUDES 1 *acute cor pulmonale (I26.Ø-)*
AHA: 2014,4Q,21
DEF: Heart-lung disease appearing in identifiable forms as chronic or acute. The chronic form of this heart-lung disease is marked by dilation, hypertrophy and failure of the right ventricle due to a disease that has affected the function of the lungs, excluding congenital or left heart diseases and is also called chronic cardiopulmonary disease. The acute form is an overload of the right ventricle from a rapid onset of pulmonary hypertension, usually arising from a pulmonary embolism.

I27.82 Chronic pulmonary embolism CC HCC
Use additional code, if applicable, for associated long-term (current) use of anticoagulants (Z79.Ø1)
EXCLUDES 1 *personal history of pulmonary embolism (Z86.711)*
AHA: 2021,2Q,9
DEF: Long-standing condition commonly associated with pulmonary hypertension in which small blood clots travel to the lungs repeatedly over many weeks, months, or years, requiring continuation of established anticoagulant or thrombolytic therapy.

I27.83 Eisenmenger's syndrome HCC
Eisenmenger's complex
(Irreversible) Eisenmenger's disease
Pulmonary hypertension with right to left shunt related to congenital heart disease
Code also underlying heart defect, if known, such as:
atrial septal defect ▶(Q21.1-)◀
Eisenmenger's defect (Q21.8)
patent ductus arteriosus (Q25.Ø)
ventricular septal defect (Q21.Ø)
DEF: Pulmonary hypertension with congenital communication between two circulations resulting in a right to left shunt. This causes reduced oxygen saturation in the arterial blood, leading to cyanosis and organ damage. Once it develops, this life-threating condition is irreversible.

I27.89 Other specified pulmonary heart diseases HCC

I27.9 Pulmonary heart disease, unspecified HCC
Chronic cardiopulmonary disease

✓4th **I28 Other diseases of pulmonary vessels**

I28.Ø Arteriovenous fistula of pulmonary vessels CC HCC
EXCLUDES 1 *congenital arteriovenous fistula (Q25.72)*

I28.1 Aneurysm of pulmonary artery CC HCC
EXCLUDES 1 *congenital aneurysm (Q25.79)*
congenital arteriovenous aneurysm (Q25.72)

I28.8 Other diseases of pulmonary vessels HCC
Pulmonary arteritis
Pulmonary endarteritis
Rupture of pulmonary vessels
Stenosis of pulmonary vessels
Stricture of pulmonary vessels

I28.9 Disease of pulmonary vessels, unspecified HCC

Other forms of heart disease (I3Ø-I5A)

✓4th **I3Ø Acute pericarditis**
INCLUDES acute mediastinopericarditis
acute myopericarditis
acute pericardial effusion
acute pleuropericarditis
acute pneumopericarditis
EXCLUDES 1 *Dressler's syndrome (I24.1)*
rheumatic pericarditis (acute) (IØ1.Ø)
viral pericarditis due to Coxsakie virus (B33.23)
DEF: Pericarditis: Inflammation affecting the pericardium, the fibroserous membrane that surrounds the heart.

I3Ø.Ø Acute nonspecific idiopathic pericarditis CC

I3Ø.1 Infective pericarditis CC
Pneumococcal pericarditis
Pneumopyopericardium
Purulent pericarditis
Pyopericarditis
Pyopericardium
Pyopneumopericardium
Staphylococcal pericarditis
Streptococcal pericarditis
Suppurative pericarditis
Viral pericarditis
Use additional code (B95-B97) to identify infectious agent

I3Ø.8 Other forms of acute pericarditis CC

I3Ø.9 Acute pericarditis, unspecified CC

✓4th **I31 Other diseases of pericardium**
EXCLUDES 1 *diseases of pericardium specified as rheumatic (IØ9.2)*
postcardiotomy syndrome (I97.Ø)
traumatic injury to pericardium (S26.-)

I31.Ø Chronic adhesive pericarditis CC
Accretio cordis
Adherent pericardium
Adhesive mediastinopericarditis

I31.1 Chronic constrictive pericarditis CC
Concretio cordis
Pericardial calcification

I31.2 Hemopericardium, not elsewhere classified CC
EXCLUDES 1 *hemopericardium as current complication following acute myocardial infarction (I23.Ø)*
▶*malignant pericardial effusion (I31.31)*◀
DEF: Presence of blood in the pericardial sac (pericardium). It can lead to potentially fatal cardiac tamponade if enough blood enters the pericardial cavity.

▲ ✓5th **I31.3 Pericardial effusion (noninflammatory)**
~~Chyloperícardium~~
EXCLUDES 1 *acute pericardial effusion (I3Ø.9)*
AHA: 2019,1Q,16

● *I31.31* ***Malignant pericardial effusion in diseases classified elsewhere*** CC
Code first underlying neoplasm (CØØ-D49)

● **I31.39 Other pericardial effusion (noninflammatory)** CC
Chylopericardium

I31.4 Cardiac tamponade CC UPD
Code first underlying cause
DEF: Life-threatening condition in which fluid or blood accumulates in the space between the muscle of the heart (myocardium) and the outer sac that covers the heart (pericardium), resulting in compression of the heart.

Cardiac Tamponade

Normal
Acute Pericardial Effusion with Cardiac Tamponade
Excessive fluid in pericardial space
Serous pericardium (visceral layer)
Fibrous pericardium
Serous pericardium (parietal layer)
Pericardial space (potential)
constricted areas

I31.8 Other specified diseases of pericardium CC
Epicardial plaques
Focal pericardial adhesions

I31.9 Disease of pericardium, unspecified CC
Pericarditis (chronic) NOS

I32 Pericarditis in diseases classified elsewhere CC
Code first underlying disease
EXCLUDES 1 *pericarditis (in):*
coxsackie (virus) (B33.23)
gonococcal (A54.83)
meningococcal (A39.53)
rheumatoid (arthritis) (MØ5.31)
syphilitic (A52.Ø6)
systemic lupus erythematosus (M32.12)
tuberculosis (A18.84)
DEF: Pericarditis: Inflammation affecting the pericardium, the fibroserous membrane that surrounds the heart.

✓4th **I33 Acute and subacute endocarditis**
EXCLUDES 1 *acute rheumatic endocarditis (IØ1.1)*
endocarditis NOS (I38)
DEF: Endocarditis: Inflammatory disease of the interior lining of the heart chamber and heart valves.

I33.Ø Acute and subacute infective endocarditis HIV MCC
Bacterial endocarditis (acute) (subacute)
Infective endocarditis (acute) (subacute) NOS
Endocarditis lenta (acute) (subacute)
Malignant endocarditis (acute) (subacute)
Purulent endocarditis (acute) (subacute)
Septic endocarditis (acute) (subacute)
Ulcerative endocarditis (acute) (subacute)
Vegetative endocarditis (acute) (subacute)
Use additional code (B95-B97) to identify infectious agent

I33.9 Acute and subacute endocarditis, unspecified HIV MCC
Acute endocarditis NOS
Acute myoendocarditis NOS
Acute periendocarditis NOS
Subacute endocarditis NOS
Subacute myoendocarditis NOS
Subacute periendocarditis NOS

✓4th **I34 Nonrheumatic mitral valve disorders**
EXCLUDES 1 *mitral valve disease (IØ5.9)*
mitral valve failure (IØ5.8)
mitral valve stenosis (IØ5.Ø)
mitral valve disorder of unspecified cause with diseases of aortic and/or tricuspid valve(s) (IØ8.-)
mitral valve disorder of unspecified cause with mitral stenosis or obstruction (IØ5.Ø)
mitral valve disorder specified as congenital (Q23.2, Q23.9)
mitral valve disorder specified as rheumatic (IØ5.-)

I34.Ø Nonrheumatic mitral (valve) insufficiency
Nonrheumatic mitral (valve) incompetence NOS
Nonrheumatic mitral (valve) regurgitation NOS
▶Code also, if applicable:◀
▶nonrheumatic mitral (valve) annulus calcification (I34.81)◀

I34.1 Nonrheumatic mitral (valve) prolapse
Floppy nonrheumatic mitral valve syndrome
EXCLUDES 1 *Marfan's syndrome (Q87.4-)*

I34.2 Nonrheumatic mitral (valve) stenosis
▶Code also, if applicable:◀
▶nonrheumatic mitral (valve) annulus calcification (I34.81)◀

▲ ✓5th **I34.8 Other nonrheumatic mitral valve disorders**

● **I34.81 Nonrheumatic mitral (valve) annulus calcification**
Nonrheumatic mitral (valve) annular calcification
Mitral (valve) annulus calcification NOS
Code also, if applicable:
nonrheumatic mitral (valve) insufficiency (I34.Ø)
nonrheumatic mitral (valve) stenosis (I34.2)

● **I34.89 Other nonrheumatic mitral valve disorders**

I34.9 Nonrheumatic mitral valve disorder, unspecified

✓4th **I35 Nonrheumatic aortic valve disorders**
EXCLUDES 1 *aortic valve disorder of unspecified cause but with diseases of mitral and/or tricuspid valve(s) (IØ8.-)*
aortic valve disorder specified as congenital (Q23.Ø, Q23.1)
aortic valve disorder specified as rheumatic (IØ6.-)
hypertrophic subaortic stenosis (I42.1)

I35.Ø Nonrheumatic aortic (valve) stenosis

I35.1 Nonrheumatic aortic (valve) insufficiency
Nonrheumatic aortic (valve) incompetence NOS
Nonrheumatic aortic (valve) regurgitation NOS

I35.2 Nonrheumatic aortic (valve) stenosis with insufficiency

I35.8 Other nonrheumatic aortic valve disorders

I35.9 Nonrheumatic aortic valve disorder, unspecified

✓4th **I36 Nonrheumatic tricuspid valve disorders**
EXCLUDES 1 *tricuspid valve disorders of unspecified cause (IØ7.-)*
tricuspid valve disorders specified as congenital (Q22.4, Q22.8, Q22.9)
tricuspid valve disorders specified as rheumatic (IØ7.-)
tricuspid valve disorders with aortic and/or mitral valve involvement (IØ8.-)

I36.Ø Nonrheumatic tricuspid (valve) stenosis

I36.1 Nonrheumatic tricuspid (valve) insufficiency
Nonrheumatic tricuspid (valve) incompetence
Nonrheumatic tricuspid (valve) regurgitation

I36.2 Nonrheumatic tricuspid (valve) stenosis with insufficiency

I36.8 Other nonrheumatic tricuspid valve disorders

I36.9 Nonrheumatic tricuspid valve disorder, unspecified

✓4th **I37 Nonrheumatic pulmonary valve disorders**
EXCLUDES 1 *pulmonary valve disorder specified as congenital (Q22.1, Q22.2, Q22.3)*
pulmonary valve disorder specified as rheumatic (IØ9.89)

I37.Ø Nonrheumatic pulmonary valve stenosis

I37.1 Nonrheumatic pulmonary valve insufficiency
Nonrheumatic pulmonary valve incompetence
Nonrheumatic pulmonary valve regurgitation

I37.2 Nonrheumatic pulmonary valve stenosis with insufficiency

I37.8 Other nonrheumatic pulmonary valve disorders

I37.9 Nonrheumatic pulmonary valve disorder, unspecified

I38 Endocarditis, valve unspecified CC

INCLUDES endocarditis (chronic) NOS
valvular incompetence NOS
valvular insufficiency NOS
valvular regurgitation NOS
valvular stenosis NOS
valvulitis (chronic) NOS

EXCLUDES 1 *congenital insufficiency of cardiac valve NOS (Q24.8)*
congenital stenosis of cardiac valve NOS (Q24.8)
endocardial fibroelastosis (I42.4)
endocarditis specified as rheumatic (IØ9.1)

DEF: Endocarditis: Inflammatory disease of the interior lining of the heart chamber and heart valves.

I39 Endocarditis and heart valve disorders in diseases classified elsewhere CC

Code first underlying disease, such as:
Q fever (A78)

EXCLUDES 1 *endocardial involvement in:*
candidiasis (B37.6)
gonococcal infection (A54.83)
Libman-Sacks disease (M32.11)
listerosis (A32.82)
meningococcal infection (A39.51)
rheumatoid arthritis (MØ5.31)
syphilis (A52.Ø3)
tuberculosis (A18.84)
typhoid fever (AØ1.Ø2)

DEF: Endocarditis: Inflammatory disease of the interior lining of the heart chamber and heart valves.

✓4th **I4Ø Acute myocarditis**

INCLUDES subacute myocarditis

EXCLUDES 1 *acute rheumatic myocarditis (IØ1.2)*

DEF: Myocarditis: Inflammation of the middle layer of the heart, which is composed of muscle tissue.

I4Ø.Ø Infective myocarditis HIV MCC
Septic myocarditis
Use additional code (B95-B97) to identify infectious agent

I4Ø.1 Isolated myocarditis HIV MCC
Fiedler's myocarditis
Giant cell myocarditis
Idiopathic myocarditis

I4Ø.8 Other acute myocarditis HIV MCC

I4Ø.9 Acute myocarditis, unspecified HIV MCC

I41 Myocarditis in diseases classified elsewhere MCC

Code first underlying disease, such as:
typhus (A75.Ø-A75.9)

EXCLUDES 1 *myocarditis (in):*
Chagas' disease (chronic) (B57.2)
acute (B57.Ø)
coxsackie (virus) infection (B33.22)
diphtheritic (A36.81)
gonococcal (A54.83)
influenzal (JØ9.X9, J1Ø.82, J11.82)
meningococcal (A39.52)
mumps (B26.82)
rheumatoid arthritis (MØ5.31)
sarcoid (D86.85)
syphilis (A52.Ø6)
toxoplasmosis (B58.81)
tuberculous (A18.84)

DEF: Myocarditis: Inflammation of the middle layer of the heart, which is composed of muscle tissue.

✓4th **I42 Cardiomyopathy**

INCLUDES myocardiopathy

Code first pre-existing cardiomyopathy complicating pregnancy and puerperium (O99.4)

EXCLUDES 2 *ischemic cardiomyopathy (I25.5)*
peripartum cardiomyopathy (O9Ø.3)
ventricular hypertrophy (I51.7)

I42.Ø Dilated cardiomyopathy CC HCC
Congestive cardiomyopathy

I42.1 Obstructive hypertrophic cardiomyopathy CC HCC
Hypertrophic subaortic stenosis (idiopathic)
DEF: Cardiomyopathy marked by left ventricle hypertrophy and an enlarged septum that result in obstructed blood flow, arrhythmias, mitral regurgitation, and sudden cardiac death.
TIP: When this condition is described as inherited, assign code Q24.8.

I42.2 Other hypertrophic cardiomyopathy CC HCC
Nonobstructive hypertrophic cardiomyopathy

I42.3 Endomyocardial (eosinophilic) disease CC HCC
Endomyocardial (tropical) fibrosis
Löffler's endocarditis

I42.4 Endocardial fibroelastosis CC HCC
Congenital cardiomyopathy
Elastomyofibrosis

I42.5 Other restrictive cardiomyopathy CC HCC
Constrictive cardiomyopathy NOS

I42.6 Alcoholic cardiomyopathy CC HCC
Code also presence of alcoholism (F1Ø.-)

I42.7 Cardiomyopathy due to drug and external agent CC HCC
Code first poisoning due to drug or toxin, if applicable (T36-T65 with fifth or sixth character 1-4 or 6)
Use additional code for adverse effect, if applicable, to identify drug (T36-T5Ø with fifth or sixth character 5)
AHA: 2021,3Q,8

I42.8 Other cardiomyopathies CC HCC

I42.9 Cardiomyopathy, unspecified CC HCC
Cardiomyopathy (primary) (secondary) NOS

I43 Cardiomyopathy in diseases classified elsewhere CC HCC

Code first underlying disease, such as:
amyloidosis (E85.-)
glycogen storage disease (E74.Ø)
gout (M1Ø.Ø-)
thyrotoxicosis (EØ5.Ø-EØ5.9-)

EXCLUDES 1 *cardiomyopathy (in):*
coxsackie (virus) (B33.24)
diphtheria (A36.81)
sarcoidosis (D86.85)
tuberculosis (A18.84)

✓4th **I44 Atrioventricular and left bundle-branch block**

I44.Ø Atrioventricular block, first degree

I44.1 Atrioventricular block, second degree
Atrioventricular block, type I and II
Möbitz block, type I and II
Second degree block, type I and II
Wenckebach's block

I44.2 Atrioventricular block, complete CC HCC
Complete heart block NOS
Third degree block
AHA: 2019,2Q,4

✓5th **I44.3 Other and unspecified atrioventricular block**
Atrioventricular block NOS

I44.3Ø Unspecified atrioventricular block

I44.39 Other atrioventricular block

I44.4 Left anterior fascicular block

I44.5 Left posterior fascicular block

✓5th **I44.6 Other and unspecified fascicular block**

I44.6Ø Unspecified fascicular block
Left bundle-branch hemiblock NOS

I44.69 Other fascicular block

I44.7 Left bundle-branch block, unspecified

Conduction Disorders

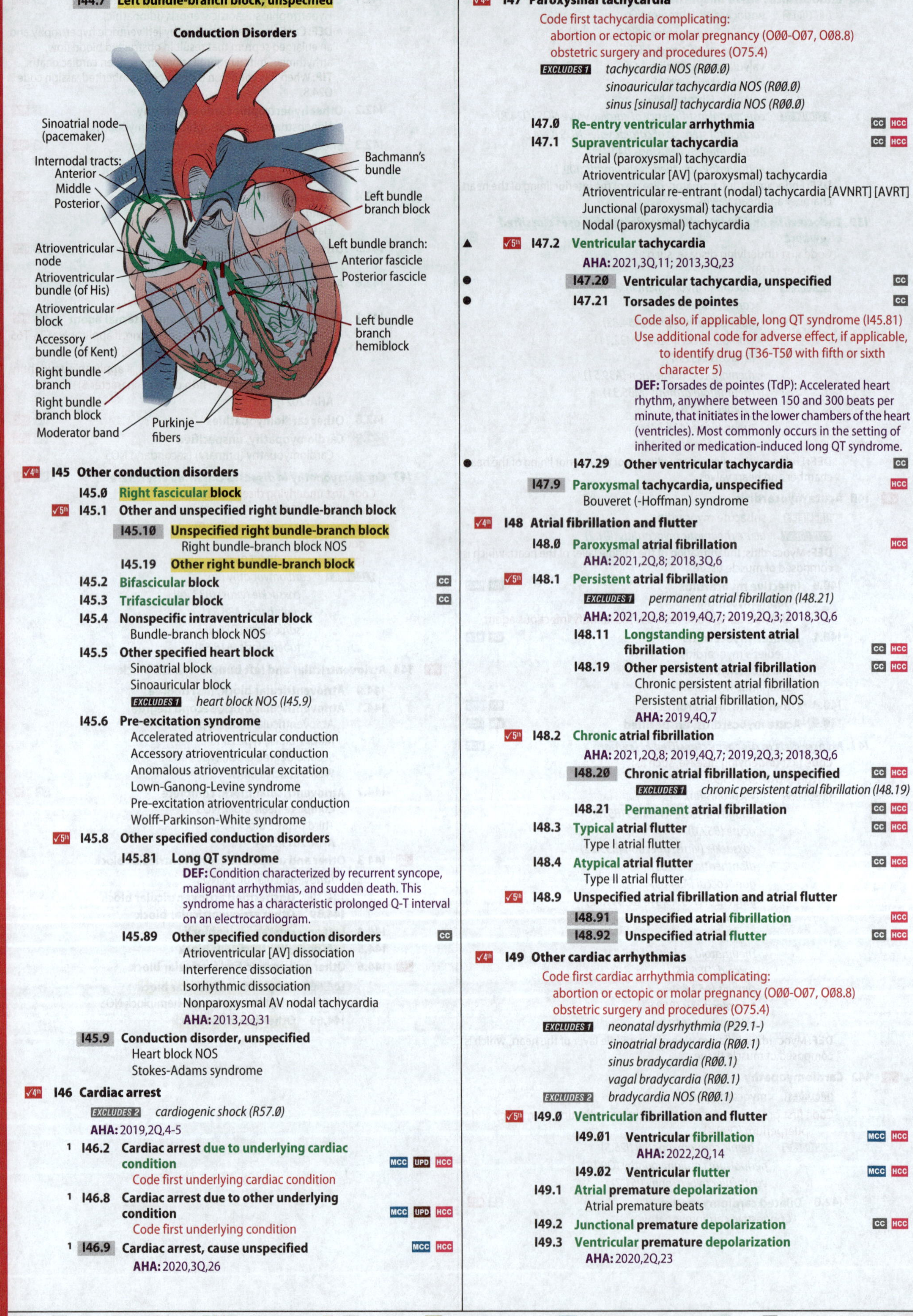

I45 Other conduction disorders (4th)

- **I45.Ø Right fascicular block**
- **I45.1 Other and unspecified right bundle-branch block** (5th)
  - **I45.1Ø Unspecified right bundle-branch block**
    - Right bundle-branch block NOS
  - **I45.19 Other right bundle-branch block**
- **I45.2 Bifascicular block** CC
- **I45.3 Trifascicular block** CC
- **I45.4 Nonspecific intraventricular block**
  - Bundle-branch block NOS
- **I45.5 Other specified heart block**
  - Sinoatrial block
  - Sinoauricular block
  - EXCLUDES 1 *heart block NOS (I45.9)*
- **I45.6 Pre-excitation syndrome**
  - Accelerated atrioventricular conduction
  - Accessory atrioventricular conduction
  - Anomalous atrioventricular excitation
  - Lown-Ganong-Levine syndrome
  - Pre-excitation atrioventricular conduction
  - Wolff-Parkinson-White syndrome
- **I45.8 Other specified conduction disorders** (5th)
  - **I45.81 Long QT syndrome**
    - **DEF:** Condition characterized by recurrent syncope, malignant arrhythmias, and sudden death. This syndrome has a characteristic prolonged Q-T interval on an electrocardiogram.
  - **I45.89 Other specified conduction disorders** CC
    - Atrioventricular [AV] dissociation
    - Interference dissociation
    - Isorhythmic dissociation
    - Nonparoxysmal AV nodal tachycardia
    - **AHA:** 2013,2Q,31
- **I45.9 Conduction disorder, unspecified**
  - Heart block NOS
  - Stokes-Adams syndrome

I46 Cardiac arrest (4th)

EXCLUDES 2 *cardiogenic shock (R57.Ø)*

AHA: 2019,2Q,4-5

- [1] **I46.2 Cardiac arrest due to underlying cardiac condition** MCC UPD HCC
  - Code first underlying cardiac condition
- [1] **I46.8 Cardiac arrest due to other underlying condition** MCC UPD HCC
  - Code first underlying condition
- [1] **I46.9 Cardiac arrest, cause unspecified** MCC HCC
  - **AHA:** 2020,3Q,26

I47 Paroxysmal tachycardia (4th)

Code first tachycardia complicating:
- abortion or ectopic or molar pregnancy (OØØ-OØ7, OØ8.8)
- obstetric surgery and procedures (O75.4)

EXCLUDES 1 *tachycardia NOS (RØØ.Ø)*
sinoauricular tachycardia NOS (RØØ.Ø)
sinus [sinusal] tachycardia NOS (RØØ.Ø)

- **I47.Ø Re-entry ventricular arrhythmia** CC HCC
- **I47.1 Supraventricular tachycardia** CC HCC
  - Atrial (paroxysmal) tachycardia
  - Atrioventricular [AV] (paroxysmal) tachycardia
  - Atrioventricular re-entrant (nodal) tachycardia [AVNRT] [AVRT]
  - Junctional (paroxysmal) tachycardia
  - Nodal (paroxysmal) tachycardia
- ▲ **I47.2 Ventricular tachycardia** (5th)
  - **AHA:** 2021,3Q,11; 2013,3Q,23
  - ● **I47.2Ø Ventricular tachycardia, unspecified** CC
  - ● **I47.21 Torsades de pointes** CC
    - Code also, if applicable, long QT syndrome (I45.81)
    - Use additional code for adverse effect, if applicable, to identify drug (T36-T5Ø with fifth or sixth character 5)
    - **DEF:** Torsades de pointes (TdP): Accelerated heart rhythm, anywhere between 150 and 300 beats per minute, that initiates in the lower chambers of the heart (ventricles). Most commonly occurs in the setting of inherited or medication-induced long QT syndrome.
  - ● **I47.29 Other ventricular tachycardia** CC
- **I47.9 Paroxysmal tachycardia, unspecified** HCC
  - Bouveret (-Hoffman) syndrome

I48 Atrial fibrillation and flutter (4th)

- **I48.Ø Paroxysmal atrial fibrillation** HCC
  - **AHA:** 2021,2Q,8; 2018,3Q,6
- **I48.1 Persistent atrial fibrillation** (5th)
  - EXCLUDES 1 *permanent atrial fibrillation (I48.21)*
  - **AHA:** 2021,2Q,8; 2019,4Q,7; 2019,2Q,3; 2018,3Q,6
  - **I48.11 Longstanding persistent atrial fibrillation** CC HCC
  - **I48.19 Other persistent atrial fibrillation** CC HCC
    - Chronic persistent atrial fibrillation
    - Persistent atrial fibrillation, NOS
    - **AHA:** 2019,4Q,7
- **I48.2 Chronic atrial fibrillation** (5th)
  - **AHA:** 2021,2Q,8; 2019,4Q,7; 2019,2Q,3; 2018,3Q,6
  - **I48.2Ø Chronic atrial fibrillation, unspecified** CC HCC
    - EXCLUDES 1 *chronic persistent atrial fibrillation (I48.19)*
  - **I48.21 Permanent atrial fibrillation** CC HCC
- **I48.3 Typical atrial flutter** CC HCC
  - Type I atrial flutter
- **I48.4 Atypical atrial flutter** CC HCC
  - Type II atrial flutter
- **I48.9 Unspecified atrial fibrillation and atrial flutter** (5th)
  - **I48.91 Unspecified atrial fibrillation** HCC
  - **I48.92 Unspecified atrial flutter** CC HCC

I49 Other cardiac arrhythmias (4th)

Code first cardiac arrhythmia complicating:
- abortion or ectopic or molar pregnancy (OØØ-OØ7, OØ8.8)
- obstetric surgery and procedures (O75.4)

EXCLUDES 1 *neonatal dysrhythmia (P29.1-)*
sinoatrial bradycardia (RØØ.1)
sinus bradycardia (RØØ.1)
vagal bradycardia (RØØ.1)

EXCLUDES 2 *bradycardia NOS (RØØ.1)*

- **I49.Ø Ventricular fibrillation and flutter** (5th)
  - **I49.Ø1 Ventricular fibrillation** MCC HCC
    - **AHA:** 2022,2Q,14
  - **I49.Ø2 Ventricular flutter** MCC HCC
- **I49.1 Atrial premature depolarization**
  - Atrial premature beats
- **I49.2 Junctional premature depolarization** CC HCC
- **I49.3 Ventricular premature depolarization**
  - **AHA:** 2020,2Q,23

I49.4 Other and unspecified premature depolarization

I49.4Ø Unspecified premature depolarization
Premature beats NOS

I49.49 Other premature depolarization
Ectopic beats
Extrasystoles
Extrasystolic arrhythmias
Premature contractions

I49.5 Sick sinus syndrome HCC
Tachycardia-bradycardia syndrome
AHA: 2019,1Q,33
TIP: The presence of a pacemaker controls but does not cure sick sinus syndrome and therefore is considered a reportable chronic condition. When a pacemaker is evaluated by a provider, this code and code Z95.0 Presence of cardiac pacemaker, should be reported, even in the absence of any notable changes or management.

I49.8 Other specified cardiac arrhythmias
Brugada syndrome
Coronary sinus rhythm disorder
Ectopic rhythm disorder
Nodal rhythm disorder

I49.9 Cardiac arrhythmia, unspecified
Arrhythmia (cardiac) NOS

I5Ø Heart failure
Code first:
heart failure complicating abortion or ectopic or molar pregnancy (OØØ-OØ7, OØ8.8)
heart failure due to hypertension (I11.Ø)
heart failure due to hypertension with chronic kidney disease (I13.-)
heart failure following surgery (I97.13-)
obstetric surgery and procedures (O75.4)
rheumatic heart failure (IØ9.81)
EXCLUDES 2 *cardiac arrest (I46.-)*
neonatal cardiac failure (P29.Ø)
AHA: 2018,4Q,67; 2018,2Q,9; 2017,1Q,47; 2014,1Q,25; 2013,2Q,33

I5Ø.1 Left ventricular failure, unspecified CC HCC
Cardiac asthma
Edema of lung with heart disease NOS
Edema of lung with heart failure
Left heart failure
Pulmonary edema with heart disease NOS
Pulmonary edema with heart failure
EXCLUDES 1 *edema of lung without heart disease or heart failure (J81.-)*
pulmonary edema without heart disease or failure (J81.-)

I5Ø.2 Systolic (congestive) heart failure
Heart failure with reduced ejection fraction [HFrEF]
Systolic left ventricular heart failure
Code also end stage heart failure, if applicable (I5Ø.84)
EXCLUDES 1 *combined systolic (congestive) and diastolic (congestive) heart failure (I5Ø.4-)*
AHA: 2020,3Q,32; 2017,1Q,46; 2016,1Q,10

I5Ø.2Ø Unspecified systolic (congestive) heart failure CC HCC
I5Ø.21 Acute systolic (congestive) heart failure MCC HCC
I5Ø.22 Chronic systolic (congestive) heart failure CC HCC
I5Ø.23 Acute on chronic systolic (congestive) heart failure MCC HCC

I5Ø.3 Diastolic (congestive) heart failure
Diastolic left ventricular heart failure
Heart failure with normal ejection fraction
Heart failure with preserved ejection fraction [HFpEF]
Code also end stage heart failure, if applicable (I5Ø.84)
EXCLUDES 1 *combined systolic (congestive) and diastolic (congestive) heart failure (I5Ø.4-)*
AHA: 2020,3Q,32; 2017,1Q,46; 2016,1Q,10

I5Ø.3Ø Unspecified diastolic (congestive) heart failure CC HCC
I5Ø.31 Acute diastolic (congestive) heart failure MCC HCC
I5Ø.32 Chronic diastolic (congestive) heart failure CC HCC
I5Ø.33 Acute on chronic diastolic (congestive) heart failure MCC HCC

I5Ø.4 Combined systolic (congestive) and diastolic (congestive) heart failure
Combined systolic and diastolic left ventricular heart failure
Heart failure with reduced ejection fraction and diastolic dysfunction
Code also end stage heart failure, if applicable (I5Ø.84)
AHA: 2017,1Q,46; 2016,1Q,10

I5Ø.4Ø Unspecified combined systolic (congestive) and diastolic (congestive) heart failure CC HCC
I5Ø.41 Acute combined systolic (congestive) and diastolic (congestive) heart failure MCC HCC
I5Ø.42 Chronic combined systolic (congestive) and diastolic (congestive) heart failure CC HCC
I5Ø.43 Acute on chronic combined systolic (congestive) and diastolic (congestive) heart failure MCC HCC

I5Ø.8 Other heart failure
AHA: 2017,4Q,15-16

I5Ø.81 Right heart failure
Right ventricular failure

I5Ø.81Ø Right heart failure, unspecified HCC
Right heart failure without mention of left heart failure
Right ventricular failure NOS

I5Ø.811 Acute right heart failure HCC
Acute isolated right heart failure
Acute (isolated) right ventricular failure

I5Ø.812 Chronic right heart failure HCC
Chronic isolated right heart failure
Chronic (isolated) right ventricular failure

I5Ø.813 Acute on chronic right heart failure HCC
Acute on chronic isolated right heart failure
Acute on chronic (isolated) right ventricular failure
Acute decompensation of chronic (isolated) right ventricular failure
Acute exacerbation of chronic (isolated) right ventricular failure

I5Ø.814 Right heart failure due to left heart failure HCC
Right ventricular failure secondary to left ventricular failure
Code also the type of left ventricular failure, if known (I5Ø.2-I5Ø.43)
EXCLUDES 1 *right heart failure with but not due to left heart failure (I5Ø.82)*

I5Ø.82 Biventricular heart failure HCC
Code also the type of left ventricular failure as systolic, diastolic, or combined, if known (I5Ø.2-I5Ø.43)

I5Ø.83 High output heart failure HCC
DEF: Occurs when the high demand for blood exceeds the capacity of a normally functioning heart to meet the demand.

I5Ø.84 End stage heart failure HCC
Stage D heart failure
Code also the type of heart failure as systolic, diastolic, or combined, if known (I5Ø.2-I5Ø.43)

I5Ø.89 Other heart failure HCC

I5Ø.9 Heart failure, unspecified HCC
Cardiac, heart or myocardial failure NOS
Congestive heart disease
Congestive heart failure NOS
EXCLUDES 2 *fluid overload unrelated to congestive heart failure (E87.7Ø)*
AHA: 2017,4Q,15-16; 2017,1Q,45-46; 2014,4Q,21; 2012,4Q,92

I51 Complications and ill-defined descriptions of heart disease

EXCLUDES 1 *any condition in I51.4-I51.9 due to hypertension (I11.-)*
any condition in I51.4-I51.9 due to hypertension and chronic kidney disease (I13.-)
heart disease specified as rheumatic (IØØ-IØ9)

I51.Ø Cardiac septal defect, acquired CC A
Acquired septal atrial defect (old)
Acquired septal auricular defect (old)
Acquired septal ventricular defect (old)
EXCLUDES 1 *cardiac septal defect as current complication following acute myocardial infarction (I23.1, I23.2)*
DEF: Abnormal communication between opposite heart chambers due to a defect of the septum. It is not present at birth.

I51.1 Rupture of chordae tendineae, not elsewhere classified MCC HCC
EXCLUDES 1 *rupture of chordae tendineae as current complication following acute myocardial infarction (I23.4)*

I51.2 Rupture of papillary muscle, not elsewhere classified MCC HCC
EXCLUDES 1 *rupture of papillary muscle as current complication following acute myocardial infarction (I23.5)*

I51.3 Intracardiac thrombosis, not elsewhere classified
Apical thrombosis (old)
Atrial thrombosis (old)
Auricular thrombosis (old)
Mural thrombosis (old)
Ventricular thrombosis (old)
EXCLUDES 1 *intracardiac thrombosis as current complication following acute myocardial infarction (I23.6)*
AHA: 2013,1Q,24

I51.4 Myocarditis, unspecified HCC
Chronic (interstitial) myocarditis
Myocardial fibrosis
Myocarditis NOS
EXCLUDES 1 *acute or subacute myocarditis (I4Ø.-)*
AHA: 2018,4Q,67; 2018,2Q,9

I51.5 Myocardial degeneration HCC
Fatty degeneration of heart or myocardium
Myocardial disease
Senile degeneration of heart or myocardium
AHA: 2018,4Q,67; 2018,2Q,9

I51.7 Cardiomegaly
Cardiac dilatation
Cardiac hypertrophy
Ventricular dilatation
AHA: 2018,4Q,67; 2018,2Q,9

I51.8 Other ill-defined heart diseases
AHA: 2018,2Q,9

I51.81 Takotsubo syndrome CC
Reversible left ventricular dysfunction following sudden emotional stress
Stress induced cardiomyopathy
Takotsubo cardiomyopathy
Transient left ventricular apical ballooning syndrome
DEF: Complex of symptoms mimicking myocardial infarct in absence of heart disease, with the majority of cases occurring in postmenopausal women. Heart muscles are temporarily weakened, and a sudden, massive surge of adrenalin stuns the heart, greatly reducing the ability to pump blood.

I51.89 Other ill-defined heart diseases
Carditis (acute)(chronic)
Pancarditis (acute)(chronic)
AHA: 2019,2Q,5; 2018,4Q,67

I51.9 Heart disease, unspecified
AHA: 2018,4Q,67; 2018,2Q,9

I52 Other heart disorders in diseases classified elsewhere
Code first underlying disease, such as:
congenital syphilis (A5Ø.5)
mucopolysaccharidosis (E76.3)
schistosomiasis (B65.Ø-B65.9)
EXCLUDES 1 *heart disease (in):*
gonococcal infection (A54.83)
meningococcal infection (A39.5Ø)
rheumatoid arthritis (MØ5.31)
syphilis (A52.Ø6)

I5A Non-ischemic myocardial injury (non-traumatic) CC
Acute (non-ischemic) myocardial injury
Chronic (non-ischemic) myocardial injury
Unspecified (non-ischemic) myocardial injury
Code first the underlying cause, if known and applicable, such as:
acute kidney failure (N17.-)
acute myocarditis (I4Ø.-)
cardiomyopathy (I42.-)
chronic kidney disease (CKD) (N18.-)
heart failure (I5Ø.-)
hypertensive urgency (I16.Ø)
nonrheumatic aortic valve disorders (I35.-)
paroxysmal tachycardia (I47.-)
pulmonary embolism (I26.-)
pulmonary hypertension (I27.Ø, I27.2-)
sepsis (A41.-)
takotsubo syndrome (I51.81)
EXCLUDES 1 *acute myocardial infarction (I21.-)*
injury of heart (S26.-)
EXCLUDES 2 *other acute ischemic heart diseases (I24.-)*
AHA: 2021,4Q,14-15

Cerebrovascular diseases (I6Ø-I69)

Use additional code to identify presence of:
alcohol abuse and dependence (F1Ø.-)
exposure to environmental tobacco smoke (Z77.22)
history of tobacco dependence (Z87.891)
hypertension (I1Ø-I16)
occupational exposure to environmental tobacco smoke (Z57.31)
tobacco dependence (F17.-)
tobacco use (Z72.Ø)
EXCLUDES 1 *traumatic intracranial hemorrhage (SØ6.-)*
AHA: 2014,3Q,5; 2012,4Q,91-92

I6Ø Nontraumatic subarachnoid hemorrhage
EXCLUDES 1 *syphilitic ruptured cerebral aneurysm (A52.Ø5)*
EXCLUDES 2 *sequelae of subarachnoid hemorrhage (I69.Ø-)*

I6Ø.Ø Nontraumatic subarachnoid hemorrhage from carotid siphon and bifurcation
I6Ø.ØØ Nontraumatic subarachnoid hemorrhage from unspecified carotid siphon and bifurcation MCC HCC
I6Ø.Ø1 Nontraumatic subarachnoid hemorrhage from right carotid siphon and bifurcation MCC HCC
I6Ø.Ø2 Nontraumatic subarachnoid hemorrhage from left carotid siphon and bifurcation MCC HCC

I6Ø.1 Nontraumatic subarachnoid hemorrhage from middle cerebral artery
I6Ø.1Ø Nontraumatic subarachnoid hemorrhage from unspecified middle cerebral artery MCC HCC
I6Ø.11 Nontraumatic subarachnoid hemorrhage from right middle cerebral artery MCC HCC
I6Ø.12 Nontraumatic subarachnoid hemorrhage from left middle cerebral artery MCC HCC

I6Ø.2 Nontraumatic subarachnoid hemorrhage from anterior communicating artery MCC HCC

I6Ø.3 Nontraumatic subarachnoid hemorrhage from posterior communicating artery
I6Ø.3Ø Nontraumatic subarachnoid hemorrhage from unspecified posterior communicating artery MCC HCC
I6Ø.31 Nontraumatic subarachnoid hemorrhage from right posterior communicating artery MCC HCC
I6Ø.32 Nontraumatic subarachnoid hemorrhage from left posterior communicating artery MCC HCC

I6Ø.4 Nontraumatic subarachnoid hemorrhage from basilar artery MCC HCC

I60.5 Nontraumatic subarachnoid hemorrhage from vertebral artery

I60.50 Nontraumatic subarachnoid hemorrhage from unspecified vertebral artery MCC HCC

I60.51 Nontraumatic subarachnoid hemorrhage from right vertebral artery MCC HCC

I60.52 Nontraumatic subarachnoid hemorrhage from left vertebral artery MCC HCC

I60.6 Nontraumatic subarachnoid hemorrhage from other intracranial arteries MCC HCC

I60.7 Nontraumatic subarachnoid hemorrhage from unspecified intracranial artery MCC HCC

Ruptured (congenital) berry aneurysm

Ruptured (congenital) cerebral aneurysm

Subarachnoid hemorrhage (nontraumatic) from cerebral artery NOS

Subarachnoid hemorrhage (nontraumatic) from communicating artery NOS

EXCLUDES 1 *berry aneurysm, nonruptured (I67.1)*

I60.8 Other nontraumatic subarachnoid hemorrhage MCC HCC

Meningeal hemorrhage

Rupture of cerebral arteriovenous malformation

I60.9 Nontraumatic subarachnoid hemorrhage, unspecified MCC HCC

I61 Nontraumatic intracerebral hemorrhage

EXCLUDES 2 *sequelae of intracerebral hemorrhage (I69.1-)*

AHA: 2017,2Q,9-10

I61.0 Nontraumatic intracerebral hemorrhage in hemisphere, subcortical MCC HCC

Deep intracerebral hemorrhage (nontraumatic)

AHA: 2016,4Q,27

I61.1 Nontraumatic intracerebral hemorrhage in hemisphere, cortical MCC HCC

Cerebral lobe hemorrhage (nontraumatic)

Superficial intracerebral hemorrhage (nontraumatic)

I61.2 Nontraumatic intracerebral hemorrhage in hemisphere, unspecified MCC HCC

I61.3 Nontraumatic intracerebral hemorrhage in brain stem MCC HCC

I61.4 Nontraumatic intracerebral hemorrhage in cerebellum MCC HCC

I61.5 Nontraumatic intracerebral hemorrhage, intraventricular MCC HCC

I61.6 Nontraumatic intracerebral hemorrhage, multiple localized MCC HCC

I61.8 Other nontraumatic intracerebral hemorrhage MCC HCC

I61.9 Nontraumatic intracerebral hemorrhage, unspecified MCC HCC

I62 Other and unspecified nontraumatic intracranial hemorrhage

EXCLUDES 2 *sequelae of intracranial hemorrhage (I69.2)*

I62.0 Nontraumatic subdural hemorrhage

I62.00 Nontraumatic subdural hemorrhage, unspecified MCC HCC

I62.01 Nontraumatic acute subdural hemorrhage MCC HCC

I62.02 Nontraumatic subacute subdural hemorrhage MCC HCC

I62.03 Nontraumatic chronic subdural hemorrhage MCC HCC

I62.1 Nontraumatic extradural hemorrhage MCC HCC

Nontraumatic epidural hemorrhage

I62.9 Nontraumatic intracranial hemorrhage, unspecified CC HCC

I63 Cerebral infarction

INCLUDES occlusion and stenosis of cerebral and precerebral arteries, resulting in cerebral infarction

Use additional code, if applicable, to identify status post administration of tPA (rtPA) in a different facility within the last 24 hours prior to admission to current facility (Z92.82)

Use additional code, if known, to indicate National Institutes of Health Stroke Scale (NIHSS) score (R29.7-)

EXCLUDES 1 *neonatal cerebral infarction (P91.82-)*

EXCLUDES 2 *sequelae of cerebral infarction (I69.3-)*

AHA: 2017,2Q,9-10; 2016,4Q,28,61-62; 2015,1Q,25; 2014,1Q,23

TIP: Weakness on one side of the body documented as secondary to stroke is synonymous with hemiparesis/hemiplegia (G81.-). Weakness of one limb documented as secondary to stroke is synonymous with monoplegia (G83.1-, G83.2-, G83.3-).

I63.0 Cerebral infarction due to thrombosis of precerebral arteries

I63.00 Cerebral infarction due to thrombosis of unspecified precerebral artery MCC HCC

I63.01 Cerebral infarction due to thrombosis of vertebral artery

I63.011 Cerebral infarction due to thrombosis of right vertebral artery MCC HCC

I63.012 Cerebral infarction due to thrombosis of left vertebral artery MCC HCC

I63.013 Cerebral infarction due to thrombosis of bilateral vertebral arteries MCC HCC

I63.019 Cerebral infarction due to thrombosis of unspecified vertebral artery MCC HCC

I63.02 Cerebral infarction due to thrombosis of basilar artery MCC HCC

I63.03 Cerebral infarction due to thrombosis of carotid artery

I63.031 Cerebral infarction due to thrombosis of right carotid artery MCC HCC

I63.032 Cerebral infarction due to thrombosis of left carotid artery MCC HCC

I63.033 Cerebral infarction due to thrombosis of bilateral carotid arteries MCC HCC

I63.039 Cerebral infarction due to thrombosis of unspecified carotid artery MCC HCC

I63.09 Cerebral infarction due to thrombosis of other precerebral artery MCC HCC

I63.1 Cerebral infarction due to embolism of precerebral arteries

I63.10 Cerebral infarction due to embolism of unspecified precerebral artery MCC HCC

I63.11 Cerebral infarction due to embolism of vertebral artery

I63.111 Cerebral infarction due to embolism of right vertebral artery MCC HCC

I63.112 Cerebral infarction due to embolism of left vertebral artery MCC HCC

I63.113 Cerebral infarction due to embolism of bilateral vertebral arteries MCC HCC

I63.119 Cerebral infarction due to embolism of unspecified vertebral artery MCC HCC

I63.12 Cerebral infarction due to embolism of basilar artery MCC HCC

I63.13 Cerebral infarction due to embolism of carotid artery

I63.131 Cerebral infarction due to embolism of right carotid artery MCC HCC

I63.132 Cerebral infarction due to embolism of left carotid artery MCC HCC

I63.133 Cerebral infarction due to embolism of bilateral carotid arteries MCC HCC

I63.139 Cerebral infarction due to embolism of unspecified carotid artery MCC HCC

I63.19 Cerebral infarction due to embolism of other precerebral artery MCC HCC

I63.2 Cerebral infarction due to unspecified occlusion or stenosis of precerebral arteries

AHA: 2020,3Q,27-28

I63.20 Cerebral infarction due to unspecified occlusion or stenosis of unspecified precerebral arteries MCC HCC

I63.21 Cerebral infarction due to unspecified occlusion or stenosis of vertebral arteries

I63.211 Cerebral infarction due to unspecified occlusion or stenosis of right vertebral artery MCC HCC

I63.212 Cerebral infarction due to unspecified occlusion or stenosis of left vertebral artery MCC HCC

I63.213 Cerebral infarction due to unspecified occlusion or stenosis of bilateral vertebral arteries MCC HCC

I63.219 Cerebral infarction due to unspecified occlusion or stenosis of unspecified vertebral artery MCC HCC

I63.22 Cerebral infarction due to unspecified occlusion or stenosis of basilar artery MCC HCC

I63.23 Cerebral infarction due to unspecified occlusion or stenosis of carotid arteries

I63.231 Cerebral infarction due to unspecified occlusion or stenosis of right carotid arteries MCC HCC

I63.232 Cerebral infarction due to unspecified occlusion or stenosis of left carotid arteries MCC HCC

I63.233 Cerebral infarction due to unspecified occlusion or stenosis of bilateral carotid arteries MCC HCC

I63.239 Cerebral infarction due to unspecified occlusion or stenosis of unspecified carotid artery MCC HCC

I63.29 Cerebral infarction due to unspecified occlusion or stenosis of other precerebral arteries MCC HCC

I63.3 Cerebral infarction due to thrombosis of cerebral arteries

I63.30 Cerebral infarction due to thrombosis of unspecified cerebral artery MCC HCC

I63.31 Cerebral infarction due to thrombosis of middle cerebral artery

I63.311 Cerebral infarction due to thrombosis of right middle cerebral artery MCC HCC

I63.312 Cerebral infarction due to thrombosis of left middle cerebral artery MCC HCC

I63.313 Cerebral infarction due to thrombosis of bilateral middle cerebral arteries MCC HCC

I63.319 Cerebral infarction due to thrombosis of unspecified middle cerebral artery MCC HCC

I63.32 Cerebral infarction due to thrombosis of anterior cerebral artery

I63.321 Cerebral infarction due to thrombosis of right anterior cerebral artery MCC HCC

I63.322 Cerebral infarction due to thrombosis of left anterior cerebral artery MCC HCC

I63.323 Cerebral infarction due to thrombosis of bilateral anterior cerebral arteries MCC HCC

I63.329 Cerebral infarction due to thrombosis of unspecified anterior cerebral artery MCC HCC

I63.33 Cerebral infarction due to thrombosis of posterior cerebral artery

I63.331 Cerebral infarction due to thrombosis of right posterior cerebral artery MCC HCC

I63.332 Cerebral infarction due to thrombosis of left posterior cerebral artery MCC HCC

I63.333 Cerebral infarction due to thrombosis of bilateral posterior cerebral arteries MCC HCC

I63.339 Cerebral infarction due to thrombosis of unspecified posterior cerebral artery MCC HCC

I63.34 Cerebral infarction due to thrombosis of cerebellar artery

I63.341 Cerebral infarction due to thrombosis of right cerebellar artery MCC HCC

I63.342 Cerebral infarction due to thrombosis of left cerebellar artery MCC HCC

I63.343 Cerebral infarction due to thrombosis of bilateral cerebellar arteries MCC HCC

I63.349 Cerebral infarction due to thrombosis of unspecified cerebellar artery MCC HCC

I63.39 Cerebral infarction due to thrombosis of other cerebral artery MCC HCC

I63.4 Cerebral infarction due to embolism of cerebral arteries

I63.40 Cerebral infarction due to embolism of unspecified cerebral artery MCC HCC

I63.41 Cerebral infarction due to embolism of middle cerebral artery

I63.411 Cerebral infarction due to embolism of right middle cerebral artery MCC HCC

I63.412 Cerebral infarction due to embolism of left middle cerebral artery MCC HCC

I63.413 Cerebral infarction due to embolism of bilateral middle cerebral arteries MCC HCC

I63.419 Cerebral infarction due to embolism of unspecified middle cerebral artery MCC HCC

I63.42 Cerebral infarction due to embolism of anterior cerebral artery

I63.421 Cerebral infarction due to embolism of right anterior cerebral artery MCC HCC

I63.422 Cerebral infarction due to embolism of left anterior cerebral artery MCC HCC

I63.423 Cerebral infarction due to embolism of bilateral anterior cerebral arteries MCC HCC

I63.429 Cerebral infarction due to embolism of unspecified anterior cerebral artery MCC HCC

I63.43 Cerebral infarction due to embolism of posterior cerebral artery

I63.431 Cerebral infarction due to embolism of right posterior cerebral artery MCC HCC

I63.432 Cerebral infarction due to embolism of left posterior cerebral artery MCC HCC

I63.433 Cerebral infarction due to embolism of bilateral posterior cerebral arteries MCC HCC

I63.439 Cerebral infarction due to embolism of unspecified posterior cerebral artery MCC HCC

I63.44 Cerebral infarction due to embolism of cerebellar artery

I63.441 Cerebral infarction due to embolism of right cerebellar artery MCC HCC

I63.442 Cerebral infarction due to embolism of left cerebellar artery MCC HCC

I63.443 Cerebral infarction due to embolism of bilateral cerebellar arteries MCC HCC

I63.449 Cerebral infarction due to embolism of unspecified cerebellar artery MCC HCC

I63.49 Cerebral infarction due to embolism of other cerebral artery MCC HCC

I63.5 Cerebral infarction due to unspecified occlusion or stenosis of cerebral arteries

I63.50 Cerebral infarction due to unspecified occlusion or stenosis of unspecified cerebral artery MCC HCC

I63.51 Cerebral infarction due to unspecified occlusion or stenosis of middle cerebral artery

I63.511 Cerebral infarction due to unspecified occlusion or stenosis of right middle cerebral artery MCC HCC

I63.512 Cerebral infarction due to unspecified occlusion or stenosis of left middle cerebral artery MCC HCC

I63.513 Cerebral infarction due to unspecified occlusion or stenosis of bilateral middle cerebral arteries MCC HCC

I63.519 Cerebral infarction due to unspecified occlusion or stenosis of unspecified middle cerebral artery MCC HCC

I63.52 Cerebral infarction due to unspecified occlusion or stenosis of anterior cerebral artery

I63.521 Cerebral infarction due to unspecified occlusion or stenosis of right anterior cerebral artery MCC HCC

I63.522 Cerebral infarction due to unspecified occlusion or stenosis of left anterior cerebral artery MCC HCC

I63.523 Cerebral infarction due to unspecified occlusion or stenosis of bilateral anterior cerebral arteries MCC HCC

I63.529 Cerebral infarction due to unspecified occlusion or stenosis of unspecified anterior cerebral artery MCC HCC

I63.53 Cerebral infarction due to unspecified occlusion or stenosis of posterior cerebral artery
- I63.531 Cerebral infarction due to unspecified occlusion or stenosis of right posterior cerebral artery MCC HCC
- I63.532 Cerebral infarction due to unspecified occlusion or stenosis of left posterior cerebral artery MCC HCC
- I63.533 Cerebral infarction due to unspecified occlusion or stenosis of bilateral posterior cerebral arteries MCC HCC
- I63.539 Cerebral infarction due to unspecified occlusion or stenosis of unspecified posterior cerebral artery MCC HCC

I63.54 Cerebral infarction due to unspecified occlusion or stenosis of cerebellar artery
- I63.541 Cerebral infarction due to unspecified occlusion or stenosis of right cerebellar artery MCC HCC
- I63.542 Cerebral infarction due to unspecified occlusion or stenosis of left cerebellar artery MCC HCC
- I63.543 Cerebral infarction due to unspecified occlusion or stenosis of bilateral cerebellar arteries MCC HCC
- I63.549 Cerebral infarction due to unspecified occlusion or stenosis of unspecified cerebellar artery MCC HCC

I63.59 Cerebral infarction due to unspecified occlusion or stenosis of other cerebral artery MCC HCC

I63.6 Cerebral infarction due to cerebral venous thrombosis, nonpyogenic MCC HCC

I63.8 Other cerebral infarction

AHA: 2018,4Q,16

- I63.81 Other cerebral infarction due to occlusion or stenosis of small artery MCC HCC
  - Lacunar infarction
  - AHA: 2020,3Q,27
- I63.89 Other cerebral infarction MCC HCC
  - AHA: 2022,1Q,25

I63.9 Cerebral infarction, unspecified MCC HCC

Stroke NOS

EXCLUDES 2 *transient cerebral ischemic attacks and related syndromes (G45.-)*

AHA: 2020,2Q,29

TIP: When provider documentation does not identify the location of an infarction, imaging reports can be used to pinpoint the location and lead to a more specific infarction code.

I65 Occlusion and stenosis of precerebral arteries, not resulting in cerebral infarction

INCLUDES embolism of precerebral artery
narrowing of precerebral artery
obstruction (complete) (partial) of precerebral artery
thrombosis of precerebral artery

EXCLUDES 1 *insufficiency, NOS, of precerebral artery (G45.-)*
insufficiency of precerebral arteries causing cerebral infarction (I63.Ø-I63.2)

AHA: 2018,2Q,9

I65.Ø Occlusion and stenosis of vertebral artery
- I65.Ø1 Occlusion and stenosis of right vertebral artery
- I65.Ø2 Occlusion and stenosis of left vertebral artery
- I65.Ø3 Occlusion and stenosis of bilateral vertebral arteries
- I65.Ø9 Occlusion and stenosis of unspecified vertebral artery

I65.1 Occlusion and stenosis of basilar artery

I65.2 Occlusion and stenosis of carotid artery

AHA: 2021,1Q,4; 2020,3Q,28

- I65.21 Occlusion and stenosis of right carotid artery
- I65.22 Occlusion and stenosis of left carotid artery
- I65.23 Occlusion and stenosis of bilateral carotid arteries
- I65.29 Occlusion and stenosis of unspecified carotid artery

I65.8 Occlusion and stenosis of other precerebral arteries

I65.9 Occlusion and stenosis of unspecified precerebral artery

Occlusion and stenosis of precerebral artery NOS

I66 Occlusion and stenosis of cerebral arteries, not resulting in cerebral infarction

INCLUDES embolism of cerebral artery
narrowing of cerebral artery
obstruction (complete) (partial) of cerebral artery
thrombosis of cerebral artery

EXCLUDES 1 *occlusion and stenosis of cerebral artery causing cerebral infarction (I63.3-I63.5)*

I66.Ø Occlusion and stenosis of middle cerebral artery
- I66.Ø1 Occlusion and stenosis of right middle cerebral artery
- I66.Ø2 Occlusion and stenosis of left middle cerebral artery
- I66.Ø3 Occlusion and stenosis of bilateral middle cerebral arteries
- I66.Ø9 Occlusion and stenosis of unspecified middle cerebral artery

I66.1 Occlusion and stenosis of anterior cerebral artery
- I66.11 Occlusion and stenosis of right anterior cerebral artery
- I66.12 Occlusion and stenosis of left anterior cerebral artery
- I66.13 Occlusion and stenosis of bilateral anterior cerebral arteries
- I66.19 Occlusion and stenosis of unspecified anterior cerebral artery

I66.2 Occlusion and stenosis of posterior cerebral artery
- I66.21 Occlusion and stenosis of right posterior cerebral artery
- I66.22 Occlusion and stenosis of left posterior cerebral artery
- I66.23 Occlusion and stenosis of bilateral posterior cerebral arteries
- I66.29 Occlusion and stenosis of unspecified posterior cerebral artery

I66.3 Occlusion and stenosis of cerebellar arteries

I66.8 Occlusion and stenosis of other cerebral arteries

Occlusion and stenosis of perforating arteries

I66.9 Occlusion and stenosis of unspecified cerebral artery

I67 Other cerebrovascular diseases

EXCLUDES 2 *sequelae of the listed conditions (I69.8)*

I67.Ø Dissection of cerebral arteries, nonruptured MCC HCC

EXCLUDES 1 *ruptured cerebral arteries (I6Ø.7)*

AHA: 2021,3Q,5

DEF: Dissecting aneurysm: Tear within an arterial wall that allows blood to accumulate between the outer and middle layers, creating a false lumen.

I67.1 Cerebral aneurysm, nonruptured
Cerebral aneurysm NOS
Cerebral arteriovenous fistula, acquired
Internal carotid artery aneurysm, intracranial portion
Internal carotid artery aneurysm, NOS
EXCLUDES 1 *congenital cerebral aneurysm, nonruptured (Q28.-)*
ruptured cerebral aneurysm (I60.7)
AHA: 2021,3Q,5
TIP: A diagnosis of dissecting aneurysm should be coded to the dissection code, I67.0. The bulging/aneurysm, although present, occurred secondary to the dissection. The dissection represents the most significant problem.

Berry Aneurysm

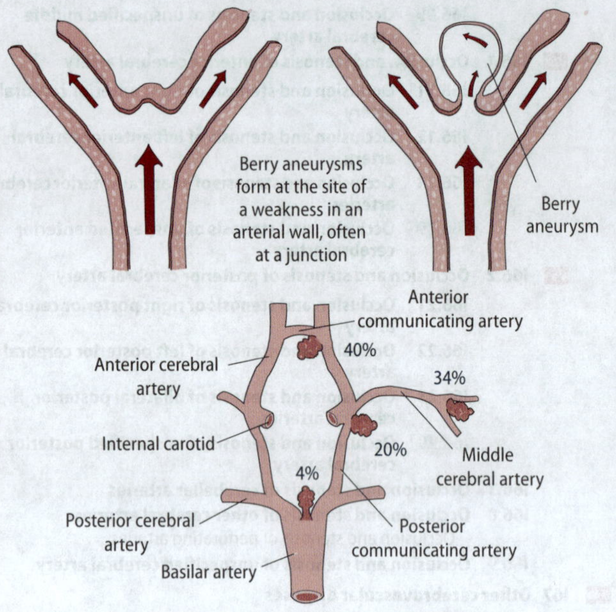

Common sites of berry aneurysms in the circle of Willis arteries

I67.2 Cerebral atherosclerosis A
Atheroma of cerebral and precerebral arteries

I67.3 Progressive vascular leukoencephalopathy HIV CC HCC
Binswanger's disease

I67.4 Hypertensive encephalopathy CC
EXCLUDES 2 *insufficiency, NOS, of precerebral arteries (G45.2)*

I67.5 Moyamoya disease CC
DEF: Cerebrovascular ischemia. Vessels occlude and rupture, causing tiny hemorrhages at the base of brain. It affects predominantly Japanese people.

I67.6 Nonpyogenic thrombosis of intracranial venous system CC
Nonpyogenic thrombosis of cerebral vein
Nonpyogenic thrombosis of intracranial venous sinus
EXCLUDES 1 *nonpyogenic thrombosis of intracranial venous system causing infarction (I63.6)*

I67.7 Cerebral arteritis, not elsewhere classified CC
Granulomatous angiitis of the nervous system
EXCLUDES 1 *allergic granulomatous angiitis (M30.1)*

√5th **I67.8 Other specified cerebrovascular diseases**

I67.81 Acute cerebrovascular insufficiency CC
Acute cerebrovascular insufficiency unspecified as to location or reversibility

I67.82 Cerebral ischemia CC
Chronic cerebral ischemia

I67.83 Posterior reversible encephalopathy syndrome HIV MCC
PRES

√6th **I67.84 Cerebral vasospasm and vasoconstriction**

I67.841 Reversible cerebrovascular vasoconstriction syndrome CC
Call-Fleming syndrome
Code first underlying condition, if applicable, such as eclampsia (O15.00-O15.9)

I67.848 Other cerebrovascular vasospasm and vasoconstriction CC

√6th **I67.85 Hereditary cerebrovascular diseases**
AHA: 2018,4Q,17

I67.850 Cerebral autosomal dominant arteriopathy with subcortical infarcts and leukoencephalopathy CC
CADASIL
Code also any associated diagnoses, such as:
epilepsy (G40.-)
stroke (I63.-)
vascular dementia (F01.-)

I67.858 Other hereditary cerebrovascular disease CC

I67.89 Other cerebrovascular disease CC

I67.9 Cerebrovascular disease, unspecified

√4th **I68 Cerebrovascular disorders in diseases classified elsewhere**

I68.0 Cerebral amyloid angiopathy
Code first underlying amyloidosis (E85.-)

I68.2 Cerebral arteritis in other diseases classified elsewhere CC
Code first underlying disease
EXCLUDES 1 *cerebral arteritis (in):*
listerosis (A32.89)
syphilis (A52.04)
systemic lupus erythematosus (M32.19)
tuberculosis (A18.89)

I68.8 Other cerebrovascular disorders in diseases classified elsewhere
Code first underlying disease
EXCLUDES 1 *syphilitic cerebral aneurysm (A52.05)*

√4th **I69 Sequelae of cerebrovascular disease**
NOTE Category I69 is to be used to indicate conditions in I60-I67 as the cause of sequelae. The "sequelae" include conditions specified as such or as residuals which may occur at any time after the onset of the causal condition
EXCLUDES 1 *personal history of cerebral infarction without residual deficit (Z86.73)*
personal history of prolonged reversible ischemic neurologic deficit (PRIND) (Z86.73)
personal history of reversible ischemic neurologcial deficit (RIND) (Z86.73)
sequelae of traumatic intracranial injury (S06.-)
AHA: 2020,2Q,29; 2017,1Q,47; 2016,4Q,28; 2015,1Q,25; 2012,4Q,106
TIP: Weakness on one side of the body (unilateral weakness) documented as secondary to old cerebrovascular disease is synonymous with hemiparesis/hemiplegia. Weakness of one limb documented as secondary to old cerebrovascular disease is synonymous with monoplegia.
TIP: For codes describing hemiplegia, hemiparesis, and monoplegia; if the documentation identifies the affected side but not whether it is the dominant or nondominant side, the default is as follows: for ambidextrous patients, the default is dominant; when the left side is affected, the default is nondominant; and when the right side is affected, the default is dominant.

√5th **I69.0 Sequelae of nontraumatic subarachnoid hemorrhage**

I69.00 Unspecified sequelae of nontraumatic subarachnoid hemorrhage

√6th **I69.01 Cognitive deficits following nontraumatic subarachnoid hemorrhage**

I69.010 Attention and concentration deficit following nontraumatic subarachnoid hemorrhage

I69.011 Memory deficit following nontraumatic subarachnoid hemorrhage

I69.012 Visuospatial deficit and spatial neglect following nontraumatic subarachnoid hemorrhage

I69.013 Psychomotor deficit following nontraumatic subarachnoid hemorrhage

I69.014 Frontal lobe and executive function deficit following nontraumatic subarachnoid hemorrhage

I69.015 Cognitive social or emotional deficit following nontraumatic subarachnoid hemorrhage

I69.018 Other symptoms and signs involving cognitive functions following nontraumatic subarachnoid hemorrhage

I69.019 Unspecified symptoms and signs involving cognitive functions following nontraumatic subarachnoid hemorrhage

I69.02 Speech and language deficits following nontraumatic subarachnoid hemorrhage

I69.020 Aphasia following nontraumatic subarachnoid hemorrhage

I69.021 Dysphasia following nontraumatic subarachnoid hemorrhage

I69.022 Dysarthria following nontraumatic subarachnoid hemorrhage

I69.023 Fluency disorder following nontraumatic subarachnoid hemorrhage

Stuttering following nontraumatic subarachnoid hemorrhage

I69.028 Other speech and language deficits following nontraumatic subarachnoid hemorrhage

I69.03 Monoplegia of upper limb following nontraumatic subarachnoid hemorrhage

AHA: 2017,1Q,47

I69.031 Monoplegia of upper limb following nontraumatic subarachnoid hemorrhage affecting right dominant side HCC

I69.032 Monoplegia of upper limb following nontraumatic subarachnoid hemorrhage affecting left dominant side HCC

I69.033 Monoplegia of upper limb following nontraumatic subarachnoid hemorrhage affecting right non-dominant side HCC

I69.034 Monoplegia of upper limb following nontraumatic subarachnoid hemorrhage affecting left non-dominant side HCC

I69.039 Monoplegia of upper limb following nontraumatic subarachnoid hemorrhage affecting unspecified side HCC

I69.04 Monoplegia of lower limb following nontraumatic subarachnoid hemorrhage

AHA: 2017,1Q,47

I69.041 Monoplegia of lower limb following nontraumatic subarachnoid hemorrhage affecting right dominant side HCC

I69.042 Monoplegia of lower limb following nontraumatic subarachnoid hemorrhage affecting left dominant side HCC

I69.043 Monoplegia of lower limb following nontraumatic subarachnoid hemorrhage affecting right non-dominant side HCC

I69.044 Monoplegia of lower limb following nontraumatic subarachnoid hemorrhage affecting left non-dominant side HCC

I69.049 Monoplegia of lower limb following nontraumatic subarachnoid hemorrhage affecting unspecified side HCC

I69.05 Hemiplegia and hemiparesis following nontraumatic subarachnoid hemorrhage

AHA: 2015,1Q,25

I69.051 Hemiplegia and hemiparesis following nontraumatic subarachnoid hemorrhage affecting right dominant side CC HCC

I69.052 Hemiplegia and hemiparesis following nontraumatic subarachnoid hemorrhage affecting left dominant side CC HCC

I69.053 Hemiplegia and hemiparesis following nontraumatic subarachnoid hemorrhage affecting right non-dominant side CC HCC

I69.054 Hemiplegia and hemiparesis following nontraumatic subarachnoid hemorrhage affecting left non-dominant side CC HCC

I69.059 Hemiplegia and hemiparesis following nontraumatic subarachnoid hemorrhage affecting unspecified side CC UNS HCC

I69.06 Other paralytic syndrome following nontraumatic subarachnoid hemorrhage

Use additional code to identify type of paralytic syndrome, such as:
- locked-in state (G83.5)
- quadriplegia (G82.5-)

EXCLUDES 1
- *hemiplegia/hemiparesis following nontraumatic subarachnoid hemorrhage (I69.05-)*
- *monoplegia of lower limb following nontraumatic subarachnoid hemorrhage (I69.04-)*
- *monoplegia of upper limb following nontraumatic subarachnoid hemorrhage (I69.03-)*

I69.061 Other paralytic syndrome following nontraumatic subarachnoid hemorrhage affecting right dominant side HCC

I69.062 Other paralytic syndrome following nontraumatic subarachnoid hemorrhage affecting left dominant side HCC

I69.063 Other paralytic syndrome following nontraumatic subarachnoid hemorrhage affecting right non-dominant side HCC

I69.064 Other paralytic syndrome following nontraumatic subarachnoid hemorrhage affecting left non-dominant side HCC

I69.065 Other paralytic syndrome following nontraumatic subarachnoid hemorrhage, bilateral HCC

I69.069 Other paralytic syndrome following nontraumatic subarachnoid hemorrhage affecting unspecified side HCC

I69.09 Other sequelae of nontraumatic subarachnoid hemorrhage

I69.090 Apraxia following nontraumatic subarachnoid hemorrhage

I69.091 Dysphagia following nontraumatic subarachnoid hemorrhage

Use additional code to identify the type of dysphagia, if known ▶(R13.11-R13.19)◀

I69.092 Facial weakness following nontraumatic subarachnoid hemorrhage

Facial droop following nontraumatic subarachnoid hemorrhage

I69.093 Ataxia following nontraumatic subarachnoid hemorrhage

I69.098 Other sequelae following nontraumatic subarachnoid hemorrhage

Alterations of sensation following nontraumatic subarachnoid hemorrhage

Disturbance of vision following nontraumatic subarachnoid hemorrhage

Use additional code to identify the sequelae

I69.1 Sequelae of nontraumatic intracerebral hemorrhage

I69.10 Unspecified sequelae of nontraumatic intracerebral hemorrhage

I69.11 Cognitive deficits following nontraumatic intracerebral hemorrhage

I69.110 Attention and concentration deficit following nontraumatic intracerebral hemorrhage

I69.111 Memory deficit following nontraumatic intracerebral hemorrhage

I69.112 Visuospatial deficit and spatial neglect following nontraumatic intracerebral hemorrhage

I69.113 Psychomotor deficit following nontraumatic intracerebral hemorrhage

I69.114 Frontal lobe and executive function deficit following nontraumatic intracerebral hemorrhage

I69.115 Cognitive social or emotional deficit following nontraumatic intracerebral hemorrhage

I69.118 Other symptoms and signs involving cognitive functions following nontraumatic intracerebral hemorrhage

Chapter 9. Diseases of the Circulatory System

I69.019–I69.118

I69.119 **Unspecified symptoms and signs involving cognitive functions following nontraumatic intracerebral hemorrhage**

✓6th **I69.12** **Speech and language deficits following nontraumatic intracerebral hemorrhage**

I69.120 **Aphasia following nontraumatic intracerebral hemorrhage**

I69.121 **Dysphasia following nontraumatic intracerebral hemorrhage**

I69.122 **Dysarthria following nontraumatic intracerebral hemorrhage**

I69.123 **Fluency disorder following nontraumatic intracerebral hemorrhage**

Stuttering following nontraumatic intracerebral hemorrhage

I69.128 **Other speech and language deficits following nontraumatic intracerebral hemorrhage**

✓6th **I69.13** **Monoplegia of upper limb following nontraumatic intracerebral hemorrhage**

AHA: 2017,1Q,47

I69.131 **Monoplegia of upper limb following nontraumatic intracerebral hemorrhage affecting right dominant side** HCC

I69.132 **Monoplegia of upper limb following nontraumatic intracerebral hemorrhage affecting left dominant side** HCC

I69.133 **Monoplegia of upper limb following nontraumatic intracerebral hemorrhage affecting right non-dominant side** HCC

I69.134 **Monoplegia of upper limb following nontraumatic intracerebral hemorrhage affecting left non-dominant side** HCC

I69.139 **Monoplegia of upper limb following nontraumatic intracerebral hemorrhage affecting unspecified side** HCC

✓6th **I69.14** **Monoplegia of lower limb following nontraumatic intracerebral hemorrhage**

AHA: 2017,1Q,47

I69.141 **Monoplegia of lower limb following nontraumatic intracerebral hemorrhage affecting right dominant side** HCC

I69.142 **Monoplegia of lower limb following nontraumatic intracerebral hemorrhage affecting left dominant side** HCC

I69.143 **Monoplegia of lower limb following nontraumatic intracerebral hemorrhage affecting right non-dominant side** HCC

I69.144 **Monoplegia of lower limb following nontraumatic intracerebral hemorrhage affecting left non-dominant side** HCC

I69.149 **Monoplegia of lower limb following nontraumatic intracerebral hemorrhage affecting unspecified side** HCC

✓6th **I69.15** **Hemiplegia and hemiparesis following nontraumatic intracerebral hemorrhage**

AHA: 2015,1Q,25

I69.151 **Hemiplegia and hemiparesis following nontraumatic intracerebral hemorrhage affecting right dominant side** CC HCC

I69.152 **Hemiplegia and hemiparesis following nontraumatic intracerebral hemorrhage affecting left dominant side** CC HCC

I69.153 **Hemiplegia and hemiparesis following nontraumatic intracerebral hemorrhage affecting right non-dominant side** CC HCC

I69.154 **Hemiplegia and hemiparesis following nontraumatic intracerebral hemorrhage affecting left non-dominant side** CC HCC

I69.159 **Hemiplegia and hemiparesis following nontraumatic intracerebral hemorrhage affecting unspecified side** CC UNS HCC

✓6th **I69.16** **Other paralytic syndrome following nontraumatic intracerebral hemorrhage**

Use additional code to identify type of paralytic syndrome, such as:
locked-in state (G83.5)
quadriplegia (G82.5-)

EXCLUDES 1 *hemiplegia/hemiparesis following nontraumatic intracerebral hemorrhage (I69.15-)*
monoplegia of lower limb following nontraumatic intracerebral hemorrhage (I69.14-)
monoplegia of upper limb following nontraumatic intracerebral hemorrhage (I69.13-)

I69.161 **Other paralytic syndrome following nontraumatic intracerebral hemorrhage affecting right dominant side** HCC

I69.162 **Other paralytic syndrome following nontraumatic intracerebral hemorrhage affecting left dominant side** HCC

I69.163 **Other paralytic syndrome following nontraumatic intracerebral hemorrhage affecting right non-dominant side** HCC

I69.164 **Other paralytic syndrome following nontraumatic intracerebral hemorrhage affecting left non-dominant side** HCC

I69.165 **Other paralytic syndrome following nontraumatic intracerebral hemorrhage, bilateral** HCC

I69.169 **Other paralytic syndrome following nontraumatic intracerebral hemorrhage affecting unspecified side** HCC

✓6th **I69.19** **Other sequelae of nontraumatic intracerebral hemorrhage**

I69.190 **Apraxia following nontraumatic intracerebral hemorrhage**

I69.191 **Dysphagia following nontraumatic intracerebral hemorrhage**

Use additional code to identify the type of dysphagia, if known
►(R13.11-R13.19)◄

I69.192 **Facial weakness following nontraumatic intracerebral hemorrhage**

Facial droop following nontraumatic intracerebral hemorrhage

I69.193 **Ataxia following nontraumatic intracerebral hemorrhage**

I69.198 **Other sequelae of nontraumatic intracerebral hemorrhage**

Alteration of sensations following nontraumatic intracerebral hemorrhage

Disturbance of vision following nontraumatic intracerebral hemorrhage

Use additional code to identify the sequelae

✓5th **I69.2** **Sequelae of other nontraumatic intracranial hemorrhage**

I69.20 **Unspecified sequelae of other nontraumatic intracranial hemorrhage**

✓6th **I69.21** **Cognitive deficits following other nontraumatic intracranial hemorrhage**

I69.210 **Attention and concentration deficit following other nontraumatic intracranial hemorrhage**

I69.211 **Memory deficit following other nontraumatic intracranial hemorrhage**

I69.212 **Visuospatial deficit and spatial neglect following other nontraumatic intracranial hemorrhage**

I69.213 **Psychomotor deficit following other nontraumatic intracranial hemorrhage**

I69.214 **Frontal lobe and executive function deficit following other nontraumatic intracranial hemorrhage**

I69.215 **Cognitive social or emotional deficit following other nontraumatic intracranial hemorrhage**

I69.218 **Other symptoms and signs involving cognitive functions following other nontraumatic intracranial hemorrhage**

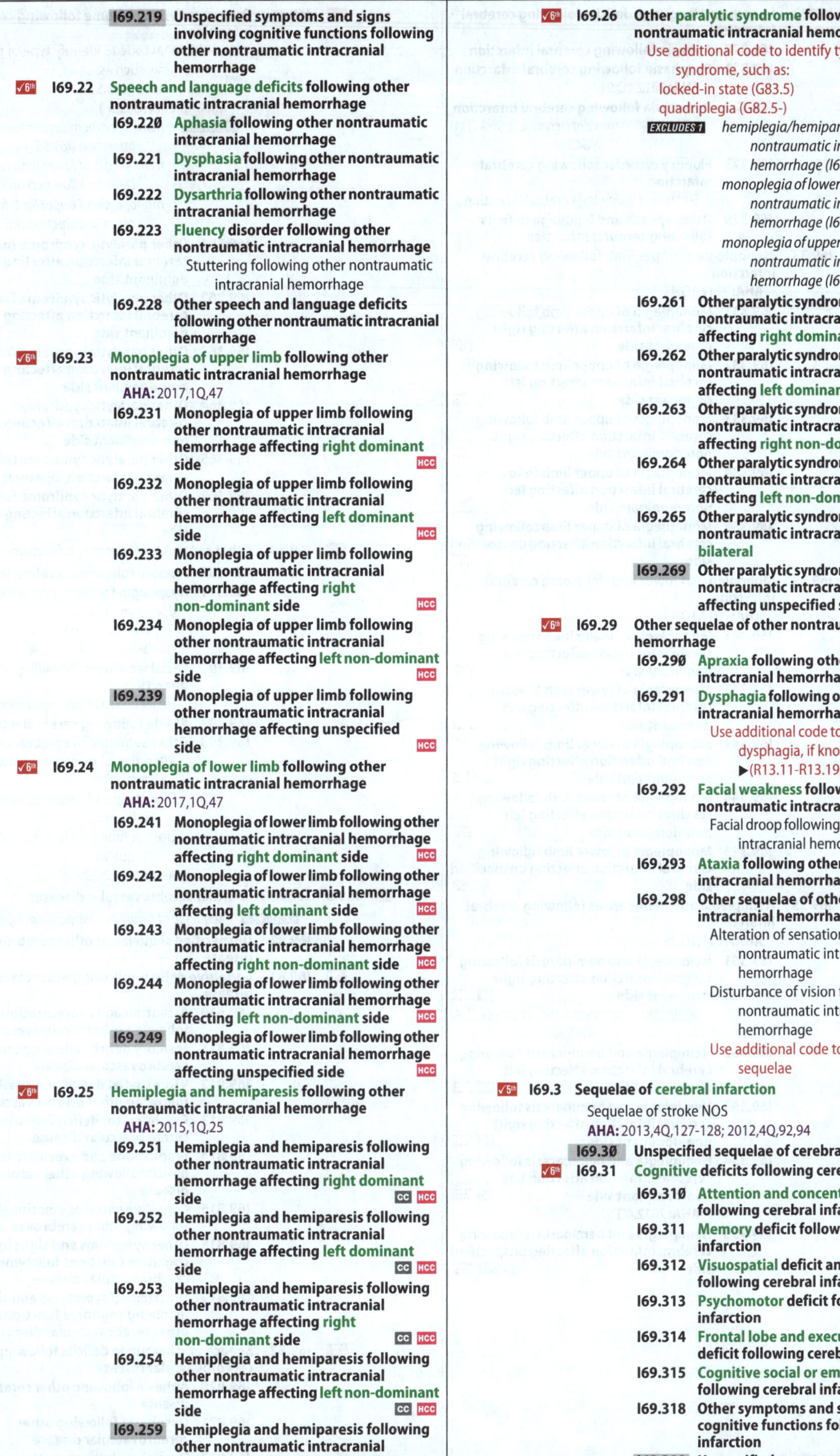

I69.219 Unspecified symptoms and signs involving cognitive functions following other nontraumatic intracranial hemorrhage

I69.22 Speech and language deficits following other nontraumatic intracranial hemorrhage
- I69.220 Aphasia following other nontraumatic intracranial hemorrhage
- I69.221 Dysphasia following other nontraumatic intracranial hemorrhage
- I69.222 Dysarthria following other nontraumatic intracranial hemorrhage
- I69.223 Fluency disorder following other nontraumatic intracranial hemorrhage
  Stuttering following other nontraumatic intracranial hemorrhage
- I69.228 Other speech and language deficits following other nontraumatic intracranial hemorrhage

I69.23 Monoplegia of upper limb following other nontraumatic intracranial hemorrhage
AHA: 2017,1Q,47
- I69.231 Monoplegia of upper limb following other nontraumatic intracranial hemorrhage affecting right dominant side HCC
- I69.232 Monoplegia of upper limb following other nontraumatic intracranial hemorrhage affecting left dominant side HCC
- I69.233 Monoplegia of upper limb following other nontraumatic intracranial hemorrhage affecting right non-dominant side HCC
- I69.234 Monoplegia of upper limb following other nontraumatic intracranial hemorrhage affecting left non-dominant side HCC
- I69.239 Monoplegia of upper limb following other nontraumatic intracranial hemorrhage affecting unspecified side HCC

I69.24 Monoplegia of lower limb following other nontraumatic intracranial hemorrhage
AHA: 2017,1Q,47
- I69.241 Monoplegia of lower limb following other nontraumatic intracranial hemorrhage affecting right dominant side HCC
- I69.242 Monoplegia of lower limb following other nontraumatic intracranial hemorrhage affecting left dominant side HCC
- I69.243 Monoplegia of lower limb following other nontraumatic intracranial hemorrhage affecting right non-dominant side HCC
- I69.244 Monoplegia of lower limb following other nontraumatic intracranial hemorrhage affecting left non-dominant side HCC
- I69.249 Monoplegia of lower limb following other nontraumatic intracranial hemorrhage affecting unspecified side HCC

I69.25 Hemiplegia and hemiparesis following other nontraumatic intracranial hemorrhage
AHA: 2015,1Q,25
- I69.251 Hemiplegia and hemiparesis following other nontraumatic intracranial hemorrhage affecting right dominant side CC HCC
- I69.252 Hemiplegia and hemiparesis following other nontraumatic intracranial hemorrhage affecting left dominant side CC HCC
- I69.253 Hemiplegia and hemiparesis following other nontraumatic intracranial hemorrhage affecting right non-dominant side CC HCC
- I69.254 Hemiplegia and hemiparesis following other nontraumatic intracranial hemorrhage affecting left non-dominant side CC HCC
- I69.259 Hemiplegia and hemiparesis following other nontraumatic intracranial hemorrhage affecting unspecified side CC UNS HCC

I69.26 Other paralytic syndrome following other nontraumatic intracranial hemorrhage
Use additional code to identify type of paralytic syndrome, such as:
locked-in state (G83.5)
quadriplegia (G82.5-)
EXCLUDES 1 *hemiplegia/hemiparesis following other nontraumatic intracranial hemorrhage (I69.25-)*
monoplegia of lower limb following other nontraumatic intracranial hemorrhage (I69.24-)
monoplegia of upper limb following other nontraumatic intracranial hemorrhage (I69.23-)
- I69.261 Other paralytic syndrome following other nontraumatic intracranial hemorrhage affecting right dominant side HCC
- I69.262 Other paralytic syndrome following other nontraumatic intracranial hemorrhage affecting left dominant side HCC
- I69.263 Other paralytic syndrome following other nontraumatic intracranial hemorrhage affecting right non-dominant side HCC
- I69.264 Other paralytic syndrome following other nontraumatic intracranial hemorrhage affecting left non-dominant side HCC
- I69.265 Other paralytic syndrome following other nontraumatic intracranial hemorrhage, bilateral HCC
- I69.269 Other paralytic syndrome following other nontraumatic intracranial hemorrhage affecting unspecified side HCC

I69.29 Other sequelae of other nontraumatic intracranial hemorrhage
- I69.290 Apraxia following other nontraumatic intracranial hemorrhage
- I69.291 Dysphagia following other nontraumatic intracranial hemorrhage
  Use additional code to identify the type of dysphagia, if known ▶(R13.11-R13.19)◀
- I69.292 Facial weakness following other nontraumatic intracranial hemorrhage
  Facial droop following other nontraumatic intracranial hemorrhage
- I69.293 Ataxia following other nontraumatic intracranial hemorrhage
- I69.298 Other sequelae of other nontraumatic intracranial hemorrhage
  Alteration of sensation following other nontraumatic intracranial hemorrhage
  Disturbance of vision following other nontraumatic intracranial hemorrhage
  Use additional code to identify the sequelae

I69.3 Sequelae of cerebral infarction
Sequelae of stroke NOS
AHA: 2013,4Q,127-128; 2012,4Q,92,94

I69.30 Unspecified sequelae of cerebral infarction

I69.31 Cognitive deficits following cerebral infarction
- I69.310 Attention and concentration deficit following cerebral infarction
- I69.311 Memory deficit following cerebral infarction
- I69.312 Visuospatial deficit and spatial neglect following cerebral infarction
- I69.313 Psychomotor deficit following cerebral infarction
- I69.314 Frontal lobe and executive function deficit following cerebral infarction
- I69.315 Cognitive social or emotional deficit following cerebral infarction
- I69.318 Other symptoms and signs involving cognitive functions following cerebral infarction
- I69.319 Unspecified symptoms and signs involving cognitive functions following cerebral infarction

✓6th I69.32 Speech and language deficits following cerebral infarction

I69.320 Aphasia following cerebral infarction

I69.321 Dysphasia following cerebral infarction

AHA: 2012,4Q,91

I69.322 Dysarthria following cerebral infarction

EXCLUDES 2 *transient ischemic attack (TIA) (G45.9)*

I69.323 Fluency disorder following cerebral infarction

Stuttering following cerebral infarction

I69.328 Other speech and language deficits following cerebral infarction

✓6th I69.33 Monoplegia of upper limb following cerebral infarction

AHA: 2017,1Q,47

I69.331 Monoplegia of upper limb following cerebral infarction affecting right dominant side HCC

I69.332 Monoplegia of upper limb following cerebral infarction affecting left dominant side HCC

I69.333 Monoplegia of upper limb following cerebral infarction affecting right non-dominant side HCC

I69.334 Monoplegia of upper limb following cerebral infarction affecting left non-dominant side HCC

I69.339 Monoplegia of upper limb following cerebral infarction affecting unspecified side HCC

✓6th I69.34 Monoplegia of lower limb following cerebral infarction

AHA: 2017,1Q,47

I69.341 Monoplegia of lower limb following cerebral infarction affecting right dominant side HCC

I69.342 Monoplegia of lower limb following cerebral infarction affecting left dominant side HCC

I69.343 Monoplegia of lower limb following cerebral infarction affecting right non-dominant side HCC

I69.344 Monoplegia of lower limb following cerebral infarction affecting left non-dominant side HCC

I69.349 Monoplegia of lower limb following cerebral infarction affecting unspecified side HCC

✓6th I69.35 Hemiplegia and hemiparesis following cerebral infarction

AHA: 2015,1Q,25

I69.351 Hemiplegia and hemiparesis following cerebral infarction affecting right dominant side CC HCC

EXCLUDES 2 *transient ischemic attack (TIA) (G45.9)*

I69.352 Hemiplegia and hemiparesis following cerebral infarction affecting left dominant side CC HCC

I69.353 Hemiplegia and hemiparesis following cerebral infarction affecting right non-dominant side CC HCC

I69.354 Hemiplegia and hemiparesis following cerebral infarction affecting left non-dominant side CC HCC

AHA: 2012,4Q,91

I69.359 Hemiplegia and hemiparesis following cerebral infarction affecting unspecified side CC UNS HCC

✓6th I69.36 Other paralytic syndrome following cerebral infarction

Use additional code to identify type of paralytic syndrome, such as:

locked-in state (G83.5)

quadriplegia (G82.5-)

EXCLUDES 1 *hemiplegia/hemiparesis following cerebral infarction (I69.35-)*

monoplegia of lower limb following cerebral infarction (I69.34-)

monoplegia of upper limb following cerebral infarction (I69.33-)

I69.361 Other paralytic syndrome following cerebral infarction affecting right dominant side HCC

I69.362 Other paralytic syndrome following cerebral infarction affecting left dominant side HCC

I69.363 Other paralytic syndrome following cerebral infarction affecting right non-dominant side HCC

I69.364 Other paralytic syndrome following cerebral infarction affecting left non-dominant side HCC

I69.365 Other paralytic syndrome following cerebral infarction, bilateral HCC

I69.369 Other paralytic syndrome following cerebral infarction affecting unspecified side HCC

✓6th I69.39 Other sequelae of cerebral infarction

I69.390 Apraxia following cerebral infarction

I69.391 Dysphagia following cerebral infarction

Use additional code to identify the type of dysphagia, if known ►(R13.11-R13.19)◄

I69.392 Facial weakness following cerebral infarction

Facial droop following cerebral infarction

I69.393 Ataxia following cerebral infarction

I69.398 Other sequelae of cerebral infarction

Alteration of sensation following cerebral infarction

Disturbance of vision following cerebral infarction

Use additional code to identify the sequelae

AHA: 2020,2Q,29

✓5th I69.8 Sequelae of other cerebrovascular diseases

EXCLUDES 1 *sequelae of traumatic intracranial injury (S06.-)*

I69.80 Unspecified sequelae of other cerebrovascular disease

✓6th I69.81 Cognitive deficits following other cerebrovascular disease

I69.810 Attention and concentration deficit following other cerebrovascular disease

I69.811 Memory deficit following other cerebrovascular disease

I69.812 Visuospatial deficit and spatial neglect following other cerebrovascular disease

I69.813 Psychomotor deficit following other cerebrovascular disease

I69.814 Frontal lobe and executive function deficit following other cerebrovascular disease

I69.815 Cognitive social or emotional deficit following other cerebrovascular disease

I69.818 Other symptoms and signs involving cognitive functions following other cerebrovascular disease

I69.819 Unspecified symptoms and signs involving cognitive functions following other cerebrovascular disease

✓6th I69.82 Speech and language deficits following other cerebrovascular disease

I69.820 Aphasia following other cerebrovascular disease

I69.821 Dysphasia following other cerebrovascular disease

I69.822 Dysarthria following other cerebrovascular disease

I69.823 Fluency disorder following other cerebrovascular disease
Stuttering following other cerebrovascular disease

I69.828 Other speech and language deficits following other cerebrovascular disease
AHA: 2019,3Q,8

√6th **I69.83 Monoplegia of upper limb following other cerebrovascular disease**
AHA: 2017,1Q,47

I69.831 Monoplegia of upper limb following other cerebrovascular disease affecting right dominant side HCC

I69.832 Monoplegia of upper limb following other cerebrovascular disease affecting left dominant side HCC

I69.833 Monoplegia of upper limb following other cerebrovascular disease affecting right non-dominant side HCC

I69.834 Monoplegia of upper limb following other cerebrovascular disease affecting left non-dominant side HCC

I69.839 Monoplegia of upper limb following other cerebrovascular disease affecting unspecified side HCC

√6th **I69.84 Monoplegia of lower limb following other cerebrovascular disease**
AHA: 2017,1Q,47

I69.841 Monoplegia of lower limb following other cerebrovascular disease affecting right dominant side HCC

I69.842 Monoplegia of lower limb following other cerebrovascular disease affecting left dominant side HCC

I69.843 Monoplegia of lower limb following other cerebrovascular disease affecting right non-dominant side HCC

I69.844 Monoplegia of lower limb following other cerebrovascular disease affecting left non-dominant side HCC

I69.849 Monoplegia of lower limb following other cerebrovascular disease affecting unspecified side HCC

√6th **I69.85 Hemiplegia and hemiparesis following other cerebrovascular disease**
AHA: 2015,1Q,25

I69.851 Hemiplegia and hemiparesis following other cerebrovascular disease affecting right dominant side CC HCC

I69.852 Hemiplegia and hemiparesis following other cerebrovascular disease affecting left dominant side CC HCC

I69.853 Hemiplegia and hemiparesis following other cerebrovascular disease affecting right non-dominant side CC HCC

I69.854 Hemiplegia and hemiparesis following other cerebrovascular disease affecting left non-dominant side CC HCC

I69.859 Hemiplegia and hemiparesis following other cerebrovascular disease affecting unspecified side CC UNS HCC

√6th **I69.86 Other paralytic syndrome following other cerebrovascular disease**
Use additional code to identify type of paralytic syndrome, such as:
locked-in state (G83.5)
quadriplegia (G82.5-)

EXCLUDES 1 *hemiplegia/hemiparesis following other cerebrovascular disease (I69.85-)*
monoplegia of lower limb following other cerebrovascular disease (I69.84-)
monoplegia of upper limb following other cerebrovascular disease (I69.83-)

I69.861 Other paralytic syndrome following other cerebrovascular disease affecting right dominant side HCC

I69.862 Other paralytic syndrome following other cerebrovascular disease affecting left dominant side HCC

I69.863 Other paralytic syndrome following other cerebrovascular disease affecting right non-dominant side HCC

I69.864 Other paralytic syndrome following other cerebrovascular disease affecting left non-dominant side HCC

I69.865 Other paralytic syndrome following other cerebrovascular disease, bilateral HCC

I69.869 Other paralytic syndrome following other cerebrovascular disease affecting unspecified side HCC

√6th **I69.89 Other sequelae of other cerebrovascular disease**

I69.890 Apraxia following other cerebrovascular disease

I69.891 Dysphagia following other cerebrovascular disease
Use additional code to identify the type of dysphagia, if known ►(R13.11-R13.19)◄

I69.892 Facial weakness following other cerebrovascular disease
Facial droop following other cerebrovascular disease

I69.893 Ataxia following other cerebrovascular disease

I69.898 Other sequelae of other cerebrovascular disease
Alteration of sensation following other cerebrovascular disease
Disturbance of vision following other cerebrovascular disease
Use additional code to identify the sequelae

√5th **I69.9 Sequelae of unspecified cerebrovascular diseases**

EXCLUDES 1 *sequelae of stroke (I69.3)*
sequelae of traumatic intracranial injury (S06.-)

I69.90 Unspecified sequelae of unspecified cerebrovascular disease

√6th **I69.91 Cognitive deficits following unspecified cerebrovascular disease**

I69.910 Attention and concentration deficit following unspecified cerebrovascular disease

I69.911 Memory deficit following unspecified cerebrovascular disease

I69.912 Visuospatial deficit and spatial neglect following unspecified cerebrovascular disease

I69.913 Psychomotor deficit following unspecified cerebrovascular disease

I69.914 Frontal lobe and executive function deficit following unspecified cerebrovascular disease

I69.915 Cognitive social or emotional deficit following unspecified cerebrovascular disease

I69.918 Other symptoms and signs involving cognitive functions following unspecified cerebrovascular disease

I69.919 Unspecified symptoms and signs involving cognitive functions following unspecified cerebrovascular disease

√6th **I69.92 Speech and language deficits following unspecified cerebrovascular disease**

I69.920 Aphasia following unspecified cerebrovascular disease

I69.921 Dysphasia following unspecified cerebrovascular disease

I69.922 Dysarthria following unspecified cerebrovascular disease

I69.923 Fluency disorder following unspecified cerebrovascular disease
Stuttering following unspecified cerebrovascular disease

I69.928 Other speech and language deficits following unspecified cerebrovascular disease

√6th **I69.93 Monoplegia of upper limb following unspecified cerebrovascular disease**
AHA: 2017,1Q,47

I69.931 Monoplegia of upper limb following unspecified cerebrovascular disease affecting right dominant side HCC

I69.932 Monoplegia of upper limb following unspecified cerebrovascular disease affecting left dominant side HCC

I69.933 Monoplegia of upper limb following unspecified cerebrovascular disease affecting right non-dominant side HCC

I69.934 Monoplegia of upper limb following unspecified cerebrovascular disease affecting left non-dominant side HCC

I69.939 Monoplegia of upper limb following unspecified cerebrovascular disease affecting unspecified side HCC

✓6th **I69.94 Monoplegia of lower limb following unspecified cerebrovascular disease**

AHA: 2017,1Q,47

I69.941 Monoplegia of lower limb following unspecified cerebrovascular disease affecting right dominant side HCC

I69.942 Monoplegia of lower limb following unspecified cerebrovascular disease affecting left dominant side HCC

I69.943 Monoplegia of lower limb following unspecified cerebrovascular disease affecting right non-dominant side HCC

I69.944 Monoplegia of lower limb following unspecified cerebrovascular disease affecting left non-dominant side HCC

I69.949 Monoplegia of lower limb following unspecified cerebrovascular disease affecting unspecified side HCC

✓6th **I69.95 Hemiplegia and hemiparesis following unspecified cerebrovascular disease**

AHA: 2015,1Q,25

I69.951 Hemiplegia and hemiparesis following unspecified cerebrovascular disease affecting right dominant side CC HCC

I69.952 Hemiplegia and hemiparesis following unspecified cerebrovascular disease affecting left dominant side CC HCC

I69.953 Hemiplegia and hemiparesis following unspecified cerebrovascular disease affecting right non-dominant side CC HCC

I69.954 Hemiplegia and hemiparesis following unspecified cerebrovascular disease affecting left non-dominant side CC HCC

I69.959 Hemiplegia and hemiparesis following unspecified cerebrovascular disease affecting unspecified side CC UNS HCC

✓6th **I69.96 Other paralytic syndrome following unspecified cerebrovascular disease**

Use additional code to identify type of paralytic syndrome, such as:
- locked-in state (G83.5)
- quadriplegia (G82.5-)

EXCLUDES 1
- *hemiplegia/hemiparesis following unspecified cerebrovascular disease (I69.95-)*
- *monoplegia of lower limb following unspecified cerebrovascular disease (I69.94-)*
- *monoplegia of upper limb following unspecified cerebrovascular disease (I69.93-)*

I69.961 Other paralytic syndrome following unspecified cerebrovascular disease affecting right dominant side HCC

I69.962 Other paralytic syndrome following unspecified cerebrovascular disease affecting left dominant side HCC

I69.963 Other paralytic syndrome following unspecified cerebrovascular disease affecting right non-dominant side HCC

I69.964 Other paralytic syndrome following unspecified cerebrovascular disease affecting left non-dominant side HCC

I69.965 Other paralytic syndrome following unspecified cerebrovascular disease, bilateral HCC

I69.969 Other paralytic syndrome following unspecified cerebrovascular disease affecting unspecified side HCC

✓6th **I69.99 Other sequelae of unspecified cerebrovascular disease**

I69.990 Apraxia following unspecified cerebrovascular disease

I69.991 Dysphagia following unspecified cerebrovascular disease

Use additional code to identify the type of dysphagia, if known ▶(R13.11-R13.19)◀

I69.992 Facial weakness following unspecified cerebrovascular disease

Facial droop following unspecified cerebrovascular disease

I69.993 Ataxia following unspecified cerebrovascular disease

I69.998 Other sequelae following unspecified cerebrovascular disease

Alteration in sensation following unspecified cerebrovascular disease

Disturbance of vision following unspecified cerebrovascular disease

Use additional code to identify the sequelae

Diseases of arteries, arterioles and capillaries (I7Ø-I79)

✓4th **I7Ø Atherosclerosis**

INCLUDES
- arterial degeneration
- arteriolosclerosis
- arteriosclerosis
- arteriosclerotic vascular disease
- arteriovascular degeneration
- atheroma
- endarteritis deformans or obliterans
- senile arteritis
- senile endarteritis
- vascular degeneration

Use additional code to identify:
- exposure to environmental tobacco smoke (Z77.22)
- history of tobacco dependence (Z87.891)
- occupational exposure to environmental tobacco smoke (Z57.31)
- tobacco dependence (F17.-)
- tobacco use (Z72.Ø)

EXCLUDES 2
- *arteriosclerotic cardiovascular disease (I25.1-)*
- *arteriosclerotic heart disease (I25.1-)*
- *atheroembolism (I75.-)*
- *cerebral atherosclerosis (I67.2)*
- *coronary atherosclerosis (I25.1-)*
- *mesenteric atherosclerosis (K55.1)*
- *precerebral atherosclerosis (I67.2)*
- *primary pulmonary atherosclerosis (I27.Ø)*

I7Ø.Ø Atherosclerosis of aorta HCC A

I7Ø.1 Atherosclerosis of renal artery HCC A

Goldblatt's kidney

EXCLUDES 2 *atherosclerosis of renal arterioles (I12.-)*

✓5th **I7Ø.2 Atherosclerosis of native arteries of the extremities**

Mönckeberg's (medial) sclerosis

Use additional code, if applicable, to identify chronic total occlusion of artery of extremity (I7Ø.92)

EXCLUDES 2 *atherosclerosis of bypass graft of extremities (I7Ø.3Ø-I7Ø.79)*

AHA: 2020,4Q,98; 2018,3Q,4; 2018,2Q,7

✓6th **I7Ø.2Ø Unspecified atherosclerosis of native arteries of extremities**

I7Ø.2Ø1 Unspecified atherosclerosis of native arteries of extremities, right leg HCC A

I7Ø.2Ø2 Unspecified atherosclerosis of native arteries of extremities, left leg HCC A

I7Ø.2Ø3 Unspecified atherosclerosis of native arteries of extremities, bilateral legs HCC A

I7Ø.2Ø8 Unspecified atherosclerosis of native arteries of extremities, other extremity HCC A

I70.209 Unspecified atherosclerosis of native arteries of extremities, unspecified extremity HCC A

I70.21 Atherosclerosis of native arteries of extremities with intermittent claudication (6th)

I70.211 Atherosclerosis of native arteries of extremities with intermittent claudication, right leg HCC A

I70.212 Atherosclerosis of native arteries of extremities with intermittent claudication, left leg HCC A

I70.213 Atherosclerosis of native arteries of extremities with intermittent claudication, bilateral legs HCC A

I70.218 Atherosclerosis of native arteries of extremities with intermittent claudication, other extremity HCC A

I70.219 Atherosclerosis of native arteries of extremities with intermittent claudication, unspecified extremity HCC A

I70.22 Atherosclerosis of native arteries of extremities with rest pain (6th)

INCLUDES any condition classifiable to I70.21-
chronic limb-threatening ischemia NOS of native arteries of extremities
chronic limb-threatening ischemia of native arteries of extremities with rest pain
critical limb ischemia NOS of native arteries of extremities
critical limb ischemia of native arteries of extremities with rest pain

I70.221 Atherosclerosis of native arteries of extremities with rest pain, right leg HCC A

I70.222 Atherosclerosis of native arteries of extremities with rest pain, left leg HCC A

I70.223 Atherosclerosis of native arteries of extremities with rest pain, bilateral legs HCC A

I70.228 Atherosclerosis of native arteries of extremities with rest pain, other extremity HCC A

I70.229 Atherosclerosis of native arteries of extremities with rest pain, unspecified extremity HCC A

I70.23 Atherosclerosis of native arteries of right leg with ulceration (6th)

INCLUDES any condition classifiable to I70.211 and I70.221
chronic limb-threatening ischemia of native arteries of right leg with ulceration
critical limb ischemia of native arteries of right leg with ulceration

Use additional code to identify severity of ulcer (L97.-)

I70.231 Atherosclerosis of native arteries of right leg with ulceration of thigh HCC A

I70.232 Atherosclerosis of native arteries of right leg with ulceration of calf HCC A

I70.233 Atherosclerosis of native arteries of right leg with ulceration of ankle HCC A

I70.234 Atherosclerosis of native arteries of right leg with ulceration of heel and midfoot HCC A

Atherosclerosis of native arteries of right leg with ulceration of plantar surface of midfoot

I70.235 Atherosclerosis of native arteries of right leg with ulceration of other part of foot HCC A

Atherosclerosis of native arteries of right leg extremities with ulceration of toe

I70.238 Atherosclerosis of native arteries of right leg with ulceration of other part of lower leg HCC A

I70.239 Atherosclerosis of native arteries of right leg with ulceration of unspecified site HCC A

I70.24 Atherosclerosis of native arteries of left leg with ulceration (6th)

INCLUDES any condition classifiable to I70.212 and I70.222
chronic limb-threatening ischemia of native arteries of left leg with ulceration
critical limb ischemia of native arteries of left leg with ulceration

Use additional code to identify severity of ulcer (L97.-)

I70.241 Atherosclerosis of native arteries of left leg with ulceration of thigh HCC A

I70.242 Atherosclerosis of native arteries of left leg with ulceration of calf HCC A

I70.243 Atherosclerosis of native arteries of left leg with ulceration of ankle HCC A

I70.244 Atherosclerosis of native arteries of left leg with ulceration of heel and midfoot HCC A

Atherosclerosis of native arteries of left leg with ulceration of plantar surface of midfoot

I70.245 Atherosclerosis of native arteries of left leg with ulceration of other part of foot HCC A

Atherosclerosis of native arteries of left leg extremities with ulceration of toe

I70.248 Atherosclerosis of native arteries of left leg with ulceration of other part of lower leg HCC A

I70.249 Atherosclerosis of native arteries of left leg with ulceration of unspecified site HCC A

I70.25 Atherosclerosis of native arteries of other extremities with ulceration HCC A

INCLUDES any condition classifiable to I70.218 and I70.228

Use additional code to identify the severity of the ulcer (L98.49-)

I70.26 Atherosclerosis of native arteries of extremities with gangrene (6th)

INCLUDES any condition classifiable to I70.21-, I70.22-, I70.23-, I70.24-, and I70.25-
chronic limb-threatening ischemia of native arteries of extremities with gangrene
critical limb ischemia of native arteries of extremities with gangrene

Use additional code to identify the severity of any ulcer (L97.-, L98.49-), if applicable

I70.261 Atherosclerosis of native arteries of extremities with gangrene, right leg CC HCC A

I70.262 Atherosclerosis of native arteries of extremities with gangrene, left leg CC HCC A

I70.263 Atherosclerosis of native arteries of extremities with gangrene, bilateral legs CC HCC A

I70.268 Atherosclerosis of native arteries of extremities with gangrene, other extremity CC HCC A

I70.269 Atherosclerosis of native arteries of extremities with gangrene, unspecified extremity CC UNS HCC A

I70.29 Other atherosclerosis of native arteries of extremities (6th)

I70.291 Other atherosclerosis of native arteries of extremities, right leg HCC A

I70.292 Other atherosclerosis of native arteries of extremities, left leg HCC A

I70.293 Other atherosclerosis of native arteries of extremities, bilateral legs HCC A

I70.298 Other atherosclerosis of native arteries of extremities, other extremity HCC A

I70.299 Other atherosclerosis of native arteries of extremities, unspecified extremity HCC A

I70.3 Atherosclerosis of unspecified type of bypass graft(s) of the extremities
Use additional code, if applicable, to identify chronic total occlusion of artery of extremity (I70.92)
EXCLUDES 1 *embolism or thrombus of bypass graft(s) of extremities (T82.8-)*
AHA: 2020,4Q,98

I70.30 Unspecified atherosclerosis of unspecified type of bypass graft(s) of the extremities
- **I70.301 Unspecified atherosclerosis of unspecified type of bypass graft(s) of the extremities, right leg** HCC A
- **I70.302 Unspecified atherosclerosis of unspecified type of bypass graft(s) of the extremities, left leg** HCC A
- **I70.303 Unspecified atherosclerosis of unspecified type of bypass graft(s) of the extremities, bilateral legs** HCC A
- **I70.308 Unspecified atherosclerosis of unspecified type of bypass graft(s) of the extremities, other extremity** HCC A
- **I70.309 Unspecified atherosclerosis of unspecified type of bypass graft(s) of the extremities, unspecified extremity** HCC A

I70.31 Atherosclerosis of unspecified type of bypass graft(s) of the extremities with intermittent claudication
- **I70.311 Atherosclerosis of unspecified type of bypass graft(s) of the extremities with intermittent claudication, right leg** HCC A
- **I70.312 Atherosclerosis of unspecified type of bypass graft(s) of the extremities with intermittent claudication, left leg** HCC A
- **I70.313 Atherosclerosis of unspecified type of bypass graft(s) of the extremities with intermittent claudication, bilateral legs** HCC A
- **I70.318 Atherosclerosis of unspecified type of bypass graft(s) of the extremities with intermittent claudication, other extremity** HCC A
- **I70.319 Atherosclerosis of unspecified type of bypass graft(s) of the extremities with intermittent claudication, unspecified extremity** HCC A

I70.32 Atherosclerosis of unspecified type of bypass graft(s) of the extremities with rest pain
INCLUDES any condition classifiable to I70.31-
chronic limb-threatening ischemia NOS of unspecified type of bypass graft(s) of the extremities
▶chronic limb-threatening ischemia of unspecified type of bypass graft(s) of the extremities with rest pain◀
critical limb ischemia NOS of unspecified type of bypass graft(s) of the extremities
critical limb ischemia of unspecified type of bypass graft(s) of the extremities with rest pain
- **I70.321 Atherosclerosis of unspecified type of bypass graft(s) of the extremities with rest pain, right leg** HCC A
- **I70.322 Atherosclerosis of unspecified type of bypass graft(s) of the extremities with rest pain, left leg** HCC A
- **I70.323 Atherosclerosis of unspecified type of bypass graft(s) of the extremities with rest pain, bilateral legs** HCC A
- **I70.328 Atherosclerosis of unspecified type of bypass graft(s) of the extremities with rest pain, other extremity** HCC A
- **I70.329 Atherosclerosis of unspecified type of bypass graft(s) of the extremities with rest pain, unspecified extremity** HCC A

I70.33 Atherosclerosis of unspecified type of bypass graft(s) of the right leg with ulceration
INCLUDES any condition classifiable to I70.311 and I70.321
chronic limb-threatening ischemia of unspecified type of bypass graft(s) of the right leg with ulceration
critical limb ischemia of unspecified type of bypass graft(s) of the right leg with ulceration
Use additional code to identify severity of ulcer (L97.-)
- **I70.331 Atherosclerosis of unspecified type of bypass graft(s) of the right leg with ulceration of thigh** CC HCC A
- **I70.332 Atherosclerosis of unspecified type of bypass graft(s) of the right leg with ulceration of calf** CC HCC A
- **I70.333 Atherosclerosis of unspecified type of bypass graft(s) of the right leg with ulceration of ankle** CC HCC A
- **I70.334 Atherosclerosis of unspecified type of bypass graft(s) of the right leg with ulceration of heel and midfoot** CC HCC A
  Atherosclerosis of unspecified type of bypass graft(s) of right leg with ulceration of plantar surface of midfoot
- **I70.335 Atherosclerosis of unspecified type of bypass graft(s) of the right leg with ulceration of other part of foot** HCC A
  Atherosclerosis of unspecified type of bypass graft(s) of the right leg with ulceration of toe
- **I70.338 Atherosclerosis of unspecified type of bypass graft(s) of the right leg with ulceration of other part of lower leg** CC HCC A
- **I70.339 Atherosclerosis of unspecified type of bypass graft(s) of the right leg with ulceration of unspecified site** CC HCC A

I70.34 Atherosclerosis of unspecified type of bypass graft(s) of the left leg with ulceration
INCLUDES any condition classifiable to I70.312 and I70.322
chronic limb-threatening ischemia of unspecified type of bypass graft(s) of the left leg with ulceration
critical limb ischemia of unspecified type of bypass graft(s) of the left leg with ulceration
Use additional code to identify severity of ulcer (L97.-)
- **I70.341 Atherosclerosis of unspecified type of bypass graft(s) of the left leg with ulceration of thigh** CC HCC A
- **I70.342 Atherosclerosis of unspecified type of bypass graft(s) of the left leg with ulceration of calf** CC HCC A
- **I70.343 Atherosclerosis of unspecified type of bypass graft(s) of the left leg with ulceration of ankle** CC HCC A
- **I70.344 Atherosclerosis of unspecified type of bypass graft(s) of the left leg with ulceration of heel and midfoot** CC HCC A
  Atherosclerosis of unspecified type of bypass graft(s) of left leg with ulceration of plantar surface of midfoot
- **I70.345 Atherosclerosis of unspecified type of bypass graft(s) of the left leg with ulceration of other part of foot** HCC A
  Atherosclerosis of unspecified type of bypass graft(s) of the left leg with ulceration of toe
- **I70.348 Atherosclerosis of unspecified type of bypass graft(s) of the left leg with ulceration of other part of lower leg** CC HCC A

I70.349 Atherosclerosis of unspecified type of bypass graft(s) of the left leg with ulceration of unspecified site CC HCC A

I70.35 Atherosclerosis of unspecified type of bypass graft(s) of other extremity with ulceration HCC A

INCLUDES any condition classifiable to I70.318 and I70.328

Use additional code to identify severity of ulcer (L98.49-)

I70.36 Atherosclerosis of unspecified type of bypass graft(s) of the extremities with gangrene

INCLUDES any condition classifiable to I70.31-, I70.32-, I70.33-, I70.34-, I70.35

chronic limb-threatening ischemia of unspecified type of bypass graft(s) of the extremities with gangrene

critical limb ischemia of unspecified type of bypass graft(s) of the extremities with gangrene

Use additional code to identify the severity of any ulcer (L97.-, L98.49-), if applicable

I70.361 Atherosclerosis of unspecified type of bypass graft(s) of the extremities with gangrene, right leg CC HCC A

I70.362 Atherosclerosis of unspecified type of bypass graft(s) of the extremities with gangrene, left leg CC HCC A

I70.363 Atherosclerosis of unspecified type of bypass graft(s) of the extremities with gangrene, bilateral legs CC HCC A

I70.368 Atherosclerosis of unspecified type of bypass graft(s) of the extremities with gangrene, other extremity CC HCC A

I70.369 Atherosclerosis of unspecified type of bypass graft(s) of the extremities with gangrene, unspecified extremity CC UNS HCC A

I70.39 Other atherosclerosis of unspecified type of bypass graft(s) of the extremities

I70.391 Other atherosclerosis of unspecified type of bypass graft(s) of the extremities, right leg HCC A

I70.392 Other atherosclerosis of unspecified type of bypass graft(s) of the extremities, left leg HCC A

I70.393 Other atherosclerosis of unspecified type of bypass graft(s) of the extremities, bilateral legs HCC A

I70.398 Other atherosclerosis of unspecified type of bypass graft(s) of the extremities, other extremity HCC A

I70.399 Other atherosclerosis of unspecified type of bypass graft(s) of the extremities, unspecified extremity HCC A

I70.4 Atherosclerosis of autologous vein bypass graft(s) of the extremities

Use additional code, if applicable, to identify chronic total occlusion of artery of extremity (I70.92)

AHA: 2020,4Q,98

I70.40 Unspecified atherosclerosis of autologous vein bypass graft(s) of the extremities

I70.401 Unspecified atherosclerosis of autologous vein bypass graft(s) of the extremities, right leg HCC A

I70.402 Unspecified atherosclerosis of autologous vein bypass graft(s) of the extremities, left leg HCC A

I70.403 Unspecified atherosclerosis of autologous vein bypass graft(s) of the extremities, bilateral legs HCC A

I70.408 Unspecified atherosclerosis of autologous vein bypass graft(s) of the extremities, other extremity HCC A

I70.409 Unspecified atherosclerosis of autologous vein bypass graft(s) of the extremities, unspecified extremity HCC A

I70.41 Atherosclerosis of autologous vein bypass graft(s) of the extremities with intermittent claudication

I70.411 Atherosclerosis of autologous vein bypass graft(s) of the extremities with intermittent claudication, right leg HCC A

I70.412 Atherosclerosis of autologous vein bypass graft(s) of the extremities with intermittent claudication, left leg HCC A

I70.413 Atherosclerosis of autologous vein bypass graft(s) of the extremities with intermittent claudication, bilateral legs HCC A

I70.418 Atherosclerosis of autologous vein bypass graft(s) of the extremities with intermittent claudication, other extremity HCC A

I70.419 Atherosclerosis of autologous vein bypass graft(s) of the extremities with intermittent claudication, unspecified extremity HCC A

I70.42 Atherosclerosis of autologous vein bypass graft(s) of the extremities with rest pain

INCLUDES any condition classifiable to I70.41-

chronic limb-threatening ischemia NOS of autologous vein bypass graft(s) of the extremities

chronic limb-threatening ischemia of autologous vein bypass graft(s) of the extremities with rest pain

critical limb ischemia NOS of autologous vein bypass graft(s) of the extremities

critical limb ischemia of autologous vein bypass graft(s) of the extremities with rest pain

I70.421 Atherosclerosis of autologous vein bypass graft(s) of the extremities with rest pain, right leg HCC A

I70.422 Atherosclerosis of autologous vein bypass graft(s) of the extremities with rest pain, left leg HCC A

I70.423 Atherosclerosis of autologous vein bypass graft(s) of the extremities with rest pain, bilateral legs HCC A

I70.428 Atherosclerosis of autologous vein bypass graft(s) of the extremities with rest pain, other extremity HCC A

I70.429 Atherosclerosis of autologous vein bypass graft(s) of the extremities with rest pain, unspecified extremity HCC A

I70.43 Atherosclerosis of autologous vein bypass graft(s) of the right leg with ulceration

INCLUDES any condition classifiable to I70.411 and I70.421

chronic limb-threatening ischemia of autologous vein bypass graft(s) of the right leg with ulceration

critical limb ischemia of autologous vein bypass graft(s) of the right leg with ulceration

Use additional code to identify severity of ulcer (L97.-)

I70.431 Atherosclerosis of autologous vein bypass graft(s) of the right leg with ulceration of thigh CC HCC A

I70.432 Atherosclerosis of autologous vein bypass graft(s) of the right leg with ulceration of calf CC HCC A

I70.433 Atherosclerosis of autologous vein bypass graft(s) of the right leg with ulceration of ankle CC HCC A

I70.434 Atherosclerosis of autologous vein bypass graft(s) of the right leg with ulceration of heel and midfoot CC HCC A

Atherosclerosis of autologous vein bypass graft(s) of right leg with ulceration of plantar surface of midfoot

I70.435 Atherosclerosis of autologous vein bypass graft(s) of the right leg with ulceration of other part of foot HCC A
Atherosclerosis of autologous vein bypass graft(s) of right leg with ulceration of toe

I70.438 Atherosclerosis of autologous vein bypass graft(s) of the right leg with ulceration of other part of lower leg CC HCC A

I70.439 Atherosclerosis of autologous vein bypass graft(s) of the right leg with unspecified site CC HCC A

✓6th I70.44 Atherosclerosis of autologous vein bypass graft(s) of the left leg with ulceration
INCLUDES any condition classifiable to I70.412 and I70.422
chronic limb-threatening ischemia of autologous vein bypass graft(s) of the left leg with ulceration
critical limb ischemia of autologous vein bypass graft(s) of the left leg with ulceration
Use additional code to identify severity of ulcer (L97.-)

I70.441 Atherosclerosis of autologous vein bypass graft(s) of the left leg with ulceration of thigh CC HCC A

I70.442 Atherosclerosis of autologous vein bypass graft(s) of the left leg with ulceration of calf CC HCC A

I70.443 Atherosclerosis of autologous vein bypass graft(s) of the left leg with ulceration of ankle CC HCC A

I70.444 Atherosclerosis of autologous vein bypass graft(s) of the left leg with ulceration of heel and midfoot CC HCC A
Atherosclerosis of autologous vein bypass graft(s) of left leg with ulceration of plantar surface of midfoot

I70.445 Atherosclerosis of autologous vein bypass graft(s) of the left leg with ulceration of other part of foot HCC A
Atherosclerosis of autologous vein bypass graft(s) of left leg with ulceration of toe

I70.448 Atherosclerosis of autologous vein bypass graft(s) of the left leg with ulceration of other part of lower leg CC HCC A

I70.449 Atherosclerosis of autologous vein bypass graft(s) of the left leg with ulceration of unspecified site CC HCC A

I70.45 Atherosclerosis of autologous vein bypass graft(s) of other extremity with ulceration HCC A
INCLUDES any condition classifiable to I70.418, I70.428, and I70.438
Use additional code to identify severity of ulcer (L98.49)

✓6th I70.46 Atherosclerosis of autologous vein bypass graft(s) of the extremities with gangrene
INCLUDES any condition classifiable to I70.41-, I70.42-, and I70.43-, I70.44-, I70.45
chronic limb-threatening ischemia of autologous vein bypass graft(s) of the extremities with gangrene
critical limb ischemia of autologous vein bypass graft(s) of the extremities with gangrene
Use additional code to identify the severity of any ulcer (L97.-, L98.49-), if applicable

I70.461 Atherosclerosis of autologous vein bypass graft(s) of the extremities with gangrene, right leg CC HCC A

I70.462 Atherosclerosis of autologous vein bypass graft(s) of the extremities with gangrene, left leg CC HCC A

I70.463 Atherosclerosis of autologous vein bypass graft(s) of the extremities with gangrene, bilateral legs CC HCC A

I70.468 Atherosclerosis of autologous vein bypass graft(s) of the extremities with gangrene, other extremity CC HCC A

I70.469 Atherosclerosis of autologous vein bypass graft(s) of the extremities with gangrene, unspecified extremity CC UNS HCC A

✓6th I70.49 Other atherosclerosis of autologous vein bypass graft(s) of the extremities

I70.491 Other atherosclerosis of autologous vein bypass graft(s) of the extremities, right leg HCC A

I70.492 Other atherosclerosis of autologous vein bypass graft(s) of the extremities, left leg HCC A

I70.493 Other atherosclerosis of autologous vein bypass graft(s) of the extremities, bilateral legs HCC A

I70.498 Other atherosclerosis of autologous vein bypass graft(s) of the extremities, other extremity HCC A

I70.499 Other atherosclerosis of autologous vein bypass graft(s) of the extremities, unspecified extremity HCC A

✓5th I70.5 Atherosclerosis of nonautologous biological bypass graft(s) of the extremities
Use additional code, if applicable, to identify chronic total occlusion of artery of extremity (I70.92)
AHA: 2020,4Q,98

✓6th I70.50 Unspecified atherosclerosis of nonautologous biological bypass graft(s) of the extremities

I70.501 Unspecified atherosclerosis of nonautologous biological bypass graft(s) of the extremities, right leg HCC A

I70.502 Unspecified atherosclerosis of nonautologous biological bypass graft(s) of the extremities, left leg HCC A

I70.503 Unspecified atherosclerosis of nonautologous biological bypass graft(s) of the extremities, bilateral legs HCC A

I70.508 Unspecified atherosclerosis of nonautologous biological bypass graft(s) of the extremities, other extremity HCC A

I70.509 Unspecified atherosclerosis of nonautologous biological bypass graft(s) of the extremities, unspecified extremity HCC A

✓6th I70.51 Atherosclerosis of nonautologous biological bypass graft(s) of the extremities intermittent claudication

I70.511 Atherosclerosis of nonautologous biological bypass graft(s) of the extremities with intermittent claudication, right leg HCC A

I70.512 Atherosclerosis of nonautologous biological bypass graft(s) of the extremities with intermittent claudication, left leg HCC A

I70.513 Atherosclerosis of nonautologous biological bypass graft(s) of the extremities with intermittent claudication, bilateral legs HCC A

I70.518 Atherosclerosis of nonautologous biological bypass graft(s) of the extremities with intermittent claudication, other extremity HCC A

I70.519 Atherosclerosis of nonautologous biological bypass graft(s) of the extremities with intermittent claudication, unspecified extremity HCC A

I70.52 Atherosclerosis of nonautologous biological bypass graft(s) of the extremities with rest pain ✓6th

INCLUDES any condition classifiable to I70.51-
chronic limb-threatening ischemia NOS of nonautologous biological bypass graft(s) of the extremities
chronic limb-threatening ischemia of nonautologous biological bypass graft(s) of the extremities with rest pain
critical limb ischemia NOS of nonautologous biological bypass graft(s) of the extremities
critical limb ischemia of nonautologous biological bypass graft(s) of the extremities with rest pain

I70.521 Atherosclerosis of nonautologous biological bypass graft(s) of the extremities with rest pain, right leg HCC A

I70.522 Atherosclerosis of nonautologous biological bypass graft(s) of the extremities with rest pain, left leg HCC A

I70.523 Atherosclerosis of nonautologous biological bypass graft(s) of the extremities with rest pain, bilateral legs HCC A

I70.528 Atherosclerosis of nonautologous biological bypass graft(s) of the extremities with rest pain, other extremity HCC A

I70.529 Atherosclerosis of nonautologous biological bypass graft(s) of the extremities with rest pain, unspecified extremity HCC A

I70.53 Atherosclerosis of nonautologous biological bypass graft(s) of the right leg with ulceration ✓6th

INCLUDES any condition classifiable to I70.511 and I70.521
chronic limb-threatening ischemia of nonautologous biological bypass graft(s) of the right leg with ulceration
critical limb ischemia of nonautologous biological bypass graft(s) of the right leg with ulceration

Use additional code to identify severity of ulcer (L97.-)

I70.531 Atherosclerosis of nonautologous biological bypass graft(s) of the right leg with ulceration of thigh CC HCC A

I70.532 Atherosclerosis of nonautologous biological bypass graft(s) of the right leg with ulceration of calf CC HCC A

I70.533 Atherosclerosis of nonautologous biological bypass graft(s) of the right leg with ulceration of ankle CC HCC A

I70.534 Atherosclerosis of nonautologous biological bypass graft(s) of the right leg with ulceration of heel and midfoot CC HCC A

Atherosclerosis of nonautologous biological bypass graft(s) of right leg with ulceration of plantar surface of midfoot

I70.535 Atherosclerosis of nonautologous biological bypass graft(s) of the right leg with ulceration of other part of foot HCC A

Atherosclerosis of nonautologous biological bypass graft(s) of the right leg with ulceration of toe

I70.538 Atherosclerosis of nonautologous biological bypass graft(s) of the right leg with ulceration of other part of lower leg CC HCC A

I70.539 Atherosclerosis of nonautologous biological bypass graft(s) of the right leg with ulceration of unspecified site CC HCC A

I70.54 Atherosclerosis of nonautologous biological bypass graft(s) of the left leg with ulceration ✓6th

INCLUDES any condition classifiable to I70.512 and I70.522
chronic limb-threatening ischemia of nonautologous biological bypass graft(s) of the left leg with ulceration
critical limb ischemia of nonautologous biological bypass graft(s) of the left leg with ulceration

Use additional code to identify severity of ulcer (L97.-)

I70.541 Atherosclerosis of nonautologous biological bypass graft(s) of the left leg with ulceration of thigh CC HCC A

I70.542 Atherosclerosis of nonautologous biological bypass graft(s) of the left leg with ulceration of calf CC HCC A

I70.543 Atherosclerosis of nonautologous biological bypass graft(s) of the left leg with ulceration of ankle CC HCC A

I70.544 Atherosclerosis of nonautologous biological bypass graft(s) of the left leg with ulceration of heel and midfoot CC HCC A

Atherosclerosis of nonautologous biological bypass graft(s) of left leg with ulceration of plantar surface of midfoot

I70.545 Atherosclerosis of nonautologous biological bypass graft(s) of the left leg with ulceration of other part of foot HCC A

Atherosclerosis of nonautologous biological bypass graft(s) of the left leg with ulceration of toe

I70.548 Atherosclerosis of nonautologous biological bypass graft(s) of the left leg with ulceration of other part of lower leg CC HCC A

I70.549 Atherosclerosis of nonautologous biological bypass graft(s) of the left leg with ulceration of unspecified site CC HCC A

I70.55 Atherosclerosis of nonautologous biological bypass graft(s) of other extremity with ulceration HCC A

INCLUDES any condition classifiable to I70.518, I70.528, and I70.538

Use additional code to identify severity of ulcer (L98.49)

I70.56 Atherosclerosis of nonautologous biological bypass graft(s) of the extremities with gangrene ✓6th

INCLUDES any condition classifiable to I70.51-, I70.52-, and I70.53-, I70.54-, I70.55
chronic limb-threatening ischemia of nonautologous biological bypass graft(s) of the extremities with gangrene
critical limb ischemia of nonautologous biological bypass graft(s) of the extremities with gangrene

Use additional code to identify the severity of any ulcer (L97.-, L98.49-), if applicable

I70.561 Atherosclerosis of nonautologous biological bypass graft(s) of the extremities with gangrene, right leg CC HCC A

I70.562 Atherosclerosis of nonautologous biological bypass graft(s) of the extremities with gangrene, left leg CC HCC A

I70.563 Atherosclerosis of nonautologous biological bypass graft(s) of the extremities with gangrene, bilateral legs CC HCC A

I70.568 Atherosclerosis of nonautologous biological bypass graft(s) of the extremities with gangrene, other extremity CC HCC A

Chapter 9. Diseases of the Circulatory System

I70.569 Atherosclerosis of nonautologous biological bypass graft(s) of the extremities with gangrene, unspecified extremity CC UNS HCC A

I70.59 Other atherosclerosis of nonautologous biological bypass graft(s) of the extremities

I70.591 Other atherosclerosis of nonautologous biological bypass graft(s) of the extremities, right leg HCC A

I70.592 Other atherosclerosis of nonautologous biological bypass graft(s) of the extremities, left leg HCC A

I70.593 Other atherosclerosis of nonautologous biological bypass graft(s) of the extremities, bilateral legs HCC A

I70.598 Other atherosclerosis of nonautologous biological bypass graft(s) of the extremities, other extremity HCC A

I70.599 Other atherosclerosis of nonautologous biological bypass graft(s) of the extremities, unspecified extremity HCC A

I70.6 Atherosclerosis of nonbiological bypass graft(s) of the extremities

Use additional code, if applicable, to identify chronic total occlusion of artery of extremity (I70.92)

AHA: 2020,4Q,98

I70.60 Unspecified atherosclerosis of nonbiological bypass graft(s) of the extremities

I70.601 Unspecified atherosclerosis of nonbiological bypass graft(s) of the extremities, right leg HCC A

I70.602 Unspecified atherosclerosis of nonbiological bypass graft(s) of the extremities, left leg HCC A

I70.603 Unspecified atherosclerosis of nonbiological bypass graft(s) of the extremities, bilateral legs HCC A

I70.608 Unspecified atherosclerosis of nonbiological bypass graft(s) of the extremities, other extremity HCC A

I70.609 Unspecified atherosclerosis of nonbiological bypass graft(s) of the extremities, unspecified extremity HCC A

I70.61 Atherosclerosis of nonbiological bypass graft(s) of the extremities with intermittent claudication

I70.611 Atherosclerosis of nonbiological bypass graft(s) of the extremities with intermittent claudication, right leg HCC A

I70.612 Atherosclerosis of nonbiological bypass graft(s) of the extremities with intermittent claudication, left leg HCC A

I70.613 Atherosclerosis of nonbiological bypass graft(s) of the extremities with intermittent claudication, bilateral legs HCC A

I70.618 Atherosclerosis of nonbiological bypass graft(s) of the extremities with intermittent claudication, other extremity HCC A

I70.619 Atherosclerosis of nonbiological bypass graft(s) of the extremities with intermittent claudication, unspecified extremity HCC A

I70.62 Atherosclerosis of nonbiological bypass graft(s) of the extremities with rest pain

INCLUDES any condition classifiable to I70.61-

chronic limb-threatening ischemia NOS of nonbiological bypass graft(s) of the extremities

chronic limb-threatening ischemia of nonbiological bypass graft(s) of the extremities with rest pain

critical limb ischemia NOS of nonbiological bypass graft(s) of the extremities

critical limb ischemia of nonbiological bypass graft(s) of the extremities with rest pain

I70.621 Atherosclerosis of nonbiological bypass graft(s) of the extremities with rest pain, right leg HCC A

I70.622 Atherosclerosis of nonbiological bypass graft(s) of the extremities with rest pain, left leg HCC A

I70.623 Atherosclerosis of nonbiological bypass graft(s) of the extremities with rest pain, bilateral legs HCC A

I70.628 Atherosclerosis of nonbiological bypass graft(s) of the extremities with rest pain, other extremity HCC A

I70.629 Atherosclerosis of nonbiological bypass graft(s) of the extremities with rest pain, unspecified extremity HCC A

I70.63 Atherosclerosis of nonbiological bypass graft(s) of the right leg with ulceration

INCLUDES any condition classifiable to I70.611 and I70.621

chronic limb-threatening ischemia of nonbiological bypass graft(s) of the right leg with ulceration

critical limb ischemia of nonbiological bypass graft(s) of the right leg with ulceration

Use additional code to identify severity of ulcer (L97.-)

I70.631 Atherosclerosis of nonbiological bypass graft(s) of the right leg with ulceration of thigh CC HCC A

I70.632 Atherosclerosis of nonbiological bypass graft(s) of the right leg with ulceration of calf CC HCC A

I70.633 Atherosclerosis of nonbiological bypass graft(s) of the right leg with ulceration of ankle CC HCC A

I70.634 Atherosclerosis of nonbiological bypass graft(s) of the right leg with ulceration of heel and midfoot CC HCC A

Atherosclerosis of nonbiological bypass graft(s) of right leg with ulceration of plantar surface of midfoot

I70.635 Atherosclerosis of nonbiological bypass graft(s) of the right leg with ulceration of other part of foot HCC A

Atherosclerosis of nonbiological bypass graft(s) of the right leg with ulceration of toe

I70.638 Atherosclerosis of nonbiological bypass graft(s) of the right leg with ulceration of other part of lower leg CC HCC A

I70.639 Atherosclerosis of nonbiological bypass graft(s) of the right leg with ulceration of unspecified site CC HCC A

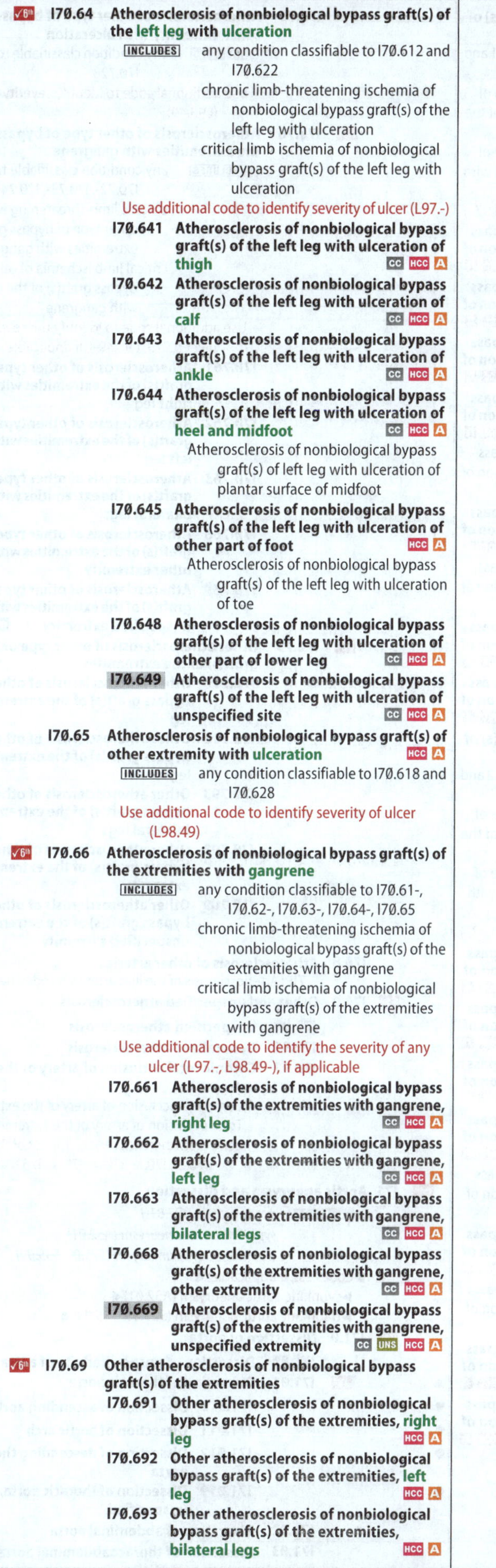

I70.64 Atherosclerosis of nonbiological bypass graft(s) of the left leg with ulceration (6th)

INCLUDES any condition classifiable to I70.612 and I70.622

chronic limb-threatening ischemia of nonbiological bypass graft(s) of the left leg with ulceration

critical limb ischemia of nonbiological bypass graft(s) of the left leg with ulceration

Use additional code to identify severity of ulcer (L97.-)

I70.641 Atherosclerosis of nonbiological bypass graft(s) of the left leg with ulceration of thigh CC HCC A

I70.642 Atherosclerosis of nonbiological bypass graft(s) of the left leg with ulceration of calf CC HCC A

I70.643 Atherosclerosis of nonbiological bypass graft(s) of the left leg with ulceration of ankle CC HCC A

I70.644 Atherosclerosis of nonbiological bypass graft(s) of the left leg with ulceration of heel and midfoot CC HCC A

Atherosclerosis of nonbiological bypass graft(s) of left leg with ulceration of plantar surface of midfoot

I70.645 Atherosclerosis of nonbiological bypass graft(s) of the left leg with ulceration of other part of foot HCC A

Atherosclerosis of nonbiological bypass graft(s) of the left leg with ulceration of toe

I70.648 Atherosclerosis of nonbiological bypass graft(s) of the left leg with ulceration of other part of lower leg CC HCC A

I70.649 Atherosclerosis of nonbiological bypass graft(s) of the left leg with ulceration of unspecified site CC HCC A

I70.65 Atherosclerosis of nonbiological bypass graft(s) of other extremity with ulceration HCC A

INCLUDES any condition classifiable to I70.618 and I70.628

Use additional code to identify severity of ulcer (L98.49)

I70.66 Atherosclerosis of nonbiological bypass graft(s) of the extremities with gangrene (6th)

INCLUDES any condition classifiable to I70.61-, I70.62-, I70.63-, I70.64-, I70.65

chronic limb-threatening ischemia of nonbiological bypass graft(s) of the extremities with gangrene

critical limb ischemia of nonbiological bypass graft(s) of the extremities with gangrene

Use additional code to identify the severity of any ulcer (L97.-, L98.49-), if applicable

I70.661 Atherosclerosis of nonbiological bypass graft(s) of the extremities with gangrene, right leg CC HCC A

I70.662 Atherosclerosis of nonbiological bypass graft(s) of the extremities with gangrene, left leg CC HCC A

I70.663 Atherosclerosis of nonbiological bypass graft(s) of the extremities with gangrene, bilateral legs CC HCC A

I70.668 Atherosclerosis of nonbiological bypass graft(s) of the extremities with gangrene, other extremity CC HCC A

I70.669 Atherosclerosis of nonbiological bypass graft(s) of the extremities with gangrene, unspecified extremity CC UNS HCC A

I70.69 Other atherosclerosis of nonbiological bypass graft(s) of the extremities (6th)

I70.691 Other atherosclerosis of nonbiological bypass graft(s) of the extremities, right leg HCC A

I70.692 Other atherosclerosis of nonbiological bypass graft(s) of the extremities, left leg HCC A

I70.693 Other atherosclerosis of nonbiological bypass graft(s) of the extremities, bilateral legs HCC A

I70.698 Other atherosclerosis of nonbiological bypass graft(s) of the extremities, other extremity HCC A

I70.699 Other atherosclerosis of nonbiological bypass graft(s) of the extremities, unspecified extremity HCC A

I70.7 Atherosclerosis of other type of bypass graft(s) of the extremities (5th)

Use additional code, if applicable, to identify chronic total occlusion of artery of extremity (I70.92)

AHA: 2020,4Q,98

I70.70 Unspecified atherosclerosis of other type of bypass graft(s) of the extremities (6th)

I70.701 Unspecified atherosclerosis of other type of bypass graft(s) of the extremities, right leg HCC A

I70.702 Unspecified atherosclerosis of other type of bypass graft(s) of the extremities, left leg HCC A

I70.703 Unspecified atherosclerosis of other type of bypass graft(s) of the extremities, bilateral legs HCC A

I70.708 Unspecified atherosclerosis of other type of bypass graft(s) of the extremities, other extremity HCC A

I70.709 Unspecified atherosclerosis of other type of bypass graft(s) of the extremities, unspecified extremity HCC A

I70.71 Atherosclerosis of other type of bypass graft(s) of the extremities with intermittent claudication (6th)

I70.711 Atherosclerosis of other type of bypass graft(s) of the extremities with intermittent claudication, right leg HCC A

I70.712 Atherosclerosis of other type of bypass graft(s) of the extremities with intermittent claudication, left leg HCC A

I70.713 Atherosclerosis of other type of bypass graft(s) of the extremities with intermittent claudication, bilateral legs HCC A

I70.718 Atherosclerosis of other type of bypass graft(s) of the extremities with intermittent claudication, other extremity HCC A

I70.719 Atherosclerosis of other type of bypass graft(s) of the extremities with intermittent claudication, unspecified extremity HCC A

I70.72 Atherosclerosis of other type of bypass graft(s) of the extremities with rest pain (6th)

INCLUDES any condition classifiable to I70.71-

chronic limb-threatening ischemia NOS of other type of bypass graft(s) of the extremities

chronic limb-threatening ischemia of other type of bypass graft(s) of the extremities with rest pain

critical limb ischemia NOS of other type of bypass graft(s) of the extremities

critical limb ischemia of other type of bypass graft(s) of the extremities with rest pain

I70.721 Atherosclerosis of other type of bypass graft(s) of the extremities with rest pain, right leg HCC A

I70.722 Atherosclerosis of other type of bypass graft(s) of the extremities with rest pain, left leg HCC A

I70.723 Atherosclerosis of other type of bypass graft(s) of the extremities with rest pain, bilateral legs HCC A

I70.728 Atherosclerosis of other type of bypass graft(s) of the extremities with rest pain, other extremity HCC A

I70.729 Atherosclerosis of other type of bypass graft(s) of the extremities with rest pain, unspecified extremity HCC A

✓6th **I70.73 Atherosclerosis of other type of bypass graft(s) of the right leg with ulceration**

INCLUDES any condition classifiable to I70.711 and I70.721

chronic limb-threatening ischemia of other type of bypass graft(s) of the right leg with ulceration

critical limb ischemia of other type of bypass graft(s) of the right leg with ulceration

Use additional code to identify severity of ulcer (L97.-)

I70.731 Atherosclerosis of other type of bypass graft(s) of the right leg with ulceration of thigh CC HCC A

I70.732 Atherosclerosis of other type of bypass graft(s) of the right leg with ulceration of calf CC HCC A

I70.733 Atherosclerosis of other type of bypass graft(s) of the right leg with ulceration of ankle CC HCC A

I70.734 Atherosclerosis of other type of bypass graft(s) of the right leg with ulceration of heel and midfoot CC HCC A

Atherosclerosis of other type of bypass graft(s) of right leg with ulceration of plantar surface of midfoot

I70.735 Atherosclerosis of other type of bypass graft(s) of the right leg with ulceration of other part of foot HCC A

Atherosclerosis of other type of bypass graft(s) of right leg with ulceration of toe

I70.738 Atherosclerosis of other type of bypass graft(s) of the right leg with ulceration of other part of lower leg CC HCC A

I70.739 Atherosclerosis of other type of bypass graft(s) of the right leg with ulceration of unspecified site CC HCC A

✓6th **I70.74 Atherosclerosis of other type of bypass graft(s) of the left leg with ulceration**

INCLUDES any condition classifiable to I70.712 and I70.722

chronic limb-threatening ischemia of other type of bypass graft(s) of the left leg with ulceration

critical limb ischemia of other type of bypass graft(s) of the left leg with ulceration

Use additional code to identify severity of ulcer (L97.-)

I70.741 Atherosclerosis of other type of bypass graft(s) of the left leg with ulceration of thigh CC HCC A

I70.742 Atherosclerosis of other type of bypass graft(s) of the left leg with ulceration of calf CC HCC A

I70.743 Atherosclerosis of other type of bypass graft(s) of the left leg with ulceration of ankle CC HCC A

I70.744 Atherosclerosis of other type of bypass graft(s) of the left leg with ulceration of heel and midfoot CC HCC A

Atherosclerosis of other type of bypass graft(s) of left leg with ulceration of plantar surface of midfoot

I70.745 Atherosclerosis of other type of bypass graft(s) of the left leg with ulceration of other part of foot HCC A

Atherosclerosis of other type of bypass graft(s) of left leg with ulceration of toe

I70.748 Atherosclerosis of other type of bypass graft(s) of the left leg with ulceration of other part of lower leg CC HCC A

I70.749 Atherosclerosis of other type of bypass graft(s) of the left leg with ulceration of unspecified site CC HCC A

I70.75 Atherosclerosis of other type of bypass graft(s) of other extremity with ulceration HCC A

INCLUDES any condition classifiable to I70.718 and I70.728

Use additional code to identify severity of ulcer (L98.49)

✓6th **I70.76 Atherosclerosis of other type of bypass graft(s) of the extremities with gangrene**

INCLUDES any condition classifiable to I70.71-, I70.72-, I70.73-, I70.74-, I70.75

chronic limb-threatening ischemia of other type of bypass graft(s) of the extremities with gangrene

critical limb ischemia of other type of bypass graft(s) of the extremities with gangrene

Use additional code to identify the severity of any ulcer (L97.-, L98.49-), if applicable

I70.761 Atherosclerosis of other type of bypass graft(s) of the extremities with gangrene, right leg CC HCC A

I70.762 Atherosclerosis of other type of bypass graft(s) of the extremities with gangrene, left leg CC HCC A

I70.763 Atherosclerosis of other type of bypass graft(s) of the extremities with gangrene, bilateral legs CC HCC A

I70.768 Atherosclerosis of other type of bypass graft(s) of the extremities with gangrene, other extremity CC HCC A

I70.769 Atherosclerosis of other type of bypass graft(s) of the extremities with gangrene, unspecified extremity CC UNS HCC A

✓6th **I70.79 Other atherosclerosis of other type of bypass graft(s) of the extremities**

I70.791 Other atherosclerosis of other type of bypass graft(s) of the extremities, right leg HCC A

I70.792 Other atherosclerosis of other type of bypass graft(s) of the extremities, left leg HCC A

I70.793 Other atherosclerosis of other type of bypass graft(s) of the extremities, bilateral legs HCC A

I70.798 Other atherosclerosis of other type of bypass graft(s) of the extremities, other extremity HCC A

I70.799 Other atherosclerosis of other type of bypass graft(s) of the extremities, unspecified extremity HCC A

I70.8 Atherosclerosis of other arteries A

TIP: Arteriosclerosis of the iliac arteries is coded here.

✓5th **I70.9 Other and unspecified atherosclerosis**

I70.90 Unspecified atherosclerosis A

I70.91 Generalized atherosclerosis A

I70.92 Chronic total occlusion of artery of the extremities CC UPD HCC A

Complete occlusion of artery of the extremities

Total occlusion of artery of the extremities

Code first atherosclerosis of arteries of the extremities (I70.2-, I70.3-, I70.4-, I70.5-, I70.6-, I70.7-)

✓4th **I71 Aortic aneurysm and dissection**

EXCLUDES 1 *aortic ectasia (I77.81-)*

syphilitic aortic aneurysm (A52.01)

traumatic aortic aneurysm (S25.09, S35.09)

▶Code first, if applicable:◀

▶syphilitic aortic aneurysm (A52.01)◀

▶traumatic aortic aneurysm (S25.09, S35.09)◀

✓5th **I71.0 Dissection of aorta**

I71.00 Dissection of unspecified site of aorta MCC HCC

▲ ✓6th **I71.01 Dissection of thoracic aorta**

● **I71.010 Dissection of ascending aorta** MCC

● **I71.011 Dissection of aortic arch** MCC

● **I71.012 Dissection of descending thoracic aorta** MCC

● **I71.019 Dissection of thoracic aorta, unspecified** MCC

I71.02 Dissection of abdominal aorta MCC HCC

I71.03 Dissection of thoracoabdominal aorta MCC HCC

▲ ✓5th **I71.1 Thoracic aortic aneurysm, ruptured**

● **I71.1Ø Thoracic aortic aneurysm, ruptured, unspecified** MCC

● **I71.11 Aneurysm of the ascending aorta, ruptured** MCC

● **I71.12 Aneurysm of the aortic arch, ruptured** MCC

● **I71.13 Aneurysm of the descending thoracic aorta, ruptured** MCC

▲ ✓5th **I71.2 Thoracic aortic aneurysm, without rupture**

● **I71.2Ø Thoracic aortic aneurysm, without rupture, unspecified**

● **I71.21 Aneurysm of the ascending aorta, without rupture**

● **I71.22 Aneurysm of the aortic arch, without rupture**

● **I71.23 Aneurysm of the descending thoracic aorta, without rupture**

▲ ✓5th **I71.3 Abdominal aortic aneurysm, ruptured**

● **I71.3Ø Abdominal aortic aneurysm, ruptured, unspecified** MCC

● **I71.31 Pararenal abdominal aortic aneurysm, ruptured** MCC

● **I71.32 Juxtarenal abdominal aortic aneurysm, ruptured** MCC

● **I71.33 Infrarenal abdominal aortic aneurysm, ruptured** MCC

▲ ✓5th **I71.4 Abdominal aortic aneurysm, without rupture**

● **I71.4Ø Abdominal aortic aneurysm, without rupture, unspecified**

● **I71.41 Pararenal abdominal aortic aneurysm, without rupture**

● **I71.42 Juxtarenal abdominal aortic aneurysm, without rupture**

● **I71.43 Infrarenal abdominal aortic aneurysm, without rupture**

▲ ✓5th **I71.5 Thoracoabdominal aortic aneurysm, ruptured**

● **I71.5Ø Thoracoabdominal aortic aneurysm, ruptured, unspecified** MCC

● **I71.51 Supraceliac aneurysm of the abdominal aorta, ruptured** MCC

● **I71.52 Paravisceral aneurysm of the abdominal aorta, ruptured** MCC

▲ ✓5th **I71.6 Thoracoabdominal aortic aneurysm, without rupture**

● **I71.6Ø Thoracoabdominal aortic aneurysm, without rupture, unspecified**

● **I71.61 Supraceliac aneurysm of the abdominal aorta, without rupture**

● **I71.62 Paravisceral aneurysm of the abdominal aorta, without rupture**

I71.8 Aortic aneurysm of unspecified site, ruptured MCC HCC

Rupture of aorta NOS

I71.9 Aortic aneurysm of unspecified site, without rupture HCC

Aneurysm of aorta

Dilatation of aorta

Hyaline necrosis of aorta

✓4th **I72 Other aneurysm**

INCLUDES aneurysm (cirsoid) (false) (ruptured)

EXCLUDES 2 *acquired aneurysm (I77.Ø)*
aneurysm (of) aorta (I71.-)
aneurysm (of) arteriovenous NOS (Q27.3-)
carotid artery dissection (I77.71)
cerebral (nonruptured) aneurysm (I67.1)
coronary aneurysm (I25.4)
coronary artery dissection (I25.42)
dissection of artery NEC (I77.79)
dissection of precerebral artery, congenital (nonruptured) (Q28.1)
heart aneurysm (I25.3)
iliac artery dissection (I77.72)
precerebral artery, congential (nonruptured) (Q28.1)
pulmonary artery aneurysm (I28.1)
renal artery dissection (I77.73)
retinal aneurysm (H35.Ø)
ruptured cerebral aneurysm (I6Ø.7)
varicose aneurysm (I77.Ø)
vertebral artery dissection (I77.74)

AHA: 2016,4Q,28-29

I72.Ø Aneurysm of carotid artery HCC

Aneurysm of common carotid artery

Aneurysm of external carotid artery

Aneurysm of internal carotid artery, extracranial portion

EXCLUDES 1 *aneurysm of internal carotid artery, intracranial portion (I67.1)*
aneurysm of internal carotid artery NOS (I67.1)

I72.1 Aneurysm of artery of upper extremity HCC

I72.2 Aneurysm of renal artery HCC

I72.3 Aneurysm of iliac artery HCC

I72.4 Aneurysm of artery of lower extremity HCC

AHA: 2019,2Q,21

I72.5 Aneurysm of other precerebral arteries HCC

Aneurysm of basilar artery (trunk)

EXCLUDES 2 *aneurysm of carotid artery (I72.Ø)*
aneurysm of vertebral artery (I72.6)
dissection of carotid artery (I77.71)
dissection of other precerebral arteries (I77.75)
dissection of vertebral artery (I77.74)

I72.6 Aneurysm of vertebral artery HCC

EXCLUDES 2 *dissection of vertebral artery (I77.74)*

I72.8 Aneurysm of other specified arteries HCC

I72.9 Aneurysm of unspecified site HCC

Aneurysm

Outer layer
Layers of muscular and elastic tissue
Inner layer
Aneurysm

✓4th **I73 Other peripheral vascular diseases**

EXCLUDES 2 *chilblains (T69.1)*
frostbite (T33-T34)
immersion hand or foot (T69.Ø-)
spasm of cerebral artery (G45.9)

AHA: 2018,4Q,87

✓5th **I73.Ø Raynaud's syndrome**

Raynaud's disease

Raynaud's phenomenon (secondary)

DEF: Constriction of the arteries of the digits caused by cold or by nerve or arterial damage and can be prompted by stress or emotion. Blood cannot reach the skin and soft tissues and the skin turns white with blue mottling.

I73.ØØ Raynaud's syndrome without gangrene

I73.Ø1 Raynaud's syndrome with gangrene CC HCC

I73.1 Thromboangiitis obliterans [Buerger's disease] HCC

DEF: Inflammatory disease of the extremity blood vessels, mainly the lower blood vessels. This disease is associated with heavy tobacco use. The arteries are more affected than veins. It occurs primarily in young men and leads to tissue ischemia and gangrene.

I73.8 Other specified peripheral vascular diseases (5th)

EXCLUDES 1 *diabetic (peripheral) angiopathy (E08-E13 with .51-.52)*

I73.81 Erythromelalgia HCC

I73.89 Other specified peripheral vascular diseases HCC

Acrocyanosis
Erythrocyanosis
Simple acroparesthesia [Schultze's type]
Vasomotor acroparesthesia [Nothnagel's type]

I73.9 Peripheral vascular disease, unspecified HCC

Intermittent claudication
Peripheral angiopathy NOS
Spasm of artery

EXCLUDES 1 *atherosclerosis of the extremities (I70.2-I70.7-)*

AHA: 2018,2Q,7

I74 Arterial embolism and thrombosis (4th)

INCLUDES embolic infarction
embolic occlusion
thrombotic infarction
thrombotic occlusion

Code first:
embolism and thrombosis complicating abortion or ectopic or molar pregnancy (O00-O07, O08.2)
embolism and thrombosis complicating pregnancy, childbirth and the puerperium (O88.-)

EXCLUDES 2 *atheroembolism (I75.-)*
basilar embolism and thrombosis (I63.0-I63.2, I65.1)
carotid embolism and thrombosis (I63.0-I63.2, I65.2)
cerebral embolism and thrombosis (I63.3-I63.5, I66.-)
coronary embolism and thrombosis (I21-I25)
mesenteric embolism and thrombosis (K55.0-)
ophthalmic embolism and thrombosis (H34.-)
precerebral embolism and thrombosis NOS (I63.0-I63.2, I65.9)
pulmonary embolism and thrombosis (I26.-)
renal embolism and thrombosis (N28.0)
retinal embolism and thrombosis (H34.-)
septic embolism and thrombosis (I76)
vertebral embolism and thrombosis (I63.0-I63.2, I65.0)

I74.0 Embolism and thrombosis of abdominal aorta (5th)

I74.01 Saddle embolus of abdominal aorta MCC HCC

I74.09 Other arterial embolism and thrombosis of abdominal aorta CC HCC

Aortic bifurcation syndrome
Aortoiliac obstruction
Leriche's syndrome

I74.1 Embolism and thrombosis of other and unspecified parts of aorta (5th)

I74.10 Embolism and thrombosis of unspecified parts of aorta CC HCC

I74.11 Embolism and thrombosis of thoracic aorta CC HCC

I74.19 Embolism and thrombosis of other parts of aorta CC HCC

I74.2 Embolism and thrombosis of arteries of the upper extremities CC HCC

I74.3 Embolism and thrombosis of arteries of the lower extremities CC HCC

I74.4 Embolism and thrombosis of arteries of extremities, unspecified CC HCC

Peripheral arterial embolism NOS

I74.5 Embolism and thrombosis of iliac artery CC HCC

I74.8 Embolism and thrombosis of other arteries CC HCC

I74.9 Embolism and thrombosis of unspecified artery CC HCC

I75 Atheroembolism (4th)

INCLUDES atherothrombotic microembolism
cholesterol embolism

I75.0 Atheroembolism of extremities (5th)

I75.01 Atheroembolism of upper extremity (6th)

I75.011 Atheroembolism of right upper extremity CC HCC

I75.012 Atheroembolism of left upper extremity CC HCC

I75.013 Atheroembolism of bilateral upper extremities CC HCC

I75.019 Atheroembolism of unspecified upper extremity CC UNS HCC

I75.02 Atheroembolism of lower extremity (6th)

I75.021 Atheroembolism of right lower extremity CC HCC

I75.022 Atheroembolism of left lower extremity CC HCC

I75.023 Atheroembolism of bilateral lower extremities CC HCC

I75.029 Atheroembolism of unspecified lower extremity CC UNS HCC

I75.8 Atheroembolism of other sites (5th)

I75.81 Atheroembolism of kidney CC HCC

Use additional code for any associated acute kidney failure and chronic kidney disease (N17.-, N18.-)

I75.89 Atheroembolism of other site CC HCC

I76 Septic arterial embolism CC UPD HCC

Code first underlying infection, such as:
infective endocarditis (I33.0)
lung abscess (J85.-)
Use additional code to identify the site of the embolism (I74.-)

EXCLUDES 2 *septic pulmonary embolism (I26.01, I26.90)*

I77 Other disorders of arteries and arterioles (4th)

EXCLUDES 2 *collagen (vascular) diseases (M30-M36)*
hypersensitivity angiitis (M31.0)
pulmonary artery (I28.-)

I77.0 Arteriovenous fistula, acquired HCC

Aneurysmal varix
Arteriovenous aneurysm, acquired

EXCLUDES 1 *arteriovenous aneurysm NOS (Q27.3-)*
presence of arteriovenous shunt (fistula) for dialysis (Z99.2)
traumatic - see injury of blood vessel by body region

EXCLUDES 2 *cerebral (I67.1)*
coronary (I25.4)

DEF: Communication between an artery and vein caused by trauma or invasive procedures.

I77.1 Stricture of artery HCC

Narrowing of artery

AHA: 2021,3Q,12

I77.2 Rupture of artery CC HCC

Erosion of artery
Fistula of artery
Ulcer of artery

EXCLUDES 1 *traumatic rupture of artery - see injury of blood vessel by body region*

I77.3 Arterial fibromuscular dysplasia HCC

Fibromuscular hyperplasia (of) carotid artery
Fibromuscular hyperplasia (of) renal artery

I77.4 Celiac artery compression syndrome CC HCC

AHA: 2021,3Q,12

I77.5 Necrosis of artery CC HCC

I77.6 Arteritis, unspecified HCC

Aortitis NOS
Endarteritis NOS

EXCLUDES 1 *arteritis or endarteritis:*
aortic arch (M31.4)
cerebral NEC (I67.7)
coronary (I25.89)
deformans (I70.-)
giant cell (M31.5, M31.6)
obliterans (I70.-)
senile (I70.-)

I77.7 Other arterial dissection (5th)

EXCLUDES 2 *dissection of aorta (I71.0-)*
dissection of coronary artery (I25.42)

AHA: 2016,4Q,28-29

I77.70 Dissection of unspecified artery MCC HCC

I77.71 Dissection of carotid artery MCC HCC

I77.72 Dissection of iliac artery MCC HCC

I77.73 Dissection of renal artery MCC HCC

I77.74 Dissection of vertebral artery MCC HCC
EXCLUDES 2 *aneurysm of vertebral artery (I72.6)*

I77.75 Dissection of other precerebral arteries MCC HCC
Dissection of basilar artery (trunk)
EXCLUDES 2 *aneurysm of carotid artery (I72.Ø)*
aneurysm of other precerebral arteries (I72.5)
aneurysm of vertebral artery (I72.6)
dissection of carotid artery (I77.71)
dissection of vertebral artery (I77.74)

I77.76 Dissection of artery of upper extremity MCC HCC

I77.77 Dissection of artery of lower extremity MCC HCC

I77.79 Dissection of other specified artery MCC HCC

I77.8 Other specified disorders of arteries and arterioles

I77.81 Aortic ectasia
Ectasis aorta
EXCLUDES 1 *aortic aneurysm and dissection ▶(I71.-)◀*

I77.810 Thoracic aortic ectasia HCC

I77.811 Abdominal aortic ectasia HCC

I77.812 Thoracoabdominal aortic ectasia HCC

I77.819 Aortic ectasia, unspecified site HCC

● **I77.82 Antineutrophilic cytoplasmic antibody [ANCA] vasculitis**
ANCA associated vasculitis
ANCA positive vasculitis
EXCLUDES 2 *eosinophilic granulomatosis with polyangiitis (M3Ø.1)*
granulomatosis with polyangiitis (M31.3-)
microscopic polyangiitis (M31.7)

I77.89 Other specified disorders of arteries and arterioles HCC
AHA: 2021,1Q,23

I77.9 Disorder of arteries and arterioles, unspecified HCC
AHA: 2021,1Q,4; 2018,2Q,7

I78 Diseases of capillaries

I78.Ø Hereditary hemorrhagic telangiectasia HCC
Rendu-Osler-Weber disease

I78.1 Nevus, non-neoplastic
Araneus nevus
Senile nevus
Spider nevus
Stellar nevus
EXCLUDES 1 *nevus NOS (D22.-)*
vascular NOS (Q82.5)
EXCLUDES 2 *blue nevus (D22.-)*
flammeus nevus (Q82.5)
hairy nevus (D22.-)
melanocytic nevus (D22.-)
pigmented nevus (D22.-)
portwine nevus (Q82.5)
sanguineous nevus (Q82.5)
strawberry nevus (Q82.5)
verrucous nevus (Q82.5)
AHA: 2019,1Q,21

I78.8 Other diseases of capillaries

I78.9 Disease of capillaries, unspecified

I79 Disorders of arteries, arterioles and capillaries in diseases classified elsewhere

I79.Ø Aneurysm of aorta in diseases classified elsewhere HCC
Code first underlying disease
EXCLUDES 1 *syphilitic aneurysm (A52.Ø1)*

I79.1 Aortitis in diseases classified elsewhere HCC
Code first underlying disease
EXCLUDES 1 *syphilitic aortitis (A52.Ø2)*

I79.8 Other disorders of arteries, arterioles and capillaries in diseases classified elsewhere HCC
Code first underlying disease, such as:
amyloidosis (E85.-)
EXCLUDES 1 *diabetic (peripheral) angiopathy (EØ8-E13 with .51-.52)*
syphilitic endarteritis (A52.Ø9)
tuberculous endarteritis (A18.89)

Diseases of veins, lymphatic vessels and lymph nodes, not elsewhere classified (I8Ø-I89)

I8Ø Phlebitis and thrombophlebitis
INCLUDES endophlebitis
inflammation, vein
periphlebitis
suppurative phlebitis
Code first:
phlebitis and thrombophlebitis complicating abortion, ectopic or molar pregnancy (OØØ-OØ7, OØ8.7)
phlebitis and thrombophlebitis complicating pregnancy, childbirth and the puerperium (O22.-, O87.-)
EXCLUDES 1 *venous embolism and thrombosis of lower extremities (I82.4-, I82.5-, I82.81-)*

I8Ø.Ø Phlebitis and thrombophlebitis of superficial vessels of lower extremities
Phlebitis and thrombophlebitis of femoropopliteal vein

I8Ø.ØØ Phlebitis and thrombophlebitis of superficial vessels of unspecified lower extremity

I8Ø.Ø1 Phlebitis and thrombophlebitis of superficial vessels of right lower extremity

I8Ø.Ø2 Phlebitis and thrombophlebitis of superficial vessels of left lower extremity

I8Ø.Ø3 Phlebitis and thrombophlebitis of superficial vessels of lower extremities, bilateral

I8Ø.1 Phlebitis and thrombophlebitis of femoral vein
Phlebitis and thrombophlebitis of common femoral vein
Phlebitis and thrombophlebitis of deep femoral vein

I8Ø.1Ø Phlebitis and thrombophlebitis of unspecified femoral vein CC UNS HCC

I8Ø.11 Phlebitis and thrombophlebitis of right femoral vein CC HCC

I8Ø.12 Phlebitis and thrombophlebitis of left femoral vein CC HCC

I8Ø.13 Phlebitis and thrombophlebitis of femoral vein, bilateral CC HCC

I8Ø.2 Phlebitis and thrombophlebitis of other and unspecified deep vessels of lower extremities

I8Ø.2Ø Phlebitis and thrombophlebitis of unspecified deep vessels of lower extremities

I8Ø.2Ø1 Phlebitis and thrombophlebitis of unspecified deep vessels of right lower extremity CC HCC

I8Ø.2Ø2 Phlebitis and thrombophlebitis of unspecified deep vessels of left lower extremity CC HCC

I8Ø.2Ø3 Phlebitis and thrombophlebitis of unspecified deep vessels of lower extremities, bilateral CC HCC

I8Ø.2Ø9 Phlebitis and thrombophlebitis of unspecified deep vessels of unspecified lower extremity CC UNS HCC

I8Ø.21 Phlebitis and thrombophlebitis of iliac vein
Phlebitis and thrombophlebitis of common iliac vein
Phlebitis and thrombophlebitis of external iliac vein
Phlebitis and thrombophlebitis of internal iliac vein

I8Ø.211 Phlebitis and thrombophlebitis of right iliac vein CC HCC

I8Ø.212 Phlebitis and thrombophlebitis of left iliac vein CC HCC

I8Ø.213 Phlebitis and thrombophlebitis of iliac vein, bilateral CC HCC

I8Ø.219 Phlebitis and thrombophlebitis of unspecified iliac vein CC UNS HCC

I8Ø.22 Phlebitis and thrombophlebitis of popliteal vein

I8Ø.221 Phlebitis and thrombophlebitis of right popliteal vein CC HCC

I8Ø.222 Phlebitis and thrombophlebitis of left popliteal vein CC HCC

I8Ø.223 Phlebitis and thrombophlebitis of popliteal vein, bilateral CC HCC

I8Ø.229 Phlebitis and thrombophlebitis of unspecified popliteal vein CC UNS HCC

I8Ø.23 Phlebitis and thrombophlebitis of tibial vein
Phlebitis and thrombophlebitis of anterior tibial vein
Phlebitis and thrombophlebitis of posterior tibial vein

I8Ø.231 Phlebitis and thrombophlebitis of right tibial vein CC HCC

I80.232 Phlebitis and thrombophlebitis of left tibial vein CC HCC

I80.233 Phlebitis and thrombophlebitis of tibial vein, bilateral CC HCC

I80.239 Phlebitis and thrombophlebitis of unspecified tibial vein CC UNS HCC

✓6th **I80.24 Phlebitis and thrombophlebitis of peroneal vein**

AHA: 2019,4Q,8

I80.241 Phlebitis and thrombophlebitis of right peroneal vein CC HCC

I80.242 Phlebitis and thrombophlebitis of left peroneal vein CC HCC

I80.243 Phlebitis and thrombophlebitis of peroneal vein, bilateral CC HCC

I80.249 Phlebitis and thrombophlebitis of unspecified peroneal vein CC UNS HCC

✓6th **I80.25 Phlebitis and thrombophlebitis of calf muscular vein**

Phlebitis and thrombophlebitis of calf muscular vein, NOS

Phlebitis and thrombophlebitis of gastrocnemial vein

Phlebitis and thrombophlebitis of soleal vein

AHA: 2019,4Q,8

I80.251 Phlebitis and thrombophlebitis of right calf muscular vein HCC

I80.252 Phlebitis and thrombophlebitis of left calf muscular vein HCC

I80.253 Phlebitis and thrombophlebitis of calf muscular vein, bilateral HCC

I80.259 Phlebitis and thrombophlebitis of unspecified calf muscular vein HCC

✓6th **I80.29 Phlebitis and thrombophlebitis of other deep vessels of lower extremities**

I80.291 Phlebitis and thrombophlebitis of other deep vessels of right lower extremity CC HCC

I80.292 Phlebitis and thrombophlebitis of other deep vessels of left lower extremity CC HCC

I80.293 Phlebitis and thrombophlebitis of other deep vessels of lower extremity, bilateral CC HCC

I80.299 Phlebitis and thrombophlebitis of other deep vessels of unspecified lower extremity CC UNS HCC

I80.3 Phlebitis and thrombophlebitis of lower extremities, unspecified

I80.8 Phlebitis and thrombophlebitis of other sites

I80.9 Phlebitis and thrombophlebitis of unspecified site

I81 Portal vein thrombosis MCC

Portal (vein) obstruction

EXCLUDES 2 *hepatic vein thrombosis (I82.0)*

phlebitis of portal vein (K75.1)

AHA: 2019,4Q,68

✓4th **I82 Other venous embolism and thrombosis**

Code first venous embolism and thrombosis complicating:

abortion, ectopic or molar pregnancy (O00-O07, O08.7)

pregnancy, childbirth and the puerperium (O22.-, O87.-)

EXCLUDES 2 *venous embolism and thrombosis (of):*

cerebral (I63.6, I67.6)

coronary (I21-I25)

intracranial and intraspinal, septic or NOS (G08)

intracranial, nonpyogenic (I67.6)

intraspinal, nonpyogenic (G95.1)

mesenteric (K55.0-)

portal (I81)

pulmonary (I26.-)

I82.0 Budd-Chiari syndrome MCC HCC

Hepatic vein thrombosis

DEF: Thrombosis or other obstruction of the hepatic veins. Symptoms include an enlarged liver, extensive collateral vessels, intractable ascites, and severe portal hypertension.

I82.1 Thrombophlebitis migrans CC

✓5th **I82.2 Embolism and thrombosis of vena cava and other thoracic veins**

✓6th **I82.21 Embolism and thrombosis of superior vena cava**

I82.210 Acute embolism and thrombosis of superior vena cava CC HCC

Embolism and thrombosis of superior vena cava NOS

I82.211 Chronic embolism and thrombosis of superior vena cava CC HCC

✓6th **I82.22 Embolism and thrombosis of inferior vena cava**

I82.220 Acute embolism and thrombosis of inferior vena cava MCC HCC

Embolism and thrombosis of inferior vena cava NOS

I82.221 Chronic embolism and thrombosis of inferior vena cava MCC HCC

✓6th **I82.29 Embolism and thrombosis of other thoracic veins**

Embolism and thrombosis of brachiocephalic (innominate) vein

I82.290 Acute embolism and thrombosis of other thoracic veins CC HCC

I82.291 Chronic embolism and thrombosis of other thoracic veins CC HCC

I82.3 Embolism and thrombosis of renal vein CC HCC

✓5th **I82.4 Acute embolism and thrombosis of deep veins of lower extremity**

✓6th **I82.40 Acute embolism and thrombosis of unspecified deep veins of lower extremity**

Deep vein thrombosis NOS

DVT NOS

EXCLUDES 1 *acute embolism and thrombosis of unspecified deep veins of distal lower extremity (I82.4Z-)*

acute embolism and thrombosis of unspecified deep veins of proximal lower extremity (I82.4Y-)

I82.401 Acute embolism and thrombosis of unspecified deep veins of right lower extremity CC H10 HCC

I82.402 Acute embolism and thrombosis of unspecified deep veins of left lower extremity CC H10 HCC

I82.403 Acute embolism and thrombosis of unspecified deep veins of lower extremity, bilateral CC H10 HCC

I82.409 Acute embolism and thrombosis of unspecified deep veins of unspecified lower extremity CC H10 UNS HCC

✓6th **I82.41 Acute embolism and thrombosis of femoral vein**

Acute embolism and thrombosis of common femoral vein

Acute embolism and thrombosis of deep femoral vein

I82.411 Acute embolism and thrombosis of right femoral vein CC H10 HCC

I82.412 Acute embolism and thrombosis of left femoral vein CC H10 HCC

I82.413 Acute embolism and thrombosis of femoral vein, bilateral CC H10 HCC

I82.419 Acute embolism and thrombosis of unspecified femoral vein CC H10 UNS HCC

✓6th **I82.42 Acute embolism and thrombosis of iliac vein**

Acute embolism and thrombosis of common iliac vein

Acute embolism and thrombosis of external iliac vein

Acute embolism and thrombosis of internal iliac vein

I82.421 Acute embolism and thrombosis of right iliac vein CC H10 HCC

I82.422 Acute embolism and thrombosis of left iliac vein CC H10 HCC

I82.423 Acute embolism and thrombosis of iliac vein, bilateral CC H10 HCC

I82.429 Acute embolism and thrombosis of unspecified iliac vein CC H10 UNS HCC

✓6th **I82.43 Acute embolism and thrombosis of popliteal vein**

I82.431 Acute embolism and thrombosis of right popliteal vein CC H10 HCC

I82.432 Acute embolism and thrombosis of left popliteal vein CC H10 HCC

I82.433 **Acute embolism and thrombosis of popliteal vein, bilateral** CC H10 HCC

I82.439 **Acute embolism and thrombosis of unspecified popliteal vein** CC H10 UNS HCC

✓6th I82.44 **Acute embolism and thrombosis of tibial vein**

Acute embolism and thrombosis of anterior tibial vein

Acute embolism and thrombosis of posterior tibial vein

I82.441 **Acute embolism and thrombosis of right tibial vein** CC H10 HCC

I82.442 **Acute embolism and thrombosis of left tibial vein** CC H10 HCC

I82.443 **Acute embolism and thrombosis of tibial vein, bilateral** CC H10 HCC

I82.449 **Acute embolism and thrombosis of unspecified tibial vein** CC H10 UNS HCC

✓6th I82.45 **Acute embolism and thrombosis of peroneal vein**

AHA: 2019,4Q,8-10

I82.451 **Acute embolism and thrombosis of right peroneal vein** CC H10 HCC

I82.452 **Acute embolism and thrombosis of left peroneal vein** CC H10 HCC

I82.453 **Acute embolism and thrombosis of peroneal vein, bilateral** CC H10 HCC

I82.459 **Acute embolism and thrombosis of unspecified peroneal vein** CC H10 UNS HCC

✓6th I82.46 **Acute embolism and thrombosis of calf muscular vein**

Acute embolism and thrombosis of calf muscular vein, NOS

Acute embolism and thrombosis of gastrocnemial vein

Acute embolism and thrombosis of soleal vein

AHA: 2019,4Q,8-10

I82.461 **Acute embolism and thrombosis of right calf muscular vein** HCC

I82.462 **Acute embolism and thrombosis of left calf muscular vein** HCC

I82.463 **Acute embolism and thrombosis of calf muscular vein, bilateral** HCC

I82.469 **Acute embolism and thrombosis of unspecified calf muscular vein** HCC

✓6th I82.49 **Acute embolism and thrombosis of other specified deep vein of lower extremity**

I82.491 **Acute embolism and thrombosis of other specified deep vein of right lower extremity** CC H10 HCC

I82.492 **Acute embolism and thrombosis of other specified deep vein of left lower extremity** CC H10 HCC

I82.493 **Acute embolism and thrombosis of other specified deep vein of lower extremity, bilateral** CC H10 HCC

I82.499 **Acute embolism and thrombosis of other specified deep vein of unspecified lower extremity** CC H10 UNS HCC

✓6th I82.4Y **Acute embolism and thrombosis of unspecified deep veins of proximal lower extremity**

Acute embolism and thrombosis of deep vein of thigh NOS

Acute embolism and thrombosis of deep vein of upper leg NOS

I82.4Y1 **Acute embolism and thrombosis of unspecified deep veins of right proximal lower extremity** CC H10 HCC

I82.4Y2 **Acute embolism and thrombosis of unspecified deep veins of left proximal lower extremity** CC H10 HCC

I82.4Y3 **Acute embolism and thrombosis of unspecified deep veins of proximal lower extremity, bilateral** CC H10 HCC

I82.4Y9 **Acute embolism and thrombosis of unspecified deep veins of unspecified proximal lower extremity** CC H10 UNS HCC

✓6th I82.4Z **Acute embolism and thrombosis of unspecified deep veins of distal lower extremity**

Acute embolism and thrombosis of deep vein of calf NOS

Acute embolism and thrombosis of deep vein of lower leg NOS

I82.4Z1 **Acute embolism and thrombosis of unspecified deep veins of right distal lower extremity** CC H10 HCC

I82.4Z2 **Acute embolism and thrombosis of unspecified deep veins of left distal lower extremity** CC H10 HCC

I82.4Z3 **Acute embolism and thrombosis of unspecified deep veins of distal lower extremity, bilateral** CC H10 HCC

I82.4Z9 **Acute embolism and thrombosis of unspecified deep veins of unspecified distal lower extremity** CC H10 UNS HCC

✓5th I82.5 **Chronic embolism and thrombosis of deep veins of lower extremity**

Use additional code, if applicable, for associated long-term (current) use of anticoagulants (Z79.01)

EXCLUDES 1 *personal history of venous embolism and thrombosis (Z86.718)*

AHA: 2020,2Q,20

✓6th I82.50 **Chronic embolism and thrombosis of unspecified deep veins of lower extremity**

EXCLUDES 1 *chronic embolism and thrombosis of unspecified deep veins of distal lower extremity (I82.5Z-)*

chronic embolism and thrombosis of unspecified deep veins of proximal lower extremity (I82.5Y-)

I82.501 **Chronic embolism and thrombosis of unspecified deep veins of right lower extremity** CC HCC

I82.502 **Chronic embolism and thrombosis of unspecified deep veins of left lower extremity** CC HCC

I82.503 **Chronic embolism and thrombosis of unspecified deep veins of lower extremity, bilateral** CC HCC

I82.509 **Chronic embolism and thrombosis of unspecified deep veins of unspecified lower extremity** CC UNS HCC

✓6th I82.51 **Chronic embolism and thrombosis of femoral vein**

Chronic embolism and thrombosis of common femoral vein

Chronic embolism and thrombosis of deep femoral vein

I82.511 **Chronic embolism and thrombosis of right femoral vein** CC HCC

I82.512 **Chronic embolism and thrombosis of left femoral vein** CC HCC

I82.513 **Chronic embolism and thrombosis of femoral vein, bilateral** CC HCC

I82.519 **Chronic embolism and thrombosis of unspecified femoral vein** CC UNS HCC

✓6th I82.52 **Chronic embolism and thrombosis of iliac vein**

Chronic embolism and thrombosis of common iliac vein

Chronic embolism and thrombosis of external iliac vein

Chronic embolism and thrombosis of internal iliac vein

I82.521 **Chronic embolism and thrombosis of right iliac vein** CC HCC

I82.522 **Chronic embolism and thrombosis of left iliac vein** CC HCC

I82.523 **Chronic embolism and thrombosis of iliac vein, bilateral** CC HCC

I82.529 **Chronic embolism and thrombosis of unspecified iliac vein** CC UNS HCC

✓6th I82.53 **Chronic embolism and thrombosis of popliteal vein**

I82.531 **Chronic embolism and thrombosis of right popliteal vein** CC HCC

I82.532 **Chronic embolism and thrombosis of left popliteal vein** CC HCC

I82.533 **Chronic embolism and thrombosis of popliteal vein, bilateral** CC HCC

I82.539 **Chronic embolism and thrombosis of unspecified popliteal vein** CC UNS HCC

✓6th **I82.54** **Chronic embolism and thrombosis of tibial vein**
- Chronic embolism and thrombosis of anterior tibial vein
- Chronic embolism and thrombosis of posterior tibial vein

I82.541 **Chronic embolism and thrombosis of right tibial vein** CC HCC

I82.542 **Chronic embolism and thrombosis of left tibial vein** CC HCC

I82.543 **Chronic embolism and thrombosis of tibial vein, bilateral** CC HCC

I82.549 **Chronic embolism and thrombosis of unspecified tibial vein** CC UNS HCC

✓6th **I82.55** **Chronic embolism and thrombosis of peroneal vein**

AHA: 2019,4Q,8-10

I82.551 **Chronic embolism and thrombosis of right peroneal vein** CC HCC

I82.552 **Chronic embolism and thrombosis of left peroneal vein** CC HCC

I82.553 **Chronic embolism and thrombosis of peroneal vein, bilateral** CC HCC

I82.559 **Chronic embolism and thrombosis of unspecified peroneal vein** CC UNS HCC

✓6th **I82.56** **Chronic embolism and thrombosis of calf muscular vein**
- Chronic embolism and thrombosis of calf muscular vein NOS
- Chronic embolism and thrombosis of gastrocnemial vein
- Chronic embolism and thrombosis of soleal vein

AHA: 2019,4Q,8-10

I82.561 **Chronic embolism and thrombosis of right calf muscular vein** HCC

I82.562 **Chronic embolism and thrombosis of left calf muscular vein** HCC

I82.563 **Chronic embolism and thrombosis of calf muscular vein, bilateral** HCC

I82.569 **Chronic embolism and thrombosis of unspecified calf muscular vein** HCC

✓6th **I82.59** **Chronic embolism and thrombosis of other specified deep vein of lower extremity**

I82.591 **Chronic embolism and thrombosis of other specified deep vein of right lower extremity** CC HCC

I82.592 **Chronic embolism and thrombosis of other specified deep vein of left lower extremity** CC HCC

I82.593 **Chronic embolism and thrombosis of other specified deep vein of lower extremity, bilateral** CC HCC

I82.599 **Chronic embolism and thrombosis of other specified deep vein of unspecified lower extremity** CC UNS HCC

✓6th **I82.5Y** **Chronic embolism and thrombosis of unspecified deep veins of proximal lower extremity**
- Chronic embolism and thrombosis of deep veins of thigh NOS
- Chronic embolism and thrombosis of deep veins of upper leg NOS

I82.5Y1 **Chronic embolism and thrombosis of unspecified deep veins of right proximal lower extremity** CC HCC

I82.5Y2 **Chronic embolism and thrombosis of unspecified deep veins of left proximal lower extremity** CC HCC

I82.5Y3 **Chronic embolism and thrombosis of unspecified deep veins of proximal lower extremity, bilateral** CC HCC

I82.5Y9 **Chronic embolism and thrombosis of unspecified deep veins of unspecified proximal lower extremity** CC UNS HCC

✓6th **I82.5Z** **Chronic embolism and thrombosis of unspecified deep veins of distal lower extremity**
- Chronic embolism and thrombosis of deep veins of calf NOS
- Chronic embolism and thrombosis of deep veins of lower leg NOS

I82.5Z1 **Chronic embolism and thrombosis of unspecified deep veins of right distal lower extremity** CC HCC

I82.5Z2 **Chronic embolism and thrombosis of unspecified deep veins of left distal lower extremity** CC HCC

I82.5Z3 **Chronic embolism and thrombosis of unspecified deep veins of distal lower extremity, bilateral** CC HCC

I82.5Z9 **Chronic embolism and thrombosis of unspecified deep veins of unspecified distal lower extremity** CC UNS HCC

✓5th **I82.6** **Acute embolism and thrombosis of veins of upper extremity**

✓6th **I82.60** **Acute embolism and thrombosis of unspecified veins of upper extremity**

I82.601 **Acute embolism and thrombosis of unspecified veins of right upper extremity** CC

I82.602 **Acute embolism and thrombosis of unspecified veins of left upper extremity** CC

I82.603 **Acute embolism and thrombosis of unspecified veins of upper extremity, bilateral** CC

I82.609 **Acute embolism and thrombosis of unspecified veins of unspecified upper extremity** CC UNS

✓6th **I82.61** **Acute embolism and thrombosis of superficial veins of upper extremity**
- Acute embolism and thrombosis of antecubital vein
- Acute embolism and thrombosis of basilic vein
- Acute embolism and thrombosis of cephalic vein

I82.611 **Acute embolism and thrombosis of superficial veins of right upper extremity** CC

I82.612 **Acute embolism and thrombosis of superficial veins of left upper extremity** CC

I82.613 **Acute embolism and thrombosis of superficial veins of upper extremity, bilateral** CC

I82.619 **Acute embolism and thrombosis of superficial veins of unspecified upper extremity** CC UNS

✓6th **I82.62** **Acute embolism and thrombosis of deep veins of upper extremity**
- Acute embolism and thrombosis of brachial vein
- Acute embolism and thrombosis of radial vein
- Acute embolism and thrombosis of ulnar vein

I82.621 **Acute embolism and thrombosis of deep veins of right upper extremity** CC HCC

I82.622 **Acute embolism and thrombosis of deep veins of left upper extremity** CC HCC

I82.623 **Acute embolism and thrombosis of deep veins of upper extremity, bilateral** CC HCC

I82.629 **Acute embolism and thrombosis of deep veins of unspecified upper extremity** CC UNS HCC

✓5th **I82.7** **Chronic embolism and thrombosis of veins of upper extremity**

Use additional code, if applicable, for associated long-term (current) use of anticoagulants (Z79.01)

EXCLUDES 1 *personal history of venous embolism and thrombosis (Z86.718)*

✓6th **I82.70** **Chronic embolism and thrombosis of unspecified veins of upper extremity**

I82.701 **Chronic embolism and thrombosis of unspecified veins of right upper extremity** CC

I82.702 **Chronic embolism and thrombosis of unspecified veins of left upper extremity** CC

I82.703 **Chronic embolism and thrombosis of unspecified veins of upper extremity, bilateral** CC

I82.709 Chronic embolism and thrombosis of unspecified veins of unspecified upper extremity CC UNS

I82.71 Chronic embolism and thrombosis of superficial veins of upper extremity
Chronic embolism and thrombosis of antecubital vein
Chronic embolism and thrombosis of basilic vein
Chronic embolism and thrombosis of cephalic vein

I82.711 Chronic embolism and thrombosis of superficial veins of right upper extremity CC

I82.712 Chronic embolism and thrombosis of superficial veins of left upper extremity CC

I82.713 Chronic embolism and thrombosis of superficial veins of upper extremity, bilateral CC

I82.719 Chronic embolism and thrombosis of superficial veins of unspecified upper extremity CC UNS

I82.72 Chronic embolism and thrombosis of deep veins of upper extremity
Chronic embolism and thrombosis of brachial vein
Chronic embolism and thrombosis of radial vein
Chronic embolism and thrombosis of ulnar vein

I82.721 Chronic embolism and thrombosis of deep veins of right upper extremity CC HCC

I82.722 Chronic embolism and thrombosis of deep veins of left upper extremity CC HCC

I82.723 Chronic embolism and thrombosis of deep veins of upper extremity, bilateral CC HCC

I82.729 Chronic embolism and thrombosis of deep veins of unspecified upper extremity CC UNS HCC

I82.A Embolism and thrombosis of axillary vein

I82.A1 Acute embolism and thrombosis of axillary vein

I82.A11 Acute embolism and thrombosis of right axillary vein CC HCC

I82.A12 Acute embolism and thrombosis of left axillary vein CC HCC

I82.A13 Acute embolism and thrombosis of axillary vein, bilateral CC HCC

I82.A19 Acute embolism and thrombosis of unspecified axillary vein CC UNS HCC

I82.A2 Chronic embolism and thrombosis of axillary vein

I82.A21 Chronic embolism and thrombosis of right axillary vein CC HCC

I82.A22 Chronic embolism and thrombosis of left axillary vein CC HCC

I82.A23 Chronic embolism and thrombosis of axillary vein, bilateral CC HCC

I82.A29 Chronic embolism and thrombosis of unspecified axillary vein CC UNS HCC

I82.B Embolism and thrombosis of subclavian vein

I82.B1 Acute embolism and thrombosis of subclavian vein

I82.B11 Acute embolism and thrombosis of right subclavian vein CC HCC

I82.B12 Acute embolism and thrombosis of left subclavian vein CC HCC

I82.B13 Acute embolism and thrombosis of subclavian vein, bilateral CC HCC

I82.B19 Acute embolism and thrombosis of unspecified subclavian vein CC UNS HCC

I82.B2 Chronic embolism and thrombosis of subclavian vein

I82.B21 Chronic embolism and thrombosis of right subclavian vein CC HCC

I82.B22 Chronic embolism and thrombosis of left subclavian vein CC HCC

I82.B23 Chronic embolism and thrombosis of subclavian vein, bilateral CC HCC

I82.B29 Chronic embolism and thrombosis of unspecified subclavian vein CC UNS HCC

I82.C Embolism and thrombosis of internal jugular vein

I82.C1 Acute embolism and thrombosis of internal jugular vein

I82.C11 Acute embolism and thrombosis of right internal jugular vein CC HCC

I82.C12 Acute embolism and thrombosis of left internal jugular vein CC HCC

I82.C13 Acute embolism and thrombosis of internal jugular vein, bilateral CC HCC

I82.C19 Acute embolism and thrombosis of unspecified internal jugular vein CC UNS HCC

I82.C2 Chronic embolism and thrombosis of internal jugular vein

I82.C21 Chronic embolism and thrombosis of right internal jugular vein CC HCC

I82.C22 Chronic embolism and thrombosis of left internal jugular vein CC HCC

I82.C23 Chronic embolism and thrombosis of internal jugular vein, bilateral CC HCC

I82.C29 Chronic embolism and thrombosis of unspecified internal jugular vein CC UNS HCC

I82.8 Embolism and thrombosis of other specified veins
Use additional code, if applicable, for associated long-term (current) use of anticoagulants (Z79.01)

I82.81 Embolism and thrombosis of superficial veins of lower extremities
Embolism and thrombosis of saphenous vein (greater) (lesser)

I82.811 Embolism and thrombosis of superficial veins of right lower extremity CC

I82.812 Embolism and thrombosis of superficial veins of left lower extremity CC

I82.813 Embolism and thrombosis of superficial veins of lower extremities, bilateral CC

I82.819 Embolism and thrombosis of superficial veins of unspecified lower extremity CC UNS

I82.89 Embolism and thrombosis of other specified veins

I82.890 Acute embolism and thrombosis of other specified veins CC

I82.891 Chronic embolism and thrombosis of other specified veins CC

I82.9 Embolism and thrombosis of unspecified vein

I82.90 Acute embolism and thrombosis of unspecified vein CC UNS
Embolism of vein NOS
Thrombosis (vein) NOS

I82.91 Chronic embolism and thrombosis of unspecified vein CC UNS

I83 Varicose veins of lower extremities

EXCLUDES 2 *varicose veins complicating pregnancy (O22.0-)*
varicose veins complicating the puerperium (O87.4)

I83.0 Varicose veins of lower extremities with ulcer
Use additional code to identify severity of ulcer (L97.-)

I83.00 Varicose veins of unspecified lower extremity with ulcer

I83.001 Varicose veins of unspecified lower extremity with ulcer of thigh HCC A

I83.002 Varicose veins of unspecified lower extremity with ulcer of calf HCC A

I83.003 Varicose veins of unspecified lower extremity with ulcer of ankle HCC A

I83.004 Varicose veins of unspecified lower extremity with ulcer of heel and midfoot HCC A
Varicose veins of unspecified lower extremity with ulcer of plantar surface of midfoot

I83.005 Varicose veins of unspecified lower extremity with ulcer other part of foot HCC A
Varicose veins of unspecified lower extremity with ulcer of toe

I83.008 Varicose veins of unspecified lower extremity with ulcer other part of lower leg HCC A

I83.009 Varicose veins of unspecified lower extremity with ulcer of unspecified site HCC A

I83.01 Varicose veins of right lower extremity with ulcer

I83.011 Varicose veins of right lower extremity with ulcer of thigh HCC A

I83.012 Varicose veins of right lower extremity with ulcer of calf HCC A

I83.013 Varicose veins of right lower extremity with ulcer of ankle HCC A

I83.014 Varicose veins of right lower extremity with ulcer of heel and midfoot HCC A

Varicose veins of right lower extremity with ulcer of plantar surface of midfoot

I83.015 Varicose veins of right lower extremity with ulcer other part of foot HCC A

Varicose veins of right lower extremity with ulcer of toe

I83.018 Varicose veins of right lower extremity with ulcer other part of lower leg HCC A

I83.019 Varicose veins of right lower extremity with ulcer of unspecified site HCC A

I83.02 Varicose veins of left lower extremity with ulcer

I83.021 Varicose veins of left lower extremity with ulcer of thigh HCC A

I83.022 Varicose veins of left lower extremity with ulcer of calf HCC A

I83.023 Varicose veins of left lower extremity with ulcer of ankle HCC A

I83.024 Varicose veins of left lower extremity with ulcer of heel and midfoot HCC A

Varicose veins of left lower extremity with ulcer of plantar surface of midfoot

I83.025 Varicose veins of left lower extremity with ulcer other part of foot HCC A

Varicose veins of left lower extremity with ulcer of toe

I83.028 Varicose veins of left lower extremity with ulcer other part of lower leg HCC A

I83.029 Varicose veins of left lower extremity with ulcer of unspecified site HCC A

I83.1 Varicose veins of lower extremities with inflammation

I83.10 Varicose veins of unspecified lower extremity with inflammation A

I83.11 Varicose veins of right lower extremity with inflammation A

I83.12 Varicose veins of left lower extremity with inflammation A

I83.2 Varicose veins of lower extremities with both ulcer and inflammation

Use additional code to identify severity of ulcer (L97.-)

I83.20 Varicose veins of unspecified lower extremity with both ulcer and inflammation

I83.201 Varicose veins of unspecified lower extremity with both ulcer of thigh and inflammation CC HCC A

I83.202 Varicose veins of unspecified lower extremity with both ulcer of calf and inflammation CC HCC A

I83.203 Varicose veins of unspecified lower extremity with both ulcer of ankle and inflammation CC HCC A

I83.204 Varicose veins of unspecified lower extremity with both ulcer of heel and midfoot and inflammation CC HCC A

Varicose veins of unspecified lower extremity with both ulcer of plantar surface of midfoot and inflammation

I83.205 Varicose veins of unspecified lower extremity with both ulcer of other part of foot and inflammation CC HCC A

Varicose veins of unspecified lower extremity with both ulcer of toe and inflammation

I83.208 Varicose veins of unspecified lower extremity with both ulcer of other part of lower extremity and inflammation CC HCC A

I83.209 Varicose veins of unspecified lower extremity with both ulcer of unspecified site and inflammation CC HCC A

I83.21 Varicose veins of right lower extremity with both ulcer and inflammation

I83.211 Varicose veins of right lower extremity with both ulcer of thigh and inflammation CC HCC A

I83.212 Varicose veins of right lower extremity with both ulcer of calf and inflammation CC HCC A

I83.213 Varicose veins of right lower extremity with both ulcer of ankle and inflammation CC HCC A

I83.214 Varicose veins of right lower extremity with both ulcer of heel and midfoot and inflammation CC HCC A

Varicose veins of right lower extremity with both ulcer of plantar surface of midfoot and inflammation

I83.215 Varicose veins of right lower extremity with both ulcer other part of foot and inflammation CC HCC A

Varicose veins of right lower extremity with both ulcer of toe and inflammation

I83.218 Varicose veins of right lower extremity with both ulcer of other part of lower extremity and inflammation CC HCC A

I83.219 Varicose veins of right lower extremity with both ulcer of unspecified site and inflammation CC HCC A

I83.22 Varicose veins of left lower extremity with both ulcer and inflammation

I83.221 Varicose veins of left lower extremity with both ulcer of thigh and inflammation CC HCC A

I83.222 Varicose veins of left lower extremity with both ulcer of calf and inflammation CC HCC A

I83.223 Varicose veins of left lower extremity with both ulcer of ankle and inflammation CC HCC A

I83.224 Varicose veins of left lower extremity with both ulcer of heel and midfoot and inflammation CC HCC A

Varicose veins of left lower extremity with both ulcer of plantar surface of midfoot and inflammation

I83.225 Varicose veins of left lower extremity with both ulcer other part of foot and inflammation CC HCC A

Varicose veins of left lower extremity with both ulcer of toe and inflammation

I83.228 Varicose veins of left lower extremity with both ulcer of other part of lower extremity and inflammation CC HCC A

I83.229 Varicose veins of left lower extremity with both ulcer of unspecified site and inflammation CC HCC A

I83.8 Varicose veins of lower extremities with other complications

I83.81 Varicose veins of lower extremities with pain

I83.811 Varicose veins of right lower extremity with pain A

I83.812 Varicose veins of left lower extremity with pain A

I83.813 Varicose veins of bilateral lower extremities with pain A

I83.819 Varicose veins of unspecified lower extremity with pain A

I83.89 Varicose veins of lower extremities with other complications

Varicose veins of lower extremities with edema

Varicose veins of lower extremities with swelling

I83.891 Varicose veins of right lower extremity with other complications A

I83.892 Varicose veins of left lower extremity with other complications A

I83.893 Varicose veins of bilateral lower extremities with other complications A

I83.899 Varicose veins of unspecified lower extremity with other complications A

I83.9 Asymptomatic varicose veins of lower extremities
Phlebectasia of lower extremities
Varicose veins of lower extremities
Varix of lower extremities

I83.90 Asymptomatic varicose veins of unspecified lower extremity A
Varicose veins NOS

I83.91 Asymptomatic varicose veins of right lower extremity A

I83.92 Asymptomatic varicose veins of left lower extremity A

I83.93 Asymptomatic varicose veins of bilateral lower extremities A

I85 Esophageal varices
Use additional code to identify:
alcohol abuse and dependence (F10.-)

I85.0 Esophageal varices
Idiopathic esophageal varices
Primary esophageal varices

I85.00 Esophageal varices without bleeding CC HCC
Esophageal varices NOS

I85.01 Esophageal varices with bleeding MCC HCC

I85.1 Secondary esophageal varices
Esophageal varices secondary to alcoholic liver disease
Esophageal varices secondary to cirrhosis of liver
Esophageal varices secondary to schistosomiasis
Esophageal varices secondary to toxic liver disease
Code first underlying disease

I85.10 Secondary esophageal varices without bleeding CC HCC

I85.11 Secondary esophageal varices with bleeding MCC HCC

I86 Varicose veins of other sites
EXCLUDES 1 *varicose veins of unspecified site (I83.9-)*
EXCLUDES 2 *retinal varices (H35.0-)*

I86.0 Sublingual varices
DEF: Distended, tortuous veins beneath the tongue.

I86.1 Scrotal varices ♂
Varicocele

I86.2 Pelvic varices

I86.3 Vulval varices ♀
EXCLUDES 1 *vulval varices complicating childbirth and the puerperium (O87.8)*
vulval varices complicating pregnancy (O22.1-)

I86.4 Gastric varices

I86.8 Varicose veins of other specified sites A
Varicose ulcer of nasal septum

I87 Other disorders of veins

I87.0 Postthrombotic syndrome
Chronic venous hypertension due to deep vein thrombosis
Postphlebitic syndrome
EXCLUDES 1 *chronic venous hypertension without deep vein thrombosis (I87.3-)*

I87.00 Postthrombotic syndrome without complications
Asymptomatic postthrombotic syndrome

I87.001 Postthrombotic syndrome without complications of right lower extremity

I87.002 Postthrombotic syndrome without complications of left lower extremity

I87.003 Postthrombotic syndrome without complications of bilateral lower extremity

I87.009 Postthrombotic syndrome without complications of unspecified extremity
Postthrombotic syndrome NOS

I87.01 Postthrombotic syndrome with ulcer
Use additional code to specify site and severity of ulcer (L97.-)

I87.011 Postthrombotic syndrome with ulcer of right lower extremity CC HCC

I87.012 Postthrombotic syndrome with ulcer of left lower extremity CC HCC

I87.013 Postthrombotic syndrome with ulcer of bilateral lower extremity CC HCC

I87.019 Postthrombotic syndrome with ulcer of unspecified lower extremity CC UNS HCC

I87.02 Postthrombotic syndrome with inflammation

I87.021 Postthrombotic syndrome with inflammation of right lower extremity

I87.022 Postthrombotic syndrome with inflammation of left lower extremity

I87.023 Postthrombotic syndrome with inflammation of bilateral lower extremity

I87.029 Postthrombotic syndrome with inflammation of unspecified lower extremity

I87.03 Postthrombotic syndrome with ulcer and inflammation
Use additional code to specify site and severity of ulcer (L97.-)

I87.031 Postthrombotic syndrome with ulcer and inflammation of right lower extremity CC HCC

I87.032 Postthrombotic syndrome with ulcer and inflammation of left lower extremity CC HCC

I87.033 Postthrombotic syndrome with ulcer and inflammation of bilateral lower extremity CC HCC

I87.039 Postthrombotic syndrome with ulcer and inflammation of unspecified lower extremity CC UNS HCC

I87.09 Postthrombotic syndrome with other complications

I87.091 Postthrombotic syndrome with other complications of right lower extremity

I87.092 Postthrombotic syndrome with other complications of left lower extremity

I87.093 Postthrombotic syndrome with other complications of bilateral lower extremity

I87.099 Postthrombotic syndrome with other complications of unspecified lower extremity

I87.1 Compression of vein CC
Stricture of vein
Vena cava syndrome (inferior) (superior)
EXCLUDES 2 *compression of pulmonary vein (I28.8)*

I87.2 Venous insufficiency (chronic) (peripheral)
Stasis dermatitis
EXCLUDES 1 *stasis dermatitis with varicose veins of lower extremities (I83.1-, I83.2-)*
DEF: Insufficient drainage of venous blood in any part of the body that results in edema or dermatosis.

I87.3 Chronic venous hypertension (idiopathic)
Stasis edema
EXCLUDES 1 *chronic venous hypertension due to deep vein thrombosis (I87.0-)*
varicose veins of lower extremities (I83.-)

I87.30 Chronic venous hypertension (idiopathic) without complications
Asymptomatic chronic venous hypertension (idiopathic)

I87.301 Chronic venous hypertension (idiopathic) without complications of right lower extremity

I87.302 Chronic venous hypertension (idiopathic) without complications of left lower extremity

I87.303 Chronic venous hypertension (idiopathic) without complications of bilateral lower extremity

I87.309 Chronic venous hypertension (idiopathic) without complications of unspecified lower extremity
Chronic venous hypertension NOS

I87.31 Chronic venous hypertension (idiopathic) with ulcer
Use additional code to specify site and severity of ulcer (L97.-)

I87.311 Chronic venous hypertension (idiopathic) with ulcer of right lower extremity CC HCC

I87.312 Chronic venous hypertension (idiopathic) with ulcer of left lower extremity CC HCC

I87.313 Chronic venous hypertension (idiopathic) with ulcer of bilateral lower extremity CC HCC

I87.319 Chronic venous hypertension (idiopathic) with ulcer of unspecified lower extremity CC UNS HCC

✓6th **I87.32 Chronic venous hypertension (idiopathic) with inflammation**

I87.321 Chronic venous hypertension (idiopathic) with inflammation of right lower extremity

I87.322 Chronic venous hypertension (idiopathic) with inflammation of left lower extremity

I87.323 Chronic venous hypertension (idiopathic) with inflammation of bilateral lower extremity

I87.329 Chronic venous hypertension (idiopathic) with inflammation of unspecified lower extremity

✓6th **I87.33 Chronic venous hypertension (idiopathic) with ulcer and inflammation**

Use additional code to specify site and severity of ulcer (L97.-)

I87.331 Chronic venous hypertension (idiopathic) with ulcer and inflammation of right lower extremity CC HCC

I87.332 Chronic venous hypertension (idiopathic) with ulcer and inflammation of left lower extremity CC HCC

I87.333 Chronic venous hypertension (idiopathic) with ulcer and inflammation of bilateral lower extremity CC HCC

I87.339 Chronic venous hypertension (idiopathic) with ulcer and inflammation of unspecified lower extremity CC UNS HCC

✓6th **I87.39 Chronic venous hypertension (idiopathic) with other complications**

I87.391 Chronic venous hypertension (idiopathic) with other complications of right lower extremity

I87.392 Chronic venous hypertension (idiopathic) with other complications of left lower extremity

I87.393 Chronic venous hypertension (idiopathic) with other complications of bilateral lower extremity

I87.399 Chronic venous hypertension (idiopathic) with other complications of unspecified lower extremity

I87.8 Other specified disorders of veins

Phlebosclerosis

Venofibrosis

I87.9 Disorder of vein, unspecified

✓4th **I88 Nonspecific lymphadenitis**

EXCLUDES 1 *acute lymphadenitis, except mesenteric (L04.-)*

enlarged lymph nodes NOS (R59.-)

human immunodeficiency virus [HIV] disease resulting in generalized lymphadenopathy (B20)

I88.0 Nonspecific mesenteric lymphadenitis

Mesenteric lymphadenitis (acute)(chronic)

I88.1 Chronic lymphadenitis, except mesenteric

Adenitis

Lymphadenitis

I88.8 Other nonspecific lymphadenitis

I88.9 Nonspecific lymphadenitis, unspecified

Lymphadenitis NOS

✓4th **I89 Other noninfective disorders of lymphatic vessels and lymph nodes**

EXCLUDES 1 *chylocele, tunica vaginalis (nonfilarial) NOS (N50.89)*

enlarged lymph nodes NOS (R59.-)

filarial chylocele (B74.-)

hereditary lymphedema (Q82.0)

I89.0 Lymphedema, not elsewhere classified

Elephantiasis (nonfilarial) NOS

Lymphangiectasis

Obliteration, lymphatic vessel

Praecox lymphedema

Secondary lymphedema

EXCLUDES 1 *postmastectomy lymphedema (I97.2)*

I89.1 Lymphangitis

Chronic lymphangitis

Lymphangitis NOS

Subacute lymphangitis

EXCLUDES 1 *acute lymphangitis (L03.-)*

I89.8 Other specified noninfective disorders of lymphatic vessels and lymph nodes

Chylocele (nonfilarial)

Chylous ascites

Chylous cyst

Lipomelanotic reticulosis

Lymph node or vessel fistula

Lymph node or vessel infarction

Lymph node or vessel rupture

I89.9 Noninfective disorder of lymphatic vessels and lymph nodes, unspecified

Disease of lymphatic vessels NOS

Other and unspecified disorders of the circulatory system (I95-I99)

✓4th **I95 Hypotension**

EXCLUDES 1 *cardiovascular collapse (R57.9) (~R57.9)*

maternal hypotension syndrome (O26.5-)

nonspecific low blood pressure reading NOS (R03.1)

I95.0 Idiopathic hypotension

I95.1 Orthostatic hypotension

Hypotension, postural

EXCLUDES 1 *neurogenic orthostatic hypotension [Shy-Drager] (G90.3)*

orthostatic hypotension due to drugs (I95.2)

I95.2 Hypotension due to drugs

Orthostatic hypotension due to drugs

Use additional code for adverse effect, if applicable, to identify drug (T36-T50 with fifth or sixth character 5)

I95.3 Hypotension of hemodialysis

Intra-dialytic hypotension

✓5th **I95.8 Other hypotension**

I95.81 Postprocedural hypotension

I95.89 Other hypotension

Chronic hypotension

I95.9 Hypotension, unspecified

I96 Gangrene, not elsewhere classified CC HCC

Gangrenous cellulitis

EXCLUDES 1 *gangrene in atherosclerosis of native arteries of the extremities (I70.26)*

gangrene in hernia (K40.1, K40.4, K41.1, K41.4, K42.1, K43.1-, K44.1, K45.1, K46.1)

gangrene in other peripheral vascular diseases (I73.-)

gangrene of certain specified sites - see Alphabetical Index

gas gangrene (A48.0)

pyoderma gangrenosum (L88)

EXCLUDES 2 *gangrene in diabetes mellitus (E08-E13 with .52)*

AHA: 2018,4Q,87; 2018,3Q,3; 2017,3Q,6; 2013,2Q,34

✓4th **I97 Intraoperative and postprocedural complications and disorders of circulatory system, not elsewhere classified**

EXCLUDES 2 *postprocedural shock (T81.1-)*

AHA: 2021,1Q,13; 2019,2Q,21

I97.0 Postcardiotomy syndrome

✓5th **I97.1 Other postprocedural cardiac functional disturbances**

EXCLUDES 2 *acute pulmonary insufficiency following thoracic surgery (J95.1)*

intraoperative cardiac functional disturbances (I97.7-)

✓6th **I97.11 Postprocedural cardiac insufficiency**

I97.110 Postprocedural cardiac insufficiency following cardiac surgery CC

I97.111 Postprocedural cardiac insufficiency following other surgery CC

✓6th **I97.12 Postprocedural cardiac arrest**

I97.120 Postprocedural cardiac arrest following cardiac surgery CC

I97.121 Postprocedural cardiac arrest following other surgery CC

I97.13 Postprocedural heart failure

Use additional code to identify the heart failure (I5Ø.-)

I97.13Ø Postprocedural heart failure following cardiac surgery CC

I97.131 Postprocedural heart failure following other surgery CC

I97.19 Other postprocedural cardiac functional disturbances

Use additional code, if applicable, to further specify disorder

I97.19Ø Other postprocedural cardiac functional disturbances following cardiac surgery CC

Use additional code, if applicable, for type 4 or type 5 myocardial infarction, to further specify disorder

AHA: 2019,2Q,33

I97.191 Other postprocedural cardiac functional disturbances following other surgery CC

I97.2 Postmastectomy lymphedema syndrome A

Elephantiasis due to mastectomy

Obliteration of lymphatic vessels

I97.3 Postprocedural hypertension

I97.4 Intraoperative hemorrhage and hematoma of a circulatory system organ or structure complicating a procedure

EXCLUDES 1 *intraoperative hemorrhage and hematoma of a circulatory system organ or structure due to accidental puncture and laceration during a procedure (I97.5-)*

EXCLUDES 2 *intraoperative cerebrovascular hemorrhage complicating a procedure (G97.3-)*

I97.41 Intraoperative hemorrhage and hematoma of a circulatory system organ or structure complicating a circulatory system procedure

I97.41Ø Intraoperative hemorrhage and hematoma of a circulatory system organ or structure complicating a cardiac catheterization CC

I97.411 Intraoperative hemorrhage and hematoma of a circulatory system organ or structure complicating a cardiac bypass CC

I97.418 Intraoperative hemorrhage and hematoma of a circulatory system organ or structure complicating other circulatory system procedure CC

I97.42 Intraoperative hemorrhage and hematoma of a circulatory system organ or structure complicating other procedure CC

AHA: 2020,1Q,19

I97.5 Accidental puncture and laceration of a circulatory system organ or structure during a procedure

EXCLUDES 2 *accidental puncture and laceration of brain during a procedure (G97.4-)*

I97.51 Accidental puncture and laceration of a circulatory system organ or structure during a circulatory system procedure CC

AHA: 2019,2Q,24

I97.52 Accidental puncture and laceration of a circulatory system organ or structure during other procedure CC

I97.6 Postprocedural hemorrhage, hematoma and seroma of a circulatory system organ or structure following a procedure

EXCLUDES 2 *postprocedural cerebrovascular hemorrhage complicating a procedure (G97.5-)*

AHA: 2016,4Q,9-10

I97.61 Postprocedural hemorrhage of a circulatory system organ or structure following a circulatory system procedure

I97.61Ø Postprocedural hemorrhage of a circulatory system organ or structure following a cardiac catheterization CC

I97.611 Postprocedural hemorrhage of a circulatory system organ or structure following cardiac bypass CC

I97.618 Postprocedural hemorrhage of a circulatory system organ or structure following other circulatory system procedure CC

I97.62 Postprocedural hemorrhage, hematoma and seroma of a circulatory system organ or structure following other procedure

I97.62Ø Postprocedural hemorrhage of a circulatory system organ or structure following other procedure CC

I97.621 Postprocedural hematoma of a circulatory system organ or structure following other procedure CC

I97.622 Postprocedural seroma of a circulatory system organ or structure following other procedure CC

I97.63 Postprocedural hematoma of a circulatory system organ or structure following a circulatory system procedure

I97.63Ø Postprocedural hematoma of a circulatory system organ or structure following a cardiac catheterization CC

I97.631 Postprocedural hematoma of a circulatory system organ or structure following cardiac bypass CC

I97.638 Postprocedural hematoma of a circulatory system organ or structure following other circulatory system procedure CC

I97.64 Postprocedural seroma of a circulatory system organ or structure following a circulatory system procedure

I97.64Ø Postprocedural seroma of a circulatory system organ or structure following a cardiac catheterization CC

I97.641 Postprocedural seroma of a circulatory system organ or structure following cardiac bypass CC

I97.648 Postprocedural seroma of a circulatory system organ or structure following other circulatory system procedure CC

I97.7 Intraoperative cardiac functional disturbances

EXCLUDES 2 *acute pulmonary insufficiency following thoracic surgery (J95.1)*
postprocedural cardiac functional disturbances (I97.1-)

I97.71 Intraoperative cardiac arrest

I97.71Ø Intraoperative cardiac arrest during cardiac surgery CC

I97.711 Intraoperative cardiac arrest during other surgery CC

I97.79 Other intraoperative cardiac functional disturbances

Use additional code, if applicable, to further specify disorder

I97.79Ø Other intraoperative cardiac functional disturbances during cardiac surgery CC

I97.791 Other intraoperative cardiac functional disturbances during other surgery CC

I97.8 Other intraoperative and postprocedural complications and disorders of the circulatory system, not elsewhere classified

Use additional code, if applicable, to further specify disorder

I97.81 Intraoperative cerebrovascular infarction

I97.81Ø Intraoperative cerebrovascular infarction during cardiac surgery CC HCC

I97.811 Intraoperative cerebrovascular infarction during other surgery CC HCC

I97.82 Postprocedural cerebrovascular infarction

I97.82Ø Postprocedural cerebrovascular infarction following cardiac surgery CC HCC

I97.821 Postprocedural cerebrovascular infarction following other surgery CC HCC

I97.88 Other intraoperative complications of the circulatory system, not elsewhere classified CC

I97.89 Other postprocedural complications and disorders of the circulatory system, not elsewhere classified CC

AHA: 2021,3Q,33; 2020,3Q,3-8; 2019,2Q,33

I99 Other and unspecified disorders of circulatory system

I99.8 Other disorder of circulatory system

AHA: 2020,4Q,98

I99.9 Unspecified disorder of circulatory system

Chapter 10. Diseases of the Respiratory System (J00–J99)

Chapter-specific Guidelines with Coding Examples

The chapter-specific guidelines from the ICD-10-CM Official Guidelines for Coding and Reporting have been provided below. Along with these guidelines are coding examples, contained in the shaded boxes, that have been developed to help illustrate the coding and/or sequencing guidance found in these guidelines.

a. Chronic obstructive pulmonary disease [COPD] and asthma

1) Acute exacerbation of chronic obstructive bronchitis and asthma

The codes in categories J44 and J45 distinguish between uncomplicated cases and those in acute exacerbation. An acute exacerbation is a worsening or a decompensation of a chronic condition. An acute exacerbation is not equivalent to an infection superimposed on a chronic condition, though an exacerbation may be triggered by an infection.

Vancomycin IV was started to treat a patient with acute pneumonia due to *Streptococcus pneumoniae*. Patient also with acute exacerbation of COPD continued on home meds.

J13 **Pneumonia due to Streptococcus pneumoniae**

J44.0 **Chronic obstructive pulmonary disease with (acute) lower respiratory infection**

J44.1 **Chronic obstructive pulmonary disease with (acute) exacerbation**

Explanation: ICD-10-CM uses combination codes to create organism-specific classifications for acute pneumonia. Category J44 codes include combination codes with severity components, which differentiate between COPD with acute lower respiratory infection (acute pneumonia), COPD with acute exacerbation, and COPD without mention of a complication (unspecified).

An acute exacerbation is a worsening or a decompensation of a chronic condition. An acute exacerbation is not equivalent to an infection superimposed on a chronic condition, though an exacerbation may be triggered by an infection, as in this example. Treatment of the pneumonia necessitated the inpatient admission. Instructional notes at J44.0 say to "code also to identify the infection," which informs the coder that another code must be assigned if applicable. Sequencing of the pneumonia and COPD exacerbation are governed by the Section II, "Selection of Principal Diagnosis," guidelines. In this case it was the pneumonia that was "chiefly responsible for occasioning the admission" with the IV vancomycin treatment.

Exacerbation of moderate persistent asthma with status asthmaticus

J45.42 **Moderate persistent asthma with status asthmaticus**

Explanation: Category J45 Asthma includes severity-specific subcategories and fifth-character codes to distinguish between uncomplicated cases, those in acute exacerbation, and those with status asthmaticus.

b. Acute respiratory failure

1) Acute respiratory failure as principal diagnosis

A code from subcategory J96.0, Acute respiratory failure, or subcategory J96.2, Acute and chronic respiratory failure, may be assigned as a principal diagnosis when it is the condition established after study to be chiefly responsible for occasioning the admission to the hospital, and the selection is supported by the Alphabetic Index and Tabular List. However, chapter-specific coding guidelines (such as obstetrics, poisoning, HIV, newborn) that provide sequencing direction take precedence.

Acute hypoxic respiratory failure due to COPD exacerbation

J96.01 **Acute respiratory failure with hypoxia**

J44.1 **Chronic obstructive pulmonary disease with (acute) exacerbation**

Explanation: Category J96 classifies respiratory failure with combination codes that designate the severity and the presence of hypoxia and hypercapnia. Code J96.01 is sequenced as the first-listed diagnosis, as the reason for the admission. Respiratory failure may be assigned as a principal diagnosis when it is the condition established after study to be chiefly responsible for occasioning the admission to the hospital and the selection is supported by the Alphabetic Index and Tabular List.

2) Acute respiratory failure as secondary diagnosis

Respiratory failure may be listed as a secondary diagnosis if it occurs after admission, or if it is present on admission, but does not meet the definition of principal diagnosis.

Acute respiratory failure due to accidental oxycodone overdose

T40.2X1A **Poisoning by other opioids, accidental (unintentional), initial encounter**

J96.00 **Acute respiratory failure, unspecified whether with hypoxia or hypercapnia**

Explanation: Respiratory failure may be assigned as a principal diagnosis when it is the condition established after study to be chiefly responsible for occasioning the admission to the hospital, and the selection is supported by the Alphabetic Index and Tabular List. However, chapter-specific coding guidelines, such as poisoning, that provide sequencing direction take precedence. When coding a poisoning or reaction to the improper use of a medication (e.g., overdose, wrong substance given or taken in error, wrong route of administration), first assign the appropriate code from categories T36–T50. Use additional code(s) for all manifestations of the poisoning. In this instance, the respiratory failure is a manifestation of the poisoning and is sequenced as a secondary diagnosis.

Acute pneumococcal pneumonia with subsequent development of acute respiratory failure

J13 **Pneumonia due to Streptococcus pneumoniae**

J96.00 **Acute respiratory failure, unspecified whether with hypoxia or hypercapnia**

Explanation: Acute respiratory failure may be listed as a secondary diagnosis if it occurs after admission, or if it is present on admission but does not meet the definition of principal diagnosis.

3) Sequencing of acute respiratory failure and another acute condition

When a patient is admitted with respiratory failure and another acute condition, (e.g., myocardial infarction, cerebrovascular accident, aspiration pneumonia), the principal diagnosis will not be the same in every situation. This applies whether the other acute condition is a respiratory or nonrespiratory condition. Selection of the principal diagnosis will be dependent on the circumstances of admission. If both the respiratory failure and the other acute condition are equally responsible for occasioning the admission to the hospital, and there are no chapter-specific sequencing rules, the guideline regarding two or more diagnoses that equally meet the definition for principal diagnosis (*Section II, C.*) may be applied in these situations.

If the documentation is not clear as to whether acute respiratory failure and another condition are equally responsible for occasioning the admission, query the provider for clarification.

Acute pneumococcal pneumonia and acute respiratory failure, both present on admission

J96.00 **Acute respiratory failure, unspecified whether with hypoxia or hypercapnia**

J13 **Pneumonia due to Streptococcus pneumoniae**

Explanation: When a patient is admitted with respiratory failure and another acute condition, such as a bacterial pneumonia, the principal diagnosis is not the same in every situation. This applies whether the other acute condition is a respiratory or nonrespiratory condition. The principal diagnosis depends on the circumstances of admission.

c. Influenza due to certain identified influenza viruses

Code only confirmed cases of influenza due to certain identified influenza viruses (category J09), and due to other identified influenza virus (category J10). This is an exception to the hospital inpatient guideline Section II, H. (Uncertain Diagnosis).

In this context, "confirmation" does not require documentation of positive laboratory testing specific for avian or other novel influenza A or other identified influenza virus. However, coding should be based on the provider's diagnostic statement that the patient has avian influenza, or other novel influenza A, for category J09, or has another particular identified strain of influenza, such as H1N1 or H3N2, but not identified as novel or variant, for category J10.

If the provider records "suspected" or "possible" or "probable" avian influenza, or novel influenza, or other identified influenza, then the appropriate influenza code from category J11, Influenza due to unidentified influenza virus, should be assigned. A code from category J09, Influenza due to certain identified influenza viruses, should not be assigned nor should a code from category J10, Influenza due to other identified influenza virus.

> Influenza due to avian influenza virus with pneumonia
>
> **J09.X1 Influenza due to identified novel influenza A virus with pneumonia**
>
> *Explanation*: Codes in category J09 Influenza due to certain identified influenza viruses should be assigned only for confirmed cases. "Confirmation" does not require positive laboratory testing of a specific influenza virus but does need to be based on the provider's diagnostic statement, which should not include terms such as "possible," "probable," or "suspected."

d. Ventilator associated pneumonia

1) Documentation of ventilator associated pneumonia

As with all procedural or postprocedural complications, code assignment is based on the provider's documentation of the relationship between the condition and the procedure.

Code J95.851, Ventilator associated pneumonia, should be assigned only when the provider has documented ventilator associated pneumonia (VAP). An additional code to identify the organism (e.g., Pseudomonas aeruginosa, code B96.5) should also be assigned. Do not assign an additional code from categories J12-J18 to identify the type of pneumonia.

Code J95.851 should not be assigned for cases where the patient has pneumonia and is on a mechanical ventilator and the provider has not specifically stated that the pneumonia is ventilator-associated pneumonia. If the documentation is unclear as to whether the patient has a pneumonia that is a complication attributable to the mechanical ventilator, query the provider.

2) Ventilator associated pneumonia develops after admission

A patient may be admitted with one type of pneumonia (e.g., code J13, Pneumonia due to Streptococcus pneumonia) and subsequently develop VAP. In this instance, the principal diagnosis would be the appropriate code from categories J12-J18 for the pneumonia diagnosed at the time of admission. Code J95.851, Ventilator associated pneumonia, would be assigned as an additional diagnosis when the provider has also documented the presence of ventilator associated pneumonia.

> Patient with pneumonia due to *Klebsiella pneumoniae* develops superimposed MRSA ventilator-associated pneumonia
>
> **J15.0 Pneumonia due to Klebsiella pneumoniae**
>
> **J95.851 Ventilator associated pneumonia**
>
> **B95.62 Methicillin resistant Staphylococcus aureus infection as the cause of diseases classified elsewhere**
>
> *Explanation*: Code assignment for ventilator-associated pneumonia is based on the provider's documentation of the relationship between the condition and the procedure and is reported only when the provider has documented ventilator-associated pneumonia (VAP).
>
> A patient may be admitted with one type of pneumonia and subsequently develop VAP. In this example, the principal diagnosis code describes the pneumonia diagnosed at the time of admission, with code J95.851 Ventilator associated pneumonia, assigned as secondary.

e. Vaping-related disorders

For patients presenting with condition(s) related to vaping, assign code U07.0, Vaping-related disorder, as the principal diagnosis. For lung injury due to vaping, assign only code U07.0. Assign additional codes for other manifestations, such as acute respiratory failure (subcategory J96.0-) or pneumonitis (code J68.0).

Associated respiratory signs and symptoms due to vaping, such as cough, shortness of breath, etc., are not coded separately, when a definitive diagnosis has been established. However, it would be appropriate to code separately any gastrointestinal symptoms, such as diarrhea and abdominal pain.

See Section I.C.1.g.1.c.i. for Pneumonia confirmed as due to COVID-19

> 23-year-old patient with history of anxiety disorder admitted with fever, dyspnea and nonproductive cough. Patient's respiratory function continued to clinically worsen, requiring intubation for suspected ARDS and required OGT suction for coffee ground hematemesis. Following extubating, patient confirmed the use of THC vaping cartridge preceding development of symptoms. Discharge diagnosis is ARDS due to EVALI and anxiety disorder.
>
> **U07.0 Vaping related disorder**
>
> **J80 Acute respiratory distress syndrome**
>
> **K92.0 Hematemesis**
>
> **F41.9 Anxiety disorder, unspecified**
>
> *Explanation:* Codes U07.0 and J80 represent the vaping-related disorder and its associated manifestation, the acute respiratory distress syndrome (ARDS). The symptoms that brought the patient in are not coded separately because these are integral to the vaping disorder and the ARDS, unlike the hematemesis (vomiting blood) a gastrointestinal symptom that is not integral to either of these conditions.

Chapter 10. Diseases of the Respiratory System (J00-J99)

NOTE When a respiratory condition is described as occurring in more than one site and is not specifically indexed, it should be classified to the lower anatomic site (e.g., tracheobronchitis to bronchitis in J40).

Use additional code, where applicable, to identify:
- exposure to environmental tobacco smoke (Z77.22)
- exposure to tobacco smoke in the perinatal period (P96.81)
- history of tobacco dependence (Z87.891)
- occupational exposure to environmental tobacco smoke (Z57.31)
- tobacco dependence (F17.-)
- tobacco use (Z72.0)

EXCLUDES 2 *certain conditions originating in the perinatal period (P04-P96)*
certain infectious and parasitic diseases (A00-B99)
complications of pregnancy, childbirth and the puerperium (O00-O9A)
congenital malformations, deformations and chromosomal abnormalities (Q00-Q99)
endocrine, nutritional and metabolic diseases (E00-E88)
injury, poisoning and certain other consequences of external causes (S00-T88)
neoplasms (C00-D49)
smoke inhalation (T59.81-)
symptoms, signs and abnormal clinical and laboratory findings, not elsewhere classified (R00-R94)

This chapter contains the following blocks:

Acute upper respiratory infections (J00-J06)

EXCLUDES 1 *chronic obstructive pulmonary disease with acute lower respiratory infection (J44.0)*

J00 Acute nasopharyngitis [common cold]
Acute rhinitis
Coryza (acute)
Infective nasopharyngitis NOS
Infective rhinitis
Nasal catarrh, acute
Nasopharyngitis NOS
EXCLUDES 1 *acute pharyngitis (J02.-)*
acute sore throat NOS (J02.9)
influenza virus with other respiratory manifestations (J09.X2, J10.1, J11.1)
pharyngitis NOS (J02.9)
rhinitis NOS (J31.0)
sore throat NOS (J02.9)
EXCLUDES 2 *allergic rhinitis (J30.1-J30.9)*
chronic pharyngitis (J31.2)
chronic rhinitis (J31.0)
chronic sore throat (J31.2)
nasopharyngitis, chronic (J31.1)
vasomotor rhinitis (J30.0)

✓4th **J01 Acute sinusitis**
INCLUDES acute abscess of sinus
acute empyema of sinus
acute infection of sinus
acute inflammation of sinus
acute suppuration of sinus
Use additional code (B95-B97) to identify infectious agent
EXCLUDES 1 *sinusitis NOS (J32.9)*
EXCLUDES 2 *chronic sinusitis (J32.0-J32.8)*

✓5th **J01.0 Acute maxillary sinusitis**
Acute antritis
J01.00 Acute maxillary sinusitis, unspecified
J01.01 Acute recurrent maxillary sinusitis

✓5th **J01.1 Acute frontal sinusitis**
J01.10 Acute frontal sinusitis, unspecified
J01.11 Acute recurrent frontal sinusitis

✓5th **J01.2 Acute ethmoidal sinusitis**
J01.20 Acute ethmoidal sinusitis, unspecified
J01.21 Acute recurrent ethmoidal sinusitis

✓5th **J01.3 Acute sphenoidal sinusitis**
J01.30 Acute sphenoidal sinusitis, unspecified
J01.31 Acute recurrent sphenoidal sinusitis

✓5th **J01.4 Acute pansinusitis**
J01.40 Acute pansinusitis, unspecified
J01.41 Acute recurrent pansinusitis

✓5th **J01.8 Other acute sinusitis**
J01.80 Other acute sinusitis
Acute sinusitis involving more than one sinus but not pansinusitis
J01.81 Other acute recurrent sinusitis
Acute recurrent sinusitis involving more than one sinus but not pansinusitis

✓5th **J01.9 Acute sinusitis, unspecified**
J01.90 Acute sinusitis, unspecified
J01.91 Acute recurrent sinusitis, unspecified

✓4th **J02 Acute pharyngitis**
INCLUDES acute sore throat
EXCLUDES 1 *acute laryngopharyngitis (J06.0)*
peritonsillar abscess (J36)
pharyngeal abscess (J39.1)
retropharyngeal abscess (J39.0)
EXCLUDES 2 *chronic pharyngitis (J31.2)*

J02.0 Streptococcal pharyngitis
Septic pharyngitis
Streptococcal sore throat
EXCLUDES 2 *scarlet fever (A38.-)*

J02.8 Acute pharyngitis due to other specified organisms
Use additional code (B95-B97) to identify infectious agent
EXCLUDES 1 *acute pharyngitis due to coxsackie virus (B08.5)*
acute pharyngitis due to gonococcus (A54.5)
acute pharyngitis due to herpes [simplex] virus (B00.2)
acute pharyngitis due to infectious mononucleosis (B27.-)
enteroviral vesicular pharyngitis (B08.5)

J02.9 Acute pharyngitis, unspecified
Gangrenous pharyngitis (acute)
Infective pharyngitis (acute) NOS
Pharyngitis (acute) NOS
Sore throat (acute) NOS
Suppurative pharyngitis (acute)
Ulcerative pharyngitis (acute)
EXCLUDES 1 *influenza virus with other respiratory manifestations (J09.X2, J10.1, J11.1)*

✓4th **J03 Acute tonsillitis**
EXCLUDES 1 *acute sore throat (J02.-)*
hypertrophy of tonsils (J35.1)
peritonsillar abscess (J36)
sore throat NOS (J02.9)
streptococcal sore throat (J02.0)
EXCLUDES 2 *chronic tonsillitis (J35.0)*

✓5th **J03.0 Streptococcal tonsillitis**
J03.00 Acute streptococcal tonsillitis, unspecified
J03.01 Acute recurrent streptococcal tonsillitis

✓5th **J03.8 Acute tonsillitis due to other specified organisms**
Use additional code (B95-B97) to identify infectious agent
EXCLUDES 1 *diphtheritic tonsillitis (A36.0)*
herpesviral pharyngotonsillitis (B00.2)
streptococcal tonsillitis (J03.0)
tuberculous tonsillitis (A15.8)
Vincent's tonsillitis (A69.1)
J03.80 Acute tonsillitis due to other specified organisms
J03.81 Acute recurrent tonsillitis due to other specified organisms

J03.9 Acute tonsillitis, unspecified
Follicular tonsillitis (acute)
Gangrenous tonsillitis (acute)
Infective tonsillitis (acute)
Tonsillitis (acute) NOS
Ulcerative tonsillitis (acute)
EXCLUDES 1 *influenza virus with other respiratory manifestations (J09.X2, J10.1, J11.1)*

J03.90 Acute tonsillitis, unspecified
J03.91 Acute recurrent tonsillitis, unspecified

J04 Acute laryngitis and tracheitis
Code also influenza, if present, such as:
influenza due to identified novel influenza A virus with other respiratory manifestations (J09.X2)
influenza due to other identified influenza virus with other respiratory manifestations (J10.1)
influenza due to unidentified influenza virus with other respiratory manifestations (J11.1)
Use additional code (B95-B97) to identify infectious agent
EXCLUDES 1 *acute obstructive laryngitis [croup] and epiglottitis (J05.-)*
EXCLUDES 2 *laryngismus (stridulus) (J38.5)*

J04.0 Acute laryngitis
Edematous laryngitis (acute)
Laryngitis (acute) NOS
Subglottic laryngitis (acute)
Suppurative laryngitis (acute)
Ulcerative laryngitis (acute)
EXCLUDES 1 *acute obstructive laryngitis (J05.0)*
EXCLUDES 2 *chronic laryngitis (J37.0)*

J04.1 Acute tracheitis
Acute viral tracheitis
Catarrhal tracheitis (acute)
Tracheitis (acute) NOS
EXCLUDES 2 *chronic tracheitis (J42)*

J04.10 Acute tracheitis without obstruction
J04.11 Acute tracheitis with obstruction MCC

J04.2 Acute laryngotracheitis
Laryngotracheitis NOS
Tracheitis (acute) with laryngitis (acute)
EXCLUDES 1 *acute obstructive laryngotracheitis (J05.0)*
EXCLUDES 2 *chronic laryngotracheitis (J37.1)*

J04.3 Supraglottitis, unspecified
J04.30 Supraglottitis, unspecified, without obstruction
J04.31 Supraglottitis, unspecified, with obstruction MCC

J05 Acute obstructive laryngitis [croup] and epiglottitis
Code also, influenza, if present, such as:
influenza due to identified novel influenza A virus with other respiratory manifestations (J09.X2)
influenza due to other identified influenza virus with other respiratory manifestations (J10.1)
influenza due to unidentified influenza virus with other respiratory manifestations (J11.1)
Use additional code (B95-B97) to identify infectious agent

J05.0 Acute obstructive laryngitis [croup]
Obstructive laryngitis (acute) NOS
Obstructive laryngotracheitis NOS
DEF: Acute laryngeal obstruction due to allergies, foreign bodies, or in the majority of cases a viral infection. Symptoms include a harsh, barking cough, hoarseness, and a persistent, high-pitched respiratory sound (stridor).

J05.1 Acute epiglottitis
EXCLUDES 2 *epiglottitis, chronic (J37.0)*

J05.10 Acute epiglottitis without obstruction CC
Epiglottitis NOS
J05.11 Acute epiglottitis with obstruction MCC

J06 Acute upper respiratory infections of multiple and unspecified sites
EXCLUDES 1 *acute respiratory infection NOS (J22)*
influenza virus with other respiratory manifestations (J09.X2, J10.1, J11.1)
streptococcal pharyngitis (J02.0)

J06.0 Acute laryngopharyngitis

J06.9 Acute upper respiratory infection, unspecified
Upper respiratory disease, acute
Upper respiratory infection NOS
Use additional code (B95-B97) to identify infectious agent, if known, such as:
respiratory syncytial virus (RSV) (B97.4)
AHA: 2020,1Q,22

Influenza and pneumonia (J09-J18)

EXCLUDES 2 *allergic or eosinophilic pneumonia (J82)*
aspiration pneumonia NOS (J69.0)
meconium pneumonia (P24.01)
neonatal aspiration pneumonia (P24.-)
pneumonia due to solids and liquids (J69.-)
congenital pneumonia (P23.9)
lipid pneumonia (J69.1)
rheumatic pneumonia (I00)
ventilator associated pneumonia (J95.851)

AHA: 2017,4Q,96
TIP: Hemoptysis (R04.2) is not customarily associated with pneumonia and may be reported separately.

J09 Influenza due to certain identified influenza viruses
EXCLUDES 1 *influenza A/H1N1 (J10.-)*
influenza due to other identified influenza virus (J10.-)
influenza due to unidentified influenza virus (J11.-)
seasonal influenza due to other identified influenza virus (J10.-)
seasonal influenza due to unidentified influenza virus (J11.-)

J09.X Influenza due to identified novel influenza A virus
Avian influenza
Bird influenza
Influenza A/H5N1
Influenza of other animal origin, not bird or swine
Swine influenza virus (viruses that normally cause infections in pigs)
AHA: 2016,3Q,10

J09.X1 Influenza due to identified novel influenza A virus with pneumonia HIV MCC
Code also, if applicable, associated:
lung abscess (J85.1)
other specified type of pneumonia

J09.X2 Influenza due to identified novel influenza A virus with other respiratory manifestations
Influenza due to identified novel influenza A virus NOS
Influenza due to identified novel influenza A virus with laryngitis
Influenza due to identified novel influenza A virus with pharyngitis
Influenza due to identified novel influenza A virus with upper respiratory symptoms
Use additional code, if applicable, for associated:
pleural effusion (J91.8)
sinusitis (J01.-)

J09.X3 Influenza due to identified novel influenza A virus with gastrointestinal manifestations
Influenza due to identified novel influenza A virus gastroenteritis
EXCLUDES 1 *'intestinal flu' [viral gastroenteritis] (A08.-)*

J09.X9 Influenza due to identified novel influenza A virus with other manifestations
Influenza due to identified novel influenza A virus with encephalopathy
Influenza due to identified novel influenza A virus with myocarditis
Influenza due to identified novel influenza A virus with otitis media
Use additional code to identify manifestation

J10 Influenza due to other identified influenza virus

INCLUDES influenza A (non-novel)
influenza B
influenza C

EXCLUDES 1 *influenza due to avian influenza virus (J09.X-)*
influenza due to swine flu (J09.X-)
influenza due to unidentifed influenza virus (J11.-)

J10.0 Influenza due to other identified influenza virus with pneumonia
Code also associated lung abscess, if applicable (J85.1)

J10.00 Influenza due to other identified influenza virus with unspecified type of pneumonia MCC

J10.01 Influenza due to other identified influenza virus with the same other identified influenza virus pneumonia MCC

J10.08 Influenza due to other identified influenza virus with other specified pneumonia HIV MCC
Code also other specified type of pneumonia

J10.1 Influenza due to other identified influenza virus with other respiratory manifestations
Influenza due to other identified influenza virus NOS
Influenza due to other identified influenza virus with laryngitis
Influenza due to other identified influenza virus with pharyngitis
Influenza due to other identified influenza virus with upper respiratory symptoms
Use additional code for associated pleural effusion, if applicable (J91.8)
Use additional code for associated sinusitis, if applicable (J01.-)
AHA: 2016,3Q,10-11

J10.2 Influenza due to other identified influenza virus with gastrointestinal manifestations
Influenza due to other identified influenza virus gastroenteritis
EXCLUDES 1 *"intestinal flu" [viral gastroenteritis] (A08.-)*

J10.8 Influenza due to other identified influenza virus with other manifestations

J10.81 Influenza due to other identified influenza virus with encephalopathy

J10.82 Influenza due to other identified influenza virus with myocarditis

J10.83 Influenza due to other identified influenza virus with otitis media
Use additional code for any associated perforated tympanic membrane (H72.-)

J10.89 Influenza due to other identified influenza virus with other manifestations
Use additional codes to identify the manifestations

J11 Influenza due to unidentified influenza virus

J11.0 Influenza due to unidentified influenza virus with pneumonia
Code also associated lung abscess, if applicable (J85.1)
AHA: 2016,3Q,11

J11.00 Influenza due to unidentified influenza virus with unspecified type of pneumonia MCC
Influenza with pneumonia NOS

J11.08 Influenza due to unidentified influenza virus with specified pneumonia MCC
Code also other specified type of pneumonia

J11.1 Influenza due to unidentified influenza virus with other respiratory manifestations
Influenza NOS
Influenzal laryngitis NOS
Influenzal pharyngitis NOS
Influenza with upper respiratory symptoms NOS
Use additional code for associated pleural effusion, if applicable (J91.8)
Use additional code for associated sinusitis, if applicable (J01.-)

J11.2 Influenza due to unidentified influenza virus with gastrointestinal manifestations
Influenza gastroenteritis NOS
EXCLUDES 1 *"intestinal flu" [viral gastroenteritis] (A08.-)*

J11.8 Influenza due to unidentified influenza virus with other manifestations

J11.81 Influenza due to unidentified influenza virus with encephalopathy
Influenzal encephalopathy NOS

J11.82 Influenza due to unidentified influenza virus with myocarditis
Influenzal myocarditis NOS

J11.83 Influenza due to unidentified influenza virus with otitis media
Influenzal otitis media NOS
Use additional code for any associated perforated tympanic membrane (H72.-)

J11.89 Influenza due to unidentified influenza virus with other manifestations
Use additional codes to identify the manifestations

J12 Viral pneumonia, not elsewhere classified

INCLUDES bronchopneumonia due to viruses other than influenza viruses
Code first associated influenza, if applicable (J09.X1, J10.0-, J11.0-)
Code also associated abscess, if applicable (J85.1)

EXCLUDES 1 *aspiration pneumonia due to anesthesia during labor and delivery (O74.0)*
aspiration pneumonia due to anesthesia during pregnancy (O29)
aspiration pneumonia due to anesthesia during puerperium (O89.0)
aspiration pneumonia due to solids and liquids (J69.-)
aspiration pneumonia NOS (J69.0)
congenital pneumonia (P23.0)
congenital rubella pneumonitis (P35.0)
interstitial pneumonia NOS (J84.9)
lipid pneumonia (J69.1)
neonatal aspiration pneumonia (P24.-)

AHA: 2020,2Q,28; 2019,1Q,35; 2018,3Q,24; 2016,3Q,15; 2013,4Q,118

J12.0 Adenoviral pneumonia MCC

J12.1 Respiratory syncytial virus pneumonia MCC
RSV pneumonia

J12.2 Parainfluenza virus pneumonia MCC

J12.3 Human metapneumovirus pneumonia HIV MCC

J12.8 Other viral pneumonia

J12.81 Pneumonia due to SARS-associated coronavirus HIV MCC
Severe acute respiratory syndrome NOS
DEF: Inflammation of the lungs with consolidation, caused by the severe adult respiratory syndrome (SARS)-associated coronavirus or SARS-CoV. This pneumonia should not be confused with that caused by SARS-CoV-2 (COVID-19).

J12.82 Pneumonia due to coronavirus disease 2019 HIV MCC UPD
Pneumonia due to 2019 novel coronavirus (SARS-CoV-2)
Pneumonia due to COVID-19
Code first COVID-19 (U07.1)
AHA: 2021,1Q,25-30,31-49

J12.89 Other viral pneumonia HIV MCC
AHA: 2021,1Q,33-34; 2020,2Q,8,11; 2020,1Q,34-36

J12.9 Viral pneumonia, unspecified HIV MCC

J13 Pneumonia due to Streptococcus pneumoniae HIV MCC HCC
Bronchopneumonia due to S. pneumoniae
Code first associated influenza, if applicable (J09.X1, J10.0-, J11.0-)
Code also associated abscess, if applicable (J85.1)

EXCLUDES 1 *congenital pneumonia due to S. pneumoniae (P23.6)*
lobar pneumonia, unspecified organism (J18.1)
pneumonia due to other streptococci (J15.3-J15.4)

AHA: 2020,2Q,28; 2019,1Q,35; 2018,3Q,24; 2016,3Q,15; 2013,4Q,118

J14 Pneumonia due to Hemophilus influenzae HIV MCC HCC
Bronchopneumonia due to H. influenzae
Code first associated influenza, if applicable (J09.X1, J10.0-, J11.0-)
Code also associated abscess, if applicable (J85.1)

EXCLUDES 1 *congenital pneumonia due to H. influenzae (P23.6)*

AHA: 2020,2Q,28; 2019,1Q,35; 2018,3Q,24; 2016,3Q,15; 2013,4Q,118

J15 Bacterial pneumonia, not elsewhere classified (4th)

INCLUDES Bronchopneumonia due to bacteria other than S. pneumoniae and H. influenzae

Code first associated influenza, if applicable (J09.X1, J10.0-, J11.0-)

Code also associated abscess, if applicable (J85.1)

EXCLUDES 1 *chlamydial pneumonia (J16.0)*
congenital pneumonia (P23.-)
Legionnaires' disease (A48.1)
spirochetal pneumonia (A69.8)

AHA: 2020,2Q,28; 2019,1Q,35; 2018,3Q,24; 2016,3Q,15; 2013,4Q,118

J15.0 Pneumonia due to Klebsiella pneumoniae HIV MCC HCC

J15.1 Pneumonia due to Pseudomonas HIV MCC HCC

J15.2 Pneumonia due to staphylococcus (5th)

J15.20 Pneumonia due to staphylococcus, unspecified HIV MCC HCC

J15.21 Pneumonia due to Staphylococcus aureus (6th)

J15.211 Pneumonia due to methicillin susceptible Staphylococcus aureus HIV MCC HCC
MSSA pneumonia
Pneumonia due to Staphylococcus aureus NOS

J15.212 Pneumonia due to methicillin resistant Staphylococcus aureus HIV MCC HCC

J15.29 Pneumonia due to other staphylococcus HIV MCC HCC

J15.3 Pneumonia due to streptococcus, group B HIV MCC HCC

J15.4 Pneumonia due to other streptococci HIV MCC HCC

EXCLUDES 1 *pneumonia due to streptococcus, group B (J15.3)*
pneumonia due to Streptococcus pneumoniae (J13)

J15.5 Pneumonia due to Escherichia coli HIV MCC HCC

J15.6 Pneumonia due to other Gram-negative bacteria HIV MCC HCC
Pneumonia due to other aerobic Gram-negative bacteria
Pneumonia due to Serratia marcescens
AHA: 2020,2Q,28

J15.7 Pneumonia due to Mycoplasma pneumoniae MCC

J15.8 Pneumonia due to other specified bacteria HIV MCC HCC

J15.9 Unspecified bacterial pneumonia HIV MCC
Pneumonia due to gram-positive bacteria

J16 Pneumonia due to other infectious organisms, not elsewhere classified (4th)

Code first associated influenza, if applicable (J09.X1, J10.0-, J11.0-)

Code also associated abscess, if applicable (J85.1)

EXCLUDES 1 *congenital pneumonia (P23.-)*
ornithosis (A70)
pneumocystosis (B59)
pneumonia NOS (J18.9)

AHA: 2020,2Q,28; 2019,1Q,35; 2018,3Q,24; 2016,3Q,15; 2013,4Q,118

J16.0 Chlamydial pneumonia MCC

J16.8 Pneumonia due to other specified infectious organisms MCC

J17 Pneumonia in diseases classified elsewhere MCC

Code first underlying disease, such as:
Q fever (A78)
rheumatic fever (I00)
schistosomiasis (B65.0-B65.9)

EXCLUDES 1 *candidial pneumonia (B37.1)*
chlamydial pneumonia (J16.0)
gonorrheal pneumonia (A54.84)
histoplasmosis pneumonia (B39.0-B39.2)
measles pneumonia (B05.2)
nocardiosis pneumonia (A43.0)
pneumocystosis (B59)
pneumonia due to Pneumocystis carinii (B59)
pneumonia due to Pneumocystis jiroveci (B59)
pneumonia in actinomycosis (A42.0)
pneumonia in anthrax (A22.1)
pneumonia in ascariasis (B77.81)
pneumonia in aspergillosis (B44.0-B44.1)
pneumonia in coccidioidomycosis (B38.0-B38.2)
pneumonia in cytomegalovirus disease (B25.0)
pneumonia in toxoplasmosis (B58.3)
rubella pneumonia (B06.81)
salmonella pneumonia (A02.22)
spirochetal infection NEC with pneumonia (A69.8)
tularemia pneumonia (A21.2)
typhoid fever with pneumonia (A01.03)
varicella pneumonia (B01.2)
whooping cough with pneumonia (A37 with fifth character 1)

AHA: 2020,2Q,28; 2019,1Q,35; 2016,3Q,15; 2013,4Q,118

J18 Pneumonia, unspecified organism (4th)

Code first associated influenza, if applicable (J09.X1, J10.0-, J11.0-)

EXCLUDES 1 *abscess of lung with pneumonia (J85.1)*
aspiration pneumonia due to anesthesia during labor and delivery (O74.0)
aspiration pneumonia due to anesthesia during pregnancy (O29)
aspiration pneumonia due to anesthesia during puerperium (O89.0)
aspiration pneumonia due to solids and liquids (J69.-)
aspiration pneumonia NOS (J69.0)
congenital pneumonia (P23.0)
drug-induced interstitial lung disorder (J70.2-J70.4)
interstitial pneumonia NOS (J84.9)
lipid pneumonia (J69.1)
neonatal aspiration pneumonia (P24.-)
pneumonitis due to external agents (J67-J70)
pneumonitis due to fumes and vapors (J68.0)
usual interstitial pneumonia (J84.178)

AHA: 2020,2Q,28; 2019,1Q,35; 2016,3Q,15; 2013,4Q,118

J18.0 Bronchopneumonia, unspecified organism MCC

EXCLUDES 1 *hypostatic bronchopneumonia (J18.2)*
lipid pneumonia (J69.1)

EXCLUDES 2 *acute bronchiolitis (J21.-)*
chronic bronchiolitis (J44.9)

J18.1 Lobar pneumonia, unspecified organism HIV MCC HCC

AHA: 2019,3Q,37; 2018,3Q,24

DEF: Lobar pneumonia is characterized by consolidated inflammation confined or localized to only one or a few lobes of the lung. The consolidation affects primarily the alveolar air spaces, unlike bronchopneumonia, which arises from the bronchi or bronchioles and affects a wide area without any localization.

TIP: Documentation of right upper lobe, left upper lobe, right lower lobe, left lower lobe, or right middle lobe pneumonia alone is not synonymous with "lobar pneumonia," nor should a diagnosis of lobar pneumonia be assumed based on an imaging report that identifies pneumonia in a specific lobe. Assign J18.1 only when the provider specifically documents "lobar pneumonia" without specifying a causal organism.

J18.2 Hypostatic pneumonia, unspecified organism CC
Hypostatic bronchopneumonia
Passive pneumonia

J18.8 Other pneumonia, unspecified organism HIV MCC

J18.9 Pneumonia, unspecified organism HIV MCC

AHA: 2020,2Q,28; 2019,3Q,15; 2019,2Q,28; 2014,3Q,4; 2013,4Q,119; 2012,4Q,94

Other acute lower respiratory infections (J20-J22)

EXCLUDES 2 *chronic obstructive pulmonary disease with acute lower respiratory infection (J44.0)*

J20 Acute bronchitis

INCLUDES acute and subacute bronchitis (with) bronchospasm
acute and subacute bronchitis (with) tracheitis
acute and subacute bronchitis (with) tracheobronchitis, acute
acute and subacute fibrinous bronchitis
acute and subacute membranous bronchitis
acute and subacute purulent bronchitis
acute and subacute septic bronchitis

EXCLUDES 1 *bronchitis NOS (J40)*
tracheobronchitis NOS (J40)

EXCLUDES 2 *acute bronchitis with bronchiectasis (J47.0)*
acute bronchitis with chronic obstructive asthma (J44.0)
acute bronchitis with chronic obstructive pulmonary disease (J44.0)
allergic bronchitis NOS (J45.909-)
bronchitis due to chemicals, fumes and vapors (J68.0)
chronic bronchitis NOS (J42)
chronic mucopurulent bronchitis (J41.1)
chronic obstructive bronchitis (J44.-)
chronic obstructive tracheobronchitis (J44.-)
chronic simple bronchitis (J41.0)
chronic tracheobronchitis (J42)

AHA: 2019,1Q,35; 2016,3Q,10,16

DEF: Acute inflammation of the main branches of the bronchial tree due to infectious or irritant agents. Symptoms include cough with a varied production of sputum, fever, substernal soreness, and lung rales. Bronchitis usually lasts three to 10 days.

J20.0 Acute bronchitis due to Mycoplasma pneumoniae

J20.1 Acute bronchitis due to Hemophilus influenzae

J20.2 Acute bronchitis due to streptococcus

J20.3 Acute bronchitis due to coxsackievirus

J20.4 Acute bronchitis due to parainfluenza virus

J20.5 Acute bronchitis due to respiratory syncytial virus
Acute bronchitis due to RSV

J20.6 Acute bronchitis due to rhinovirus

J20.7 Acute bronchitis due to echovirus

J20.8 Acute bronchitis due to other specified organisms
AHA: 2020,1Q,34-36
TIP: Assign as a secondary code for a patient with acute bronchitis confirmed as due to COVID-19; assign U07.1 as the principal or first-listed code.

J20.9 Acute bronchitis, unspecified

J21 Acute bronchiolitis

INCLUDES acute bronchiolitis with bronchospasm

EXCLUDES 2 *respiratory bronchiolitis interstitial lung disease (J84.115)*

J21.0 Acute bronchiolitis due to respiratory syncytial virus CC
Acute bronchiolitis due to RSV

J21.1 Acute bronchiolitis due to human metapneumovirus CC

J21.8 Acute bronchiolitis due to other specified organisms CC

J21.9 Acute bronchiolitis, unspecified CC
Bronchiolitis (acute)
EXCLUDES 1 *chronic bronchiolitis (J44.-)*

J22 Unspecified acute lower respiratory infection
Acute (lower) respiratory (tract) infection NOS
EXCLUDES 1 *upper respiratory infection (acute) (J06.9)*
AHA: 2020,1Q,22,34-36
TIP: Assign as a secondary code for a patient with a respiratory infection specified as acute or lower that is documented as being associated with COVID-19; assign U07.1 as the principal or first-listed code. If the respiratory infection documentation does not specify acute or lower, assign J98.8.

Other diseases of upper respiratory tract (J30-J39)

J30 Vasomotor and allergic rhinitis

INCLUDES spasmodic rhinorrhea

EXCLUDES 1 *allergic rhinitis with asthma (bronchial) (J45.909)*
rhinitis NOS (J31.0)

J30.0 Vasomotor rhinitis
DEF: Noninfectious and nonallergic type of rhinitis for which the cause is often unknown. Symptoms often mimic those of allergic rhinitis with a diagnosis of vasomotor rhinitis typically made after ruling out allergens as the cause.

J30.1 Allergic rhinitis due to pollen
Allergy NOS due to pollen
Hay fever
Pollinosis

J30.2 Other seasonal allergic rhinitis

J30.5 Allergic rhinitis due to food

J30.8 Other allergic rhinitis

J30.81 Allergic rhinitis due to animal (cat) (dog) hair and dander

J30.89 Other allergic rhinitis
Perennial allergic rhinitis

J30.9 Allergic rhinitis, unspecified

J31 Chronic rhinitis, nasopharyngitis and pharyngitis

Use additional code to identify:
exposure to environmental tobacco smoke (Z77.22)
exposure to tobacco smoke in the perinatal period (P96.81)
history of tobacco dependence (Z87.891)
occupational exposure to environmental tobacco smoke (Z57.31)
tobacco dependence (F17.-)
tobacco use (Z72.0)

J31.0 Chronic rhinitis
Atrophic rhinitis (chronic)
Granulomatous rhinitis (chronic)
Hypertrophic rhinitis (chronic)
Obstructive rhinitis (chronic)
Ozena
Purulent rhinitis (chronic)
Rhinitis (chronic) NOS
Ulcerative rhinitis (chronic)
EXCLUDES 1 *allergic rhinitis (J30.1-J30.9)*
vasomotor rhinitis (J30.0)
DEF: Persistent inflammation of the mucous membranes of the nose, characterized by a postnasal drip.

J31.1 Chronic nasopharyngitis
EXCLUDES 2 *acute nasopharyngitis (J00)*
DEF: Persistent inflammation of the mucous membranes extending from the nares to the pharynx. It is characterized by constant irritation in the nasopharynx and postnasal drip.

J31.2 Chronic pharyngitis
Atrophic pharyngitis (chronic)
Chronic sore throat
Granular pharyngitis (chronic)
Hypertrophic pharyngitis (chronic)
EXCLUDES 2 *acute pharyngitis (J02.9)*

J32 Chronic sinusitis

INCLUDES sinus abscess
sinus empyema
sinus infection
sinus suppuration

Use additional code to identify:
exposure to environmental tobacco smoke (Z77.22)
exposure to tobacco smoke in the perinatal period (P96.81)
history of tobacco dependence (Z87.891)
infectious agent (B95-B97)
occupational exposure to environmental tobacco smoke (Z57.31)
tobacco dependence (F17.-)
tobacco use (Z72.0)

EXCLUDES 2 *acute sinusitis (J01.-)*

J32.0 Chronic maxillary sinusitis
Antritis (chronic)
Maxillary sinusitis NOS

J32.1 Chronic frontal sinusitis
Frontal sinusitis NOS

J32.2 Chronic ethmoidal sinusitis
Ethmoidal sinusitis NOS
EXCLUDES 1 *Woakes' ethmoiditis (J33.1)*

J32.3 Chronic sphenoidal sinusitis
Sphenoidal sinusitis NOS

J32.4 Chronic pansinusitis
Pansinusitis NOS

J32.8 Other chronic sinusitis
Sinusitis (chronic) involving more than one sinus but not pansinusitis

J32.9 Chronic sinusitis, unspecified
Sinusitis (chronic) NOS

J33 Nasal polyp
Use additional code to identify:
exposure to environmental tobacco smoke (Z77.22)
exposure to tobacco smoke in the perinatal period (P96.81)
history of tobacco dependence (Z87.891)
occupational exposure to environmental tobacco smoke (Z57.31)
tobacco dependence (F17.-)
tobacco use (Z72.Ø)
EXCLUDES 1 *adenomatous polyps (D14.Ø)*

J33.Ø Polyp of nasal cavity
Choanal polyp
Nasopharyngeal polyp

J33.1 Polypoid sinus degeneration
Woakes' syndrome or ethmoiditis

J33.8 Other polyp of sinus
Accessory polyp of sinus
Ethmoidal polyp of sinus
Maxillary polyp of sinus
Sphenoidal polyp of sinus

J33.9 Nasal polyp, unspecified

J34 Other and unspecified disorders of nose and nasal sinuses
EXCLUDES 2 *varicose ulcer of nasal septum (I86.8)*

J34.Ø Abscess, furuncle and carbuncle of nose
Cellulitis of nose
Necrosis of nose
Ulceration of nose

J34.1 Cyst and mucocele of nose and nasal sinus

J34.2 Deviated nasal septum
Deflection or deviation of septum (nasal) (acquired)
EXCLUDES 1 *congenital deviated nasal septum (Q67.4)*
DEF: Condition in which the nasal septum, a thin wall composed of cartilage and bone that separates the two nostrils, is crooked or displaced from the midline.

J34.3 Hypertrophy of nasal turbinates
DEF: Overgrowth of bones within the nasal turbinate, which are ridges of bone and soft tissue that project from the sidewalls of the nasal passages. Hypertrophy can cause obstruction of the nasal passages.

J34.8 Other specified disorders of nose and nasal sinuses

J34.81 Nasal mucositis (ulcerative)
Code also type of associated therapy, such as:
antineoplastic and immunosuppressive drugs (T45.1X-)
radiological procedure and radiotherapy (Y84.2)
EXCLUDES 2 *gastrointestinal mucositis (ulcerative) (K92.81)*
mucositis (ulcerative) of vagina and vulva (N76.81)
oral mucositis (ulcerative) (K12.3-)

J34.89 Other specified disorders of nose and nasal sinuses
Perforation of nasal septum NOS
Rhinolith

J34.9 Unspecified disorder of nose and nasal sinuses

J35 Chronic diseases of tonsils and adenoids
Use additional code to identify:
exposure to environmental tobacco smoke (Z77.22)
exposure to tobacco smoke in the perinatal period (P96.81)
history of tobacco dependence (Z87.891)
occupational exposure to environmental tobacco smoke (Z57.31)
tobacco dependence (F17.-)
tobacco use (Z72.Ø)

J35.Ø Chronic tonsillitis and adenoiditis
EXCLUDES 2 *acute tonsillitis (JØ3.-)*

J35.Ø1 Chronic tonsillitis

J35.Ø2 Chronic adenoiditis

J35.Ø3 Chronic tonsillitis and adenoiditis

J35.1 Hypertrophy of tonsils
Enlargement of tonsils
EXCLUDES 1 *hypertrophy of tonsils with tonsillitis (J35.Ø-)*

J35.2 Hypertrophy of adenoids
Enlargement of adenoids
EXCLUDES 1 *hypertrophy of adenoids with adenoiditis (J35.Ø-)*

J35.3 Hypertrophy of tonsils with hypertrophy of adenoids
EXCLUDES 1 *hypertrophy of tonsils and adenoids with tonsillitis and adenoiditis (J35.Ø3)*

J35.8 Other chronic diseases of tonsils and adenoids
Adenoid vegetations
Amygdalolith
Calculus, tonsil
Cicatrix of tonsil (and adenoid)
Tonsillar tag
Ulcer of tonsil

J35.9 Chronic disease of tonsils and adenoids, unspecified
Disease (chronic) of tonsils and adenoids NOS

J36 Peritonsillar abscess CC
INCLUDES abscess of tonsil
peritonsillar cellulitis
quinsy
Use additional code (B95-B97) to identify infectious agent
EXCLUDES 1 *acute tonsillitis (JØ3.-)*
chronic tonsillitis (J35.Ø)
retropharyngeal abscess (J39.Ø)
tonsillitis NOS (JØ3.9-)

J37 Chronic laryngitis and laryngotracheitis
Use additional code to identify:
exposure to environmental tobacco smoke (Z77.22)
exposure to tobacco smoke in the perinatal period (P96.81)
history of tobacco dependence (Z87.891)
infectious agent (B95-B97)
occupational exposure to environmental tobacco smoke (Z57.31)
tobacco dependence (F17.-)
tobacco use (Z72.Ø)

J37.Ø Chronic laryngitis
Catarrhal laryngitis
Hypertrophic laryngitis
Sicca laryngitis
EXCLUDES 2 *acute laryngitis (JØ4.Ø)*
obstructive (acute) laryngitis (JØ5.Ø)

J37.1 Chronic laryngotracheitis
Laryngitis, chronic, with tracheitis (chronic)
Tracheitis, chronic, with laryngitis
EXCLUDES 1 *chronic tracheitis (J42)*
EXCLUDES 2 *acute laryngotracheitis (JØ4.2)*
acute tracheitis (JØ4.1)

J38 Diseases of vocal cords and larynx, not elsewhere classified
Use additional code to identify:
exposure to environmental tobacco smoke (Z77.22)
exposure to tobacco smoke in the perinatal period (P96.81)
history of tobacco dependence (Z87.891)
occupational exposure to environmental tobacco smoke (Z57.31)
tobacco dependence (F17.-)
tobacco use (Z72.Ø)
EXCLUDES 1 *congenital laryngeal stridor (P28.89)*
obstructive laryngitis (acute) (JØ5.Ø)
postprocedural subglottic stenosis (J95.5)
stridor (RØ6.1)
ulcerative laryngitis (JØ4.Ø)

J38.Ø Paralysis of vocal cords and larynx
Laryngoplegia
Paralysis of glottis

J38.ØØ Paralysis of vocal cords and larynx, unspecified

J38.Ø1 Paralysis of vocal cords and larynx, unilateral

J38.Ø2 Paralysis of vocal cords and larynx, bilateral

J38.1 Polyp of vocal cord and larynx
EXCLUDES 1 *adenomatous polyps (D14.1)*

J38.2 Nodules of vocal cords
Chorditis (fibrinous)(nodosa)(tuberosa)
Singer's nodes
Teacher's nodes

J38.3 Other diseases of vocal cords
Abscess of vocal cords
Cellulitis of vocal cords
Granuloma of vocal cords
Leukokeratosis of vocal cords
Leukoplakia of vocal cords

J38.4 Edema of larynx
Edema (of) glottis
Subglottic edema
Supraglottic edema
EXCLUDES 1 *acute obstructive laryngitis [croup] (J05.0)*
edematous laryngitis (J04.0)

J38.5 Laryngeal spasm
Laryngismus (stridulus)

J38.6 Stenosis of larynx

J38.7 Other diseases of larynx
Abscess of larynx
Cellulitis of larynx
Disease of larynx NOS
Necrosis of larynx
Pachyderma of larynx
Perichondritis of larynx
Ulcer of larynx

J39 Other diseases of upper respiratory tract (4th)
EXCLUDES 1 *acute respiratory infection NOS (J22)*
acute upper respiratory infection (J06.9)
upper respiratory inflammation due to chemicals, gases, fumes or vapors (J68.2)

J39.0 Retropharyngeal and parapharyngeal abscess CC
Peripharyngeal abscess
EXCLUDES 1 *peritonsillar abscess (J36)*
DEF: Purulent infection behind the pharynx and the front of the precerebral fascia, characterized by neck stiffness, cervical lymphadenopathy, sore throat, fever, and stridor.

J39.1 Other abscess of pharynx CC
Cellulitis of pharynx
Nasopharyngeal abscess

J39.2 Other diseases of pharynx
Cyst of pharynx
Edema of pharynx
EXCLUDES 2 *chronic pharyngitis (J31.2)*
ulcerative pharyngitis (J02.9)

J39.3 Upper respiratory tract hypersensitivity reaction, site unspecified
EXCLUDES 1 *hypersensitivity reaction of upper respiratory tract, such as:*
extrinsic allergic alveolitis (J67.9)
pneumoconiosis (J60-J67.9)

J39.8 Other specified diseases of upper respiratory tract

J39.9 Disease of upper respiratory tract, unspecified

Chronic lower respiratory diseases (J40-J47)

EXCLUDES 1 *bronchitis due to chemicals, gases, fumes and vapors (J68.0)*
EXCLUDES 2 *cystic fibrosis (E84.-)*

J40 Bronchitis, not specified as acute or chronic
Bronchitis NOS
Bronchitis with tracheitis NOS
Catarrhal bronchitis
Tracheobronchitis NOS
Use additional code to identify:
exposure to environmental tobacco smoke (Z77.22)
exposure to tobacco smoke in the perinatal period (P96.81)
history of tobacco dependence (Z87.891)
occupational exposure to environmental tobacco smoke (Z57.31)
tobacco dependence (F17.-)
tobacco use (Z72.0)
EXCLUDES 1 *acute bronchitis (J20.-)*
allergic bronchitis NOS (J45.909-)
asthmatic bronchitis NOS (J45.9-)
bronchitis due to chemicals, gases, fumes and vapors (J68.0)
AHA: 2020,1Q,34-36
TIP: Assign as a secondary code for a patient with bronchitis of unspecified acuity due to COVID-19; assign U07.1 as the principal or first-listed code.

J41 Simple and mucopurulent chronic bronchitis (4th)
Use additional code to identify:
exposure to environmental tobacco smoke (Z77.22)
exposure to tobacco smoke in the perinatal period (P96.81)
history of tobacco dependence (Z87.891)
occupational exposure to environmental tobacco smoke (Z57.31)
tobacco dependence (F17.-)
tobacco use (Z72.0)
EXCLUDES 1 *chronic bronchitis NOS (J42)*
chronic obstructive bronchitis (J44.-)

J41.0 Simple chronic bronchitis HCC
J41.1 Mucopurulent chronic bronchitis HCC
J41.8 Mixed simple and mucopurulent chronic bronchitis HCC

J42 Unspecified chronic bronchitis HCC
Chronic bronchitis NOS
Chronic tracheitis
Chronic tracheobronchitis
Use additional code to identify:
exposure to environmental tobacco smoke (Z77.22)
exposure to tobacco smoke in the perinatal period (P96.81)
history of tobacco dependence (Z87.891)
occupational exposure to environmental tobacco smoke (Z57.31)
tobacco dependence (F17.-)
tobacco use (Z72.0)
EXCLUDES 1 *chronic asthmatic bronchitis (J44.-)*
chronic bronchitis with airways obstruction (J44.-)
chronic emphysematous bronchitis (J44.-)
chronic obstructive pulmonary disease NOS (J44.9)
simple and mucopurulent chronic bronchitis (J41.-)

4th J43 Emphysema

Use additional code to identify:
- exposure to environmental tobacco smoke (Z77.22)
- history of tobacco dependence (Z87.891)
- occupational exposure to environmental tobacco smoke (Z57.31)
- tobacco dependence (F17.-)
- tobacco use (Z72.Ø)

EXCLUDES 1 *compensatory emphysema (J98.3)*
emphysema due to inhalation of chemicals, gases, fumes or vapors (J68.4)
emphysema with chronic (obstructive) bronchitis (J44.-)
emphysematous (obstructive) bronchitis (J44.-)
interstitial emphysema (J98.2)
mediastinal emphysema (J98.2)
neonatal interstitial emphysema (P25.Ø)
surgical (subcutaneous) emphysema (T81.82)

EXCLUDES 2 *traumatic subcutaneous emphysema (T79.7)*

DEF: Pathological condition in which there is destructive enlargement of the air sacs in the lungs resulting in damage and lack of elasticity to the alveolar walls, commonly seen in long-term smokers.

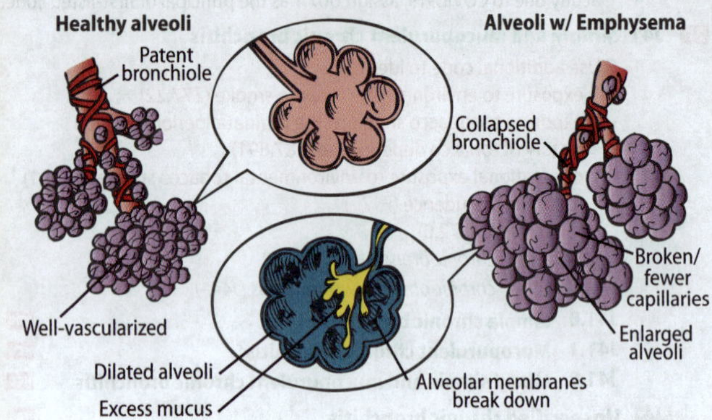

J43.Ø Unilateral pulmonary emphysema [MacLeod's syndrome] HCC
- Swyer-James syndrome
- Unilateral emphysema
- Unilateral hyperlucent lung
- Unilateral pulmonary artery functional hypoplasia
- Unilateral transparency of lung

J43.1 Panlobular emphysema HCC
- Panacinar emphysema

J43.2 Centrilobular emphysema HCC

J43.8 Other emphysema HCC

J43.9 Emphysema, unspecified HCC
- Bullous emphysema (lung)(pulmonary)
- Emphysema (lung)(pulmonary) NOS
- Emphysematous bleb
- Vesicular emphysema (lung)(pulmonary)

AHA: 2019,1Q,34-36; 2017,4Q,97-98

4th J44 Other chronic obstructive pulmonary disease

INCLUDES asthma with chronic obstructive pulmonary disease
chronic asthmatic (obstructive) bronchitis
chronic bronchitis with airway obstruction
chronic bronchitis with emphysema
chronic emphysematous bronchitis
chronic obstructive asthma
chronic obstructive bronchitis
chronic obstructive tracheobronchitis

Code also type of asthma, if applicable (J45.-)

Use additional code to identify:
- exposure to environmental tobacco smoke (Z77.22)
- history of tobacco dependence (Z87.891)
- occupational exposure to environmental tobacco smoke (Z57.31)
- tobacco dependence (F17.-)
- tobacco use (Z72.Ø)

EXCLUDES 1 *bronchiectasis (J47.-)*
chronic bronchitis NOS (J42)
chronic simple and mucopurulent bronchitis (J41.-)
chronic tracheitis (J42)
chronic tracheobronchitis (J42)
emphysema without chronic bronchitis (J43.-)

AHA: 2019,1Q,34-36; 2017,4Q,97-98; 2017,1Q,25-26; 2016,3Q,15-16; 2013,4Q,109

J44.Ø Chronic obstructive pulmonary disease with (acute) lower respiratory infection CC HCC

Code also to identify the infection

AHA: 2019,1Q,35; 2017,4Q,96; 2017,1Q,24-25

TIP: Do not assign when only aspiration pneumonia is present. Aspiration pneumonia is not classified as a respiratory infection.

J44.1 Chronic obstructive pulmonary disease with (acute) exacerbation CC HCC
- Decompensated COPD
- Decompensated COPD with (acute) exacerbation

EXCLUDES 2 *chronic obstructive pulmonary disease [COPD] with acute bronchitis (J44.Ø)*
lung diseases due to external agents (J6Ø-J7Ø)

AHA: 2019,1Q,34; 2017,4Q,96; 2017,1Q,26; 2016,1Q,36

TIP: Exacerbation of COPD should not be assumed based upon worsening of a concomitant respiratory disease or when COPD is described as end-stage.

J44.9 Chronic obstructive pulmonary disease, unspecified HCC
- Chronic obstructive airway disease NOS
- Chronic obstructive lung disease NOS

EXCLUDES 2 *lung diseases due to external agents (J6Ø-J7Ø)*

AHA: 2019,1Q,36; 2017,4Q,96-97; 2016,1Q,36; 2014,4Q,21; 2013,4Q,109

J45 Asthma

INCLUDES allergic (predominantly) asthma
allergic bronchitis NOS
allergic rhinitis with asthma
atopic asthma
extrinsic allergic asthma
hay fever with asthma
idiosyncratic asthma
intrinsic nonallergic asthma
nonallergic asthma

Use additional code to identify:
eosinophilic asthma (J82.83)
exposure to environmental tobacco smoke (Z77.22)
exposure to tobacco smoke in the perinatal period (P96.81)
history of tobacco dependence (Z87.891)
occupational exposure to environmental tobacco smoke (Z57.31)
tobacco dependence (F17.-)
tobacco use (Z72.Ø)

EXCLUDES 1 *detergent asthma (J69.8)*
~~eosinophilic asthma (J82)~~
miner's asthma (J6Ø)
wheezing NOS (RØ6.2)
wood asthma (J67.8)

EXCLUDES 2 *asthma with chronic obstructive pulmonary disease (J44.9)*
chronic asthmatic (obstructive) bronchitis (J44.9)
chronic obstructive asthma (J44.9)

AHA: 2019,1Q,36; 2017,1Q,25-26; 2012,4Q,99

DEF: Status asthmaticus: Severe, intractable episode of asthma that is unresponsive to normal therapeutic measures.

J45.2 Mild intermittent asthma

J45.2Ø Mild intermittent asthma, uncomplicated
Mild intermittent asthma NOS

J45.21 Mild intermittent asthma with (acute) exacerbation CC

J45.22 Mild intermittent asthma with status asthmaticus CC

J45.3 Mild persistent asthma

J45.3Ø Mild persistent asthma, uncomplicated
Mild persistent asthma NOS

J45.31 Mild persistent asthma with (acute) exacerbation CC
AHA: 2016,1Q,35

J45.32 Mild persistent asthma with status asthmaticus CC

J45.4 Moderate persistent asthma

J45.4Ø Moderate persistent asthma, uncomplicated
Moderate persistent asthma NOS

J45.41 Moderate persistent asthma with (acute) exacerbation CC
AHA: 2017,1Q,26

J45.42 Moderate persistent asthma with status asthmaticus CC

J45.5 Severe persistent asthma

J45.5Ø Severe persistent asthma, uncomplicated
Severe persistent asthma NOS

J45.51 Severe persistent asthma with (acute) exacerbation CC

J45.52 Severe persistent asthma with status asthmaticus CC

J45.9 Other and unspecified asthma

J45.9Ø Unspecified asthma
Asthmatic bronchitis NOS
Childhood asthma NOS
Late onset asthma
AHA: 2017,4Q,96; 2017,1Q,25

J45.9Ø1 Unspecified asthma with (acute) exacerbation CC

J45.9Ø2 Unspecified asthma with status asthmaticus CC

J45.9Ø9 Unspecified asthma, uncomplicated
Asthma NOS
EXCLUDES 2 *lung diseases due to external agents (J6Ø-J7Ø)*
AHA: 2017,1Q,25

J45.99 Other asthma

J45.99Ø Exercise induced bronchospasm

J45.991 Cough variant asthma

J45.998 Other asthma

J47 Bronchiectasis

INCLUDES bronchiolectasis

Use additional code to identify:
exposure to environmental tobacco smoke (Z77.22)
exposure to tobacco smoke in the perinatal period (P96.81)
history of tobacco dependence (Z87.891)
occupational exposure to environmental tobacco smoke (Z57.31)
tobacco dependence (F17.-)
tobacco use (Z72.Ø)

EXCLUDES 1 *congenital bronchiectasis (Q33.4)*
tuberculous bronchiectasis (current disease) (A15.Ø)

DEF: Dilation of the bronchi with mucus production and persistent cough due to infection or chronic conditions that causes diminished lung capacity and frequent infections of the lung.

J47.Ø Bronchiectasis with acute lower respiratory infection CC HCC
Bronchiectasis with acute bronchitis
Code also to identify infection, if applicable

J47.1 Bronchiectasis with (acute) exacerbation CC HCC
AHA: 2021,1Q,23

J47.9 Bronchiectasis, uncomplicated HCC
Bronchiectasis NOS

Lung diseases due to external agents (J6Ø-J7Ø)

EXCLUDES 2 *asthma (J45.-)*
malignant neoplasm of bronchus and lung (C34.-)

DEF: Pneumoconiosis: Condition caused by inhaling inorganic dust particles, typically associated with occupations that require regular exposure to mineral dusts. A form of interstitial lung disease that contributes to the inflammation of the air sacs, causing the lung tissue to harden.

J6Ø Coalworker's pneumoconiosis HCC A
Anthracosilicosis
Anthracosis
Black lung disease
Coalworker's lung
EXCLUDES 1 *coalworker pneumoconiosis with tuberculosis, any type in A15 (J65)*

J61 Pneumoconiosis due to asbestos and other mineral fibers HCC A
Asbestosis
EXCLUDES 1 *pleural plaque with asbestosis (J92.Ø)*
pneumoconiosis with tuberculosis, any type in A15 (J65)

J62 Pneumoconiosis due to dust containing silica

INCLUDES silicotic fibrosis (massive) of lung

EXCLUDES 1 *pneumoconiosis with tuberculosis, any type in A15 (J65)*

J62.Ø Pneumoconiosis due to talc dust HCC

J62.8 Pneumoconiosis due to other dust containing silica HCC
Silicosis NOS

J63 Pneumoconiosis due to other inorganic dusts

EXCLUDES 1 *pneumoconiosis with tuberculosis, any type in A15 (J65)*

J63.Ø Aluminosis (of lung) HCC

J63.1 Bauxite fibrosis (of lung) HCC

J63.2 Berylliosis HCC

J63.3 Graphite fibrosis (of lung) HCC

J63.4 Siderosis HCC
AHA: 2019,3Q,8

J63.5 Stannosis HCC

J63.6 Pneumoconiosis due to other specified inorganic dusts HCC

J64 Unspecified pneumoconiosis HCC
EXCLUDES 1 *pneumonoconiosis with tuberculosis, any type in A15 (J65)*

J65 Pneumoconiosis associated with tuberculosis HCC
Any condition in J6Ø-J64 with tuberculosis, any type in A15
Silicotuberculosis

J66 Airway disease due to specific organic dust

EXCLUDES 2 *allergic alveolitis (J67.-)*
asbestosis (J61)
bagassosis (J67.1)
farmer's lung (J67.0)
hypersensitivity pneumonitis due to organic dust (J67.-)
reactive airways dysfunction syndrome (J68.3)

J66.0 Byssinosis HCC
Airway disease due to cotton dust

J66.1 Flax-dressers' disease HCC

J66.2 Cannabinosis HCC

J66.8 Airway disease due to other specific organic dusts HCC

J67 Hypersensitivity pneumonitis due to organic dust

INCLUDES allergic alveolitis and pneumonitis due to inhaled organic dust and particles of fungal, actinomycetic or other origin

EXCLUDES 1 *pneumonitis due to inhalation of chemicals, gases, fumes or vapors (J68.0)*

J67.0 Farmer's lung HCC
Harvester's lung
Haymaker's lung
Moldy hay disease

J67.1 Bagassosis HCC
Bagasse disease
Bagasse pneumonitis

J67.2 Bird fancier's lung HCC
Budgerigar fancier's disease or lung
Pigeon fancier's disease or lung

J67.3 Suberosis HCC
Corkhandler's disease or lung
Corkworker's disease or lung

J67.4 Maltworker's lung HCC
Alveolitis due to Aspergillus clavatus

J67.5 Mushroom-worker's lung HCC

J67.6 Maple-bark-stripper's lung HCC
Alveolitis due to Cryptostroma corticale
Cryptostromosis

J67.7 Air conditioner and humidifier lung CC HCC
Allergic alveolitis due to fungal, thermophilic actinomycetes and other organisms growing in ventilation [air conditioning] systems

J67.8 Hypersensitivity pneumonitis due to other organic dusts CC HCC
Cheese-washer's lung
Coffee-worker's lung
Fish-meal worker's lung
Furrier's lung
Sequoiosis

J67.9 Hypersensitivity pneumonitis due to unspecified organic dust CC HCC
Allergic alveolitis (extrinsic) NOS
Hypersensitivity pneumonitis NOS

J68 Respiratory conditions due to inhalation of chemicals, gases, fumes and vapors

Code first (T51-T65) to identify cause
Use additional code to identify associated respiratory conditions, such as:
acute respiratory failure (J96.0-)

J68.0 Bronchitis and pneumonitis due to chemicals, gases, fumes and vapors CC HCC
Chemical bronchitis (acute)
AHA: 2019,2Q,31

J68.1 Pulmonary edema due to chemicals, gases, fumes and vapors MCC HCC
Chemical pulmonary edema (acute) (chronic)
EXCLUDES 1 *pulmonary edema (acute) (chronic) NOS (J81.-)*

J68.2 Upper respiratory inflammation due to chemicals, gases, fumes and vapors, not elsewhere classified HCC

J68.3 Other acute and subacute respiratory conditions due to chemicals, gases, fumes and vapors HCC
Reactive airways dysfunction syndrome

J68.4 Chronic respiratory conditions due to chemicals, gases, fumes and vapors HCC
Emphysema (diffuse) (chronic) due to inhalation of chemicals, gases, fumes and vapors
Obliterative bronchiolitis (chronic) (subacute) due to inhalation of chemicals, gases, fumes and vapors
Pulmonary fibrosis (chronic) due to inhalation of chemicals, gases, fumes and vapors
EXCLUDES 1 *chronic pulmonary edema due to chemicals, gases, fumes and vapors (J68.1)*

J68.8 Other respiratory conditions due to chemicals, gases, fumes and vapors HCC

J68.9 Unspecified respiratory condition due to chemicals, gases, fumes and vapors HCC

J69 Pneumonitis due to solids and liquids

EXCLUDES 1 *neonatal aspiration syndromes (P24.-)*
postprocedural pneumonitis (J95.4)

AHA: 2017,1Q,24

DEF: Pneumonitis: Noninfectious inflammation of the walls of the alveoli in the lung tissue due to inhalation of food, vomit, oils, essences, or other solids or liquids.

J69.0 Pneumonitis due to inhalation of food and vomit MCC HCC
Aspiration pneumonia NOS
Aspiration pneumonia (due to) food (regurgitated)
Aspiration pneumonia (due to) gastric secretions
Aspiration pneumonia (due to) milk
Aspiration pneumonia (due to) vomit
Code also any associated foreign body in respiratory tract (T17.-)
EXCLUDES 1 *chemical pneumonitis due to anesthesia (J95.4)*
obstetric aspiration pneumonitis (O74.0)
AHA: 2020,2Q,11,28; 2019,3Q,17; 2019,2Q,6,31

J69.1 Pneumonitis due to inhalation of oils and essences MCC HCC
Exogenous lipoid pneumonia
Lipid pneumonia NOS
Code first (T51-T65) to identify substance
EXCLUDES 1 *endogenous lipoid pneumonia (J84.89)*

J69.8 Pneumonitis due to inhalation of other solids and liquids MCC HCC
Pneumonitis due to aspiration of blood
Pneumonitis due to aspiration of detergent
Code first (T51-T65) to identify substance

J70 Respiratory conditions due to other external agents

J70.0 Acute pulmonary manifestations due to radiation CC HCC
Radiation pneumonitis
Use additional code (W88-W90, X39.0-) to identify the external cause

J70.1 Chronic and other pulmonary manifestations due to radiation CC HCC
Fibrosis of lung following radiation
Use additional code (W88-W90, X39.0-) to identify the external cause

J70.2 Acute drug-induced interstitial lung disorders HCC
Use additional code for adverse effect, if applicable, to identify drug (T36-T50 with fifth or sixth character 5)
EXCLUDES 1 *interstitial pneumonia NOS (J84.9)*
lymphoid interstitial pneumonia (J84.2)
AHA: 2019,2Q,28

J70.3 Chronic drug-induced interstitial lung disorders HCC
Use additional code for adverse effect, if applicable, to identify drug (T36-T50 with fifth or sixth character 5)
EXCLUDES 1 *interstitial pneumonia NOS (J84.9)*
lymphoid interstitial pneumonia (J84.2)

J70.4 Drug-induced interstitial lung disorders, unspecified HCC
Use additional code for adverse effect, if applicable, to identify drug (T36-T50 with fifth or sixth character 5)
EXCLUDES 1 *interstitial pneumonia NOS (J84.9)*
lymphoid interstitial pneumonia (J84.2)
AHA: 2019,2Q,28

J70.5 Respiratory conditions due to smoke inhalation HCC
Code first smoke inhalation (T59.81-)
EXCLUDES 2 *smoke inhalation due to chemicals, gases, fumes and vapors (J68.9)*
AHA: 2013,4Q,121

J70.8 Respiratory conditions due to other specified external agents HCC
Code first (T51-T65) to identify the external agent

J70.9 Respiratory conditions due to unspecified external agent HCC
Code first (T51-T65) to identify the external agent

Other respiratory diseases principally affecting the interstitium (J80-J84)

J80 Acute respiratory distress syndrome MCC HCC
Acute respiratory distress syndrome in adult or child
Adult hyaline membrane disease
EXCLUDES 1 *respiratory distress syndrome in newborn (perinatal) (P22.0)*
AHA: 2021,1Q,23; 2020,4Q,96; 2020,1Q,34-36; 2017,1Q,26
DEF: Lung inflammation or injury resulting in a build-up of fluid in the air sacs, preventing the passage of oxygen from the air into the bloodstream.
TIP: Assign as a secondary code for a patient with acute respiratory distress syndrome (ARDS) due to COVID-19; assign code U07.1 as the principal or first-listed code.

J81 Pulmonary edema (4th)
Use additional code to identify:
exposure to environmental tobacco smoke (Z77.22)
history of tobacco dependence (Z87.891)
occupational exposure to environmental tobacco smoke (Z57.31)
tobacco dependence (F17.-)
tobacco use (Z72.0)
EXCLUDES 1 *chemical (acute) pulmonary edema (J68.1)*
hypostatic pneumonia (J18.2)
passive pneumonia (J18.2)
pulmonary edema due to external agents (J60-J70)
pulmonary edema with heart disease NOS (I50.1)
pulmonary edema with heart failure (I50.1)
DEF: Accumulation of fluid in the air sacs of the lungs, making it difficult to breathe.

J81.0 Acute pulmonary edema MCC HCC
Acute edema of lung
AHA: 2020,3Q,27

J81.1 Chronic pulmonary edema CC
Pulmonary congestion (chronic) (passive)
Pulmonary edema NOS

J82 Pulmonary eosinophilia, not elsewhere classified (4th)
EXCLUDES 2 *pulmonary eosinophilia due to aspergillosis (B44.-)*
pulmonary eosinophilia due to drugs (J70.2-J70.4)
pulmonary eosinophilia due to specified parasitic infection (B50-B83)
pulmonary eosinophilia due to systemic connective tissue disorders (M30-M36)
pulmonary infiltrate NOS (R91.8)
DEF: Infiltration of eosinophils (white blood cells of the immune system) into the parenchyma of the lungs, resulting in cough, fever, and dyspnea.

J82.8 Pulmonary eosinophilia, not elsewhere classified (5th)
AHA: 2020,4Q,25-27

J82.81 Chronic eosinophilic pneumonia CC HCC
Eosinophilic pneumonia, NOS

J82.82 Acute eosinophilic pneumonia CC

J82.83 Eosinophilic asthma CC
Code first asthma, by type, such as:
mild intermittent asthma (J45.2-)
mild persistent asthma (J45.3-)
moderate persistent asthma (J45.4-)
severe persistent asthma (J45.5-)

J82.89 Other pulmonary eosinophilia, not elsewhere classified CC HCC
Allergic pneumonia
Löffler's pneumonia
Tropical (pulmonary) eosinophilia NOS

J84 Other interstitial pulmonary diseases (4th)
EXCLUDES 1 *drug-induced interstitial lung disorders (J70.2-J70.4)*
interstitial emphysema (J98.2)
EXCLUDES 2 *lung diseases due to external agents (J60-J70)*
DEF: Interstitial: Within the small spaces or gaps occurring in tissue or organs.

J84.0 Alveolar and parieto-alveolar conditions (5th)

J84.01 Alveolar proteinosis CC HCC
DEF: Reduced ventilation due to proteinaceous deposits on alveoli. Symptoms include dyspnea, cough, chest pain, weakness, weight loss, and hemoptysis.

J84.02 Pulmonary alveolar microlithiasis CC HCC

J84.03 Idiopathic pulmonary hemosiderosis CC HCC
Essential brown induration of lung
Code first underlying disease, such as:
disorders of iron metabolism (E83.1-)
EXCLUDES 1 *acute idiopathic pulmonary hemorrhage in infants [AIPHI] (R04.81)*
DEF: Fibrosis of the alveolar walls marked by abnormal accumulation of iron as hemosiderin in the lungs. It primarily affects children and symptoms include anemia, fluid in the lungs, and blood in the sputum. Etiology is unknown.

J84.09 Other alveolar and parieto-alveolar conditions CC HCC

J84.1 Other interstitial pulmonary diseases with fibrosis (5th)
EXCLUDES 1 *pulmonary fibrosis (chronic) due to inhalation of chemicals, gases, fumes or vapors (J68.4)*
pulmonary fibrosis (chronic) following radiation (J70.1)

J84.10 Pulmonary fibrosis, unspecified HCC
Capillary fibrosis of lung
Cirrhosis of lung (chronic) NOS
Fibrosis of lung (atrophic) (chronic) (confluent) (massive) (perialveolar) (peribronchial) NOS
Induration of lung (chronic) NOS
Postinflammatory pulmonary fibrosis

J84.11 Idiopathic interstitial pneumonia (6th)
EXCLUDES 1 *lymphoid interstitial pneumonia (J84.2)*
pneumocystis pneumonia (B59)

J84.111 Idiopathic interstitial pneumonia, not otherwise specified HCC

J84.112 Idiopathic pulmonary fibrosis HCC
Cryptogenic fibrosing alveolitis
Idiopathic fibrosing alveolitis

J84.113 Idiopathic non-specific interstitial pneumonitis HCC
EXCLUDES 1 *non-specific interstitial pneumonia NOS, or due to known underlying cause (J84.89)*

J84.114 Acute interstitial pneumonitis CC HCC
Hamman-Rich syndrome
EXCLUDES 1 *pneumocystis pneumonia (B59)*

J84.115 Respiratory bronchiolitis interstitial lung disease HCC

J84.116 Cryptogenic organizing pneumonia CC HCC
EXCLUDES 1 *organizing pneumonia NOS, or due to known underlying cause (J84.89)*

J84.117 Desquamative interstitial pneumonia CC HCC

Chapter 10. Diseases of the Respiratory System

J70.8–J84.117

✓6th **J84.17 Other interstitial pulmonary diseases with fibrosis in diseases classified elsewhere**
AHA: 2020,4Q,27-28

J84.17Ø Interstitial lung disease with progressive fibrotic phenotype in diseases classified elsewhere HCC
Progressive fibrotic interstitial lung disease
Code first underlying disease, such as:
lung diseases due to external agents (J6Ø-J7Ø)
rheumatoid arthritis (MØ5.ØØ-MØ6.9)
sarcoidosis (D86)
systemic connective tissue disorders (M3Ø-M36)

J84.178 Other interstitial pulmonary diseases with fibrosis in diseases classified elsewhere HCC
Interstitial pneumonia (nonspecific) (usual) due to collagen vascular disease
Interstitial pneumonia (nonspecific) (usual) in diseases classified elsewhere
Organizing pneumonia due to collagen vascular disease
Organizing pneumonia in diseases classified elsewhere
Code first underlying disease, such as:
progressive systemic sclerosis (M34.Ø)
rheumatoid arthritis (MØ5.ØØ-MØ6.9)
systemic lupus erythematosis (M32.Ø-M32.9)

J84.2 Lymphoid interstitial pneumonia CC HCC
Lymphoid interstitial pneumonitis

✓5th **J84.8 Other specified interstitial pulmonary diseases**
EXCLUDES 1 *exogenous lipoid pneumonia (J69.1)*
unspecified lipoid pneumonia (J69.1)

J84.81 Lymphangioleiomyomatosis MCC HCC
Lymphangiomyomatosis

J84.82 Adult pulmonary Langerhans cell histiocytosis CC HCC A
Adult PLCH

J84.83 Surfactant mutations of the lung MCC HCC
DEF: Genetic disorder resulting in insufficient secretion of a complex mixture of phospholipids and proteins that reduce surface tension in the alveoli following the onset of breathing to facilitate lung expansion in the newborn. It is the leading indication for pediatric lung transplantation.

✓6th **J84.84 Other interstitial lung diseases of childhood**

J84.841 Neuroendocrine cell hyperplasia of infancy MCC HCC

J84.842 Pulmonary interstitial glycogenosis MCC HCC

J84.843 Alveolar capillary dysplasia with vein misalignment MCC HCC

J84.848 Other interstitial lung diseases of childhood MCC HCC

J84.89 Other specified interstitial pulmonary diseases HCC
Endogenous lipoid pneumonia
Interstitial pneumonitis
Non-specific interstitial pneumonitis NOS
Organizing pneumonia NOS
Code first, if applicable:
poisoning due to drug or toxin (T51-T65 with fifth or sixth character to indicate intent), for toxic pneumonopathy
underlying cause of pneumonopathy, if known
Use additional code, for adverse effect, to identify drug (T36-T5Ø with fifth or sixth character 5), if drug-induced
EXCLUDES 1 *cryptogenic organizing pneumonia (J84.116)*
idiopathic non-specific interstitial pneumonitis (J84.113)
lymphoid interstitial pneumonia (J84.2)
lipoid pneumonia, exogenous or unspecified (J69.1)
AHA: 2021,4Q,106; 2021,1Q,48; 2019,2Q,28

J84.9 Interstitial pulmonary disease, unspecified CC HCC
Interstitial pneumonia NOS

Suppurative and necrotic conditions of the lower respiratory tract (J85-J86)

✓4th **J85 Abscess of lung and mediastinum**
Use additional code (B95-B97) to identify infectious agent

J85.Ø Gangrene and necrosis of lung MCC HCC

J85.1 Abscess of lung with pneumonia MCC HCC
Code also the type of pneumonia

J85.2 Abscess of lung without pneumonia MCC HCC
Abscess of lung NOS

J85.3 Abscess of mediastinum MCC HCC

✓4th **J86 Pyothorax**
Use additional code (B95-B97) to identify infectious agent
EXCLUDES 1 *abscess of lung (J85.-)*
pyothorax due to tuberculosis (A15.6)
DEF: Collection of pus in the pleural space that is commonly caused by an infection that spreads from the lung, such as bacterial pneumonia or a lung abscess.

J86.Ø Pyothorax with fistula MCC HCC
Bronchocutaneous fistula
Bronchopleural fistula
Hepatopleural fistula
Mediastinal fistula
Pleural fistula
Thoracic fistula
Any condition classifiable to J86.9 with fistula
DEF: Purulent infection of the respiratory cavity, with communication from a cavity to another structure.

J86.9 Pyothorax without fistula MCC HCC
Abscess of pleura
Abscess of thorax
Empyema (chest) (lung) (pleura)
Fibrinopurulent pleurisy
Purulent pleurisy
Pyopneumothorax
Septic pleurisy
Seropurulent pleurisy
Suppurative pleurisy

Other diseases of the pleura (J9Ø-J94)

J9Ø Pleural effusion, not elsewhere classified CC
Encysted pleurisy
Pleural effusion NOS
Pleurisy with effusion (exudative) (serous)
EXCLUDES 1 *chylous (pleural) effusion (J94.Ø)*
malignant pleural effusion (J91.Ø)
pleurisy NOS (RØ9.1)
tuberculous pleural effusion (A15.6)
DEF: Collection of lymph and other fluid within the pleural space.

✓4th **J91 Pleural effusion in conditions classified elsewhere**
EXCLUDES 2 *pleural effusion in heart failure (I5Ø.-)*
pleural effusion in systemic lupus erythematosus (M32.13)
DEF: Collection of lymph and other fluid within the pleural space.

J91.Ø Malignant pleural effusion CC
Code first underlying neoplasm ►(CØØ-D49)◄

J91.8 Pleural effusion in other conditions classified elsewhere CC
Code first underlying disease, such as:
filariasis (B74.Ø-B74.9)
influenza (JØ9.X2, J1Ø.1, J11.1)
AHA: 2015,2Q,15
TIP: Assign this code as a secondary diagnosis to congestive heart failure (I5Ø.-) only if pleural effusion is specifically evaluated or treated.

Pleural Effusion

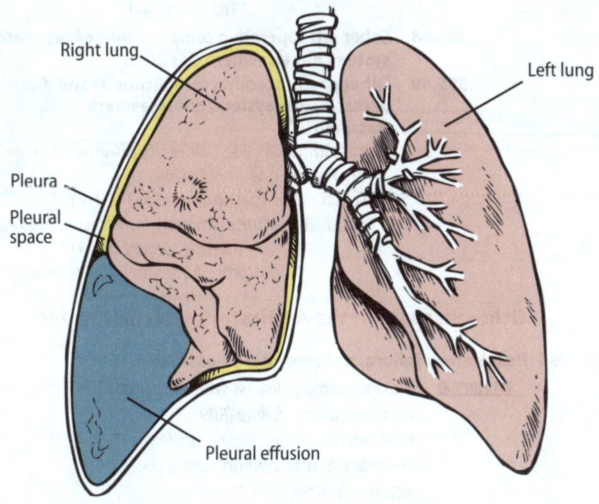

J92 Pleural plaque (4th)
INCLUDES pleural thickening
DEF: Areas of fibrous thickening that form on the parietal or visceral pleura, the membranes that line the ribs and lungs.
J92.Ø Pleural plaque with presence of asbestos
J92.9 Pleural plaque without asbestos
Pleural plaque NOS

J93 Pneumothorax and air leak (4th)
EXCLUDES 1 *congenital or perinatal pneumothorax (P25.1)*
postprocedural air leak (J95.812)
postprocedural pneumothorax (J95.811)
pyopneumothorax (J86.-)
traumatic pneumothorax (S27.Ø)
tuberculous (current disease) pneumothorax (A15.-)
DEF: Pneumothorax: Lung displacement due to abnormal leakage of air or gas that is trapped in the pleural space formed by the membrane that encloses the lungs and lines the thoracic cavity.
J93.Ø Spontaneous tension pneumothorax MCC
DEF: Leaking air from the lung into the lining, causing collapse.
J93.1 Other spontaneous pneumothorax (5th)
J93.11 Primary spontaneous pneumothorax CC
J93.12 Secondary spontaneous pneumothorax CC UPD
Code first underlying condition, such as:
catamenial pneumothorax due to endometriosis ▶(N8Ø.B-)◀
cystic fibrosis (E84.-)
eosinophilic pneumonia (J82)
lymphangioleiomyomatosis (J84.81)
malignant neoplasm of bronchus and lung (C34.-)
Marfan's syndrome (Q87.4)
pneumonia due to Pneumocystis carinii (B59)
secondary malignant neoplasm of lung (C78.Ø-)
spontaneous rupture of the esophagus (K22.3)
J93.8 Other pneumothorax and air leak (5th)
J93.81 Chronic pneumothorax CC
J93.82 Other air leak CC
Persistent air leak
J93.83 Other pneumothorax CC
Acute pneumothorax
Spontaneous pneumothorax NOS
AHA: 2020,3Q,9-10
J93.9 Pneumothorax, unspecified CC
Pneumothorax NOS

J94 Other pleural conditions (4th)
EXCLUDES 1 *pleurisy NOS (RØ9.1)*
traumatic hemopneumothorax (S27.2)
traumatic hemothorax (S27.1)
tuberculous pleural conditions (current disease) (A15.-)
J94.Ø Chylous effusion CC
Chyliform effusion
DEF: Fluid within the pleural space due to the leaking of lymph contents into the space, usually as a result of thoracic duct damage or injury or mediastinal lymphoma.
J94.1 Fibrothorax
DEF: Fibrosis within the pleural lining of the lungs commonly seen as a stiff layer surrounding the lung typically attributed to traumatic hemothorax or pleural effusion.
J94.2 Hemothorax CC
Hemopneumothorax
J94.8 Other specified pleural conditions CC
Hydropneumothorax
Hydrothorax
AHA: 2021,1Q,48
J94.9 Pleural condition, unspecified

Intraoperative and postprocedural complications and disorders of respiratory system, not elsewhere classified (J95)

J95 Intraoperative and postprocedural complications and disorders of respiratory system, not elsewhere classified (4th)
EXCLUDES 2 *aspiration pneumonia (J69.-)*
emphysema (subcutaneous) resulting from a procedure (T81.82)
hypostatic pneumonia (J18.2)
pulmonary manifestations due to radiation (J7Ø.Ø-J7Ø.1)
J95.Ø Tracheostomy complications (5th)
DEF: Tracheostomy: Formation of a tracheal opening on the neck surface with tube insertion to allow for respiration in cases of obstruction or decreased patency. A tracheostomy may be planned or performed on an emergency basis for temporary or long-term use.
J95.ØØ Unspecified tracheostomy complication CC HCC
J95.Ø1 Hemorrhage from tracheostomy stoma CC HCC
J95.Ø2 Infection of tracheostomy stoma CC HCC
Use additional code to identify type of infection, such as:
cellulitis of neck (LØ3.221)
sepsis (A4Ø, A41.-)
J95.Ø3 Malfunction of tracheostomy stoma CC HCC
Mechanical complication of tracheostomy stoma
Obstruction of tracheostomy airway
Tracheal stenosis due to tracheostomy
J95.Ø4 Tracheo-esophageal fistula following tracheostomy CC HCC
J95.Ø9 Other tracheostomy complication CC HCC
J95.1 Acute pulmonary insufficiency following thoracic surgery MCC HCC
EXCLUDES 2 *functional disturbances following cardiac surgery (I97.Ø, I97.1-)*
J95.2 Acute pulmonary insufficiency following nonthoracic surgery MCC HCC
EXCLUDES 2 *functional disturbances following cardiac surgery (I97.Ø, I97.1-)*
J95.3 Chronic pulmonary insufficiency following surgery MCC HCC
EXCLUDES 2 *functional disturbances following cardiac surgery (I97.Ø, I97.1-)*
J95.4 Chemical pneumonitis due to anesthesia CC
Mendelson's syndrome
Postprocedural aspiration pneumonia
Use additional code for adverse effect, if applicable, to identify drug (T41.- with fifth or sixth character 5)
EXCLUDES 1 *aspiration pneumonitis due to anesthesia complicating labor and delivery (O74.Ø)*
aspiration pneumonitis due to anesthesia complicating pregnancy (O29)
aspiration pneumonitis due to anesthesia complicating the puerperium (O89.Ø1)
J95.5 Postprocedural subglottic stenosis CC

√5th **J95.6 Intraoperative hemorrhage and hematoma of a respiratory system organ or structure complicating a procedure**
EXCLUDES 1 *intraoperative hemorrhage and hematoma of a respiratory system organ or structure due to accidental puncture and laceration during procedure (J95.7-)*

J95.61 Intraoperative hemorrhage and hematoma of a respiratory system organ or structure complicating a respiratory system procedure CC

J95.62 Intraoperative hemorrhage and hematoma of a respiratory system organ or structure complicating other procedure CC

√5th **J95.7 Accidental puncture and laceration of a respiratory system organ or structure during a procedure**
EXCLUDES 2 *postprocedural pneumothorax (J95.811)*

J95.71 Accidental puncture and laceration of a respiratory system organ or structure during a respiratory system procedure CC

J95.72 Accidental puncture and laceration of a respiratory system organ or structure during other procedure CC

√5th **J95.8 Other intraoperative and postprocedural complications and disorders of respiratory system, not elsewhere classified**
AHA: 2016,4Q,9-10

√6th **J95.81 Postprocedural pneumothorax and air leak**

J95.811 Postprocedural pneumothorax CC H14
AHA: 2021,1Q,48

J95.812 Postprocedural air leak CC

√6th **J95.82 Postprocedural respiratory failure**
EXCLUDES 1 *respiratory failure in other conditions (J96.-)*

J95.821 Acute postprocedural respiratory failure MCC HCC
Postprocedural respiratory failure NOS

J95.822 Acute and chronic postprocedural respiratory failure MCC HCC

√6th **J95.83 Postprocedural hemorrhage of a respiratory system organ or structure following a procedure**

J95.830 Postprocedural hemorrhage of a respiratory system organ or structure following a respiratory system procedure CC

J95.831 Postprocedural hemorrhage of a respiratory system organ or structure following other procedure CC

J95.84 Transfusion-related acute lung injury (TRALI) CC
DEF: Relatively rare, but serious, pulmonary complication of blood transfusion, with acute respiratory distress, noncardiogenic pulmonary edema, cyanosis, hypoxemia, hypotension, fever, and chills.

√6th **J95.85 Complication of respirator [ventilator]**

J95.850 Mechanical complication of respirator CC HCC
EXCLUDES 1 *encounter for respirator [ventilator] dependence during power failure (Z99.12)*

J95.851 Ventilator associated pneumonia CC HCC
Ventilator associated pneumonitis
Use additional code to identify the organism, if known (B95.-, B96.-, B97.-)
EXCLUDES 1 *ventilator lung in newborn (P27.8)*
AHA: 2020,2Q,17; 2017,1Q,25

J95.859 Other complication of respirator [ventilator] CC HCC
AHA: 2021,1Q,48

√6th **J95.86 Postprocedural hematoma and seroma of a respiratory system organ or structure following a procedure**

J95.860 Postprocedural hematoma of a respiratory system organ or structure following a respiratory system procedure CC

J95.861 Postprocedural hematoma of a respiratory system organ or structure following other procedure CC

J95.862 Postprocedural seroma of a respiratory system organ or structure following a respiratory system procedure CC

J95.863 Postprocedural seroma of a respiratory system organ or structure following other procedure CC

● **J95.87 Transfusion-associated dyspnea (TAD)** CC
EXCLUDES 1 *transfusion associated circulatory overload (TACO) (E87.71)*
transfusion-related acute lung injury (TRALI) (J95.84)

J95.88 Other intraoperative complications of respiratory system, not elsewhere classified CC

J95.89 Other postprocedural complications and disorders of respiratory system, not elsewhere classified CC
Use additional code to identify disorder, such as:
aspiration pneumonia (J69.-)
bacterial or viral pneumonia (J12-J18)
EXCLUDES 2 *acute pulmonary insufficiency following thoracic surgery (J95.1)*
postprocedural subglottic stenosis (J95.5)

Other diseases of the respiratory system (J96-J99)

√4th **J96 Respiratory failure, not elsewhere classified**
EXCLUDES 1 *acute respiratory distress syndrome (J80)*
cardiorespiratory failure (R09.2)
newborn respiratory distress syndrome (P22.0)
postprocedural respiratory failure (J95.82-)
respiratory arrest (R09.2)
respiratory arrest of newborn (P28.81)
respiratory failure of newborn (P28.5)
AHA: 2021,1Q,27,44-45; 2020,4Q,96

√5th **J96.0 Acute respiratory failure**

J96.00 Acute respiratory failure, unspecified whether with hypoxia or hypercapnia MCC HCC
AHA: 2016,3Q,14; 2013,4Q,121

J96.01 Acute respiratory failure with hypoxia MCC HCC
AHA: 2020,3Q,12

J96.02 Acute respiratory failure with hypercapnia MCC HCC
▶Acute respiratory acidosis◀

√5th **J96.1 Chronic respiratory failure**

J96.10 Chronic respiratory failure, unspecified whether with hypoxia or hypercapnia CC HCC
AHA: 2016,1Q,38; 2015,1Q,21

J96.11 Chronic respiratory failure with hypoxia CC HCC
AHA: 2013,4Q,129

J96.12 Chronic respiratory failure with hypercapnia CC HCC
▶Chronic respiratory acidosis◀

√5th **J96.2 Acute and chronic respiratory failure**
Acute on chronic respiratory failure

J96.20 Acute and chronic respiratory failure, unspecified whether with hypoxia or hypercapnia MCC HCC

J96.21 Acute and chronic respiratory failure with hypoxia MCC HCC

J96.22 Acute and chronic respiratory failure with hypercapnia MCC HCC

√5th **J96.9 Respiratory failure, unspecified**

J96.90 Respiratory failure, unspecified, unspecified whether with hypoxia or hypercapnia MCC HCC

J96.91 Respiratory failure, unspecified with hypoxia MCC HCC

J96.92 Respiratory failure, unspecified with hypercapnia MCC HCC

J98 Other respiratory disorders

Use additional code to identify:
- exposure to environmental tobacco smoke (Z77.22)
- exposure to tobacco smoke in the perinatal period (P96.81)
- history of tobacco dependence (Z87.891)
- occupational exposure to environmental tobacco smoke (Z57.31)
- tobacco dependence (F17.-)
- tobacco use (Z72.Ø)

EXCLUDES 1 *newborn apnea ▶(P28.4-)◀*
newborn sleep apnea ▶(P28.3-)◀

EXCLUDES 2 *apnea NOS (RØ6.81)*
sleep apnea (G47.3-)

J98.Ø Diseases of bronchus, not elsewhere classified

J98.Ø1 Acute bronchospasm

EXCLUDES 1 *acute bronchiolitis with bronchospasm (J21.-)*
acute bronchitis with bronchospasm (J2Ø.-)
asthma (J45.-)
exercise induced bronchospasm (J45.99Ø)

J98.Ø9 Other diseases of bronchus, not elsewhere classified

Broncholithiasis
Calcification of bronchus
Stenosis of bronchus
Tracheobronchial collapse
Tracheobronchial dyskinesia
Ulcer of bronchus

J98.1 Pulmonary collapse

EXCLUDES 1 *therapeutic collapse of lung status (Z98.3)*

J98.11 Atelectasis CC

EXCLUDES 1 *newborn atelectasis*
tuberculous atelectasis (current disease) (A15)

DEF: Collapse of lung tissue affecting part or all of one lung, preventing normal oxygen absorption to healthy tissues.

J98.19 Other pulmonary collapse CC

J98.2 Interstitial emphysema HCC

Mediastinal emphysema

EXCLUDES 1 *emphysema NOS (J43.9)*
emphysema in newborn (P25.Ø)
surgical emphysema (subcutaneous) (T81.82)
traumatic subcutaneous emphysema (T79.7)

J98.3 Compensatory emphysema HCC

DEF: Distention of all or part of the lung caused by disease processes or surgical intervention that decreased volume in another part of the lung, causing an overcompensation reaction. Compensatory emphysema occurs in association with pneumonias, pleural effusions, atelectasis, empyema, and pneumothorax.

J98.4 Other disorders of lung

Calcification of lung
Cystic lung disease (acquired)
Lung disease NOS
Pulmolithiasis

EXCLUDES 1 *acute interstitial pneumonitis (J84.114)*
pulmonary insufficiency following surgery (J95.1-J95.2)

J98.5 Diseases of mediastinum, not elsewhere classified

EXCLUDES 2 *abscess of mediastinum (J85.3)*

AHA: 2016,4Q,29

J98.51 Mediastinitis MCC H8

Code first underlying condition, if applicable, such as postoperative mediastinitis (T81.-)

J98.59 Other diseases of mediastinum, not elsewhere classified MCC H8

Fibrosis of mediastinum
Hernia of mediastinum
Retraction of mediastinum

J98.6 Disorders of diaphragm

Diaphragmatitis
Paralysis of diaphragm
Relaxation of diaphragm

EXCLUDES 1 *congenital malformation of diaphragm NEC (Q79.1)*
congenital diaphragmatic hernia (Q79.Ø)

EXCLUDES 2 *diaphragmatic hernia (K44.-)*

J98.8 Other specified respiratory disorders

AHA: 2020,1Q,34-36

TIP: Assign as a secondary code for a patient with a respiratory infection that is not further specified but is documented as being associated with COVID-19; assign U07.1 as the principal or first-listed code. If the respiratory infection documentation specifies acute or lower respiratory infection (NOS), assign J22 instead.

J98.9 Respiratory disorder, unspecified

Respiratory disease (chronic) NOS

J99 Respiratory disorders in diseases classified elsewhere HCC

Code first underlying disease, such as:
- amyloidosis (E85.-)
- ankylosing spondylitis (M45)
- congenital syphilis (A5Ø.5)
- cryoglobulinemia (D89.1)
- early congenital syphilis (A5Ø.Ø)
- plasminogen deficiency (E88.Ø2)
- schistosomiasis (B65.Ø-B65.9)

EXCLUDES 1 *respiratory disorders in:*
- *amebiasis (AØ6.5)*
- *blastomycosis (B4Ø.Ø-B4Ø.2)*
- *candidiasis (B37.1)*
- *coccidioidomycosis (B38.Ø-B38.2)*
- *cystic fibrosis with pulmonary manifestations (E84.Ø)*
- *dermatomyositis (M33.Ø1, M33.11)*
- *histoplasmosis (B39.Ø-B39.2)*
- *late syphilis (A52.72, A52.73)*
- *polymyositis (M33.21)*
- *Sjögren syndrome (M35.Ø2)*
- *systemic lupus erythematosus (M32.13)*
- *systemic sclerosis (M34.81)*
- *Wegener's granulomatosis (M31.3Ø-M31.31)*

Chapter 11. Diseases of the Digestive System (KØØ–K95)

Chapter-specific Guidelines with Coding Examples
Reserved for future guideline expansion.

Chapter 11. Diseases of the Digestive System (KØØ-K95)

EXCLUDES 2 *certain conditions originating in the perinatal period (PØ4-P96)*
certain infectious and parasitic diseases (AØØ-B99)
complications of pregnancy, childbirth and the puerperium (OØØ-O9A)
congenital malformations, deformations and chromosomal abnormalities (QØØ-Q99)
endocrine, nutritional and metabolic diseases (EØØ-E88)
injury, poisoning and certain other consequences of external causes (SØØ-T88)
neoplasms (CØØ-D49)
symptoms, signs and abnormal clinical and laboratory findings, not elsewhere classified (RØØ-R94)

This chapter contains the following blocks:

KØØ-K14 Diseases of oral cavity and salivary glands
K2Ø-K31 Diseases of esophagus, stomach and duodenum
K35-K38 Diseases of appendix
K4Ø-K46 Hernia
K5Ø-K52 Noninfective enteritis and colitis
K55-K64 Other diseases of intestines
K65-K68 Diseases of peritoneum and retroperitoneum
K7Ø-K77 Diseases of liver
K8Ø-K87 Disorders of gallbladder, biliary tract and pancreas
K9Ø-K95 Other diseases of the digestive system

Diseases of oral cavity and salivary glands (KØØ-K14)

✓4th **KØØ Disorders of tooth development and eruption**

EXCLUDES 2 *embedded and impacted teeth (KØ1.-)*

KØØ.Ø Anodontia
Hypodontia
Oligodontia
EXCLUDES 1 *acquired absence of teeth (KØ8.1-)*
DEF: Partial or complete absence of teeth due to a congenital defect involving the tooth bud.

KØØ.1 Supernumerary teeth
Distomolar
Fourth molar
Mesiodens
Paramolar
Supplementary teeth
EXCLUDES 2 *supernumerary roots (KØØ.2)*

KØØ.2 Abnormalities of size and form of teeth
Concrescence of teeth
Fusion of teeth
Gemination of teeth
Dens evaginatus
Dens in dente
Dens invaginatus
Enamel pearls
Macrodontia
Microdontia
Peg-shaped [conical] teeth
Supernumerary roots
Taurodontism
Tuberculum paramolare
EXCLUDES 1 *abnormalities of teeth due to congenital syphilis (A5Ø.5)*
tuberculum Carabelli, which is regarded as a normal variation and should not be coded

KØØ.3 Mottled teeth
Dental fluorosis
Mottling of enamel
Nonfluoride enamel opacities
EXCLUDES 2 *deposits [accretions] on teeth (KØ3.6)*

KØØ.4 Disturbances in tooth formation
Aplasia and hypoplasia of cementum
Dilaceration of tooth
Enamel hypoplasia (neonatal) (postnatal) (prenatal)
Regional odontodysplasia
Turner's tooth
EXCLUDES 1 *Hutchinson's teeth and mulberry molars in congenital syphilis (A5Ø.5)*
EXCLUDES 2 *mottled teeth (KØØ.3)*

KØØ.5 Hereditary disturbances in tooth structure, not elsewhere classified
Amelogenesis imperfecta
Dentinogenesis imperfecta
Odontogenesis imperfecta
Dentinal dysplasia
Shell teeth

KØØ.6 Disturbances in tooth eruption
Dentia praecox
Natal tooth
Neonatal tooth
Premature eruption of tooth
Premature shedding of primary [deciduous] tooth
Prenatal teeth
Retained [persistent] primary tooth
EXCLUDES 2 *embedded and impacted teeth (KØ1.-)*

KØØ.7 Teething syndrome

KØØ.8 Other disorders of tooth development
Color changes during tooth formation
Intrinsic staining of teeth NOS
EXCLUDES 2 *posteruptive color changes (KØ3.7)*

KØØ.9 Disorder of tooth development, unspecified
Disorder of odontogenesis NOS

✓4th **KØ1 Embedded and impacted teeth**

EXCLUDES 1 *abnormal position of fully erupted teeth (M26.3-)*

KØ1.Ø Embedded teeth

KØ1.1 Impacted teeth

✓4th **KØ2 Dental caries**

INCLUDES caries of dentine
dental cavities
early childhood caries
pre-eruptive caries
recurrent caries (dentino enamel junction) (enamel) (to the pulp)
tooth decay

Tooth Anatomy

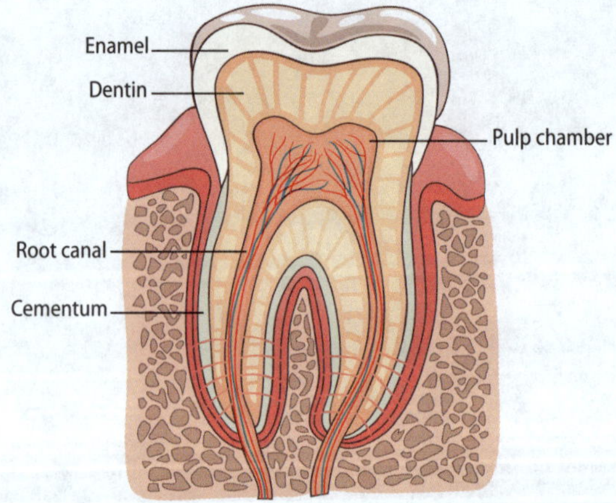

KØ2.3 Arrested dental caries
Arrested coronal and root caries

✓5th **KØ2.5 Dental caries on pit and fissure surface**
Dental caries on chewing surface of tooth

KØ2.51 Dental caries on pit and fissure surface limited to enamel
White spot lesions [initial caries] on pit and fissure surface of tooth

KØ2.52 Dental caries on pit and fissure surface penetrating into dentin
Primary dental caries, cervical origin

KØ2.53 Dental caries on pit and fissure surface penetrating into pulp

✓5th **KØ2.6 Dental caries on smooth surface**

KØ2.61 Dental caries on smooth surface limited to enamel
White spot lesions [initial caries] on smooth surface of tooth

KØ2.62 Dental caries on smooth surface penetrating into dentin

KØ2.63 Dental caries on smooth surface penetrating into pulp

KØ2.7 Dental root caries

KØ2.9 Dental caries, unspecified

KØ3 Other diseases of hard tissues of teeth

EXCLUDES 2 *bruxism (F45.8)*
dental caries (KØ2.-)
teeth-grinding NOS (F45.8)

KØ3.Ø Excessive attrition of teeth
Approximal wear of teeth
Occlusal wear of teeth
DEF: Attrition: In dentistry, wearing away or erosion of tooth surface from abrasive food or grinding teeth.

KØ3.1 Abrasion of teeth
Dentifrice abrasion of teeth
Habitual abrasion of teeth
Occupational abrasion of teeth
Ritual abrasion of teeth
Traditional abrasion of teeth
Wedge defect NOS

KØ3.2 Erosion of teeth
Erosion of teeth due to diet
Erosion of teeth due to drugs and medicaments
Erosion of teeth due to persistent vomiting
Erosion of teeth NOS
Idiopathic erosion of teeth
Occupational erosion of teeth

KØ3.3 Pathological resorption of teeth
Internal granuloma of pulp
Resorption of teeth (external)

KØ3.4 Hypercementosis
Cementation hyperplasia

KØ3.5 Ankylosis of teeth

KØ3.6 Deposits [accretions] on teeth
Betel deposits [accretions] on teeth
Black deposits [accretions] on teeth
Extrinsic staining of teeth NOS
Green deposits [accretions] on teeth
Materia alba deposits [accretions] on teeth
Orange deposits [accretions] on teeth
Staining of teeth NOS
Subgingival dental calculus
Supragingival dental calculus
Tobacco deposits [accretions] on teeth

KØ3.7 Posteruptive color changes of dental hard tissues
EXCLUDES 2 *deposits [accretions] on teeth (KØ3.6)*

KØ3.8 Other specified diseases of hard tissues of teeth

KØ3.81 Cracked tooth
EXCLUDES 1 *asymptomatic craze lines in enamel - omit code*
broken or fractured tooth due to trauma (SØ2.5)

KØ3.89 Other specified diseases of hard tissues of teeth

KØ3.9 Disease of hard tissues of teeth, unspecified

KØ4 Diseases of pulp and periapical tissues
AHA: 2016,4Q,29-30

KØ4.Ø Pulpitis
Acute pulpitis
Chronic (hyperplastic) (ulcerative) pulpitis

KØ4.Ø1 Reversible pulpitis CC

KØ4.Ø2 Irreversible pulpitis CC

KØ4.1 Necrosis of pulp
Pulpal gangrene

KØ4.2 Pulp degeneration
Denticles
Pulpal calcifications
Pulpal stones

KØ4.3 Abnormal hard tissue formation in pulp
Secondary or irregular dentine

KØ4.4 Acute apical periodontitis of pulpal origin CC
Acute apical periodontitis NOS
EXCLUDES 1 *acute periodontitis (KØ5.2-)*
DEF: Severe inflammation of the area surrounding the tip of a tooth's root that is often secondary to infection or trauma.

KØ4.5 Chronic apical periodontitis
Apical or periapical granuloma
Apical periodontitis NOS
EXCLUDES 1 *chronic periodontitis (KØ5.3-)*

KØ4.6 Periapical abscess with sinus
Dental abscess with sinus
Dentoalveolar abscess with sinus

KØ4.7 Periapical abscess without sinus
Dental abscess without sinus
Dentoalveolar abscess without sinus

KØ4.8 Radicular cyst
Apical (periodontal) cyst
Periapical cyst
Residual radicular cyst
EXCLUDES 2 *lateral periodontal cyst (KØ9.Ø)*
DEF: Most common odontogenic cyst in tissue around the tooth apex due to chronic inflammation of dental pulp.

KØ4.9 Other and unspecified diseases of pulp and periapical tissues

KØ4.9Ø Unspecified diseases of pulp and periapical tissues

KØ4.99 Other diseases of pulp and periapical tissues

KØ5 Gingivitis and periodontal diseases
Use additional code to identify:
alcohol abuse and dependence (F1Ø.-)
exposure to environmental tobacco smoke (Z77.22)
exposure to tobacco smoke in the perinatal period (P96.81)
history of tobacco dependence (Z87.891)
occupational exposure to environmental tobacco smoke (Z57.31)
tobacco dependence (F17.-)
tobacco use (Z72.Ø)
AHA: 2016,4Q,29-30

KØ5.Ø Acute gingivitis
EXCLUDES 1 *acute necrotizing ulcerative gingivitis (A69.1)*
herpesviral [herpes simplex] gingivostomatitis (BØØ.2)

KØ5.ØØ Acute gingivitis, plaque induced
Acute gingivitis NOS
Plaque induced gingival disease

KØ5.Ø1 Acute gingivitis, non-plaque induced

KØ5.1 Chronic gingivitis
Desquamative gingivitis (chronic)
Gingivitis (chronic) NOS
Hyperplastic gingivitis (chronic)
Pregnancy associated gingivitis
Simple marginal gingivitis (chronic)
Ulcerative gingivitis (chronic)
Code first, if applicable, diseases of the digestive system complicating pregnacy (O99.61-)

KØ5.1Ø Chronic gingivitis, plaque induced
Chronic gingivitis NOS
Gingivitis NOS

KØ5.11 Chronic gingivitis, non-plaque induced

KØ5.2 Aggressive periodontitis
Acute pericoronitis
EXCLUDES 1 *acute apical periodontitis (KØ4.4)*
periapical abscess (KØ4.7)
periapical abscess with sinus (KØ4.6)

KØ5.2Ø Aggressive periodontitis, unspecified

KØ5.21 Aggressive periodontitis, localized
Periodontal abscess

KØ5.211 Aggressive periodontitis, localized, slight

KØ5.212 Aggressive periodontitis, localized, moderate

KØ5.213 Aggressive periodontitis, localized, severe

KØ5.219 Aggressive periodontitis, localized, unspecified severity

KØ5.22 Aggressive periodontitis, generalized

KØ5.221 Aggressive periodontitis, generalized, slight

KØ5.222 Aggressive periodontitis, generalized, moderate

KØ5.223 Aggressive periodontitis, generalized, severe

KØ5.229 Aggressive periodontitis, generalized, unspecified severity

K05.3 Chronic periodontitis
Chronic pericoronitis
Complex periodontitis
Periodontitis NOS
Simplex periodontitis
EXCLUDES 1 *chronic apical periodontitis (K04.5)*

K05.30 Chronic periodontitis, unspecified

K05.31 Chronic periodontitis, localized

K05.311 Chronic periodontitis, localized, slight

K05.312 Chronic periodontitis, localized, moderate

K05.313 Chronic periodontitis, localized, severe

K05.319 Chronic periodontitis, localized, unspecified severity

K05.32 Chronic periodontitis, generalized

K05.321 Chronic periodontitis, generalized, slight

K05.322 Chronic periodontitis, generalized, moderate

K05.323 Chronic periodontitis, generalized, severe

K05.329 Chronic periodontitis, generalized, unspecified

K05.4 Periodontosis
Juvenile periodontosis

K05.5 Other periodontal diseases
Combined periodontic-endodontic lesion
Narrow gingival width (of periodontal soft tissue)
EXCLUDES 2 *leukoplakia of gingiva (K13.21)*

K05.6 Periodontal disease, unspecified

K06 Other disorders of gingiva and edentulous alveolar ridge
EXCLUDES 2 *acute gingivitis (K05.0)*
atrophy of edentulous alveolar ridge (K08.2)
chronic gingivitis (K05.1)
gingivitis NOS (K05.1)
AHA: 2016,4Q,29-30

K06.0 Gingival recession
Gingival recession (postinfective) (postprocedural)
AHA: 2017,4Q,16

K06.01 Gingival recession, localized

K06.010 Localized gingival recession, unspecified
Localized gingival recession, NOS

K06.011 Localized gingival recession, minimal

K06.012 Localized gingival recession, moderate

K06.013 Localized gingival recession, severe

K06.02 Gingival recession, generalized

K06.020 Generalized gingival recession, unspecified
Generalized gingival recession, NOS

K06.021 Generalized gingival recession, minimal

K06.022 Generalized gingival recession, moderate

K06.023 Generalized gingival recession, severe

K06.1 Gingival enlargement
Gingival fibromatosis

K06.2 Gingival and edentulous alveolar ridge lesions associated with trauma
Irritative hyperplasia of edentulous ridge [denture hyperplasia]
Use additional code (Chapter 20) to identify external cause or denture status (Z97.2)

K06.3 Horizontal alveolar bone loss

K06.8 Other specified disorders of gingiva and edentulous alveolar ridge
Fibrous epulis
Flabby alveolar ridge
Giant cell epulis
Peripheral giant cell granuloma of gingiva
Pyogenic granuloma of gingiva
Vertical ridge deficiency
EXCLUDES 2 *gingival cyst (K09.0)*

K06.9 Disorder of gingiva and edentulous alveolar ridge, unspecified

K08 Other disorders of teeth and supporting structures
EXCLUDES 2 *dentofacial anomalies [including malocclusion] (M26.-)*
disorders of jaw (M27.-)
AHA: 2016,4Q,29-30

K08.0 Exfoliation of teeth due to systemic causes
Code also underlying systemic condition

K08.1 Complete loss of teeth
Acquired loss of teeth, complete
EXCLUDES 1 *congenital absence of teeth (K00.0)*
exfoliation of teeth due to systemic causes (K08.0)
partial loss of teeth (K08.4-)

K08.10 Complete loss of teeth, unspecified cause

K08.101 Complete loss of teeth, unspecified cause, class I

K08.102 Complete loss of teeth, unspecified cause, class II

K08.103 Complete loss of teeth, unspecified cause, class III

K08.104 Complete loss of teeth, unspecified cause, class IV

K08.109 Complete loss of teeth, unspecified cause, unspecified class
Edentulism NOS

K08.11 Complete loss of teeth due to trauma

K08.111 Complete loss of teeth due to trauma, class I

K08.112 Complete loss of teeth due to trauma, class II

K08.113 Complete loss of teeth due to trauma, class III

K08.114 Complete loss of teeth due to trauma, class IV

K08.119 Complete loss of teeth due to trauma, unspecified class

K08.12 Complete loss of teeth due to periodontal diseases

K08.121 Complete loss of teeth due to periodontal diseases, class I

K08.122 Complete loss of teeth due to periodontal diseases, class II

K08.123 Complete loss of teeth due to periodontal diseases, class III

K08.124 Complete loss of teeth due to periodontal diseases, class IV

K08.129 Complete loss of teeth due to periodontal diseases, unspecified class

K08.13 Complete loss of teeth due to caries

K08.131 Complete loss of teeth due to caries, class I

K08.132 Complete loss of teeth due to caries, class II

K08.133 Complete loss of teeth due to caries, class III

K08.134 Complete loss of teeth due to caries, class IV

K08.139 Complete loss of teeth due to caries, unspecified class

K08.19 Complete loss of teeth due to other specified cause

K08.191 Complete loss of teeth due to other specified cause, class I

K08.192 Complete loss of teeth due to other specified cause, class II

K08.193 Complete loss of teeth due to other specified cause, class III

K08.194 Complete loss of teeth due to other specified cause, class IV

K08.199 Complete loss of teeth due to other specified cause, unspecified class

K08.2 Atrophy of edentulous alveolar ridge

K08.20 Unspecified atrophy of edentulous alveolar ridge
Atrophy of the mandible NOS
Atrophy of the maxilla NOS

K08.21 Minimal atrophy of the mandible
Minimal atrophy of the edentulous mandible

K08.22 Moderate atrophy of the mandible
Moderate atrophy of the edentulous mandible

K08.23 Severe atrophy of the mandible
Severe atrophy of the edentulous mandible

K08.24 Minimal atrophy of maxilla
Minimal atrophy of the edentulous maxilla

K08.25 Moderate atrophy of the maxilla
Moderate atrophy of the edentulous maxilla

K08.26 Severe atrophy of the maxilla
Severe atrophy of the edentulous maxilla

K08.3 Retained dental root

K08.4 Partial loss of teeth
Acquired loss of teeth, partial
EXCLUDES 1 *complete loss of teeth (K08.1-)*
congenital absence of teeth (K00.0)
EXCLUDES 2 *exfoliation of teeth due to systemic causes (K08.0)*

K08.40 Partial loss of teeth, unspecified cause
K08.401 Partial loss of teeth, unspecified cause, class I
K08.402 Partial loss of teeth, unspecified cause, class II
K08.403 Partial loss of teeth, unspecified cause, class III
K08.404 Partial loss of teeth, unspecified cause, class IV
K08.409 Partial loss of teeth, unspecified cause, unspecified class
Tooth extraction status NOS

K08.41 Partial loss of teeth due to trauma
K08.411 Partial loss of teeth due to trauma, class I
K08.412 Partial loss of teeth due to trauma, class II
K08.413 Partial loss of teeth due to trauma, class III
K08.414 Partial loss of teeth due to trauma, class IV
K08.419 Partial loss of teeth due to trauma, unspecified class

K08.42 Partial loss of teeth due to periodontal diseases
K08.421 Partial loss of teeth due to periodontal diseases, class I
K08.422 Partial loss of teeth due to periodontal diseases, class II
K08.423 Partial loss of teeth due to periodontal diseases, class III
K08.424 Partial loss of teeth due to periodontal diseases, class IV
K08.429 Partial loss of teeth due to periodontal diseases, unspecified class

K08.43 Partial loss of teeth due to caries
K08.431 Partial loss of teeth due to caries, class I
K08.432 Partial loss of teeth due to caries, class II
K08.433 Partial loss of teeth due to caries, class III
K08.434 Partial loss of teeth due to caries, class IV
K08.439 Partial loss of teeth due to caries, unspecified class

K08.49 Partial loss of teeth due to other specified cause
K08.491 Partial loss of teeth due to other specified cause, class I
K08.492 Partial loss of teeth due to other specified cause, class II
K08.493 Partial loss of teeth due to other specified cause, class III
K08.494 Partial loss of teeth due to other specified cause, class IV
K08.499 Partial loss of teeth due to other specified cause, unspecified class

K08.5 Unsatisfactory restoration of tooth
Defective bridge, crown, filling
Defective dental restoration
EXCLUDES 1 *dental restoration status (Z98.811)*
EXCLUDES 2 *endosseous dental implant failure (M27.6-)*
unsatisfactory endodontic treatment (M27.5-)

K08.50 Unsatisfactory restoration of tooth, unspecified
Defective dental restoration NOS

K08.51 Open restoration margins of tooth
Dental restoration failure of marginal integrity
Open margin on tooth restoration
Poor gingival margin to tooth restoration

K08.52 Unrepairable overhanging of dental restorative materials
Overhanging of tooth restoration

K08.53 Fractured dental restorative material
EXCLUDES 1 *cracked tooth (K03.81)*
traumatic fracture of tooth (S02.5)
K08.530 Fractured dental restorative material without loss of material
K08.531 Fractured dental restorative material with loss of material
K08.539 Fractured dental restorative material, unspecified

K08.54 Contour of existing restoration of tooth biologically incompatible with oral health
Dental restoration failure of periodontal anatomical integrity
Unacceptable contours of existing restoration of tooth
Unacceptable morphology of existing restoration of tooth

K08.55 Allergy to existing dental restorative material
Use additional code to identify the specific type of allergy

K08.56 Poor aesthetic of existing restoration of tooth
Dental restoration aesthetically inadequate or displeasing

K08.59 Other unsatisfactory restoration of tooth
Other defective dental restoration

K08.8 Other specified disorders of teeth and supporting structures
K08.81 Primary occlusal trauma
K08.82 Secondary occlusal trauma
K08.89 Other specified disorders of teeth and supporting structures
Enlargement of alveolar ridge NOS
Insufficient anatomic crown height
Insufficient clinical crown length
Irregular alveolar process
Toothache NOS

K08.9 Disorder of teeth and supporting structures, unspecified

K09 Cysts of oral region, not elsewhere classified
INCLUDES lesions showing histological features both of aneurysmal cyst and of another fibro-osseous lesion
EXCLUDES 2 *cysts of jaw (M27.0-, M27.4-)*
radicular cyst (K04.8)

K09.0 Developmental odontogenic cysts
Dentigerous cyst
Eruption cyst
Follicular cyst
Gingival cyst
Lateral periodontal cyst
Primordial cyst
EXCLUDES 2 *keratocysts (D16.4, D16.5)*
odontogenic keratocystic tumors (D16.4, D16.5)

K09.1 Developmental (nonodontogenic) cysts of oral region
Cyst (of) incisive canal
Cyst (of) palatine of papilla
Globulomaxillary cyst
Median palatal cyst
Nasoalveolar cyst
Nasolabial cyst
Nasopalatine duct cyst

K09.8 Other cysts of oral region, not elsewhere classified
Dermoid cyst
Epidermoid cyst
Lymphoepithelial cyst
Epstein's pearl

K09.9 Cyst of oral region, unspecified

K11 Diseases of salivary glands
Use additional code to identify:
alcohol abuse and dependence (F10.-)
exposure to environmental tobacco smoke (Z77.22)
exposure to tobacco smoke in the perinatal period (P96.81)
history of tobacco dependence (Z87.891)
occupational exposure to environmental tobacco smoke (Z57.31)
tobacco dependence (F17.-)
tobacco use (Z72.0)

K11.0 Atrophy of salivary gland
K11.1 Hypertrophy of salivary gland
DEF: Overgrowth of or enlarged salivary gland tissue caused by infection, salivary duct blockage, autoimmune diseases, and benign and malignant tumors.

K11.2 Sialoadenitis
Parotitis
EXCLUDES 1 *epidemic parotitis (B26.-)*
mumps (B26.-)
uveoparotid fever [Heerfordt] (D86.89)
DEF: Inflammation of the salivary gland.
K11.20 Sialoadenitis, unspecified

K11.21 Acute sialoadenitis
EXCLUDES 1 *acute recurrent sialoadenitis (K11.22)*

K11.22 Acute recurrent sialoadenitis

K11.23 Chronic sialoadenitis

K11.3 Abscess of salivary gland CC

K11.4 Fistula of salivary gland CC
EXCLUDES 1 *congenital fistula of salivary gland (Q38.4)*

K11.5 Sialolithiasis
Calculus of salivary gland or duct
Stone of salivary gland or duct

K11.6 Mucocele of salivary gland
Mucous extravasation cyst of salivary gland
Mucous retention cyst of salivary gland
Ranula

K11.7 Disturbances of salivary secretion
Hypoptyalism
Ptyalism
Xerostomia
EXCLUDES 2 *dry mouth NOS (R68.2)*

K11.8 Other diseases of salivary glands
Benign lymphoepithelial lesion of salivary gland
Mikulicz' disease
Necrotizing sialometaplasia
Sialectasia
Stenosis of salivary duct
Stricture of salivary duct
EXCLUDES 1 *Sjögren syndrome (M35.Ø-)*

K11.9 Disease of salivary gland, unspecified
Sialoadenopathy NOS

✓4th K12 Stomatitis and related lesions
Use additional code to identify:
alcohol abuse and dependence (F1Ø.-)
exposure to environmental tobacco smoke (Z77.22)
exposure to tobacco smoke in the perinatal period (P96.81)
history of tobacco dependence (Z87.891)
occupational exposure to environmental tobacco smoke (Z57.31)
tobacco dependence (F17.-)
tobacco use (Z72.Ø)
EXCLUDES 1 *cancrum oris (A69.Ø)*
cheilitis (K13.Ø)
gangrenous stomatitis (A69.Ø)
herpesviral [herpes simplex] gingivostomatitis (BØØ.2)
noma (A69.Ø)

K12.Ø Recurrent oral aphthae
Aphthous stomatitis (major) (minor)
Bednar's aphthae
Periadenitis mucosa necrotica recurrens
Recurrent aphthous ulcer
Stomatitis herpetiformis
DEF: Disorder of unknown etiology with small oval or round painful ulcers of the mouth marked by a grayish exudate and a red halo effect.

K12.1 Other forms of stomatitis
Stomatitis NOS
Denture stomatitis
Ulcerative stomatitis
Vesicular stomatitis
EXCLUDES 1 *acute necrotizing ulcerative stomatitis (A69.1)*
Vincent's stomatitis (A69.1)

K12.2 Cellulitis and abscess of mouth CC
Cellulitis of mouth (floor)
Submandibular abscess
EXCLUDES 2 *abscess of salivary gland (K11.3)*
abscess of tongue (K14.Ø)
periapical abscess (KØ4.6-KØ4.7)
periodontal abscess (KØ5.21)
peritonsillar abscess (J36)

✓5th K12.3 Oral mucositis (ulcerative)
Mucositis (oral) (oropharyneal)
EXCLUDES 2 *gastrointestinal mucositis (ulcerative) (K92.81)*
mucositis (ulcerative) of vagina and vulva (N76.81)
nasal mucositis (ulcerative) (J34.81)

K12.3Ø Oral mucositis (ulcerative), unspecified

K12.31 Oral mucositis (ulcerative) due to antineoplastic therapy
Use additional code for adverse effect, if applicable, to identify antineoplastic and immunosuppressive drugs (T45.1X5)
Use additional code for other antineoplastic therapy, such as:
radiological procedure and radiotherapy (Y84.2)

K12.32 Oral mucositis (ulcerative) due to other drugs
Use additional code for adverse effect, if applicable, to identify drug (T36-T5Ø with fifth or sixth character 5)

K12.33 Oral mucositis (ulcerative) due to radiation
Use additional external cause code (W88-W9Ø, X39.Ø-) to identify cause

K12.39 Other oral mucositis (ulcerative)
Viral oral mucositis (ulcerative)

✓4th K13 Other diseases of lip and oral mucosa
INCLUDES epithelial disturbances of tongue
Use additional code to identify:
alcohol abuse and dependence (F1Ø.-)
exposure to environmental tobacco smoke (Z77.22)
exposure to tobacco smoke in the perinatal period (P96.81)
history of tobacco dependence (Z87.891)
occupational exposure to environmental tobacco smoke (Z57.31)
tobacco dependence (F17.-)
tobacco use (Z72.Ø)
EXCLUDES 2 *certain disorders of gingiva and edentulous alveolar ridge (KØ5-KØ6)*
cysts of oral region (KØ9.-)
diseases of tongue (K14.-)
stomatitis and related lesions (K12.-)

K13.Ø Diseases of lips
Abscess of lips
Angular cheilitis
Cellulitis of lips
Cheilitis NOS
Cheilodynia
Cheilosis
Exfoliative cheilitis
Fistula of lips
Glandular cheilitis
Hypertrophy of lips
Perlèche NEC
EXCLUDES 1 *ariboflavinosis (E53.Ø)*
cheilitis due to radiation-related disorders (L55-L59)
congenital fistula of lips (Q38.Ø)
congenital hypertrophy of lips (Q18.6)
perlèche due to candidiasis (B37.83)
perlèche due to riboflavin deficiency (E53.Ø)

K13.1 Cheek and lip biting

✓5th K13.2 Leukoplakia and other disturbances of oral epithelium, including tongue
EXCLUDES 1 *carcinoma in situ of oral epithelium (DØØ.Ø-)*
hairy leukoplakia (K13.3)
DEF: Leukoplakia: Thickened white patches or lesions appearing on a mucous membrane, such as oral mucosa or tongue.

K13.21 Leukoplakia of oral mucosa, including tongue
Leukokeratosis of oral mucosa
Leukoplakia of gingiva, lips, tongue
EXCLUDES 1 *hairy leukoplakia (K13.3)*
leukokeratosis nicotina palati (K13.24)

K13.22 Minimal keratinized residual ridge mucosa
Minimal keratinization of alveolar ridge mucosa

K13.23 Excessive keratinized residual ridge mucosa
Excessive keratinization of alveolar ridge mucosa

K13.24 Leukokeratosis nicotina palati
Smoker's palate

K13.29 Other disturbances of oral epithelium, including tongue
Erythroplakia of mouth or tongue
Focal epithelial hyperplasia of mouth or tongue
Leukoedema of mouth or tongue
Other oral epithelium disturbances

K13.3 Hairy leukoplakia

K13.4 Granuloma and granuloma-like lesions of oral mucosa
Eosinophilic granuloma
Granuloma pyogenicum
Verrucous xanthoma

K13.5 Oral submucous fibrosis
Submucous fibrosis of tongue

K13.6 Irritative hyperplasia of oral mucosa
EXCLUDES 2 *irritative hyperplasia of edentulous ridge [denture hyperplasia] (KØ6.2)*

K13.7 Other and unspecified lesions of oral mucosa

K13.7Ø Unspecified lesions of oral mucosa

K13.79 Other lesions of oral mucosa
Focal oral mucinosis
AHA: 2022,2Q,7

K14 Diseases of tongue
Use additional code to identify:
alcohol abuse and dependence (F1Ø.-)
exposure to environmental tobacco smoke (Z77.22)
history of tobacco dependence (Z87.891)
occupational exposure to environmental tobacco smoke (Z57.31)
tobacco dependence (F17.-)
tobacco use (Z72.Ø)
EXCLUDES 2 *erythroplakia (K13.29)*
focal epithelial hyperplasia (K13.29)
leukedema of tongue (K13.29)
leukoplakia of tongue (K13.21)
hairy leukoplakia (K13.3)
macroglossia (congenital) (Q38.2)
submucous fibrosis of tongue (K13.5)

K14.Ø Glossitis
Abscess of tongue
Ulceration (traumatic) of tongue
EXCLUDES 1 *atrophic glossitis (K14.4)*
DEF: Inflammation and swelling of the tongue that may be associated with infection, adverse drug reactions, smoking, or injury.

K14.1 Geographic tongue
Benign migratory glossitis
Glossitis areata exfoliativa

K14.2 Median rhomboid glossitis

K14.3 Hypertrophy of tongue papillae
Black hairy tongue
Coated tongue
Hypertrophy of foliate papillae
Lingua villosa nigra

K14.4 Atrophy of tongue papillae
Atrophic glossitis

K14.5 Plicated tongue
Fissured tongue
Furrowed tongue
Scrotal tongue
EXCLUDES 1 *fissured tongue, congenital (Q38.3)*

K14.6 Glossodynia
Glossopyrosis
Painful tongue

K14.8 Other diseases of tongue
Atrophy of tongue
Crenated tongue
Enlargement of tongue
Glossocele
Glossoptosis
Hypertrophy of tongue

K14.9 Disease of tongue, unspecified
Glossopathy NOS

Diseases of esophagus, stomach and duodenum (K2Ø-K31)

EXCLUDES 2 *hiatus hernia (K44.-)*

K2Ø Esophagitis
Use additional code to identify:
alcohol abuse and dependence (F1Ø.-)
EXCLUDES 1 *erosion of esophagus (K22.1-)*
esophagitis with gastro-esophageal reflux disease (K21.Ø-)
reflux esophagitis (K21.Ø-)
ulcerative esophagitis (K22.1-)
EXCLUDES 2 *eosinophilic gastritis or gastroenteritis (K52.81)*

K2Ø.Ø Eosinophilic esophagitis
AHA: 2020,4Q,9

K2Ø.8 Other esophagitis
AHA: 2020,4Q,28-29

K2Ø.8Ø Other esophagitis without bleeding
Abscess of esophagus
Other esophagitis NOS

K2Ø.81 Other esophagitis with bleeding MCC

K2Ø.9 Esophagitis, unspecified
AHA: 2020,4Q,28-29

K2Ø.9Ø Esophagitis, unspecified without bleeding
Esophagitis NOS

K2Ø.91 Esophagitis, unspecified with bleeding MCC

K21 Gastro-esophageal reflux disease
EXCLUDES 1 *newborn esophageal reflux (P78.83)*

K21.Ø Gastro-esophageal reflux disease with esophagitis
AHA: 2020,4Q,28-29

K21.ØØ Gastro-esophageal reflux disease with esophagitis, without bleeding
Reflux esophagitis

K21.Ø1 Gastro-esophageal reflux disease with esophagitis, with bleeding MCC

K21.9 Gastro-esophageal reflux disease without esophagitis
Esophageal reflux NOS
AHA: 2016,1Q,18

K22 Other diseases of esophagus
EXCLUDES 2 *esophageal varices (I85.-)*

K22.Ø Achalasia of cardia
Achalasia NOS
Cardiospasm
EXCLUDES 1 *congenital cardiospasm (Q39.5)*
DEF: Esophageal motility disorder that is caused by absence of the esophageal peristalsis and impaired relaxation of the lower esophageal sphincter. It is characterized by dysphagia, regurgitation, and heartburn.

K22.1 Ulcer of esophagus
Barrett's ulcer
Erosion of esophagus
Fungal ulcer of esophagus
Peptic ulcer of esophagus
Ulcer of esophagus due to ingestion of chemicals
Ulcer of esophagus due to ingestion of drugs and medicaments
Ulcerative esophagitis
Code first poisoning due to drug or toxin, if applicable (T36-T65 with fifth or sixth character 1-4 or 6)
Use additional code for adverse effect, if applicable, to identify drug (T36-T5Ø with fifth or sixth character 5)
EXCLUDES 1 *Barrett's esophagus (K22.7-)*
AHA: 2018,3Q,22; 2017,3Q,27
TIP: Assign a code for "with bleeding" when an esophageal ulcer and bleeding (hematemesis) are documented. The ICD-10-CM classification assumes the two are related without the provider linking the two conditions. Evidence of bleeding during a procedure is not required.

K22.1Ø Ulcer of esophagus without bleeding CC
Ulcer of esophagus NOS

K22.11 Ulcer of esophagus with bleeding MCC
EXCLUDES 2 *bleeding esophageal varices (I85.Ø1, I85.11)*
TIP: For bleeding esophageal ulcers resulting from anticoagulant therapy, assign this code, code D68.32 Hemorrhagic disorder due to extrinsic circulating anticoagulant, and adverse effect code T45.515- with the appropriate seventh character. Either code K22.11 or D68.32 may be sequenced first, depending on the circumstances of admission.

K22.2 Esophageal obstruction
Compression of esophagus
Constriction of esophagus
Stenosis of esophagus
Stricture of esophagus
EXCLUDES 1 *congenital stenosis or stricture of esophagus (Q39.3)*

K22.3 Perforation of esophagus MCC
Rupture of esophagus
EXCLUDES 1 *traumatic perforation of (thoracic) esophagus (S27.8-)*

K22.4 Dyskinesia of esophagus
Corkscrew esophagus
Diffuse esophageal spasm
Spasm of esophagus
EXCLUDES 1 *cardiospasm (K22.Ø)*

K22.5 Diverticulum of esophagus, acquired
Esophageal pouch, acquired
EXCLUDES 1 *diverticulum of esophagus (congenital) (Q39.6)*

K22.6 Gastro-esophageal laceration-hemorrhage syndrome MCC
Mallory-Weiss syndrome

5th **K22.7 Barrett's esophagus**
Barrett's disease
Barrett's syndrome
EXCLUDES 1 *Barrett's ulcer (K22.1)*
malignant neoplasm of esophagus (C15.-)
DEF: Metaplastic disorder in which specialized columnar epithelial cells replace the normal squamous epithelial cells. Secondary to chronic gastroesophageal reflux damage to the mucosa, this disorder increases the risk of developing adenocarcinoma.

K22.7Ø Barrett's esophagus without dysplasia
Barrett's esophagus NOS

6th **K22.71 Barrett's esophagus with dysplasia**

K22.71Ø Barrett's esophagus with low grade dysplasia

K22.711 Barrett's esophagus with high grade dysplasia

K22.719 Barrett's esophagus with dysplasia, unspecified

5th **K22.8 Other specified diseases of esophagus**
EXCLUDES 2 *esophageal varices (I85.-)*
Paterson-Kelly syndrome (D5Ø.1)
AHA: 2021,4Q,15; 2020,1Q,16

K22.81 Esophageal polyp
EXCLUDES 1 *benign neoplasm of esophagus (D13.Ø)*

K22.82 Esophagogastric junction polyp
EXCLUDES 1 *benign neoplasm of stomach (D13.1)*

K22.89 Other specified disease of esophagus
Hemorrhage of esophagus NOS

K22.9 Disease of esophagus, unspecified

K23 Disorders of esophagus in diseases classified elsewhere
Code first underlying disease, such as:
congenital syphilis (A5Ø.5)
EXCLUDES 1 *late syphilis (A52.79)*
megaesophagus due to Chagas' disease (B57.31)
tuberculosis (A18.83)

4th **K25 Gastric ulcer**
INCLUDES erosion (acute) of stomach
pylorus ulcer (peptic)
stomach ulcer (peptic)
Use additional code to identify:
alcohol abuse and dependence (F1Ø.-)
EXCLUDES 1 *acute gastritis (K29.Ø-)*
peptic ulcer NOS (K27.-)
AHA: 2021,1Q,9,11; 2017,3Q,27
TIP: Assign a code for "with hemorrhage" when a gastric ulcer and GI bleeding are documented. The ICD-10-CM classification assumes the two are related without the provider linking the two conditions. Evidence of bleeding during a procedure is not required.
TIP: For bleeding ulcers resulting from anticoagulant therapy, assign the appropriate "with hemorrhage" ulcer code from this category, code D68.32 Hemorrhagic disorder due to extrinsic circulating anticoagulant, and adverse effect code T45.515- with the appropriate seventh character. Either the bleeding ulcer code or code D68.32 may be sequenced first, depending on the circumstances of admission.

K25.Ø Acute gastric ulcer with hemorrhage MCC
K25.1 Acute gastric ulcer with perforation MCC HCC
K25.2 Acute gastric ulcer with both hemorrhage and perforation MCC HCC
K25.3 Acute gastric ulcer without hemorrhage or perforation CC
K25.4 Chronic or unspecified gastric ulcer with hemorrhage MCC
K25.5 Chronic or unspecified gastric ulcer with perforation MCC HCC
K25.6 Chronic or unspecified gastric ulcer with both hemorrhage and perforation MCC HCC
K25.7 Chronic gastric ulcer without hemorrhage or perforation
K25.9 Gastric ulcer, unspecified as acute or chronic, without hemorrhage or perforation

Gastrointestinal Ulcers

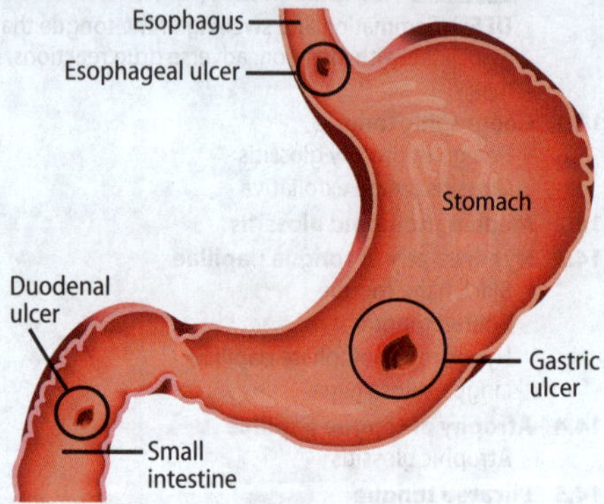

4th **K26 Duodenal ulcer**
INCLUDES erosion (acute) of duodenum
duodenum ulcer (peptic)
postpyloric ulcer (peptic)
Use additional code to identify:
alcohol abuse and dependence (F1Ø.-)
EXCLUDES 1 *peptic ulcer NOS (K27.-)*
AHA: 2017,3Q,27
TIP: Assign a code for "with hemorrhage" when a duodenal ulcer and GI bleeding are documented. The ICD-10-CM classification assumes the two are related without the provider linking the two conditions. Evidence of bleeding during a procedure is not required.
TIP: For bleeding ulcers resulting from anticoagulant therapy, assign the appropriate "with hemorrhage" ulcer code from this category, code D68.32 Hemorrhagic disorder due to extrinsic circulating anticoagulant, and adverse effect code T45.515- with the appropriate seventh character. Either the bleeding ulcer code or code D68.32 may be sequenced first, depending on the circumstances of admission.

K26.Ø Acute duodenal ulcer with hemorrhage MCC
K26.1 Acute duodenal ulcer with perforation MCC HCC
K26.2 Acute duodenal ulcer with both hemorrhage and perforation MCC HCC
K26.3 Acute duodenal ulcer without hemorrhage or perforation CC
K26.4 Chronic or unspecified duodenal ulcer with hemorrhage MCC
AHA: 2016,1Q,14

K26.5 Chronic or unspecified duodenal ulcer with perforation MCC HCC

K26.6 Chronic or unspecified duodenal ulcer with both hemorrhage and perforation MCC HCC

K26.7 Chronic duodenal ulcer without hemorrhage or perforation

K26.9 Duodenal ulcer, unspecified as acute or chronic, without hemorrhage or perforation

✓4th K27 Peptic ulcer, site unspecified

INCLUDES gastroduodenal ulcer NOS
peptic ulcer NOS

Use additional code to identify:
alcohol abuse and dependence (F1Ø.-)

EXCLUDES 1 *peptic ulcer of newborn (P78.82)*

AHA: 2017,3Q,27

TIP: Assign a code for "with hemorrhage" when a peptic ulcer and GI bleeding are documented. The ICD-10-CM classification assumes the two are related without the provider linking the two conditions. Evidence of bleeding during a procedure is not required.

TIP: For bleeding ulcers resulting from anticoagulant therapy, assign the appropriate "with hemorrhage" ulcer code from this category, code D68.32 Hemorrhagic disorder due to extrinsic circulating anticoagulant, and adverse effect code T45.515- with the appropriate seventh character. Either the bleeding ulcer code or code D68.32 may be sequenced first, depending on the circumstances of admission.

K27.Ø Acute peptic ulcer, site unspecified, with hemorrhage MCC

K27.1 Acute peptic ulcer, site unspecified, with perforation MCC HCC

K27.2 Acute peptic ulcer, site unspecified, with both hemorrhage and perforation MCC HCC

K27.3 Acute peptic ulcer, site unspecified, without hemorrhage or perforation CC

K27.4 Chronic or unspecified peptic ulcer, site unspecified, with hemorrhage MCC

K27.5 Chronic or unspecified peptic ulcer, site unspecified, with perforation MCC HCC

K27.6 Chronic or unspecified peptic ulcer, site unspecified, with both hemorrhage and perforation MCC HCC

K27.7 Chronic peptic ulcer, site unspecified, without hemorrhage or perforation

K27.9 Peptic ulcer, site unspecified, unspecified as acute or chronic, without hemorrhage or perforation

✓4th K28 Gastrojejunal ulcer

INCLUDES anastomotic ulcer (peptic) or erosion
gastrocolic ulcer (peptic) or erosion
gastrointestinal ulcer (peptic) or erosion
gastrojejunal ulcer (peptic) or erosion
jejunal ulcer (peptic) or erosion
marginal ulcer (peptic) or erosion
stomal ulcer (peptic) or erosion

Use additional code to identify:
alcohol abuse and dependence (F1Ø.-)

EXCLUDES 1 *primary ulcer of small intestine (K63.3)*

AHA: 2017,3Q,27

TIP: Assign a code for "with hemorrhage" when a gastrojejunal ulcer and GI bleeding are documented. The ICD-10-CM classification assumes the two are related without the provider linking the two conditions. Evidence of bleeding during a procedure is not required.

TIP: For bleeding ulcers resulting from anticoagulant therapy, assign the appropriate "with hemorrhage" ulcer code from this category, code D68.32 Hemorrhagic disorder due to extrinsic circulating anticoagulant, and adverse effect code T45.515- with the appropriate seventh character. Either the bleeding ulcer code or code D68.32 may be sequenced first, depending on the circumstances of admission.

K28.Ø Acute gastrojejunal ulcer with hemorrhage MCC

K28.1 Acute gastrojejunal ulcer with perforation MCC HCC

K28.2 Acute gastrojejunal ulcer with both hemorrhage and perforation MCC HCC

K28.3 Acute gastrojejunal ulcer without hemorrhage or perforation CC

K28.4 Chronic or unspecified gastrojejunal ulcer with hemorrhage MCC

K28.5 Chronic or unspecified gastrojejunal ulcer with perforation MCC HCC

K28.6 Chronic or unspecified gastrojejunal ulcer with both hemorrhage and perforation MCC HCC

K28.7 Chronic gastrojejunal ulcer without hemorrhage or perforation

K28.9 Gastrojejunal ulcer, unspecified as acute or chronic, without hemorrhage or perforation

✓4th K29 Gastritis and duodenitis

EXCLUDES 1 *eosinophilic gastritis or gastroenteritis (K52.81)*
Zollinger-Ellison syndrome (E16.4)

AHA: 2018,3Q,22

TIP: Assign a code for "with bleeding" when gastritis or duodenitis and GI bleeding are documented. The ICD-10-CM classification assumes the two are related without the provider linking the two conditions. Evidence of bleeding during a procedure is not required.

TIP: For bleeding ulcers resulting from anticoagulant therapy, assign the appropriate "with hemorrhage" ulcer code from this category, code D68.32 Hemorrhagic disorder due to extrinsic circulating anticoagulant, and adverse effect code T45.515- with the appropriate seventh character. Either the bleeding ulcer code or code D68.32 may be sequenced first, depending on the circumstances of admission.

✓5th K29.Ø Acute gastritis

Use additional code to identify:
alcohol abuse and dependence (F1Ø.-)

EXCLUDES 1 *erosion (acute) of stomach (K25.-)*

K29.ØØ Acute gastritis without bleeding

K29.Ø1 Acute gastritis with bleeding MCC

✓5th K29.2 Alcoholic gastritis

Use additional code to identify:
alcohol abuse and dependence (F1Ø.-)

K29.2Ø Alcoholic gastritis without bleeding

K29.21 Alcoholic gastritis with bleeding MCC

✓5th K29.3 Chronic superficial gastritis

K29.3Ø Chronic superficial gastritis without bleeding

K29.31 Chronic superficial gastritis with bleeding MCC

✓5th K29.4 Chronic atrophic gastritis

Gastric atrophy

K29.4Ø Chronic atrophic gastritis without bleeding

K29.41 Chronic atrophic gastritis with bleeding MCC

✓5th K29.5 Unspecified chronic gastritis

Chronic antral gastritis
Chronic fundal gastritis

K29.5Ø Unspecified chronic gastritis without bleeding

K29.51 Unspecified chronic gastritis with bleeding MCC

✓5th K29.6 Other gastritis

Giant hypertrophic gastritis
Granulomatous gastritis
Ménétrier's disease

K29.6Ø Other gastritis without bleeding

K29.61 Other gastritis with bleeding MCC

✓5th K29.7 Gastritis, unspecified

K29.7Ø Gastritis, unspecified, without bleeding

K29.71 Gastritis, unspecified, with bleeding MCC

✓5th K29.8 Duodenitis

K29.8Ø Duodenitis without bleeding

K29.81 Duodenitis with bleeding MCC

✓5th K29.9 Gastroduodenitis, unspecified

K29.9Ø Gastroduodenitis, unspecified, without bleeding

K29.91 Gastroduodenitis, unspecified, with bleeding MCC

K3Ø Functional dyspepsia

Indigestion

EXCLUDES 1 *dyspepsia NOS (R1Ø.13)*
heartburn (R12)
nervous dyspepsia (F45.8)
neurotic dyspepsia (F45.8)
psychogenic dyspepsia (F45.8)

✓4th K31 Other diseases of stomach and duodenum

INCLUDES functional disorders of stomach

EXCLUDES 2 *diabetic gastroparesis (EØ8.43, EØ9.43, E1Ø.43, E11.43, E13.43)*
diverticulum of duodenum (K57.ØØ-K57.13)

K31.Ø Acute dilatation of stomach CC

Acute distention of stomach

K31.1 Adult hypertrophic pyloric stenosis CC A

Pyloric stenosis NOS

EXCLUDES 1 *congenital or infantile pyloric stenosis (Q4Ø.Ø)*

K31.2 Hourglass stricture and stenosis of stomach

EXCLUDES 1 *congenital hourglass stomach (Q4Ø.2)*
hourglass contraction of stomach (K31.89)

K31.3 Pylorospasm, not elsewhere classified
EXCLUDES 1 *congenital or infantile pylorospasm (Q40.0)*
neurotic pylorospasm (F45.8)
psychogenic pylorospasm (F45.8)

K31.4 Gastric diverticulum
EXCLUDES 1 *congenital diverticulum of stomach (Q40.2)*

K31.5 Obstruction of duodenum CC
Constriction of duodenum
Duodenal ileus (chronic)
Stenosis of duodenum
Stricture of duodenum
Volvulus of duodenum
EXCLUDES 1 *congenital stenosis of duodenum (Q41.0)*

K31.6 Fistula of stomach and duodenum CC
Gastrocolic fistula
Gastrojejunocolic fistula

K31.7 Polyp of stomach and duodenum
EXCLUDES 1 *adenomatous polyp of stomach (D13.1)*
AHA: 2020,1Q,16

5th **K31.8 Other specified diseases of stomach and duodenum**

6th **K31.81 Angiodysplasia of stomach and duodenum**
TIP: Assign a code for "with bleeding" when angiodysplasia of the stomach or the duodenum and GI bleeding are documented. The ICD-10-CM classification assumes the two are related without the provider linking the two conditions. Evidence of bleeding during a procedure is not required.

K31.811 Angiodysplasia of stomach and duodenum with bleeding MCC

K31.819 Angiodysplasia of stomach and duodenum without bleeding
Angiodysplasia of stomach and duodenum NOS

K31.82 Dieulafoy lesion (hemorrhagic) of stomach and duodenum MCC
EXCLUDES 2 *Dieulafoy lesion of intestine (K63.81)*
DEF: Abnormally large submucosal artery protruding through a defect in the stomach mucosa or intestines that can cause massive and life-threatening hemorrhaging.

K31.83 Achlorhydria
DEF: Absence of hydrochloric acid in gastric secretions due to gastric mucosa atrophy. Achlorhydria is unresponsive to histamines.

K31.84 Gastroparesis
Gastroparalysis
Code first underlying disease, if known, such as:
anorexia nervosa (F50.0-)
diabetes mellitus (E08.43, E09.43, E10.43, E11.43, E13.43)
scleroderma (M34.-)
AHA: 2013,4Q,114

K31.89 Other diseases of stomach and duodenum
AHA: 2020,1Q,15; 2017,1Q,28

UNS **K31.9 Disease of stomach and duodenum, unspecified**

5th **K31.A Gastric intestinal metaplasia**
AHA: 2021,4Q,15-16

UNS **K31.A0 Gastric intestinal metaplasia, unspecified**
Gastric intestinal metaplasia indefinite for dysplasia
Gastric intestinal metaplasia NOS

6th **K31.A1 Gastric intestinal metaplasia without dysplasia**

K31.A11 Gastric intestinal metaplasia without dysplasia, involving the antrum

K31.A12 Gastric intestinal metaplasia without dysplasia, involving the body (corpus)

K31.A13 Gastric intestinal metaplasia without dysplasia, involving the fundus

K31.A14 Gastric intestinal metaplasia without dysplasia, involving the cardia

K31.A15 Gastric intestinal metaplasia without dysplasia, involving multiple sites

UNS **K31.A19 Gastric intestinal metaplasia without dysplasia, unspecified site**

6th **K31.A2 Gastric intestinal metaplasia with dysplasia**

K31.A21 Gastric intestinal metaplasia with low grade dysplasia

K31.A22 Gastric intestinal metaplasia with high grade dysplasia

UNS **K31.A29 Gastric intestinal metaplasia with dysplasia, unspecified**

Diseases of appendix (K35-K38)

4th **K35 Acute appendicitis**
AHA: 2018,4Q,17-18

5th **K35.2 Acute appendicitis with generalized peritonitis**
Appendicitis (acute) with generalized (diffuse) peritonitis following rupture or perforation of appendix

K35.20 Acute appendicitis with generalized peritonitis, without abscess CC
(Acute) appendicitis with generalized peritonitis NOS

K35.21 Acute appendicitis with generalized peritonitis, with abscess MCC

5th **K35.3 Acute appendicitis with localized peritonitis**

K35.30 Acute appendicitis with localized peritonitis, without perforation or gangrene CC
Acute appendicitis with localized peritonitis NOS

K35.31 Acute appendicitis with localized peritonitis and gangrene, without perforation CC

▲ **K35.32 Acute appendicitis with perforation, localized peritonitis, and gangrene, without abscess** MCC
(Acute) appendicitis with perforation NOS
Perforated appendix NOS
Ruptured appendix (with localized peritonitis) NOS
AHA: 2020,1Q,16

▲ **K35.33 Acute appendicitis with perforation, localized peritonitis, and gangrene, with abscess** MCC
(Acute) appendicitis with (peritoneal) abscess NOS
Ruptured appendix with localized peritonitis and abscess

5th **K35.8 Other and unspecified acute appendicitis**

UNS **K35.80 Unspecified acute appendicitis** CC
Acute appendicitis NOS
Acute appendicitis without (localized) (generalized) peritonitis

6th **K35.89 Other acute appendicitis**
AHA: 2020,1Q,16

K35.890 Other acute appendicitis without perforation or gangrene CC

K35.891 Other acute appendicitis without perforation, with gangrene CC
(Acute) appendicitis with gangrene NOS

K36 Other appendicitis
Chronic appendicitis
Recurrent appendicitis

UNS **K37 Unspecified appendicitis**
EXCLUDES 1 *unspecified appendicitis with peritonitis (K35.2-, K35.3-)*

4th **K38 Other diseases of appendix**

K38.0 Hyperplasia of appendix

K38.1 Appendicular concretions
Fecalith of appendix
Stercolith of appendix

K38.2 Diverticulum of appendix

K38.3 Fistula of appendix

K38.8 Other specified diseases of appendix
Intussusception of appendix

UNS **K38.9 Disease of appendix, unspecified**

Hernia (K4Ø-K46)

NOTE Hernia with both gangrene and obstruction is classified to hernia with gangrene.

INCLUDES acquired hernia
congenital [except diaphragmatic or hiatus] hernia
recurrent hernia

AHA: 2021,3Q,30-31

TIP: Do not assign a code for bilateral hernia when the right and left sides have differing pathology. For example, two codes would be assigned for bilateral femoral hernia in which the left side is incarcerated (with obstruction) but the right side is not incarcerated; the code for bilateral would not apply in this case.

✓4th K4Ø Inguinal hernia

INCLUDES bubonocele
direct inguinal hernia
double inguinal hernia
indirect inguinal hernia
inguinal hernia NOS
oblique inguinal hernia
scrotal hernia

DEF: Within the groin region.

✓5th K4Ø.Ø Bilateral inguinal hernia, with obstruction, without gangrene
Inguinal hernia (bilateral) causing obstruction without gangrene
Incarcerated inguinal hernia (bilateral) without gangrene
Irreducible inguinal hernia (bilateral) without gangrene
Strangulated inguinal hernia (bilateral) without gangrene

K4Ø.ØØ Bilateral inguinal hernia, with obstruction, without gangrene, not specified as recurrent CC
Bilateral inguinal hernia, with obstruction, without gangrene NOS

K4Ø.Ø1 Bilateral inguinal hernia, with obstruction, without gangrene, recurrent CC

✓5th K4Ø.1 Bilateral inguinal hernia, with gangrene

K4Ø.1Ø Bilateral inguinal hernia, with gangrene, not specified as recurrent MCC
Bilateral inguinal hernia, with gangrene NOS

K4Ø.11 Bilateral inguinal hernia, with gangrene, recurrent MCC

✓5th K4Ø.2 Bilateral inguinal hernia, without obstruction or gangrene

K4Ø.2Ø Bilateral inguinal hernia, without obstruction or gangrene, not specified as recurrent
Bilateral inguinal hernia NOS

K4Ø.21 Bilateral inguinal hernia, without obstruction or gangrene, recurrent

✓5th K4Ø.3 Unilateral inguinal hernia, with obstruction, without gangrene
Inguinal hernia (unilateral) causing obstruction without gangrene
Incarcerated inguinal hernia (unilateral) without gangrene
Irreducible inguinal hernia (unilateral) without gangrene
Strangulated inguinal hernia (unilateral) without gangrene

K4Ø.3Ø Unilateral inguinal hernia, with obstruction, without gangrene, not specified as recurrent CC
Inguinal hernia, with obstruction NOS
Unilateral inguinal hernia, with obstruction, without gangrene NOS

K4Ø.31 Unilateral inguinal hernia, with obstruction, without gangrene, recurrent CC

✓5th K4Ø.4 Unilateral inguinal hernia, with gangrene

K4Ø.4Ø Unilateral inguinal hernia, with gangrene, not specified as recurrent MCC
Inguinal hernia with gangrene NOS
Unilateral inguinal hernia with gangrene NOS

K4Ø.41 Unilateral inguinal hernia, with gangrene, recurrent MCC

✓5th K4Ø.9 Unilateral inguinal hernia, without obstruction or gangrene

K4Ø.9Ø Unilateral inguinal hernia, without obstruction or gangrene, not specified as recurrent
Inguinal hernia NOS
Unilateral inguinal hernia NOS

K4Ø.91 Unilateral inguinal hernia, without obstruction or gangrene, recurrent

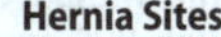

Hernia Sites

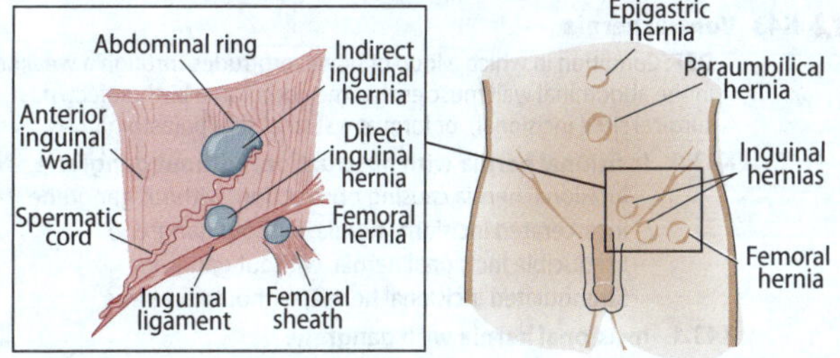

✓4th K41 Femoral hernia

✓5th K41.Ø Bilateral femoral hernia, with obstruction, without gangrene
Femoral hernia (bilateral) causing obstruction, without gangrene
Incarcerated femoral hernia (bilateral), without gangrene
Irreducible femoral hernia (bilateral), without gangrene
Strangulated femoral hernia (bilateral), without gangrene

K41.ØØ Bilateral femoral hernia, with obstruction, without gangrene, not specified as recurrent CC
Bilateral femoral hernia, with obstruction, without gangrene NOS

K41.Ø1 Bilateral femoral hernia, with obstruction, without gangrene, recurrent CC

✓5th K41.1 Bilateral femoral hernia, with gangrene

K41.1Ø Bilateral femoral hernia, with gangrene, not specified as recurrent MCC
Bilateral femoral hernia, with gangrene NOS

K41.11 Bilateral femoral hernia, with gangrene, recurrent MCC

✓5th K41.2 Bilateral femoral hernia, without obstruction or gangrene

K41.2Ø Bilateral femoral hernia, without obstruction or gangrene, not specified as recurrent
Bilateral femoral hernia NOS

K41.21 Bilateral femoral hernia, without obstruction or gangrene, recurrent

✓5th K41.3 Unilateral femoral hernia, with obstruction, without gangrene
Femoral hernia (unilateral) causing obstruction, without gangrene
Incarcerated femoral hernia (unilateral), without gangrene
Irreducible femoral hernia (unilateral), without gangrene
Strangulated femoral hernia (unilateral), without gangrene

K41.3Ø Unilateral femoral hernia, with obstruction, without gangrene, not specified as recurrent CC
Femoral hernia, with obstruction NOS
Unilateral femoral hernia, with obstruction NOS

K41.31 Unilateral femoral hernia, with obstruction, without gangrene, recurrent CC

✓5th K41.4 Unilateral femoral hernia, with gangrene

K41.4Ø Unilateral femoral hernia, with gangrene, not specified as recurrent MCC
Femoral hernia, with gangrene NOS
Unilateral femoral hernia, with gangrene NOS

K41.41 Unilateral femoral hernia, with gangrene, recurrent MCC

✓5th K41.9 Unilateral femoral hernia, without obstruction or gangrene

K41.9Ø Unilateral femoral hernia, without obstruction or gangrene, not specified as recurrent
Femoral hernia NOS
Unilateral femoral hernia NOS

K41.91 Unilateral femoral hernia, without obstruction or gangrene, recurrent

✓4th K42 Umbilical hernia

INCLUDES paraumbilical hernia

EXCLUDES 1 *omphalocele (Q79.2)*

K42.Ø Umbilical hernia with obstruction, without gangrene CC
Umbilical hernia causing obstruction, without gangrene
Incarcerated umbilical hernia, without gangrene
Irreducible umbilical hernia, without gangrene
Strangulated umbilical hernia, without gangrene

K42.1 Umbilical hernia with gangrene MCC
Gangrenous umbilical hernia

K42.9 Umbilical hernia without obstruction or gangrene
Umbilical hernia NOS

K43 Ventral hernia

DEF: Condition in which a loop of bowel protrudes through a weakness in the abdominal wall muscles that may occur as a birth defect, past surgical site (incisional), or form at a stomal site (parastomal).

K43.Ø Incisional hernia with obstruction, without gangrene CC
Incisional hernia causing obstruction, without gangrene
Incarcerated incisional hernia, without gangrene
Irreducible incisional hernia, without gangrene
Strangulated incisional hernia, without gangrene

K43.1 Incisional hernia with gangrene MCC
Gangrenous incisional hernia
AHA: 2020,2Q,22

K43.2 Incisional hernia without obstruction or gangrene
Incisional hernia NOS

K43.3 Parastomal hernia with obstruction, without gangrene CC
Incarcerated parastomal hernia, without gangrene
Irreducible parastomal hernia, without gangrene
Parastomal hernia causing obstruction, without gangrene
Strangulated parastomal hernia, without gangrene

K43.4 Parastomal hernia with gangrene MCC
Gangrenous parastomal hernia

K43.5 Parastomal hernia without obstruction or gangrene
Parastomal hernia NOS

K43.6 Other and unspecified ventral hernia with obstruction, without gangrene CC
Epigastric hernia causing obstruction, without gangrene
Hypogastric hernia causing obstruction, without gangrene
Incarcerated epigastric hernia without gangrene
Incarcerated hypogastric hernia without gangrene
Incarcerated midline hernia without gangrene
Incarcerated spigelian hernia without gangrene
Incarcerated subxiphoid hernia without gangrene
Irreducible epigastric hernia without gangrene
Irreducible hypogastric hernia without gangrene
Irreducible midline hernia without gangrene
Irreducible spigelian hernia without gangrene
Irreducible subxiphoid hernia without gangrene
Midline hernia causing obstruction, without gangrene
Spigelian hernia causing obstruction, without gangrene
Strangulated epigastric hernia without gangrene
Strangulated hypogastric hernia without gangrene
Strangulated midline hernia without gangrene
Strangulated spigelian hernia without gangrene
Strangulated subxiphoid hernia without gangrene
Subxiphoid hernia causing obstruction, without gangrene

K43.7 Other and unspecified ventral hernia with gangrene MCC
Any condition listed under K43.6 specified as gangrenous

K43.9 Ventral hernia without obstruction or gangrene
Epigastric hernia
Ventral hernia NOS

K44 Diaphragmatic hernia

INCLUDES hiatus hernia (esophageal) (sliding)
paraesophageal hernia

EXCLUDES 1 *congenital diaphragmatic hernia (Q79.Ø)*
congenital hiatus hernia (Q4Ø.1)

DEF: Protrusion of an abdominal organ, usually the stomach, through the esophageal opening within the diaphragm and occurring in two types: the sliding hiatal hernia and the paraesophageal hernia.

Hiatal Hernia

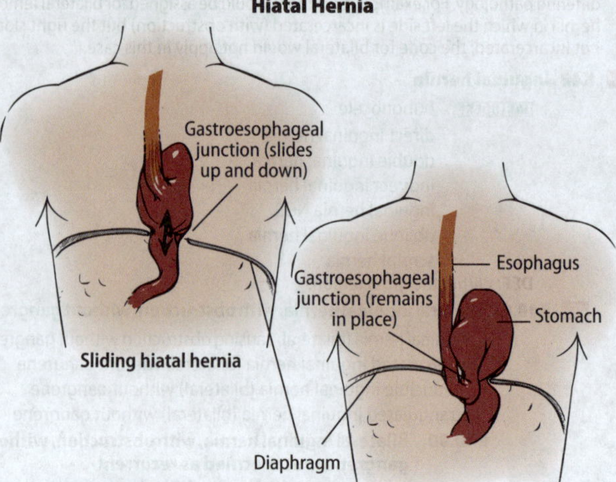

K44.Ø Diaphragmatic hernia with obstruction, without gangrene CC
Diaphragmatic hernia causing obstruction
Incarcerated diaphragmatic hernia
Irreducible diaphragmatic hernia
Strangulated diaphragmatic hernia
AHA: 2022,2Q,13

K44.1 Diaphragmatic hernia with gangrene MCC
Gangrenous diaphragmatic hernia

K44.9 Diaphragmatic hernia without obstruction or gangrene
Diaphragmatic hernia NOS

K45 Other abdominal hernia

INCLUDES abdominal hernia, specified site NEC
lumbar hernia
obturator hernia
pudendal hernia
retroperitoneal hernia
sciatic hernia

K45.Ø Other specified abdominal hernia with obstruction, without gangrene CC
Other specified abdominal hernia causing obstruction
Other specified incarcerated abdominal hernia
Other specified irreducible abdominal hernia
Other specified strangulated abdominal hernia

K45.1 Other specified abdominal hernia with gangrene MCC
Any condition listed under K45 specified as gangrenous

K45.8 Other specified abdominal hernia without obstruction or gangrene

K46 Unspecified abdominal hernia

INCLUDES enterocele
epiplocele
hernia NOS
interstitial hernia
intestinal hernia
intra-abdominal hernia

EXCLUDES 1 *vaginal enterocele (N81.5)*

K46.Ø Unspecified abdominal hernia with obstruction, without gangrene CC
Unspecified abdominal hernia causing obstruction
Unspecified incarcerated abdominal hernia
Unspecified irreducible abdominal hernia
Unspecified strangulated abdominal hernia

K46.1 Unspecified abdominal hernia with gangrene MCC
Any condition listed under K46 specified as gangrenous

K46.9 Unspecified abdominal hernia without obstruction or gangrene
Abdominal hernia NOS

Noninfective enteritis and colitis (K5Ø-K52)

INCLUDES noninfective inflammatory bowel disease
EXCLUDES 1 *irritable bowel syndrome (K58.-)*
megacolon (K59.3-)

K5Ø Crohn's disease [regional enteritis]
INCLUDES granulomatous enteritis
Use additional code to identify manifestations, such as:
pyoderma gangrenosum (L88)
EXCLUDES 1 *ulcerative colitis (K51.-)*
AHA: 2019,3Q,5; 2012,4Q,104
DEF: Chronic inflammation of the gastrointestinal tract characterized by chronic granulomatous disease, most commonly affecting the intestines and the terminal ileum.

K5Ø.Ø Crohn's disease of small intestine
Crohn's disease [regional enteritis] of duodenum
Crohn's disease [regional enteritis] of ileum
Crohn's disease [regional enteritis] of jejunum
Regional ileitis
Terminal ileitis
EXCLUDES 1 *Crohn's disease of both small and large intestine (K5Ø.8-)*

K5Ø.ØØ Crohn's disease of small intestine without complications CC HCC
K5Ø.Ø1 Crohn's disease of small intestine with complications
K5Ø.Ø11 Crohn's disease of small intestine with rectal bleeding CC HCC
K5Ø.Ø12 Crohn's disease of small intestine with intestinal obstruction CC HCC
K5Ø.Ø13 Crohn's disease of small intestine with fistula CC HCC
K5Ø.Ø14 Crohn's disease of small intestine with abscess CC HCC
AHA: 2012,4Q,104
K5Ø.Ø18 Crohn's disease of small intestine with other complication CC HCC
K5Ø.Ø19 Crohn's disease of small intestine with unspecified complications CC HCC

K5Ø.1 Crohn's disease of large intestine
Crohn's disease [regional enteritis] of colon
Crohn's disease [regional enteritis] of large bowel
Crohn's disease [regional enteritis] of rectum
Granulomatous colitis
Regional colitis
EXCLUDES 1 *Crohn's disease of both small and large intestine (K5Ø.8)*

K5Ø.1Ø Crohn's disease of large intestine without complications CC HCC
K5Ø.11 Crohn's disease of large intestine with complications
K5Ø.111 Crohn's disease of large intestine with rectal bleeding CC HCC
K5Ø.112 Crohn's disease of large intestine with intestinal obstruction CC HCC
K5Ø.113 Crohn's disease of large intestine with fistula CC HCC
K5Ø.114 Crohn's disease of large intestine with abscess CC HCC
K5Ø.118 Crohn's disease of large intestine with other complication CC HCC
K5Ø.119 Crohn's disease of large intestine with unspecified complications CC HCC

K5Ø.8 Crohn's disease of both small and large intestine
K5Ø.8Ø Crohn's disease of both small and large intestine without complications CC HCC
K5Ø.81 Crohn's disease of both small and large intestine with complications
K5Ø.811 Crohn's disease of both small and large intestine with rectal bleeding CC HCC
K5Ø.812 Crohn's disease of both small and large intestine with intestinal obstruction CC HCC
K5Ø.813 Crohn's disease of both small and large intestine with fistula CC HCC
K5Ø.814 Crohn's disease of both small and large intestine with abscess CC HCC
K5Ø.818 Crohn's disease of both small and large intestine with other complication CC HCC
K5Ø.819 Crohn's disease of both small and large intestine with unspecified complications CC HCC

K5Ø.9 Crohn's disease, unspecified
K5Ø.9Ø Crohn's disease, unspecified, without complications CC HCC
Crohn's disease NOS
Regional enteritis NOS
K5Ø.91 Crohn's disease, unspecified, with complications
K5Ø.911 Crohn's disease, unspecified, with rectal bleeding CC HCC
K5Ø.912 Crohn's disease, unspecified, with intestinal obstruction CC HCC
K5Ø.913 Crohn's disease, unspecified, with fistula CC HCC
K5Ø.914 Crohn's disease, unspecified, with abscess CC HCC
K5Ø.918 Crohn's disease, unspecified, with other complication CC HCC
K5Ø.919 Crohn's disease, unspecified, with unspecified complications CC HCC

K51 Ulcerative colitis
Use additional code to identify manifestations, such as:
pyoderma gangrenosum (L88)
EXCLUDES 1 *Crohn's disease [regional enteritis] (K5Ø.-)*

K51.Ø Ulcerative (chronic) pancolitis
Backwash ileitis
K51.ØØ Ulcerative (chronic) pancolitis without complications CC HCC
Ulcerative (chronic) pancolitis NOS
K51.Ø1 Ulcerative (chronic) pancolitis with complications
K51.Ø11 Ulcerative (chronic) pancolitis with rectal bleeding CC HCC
K51.Ø12 Ulcerative (chronic) pancolitis with intestinal obstruction CC HCC
K51.Ø13 Ulcerative (chronic) pancolitis with fistula CC HCC
K51.Ø14 Ulcerative (chronic) pancolitis with abscess CC HCC
K51.Ø18 Ulcerative (chronic) pancolitis with other complication CC HCC
K51.Ø19 Ulcerative (chronic) pancolitis with unspecified complications CC HCC

K51.2 Ulcerative (chronic) proctitis
K51.2Ø Ulcerative (chronic) proctitis without complications CC HCC
Ulcerative (chronic) proctitis NOS
K51.21 Ulcerative (chronic) proctitis with complications
K51.211 Ulcerative (chronic) proctitis with rectal bleeding CC HCC
K51.212 Ulcerative (chronic) proctitis with intestinal obstruction CC HCC
K51.213 Ulcerative (chronic) proctitis with fistula CC HCC
K51.214 Ulcerative (chronic) proctitis with abscess CC HCC
K51.218 Ulcerative (chronic) proctitis with other complication CC HCC
K51.219 Ulcerative (chronic) proctitis with unspecified complications CC HCC

K51.3 Ulcerative (chronic) rectosigmoiditis
K51.3Ø Ulcerative (chronic) rectosigmoiditis without complications CC HCC
Ulcerative (chronic) rectosigmoiditis NOS
K51.31 Ulcerative (chronic) rectosigmoiditis with complications
K51.311 Ulcerative (chronic) rectosigmoiditis with rectal bleeding CC HCC
K51.312 Ulcerative (chronic) rectosigmoiditis with intestinal obstruction CC HCC
K51.313 Ulcerative (chronic) rectosigmoiditis with fistula CC HCC

K51.314 Ulcerative (chronic) rectosigmoiditis with abscess CC HCC

K51.318 Ulcerative (chronic) rectosigmoiditis with other complication CC HCC

K51.319 Ulcerative (chronic) rectosigmoiditis with unspecified complications CC HCC

K51.4 Inflammatory polyps of colon

EXCLUDES 1 *adenomatous polyp of colon (D12.6)*
polyposis of colon (D12.6)
polyps of colon NOS (K63.5)

K51.40 Inflammatory polyps of colon without complications CC HCC

Inflammatory polyps of colon NOS

K51.41 Inflammatory polyps of colon with complications

K51.411 Inflammatory polyps of colon with rectal bleeding CC HCC

K51.412 Inflammatory polyps of colon with intestinal obstruction CC HCC

K51.413 Inflammatory polyps of colon with fistula CC HCC

K51.414 Inflammatory polyps of colon with abscess CC HCC

K51.418 Inflammatory polyps of colon with other complication CC HCC

K51.419 Inflammatory polyps of colon with unspecified complications CC HCC

K51.5 Left sided colitis

Left hemicolitis

K51.50 Left sided colitis without complications CC HCC

Left sided colitis NOS

K51.51 Left sided colitis with complications

K51.511 Left sided colitis with rectal bleeding CC HCC

K51.512 Left sided colitis with intestinal obstruction CC HCC

K51.513 Left sided colitis with fistula CC HCC

K51.514 Left sided colitis with abscess CC HCC

K51.518 Left sided colitis with other complication CC HCC

K51.519 Left sided colitis with unspecified complications CC HCC

K51.8 Other ulcerative colitis

K51.80 Other ulcerative colitis without complications CC HCC

K51.81 Other ulcerative colitis with complications

K51.811 Other ulcerative colitis with rectal bleeding CC HCC

K51.812 Other ulcerative colitis with intestinal obstruction CC HCC

K51.813 Other ulcerative colitis with fistula CC HCC

K51.814 Other ulcerative colitis with abscess CC HCC

K51.818 Other ulcerative colitis with other complication CC HCC

K51.819 Other ulcerative colitis with unspecified complications CC HCC

K51.9 Ulcerative colitis, unspecified

K51.90 Ulcerative colitis, unspecified, without complications CC HCC

K51.91 Ulcerative colitis, unspecified, with complications

K51.911 Ulcerative colitis, unspecified with rectal bleeding CC HCC

K51.912 Ulcerative colitis, unspecified with intestinal obstruction CC HCC

K51.913 Ulcerative colitis, unspecified with fistula CC HCC

K51.914 Ulcerative colitis, unspecified with abscess CC HCC

K51.918 Ulcerative colitis, unspecified with other complication CC HCC

K51.919 Ulcerative colitis, unspecified with unspecified complications CC HCC

K52 Other and unspecified noninfective gastroenteritis and colitis

AHA: 2016,4Q,30-31

K52.0 Gastroenteritis and colitis due to radiation CC

K52.1 Toxic gastroenteritis and colitis CC

Drug-induced gastroenteritis and colitis

Code first (T51-T65) to identify toxic agent

Use additional code for adverse effect, if applicable, to identify drug (T36-T50 with fifth or sixth character 5)

AHA: 2019,1Q,17

K52.2 Allergic and dietetic gastroenteritis and colitis

Food hypersensitivity gastroenteritis or colitis

Use additional code to identify type of food allergy (Z91.01-, Z91.02-)

EXCLUDES 2 *allergic eosinophilic colitis (K52.82)*
allergic eosinophilic esophagitis (K20.0)
allergic eosinophilic gastritis (K52.81)
allergic eosinophilic gastroenteritis (K52.81)

DEF: True immunoglobulin E (IgE)-mediated allergic reaction of the lining of the stomach, intestines, or colon to food proteins. It causes nausea, vomiting, diarrhea, and abdominal cramping.

K52.21 Food protein-induced enterocolitis syndrome

FPIES

Use additional code for hypovolemic shock, if present (R57.1)

K52.22 Food protein-induced enteropathy

K52.29 Other allergic and dietetic gastroenteritis and colitis

Allergic proctocolitis
Food hypersensitivity gastroenteritis or colitis
Food-induced eosinophilic proctocolitis
Food protein-induced proctocolitis
Immediate gastrointestinal hypersensitivity
Milk protein-induced proctocolitis

K52.3 Indeterminate colitis

Colonic inflammatory bowel disease unclassified (IBDU)

EXCLUDES 1 *unspecified colitis (K52.9)*

K52.8 Other specified noninfective gastroenteritis and colitis

K52.81 Eosinophilic gastritis or gastroenteritis

Eosinophilic enteritis

EXCLUDES 2 *eosinophilic esophagitis (K20.0)*

DEF: Disorder involving the accumulation of eosinophil in the lining of the stomach or multiple levels of the gastrointestinal tract, but without a known cause such as connective tissue disease, drug reaction, malignancy, or parasitic infection.

K52.82 Eosinophilic colitis

EXCLUDES 2 *allergic proctocolitis (K52.29)*
food-induced eosinophilic proctocolitis (K52.29)
food protein-induced enterocolitis syndrome (FPIES) (K52.21)
food protein-induced proctocolitis (K52.29)
milk protein-induced proctocolitis (K52.29)

DEF: Disorder involving the accumulation of eosinophil in the tissues lining the colon, but without a known cause such as connective tissue disease, drug reaction, malignancy, or parasitic infection. The resultant inflammation may cause extreme abdominal pain, diarrhea, or bloody stool.

K52.83 Microscopic colitis

K52.831 Collagenous colitis

K52.832 Lymphocytic colitis

K52.838 Other microscopic colitis

K52.839 Microscopic colitis, unspecified

K52.89 Other specified noninfective gastroenteritis and colitis

AHA: 2019,1Q,20

K52.9 Noninfective gastroenteritis and colitis, unspecified

Colitis NOS
Enteritis NOS
Gastroenteritis NOS
Ileitis NOS
Jejunitis NOS
Sigmoiditis NOS

EXCLUDES 1 *diarrhea NOS (R19.7)*
functional diarrhea (K59.1)
infectious gastroenteritis and colitis NOS (A09)
neonatal diarrhea (noninfective) (P78.3)
psychogenic diarrhea (F45.8)

AHA: 2021,3Q,3

Other diseases of intestines (K55-K64)

K55 Vascular disorders of intestine

EXCLUDES 1 *necrotizing enterocolitis of newborn (P77.-)*

AHA: 2016,4Q,32

K55.0 Acute vascular disorders of intestine

Infarction of appendices epiploicae
Mesenteric (artery) (vein) embolism
Mesenteric (artery) (vein) infarction
Mesenteric (artery) (vein) thrombosis

AHA: 2019,4Q,68

K55.01 Acute (reversible) ischemia of small intestine

K55.011 Focal (segmental) acute (reversible) ischemia of small intestine MCC HCC

K55.012 Diffuse acute (reversible) ischemia of small intestine MCC HCC

K55.019 Acute (reversible) ischemia of small intestine, extent unspecified MCC HCC

K55.02 Acute infarction of small intestine

Gangrene of small intestine
Necrosis of small intestine

K55.021 Focal (segmental) acute infarction of small intestine MCC HCC

K55.022 Diffuse acute infarction of small intestine MCC HCC

K55.029 Acute infarction of small intestine, extent unspecified MCC HCC

K55.03 Acute (reversible) ischemia of large intestine

Acute fulminant ischemic colitis
Subacute ischemic colitis

K55.031 Focal (segmental) acute (reversible) ischemia of large intestine MCC HCC

K55.032 Diffuse acute (reversible) ischemia of large intestine MCC HCC

K55.039 Acute (reversible) ischemia of large intestine, extent unspecified MCC HCC

AHA: 2019,4Q,68

K55.04 Acute infarction of large intestine

Gangrene of large intestine
Necrosis of large intestine

K55.041 Focal (segmental) acute infarction of large intestine MCC HCC

K55.042 Diffuse acute infarction of large intestine MCC HCC

K55.049 Acute infarction of large intestine, extent unspecified MCC HCC

K55.05 Acute (reversible) ischemia of intestine, part unspecified

K55.051 Focal (segmental) acute (reversible) ischemia of intestine, part unspecified MCC HCC

K55.052 Diffuse acute (reversible) ischemia of intestine, part unspecified MCC HCC

K55.059 Acute (reversible) ischemia of intestine, part and extent unspecified MCC HCC

K55.06 Acute infarction of intestine, part unspecified

Acute intestinal infarction
Gangrene of intestine
Necrosis of intestine

K55.061 Focal (segmental) acute infarction of intestine, part unspecified MCC HCC

K55.062 Diffuse acute infarction of intestine, part unspecified MCC HCC

K55.069 Acute infarction of intestine, part and extent unspecified MCC HCC

K55.1 Chronic vascular disorders of intestine CC HCC

Chronic ischemic colitis
Chronic ischemic enteritis
Chronic ischemic enterocolitis
Ischemic stricture of intestine
Mesenteric atherosclerosis
Mesenteric vascular insufficiency

K55.2 Angiodysplasia of colon

AHA: 2018,3Q,21

TIP: Assign a code for "with hemorrhage" when angiodysplasia and GI bleeding are documented. The ICD-10-CM classification assumes the two are related without the provider linking the two conditions. Evidence of bleeding during a procedure is not required.

K55.20 Angiodysplasia of colon without hemorrhage

K55.21 Angiodysplasia of colon with hemorrhage MCC

DEF: Small vascular abnormalities due to fragile blood vessels in the colon, resulting in blood loss from the gastrointestinal (GI) tract.

K55.3 Necrotizing enterocolitis

EXCLUDES 1 *necrotizing enterocolitis of newborn (P77.-)*

EXCLUDES 2 *necrotizing enterocolitis due to Clostridium difficile (A04.7-)*

K55.30 Necrotizing enterocolitis, unspecified MCC HCC

Necrotizing enterocolitis, NOS

K55.31 Stage 1 necrotizing enterocolitis MCC HCC

Necrotizing enterocolitis without pneumatosis, without perforation

K55.32 Stage 2 necrotizing enterocolitis MCC HCC

Necrotizing enterocolitis with pneumatosis, without perforation

K55.33 Stage 3 necrotizing enterocolitis MCC HCC

Necrotizing enterocolitis with perforation
Necrotizing enterocolitis with pneumatosis and perforation

K55.8 Other vascular disorders of intestine CC HCC

K55.9 Vascular disorder of intestine, unspecified CC HCC

Ischemic colitis
Ischemic enteritis
Ischemic enterocolitis

K56 Paralytic ileus and intestinal obstruction without hernia

EXCLUDES 1 *congenital stricture or stenosis of intestine (Q41-Q42)*
cystic fibrosis with meconium ileus (E84.11)
ischemic stricture of intestine (K55.1)
meconium ileus NOS (P76.0)
neonatal intestinal obstructions classifiable to P76.-
obstruction of duodenum (K31.5)
postprocedural intestinal obstruction (K91.3-)

EXCLUDES 2 *stenosis of anus or rectum (K62.4)*

K56.0 Paralytic ileus CC HCC

Paralysis of bowel
Paralysis of colon
Paralysis of intestine

EXCLUDES 1 *gallstone ileus (K56.3)*
ileus NOS (K56.7)
obstructive ileus NOS (K56.69-)

DEF: Intestinal obstruction due to paralysis of bowel motility or peristalsis.

K56.1 Intussusception CC HCC

Intussusception or invagination of bowel
Intussusception or invagination of colon
Intussusception or invagination of intestine
Intussusception or invagination of rectum

EXCLUDES 2 *intussusception of appendix (K38.8)*

DEF: Intestinal obstruction due to prolapse of a bowel section into an adjacent section. It occurs primarily in children and symptoms include acute abdominal pain, vomiting, and passage of blood and mucus from the rectum.

K56.2 Volvulus MCC HCC
- Strangulation of colon or intestine
- Torsion of colon or intestine
- Twist of colon or intestine

EXCLUDES 2 *volvulus of duodenum (K31.5)*

DEF: Twisting, knotting, or entanglement of the bowel on itself that may quickly compromise oxygen supply to the intestinal tissues. A volvulus usually occurs at the sigmoid and ileocecal areas of the intestines.

Volvulus

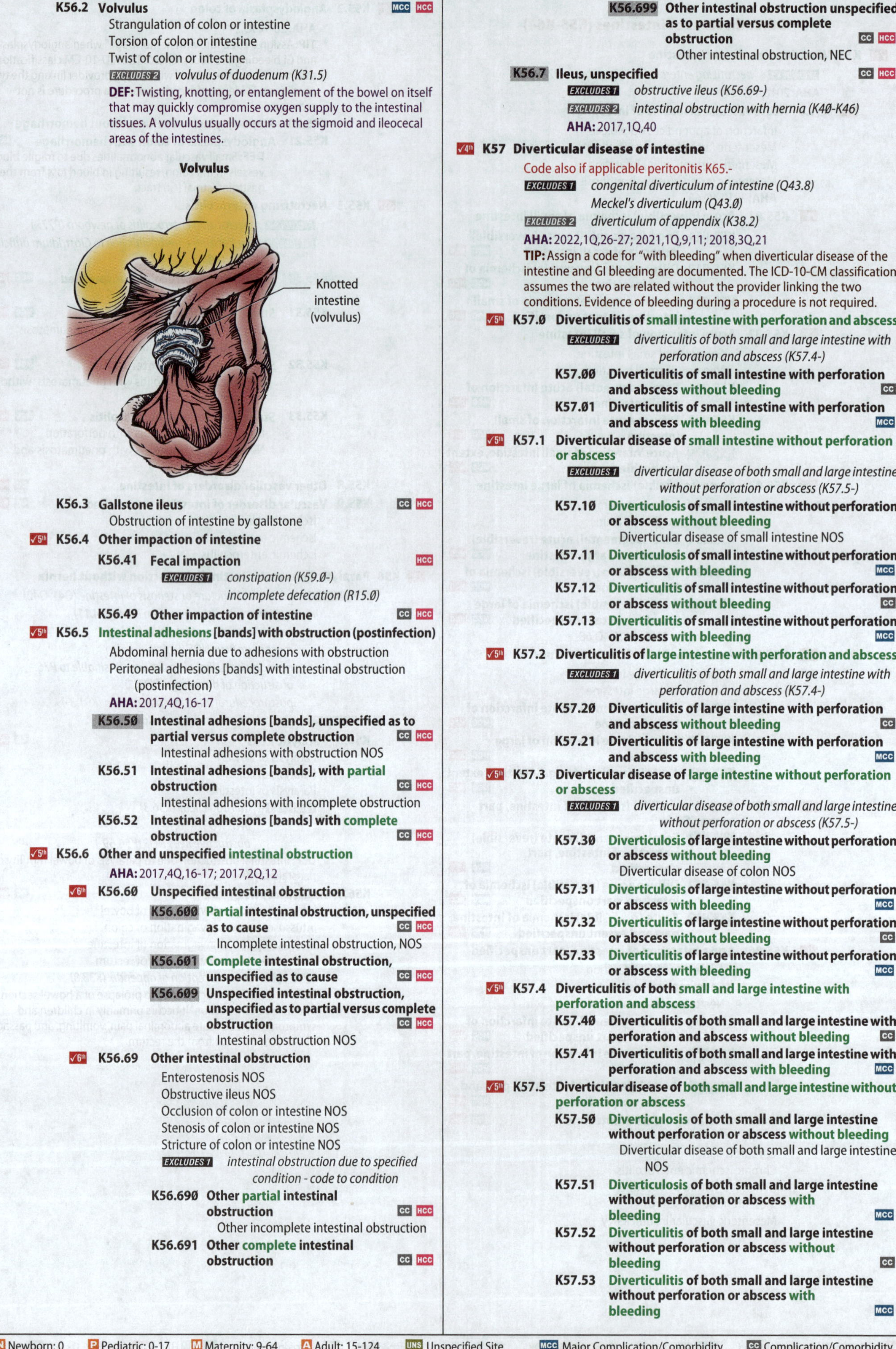

K56.3 Gallstone ileus CC HCC
- Obstruction of intestine by gallstone

✓5th **K56.4 Other impaction of intestine**

K56.41 Fecal impaction HCC

EXCLUDES 1 *constipation (K59.Ø-)*
incomplete defecation (R15.Ø)

K56.49 Other impaction of intestine CC HCC

✓5th **K56.5 Intestinal adhesions [bands] with obstruction (postinfection)**
- Abdominal hernia due to adhesions with obstruction
- Peritoneal adhesions [bands] with intestinal obstruction (postinfection)

AHA: 2017,4Q,16-17

K56.5Ø Intestinal adhesions [bands], unspecified as to partial versus complete obstruction CC HCC
- Intestinal adhesions with obstruction NOS

K56.51 Intestinal adhesions [bands], with partial obstruction CC HCC
- Intestinal adhesions with incomplete obstruction

K56.52 Intestinal adhesions [bands] with complete obstruction CC HCC

✓5th **K56.6 Other and unspecified intestinal obstruction**

AHA: 2017,4Q,16-17; 2017,2Q,12

✓6th **K56.6Ø Unspecified intestinal obstruction**

K56.6ØØ Partial intestinal obstruction, unspecified as to cause CC HCC
- Incomplete intestinal obstruction, NOS

K56.6Ø1 Complete intestinal obstruction, unspecified as to cause CC HCC

K56.6Ø9 Unspecified intestinal obstruction, unspecified as to partial versus complete obstruction CC HCC
- Intestinal obstruction NOS

✓6th **K56.69 Other intestinal obstruction**
- Enterostenosis NOS
- Obstructive ileus NOS
- Occlusion of colon or intestine NOS
- Stenosis of colon or intestine NOS
- Stricture of colon or intestine NOS

EXCLUDES 1 *intestinal obstruction due to specified condition - code to condition*

K56.69Ø Other partial intestinal obstruction CC HCC
- Other incomplete intestinal obstruction

K56.691 Other complete intestinal obstruction CC HCC

K56.699 Other intestinal obstruction unspecified as to partial versus complete obstruction CC HCC
- Other intestinal obstruction, NEC

K56.7 Ileus, unspecified CC HCC

EXCLUDES 1 *obstructive ileus (K56.69-)*

EXCLUDES 2 *intestinal obstruction with hernia (K4Ø-K46)*

AHA: 2017,1Q,40

✓4th **K57 Diverticular disease of intestine**

Code also if applicable peritonitis K65.-

EXCLUDES 1 *congenital diverticulum of intestine (Q43.8)*
Meckel's diverticulum (Q43.Ø)

EXCLUDES 2 *diverticulum of appendix (K38.2)*

AHA: 2022,1Q,26-27; 2021,1Q,9,11; 2018,3Q,21

TIP: Assign a code for "with bleeding" when diverticular disease of the intestine and GI bleeding are documented. The ICD-10-CM classification assumes the two are related without the provider linking the two conditions. Evidence of bleeding during a procedure is not required.

✓5th **K57.Ø Diverticulitis of small intestine with perforation and abscess**

EXCLUDES 1 *diverticulitis of both small and large intestine with perforation and abscess (K57.4-)*

K57.ØØ Diverticulitis of small intestine with perforation and abscess without bleeding CC

K57.Ø1 Diverticulitis of small intestine with perforation and abscess with bleeding MCC

✓5th **K57.1 Diverticular disease of small intestine without perforation or abscess**

EXCLUDES 1 *diverticular disease of both small and large intestine without perforation or abscess (K57.5-)*

K57.1Ø Diverticulosis of small intestine without perforation or abscess without bleeding
- Diverticular disease of small intestine NOS

K57.11 Diverticulosis of small intestine without perforation or abscess with bleeding MCC

K57.12 Diverticulitis of small intestine without perforation or abscess without bleeding CC

K57.13 Diverticulitis of small intestine without perforation or abscess with bleeding MCC

✓5th **K57.2 Diverticulitis of large intestine with perforation and abscess**

EXCLUDES 1 *diverticulitis of both small and large intestine with perforation and abscess (K57.4-)*

K57.2Ø Diverticulitis of large intestine with perforation and abscess without bleeding CC

K57.21 Diverticulitis of large intestine with perforation and abscess with bleeding MCC

✓5th **K57.3 Diverticular disease of large intestine without perforation or abscess**

EXCLUDES 1 *diverticular disease of both small and large intestine without perforation or abscess (K57.5-)*

K57.3Ø Diverticulosis of large intestine without perforation or abscess without bleeding
- Diverticular disease of colon NOS

K57.31 Diverticulosis of large intestine without perforation or abscess with bleeding MCC

K57.32 Diverticulitis of large intestine without perforation or abscess without bleeding CC

K57.33 Diverticulitis of large intestine without perforation or abscess with bleeding MCC

✓5th **K57.4 Diverticulitis of both small and large intestine with perforation and abscess**

K57.4Ø Diverticulitis of both small and large intestine with perforation and abscess without bleeding CC

K57.41 Diverticulitis of both small and large intestine with perforation and abscess with bleeding MCC

✓5th **K57.5 Diverticular disease of both small and large intestine without perforation or abscess**

K57.5Ø Diverticulosis of both small and large intestine without perforation or abscess without bleeding
- Diverticular disease of both small and large intestine NOS

K57.51 Diverticulosis of both small and large intestine without perforation or abscess with bleeding MCC

K57.52 Diverticulitis of both small and large intestine without perforation or abscess without bleeding CC

K57.53 Diverticulitis of both small and large intestine without perforation or abscess with bleeding MCC

K57.8 Diverticulitis of intestine, part unspecified, with perforation and abscess

K57.80 Diverticulitis of intestine, part unspecified, with perforation and abscess without bleeding CC

K57.81 Diverticulitis of intestine, part unspecified, with perforation and abscess with bleeding MCC

K57.9 Diverticular disease of intestine, part unspecified, without perforation or abscess

K57.90 Diverticulosis of intestine, part unspecified, without perforation or abscess without bleeding
Diverticular disease of intestine NOS

K57.91 Diverticulosis of intestine, part unspecified, without perforation or abscess with bleeding MCC

K57.92 Diverticulitis of intestine, part unspecified, without perforation or abscess without bleeding CC

K57.93 Diverticulitis of intestine, part unspecified, without perforation or abscess with bleeding MCC

K58 Irritable bowel syndrome
INCLUDES irritable colon
spastic colon
AHA: 2016,4Q,32-33

K58.Ø Irritable bowel syndrome with diarrhea

K58.1 Irritable bowel syndrome with constipation

K58.2 Mixed irritable bowel syndrome

K58.8 Other irritable bowel syndrome

K58.9 Irritable bowel syndrome without diarrhea
Irritable bowel syndrome NOS

K59 Other functional intestinal disorders
EXCLUDES 1 *change in bowel habit NOS (R19.4)*
intestinal malabsorption (K9Ø.-)
psychogenic intestinal disorders (F45.8)
EXCLUDES 2 *functional disorders of stomach (K31.-)*

K59.Ø Constipation
EXCLUDES 1 *fecal impaction (K56.41)*
incomplete defecation (R15.Ø)
AHA: 2016,4Q,33

K59.ØØ Constipation, unspecified

K59.Ø1 Slow transit constipation
DEF: Delay in the transit of fecal material through the colon secondary to smooth muscle dysfunction or decreased peristaltic contractions along the colon.

K59.Ø2 Outlet dysfunction constipation

K59.Ø3 Drug induced constipation
Use additional code for adverse effect, if applicable, to identify drug (T36-T5Ø with fifth or sixth character 5)

K59.Ø4 Chronic idiopathic constipation
Functional constipation

K59.Ø9 Other constipation
Chronic constipation

K59.1 Functional diarrhea
EXCLUDES 1 *diarrhea NOS (R19.7)*
irritable bowel syndrome with diarrhea (K58.Ø)

K59.2 Neurogenic bowel, not elsewhere classified CC
DEF: Disorder of bowel due to a spinal cord lesion because of injury or as a complication of conditions such as multiple sclerosis (MS) or spina bifida. Loss of bowel control is the primary symptom, manifested as constipation or bowel incontinence.

K59.3 Megacolon, not elsewhere classified
Dilatation of colon
Code first, if applicable (T51-T65) to identify toxic agent
EXCLUDES 1 *congenital megacolon (aganglionic) (Q43.1)*
megacolon (due to) (in) Chagas' disease (B57.32)
megacolon (due to) (in) Clostridium difficile (AØ4.7-)
megacolon (due to) (in) Hirschsprung's disease (Q43.1)
AHA: 2016,4Q,33-34

K59.31 Toxic megacolon CC HCC

K59.39 Other megacolon CC
Megacolon NOS

K59.4 Anal spasm
Proctalgia fugax

K59.8 Other specified functional intestinal disorders
AHA: 2020,4Q,29-30

K59.81 Ogilvie syndrome
Acute colonic pseudo-obstruction (ACPO)

K59.89 Other specified functional intestinal disorders
Atony of colon
Pseudo-obstruction (acute) (chronic) of intestine

K59.9 Functional intestinal disorder, unspecified

K6Ø Fissure and fistula of anal and rectal regions
EXCLUDES 1 *fissure and fistula of anal and rectal regions with abscess or cellulitis (K61.-)*
EXCLUDES 2 *anal sphincter tear (healed) (nontraumatic) (old) (K62.81)*

K6Ø.Ø Acute anal fissure

K6Ø.1 Chronic anal fissure

K6Ø.2 Anal fissure, unspecified

K6Ø.3 Anal fistula

K6Ø.4 Rectal fistula
Fistula of rectum to skin
EXCLUDES 1 *rectovaginal fistula (N82.3)*
vesicorectal fistual (N32.1)

K6Ø.5 Anorectal fistula

K61 Abscess of anal and rectal regions
INCLUDES abscess of anal and rectal regions
cellulitis of anal and rectal regions

K61.Ø Anal abscess CC
Perianal abscess
EXCLUDES 2 *intrasphincteric abscess (K61.4)*

K61.1 Rectal abscess CC
Perirectal abscess
EXCLUDES 1 *ischiorectal abscess (K61.39)*
AHA: 2012,4Q,104

K61.2 Anorectal abscess CC

K61.3 Ischiorectal abscess
AHA: 2018,4Q,19

K61.31 Horseshoe abscess

K61.39 Other ischiorectal abscess
Abscess of ischiorectal fossa
Ischiorectal abscess, NOS

K61.4 Intrasphincteric abscess CC
Intersphincteric abscess

K61.5 Supralevator abscess
AHA: 2018,4Q,19

K62 Other diseases of anus and rectum
INCLUDES anal canal
EXCLUDES 2 *colostomy and enterostomy malfunction (K94.Ø-, K94.1-)*
fecal incontinence (R15.-)
hemorrhoids (K64.-)

K62.Ø Anal polyp

K62.1 Rectal polyp
EXCLUDES 1 *adenomatous polyp (D12.8)*
AHA: 2018,1Q,6

K62.2 Anal prolapse
Prolapse of anal canal

K62.3 Rectal prolapse
Prolapse of rectal mucosa

K62.4 Stenosis of anus and rectum
Stricture of anus (sphincter)
AHA: 2019,2Q,13

K62.5 Hemorrhage of anus and rectum CC
EXCLUDES 1 *gastrointestinal bleeding NOS (K92.2)*
melena (K92.1)
neonatal rectal hemorrhage (P54.2)
AHA: 2019,1Q,21

K62.6 Ulcer of anus and rectum CC
Solitary ulcer of anus and rectum
Stercoral ulcer of anus and rectum
EXCLUDES 1 *fissure and fistula of anus and rectum (K6Ø.-)*
ulcerative colitis (K51.-)

K62.7 Radiation proctitis
Use additional code to identify the type of radiation (W88.-) or radiation therapy (Y84.2)
AHA: 2019,1Q,21

K62.8 Other specified diseases of anus and rectum

EXCLUDES 2 *ulcerative proctitis (K51.2)*

K62.81 Anal sphincter tear (healed) (nontraumatic) (old)

Tear of anus, nontraumatic

Use additional code for any associated fecal incontinence (R15.-)

EXCLUDES 2 *anal fissure (K6Ø.-)*
anal sphincter tear (healed) (old) complicating delivery (O34.7-)
traumatic tear of anal sphincter (S31.831)

K62.82 Dysplasia of anus

Anal intraepithelial neoplasia I and II (AIN I and II) (histologically confirmed)

Dysplasia of anus NOS

Mild and moderate dysplasia of anus (histologically confirmed)

EXCLUDES 1 *abnormal results from anal cytologic examination without histologic confirmation (R85.61-)*
anal intraepithelial neoplasia III (DØ1.3)
carcinoma in situ of anus (DØ1.3)
HGSIL of anus (R85.613)
severe dysplasia of anus (DØ1.3)

K62.89 Other specified diseases of anus and rectum

Proctitis NOS

Use additional code for any associated fecal incontinence (R15.-)

K62.9 Disease of anus and rectum, unspecified

K63 Other diseases of intestine

K63.Ø Abscess of intestine CC

EXCLUDES 1 *abscess of intestine with Crohn's disease (K5Ø.Ø14, K5Ø.114, K5Ø.814, K5Ø.914)*
abscess of intestine with diverticular disease (K57.Ø, K57.2, K57.4, K57.8)
abscess of intestine with ulcerative colitis (K51.Ø14, K51.214, K51.314, K51.414, K51.514, K51.814, K51.914)

EXCLUDES 2 *abscess of anal and rectal regions (K61.-)*
abscess of appendix (K35.3-)

K63.1 Perforation of intestine (nontraumatic) MCC HCC

Perforation (nontraumatic) of rectum

EXCLUDES 1 *perforation (nontraumatic) of duodenum (K26.-)*
perforation (nontraumatic) of intestine with diverticular disease (K57.Ø, K57.2, K57.4, K57.8)

EXCLUDES 2 *perforation (nontraumatic) of appendix (K35.2-, K35.3-)*

AHA: 2020,2Q,22

K63.2 Fistula of intestine CC

EXCLUDES 1 *fistula of duodenum (K31.6)*
fistula of intestine with Crohn's disease (K5Ø.Ø13, K5Ø.113, K5Ø.813, K5Ø.913)
fistula of intestine with ulcerative colitis (K51.Ø13, K51.213, K51.313, K51.413, K51.513, K51.813, K51.913)

EXCLUDES 2 *fistula of anal and rectal regions (K6Ø.-)*
fistula of appendix (K38.3)
intestinal-genital fistula, female (N82.2-N82.4)
vesicointestinal fistula (N32.1)

AHA: 2017,3Q,4

K63.3 Ulcer of intestine CC

Primary ulcer of small intestine

EXCLUDES 1 *duodenal ulcer (K26.-)*
gastrointestinal ulcer (K28.-)
gastrojejunal ulcer (K28.-)
jejunal ulcer (K28.-)
peptic ulcer, site unspecified (K27.-)
ulcer of intestine with perforation (K63.1)
ulcer of anus or rectum (K62.6)
ulcerative colitis (K51.-)

K63.4 Enteroptosis

K63.5 Polyp of colon

EXCLUDES 1 *adenomatous polyp of colon (D12.-)*
inflammatory polyp of colon (K51.4-)
polyposis of colon (D12.6)

AHA: 2019,1Q,33; 2018,2Q,14; 2017,1Q,15; 2015,2Q,14

TIP: Assign this code when documentation states hyperplastic colon polyp regardless of the site in the colon. Slow-growing, hyperplastic polyps are not precancerous and are classified differently from benign or adenomatous polyps.

K63.8 Other specified diseases of intestine

K63.81 Dieulafoy lesion of intestine MCC

EXCLUDES 2 *Dieulafoy lesion of stomach and duodenum (K31.82)*

DEF: Abnormally large submucosal artery protruding through a defect in the stomach mucosa or intestines that can cause massive and life-threatening hemorrhaging.

K63.89 Other specified diseases of intestine

AHA: 2013,2Q,31

K63.9 Disease of intestine, unspecified

K64 Hemorrhoids and perianal venous thrombosis

INCLUDES piles

EXCLUDES 1 *hemorrhoids complicating childbirth and the puerperium (O87.2)*
hemorrhoids complicating pregnancy (O22.4)

Hemorrhoids

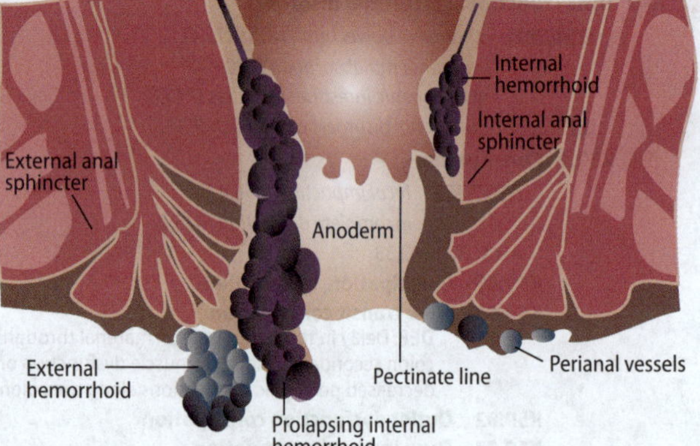

K64.Ø First degree hemorrhoids

Grade/stage I hemorrhoids

Hemorrhoids (bleeding) without prolapse outside of anal canal

K64.1 Second degree hemorrhoids

Grade/stage II hemorrhoids

Hemorrhoids (bleeding) that prolapse with straining, but retract spontaneously

K64.2 Third degree hemorrhoids

Grade/stage III hemorrhoids

Hemorrhoids (bleeding) that prolapse with straining and require manual replacement back inside anal canal

K64.3 Fourth degree hemorrhoids

Grade/stage IV hemorrhoids

Hemorrhoids (bleeding) with prolapsed tissue that cannot be manually replaced

K64.4 Residual hemorrhoidal skin tags

External hemorrhoids, NOS

Skin tags of anus

K64.5 Perianal venous thrombosis

External hemorrhoids with thrombosis

Perianal hematoma

Thrombosed hemorrhoids NOS

K64.8 Other hemorrhoids

Internal hemorrhoids, without mention of degree

Prolapsed hemorrhoids, degree not specified

K64.9 Unspecified hemorrhoids

Hemorrhoids (bleeding) NOS

Hemorrhoids (bleeding) without mention of degree

Diseases of peritoneum and retroperitoneum (K65-K68)

K65 Peritonitis

Use additional code (B95-B97), to identify infectious agent, if known
Code also if applicable diverticular disease of intestine (K57.-)

EXCLUDES 1 *acute appendicitis with generalized peritonitis (K35.2-)*
aseptic peritonitis (T81.6)
benign paroxysmal peritonitis (E85.Ø)
chemical peritonitis (T81.6)
gonococcal peritonitis (A54.85)
neonatal peritonitis (P78.Ø-P78.1)
pelvic peritonitis, female (N73.3-N73.5)
periodic familial peritonitis (E85.Ø)
peritonitis due to talc or other foreign substance (T81.6)
peritonitis in chlamydia (A74.81)
peritonitis in diphtheria (A36.89)
peritonitis in syphilis (late) (A52.74)
peritonitis in tuberculosis (A18.31)
peritonitis with or following abortion or ectopic or molar pregnancy (OØØ-OØ7, OØ8.Ø)
peritonitis with or following appendicitis (K35.-)
puerperal peritonitis (O85)
retroperitoneal infections (K68.-)

K65.Ø Generalized (acute) peritonitis MCC HCC
Pelvic peritonitis (acute), male
Subphrenic peritonitis (acute)
Suppurative peritonitis (acute)

K65.1 Peritoneal abscess MCC HCC
Abdominopelvic abscess
Abscess (of) omentum
Abscess (of) peritoneum
Mesenteric abscess
Retrocecal abscess
Subdiaphragmatic abscess
Subhepatic abscess
Subphrenic abscess
AHA: 2022,1Q,26; 2019,1Q,15

K65.2 Spontaneous bacterial peritonitis MCC HCC
EXCLUDES 1 *bacterial peritonitis NOS (K65.9)*

K65.3 Choleperitonitis MCC HCC
Peritonitis due to bile
DEF: Inflammation of the peritoneum due to leakage of bile into the peritoneal cavity resulting from rupture of the bile passages or gallbladder.

K65.4 Sclerosing mesenteritis CC HCC
Fat necrosis of peritoneum
(Idiopathic) sclerosing mesenteric fibrosis
Mesenteric lipodystrophy
Mesenteric panniculitis
Retractile mesenteritis

K65.8 Other peritonitis MCC HCC
Chronic proliferative peritonitis
Peritonitis due to urine

K65.9 Peritonitis, unspecified MCC HCC
Bacterial peritonitis NOS
AHA: 2022,1Q,27; 2013,2Q,31

K66 Other disorders of peritoneum

EXCLUDES 2 *ascites (R18.-)*
peritoneal effusion (chronic) (R18.8)

K66.Ø Peritoneal adhesions (postprocedural) (postinfection)
Adhesions (of) abdominal (wall)
Adhesions (of) diaphragm
Adhesions (of) intestine
Adhesions (of) male pelvis
Adhesions (of) omentum
Adhesions (of) stomach
Adhesive bands
Mesenteric adhesions
EXCLUDES 1 *female pelvic adhesions [bands] (N73.6)*
peritoneal adhesions with intestinal obstruction (K56.5-)

K66.1 Hemoperitoneum MCC
EXCLUDES 1 *traumatic hemoperitoneum (S36.8-)*
AHA: 2022,1Q,22-23

K66.8 Other specified disorders of peritoneum

K66.9 Disorder of peritoneum, unspecified

K67 Disorders of peritoneum in infectious diseases classified elsewhere MCC HCC

Code first underlying disease, such as:
congenital syphilis (A5Ø.Ø)
helminthiasis (B65.Ø-B83.9)

EXCLUDES 1 *peritonitis in chlamydia (A74.81)*
peritonitis in diphtheria (A36.89)
peritonitis in gonococcal (A54.85)
peritonitis in syphilis (late) (A52.74)
peritonitis in tuberculosis (A18.31)

K68 Disorders of retroperitoneum

K68.1 Retroperitoneal abscess

K68.11 Postprocedural retroperitoneal abscess CC H11 H12 H13
EXCLUDES 2 *infection following procedure (T81.4-)*

K68.12 Psoas muscle abscess MCC HCC

K68.19 Other retroperitoneal abscess MCC HCC
AHA: 2019,1Q,15
TIP: This code should be used for a diagnosis of internal presacral abscess. If an intra-abdominal abscess is also present, code K65.1 can also be assigned; sequencing depends on the circumstances of admission.

K68.9 Other disorders of retroperitoneum MCC

Diseases of liver (K7Ø-K77)

EXCLUDES 1 *jaundice NOS (R17)*
EXCLUDES 2 *hemochromatosis (E83.11-)*
Reye's syndrome (G93.7)
viral hepatitis (B15-B19)
Wilson's disease (E83.Ø)

K7Ø Alcoholic liver disease

Use additional code to identify:
alcohol abuse and dependence (F1Ø.-)

K7Ø.Ø Alcoholic fatty liver A

K7Ø.1 Alcoholic hepatitis

K7Ø.1Ø Alcoholic hepatitis without ascites A

K7Ø.11 Alcoholic hepatitis with ascites A

K7Ø.2 Alcoholic fibrosis and sclerosis of liver A

K7Ø.3 Alcoholic cirrhosis of liver
Alcoholic cirrhosis NOS

K7Ø.3Ø Alcoholic cirrhosis of liver without ascites HCC A

K7Ø.31 Alcoholic cirrhosis of liver with ascites HCC A
AHA: 2018,1Q,4

K7Ø.4 Alcoholic hepatic failure
Acute alcoholic hepatic failure
Alcoholic hepatic failure NOS
Chronic alcoholic hepatic failure
Subacute alcoholic hepatic failure

K7Ø.4Ø Alcoholic hepatic failure without coma HCC A

K7Ø.41 Alcoholic hepatic failure with coma MCC HCC A

K7Ø.9 Alcoholic liver disease, unspecified HCC A

K71 Toxic liver disease

INCLUDES drug-induced idiosyncratic (unpredictable) liver disease
drug-induced toxic (predictable) liver disease

Code first poisoning due to drug or toxin, if applicable (T36-T65 with fifth or sixth character 1-4 or 6)
Use additional code for adverse effect, if applicable, to identify drug (T36-T5Ø with fifth or sixth character 5)

EXCLUDES 2 *alcoholic liver disease (K7Ø.-)*
Budd-Chiari syndrome (I82.Ø)

K71.Ø Toxic liver disease with cholestasis
Cholestasis with hepatocyte injury
"Pure" cholestasis

K71.1 Toxic liver disease with hepatic necrosis
Hepatic failure (acute) (chronic) due to drugs

K71.1Ø Toxic liver disease with hepatic necrosis, without coma

K71.11 Toxic liver disease with hepatic necrosis, with coma MCC HCC

K71.2 Toxic liver disease with acute hepatitis

K71.3 Toxic liver disease with chronic persistent hepatitis

K71.4 Toxic liver disease with chronic lobular hepatitis

K71.5 Toxic liver disease with chronic active hepatitis
Toxic liver disease with lupoid hepatitis
K71.50 Toxic liver disease with chronic active hepatitis without ascites
K71.51 Toxic liver disease with chronic active hepatitis with ascites
AHA: 2018,1Q,4
K71.6 Toxic liver disease with hepatitis, not elsewhere classified
K71.7 Toxic liver disease with fibrosis and cirrhosis of liver
K71.8 Toxic liver disease with other disorders of liver
Toxic liver disease with focal nodular hyperplasia
Toxic liver disease with hepatic granulomas
Toxic liver disease with peliosis hepatis
Toxic liver disease with veno-occlusive disease of liver
K71.9 Toxic liver disease, unspecified

K72 Hepatic failure, not elsewhere classified
INCLUDES fulminant hepatitis NEC, with hepatic failure
hepatic encephalopathy NOS
liver (cell) necrosis with hepatic failure
malignant hepatitis NEC, with hepatic failure
yellow liver atrophy or dystrophy
EXCLUDES 1 *alcoholic hepatic failure (K70.4)*
hepatic failure with toxic liver disease (K71.1-)
icterus of newborn (P55-P59)
postprocedural hepatic failure (K91.82)
EXCLUDES 2 *hepatic failure complicating abortion or ectopic or molar pregnancy (O00-O07, O08.8)*
hepatic failure complicating pregnancy, childbirth and the puerperium (O26.6-)
viral hepatitis with hepatic coma (B15-B19)
AHA: 2017,1Q,41
K72.0 Acute and subacute hepatic failure
Acute non-viral hepatitis NOS
AHA: 2015,2Q,17; 2014,2Q,13
K72.00 Acute and subacute hepatic failure without coma MCC
AHA: 2021,1Q,13
K72.01 Acute and subacute hepatic failure with coma MCC HCC
K72.1 Chronic hepatic failure
End stage liver disease
K72.10 Chronic hepatic failure without coma HCC
AHA: 2021,1Q,13
K72.11 Chronic hepatic failure with coma MCC HCC
K72.9 Hepatic failure, unspecified
K72.90 Hepatic failure, unspecified without coma HCC
AHA: 2022,1Q,52; 2018,4Q,20; 2016,2Q,35
K72.91 Hepatic failure, unspecified with coma MCC HCC
Hepatic coma NOS

K73 Chronic hepatitis, not elsewhere classified
EXCLUDES 1 *alcoholic hepatitis (chronic) (K70.1-)*
drug-induced hepatitis (chronic) (K71.-)
granulomatous hepatitis (chronic) NEC (K75.3)
reactive, nonspecific hepatitis (chronic) (K75.2)
viral hepatitis (chronic) (B15-B19)
K73.0 Chronic persistent hepatitis, not elsewhere classified HCC
K73.1 Chronic lobular hepatitis, not elsewhere classified HCC
K73.2 Chronic active hepatitis, not elsewhere classified HCC
K73.8 Other chronic hepatitis, not elsewhere classified HCC
K73.9 Chronic hepatitis, unspecified HCC

K74 Fibrosis and cirrhosis of liver
Code also, if applicable, viral hepatitis (acute) (chronic) (B15-B19)
EXCLUDES 1 *alcoholic cirrhosis (of liver) (K70.3)*
alcoholic fibrosis of liver (K70.2)
cardiac sclerosis of liver (K76.1)
cirrhosis (of liver) with toxic liver disease (K71.7)
congenital cirrhosis (of liver) (P78.81)
pigmentary cirrhosis (of liver) (E83.110)
K74.0 Hepatic fibrosis
Code first underlying liver disease, such as:
nonalcoholic steatohepatitis (NASH) (K75.81)
AHA: 2020,4Q,30-31
K74.00 Hepatic fibrosis, unspecified UPD
K74.01 Hepatic fibrosis, early fibrosis UPD
Hepatic fibrosis, stage F1 or stage F2
K74.02 Hepatic fibrosis, advanced fibrosis UPD
Hepatic fibrosis, stage F3
EXCLUDES 1 *cirrhosis of liver (K74.6-)*
hepatic fibrosis, stage F4 (K74.6-)
K74.1 Hepatic sclerosis
K74.2 Hepatic fibrosis with hepatic sclerosis
K74.3 Primary biliary cirrhosis HCC
Chronic nonsuppurative destructive cholangitis
Primary biliary cholangitis
EXCLUDES 2 *primary sclerosing cholangitis (K83.01)*
K74.4 Secondary biliary cirrhosis HCC
K74.5 Biliary cirrhosis, unspecified HCC
K74.6 Other and unspecified cirrhosis of liver
AHA: 2020,4Q,30-31
K74.60 Unspecified cirrhosis of liver HCC
Cirrhosis (of liver) NOS
AHA: 2018,1Q,4
K74.69 Other cirrhosis of liver HCC
Cryptogenic cirrhosis (of liver)
Macronodular cirrhosis (of liver)
Micronodular cirrhosis (of liver)
Mixed type cirrhosis (of liver)
Portal cirrhosis (of liver)
Postnecrotic cirrhosis (of liver)

K75 Other inflammatory liver diseases
EXCLUDES 2 *toxic liver disease (K71.-)*
K75.0 Abscess of liver MCC
Cholangitic hepatic abscess
Hematogenic hepatic abscess
Hepatic abscess NOS
Lymphogenic hepatic abscess
Pylephlebitic hepatic abscess
EXCLUDES 1 *amebic liver abscess (A06.4)*
cholangitis without liver abscess (K83.09)
pylephlebitis without liver abscess (K75.1)
EXCLUDES 2 *acute or subacute hepatitis NOS (B17.9)*
acute or subacute non-viral hepatitis (K72.0)
chronic hepatitis NEC (K73.8)
K75.1 Phlebitis of portal vein MCC
Pylephlebitis
EXCLUDES 1 *pylephlebitic liver abscess (K75.0)*
DEF: Inflammation of the portal vein or branches due to diverticulitis, perforated appendicitis, or peritonitis. Symptoms include fever, chills, jaundice, sweating, and abscess in various body parts.
K75.2 Nonspecific reactive hepatitis
EXCLUDES 1 *acute or subacute hepatitis (K72.0-)*
chronic hepatitis NEC (K73.-)
viral hepatitis (B15-B19)
K75.3 Granulomatous hepatitis, not elsewhere classified
EXCLUDES 1 *acute or subacute hepatitis (K72.0-)*
chronic hepatitis NEC (K73.-)
viral hepatitis (B15-B19)
K75.4 Autoimmune hepatitis HCC
Lupoid hepatitis NEC
K75.8 Other specified inflammatory liver diseases
K75.81 Nonalcoholic steatohepatitis (NASH)
Use additional code, if applicable, hepatic fibrosis (K74.0-)
K75.89 Other specified inflammatory liver diseases
K75.9 Inflammatory liver disease, unspecified
Hepatitis NOS
EXCLUDES 1 *acute or subacute hepatitis (K72.0-)*
chronic hepatitis NEC (K73.-)
viral hepatitis (B15-B19)
AHA: 2015,2Q,17

K76 Other diseases of liver
EXCLUDES 2 *alcoholic liver disease (K70.-)*
amyloid degeneration of liver (E85.-)
cystic disease of liver (congenital) (Q44.6)
hepatic vein thrombosis (I82.0)
hepatomegaly NOS (R16.0)
pigmentary cirrhosis (of liver) (E83.110)
portal vein thrombosis (I81)
toxic liver disease (K71.-)

K76.0 Fatty (change of) liver, not elsewhere classified
Nonalcoholic fatty liver disease (NAFLD)
EXCLUDES 1 *nonalcoholic steatohepatitis (NASH) (K75.81)*

K76.1 Chronic passive congestion of liver
Cardiac cirrhosis
Cardiac sclerosis

K76.2 Central hemorrhagic necrosis of liver MCC
EXCLUDES 1 *liver necrosis with hepatic failure (K72.-)*

K76.3 Infarction of liver MCC

K76.4 Peliosis hepatis
Hepatic angiomatosis

K76.5 Hepatic veno-occlusive disease
EXCLUDES 1 *Budd-Chiari syndrome (I82.0)*

K76.6 Portal hypertension CC HCC
Use additional code for any associated complications, such as:
portal hypertensive gastropathy (K31.89)
AHA: 2020,1Q,15

K76.7 Hepatorenal syndrome MCC HCC
EXCLUDES 1 *hepatorenal syndrome following labor and delivery (O90.4)*
postprocedural hepatorenal syndrome (K91.83)

K76.8 Other specified diseases of liver

K76.81 Hepatopulmonary syndrome UPD HCC
Code first underlying liver disease, such as:
alcoholic cirrhosis of liver (K70.3-)
cirrhosis of liver without mention of alcohol (K74.6-)

● **K76.82 Hepatic encephalopathy**
Hepatic encephalopathy, NOS
Hepatic encephalopathy without coma
Hepatocerebral intoxication
Portal-systemic encephalopathy
Code also underlying liver disease, such as:
acute and subacute hepatic failure without coma (K72.00)
alcoholic hepatic failure without coma (K70.40)
chronic hepatic failure without coma (K72.10)
hepatic failure with toxic liver disease without coma (K71.10)
hepatic failure without coma (K72.90)
icterus of newborn (P55-P59)
postprocedural hepatic failure (K91.82)
viral hepatitis without hepatic coma (B15.9, B16.1, B16.9, B17.10, B19.10, B19.20, B19.9)
EXCLUDES 1 *acute and subacute hepatic failure with coma (K72.01)*
alcoholic hepatic failure with coma (K70.41)
chronic hepatic failure with coma (K72.11)
hepatic failure with coma (K72.91)

K76.89 Other specified diseases of liver
Cyst (simple) of liver
Focal nodular hyperplasia of liver
Hepatoptosis

K76.9 Liver disease, unspecified

K77 Liver disorders in diseases classified elsewhere CC
Code first underlying disease, such as:
amyloidosis (E85.-)
congenital syphilis (A50.0, A50.5)
congenital toxoplasmosis (P37.1)
infectious mononucleosis with liver disease ▶(B27.0-B27.9 with fifth character 9)◀
schistosomiasis (B65.0-B65.9)
EXCLUDES 1 *alcoholic hepatitis (K70.1-)*
alcoholic liver disease (K70.-)
cytomegaloviral hepatitis (B25.1)
herpesviral [herpes simplex] hepatitis (B00.81)
mumps hepatitis (B26.81)
sarcoidosis with liver disease (D86.89)
secondary syphilis with liver disease (A51.45)
syphilis (late) with liver disease (A52.74)
toxoplasmosis (acquired) hepatitis (B58.1)
tuberculosis with liver disease (A18.83)

Disorders of gallbladder, biliary tract and pancreas (K80-K87)

K80 Cholelithiasis
EXCLUDES 1 *retained cholelithiasis following cholecystectomy (K91.86)*
AHA: 2018,4Q,20
DEF: Presence or formation of concretions (calculi or "gallstones") in the gallbladder. The stones contain cholesterol, calcium carbonate, or calcium bilirubinate in pure forms or in various combinations.

Cholelithiasis

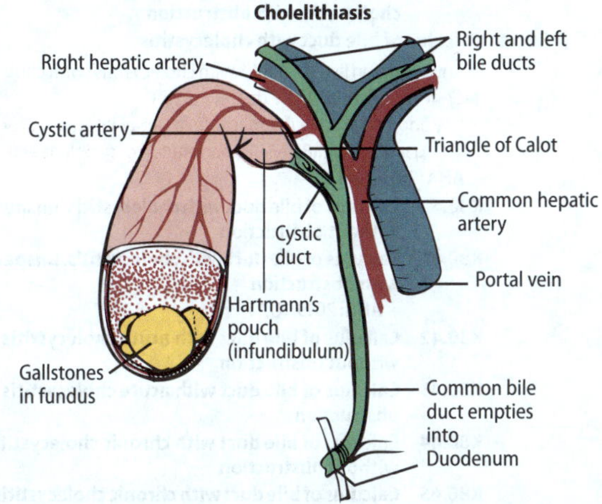

K80.0 Calculus of gallbladder with acute cholecystitis
Any condition listed in K80.2 with acute cholecystitis
Use additional code if applicable for associated gangrene of gallbladder (K82.A1), or perforation of gallbladder (K82.A2)

K80.00 Calculus of gallbladder with acute cholecystitis without obstruction CC

K80.01 Calculus of gallbladder with acute cholecystitis with obstruction CC

K80.1 Calculus of gallbladder with other cholecystitis
Use additional code if applicable for associated gangrene of gallbladder (K82.A1), or perforation of gallbladder (K82.A2)

K80.10 Calculus of gallbladder with chronic cholecystitis without obstruction CC
Cholelithiasis with cholecystitis NOS

K80.11 Calculus of gallbladder with chronic cholecystitis with obstruction CC

K80.12 Calculus of gallbladder with acute and chronic cholecystitis without obstruction CC

K80.13 Calculus of gallbladder with acute and chronic cholecystitis with obstruction CC

K80.18 Calculus of gallbladder with other cholecystitis without obstruction CC

K80.19 Calculus of gallbladder with other cholecystitis with obstruction CC

K80.2 Calculus of gallbladder without cholecystitis
Cholecystolithiasis without cholecystitis
Cholelithiasis (without cholecystitis)
Colic (recurrent) of gallbladder (without cholecystitis)
Gallstone (impacted) of cystic duct (without cholecystitis)
Gallstone (impacted) of gallbladder (without cholecystitis)

K80.20 Calculus of gallbladder without cholecystitis without obstruction

K80.21 Calculus of gallbladder without cholecystitis with obstruction CC

K80.3 Calculus of bile duct with cholangitis
Any condition listed in K80.5 with cholangitis
DEF: Cholangitis: Inflammation of the bile ducts.

K80.30 Calculus of bile duct with cholangitis, unspecified, without obstruction CC

K80.31 Calculus of bile duct with cholangitis, unspecified, with obstruction CC

K80.32 Calculus of bile duct with acute cholangitis without obstruction CC

K80.33 Calculus of bile duct with acute cholangitis with obstruction CC

K80.34 Calculus of bile duct with chronic cholangitis without obstruction CC

K80.35 Calculus of bile duct with chronic cholangitis with obstruction CC

K80.36 Calculus of bile duct with acute and chronic cholangitis without obstruction CC

K80.37 Calculus of bile duct with acute and chronic cholangitis with obstruction CC

K80.4 Calculus of bile duct with cholecystitis
Any condition listed in K80.5 with cholecystitis (with cholangitis)
▶Code also fistula of bile duct◀ (K83.3)
Use additional code if applicable for associated gangrene of gallbladder (K82.A1), or perforation of gallbladder (K82.A2)
AHA: 2019,1Q,17

K80.40 Calculus of bile duct with cholecystitis, unspecified, without obstruction CC

K80.41 Calculus of bile duct with cholecystitis, unspecified, with obstruction CC
AHA: 2019,1Q,17

K80.42 Calculus of bile duct with acute cholecystitis without obstruction CC

K80.43 Calculus of bile duct with acute cholecystitis with obstruction CC

K80.44 Calculus of bile duct with chronic cholecystitis without obstruction CC

K80.45 Calculus of bile duct with chronic cholecystitis with obstruction CC

K80.46 Calculus of bile duct with acute and chronic cholecystitis without obstruction CC

K80.47 Calculus of bile duct with acute and chronic cholecystitis with obstruction CC

K80.5 Calculus of bile duct without cholangitis or cholecystitis
Choledocholithiasis (without cholangitis or cholecystitis)
Gallstone (impacted) of bile duct NOS (without cholangitis or cholecystitis)
Gallstone (impacted) of common duct (without cholangitis or cholecystitis)
Gallstone (impacted) of hepatic duct (without cholangitis or cholecystitis)
Hepatic cholelithiasis (without cholangitis or cholecystitis)
Hepatic colic (recurrent) (without cholangitis or cholecystitis)
DEF: Cholangitis: Inflammation of the bile ducts.

K80.50 Calculus of bile duct without cholangitis or cholecystitis without obstruction

K80.51 Calculus of bile duct without cholangitis or cholecystitis with obstruction CC

K80.6 Calculus of gallbladder and bile duct with cholecystitis
Use additional code if applicable for associated gangrene of gallbladder (K82.A1), or perforation of gallbladder (K82.A2)

K80.60 Calculus of gallbladder and bile duct with cholecystitis, unspecified, without obstruction CC

K80.61 Calculus of gallbladder and bile duct with cholecystitis, unspecified, with obstruction CC

K80.62 Calculus of gallbladder and bile duct with acute cholecystitis without obstruction CC

K80.63 Calculus of gallbladder and bile duct with acute cholecystitis with obstruction CC

K80.64 Calculus of gallbladder and bile duct with chronic cholecystitis without obstruction CC

K80.65 Calculus of gallbladder and bile duct with chronic cholecystitis with obstruction CC

K80.66 Calculus of gallbladder and bile duct with acute and chronic cholecystitis without obstruction CC

K80.67 Calculus of gallbladder and bile duct with acute and chronic cholecystitis with obstruction MCC

K80.7 Calculus of gallbladder and bile duct without cholecystitis

K80.70 Calculus of gallbladder and bile duct without cholecystitis without obstruction

K80.71 Calculus of gallbladder and bile duct without cholecystitis with obstruction CC

K80.8 Other cholelithiasis

K80.80 Other cholelithiasis without obstruction

K80.81 Other cholelithiasis with obstruction CC

K81 Cholecystitis
Use additional code if applicable for associated gangrene of gallbladder (K82.A1), or perforation of gallbladder (K82.A2)
EXCLUDES 1 *cholecystitis with cholelithiasis (K80.-)*
AHA: 2018,4Q,20

K81.0 Acute cholecystitis CC
Abscess of gallbladder
Angiocholecystitis
Emphysematous (acute) cholecystitis
Empyema of gallbladder
Gangrene of gallbladder
Gangrenous cholecystitis
Suppurative cholecystitis

K81.1 Chronic cholecystitis

K81.2 Acute cholecystitis with chronic cholecystitis CC

K81.9 Cholecystitis, unspecified

K82 Other diseases of gallbladder
EXCLUDES 1 *nonvisualization of gallbladder (R93.2)*
postcholecystectomy syndrome (K91.5)

K82.0 Obstruction of gallbladder CC
Occlusion of cystic duct or gallbladder without cholelithiasis
Stenosis of cystic duct or gallbladder without cholelithiasis
Stricture of cystic duct or gallbladder without cholelithiasis
EXCLUDES 1 *obstruction of gallbladder with cholelithiasis (K80.-)*

K82.1 Hydrops of gallbladder CC
Mucocele of gallbladder

K82.2 Perforation of gallbladder MCC
Rupture of cystic duct or gallbladder
EXCLUDES 1 *perforation of gallbladder in cholecystitis (K82.A2)*

K82.3 Fistula of gallbladder CC
Cholecystocolic fistula
Cholecystoduodenal fistula

K82.4 Cholesterolosis of gallbladder
Strawberry gallbladder
EXCLUDES 1 *cholesterolosis of gallbladder with cholecystitis (K81.-)*
cholesterolosis of gallbladder with cholelithiasis (K80.-)

K82.8 Other specified diseases of gallbladder
Adhesions of cystic duct or gallbladder
Atrophy of cystic duct or gallbladder
Cyst of cystic duct or gallbladder
Dyskinesia of cystic duct or gallbladder
Hypertrophy of cystic duct or gallbladder
Nonfunctioning of cystic duct or gallbladder
Ulcer of cystic duct or gallbladder

K82.9 Disease of gallbladder, unspecified

K82.A Disorders of gallbladder in diseases classified elsewhere
Code first the type of cholecystitis (K81.-), or cholelithiasis with cholecystitis (K80.00-K80.19, K80.40-K80.47, K80.60-K80.67)
AHA: 2018,4Q,19-20

K82.A1 Gangrene of gallbladder in cholecystitis

K82.A2 Perforation of gallbladder in cholecystitis CC

K83 Other diseases of biliary tract
EXCLUDES 1 *postcholecystectomy syndrome (K91.5)*
EXCLUDES 2 *conditions involving the gallbladder (K81-K82)*
conditions involving the cystic duct (K81-K82)

K83.Ø Cholangitis
EXCLUDES 1 *cholangitic liver abscess (K75.Ø)*
cholangitis with choledocholithiasis (K8Ø.3-, K8Ø.4-)
EXCLUDES 2 *chronic nonsuppurative destructive cholangitis (K74.3)*
primary biliary cholangitis (K74.3)
primary biliary cirrhosis (K74.3)
AHA: 2018,4Q,20

K83.Ø1 Primary sclerosing cholangitis CC
K83.Ø9 Other cholangitis CC
Ascending cholangitis
Cholangitis NOS
Primary cholangitis
Recurrent cholangitis
Sclerosing cholangitis
Secondary cholangitis
Stenosing cholangitis
Suppurative cholangitis

K83.1 Obstruction of bile duct MCC
Occlusion of bile duct without cholelithiasis
Stenosis of bile duct without cholelithiasis
Stricture of bile duct without cholelithiasis
EXCLUDES 1 *congenital obstruction of bile duct (Q44.3)*
obstruction of bile duct with cholelithiasis (K8Ø.-)
AHA: 2016,1Q,18

K83.2 Perforation of bile duct MCC
Rupture of bile duct

K83.3 Fistula of bile duct CC
Choledochoduodenal fistula
AHA: 2019,1Q,17

K83.4 Spasm of sphincter of Oddi
K83.5 Biliary cyst
K83.8 Other specified diseases of biliary tract
Adhesions of biliary tract
Atrophy of biliary tract
Hypertrophy of biliary tract
Ulcer of biliary tract

K83.9 Disease of biliary tract, unspecified

K85 Acute pancreatitis
INCLUDES acute (recurrent) pancreatitis
subacute pancreatitis
AHA: 2016,4Q,34

K85.Ø Idiopathic acute pancreatitis
K85.ØØ Idiopathic acute pancreatitis without necrosis or infection MCC
K85.Ø1 Idiopathic acute pancreatitis with uninfected necrosis MCC
K85.Ø2 Idiopathic acute pancreatitis with infected necrosis MCC

K85.1 Biliary acute pancreatitis
Gallstone pancreatitis
K85.1Ø Biliary acute pancreatitis without necrosis or infection MCC
K85.11 Biliary acute pancreatitis with uninfected necrosis MCC
K85.12 Biliary acute pancreatitis with infected necrosis MCC

K85.2 Alcohol induced acute pancreatitis
EXCLUDES 2 *alcohol induced chronic pancreatitis (K86.Ø)*
K85.2Ø Alcohol induced acute pancreatitis without necrosis or infection MCC
AHA: 2020,1Q,9
K85.21 Alcohol induced acute pancreatitis with uninfected necrosis MCC
K85.22 Alcohol induced acute pancreatitis with infected necrosis MCC

K85.3 Drug induced acute pancreatitis
Use additional code for adverse effect, if applicable, to identify drug (T36-T5Ø with fifth or sixth character 5)
Use additional code to identify drug abuse and dependence (F11.- F17.-)
K85.3Ø Drug induced acute pancreatitis without necrosis or infection MCC
K85.31 Drug induced acute pancreatitis with uninfected necrosis MCC
K85.32 Drug induced acute pancreatitis with infected necrosis MCC

K85.8 Other acute pancreatitis
K85.8Ø Other acute pancreatitis without necrosis or infection MCC
K85.81 Other acute pancreatitis with uninfected necrosis MCC
K85.82 Other acute pancreatitis with infected necrosis MCC

K85.9 Acute pancreatitis, unspecified
Pancreatitis NOS
K85.9Ø Acute pancreatitis without necrosis or infection, unspecified MCC
K85.91 Acute pancreatitis with uninfected necrosis, unspecified MCC
K85.92 Acute pancreatitis with infected necrosis, unspecified MCC

K86 Other diseases of pancreas
EXCLUDES 2 *fibrocystic disease of pancreas (E84.-)*
islet cell tumor (of pancreas) (D13.7)
pancreatic steatorrhea (K9Ø.3)

K86.Ø Alcohol-induced chronic pancreatitis CC HCC
Use additional code to identify:
alcohol abuse and dependence (F1Ø.-)
Code also exocrine pancreatic insufficiency (K86.81)
EXCLUDES 2 *alcohol induced acute pancreatitis (K85.2-)*

K86.1 Other chronic pancreatitis CC HCC
Chronic pancreatitis NOS
Infectious chronic pancreatitis
Recurrent chronic pancreatitis
Relapsing chronic pancreatitis
Code also exocrine pancreatic insufficiency (K86.81)

K86.2 Cyst of pancreas CC
K86.3 Pseudocyst of pancreas CC
K86.8 Other specified diseases of pancreas
AHA: 2016,4Q,34-35
K86.81 Exocrine pancreatic insufficiency
K86.89 Other specified diseases of pancreas
Aseptic pancreatic necrosis, unrelated to acute pancreatitis
Atrophy of pancreas
Calculus of pancreas
Cirrhosis of pancreas
Fibrosis of pancreas
Pancreatic fat necrosis, unrelated to acute pancreatitis
Pancreatic infantilism
Pancreatic necrosis NOS, unrelated to acute pancreatitis

K86.9 Disease of pancreas, unspecified

K87 Disorders of gallbladder, biliary tract and pancreas in diseases classified elsewhere
Code first underlying disease
EXCLUDES 1 *cytomegaloviral pancreatitis (B25.2)*
mumps pancreatitis (B26.3)
syphilitic gallbladder (A52.74)
syphilitic pancreas (A52.74)
tuberculosis of gallbladder (A18.83)
tuberculosis of pancreas (A18.83)

Chapter 11. Diseases of the Digestive System
K83–K87

Other diseases of the digestive system (K90-K95)

K90 Intestinal malabsorption

EXCLUDES 1 *intestinal malabsorption following gastrointestinal surgery (K91.2)*

AHA: 2017,4Q,108

K90.0 Celiac disease
Celiac disease with steatorrhea
Celiac gluten-sensitive enteropathy
Nontropical sprue
Use additional code for associated disorders including:
dermatitis herpetiformis (L13.0)
gluten ataxia (G32.81)
Code also exocrine pancreatic insufficiency (K86.81)
DEF: Malabsorption syndrome due to gluten consumption. Symptoms include fetid, bulky, frothy, oily stools; a distended abdomen; gas; asthenia; electrolyte depletion; and vitamin B, D, and K deficiency.

K90.1 Tropical sprue CC
Sprue NOS
Tropical steatorrhea

K90.2 Blind loop syndrome, not elsewhere classified CC
Blind loop syndrome NOS
EXCLUDES 1 *congenital blind loop syndrome (Q43.8)*
postsurgical blind loop syndrome (K91.2)

K90.3 Pancreatic steatorrhea CC

K90.4 Other malabsorption due to intolerance
EXCLUDES 2 *celiac gluten-sensitive enteropathy (K90.0)*
lactose intolerance (E73.-)
AHA: 2016,4Q,35-36

K90.41 Non-celiac gluten sensitivity CC
Gluten sensitivity NOS
Non-celiac gluten sensitive enteropathy

K90.49 Malabsorption due to intolerance, not elsewhere classified CC
Malabsorption due to intolerance to carbohydrate
Malabsorption due to intolerance to fat
Malabsorption due to intolerance to protein
Malabsorption due to intolerance to starch

K90.8 Other intestinal malabsorption

K90.81 Whipple's disease CC

K90.89 Other intestinal malabsorption CC

K90.9 Intestinal malabsorption, unspecified CC

K91 Intraoperative and postprocedural complications and disorders of digestive system, not elsewhere classified

EXCLUDES 2 *complications of artificial opening of digestive system (K94.-)*
complications of bariatric procedures (K95.-)
gastrojejunal ulcer (K28.-)
postprocedural (radiation) retroperitoneal abscess (K68.11)
radiation colitis (K52.0)
radiation gastroenteritis (K52.0)
radiation proctitis (K62.7)

AHA: 2016,4Q,9-10

K91.0 Vomiting following gastrointestinal surgery

K91.1 Postgastric surgery syndromes
Dumping syndrome
Postgastrectomy syndrome
Postvagotomy syndrome

K91.2 Postsurgical malabsorption, not elsewhere classified CC
Postsurgical blind loop syndrome
EXCLUDES 1 *malabsorption osteomalacia in adults (M83.2)*
malabsorption osteoporosis, postsurgical (M80.8-, M81.8)

K91.3 Postprocedural intestinal obstruction
AHA: 2017,4Q,16-17; 2017,1Q,40

K91.30 Postprocedural intestinal obstruction, unspecified as to partial versus complete CC
Postprocedural intestinal obstruction NOS

K91.31 Postprocedural partial intestinal obstruction CC
Postprocedural incomplete intestinal obstruction

K91.32 Postprocedural complete intestinal obstruction CC

K91.5 Postcholecystectomy syndrome

K91.6 Intraoperative hemorrhage and hematoma of a digestive system organ or structure complicating a procedure
EXCLUDES 1 *intraoperative hemorrhage and hematoma of a digestive system organ or structure due to accidental puncture and laceration during a procedure (K91.7-)*

K91.61 Intraoperative hemorrhage and hematoma of a digestive system organ or structure complicating a digestive system procedure CC
AHA: 2020,1Q,19

K91.62 Intraoperative hemorrhage and hematoma of a digestive system organ or structure complicating other procedure CC

K91.7 Accidental puncture and laceration of a digestive system organ or structure during a procedure
AHA: 2022,1Q,51

K91.71 Accidental puncture and laceration of a digestive system organ or structure during a digestive system procedure CC
AHA: 2021,2Q,11

K91.72 Accidental puncture and laceration of a digestive system organ or structure during other procedure CC
AHA: 2019,2Q,23

K91.8 Other intraoperative and postprocedural complications and disorders of digestive system

K91.81 Other intraoperative complications of digestive system CC

K91.82 Postprocedural hepatic failure CC

K91.83 Postprocedural hepatorenal syndrome CC

K91.84 Postprocedural hemorrhage of a digestive system organ or structure following a procedure

K91.840 Postprocedural hemorrhage of a digestive system organ or structure following a digestive system procedure CC
AHA: 2016,1Q,15

K91.841 Postprocedural hemorrhage of a digestive system organ or structure following other procedure CC

K91.85 Complications of intestinal pouch

K91.850 Pouchitis CC HCC
Inflammation of internal ileoanal pouch
DEF: Inflammatory complication of an existing surgically created ileoanal pouch, resulting in multiple GI complaints, including diarrhea, abdominal pain, rectal bleeding, fecal urgency, or incontinence.

K91.858 Other complications of intestinal pouch CC HCC
AHA: 2019,2Q,13

K91.86 Retained cholelithiasis following cholecystectomy CC

K91.87 Postprocedural hematoma and seroma of a digestive system organ or structure following a procedure

K91.870 Postprocedural hematoma of a digestive system organ or structure following a digestive system procedure CC
AHA: 2022,1Q,24

K91.871 Postprocedural hematoma of a digestive system organ or structure following other procedure CC

K91.872 Postprocedural seroma of a digestive system organ or structure following a digestive system procedure CC

K91.873 Postprocedural seroma of a digestive system organ or structure following other procedure CC

K91.89 Other postprocedural complications and disorders of digestive system CC
Use additional code, if applicable, to further specify disorder
EXCLUDES 2 *postprocedural retroperitoneal abscess (K68.11)*
AHA: 2020,2Q,22; 2017,1Q,40

K92 Other diseases of digestive system

EXCLUDES 1 *neonatal gastrointestinal hemorrhage (P54.0-P54.3)*

K92.0 Hematemesis CC

K92.1 Melena CC

EXCLUDES 1 *occult blood in feces (R19.5)*

K92.2 Gastrointestinal hemorrhage, unspecified CC

Gastric hemorrhage NOS

Intestinal hemorrhage NOS

EXCLUDES 1 *acute hemorrhagic gastritis (K29.01)*
hemorrhage of anus and rectum (K62.5)
angiodysplasia of stomach with hemorrhage (K31.811)
diverticular disease with hemorrhage (K57.-)
gastritis and duodenitis with hemorrhage (K29.-)
peptic ulcer with hemorrhage (K25-K28)

AHA: 2021,1Q,11

✓5th **K92.8 Other specified diseases of the digestive system**

K92.81 Gastrointestinal mucositis (ulcerative) CC

Code also type of associated therapy, such as:
antineoplastic and immunosuppressive drugs (T45.1X-)
radiological procedure and radiotherapy (Y84.2)

EXCLUDES 2 *mucositis (ulcerative) of vagina and vulva (N76.81)*
nasal mucositis (ulcerative) (J34.81)
oral mucositis (ulcerative) (K12.3-)

K92.89 Other specified diseases of the digestive system

K92.9 Disease of digestive system, unspecified

✓4th **K94 Complications of artificial openings of the digestive system**

✓5th **K94.0 Colostomy complications**

K94.00 Colostomy complication, unspecified HCC

K94.01 Colostomy hemorrhage CC HCC

K94.02 Colostomy infection CC HCC

Use additional code to specify type of infection, such as:
cellulitis of abdominal wall (L03.311)
sepsis (A40.-, A41.-)

K94.03 Colostomy malfunction CC HCC

Mechanical complication of colostomy

K94.09 Other complications of colostomy CC HCC

✓5th **K94.1 Enterostomy complications**

K94.10 Enterostomy complication, unspecified HCC

K94.11 Enterostomy hemorrhage CC HCC

K94.12 Enterostomy infection CC HCC

Use additional code to specify type of infection, such as:
cellulitis of abdominal wall (L03.311)
sepsis (A40.-, A41.-)

K94.13 Enterostomy malfunction CC HCC

Mechanical complication of enterostomy

K94.19 Other complications of enterostomy CC HCC

✓5th **K94.2 Gastrostomy complications**

K94.20 Gastrostomy complication, unspecified HCC

K94.21 Gastrostomy hemorrhage HCC

K94.22 Gastrostomy infection CC HCC

Use additional code to specify type of infection, such as:
cellulitis of abdominal wall (L03.311)
sepsis (A40.-, A41.-)

K94.23 Gastrostomy malfunction CC HCC

Mechanical complication of gastrostomy

AHA: 2019,1Q,26

K94.29 Other complications of gastrostomy HCC

✓5th **K94.3 Esophagostomy complications**

K94.30 Esophagostomy complications, unspecified CC HCC

K94.31 Esophagostomy hemorrhage CC HCC

K94.32 Esophagostomy infection CC HCC

Use additional code to identify the infection

K94.33 Esophagostomy malfunction CC HCC

Mechanical complication of esophagostomy

K94.39 Other complications of esophagostomy CC HCC

✓4th **K95 Complications of bariatric procedures**

✓5th **K95.0 Complications of gastric band procedure**

K95.01 Infection due to gastric band procedure CC H11

Use additional code to specify type of infection or organism, such as:
bacterial and viral infectious agents (B95.-, B96.-)
cellulitis of abdominal wall (L03.311)
sepsis (A40.-, A41.-)

K95.09 Other complications of gastric band procedure CC

Use additional code, if applicable, to further specify complication

✓5th **K95.8 Complications of other bariatric procedure**

EXCLUDES 1 *complications of gastric band surgery (K95.0-)*

K95.81 Infection due to other bariatric procedure CC H11

Use additional code to specify type of infection or organism, such as:
bacterial and viral infectious agents (B95.-, B96.-)
cellulitis of abdominal wall (L03.311)
sepsis (A40.-, A41.-)

K95.89 Other complications of other bariatric procedure CC

Use additional code, if applicable, to further specify complication

Chapter 12. Diseases of the Skin and Subcutaneous Tissue (LØØ–L99)

Chapter-specific Guidelines with Coding Examples

The chapter-specific guidelines from the ICD-10-CM Official Guidelines for Coding and Reporting have been provided below. Along with these guidelines are coding examples, contained in the shaded boxes, that have been developed to help illustrate the coding and/or sequencing guidance found in these guidelines.

a. Pressure ulcer stage codes

1) Pressure ulcer stages

Codes in category L89, Pressure ulcer, identify the site and stage of the pressure ulcer.

The ICD-10-CM classifies pressure ulcer stages based on severity, which is designated by stages 1-4, deep tissue pressure injury, unspecified stage, and unstageable.

Assign as many codes from category L89 as needed to identify all the pressure ulcers the patient has, if applicable.

See Section I.B.14. for pressure ulcer stage documentation by clinicians other than patient's provider

> Nursing notes: Dressings changed daily on stage 4 ulcer on heel and stage 2 ulcer on elbow
>
> Discharge summary: Pressure ulcers on right heel and left elbow
>
> **L89.614 Pressure ulcer of right heel, stage 4**
>
> **L89.Ø22 Pressure ulcer of left elbow, stage 2**
>
> *Explanation:* Right heel and left elbow pressure ulcers were documented by the patient's provider in the discharge summary. Although the stage of these ulcers was not included in the provider's diagnostic statement, it is appropriate to code the stage from documentation from other clinicians involved in the patient's care, such as the nurse's notes, according to section I.B.14. Combination codes from category L89 Pressure ulcer, identify the site of the pressure ulcer as well as the stage. Assign as many codes from category L89 as needed to identify all the pressure ulcers the patient has.

2) Unstageable pressure ulcers

Assignment of the code for unstageable pressure ulcer (L89.--Ø) should be based on the clinical documentation. These codes are used for pressure ulcers whose stage cannot be clinically determined (e.g., the ulcer is covered by eschar or has been treated with a skin or muscle graft). This code should not be confused with the codes for unspecified stage (L89.--9). When there is no documentation regarding the stage of the pressure ulcer, assign the appropriate code for unspecified stage (L89.--9).

> Pressure ulcer of the right lower back documented as unstageable due to the presence of thick eschar covering the ulcer
>
> **L89.13Ø Pressure ulcer of right lower back, unstageable**
>
> *Explanation:* Codes for unstageable pressure ulcers are assigned when the stage cannot be clinically determined (e.g., the ulcer is covered by eschar or has been treated with a skin or muscle graft).

If during an encounter, the stage of an unstageable pressure ulcer is revealed after debridement, assign only the code for the stage revealed following debridement.

3) Documented pressure ulcer stage

Assignment of the pressure ulcer stage code should be guided by clinical documentation of the stage or documentation of the terms found in the Alphabetic Index. For clinical terms describing the stage that are not found in the Alphabetic Index, and there is no documentation of the stage, the provider should be queried.

> Left heel pressure ulcer with partial thickness skin loss involving the dermis
>
> **L89.622 Pressure ulcer of left heel, stage 2**
>
> *Explanation:* Code assignment for the pressure ulcer stage should be guided by either the clinical documentation of the stage or the documentation of terms found in the Alphabetic Index. The clinical documentation describing the left heel pressure ulcer "partial thickness skin loss involving the dermis" matches the ICD-10-CM index parenthetical description for stage 2 "(abrasion, blister, partial thickness skin loss involving epidermis and/or dermis)."

4) Patients admitted with pressure ulcers documented as healed

No code is assigned if the documentation states that the pressure ulcer is completely healed at the time of admission.

5) Pressure ulcers documented as healing

Pressure ulcers described as healing should be assigned the appropriate pressure ulcer stage code based on the documentation in the medical record. If the documentation does not provide information about the stage of the healing pressure ulcer, assign the appropriate code for unspecified stage.

If the documentation is unclear as to whether the patient has a current (new) pressure ulcer or if the patient is being treated for a healing pressure ulcer, query the provider.

For ulcers that were present on admission but healed at the time of discharge, assign the code for the site and stage of the pressure ulcer at the time of admission.

> H & P noted healing stage 2 sacral pressure ulcer. Resolved at time of discharge summary.
>
> **L89.152 Pressure ulcer of sacral region, stage 2**
>
> *Explanation:* Although completely healed upon discharge, the pressure ulcer required observation and/or treatment and should be coded based on the site and stage upon admission.

6) Patient admitted with pressure ulcer evolving into another stage during the admission

If a patient is admitted to an inpatient hospital with a pressure ulcer at one stage and it progresses to a higher stage, two separate codes should be assigned: one code for the site and stage of the ulcer on admission and a second code for the same ulcer site and the highest stage reported during the stay.

> Stage 3 right hip pressure ulcer worsened during admission to a stage 4
>
> **L89.213 Pressure ulcer of right hip, stage 3**
>
> **L89.214 Pressure ulcer of right hip, stage 4**
>
> *Explanation:* A pressure ulcer that progresses from a lower stage to a higher stage is assigned two codes, one for the documented stage upon admission and one for the documented stage at discharge.

7) Pressure-induced deep tissue damage

For pressure-induced deep tissue damage or deep tissue pressure injury, assign only the appropriate code for pressure-induced deep tissue damage (L89.--6).

b. Non-pressure chronic ulcers

1) Patients admitted with non-pressure ulcers documented as healed

No code is assigned if the documentation states that the non-pressure ulcer is completely healed at the time of admission.

2) Non-pressure ulcers documented as healing

Non-pressure ulcers described as healing should be assigned the appropriate non-pressure ulcer code based on the documentation in the medical record. If the documentation does not provide information about the severity of the healing non-pressure ulcer, assign the appropriate code for unspecified severity.

If the documentation is unclear as to whether the patient has a current (new) non-pressure ulcer or if the patient is being treated for a healing non-pressure ulcer, query the provider.

For ulcers that were present on admission but healed at the time of discharge, assign the code for the site and severity of the non-pressure ulcer at the time of admission.

> Admission diagnosis: Chronic ulcer, fat layer exposed, on left ankle
>
> Discharge diagnosis: Resolution of ulcer on the left ankle
>
> **L97.322 Non-pressure chronic ulcer of left ankle with fat layer exposed**
>
> *Explanation:* Although the ulcer was documented as resolved (healed) at discharge, a code representing the site and severity of the ulcer upon admission should be appended.

3) Patient admitted with non-pressure ulcer that progresses to another severity level during the admission

If a patient is admitted to an inpatient hospital with a non-pressure ulcer at one severity level and it progresses to a higher severity level, two separate codes should be assigned: one code for the site and severity level of the ulcer on admission and a second code for the same ulcer site and the highest severity level reported during the stay.

See Section I.B.14. for pressure ulcer stage documentation by clinicians other than patient's provider

Chapter 12. Diseases of the Skin and Subcutaneous Tissue (LØØ-L99)

EXCLUDES 2 *certain conditions originating in the perinatal period (PØ4-P96)*
certain infectious and parasitic diseases (AØØ-B99)
complications of pregnancy, childbirth and the puerperium (OØØ-O9A)
congenital malformations, deformations, and chromosomal abnormalities (QØØ-Q99)
endocrine, nutritional and metabolic diseases (EØØ-E88)
lipomelanotic reticulosis (I89.8)
neoplasms (CØØ-D49)
symptoms, signs and abnormal clinical and laboratory findings, not elsewhere classified (RØØ-R94)
systemic connective tissue disorders (M3Ø-M36)
viral warts (BØ7.-)

AHA: 2022,2Q,7

This chapter contains the following blocks:

- LØØ-LØ8 Infections of the skin and subcutaneous tissue
- L1Ø-L14 Bullous disorders
- L2Ø-L3Ø Dermatitis and eczema
- L4Ø-L45 Papulosquamous disorders
- L49-L54 Urticaria and erythema
- L55-L59 Radiation-related disorders of the skin and subcutaneous tissue
- L6Ø-L75 Disorders of skin appendages
- L76 Intraoperative and postprocedural complications of skin and subcutaneous tissue
- L8Ø-L99 Other disorders of the skin and subcutaneous tissue

Infections of the skin and subcutaneous tissue (LØØ-LØ8)

Use additional code (B95-B97) to identify infectious agent

EXCLUDES 2 *hordeolum (HØØ.Ø)*
infective dermatitis (L3Ø.3)
local infections of skin classified in Chapter 1
lupus panniculitis (L93.2)
panniculitis NOS (M79.3)
panniculitis of neck and back (M54.Ø-)
perlèche NOS (K13.Ø)
perlèche due to candidiasis (B37.Ø)
perlèche due to riboflavin deficiency (E53.Ø)
pyogenic granuloma (L98.Ø)
relapsing panniculitis [Weber-Christian] (M35.6)
viral warts (BØ7.-)
zoster (BØ2.-)

LØØ Staphylococcal scalded skin syndrome
Ritter's disease
Use additional code to identify percentage of skin exfoliation (L49.-)
EXCLUDES 1 *bullous impetigo (LØ1.Ø3)*
pemphigus neonatorum (LØ1.Ø3)
toxic epidermal necrolysis [Lyell] (L51.2)
DEF: Infectious skin disease of children younger than 5 years marked by eruptions ranging from a few localized blisters to widespread, easily ruptured, fine vesicles and bullae affecting almost the entire body. It results in exfoliation of large planes of skin and leaves raw areas.

√4th **LØ1 Impetigo**
EXCLUDES 1 *impetigo herpetiformis (L4Ø.1)*
DEF: Acute, superficial, highly contagious skin infection commonly occurring in children. Skin lesions usually appear on the face and consist of vesicles and bullae that burst and form yellow crusts.

√5th **LØ1.Ø Impetigo**
Impetigo contagiosa
Impetigo vulgaris

LØ1.ØØ Impetigo, unspecified (UNS)
Impetigo NOS

LØ1.Ø1 Non-bullous impetigo

LØ1.Ø2 Bockhart's impetigo
Impetigo follicularis
Perifolliculitis NOS
Superficial pustular perifolliculitis
DEF: Superficial inflammation of the hair follicles commonly caused by *Staphylococcus aureus* that manifests as rounded, sphere-shaped, pustular eruptions in the areas of the scalp, beard, underarms, extremities, and buttocks.

LØ1.Ø3 Bullous impetigo
Impetigo neonatorum
Pemphigus neonatorum

LØ1.Ø9 Other impetigo
Ulcerative impetigo

LØ1.1 Impetiginization of other dermatoses

√4th **LØ2 Cutaneous abscess, furuncle and carbuncle**
Use additional code to identify organism (B95-B96)
EXCLUDES 2 *abscess of anus and rectal regions (K61.-)*
abscess of female genital organs (external) (N76.4)
abscess of male genital organs (external) (N48.2, N49.-)
DEF: Carbuncle: Infection of the skin that arises from a collection of interconnected infected boils or furuncles, usually from hair follicles infected by *Staphylococcus*. This condition can produce pus and form drainage cavities.
DEF: Furuncle: Inflamed, painful abscess, cyst, or nodule on the skin caused by bacteria, often *Staphylococcus*, entering along the hair follicle.

√5th **LØ2.Ø Cutaneous abscess, furuncle and carbuncle of face**
EXCLUDES 2 *abscess of ear, external (H6Ø.Ø)*
abscess of eyelid (HØØ.Ø)
abscess of head [any part, except face] (LØ2.8)
abscess of lacrimal gland (HØ4.Ø)
abscess of lacrimal passages (HØ4.3)
abscess of mouth (K12.2)
abscess of nose (J34.Ø)
abscess of orbit (HØ5.Ø)
submandibular abscess (K12.2)

LØ2.Ø1 Cutaneous abscess of face CC

LØ2.Ø2 Furuncle of face
Boil of face
Folliculitis of face

LØ2.Ø3 Carbuncle of face

√5th **LØ2.1 Cutaneous abscess, furuncle and carbuncle of neck**

LØ2.11 Cutaneous abscess of neck CC

LØ2.12 Furuncle of neck
Boil of neck
Folliculitis of neck

LØ2.13 Carbuncle of neck

√5th **LØ2.2 Cutaneous abscess, furuncle and carbuncle of trunk**
EXCLUDES 1 *non-newborn omphalitis (LØ8.82)*
omphalitis of newborn (P38.-)
EXCLUDES 2 *abscess of breast (N61.1)*
abscess of buttocks (LØ2.3)
abscess of female external genital organs (N76.4)
abscess of hip (LØ2.4)
abscess of male external genital organs (N48.2, N49.-)

√6th **LØ2.21 Cutaneous abscess of trunk**
- **LØ2.211 Cutaneous abscess of abdominal wall** CC
- **LØ2.212 Cutaneous abscess of back [any part, except buttock]** CC
- **LØ2.213 Cutaneous abscess of chest wall** CC
- **LØ2.214 Cutaneous abscess of groin** CC
- **LØ2.215 Cutaneous abscess of perineum** CC
- **LØ2.216 Cutaneous abscess of umbilicus** CC
- **LØ2.219 Cutaneous abscess of trunk, unspecified** (UNS) CC

√6th **LØ2.22 Furuncle of trunk**
Boil of trunk
Folliculitis of trunk
- **LØ2.221 Furuncle of abdominal wall**
- **LØ2.222 Furuncle of back [any part, except buttock]**
- **LØ2.223 Furuncle of chest wall**
- **LØ2.224 Furuncle of groin**
- **LØ2.225 Furuncle of perineum**
- **LØ2.226 Furuncle of umbilicus**
- **LØ2.229 Furuncle of trunk, unspecified** (UNS)

√6th **LØ2.23 Carbuncle of trunk**
- **LØ2.231 Carbuncle of abdominal wall**
- **LØ2.232 Carbuncle of back [any part, except buttock]**
- **LØ2.233 Carbuncle of chest wall**
- **LØ2.234 Carbuncle of groin**
- **LØ2.235 Carbuncle of perineum**
- **LØ2.236 Carbuncle of umbilicus**
- **LØ2.239 Carbuncle of trunk, unspecified** (UNS)

√5th **LØ2.3 Cutaneous abscess, furuncle and carbuncle of buttock**
EXCLUDES 1 *pilonidal cyst with abscess (LØ5.Ø1)*

LØ2.31 Cutaneous abscess of buttock CC
Cutaneous abscess of gluteal region

L02.32 Furuncle of buttock
Boil of buttock
Folliculitis of buttock
Furuncle of gluteal region

L02.33 Carbuncle of buttock
Carbuncle of gluteal region

L02.4 Cutaneous abscess, furuncle and carbuncle of limb
EXCLUDES 2 *cutaneous abscess, furuncle and carbuncle of groin (L02.214, L02.224, L02.234)*
cutaneous abscess, furuncle and carbuncle of hand (L02.5-)
cutaneous abscess, furuncle and carbuncle of foot (L02.6-)

L02.41 Cutaneous abscess of limb
L02.411 Cutaneous abscess of right axilla CC
L02.412 Cutaneous abscess of left axilla CC
L02.413 Cutaneous abscess of right upper limb CC
L02.414 Cutaneous abscess of left upper limb CC
L02.415 Cutaneous abscess of right lower limb CC
L02.416 Cutaneous abscess of left lower limb CC
L02.419 Cutaneous abscess of limb, unspecified CC UNS

L02.42 Furuncle of limb
Boil of limb
Folliculitis of limb
L02.421 Furuncle of right axilla
L02.422 Furuncle of left axilla
L02.423 Furuncle of right upper limb
L02.424 Furuncle of left upper limb
L02.425 Furuncle of right lower limb
L02.426 Furuncle of left lower limb
L02.429 Furuncle of limb, unspecified

L02.43 Carbuncle of limb
L02.431 Carbuncle of right axilla
L02.432 Carbuncle of left axilla
L02.433 Carbuncle of right upper limb
L02.434 Carbuncle of left upper limb
L02.435 Carbuncle of right lower limb
L02.436 Carbuncle of left lower limb
L02.439 Carbuncle of limb, unspecified

L02.5 Cutaneous abscess, furuncle and carbuncle of hand

L02.51 Cutaneous abscess of hand
L02.511 Cutaneous abscess of right hand CC
L02.512 Cutaneous abscess of left hand CC
L02.519 Cutaneous abscess of unspecified hand CC UNS

L02.52 Furuncle hand
Boil of hand
Folliculitis of hand
L02.521 Furuncle right hand
L02.522 Furuncle left hand
L02.529 Furuncle unspecified hand

L02.53 Carbuncle of hand
L02.531 Carbuncle of right hand
L02.532 Carbuncle of left hand
L02.539 Carbuncle of unspecified hand

L02.6 Cutaneous abscess, furuncle and carbuncle of foot

L02.61 Cutaneous abscess of foot
L02.611 Cutaneous abscess of right foot CC
L02.612 Cutaneous abscess of left foot CC
L02.619 Cutaneous abscess of unspecified foot CC UNS

L02.62 Furuncle of foot
Boil of foot
Folliculitis of foot
L02.621 Furuncle of right foot
L02.622 Furuncle of left foot
L02.629 Furuncle of unspecified foot

L02.63 Carbuncle of foot
L02.631 Carbuncle of right foot
L02.632 Carbuncle of left foot
L02.639 Carbuncle of unspecified foot

L02.8 Cutaneous abscess, furuncle and carbuncle of other sites

L02.81 Cutaneous abscess of other sites
L02.811 Cutaneous abscess of head [any part, except face] CC
L02.818 Cutaneous abscess of other sites CC

L02.82 Furuncle of other sites
Boil of other sites
Folliculitis of other sites
L02.821 Furuncle of head [any part, except face]
L02.828 Furuncle of other sites

L02.83 Carbuncle of other sites
L02.831 Carbuncle of head [any part, except face]
L02.838 Carbuncle of other sites

L02.9 Cutaneous abscess, furuncle and carbuncle, unspecified
L02.91 Cutaneous abscess, unspecified CC
L02.92 Furuncle, unspecified
Boil NOS
Furunculosis NOS
L02.93 Carbuncle, unspecified

L03 Cellulitis and acute lymphangitis
EXCLUDES 2 *cellulitis of anal and rectal region (K61.-)*
cellulitis of external auditory canal (H60.1)
cellulitis of eyelid (H00.0)
cellulitis of female external genital organs (N76.4)
cellulitis of lacrimal apparatus (H04.3)
cellulitis of male external genital organs (N48.2, N49.-)
cellulitis of mouth (K12.2)
cellulitis of nose (J34.0)
eosinophilic cellulitis [Wells] (L98.3)
febrile neutrophilic dermatosis [Sweet] (L98.2)
lymphangitis (chronic) (subacute) (I89.1)

AHA: 2017,4Q,100
DEF: Cellulitis: Infection of the skin and subcutaneous tissues, most often caused by *Staphylococcus* or *Streptococcus* bacteria secondary to a cutaneous lesion. Progression of the inflammation may lead to abscess and tissue death, or even systemic infection-like bacteremia.
DEF: Lymphangitis: Inflammation of the lymph channels most often caused by *Streptococcus*.

L03.0 Cellulitis and acute lymphangitis of finger and toe
Infection of nail
Onychia
Paronychia
Perionychia

L03.01 Cellulitis of finger
Felon
Whitlow
EXCLUDES 1 *herpetic whitlow (B00.89)*
DEF: Felon: Superficial bacterial skin infection at the tip of the finger.
L03.011 Cellulitis of right finger
L03.012 Cellulitis of left finger
L03.019 Cellulitis of unspecified finger

L03.02 Acute lymphangitis of finger
Hangnail with lymphangitis of finger
L03.021 Acute lymphangitis of right finger
L03.022 Acute lymphangitis of left finger
L03.029 Acute lymphangitis of unspecified finger

L03.03 Cellulitis of toe
L03.031 Cellulitis of right toe
L03.032 Cellulitis of left toe
L03.039 Cellulitis of unspecified toe

L03.04 Acute lymphangitis of toe
Hangnail with lymphangitis of toe
L03.041 Acute lymphangitis of right toe
L03.042 Acute lymphangitis of left toe
L03.049 Acute lymphangitis of unspecified toe

L03.1 Cellulitis and acute lymphangitis of other parts of limb

L03.11 Cellulitis of other parts of limb
EXCLUDES 2 *cellulitis of fingers (L03.01-)*
cellulitis of toes (L03.03-)
groin (L03.314)
L03.111 Cellulitis of right axilla CC
L03.112 Cellulitis of left axilla CC
L03.113 Cellulitis of right upper limb CC
L03.114 Cellulitis of left upper limb CC

LØ3.115 Cellulitis of right lower limb CC

LØ3.116 Cellulitis of left lower limb CC

LØ3.119 Cellulitis of unspecified part of limb CC UNS

LØ3.12 Acute lymphangitis of other parts of limb

EXCLUDES 2 *acute lymphangitis of fingers (LØ3.2-)*
acute lymphangitis of groin (LØ3.324)
acute lymphangitis of toes (LØ3.Ø4-)

LØ3.121 Acute lymphangitis of right axilla CC

LØ3.122 Acute lymphangitis of left axilla CC

LØ3.123 Acute lymphangitis of right upper limb CC

LØ3.124 Acute lymphangitis of left upper limb CC

LØ3.125 Acute lymphangitis of right lower limb CC

LØ3.126 Acute lymphangitis of left lower limb CC

LØ3.129 Acute lymphangitis of unspecified part of limb CC UNS

LØ3.2 Cellulitis and acute lymphangitis of face and neck

LØ3.21 Cellulitis and acute lymphangitis of face

LØ3.211 Cellulitis of face CC

EXCLUDES 2 *abscess of orbit (HØ5.Ø1-)*
cellulitis of ear (H6Ø.1-)
cellulitis of eyelid (HØØ.Ø-)
cellulitis of head (LØ3.81)
cellulitis of lacrimal apparatus (HØ4.3)
cellulitis of lip (K13.Ø)
cellulitis of mouth (K12.2)
cellulitis of nose (internal) (J34.Ø)
cellulitis of orbit (HØ5.Ø1-)
cellulitis of scalp (LØ3.81)

AHA: 2013,4Q,123

LØ3.212 Acute lymphangitis of face CC

LØ3.213 Periorbital cellulitis CC

Preseptal cellulitis

AHA: 2016,4Q,36

LØ3.22 Cellulitis and acute lymphangitis of neck

LØ3.221 Cellulitis of neck CC

LØ3.222 Acute lymphangitis of neck CC

LØ3.3 Cellulitis and acute lymphangitis of trunk

LØ3.31 Cellulitis of trunk

EXCLUDES 2 *cellulitis of anal and rectal regions (K61.-)*
cellulitis of breast NOS (N61.Ø)
cellulitis of female external genital organs (N76.4)
cellulitis of male external genital organs (N48.2, N49.-)
omphalitis of newborn (P38.-)
puerperal cellulitis of breast (O91.2)

LØ3.311 Cellulitis of abdominal wall CC

EXCLUDES 2 *cellulitis of umbilicus (LØ3.316)*
cellulitis of groin (LØ3.314)

LØ3.312 Cellulitis of back [any part except buttock] CC

LØ3.313 Cellulitis of chest wall CC

LØ3.314 Cellulitis of groin CC

LØ3.315 Cellulitis of perineum CC

LØ3.316 Cellulitis of umbilicus CC

LØ3.317 Cellulitis of buttock CC

LØ3.319 Cellulitis of trunk, unspecified CC

LØ3.32 Acute lymphangitis of trunk

LØ3.321 Acute lymphangitis of abdominal wall CC

LØ3.322 Acute lymphangitis of back [any part except buttock] CC

LØ3.323 Acute lymphangitis of chest wall CC

LØ3.324 Acute lymphangitis of groin CC

LØ3.325 Acute lymphangitis of perineum CC

LØ3.326 Acute lymphangitis of umbilicus CC

LØ3.327 Acute lymphangitis of buttock CC

LØ3.329 Acute lymphangitis of trunk, unspecified CC

LØ3.8 Cellulitis and acute lymphangitis of other sites

LØ3.81 Cellulitis of other sites

LØ3.811 Cellulitis of head [any part, except face] CC

Cellulitis of scalp

EXCLUDES 2 *cellulitis of face (LØ3.211)*

LØ3.818 Cellulitis of other sites CC

LØ3.89 Acute lymphangitis of other sites

LØ3.891 Acute lymphangitis of head [any part, except face] CC

LØ3.898 Acute lymphangitis of other sites CC

LØ3.9 Cellulitis and acute lymphangitis, unspecified

LØ3.9Ø Cellulitis, unspecified CC

LØ3.91 Acute lymphangitis, unspecified CC

EXCLUDES 1 *lymphangitis NOS (I89.1)*

LØ4 Acute lymphadenitis

INCLUDES abscess (acute) of lymph nodes, except mesenteric
acute lymphadenitis, except mesenteric

EXCLUDES 1 *chronic or subacute lymphadenitis, except mesenteric (I88.1)*
enlarged lymph nodes (R59.-)
human immunodeficiency virus [HIV] disease resulting in generalized lymphadenopathy (B2Ø)
lymphadenitis NOS (I88.9)
nonspecific mesenteric lymphadenitis (I88.Ø)

DEF: Inflammation or enlargement of the lymph nodes.

LØ4.Ø Acute lymphadenitis of face, head and neck

LØ4.1 Acute lymphadenitis of trunk

LØ4.2 Acute lymphadenitis of upper limb

Acute lymphadenitis of axilla
Acute lymphadenitis of shoulder

LØ4.3 Acute lymphadenitis of lower limb

Acute lymphadenitis of hip

EXCLUDES 2 *acute lymphadenitis of groin (LØ4.1)*

LØ4.8 Acute lymphadenitis of other sites

LØ4.9 Acute lymphadenitis, unspecified

LØ5 Pilonidal cyst and sinus

DEF: Pilonidal cyst: Sac or sinus cavity of trapped epithelial tissues in the sacrococcygeal region, usually associated with ingrown hair.

DEF: Pilonidal sinus: Fistula, tract, or channel that extends from an infected area of ingrown hair to another site within the skin or out to the skin surface.

Pilonidal Cyst

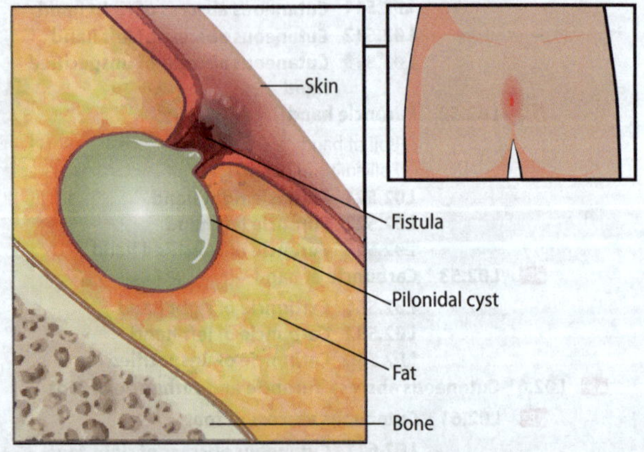

LØ5.Ø Pilonidal cyst and sinus with abscess

LØ5.Ø1 Pilonidal cyst with abscess CC

Pilonidal abscess
Pilonidal dimple with abscess
Postanal dimple with abscess

EXCLUDES 2 *congenital sacral dimple (Q82.6)*
parasacral dimple (Q82.6)

LØ5.Ø2 Pilonidal sinus with abscess CC

Coccygeal fistula with abscess
Coccygeal sinus with abscess
Pilonidal fistula with abscess

L05.9 Pilonidal cyst and sinus without abscess

L05.91 Pilonidal cyst without abscess
Pilonidal dimple
Postanal dimple
Pilonidal cyst NOS
EXCLUDES 2 *congenital sacral dimple (Q82.6)*
parasacral dimple (Q82.6)

L05.92 Pilonidal sinus without abscess
Coccygeal fistula
Coccygeal sinus without abscess
Pilonidal fistula

L08 Other local infections of skin and subcutaneous tissue

L08.0 Pyoderma
Dermatitis gangrenosa
Purulent dermatitis
Septic dermatitis
Suppurative dermatitis
EXCLUDES 1 *pyoderma gangrenosum (L88)*
pyoderma vegetans (L08.81)
DEF: Any superficial skin disease commonly characterized by the discharging of pus not attributed to another condition.

L08.1 Erythrasma HIV CC
DEF: Chronic, superficial skin infection of brown scaly patches, commonly found in skin folds most prevalent in the overweight or diabetic population.

L08.8 Other specified local infections of the skin and subcutaneous tissue

L08.81 Pyoderma vegetans
EXCLUDES 1 *pyoderma gangrenosum (L88)*
pyoderma NOS (L08.0)

L08.82 Omphalitis not of newborn
EXCLUDES 1 *omphalitis of newborn (P38.-)*

L08.89 Other specified local infections of the skin and subcutaneous tissue

L08.9 Local infection of the skin and subcutaneous tissue, unspecified

Bullous disorders (L10-L14)

EXCLUDES 1 *benign familial pemphigus [Hailey-Hailey] (Q82.8)*
staphylococcal scalded skin syndrome (L00)
toxic epidermal necrolysis [Lyell] (L51.2)

L10 Pemphigus
EXCLUDES 1 *pemphigus neonatorum (L01.03)*

L10.0 Pemphigus vulgaris CC
L10.1 Pemphigus vegetans CC
L10.2 Pemphigus foliaceous CC
L10.3 Brazilian pemphigus [fogo selvagem] CC
L10.4 Pemphigus erythematosus CC
Senear-Usher syndrome
L10.5 Drug-induced pemphigus CC
Use additional code for adverse effect, if applicable, to identify drug (T36-T50 with fifth or sixth character 5)

L10.8 Other pemphigus
L10.81 Paraneoplastic pemphigus CC
L10.89 Other pemphigus CC
L10.9 Pemphigus, unspecified CC

L11 Other acantholytic disorders

L11.0 Acquired keratosis follicularis
EXCLUDES 1 *keratosis follicularis (congenital) [Darier-White] (Q82.8)*
AHA: 2021,3Q,10
L11.1 Transient acantholytic dermatosis [Grover]
L11.8 Other specified acantholytic disorders
L11.9 Acantholytic disorder, unspecified

L12 Pemphigoid
EXCLUDES 1 *herpes gestationis (O26.4-)*
impetigo herpetiformis (L40.1)

L12.0 Bullous pemphigoid CC
L12.1 Cicatricial pemphigoid
Benign mucous membrane pemphigoid
DEF: Chronic autoimmune disease characterized by subepidermal blistering lesions of the mucosa, including the conjunctiva. It is seen predominantly in the elderly and produces adhesions and scarring.

L12.2 Chronic bullous disease of childhood P
Juvenile dermatitis herpetiformis

L12.3 Acquired epidermolysis bullosa
EXCLUDES 1 *epidermolysis bullosa (congenital) (Q81.-)*
L12.30 Acquired epidermolysis bullosa, unspecified CC HCC
L12.31 Epidermolysis bullosa due to drug CC HCC
Use additional code for adverse effect, if applicable, to identify drug (T36-T50 with fifth or sixth character 5)
L12.35 Other acquired epidermolysis bullosa CC HCC

L12.8 Other pemphigoid CC
L12.9 Pemphigoid, unspecified CC

L13 Other bullous disorders

L13.0 Dermatitis herpetiformis
Duhring's disease
Hydroa herpetiformis
EXCLUDES 1 *juvenile dermatitis herpetiformis (L12.2)*
senile dermatitis herpetiformis (L12.0)
DEF: Skin disease to which people are genetically predisposed resulting from an immunological response to gluten. Dermatitis herpetiformis is an extremely pruritic eruption of various lesions that frequently heal, leaving hyperpigmentation or hypopigmentation and occasionally scarring. It is usually associated with asymptomatic gluten-sensitive enteropathy.

L13.1 Subcorneal pustular dermatitis
Sneddon-Wilkinson disease
L13.8 Other specified bullous disorders
L13.9 Bullous disorder, unspecified

L14 Bullous disorders in diseases classified elsewhere
Code first underlying disease

Dermatitis and eczema (L20-L30)

NOTE In this block the terms dermatitis and eczema are used synonymously and interchangeably.

EXCLUDES 2 *chronic (childhood) granulomatous disease (D71)*
dermatitis gangrenosa (L08.0)
dermatitis herpetiformis (L13.0)
dry skin dermatitis (L85.3)
factitial dermatitis (L98.1)
perioral dermatitis (L71.0)
radiation-related disorders of the skin and subcutaneous tissue (L55-L59)
stasis dermatitis (I87.2)

L20 Atopic dermatitis

L20.0 Besnier's prurigo

L20.8 Other atopic dermatitis
EXCLUDES 2 *circumscribed neurodermatitis (L28.0)*
L20.81 Atopic neurodermatitis
Diffuse neurodermatitis
L20.82 Flexural eczema
L20.83 Infantile (acute) (chronic) eczema P
L20.84 Intrinsic (allergic) eczema
L20.89 Other atopic dermatitis

L20.9 Atopic dermatitis, unspecified

L21 Seborrheic dermatitis
EXCLUDES 2 *infective dermatitis (L30.3)*
seborrheic keratosis (L82.-)

L21.0 Seborrhea capitis
Cradle cap
AHA: 2018,1Q,6
TIP: Assign for dandruff in an adult patient.
L21.1 Seborrheic infantile dermatitis P
L21.8 Other seborrheic dermatitis
L21.9 Seborrheic dermatitis, unspecified
Seborrhea NOS

L22 Diaper dermatitis
Diaper erythema
Diaper rash
Psoriasiform diaper rash
AHA: 2021,4Q,18

L23 Allergic contact dermatitis

EXCLUDES 1 *allergy NOS (T78.4Ø)*
contact dermatitis NOS (L25.9)
dermatitis NOS (L3Ø.9)

EXCLUDES 2 *dermatitis due to substances taken internally (L27.-)*
dermatitis of eyelid (HØ1.1-)
diaper dermatitis (L22)
eczema of external ear (H6Ø.5-)
irritant contact dermatitis (L24.-)
perioral dermatitis (L71.Ø)
radiation-related disorders of the skin and subcutaneous tissue (L55-L59)

L23.Ø Allergic contact dermatitis due to metals
Allergic contact dermatitis due to chromium
Allergic contact dermatitis due to nickel

L23.1 Allergic contact dermatitis due to adhesives

L23.2 Allergic contact dermatitis due to cosmetics

L23.3 Allergic contact dermatitis due to drugs in contact with skin
Use additional code for adverse effect, if applicable, to identify drug (T36-T5Ø with fifth or sixth character 5)
EXCLUDES 2 *dermatitis due to ingested drugs and medicaments (L27.Ø-L27.1)*

L23.4 Allergic contact dermatitis due to dyes

L23.5 Allergic contact dermatitis due to other chemical products
Allergic contact dermatitis due to cement
Allergic contact dermatitis due to insecticide
Allergic contact dermatitis due to plastic
Allergic contact dermatitis due to rubber

L23.6 Allergic contact dermatitis due to food in contact with the skin
EXCLUDES 2 *dermatitis due to ingested food (L27.2)*

L23.7 Allergic contact dermatitis due to plants, except food
EXCLUDES 2 *allergy NOS due to pollen (J3Ø.1)*

L23.8 Allergic contact dermatitis due to other agents

L23.81 Allergic contact dermatitis due to animal (cat) (dog) dander
Allergic contact dermatitis due to animal (cat) (dog) hair

L23.89 Allergic contact dermatitis due to other agents

L23.9 Allergic contact dermatitis, unspecified cause
Allergic contact eczema NOS

L24 Irritant contact dermatitis

EXCLUDES 1 *allergy NOS (T78.4Ø)*
contact dermatitis NOS (L25.9)
dermatitis NOS (L3Ø.9)

EXCLUDES 2 *allergic contact dermatitis (L23.-)*
dermatitis due to substances taken internally (L27.-)
dermatitis of eyelid (HØ1.1-)
diaper dermatitis (L22)
eczema of external ear (H6Ø.5-)
perioral dermatitis (L71.Ø)
radiation-related disorders of the skin and subcutaneous tissue (L55-L59)

L24.Ø Irritant contact dermatitis due to detergents

L24.1 Irritant contact dermatitis due to oils and greases

L24.2 Irritant contact dermatitis due to solvents
Irritant contact dermatitis due to chlorocompound
Irritant contact dermatitis due to cyclohexane
Irritant contact dermatitis due to ester
Irritant contact dermatitis due to glycol
Irritant contact dermatitis due to hydrocarbon
Irritant contact dermatitis due to ketone

L24.3 Irritant contact dermatitis due to cosmetics

L24.4 Irritant contact dermatitis due to drugs in contact with skin
Use additional code for adverse effect, if applicable, to identify drug (T36-T5Ø with fifth or sixth character 5)

L24.5 Irritant contact dermatitis due to other chemical products
Irritant contact dermatitis due to cement
Irritant contact dermatitis due to insecticide
Irritant contact dermatitis due to plastic
Irritant contact dermatitis due to rubber

L24.6 Irritant contact dermatitis due to food in contact with skin
EXCLUDES 2 *dermatitis due to ingested food (L27.2)*

L24.7 Irritant contact dermatitis due to plants, except food
EXCLUDES 2 *allergy NOS to pollen (J3Ø.1)*

L24.8 Irritant contact dermatitis due to other agents

L24.81 Irritant contact dermatitis due to metals
Irritant contact dermatitis due to chromium
Irritant contact dermatitis due to nickel

L24.89 Irritant contact dermatitis due to other agents
Irritant contact dermatitis due to dyes

L24.9 Irritant contact dermatitis, unspecified cause
Irritant contact eczema NOS

L24.A Irritant contact dermatitis due to friction or contact with body fluids
EXCLUDES 1 *irritant contact dermatitis related to stoma or fistula (L24.B-)*
EXCLUDES 2 *erythema intertrigo (L3Ø.4)*
AHA: 2021,4Q,16-18

L24.AØ Irritant contact dermatitis due to friction or contact with body fluids, unspecified

L24.A1 Irritant contact dermatitis due to saliva

L24.A2 Irritant contact dermatitis due to fecal, urinary or dual incontinence
EXCLUDES 1 *diaper dermatitis (L22)*

L24.A9 Irritant contact dermatitis due friction or contact with other specified body fluids
Irritant contact dermatitis related to endotracheal tube
Wound fluids, exudate

L24.B Irritant contact dermatitis related to stoma or fistula
Use additional code to identify any artificial opening status (Z93.-), if applicable, for contact dermatitis related to stoma secretions
AHA: 2021,4Q,16-18

L24.BØ Irritant contact dermatitis related to unspecified stoma or fistula
Irritant contact dermatitis related to fistula NOS
Irritant contact dermatitis related to stoma NOS

L24.B1 Irritant contact dermatitis related to digestive stoma or fistula
Irritant contact dermatitis related to gastrostomy
Irritant contact dermatitis related to jejunostomy
Irritant contact dermatitis related to saliva or spit fistula

L24.B2 Irritant contact dermatitis related to respiratory stoma or fistula
Irritant contact dermatitis related to tracheostomy

L24.B3 Irritant contact dermatitis related to fecal or urinary stoma or fistula
Irritant contact dermatitis related to colostomy
Irritant contact dermatitis related to enterocutaneous fistula
Irritant contact dermatitis related to ileostomy

L25 Unspecified contact dermatitis

EXCLUDES 1 *allergic contact dermatitis (L23.-)*
allergy NOS (T78.4Ø)
dermatitis NOS (L3Ø.9)
irritant contact dermatitis (L24.-)

EXCLUDES 2 *dermatitis due to ingested substances (L27.-)*
dermatitis of eyelid (HØ1.1-)
eczema of external ear (H6Ø.5-)
perioral dermatitis (L71.Ø)
radiation-related disorders of the skin and subcutaneous tissue (L55-L59)

L25.Ø Unspecified contact dermatitis due to cosmetics

L25.1 Unspecified contact dermatitis due to drugs in contact with skin
Use additional code for adverse effect, if applicable, to identify drug (T36-T5Ø with fifth or sixth character 5)
EXCLUDES 2 *dermatitis due to ingested drugs and medicaments (L27.Ø-L27.1)*

L25.2 Unspecified contact dermatitis due to dyes

L25.3 Unspecified contact dermatitis due to other chemical products
Unspecified contact dermatitis due to cement
Unspecified contact dermatitis due to insecticide

L25.4 Unspecified contact dermatitis due to food in contact with skin
EXCLUDES 2 *dermatitis due to ingested food (L27.2)*

L25.5 Unspecified contact dermatitis due to plants, except food
EXCLUDES 1 *nettle rash (L50.9)*
EXCLUDES 2 *allergy NOS due to pollen (J30.1)*

L25.8 Unspecified contact dermatitis due to other agents

L25.9 Unspecified contact dermatitis, unspecified cause
Contact dermatitis (occupational) NOS
Contact eczema (occupational) NOS

L26 Exfoliative dermatitis
Hebra's pityriasis
EXCLUDES 1 *Ritter's disease (L00)*

L27 Dermatitis due to substances taken internally
EXCLUDES 1 *allergy NOS (T78.40)*
EXCLUDES 2 *adverse food reaction, except dermatitis (T78.0-T78.1)*
contact dermatitis (L23-L25)
drug photoallergic response (L56.1)
drug phototoxic response (L56.0)
urticaria (L50.-)

L27.0 Generalized skin eruption due to drugs and medicaments taken internally
Use additional code for adverse effect, if applicable, to identify drug (T36-T50 with fifth or sixth character 5)

L27.1 Localized skin eruption due to drugs and medicaments taken internally
Use additional code for adverse effect, if applicable, to identify drug (T36-T50 with fifth or sixth character 5)

L27.2 Dermatitis due to ingested food
EXCLUDES 2 *dermatitis due to food in contact with skin (L23.6, L24.6, L25.4)*

L27.8 Dermatitis due to other substances taken internally

L27.9 Dermatitis due to unspecified substance taken internally

L28 Lichen simplex chronicus and prurigo

L28.0 Lichen simplex chronicus
Circumscribed neurodermatitis
Lichen NOS

L28.1 Prurigo nodularis

L28.2 Other prurigo
Prurigo NOS
Prurigo Hebra
Prurigo mitis
Urticaria papulosa

L29 Pruritus
EXCLUDES 1 *neurotic excoriation (L98.1)*
psychogenic pruritus (F45.8)

L29.0 Pruritus ani

L29.1 Pruritus scroti ♂

L29.2 Pruritus vulvae ♀

L29.3 Anogenital pruritus, unspecified

L29.8 Other pruritus

L29.9 Pruritus, unspecified
Itch NOS

L30 Other and unspecified dermatitis
EXCLUDES 2 *contact dermatitis (L23-L25)*
dry skin dermatitis (L85.3)
small plaque parapsoriasis (L41.3)
stasis dermatitis (I87.2)

L30.0 Nummular dermatitis

L30.1 Dyshidrosis [pompholyx]

L30.2 Cutaneous autosensitization
Candidid [levurid]
Dermatophytid
Eczematid

L30.3 Infective dermatitis
Infectious eczematoid dermatitis

L30.4 Erythema intertrigo

L30.5 Pityriasis alba
AHA: 2018,1Q,6

L30.8 Other specified dermatitis

L30.9 Dermatitis, unspecified
Eczema NOS

Papulosquamous disorders (L40-L45)

L40 Psoriasis
DEF: Chronic autoimmune condition that speeds up skin cell growth, causing excessive immature skin cells to form raised, rounded erythematous lesions covered by dry, silvery scaling patches. Most commonly found on the scalp, elbows, knees, hands, feet, and genitals, it can also affect the joints with stiffness and swelling.

L40.0 Psoriasis vulgaris
Nummular psoriasis
Plaque psoriasis

L40.1 Generalized pustular psoriasis
Impetigo herpetiformis
Von Zumbusch's disease

L40.2 Acrodermatitis continua

L40.3 Pustulosis palmaris et plantaris

L40.4 Guttate psoriasis

L40.5 Arthropathic psoriasis

L40.50 Arthropathic psoriasis, unspecified HCC

L40.51 Distal interphalangeal psoriatic arthropathy HCC

L40.52 Psoriatic arthritis mutilans HCC

L40.53 Psoriatic spondylitis HCC

L40.54 Psoriatic juvenile arthropathy HCC

L40.59 Other psoriatic arthropathy HCC

L40.8 Other psoriasis
Flexural psoriasis

L40.9 Psoriasis, unspecified

L41 Parapsoriasis
EXCLUDES 1 *poikiloderma vasculare atrophicans (L94.5)*

L41.0 Pityriasis lichenoides et varioliformis acuta
Mucha-Habermann disease

L41.1 Pityriasis lichenoides chronica

L41.3 Small plaque parapsoriasis

L41.4 Large plaque parapsoriasis

L41.5 Retiform parapsoriasis

L41.8 Other parapsoriasis

L41.9 Parapsoriasis, unspecified

L42 Pityriasis rosea

L43 Lichen planus
EXCLUDES 1 *lichen planopilaris (L66.1)*

L43.0 Hypertrophic lichen planus

L43.1 Bullous lichen planus

L43.2 Lichenoid drug reaction
Use additional code for adverse effect, if applicable, to identify drug (T36-T50 with fifth or sixth character 5)

L43.3 Subacute (active) lichen planus
Lichen planus tropicus

L43.8 Other lichen planus

L43.9 Lichen planus, unspecified

L44 Other papulosquamous disorders

L44.0 Pityriasis rubra pilaris

L44.1 Lichen nitidus
DEF: Chronic, inflammatory, asymptomatic skin disorder, characterized by numerous glistening, flat-topped, discrete, skin-colored micropapules, most often on the penis, lower abdomen, inner thighs, wrists, forearms, breasts, and buttocks.

L44.2 Lichen striatus

L44.3 Lichen ruber moniliformis

L44.4 Infantile papular acrodermatitis [Gianotti-Crosti] P

L44.8 Other specified papulosquamous disorders

L44.9 Papulosquamous disorder, unspecified

L45 Papulosquamous disorders in diseases classified elsewhere
Code first underlying disease

Urticaria and erythema (L49-L54)

EXCLUDES 1 *Lyme disease (A69.2-)*
rosacea (L71.-)

L49 Exfoliation due to erythematous conditions according to extent of body surface involved

Code first erythematous condition causing exfoliation, such as:
- Ritter's disease (LØØ)
- (Staphylococcal) scalded skin syndrome (LØØ)
- Stevens-Johnson syndrome (L51.1)
- Stevens-Johnson syndrome-toxic epidermal necrolysis overlap syndrome (L51.3)
- toxic epidermal necrolysis (L51.2)

DEF: Exfoliation: Falling or sloughing off skin in layers.

L49.Ø Exfoliation due to erythematous condition involving less than 1Ø percent of body surface UPD
Exfoliation due to erythematous condition NOS

L49.1 Exfoliation due to erythematous condition involving 1Ø-19 percent of body surface UPD

L49.2 Exfoliation due to erythematous condition involving 2Ø-29 percent of body surface UPD

L49.3 Exfoliation due to erythematous condition involving 3Ø-39 percent of body surface CC UPD

L49.4 Exfoliation due to erythematous condition involving 4Ø-49 percent of body surface CC UPD

L49.5 Exfoliation due to erythematous condition involving 5Ø-59 percent of body surface CC UPD

L49.6 Exfoliation due to erythematous condition involving 6Ø-69 percent of body surface CC UPD

L49.7 Exfoliation due to erythematous condition involving 7Ø-79 percent of body surface CC UPD

L49.8 Exfoliation due to erythematous condition involving 8Ø-89 percent of body surface CC UPD

L49.9 Exfoliation due to erythematous condition involving 9Ø or more percent of body surface CC UPD

L5Ø Urticaria

EXCLUDES 1 *allergic contact dermatitis (L23.-)*
angioneurotic edema (T78.3)
giant urticaria (T78.3)
hereditary angio-edema (D84.1)
Quincke's edema (T78.3)
serum urticaria (T8Ø.6-)
solar urticaria (L56.3)
urticaria neonatorum (P83.8)
urticaria papulosa (L28.2)
urticaria pigmentosa (D47.Ø1)

DEF: Eruption of itching edema of the skin. ***Synonym(s):*** *hives.*

L5Ø.Ø Allergic urticaria

L5Ø.1 Idiopathic urticaria

L5Ø.2 Urticaria due to cold and heat
EXCLUDES 2 *familial cold urticaria (MØ4.2)*

L5Ø.3 Dermatographic urticaria

L5Ø.4 Vibratory urticaria

L5Ø.5 Cholinergic urticaria

L5Ø.6 Contact urticaria

L5Ø.8 Other urticaria
Chronic urticaria
Recurrent periodic urticaria

L5Ø.9 Urticaria, unspecified

L51 Erythema multiforme

Use additional code for adverse effect, if applicable, to identify drug (T36-T5Ø with fifth or sixth character 5)

Use additional code to identify associated manifestations, such as:
- arthropathy associated with dermatological disorders (M14.8-)
- conjunctival edema (H11.42)
- conjunctivitis (H1Ø.22-)
- corneal scars and opacities (H17.-)
- corneal ulcer (H16.Ø-)
- edema of eyelid (HØ2.84-)
- inflammation of eyelid (HØ1.8)
- keratoconjunctivitis sicca (H16.22-)
- mechanical lagophthalmos (HØ2.22-)
- stomatitis (K12.-)
- symblepharon (H11.23-)

Use additional code to identify percentage of skin exfoliation (L49.-)

EXCLUDES 1 *staphylococcal scalded skin syndrome (LØØ)*
Ritter's disease (LØØ)

DEF: Acute complex of symptoms with a varied pattern of skin eruptions, such as macular, bullous, papular, nodose, or vesicular lesions on the neck, face, and legs. Erythema (redness of skin and mucous membranes) multiforme (multiple forms) is a hypersensitivity (allergic) reaction that can occur at any age but primarily affects children or young adults.

L51.Ø Nonbullous erythema multiforme

L51.1 Stevens-Johnson syndrome CC HCC

L51.2 Toxic epidermal necrolysis [Lyell] CC HCC

L51.3 Stevens-Johnson syndrome-toxic epidermal necrolysis overlap syndrome CC HCC
SJS-TEN overlap syndrome

L51.8 Other erythema multiforme

L51.9 Erythema multiforme, unspecified
Erythema iris
Erythema multiforme major NOS
Erythema multiforme minor NOS
Herpes iris

L52 Erythema nodosum

EXCLUDES 1 *tuberculous erythema nodosum (A18.4)*

DEF: Form of panniculitis (inflammation of the fat layer beneath the skin) most often occurring in women. Commonly seen as a hypersensitivity reaction to infections, drugs, sarcoidosis, and specific enteropathies. The acute stage is associated with fever, malaise, and arthralgia. The lesions are pink to blue in color as tender nodules and are found on the front of the legs below the knees.

L53 Other erythematous conditions

EXCLUDES 1 *erythema ab igne (L59.Ø)*
erythema due to external agents in contact with skin (L23-L25)
erythema intertrigo (L3Ø.4)

L53.Ø Toxic erythema CC
Code first poisoning due to drug or toxin, if applicable (T36-T65 with fifth or sixth character 1-4 or 6)
Use additional code for adverse effect, if applicable, to identify drug (T36-T5Ø with fifth or sixth character 5)
EXCLUDES 1 *neonatal erythema toxicum (P83.1)*

L53.1 Erythema annulare centrifugum CC

L53.2 Erythema marginatum CC

L53.3 Other chronic figurate erythema CC

L53.8 Other specified erythematous conditions

L53.9 Erythematous condition, unspecified
Erythema NOS
Erythroderma NOS

L54 Erythema in diseases classified elsewhere
Code first underlying disease

Radiation-related disorders of the skin and subcutaneous tissue (L55-L59)

L55 Sunburn

L55.Ø Sunburn of first degree

L55.1 Sunburn of second degree

L55.2 Sunburn of third degree

L55.9 Sunburn, unspecified

✓4th L56 Other acute skin changes due to ultraviolet radiation

Use additional code to identify the source of the ultraviolet radiation (W89, X32)

L56.Ø Drug phototoxic response

Use additional code for adverse effect, if applicable, to identify drug (T36-T5Ø with fifth or sixth character 5)

L56.1 Drug photoallergic response

Use additional code for adverse effect, if applicable, to identify drug (T36-T5Ø with fifth or sixth character 5)

L56.2 Photocontact dermatitis [berloque dermatitis]

L56.3 Solar urticaria

L56.4 Polymorphous light eruption

L56.5 Disseminated superficial actinic porokeratosis (DSAP)

DEF: Autosomal dominant skin condition occurring in sun-exposed areas of the skin (particularly the arms and legs), characterized by superficial annular, keratotic, brownish-red spots or thickenings with depressed centers and sharp, ridged borders. It may evolve into squamous cell carcinoma.

L56.8 Other specified acute skin changes due to ultraviolet radiation

L56.9 Acute skin change due to ultraviolet radiation, unspecified

✓4th L57 Skin changes due to chronic exposure to nonionizing radiation

Use additional code to identify the source of the ultraviolet radiation (W89), or other nonionizing radiation (W9Ø)

L57.Ø Actinic keratosis

Keratosis NOS

Senile keratosis

Solar keratosis

L57.1 Actinic reticuloid

L57.2 Cutis rhomboidalis nuchae

L57.3 Poikiloderma of Civatte

L57.4 Cutis laxa senilis

Elastosis senilis

L57.5 Actinic granuloma

L57.8 Other skin changes due to chronic exposure to nonionizing radiation

Farmer's skin

Sailor's skin

Solar dermatitis

L57.9 Skin changes due to chronic exposure to nonionizing radiation, unspecified

✓4th L58 Radiodermatitis

Use additional code to identify the source of the radiation (W88, W9Ø)

L58.Ø Acute radiodermatitis

L58.1 Chronic radiodermatitis

L58.9 Radiodermatitis, unspecified

✓4th L59 Other disorders of skin and subcutaneous tissue related to radiation

L59.Ø Erythema ab igne [dermatitis ab igne]

L59.8 Other specified disorders of the skin and subcutaneous tissue related to radiation

AHA: 2017,1Q,33

L59.9 Disorder of the skin and subcutaneous tissue related to radiation, unspecified

Disorders of skin appendages (L6Ø-L75)

EXCLUDES 1 *congenital malformations of integument (Q84.-)*

✓4th L6Ø Nail disorders

EXCLUDES 2 *clubbing of nails (R68.3)*

onychia and paronychia (LØ3.Ø-)

Nail Disorders

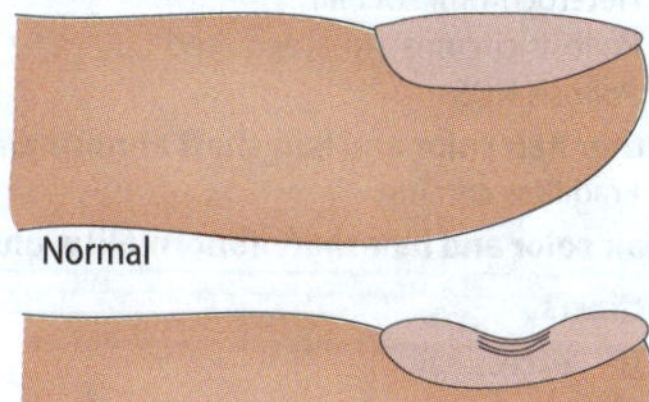

Normal

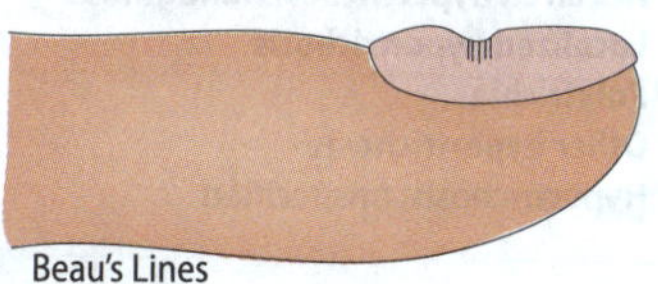

Koilonychia

Beau's Lines

L6Ø.Ø Ingrowing nail

L6Ø.1 Onycholysis

L6Ø.2 Onychogryphosis

L6Ø.3 Nail dystrophy

L6Ø.4 Beau's lines

L6Ø.5 Yellow nail syndrome

L6Ø.8 Other nail disorders

L6Ø.9 Nail disorder, unspecified

L62 Nail disorders in diseases classified elsewhere

Code first underlying disease, such as: pachydermoperiostosis (M89.4-)

✓4th L63 Alopecia areata

L63.Ø Alopecia (capitis) totalis

L63.1 Alopecia universalis

L63.2 Ophiasis

L63.8 Other alopecia areata

L63.9 Alopecia areata, unspecified

✓4th L64 Androgenic alopecia

INCLUDES male-pattern baldness

L64.Ø Drug-induced androgenic alopecia

Use additional code for adverse effect, if applicable, to identify drug (T36-T5Ø with fifth or sixth character 5)

L64.8 Other androgenic alopecia

L64.9 Androgenic alopecia, unspecified

✓4th L65 Other nonscarring hair loss

Use additional code for adverse effect, if applicable, to identify drug (T36-T5Ø with fifth or sixth character 5)

EXCLUDES 1 *trichotillomania (F63.3)*

L65.Ø Telogen effluvium

DEF: Form of nonscarring alopecia characterized by shedding of hair from premature telogen development in follicles due to stress, including shock, childbirth, surgery, drugs, or weight loss.

L65.1 Anagen effluvium

L65.2 Alopecia mucinosa

L65.8 Other specified nonscarring hair loss

L65.9 Nonscarring hair loss, unspecified

Alopecia NOS

✓4th L66 Cicatricial alopecia [scarring hair loss]

L66.Ø Pseudopelade

L66.1 Lichen planopilaris

Follicular lichen planus

L66.2 Folliculitis decalvans

L66.3 Perifolliculitis capitis abscedens

L66.4 Folliculitis ulerythematosa reticulata

L66.8 Other cicatricial alopecia

AHA: 2015,1Q,19

L66.9 Cicatricial alopecia, unspecified

L67 Hair color and hair shaft abnormalities

EXCLUDES 1 *monilethrix (Q84.1)*
pili annulati (Q84.1)
telogen effluvium (L65.Ø)

L67.Ø Trichorrhexis nodosa

L67.1 Variations in hair color
Canities
Greyness, hair (premature)
Heterochromia of hair
Poliosis circumscripta, acquired
Poliosis NOS

L67.8 Other hair color and hair shaft abnormalities
Fragilitas crinium

L67.9 Hair color and hair shaft abnormality, unspecified

L68 Hypertrichosis

INCLUDES excess hair
EXCLUDES 1 *congenital hypertrichosis (Q84.2)*
persistent lanugo (Q84.2)

L68.Ø Hirsutism
L68.1 Acquired hypertrichosis lanuginosa
L68.2 Localized hypertrichosis
L68.3 Polytrichia
L68.8 Other hypertrichosis
L68.9 Hypertrichosis, unspecified

L7Ø Acne

EXCLUDES 2 *acne keloid (L73.Ø)*

L7Ø.Ø Acne vulgaris
L7Ø.1 Acne conglobata
L7Ø.2 Acne varioliformis
Acne necrotica miliaris
DEF: Rare form of acne characterized by development of persistent brown papulopustules followed by scar formation. This type of acne usually presents on the brow and temporoparietal part of the scalp.

L7Ø.3 Acne tropica
L7Ø.4 Infantile acne P
L7Ø.5 Acné excoriée
Acné excoriée des jeunes filles
Picker's acne
L7Ø.8 Other acne
L7Ø.9 Acne, unspecified

L71 Rosacea

Use additional code for adverse effect, if applicable, to identify drug (T36-T5Ø with fifth or sixth character 5)

L71.Ø Perioral dermatitis
L71.1 Rhinophyma
L71.8 Other rosacea
AHA: 2018,4Q,15
L71.9 Rosacea, unspecified

L72 Follicular cysts of skin and subcutaneous tissue

L72.Ø Epidermal cyst
L72.1 Pilar and trichodermal cyst
L72.11 Pilar cyst
L72.12 Trichodermal cyst
Trichilemmal (proliferating) cyst
L72.2 Steatocystoma multiplex
L72.3 Sebaceous cyst
EXCLUDES 2 *pilar cyst (L72.11)*
trichilemmal (proliferating) cyst (L72.12)
L72.8 Other follicular cysts of the skin and subcutaneous tissue
L72.9 Follicular cyst of the skin and subcutaneous tissue, unspecified

L73 Other follicular disorders

L73.Ø Acne keloid
L73.1 Pseudofolliculitis barbae
L73.2 Hidradenitis suppurativa
L73.8 Other specified follicular disorders
Sycosis barbae
L73.9 Follicular disorder, unspecified

L74 Eccrine sweat disorders

EXCLUDES 2 *generalized hyperhidrosis (R61)*

DEF: Eccrine sweat glands: Glands found in the dermal and hypodermal layer of the skin throughout the body, particularly on the forehead, scalp, axillae, palms, and soles. These glands produce watery and neutral or slightly acidic sweat.

L74.Ø Miliaria rubra
L74.1 Miliaria crystallina
L74.2 Miliaria profunda
Miliaria tropicalis
L74.3 Miliaria, unspecified
L74.4 Anhidrosis
Hypohidrosis
DEF: Inability to sweat normally. When the body can't cool itself through perspiration it can lead to heatstroke, a life-threatening condition.
L74.5 Focal hyperhidrosis
L74.51 Primary focal hyperhidrosis
L74.51Ø Primary focal hyperhidrosis, axilla
L74.511 Primary focal hyperhidrosis, face
L74.512 Primary focal hyperhidrosis, palms
L74.513 Primary focal hyperhidrosis, soles
L74.519 Primary focal hyperhidrosis, unspecified
L74.52 Secondary focal hyperhidrosis
Frey's syndrome
L74.8 Other eccrine sweat disorders
L74.9 Eccrine sweat disorder, unspecified
Sweat gland disorder NOS

L75 Apocrine sweat disorders

EXCLUDES 1 *dyshidrosis (L3Ø.1)*
hidradenitis suppurativa (L73.2)

DEF: Apocrine sweat glands: Found in the axilla, areola, and circumanal region, these glands begin to function in puberty and produce viscid milky secretions in response to external stimuli.

L75.Ø Bromhidrosis
L75.1 Chromhidrosis
L75.2 Apocrine miliaria
Fox-Fordyce disease
DEF: Chronic, usually pruritic disease evidenced by small follicular papular eruptions, especially in the axillary and pubic areas. Apocrine miliaria develops from the closure and rupture of the affected apocrine glands' intraepidermal portion of the ducts.
L75.8 Other apocrine sweat disorders
L75.9 Apocrine sweat disorder, unspecified

Intraoperative and postprocedural complications of skin and subcutaneous tissue (L76)

L76 Intraoperative and postprocedural complications of skin and subcutaneous tissue

AHA: 2016,4Q,9-10

L76.Ø Intraoperative hemorrhage and hematoma of skin and subcutaneous tissue complicating a procedure
EXCLUDES 1 *intraoperative hemorrhage and hematoma of skin and subcutaneous tissue due to accidental puncture and laceration during a procedure (L76.1-)*
L76.Ø1 Intraoperative hemorrhage and hematoma of skin and subcutaneous tissue complicating a dermatologic procedure CC
L76.Ø2 Intraoperative hemorrhage and hematoma of skin and subcutaneous tissue complicating other procedure CC

L76.1 Accidental puncture and laceration of skin and subcutaneous tissue during a procedure
L76.11 Accidental puncture and laceration of skin and subcutaneous tissue during a dermatologic procedure CC
L76.12 Accidental puncture and laceration of skin and subcutaneous tissue during other procedure CC

L76.2 Postprocedural hemorrhage of skin and subcutaneous tissue following a procedure
L76.21 Postprocedural hemorrhage of skin and subcutaneous tissue following a dermatologic procedure CC
L76.22 Postprocedural hemorrhage of skin and subcutaneous tissue following other procedure CC

✓5th **L76.3 Postprocedural hematoma and seroma of skin and subcutaneous tissue following a procedure**

L76.31 Postprocedural hematoma of skin and subcutaneous tissue following a dermatologic procedure CC

L76.32 Postprocedural hematoma of skin and subcutaneous tissue following other procedure CC

L76.33 Postprocedural seroma of skin and subcutaneous tissue following a dermatologic procedure CC

L76.34 Postprocedural seroma of skin and subcutaneous tissue following other procedure CC

✓5th **L76.8 Other intraoperative and postprocedural complications of skin and subcutaneous tissue**

Use additional code, if applicable, to further specify disorder

L76.81 Other intraoperative complications of skin and subcutaneous tissue

L76.82 Other postprocedural complications of skin and subcutaneous tissue

AHA: 2017,3Q,6

Other disorders of the skin and subcutaneous tissue (L80-L99)

L80 Vitiligo

EXCLUDES 2 *vitiligo of eyelids (H02.73-)*
vitiligo of vulva (N90.89)

DEF: Persistent, progressive development of nonpigmented white patches on otherwise normal skin.

✓4th **L81 Other disorders of pigmentation**

EXCLUDES 1 *birthmark NOS (Q82.5)*
Peutz-Jeghers syndrome ►(Q85.89)◄

EXCLUDES 2 *nevus - see Alphabetical Index*

L81.0 Postinflammatory hyperpigmentation

L81.1 Chloasma

L81.2 Freckles

L81.3 Café au lait spots

L81.4 Other melanin hyperpigmentation
Lentigo

L81.5 Leukoderma, not elsewhere classified

L81.6 Other disorders of diminished melanin formation

L81.7 Pigmented purpuric dermatosis
Angioma serpiginosum

L81.8 Other specified disorders of pigmentation
Iron pigmentation
Tattoo pigmentation

L81.9 Disorder of pigmentation, unspecified

✓4th **L82 Seborrheic keratosis**

INCLUDES basal cell papilloma
dermatosis papulosa nigra
Leser-Trélat disease

EXCLUDES 2 *seborrheic dermatitis (L21.-)*

DEF: Common, benign, noninvasive, lightly pigmented, warty growth composed of basaloid cells that usually appear at middle age as soft, easily crumbling plaques on the face, trunk, and extremities.

L82.0 Inflamed seborrheic keratosis
AHA: 2021,3Q,10

L82.1 Other seborrheic keratosis
Seborrheic keratosis NOS

L83 Acanthosis nigricans
Confluent and reticulated papillomatosis

DEF: Diffuse, velvety hyperplasia of the spinous skin layer of the axilla and other body folds marked by gray, brown, or black pigmentation. In adult form, it is often associated with malignant acanthosis nigricans in a benign, nevoid form relatively generalized.

L84 Corns and callosities
Callus
Clavus

✓4th **L85 Other epidermal thickening**

EXCLUDES 2 *hypertrophic disorders of the skin (L91.-)*

L85.0 Acquired ichthyosis
EXCLUDES 1 *congenital ichthyosis (Q80.-)*

L85.1 Acquired keratosis [keratoderma] palmaris et plantaris
EXCLUDES 1 *inherited keratosis palmaris et plantaris (Q82.8)*

L85.2 Keratosis punctata (palmaris et plantaris)

L85.3 Xerosis cutis
Dry skin dermatitis

L85.8 Other specified epidermal thickening
Cutaneous horn

L85.9 Epidermal thickening, unspecified

L86 Keratoderma in diseases classified elsewhere

Code first underlying disease, such as:
Reiter's disease (M02.3-)

EXCLUDES 1 *gonococcal keratoderma (A54.89)*
gonococcal keratosis (A54.89)
keratoderma due to vitamin A deficiency (E50.8)
keratosis due to vitamin A deficiency (E50.8)
xeroderma due to vitamin A deficiency (E50.8)

✓4th **L87 Transepidermal elimination disorders**

EXCLUDES 1 *granuloma annulare (perforating) (L92.0)*

L87.0 Keratosis follicularis et parafollicularis in cutem penetrans
Hyperkeratosis follicularis penetrans
Kyrle disease

L87.1 Reactive perforating collagenosis

L87.2 Elastosis perforans serpiginosa

L87.8 Other transepidermal elimination disorders

L87.9 Transepidermal elimination disorder, unspecified

L88 Pyoderma gangrenosum CC
Phagedenic pyoderma

EXCLUDES 1 *dermatitis gangrenosa (L08.0)*

DEF: Persistent debilitating skin disease characterized by irregular, boggy, blue-red ulcerations, with central healing and undermined edges.

✓4th **L89 Pressure ulcer**

INCLUDES bed sore
decubitus ulcer
plaster ulcer
pressure area
pressure sore

Code first any associated gangrene (I96)

EXCLUDES 2 *decubitus (trophic) ulcer of cervix (uteri) (N86)*
diabetic ulcers (E08.621, E08.622, E09.621, E09.622, E10.621, E10.622, E11.621, E11.622, E13.621, E13.622)
non-pressure chronic ulcer of skin (L97.-)
skin infections (L00-L08)
varicose ulcer (I83.0, I83.2)

AHA: 2022,2Q,8; 2021,1Q,24; 2019,4Q,10-11,54; 2018,4Q,69; 2018,3Q,3; 2018,2Q,21; 2017,4Q,109; 2017,1Q,49; 2016,4Q,143

TIP: The stage of a diagnosed pressure ulcer can be based on documentation from clinicians who are not the patient's provider.

Four Stages of Pressure Ulcer

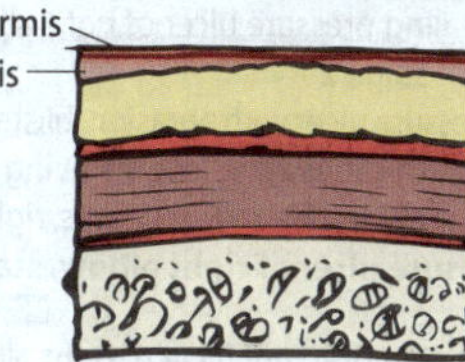

Stage 1
Persistent focal edema

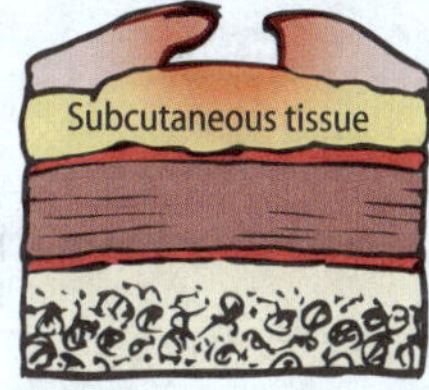

Stage 2
Abrasion, blister, partial thickness skin loss involving epidermis and/or dermis

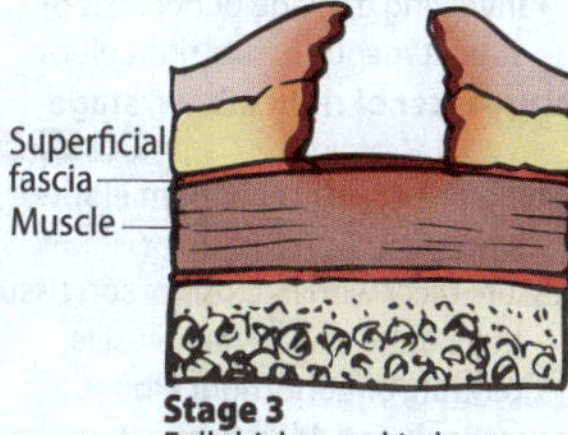

Stage 3
Full thickness skin loss involving damage or necrosis of subcutaneous tissue

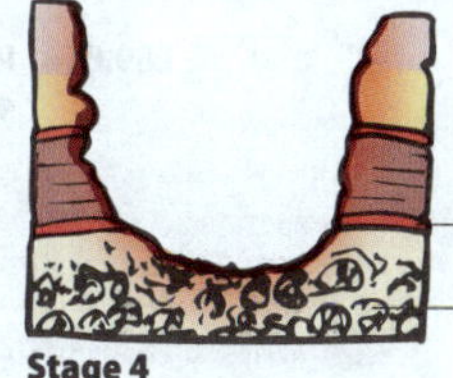

Stage 4
Necrosis of soft tissues through to underlying muscle, tendon, or bone

✓5th **L89.0 Pressure ulcer of elbow**

✓6th **L89.00 Pressure ulcer of unspecified elbow**

L89.000 Pressure ulcer of unspecified elbow, unstageable HCC

L89.001 Pressure ulcer of unspecified elbow, stage 1
Healing pressure ulcer of unspecified elbow, stage 1
Pressure pre-ulcer skin changes limited to persistent focal edema, unspecified elbow

L89.002 Pressure ulcer of unspecified elbow, stage 2 HCC
Healing pressure ulcer of unspecified elbow, stage 2
Pressure ulcer with abrasion, blister, partial thickness skin loss involving epidermis and/or dermis, unspecified elbow

L89.003 Pressure ulcer of unspecified elbow, stage 3 MCC H4 UNS HCC
Healing pressure ulcer of unspecified elbow, stage 3
Pressure ulcer with full thickness skin loss involving damage or necrosis of subcutaneous tissue, unspecified elbow

L89.004 Pressure ulcer of unspecified elbow, stage 4 MCC H4 UNS HCC
Healing pressure ulcer of unspecified elbow, stage 4
Pressure ulcer with necrosis of soft tissues through to underlying muscle, tendon, or bone, unspecified elbow

L89.006 Pressure-induced deep tissue damage of unspecified elbow

L89.009 Pressure ulcer of unspecified elbow, unspecified stage
Healing pressure ulcer of elbow NOS
Healing pressure ulcer of unspecified elbow, unspecified stage

✓6th **L89.01 Pressure ulcer of right elbow**

L89.010 Pressure ulcer of right elbow, unstageable HCC

L89.011 Pressure ulcer of right elbow, stage 1
Healing pressure ulcer of right elbow, stage 1
Pressure pre-ulcer skin changes limited to persistent focal edema, right elbow

L89.012 Pressure ulcer of right elbow, stage 2 HCC
Healing pressure ulcer of right elbow, stage 2
Pressure ulcer with abrasion, blister, partial thickness skin loss involving epidermis and/or dermis, right elbow

L89.013 Pressure ulcer of right elbow, stage 3 MCC H4 HCC
Healing pressure ulcer of right elbow, stage 3
Pressure ulcer with full thickness skin loss involving damage or necrosis of subcutaneous tissue, right elbow

L89.014 Pressure ulcer of right elbow, stage 4 MCC H4 HCC
Healing pressure ulcer of right elbow, stage 4
Pressure ulcer with necrosis of soft tissues through to underlying muscle, tendon, or bone, right elbow

L89.016 Pressure-induced deep tissue damage of right elbow

L89.019 Pressure ulcer of right elbow, unspecified stage
Healing pressure ulcer of right elbow NOS

✓6th **L89.02 Pressure ulcer of left elbow**

L89.020 Pressure ulcer of left elbow, unstageable HCC

L89.021 Pressure ulcer of left elbow, stage 1
Healing pressure ulcer of left elbow, stage 1
Pressure pre-ulcer skin changes limited to persistent focal edema, left elbow

L89.022 Pressure ulcer of left elbow, stage 2 HCC
Healing pressure ulcer of left elbow, stage 2
Pressure ulcer with abrasion, blister, partial thickness skin loss involving epidermis and/or dermis, left elbow

L89.023 Pressure ulcer of left elbow, stage 3 MCC H4 HCC
Healing pressure ulcer of left elbow, stage 3
Pressure ulcer with full thickness skin loss involving damage or necrosis of subcutaneous tissue, left elbow

L89.024 Pressure ulcer of left elbow, stage 4 MCC H4 HCC
Healing pressure ulcer of left elbow, stage 4
Pressure ulcer with necrosis of soft tissues through to underlying muscle, tendon, or bone, left elbow

L89.026 Pressure-induced deep tissue damage of left elbow

L89.029 Pressure ulcer of left elbow, unspecified stage
Healing pressure ulcer of left elbow NOS

✓5th **L89.1 Pressure ulcer of back**

✓6th **L89.10 Pressure ulcer of unspecified part of back**

L89.100 Pressure ulcer of unspecified part of back, unstageable HCC

L89.101 Pressure ulcer of unspecified part of back, stage 1
Healing pressure ulcer of unspecified part of back, stage 1
Pressure pre-ulcer skin changes limited to persistent focal edema, unspecified part of back

L89.102 Pressure ulcer of unspecified part of back, stage 2 HCC
Healing pressure ulcer of unspecified part of back, stage 2
Pressure ulcer with abrasion, blister, partial thickness skin loss involving epidermis and/or dermis, unspecified part of back

L89.103 Pressure ulcer of unspecified part of back, stage 3 MCC H4 HCC
Healing pressure ulcer of unspecified part of back, stage 3
Pressure ulcer with full thickness skin loss involving damage or necrosis of subcutaneous tissue, unspecified part of back

L89.104 Pressure ulcer of unspecified part of back, stage 4 MCC H4 HCC
Healing pressure ulcer of unspecified part of back, stage 4
Pressure ulcer with necrosis of soft tissues through to underlying muscle, tendon, or bone, unspecified part of back

L89.106 Pressure-induced deep tissue damage of unspecified part of back

L89.109 Pressure ulcer of unspecified part of back, unspecified stage
Healing pressure ulcer of unspecified part of back NOS
Healing pressure ulcer of unspecified part of back, unspecified stage

✓6th **L89.11 Pressure ulcer of right upper back**
Pressure ulcer of right shoulder blade

L89.110 Pressure ulcer of right upper back, unstageable HCC

L89.111 Pressure ulcer of right upper back, stage 1
Healing pressure ulcer of right upper back, stage 1
Pressure pre-ulcer skin changes limited to persistent focal edema, right upper back

L89.112 Pressure ulcer of right upper back, stage 2 HCC
Healing pressure ulcer of right upper back, stage 2
Pressure ulcer with abrasion, blister, partial thickness skin loss involving epidermis and/or dermis, right upper back

L89.113 Pressure ulcer of right upper back, stage 3 MCC H4 HCC
Healing pressure ulcer of right upper back, stage 3
Pressure ulcer with full thickness skin loss involving damage or necrosis of subcutaneous tissue, right upper back

L89.114 Pressure ulcer of right upper back, stage 4 MCC H4 HCC
Healing pressure ulcer of right upper back, stage 4
Pressure ulcer with necrosis of soft tissues through to underlying muscle, tendon, or bone, right upper back

L89.116 Pressure-induced deep tissue damage of right upper back

L89.119 Pressure ulcer of right upper back, unspecified stage
Healing pressure ulcer of right upper back NOS
Healing pressure ulcer of right upper back, unspecified stage

✓6th **L89.12 Pressure ulcer of left upper back**
Pressure ulcer of left shoulder blade

L89.120 Pressure ulcer of left upper back, unstageable HCC

L89.121 Pressure ulcer of left upper back, stage 1
Healing pressure ulcer of left upper back, stage 1
Pressure pre-ulcer skin changes limited to persistent focal edema, left upper back

L89.122 Pressure ulcer of left upper back, stage 2 HCC
Healing pressure ulcer of left upper back, stage 2
Pressure ulcer with abrasion, blister, partial thickness skin loss involving epidermis and/or dermis, left upper back

L89.123 Pressure ulcer of left upper back, stage 3 MCC H4 HCC
Healing pressure ulcer of left upper back, stage 3
Pressure ulcer with full thickness skin loss involving damage or necrosis of subcutaneous tissue, left upper back

L89.124 Pressure ulcer of left upper back, stage 4 MCC H4 HCC
Healing pressure ulcer of left upper back, stage 4
Pressure ulcer with necrosis of soft tissues through to underlying muscle, tendon, or bone, left upper back

L89.126 Pressure-induced deep tissue damage of left upper back

L89.129 Pressure ulcer of left upper back, unspecified stage
Healing pressure ulcer of left upper back NOS
Healing pressure ulcer of left upper back, unspecified stage

✓6th **L89.13 Pressure ulcer of right lower back**

L89.130 Pressure ulcer of right lower back, unstageable HCC

L89.131 Pressure ulcer of right lower back, stage 1
Healing pressure ulcer of right lower back, stage 1
Pressure pre-ulcer skin changes limited to persistent focal edema, right lower back

L89.132 Pressure ulcer of right lower back, stage 2 HCC
Healing pressure ulcer of right lower back, stage 2
Pressure ulcer with abrasion, blister, partial thickness skin loss involving epidermis and/or dermis, right lower back

L89.133 Pressure ulcer of right lower back, stage 3 MCC H4 HCC
Healing pressure ulcer of right lower back, stage 3
Pressure ulcer with full thickness skin loss involving damage or necrosis of subcutaneous tissue, right lower back

L89.134 Pressure ulcer of right lower back, stage 4 MCC H4 HCC
Healing pressure ulcer of right lower back, stage 4
Pressure ulcer with necrosis of soft tissues through to underlying muscle, tendon, or bone, right lower back

L89.136 Pressure-induced deep tissue damage of right lower back

L89.139 Pressure ulcer of right lower back, unspecified stage
Healing pressure ulcer of right lower back NOS
Healing pressure ulcer of right lower back, unspecified stage

✓6th **L89.14 Pressure ulcer of left lower back**

L89.140 Pressure ulcer of left lower back, unstageable HCC

L89.141 Pressure ulcer of left lower back, stage 1
Healing pressure ulcer of left lower back, stage 1
Pressure pre-ulcer skin changes limited to persistent focal edema, left lower back

L89.142 Pressure ulcer of left lower back, stage 2 HCC
Healing pressure ulcer of left lower back, stage 2
Pressure ulcer with abrasion, blister, partial thickness skin loss involving epidermis and/or dermis, left lower back

L89.143 Pressure ulcer of left lower back, stage 3 MCC H4 HCC
Healing pressure ulcer of left lower back, stage 3
Pressure ulcer with full thickness skin loss involving damage or necrosis of subcutaneous tissue, left lower back

L89.144 Pressure ulcer of left lower back, stage 4 MCC H4 HCC
Healing pressure ulcer of left lower back, stage 4
Pressure ulcer with necrosis of soft tissues through to underlying muscle, tendon, or bone, left lower back

L89.146 Pressure-induced deep tissue damage of left lower back

L89.149 Pressure ulcer of left lower back, unspecified stage
Healing pressure ulcer of left lower back NOS
Healing pressure ulcer of left lower back, unspecified stage

✓6th **L89.15 Pressure ulcer of sacral region**
Pressure ulcer of coccyx
Pressure ulcer of tailbone
AHA: 2021,3Q,10

L89.150 Pressure ulcer of sacral region, unstageable HCC

L89.151 Pressure ulcer of sacral region, stage 1
Healing pressure ulcer of sacral region, stage 1
Pressure pre-ulcer skin changes limited to persistent focal edema, sacral region

L89.152 Pressure ulcer of sacral region, stage 2 HCC
Healing pressure ulcer of sacral region, stage 2
Pressure ulcer with abrasion, blister, partial thickness skin loss involving epidermis and/or dermis, sacral region

L89.153 Pressure ulcer of sacral region, stage 3 MCC H4 HCC
Healing pressure ulcer of sacral region, stage 3
Pressure ulcer with full thickness skin loss involving damage or necrosis of subcutaneous tissue, sacral region

L89.154 Pressure ulcer of sacral region, stage 4 MCC H4 HCC
Healing pressure ulcer of sacral region, stage 4
Pressure ulcer with necrosis of soft tissues through to underlying muscle, tendon, or bone, sacral region
AHA: 2022,2Q,8

L89.156 Pressure-induced deep tissue damage of sacral region

L89.159 Pressure ulcer of sacral region, unspecified stage
Healing pressure ulcer of sacral region NOS
Healing pressure ulcer of sacral region, unspecified stage

✓5th **L89.2 Pressure ulcer of hip**

✓6th **L89.20 Pressure ulcer of unspecified hip**

L89.200 Pressure ulcer of unspecified hip, unstageable HCC

L89.201 Pressure ulcer of unspecified hip, stage 1
Healing pressure ulcer of unspecified hip back, stage 1
Pressure pre-ulcer skin changes limited to persistent focal edema, unspecified hip

L89.202 Pressure ulcer of unspecified hip, stage 2 HCC
Healing pressure ulcer of unspecified hip, stage 2
Pressure ulcer with abrasion, blister, partial thickness skin loss involving epidermis and/or dermis, unspecified hip

L89.203 Pressure ulcer of unspecified hip, stage 3 MCC H4 UNS HCC
Healing pressure ulcer of unspecified hip, stage 3
Pressure ulcer with full thickness skin loss involving damage or necrosis of subcutaneous tissue, unspecified hip

L89.204 Pressure ulcer of unspecified hip, stage 4 MCC H4 UNS HCC
Healing pressure ulcer of unspecified hip, stage 4
Pressure ulcer with necrosis of soft tissues through to underlying muscle, tendon, or bone, unspecified hip

L89.206 Pressure-induced deep tissue damage of unspecified hip

L89.209 Pressure ulcer of unspecified hip, unspecified stage
Healing pressure ulcer of unspecified hip NOS
Healing pressure ulcer of unspecified hip, unspecified stage

✓6th **L89.21 Pressure ulcer of right hip**

L89.210 Pressure ulcer of right hip, unstageable HCC

L89.211 Pressure ulcer of right hip, stage 1
Healing pressure ulcer of right hip back, stage 1
Pressure pre-ulcer skin changes limited to persistent focal edema, right hip

L89.212 Pressure ulcer of right hip, stage 2 HCC
Healing pressure ulcer of right hip, stage 2
Pressure ulcer with abrasion, blister, partial thickness skin loss involving epidermis and/or dermis, right hip

L89.213 Pressure ulcer of right hip, stage 3 MCC H4 HCC
Healing pressure ulcer of right hip, stage 3
Pressure ulcer with full thickness skin loss involving damage or necrosis of subcutaneous tissue, right hip

L89.214 Pressure ulcer of right hip, stage 4 MCC H4 HCC
Healing pressure ulcer of right hip, stage 4
Pressure ulcer with necrosis of soft tissues through to underlying muscle, tendon, or bone, right hip

L89.216 Pressure-induced deep tissue damage of right hip

L89.219 Pressure ulcer of right hip, unspecified stage
Healing pressure ulcer of right hip NOS
Healing pressure ulcer of right hip, unspecified stage

✓6th **L89.22 Pressure ulcer of left hip**

L89.220 Pressure ulcer of left hip, unstageable HCC

L89.221 Pressure ulcer of left hip, stage 1
Healing pressure ulcer of left hip back, stage 1
Pressure pre-ulcer skin changes limited to persistent focal edema, left hip

L89.222 Pressure ulcer of left hip, stage 2 HCC
Healing pressure ulcer of left hip, stage 2
Pressure ulcer with abrasion, blister, partial thickness skin loss involving epidermis and/or dermis, left hip

L89.223 Pressure ulcer of left hip, stage 3 MCC H4 HCC
Healing pressure ulcer of left hip, stage 3
Pressure ulcer with full thickness skin loss involving damage or necrosis of subcutaneous tissue, left hip

L89.224 Pressure ulcer of left hip, stage 4 MCC H4 HCC
Healing pressure ulcer of left hip, stage 4
Pressure ulcer with necrosis of soft tissues through to underlying muscle, tendon, or bone, left hip

L89.226 Pressure-induced deep tissue damage of left hip

L89.229 Pressure ulcer of left hip, unspecified stage
Healing pressure ulcer of left hip NOS
Healing pressure ulcer of left hip, unspecified stage

✓5th **L89.3 Pressure ulcer of buttock**
AHA: 2021,3Q,10

✓6th **L89.30 Pressure ulcer of unspecified buttock**

L89.300 Pressure ulcer of unspecified buttock, unstageable HCC

Chapter 12. Diseases of the Skin and Subcutaneous Tissue
L89.15–L89.300

L89.301 Pressure ulcer of unspecified buttock, stage 1
Healing pressure ulcer of unspecified buttock, stage 1
Pressure pre-ulcer skin changes limited to persistent focal edema, unspecified buttock

L89.302 Pressure ulcer of unspecified buttock, stage 2 HCC
Healing pressure ulcer of unspecified buttock, stage 2
Pressure ulcer with abrasion, blister, partial thickness skin loss involving epidermis and/or dermis, unspecified buttock

L89.303 Pressure ulcer of unspecified buttock, stage 3 MCC H4 UNS HCC
Healing pressure ulcer of unspecified buttock, stage 3
Pressure ulcer with full thickness skin loss involving damage or necrosis of subcutaneous tissue, unspecified buttock

L89.304 Pressure ulcer of unspecified buttock, stage 4 MCC H4 UNS HCC
Healing pressure ulcer of unspecified buttock, stage 4
Pressure ulcer with necrosis of soft tissues through to underlying muscle, tendon, or bone, unspecified buttock

L89.306 Pressure-induced deep tissue damage of unspecified buttock

L89.309 Pressure ulcer of unspecified buttock, unspecified stage
Healing pressure ulcer of unspecified buttock NOS
Healing pressure ulcer of unspecified buttock, unspecified stage

✓6th **L89.31 Pressure ulcer of right buttock**

L89.310 Pressure ulcer of right buttock, unstageable HCC

L89.311 Pressure ulcer of right buttock, stage 1
Healing pressure ulcer of right buttock, stage 1
Pressure pre-ulcer skin changes limited to persistent focal edema, right buttock

L89.312 Pressure ulcer of right buttock, stage 2 HCC
Healing pressure ulcer of right buttock, stage 2
Pressure ulcer with abrasion, blister, partial thickness skin loss involving epidermis and/or dermis, right buttock

L89.313 Pressure ulcer of right buttock, stage 3 MCC H4 HCC
Healing pressure ulcer of right buttock, stage 3
Pressure ulcer with full thickness skin loss involving damage or necrosis of subcutaneous tissue, right buttock

L89.314 Pressure ulcer of right buttock, stage 4 MCC H4 HCC
Healing pressure ulcer of right buttock, stage 4
Pressure ulcer with necrosis of soft tissues through to underlying muscle, tendon, or bone, right buttock

L89.316 Pressure-induced deep tissue damage of right buttock

L89.319 Pressure ulcer of right buttock, unspecified stage
Healing pressure ulcer of right buttock NOS
Healing pressure ulcer of right buttock, unspecified stage

✓6th **L89.32 Pressure ulcer of left buttock**

L89.320 Pressure ulcer of left buttock, unstageable HCC

L89.321 Pressure ulcer of left buttock, stage 1
Healing pressure ulcer of left buttock, stage 1
Pressure pre-ulcer skin changes limited to persistent focal edema, left buttock

L89.322 Pressure ulcer of left buttock, stage 2 HCC
Healing pressure ulcer of left buttock, stage 2
Pressure ulcer with abrasion, blister, partial thickness skin loss involving epidermis and/or dermis, left buttock

L89.323 Pressure ulcer of left buttock, stage 3 MCC H4 HCC
Healing pressure ulcer of left buttock, stage 3
Pressure ulcer with full thickness skin loss involving damage or necrosis of subcutaneous tissue, left buttock

L89.324 Pressure ulcer of left buttock, stage 4 MCC H4 HCC
Healing pressure ulcer of left buttock, stage 4
Pressure ulcer with necrosis of soft tissues through to underlying muscle, tendon, or bone, left buttock

L89.326 Pressure-induced deep tissue damage of left buttock

L89.329 Pressure ulcer of left buttock, unspecified stage
Healing pressure ulcer of left buttock NOS
Healing pressure ulcer of left buttock, unspecified stage

✓5th **L89.4 Pressure ulcer of contiguous site of back, buttock and hip**

L89.40 Pressure ulcer of contiguous site of back, buttock and hip, unspecified stage
Healing pressure ulcer of contiguous site of back, buttock and hip NOS
Healing pressure ulcer of contiguous site of back, buttock and hip, unspecified stage

L89.41 Pressure ulcer of contiguous site of back, buttock and hip, stage 1
Healing pressure ulcer of contiguous site of back, buttock and hip, stage 1
Pressure pre-ulcer skin changes limited to persistent focal edema, contiguous site of back, buttock and hip

L89.42 Pressure ulcer of contiguous site of back, buttock and hip, stage 2 HCC
Healing pressure ulcer of contiguous site of back, buttock and hip, stage 2
Pressure ulcer with abrasion, blister, partial thickness skin loss involving epidermis and/or dermis, contiguous site of back, buttock and hip

L89.43 Pressure ulcer of contiguous site of back, buttock and hip, stage 3 MCC H4 HCC
Healing pressure ulcer of contiguous site of back, buttock and hip, stage 3
Pressure ulcer with full thickness skin loss involving damage or necrosis of subcutaneous tissue, contiguous site of back, buttock and hip

L89.44 Pressure ulcer of contiguous site of back, buttock and hip, stage 4 MCC H4 HCC
Healing pressure ulcer of contiguous site of back, buttock and hip, stage 4
Pressure ulcer with necrosis of soft tissues through to underlying muscle, tendon, or bone, contiguous site of back, buttock and hip

L89.45 Pressure ulcer of contiguous site of back, buttock and hip, unstageable HCC

L89.46 Pressure-induced deep tissue damage of contiguous site of back, buttock and hip

✓5th **L89.5 Pressure ulcer of ankle**

✓6th **L89.50 Pressure ulcer of unspecified ankle**

L89.500 Pressure ulcer of unspecified ankle, unstageable HCC

Chapter 12. Diseases of the Skin and Subcutaneous Tissue

L89.301–L89.500

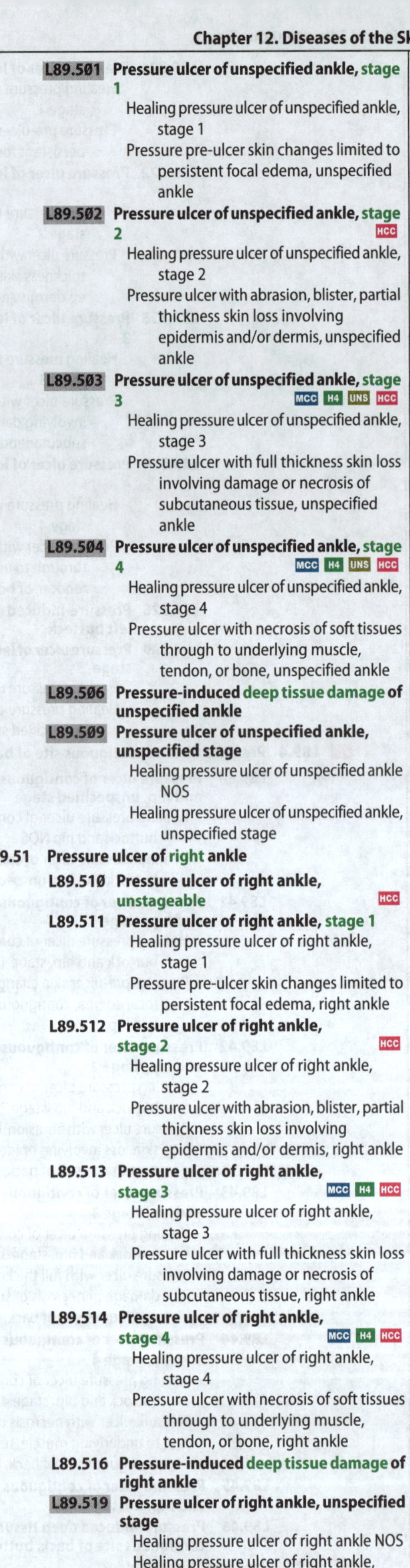

L89.501 Pressure ulcer of unspecified ankle, stage 1
Healing pressure ulcer of unspecified ankle, stage 1
Pressure pre-ulcer skin changes limited to persistent focal edema, unspecified ankle

L89.502 Pressure ulcer of unspecified ankle, stage 2 HCC
Healing pressure ulcer of unspecified ankle, stage 2
Pressure ulcer with abrasion, blister, partial thickness skin loss involving epidermis and/or dermis, unspecified ankle

L89.503 Pressure ulcer of unspecified ankle, stage 3 MCC H4 UNS HCC
Healing pressure ulcer of unspecified ankle, stage 3
Pressure ulcer with full thickness skin loss involving damage or necrosis of subcutaneous tissue, unspecified ankle

L89.504 Pressure ulcer of unspecified ankle, stage 4 MCC H4 UNS HCC
Healing pressure ulcer of unspecified ankle, stage 4
Pressure ulcer with necrosis of soft tissues through to underlying muscle, tendon, or bone, unspecified ankle

L89.506 Pressure-induced deep tissue damage of unspecified ankle

L89.509 Pressure ulcer of unspecified ankle, unspecified stage
Healing pressure ulcer of unspecified ankle NOS
Healing pressure ulcer of unspecified ankle, unspecified stage

✓6th **L89.51 Pressure ulcer of right ankle**

L89.510 Pressure ulcer of right ankle, unstageable HCC

L89.511 Pressure ulcer of right ankle, stage 1
Healing pressure ulcer of right ankle, stage 1
Pressure pre-ulcer skin changes limited to persistent focal edema, right ankle

L89.512 Pressure ulcer of right ankle, stage 2 HCC
Healing pressure ulcer of right ankle, stage 2
Pressure ulcer with abrasion, blister, partial thickness skin loss involving epidermis and/or dermis, right ankle

L89.513 Pressure ulcer of right ankle, stage 3 MCC H4 HCC
Healing pressure ulcer of right ankle, stage 3
Pressure ulcer with full thickness skin loss involving damage or necrosis of subcutaneous tissue, right ankle

L89.514 Pressure ulcer of right ankle, stage 4 MCC H4 HCC
Healing pressure ulcer of right ankle, stage 4
Pressure ulcer with necrosis of soft tissues through to underlying muscle, tendon, or bone, right ankle

L89.516 Pressure-induced deep tissue damage of right ankle

L89.519 Pressure ulcer of right ankle, unspecified stage
Healing pressure ulcer of right ankle NOS
Healing pressure ulcer of right ankle, unspecified stage

✓6th **L89.52 Pressure ulcer of left ankle**

L89.520 Pressure ulcer of left ankle, unstageable HCC

L89.521 Pressure ulcer of left ankle, stage 1
Healing pressure ulcer of left ankle, stage 1
Pressure pre-ulcer skin changes limited to persistent focal edema, left ankle

L89.522 Pressure ulcer of left ankle, stage 2 HCC
Healing pressure ulcer of left ankle, stage 2
Pressure ulcer with abrasion, blister, partial thickness skin loss involving epidermis and/or dermis, left ankle

L89.523 Pressure ulcer of left ankle, stage 3 MCC H4 HCC
Healing pressure ulcer of left ankle, stage 3
Pressure ulcer with full thickness skin loss involving damage or necrosis of subcutaneous tissue, left ankle

L89.524 Pressure ulcer of left ankle, stage 4 MCC H4 HCC
Healing pressure ulcer of left ankle, stage 4
Pressure ulcer with necrosis of soft tissues through to underlying muscle, tendon, or bone, left ankle

L89.526 Pressure-induced deep tissue damage of left ankle

L89.529 Pressure ulcer of left ankle, unspecified stage
Healing pressure ulcer of left ankle NOS
Healing pressure ulcer of left ankle, unspecified stage

✓5th **L89.6 Pressure ulcer of heel**

✓6th **L89.60 Pressure ulcer of unspecified heel**

L89.600 Pressure ulcer of unspecified heel, unstageable HCC

L89.601 Pressure ulcer of unspecified heel, stage 1
Healing pressure ulcer of unspecified heel, stage 1
Pressure pre-ulcer skin changes limited to persistent focal edema, unspecified heel

L89.602 Pressure ulcer of unspecified heel, stage 2 HCC
Healing pressure ulcer of unspecified heel, stage 2
Pressure ulcer with abrasion, blister, partial thickness skin loss involving epidermis and/or dermis, unspecified heel

L89.603 Pressure ulcer of unspecified heel, stage 3 MCC H4 UNS HCC
Healing pressure ulcer of unspecified heel, stage 3
Pressure ulcer with full thickness skin loss involving damage or necrosis of subcutaneous tissue, unspecified heel

L89.604 Pressure ulcer of unspecified heel, stage 4 MCC H4 UNS HCC
Healing pressure ulcer of unspecified heel, stage 4
Pressure ulcer with necrosis of soft tissues through to underlying muscle, tendon, or bone, unspecified heel

L89.606 Pressure-induced deep tissue damage of unspecified heel

L89.609 Pressure ulcer of unspecified heel, unspecified stage
Healing pressure ulcer of unspecified heel NOS
Healing pressure ulcer of unspecified heel, unspecified stage

✓6th **L89.61 Pressure ulcer of right heel**

L89.610 Pressure ulcer of right heel, unstageable HCC

L89.611 Pressure ulcer of right heel, stage 1
Healing pressure ulcer of right heel, stage 1
Pressure pre-ulcer skin changes limited to persistent focal edema, right heel

L89.612 Pressure ulcer of right heel, stage 2 HCC
Healing pressure ulcer of right heel, stage 2
Pressure ulcer with abrasion, blister, partial thickness skin loss involving epidermis and/or dermis, right heel

L89.613 Pressure ulcer of right heel, stage 3 MCC H4 HCC
Healing pressure ulcer of right heel, stage 3
Pressure ulcer with full thickness skin loss involving damage or necrosis of subcutaneous tissue, right heel

L89.614 Pressure ulcer of right heel, stage 4 MCC H4 HCC
Healing pressure ulcer of right heel, stage 4
Pressure ulcer with necrosis of soft tissues through to underlying muscle, tendon, or bone, right heel

L89.616 Pressure-induced deep tissue damage of right heel

L89.619 Pressure ulcer of right heel, unspecified stage
Healing pressure ulcer of right heel NOS
Healing pressure ulcer of right heel, unspecified stage

L89.62 Pressure ulcer of left heel

L89.620 Pressure ulcer of left heel, unstageable HCC

L89.621 Pressure ulcer of left heel, stage 1
Healing pressure ulcer of left heel, stage 1
Pressure pre-ulcer skin changes limited to persistent focal edema, left heel

L89.622 Pressure ulcer of left heel, stage 2 HCC
Healing pressure ulcer of left heel, stage 2
Pressure ulcer with abrasion, blister, partial thickness skin loss involving epidermis and/or dermis, left heel

L89.623 Pressure ulcer of left heel, stage 3 MCC H4 HCC
Healing pressure ulcer of left heel, stage 3
Pressure ulcer with full thickness skin loss involving damage or necrosis of subcutaneous tissue, left heel

L89.624 Pressure ulcer of left heel, stage 4 MCC H4 HCC
Healing pressure ulcer of left heel, stage 4
Pressure ulcer with necrosis of soft tissues through to underlying muscle, tendon, or bone, left heel

L89.626 Pressure-induced deep tissue damage of left heel

L89.629 Pressure ulcer of left heel, unspecified stage
Healing pressure ulcer of left heel NOS
Healing pressure ulcer of left heel, unspecified stage

L89.8 Pressure ulcer of other site

L89.81 Pressure ulcer of head
Pressure ulcer of face

L89.810 Pressure ulcer of head, unstageable HCC

L89.811 Pressure ulcer of head, stage 1
Healing pressure ulcer of head, stage 1
Pressure pre-ulcer skin changes limited to persistent focal edema, head

L89.812 Pressure ulcer of head, stage 2 HCC
Healing pressure ulcer of head, stage 2
Pressure ulcer with abrasion, blister, partial thickness skin loss involving epidermis and/or dermis, head

L89.813 Pressure ulcer of head, stage 3 MCC H4 HCC
Healing pressure ulcer of head, stage 3
Pressure ulcer with full thickness skin loss involving damage or necrosis of subcutaneous tissue, head

L89.814 Pressure ulcer of head, stage 4 MCC H4 HCC
Healing pressure ulcer of head, stage 4
Pressure ulcer with necrosis of soft tissues through to underlying muscle, tendon, or bone, head

L89.816 Pressure-induced deep tissue damage of head

L89.819 Pressure ulcer of head, unspecified stage
Healing pressure ulcer of head NOS
Healing pressure ulcer of head, unspecified stage

L89.89 Pressure ulcer of other site

L89.890 Pressure ulcer of other site, unstageable HCC

L89.891 Pressure ulcer of other site, stage 1
Healing pressure ulcer of other site, stage 1
Pressure pre-ulcer skin changes limited to persistent focal edema, other site

L89.892 Pressure ulcer of other site, stage 2 HCC
Healing pressure ulcer of other site, stage 2
Pressure ulcer with abrasion, blister, partial thickness skin loss involving epidermis and/or dermis, other site

L89.893 Pressure ulcer of other site, stage 3 MCC H4 HCC
Healing pressure ulcer of other site, stage 3
Pressure ulcer with full thickness skin loss involving damage or necrosis of subcutaneous tissue, other site

L89.894 Pressure ulcer of other site, stage 4 MCC H4 HCC
Healing pressure ulcer of other site, stage 4
Pressure ulcer with necrosis of soft tissues through to underlying muscle, tendon, or bone, other site

L89.896 Pressure-induced deep tissue damage of other site

L89.899 Pressure ulcer of other site, unspecified stage
Healing pressure ulcer of other site NOS
Healing pressure ulcer of other site, unspecified stage

L89.9 Pressure ulcer of unspecified site

L89.90 Pressure ulcer of unspecified site, unspecified stage
Healing pressure ulcer of unspecified site NOS
Healing pressure ulcer of unspecified site, unspecified stage

L89.91 Pressure ulcer of unspecified site, stage 1
Healing pressure ulcer of unspecified site, stage 1
Pressure pre-ulcer skin changes limited to persistent focal edema, unspecified site

L89.92 Pressure ulcer of unspecified site, stage 2 HCC
Healing pressure ulcer of unspecified site, stage 2
Pressure ulcer with abrasion, blister, partial thickness skin loss involving epidermis and/or dermis, unspecified site

L89.93 Pressure ulcer of unspecified site, stage 3 MCC H4 HCC
Healing pressure ulcer of unspecified site, stage 3
Pressure ulcer with full thickness skin loss involving damage or necrosis of subcutaneous tissue, unspecified site

L89.94 Pressure ulcer of unspecified site, stage 4 MCC H4 HCC
Healing pressure ulcer of unspecified site, stage 4
Pressure ulcer with necrosis of soft tissues through to underlying muscle, tendon, or bone, unspecified site

L89.95 Pressure ulcer of unspecified site, unstageable HCC

L89.96 Pressure-induced deep tissue damage of unspecified site

L90 Atrophic disorders of skin

L90.0 Lichen sclerosus et atrophicus

EXCLUDES 2 *lichen sclerosus of external female genital organs (N90.4)*
lichen sclerosus of external male genital organs (N48.0)

L90.1 Anetoderma of Schweninger-Buzzi

L90.2 Anetoderma of Jadassohn-Pellizzari

L90.3 Atrophoderma of Pasini and Pierini

L90.4 Acrodermatitis chronica atrophicans

L90.5 Scar conditions and fibrosis of skin

Adherent scar (skin)
Cicatrix
Disfigurement of skin due to scar
Fibrosis of skin NOS
Scar NOS

EXCLUDES 2 *hypertrophic scar (L91.0)*
keloid scar (L91.0)

AHA: 2016,2Q,5; 2015,1Q,19

L90.6 Striae atrophicae

L90.8 Other atrophic disorders of skin

L90.9 Atrophic disorder of skin, unspecified

L91 Hypertrophic disorders of skin

L91.0 Hypertrophic scar

Keloid
Keloid scar

EXCLUDES 2 *acne keloid (L73.0)*
scar NOS (L90.5)

DEF: Overgrowth of scar tissue due to excess amounts of collagen during connective tissue repair, occurring mainly on the upper trunk and face.

L91.8 Other hypertrophic disorders of the skin

L91.9 Hypertrophic disorder of the skin, unspecified

L92 Granulomatous disorders of skin and subcutaneous tissue

EXCLUDES 2 *actinic granuloma (L57.5)*

L92.0 Granuloma annulare

Perforating granuloma annulare

L92.1 Necrobiosis lipoidica, not elsewhere classified

EXCLUDES 1 *necrobiosis lipoidica associated with diabetes mellitus (E08-E13 with .620)*

L92.2 Granuloma faciale [eosinophilic granuloma of skin]

L92.3 Foreign body granuloma of the skin and subcutaneous tissue

Use additional code to identify the type of retained foreign body (Z18.-)

L92.8 Other granulomatous disorders of the skin and subcutaneous tissue

L92.9 Granulomatous disorder of the skin and subcutaneous tissue, unspecified

EXCLUDES 2 *umbilical granuloma (P83.81)*

AHA: 2017,4Q,21-22

L93 Lupus erythematosus

Use additional code for adverse effect, if applicable, to identify drug (T36-T50 with fifth or sixth character 5)

EXCLUDES 1 *lupus exedens (A18.4)*
lupus vulgaris (A18.4)
scleroderma (M34.-)
systemic lupus erythematosus (M32.-)

DEF: Inflammatory, autoimmune skin condition in which the body's autoimmune system attacks healthy tissue of the integumentary system.

L93.0 Discoid lupus erythematosus

Lupus erythematosus NOS

L93.1 Subacute cutaneous lupus erythematosus

L93.2 Other local lupus erythematosus

Lupus erythematosus profundus
Lupus panniculitis

L94 Other localized connective tissue disorders

EXCLUDES 1 *systemic connective tissue disorders (M30-M36)*

L94.0 Localized scleroderma [morphea]

Circumscribed scleroderma

L94.1 Linear scleroderma

En coup de sabre lesion

L94.2 Calcinosis cutis

L94.3 Sclerodactyly

L94.4 Gottron's papules

L94.5 Poikiloderma vasculare atrophicans

L94.6 Ainhum

L94.8 Other specified localized connective tissue disorders

L94.9 Localized connective tissue disorder, unspecified

L95 Vasculitis limited to skin, not elsewhere classified

EXCLUDES 1 *angioma serpiginosum (L81.7)*
Henoch(-Schönlein) purpura (D69.0)
hypersensitivity angiitis (M31.0)
lupus panniculitis (L93.2)
panniculitis NOS (M79.3)
panniculitis of neck and back (M54.0-)
polyarteritis nodosa (M30.0)
relapsing panniculitis (M35.6)
rheumatoid vasculitis (M05.2)
serum sickness (T80.6-)
urticaria (L50.-)
Wegener's granulomatosis (M31.3-)

L95.0 Livedoid vasculitis

Atrophie blanche (en plaque)

L95.1 Erythema elevatum diutinum

L95.8 Other vasculitis limited to the skin

L95.9 Vasculitis limited to the skin, unspecified

L97 Non-pressure chronic ulcer of lower limb, not elsewhere classified

INCLUDES chronic ulcer of skin of lower limb NOS
non-healing ulcer of skin
non-infected sinus of skin
trophic ulcer NOS
tropical ulcer NOS
ulcer of skin of lower limb NOS

Code first any associated underlying condition, such as:
any associated gangrene (I96)
atherosclerosis of the lower extremities (I70.23-, I70.24-, I70.33-, I70.34-, I70.43-, I70.44-, I70.53-, I70.54-, I70.63-, I70.64-, I70.73-, I70.74-)
chronic venous hypertension (I87.31-, I87.33-)
diabetic ulcers (E08.621, E08.622, E09.621, E09.622, E10.621, E10.622, E11.621, E11.622, E13.621, E13.622)
postphlebitic syndrome (I87.01-, I87.03-)
postthrombotic syndrome (I87.01-, I87.03-)
varicose ulcer (I83.0-, I83.2-)

EXCLUDES 2 *pressure ulcer (pressure area) (L89.-)*
skin infections (L00-L08)
specific infections classified to A00-B99

AHA: 2021,1Q,7; 2020,2Q,19; 2018,4Q,69; 2017,4Q,17

TIP: The depth and/or severity of a diagnosed nonpressure ulcer can be determined based on medical record documentation from clinicians who are not the patient's provider.

TIP: Assign a code from this category/subcategory for nonpressure ulcers documented as acute.

L97.1 Non-pressure chronic ulcer of thigh

L97.10 Non-pressure chronic ulcer of unspecified thigh

L97.101 Non-pressure chronic ulcer of unspecified thigh limited to breakdown of skin CC UNS HCC

L97.102 Non-pressure chronic ulcer of unspecified thigh with fat layer exposed CC UNS HCC

L97.103 Non-pressure chronic ulcer of unspecified thigh with necrosis of muscle CC UNS HCC

L97.104 Non-pressure chronic ulcer of unspecified thigh with necrosis of bone CC UNS HCC

L97.105 Non-pressure chronic ulcer of unspecified thigh with muscle involvement without evidence of necrosis CC UNS HCC

L97.106 Non-pressure chronic ulcer of unspecified thigh with bone involvement without evidence of necrosis CC UNS HCC

L97.108 Non-pressure chronic ulcer of unspecified thigh with other specified severity CC UNS HCC

L97.109 Non-pressure chronic ulcer of unspecified thigh with unspecified severity CC UNS HCC

L97.11 Non-pressure chronic ulcer of right thigh

L97.111 Non-pressure chronic ulcer of right thigh limited to breakdown of skin CC HCC

L97.112 Non-pressure chronic ulcer of right thigh with fat layer exposed CC HCC
L97.113 Non-pressure chronic ulcer of right thigh with necrosis of muscle CC HCC
L97.114 Non-pressure chronic ulcer of right thigh with necrosis of bone CC HCC
L97.115 Non-pressure chronic ulcer of right thigh with muscle involvement without evidence of necrosis CC HCC
L97.116 Non-pressure chronic ulcer of right thigh with bone involvement without evidence of necrosis CC HCC
L97.118 Non-pressure chronic ulcer of right thigh with other specified severity CC HCC
L97.119 Non-pressure chronic ulcer of right thigh with unspecified severity CC HCC

6th L97.12 Non-pressure chronic ulcer of left thigh
L97.121 Non-pressure chronic ulcer of left thigh limited to breakdown of skin CC HCC
L97.122 Non-pressure chronic ulcer of left thigh with fat layer exposed CC HCC
L97.123 Non-pressure chronic ulcer of left thigh with necrosis of muscle CC HCC
L97.124 Non-pressure chronic ulcer of left thigh with necrosis of bone CC HCC
L97.125 Non-pressure chronic ulcer of left thigh with muscle involvement without evidence of necrosis CC HCC
L97.126 Non-pressure chronic ulcer of left thigh with bone involvement without evidence of necrosis CC HCC
L97.128 Non-pressure chronic ulcer of left thigh with other specified severity CC HCC
L97.129 Non-pressure chronic ulcer of left thigh with unspecified severity CC HCC

5th L97.2 Non-pressure chronic ulcer of calf

6th L97.20 Non-pressure chronic ulcer of unspecified calf
L97.201 Non-pressure chronic ulcer of unspecified calf limited to breakdown of skin CC UNS HCC
L97.202 Non-pressure chronic ulcer of unspecified calf with fat layer exposed CC UNS HCC
L97.203 Non-pressure chronic ulcer of unspecified calf with necrosis of muscle CC UNS HCC
L97.204 Non-pressure chronic ulcer of unspecified calf with necrosis of bone CC UNS HCC
L97.205 Non-pressure chronic ulcer of unspecified calf with muscle involvement without evidence of necrosis CC UNS HCC
L97.206 Non-pressure chronic ulcer of unspecified calf with bone involvement without evidence of necrosis CC UNS HCC
L97.208 Non-pressure chronic ulcer of unspecified calf with other specified severity CC UNS HCC
L97.209 Non-pressure chronic ulcer of unspecified calf with unspecified severity CC UNS HCC

6th L97.21 Non-pressure chronic ulcer of right calf
L97.211 Non-pressure chronic ulcer of right calf limited to breakdown of skin CC HCC
L97.212 Non-pressure chronic ulcer of right calf with fat layer exposed CC HCC
L97.213 Non-pressure chronic ulcer of right calf with necrosis of muscle CC HCC
L97.214 Non-pressure chronic ulcer of right calf with necrosis of bone CC HCC
L97.215 Non-pressure chronic ulcer of right calf with muscle involvement without evidence of necrosis CC HCC
L97.216 Non-pressure chronic ulcer of right calf with bone involvement without evidence of necrosis CC HCC
L97.218 Non-pressure chronic ulcer of right calf with other specified severity CC HCC
L97.219 Non-pressure chronic ulcer of right calf with unspecified severity CC HCC

6th L97.22 Non-pressure chronic ulcer of left calf
L97.221 Non-pressure chronic ulcer of left calf limited to breakdown of skin CC HCC
L97.222 Non-pressure chronic ulcer of left calf with fat layer exposed CC HCC
L97.223 Non-pressure chronic ulcer of left calf with necrosis of muscle CC HCC
L97.224 Non-pressure chronic ulcer of left calf with necrosis of bone CC HCC
L97.225 Non-pressure chronic ulcer of left calf with muscle involvement without evidence of necrosis CC HCC
L97.226 Non-pressure chronic ulcer of left calf with bone involvement without evidence of necrosis CC HCC
L97.228 Non-pressure chronic ulcer of left calf with other specified severity CC HCC
L97.229 Non-pressure chronic ulcer of left calf with unspecified severity CC HCC

5th L97.3 Non-pressure chronic ulcer of ankle

6th L97.30 Non-pressure chronic ulcer of unspecified ankle
L97.301 Non-pressure chronic ulcer of unspecified ankle limited to breakdown of skin CC UNS HCC
L97.302 Non-pressure chronic ulcer of unspecified ankle with fat layer exposed CC UNS HCC
L97.303 Non-pressure chronic ulcer of unspecified ankle with necrosis of muscle CC UNS HCC
L97.304 Non-pressure chronic ulcer of unspecified ankle with necrosis of bone CC UNS HCC
L97.305 Non-pressure chronic ulcer of unspecified ankle with muscle involvement without evidence of necrosis CC UNS HCC
L97.306 Non-pressure chronic ulcer of unspecified ankle with bone involvement without evidence of necrosis CC UNS HCC
L97.308 Non-pressure chronic ulcer of unspecified ankle with other specified severity CC UNS HCC
L97.309 Non-pressure chronic ulcer of unspecified ankle with unspecified severity CC UNS HCC

6th L97.31 Non-pressure chronic ulcer of right ankle
L97.311 Non-pressure chronic ulcer of right ankle limited to breakdown of skin CC HCC
L97.312 Non-pressure chronic ulcer of right ankle with fat layer exposed CC HCC
L97.313 Non-pressure chronic ulcer of right ankle with necrosis of muscle CC HCC
L97.314 Non-pressure chronic ulcer of right ankle with necrosis of bone CC HCC
L97.315 Non-pressure chronic ulcer of right ankle with muscle involvement without evidence of necrosis CC HCC
L97.316 Non-pressure chronic ulcer of right ankle with bone involvement without evidence of necrosis CC HCC
L97.318 Non-pressure chronic ulcer of right ankle with other specified severity CC HCC
L97.319 Non-pressure chronic ulcer of right ankle with unspecified severity CC HCC

6th L97.32 Non-pressure chronic ulcer of left ankle
L97.321 Non-pressure chronic ulcer of left ankle limited to breakdown of skin CC HCC
L97.322 Non-pressure chronic ulcer of left ankle with fat layer exposed CC HCC
L97.323 Non-pressure chronic ulcer of left ankle with necrosis of muscle CC HCC
L97.324 Non-pressure chronic ulcer of left ankle with necrosis of bone CC HCC
L97.325 Non-pressure chronic ulcer of left ankle with muscle involvement without evidence of necrosis CC HCC
L97.326 Non-pressure chronic ulcer of left ankle with bone involvement without evidence of necrosis CC HCC
L97.328 Non-pressure chronic ulcer of left ankle with other specified severity CC HCC
L97.329 Non-pressure chronic ulcer of left ankle with unspecified severity CC HCC

L97.4 Non-pressure chronic ulcer of heel and midfoot
Non-pressure chronic ulcer of plantar surface of midfoot

L97.40 Non-pressure chronic ulcer of unspecified heel and midfoot
L97.401 Non-pressure chronic ulcer of unspecified heel and midfoot limited to breakdown of skin CC UNS HCC
L97.402 Non-pressure chronic ulcer of unspecified heel and midfoot with fat layer exposed CC UNS HCC
L97.403 Non-pressure chronic ulcer of unspecified heel and midfoot with necrosis of muscle CC UNS HCC
L97.404 Non-pressure chronic ulcer of unspecified heel and midfoot with necrosis of bone CC UNS HCC
L97.405 Non-pressure chronic ulcer of unspecified heel and midfoot with muscle involvement without evidence of necrosis CC UNS HCC
L97.406 Non-pressure chronic ulcer of unspecified heel and midfoot with bone involvement without evidence of necrosis CC UNS HCC
L97.408 Non-pressure chronic ulcer of unspecified heel and midfoot with other specified severity CC UNS HCC
L97.409 Non-pressure chronic ulcer of unspecified heel and midfoot with unspecified severity CC UNS HCC

L97.41 Non-pressure chronic ulcer of right heel and midfoot
L97.411 Non-pressure chronic ulcer of right heel and midfoot limited to breakdown of skin CC HCC
L97.412 Non-pressure chronic ulcer of right heel and midfoot with fat layer exposed CC HCC
AHA: 2020,2Q,19
L97.413 Non-pressure chronic ulcer of right heel and midfoot with necrosis of muscle CC HCC
L97.414 Non-pressure chronic ulcer of right heel and midfoot with necrosis of bone CC HCC
L97.415 Non-pressure chronic ulcer of right heel and midfoot with muscle involvement without evidence of necrosis CC HCC
L97.416 Non-pressure chronic ulcer of right heel and midfoot with bone involvement without evidence of necrosis CC HCC
L97.418 Non-pressure chronic ulcer of right heel and midfoot with other specified severity CC HCC
L97.419 Non-pressure chronic ulcer of right heel and midfoot with unspecified severity CC HCC

L97.42 Non-pressure chronic ulcer of left heel and midfoot
L97.421 Non-pressure chronic ulcer of left heel and midfoot limited to breakdown of skin CC HCC
AHA: 2016,1Q,12
L97.422 Non-pressure chronic ulcer of left heel and midfoot with fat layer exposed CC HCC
AHA: 2020,2Q,19
L97.423 Non-pressure chronic ulcer of left heel and midfoot with necrosis of muscle CC HCC
L97.424 Non-pressure chronic ulcer of left heel and midfoot with necrosis of bone CC HCC
L97.425 Non-pressure chronic ulcer of left heel and midfoot with muscle involvement without evidence of necrosis CC HCC
L97.426 Non-pressure chronic ulcer of left heel and midfoot with bone involvement without evidence of necrosis CC HCC
L97.428 Non-pressure chronic ulcer of left heel and midfoot with other specified severity CC HCC
L97.429 Non-pressure chronic ulcer of left heel and midfoot with unspecified severity CC HCC

L97.5 Non-pressure chronic ulcer of other part of foot
Non-pressure chronic ulcer of toe

L97.50 Non-pressure chronic ulcer of other part of unspecified foot
L97.501 Non-pressure chronic ulcer of other part of unspecified foot limited to breakdown of skin HCC
L97.502 Non-pressure chronic ulcer of other part of unspecified foot with fat layer exposed HCC
L97.503 Non-pressure chronic ulcer of other part of unspecified foot with necrosis of muscle HCC
L97.504 Non-pressure chronic ulcer of other part of unspecified foot with necrosis of bone HCC
L97.505 Non-pressure chronic ulcer of other part of unspecified foot with muscle involvement without evidence of necrosis CC HCC
L97.506 Non-pressure chronic ulcer of other part of unspecified foot with bone involvement without evidence of necrosis CC HCC
L97.508 Non-pressure chronic ulcer of other part of unspecified foot with other specified severity CC HCC
L97.509 Non-pressure chronic ulcer of other part of unspecified foot with unspecified severity HCC

L97.51 Non-pressure chronic ulcer of other part of right foot
AHA: 2020,1Q,12
L97.511 Non-pressure chronic ulcer of other part of right foot limited to breakdown of skin HCC
L97.512 Non-pressure chronic ulcer of other part of right foot with fat layer exposed HCC
AHA: 2020,2Q,19
L97.513 Non-pressure chronic ulcer of other part of right foot with necrosis of muscle HCC
L97.514 Non-pressure chronic ulcer of other part of right foot with necrosis of bone HCC
L97.515 Non-pressure chronic ulcer of other part of right foot with muscle involvement without evidence of necrosis CC HCC
L97.516 Non-pressure chronic ulcer of other part of right foot with bone involvement without evidence of necrosis CC HCC
L97.518 Non-pressure chronic ulcer of other part of right foot with other specified severity CC HCC
L97.519 Non-pressure chronic ulcer of other part of right foot with unspecified severity HCC

L97.52 Non-pressure chronic ulcer of other part of left foot
AHA: 2020,1Q,12
L97.521 Non-pressure chronic ulcer of other part of left foot limited to breakdown of skin HCC
L97.522 Non-pressure chronic ulcer of other part of left foot with fat layer exposed HCC
AHA: 2020,2Q,19
L97.523 Non-pressure chronic ulcer of other part of left foot with necrosis of muscle HCC
L97.524 Non-pressure chronic ulcer of other part of left foot with necrosis of bone HCC
L97.525 Non-pressure chronic ulcer of other part of left foot with muscle involvement without evidence of necrosis CC HCC
L97.526 Non-pressure chronic ulcer of other part of left foot with bone involvement without evidence of necrosis CC HCC
L97.528 Non-pressure chronic ulcer of other part of left foot with other specified severity CC HCC

L97.529 Non-pressure chronic ulcer of other part of left foot with unspecified severity HCC

L97.8 Non-pressure chronic ulcer of other part of lower leg

L97.80 Non-pressure chronic ulcer of other part of unspecified lower leg

L97.801 Non-pressure chronic ulcer of other part of unspecified lower leg limited to breakdown of skin CC HCC

L97.802 Non-pressure chronic ulcer of other part of unspecified lower leg with fat layer exposed CC HCC

L97.803 Non-pressure chronic ulcer of other part of unspecified lower leg with necrosis of muscle CC HCC

L97.804 Non-pressure chronic ulcer of other part of unspecified lower leg with necrosis of bone CC HCC

L97.805 Non-pressure chronic ulcer of other part of unspecified lower leg with muscle involvement without evidence of necrosis CC HCC

L97.806 Non-pressure chronic ulcer of other part of unspecified lower leg with bone involvement without evidence of necrosis CC HCC

L97.808 Non-pressure chronic ulcer of other part of unspecified lower leg with other specified severity CC HCC

L97.809 Non-pressure chronic ulcer of other part of unspecified lower leg with unspecified severity CC HCC

L97.81 Non-pressure chronic ulcer of other part of right lower leg

L97.811 Non-pressure chronic ulcer of other part of right lower leg limited to breakdown of skin CC HCC

L97.812 Non-pressure chronic ulcer of other part of right lower leg with fat layer exposed CC HCC

L97.813 Non-pressure chronic ulcer of other part of right lower leg with necrosis of muscle CC HCC

L97.814 Non-pressure chronic ulcer of other part of right lower leg with necrosis of bone CC HCC

L97.815 Non-pressure chronic ulcer of other part of right lower leg with muscle involvement without evidence of necrosis CC HCC

L97.816 Non-pressure chronic ulcer of other part of right lower leg with bone involvement without evidence of necrosis CC HCC

L97.818 Non-pressure chronic ulcer of other part of right lower leg with other specified severity CC HCC

L97.819 Non-pressure chronic ulcer of other part of right lower leg with unspecified severity CC HCC

L97.82 Non-pressure chronic ulcer of other part of left lower leg

L97.821 Non-pressure chronic ulcer of other part of left lower leg limited to breakdown of skin CC HCC

L97.822 Non-pressure chronic ulcer of other part of left lower leg with fat layer exposed CC HCC

L97.823 Non-pressure chronic ulcer of other part of left lower leg with necrosis of muscle CC HCC

L97.824 Non-pressure chronic ulcer of other part of left lower leg with necrosis of bone CC HCC

L97.825 Non-pressure chronic ulcer of other part of left lower leg with muscle involvement without evidence of necrosis CC HCC

L97.826 Non-pressure chronic ulcer of other part of left lower leg with bone involvement without evidence of necrosis CC HCC

L97.828 Non-pressure chronic ulcer of other part of left lower leg with other specified severity CC HCC

L97.829 Non-pressure chronic ulcer of other part of left lower leg with unspecified severity CC HCC

L97.9 Non-pressure chronic ulcer of unspecified part of lower leg

L97.90 Non-pressure chronic ulcer of unspecified part of unspecified lower leg

L97.901 Non-pressure chronic ulcer of unspecified part of unspecified lower leg limited to breakdown of skin CC UNS HCC

L97.902 Non-pressure chronic ulcer of unspecified part of unspecified lower leg with fat layer exposed CC UNS HCC

L97.903 Non-pressure chronic ulcer of unspecified part of unspecified lower leg with necrosis of muscle CC UNS HCC

L97.904 Non-pressure chronic ulcer of unspecified part of unspecified lower leg with necrosis of bone CC UNS HCC

L97.905 Non-pressure chronic ulcer of unspecified part of unspecified lower leg with muscle involvement without evidence of necrosis CC UNS HCC

L97.906 Non-pressure chronic ulcer of unspecified part of unspecified lower leg with bone involvement without evidence of necrosis CC UNS HCC

L97.908 Non-pressure chronic ulcer of unspecified part of unspecified lower leg with other specified severity CC UNS HCC

L97.909 Non-pressure chronic ulcer of unspecified part of unspecified lower leg with unspecified severity CC UNS HCC

L97.91 Non-pressure chronic ulcer of unspecified part of right lower leg

L97.911 Non-pressure chronic ulcer of unspecified part of right lower leg limited to breakdown of skin CC HCC

L97.912 Non-pressure chronic ulcer of unspecified part of right lower leg with fat layer exposed CC HCC

L97.913 Non-pressure chronic ulcer of unspecified part of right lower leg with necrosis of muscle CC HCC

L97.914 Non-pressure chronic ulcer of unspecified part of right lower leg with necrosis of bone CC HCC

L97.915 Non-pressure chronic ulcer of unspecified part of right lower leg with muscle involvement without evidence of necrosis CC HCC

L97.916 Non-pressure chronic ulcer of unspecified part of right lower leg with bone involvement without evidence of necrosis CC HCC

L97.918 Non-pressure chronic ulcer of unspecified part of right lower leg with other specified severity CC HCC

L97.919 Non-pressure chronic ulcer of unspecified part of right lower leg with unspecified severity CC HCC

L97.92 Non-pressure chronic ulcer of unspecified part of left lower leg

L97.921 Non-pressure chronic ulcer of unspecified part of left lower leg limited to breakdown of skin CC HCC

L97.922 Non-pressure chronic ulcer of unspecified part of left lower leg with fat layer exposed CC HCC

L97.923 Non-pressure chronic ulcer of unspecified part of left lower leg with necrosis of muscle CC HCC

L97.924 Non-pressure chronic ulcer of unspecified part of left lower leg with necrosis of bone CC HCC

L97.925 Non-pressure chronic ulcer of unspecified part of left lower leg with muscle involvement without evidence of necrosis CC HCC

L97.926 Non-pressure chronic ulcer of unspecified part of left lower leg with bone involvement without evidence of necrosis CC HCC

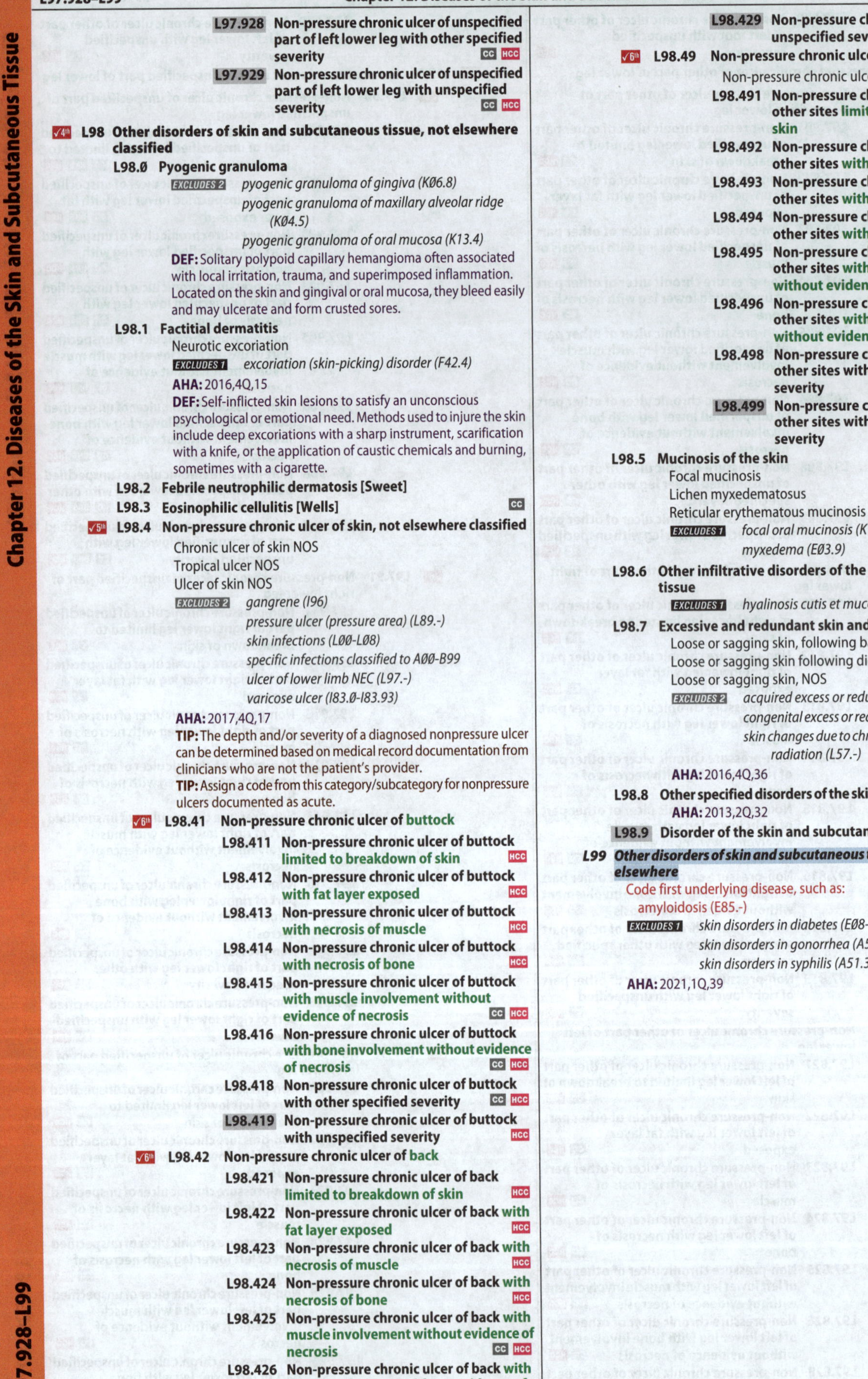

L97.928 **Non-pressure chronic ulcer of unspecified part of left lower leg with other specified severity** CC HCC

L97.929 **Non-pressure chronic ulcer of unspecified part of left lower leg with unspecified severity** CC HCC

✓4th **L98 Other disorders of skin and subcutaneous tissue, not elsewhere classified**

L98.Ø Pyogenic granuloma

EXCLUDES 2 *pyogenic granuloma of gingiva (KØ6.8)*
pyogenic granuloma of maxillary alveolar ridge (KØ4.5)
pyogenic granuloma of oral mucosa (K13.4)

DEF: Solitary polypoid capillary hemangioma often associated with local irritation, trauma, and superimposed inflammation. Located on the skin and gingival or oral mucosa, they bleed easily and may ulcerate and form crusted sores.

L98.1 Factitial dermatitis

Neurotic excoriation

EXCLUDES 1 *excoriation (skin-picking) disorder (F42.4)*

AHA: 2016,4Q,15

DEF: Self-inflicted skin lesions to satisfy an unconscious psychological or emotional need. Methods used to injure the skin include deep excoriations with a sharp instrument, scarification with a knife, or the application of caustic chemicals and burning, sometimes with a cigarette.

L98.2 Febrile neutrophilic dermatosis [Sweet]

L98.3 Eosinophilic cellulitis [Wells] CC

✓5th **L98.4 Non-pressure chronic ulcer of skin, not elsewhere classified**

Chronic ulcer of skin NOS
Tropical ulcer NOS
Ulcer of skin NOS

EXCLUDES 2 *gangrene (I96)*
pressure ulcer (pressure area) (L89.-)
skin infections (LØØ-LØ8)
specific infections classified to AØØ-B99
ulcer of lower limb NEC (L97.-)
varicose ulcer (I83.Ø-I83.93)

AHA: 2017,4Q,17

TIP: The depth and/or severity of a diagnosed nonpressure ulcer can be determined based on medical record documentation from clinicians who are not the patient's provider.

TIP: Assign a code from this category/subcategory for nonpressure ulcers documented as acute.

✓6th **L98.41 Non-pressure chronic ulcer of buttock**

L98.411 Non-pressure chronic ulcer of buttock limited to breakdown of skin HCC

L98.412 Non-pressure chronic ulcer of buttock with fat layer exposed HCC

L98.413 Non-pressure chronic ulcer of buttock with necrosis of muscle HCC

L98.414 Non-pressure chronic ulcer of buttock with necrosis of bone HCC

L98.415 Non-pressure chronic ulcer of buttock with muscle involvement without evidence of necrosis CC HCC

L98.416 Non-pressure chronic ulcer of buttock with bone involvement without evidence of necrosis CC HCC

L98.418 Non-pressure chronic ulcer of buttock with other specified severity CC HCC

L98.419 Non-pressure chronic ulcer of buttock with unspecified severity HCC

✓6th **L98.42 Non-pressure chronic ulcer of back**

L98.421 Non-pressure chronic ulcer of back limited to breakdown of skin HCC

L98.422 Non-pressure chronic ulcer of back with fat layer exposed HCC

L98.423 Non-pressure chronic ulcer of back with necrosis of muscle HCC

L98.424 Non-pressure chronic ulcer of back with necrosis of bone HCC

L98.425 Non-pressure chronic ulcer of back with muscle involvement without evidence of necrosis CC HCC

L98.426 Non-pressure chronic ulcer of back with bone involvement without evidence of necrosis CC HCC

L98.428 Non-pressure chronic ulcer of back with other specified severity CC HCC

L98.429 Non-pressure chronic ulcer of back with unspecified severity HCC

✓6th **L98.49 Non-pressure chronic ulcer of skin of other sites**

Non-pressure chronic ulcer of skin NOS

L98.491 Non-pressure chronic ulcer of skin of other sites limited to breakdown of skin HCC

L98.492 Non-pressure chronic ulcer of skin of other sites with fat layer exposed HCC

L98.493 Non-pressure chronic ulcer of skin of other sites with necrosis of muscle HCC

L98.494 Non-pressure chronic ulcer of skin of other sites with necrosis of bone HCC

L98.495 Non-pressure chronic ulcer of skin of other sites with muscle involvement without evidence of necrosis CC HCC

L98.496 Non-pressure chronic ulcer of skin of other sites with bone involvement without evidence of necrosis CC HCC

L98.498 Non-pressure chronic ulcer of skin of other sites with other specified severity CC HCC

L98.499 Non-pressure chronic ulcer of skin of other sites with unspecified severity HCC

L98.5 Mucinosis of the skin

Focal mucinosis
Lichen myxedematosus
Reticular erythematous mucinosis

EXCLUDES 1 *focal oral mucinosis (K13.79)*
myxedema (EØ3.9)

L98.6 Other infiltrative disorders of the skin and subcutaneous tissue

EXCLUDES 1 *hyalinosis cutis et mucosae (E78.89)*

L98.7 Excessive and redundant skin and subcutaneous tissue

Loose or sagging skin, following bariatric surgery weight loss
Loose or sagging skin following dietary weight loss
Loose or sagging skin, NOS

EXCLUDES 2 *acquired excess or redundant skin of eyelid (HØ2.3-)*
congenital excess or redundant skin of eyelid (Q1Ø.3)
skin changes due to chronic exposure to nonionizing radiation (L57.-)

AHA: 2016,4Q,36

L98.8 Other specified disorders of the skin and subcutaneous tissue

AHA: 2013,2Q,32

L98.9 Disorder of the skin and subcutaneous tissue, unspecified

L99 Other disorders of skin and subcutaneous tissue in diseases classified elsewhere

Code first underlying disease, such as:
amyloidosis (E85.-)

EXCLUDES 1 *skin disorders in diabetes (EØ8-E13 with .62-)*
skin disorders in gonorrhea (A54.89)
skin disorders in syphilis (A51.31, A52.79)

AHA: 2021,1Q,39

Chapter 13. Diseases of the Musculoskeletal System and Connective Tissue (MØØ–M99)

Chapter-specific Guidelines with Coding Examples

The chapter-specific guidelines from the ICD-10-CM Official Guidelines for Coding and Reporting have been provided below. Along with these guidelines are coding examples, contained in the shaded boxes, that have been developed to help illustrate the coding and/or sequencing guidance found in these guidelines.

a. Site and laterality

Most of the codes within Chapter 13 have site and laterality designations. The site represents the bone, joint or the muscle involved. For some conditions where more than one bone, joint or muscle is usually involved, such as osteoarthritis, there is a "multiple sites" code available. For categories where no multiple site code is provided and more than one bone, joint or muscle is involved, multiple codes should be used to indicate the different sites involved.

> Rheumatoid arthritis of multiple sites without rheumatoid factor
>
> **MØ6.Ø9 Rheumatoid arthritis without rheumatoid factor, multiple sites**
>
> *Explanation:* For some conditions where more than one bone, joint or muscle is usually involved, such as rheumatoid arthritis, there is a "multiple sites" code available.

> Osteomyelitis of the fourth thoracic and second lumbar vertebrae
>
> **M46.24 Osteomyelitis of vertebra, thoracic region**
>
> **M46.26 Osteomyelitis of vertebra, lumbar region**
>
> *Explanation:* For categories without a multiple site code and more than one bone, joint, or muscle is involved, multiple codes should be used to indicate the different sites involved.

1) Bone versus joint

For certain conditions, the bone may be affected at the upper or lower end, (e.g., avascular necrosis of bone, M87, Osteoporosis, M8Ø, M81). Though the portion of the bone affected may be at the joint, the site designation will be the bone, not the joint.

> Idiopathic avascular necrosis of the femoral head of the left hip joint
>
> **M87.Ø52 Idiopathic aseptic necrosis of left femur**
>
> *Explanation:* For certain conditions such as avascular necrosis, the bone may be affected at the joint, but the site designation is the bone, not the joint.

b. Acute traumatic versus chronic or recurrent musculoskeletal conditions

Many musculoskeletal conditions are a result of previous injury or trauma to a site, or are recurrent conditions. Bone, joint or muscle conditions that are the result of a healed injury are usually found in chapter 13. Recurrent bone, joint or muscle conditions are also usually found in chapter 13. Any current, acute injury should be coded to the appropriate injury code from chapter 19. Chronic or recurrent conditions should generally be coded with a code from chapter 13. If it is difficult to determine from the documentation in the record which code is best to describe a condition, query the provider.

> Acute traumatic bucket-handle tear of right medial meniscus
>
> **S83.211A Bucket-handle tear of medial meniscus, current injury, right knee, initial encounter**
>
> *Explanation:* Any current, acute injury is not coded in chapter 13. It should instead be coded to the appropriate injury code from chapter 19.

> Old bucket-handle tear of right medial meniscus
>
> **M23.2Ø3 Derangement of unspecified medial meniscus due to old tear or injury, right knee**
>
> *Explanation:* Chronic or recurrent conditions should generally be coded with a code from chapter 13.

c. Coding of pathologic fractures

7th character A is for use as long as the patient is receiving active treatment for the fracture. Examples of active treatment are: surgical treatment, emergency department encounter, evaluation and continuing treatment by the same or a different physician. While the patient may be seen by a new or different provider over the course of treatment for a pathological fracture, assignment of the 7th character is based on whether the patient is undergoing active treatment and not whether the provider is seeing the patient for the first time.

> Patient admitted for repair of pathologic fracture of left foot, unknown cause. The surgery will be performed by his orthopedic specialist who he has been seeing for this fracture for the past month.
>
> **M84.475A Pathological fracture, left foot, initial encounter for fracture**
>
> *Explanation:* Seventh character A is for use as long as the patient is receiving active treatment for a pathologic fracture. Examples of active treatment are surgical treatment, emergency department encounter, evaluation, and continuing treatment by the same or a different physician.
>
> The seventh character is based on whether the patient is undergoing active treatment such as surgery, and not whether the provider is seeing the patient for the first time.

7th character D is to be used for encounters after the patient has completed active treatment for the fracture and is receiving routine care for the fracture during the healing or recovery phase. The other 7th characters, listed under each subcategory in the Tabular List, are to be used for subsequent encounters for treatment of problems associated with the healing, such as malunions, nonunions, and sequelae.

Care for complications of surgical treatment for fracture repairs during the healing or recovery phase should be coded with the appropriate complication codes.

See Section I.C.19. Coding of traumatic fractures.

d. Osteoporosis

Osteoporosis is a systemic condition, meaning that all bones of the musculoskeletal system are affected. Therefore, site is not a component of the codes under category M81, Osteoporosis without current pathological fracture. The site codes under category M8Ø, Osteoporosis with current pathological fracture, identify the site of the fracture, not the osteoporosis.

1) Osteoporosis without pathological fracture

Category M81, Osteoporosis without current pathological fracture, is for use for patients with osteoporosis who do not currently have a pathologic fracture due to the osteoporosis, even if they have had a fracture in the past. For patients with a history of osteoporosis fractures, status code Z87.31Ø, Personal history of (healed) osteoporosis fracture, should follow the code from M81.

> Age-related osteoporosis with healed osteoporotic fracture of the lumbar vertebra
>
> **M81.Ø Age-related osteoporosis without current pathological fracture**
>
> **Z87.31Ø Personal history of (healed) osteoporosis fracture**
>
> *Explanation:* Category M81 is used for patients with osteoporosis who do not currently have a pathologic fracture due to the osteoporosis. To report a previous (healed) fracture, status code Z87.31Ø Personal history of (healed) osteoporosis fracture, should follow the code from M81.

2) Osteoporosis with current pathological fracture

Category M8Ø, Osteoporosis with current pathological fracture, is for patients who have a current pathologic fracture at the time of an encounter. The codes under M8Ø identify the site of the fracture. A code from category M8Ø, not a traumatic fracture code, should be used for any patient with known osteoporosis who suffers a fracture, even if the patient had a minor fall or trauma, if that fall or trauma would not usually break a normal, healthy bone.

> Disuse osteoporosis with current fracture of right shoulder sustained lifting a grocery bag, initial encounter
>
> **M8Ø.811A Other osteoporosis with current pathological fracture, right shoulder, initial encounter for fracture**
>
> *Explanation:* A code from category M8Ø, not a traumatic fracture code, should be used for any patient with known osteoporosis who suffers a fracture, even if the patient had a minor fall or trauma, if that fall or trauma would not usually break a normal, healthy bone.

e. Multisystem inflammatory syndrome

See Section I.C.1.g.1.l. for Multisystem Inflammatory Syndrome

Muscle/Tendon Table

ICD-10-CM categorizes certain muscles and tendons in the upper and lower extremities by their action (e.g., extension, flexion), their anatomical location (e.g., posterior, anterior), and/or whether they are intrinsic or extrinsic to a certain anatomical area. The Muscle/Tendon Table is provided at the beginning of chapters 13 and 19 as a resource to help users when code selection depends on one or more of these characteristics. Please note that this table is not all-inclusive, and proper code assignment should be based on the provider's documentation.

Body Region	Muscle	Extensor Tendon	Flexor Tendon	Other Tendon
Shoulder				
	Deltoid	Posterior deltoid	Anterior deltoid	
	Rotator cuff			
	Infraspinatus			Infraspinatus
	Subscapularis			Subscapularis
	Supraspinatus			Supraspinatus
	Teres minor			Teres minor
	Teres major	Teres major		
Upper arm				
	Anterior muscles			
	Biceps brachii — long head		Biceps brachii — long head	
	Biceps brachii — short head		Biceps brachii — short head	
	Brachialis		Brachialis	
	Coracobrachialis		Coracobrachialis	
	Posterior muscles			
	Triceps brachii	Triceps brachii		
Forearm				
	Anterior muscles			
	Flexors			
	Deep			
	Flexor digitorum profundus		Flexor digitorum profundus	
	Flexor pollicis longus		Flexor pollicis longus	
	Intermediate			
	Flexor digitorum superficialis		Flexor digitorum superficialis	
	Superficial			
	Flexor carpi radialis		Flexor carpi radialis	
	Flexor carpi ulnaris		Flexor carpi ulnaris	
	Palmaris longus		Palmaris longus	
	Pronators			
	Pronator quadratus			Pronator quadratus
	Pronator teres			Pronator teres
	Posterior muscles			
	Extensors			
	Deep			
	Abductor pollicis longus			Abductor pollicis longus
	Extensor indicis	Extensor indicis		
	Extensor pollicis brevis	Extensor pollicis brevis		
	Extensor pollicis longus	Extensor pollicis longus		
	Superficial			
	Brachioradialis			Brachioradialis
	Extensor carpi radialis brevis	Extensor carpi radialis brevis		
	Extensor carpi radialis longus	Extensor carpi radialis longus		
	Extensor carpi ulnaris	Extensor carpi ulnaris		
	Extensor digiti minimi	Extensor digiti minimi		
	Extensor digitorum	Extensor digitorum		
	Anconeus	Anconeus		
	Supinator			Supinator

Body Region	Muscle	Extensor Tendon	Flexor Tendon	Other Tendon
Hand				
Extrinsic — attach to a site in the forearm as well as a site in the hand with action related to hand movement at the wrist				
	Extensor carpi radialis brevis	Extensor carpi radialis brevis		
	Extensor carpi radialis longus	Extensor carpi radialis longus		
	Extensor carpi ulnaris	Extensor carpi ulnaris		
	Flexor carpi radialis		Flexor carpi radialis	
	Flexor carpi ulnaris		Flexor carpi ulnaris	
	Flexor digitorum superficialis		Flexor digitorum superficialis	
	Palmaris longus		Palmaris longus	
Extrinsic — attach to a site in the forearm as well as a site in the hand with action in the hand related to finger movement				
	Adductor pollicis longus			Adductor pollicis longus
	Extensor digiti minimi	Extensor digiti minimi		
	Extensor digitorum	Extensor digitorum		
	Extensor indicis	Extensor indicis		
	Flexor digitorum profundus		Flexor digitorum profundus	
	Flexor digitorum superficialis		Flexor digitorum superficialis	
Extrinsic — attach to a site in the forearm as well as a site in the hand with action in the hand related to thumb movement				
	Extensor pollicis brevis	Extensor pollicis brevis		
	Extensor pollicis longus	Extensor pollicis longus		
	Flexor pollicis longus		Flexor pollicis longus	
Intrinsic — found within the hand only				
	Adductor pollicis			Adductor pollicis
	Dorsal interossei	Dorsal interossei	Dorsal interossei	
	Lumbricals	Lumbricals	Lumbricals	
	Palmaris brevis			Palmaris brevis
	Palmar interossei	Palmar interossei	Palmar interossei	
	Hypothenar muscles			
	Abductor digiti minimi			Abductor digiti minimi
	Flexor digiti minimi brevis		Flexor digiti minimi brevis	
	Opponens digiti minimi		Opponens digiti minimi	
	Thenar muscles			
	Abductor pollicis brevis			Abductor pollicis brevis
	Flexor pollicis brevis		Flexor pollicis brevis	
	Opponens pollicis		Opponens pollicis	
Thigh				
	Anterior muscles			
	Iliopsoas		Iliopsoas	
	Pectineus		Pectineus	
	Quadriceps	Quadriceps		
	Rectus femoris	Rectus femoris — Extends knee	Rectus femoris — Flexes hip	
	Vastus intermedius	Vastus intermedius		
	Vastus lateralis	Vastus lateralis		
	Vastus medialis	Vastus medialis		
	Sartorius		Sartorius	
	Medial muscles			
	Adductor brevis			Adductor brevis
	Adductor longus			Adductor longus
	Adductor magnus			Adductor magnus
	Gracilis			Gracilis
	Obturator externus			Obturator externus
	Posterior muscles			
	Hamstring	Hamstring — Extends hip	Hamstring — Flexes knee	
	Biceps femoris	Biceps femoris	Biceps femoris	
	Semimembranosus	Semimembranosus	Semimembranosus	
	Semitendinosus	Semitendinosus	Semitendinosus	

Body Region	Muscle	Extensor Tendon	Flexor Tendon	Other Tendon
Lower leg				
	Anterior muscles			
	Extensor digitorum longus	Extensor digitorum longus		
	Extensor hallucis longus	Extensor hallucis longus		
	Fibularis (peroneus) tertius	Fibularis (peroneus) tertius		
	Tibialis anterior	Tibialis anterior		Tibialis anterior
	Lateral muscles			
	Fibularis (peroneus) brevis		Fibularis (peroneus) brevis	
	Fibularis (peroneus) longus		Fibularis (peroneus) longus	
	Posterior muscles			
	Deep			
	Flexor digitorum longus		Flexor digitorum longus	
	Flexor hallucis longus		Flexor hallucis longus	
	Popliteus		Popliteus	
	Tibialis posterior		Tibialis posterior	
	Superficial			
	Gastrocnemius		Gastrocnemius	
	Plantaris		Plantaris	
	Soleus		Soleus	
				Calcaneal (Achilles)
Ankle/Foot				
Extrinsic — attach to a site in the lower leg as well as a site in the foot with action related to foot movement at the ankle				
	Plantaris		Plantaris	
	Soleus		Soleus	
	Tibialis anterior	Tibialis anterior		
	Tibialis posterior		Tibialis posterior	
Extrinsic — attach to a site in the lower leg as well as a site in the foot with action in the foot related to toe movement				
	Extensor digitorum longus	Extensor digitorum longus		
	Extensor hallucis longus	Extensor hallucis longus		
	Flexor digitorum longus		Flexor digitorum longus	
	Flexor hallucis longus		Flexor hallucis longus	
Intrinsic — found within the ankle/foot only				
	Dorsal muscles			
	Extensor digitorum brevis	Extensor digitorum brevis		
	Extensor hallucis brevis	Extensor hallucis brevis		
	Plantar muscles			
	Abductor digiti minimi		Abductor digiti minimi	
	Abductor hallucis		Abductor hallucis	
	Dorsal interossei	Dorsal interossei	Dorsal interossei	
	Flexor digiti minimi brevis		Flexor digiti minimi brevis	
	Flexor digitorum brevis		Flexor digitorum brevis	
	Flexor hallucis brevis		Flexor hallucis brevis	
	Lumbricals	Lumbricals	Lumbricals	
	Quadratus plantae		Quadratus plantae	
	Plantar interossei	Plantar interossei	Plantar interossei	

Chapter 13. Diseases of the Musculoskeletal System and Connective Tissue (M00-M99)

NOTE Use an external cause code following the code for the musculoskeletal condition, if applicable, to identify the cause of the musculoskeletal condition

EXCLUDES 2 *arthropathic psoriasis (L40.5-)*
certain conditions originating in the perinatal period (P04-P96)
certain infectious and parasitic diseases (A00-B99)
compartment syndrome (traumatic) (T79.A-)
complications of pregnancy, childbirth and the puerperium (O00-O9A)
congenital malformations, deformations, and chromosomal abnormalities (Q00-Q99)
endocrine, nutritional and metabolic diseases (E00-E88)
injury, poisoning and certain other consequences of external causes (S00-T88)
neoplasms (C00-D49)
symptoms, signs and abnormal clinical and laboratory findings, not elsewhere classified (R00-R94)

This chapter contains the following blocks:

M00-M02 Infectious arthropathies
M04 Autoinflammatory syndromes
M05-M14 Inflammatory polyarthropathies
M15-M19 Osteoarthritis
M20-M25 Other joint disorders
M26-M27 Dentofacial anomalies [including malocclusion] and other disorders of jaw
M30-M36 Systemic connective tissue disorders
M40-M43 Deforming dorsopathies
M45-M49 Spondylopathies
M50-M54 Other dorsopathies
M60-M63 Disorders of muscles
M65-M67 Disorders of synovium and tendon
M70-M79 Other soft tissue disorders
M80-M85 Disorders of bone density and structure
M86-M90 Other osteopathies
M91-M94 Chondropathies
M95 Other disorders of the musculoskeletal system and connective tissue
M96 Intraoperative and postprocedural complications and disorders of musculoskeletal system, not elsewhere classified
M97 Periprosthetic fracture around internal prosthetic joint
M99 Biomechanical lesions, not elsewhere classified

ARTHROPATHIES (M00-M25)

INCLUDES disorders affecting predominantly peripheral (limb) joints

Infectious arthropathies (M00-M02)

NOTE This block comprises arthropathies due to microbiological agents. Distinction is made between the following types of etiological relationship:

a) direct infection of joint, where organisms invade synovial tissue and microbial antigen is present in the joint;

b) indirect infection, which may be of two types: a reactive arthropathy, where microbial infection of the body is established but neither organisms nor antigens can be identified in the joint, and a postinfective arthropathy, where microbial antigen is present but recovery of an organism is inconstant and evidence of local multiplication is lacking.

AHA: 2019,3Q,16

✓4th **M00 Pyogenic arthritis**

EXCLUDES 2 *infection and inflammatory reaction due to internal joint prosthesis (T84.5-)*

AHA: 2022,1Q,31

DEF: Pyogenic: Relating to or involving pus production, often referred to as suppurative or purulent.

✓5th **M00.0 Staphylococcal arthritis and polyarthritis**

Use additional code (B95.61-B95.8) to identify bacterial agent

M00.00 Staphylococcal arthritis, unspecified joint CC UNS HCC

✓6th **M00.01 Staphylococcal arthritis, shoulder**

M00.011 Staphylococcal arthritis, right shoulder CC HCC

M00.012 Staphylococcal arthritis, left shoulder CC HCC

M00.019 Staphylococcal arthritis, unspecified shoulder CC UNS HCC

✓6th **M00.02 Staphylococcal arthritis, elbow**

M00.021 Staphylococcal arthritis, right elbow CC HCC

M00.022 Staphylococcal arthritis, left elbow CC HCC

M00.029 Staphylococcal arthritis, unspecified elbow CC UNS HCC

✓6th **M00.03 Staphylococcal arthritis, wrist**

Staphylococcal arthritis of carpal bones

M00.031 Staphylococcal arthritis, right wrist CC HCC

M00.032 Staphylococcal arthritis, left wrist CC HCC

M00.039 Staphylococcal arthritis, unspecified wrist CC UNS HCC

✓6th **M00.04 Staphylococcal arthritis, hand**

Staphylococcal arthritis of metacarpus and phalanges

M00.041 Staphylococcal arthritis, right hand CC HCC

M00.042 Staphylococcal arthritis, left hand CC HCC

M00.049 Staphylococcal arthritis, unspecified hand CC UNS HCC

✓6th **M00.05 Staphylococcal arthritis, hip**

M00.051 Staphylococcal arthritis, right hip CC HCC

M00.052 Staphylococcal arthritis, left hip CC HCC

M00.059 Staphylococcal arthritis, unspecified hip CC UNS HCC

✓6th **M00.06 Staphylococcal arthritis, knee**

M00.061 Staphylococcal arthritis, right knee CC HCC

M00.062 Staphylococcal arthritis, left knee CC HCC

M00.069 Staphylococcal arthritis, unspecified knee CC UNS HCC

✓6th **M00.07 Staphylococcal arthritis, ankle and foot**

Staphylococcal arthritis, tarsus, metatarsus and phalanges

M00.071 Staphylococcal arthritis, right ankle and foot CC HCC

M00.072 Staphylococcal arthritis, left ankle and foot CC HCC

M00.079 Staphylococcal arthritis, unspecified ankle and foot CC UNS HCC

M00.08 Staphylococcal arthritis, vertebrae CC HCC

M00.09 Staphylococcal polyarthritis CC HCC

✓5th **M00.1 Pneumococcal arthritis and polyarthritis**

M00.10 Pneumococcal arthritis, unspecified joint CC UNS HCC

✓6th **M00.11 Pneumococcal arthritis, shoulder**

M00.111 Pneumococcal arthritis, right shoulder CC HCC

M00.112 Pneumococcal arthritis, left shoulder CC HCC

M00.119 Pneumococcal arthritis, unspecified shoulder CC UNS HCC

✓6th **M00.12 Pneumococcal arthritis, elbow**

M00.121 Pneumococcal arthritis, right elbow CC HCC

M00.122 Pneumococcal arthritis, left elbow CC HCC

M00.129 Pneumococcal arthritis, unspecified elbow CC UNS HCC

✓6th **M00.13 Pneumococcal arthritis, wrist**

Pneumococcal arthritis of carpal bones

M00.131 Pneumococcal arthritis, right wrist CC HCC

M00.132 Pneumococcal arthritis, left wrist CC HCC

M00.139 Pneumococcal arthritis, unspecified wrist CC UNS HCC

✓6th **M00.14 Pneumococcal arthritis, hand**

Pneumococcal arthritis of metacarpus and phalanges

M00.141 Pneumococcal arthritis, right hand CC HCC

M00.142 Pneumococcal arthritis, left hand CC HCC

M00.149 Pneumococcal arthritis, unspecified hand CC UNS HCC

M00.15 Pneumococcal arthritis, hip
M00.151 Pneumococcal arthritis, right hip CC HCC
M00.152 Pneumococcal arthritis, left hip CC HCC
M00.159 Pneumococcal arthritis, unspecified hip CC UNS HCC
M00.16 Pneumococcal arthritis, knee
M00.161 Pneumococcal arthritis, right knee CC HCC
M00.162 Pneumococcal arthritis, left knee CC HCC
M00.169 Pneumococcal arthritis, unspecified knee CC UNS HCC
M00.17 Pneumococcal arthritis, ankle and foot
Pneumococcal arthritis, tarsus, metatarsus and phalanges
M00.171 Pneumococcal arthritis, right ankle and foot CC HCC
M00.172 Pneumococcal arthritis, left ankle and foot CC HCC
M00.179 Pneumococcal arthritis, unspecified ankle and foot CC UNS HCC
M00.18 Pneumococcal arthritis, vertebrae CC HCC
M00.19 Pneumococcal polyarthritis CC HCC
M00.2 Other streptococcal arthritis and polyarthritis
Use additional code (B95.0-B95.2, B95.4-B95.5) to identify bacterial agent
M00.20 Other streptococcal arthritis, unspecified joint CC UNS HCC
M00.21 Other streptococcal arthritis, shoulder
M00.211 Other streptococcal arthritis, right shoulder CC HCC
M00.212 Other streptococcal arthritis, left shoulder CC HCC
M00.219 Other streptococcal arthritis, unspecified shoulder CC UNS HCC
M00.22 Other streptococcal arthritis, elbow
M00.221 Other streptococcal arthritis, right elbow CC HCC
M00.222 Other streptococcal arthritis, left elbow CC HCC
M00.229 Other streptococcal arthritis, unspecified elbow CC UNS HCC
M00.23 Other streptococcal arthritis, wrist
Other streptococcal arthritis of carpal bones
M00.231 Other streptococcal arthritis, right wrist CC HCC
M00.232 Other streptococcal arthritis, left wrist CC HCC
M00.239 Other streptococcal arthritis, unspecified wrist CC UNS HCC
M00.24 Other streptococcal arthritis, hand
Other streptococcal arthritis metacarpus and phalanges
M00.241 Other streptococcal arthritis, right hand CC HCC
M00.242 Other streptococcal arthritis, left hand CC HCC
M00.249 Other streptococcal arthritis, unspecified hand CC UNS HCC
M00.25 Other streptococcal arthritis, hip
M00.251 Other streptococcal arthritis, right hip CC HCC
M00.252 Other streptococcal arthritis, left hip CC HCC
M00.259 Other streptococcal arthritis, unspecified hip CC UNS HCC
M00.26 Other streptococcal arthritis, knee
M00.261 Other streptococcal arthritis, right knee CC HCC
M00.262 Other streptococcal arthritis, left knee CC HCC
M00.269 Other streptococcal arthritis, unspecified knee CC UNS HCC
M00.27 Other streptococcal arthritis, ankle and foot
Other streptococcal arthritis, tarsus, metatarsus and phalanges
M00.271 Other streptococcal arthritis, right ankle and foot CC HCC
M00.272 Other streptococcal arthritis, left ankle and foot CC HCC
M00.279 Other streptococcal arthritis, unspecified ankle and foot CC UNS HCC
M00.28 Other streptococcal arthritis, vertebrae CC HCC
M00.29 Other streptococcal polyarthritis CC HCC
M00.8 Arthritis and polyarthritis due to other bacteria
Use additional code (B96) to identify bacteria
M00.80 Arthritis due to other bacteria, unspecified joint CC UNS HCC
M00.81 Arthritis due to other bacteria, shoulder
M00.811 Arthritis due to other bacteria, right shoulder CC HCC
M00.812 Arthritis due to other bacteria, left shoulder CC HCC
M00.819 Arthritis due to other bacteria, unspecified shoulder CC UNS HCC
M00.82 Arthritis due to other bacteria, elbow
M00.821 Arthritis due to other bacteria, right elbow CC HCC
M00.822 Arthritis due to other bacteria, left elbow CC HCC
M00.829 Arthritis due to other bacteria, unspecified elbow CC UNS HCC
M00.83 Arthritis due to other bacteria, wrist
Arthritis due to other bacteria, carpal bones
M00.831 Arthritis due to other bacteria, right wrist CC HCC
M00.832 Arthritis due to other bacteria, left wrist CC HCC
M00.839 Arthritis due to other bacteria, unspecified wrist CC UNS HCC
M00.84 Arthritis due to other bacteria, hand
Arthritis due to other bacteria, metacarpus and phalanges
M00.841 Arthritis due to other bacteria, right hand CC HCC
M00.842 Arthritis due to other bacteria, left hand CC HCC
M00.849 Arthritis due to other bacteria, unspecified hand CC UNS HCC
M00.85 Arthritis due to other bacteria, hip
M00.851 Arthritis due to other bacteria, right hip CC HCC
M00.852 Arthritis due to other bacteria, left hip CC HCC
M00.859 Arthritis due to other bacteria, unspecified hip CC UNS HCC
M00.86 Arthritis due to other bacteria, knee
AHA: 2019,3Q,16
M00.861 Arthritis due to other bacteria, right knee CC HCC
M00.862 Arthritis due to other bacteria, left knee CC HCC
M00.869 Arthritis due to other bacteria, unspecified knee CC UNS HCC
M00.87 Arthritis due to other bacteria, ankle and foot
Arthritis due to other bacteria, tarsus, metatarsus, and phalanges
M00.871 Arthritis due to other bacteria, right ankle and foot CC HCC
M00.872 Arthritis due to other bacteria, left ankle and foot CC HCC
M00.879 Arthritis due to other bacteria, unspecified ankle and foot CC UNS HCC
M00.88 Arthritis due to other bacteria, vertebrae CC HCC
M00.89 Polyarthritis due to other bacteria CC HCC
M00.9 Pyogenic arthritis, unspecified CC HCC
Infective arthritis NOS

N Newborn: 0 P Pediatric: 0-17 M Maternity: 9-64 A Adult: 15-124 UNS Unspecified Site MCC Major Complication/Comorbidity CC Complication/Comorbidity

M01 Direct infections of joint in infectious and parasitic diseases classified elsewhere

Code first underlying disease, such as:
- leprosy [Hansen's disease] (A30.-)
- mycoses (B35-B49)
- O'nyong-nyong fever (A92.1)
- paratyphoid fever (A01.1-A01.4)

EXCLUDES 1
- *arthropathy in Lyme disease (A69.23)*
- *gonococcal arthritis (A54.42)*
- *meningococcal arthritis (A39.83)*
- *mumps arthritis (B26.85)*
- *postinfective arthropathy (M02.-)*
- *postmeningococcal arthritis (A39.84)*
- *reactive arthritis (M02.3)*
- *rubella arthritis (B06.82)*
- *sarcoidosis arthritis (D86.86)*
- *typhoid fever arthritis (A01.04)*
- *tuberculosis arthritis (A18.01-A18.02)*

M01.X Direct infection of joint in infectious and parasitic diseases classified elsewhere

M01.X0 Direct infection of unspecified joint in infectious and parasitic diseases classified elsewhere CC UNS HCC

M01.X1 Direct infection of shoulder joint in infectious and parasitic diseases classified elsewhere

M01.X11 Direct infection of right shoulder in infectious and parasitic diseases classified elsewhere CC HCC

M01.X12 Direct infection of left shoulder in infectious and parasitic diseases classified elsewhere CC HCC

M01.X19 Direct infection of unspecified shoulder in infectious and parasitic diseases classified elsewhere CC UNS HCC

M01.X2 Direct infection of elbow in infectious and parasitic diseases classified elsewhere

M01.X21 Direct infection of right elbow in infectious and parasitic diseases classified elsewhere CC HCC

M01.X22 Direct infection of left elbow in infectious and parasitic diseases classified elsewhere CC HCC

M01.X29 Direct infection of unspecified elbow in infectious and parasitic diseases classified elsewhere CC UNS HCC

M01.X3 Direct infection of wrist in infectious and parasitic diseases classified elsewhere

Direct infection of carpal bones in infectious and parasitic diseases classified elsewhere

M01.X31 Direct infection of right wrist in infectious and parasitic diseases classified elsewhere CC HCC

M01.X32 Direct infection of left wrist in infectious and parasitic diseases classified elsewhere CC HCC

M01.X39 Direct infection of unspecified wrist in infectious and parasitic diseases classified elsewhere CC UNS HCC

M01.X4 Direct infection of hand in infectious and parasitic diseases classified elsewhere

Direct infection of metacarpus and phalanges in infectious and parasitic diseases classified elsewhere

M01.X41 Direct infection of right hand in infectious and parasitic diseases classified elsewhere CC HCC

M01.X42 Direct infection of left hand in infectious and parasitic diseases classified elsewhere CC HCC

M01.X49 Direct infection of unspecified hand in infectious and parasitic diseases classified elsewhere CC UNS HCC

M01.X5 Direct infection of hip in infectious and parasitic diseases classified elsewhere

M01.X51 Direct infection of right hip in infectious and parasitic diseases classified elsewhere CC HCC

M01.X52 Direct infection of left hip in infectious and parasitic diseases classified elsewhere CC HCC

M01.X59 Direct infection of unspecified hip in infectious and parasitic diseases classified elsewhere CC UNS HCC

M01.X6 Direct infection of knee in infectious and parasitic diseases classified elsewhere

M01.X61 Direct infection of right knee in infectious and parasitic diseases classified elsewhere CC HCC

M01.X62 Direct infection of left knee in infectious and parasitic diseases classified elsewhere CC HCC

M01.X69 Direct infection of unspecified knee in infectious and parasitic diseases classified elsewhere CC UNS HCC

M01.X7 Direct infection of ankle and foot in infectious and parasitic diseases classified elsewhere

Direct infection of tarsus, metatarsus and phalanges in infectious and parasitic diseases classified elsewhere

M01.X71 Direct infection of right ankle and foot in infectious and parasitic diseases classified elsewhere CC HCC

M01.X72 Direct infection of left ankle and foot in infectious and parasitic diseases classified elsewhere CC HCC

M01.X79 Direct infection of unspecified ankle and foot in infectious and parasitic diseases classified elsewhere CC UNS HCC

M01.X8 Direct infection of vertebrae in infectious and parasitic diseases classified elsewhere CC HCC

M01.X9 Direct infection of multiple joints in infectious and parasitic diseases classified elsewhere CC HCC

M02 Postinfective and reactive arthropathies

Code first underlying disease, such as:
- congenital syphilis [Clutton's joints] (A50.5)
- enteritis due to Yersinia enterocolitica (A04.6)
- infective endocarditis (I33.0)
- viral hepatitis (B15-B19)

EXCLUDES 1
- *Behçet's disease (M35.2)*
- *direct infections of joint in infectious and parasitic diseases classified elsewhere (M01.-)*
- *mumps arthritis (B26.85)*
- *postmeningococcal arthritis (A39.84)*
- *rheumatic fever (I00)*
- *rubella arthritis (B06.82)*
- *syphilis arthritis (late) (A52.77)*
- *tabetic arthropathy [Charcôt's] (A52.16)*

M02.0 Arthropathy following intestinal bypass

M02.00 Arthropathy following intestinal bypass, unspecified site

M02.01 Arthropathy following intestinal bypass, shoulder

M02.011 Arthropathy following intestinal bypass, right shoulder

M02.012 Arthropathy following intestinal bypass, left shoulder

M02.019 Arthropathy following intestinal bypass, unspecified shoulder

M02.02 Arthropathy following intestinal bypass, elbow

M02.021 Arthropathy following intestinal bypass, right elbow

M02.022 Arthropathy following intestinal bypass, left elbow

M02.029 Arthropathy following intestinal bypass, unspecified elbow

M02.03 Arthropathy following intestinal bypass, wrist

Arthropathy following intestinal bypass, carpal bones

M02.031 Arthropathy following intestinal bypass, right wrist

M02.032 Arthropathy following intestinal bypass, left wrist

M02.039 Arthropathy following intestinal bypass, unspecified wrist

M02.04 Arthropathy following intestinal bypass, hand

Arthropathy following intestinal bypass, metacarpals and phalanges

M02.041 Arthropathy following intestinal bypass, right hand

M02.042 Arthropathy following intestinal bypass, left hand

MØ2.Ø49 Arthropathy following intestinal bypass, unspecified hand

✓6th **MØ2.Ø5** Arthropathy following intestinal bypass, hip

MØ2.Ø51 Arthropathy following intestinal bypass, right hip

MØ2.Ø52 Arthropathy following intestinal bypass, left hip

MØ2.Ø59 Arthropathy following intestinal bypass, unspecified hip

✓6th **MØ2.Ø6** Arthropathy following intestinal bypass, knee

MØ2.Ø61 Arthropathy following intestinal bypass, right knee

MØ2.Ø62 Arthropathy following intestinal bypass, left knee

MØ2.Ø69 Arthropathy following intestinal bypass, unspecified knee

✓6th **MØ2.Ø7** Arthropathy following intestinal bypass, ankle and foot

Arthropathy following intestinal bypass, tarsus, metatarsus and phalanges

MØ2.Ø71 Arthropathy following intestinal bypass, right ankle and foot

MØ2.Ø72 Arthropathy following intestinal bypass, left ankle and foot

MØ2.Ø79 Arthropathy following intestinal bypass, unspecified ankle and foot

MØ2.Ø8 Arthropathy following intestinal bypass, vertebrae

MØ2.Ø9 Arthropathy following intestinal bypass, multiple sites

✓5th **MØ2.1** Postdysenteric arthropathy

MØ2.1Ø Postdysenteric arthropathy, unspecified site CC UNS HCC

✓6th **MØ2.11** Postdysenteric arthropathy, shoulder

MØ2.111 Postdysenteric arthropathy, right shoulder CC HCC

MØ2.112 Postdysenteric arthropathy, left shoulder CC HCC

MØ2.119 Postdysenteric arthropathy, unspecified shoulder CC UNS HCC

✓6th **MØ2.12** Postdysenteric arthropathy, elbow

MØ2.121 Postdysenteric arthropathy, right elbow CC HCC

MØ2.122 Postdysenteric arthropathy, left elbow CC HCC

MØ2.129 Postdysenteric arthropathy, unspecified elbow CC UNS HCC

✓6th **MØ2.13** Postdysenteric arthropathy, wrist

Postdysenteric arthropathy, carpal bones

MØ2.131 Postdysenteric arthropathy, right wrist CC HCC

MØ2.132 Postdysenteric arthropathy, left wrist CC HCC

MØ2.139 Postdysenteric arthropathy, unspecified wrist CC UNS HCC

✓6th **MØ2.14** Postdysenteric arthropathy, hand

Postdysenteric arthropathy, metacarpus and phalanges

MØ2.141 Postdysenteric arthropathy, right hand CC HCC

MØ2.142 Postdysenteric arthropathy, left hand CC HCC

MØ2.149 Postdysenteric arthropathy, unspecified hand CC UNS HCC

✓6th **MØ2.15** Postdysenteric arthropathy, hip

MØ2.151 Postdysenteric arthropathy, right hip CC HCC

MØ2.152 Postdysenteric arthropathy, left hip CC HCC

MØ2.159 Postdysenteric arthropathy, unspecified hip CC UNS HCC

✓6th **MØ2.16** Postdysenteric arthropathy, knee

MØ2.161 Postdysenteric arthropathy, right knee CC HCC

MØ2.162 Postdysenteric arthropathy, left knee CC HCC

MØ2.169 Postdysenteric arthropathy, unspecified knee CC UNS HCC

✓6th **MØ2.17** Postdysenteric arthropathy, ankle and foot

Postdysenteric arthropathy, tarsus, metatarsus and phalanges

MØ2.171 Postdysenteric arthropathy, right ankle and foot CC HCC

MØ2.172 Postdysenteric arthropathy, left ankle and foot CC HCC

MØ2.179 Postdysenteric arthropathy, unspecified ankle and foot CC UNS HCC

MØ2.18 Postdysenteric arthropathy, vertebrae CC HCC

MØ2.19 Postdysenteric arthropathy, multiple sites CC HCC

✓5th **MØ2.2** Postimmunization arthropathy

MØ2.2Ø Postimmunization arthropathy, unspecified site

✓6th **MØ2.21** Postimmunization arthropathy, shoulder

MØ2.211 Postimmunization arthropathy, right shoulder

MØ2.212 Postimmunization arthropathy, left shoulder

MØ2.219 Postimmunization arthropathy, unspecified shoulder

✓6th **MØ2.22** Postimmunization arthropathy, elbow

MØ2.221 Postimmunization arthropathy, right elbow

MØ2.222 Postimmunization arthropathy, left elbow

MØ2.229 Postimmunization arthropathy, unspecified elbow

✓6th **MØ2.23** Postimmunization arthropathy, wrist

Postimmunization arthropathy, carpal bones

MØ2.231 Postimmunization arthropathy, right wrist

MØ2.232 Postimmunization arthropathy, left wrist

MØ2.239 Postimmunization arthropathy, unspecified wrist

✓6th **MØ2.24** Postimmunization arthropathy, hand

Postimmunization arthropathy, metacarpus and phalanges

MØ2.241 Postimmunization arthropathy, right hand

MØ2.242 Postimmunization arthropathy, left hand

MØ2.249 Postimmunization arthropathy, unspecified hand

✓6th **MØ2.25** Postimmunization arthropathy, hip

MØ2.251 Postimmunization arthropathy, right hip

MØ2.252 Postimmunization arthropathy, left hip

MØ2.259 Postimmunization arthropathy, unspecified hip

✓6th **MØ2.26** Postimmunization arthropathy, knee

MØ2.261 Postimmunization arthropathy, right knee

MØ2.262 Postimmunization arthropathy, left knee

MØ2.269 Postimmunization arthropathy, unspecified knee

✓6th **MØ2.27** Postimmunization arthropathy, ankle and foot

Postimmunization arthropathy, tarsus, metatarsus and phalanges

MØ2.271 Postimmunization arthropathy, right ankle and foot

MØ2.272 Postimmunization arthropathy, left ankle and foot

MØ2.279 Postimmunization arthropathy, unspecified ankle and foot

MØ2.28 Postimmunization arthropathy, vertebrae

MØ2.29 Postimmunization arthropathy, multiple sites

✓5th **MØ2.3** Reiter's disease

Reactive arthritis

DEF: Arthritis, iridocyclitis, and urethritis, sometimes with diarrhea. While symptoms may recur, arthritis is constant.

MØ2.3Ø Reiter's disease, unspecified site CC UNS HCC

✓6th **MØ2.31** Reiter's disease, shoulder

MØ2.311 Reiter's disease, right shoulder CC HCC

MØ2.312 Reiter's disease, left shoulder CC HCC

MØ2.319 Reiter's disease, unspecified shoulder CC UNS HCC

✓6th **MØ2.32** Reiter's disease, elbow

MØ2.321 Reiter's disease, right elbow CC HCC

MØ2.322 Reiter's disease, left elbow CC HCC

M02.329 Reiter's disease, unspecified elbow CC UNS HCC

M02.33 Reiter's disease, wrist
Reiter's disease, carpal bones
M02.331 Reiter's disease, right wrist CC HCC
M02.332 Reiter's disease, left wrist CC HCC
M02.339 Reiter's disease, unspecified wrist CC UNS HCC

M02.34 Reiter's disease, hand
Reiter's disease, metacarpus and phalanges
M02.341 Reiter's disease, right hand CC HCC
M02.342 Reiter's disease, left hand CC HCC
M02.349 Reiter's disease, unspecified hand CC UNS HCC

M02.35 Reiter's disease, hip
M02.351 Reiter's disease, right hip CC HCC
M02.352 Reiter's disease, left hip CC HCC
M02.359 Reiter's disease, unspecified hip CC UNS HCC

M02.36 Reiter's disease, knee
M02.361 Reiter's disease, right knee CC HCC
M02.362 Reiter's disease, left knee CC HCC
M02.369 Reiter's disease, unspecified knee CC UNS HCC

M02.37 Reiter's disease, ankle and foot
Reiter's disease, tarsus, metatarsus and phalanges
M02.371 Reiter's disease, right ankle and foot CC HCC
M02.372 Reiter's disease, left ankle and foot CC HCC
M02.379 Reiter's disease, unspecified ankle and foot CC UNS HCC

M02.38 Reiter's disease, vertebrae CC HCC
M02.39 Reiter's disease, multiple sites CC HCC

M02.8 Other reactive arthropathies
M02.80 Other reactive arthropathies, unspecified site CC UNS HCC

M02.81 Other reactive arthropathies, shoulder
M02.811 Other reactive arthropathies, right shoulder CC HCC
M02.812 Other reactive arthropathies, left shoulder CC HCC
M02.819 Other reactive arthropathies, unspecified shoulder CC UNS HCC

M02.82 Other reactive arthropathies, elbow
M02.821 Other reactive arthropathies, right elbow CC HCC
M02.822 Other reactive arthropathies, left elbow CC HCC
M02.829 Other reactive arthropathies, unspecified elbow CC UNS HCC

M02.83 Other reactive arthropathies, wrist
Other reactive arthropathies, carpal bones
M02.831 Other reactive arthropathies, right wrist CC HCC
M02.832 Other reactive arthropathies, left wrist CC HCC
M02.839 Other reactive arthropathies, unspecified wrist CC UNS HCC

M02.84 Other reactive arthropathies, hand
Other reactive arthropathies, metacarpus and phalanges
M02.841 Other reactive arthropathies, right hand CC HCC
M02.842 Other reactive arthropathies, left hand CC HCC
M02.849 Other reactive arthropathies, unspecified hand CC UNS HCC

M02.85 Other reactive arthropathies, hip
M02.851 Other reactive arthropathies, right hip CC HCC
M02.852 Other reactive arthropathies, left hip CC HCC
M02.859 Other reactive arthropathies, unspecified hip CC UNS HCC

M02.86 Other reactive arthropathies, knee
M02.861 Other reactive arthropathies, right knee CC HCC
M02.862 Other reactive arthropathies, left knee CC HCC
M02.869 Other reactive arthropathies, unspecified knee CC UNS HCC

M02.87 Other reactive arthropathies, ankle and foot
Other reactive arthropathies, tarsus, metatarsus and phalanges
M02.871 Other reactive arthropathies, right ankle and foot CC HCC
M02.872 Other reactive arthropathies, left ankle and foot CC HCC
M02.879 Other reactive arthropathies, unspecified ankle and foot CC UNS HCC

M02.88 Other reactive arthropathies, vertebrae CC HCC
M02.89 Other reactive arthropathies, multiple sites CC HCC

M02.9 Reactive arthropathy, unspecified HCC

Autoinflammatory syndromes (M04)

M04 Autoinflammatory syndromes
EXCLUDES 2 *Crohn's disease (K50.-)*
AHA: 2016,4Q,37

M04.1 Periodic fever syndromes HCC
Familial Mediterranean fever
Hyperimmunoglobin D syndrome
Mevalonate kinase deficiency
Tumor necrosis factor receptor associated periodic syndrome [TRAPS]

M04.2 Cryopyrin-associated periodic syndromes HCC
Chronic infantile neurological, cutaneous and articular syndrome [CINCA]
Familial cold autoinflammatory syndrome
Familial cold urticaria
Muckle-Wells syndrome
Neonatal onset multisystemic inflammatory disorder [NOMID]

M04.8 Other autoinflammatory syndromes HCC
Blau syndrome
Deficiency of interleukin 1 receptor antagonist [DIRA]
Majeed syndrome
Periodic fever, aphthous stomatitis, pharyngitis, and adenopathy syndrome [PFAPA]
Pyogenic arthritis, pyoderma gangrenosum, and acne syndrome [PAPA]

M04.9 Autoinflammatory syndrome, unspecified HCC

Inflammatory polyarthropathies (M05-M14)

M05 Rheumatoid arthritis with rheumatoid factor
EXCLUDES 1 *rheumatic fever (I00)*
juvenile rheumatoid arthritis (M08.-)
rheumatoid arthritis of spine (M45.-)
AHA: 2020,4Q,31-32
DEF: Rheumatoid arthritis: Autoimmune systemic disease that causes chronic inflammation of the joints and other areas of the body, manifested by inflammatory changes in articular structures and synovial membranes, atrophy, and loss in bone density.

M05.0 Felty's syndrome
Rheumatoid arthritis with splenoadenomegaly and leukopenia
M05.00 Felty's syndrome, unspecified site HCC

M05.01 Felty's syndrome, shoulder
M05.011 Felty's syndrome, right shoulder HCC
M05.012 Felty's syndrome, left shoulder HCC
M05.019 Felty's syndrome, unspecified shoulder HCC

M05.02 Felty's syndrome, elbow
M05.021 Felty's syndrome, right elbow HCC
M05.022 Felty's syndrome, left elbow HCC
M05.029 Felty's syndrome, unspecified elbow HCC

M05.03 Felty's syndrome, wrist
Felty's syndrome, carpal bones
M05.031 Felty's syndrome, right wrist HCC
M05.032 Felty's syndrome, left wrist HCC

MØ5.Ø39 Felty's syndrome, unspecified wrist HCC
MØ5.Ø4 Felty's syndrome, hand
Felty's syndrome, metacarpus and phalanges
MØ5.Ø41 Felty's syndrome, right hand HCC
MØ5.Ø42 Felty's syndrome, left hand HCC
MØ5.Ø49 Felty's syndrome, unspecified hand HCC
MØ5.Ø5 Felty's syndrome, hip
MØ5.Ø51 Felty's syndrome, right hip HCC
MØ5.Ø52 Felty's syndrome, left hip HCC
MØ5.Ø59 Felty's syndrome, unspecified hip HCC
MØ5.Ø6 Felty's syndrome, knee
MØ5.Ø61 Felty's syndrome, right knee HCC
MØ5.Ø62 Felty's syndrome, left knee HCC
MØ5.Ø69 Felty's syndrome, unspecified knee HCC
MØ5.Ø7 Felty's syndrome, ankle and foot
Felty's syndrome, tarsus, metatarsus and phalanges
MØ5.Ø71 Felty's syndrome, right ankle and foot HCC
MØ5.Ø72 Felty's syndrome, left ankle and foot HCC
MØ5.Ø79 Felty's syndrome, unspecified ankle and foot HCC
MØ5.Ø9 Felty's syndrome, multiple sites HCC
MØ5.1 Rheumatoid lung disease with rheumatoid arthritis
MØ5.1Ø Rheumatoid lung disease with rheumatoid arthritis of unspecified site HCC
MØ5.11 Rheumatoid lung disease with rheumatoid arthritis of shoulder
MØ5.111 Rheumatoid lung disease with rheumatoid arthritis of right shoulder HCC
MØ5.112 Rheumatoid lung disease with rheumatoid arthritis of left shoulder HCC
MØ5.119 Rheumatoid lung disease with rheumatoid arthritis of unspecified shoulder HCC
MØ5.12 Rheumatoid lung disease with rheumatoid arthritis of elbow
MØ5.121 Rheumatoid lung disease with rheumatoid arthritis of right elbow HCC
MØ5.122 Rheumatoid lung disease with rheumatoid arthritis of left elbow HCC
MØ5.129 Rheumatoid lung disease with rheumatoid arthritis of unspecified elbow HCC
MØ5.13 Rheumatoid lung disease with rheumatoid arthritis of wrist
Rheumatoid lung disease with rheumatoid arthritis, carpal bones
MØ5.131 Rheumatoid lung disease with rheumatoid arthritis of right wrist HCC
MØ5.132 Rheumatoid lung disease with rheumatoid arthritis of left wrist HCC
MØ5.139 Rheumatoid lung disease with rheumatoid arthritis of unspecified wrist HCC
MØ5.14 Rheumatoid lung disease with rheumatoid arthritis of hand
Rheumatoid lung disease with rheumatoid arthritis, metacarpus and phalanges
MØ5.141 Rheumatoid lung disease with rheumatoid arthritis of right hand HCC
MØ5.142 Rheumatoid lung disease with rheumatoid arthritis of left hand HCC
MØ5.149 Rheumatoid lung disease with rheumatoid arthritis of unspecified hand HCC
MØ5.15 Rheumatoid lung disease with rheumatoid arthritis of hip
MØ5.151 Rheumatoid lung disease with rheumatoid arthritis of right hip HCC
MØ5.152 Rheumatoid lung disease with rheumatoid arthritis of left hip HCC
MØ5.159 Rheumatoid lung disease with rheumatoid arthritis of unspecified hip HCC
MØ5.16 Rheumatoid lung disease with rheumatoid arthritis of knee
MØ5.161 Rheumatoid lung disease with rheumatoid arthritis of right knee HCC
MØ5.162 Rheumatoid lung disease with rheumatoid arthritis of left knee HCC
MØ5.169 Rheumatoid lung disease with rheumatoid arthritis of unspecified knee HCC
MØ5.17 Rheumatoid lung disease with rheumatoid arthritis of ankle and foot
Rheumatoid lung disease with rheumatoid arthritis, tarsus, metatarsus and phalanges
MØ5.171 Rheumatoid lung disease with rheumatoid arthritis of right ankle and foot HCC
MØ5.172 Rheumatoid lung disease with rheumatoid arthritis of left ankle and foot HCC
MØ5.179 Rheumatoid lung disease with rheumatoid arthritis of unspecified ankle and foot HCC
MØ5.19 Rheumatoid lung disease with rheumatoid arthritis of multiple sites HCC
MØ5.2 Rheumatoid vasculitis with rheumatoid arthritis
MØ5.2Ø Rheumatoid vasculitis with rheumatoid arthritis of unspecified site HCC
MØ5.21 Rheumatoid vasculitis with rheumatoid arthritis of shoulder
MØ5.211 Rheumatoid vasculitis with rheumatoid arthritis of right shoulder HCC
MØ5.212 Rheumatoid vasculitis with rheumatoid arthritis of left shoulder HCC
MØ5.219 Rheumatoid vasculitis with rheumatoid arthritis of unspecified shoulder HCC
MØ5.22 Rheumatoid vasculitis with rheumatoid arthritis of elbow
MØ5.221 Rheumatoid vasculitis with rheumatoid arthritis of right elbow HCC
MØ5.222 Rheumatoid vasculitis with rheumatoid arthritis of left elbow HCC
MØ5.229 Rheumatoid vasculitis with rheumatoid arthritis of unspecified elbow HCC
MØ5.23 Rheumatoid vasculitis with rheumatoid arthritis of wrist
Rheumatoid vasculitis with rheumatoid arthritis, carpal bones
MØ5.231 Rheumatoid vasculitis with rheumatoid arthritis of right wrist HCC
MØ5.232 Rheumatoid vasculitis with rheumatoid arthritis of left wrist HCC
MØ5.239 Rheumatoid vasculitis with rheumatoid arthritis of unspecified wrist HCC
MØ5.24 Rheumatoid vasculitis with rheumatoid arthritis of hand
Rheumatoid vasculitis with rheumatoid arthritis, metacarpus and phalanges
MØ5.241 Rheumatoid vasculitis with rheumatoid arthritis of right hand HCC
MØ5.242 Rheumatoid vasculitis with rheumatoid arthritis of left hand HCC
MØ5.249 Rheumatoid vasculitis with rheumatoid arthritis of unspecified hand HCC
MØ5.25 Rheumatoid vasculitis with rheumatoid arthritis of hip
MØ5.251 Rheumatoid vasculitis with rheumatoid arthritis of right hip HCC
MØ5.252 Rheumatoid vasculitis with rheumatoid arthritis of left hip HCC
MØ5.259 Rheumatoid vasculitis with rheumatoid arthritis of unspecified hip HCC
MØ5.26 Rheumatoid vasculitis with rheumatoid arthritis of knee
MØ5.261 Rheumatoid vasculitis with rheumatoid arthritis of right knee HCC
MØ5.262 Rheumatoid vasculitis with rheumatoid arthritis of left knee HCC

M05.269 Rheumatoid vasculitis with rheumatoid arthritis of unspecified knee HCC

M05.27 Rheumatoid vasculitis with rheumatoid arthritis of ankle and foot
Rheumatoid vasculitis with rheumatoid arthritis, tarsus, metatarsus and phalanges

M05.271 Rheumatoid vasculitis with rheumatoid arthritis of right ankle and foot HCC

M05.272 Rheumatoid vasculitis with rheumatoid arthritis of left ankle and foot HCC

M05.279 Rheumatoid vasculitis with rheumatoid arthritis of unspecified ankle and foot HCC

M05.29 Rheumatoid vasculitis with rheumatoid arthritis of multiple sites HCC

M05.3 Rheumatoid heart disease with rheumatoid arthritis
Rheumatoid carditis
Rheumatoid endocarditis
Rheumatoid myocarditis
Rheumatoid pericarditis

M05.30 Rheumatoid heart disease with rheumatoid arthritis of unspecified site HCC

M05.31 Rheumatoid heart disease with rheumatoid arthritis of shoulder

M05.311 Rheumatoid heart disease with rheumatoid arthritis of right shoulder HCC

M05.312 Rheumatoid heart disease with rheumatoid arthritis of left shoulder HCC

M05.319 Rheumatoid heart disease with rheumatoid arthritis of unspecified shoulder HCC

M05.32 Rheumatoid heart disease with rheumatoid arthritis of elbow

M05.321 Rheumatoid heart disease with rheumatoid arthritis of right elbow HCC

M05.322 Rheumatoid heart disease with rheumatoid arthritis of left elbow HCC

M05.329 Rheumatoid heart disease with rheumatoid arthritis of unspecified elbow HCC

M05.33 Rheumatoid heart disease with rheumatoid arthritis of wrist
Rheumatoid heart disease with rheumatoid arthritis, carpal bones

M05.331 Rheumatoid heart disease with rheumatoid arthritis of right wrist HCC

M05.332 Rheumatoid heart disease with rheumatoid arthritis of left wrist HCC

M05.339 Rheumatoid heart disease with rheumatoid arthritis of unspecified wrist HCC

M05.34 Rheumatoid heart disease with rheumatoid arthritis of hand
Rheumatoid heart disease with rheumatoid arthritis, metacarpus and phalanges

M05.341 Rheumatoid heart disease with rheumatoid arthritis of right hand HCC

M05.342 Rheumatoid heart disease with rheumatoid arthritis of left hand HCC

M05.349 Rheumatoid heart disease with rheumatoid arthritis of unspecified hand HCC

M05.35 Rheumatoid heart disease with rheumatoid arthritis of hip

M05.351 Rheumatoid heart disease with rheumatoid arthritis of right hip HCC

M05.352 Rheumatoid heart disease with rheumatoid arthritis of left hip HCC

M05.359 Rheumatoid heart disease with rheumatoid arthritis of unspecified hip HCC

M05.36 Rheumatoid heart disease with rheumatoid arthritis of knee

M05.361 Rheumatoid heart disease with rheumatoid arthritis of right knee HCC

M05.362 Rheumatoid heart disease with rheumatoid arthritis of left knee HCC

M05.369 Rheumatoid heart disease with rheumatoid arthritis of unspecified knee HCC

M05.37 Rheumatoid heart disease with rheumatoid arthritis of ankle and foot
Rheumatoid heart disease with rheumatoid arthritis, tarsus, metatarsus and phalanges

M05.371 Rheumatoid heart disease with rheumatoid arthritis of right ankle and foot HCC

M05.372 Rheumatoid heart disease with rheumatoid arthritis of left ankle and foot HCC

M05.379 Rheumatoid heart disease with rheumatoid arthritis of unspecified ankle and foot HCC

M05.39 Rheumatoid heart disease with rheumatoid arthritis of multiple sites HCC

M05.4 Rheumatoid myopathy with rheumatoid arthritis

M05.40 Rheumatoid myopathy with rheumatoid arthritis of unspecified site CC UNS HCC

M05.41 Rheumatoid myopathy with rheumatoid arthritis of shoulder

M05.411 Rheumatoid myopathy with rheumatoid arthritis of right shoulder CC HCC

M05.412 Rheumatoid myopathy with rheumatoid arthritis of left shoulder CC HCC

M05.419 Rheumatoid myopathy with rheumatoid arthritis of unspecified shoulder CC UNS HCC

M05.42 Rheumatoid myopathy with rheumatoid arthritis of elbow

M05.421 Rheumatoid myopathy with rheumatoid arthritis of right elbow CC HCC

M05.422 Rheumatoid myopathy with rheumatoid arthritis of left elbow CC HCC

M05.429 Rheumatoid myopathy with rheumatoid arthritis of unspecified elbow CC UNS HCC

M05.43 Rheumatoid myopathy with rheumatoid arthritis of wrist
Rheumatoid myopathy with rheumatoid arthritis, carpal bones

M05.431 Rheumatoid myopathy with rheumatoid arthritis of right wrist CC HCC

M05.432 Rheumatoid myopathy with rheumatoid arthritis of left wrist CC HCC

M05.439 Rheumatoid myopathy with rheumatoid arthritis of unspecified wrist CC UNS HCC

M05.44 Rheumatoid myopathy with rheumatoid arthritis of hand
Rheumatoid myopathy with rheumatoid arthritis, metacarpus and phalanges

M05.441 Rheumatoid myopathy with rheumatoid arthritis of right hand CC HCC

M05.442 Rheumatoid myopathy with rheumatoid arthritis of left hand CC HCC

M05.449 Rheumatoid myopathy with rheumatoid arthritis of unspecified hand CC UNS HCC

M05.45 Rheumatoid myopathy with rheumatoid arthritis of hip

M05.451 Rheumatoid myopathy with rheumatoid arthritis of right hip CC HCC

M05.452 Rheumatoid myopathy with rheumatoid arthritis of left hip CC HCC

M05.459 Rheumatoid myopathy with rheumatoid arthritis of unspecified hip CC UNS HCC

M05.46 Rheumatoid myopathy with rheumatoid arthritis of knee

M05.461 Rheumatoid myopathy with rheumatoid arthritis of right knee CC HCC

M05.462 Rheumatoid myopathy with rheumatoid arthritis of left knee CC HCC

M05.469 Rheumatoid myopathy with rheumatoid arthritis of unspecified knee CC UNS HCC

MØ5.47 Rheumatoid myopathy with rheumatoid arthritis of ankle and foot
Rheumatoid myopathy with rheumatoid arthritis, tarsus, metatarsus and phalanges
MØ5.471 Rheumatoid myopathy with rheumatoid arthritis of right ankle and foot CC HCC
MØ5.472 Rheumatoid myopathy with rheumatoid arthritis of left ankle and foot CC HCC
MØ5.479 Rheumatoid myopathy with rheumatoid arthritis of unspecified ankle and foot CC UNS HCC
MØ5.49 Rheumatoid myopathy with rheumatoid arthritis of multiple sites CC HCC

MØ5.5 Rheumatoid polyneuropathy with rheumatoid arthritis
MØ5.50 Rheumatoid polyneuropathy with rheumatoid arthritis of unspecified site HCC
MØ5.51 Rheumatoid polyneuropathy with rheumatoid arthritis of shoulder
MØ5.511 Rheumatoid polyneuropathy with rheumatoid arthritis of right shoulder HCC
MØ5.512 Rheumatoid polyneuropathy with rheumatoid arthritis of left shoulder HCC
MØ5.519 Rheumatoid polyneuropathy with rheumatoid arthritis of unspecified shoulder HCC
MØ5.52 Rheumatoid polyneuropathy with rheumatoid arthritis of elbow
MØ5.521 Rheumatoid polyneuropathy with rheumatoid arthritis of right elbow HCC
MØ5.522 Rheumatoid polyneuropathy with rheumatoid arthritis of left elbow HCC
MØ5.529 Rheumatoid polyneuropathy with rheumatoid arthritis of unspecified elbow HCC
MØ5.53 Rheumatoid polyneuropathy with rheumatoid arthritis of wrist
Rheumatoid polyneuropathy with rheumatoid arthritis, carpal bones
MØ5.531 Rheumatoid polyneuropathy with rheumatoid arthritis of right wrist HCC
MØ5.532 Rheumatoid polyneuropathy with rheumatoid arthritis of left wrist HCC
MØ5.539 Rheumatoid polyneuropathy with rheumatoid arthritis of unspecified wrist HCC
MØ5.54 Rheumatoid polyneuropathy with rheumatoid arthritis of hand
Rheumatoid polyneuropathy with rheumatoid arthritis, metacarpus and phalanges
MØ5.541 Rheumatoid polyneuropathy with rheumatoid arthritis of right hand HCC
MØ5.542 Rheumatoid polyneuropathy with rheumatoid arthritis of left hand HCC
MØ5.549 Rheumatoid polyneuropathy with rheumatoid arthritis of unspecified hand HCC
MØ5.55 Rheumatoid polyneuropathy with rheumatoid arthritis of hip
MØ5.551 Rheumatoid polyneuropathy with rheumatoid arthritis of right hip HCC
MØ5.552 Rheumatoid polyneuropathy with rheumatoid arthritis of left hip HCC
MØ5.559 Rheumatoid polyneuropathy with rheumatoid arthritis of unspecified hip HCC
MØ5.56 Rheumatoid polyneuropathy with rheumatoid arthritis of knee
MØ5.561 Rheumatoid polyneuropathy with rheumatoid arthritis of right knee HCC
MØ5.562 Rheumatoid polyneuropathy with rheumatoid arthritis of left knee HCC
MØ5.569 Rheumatoid polyneuropathy with rheumatoid arthritis of unspecified knee HCC
MØ5.57 Rheumatoid polyneuropathy with rheumatoid arthritis of ankle and foot
Rheumatoid polyneuropathy with rheumatoid arthritis, tarsus, metatarsus and phalanges
MØ5.571 Rheumatoid polyneuropathy with rheumatoid arthritis of right ankle and foot HCC
MØ5.572 Rheumatoid polyneuropathy with rheumatoid arthritis of left ankle and foot HCC
MØ5.579 Rheumatoid polyneuropathy with rheumatoid arthritis of unspecified ankle and foot HCC
MØ5.59 Rheumatoid polyneuropathy with rheumatoid arthritis of multiple sites HCC

MØ5.6 Rheumatoid arthritis with involvement of other organs and systems
MØ5.60 Rheumatoid arthritis of unspecified site with involvement of other organs and systems HCC
MØ5.61 Rheumatoid arthritis of shoulder with involvement of other organs and systems
MØ5.611 Rheumatoid arthritis of right shoulder with involvement of other organs and systems HCC
MØ5.612 Rheumatoid arthritis of left shoulder with involvement of other organs and systems HCC
MØ5.619 Rheumatoid arthritis of unspecified shoulder with involvement of other organs and systems HCC
MØ5.62 Rheumatoid arthritis of elbow with involvement of other organs and systems
MØ5.621 Rheumatoid arthritis of right elbow with involvement of other organs and systems HCC
MØ5.622 Rheumatoid arthritis of left elbow with involvement of other organs and systems HCC
MØ5.629 Rheumatoid arthritis of unspecified elbow with involvement of other organs and systems HCC
MØ5.63 Rheumatoid arthritis of wrist with involvement of other organs and systems
Rheumatoid arthritis of carpal bones with involvement of other organs and systems
MØ5.631 Rheumatoid arthritis of right wrist with involvement of other organs and systems HCC
MØ5.632 Rheumatoid arthritis of left wrist with involvement of other organs and systems HCC
MØ5.639 Rheumatoid arthritis of unspecified wrist with involvement of other organs and systems HCC
MØ5.64 Rheumatoid arthritis of hand with involvement of other organs and systems
Rheumatoid arthritis of metacarpus and phalanges with involvement of other organs and systems
MØ5.641 Rheumatoid arthritis of right hand with involvement of other organs and systems HCC
MØ5.642 Rheumatoid arthritis of left hand with involvement of other organs and systems HCC
MØ5.649 Rheumatoid arthritis of unspecified hand with involvement of other organs and systems HCC
MØ5.65 Rheumatoid arthritis of hip with involvement of other organs and systems
MØ5.651 Rheumatoid arthritis of right hip with involvement of other organs and systems HCC
MØ5.652 Rheumatoid arthritis of left hip with involvement of other organs and systems HCC
MØ5.659 Rheumatoid arthritis of unspecified hip with involvement of other organs and systems HCC
MØ5.66 Rheumatoid arthritis of knee with involvement of other organs and systems
MØ5.661 Rheumatoid arthritis of right knee with involvement of other organs and systems HCC

M05.662 Rheumatoid arthritis of left knee with involvement of other organs and systems HCC

M05.669 Rheumatoid arthritis of unspecified knee with involvement of other organs and systems HCC

6th M05.67 Rheumatoid arthritis of ankle and foot with involvement of other organs and systems

Rheumatoid arthritis of tarsus, metatarsus and phalanges with involvement of other organs and systems

M05.671 Rheumatoid arthritis of right ankle and foot with involvement of other organs and systems HCC

M05.672 Rheumatoid arthritis of left ankle and foot with involvement of other organs and systems HCC

M05.679 Rheumatoid arthritis of unspecified ankle and foot with involvement of other organs and systems HCC

M05.69 Rheumatoid arthritis of multiple sites with involvement of other organs and systems HCC

5th M05.7 Rheumatoid arthritis with rheumatoid factor without organ or systems involvement

M05.70 Rheumatoid arthritis with rheumatoid factor of unspecified site without organ or systems involvement HCC

6th M05.71 Rheumatoid arthritis with rheumatoid factor of shoulder without organ or systems involvement

M05.711 Rheumatoid arthritis with rheumatoid factor of right shoulder without organ or systems involvement HCC

M05.712 Rheumatoid arthritis with rheumatoid factor of left shoulder without organ or systems involvement HCC

M05.719 Rheumatoid arthritis with rheumatoid factor of unspecified shoulder without organ or systems involvement HCC

6th M05.72 Rheumatoid arthritis with rheumatoid factor of elbow without organ or systems involvement

M05.721 Rheumatoid arthritis with rheumatoid factor of right elbow without organ or systems involvement HCC

M05.722 Rheumatoid arthritis with rheumatoid factor of left elbow without organ or systems involvement HCC

M05.729 Rheumatoid arthritis with rheumatoid factor of unspecified elbow without organ or systems involvement HCC

6th M05.73 Rheumatoid arthritis with rheumatoid factor of wrist without organ or systems involvement

M05.731 Rheumatoid arthritis with rheumatoid factor of right wrist without organ or systems involvement HCC

M05.732 Rheumatoid arthritis with rheumatoid factor of left wrist without organ or systems involvement HCC

M05.739 Rheumatoid arthritis with rheumatoid factor of unspecified wrist without organ or systems involvement HCC

6th M05.74 Rheumatoid arthritis with rheumatoid factor of hand without organ or systems involvement

M05.741 Rheumatoid arthritis with rheumatoid factor of right hand without organ or systems involvement HCC

M05.742 Rheumatoid arthritis with rheumatoid factor of left hand without organ or systems involvement HCC

M05.749 Rheumatoid arthritis with rheumatoid factor of unspecified hand without organ or systems involvement HCC

6th M05.75 Rheumatoid arthritis with rheumatoid factor of hip without organ or systems involvement

M05.751 Rheumatoid arthritis with rheumatoid factor of right hip without organ or systems involvement HCC

M05.752 Rheumatoid arthritis with rheumatoid factor of left hip without organ or systems involvement HCC

M05.759 Rheumatoid arthritis with rheumatoid factor of unspecified hip without organ or systems involvement HCC

6th M05.76 Rheumatoid arthritis with rheumatoid factor of knee without organ or systems involvement

M05.761 Rheumatoid arthritis with rheumatoid factor of right knee without organ or systems involvement HCC

M05.762 Rheumatoid arthritis with rheumatoid factor of left knee without organ or systems involvement HCC

M05.769 Rheumatoid arthritis with rheumatoid factor of unspecified knee without organ or systems involvement HCC

6th M05.77 Rheumatoid arthritis with rheumatoid factor of ankle and foot without organ or systems involvement

M05.771 Rheumatoid arthritis with rheumatoid factor of right ankle and foot without organ or systems involvement HCC

M05.772 Rheumatoid arthritis with rheumatoid factor of left ankle and foot without organ or systems involvement HCC

M05.779 Rheumatoid arthritis with rheumatoid factor of unspecified ankle and foot without organ or systems involvement HCC

M05.79 Rheumatoid arthritis with rheumatoid factor of multiple sites without organ or systems involvement HCC

M05.7A Rheumatoid arthritis with rheumatoid factor of other specified site without organ or systems involvement HCC

5th M05.8 Other rheumatoid arthritis with rheumatoid factor

M05.80 Other rheumatoid arthritis with rheumatoid factor of unspecified site HCC

6th M05.81 Other rheumatoid arthritis with rheumatoid factor of shoulder

M05.811 Other rheumatoid arthritis with rheumatoid factor of right shoulder HCC

M05.812 Other rheumatoid arthritis with rheumatoid factor of left shoulder HCC

M05.819 Other rheumatoid arthritis with rheumatoid factor of unspecified shoulder HCC

6th M05.82 Other rheumatoid arthritis with rheumatoid factor of elbow

M05.821 Other rheumatoid arthritis with rheumatoid factor of right elbow HCC

M05.822 Other rheumatoid arthritis with rheumatoid factor of left elbow HCC

M05.829 Other rheumatoid arthritis with rheumatoid factor of unspecified elbow HCC

6th M05.83 Other rheumatoid arthritis with rheumatoid factor of wrist

M05.831 Other rheumatoid arthritis with rheumatoid factor of right wrist HCC

M05.832 Other rheumatoid arthritis with rheumatoid factor of left wrist HCC

M05.839 Other rheumatoid arthritis with rheumatoid factor of unspecified wrist HCC

6th M05.84 Other rheumatoid arthritis with rheumatoid factor of hand

M05.841 Other rheumatoid arthritis with rheumatoid factor of right hand HCC

M05.842 Other rheumatoid arthritis with rheumatoid factor of left hand HCC

M05.849 Other rheumatoid arthritis with rheumatoid factor of unspecified hand HCC

6th M05.85 Other rheumatoid arthritis with rheumatoid factor of hip

M05.851 Other rheumatoid arthritis with rheumatoid factor of right hip HCC

M05.852 Other rheumatoid arthritis with rheumatoid factor of left hip HCC

M05.859 Other rheumatoid arthritis with rheumatoid factor of unspecified hip HCC

M05.86 Other rheumatoid arthritis with rheumatoid factor of knee
- **M05.861 Other rheumatoid arthritis with rheumatoid factor of right knee** HCC
- **M05.862 Other rheumatoid arthritis with rheumatoid factor of left knee** HCC
- **M05.869 Other rheumatoid arthritis with rheumatoid factor of unspecified knee** HCC

M05.87 Other rheumatoid arthritis with rheumatoid factor of ankle and foot
- **M05.871 Other rheumatoid arthritis with rheumatoid factor of right ankle and foot** HCC
- **M05.872 Other rheumatoid arthritis with rheumatoid factor of left ankle and foot** HCC
- **M05.879 Other rheumatoid arthritis with rheumatoid factor of unspecified ankle and foot** HCC

M05.89 Other rheumatoid arthritis with rheumatoid factor of multiple sites HCC

M05.8A Other rheumatoid arthritis with rheumatoid factor of other specified site HCC

M05.9 Rheumatoid arthritis with rheumatoid factor, unspecified HCC

M06 Other rheumatoid arthritis

AHA: 2020,4Q,31-32

DEF: Rheumatoid arthritis: Autoimmune systemic disease that causes chronic inflammation of the joints and other areas of the body, manifested by inflammatory changes in articular structures and synovial membranes, atrophy, and loss in bone density.

M06.0 Rheumatoid arthritis without rheumatoid factor

M06.00 Rheumatoid arthritis without rheumatoid factor, unspecified site HCC

M06.01 Rheumatoid arthritis without rheumatoid factor, shoulder
- **M06.011 Rheumatoid arthritis without rheumatoid factor, right shoulder** HCC
- **M06.012 Rheumatoid arthritis without rheumatoid factor, left shoulder** HCC
- **M06.019 Rheumatoid arthritis without rheumatoid factor, unspecified shoulder** HCC

M06.02 Rheumatoid arthritis without rheumatoid factor, elbow
- **M06.021 Rheumatoid arthritis without rheumatoid factor, right elbow** HCC
- **M06.022 Rheumatoid arthritis without rheumatoid factor, left elbow** HCC
- **M06.029 Rheumatoid arthritis without rheumatoid factor, unspecified elbow** HCC

M06.03 Rheumatoid arthritis without rheumatoid factor, wrist
- **M06.031 Rheumatoid arthritis without rheumatoid factor, right wrist** HCC
- **M06.032 Rheumatoid arthritis without rheumatoid factor, left wrist** HCC
- **M06.039 Rheumatoid arthritis without rheumatoid factor, unspecified wrist** HCC

M06.04 Rheumatoid arthritis without rheumatoid factor, hand
- **M06.041 Rheumatoid arthritis without rheumatoid factor, right hand** HCC
- **M06.042 Rheumatoid arthritis without rheumatoid factor, left hand** HCC
- **M06.049 Rheumatoid arthritis without rheumatoid factor, unspecified hand** HCC

M06.05 Rheumatoid arthritis without rheumatoid factor, hip
- **M06.051 Rheumatoid arthritis without rheumatoid factor, right hip** HCC
- **M06.052 Rheumatoid arthritis without rheumatoid factor, left hip** HCC
- **M06.059 Rheumatoid arthritis without rheumatoid factor, unspecified hip** HCC

M06.06 Rheumatoid arthritis without rheumatoid factor, knee
- **M06.061 Rheumatoid arthritis without rheumatoid factor, right knee** HCC
- **M06.062 Rheumatoid arthritis without rheumatoid factor, left knee** HCC
- **M06.069 Rheumatoid arthritis without rheumatoid factor, unspecified knee** HCC

M06.07 Rheumatoid arthritis without rheumatoid factor, ankle and foot
- **M06.071 Rheumatoid arthritis without rheumatoid factor, right ankle and foot** HCC
- **M06.072 Rheumatoid arthritis without rheumatoid factor, left ankle and foot** HCC
- **M06.079 Rheumatoid arthritis without rheumatoid factor, unspecified ankle and foot** HCC

M06.08 Rheumatoid arthritis without rheumatoid factor, vertebrae HCC

M06.09 Rheumatoid arthritis without rheumatoid factor, multiple sites HCC

M06.0A Rheumatoid arthritis without rheumatoid factor, other specified site HCC

M06.1 Adult-onset Still's disease HCC A

EXCLUDES 1 *Still's disease NOS (M08.2-)*

DEF: Type of systemic arthritis characterized by a transient rash and spiking fevers. This condition may resolve or develop into a chronic condition and may affect internal organs, as well as joints.

Synonym(s): *AOSD*

M06.2 Rheumatoid bursitis

M06.20 Rheumatoid bursitis, unspecified site HCC

M06.21 Rheumatoid bursitis, shoulder
- **M06.211 Rheumatoid bursitis, right shoulder** HCC
- **M06.212 Rheumatoid bursitis, left shoulder** HCC
- **M06.219 Rheumatoid bursitis, unspecified shoulder** HCC

M06.22 Rheumatoid bursitis, elbow
- **M06.221 Rheumatoid bursitis, right elbow** HCC
- **M06.222 Rheumatoid bursitis, left elbow** HCC
- **M06.229 Rheumatoid bursitis, unspecified elbow** HCC

M06.23 Rheumatoid bursitis, wrist
- **M06.231 Rheumatoid bursitis, right wrist** HCC
- **M06.232 Rheumatoid bursitis, left wrist** HCC
- **M06.239 Rheumatoid bursitis, unspecified wrist** HCC

M06.24 Rheumatoid bursitis, hand
- **M06.241 Rheumatoid bursitis, right hand** HCC
- **M06.242 Rheumatoid bursitis, left hand** HCC
- **M06.249 Rheumatoid bursitis, unspecified hand** HCC

M06.25 Rheumatoid bursitis, hip
- **M06.251 Rheumatoid bursitis, right hip** HCC
- **M06.252 Rheumatoid bursitis, left hip** HCC
- **M06.259 Rheumatoid bursitis, unspecified hip** HCC

M06.26 Rheumatoid bursitis, knee
- **M06.261 Rheumatoid bursitis, right knee** HCC
- **M06.262 Rheumatoid bursitis, left knee** HCC
- **M06.269 Rheumatoid bursitis, unspecified knee** HCC

M06.27 Rheumatoid bursitis, ankle and foot
- **M06.271 Rheumatoid bursitis, right ankle and foot** HCC
- **M06.272 Rheumatoid bursitis, left ankle and foot** HCC
- **M06.279 Rheumatoid bursitis, unspecified ankle and foot** HCC

M06.28 Rheumatoid bursitis, vertebrae HCC

M06.29 Rheumatoid bursitis, multiple sites HCC

M06.3 Rheumatoid nodule

M06.30 Rheumatoid nodule, unspecified site HCC

M06.31 Rheumatoid nodule, shoulder
- **M06.311 Rheumatoid nodule, right shoulder** HCC
- **M06.312 Rheumatoid nodule, left shoulder** HCC
- **M06.319 Rheumatoid nodule, unspecified shoulder** HCC

M06.32 Rheumatoid nodule, elbow
- **M06.321 Rheumatoid nodule, right elbow** HCC
- **M06.322 Rheumatoid nodule, left elbow** HCC

M06.329 Rheumatoid nodule, unspecified elbow HCC
M06.33 Rheumatoid nodule, wrist
M06.331 Rheumatoid nodule, right wrist HCC
M06.332 Rheumatoid nodule, left wrist HCC
M06.339 Rheumatoid nodule, unspecified wrist HCC
M06.34 Rheumatoid nodule, hand
M06.341 Rheumatoid nodule, right hand HCC
M06.342 Rheumatoid nodule, left hand HCC
M06.349 Rheumatoid nodule, unspecified hand HCC
M06.35 Rheumatoid nodule, hip
M06.351 Rheumatoid nodule, right hip HCC
M06.352 Rheumatoid nodule, left hip HCC
M06.359 Rheumatoid nodule, unspecified hip HCC
M06.36 Rheumatoid nodule, knee
M06.361 Rheumatoid nodule, right knee HCC
M06.362 Rheumatoid nodule, left knee HCC
M06.369 Rheumatoid nodule, unspecified knee HCC
M06.37 Rheumatoid nodule, ankle and foot
M06.371 Rheumatoid nodule, right ankle and foot HCC
M06.372 Rheumatoid nodule, left ankle and foot HCC
M06.379 Rheumatoid nodule, unspecified ankle and foot HCC
M06.38 Rheumatoid nodule, vertebrae HCC
M06.39 Rheumatoid nodule, multiple sites HCC
M06.4 Inflammatory polyarthropathy HCC

EXCLUDES 1 *polyarthritis NOS (M13.0)*

M06.8 Other specified rheumatoid arthritis
M06.80 Other specified rheumatoid arthritis, unspecified site HCC
M06.81 Other specified rheumatoid arthritis, shoulder
M06.811 Other specified rheumatoid arthritis, right shoulder HCC
M06.812 Other specified rheumatoid arthritis, left shoulder HCC
M06.819 Other specified rheumatoid arthritis, unspecified shoulder HCC
M06.82 Other specified rheumatoid arthritis, elbow
M06.821 Other specified rheumatoid arthritis, right elbow HCC
M06.822 Other specified rheumatoid arthritis, left elbow HCC
M06.829 Other specified rheumatoid arthritis, unspecified elbow HCC
M06.83 Other specified rheumatoid arthritis, wrist
M06.831 Other specified rheumatoid arthritis, right wrist HCC
M06.832 Other specified rheumatoid arthritis, left wrist HCC
M06.839 Other specified rheumatoid arthritis, unspecified wrist HCC
M06.84 Other specified rheumatoid arthritis, hand
M06.841 Other specified rheumatoid arthritis, right hand HCC
M06.842 Other specified rheumatoid arthritis, left hand HCC
M06.849 Other specified rheumatoid arthritis, unspecified hand HCC
M06.85 Other specified rheumatoid arthritis, hip
M06.851 Other specified rheumatoid arthritis, right hip HCC
M06.852 Other specified rheumatoid arthritis, left hip HCC
M06.859 Other specified rheumatoid arthritis, unspecified hip HCC
M06.86 Other specified rheumatoid arthritis, knee
M06.861 Other specified rheumatoid arthritis, right knee HCC
M06.862 Other specified rheumatoid arthritis, left knee HCC
M06.869 Other specified rheumatoid arthritis, unspecified knee HCC
M06.87 Other specified rheumatoid arthritis, ankle and foot
M06.871 Other specified rheumatoid arthritis, right ankle and foot HCC
M06.872 Other specified rheumatoid arthritis, left ankle and foot HCC
M06.879 Other specified rheumatoid arthritis, unspecified ankle and foot HCC
M06.88 Other specified rheumatoid arthritis, vertebrae HCC
M06.89 Other specified rheumatoid arthritis, multiple sites HCC
M06.8A Other specified rheumatoid arthritis, other specified site HCC
M06.9 Rheumatoid arthritis, unspecified HCC

M07 Enteropathic arthropathies

Code also associated enteropathy, such as:
regional enteritis [Crohn's disease] (K50.-)
ulcerative colitis (K51.-)

EXCLUDES 1 *psoriatic arthropathies (L40.5-)*

M07.6 Enteropathic arthropathies
M07.60 Enteropathic arthropathies, unspecified site
M07.61 Enteropathic arthropathies, shoulder
M07.611 Enteropathic arthropathies, right shoulder
M07.612 Enteropathic arthropathies, left shoulder
M07.619 Enteropathic arthropathies, unspecified shoulder
M07.62 Enteropathic arthropathies, elbow
M07.621 Enteropathic arthropathies, right elbow
M07.622 Enteropathic arthropathies, left elbow
M07.629 Enteropathic arthropathies, unspecified elbow
M07.63 Enteropathic arthropathies, wrist
M07.631 Enteropathic arthropathies, right wrist
M07.632 Enteropathic arthropathies, left wrist
M07.639 Enteropathic arthropathies, unspecified wrist
M07.64 Enteropathic arthropathies, hand
M07.641 Enteropathic arthropathies, right hand
M07.642 Enteropathic arthropathies, left hand
M07.649 Enteropathic arthropathies, unspecified hand
M07.65 Enteropathic arthropathies, hip
M07.651 Enteropathic arthropathies, right hip
M07.652 Enteropathic arthropathies, left hip
M07.659 Enteropathic arthropathies, unspecified hip
M07.66 Enteropathic arthropathies, knee
M07.661 Enteropathic arthropathies, right knee
M07.662 Enteropathic arthropathies, left knee
M07.669 Enteropathic arthropathies, unspecified knee
M07.67 Enteropathic arthropathies, ankle and foot
M07.671 Enteropathic arthropathies, right ankle and foot
M07.672 Enteropathic arthropathies, left ankle and foot
M07.679 Enteropathic arthropathies, unspecified ankle and foot
M07.68 Enteropathic arthropathies, vertebrae
M07.69 Enteropathic arthropathies, multiple sites

M08 Juvenile arthritis

Code also any associated underlying condition, such as:
regional enteritis [Crohn's disease] (K50.-)
ulcerative colitis (K51.-)

EXCLUDES 1 *arthropathy in Whipple's disease (M14.8)*
Felty's syndrome (M05.0)
juvenile dermatomyositis (M33.0-)
psoriatic juvenile arthropathy (L40.54)

AHA: 2020,4Q,31-32

M08.0 Unspecified juvenile rheumatoid arthritis
Juvenile rheumatoid arthritis with or without rheumatoid factor
M08.00 Unspecified juvenile rheumatoid arthritis of unspecified site HCC

✓6th **MØ8.Ø1 Unspecified juvenile rheumatoid arthritis, shoulder**
- **MØ8.Ø11 Unspecified juvenile rheumatoid arthritis, right shoulder** HCC
- **MØ8.Ø12 Unspecified juvenile rheumatoid arthritis, left shoulder** HCC
- **MØ8.Ø19 Unspecified juvenile rheumatoid arthritis, unspecified shoulder** HCC

✓6th **MØ8.Ø2 Unspecified juvenile rheumatoid arthritis of elbow**
- **MØ8.Ø21 Unspecified juvenile rheumatoid arthritis, right elbow** HCC
- **MØ8.Ø22 Unspecified juvenile rheumatoid arthritis, left elbow** HCC
- **MØ8.Ø29 Unspecified juvenile rheumatoid arthritis, unspecified elbow** HCC

✓6th **MØ8.Ø3 Unspecified juvenile rheumatoid arthritis, wrist**
- **MØ8.Ø31 Unspecified juvenile rheumatoid arthritis, right wrist** HCC
- **MØ8.Ø32 Unspecified juvenile rheumatoid arthritis, left wrist** HCC
- **MØ8.Ø39 Unspecified juvenile rheumatoid arthritis, unspecified wrist** HCC

✓6th **MØ8.Ø4 Unspecified juvenile rheumatoid arthritis, hand**
- **MØ8.Ø41 Unspecified juvenile rheumatoid arthritis, right hand** HCC
- **MØ8.Ø42 Unspecified juvenile rheumatoid arthritis, left hand** HCC
- **MØ8.Ø49 Unspecified juvenile rheumatoid arthritis, unspecified hand** HCC

✓6th **MØ8.Ø5 Unspecified juvenile rheumatoid arthritis, hip**
- **MØ8.Ø51 Unspecified juvenile rheumatoid arthritis, right hip** HCC
- **MØ8.Ø52 Unspecified juvenile rheumatoid arthritis, left hip** HCC
- **MØ8.Ø59 Unspecified juvenile rheumatoid arthritis, unspecified hip** HCC

✓6th **MØ8.Ø6 Unspecified juvenile rheumatoid arthritis, knee**
- **MØ8.Ø61 Unspecified juvenile rheumatoid arthritis, right knee** HCC
- **MØ8.Ø62 Unspecified juvenile rheumatoid arthritis, left knee** HCC
- **MØ8.Ø69 Unspecified juvenile rheumatoid arthritis, unspecified knee** HCC

✓6th **MØ8.Ø7 Unspecified juvenile rheumatoid arthritis, ankle and foot**
- **MØ8.Ø71 Unspecified juvenile rheumatoid arthritis, right ankle and foot** HCC
- **MØ8.Ø72 Unspecified juvenile rheumatoid arthritis, left ankle and foot** HCC
- **MØ8.Ø79 Unspecified juvenile rheumatoid arthritis, unspecified ankle and foot** HCC

MØ8.Ø8 Unspecified juvenile rheumatoid arthritis, vertebrae HCC

MØ8.Ø9 Unspecified juvenile rheumatoid arthritis, multiple sites HCC

MØ8.ØA Unspecified juvenile rheumatoid arthritis, other specified site HCC

MØ8.1 Juvenile ankylosing spondylitis HCC

EXCLUDES 1 *ankylosing spondylitis in adults (M45.Ø-)*

✓5th **MØ8.2 Juvenile rheumatoid arthritis with systemic onset**

Still's disease NOS

EXCLUDES 1 *adult-onset Still's disease (MØ6.1-)*

DEF: Systemic juvenile rheumatoid arthritis characterized by a transient rash and spiking fevers that may affect internal organs, as well as joints.

MØ8.2Ø Juvenile rheumatoid arthritis with systemic onset, unspecified site HCC

✓6th **MØ8.21 Juvenile rheumatoid arthritis with systemic onset, shoulder**
- **MØ8.211 Juvenile rheumatoid arthritis with systemic onset, right shoulder** HCC
- **MØ8.212 Juvenile rheumatoid arthritis with systemic onset, left shoulder** HCC
- **MØ8.219 Juvenile rheumatoid arthritis with systemic onset, unspecified shoulder** HCC

✓6th **MØ8.22 Juvenile rheumatoid arthritis with systemic onset, elbow**
- **MØ8.221 Juvenile rheumatoid arthritis with systemic onset, right elbow** HCC
- **MØ8.222 Juvenile rheumatoid arthritis with systemic onset, left elbow** HCC
- **MØ8.229 Juvenile rheumatoid arthritis with systemic onset, unspecified elbow** HCC

✓6th **MØ8.23 Juvenile rheumatoid arthritis with systemic onset, wrist**
- **MØ8.231 Juvenile rheumatoid arthritis with systemic onset, right wrist** HCC
- **MØ8.232 Juvenile rheumatoid arthritis with systemic onset, left wrist** HCC
- **MØ8.239 Juvenile rheumatoid arthritis with systemic onset, unspecified wrist** HCC

✓6th **MØ8.24 Juvenile rheumatoid arthritis with systemic onset, hand**
- **MØ8.241 Juvenile rheumatoid arthritis with systemic onset, right hand** HCC
- **MØ8.242 Juvenile rheumatoid arthritis with systemic onset, left hand** HCC
- **MØ8.249 Juvenile rheumatoid arthritis with systemic onset, unspecified hand** HCC

✓6th **MØ8.25 Juvenile rheumatoid arthritis with systemic onset, hip**
- **MØ8.251 Juvenile rheumatoid arthritis with systemic onset, right hip** HCC
- **MØ8.252 Juvenile rheumatoid arthritis with systemic onset, left hip** HCC
- **MØ8.259 Juvenile rheumatoid arthritis with systemic onset, unspecified hip** HCC

✓6th **MØ8.26 Juvenile rheumatoid arthritis with systemic onset, knee**
- **MØ8.261 Juvenile rheumatoid arthritis with systemic onset, right knee** HCC
- **MØ8.262 Juvenile rheumatoid arthritis with systemic onset, left knee** HCC
- **MØ8.269 Juvenile rheumatoid arthritis with systemic onset, unspecified knee** HCC

✓6th **MØ8.27 Juvenile rheumatoid arthritis with systemic onset, ankle and foot**
- **MØ8.271 Juvenile rheumatoid arthritis with systemic onset, right ankle and foot** HCC
- **MØ8.272 Juvenile rheumatoid arthritis with systemic onset, left ankle and foot** HCC
- **MØ8.279 Juvenile rheumatoid arthritis with systemic onset, unspecified ankle and foot** HCC

MØ8.28 Juvenile rheumatoid arthritis with systemic onset, vertebrae HCC

MØ8.29 Juvenile rheumatoid arthritis with systemic onset, multiple sites HCC

MØ8.2A Juvenile rheumatoid arthritis with systemic onset, other specified site HCC

MØ8.3 Juvenile rheumatoid polyarthritis (seronegative) HCC

✓5th **MØ8.4 Pauciarticular juvenile rheumatoid arthritis**

MØ8.4Ø Pauciarticular juvenile rheumatoid arthritis, unspecified site HCC

✓6th **MØ8.41 Pauciarticular juvenile rheumatoid arthritis, shoulder**
- **MØ8.411 Pauciarticular juvenile rheumatoid arthritis, right shoulder** HCC
- **MØ8.412 Pauciarticular juvenile rheumatoid arthritis, left shoulder** HCC
- **MØ8.419 Pauciarticular juvenile rheumatoid arthritis, unspecified shoulder** HCC

✓6th **MØ8.42 Pauciarticular juvenile rheumatoid arthritis, elbow**
- **MØ8.421 Pauciarticular juvenile rheumatoid arthritis, right elbow** HCC
- **MØ8.422 Pauciarticular juvenile rheumatoid arthritis, left elbow** HCC
- **MØ8.429 Pauciarticular juvenile rheumatoid arthritis, unspecified elbow** HCC

✓6th **MØ8.43 Pauciarticular juvenile rheumatoid arthritis, wrist**
- **MØ8.431 Pauciarticular juvenile rheumatoid arthritis, right wrist** HCC
- **MØ8.432 Pauciarticular juvenile rheumatoid arthritis, left wrist** HCC
- **MØ8.439 Pauciarticular juvenile rheumatoid arthritis, unspecified wrist** HCC

M08.44 Pauciarticular juvenile rheumatoid arthritis, hand
- **M08.441 Pauciarticular juvenile rheumatoid arthritis, right hand** HCC
- **M08.442 Pauciarticular juvenile rheumatoid arthritis, left hand** HCC
- **M08.449 Pauciarticular juvenile rheumatoid arthritis, unspecified hand** HCC

M08.45 Pauciarticular juvenile rheumatoid arthritis, hip
- **M08.451 Pauciarticular juvenile rheumatoid arthritis, right hip** HCC
- **M08.452 Pauciarticular juvenile rheumatoid arthritis, left hip** HCC
- **M08.459 Pauciarticular juvenile rheumatoid arthritis, unspecified hip** HCC

M08.46 Pauciarticular juvenile rheumatoid arthritis, knee
- **M08.461 Pauciarticular juvenile rheumatoid arthritis, right knee** HCC
- **M08.462 Pauciarticular juvenile rheumatoid arthritis, left knee** HCC
- **M08.469 Pauciarticular juvenile rheumatoid arthritis, unspecified knee** HCC

M08.47 Pauciarticular juvenile rheumatoid arthritis, ankle and foot
- **M08.471 Pauciarticular juvenile rheumatoid arthritis, right ankle and foot** HCC
- **M08.472 Pauciarticular juvenile rheumatoid arthritis, left ankle and foot** HCC
- **M08.479 Pauciarticular juvenile rheumatoid arthritis, unspecified ankle and foot** HCC

M08.48 Pauciarticular juvenile rheumatoid arthritis, vertebrae HCC

M08.4A Pauciarticular juvenile rheumatoid arthritis, other specified site HCC

M08.8 Other juvenile arthritis

M08.80 Other juvenile arthritis, unspecified site HCC

M08.81 Other juvenile arthritis, shoulder
- **M08.811 Other juvenile arthritis, right shoulder** HCC
- **M08.812 Other juvenile arthritis, left shoulder** HCC
- **M08.819 Other juvenile arthritis, unspecified shoulder** HCC

M08.82 Other juvenile arthritis, elbow
- **M08.821 Other juvenile arthritis, right elbow** HCC
- **M08.822 Other juvenile arthritis, left elbow** HCC
- **M08.829 Other juvenile arthritis, unspecified elbow** HCC

M08.83 Other juvenile arthritis, wrist
- **M08.831 Other juvenile arthritis, right wrist** HCC
- **M08.832 Other juvenile arthritis, left wrist** HCC
- **M08.839 Other juvenile arthritis, unspecified wrist** HCC

M08.84 Other juvenile arthritis, hand
- **M08.841 Other juvenile arthritis, right hand** HCC
- **M08.842 Other juvenile arthritis, left hand** HCC
- **M08.849 Other juvenile arthritis, unspecified hand** HCC

M08.85 Other juvenile arthritis, hip
- **M08.851 Other juvenile arthritis, right hip** HCC
- **M08.852 Other juvenile arthritis, left hip** HCC
- **M08.859 Other juvenile arthritis, unspecified hip** HCC

M08.86 Other juvenile arthritis, knee
- **M08.861 Other juvenile arthritis, right knee** HCC
- **M08.862 Other juvenile arthritis, left knee** HCC
- **M08.869 Other juvenile arthritis, unspecified knee** HCC

M08.87 Other juvenile arthritis, ankle and foot
- **M08.871 Other juvenile arthritis, right ankle and foot** HCC
- **M08.872 Other juvenile arthritis, left ankle and foot** HCC
- **M08.879 Other juvenile arthritis, unspecified ankle and foot** HCC

M08.88 Other juvenile arthritis, other specified site HCC
Other juvenile arthritis, vertebrae

M08.89 Other juvenile arthritis, multiple sites HCC

M08.9 Juvenile arthritis, unspecified

EXCLUDES 1 *juvenile rheumatoid arthritis, unspecified (M08.0-)*

M08.90 Juvenile arthritis, unspecified, unspecified site HCC

M08.91 Juvenile arthritis, unspecified, shoulder
- **M08.911 Juvenile arthritis, unspecified, right shoulder** HCC
- **M08.912 Juvenile arthritis, unspecified, left shoulder** HCC
- **M08.919 Juvenile arthritis, unspecified, unspecified shoulder** HCC

M08.92 Juvenile arthritis, unspecified, elbow
- **M08.921 Juvenile arthritis, unspecified, right elbow** HCC
- **M08.922 Juvenile arthritis, unspecified, left elbow** HCC
- **M08.929 Juvenile arthritis, unspecified, unspecified elbow** HCC

M08.93 Juvenile arthritis, unspecified, wrist
- **M08.931 Juvenile arthritis, unspecified, right wrist** HCC
- **M08.932 Juvenile arthritis, unspecified, left wrist** HCC
- **M08.939 Juvenile arthritis, unspecified, unspecified wrist** HCC

M08.94 Juvenile arthritis, unspecified, hand
- **M08.941 Juvenile arthritis, unspecified, right hand** HCC
- **M08.942 Juvenile arthritis, unspecified, left hand** HCC
- **M08.949 Juvenile arthritis, unspecified, unspecified hand** HCC

M08.95 Juvenile arthritis, unspecified, hip
- **M08.951 Juvenile arthritis, unspecified, right hip** HCC
- **M08.952 Juvenile arthritis, unspecified, left hip** HCC
- **M08.959 Juvenile arthritis, unspecified, unspecified hip** HCC

M08.96 Juvenile arthritis, unspecified, knee
- **M08.961 Juvenile arthritis, unspecified, right knee** HCC
- **M08.962 Juvenile arthritis, unspecified, left knee** HCC
- **M08.969 Juvenile arthritis, unspecified, unspecified knee** HCC

M08.97 Juvenile arthritis, unspecified, ankle and foot
- **M08.971 Juvenile arthritis, unspecified, right ankle and foot** HCC
- **M08.972 Juvenile arthritis, unspecified, left ankle and foot** HCC
- **M08.979 Juvenile arthritis, unspecified, unspecified ankle and foot** HCC

M08.98 Juvenile arthritis, unspecified, vertebrae HCC

M08.99 Juvenile arthritis, unspecified, multiple sites HCC

M08.9A Juvenile arthritis, unspecified, other specified site HCC

M1A Chronic gout

Use additional code to identify:
- autonomic neuropathy in diseases classified elsewhere (G99.Ø)
- calculus of urinary tract in diseases classified elsewhere (N22)
- cardiomyopathy in diseases classified elsewhere (I43)
- disorders of external ear in diseases classified elsewhere (H61.1-, H62.8-)
- disorders of iris and ciliary body in diseases classified elsewhere (H22)
- glomerular disorders in diseases classified elsewhere (NØ8)

EXCLUDES 1 *gout NOS (M1Ø.-)*

EXCLUDES 2 *acute gout (M1Ø.-)*

The appropriate 7th character is to be added to each code from category M1A.
- Ø without tophus (tophi)
- 1 with tophus (tophi)

M1A.Ø Idiopathic chronic gout
Chronic gouty bursitis
Primary chronic gout

M1A.ØØ Idiopathic chronic gout, unspecified site
M1A.Ø1 Idiopathic chronic gout, shoulder
M1A.Ø11 Idiopathic chronic gout, right shoulder
M1A.Ø12 Idiopathic chronic gout, left shoulder
M1A.Ø19 Idiopathic chronic gout, unspecified shoulder
M1A.Ø2 Idiopathic chronic gout, elbow
M1A.Ø21 Idiopathic chronic gout, right elbow
M1A.Ø22 Idiopathic chronic gout, left elbow
M1A.Ø29 Idiopathic chronic gout, unspecified elbow
M1A.Ø3 Idiopathic chronic gout, wrist
M1A.Ø31 Idiopathic chronic gout, right wrist
M1A.Ø32 Idiopathic chronic gout, left wrist
M1A.Ø39 Idiopathic chronic gout, unspecified wrist
M1A.Ø4 Idiopathic chronic gout, hand
M1A.Ø41 Idiopathic chronic gout, right hand
M1A.Ø42 Idiopathic chronic gout, left hand
M1A.Ø49 Idiopathic chronic gout, unspecified hand
M1A.Ø5 Idiopathic chronic gout, hip
M1A.Ø51 Idiopathic chronic gout, right hip
M1A.Ø52 Idiopathic chronic gout, left hip
M1A.Ø59 Idiopathic chronic gout, unspecified hip
M1A.Ø6 Idiopathic chronic gout, knee
M1A.Ø61 Idiopathic chronic gout, right knee
M1A.Ø62 Idiopathic chronic gout, left knee
M1A.Ø69 Idiopathic chronic gout, unspecified knee
M1A.Ø7 Idiopathic chronic gout, ankle and foot
M1A.Ø71 Idiopathic chronic gout, right ankle and foot
M1A.Ø72 Idiopathic chronic gout, left ankle and foot
M1A.Ø79 Idiopathic chronic gout, unspecified ankle and foot
M1A.Ø8 Idiopathic chronic gout, vertebrae
M1A.Ø9 Idiopathic chronic gout, multiple sites

M1A.1 Lead-induced chronic gout
Code first toxic effects of lead and its compounds (T56.Ø-)

M1A.1Ø Lead-induced chronic gout, unspecified site
M1A.11 Lead-induced chronic gout, shoulder
M1A.111 Lead-induced chronic gout, right shoulder
M1A.112 Lead-induced chronic gout, left shoulder
M1A.119 Lead-induced chronic gout, unspecified shoulder
M1A.12 Lead-induced chronic gout, elbow
M1A.121 Lead-induced chronic gout, right elbow
M1A.122 Lead-induced chronic gout, left elbow
M1A.129 Lead-induced chronic gout, unspecified elbow
M1A.13 Lead-induced chronic gout, wrist
M1A.131 Lead-induced chronic gout, right wrist
M1A.132 Lead-induced chronic gout, left wrist
M1A.139 Lead-induced chronic gout, unspecified wrist
M1A.14 Lead-induced chronic gout, hand
M1A.141 Lead-induced chronic gout, right hand
M1A.142 Lead-induced chronic gout, left hand
M1A.149 Lead-induced chronic gout, unspecified hand
M1A.15 Lead-induced chronic gout, hip
M1A.151 Lead-induced chronic gout, right hip
M1A.152 Lead-induced chronic gout, left hip
M1A.159 Lead-induced chronic gout, unspecified hip
M1A.16 Lead-induced chronic gout, knee
M1A.161 Lead-induced chronic gout, right knee
M1A.162 Lead-induced chronic gout, left knee
M1A.169 Lead-induced chronic gout, unspecified knee
M1A.17 Lead-induced chronic gout, ankle and foot
M1A.171 Lead-induced chronic gout, right ankle and foot
M1A.172 Lead-induced chronic gout, left ankle and foot
M1A.179 Lead-induced chronic gout, unspecified ankle and foot
M1A.18 Lead-induced chronic gout, vertebrae
M1A.19 Lead-induced chronic gout, multiple sites

M1A.2 Drug-induced chronic gout
Use additional code for adverse effect, if applicable, to identify drug (T36-T5Ø with fifth or sixth character 5)

M1A.2Ø Drug-induced chronic gout, unspecified site
M1A.21 Drug-induced chronic gout, shoulder
M1A.211 Drug-induced chronic gout, right shoulder
M1A.212 Drug-induced chronic gout, left shoulder
M1A.219 Drug-induced chronic gout, unspecified shoulder
M1A.22 Drug-induced chronic gout, elbow
M1A.221 Drug-induced chronic gout, right elbow
M1A.222 Drug-induced chronic gout, left elbow
M1A.229 Drug-induced chronic gout, unspecified elbow
M1A.23 Drug-induced chronic gout, wrist
M1A.231 Drug-induced chronic gout, right wrist
M1A.232 Drug-induced chronic gout, left wrist
M1A.239 Drug-induced chronic gout, unspecified wrist
M1A.24 Drug-induced chronic gout, hand
M1A.241 Drug-induced chronic gout, right hand
M1A.242 Drug-induced chronic gout, left hand
M1A.249 Drug-induced chronic gout, unspecified hand
M1A.25 Drug-induced chronic gout, hip
M1A.251 Drug-induced chronic gout, right hip
M1A.252 Drug-induced chronic gout, left hip
M1A.259 Drug-induced chronic gout, unspecified hip
M1A.26 Drug-induced chronic gout, knee
M1A.261 Drug-induced chronic gout, right knee
M1A.262 Drug-induced chronic gout, left knee
M1A.269 Drug-induced chronic gout, unspecified knee
M1A.27 Drug-induced chronic gout, ankle and foot
M1A.271 Drug-induced chronic gout, right ankle and foot
M1A.272 Drug-induced chronic gout, left ankle and foot
M1A.279 Drug-induced chronic gout, unspecified ankle and foot
M1A.28 Drug-induced chronic gout, vertebrae
M1A.29 Drug-induced chronic gout, multiple sites

M1A.3 Chronic gout due to renal impairment
Code first associated renal disease
M1A.30 Chronic gout due to renal impairment, unspecified site
M1A.31 Chronic gout due to renal impairment, shoulder
M1A.311 Chronic gout due to renal impairment, right shoulder
M1A.312 Chronic gout due to renal impairment, left shoulder
M1A.319 Chronic gout due to renal impairment, unspecified shoulder
M1A.32 Chronic gout due to renal impairment, elbow
M1A.321 Chronic gout due to renal impairment, right elbow
M1A.322 Chronic gout due to renal impairment, left elbow
M1A.329 Chronic gout due to renal impairment, unspecified elbow
M1A.33 Chronic gout due to renal impairment, wrist
M1A.331 Chronic gout due to renal impairment, right wrist
M1A.332 Chronic gout due to renal impairment, left wrist
M1A.339 Chronic gout due to renal impairment, unspecified wrist
M1A.34 Chronic gout due to renal impairment, hand
M1A.341 Chronic gout due to renal impairment, right hand
M1A.342 Chronic gout due to renal impairment, left hand
M1A.349 Chronic gout due to renal impairment, unspecified hand
M1A.35 Chronic gout due to renal impairment, hip
M1A.351 Chronic gout due to renal impairment, right hip
M1A.352 Chronic gout due to renal impairment, left hip
M1A.359 Chronic gout due to renal impairment, unspecified hip
M1A.36 Chronic gout due to renal impairment, knee
M1A.361 Chronic gout due to renal impairment, right knee
M1A.362 Chronic gout due to renal impairment, left knee
M1A.369 Chronic gout due to renal impairment, unspecified knee
M1A.37 Chronic gout due to renal impairment, ankle and foot
M1A.371 Chronic gout due to renal impairment, right ankle and foot
M1A.372 Chronic gout due to renal impairment, left ankle and foot
M1A.379 Chronic gout due to renal impairment, unspecified ankle and foot
M1A.38 Chronic gout due to renal impairment, vertebrae
M1A.39 Chronic gout due to renal impairment, multiple sites

M1A.4 Other secondary chronic gout
Code first associated condition
M1A.40 Other secondary chronic gout, unspecified site
M1A.41 Other secondary chronic gout, shoulder
M1A.411 Other secondary chronic gout, right shoulder
M1A.412 Other secondary chronic gout, left shoulder
M1A.419 Other secondary chronic gout, unspecified shoulder
M1A.42 Other secondary chronic gout, elbow
M1A.421 Other secondary chronic gout, right elbow
M1A.422 Other secondary chronic gout, left elbow
M1A.429 Other secondary chronic gout, unspecified elbow
M1A.43 Other secondary chronic gout, wrist
M1A.431 Other secondary chronic gout, right wrist
M1A.432 Other secondary chronic gout, left wrist
M1A.439 Other secondary chronic gout, unspecified wrist
M1A.44 Other secondary chronic gout, hand
M1A.441 Other secondary chronic gout, right hand
M1A.442 Other secondary chronic gout, left hand
M1A.449 Other secondary chronic gout, unspecified hand
M1A.45 Other secondary chronic gout, hip
M1A.451 Other secondary chronic gout, right hip
M1A.452 Other secondary chronic gout, left hip
M1A.459 Other secondary chronic gout, unspecified hip
M1A.46 Other secondary chronic gout, knee
M1A.461 Other secondary chronic gout, right knee
M1A.462 Other secondary chronic gout, left knee
M1A.469 Other secondary chronic gout, unspecified knee
M1A.47 Other secondary chronic gout, ankle and foot
M1A.471 Other secondary chronic gout, right ankle and foot
M1A.472 Other secondary chronic gout, left ankle and foot
M1A.479 Other secondary chronic gout, unspecified ankle and foot
M1A.48 Other secondary chronic gout, vertebrae
M1A.49 Other secondary chronic gout, multiple sites
M1A.9 Chronic gout, unspecified

M1Ø Gout
Acute gout
Gout attack
Gout flare
Podagra
Use additional code to identify:
autonomic neuropathy in diseases classified elsewhere (G99.Ø)
calculus of urinary tract in diseases classified elsewhere (N22)
cardiomyopathy in diseases classified elsewhere (I43)
disorders of external ear in diseases classified elsewhere (H61.1-, H62.8-)
disorders of iris and ciliary body in diseases classified elsewhere (H22)
glomerular disorders in diseases classified elsewhere (NØ8)
EXCLUDES 2 *chronic gout (M1A.-)*
DEF: Purine and pyrimidine metabolic disorders, manifested by hyperuricemia and recurrent acute inflammatory arthritis. Monosodium urate or monohydrate crystals may be deposited in and around the joints, leading to joint destruction and severe crippling.

M1Ø.Ø Idiopathic gout
Gouty bursitis
Primary gout
M1Ø.ØØ Idiopathic gout, unspecified site
M1Ø.Ø1 Idiopathic gout, shoulder
M1Ø.Ø11 Idiopathic gout, right shoulder
M1Ø.Ø12 Idiopathic gout, left shoulder
M1Ø.Ø19 Idiopathic gout, unspecified shoulder
M1Ø.Ø2 Idiopathic gout, elbow
M1Ø.Ø21 Idiopathic gout, right elbow
M1Ø.Ø22 Idiopathic gout, left elbow
M1Ø.Ø29 Idiopathic gout, unspecified elbow
M1Ø.Ø3 Idiopathic gout, wrist
M1Ø.Ø31 Idiopathic gout, right wrist
M1Ø.Ø32 Idiopathic gout, left wrist
M1Ø.Ø39 Idiopathic gout, unspecified wrist
M1Ø.Ø4 Idiopathic gout, hand
M1Ø.Ø41 Idiopathic gout, right hand
M1Ø.Ø42 Idiopathic gout, left hand
M1Ø.Ø49 Idiopathic gout, unspecified hand
M1Ø.Ø5 Idiopathic gout, hip
M1Ø.Ø51 Idiopathic gout, right hip
M1Ø.Ø52 Idiopathic gout, left hip
M1Ø.Ø59 Idiopathic gout, unspecified hip
M1Ø.Ø6 Idiopathic gout, knee
M1Ø.Ø61 Idiopathic gout, right knee
M1Ø.Ø62 Idiopathic gout, left knee
M1Ø.Ø69 Idiopathic gout, unspecified knee
M1Ø.Ø7 Idiopathic gout, ankle and foot
M1Ø.Ø71 Idiopathic gout, right ankle and foot
M1Ø.Ø72 Idiopathic gout, left ankle and foot

M10.079 Idiopathic gout, unspecified ankle and foot
M10.08 Idiopathic gout, vertebrae
M10.09 Idiopathic gout, multiple sites

M10.1 Lead-induced gout
Code first toxic effects of lead and its compounds (T56.0-)
M10.10 Lead-induced gout, unspecified site
M10.11 Lead-induced gout, shoulder
M10.111 Lead-induced gout, right shoulder
M10.112 Lead-induced gout, left shoulder
M10.119 Lead-induced gout, unspecified shoulder
M10.12 Lead-induced gout, elbow
M10.121 Lead-induced gout, right elbow
M10.122 Lead-induced gout, left elbow
M10.129 Lead-induced gout, unspecified elbow
M10.13 Lead-induced gout, wrist
M10.131 Lead-induced gout, right wrist
M10.132 Lead-induced gout, left wrist
M10.139 Lead-induced gout, unspecified wrist
M10.14 Lead-induced gout, hand
M10.141 Lead-induced gout, right hand
M10.142 Lead-induced gout, left hand
M10.149 Lead-induced gout, unspecified hand
M10.15 Lead-induced gout, hip
M10.151 Lead-induced gout, right hip
M10.152 Lead-induced gout, left hip
M10.159 Lead-induced gout, unspecified hip
M10.16 Lead-induced gout, knee
M10.161 Lead-induced gout, right knee
M10.162 Lead-induced gout, left knee
M10.169 Lead-induced gout, unspecified knee
M10.17 Lead-induced gout, ankle and foot
M10.171 Lead-induced gout, right ankle and foot
M10.172 Lead-induced gout, left ankle and foot
M10.179 Lead-induced gout, unspecified ankle and foot
M10.18 Lead-induced gout, vertebrae
M10.19 Lead-induced gout, multiple sites

M10.2 Drug-induced gout
Use additional code for adverse effect, if applicable, to identify drug (T36-T50 with fifth or sixth character 5)
M10.20 Drug-induced gout, unspecified site
M10.21 Drug-induced gout, shoulder
M10.211 Drug-induced gout, right shoulder
M10.212 Drug-induced gout, left shoulder
M10.219 Drug-induced gout, unspecified shoulder
M10.22 Drug-induced gout, elbow
M10.221 Drug-induced gout, right elbow
M10.222 Drug-induced gout, left elbow
M10.229 Drug-induced gout, unspecified elbow
M10.23 Drug-induced gout, wrist
M10.231 Drug-induced gout, right wrist
M10.232 Drug-induced gout, left wrist
M10.239 Drug-induced gout, unspecified wrist
M10.24 Drug-induced gout, hand
M10.241 Drug-induced gout, right hand
M10.242 Drug-induced gout, left hand
M10.249 Drug-induced gout, unspecified hand
M10.25 Drug-induced gout, hip
M10.251 Drug-induced gout, right hip
M10.252 Drug-induced gout, left hip
M10.259 Drug-induced gout, unspecified hip
M10.26 Drug-induced gout, knee
M10.261 Drug-induced gout, right knee
M10.262 Drug-induced gout, left knee
M10.269 Drug-induced gout, unspecified knee
M10.27 Drug-induced gout, ankle and foot
M10.271 Drug-induced gout, right ankle and foot
M10.272 Drug-induced gout, left ankle and foot
M10.279 Drug-induced gout, unspecified ankle and foot
M10.28 Drug-induced gout, vertebrae
M10.29 Drug-induced gout, multiple sites

M10.3 Gout due to renal impairment
Code first associated renal disease
M10.30 Gout due to renal impairment, unspecified site
M10.31 Gout due to renal impairment, shoulder
M10.311 Gout due to renal impairment, right shoulder
M10.312 Gout due to renal impairment, left shoulder
M10.319 Gout due to renal impairment, unspecified shoulder
M10.32 Gout due to renal impairment, elbow
M10.321 Gout due to renal impairment, right elbow
M10.322 Gout due to renal impairment, left elbow
M10.329 Gout due to renal impairment, unspecified elbow
M10.33 Gout due to renal impairment, wrist
M10.331 Gout due to renal impairment, right wrist
M10.332 Gout due to renal impairment, left wrist
M10.339 Gout due to renal impairment, unspecified wrist
M10.34 Gout due to renal impairment, hand
M10.341 Gout due to renal impairment, right hand
M10.342 Gout due to renal impairment, left hand
M10.349 Gout due to renal impairment, unspecified hand
M10.35 Gout due to renal impairment, hip
M10.351 Gout due to renal impairment, right hip
M10.352 Gout due to renal impairment, left hip
M10.359 Gout due to renal impairment, unspecified hip
M10.36 Gout due to renal impairment, knee
M10.361 Gout due to renal impairment, right knee
M10.362 Gout due to renal impairment, left knee
M10.369 Gout due to renal impairment, unspecified knee
M10.37 Gout due to renal impairment, ankle and foot
M10.371 Gout due to renal impairment, right ankle and foot
M10.372 Gout due to renal impairment, left ankle and foot
M10.379 Gout due to renal impairment, unspecified ankle and foot
M10.38 Gout due to renal impairment, vertebrae
M10.39 Gout due to renal impairment, multiple sites

M10.4 Other secondary gout
Code first associated condition
M10.40 Other secondary gout, unspecified site
M10.41 Other secondary gout, shoulder
M10.411 Other secondary gout, right shoulder
M10.412 Other secondary gout, left shoulder
M10.419 Other secondary gout, unspecified shoulder
M10.42 Other secondary gout, elbow
M10.421 Other secondary gout, right elbow
M10.422 Other secondary gout, left elbow
M10.429 Other secondary gout, unspecified elbow
M10.43 Other secondary gout, wrist
M10.431 Other secondary gout, right wrist
M10.432 Other secondary gout, left wrist
M10.439 Other secondary gout, unspecified wrist
M10.44 Other secondary gout, hand
M10.441 Other secondary gout, right hand
M10.442 Other secondary gout, left hand
M10.449 Other secondary gout, unspecified hand
M10.45 Other secondary gout, hip
M10.451 Other secondary gout, right hip
M10.452 Other secondary gout, left hip
M10.459 Other secondary gout, unspecified hip
M10.46 Other secondary gout, knee
M10.461 Other secondary gout, right knee
M10.462 Other secondary gout, left knee
M10.469 Other secondary gout, unspecified knee
M10.47 Other secondary gout, ankle and foot
M10.471 Other secondary gout, right ankle and foot
M10.472 Other secondary gout, left ankle and foot

M10.479 Other secondary gout, unspecified ankle and foot
M10.48 Other secondary gout, vertebrae
M10.49 Other secondary gout, multiple sites
M10.9 Gout, unspecified
Gout NOS

M11 Other crystal arthropathies

M11.0 Hydroxyapatite deposition disease
DEF: Disease caused by deposits of calcium phosphate crystals in the soft tissues close to the joint (especially tendons) or in the joints. These calcifications can be mono or polyarticular and can cause destruction of the joint involved.
M11.00 Hydroxyapatite deposition disease, unspecified site
M11.01 Hydroxyapatite deposition disease, shoulder
M11.011 Hydroxyapatite deposition disease, right shoulder
M11.012 Hydroxyapatite deposition disease, left shoulder
M11.019 Hydroxyapatite deposition disease, unspecified shoulder
M11.02 Hydroxyapatite deposition disease, elbow
M11.021 Hydroxyapatite deposition disease, right elbow
M11.022 Hydroxyapatite deposition disease, left elbow
M11.029 Hydroxyapatite deposition disease, unspecified elbow
M11.03 Hydroxyapatite deposition disease, wrist
M11.031 Hydroxyapatite deposition disease, right wrist
M11.032 Hydroxyapatite deposition disease, left wrist
M11.039 Hydroxyapatite deposition disease, unspecified wrist
M11.04 Hydroxyapatite deposition disease, hand
M11.041 Hydroxyapatite deposition disease, right hand
M11.042 Hydroxyapatite deposition disease, left hand
M11.049 Hydroxyapatite deposition disease, unspecified hand
M11.05 Hydroxyapatite deposition disease, hip
M11.051 Hydroxyapatite deposition disease, right hip
M11.052 Hydroxyapatite deposition disease, left hip
M11.059 Hydroxyapatite deposition disease, unspecified hip
M11.06 Hydroxyapatite deposition disease, knee
M11.061 Hydroxyapatite deposition disease, right knee
M11.062 Hydroxyapatite deposition disease, left knee
M11.069 Hydroxyapatite deposition disease, unspecified knee
M11.07 Hydroxyapatite deposition disease, ankle and foot
M11.071 Hydroxyapatite deposition disease, right ankle and foot
M11.072 Hydroxyapatite deposition disease, left ankle and foot
M11.079 Hydroxyapatite deposition disease, unspecified ankle and foot
M11.08 Hydroxyapatite deposition disease, vertebrae
M11.09 Hydroxyapatite deposition disease, multiple sites

M11.1 Familial chondrocalcinosis
M11.10 Familial chondrocalcinosis, unspecified site
M11.11 Familial chondrocalcinosis, shoulder
M11.111 Familial chondrocalcinosis, right shoulder
M11.112 Familial chondrocalcinosis, left shoulder
M11.119 Familial chondrocalcinosis, unspecified shoulder
M11.12 Familial chondrocalcinosis, elbow
M11.121 Familial chondrocalcinosis, right elbow
M11.122 Familial chondrocalcinosis, left elbow
M11.129 Familial chondrocalcinosis, unspecified elbow
M11.13 Familial chondrocalcinosis, wrist
M11.131 Familial chondrocalcinosis, right wrist
M11.132 Familial chondrocalcinosis, left wrist
M11.139 Familial chondrocalcinosis, unspecified wrist
M11.14 Familial chondrocalcinosis, hand
M11.141 Familial chondrocalcinosis, right hand
M11.142 Familial chondrocalcinosis, left hand
M11.149 Familial chondrocalcinosis, unspecified hand
M11.15 Familial chondrocalcinosis, hip
M11.151 Familial chondrocalcinosis, right hip
M11.152 Familial chondrocalcinosis, left hip
M11.159 Familial chondrocalcinosis, unspecified hip
M11.16 Familial chondrocalcinosis, knee
M11.161 Familial chondrocalcinosis, right knee
M11.162 Familial chondrocalcinosis, left knee
M11.169 Familial chondrocalcinosis, unspecified knee
M11.17 Familial chondrocalcinosis, ankle and foot
M11.171 Familial chondrocalcinosis, right ankle and foot
M11.172 Familial chondrocalcinosis, left ankle and foot
M11.179 Familial chondrocalcinosis, unspecified ankle and foot
M11.18 Familial chondrocalcinosis, vertebrae
M11.19 Familial chondrocalcinosis, multiple sites

M11.2 Other chondrocalcinosis
Chondrocalcinosis NOS
AHA: 2018,3Q,20
TIP: Pseudogout is captured with codes in this subcategory.
M11.20 Other chondrocalcinosis, unspecified site
M11.21 Other chondrocalcinosis, shoulder
M11.211 Other chondrocalcinosis, right shoulder
M11.212 Other chondrocalcinosis, left shoulder
M11.219 Other chondrocalcinosis, unspecified shoulder
M11.22 Other chondrocalcinosis, elbow
M11.221 Other chondrocalcinosis, right elbow
M11.222 Other chondrocalcinosis, left elbow
M11.229 Other chondrocalcinosis, unspecified elbow
M11.23 Other chondrocalcinosis, wrist
M11.231 Other chondrocalcinosis, right wrist
M11.232 Other chondrocalcinosis, left wrist
M11.239 Other chondrocalcinosis, unspecified wrist
M11.24 Other chondrocalcinosis, hand
M11.241 Other chondrocalcinosis, right hand
M11.242 Other chondrocalcinosis, left hand
M11.249 Other chondrocalcinosis, unspecified hand
M11.25 Other chondrocalcinosis, hip
M11.251 Other chondrocalcinosis, right hip
M11.252 Other chondrocalcinosis, left hip
M11.259 Other chondrocalcinosis, unspecified hip
M11.26 Other chondrocalcinosis, knee
M11.261 Other chondrocalcinosis, right knee
M11.262 Other chondrocalcinosis, left knee
M11.269 Other chondrocalcinosis, unspecified knee
M11.27 Other chondrocalcinosis, ankle and foot
M11.271 Other chondrocalcinosis, right ankle and foot
M11.272 Other chondrocalcinosis, left ankle and foot
M11.279 Other chondrocalcinosis, unspecified ankle and foot
M11.28 Other chondrocalcinosis, vertebrae
M11.29 Other chondrocalcinosis, multiple sites

M11.8 Other specified crystal arthropathies
M11.80 Other specified crystal arthropathies, unspecified site
M11.81 Other specified crystal arthropathies, shoulder
M11.811 Other specified crystal arthropathies, right shoulder
M11.812 Other specified crystal arthropathies, left shoulder

M11.819 Other specified crystal arthropathies, unspecified shoulder
M11.82 Other specified crystal arthropathies, elbow
M11.821 Other specified crystal arthropathies, right elbow
M11.822 Other specified crystal arthropathies, left elbow
M11.829 Other specified crystal arthropathies, unspecified elbow
M11.83 Other specified crystal arthropathies, wrist
M11.831 Other specified crystal arthropathies, right wrist
M11.832 Other specified crystal arthropathies, left wrist
M11.839 Other specified crystal arthropathies, unspecified wrist
M11.84 Other specified crystal arthropathies, hand
M11.841 Other specified crystal arthropathies, right hand
M11.842 Other specified crystal arthropathies, left hand
M11.849 Other specified crystal arthropathies, unspecified hand
M11.85 Other specified crystal arthropathies, hip
M11.851 Other specified crystal arthropathies, right hip
M11.852 Other specified crystal arthropathies, left hip
M11.859 Other specified crystal arthropathies, unspecified hip
M11.86 Other specified crystal arthropathies, knee
M11.861 Other specified crystal arthropathies, right knee
M11.862 Other specified crystal arthropathies, left knee
M11.869 Other specified crystal arthropathies, unspecified knee
M11.87 Other specified crystal arthropathies, ankle and foot
M11.871 Other specified crystal arthropathies, right ankle and foot
M11.872 Other specified crystal arthropathies, left ankle and foot
M11.879 Other specified crystal arthropathies, unspecified ankle and foot
M11.88 Other specified crystal arthropathies, vertebrae
M11.89 Other specified crystal arthropathies, multiple sites
M11.9 Crystal arthropathy, unspecified

M12 Other and unspecified arthropathy

EXCLUDES 1 *arthrosis (M15-M19)*
cricoarytenoid arthropathy (J38.7)

M12.Ø Chronic postrheumatic arthropathy [Jaccoud]
M12.ØØ Chronic postrheumatic arthropathy [Jaccoud], unspecified site HCC
M12.Ø1 Chronic postrheumatic arthropathy [Jaccoud], shoulder
M12.Ø11 Chronic postrheumatic arthropathy [Jaccoud], right shoulder HCC
M12.Ø12 Chronic postrheumatic arthropathy [Jaccoud], left shoulder HCC
M12.Ø19 Chronic postrheumatic arthropathy [Jaccoud], unspecified shoulder HCC
M12.Ø2 Chronic postrheumatic arthropathy [Jaccoud], elbow
M12.Ø21 Chronic postrheumatic arthropathy [Jaccoud], right elbow HCC
M12.Ø22 Chronic postrheumatic arthropathy [Jaccoud], left elbow HCC
M12.Ø29 Chronic postrheumatic arthropathy [Jaccoud], unspecified elbow HCC
M12.Ø3 Chronic postrheumatic arthropathy [Jaccoud], wrist
M12.Ø31 Chronic postrheumatic arthropathy [Jaccoud], right wrist HCC
M12.Ø32 Chronic postrheumatic arthropathy [Jaccoud], left wrist HCC
M12.Ø39 Chronic postrheumatic arthropathy [Jaccoud], unspecified wrist HCC
M12.Ø4 Chronic postrheumatic arthropathy [Jaccoud], hand
M12.Ø41 Chronic postrheumatic arthropathy [Jaccoud], right hand HCC
M12.Ø42 Chronic postrheumatic arthropathy [Jaccoud], left hand HCC
M12.Ø49 Chronic postrheumatic arthropathy [Jaccoud], unspecified hand HCC
M12.Ø5 Chronic postrheumatic arthropathy [Jaccoud], hip
M12.Ø51 Chronic postrheumatic arthropathy [Jaccoud], right hip HCC
M12.Ø52 Chronic postrheumatic arthropathy [Jaccoud], left hip HCC
M12.Ø59 Chronic postrheumatic arthropathy [Jaccoud], unspecified hip HCC
M12.Ø6 Chronic postrheumatic arthropathy [Jaccoud], knee
M12.Ø61 Chronic postrheumatic arthropathy [Jaccoud], right knee HCC
M12.Ø62 Chronic postrheumatic arthropathy [Jaccoud], left knee HCC
M12.Ø69 Chronic postrheumatic arthropathy [Jaccoud], unspecified knee HCC
M12.Ø7 Chronic postrheumatic arthropathy [Jaccoud], ankle and foot
M12.Ø71 Chronic postrheumatic arthropathy [Jaccoud], right ankle and foot HCC
M12.Ø72 Chronic postrheumatic arthropathy [Jaccoud], left ankle and foot HCC
M12.Ø79 Chronic postrheumatic arthropathy [Jaccoud], unspecified ankle and foot HCC
M12.Ø8 Chronic postrheumatic arthropathy [Jaccoud], other specified site HCC
Chronic postrheumatic arthropathy [Jaccoud], vertebrae
M12.Ø9 Chronic postrheumatic arthropathy [Jaccoud], multiple sites HCC

M12.1 Kaschin-Beck disease
Osteochondroarthrosis deformans endemica
M12.1Ø Kaschin-Beck disease, unspecified site
M12.11 Kaschin-Beck disease, shoulder
M12.111 Kaschin-Beck disease, right shoulder
M12.112 Kaschin-Beck disease, left shoulder
M12.119 Kaschin-Beck disease, unspecified shoulder
M12.12 Kaschin-Beck disease, elbow
M12.121 Kaschin-Beck disease, right elbow
M12.122 Kaschin-Beck disease, left elbow
M12.129 Kaschin-Beck disease, unspecified elbow
M12.13 Kaschin-Beck disease, wrist
M12.131 Kaschin-Beck disease, right wrist
M12.132 Kaschin-Beck disease, left wrist
M12.139 Kaschin-Beck disease, unspecified wrist
M12.14 Kaschin-Beck disease, hand
M12.141 Kaschin-Beck disease, right hand
M12.142 Kaschin-Beck disease, left hand
M12.149 Kaschin-Beck disease, unspecified hand
M12.15 Kaschin-Beck disease, hip
M12.151 Kaschin-Beck disease, right hip
M12.152 Kaschin-Beck disease, left hip
M12.159 Kaschin-Beck disease, unspecified hip
M12.16 Kaschin-Beck disease, knee
M12.161 Kaschin-Beck disease, right knee
M12.162 Kaschin-Beck disease, left knee
M12.169 Kaschin-Beck disease, unspecified knee
M12.17 Kaschin-Beck disease, ankle and foot
M12.171 Kaschin-Beck disease, right ankle and foot
M12.172 Kaschin-Beck disease, left ankle and foot
M12.179 Kaschin-Beck disease, unspecified ankle and foot
M12.18 Kaschin-Beck disease, vertebrae
M12.19 Kaschin-Beck disease, multiple sites

M12.2 Villonodular synovitis (pigmented)
M12.2Ø Villonodular synovitis (pigmented), unspecified site

M12.21 Villonodular synovitis (pigmented), shoulder
M12.211 Villonodular synovitis (pigmented), right shoulder
M12.212 Villonodular synovitis (pigmented), left shoulder
M12.219 Villonodular synovitis (pigmented), unspecified shoulder
M12.22 Villonodular synovitis (pigmented), elbow
M12.221 Villonodular synovitis (pigmented), right elbow
M12.222 Villonodular synovitis (pigmented), left elbow
M12.229 Villonodular synovitis (pigmented), unspecified elbow
M12.23 Villonodular synovitis (pigmented), wrist
M12.231 Villonodular synovitis (pigmented), right wrist
M12.232 Villonodular synovitis (pigmented), left wrist
M12.239 Villonodular synovitis (pigmented), unspecified wrist
M12.24 Villonodular synovitis (pigmented), hand
M12.241 Villonodular synovitis (pigmented), right hand
M12.242 Villonodular synovitis (pigmented), left hand
M12.249 Villonodular synovitis (pigmented), unspecified hand
M12.25 Villonodular synovitis (pigmented), hip
M12.251 Villonodular synovitis (pigmented), right hip
M12.252 Villonodular synovitis (pigmented), left hip
M12.259 Villonodular synovitis (pigmented), unspecified hip
M12.26 Villonodular synovitis (pigmented), knee
M12.261 Villonodular synovitis (pigmented), right knee
M12.262 Villonodular synovitis (pigmented), left knee
M12.269 Villonodular synovitis (pigmented), unspecified knee
M12.27 Villonodular synovitis (pigmented), ankle and foot
M12.271 Villonodular synovitis (pigmented), right ankle and foot
M12.272 Villonodular synovitis (pigmented), left ankle and foot
M12.279 Villonodular synovitis (pigmented), unspecified ankle and foot
M12.28 Villonodular synovitis (pigmented), other specified site
Villonodular synovitis (pigmented), vertebrae
M12.29 Villonodular synovitis (pigmented), multiple sites

M12.3 Palindromic rheumatism
DEF: Sudden and recurring attacks of moderate to severe joint pain and swelling generally occurring in the hands or feet of unknown etiology. After the attack subsides, the joints appear normal again.
M12.30 Palindromic rheumatism, unspecified site
M12.31 Palindromic rheumatism, shoulder
M12.311 Palindromic rheumatism, right shoulder
M12.312 Palindromic rheumatism, left shoulder
M12.319 Palindromic rheumatism, unspecified shoulder
M12.32 Palindromic rheumatism, elbow
M12.321 Palindromic rheumatism, right elbow
M12.322 Palindromic rheumatism, left elbow
M12.329 Palindromic rheumatism, unspecified elbow
M12.33 Palindromic rheumatism, wrist
M12.331 Palindromic rheumatism, right wrist
M12.332 Palindromic rheumatism, left wrist
M12.339 Palindromic rheumatism, unspecified wrist
M12.34 Palindromic rheumatism, hand
M12.341 Palindromic rheumatism, right hand
M12.342 Palindromic rheumatism, left hand
M12.349 Palindromic rheumatism, unspecified hand
M12.35 Palindromic rheumatism, hip
M12.351 Palindromic rheumatism, right hip
M12.352 Palindromic rheumatism, left hip
M12.359 Palindromic rheumatism, unspecified hip
M12.36 Palindromic rheumatism, knee
M12.361 Palindromic rheumatism, right knee
M12.362 Palindromic rheumatism, left knee
M12.369 Palindromic rheumatism, unspecified knee
M12.37 Palindromic rheumatism, ankle and foot
M12.371 Palindromic rheumatism, right ankle and foot
M12.372 Palindromic rheumatism, left ankle and foot
M12.379 Palindromic rheumatism, unspecified ankle and foot
M12.38 Palindromic rheumatism, other specified site
Palindromic rheumatism, vertebrae
M12.39 Palindromic rheumatism, multiple sites

M12.4 Intermittent hydrarthrosis
M12.40 Intermittent hydrarthrosis, unspecified site
M12.41 Intermittent hydrarthrosis, shoulder
M12.411 Intermittent hydrarthrosis, right shoulder
M12.412 Intermittent hydrarthrosis, left shoulder
M12.419 Intermittent hydrarthrosis, unspecified shoulder
M12.42 Intermittent hydrarthrosis, elbow
M12.421 Intermittent hydrarthrosis, right elbow
M12.422 Intermittent hydrarthrosis, left elbow
M12.429 Intermittent hydrarthrosis, unspecified elbow
M12.43 Intermittent hydrarthrosis, wrist
M12.431 Intermittent hydrarthrosis, right wrist
M12.432 Intermittent hydrarthrosis, left wrist
M12.439 Intermittent hydrarthrosis, unspecified wrist
M12.44 Intermittent hydrarthrosis, hand
M12.441 Intermittent hydrarthrosis, right hand
M12.442 Intermittent hydrarthrosis, left hand
M12.449 Intermittent hydrarthrosis, unspecified hand
M12.45 Intermittent hydrarthrosis, hip
M12.451 Intermittent hydrarthrosis, right hip
M12.452 Intermittent hydrarthrosis, left hip
M12.459 Intermittent hydrarthrosis, unspecified hip
M12.46 Intermittent hydrarthrosis, knee
M12.461 Intermittent hydrarthrosis, right knee
M12.462 Intermittent hydrarthrosis, left knee
M12.469 Intermittent hydrarthrosis, unspecified knee
M12.47 Intermittent hydrarthrosis, ankle and foot
M12.471 Intermittent hydrarthrosis, right ankle and foot
M12.472 Intermittent hydrarthrosis, left ankle and foot
M12.479 Intermittent hydrarthrosis, unspecified ankle and foot
M12.48 Intermittent hydrarthrosis, other site
M12.49 Intermittent hydrarthrosis, multiple sites

M12.5 Traumatic arthropathy
EXCLUDES 1
current injury-see Alphabetic Index
post-traumatic osteoarthritis of first carpometacarpal joint (M18.2-M18.3)
post-traumatic osteoarthritis of hip (M16.4-M16.5)
post-traumatic osteoarthritis of knee (M17.2-M17.3)
post-traumatic osteoarthritis NOS (M19.1-)
post-traumatic osteoarthritis of other single joints (M19.1-)
AHA: 2015,1Q,17
M12.50 Traumatic arthropathy, unspecified site
M12.51 Traumatic arthropathy, shoulder
M12.511 Traumatic arthropathy, right shoulder
M12.512 Traumatic arthropathy, left shoulder
M12.519 Traumatic arthropathy, unspecified shoulder

M12.52 Traumatic arthropathy, elbow
- **M12.521 Traumatic arthropathy, right elbow**
- **M12.522 Traumatic arthropathy, left elbow**
- **M12.529 Traumatic arthropathy, unspecified elbow**

M12.53 Traumatic arthropathy, wrist
- **M12.531 Traumatic arthropathy, right wrist**
- **M12.532 Traumatic arthropathy, left wrist**
- **M12.539 Traumatic arthropathy, unspecified wrist**

M12.54 Traumatic arthropathy, hand
- **M12.541 Traumatic arthropathy, right hand**
- **M12.542 Traumatic arthropathy, left hand**
- **M12.549 Traumatic arthropathy, unspecified hand**

M12.55 Traumatic arthropathy, hip
- **M12.551 Traumatic arthropathy, right hip**
- **M12.552 Traumatic arthropathy, left hip**
- **M12.559 Traumatic arthropathy, unspecified hip**

M12.56 Traumatic arthropathy, knee
- **M12.561 Traumatic arthropathy, right knee**
- **M12.562 Traumatic arthropathy, left knee**
- **M12.569 Traumatic arthropathy, unspecified knee**

M12.57 Traumatic arthropathy, ankle and foot
- **M12.571 Traumatic arthropathy, right ankle and foot**
- **M12.572 Traumatic arthropathy, left ankle and foot**
- **M12.579 Traumatic arthropathy, unspecified ankle and foot**

M12.58 Traumatic arthropathy, other specified site
Traumatic arthropathy, vertebrae

M12.59 Traumatic arthropathy, multiple sites

M12.8 Other specific arthropathies, not elsewhere classified
Transient arthropathy

M12.80 Other specific arthropathies, not elsewhere classified, unspecified site

M12.81 Other specific arthropathies, not elsewhere classified, shoulder
- **M12.811 Other specific arthropathies, not elsewhere classified, right shoulder**
- **M12.812 Other specific arthropathies, not elsewhere classified, left shoulder**
- **M12.819 Other specific arthropathies, not elsewhere classified, unspecified shoulder**

M12.82 Other specific arthropathies, not elsewhere classified, elbow
- **M12.821 Other specific arthropathies, not elsewhere classified, right elbow**
- **M12.822 Other specific arthropathies, not elsewhere classified, left elbow**
- **M12.829 Other specific arthropathies, not elsewhere classified, unspecified elbow**

M12.83 Other specific arthropathies, not elsewhere classified, wrist
- **M12.831 Other specific arthropathies, not elsewhere classified, right wrist**
- **M12.832 Other specific arthropathies, not elsewhere classified, left wrist**
- **M12.839 Other specific arthropathies, not elsewhere classified, unspecified wrist**

M12.84 Other specific arthropathies, not elsewhere classified, hand
- **M12.841 Other specific arthropathies, not elsewhere classified, right hand**
- **M12.842 Other specific arthropathies, not elsewhere classified, left hand**
- **M12.849 Other specific arthropathies, not elsewhere classified, unspecified hand**

M12.85 Other specific arthropathies, not elsewhere classified, hip
- **M12.851 Other specific arthropathies, not elsewhere classified, right hip**
- **M12.852 Other specific arthropathies, not elsewhere classified, left hip**
- **M12.859 Other specific arthropathies, not elsewhere classified, unspecified hip**

M12.86 Other specific arthropathies, not elsewhere classified, knee
- **M12.861 Other specific arthropathies, not elsewhere classified, right knee**
- **M12.862 Other specific arthropathies, not elsewhere classified, left knee**
- **M12.869 Other specific arthropathies, not elsewhere classified, unspecified knee**

M12.87 Other specific arthropathies, not elsewhere classified, ankle and foot
- **M12.871 Other specific arthropathies, not elsewhere classified, right ankle and foot**
- **M12.872 Other specific arthropathies, not elsewhere classified, left ankle and foot**
- **M12.879 Other specific arthropathies, not elsewhere classified, unspecified ankle and foot**

M12.88 Other specific arthropathies, not elsewhere classified, other specified site
Other specific arthropathies, not elsewhere classified, vertebrae

M12.89 Other specific arthropathies, not elsewhere classified, multiple sites

M12.9 Arthropathy, unspecified

M13 Other arthritis

EXCLUDES 1 *arthrosis (M15-M19)*
osteoarthritis (M15-M19)

M13.0 Polyarthritis, unspecified

M13.1 Monoarthritis, not elsewhere classified

M13.10 Monoarthritis, not elsewhere classified, unspecified site

M13.11 Monoarthritis, not elsewhere classified, shoulder
- **M13.111 Monoarthritis, not elsewhere classified, right shoulder**
- **M13.112 Monoarthritis, not elsewhere classified, left shoulder**
- **M13.119 Monoarthritis, not elsewhere classified, unspecified shoulder**

M13.12 Monoarthritis, not elsewhere classified, elbow
- **M13.121 Monoarthritis, not elsewhere classified, right elbow**
- **M13.122 Monoarthritis, not elsewhere classified, left elbow**
- **M13.129 Monoarthritis, not elsewhere classified, unspecified elbow**

M13.13 Monoarthritis, not elsewhere classified, wrist
- **M13.131 Monoarthritis, not elsewhere classified, right wrist**
- **M13.132 Monoarthritis, not elsewhere classified, left wrist**
- **M13.139 Monoarthritis, not elsewhere classified, unspecified wrist**

M13.14 Monoarthritis, not elsewhere classified, hand
- **M13.141 Monoarthritis, not elsewhere classified, right hand**
- **M13.142 Monoarthritis, not elsewhere classified, left hand**
- **M13.149 Monoarthritis, not elsewhere classified, unspecified hand**

M13.15 Monoarthritis, not elsewhere classified, hip
- **M13.151 Monoarthritis, not elsewhere classified, right hip**
- **M13.152 Monoarthritis, not elsewhere classified, left hip**
- **M13.159 Monoarthritis, not elsewhere classified, unspecified hip**

M13.16 Monoarthritis, not elsewhere classified, knee
- **M13.161 Monoarthritis, not elsewhere classified, right knee**
- **M13.162 Monoarthritis, not elsewhere classified, left knee**
- **M13.169 Monoarthritis, not elsewhere classified, unspecified knee**

M13.17 Monoarthritis, not elsewhere classified, ankle and foot
- **M13.171 Monoarthritis, not elsewhere classified, right ankle and foot**
- **M13.172 Monoarthritis, not elsewhere classified, left ankle and foot**
- **M13.179 Monoarthritis, not elsewhere classified, unspecified ankle and foot**

✓5th **M13.8 Other specified arthritis**
Allergic arthritis
EXCLUDES 1 *osteoarthritis (M15-M19)*
M13.80 Other specified arthritis, unspecified site
✓6th **M13.81 Other specified arthritis, shoulder**
M13.811 Other specified arthritis, right shoulder
M13.812 Other specified arthritis, left shoulder
M13.819 Other specified arthritis, unspecified shoulder
✓6th **M13.82 Other specified arthritis, elbow**
M13.821 Other specified arthritis, right elbow
M13.822 Other specified arthritis, left elbow
M13.829 Other specified arthritis, unspecified elbow
✓6th **M13.83 Other specified arthritis, wrist**
M13.831 Other specified arthritis, right wrist
M13.832 Other specified arthritis, left wrist
M13.839 Other specified arthritis, unspecified wrist
✓6th **M13.84 Other specified arthritis, hand**
M13.841 Other specified arthritis, right hand
M13.842 Other specified arthritis, left hand
M13.849 Other specified arthritis, unspecified hand
✓6th **M13.85 Other specified arthritis, hip**
M13.851 Other specified arthritis, right hip
M13.852 Other specified arthritis, left hip
M13.859 Other specified arthritis, unspecified hip
✓6th **M13.86 Other specified arthritis, knee**
M13.861 Other specified arthritis, right knee
M13.862 Other specified arthritis, left knee
M13.869 Other specified arthritis, unspecified knee
✓6th **M13.87 Other specified arthritis, ankle and foot**
M13.871 Other specified arthritis, right ankle and foot
M13.872 Other specified arthritis, left ankle and foot
M13.879 Other specified arthritis, unspecified ankle and foot
M13.88 Other specified arthritis, other site
M13.89 Other specified arthritis, multiple sites

✓4th **M14 Arthropathies in other diseases classified elsewhere**
EXCLUDES 1 *arthropathy in:*
diabetes mellitus (E08-E13 with .61-)
hematological disorders (M36.2-M36.3)
hypersensitivity reactions (M36.4)
neoplastic disease (M36.1)
neurosyphillis (A52.16)
sarcoidosis (D86.86)
enteropathic arthropathies (M07.-)
juvenile psoriatic arthropathy (L40.54)
lipoid dermatoarthritis (E78.81)

✓5th **M14.6 Charcôt's joint**
Neuropathic arthropathy
EXCLUDES 1 *Charcôt's joint in diabetes mellitus (E08-E13 with .610)*
Charcôt's joint in tabes dorsalis (A52.16)
DEF: Progressive neurologic arthropathy in which chronic degeneration of joints in the weight-bearing areas with peripheral hypertrophy occurs as a complication of a neuropathy disorder. Supporting structures relax from a loss of sensation resulting in chronic joint instability.
M14.60 Charcôt's joint, unspecified site
✓6th **M14.61 Charcôt's joint, shoulder**
M14.611 Charcôt's joint, right shoulder
M14.612 Charcôt's joint, left shoulder
M14.619 Charcôt's joint, unspecified shoulder
✓6th **M14.62 Charcôt's joint, elbow**
M14.621 Charcôt's joint, right elbow
M14.622 Charcôt's joint, left elbow
M14.629 Charcôt's joint, unspecified elbow
✓6th **M14.63 Charcôt's joint, wrist**
M14.631 Charcôt's joint, right wrist
M14.632 Charcôt's joint, left wrist
M14.639 Charcôt's joint, unspecified wrist
✓6th **M14.64 Charcôt's joint, hand**
M14.641 Charcôt's joint, right hand
M14.642 Charcôt's joint, left hand
M14.649 Charcôt's joint, unspecified hand
✓6th **M14.65 Charcôt's joint, hip**
M14.651 Charcôt's joint, right hip
M14.652 Charcôt's joint, left hip
M14.659 Charcôt's joint, unspecified hip
✓6th **M14.66 Charcôt's joint, knee**
M14.661 Charcôt's joint, right knee
M14.662 Charcôt's joint, left knee
M14.669 Charcôt's joint, unspecified knee
✓6th **M14.67 Charcôt's joint, ankle and foot**
M14.671 Charcôt's joint, right ankle and foot
M14.672 Charcôt's joint, left ankle and foot
M14.679 Charcôt's joint, unspecified ankle and foot
M14.68 Charcôt's joint, vertebrae
M14.69 Charcôt's joint, multiple sites

✓5th **M14.8 Arthropathies in other specified diseases classified elsewhere**
Code first underlying disease, such as:
amyloidosis (E85.-)
erythema multiforme (L51.-)
erythema nodosum (L52)
hemochromatosis (E83.11-)
hyperparathyroidism (E21.-)
hypothyroidism (E00-E03)
sickle-cell disorders (D57.-)
thyrotoxicosis [hyperthyroidism] (E05.-)
Whipple's disease (K90.81)
M14.80 Arthropathies in other specified diseases classified elsewhere, unspecified site
✓6th **M14.81 Arthropathies in other specified diseases classified elsewhere, shoulder**
M14.811 Arthropathies in other specified diseases classified elsewhere, right shoulder
M14.812 Arthropathies in other specified diseases classified elsewhere, left shoulder
M14.819 Arthropathies in other specified diseases classified elsewhere, unspecified shoulder
✓6th **M14.82 Arthropathies in other specified diseases classified elsewhere, elbow**
M14.821 Arthropathies in other specified diseases classified elsewhere, right elbow
M14.822 Arthropathies in other specified diseases classified elsewhere, left elbow
M14.829 Arthropathies in other specified diseases classified elsewhere, unspecified elbow
✓6th **M14.83 Arthropathies in other specified diseases classified elsewhere, wrist**
M14.831 Arthropathies in other specified diseases classified elsewhere, right wrist
M14.832 Arthropathies in other specified diseases classified elsewhere, left wrist
M14.839 Arthropathies in other specified diseases classified elsewhere, unspecified wrist
✓6th **M14.84 Arthropathies in other specified diseases classified elsewhere, hand**
M14.841 Arthropathies in other specified diseases classified elsewhere, right hand
M14.842 Arthropathies in other specified diseases classified elsewhere, left hand
M14.849 Arthropathies in other specified diseases classified elsewhere, unspecified hand
✓6th **M14.85 Arthropathies in other specified diseases classified elsewhere, hip**
M14.851 Arthropathies in other specified diseases classified elsewhere, right hip
M14.852 Arthropathies in other specified diseases classified elsewhere, left hip
M14.859 Arthropathies in other specified diseases classified elsewhere, unspecified hip
✓6th **M14.86 Arthropathies in other specified diseases classified elsewhere, knee**
M14.861 Arthropathies in other specified diseases classified elsewhere, right knee
M14.862 Arthropathies in other specified diseases classified elsewhere, left knee
M14.869 Arthropathies in other specified diseases classified elsewhere, unspecified knee

6th **M14.87 Arthropathies in other specified diseases classified elsewhere, ankle and foot**

M14.871 Arthropathies in other specified diseases classified elsewhere, right ankle and foot

M14.872 Arthropathies in other specified diseases classified elsewhere, left ankle and foot

M14.879 Arthropathies in other specified diseases classified elsewhere, unspecified ankle and foot

M14.88 Arthropathies in other specified diseases classified elsewhere, vertebrae

M14.89 Arthropathies in other specified diseases classified elsewhere, multiple sites

Osteoarthritis (M15-M19)

EXCLUDES 2 *osteoarthritis of spine (M47.-)*

AHA: 2020,2Q,14; 2016,4Q,147

TIP: Assign a primary osteoarthritis code when the site of the osteoarthritis is documented but the type of osteoarthritis — primary, secondary, generalized, or post-traumatic — is not documented. Primary is considered the default.

4th **M15 Polyosteoarthritis**

INCLUDES arthritis of multiple sites

EXCLUDES 1 *bilateral involvement of single joint (M16-M19)*

M15.0 Primary generalized (osteo)arthritis

M15.1 Heberden's nodes (with arthropathy)
Interphalangeal distal osteoarthritis

M15.2 Bouchard's nodes (with arthropathy)
Juxtaphalangeal distal osteoarthritis

M15.3 Secondary multiple arthritis
Post-traumatic polyosteoarthritis

M15.4 Erosive (osteo)arthritis

M15.8 Other polyosteoarthritis

M15.9 Polyosteoarthritis, unspecified
Generalized osteoarthritis NOS

4th **M16 Osteoarthritis of hip**

AHA: 2016,4Q,146

M16.0 Bilateral primary osteoarthritis of hip
AHA: 2018,2Q,15

5th **M16.1 Unilateral primary osteoarthritis of hip**
Primary osteoarthritis of hip NOS
AHA: 2018,2Q,15

M16.10 Unilateral primary osteoarthritis, unspecified hip

M16.11 Unilateral primary osteoarthritis, right hip

M16.12 Unilateral primary osteoarthritis, left hip

M16.2 Bilateral osteoarthritis resulting from hip dysplasia

5th **M16.3 Unilateral osteoarthritis resulting from hip dysplasia**
Dysplastic osteoarthritis of hip NOS

M16.30 Unilateral osteoarthritis resulting from hip dysplasia, unspecified hip

M16.31 Unilateral osteoarthritis resulting from hip dysplasia, right hip

M16.32 Unilateral osteoarthritis resulting from hip dysplasia, left hip

M16.4 Bilateral post-traumatic osteoarthritis of hip

5th **M16.5 Unilateral post-traumatic osteoarthritis of hip**
Post-traumatic osteoarthritis of hip NOS

M16.50 Unilateral post-traumatic osteoarthritis, unspecified hip

M16.51 Unilateral post-traumatic osteoarthritis, right hip

M16.52 Unilateral post-traumatic osteoarthritis, left hip

M16.6 Other bilateral secondary osteoarthritis of hip

M16.7 Other unilateral secondary osteoarthritis of hip
Secondary osteoarthritis of hip NOS

M16.9 Osteoarthritis of hip, unspecified

4th **M17 Osteoarthritis of knee**

AHA: 2016,4Q,146-147

M17.0 Bilateral primary osteoarthritis of knee
AHA: 2018,2Q,15

5th **M17.1 Unilateral primary osteoarthritis of knee**
Primary osteoarthritis of knee NOS
AHA: 2018,2Q,15

M17.10 Unilateral primary osteoarthritis, unspecified knee

M17.11 Unilateral primary osteoarthritis, right knee

M17.12 Unilateral primary osteoarthritis, left knee

M17.2 Bilateral post-traumatic osteoarthritis of knee

5th **M17.3 Unilateral post-traumatic osteoarthritis of knee**
Post-traumatic osteoarthritis of knee NOS

M17.30 Unilateral post-traumatic osteoarthritis, unspecified knee

M17.31 Unilateral post-traumatic osteoarthritis, right knee

M17.32 Unilateral post-traumatic osteoarthritis, left knee

M17.4 Other bilateral secondary osteoarthritis of knee

M17.5 Other unilateral secondary osteoarthritis of knee
Secondary osteoarthritis of knee NOS

M17.9 Osteoarthritis of knee, unspecified

4th **M18 Osteoarthritis of first carpometacarpal joint**

M18.0 Bilateral primary osteoarthritis of first carpometacarpal joints

5th **M18.1 Unilateral primary osteoarthritis of first carpometacarpal joint**
Primary osteoarthritis of first carpometacarpal joint NOS

M18.10 Unilateral primary osteoarthritis of first carpometacarpal joint, unspecified hand

M18.11 Unilateral primary osteoarthritis of first carpometacarpal joint, right hand

M18.12 Unilateral primary osteoarthritis of first carpometacarpal joint, left hand

M18.2 Bilateral post-traumatic osteoarthritis of first carpometacarpal joints

5th **M18.3 Unilateral post-traumatic osteoarthritis of first carpometacarpal joint**
Post-traumatic osteoarthritis of first carpometacarpal joint NOS

M18.30 Unilateral post-traumatic osteoarthritis of first carpometacarpal joint, unspecified hand

M18.31 Unilateral post-traumatic osteoarthritis of first carpometacarpal joint, right hand

M18.32 Unilateral post-traumatic osteoarthritis of first carpometacarpal joint, left hand

M18.4 Other bilateral secondary osteoarthritis of first carpometacarpal joints

5th **M18.5 Other unilateral secondary osteoarthritis of first carpometacarpal joint**
Secondary osteoarthritis of first carpometacarpal joint NOS

M18.50 Other unilateral secondary osteoarthritis of first carpometacarpal joint, unspecified hand

M18.51 Other unilateral secondary osteoarthritis of first carpometacarpal joint, right hand

M18.52 Other unilateral secondary osteoarthritis of first carpometacarpal joint, left hand

M18.9 Osteoarthritis of first carpometacarpal joint, unspecified

4th **M19 Other and unspecified osteoarthritis**

EXCLUDES 1 *polyarthritis (M15.-)*

EXCLUDES 2 *arthrosis of spine (M47.-)*
hallux rigidus (M20.2)
osteoarthritis of spine (M47.-)

AHA: 2020,4Q,31-32

5th **M19.0 Primary osteoarthritis of other joints**
AHA: 2018,2Q,15; 2016,4Q,145

6th **M19.01 Primary osteoarthritis, shoulder**

M19.011 Primary osteoarthritis, right shoulder

M19.012 Primary osteoarthritis, left shoulder

M19.019 Primary osteoarthritis, unspecified shoulder

6th **M19.02 Primary osteoarthritis, elbow**

M19.021 Primary osteoarthritis, right elbow

M19.022 Primary osteoarthritis, left elbow

M19.029 Primary osteoarthritis, unspecified elbow

6th **M19.03 Primary osteoarthritis, wrist**

M19.031 Primary osteoarthritis, right wrist

M19.032 Primary osteoarthritis, left wrist

M19.039 Primary osteoarthritis, unspecified wrist

6th **M19.04 Primary osteoarthritis, hand**

EXCLUDES 2 *primary osteoarthritis of first carpometacarpal joint (M18.0-, M18.1-)*

M19.041 Primary osteoarthritis, right hand

M19.042 Primary osteoarthritis, left hand

M19.049 Primary osteoarthritis, unspecified hand

6th **M19.07 Primary osteoarthritis ankle and foot**

M19.071 Primary osteoarthritis, right ankle and foot

M19.072 Primary osteoarthritis, left ankle and foot

M19.079 Primary osteoarthritis, unspecified ankle and foot

M19.09 Primary osteoarthritis, other specified site

M19.1 Post-traumatic osteoarthritis of other joints

M19.11 Post-traumatic osteoarthritis, shoulder

M19.111 Post-traumatic osteoarthritis, right shoulder

M19.112 Post-traumatic osteoarthritis, left shoulder

M19.119 Post-traumatic osteoarthritis, unspecified shoulder

M19.12 Post-traumatic osteoarthritis, elbow

M19.121 Post-traumatic osteoarthritis, right elbow

M19.122 Post-traumatic osteoarthritis, left elbow

M19.129 Post-traumatic osteoarthritis, unspecified elbow

M19.13 Post-traumatic osteoarthritis, wrist

M19.131 Post-traumatic osteoarthritis, right wrist

M19.132 Post-traumatic osteoarthritis, left wrist

M19.139 Post-traumatic osteoarthritis, unspecified wrist

M19.14 Post-traumatic osteoarthritis, hand

EXCLUDES 2 *post-traumatic osteoarthritis of first carpometacarpal joint (M18.2-, M18.3-)*

M19.141 Post-traumatic osteoarthritis, right hand

M19.142 Post-traumatic osteoarthritis, left hand

M19.149 Post-traumatic osteoarthritis, unspecified hand

M19.17 Post-traumatic osteoarthritis, ankle and foot

M19.171 Post-traumatic osteoarthritis, right ankle and foot

M19.172 Post-traumatic osteoarthritis, left ankle and foot

M19.179 Post-traumatic osteoarthritis, unspecified ankle and foot

M19.19 Post-traumatic osteoarthritis, other specified site

M19.2 Secondary osteoarthritis of other joints

M19.21 Secondary osteoarthritis, shoulder

M19.211 Secondary osteoarthritis, right shoulder

M19.212 Secondary osteoarthritis, left shoulder

M19.219 Secondary osteoarthritis, unspecified shoulder

M19.22 Secondary osteoarthritis, elbow

M19.221 Secondary osteoarthritis, right elbow

M19.222 Secondary osteoarthritis, left elbow

M19.229 Secondary osteoarthritis, unspecified elbow

M19.23 Secondary osteoarthritis, wrist

M19.231 Secondary osteoarthritis, right wrist

M19.232 Secondary osteoarthritis, left wrist

M19.239 Secondary osteoarthritis, unspecified wrist

M19.24 Secondary osteoarthritis, hand

M19.241 Secondary osteoarthritis, right hand

M19.242 Secondary osteoarthritis, left hand

M19.249 Secondary osteoarthritis, unspecified hand

M19.27 Secondary osteoarthritis, ankle and foot

M19.271 Secondary osteoarthritis, right ankle and foot

M19.272 Secondary osteoarthritis, left ankle and foot

M19.279 Secondary osteoarthritis, unspecified ankle and foot

M19.29 Secondary osteoarthritis, other specified site

M19.9 Osteoarthritis, unspecified site

TIP: Assign M19.90 when neither the site nor the type of osteoarthritis — primary, secondary, or post-traumatic — is documented.

M19.90 Unspecified osteoarthritis, unspecified site

Arthrosis NOS

Arthritis NOS

Osteoarthritis NOS

AHA: 2016,4Q,145-147

M19.91 Primary osteoarthritis, unspecified site

Primary osteoarthritis NOS

M19.92 Post-traumatic osteoarthritis, unspecified site

Post-traumatic osteoarthritis NOS

M19.93 Secondary osteoarthritis, unspecified site

Secondary osteoarthritis NOS

Other joint disorders (M20-M25)

EXCLUDES 2 *joints of the spine (M40-M54)*

M20 Acquired deformities of fingers and toes

EXCLUDES 1 *acquired absence of fingers and toes (Z89.-)*
congenital absence of fingers and toes (Q71.3-, Q72.3-)
congenital deformities and malformations of fingers and toes (Q66.-, Q68-Q70, Q74.-)

M20.0 Deformity of finger(s)

EXCLUDES 1 *clubbing of fingers (R68.3)*
palmar fascial fibromatosis [Dupuytren] (M72.0)
trigger finger (M65.3)

M20.00 Unspecified deformity of finger(s)

M20.001 Unspecified deformity of right finger(s)

M20.002 Unspecified deformity of left finger(s)

M20.009 Unspecified deformity of unspecified finger(s)

M20.01 Mallet finger

M20.011 Mallet finger of right finger(s)

M20.012 Mallet finger of left finger(s)

M20.019 Mallet finger of unspecified finger(s)

M20.02 Boutonnière deformity

DEF: Deformity of the finger caused by flexion of the proximal interphalangeal joint and hyperextension of the distal joint. The deformity results from rheumatoid arthritis, osteoarthritis, or injury.

M20.021 Boutonnière deformity of right finger(s)

M20.022 Boutonnière deformity of left finger(s)

M20.029 Boutonnière deformity of unspecified finger(s)

M20.03 Swan-neck deformity

DEF: Flexed distal and hyperextended proximal interphalangeal joint most commonly caused by rheumatoid arthritis.

M20.031 Swan-neck deformity of right finger(s)

M20.032 Swan-neck deformity of left finger(s)

M20.039 Swan-neck deformity of unspecified finger(s)

M20.09 Other deformity of finger(s)

M20.091 Other deformity of right finger(s)

M20.092 Other deformity of left finger(s)

M20.099 Other deformity of finger(s), unspecified finger(s)

M20.1 Hallux valgus (acquired)

EXCLUDES 2 *bunion (M21.6-)*

AHA: 2016,4Q,38

DEF: Deformity in which the great toe deviates toward the other toes and may even be positioned over or under the second toe.

Hallux Valgus

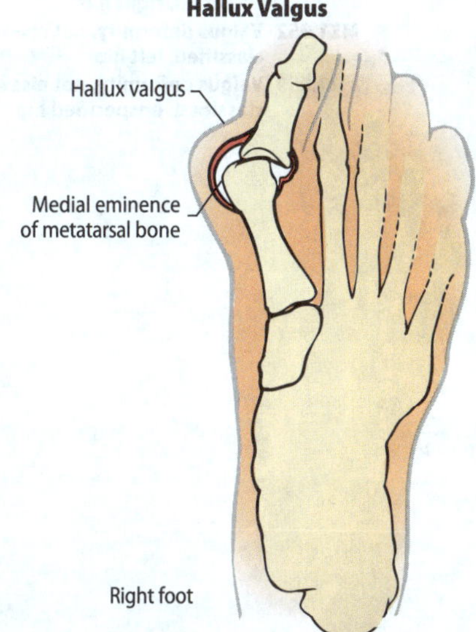

M20.10 Hallux valgus (acquired), unspecified foot

M20.11 Hallux valgus (acquired), right foot
M20.12 Hallux valgus (acquired), left foot

M20.2 Hallux rigidus
M20.20 Hallux rigidus, unspecified foot
M20.21 Hallux rigidus, right foot
M20.22 Hallux rigidus, left foot

M20.3 Hallux varus (acquired)
DEF: Deformity in which the great toe deviates away from the other toes.
M20.30 Hallux varus (acquired), unspecified foot
M20.31 Hallux varus (acquired), right foot
M20.32 Hallux varus (acquired), left foot

M20.4 Other hammer toe(s) (acquired)
M20.40 Other hammer toe(s) (acquired), unspecified foot
M20.41 Other hammer toe(s) (acquired), right foot
M20.42 Other hammer toe(s) (acquired), left foot

M20.5 Other deformities of toe(s) (acquired)
M20.5X Other deformities of toe(s) (acquired)
M20.5X1 Other deformities of toe(s) (acquired), right foot
M20.5X2 Other deformities of toe(s) (acquired), left foot
M20.5X9 Other deformities of toe(s) (acquired), unspecified foot

M20.6 Acquired deformities of toe(s), unspecified
M20.60 Acquired deformities of toe(s), unspecified, unspecified foot
M20.61 Acquired deformities of toe(s), unspecified, right foot
M20.62 Acquired deformities of toe(s), unspecified, left foot

M21 Other acquired deformities of limbs
EXCLUDES 1 *acquired absence of limb (Z89.-)*
congenital absence of limbs (Q71-Q73)
congenital deformities and malformations of limbs (Q65-Q66, Q68-Q74)
EXCLUDES 2 *acquired deformities of fingers or toes (M20.-)*
coxa plana (M91.2)

M21.0 Valgus deformity, not elsewhere classified
EXCLUDES 1 *metatarsus valgus (Q66.6)*
talipes calcaneovalgus (Q66.4-)
M21.00 Valgus deformity, not elsewhere classified, unspecified site
M21.02 Valgus deformity, not elsewhere classified, elbow
Cubitus valgus
M21.021 Valgus deformity, not elsewhere classified, right elbow
M21.022 Valgus deformity, not elsewhere classified, left elbow
M21.029 Valgus deformity, not elsewhere classified, unspecified elbow
M21.05 Valgus deformity, not elsewhere classified, hip
M21.051 Valgus deformity, not elsewhere classified, right hip
M21.052 Valgus deformity, not elsewhere classified, left hip
M21.059 Valgus deformity, not elsewhere classified, unspecified hip
M21.06 Valgus deformity, not elsewhere classified, knee
Genu valgum
Knock knee
DEF: Genu valga/valgum: Condition in which the thighs slant inward, causing the knees to be angled abnormally close together, leaving the space between the ankles wider than normal.

Genu Valga (knock-knee)

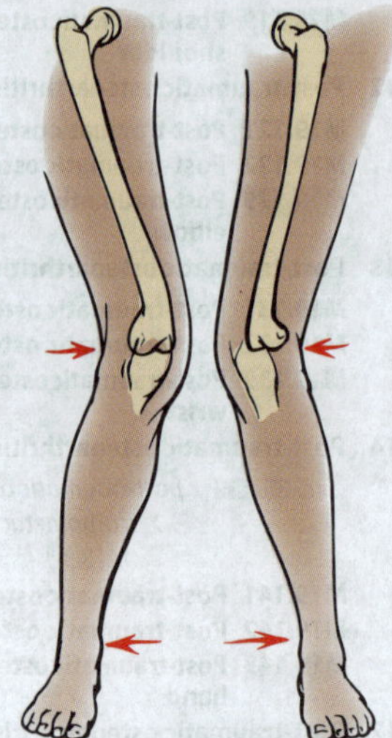

M21.061 Valgus deformity, not elsewhere classified, right knee
M21.062 Valgus deformity, not elsewhere classified, left knee
M21.069 Valgus deformity, not elsewhere classified, unspecified knee
M21.07 Valgus deformity, not elsewhere classified, ankle
M21.071 Valgus deformity, not elsewhere classified, right ankle
M21.072 Valgus deformity, not elsewhere classified, left ankle
M21.079 Valgus deformity, not elsewhere classified, unspecified ankle

M21.1 Varus deformity, not elsewhere classified
EXCLUDES 1 *metatarsus varus (Q66.22-)*
tibia vara (M92.51-)
M21.10 Varus deformity, not elsewhere classified, unspecified site
M21.12 Varus deformity, not elsewhere classified, elbow
Cubitus varus, elbow
M21.121 Varus deformity, not elsewhere classified, right elbow
M21.122 Varus deformity, not elsewhere classified, left elbow
M21.129 Varus deformity, not elsewhere classified, unspecified elbow
M21.15 Varus deformity, not elsewhere classified, hip
M21.151 Varus deformity, not elsewhere classified, right hip
M21.152 Varus deformity, not elsewhere classified, left hip
M21.159 Varus deformity, not elsewhere classified, unspecified

✓6th **M21.16 Varus deformity, not elsewhere classified, knee**
Bow leg
Genu varum
DEF: Genu varus/varum: Condition in which the thighs and/or legs are bowed in an outward curve with an abnormally increased space between the knees.

Genu Varus (bowleg)

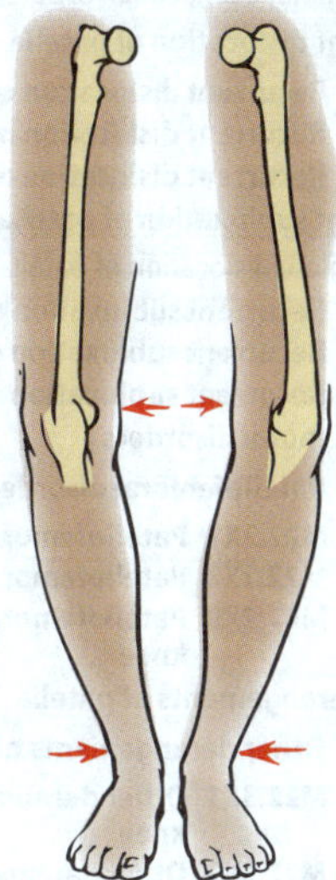

M21.161 Varus deformity, not elsewhere classified, right knee
M21.162 Varus deformity, not elsewhere classified, left knee
M21.169 Varus deformity, not elsewhere classified, unspecified knee

✓6th **M21.17 Varus deformity, not elsewhere classified, ankle**
M21.171 Varus deformity, not elsewhere classified, right ankle
M21.172 Varus deformity, not elsewhere classified, left ankle
M21.179 Varus deformity, not elsewhere classified, unspecified ankle

✓5th **M21.2 Flexion deformity**
M21.20 Flexion deformity, unspecified site

✓6th **M21.21 Flexion deformity, shoulder**
M21.211 Flexion deformity, right shoulder
M21.212 Flexion deformity, left shoulder
M21.219 Flexion deformity, unspecified shoulder

✓6th **M21.22 Flexion deformity, elbow**
M21.221 Flexion deformity, right elbow
M21.222 Flexion deformity, left elbow
M21.229 Flexion deformity, unspecified elbow

✓6th **M21.23 Flexion deformity, wrist**
M21.231 Flexion deformity, right wrist
M21.232 Flexion deformity, left wrist
M21.239 Flexion deformity, unspecified wrist

✓6th **M21.24 Flexion deformity, finger joints**
M21.241 Flexion deformity, right finger joints
M21.242 Flexion deformity, left finger joints
M21.249 Flexion deformity, unspecified finger joints

✓6th **M21.25 Flexion deformity, hip**
M21.251 Flexion deformity, right hip
M21.252 Flexion deformity, left hip
M21.259 Flexion deformity, unspecified hip

✓6th **M21.26 Flexion deformity, knee**
M21.261 Flexion deformity, right knee
M21.262 Flexion deformity, left knee
M21.269 Flexion deformity, unspecified knee

✓6th **M21.27 Flexion deformity, ankle and toes**
M21.271 Flexion deformity, right ankle and toes
M21.272 Flexion deformity, left ankle and toes
M21.279 Flexion deformity, unspecified ankle and toes

✓5th **M21.3 Wrist or foot drop (acquired)**

✓6th **M21.33 Wrist drop (acquired)**
M21.331 Wrist drop, right wrist
M21.332 Wrist drop, left wrist
M21.339 Wrist drop, unspecified wrist

✓6th **M21.37 Foot drop (acquired)**
M21.371 Foot drop, right foot
M21.372 Foot drop, left foot
M21.379 Foot drop, unspecified foot

✓5th **M21.4 Flat foot [pes planus] (acquired)**
EXCLUDES 1 *congenital pes planus (Q66.5-)*
M21.40 Flat foot [pes planus] (acquired), unspecified foot
M21.41 Flat foot [pes planus] (acquired), right foot
M21.42 Flat foot [pes planus] (acquired), left foot

✓5th **M21.5 Acquired clawhand, clubhand, clawfoot and clubfoot**
EXCLUDES 1 *clubfoot, not specified as acquired (Q66.89)*

✓6th **M21.51 Acquired clawhand**
M21.511 Acquired clawhand, right hand
M21.512 Acquired clawhand, left hand
M21.519 Acquired clawhand, unspecified hand

✓6th **M21.52 Acquired clubhand**
M21.521 Acquired clubhand, right hand
M21.522 Acquired clubhand, left hand
M21.529 Acquired clubhand, unspecified hand

✓6th **M21.53 Acquired clawfoot**
DEF: High foot arch with hyperextended toes at the metatarsophalangeal joint and flexed toes at the distal joints.
M21.531 Acquired clawfoot, right foot
M21.532 Acquired clawfoot, left foot
M21.539 Acquired clawfoot, unspecified foot

✓6th **M21.54 Acquired clubfoot**
DEF: Acquired anomaly of the foot with the heel elevated and rotated outward and the toes pointing inward.
M21.541 Acquired clubfoot, right foot
M21.542 Acquired clubfoot, left foot
M21.549 Acquired clubfoot, unspecified foot

✓5th **M21.6 Other acquired deformities of foot**
EXCLUDES 2 *deformities of toe (acquired) (M20.1-M20.6-)*
AHA: 2016,4Q,38

✓6th **M21.61 Bunion**
M21.611 Bunion of right foot
M21.612 Bunion of left foot
M21.619 Bunion of unspecified foot

✓6th **M21.62 Bunionette**
M21.621 Bunionette of right foot
M21.622 Bunionette of left foot
M21.629 Bunionette of unspecified foot

✓6th **M21.6X Other acquired deformities of foot**
M21.6X1 Other acquired deformities of right foot
M21.6X2 Other acquired deformities of left foot
M21.6X9 Other acquired deformities of unspecified foot

✓5th **M21.7 Unequal limb length (acquired)**
NOTE The site used should correspond to the shorter limb
M21.70 Unequal limb length (acquired), unspecified site

✓6th **M21.72 Unequal limb length (acquired), humerus**
M21.721 Unequal limb length (acquired), right humerus
M21.722 Unequal limb length (acquired), left humerus
M21.729 Unequal limb length (acquired), unspecified humerus

✓6th **M21.73 Unequal limb length (acquired), ulna and radius**
M21.731 Unequal limb length (acquired), right ulna
M21.732 Unequal limb length (acquired), left ulna
M21.733 Unequal limb length (acquired), right radius
M21.734 Unequal limb length (acquired), left radius
M21.739 Unequal limb length (acquired), unspecified ulna and radius

M21.75 Unequal limb length (acquired), femur
- **M21.751 Unequal limb length (acquired), right femur**
- **M21.752 Unequal limb length (acquired), left femur**
- **M21.759 Unequal limb length (acquired), unspecified femur**

M21.76 Unequal limb length (acquired), tibia and fibula
- **M21.761 Unequal limb length (acquired), right tibia**
- **M21.762 Unequal limb length (acquired), left tibia**
- **M21.763 Unequal limb length (acquired), right fibula**
- **M21.764 Unequal limb length (acquired), left fibula**
- **M21.769 Unequal limb length (acquired), unspecified tibia and fibula**

M21.8 Other specified acquired deformities of limbs

EXCLUDES 2 *coxa plana (M91.2)*

- **M21.80 Other specified acquired deformities of unspecified limb**

M21.82 Other specified acquired deformities of upper arm
- **M21.821 Other specified acquired deformities of right upper arm**
- **M21.822 Other specified acquired deformities of left upper arm**
- **M21.829 Other specified acquired deformities of unspecified upper arm**

M21.83 Other specified acquired deformities of forearm
- **M21.831 Other specified acquired deformities of right forearm**
- **M21.832 Other specified acquired deformities of left forearm**
- **M21.839 Other specified acquired deformities of unspecified forearm**

M21.85 Other specified acquired deformities of thigh
- **M21.851 Other specified acquired deformities of right thigh**
- **M21.852 Other specified acquired deformities of left thigh**
- **M21.859 Other specified acquired deformities of unspecified thigh**

M21.86 Other specified acquired deformities of lower leg
- **M21.861 Other specified acquired deformities of right lower leg**
- **M21.862 Other specified acquired deformities of left lower leg**
- **M21.869 Other specified acquired deformities of unspecified lower leg**

M21.9 Unspecified acquired deformity of limb and hand
- **M21.90 Unspecified acquired deformity of unspecified limb**

M21.92 Unspecified acquired deformity of upper arm
- **M21.921 Unspecified acquired deformity of right upper arm**
- **M21.922 Unspecified acquired deformity of left upper arm**
- **M21.929 Unspecified acquired deformity of unspecified upper arm**

M21.93 Unspecified acquired deformity of forearm
- **M21.931 Unspecified acquired deformity of right forearm**
- **M21.932 Unspecified acquired deformity of left forearm**
- **M21.939 Unspecified acquired deformity of unspecified forearm**

M21.94 Unspecified acquired deformity of hand
- **M21.941 Unspecified acquired deformity of hand, right hand**
- **M21.942 Unspecified acquired deformity of hand, left hand**
- **M21.949 Unspecified acquired deformity of hand, unspecified hand**

M21.95 Unspecified acquired deformity of thigh
- **M21.951 Unspecified acquired deformity of right thigh**
- **M21.952 Unspecified acquired deformity of left thigh**
- **M21.959 Unspecified acquired deformity of unspecified thigh**

M21.96 Unspecified acquired deformity of lower leg
- **M21.961 Unspecified acquired deformity of right lower leg**
- **M21.962 Unspecified acquired deformity of left lower leg**
- **M21.969 Unspecified acquired deformity of unspecified lower leg**

M22 Disorder of patella

EXCLUDES 2 *traumatic dislocation of patella (S83.0-)*

M22.0 Recurrent dislocation of patella
- **M22.00 Recurrent dislocation of patella, unspecified knee**
- **M22.01 Recurrent dislocation of patella, right knee**
- **M22.02 Recurrent dislocation of patella, left knee**

M22.1 Recurrent subluxation of patella

Incomplete dislocation of patella

- **M22.10 Recurrent subluxation of patella, unspecified knee**
- **M22.11 Recurrent subluxation of patella, right knee**
- **M22.12 Recurrent subluxation of patella, left knee**

M22.2 Patellofemoral disorders

M22.2X Patellofemoral disorders
- **M22.2X1 Patellofemoral disorders, right knee**
- **M22.2X2 Patellofemoral disorders, left knee**
- **M22.2X9 Patellofemoral disorders, unspecified knee**

M22.3 Other derangements of patella

M22.3X Other derangements of patella
- **M22.3X1 Other derangements of patella, right knee**
- **M22.3X2 Other derangements of patella, left knee**
- **M22.3X9 Other derangements of patella, unspecified knee**

M22.4 Chondromalacia patellae
- **M22.40 Chondromalacia patellae, unspecified knee**
- **M22.41 Chondromalacia patellae, right knee**
- **M22.42 Chondromalacia patellae, left knee**

M22.8 Other disorders of patella

M22.8X Other disorders of patella
- **M22.8X1 Other disorders of patella, right knee**
- **M22.8X2 Other disorders of patella, left knee**
- **M22.8X9 Other disorders of patella, unspecified knee**

M22.9 Unspecified disorder of patella
- **M22.90 Unspecified disorder of patella, unspecified knee**
- **M22.91 Unspecified disorder of patella, right knee**
- **M22.92 Unspecified disorder of patella, left knee**

M23 Internal derangement of knee

EXCLUDES 1 *ankylosis (M24.66)*
deformity of knee (M21.-)
osteochondritis dissecans (M93.2)

EXCLUDES 2 *current injury - see injury of knee and lower leg (S80-S89)*
recurrent dislocation or subluxation of joints (M24.4)
recurrent dislocation or subluxation of patella (M22.0-M22.1)

M23.0 Cystic meniscus

M23.00 Cystic meniscus, unspecified meniscus

Cystic meniscus, unspecified lateral meniscus
Cystic meniscus, unspecified medial meniscus

- **M23.000 Cystic meniscus, unspecified lateral meniscus, right knee**
- **M23.001 Cystic meniscus, unspecified lateral meniscus, left knee**
- **M23.002 Cystic meniscus, unspecified lateral meniscus, unspecified knee**
- **M23.003 Cystic meniscus, unspecified medial meniscus, right knee**
- **M23.004 Cystic meniscus, unspecified medial meniscus, left knee**
- **M23.005 Cystic meniscus, unspecified medial meniscus, unspecified knee**
- **M23.006 Cystic meniscus, unspecified meniscus, right knee**
- **M23.007 Cystic meniscus, unspecified meniscus, left knee**
- **M23.009 Cystic meniscus, unspecified meniscus, unspecified knee**

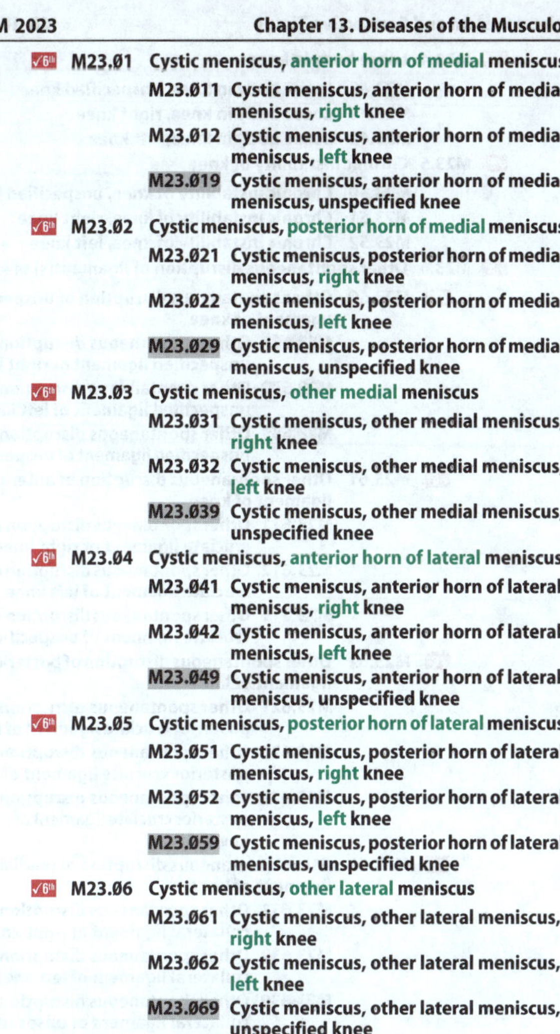

✓6th **M23.01 Cystic meniscus, anterior horn of medial meniscus**

M23.011 Cystic meniscus, anterior horn of medial meniscus, right knee

M23.012 Cystic meniscus, anterior horn of medial meniscus, left knee

M23.019 Cystic meniscus, anterior horn of medial meniscus, unspecified knee

✓6th **M23.02 Cystic meniscus, posterior horn of medial meniscus**

M23.021 Cystic meniscus, posterior horn of medial meniscus, right knee

M23.022 Cystic meniscus, posterior horn of medial meniscus, left knee

M23.029 Cystic meniscus, posterior horn of medial meniscus, unspecified knee

✓6th **M23.03 Cystic meniscus, other medial meniscus**

M23.031 Cystic meniscus, other medial meniscus, right knee

M23.032 Cystic meniscus, other medial meniscus, left knee

M23.039 Cystic meniscus, other medial meniscus, unspecified knee

✓6th **M23.04 Cystic meniscus, anterior horn of lateral meniscus**

M23.041 Cystic meniscus, anterior horn of lateral meniscus, right knee

M23.042 Cystic meniscus, anterior horn of lateral meniscus, left knee

M23.049 Cystic meniscus, anterior horn of lateral meniscus, unspecified knee

✓6th **M23.05 Cystic meniscus, posterior horn of lateral meniscus**

M23.051 Cystic meniscus, posterior horn of lateral meniscus, right knee

M23.052 Cystic meniscus, posterior horn of lateral meniscus, left knee

M23.059 Cystic meniscus, posterior horn of lateral meniscus, unspecified knee

✓6th **M23.06 Cystic meniscus, other lateral meniscus**

M23.061 Cystic meniscus, other lateral meniscus, right knee

M23.062 Cystic meniscus, other lateral meniscus, left knee

M23.069 Cystic meniscus, other lateral meniscus, unspecified knee

✓5th **M23.2 Derangement of meniscus due to old tear or injury**

Old bucket-handle tear

AHA: 2019,2Q,26

Derangement of Meniscus

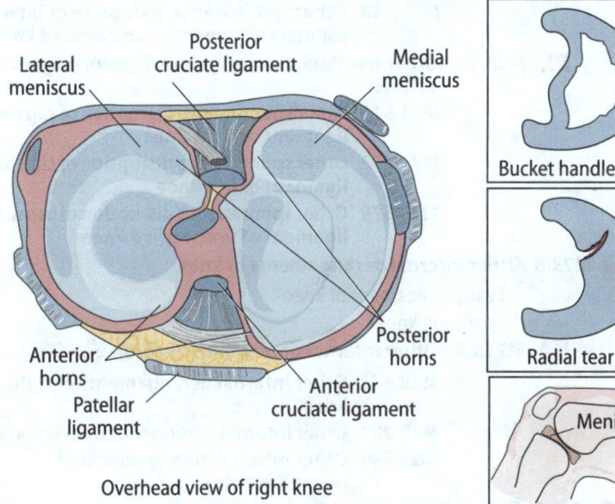

✓6th **M23.20 Derangement of unspecified meniscus due to old tear or injury**

Derangement of unspecified lateral meniscus due to old tear or injury

Derangement of unspecified medial meniscus due to old tear or injury

M23.200 Derangement of unspecified lateral meniscus due to old tear or injury, right knee

M23.201 Derangement of unspecified lateral meniscus due to old tear or injury, left knee

M23.202 Derangement of unspecified lateral meniscus due to old tear or injury, unspecified knee

M23.203 Derangement of unspecified medial meniscus due to old tear or injury, right knee

M23.204 Derangement of unspecified medial meniscus due to old tear or injury, left knee

M23.205 Derangement of unspecified medial meniscus due to old tear or injury, unspecified knee

M23.206 Derangement of unspecified meniscus due to old tear or injury, right knee

M23.207 Derangement of unspecified meniscus due to old tear or injury, left knee

M23.209 Derangement of unspecified meniscus due to old tear or injury, unspecified knee

✓6th **M23.21 Derangement of anterior horn of medial meniscus due to old tear or injury**

M23.211 Derangement of anterior horn of medial meniscus due to old tear or injury, right knee

M23.212 Derangement of anterior horn of medial meniscus due to old tear or injury, left knee

M23.219 Derangement of anterior horn of medial meniscus due to old tear or injury, unspecified knee

✓6th **M23.22 Derangement of posterior horn of medial meniscus due to old tear or injury**

M23.221 Derangement of posterior horn of medial meniscus due to old tear or injury, right knee

M23.222 Derangement of posterior horn of medial meniscus due to old tear or injury, left knee

M23.229 Derangement of posterior horn of medial meniscus due to old tear or injury, unspecified knee

✓6th **M23.23 Derangement of other medial meniscus due to old tear or injury**

M23.231 Derangement of other medial meniscus due to old tear or injury, right knee

M23.232 Derangement of other medial meniscus due to old tear or injury, left knee

M23.239 Derangement of other medial meniscus due to old tear or injury, unspecified knee

✓6th **M23.24 Derangement of anterior horn of lateral meniscus due to old tear or injury**

M23.241 Derangement of anterior horn of lateral meniscus due to old tear or injury, right knee

M23.242 Derangement of anterior horn of lateral meniscus due to old tear or injury, left knee

M23.249 Derangement of anterior horn of lateral meniscus due to old tear or injury, unspecified knee

✓6th **M23.25 Derangement of posterior horn of lateral meniscus due to old tear or injury**

M23.251 Derangement of posterior horn of lateral meniscus due to old tear or injury, right knee

M23.252 Derangement of posterior horn of lateral meniscus due to old tear or injury, left knee

M23.259 Derangement of posterior horn of lateral meniscus due to old tear or injury, unspecified knee

✓6th **M23.26 Derangement of other lateral meniscus due to old tear or injury**

M23.261 Derangement of other lateral meniscus due to old tear or injury, right knee

M23.262 Derangement of other lateral meniscus due to old tear or injury, left knee

M23.269 Derangement of other lateral meniscus due to old tear or injury, unspecified knee

M23.3 Other meniscus derangements
- Degenerate meniscus
- Detached meniscus
- Retained meniscus

M23.30 Other meniscus derangements, unspecified meniscus
- Other meniscus derangements, unspecified lateral meniscus
- Other meniscus derangements, unspecified medial meniscus

M23.300 Other meniscus derangements, unspecified lateral meniscus, right knee
M23.301 Other meniscus derangements, unspecified lateral meniscus, left knee
M23.302 Other meniscus derangements, unspecified lateral meniscus, unspecified knee
M23.303 Other meniscus derangements, unspecified medial meniscus, right knee
M23.304 Other meniscus derangements, unspecified medial meniscus, left knee
M23.305 Other meniscus derangements, unspecified medial meniscus, unspecified knee
M23.306 Other meniscus derangements, unspecified meniscus, right knee
M23.307 Other meniscus derangements, unspecified meniscus, left knee
M23.309 Other meniscus derangements, unspecified meniscus, unspecified knee

M23.31 Other meniscus derangements, anterior horn of medial meniscus
M23.311 Other meniscus derangements, anterior horn of medial meniscus, right knee
M23.312 Other meniscus derangements, anterior horn of medial meniscus, left knee
M23.319 Other meniscus derangements, anterior horn of medial meniscus, unspecified knee

M23.32 Other meniscus derangements, posterior horn of medial meniscus
M23.321 Other meniscus derangements, posterior horn of medial meniscus, right knee
M23.322 Other meniscus derangements, posterior horn of medial meniscus, left knee
M23.329 Other meniscus derangements, posterior horn of medial meniscus, unspecified knee

M23.33 Other meniscus derangements, other medial meniscus
M23.331 Other meniscus derangements, other medial meniscus, right knee
M23.332 Other meniscus derangements, other medial meniscus, left knee
M23.339 Other meniscus derangements, other medial meniscus, unspecified knee

M23.34 Other meniscus derangements, anterior horn of lateral meniscus
M23.341 Other meniscus derangements, anterior horn of lateral meniscus, right knee
M23.342 Other meniscus derangements, anterior horn of lateral meniscus, left knee
M23.349 Other meniscus derangements, anterior horn of lateral meniscus, unspecified knee

M23.35 Other meniscus derangements, posterior horn of lateral meniscus
M23.351 Other meniscus derangements, posterior horn of lateral meniscus, right knee
M23.352 Other meniscus derangements, posterior horn of lateral meniscus, left knee
M23.359 Other meniscus derangements, posterior horn of lateral meniscus, unspecified knee

M23.36 Other meniscus derangements, other lateral meniscus
M23.361 Other meniscus derangements, other lateral meniscus, right knee
M23.362 Other meniscus derangements, other lateral meniscus, left knee
M23.369 Other meniscus derangements, other lateral meniscus, unspecified knee

M23.4 Loose body in knee
M23.40 Loose body in knee, unspecified knee
M23.41 Loose body in knee, right knee
M23.42 Loose body in knee, left knee

M23.5 Chronic instability of knee
M23.50 Chronic instability of knee, unspecified knee
M23.51 Chronic instability of knee, right knee
M23.52 Chronic instability of knee, left knee

M23.6 Other spontaneous disruption of ligament(s) of knee

M23.60 Other spontaneous disruption of unspecified ligament of knee
M23.601 Other spontaneous disruption of unspecified ligament of right knee
M23.602 Other spontaneous disruption of unspecified ligament of left knee
M23.609 Other spontaneous disruption of unspecified ligament of unspecified knee

M23.61 Other spontaneous disruption of anterior cruciate ligament of knee
M23.611 Other spontaneous disruption of anterior cruciate ligament of right knee
M23.612 Other spontaneous disruption of anterior cruciate ligament of left knee
M23.619 Other spontaneous disruption of anterior cruciate ligament of unspecified knee

M23.62 Other spontaneous disruption of posterior cruciate ligament of knee
M23.621 Other spontaneous disruption of posterior cruciate ligament of right knee
M23.622 Other spontaneous disruption of posterior cruciate ligament of left knee
M23.629 Other spontaneous disruption of posterior cruciate ligament of unspecified knee

M23.63 Other spontaneous disruption of medial collateral ligament of knee
M23.631 Other spontaneous disruption of medial collateral ligament of right knee
M23.632 Other spontaneous disruption of medial collateral ligament of left knee
M23.639 Other spontaneous disruption of medial collateral ligament of unspecified knee

M23.64 Other spontaneous disruption of lateral collateral ligament of knee
M23.641 Other spontaneous disruption of lateral collateral ligament of right knee
M23.642 Other spontaneous disruption of lateral collateral ligament of left knee
M23.649 Other spontaneous disruption of lateral collateral ligament of unspecified knee

M23.67 Other spontaneous disruption of capsular ligament of knee
M23.671 Other spontaneous disruption of capsular ligament of right knee
M23.672 Other spontaneous disruption of capsular ligament of left knee
M23.679 Other spontaneous disruption of capsular ligament of unspecified knee

M23.8 Other internal derangements of knee
- Laxity of ligament of knee
- Snapping knee

M23.8X Other internal derangements of knee
M23.8X1 Other internal derangements of right knee
M23.8X2 Other internal derangements of left knee
M23.8X9 Other internal derangements of unspecified knee

M23.9 Unspecified internal derangement of knee
M23.90 Unspecified internal derangement of unspecified knee
M23.91 Unspecified internal derangement of right knee
M23.92 Unspecified internal derangement of left knee

M24 Other specific joint derangements

EXCLUDES 1 *current injury - see injury of joint by body region*

EXCLUDES 2 *ganglion (M67.4)*
snapping knee (M23.8-)
temporomandibular joint disorders (M26.6-)

AHA: 2020,4Q,31-32

M24.0 Loose body in joint

EXCLUDES 2 *loose body in knee (M23.4)*

M24.00 Loose body in unspecified joint
M24.01 Loose body in shoulder
- **M24.011** Loose body in right shoulder
- **M24.012** Loose body in left shoulder
- **M24.019** Loose body in unspecified shoulder

M24.02 Loose body in elbow
- **M24.021** Loose body in right elbow
- **M24.022** Loose body in left elbow
- **M24.029** Loose body in unspecified elbow

M24.03 Loose body in wrist
- **M24.031** Loose body in right wrist
- **M24.032** Loose body in left wrist
- **M24.039** Loose body in unspecified wrist

M24.04 Loose body in finger joints
- **M24.041** Loose body in right finger joint(s)
- **M24.042** Loose body in left finger joint(s)
- **M24.049** Loose body in unspecified finger joint(s)

M24.05 Loose body in hip
- **M24.051** Loose body in right hip
- **M24.052** Loose body in left hip
- **M24.059** Loose body in unspecified hip

M24.07 Loose body in ankle and toe joints
- **M24.071** Loose body in right ankle
- **M24.072** Loose body in left ankle
- **M24.073** Loose body in unspecified ankle
- **M24.074** Loose body in right toe joint(s)
- **M24.075** Loose body in left toe joint(s)
- **M24.076** Loose body in unspecified toe joints

M24.08 Loose body, other site

M24.1 Other articular cartilage disorders

EXCLUDES 2 *chondrocalcinosis (M11.1, M11.2-)*
internal derangement of knee (M23.-)
metastatic calcification (E83.5)
ochronosis (E70.2)

M24.10 Other articular cartilage disorders, unspecified site
M24.11 Other articular cartilage disorders, shoulder
- **M24.111** Other articular cartilage disorders, right shoulder
- **M24.112** Other articular cartilage disorders, left shoulder
- **M24.119** Other articular cartilage disorders, unspecified shoulder

M24.12 Other articular cartilage disorders, elbow
- **M24.121** Other articular cartilage disorders, right elbow
- **M24.122** Other articular cartilage disorders, left elbow
- **M24.129** Other articular cartilage disorders, unspecified elbow

M24.13 Other articular cartilage disorders, wrist
- **M24.131** Other articular cartilage disorders, right wrist
- **M24.132** Other articular cartilage disorders, left wrist
- **M24.139** Other articular cartilage disorders, unspecified wrist

M24.14 Other articular cartilage disorders, hand
- **M24.141** Other articular cartilage disorders, right hand
- **M24.142** Other articular cartilage disorders, left hand
- **M24.149** Other articular cartilage disorders, unspecified hand

M24.15 Other articular cartilage disorders, hip
- **M24.151** Other articular cartilage disorders, right hip
- **M24.152** Other articular cartilage disorders, left hip
- **M24.159** Other articular cartilage disorders, unspecified hip

M24.17 Other articular cartilage disorders, ankle and foot
- **M24.171** Other articular cartilage disorders, right ankle
- **M24.172** Other articular cartilage disorders, left ankle
- **M24.173** Other articular cartilage disorders, unspecified ankle
- **M24.174** Other articular cartilage disorders, right foot
- **M24.175** Other articular cartilage disorders, left foot
- **M24.176** Other articular cartilage disorders, unspecified foot

M24.19 Other articular cartilage disorders, other specified site

M24.2 Disorder of ligament

Instability secondary to old ligament injury
Ligamentous laxity NOS

EXCLUDES 1 *familial ligamentous laxity (M35.7)*

EXCLUDES 2 *internal derangement of knee (M23.5-M23.8X9)*

M24.20 Disorder of ligament, unspecified site
M24.21 Disorder of ligament, shoulder
- **M24.211** Disorder of ligament, right shoulder
- **M24.212** Disorder of ligament, left shoulder
- **M24.219** Disorder of ligament, unspecified shoulder

M24.22 Disorder of ligament, elbow
- **M24.221** Disorder of ligament, right elbow
- **M24.222** Disorder of ligament, left elbow
- **M24.229** Disorder of ligament, unspecified elbow

M24.23 Disorder of ligament, wrist
- **M24.231** Disorder of ligament, right wrist
- **M24.232** Disorder of ligament, left wrist
- **M24.239** Disorder of ligament, unspecified wrist

M24.24 Disorder of ligament, hand
- **M24.241** Disorder of ligament, right hand
- **M24.242** Disorder of ligament, left hand
- **M24.249** Disorder of ligament, unspecified hand

M24.25 Disorder of ligament, hip
- **M24.251** Disorder of ligament, right hip
- **M24.252** Disorder of ligament, left hip
- **M24.259** Disorder of ligament, unspecified hip

M24.27 Disorder of ligament, ankle and foot
- **M24.271** Disorder of ligament, right ankle
- **M24.272** Disorder of ligament, left ankle
- **M24.273** Disorder of ligament, unspecified ankle
- **M24.274** Disorder of ligament, right foot
- **M24.275** Disorder of ligament, left foot
- **M24.276** Disorder of ligament, unspecified foot

M24.28 Disorder of ligament, vertebrae
M24.29 Disorder of ligament, other specified site

M24.3 Pathological dislocation of joint, not elsewhere classified

EXCLUDES 1 *congenital dislocation or displacement of joint - see congenital malformations and deformations of the musculoskeletal system (Q65-Q79)*
current injury - see injury of joints and ligaments by body region
recurrent dislocation of joint (M24.4-)

M24.30 Pathological dislocation of unspecified joint, not elsewhere classified
M24.31 Pathological dislocation of shoulder, not elsewhere classified
- **M24.311** Pathological dislocation of right shoulder, not elsewhere classified
- **M24.312** Pathological dislocation of left shoulder, not elsewhere classified
- **M24.319** Pathological dislocation of unspecified shoulder, not elsewhere classified

M24.32 Pathological dislocation of elbow, not elsewhere classified
- **M24.321** Pathological dislocation of right elbow, not elsewhere classified
- **M24.322** Pathological dislocation of left elbow, not elsewhere classified
- **M24.329** Pathological dislocation of unspecified elbow, not elsewhere classified

6th **M24.33 Pathological dislocation of wrist, not elsewhere classified**
- **M24.331 Pathological dislocation of right wrist, not elsewhere classified**
- **M24.332 Pathological dislocation of left wrist, not elsewhere classified**
- **M24.339 Pathological dislocation of unspecified wrist, not elsewhere classified**

6th **M24.34 Pathological dislocation of hand, not elsewhere classified**
- **M24.341 Pathological dislocation of right hand, not elsewhere classified**
- **M24.342 Pathological dislocation of left hand, not elsewhere classified**
- **M24.349 Pathological dislocation of unspecified hand, not elsewhere classified**

6th **M24.35 Pathological dislocation of hip, not elsewhere classified**
AHA: 2022,1Q,32
- **M24.351 Pathological dislocation of right hip, not elsewhere classified**
- **M24.352 Pathological dislocation of left hip, not elsewhere classified**
- **M24.359 Pathological dislocation of unspecified hip, not elsewhere classified**

6th **M24.36 Pathological dislocation of knee, not elsewhere classified**
- **M24.361 Pathological dislocation of right knee, not elsewhere classified**
- **M24.362 Pathological dislocation of left knee, not elsewhere classified**
- **M24.369 Pathological dislocation of unspecified knee, not elsewhere classified**

6th **M24.37 Pathological dislocation of ankle and foot, not elsewhere classified**
- **M24.371 Pathological dislocation of right ankle, not elsewhere classified**
- **M24.372 Pathological dislocation of left ankle, not elsewhere classified**
- **M24.373 Pathological dislocation of unspecified ankle, not elsewhere classified**
- **M24.374 Pathological dislocation of right foot, not elsewhere classified**
- **M24.375 Pathological dislocation of left foot, not elsewhere classified**
- **M24.376 Pathological dislocation of unspecified foot, not elsewhere classified**

M24.39 Pathological dislocation of other specified joint, not elsewhere classified

5th **M24.4 Recurrent dislocation of joint**
Recurrent subluxation of joint
EXCLUDES 2 *recurrent dislocation of patella (M22.Ø-M22.1)*
recurrent vertebral dislocation (M43.3-, M43.4, M43.5-)

M24.4Ø Recurrent dislocation, unspecified joint

6th **M24.41 Recurrent dislocation, shoulder**
- **M24.411 Recurrent dislocation, right shoulder**
- **M24.412 Recurrent dislocation, left shoulder**
- **M24.419 Recurrent dislocation, unspecified shoulder**

6th **M24.42 Recurrent dislocation, elbow**
- **M24.421 Recurrent dislocation, right elbow**
- **M24.422 Recurrent dislocation, left elbow**
- **M24.429 Recurrent dislocation, unspecified elbow**

6th **M24.43 Recurrent dislocation, wrist**
- **M24.431 Recurrent dislocation, right wrist**
- **M24.432 Recurrent dislocation, left wrist**
- **M24.439 Recurrent dislocation, unspecified wrist**

6th **M24.44 Recurrent dislocation, hand and finger(s)**
- **M24.441 Recurrent dislocation, right hand**
- **M24.442 Recurrent dislocation, left hand**
- **M24.443 Recurrent dislocation, unspecified hand**
- **M24.444 Recurrent dislocation, right finger**
- **M24.445 Recurrent dislocation, left finger**
- **M24.446 Recurrent dislocation, unspecified finger**

6th **M24.45 Recurrent dislocation, hip**
- **M24.451 Recurrent dislocation, right hip**
- **M24.452 Recurrent dislocation, left hip**
- **M24.459 Recurrent dislocation, unspecified hip**

6th **M24.46 Recurrent dislocation, knee**
- **M24.461 Recurrent dislocation, right knee**
- **M24.462 Recurrent dislocation, left knee**
- **M24.469 Recurrent dislocation, unspecified knee**

6th **M24.47 Recurrent dislocation, ankle, foot and toes**
- **M24.471 Recurrent dislocation, right ankle**
- **M24.472 Recurrent dislocation, left ankle**
- **M24.473 Recurrent dislocation, unspecified ankle**
- **M24.474 Recurrent dislocation, right foot**
- **M24.475 Recurrent dislocation, left foot**
- **M24.476 Recurrent dislocation, unspecified foot**
- **M24.477 Recurrent dislocation, right toe(s)**
- **M24.478 Recurrent dislocation, left toe(s)**
- **M24.479 Recurrent dislocation, unspecified toe(s)**

M24.49 Recurrent dislocation, other specified joint

5th **M24.5 Contracture of joint**
EXCLUDES 1 *contracture of muscle without contracture of joint (M62.4-)*
contracture of tendon (sheath) without contracture of joint (M62.4-)
Dupuytren's contracture (M72.Ø)
EXCLUDES 2 *acquired deformities of limbs (M2Ø-M21)*
AHA: 2016,2Q,6

M24.5Ø Contracture, unspecified joint

6th **M24.51 Contracture, shoulder**
- **M24.511 Contracture, right shoulder**
- **M24.512 Contracture, left shoulder**
- **M24.519 Contracture, unspecified shoulder**

6th **M24.52 Contracture, elbow**
- **M24.521 Contracture, right elbow**
- **M24.522 Contracture, left elbow**
- **M24.529 Contracture, unspecified elbow**

6th **M24.53 Contracture, wrist**
- **M24.531 Contracture, right wrist**
- **M24.532 Contracture, left wrist**
- **M24.539 Contracture, unspecified wrist**

6th **M24.54 Contracture, hand**
- **M24.541 Contracture, right hand**
- **M24.542 Contracture, left hand**
- **M24.549 Contracture, unspecified hand**

6th **M24.55 Contracture, hip**
- **M24.551 Contracture, right hip**
- **M24.552 Contracture, left hip**
- **M24.559 Contracture, unspecified hip**

6th **M24.56 Contracture, knee**
- **M24.561 Contracture, right knee**
- **M24.562 Contracture, left knee**
- **M24.569 Contracture, unspecified knee**

6th **M24.57 Contracture, ankle and foot**
- **M24.571 Contracture, right ankle**
- **M24.572 Contracture, left ankle**
- **M24.573 Contracture, unspecified ankle**
- **M24.574 Contracture, right foot**
- **M24.575 Contracture, left foot**
- **M24.576 Contracture, unspecified foot**

M24.59 Contracture, other specified joint

5th **M24.6 Ankylosis of joint**
EXCLUDES 1 *stiffness of joint without ankylosis (M25.6-)*
EXCLUDES 2 *spine (M43.2-)*
DEF: Ankylosis: Abnormal union or fusion of bones in a joint, which is normally moveable.

M24.6Ø Ankylosis, unspecified joint

6th **M24.61 Ankylosis, shoulder**
- **M24.611 Ankylosis, right shoulder**
- **M24.612 Ankylosis, left shoulder**
- **M24.619 Ankylosis, unspecified shoulder**

6th **M24.62 Ankylosis, elbow**
- **M24.621 Ankylosis, right elbow**
- **M24.622 Ankylosis, left elbow**
- **M24.629 Ankylosis, unspecified elbow**

6th **M24.63 Ankylosis, wrist**
- **M24.631 Ankylosis, right wrist**
- **M24.632 Ankylosis, left wrist**
- **M24.639 Ankylosis, unspecified wrist**

M24.64 Ankylosis, hand
M24.641 Ankylosis, right hand
M24.642 Ankylosis, left hand
M24.649 Ankylosis, unspecified hand
M24.65 Ankylosis, hip
M24.651 Ankylosis, right hip
M24.652 Ankylosis, left hip
M24.659 Ankylosis, unspecified hip
M24.66 Ankylosis, knee
M24.661 Ankylosis, right knee
M24.662 Ankylosis, left knee
M24.669 Ankylosis, unspecified knee
M24.67 Ankylosis, ankle and foot
M24.671 Ankylosis, right ankle
M24.672 Ankylosis, left ankle
M24.673 Ankylosis, unspecified ankle
M24.674 Ankylosis, right foot
M24.675 Ankylosis, left foot
M24.676 Ankylosis, unspecified foot
M24.69 Ankylosis, other specified joint

M24.7 Protrusio acetabuli

DEF: Intrapelvic protrusion of the acetabulum characterized by the sinking of the floor of the acetabulum, causing the femoral head to protrude. It limits hip movement and is of unknown etiology. ***Synonym(s):*** *Otto's pelvis.*

M24.8 Other specific joint derangements, not elsewhere classified

EXCLUDES 2 *iliotibial band syndrome (M76.3)*

M24.80 Other specific joint derangements of unspecified joint, not elsewhere classified
M24.81 Other specific joint derangements of shoulder, not elsewhere classified
M24.811 Other specific joint derangements of right shoulder, not elsewhere classified
M24.812 Other specific joint derangements of left shoulder, not elsewhere classified
M24.819 Other specific joint derangements of unspecified shoulder, not elsewhere classified
M24.82 Other specific joint derangements of elbow, not elsewhere classified
M24.821 Other specific joint derangements of right elbow, not elsewhere classified
M24.822 Other specific joint derangements of left elbow, not elsewhere classified
M24.829 Other specific joint derangements of unspecified elbow, not elsewhere classified
M24.83 Other specific joint derangements of wrist, not elsewhere classified
M24.831 Other specific joint derangements of right wrist, not elsewhere classified
M24.832 Other specific joint derangements of left wrist, not elsewhere classified
M24.839 Other specific joint derangements of unspecified wrist, not elsewhere classified
M24.84 Other specific joint derangements of hand, not elsewhere classified
M24.841 Other specific joint derangements of right hand, not elsewhere classified
M24.842 Other specific joint derangements of left hand, not elsewhere classified
M24.849 Other specific joint derangements of unspecified hand, not elsewhere classified
M24.85 Other specific joint derangements of hip, not elsewhere classified

Irritable hip

M24.851 Other specific joint derangements of right hip, not elsewhere classified
M24.852 Other specific joint derangements of left hip, not elsewhere classified
M24.859 Other specific joint derangements of unspecified hip, not elsewhere classified
M24.87 Other specific joint derangements of ankle and foot, not elsewhere classified
M24.871 Other specific joint derangements of right ankle, not elsewhere classified
M24.872 Other specific joint derangements of left ankle, not elsewhere classified
M24.873 Other specific joint derangements of unspecified ankle, not elsewhere classified
M24.874 Other specific joint derangements of right foot, not elsewhere classified
M24.875 Other specific joint derangements left foot, not elsewhere classified
M24.876 Other specific joint derangements of unspecified foot, not elsewhere classified
M24.89 Other specific joint derangement of other specified joint, not elsewhere classified

M24.9 Joint derangement, unspecified

M25 Other joint disorder, not elsewhere classified

EXCLUDES 2 *abnormality of gait and mobility (R26.-)*
acquired deformities of limb (M20-M21)
calcification of bursa (M71.4-)
calcification of shoulder (joint) (M75.3)
calcification of tendon (M65.2-)
difficulty in walking (R26.2)
temporomandibular joint disorder (M26.6-)

AHA: 2020,4Q,31-32

M25.0 Hemarthrosis

EXCLUDES 1 *current injury - see injury of joint by body region*
hemophilic arthropathy (M36.2)

M25.00 Hemarthrosis, unspecified joint CC UNS
M25.01 Hemarthrosis, shoulder
M25.011 Hemarthrosis, right shoulder CC
M25.012 Hemarthrosis, left shoulder CC
M25.019 Hemarthrosis, unspecified shoulder CC UNS
M25.02 Hemarthrosis, elbow
M25.021 Hemarthrosis, right elbow CC
M25.022 Hemarthrosis, left elbow CC
M25.029 Hemarthrosis, unspecified elbow CC UNS
M25.03 Hemarthrosis, wrist
M25.031 Hemarthrosis, right wrist CC
M25.032 Hemarthrosis, left wrist CC
M25.039 Hemarthrosis, unspecified wrist CC UNS
M25.04 Hemarthrosis, hand
M25.041 Hemarthrosis, right hand CC
M25.042 Hemarthrosis, left hand CC
M25.049 Hemarthrosis, unspecified hand CC UNS
M25.05 Hemarthrosis, hip
M25.051 Hemarthrosis, right hip CC
M25.052 Hemarthrosis, left hip CC
M25.059 Hemarthrosis, unspecified hip CC UNS
M25.06 Hemarthrosis, knee
M25.061 Hemarthrosis, right knee CC
M25.062 Hemarthrosis, left knee CC
M25.069 Hemarthrosis, unspecified knee CC UNS
M25.07 Hemarthrosis, ankle and foot
M25.071 Hemarthrosis, right ankle CC
M25.072 Hemarthrosis, left ankle CC
M25.073 Hemarthrosis, unspecified ankle CC UNS
M25.074 Hemarthrosis, right foot CC
M25.075 Hemarthrosis, left foot CC
M25.076 Hemarthrosis, unspecified foot CC UNS
M25.08 Hemarthrosis, other specified site CC

Hemarthrosis, vertebrae

M25.1 Fistula of joint

M25.10 Fistula, unspecified joint
M25.11 Fistula, shoulder
M25.111 Fistula, right shoulder
M25.112 Fistula, left shoulder
M25.119 Fistula, unspecified shoulder
M25.12 Fistula, elbow
M25.121 Fistula, right elbow
M25.122 Fistula, left elbow
M25.129 Fistula, unspecified elbow

M25.13 Fistula, wrist
- **M25.131 Fistula, right wrist**
- **M25.132 Fistula, left wrist**
- **M25.139 Fistula, unspecified wrist**

M25.14 Fistula, hand
- **M25.141 Fistula, right hand**
- **M25.142 Fistula, left hand**
- **M25.149 Fistula, unspecified hand**

M25.15 Fistula, hip
- **M25.151 Fistula, right hip**
- **M25.152 Fistula, left hip**
- **M25.159 Fistula, unspecified hip**

M25.16 Fistula, knee
- **M25.161 Fistula, right knee**
- **M25.162 Fistula, left knee**
- **M25.169 Fistula, unspecified knee**

M25.17 Fistula, ankle and foot
- **M25.171 Fistula, right ankle**
- **M25.172 Fistula, left ankle**
- **M25.173 Fistula, unspecified ankle**
- **M25.174 Fistula, right foot**
- **M25.175 Fistula, left foot**
- **M25.176 Fistula, unspecified foot**

M25.18 Fistula, other specified site
Fistula, vertebrae

M25.2 Flail joint

DEF: Hinged joint that exhibits an abnormal or excessive degree of range and mobility.

M25.20 Flail joint, unspecified joint

M25.21 Flail joint, shoulder
- **M25.211 Flail joint, right shoulder**
- **M25.212 Flail joint, left shoulder**
- **M25.219 Flail joint, unspecified shoulder**

M25.22 Flail joint, elbow
- **M25.221 Flail joint, right elbow**
- **M25.222 Flail joint, left elbow**
- **M25.229 Flail joint, unspecified elbow**

M25.23 Flail joint, wrist
- **M25.231 Flail joint, right wrist**
- **M25.232 Flail joint, left wrist**
- **M25.239 Flail joint, unspecified wrist**

M25.24 Flail joint, hand
- **M25.241 Flail joint, right hand**
- **M25.242 Flail joint, left hand**
- **M25.249 Flail joint, unspecified hand**

M25.25 Flail joint, hip
- **M25.251 Flail joint, right hip**
- **M25.252 Flail joint, left hip**
- **M25.259 Flail joint, unspecified hip**

M25.26 Flail joint, knee
- **M25.261 Flail joint, right knee**
- **M25.262 Flail joint, left knee**
- **M25.269 Flail joint, unspecified knee**

M25.27 Flail joint, ankle and foot
- **M25.271 Flail joint, right ankle and foot**
- **M25.272 Flail joint, left ankle and foot**
- **M25.279 Flail joint, unspecified ankle and foot**

M25.28 Flail joint, other site

M25.3 Other instability of joint

EXCLUDES 1 *instability of joint secondary to old ligament injury (M24.2-)*
instability of joint secondary to removal of joint prosthesis (M96.8-)

EXCLUDES 2 *spinal instabilities (M53.2-)*

M25.30 Other instability, unspecified joint

M25.31 Other instability, shoulder
- **M25.311 Other instability, right shoulder**
- **M25.312 Other instability, left shoulder**
- **M25.319 Other instability, unspecified shoulder**

M25.32 Other instability, elbow
- **M25.321 Other instability, right elbow**
- **M25.322 Other instability, left elbow**
- **M25.329 Other instability, unspecified elbow**

M25.33 Other instability, wrist
- **M25.331 Other instability, right wrist**
- **M25.332 Other instability, left wrist**
- **M25.339 Other instability, unspecified wrist**

M25.34 Other instability, hand
- **M25.341 Other instability, right hand**
- **M25.342 Other instability, left hand**
- **M25.349 Other instability, unspecified hand**

M25.35 Other instability, hip
- **M25.351 Other instability, right hip**
- **M25.352 Other instability, left hip**
- **M25.359 Other instability, unspecified hip**

M25.36 Other instability, knee
- **M25.361 Other instability, right knee**
- **M25.362 Other instability, left knee**
- **M25.369 Other instability, unspecified knee**

M25.37 Other instability, ankle and foot
- **M25.371 Other instability, right ankle**
- **M25.372 Other instability, left ankle**
- **M25.373 Other instability, unspecified ankle**
- **M25.374 Other instability, right foot**
- **M25.375 Other instability, left foot**
- **M25.376 Other instability, unspecified foot**

M25.39 Other instability, other specified joint

M25.4 Effusion of joint

EXCLUDES 1 *hydrarthrosis in yaws (A66.6)*
intermittent hydrarthrosis (M12.4-)
other infective (teno)synovitis (M65.1-)

M25.40 Effusion, unspecified joint

M25.41 Effusion, shoulder
- **M25.411 Effusion, right shoulder**
- **M25.412 Effusion, left shoulder**
- **M25.419 Effusion, unspecified shoulder**

M25.42 Effusion, elbow
- **M25.421 Effusion, right elbow**
- **M25.422 Effusion, left elbow**
- **M25.429 Effusion, unspecified elbow**

M25.43 Effusion, wrist
- **M25.431 Effusion, right wrist**
- **M25.432 Effusion, left wrist**
- **M25.439 Effusion, unspecified wrist**

M25.44 Effusion, hand
- **M25.441 Effusion, right hand**
- **M25.442 Effusion, left hand**
- **M25.449 Effusion, unspecified hand**

M25.45 Effusion, hip
- **M25.451 Effusion, right hip**
- **M25.452 Effusion, left hip**
- **M25.459 Effusion, unspecified hip**

M25.46 Effusion, knee
- **M25.461 Effusion, right knee**
- **M25.462 Effusion, left knee**
- **M25.469 Effusion, unspecified knee**

M25.47 Effusion, ankle and foot
- **M25.471 Effusion, right ankle**
- **M25.472 Effusion, left ankle**
- **M25.473 Effusion, unspecified ankle**
- **M25.474 Effusion, right foot**
- **M25.475 Effusion, left foot**
- **M25.476 Effusion, unspecified foot**

M25.48 Effusion, other site

M25.5 Pain in joint

EXCLUDES 2 *pain in hand (M79.64-)*
pain in fingers (M79.64-)
pain in foot (M79.67-)
pain in limb (M79.6-)
pain in toes (M79.67-)

M25.50 Pain in unspecified joint

M25.51 Pain in shoulder
- **M25.511 Pain in right shoulder**
- **M25.512 Pain in left shoulder**
- **M25.519 Pain in unspecified shoulder**

M25.52 Pain in elbow
- **M25.521 Pain in right elbow**
- **M25.522 Pain in left elbow**
- **M25.529 Pain in unspecified elbow**

M25.53 Pain in wrist
M25.531 Pain in right wrist
M25.532 Pain in left wrist
M25.539 Pain in unspecified wrist
M25.54 Pain in joints of hand
AHA: 2016,4Q,38
M25.541 Pain in joints of right hand
M25.542 Pain in joints of left hand
M25.549 Pain in joints of unspecified hand
Pain in joints of hand NOS
M25.55 Pain in hip
M25.551 Pain in right hip
M25.552 Pain in left hip
M25.559 Pain in unspecified hip
M25.56 Pain in knee
M25.561 Pain in right knee
M25.562 Pain in left knee
M25.569 Pain in unspecified knee
M25.57 Pain in ankle and joints of foot
M25.571 Pain in right ankle and joints of right foot
M25.572 Pain in left ankle and joints of left foot
M25.579 Pain in unspecified ankle and joints of unspecified foot
M25.59 Pain in other specified joint
M25.6 Stiffness of joint, not elsewhere classified
EXCLUDES 1 *ankylosis of joint (M24.6-)*
contracture of joint (M24.5-)
M25.60 Stiffness of unspecified joint, not elsewhere classified
M25.61 Stiffness of shoulder, not elsewhere classified
M25.611 Stiffness of right shoulder, not elsewhere classified
M25.612 Stiffness of left shoulder, not elsewhere classified
M25.619 Stiffness of unspecified shoulder, not elsewhere classified
M25.62 Stiffness of elbow, not elsewhere classified
M25.621 Stiffness of right elbow, not elsewhere classified
M25.622 Stiffness of left elbow, not elsewhere classified
M25.629 Stiffness of unspecified elbow, not elsewhere classified
M25.63 Stiffness of wrist, not elsewhere classified
M25.631 Stiffness of right wrist, not elsewhere classified
M25.632 Stiffness of left wrist, not elsewhere classified
M25.639 Stiffness of unspecified wrist, not elsewhere classified
M25.64 Stiffness of hand, not elsewhere classified
M25.641 Stiffness of right hand, not elsewhere classified
M25.642 Stiffness of left hand, not elsewhere classified
M25.649 Stiffness of unspecified hand, not elsewhere classified
M25.65 Stiffness of hip, not elsewhere classified
M25.651 Stiffness of right hip, not elsewhere classified
M25.652 Stiffness of left hip, not elsewhere classified
M25.659 Stiffness of unspecified hip, not elsewhere classified
M25.66 Stiffness of knee, not elsewhere classified
M25.661 Stiffness of right knee, not elsewhere classified
M25.662 Stiffness of left knee, not elsewhere classified
M25.669 Stiffness of unspecified knee, not elsewhere classified
M25.67 Stiffness of ankle and foot, not elsewhere classified
M25.671 Stiffness of right ankle, not elsewhere classified
M25.672 Stiffness of left ankle, not elsewhere classified
M25.673 Stiffness of unspecified ankle, not elsewhere classified
M25.674 Stiffness of right foot, not elsewhere classified
M25.675 Stiffness of left foot, not elsewhere classified
M25.676 Stiffness of unspecified foot, not elsewhere classified
M25.69 Stiffness of other specified joint, not elsewhere classified
M25.7 Osteophyte
M25.70 Osteophyte, unspecified joint
M25.71 Osteophyte, shoulder
M25.711 Osteophyte, right shoulder
M25.712 Osteophyte, left shoulder
M25.719 Osteophyte, unspecified shoulder
M25.72 Osteophyte, elbow
M25.721 Osteophyte, right elbow
M25.722 Osteophyte, left elbow
M25.729 Osteophyte, unspecified elbow
M25.73 Osteophyte, wrist
M25.731 Osteophyte, right wrist
M25.732 Osteophyte, left wrist
M25.739 Osteophyte, unspecified wrist
M25.74 Osteophyte, hand
M25.741 Osteophyte, right hand
M25.742 Osteophyte, left hand
M25.749 Osteophyte, unspecified hand
M25.75 Osteophyte, hip
M25.751 Osteophyte, right hip
M25.752 Osteophyte, left hip
M25.759 Osteophyte, unspecified hip
M25.76 Osteophyte, knee
M25.761 Osteophyte, right knee
M25.762 Osteophyte, left knee
M25.769 Osteophyte, unspecified knee
M25.77 Osteophyte, ankle and foot
M25.771 Osteophyte, right ankle
M25.772 Osteophyte, left ankle
M25.773 Osteophyte, unspecified ankle
M25.774 Osteophyte, right foot
M25.775 Osteophyte, left foot
M25.776 Osteophyte, unspecified foot
M25.78 Osteophyte, vertebrae
M25.8 Other specified joint disorders
M25.80 Other specified joint disorders, unspecified joint
M25.81 Other specified joint disorders, shoulder
M25.811 Other specified joint disorders, right shoulder
M25.812 Other specified joint disorders, left shoulder
M25.819 Other specified joint disorders, unspecified shoulder
M25.82 Other specified joint disorders, elbow
M25.821 Other specified joint disorders, right elbow
M25.822 Other specified joint disorders, left elbow
M25.829 Other specified joint disorders, unspecified elbow
M25.83 Other specified joint disorders, wrist
M25.831 Other specified joint disorders, right wrist
M25.832 Other specified joint disorders, left wrist
M25.839 Other specified joint disorders, unspecified wrist
M25.84 Other specified joint disorders, hand
M25.841 Other specified joint disorders, right hand
M25.842 Other specified joint disorders, left hand
M25.849 Other specified joint disorders, unspecified hand
M25.85 Other specified joint disorders, hip
AHA: 2014,4Q,25
M25.851 Other specified joint disorders, right hip
M25.852 Other specified joint disorders, left hip
M25.859 Other specified joint disorders, unspecified hip
M25.86 Other specified joint disorders, knee
M25.861 Other specified joint disorders, right knee
M25.862 Other specified joint disorders, left knee

M25.869 Other specified joint disorders, unspecified knee
M25.87 Other specified joint disorders, ankle and foot
M25.871 Other specified joint disorders, right ankle and foot
M25.872 Other specified joint disorders, left ankle and foot
M25.879 Other specified joint disorders, unspecified ankle and foot
M25.9 Joint disorder, unspecified

Dentofacial anomalies [including malocclusion] and other disorders of jaw (M26-M27)

EXCLUDES 1 *hemifacial atrophy or hypertrophy (Q67.4)*
unilateral condylar hyperplasia or hypoplasia (M27.8)

M26 Dentofacial anomalies [including malocclusion]

M26.0 Major anomalies of jaw size
EXCLUDES 1 *acromegaly (E22.0)*
Robin's syndrome (Q87.0)
M26.00 Unspecified anomaly of jaw size
M26.01 Maxillary hyperplasia
M26.02 Maxillary hypoplasia
AHA: 2014,3Q,23
M26.03 Mandibular hyperplasia
M26.04 Mandibular hypoplasia
M26.05 Macrogenia
M26.06 Microgenia
M26.07 Excessive tuberosity of jaw
Entire maxillary tuberosity
M26.09 Other specified anomalies of jaw size

M26.1 Anomalies of jaw-cranial base relationship
M26.10 Unspecified anomaly of jaw-cranial base relationship
M26.11 Maxillary asymmetry
M26.12 Other jaw asymmetry
M26.19 Other specified anomalies of jaw-cranial base relationship
AHA: 2020,1Q,21

M26.2 Anomalies of dental arch relationship
M26.20 Unspecified anomaly of dental arch relationship
M26.21 Malocclusion, Angle's class
M26.211 Malocclusion, Angle's class I
Neutro-occlusion
M26.212 Malocclusion, Angle's class II
Disto-occlusion Division I
Disto-occlusion Division II
M26.213 Malocclusion, Angle's class III
Mesio-occlusion
M26.219 Malocclusion, Angle's class, unspecified
M26.22 Open occlusal relationship
M26.220 Open anterior occlusal relationship
Anterior open bite
M26.221 Open posterior occlusal relationship
Posterior open bite
M26.23 Excessive horizontal overlap
Excessive horizontal overjet
M26.24 Reverse articulation
Crossbite (anterior) (posterior)
M26.25 Anomalies of interarch distance
M26.29 Other anomalies of dental arch relationship
Midline deviation of dental arch
Overbite (excessive) deep
Overbite (excessive) horizontal
Overbite (excessive) vertical
Posterior lingual occlusion of mandibular teeth

M26.3 Anomalies of tooth position of fully erupted tooth or teeth
EXCLUDES 2 *embedded and impacted teeth (K01.-)*
M26.30 Unspecified anomaly of tooth position of fully erupted tooth or teeth
Abnormal spacing of fully erupted tooth or teeth NOS
Displacement of fully erupted tooth or teeth NOS
Transposition of fully erupted tooth or teeth NOS
M26.31 Crowding of fully erupted teeth
M26.32 Excessive spacing of fully erupted teeth
Diastema of fully erupted tooth or teeth NOS
M26.33 Horizontal displacement of fully erupted tooth or teeth
Tipped tooth or teeth
Tipping of fully erupted tooth
M26.34 Vertical displacement of fully erupted tooth or teeth
Extruded tooth
Infraeruption of tooth or teeth
Supraeruption of tooth or teeth
M26.35 Rotation of fully erupted tooth or teeth
M26.36 Insufficient interocclusal distance of fully erupted teeth (ridge)
Lack of adequate intermaxillary vertical dimension of fully erupted teeth
M26.37 Excessive interocclusal distance of fully erupted teeth
Excessive intermaxillary vertical dimension of fully erupted teeth
Loss of occlusal vertical dimension of fully erupted teeth
M26.39 Other anomalies of tooth position of fully erupted tooth or teeth

M26.4 Malocclusion, unspecified

M26.5 Dentofacial functional abnormalities
EXCLUDES 1 *bruxism (F45.8)*
teeth-grinding NOS (F45.8)
M26.50 Dentofacial functional abnormalities, unspecified
M26.51 Abnormal jaw closure
M26.52 Limited mandibular range of motion
M26.53 Deviation in opening and closing of the mandible
M26.54 Insufficient anterior guidance
Insufficient anterior occlusal guidance
M26.55 Centric occlusion maximum intercuspation discrepancy
EXCLUDES 1 *centric occlusion NOS (M26.59)*
M26.56 Non-working side interference
Balancing side interference
M26.57 Lack of posterior occlusal support
M26.59 Other dentofacial functional abnormalities
Centric occlusion (of teeth) NOS
Malocclusion due to abnormal swallowing
Malocclusion due to mouth breathing
Malocclusion due to tongue, lip or finger habits

M26.6 Temporomandibular joint disorders
EXCLUDES 2 *current temporomandibular joint dislocation (S03.0)*
current temporomandibular joint sprain (S03.4)
AHA: 2016,4Q,38-39

Temporomandibular Joint

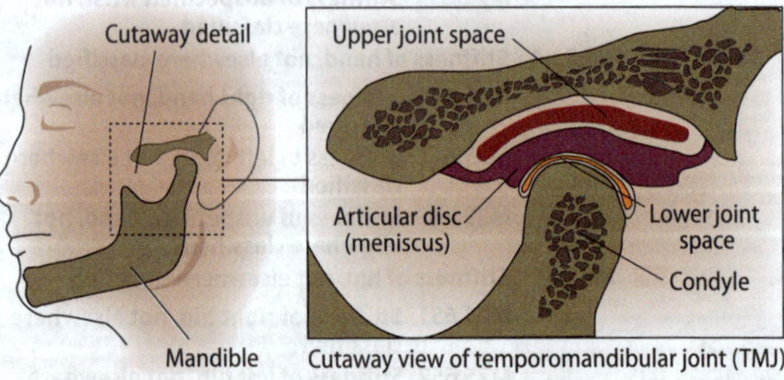

Cutaway view of temporomandibular joint (TMJ)

M26.60 Temporomandibular joint disorder, unspecified
M26.601 Right temporomandibular joint disorder, unspecified
M26.602 Left temporomandibular joint disorder, unspecified
M26.603 Bilateral temporomandibular joint disorder, unspecified
M26.609 Unspecified temporomandibular joint disorder, unspecified side
Temporomandibular joint disorder NOS
M26.61 Adhesions and ankylosis of temporomandibular joint
M26.611 Adhesions and ankylosis of right temporomandibular joint
M26.612 Adhesions and ankylosis of left temporomandibular joint

M26.613 Adhesions and ankylosis of bilateral temporomandibular joint
M26.619 Adhesions and ankylosis of temporomandibular joint, unspecified side
M26.62 Arthralgia of temporomandibular joint
M26.621 Arthralgia of right temporomandibular joint
M26.622 Arthralgia of left temporomandibular joint
M26.623 Arthralgia of bilateral temporomandibular joint
M26.629 Arthralgia of temporomandibular joint, unspecified side
M26.63 Articular disc disorder of temporomandibular joint
M26.631 Articular disc disorder of right temporomandibular joint
M26.632 Articular disc disorder of left temporomandibular joint
M26.633 Articular disc disorder of bilateral temporomandibular joint
M26.639 Articular disc disorder of temporomandibular joint, unspecified side
M26.64 Arthritis of temporomandibular joint
AHA: 2020,4Q,32
M26.641 Arthritis of right temporomandibular joint
M26.642 Arthritis of left temporomandibular joint
M26.643 Arthritis of bilateral temporomandibular joint
M26.649 Arthritis of unspecified temporomandibular joint
M26.65 Arthropathy of temporomandibular joint
AHA: 2020,4Q,32
M26.651 Arthropathy of right temporomandibular joint
M26.652 Arthropathy of left temporomandibular joint
M26.653 Arthropathy of bilateral temporomandibular joint
M26.659 Arthropathy of unspecified temporomandibular joint
M26.69 Other specified disorders of temporomandibular joint
M26.7 Dental alveolar anomalies
M26.70 Unspecified alveolar anomaly
M26.71 Alveolar maxillary hyperplasia
M26.72 Alveolar mandibular hyperplasia
M26.73 Alveolar maxillary hypoplasia
M26.74 Alveolar mandibular hypoplasia
M26.79 Other specified alveolar anomalies
M26.8 Other dentofacial anomalies
M26.81 Anterior soft tissue impingement
Anterior soft tissue impingement on teeth
M26.82 Posterior soft tissue impingement
Posterior soft tissue impingement on teeth
M26.89 Other dentofacial anomalies
M26.9 Dentofacial anomaly, unspecified
M27 Other diseases of jaws
M27.0 Developmental disorders of jaws
Latent bone cyst of jaw
Stafne's cyst
Torus mandibularis
Torus palatinus
M27.1 Giant cell granuloma, central
Giant cell granuloma NOS
EXCLUDES 1 *peripheral giant cell granuloma (K06.8)*
M27.2 Inflammatory conditions of jaws
Osteitis of jaw(s)
Osteomyelitis (neonatal) jaw(s)
Osteoradionecrosis jaw(s)
Periostitis jaw(s)
Sequestrum of jaw bone
Use additional code (W88-W90, X39.0) to identify radiation, if radiation-induced
EXCLUDES 2 *osteonecrosis of jaw due to drug (M87.180)*
M27.3 Alveolitis of jaws
Alveolar osteitis
Dry socket
M27.4 Other and unspecified cysts of jaw
EXCLUDES 1 *cysts of oral region (K09.-)*
latent bone cyst of jaw (M27.0)
Stafne's cyst (M27.0)
M27.40 Unspecified cyst of jaw
Cyst of jaw NOS
M27.49 Other cysts of jaw
Aneurysmal cyst of jaw
Hemorrhagic cyst of jaw
Traumatic cyst of jaw
M27.5 Periradicular pathology associated with previous endodontic treatment
M27.51 Perforation of root canal space due to endodontic treatment
M27.52 Endodontic overfill
M27.53 Endodontic underfill
M27.59 Other periradicular pathology associated with previous endodontic treatment
M27.6 Endosseous dental implant failure
M27.61 Osseointegration failure of dental implant
Hemorrhagic complications of dental implant placement
Iatrogenic osseointegration failure of dental implant
Osseointegration failure of dental implant due to complications of systemic disease
Osseointegration failure of dental implant due to poor bone quality
Pre-integration failure of dental implant NOS
Pre-osseointegration failure of dental implant
M27.62 Post-osseointegration biological failure of dental implant
Failure of dental implant due to lack of attached gingiva
Failure of dental implant due to occlusal trauma (caused by poor prosthetic design)
Failure of dental implant due to parafunctional habits
Failure of dental implant due to periodontal infection (peri-implantitis)
Failure of dental implant due to poor oral hygiene
Iatrogenic post-osseointegration failure of dental implant
Post-osseointegration failure of dental implant due to complications of systemic disease
M27.63 Post-osseointegration mechanical failure of dental implant
Failure of dental prosthesis causing loss of dental implant
Fracture of dental implant
EXCLUDES 2 *cracked tooth (K03.81)*
fractured dental restorative material with loss of material (K08.531)
fractured dental restorative material without loss of material (K08.530)
fractured tooth (S02.5)
M27.69 Other endosseous dental implant failure
Dental implant failure NOS
M27.8 Other specified diseases of jaws
Cherubism
Exostosis
Fibrous dysplasia
Unilateral condylar hyperplasia
Unilateral condylar hypoplasia
EXCLUDES 1 *jaw pain (R68.84)*
M27.9 Disease of jaws, unspecified

Systemic connective tissue disorders (M30-M36)

INCLUDES autoimmune disease NOS
collagen (vascular) disease NOS
systemic autoimmune disease
systemic collagen (vascular) disease

EXCLUDES 1 *autoimmune disease, single organ or single cell-type-code to relevant condition category*

M30 Polyarteritis nodosa and related conditions
EXCLUDES 1 *microscopic polyarteritis (M31.7)*

M30.0 Polyarteritis nodosa CC HCC
M30.1 Polyarteritis with lung involvement [Churg-Strauss] CC HCC
Allergic granulomatous angiitis
Eosinophilic granulomatosis with polyangiitis [EGPA]
AHA: 2021,1Q,23
M30.2 Juvenile polyarteritis CC HCC
M30.3 Mucocutaneous lymph node syndrome [Kawasaki] CC HCC
M30.8 Other conditions related to polyarteritis nodosa CC HCC
Polyangiitis overlap syndrome

M31 Other necrotizing vasculopathies
M31.0 Hypersensitivity angiitis CC HCC
Goodpasture's syndrome
M31.1 Thrombotic microangiopathy
AHA: 2021,4Q,19
M31.10 Thrombotic microangiopathy, unspecified MCC HCC
M31.11 Hematopoietic stem cell transplantation-associated thrombotic microangiopathy [HSCT-TMA] MCC HCC
Transplant-associated thrombotic microangiopathy [TA-TMA]
Code first if applicable:
complications of bone marrow transplant (T86.0-)
complications of stem cell transplant (T86.5)
Use additional code to identify specific organ dysfunction, such as:
acute kidney failure (N17.-)
acute respiratory distress syndrome (J80)
capillary leak syndrome (I78.8)
diffuse alveolar hemorrhage (R04.89)
encephalopathy (metabolic) (septic) (G93.41)
fluid overload, unspecified (E87.70)
graft versus host disease (D89.81-)
hemolytic uremic syndrome ▶(D59.3-)◀
hepatic failure (K72.-)
hepatic veno-occlusive disease (K76.5)
idiopathic interstitial pneumonia (J84.11-)
sinusoidal obstruction syndrome (K76.5)
M31.19 Other thrombotic microangiopathy MCC HCC
Thrombotic thrombocytopenic purpura
M31.2 Lethal midline granuloma CC HCC
M31.3 Wegener's granulomatosis
Granulomatosis with polyangiitis
Necrotizing respiratory granulomatosis
AHA: 2021,1Q,23
M31.30 Wegener's granulomatosis without renal involvement CC HCC
Wegener's granulomatosis NOS
AHA: 2021,2Q,10
M31.31 Wegener's granulomatosis with renal involvement CC HCC
M31.4 Aortic arch syndrome [Takayasu] CC HCC
M31.5 Giant cell arteritis with polymyalgia rheumatica HCC
M31.6 Other giant cell arteritis HCC
M31.7 Microscopic polyangiitis CC HCC
Microscopic polyarteritis
EXCLUDES 1 *polyarteritis nodosa (M30.0)*
AHA: 2021,1Q,23
M31.8 Other specified necrotizing vasculopathies CC HCC
Hypocomplementemic vasculitis
Septic vasculitis
M31.9 Necrotizing vasculopathy, unspecified CC HCC

M32 Systemic lupus erythematosus (SLE)
EXCLUDES 1 *lupus erythematosus (discoid) (NOS) (L93.0)*
AHA: 2020,4Q,11; 2018,3Q,14
TIP: There is no default code for "lupus NOS." Query the provider for the specific type of lupus in order to assign the appropriate code.
M32.0 Drug-induced systemic lupus erythematosus HCC
Use additional code for adverse effect, if applicable, to identify drug (T36-T50 with fifth or sixth character 5)
M32.1 Systemic lupus erythematosus with organ or system involvement
M32.10 Systemic lupus erythematosus, organ or system involvement unspecified HCC
M32.11 Endocarditis in systemic lupus erythematosus CC HCC
Libman-Sacks disease
M32.12 Pericarditis in systemic lupus erythematosus CC HCC
Lupus pericarditis
M32.13 Lung involvement in systemic lupus erythematosus HCC
Pleural effusion due to systemic lupus erythematosus
M32.14 Glomerular disease in systemic lupus erythematosus HCC
Lupus renal disease NOS
AHA: 2013,4Q,125
M32.15 Tubulo-interstitial nephropathy in systemic lupus erythematosus HCC
M32.19 Other organ or system involvement in systemic lupus erythematosus HCC
M32.8 Other forms of systemic lupus erythematosus HCC
M32.9 Systemic lupus erythematosus, unspecified HCC
SLE NOS
Systemic lupus erythematosus NOS
Systemic lupus erythematosus without organ involvement

M33 Dermatopolymyositis
AHA: 2017,4Q,18
M33.0 Juvenile dermatomyositis
M33.00 Juvenile dermatomyositis, organ involvement unspecified CC HCC
M33.01 Juvenile dermatomyositis with respiratory involvement CC HCC
M33.02 Juvenile dermatomyositis with myopathy CC HCC
M33.03 Juvenile dermatomyositis without myopathy CC HCC
M33.09 Juvenile dermatomyositis with other organ involvement CC HCC
M33.1 Other dermatomyositis
Adult dermatomyositis
M33.10 Other dermatomyositis, organ involvement unspecified CC HCC
M33.11 Other dermatomyositis with respiratory involvement CC HCC
M33.12 Other dermatomyositis with myopathy CC HCC
M33.13 Other dermatomyositis without myopathy CC HCC
Dermatomyositis NOS
M33.19 Other dermatomyositis with other organ involvement CC HCC
M33.2 Polymyositis
M33.20 Polymyositis, organ involvement unspecified CC HCC
M33.21 Polymyositis with respiratory involvement CC HCC
M33.22 Polymyositis with myopathy CC HCC
M33.29 Polymyositis with other organ involvement CC HCC
M33.9 Dermatopolymyositis, unspecified
M33.90 Dermatopolymyositis, unspecified, organ involvement unspecified CC HCC
M33.91 Dermatopolymyositis, unspecified with respiratory involvement CC HCC
M33.92 Dermatopolymyositis, unspecified with myopathy CC HCC
M33.93 Dermatopolymyositis, unspecified without myopathy CC HCC

M33.99 Dermatopolymyositis, unspecified with other organ involvement CC HCC

M34 Systemic sclerosis [scleroderma]
EXCLUDES 1 *circumscribed scleroderma (L94.Ø)*
neonatal scleroderma (P83.88)

M34.Ø Progressive systemic sclerosis HCC

M34.1 CR(E)ST syndrome HCC
Combination of calcinosis, Raynaud's phenomenon, esophageal dysfunction, sclerodactyly, telangiectasia

M34.2 Systemic sclerosis induced by drug and chemical HCC
Code first poisoning due to drug or toxin, if applicable (T36-T65 with fifth or sixth character 1-4 or 6)
Use additional code for adverse effect, if applicable, to identify drug (T36-T5Ø with fifth or sixth character 5)

M34.8 Other forms of systemic sclerosis

M34.81 Systemic sclerosis with lung involvement CC HCC
Code also if applicable:
other interstitial pulmonary diseases (J84.89)
secondary pulmonary arterial hypertension (I27.21)

M34.82 Systemic sclerosis with myopathy CC HCC

M34.83 Systemic sclerosis with polyneuropathy HCC

M34.89 Other systemic sclerosis HCC

M34.9 Systemic sclerosis, unspecified HCC

M35 Other systemic involvement of connective tissue
EXCLUDES 1 *reactive perforating collagenosis (L87.1)*

M35.Ø Sjögren syndrome
Sicca syndrome
Use additional code to identify associated manifestations
EXCLUDES 1 *dry mouth, unspecified (R68.2)*
AHA: 2021,4Q,20
DEF: Autoimmune disease associated with keratoconjunctivitis, laryngopharyngitis, rhinitis, dry mouth, enlarged parotid gland, and chronic polyarthritis.

M35.ØØ Sjögren syndrome, unspecified HCC

M35.Ø1 Sjögren syndrome with keratoconjunctivitis HCC

M35.Ø2 Sjögren syndrome with lung involvement HCC

M35.Ø3 Sjögren syndrome with myopathy CC HCC

M35.Ø4 Sjögren syndrome with tubulo-interstitial nephropathy HCC
Renal tubular acidosis in sicca syndrome

M35.Ø5 Sjögren syndrome with inflammatory arthritis HCC

M35.Ø6 Sjögren syndrome with peripheral nervous system involvement HCC

M35.Ø7 Sjögren syndrome with central nervous system involvement CC HCC

M35.Ø8 Sjögren syndrome with gastrointestinal involvement HCC

M35.ØA Sjögren syndrome with glomerular disease HCC

M35.ØB Sjögren syndrome with vasculitis HCC

M35.ØC Sjögren syndrome with dental involvement HCC

M35.Ø9 Sjögren syndrome with other organ involvement HCC

M35.1 Other overlap syndromes CC HCC
Mixed connective tissue disease
EXCLUDES 1 *polyangiitis overlap syndrome (M3Ø.8)*

M35.2 Behçet's disease CC HCC

M35.3 Polymyalgia rheumatica HCC
EXCLUDES 1 *polymyalgia rheumatica with giant cell arteritis (M31.5)*

M35.4 Diffuse (eosinophilic) fasciitis

M35.5 Multifocal fibrosclerosis CC HCC

M35.6 Relapsing panniculitis [Weber-Christian]
EXCLUDES 1 *lupus panniculitis (L93.2)*
panniculitis NOS (M79.3-)

M35.7 Hypermobility syndrome
Familial ligamentous laxity
EXCLUDES 1 *ligamentous laxity, NOS (M24.2-)*
EXCLUDES 2 *Ehlers-Danlos syndromes (Q79.6-)*

M35.8 Other specified systemic involvement of connective tissue
AHA: 2021,1Q,36; 2020,3Q,13-14

M35.81 Multisystem inflammatory syndrome CC HCC
MIS-A
MIS-C
Multisystem inflammatory syndrome in adults
Multisystem inflammatory syndrome in children
Pediatric inflammatory multisystem syndrome
PIMS
Code first, if applicable, COVID-19 (UØ7.1)
Code also any associated complications such as:
acute hepatic failure (K72.Ø-)
acute kidney failure (N17.-)
acute myocarditis (I4Ø.-)
acute respiratory distress syndrome (J8Ø)
cardiac arrhythmia (I47-I49.-)
pneumonia due to COVID-19 (J12.82)
severe sepsis (R65.2-)
viral cardiomyopathy (B33.24)
viral pericarditis (B33.23)
Use additional code, if applicable, for:
exposure to COVID-19 or SARS-CoV-2 infection (Z2Ø.822)
personal history of COVID-19 (Z86.16)
post COVID-19 condition (UØ9.9)
AHA: 2021,4Q,102; 2021,1Q,29,36,41
DEF: Hyperinflammatory condition that seems to be largely associated with past or present coronavirus disease 2019 (COVID-19) infection. Predominantly occurring in children, with less frequent occurrences in adults, symptoms often include fever, laboratory evidence of inflammation, and evidence of clinically severe illness requiring hospitalization with multisystem (two or more) organ involvement. ***Synonym(s):*** *MIS, MIS-C.*

M35.89 Other specified systemic involvement of connective tissue CC HCC

M35.9 Systemic involvement of connective tissue, unspecified HCC
Autoimmune disease (systemic) NOS
Collagen (vascular) disease NOS

M36 Systemic disorders of connective tissue in diseases classified elsewhere
EXCLUDES 2 *arthropathies in diseases classified elsewhere (M14.-)*

M36.Ø Dermato(poly)myositis in neoplastic disease CC HCC
Code first underlying neoplasm (CØØ-D49)

M36.1 Arthropathy in neoplastic disease
Code first underlying neoplasm, such as:
leukemia (C91-C95)
malignant histiocytosis (C96.A)
multiple myeloma (C9Ø.Ø)

M36.2 Hemophilic arthropathy
Hemarthrosis in hemophilic arthropathy
Code first underlying disease, such as:
factor VIII deficiency (D66)
with vascular defect ►(D68.Ø-)◄
factor IX deficiency (D67)
hemophilia (classical) (D66)
hemophilia B (D67)
hemophilia C (D68.1)

M36.3 Arthropathy in other blood disorders

M36.4 Arthropathy in hypersensitivity reactions classified elsewhere
Code first underlying disease, such as:
Henoch (-Schönlein) purpura (D69.Ø)
serum sickness (T8Ø.6-)

M36.8 Systemic disorders of connective tissue in other diseases classified elsewhere HCC
Code first underlying disease, such as:
alkaptonuria (E7Ø.2)
hypogammaglobulinemia (D8Ø.-)
ochronosis (E7Ø.2)

DORSOPATHIES (M40-M54)

Deforming dorsopathies (M40-M43)

M40 Kyphosis and lordosis

Code first underlying disease

EXCLUDES 1 *congenital kyphosis and lordosis (Q76.4)*
kyphoscoliosis (M41.-)
postprocedural kyphosis and lordosis (M96.-)

Kyphosis and Lordosis

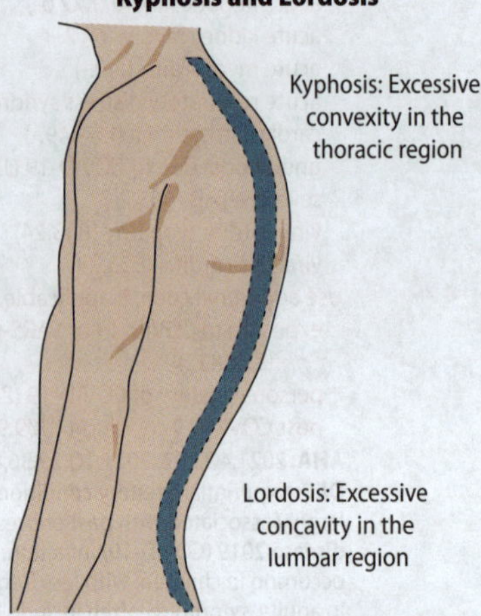

M40.0 Postural kyphosis

EXCLUDES 1 *osteochondrosis of spine (M42.-)*

- **M40.00** Postural kyphosis, site unspecified
- **M40.03** Postural kyphosis, cervicothoracic region
- **M40.04** Postural kyphosis, thoracic region
- **M40.05** Postural kyphosis, thoracolumbar region

M40.1 Other secondary kyphosis

- **M40.10** Other secondary kyphosis, site unspecified UPD
- **M40.12** Other secondary kyphosis, cervical region UPD
- **M40.13** Other secondary kyphosis, cervicothoracic region UPD
- **M40.14** Other secondary kyphosis, thoracic region UPD
- **M40.15** Other secondary kyphosis, thoracolumbar region UPD

M40.2 Other and unspecified kyphosis

M40.20 Unspecified kyphosis

- **M40.202** Unspecified kyphosis, cervical region
- **M40.203** Unspecified kyphosis, cervicothoracic region
- **M40.204** Unspecified kyphosis, thoracic region
- **M40.205** Unspecified kyphosis, thoracolumbar region
- **M40.209** Unspecified kyphosis, site unspecified

M40.29 Other kyphosis

- **M40.292** Other kyphosis, cervical region
- **M40.293** Other kyphosis, cervicothoracic region
- **M40.294** Other kyphosis, thoracic region
- **M40.295** Other kyphosis, thoracolumbar region
- **M40.299** Other kyphosis, site unspecified

M40.3 Flatback syndrome

- **M40.30** Flatback syndrome, site unspecified
- **M40.35** Flatback syndrome, thoracolumbar region
- **M40.36** Flatback syndrome, lumbar region
- **M40.37** Flatback syndrome, lumbosacral region

M40.4 Postural lordosis

Acquired lordosis

- **M40.40** Postural lordosis, site unspecified
- **M40.45** Postural lordosis, thoracolumbar region
- **M40.46** Postural lordosis, lumbar region
- **M40.47** Postural lordosis, lumbosacral region

M40.5 Lordosis, unspecified

- **M40.50** Lordosis, unspecified, site unspecified
- **M40.55** Lordosis, unspecified, thoracolumbar region
- **M40.56** Lordosis, unspecified, lumbar region
- **M40.57** Lordosis, unspecified, lumbosacral region

M41 Scoliosis

INCLUDES kyphoscoliosis

EXCLUDES 1 *congenital scoliosis due to bony malformation (Q76.3)*
congenital scoliosis NOS (Q67.5)
kyphoscoliotic heart disease (I27.1)
postural congenital scoliosis (Q67.5)

EXCLUDES 2 *postprocedural scoliosis (M96.-)*

AHA: 2022,1Q,30

Scoliosis

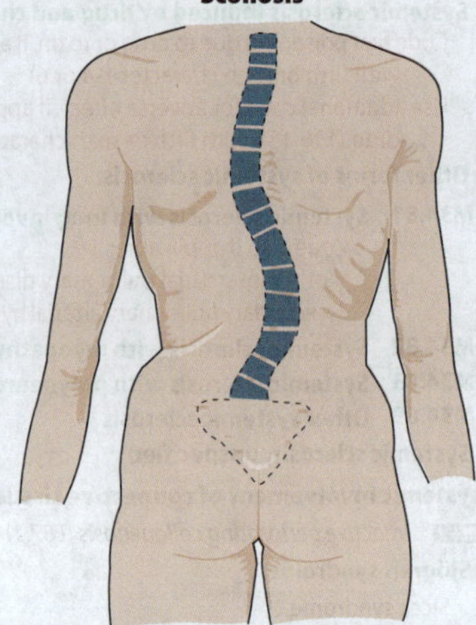

Lateral curvature of spine

M41.0 Infantile idiopathic scoliosis

AHA: 2014,4Q,26

- **M41.00** Infantile idiopathic scoliosis, site unspecified
- **M41.02** Infantile idiopathic scoliosis, cervical region
- **M41.03** Infantile idiopathic scoliosis, cervicothoracic region
- **M41.04** Infantile idiopathic scoliosis, thoracic region
- **M41.05** Infantile idiopathic scoliosis, thoracolumbar region
- **M41.06** Infantile idiopathic scoliosis, lumbar region
- **M41.07** Infantile idiopathic scoliosis, lumbosacral region
- **M41.08** Infantile idiopathic scoliosis, sacral and sacrococcygeal region

M41.1 Juvenile and adolescent idiopathic scoliosis

M41.11 Juvenile idiopathic scoliosis

AHA: 2014,4Q,28

- **M41.112** Juvenile idiopathic scoliosis, cervical region
- **M41.113** Juvenile idiopathic scoliosis, cervicothoracic region
- **M41.114** Juvenile idiopathic scoliosis, thoracic region
- **M41.115** Juvenile idiopathic scoliosis, thoracolumbar region
- **M41.116** Juvenile idiopathic scoliosis, lumbar region
- **M41.117** Juvenile idiopathic scoliosis, lumbosacral region
- **M41.119** Juvenile idiopathic scoliosis, site unspecified

M41.12 Adolescent scoliosis

- **M41.122** Adolescent idiopathic scoliosis, cervical region
- **M41.123** Adolescent idiopathic scoliosis, cervicothoracic region
- **M41.124** Adolescent idiopathic scoliosis, thoracic region
- **M41.125** Adolescent idiopathic scoliosis, thoracolumbar region
- **M41.126** Adolescent idiopathic scoliosis, lumbar region
- **M41.127** Adolescent idiopathic scoliosis, lumbosacral region
- **M41.129** Adolescent idiopathic scoliosis, site unspecified

M41.2 Other idiopathic scoliosis

- **M41.20** Other idiopathic scoliosis, site unspecified
- **M41.22** Other idiopathic scoliosis, cervical region
- **M41.23** Other idiopathic scoliosis, cervicothoracic region

M41.24 Other idiopathic scoliosis, thoracic region
M41.25 Other idiopathic scoliosis, thoracolumbar region
M41.26 Other idiopathic scoliosis, lumbar region
M41.27 Other idiopathic scoliosis, lumbosacral region

√5th M41.3 Thoracogenic scoliosis

M41.30 Thoracogenic scoliosis, site unspecified
M41.34 Thoracogenic scoliosis, thoracic region
M41.35 Thoracogenic scoliosis, thoracolumbar region

√5th M41.4 Neuromuscular scoliosis

Scoliosis secondary to cerebral palsy, Friedreich's ataxia, poliomyelitis and other neuromuscular disorders

Code also underlying condition

AHA: 2014,4Q,27

M41.40 Neuromuscular scoliosis, site unspecified
M41.41 Neuromuscular scoliosis, occipito-atlanto-axial region
M41.42 Neuromuscular scoliosis, cervical region
M41.43 Neuromuscular scoliosis, cervicothoracic region
M41.44 Neuromuscular scoliosis, thoracic region
M41.45 Neuromuscular scoliosis, thoracolumbar region
M41.46 Neuromuscular scoliosis, lumbar region
M41.47 Neuromuscular scoliosis, lumbosacral region

√5th M41.5 Other secondary scoliosis

Code first underlying disease

AHA: 2019,1Q,19

M41.50 Other secondary scoliosis, site unspecified UPD
M41.52 Other secondary scoliosis, cervical region UPD
M41.53 Other secondary scoliosis, cervicothoracic region UPD
M41.54 Other secondary scoliosis, thoracic region UPD
M41.55 Other secondary scoliosis, thoracolumbar region UPD
M41.56 Other secondary scoliosis, lumbar region UPD
M41.57 Other secondary scoliosis, lumbosacral region UPD

√5th M41.8 Other forms of scoliosis

AHA: 2022,1Q,30

M41.80 Other forms of scoliosis, site unspecified
M41.82 Other forms of scoliosis, cervical region
M41.83 Other forms of scoliosis, cervicothoracic region
M41.84 Other forms of scoliosis, thoracic region
M41.85 Other forms of scoliosis, thoracolumbar region
M41.86 Other forms of scoliosis, lumbar region
M41.87 Other forms of scoliosis, lumbosacral region

M41.9 Scoliosis, unspecified

AHA: 2022,1Q,30

√4th M42 Spinal osteochondrosis

√5th M42.0 Juvenile osteochondrosis of spine

Calvé's disease
Scheuermann's disease

EXCLUDES 1 *postural kyphosis (M40.0)*

M42.00 Juvenile osteochondrosis of spine, site unspecified
M42.01 Juvenile osteochondrosis of spine, occipito-atlanto-axial region
M42.02 Juvenile osteochondrosis of spine, cervical region
M42.03 Juvenile osteochondrosis of spine, cervicothoracic region
M42.04 Juvenile osteochondrosis of spine, thoracic region
M42.05 Juvenile osteochondrosis of spine, thoracolumbar region
M42.06 Juvenile osteochondrosis of spine, lumbar region
M42.07 Juvenile osteochondrosis of spine, lumbosacral region
M42.08 Juvenile osteochondrosis of spine, sacral and sacrococcygeal region
M42.09 Juvenile osteochondrosis of spine, multiple sites in spine

√5th M42.1 Adult osteochondrosis of spine

M42.10 Adult osteochondrosis of spine, site unspecified A
M42.11 Adult osteochondrosis of spine, occipito-atlanto-axial region A
M42.12 Adult osteochondrosis of spine, cervical region A
M42.13 Adult osteochondrosis of spine, cervicothoracic region A
M42.14 Adult osteochondrosis of spine, thoracic region A
M42.15 Adult osteochondrosis of spine, thoracolumbar region A
M42.16 Adult osteochondrosis of spine, lumbar region A
M42.17 Adult osteochondrosis of spine, lumbosacral region A
M42.18 Adult osteochondrosis of spine, sacral and sacrococcygeal region A
M42.19 Adult osteochondrosis of spine, multiple sites in spine A

M42.9 Spinal osteochondrosis, unspecified

√4th M43 Other deforming dorsopathies

EXCLUDES 1 *congenital spondylolysis and spondylolisthesis (Q76.2)*
hemivertebra (Q76.3-Q76.4)
Klippel-Feil syndrome (Q76.1)
lumbarization and sacralization (Q76.4)
platyspondylisis (Q76.4)
spina bifida occulta (Q76.0)
spinal curvature in osteoporosis (M80.-)
spinal curvature in Paget's disease of bone [osteitis deformans] (M88.-)

√5th M43.0 Spondylolysis

EXCLUDES 1 *congenital spondylolysis (Q76.2)*
spondylolisthesis (M43.1)

M43.00 Spondylolysis, site unspecified
M43.01 Spondylolysis, occipito-atlanto-axial region
M43.02 Spondylolysis, cervical region
M43.03 Spondylolysis, cervicothoracic region
M43.04 Spondylolysis, thoracic region
M43.05 Spondylolysis, thoracolumbar region
M43.06 Spondylolysis, lumbar region
M43.07 Spondylolysis, lumbosacral region
M43.08 Spondylolysis, sacral and sacrococcygeal region
M43.09 Spondylolysis, multiple sites in spine

√5th M43.1 Spondylolisthesis

EXCLUDES 1 *acute traumatic of lumbosacral region (S33.1)*
acute traumatic of sites other than lumbosacral - code to Fracture, vertebra, by region
congenital spondylolisthesis (Q76.2)

AHA: 2020,2Q,21; 2018,3Q,18

TIP: Code also any associated radiculopathy (M54.1-) and/or myelopathy (G99.2).

M43.10 Spondylolisthesis, site unspecified
M43.11 Spondylolisthesis, occipito-atlanto-axial region
M43.12 Spondylolisthesis, cervical region
M43.13 Spondylolisthesis, cervicothoracic region
M43.14 Spondylolisthesis, thoracic region
M43.15 Spondylolisthesis, thoracolumbar region
M43.16 Spondylolisthesis, lumbar region
M43.17 Spondylolisthesis, lumbosacral region
M43.18 Spondylolisthesis, sacral and sacrococcygeal region
M43.19 Spondylolisthesis, multiple sites in spine

√5th M43.2 Fusion of spine

Ankylosis of spinal joint

EXCLUDES 1 *ankylosing spondylitis (M45.0-)*
congenital fusion of spine (Q76.4)

EXCLUDES 2 *arthrodesis status (Z98.1)*
pseudoarthrosis after fusion or arthrodesis (M96.0)

M43.20 Fusion of spine, site unspecified
M43.21 Fusion of spine, occipito-atlanto-axial region
M43.22 Fusion of spine, cervical region
M43.23 Fusion of spine, cervicothoracic region
M43.24 Fusion of spine, thoracic region
M43.25 Fusion of spine, thoracolumbar region
M43.26 Fusion of spine, lumbar region
M43.27 Fusion of spine, lumbosacral region
M43.28 Fusion of spine, sacral and sacrococcygeal region

M43.3 Recurrent atlantoaxial dislocation with myelopathy
M43.4 Other recurrent atlantoaxial dislocation

M43.5 Other recurrent vertebral dislocation

EXCLUDES 1 *biomechanical lesions NEC (M99.-)*

M43.5X Other recurrent vertebral dislocation

M43.5X2 Other recurrent vertebral dislocation, cervical region

M43.5X3 Other recurrent vertebral dislocation, cervicothoracic region

M43.5X4 Other recurrent vertebral dislocation, thoracic region

M43.5X5 Other recurrent vertebral dislocation, thoracolumbar region

M43.5X6 Other recurrent vertebral dislocation, lumbar region

M43.5X7 Other recurrent vertebral dislocation, lumbosacral region

M43.5X8 Other recurrent vertebral dislocation, sacral and sacrococcygeal region

M43.5X9 Other recurrent vertebral dislocation, site unspecified

M43.6 Torticollis

EXCLUDES 1 *congenital (sternomastoid) torticollis (Q68.0)*
current injury - see Injury, of spine, by body region
ocular torticollis (R29.891)
psychogenic torticollis (F45.8)
spasmodic torticollis (G24.3)
torticollis due to birth injury (P15.2)

DEF: Twisted, unnatural position of the neck due to contracted cervical muscles that pull the head to one side.

M43.8 Other specified deforming dorsopathies

EXCLUDES 2 *kyphosis and lordosis (M40.-)*
scoliosis (M41.-)

M43.8X Other specified deforming dorsopathies

M43.8X1 Other specified deforming dorsopathies, occipito-atlanto-axial region

M43.8X2 Other specified deforming dorsopathies, cervical region

M43.8X3 Other specified deforming dorsopathies, cervicothoracic region

M43.8X4 Other specified deforming dorsopathies, thoracic region

M43.8X5 Other specified deforming dorsopathies, thoracolumbar region

M43.8X6 Other specified deforming dorsopathies, lumbar region

M43.8X7 Other specified deforming dorsopathies, lumbosacral region

M43.8X8 Other specified deforming dorsopathies, sacral and sacrococcygeal region

M43.8X9 Other specified deforming dorsopathies, site unspecified

M43.9 Deforming dorsopathy, unspecified

Curvature of spine NOS

Spondylopathies (M45-M49)

M45 Ankylosing spondylitis

Rheumatoid arthritis of spine

EXCLUDES 1 *arthropathy in Reiter's disease (M02.3-)*
juvenile (ankylosing) spondylitis (M08.1)

EXCLUDES 2 *Behçet's disease (M35.2)*

M45.0 Ankylosing spondylitis of multiple sites in spine HCC

M45.1 Ankylosing spondylitis of occipito-atlanto-axial region HCC

M45.2 Ankylosing spondylitis of cervical region HCC

M45.3 Ankylosing spondylitis of cervicothoracic region HCC

M45.4 Ankylosing spondylitis of thoracic region HCC

M45.5 Ankylosing spondylitis of thoracolumbar region HCC

M45.6 Ankylosing spondylitis lumbar region HCC

M45.7 Ankylosing spondylitis of lumbosacral region HCC

M45.8 Ankylosing spondylitis sacral and sacrococcygeal region HCC

M45.9 Ankylosing spondylitis of unspecified sites in spine HCC

M45.A Non-radiographic axial spondyloarthritis

AHA: 2021,4Q,21-22

M45.A0 Non-radiographic axial spondyloarthritis of unspecified sites in spine HCC

M45.A1 Non-radiographic axial spondyloarthritis of occipito-atlanto-axial region HCC

M45.A2 Non-radiographic axial spondyloarthritis of cervical region HCC

M45.A3 Non-radiographic axial spondyloarthritis of cervicothoracic region HCC

M45.A4 Non-radiographic axial spondyloarthritis of thoracic region HCC

M45.A5 Non-radiographic axial spondyloarthritis of thoracolumbar region HCC

M45.A6 Non-radiographic axial spondyloarthritis of lumbar region HCC

M45.A7 Non-radiographic axial spondyloarthritis of lumbosacral region HCC

M45.A8 Non-radiographic axial spondyloarthritis of sacral and sacrococcygeal region HCC

M45.AB Non-radiographic axial spondyloarthritis of multiple sites in spine HCC

M46 Other inflammatory spondylopathies

M46.0 Spinal enthesopathy

Disorder of ligamentous or muscular attachments of spine

M46.00 Spinal enthesopathy, site unspecified HCC

M46.01 Spinal enthesopathy, occipito-atlanto-axial region HCC

M46.02 Spinal enthesopathy, cervical region HCC

M46.03 Spinal enthesopathy, cervicothoracic region HCC

M46.04 Spinal enthesopathy, thoracic region HCC

M46.05 Spinal enthesopathy, thoracolumbar region HCC

M46.06 Spinal enthesopathy, lumbar region HCC

M46.07 Spinal enthesopathy, lumbosacral region HCC

M46.08 Spinal enthesopathy, sacral and sacrococcygeal region HCC

M46.09 Spinal enthesopathy, multiple sites in spine HCC

M46.1 Sacroiliitis, not elsewhere classified HCC

AHA: 2020,2Q,14

DEF: Inflammation of the sacroiliac joint (situated at the juncture of the sacrum and hip). Symptoms include pain in the buttocks or lower back that can extend down one or both legs.

M46.2 Osteomyelitis of vertebra

M46.20 Osteomyelitis of vertebra, site unspecified CC UNS HCC

M46.21 Osteomyelitis of vertebra, occipito-atlanto-axial region CC HCC

M46.22 Osteomyelitis of vertebra, cervical region CC HCC

M46.23 Osteomyelitis of vertebra, cervicothoracic region CC HCC

M46.24 Osteomyelitis of vertebra, thoracic region CC HCC

M46.25 Osteomyelitis of vertebra, thoracolumbar region CC HCC

M46.26 Osteomyelitis of vertebra, lumbar region CC HCC

M46.27 Osteomyelitis of vertebra, lumbosacral region CC HCC

M46.28 Osteomyelitis of vertebra, sacral and sacrococcygeal region CC HCC

M46.3 Infection of intervertebral disc (pyogenic)

Use additional code (B95-B97) to identify infectious agent

M46.30 Infection of intervertebral disc (pyogenic), site unspecified CC UNS HCC

M46.31 Infection of intervertebral disc (pyogenic), occipito-atlanto-axial region CC HCC

M46.32 Infection of intervertebral disc (pyogenic), cervical region CC HCC

M46.33 Infection of intervertebral disc (pyogenic), cervicothoracic region CC HCC

M46.34 Infection of intervertebral disc (pyogenic), thoracic region CC HCC

M46.35 Infection of intervertebral disc (pyogenic), thoracolumbar region CC HCC

M46.36 Infection of intervertebral disc (pyogenic), lumbar region CC HCC

M46.37 Infection of intervertebral disc (pyogenic), lumbosacral region CC HCC

M46.38 Infection of intervertebral disc (pyogenic), sacral and sacrococcygeal region CC HCC

M46.39 Infection of intervertebral disc (pyogenic), multiple sites in spine CC HCC

M46.4 Discitis, unspecified

M46.40 Discitis, unspecified, site unspecified

N Newborn: 0 P Pediatric: 0-17 M Maternity: 9-64 A Adult: 15-124 UNS Unspecified Site MCC Major Complication/Comorbidity CC Complication/Comorbidity

M46.41 Discitis, unspecified, occipito-atlanto-axial region
M46.42 Discitis, unspecified, cervical region
M46.43 Discitis, unspecified, cervicothoracic region
M46.44 Discitis, unspecified, thoracic region
M46.45 Discitis, unspecified, thoracolumbar region
M46.46 Discitis, unspecified, lumbar region
M46.47 Discitis, unspecified, lumbosacral region
M46.48 Discitis, unspecified, sacral and sacrococcygeal region
M46.49 Discitis, unspecified, multiple sites in spine

M46.5 Other infective spondylopathies
M46.50 Other infective spondylopathies, site unspecified HCC
M46.51 Other infective spondylopathies, occipito-atlanto-axial region HCC
M46.52 Other infective spondylopathies, cervical region HCC
M46.53 Other infective spondylopathies, cervicothoracic region HCC
M46.54 Other infective spondylopathies, thoracic region HCC
M46.55 Other infective spondylopathies, thoracolumbar region HCC
M46.56 Other infective spondylopathies, lumbar region HCC
M46.57 Other infective spondylopathies, lumbosacral region HCC
M46.58 Other infective spondylopathies, sacral and sacrococcygeal region HCC
M46.59 Other infective spondylopathies, multiple sites in spine HCC

M46.8 Other specified inflammatory spondylopathies
M46.80 Other specified inflammatory spondylopathies, site unspecified HCC
M46.81 Other specified inflammatory spondylopathies, occipito-atlanto-axial region HCC
M46.82 Other specified inflammatory spondylopathies, cervical region HCC
M46.83 Other specified inflammatory spondylopathies, cervicothoracic region HCC
M46.84 Other specified inflammatory spondylopathies, thoracic region HCC
M46.85 Other specified inflammatory spondylopathies, thoracolumbar region HCC
M46.86 Other specified inflammatory spondylopathies, lumbar region HCC
M46.87 Other specified inflammatory spondylopathies, lumbosacral region HCC
M46.88 Other specified inflammatory spondylopathies, sacral and sacrococcygeal region HCC
M46.89 Other specified inflammatory spondylopathies, multiple sites in spine HCC

M46.9 Unspecified inflammatory spondylopathy
M46.90 Unspecified inflammatory spondylopathy, site unspecified HCC
M46.91 Unspecified inflammatory spondylopathy, occipito-atlanto-axial region HCC
M46.92 Unspecified inflammatory spondylopathy, cervical region HCC
AHA: 2019,3Q,10
M46.93 Unspecified inflammatory spondylopathy, cervicothoracic region HCC
M46.94 Unspecified inflammatory spondylopathy, thoracic region HCC
M46.95 Unspecified inflammatory spondylopathy, thoracolumbar region HCC
M46.96 Unspecified inflammatory spondylopathy, lumbar region HCC
M46.97 Unspecified inflammatory spondylopathy, lumbosacral region HCC
M46.98 Unspecified inflammatory spondylopathy, sacral and sacrococcygeal region HCC
M46.99 Unspecified inflammatory spondylopathy, multiple sites in spine HCC

M47 Spondylosis
INCLUDES arthrosis or osteoarthritis of spine
degeneration of facet joints
AHA: 2020,1Q,17; 2019,3Q,10-11; 2016,4Q,147

M47.0 Anterior spinal and vertebral artery compression syndromes
M47.01 Anterior spinal artery compression syndromes
M47.011 Anterior spinal artery compression syndromes, occipito-atlanto-axial region CC
M47.012 Anterior spinal artery compression syndromes, cervical region CC
M47.013 Anterior spinal artery compression syndromes, cervicothoracic region CC
M47.014 Anterior spinal artery compression syndromes, thoracic region CC
M47.015 Anterior spinal artery compression syndromes, thoracolumbar region CC
M47.016 Anterior spinal artery compression syndromes, lumbar region CC
M47.019 Anterior spinal artery compression syndromes, site unspecified CC UNS
M47.02 Vertebral artery compression syndromes
M47.021 Vertebral artery compression syndromes, occipito-atlanto-axial region CC
M47.022 Vertebral artery compression syndromes, cervical region CC
M47.029 Vertebral artery compression syndromes, site unspecified CC UNS

M47.1 Other spondylosis with myelopathy
Spondylogenic compression of spinal cord
EXCLUDES 1 *vertebral subluxation (M43.3-M43.5X9)*
AHA: 2020,1Q,17
M47.10 Other spondylosis with myelopathy, site unspecified CC UNS
M47.11 Other spondylosis with myelopathy, occipito-atlanto-axial region CC
M47.12 Other spondylosis with myelopathy, cervical region CC
M47.13 Other spondylosis with myelopathy, cervicothoracic region CC
M47.14 Other spondylosis with myelopathy, thoracic region CC
M47.15 Other spondylosis with myelopathy, thoracolumbar region CC
M47.16 Other spondylosis with myelopathy, lumbar region CC

M47.2 Other spondylosis with radiculopathy
AHA: 2020,1Q,17
M47.20 Other spondylosis with radiculopathy, site unspecified
M47.21 Other spondylosis with radiculopathy, occipito-atlanto-axial region
M47.22 Other spondylosis with radiculopathy, cervical region
M47.23 Other spondylosis with radiculopathy, cervicothoracic region
M47.24 Other spondylosis with radiculopathy, thoracic region
M47.25 Other spondylosis with radiculopathy, thoracolumbar region
M47.26 Other spondylosis with radiculopathy, lumbar region
M47.27 Other spondylosis with radiculopathy, lumbosacral region
M47.28 Other spondylosis with radiculopathy, sacral and sacrococcygeal region

M47.8 Other spondylosis
M47.81 Spondylosis without myelopathy or radiculopathy
AHA: 2019,3Q,10-11; 2018,2Q,14
M47.811 Spondylosis without myelopathy or radiculopathy, occipito-atlanto-axial region
M47.812 Spondylosis without myelopathy or radiculopathy, cervical region
M47.813 Spondylosis without myelopathy or radiculopathy, cervicothoracic region
M47.814 Spondylosis without myelopathy or radiculopathy, thoracic region

M47.815 Spondylosis without myelopathy or radiculopathy, thoracolumbar region
M47.816 Spondylosis without myelopathy or radiculopathy, lumbar region
M47.817 Spondylosis without myelopathy or radiculopathy, lumbosacral region
M47.818 Spondylosis without myelopathy or radiculopathy, sacral and sacrococcygeal region
M47.819 Spondylosis without myelopathy or radiculopathy, site unspecified

✓6th **M47.89 Other spondylosis**
M47.891 Other spondylosis, occipito-atlanto-axial region
M47.892 Other spondylosis, cervical region
M47.893 Other spondylosis, cervicothoracic region
M47.894 Other spondylosis, thoracic region
M47.895 Other spondylosis, thoracolumbar region
M47.896 Other spondylosis, lumbar region
M47.897 Other spondylosis, lumbosacral region
M47.898 Other spondylosis, sacral and sacrococcygeal region
M47.899 Other spondylosis, site unspecified

M47.9 Spondylosis, unspecified

✓4th **M48 Other spondylopathies**

✓5th **M48.Ø Spinal stenosis**
Caudal stenosis
AHA: 2020,1Q,17; 2018,3Q,18-19
TIP: Code also any associated radiculopathy (M54.1-) and/or myelopathy (G99.2).
M48.ØØ Spinal stenosis, site unspecified
M48.Ø1 Spinal stenosis, occipito-atlanto-axial region
M48.Ø2 Spinal stenosis, cervical region
M48.Ø3 Spinal stenosis, cervicothoracic region
M48.Ø4 Spinal stenosis, thoracic region
M48.Ø5 Spinal stenosis, thoracolumbar region
✓6th **M48.Ø6 Spinal stenosis, lumbar region**
AHA: 2018,3Q,19; 2017,4Q,18-19
M48.Ø61 Spinal stenosis, lumbar region without neurogenic claudication
Spinal stenosis, lumbar region NOS
M48.Ø62 Spinal stenosis, lumbar region with neurogenic claudication
M48.Ø7 Spinal stenosis, lumbosacral region
M48.Ø8 Spinal stenosis, sacral and sacrococcygeal region

✓5th **M48.1 Ankylosing hyperostosis [Forestier]**
Diffuse idiopathic skeletal hyperostosis [DISH]
M48.1Ø Ankylosing hyperostosis [Forestier], site unspecified
M48.11 Ankylosing hyperostosis [Forestier], occipito-atlanto-axial region
M48.12 Ankylosing hyperostosis [Forestier], cervical region
M48.13 Ankylosing hyperostosis [Forestier], cervicothoracic region
M48.14 Ankylosing hyperostosis [Forestier], thoracic region
M48.15 Ankylosing hyperostosis [Forestier], thoracolumbar region
M48.16 Ankylosing hyperostosis [Forestier], lumbar region
M48.17 Ankylosing hyperostosis [Forestier], lumbosacral region
M48.18 Ankylosing hyperostosis [Forestier], sacral and sacrococcygeal region
M48.19 Ankylosing hyperostosis [Forestier], multiple sites in spine

✓5th **M48.2 Kissing spine**
M48.2Ø Kissing spine, site unspecified
M48.21 Kissing spine, occipito-atlanto-axial region
M48.22 Kissing spine, cervical region
M48.23 Kissing spine, cervicothoracic region
M48.24 Kissing spine, thoracic region
M48.25 Kissing spine, thoracolumbar region
M48.26 Kissing spine, lumbar region
M48.27 Kissing spine, lumbosacral region

✓5th **M48.3 Traumatic spondylopathy**
M48.3Ø Traumatic spondylopathy, site unspecified CC UNS
M48.31 Traumatic spondylopathy, occipito-atlanto-axial region CC
M48.32 Traumatic spondylopathy, cervical region CC
M48.33 Traumatic spondylopathy, cervicothoracic region CC
M48.34 Traumatic spondylopathy, thoracic region CC
M48.35 Traumatic spondylopathy, thoracolumbar region CC
M48.36 Traumatic spondylopathy, lumbar region CC
M48.37 Traumatic spondylopathy, lumbosacral region CC
M48.38 Traumatic spondylopathy, sacral and sacrococcygeal region CC

✓5th **M48.4 Fatigue fracture of vertebra**
Stress fracture of vertebra
EXCLUDES 1 *pathological fracture NOS (M84.4-)*
pathological fracture of vertebra due to neoplasm (M84.58)
pathological fracture of vertebra due to osteoporosis (M8Ø.-)
pathological fracture of vertebra due to other diagnosis (M84.68)
traumatic fracture of vertebrae (S12.Ø-S12.3-, S22.Ø-, S32.Ø-)

The appropriate 7th character is to be added to each code from subcategory M48.4.
A initial encounter for fracture
D subsequent encounter for fracture with routine healing
G subsequent encounter for fracture with delayed healing
S sequela of fracture

✓x7th **M48.4Ø Fatigue fracture of vertebra, site unspecified**
✓x7th **M48.41 Fatigue fracture of vertebra, occipito-atlanto-axial region**
✓x7th **M48.42 Fatigue fracture of vertebra, cervical region**
✓x7th **M48.43 Fatigue fracture of vertebra, cervicothoracic region**
✓x7th **M48.44 Fatigue fracture of vertebra, thoracic region**
✓x7th **M48.45 Fatigue fracture of vertebra, thoracolumbar region**
✓x7th **M48.46 Fatigue fracture of vertebra, lumbar region**
✓x7th **M48.47 Fatigue fracture of vertebra, lumbosacral region**
✓x7th **M48.48 Fatigue fracture of vertebra, sacral and sacrococcygeal region**

✓5th **M48.5 Collapsed vertebra, not elsewhere classified**
Collapsed vertebra NOS
Compression fracture of vertebra NOS
Wedging of vertebra NOS
EXCLUDES 1 *current injury - see Injury of spine, by body region*
fatigue fracture of vertebra (M48.4)
pathological fracture NOS (M84.4-)
pathological fracture of vertebra due to neoplasm (M84.58)
pathological fracture of vertebra due to osteoporosis (M8Ø.-)
pathological fracture of vertebra due to other diagnosis (M84.68)
stress fracture of vertebra (M48.4-)
traumatic fracture of vertebra (S12.-, S22.-, S32.-)

The appropriate 7th character is to be added to each code from subcategory M48.5.
A initial encounter for fracture
D subsequent encounter for fracture with routine healing
G subsequent encounter for fracture with delayed healing
S sequela of fracture

6 ✓x7th **M48.5Ø Collapsed vertebra, not elsewhere classified, site unspecified** CC UNS HCC
6 ✓x7th **M48.51 Collapsed vertebra, not elsewhere classified, occipito-atlanto-axial region** CC HCC
6 ✓x7th **M48.52 Collapsed vertebra, not elsewhere classified, cervical region** CC HCC
6 ✓x7th **M48.53 Collapsed vertebra, not elsewhere classified, cervicothoracic region** CC HCC
6 ✓x7th **M48.54 Collapsed vertebra, not elsewhere classified, thoracic region** CC HCC
6 ✓x7th **M48.55 Collapsed vertebra, not elsewhere classified, thoracolumbar region** CC HCC
6 ✓x7th **M48.56 Collapsed vertebra, not elsewhere classified, lumbar region** CC HCC

6 ✓x7th **M48.57 Collapsed vertebra, not elsewhere classified, lumbosacral region** CC HCC

6 ✓x7th **M48.58 Collapsed vertebra, not elsewhere classified, sacral and sacrococcygeal region** CC HCC

✓5th **M48.8 Other specified spondylopathies**

Ossification of posterior longitudinal ligament

✓6th **M48.8X Other specified spondylopathies**

M48.8X1 Other specified spondylopathies, occipito-atlanto-axial region HCC

M48.8X2 Other specified spondylopathies, cervical region HCC

M48.8X3 Other specified spondylopathies, cervicothoracic region HCC

M48.8X4 Other specified spondylopathies, thoracic region HCC

M48.8X5 Other specified spondylopathies, thoracolumbar region HCC

M48.8X6 Other specified spondylopathies, lumbar region HCC

M48.8X7 Other specified spondylopathies, lumbosacral region HCC

M48.8X8 Other specified spondylopathies, sacral and sacrococcygeal region HCC

M48.8X9 Other specified spondylopathies, site unspecified HCC

M48.9 Spondylopathy, unspecified

✓4th **M49 Spondylopathies in diseases classified elsewhere**

INCLUDES curvature of spine in diseases classified elsewhere
deformity of spine in diseases classified elsewhere
kyphosis in diseases classified elsewhere
scoliosis in diseases classified elsewhere
spondylopathy in diseases classified elsewhere

Code first underlying disease, such as:
brucellosis (A23.-)
Charcôt-Marie-Tooth disease (G60.0)
enterobacterial infections (A01-A04)
osteitis fibrosa cystica (E21.0)

EXCLUDES 1 *curvature of spine in tuberculosis [Pott's] (A18.01)*
enteropathic arthropathies (M07.-)
gonococcal spondylitis (A54.41)
neuropathic spondylopathy in syringomyelia (G95.0)
neuropathic spondylopathy in tabes dorsalis (A52.11)
neuropathic [tabes dorsalis] spondylitis (A52.11)
nonsyphilitic neuropathic spondylopathy NEC (G98.0)
spondylitis in syphilis (acquired) (A52.77)
tuberculous spondylitis (A18.01)
typhoid fever spondylitis (A01.05)

✓5th **M49.8 Spondylopathy in diseases classified elsewhere**

M49.80 Spondylopathy in diseases classified elsewhere, site unspecified HCC

M49.81 Spondylopathy in diseases classified elsewhere, occipito-atlanto-axial region HCC

M49.82 Spondylopathy in diseases classified elsewhere, cervical region HCC

M49.83 Spondylopathy in diseases classified elsewhere, cervicothoracic region HCC

M49.84 Spondylopathy in diseases classified elsewhere, thoracic region HCC

M49.85 Spondylopathy in diseases classified elsewhere, thoracolumbar region HCC

M49.86 Spondylopathy in diseases classified elsewhere, lumbar region HCC

M49.87 Spondylopathy in diseases classified elsewhere, lumbosacral region HCC

M49.88 Spondylopathy in diseases classified elsewhere, sacral and sacrococcygeal region HCC

M49.89 Spondylopathy in diseases classified elsewhere, multiple sites in spine HCC

Other dorsopathies (M50-M54)

EXCLUDES 1 *current injury - see injury of spine by body region*
discitis NOS (M46.4-)

✓4th **M50 Cervical disc disorders**

NOTE Code to the most superior level of disorder

INCLUDES cervicothoracic disc disorders
cervicothoracic disc disorders with cervicalgia

AHA: 2016,4Q,39-40; 2016,1Q,17

✓5th **M50.0 Cervical disc disorder with myelopathy**

AHA: 2018,3Q,19

M50.00 Cervical disc disorder with myelopathy, unspecified cervical region CC UNS

M50.01 Cervical disc disorder with myelopathy, high cervical region CC

C2-C3 disc disorder with myelopathy
C3-C4 disc disorder with myelopathy

✓6th **M50.02 Cervical disc disorder with myelopathy, mid-cervical region**

M50.020 Cervical disc disorder with myelopathy, mid-cervical region, unspecified level CC UNS

M50.021 Cervical disc disorder at C4-C5 level with myelopathy CC

C4-C5 disc disorder with myelopathy

M50.022 Cervical disc disorder at C5-C6 level with myelopathy CC

C5-C6 disc disorder with myelopathy

M50.023 Cervical disc disorder at C6-C7 level with myelopathy CC

C6-C7 disc disorder with myelopathy

M50.03 Cervical disc disorder with myelopathy, cervicothoracic region CC

C7-T1 disc disorder with myelopathy

✓5th **M50.1 Cervical disc disorder with radiculopathy**

EXCLUDES 2 *brachial radiculitis NOS (M54.13)*

AHA: 2018,3Q,19

M50.10 Cervical disc disorder with radiculopathy, unspecified cervical region

M50.11 Cervical disc disorder with radiculopathy, high cervical region

C2-C3 disc disorder with radiculopathy
C3 radiculopathy due to disc disorder
C3-C4 disc disorder with radiculopathy
C4 radiculopathy due to disc disorder

✓6th **M50.12 Cervical disc disorder with radiculopathy, mid-cervical region**

M50.120 Mid-cervical disc disorder, unspecified level

M50.121 Cervical disc disorder at C4-C5 level with radiculopathy

C4-C5 disc disorder with radiculopathy
C5 radiculopathy due to disc disorder

M50.122 Cervical disc disorder at C5-C6 level with radiculopathy

C5-C6 disc disorder with radiculopathy
C6 radiculopathy due to disc disorder

M50.123 Cervical disc disorder at C6-C7 level with radiculopathy

C6-C7 disc disorder with radiculopathy
C7 radiculopathy due to disc disorder

M50.13 Cervical disc disorder with radiculopathy, cervicothoracic region

C7-T1 disc disorder with radiculopathy
C8 radiculopathy due to disc disorder

✓5th **M50.2 Other cervical disc displacement**

M50.20 Other cervical disc displacement, unspecified cervical region

M50.21 Other cervical disc displacement, high cervical region

Other C2-C3 cervical disc displacement
Other C3-C4 cervical disc displacement

✓6th **M50.22 Other cervical disc displacement, mid-cervical region**

M50.220 Other cervical disc displacement, mid-cervical region, unspecified level

Chapter 13. Diseases of the Musculoskeletal System and Connective Tissue

M48.57–M50.220

M5Ø.221 Other cervical disc displacement at C4-C5 level
Other C4-C5 cervical disc displacement

M5Ø.222 Other cervical disc displacement at C5-C6 level
Other C5-C6 cervical disc displacement

M5Ø.223 Other cervical disc displacement at C6-C7 level
Other C6-C7 cervical disc displacement

M5Ø.23 Other cervical disc displacement, cervicothoracic region
Other C7-T1 cervical disc displacement

✓5th **M5Ø.3 Other cervical disc degeneration**

M5Ø.3Ø Other cervical disc degeneration, unspecified cervical region

M5Ø.31 Other cervical disc degeneration, high cervical region
Other C2-C3 cervical disc degeneration
Other C3-C4 cervical disc degeneration

✓6th **M5Ø.32 Other cervical disc degeneration, mid-cervical region**

M5Ø.32Ø Other cervical disc degeneration, mid-cervical region, unspecified level

M5Ø.321 Other cervical disc degeneration at C4-C5 level
Other C4-C5 cervical disc degeneration

M5Ø.322 Other cervical disc degeneration at C5-C6 level
Other C5-C6 cervical disc degeneration

M5Ø.323 Other cervical disc degeneration at C6-C7 level
Other C6-C7 cervical disc degeneration

M5Ø.33 Other cervical disc degeneration, cervicothoracic region
Other C7-T1 cervical disc degeneration

✓5th **M5Ø.8 Other cervical disc disorders**

M5Ø.8Ø Other cervical disc disorders, unspecified cervical region

M5Ø.81 Other cervical disc disorders, high cervical region
Other C2-C3 cervical disc disorders
Other C3-C4 cervical disc disorders

✓6th **M5Ø.82 Other cervical disc disorders, mid-cervical region**

M5Ø.82Ø Other cervical disc disorders, mid-cervical region, unspecified level

M5Ø.821 Other cervical disc disorders at C4-C5 level
Other C4-C5 cervical disc disorders

M5Ø.822 Other cervical disc disorders at C5-C6 level
Other C5-C6 cervical disc disorders

M5Ø.823 Other cervical disc disorders at C6-C7 level
Other C6-C7 cervical disc disorders

M5Ø.83 Other cervical disc disorders, cervicothoracic region
Other C7-T1 cervical disc disorders

✓5th **M5Ø.9 Cervical disc disorder, unspecified**

M5Ø.9Ø Cervical disc disorder, unspecified, unspecified cervical region

M5Ø.91 Cervical disc disorder, unspecified, high cervical region
C2-C3 cervical disc disorder, unspecified
C3-C4 cervical disc disorder, unspecified

✓6th **M5Ø.92 Cervical disc disorder, unspecified, mid-cervical region**

M5Ø.92Ø Unspecified cervical disc disorder, mid-cervical region, unspecified level

M5Ø.921 Unspecified cervical disc disorder at C4-C5 level
Unspecified C4-C5 cervical disc disorder

M5Ø.922 Unspecified cervical disc disorder at C5-C6 level
Unspecified C5-C6 cervical disc disorder

M5Ø.923 Unspecified cervical disc disorder at C6-C7 level
Unspecified C6-C7 cervical disc disorder

M5Ø.93 Cervical disc disorder, unspecified, cervicothoracic region
C7-T1 cervical disc disorder, unspecified

✓4th **M51 Thoracic, thoracolumbar, and lumbosacral intervertebral disc disorders**

EXCLUDES 2 *cervical and cervicothoracic disc disorders (M5Ø.-)*
sacral and sacrococcygeal disorders (M53.3)

✓5th **M51.Ø Thoracic, thoracolumbar and lumbosacral intervertebral disc disorders with myelopathy**

M51.Ø4 Intervertebral disc disorders with myelopathy, thoracic region CC

M51.Ø5 Intervertebral disc disorders with myelopathy, thoracolumbar region CC

M51.Ø6 Intervertebral disc disorders with myelopathy, lumbar region CC

✓5th **M51.1 Thoracic, thoracolumbar and lumbosacral intervertebral disc disorders with radiculopathy**
Sciatica due to intervertebral disc disorder
EXCLUDES 1 *lumbar radiculitis NOS (M54.16)*
sciatica NOS (M54.3)
AHA: 2018,3Q,18

M51.14 Intervertebral disc disorders with radiculopathy, thoracic region

M51.15 Intervertebral disc disorders with radiculopathy, thoracolumbar region

M51.16 Intervertebral disc disorders with radiculopathy, lumbar region

M51.17 Intervertebral disc disorders with radiculopathy, lumbosacral region

✓5th **M51.2 Other thoracic, thoracolumbar and lumbosacral intervertebral disc displacement**
Lumbago due to displacement of intervertebral disc
AHA: 2022,1Q,26

Displacement Intervertebral Disc

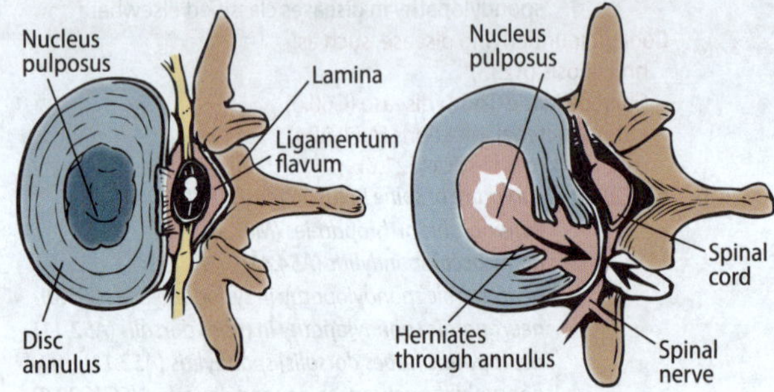

M51.24 Other intervertebral disc displacement, thoracic region

M51.25 Other intervertebral disc displacement, thoracolumbar region

M51.26 Other intervertebral disc displacement, lumbar region

M51.27 Other intervertebral disc displacement, lumbosacral region

✓5th **M51.3 Other thoracic, thoracolumbar and lumbosacral intervertebral disc degeneration**
AHA: 2022,1Q,26; 2018,2Q,15; 2013,3Q,22

M51.34 Other intervertebral disc degeneration, thoracic region

M51.35 Other intervertebral disc degeneration, thoracolumbar region

M51.36 Other intervertebral disc degeneration, lumbar region

M51.37 Other intervertebral disc degeneration, lumbosacral region

✓5th **M51.4 Schmorl's nodes**
DEF: Irregular bone defect in the margin of the vertebral body that causes herniation into the end plate of the vertebral body.

M51.44 Schmorl's nodes, thoracic region

M51.45 Schmorl's nodes, thoracolumbar region

M51.46 Schmorl's nodes, lumbar region

M51.47 Schmorl's nodes, lumbosacral region

✓5th **M51.8 Other thoracic, thoracolumbar and lumbosacral intervertebral disc disorders**

M51.84 Other intervertebral disc disorders, thoracic region

M51.85 Other intervertebral disc disorders, thoracolumbar region

M51.86 Other intervertebral disc disorders, lumbar region

M51.87 Other intervertebral disc disorders, lumbosacral region

M51.9 Unspecified thoracic, thoracolumbar and lumbosacral intervertebral disc disorder

● M51.A Other lumbar and lumbosacral annulus fibrosus disc defects

● M51.A0 Intervertebral annulus fibrosus defect, lumbar region, unspecified size
Code first, if applicable, lumbar disc herniation (M51.06, M51.16, M51.26)

● M51.A1 Intervertebral annulus fibrosus defect, small, lumbar region
Code first, if applicable, lumbar disc herniation (M51.06, M51.16, M51.26)

● M51.A2 Intervertebral annulus fibrosus defect, large, lumbar region
Code first, if applicable, lumbar disc herniation (M51.06, M51.16, M51.26)

● M51.A3 Intervertebral annulus fibrosus defect, lumbosacral region, unspecified size
Code first, if applicable, lumbosacral disc herniation (M51.17, M51.27)

● M51.A4 Intervertebral annulus fibrosus defect, small, lumbosacral region
Code first, if applicable, lumbosacral disc herniation (M51.17, M51.27)

● M51.A5 Intervertebral annulus fibrosus defect, large, lumbosacral region
Code first, if applicable, lumbosacral disc herniation (M51.17, M51.27)

M53 Other and unspecified dorsopathies, not elsewhere classified

M53.0 Cervicocranial syndrome
Posterior cervical sympathetic syndrome

M53.1 Cervicobrachial syndrome
EXCLUDES 2 *cervical disc disorder (M50.-)*
thoracic outlet syndrome (G54.0)

M53.2 Spinal instabilities

M53.2X Spinal instabilities

M53.2X1 Spinal instabilities, occipito-atlanto-axial region
M53.2X2 Spinal instabilities, cervical region
M53.2X3 Spinal instabilities, cervicothoracic region
M53.2X4 Spinal instabilities, thoracic region
M53.2X5 Spinal instabilities, thoracolumbar region
M53.2X6 Spinal instabilities, lumbar region
M53.2X7 Spinal instabilities, lumbosacral region
M53.2X8 Spinal instabilities, sacral and sacrococcygeal region
M53.2X9 Spinal instabilities, site unspecified

M53.3 Sacrococcygeal disorders, not elsewhere classified
Coccygodynia

M53.8 Other specified dorsopathies

M53.80 Other specified dorsopathies, site unspecified
M53.81 Other specified dorsopathies, occipito-atlanto-axial region
M53.82 Other specified dorsopathies, cervical region
M53.83 Other specified dorsopathies, cervicothoracic region
M53.84 Other specified dorsopathies, thoracic region
M53.85 Other specified dorsopathies, thoracolumbar region
M53.86 Other specified dorsopathies, lumbar region
M53.87 Other specified dorsopathies, lumbosacral region
M53.88 Other specified dorsopathies, sacral and sacrococcygeal region

M53.9 Dorsopathy, unspecified

M54 Dorsalgia
EXCLUDES 1 *psychogenic dorsalgia (F45.41)*

M54.0 Panniculitis affecting regions of neck and back
EXCLUDES 1 *lupus panniculitis (L93.2)*
panniculitis NOS (M79.3)
relapsing [Weber-Christian] panniculitis (M35.6)

M54.00 Panniculitis affecting regions of neck and back, site unspecified
M54.01 Panniculitis affecting regions of neck and back, occipito-atlanto-axial region
M54.02 Panniculitis affecting regions of neck and back, cervical region
M54.03 Panniculitis affecting regions of neck and back, cervicothoracic region
M54.04 Panniculitis affecting regions of neck and back, thoracic region
M54.05 Panniculitis affecting regions of neck and back, thoracolumbar region
M54.06 Panniculitis affecting regions of neck and back, lumbar region
M54.07 Panniculitis affecting regions of neck and back, lumbosacral region
M54.08 Panniculitis affecting regions of neck and back, sacral and sacrococcygeal region
M54.09 Panniculitis affecting regions, neck and back, multiple sites in spine

M54.1 Radiculopathy
Brachial neuritis or radiculitis NOS
Lumbar neuritis or radiculitis NOS
Lumbosacral neuritis or radiculitis NOS
Thoracic neuritis or radiculitis NOS
Radiculitis NOS
EXCLUDES 1 *neuralgia and neuritis NOS (M79.2)*
radiculopathy with cervical disc disorder (M50.1)
radiculopathy with lumbar and other intervertebral disc disorder (M51.1-)
radiculopathy with spondylosis (M47.2-)

AHA: 2018,3Q,18

TIP: A code from this subcategory can be used in addition to a spondylolisthesis code (M43.1-) or a spinal stenosis code (M48.0-) when either condition is documented as the cause of the radiculopathy.

M54.10 Radiculopathy, site unspecified
M54.11 Radiculopathy, occipito-atlanto-axial region
M54.12 Radiculopathy, cervical region
M54.13 Radiculopathy, cervicothoracic region
M54.14 Radiculopathy, thoracic region
M54.15 Radiculopathy, thoracolumbar region
M54.16 Radiculopathy, lumbar region
M54.17 Radiculopathy, lumbosacral region
M54.18 Radiculopathy, sacral and sacrococcygeal region

M54.2 Cervicalgia
EXCLUDES 1 *cervicalgia due to intervertebral cervical disc disorder (M50.-)*

M54.3 Sciatica
EXCLUDES 1 *lesion of sciatic nerve (G57.0)*
sciatica due to intervertebral disc disorder (M51.1-)
sciatica with lumbago (M54.4-)

M54.30 Sciatica, unspecified side
M54.31 Sciatica, right side
M54.32 Sciatica, left side

M54.4 Lumbago with sciatica
EXCLUDES 1 *lumbago with sciatica due to intervertebral disc disorder (M51.1-)*

AHA: 2016,2Q,7

M54.40 Lumbago with sciatica, unspecified side
M54.41 Lumbago with sciatica, right side
M54.42 Lumbago with sciatica, left side

M54.5 Low back pain
EXCLUDES 1 *low back strain (S39.012)*
lumbago due to intervertebral disc displacement (M51.2-)
lumbago with sciatica (M54.4-)

AHA: 2021,4Q,22

M54.50 Low back pain, unspecified
Loin pain
Lumbago NOS

M54.51 Vertebrogenic low back pain
Low back vertebral endplate pain

M54.59 Other low back pain

M54.6 Pain in thoracic spine
EXCLUDES 1 *pain in thoracic spine due to intervertebral disc disorder (M51.-)*

M54.8 Other dorsalgia
EXCLUDES 1 *dorsalgia in thoracic region (M54.6)*
low back pain (M54.5-)

M54.81 Occipital neuralgia
M54.89 Other dorsalgia

M54.9 Dorsalgia, unspecified
Backache NOS
Back pain NOS

SOFT TISSUE DISORDERS (M60-M79)

Disorders of muscles (M60-M63)

EXCLUDES 1 *dermatopolymyositis (M33.-)*
muscular dystrophies and myopathies (G71-G72)
myopathy in amyloidosis (E85.-)
myopathy in polyarteritis nodosa (M30.0)
myopathy in rheumatoid arthritis (M05.32)
myopathy in scleroderma (M34.-)
myopathy in Sjögren's syndrome (M35.03)
myopathy in systemic lupus erythematosus (M32.-)
EXCLUDES 2 ▶*muscular dystrophies and myopathies (G71-G72)*◀

4th M60 Myositis
EXCLUDES 2 *inclusion body myositis [IBM] (G72.41)*

5th M60.0 Infective myositis
Tropical pyomyositis
Use additional code (B95-B97) to identify infectious agent

6th M60.00 Infective myositis, unspecified site
M60.000 Infective myositis, unspecified right arm CC
Infective myositis, right upper limb NOS
M60.001 Infective myositis, unspecified left arm CC
Infective myositis, left upper limb NOS
M60.002 Infective myositis, unspecified arm CC UNS
Infective myositis, upper limb NOS
M60.003 Infective myositis, unspecified right leg CC
Infective myositis, right lower limb NOS
M60.004 Infective myositis, unspecified left leg CC
Infective myositis, left lower limb NOS
M60.005 Infective myositis, unspecified leg CC UNS
Infective myositis, lower limb NOS
M60.009 Infective myositis, unspecified site CC UNS

6th M60.01 Infective myositis, shoulder
M60.011 Infective myositis, right shoulder CC
M60.012 Infective myositis, left shoulder CC
M60.019 Infective myositis, unspecified shoulder CC UNS

6th M60.02 Infective myositis, upper arm
M60.021 Infective myositis, right upper arm CC
M60.022 Infective myositis, left upper arm CC
M60.029 Infective myositis, unspecified upper arm CC UNS

6th M60.03 Infective myositis, forearm
M60.031 Infective myositis, right forearm CC
M60.032 Infective myositis, left forearm CC
M60.039 Infective myositis, unspecified forearm CC UNS

6th M60.04 Infective myositis, hand and fingers
M60.041 Infective myositis, right hand CC
M60.042 Infective myositis, left hand CC
M60.043 Infective myositis, unspecified hand CC UNS
M60.044 Infective myositis, right finger(s) CC
M60.045 Infective myositis, left finger(s) CC
M60.046 Infective myositis, unspecified finger(s) CC UNS

6th M60.05 Infective myositis, thigh
M60.051 Infective myositis, right thigh CC
M60.052 Infective myositis, left thigh CC
M60.059 Infective myositis, unspecified thigh CC UNS

6th M60.06 Infective myositis, lower leg
M60.061 Infective myositis, right lower leg CC
M60.062 Infective myositis, left lower leg CC
M60.069 Infective myositis, unspecified lower leg CC UNS

6th M60.07 Infective myositis, ankle, foot and toes
M60.070 Infective myositis, right ankle CC
M60.071 Infective myositis, left ankle CC
M60.072 Infective myositis, unspecified ankle CC UNS
M60.073 Infective myositis, right foot CC
M60.074 Infective myositis, left foot CC
M60.075 Infective myositis, unspecified foot CC UNS
M60.076 Infective myositis, right toe(s) CC
M60.077 Infective myositis, left toe(s) CC
M60.078 Infective myositis, unspecified toe(s) CC UNS

M60.08 Infective myositis, other site CC
M60.09 Infective myositis, multiple sites CC

5th M60.1 Interstitial myositis
M60.10 Interstitial myositis of unspecified site

6th M60.11 Interstitial myositis, shoulder
M60.111 Interstitial myositis, right shoulder
M60.112 Interstitial myositis, left shoulder
M60.119 Interstitial myositis, unspecified shoulder

6th M60.12 Interstitial myositis, upper arm
M60.121 Interstitial myositis, right upper arm
M60.122 Interstitial myositis, left upper arm
M60.129 Interstitial myositis, unspecified upper arm

6th M60.13 Interstitial myositis, forearm
M60.131 Interstitial myositis, right forearm
M60.132 Interstitial myositis, left forearm
M60.139 Interstitial myositis, unspecified forearm

6th M60.14 Interstitial myositis, hand
M60.141 Interstitial myositis, right hand
M60.142 Interstitial myositis, left hand
M60.149 Interstitial myositis, unspecified hand

6th M60.15 Interstitial myositis, thigh
M60.151 Interstitial myositis, right thigh
M60.152 Interstitial myositis, left thigh
M60.159 Interstitial myositis, unspecified thigh

6th M60.16 Interstitial myositis, lower leg
M60.161 Interstitial myositis, right lower leg
M60.162 Interstitial myositis, left lower leg
M60.169 Interstitial myositis, unspecified lower leg

6th M60.17 Interstitial myositis, ankle and foot
M60.171 Interstitial myositis, right ankle and foot
M60.172 Interstitial myositis, left ankle and foot
M60.179 Interstitial myositis, unspecified ankle and foot

M60.18 Interstitial myositis, other site
M60.19 Interstitial myositis, multiple sites

5th M60.2 Foreign body granuloma of soft tissue, not elsewhere classified
Use additional code to identify the type of retained foreign body (Z18.-)
EXCLUDES 1 *foreign body granuloma of skin and subcutaneous tissue (L92.3)*

M60.20 Foreign body granuloma of soft tissue, not elsewhere classified, unspecified site

6th M60.21 Foreign body granuloma of soft tissue, not elsewhere classified, shoulder
M60.211 Foreign body granuloma of soft tissue, not elsewhere classified, right shoulder
M60.212 Foreign body granuloma of soft tissue, not elsewhere classified, left shoulder
M60.219 Foreign body granuloma of soft tissue, not elsewhere classified, unspecified shoulder

6th M60.22 Foreign body granuloma of soft tissue, not elsewhere classified, upper arm
M60.221 Foreign body granuloma of soft tissue, not elsewhere classified, right upper arm
M60.222 Foreign body granuloma of soft tissue, not elsewhere classified, left upper arm
M60.229 Foreign body granuloma of soft tissue, not elsewhere classified, unspecified upper arm

M60.23 Foreign body granuloma of soft tissue, not elsewhere classified, forearm
M60.231 Foreign body granuloma of soft tissue, not elsewhere classified, right forearm
M60.232 Foreign body granuloma of soft tissue, not elsewhere classified, left forearm
M60.239 Foreign body granuloma of soft tissue, not elsewhere classified, unspecified forearm
M60.24 Foreign body granuloma of soft tissue, not elsewhere classified, hand
M60.241 Foreign body granuloma of soft tissue, not elsewhere classified, right hand
M60.242 Foreign body granuloma of soft tissue, not elsewhere classified, left hand
M60.249 Foreign body granuloma of soft tissue, not elsewhere classified, unspecified hand
M60.25 Foreign body granuloma of soft tissue, not elsewhere classified, thigh
M60.251 Foreign body granuloma of soft tissue, not elsewhere classified, right thigh
M60.252 Foreign body granuloma of soft tissue, not elsewhere classified, left thigh
M60.259 Foreign body granuloma of soft tissue, not elsewhere classified, unspecified thigh
M60.26 Foreign body granuloma of soft tissue, not elsewhere classified, lower leg
M60.261 Foreign body granuloma of soft tissue, not elsewhere classified, right lower leg
M60.262 Foreign body granuloma of soft tissue, not elsewhere classified, left lower leg
M60.269 Foreign body granuloma of soft tissue, not elsewhere classified, unspecified lower leg
M60.27 Foreign body granuloma of soft tissue, not elsewhere classified, ankle and foot
M60.271 Foreign body granuloma of soft tissue, not elsewhere classified, right ankle and foot
M60.272 Foreign body granuloma of soft tissue, not elsewhere classified, left ankle and foot
M60.279 Foreign body granuloma of soft tissue, not elsewhere classified, unspecified ankle and foot
M60.28 Foreign body granuloma of soft tissue, not elsewhere classified, other site
M60.8 Other myositis
M60.80 Other myositis, unspecified site
M60.81 Other myositis shoulder
M60.811 Other myositis, right shoulder
M60.812 Other myositis, left shoulder
M60.819 Other myositis, unspecified shoulder
M60.82 Other myositis, upper arm
M60.821 Other myositis, right upper arm
M60.822 Other myositis, left upper arm
M60.829 Other myositis, unspecified upper arm
M60.83 Other myositis, forearm
M60.831 Other myositis, right forearm
M60.832 Other myositis, left forearm
M60.839 Other myositis, unspecified forearm
M60.84 Other myositis, hand
M60.841 Other myositis, right hand
M60.842 Other myositis, left hand
M60.849 Other myositis, unspecified hand
M60.85 Other myositis, thigh
M60.851 Other myositis, right thigh
M60.852 Other myositis, left thigh
M60.859 Other myositis, unspecified thigh
M60.86 Other myositis, lower leg
M60.861 Other myositis, right lower leg
M60.862 Other myositis, left lower leg
M60.869 Other myositis, unspecified lower leg
M60.87 Other myositis, ankle and foot
M60.871 Other myositis, right ankle and foot
M60.872 Other myositis, left ankle and foot
M60.879 Other myositis, unspecified ankle and foot
M60.88 Other myositis, other site
M60.89 Other myositis, multiple sites
M60.9 Myositis, unspecified

M61 Calcification and ossification of muscle
M61.0 Myositis ossificans traumatica
M61.00 Myositis ossificans traumatica, unspecified site
M61.01 Myositis ossificans traumatica, shoulder
M61.011 Myositis ossificans traumatica, right shoulder
M61.012 Myositis ossificans traumatica, left shoulder
M61.019 Myositis ossificans traumatica, unspecified shoulder
M61.02 Myositis ossificans traumatica, upper arm
M61.021 Myositis ossificans traumatica, right upper arm
M61.022 Myositis ossificans traumatica, left upper arm
M61.029 Myositis ossificans traumatica, unspecified upper arm
M61.03 Myositis ossificans traumatica, forearm
M61.031 Myositis ossificans traumatica, right forearm
M61.032 Myositis ossificans traumatica, left forearm
M61.039 Myositis ossificans traumatica, unspecified forearm
M61.04 Myositis ossificans traumatica, hand
M61.041 Myositis ossificans traumatica, right hand
M61.042 Myositis ossificans traumatica, left hand
M61.049 Myositis ossificans traumatica, unspecified hand
M61.05 Myositis ossificans traumatica, thigh
M61.051 Myositis ossificans traumatica, right thigh
M61.052 Myositis ossificans traumatica, left thigh
M61.059 Myositis ossificans traumatica, unspecified thigh
M61.06 Myositis ossificans traumatica, lower leg
M61.061 Myositis ossificans traumatica, right lower leg
M61.062 Myositis ossificans traumatica, left lower leg
M61.069 Myositis ossificans traumatica, unspecified lower leg
M61.07 Myositis ossificans traumatica, ankle and foot
M61.071 Myositis ossificans traumatica, right ankle and foot
M61.072 Myositis ossificans traumatica, left ankle and foot
M61.079 Myositis ossificans traumatica, unspecified ankle and foot
M61.08 Myositis ossificans traumatica, other site
M61.09 Myositis ossificans traumatica, multiple sites
M61.1 Myositis ossificans progressiva
Fibrodysplasia ossificans progressiva
M61.10 Myositis ossificans progressiva, unspecified site
M61.11 Myositis ossificans progressiva, shoulder
M61.111 Myositis ossificans progressiva, right shoulder
M61.112 Myositis ossificans progressiva, left shoulder
M61.119 Myositis ossificans progressiva, unspecified shoulder
M61.12 Myositis ossificans progressiva, upper arm
M61.121 Myositis ossificans progressiva, right upper arm
M61.122 Myositis ossificans progressiva, left upper arm
M61.129 Myositis ossificans progressiva, unspecified arm
M61.13 Myositis ossificans progressiva, forearm
M61.131 Myositis ossificans progressiva, right forearm
M61.132 Myositis ossificans progressiva, left forearm
M61.139 Myositis ossificans progressiva, unspecified forearm

√6th M61.14 Myositis ossificans progressiva, hand and finger(s)
M61.141 Myositis ossificans progressiva, right hand
M61.142 Myositis ossificans progressiva, left hand
M61.143 Myositis ossificans progressiva, unspecified hand
M61.144 Myositis ossificans progressiva, right finger(s)
M61.145 Myositis ossificans progressiva, left finger(s)
M61.146 Myositis ossificans progressiva, unspecified finger(s)

√6th M61.15 Myositis ossificans progressiva, thigh
M61.151 Myositis ossificans progressiva, right thigh
M61.152 Myositis ossificans progressiva, left thigh
M61.159 Myositis ossificans progressiva, unspecified thigh

√6th M61.16 Myositis ossificans progressiva, lower leg
M61.161 Myositis ossificans progressiva, right lower leg
M61.162 Myositis ossificans progressiva, left lower leg
M61.169 Myositis ossificans progressiva, unspecified lower leg

√6th M61.17 Myositis ossificans progressiva, ankle, foot and toe(s)
M61.171 Myositis ossificans progressiva, right ankle
M61.172 Myositis ossificans progressiva, left ankle
M61.173 Myositis ossificans progressiva, unspecified ankle
M61.174 Myositis ossificans progressiva, right foot
M61.175 Myositis ossificans progressiva, left foot
M61.176 Myositis ossificans progressiva, unspecified foot
M61.177 Myositis ossificans progressiva, right toe(s)
M61.178 Myositis ossificans progressiva, left toe(s)
M61.179 Myositis ossificans progressiva, unspecified toe(s)

M61.18 Myositis ossificans progressiva, other site
M61.19 Myositis ossificans progressiva, multiple sites

√5th M61.2 Paralytic calcification and ossification of muscle
Myositis ossificans associated with quadriplegia or paraplegia

M61.20 Paralytic calcification and ossification of muscle, unspecified site

√6th M61.21 Paralytic calcification and ossification of muscle, shoulder
M61.211 Paralytic calcification and ossification of muscle, right shoulder
M61.212 Paralytic calcification and ossification of muscle, left shoulder
M61.219 Paralytic calcification and ossification of muscle, unspecified shoulder

√6th M61.22 Paralytic calcification and ossification of muscle, upper arm
M61.221 Paralytic calcification and ossification of muscle, right upper arm
M61.222 Paralytic calcification and ossification of muscle, left upper arm
M61.229 Paralytic calcification and ossification of muscle, unspecified upper arm

√6th M61.23 Paralytic calcification and ossification of muscle, forearm
M61.231 Paralytic calcification and ossification of muscle, right forearm
M61.232 Paralytic calcification and ossification of muscle, left forearm
M61.239 Paralytic calcification and ossification of muscle, unspecified forearm

√6th M61.24 Paralytic calcification and ossification of muscle, hand
M61.241 Paralytic calcification and ossification of muscle, right hand
M61.242 Paralytic calcification and ossification of muscle, left hand
M61.249 Paralytic calcification and ossification of muscle, unspecified hand

√6th M61.25 Paralytic calcification and ossification of muscle, thigh
M61.251 Paralytic calcification and ossification of muscle, right thigh
M61.252 Paralytic calcification and ossification of muscle, left thigh
M61.259 Paralytic calcification and ossification of muscle, unspecified thigh

√6th M61.26 Paralytic calcification and ossification of muscle, lower leg
M61.261 Paralytic calcification and ossification of muscle, right lower leg
M61.262 Paralytic calcification and ossification of muscle, left lower leg
M61.269 Paralytic calcification and ossification of muscle, unspecified lower leg

√6th M61.27 Paralytic calcification and ossification of muscle, ankle and foot
M61.271 Paralytic calcification and ossification of muscle, right ankle and foot
M61.272 Paralytic calcification and ossification of muscle, left ankle and foot
M61.279 Paralytic calcification and ossification of muscle, unspecified ankle and foot

M61.28 Paralytic calcification and ossification of muscle, other site
M61.29 Paralytic calcification and ossification of muscle, multiple sites

√5th M61.3 Calcification and ossification of muscles associated with burns
Myositis ossificans associated with burns

M61.30 Calcification and ossification of muscles associated with burns, unspecified site

√6th M61.31 Calcification and ossification of muscles associated with burns, shoulder
M61.311 Calcification and ossification of muscles associated with burns, right shoulder
M61.312 Calcification and ossification of muscles associated with burns, left shoulder
M61.319 Calcification and ossification of muscles associated with burns, unspecified shoulder

√6th M61.32 Calcification and ossification of muscles associated with burns, upper arm
M61.321 Calcification and ossification of muscles associated with burns, right upper arm
M61.322 Calcification and ossification of muscles associated with burns, left upper arm
M61.329 Calcification and ossification of muscles associated with burns, unspecified upper arm

√6th M61.33 Calcification and ossification of muscles associated with burns, forearm
M61.331 Calcification and ossification of muscles associated with burns, right forearm
M61.332 Calcification and ossification of muscles associated with burns, left forearm
M61.339 Calcification and ossification of muscles associated with burns, unspecified forearm

√6th M61.34 Calcification and ossification of muscles associated with burns, hand
M61.341 Calcification and ossification of muscles associated with burns, right hand
M61.342 Calcification and ossification of muscles associated with burns, left hand
M61.349 Calcification and ossification of muscles associated with burns, unspecified hand

√6th M61.35 Calcification and ossification of muscles associated with burns, thigh
M61.351 Calcification and ossification of muscles associated with burns, right thigh
M61.352 Calcification and ossification of muscles associated with burns, left thigh
M61.359 Calcification and ossification of muscles associated with burns, unspecified thigh

√6th M61.36 Calcification and ossification of muscles associated with burns, lower leg
M61.361 Calcification and ossification of muscles associated with burns, right lower leg
M61.362 Calcification and ossification of muscles associated with burns, left lower leg

M61.369 Calcification and ossification of muscles associated with burns, unspecified lower leg

M61.37 Calcification and ossification of muscles associated with burns, ankle and foot

M61.371 Calcification and ossification of muscles associated with burns, right ankle and foot

M61.372 Calcification and ossification of muscles associated with burns, left ankle and foot

M61.379 Calcification and ossification of muscles associated with burns, unspecified ankle and foot

M61.38 Calcification and ossification of muscles associated with burns, other site

M61.39 Calcification and ossification of muscles associated with burns, multiple sites

M61.4 Other calcification of muscle

EXCLUDES 1 *calcific tendinitis NOS (M65.2-)*
calcific tendinitis of shoulder (M75.3)

M61.4Ø Other calcification of muscle, unspecified site

M61.41 Other calcification of muscle, shoulder

M61.411 Other calcification of muscle, right shoulder

M61.412 Other calcification of muscle, left shoulder

M61.419 Other calcification of muscle, unspecified shoulder

M61.42 Other calcification of muscle, upper arm

M61.421 Other calcification of muscle, right upper arm

M61.422 Other calcification of muscle, left upper arm

M61.429 Other calcification of muscle, unspecified upper arm

M61.43 Other calcification of muscle, forearm

M61.431 Other calcification of muscle, right forearm

M61.432 Other calcification of muscle, left forearm

M61.439 Other calcification of muscle, unspecified forearm

M61.44 Other calcification of muscle, hand

M61.441 Other calcification of muscle, right hand

M61.442 Other calcification of muscle, left hand

M61.449 Other calcification of muscle, unspecified hand

M61.45 Other calcification of muscle, thigh

M61.451 Other calcification of muscle, right thigh

M61.452 Other calcification of muscle, left thigh

M61.459 Other calcification of muscle, unspecified thigh

M61.46 Other calcification of muscle, lower leg

M61.461 Other calcification of muscle, right lower leg

M61.462 Other calcification of muscle, left lower leg

M61.469 Other calcification of muscle, unspecified lower leg

M61.47 Other calcification of muscle, ankle and foot

M61.471 Other calcification of muscle, right ankle and foot

M61.472 Other calcification of muscle, left ankle and foot

M61.479 Other calcification of muscle, unspecified ankle and foot

M61.48 Other calcification of muscle, other site

M61.49 Other calcification of muscle, multiple sites

M61.5 Other ossification of muscle

M61.5Ø Other ossification of muscle, unspecified site

M61.51 Other ossification of muscle, shoulder

M61.511 Other ossification of muscle, right shoulder

M61.512 Other ossification of muscle, left shoulder

M61.519 Other ossification of muscle, unspecified shoulder

M61.52 Other ossification of muscle, upper arm

M61.521 Other ossification of muscle, right upper arm

M61.522 Other ossification of muscle, left upper arm

M61.529 Other ossification of muscle, unspecified upper arm

M61.53 Other ossification of muscle, forearm

M61.531 Other ossification of muscle, right forearm

M61.532 Other ossification of muscle, left forearm

M61.539 Other ossification of muscle, unspecified forearm

M61.54 Other ossification of muscle, hand

M61.541 Other ossification of muscle, right hand

M61.542 Other ossification of muscle, left hand

M61.549 Other ossification of muscle, unspecified hand

M61.55 Other ossification of muscle, thigh

M61.551 Other ossification of muscle, right thigh

M61.552 Other ossification of muscle, left thigh

M61.559 Other ossification of muscle, unspecified thigh

M61.56 Other ossification of muscle, lower leg

M61.561 Other ossification of muscle, right lower leg

M61.562 Other ossification of muscle, left lower leg

M61.569 Other ossification of muscle, unspecified lower leg

M61.57 Other ossification of muscle, ankle and foot

M61.571 Other ossification of muscle, right ankle and foot

M61.572 Other ossification of muscle, left ankle and foot

M61.579 Other ossification of muscle, unspecified ankle and foot

M61.58 Other ossification of muscle, other site

M61.59 Other ossification of muscle, multiple sites

M61.9 Calcification and ossification of muscle, unspecified

M62 Other disorders of muscle

EXCLUDES 1 *alcoholic myopathy (G72.1)*
cramp and spasm (R25.2)
drug-induced myopathy (G72.Ø)
myalgia (M79.1-)
stiff-man syndrome (G25.82)

EXCLUDES 2 *nontraumatic hematoma of muscle (M79.81)*

M62.Ø Separation of muscle (nontraumatic)

Diastasis of muscle

EXCLUDES 1 *diastasis recti complicating pregnancy, labor and delivery (O71.8)*
traumatic separation of muscle - see strain of muscle by body region

M62.ØØ Separation of muscle (nontraumatic), unspecified site

M62.Ø1 Separation of muscle (nontraumatic), shoulder

M62.Ø11 Separation of muscle (nontraumatic), right shoulder

M62.Ø12 Separation of muscle (nontraumatic), left shoulder

M62.Ø19 Separation of muscle (nontraumatic), unspecified shoulder

M62.Ø2 Separation of muscle (nontraumatic), upper arm

M62.Ø21 Separation of muscle (nontraumatic), right upper arm

M62.Ø22 Separation of muscle (nontraumatic), left upper arm

M62.Ø29 Separation of muscle (nontraumatic), unspecified upper arm

M62.Ø3 Separation of muscle (nontraumatic), forearm

M62.Ø31 Separation of muscle (nontraumatic), right forearm

M62.Ø32 Separation of muscle (nontraumatic), left forearm

M62.Ø39 Separation of muscle (nontraumatic), unspecified forearm

M62.Ø4 Separation of muscle (nontraumatic), hand

M62.Ø41 Separation of muscle (nontraumatic), right hand

M62.Ø42 Separation of muscle (nontraumatic), left hand

M62.049 Separation of muscle (nontraumatic), unspecified hand

M62.05 Separation of muscle (nontraumatic), thigh

M62.051 Separation of muscle (nontraumatic), right thigh

M62.052 Separation of muscle (nontraumatic), left thigh

M62.059 Separation of muscle (nontraumatic), unspecified thigh

M62.06 Separation of muscle (nontraumatic), lower leg

M62.061 Separation of muscle (nontraumatic), right lower leg

M62.062 Separation of muscle (nontraumatic), left lower leg

M62.069 Separation of muscle (nontraumatic), unspecified lower leg

M62.07 Separation of muscle (nontraumatic), ankle and foot

M62.071 Separation of muscle (nontraumatic), right ankle and foot

M62.072 Separation of muscle (nontraumatic), left ankle and foot

M62.079 Separation of muscle (nontraumatic), unspecified ankle and foot

M62.08 Separation of muscle (nontraumatic), other site

M62.1 Other rupture of muscle (nontraumatic)

EXCLUDES 1 *traumatic rupture of muscle - see strain of muscle by body region*

EXCLUDES 2 *rupture of tendon (M66.-)*

M62.10 Other rupture of muscle (nontraumatic), unspecified site

M62.11 Other rupture of muscle (nontraumatic), shoulder

M62.111 Other rupture of muscle (nontraumatic), right shoulder

M62.112 Other rupture of muscle (nontraumatic), left shoulder

M62.119 Other rupture of muscle (nontraumatic), unspecified shoulder

M62.12 Other rupture of muscle (nontraumatic), upper arm

M62.121 Other rupture of muscle (nontraumatic), right upper arm

M62.122 Other rupture of muscle (nontraumatic), left upper arm

M62.129 Other rupture of muscle (nontraumatic), unspecified upper arm

M62.13 Other rupture of muscle (nontraumatic), forearm

M62.131 Other rupture of muscle (nontraumatic), right forearm

M62.132 Other rupture of muscle (nontraumatic), left forearm

M62.139 Other rupture of muscle (nontraumatic), unspecified forearm

M62.14 Other rupture of muscle (nontraumatic), hand

M62.141 Other rupture of muscle (nontraumatic), right hand

M62.142 Other rupture of muscle (nontraumatic), left hand

M62.149 Other rupture of muscle (nontraumatic), unspecified hand

M62.15 Other rupture of muscle (nontraumatic), thigh

M62.151 Other rupture of muscle (nontraumatic), right thigh

M62.152 Other rupture of muscle (nontraumatic), left thigh

M62.159 Other rupture of muscle (nontraumatic), unspecified thigh

M62.16 Other rupture of muscle (nontraumatic), lower leg

M62.161 Other rupture of muscle (nontraumatic), right lower leg

M62.162 Other rupture of muscle (nontraumatic), left lower leg

M62.169 Other rupture of muscle (nontraumatic), unspecified lower leg

M62.17 Other rupture of muscle (nontraumatic), ankle and foot

M62.171 Other rupture of muscle (nontraumatic), right ankle and foot

M62.172 Other rupture of muscle (nontraumatic), left ankle and foot

M62.179 Other rupture of muscle (nontraumatic), unspecified ankle and foot

M62.18 Other rupture of muscle (nontraumatic), other site

M62.2 Nontraumatic ischemic infarction of muscle

EXCLUDES 1 *compartment syndrome (traumatic) (T79.A-)*
nontraumatic compartment syndrome (M79.A-)
rhabdomyolysis (M62.82)
traumatic ischemia of muscle (T79.6)
Volkmann's ischemic contracture (T79.6)

M62.20 Nontraumatic ischemic infarction of muscle, unspecified site

M62.21 Nontraumatic ischemic infarction of muscle, shoulder

M62.211 Nontraumatic ischemic infarction of muscle, right shoulder

M62.212 Nontraumatic ischemic infarction of muscle, left shoulder

M62.219 Nontraumatic ischemic infarction of muscle, unspecified shoulder

M62.22 Nontraumatic ischemic infarction of muscle, upper arm

M62.221 Nontraumatic ischemic infarction of muscle, right upper arm

M62.222 Nontraumatic ischemic infarction of muscle, left upper arm

M62.229 Nontraumatic ischemic infarction of muscle, unspecified upper arm

M62.23 Nontraumatic ischemic infarction of muscle, forearm

M62.231 Nontraumatic ischemic infarction of muscle, right forearm

M62.232 Nontraumatic ischemic infarction of muscle, left forearm

M62.239 Nontraumatic ischemic infarction of muscle, unspecified forearm

M62.24 Nontraumatic ischemic infarction of muscle, hand

M62.241 Nontraumatic ischemic infarction of muscle, right hand

M62.242 Nontraumatic ischemic infarction of muscle, left hand

M62.249 Nontraumatic ischemic infarction of muscle, unspecified hand

M62.25 Nontraumatic ischemic infarction of muscle, thigh

M62.251 Nontraumatic ischemic infarction of muscle, right thigh

M62.252 Nontraumatic ischemic infarction of muscle, left thigh

M62.259 Nontraumatic ischemic infarction of muscle, unspecified thigh

M62.26 Nontraumatic ischemic infarction of muscle, lower leg

M62.261 Nontraumatic ischemic infarction of muscle, right lower leg

M62.262 Nontraumatic ischemic infarction of muscle, left lower leg

M62.269 Nontraumatic ischemic infarction of muscle, unspecified lower leg

M62.27 Nontraumatic ischemic infarction of muscle, ankle and foot

M62.271 Nontraumatic ischemic infarction of muscle, right ankle and foot

M62.272 Nontraumatic ischemic infarction of muscle, left ankle and foot

M62.279 Nontraumatic ischemic infarction of muscle, unspecified ankle and foot

M62.28 Nontraumatic ischemic infarction of muscle, other site

M62.3 Immobility syndrome (paraplegic)

M62.4 Contracture of muscle

Contracture of tendon (sheath)

EXCLUDES 1 *contracture of joint (M24.5-)*

M62.40 Contracture of muscle, unspecified site

M62.41 Contracture of muscle, shoulder

M62.411 Contracture of muscle, right shoulder

M62.412 Contracture of muscle, left shoulder

M62.419 Contracture of muscle, unspecified shoulder

M62.42 Contracture of muscle, upper arm

M62.421 Contracture of muscle, right upper arm

M62.422 Contracture of muscle, left upper arm

M62.429 Contracture of muscle, unspecified upper arm

M62.43 Contracture of muscle, forearm
- M62.431 Contracture of muscle, right forearm
- M62.432 Contracture of muscle, left forearm
- M62.439 Contracture of muscle, unspecified forearm

M62.44 Contracture of muscle, hand
- M62.441 Contracture of muscle, right hand
- M62.442 Contracture of muscle, left hand
- M62.449 Contracture of muscle, unspecified hand

M62.45 Contracture of muscle, thigh
- M62.451 Contracture of muscle, right thigh
- M62.452 Contracture of muscle, left thigh
- M62.459 Contracture of muscle, unspecified thigh

M62.46 Contracture of muscle, lower leg
- M62.461 Contracture of muscle, right lower leg
- M62.462 Contracture of muscle, left lower leg
- M62.469 Contracture of muscle, unspecified lower leg

M62.47 Contracture of muscle, ankle and foot
- M62.471 Contracture of muscle, right ankle and foot
- M62.472 Contracture of muscle, left ankle and foot
- M62.479 Contracture of muscle, unspecified ankle and foot

M62.48 Contracture of muscle, other site

M62.49 Contracture of muscle, multiple sites

M62.5 Muscle wasting and atrophy, not elsewhere classified

Disuse atrophy NEC

EXCLUDES 1 *neuralgic amyotrophy (G54.5)*
progressive muscular atrophy (G12.21)
sarcopenia (M62.84)

EXCLUDES 2 *pelvic muscle wasting (N81.84)*

M62.50 Muscle wasting and atrophy, not elsewhere classified, unspecified site

M62.51 Muscle wasting and atrophy, not elsewhere classified, shoulder
- M62.511 Muscle wasting and atrophy, not elsewhere classified, right shoulder
- M62.512 Muscle wasting and atrophy, not elsewhere classified, left shoulder
- M62.519 Muscle wasting and atrophy, not elsewhere classified, unspecified shoulder

M62.52 Muscle wasting and atrophy, not elsewhere classified, upper arm
- M62.521 Muscle wasting and atrophy, not elsewhere classified, right upper arm
- M62.522 Muscle wasting and atrophy, not elsewhere classified, left upper arm
- M62.529 Muscle wasting and atrophy, not elsewhere classified, unspecified upper arm

M62.53 Muscle wasting and atrophy, not elsewhere classified, forearm
- M62.531 Muscle wasting and atrophy, not elsewhere classified, right forearm
- M62.532 Muscle wasting and atrophy, not elsewhere classified, left forearm
- M62.539 Muscle wasting and atrophy, not elsewhere classified, unspecified forearm

M62.54 Muscle wasting and atrophy, not elsewhere classified, hand
- M62.541 Muscle wasting and atrophy, not elsewhere classified, right hand
- M62.542 Muscle wasting and atrophy, not elsewhere classified, left hand
- M62.549 Muscle wasting and atrophy, not elsewhere classified, unspecified hand

M62.55 Muscle wasting and atrophy, not elsewhere classified, thigh
- M62.551 Muscle wasting and atrophy, not elsewhere classified, right thigh
- M62.552 Muscle wasting and atrophy, not elsewhere classified, left thigh
- M62.559 Muscle wasting and atrophy, not elsewhere classified, unspecified thigh

M62.56 Muscle wasting and atrophy, not elsewhere classified, lower leg
- M62.561 Muscle wasting and atrophy, not elsewhere classified, right lower leg
- M62.562 Muscle wasting and atrophy, not elsewhere classified, left lower leg
- M62.569 Muscle wasting and atrophy, not elsewhere classified, unspecified lower leg

M62.57 Muscle wasting and atrophy, not elsewhere classified, ankle and foot
- M62.571 Muscle wasting and atrophy, not elsewhere classified, right ankle and foot
- M62.572 Muscle wasting and atrophy, not elsewhere classified, left ankle and foot
- M62.579 Muscle wasting and atrophy, not elsewhere classified, unspecified ankle and foot

M62.58 Muscle wasting and atrophy, not elsewhere classified, other site

M62.59 Muscle wasting and atrophy, not elsewhere classified, multiple sites

● M62.5A Muscle wasting and atrophy, not elsewhere classified, back
- ● M62.5A0 Muscle wasting and atrophy, not elsewhere classified, back, cervical
- ● M62.5A1 Muscle wasting and atrophy, not elsewhere classified, back, thoracic
- ● M62.5A2 Muscle wasting and atrophy, not elsewhere classified, back, lumbosacral
- ● M62.5A9 Muscle wasting and atrophy, not elsewhere classified, back, unspecified level

M62.8 Other specified disorders of muscle

EXCLUDES 2 *nontraumatic hematoma of muscle (M79.81)*

M62.81 Muscle weakness (generalized)

EXCLUDES 1 *muscle weakness in sarcopenia (M62.84)*

M62.82 Rhabdomyolysis CC

EXCLUDES 1 *traumatic rhabdomyolysis (T79.6)*

AHA: 2019,2Q,12

DEF: Rapid disintegration or destruction of skeletal muscle caused by direct or indirect injury, resulting in the excretion of muscle protein myoglobin into the urine.

M62.83 Muscle spasm
- M62.830 Muscle spasm of back
- M62.831 Muscle spasm of calf
  Charley-horse
- M62.838 Other muscle spasm

M62.84 Sarcopenia

Age-related sarcopenia

Code first underlying disease, if applicable, such as:
- disorders of myoneural junction and muscle disease in diseases classified elsewhere (G73.-)
- other and unspecified myopathies (G72.-)
- primary disorders of muscles (G71.-)

AHA: 2016,4Q,41

M62.89 Other specified disorders of muscle

Muscle (sheath) hernia

M62.9 Disorder of muscle, unspecified

M63 Disorders of muscle in diseases classified elsewhere

Code first underlying disease, such as:
- leprosy (A30.-)
- neoplasm (C49.-, C79.89, D21.-, D48.1)
- schistosomiasis (B65.-)
- trichinellosis (B75)

EXCLUDES 1 *myopathy in cysticercosis (B69.81)*
myopathy in endocrine diseases (G73.7)
myopathy in metabolic diseases (G73.7)
myopathy in sarcoidosis (D86.87)
myopathy in secondary syphilis (A51.49)
myopathy in syphilis (late) (A52.78)
myopathy in toxoplasmosis (B58.82)
myopathy in tuberculosis (A18.09)

M63.8 Disorders of muscle in diseases classified elsewhere

M63.80 Disorders of muscle in diseases classified elsewhere, unspecified site

- ✓6th **M63.81 Disorders of muscle in diseases classified elsewhere, shoulder**
  - *M63.811 Disorders of muscle in diseases classified elsewhere, right shoulder*
  - *M63.812 Disorders of muscle in diseases classified elsewhere, left shoulder*
  - *M63.819 Disorders of muscle in diseases classified elsewhere, unspecified shoulder*
- ✓6th **M63.82 Disorders of muscle in diseases classified elsewhere, upper arm**
  - *M63.821 Disorders of muscle in diseases classified elsewhere, right upper arm*
  - *M63.822 Disorders of muscle in diseases classified elsewhere, left upper arm*
  - *M63.829 Disorders of muscle in diseases classified elsewhere, unspecified upper arm*
- ✓6th **M63.83 Disorders of muscle in diseases classified elsewhere, forearm**
  - *M63.831 Disorders of muscle in diseases classified elsewhere, right forearm*
  - *M63.832 Disorders of muscle in diseases classified elsewhere, left forearm*
  - *M63.839 Disorders of muscle in diseases classified elsewhere, unspecified forearm*
- ✓6th **M63.84 Disorders of muscle in diseases classified elsewhere, hand**
  - *M63.841 Disorders of muscle in diseases classified elsewhere, right hand*
  - *M63.842 Disorders of muscle in diseases classified elsewhere, left hand*
  - *M63.849 Disorders of muscle in diseases classified elsewhere, unspecified hand*
- ✓6th **M63.85 Disorders of muscle in diseases classified elsewhere, thigh**
  - *M63.851 Disorders of muscle in diseases classified elsewhere, right thigh*
  - *M63.852 Disorders of muscle in diseases classified elsewhere, left thigh*
  - *M63.859 Disorders of muscle in diseases classified elsewhere, unspecified thigh*
- ✓6th **M63.86 Disorders of muscle in diseases classified elsewhere, lower leg**
  - *M63.861 Disorders of muscle in diseases classified elsewhere, right lower leg*
  - *M63.862 Disorders of muscle in diseases classified elsewhere, left lower leg*
  - *M63.869 Disorders of muscle in diseases classified elsewhere, unspecified lower leg*
- ✓6th **M63.87 Disorders of muscle in diseases classified elsewhere, ankle and foot**
  - *M63.871 Disorders of muscle in diseases classified elsewhere, right ankle and foot*
  - *M63.872 Disorders of muscle in diseases classified elsewhere, left ankle and foot*
  - *M63.879 Disorders of muscle in diseases classified elsewhere, unspecified ankle and foot*
- *M63.88 Disorders of muscle in diseases classified elsewhere, other site*
- *M63.89 Disorders of muscle in diseases classified elsewhere, multiple sites*

Disorders of synovium and tendon (M65-M67)

✓4th **M65 Synovitis and tenosynovitis**

EXCLUDES 1 *chronic crepitant synovitis of hand and wrist (M7Ø.Ø-)*
current injury - see injury of ligament or tendon by body region
soft tissue disorders related to use, overuse and pressure (M7Ø.-)

- ✓5th **M65.Ø Abscess of tendon sheath**
  - Use additional code (B95-B96) to identify bacterial agent.
  - **M65.ØØ Abscess of tendon sheath, unspecified site**
  - ✓6th **M65.Ø1 Abscess of tendon sheath, shoulder**
    - **M65.Ø11 Abscess of tendon sheath, right shoulder**
    - **M65.Ø12 Abscess of tendon sheath, left shoulder**
    - **M65.Ø19 Abscess of tendon sheath, unspecified shoulder**
  - ✓6th **M65.Ø2 Abscess of tendon sheath, upper arm**
    - **M65.Ø21 Abscess of tendon sheath, right upper arm**
    - **M65.Ø22 Abscess of tendon sheath, left upper arm**
    - **M65.Ø29 Abscess of tendon sheath, unspecified upper arm**
  - ✓6th **M65.Ø3 Abscess of tendon sheath, forearm**
    - **M65.Ø31 Abscess of tendon sheath, right forearm**
    - **M65.Ø32 Abscess of tendon sheath, left forearm**
    - **M65.Ø39 Abscess of tendon sheath, unspecified forearm**
  - ✓6th **M65.Ø4 Abscess of tendon sheath, hand**
    - **M65.Ø41 Abscess of tendon sheath, right hand**
    - **M65.Ø42 Abscess of tendon sheath, left hand**
    - **M65.Ø49 Abscess of tendon sheath, unspecified hand**
  - ✓6th **M65.Ø5 Abscess of tendon sheath, thigh**
    - **M65.Ø51 Abscess of tendon sheath, right thigh**
    - **M65.Ø52 Abscess of tendon sheath, left thigh**
    - **M65.Ø59 Abscess of tendon sheath, unspecified thigh**
  - ✓6th **M65.Ø6 Abscess of tendon sheath, lower leg**
    - **M65.Ø61 Abscess of tendon sheath, right lower leg**
    - **M65.Ø62 Abscess of tendon sheath, left lower leg**
    - **M65.Ø69 Abscess of tendon sheath, unspecified lower leg**
  - ✓6th **M65.Ø7 Abscess of tendon sheath, ankle and foot**
    - **M65.Ø71 Abscess of tendon sheath, right ankle and foot**
    - **M65.Ø72 Abscess of tendon sheath, left ankle and foot**
    - **M65.Ø79 Abscess of tendon sheath, unspecified ankle and foot**
  - **M65.Ø8 Abscess of tendon sheath, other site**
- ✓5th **M65.1 Other infective (teno)synovitis**
  - **M65.1Ø Other infective (teno)synovitis, unspecified site**
  - ✓6th **M65.11 Other infective (teno)synovitis, shoulder**
    - **M65.111 Other infective (teno)synovitis, right shoulder**
    - **M65.112 Other infective (teno)synovitis, left shoulder**
    - **M65.119 Other infective (teno)synovitis, unspecified shoulder**
  - ✓6th **M65.12 Other infective (teno)synovitis, elbow**
    - **M65.121 Other infective (teno)synovitis, right elbow**
    - **M65.122 Other infective (teno)synovitis, left elbow**
    - **M65.129 Other infective (teno)synovitis, unspecified elbow**
  - ✓6th **M65.13 Other infective (teno)synovitis, wrist**
    - **M65.131 Other infective (teno)synovitis, right wrist**
    - **M65.132 Other infective (teno)synovitis, left wrist**
    - **M65.139 Other infective (teno)synovitis, unspecified wrist**
  - ✓6th **M65.14 Other infective (teno)synovitis, hand**
    - **M65.141 Other infective (teno)synovitis, right hand**
    - **M65.142 Other infective (teno)synovitis, left hand**
    - **M65.149 Other infective (teno)synovitis, unspecified hand**
  - ✓6th **M65.15 Other infective (teno)synovitis, hip**
    - **M65.151 Other infective (teno)synovitis, right hip**
    - **M65.152 Other infective (teno)synovitis, left hip**
    - **M65.159 Other infective (teno)synovitis, unspecified hip**
  - ✓6th **M65.16 Other infective (teno)synovitis, knee**
    - **M65.161 Other infective (teno)synovitis, right knee**
    - **M65.162 Other infective (teno)synovitis, left knee**
    - **M65.169 Other infective (teno)synovitis, unspecified knee**
  - ✓6th **M65.17 Other infective (teno)synovitis, ankle and foot**
    - **M65.171 Other infective (teno)synovitis, right ankle and foot**
    - **M65.172 Other infective (teno)synovitis, left ankle and foot**
    - **M65.179 Other infective (teno)synovitis, unspecified ankle and foot**
  - **M65.18 Other infective (teno)synovitis, other site**
  - **M65.19 Other infective (teno)synovitis, multiple sites**
- ✓5th **M65.2 Calcific tendinitis**
  - EXCLUDES 1 *tendinitis as classified in M75-M77*
    calcified tendinitis of shoulder (M75.3)
  - **M65.2Ø Calcific tendinitis, unspecified site**

M65.22 Calcific tendinitis, upper arm
M65.221 Calcific tendinitis, right upper arm
M65.222 Calcific tendinitis, left upper arm
M65.229 Calcific tendinitis, unspecified upper arm
M65.23 Calcific tendinitis, forearm
M65.231 Calcific tendinitis, right forearm
M65.232 Calcific tendinitis, left forearm
M65.239 Calcific tendinitis, unspecified forearm
M65.24 Calcific tendinitis, hand
M65.241 Calcific tendinitis, right hand
M65.242 Calcific tendinitis, left hand
M65.249 Calcific tendinitis, unspecified hand
M65.25 Calcific tendinitis, thigh
M65.251 Calcific tendinitis, right thigh
M65.252 Calcific tendinitis, left thigh
M65.259 Calcific tendinitis, unspecified thigh
M65.26 Calcific tendinitis, lower leg
M65.261 Calcific tendinitis, right lower leg
M65.262 Calcific tendinitis, left lower leg
M65.269 Calcific tendinitis, unspecified lower leg
M65.27 Calcific tendinitis, ankle and foot
M65.271 Calcific tendinitis, right ankle and foot
M65.272 Calcific tendinitis, left ankle and foot
M65.279 Calcific tendinitis, unspecified ankle and foot
M65.28 Calcific tendinitis, other site
M65.29 Calcific tendinitis, multiple sites
M65.3 Trigger finger
Nodular tendinous disease
M65.3Ø Trigger finger, unspecified finger
M65.31 Trigger thumb
M65.311 Trigger thumb, right thumb
M65.312 Trigger thumb, left thumb
M65.319 Trigger thumb, unspecified thumb
M65.32 Trigger finger, index finger
M65.321 Trigger finger, right index finger
M65.322 Trigger finger, left index finger
M65.329 Trigger finger, unspecified index finger
M65.33 Trigger finger, middle finger
M65.331 Trigger finger, right middle finger
M65.332 Trigger finger, left middle finger
M65.339 Trigger finger, unspecified middle finger
M65.34 Trigger finger, ring finger
M65.341 Trigger finger, right ring finger
M65.342 Trigger finger, left ring finger
M65.349 Trigger finger, unspecified ring finger
M65.35 Trigger finger, little finger
M65.351 Trigger finger, right little finger
M65.352 Trigger finger, left little finger
M65.359 Trigger finger, unspecified little finger
M65.4 Radial styloid tenosynovitis [de Quervain]
M65.8 Other synovitis and tenosynovitis
M65.8Ø Other synovitis and tenosynovitis, unspecified site
M65.81 Other synovitis and tenosynovitis, shoulder
M65.811 Other synovitis and tenosynovitis, right shoulder
M65.812 Other synovitis and tenosynovitis, left shoulder
M65.819 Other synovitis and tenosynovitis, unspecified shoulder
M65.82 Other synovitis and tenosynovitis, upper arm
M65.821 Other synovitis and tenosynovitis, right upper arm
M65.822 Other synovitis and tenosynovitis, left upper arm
M65.829 Other synovitis and tenosynovitis, unspecified upper arm
M65.83 Other synovitis and tenosynovitis, forearm
M65.831 Other synovitis and tenosynovitis, right forearm
M65.832 Other synovitis and tenosynovitis, left forearm
M65.839 Other synovitis and tenosynovitis, unspecified forearm
M65.84 Other synovitis and tenosynovitis, hand
M65.841 Other synovitis and tenosynovitis, right hand
M65.842 Other synovitis and tenosynovitis, left hand
M65.849 Other synovitis and tenosynovitis, unspecified hand
M65.85 Other synovitis and tenosynovitis, thigh
M65.851 Other synovitis and tenosynovitis, right thigh
M65.852 Other synovitis and tenosynovitis, left thigh
M65.859 Other synovitis and tenosynovitis, unspecified thigh
M65.86 Other synovitis and tenosynovitis, lower leg
M65.861 Other synovitis and tenosynovitis, right lower leg
M65.862 Other synovitis and tenosynovitis, left lower leg
M65.869 Other synovitis and tenosynovitis, unspecified lower leg
M65.87 Other synovitis and tenosynovitis, ankle and foot
M65.871 Other synovitis and tenosynovitis, right ankle and foot
M65.872 Other synovitis and tenosynovitis, left ankle and foot
M65.879 Other synovitis and tenosynovitis, unspecified ankle and foot
M65.88 Other synovitis and tenosynovitis, other site
M65.89 Other synovitis and tenosynovitis, multiple sites
M65.9 Synovitis and tenosynovitis, unspecified

M66 Spontaneous rupture of synovium and tendon
INCLUDES rupture that occurs when a normal force is applied to tissues that are inferred to have less than normal strength
EXCLUDES 2 *rotator cuff syndrome (M75.1-)*
rupture where an abnormal force is applied to normal tissue - see injury of tendon by body region
M66.Ø Rupture of popliteal cyst
M66.1 Rupture of synovium
Rupture of synovial cyst
EXCLUDES 2 *rupture of popliteal cyst (M66.Ø)*
M66.1Ø Rupture of synovium, unspecified joint
M66.11 Rupture of synovium, shoulder
M66.111 Rupture of synovium, right shoulder
M66.112 Rupture of synovium, left shoulder
M66.119 Rupture of synovium, unspecified shoulder
M66.12 Rupture of synovium, elbow
M66.121 Rupture of synovium, right elbow
M66.122 Rupture of synovium, left elbow
M66.129 Rupture of synovium, unspecified elbow
M66.13 Rupture of synovium, wrist
M66.131 Rupture of synovium, right wrist
M66.132 Rupture of synovium, left wrist
M66.139 Rupture of synovium, unspecified wrist
M66.14 Rupture of synovium, hand and fingers
M66.141 Rupture of synovium, right hand
M66.142 Rupture of synovium, left hand
M66.143 Rupture of synovium, unspecified hand
M66.144 Rupture of synovium, right finger(s)
M66.145 Rupture of synovium, left finger(s)
M66.146 Rupture of synovium, unspecified finger(s)
M66.15 Rupture of synovium, hip
M66.151 Rupture of synovium, right hip
M66.152 Rupture of synovium, left hip
M66.159 Rupture of synovium, unspecified hip
M66.17 Rupture of synovium, ankle, foot and toes
M66.171 Rupture of synovium, right ankle
M66.172 Rupture of synovium, left ankle
M66.173 Rupture of synovium, unspecified ankle
M66.174 Rupture of synovium, right foot
M66.175 Rupture of synovium, left foot
M66.176 Rupture of synovium, unspecified foot
M66.177 Rupture of synovium, right toe(s)
M66.178 Rupture of synovium, left toe(s)

M66.179 Rupture of synovium, unspecified toe(s)
M66.18 Rupture of synovium, other site
M66.2 Spontaneous rupture of extensor tendons
TIP: Refer to the Muscle/Tendon table at the beginning of this chapter.
M66.20 Spontaneous rupture of extensor tendons, unspecified site
M66.21 Spontaneous rupture of extensor tendons, shoulder
M66.211 Spontaneous rupture of extensor tendons, right shoulder
M66.212 Spontaneous rupture of extensor tendons, left shoulder
M66.219 Spontaneous rupture of extensor tendons, unspecified shoulder
M66.22 Spontaneous rupture of extensor tendons, upper arm
M66.221 Spontaneous rupture of extensor tendons, right upper arm
M66.222 Spontaneous rupture of extensor tendons, left upper arm
M66.229 Spontaneous rupture of extensor tendons, unspecified upper arm
M66.23 Spontaneous rupture of extensor tendons, forearm
M66.231 Spontaneous rupture of extensor tendons, right forearm
M66.232 Spontaneous rupture of extensor tendons, left forearm
M66.239 Spontaneous rupture of extensor tendons, unspecified forearm
M66.24 Spontaneous rupture of extensor tendons, hand
M66.241 Spontaneous rupture of extensor tendons, right hand
M66.242 Spontaneous rupture of extensor tendons, left hand
M66.249 Spontaneous rupture of extensor tendons, unspecified hand
M66.25 Spontaneous rupture of extensor tendons, thigh
M66.251 Spontaneous rupture of extensor tendons, right thigh
M66.252 Spontaneous rupture of extensor tendons, left thigh
M66.259 Spontaneous rupture of extensor tendons, unspecified thigh
M66.26 Spontaneous rupture of extensor tendons, lower leg
M66.261 Spontaneous rupture of extensor tendons, right lower leg
M66.262 Spontaneous rupture of extensor tendons, left lower leg
M66.269 Spontaneous rupture of extensor tendons, unspecified lower leg
M66.27 Spontaneous rupture of extensor tendons, ankle and foot
M66.271 Spontaneous rupture of extensor tendons, right ankle and foot
M66.272 Spontaneous rupture of extensor tendons, left ankle and foot
M66.279 Spontaneous rupture of extensor tendons, unspecified ankle and foot
M66.28 Spontaneous rupture of extensor tendons, other site
M66.29 Spontaneous rupture of extensor tendons, multiple sites
M66.3 Spontaneous rupture of flexor tendons
TIP: Refer to the Muscle/Tendon table at the beginning of this chapter.
M66.30 Spontaneous rupture of flexor tendons, unspecified site
M66.31 Spontaneous rupture of flexor tendons, shoulder
M66.311 Spontaneous rupture of flexor tendons, right shoulder
M66.312 Spontaneous rupture of flexor tendons, left shoulder
M66.319 Spontaneous rupture of flexor tendons, unspecified shoulder
M66.32 Spontaneous rupture of flexor tendons, upper arm
M66.321 Spontaneous rupture of flexor tendons, right upper arm
M66.322 Spontaneous rupture of flexor tendons, left upper arm
M66.329 Spontaneous rupture of flexor tendons, unspecified upper arm
M66.33 Spontaneous rupture of flexor tendons, forearm
M66.331 Spontaneous rupture of flexor tendons, right forearm
M66.332 Spontaneous rupture of flexor tendons, left forearm
M66.339 Spontaneous rupture of flexor tendons, unspecified forearm
M66.34 Spontaneous rupture of flexor tendons, hand
M66.341 Spontaneous rupture of flexor tendons, right hand
M66.342 Spontaneous rupture of flexor tendons, left hand
M66.349 Spontaneous rupture of flexor tendons, unspecified hand
M66.35 Spontaneous rupture of flexor tendons, thigh
M66.351 Spontaneous rupture of flexor tendons, right thigh
M66.352 Spontaneous rupture of flexor tendons, left thigh
M66.359 Spontaneous rupture of flexor tendons, unspecified thigh
M66.36 Spontaneous rupture of flexor tendons, lower leg
M66.361 Spontaneous rupture of flexor tendons, right lower leg
M66.362 Spontaneous rupture of flexor tendons, left lower leg
M66.369 Spontaneous rupture of flexor tendons, unspecified lower leg
M66.37 Spontaneous rupture of flexor tendons, ankle and foot
M66.371 Spontaneous rupture of flexor tendons, right ankle and foot
M66.372 Spontaneous rupture of flexor tendons, left ankle and foot
M66.379 Spontaneous rupture of flexor tendons, unspecified ankle and foot
M66.38 Spontaneous rupture of flexor tendons, other site
M66.39 Spontaneous rupture of flexor tendons, multiple sites
M66.8 Spontaneous rupture of other tendons
TIP: Refer to the Muscle/Tendon table at the beginning of this chapter.
M66.80 Spontaneous rupture of other tendons, unspecified site
M66.81 Spontaneous rupture of other tendons, shoulder
M66.811 Spontaneous rupture of other tendons, right shoulder
M66.812 Spontaneous rupture of other tendons, left shoulder
M66.819 Spontaneous rupture of other tendons, unspecified shoulder
M66.82 Spontaneous rupture of other tendons, upper arm
M66.821 Spontaneous rupture of other tendons, right upper arm
M66.822 Spontaneous rupture of other tendons, left upper arm
M66.829 Spontaneous rupture of other tendons, unspecified upper arm
M66.83 Spontaneous rupture of other tendons, forearm
M66.831 Spontaneous rupture of other tendons, right forearm
M66.832 Spontaneous rupture of other tendons, left forearm
M66.839 Spontaneous rupture of other tendons, unspecified forearm
M66.84 Spontaneous rupture of other tendons, hand
M66.841 Spontaneous rupture of other tendons, right hand
M66.842 Spontaneous rupture of other tendons, left hand
M66.849 Spontaneous rupture of other tendons, unspecified hand
M66.85 Spontaneous rupture of other tendons, thigh
M66.851 Spontaneous rupture of other tendons, right thigh
M66.852 Spontaneous rupture of other tendons, left thigh

M66.859 Spontaneous rupture of other tendons, unspecified thigh

✓6th M66.86 Spontaneous rupture of other tendons, lower leg

M66.861 Spontaneous rupture of other tendons, right lower leg

M66.862 Spontaneous rupture of other tendons, left lower leg

M66.869 Spontaneous rupture of other tendons, unspecified lower leg

✓6th M66.87 Spontaneous rupture of other tendons, ankle and foot

M66.871 Spontaneous rupture of other tendons, right ankle and foot

M66.872 Spontaneous rupture of other tendons, left ankle and foot

M66.879 Spontaneous rupture of other tendons, unspecified ankle and foot

M66.88 Spontaneous rupture of other tendons, other sites

M66.89 Spontaneous rupture of other tendons, multiple sites

M66.9 Spontaneous rupture of unspecified tendon

Rupture at musculotendinous junction, nontraumatic

✓4th **M67 Other disorders of synovium and tendon**

EXCLUDES 1 *palmar fascial fibromatosis [Dupuytren] (M72.Ø)*
tendinitis NOS (M77.9-)
xanthomatosis localized to tendons (E78.2)

✓5th M67.Ø Short Achilles tendon (acquired)

M67.ØØ Short Achilles tendon (acquired), unspecified ankle

M67.Ø1 Short Achilles tendon (acquired), right ankle

M67.Ø2 Short Achilles tendon (acquired), left ankle

✓5th M67.2 Synovial hypertrophy, not elsewhere classified

EXCLUDES 1 *villonodular synovitis (pigmented) (M12.2-)*

M67.2Ø Synovial hypertrophy, not elsewhere classified, unspecified site

✓6th M67.21 Synovial hypertrophy, not elsewhere classified, shoulder

M67.211 Synovial hypertrophy, not elsewhere classified, right shoulder

M67.212 Synovial hypertrophy, not elsewhere classified, left shoulder

M67.219 Synovial hypertrophy, not elsewhere classified, unspecified shoulder

✓6th M67.22 Synovial hypertrophy, not elsewhere classified, upper arm

M67.221 Synovial hypertrophy, not elsewhere classified, right upper arm

M67.222 Synovial hypertrophy, not elsewhere classified, left upper arm

M67.229 Synovial hypertrophy, not elsewhere classified, unspecified upper arm

✓6th M67.23 Synovial hypertrophy, not elsewhere classified, forearm

M67.231 Synovial hypertrophy, not elsewhere classified, right forearm

M67.232 Synovial hypertrophy, not elsewhere classified, left forearm

M67.239 Synovial hypertrophy, not elsewhere classified, unspecified forearm

✓6th M67.24 Synovial hypertrophy, not elsewhere classified, hand

M67.241 Synovial hypertrophy, not elsewhere classified, right hand

M67.242 Synovial hypertrophy, not elsewhere classified, left hand

M67.249 Synovial hypertrophy, not elsewhere classified, unspecified hand

✓6th M67.25 Synovial hypertrophy, not elsewhere classified, thigh

M67.251 Synovial hypertrophy, not elsewhere classified, right thigh

M67.252 Synovial hypertrophy, not elsewhere classified, left thigh

M67.259 Synovial hypertrophy, not elsewhere classified, unspecified thigh

✓6th M67.26 Synovial hypertrophy, not elsewhere classified, lower leg

M67.261 Synovial hypertrophy, not elsewhere classified, right lower leg

M67.262 Synovial hypertrophy, not elsewhere classified, left lower leg

M67.269 Synovial hypertrophy, not elsewhere classified, unspecified lower leg

✓6th M67.27 Synovial hypertrophy, not elsewhere classified, ankle and foot

M67.271 Synovial hypertrophy, not elsewhere classified, right ankle and foot

M67.272 Synovial hypertrophy, not elsewhere classified, left ankle and foot

M67.279 Synovial hypertrophy, not elsewhere classified, unspecified ankle and foot

M67.28 Synovial hypertrophy, not elsewhere classified, other site

M67.29 Synovial hypertrophy, not elsewhere classified, multiple sites

✓5th M67.3 Transient synovitis

Toxic synovitis

EXCLUDES 1 *palindromic rheumatism (M12.3-)*

M67.3Ø Transient synovitis, unspecified site

✓6th M67.31 Transient synovitis, shoulder

M67.311 Transient synovitis, right shoulder

M67.312 Transient synovitis, left shoulder

M67.319 Transient synovitis, unspecified shoulder

✓6th M67.32 Transient synovitis, elbow

M67.321 Transient synovitis, right elbow

M67.322 Transient synovitis, left elbow

M67.329 Transient synovitis, unspecified elbow

✓6th M67.33 Transient synovitis, wrist

M67.331 Transient synovitis, right wrist

M67.332 Transient synovitis, left wrist

M67.339 Transient synovitis, unspecified wrist

✓6th M67.34 Transient synovitis, hand

M67.341 Transient synovitis, right hand

M67.342 Transient synovitis, left hand

M67.349 Transient synovitis, unspecified hand

✓6th M67.35 Transient synovitis, hip

M67.351 Transient synovitis, right hip

M67.352 Transient synovitis, left hip

M67.359 Transient synovitis, unspecified hip

✓6th M67.36 Transient synovitis, knee

M67.361 Transient synovitis, right knee

M67.362 Transient synovitis, left knee

M67.369 Transient synovitis, unspecified knee

✓6th M67.37 Transient synovitis, ankle and foot

M67.371 Transient synovitis, right ankle and foot

M67.372 Transient synovitis, left ankle and foot

M67.379 Transient synovitis, unspecified ankle and foot

M67.38 Transient synovitis, other site

M67.39 Transient synovitis, multiple sites

✓5th M67.4 Ganglion

Ganglion of joint or tendon (sheath)

EXCLUDES 1 *ganglion in yaws (A66.6)*

EXCLUDES 2 *cyst of bursa (M71.2-M71.3)*
cyst of synovium (M71.2-M71.3)

DEF: Fluid-filled, benign cyst appearing on a tendon sheath or aponeurosis, frequently connecting to an underlying joint.

M67.4Ø Ganglion, unspecified site

✓6th M67.41 Ganglion, shoulder

M67.411 Ganglion, right shoulder

M67.412 Ganglion, left shoulder

M67.419 Ganglion, unspecified shoulder

✓6th M67.42 Ganglion, elbow

M67.421 Ganglion, right elbow

M67.422 Ganglion, left elbow

M67.429 Ganglion, unspecified elbow

✓6th **M67.43 Ganglion, wrist**

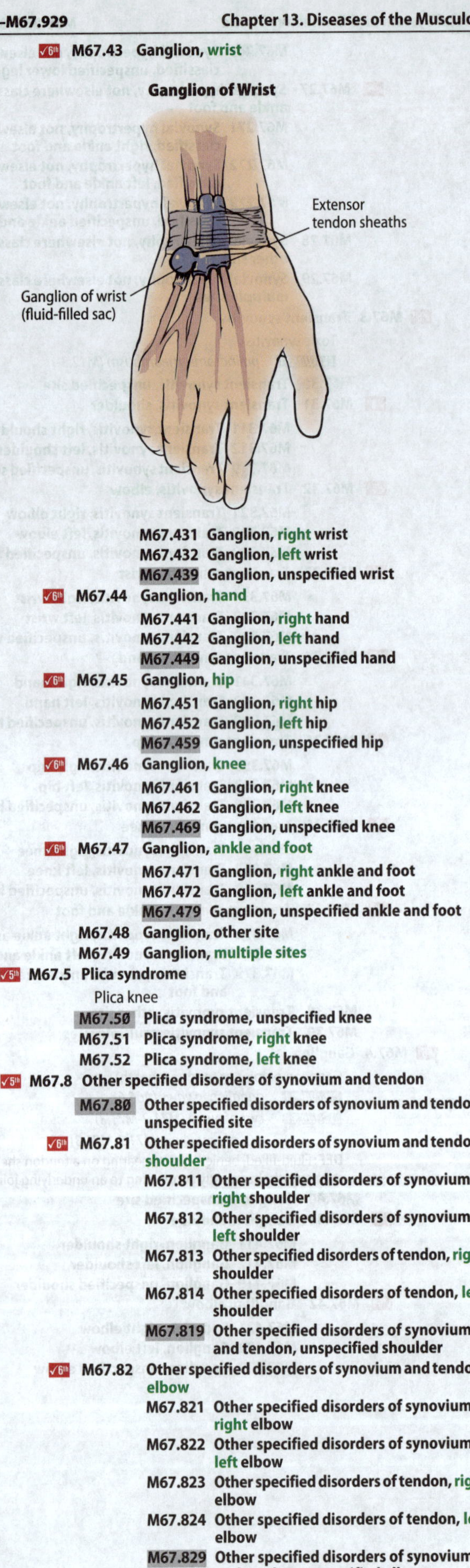

M67.431 Ganglion, right wrist
M67.432 Ganglion, left wrist
M67.439 Ganglion, unspecified wrist

✓6th **M67.44 Ganglion, hand**
M67.441 Ganglion, right hand
M67.442 Ganglion, left hand
M67.449 Ganglion, unspecified hand

✓6th **M67.45 Ganglion, hip**
M67.451 Ganglion, right hip
M67.452 Ganglion, left hip
M67.459 Ganglion, unspecified hip

✓6th **M67.46 Ganglion, knee**
M67.461 Ganglion, right knee
M67.462 Ganglion, left knee
M67.469 Ganglion, unspecified knee

✓6th **M67.47 Ganglion, ankle and foot**
M67.471 Ganglion, right ankle and foot
M67.472 Ganglion, left ankle and foot
M67.479 Ganglion, unspecified ankle and foot

M67.48 Ganglion, other site
M67.49 Ganglion, multiple sites

✓5th **M67.5 Plica syndrome**
Plica knee
M67.5Ø Plica syndrome, unspecified knee
M67.51 Plica syndrome, right knee
M67.52 Plica syndrome, left knee

✓5th **M67.8 Other specified disorders of synovium and tendon**
M67.8Ø Other specified disorders of synovium and tendon, unspecified site

✓6th **M67.81 Other specified disorders of synovium and tendon, shoulder**
M67.811 Other specified disorders of synovium, right shoulder
M67.812 Other specified disorders of synovium, left shoulder
M67.813 Other specified disorders of tendon, right shoulder
M67.814 Other specified disorders of tendon, left shoulder
M67.819 Other specified disorders of synovium and tendon, unspecified shoulder

✓6th **M67.82 Other specified disorders of synovium and tendon, elbow**
M67.821 Other specified disorders of synovium, right elbow
M67.822 Other specified disorders of synovium, left elbow
M67.823 Other specified disorders of tendon, right elbow
M67.824 Other specified disorders of tendon, left elbow
M67.829 Other specified disorders of synovium and tendon, unspecified elbow

✓6th **M67.83 Other specified disorders of synovium and tendon, wrist**
M67.831 Other specified disorders of synovium, right wrist
M67.832 Other specified disorders of synovium, left wrist
M67.833 Other specified disorders of tendon, right wrist
M67.834 Other specified disorders of tendon, left wrist
M67.839 Other specified disorders of synovium and tendon, unspecified wrist

✓6th **M67.84 Other specified disorders of synovium and tendon, hand**
M67.841 Other specified disorders of synovium, right hand
M67.842 Other specified disorders of synovium, left hand
M67.843 Other specified disorders of tendon, right hand
M67.844 Other specified disorders of tendon, left hand
M67.849 Other specified disorders of synovium and tendon, unspecified hand

✓6th **M67.85 Other specified disorders of synovium and tendon, hip**
M67.851 Other specified disorders of synovium, right hip
M67.852 Other specified disorders of synovium, left hip
M67.853 Other specified disorders of tendon, right hip
M67.854 Other specified disorders of tendon, left hip
M67.859 Other specified disorders of synovium and tendon, unspecified hip

✓6th **M67.86 Other specified disorders of synovium and tendon, knee**
M67.861 Other specified disorders of synovium, right knee
M67.862 Other specified disorders of synovium, left knee
M67.863 Other specified disorders of tendon, right knee
M67.864 Other specified disorders of tendon, left knee
M67.869 Other specified disorders of synovium and tendon, unspecified knee

✓6th **M67.87 Other specified disorders of synovium and tendon, ankle and foot**
M67.871 Other specified disorders of synovium, right ankle and foot
M67.872 Other specified disorders of synovium, left ankle and foot
M67.873 Other specified disorders of tendon, right ankle and foot
M67.874 Other specified disorders of tendon, left ankle and foot
M67.879 Other specified disorders of synovium and tendon, unspecified ankle and foot

M67.88 Other specified disorders of synovium and tendon, other site
M67.89 Other specified disorders of synovium and tendon, multiple sites

✓5th **M67.9 Unspecified disorder of synovium and tendon**
M67.9Ø Unspecified disorder of synovium and tendon, unspecified site

✓6th **M67.91 Unspecified disorder of synovium and tendon, shoulder**
M67.911 Unspecified disorder of synovium and tendon, right shoulder
M67.912 Unspecified disorder of synovium and tendon, left shoulder
M67.919 Unspecified disorder of synovium and tendon, unspecified shoulder

✓6th **M67.92 Unspecified disorder of synovium and tendon, upper arm**
M67.921 Unspecified disorder of synovium and tendon, right upper arm
M67.922 Unspecified disorder of synovium and tendon, left upper arm
M67.929 Unspecified disorder of synovium and tendon, unspecified upper arm

M67.93 Unspecified disorder of synovium and tendon, forearm
- M67.931 Unspecified disorder of synovium and tendon, right forearm
- M67.932 Unspecified disorder of synovium and tendon, left forearm
- M67.939 Unspecified disorder of synovium and tendon, unspecified forearm

M67.94 Unspecified disorder of synovium and tendon, hand
- M67.941 Unspecified disorder of synovium and tendon, right hand
- M67.942 Unspecified disorder of synovium and tendon, left hand
- M67.949 Unspecified disorder of synovium and tendon, unspecified hand

M67.95 Unspecified disorder of synovium and tendon, thigh
- M67.951 Unspecified disorder of synovium and tendon, right thigh
- M67.952 Unspecified disorder of synovium and tendon, left thigh
- M67.959 Unspecified disorder of synovium and tendon, unspecified thigh

M67.96 Unspecified disorder of synovium and tendon, lower leg
- M67.961 Unspecified disorder of synovium and tendon, right lower leg
- M67.962 Unspecified disorder of synovium and tendon, left lower leg
- M67.969 Unspecified disorder of synovium and tendon, unspecified lower leg

M67.97 Unspecified disorder of synovium and tendon, ankle and foot
- M67.971 Unspecified disorder of synovium and tendon, right ankle and foot
- M67.972 Unspecified disorder of synovium and tendon, left ankle and foot
- M67.979 Unspecified disorder of synovium and tendon, unspecified ankle and foot

M67.98 Unspecified disorder of synovium and tendon, other site

M67.99 Unspecified disorder of synovium and tendon, multiple sites

Other soft tissue disorders (M70-M79)

M70 Soft tissue disorders related to use, overuse and pressure

INCLUDES soft tissue disorders of occupational origin

Use additional external cause code to identify activity causing disorder (Y93.-)

EXCLUDES 1 *bursitis NOS (M71.9-)*

EXCLUDES 2 *bursitis of shoulder (M75.5)*
enthesopathies (M76-M77)
pressure ulcer (pressure area) (L89.-)

M70.0 Crepitant synovitis (acute) (chronic) of hand and wrist

M70.03 Crepitant synovitis (acute) (chronic), wrist
- M70.031 Crepitant synovitis (acute) (chronic), right wrist
- M70.032 Crepitant synovitis (acute) (chronic), left wrist
- M70.039 Crepitant synovitis (acute) (chronic), unspecified wrist

M70.04 Crepitant synovitis (acute) (chronic), hand
- M70.041 Crepitant synovitis (acute) (chronic), right hand
- M70.042 Crepitant synovitis (acute) (chronic), left hand
- M70.049 Crepitant synovitis (acute) (chronic), unspecified hand

M70.1 Bursitis of hand
- M70.10 Bursitis, unspecified hand
- M70.11 Bursitis, right hand
- M70.12 Bursitis, left hand

M70.2 Olecranon bursitis
- M70.20 Olecranon bursitis, unspecified elbow
- M70.21 Olecranon bursitis, right elbow
- M70.22 Olecranon bursitis, left elbow

M70.3 Other bursitis of elbow
- M70.30 Other bursitis of elbow, unspecified elbow
- M70.31 Other bursitis of elbow, right elbow
- M70.32 Other bursitis of elbow, left elbow

M70.4 Prepatellar bursitis
- M70.40 Prepatellar bursitis, unspecified knee
- M70.41 Prepatellar bursitis, right knee
- M70.42 Prepatellar bursitis, left knee

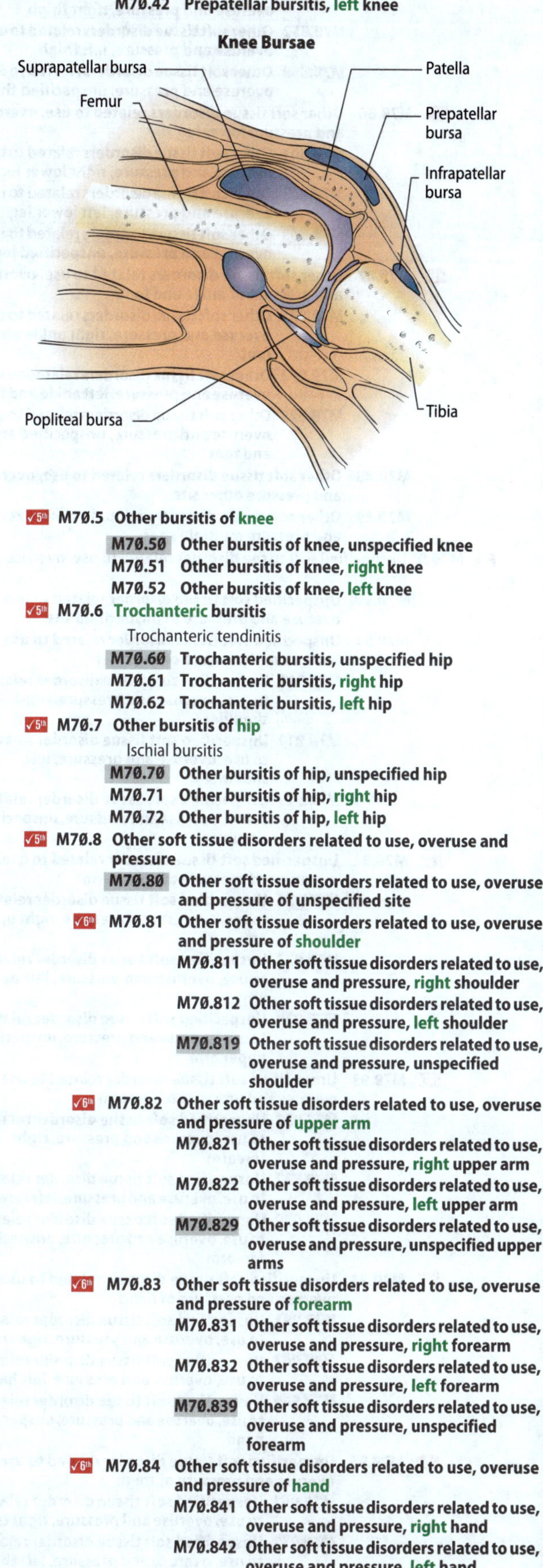

M70.5 Other bursitis of knee
- M70.50 Other bursitis of knee, unspecified knee
- M70.51 Other bursitis of knee, right knee
- M70.52 Other bursitis of knee, left knee

M70.6 Trochanteric bursitis

Trochanteric tendinitis
- M70.60 Trochanteric bursitis, unspecified hip
- M70.61 Trochanteric bursitis, right hip
- M70.62 Trochanteric bursitis, left hip

M70.7 Other bursitis of hip

Ischial bursitis
- M70.70 Other bursitis of hip, unspecified hip
- M70.71 Other bursitis of hip, right hip
- M70.72 Other bursitis of hip, left hip

M70.8 Other soft tissue disorders related to use, overuse and pressure

M70.80 Other soft tissue disorders related to use, overuse and pressure of unspecified site

M70.81 Other soft tissue disorders related to use, overuse and pressure of shoulder
- M70.811 Other soft tissue disorders related to use, overuse and pressure, right shoulder
- M70.812 Other soft tissue disorders related to use, overuse and pressure, left shoulder
- M70.819 Other soft tissue disorders related to use, overuse and pressure, unspecified shoulder

M70.82 Other soft tissue disorders related to use, overuse and pressure of upper arm
- M70.821 Other soft tissue disorders related to use, overuse and pressure, right upper arm
- M70.822 Other soft tissue disorders related to use, overuse and pressure, left upper arm
- M70.829 Other soft tissue disorders related to use, overuse and pressure, unspecified upper arms

M70.83 Other soft tissue disorders related to use, overuse and pressure of forearm
- M70.831 Other soft tissue disorders related to use, overuse and pressure, right forearm
- M70.832 Other soft tissue disorders related to use, overuse and pressure, left forearm
- M70.839 Other soft tissue disorders related to use, overuse and pressure, unspecified forearm

M70.84 Other soft tissue disorders related to use, overuse and pressure of hand
- M70.841 Other soft tissue disorders related to use, overuse and pressure, right hand
- M70.842 Other soft tissue disorders related to use, overuse and pressure, left hand

M70.849 Other soft tissue disorders related to use, overuse and pressure, unspecified hand

M70.85 Other soft tissue disorders related to use, overuse and pressure of thigh

M70.851 Other soft tissue disorders related to use, overuse and pressure, right thigh

M70.852 Other soft tissue disorders related to use, overuse and pressure, left thigh

M70.859 Other soft tissue disorders related to use, overuse and pressure, unspecified thigh

M70.86 Other soft tissue disorders related to use, overuse and pressure lower leg

M70.861 Other soft tissue disorders related to use, overuse and pressure, right lower leg

M70.862 Other soft tissue disorders related to use, overuse and pressure, left lower leg

M70.869 Other soft tissue disorders related to use, overuse and pressure, unspecified leg

M70.87 Other soft tissue disorders related to use, overuse and pressure of ankle and foot

M70.871 Other soft tissue disorders related to use, overuse and pressure, right ankle and foot

M70.872 Other soft tissue disorders related to use, overuse and pressure, left ankle and foot

M70.879 Other soft tissue disorders related to use, overuse and pressure, unspecified ankle and foot

M70.88 Other soft tissue disorders related to use, overuse and pressure other site

M70.89 Other soft tissue disorders related to use, overuse and pressure multiple sites

M70.9 Unspecified soft tissue disorder related to use, overuse and pressure

M70.90 Unspecified soft tissue disorder related to use, overuse and pressure of unspecified site

M70.91 Unspecified soft tissue disorder related to use, overuse and pressure of shoulder

M70.911 Unspecified soft tissue disorder related to use, overuse and pressure, right shoulder

M70.912 Unspecified soft tissue disorder related to use, overuse and pressure, left shoulder

M70.919 Unspecified soft tissue disorder related to use, overuse and pressure, unspecified shoulder

M70.92 Unspecified soft tissue disorder related to use, overuse and pressure of upper arm

M70.921 Unspecified soft tissue disorder related to use, overuse and pressure, right upper arm

M70.922 Unspecified soft tissue disorder related to use, overuse and pressure, left upper arm

M70.929 Unspecified soft tissue disorder related to use, overuse and pressure, unspecified upper arm

M70.93 Unspecified soft tissue disorder related to use, overuse and pressure of forearm

M70.931 Unspecified soft tissue disorder related to use, overuse and pressure, right forearm

M70.932 Unspecified soft tissue disorder related to use, overuse and pressure, left forearm

M70.939 Unspecified soft tissue disorder related to use, overuse and pressure, unspecified forearm

M70.94 Unspecified soft tissue disorder related to use, overuse and pressure of hand

M70.941 Unspecified soft tissue disorder related to use, overuse and pressure, right hand

M70.942 Unspecified soft tissue disorder related to use, overuse and pressure, left hand

M70.949 Unspecified soft tissue disorder related to use, overuse and pressure, unspecified hand

M70.95 Unspecified soft tissue disorder related to use, overuse and pressure of thigh

M70.951 Unspecified soft tissue disorder related to use, overuse and pressure, right thigh

M70.952 Unspecified soft tissue disorder related to use, overuse and pressure, left thigh

M70.959 Unspecified soft tissue disorder related to use, overuse and pressure, unspecified thigh

M70.96 Unspecified soft tissue disorder related to use, overuse and pressure lower leg

M70.961 Unspecified soft tissue disorder related to use, overuse and pressure, right lower leg

M70.962 Unspecified soft tissue disorder related to use, overuse and pressure, left lower leg

M70.969 Unspecified soft tissue disorder related to use, overuse and pressure, unspecified lower leg

M70.97 Unspecified soft tissue disorder related to use, overuse and pressure of ankle and foot

M70.971 Unspecified soft tissue disorder related to use, overuse and pressure, right ankle and foot

M70.972 Unspecified soft tissue disorder related to use, overuse and pressure, left ankle and foot

M70.979 Unspecified soft tissue disorder related to use, overuse and pressure, unspecified ankle and foot

M70.98 Unspecified soft tissue disorder related to use, overuse and pressure other

M70.99 Unspecified soft tissue disorder related to use, overuse and pressure multiple sites

M71 Other bursopathies

EXCLUDES 1 *bunion (M20.1)*
bursitis related to use, overuse or pressure (M70.-)
enthesopathies (M76-M77)

M71.0 Abscess of bursa

Use additional code (B95.-, B96.-) to identify causative organism

M71.00 Abscess of bursa, unspecified site

M71.01 Abscess of bursa, shoulder

M71.011 Abscess of bursa, right shoulder

M71.012 Abscess of bursa, left shoulder

M71.019 Abscess of bursa, unspecified shoulder

M71.02 Abscess of bursa, elbow

M71.021 Abscess of bursa, right elbow

M71.022 Abscess of bursa, left elbow

M71.029 Abscess of bursa, unspecified elbow

M71.03 Abscess of bursa, wrist

M71.031 Abscess of bursa, right wrist

M71.032 Abscess of bursa, left wrist

M71.039 Abscess of bursa, unspecified wrist

M71.04 Abscess of bursa, hand

M71.041 Abscess of bursa, right hand

M71.042 Abscess of bursa, left hand

M71.049 Abscess of bursa, unspecified hand

M71.05 Abscess of bursa, hip

M71.051 Abscess of bursa, right hip

M71.052 Abscess of bursa, left hip

M71.059 Abscess of bursa, unspecified hip

M71.06 Abscess of bursa, knee

M71.061 Abscess of bursa, right knee

M71.062 Abscess of bursa, left knee

M71.069 Abscess of bursa, unspecified knee

M71.07 Abscess of bursa, ankle and foot

M71.071 Abscess of bursa, right ankle and foot

M71.072 Abscess of bursa, left ankle and foot

M71.079 Abscess of bursa, unspecified ankle and foot

M71.08 Abscess of bursa, other site

M71.09 Abscess of bursa, multiple sites

M71.1 Other infective bursitis

Use additional code (B95.-, B96.-) to identify causative organism

M71.10 Other infective bursitis, unspecified site

M71.11 Other infective bursitis, shoulder

M71.111 Other infective bursitis, right shoulder

M71.112 Other infective bursitis, left shoulder

M71.119 Other infective bursitis, unspecified shoulder

M71.12 Other infective bursitis, elbow

M71.121 Other infective bursitis, right elbow

M71.122 Other infective bursitis, left elbow

M71.129 Other infective bursitis, unspecified elbow
M71.13 Other infective bursitis, wrist
M71.131 Other infective bursitis, right wrist
M71.132 Other infective bursitis, left wrist
M71.139 Other infective bursitis, unspecified wrist
M71.14 Other infective bursitis, hand
M71.141 Other infective bursitis, right hand
M71.142 Other infective bursitis, left hand
M71.149 Other infective bursitis, unspecified hand
M71.15 Other infective bursitis, hip
M71.151 Other infective bursitis, right hip
M71.152 Other infective bursitis, left hip
M71.159 Other infective bursitis, unspecified hip
M71.16 Other infective bursitis, knee
M71.161 Other infective bursitis, right knee
M71.162 Other infective bursitis, left knee
M71.169 Other infective bursitis, unspecified knee
M71.17 Other infective bursitis, ankle and foot
M71.171 Other infective bursitis, right ankle and foot
M71.172 Other infective bursitis, left ankle and foot
M71.179 Other infective bursitis, unspecified ankle and foot
M71.18 Other infective bursitis, other site
M71.19 Other infective bursitis, multiple sites
M71.2 Synovial cyst of popliteal space [Baker]
EXCLUDES 1 *synovial cyst of popliteal space with rupture (M66.Ø)*
DEF: Sac filled with clear synovial fluid in adults, usually secondary to disease inside the joint, located on the back of the knee in the popliteal fossa area. In children, the cyst usually represents a ganglion of one of the tendons in the knee.

Baker's Cyst

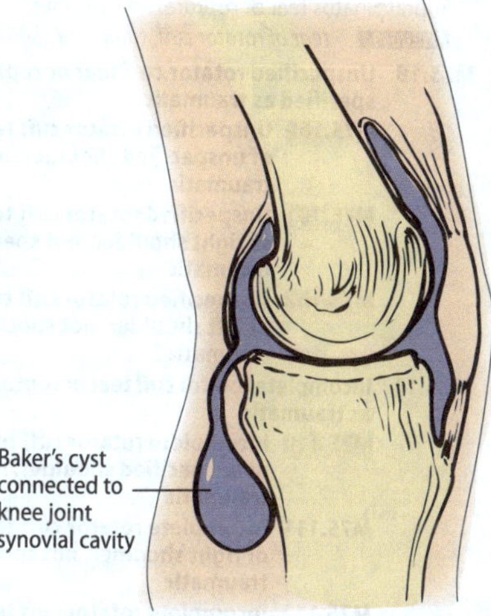

M71.2Ø Synovial cyst of popliteal space [Baker], unspecified knee
M71.21 Synovial cyst of popliteal space [Baker], right knee
M71.22 Synovial cyst of popliteal space [Baker], left knee
M71.3 Other bursal cyst
Synovial cyst NOS
EXCLUDES 1 *synovial cyst with rupture (M66.1-)*
M71.3Ø Other bursal cyst, unspecified site
M71.31 Other bursal cyst, shoulder
M71.311 Other bursal cyst, right shoulder
M71.312 Other bursal cyst, left shoulder
M71.319 Other bursal cyst, unspecified shoulder
M71.32 Other bursal cyst, elbow
M71.321 Other bursal cyst, right elbow
M71.322 Other bursal cyst, left elbow
M71.329 Other bursal cyst, unspecified elbow
M71.33 Other bursal cyst, wrist
M71.331 Other bursal cyst, right wrist
M71.332 Other bursal cyst, left wrist
M71.339 Other bursal cyst, unspecified wrist
M71.34 Other bursal cyst, hand
M71.341 Other bursal cyst, right hand
M71.342 Other bursal cyst, left hand
M71.349 Other bursal cyst, unspecified hand
M71.35 Other bursal cyst, hip
M71.351 Other bursal cyst, right hip
M71.352 Other bursal cyst, left hip
M71.359 Other bursal cyst, unspecified hip
M71.37 Other bursal cyst, ankle and foot
M71.371 Other bursal cyst, right ankle and foot
M71.372 Other bursal cyst, left ankle and foot
M71.379 Other bursal cyst, unspecified ankle and foot
M71.38 Other bursal cyst, other site
M71.39 Other bursal cyst, multiple sites
M71.4 Calcium deposit in bursa
EXCLUDES 2 *calcium deposit in bursa of shoulder (M75.3)*
M71.4Ø Calcium deposit in bursa, unspecified site
M71.42 Calcium deposit in bursa, elbow
M71.421 Calcium deposit in bursa, right elbow
M71.422 Calcium deposit in bursa, left elbow
M71.429 Calcium deposit in bursa, unspecified elbow
M71.43 Calcium deposit in bursa, wrist
M71.431 Calcium deposit in bursa, right wrist
M71.432 Calcium deposit in bursa, left wrist
M71.439 Calcium deposit in bursa, unspecified wrist
M71.44 Calcium deposit in bursa, hand
M71.441 Calcium deposit in bursa, right hand
M71.442 Calcium deposit in bursa, left hand
M71.449 Calcium deposit in bursa, unspecified hand
M71.45 Calcium deposit in bursa, hip
M71.451 Calcium deposit in bursa, right hip
M71.452 Calcium deposit in bursa, left hip
M71.459 Calcium deposit in bursa, unspecified hip
M71.46 Calcium deposit in bursa, knee
M71.461 Calcium deposit in bursa, right knee
M71.462 Calcium deposit in bursa, left knee
M71.469 Calcium deposit in bursa, unspecified knee
M71.47 Calcium deposit in bursa, ankle and foot
M71.471 Calcium deposit in bursa, right ankle and foot
M71.472 Calcium deposit in bursa, left ankle and foot
M71.479 Calcium deposit in bursa, unspecified ankle and foot
M71.48 Calcium deposit in bursa, other site
M71.49 Calcium deposit in bursa, multiple sites
M71.5 Other bursitis, not elsewhere classified
EXCLUDES 1 *bursitis NOS (M71.9-)*
EXCLUDES 2 *bursitis of shoulder (M75.5)*
bursitis of tibial collateral [Pellegrini-Stieda] (M76.4-)
M71.5Ø Other bursitis, not elsewhere classified, unspecified site
M71.52 Other bursitis, not elsewhere classified, elbow
M71.521 Other bursitis, not elsewhere classified, right elbow
M71.522 Other bursitis, not elsewhere classified, left elbow
M71.529 Other bursitis, not elsewhere classified, unspecified elbow
M71.53 Other bursitis, not elsewhere classified, wrist
M71.531 Other bursitis, not elsewhere classified, right wrist
M71.532 Other bursitis, not elsewhere classified, left wrist
M71.539 Other bursitis, not elsewhere classified, unspecified wrist
M71.54 Other bursitis, not elsewhere classified, hand
M71.541 Other bursitis, not elsewhere classified, right hand
M71.542 Other bursitis, not elsewhere classified, left hand

M71.549 **Other bursitis, not elsewhere classified, unspecified hand**

M71.55 **Other bursitis, not elsewhere classified, hip**

M71.551 **Other bursitis, not elsewhere classified, right hip**

M71.552 **Other bursitis, not elsewhere classified, left hip**

M71.559 **Other bursitis, not elsewhere classified, unspecified hip**

M71.56 **Other bursitis, not elsewhere classified, knee**

M71.561 **Other bursitis, not elsewhere classified, right knee**

M71.562 **Other bursitis, not elsewhere classified, left knee**

M71.569 **Other bursitis, not elsewhere classified, unspecified knee**

M71.57 **Other bursitis, not elsewhere classified, ankle and foot**

M71.571 **Other bursitis, not elsewhere classified, right ankle and foot**

M71.572 **Other bursitis, not elsewhere classified, left ankle and foot**

M71.579 **Other bursitis, not elsewhere classified, unspecified ankle and foot**

M71.58 **Other bursitis, not elsewhere classified, other site**

M71.8 **Other specified bursopathies**

M71.8Ø **Other specified bursopathies, unspecified site**

M71.81 **Other specified bursopathies, shoulder**

M71.811 **Other specified bursopathies, right shoulder**

M71.812 **Other specified bursopathies, left shoulder**

M71.819 **Other specified bursopathies, unspecified shoulder**

M71.82 **Other specified bursopathies, elbow**

M71.821 **Other specified bursopathies, right elbow**

M71.822 **Other specified bursopathies, left elbow**

M71.829 **Other specified bursopathies, unspecified elbow**

M71.83 **Other specified bursopathies, wrist**

M71.831 **Other specified bursopathies, right wrist**

M71.832 **Other specified bursopathies, left wrist**

M71.839 **Other specified bursopathies, unspecified wrist**

M71.84 **Other specified bursopathies, hand**

M71.841 **Other specified bursopathies, right hand**

M71.842 **Other specified bursopathies, left hand**

M71.849 **Other specified bursopathies, unspecified hand**

M71.85 **Other specified bursopathies, hip**

M71.851 **Other specified bursopathies, right hip**

M71.852 **Other specified bursopathies, left hip**

M71.859 **Other specified bursopathies, unspecified hip**

M71.86 **Other specified bursopathies, knee**

M71.861 **Other specified bursopathies, right knee**

M71.862 **Other specified bursopathies, left knee**

M71.869 **Other specified bursopathies, unspecified knee**

M71.87 **Other specified bursopathies, ankle and foot**

M71.871 **Other specified bursopathies, right ankle and foot**

M71.872 **Other specified bursopathies, left ankle and foot**

M71.879 **Other specified bursopathies, unspecified ankle and foot**

M71.88 **Other specified bursopathies, other site**

M71.89 **Other specified bursopathies, multiple sites**

M71.9 **Bursopathy, unspecified**

Bursitis NOS

M72 **Fibroblastic disorders**

EXCLUDES 2 *retroperitoneal fibromatosis (D48.3)*

M72.Ø **Palmar fascial fibromatosis [Dupuytren]** A

DEF: Dupuytren's contracture: Flexion deformity of a finger, due to shortened, thickened fibrosing of palmar fascia. The cause is unknown, but it is associated with long-standing epilepsy.

M72.1 **Knuckle pads**

M72.2 **Plantar fascial fibromatosis**

Plantar fasciitis

DEF: Rapid-growing and multiplanar nodular swellings and pain in the foot that is not associated with contractures.

M72.4 **Pseudosarcomatous fibromatosis**

Nodular fasciitis

M72.6 **Necrotizing fasciitis** MCC HCC

Use additional code (B95.-, B96.-) to identify causative organism

M72.8 **Other fibroblastic disorders**

Abscess of fascia

Fasciitis NEC

Other infective fasciitis

Use additional code to (B95.-, B96.-) identify causative organism

EXCLUDES 1 *diffuse (eosinophilic) fasciitis (M35.4)*

necrotizing fasciitis (M72.6)

nodular fasciitis (M72.4)

perirenal fasciitis NOS (N13.5)

perirenal fasciitis with infection (N13.6)

plantar fasciitis (M72.2)

M72.9 **Fibroblastic disorder, unspecified**

Fasciitis NOS

Fibromatosis NOS

M75 **Shoulder lesions**

EXCLUDES 2 *shoulder-hand syndrome (M89.Ø-)*

M75.Ø **Adhesive capsulitis of shoulder**

Frozen shoulder

Periarthritis of shoulder

AHA: 2015,2Q,23

M75.ØØ **Adhesive capsulitis of unspecified shoulder**

M75.Ø1 **Adhesive capsulitis of right shoulder**

M75.Ø2 **Adhesive capsulitis of left shoulder**

M75.1 **Rotator cuff tear or rupture, not specified as traumatic**

Rotator cuff syndrome

Supraspinatus syndrome

Supraspinatus tear or rupture, not specified as traumatic

EXCLUDES 1 *tear of rotator cuff, traumatic (S46.Ø1-)*

M75.1Ø **Unspecified rotator cuff tear or rupture, not specified as traumatic**

M75.1ØØ **Unspecified rotator cuff tear or rupture of unspecified shoulder, not specified as traumatic**

M75.1Ø1 **Unspecified rotator cuff tear or rupture of right shoulder, not specified as traumatic**

M75.1Ø2 **Unspecified rotator cuff tear or rupture of left shoulder, not specified as traumatic**

M75.11 **Incomplete rotator cuff tear or rupture not specified as traumatic**

M75.11Ø **Incomplete rotator cuff tear or rupture of unspecified shoulder, not specified as traumatic**

M75.111 **Incomplete rotator cuff tear or rupture of right shoulder, not specified as traumatic**

M75.112 **Incomplete rotator cuff tear or rupture of left shoulder, not specified as traumatic**

M75.12 **Complete rotator cuff tear or rupture not specified as traumatic**

M75.12Ø **Complete rotator cuff tear or rupture of unspecified shoulder, not specified as traumatic**

M75.121 **Complete rotator cuff tear or rupture of right shoulder, not specified as traumatic**

M75.122 **Complete rotator cuff tear or rupture of left shoulder, not specified as traumatic**

M75.2 **Bicipital tendinitis**

M75.2Ø **Bicipital tendinitis, unspecified shoulder**

M75.21 **Bicipital tendinitis, right shoulder**

M75.22 **Bicipital tendinitis, left shoulder**

M75.3 **Calcific tendinitis of shoulder**

Calcified bursa of shoulder

M75.3Ø **Calcific tendinitis of unspecified shoulder**

M75.31 **Calcific tendinitis of right shoulder**

M75.32 **Calcific tendinitis of left shoulder**

M75.4 **Impingement syndrome of shoulder**

M75.4Ø **Impingement syndrome of unspecified shoulder**

M75.41 Impingement syndrome of right shoulder
M75.42 Impingement syndrome of left shoulder

M75.5 Bursitis of shoulder
M75.50 Bursitis of unspecified shoulder
M75.51 Bursitis of right shoulder
M75.52 Bursitis of left shoulder

M75.8 Other shoulder lesions
M75.80 Other shoulder lesions, unspecified shoulder
M75.81 Other shoulder lesions, right shoulder
M75.82 Other shoulder lesions, left shoulder

M75.9 Shoulder lesion, unspecified
M75.90 Shoulder lesion, unspecified, unspecified shoulder
M75.91 Shoulder lesion, unspecified, right shoulder
M75.92 Shoulder lesion, unspecified, left shoulder

M76 Enthesopathies, lower limb, excluding foot

EXCLUDES 2 *bursitis due to use, overuse and pressure (M7Ø.-)*
enthesopathies of ankle and foot (M77.5-)

M76.Ø Gluteal tendinitis
M76.ØØ Gluteal tendinitis, unspecified hip
M76.Ø1 Gluteal tendinitis, right hip
M76.Ø2 Gluteal tendinitis, left hip

M76.1 Psoas tendinitis
M76.1Ø Psoas tendinitis, unspecified hip
M76.11 Psoas tendinitis, right hip
M76.12 Psoas tendinitis, left hip

M76.2 Iliac crest spur
M76.2Ø Iliac crest spur, unspecified hip
M76.21 Iliac crest spur, right hip
M76.22 Iliac crest spur, left hip

M76.3 Iliotibial band syndrome
M76.3Ø Iliotibial band syndrome, unspecified leg
M76.31 Iliotibial band syndrome, right leg
M76.32 Iliotibial band syndrome, left leg

M76.4 Tibial collateral bursitis [Pellegrini-Stieda]
M76.4Ø Tibial collateral bursitis [Pellegrini-Stieda], unspecified leg
M76.41 Tibial collateral bursitis [Pellegrini-Stieda], right leg
M76.42 Tibial collateral bursitis [Pellegrini-Stieda], left leg

M76.5 Patellar tendinitis
M76.5Ø Patellar tendinitis, unspecified knee
M76.51 Patellar tendinitis, right knee
M76.52 Patellar tendinitis, left knee

M76.6 Achilles tendinitis
Achilles bursitis
M76.6Ø Achilles tendinitis, unspecified leg
M76.61 Achilles tendinitis, right leg
M76.62 Achilles tendinitis, left leg

M76.7 Peroneal tendinitis
M76.7Ø Peroneal tendinitis, unspecified leg
M76.71 Peroneal tendinitis, right leg
M76.72 Peroneal tendinitis, left leg

M76.8 Other specified enthesopathies of lower limb, excluding foot
M76.81 Anterior tibial syndrome
M76.811 Anterior tibial syndrome, right leg
M76.812 Anterior tibial syndrome, left leg
M76.819 Anterior tibial syndrome, unspecified leg
M76.82 Posterior tibial tendinitis
M76.821 Posterior tibial tendinitis, right leg
M76.822 Posterior tibial tendinitis, left leg
M76.829 Posterior tibial tendinitis, unspecified leg
M76.89 Other specified enthesopathies of lower limb, excluding foot
M76.891 Other specified enthesopathies of right lower limb, excluding foot
M76.892 Other specified enthesopathies of left lower limb, excluding foot
M76.899 Other specified enthesopathies of unspecified lower limb, excluding foot

M76.9 Unspecified enthesopathy, lower limb, excluding foot

M77 Other enthesopathies

EXCLUDES 1 *bursitis NOS (M71.9-)*
EXCLUDES 2 *bursitis due to use, overuse and pressure (M7Ø.-)*
osteophyte (M25.7)
spinal enthesopathy (M46.Ø-)

M77.Ø Medial epicondylitis
M77.ØØ Medial epicondylitis, unspecified elbow
M77.Ø1 Medial epicondylitis, right elbow
M77.Ø2 Medial epicondylitis, left elbow

M77.1 Lateral epicondylitis
Tennis elbow
M77.1Ø Lateral epicondylitis, unspecified elbow
M77.11 Lateral epicondylitis, right elbow
M77.12 Lateral epicondylitis, left elbow

M77.2 Periarthritis of wrist
M77.2Ø Periarthritis, unspecified wrist
M77.21 Periarthritis, right wrist
M77.22 Periarthritis, left wrist

M77.3 Calcaneal spur
DEF: Overgrowth of calcaneus bone on the underside of the heel that causes pain on walking. Calcaneal spur is due to a chronic avulsion injury of the plantar fascia from the calcaneus.
M77.3Ø Calcaneal spur, unspecified foot
M77.31 Calcaneal spur, right foot
M77.32 Calcaneal spur, left foot

M77.4 Metatarsalgia
EXCLUDES 1 *Morton's metatarsalgia (G57.6)*
M77.4Ø Metatarsalgia, unspecified foot
M77.41 Metatarsalgia, right foot
M77.42 Metatarsalgia, left foot

M77.5 Other enthesopathy of foot and ankle
M77.5Ø Other enthesopathy of unspecified foot and ankle
M77.51 Other enthesopathy of right foot and ankle
M77.52 Other enthesopathy of left foot and ankle

M77.8 Other enthesopathies, not elsewhere classified

M77.9 Enthesopathy, unspecified
Bone spur NOS
Capsulitis NOS
Periarthritis NOS
Tendinitis NOS

M79 Other and unspecified soft tissue disorders, not elsewhere classified

EXCLUDES 1 *psychogenic rheumatism (F45.8)*
soft tissue pain, psychogenic (F45.41)

M79.Ø Rheumatism, unspecified
EXCLUDES 1 *fibromyalgia (M79.7)*
palindromic rheumatism (M12.3-)

M79.1 Myalgia
Myofascial pain syndrome
EXCLUDES 1 *fibromyalgia (M79.7)*
myositis (M6Ø.-)
AHA: 2018,4Q,21
M79.1Ø Myalgia, unspecified site
M79.11 Myalgia of mastication muscle
M79.12 Myalgia of auxiliary muscles, head and neck
M79.18 Myalgia, other site

M79.2 Neuralgia and neuritis, unspecified
EXCLUDES 1 *brachial radiculitis NOS (M54.1)*
lumbosacral radiculitis NOS (M54.1)
mononeuropathies (G56-G58)
radiculitis NOS (M54.1)
sciatica (M54.3-M54.4)
TIP: Assign for documented neuropathic pain.

M79.3 Panniculitis, unspecified
EXCLUDES 1 *lupus panniculitis (L93.2)*
neck and back panniculitis (M54.Ø-)
relapsing [Weber-Christian] panniculitis (M35.6)

M79.4 Hypertrophy of (infrapatellar) fat pad

M79.5 Residual foreign body in soft tissue
EXCLUDES 1 *foreign body granuloma of skin and subcutaneous tissue (L92.3)*
foreign body granuloma of soft tissue (M6Ø.2-)

√5th **M79.6 Pain in limb, hand, foot, fingers and toes**
EXCLUDES 2 *pain in joint (M25.5-)*

√6th **M79.60 Pain in limb, unspecified**
M79.601 Pain in right arm
Pain in right upper limb NOS
M79.602 Pain in left arm
Pain in left upper limb NOS
M79.603 Pain in arm, unspecified
Pain in upper limb NOS
M79.604 Pain in right leg
Pain in right lower limb NOS
M79.605 Pain in left leg
Pain in left lower limb NOS
M79.606 Pain in leg, unspecified
Pain in lower limb NOS
M79.609 Pain in unspecified limb
Pain in limb NOS

√6th **M79.62 Pain in upper arm**
Pain in axillary region
M79.621 Pain in right upper arm
M79.622 Pain in left upper arm
M79.629 Pain in unspecified upper arm

√6th **M79.63 Pain in forearm**
M79.631 Pain in right forearm
M79.632 Pain in left forearm
M79.639 Pain in unspecified forearm

√6th **M79.64 Pain in hand and fingers**
M79.641 Pain in right hand
M79.642 Pain in left hand
M79.643 Pain in unspecified hand
M79.644 Pain in right finger(s)
M79.645 Pain in left finger(s)
M79.646 Pain in unspecified finger(s)

√6th **M79.65 Pain in thigh**
M79.651 Pain in right thigh
M79.652 Pain in left thigh
M79.659 Pain in unspecified thigh

√6th **M79.66 Pain in lower leg**
M79.661 Pain in right lower leg
M79.662 Pain in left lower leg
M79.669 Pain in unspecified lower leg

√6th **M79.67 Pain in foot and toes**
M79.671 Pain in right foot
M79.672 Pain in left foot
M79.673 Pain in unspecified foot
M79.674 Pain in right toe(s)
M79.675 Pain in left toe(s)
M79.676 Pain in unspecified toe(s)

M79.7 Fibromyalgia
Fibromyositis
Fibrositis
Myofibrositis

√5th **M79.A Nontraumatic compartment syndrome**
Code first, if applicable, associated postprocedural complication
EXCLUDES 1 *compartment syndrome NOS (T79.A-)*
fibromyalgia (M79.7)
nontraumatic ischemic infarction of muscle (M62.2-)
traumatic compartment syndrome (T79.A-)

√6th **M79.A1 Nontraumatic compartment syndrome of upper extremity**
Nontraumatic compartment syndrome of shoulder, arm, forearm, wrist, hand, and fingers
M79.A11 Nontraumatic compartment syndrome of right upper extremity CC
M79.A12 Nontraumatic compartment syndrome of left upper extremity CC
M79.A19 Nontraumatic compartment syndrome of unspecified upper extremity CC UNS

√6th **M79.A2 Nontraumatic compartment syndrome of lower extremity**
Nontraumatic compartment syndrome of hip, buttock, thigh, leg, foot, and toes
M79.A21 Nontraumatic compartment syndrome of right lower extremity CC
M79.A22 Nontraumatic compartment syndrome of left lower extremity CC
M79.A29 Nontraumatic compartment syndrome of unspecified lower extremity CC UNS

M79.A3 Nontraumatic compartment syndrome of abdomen CC
M79.A9 Nontraumatic compartment syndrome of other sites CC

√5th **M79.8 Other specified soft tissue disorders**
M79.81 Nontraumatic hematoma of soft tissue
Nontraumatic hematoma of muscle
Nontraumatic seroma of muscle and soft tissue
M79.89 Other specified soft tissue disorders
Polyalgia

M79.9 Soft tissue disorder, unspecified

OSTEOPATHIES AND CHONDROPATHIES (M80-M94)

Disorders of bone density and structure (M80-M85)

√4th **M80 Osteoporosis with current pathological fracture**
INCLUDES osteoporosis with current fragility fracture
Use additional code to identify major osseous defect, if applicable (M89.7-)
EXCLUDES 1 *collapsed vertebra NOS (M48.5)*
pathological fracture NOS (M84.4)
wedging of vertebra NOS (M48.5)
EXCLUDES 2 *personal history of (healed) osteoporosis fracture (Z87.310)*
AHA: 2018,2Q,12
TIP: The site codes in this category identify the site of the fracture, not the site of the osteoporosis.

The appropriate 7th character is to be added to each code from category M80:
A initial encounter for fracture
D subsequent encounter for fracture with routine healing
G subsequent encounter for fracture with delayed healing
K subsequent encounter for fracture with nonunion
P subsequent encounter for fracture with malunion
S sequela

√5th **M80.0 Age-related osteoporosis with current pathological fracture**
Involutional osteoporosis with current pathological fracture
Osteoporosis NOS with current pathological fracture
Postmenopausal osteoporosis with current pathological fracture
Senile osteoporosis with current pathological fracture

3 √x7th **M80.00 Age-related osteoporosis with current pathological fracture, unspecified site** CC UNS A

√6th **M80.01 Age-related osteoporosis with current pathological fracture, shoulder**
3 √7th **M80.011 Age-related osteoporosis with current pathological fracture, right shoulder** CC A
3 √7th **M80.012 Age-related osteoporosis with current pathological fracture, left shoulder** CC A
3 √7th **M80.019 Age-related osteoporosis with current pathological fracture, unspecified shoulder** CC UNS A

√6th **M80.02 Age-related osteoporosis with current pathological fracture, humerus**
3 √7th **M80.021 Age-related osteoporosis with current pathological fracture, right humerus** CC A
3 √7th **M80.022 Age-related osteoporosis with current pathological fracture, left humerus** CC A
3 √7th **M80.029 Age-related osteoporosis with current pathological fracture, unspecified humerus** CC UNS A

√6th **M80.03 Age-related osteoporosis with current pathological fracture, forearm**
Age-related osteoporosis with current pathological fracture of wrist
3 √7th **M80.031 Age-related osteoporosis with current pathological fracture, right forearm** CC A
3 √7th **M80.032 Age-related osteoporosis with current pathological fracture, left forearm** CC A
3 √7th **M80.039 Age-related osteoporosis with current pathological fracture, unspecified forearm** CC UNS A

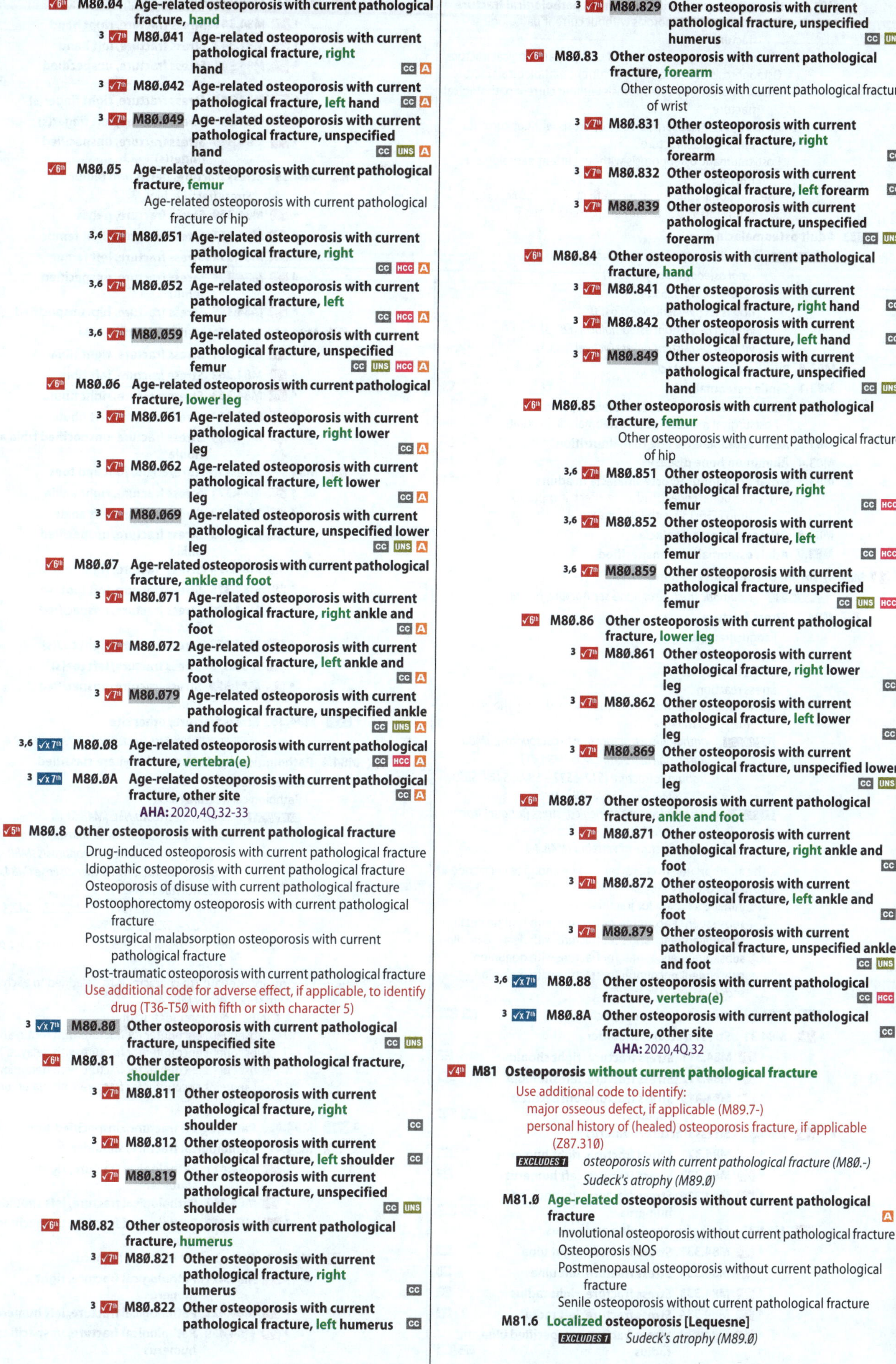

M80.04 Age-related osteoporosis with current pathological fracture, hand
- M80.041 Age-related osteoporosis with current pathological fracture, right hand CC A
- M80.042 Age-related osteoporosis with current pathological fracture, left hand CC A
- M80.049 Age-related osteoporosis with current pathological fracture, unspecified hand CC UNS A

M80.05 Age-related osteoporosis with current pathological fracture, femur
Age-related osteoporosis with current pathological fracture of hip
- M80.051 Age-related osteoporosis with current pathological fracture, right femur CC HCC A
- M80.052 Age-related osteoporosis with current pathological fracture, left femur CC HCC A
- M80.059 Age-related osteoporosis with current pathological fracture, unspecified femur CC UNS HCC A

M80.06 Age-related osteoporosis with current pathological fracture, lower leg
- M80.061 Age-related osteoporosis with current pathological fracture, right lower leg CC A
- M80.062 Age-related osteoporosis with current pathological fracture, left lower leg CC A
- M80.069 Age-related osteoporosis with current pathological fracture, unspecified lower leg CC UNS A

M80.07 Age-related osteoporosis with current pathological fracture, ankle and foot
- M80.071 Age-related osteoporosis with current pathological fracture, right ankle and foot CC A
- M80.072 Age-related osteoporosis with current pathological fracture, left ankle and foot CC A
- M80.079 Age-related osteoporosis with current pathological fracture, unspecified ankle and foot CC UNS A

M80.08 Age-related osteoporosis with current pathological fracture, vertebra(e) CC HCC A

M80.0A Age-related osteoporosis with current pathological fracture, other site CC A
AHA: 2020,4Q,32-33

M80.8 Other osteoporosis with current pathological fracture
Drug-induced osteoporosis with current pathological fracture
Idiopathic osteoporosis with current pathological fracture
Osteoporosis of disuse with current pathological fracture
Postoophorectomy osteoporosis with current pathological fracture
Postsurgical malabsorption osteoporosis with current pathological fracture
Post-traumatic osteoporosis with current pathological fracture
Use additional code for adverse effect, if applicable, to identify drug (T36-T50 with fifth or sixth character 5)

M80.80 Other osteoporosis with current pathological fracture, unspecified site CC UNS

M80.81 Other osteoporosis with pathological fracture, shoulder
- M80.811 Other osteoporosis with current pathological fracture, right shoulder CC
- M80.812 Other osteoporosis with current pathological fracture, left shoulder CC
- M80.819 Other osteoporosis with current pathological fracture, unspecified shoulder CC UNS

M80.82 Other osteoporosis with current pathological fracture, humerus
- M80.821 Other osteoporosis with current pathological fracture, right humerus CC
- M80.822 Other osteoporosis with current pathological fracture, left humerus CC
- M80.829 Other osteoporosis with current pathological fracture, unspecified humerus CC UNS

M80.83 Other osteoporosis with current pathological fracture, forearm
Other osteoporosis with current pathological fracture of wrist
- M80.831 Other osteoporosis with current pathological fracture, right forearm CC
- M80.832 Other osteoporosis with current pathological fracture, left forearm CC
- M80.839 Other osteoporosis with current pathological fracture, unspecified forearm CC UNS

M80.84 Other osteoporosis with current pathological fracture, hand
- M80.841 Other osteoporosis with current pathological fracture, right hand CC
- M80.842 Other osteoporosis with current pathological fracture, left hand CC
- M80.849 Other osteoporosis with current pathological fracture, unspecified hand CC UNS

M80.85 Other osteoporosis with current pathological fracture, femur
Other osteoporosis with current pathological fracture of hip
- M80.851 Other osteoporosis with current pathological fracture, right femur CC HCC
- M80.852 Other osteoporosis with current pathological fracture, left femur CC HCC
- M80.859 Other osteoporosis with current pathological fracture, unspecified femur CC UNS HCC

M80.86 Other osteoporosis with current pathological fracture, lower leg
- M80.861 Other osteoporosis with current pathological fracture, right lower leg CC
- M80.862 Other osteoporosis with current pathological fracture, left lower leg CC
- M80.869 Other osteoporosis with current pathological fracture, unspecified lower leg CC UNS

M80.87 Other osteoporosis with current pathological fracture, ankle and foot
- M80.871 Other osteoporosis with current pathological fracture, right ankle and foot CC
- M80.872 Other osteoporosis with current pathological fracture, left ankle and foot CC
- M80.879 Other osteoporosis with current pathological fracture, unspecified ankle and foot CC UNS

M80.88 Other osteoporosis with current pathological fracture, vertebra(e) CC HCC

M80.8A Other osteoporosis with current pathological fracture, other site CC
AHA: 2020,4Q,32

M81 Osteoporosis without current pathological fracture
Use additional code to identify:
major osseous defect, if applicable (M89.7-)
personal history of (healed) osteoporosis fracture, if applicable (Z87.310)

EXCLUDES 1 *osteoporosis with current pathological fracture (M80.-)*
Sudeck's atrophy (M89.0)

M81.0 Age-related osteoporosis without current pathological fracture A
Involutional osteoporosis without current pathological fracture
Osteoporosis NOS
Postmenopausal osteoporosis without current pathological fracture
Senile osteoporosis without current pathological fracture

M81.6 Localized osteoporosis [Lequesne]
EXCLUDES 1 *Sudeck's atrophy (M89.0)*

M81.8 Other osteoporosis without current pathological fracture
Drug-induced osteoporosis without current pathological fracture
Idiopathic osteoporosis without current pathological fracture
Osteoporosis of disuse without current pathological fracture
Postoophorectomy osteoporosis without current pathological fracture
Postsurgical malabsorption osteoporosis without current pathological fracture
Post-traumatic osteoporosis without current pathological fracture
Use additional code for adverse effect, if applicable, to identify drug (T36-T5Ø with fifth or sixth character 5)

4th M83 Adult osteomalacia
EXCLUDES 1 *infantile and juvenile osteomalacia (E55.Ø)*
renal osteodystrophy (N25.Ø)
rickets (active) (E55.Ø)
rickets (active) sequelae (E64.3)
vitamin D-resistant osteomalacia (E83.3)
vitamin D-resistant rickets (active) (E83.3)

M83.Ø Puerperal osteomalacia M ♀
M83.1 Senile osteomalacia A
M83.2 Adult osteomalacia due to malabsorption A
Postsurgical malabsorption osteomalacia in adults
M83.3 Adult osteomalacia due to malnutrition A
M83.4 Aluminum bone disease
M83.5 Other drug-induced osteomalacia in adults A
Use additional code for adverse effect, if applicable, to identify drug (T36-T5Ø with fifth or sixth character 5)
M83.8 Other adult osteomalacia A
M83.9 Adult osteomalacia, unspecified A

4th M84 Disorder of continuity of bone
EXCLUDES 2 *traumatic fracture of bone-see fracture, by site*

5th M84.3 Stress fracture
Fatigue fracture
March fracture
Stress fracture NOS
Stress reaction
Use additional external cause code(s) to identify the cause of the stress fracture
EXCLUDES 1 *pathological fracture due to osteoporosis (M8Ø.-)*
pathological fracture NOS (M84.4.-)
traumatic fracture (S12.-, S22.-, S32.-, S42.-, S52.-, S62.-, S72.-, S82.-, S92.-)
EXCLUDES 2 *personal history of (healed) stress (fatigue) fracture (Z87.312)*
stress fracture of vertebra (M48.4-)

The appropriate 7th character is to be added to each code from subcategory M84.3.
A initial encounter for fracture
D subsequent encounter for fracture with routine healing
G subsequent encounter for fracture with delayed healing
K subsequent encounter for fracture with nonunion
P subsequent encounter for fracture with malunion
S sequela

4 x7th **M84.3Ø Stress fracture, unspecified site** CC UNS
6th **M84.31 Stress fracture, shoulder**
4 7th **M84.311 Stress fracture, right shoulder** CC
4 7th **M84.312 Stress fracture, left shoulder** CC
4 7th **M84.319 Stress fracture, unspecified shoulder** CC UNS
6th **M84.32 Stress fracture, humerus**
4 7th **M84.321 Stress fracture, right humerus** CC
4 7th **M84.322 Stress fracture, left humerus** CC
4 7th **M84.329 Stress fracture, unspecified humerus** CC UNS
6th **M84.33 Stress fracture, ulna and radius**
4 7th **M84.331 Stress fracture, right ulna** CC
4 7th **M84.332 Stress fracture, left ulna** CC
4 7th **M84.333 Stress fracture, right radius** CC
4 7th **M84.334 Stress fracture, left radius** CC
4 7th **M84.339 Stress fracture, unspecified ulna and radius** CC UNS
6th **M84.34 Stress fracture, hand and fingers**
4 7th **M84.341 Stress fracture, right hand** CC
4 7th **M84.342 Stress fracture, left hand** CC
4 7th **M84.343 Stress fracture, unspecified hand** CC UNS
4 7th **M84.344 Stress fracture, right finger(s)** CC
4 7th **M84.345 Stress fracture, left finger(s)** CC
4 7th **M84.346 Stress fracture, unspecified finger(s)** CC UNS
6th **M84.35 Stress fracture, pelvis and femur**
Stress fracture, hip
4 7th **M84.35Ø Stress fracture, pelvis** CC
4 7th **M84.351 Stress fracture, right femur** CC
4 7th **M84.352 Stress fracture, left femur** CC
4 7th **M84.353 Stress fracture, unspecified femur** CC UNS
4 7th **M84.359 Stress fracture, hip, unspecified** CC
6th **M84.36 Stress fracture, tibia and fibula**
4 7th **M84.361 Stress fracture, right tibia** CC
4 7th **M84.362 Stress fracture, left tibia** CC
4 7th **M84.363 Stress fracture, right fibula** CC
4 7th **M84.364 Stress fracture, left fibula** CC
4 7th **M84.369 Stress fracture, unspecified tibia and fibula** CC UNS
6th **M84.37 Stress fracture, ankle, foot and toes**
4 7th **M84.371 Stress fracture, right ankle** CC
4 7th **M84.372 Stress fracture, left ankle** CC
4 7th **M84.373 Stress fracture, unspecified ankle** CC UNS
4 7th **M84.374 Stress fracture, right foot** CC
4 7th **M84.375 Stress fracture, left foot** CC
4 7th **M84.376 Stress fracture, unspecified foot** CC UNS
4 7th **M84.377 Stress fracture, right toe(s)** CC
4 7th **M84.378 Stress fracture, left toe(s)** CC
4 7th **M84.379 Stress fracture, unspecified toe(s)** CC UNS
4 x7th **M84.38 Stress fracture, other site** CC
EXCLUDES 2 *stress fracture of vertebra (M48.4-)*

5th M84.4 Pathological fracture, not elsewhere classified
Chronic fracture
Pathological fracture NOS
EXCLUDES 1 *collapsed vertebra NEC (M48.5)*
pathological fracture in neoplastic disease (M84.5-)
pathological fracture in osteoporosis (M8Ø.-)
pathological fracture in other disease (M84.6-)
stress fracture (M84.3-)
traumatic fracture (S12.-, S22.-, S32.-, S42.-, S52.-, S62.-, S72.-, S82.-, S92.-)
EXCLUDES 2 *personal history of (healed) pathological fracture (Z87.311)*

The appropriate 7th character is to be added to each code from subcategory M84.4.
A initial encounter for fracture
D subsequent encounter for fracture with routine healing
G subsequent encounter for fracture with delayed healing
K subsequent encounter for fracture with nonunion
P subsequent encounter for fracture with malunion
S sequela

3 x7th **M84.4Ø Pathological fracture, unspecified site** CC UNS
6th **M84.41 Pathological fracture, shoulder**
3 7th **M84.411 Pathological fracture, right shoulder** CC
3 7th **M84.412 Pathological fracture, left shoulder** CC
3 7th **M84.419 Pathological fracture, unspecified shoulder** CC UNS
6th **M84.42 Pathological fracture, humerus**
3 7th **M84.421 Pathological fracture, right humerus** CC
3 7th **M84.422 Pathological fracture, left humerus** CC
3 7th **M84.429 Pathological fracture, unspecified humerus** CC UNS

M84.43 Pathological fracture, ulna and radius
- M84.431 Pathological fracture, right ulna CC
- M84.432 Pathological fracture, left ulna CC
- M84.433 Pathological fracture, right radius CC
- M84.434 Pathological fracture, left radius CC
- M84.439 Pathological fracture, unspecified ulna and radius CC UNS

M84.44 Pathological fracture, hand and fingers
- M84.441 Pathological fracture, right hand CC
- M84.442 Pathological fracture, left hand CC
- M84.443 Pathological fracture, unspecified hand CC UNS
- M84.444 Pathological fracture, right finger(s) CC
- M84.445 Pathological fracture, left finger(s) CC
- M84.446 Pathological fracture, unspecified finger(s) CC UNS

M84.45 Pathological fracture, femur and pelvis

AHA: 2016,4Q,43
- M84.451 Pathological fracture, right femur CC HCC
- M84.452 Pathological fracture, left femur CC HCC
- M84.453 Pathological fracture, unspecified femur CC UNS HCC
- M84.454 Pathological fracture, pelvis CC
- M84.459 Pathological fracture, hip, unspecified CC HCC

M84.46 Pathological fracture, tibia and fibula
- M84.461 Pathological fracture, right tibia CC
- M84.462 Pathological fracture, left tibia CC
- M84.463 Pathological fracture, right fibula CC
- M84.464 Pathological fracture, left fibula CC
- M84.469 Pathological fracture, unspecified tibia and fibula CC UNS

M84.47 Pathological fracture, ankle, foot and toes
- M84.471 Pathological fracture, right ankle CC
- M84.472 Pathological fracture, left ankle CC
- M84.473 Pathological fracture, unspecified ankle CC UNS
- M84.474 Pathological fracture, right foot CC
- M84.475 Pathological fracture, left foot CC
- M84.476 Pathological fracture, unspecified foot CC UNS
- M84.477 Pathological fracture, right toe(s) CC
- M84.478 Pathological fracture, left toe(s) CC
- M84.479 Pathological fracture, unspecified toe(s) CC UNS

M84.48 Pathological fracture, other site CC

M84.5 Pathological fracture in neoplastic disease

Code also underlying neoplasm

The appropriate 7th character is to be added to each code from subcategory M84.5.
- A initial encounter for fracture
- D subsequent encounter for fracture with routine healing
- G subsequent encounter for fracture with delayed healing
- K subsequent encounter for fracture with nonunion
- P subsequent encounter for fracture with malunion
- S sequela

M84.50 Pathological fracture in neoplastic disease, unspecified site CC UNS

M84.51 Pathological fracture in neoplastic disease, shoulder
- M84.511 Pathological fracture in neoplastic disease, right shoulder CC
- M84.512 Pathological fracture in neoplastic disease, left shoulder CC
- M84.519 Pathological fracture in neoplastic disease, unspecified shoulder CC UNS

M84.52 Pathological fracture in neoplastic disease, humerus
- M84.521 Pathological fracture in neoplastic disease, right humerus CC
- M84.522 Pathological fracture in neoplastic disease, left humerus CC
- M84.529 Pathological fracture in neoplastic disease, unspecified humerus CC UNS

M84.53 Pathological fracture in neoplastic disease, ulna and radius
- M84.531 Pathological fracture in neoplastic disease, right ulna CC
- M84.532 Pathological fracture in neoplastic disease, left ulna CC
- M84.533 Pathological fracture in neoplastic disease, right radius CC
- M84.534 Pathological fracture in neoplastic disease, left radius CC
- M84.539 Pathological fracture in neoplastic disease, unspecified ulna and radius CC UNS

M84.54 Pathological fracture in neoplastic disease, hand
- M84.541 Pathological fracture in neoplastic disease, right hand CC
- M84.542 Pathological fracture in neoplastic disease, left hand CC
- M84.549 Pathological fracture in neoplastic disease, unspecified hand CC UNS

M84.55 Pathological fracture in neoplastic disease, pelvis and femur
- M84.550 Pathological fracture in neoplastic disease, pelvis CC
- M84.551 Pathological fracture in neoplastic disease, right femur CC HCC
- M84.552 Pathological fracture in neoplastic disease, left femur CC HCC
- M84.553 Pathological fracture in neoplastic disease, unspecified femur CC UNS HCC
- M84.559 Pathological fracture in neoplastic disease, hip, unspecified CC UNS HCC

M84.56 Pathological fracture in neoplastic disease, tibia and fibula
- M84.561 Pathological fracture in neoplastic disease, right tibia CC
- M84.562 Pathological fracture in neoplastic disease, left tibia CC
- M84.563 Pathological fracture in neoplastic disease, right fibula CC
- M84.564 Pathological fracture in neoplastic disease, left fibula CC
- M84.569 Pathological fracture in neoplastic disease, unspecified tibia and fibula CC UNS

M84.57 Pathological fracture in neoplastic disease, ankle and foot
- M84.571 Pathological fracture in neoplastic disease, right ankle CC
- M84.572 Pathological fracture in neoplastic disease, left ankle CC
- M84.573 Pathological fracture in neoplastic disease, unspecified ankle CC UNS
- M84.574 Pathological fracture in neoplastic disease, right foot CC
- M84.575 Pathological fracture in neoplastic disease, left foot CC
- M84.576 Pathological fracture in neoplastic disease, unspecified foot CC UNS

M84.58 Pathological fracture in neoplastic disease, other specified site CC

Pathological fracture in neoplastic disease, vertebrae

M84.6 Pathological fracture in other disease

Code also underlying condition

EXCLUDES 1 *pathological fracture in osteoporosis (M80.-)*

The appropriate 7th character is to be added to each code from subcategory M84.6.
- A initial encounter for fracture
- D subsequent encounter for fracture with routine healing
- G subsequent encounter for fracture with delayed healing
- K subsequent encounter for fracture with nonunion
- P subsequent encounter for fracture with malunion
- S sequela

M84.60 Pathological fracture in other disease, unspecified site CC UNS

M84.61 Pathological fracture in other disease, shoulder
- 3 **M84.611** Pathological fracture in other disease, right shoulder CC
- 3 **M84.612** Pathological fracture in other disease, left shoulder CC
- 3 **M84.619** Pathological fracture in other disease, unspecified shoulder CC UNS

M84.62 Pathological fracture in other disease, humerus
- 3 **M84.621** Pathological fracture in other disease, right humerus CC
- 3 **M84.622** Pathological fracture in other disease, left humerus CC
- 3 **M84.629** Pathological fracture in other disease, unspecified humerus CC UNS

M84.63 Pathological fracture in other disease, ulna and radius
- 3 **M84.631** Pathological fracture in other disease, right ulna CC
- 3 **M84.632** Pathological fracture in other disease, left ulna CC
- 3 **M84.633** Pathological fracture in other disease, right radius CC
- 3 **M84.634** Pathological fracture in other disease, left radius CC
- 3 **M84.639** Pathological fracture in other disease, unspecified ulna and radius CC UNS

M84.64 Pathological fracture in other disease, hand
- 3 **M84.641** Pathological fracture in other disease, right hand CC
- 3 **M84.642** Pathological fracture in other disease, left hand CC
- 3 **M84.649** Pathological fracture in other disease, unspecified hand CC UNS

M84.65 Pathological fracture in other disease, pelvis and femur
- 3 **M84.650** Pathological fracture in other disease, pelvis CC
- 3,6 **M84.651** Pathological fracture in other disease, right femur CC HCC
- 3,6 **M84.652** Pathological fracture in other disease, left femur CC HCC
- 3,6 **M84.653** Pathological fracture in other disease, unspecified femur CC UNS HCC
- 3,6 **M84.659** Pathological fracture in other disease, hip, unspecified CC HCC

M84.66 Pathological fracture in other disease, tibia and fibula
- 3 **M84.661** Pathological fracture in other disease, right tibia CC
- 3 **M84.662** Pathological fracture in other disease, left tibia CC
- 3 **M84.663** Pathological fracture in other disease, right fibula CC
- 3 **M84.664** Pathological fracture in other disease, left fibula CC
- 3 **M84.669** Pathological fracture in other disease, unspecified tibia and fibula CC UNS

M84.67 Pathological fracture in other disease, ankle and foot
- 3 **M84.671** Pathological fracture in other disease, right ankle CC
- 3 **M84.672** Pathological fracture in other disease, left ankle CC
- 3 **M84.673** Pathological fracture in other disease, unspecified ankle CC UNS
- 3 **M84.674** Pathological fracture in other disease, right foot CC
- 3 **M84.675** Pathological fracture in other disease, left foot CC
- 3 **M84.676** Pathological fracture in other disease, unspecified foot CC UNS

3 **M84.68 Pathological fracture in other disease, other site** CC

M84.7 Nontraumatic fracture, not elsewhere classified

M84.75 Atypical femoral fracture

AHA: 2016,4Q,41-42

The appropriate 7th character is to be added to each code from M84.75.
- A initial encounter for fracture
- D subsequent encounter for fracture with routine healing
- G subsequent encounter for fracture with delayed healing
- K subsequent encounter for fracture with nonunion
- P subsequent encounter for fracture with malunion
- S sequela

- 3 **M84.750** Atypical femoral fracture, unspecified CC
- 3 **M84.751** Incomplete atypical femoral fracture, right leg CC
- 3 **M84.752** Incomplete atypical femoral fracture, left leg CC
- 3 **M84.753** Incomplete atypical femoral fracture, unspecified leg CC UNS
- 3,6 **M84.754** Complete transverse atypical femoral fracture, right leg CC HCC
- 3,6 **M84.755** Complete transverse atypical femoral fracture, left leg CC HCC
- 3,6 **M84.756** Complete transverse atypical femoral fracture, unspecified leg CC UNS HCC
- 3,6 **M84.757** Complete oblique atypical femoral fracture, right leg CC HCC
- 3,6 **M84.758** Complete oblique atypical femoral fracture, left leg CC HCC
- 3,6 **M84.759** Complete oblique atypical femoral fracture, unspecified leg CC UNS HCC

M84.8 Other disorders of continuity of bone

M84.80 Other disorders of continuity of bone, unspecified site

M84.81 Other disorders of continuity of bone, shoulder
- **M84.811** Other disorders of continuity of bone, right shoulder
- **M84.812** Other disorders of continuity of bone, left shoulder
- **M84.819** Other disorders of continuity of bone, unspecified shoulder

M84.82 Other disorders of continuity of bone, humerus
- **M84.821** Other disorders of continuity of bone, right humerus
- **M84.822** Other disorders of continuity of bone, left humerus
- **M84.829** Other disorders of continuity of bone, unspecified humerus

M84.83 Other disorders of continuity of bone, ulna and radius
- **M84.831** Other disorders of continuity of bone, right ulna
- **M84.832** Other disorders of continuity of bone, left ulna
- **M84.833** Other disorders of continuity of bone, right radius
- **M84.834** Other disorders of continuity of bone, left radius
- **M84.839** Other disorders of continuity of bone, unspecified ulna and radius

M84.84 Other disorders of continuity of bone, hand
- **M84.841** Other disorders of continuity of bone, right hand
- **M84.842** Other disorders of continuity of bone, left hand
- **M84.849** Other disorders of continuity of bone, unspecified hand

M84.85 Other disorders of continuity of bone, pelvic region and thigh
- **M84.851** Other disorders of continuity of bone, right pelvic region and thigh
- **M84.852** Other disorders of continuity of bone, left pelvic region and thigh
- **M84.859** Other disorders of continuity of bone, unspecified pelvic region and thigh

M84.86 Other disorders of continuity of bone, tibia and fibula
M84.861 Other disorders of continuity of bone, right tibia
M84.862 Other disorders of continuity of bone, left tibia
M84.863 Other disorders of continuity of bone, right fibula
M84.864 Other disorders of continuity of bone, left fibula
M84.869 Other disorders of continuity of bone, unspecified tibia and fibula
M84.87 Other disorders of continuity of bone, ankle and foot
M84.871 Other disorders of continuity of bone, right ankle and foot
M84.872 Other disorders of continuity of bone, left ankle and foot
M84.879 Other disorders of continuity of bone, unspecified ankle and foot
M84.88 Other disorders of continuity of bone, other site
M84.9 Disorder of continuity of bone, unspecified

M85 Other disorders of bone density and structure

EXCLUDES 1 *osteogenesis imperfecta (Q78.Ø)*
osteopetrosis (Q78.2)
osteopoikilosis (Q78.8)
polyostotic fibrous dysplasia (Q78.1)

M85.Ø Fibrous dysplasia (monostotic)
EXCLUDES 2 *fibrous dysplasia of jaw (M27.8)*
M85.ØØ Fibrous dysplasia (monostotic), unspecified site
M85.Ø1 Fibrous dysplasia (monostotic), shoulder
M85.Ø11 Fibrous dysplasia (monostotic), right shoulder
M85.Ø12 Fibrous dysplasia (monostotic), left shoulder
M85.Ø19 Fibrous dysplasia (monostotic), unspecified shoulder
M85.Ø2 Fibrous dysplasia (monostotic), upper arm
M85.Ø21 Fibrous dysplasia (monostotic), right upper arm
M85.Ø22 Fibrous dysplasia (monostotic), left upper arm
M85.Ø29 Fibrous dysplasia (monostotic), unspecified upper arm
M85.Ø3 Fibrous dysplasia (monostotic), forearm
M85.Ø31 Fibrous dysplasia (monostotic), right forearm
M85.Ø32 Fibrous dysplasia (monostotic), left forearm
M85.Ø39 Fibrous dysplasia (monostotic), unspecified forearm
M85.Ø4 Fibrous dysplasia (monostotic), hand
M85.Ø41 Fibrous dysplasia (monostotic), right hand
M85.Ø42 Fibrous dysplasia (monostotic), left hand
M85.Ø49 Fibrous dysplasia (monostotic), unspecified hand
M85.Ø5 Fibrous dysplasia (monostotic), thigh
M85.Ø51 Fibrous dysplasia (monostotic), right thigh
M85.Ø52 Fibrous dysplasia (monostotic), left thigh
M85.Ø59 Fibrous dysplasia (monostotic), unspecified thigh
M85.Ø6 Fibrous dysplasia (monostotic), lower leg
M85.Ø61 Fibrous dysplasia (monostotic), right lower leg
M85.Ø62 Fibrous dysplasia (monostotic), left lower leg
M85.Ø69 Fibrous dysplasia (monostotic), unspecified lower leg
M85.Ø7 Fibrous dysplasia (monostotic), ankle and foot
M85.Ø71 Fibrous dysplasia (monostotic), right ankle and foot
M85.Ø72 Fibrous dysplasia (monostotic), left ankle and foot
M85.Ø79 Fibrous dysplasia (monostotic), unspecified ankle and foot
M85.Ø8 Fibrous dysplasia (monostotic), other site
M85.Ø9 Fibrous dysplasia (monostotic), multiple sites

M85.1 Skeletal fluorosis
M85.1Ø Skeletal fluorosis, unspecified site
M85.11 Skeletal fluorosis, shoulder
M85.111 Skeletal fluorosis, right shoulder
M85.112 Skeletal fluorosis, left shoulder
M85.119 Skeletal fluorosis, unspecified shoulder
M85.12 Skeletal fluorosis, upper arm
M85.121 Skeletal fluorosis, right upper arm
M85.122 Skeletal fluorosis, left upper arm
M85.129 Skeletal fluorosis, unspecified upper arm
M85.13 Skeletal fluorosis, forearm
M85.131 Skeletal fluorosis, right forearm
M85.132 Skeletal fluorosis, left forearm
M85.139 Skeletal fluorosis, unspecified forearm
M85.14 Skeletal fluorosis, hand
M85.141 Skeletal fluorosis, right hand
M85.142 Skeletal fluorosis, left hand
M85.149 Skeletal fluorosis, unspecified hand
M85.15 Skeletal fluorosis, thigh
M85.151 Skeletal fluorosis, right thigh
M85.152 Skeletal fluorosis, left thigh
M85.159 Skeletal fluorosis, unspecified thigh
M85.16 Skeletal fluorosis, lower leg
M85.161 Skeletal fluorosis, right lower leg
M85.162 Skeletal fluorosis, left lower leg
M85.169 Skeletal fluorosis, unspecified lower leg
M85.17 Skeletal fluorosis, ankle and foot
M85.171 Skeletal fluorosis, right ankle and foot
M85.172 Skeletal fluorosis, left ankle and foot
M85.179 Skeletal fluorosis, unspecified ankle and foot
M85.18 Skeletal fluorosis, other site
M85.19 Skeletal fluorosis, multiple sites
M85.2 Hyperostosis of skull
DEF: Abnormal bone growth on the inner aspect of the cranial bones.
M85.3 Osteitis condensans
M85.3Ø Osteitis condensans, unspecified site
M85.31 Osteitis condensans, shoulder
M85.311 Osteitis condensans, right shoulder
M85.312 Osteitis condensans, left shoulder
M85.319 Osteitis condensans, unspecified shoulder
M85.32 Osteitis condensans, upper arm
M85.321 Osteitis condensans, right upper arm
M85.322 Osteitis condensans, left upper arm
M85.329 Osteitis condensans, unspecified upper arm
M85.33 Osteitis condensans, forearm
M85.331 Osteitis condensans, right forearm
M85.332 Osteitis condensans, left forearm
M85.339 Osteitis condensans, unspecified forearm
M85.34 Osteitis condensans, hand
M85.341 Osteitis condensans, right hand
M85.342 Osteitis condensans, left hand
M85.349 Osteitis condensans, unspecified hand
M85.35 Osteitis condensans, thigh
M85.351 Osteitis condensans, right thigh
M85.352 Osteitis condensans, left thigh
M85.359 Osteitis condensans, unspecified thigh
M85.36 Osteitis condensans, lower leg
M85.361 Osteitis condensans, right lower leg
M85.362 Osteitis condensans, left lower leg
M85.369 Osteitis condensans, unspecified lower leg
M85.37 Osteitis condensans, ankle and foot
M85.371 Osteitis condensans, right ankle and foot
M85.372 Osteitis condensans, left ankle and foot
M85.379 Osteitis condensans, unspecified ankle and foot
M85.38 Osteitis condensans, other site
M85.39 Osteitis condensans, multiple sites
M85.4 Solitary bone cyst
EXCLUDES 2 *solitary cyst of jaw (M27.4)*
M85.4Ø Solitary bone cyst, unspecified site

M85.41 Solitary bone cyst, shoulder
- **M85.411 Solitary bone cyst, right shoulder**
- **M85.412 Solitary bone cyst, left shoulder**
- **M85.419 Solitary bone cyst, unspecified shoulder**

M85.42 Solitary bone cyst, humerus
- **M85.421 Solitary bone cyst, right humerus**
- **M85.422 Solitary bone cyst, left humerus**
- **M85.429 Solitary bone cyst, unspecified humerus**

M85.43 Solitary bone cyst, ulna and radius
- **M85.431 Solitary bone cyst, right ulna and radius**
- **M85.432 Solitary bone cyst, left ulna and radius**
- **M85.439 Solitary bone cyst, unspecified ulna and radius**

M85.44 Solitary bone cyst, hand
- **M85.441 Solitary bone cyst, right hand**
- **M85.442 Solitary bone cyst, left hand**
- **M85.449 Solitary bone cyst, unspecified hand**

M85.45 Solitary bone cyst, pelvis
- **M85.451 Solitary bone cyst, right pelvis**
- **M85.452 Solitary bone cyst, left pelvis**
- **M85.459 Solitary bone cyst, unspecified pelvis**

M85.46 Solitary bone cyst, tibia and fibula
- **M85.461 Solitary bone cyst, right tibia and fibula**
- **M85.462 Solitary bone cyst, left tibia and fibula**
- **M85.469 Solitary bone cyst, unspecified tibia and fibula**

M85.47 Solitary bone cyst, ankle and foot
- **M85.471 Solitary bone cyst, right ankle and foot**
- **M85.472 Solitary bone cyst, left ankle and foot**
- **M85.479 Solitary bone cyst, unspecified ankle and foot**

M85.48 Solitary bone cyst, other site

M85.5 Aneurysmal bone cyst

EXCLUDES 2 *aneurysmal cyst of jaw (M27.4)*

DEF: Solitary bone lesion that bulges into the periosteum and is marked by a calcified rim.

M85.50 Aneurysmal bone cyst, unspecified site

M85.51 Aneurysmal bone cyst, shoulder
- **M85.511 Aneurysmal bone cyst, right shoulder**
- **M85.512 Aneurysmal bone cyst, left shoulder**
- **M85.519 Aneurysmal bone cyst, unspecified shoulder**

M85.52 Aneurysmal bone cyst, upper arm
- **M85.521 Aneurysmal bone cyst, right upper arm**
- **M85.522 Aneurysmal bone cyst, left upper arm**
- **M85.529 Aneurysmal bone cyst, unspecified upper arm**

M85.53 Aneurysmal bone cyst, forearm
- **M85.531 Aneurysmal bone cyst, right forearm**
- **M85.532 Aneurysmal bone cyst, left forearm**
- **M85.539 Aneurysmal bone cyst, unspecified forearm**

M85.54 Aneurysmal bone cyst, hand
- **M85.541 Aneurysmal bone cyst, right hand**
- **M85.542 Aneurysmal bone cyst, left hand**
- **M85.549 Aneurysmal bone cyst, unspecified hand**

M85.55 Aneurysmal bone cyst, thigh
- **M85.551 Aneurysmal bone cyst, right thigh**
- **M85.552 Aneurysmal bone cyst, left thigh**
- **M85.559 Aneurysmal bone cyst, unspecified thigh**

M85.56 Aneurysmal bone cyst, lower leg
- **M85.561 Aneurysmal bone cyst, right lower leg**
- **M85.562 Aneurysmal bone cyst, left lower leg**
- **M85.569 Aneurysmal bone cyst, unspecified lower leg**

M85.57 Aneurysmal bone cyst, ankle and foot
- **M85.571 Aneurysmal bone cyst, right ankle and foot**
- **M85.572 Aneurysmal bone cyst, left ankle and foot**
- **M85.579 Aneurysmal bone cyst, unspecified ankle and foot**

M85.58 Aneurysmal bone cyst, other site

M85.59 Aneurysmal bone cyst, multiple sites

M85.6 Other cyst of bone

EXCLUDES 1 *cyst of jaw NEC (M27.4)*
osteitis fibrosa cystica generalisata [von Recklinghausen's disease of bone] (E21.0)

M85.60 Other cyst of bone, unspecified site

M85.61 Other cyst of bone, shoulder
- **M85.611 Other cyst of bone, right shoulder**
- **M85.612 Other cyst of bone, left shoulder**
- **M85.619 Other cyst of bone, unspecified shoulder**

M85.62 Other cyst of bone, upper arm
- **M85.621 Other cyst of bone, right upper arm**
- **M85.622 Other cyst of bone, left upper arm**
- **M85.629 Other cyst of bone, unspecified upper arm**

M85.63 Other cyst of bone, forearm
- **M85.631 Other cyst of bone, right forearm**
- **M85.632 Other cyst of bone, left forearm**
- **M85.639 Other cyst of bone, unspecified forearm**

M85.64 Other cyst of bone, hand
- **M85.641 Other cyst of bone, right hand**
- **M85.642 Other cyst of bone, left hand**
- **M85.649 Other cyst of bone, unspecified hand**

M85.65 Other cyst of bone, thigh
- **M85.651 Other cyst of bone, right thigh**
- **M85.652 Other cyst of bone, left thigh**
- **M85.659 Other cyst of bone, unspecified thigh**

M85.66 Other cyst of bone, lower leg
- **M85.661 Other cyst of bone, right lower leg**
- **M85.662 Other cyst of bone, left lower leg**
- **M85.669 Other cyst of bone, unspecified lower leg**

M85.67 Other cyst of bone, ankle and foot
- **M85.671 Other cyst of bone, right ankle and foot**
- **M85.672 Other cyst of bone, left ankle and foot**
- **M85.679 Other cyst of bone, unspecified ankle and foot**

M85.68 Other cyst of bone, other site

M85.69 Other cyst of bone, multiple sites

M85.8 Other specified disorders of bone density and structure

Hyperostosis of bones, except skull
Osteosclerosis, acquired

EXCLUDES 1 *diffuse idiopathic skeletal hyperostosis [DISH] (M48.1)*
osteosclerosis congenita (Q77.4)
osteosclerosis fragilitas (generalista) (Q78.2)
osteosclerosis myelofibrosis (D75.81)

M85.80 Other specified disorders of bone density and structure, unspecified site

M85.81 Other specified disorders of bone density and structure, shoulder
- **M85.811 Other specified disorders of bone density and structure, right shoulder**
- **M85.812 Other specified disorders of bone density and structure, left shoulder**
- **M85.819 Other specified disorders of bone density and structure, unspecified shoulder**

M85.82 Other specified disorders of bone density and structure, upper arm
- **M85.821 Other specified disorders of bone density and structure, right upper arm**
- **M85.822 Other specified disorders of bone density and structure, left upper arm**
- **M85.829 Other specified disorders of bone density and structure, unspecified upper arm**

M85.83 Other specified disorders of bone density and structure, forearm
- **M85.831 Other specified disorders of bone density and structure, right forearm**
- **M85.832 Other specified disorders of bone density and structure, left forearm**
- **M85.839 Other specified disorders of bone density and structure, unspecified forearm**

M85.84 Other specified disorders of bone density and structure, hand
- **M85.841 Other specified disorders of bone density and structure, right hand**
- **M85.842 Other specified disorders of bone density and structure, left hand**
- **M85.849 Other specified disorders of bone density and structure, unspecified hand**

M85.85 Other specified disorders of bone density and structure, thigh
M85.851 Other specified disorders of bone density and structure, right thigh
M85.852 Other specified disorders of bone density and structure, left thigh
M85.859 Other specified disorders of bone density and structure, unspecified thigh
M85.86 Other specified disorders of bone density and structure, lower leg
M85.861 Other specified disorders of bone density and structure, right lower leg
M85.862 Other specified disorders of bone density and structure, left lower leg
M85.869 Other specified disorders of bone density and structure, unspecified lower leg
M85.87 Other specified disorders of bone density and structure, ankle and foot
M85.871 Other specified disorders of bone density and structure, right ankle and foot
M85.872 Other specified disorders of bone density and structure, left ankle and foot
M85.879 Other specified disorders of bone density and structure, unspecified ankle and foot
M85.88 Other specified disorders of bone density and structure, other site
M85.89 Other specified disorders of bone density and structure, multiple sites
M85.9 Disorder of bone density and structure, unspecified
AHA: 2021,3Q,11

Other osteopathies (M86-M9Ø)

EXCLUDES 1 *postprocedural osteopathies (M96.-)*

M86 Osteomyelitis

Use additional code (B95-B97) to identify infectious agent
Use additional code to identify major osseous defect, if applicable (M89.7-)

EXCLUDES 1 *osteomyelitis due to:*
echinococcus (B67.2)
gonococcus (A54.43)
salmonella (AØ2.24)

EXCLUDES 2 *ostemyelitis of:*
orbit (HØ5.Ø-)
petrous bone (H7Ø.2-)
vertebra (M46.2-)

M86.Ø Acute hematogenous osteomyelitis
M86.ØØ Acute hematogenous osteomyelitis, unspecified site CC UNS HCC
M86.Ø1 Acute hematogenous osteomyelitis, shoulder
M86.Ø11 Acute hematogenous osteomyelitis, right shoulder CC HCC
M86.Ø12 Acute hematogenous osteomyelitis, left shoulder CC HCC
M86.Ø19 Acute hematogenous osteomyelitis, unspecified shoulder CC UNS HCC
M86.Ø2 Acute hematogenous osteomyelitis, humerus
M86.Ø21 Acute hematogenous osteomyelitis, right humerus CC HCC
M86.Ø22 Acute hematogenous osteomyelitis, left humerus CC HCC
M86.Ø29 Acute hematogenous osteomyelitis, unspecified humerus CC UNS HCC
M86.Ø3 Acute hematogenous osteomyelitis, radius and ulna
M86.Ø31 Acute hematogenous osteomyelitis, right radius and ulna CC HCC
M86.Ø32 Acute hematogenous osteomyelitis, left radius and ulna CC HCC
M86.Ø39 Acute hematogenous osteomyelitis, unspecified radius and ulna CC UNS HCC
M86.Ø4 Acute hematogenous osteomyelitis, hand
M86.Ø41 Acute hematogenous osteomyelitis, right hand CC HCC
M86.Ø42 Acute hematogenous osteomyelitis, left hand CC HCC
M86.Ø49 Acute hematogenous osteomyelitis, unspecified hand CC UNS HCC
M86.Ø5 Acute hematogenous osteomyelitis, femur
M86.Ø51 Acute hematogenous osteomyelitis, right femur CC HCC
M86.Ø52 Acute hematogenous osteomyelitis, left femur CC HCC
M86.Ø59 Acute hematogenous osteomyelitis, unspecified femur CC UNS HCC
M86.Ø6 Acute hematogenous osteomyelitis, tibia and fibula
M86.Ø61 Acute hematogenous osteomyelitis, right tibia and fibula CC HCC
M86.Ø62 Acute hematogenous osteomyelitis, left tibia and fibula CC HCC
M86.Ø69 Acute hematogenous osteomyelitis, unspecified tibia and fibula CC UNS HCC
M86.Ø7 Acute hematogenous osteomyelitis, ankle and foot
M86.Ø71 Acute hematogenous osteomyelitis, right ankle and foot CC HCC
M86.Ø72 Acute hematogenous osteomyelitis, left ankle and foot CC HCC
M86.Ø79 Acute hematogenous osteomyelitis, unspecified ankle and foot CC UNS HCC
M86.Ø8 Acute hematogenous osteomyelitis, other sites CC HCC
M86.Ø9 Acute hematogenous osteomyelitis, multiple sites CC HCC
M86.1 Other acute osteomyelitis
M86.1Ø Other acute osteomyelitis, unspecified site CC UNS HCC
M86.11 Other acute osteomyelitis, shoulder
M86.111 Other acute osteomyelitis, right shoulder CC HCC
M86.112 Other acute osteomyelitis, left shoulder CC HCC
M86.119 Other acute osteomyelitis, unspecified shoulder CC UNS HCC
M86.12 Other acute osteomyelitis, humerus
M86.121 Other acute osteomyelitis, right humerus CC HCC
M86.122 Other acute osteomyelitis, left humerus CC HCC
M86.129 Other acute osteomyelitis, unspecified humerus CC UNS HCC
M86.13 Other acute osteomyelitis, radius and ulna
M86.131 Other acute osteomyelitis, right radius and ulna CC HCC
M86.132 Other acute osteomyelitis, left radius and ulna CC HCC
M86.139 Other acute osteomyelitis, unspecified radius and ulna CC UNS HCC
M86.14 Other acute osteomyelitis, hand
M86.141 Other acute osteomyelitis, right hand CC HCC
M86.142 Other acute osteomyelitis, left hand CC HCC
M86.149 Other acute osteomyelitis, unspecified hand CC UNS HCC
M86.15 Other acute osteomyelitis, femur
M86.151 Other acute osteomyelitis, right femur CC HCC
M86.152 Other acute osteomyelitis, left femur CC HCC
M86.159 Other acute osteomyelitis, unspecified femur CC UNS HCC
M86.16 Other acute osteomyelitis, tibia and fibula
M86.161 Other acute osteomyelitis, right tibia and fibula CC HCC
M86.162 Other acute osteomyelitis, left tibia and fibula CC HCC
M86.169 Other acute osteomyelitis, unspecified tibia and fibula CC UNS HCC
M86.17 Other acute osteomyelitis, ankle and foot
AHA: 2020,1Q,12
M86.171 Other acute osteomyelitis, right ankle and foot CC HCC
M86.172 Other acute osteomyelitis, left ankle and foot CC HCC

- **M86.179** Other acute osteomyelitis, unspecified ankle and foot CC UNS HCC
- **M86.18** Other acute osteomyelitis, other site CC HCC
- **M86.19** Other acute osteomyelitis, multiple sites CC HCC

✓5th M86.2 Subacute osteomyelitis

- **M86.2Ø** Subacute osteomyelitis, unspecified site CC UNS HCC
- ✓6th **M86.21** Subacute osteomyelitis, shoulder
  - **M86.211** Subacute osteomyelitis, right shoulder CC HCC
  - **M86.212** Subacute osteomyelitis, left shoulder CC HCC
  - **M86.219** Subacute osteomyelitis, unspecified shoulder CC UNS HCC
- ✓6th **M86.22** Subacute osteomyelitis, humerus
  - **M86.221** Subacute osteomyelitis, right humerus CC HCC
  - **M86.222** Subacute osteomyelitis, left humerus CC HCC
  - **M86.229** Subacute osteomyelitis, unspecified humerus CC UNS HCC
- ✓6th **M86.23** Subacute osteomyelitis, radius and ulna
  - **M86.231** Subacute osteomyelitis, right radius and ulna CC HCC
  - **M86.232** Subacute osteomyelitis, left radius and ulna CC HCC
  - **M86.239** Subacute osteomyelitis, unspecified radius and ulna CC UNS HCC
- ✓6th **M86.24** Subacute osteomyelitis, hand
  - **M86.241** Subacute osteomyelitis, right hand CC HCC
  - **M86.242** Subacute osteomyelitis, left hand CC HCC
  - **M86.249** Subacute osteomyelitis, unspecified hand CC UNS HCC
- ✓6th **M86.25** Subacute osteomyelitis, femur
  - **M86.251** Subacute osteomyelitis, right femur CC HCC
  - **M86.252** Subacute osteomyelitis, left femur CC HCC
  - **M86.259** Subacute osteomyelitis, unspecified femur CC UNS HCC
- ✓6th **M86.26** Subacute osteomyelitis, tibia and fibula
  - **M86.261** Subacute osteomyelitis, right tibia and fibula CC HCC
  - **M86.262** Subacute osteomyelitis, left tibia and fibula CC HCC
  - **M86.269** Subacute osteomyelitis, unspecified tibia and fibula CC UNS HCC
- ✓6th **M86.27** Subacute osteomyelitis, ankle and foot
  - **M86.271** Subacute osteomyelitis, right ankle and foot CC HCC
  - **M86.272** Subacute osteomyelitis, left ankle and foot CC HCC
  - **M86.279** Subacute osteomyelitis, unspecified ankle and foot CC UNS HCC
- **M86.28** Subacute osteomyelitis, other site CC HCC
- **M86.29** Subacute osteomyelitis, multiple sites CC HCC

✓5th M86.3 Chronic multifocal osteomyelitis

- **M86.3Ø** Chronic multifocal osteomyelitis, unspecified site CC UNS HCC
- ✓6th **M86.31** Chronic multifocal osteomyelitis, shoulder
  - **M86.311** Chronic multifocal osteomyelitis, right shoulder CC HCC
  - **M86.312** Chronic multifocal osteomyelitis, left shoulder CC HCC
  - **M86.319** Chronic multifocal osteomyelitis, unspecified shoulder CC UNS HCC
- ✓6th **M86.32** Chronic multifocal osteomyelitis, humerus
  - **M86.321** Chronic multifocal osteomyelitis, right humerus CC HCC
  - **M86.322** Chronic multifocal osteomyelitis, left humerus CC HCC
  - **M86.329** Chronic multifocal osteomyelitis, unspecified humerus CC UNS HCC
- ✓6th **M86.33** Chronic multifocal osteomyelitis, radius and ulna
  - **M86.331** Chronic multifocal osteomyelitis, right radius and ulna CC HCC
  - **M86.332** Chronic multifocal osteomyelitis, left radius and ulna CC HCC
  - **M86.339** Chronic multifocal osteomyelitis, unspecified radius and ulna CC UNS HCC
- ✓6th **M86.34** Chronic multifocal osteomyelitis, hand
  - **M86.341** Chronic multifocal osteomyelitis, right hand CC HCC
  - **M86.342** Chronic multifocal osteomyelitis, left hand CC HCC
  - **M86.349** Chronic multifocal osteomyelitis, unspecified hand CC UNS HCC
- ✓6th **M86.35** Chronic multifocal osteomyelitis, femur
  - **M86.351** Chronic multifocal osteomyelitis, right femur CC HCC
  - **M86.352** Chronic multifocal osteomyelitis, left femur CC HCC
  - **M86.359** Chronic multifocal osteomyelitis, unspecified femur CC UNS HCC
- ✓6th **M86.36** Chronic multifocal osteomyelitis, tibia and fibula
  - **M86.361** Chronic multifocal osteomyelitis, right tibia and fibula CC HCC
  - **M86.362** Chronic multifocal osteomyelitis, left tibia and fibula CC HCC
  - **M86.369** Chronic multifocal osteomyelitis, unspecified tibia and fibula CC UNS HCC
- ✓6th **M86.37** Chronic multifocal osteomyelitis, ankle and foot
  - **M86.371** Chronic multifocal osteomyelitis, right ankle and foot CC HCC
  - **M86.372** Chronic multifocal osteomyelitis, left ankle and foot CC HCC
  - **M86.379** Chronic multifocal osteomyelitis, unspecified ankle and foot CC UNS HCC
- **M86.38** Chronic multifocal osteomyelitis, other site CC HCC
- **M86.39** Chronic multifocal osteomyelitis, multiple sites CC HCC

✓5th M86.4 Chronic osteomyelitis with draining sinus

- **M86.4Ø** Chronic osteomyelitis with draining sinus, unspecified site CC UNS HCC
- ✓6th **M86.41** Chronic osteomyelitis with draining sinus, shoulder
  - **M86.411** Chronic osteomyelitis with draining sinus, right shoulder CC HCC
  - **M86.412** Chronic osteomyelitis with draining sinus, left shoulder CC HCC
  - **M86.419** Chronic osteomyelitis with draining sinus, unspecified shoulder CC UNS HCC
- ✓6th **M86.42** Chronic osteomyelitis with draining sinus, humerus
  - **M86.421** Chronic osteomyelitis with draining sinus, right humerus CC HCC
  - **M86.422** Chronic osteomyelitis with draining sinus, left humerus CC HCC
  - **M86.429** Chronic osteomyelitis with draining sinus, unspecified humerus CC UNS HCC
- ✓6th **M86.43** Chronic osteomyelitis with draining sinus, radius and ulna
  - **M86.431** Chronic osteomyelitis with draining sinus, right radius and ulna CC HCC
  - **M86.432** Chronic osteomyelitis with draining sinus, left radius and ulna CC HCC
  - **M86.439** Chronic osteomyelitis with draining sinus, unspecified radius and ulna CC UNS HCC
- ✓6th **M86.44** Chronic osteomyelitis with draining sinus, hand
  - **M86.441** Chronic osteomyelitis with draining sinus, right hand CC HCC
  - **M86.442** Chronic osteomyelitis with draining sinus, left hand CC HCC
  - **M86.449** Chronic osteomyelitis with draining sinus, unspecified hand CC UNS HCC
- ✓6th **M86.45** Chronic osteomyelitis with draining sinus, femur
  - **M86.451** Chronic osteomyelitis with draining sinus, right femur CC HCC

M86.452 Chronic osteomyelitis with draining sinus, left femur CC HCC

M86.459 Chronic osteomyelitis with draining sinus, unspecified femur CC UNS HCC

✓6th M86.46 Chronic osteomyelitis with draining sinus, tibia and fibula

M86.461 Chronic osteomyelitis with draining sinus, right tibia and fibula CC HCC

M86.462 Chronic osteomyelitis with draining sinus, left tibia and fibula CC HCC

M86.469 Chronic osteomyelitis with draining sinus, unspecified tibia and fibula CC UNS HCC

✓6th M86.47 Chronic osteomyelitis with draining sinus, ankle and foot

M86.471 Chronic osteomyelitis with draining sinus, right ankle and foot CC HCC

M86.472 Chronic osteomyelitis with draining sinus, left ankle and foot CC HCC

M86.479 Chronic osteomyelitis with draining sinus, unspecified ankle and foot CC UNS HCC

M86.48 Chronic osteomyelitis with draining sinus, other site CC HCC

M86.49 Chronic osteomyelitis with draining sinus, multiple sites CC HCC

✓5th M86.5 Other chronic hematogenous osteomyelitis

M86.50 Other chronic hematogenous osteomyelitis, unspecified site CC UNS HCC

✓6th M86.51 Other chronic hematogenous osteomyelitis, shoulder

M86.511 Other chronic hematogenous osteomyelitis, right shoulder CC HCC

M86.512 Other chronic hematogenous osteomyelitis, left shoulder CC HCC

M86.519 Other chronic hematogenous osteomyelitis, unspecified shoulder CC UNS HCC

✓6th M86.52 Other chronic hematogenous osteomyelitis, humerus

M86.521 Other chronic hematogenous osteomyelitis, right humerus CC HCC

M86.522 Other chronic hematogenous osteomyelitis, left humerus CC HCC

M86.529 Other chronic hematogenous osteomyelitis, unspecified humerus CC UNS HCC

✓6th M86.53 Other chronic hematogenous osteomyelitis, radius and ulna

M86.531 Other chronic hematogenous osteomyelitis, right radius and ulna CC HCC

M86.532 Other chronic hematogenous osteomyelitis, left radius and ulna CC HCC

M86.539 Other chronic hematogenous osteomyelitis, unspecified radius and ulna CC UNS HCC

✓6th M86.54 Other chronic hematogenous osteomyelitis, hand

M86.541 Other chronic hematogenous osteomyelitis, right hand CC HCC

M86.542 Other chronic hematogenous osteomyelitis, left hand CC HCC

M86.549 Other chronic hematogenous osteomyelitis, unspecified hand CC UNS HCC

✓6th M86.55 Other chronic hematogenous osteomyelitis, femur

M86.551 Other chronic hematogenous osteomyelitis, right femur CC HCC

M86.552 Other chronic hematogenous osteomyelitis, left femur CC HCC

M86.559 Other chronic hematogenous osteomyelitis, unspecified femur CC UNS HCC

✓6th M86.56 Other chronic hematogenous osteomyelitis, tibia and fibula

M86.561 Other chronic hematogenous osteomyelitis, right tibia and fibula CC HCC

M86.562 Other chronic hematogenous osteomyelitis, left tibia and fibula CC HCC

M86.569 Other chronic hematogenous osteomyelitis, unspecified tibia and fibula CC UNS HCC

AHA: 2022,1Q,7

✓6th M86.57 Other chronic hematogenous osteomyelitis, ankle and foot

M86.571 Other chronic hematogenous osteomyelitis, right ankle and foot CC HCC

M86.572 Other chronic hematogenous osteomyelitis, left ankle and foot CC HCC

M86.579 Other chronic hematogenous osteomyelitis, unspecified ankle and foot CC UNS HCC

M86.58 Other chronic hematogenous osteomyelitis, other site CC HCC

M86.59 Other chronic hematogenous osteomyelitis, multiple sites CC HCC

✓5th M86.6 Other chronic osteomyelitis

M86.60 Other chronic osteomyelitis, unspecified site CC UNS HCC

✓6th M86.61 Other chronic osteomyelitis, shoulder

M86.611 Other chronic osteomyelitis, right shoulder CC HCC

M86.612 Other chronic osteomyelitis, left shoulder CC HCC

M86.619 Other chronic osteomyelitis, unspecified shoulder CC UNS HCC

✓6th M86.62 Other chronic osteomyelitis, humerus

M86.621 Other chronic osteomyelitis, right humerus CC HCC

M86.622 Other chronic osteomyelitis, left humerus CC HCC

M86.629 Other chronic osteomyelitis, unspecified humerus CC UNS HCC

✓6th M86.63 Other chronic osteomyelitis, radius and ulna

M86.631 Other chronic osteomyelitis, right radius and ulna CC HCC

M86.632 Other chronic osteomyelitis, left radius and ulna CC HCC

M86.639 Other chronic osteomyelitis, unspecified radius and ulna CC UNS HCC

✓6th M86.64 Other chronic osteomyelitis, hand

M86.641 Other chronic osteomyelitis, right hand CC HCC

M86.642 Other chronic osteomyelitis, left hand CC HCC

M86.649 Other chronic osteomyelitis, unspecified hand CC UNS HCC

✓6th M86.65 Other chronic osteomyelitis, thigh

M86.651 Other chronic osteomyelitis, right thigh CC HCC

M86.652 Other chronic osteomyelitis, left thigh CC HCC

M86.659 Other chronic osteomyelitis, unspecified thigh CC UNS HCC

✓6th M86.66 Other chronic osteomyelitis, tibia and fibula

M86.661 Other chronic osteomyelitis, right tibia and fibula CC HCC

M86.662 Other chronic osteomyelitis, left tibia and fibula CC HCC

M86.669 Other chronic osteomyelitis, unspecified tibia and fibula CC UNS HCC

✓6th M86.67 Other chronic osteomyelitis, ankle and foot

M86.671 Other chronic osteomyelitis, right ankle and foot CC HCC

AHA: 2016,1Q,13

M86.672 Other chronic osteomyelitis, left ankle and foot CC HCC

M86.679 Other chronic osteomyelitis, unspecified ankle and foot CC UNS HCC

M86.68 Other chronic osteomyelitis, other site CC HCC

M86.69 Other chronic osteomyelitis, multiple sites CC HCC

M86.8 Other osteomyelitis (5th)
Brodie's abscess
AHA: 2022,1Q,31

M86.8X Other osteomyelitis (6th)

M86.8X0 Other osteomyelitis, multiple sites CC HCC
M86.8X1 Other osteomyelitis, shoulder CC HCC
M86.8X2 Other osteomyelitis, upper arm CC HCC
M86.8X3 Other osteomyelitis, forearm CC HCC
M86.8X4 Other osteomyelitis, hand CC HCC
M86.8X5 Other osteomyelitis, thigh CC HCC
M86.8X6 Other osteomyelitis, lower leg CC HCC
M86.8X7 Other osteomyelitis, ankle and foot CC HCC
M86.8X8 Other osteomyelitis, other site CC HCC
M86.8X9 Other osteomyelitis, unspecified sites CC UNS HCC

M86.9 Osteomyelitis, unspecified CC HCC
Infection of bone NOS
Periostitis without osteomyelitis

M87 Osteonecrosis (4th)
INCLUDES avascular necrosis of bone
Use additional code to identify major osseous defect, if applicable (M89.7-)
EXCLUDES 1 *juvenile osteonecrosis (M91-M92)*
osteochondropathies (M90-M93)

M87.0 Idiopathic aseptic necrosis of bone (5th)

M87.00 Idiopathic aseptic necrosis of unspecified bone CC UNS HCC

M87.01 Idiopathic aseptic necrosis of shoulder (6th)
Idiopathic aseptic necrosis of clavicle and scapula

M87.011 Idiopathic aseptic necrosis of right shoulder CC HCC
M87.012 Idiopathic aseptic necrosis of left shoulder CC HCC
M87.019 Idiopathic aseptic necrosis of unspecified shoulder CC UNS HCC

M87.02 Idiopathic aseptic necrosis of humerus (6th)

M87.021 Idiopathic aseptic necrosis of right humerus CC HCC
M87.022 Idiopathic aseptic necrosis of left humerus CC HCC
M87.029 Idiopathic aseptic necrosis of unspecified humerus CC UNS HCC

M87.03 Idiopathic aseptic necrosis of radius, ulna and carpus (6th)

M87.031 Idiopathic aseptic necrosis of right radius CC HCC
M87.032 Idiopathic aseptic necrosis of left radius CC HCC
M87.033 Idiopathic aseptic necrosis of unspecified radius CC UNS HCC
M87.034 Idiopathic aseptic necrosis of right ulna CC HCC
M87.035 Idiopathic aseptic necrosis of left ulna CC HCC
M87.036 Idiopathic aseptic necrosis of unspecified ulna CC UNS HCC
M87.037 Idiopathic aseptic necrosis of right carpus CC HCC
M87.038 Idiopathic aseptic necrosis of left carpus CC HCC
M87.039 Idiopathic aseptic necrosis of unspecified carpus CC UNS HCC

M87.04 Idiopathic aseptic necrosis of hand and fingers (6th)
Idiopathic aseptic necrosis of metacarpals and phalanges of hands

M87.041 Idiopathic aseptic necrosis of right hand CC HCC
M87.042 Idiopathic aseptic necrosis of left hand CC HCC
M87.043 Idiopathic aseptic necrosis of unspecified hand CC UNS HCC
M87.044 Idiopathic aseptic necrosis of right finger(s) CC HCC
M87.045 Idiopathic aseptic necrosis of left finger(s) CC HCC
M87.046 Idiopathic aseptic necrosis of unspecified finger(s) CC UNS HCC

M87.05 Idiopathic aseptic necrosis of pelvis and femur (6th)

M87.050 Idiopathic aseptic necrosis of pelvis CC HCC
M87.051 Idiopathic aseptic necrosis of right femur CC HCC
M87.052 Idiopathic aseptic necrosis of left femur CC HCC
M87.059 Idiopathic aseptic necrosis of unspecified femur CC UNS HCC

M87.06 Idiopathic aseptic necrosis of tibia and fibula (6th)

M87.061 Idiopathic aseptic necrosis of right tibia CC HCC
M87.062 Idiopathic aseptic necrosis of left tibia CC HCC
M87.063 Idiopathic aseptic necrosis of unspecified tibia CC UNS HCC
M87.064 Idiopathic aseptic necrosis of right fibula CC HCC
M87.065 Idiopathic aseptic necrosis of left fibula CC HCC
M87.066 Idiopathic aseptic necrosis of unspecified fibula CC UNS HCC

M87.07 Idiopathic aseptic necrosis of ankle, foot and toes (6th)
Idiopathic aseptic necrosis of metatarsus, tarsus, and phalanges of toes

M87.071 Idiopathic aseptic necrosis of right ankle CC HCC
M87.072 Idiopathic aseptic necrosis of left ankle CC HCC
M87.073 Idiopathic aseptic necrosis of unspecified ankle CC UNS HCC
M87.074 Idiopathic aseptic necrosis of right foot CC HCC
M87.075 Idiopathic aseptic necrosis of left foot CC HCC
M87.076 Idiopathic aseptic necrosis of unspecified foot CC UNS HCC
M87.077 Idiopathic aseptic necrosis of right toe(s) CC HCC
M87.078 Idiopathic aseptic necrosis of left toe(s) CC HCC
M87.079 Idiopathic aseptic necrosis of unspecified toe(s) CC UNS HCC

M87.08 Idiopathic aseptic necrosis of bone, other site CC HCC

M87.09 Idiopathic aseptic necrosis of bone, multiple sites CC HCC

M87.1 Osteonecrosis due to drugs (5th)
Use additional code for adverse effect, if applicable, to identify drug (T36-T50 with fifth or sixth character 5)

M87.10 Osteonecrosis due to drugs, unspecified bone CC UNS HCC

M87.11 Osteonecrosis due to drugs, shoulder (6th)

M87.111 Osteonecrosis due to drugs, right shoulder CC HCC
M87.112 Osteonecrosis due to drugs, left shoulder CC HCC
M87.119 Osteonecrosis due to drugs, unspecified shoulder CC UNS HCC

M87.12 Osteonecrosis due to drugs, humerus (6th)

M87.121 Osteonecrosis due to drugs, right humerus CC HCC
M87.122 Osteonecrosis due to drugs, left humerus CC HCC
M87.129 Osteonecrosis due to drugs, unspecified humerus CC UNS HCC

M87.13 Osteonecrosis due to drugs of radius, ulna and carpus (6th)

M87.131 Osteonecrosis due to drugs of right radius CC HCC
M87.132 Osteonecrosis due to drugs of left radius CC HCC
M87.133 Osteonecrosis due to drugs of unspecified radius CC UNS HCC
M87.134 Osteonecrosis due to drugs of right ulna CC HCC

M87.135 Osteonecrosis due to drugs of left ulna CC HCC

M87.136 Osteonecrosis due to drugs of unspecified ulna CC UNS HCC

M87.137 Osteonecrosis due to drugs of right carpus CC HCC

M87.138 Osteonecrosis due to drugs of left carpus CC HCC

M87.139 Osteonecrosis due to drugs of unspecified carpus CC UNS HCC

✓6th M87.14 Osteonecrosis due to drugs, hand and fingers

M87.141 Osteonecrosis due to drugs, right hand CC HCC

M87.142 Osteonecrosis due to drugs, left hand CC HCC

M87.143 Osteonecrosis due to drugs, unspecified hand CC UNS HCC

M87.144 Osteonecrosis due to drugs, right finger(s) CC HCC

M87.145 Osteonecrosis due to drugs, left finger(s) CC HCC

M87.146 Osteonecrosis due to drugs, unspecified finger(s) CC UNS HCC

✓6th M87.15 Osteonecrosis due to drugs, pelvis and femur

M87.150 Osteonecrosis due to drugs, pelvis CC HCC

M87.151 Osteonecrosis due to drugs, right femur CC HCC

M87.152 Osteonecrosis due to drugs, left femur CC HCC

M87.159 Osteonecrosis due to drugs, unspecified femur CC UNS HCC

✓6th M87.16 Osteonecrosis due to drugs, tibia and fibula

M87.161 Osteonecrosis due to drugs, right tibia CC HCC

M87.162 Osteonecrosis due to drugs, left tibia CC HCC

M87.163 Osteonecrosis due to drugs, unspecified tibia CC UNS HCC

M87.164 Osteonecrosis due to drugs, right fibula CC HCC

M87.165 Osteonecrosis due to drugs, left fibula CC HCC

M87.166 Osteonecrosis due to drugs, unspecified fibula CC UNS HCC

✓6th M87.17 Osteonecrosis due to drugs, ankle, foot and toes

M87.171 Osteonecrosis due to drugs, right ankle CC HCC

M87.172 Osteonecrosis due to drugs, left ankle CC HCC

M87.173 Osteonecrosis due to drugs, unspecified ankle CC UNS HCC

M87.174 Osteonecrosis due to drugs, right foot CC HCC

M87.175 Osteonecrosis due to drugs, left foot CC HCC

M87.176 Osteonecrosis due to drugs, unspecified foot CC UNS HCC

M87.177 Osteonecrosis due to drugs, right toe(s) CC HCC

M87.178 Osteonecrosis due to drugs, left toe(s) CC HCC

M87.179 Osteonecrosis due to drugs, unspecified toe(s) CC UNS HCC

✓6th M87.18 Osteonecrosis due to drugs, other site

M87.180 Osteonecrosis due to drugs, jaw CC HCC

M87.188 Osteonecrosis due to drugs, other site CC HCC

M87.19 Osteonecrosis due to drugs, multiple sites CC HCC

✓5th M87.2 Osteonecrosis due to previous trauma

M87.20 Osteonecrosis due to previous trauma, unspecified bone CC UNS HCC

✓6th M87.21 Osteonecrosis due to previous trauma, shoulder

M87.211 Osteonecrosis due to previous trauma, right shoulder CC HCC

M87.212 Osteonecrosis due to previous trauma, left shoulder CC HCC

M87.219 Osteonecrosis due to previous trauma, unspecified shoulder CC UNS HCC

✓6th M87.22 Osteonecrosis due to previous trauma, humerus

M87.221 Osteonecrosis due to previous trauma, right humerus CC HCC

M87.222 Osteonecrosis due to previous trauma, left humerus CC HCC

M87.229 Osteonecrosis due to previous trauma, unspecified humerus CC UNS HCC

✓6th M87.23 Osteonecrosis due to previous trauma of radius, ulna and carpus

M87.231 Osteonecrosis due to previous trauma of right radius CC HCC

M87.232 Osteonecrosis due to previous trauma of left radius CC HCC

M87.233 Osteonecrosis due to previous trauma of unspecified radius CC UNS HCC

M87.234 Osteonecrosis due to previous trauma of right ulna CC HCC

M87.235 Osteonecrosis due to previous trauma of left ulna CC HCC

M87.236 Osteonecrosis due to previous trauma of unspecified ulna CC UNS HCC

M87.237 Osteonecrosis due to previous trauma of right carpus CC HCC

M87.238 Osteonecrosis due to previous trauma of left carpus CC HCC

M87.239 Osteonecrosis due to previous trauma of unspecified carpus CC UNS HCC

✓6th M87.24 Osteonecrosis due to previous trauma, hand and fingers

M87.241 Osteonecrosis due to previous trauma, right hand CC HCC

M87.242 Osteonecrosis due to previous trauma, left hand CC HCC

M87.243 Osteonecrosis due to previous trauma, unspecified hand CC UNS HCC

M87.244 Osteonecrosis due to previous trauma, right finger(s) CC HCC

M87.245 Osteonecrosis due to previous trauma, left finger(s) CC HCC

M87.246 Osteonecrosis due to previous trauma, unspecified finger(s) CC UNS HCC

✓6th M87.25 Osteonecrosis due to previous trauma, pelvis and femur

M87.250 Osteonecrosis due to previous trauma, pelvis CC HCC

M87.251 Osteonecrosis due to previous trauma, right femur CC HCC

M87.252 Osteonecrosis due to previous trauma, left femur CC HCC

M87.256 Osteonecrosis due to previous trauma, unspecified femur CC UNS HCC

✓6th M87.26 Osteonecrosis due to previous trauma, tibia and fibula

M87.261 Osteonecrosis due to previous trauma, right tibia CC HCC

M87.262 Osteonecrosis due to previous trauma, left tibia CC HCC

M87.263 Osteonecrosis due to previous trauma, unspecified tibia CC UNS HCC

M87.264 Osteonecrosis due to previous trauma, right fibula CC HCC

M87.265 Osteonecrosis due to previous trauma, left fibula CC HCC

M87.266 Osteonecrosis due to previous trauma, unspecified fibula CC UNS HCC

✓6th M87.27 Osteonecrosis due to previous trauma, ankle, foot and toes

M87.271 Osteonecrosis due to previous trauma, right ankle CC HCC

M87.272 Osteonecrosis due to previous trauma, left ankle CC HCC

M87.273 Osteonecrosis due to previous trauma, unspecified ankle CC UNS HCC

M87.274 Osteonecrosis due to previous trauma, right foot CC HCC

M87.275 Osteonecrosis due to previous trauma, left foot CC HCC

M87.276 Osteonecrosis due to previous trauma, unspecified foot CC UNS HCC

M87.277 Osteonecrosis due to previous trauma, right toe(s) CC HCC

M87.278 Osteonecrosis due to previous trauma, left toe(s) CC HCC

M87.279 Osteonecrosis due to previous trauma, unspecified toe(s) CC UNS HCC

M87.28 Osteonecrosis due to previous trauma, other site CC HCC

M87.29 Osteonecrosis due to previous trauma, multiple sites CC HCC

✓5th M87.3 Other secondary osteonecrosis

M87.30 Other secondary osteonecrosis, unspecified bone CC UNS HCC

✓6th M87.31 Other secondary osteonecrosis, shoulder

M87.311 Other secondary osteonecrosis, right shoulder CC HCC

M87.312 Other secondary osteonecrosis, left shoulder CC HCC

M87.319 Other secondary osteonecrosis, unspecified shoulder CC UNS HCC

✓6th M87.32 Other secondary osteonecrosis, humerus

M87.321 Other secondary osteonecrosis, right humerus CC HCC

M87.322 Other secondary osteonecrosis, left humerus CC HCC

M87.329 Other secondary osteonecrosis, unspecified humerus CC UNS HCC

✓6th M87.33 Other secondary osteonecrosis of radius, ulna and carpus

M87.331 Other secondary osteonecrosis of right radius CC HCC

M87.332 Other secondary osteonecrosis of left radius CC HCC

M87.333 Other secondary osteonecrosis of unspecified radius CC UNS HCC

M87.334 Other secondary osteonecrosis of right ulna CC HCC

M87.335 Other secondary osteonecrosis of left ulna CC HCC

M87.336 Other secondary osteonecrosis of unspecified ulna CC UNS HCC

M87.337 Other secondary osteonecrosis of right carpus CC HCC

M87.338 Other secondary osteonecrosis of left carpus CC HCC

M87.339 Other secondary osteonecrosis of unspecified carpus CC UNS HCC

✓6th M87.34 Other secondary osteonecrosis, hand and fingers

M87.341 Other secondary osteonecrosis, right hand CC HCC

M87.342 Other secondary osteonecrosis, left hand CC HCC

M87.343 Other secondary osteonecrosis, unspecified hand CC UNS HCC

M87.344 Other secondary osteonecrosis, right finger(s) CC HCC

M87.345 Other secondary osteonecrosis, left finger(s) CC HCC

M87.346 Other secondary osteonecrosis, unspecified finger(s) CC UNS HCC

✓6th M87.35 Other secondary osteonecrosis, pelvis and femur

M87.350 Other secondary osteonecrosis, pelvis CC HCC

M87.351 Other secondary osteonecrosis, right femur CC HCC

M87.352 Other secondary osteonecrosis, left femur CC HCC

M87.353 Other secondary osteonecrosis, unspecified femur CC UNS HCC

✓6th M87.36 Other secondary osteonecrosis, tibia and fibula

M87.361 Other secondary osteonecrosis, right tibia CC HCC

M87.362 Other secondary osteonecrosis, left tibia CC HCC

M87.363 Other secondary osteonecrosis, unspecified tibia CC UNS HCC

M87.364 Other secondary osteonecrosis, right fibula CC HCC

M87.365 Other secondary osteonecrosis, left fibula CC HCC

M87.366 Other secondary osteonecrosis, unspecified fibula CC UNS HCC

✓6th M87.37 Other secondary osteonecrosis, ankle and foot

M87.371 Other secondary osteonecrosis, right ankle CC HCC

M87.372 Other secondary osteonecrosis, left ankle CC HCC

M87.373 Other secondary osteonecrosis, unspecified ankle CC UNS HCC

M87.374 Other secondary osteonecrosis, right foot CC HCC

M87.375 Other secondary osteonecrosis, left foot CC HCC

M87.376 Other secondary osteonecrosis, unspecified foot CC UNS HCC

M87.377 Other secondary osteonecrosis, right toe(s) CC HCC

M87.378 Other secondary osteonecrosis, left toe(s) CC HCC

M87.379 Other secondary osteonecrosis, unspecified toe(s) CC UNS HCC

M87.38 Other secondary osteonecrosis, other site CC HCC

M87.39 Other secondary osteonecrosis, multiple sites CC HCC

✓5th M87.8 Other osteonecrosis

M87.80 Other osteonecrosis, unspecified bone CC UNS HCC

✓6th M87.81 Other osteonecrosis, shoulder

M87.811 Other osteonecrosis, right shoulder CC HCC

M87.812 Other osteonecrosis, left shoulder CC HCC

M87.819 Other osteonecrosis, unspecified shoulder CC UNS HCC

✓6th M87.82 Other osteonecrosis, humerus

M87.821 Other osteonecrosis, right humerus CC HCC

M87.822 Other osteonecrosis, left humerus CC HCC

M87.829 Other osteonecrosis, unspecified humerus CC UNS HCC

✓6th M87.83 Other osteonecrosis of radius, ulna and carpus

M87.831 Other osteonecrosis of right radius CC HCC

M87.832 Other osteonecrosis of left radius CC HCC

M87.833 Other osteonecrosis of unspecified radius CC UNS HCC

M87.834 Other osteonecrosis of right ulna CC HCC

M87.835 Other osteonecrosis of left ulna CC HCC

M87.836 Other osteonecrosis of unspecified ulna CC UNS HCC

M87.837 Other osteonecrosis of right carpus CC HCC

M87.838 Other osteonecrosis of left carpus CC HCC

M87.839 Other osteonecrosis of unspecified carpus CC UNS HCC

✓6th M87.84 Other osteonecrosis, hand and fingers

M87.841 Other osteonecrosis, right hand CC HCC

M87.842 Other osteonecrosis, left hand CC HCC

M87.843 Other osteonecrosis, unspecified hand CC UNS HCC

M87.844 Other osteonecrosis, right finger(s) CC HCC

M87.845 Other osteonecrosis, left finger(s) CC HCC

M87.849 Other osteonecrosis, unspecified finger(s) CC UNS HCC

✓6th M87.85 Other osteonecrosis, pelvis and femur

M87.850 Other osteonecrosis, pelvis CC HCC

M87.851 Other osteonecrosis, right femur CC HCC

M87.852 Other osteonecrosis, left femur CC HCC

N Newborn: 0 P Pediatric: 0-17 M Maternity: 9-64 A Adult: 15-124 UNS Unspecified Site MCC Major Complication/Comorbidity CC Complication/Comorbidity

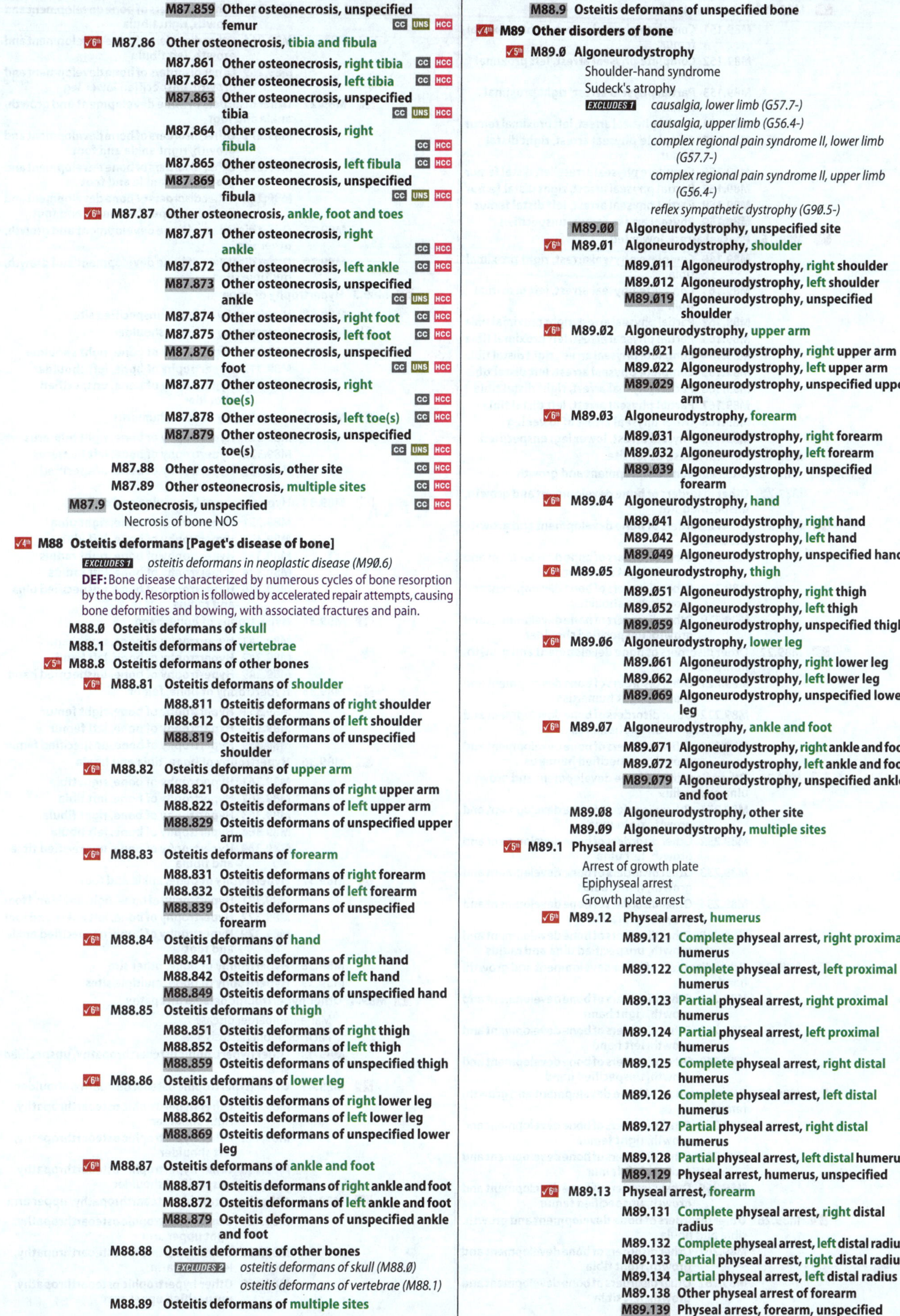

M87.859 Other osteonecrosis, unspecified femur CC UNS HCC

M87.86 Other osteonecrosis, tibia and fibula
- M87.861 Other osteonecrosis, right tibia CC HCC
- M87.862 Other osteonecrosis, left tibia CC HCC
- M87.863 Other osteonecrosis, unspecified tibia CC UNS HCC
- M87.864 Other osteonecrosis, right fibula CC HCC
- M87.865 Other osteonecrosis, left fibula CC HCC
- M87.869 Other osteonecrosis, unspecified fibula CC UNS HCC

M87.87 Other osteonecrosis, ankle, foot and toes
- M87.871 Other osteonecrosis, right ankle CC HCC
- M87.872 Other osteonecrosis, left ankle CC HCC
- M87.873 Other osteonecrosis, unspecified ankle CC UNS HCC
- M87.874 Other osteonecrosis, right foot CC HCC
- M87.875 Other osteonecrosis, left foot CC HCC
- M87.876 Other osteonecrosis, unspecified foot CC UNS HCC
- M87.877 Other osteonecrosis, right toe(s) CC HCC
- M87.878 Other osteonecrosis, left toe(s) CC HCC
- M87.879 Other osteonecrosis, unspecified toe(s) CC UNS HCC

M87.88 Other osteonecrosis, other site CC HCC

M87.89 Other osteonecrosis, multiple sites CC HCC

M87.9 Osteonecrosis, unspecified CC HCC
Necrosis of bone NOS

M88 Osteitis deformans [Paget's disease of bone]

EXCLUDES 1 *osteitis deformans in neoplastic disease (M90.6)*

DEF: Bone disease characterized by numerous cycles of bone resorption by the body. Resorption is followed by accelerated repair attempts, causing bone deformities and bowing, with associated fractures and pain.

M88.0 Osteitis deformans of skull

M88.1 Osteitis deformans of vertebrae

M88.8 Osteitis deformans of other bones

M88.81 Osteitis deformans of shoulder
- M88.811 Osteitis deformans of right shoulder
- M88.812 Osteitis deformans of left shoulder
- M88.819 Osteitis deformans of unspecified shoulder

M88.82 Osteitis deformans of upper arm
- M88.821 Osteitis deformans of right upper arm
- M88.822 Osteitis deformans of left upper arm
- M88.829 Osteitis deformans of unspecified upper arm

M88.83 Osteitis deformans of forearm
- M88.831 Osteitis deformans of right forearm
- M88.832 Osteitis deformans of left forearm
- M88.839 Osteitis deformans of unspecified forearm

M88.84 Osteitis deformans of hand
- M88.841 Osteitis deformans of right hand
- M88.842 Osteitis deformans of left hand
- M88.849 Osteitis deformans of unspecified hand

M88.85 Osteitis deformans of thigh
- M88.851 Osteitis deformans of right thigh
- M88.852 Osteitis deformans of left thigh
- M88.859 Osteitis deformans of unspecified thigh

M88.86 Osteitis deformans of lower leg
- M88.861 Osteitis deformans of right lower leg
- M88.862 Osteitis deformans of left lower leg
- M88.869 Osteitis deformans of unspecified lower leg

M88.87 Osteitis deformans of ankle and foot
- M88.871 Osteitis deformans of right ankle and foot
- M88.872 Osteitis deformans of left ankle and foot
- M88.879 Osteitis deformans of unspecified ankle and foot

M88.88 Osteitis deformans of other bones

EXCLUDES 2 *osteitis deformans of skull (M88.0)*
osteitis deformans of vertebrae (M88.1)

M88.89 Osteitis deformans of multiple sites

M88.9 Osteitis deformans of unspecified bone

M89 Other disorders of bone

M89.0 Algoneurodystrophy
Shoulder-hand syndrome
Sudeck's atrophy

EXCLUDES 1 *causalgia, lower limb (G57.7-)*
causalgia, upper limb (G56.4-)
complex regional pain syndrome II, lower limb (G57.7-)
complex regional pain syndrome II, upper limb (G56.4-)
reflex sympathetic dystrophy (G90.5-)

M89.00 Algoneurodystrophy, unspecified site

M89.01 Algoneurodystrophy, shoulder
- M89.011 Algoneurodystrophy, right shoulder
- M89.012 Algoneurodystrophy, left shoulder
- M89.019 Algoneurodystrophy, unspecified shoulder

M89.02 Algoneurodystrophy, upper arm
- M89.021 Algoneurodystrophy, right upper arm
- M89.022 Algoneurodystrophy, left upper arm
- M89.029 Algoneurodystrophy, unspecified upper arm

M89.03 Algoneurodystrophy, forearm
- M89.031 Algoneurodystrophy, right forearm
- M89.032 Algoneurodystrophy, left forearm
- M89.039 Algoneurodystrophy, unspecified forearm

M89.04 Algoneurodystrophy, hand
- M89.041 Algoneurodystrophy, right hand
- M89.042 Algoneurodystrophy, left hand
- M89.049 Algoneurodystrophy, unspecified hand

M89.05 Algoneurodystrophy, thigh
- M89.051 Algoneurodystrophy, right thigh
- M89.052 Algoneurodystrophy, left thigh
- M89.059 Algoneurodystrophy, unspecified thigh

M89.06 Algoneurodystrophy, lower leg
- M89.061 Algoneurodystrophy, right lower leg
- M89.062 Algoneurodystrophy, left lower leg
- M89.069 Algoneurodystrophy, unspecified lower leg

M89.07 Algoneurodystrophy, ankle and foot
- M89.071 Algoneurodystrophy, right ankle and foot
- M89.072 Algoneurodystrophy, left ankle and foot
- M89.079 Algoneurodystrophy, unspecified ankle and foot

M89.08 Algoneurodystrophy, other site

M89.09 Algoneurodystrophy, multiple sites

M89.1 Physeal arrest
Arrest of growth plate
Epiphyseal arrest
Growth plate arrest

M89.12 Physeal arrest, humerus
- M89.121 Complete physeal arrest, right proximal humerus
- M89.122 Complete physeal arrest, left proximal humerus
- M89.123 Partial physeal arrest, right proximal humerus
- M89.124 Partial physeal arrest, left proximal humerus
- M89.125 Complete physeal arrest, right distal humerus
- M89.126 Complete physeal arrest, left distal humerus
- M89.127 Partial physeal arrest, right distal humerus
- M89.128 Partial physeal arrest, left distal humerus
- M89.129 Physeal arrest, humerus, unspecified

M89.13 Physeal arrest, forearm
- M89.131 Complete physeal arrest, right distal radius
- M89.132 Complete physeal arrest, left distal radius
- M89.133 Partial physeal arrest, right distal radius
- M89.134 Partial physeal arrest, left distal radius
- M89.138 Other physeal arrest of forearm
- M89.139 Physeal arrest, forearm, unspecified

✓6th M89.15 Physeal arrest, femur
M89.151 Complete physeal arrest, right proximal femur
M89.152 Complete physeal arrest, left proximal femur
M89.153 Partial physeal arrest, right proximal femur
M89.154 Partial physeal arrest, left proximal femur
M89.155 Complete physeal arrest, right distal femur
M89.156 Complete physeal arrest, left distal femur
M89.157 Partial physeal arrest, right distal femur
M89.158 Partial physeal arrest, left distal femur
M89.159 Physeal arrest, femur, unspecified
✓6th M89.16 Physeal arrest, lower leg
M89.160 Complete physeal arrest, right proximal tibia
M89.161 Complete physeal arrest, left proximal tibia
M89.162 Partial physeal arrest, right proximal tibia
M89.163 Partial physeal arrest, left proximal tibia
M89.164 Complete physeal arrest, right distal tibia
M89.165 Complete physeal arrest, left distal tibia
M89.166 Partial physeal arrest, right distal tibia
M89.167 Partial physeal arrest, left distal tibia
M89.168 Other physeal arrest of lower leg
M89.169 Physeal arrest, lower leg, unspecified
M89.18 Physeal arrest, other site
✓5th M89.2 Other disorders of bone development and growth
M89.20 Other disorders of bone development and growth, unspecified site
✓6th M89.21 Other disorders of bone development and growth, shoulder
M89.211 Other disorders of bone development and growth, right shoulder
M89.212 Other disorders of bone development and growth, left shoulder
M89.219 Other disorders of bone development and growth, unspecified shoulder
✓6th M89.22 Other disorders of bone development and growth, humerus
M89.221 Other disorders of bone development and growth, right humerus
M89.222 Other disorders of bone development and growth, left humerus
M89.229 Other disorders of bone development and growth, unspecified humerus
✓6th M89.23 Other disorders of bone development and growth, ulna and radius
M89.231 Other disorders of bone development and growth, right ulna
M89.232 Other disorders of bone development and growth, left ulna
M89.233 Other disorders of bone development and growth, right radius
M89.234 Other disorders of bone development and growth, left radius
M89.239 Other disorders of bone development and growth, unspecified ulna and radius
✓6th M89.24 Other disorders of bone development and growth, hand
M89.241 Other disorders of bone development and growth, right hand
M89.242 Other disorders of bone development and growth, left hand
M89.249 Other disorders of bone development and growth, unspecified hand
✓6th M89.25 Other disorders of bone development and growth, femur
M89.251 Other disorders of bone development and growth, right femur
M89.252 Other disorders of bone development and growth, left femur
M89.259 Other disorders of bone development and growth, unspecified femur
✓6th M89.26 Other disorders of bone development and growth, tibia and fibula
M89.261 Other disorders of bone development and growth, right tibia
M89.262 Other disorders of bone development and growth, left tibia
M89.263 Other disorders of bone development and growth, right fibula
M89.264 Other disorders of bone development and growth, left fibula
M89.269 Other disorders of bone development and growth, unspecified lower leg
✓6th M89.27 Other disorders of bone development and growth, ankle and foot
M89.271 Other disorders of bone development and growth, right ankle and foot
M89.272 Other disorders of bone development and growth, left ankle and foot
M89.279 Other disorders of bone development and growth, unspecified ankle and foot
M89.28 Other disorders of bone development and growth, other site
M89.29 Other disorders of bone development and growth, multiple sites
✓5th M89.3 Hypertrophy of bone
M89.30 Hypertrophy of bone, unspecified site
✓6th M89.31 Hypertrophy of bone, shoulder
M89.311 Hypertrophy of bone, right shoulder
M89.312 Hypertrophy of bone, left shoulder
M89.319 Hypertrophy of bone, unspecified shoulder
✓6th M89.32 Hypertrophy of bone, humerus
M89.321 Hypertrophy of bone, right humerus
M89.322 Hypertrophy of bone, left humerus
M89.329 Hypertrophy of bone, unspecified humerus
✓6th M89.33 Hypertrophy of bone, ulna and radius
M89.331 Hypertrophy of bone, right ulna
M89.332 Hypertrophy of bone, left ulna
M89.333 Hypertrophy of bone, right radius
M89.334 Hypertrophy of bone, left radius
M89.339 Hypertrophy of bone, unspecified ulna and radius
✓6th M89.34 Hypertrophy of bone, hand
M89.341 Hypertrophy of bone, right hand
M89.342 Hypertrophy of bone, left hand
M89.349 Hypertrophy of bone, unspecified hand
✓6th M89.35 Hypertrophy of bone, femur
M89.351 Hypertrophy of bone, right femur
M89.352 Hypertrophy of bone, left femur
M89.359 Hypertrophy of bone, unspecified femur
✓6th M89.36 Hypertrophy of bone, tibia and fibula
M89.361 Hypertrophy of bone, right tibia
M89.362 Hypertrophy of bone, left tibia
M89.363 Hypertrophy of bone, right fibula
M89.364 Hypertrophy of bone, left fibula
M89.369 Hypertrophy of bone, unspecified tibia and fibula
✓6th M89.37 Hypertrophy of bone, ankle and foot
M89.371 Hypertrophy of bone, right ankle and foot
M89.372 Hypertrophy of bone, left ankle and foot
M89.379 Hypertrophy of bone, unspecified ankle and foot
M89.38 Hypertrophy of bone, other site
M89.39 Hypertrophy of bone, multiple sites
✓5th M89.4 Other hypertrophic osteoarthropathy
Marie-Bamberger disease
Pachydermoperiostosis
M89.40 Other hypertrophic osteoarthropathy, unspecified site
✓6th M89.41 Other hypertrophic osteoarthropathy, shoulder
M89.411 Other hypertrophic osteoarthropathy, right shoulder
M89.412 Other hypertrophic osteoarthropathy, left shoulder
M89.419 Other hypertrophic osteoarthropathy, unspecified shoulder
✓6th M89.42 Other hypertrophic osteoarthropathy, upper arm
M89.421 Other hypertrophic osteoarthropathy, right upper arm
M89.422 Other hypertrophic osteoarthropathy, left upper arm
M89.429 Other hypertrophic osteoarthropathy, unspecified upper arm

M89.43 Other hypertrophic osteoarthropathy, forearm
- M89.431 Other hypertrophic osteoarthropathy, right forearm
- M89.432 Other hypertrophic osteoarthropathy, left forearm
- M89.439 Other hypertrophic osteoarthropathy, unspecified forearm

M89.44 Other hypertrophic osteoarthropathy, hand
- M89.441 Other hypertrophic osteoarthropathy, right hand
- M89.442 Other hypertrophic osteoarthropathy, left hand
- M89.449 Other hypertrophic osteoarthropathy, unspecified hand

M89.45 Other hypertrophic osteoarthropathy, thigh
- M89.451 Other hypertrophic osteoarthropathy, right thigh
- M89.452 Other hypertrophic osteoarthropathy, left thigh
- M89.459 Other hypertrophic osteoarthropathy, unspecified thigh

M89.46 Other hypertrophic osteoarthropathy, lower leg
- M89.461 Other hypertrophic osteoarthropathy, right lower leg
- M89.462 Other hypertrophic osteoarthropathy, left lower leg
- M89.469 Other hypertrophic osteoarthropathy, unspecified lower leg

M89.47 Other hypertrophic osteoarthropathy, ankle and foot
- M89.471 Other hypertrophic osteoarthropathy, right ankle and foot
- M89.472 Other hypertrophic osteoarthropathy, left ankle and foot
- M89.479 Other hypertrophic osteoarthropathy, unspecified ankle and foot

M89.48 Other hypertrophic osteoarthropathy, other site

M89.49 Other hypertrophic osteoarthropathy, multiple sites

M89.5 Osteolysis

Use additional code to identify major osseous defect, if applicable (M89.7-)

EXCLUDES 2 *periprosthetic osteolysis of internal prosthetic joint (T84.05-)*

M89.50 Osteolysis, unspecified site

M89.51 Osteolysis, shoulder
- M89.511 Osteolysis, right shoulder
- M89.512 Osteolysis, left shoulder
- M89.519 Osteolysis, unspecified shoulder

M89.52 Osteolysis, upper arm
- M89.521 Osteolysis, right upper arm
- M89.522 Osteolysis, left upper arm
- M89.529 Osteolysis, unspecified upper arm

M89.53 Osteolysis, forearm
- M89.531 Osteolysis, right forearm
- M89.532 Osteolysis, left forearm
- M89.539 Osteolysis, unspecified forearm

M89.54 Osteolysis, hand
- M89.541 Osteolysis, right hand
- M89.542 Osteolysis, left hand
- M89.549 Osteolysis, unspecified hand

M89.55 Osteolysis, thigh
- M89.551 Osteolysis, right thigh
- M89.552 Osteolysis, left thigh
- M89.559 Osteolysis, unspecified thigh

M89.56 Osteolysis, lower leg
- M89.561 Osteolysis, right lower leg
- M89.562 Osteolysis, left lower leg
- M89.569 Osteolysis, unspecified lower leg

M89.57 Osteolysis, ankle and foot
- M89.571 Osteolysis, right ankle and foot
- M89.572 Osteolysis, left ankle and foot
- M89.579 Osteolysis, unspecified ankle and foot

M89.58 Osteolysis, other site

M89.59 Osteolysis, multiple sites

M89.6 Osteopathy after poliomyelitis

Use additional code (B91) to identify previous poliomyelitis

EXCLUDES 1 *postpolio syndrome (G14)*

M89.60 Osteopathy after poliomyelitis, unspecified site HCC

M89.61 Osteopathy after poliomyelitis, shoulder
- M89.611 Osteopathy after poliomyelitis, right shoulder HCC
- M89.612 Osteopathy after poliomyelitis, left shoulder HCC
- M89.619 Osteopathy after poliomyelitis, unspecified shoulder HCC

M89.62 Osteopathy after poliomyelitis, upper arm
- M89.621 Osteopathy after poliomyelitis, right upper arm HCC
- M89.622 Osteopathy after poliomyelitis, left upper arm HCC
- M89.629 Osteopathy after poliomyelitis, unspecified upper arm HCC

M89.63 Osteopathy after poliomyelitis, forearm
- M89.631 Osteopathy after poliomyelitis, right forearm HCC
- M89.632 Osteopathy after poliomyelitis, left forearm HCC
- M89.639 Osteopathy after poliomyelitis, unspecified forearm HCC

M89.64 Osteopathy after poliomyelitis, hand
- M89.641 Osteopathy after poliomyelitis, right hand HCC
- M89.642 Osteopathy after poliomyelitis, left hand HCC
- M89.649 Osteopathy after poliomyelitis, unspecified hand HCC

M89.65 Osteopathy after poliomyelitis, thigh
- M89.651 Osteopathy after poliomyelitis, right thigh HCC
- M89.652 Osteopathy after poliomyelitis, left thigh HCC
- M89.659 Osteopathy after poliomyelitis, unspecified thigh HCC

M89.66 Osteopathy after poliomyelitis, lower leg
- M89.661 Osteopathy after poliomyelitis, right lower leg HCC
- M89.662 Osteopathy after poliomyelitis, left lower leg HCC
- M89.669 Osteopathy after poliomyelitis, unspecified lower leg HCC

M89.67 Osteopathy after poliomyelitis, ankle and foot
- M89.671 Osteopathy after poliomyelitis, right ankle and foot HCC
- M89.672 Osteopathy after poliomyelitis, left ankle and foot HCC
- M89.679 Osteopathy after poliomyelitis, unspecified ankle and foot HCC

M89.68 Osteopathy after poliomyelitis, other site HCC

M89.69 Osteopathy after poliomyelitis, multiple sites HCC

M89.7 Major osseous defect

Code first underlying disease, if known, such as:
- aseptic necrosis of bone (M87.-)
- malignant neoplasm of bone (C40.-)
- osteolysis (M89.5)
- osteomyelitis (M86.-)
- osteonecrosis (M87.-)
- osteoporosis (M80.-, M81.-)
- periprosthetic osteolysis (T84.05-)

M89.70 Major osseous defect, unspecified site

M89.71 Major osseous defect, shoulder region

Major osseous defect clavicle or scapula
- M89.711 Major osseous defect, right shoulder region
- M89.712 Major osseous defect, left shoulder region
- M89.719 Major osseous defect, unspecified shoulder region

M89.72 Major osseous defect, humerus
- M89.721 Major osseous defect, right humerus
- M89.722 Major osseous defect, left humerus

M89.729 Major osseous defect, unspecified humerus

M89.73 Major osseous defect, forearm
Major osseous defect of radius and ulna
M89.731 Major osseous defect, right forearm
M89.732 Major osseous defect, left forearm
M89.739 Major osseous defect, unspecified forearm

M89.74 Major osseous defect, hand
Major osseous defect of carpus, fingers, metacarpus
M89.741 Major osseous defect, right hand
M89.742 Major osseous defect, left hand
M89.749 Major osseous defect, unspecified hand

M89.75 Major osseous defect, pelvic region and thigh
Major osseous defect of femur and pelvis
M89.751 Major osseous defect, right pelvic region and thigh
M89.752 Major osseous defect, left pelvic region and thigh
M89.759 Major osseous defect, unspecified pelvic region and thigh

M89.76 Major osseous defect, lower leg
Major osseous defect of fibula and tibia
M89.761 Major osseous defect, right lower leg
M89.762 Major osseous defect, left lower leg
M89.769 Major osseous defect, unspecified lower leg

M89.77 Major osseous defect, ankle and foot
Major osseous defect of metatarsus, tarsus, toes
M89.771 Major osseous defect, right ankle and foot
M89.772 Major osseous defect, left ankle and foot
M89.779 Major osseous defect, unspecified ankle and foot

M89.78 Major osseous defect, other site
M89.79 Major osseous defect, multiple sites

M89.8 Other specified disorders of bone
Infantile cortical hyperostoses
Post-traumatic subperiosteal ossification
AHA: 2022,2Q,10

M89.8X Other specified disorders of bone
M89.8X0 Other specified disorders of bone, multiple sites
M89.8X1 Other specified disorders of bone, shoulder
M89.8X2 Other specified disorders of bone, upper arm
M89.8X3 Other specified disorders of bone, forearm
AHA: 2019,3Q,9
M89.8X4 Other specified disorders of bone, hand
M89.8X5 Other specified disorders of bone, thigh
M89.8X6 Other specified disorders of bone, lower leg
M89.8X7 Other specified disorders of bone, ankle and foot
M89.8X8 Other specified disorders of bone, other site
M89.8X9 Other specified disorders of bone, unspecified site

M89.9 Disorder of bone, unspecified

M90 Osteopathies in diseases classified elsewhere

EXCLUDES 1 *osteochondritis, osteomyelitis, and osteopathy (in):*
cryptococcosis (B45.3)
diabetes mellitus (E08-E13 with .69-)
gonococcal (A54.43)
neurogenic syphilis (A52.11)
renal osteodystrophy (N25.0)
salmonellosis (A02.24)
secondary syphilis (A51.46)
syphilis (late) (A52.77)

M90.5 Osteonecrosis in diseases classified elsewhere
Code first underlying disease, such as:
caisson disease (T70.3)
hemoglobinopathy (D50-D64)

M90.50 Osteonecrosis in diseases classified elsewhere, unspecified site CC UNS HCC

M90.51 Osteonecrosis in diseases classified elsewhere, shoulder
M90.511 Osteonecrosis in diseases classified elsewhere, right shoulder CC HCC
M90.512 Osteonecrosis in diseases classified elsewhere, left shoulder CC HCC
M90.519 Osteonecrosis in diseases classified elsewhere, unspecified shoulder CC UNS HCC

M90.52 Osteonecrosis in diseases classified elsewhere, upper arm
M90.521 Osteonecrosis in diseases classified elsewhere, right upper arm CC HCC
M90.522 Osteonecrosis in diseases classified elsewhere, left upper arm CC HCC
M90.529 Osteonecrosis in diseases classified elsewhere, unspecified upper arm CC UNS HCC

M90.53 Osteonecrosis in diseases classified elsewhere, forearm
M90.531 Osteonecrosis in diseases classified elsewhere, right forearm CC HCC
M90.532 Osteonecrosis in diseases classified elsewhere, left forearm CC HCC
M90.539 Osteonecrosis in diseases classified elsewhere, unspecified forearm CC UNS HCC

M90.54 Osteonecrosis in diseases classified elsewhere, hand
M90.541 Osteonecrosis in diseases classified elsewhere, right hand CC HCC
M90.542 Osteonecrosis in diseases classified elsewhere, left hand CC HCC
M90.549 Osteonecrosis in diseases classified elsewhere, unspecified hand CC UNS HCC

M90.55 Osteonecrosis in diseases classified elsewhere, thigh
M90.551 Osteonecrosis in diseases classified elsewhere, right thigh CC HCC
M90.552 Osteonecrosis in diseases classified elsewhere, left thigh CC HCC
M90.559 Osteonecrosis in diseases classified elsewhere, unspecified thigh CC UNS HCC

M90.56 Osteonecrosis in diseases classified elsewhere, lower leg
M90.561 Osteonecrosis in diseases classified elsewhere, right lower leg CC HCC
M90.562 Osteonecrosis in diseases classified elsewhere, left lower leg CC HCC
M90.569 Osteonecrosis in diseases classified elsewhere, unspecified lower leg CC UNS HCC

M90.57 Osteonecrosis in diseases classified elsewhere, ankle and foot
M90.571 Osteonecrosis in diseases classified elsewhere, right ankle and foot CC HCC
M90.572 Osteonecrosis in diseases classified elsewhere, left ankle and foot CC HCC
M90.579 Osteonecrosis in diseases classified elsewhere, unspecified ankle and foot CC UNS HCC

M90.58 Osteonecrosis in diseases classified elsewhere, other site CC HCC
M90.59 Osteonecrosis in diseases classified elsewhere, multiple sites CC HCC

M90.6 Osteitis deformans in neoplastic diseases
Osteitis deformans in malignant neoplasm of bone
Code first the neoplasm (C40.-, C41.-)
EXCLUDES 1 *osteitis deformans [Paget's disease of bone] (M88.-)*

M90.60 Osteitis deformans in neoplastic diseases, unspecified site

M90.61 Osteitis deformans in neoplastic diseases, shoulder
M90.611 Osteitis deformans in neoplastic diseases, right shoulder
M90.612 Osteitis deformans in neoplastic diseases, left shoulder
M90.619 Osteitis deformans in neoplastic diseases, unspecified shoulder

M90.62 Osteitis deformans in neoplastic diseases, upper arm
- M90.621 *Osteitis deformans in neoplastic diseases, right upper arm*
- M90.622 *Osteitis deformans in neoplastic diseases, left upper arm*
- M90.629 *Osteitis deformans in neoplastic diseases, unspecified upper arm*

M90.63 Osteitis deformans in neoplastic diseases, forearm
- M90.631 *Osteitis deformans in neoplastic diseases, right forearm*
- M90.632 *Osteitis deformans in neoplastic diseases, left forearm*
- M90.639 *Osteitis deformans in neoplastic diseases, unspecified forearm*

M90.64 Osteitis deformans in neoplastic diseases, hand
- M90.641 *Osteitis deformans in neoplastic diseases, right hand*
- M90.642 *Osteitis deformans in neoplastic diseases, left hand*
- M90.649 *Osteitis deformans in neoplastic diseases, unspecified hand*

M90.65 Osteitis deformans in neoplastic diseases, thigh
- M90.651 *Osteitis deformans in neoplastic diseases, right thigh*
- M90.652 *Osteitis deformans in neoplastic diseases, left thigh*
- M90.659 *Osteitis deformans in neoplastic diseases, unspecified thigh*

M90.66 Osteitis deformans in neoplastic diseases, lower leg
- M90.661 *Osteitis deformans in neoplastic diseases, right lower leg*
- M90.662 *Osteitis deformans in neoplastic diseases, left lower leg*
- M90.669 *Osteitis deformans in neoplastic diseases, unspecified lower leg*

M90.67 Osteitis deformans in neoplastic diseases, ankle and foot
- M90.671 *Osteitis deformans in neoplastic diseases, right ankle and foot*
- M90.672 *Osteitis deformans in neoplastic diseases, left ankle and foot*
- M90.679 *Osteitis deformans in neoplastic diseases, unspecified ankle and foot*

M90.68 *Osteitis deformans in neoplastic diseases, other site*

M90.69 *Osteitis deformans in neoplastic diseases, multiple sites*

M90.8 Osteopathy in diseases classified elsewhere

Code first underlying disease, such as:
- rickets (E55.0)
- vitamin-D-resistant rickets (E83.3)

M90.80 *Osteopathy in diseases classified elsewhere, unspecified site*

M90.81 Osteopathy in diseases classified elsewhere, shoulder
- M90.811 *Osteopathy in diseases classified elsewhere, right shoulder*
- M90.812 *Osteopathy in diseases classified elsewhere, left shoulder*
- M90.819 *Osteopathy in diseases classified elsewhere, unspecified shoulder*

M90.82 Osteopathy in diseases classified elsewhere, upper arm
- M90.821 *Osteopathy in diseases classified elsewhere, right upper arm*
- M90.822 *Osteopathy in diseases classified elsewhere, left upper arm*
- M90.829 *Osteopathy in diseases classified elsewhere, unspecified upper arm*

M90.83 Osteopathy in diseases classified elsewhere, forearm
- M90.831 *Osteopathy in diseases classified elsewhere, right forearm*
- M90.832 *Osteopathy in diseases classified elsewhere, left forearm*
- M90.839 *Osteopathy in diseases classified elsewhere, unspecified forearm*

M90.84 Osteopathy in diseases classified elsewhere, hand
- M90.841 *Osteopathy in diseases classified elsewhere, right hand*
- M90.842 *Osteopathy in diseases classified elsewhere, left hand*
- M90.849 *Osteopathy in diseases classified elsewhere, unspecified hand*

M90.85 Osteopathy in diseases classified elsewhere, thigh
- M90.851 *Osteopathy in diseases classified elsewhere, right thigh*
- M90.852 *Osteopathy in diseases classified elsewhere, left thigh*
- M90.859 *Osteopathy in diseases classified elsewhere, unspecified thigh*

M90.86 Osteopathy in diseases classified elsewhere, lower leg
- M90.861 *Osteopathy in diseases classified elsewhere, right lower leg*
- M90.862 *Osteopathy in diseases classified elsewhere, left lower leg*
- M90.869 *Osteopathy in diseases classified elsewhere, unspecified lower leg*

M90.87 Osteopathy in diseases classified elsewhere, ankle and foot
- M90.871 *Osteopathy in diseases classified elsewhere, right ankle and foot*
- M90.872 *Osteopathy in diseases classified elsewhere, left ankle and foot*
- M90.879 *Osteopathy in diseases classified elsewhere, unspecified ankle and foot*

M90.88 *Osteopathy in diseases classified elsewhere, other site*

M90.89 *Osteopathy in diseases classified elsewhere, multiple sites*

Chondropathies (M91-M94)

EXCLUDES 1 *postprocedural chondropathies (M96.-)*

M91 Juvenile osteochondrosis of hip and pelvis

EXCLUDES 1 *slipped upper femoral epiphysis (nontraumatic) ►(M93.0-)◄*

M91.0 Juvenile osteochondrosis of pelvis
- Osteochondrosis (juvenile) of acetabulum
- Osteochondrosis (juvenile) of iliac crest [Buchanan]
- Osteochondrosis (juvenile) of ischiopubic synchondrosis [van Neck]
- Osteochondrosis (juvenile) of symphysis pubis [Pierson]

M91.1 Juvenile osteochondrosis of head of femur [Legg-Calvé-Perthes]
- M91.10 Juvenile osteochondrosis of head of femur [Legg-Calvé-Perthes], unspecified leg
- M91.11 Juvenile osteochondrosis of head of femur [Legg-Calvé-Perthes], right leg
- M91.12 Juvenile osteochondrosis of head of femur [Legg-Calvé-Perthes], left leg

M91.2 Coxa plana

Hip deformity due to previous juvenile osteochondrosis
- M91.20 Coxa plana, unspecified hip
- M91.21 Coxa plana, right hip
- M91.22 Coxa plana, left hip

M91.3 Pseudocoxalgia
- M91.30 Pseudocoxalgia, unspecified hip
- M91.31 Pseudocoxalgia, right hip
- M91.32 Pseudocoxalgia, left hip

M91.4 Coxa magna
- M91.40 Coxa magna, unspecified hip
- M91.41 Coxa magna, right hip
- M91.42 Coxa magna, left hip

M91.8 Other juvenile osteochondrosis of hip and pelvis

Juvenile osteochondrosis after reduction of congenital dislocation of hip
- M91.80 Other juvenile osteochondrosis of hip and pelvis, unspecified leg
- M91.81 Other juvenile osteochondrosis of hip and pelvis, right leg
- M91.82 Other juvenile osteochondrosis of hip and pelvis, left leg

M91.9 Juvenile osteochondrosis of hip and pelvis, unspecified
- M91.90 Juvenile osteochondrosis of hip and pelvis, unspecified, unspecified leg
- M91.91 Juvenile osteochondrosis of hip and pelvis, unspecified, right leg
- M91.92 Juvenile osteochondrosis of hip and pelvis, unspecified, left leg

M92 Other juvenile osteochondrosis

M92.0 Juvenile osteochondrosis of humerus
Osteochondrosis (juvenile) of capitulum of humerus [Panner]
Osteochondrosis (juvenile) of head of humerus [Haas]
M92.00 Juvenile osteochondrosis of humerus, unspecified arm
M92.01 Juvenile osteochondrosis of humerus, right arm
M92.02 Juvenile osteochondrosis of humerus, left arm

M92.1 Juvenile osteochondrosis of radius and ulna
Osteochondrosis (juvenile) of lower ulna [Burns]
Osteochondrosis (juvenile) of radial head [Brailsford]
M92.10 Juvenile osteochondrosis of radius and ulna, unspecified arm
M92.11 Juvenile osteochondrosis of radius and ulna, right arm
M92.12 Juvenile osteochondrosis of radius and ulna, left arm

M92.2 Juvenile osteochondrosis, hand
M92.20 Unspecified juvenile osteochondrosis, hand
M92.201 Unspecified juvenile osteochondrosis, right hand
M92.202 Unspecified juvenile osteochondrosis, left hand
M92.209 Unspecified juvenile osteochondrosis, unspecified hand
M92.21 Osteochondrosis (juvenile) of carpal lunate [Kienböck]
M92.211 Osteochondrosis (juvenile) of carpal lunate [Kienböck], right hand
M92.212 Osteochondrosis (juvenile) of carpal lunate [Kienböck], left hand
M92.219 Osteochondrosis (juvenile) of carpal lunate [Kienböck], unspecified hand
M92.22 Osteochondrosis (juvenile) of metacarpal heads [Mauclaire]
M92.221 Osteochondrosis (juvenile) of metacarpal heads [Mauclaire], right hand
M92.222 Osteochondrosis (juvenile) of metacarpal heads [Mauclaire], left hand
M92.229 Osteochondrosis (juvenile) of metacarpal heads [Mauclaire], unspecified hand
M92.29 Other juvenile osteochondrosis, hand
M92.291 Other juvenile osteochondrosis, right hand
M92.292 Other juvenile osteochondrosis, left hand
M92.299 Other juvenile osteochondrosis, unspecified hand

M92.3 Other juvenile osteochondrosis, upper limb
M92.30 Other juvenile osteochondrosis, unspecified upper limb
M92.31 Other juvenile osteochondrosis, right upper limb
M92.32 Other juvenile osteochondrosis, left upper limb

M92.4 Juvenile osteochondrosis of patella
Osteochondrosis (juvenile) of primary patellar center [Köhler]
Osteochondrosis (juvenile) of secondary patellar centre [Sinding Larsen]
M92.40 Juvenile osteochondrosis of patella, unspecified knee
M92.41 Juvenile osteochondrosis of patella, right knee
M92.42 Juvenile osteochondrosis of patella, left knee

M92.5 Juvenile osteochondrosis of tibia and fibula
AHA: 2020,4Q,33-34
M92.50 Unspecified juvenile osteochondrosis of tibia and fibula
M92.501 Unspecified juvenile osteochondrosis, right leg
M92.502 Unspecified juvenile osteochondrosis, left leg
M92.503 Unspecified juvenile osteochondrosis, bilateral leg
M92.509 Unspecified juvenile osteochondrosis, unspecified leg
M92.51 Juvenile osteochondrosis of proximal tibia
Blount disease
Tibia vara
M92.511 Juvenile osteochondrosis of proximal tibia, right leg
M92.512 Juvenile osteochondrosis of proximal tibia, left leg
M92.513 Juvenile osteochondrosis of proximal tibia, bilateral
M92.519 Juvenile osteochondrosis of proximal tibia, unspecified leg
M92.52 Juvenile osteochondrosis of tibia tubercle
Osgood-Schlatter disease
M92.521 Juvenile osteochondrosis of tibia tubercle, right leg
M92.522 Juvenile osteochondrosis of tibia tubercle, left leg
M92.523 Juvenile osteochondrosis of tibia tubercle, bilateral
M92.529 Juvenile osteochondrosis of tibia tubercle, unspecified leg
M92.59 Other juvenile osteochondrosis of tibia and fibula
M92.591 Other juvenile osteochondrosis of tibia and fibula, right leg
M92.592 Other juvenile osteochondrosis of tibia and fibula, left leg
M92.593 Other juvenile osteochondrosis of tibia and fibula, bilateral
M92.599 Other juvenile osteochondrosis of tibia and fibula, unspecified leg

M92.6 Juvenile osteochondrosis of tarsus
Osteochondrosis (juvenile) of calcaneum [Sever]
Osteochondrosis (juvenile) of os tibiale externum [Haglund]
Osteochondrosis (juvenile) of talus [Diaz]
Osteochondrosis (juvenile) of tarsal navicular [Köhler]
M92.60 Juvenile osteochondrosis of tarsus, unspecified ankle
M92.61 Juvenile osteochondrosis of tarsus, right ankle
M92.62 Juvenile osteochondrosis of tarsus, left ankle

M92.7 Juvenile osteochondrosis of metatarsus
Osteochondrosis (juvenile) of fifth metatarsus [Iselin]
Osteochondrosis (juvenile) of second metatarsus [Freiberg]
M92.70 Juvenile osteochondrosis of metatarsus, unspecified foot
M92.71 Juvenile osteochondrosis of metatarsus, right foot
M92.72 Juvenile osteochondrosis of metatarsus, left foot

M92.8 Other specified juvenile osteochondrosis
Calcaneal apophysitis
DEF: Calcaneal apophysitis: Inflammation of the calcaneus at the point of Achilles tendon insertion usually occurring in boys ages 8 to 14. Pain, tenderness, and localized swelling are present.

M92.9 Juvenile osteochondrosis, unspecified
Juvenile apophysitis NOS
Juvenile epiphysitis NOS
Juvenile osteochondritis NOS
Juvenile osteochondrosis NOS

M93 Other osteochondropathies
EXCLUDES 2 *osteochondrosis of spine (M42.-)*

M93.0 Slipped upper femoral epiphysis (nontraumatic)
▶Slipped capital femoral epiphysis (SCFE)◀
▶Slipped upper femoral epiphysis (SUFE)◀
Use additional code for associated chondrolysis (M94.3)
M93.00 Unspecified slipped upper femoral epiphysis (nontraumatic)
M93.001 Unspecified slipped upper femoral epiphysis (nontraumatic), right hip
M93.002 Unspecified slipped upper femoral epiphysis (nontraumatic), left hip
M93.003 Unspecified slipped upper femoral epiphysis (nontraumatic), unspecified hip
● **M93.004 Unspecified slipped upper femoral epiphysis (nontraumatic), bilateral hips**
▲ **M93.01 Acute slipped upper femoral epiphysis, stable (nontraumatic)**
▲ **M93.011 Acute slipped upper femoral epiphysis, stable (nontraumatic), right hip**
▲ **M93.012 Acute slipped upper femoral epiphysis, stable (nontraumatic), left hip**
▲ **M93.013 Acute slipped upper femoral epiphysis, stable (nontraumatic), unspecified hip**
● **M93.014 Acute slipped upper femoral epiphysis, stable (nontraumatic), bilateral hips**
▲ **M93.02 Chronic slipped upper femoral epiphysis, stable (nontraumatic)**
▲ **M93.021 Chronic slipped upper femoral epiphysis, stable (nontraumatic), right hip**

▲ M93.022 Chronic slipped upper femoral epiphysis, stable (nontraumatic), left hip
▲ M93.023 Chronic slipped upper femoral epiphysis, stable (nontraumatic), unspecified hip
● M93.024 Chronic slipped upper femoral epiphysis, stable (nontraumatic), bilateral hips
▲ M93.03 Acute on chronic slipped upper femoral epiphysis, stable (nontraumatic)
▲ M93.031 Acute on chronic slipped upper femoral epiphysis, stable (nontraumatic), right hip
▲ M93.032 Acute on chronic slipped upper femoral epiphysis, stable (nontraumatic), left hip
▲ M93.033 Acute on chronic slipped upper femoral epiphysis, stable (nontraumatic), unspecified hip
● M93.034 Acute on chronic slipped upper femoral epiphysis, stable (nontraumatic), bilateral hips
● M93.04 Acute slipped upper femoral epiphysis, unstable (nontraumatic)
● M93.041 Acute slipped upper femoral epiphysis, unstable (nontraumatic), right hip
● M93.042 Acute slipped upper femoral epiphysis, unstable (nontraumatic), left hip
● M93.043 Acute slipped upper femoral epiphysis, unstable (nontraumatic), unspecified hip
● M93.044 Acute slipped upper femoral epiphysis, unstable (nontraumatic), bilateral hips
● M93.05 Acute on chronic slipped upper femoral epiphysis, unstable (nontraumatic)
● M93.051 Acute on chronic slipped upper femoral epiphysis, unstable (nontraumatic), right hip
● M93.052 Acute on chronic slipped upper femoral epiphysis, unstable (nontraumatic), left hip
● M93.053 Acute on chronic slipped upper femoral epiphysis, unstable (nontraumatic), unspecified hip
● M93.054 Acute on chronic slipped upper femoral epiphysis, unstable (nontraumatic), bilateral hips
● M93.06 Acute slipped upper femoral epiphysis, unspecified stability (nontraumatic)
● M93.061 Acute slipped upper femoral epiphysis, unspecified stability (nontraumatic), right hip
● M93.062 Acute slipped upper femoral epiphysis, unspecified stability (nontraumatic), left hip
● M93.063 Acute slipped upper femoral epiphysis, unspecified stability (nontraumatic), unspecified hip
● M93.064 Acute slipped upper femoral epiphysis, unspecified stability (nontraumatic), bilateral hips
● M93.07 Acute on chronic slipped upper femoral epiphysis, unspecified stability (nontraumatic)
● M93.071 Acute on chronic slipped upper femoral epiphysis, unspecified stability (nontraumatic), right hip
● M93.072 Acute on chronic slipped upper femoral epiphysis, unspecified stability (nontraumatic), left hip
● M93.073 Acute on chronic slipped upper femoral epiphysis, unspecified stability (nontraumatic), unspecified hip
● M93.074 Acute on chronic slipped upper femoral epiphysis, unspecified stability (nontraumatic), bilateral hips

M93.1 Kienböck's disease of adults A
Adult osteochondrosis of carpal lunates

M93.2 Osteochondritis dissecans
DEF: Avascular necrosis caused by lack of blood flow to the bone and cartilage of a joint causing the bone to die. This can result in splinters or pieces of cartilage breaking off in the joint.
M93.20 Osteochondritis dissecans of unspecified site
M93.21 Osteochondritis dissecans of shoulder
M93.211 Osteochondritis dissecans, right shoulder
M93.212 Osteochondritis dissecans, left shoulder
M93.219 Osteochondritis dissecans, unspecified shoulder
M93.22 Osteochondritis dissecans of elbow
M93.221 Osteochondritis dissecans, right elbow
M93.222 Osteochondritis dissecans, left elbow
M93.229 Osteochondritis dissecans, unspecified elbow
M93.23 Osteochondritis dissecans of wrist
M93.231 Osteochondritis dissecans, right wrist
M93.232 Osteochondritis dissecans, left wrist
M93.239 Osteochondritis dissecans, unspecified wrist
M93.24 Osteochondritis dissecans of joints of hand
M93.241 Osteochondritis dissecans, joints of right hand
M93.242 Osteochondritis dissecans, joints of left hand
M93.249 Osteochondritis dissecans, joints of unspecified hand
M93.25 Osteochondritis dissecans of hip
M93.251 Osteochondritis dissecans, right hip
M93.252 Osteochondritis dissecans, left hip
M93.259 Osteochondritis dissecans, unspecified hip
M93.26 Osteochondritis dissecans knee
M93.261 Osteochondritis dissecans, right knee
M93.262 Osteochondritis dissecans, left knee
M93.269 Osteochondritis dissecans, unspecified knee
M93.27 Osteochondritis dissecans of ankle and joints of foot
M93.271 Osteochondritis dissecans, right ankle and joints of right foot
M93.272 Osteochondritis dissecans, left ankle and joints of left foot
M93.279 Osteochondritis dissecans, unspecified ankle and joints of foot
M93.28 Osteochondritis dissecans other site
M93.29 Osteochondritis dissecans multiple sites

M93.8 Other specified osteochondropathies
M93.80 Other specified osteochondropathies of unspecified site
M93.81 Other specified osteochondropathies of shoulder
M93.811 Other specified osteochondropathies, right shoulder
M93.812 Other specified osteochondropathies, left shoulder
M93.819 Other specified osteochondropathies, unspecified shoulder
M93.82 Other specified osteochondropathies of upper arm
M93.821 Other specified osteochondropathies, right upper arm
M93.822 Other specified osteochondropathies, left upper arm
M93.829 Other specified osteochondropathies, unspecified upper arm
M93.83 Other specified osteochondropathies of forearm
M93.831 Other specified osteochondropathies, right forearm
M93.832 Other specified osteochondropathies, left forearm
M93.839 Other specified osteochondropathies, unspecified forearm
M93.84 Other specified osteochondropathies of hand
M93.841 Other specified osteochondropathies, right hand
M93.842 Other specified osteochondropathies, left hand
M93.849 Other specified osteochondropathies, unspecified hand
M93.85 Other specified osteochondropathies of thigh
M93.851 Other specified osteochondropathies, right thigh
M93.852 Other specified osteochondropathies, left thigh
M93.859 Other specified osteochondropathies, unspecified thigh
M93.86 Other specified osteochondropathies lower leg
M93.861 Other specified osteochondropathies, right lower leg

M93.862 **Other specified osteochondropathies, left lower leg**

M93.869 **Other specified osteochondropathies, unspecified lower leg**

✓6th **M93.87** **Other specified osteochondropathies of ankle and foot**

M93.871 **Other specified osteochondropathies, right ankle and foot**

M93.872 **Other specified osteochondropathies, left ankle and foot**

M93.879 **Other specified osteochondropathies, unspecified ankle and foot**

M93.88 **Other specified osteochondropathies other site**

M93.89 **Other specified osteochondropathies multiple sites**

✓5th **M93.9** **Osteochondropathy, unspecified**

Apophysitis NOS
Epiphysitis NOS
Osteochondritis NOS
Osteochondrosis NOS

M93.90 **Osteochondropathy, unspecified of unspecified site**

✓6th **M93.91** **Osteochondropathy, unspecified of shoulder**

M93.911 **Osteochondropathy, unspecified, right shoulder**

M93.912 **Osteochondropathy, unspecified, left shoulder**

M93.919 **Osteochondropathy, unspecified, unspecified shoulder**

✓6th **M93.92** **Osteochondropathy, unspecified of upper arm**

M93.921 **Osteochondropathy, unspecified, right upper arm**

M93.922 **Osteochondropathy, unspecified, left upper arm**

M93.929 **Osteochondropathy, unspecified, unspecified upper arm**

✓6th **M93.93** **Osteochondropathy, unspecified of forearm**

M93.931 **Osteochondropathy, unspecified, right forearm**

M93.932 **Osteochondropathy, unspecified, left forearm**

M93.939 **Osteochondropathy, unspecified, unspecified forearm**

✓6th **M93.94** **Osteochondropathy, unspecified of hand**

M93.941 **Osteochondropathy, unspecified, right hand**

M93.942 **Osteochondropathy, unspecified, left hand**

M93.949 **Osteochondropathy, unspecified, unspecified hand**

✓6th **M93.95** **Osteochondropathy, unspecified of thigh**

M93.951 **Osteochondropathy, unspecified, right thigh**

M93.952 **Osteochondropathy, unspecified, left thigh**

M93.959 **Osteochondropathy, unspecified, unspecified thigh**

✓6th **M93.96** **Osteochondropathy, unspecified lower leg**

M93.961 **Osteochondropathy, unspecified, right lower leg**

M93.962 **Osteochondropathy, unspecified, left lower leg**

M93.969 **Osteochondropathy, unspecified, unspecified lower leg**

✓6th **M93.97** **Osteochondropathy, unspecified of ankle and foot**

M93.971 **Osteochondropathy, unspecified, right ankle and foot**

M93.972 **Osteochondropathy, unspecified, left ankle and foot**

M93.979 **Osteochondropathy, unspecified, unspecified ankle and foot**

M93.98 **Osteochondropathy, unspecified other site**

M93.99 **Osteochondropathy, unspecified multiple sites**

✓4th **M94** **Other disorders of cartilage**

M94.0 **Chondrocostal junction syndrome [Tietze]**

Costochondritis

M94.1 **Relapsing polychondritis**

✓5th **M94.2** **Chondromalacia**

EXCLUDES 1 *chondromalacia patellae (M22.4)*

M94.20 **Chondromalacia, unspecified site**

✓6th **M94.21** **Chondromalacia, shoulder**

M94.211 **Chondromalacia, right shoulder**

M94.212 **Chondromalacia, left shoulder**

M94.219 **Chondromalacia, unspecified shoulder**

✓6th **M94.22** **Chondromalacia, elbow**

M94.221 **Chondromalacia, right elbow**

M94.222 **Chondromalacia, left elbow**

M94.229 **Chondromalacia, unspecified elbow**

✓6th **M94.23** **Chondromalacia, wrist**

M94.231 **Chondromalacia, right wrist**

M94.232 **Chondromalacia, left wrist**

M94.239 **Chondromalacia, unspecified wrist**

✓6th **M94.24** **Chondromalacia, joints of hand**

M94.241 **Chondromalacia, joints of right hand**

M94.242 **Chondromalacia, joints of left hand**

M94.249 **Chondromalacia, joints of unspecified hand**

✓6th **M94.25** **Chondromalacia, hip**

M94.251 **Chondromalacia, right hip**

M94.252 **Chondromalacia, left hip**

M94.259 **Chondromalacia, unspecified hip**

✓6th **M94.26** **Chondromalacia, knee**

M94.261 **Chondromalacia, right knee**

M94.262 **Chondromalacia, left knee**

M94.269 **Chondromalacia, unspecified knee**

✓6th **M94.27** **Chondromalacia, ankle and joints of foot**

M94.271 **Chondromalacia, right ankle and joints of right foot**

M94.272 **Chondromalacia, left ankle and joints of left foot**

M94.279 **Chondromalacia, unspecified ankle and joints of foot**

M94.28 **Chondromalacia, other site**

M94.29 **Chondromalacia, multiple sites**

✓5th **M94.3** **Chondrolysis**

Code first any associated slipped upper femoral epiphysis (nontraumatic) (M93.0-)

✓6th **M94.35** **Chondrolysis, hip**

M94.351 **Chondrolysis, right hip**

M94.352 **Chondrolysis, left hip**

M94.359 **Chondrolysis, unspecified hip**

✓5th **M94.8** **Other specified disorders of cartilage**

✓6th **M94.8X** **Other specified disorders of cartilage**

M94.8X0 **Other specified disorders of cartilage, multiple sites**

M94.8X1 **Other specified disorders of cartilage, shoulder**

M94.8X2 **Other specified disorders of cartilage, upper arm**

M94.8X3 **Other specified disorders of cartilage, forearm**

M94.8X4 **Other specified disorders of cartilage, hand**

M94.8X5 **Other specified disorders of cartilage, thigh**

M94.8X6 **Other specified disorders of cartilage, lower leg**

M94.8X7 **Other specified disorders of cartilage, ankle and foot**

M94.8X8 **Other specified disorders of cartilage, other site**

M94.8X9 **Other specified disorders of cartilage, unspecified sites**

M94.9 **Disorder of cartilage, unspecified**

Other disorders of the musculoskeletal system and connective tissue (M95)

M95 Other acquired deformities of musculoskeletal system and connective tissue

EXCLUDES 2 *acquired absence of limbs and organs (Z89-Z90)*
acquired deformities of limbs (M20-M21)
congenital malformations and deformations of the musculoskeletal system (Q65-Q79)
deforming dorsopathies (M40-M43)
dentofacial anomalies [including malocclusion] (M26.-)
postprocedural musculoskeletal disorders (M96.-)

M95.0 Acquired deformity of nose
EXCLUDES 2 *deviated nasal septum (J34.2)*

M95.1 Cauliflower ear
EXCLUDES 2 *other acquired deformities of ear (H61.1)*
DEF: Acquired deformity of the external ear due to injury or subsequent perichondritis.

M95.10 Cauliflower ear, unspecified ear
M95.11 Cauliflower ear, right ear
M95.12 Cauliflower ear, left ear

M95.2 Other acquired deformity of head
AHA: 2022,1Q,34

M95.3 Acquired deformity of neck

M95.4 Acquired deformity of chest and rib
AHA: 2022,2Q,14; 2014,4Q,26-27

M95.5 Acquired deformity of pelvis
EXCLUDES 1 *maternal care for known or suspected disproportion (O33.-)*

M95.8 Other specified acquired deformities of musculoskeletal system

M95.9 Acquired deformity of musculoskeletal system, unspecified

Intraoperative and postprocedural complications and disorders of musculoskeletal system, not elsewhere classified (M96)

M96 Intraoperative and postprocedural complications and disorders of musculoskeletal system, not elsewhere classified

EXCLUDES 2 *arthropathy following intestinal bypass (M02.0-)*
complications of internal orthopedic prosthetic devices, implants and grafts (T84.-)
disorders associated with osteoporosis (M80)
periprosthetic fracture around internal prosthetic joint (M97.-)
presence of functional implants and other devices (Z96-Z97)

M96.0 Pseudarthrosis after fusion or arthrodesis CC
M96.1 Postlaminectomy syndrome, not elsewhere classified
M96.2 Postradiation kyphosis
M96.3 Postlaminectomy kyphosis
M96.4 Postsurgical lordosis
M96.5 Postradiation scoliosis

M96.6 Fracture of bone following insertion of orthopedic implant, joint prosthesis, or bone plate
Intraoperative fracture of bone during insertion of orthopedic implant, joint prosthesis, or bone plate
EXCLUDES 2 *complication of internal orthopedic devices, implants or grafts (T84.-)*

M96.62 Fracture of humerus following insertion of orthopedic implant, joint prosthesis, or bone plate
M96.621 Fracture of humerus following insertion of orthopedic implant, joint prosthesis, or bone plate, right arm CC HCC
M96.622 Fracture of humerus following insertion of orthopedic implant, joint prosthesis, or bone plate, left arm CC HCC
M96.629 Fracture of humerus following insertion of orthopedic implant, joint prosthesis, or bone plate, unspecified arm CC UNS HCC

M96.63 Fracture of radius or ulna following insertion of orthopedic implant, joint prosthesis, or bone plate
M96.631 Fracture of radius or ulna following insertion of orthopedic implant, joint prosthesis, or bone plate, right arm CC HCC
M96.632 Fracture of radius or ulna following insertion of orthopedic implant, joint prosthesis, or bone plate, left arm CC HCC
M96.639 Fracture of radius or ulna following insertion of orthopedic implant, joint prosthesis, or bone plate, unspecified arm CC UNS HCC

M96.65 Fracture of pelvis following insertion of orthopedic implant, joint prosthesis, or bone plate CC HCC

M96.66 Fracture of femur following insertion of orthopedic implant, joint prosthesis, or bone plate
M96.661 Fracture of femur following insertion of orthopedic implant, joint prosthesis, or bone plate, right leg CC HCC
M96.662 Fracture of femur following insertion of orthopedic implant, joint prosthesis, or bone plate, left leg CC HCC
M96.669 Fracture of femur following insertion of orthopedic implant, joint prosthesis, or bone plate, unspecified leg CC UNS HCC

M96.67 Fracture of tibia or fibula following insertion of orthopedic implant, joint prosthesis, or bone plate
M96.671 Fracture of tibia or fibula following insertion of orthopedic implant, joint prosthesis, or bone plate, right leg CC HCC
M96.672 Fracture of tibia or fibula following insertion of orthopedic implant, joint prosthesis, or bone plate, left leg CC HCC
M96.679 Fracture of tibia or fibula following insertion of orthopedic implant, joint prosthesis, or bone plate, unspecified leg CC UNS HCC

M96.69 Fracture of other bone following insertion of orthopedic implant, joint prosthesis, or bone plate CC HCC

M96.8 Other intraoperative and postprocedural complications and disorders of musculoskeletal system, not elsewhere classified
AHA: 2016,4Q,9-10

M96.81 Intraoperative hemorrhage and hematoma of a musculoskeletal structure complicating a procedure
EXCLUDES 1 *intraoperative hemorrhage and hematoma of a musculoskeletal structure due to accidental puncture and laceration during a procedure (M96.82-)*
M96.810 Intraoperative hemorrhage and hematoma of a musculoskeletal structure complicating a musculoskeletal system procedure CC
M96.811 Intraoperative hemorrhage and hematoma of a musculoskeletal structure complicating other procedure CC

M96.82 Accidental puncture and laceration of a musculoskeletal structure during a procedure
M96.820 Accidental puncture and laceration of a musculoskeletal structure during a musculoskeletal system procedure CC
M96.821 Accidental puncture and laceration of a musculoskeletal structure during other procedure CC

M96.83 Postprocedural hemorrhage of a musculoskeletal structure following a procedure
M96.830 Postprocedural hemorrhage of a musculoskeletal structure following a musculoskeletal system procedure CC
M96.831 Postprocedural hemorrhage of a musculoskeletal structure following other procedure CC

M96.84 Postprocedural hematoma and seroma of a musculoskeletal structure following a procedure
M96.840 Postprocedural hematoma of a musculoskeletal structure following a musculoskeletal system procedure CC
M96.841 Postprocedural hematoma of a musculoskeletal structure following other procedure CC
AHA: 2016,4Q,10
M96.842 Postprocedural seroma of a musculoskeletal structure following a musculoskeletal system procedure CC

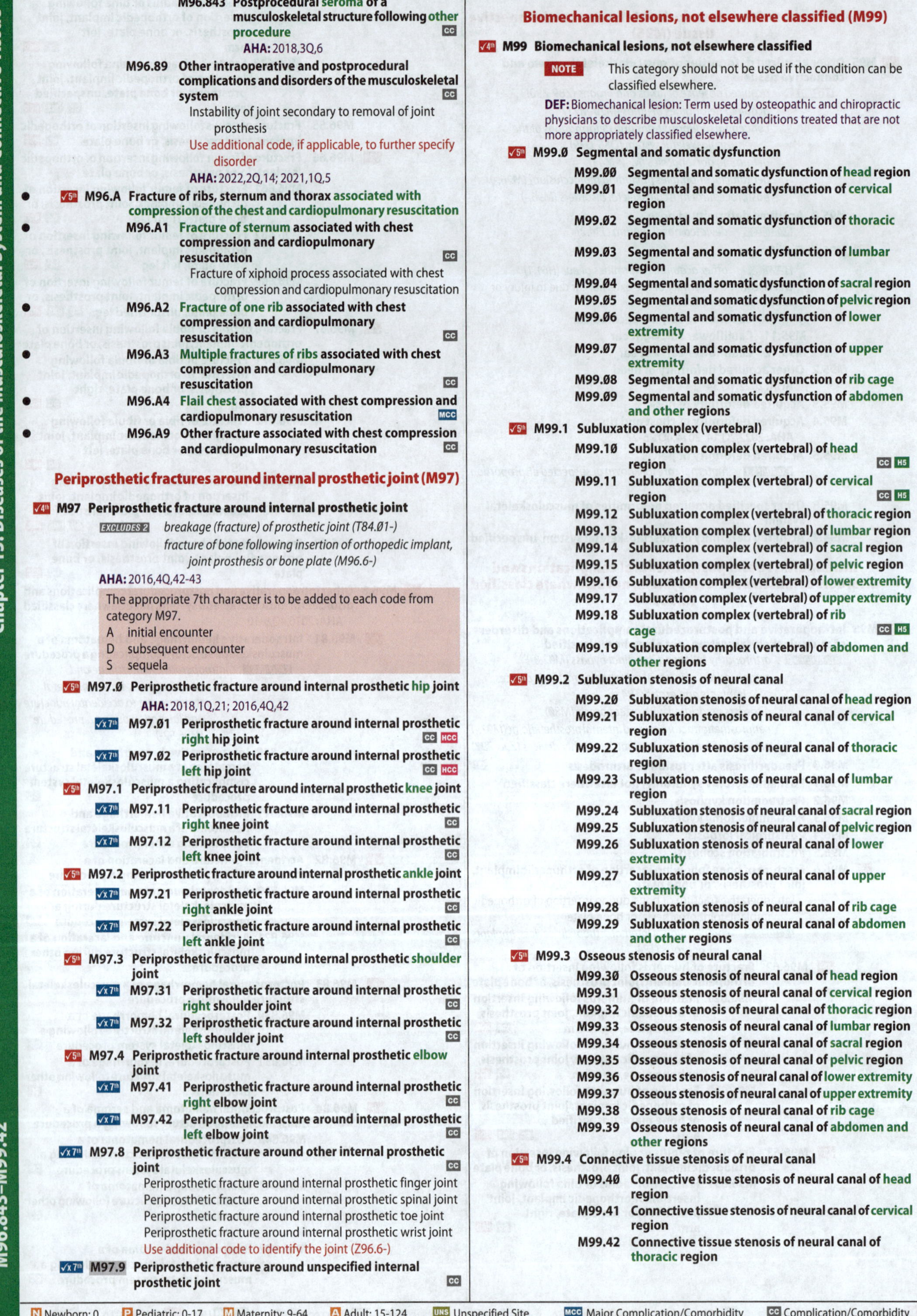

M96.843 Postprocedural seroma of a musculoskeletal structure following other procedure CC
AHA: 2018,3Q,6

M96.89 Other intraoperative and postprocedural complications and disorders of the musculoskeletal system CC
Instability of joint secondary to removal of joint prosthesis
Use additional code, if applicable, to further specify disorder
AHA: 2022,2Q,14; 2021,1Q,5

● **M96.A Fracture of ribs, sternum and thorax associated with compression of the chest and cardiopulmonary resuscitation**

● **M96.A1 Fracture of sternum associated with chest compression and cardiopulmonary resuscitation** CC
Fracture of xiphoid process associated with chest compression and cardiopulmonary resuscitation

● **M96.A2 Fracture of one rib associated with chest compression and cardiopulmonary resuscitation** CC

● **M96.A3 Multiple fractures of ribs associated with chest compression and cardiopulmonary resuscitation** CC

● **M96.A4 Flail chest associated with chest compression and cardiopulmonary resuscitation** MCC

● **M96.A9 Other fracture associated with chest compression and cardiopulmonary resuscitation** CC

Periprosthetic fractures around internal prosthetic joint (M97)

M97 Periprosthetic fracture around internal prosthetic joint
EXCLUDES 2 *breakage (fracture) of prosthetic joint (T84.01-)*
fracture of bone following insertion of orthopedic implant, joint prosthesis or bone plate (M96.6-)
AHA: 2016,4Q,42-43

The appropriate 7th character is to be added to each code from category M97.
A initial encounter
D subsequent encounter
S sequela

M97.0 Periprosthetic fracture around internal prosthetic hip joint
AHA: 2018,1Q,21; 2016,4Q,42

M97.01 Periprosthetic fracture around internal prosthetic right hip joint CC HCC

M97.02 Periprosthetic fracture around internal prosthetic left hip joint CC HCC

M97.1 Periprosthetic fracture around internal prosthetic knee joint

M97.11 Periprosthetic fracture around internal prosthetic right knee joint CC

M97.12 Periprosthetic fracture around internal prosthetic left knee joint CC

M97.2 Periprosthetic fracture around internal prosthetic ankle joint

M97.21 Periprosthetic fracture around internal prosthetic right ankle joint CC

M97.22 Periprosthetic fracture around internal prosthetic left ankle joint CC

M97.3 Periprosthetic fracture around internal prosthetic shoulder joint

M97.31 Periprosthetic fracture around internal prosthetic right shoulder joint CC

M97.32 Periprosthetic fracture around internal prosthetic left shoulder joint CC

M97.4 Periprosthetic fracture around internal prosthetic elbow joint

M97.41 Periprosthetic fracture around internal prosthetic right elbow joint CC

M97.42 Periprosthetic fracture around internal prosthetic left elbow joint CC

M97.8 Periprosthetic fracture around other internal prosthetic joint CC
Periprosthetic fracture around internal prosthetic finger joint
Periprosthetic fracture around internal prosthetic spinal joint
Periprosthetic fracture around internal prosthetic toe joint
Periprosthetic fracture around internal prosthetic wrist joint
Use additional code to identify the joint (Z96.6-)

M97.9 Periprosthetic fracture around unspecified internal prosthetic joint CC

Biomechanical lesions, not elsewhere classified (M99)

M99 Biomechanical lesions, not elsewhere classified
NOTE This category should not be used if the condition can be classified elsewhere.
DEF: Biomechanical lesion: Term used by osteopathic and chiropractic physicians to describe musculoskeletal conditions treated that are not more appropriately classified elsewhere.

M99.0 Segmental and somatic dysfunction
M99.00 Segmental and somatic dysfunction of head region
M99.01 Segmental and somatic dysfunction of cervical region
M99.02 Segmental and somatic dysfunction of thoracic region
M99.03 Segmental and somatic dysfunction of lumbar region
M99.04 Segmental and somatic dysfunction of sacral region
M99.05 Segmental and somatic dysfunction of pelvic region
M99.06 Segmental and somatic dysfunction of lower extremity
M99.07 Segmental and somatic dysfunction of upper extremity
M99.08 Segmental and somatic dysfunction of rib cage
M99.09 Segmental and somatic dysfunction of abdomen and other regions

M99.1 Subluxation complex (vertebral)
M99.10 Subluxation complex (vertebral) of head region CC H5
M99.11 Subluxation complex (vertebral) of cervical region CC H5
M99.12 Subluxation complex (vertebral) of thoracic region
M99.13 Subluxation complex (vertebral) of lumbar region
M99.14 Subluxation complex (vertebral) of sacral region
M99.15 Subluxation complex (vertebral) of pelvic region
M99.16 Subluxation complex (vertebral) of lower extremity
M99.17 Subluxation complex (vertebral) of upper extremity
M99.18 Subluxation complex (vertebral) of rib cage CC H5
M99.19 Subluxation complex (vertebral) of abdomen and other regions

M99.2 Subluxation stenosis of neural canal
M99.20 Subluxation stenosis of neural canal of head region
M99.21 Subluxation stenosis of neural canal of cervical region
M99.22 Subluxation stenosis of neural canal of thoracic region
M99.23 Subluxation stenosis of neural canal of lumbar region
M99.24 Subluxation stenosis of neural canal of sacral region
M99.25 Subluxation stenosis of neural canal of pelvic region
M99.26 Subluxation stenosis of neural canal of lower extremity
M99.27 Subluxation stenosis of neural canal of upper extremity
M99.28 Subluxation stenosis of neural canal of rib cage
M99.29 Subluxation stenosis of neural canal of abdomen and other regions

M99.3 Osseous stenosis of neural canal
M99.30 Osseous stenosis of neural canal of head region
M99.31 Osseous stenosis of neural canal of cervical region
M99.32 Osseous stenosis of neural canal of thoracic region
M99.33 Osseous stenosis of neural canal of lumbar region
M99.34 Osseous stenosis of neural canal of sacral region
M99.35 Osseous stenosis of neural canal of pelvic region
M99.36 Osseous stenosis of neural canal of lower extremity
M99.37 Osseous stenosis of neural canal of upper extremity
M99.38 Osseous stenosis of neural canal of rib cage
M99.39 Osseous stenosis of neural canal of abdomen and other regions

M99.4 Connective tissue stenosis of neural canal
M99.40 Connective tissue stenosis of neural canal of head region
M99.41 Connective tissue stenosis of neural canal of cervical region
M99.42 Connective tissue stenosis of neural canal of thoracic region

N Newborn: 0 P Pediatric: 0-17 M Maternity: 9-64 A Adult: 15-124 UNS Unspecified Site MCC Major Complication/Comorbidity CC Complication/Comorbidity

M99.43 Connective tissue stenosis of neural canal of lumbar region
M99.44 Connective tissue stenosis of neural canal of sacral region
M99.45 Connective tissue stenosis of neural canal of pelvic region
M99.46 Connective tissue stenosis of neural canal of lower extremity
M99.47 Connective tissue stenosis of neural canal of upper extremity
M99.48 Connective tissue stenosis of neural canal of rib cage
M99.49 Connective tissue stenosis of neural canal of abdomen and other regions

M99.5 Intervertebral disc stenosis of neural canal
M99.50 Intervertebral disc stenosis of neural canal of head region
M99.51 Intervertebral disc stenosis of neural canal of cervical region
M99.52 Intervertebral disc stenosis of neural canal of thoracic region
M99.53 Intervertebral disc stenosis of neural canal of lumbar region
M99.54 Intervertebral disc stenosis of neural canal of sacral region
M99.55 Intervertebral disc stenosis of neural canal of pelvic region
M99.56 Intervertebral disc stenosis of neural canal of lower extremity
M99.57 Intervertebral disc stenosis of neural canal of upper extremity
M99.58 Intervertebral disc stenosis of neural canal of rib cage
M99.59 Intervertebral disc stenosis of neural canal of abdomen and other regions

M99.6 Osseous and subluxation stenosis of intervertebral foramina
M99.60 Osseous and subluxation stenosis of intervertebral foramina of head region
M99.61 Osseous and subluxation stenosis of intervertebral foramina of cervical region
M99.62 Osseous and subluxation stenosis of intervertebral foramina of thoracic region
M99.63 Osseous and subluxation stenosis of intervertebral foramina of lumbar region
M99.64 Osseous and subluxation stenosis of intervertebral foramina of sacral region
M99.65 Osseous and subluxation stenosis of intervertebral foramina of pelvic region
M99.66 Osseous and subluxation stenosis of intervertebral foramina of lower extremity
M99.67 Osseous and subluxation stenosis of intervertebral foramina of upper extremity
M99.68 Osseous and subluxation stenosis of intervertebral foramina of rib cage
M99.69 Osseous and subluxation stenosis of intervertebral foramina of abdomen and other regions

M99.7 Connective tissue and disc stenosis of intervertebral foramina
M99.70 Connective tissue and disc stenosis of intervertebral foramina of head region
M99.71 Connective tissue and disc stenosis of intervertebral foramina of cervical region
M99.72 Connective tissue and disc stenosis of intervertebral foramina of thoracic region
M99.73 Connective tissue and disc stenosis of intervertebral foramina of lumbar region
M99.74 Connective tissue and disc stenosis of intervertebral foramina of sacral region
M99.75 Connective tissue and disc stenosis of intervertebral foramina of pelvic region
M99.76 Connective tissue and disc stenosis of intervertebral foramina of lower extremity
M99.77 Connective tissue and disc stenosis of intervertebral foramina of upper extremity
M99.78 Connective tissue and disc stenosis of intervertebral foramina of rib cage
M99.79 Connective tissue and disc stenosis of intervertebral foramina of abdomen and other regions

M99.8 Other biomechanical lesions
M99.80 Other biomechanical lesions of head region
M99.81 Other biomechanical lesions of cervical region
M99.82 Other biomechanical lesions of thoracic region
M99.83 Other biomechanical lesions of lumbar region
M99.84 Other biomechanical lesions of sacral region
M99.85 Other biomechanical lesions of pelvic region
M99.86 Other biomechanical lesions of lower extremity
M99.87 Other biomechanical lesions of upper extremity
M99.88 Other biomechanical lesions of rib cage
M99.89 Other biomechanical lesions of abdomen and other regions

M99.9 Biomechanical lesion, unspecified

Chapter 14. Diseases of Genitourinary System (NØØ–N99)

Chapter-specific Guidelines with Coding Examples

The chapter-specific guidelines from the ICD-10-CM Official Guidelines for Coding and Reporting have been provided below. Along with these guidelines are coding examples, contained in the shaded boxes, that have been developed to help illustrate the coding and/or sequencing guidance found in these guidelines.

a. Chronic kidney disease

1) Stages of chronic kidney disease (CKD)

The ICD-10-CM classifies CKD based on severity. The severity of CKD is designated by stages 1-5. Stage 2, code N18.2, equates to mild CKD; stage 3, codes N18.3Ø-N18.32, equate to moderate CKD; and stage 4, code N18.4, equates to severe CKD. Code N18.6, End stage renal disease (ESRD), is assigned when the provider has documented end-stage renal disease (ESRD).

If both a stage of CKD and ESRD are documented, assign code N18.6 only.

Stage 5 chronic kidney disease with ESRD requiring chronic dialysis

N18.6 **End stage renal disease**

Z99.2 **Dependence on renal dialysis**

Explanation: The diagnostic statement indicates the patient has chronic kidney disease, documented both as stage 5 and as ESRD requiring chronic dialysis. Code N18.6 End stage renal disease (ESRD), is assigned when the provider has documented end-stage-renal disease (ESRD). If both a stage of CKD and ESRD are documented, assign code N18.6 only.

2) Chronic kidney disease and kidney transplant status

Patients who have undergone kidney transplant may still have some form of chronic kidney disease (CKD) because the kidney transplant may not fully restore kidney function. Therefore, the presence of CKD alone does not constitute a transplant complication. Assign the appropriate N18 code for the patient's stage of CKD and code Z94.Ø, Kidney transplant status. If a transplant complication such as failure or rejection or other transplant complication is documented, see section I.C.19.g for information on coding complications of a kidney transplant. If the documentation is unclear as to whether the patient has a complication of the transplant, query the provider.

Patient with residual chronic kidney disease stage 1 after kidney transplant

N18.1 **Chronic kidney disease, stage 1**

Z94.Ø **Kidney transplant status**

Explanation: Patients who have undergone kidney transplant may still have some form of chronic kidney disease (CKD) because the kidney transplant may not fully restore kidney function. The presence of CKD alone does not constitute a transplant complication. Assign the appropriate N18 code for the patient's stage of CKD and code Z94.Ø Kidney transplant status.

3) Chronic kidney disease with other conditions

Patients with CKD may also suffer from other serious conditions, most commonly diabetes mellitus and hypertension. The sequencing of the CKD code in relationship to codes for other contributing conditions is based on the conventions in the Tabular List.

See I.C.9. Hypertensive chronic kidney disease.

See I.C.19. Chronic kidney disease and kidney transplant complications.

Type 1 diabetic chronic kidney disease, stage 2

E1Ø.22 **Type 1 diabetes mellitus with diabetic chronic kidney disease**

N18.2 **Chronic kidney disease, stage 2 (mild)**

Explanation: Patients with CKD may also suffer from other serious conditions such as diabetes mellitus. The sequencing of the CKD code in relationship to codes for other contributing conditions is based on the conventions in the Tabular List. Diabetic CKD code E1Ø.22 includes an instructional note to "Use additional code to identify stage of chronic kidney disease (N18.1–N18.6)," thus providing sequencing direction.

Chapter 14. Diseases of the Genitourinary System (N00-N99)

EXCLUDES 2 *certain conditions originating in the perinatal period (P04-P96)*
certain infectious and parasitic diseases (A00-B99)
complications of pregnancy, childbirth and the puerperium (O00-O9A)
congenital malformations, deformations and chromosomal abnormalities (Q00-Q99)
endocrine, nutritional and metabolic diseases (E00-E88)
injury, poisoning and certain other consequences of external causes (S00-T88)
neoplasms (C00-D49)
symptoms, signs and abnormal clinical and laboratory findings, not elsewhere classified (R00-R94)

This chapter contains the following blocks:

- N00-N08 Glomerular diseases
- N10-N16 Renal tubulo-interstitial diseases
- N17-N19 Acute kidney failure and chronic kidney disease
- N20-N23 Urolithiasis
- N25-N29 Other disorders of kidney and ureter
- N30-N39 Other diseases of the urinary system
- N40-N53 Diseases of male genital organs
- N60-N65 Disorders of breast
- N70-N77 Inflammatory diseases of female pelvic organs
- N80-N98 Noninflammatory disorders of female genital tract
- N99 Intraoperative and postprocedural complications and disorders of genitourinary system, not elsewhere classified

Glomerular diseases (N00-N08)

Code also any associated kidney failure (N17-N19).

EXCLUDES 1 *hypertensive chronic kidney disease (I12.-)*

AHA: 2020,4Q,34-35

DEF: Glomeruli: Clusters of microscopic blood vessels located within the kidneys containing small pores through which waste products are filtered from the blood and urine is formed.

DEF: Glomerulonephritis: Disease of the kidney with diffuse inflammation of the capillary loops of the glomeruli.

✓4th N00 Acute nephritic syndrome

INCLUDES acute glomerular disease
acute glomerulonephritis
acute nephritis

EXCLUDES 1 *acute tubulo-interstitial nephritis (N10)*
nephritic syndrome NOS (N05.-)

AHA: 2021,1Q,23

N00.0 Acute nephritic syndrome with minor glomerular abnormality MCC
Acute nephritic syndrome with minimal change lesion

N00.1 Acute nephritic syndrome with focal and segmental glomerular lesions MCC
Acute nephritic syndrome with focal and segmental hyalinosis
Acute nephritic syndrome with focal and segmental sclerosis
Acute nephritic syndrome with focal glomerulonephritis

N00.2 Acute nephritic syndrome with diffuse membranous glomerulonephritis MCC

N00.3 Acute nephritic syndrome with diffuse mesangial proliferative glomerulonephritis MCC

N00.4 Acute nephritic syndrome with diffuse endocapillary proliferative glomerulonephritis MCC

N00.5 Acute nephritic syndrome with diffuse mesangiocapillary glomerulonephritis MCC
Acute nephritic syndrome with membranoproliferative glomerulonephritis, types 1 and 3, or NOS

EXCLUDES 1 *acute nephritic syndrome with C3 glomerulonephritis (N00.A)*
acute nephritic syndrome with C3 glomerulopathy (N00.A)

N00.6 Acute nephritic syndrome with dense deposit disease MCC
Acute nephritic syndrome with C3 glomerulopathy with dense deposit disease
Acute nephritic syndrome with membranoproliferative glomerulonephritis, type 2

N00.7 Acute nephritic syndrome with diffuse crescentic glomerulonephritis MCC
Acute nephritic syndrome with extracapillary glomerulonephritis

N00.8 Acute nephritic syndrome with other morphologic changes MCC
Acute nephritic syndrome with proliferative glomerulonephritis NOS

N00.9 Acute nephritic syndrome with unspecified morphologic changes MCC

N00.A Acute nephritic syndrome with C3 glomerulonephritis MCC
Acute nephritic syndrome with C3 glomerulopathy, NOS

EXCLUDES 1 *acute nephritic syndrome (with C3 glomerulopathy) with dense deposit disease (N00.6)*

✓4th N01 Rapidly progressive nephritic syndrome

INCLUDES rapidly progressive glomerular disease
rapidly progressive glomerulonephritis
rapidly progressive nephritis

EXCLUDES 1 *nephritic syndrome NOS (N05.-)*

AHA: 2021,1Q,23

N01.0 Rapidly progressive nephritic syndrome with minor glomerular abnormality MCC
Rapidly progressive nephritic syndrome with minimal change lesion

N01.1 Rapidly progressive nephritic syndrome with focal and segmental glomerular lesions MCC
Rapidly progressive nephritic syndrome with focal and segmental hyalinosis
Rapidly progressive nephritic syndrome with focal and segmental sclerosis
Rapidly progressive nephritic syndrome with focal glomerulonephritis

N01.2 Rapidly progressive nephritic syndrome with diffuse membranous glomerulonephritis MCC

N01.3 Rapidly progressive nephritic syndrome with diffuse mesangial proliferative glomerulonephritis MCC

N01.4 Rapidly progressive nephritic syndrome with diffuse endocapillary proliferative glomerulonephritis MCC

N01.5 Rapidly progressive nephritic syndrome with diffuse mesangiocapillary glomerulonephritis MCC
Rapidly progressive nephritic syndrome with membranoproliferative glomerulonephritis, types 1 and 3, or NOS

EXCLUDES 1 *rapidly progressive nephritic syndrome with C3 glomerulonephritis (N01.A)*
rapidly progressive nephritic syndrome with C3 glomerulopathy (N01.A)

N01.6 Rapidly progressive nephritic syndrome with dense deposit disease MCC
Rapidly progressive nephritic syndrome with C3 glomerulopathy with dense deposit disease
Rapidly progressive nephritic syndrome with membranoproliferative glomerulonephritis, type 2

N01.7 Rapidly progressive nephritic syndrome with diffuse crescentic glomerulonephritis MCC
Rapidly progressive nephritic syndrome with extracapillary glomerulonephritis

N01.8 Rapidly progressive nephritic syndrome with other morphologic changes MCC
Rapidly progressive nephritic syndrome with proliferative glomerulonephritis NOS

N01.9 Rapidly progressive nephritic syndrome with unspecified morphologic changes MCC

N01.A Rapidly progressive nephritic syndrome with C3 glomerulonephritis MCC
Rapidly progressive nephritic syndrome with C3 glomerulopathy, NOS

EXCLUDES 1 *rapidly progressive nephritic syndrome (with C3 glomerulopathy) with dense deposit disease (N01.6)*

✓4th N02 Recurrent and persistent hematuria

EXCLUDES 1 *acute cystitis with hematuria (N30.01)*
hematuria NOS (R31.9)
hematuria not associated with specified morphologic lesions (R31.-)

N02.0 Recurrent and persistent hematuria with minor glomerular abnormality CC
Recurrent and persistent hematuria with minimal change lesion

NØ2.1 Recurrent and persistent hematuria with focal and segmental glomerular lesions CC
Recurrent and persistent hematuria with focal and segmental hyalinosis
Recurrent and persistent hematuria with focal and segmental sclerosis
Recurrent and persistent hematuria with focal glomerulonephritis

NØ2.2 Recurrent and persistent hematuria with diffuse membranous glomerulonephritis CC

NØ2.3 Recurrent and persistent hematuria with diffuse mesangial proliferative glomerulonephritis CC

NØ2.4 Recurrent and persistent hematuria with diffuse endocapillary proliferative glomerulonephritis CC

NØ2.5 Recurrent and persistent hematuria with diffuse mesangiocapillary glomerulonephritis CC
Recurrent and persistent hematuria with membranoproliferative glomerulonephritis, types 1 and 3, or NOS
EXCLUDES 1 *recurrent and persistent hematuria with C3 glomerulonephritis (NØ2.A)*
recurrent and persistent hematuria with C3 glomerulopathy (NØ2.A)

NØ2.6 Recurrent and persistent hematuria with dense deposit disease CC
Recurrent and persistent hematuria with C3 glomerulopathy with dense deposit disease
Recurrent and persistent hematuria with membranoproliferative glomerulonephritis, type 2

NØ2.7 Recurrent and persistent hematuria with diffuse crescentic glomerulonephritis CC
Recurrent and persistent hematuria with extracapillary glomerulonephritis

NØ2.8 Recurrent and persistent hematuria with other morphologic changes CC
Recurrent and persistent hematuria with proliferative glomerulonephritis NOS

NØ2.9 Recurrent and persistent hematuria with unspecified morphologic changes CC
AHA: 2017,2Q,5

NØ2.A Recurrent and persistent hematuria with C3 glomerulonephritis CC
Recurrent and persistent hematuria with C3 glomerulopathy
EXCLUDES 1 *recurrent and persistent hematuria (with C3 glomerulopathy) with dense deposit disease (NØ2.6)*

✓4th NØ3 Chronic nephritic syndrome

INCLUDES chronic glomerular disease
chronic glomerulonephritis
chronic nephritis

EXCLUDES 1 *chronic tubulo-interstitial nephritis (N11.-)*
diffuse sclerosing glomerulonephritis (NØ5.8-)
nephritic syndrome NOS (NØ5.-)

AHA: 2021,1Q,23

DEF: Slow, progressive type of nephritis characterized by inflammation of the capillary loops in the glomeruli of the kidney, which leads to renal failure.

NØ3.Ø Chronic nephritic syndrome with minor glomerular abnormality CC
Chronic nephritic syndrome with minimal change lesion

NØ3.1 Chronic nephritic syndrome with focal and segmental glomerular lesions CC
Chronic nephritic syndrome with focal and segmental hyalinosis
Chronic nephritic syndrome with focal and segmental sclerosis
Chronic nephritic syndrome with focal glomerulonephritis

NØ3.2 Chronic nephritic syndrome with diffuse membranous glomerulonephritis CC

NØ3.3 Chronic nephritic syndrome with diffuse mesangial proliferative glomerulonephritis CC

NØ3.4 Chronic nephritic syndrome with diffuse endocapillary proliferative glomerulonephritis CC

NØ3.5 Chronic nephritic syndrome with diffuse mesangiocapillary glomerulonephritis CC
Chronic nephritic syndrome with membranoproliferative glomerulonephritis, types 1 and 3, or NOS
EXCLUDES 1 *chronic nephritic syndrome with C3 glomerulonephritis (NØ3.A)*
chronic nephritic syndrome with C3 glomerulopathy (NØ3.A)

NØ3.6 Chronic nephritic syndrome with dense deposit disease CC
Chronic nephritic syndrome with C3 glomerulopathy with dense deposit disease
Chronic nephritic syndrome with membranoproliferative glomerulonephritis, type 2

NØ3.7 Chronic nephritic syndrome with diffuse crescentic glomerulonephritis CC
Chronic nephritic syndrome with extracapillary glomerulonephritis

NØ3.8 Chronic nephritic syndrome with other morphologic changes CC
Chronic nephritic syndrome with proliferative glomerulonephritis NOS

NØ3.9 Chronic nephritic syndrome with unspecified morphologic changes CC

NØ3.A Chronic nephritic syndrome with C3 glomerulonephritis CC
Chronic nephritic syndrome with C3 glomerulopathy
EXCLUDES 1 *chronic nephritic syndrome (with C3 glomerulopathy) with dense deposit disease (NØ3.6)*

✓4th NØ4 Nephrotic syndrome

INCLUDES congenital nephrotic syndrome
lipoid nephrosis

NØ4.Ø Nephrotic syndrome with minor glomerular abnormality CC
Nephrotic syndrome with minimal change lesion

NØ4.1 Nephrotic syndrome with focal and segmental glomerular lesions CC
Nephrotic syndrome with focal and segmental hyalinosis
Nephrotic syndrome with focal and segmental sclerosis
Nephrotic syndrome with focal glomerulonephritis

NØ4.2 Nephrotic syndrome with diffuse membranous glomerulonephritis CC

NØ4.3 Nephrotic syndrome with diffuse mesangial proliferative glomerulonephritis CC

NØ4.4 Nephrotic syndrome with diffuse endocapillary proliferative glomerulonephritis CC

NØ4.5 Nephrotic syndrome with diffuse mesangiocapillary glomerulonephritis CC
Nephrotic syndrome with membranoproliferative glomerulonephritis, types 1 and 3, or NOS
EXCLUDES 1 *nephrotic syndrome with C3 glomerulonephritis (NØ4.A)*
nephrotic syndrome with C3 glomerulopathy (NØ4.A)

NØ4.6 Nephrotic syndrome with dense deposit disease CC
Nephrotic syndrome with C3 glomerulopathy with dense deposit disease
Nephrotic syndrome with membranoproliferative glomerulonephritis, type 2

NØ4.7 Nephrotic syndrome with diffuse crescentic glomerulonephritis CC
Nephrotic syndrome with extracapillary glomerulonephritis

NØ4.8 Nephrotic syndrome with other morphologic changes CC
Nephrotic syndrome with proliferative glomerulonephritis NOS

NØ4.9 Nephrotic syndrome with unspecified morphologic changes CC

NØ4.A Nephrotic syndrome with C3 glomerulonephritis CC
Nephrotic syndrome with C3 glomerulopathy
EXCLUDES 1 *nephrotic syndrome (with C3 glomerulopathy) with dense deposit disease (NØ4.6)*

NØ5 Unspecified nephritic syndrome

INCLUDES glomerular disease NOS
glomerulonephritis NOS
nephritis NOS
nephropathy NOS and renal disease NOS with morphological lesion specified in .Ø-.8

EXCLUDES 1 *nephropathy NOS with no stated morphological lesion (N28.9)*
renal disease NOS with no stated morphological lesion (N28.9)
tubulo-interstitial nephritis NOS (N12)

NØ5.Ø Unspecified nephritic syndrome with minor glomerular abnormality
Unspecified nephritic syndrome with minimal change lesion

NØ5.1 Unspecified nephritic syndrome with focal and segmental glomerular lesions
Unspecified nephritic syndrome with focal and segmental hyalinosis
Unspecified nephritic syndrome with focal and segmental sclerosis
Unspecified nephritic syndrome with focal glomerulonephritis

NØ5.2 Unspecified nephritic syndrome with diffuse membranous glomerulonephritis CC

NØ5.3 Unspecified nephritic syndrome with diffuse mesangial proliferative glomerulonephritis CC

NØ5.4 Unspecified nephritic syndrome with diffuse endocapillary proliferative glomerulonephritis CC

NØ5.5 Unspecified nephritic syndrome with diffuse mesangiocapillary glomerulonephritis CC
Unspecified nephritic syndrome with membranoproliferative glomerulonephritis, types 1 and 3, or NOS

EXCLUDES 1 *unspecified nephritic syndrome with C3 glomerulonephritis (NØ5.A)*
unspecified nephritic syndrome with C3 glomerulopathy (NØ5.A)

NØ5.6 Unspecified nephritic syndrome with dense deposit disease
Unspecified nephritic syndrome with C3 glomerulopathy with dense deposit disease
Unspecified nephritic syndrome with membranoproliferative glomerulonephritis, type 2

NØ5.7 Unspecified nephritic syndrome with diffuse crescentic glomerulonephritis
Unspecified nephritic syndrome with extracapillary glomerulonephritis

NØ5.8 Unspecified nephritic syndrome with other morphologic changes
Unspecified nephritic syndrome with proliferative glomerulonephritis NOS

NØ5.9 Unspecified nephritic syndrome with unspecified morphologic changes

NØ5.A Unspecified nephritic syndrome with C3 glomerulonephritis CC
Unspecified nephritic syndrome with C3 glomerulopathy

EXCLUDES 1 *unspecified nephritic syndrome (with C3 glomerulopathy) with dense deposit disease (NØ5.6)*

NØ6 Isolated proteinuria with specified morphological lesion

EXCLUDES 1 *proteinuria not associated with specific morphologic lesions (R8Ø.Ø)*

NØ6.Ø Isolated proteinuria with minor glomerular abnormality
Isolated proteinuria with minimal change lesion

NØ6.1 Isolated proteinuria with focal and segmental glomerular lesions
Isolated proteinuria with focal and segmental hyalinosis
Isolated proteinuria with focal and segmental sclerosis
Isolated proteinuria with focal glomerulonephritis

NØ6.2 Isolated proteinuria with diffuse membranous glomerulonephritis CC

NØ6.3 Isolated proteinuria with diffuse mesangial proliferative glomerulonephritis CC

NØ6.4 Isolated proteinuria with diffuse endocapillary proliferative glomerulonephritis CC

NØ6.5 Isolated proteinuria with diffuse mesangiocapillary glomerulonephritis CC
Isolated proteinuria with membranoproliferative glomerulonephritis, types 1 and 3, or NOS

EXCLUDES 1 *isolated proteinuria with C3 glomerulonephritis (NØ6.A)*
isolated proteinuria with C3 glomerulopathy (NØ6.A)

NØ6.6 Isolated proteinuria with dense deposit disease
Isolated proteinuria with C3 glomerulopathy with dense deposit disease
Isolated proteinuria with membranoproliferative glomerulonephritis, type 2

NØ6.7 Isolated proteinuria with diffuse crescentic glomerulonephritis
Isolated proteinuria with extracapillary glomerulonephritis

NØ6.8 Isolated proteinuria with other morphologic lesion
Isolated proteinuria with proliferative glomerulonephritis NOS

NØ6.9 Isolated proteinuria with unspecified morphologic lesion

NØ6.A Isolated proteinuria with C3 glomerulonephritis CC
Isolated proteinuria with C3 glomerulopathy

EXCLUDES 1 *isolated proteinuria (with C3 glomerulopathy) with dense deposit disease (NØ6.6)*

NØ7 Hereditary nephropathy, not elsewhere classified

EXCLUDES 2 *Alport's syndrome (Q87.81-)*
hereditary amyloid nephropathy (E85.-)
nail patella syndrome (Q87.2)
non-neuropathic heredofamilial amyloidosis (E85.-)

NØ7.Ø Hereditary nephropathy, not elsewhere classified with minor glomerular abnormality
Hereditary nephropathy, not elsewhere classified with minimal change lesion

NØ7.1 Hereditary nephropathy, not elsewhere classified with focal and segmental glomerular lesions
Hereditary nephropathy, not elsewhere classified with focal and segmental hyalinosis
Hereditary nephropathy, not elsewhere classified with focal and segmental sclerosis
Hereditary nephropathy, not elsewhere classified with focal glomerulonephritis

NØ7.2 Hereditary nephropathy, not elsewhere classified with diffuse membranous glomerulonephritis CC

NØ7.3 Hereditary nephropathy, not elsewhere classified with diffuse mesangial proliferative glomerulonephritis CC

NØ7.4 Hereditary nephropathy, not elsewhere classified with diffuse endocapillary proliferative glomerulonephritis CC

NØ7.5 Hereditary nephropathy, not elsewhere classified with diffuse mesangiocapillary glomerulonephritis CC
Hereditary nephropathy, not elsewhere classified with membranoproliferative glomerulonephritis, types 1 and 3, or NOS

EXCLUDES 1 *hereditary nephropathy, not elsewhere classified with C3 glomerulonephritis (NØ7.A)*
hereditary nephropathy, not elsewhere classified with C3 glomerulopathy (NØ7.A)

NØ7.6 Hereditary nephropathy, not elsewhere classified with dense deposit disease
Hereditary nephropathy, not elsewhere classified with C3 glomerulopathy with dense deposit disease
Hereditary nephropathy, not elsewhere classified with membranoproliferative glomerulonephritis, type 2

NØ7.7 Hereditary nephropathy, not elsewhere classified with diffuse crescentic glomerulonephritis
Hereditary nephropathy, not elsewhere classified with extracapillary glomerulonephritis

NØ7.8 Hereditary nephropathy, not elsewhere classified with other morphologic lesions
Hereditary nephropathy, not elsewhere classified with proliferative glomerulonephritis NOS

NØ7.9 Hereditary nephropathy, not elsewhere classified with unspecified morphologic lesions

NØ7.A Hereditary nephropathy, not elsewhere classified with C3 glomerulonephritis CC
Hereditary nephropathy, not elsewhere classified with C3 glomerulopathy

EXCLUDES 1 *hereditary nephropathy, not elsewhere classified (with C3 glomerulopathy) with dense deposit disease (NØ7.6)*

N Newborn: 0 P Pediatric: 0-17 M Maternity: 9-64 A Adult: 15-124 UNS Unspecified Site MCC Major Complication/Comorbidity CC Complication/Comorbidity

N08 Glomerular disorders in diseases classified elsewhere
Glomerulonephritis
Nephritis
Nephropathy
Code first underlying disease, such as:
amyloidosis (E85.-)
congenital syphilis (A50.5)
cryoglobulinemia (D89.1)
disseminated intravascular coagulation (D65)
gout (M1A.-, M10.-)
microscopic polyangiitis (M31.7)
multiple myeloma (C90.0-)
sepsis (A40.0-A41.9)
sickle-cell disease (D57.0-D57.8)
EXCLUDES 1 *glomerulonephritis, nephritis and nephropathy (in):*
antiglomerular basement membrane disease (M31.0)
diabetes (E08-E13 with .21)
gonococcal (A54.21)
Goodpasture's syndrome (M31.0)
hemolytic-uremic syndrome ►(D59.3-)◄
lupus (M32.14)
mumps (B26.83)
syphilis (A52.75)
systemic lupus erythematosus (M32.14)
Wegener's granulomatosis (M31.31)
pyelonephritis in diseases classified elsewhere (N16)
renal tubulo-interstitial disorders classified elsewhere (N16)

Renal tubulo-interstitial diseases (N10-N16)

INCLUDES pyelonephritis
EXCLUDES 1 *pyeloureteritis cystica (N28.85)*

N10 Acute pyelonephritis CC H6
Acute infectious interstitial nephritis
Acute pyelitis
Acute tubulo-interstitial nephritis
Hemoglobin nephrosis
Myoglobin nephrosis
Use additional code (B95-B97), to identify infectious agent
AHA: 2020,3Q,25; 2019,3Q,13

✓4th **N11 Chronic tubulo-interstitial nephritis**
INCLUDES chronic infectious interstitial nephritis
chronic pyelitis
chronic pyelonephritis
Use additional code (B95-B97), to identify infectious agent

N11.0 Nonobstructive reflux-associated chronic pyelonephritis
Pyelonephritis (chronic) associated with (vesicoureteral) reflux
EXCLUDES 1 *vesicoureteral reflux NOS (N13.70)*

N11.1 Chronic obstructive pyelonephritis CC
Pyelonephritis (chronic) associated with anomaly of pelviureteric junction
Pyelonephritis (chronic) associated with anomaly of pyeloureteric junction
Pyelonephritis (chronic) associated with crossing of vessel
Pyelonephritis (chronic) associated with kinking of ureter
Pyelonephritis (chronic) associated with obstruction of ureter
Pyelonephritis (chronic) associated with stricture of pelviureteric junction
Pyelonephritis (chronic) associated with stricture of ureter
EXCLUDES 1 *calculous pyelonephritis (N20.9)*
obstructive uropathy (N13.-)

N11.8 Other chronic tubulo-interstitial nephritis CC
Nonobstructive chronic pyelonephritis NOS

N11.9 Chronic tubulo-interstitial nephritis, unspecified CC H6
Chronic interstitial nephritis NOS
Chronic pyelitis NOS
Chronic pyelonephritis NOS

N12 Tubulo-interstitial nephritis, not specified as acute or chronic CC H6
Interstitial nephritis NOS
Pyelitis NOS
Pyelonephritis NOS
EXCLUDES 1 *calculous pyelonephritis (N20.9)*

✓4th **N13 Obstructive and reflux uropathy**
EXCLUDES 2 *calculus of kidney and ureter without hydronephrosis (N20.-)*
congenital obstructive defects of renal pelvis and ureter (Q62.0-Q62.3)
hydronephrosis with ureteropelvic junction obstruction (Q62.11)
obstructive pyelonephritis (N11.1)
DEF: Hydronephrosis: Distension of the kidney caused by an accumulation of urine that cannot flow out due to an obstruction that may be caused by conditions such as kidney stones or vesicoureteral reflux.

N13.0 Hydronephrosis with ureteropelvic junction obstruction CC
Hydronephrosis due to acquired occlusion of ureteropelvic junction
EXCLUDES 2 *hydronephrosis with ureteropelvic junction obstruction due to calculus (N13.2)*
AHA: 2016,4Q,43

Hydronephrosis/UPJ Obstruction

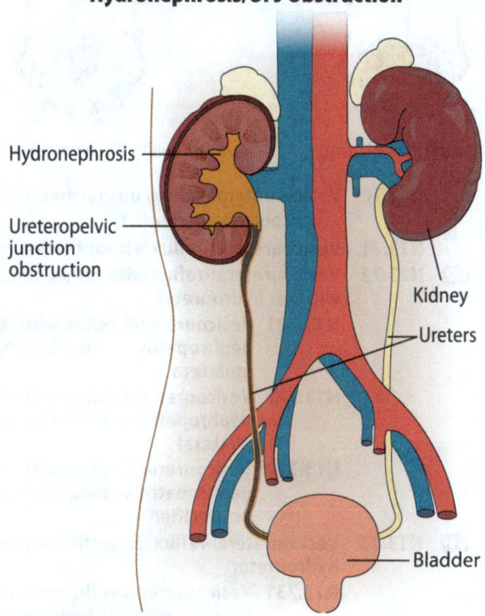

N13.1 Hydronephrosis with ureteral stricture, not elsewhere classified CC
EXCLUDES 1 *hydronephrosis with ureteral stricture with infection (N13.6)*

N13.2 Hydronephrosis with renal and ureteral calculous obstruction CC
EXCLUDES 1 *hydronephrosis with renal and ureteral calculous obstruction with infection (N13.6)*

✓5th **N13.3 Other and unspecified hydronephrosis**
EXCLUDES 1 *hydronephrosis with infection (N13.6)*

N13.30 Unspecified hydronephrosis CC

N13.39 Other hydronephrosis CC

N13.4 Hydroureter CC
EXCLUDES 1 *congenital hydroureter (Q62.3-)*
hydroureter with infection (N13.6)
vesicoureteral-reflux with hydroureter (N13.73-)
DEF: Abnormal enlargement or distension of the ureter with water or urine caused by an obstruction.

N13.5 Crossing vessel and stricture of ureter without hydronephrosis
Kinking and stricture of ureter without hydronephrosis
EXCLUDES 1 *crossing vessel and stricture of ureter without hydronephrosis with infection (N13.6)*

N13.6 Pyonephrosis CC H6
Conditions in N13.0-N13.5 with infection
Obstructive uropathy with infection
Use additional code (B95-B97), to identify infectious agent
AHA: 2018,2Q,21

✓5th **N13.7 Vesicoureteral-reflux**

EXCLUDES 1 *reflux-associated pyelonephritis (N11.0)*

DEF: Urine passage from the bladder flows backward up into the ureter and kidneys that can lead to bacterial infection and an increase in hydrostatic pressure, causing kidney damage.

Vesicoureteral Reflux

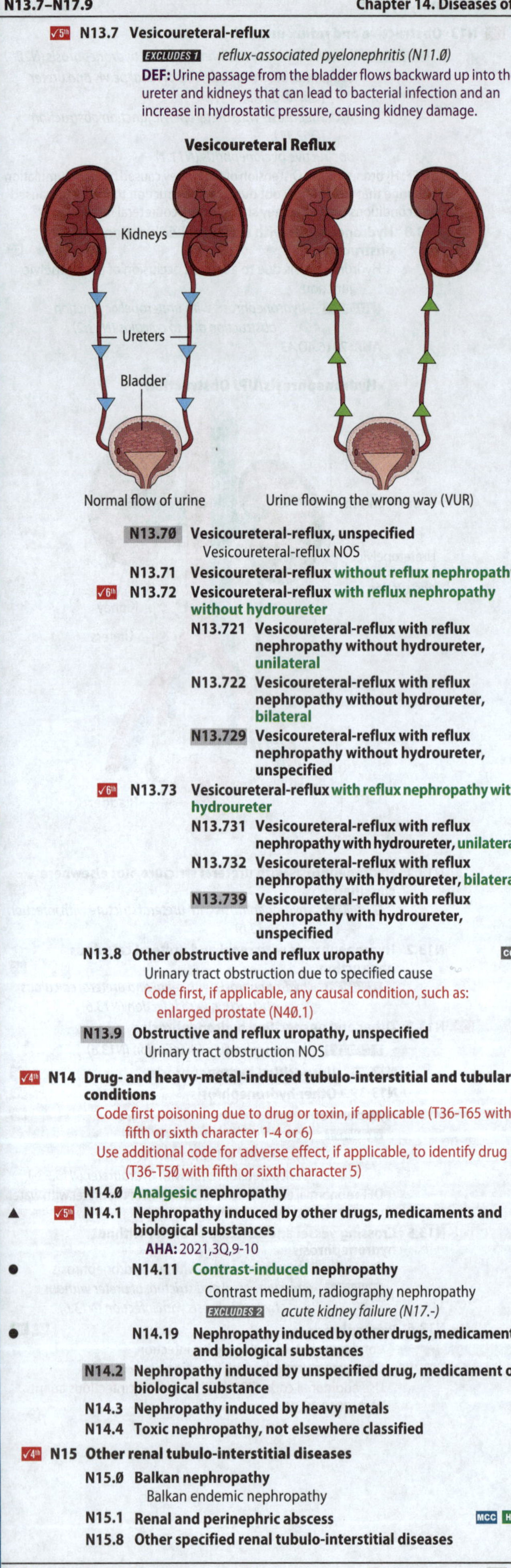

N13.70 Vesicoureteral-reflux, unspecified
Vesicoureteral-reflux NOS

N13.71 Vesicoureteral-reflux without reflux nephropathy

✓6th **N13.72 Vesicoureteral-reflux with reflux nephropathy without hydroureter**

N13.721 Vesicoureteral-reflux with reflux nephropathy without hydroureter, unilateral

N13.722 Vesicoureteral-reflux with reflux nephropathy without hydroureter, bilateral

N13.729 Vesicoureteral-reflux with reflux nephropathy without hydroureter, unspecified

✓6th **N13.73 Vesicoureteral-reflux with reflux nephropathy with hydroureter**

N13.731 Vesicoureteral-reflux with reflux nephropathy with hydroureter, unilateral

N13.732 Vesicoureteral-reflux with reflux nephropathy with hydroureter, bilateral

N13.739 Vesicoureteral-reflux with reflux nephropathy with hydroureter, unspecified

N13.8 Other obstructive and reflux uropathy CC
Urinary tract obstruction due to specified cause
Code first, if applicable, any causal condition, such as:
enlarged prostate (N40.1)

N13.9 Obstructive and reflux uropathy, unspecified
Urinary tract obstruction NOS

✓4th **N14 Drug- and heavy-metal-induced tubulo-interstitial and tubular conditions**
Code first poisoning due to drug or toxin, if applicable (T36-T65 with fifth or sixth character 1-4 or 6)
Use additional code for adverse effect, if applicable, to identify drug (T36-T50 with fifth or sixth character 5)

N14.0 Analgesic nephropathy

▲ ✓5th **N14.1 Nephropathy induced by other drugs, medicaments and biological substances**
AHA: 2021,3Q,9-10

● **N14.11 Contrast-induced nephropathy**
Contrast medium, radiography nephropathy
EXCLUDES 2 *acute kidney failure (N17.-)*

● **N14.19 Nephropathy induced by other drugs, medicaments and biological substances**

N14.2 Nephropathy induced by unspecified drug, medicament or biological substance

N14.3 Nephropathy induced by heavy metals

N14.4 Toxic nephropathy, not elsewhere classified

✓4th **N15 Other renal tubulo-interstitial diseases**

N15.0 Balkan nephropathy
Balkan endemic nephropathy

N15.1 Renal and perinephric abscess MCC H6

N15.8 Other specified renal tubulo-interstitial diseases

N15.9 Renal tubulo-interstitial disease, unspecified
Infection of kidney NOS
EXCLUDES 1 *urinary tract infection NOS (N39.0)*

N16 Renal tubulo-interstitial disorders in diseases classified elsewhere
Pyelonephritis
Tubulo-interstitial nephritis
Code first underlying disease, such as:
brucellosis (A23.0-A23.9)
cryoglobulinemia (D89.1)
glycogen storage disease (E74.0)
leukemia (C91-C95)
lymphoma (C81.0-C85.9, C96.0-C96.9)
multiple myeloma (C90.0-)
sepsis (A40.0-A41.9)
Wilson's disease (E83.0)

EXCLUDES 1 *diphtheritic pyelonephritis and tubulo-interstitial nephritis (A36.84)*
pyelonephritis and tubulo-interstitial nephritis in candidiasis (B37.49)
pyelonephritis and tubulo-interstitial nephritis in cystinosis (E72.04)
pyelonephritis and tubulo-interstitial nephritis in salmonella infection (A02.25)
pyelonephritis and tubulo-interstitial nephritis in sarcoidosis (D86.84)
pyelonephritis and tubulo-interstitial nephritis in Sjögren syndrome (M35.04)
pyelonephritis and tubulo-interstitial nephritis in systemic lupus erythematosus (M32.15)
pyelonephritis and tubulo-interstitial nephritis in toxoplasmosis (B58.83)
renal tubular degeneration in diabetes (E08-E13 with .29)
syphilitic pyelonephritis and tubulo-interstitial nephritis (A52.75)

Acute kidney failure and chronic kidney disease (N17-N19)

EXCLUDES 2 *congenital renal failure (P96.0)*
drug- and heavy-metal-induced tubulo-interstitial and tubular conditions (N14.-)
extrarenal uremia (R39.2)
hemolytic-uremic syndrome ▶(D59.3-)◀
hepatorenal syndrome (K76.7)
postpartum hepatorenal syndrome (O90.4)
posttraumatic renal failure (T79.5)
prerenal uremia (R39.2)
renal failure complicating abortion or ectopic or molar pregnancy (O00-O07, O08.4)
renal failure following labor and delivery (O90.4)
renal failure postprocedural (N99.0)

✓4th **N17 Acute kidney failure**
Code also associated underlying condition
EXCLUDES 1 *posttraumatic renal failure (T79.5)*
AHA: 2020,3Q,22; 2019,2Q,7; 2019,1Q,12; 2013,4Q,124

N17.0 Acute kidney failure with tubular necrosis MCC HCC
Acute tubular necrosis
Renal tubular necrosis
Tubular necrosis NOS
AHA: 2021,3Q,10

N17.1 Acute kidney failure with acute cortical necrosis MCC HCC
Acute cortical necrosis
Cortical necrosis NOS
Renal cortical necrosis

N17.2 Acute kidney failure with medullary necrosis MCC HCC
Medullary [papillary] necrosis NOS
Acute medullary [papillary] necrosis
Renal medullary [papillary] necrosis

N17.8 Other acute kidney failure CC HCC

N17.9 Acute kidney failure, unspecified CC HCC
Acute kidney injury (nontraumatic)
EXCLUDES 2 *traumatic kidney injury (S37.0-)*

N18 Chronic kidney disease (CKD)
Code first any associated:
diabetic chronic kidney disease (EØ8.22, EØ9.22, E1Ø.22, E11.22, E13.22)
hypertensive chronic kidney disease (I12.-, I13.-)
Use additional code to identify kidney transplant status, if applicable, (Z94.Ø)
AHA: 2019,3Q,3; 2018,4Q,88; 2013,1Q,24

N18.1 Chronic kidney disease, stage 1
N18.2 Chronic kidney disease, stage 2 (mild)
N18.3 Chronic kidney disease, stage 3 (moderate)
AHA: 2020,4Q,35
N18.3Ø Chronic kidney disease, stage 3 unspecified HCC
N18.31 Chronic kidney disease, stage 3a HCC
N18.32 Chronic kidney disease, stage 3b HCC
N18.4 Chronic kidney disease, stage 4 (severe) CC HCC
N18.5 Chronic kidney disease, stage 5 CC HCC
EXCLUDES 1 *chronic kidney disease, stage 5 requiring chronic dialysis (N18.6)*
DEF: End-stage renal disease (ESRD) with a GFR value of 15 ml/min or less not yet requiring chronic dialysis.
TIP: When both ESRD and CKD 5 are documented, code only for ESRD.
N18.6 End stage renal disease MCC HCC
Chronic kidney disease requiring chronic dialysis
Use additional code to identify dialysis status (Z99.2)
AHA: 2016,3Q,22; 2016,1Q,12; 2013,4Q,124-125
TIP: When both ESRD and CKD 5 are documented, code only for ESRD.
N18.9 Chronic kidney disease, unspecified
Chronic renal disease
Chronic renal failure NOS
Chronic renal insufficiency
Chronic uremia NOS
Diffuse sclerosing glomerulonephritis NOS

N19 Unspecified kidney failure
Uremia NOS
EXCLUDES 1 *acute kidney failure (N17.-)*
chronic kidney disease (N18.-)
chronic uremia (N18.9)
extrarenal uremia (R39.2)
prerenal uremia (R39.2)
renal insufficiency (acute) (N28.9)
uremia of newborn (P96.Ø)

Urolithiasis (N2Ø-N23)

AHA: 2017,1Q,5; 2015,2Q,8
TIP: Codes from this code block can be assigned based on the diagnosis listed in a radiology report when authenticated by a radiologist and available at the time of code assignment.

N2Ø Calculus of kidney and ureter
Calculous pyelonephritis
EXCLUDES 1 *nephrocalcinosis (E83.5)*
that with hydronephrosis (N13.2)
AHA: 2019,3Q,13
N2Ø.Ø Calculus of kidney
Nephrolithiasis NOS
Renal calculus
Renal stone
Staghorn calculus
Stone in kidney
AHA: 2019,3Q,13
N2Ø.1 Calculus of ureter CC
Calculus of the ureteropelvic junction
Ureteric stone
AHA: 2016,3Q,22
N2Ø.2 Calculus of kidney with calculus of ureter CC
N2Ø.9 Urinary calculus, unspecified

N21 Calculus of lower urinary tract
INCLUDES calculus of lower urinary tract with cystitis and urethritis
N21.Ø Calculus in bladder
Calculus in diverticulum of bladder
Urinary bladder stone
EXCLUDES 2 *staghorn calculus (N2Ø.Ø)*
N21.1 Calculus in urethra
EXCLUDES 2 *calculus of prostate (N42.Ø)*
N21.8 Other lower urinary tract calculus
N21.9 Calculus of lower urinary tract, unspecified
EXCLUDES 1 *calculus of urinary tract NOS (N2Ø.9)*

N22 Calculus of urinary tract in diseases classified elsewhere
Code first underlying disease, such as:
gout (M1A.-, M1Ø.-)
schistosomiasis (B65.Ø-B65.9)

N23 Unspecified renal colic

Other disorders of kidney and ureter (N25-N29)

EXCLUDES 2 *disorders of kidney and ureter with urolithiasis (N2Ø-N23)*

N25 Disorders resulting from impaired renal tubular function
N25.Ø Renal osteodystrophy
Azotemic osteodystrophy
Phosphate-losing tubular disorders
Renal rickets
Renal short stature
EXCLUDES 2 *metabolic disorders classifiable to E7Ø-E88*
DEF: Various bone diseases occurring when kidney function is impaired or fails. Abnormal levels of phosphorous and calcium can lead to osteomalacia, osteoporosis, or osteosclerosis.
N25.1 Nephrogenic diabetes insipidus CC HCC
EXCLUDES 1 *diabetes insipidus NOS (E23.2)*
DEF: Type of diabetes due to the inability of renal tubules to reabsorb water back into the body. It is not responsive to vasopressin (antidiuretic hormone) and it is characterized by excessive thirst and excessive urine production. It may develop into chronic renal insufficiency.
N25.8 Other disorders resulting from impaired renal tubular function
N25.81 Secondary hyperparathyroidism of renal origin CC HCC
EXCLUDES 1 *secondary hyperparathyroidism, non-renal (E21.1)*
EXCLUDES 2 *metabolic disorders classifiable to E7Ø-E88*
DEF: Parathyroid dysfunction caused by chronic renal failure. Phosphate clearance and vitamin D production is impaired resulting in lowered calcium blood levels and an excessive production of parathyroid hormone.
N25.89 Other disorders resulting from impaired renal tubular function
Hypokalemic nephropathy
Lightwood-Albright syndrome
Renal tubular acidosis NOS
N25.9 Disorder resulting from impaired renal tubular function, unspecified

N26 Unspecified contracted kidney
EXCLUDES 1 *contracted kidney due to hypertension (I12.-)*
diffuse sclerosing glomerulonephritis (NØ5.8.-)
hypertensive nephrosclerosis (arteriolar) (arteriosclerotic) (I12.-)
small kidney of unknown cause (N27.-)
N26.1 Atrophy of kidney (terminal)
N26.2 Page kidney
N26.9 Renal sclerosis, unspecified

N27 Small kidney of unknown cause
INCLUDES oligonephronia
N27.Ø Small kidney, unilateral
N27.1 Small kidney, bilateral
N27.9 Small kidney, unspecified

N28 Other disorders of kidney and ureter, not elsewhere classified
N28.Ø Ischemia and infarction of kidney CC HCC
Renal artery embolism
Renal artery obstruction
Renal artery occlusion
Renal artery thrombosis
Renal infarct
EXCLUDES 1 *atherosclerosis of renal artery (extrarenal part) (I7Ø.1)*
congenital stenosis of renal artery (Q27.1)
Goldblatt's kidney (I7Ø.1)

N28.1 Cyst of kidney, acquired
Cyst (multiple) (solitary) of kidney (acquired)
EXCLUDES 1 *cystic kidney disease (congenital) (Q61.-)*

✓5th **N28.8 Other specified disorders of kidney and ureter**
EXCLUDES 1 *hydroureter (N13.4)*
ureteric stricture with hydronephrosis (N13.1)
ureteric stricture without hydronephrosis (N13.5)

N28.81 Hypertrophy of kidney
N28.82 Megaloureter
N28.83 Nephroptosis
N28.84 Pyelitis cystica CC H6
N28.85 Pyeloureteritis cystica CC H6
N28.86 Ureteritis cystica CC H6
N28.89 Other specified disorders of kidney and ureter

N28.9 Disorder of kidney and ureter, unspecified
Nephropathy NOS
Renal disease (acute) NOS
Renal insufficiency (acute)
EXCLUDES 1 *chronic renal insufficiency (N18.9)*
unspecified nephritic syndrome (NØ5.-)
AHA: 2016,1Q,13

N29 Other disorders of kidney and ureter in diseases classified elsewhere
Code first underlying disease, such as:
amyloidosis (E85.-)
nephrocalcinosis (E83.5)
schistosomiasis (B65.Ø-B65.9)
EXCLUDES 1 *disorders of kidney and ureter in:*
cystinosis (E72.Ø)
gonorrhea (A54.21)
syphilis (A52.75)
tuberculosis (A18.11)

Other diseases of the urinary system (N3Ø-N39)

EXCLUDES 2 *urinary infection (complicating):*
abortion or ectopic or molar pregnancy (OØØ-OØ7, OØ8.8)
pregnancy, childbirth and the puerperium (O23.-, O75.3, O86.2-)

✓4th **N3Ø Cystitis**
Use additional code to identify infectious agent (B95-B97)
EXCLUDES 1 *prostatocystitis (N41.3)*
AHA: 2017,1Q,6
DEF: Inflammation of the urinary bladder. Symptoms include dysuria, frequency of urination, urgency, and hematuria.

✓5th **N3Ø.Ø Acute cystitis**
EXCLUDES 1 *irradiation cystitis (N3Ø.4-)*
trigonitis (N3Ø.3-)

N3Ø.ØØ Acute cystitis without hematuria CC H6
N3Ø.Ø1 Acute cystitis with hematuria CC H6

✓5th **N3Ø.1 Interstitial cystitis (chronic)**
N3Ø.1Ø Interstitial cystitis (chronic) without hematuria
N3Ø.11 Interstitial cystitis (chronic) with hematuria

✓5th **N3Ø.2 Other chronic cystitis**
N3Ø.2Ø Other chronic cystitis without hematuria
N3Ø.21 Other chronic cystitis with hematuria

✓5th **N3Ø.3 Trigonitis**
Urethrotrigonitis
N3Ø.3Ø Trigonitis without hematuria
N3Ø.31 Trigonitis with hematuria

✓5th **N3Ø.4 Irradiation cystitis**
N3Ø.4Ø Irradiation cystitis without hematuria CC
N3Ø.41 Irradiation cystitis with hematuria CC

✓5th **N3Ø.8 Other cystitis**
Abscess of bladder
N3Ø.8Ø Other cystitis without hematuria
N3Ø.81 Other cystitis with hematuria

✓5th **N3Ø.9 Cystitis, unspecified**
N3Ø.9Ø Cystitis, unspecified without hematuria
N3Ø.91 Cystitis, unspecified with hematuria

✓4th **N31 Neuromuscular dysfunction of bladder, not elsewhere classified**
Use additional code to identify any associated urinary incontinence (N39.3-N39.4-)
EXCLUDES 1 *cord bladder NOS (G95.89)*
neurogenic bladder due to cauda equina syndrome (G83.4)
neuromuscular dysfunction due to spinal cord lesion (G95.89)

N31.Ø Uninhibited neuropathic bladder, not elsewhere classified
N31.1 Reflex neuropathic bladder, not elsewhere classified
N31.2 Flaccid neuropathic bladder, not elsewhere classified
Atonic (motor) (sensory) neuropathic bladder
Autonomous neuropathic bladder
Nonreflex neuropathic bladder
N31.8 Other neuromuscular dysfunction of bladder
N31.9 Neuromuscular dysfunction of bladder, unspecified
Neurogenic bladder dysfunction NOS

✓4th **N32 Other disorders of bladder**
EXCLUDES 2 *calculus of bladder (N21.Ø)*
cystocele (N81.1-)
hernia or prolapse of bladder, female (N81.1-)

N32.Ø Bladder-neck obstruction
Bladder-neck stenosis (acquired)
EXCLUDES 1 *congenital bladder-neck obstruction (Q64.3-)*
DEF: Bladder outlet and vesicourethral obstruction that occurs as a consequence of benign prostatic hypertrophy or prostatic cancer. It may also occur in either sex due to strictures, radiation, cystoscopy, catheterization, injury, infection, blood clots, bladder cancer, impaction, or other disease that compresses the bladder neck.

N32.1 Vesicointestinal fistula CC
Vesicorectal fistula

N32.2 Vesical fistula, not elsewhere classified CC
EXCLUDES 1 *fistula between bladder and female genital tract (N82.Ø-N82.1)*

N32.3 Diverticulum of bladder
EXCLUDES 1 *congenital diverticulum of bladder (Q64.6)*
diverticulitis of bladder (N3Ø.8-)

✓5th **N32.8 Other specified disorders of bladder**
N32.81 Overactive bladder
Detrusor muscle hyperactivity
EXCLUDES 1 *frequent urination due to specified bladder condition — code to condition*
DEF: Sudden involuntary contractions of the muscular wall of the bladder that results in a sudden, strong urge to urinate.
N32.89 Other specified disorders of bladder
Bladder hemorrhage
Bladder hypertrophy
Calcified bladder
Contracted bladder

N32.9 Bladder disorder, unspecified

N33 Bladder disorders in diseases classified elsewhere
Code first underlying disease, such as:
schistosomiasis (B65.Ø-B65.9)
EXCLUDES 1 *bladder disorder in syphilis (A52.76)*
bladder disorder in tuberculosis (A18.12)
candidal cystitis (B37.41)
chlamydial cystitis (A56.Ø1)
cystitis in gonorrhea (A54.Ø1)
cystitis in neurogenic bladder (N31.-)
diphtheritic cystitis (A36.85)
neurogenic bladder (N31.-)
syphilitic cystitis (A52.76)
trichomonal cystitis (A59.Ø3)

N34 Urethritis and urethral syndrome
Use additional code (B95-B97), to identify infectious agent
EXCLUDES 2 *Reiter's disease (MØ2.3-)*
urethritis in diseases with a predominantly sexual mode of transmission (A5Ø-A64)
urethrotrigonitis (N3Ø.3-)
AHA: 2017,1Q,6

N34.Ø Urethral abscess CC H6
Abscess (of) Cowper's gland
Abscess (of) Littré's gland
Abscess (of) urethral (gland)
Periurethral abscess
EXCLUDES 1 *urethral caruncle (N36.2)*

N34.1 Nonspecific urethritis
Nongonococcal urethritis
Nonvenereal urethritis

N34.2 Other urethritis
Meatitis, urethral
Postmenopausal urethritis
Ulcer of urethra (meatus)
Urethritis NOS

N34.3 Urethral syndrome, unspecified

N35 Urethral stricture
EXCLUDES 1 *congenital urethral stricture (Q64.3-)*
postprocedural urethral stricture (N99.1-)
AHA: 2018,4Q,21-22

N35.Ø Post-traumatic urethral stricture
Urethral stricture due to injury
EXCLUDES 1 *postprocedural urethral stricture (N99.1-)*

N35.Ø1 Post-traumatic urethral stricture, male
N35.Ø1Ø Post-traumatic urethral stricture, male, meatal ♂
N35.Ø11 Post-traumatic bulbous urethral stricture ♂
N35.Ø12 Post-traumatic membranous urethral stricture ♂
N35.Ø13 Post-traumatic anterior urethral stricture ♂
N35.Ø14 Post-traumatic urethral stricture, male, unspecified ♂
N35.Ø16 Post-traumatic urethral stricture, male, overlapping sites ♂

N35.Ø2 Post-traumatic urethral stricture, female
N35.Ø21 Urethral stricture due to childbirth ♀
N35.Ø28 Other post-traumatic urethral stricture, female ♀

N35.1 Postinfective urethral stricture, not elsewhere classified
EXCLUDES 1 *gonococcal urethral stricture (A54.Ø1)*
syphilitic urethral stricture (A52.76)
urethral stricture associated with schistosomiasis (B65.-, N29)

N35.11 Postinfective urethral stricture, not elsewhere classified, male
N35.111 Postinfective urethral stricture, not elsewhere classified, male, meatal ♂
N35.112 Postinfective bulbous urethral stricture, not elsewhere classified, male ♂
N35.113 Postinfective membranous urethral stricture, not elsewhere classified, male ♂
N35.114 Postinfective anterior urethral stricture, not elsewhere classified, male ♂
N35.116 Postinfective urethral stricture, not elsewhere classified, male, overlapping sites ♂
N35.119 Postinfective urethral stricture, not elsewhere classified, male, unspecified ♂

N35.12 Postinfective urethral stricture, not elsewhere classified, female ♀

N35.8 Other urethral stricture
EXCLUDES 1 *postprocedural urethral stricture (N99.1-)*

N35.81 Other urethral stricture, male
N35.811 Other urethral stricture, male, meatal ♂
N35.812 Other urethral bulbous stricture, male ♂
N35.813 Other membranous urethral stricture, male ♂
N35.814 Other anterior urethral stricture, male ♂
N35.816 Other urethral stricture, male, overlapping sites ♂
N35.819 Other urethral stricture, male, unspecified site ♂

N35.82 Other urethral stricture, female ♀

N35.9 Urethral stricture, unspecified

N35.91 Urethral stricture, unspecified, male
N35.911 Unspecified urethral stricture, male, meatal ♂
N35.912 Unspecified bulbous urethral stricture, male ♂
N35.913 Unspecified membranous urethral stricture, male ♂
N35.914 Unspecified anterior urethral stricture, male ♂
N35.916 Unspecified urethral stricture, male, overlapping sites ♂
N35.919 Unspecified urethral stricture, male, unspecified site ♂
Pinhole meatus NOS
Urethral stricture NOS

N35.92 Unspecified urethral stricture, female ♀

N36 Other disorders of urethra

N36.Ø Urethral fistula CC
Urethroperineal fistula
Urethrorectal fistula
Urinary fistula NOS
EXCLUDES 1 *urethroscrotal fistula (N5Ø.89)*
urethrovaginal fistula (N82.1)
urethrovesicovaginal fistula (N82.1)

N36.1 Urethral diverticulum

N36.2 Urethral caruncle

N36.4 Urethral functional and muscular disorders
Use additional code to identify associated urinary stress incontinence (N39.3)
N36.41 Hypermobility of urethra
N36.42 Intrinsic sphincter deficiency (ISD)
N36.43 Combined hypermobility of urethra and intrinsic sphincter deficiency
N36.44 Muscular disorders of urethra
Bladder sphincter dyssynergy

N36.5 Urethral false passage

N36.8 Other specified disorders of urethra
EXCLUDES 1 *congenital urethrocele (Q64.7)*
female urethrocele (N81.Ø)
AHA: 2022,2Q,7

N36.9 Urethral disorder, unspecified

N37 Urethral disorders in diseases classified elsewhere
Code first underlying disease
EXCLUDES 1 *urethritis (in):*
candidal infection (B37.41)
chlamydial (A56.Ø1)
gonorrhea (A54.Ø1)
syphilis (A52.76)
trichomonal infection (A59.Ø3)
tuberculosis (A18.13)

✓4th N39 Other disorders of urinary system

EXCLUDES 2 *hematuria NOS (R31.-)*
recurrent or persistent hematuria (NØ2.-)
recurrent or persistent hematuria with specified morphological lesion (NØ2.-)
proteinuria NOS (R8Ø.-)

N39.Ø Urinary tract infection, site not specified CC H6
Use additional code (B95-B97), to identify infectious agent
EXCLUDES 1 *candidiasis of urinary tract (B37.4-)*
neonatal urinary tract infection (P39.3)
pyuria (R82.81)
urinary tract infection of specified site, such as:
cystitis (N3Ø.-)
urethritis (N34.-)
AHA: 2019,3Q,17; 2018,2Q,21,22; 2018,1Q,16; 2017,1Q,6; 2012,4Q,94

N39.3 Stress incontinence (female) (male)
Code also any associated overactive bladder (N32.81)
EXCLUDES 1 *mixed incontinence (N39.46)*

✓5th N39.4 Other specified urinary incontinence
Code also any associated overactive bladder (N32.81)
EXCLUDES 1 *enuresis NOS (R32)*
functional urinary incontinence (R39.81)
urinary incontinence associated with cognitive impairment (R39.81)
urinary incontinence NOS (R32)
urinary incontinence of nonorganic origin (F98.Ø)

N39.41 Urge incontinence
EXCLUDES 1 *mixed incontinence (N39.46)*

N39.42 Incontinence without sensory awareness
Insensible (urinary) incontinence

N39.43 Post-void dribbling

N39.44 Nocturnal enuresis
EXCLUDES 2 *nocturnal polyuria (R35.81)*

N39.45 Continuous leakage

N39.46 Mixed incontinence
Urge and stress incontinence

✓6th N39.49 Other specified urinary incontinence
AHA: 2016,4Q,44

N39.49Ø Overflow incontinence

N39.491 Coital incontinence

N39.492 Postural (urinary) incontinence

N39.498 Other specified urinary incontinence
Reflex incontinence
Total incontinence

N39.8 Other specified disorders of urinary system

N39.9 Disorder of urinary system, unspecified

Diseases of male genital organs (N4Ø-N53)

✓4th N4Ø Benign prostatic hyperplasia

INCLUDES adenofibromatous hypertrophy of prostate
benign hypertrophy of the prostate
benign prostatic hypertrophy
BPH
enlarged prostate
nodular prostate
polyp of prostate

EXCLUDES 1 *benign neoplasms of prostate (adenoma, benign) (fibroadenoma) (fibroma) (myoma) (D29.1)*
EXCLUDES 2 *malignant neoplasm of prostate (C61)*

DEF: Enlargement of the prostate gland due to an abnormal proliferation of fibrostromal tissue in the paraurethral glands. This condition causes impingement of the urethra resulting in obstructed urinary flow.

N4Ø.Ø Benign prostatic hyperplasia without lower urinary tract symptoms A ♂
Enlarged prostate NOS
Enlarged prostate without LUTS

N4Ø.1 Benign prostatic hyperplasia with lower urinary tract symptoms A ♂
Enlarged prostate with LUTS
Use additional code for associated symptoms, when specified:
incomplete bladder emptying (R39.14)
nocturia (R35.1)
straining on urination (R39.16)
urinary frequency (R35.Ø)
urinary hesitancy (R39.11)
urinary incontinence (N39.4-)
urinary obstruction (N13.8)
urinary retention (R33.8)
urinary urgency (R39.15)
weak urinary stream (R39.12)
AHA: 2018,4Q,55

N4Ø.2 Nodular prostate without lower urinary tract symptoms A ♂
Nodular prostate without LUTS

N4Ø.3 Nodular prostate with lower urinary tract symptoms A ♂
Use additional code for associated symptoms, when specified:
incomplete bladder emptying (R39.14)
nocturia (R35.1)
straining on urination (R39.16)
urinary frequency (R35.Ø)
urinary hesitancy (R39.11)
urinary incontinence (N39.4-)
urinary obstruction (N13.8)
urinary retention (R33.8)
urinary urgency (R39.15)
weak urinary stream (R39.12)

✓4th N41 Inflammatory diseases of prostate
Use additional code (B95-B97), to identify infectious agent

N41.Ø Acute prostatitis CC A ♂

N41.1 Chronic prostatitis A ♂

N41.2 Abscess of prostate CC A ♂

N41.3 Prostatocystitis A ♂

N41.4 Granulomatous prostatitis A ♂

N41.8 Other inflammatory diseases of prostate A ♂

N41.9 Inflammatory disease of prostate, unspecified A ♂
Prostatitis NOS

✓4th N42 Other and unspecified disorders of prostate

N42.Ø Calculus of prostate A ♂
Prostatic stone
DEF: Formation of a small, solid stone often composed of calcium carbonate or calcium phosphate in the prostate gland.

N42.1 Congestion and hemorrhage of prostate A ♂
EXCLUDES 1 *enlarged prostate (N4Ø.-)*
hematuria (R31.-)
hyperplasia of prostate (N4Ø.-)
inflammatory diseases of prostate (N41.-)

✓5th N42.3 Dysplasia of prostate
AHA: 2016,4Q,44

N42.3Ø Unspecified dysplasia of prostate ♂

N42.31 Prostatic intraepithelial neoplasia ♂
PIN
Prostatic intraepithelial neoplasia I (PIN I)
Prostatic intraepithelial neoplasia II (PIN II)
EXCLUDES 1 *prostatic intraepithelial neoplasia III (PIN III) (DØ7.5)*
DEF: Abnormality of shape and size of the intraepithelial tissues of the prostate. It is a premalignant condition characterized by stalks and absence of a basilar cell layer.

N42.32 Atypical small acinar proliferation of prostate ♂

N42.39 Other dysplasia of prostate ♂

✓5th N42.8 Other specified disorders of prostate

N42.81 Prostatodynia syndrome A ♂
Painful prostate syndrome

N42.82 Prostatosis syndrome A ♂

N42.83 Cyst of prostate A ♂

N42.89 Other specified disorders of prostate A ♂

N42.9 Disorder of prostate, unspecified A ♂

N43 Hydrocele and spermatocele

INCLUDES hydrocele of spermatic cord, testis or tunica vaginalis

EXCLUDES 1 *congenital hydrocele (P83.5)*

DEF: Hydrocele: Serous fluid that collects in the tunica vaginalis of the scrotum along the spermatic cord in males.

N43.0 Encysted hydrocele ♂

N43.1 Infected hydrocele CC ♂

Use additional code (B95-B97), to identify infectious agent

N43.2 Other hydrocele ♂

Hydrocele

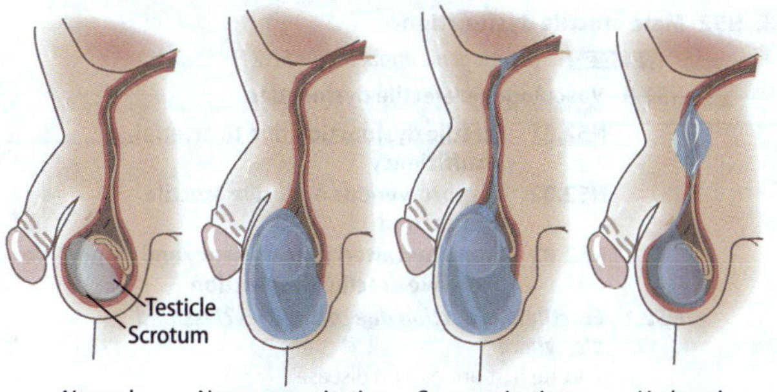

Testicle
Scrotum
Normal
Noncommunicating hydrocele
Communicating hydrocele
Hydrocele of the cord

N43.3 Hydrocele, unspecified ♂

N43.4 Spermatocele of epididymis

Spermatic cyst

DEF: Spermatocele: Noncancerous accumulation of fluid and dead sperm cells normally located at the head of the epididymis that exhibits itself as a hard, smooth scrotal mass and do not normally require treatment unless they become enlarged or cause pain.

N43.40 Spermatocele of epididymis, unspecified ♂

N43.41 Spermatocele of epididymis, single ♂

N43.42 Spermatocele of epididymis, multiple ♂

N44 Noninflammatory disorders of testis

N44.0 Torsion of testis

N44.00 Torsion of testis, unspecified CC ♂

N44.01 Extravaginal torsion of spermatic cord CC ♂

DEF: Torsion of the spermatic cord just below the tunica vaginalis attachments.

N44.02 Intravaginal torsion of spermatic cord CC ♂

Torsion of spermatic cord NOS

N44.03 Torsion of appendix testis CC ♂

N44.04 Torsion of appendix epididymis CC ♂

N44.1 Cyst of tunica albuginea testis ♂

N44.2 Benign cyst of testis ♂

N44.8 Other noninflammatory disorders of the testis ♂

N45 Orchitis and epididymitis

Use additional code (B95-B97), to identify infectious agent

N45.1 Epididymitis ♂

N45.2 Orchitis ♂

N45.3 Epididymo-orchitis ♂

N45.4 Abscess of epididymis or testis CC ♂

N46 Male infertility

EXCLUDES 1 *vasectomy status (Z98.52)*

N46.0 Azoospermia

Absolute male infertility
Male infertility due to germinal (cell) aplasia
Male infertility due to spermatogenic arrest (complete)

DEF: Failure of the development of sperm or the absence of sperm in semen.

N46.01 Organic azoospermia A ♂

Azoospermia NOS

N46.02 Azoospermia due to extratesticular causes

Code also associated cause

N46.021 Azoospermia due to drug therapy A ♂

N46.022 Azoospermia due to infection A ♂

N46.023 Azoospermia due to obstruction of efferent ducts A ♂

N46.024 Azoospermia due to radiation A ♂

N46.025 Azoospermia due to systemic disease A ♂

N46.029 Azoospermia due to other extratesticular causes A ♂

N46.1 Oligospermia

Male infertility due to germinal cell desquamation
Male infertility due to hypospermatogenesis
Male infertility due to incomplete spermatogenic arrest

DEF: Insufficient production of sperm in semen.

N46.11 Organic oligospermia A ♂

Oligospermia NOS

N46.12 Oligospermia due to extratesticular causes

Code also associated cause

N46.121 Oligospermia due to drug therapy A ♂

N46.122 Oligospermia due to infection A ♂

N46.123 Oligospermia due to obstruction of efferent ducts A ♂

N46.124 Oligospermia due to radiation A ♂

N46.125 Oligospermia due to systemic disease A ♂

N46.129 Oligospermia due to other extratesticular causes A ♂

N46.8 Other male infertility A ♂

N46.9 Male infertility, unspecified A ♂

N47 Disorders of prepuce

N47.0 Adherent prepuce, newborn N ♂

N47.1 Phimosis ♂

DEF: Condition in which the foreskin is contracted and cannot be drawn back behind the glans penis.

N47.2 Paraphimosis ♂

N47.3 Deficient foreskin ♂

N47.4 Benign cyst of prepuce ♂

N47.5 Adhesions of prepuce and glans penis ♂

N47.6 Balanoposthitis ♂

Use additional code (B95-B97), to identify infectious agent

EXCLUDES 1 *balanitis (N48.1)*

N47.7 Other inflammatory diseases of prepuce ♂

Use additional code (B95-B97), to identify infectious agent

N47.8 Other disorders of prepuce ♂

N48 Other disorders of penis

N48.0 Leukoplakia of penis ♂

Balanitis xerotica obliterans
Kraurosis of penis
Lichen sclerosus of external male genital organs

EXCLUDES 1 *carcinoma in situ of penis (D07.4)*

N48.1 Balanitis ♂

Use additional code (B95-B97), to identify infectious agent

EXCLUDES 1 *amebic balanitis (A06.8)*
balanitis xerotica obliterans (N48.0)
candidal balanitis (B37.42)
gonococcal balanitis (A54.23)
herpesviral [herpes simplex] balanitis (A60.01)

DEF: Inflammation of the glans penis, most often affecting uncircumcised males.

N48.2 Other inflammatory disorders of penis

Use additional code (B95-B97), to identify infectious agent

EXCLUDES 1 *balanitis (N48.1)*
balanitis xerotica obliterans (N48.0)
balanoposthitis (N47.6)

N48.21 Abscess of corpus cavernosum and penis ♂

N48.22 Cellulitis of corpus cavernosum and penis ♂

N48.29 Other inflammatory disorders of penis ♂

N48.3 Priapism

Painful erection

Code first underlying cause

N48.30 Priapism, unspecified CC ♂

N48.31 Priapism due to trauma CC ♂

N48.32 Priapism due to disease classified elsewhere CC ♂

N48.33 Priapism, drug-induced CC ♂

N48.39 Other priapism CC ♂

N48.5 Ulcer of penis ♂

N48.6 Induration penis plastica ♂
Peyronie's disease
Plastic induration of penis

N48.8 Other specified disorders of penis

N48.81 Thrombosis of superficial vein of penis ♂

N48.82 Acquired torsion of penis ♂
Acquired torsion of penis NOS
EXCLUDES 1 *congenital torsion of penis (Q55.63)*

N48.83 Acquired buried penis ♂
EXCLUDES 1 *congenital hidden penis (Q55.64)*

N48.89 Other specified disorders of penis ♂

N48.9 Disorder of penis, unspecified ♂

N49 Inflammatory disorders of male genital organs, not elsewhere classified
Use additional code (B95-B97), to identify infectious agent
EXCLUDES 1 *inflammation of penis (N48.1, N48.2-)*
orchitis and epididymitis (N45.-)

N49.0 Inflammatory disorders of seminal vesicle ♂
Vesiculitis NOS

N49.1 Inflammatory disorders of spermatic cord, tunica vaginalis and vas deferens ♂
Vasitis

N49.2 Inflammatory disorders of scrotum ♂

N49.3 Fournier gangrene ♂
AHA: 2020,2Q,18

N49.8 Inflammatory disorders of other specified male genital organs ♂
Inflammation of multiple sites in male genital organs

N49.9 Inflammatory disorder of unspecified male genital organ ♂
Abscess of unspecified male genital organ
Boil of unspecified male genital organ
Carbuncle of unspecified male genital organ
Cellulitis of unspecified male genital organ

N50 Other and unspecified disorders of male genital organs
EXCLUDES 2 *torsion of testis (N44.0-)*

N50.0 Atrophy of testis ♂

N50.1 Vascular disorders of male genital organs ♂
Hematocele, NOS, of male genital organs
Hemorrhage of male genital organs
Thrombosis of male genital organs

N50.3 Cyst of epididymis ♂

N50.8 Other specified disorders of male genital organs
AHA: 2016,4Q,45

N50.81 Testicular pain

N50.811 Right testicular pain ♂

N50.812 Left testicular pain ♂

N50.819 Testicular pain, unspecified ♂

N50.82 Scrotal pain ♂

N50.89 Other specified disorders of the male genital organs ♂
Atrophy of scrotum, seminal vesicle, spermatic cord, tunica vaginalis and vas deferens
Chylocele, tunica vaginalis (nonfilarial) NOS
Edema of scrotum, seminal vesicle, spermatic cord, tunica vaginalis and vas deferens
Hypertrophy of scrotum, seminal vesicle, spermatic cord, tunica vaginalis and vas deferens
Stricture of spermatic cord, tunica vaginalis, and vas deferens
Ulcer of scrotum, seminal vesicle, spermatic cord, testis, tunica vaginalis and vas deferens
Urethroscrotal fistula

N50.9 Disorder of male genital organs, unspecified ♂

N51 Disorders of male genital organs in diseases classified elsewhere ♂
Code first underlying disease, such as:
filariasis (B74.0-B74.9)
EXCLUDES 1 *amebic balanitis (A06.8)*
candidal balanitis (B37.42)
gonococcal balanitis (A54.23)
gonococcal prostatitis (A54.22)
herpesviral [herpes simplex] balanitis (A60.01)
trichomonal prostatitis (A59.02)
tuberculous prostatitis (A18.14)

N52 Male erectile dysfunction
EXCLUDES 1 *psychogenic impotence (F52.21)*

N52.0 Vasculogenic erectile dysfunction

N52.01 Erectile dysfunction due to arterial insufficiency A ♂

N52.02 Corporo-venous occlusive erectile dysfunction A ♂

N52.03 Combined arterial insufficiency and corporo-venous occlusive erectile dysfunction A ♂

N52.1 Erectile dysfunction due to diseases classified elsewhere A ♂
Code first underlying disease

N52.2 Drug-induced erectile dysfunction A ♂

N52.3 Postprocedural erectile dysfunction
AHA: 2016,4Q,45

N52.31 Erectile dysfunction following radical prostatectomy A ♂

N52.32 Erectile dysfunction following radical cystectomy A ♂

N52.33 Erectile dysfunction following urethral surgery A ♂

N52.34 Erectile dysfunction following simple prostatectomy A ♂

N52.35 Erectile dysfunction following radiation therapy A ♂

N52.36 Erectile dysfunction following interstitial seed therapy A ♂

N52.37 Erectile dysfunction following prostate ablative therapy A ♂
Erectile dysfunction following cryotherapy
Erectile dysfunction following other prostate ablative therapies
Erectile dysfunction following ultrasound ablative therapies

N52.39 Other and unspecified postprocedural erectile dysfunction A ♂

N52.8 Other male erectile dysfunction A ♂

N52.9 Male erectile dysfunction, unspecified A ♂
Impotence NOS

N53 Other male sexual dysfunction
EXCLUDES 1 *psychogenic sexual dysfunction (F52.-)*

N53.1 Ejaculatory dysfunction
EXCLUDES 1 *premature ejaculation (F52.4)*

N53.11 Retarded ejaculation ♂

N53.12 Painful ejaculation ♂

N53.13 Anejaculatory orgasm ♂

N53.14 Retrograde ejaculation ♂
DEF: Form of male sexual dysfunction in which the semen enters the bladder instead of going out through the urethra during ejaculation.

N53.19 Other ejaculatory dysfunction ♂
Ejaculatory dysfunction NOS

N53.8 Other male sexual dysfunction ♂

N53.9 Unspecified male sexual dysfunction ♂

Disorders of breast (N60-N65)

EXCLUDES 1 *disorders of breast associated with childbirth (O91-O92)*

N60 Benign mammary dysplasia
INCLUDES fibrocystic mastopathy

N60.0 Solitary cyst of breast
Cyst of breast

N60.01 Solitary cyst of right breast

N60.02 Solitary cyst of left breast

N60.09 Solitary cyst of unspecified breast

N6Ø.1 Diffuse cystic mastopathy
Cystic breast
Fibrocystic disease of breast
EXCLUDES 1 *diffuse cystic mastopathy with epithelial proliferation (N6Ø.3-)*
N6Ø.11 Diffuse cystic mastopathy of right breast A
N6Ø.12 Diffuse cystic mastopathy of left breast A
N6Ø.19 Diffuse cystic mastopathy of unspecified breast A

N6Ø.2 Fibroadenosis of breast
Adenofibrosis of breast
EXCLUDES 2 *fibroadenoma of breast (D24.-)*
N6Ø.21 Fibroadenosis of right breast
N6Ø.22 Fibroadenosis of left breast
N6Ø.29 Fibroadenosis of unspecified breast

N6Ø.3 Fibrosclerosis of breast
Cystic mastopathy with epithelial proliferation
N6Ø.31 Fibrosclerosis of right breast
N6Ø.32 Fibrosclerosis of left breast
N6Ø.39 Fibrosclerosis of unspecified breast

N6Ø.4 Mammary duct ectasia
N6Ø.41 Mammary duct ectasia of right breast
N6Ø.42 Mammary duct ectasia of left breast
N6Ø.49 Mammary duct ectasia of unspecified breast

N6Ø.8 Other benign mammary dysplasias
N6Ø.81 Other benign mammary dysplasias of right breast
N6Ø.82 Other benign mammary dysplasias of left breast
N6Ø.89 Other benign mammary dysplasias of unspecified breast

N6Ø.9 Unspecified benign mammary dysplasia
N6Ø.91 Unspecified benign mammary dysplasia of right breast
N6Ø.92 Unspecified benign mammary dysplasia of left breast
N6Ø.99 Unspecified benign mammary dysplasia of unspecified breast

N61 Inflammatory disorders of breast
EXCLUDES 1 *inflammatory carcinoma of breast (C5Ø.9)*
inflammatory disorder of breast associated with childbirth (O91.-)
neonatal infective mastitis (P39.Ø)
thrombophlebitis of breast [Mondor's disease] (I8Ø.8)

N61.Ø Mastitis without abscess
Infective mastitis (acute) (nonpuerperal) (subacute)
Mastitis (acute) (nonpuerperal) (subacute) NOS
Cellulitis (acute) (nonpuerperal) (subacute) of breast NOS
Cellulitis (acute) (nonpuerperal) (subacute) of nipple NOS

N61.1 Abscess of the breast and nipple
Abscess (acute) (chronic) (nonpuerperal) of areola
Abscess (acute) (chronic) (nonpuerperal) of breast
Carbuncle of breast
Mastitis with abscess

N61.2 Granulomatous mastitis
AHA: 2020,4Q,35
N61.2Ø Granulomatous mastitis, unspecified breast
N61.21 Granulomatous mastitis, right breast
N61.22 Granulomatous mastitis, left breast
N61.23 Granulomatous mastitis, bilateral breast

N62 Hypertrophy of breast
Gynecomastia
Hypertrophy of breast NOS
Massive pubertal hypertrophy of breast
EXCLUDES 1 *breast engorgement of newborn (P83.4)*
disproportion of reconstructed breast (N65.1)

N63 Unspecified lump in breast
Nodule(s) NOS in breast
AHA: 2019,4Q,12; 2017,4Q,19
N63.Ø Unspecified lump in unspecified breast

N63.1 Unspecified lump in the right breast
N63.1Ø Unspecified lump in the right breast, unspecified quadrant
N63.11 Unspecified lump in the right breast, upper outer quadrant
N63.12 Unspecified lump in the right breast, upper inner quadrant
N63.13 Unspecified lump in the right breast, lower outer quadrant
N63.14 Unspecified lump in the right breast, lower inner quadrant
N63.15 Unspecified lump in the right breast, overlapping quadrants

N63.2 Unspecified lump in the left breast
N63.2Ø Unspecified lump in the left breast, unspecified quadrant
N63.21 Unspecified lump in the left breast, upper outer quadrant
N63.22 Unspecified lump in the left breast, upper inner quadrant
N63.23 Unspecified lump in the left breast, lower outer quadrant
N63.24 Unspecified lump in the left breast, lower inner quadrant
N63.25 Unspecified lump in the left breast, overlapping quadrants

N63.3 Unspecified lump in axillary tail
N63.31 Unspecified lump in axillary tail of the right breast
N63.32 Unspecified lump in axillary tail of the left breast

N63.4 Unspecified lump in breast, subareolar
N63.41 Unspecified lump in right breast, subareolar
N63.42 Unspecified lump in left breast, subareolar

N64 Other disorders of breast
EXCLUDES 2 *mechanical complication of breast prosthesis and implant (T85.4-)*
N64.Ø Fissure and fistula of nipple
N64.1 Fat necrosis of breast UPD
Fat necrosis (segmental) of breast
Code first breast necrosis due to breast graft (T85.898)
N64.2 Atrophy of breast
N64.3 Galactorrhea not associated with childbirth
N64.4 Mastodynia

N64.5 Other signs and symptoms in breast
EXCLUDES 2 *abnormal findings on diagnostic imaging of breast (R92.-)*
N64.51 Induration of breast
N64.52 Nipple discharge
EXCLUDES 1 *abnormal findings in nipple discharge (R89.-)*
N64.53 Retraction of nipple
N64.59 Other signs and symptoms in breast

N64.8 Other specified disorders of breast
N64.81 Ptosis of breast A
EXCLUDES 1 *ptosis of native breast in relation to reconstructed breast (N65.1)*
N64.82 Hypoplasia of breast A
Micromastia
EXCLUDES 1 *congenital absence of breast (Q83.Ø)*
hypoplasia of native breast in relation to reconstructed breast (N65.1)
N64.89 Other specified disorders of breast
Galactocele
Subinvolution of breast (postlactational)
AHA: 2019,1Q,32; 2018,1Q,3
N64.9 Disorder of breast, unspecified

N65 Deformity and disproportion of reconstructed breast
N65.Ø Deformity of reconstructed breast A
Contour irregularity in reconstructed breast
Excess tissue in reconstructed breast
Misshapen reconstructed breast
N65.1 Disproportion of reconstructed breast A
Breast asymmetry between native breast and reconstructed breast
Disproportion between native breast and reconstructed breast

Chapter 14. Diseases of the Genitourinary System

N6Ø.1–N65.1

Inflammatory diseases of female pelvic organs (N70-N77)

EXCLUDES 1 *inflammatory diseases of female pelvic organs complicating:*
abortion or ectopic or molar pregnancy (O00-O07, O08.0)
pregnancy, childbirth and the puerperium (O23.-, O75.3, O85, O86.-)

N70 Salpingitis and oophoritis
INCLUDES abscess (of) fallopian tube
abscess (of) ovary
pyosalpinx
salpingo-oophoritis
tubo-ovarian abscess
tubo-ovarian inflammatory disease
Use additional code (B95-B97), to identify infectious agent
EXCLUDES 1 *gonococcal infection (A54.24)*
tuberculous infection (A18.17)

N70.0 Acute salpingitis and oophoritis
N70.01 Acute salpingitis CC ♀
N70.02 Acute oophoritis CC ♀
N70.03 Acute salpingitis and oophoritis CC ♀

N70.1 Chronic salpingitis and oophoritis
Hydrosalpinx
N70.11 Chronic salpingitis ♀
N70.12 Chronic oophoritis ♀
N70.13 Chronic salpingitis and oophoritis ♀

N70.9 Salpingitis and oophoritis, unspecified
N70.91 Salpingitis, unspecified ♀
N70.92 Oophoritis, unspecified ♀
N70.93 Salpingitis and oophoritis, unspecified ♀

N71 Inflammatory disease of uterus, except cervix
INCLUDES endo (myo) metritis
metritis
myometritis
pyometra
uterine abscess
Use additional code (B95-B97), to identify infectious agent
EXCLUDES 1 *hyperplastic endometritis (N85.0-)*
infection of uterus following delivery (O85, O86.-)

N71.0 Acute inflammatory disease of uterus CC ♀
N71.1 Chronic inflammatory disease of uterus ♀
N71.9 Inflammatory disease of uterus, unspecified ♀

N72 Inflammatory disease of cervix uteri ♀
INCLUDES cervicitis (with or without erosion or ectropion)
endocervicitis (with or without erosion or ectropion)
exocervicitis (with or without erosion or ectropion)
Use additional code (B95-B97), to identify infectious agent
EXCLUDES 1 *erosion and ectropion of cervix without cervicitis (N86)*

N73 Other female pelvic inflammatory diseases
Use additional code (B95-B97), to identify infectious agent

N73.0 Acute parametritis and pelvic cellulitis CC ♀
Abscess of broad ligament
Abscess of parametrium
Pelvic cellulitis, female
DEF: Parametritis: Inflammation of the parametrium.

N73.1 Chronic parametritis and pelvic cellulitis ♀
Any condition in N73.0 specified as chronic
EXCLUDES 1 *tuberculous parametritis and pelvic cellulitis (A18.17)*

N73.2 Unspecified parametritis and pelvic cellulitis ♀
Any condition in N73.0 unspecified whether acute or chronic

N73.3 Female acute pelvic peritonitis MCC ♀

N73.4 Female chronic pelvic peritonitis CC ♀
EXCLUDES 1 *tuberculous pelvic (female) peritonitis (A18.17)*

N73.5 Female pelvic peritonitis, unspecified ♀

N73.6 Female pelvic peritoneal adhesions (postinfective) ♀
EXCLUDES 2 *postprocedural pelvic peritoneal adhesions (N99.4)*
AHA: 2014,1Q,6

N73.8 Other specified female pelvic inflammatory diseases ♀

N73.9 Female pelvic inflammatory disease, unspecified ♀
Female pelvic infection or inflammation NOS

N74 Female pelvic inflammatory disorders in diseases classified elsewhere ♀
Code first underlying disease
EXCLUDES 1 *chlamydial cervicitis (A56.02)*
chlamydial pelvic inflammatory disease (A56.11)
gonococcal cervicitis (A54.03)
gonococcal pelvic inflammatory disease (A54.24)
herpesviral [herpes simplex] cervicitis (A60.03)
herpesviral [herpes simplex] pelvic inflammatory disease (A60.09)
syphilitic cervicitis (A52.76)
syphilitic pelvic inflammatory disease (A52.76)
trichomonal cervicitis (A59.09)
tuberculous cervicitis (A18.16)
tuberculous pelvic inflammatory disease (A18.17)

N75 Diseases of Bartholin's gland
DEF: Bartholin's gland: Mucous-producing gland found in the vestibular bulbs on either side of the vaginal orifice and connected to the mucosal membrane at the opening by a duct.

N75.0 Cyst of Bartholin's gland ♀
N75.1 Abscess of Bartholin's gland CC ♀
N75.8 Other diseases of Bartholin's gland ♀
Bartholinitis
N75.9 Disease of Bartholin's gland, unspecified ♀

N76 Other inflammation of vagina and vulva
Use additional code (B95-B97), to identify infectious agent
EXCLUDES 2 *senile (atrophic) vaginitis (N95.2)*
vulvar vestibulitis (N94.810)

N76.0 Acute vaginitis ♀
Acute vulvovaginitis
Vaginitis NOS
Vulvovaginitis NOS

N76.1 Subacute and chronic vaginitis ♀
Chronic vulvovaginitis
Subacute vulvovaginitis

N76.2 Acute vulvitis ♀
Vulvitis NOS

N76.3 Subacute and chronic vulvitis ♀

N76.4 Abscess of vulva CC ♀
Furuncle of vulva

N76.5 Ulceration of vagina ♀

N76.6 Ulceration of vulva ♀

N76.8 Other specified inflammation of vagina and vulva

N76.81 Mucositis (ulcerative) of vagina and vulva CC ♀
Code also type of associated therapy, such as:
antineoplastic and immunosuppressive drugs (T45.1X-)
radiological procedure and radiotherapy (Y84.2)
EXCLUDES 2 *gastrointestinal mucositis (ulcerative) (K92.81)*
nasal mucositis (ulcerative) (J34.81)
oral mucositis (ulcerative) (K12.3-)

● **N76.82 Fournier disease of vagina and vulva** ♀
Fournier gangrene of vagina and vulva
Code also, if applicable, diabetes mellitus (E08-E13 with .9)
EXCLUDES 1 *gangrene in diabetes mellitus (E08-E13 with .52)*

N76.89 Other specified inflammation of vagina and vulva ♀

N77 Vulvovaginal ulceration and inflammation in diseases classified elsewhere

N77.0 Ulceration of vulva in diseases classified elsewhere ♀
Code first underlying disease, such as:
Behçet's disease (M35.2)
EXCLUDES 1 *ulceration of vulva in gonococcal infection (A54.02)*
ulceration of vulva in herpesviral [herpes simplex] infection (A60.04)
ulceration of vulva in syphilis (A51.0)
ulceration of vulva in tuberculosis (A18.18)

N77.1 ***Vaginitis, vulvitis and vulvovaginitis in diseases classified elsewhere*** ♀
Code first underlying disease, such as:
pinworm (B80)
EXCLUDES 1 *candidal vulvovaginitis ►(B37.3-)◄*
chlamydial vulvovaginitis (A56.02)
gonococcal vulvovaginitis (A54.02)
herpesviral [herpes simplex] vulvovaginitis (A60.04)
trichomonal vulvovaginitis (A59.01)
tuberculous vulvovaginitis (A18.18)
vulvovaginitis in early syphilis (A51.0)
vulvovaginitis in late syphilis (A52.76)

Noninflammatory disorders of female genital tract (N80-N98)

N80 Endometriosis
DEF: Aberrant uterine mucosal tissue appearing in areas of the pelvic cavity outside of its normal location, lining the uterus, and inflaming surrounding tissues often resulting in infertility or spontaneous abortion.

▲ **N80.0 Endometriosis of uterus**
Adenomyosis
►Endometriosis of the cervix◄
EXCLUDES 1 *stromal endometriosis (D39.0)*

● **N80.00 Endometriosis of the uterus, unspecified** ♀
● **N80.01 Superficial endometriosis of the uterus** ♀
● **N80.02 Deep endometriosis of the uterus** ♀
Deep retrocervical endometriosis
● **N80.03 Adenomyosis of the uterus** ♀
Adenomyosis NOS

▲ **N80.1 Endometriosis of ovary**
● **N80.10 Endometriosis of ovary, unspecified depth**
● **N80.101 Endometriosis of right ovary, unspecified depth** ♀
● **N80.102 Endometriosis of left ovary, unspecified depth** ♀
● **N80.103 Endometriosis of bilateral ovaries, unspecified depth** ♀
● **N80.109 Endometriosis of ovary, unspecified side, unspecified depth** ♀
Endometriosis of ovary NOS
● **N80.11 Superficial endometriosis of the ovary**
● **N80.111 Superficial endometriosis of right ovary** ♀
● **N80.112 Superficial endometriosis of left ovary** ♀
● **N80.113 Superficial endometriosis of bilateral ovaries** ♀
● **N80.119 Superficial endometriosis of ovary, unspecified ovary** ♀
● **N80.12 Deep endometriosis of ovary**
Deep ovarian endometriosis
Endometrioma
● **N80.121 Deep endometriosis of right ovary** ♀
● **N80.122 Deep endometriosis of left ovary** ♀
● **N80.123 Deep endometriosis of bilateral ovaries** ♀
● **N80.129 Deep endometriosis of ovary, unspecified ovary** ♀

▲ **N80.2 Endometriosis of fallopian tube**
● **N80.20 Endometriosis of fallopian tube, unspecified depth**
● **N80.201 Endometriosis of right fallopian tube, unspecified depth** ♀
● **N80.202 Endometriosis of left fallopian tube, unspecified depth** ♀
● **N80.203 Endometriosis of bilateral fallopian tubes, unspecified depth** ♀
● **N80.209 Endometriosis of unspecified fallopian tube, unspecified depth** ♀
Endometriosis fallopian tube NOS
● **N80.21 Superficial endometriosis of fallopian tube**
● **N80.211 Superficial endometriosis of right fallopian tube** ♀
● **N80.212 Superficial endometriosis of left fallopian tube** ♀
● **N80.213 Superficial endometriosis of bilateral fallopian tubes** ♀
● **N80.219 Superficial endometriosis of unspecified fallopian tube** ♀
● **N80.22 Deep endometriosis of the fallopian tube**
Deep endometriosis involving muscular wall of fallopian tube
● **N80.221 Deep endometriosis of right fallopian tube** ♀
● **N80.222 Deep endometriosis of left fallopian tube** ♀
● **N80.223 Deep endometriosis of bilateral fallopian tubes** ♀
● **N80.229 Deep endometriosis of unspecified fallopian tube** ♀

▲ **N80.3 Endometriosis of pelvic peritoneum**
● **N80.30 Endometriosis of pelvic peritoneum, unspecified** ♀
Endometriosis of the retroperitoneum NOS
● **N80.31 Endometriosis of the anterior cul-de-sac**
● **N80.311 Superficial endometriosis of the anterior cul-de-sac** ♀
● **N80.312 Deep endometriosis of the anterior cul-de-sac** ♀
● **N80.319 Endometriosis of the anterior cul-de-sac, unspecified depth** ♀
Endometriosis of the anterior cul-de-sac NOS
● **N80.32 Endometriosis of the posterior cul-de-sac**
● **N80.321 Superficial endometriosis of the posterior cul-de-sac** ♀
● **N80.322 Deep endometriosis of the posterior cul-de-sac** ♀
● **N80.329 Endometriosis of the posterior cul-de-sac, unspecified depth** ♀
Endometriosis of the posterior cul-de-sac NOS
● **N80.33 Superficial endometriosis of the pelvic sidewall**
● **N80.331 Superficial endometriosis of the right pelvic sidewall** ♀
● **N80.332 Superficial endometriosis of the left pelvic sidewall** ♀
● **N80.333 Superficial endometriosis of bilateral pelvic sidewall** ♀
● **N80.339 Superficial endometriosis of pelvic sidewall, unspecified side** ♀
● **N80.34 Deep endometriosis of the pelvic sidewall**
● **N80.341 Deep endometriosis of the right pelvic sidewall** ♀
● **N80.342 Deep endometriosis of the left pelvic sidewall** ♀
● **N80.343 Deep endometriosis of the bilateral pelvic sidewall** ♀
● **N80.349 Deep endometriosis of the pelvic sidewall, unspecified side** ♀
● **N80.35 Endometriosis of the pelvic sidewall, unspecified depth**
● **N80.351 Endometriosis of the right pelvic sidewall, unspecified depth** ♀
● **N80.352 Endometriosis of the left pelvic sidewall, unspecified depth** ♀
● **N80.353 Endometriosis of bilateral pelvic sidewall, unspecified depth** ♀
● **N80.359 Endometriosis of pelvic sidewall, unspecified side, unspecified depth** ♀
Endometriosis of the pelvic sidewall NOS
● **N80.36 Superficial endometriosis of the pelvic brim**
● **N80.361 Superficial endometriosis of the right pelvic brim** ♀
● **N80.362 Superficial endometriosis of the left pelvic brim** ♀
● **N80.363 Superficial endometriosis of bilateral pelvic brim** ♀
● **N80.369 Superficial endometriosis of the pelvic brim, unspecified side** ♀
● **N80.37 Deep endometriosis of the pelvic brim**
● **N80.371 Deep endometriosis of the right pelvic brim** ♀
● **N80.372 Deep endometriosis of the left pelvic brim** ♀

- N80.373 Deep endometriosis of bilateral pelvic brim ♀
- N80.379 Deep endometriosis of the pelvic brim, unspecified side ♀
- N80.38 Endometriosis of the pelvic brim, unspecified depth
  - N80.381 Endometriosis of the right pelvic brim, unspecified depth ♀
  - N80.382 Endometriosis of the left pelvic brim, unspecified depth ♀
  - N80.383 Endometriosis of bilateral pelvic brim, unspecified depth ♀
  - N80.389 Endometriosis of the pelvic brim, unspecified side, unspecified depth ♀
    Endometriosis of the pelvic brim NOS
- N80.3A Superficial endometriosis of the uterosacral ligament(s)
  - N80.3A1 Superficial endometriosis of the right uterosacral ligament ♀
  - N80.3A2 Superficial endometriosis of the left uterosacral ligament ♀
  - N80.3A3 Superficial endometriosis of the bilateral uterosacral ligament(s) ♀
  - N80.3A9 Superficial endometriosis of the uterosacral ligament(s), unspecified side ♀
- N80.3B Deep endometriosis of the uterosacral ligament(s)
  - N80.3B1 Deep endometriosis of the right uterosacral ligament ♀
  - N80.3B2 Deep endometriosis of the left uterosacral ligament ♀
  - N80.3B3 Deep endometriosis of bilateral uterosacral ligament(s) ♀
  - N80.3B9 Deep endometriosis of the uterosacral ligament(s), unspecified side ♀
- N80.3C Endometriosis of the uterosacral ligament(s), unspecified depth
  - N80.3C1 Endometriosis of the right uterosacral ligament, unspecified depth ♀
  - N80.3C2 Endometriosis of the left uterosacral ligament, unspecified depth ♀
  - N80.3C3 Endometriosis of bilateral uterosacral ligament(s), unspecified depth ♀
  - N80.3C9 Endometriosis of the uterosacral ligament(s), unspecified side, unspecified depth ♀
    Endometriosis of the uterosacral ligament(s) NOS
- N80.39 Endometriosis of other pelvic peritoneum
  - N80.391 Superficial endometriosis of the pelvic peritoneum, other specified sites ♀
  - N80.392 Deep endometriosis of the pelvic peritoneum, other specified sites ♀
  - N80.399 Endometriosis of the pelvic peritoneum, other specified sites, unspecified depth ♀
- N80.4 Endometriosis of rectovaginal septum and vagina
  - N80.40 Endometriosis of rectovaginal septum, unspecified involvement of vagina ♀
    Endometriosis of the rectovaginal septum, NOS
  - N80.41 Endometriosis of rectovaginal septum without involvement of vagina ♀
  - N80.42 Endometriosis of rectovaginal septum with involvement of vagina ♀
- N80.5 Endometriosis of intestine
  - N80.50 Endometriosis of intestine, unspecified ♀
  - N80.51 Endometriosis of the rectum
    - N80.511 Superficial endometriosis of the rectum ♀
    - N80.512 Deep endometriosis of the rectum ♀
      Deep endometriosis of the rectum, multifocal
    - N80.519 Endometriosis of the rectum, unspecified depth ♀
      Endometriosis of the rectum NOS
  - N80.52 Endometriosis of the sigmoid colon
    - N80.521 Superficial endometriosis of the sigmoid colon ♀
    - N80.522 Deep endometriosis of the sigmoid colon ♀
    - N80.529 Endometriosis of the sigmoid colon, unspecified depth ♀
      Endometriosis of the sigmoid colon NOS
  - N80.53 Endometriosis of the cecum
    - N80.531 Superficial endometriosis of the cecum ♀
    - N80.532 Deep endometriosis of the cecum ♀
    - N80.539 Endometriosis of the cecum, unspecified depth ♀
      Endometriosis of the cecum NOS
  - N80.54 Endometriosis of the appendix
    - N80.541 Superficial endometriosis of the appendix ♀
    - N80.542 Deep endometriosis of the appendix ♀
    - N80.549 Endometriosis of the appendix, unspecified depth ♀
      Endometriosis of the appendix NOS
  - N80.55 Endometriosis of other parts of the colon
    Endometriosis of descending colon
    Endometriosis of transverse colon
    - N80.551 Superficial endometriosis of other parts of the colon ♀
    - N80.552 Deep endometriosis of other parts of the colon ♀
    - N80.559 Endometriosis of other parts of the colon, unspecified depth ♀
      Endometriosis of colon NOS
  - N80.56 Endometriosis of the small intestine
    - N80.561 Superficial endometriosis of the small intestine ♀
    - N80.562 Deep endometriosis of the small intestine ♀
      Deep endometriosis of the small intestine, multifocal
    - N80.569 Endometriosis of the small intestine, unspecified depth ♀
      Endometriosis of the small intestine NOS
- N80.6 Endometriosis in cutaneous scar ♀
- N80.A Endometriosis of bladder and ureters
  - N80.A0 Endometriosis of bladder, unspecified depth ♀
    Endometriosis of bladder NOS
  - N80.A1 Superficial endometriosis of bladder ♀
  - N80.A2 Deep endometriosis of bladder ♀
  - N80.A4 Superficial endometriosis of ureter
    Extrinsic endometriosis of ureter
    Code also, if applicable, obstructive and reflux uropathy (N13.-)
    - N80.A41 Superficial endometriosis of right ureter ♀
    - N80.A42 Superficial endometriosis of left ureter ♀
    - N80.A43 Superficial endometriosis of bilateral ureters ♀
    - N80.A49 Superficial endometriosis of unspecified ureter ♀
  - N80.A5 Deep endometriosis of ureter
    Intrinsic endometriosis of ureter
    Code also, if applicable, obstructive and reflux uropathy (N13.-)
    - N80.A51 Deep endometriosis of right ureter ♀
    - N80.A52 Deep endometriosis of left ureter ♀
    - N80.A53 Deep endometriosis of bilateral ureters ♀
    - N80.A59 Deep endometriosis of unspecified ureter ♀
  - N80.A6 Endometriosis of ureter, unspecified depth
    Code also, if applicable, obstructive and reflux uropathy (N13.-)
    - N80.A61 Endometriosis of right ureter, unspecified depth ♀
    - N80.A62 Endometriosis of left ureter, unspecified depth ♀
    - N80.A63 Endometriosis of bilateral ureters, unspecified depth ♀
    - N80.A69 Endometriosis of unspecified ureter, unspecified depth ♀

● ✓5th **N8Ø.B Endometriosis of cardiothoracic space**

Endometriosis of thorax

Code also, if applicable:

catamenial hemothorax (J94.2)

catamenial pneumothorax (J93.12)

● **N8Ø.B1 Endometriosis of pleura** ♀

● **N8Ø.B2 Endometriosis of lung** ♀

● ✓6th **N8Ø.B3 Endometriosis of diaphragm**

● **N8Ø.B31 Superficial endometriosis of diaphragm** ♀

● **N8Ø.B32 Deep endometriosis of diaphragm** ♀

● **N8Ø.B39 Endometriosis of diaphragm, unspecified depth** ♀

Endometriosis of the diaphragm NOS

● **N8Ø.B4 Endometriosis of the pericardial space** ♀

● **N8Ø.B5 Endometriosis of the mediastinal space** ♀

● **N8Ø.B6 Endometriosis of cardiothoracic space** ♀

● ✓5th **N8Ø.C Endometriosis of the abdomen**

● **N8Ø.CØ Endometriosis of the abdomen, unspecified** ♀

Endometriosis of the abdomen NOS

● ✓6th **N8Ø.C1 Endometriosis of the anterior abdominal wall**

● **N8Ø.C1Ø Endometriosis of the anterior abdominal wall, subcutaneous tissue** ♀

● **N8Ø.C11 Endometriosis of the anterior abdominal wall, fascia and muscular layers** ♀

● **N8Ø.C19 Endometriosis of the anterior abdominal wall, unspecified depth** ♀

Endometriosis of the anterior abdominal wall NOS

● **N8Ø.C2 Endometriosis of the umbilicus** ♀

● **N8Ø.C3 Endometriosis of the inguinal canal** ♀

● **N8Ø.C4 Endometriosis of extra-pelvic abdominal peritoneum** ♀

● **N8Ø.C9 Endometriosis of other site of abdomen** ♀

● ✓5th **N8Ø.D Endometriosis of the pelvic nerves**

Endometriosis of the nerves of the retroperitoneum

● **N8Ø.DØ Endometriosis of the pelvic nerves, unspecified** ♀

Endometriosis of nerve of the retroperitoneum, NOS

● **N8Ø.D1 Endometriosis of the sacral splanchnic nerves** ♀

Endometriosis of the pelvic splanchnic nerves

● **N8Ø.D2 Endometriosis of the sacral nerve roots** ♀

● **N8Ø.D3 Endometriosis of the obturator nerve** ♀

● **N8Ø.D4 Endometriosis of the sciatic nerve** ♀

● **N8Ø.D5 Endometriosis of the pudendal nerve** ♀

● **N8Ø.D6 Endometriosis of the femoral nerve** ♀

● **N8Ø.D9 Endometriosis of other pelvic nerve** ♀

Endometriosis of the other nerves of the retroperitoneum

N8Ø.8 Other endometriosis ♀

▶Endometriosis of other site◀

N8Ø.9 Endometriosis, unspecified ♀

✓4th **N81 Female genital prolapse**

EXCLUDES 1 *genital prolapse complicating pregnancy, labor or delivery (O34.5-)*

prolapse and hernia of ovary and fallopian tube (N83.4-)

prolapse of vaginal vault after hysterectomy (N99.3)

Types of Pelvic Organ Prolapse

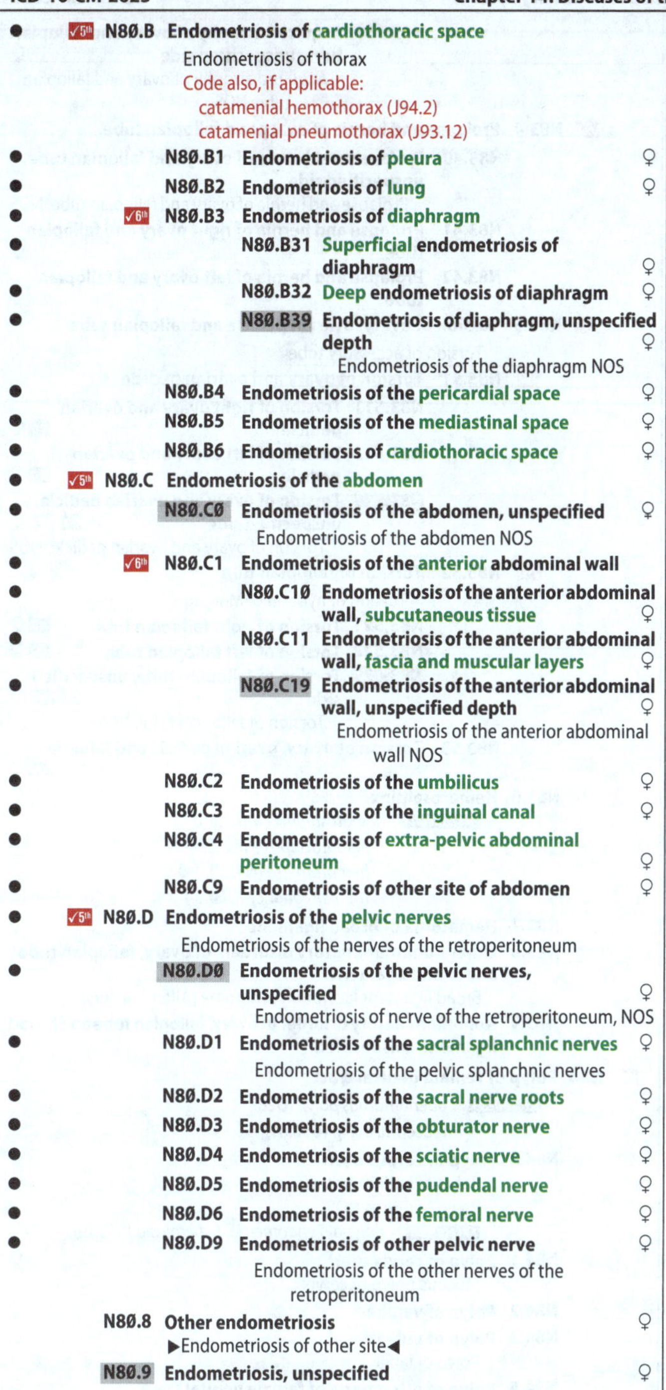

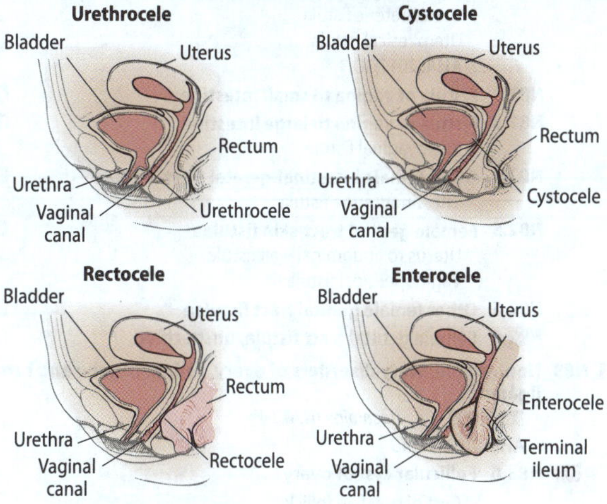

N81.Ø Urethrocele ♀

EXCLUDES 1 *urethrocele with cystocele (N81.1-)*

urethrocele with prolapse of uterus (N81.2-N81.4)

✓5th **N81.1 Cystocele**

Cystocele with urethrocele

Cystourethrocele

EXCLUDES 1 *cystocele with prolapse of uterus (N81.2-N81.4)*

N81.1Ø Cystocele, unspecified ♀

Prolapse of (anterior) vaginal wall NOS

N81.11 Cystocele, midline ♀

N81.12 Cystocele, lateral ♀

Paravaginal cystocele

DEF: Detachment of the lateral support connections of the vagina at the arcus tendineus fasciae pelvis (ATFP) that results in bladder drop. The bladder herniates into the vagina laterally.

N81.2 Incomplete uterovaginal prolapse ♀

First degree uterine prolapse

Prolapse of cervix NOS

Second degree uterine prolapse

EXCLUDES 1 *cervical stump prolapse (N81.85)*

N81.3 Complete uterovaginal prolapse ♀

Procidentia (uteri) NOS

Third degree uterine prolapse

N81.4 Uterovaginal prolapse, unspecified ♀

Prolapse of uterus NOS

N81.5 Vaginal enterocele ♀

EXCLUDES 1 *enterocele with prolapse of uterus (N81.2-N81.4)*

N81.6 Rectocele ♀

Prolapse of posterior vaginal wall

Use additional code for any associated fecal incontinence, if applicable (R15.-)

EXCLUDES 2 *perineocele (N81.81)*

rectal prolapse (K62.3)

rectocele with prolapse of uterus (N81.2-N81.4)

✓5th **N81.8 Other female genital prolapse**

N81.81 Perineocele ♀

N81.82 Incompetence or weakening of pubocervical tissue ♀

N81.83 Incompetence or weakening of rectovaginal tissue ♀

N81.84 Pelvic muscle wasting ♀

Disuse atrophy of pelvic muscles and anal sphincter

N81.85 Cervical stump prolapse ♀

N81.89 Other female genital prolapse ♀

Deficient perineum

Old laceration of muscles of pelvic floor

N81.9 Female genital prolapse, unspecified ♀

✓4th N82 Fistulae involving female genital tract

EXCLUDES 1 *vesicointestinal fistulae (N32.1)*

N82.Ø Vesicovaginal fistula CC ♀

N82.1 Other female urinary-genital tract fistulae CC ♀

Cervicovesical fistula

Ureterovaginal fistula

Urethrovaginal fistula

Uteroureteric fistula

Uterovesical fistula

AHA: 2017,3Q,3

N82.2 Fistula of vagina to small intestine CC ♀

N82.3 Fistula of vagina to large intestine CC ♀

Rectovaginal fistula

N82.4 Other female intestinal-genital tract fistulae CC ♀

Intestinouterine fistula

N82.5 Female genital tract-skin fistulae CC ♀

Uterus to abdominal wall fistula

Vaginoperineal fistula

N82.8 Other female genital tract fistulae CC ♀

N82.9 Female genital tract fistula, unspecified CC ♀

✓4th N83 Noninflammatory disorders of ovary, fallopian tube and broad ligament

EXCLUDES 2 *hydrosalpinx (N7Ø.1-)*

AHA: 2016,4Q,46

✓5th N83.Ø Follicular cyst of ovary

Cyst of graafian follicle

Hemorrhagic follicular cyst (of ovary)

N83.ØØ Follicular cyst of ovary, unspecified side ♀

N83.Ø1 Follicular cyst of right ovary ♀

N83.Ø2 Follicular cyst of left ovary ♀

✓5th N83.1 Corpus luteum cyst

Hemorrhagic corpus luteum cyst

AHA: 2022,1Q,23

N83.1Ø Corpus luteum cyst of ovary, unspecified side ♀

N83.11 Corpus luteum cyst of right ovary ♀

N83.12 Corpus luteum cyst of left ovary ♀

✓5th N83.2 Other and unspecified ovarian cysts

EXCLUDES 1 *developmental ovarian cyst (Q5Ø.1)*
neoplastic ovarian cyst (D27.-)
polycystic ovarian syndrome (E28.2)
Stein-Leventhal syndrome (E28.2)

AHA: 2022,1Q,23

✓6th N83.2Ø Unspecified ovarian cysts

N83.2Ø1 Unspecified ovarian cyst, right side ♀

N83.2Ø2 Unspecified ovarian cyst, left side ♀

N83.2Ø9 Unspecified ovarian cyst, unspecified side ♀

Ovarian cyst, NOS

✓6th N83.29 Other ovarian cysts

Retention cyst of ovary

Simple cyst of ovary

N83.291 Other ovarian cyst, right side ♀

N83.292 Other ovarian cyst, left side ♀

N83.299 Other ovarian cyst, unspecified side ♀

✓5th N83.3 Acquired atrophy of ovary and fallopian tube

✓6th N83.31 Acquired atrophy of ovary

N83.311 Acquired atrophy of right ovary ♀

N83.312 Acquired atrophy of left ovary ♀

N83.319 Acquired atrophy of ovary, unspecified side ♀

Acquired atrophy of ovary, NOS

✓6th N83.32 Acquired atrophy of fallopian tube

N83.321 Acquired atrophy of right fallopian tube ♀

N83.322 Acquired atrophy of left fallopian tube ♀

N83.329 Acquired atrophy of fallopian tube, unspecified side ♀

Acquired atrophy of fallopian tube, NOS

✓6th N83.33 Acquired atrophy of ovary and fallopian tube

N83.331 Acquired atrophy of right ovary and fallopian tube ♀

N83.332 Acquired atrophy of left ovary and fallopian tube ♀

N83.339 Acquired atrophy of ovary and fallopian tube, unspecified side ♀

Acquired atrophy of ovary and fallopian tube, NOS

✓5th N83.4 Prolapse and hernia of ovary and fallopian tube

N83.4Ø Prolapse and hernia of ovary and fallopian tube, unspecified side ♀

Prolapse and hernia of ovary and fallopian tube, NOS

N83.41 Prolapse and hernia of right ovary and fallopian tube ♀

N83.42 Prolapse and hernia of left ovary and fallopian tube ♀

✓5th N83.5 Torsion of ovary, ovarian pedicle and fallopian tube

Torsion of accessory tube

✓6th N83.51 Torsion of ovary and ovarian pedicle

N83.511 Torsion of right ovary and ovarian pedicle CC ♀

N83.512 Torsion of left ovary and ovarian pedicle CC ♀

N83.519 Torsion of ovary and ovarian pedicle, unspecified side CC UNS ♀

Torsion of ovary and ovarian pedicle, NOS

✓6th N83.52 Torsion of fallopian tube

Torsion of hydatid of Morgagni

N83.521 Torsion of right fallopian tube CC ♀

N83.522 Torsion of left fallopian tube CC ♀

N83.529 Torsion of fallopian tube, unspecified side CC UNS ♀

Torsion of fallopian tube, NOS

N83.53 Torsion of ovary, ovarian pedicle and fallopian tube CC ♀

N83.6 Hematosalpinx ♀

EXCLUDES 1 *hematosalpinx (with) (in):*
hematocolpos (N89.7)
hematometra (N85.7)
tubal pregnancy (OØØ.1-)

N83.7 Hematoma of broad ligament ♀

N83.8 Other noninflammatory disorders of ovary, fallopian tube and broad ligament ♀

Broad ligament laceration syndrome [Allen-Masters]

N83.9 Noninflammatory disorder of ovary, fallopian tube and broad ligament, unspecified ♀

✓4th N84 Polyp of female genital tract

EXCLUDES 1 *adenomatous polyp (D28.-)*
placental polyp (O9Ø.89)

N84.Ø Polyp of corpus uteri ♀

Polyp of endometrium

Polyp of uterus NOS

EXCLUDES 1 *polypoid endometrial hyperplasia (N85.Ø-)*

N84.1 Polyp of cervix uteri ♀

Mucous polyp of cervix

N84.2 Polyp of vagina ♀

N84.3 Polyp of vulva ♀

Polyp of labia

N84.8 Polyp of other parts of female genital tract ♀

N84.9 Polyp of female genital tract, unspecified ♀

✓4th N85 Other noninflammatory disorders of uterus, except cervix

EXCLUDES 1 *endometriosis (N8Ø.-)*
inflammatory diseases of uterus (N71.-)
noninflammatory disorders of cervix, except malposition (N86-N88)
polyp of corpus uteri (N84.Ø)
uterine prolapse (N81.-)

✓5th N85.Ø Endometrial hyperplasia

N85.ØØ Endometrial hyperplasia, unspecified ♀

Hyperplasia (adenomatous) (cystic) (glandular) of endometrium

Hyperplastic endometritis

N85.Ø1 Benign endometrial hyperplasia ♀

Endometrial hyperplasia (complex) (simple) without atypia

N85.02 Endometrial intraepithelial neoplasia [EIN] ♀
Endometrial hyperplasia with atypia
EXCLUDES 1 *malignant neoplasm of endometrium (with endometrial intraepithelial neoplasia [EIN]) (C54.1)*

N85.2 Hypertrophy of uterus ♀
Bulky or enlarged uterus
EXCLUDES 1 *puerperal hypertrophy of uterus (O90.89)*

N85.3 Subinvolution of uterus ♀
EXCLUDES 1 *puerperal subinvolution of uterus (O90.89)*

N85.4 Malposition of uterus ♀
Anteversion of uterus
Retroflexion of uterus
Retroversion of uterus
EXCLUDES 1 *malposition of uterus complicating pregnancy, labor or delivery (O34.5-, O65.5)*

N85.5 Inversion of uterus ♀
EXCLUDES 1 *current obstetric trauma (O71.2)*
postpartum inversion of uterus (O71.2)
DEF: Abnormality in which the uterus turns inside out.

Inversion of Uterus

N85.6 Intrauterine synechiae ♀

N85.7 Hematometra ♀
Hematosalpinx with hematometra
EXCLUDES 1 *hematometra with hematocolpos (N89.7)*
DEF: Accumulation of blood within the uterus.

N85.8 Other specified noninflammatory disorders of uterus ♀
Atrophy of uterus, acquired
Fibrosis of uterus NOS

N85.9 Noninflammatory disorder of uterus, unspecified ♀
Disorder of uterus NOS

● **N85.A Isthmocele**
Isthmocele (non-pregnant state)
Code also any associated conditions such as:
abnormal uterine and vaginal bleeding, unspecified (N93.9)
female infertility of uterine origin (N97.2)
pelvic and perineal pain (R10.2)
EXCLUDES 1 *maternal care for cesarean scar defect (isthmocele) (O34.22)*

N86 Erosion and ectropion of cervix uteri ♀
Decubitus (trophic) ulcer of cervix
Eversion of cervix
EXCLUDES 1 *erosion and ectropion of cervix with cervicitis (N72)*

N87 Dysplasia of cervix uteri
EXCLUDES 1 *abnormal results from cervical cytologic examination without histologic confirmation (R87.61-)*
carcinoma in situ of cervix uteri (D06.-)
cervical intraepithelial neoplasia III [CIN III] (D06.-)
HGSIL of cervix (R87.613)
severe dysplasia of cervix uteri (D06.-)

N87.0 Mild cervical dysplasia ♀
Cervical intraepithelial neoplasia I [CIN I]

N87.1 Moderate cervical dysplasia ♀
Cervical intraepithelial neoplasia II [CIN II]

N87.9 Dysplasia of cervix uteri, unspecified ♀
Anaplasia of cervix
Cervical atypism
Cervical dysplasia NOS

N88 Other noninflammatory disorders of cervix uteri
EXCLUDES 2 *inflammatory disease of cervix (N72)*
polyp of cervix (N84.1)

N88.0 Leukoplakia of cervix uteri ♀

N88.1 Old laceration of cervix uteri ♀
Adhesions of cervix
EXCLUDES 1 *current obstetric trauma (O71.3)*

N88.2 Stricture and stenosis of cervix uteri ♀
EXCLUDES 1 *stricture and stenosis of cervix uteri complicating labor (O65.5)*

N88.3 Incompetence of cervix uteri ♀
Investigation and management of (suspected) cervical incompetence in a nonpregnant woman
EXCLUDES 1 *cervical incompetence complicating pregnancy (O34.3-)*
DEF: Inadequate functioning of the cervix marked by abnormal widening during pregnancy and causing premature birth or miscarriage.

N88.4 Hypertrophic elongation of cervix uteri ♀

N88.8 Other specified noninflammatory disorders of cervix uteri ♀
EXCLUDES 1 *current obstetric trauma (O71.3)*

N88.9 Noninflammatory disorder of cervix uteri, unspecified ♀

N89 Other noninflammatory disorders of vagina
EXCLUDES 1 *abnormal results from vaginal cytologic examination without histologic confirmation (R87.62-)*
carcinoma in situ of vagina (D07.2)
HGSIL of vagina (R87.623)
inflammation of vagina (N76.-)
senile (atrophic) vaginitis (N95.2)
severe dysplasia of vagina (D07.2)
trichomonal leukorrhea (A59.00)
vaginal intraepithelial neoplasia [VAIN], grade III (D07.2)

N89.0 Mild vaginal dysplasia ♀
Vaginal intraepithelial neoplasia [VAIN], grade I

N89.1 Moderate vaginal dysplasia ♀
Vaginal intraepithelial neoplasia [VAIN], grade II

N89.3 Dysplasia of vagina, unspecified ♀

N89.4 Leukoplakia of vagina ♀

N89.5 Stricture and atresia of vagina ♀
Vaginal adhesions
Vaginal stenosis
EXCLUDES 1 *congenital atresia or stricture (Q52.4)*
postprocedural adhesions of vagina (N99.2)

N89.6 Tight hymenal ring ♀
Rigid hymen
Tight introitus
EXCLUDES 1 *imperforate hymen (Q52.3)*

N89.7 Hematocolpos ♀
Hematocolpos with hematometra or hematosalpinx
AHA: 2016,4Q,58

N89.8 Other specified noninflammatory disorders of vagina ♀
Leukorrhea NOS
Old vaginal laceration
Pessary ulcer of vagina
EXCLUDES 1 *current obstetric trauma (O70.-, O71.4, O71.7-O71.8)*
old laceration involving muscles of pelvic floor (N81.8)

N89.9 Noninflammatory disorder of vagina, unspecified ♀

N90 Other noninflammatory disorders of vulva and perineum
EXCLUDES 1 *anogenital (venereal) warts (A63.0)*
carcinoma in situ of vulva (D07.1)
condyloma acuminatum (A63.0)
current obstetric trauma (O70.-, O71.7-O71.8)
inflammation of vulva (N76.-)
severe dysplasia of vulva (D07.1)
vulvar intraepithelial neoplasm III [VIN III] (D07.1)

N90.0 Mild vulvar dysplasia ♀
Vulvar intraepithelial neoplasia [VIN], grade I

N90.1 Moderate vulvar dysplasia ♀
Vulvar intraepithelial neoplasia [VIN], grade II

N90.3 Dysplasia of vulva, unspecified ♀

N90.4 Leukoplakia of vulva ♀
Dystrophy of vulva
Kraurosis of vulva
Lichen sclerosus of external female genital organs

N90.5 Atrophy of vulva ♀
Stenosis of vulva

N90.6 Hypertrophy of vulva
AHA: 2016,4Q,46

N90.60 Unspecified hypertrophy of vulva ♀
Unspecified hypertrophy of labia

N90.61 Childhood asymmetric labium majus enlargement ♀
CALME

N90.69 Other specified hypertrophy of vulva ♀
Other specified hypertrophy of labia

N90.7 Vulvar cyst ♀

N90.8 Other specified noninflammatory disorders of vulva and perineum

N90.81 Female genital mutilation status
Female genital cutting status

N90.810 Female genital mutilation status, unspecified ♀
Female genital cutting status, unspecified
Female genital mutilation status NOS

N90.811 Female genital mutilation Type I status ♀
Clitorectomy status
Female genital cutting Type I status

N90.812 Female genital mutilation Type II status ♀
Clitorectomy with excision of labia minora status
Female genital cutting Type II status

N90.813 Female genital mutilation Type III status ♀
Female genital cutting Type III status
Infibulation status

N90.818 Other female genital mutilation status ♀
Female genital cutting Type IV status
Female genital mutilation Type IV status
Other female genital cutting status

N90.89 Other specified noninflammatory disorders of vulva and perineum ♀
Adhesions of vulva
Hypertrophy of clitoris

N90.9 Noninflammatory disorder of vulva and perineum, unspecified ♀

N91 Absent, scanty and rare menstruation
EXCLUDES 1 *ovarian dysfunction (E28.-)*

N91.0 Primary amenorrhea ♀
N91.1 Secondary amenorrhea ♀
N91.2 Amenorrhea, unspecified ♀
N91.3 Primary oligomenorrhea ♀
N91.4 Secondary oligomenorrhea ♀
N91.5 Oligomenorrhea, unspecified ♀
Hypomenorrhea NOS

N92 Excessive, frequent and irregular menstruation
EXCLUDES 1 *postmenopausal bleeding (N95.0)*
precocious puberty (menstruation) (E30.1)

N92.0 Excessive and frequent menstruation with regular cycle ♀
Heavy periods NOS
Menorrhagia NOS
Polymenorrhea

N92.1 Excessive and frequent menstruation with irregular cycle ♀
Irregular intermenstrual bleeding
Irregular, shortened intervals between menstrual bleeding
Menometrorrhagia
Metrorrhagia

N92.2 Excessive menstruation at puberty P ♀
Excessive bleeding associated with onset of menstrual periods
Pubertal menorrhagia
Puberty bleeding

N92.3 Ovulation bleeding ♀
Regular intermenstrual bleeding

N92.4 Excessive bleeding in the premenopausal period ♀
Climacteric menorrhagia or metrorrhagia
Menopausal menorrhagia or metrorrhagia
Perimenopausal bleeding
Perimenopausal menorrhagia or metrorrhagia
Preclimacteric menorrhagia or metrorrhagia
Premenopausal menorrhagia or metrorrhagia

N92.5 Other specified irregular menstruation ♀

N92.6 Irregular menstruation, unspecified ♀
Irregular bleeding NOS
Irregular periods NOS
EXCLUDES 1 *irregular menstruation with:*
lengthened intervals or scanty bleeding (N91.3-N91.5)
shortened intervals or excessive bleeding (N92.1)

N93 Other abnormal uterine and vaginal bleeding
EXCLUDES 1 *neonatal vaginal hemorrhage (P54.6)*
precocious puberty (menstruation) (E30.1)
pseudomenses (P54.6)

N93.0 Postcoital and contact bleeding ♀

N93.1 Pre-pubertal vaginal bleeding ♀
AHA: 2016,4Q,47

N93.8 Other specified abnormal uterine and vaginal bleeding ♀
Dysfunctional or functional uterine or vaginal bleeding NOS

N93.9 Abnormal uterine and vaginal bleeding, unspecified ♀

N94 Pain and other conditions associated with female genital organs and menstrual cycle

N94.0 Mittelschmerz ♀
DEF: One-sided, lower abdominal pain occurring between menstrual periods that is associated with ovulation.

N94.1 Dyspareunia
EXCLUDES 1 *psychogenic dyspareunia (F52.6)*
AHA: 2016,4Q,47

N94.10 Unspecified dyspareunia ♀
N94.11 Superficial (introital) dyspareunia ♀
N94.12 Deep dyspareunia ♀
N94.19 Other specified dyspareunia ♀

N94.2 Vaginismus ♀
EXCLUDES 1 *psychogenic vaginismus (F52.5)*
DEF: Spontaneous contractions of the muscles surrounding the vagina, causing it to constrict or close.

N94.3 Premenstrual tension syndrome ♀
Code also associated menstrual migraine (G43.82-, G43.83-)
EXCLUDES 1 *premenstrual dysphoric disorder (F32.81)*

N94.4 Primary dysmenorrhea ♀
N94.5 Secondary dysmenorrhea ♀
N94.6 Dysmenorrhea, unspecified ♀
EXCLUDES 1 *psychogenic dysmenorrhea (F45.8)*

N94.8 Other specified conditions associated with female genital organs and menstrual cycle

N94.81 Vulvodynia
N94.810 Vulvar vestibulitis ♀
N94.818 Other vulvodynia ♀
N94.819 Vulvodynia, unspecified ♀
Vulvodynia NOS

N94.89 Other specified conditions associated with female genital organs and menstrual cycle ♀
DEF: Hydrocele: Serous fluid that collects in the canal of Nuck in females.

N94.9 Unspecified condition associated with female genital organs and menstrual cycle ♀

N95 Menopausal and other perimenopausal disorders
Menopausal and other perimenopausal disorders due to naturally occurring (age-related) menopause and perimenopause
EXCLUDES 1 *excessive bleeding in the premenopausal period (N92.4)*
menopausal and perimenopausal disorders due to artificial or premature menopause (E89.4-, E28.31-)
premature menopause (E28.31-)
EXCLUDES 2 *postmenopausal osteoporosis (M81.Ø-)*
postmenopausal osteoporosis with current pathological fracture (M8Ø.Ø-)
postmenopausal urethritis (N34.2)

N95.Ø Postmenopausal bleeding ♀
N95.1 Menopausal and female climacteric states ♀
Symptoms such as flushing, sleeplessness, headache, lack of concentration, associated with natural (age-related) menopause
Use additional code for associated symptoms
EXCLUDES 1 *asymptomatic menopausal state (Z78.Ø)*
symptoms associated with artificial menopause (E89.41)
symptoms associated with premature menopause (E28.31Ø)
N95.2 Postmenopausal atrophic vaginitis ♀
Senile (atrophic) vaginitis
N95.8 Other specified menopausal and perimenopausal disorders ♀
N95.9 Unspecified menopausal and perimenopausal disorder ♀

N96 Recurrent pregnancy loss ♀
Investigation or care in a nonpregnant woman with history of recurrent pregnancy loss
EXCLUDES 1 *recurrent pregnancy loss with current pregnancy (O26.2-)*

N97 Female infertility
INCLUDES inability to achieve a pregnancy
sterility, female NOS
EXCLUDES 2 *female infertility associated with:*
hypopituitarism (E23.Ø)
Stein-Leventhal syndrome (E28.2)
incompetence of cervix uteri (N88.3)
DEF: Infertility: Inability to conceive for at least one year with regular intercourse.
DEF: Primary infertility: Infertility occurring in patients who have never conceived.
DEF: Secondary infertility: Infertility occurring in patients who have previously conceived.

N97.Ø Female infertility associated with anovulation ♀
AHA: 2022,2Q,16
N97.1 Female infertility of tubal origin ♀
Female infertility associated with congenital anomaly of tube
Female infertility due to tubal block
Female infertility due to tubal occlusion
Female infertility due to tubal stenosis
N97.2 Female infertility of uterine origin ♀
Female infertility associated with congenital anomaly of uterus
Female infertility due to nonimplantation of ovum
N97.8 Female infertility of other origin ♀
AHA: 2022,2Q,15
N97.9 Female infertility, unspecified ♀

N98 Complications associated with artificial fertilization
N98.Ø Infection associated with artificial insemination CC ♀
N98.1 Hyperstimulation of ovaries CC ♀
Hyperstimulation of ovaries NOS
Hyperstimulation of ovaries associated with induced ovulation
N98.2 Complications of attempted introduction of fertilized ovum following in vitro fertilization CC ♀
N98.3 Complications of attempted introduction of embryo in embryo transfer CC ♀
N98.8 Other complications associated with artificial fertilization CC ♀
N98.9 Complication associated with artificial fertilization, unspecified CC ♀

Intraoperative and postprocedural complications and disorders of genitourinary system, not elsewhere classified (N99)

N99 Intraoperative and postprocedural complications and disorders of genitourinary system, not elsewhere classified
EXCLUDES 2 *irradiation cystitis (N3Ø.4-)*
postoophorectomy osteoporosis with current pathological fracture (M8Ø.8-)
postoophorectomy osteoporosis without current pathological fracture (M81.8)

N99.Ø Postprocedural (acute) (chronic) kidney failure
Use additional code to type of kidney disease
N99.1 Postprocedural urethral stricture
Postcatheterization urethral stricture
N99.11 Postprocedural urethral stricture, male
AHA: 2016,4Q,47-48
N99.11Ø Postprocedural urethral stricture, male, meatal ♂
N99.111 Postprocedural bulbous urethral stricture, male ♂
N99.112 Postprocedural membranous urethral stricture, male ♂
N99.113 Postprocedural anterior bulbous urethral stricture, male ♂
N99.114 Postprocedural urethral stricture, male, unspecified ♂
N99.115 Postprocedural fossa navicularis urethral stricture ♂
N99.116 Postprocedural urethral stricture, male, overlapping sites ♂
N99.12 Postprocedural urethral stricture, female ♀
N99.2 Postprocedural adhesions of vagina ♀
N99.3 Prolapse of vaginal vault after hysterectomy ♀
N99.4 Postprocedural pelvic peritoneal adhesions
EXCLUDES 2 *pelvic peritoneal adhesions NOS (N73.6)*
postinfective pelvic peritoneal adhesions (N73.6)
N99.5 Complications of stoma of urinary tract
EXCLUDES 2 *mechanical complication of urinary catheter (T83.Ø-)*
AHA: 2016,4Q,48
N99.51 Complication of cystostomy
N99.51Ø Cystostomy hemorrhage CC HCC
N99.511 Cystostomy infection CC HCC
N99.512 Cystostomy malfunction CC HCC
N99.518 Other cystostomy complication CC HCC
N99.52 Complication of incontinent external stoma of urinary tract
N99.52Ø Hemorrhage of incontinent external stoma of urinary tract HCC
N99.521 Infection of incontinent external stoma of urinary tract HCC
N99.522 Malfunction of incontinent external stoma of urinary tract HCC
N99.523 Herniation of incontinent stoma of urinary tract HCC
N99.524 Stenosis of incontinent stoma of urinary tract HCC
N99.528 Other complication of incontinent external stoma of urinary tract HCC
N99.53 Complication of continent stoma of urinary tract
N99.53Ø Hemorrhage of continent stoma of urinary tract HCC
N99.531 Infection of continent stoma of urinary tract HCC
N99.532 Malfunction of continent stoma of urinary tract HCC
N99.533 Herniation of continent stoma of urinary tract HCC
N99.534 Stenosis of continent stoma of urinary tract HCC
N99.538 Other complication of continent stoma of urinary tract HCC

√5th **N99.6 Intraoperative hemorrhage and hematoma of a genitourinary system organ or structure complicating a procedure**

EXCLUDES 1 *intraoperative hemorrhage and hematoma of a genitourinary system organ or structure due to accidental puncture or laceration during a procedure (N99.7-)*

N99.61 Intraoperative hemorrhage and hematoma of a genitourinary system organ or structure complicating a genitourinary system procedure CC

N99.62 Intraoperative hemorrhage and hematoma of a genitourinary system organ or structure complicating other procedure CC

√5th **N99.7 Accidental puncture and laceration of a genitourinary system organ or structure during a procedure**

N99.71 Accidental puncture and laceration of a genitourinary system organ or structure during a genitourinary system procedure CC

N99.72 Accidental puncture and laceration of a genitourinary system organ or structure during other procedure CC

√5th **N99.8 Other intraoperative and postprocedural complications and disorders of genitourinary system**

AHA: 2016,4Q,9-10

N99.81 Other intraoperative complications of genitourinary system

√6th **N99.82 Postprocedural hemorrhage of a genitourinary system organ or structure following a procedure**

N99.820 Postprocedural hemorrhage of a genitourinary system organ or structure following a genitourinary system procedure CC

N99.821 Postprocedural hemorrhage of a genitourinary system organ or structure following other procedure CC

N99.83 Residual ovary syndrome ♀

√6th **N99.84 Postprocedural hematoma and seroma of a genitourinary system organ or structure following a procedure**

N99.840 Postprocedural hematoma of a genitourinary system organ or structure following a genitourinary system procedure CC

N99.841 Postprocedural hematoma of a genitourinary system organ or structure following other procedure CC

N99.842 Postprocedural seroma of a genitourinary system organ or structure following a genitourinary system procedure CC

N99.843 Postprocedural seroma of a genitourinary system organ or structure following other procedure CC

N99.85 Post endometrial ablation syndrome ♀

AHA: 2019,4Q,12

N99.89 Other postprocedural complications and disorders of genitourinary system

Chapter 15. Pregnancy, Childbirth and the Puerperium (O00–O9A)

Chapter-specific Guidelines with Coding Examples

The chapter-specific guidelines from the ICD-10-CM Official Guidelines for Coding and Reporting have been provided below. Along with these guidelines are coding examples, contained in the shaded boxes, that have been developed to help illustrate the coding and/or sequencing guidance found in these guidelines.

a. General rules for obstetric cases

1) Codes from Chapter 15 and sequencing priority

Obstetric cases require codes from chapter 15, codes in the range O00-O9A, Pregnancy, Childbirth, and the Puerperium. Chapter 15 codes have sequencing priority over codes from other chapters. Additional codes from other chapters may be used in conjunction with chapter 15 codes to further specify conditions. Should the provider document that the pregnancy is incidental to the encounter, then code Z33.1, Pregnant state, incidental, should be used in place of any chapter 15 codes. It is the provider's responsibility to state that the condition being treated is not affecting the pregnancy.

Pregnant patient at 25 weeks' gestation admitted for bladder abscess

O23.12	**Infections of bladder in pregnancy, second trimester**
N30.80	**Other cystitis without hematuria**
Z3A.25	**25 weeks gestation of pregnancy**

Explanation: The documentation does not indicate that the pregnancy is incidental or in any way unaffected by the bladder abscess; therefore, an obstetrics code should be sequenced first. An additional code was provided to identify the specific bladder condition as this information is not called out specifically in the obstetrics code.

2) Chapter 15 codes used only on the maternal record

Chapter 15 codes are to be used only on the maternal record, never on the record of the newborn.

3) Final character for trimester

The majority of codes in Chapter 15 have a final character indicating the trimester of pregnancy. The timeframes for the trimesters are indicated at the beginning of the chapter. If trimester is not a component of a code, it is because the condition always occurs in a specific trimester, or the concept of trimester of pregnancy is not applicable. Certain codes have characters for only certain trimesters because the condition does not occur in all trimesters, but it may occur in more than just one.

Assignment of the final character for trimester should be based on the provider's documentation of the trimester (or number of weeks) for the current admission/encounter. This applies to the assignment of trimester for pre-existing conditions as well as those that develop during or are due to the pregnancy. The provider's documentation of the number of weeks may be used to assign the appropriate code identifying the trimester.

Whenever delivery occurs during the current admission, and there is an "in childbirth" option for the obstetric complication being coded, the "in childbirth" code should be assigned. When the classification does not provide an obstetric code with an "in childbirth" option, it is appropriate to assign a code describing the current trimester.

Pregnant patient at 21 weeks' gestation admitted with excessive vomiting

O21.2	**Late vomiting of pregnancy**
Z3A.21	**21 weeks gestation of pregnancy**

Explanation: Category O21 classifies vomiting in pregnancy. Although code selection is based on whether the vomiting is before or after 20 completed weeks, these codes are not further classified by trimester. If vomiting only in the second trimester was documented, the provider should be queried for the specific week of gestation, as this will affect code selection.

4) Selection of trimester for inpatient admissions that encompass more than one trimester

In instances when a patient is admitted to a hospital for complications of pregnancy during one trimester and remains in the hospital into a subsequent trimester, the trimester character for the antepartum complication code should be assigned on the basis of the trimester when the complication developed, not the trimester of the discharge. If the condition developed prior to the current admission/encounter or represents a pre-existing condition, the trimester character for the trimester at the time of the admission/encounter should be assigned.

Patient admitted at 27 6/7 weeks' gestation for hemorrhaging from partial placenta previa; three days after admission at 28 1/7 weeks' gestation, she developed gestational hypertension

O44.32	**Partial placenta previa with hemorrhage, second trimester**
O13.3	**Gestational [pregnancy-induced] hypertension without significant proteinuria, third trimester**
Z3A.27	**27 weeks gestation of pregnancy**

Explanation: The patient presented with hemorrhaging from partial placenta previa while still in her 27th week, which falls within the second trimester. The gestational hypertension did not occur until three days after admission, putting the patient in her 28th week of pregnancy or what is considered to be the third trimester. The weeks of gestation captured by a code from category Z3A should represent only the gestational weeks upon admission.

5) Unspecified trimester

Each category that includes codes for trimester has a code for "unspecified trimester." The "unspecified trimester" code should rarely be used, such as when the documentation in the record is insufficient to determine the trimester and it is not possible to obtain clarification.

6) 7th character for fetus identification

Where applicable, a 7th character is to be assigned for certain categories (O31, O32, O33.3 - O33.6, O35, O36, O40, O41, O60.1, O60.2, O64, and O69) to identify the fetus for which the complication code applies.

Assign 7th character "0":

- For single gestations
- When the documentation in the record is insufficient to determine the fetus affected and it is not possible to obtain clarification.
- When it is not possible to clinically determine which fetus is affected.

7) Completed weeks of gestation

In ICD-10-CM, "completed" weeks of gestation refers to full weeks. For example, if the provider documents gestation at 39 weeks and 6 days, the code for 39 weeks of gestation should be assigned, as the patient has not yet reached 40 completed weeks.

b. Selection of OB principal or first-listed diagnosis

1) Routine outpatient prenatal visits

For routine outpatient prenatal visits when no complications are present, a code from category Z34, Encounter for supervision of normal pregnancy, should be used as the first-listed diagnosis. These codes should not be used in conjunction with chapter 15 codes.

2) Supervision of high-risk pregnancy

Codes from category O09, Supervision of high-risk pregnancy, are intended for use only during the prenatal period. For complications during the labor or delivery episode as a result of a high-risk pregnancy, assign the applicable complication codes from Chapter 15. If there are no complications during the labor or delivery episode, assign code O80, Encounter for full-term uncomplicated delivery.

For routine prenatal outpatient visits for patients with high-risk pregnancies, a code from category O09, Supervision of high-risk pregnancy, should be used as the first-listed diagnosis. Secondary chapter 15 codes may be used in conjunction with these codes if appropriate.

36-year-old with history of preterm labor admitted in labor with second child at 39 weeks' gestation, delivered healthy baby without complications

O80	**Encounter for full-term uncomplicated delivery**
Z3A.39	**39 weeks gestation of pregnancy**
Z37.0	**Single live birth**

Explanation: Although this patient is over 35 and having her second child (elderly multigravida) and has a history of preterm labor with her first child, no codes from category O09.- should be appended. In the absence of any other complications noted during the encounter, code O80 is the most appropriate code to describe the principal diagnosis.

3) Episodes when no delivery occurs

In episodes when no delivery occurs, the principal diagnosis should correspond to the principal complication of the pregnancy which necessitated the encounter. Should more than one complication exist, all of which are treated or monitored, any of the complication codes may be sequenced first.

4) When a delivery occurs

When an obstetric patient is admitted and delivers during that admission, the condition that prompted the admission should be sequenced as the principal diagnosis. If multiple conditions prompted the admission, sequence the one most related to the delivery as the principal diagnosis. A code for any complication of the delivery should be assigned as an additional diagnosis. In cases of cesarean delivery, if the patient was admitted with a condition that resulted in the performance of a cesarean procedure, that condition should be selected as the principal diagnosis. If the reason for the admission was unrelated to the condition resulting in the cesarean delivery, the condition related to the reason for the admission should be selected as the principal diagnosis.

Maternal patient with diet-controlled gestational diabetes was admitted at 38 weeks' gestation in obstructed labor due to footling presentation; cesarean performed for the malpresentation

O64.8XXØ	**Obstructed labor due to other malposition and malpresentation, not applicable or unspecified**
O24.42Ø	**Gestational diabetes mellitus in childbirth, diet controlled**
Z3A.38	**38 weeks gestation of pregnancy**
Z37.Ø	**Single live birth**

Explanation: The obstructed labor necessitated the cesarean procedure.

At 39 weeks' gestation, a maternal patient presents with hemorrhage with coagulation defect; the next day the patient goes into labor and eventually delivers via cesarean section due to arrested active phase of labor

O46.ØØ3	**Antepartum hemorrhage with coagulation defect, unspecified, third trimester**
O62.1	**Secondary uterine inertia**
Z3A.39	**39 weeks gestation of pregnancy**
Z37.Ø	**Single live birth**

Explanation: The patient was admitted because of the antepartum hemorrhage with coagulation defect. The arrested active phase, although the reason for the cesarean delivery, did not develop until later into the stay.

5) Outcome of delivery

A code from category Z37, Outcome of delivery, should be included on every maternal record when a delivery has occurred. These codes are not to be used on subsequent records or on the newborn record.

c. Pre-existing conditions versus conditions due to the pregnancy

Certain categories in Chapter 15 distinguish between conditions of the mother that existed prior to pregnancy (pre-existing) and those that are a direct result of pregnancy. When assigning codes from Chapter 15, it is important to assess if a condition was pre-existing prior to pregnancy or developed during or due to the pregnancy in order to assign the correct code.

Categories that do not distinguish between pre-existing and pregnancy-related conditions may be used for either. It is acceptable to use codes specifically for the puerperium with codes complicating pregnancy and childbirth if a condition arises postpartum during the delivery encounter.

d. Pre-existing hypertension in pregnancy

Category O1Ø, Pre-existing hypertension complicating pregnancy, childbirth and the puerperium, includes codes for hypertensive heart and hypertensive chronic kidney disease. When assigning one of the O1Ø codes that includes hypertensive heart disease or hypertensive chronic kidney disease, it is necessary to add a secondary code from the appropriate hypertension category to specify the type of heart failure or chronic kidney disease.

See Section I.C.9. Hypertension.

e. Fetal conditions affecting the management of the mother

1) Codes from categories O35 and O36

Codes from categories O35, Maternal care for known or suspected fetal abnormality and damage, and O36, Maternal care for other fetal problems, are assigned only when the fetal condition is actually responsible for modifying the management of the mother, i.e., by requiring diagnostic studies, additional observation, special care, or termination of pregnancy. The fact that the fetal condition exists does not justify assigning a code from this series to the mother's record.

A patient is seen in ED for spotting 15 weeks into her pregnancy; the doctors also suspect fetal hydrocephalus.

O26.852	**Spotting complicating pregnancy, second trimester**
Z3A.15	**15 weeks gestation of pregnancy**

Explanation: Whether the fetal hydrocephalus was suspected or confirmed, an additional code is not warranted for this condition as the documentation does not indicate that this fetal condition is in any way altering the management of the mother or complicating her pregnancy.

2) In utero surgery

In cases when surgery is performed on the fetus, a diagnosis code from category O35, Maternal care for known or suspected fetal abnormality and damage, should be assigned identifying the fetal condition. Assign the appropriate procedure code for the procedure performed.

No code from Chapter 16, the perinatal codes, should be used on the mother's record to identify fetal conditions. Surgery performed in utero on a fetus is still to be coded as an obstetric encounter.

f. HIV infection in pregnancy, childbirth and the puerperium

During pregnancy, childbirth or the puerperium, a patient admitted because of an HIV-related illness should receive a principal diagnosis from subcategory O98.7-, Human immunodeficiency [HIV] disease complicating pregnancy, childbirth and the puerperium, followed by the code(s) for the HIV-related illness(es).

Patients with asymptomatic HIV infection status admitted during pregnancy, childbirth, or the puerperium should receive codes of O98.7- and Z21, Asymptomatic human immunodeficiency virus [HIV] infection status.

A previously asymptomatic HIV patient who is 13 weeks pregnant is admitted with oral thrush.

O98.711	**Human immunodeficiency virus [HIV] disease complicating pregnancy, first trimester**
B2Ø	**Human immunodeficiency virus [HIV] disease**
B37.Ø	**Candidal stomatitis**
Z3A.13	**13 weeks gestation of pregnancy**

Explanation: Because oral thrush is an HIV-related condition, this patient is now considered to have HIV disease. An obstetrics code indicating that HIV is complicating the pregnancy is coded first, followed by B2Ø for HIV disease as well as a code for the oral thrush.

g. Diabetes mellitus in pregnancy

Diabetes mellitus is a significant complicating factor in pregnancy. Pregnant patients who are diabetic should be assigned a code from category O24, Diabetes mellitus in pregnancy, childbirth, and the puerperium, first, followed by the appropriate diabetes code(s) (EØ8-E13) from Chapter 4.

h. Long term use of insulin and oral hypoglycemics

See section I.C.4.a.3 for information on the long-term use of insulin and oral hypoglycemics.

i. Gestational (pregnancy induced) diabetes

Gestational (pregnancy induced) diabetes can occur during the second and third trimester of pregnancy in patients who were not diabetic prior to pregnancy. Gestational diabetes can cause complications in the pregnancy similar to those of pre-existing diabetes mellitus. It also puts the patient at greater risk of developing diabetes after the pregnancy.

Codes for gestational diabetes are in subcategory O24.4, Gestational diabetes mellitus. No other code from category O24, Diabetes mellitus in pregnancy, childbirth, and the puerperium, should be used with a code from O24.4.

The codes under subcategory O24.4 include diet controlled, insulin controlled, and controlled by oral hypoglycemic drugs. If a patient with gestational diabetes is treated with both diet and insulin, only the code for insulin-controlled is required. If a patient with gestational diabetes is treated with both diet and oral hypoglycemic medications, only the code for "controlled by oral hypoglycemic drugs" is required. Codes Z79.4, Long-term (current) use of insulin, Z79.84, Long-term (current) use of oral hypoglycemic drugs, **and Z79.85, Long-term (current) use of injectable non-insulin antidiabetic drugs,** should not be assigned with codes from subcategory O24.4.

An abnormal glucose tolerance in pregnancy is assigned a code from subcategory O99.81, Abnormal glucose complicating pregnancy, childbirth, and the puerperium.

Patient at 39 weeks term pregnancy with gestational diabetes was admitted in labor and delivered a healthy newborn. Patient is on a diabetic diet with daily metformin.

O24.425	**Gestational diabetes mellitus in childbirth, controlled by oral hypoglycemic drugs**
Z3A.39	**39 weeks gestation of pregnancy**
Z37.Ø	**Single live birth**

Explanation: When the patient is admitted for delivery and the patient's gestational diabetes is controlled by both diet and oral hypoglycemic medications, only the combination code in subcategory O24.4- Gestational diabetes mellitus, is reported. No code is added for diet controlled diabetes, and no Z code for long-term use of oral hypoglycemics is reported with the O24.4 combination codes.

j. Sepsis and septic shock complicating abortion, pregnancy, childbirth and the puerperium

When assigning a chapter 15 code for sepsis complicating abortion, pregnancy, childbirth, and the puerperium, a code for the specific type of infection should be assigned as an additional diagnosis. If severe sepsis is present, a code from subcategory R65.2, Severe sepsis, and code(s) for associated organ dysfunction(s) should also be assigned as additional diagnoses.

Patient is seen several days after a miscarriage with sepsis; cultures return MSSA

OØ3.87	**Sepsis following complete or unspecified spontaneous abortion**
B95.61	**Methicillin susceptible Staphylococcus aureus infection as the cause of diseases classified elsewhere**

Explanation: The type of infection that caused this patient to become septic was methicillin susceptible *Staphylococcus aureus* (MSSA), which as a secondary code helps capture all aspects related to this patient's septic condition.

k. Puerperal sepsis

Code O85, Puerperal sepsis, should be assigned with a secondary code to identify the causal organism (e.g., for a bacterial infection, assign a code from category B95-B96, Bacterial infections in conditions classified elsewhere). A code from category A4Ø, Streptococcal sepsis, or A41, Other sepsis, should not be used for puerperal sepsis. If applicable, use additional codes to identify severe sepsis (R65.2-) and any associated acute organ dysfunction.

Code O85 should not be assigned for sepsis following an obstetrical procedure (See Section I.C.1.d.5.b., Sepsis due to a postprocedural infection).

l. Alcohol, tobacco and drug use during pregnancy, childbirth and the puerperium

1) Alcohol use during pregnancy, childbirth and the puerperium

Codes under subcategory O99.31, Alcohol use complicating pregnancy, childbirth, and the puerperium, should be assigned for any pregnancy case when a patient uses alcohol during the pregnancy or postpartum. A secondary code from category F1Ø, Alcohol related disorders, should also be assigned to identify manifestations of the alcohol use.

2) Tobacco use during pregnancy, childbirth and the puerperium

Codes under subcategory O99.33, Smoking (tobacco) complicating pregnancy, childbirth, and the puerperium, should be assigned for any pregnancy case when a patient uses any type of tobacco product during the pregnancy or postpartum.

A secondary code from category F17, Nicotine dependence, should also be assigned to identify the type of nicotine dependence.

3) Drug use during pregnancy, childbirth and the puerperium

Codes under subcategory O99.32, Drug use complicating pregnancy, childbirth, and the puerperium, should be assigned for any pregnancy case when a patient uses drugs during the pregnancy or postpartum. This can involve illegal drugs, or inappropriate use or abuse of prescription drugs. Secondary code(s) from categories F11-F16 and F18-F19 should also be assigned to identify manifestations of the drug use.

m. Poisoning, toxic effects, adverse effects and underdosing in a pregnant patient

A code from subcategory O9A.2, Injury, poisoning and certain other consequences of external causes complicating pregnancy, childbirth, and the puerperium, should be sequenced first, followed by the appropriate injury, poisoning, toxic effect, adverse effect or underdosing code, and then the additional code(s) that specifies the condition caused by the poisoning, toxic effect, adverse effect or underdosing.

See Section I.C.19. Adverse effects, poisoning, underdosing and toxic effects.

Patient admitted with accidental carbon monoxide poisoning from a gas heating implement; the patient is 18 weeks' pregnant

O9A.212	**Injury, poisoning and certain other consequences of external causes complicating pregnancy, second trimester**
T58.11XA	**Toxic effect of carbon monoxide from utility gas, accidental (unintentional), initial encounter**
Z3A.18	**18 weeks gestation of pregnancy**

Explanation: Although the carbon monoxide poisoning is the reason the patient was admitted, a code from the obstetrics chapter must be sequenced first. Chapter 15 codes have sequencing priority over codes from other chapters.

n. Normal delivery, code O8Ø

1) Encounter for full term uncomplicated delivery

Code O8Ø should be assigned when a patient is admitted for a full-term normal delivery and delivers a single, healthy infant without any complications antepartum, during the delivery, or postpartum during the delivery episode. Code O8Ø is always a principal diagnosis. It is not to be used if any other code from chapter 15 is needed to describe a current complication of the antenatal, delivery, or postnatal period. Additional codes from other chapters may be used with code O8Ø if they are not related to or are in any way complicating the pregnancy.

2) Uncomplicated delivery with resolved antepartum complication

Code O8Ø may be used if the patient had a complication at some point during the pregnancy, but the complication is not present at the time of the admission for delivery.

Patient presents in labor at 39 weeks' gestation and delivers a healthy newborn; patient had abnormal glucose levels in her first trimester, which have since resolved

O8Ø	**Encounter for full-term uncomplicated delivery**
Z37.Ø	**Single live birth**

Explanation: The abnormal glucose levels during the first trimester cannot be coded if they are not affecting the patient's current trimester. Without additional complications associated with the pregnancy, fetus, or mother, code O8Ø is appropriate.

3) Outcome of delivery for O8Ø

Z37.Ø, Single live birth, is the only outcome of delivery code appropriate for use with O8Ø.

o. The peripartum and postpartum periods

1) Peripartum and postpartum periods

The postpartum period begins immediately after delivery and continues for six weeks following delivery. The peripartum period is defined as the last month of pregnancy to five months postpartum.

2) Peripartum and postpartum complication

A postpartum complication is any complication occurring within the six-week period.

3) Pregnancy-related complications after 6-week period

Chapter 15 codes may also be used to describe pregnancy-related complications after the peripartum or postpartum period if the provider documents that a condition is pregnancy related.

Patient admitted for varicose veins. She had a baby boy three months ago; the varicose veins started to appear one month ago. The doctor attributes the patient's pregnancy as the cause of the varicose veins, which continue to be painful and bother the patient. She is seeking surgical relief.

O87.4 **Varicose veins of the lower extremity in the puerperium**

Explanation: Although the varicose veins occurred several months after the delivery of the newborn, the doctor attributed the varicose veins to pregnancy and therefore a code from chapter 15 is appropriate.

4) Admission for routine postpartum care following delivery outside hospital

When the mother delivers outside the hospital prior to admission and is admitted for routine postpartum care and no complications are noted, code Z39.Ø, Encounter for care and examination of mother immediately after delivery, should be assigned as the principal diagnosis.

5) Pregnancy associated cardiomyopathy

Pregnancy associated cardiomyopathy, code O9Ø.3, is unique in that it may be diagnosed in the third trimester of pregnancy but may continue to progress months after delivery. For this reason, it is referred to as peripartum cardiomyopathy. Code O9Ø.3 is only for use when the cardiomyopathy develops as a result of pregnancy in a patient who did not have pre-existing heart disease.

p. Code O94, Sequelae of complication of pregnancy, childbirth, and the puerperium

1) Code O94

Code O94, Sequelae of complication of pregnancy, childbirth, and the puerperium, is for use in those cases when an initial complication of a pregnancy develops a sequela or sequelae requiring care or treatment at a future date.

2) After the initial postpartum period

This code may be used at any time after the initial postpartum period.

3) Sequencing of code O94

This code, like all sequela codes, is to be sequenced following the code describing the sequelae of the complication.

q. Termination of pregnancy and spontaneous abortions

1) Abortion with liveborn fetus

When an attempted termination of pregnancy results in a liveborn fetus, assign code Z33.2, Encounter for elective termination of pregnancy and a code from category Z37, Outcome of Delivery.

2) Retained products of conception following an abortion

Subsequent encounters for retained products of conception following a spontaneous abortion or elective termination of pregnancy, without complications are assigned OØ3.4, Incomplete spontaneous, abortion without complication, or code OØ7.4, Failed attempted termination of pregnancy without complication. This advice is appropriate even when the patient was discharged previously with a discharge diagnosis of complete abortion. If the patient has a specific complication associated with the spontaneous abortion or elective termination of pregnancy in addition to retained products of conception, assign the appropriate complication code (e.g., OØ3.-, OØ4.-, OØ7.-) instead of code OØ3.4 or OØ7.4.

Patient was seen two days ago for complete spontaneous abortion but returns today for urinary tract infection (UTI) with ultrasound showing retained products of conception

OØ3.38 **Urinary tract infection following incomplete spontaneous abortion**

Explanation: Although the diagnosis from the patient's previous stay indicated that the patient had a complete abortion, it is now determined that there were actually retained products of conception (POC). An abortion with retained POC is considered incomplete and in this case resulted in the patient developing a UTI.

3) Complications leading to abortion

Codes from Chapter 15 may be used as additional codes to identify any documented complications of the pregnancy in conjunction with codes in categories in OØ4, OØ7 and OØ8.

4) Hemorrhage following elective abortion

For hemorrhage post elective abortion, assign code OØ4.6, Delayed or excessive hemorrhage following (induced) termination of pregnancy. Do not assign code O72.1, Other immediate postpartum hemorrhage, as this code should not be assigned for post abortion conditions. Do not assign code Z33.2, Encounter for elective termination of pregnancy, when the patient experiences a complication post elective abortion.

r. Abuse in a pregnant patient

For suspected or confirmed cases of abuse of a pregnant patient, a code(s) from subcategories O9A.3, Physical abuse complicating pregnancy, childbirth, and the puerperium, O9A.4, Sexual abuse complicating pregnancy, childbirth, and the puerperium, and O9A.5, Psychological abuse complicating pregnancy, childbirth, and the puerperium, should be sequenced first, followed by the appropriate codes (if applicable) to identify any associated current injury due to physical abuse, sexual abuse, and the perpetrator of abuse.

See Section I.C.19. Adult and child abuse, neglect and other maltreatment.

s. COVID-19 infection in pregnancy, childbirth, and the puerperium

During pregnancy, childbirth or the puerperium, when COVID-19 is the reason for admission/encounter , code O98.5-, Other viral diseases complicating pregnancy, childbirth and the puerperium, should be sequenced as the principal/first-listed diagnosis, and code UØ7.1, COVID-19, and the appropriate codes for associated manifestation(s) should be assigned as additional diagnoses. Codes from Chapter 15 always take sequencing priority.

If the reason for admission/encounter is unrelated to COVID-19 but the patient tests positive for COVID-19 during the admission/encounter, the appropriate code for the reason for admission/encounter should be sequenced as the principal/first-listed diagnosis, and codes O98.5- and UØ7.1, as well as the appropriate codes for associated COVID-19 manifestations, should be assigned as additional diagnoses.

Patient admitted in labor at 39 weeks' gestation and delivered a healthy newborn. Prenatal care consisted of some hyperemesis early in the pregnancy that has since resolved. No complications encountered during or following delivery. As per hospital protocol, during the pandemic, all patients are to be screened for COVID-19, and the patient tested positive. She remains asymptomatic, will be sent home to quarantine for 14 days.

O98.52 **Other viral diseases complicating childbirth**

UØ7.1 **COVID-19**

Z3A.39 **39 weeks gestation of pregnancy**

Z37.Ø **Single live birth**

Explanation: No code is assigned for the hyperemesis as it resolved prior to this admission. Per guideline I.C.1.g.1.f, a screening code is generally not appropriate during the pandemic phase of COVID-19. Most hospitals screen their patients upon admission to the hospital to ensure proper protocols are in place for monitoring and treating those patients who do test positive for the disease. A positive test result alone is confirmation of the disease, according to guideline I.C.1.g.1.a, and code UØ7.1 should be assigned. A claim for any patient admitted during pregnancy, childbirth, or the puerperium and who tests positive or is treated for COVID-19 should have a code from subcategory O98.5- sequenced first, followed by code UØ7.1. As the patient was asymptomatic, no additional codes are assigned to represent any manifestation of the COVID-19 infection.

Chapter 15. Pregnancy, Childbirth and the Puerperium (O00-O9A)

NOTE CODES FROM THIS CHAPTER ARE FOR USE ONLY ON MATERNAL RECORDS, NEVER ON NEWBORN RECORDS

Codes from this chapter are for use for conditions related to or aggravated by the pregnancy, childbirth, or by the puerperium (maternal causes or obstetric causes)

NOTE Trimesters are counted from the first day of the last menstrual period. They are defined as follows:

1st trimester- less than 14 weeks 0 days

2nd trimester- 14 weeks 0 days to less than 28 weeks 0 days

3rd trimester- 28 weeks 0 days until delivery

Use additional code from category Z3A, Weeks of gestation, to identify the specific week of the pregnancy, if known.

EXCLUDES 1 *supervision of normal pregnancy (Z34.-)*

EXCLUDES 2 *mental and behavioral disorders associated with the puerperium (F53.-)*
obstetrical tetanus (A34)
postpartum necrosis of pituitary gland (E23.0)
puerperal osteomalacia (M83.0)

AHA: 2016,1Q,3-5; 2014,3Q,17

This chapter contains the following blocks:

- O00-O08 Pregnancy with abortive outcome
- O09 Supervision of high risk pregnancy
- O10-O16 Edema, proteinuria and hypertensive disorders in pregnancy, childbirth and the puerperium
- O20-O29 Other maternal disorders predominantly related to pregnancy
- O30-O48 Maternal care related to the fetus and amniotic cavity and possible delivery problems
- O60-O77 Complications of labor and delivery
- O80-O82 Encounter for delivery
- O85-O92 Complications predominantly related to the puerperium
- O94-O9A Other obstetric conditions, not elsewhere classified

Pregnancy with abortive outcome (O00-O08)

EXCLUDES 1 *continuing pregnancy in multiple gestation after abortion of one fetus or more (O31.1-, O31.3-)*

TIP: Do not assign a code from category Z3A with codes in this code block.

✓4th O00 Ectopic pregnancy

INCLUDES ruptured ectopic pregnancy

Use additional code from category O08 to identify any associated complication

AHA: 2016,4Q,48-50; 2014,3Q,17

DEF: Implantation of a fertilized egg outside the uterus, usually in the fallopian tube or abdomen that requires emergency treatment.

✓5th O00.0 Abdominal pregnancy

EXCLUDES 1 *maternal care for viable fetus in abdominal pregnancy (O36.7-)*

O00.00 Abdominal pregnancy without intrauterine pregnancy CC M ♀
Abdominal pregnancy NOS

O00.01 Abdominal pregnancy with intrauterine pregnancy CC M ♀

✓5th O00.1 Tubal pregnancy
Fallopian pregnancy
Rupture of (fallopian) tube due to pregnancy
Tubal abortion
AHA: 2017,4Q,20

✓6th O00.10 Tubal pregnancy without intrauterine pregnancy
Tubal pregnancy NOS

O00.101 Right tubal pregnancy without intrauterine pregnancy CC M ♀

O00.102 Left tubal pregnancy without intrauterine pregnancy CC M ♀

O00.109 Unspecified tubal pregnancy without intrauterine pregnancy CC UNS M ♀

✓6th O00.11 Tubal pregnancy with intrauterine pregnancy

O00.111 Right tubal pregnancy with intrauterine pregnancy CC M ♀

O00.112 Left tubal pregnancy with intrauterine pregnancy CC M ♀

O00.119 Unspecified tubal pregnancy with intrauterine pregnancy CC UNS M ♀

✓5th O00.2 Ovarian pregnancy
AHA: 2017,4Q,20

✓6th O00.20 Ovarian pregnancy without intrauterine pregnancy
Ovarian pregnancy NOS

O00.201 Right ovarian pregnancy without intrauterine pregnancy CC M ♀

O00.202 Left ovarian pregnancy without intrauterine pregnancy CC M ♀

O00.209 Unspecified ovarian pregnancy without intrauterine pregnancy CC UNS M ♀

✓6th O00.21 Ovarian pregnancy with intrauterine pregnancy

O00.211 Right ovarian pregnancy with intrauterine pregnancy CC M ♀

O00.212 Left ovarian pregnancy with intrauterine pregnancy CC M ♀

O00.219 Unspecified ovarian pregnancy with intrauterine pregnancy CC UNS M ♀

✓5th O00.8 Other ectopic pregnancy
Cervical pregnancy
Cornual pregnancy
Intraligamentous pregnancy
Mural pregnancy

O00.80 Other ectopic pregnancy without intrauterine pregnancy CC M ♀
Other ectopic pregnancy NOS

O00.81 Other ectopic pregnancy with intrauterine pregnancy CC M ♀

✓5th O00.9 Ectopic pregnancy, unspecified

O00.90 Unspecified ectopic pregnancy without intrauterine pregnancy CC M ♀
Ectopic pregnancy NOS

O00.91 Unspecified ectopic pregnancy with intrauterine pregnancy CC M ♀

✓4th O01 Hydatidiform mole

Use additional code from category O08 to identify any associated complication

EXCLUDES 1 *chorioadenoma (destruens) (D39.2)*
malignant hydatidiform mole (D39.2)

AHA: 2014,3Q,17

DEF: Abnormal product of pregnancy, marked by a mass of cysts resembling a bunch of grapes due to chorionic villi proliferation and dissolution. It must be surgically removed.

O01.0 Classical hydatidiform mole M ♀
Complete hydatidiform mole

O01.1 Incomplete and partial hydatidiform mole M ♀

O01.9 Hydatidiform mole, unspecified M ♀
Trophoblastic disease NOS
Vesicular mole NOS

✓4th O02 Other abnormal products of conception

Use additional code from category O08 to identify any associated complication

EXCLUDES 1 *papyraceous fetus (O31.0-)*

AHA: 2014,3Q,17

O02.0 Blighted ovum and nonhydatidiform mole M ♀
Carneous mole
Fleshy mole
Intrauterine mole NOS
Molar pregnancy NEC
Pathological ovum

O02.1 Missed abortion M ♀
Early fetal death, before completion of 20 weeks of gestation, with retention of dead fetus

EXCLUDES 1 *failed induced abortion (O07.-)*
fetal death (intrauterine) (late) (O36.4)
missed abortion with blighted ovum (O02.0)
missed abortion with hydatidiform mole (O01.-)
missed abortion with nonhydatidiform (O02.0)
missed abortion with other abnormal products of conception (O02.8-)
missed delivery (O36.4)
stillbirth (P95)

AHA: 2022,2Q,3; 2019,3Q,11

O02.8 Other specified abnormal products of conception

EXCLUDES 1 *abnormal products of conception with blighted ovum (O02.0)*
abnormal products of conception with hydatidiform mole (O01.-)
abnormal products of conception with nonhydatidiform mole (O02.0)

O02.81 Inappropriate change in quantitative human chorionic gonadotropin (hCG) in early pregnancy M ♀

Biochemical pregnancy
Chemical pregnancy
Inappropriate level of quantitative human chorionic gonadotropin (hCG) for gestational age in early pregnancy

O02.89 Other abnormal products of conception M ♀

O02.9 Abnormal product of conception, unspecified M ♀

O03 Spontaneous abortion

NOTE Incomplete abortion includes retained products of conception following spontaneous abortion

INCLUDES miscarriage

O03.0 Genital tract and pelvic infection following incomplete spontaneous abortion CC M ♀

Endometritis following incomplete spontaneous abortion
Oophoritis following incomplete spontaneous abortion
Parametritis following incomplete spontaneous abortion
Pelvic peritonitis following incomplete spontaneous abortion
Salpingitis following incomplete spontaneous abortion
Salpingo-oophoritis following incomplete spontaneous abortion

EXCLUDES 1 *sepsis following incomplete spontaneous abortion (O03.37)*
urinary tract infection following incomplete spontaneous abortion (O03.38)

O03.1 Delayed or excessive hemorrhage following incomplete spontaneous abortion M ♀

Afibrinogenemia following incomplete spontaneous abortion
Defibrination syndrome following incomplete spontaneous abortion
Hemolysis following incomplete spontaneous abortion
Intravascular coagulation following incomplete spontaneous abortion

AHA: 2022,1Q,19

O03.2 Embolism following incomplete spontaneous abortion MCC M ♀

Air embolism following incomplete spontaneous abortion
Amniotic fluid embolism following incomplete spontaneous abortion
Blood-clot embolism following incomplete spontaneous abortion
Embolism NOS following incomplete spontaneous abortion
Fat embolism following incomplete spontaneous abortion
Pulmonary embolism following incomplete spontaneous abortion
Pyemic embolism following incomplete spontaneous abortion
Septic or septicopyemic embolism following incomplete spontaneous abortion
Soap embolism following incomplete spontaneous abortion

O03.3 Other and unspecified complications following incomplete spontaneous abortion

O03.30 Unspecified complication following incomplete spontaneous abortion CC M ♀

O03.31 Shock following incomplete spontaneous abortion MCC M ♀

Circulatory collapse following incomplete spontaneous abortion
Shock (postprocedural) following incomplete spontaneous abortion

EXCLUDES 1 *shock due to infection following incomplete spontaneous abortion (O03.37)*

O03.32 Renal failure following incomplete spontaneous abortion MCC M ♀

Kidney failure (acute) following incomplete spontaneous abortion
Oliguria following incomplete spontaneous abortion
Renal shutdown following incomplete spontaneous abortion
Renal tubular necrosis following incomplete spontaneous abortion
Uremia following incomplete spontaneous abortion

O03.33 Metabolic disorder following incomplete spontaneous abortion CC M ♀

O03.34 Damage to pelvic organs following incomplete spontaneous abortion CC M ♀

Laceration, perforation, tear or chemical damage of bladder following incomplete spontaneous abortion
Laceration, perforation, tear or chemical damage of bowel following incomplete spontaneous abortion
Laceration, perforation, tear or chemical damage of broad ligament following incomplete spontaneous abortion
Laceration, perforation, tear or chemical damage of cervix following incomplete spontaneous abortion
Laceration, perforation, tear or chemical damage of periurethral tissue following incomplete spontaneous abortion
Laceration, perforation, tear or chemical damage of uterus following incomplete spontaneous abortion
Laceration, perforation, tear or chemical damage of vagina following incomplete spontaneous abortion

O03.35 Other venous complications following incomplete spontaneous abortion CC M ♀

O03.36 Cardiac arrest following incomplete spontaneous abortion CC M ♀

O03.37 Sepsis following incomplete spontaneous abortion CC M ♀

Use additional code to identify infectious agent (B95-B97)
Use additional code to identify severe sepsis, if applicable (R65.2-)

EXCLUDES 1 *septic or septicopyemic embolism following incomplete spontaneous abortion (O03.2)*

O03.38 Urinary tract infection following incomplete spontaneous abortion CC M ♀

Cystitis following incomplete spontaneous abortion

O03.39 Incomplete spontaneous abortion with other complications CC M ♀

O03.4 Incomplete spontaneous abortion without complication M ♀

O03.5 Genital tract and pelvic infection following complete or unspecified spontaneous abortion CC M ♀

Endometritis following complete or unspecified spontaneous abortion
Oophoritis following complete or unspecified spontaneous abortion
Parametritis following complete or unspecified spontaneous abortion
Pelvic peritonitis following complete or unspecified spontaneous abortion
Salpingitis following complete or unspecified spontaneous abortion
Salpingo-oophoritis following complete or unspecified spontaneous abortion

EXCLUDES 1 *sepsis following complete or unspecified spontaneous abortion (O03.87)*
urinary tract infection following complete or unspecified spontaneous abortion (O03.88)

O03.6 Delayed or excessive hemorrhage following complete or unspecified spontaneous abortion M ♀
- Afibrinogenemia following complete or unspecified spontaneous abortion
- Defibrination syndrome following complete or unspecified spontaneous abortion
- Hemolysis following complete or unspecified spontaneous abortion
- Intravascular coagulation following complete or unspecified spontaneous abortion

AHA: 2022,1Q,19

O03.7 Embolism following complete or unspecified spontaneous abortion CC M ♀
- Air embolism following complete or unspecified spontaneous abortion
- Amniotic fluid embolism following complete or unspecified spontaneous abortion
- Blood-clot embolism following complete or unspecified spontaneous abortion
- Embolism NOS following complete or unspecified spontaneous abortion
- Fat embolism following complete or unspecified spontaneous abortion
- Pulmonary embolism following complete or unspecified spontaneous abortion
- Pyemic embolism following complete or unspecified spontaneous abortion
- Septic or septicopyemic embolism following complete or unspecified spontaneous abortion
- Soap embolism following complete or unspecified spontaneous abortion

5th **O03.8 Other and unspecified complications following complete or unspecified spontaneous abortion**

O03.80 Unspecified complication following complete or unspecified spontaneous abortion CC M ♀

O03.81 Shock following complete or unspecified spontaneous abortion MCC M ♀
- Circulatory collapse following complete or unspecified spontaneous abortion
- Shock (postprocedural) following complete or unspecified spontaneous abortion

EXCLUDES 1 *shock due to infection following complete or unspecified spontaneous abortion (O03.87)*

O03.82 Renal failure following complete or unspecified spontaneous abortion MCC M ♀
- Kidney failure (acute) following complete or unspecified spontaneous abortion
- Oliguria following complete or unspecified spontaneous abortion
- Renal shutdown following complete or unspecified spontaneous abortion
- Renal tubular necrosis following complete or unspecified spontaneous abortion
- Uremia following complete or unspecified spontaneous abortion

O03.83 Metabolic disorder following complete or unspecified spontaneous abortion CC M ♀

O03.84 Damage to pelvic organs following complete or unspecified spontaneous abortion CC M ♀
- Laceration, perforation, tear or chemical damage of bladder following complete or unspecified spontaneous abortion
- Laceration, perforation, tear or chemical damage of bowel following complete or unspecified spontaneous abortion
- Laceration, perforation, tear or chemical damage of broad ligament following complete or unspecified spontaneous abortion
- Laceration, perforation, tear or chemical damage of cervix following complete or unspecified spontaneous abortion
- Laceration, perforation, tear or chemical damage of periurethral tissue following complete or unspecified spontaneous abortion
- Laceration, perforation, tear or chemical damage of uterus following complete or unspecified spontaneous abortion
- Laceration, perforation, tear or chemical damage of vagina following complete or unspecified spontaneous abortion

O03.85 Other venous complications following complete or unspecified spontaneous abortion CC M ♀

O03.86 Cardiac arrest following complete or unspecified spontaneous abortion CC M ♀

O03.87 Sepsis following complete or unspecified spontaneous abortion CC M ♀

Use additional code to identify infectious agent (B95-B97)

Use additional code to identify severe sepsis, if applicable (R65.2-)

EXCLUDES 1 *septic or septicopyemic embolism following complete or unspecified spontaneous abortion (O03.7)*

O03.88 Urinary tract infection following complete or unspecified spontaneous abortion CC M ♀
- Cystitis following complete or unspecified spontaneous abortion

O03.89 Complete or unspecified spontaneous abortion with other complications CC M ♀

O03.9 Complete or unspecified spontaneous abortion without complication M ♀
- Miscarriage NOS
- Spontaneous abortion NOS

4th **O04 Complications following (induced) termination of pregnancy**

INCLUDES complications following (induced) termination of pregnancy

EXCLUDES 1 *encounter for elective termination of pregnancy, uncomplicated (Z33.2)*
failed attempted termination of pregnancy (O07.-)

O04.5 Genital tract and pelvic infection following (induced) termination of pregnancy CC M ♀
- Endometritis following (induced) termination of pregnancy
- Oophoritis following (induced) termination of pregnancy
- Parametritis following (induced) termination of pregnancy
- Pelvic peritonitis following (induced) termination of pregnancy
- Salpingitis following (induced) termination of pregnancy
- Salpingo-oophoritis following (induced) termination of pregnancy

EXCLUDES 1 *sepsis following (induced) termination of pregnancy (O04.87)*
urinary tract infection following (induced) termination of pregnancy (O04.88)

O04.6 Delayed or excessive hemorrhage following (induced) termination of pregnancy M ♀
- Afibrinogenemia following (induced) termination of pregnancy
- Defibrination syndrome following (induced) termination of pregnancy
- Hemolysis following (induced) termination of pregnancy
- Intravascular coagulation following (induced) termination of pregnancy

AHA: 2019,3Q,11

Chapter 15. Pregnancy, Childbirth and the Puerperium

O03.6–O04.6

O04.7 Embolism following (induced) termination of pregnancy MCC M ♀
- Air embolism following (induced) termination of pregnancy
- Amniotic fluid embolism following (induced) termination of pregnancy
- Blood-clot embolism following (induced) termination of pregnancy
- Embolism NOS following (induced) termination of pregnancy
- Fat embolism following (induced) termination of pregnancy
- Pulmonary embolism following (induced) termination of pregnancy
- Pyemic embolism following (induced) termination of pregnancy
- Septic or septicopyemic embolism following (induced) termination of pregnancy
- Soap embolism following (induced) termination of pregnancy

✓5th **O04.8 (Induced) termination of pregnancy with other and unspecified complications**

O04.80 (Induced) termination of pregnancy with unspecified complications CC M ♀

O04.81 Shock following (induced) termination of pregnancy MCC M ♀
- Circulatory collapse following (induced) termination of pregnancy
- Shock (postprocedural) following (induced) termination of pregnancy

EXCLUDES 1 *shock due to infection following (induced) termination of pregnancy (O04.87)*

O04.82 Renal failure following (induced) termination of pregnancy MCC M ♀
- Kidney failure (acute) following (induced) termination of pregnancy
- Oliguria following (induced) termination of pregnancy
- Renal shutdown following (induced) termination of pregnancy
- Renal tubular necrosis following (induced) termination of pregnancy
- Uremia following (induced) termination of pregnancy

O04.83 Metabolic disorder following (induced) termination of pregnancy CC M ♀

O04.84 Damage to pelvic organs following (induced) termination of pregnancy CC M ♀
- Laceration, perforation, tear or chemical damage of bladder following (induced) termination of pregnancy
- Laceration, perforation, tear or chemical damage of bowel following (induced) termination of pregnancy
- Laceration, perforation, tear or chemical damage of broad ligament following (induced) termination of pregnancy
- Laceration, perforation, tear or chemical damage of cervix following (induced) termination of pregnancy
- Laceration, perforation, tear or chemical damage of periurethral tissue following (induced) termination of pregnancy
- Laceration, perforation, tear or chemical damage of uterus following (induced) termination of pregnancy
- Laceration, perforation, tear or chemical damage of vagina following (induced) termination of pregnancy

O04.85 Other venous complications following (induced) termination of pregnancy CC M ♀

O04.86 Cardiac arrest following (induced) termination of pregnancy CC M ♀

O04.87 Sepsis following (induced) termination of pregnancy CC M ♀

Use additional code to identify infectious agent (B95-B97)

Use additional code to identify severe sepsis, if applicable (R65.2-)

EXCLUDES 1 *septic or septicopyemic embolism following (induced) termination of pregnancy (O04.7)*

O04.88 Urinary tract infection following (induced) termination of pregnancy CC M ♀
- Cystitis following (induced) termination of pregnancy

O04.89 (Induced) termination of pregnancy with other complications CC M ♀

✓4th **O07 Failed attempted termination of pregnancy**

INCLUDES failure of attempted induction of termination of pregnancy
incomplete elective abortion

EXCLUDES 1 *incomplete spontaneous abortion (O03.0-)*

O07.0 Genital tract and pelvic infection following failed attempted termination of pregnancy CC M ♀
- Endometritis following failed attempted termination of pregnancy
- Oophoritis following failed attempted termination of pregnancy
- Parametritis following failed attempted termination of pregnancy
- Pelvic peritonitis following failed attempted termination of pregnancy
- Salpingitis following failed attempted termination of pregnancy
- Salpingo-oophoritis following failed attempted termination of pregnancy

EXCLUDES 1 *sepsis following failed attempted termination of pregnancy (O07.37)*
urinary tract infection following failed attempted termination of pregnancy (O07.38)

O07.1 Delayed or excessive hemorrhage following failed attempted termination of pregnancy CC M ♀
- Afibrinogenemia following failed attempted termination of pregnancy
- Defibrination syndrome following failed attempted termination of pregnancy
- Hemolysis following failed attempted termination of pregnancy
- Intravascular coagulation following failed attempted termination of pregnancy

O07.2 Embolism following failed attempted termination of pregnancy MCC M ♀
- Air embolism following failed attempted termination of pregnancy
- Amniotic fluid embolism following failed attempted termination of pregnancy
- Blood-clot embolism following failed attempted termination of pregnancy
- Embolism NOS following failed attempted termination of pregnancy
- Fat embolism following failed attempted termination of pregnancy
- Pulmonary embolism following failed attempted termination of pregnancy
- Pyemic embolism following failed attempted termination of pregnancy
- Septic or septicopyemic embolism following failed attempted termination of pregnancy
- Soap embolism following failed attempted termination of pregnancy

✓5th **O07.3 Failed attempted termination of pregnancy with other and unspecified complications**

O07.30 Failed attempted termination of pregnancy with unspecified complications CC M ♀

O07.31 Shock following failed attempted termination of pregnancy MCC M ♀
- Circulatory collapse following failed attempted termination of pregnancy
- Shock (postprocedural) following failed attempted termination of pregnancy

EXCLUDES 1 *shock due to infection following failed attempted termination of pregnancy (O07.37)*

O07.32 Renal failure following failed attempted termination of pregnancy MCC M ♀
- Kidney failure (acute) following failed attempted termination of pregnancy
- Oliguria following failed attempted termination of pregnancy
- Renal shutdown following failed attempted termination of pregnancy
- Renal tubular necrosis following failed attempted termination of pregnancy
- Uremia following failed attempted termination of pregnancy

O07.33 Metabolic disorder following failed attempted termination of pregnancy CC M ♀

O07.34 Damage to pelvic organs following failed attempted termination of pregnancy CC M ♀
Laceration, perforation, tear or chemical damage of bladder following failed attempted termination of pregnancy
Laceration, perforation, tear or chemical damage of bowel following failed attempted termination of pregnancy
Laceration, perforation, tear or chemical damage of broad ligament following failed attempted termination of pregnancy
Laceration, perforation, tear or chemical damage of cervix following failed attempted termination of pregnancy
Laceration, perforation, tear or chemical damage of periurethral tissue following failed attempted termination of pregnancy
Laceration, perforation, tear or chemical damage of uterus following failed attempted termination of pregnancy
Laceration, perforation, tear or chemical damage of vagina following failed attempted termination of pregnancy

O07.35 Other venous complications following failed attempted termination of pregnancy CC M ♀

O07.36 Cardiac arrest following failed attempted termination of pregnancy CC M ♀

O07.37 Sepsis following failed attempted termination of pregnancy CC M ♀
Use additional code (B95-B97), to identify infectious agent
Use additional code (R65.2-) to identify severe sepsis, if applicable
EXCLUDES 1 *septic or septicopyemic embolism following failed attempted termination of pregnancy (O07.2)*

O07.38 Urinary tract infection following failed attempted termination of pregnancy CC M ♀
Cystitis following failed attempted termination of pregnancy

O07.39 Failed attempted termination of pregnancy with other complications CC M ♀

O07.4 Failed attempted termination of pregnancy without complication M ♀

O08 Complications following ectopic and molar pregnancy (4th)
This category is for use with categories O00-O02 to identify any associated complications

O08.0 Genital tract and pelvic infection following ectopic and molar pregnancy CC M ♀
Endometritis following ectopic and molar pregnancy
Oophoritis following ectopic and molar pregnancy
Parametritis following ectopic and molar pregnancy
Pelvic peritonitis following ectopic and molar pregnancy
Salpingitis following ectopic and molar pregnancy
Salpingo-oophoritis following ectopic and molar pregnancy
EXCLUDES 1 *sepsis following ectopic and molar pregnancy (O08.82)*
urinary tract infection (O08.83)

O08.1 Delayed or excessive hemorrhage following ectopic and molar pregnancy CC M ♀
Afibrinogenemia following ectopic and molar pregnancy
Defibrination syndrome following ectopic and molar pregnancy
Hemolysis following ectopic and molar pregnancy
Intravascular coagulation following ectopic and molar pregnancy
EXCLUDES 1 *delayed or excessive hemorrhage due to incomplete abortion (O03.1)*

O08.2 Embolism following ectopic and molar pregnancy MCC M ♀
Air embolism following ectopic and molar pregnancy
Amniotic fluid embolism following ectopic and molar pregnancy
Blood-clot embolism following ectopic and molar pregnancy
Embolism NOS following ectopic and molar pregnancy
Fat embolism following ectopic and molar pregnancy
Pulmonary embolism following ectopic and molar pregnancy
Pyemic embolism following ectopic and molar pregnancy
Septic or septicopyemic embolism following ectopic and molar pregnancy
Soap embolism following ectopic and molar pregnancy

O08.3 Shock following ectopic and molar pregnancy MCC M ♀
Circulatory collapse following ectopic and molar pregnancy
Shock (postprocedural) following ectopic and molar pregnancy
EXCLUDES 1 *shock due to infection following ectopic and molar pregnancy (O08.82)*

O08.4 Renal failure following ectopic and molar pregnancy MCC M ♀
Kidney failure (acute) following ectopic and molar pregnancy
Oliguria following ectopic and molar pregnancy
Renal shutdown following ectopic and molar pregnancy
Renal tubular necrosis following ectopic and molar pregnancy
Uremia following ectopic and molar pregnancy

O08.5 Metabolic disorders following an ectopic and molar pregnancy CC M ♀

O08.6 Damage to pelvic organs and tissues following an ectopic and molar pregnancy CC M ♀
Laceration, perforation, tear or chemical damage of bladder following an ectopic and molar pregnancy
Laceration, perforation, tear or chemical damage of bowel following an ectopic and molar pregnancy
Laceration, perforation, tear or chemical damage of broad ligament following an ectopic and molar pregnancy
Laceration, perforation, tear or chemical damage of cervix following an ectopic and molar pregnancy
Laceration, perforation, tear or chemical damage of periurethral tissue following an ectopic and molar pregnancy
Laceration, perforation, tear or chemical damage of uterus following an ectopic and molar pregnancy
Laceration, perforation, tear or chemical damage of vagina following an ectopic and molar pregnancy

O08.7 Other venous complications following an ectopic and molar pregnancy CC M ♀

O08.8 Other complications following an ectopic and molar pregnancy (5th)

O08.81 Cardiac arrest following an ectopic and molar pregnancy CC M ♀

O08.82 Sepsis following ectopic and molar pregnancy CC M ♀
Use additional code (B95-B97), to identify infectious agent
Use additional code (R65.2-) to identify severe sepsis, if applicable
EXCLUDES 1 *septic or septicopyemic embolism following ectopic and molar pregnancy (O08.2)*

O08.83 Urinary tract infection following an ectopic and molar pregnancy CC M ♀
Cystitis following an ectopic and molar pregnancy

O08.89 Other complications following an ectopic and molar pregnancy CC M ♀

O08.9 Unspecified complication following an ectopic and molar pregnancy CC M ♀

Supervision of high risk pregnancy (O09)

O09 Supervision of high risk pregnancy (4th)
AHA: 2019,3Q,5; 2016,4Q,48-50,150

O09.0 Supervision of pregnancy with history of infertility (5th)

O09.00 Supervision of pregnancy with history of infertility, unspecified trimester UPD M ♀

O09.01 Supervision of pregnancy with history of infertility, first trimester UPD M ♀

O09.02 Supervision of pregnancy with history of infertility, second trimester UPD M ♀

O09.03 Supervision of pregnancy with history of infertility, third trimester UPD M ♀

O09.1 Supervision of pregnancy with history of ectopic pregnancy

O09.10 Supervision of pregnancy with history of ectopic pregnancy, unspecified trimester UPD M ♀

O09.11 Supervision of pregnancy with history of ectopic pregnancy, first trimester UPD M ♀

O09.12 Supervision of pregnancy with history of ectopic pregnancy, second trimester UPD M ♀

O09.13 Supervision of pregnancy with history of ectopic pregnancy, third trimester UPD M ♀

O09.A Supervision of pregnancy with history of molar pregnancy

DEF: Molar pregnancy: Trophoblastic neoplasm that mimics pregnancy by proliferating from a pathologic ovum and resulting only in a mass of cysts resembling grapes, 80 percent of which are benign, but require surgical removal.

O09.A0 Supervision of pregnancy with history of molar pregnancy, unspecified trimester UPD M ♀

O09.A1 Supervision of pregnancy with history of molar pregnancy, first trimester UPD M ♀

O09.A2 Supervision of pregnancy with history of molar pregnancy, second trimester UPD M ♀

O09.A3 Supervision of pregnancy with history of molar pregnancy, third trimester UPD M ♀

O09.2 Supervision of pregnancy with other poor reproductive or obstetric history

EXCLUDES 2 *pregnancy care for patient with history of recurrent pregnancy loss (O26.2-)*

O09.21 Supervision of pregnancy with history of pre-term labor

O09.211 Supervision of pregnancy with history of pre-term labor, first trimester UPD M ♀

O09.212 Supervision of pregnancy with history of pre-term labor, second trimester UPD M ♀

O09.213 Supervision of pregnancy with history of pre-term labor, third trimester UPD M ♀

O09.219 Supervision of pregnancy with history of pre-term labor, unspecified trimester UPD M ♀

O09.29 Supervision of pregnancy with other poor reproductive or obstetric history

Supervision of pregnancy with history of neonatal death

Supervision of pregnancy with history of stillbirth

O09.291 Supervision of pregnancy with other poor reproductive or obstetric history, first trimester UPD M ♀

O09.292 Supervision of pregnancy with other poor reproductive or obstetric history, second trimester UPD M ♀

O09.293 Supervision of pregnancy with other poor reproductive or obstetric history, third trimester UPD M ♀

O09.299 Supervision of pregnancy with other poor reproductive or obstetric history, unspecified trimester UPD M ♀

O09.3 Supervision of pregnancy with insufficient antenatal care

Supervision of concealed pregnancy

Supervision of hidden pregnancy

O09.30 Supervision of pregnancy with insufficient antenatal care, unspecified trimester UPD M ♀

O09.31 Supervision of pregnancy with insufficient antenatal care, first trimester UPD M ♀

O09.32 Supervision of pregnancy with insufficient antenatal care, second trimester UPD M ♀

O09.33 Supervision of pregnancy with insufficient antenatal care, third trimester UPD M ♀

O09.4 Supervision of pregnancy with grand multiparity

O09.40 Supervision of pregnancy with grand multiparity, unspecified trimester UPD M ♀

O09.41 Supervision of pregnancy with grand multiparity, first trimester UPD M ♀

O09.42 Supervision of pregnancy with grand multiparity, second trimester UPD M ♀

O09.43 Supervision of pregnancy with grand multiparity, third trimester UPD M ♀

O09.5 Supervision of elderly primigravida and multigravida

Pregnancy for a female 35 years and older at expected date of delivery

O09.51 Supervision of elderly primigravida

O09.511 Supervision of elderly primigravida, first trimester UPD M ♀

O09.512 Supervision of elderly primigravida, second trimester UPD M ♀

O09.513 Supervision of elderly primigravida, third trimester UPD M ♀

O09.519 Supervision of elderly primigravida, unspecified trimester UPD M ♀

O09.52 Supervision of elderly multigravida

O09.521 Supervision of elderly multigravida, first trimester UPD M ♀

O09.522 Supervision of elderly multigravida, second trimester UPD M ♀

O09.523 Supervision of elderly multigravida, third trimester UPD M ♀

O09.529 Supervision of elderly multigravida, unspecified trimester UPD M ♀

O09.6 Supervision of young primigravida and multigravida

Supervision of pregnancy for a female less than 16 years old at expected date of delivery

O09.61 Supervision of young primigravida

O09.611 Supervision of young primigravida, first trimester UPD M ♀

O09.612 Supervision of young primigravida, second trimester UPD M ♀

O09.613 Supervision of young primigravida, third trimester UPD M ♀

O09.619 Supervision of young primigravida, unspecified trimester UPD M ♀

O09.62 Supervision of young multigravida

O09.621 Supervision of young multigravida, first trimester UPD M ♀

O09.622 Supervision of young multigravida, second trimester UPD M ♀

O09.623 Supervision of young multigravida, third trimester UPD M ♀

O09.629 Supervision of young multigravida, unspecified trimester UPD M ♀

O09.7 Supervision of high risk pregnancy due to social problems

O09.70 Supervision of high risk pregnancy due to social problems, unspecified trimester UPD M ♀

O09.71 Supervision of high risk pregnancy due to social problems, first trimester UPD M ♀

O09.72 Supervision of high risk pregnancy due to social problems, second trimester UPD M ♀

O09.73 Supervision of high risk pregnancy due to social problems, third trimester UPD M ♀

O09.8 Supervision of other high risk pregnancies

O09.81 Supervision of pregnancy resulting from assisted reproductive technology

Supervision of pregnancy resulting from in-vitro fertilization

EXCLUDES 2 *gestational carrier status (Z33.3)*

O09.811 Supervision of pregnancy resulting from assisted reproductive technology, first trimester UPD M ♀

O09.812 Supervision of pregnancy resulting from assisted reproductive technology, second trimester UPD M ♀

O09.813 Supervision of pregnancy resulting from assisted reproductive technology, third trimester UPD M ♀

O09.819 Supervision of pregnancy resulting from assisted reproductive technology, unspecified trimester UPD M ♀

O09.82 Supervision of pregnancy with history of in utero procedure during previous pregnancy

O09.821 Supervision of pregnancy with history of in utero procedure during previous pregnancy, first trimester UPD M ♀

O09.822 Supervision of pregnancy with history of in utero procedure during previous pregnancy, second trimester UPD M ♀

O09.823 Supervision of pregnancy with history of in utero procedure during previous pregnancy, third trimester UPD M ♀

O09.829 Supervision of pregnancy with history of in utero procedure during previous pregnancy, unspecified trimester UPD M ♀

EXCLUDES 1 *supervision of pregnancy affected by in utero procedure during current pregnancy (O35.7)*

✓6th **O09.89 Supervision of other high risk pregnancies**

O09.891 Supervision of other high risk pregnancies, first trimester UPD M ♀

O09.892 Supervision of other high risk pregnancies, second trimester UPD M ♀

O09.893 Supervision of other high risk pregnancies, third trimester UPD M ♀

O09.899 Supervision of other high risk pregnancies, unspecified trimester UPD M ♀

✓5th **O09.9 Supervision of high risk pregnancy, unspecified**

O09.90 Supervision of high risk pregnancy, unspecified, unspecified trimester UPD M ♀

O09.91 Supervision of high risk pregnancy, unspecified, first trimester UPD M ♀

O09.92 Supervision of high risk pregnancy, unspecified, second trimester UPD M ♀

O09.93 Supervision of high risk pregnancy, unspecified, third trimester UPD M ♀

Edema, proteinuria and hypertensive disorders in pregnancy, childbirth and the puerperium (O10-O16)

AHA: 2016,4Q,50

✓4th **O10 Pre-existing hypertension complicating pregnancy, childbirth and the puerperium**

INCLUDES pre-existing hypertension with pre-existing proteinuria complicating pregnancy, childbirth and the puerperium

EXCLUDES 2 *pre-existing hypertension with superimposed pre-eclampsia complicating pregnancy, childbirth and the puerperium (O11.-)*

✓5th **O10.0 Pre-existing essential hypertension complicating pregnancy, childbirth and the puerperium**

Any condition in I10 specified as a reason for obstetric care during pregnancy, childbirth or the puerperium

✓6th **O10.01 Pre-existing essential hypertension complicating pregnancy**

O10.011 Pre-existing essential hypertension complicating pregnancy, first trimester CC M ♀

O10.012 Pre-existing essential hypertension complicating pregnancy, second trimester CC M ♀

O10.013 Pre-existing essential hypertension complicating pregnancy, third trimester CC M ♀

O10.019 Pre-existing essential hypertension complicating pregnancy, unspecified trimester M ♀

O10.02 Pre-existing essential hypertension complicating childbirth CC M ♀

O10.03 Pre-existing essential hypertension complicating the puerperium M ♀

✓5th **O10.1 Pre-existing hypertensive heart disease complicating pregnancy, childbirth and the puerperium**

Any condition in I11 specified as a reason for obstetric care during pregnancy, childbirth or the puerperium

Use additional code from I11 to identify the type of hypertensive heart disease

✓6th **O10.11 Pre-existing hypertensive heart disease complicating pregnancy**

O10.111 Pre-existing hypertensive heart disease complicating pregnancy, first trimester M ♀

O10.112 Pre-existing hypertensive heart disease complicating pregnancy, second trimester M ♀

O10.113 Pre-existing hypertensive heart disease complicating pregnancy, third trimester M ♀

O10.119 Pre-existing hypertensive heart disease complicating pregnancy, unspecified trimester M ♀

O10.12 Pre-existing hypertensive heart disease complicating childbirth M ♀

O10.13 Pre-existing hypertensive heart disease complicating the puerperium M ♀

✓5th **O10.2 Pre-existing hypertensive chronic kidney disease complicating pregnancy, childbirth and the puerperium**

Any condition in I12 specified as a reason for obstetric care during pregnancy, childbirth or the puerperium

Use additional code from I12 to identify the type of hypertensive chronic kidney disease

✓6th **O10.21 Pre-existing hypertensive chronic kidney disease complicating pregnancy**

O10.211 Pre-existing hypertensive chronic kidney disease complicating pregnancy, first trimester M ♀

O10.212 Pre-existing hypertensive chronic kidney disease complicating pregnancy, second trimester M ♀

O10.213 Pre-existing hypertensive chronic kidney disease complicating pregnancy, third trimester M ♀

O10.219 Pre-existing hypertensive chronic kidney disease complicating pregnancy, unspecified trimester M ♀

O10.22 Pre-existing hypertensive chronic kidney disease complicating childbirth M ♀

O10.23 Pre-existing hypertensive chronic kidney disease complicating the puerperium M ♀

✓5th **O10.3 Pre-existing hypertensive heart and chronic kidney disease complicating pregnancy, childbirth and the puerperium**

Any condition in I13 specified as a reason for obstetric care during pregnancy, childbirth or the puerperium

Use additional code from I13 to identify the type of hypertensive heart and chronic kidney disease

✓6th **O10.31 Pre-existing hypertensive heart and chronic kidney disease complicating pregnancy**

O10.311 Pre-existing hypertensive heart and chronic kidney disease complicating pregnancy, first trimester M ♀

O10.312 Pre-existing hypertensive heart and chronic kidney disease complicating pregnancy, second trimester M ♀

O10.313 Pre-existing hypertensive heart and chronic kidney disease complicating pregnancy, third trimester M ♀

O10.319 Pre-existing hypertensive heart and chronic kidney disease complicating pregnancy, unspecified trimester M ♀

O10.32 Pre-existing hypertensive heart and chronic kidney disease complicating childbirth M ♀

O10.33 Pre-existing hypertensive heart and chronic kidney disease complicating the puerperium M ♀

✓5th **O10.4 Pre-existing secondary hypertension complicating pregnancy, childbirth and the puerperium**

Any condition in I15 specified as a reason for obstetric care during pregnancy, childbirth or the puerperium

Use additional code from I15 to identify the type of secondary hypertension

✓6th **O10.41 Pre-existing secondary hypertension complicating pregnancy**

O10.411 Pre-existing secondary hypertension complicating pregnancy, first trimester CC M ♀

O10.412 Pre-existing secondary hypertension complicating pregnancy, second trimester CC M ♀

O10.413 Pre-existing secondary hypertension complicating pregnancy, third trimester CC M ♀

O10.419 Pre-existing secondary hypertension complicating pregnancy, unspecified trimester M ♀

O10.42 Pre-existing secondary hypertension complicating childbirth MCC M ♀

O10.43 Pre-existing secondary hypertension complicating the puerperium CC M ♀

O10.9 Unspecified pre-existing hypertension complicating pregnancy, childbirth and the puerperium

O10.91 Unspecified pre-existing hypertension complicating pregnancy

O10.911 Unspecified pre-existing hypertension complicating pregnancy, first trimester CC M ♀

O10.912 Unspecified pre-existing hypertension complicating pregnancy, second trimester CC M ♀

O10.913 Unspecified pre-existing hypertension complicating pregnancy, third trimester CC M ♀

O10.919 Unspecified pre-existing hypertension complicating pregnancy, unspecified trimester M ♀

O10.92 Unspecified pre-existing hypertension complicating childbirth CC M ♀

O10.93 Unspecified pre-existing hypertension complicating the puerperium M ♀

O11 Pre-existing hypertension with pre-eclampsia

INCLUDES conditions in O10 complicated by pre-eclampsia
pre-eclampsia superimposed pre-existing in hypertension

Use additional code from O10 to identify the type of hypertension

DEF: Complication of pregnancy manifesting in the development of borderline hypertension, protein in the urine, and unresponsive swelling between the 20th week of pregnancy and the end of the first week following birth in mild to moderate cases. Severe preeclampsia presents with hypertension, associated with marked swelling, proteinuria, abdominal pain, and/or visual changes.

O11.1 Pre-existing hypertension with pre-eclampsia, first trimester MCC M ♀

O11.2 Pre-existing hypertension with pre-eclampsia, second trimester MCC M ♀

O11.3 Pre-existing hypertension with pre-eclampsia, third trimester MCC M ♀

O11.4 Pre-existing hypertension with pre-eclampsia, complicating childbirth M ♀

O11.5 Pre-existing hypertension with pre-eclampsia, complicating the puerperium M ♀

O11.9 Pre-existing hypertension with pre-eclampsia, unspecified trimester M ♀

O12 Gestational [pregnancy-induced] edema and proteinuria without hypertension

O12.0 Gestational edema

O12.00 Gestational edema, unspecified trimester M ♀

O12.01 Gestational edema, first trimester M ♀

O12.02 Gestational edema, second trimester M ♀

O12.03 Gestational edema, third trimester M ♀

O12.04 Gestational edema, complicating childbirth M ♀

O12.05 Gestational edema, complicating the puerperium M ♀

O12.1 Gestational proteinuria

O12.10 Gestational proteinuria, unspecified trimester M ♀

O12.11 Gestational proteinuria, first trimester CC M ♀

O12.12 Gestational proteinuria, second trimester CC M ♀

O12.13 Gestational proteinuria, third trimester CC M ♀

O12.14 Gestational proteinuria, complicating childbirth M ♀

O12.15 Gestational proteinuria, complicating the puerperium M ♀

O12.2 Gestational edema with proteinuria

O12.20 Gestational edema with proteinuria, unspecified trimester M ♀

O12.21 Gestational edema with proteinuria, first trimester CC M ♀

O12.22 Gestational edema with proteinuria, second trimester CC M ♀

O12.23 Gestational edema with proteinuria, third trimester CC M ♀

O12.24 Gestational edema with proteinuria, complicating childbirth M ♀

O12.25 Gestational edema with proteinuria, complicating the puerperium M ♀

O13 Gestational [pregnancy-induced] hypertension without significant proteinuria

INCLUDES gestational hypertension NOS
transient hypertension of pregnancy

AHA: 2016,1Q,5

O13.1 Gestational [pregnancy-induced] hypertension without significant proteinuria, first trimester M ♀

O13.2 Gestational [pregnancy-induced] hypertension without significant proteinuria, second trimester M ♀

O13.3 Gestational [pregnancy-induced] hypertension without significant proteinuria, third trimester M ♀

O13.4 Gestational [pregnancy-induced] hypertension without significant proteinuria, complicating childbirth M ♀

O13.5 Gestational [pregnancy-induced] hypertension without significant proteinuria, complicating the puerperium M ♀

O13.9 Gestational [pregnancy-induced] hypertension without significant proteinuria, unspecified trimester M ♀

O14 Pre-eclampsia

EXCLUDES 1 *pre-existing hypertension with pre-eclampsia (O11)*

DEF: Complication of pregnancy manifesting in the development of borderline hypertension, protein in the urine, and unresponsive swelling between the 20th week of pregnancy and the end of the first week following birth in mild to moderate cases. Severe preeclampsia presents with hypertension, associated with marked swelling, proteinuria, abdominal pain, and/or visual changes.

O14.0 Mild to moderate pre-eclampsia

AHA: 2019,3Q,12; 2019,2Q,8

O14.00 Mild to moderate pre-eclampsia, unspecified trimester M ♀

O14.02 Mild to moderate pre-eclampsia, second trimester CC M ♀

O14.03 Mild to moderate pre-eclampsia, third trimester CC M ♀

O14.04 Mild to moderate pre-eclampsia, complicating childbirth M ♀

AHA: 2019,2Q,8

O14.05 Mild to moderate pre-eclampsia, complicating the puerperium M ♀

O14.1 Severe pre-eclampsia

EXCLUDES 1 *HELLP syndrome (O14.2-)*

AHA: 2019,3Q,12

O14.10 Severe pre-eclampsia, unspecified trimester M ♀

O14.12 Severe pre-eclampsia, second trimester MCC M ♀

O14.13 Severe pre-eclampsia, third trimester MCC M ♀

O14.14 Severe pre-eclampsia complicating childbirth M ♀

O14.15 Severe pre-eclampsia, complicating the puerperium M ♀

O14.2 HELLP syndrome

Severe pre-eclampsia with hemolysis, elevated liver enzymes and low platelet count (HELLP)

AHA: 2019,3Q,12

O14.20 HELLP syndrome (HELLP), unspecified trimester M ♀

O14.22 HELLP syndrome (HELLP), second trimester MCC M ♀

O14.23 HELLP syndrome (HELLP), third trimester MCC M ♀

O14.24 HELLP syndrome, complicating childbirth M ♀

O14.25 HELLP syndrome, complicating the puerperium M ♀

O14.9 Unspecified pre-eclampsia

O14.90 Unspecified pre-eclampsia, unspecified trimester M ♀

O14.92 Unspecified pre-eclampsia, second trimester CC M ♀

O14.93 Unspecified pre-eclampsia, third trimester CC M ♀

O14.94 Unspecified pre-eclampsia, complicating childbirth M ♀

O14.95 Unspecified pre-eclampsia, complicating the puerperium M ♀

O15 Eclampsia

INCLUDES convulsions following conditions in O1Ø-O14 and O16

DEF: Tetany and toxemia producing seizure activity or coma in a pregnant patient who most often has presented with prior preeclampsia (i.e., hypertension, albuminuria, and edema).

O15.Ø Eclampsia complicating pregnancy

O15.ØØ Eclampsia complicating pregnancy, unspecified trimester M ♀

O15.Ø2 Eclampsia complicating pregnancy, second trimester MCC M ♀

O15.Ø3 Eclampsia complicating pregnancy, third trimester MCC M ♀

O15.1 Eclampsia complicating labor MCC M ♀

O15.2 Eclampsia complicating the puerperium MCC M ♀

O15.9 Eclampsia, unspecified as to time period M ♀

Eclampsia NOS

O16 Unspecified maternal hypertension

O16.1 Unspecified maternal hypertension, first trimester CC M ♀

O16.2 Unspecified maternal hypertension, second trimester CC M ♀

O16.3 Unspecified maternal hypertension, third trimester CC M ♀

O16.4 Unspecified maternal hypertension, complicating childbirth M ♀

O16.5 Unspecified maternal hypertension, complicating the puerperium M ♀

O16.9 Unspecified maternal hypertension, unspecified trimester M ♀

Other maternal disorders predominantly related to pregnancy (O2Ø-O29)

EXCLUDES 2 *maternal care related to the fetus and amniotic cavity and possible delivery problems (O3Ø-O48)*

maternal diseases classifiable elsewhere but complicating pregnancy, labor and delivery, and the puerperium (O98-O99)

O2Ø Hemorrhage in early pregnancy

INCLUDES hemorrhage before completion of 2Ø weeks gestation

EXCLUDES 1 *pregnancy with abortive outcome (OØØ-OØ8)*

O2Ø.Ø Threatened abortion CC M ♀

Hemorrhage specified as due to threatened abortion

DEF: Bloody discharge during pregnancy. The cervix may be dilated and pregnancy threatened, but the pregnancy is not terminated.

O2Ø.8 Other hemorrhage in early pregnancy M ♀

O2Ø.9 Hemorrhage in early pregnancy, unspecified CC M ♀

O21 Excessive vomiting in pregnancy

O21.Ø Mild hyperemesis gravidarum M ♀

Hyperemesis gravidarum, mild or unspecified, starting before the end of the 2Øth week of gestation

O21.1 Hyperemesis gravidarum with metabolic disturbance M ♀

Hyperemesis gravidarum, starting before the end of the 2Øth week of gestation, with metabolic disturbance such as carbohydrate depletion

Hyperemesis gravidarum, starting before the end of the 2Øth week of gestation, with metabolic disturbance such as dehydration

Hyperemesis gravidarum, starting before the end of the 2Øth week of gestation, with metabolic disturbance such as electrolyte imbalance

O21.2 Late vomiting of pregnancy M ♀

Excessive vomiting starting after 2Ø completed weeks of gestation

O21.8 Other vomiting complicating pregnancy M ♀

Vomiting due to diseases classified elsewhere, complicating pregnancy

Use additional code, to identify cause

O21.9 Vomiting of pregnancy, unspecified M ♀

O22 Venous complications and hemorrhoids in pregnancy

EXCLUDES 1 *venous complications of:*

abortion NOS (OØ3.9)

ectopic or molar pregnancy (OØ8.7)

failed attempted abortion (OØ7.35)

induced abortion (OØ4.85)

spontaneous abortion (OØ3.89)

EXCLUDES 2 *obstetric pulmonary embolism (O88.-)*

venous complications and hemorrhoids of childbirth and the puerperium (O87.-)

O22.Ø Varicose veins of lower extremity in pregnancy

Varicose veins NOS in pregnancy

DEF: Distended, tortuous veins of the lower extremities associated with pregnancy.

O22.ØØ Varicose veins of lower extremity in pregnancy, unspecified trimester M ♀

O22.Ø1 Varicose veins of lower extremity in pregnancy, first trimester M ♀

O22.Ø2 Varicose veins of lower extremity in pregnancy, second trimester M ♀

O22.Ø3 Varicose veins of lower extremity in pregnancy, third trimester M ♀

O22.1 Genital varices in pregnancy

Perineal varices in pregnancy

Vaginal varices in pregnancy

Vulval varices in pregnancy

O22.1Ø Genital varices in pregnancy, unspecified trimester M ♀

O22.11 Genital varices in pregnancy, first trimester M ♀

O22.12 Genital varices in pregnancy, second trimester M ♀

O22.13 Genital varices in pregnancy, third trimester M ♀

O22.2 Superficial thrombophlebitis in pregnancy

Phlebitis in pregnancy NOS

Thrombophlebitis of legs in pregnancy

Thrombosis in pregnancy NOS

Use additional code to identify the superficial thrombophlebitis (I8Ø.Ø-)

O22.2Ø Superficial thrombophlebitis in pregnancy, unspecified trimester CC M ♀

O22.21 Superficial thrombophlebitis in pregnancy, first trimester CC M ♀

O22.22 Superficial thrombophlebitis in pregnancy, second trimester CC M ♀

O22.23 Superficial thrombophlebitis in pregnancy, third trimester CC M ♀

O22.3 Deep phlebothrombosis in pregnancy

Deep vein thrombosis, antepartum

Use additional code to identify the deep vein thrombosis (I82.4-, I82.5-, I82.62-, I82.72-)

Use additional code, if applicable, for associated long-term (current) use of anticoagulants (Z79.Ø1)

O22.3Ø Deep phlebothrombosis in pregnancy, unspecified trimester CC M ♀

O22.31 Deep phlebothrombosis in pregnancy, first trimester MCC M ♀

O22.32 Deep phlebothrombosis in pregnancy, second trimester MCC M ♀

O22.33 Deep phlebothrombosis in pregnancy, third trimester MCC M ♀

O22.4 Hemorrhoids in pregnancy

O22.4Ø Hemorrhoids in pregnancy, unspecified trimester CC M ♀

O22.41 Hemorrhoids in pregnancy, first trimester CC M ♀

O22.42 Hemorrhoids in pregnancy, second trimester CC M ♀

O22.43 Hemorrhoids in pregnancy, third trimester CC M ♀

O22.5 Cerebral venous thrombosis in pregnancy

Cerebrovenous sinus thrombosis in pregnancy

O22.5Ø Cerebral venous thrombosis in pregnancy, unspecified trimester CC M ♀

O22.51 Cerebral venous thrombosis in pregnancy, first trimester CC M ♀

O22.52 Cerebral venous thrombosis in pregnancy, second trimester CC M ♀

O22.53 Cerebral venous thrombosis in pregnancy, third trimester CC M ♀

5th **O22.8 Other venous complications in pregnancy**

6th **O22.8X Other venous complications in pregnancy**

O22.8X1 Other venous complications in pregnancy, first trimester CC M ♀

O22.8X2 Other venous complications in pregnancy, second trimester CC M ♀

O22.8X3 Other venous complications in pregnancy, third trimester CC M ♀

O22.8X9 Other venous complications in pregnancy, unspecified trimester CC M ♀

5th **O22.9 Venous complication in pregnancy, unspecified**

Gestational phlebitis NOS
Gestational phlebopathy NOS
Gestational thrombosis NOS

O22.9Ø Venous complication in pregnancy, unspecified, unspecified trimester CC M ♀

O22.91 Venous complication in pregnancy, unspecified, first trimester M ♀

O22.92 Venous complication in pregnancy, unspecified, second trimester M ♀

O22.93 Venous complication in pregnancy, unspecified, third trimester M ♀

4th **O23 Infections of genitourinary tract in pregnancy**

Use additional code to identify organism (B95.-, B96.-)

EXCLUDES 2 *gonococcal infections complicating pregnancy, childbirth and the puerperium (O98.2)*
infections with a predominantly sexual mode of transmission NOS complicating pregnancy, childbirth and the puerperium (O98.3)
syphilis complicating pregnancy, childbirth and the puerperium (O98.1)
tuberculosis of genitourinary system complicating pregnancy, childbirth and the puerperium (O98.Ø)
venereal disease NOS complicating pregnancy, childbirth and the puerperium (O98.3)

AHA: 2018,2Q,20

5th **O23.Ø Infections of kidney in pregnancy**

Pyelonephritis in pregnancy

O23.ØØ Infections of kidney in pregnancy, unspecified trimester M ♀

O23.Ø1 Infections of kidney in pregnancy, first trimester CC M ♀

O23.Ø2 Infections of kidney in pregnancy, second trimester CC M ♀

O23.Ø3 Infections of kidney in pregnancy, third trimester CC M ♀

5th **O23.1 Infections of bladder in pregnancy**

O23.1Ø Infections of bladder in pregnancy, unspecified trimester M ♀

O23.11 Infections of bladder in pregnancy, first trimester CC M ♀

O23.12 Infections of bladder in pregnancy, second trimester CC M ♀

O23.13 Infections of bladder in pregnancy, third trimester CC M ♀

5th **O23.2 Infections of urethra in pregnancy**

O23.2Ø Infections of urethra in pregnancy, unspecified trimester M ♀

O23.21 Infections of urethra in pregnancy, first trimester CC M ♀

O23.22 Infections of urethra in pregnancy, second trimester CC M ♀

O23.23 Infections of urethra in pregnancy, third trimester CC M ♀

5th **O23.3 Infections of other parts of urinary tract in pregnancy**

O23.3Ø Infections of other parts of urinary tract in pregnancy, unspecified trimester M ♀

O23.31 Infections of other parts of urinary tract in pregnancy, first trimester CC M ♀

O23.32 Infections of other parts of urinary tract in pregnancy, second trimester CC M ♀

O23.33 Infections of other parts of urinary tract in pregnancy, third trimester CC M ♀

5th **O23.4 Unspecified infection of urinary tract in pregnancy**

O23.4Ø Unspecified infection of urinary tract in pregnancy, unspecified trimester M ♀

O23.41 Unspecified infection of urinary tract in pregnancy, first trimester CC M ♀

O23.42 Unspecified infection of urinary tract in pregnancy, second trimester CC M ♀

O23.43 Unspecified infection of urinary tract in pregnancy, third trimester CC M ♀

5th **O23.5 Infections of the genital tract in pregnancy**

6th **O23.51 Infection of cervix in pregnancy**

O23.511 Infections of cervix in pregnancy, first trimester CC M ♀

O23.512 Infections of cervix in pregnancy, second trimester CC M ♀

O23.513 Infections of cervix in pregnancy, third trimester CC M ♀

O23.519 Infections of cervix in pregnancy, unspecified trimester M ♀

6th **O23.52 Salpingo-oophoritis in pregnancy**

Oophoritis in pregnancy
Salpingitis in pregnancy

O23.521 Salpingo-oophoritis in pregnancy, first trimester CC M ♀

O23.522 Salpingo-oophoritis in pregnancy, second trimester CC M ♀

O23.523 Salpingo-oophoritis in pregnancy, third trimester CC M ♀

O23.529 Salpingo-oophoritis in pregnancy, unspecified trimester M ♀

6th **O23.59 Infection of other part of genital tract in pregnancy**

AHA: 2022,1Q,20

O23.591 Infection of other part of genital tract in pregnancy, first trimester CC M ♀

O23.592 Infection of other part of genital tract in pregnancy, second trimester CC M ♀

O23.593 Infection of other part of genital tract in pregnancy, third trimester CC M ♀

O23.599 Infection of other part of genital tract in pregnancy, unspecified trimester M ♀

5th **O23.9 Unspecified genitourinary tract infection in pregnancy**

Genitourinary tract infection in pregnancy NOS

O23.9Ø Unspecified genitourinary tract infection in pregnancy, unspecified trimester M ♀

O23.91 Unspecified genitourinary tract infection in pregnancy, first trimester CC M ♀

O23.92 Unspecified genitourinary tract infection in pregnancy, second trimester CC M ♀

O23.93 Unspecified genitourinary tract infection in pregnancy, third trimester CC M ♀

4th **O24 Diabetes mellitus in pregnancy, childbirth and the puerperium**

5th **O24.Ø Pre-existing type 1 diabetes mellitus, in pregnancy, childbirth and the puerperium**

Juvenile onset diabetes mellitus, in pregnancy, childbirth and the puerperium
Ketosis-prone diabetes mellitus in pregnancy, childbirth and the puerperium

Use additional code from category E1Ø to further identify any manifestations

6th **O24.Ø1 Pre-existing type 1 diabetes mellitus, in pregnancy**

O24.Ø11 Pre-existing type 1 diabetes mellitus, in pregnancy, first trimester CC M ♀

O24.Ø12 Pre-existing type 1 diabetes mellitus, in pregnancy, second trimester CC M ♀

O24.Ø13 Pre-existing type 1 diabetes mellitus, in pregnancy, third trimester CC M ♀

O24.Ø19 Pre-existing type 1 diabetes mellitus, in pregnancy, unspecified trimester CC M ♀

O24.Ø2 Pre-existing type 1 diabetes mellitus, in childbirth MCC M ♀

O24.Ø3 Pre-existing type 1 diabetes mellitus, in the puerperium CC M ♀

O24.1 Pre-existing type 2 diabetes mellitus, in pregnancy, childbirth and the puerperium
Insulin-resistant diabetes mellitus in pregnancy, childbirth and the puerperium
Use additional code (for):
from category E11 to further identify any manifestations
long-term (current) use of insulin (Z79.4)

O24.11 Pre-existing type 2 diabetes mellitus, in pregnancy
- **O24.111 Pre-existing type 2 diabetes mellitus, in pregnancy, first trimester** CC M ♀
- **O24.112 Pre-existing type 2 diabetes mellitus, in pregnancy, second trimester** CC M ♀
- **O24.113 Pre-existing type 2 diabetes mellitus, in pregnancy, third trimester** CC M ♀
- **O24.119 Pre-existing type 2 diabetes mellitus, in pregnancy, unspecified trimester** CC M ♀

O24.12 Pre-existing type 2 diabetes mellitus, in childbirth MCC M ♀

O24.13 Pre-existing type 2 diabetes mellitus, in the puerperium CC M ♀

O24.3 Unspecified pre-existing diabetes mellitus in pregnancy, childbirth and the puerperium
Use additional code (for):
from category E11 to further identify any manifestation
long-term (current) use of insulin (Z79.4)

O24.31 Unspecified pre-existing diabetes mellitus in pregnancy
- **O24.311 Unspecified pre-existing diabetes mellitus in pregnancy, first trimester** CC M ♀
- **O24.312 Unspecified pre-existing diabetes mellitus in pregnancy, second trimester** CC M ♀
- **O24.313 Unspecified pre-existing diabetes mellitus in pregnancy, third trimester** CC M ♀
- **O24.319 Unspecified pre-existing diabetes mellitus in pregnancy, unspecified trimester** CC M ♀

O24.32 Unspecified pre-existing diabetes mellitus in childbirth MCC M ♀

O24.33 Unspecified pre-existing diabetes mellitus in the puerperium CC M ♀

O24.4 Gestational diabetes mellitus
Diabetes mellitus arising in pregnancy
Gestational diabetes mellitus NOS
AHA: 2020,3Q,30; 2016,4Q,50; 2015,4Q,34

O24.41 Gestational diabetes mellitus in pregnancy
- **O24.410 Gestational diabetes mellitus in pregnancy, diet controlled** M ♀
- **O24.414 Gestational diabetes mellitus in pregnancy, insulin controlled** M ♀
- **O24.415 Gestational diabetes mellitus in pregnancy, controlled by oral hypoglycemic drugs** M ♀
  Gestational diabetes mellitus in pregnancy, controlled by oral antidiabetic drugs
- **O24.419 Gestational diabetes mellitus in pregnancy, unspecified control** M ♀

O24.42 Gestational diabetes mellitus in childbirth
AHA: 2016,1Q,5
- **O24.420 Gestational diabetes mellitus in childbirth, diet controlled** M ♀
- **O24.424 Gestational diabetes mellitus in childbirth, insulin controlled** M ♀
- **O24.425 Gestational diabetes mellitus in childbirth, controlled by oral hypoglycemic drugs** M ♀
  Gestational diabetes mellitus in childbirth, controlled by oral antidiabetic drugs
- **O24.429 Gestational diabetes mellitus in childbirth, unspecified control** M ♀

O24.43 Gestational diabetes mellitus in the puerperium
- **O24.430 Gestational diabetes mellitus in the puerperium, diet controlled** M ♀
- **O24.434 Gestational diabetes mellitus in the puerperium, insulin controlled** M ♀
- **O24.435 Gestational diabetes mellitus in puerperium, controlled by oral hypoglycemic drugs** M ♀
  Gestational diabetes mellitus in puerperium, controlled by oral antidiabetic drugs
- **O24.439 Gestational diabetes mellitus in the puerperium, unspecified control** M ♀

O24.8 Other pre-existing diabetes mellitus in pregnancy, childbirth, and the puerperium
Use additional code (for):
from categories E08, E09 and E13 to further identify any manifestation
long-term (current) use of insulin (Z79.4)

O24.81 Other pre-existing diabetes mellitus in pregnancy
- **O24.811 Other pre-existing diabetes mellitus in pregnancy, first trimester** CC M ♀
- **O24.812 Other pre-existing diabetes mellitus in pregnancy, second trimester** CC M ♀
- **O24.813 Other pre-existing diabetes mellitus in pregnancy, third trimester** CC M ♀
- **O24.819 Other pre-existing diabetes mellitus in pregnancy, unspecified trimester** CC M ♀

O24.82 Other pre-existing diabetes mellitus in childbirth MCC M ♀

O24.83 Other pre-existing diabetes mellitus in the puerperium CC M ♀

O24.9 Unspecified diabetes mellitus in pregnancy, childbirth and the puerperium
Use additional code for long-term (current) use of insulin (Z79.4)

O24.91 Unspecified diabetes mellitus in pregnancy
- **O24.911 Unspecified diabetes mellitus in pregnancy, first trimester** CC M ♀
- **O24.912 Unspecified diabetes mellitus in pregnancy, second trimester** CC M ♀
- **O24.913 Unspecified diabetes mellitus in pregnancy, third trimester** CC M ♀
- **O24.919 Unspecified diabetes mellitus in pregnancy, unspecified trimester** CC M ♀

O24.92 Unspecified diabetes mellitus in childbirth M ♀

O24.93 Unspecified diabetes mellitus in the puerperium CC M ♀

O25 Malnutrition in pregnancy, childbirth and the puerperium

O25.1 Malnutrition in pregnancy
- **O25.10 Malnutrition in pregnancy, unspecified trimester** M ♀
- **O25.11 Malnutrition in pregnancy, first trimester** M ♀
- **O25.12 Malnutrition in pregnancy, second trimester** M ♀
- **O25.13 Malnutrition in pregnancy, third trimester** M ♀

O25.2 Malnutrition in childbirth M ♀

O25.3 Malnutrition in the puerperium M ♀

O26 Maternal care for other conditions predominantly related to pregnancy

O26.0 Excessive weight gain in pregnancy
EXCLUDES 2 *gestational edema (O12.0, O12.2)*
- **O26.00 Excessive weight gain in pregnancy, unspecified trimester** M ♀
- **O26.01 Excessive weight gain in pregnancy, first trimester** M ♀
- **O26.02 Excessive weight gain in pregnancy, second trimester** M ♀
- **O26.03 Excessive weight gain in pregnancy, third trimester** M ♀

O26.1 Low weight gain in pregnancy
- **O26.10 Low weight gain in pregnancy, unspecified trimester** M ♀
- **O26.11 Low weight gain in pregnancy, first trimester** M ♀
- **O26.12 Low weight gain in pregnancy, second trimester** M ♀
- **O26.13 Low weight gain in pregnancy, third trimester** M ♀

O26.2 Pregnancy care for patient with recurrent pregnancy loss
- **O26.20 Pregnancy care for patient with recurrent pregnancy loss, unspecified trimester** M ♀

O26.21 Pregnancy care for patient with recurrent pregnancy loss, first trimester M♀

O26.22 Pregnancy care for patient with recurrent pregnancy loss, second trimester M♀

O26.23 Pregnancy care for patient with recurrent pregnancy loss, third trimester M♀

5th **O26.3 Retained intrauterine contraceptive device in pregnancy**

O26.30 Retained intrauterine contraceptive device in pregnancy, unspecified trimester M♀

O26.31 Retained intrauterine contraceptive device in pregnancy, first trimester M♀

O26.32 Retained intrauterine contraceptive device in pregnancy, second trimester M♀

O26.33 Retained intrauterine contraceptive device in pregnancy, third trimester M♀

5th **O26.4 Herpes gestationis**

DEF: Rare skin disorder of unknown origin that appears on the abdomen in the second and third trimester as intensely itchy blisters that spread to other sites.

O26.40 Herpes gestationis, unspecified trimester M♀

O26.41 Herpes gestationis, first trimester M♀

O26.42 Herpes gestationis, second trimester M♀

O26.43 Herpes gestationis, third trimester M♀

5th **O26.5 Maternal hypotension syndrome**

Supine hypotensive syndrome

O26.50 Maternal hypotension syndrome, unspecified trimester M♀

O26.51 Maternal hypotension syndrome, first trimester M♀

O26.52 Maternal hypotension syndrome, second trimester M♀

O26.53 Maternal hypotension syndrome, third trimester M♀

5th **O26.6 Liver and biliary tract disorders in pregnancy, childbirth and the puerperium**

Use additional code to identify the specific disorder

EXCLUDES 2 *hepatorenal syndrome following labor and delivery (O90.4)*

6th **O26.61 Liver and biliary tract disorders in pregnancy**

O26.611 Liver and biliary tract disorders in pregnancy, first trimester CC M♀

O26.612 Liver and biliary tract disorders in pregnancy, second trimester CC M♀

O26.613 Liver and biliary tract disorders in pregnancy, third trimester CC M♀

O26.619 Liver and biliary tract disorders in pregnancy, unspecified trimester M♀

O26.62 Liver and biliary tract disorders in childbirth CC M♀

O26.63 Liver and biliary tract disorders in the puerperium M♀

5th **O26.7 Subluxation of symphysis (pubis) in pregnancy, childbirth and the puerperium**

EXCLUDES 1 *traumatic separation of symphysis (pubis) during childbirth (O71.6)*

6th **O26.71 Subluxation of symphysis (pubis) in pregnancy**

O26.711 Subluxation of symphysis (pubis) in pregnancy, first trimester M♀

O26.712 Subluxation of symphysis (pubis) in pregnancy, second trimester M♀

O26.713 Subluxation of symphysis (pubis) in pregnancy, third trimester M♀

O26.719 Subluxation of symphysis (pubis) in pregnancy, unspecified trimester M♀

O26.72 Subluxation of symphysis (pubis) in childbirth M♀

O26.73 Subluxation of symphysis (pubis) in the puerperium M♀

5th **O26.8 Other specified pregnancy related conditions**

6th **O26.81 Pregnancy related exhaustion and fatigue**

O26.811 Pregnancy related exhaustion and fatigue, first trimester M♀

O26.812 Pregnancy related exhaustion and fatigue, second trimester M♀

O26.813 Pregnancy related exhaustion and fatigue, third trimester M♀

O26.819 Pregnancy related exhaustion and fatigue, unspecified trimester M♀

6th **O26.82 Pregnancy related peripheral neuritis**

O26.821 Pregnancy related peripheral neuritis, first trimester M♀

O26.822 Pregnancy related peripheral neuritis, second trimester M♀

O26.823 Pregnancy related peripheral neuritis, third trimester M♀

O26.829 Pregnancy related peripheral neuritis, unspecified trimester M♀

6th **O26.83 Pregnancy related renal disease**

Use additional code to identify the specific disorder

O26.831 Pregnancy related renal disease, first trimester CC M♀

O26.832 Pregnancy related renal disease, second trimester CC M♀

O26.833 Pregnancy related renal disease, third trimester CC M♀

O26.839 Pregnancy related renal disease, unspecified trimester M♀

6th **O26.84 Uterine size-date discrepancy complicating pregnancy**

EXCLUDES 1 *encounter for suspected problem with fetal growth ruled out (Z03.74)*

O26.841 Uterine size-date discrepancy, first trimester M♀

O26.842 Uterine size-date discrepancy, second trimester M♀

O26.843 Uterine size-date discrepancy, third trimester M♀

O26.849 Uterine size-date discrepancy, unspecified trimester M♀

6th **O26.85 Spotting complicating pregnancy**

O26.851 Spotting complicating pregnancy, first trimester M♀

O26.852 Spotting complicating pregnancy, second trimester M♀

O26.853 Spotting complicating pregnancy, third trimester M♀

O26.859 Spotting complicating pregnancy, unspecified trimester M♀

O26.86 Pruritic urticarial papules and plaques of pregnancy (PUPPP) M♀

Polymorphic eruption of pregnancy

6th **O26.87 Cervical shortening**

EXCLUDES 1 *encounter for suspected cervical shortening ruled out (Z03.75)*

DEF: Cervix that has shortened to less than 25 mm before the 24th week of pregnancy. A shortened cervix is a warning sign for impending premature delivery and is treated by cervical cerclage placement or progesterone.

O26.872 Cervical shortening, second trimester CC M♀

O26.873 Cervical shortening, third trimester CC M♀

O26.879 Cervical shortening, unspecified trimester CC M♀

6th **O26.89 Other specified pregnancy related conditions**

AHA: 2015,3Q,40

O26.891 Other specified pregnancy related conditions, first trimester M♀

O26.892 Other specified pregnancy related conditions, second trimester M♀

O26.893 Other specified pregnancy related conditions, third trimester M♀

O26.899 Other specified pregnancy related conditions, unspecified trimester M♀

5th **O26.9 Pregnancy related conditions, unspecified**

O26.90 Pregnancy related conditions, unspecified, unspecified trimester M♀

O26.91 Pregnancy related conditions, unspecified, first trimester M♀

O26.92 Pregnancy related conditions, unspecified, second trimester M♀

O26.93 Pregnancy related conditions, unspecified, third trimester M♀

O28 Abnormal findings on antenatal screening of mother

EXCLUDES 1 *diagnostic findings classified elsewhere - see Alphabetical Index*

O28.Ø Abnormal hematological finding on antenatal screening of mother M ♀

O28.1 Abnormal biochemical finding on antenatal screening of mother M ♀

O28.2 Abnormal cytological finding on antenatal screening of mother M ♀

O28.3 Abnormal ultrasonic finding on antenatal screening of mother M ♀

O28.4 Abnormal radiological finding on antenatal screening of mother M ♀

O28.5 Abnormal chromosomal and genetic finding on antenatal screening of mother M ♀

O28.8 Other abnormal findings on antenatal screening of mother M ♀

O28.9 Unspecified abnormal findings on antenatal screening of mother M ♀

O29 Complications of anesthesia during pregnancy

INCLUDES maternal complications arising from the administration of a general, regional or local anesthetic, analgesic or other sedation during pregnancy

Use additional code, if necessary, to identify the complication

EXCLUDES 2 *complications of anesthesia during labor and delivery (O74.-)*
complications of anesthesia during the puerperium (O89.-)

O29.Ø Pulmonary complications of anesthesia during pregnancy

O29.Ø1 Aspiration pneumonitis due to anesthesia during pregnancy

Inhalation of stomach contents or secretions NOS due to anesthesia during pregnancy

Mendelson's syndrome due to anesthesia during pregnancy

O29.Ø11 Aspiration pneumonitis due to anesthesia during pregnancy, first trimester M ♀

O29.Ø12 Aspiration pneumonitis due to anesthesia during pregnancy, second trimester M ♀

O29.Ø13 Aspiration pneumonitis due to anesthesia during pregnancy, third trimester M ♀

O29.Ø19 Aspiration pneumonitis due to anesthesia during pregnancy, unspecified trimester M ♀

O29.Ø2 Pressure collapse of lung due to anesthesia during pregnancy

O29.Ø21 Pressure collapse of lung due to anesthesia during pregnancy, first trimester M ♀

O29.Ø22 Pressure collapse of lung due to anesthesia during pregnancy, second trimester M ♀

O29.Ø23 Pressure collapse of lung due to anesthesia during pregnancy, third trimester M ♀

O29.Ø29 Pressure collapse of lung due to anesthesia during pregnancy, unspecified trimester M ♀

O29.Ø9 Other pulmonary complications of anesthesia during pregnancy

O29.Ø91 Other pulmonary complications of anesthesia during pregnancy, first trimester M ♀

O29.Ø92 Other pulmonary complications of anesthesia during pregnancy, second trimester M ♀

O29.Ø93 Other pulmonary complications of anesthesia during pregnancy, third trimester M ♀

O29.Ø99 Other pulmonary complications of anesthesia during pregnancy, unspecified trimester M ♀

O29.1 Cardiac complications of anesthesia during pregnancy

O29.11 Cardiac arrest due to anesthesia during pregnancy

O29.111 Cardiac arrest due to anesthesia during pregnancy, first trimester M ♀

O29.112 Cardiac arrest due to anesthesia during pregnancy, second trimester M ♀

O29.113 Cardiac arrest due to anesthesia during pregnancy, third trimester M ♀

O29.119 Cardiac arrest due to anesthesia during pregnancy, unspecified trimester M ♀

O29.12 Cardiac failure due to anesthesia during pregnancy

O29.121 Cardiac failure due to anesthesia during pregnancy, first trimester M ♀

O29.122 Cardiac failure due to anesthesia during pregnancy, second trimester M ♀

O29.123 Cardiac failure due to anesthesia during pregnancy, third trimester M ♀

O29.129 Cardiac failure due to anesthesia during pregnancy, unspecified trimester M ♀

O29.19 Other cardiac complications of anesthesia during pregnancy

O29.191 Other cardiac complications of anesthesia during pregnancy, first trimester M ♀

O29.192 Other cardiac complications of anesthesia during pregnancy, second trimester M ♀

O29.193 Other cardiac complications of anesthesia during pregnancy, third trimester M ♀

O29.199 Other cardiac complications of anesthesia during pregnancy, unspecified trimester M ♀

O29.2 Central nervous system complications of anesthesia during pregnancy

O29.21 Cerebral anoxia due to anesthesia during pregnancy

O29.211 Cerebral anoxia due to anesthesia during pregnancy, first trimester M ♀

O29.212 Cerebral anoxia due to anesthesia during pregnancy, second trimester M ♀

O29.213 Cerebral anoxia due to anesthesia during pregnancy, third trimester M ♀

O29.219 Cerebral anoxia due to anesthesia during pregnancy, unspecified trimester M ♀

O29.29 Other central nervous system complications of anesthesia during pregnancy

O29.291 Other central nervous system complications of anesthesia during pregnancy, first trimester M ♀

O29.292 Other central nervous system complications of anesthesia during pregnancy, second trimester M ♀

O29.293 Other central nervous system complications of anesthesia during pregnancy, third trimester M ♀

O29.299 Other central nervous system complications of anesthesia during pregnancy, unspecified trimester M ♀

O29.3 Toxic reaction to local anesthesia during pregnancy

O29.3X Toxic reaction to local anesthesia during pregnancy

O29.3X1 Toxic reaction to local anesthesia during pregnancy, first trimester M ♀

O29.3X2 Toxic reaction to local anesthesia during pregnancy, second trimester M ♀

O29.3X3 Toxic reaction to local anesthesia during pregnancy, third trimester M ♀

O29.3X9 Toxic reaction to local anesthesia during pregnancy, unspecified trimester M ♀

O29.4 Spinal and epidural anesthesia induced headache during pregnancy

O29.4Ø Spinal and epidural anesthesia induced headache during pregnancy, unspecified trimester M ♀

O29.41 Spinal and epidural anesthesia induced headache during pregnancy, first trimester M ♀

O29.42 Spinal and epidural anesthesia induced headache during pregnancy, second trimester M ♀

O29.43 Spinal and epidural anesthesia induced headache during pregnancy, third trimester M ♀

O29.5 Other complications of spinal and epidural anesthesia during pregnancy

O29.5X Other complications of spinal and epidural anesthesia during pregnancy

O29.5X1 Other complications of spinal and epidural anesthesia during pregnancy, first trimester M ♀

O29.5X2 Other complications of spinal and epidural anesthesia during pregnancy, second trimester M ♀

O29.5X3 Other complications of spinal and epidural anesthesia during pregnancy, third trimester M ♀

O29.5X9 Other complications of spinal and epidural anesthesia during pregnancy, unspecified trimester M ♀

✓5th **O29.6 Failed or difficult intubation for anesthesia during pregnancy**

O29.60 Failed or difficult intubation for anesthesia during pregnancy, unspecified trimester M ♀

O29.61 Failed or difficult intubation for anesthesia during pregnancy, first trimester M ♀

O29.62 Failed or difficult intubation for anesthesia during pregnancy, second trimester M ♀

O29.63 Failed or difficult intubation for anesthesia during pregnancy, third trimester M ♀

✓5th **O29.8 Other complications of anesthesia during pregnancy**

✓6th **O29.8X Other complications of anesthesia during pregnancy**

O29.8X1 Other complications of anesthesia during pregnancy, first trimester M ♀

O29.8X2 Other complications of anesthesia during pregnancy, second trimester M ♀

O29.8X3 Other complications of anesthesia during pregnancy, third trimester M ♀

O29.8X9 Other complications of anesthesia during pregnancy, unspecified trimester M ♀

✓5th **O29.9 Unspecified complication of anesthesia during pregnancy**

O29.90 Unspecified complication of anesthesia during pregnancy, unspecified trimester M ♀

O29.91 Unspecified complication of anesthesia during pregnancy, first trimester M ♀

O29.92 Unspecified complication of anesthesia during pregnancy, second trimester M ♀

O29.93 Unspecified complication of anesthesia during pregnancy, third trimester M ♀

Maternal care related to the fetus and amniotic cavity and possible delivery problems (O30-O48)

✓4th **O30 Multiple gestation**

Code also any complications specific to multiple gestation

AHA: 2016,4Q,51

✓5th **O30.0 Twin pregnancy**

✓6th **O30.00 Twin pregnancy, unspecified number of placenta and unspecified number of amniotic sacs**

O30.001 Twin pregnancy, unspecified number of placenta and unspecified number of amniotic sacs, first trimester M ♀

O30.002 Twin pregnancy, unspecified number of placenta and unspecified number of amniotic sacs, second trimester M ♀

O30.003 Twin pregnancy, unspecified number of placenta and unspecified number of amniotic sacs, third trimester M ♀

O30.009 Twin pregnancy, unspecified number of placenta and unspecified number of amniotic sacs, unspecified trimester M ♀

✓6th **O30.01 Twin pregnancy, monochorionic/monoamniotic**

Twin pregnancy, one placenta, one amniotic sac

EXCLUDES 1 *conjoined twins (O30.02-)*

O30.011 Twin pregnancy, monochorionic/monoamniotic, first trimester M ♀

O30.012 Twin pregnancy, monochorionic/monoamniotic, second trimester M ♀

O30.013 Twin pregnancy, monochorionic/monoamniotic, third trimester M ♀

O30.019 Twin pregnancy, monochorionic/monoamniotic, unspecified trimester M ♀

✓6th **O30.02 Conjoined twin pregnancy**

O30.021 Conjoined twin pregnancy, first trimester M ♀

O30.022 Conjoined twin pregnancy, second trimester M ♀

O30.023 Conjoined twin pregnancy, third trimester M ♀

O30.029 Conjoined twin pregnancy, unspecified trimester M ♀

✓6th **O30.03 Twin pregnancy, monochorionic/diamniotic**

Twin pregnancy, one placenta, two amniotic sacs

O30.031 Twin pregnancy, monochorionic/diamniotic, first trimester M ♀

O30.032 Twin pregnancy, monochorionic/diamniotic, second trimester M ♀

O30.033 Twin pregnancy, monochorionic/diamniotic, third trimester M ♀

O30.039 Twin pregnancy, monochorionic/diamniotic, unspecified trimester M ♀

✓6th **O30.04 Twin pregnancy, dichorionic/diamniotic**

Twin pregnancy, two placentae, two amniotic sacs

O30.041 Twin pregnancy, dichorionic/diamniotic, first trimester M ♀

O30.042 Twin pregnancy, dichorionic/diamniotic, second trimester M ♀

O30.043 Twin pregnancy, dichorionic/diamniotic, third trimester M ♀

O30.049 Twin pregnancy, dichorionic/diamniotic, unspecified trimester M ♀

✓6th **O30.09 Twin pregnancy, unable to determine number of placenta and number of amniotic sacs**

O30.091 Twin pregnancy, unable to determine number of placenta and number of amniotic sacs, first trimester M ♀

O30.092 Twin pregnancy, unable to determine number of placenta and number of amniotic sacs, second trimester M ♀

O30.093 Twin pregnancy, unable to determine number of placenta and number of amniotic sacs, third trimester M ♀

O30.099 Twin pregnancy, unable to determine number of placenta and number of amniotic sacs, unspecified trimester M ♀

✓5th **O30.1 Triplet pregnancy**

✓6th **O30.10 Triplet pregnancy, unspecified number of placenta and unspecified number of amniotic sacs**

AHA: 2016,2Q,8

O30.101 Triplet pregnancy, unspecified number of placenta and unspecified number of amniotic sacs, first trimester CC M ♀

O30.102 Triplet pregnancy, unspecified number of placenta and unspecified number of amniotic sacs, second trimester CC M ♀

O30.103 Triplet pregnancy, unspecified number of placenta and unspecified number of amniotic sacs, third trimester CC M ♀

O30.109 Triplet pregnancy, unspecified number of placenta and unspecified number of amniotic sacs, unspecified trimester M ♀

✓6th **O30.11 Triplet pregnancy with two or more monochorionic fetuses**

O30.111 Triplet pregnancy with two or more monochorionic fetuses, first trimester CC M ♀

O30.112 Triplet pregnancy with two or more monochorionic fetuses, second trimester CC M ♀

O30.113 Triplet pregnancy with two or more monochorionic fetuses, third trimester CC M ♀

O30.119 Triplet pregnancy with two or more monochorionic fetuses, unspecified trimester M ♀

✓6th **O30.12 Triplet pregnancy with two or more monoamniotic fetuses**

O30.121 Triplet pregnancy with two or more monoamniotic fetuses, first trimester CC M ♀

O30.122 Triplet pregnancy with two or more monoamniotic fetuses, second trimester CC M ♀

O30.123 Triplet pregnancy with two or more monoamniotic fetuses, third trimester CC M ♀

O30.129 Triplet pregnancy with two or more monoamniotic fetuses, unspecified trimester M ♀

✓6th O30.13 Triplet pregnancy, trichorionic/triamniotic

AHA: 2018,4Q,22

O30.131 Triplet pregnancy, trichorionic/triamniotic, first trimester CC M ♀

O30.132 Triplet pregnancy, trichorionic/triamniotic, second trimester CC M ♀

O30.133 Triplet pregnancy, trichorionic/triamniotic, third trimester CC M ♀

O30.139 Triplet pregnancy, trichorionic/triamniotic, unspecified trimester M ♀

✓6th O30.19 Triplet pregnancy, unable to determine number of placenta and number of amniotic sacs

O30.191 Triplet pregnancy, unable to determine number of placenta and number of amniotic sacs, first trimester CC M ♀

O30.192 Triplet pregnancy, unable to determine number of placenta and number of amniotic sacs, second trimester CC M ♀

O30.193 Triplet pregnancy, unable to determine number of placenta and number of amniotic sacs, third trimester CC M ♀

O30.199 Triplet pregnancy, unable to determine number of placenta and number of amniotic sacs, unspecified trimester M ♀

✓5th O30.2 Quadruplet pregnancy

✓6th O30.20 Quadruplet pregnancy, unspecified number of placenta and unspecified number of amniotic sacs

O30.201 Quadruplet pregnancy, unspecified number of placenta and unspecified number of amniotic sacs, first trimester CC M ♀

O30.202 Quadruplet pregnancy, unspecified number of placenta and unspecified number of amniotic sacs, second trimester CC M ♀

O30.203 Quadruplet pregnancy, unspecified number of placenta and unspecified number of amniotic sacs, third trimester CC M ♀

O30.209 Quadruplet pregnancy, unspecified number of placenta and unspecified number of amniotic sacs, unspecified trimester M ♀

✓6th O30.21 Quadruplet pregnancy with two or more monochorionic fetuses

O30.211 Quadruplet pregnancy with two or more monochorionic fetuses, first trimester CC M ♀

O30.212 Quadruplet pregnancy with two or more monochorionic fetuses, second trimester CC M ♀

O30.213 Quadruplet pregnancy with two or more monochorionic fetuses, third trimester CC M ♀

O30.219 Quadruplet pregnancy with two or more monochorionic fetuses, unspecified trimester M ♀

✓6th O30.22 Quadruplet pregnancy with two or more monoamniotic fetuses

O30.221 Quadruplet pregnancy with two or more monoamniotic fetuses, first trimester CC M ♀

O30.222 Quadruplet pregnancy with two or more monoamniotic fetuses, second trimester CC M ♀

O30.223 Quadruplet pregnancy with two or more monoamniotic fetuses, third trimester CC M ♀

O30.229 Quadruplet pregnancy with two or more monoamniotic fetuses, unspecified trimester M ♀

✓6th O30.23 Quadruplet pregnancy, quadrachorionic/quadra-amniotic

AHA: 2018,4Q,22

O30.231 Quadruplet pregnancy, quadrachorionic/quadra-amniotic, first trimester CC M ♀

O30.232 Quadruplet pregnancy, quadrachorionic/quadra-amniotic, second trimester CC M ♀

O30.233 Quadruplet pregnancy, quadrachorionic/quadra-amniotic, third trimester CC M ♀

O30.239 Quadruplet pregnancy, quadrachorionic/quadra-amniotic, unspecified trimester M ♀

✓6th O30.29 Quadruplet pregnancy, unable to determine number of placenta and number of amniotic sacs

O30.291 Quadruplet pregnancy, unable to determine number of placenta and number of amniotic sacs, first trimester CC M ♀

O30.292 Quadruplet pregnancy, unable to determine number of placenta and number of amniotic sacs, second trimester CC M ♀

O30.293 Quadruplet pregnancy, unable to determine number of placenta and number of amniotic sacs, third trimester CC M ♀

O30.299 Quadruplet pregnancy, unable to determine number of placenta and number of amniotic sacs, unspecified trimester M ♀

✓5th O30.8 Other specified multiple gestation

Multiple gestation pregnancy greater then quadruplets

✓6th O30.80 Other specified multiple gestation, unspecified number of placenta and unspecified number of amniotic sacs

O30.801 Other specified multiple gestation, unspecified number of placenta and unspecified number of amniotic sacs, first trimester CC M ♀

O30.802 Other specified multiple gestation, unspecified number of placenta and unspecified number of amniotic sacs, second trimester CC M ♀

O30.803 Other specified multiple gestation, unspecified number of placenta and unspecified number of amniotic sacs, third trimester CC M ♀

O30.809 Other specified multiple gestation, unspecified number of placenta and unspecified number of amniotic sacs, unspecified trimester M ♀

✓6th O30.81 Other specified multiple gestation with two or more monochorionic fetuses

O30.811 Other specified multiple gestation with two or more monochorionic fetuses, first trimester CC M ♀

O30.812 Other specified multiple gestation with two or more monochorionic fetuses, second trimester CC M ♀

O30.813 Other specified multiple gestation with two or more monochorionic fetuses, third trimester CC M ♀

O30.819 Other specified multiple gestation with two or more monochorionic fetuses, unspecified trimester M ♀

✓6th O30.82 Other specified multiple gestation with two or more monoamniotic fetuses

O30.821 Other specified multiple gestation with two or more monoamniotic fetuses, first trimester CC M ♀

O30.822 Other specified multiple gestation with two or more monoamniotic fetuses, second trimester CC M ♀

O30.823 Other specified multiple gestation with two or more monoamniotic fetuses, third trimester CC M ♀

O30.829 Other specified multiple gestation with two or more monoamniotic fetuses, unspecified trimester M ♀

O30.83 Other specified multiple gestation, number of chorions and amnions are both equal to the number of fetuses

Pentachorionic, penta-amniotic pregnancy (quintuplets)

Hexachorionic, hexa-amniotic pregnancy (sextuplets)

Heptachorionic, hepta-amniotic pregnancy (septuplets)

AHA: 2018,4Q,22

O30.831 Other specified multiple gestation, number of chorions and amnions are both equal to the number of fetuses, first trimester CC M ♀

O30.832 Other specified multiple gestation, number of chorions and amnions are both equal to the number of fetuses, second trimester CC M ♀

O30.833 Other specified multiple gestation, number of chorions and amnions are both equal to the number of fetuses, third trimester CC M ♀

O30.839 Other specified multiple gestation, number of chorions and amnions are both equal to the number of fetuses, unspecified trimester M ♀

O30.89 Other specified multiple gestation, unable to determine number of placenta and number of amniotic sacs

O30.891 Other specified multiple gestation, unable to determine number of placenta and number of amniotic sacs, first trimester CC M ♀

O30.892 Other specified multiple gestation, unable to determine number of placenta and number of amniotic sacs, second trimester CC M ♀

O30.893 Other specified multiple gestation, unable to determine number of placenta and number of amniotic sacs, third trimester CC M ♀

O30.899 Other specified multiple gestation, unable to determine number of placenta and number of amniotic sacs, unspecified trimester M ♀

O30.9 Multiple gestation, unspecified

Multiple pregnancy NOS

O30.90 Multiple gestation, unspecified, unspecified trimester M ♀

O30.91 Multiple gestation, unspecified, first trimester M ♀

O30.92 Multiple gestation, unspecified, second trimester M ♀

O30.93 Multiple gestation, unspecified, third trimester M ♀

O31 Complications specific to multiple gestation

EXCLUDES 2 *delayed delivery of second twin, triplet, etc. (O63.2)*
malpresentation of one fetus or more (O32.9)
placental transfusion syndromes (O43.0-)

AHA: 2012,4Q,107

One of the following 7th characters is to be assigned to each code under category O31. 7th character 0 is for single gestations and multiple gestations where the fetus is unspecified. 7th characters 1 through 9 are for cases of multiple gestations to identify the fetus for which the code applies. The appropriate code from category O30, Multiple gestation, must also be assigned when assigning a code from category O31 that has a 7th character of 1 through 9.

0 not applicable or unspecified
1 fetus 1
2 fetus 2
3 fetus 3
4 fetus 4
5 fetus 5
9 other fetus

O31.0 Papyraceous fetus

Fetus compressus

DEF: Fetus that has died, but remains in utero for weeks before delivery, becoming compacted and mummified in appearance, with skin resembling parchment. Occurs most commonly in multigestational pregnancies. ***Synonym(s):*** *paper doll fetus.*

O31.00 Papyraceous fetus, unspecified trimester M ♀

O31.01 Papyraceous fetus, first trimester M ♀

O31.02 Papyraceous fetus, second trimester M ♀

O31.03 Papyraceous fetus, third trimester M ♀

O31.1 Continuing pregnancy after spontaneous abortion of one fetus or more

O31.10 Continuing pregnancy after spontaneous abortion of one fetus or more, unspecified trimester M ♀

O31.11 Continuing pregnancy after spontaneous abortion of one fetus or more, first trimester M ♀

O31.12 Continuing pregnancy after spontaneous abortion of one fetus or more, second trimester M ♀

O31.13 Continuing pregnancy after spontaneous abortion of one fetus or more, third trimester M ♀

O31.2 Continuing pregnancy after intrauterine death of one fetus or more

O31.20 Continuing pregnancy after intrauterine death of one fetus or more, unspecified trimester M ♀

O31.21 Continuing pregnancy after intrauterine death of one fetus or more, first trimester M ♀

O31.22 Continuing pregnancy after intrauterine death of one fetus or more, second trimester M ♀

O31.23 Continuing pregnancy after intrauterine death of one fetus or more, third trimester M ♀

O31.3 Continuing pregnancy after elective fetal reduction of one fetus or more

Continuing pregnancy after selective termination of one fetus or more

O31.30 Continuing pregnancy after elective fetal reduction of one fetus or more, unspecified trimester M ♀

O31.31 Continuing pregnancy after elective fetal reduction of one fetus or more, first trimester M ♀

O31.32 Continuing pregnancy after elective fetal reduction of one fetus or more, second trimester M ♀

O31.33 Continuing pregnancy after elective fetal reduction of one fetus or more, third trimester M ♀

O31.8 Other complications specific to multiple gestation

O31.8X Other complications specific to multiple gestation

O31.8X1 Other complications specific to multiple gestation, first trimester CC M ♀

O31.8X2 Other complications specific to multiple gestation, second trimester CC M ♀

O31.8X3 Other complications specific to multiple gestation, third trimester CC M ♀

O31.8X9 Other complications specific to multiple gestation, unspecified trimester CC M ♀

✓4th O32 Maternal care for malpresentation of fetus

INCLUDES the listed conditions as a reason for observation, hospitalization or other obstetric care of the mother, or for cesarean delivery before onset of labor

EXCLUDES 1 *malpresentation of fetus with obstructed labor (O64.-)*

AHA: 2012,4Q,107

One of the following 7th characters is to be assigned to each code under category O32. 7th character Ø is for single gestations and multiple gestations where the fetus is unspecified. 7th characters 1 through 9 are for cases of multiple gestations to identify the fetus for which the code applies. The appropriate code from category O3Ø, Multiple gestation, must also be assigned when assigning a code from category O32 that has a 7th character of 1 through 9.
- Ø not applicable or unspecified
- 1 fetus 1
- 2 fetus 2
- 3 fetus 3
- 4 fetus 4
- 5 fetus 5
- 9 other fetus

Fetal Malpresentation

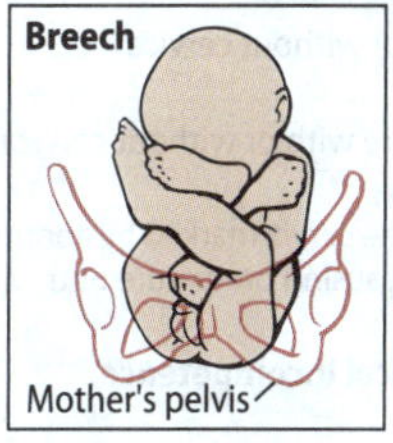

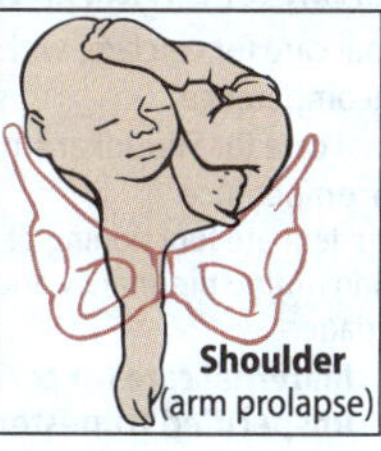

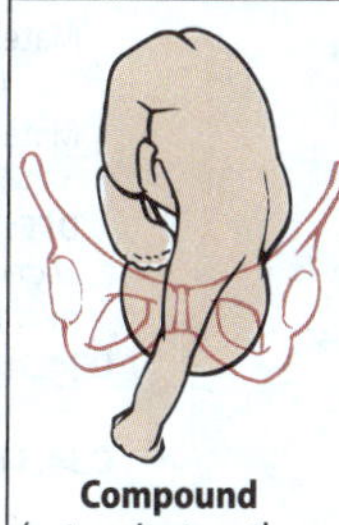

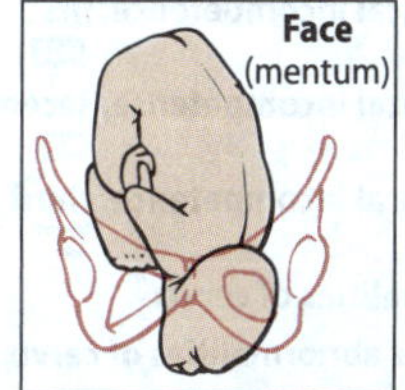

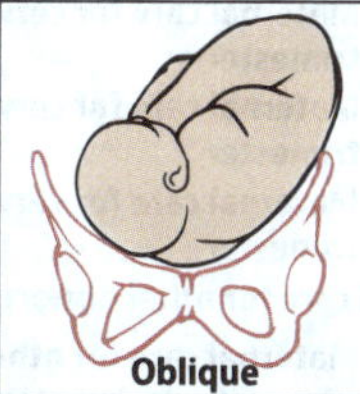

✓x7th **O32.Ø Maternal care for unstable lie** M♀

✓x7th **O32.1 Maternal care for breech presentation** M♀

Maternal care for buttocks presentation
Maternal care for complete breech
Maternal care for frank breech

EXCLUDES 1 *footling presentation (O32.8)*
incomplete breech (O32.8)

DEF: Fetus presentation in a longitudinal lie with the buttocks or feet closest to birth canal that may require external cephalic version or cesarean delivery.

✓x7th **O32.2 Maternal care for transverse and oblique lie** M♀

Maternal care for oblique presentation
Maternal care for transverse presentation

✓x7th **O32.3 Maternal care for face, brow and chin presentation** M♀

✓x7th **O32.4 Maternal care for high head at term** M♀

Maternal care for failure of head to enter pelvic brim

✓x7th **O32.6 Maternal care for compound presentation** M♀

✓x7th **O32.8 Maternal care for other malpresentation of fetus** M♀

Maternal care for footling presentation
Maternal care for incomplete breech

✓x7th **O32.9 Maternal care for malpresentation of fetus, unspecified** M♀

✓4th O33 Maternal care for disproportion

INCLUDES the listed conditions as a reason for observation, hospitalization or other obstetric care of the mother, or for cesarean delivery before onset of labor

EXCLUDES 1 *disproportion with obstructed labor (O65-O66)*

O33.Ø Maternal care for disproportion due to deformity of maternal pelvic bones CC M♀

Maternal care for disproportion due to pelvic deformity causing disproportion NOS

O33.1 Maternal care for disproportion due to generally contracted pelvis M♀

Maternal care for disproportion due to contracted pelvis NOS causing disproportion

O33.2 Maternal care for disproportion due to inlet contraction of pelvis M♀

Maternal care for disproportion due to inlet contraction (pelvis) causing disproportion

✓x7th **O33.3 Maternal care for disproportion due to outlet contraction of pelvis** M♀

Maternal care for disproportion due to mid-cavity contraction (pelvis)
Maternal care for disproportion due to outlet contraction (pelvis)

One of the following 7th characters is to be assigned to code O33.3. 7th character Ø is for single gestations and multiple gestations where the fetus is unspecified. 7th characters 1 through 9 are for cases of multiple gestations to identify the fetus for which the code applies. The appropriate code from category O3Ø, Multiple gestation, must also be assigned when assigning code O33.3 with a 7th character of 1 through 9.
- Ø not applicable or unspecified
- 1 fetus 1
- 2 fetus 2
- 3 fetus 3
- 4 fetus 4
- 5 fetus 5
- 9 other fetus

✓x7th **O33.4 Maternal care for disproportion of mixed maternal and fetal origin** M♀

One of the following 7th characters is to be assigned to code O33.4. 7th character Ø is for single gestations and multiple gestations where the fetus is unspecified. 7th characters 1 through 9 are for cases of multiple gestations to identify the fetus for which the code applies. The appropriate code from category O3Ø, Multiple gestation, must also be assigned when assigning code O33.4 with a 7th character of 1 through 9.
- Ø not applicable or unspecified
- 1 fetus 1
- 2 fetus 2
- 3 fetus 3
- 4 fetus 4
- 5 fetus 5
- 9 other fetus

✓x7th **O33.5 Maternal care for disproportion due to unusually large fetus** M♀

Maternal care for disproportion due to disproportion of fetal origin with normally formed fetus
Maternal care for disproportion due to fetal disproportion NOS

One of the following 7th characters is to be assigned to code O33.5. 7th character Ø is for single gestations and multiple gestations where the fetus is unspecified. 7th characters 1 through 9 are for cases of multiple gestations to identify the fetus for which the code applies. The appropriate code from category O3Ø, Multiple gestation, must also be assigned when assigning code O33.5 with a 7th character of 1 through 9.
- Ø not applicable or unspecified
- 1 fetus 1
- 2 fetus 2
- 3 fetus 3
- 4 fetus 4
- 5 fetus 5
- 9 other fetus

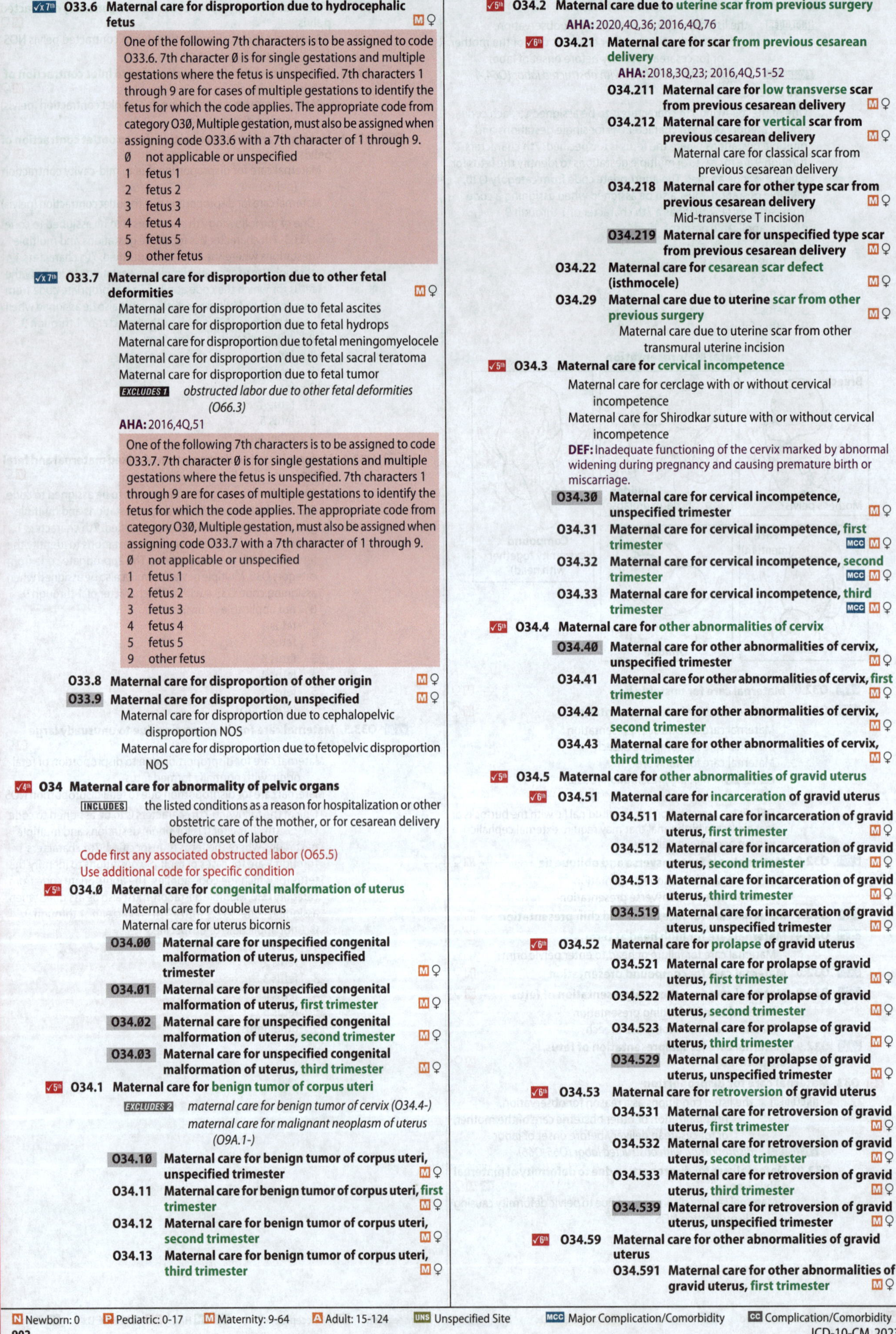

O33.6 Maternal care for disproportion due to hydrocephalic fetus M ♀

One of the following 7th characters is to be assigned to code O33.6. 7th character Ø is for single gestations and multiple gestations where the fetus is unspecified. 7th characters 1 through 9 are for cases of multiple gestations to identify the fetus for which the code applies. The appropriate code from category O3Ø, Multiple gestation, must also be assigned when assigning code O33.6 with a 7th character of 1 through 9.
- Ø not applicable or unspecified
- 1 fetus 1
- 2 fetus 2
- 3 fetus 3
- 4 fetus 4
- 5 fetus 5
- 9 other fetus

O33.7 Maternal care for disproportion due to other fetal deformities M ♀

Maternal care for disproportion due to fetal ascites
Maternal care for disproportion due to fetal hydrops
Maternal care for disproportion due to fetal meningomyelocele
Maternal care for disproportion due to fetal sacral teratoma
Maternal care for disproportion due to fetal tumor

EXCLUDES 1 *obstructed labor due to other fetal deformities (O66.3)*

AHA: 2016,4Q,51

One of the following 7th characters is to be assigned to code O33.7. 7th character Ø is for single gestations and multiple gestations where the fetus is unspecified. 7th characters 1 through 9 are for cases of multiple gestations to identify the fetus for which the code applies. The appropriate code from category O3Ø, Multiple gestation, must also be assigned when assigning code O33.7 with a 7th character of 1 through 9.
- Ø not applicable or unspecified
- 1 fetus 1
- 2 fetus 2
- 3 fetus 3
- 4 fetus 4
- 5 fetus 5
- 9 other fetus

O33.8 Maternal care for disproportion of other origin M ♀

O33.9 Maternal care for disproportion, unspecified M ♀

Maternal care for disproportion due to cephalopelvic disproportion NOS
Maternal care for disproportion due to fetopelvic disproportion NOS

O34 Maternal care for abnormality of pelvic organs

INCLUDES the listed conditions as a reason for hospitalization or other obstetric care of the mother, or for cesarean delivery before onset of labor

Code first any associated obstructed labor (O65.5)
Use additional code for specific condition

O34.Ø Maternal care for congenital malformation of uterus

Maternal care for double uterus
Maternal care for uterus bicornis

O34.ØØ Maternal care for unspecified congenital malformation of uterus, unspecified trimester M ♀

O34.Ø1 Maternal care for unspecified congenital malformation of uterus, first trimester M ♀

O34.Ø2 Maternal care for unspecified congenital malformation of uterus, second trimester M ♀

O34.Ø3 Maternal care for unspecified congenital malformation of uterus, third trimester M ♀

O34.1 Maternal care for benign tumor of corpus uteri

EXCLUDES 2 *maternal care for benign tumor of cervix (O34.4-)*
maternal care for malignant neoplasm of uterus (O9A.1-)

O34.1Ø Maternal care for benign tumor of corpus uteri, unspecified trimester M ♀

O34.11 Maternal care for benign tumor of corpus uteri, first trimester M ♀

O34.12 Maternal care for benign tumor of corpus uteri, second trimester M ♀

O34.13 Maternal care for benign tumor of corpus uteri, third trimester M ♀

O34.2 Maternal care due to uterine scar from previous surgery

AHA: 2020,4Q,36; 2016,4Q,76

O34.21 Maternal care for scar from previous cesarean delivery

AHA: 2018,3Q,23; 2016,4Q,51-52

O34.211 Maternal care for low transverse scar from previous cesarean delivery M ♀

O34.212 Maternal care for vertical scar from previous cesarean delivery M ♀

Maternal care for classical scar from previous cesarean delivery

O34.218 Maternal care for other type scar from previous cesarean delivery M ♀

Mid-transverse T incision

O34.219 Maternal care for unspecified type scar from previous cesarean delivery M ♀

O34.22 Maternal care for cesarean scar defect (isthmocele) M ♀

O34.29 Maternal care due to uterine scar from other previous surgery M ♀

Maternal care due to uterine scar from other transmural uterine incision

O34.3 Maternal care for cervical incompetence

Maternal care for cerclage with or without cervical incompetence
Maternal care for Shirodkar suture with or without cervical incompetence

DEF: Inadequate functioning of the cervix marked by abnormal widening during pregnancy and causing premature birth or miscarriage.

O34.3Ø Maternal care for cervical incompetence, unspecified trimester M ♀

O34.31 Maternal care for cervical incompetence, first trimester MCC M ♀

O34.32 Maternal care for cervical incompetence, second trimester MCC M ♀

O34.33 Maternal care for cervical incompetence, third trimester MCC M ♀

O34.4 Maternal care for other abnormalities of cervix

O34.4Ø Maternal care for other abnormalities of cervix, unspecified trimester M ♀

O34.41 Maternal care for other abnormalities of cervix, first trimester M ♀

O34.42 Maternal care for other abnormalities of cervix, second trimester M ♀

O34.43 Maternal care for other abnormalities of cervix, third trimester M ♀

O34.5 Maternal care for other abnormalities of gravid uterus

O34.51 Maternal care for incarceration of gravid uterus

O34.511 Maternal care for incarceration of gravid uterus, first trimester M ♀

O34.512 Maternal care for incarceration of gravid uterus, second trimester M ♀

O34.513 Maternal care for incarceration of gravid uterus, third trimester M ♀

O34.519 Maternal care for incarceration of gravid uterus, unspecified trimester M ♀

O34.52 Maternal care for prolapse of gravid uterus

O34.521 Maternal care for prolapse of gravid uterus, first trimester M ♀

O34.522 Maternal care for prolapse of gravid uterus, second trimester M ♀

O34.523 Maternal care for prolapse of gravid uterus, third trimester M ♀

O34.529 Maternal care for prolapse of gravid uterus, unspecified trimester M ♀

O34.53 Maternal care for retroversion of gravid uterus

O34.531 Maternal care for retroversion of gravid uterus, first trimester M ♀

O34.532 Maternal care for retroversion of gravid uterus, second trimester M ♀

O34.533 Maternal care for retroversion of gravid uterus, third trimester M ♀

O34.539 Maternal care for retroversion of gravid uterus, unspecified trimester M ♀

O34.59 Maternal care for other abnormalities of gravid uterus

O34.591 Maternal care for other abnormalities of gravid uterus, first trimester M ♀

O34.592 Maternal care for other abnormalities of gravid uterus, second trimester M♀

O34.593 Maternal care for other abnormalities of gravid uterus, third trimester M♀

O34.599 Maternal care for other abnormalities of gravid uterus, unspecified trimester M♀

O34.6 Maternal care for abnormality of vagina

EXCLUDES 2 *maternal care for vaginal varices in pregnancy (O22.1-)*

O34.60 Maternal care for abnormality of vagina, unspecified trimester M♀

O34.61 Maternal care for abnormality of vagina, first trimester M♀

O34.62 Maternal care for abnormality of vagina, second trimester M♀

O34.63 Maternal care for abnormality of vagina, third trimester M♀

O34.7 Maternal care for abnormality of vulva and perineum

EXCLUDES 2 *maternal care for perineal and vulval varices in pregnancy (O22.1-)*

O34.70 Maternal care for abnormality of vulva and perineum, unspecified trimester M♀

O34.71 Maternal care for abnormality of vulva and perineum, first trimester M♀

O34.72 Maternal care for abnormality of vulva and perineum, second trimester M♀

O34.73 Maternal care for abnormality of vulva and perineum, third trimester M♀

O34.8 Maternal care for other abnormalities of pelvic organs

O34.80 Maternal care for other abnormalities of pelvic organs, unspecified trimester M♀

O34.81 Maternal care for other abnormalities of pelvic organs, first trimester M♀

O34.82 Maternal care for other abnormalities of pelvic organs, second trimester M♀

O34.83 Maternal care for other abnormalities of pelvic organs, third trimester M♀

O34.9 Maternal care for abnormality of pelvic organ, unspecified

O34.90 Maternal care for abnormality of pelvic organ, unspecified, unspecified trimester M♀

O34.91 Maternal care for abnormality of pelvic organ, unspecified, first trimester M♀

O34.92 Maternal care for abnormality of pelvic organ, unspecified, second trimester M♀

O34.93 Maternal care for abnormality of pelvic organ, unspecified, third trimester M♀

O35 Maternal care for known or suspected fetal abnormality and damage

INCLUDES the listed conditions in the fetus as a reason for hospitalization or other obstetric care to the mother, or for termination of pregnancy

Code also any associated maternal condition

EXCLUDES 1 *encounter for suspected maternal and fetal conditions ruled out (Z03.7-)*

One of the following 7th characters is to be assigned to each code under category O35. 7th character 0 is for single gestations and multiple gestations where the fetus is unspecified. 7th characters 1 through 9 are for cases of multiple gestations to identify the fetus for which the code applies. The appropriate code from category O30, Multiple gestation, must also be assigned when assigning a code from category O35 that has a 7th character of 1 through 9.

0 not applicable or unspecified
1 fetus 1
2 fetus 2
3 fetus 3
4 fetus 4
5 fetus 5
9 other fetus

O35.0 Maternal care for (suspected) central nervous system malformation in fetus

~~Maternal care for fetal anencephaly~~
~~Maternal care for fetal hydrocephalus~~
~~Maternal care for fetal spina bifida~~

EXCLUDES 2 *chromosomal abnormality in fetus ▶(O35.1-)◀*

● **O35.00 Maternal care for (suspected) central nervous system malformation or damage in fetus, unspecified** M♀

● **O35.01 Maternal care for (suspected) central nervous system malformation or damage in fetus, agenesis of the corpus callosum** M♀

● **O35.02 Maternal care for (suspected) central nervous system malformation or damage in fetus, anencephaly** M♀

● **O35.03 Maternal care for (suspected) central nervous system malformation or damage in fetus, choroid plexus cysts** M♀

● **O35.04 Maternal care for (suspected) central nervous system malformation or damage in fetus, encephalocele** M♀

● **O35.05 Maternal care for (suspected) central nervous system malformation or damage in fetus, holoprosencephaly** M♀

● **O35.06 Maternal care for (suspected) central nervous system malformation or damage in fetus, hydrocephaly** M♀

Maternal care for fetal hydrocephalus

● **O35.07 Maternal care for (suspected) central nervous system malformation or damage in fetus, microcephaly** M♀

● **O35.08 Maternal care for (suspected) central nervous system malformation or damage in fetus, spina bifida** M♀

● **O35.09 Maternal care for (suspected) other central nervous system malformation or damage in fetus** M♀

O35.1 Maternal care for (suspected) chromosomal abnormality in fetus

● **O35.10 Maternal care for (suspected) chromosomal abnormality in fetus, unspecified** M♀

● **O35.11 Maternal care for (suspected) chromosomal abnormality in fetus, Trisomy 13** M♀

● **O35.12 Maternal care for (suspected) chromosomal abnormality in fetus, Trisomy 18** M♀

● **O35.13 Maternal care for (suspected) chromosomal abnormality in fetus, Trisomy 21** M♀

● **O35.14 Maternal care for (suspected) chromosomal abnormality in fetus, Turner Syndrome** M♀

● **O35.15 Maternal care for (suspected) chromosomal abnormality in fetus, sex chromosome abnormality** M♀

● **O35.19 Maternal care for (suspected) chromosomal abnormality in fetus, other chromosomal abnormality** M♀

● **O35.A Maternal care for other (suspected) fetal abnormality and damage, fetal facial anomalies** M♀

● **O35.B Maternal care for other (suspected) fetal abnormality and damage, fetal cardiac anomalies** M♀

● **O35.C Maternal care for other (suspected) fetal abnormality and damage, fetal pulmonary anomalies** M♀

● **O35.D Maternal care for other (suspected) fetal abnormality and damage, fetal gastrointestinal anomalies** M♀

● **O35.E Maternal care for other (suspected) fetal abnormality and damage, fetal genitourinary anomalies** M♀

● **O35.F Maternal care for other (suspected) fetal abnormality and damage, fetal musculoskeletal anomalies of trunk** M♀

EXCLUDES 2 *maternal care for other (suspected) fetal abnormality and damage, fetal lower extremities anomalies (O35.H)*
maternal care for other (suspected) fetal abnormality and damage, fetal upper extremities anomalies (O35.G)

● **O35.G Maternal care for other (suspected) fetal abnormality and damage, fetal upper extremities anomalies** M♀

● **O35.H Maternal care for other (suspected) fetal abnormality and damage, fetal lower extremities anomalies** M♀

O35.2 Maternal care for (suspected) hereditary disease in fetus M♀

EXCLUDES 2 *chromosomal abnormality in fetus ▶(O35.1-)◀*

O35.3 Maternal care for (suspected) damage to fetus from viral disease in mother M♀

Maternal care for damage to fetus from maternal cytomegalovirus infection
Maternal care for damage to fetus from maternal rubella

O35.4 Maternal care for (suspected) damage to fetus from alcohol M♀

O35.5 Maternal care for (suspected) damage to fetus by drugs M ♀
Maternal care for damage to fetus from drug addiction

O35.6 Maternal care for (suspected) damage to fetus by radiation M ♀

O35.7 Maternal care for (suspected) damage to fetus by other medical procedures M ♀
Maternal care for damage to fetus by amniocentesis
Maternal care for damage to fetus by biopsy procedures
Maternal care for damage to fetus by hematological investigation
Maternal care for damage to fetus by intrauterine contraceptive device
Maternal care for damage to fetus by intrauterine surgery

O35.8 Maternal care for other (suspected) fetal abnormality and damage M ♀
Maternal care for damage to fetus from maternal listeriosis
Maternal care for damage to fetus from maternal toxoplasmosis

O35.9 Maternal care for (suspected) fetal abnormality and damage, unspecified M ♀

O36 Maternal care for other fetal problems

INCLUDES the listed conditions in the fetus as a reason for hospitalization or other obstetric care of the mother, or for termination of pregnancy

EXCLUDES 1 *encounter for suspected maternal and fetal conditions ruled out (Z03.7-)*
placental transfusion syndromes (O43.0-)

EXCLUDES 2 *labor and delivery complicated by fetal stress (O77.-)*

AHA: 2015,3Q,40

One of the following 7th characters is to be assigned to each code under category O36. 7th character 0 is for single gestations and multiple gestations where the fetus is unspecified. 7th characters 1 through 9 are for cases of multiple gestations to identify the fetus for which the code applies. The appropriate code from category O30, Multiple gestation, must also be assigned when assigning a code from category O36 that has a 7th character of 1 through 9.
- 0 not applicable or unspecified
- 1 fetus 1
- 2 fetus 2
- 3 fetus 3
- 4 fetus 4
- 5 fetus 5
- 9 other fetus

O36.0 Maternal care for rhesus isoimmunization
Maternal care for Rh incompatibility (with hydrops fetalis)

O36.01 Maternal care for anti-D [Rh] antibodies
AHA: 2014,4Q,17

O36.011 Maternal care for anti-D [Rh] antibodies, first trimester CC M ♀

O36.012 Maternal care for anti-D [Rh] antibodies, second trimester CC M ♀

O36.013 Maternal care for anti-D [Rh] antibodies, third trimester CC M ♀

O36.019 Maternal care for anti-D [Rh] antibodies, unspecified trimester M ♀

O36.09 Maternal care for other rhesus isoimmunization

O36.091 Maternal care for other rhesus isoimmunization, first trimester CC M ♀

O36.092 Maternal care for other rhesus isoimmunization, second trimester CC M ♀

O36.093 Maternal care for other rhesus isoimmunization, third trimester CC M ♀

O36.099 Maternal care for other rhesus isoimmunization, unspecified trimester M ♀

O36.1 Maternal care for other isoimmunization
Maternal care for ABO isoimmunization

O36.11 Maternal care for Anti-A sensitization
Maternal care for isoimmunization NOS (with hydrops fetalis)

O36.111 Maternal care for Anti-A sensitization, first trimester M ♀

O36.112 Maternal care for Anti-A sensitization, second trimester M ♀

O36.113 Maternal care for Anti-A sensitization, third trimester M ♀

O36.119 Maternal care for Anti-A sensitization, unspecified trimester M ♀

O36.19 Maternal care for other isoimmunization
Maternal care for Anti-B sensitization

O36.191 Maternal care for other isoimmunization, first trimester M ♀

O36.192 Maternal care for other isoimmunization, second trimester M ♀

O36.193 Maternal care for other isoimmunization, third trimester M ♀

O36.199 Maternal care for other isoimmunization, unspecified trimester M ♀

O36.2 Maternal care for hydrops fetalis
Maternal care for hydrops fetalis NOS
Maternal care for hydrops fetalis not associated with isoimmunization

EXCLUDES 1 *hydrops fetalis associated with ABO isoimmunization (O36.1-)*
hydrops fetalis associated with rhesus isoimmunization (O36.0-)

DEF: Hydrops fetalis: Abnormal fluid buildup in at least two of the following fetal organ spaces: the skin (edema), abdomen (ascites), around the heart (pericardia effusion), and around the lung (pleural effusion). Fluid accumulation may also occur in the mother as polyhydramnios and edema of the placenta.

O36.20 Maternal care for hydrops fetalis, unspecified trimester M ♀

O36.21 Maternal care for hydrops fetalis, first trimester M ♀

O36.22 Maternal care for hydrops fetalis, second trimester M ♀

O36.23 Maternal care for hydrops fetalis, third trimester M ♀

O36.4 Maternal care for intrauterine death CC M ♀
Maternal care for intrauterine fetal death NOS
Maternal care for intrauterine fetal death after completion of 20 weeks of gestation
Maternal care for late fetal death
Maternal care for missed delivery

EXCLUDES 1 *missed abortion (O02.1)*
stillbirth (P95)

AHA: 2022,2Q,3

O36.5 Maternal care for known or suspected poor fetal growth

O36.51 Maternal care for known or suspected placental insufficiency

O36.511 Maternal care for known or suspected placental insufficiency, first trimester M ♀

O36.512 Maternal care for known or suspected placental insufficiency, second trimester M ♀

O36.513 Maternal care for known or suspected placental insufficiency, third trimester M ♀

O36.519 Maternal care for known or suspected placental insufficiency, unspecified trimester M ♀

O36.59 Maternal care for other known or suspected poor fetal growth
Maternal care for known or suspected light-for-dates NOS
Maternal care for known or suspected small-for-dates NOS

O36.591 Maternal care for other known or suspected poor fetal growth, first trimester M ♀

O36.592 Maternal care for other known or suspected poor fetal growth, second trimester M ♀

O36.593 Maternal care for other known or suspected poor fetal growth, third trimester M ♀

O36.599 Maternal care for other known or suspected poor fetal growth, unspecified trimester M ♀

O36.6 **Maternal care for excessive fetal growth**
Maternal care for known or suspected large-for-dates
O36.60 **Maternal care for excessive fetal growth, unspecified trimester** M ♀
O36.61 **Maternal care for excessive fetal growth, first trimester** M ♀
O36.62 **Maternal care for excessive fetal growth, second trimester** M ♀
O36.63 **Maternal care for excessive fetal growth, third trimester** M ♀
O36.7 **Maternal care for viable fetus in abdominal pregnancy**
O36.70 **Maternal care for viable fetus in abdominal pregnancy, unspecified trimester** M ♀
O36.71 **Maternal care for viable fetus in abdominal pregnancy, first trimester** M ♀
O36.72 **Maternal care for viable fetus in abdominal pregnancy, second trimester** M ♀
O36.73 **Maternal care for viable fetus in abdominal pregnancy, third trimester** M ♀
O36.8 **Maternal care for other specified fetal problems**
O36.80 **Pregnancy with inconclusive fetal viability** UPD M ♀
Encounter to determine fetal viability of pregnancy
AHA: 2019,2Q,29
O36.81 **Decreased fetal movements**
O36.812 **Decreased fetal movements, second trimester** M ♀
O36.813 **Decreased fetal movements, third trimester** M ♀
O36.819 **Decreased fetal movements, unspecified trimester** M ♀
O36.82 **Fetal anemia and thrombocytopenia**
O36.821 **Fetal anemia and thrombocytopenia, first trimester** M ♀
O36.822 **Fetal anemia and thrombocytopenia, second trimester** M ♀
O36.823 **Fetal anemia and thrombocytopenia, third trimester** M ♀
O36.829 **Fetal anemia and thrombocytopenia, unspecified trimester** M ♀
O36.83 **Maternal care for abnormalities of the fetal heart rate or rhythm**
Maternal care for depressed fetal heart rate tones
Maternal care for fetal bradycardia
Maternal care for fetal heart rate abnormal variability
Maternal care for fetal heart rate decelerations
Maternal care for fetal heart rate irregularity
Maternal care for fetal tachycardia
Maternal care for non-reassuring fetal heart rate or rhythm
AHA: 2017,4Q,20
TIP: Assign for documented fetal tachycardia, bradycardia, decelerations, or loss of variability detected during antenatal testing.
O36.831 **Maternal care for abnormalities of the fetal heart rate or rhythm, first trimester** M ♀
O36.832 **Maternal care for abnormalities of the fetal heart rate or rhythm, second trimester** M ♀
O36.833 **Maternal care for abnormalities of the fetal heart rate or rhythm, third trimester** M ♀
O36.839 **Maternal care for abnormalities of the fetal heart rate or rhythm, unspecified trimester** M ♀
O36.89 **Maternal care for other specified fetal problems**
O36.891 **Maternal care for other specified fetal problems, first trimester** M ♀
O36.892 **Maternal care for other specified fetal problems, second trimester** M ♀
O36.893 **Maternal care for other specified fetal problems, third trimester** M ♀
O36.899 **Maternal care for other specified fetal problems, unspecified trimester** M ♀
O36.9 **Maternal care for fetal problem, unspecified**
O36.90 **Maternal care for fetal problem, unspecified, unspecified trimester** M ♀
O36.91 **Maternal care for fetal problem, unspecified, first trimester** M ♀
O36.92 **Maternal care for fetal problem, unspecified, second trimester** M ♀
O36.93 **Maternal care for fetal problem, unspecified, third trimester** M ♀

O40 **Polyhydramnios**
INCLUDES hydramnios
EXCLUDES 1 *encounter for suspected maternal and fetal conditions ruled out (Z03.7-)*
AHA: 2016,1Q,4
DEF: Excess amniotic fluid surrounding the fetus, typically defined as a total fluid volume of greater than 24 cm.

One of the following 7th characters is to be assigned to each code under category O40. 7th character 0 is for single gestations and multiple gestations where the fetus is unspecified. 7th characters 1 through 9 are for cases of multiple gestations to identify the fetus for which the code applies. The appropriate code from category O30, Multiple gestation, must also be assigned when assigning a code from category O40 that has a 7th character of 1 through 9.
0 not applicable or unspecified
1 fetus 1
2 fetus 2
3 fetus 3
4 fetus 4
5 fetus 5
9 other fetus

O40.1 **Polyhydramnios, first trimester** M ♀
O40.2 **Polyhydramnios, second trimester** M ♀
O40.3 **Polyhydramnios, third trimester** M ♀
O40.9 **Polyhydramnios, unspecified trimester** M ♀

O41 **Other disorders of amniotic fluid and membranes**
EXCLUDES 1 *encounter for suspected maternal and fetal conditions ruled out (Z03.7-)*

One of the following 7th characters is to be assigned to each code under category O41. 7th character 0 is for single gestations and multiple gestations where the fetus is unspecified. 7th characters 1 through 9 are for cases of multiple gestations to identify the fetus for which the code applies. The appropriate code from category O30, Multiple gestation, must also be assigned when assigning a code from category O41 that has a 7th character of 1 through 9.
0 not applicable or unspecified
1 fetus 1
2 fetus 2
3 fetus 3
4 fetus 4
5 fetus 5
9 other fetus

O41.0 **Oligohydramnios**
Oligohydramnios without rupture of membranes
DEF: Low amniotic fluid, occurring most frequently in the last trimester.
O41.00 **Oligohydramnios, unspecified trimester** M ♀
O41.01 **Oligohydramnios, first trimester** CC M ♀
O41.02 **Oligohydramnios, second trimester** CC M ♀
O41.03 **Oligohydramnios, third trimester** CC M ♀
O41.1 **Infection of amniotic sac and membranes**
O41.10 **Infection of amniotic sac and membranes, unspecified**
O41.101 **Infection of amniotic sac and membranes, unspecified, first trimester** MCC M ♀
O41.102 **Infection of amniotic sac and membranes, unspecified, second trimester** MCC M ♀
O41.103 **Infection of amniotic sac and membranes, unspecified, third trimester** MCC M ♀
O41.109 **Infection of amniotic sac and membranes, unspecified, unspecified trimester** M ♀
O41.12 **Chorioamnionitis**
AHA: 2019,2Q,34
O41.121 **Chorioamnionitis, first trimester** MCC M ♀
O41.122 **Chorioamnionitis, second trimester** MCC M ♀

O41.123 Chorioamnionitis, third trimester MCC M ♀

O41.129 Chorioamnionitis, unspecified trimester M ♀

O41.14 Placentitis

O41.141 Placentitis, first trimester MCC M ♀

O41.142 Placentitis, second trimester MCC M ♀

O41.143 Placentitis, third trimester MCC M ♀

O41.149 Placentitis, unspecified trimester M ♀

O41.8 Other specified disorders of amniotic fluid and membranes

O41.8X Other specified disorders of amniotic fluid and membranes

O41.8X1 Other specified disorders of amniotic fluid and membranes, first trimester M ♀

O41.8X2 Other specified disorders of amniotic fluid and membranes, second trimester M ♀

O41.8X3 Other specified disorders of amniotic fluid and membranes, third trimester M ♀

O41.8X9 Other specified disorders of amniotic fluid and membranes, unspecified trimester M ♀

O41.9 Disorder of amniotic fluid and membranes, unspecified

O41.90 Disorder of amniotic fluid and membranes, unspecified, unspecified trimester M ♀

O41.91 Disorder of amniotic fluid and membranes, unspecified, first trimester M ♀

O41.92 Disorder of amniotic fluid and membranes, unspecified, second trimester M ♀

O41.93 Disorder of amniotic fluid and membranes, unspecified, third trimester M ♀

O42 Premature rupture of membranes

AHA: 2016,1Q,3

O42.0 Premature rupture of membranes, onset of labor within 24 hours of rupture

O42.00 Premature rupture of membranes, onset of labor within 24 hours of rupture, unspecified weeks of gestation M ♀

O42.01 Preterm premature rupture of membranes, onset of labor within 24 hours of rupture

Premature rupture of membranes before 37 completed weeks of gestation

O42.011 Preterm premature rupture of membranes, onset of labor within 24 hours of rupture, first trimester M ♀

O42.012 Preterm premature rupture of membranes, onset of labor within 24 hours of rupture, second trimester M ♀

O42.013 Preterm premature rupture of membranes, onset of labor within 24 hours of rupture, third trimester M ♀

O42.019 Preterm premature rupture of membranes, onset of labor within 24 hours of rupture, unspecified trimester M ♀

O42.02 Full-term premature rupture of membranes, onset of labor within 24 hours of rupture M ♀

Premature rupture of membranes at or after 37 completed weeks of gestation, onset of labor within 24 hours of rupture

O42.1 Premature rupture of membranes, onset of labor more than 24 hours following rupture

AHA: 2016,1Q,5

O42.10 Premature rupture of membranes, onset of labor more than 24 hours following rupture, unspecified weeks of gestation M ♀

O42.11 Preterm premature rupture of membranes, onset of labor more than 24 hours following rupture

Premature rupture of membranes before 37 completed weeks of gestation

O42.111 Preterm premature rupture of membranes, onset of labor more than 24 hours following rupture, first trimester M ♀

O42.112 Preterm premature rupture of membranes, onset of labor more than 24 hours following rupture, second trimester M ♀

O42.113 Preterm premature rupture of membranes, onset of labor more than 24 hours following rupture, third trimester M ♀

O42.119 Preterm premature rupture of membranes, onset of labor more than 24 hours following rupture, unspecified trimester M ♀

O42.12 Full-term premature rupture of membranes, onset of labor more than 24 hours following rupture M ♀

Premature rupture of membranes at or after 37 completed weeks of gestation, onset of labor more than 24 hours following rupture

O42.9 Premature rupture of membranes, unspecified as to length of time between rupture and onset of labor

O42.90 Premature rupture of membranes, unspecified as to length of time between rupture and onset of labor, unspecified weeks of gestation M ♀

O42.91 Preterm premature rupture of membranes, unspecified as to length of time between rupture and onset of labor

Premature rupture of membranes before 37 completed weeks of gestation

O42.911 Preterm premature rupture of membranes, unspecified as to length of time between rupture and onset of labor, first trimester M ♀

O42.912 Preterm premature rupture of membranes, unspecified as to length of time between rupture and onset of labor, second trimester M ♀

O42.913 Preterm premature rupture of membranes, unspecified as to length of time between rupture and onset of labor, third trimester M ♀

O42.919 Preterm premature rupture of membranes, unspecified as to length of time between rupture and onset of labor, unspecified trimester M ♀

O42.92 Full-term premature rupture of membranes, unspecified as to length of time between rupture and onset of labor M ♀

Premature rupture of membranes at or after 37 completed weeks of gestation, unspecified as to length of time between rupture and onset of labor

O43 Placental disorders

EXCLUDES 2 *maternal care for poor fetal growth due to placental insufficiency (O36.5-)*
placenta previa (O44.-)
placental polyp (O90.89)
placentitis (O41.14-)
premature separation of placenta [abruptio placentae] (O45.-)

O43.0 Placental transfusion syndromes

O43.01 Fetomaternal placental transfusion syndrome

Maternofetal placental transfusion syndrome

O43.011 Fetomaternal placental transfusion syndrome, first trimester M ♀

O43.012 Fetomaternal placental transfusion syndrome, second trimester M ♀

O43.013 Fetomaternal placental transfusion syndrome, third trimester M ♀

O43.019 Fetomaternal placental transfusion syndrome, unspecified trimester M ♀

✓6th **O43.Ø2 Fetus-to-fetus placental transfusion syndrome**

DEF: Condition in which an imbalance in amniotic fluid occurs due to uneven blood flow between twins sharing a placenta.

Twin to Twin Transfusion Syndrome (TTTS)

Healthy twins Twins with TTTS

- **O43.Ø21 Fetus-to-fetus placental transfusion syndrome, first trimester** M ♀
- **O43.Ø22 Fetus-to-fetus placental transfusion syndrome, second trimester** M ♀
- **O43.Ø23 Fetus-to-fetus placental transfusion syndrome, third trimester** M ♀
- **O43.Ø29 Fetus-to-fetus placental transfusion syndrome, unspecified trimester** M ♀

✓5th **O43.1 Malformation of placenta**

✓6th **O43.1Ø Malformation of placenta, unspecified**

Abnormal placenta NOS

- **O43.1Ø1 Malformation of placenta, unspecified, first trimester** M ♀
- **O43.1Ø2 Malformation of placenta, unspecified, second trimester** M ♀
- **O43.1Ø3 Malformation of placenta, unspecified, third trimester** M ♀
- **O43.1Ø9 Malformation of placenta, unspecified, unspecified trimester** M ♀

✓6th **O43.11 Circumvallate placenta**

- **O43.111 Circumvallate placenta, first trimester** M ♀
- **O43.112 Circumvallate placenta, second trimester** M ♀
- **O43.113 Circumvallate placenta, third trimester** M ♀
- **O43.119 Circumvallate placenta, unspecified trimester** M ♀

✓6th **O43.12 Velamentous insertion of umbilical cord**

- **O43.121 Velamentous insertion of umbilical cord, first trimester** M ♀
- **O43.122 Velamentous insertion of umbilical cord, second trimester** M ♀
- **O43.123 Velamentous insertion of umbilical cord, third trimester** M ♀
- **O43.129 Velamentous insertion of umbilical cord, unspecified trimester** M ♀

✓6th **O43.19 Other malformation of placenta**

- **O43.191 Other malformation of placenta, first trimester** M ♀
- **O43.192 Other malformation of placenta, second trimester** M ♀
- **O43.193 Other malformation of placenta, third trimester** M ♀
- **O43.199 Other malformation of placenta, unspecified trimester** M ♀

✓5th **O43.2 Morbidly adherent placenta**

Code also associated third stage postpartum hemorrhage, if applicable (O72.Ø)

EXCLUDES 1 *retained placenta (O73.-)*

✓6th **O43.21 Placenta accreta**

DEF: Condition where the placenta adheres too deeply to the uterine wall; often associated with placenta previa.

- **O43.211 Placenta accreta, first trimester** M ♀
- **O43.212 Placenta accreta, second trimester** M ♀
- **O43.213 Placenta accreta, third trimester** M ♀
- **O43.219 Placenta accreta, unspecified trimester** M ♀

✓6th **O43.22 Placenta increta**

AHA: 2022,1Q,20

DEF: Condition where the placenta adheres too deeply to the uterine wall and penetrates the muscle; often associated with placenta previa.

- **O43.221 Placenta increta, first trimester** M ♀
- **O43.222 Placenta increta, second trimester** M ♀
- **O43.223 Placenta increta, third trimester** M ♀
- **O43.229 Placenta increta, unspecified trimester** M ♀

✓6th **O43.23 Placenta percreta**

DEF: Condition where the placenta attaches through the uterine muscle and may invade other organs, resulting in antenatal complications, premature delivery, retention of all or a portion of the placenta, or postpartum bleeding.

- **O43.231 Placenta percreta, first trimester** M ♀
- **O43.232 Placenta percreta, second trimester** M ♀
- **O43.233 Placenta percreta, third trimester** M ♀
- **O43.239 Placenta percreta, unspecified trimester** M ♀

✓5th **O43.8 Other placental disorders**

✓6th **O43.81 Placental infarction**

- **O43.811 Placental infarction, first trimester** M ♀
- **O43.812 Placental infarction, second trimester** M ♀
- **O43.813 Placental infarction, third trimester** M ♀
- **O43.819 Placental infarction, unspecified trimester** M ♀

✓6th **O43.89 Other placental disorders**

Placental dysfunction

- **O43.891 Other placental disorders, first trimester** M ♀
- **O43.892 Other placental disorders, second trimester** M ♀
- **O43.893 Other placental disorders, third trimester** M ♀
- **O43.899 Other placental disorders, unspecified trimester** M ♀

✓5th **O43.9 Unspecified placental disorder**

- **O43.9Ø Unspecified placental disorder, unspecified trimester** M ♀
- **O43.91 Unspecified placental disorder, first trimester** M ♀
- **O43.92 Unspecified placental disorder, second trimester** M ♀
- **O43.93 Unspecified placental disorder, third trimester** M ♀

✓4th **O44 Placenta previa**

AHA: 2016,4Q,52-53

DEF: Placenta implanted in the lower segment of the uterus, which commonly causes hemorrhage in the last trimester of pregnancy.

✓5th **O44.Ø Complete placenta previa NOS or without hemorrhage**

Placenta previa NOS

- **O44.ØØ Complete placenta previa NOS or without hemorrhage, unspecified trimester** M ♀
- **O44.Ø1 Complete placenta previa NOS or without hemorrhage, first trimester** CC M ♀
- **O44.Ø2 Complete placenta previa NOS or without hemorrhage, second trimester** CC M ♀
- **O44.Ø3 Complete placenta previa NOS or without hemorrhage, third trimester** CC M ♀

✓5th **O44.1 Complete placenta previa with hemorrhage**

EXCLUDES 1 *labor and delivery complicated by hemorrhage from vasa previa (O69.4)*

- **O44.1Ø Complete placenta previa with hemorrhage, unspecified trimester** M ♀
- **O44.11 Complete placenta previa with hemorrhage, first trimester** MCC M ♀

O44.12 Complete placenta previa with hemorrhage, second trimester MCC M ♀

O44.13 Complete placenta previa with hemorrhage, third trimester MCC M ♀

O44.2 Partial placenta previa without hemorrhage

Marginal placenta previa, NOS or without hemorrhage

O44.2Ø Partial placenta previa NOS or without hemorrhage, unspecified trimester M ♀

O44.21 Partial placenta previa NOS or without hemorrhage, first trimester CC M ♀

O44.22 Partial placenta previa NOS or without hemorrhage, second trimester CC M ♀

O44.23 Partial placenta previa NOS or without hemorrhage, third trimester CC M ♀

O44.3 Partial placenta previa with hemorrhage

Marginal placenta previa with hemorrhage

O44.3Ø Partial placenta previa with hemorrhage, unspecified trimester M ♀

O44.31 Partial placenta previa with hemorrhage, first trimester MCC M ♀

O44.32 Partial placenta previa with hemorrhage, second trimester MCC M ♀

O44.33 Partial placenta previa with hemorrhage, third trimester MCC M ♀

O44.4 Low lying placenta NOS or without hemorrhage

Low implantation of placenta NOS or without hemorrhage

O44.4Ø Low lying placenta NOS or without hemorrhage, unspecified trimester M ♀

O44.41 Low lying placenta NOS or without hemorrhage, first trimester CC M ♀

O44.42 Low lying placenta NOS or without hemorrhage, second trimester CC M ♀

O44.43 Low lying placenta NOS or without hemorrhage, third trimester CC M ♀

O44.5 Low lying placenta with hemorrhage

Low implantation of placenta with hemorrhage

O44.5Ø Low lying placenta with hemorrhage, unspecified trimester M ♀

O44.51 Low lying placenta with hemorrhage, first trimester MCC M ♀

O44.52 Low lying placenta with hemorrhage, second trimester MCC M ♀

O44.53 Low lying placenta with hemorrhage, third trimester MCC M ♀

O45 Premature separation of placenta [abruptio placentae]

O45.Ø Premature separation of placenta with coagulation defect

O45.ØØ Premature separation of placenta with coagulation defect, unspecified

O45.ØØ1 Premature separation of placenta with coagulation defect, unspecified, first trimester MCC M ♀

O45.ØØ2 Premature separation of placenta with coagulation defect, unspecified, second trimester MCC M ♀

O45.ØØ3 Premature separation of placenta with coagulation defect, unspecified, third trimester MCC M ♀

O45.ØØ9 Premature separation of placenta with coagulation defect, unspecified, unspecified trimester M ♀

O45.Ø1 Premature separation of placenta with afibrinogenemia

Premature separation of placenta with hypofibrinogenemia

O45.Ø11 Premature separation of placenta with afibrinogenemia, first trimester MCC M ♀

O45.Ø12 Premature separation of placenta with afibrinogenemia, second trimester MCC M ♀

O45.Ø13 Premature separation of placenta with afibrinogenemia, third trimester MCC M ♀

O45.Ø19 Premature separation of placenta with afibrinogenemia, unspecified trimester M ♀

O45.Ø2 Premature separation of placenta with disseminated intravascular coagulation

O45.Ø21 Premature separation of placenta with disseminated intravascular coagulation, first trimester MCC M ♀

O45.Ø22 Premature separation of placenta with disseminated intravascular coagulation, second trimester MCC M ♀

O45.Ø23 Premature separation of placenta with disseminated intravascular coagulation, third trimester MCC M ♀

O45.Ø29 Premature separation of placenta with disseminated intravascular coagulation, unspecified trimester M ♀

O45.Ø9 Premature separation of placenta with other coagulation defect

O45.Ø91 Premature separation of placenta with other coagulation defect, first trimester MCC M ♀

O45.Ø92 Premature separation of placenta with other coagulation defect, second trimester MCC M ♀

O45.Ø93 Premature separation of placenta with other coagulation defect, third trimester MCC M ♀

O45.Ø99 Premature separation of placenta with other coagulation defect, unspecified trimester M ♀

O45.8 Other premature separation of placenta

O45.8X Other premature separation of placenta

O45.8X1 Other premature separation of placenta, first trimester MCC M ♀

O45.8X2 Other premature separation of placenta, second trimester MCC M ♀

O45.8X3 Other premature separation of placenta, third trimester MCC M ♀

O45.8X9 Other premature separation of placenta, unspecified trimester M ♀

O45.9 Premature separation of placenta, unspecified

Abruptio placentae NOS

O45.9Ø Premature separation of placenta, unspecified, unspecified trimester M ♀

O45.91 Premature separation of placenta, unspecified, first trimester MCC M ♀

O45.92 Premature separation of placenta, unspecified, second trimester MCC M ♀

O45.93 Premature separation of placenta, unspecified, third trimester MCC M ♀

O46 Antepartum hemorrhage, not elsewhere classified

EXCLUDES 1 *hemorrhage in early pregnancy (O2Ø.-)*
intrapartum hemorrhage NEC (O67.-)
placenta previa (O44.-)
premature separation of placenta [abruptio placentae] (O45.-)

DEF: Uterine hemorrhage prior to delivery that is not related to placenta previa or abruptio placentae.

O46.Ø Antepartum hemorrhage with coagulation defect

O46.ØØ Antepartum hemorrhage with coagulation defect, unspecified

O46.ØØ1 Antepartum hemorrhage with coagulation defect, unspecified, first trimester MCC M ♀

O46.ØØ2 Antepartum hemorrhage with coagulation defect, unspecified, second trimester MCC M ♀

O46.ØØ3 Antepartum hemorrhage with coagulation defect, unspecified, third trimester MCC M ♀

O46.ØØ9 Antepartum hemorrhage with coagulation defect, unspecified, unspecified trimester M ♀

O46.Ø1 Antepartum hemorrhage with afibrinogenemia

Antepartum hemorrhage with hypofibrinogenemia

O46.Ø11 Antepartum hemorrhage with afibrinogenemia, first trimester MCC M ♀

O46.Ø12 Antepartum hemorrhage with afibrinogenemia, second trimester MCC M ♀

O46.Ø13 **Antepartum hemorrhage with afibrinogenemia, third trimester** MCC M ♀

O46.Ø19 **Antepartum hemorrhage with afibrinogenemia, unspecified trimester** M ♀

✓6th O46.Ø2 **Antepartum hemorrhage with disseminated intravascular coagulation**

O46.Ø21 **Antepartum hemorrhage with disseminated intravascular coagulation, first trimester** MCC M ♀

O46.Ø22 **Antepartum hemorrhage with disseminated intravascular coagulation, second trimester** MCC M ♀

O46.Ø23 **Antepartum hemorrhage with disseminated intravascular coagulation, third trimester** MCC M ♀

O46.Ø29 **Antepartum hemorrhage with disseminated intravascular coagulation, unspecified trimester** M ♀

✓6th O46.Ø9 **Antepartum hemorrhage with other coagulation defect**

O46.Ø91 **Antepartum hemorrhage with other coagulation defect, first trimester** MCC M ♀

O46.Ø92 **Antepartum hemorrhage with other coagulation defect, second trimester** MCC M ♀

O46.Ø93 **Antepartum hemorrhage with other coagulation defect, third trimester** MCC M ♀

O46.Ø99 **Antepartum hemorrhage with other coagulation defect, unspecified trimester** M ♀

✓5th O46.8 **Other antepartum hemorrhage**

✓6th O46.8X **Other antepartum hemorrhage**

O46.8X1 **Other antepartum hemorrhage, first trimester** M ♀

O46.8X2 **Other antepartum hemorrhage, second trimester** M ♀

O46.8X3 **Other antepartum hemorrhage, third trimester** M ♀

O46.8X9 **Other antepartum hemorrhage, unspecified trimester** M ♀

✓5th O46.9 **Antepartum hemorrhage, unspecified**

O46.9Ø **Antepartum hemorrhage, unspecified, unspecified trimester** M ♀

O46.91 **Antepartum hemorrhage, unspecified, first trimester** M ♀

O46.92 **Antepartum hemorrhage, unspecified, second trimester** M ♀

O46.93 **Antepartum hemorrhage, unspecified, third trimester** M ♀

✓4th O47 **False labor**

INCLUDES Braxton Hicks contractions
threatened labor

EXCLUDES 1 *preterm labor (O6Ø.-)*

AHA: 2021,1Q,10

✓5th O47.Ø **False labor before 37 completed weeks of gestation**

O47.ØØ **False labor before 37 completed weeks of gestation, unspecified trimester** M ♀

O47.Ø2 **False labor before 37 completed weeks of gestation, second trimester** CC M ♀

O47.Ø3 **False labor before 37 completed weeks of gestation, third trimester** CC M ♀

O47.1 **False labor at or after 37 completed weeks of gestation** CC M ♀

O47.9 **False labor, unspecified** M ♀

✓4th O48 **Late pregnancy**

AHA: 2022,2Q,3

O48.Ø **Post-term pregnancy** M ♀

Pregnancy over 4Ø completed weeks to 42 completed weeks gestation

O48.1 **Prolonged pregnancy** M ♀

Pregnancy which has advanced beyond 42 completed weeks gestation

AHA: 2016,1Q,5

Complications of labor and delivery (O6Ø-O77)

✓4th O6Ø **Preterm labor**

INCLUDES onset (spontaneous) of labor before 37 completed weeks of gestation

EXCLUDES 1 *false labor (O47.Ø-)*
threatened labor NOS (O47.Ø-)

✓5th O6Ø.Ø **Preterm labor without delivery**

O6Ø.ØØ **Preterm labor without delivery, unspecified trimester** M ♀

O6Ø.Ø2 **Preterm labor without delivery, second trimester** MCC M ♀

O6Ø.Ø3 **Preterm labor without delivery, third trimester** MCC M ♀

✓5th O6Ø.1 **Preterm labor with preterm delivery**

AHA: 2016,2Q,10

One of the following 7th characters is to be assigned to each code under subcategory O6Ø.1. 7th character Ø is for single gestations and multiple gestations where the fetus is unspecified. 7th characters 1 through 9 are for cases of multiple gestations to identify the fetus for which the code applies. The appropriate code from category O3Ø, Multiple gestation, must also be assigned when assigning a code from subcategory O6Ø.1 that has a 7th character of 1 through 9.
Ø not applicable or unspecified
1 fetus 1
2 fetus 2
3 fetus 3
4 fetus 4
5 fetus 5
9 other fetus

✓x7th O6Ø.1Ø **Preterm labor with preterm delivery, unspecified trimester** CC M ♀

Preterm labor with delivery NOS

✓x7th O6Ø.12 **Preterm labor second trimester with preterm delivery second trimester** MCC M ♀

✓x7th O6Ø.13 **Preterm labor second trimester with preterm delivery third trimester** MCC M ♀

✓x7th O6Ø.14 **Preterm labor third trimester with preterm delivery third trimester** MCC M ♀

✓5th O6Ø.2 **Term delivery with preterm labor**

One of the following 7th characters is to be assigned to each code under subcategory O6Ø.2. 7th character Ø is for single gestations and multiple gestations where the fetus is unspecified. 7th characters 1 through 9 are for cases of multiple gestations to identify the fetus for which the code applies. The appropriate code from category O3Ø, Multiple gestation, must also be assigned when assigning a code from subcategory O6Ø.2 that has a 7th character of 1 through 9.
Ø not applicable or unspecified
1 fetus 1
2 fetus 2
3 fetus 3
4 fetus 4
5 fetus 5
9 other fetus

✓x7th O6Ø.2Ø **Term delivery with preterm labor, unspecified trimester** CC M ♀

✓x7th O6Ø.22 **Term delivery with preterm labor, second trimester** MCC M ♀

✓x7th O6Ø.23 **Term delivery with preterm labor, third trimester** MCC M ♀

✓4th O61 **Failed induction of labor**

O61.Ø **Failed medical induction of labor** M ♀

Failed induction (of labor) by oxytocin
Failed induction (of labor) by prostaglandins

O61.1 **Failed instrumental induction of labor** M ♀

Failed mechanical induction (of labor)
Failed surgical induction (of labor)

O61.8 **Other failed induction of labor** M ♀

O61.9 **Failed induction of labor, unspecified** M ♀

O62 Abnormalities of forces of labor

DEF: Uterine inertia: Weak or poorly coordinated contractions of the uterus during labor.

O62.0 Primary inadequate contractions M ♀
- Failure of cervical dilatation
- Primary hypotonic uterine dysfunction
- Uterine inertia during latent phase of labor

O62.1 Secondary uterine inertia M ♀
- Arrested active phase of labor
- Secondary hypotonic uterine dysfunction

O62.2 Other uterine inertia M ♀
- Atony of uterus without hemorrhage
- Atony of uterus NOS
- Desultory labor
- Hypotonic uterine dysfunction NOS
- Irregular labor
- Poor contractions
- Slow slope active phase of labor
- Uterine inertia NOS

EXCLUDES 1 *atony of uterus with hemorrhage (postpartum) (O72.1)*
postpartum atony of uterus without hemorrhage (O75.89)

DEF: Uterine atony: Failure of the uterine muscles to contract after the fetus and placenta are delivered.

O62.3 Precipitate labor M ♀

DEF: Rapid labor with delivery occurring in three hours or less from the onset of contractions.

O62.4 Hypertonic, incoordinate, and prolonged uterine contractions M ♀
- Cervical spasm
- Contraction ring dystocia
- Dyscoordinate labor
- Hour-glass contraction of uterus
- Hypertonic uterine dysfunction
- Incoordinate uterine action
- Tetanic contractions
- Uterine dystocia NOS
- Uterine spasm

EXCLUDES 1 *dystocia (fetal) (maternal) NOS (O66.9)*

O62.8 Other abnormalities of forces of labor M ♀

O62.9 Abnormality of forces of labor, unspecified M ♀

O63 Long labor

O63.0 Prolonged first stage (of labor) M ♀

O63.1 Prolonged second stage (of labor) M ♀

O63.2 Delayed delivery of second twin, triplet, etc. M ♀

O63.9 Long labor, unspecified CC M ♀
- Prolonged labor NOS

O64 Obstructed labor due to malposition and malpresentation of fetus

One of the following 7th characters is to be assigned to each code under category O64. 7th character 0 is for single gestations and multiple gestations where the fetus is unspecified. 7th characters 1 through 9 are for cases of multiple gestations to identify the fetus for which the code applies. The appropriate code from category O30, Multiple gestation, must also be assigned when assigning a code from category O64 that has a 7th character of 1 through 9.

- 0 not applicable or unspecified
- 1 fetus 1
- 2 fetus 2
- 3 fetus 3
- 4 fetus 4
- 5 fetus 5
- 9 other fetus

Fetal Malposition

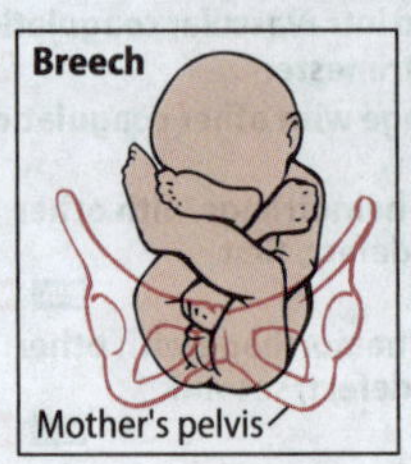

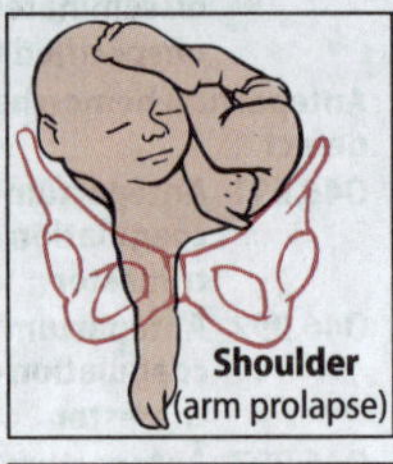

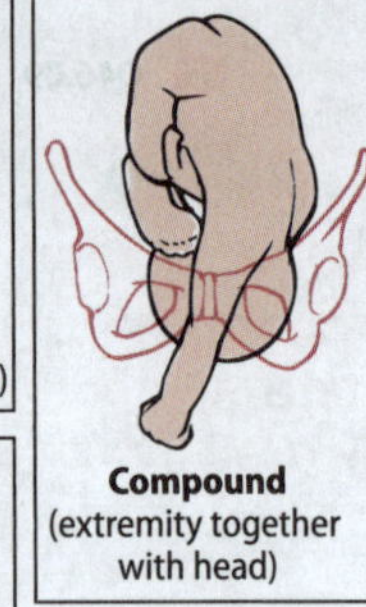

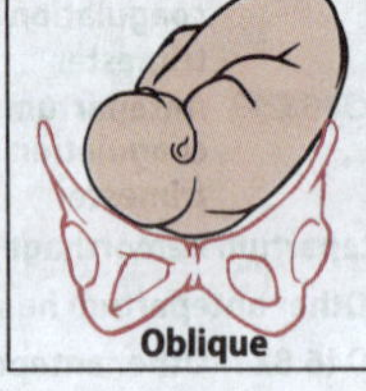

O64.0 Obstructed labor due to incomplete rotation of fetal head M ♀
- Deep transverse arrest
- Obstructed labor due to persistent occipitoiliac (position)
- Obstructed labor due to persistent occipitoposterior (position)
- Obstructed labor due to persistent occipitosacral (position)
- Obstructed labor due to persistent occipitotransverse (position)

O64.1 Obstructed labor due to breech presentation M ♀
- Obstructed labor due to buttocks presentation
- Obstructed labor due to complete breech presentation
- Obstructed labor due to frank breech presentation

O64.2 Obstructed labor due to face presentation M ♀
- Obstructed labor due to chin presentation

O64.3 Obstructed labor due to brow presentation M ♀

O64.4 Obstructed labor due to shoulder presentation M ♀
- Prolapsed arm

EXCLUDES 1 *impacted shoulders (O66.0)*
shoulder dystocia (O66.0)

O64.5 Obstructed labor due to compound presentation M ♀

O64.8 Obstructed labor due to other malposition and malpresentation M ♀
- Obstructed labor due to footling presentation
- Obstructed labor due to incomplete breech presentation

O64.9 Obstructed labor due to malposition and malpresentation, unspecified M ♀

O65 Obstructed labor due to maternal pelvic abnormality

O65.0 Obstructed labor due to deformed pelvis M ♀

O65.1 Obstructed labor due to generally contracted pelvis M ♀

O65.2 Obstructed labor due to pelvic inlet contraction M ♀

O65.3 Obstructed labor due to pelvic outlet and mid-cavity contraction M ♀

O65.4 Obstructed labor due to fetopelvic disproportion, unspecified M ♀

EXCLUDES 1 *dystocia due to abnormality of fetus (O66.2-O66.3)*

O65.5 Obstructed labor due to abnormality of maternal pelvic organs M ♀
- Obstructed labor due to conditions listed in O34.-

Use additional code to identify abnormality of pelvic organs O34.-

O65.8 Obstructed labor due to other maternal pelvic abnormalities M ♀

O65.9 Obstructed labor due to maternal pelvic abnormality, unspecified M ♀

O66 Other obstructed labor

O66.0 Obstructed labor due to shoulder dystocia M ♀
Impacted shoulders
DEF: Obstructed labor due to impacted fetal shoulders. It is an emergency condition that may require cesarean section, forceps delivery, vacuum extraction, or symphysiotomy.

O66.1 Obstructed labor due to locked twins M ♀

O66.2 Obstructed labor due to unusually large fetus M ♀

O66.3 Obstructed labor due to other abnormalities of fetus M ♀
Dystocia due to fetal ascites
Dystocia due to fetal hydrops
Dystocia due to fetal meningomyelocele
Dystocia due to fetal sacral teratoma
Dystocia due to fetal tumor
Dystocia due to hydrocephalic fetus
Use additional code to identify cause of obstruction

O66.4 Failed trial of labor

O66.40 Failed trial of labor, unspecified M ♀

O66.41 Failed attempted vaginal birth after previous cesarean delivery M ♀
Code first rupture of uterus, if applicable (O71.0-, O71.1)

O66.5 Attempted application of vacuum extractor and forceps M ♀
Attempted application of vacuum or forceps, with subsequent delivery by forceps or cesarean delivery

O66.6 Obstructed labor due to other multiple fetuses M ♀

O66.8 Other specified obstructed labor M ♀
Use additional code to identify cause of obstruction

O66.9 Obstructed labor, unspecified M ♀
Dystocia NOS
Fetal dystocia NOS
Maternal dystocia NOS

O67 Labor and delivery complicated by intrapartum hemorrhage, not elsewhere classified

EXCLUDES 1 *antepartum hemorrhage NEC (O46.-)*
placenta previa (O44.-)
premature separation of placenta [abruptio placentae] (O45.-)

EXCLUDES 2 *postpartum hemorrhage (O72.-)*

O67.0 Intrapartum hemorrhage with coagulation defect MCC M ♀
Intrapartum hemorrhage (excessive) associated with afibrinogenemia
Intrapartum hemorrhage (excessive) associated with disseminated intravascular coagulation
Intrapartum hemorrhage (excessive) associated with hyperfibrinolysis
Intrapartum hemorrhage (excessive) associated with hypofibrinogenemia

O67.8 Other intrapartum hemorrhage M ♀
Excessive intrapartum hemorrhage

O67.9 Intrapartum hemorrhage, unspecified M ♀

O68 Labor and delivery complicated by abnormality of fetal acid-base balance CC M ♀
Fetal acidemia complicating labor and delivery
Fetal acidosis complicating labor and delivery
Fetal alkalosis complicating labor and delivery
Fetal metabolic acidemia complicating labor and delivery

EXCLUDES 1 *fetal stress NOS (O77.9)*
labor and delivery complicated by electrocardiographic evidence of fetal stress (O77.8)
labor and delivery complicated by ultrasonic evidence of fetal stress (O77.8)

EXCLUDES 2 *abnormality in fetal heart rate or rhythm (O76)*
labor and delivery complicated by meconium in amniotic fluid (O77.0)

O69 Labor and delivery complicated by umbilical cord complications
AHA: 2016,1Q,5

One of the following 7th characters is to be assigned to each code under category O69. 7th character 0 is for single gestations and multiple gestations where the fetus is unspecified. 7th characters 1 through 9 are for cases of multiple gestations to identify the fetus for which the code applies. The appropriate code from category O30, Multiple gestation, must also be assigned when assigning a code from category O69 that has a 7th character of 1 through 9.
0 not applicable or unspecified
1 fetus 1
2 fetus 2
3 fetus 3
4 fetus 4
5 fetus 5
9 other fetus

O69.0 Labor and delivery complicated by prolapse of cord M ♀
DEF: Abnormal presentation of the fetus marked by a protruding umbilical cord during labor. It can cause fetal death.

O69.1 Labor and delivery complicated by cord around neck, with compression M ♀
EXCLUDES 1 *labor and delivery complicated by cord around neck, without compression (O69.81)*

O69.2 Labor and delivery complicated by other cord entanglement, with compression M ♀
Labor and delivery complicated by compression of cord NOS
Labor and delivery complicated by entanglement of cords of twins in monoamniotic sac
Labor and delivery complicated by knot in cord
EXCLUDES 1 *labor and delivery complicated by other cord entanglement, without compression (O69.82)*

O69.3 Labor and delivery complicated by short cord M ♀

O69.4 Labor and delivery complicated by vasa previa M ♀
Labor and delivery complicated by hemorrhage from vasa previa

O69.5 Labor and delivery complicated by vascular lesion of cord M ♀
Labor and delivery complicated by cord bruising
Labor and delivery complicated by cord hematoma
Labor and delivery complicated by thrombosis of umbilical vessels

O69.8 Labor and delivery complicated by other cord complications

O69.81 Labor and delivery complicated by cord around neck, without compression M ♀
AHA: 2016,1Q,5

O69.82 Labor and delivery complicated by other cord entanglement, without compression M ♀

O69.89 Labor and delivery complicated by other cord complications M ♀

O69.9 Labor and delivery complicated by cord complication, unspecified M ♀

O70 Perineal laceration during delivery

INCLUDES episiotomy extended by laceration

EXCLUDES 1 *obstetric high vaginal laceration alone (O71.4)*

AHA: 2016,2Q,34; 2016,1Q,3-4,5

O70.0 First degree perineal laceration during delivery M ♀
Perineal laceration, rupture or tear involving fourchette during delivery
Perineal laceration, rupture or tear involving labia during delivery
Perineal laceration, rupture or tear involving skin during delivery
Perineal laceration, rupture or tear involving vagina during delivery
Perineal laceration, rupture or tear involving vulva during delivery
Slight perineal laceration, rupture or tear during delivery

O70.1 Second degree perineal laceration during delivery M ♀
Perineal laceration, rupture or tear during delivery as in O70.0, also involving pelvic floor
Perineal laceration, rupture or tear during delivery as in O70.0, also involving perineal muscles
Perineal laceration, rupture or tear during delivery as in O70.0, also involving vaginal muscles
EXCLUDES 1 *perineal laceration involving anal sphincter (O70.2)*

O70.2 Third degree perineal laceration during delivery
Perineal laceration, rupture or tear during delivery as in O70.1, also involving anal sphincter
Perineal laceration, rupture or tear during delivery as in O70.1, also involving rectovaginal septum
Perineal laceration, rupture or tear during delivery as in O70.1, also involving sphincter NOS
EXCLUDES 1 *anal sphincter tear during delivery without third degree perineal laceration (O70.4)*
perineal laceration involving anal or rectal mucosa (O70.3)
AHA: 2016,4Q,53-54

O70.20 Third degree perineal laceration during delivery, unspecified CC M ♀

O70.21 Third degree perineal laceration during delivery, IIIa CC M ♀
Third degree perineal laceration during delivery with less than 50% of external anal sphincter (EAS) thickness torn

O70.22 Third degree perineal laceration during delivery, IIIb CC M ♀
Third degree perineal laceration during delivery with more than 50% external anal sphincter (EAS) thickness torn

O70.23 Third degree perineal laceration during delivery, IIIc CC M ♀
Third degree perineal laceration during delivery with both external anal sphincter (EAS) and internal anal sphincter (IAS) torn

O70.3 Fourth degree perineal laceration during delivery CC M ♀
Perineal laceration, rupture or tear during delivery as in O70.2, also involving anal mucosa
Perineal laceration, rupture or tear during delivery as in O70.2, also involving rectal mucosa

O70.4 Anal sphincter tear complicating delivery, not associated with third degree laceration CC M ♀
EXCLUDES 1 *anal sphincter tear with third degree perineal laceration (O70.2)*

O70.9 Perineal laceration during delivery, unspecified M ♀

O71 Other obstetric trauma
INCLUDES obstetric damage from instruments

O71.0 Rupture of uterus (spontaneous) before onset of labor
EXCLUDES 1 *disruption of (current) cesarean delivery wound (O90.0)*
laceration of uterus, NEC (O71.81)

O71.00 Rupture of uterus before onset of labor, unspecified trimester M ♀

O71.02 Rupture of uterus before onset of labor, second trimester MCC M ♀

O71.03 Rupture of uterus before onset of labor, third trimester MCC M ♀

O71.1 Rupture of uterus during labor MCC M ♀
Rupture of uterus not stated as occurring before onset of labor
EXCLUDES 1 *disruption of cesarean delivery wound (O90.0)*
laceration of uterus, NEC (O71.81)

O71.2 Postpartum inversion of uterus CC M ♀

O71.3 Obstetric laceration of cervix CC M ♀
Annular detachment of cervix

O71.4 Obstetric high vaginal laceration alone CC M ♀
Laceration of vaginal wall without perineal laceration
EXCLUDES 1 *obstetric high vaginal laceration with perineal laceration (O70.-)*
AHA: 2016,1Q,5

O71.5 Other obstetric injury to pelvic organs CC M ♀
Obstetric injury to bladder
Obstetric injury to urethra
EXCLUDES 2 *obstetric periurethral trauma (O71.82)*
AHA: 2014,4Q,18

O71.6 Obstetric damage to pelvic joints and ligaments CC M ♀
Obstetric avulsion of inner symphyseal cartilage
Obstetric damage to coccyx
Obstetric traumatic separation of symphysis (pubis)

O71.7 Obstetric hematoma of pelvis CC M ♀
Obstetric hematoma of perineum
Obstetric hematoma of vagina
Obstetric hematoma of vulva

O71.8 Other specified obstetric trauma

O71.81 Laceration of uterus, not elsewhere classified M ♀

O71.82 Other specified trauma to perineum and vulva M ♀
Obstetric periurethral trauma
AHA: 2016,1Q,4; 2014,4Q,18

O71.89 Other specified obstetric trauma M ♀

O71.9 Obstetric trauma, unspecified M ♀

O72 Postpartum hemorrhage
INCLUDES hemorrhage after delivery of fetus or infant

O72.0 Third-stage hemorrhage CC M ♀
Hemorrhage associated with retained, trapped or adherent placenta
Retained placenta NOS
Code also type of adherent placenta (O43.2-)
AHA: 2019,3Q,11

O72.1 Other immediate postpartum hemorrhage CC M ♀
Hemorrhage following delivery of placenta
Postpartum hemorrhage (atonic) NOS
Uterine atony with hemorrhage
EXCLUDES 1 *uterine atony NOS (O62.2)*
uterine atony without hemorrhage (O62.2)
postpartum atony of uterus without hemorrhage (O75.89)
AHA: 2016,1Q,4
DEF: Uterine atony: Failure of the uterine muscles to contract after the fetus and placenta are delivered.

O72.2 Delayed and secondary postpartum hemorrhage CC M ♀
Hemorrhage associated with retained portions of placenta or membranes after the first 24 hours following delivery of placenta
Retained products of conception NOS, following delivery

O72.3 Postpartum coagulation defects M ♀
Postpartum afibrinogenemia
Postpartum fibrinolysis

O73 Retained placenta and membranes, without hemorrhage
EXCLUDES 1 *placenta accreta (O43.21-)*
placenta increta (O43.22-)
placenta percreta (O43.23-)
DEF: Postpartum condition resulting from failure to expel placental membrane tissues due to failed contractions of the uterine wall.

O73.0 Retained placenta without hemorrhage M ♀
Adherent placenta, without hemorrhage
Trapped placenta without hemorrhage

O73.1 Retained portions of placenta and membranes, without hemorrhage M ♀
Retained products of conception following delivery, without hemorrhage

O74 Complications of anesthesia during labor and delivery
INCLUDES maternal complications arising from the administration of a general, regional or local anesthetic, analgesic or other sedation during labor and delivery
Use additional code, if applicable, to identify specific complication

O74.0 Aspiration pneumonitis due to anesthesia during labor and delivery M ♀
Inhalation of stomach contents or secretions NOS due to anesthesia during labor and delivery
Mendelson's syndrome due to anesthesia during labor and delivery

O74.1 Other pulmonary complications of anesthesia during labor and delivery M ♀

O74.2 Cardiac complications of anesthesia during labor and delivery M ♀

O74.3 Central nervous system complications of anesthesia during labor and delivery M ♀

O74.4 Toxic reaction to local anesthesia during labor and delivery M ♀

O74.5 Spinal and epidural anesthesia-induced headache during labor and delivery M ♀

O74.6 Other complications of spinal and epidural anesthesia during labor and delivery M ♀

N Newborn: 0 P Pediatric: 0-17 M Maternity: 9-64 A Adult: 15-124 UNS Unspecified Site MCC Major Complication/Comorbidity CC Complication/Comorbidity

O74.7 Failed or difficult intubation for anesthesia during labor and delivery M♀

O74.8 Other complications of anesthesia during labor and delivery M♀

O74.9 Complication of anesthesia during labor and delivery, unspecified M♀

O75 Other complications of labor and delivery, not elsewhere classified

EXCLUDES 2 *puerperal (postpartum) infection (O86.-)*
puerperal (postpartum) sepsis (O85)

O75.0 Maternal distress during labor and delivery M♀

O75.1 Shock during or following labor and delivery MCC M♀
Obstetric shock following labor and delivery

O75.2 Pyrexia during labor, not elsewhere classified CC M♀

O75.3 Other infection during labor MCC M♀
Sepsis during labor
Use additional code (B95-B97), to identify infectious agent

O75.4 Other complications of obstetric surgery and procedures M♀
Cardiac arrest following obstetric surgery or procedures
Cardiac failure following obstetric surgery or procedures
Cerebral anoxia following obstetric surgery or procedures
Pulmonary edema following obstetric surgery or procedures
Use additional code to identify specific complication

EXCLUDES 2 *complications of anesthesia during labor and delivery (O74.-)*
disruption of obstetrical (surgical) wound (O90.0-O90.1)
hematoma of obstetrical (surgical) wound (O90.2)
infection of obstetrical (surgical) wound (O86.0-)

O75.5 Delayed delivery after artificial rupture of membranes M♀

O75.8 Other specified complications of labor and delivery

O75.81 Maternal exhaustion complicating labor and delivery M♀

O75.82 Onset (spontaneous) of labor after 37 completed weeks of gestation but before 39 completed weeks gestation, with delivery by (planned) cesarean section M♀
Delivery by (planned) cesarean section occurring after 37 completed weeks of gestation but before 39 completed weeks gestation due to (spontaneous) onset of labor
Code first to specify reason for planned cesarean section such as:
cephalopelvic disproportion (normally formed fetus) (O33.9)
previous cesarean delivery (O34.21)
AHA: 2022,2Q,3

O75.89 Other specified complications of labor and delivery M♀

O75.9 Complication of labor and delivery, unspecified M♀

O76 Abnormality in fetal heart rate and rhythm complicating labor and delivery M♀
Depressed fetal heart rate tones complicating labor and delivery
Fetal bradycardia complicating labor and delivery
Fetal heart rate decelerations complicating labor and delivery
Fetal heart rate irregularity complicating labor and delivery
Fetal heart rate abnormal variability complicating labor and delivery
Fetal tachycardia complicating labor and delivery
Non-reassuring fetal heart rate or rhythm complicating labor and delivery

EXCLUDES 1 *fetal stress NOS (O77.9)*
labor and delivery complicated by electrocardiographic evidence of fetal stress (O77.8)
labor and delivery complicated by ultrasonic evidence of fetal stress (O77.8)

EXCLUDES 2 *fetal metabolic acidemia (O68)*
other fetal stress (O77.0-O77.1)

AHA: 2013,4Q,118

O77 Other fetal stress complicating labor and delivery

O77.0 Labor and delivery complicated by meconium in amniotic fluid M♀
AHA: 2022,2Q,16; 2013,4Q,117-118

O77.1 Fetal stress in labor or delivery due to drug administration M♀

O77.8 Labor and delivery complicated by other evidence of fetal stress M♀
Labor and delivery complicated by electrocardiographic evidence of fetal stress
Labor and delivery complicated by ultrasonic evidence of fetal stress

EXCLUDES 1 *abnormality of fetal acid-base balance (O68)*
abnormality in fetal heart rate or rhythm (O76)
fetal metabolic acidemia (O68)

O77.9 Labor and delivery complicated by fetal stress, unspecified M♀

EXCLUDES 1 *abnormality of fetal acid-base balance (O68)*
abnormality in fetal heart rate or rhythm (O76)
fetal metabolic acidemia (O68)

Encounter for delivery (O80-O82)

O80 Encounter for full-term uncomplicated delivery M♀

NOTE Delivery requiring minimal or no assistance, with or without episiotomy, without fetal manipulation [e.g., rotation version] or instrumentation [forceps] of a spontaneous, cephalic, vaginal, full-term, single, live-born infant. This code is for use as a single diagnosis code and is not to be used with any other code from chapter 15.

Use additional code to indicate outcome of delivery (Z37.0)
AHA: 2016,4Q,150; 2014,2Q,9

O82 Encounter for cesarean delivery without indication M♀
Use additional code to indicate outcome of delivery (Z37.0)

Complications predominantly related to the puerperium (O85-O92)

EXCLUDES 2 *mental and behavioral disorders associated with the puerperium (F53.-)*
obstetrical tetanus (A34)
puerperal osteomalacia (M83.0)

O85 Puerperal sepsis MCC M♀
Postpartum sepsis
Puerperal peritonitis
Puerperal pyemia
Use additional code (B95-B97), to identify infectious agent
Use additional code (R65.2-) to identify severe sepsis, if applicable

EXCLUDES 1 *fever of unknown origin following delivery (O86.4)*
genital tract infection following delivery (O86.1-)
obstetric pyemic and septic embolism (O88.3-)
puerperal septic thrombophlebitis (O86.81)
urinary tract infection following delivery (O86.2-)

EXCLUDES 2 *sepsis during labor (O75.3)*

AHA: 2022,2Q,5; 2020,2Q,32; 2019,2Q,39; 2018,4Q,23

O86 Other puerperal infections
Use additional code (B95-B97), to identify infectious agent

EXCLUDES 2 *infection during labor (O75.3)*
obstetrical tetanus (A34)

O86.0 Infection of obstetric surgical wound
Infected cesarean delivery wound following delivery
Infected perineal repair following delivery

EXCLUDES 1 *complications of procedures, not elsewhere classified (T81.4-)*
postprocedural fever NOS (R50.82)
postprocedural retroperitoneal abscess (K68.11)

AHA: 2020,2Q,32; 2018,4Q,22-23,62

O86.00 Infection of obstetric surgical wound, unspecified M♀

O86.01 Infection of obstetric surgical wound, superficial incisional site M♀
Subcutaneous abscess following an obstetrical procedure
Stitch abscess following an obstetrical procedure

O86.02 Infection of obstetric surgical wound, deep incisional site M♀
Intramuscular abscess following an obstetrical procedure
Sub-fascial abscess following an obstetrical procedure
AHA: 2020,2Q,32

O86.03 Infection of obstetric surgical wound, organ and space site M ♀
Intraabdominal abscess following an obstetrical procedure
Subphrenic abscess following an obstetrical procedure

O86.04 Sepsis following an obstetrical procedure MCC M ♀
Use additional code to identify the sepsis
AHA: 2020,2Q,32; 2019,2Q,39

O86.09 Infection of obstetric surgical wound, other surgical site M ♀

5th **O86.1 Other infection of genital tract following delivery**

O86.11 Cervicitis following delivery CC M ♀
O86.12 Endometritis following delivery CC M ♀
O86.13 Vaginitis following delivery CC M ♀
O86.19 Other infection of genital tract following delivery CC M ♀

5th **O86.2 Urinary tract infection following delivery**

O86.20 Urinary tract infection following delivery, unspecified CC M ♀
Puerperal urinary tract infection NOS
AHA: 2022,2Q,5

O86.21 Infection of kidney following delivery CC M ♀
O86.22 Infection of bladder following delivery CC M ♀
Infection of urethra following delivery
O86.29 Other urinary tract infection following delivery CC M ♀

O86.4 Pyrexia of unknown origin following delivery CC M ♀
Puerperal infection NOS following delivery
Puerperal pyrexia NOS following delivery
EXCLUDES 2 *pyrexia during labor (O75.2)*
DEF: Fever of unknown origin experienced by the mother after childbirth.

5th **O86.8 Other specified puerperal infections**

O86.81 Puerperal septic thrombophlebitis MCC M ♀
O86.89 Other specified puerperal infections MCC M ♀

4th **O87 Venous complications and hemorrhoids in the puerperium**
INCLUDES venous complications in labor, delivery and the puerperium
EXCLUDES 2 *obstetric embolism (O88.-)*
puerperal septic thrombophlebitis (O86.81)
venous complications in pregnancy (O22.-)

O87.0 Superficial thrombophlebitis in the puerperium CC M ♀
Puerperal phlebitis NOS
Puerperal thrombosis NOS

O87.1 Deep phlebothrombosis in the puerperium MCC M ♀
Deep vein thrombosis, postpartum
Pelvic thrombophlebitis, postpartum
Use additional code to identify the deep vein thrombosis (I82.4-, I82.5-, I82.62-, I82.72-)
Use additional code, if applicable, for associated long-term (current) use of anticoagulants (Z79.01)

O87.2 Hemorrhoids in the puerperium CC M ♀
O87.3 Cerebral venous thrombosis in the puerperium CC M ♀
Cerebrovenous sinus thrombosis in the puerperium
O87.4 Varicose veins of lower extremity in the puerperium M ♀
O87.8 Other venous complications in the puerperium CC M ♀
Genital varices in the puerperium
O87.9 Venous complication in the puerperium, unspecified M ♀
Puerperal phlebopathy NOS

4th **O88 Obstetric embolism**
EXCLUDES 1 *embolism complicating abortion NOS (O03.2)*
embolism complicating ectopic or molar pregnancy (O08.2)
embolism complicating failed attempted abortion (O07.2)
embolism complicating induced abortion (O04.7)
embolism complicating spontaneous abortion (O03.2, O03.7)

5th **O88.0 Obstetric air embolism**
DEF: Sudden blocking of the pulmonary artery or right ventricle with air or nitrogen bubbles.

6th **O88.01 Obstetric air embolism in pregnancy**

O88.011 Air embolism in pregnancy, first trimester MCC M ♀
O88.012 Air embolism in pregnancy, second trimester MCC M ♀
O88.013 Air embolism in pregnancy, third trimester MCC M ♀
O88.019 Air embolism in pregnancy, unspecified trimester M ♀

O88.02 Air embolism in childbirth MCC M ♀
O88.03 Air embolism in the puerperium MCC M ♀

5th **O88.1 Amniotic fluid embolism**
Anaphylactoid syndrome in pregnancy

6th **O88.11 Amniotic fluid embolism in pregnancy**

O88.111 Amniotic fluid embolism in pregnancy, first trimester MCC M ♀
O88.112 Amniotic fluid embolism in pregnancy, second trimester MCC M ♀
O88.113 Amniotic fluid embolism in pregnancy, third trimester MCC M ♀
O88.119 Amniotic fluid embolism in pregnancy, unspecified trimester M ♀

O88.12 Amniotic fluid embolism in childbirth MCC M ♀
O88.13 Amniotic fluid embolism in the puerperium MCC M ♀

5th **O88.2 Obstetric thromboembolism**

6th **O88.21 Thromboembolism in pregnancy**
Obstetric (pulmonary) embolism NOS

O88.211 Thromboembolism in pregnancy, first trimester MCC M ♀
O88.212 Thromboembolism in pregnancy, second trimester MCC M ♀
O88.213 Thromboembolism in pregnancy, third trimester MCC M ♀
O88.219 Thromboembolism in pregnancy, unspecified trimester M ♀

O88.22 Thromboembolism in childbirth MCC M ♀
O88.23 Thromboembolism in the puerperium MCC M ♀
Puerperal (pulmonary) embolism NOS

5th **O88.3 Obstetric pyemic and septic embolism**

6th **O88.31 Pyemic and septic embolism in pregnancy**

O88.311 Pyemic and septic embolism in pregnancy, first trimester MCC M ♀
O88.312 Pyemic and septic embolism in pregnancy, second trimester MCC M ♀
O88.313 Pyemic and septic embolism in pregnancy, third trimester MCC M ♀
O88.319 Pyemic and septic embolism in pregnancy, unspecified trimester CC M ♀

O88.32 Pyemic and septic embolism in childbirth MCC M ♀
O88.33 Pyemic and septic embolism in the puerperium MCC M ♀

5th **O88.8 Other obstetric embolism**
Obstetric fat embolism

6th **O88.81 Other embolism in pregnancy**

O88.811 Other embolism in pregnancy, first trimester MCC M ♀
O88.812 Other embolism in pregnancy, second trimester MCC M ♀
O88.813 Other embolism in pregnancy, third trimester MCC M ♀
O88.819 Other embolism in pregnancy, unspecified trimester M ♀

O88.82 Other embolism in childbirth MCC M ♀
O88.83 Other embolism in the puerperium MCC M ♀

4th **O89 Complications of anesthesia during the puerperium**
INCLUDES maternal complications arising from the administration of a general, regional or local anesthetic, analgesic or other sedation during the puerperium
Use additional code, if applicable, to identify specific complication

5th **O89.0 Pulmonary complications of anesthesia during the puerperium**

O89.01 Aspiration pneumonitis due to anesthesia during the puerperium M ♀
Inhalation of stomach contents or secretions NOS due to anesthesia during the puerperium
Mendelson's syndrome due to anesthesia during the puerperium

O89.09 Other pulmonary complications of anesthesia during the puerperium M ♀

O89.1 Cardiac complications of anesthesia during the puerperium M♀

O89.2 Central nervous system complications of anesthesia during the puerperium M♀

O89.3 Toxic reaction to local anesthesia during the puerperium M♀

O89.4 Spinal and epidural anesthesia-induced headache during the puerperium M♀

O89.5 Other complications of spinal and epidural anesthesia during the puerperium M♀

O89.6 Failed or difficult intubation for anesthesia during the puerperium M♀

O89.8 Other complications of anesthesia during the puerperium M♀

O89.9 Complication of anesthesia during the puerperium, unspecified M♀

✓4th O90 Complications of the puerperium, not elsewhere classified

O90.0 Disruption of cesarean delivery wound M♀
Dehiscence of cesarean delivery wound
EXCLUDES 1 *rupture of uterus (spontaneous) before onset of labor (O71.0-)*
rupture of uterus during labor (O71.1)

O90.1 Disruption of perineal obstetric wound M♀
Disruption of wound of episiotomy
Disruption of wound of perineal laceration
Secondary perineal tear

O90.2 Hematoma of obstetric wound M♀

O90.3 Peripartum cardiomyopathy MCC M♀
Conditions in I42- arising during pregnancy and the puerperium
EXCLUDES 1 *pre-existing heart disease complicating pregnancy and the puerperium (O99.4-)*
DEF: Any structural or functional abnormality of the ventricular myocardium. It is a noninflammatory disease of obscure or unknown etiology with onset during the postpartum period.

O90.4 Postpartum acute kidney failure MCC M♀
Hepatorenal syndrome following labor and delivery

O90.5 Postpartum thyroiditis M♀

O90.6 Postpartum mood disturbance M♀
Postpartum blues
Postpartum dysphoria
Postpartum sadness
EXCLUDES 1 *postpartum depression (F53.0)*
puerperal psychosis (F53.1)

✓5th O90.8 Other complications of the puerperium, not elsewhere classified

O90.81 Anemia of the puerperium M♀
Postpartum anemia NOS
EXCLUDES 1 *pre-existing anemia complicating the puerperium (O99.03)*
AHA: 2019,3Q,11

O90.89 Other complications of the puerperium, not elsewhere classified M♀
Placental polyp

O90.9 Complication of the puerperium, unspecified M♀

✓4th O91 Infections of breast associated with pregnancy, the puerperium and lactation
Use additional code to identify infection

✓5th O91.0 Infection of nipple associated with pregnancy, the puerperium and lactation

✓6th O91.01 Infection of nipple associated with pregnancy
Gestational abscess of nipple

O91.011 Infection of nipple associated with pregnancy, first trimester M♀

O91.012 Infection of nipple associated with pregnancy, second trimester M♀

O91.013 Infection of nipple associated with pregnancy, third trimester M♀

O91.019 Infection of nipple associated with pregnancy, unspecified trimester M♀

O91.02 Infection of nipple associated with the puerperium M♀
Puerperal abscess of nipple

O91.03 Infection of nipple associated with lactation M♀
Abscess of nipple associated with lactation

✓5th O91.1 Abscess of breast associated with pregnancy, the puerperium and lactation

✓6th O91.11 Abscess of breast associated with pregnancy
Gestational mammary abscess
Gestational purulent mastitis
Gestational subareolar abscess

O91.111 Abscess of breast associated with pregnancy, first trimester M♀

O91.112 Abscess of breast associated with pregnancy, second trimester M♀

O91.113 Abscess of breast associated with pregnancy, third trimester M♀

O91.119 Abscess of breast associated with pregnancy, unspecified trimester M♀

O91.12 Abscess of breast associated with the puerperium M♀
Puerperal mammary abscess
Puerperal purulent mastitis
Puerperal subareolar abscess

O91.13 Abscess of breast associated with lactation M♀
Mammary abscess associated with lactation
Purulent mastitis associated with lactation
Subareolar abscess associated with lactation

✓5th O91.2 Nonpurulent mastitis associated with pregnancy, the puerperium and lactation

✓6th O91.21 Nonpurulent mastitis associated with pregnancy
Gestational interstitial mastitis
Gestational lymphangitis of breast
Gestational mastitis NOS
Gestational parenchymatous mastitis

O91.211 Nonpurulent mastitis associated with pregnancy, first trimester M♀

O91.212 Nonpurulent mastitis associated with pregnancy, second trimester M♀

O91.213 Nonpurulent mastitis associated with pregnancy, third trimester M♀

O91.219 Nonpurulent mastitis associated with pregnancy, unspecified trimester M♀

O91.22 Nonpurulent mastitis associated with the puerperium M♀
Puerperal interstitial mastitis
Puerperal lymphangitis of breast
Puerperal mastitis NOS
Puerperal parenchymatous mastitis

O91.23 Nonpurulent mastitis associated with lactation M♀
Interstitial mastitis associated with lactation
Lymphangitis of breast associated with lactation
Mastitis NOS associated with lactation
Parenchymatous mastitis associated with lactation

✓4th O92 Other disorders of breast and disorders of lactation associated with pregnancy and the puerperium

✓5th O92.0 Retracted nipple associated with pregnancy, the puerperium, and lactation

✓6th O92.01 Retracted nipple associated with pregnancy

O92.011 Retracted nipple associated with pregnancy, first trimester M♀

O92.012 Retracted nipple associated with pregnancy, second trimester M♀

O92.013 Retracted nipple associated with pregnancy, third trimester M♀

O92.019 Retracted nipple associated with pregnancy, unspecified trimester M♀

O92.02 Retracted nipple associated with the puerperium M♀

O92.03 Retracted nipple associated with lactation M♀

✓5th O92.1 Cracked nipple associated with pregnancy, the puerperium, and lactation
Fissure of nipple, gestational or puerperal

✓6th O92.11 Cracked nipple associated with pregnancy

O92.111 Cracked nipple associated with pregnancy, first trimester M♀

O92.112 Cracked nipple associated with pregnancy, second trimester M♀

O92.113 Cracked nipple associated with pregnancy, third trimester M♀

O92.119 Cracked nipple associated with pregnancy, unspecified trimester M♀

O92.12 Cracked nipple associated with the puerperium M ♀

O92.13 Cracked nipple associated with lactation M ♀

5th **O92.2 Other and unspecified disorders of breast associated with pregnancy and the puerperium**

O92.20 Unspecified disorder of breast associated with pregnancy and the puerperium M ♀

O92.29 Other disorders of breast associated with pregnancy and the puerperium M ♀

O92.3 Agalactia M ♀

Primary agalactia

EXCLUDES 1 *elective agalactia (O92.5)*
secondary agalactia (O92.5)
therapeutic agalactia (O92.5)

DEF: Absence of milk secretion in a female after delivery.

O92.4 Hypogalactia M ♀

O92.5 Suppressed lactation M ♀

Elective agalactia
Secondary agalactia
Therapeutic agalactia

EXCLUDES 1 *primary agalactia (O92.3)*

O92.6 Galactorrhea M ♀

DEF: Excessive or persistent milk secretion by the breast that may occur in the absence of nursing.

5th **O92.7 Other and unspecified disorders of lactation**

O92.70 Unspecified disorders of lactation M ♀

O92.79 Other disorders of lactation M ♀

Puerperal galactocele

Other obstetric conditions, not elsewhere classified (O94-O9A)

O94 Sequelae of complication of pregnancy, childbirth, and the puerperium UPD M ♀

NOTE This category is to be used to indicate conditions in O00-O77.-, O85-O94 and O98-O9A.- as the cause of late effects. The sequelae include conditions specified as such, or as late effects, which may occur at any time after the puerperium

Code first condition resulting from (sequela) of complication of pregnancy, childbirth, and the puerperium

4th **O98 Maternal infectious and parasitic diseases classifiable elsewhere but complicating pregnancy, childbirth and the puerperium**

INCLUDES the listed conditions when complicating the pregnant state, when aggravated by the pregnancy, or as a reason for obstetric care

Use additional code (Chapter 1), to identify specific infectious or parasitic disease

EXCLUDES 2 *herpes gestationis (O26.4-)*
infectious carrier state (O99.82-, O99.83-)
obstetrical tetanus (A34)
puerperal infection (O86.-)
puerperal sepsis (O85)
when the reason for maternal care is that the disease is known or suspected to have affected the fetus (O35-O36)

5th **O98.0 Tuberculosis complicating pregnancy, childbirth and the puerperium**

Conditions in A15-A19

6th **O98.01 Tuberculosis complicating pregnancy**

O98.011 Tuberculosis complicating pregnancy, first trimester CC M ♀

O98.012 Tuberculosis complicating pregnancy, second trimester CC M ♀

O98.013 Tuberculosis complicating pregnancy, third trimester CC M ♀

O98.019 Tuberculosis complicating pregnancy, unspecified trimester M ♀

O98.02 Tuberculosis complicating childbirth CC M ♀

O98.03 Tuberculosis complicating the puerperium CC M ♀

5th **O98.1 Syphilis complicating pregnancy, childbirth and the puerperium**

Conditions in A50-A53

6th **O98.11 Syphilis complicating pregnancy**

O98.111 Syphilis complicating pregnancy, first trimester CC M ♀

O98.112 Syphilis complicating pregnancy, second trimester CC M ♀

O98.113 Syphilis complicating pregnancy, third trimester CC M ♀

O98.119 Syphilis complicating pregnancy, unspecified trimester M ♀

O98.12 Syphilis complicating childbirth CC M ♀

O98.13 Syphilis complicating the puerperium CC M ♀

5th **O98.2 Gonorrhea complicating pregnancy, childbirth and the puerperium**

Conditions in A54.-

6th **O98.21 Gonorrhea complicating pregnancy**

O98.211 Gonorrhea complicating pregnancy, first trimester CC M ♀

O98.212 Gonorrhea complicating pregnancy, second trimester CC M ♀

O98.213 Gonorrhea complicating pregnancy, third trimester CC M ♀

O98.219 Gonorrhea complicating pregnancy, unspecified trimester M ♀

O98.22 Gonorrhea complicating childbirth CC M ♀

O98.23 Gonorrhea complicating the puerperium CC M ♀

5th **O98.3 Other infections with a predominantly sexual mode of transmission complicating pregnancy, childbirth and the puerperium**

Conditions in A55-A64

AHA: 2020,1Q,20

6th **O98.31 Other infections with a predominantly sexual mode of transmission complicating pregnancy**

O98.311 Other infections with a predominantly sexual mode of transmission complicating pregnancy, first trimester CC M ♀

O98.312 Other infections with a predominantly sexual mode of transmission complicating pregnancy, second trimester CC M ♀

O98.313 Other infections with a predominantly sexual mode of transmission complicating pregnancy, third trimester CC M ♀

O98.319 Other infections with a predominantly sexual mode of transmission complicating pregnancy, unspecified trimester M ♀

O98.32 Other infections with a predominantly sexual mode of transmission complicating childbirth CC M ♀

O98.33 Other infections with a predominantly sexual mode of transmission complicating the puerperium CC M ♀

5th **O98.4 Viral hepatitis complicating pregnancy, childbirth and the puerperium**

Conditions in B15-B19

6th **O98.41 Viral hepatitis complicating pregnancy**

O98.411 Viral hepatitis complicating pregnancy, first trimester CC M ♀

O98.412 Viral hepatitis complicating pregnancy, second trimester CC M ♀

O98.413 Viral hepatitis complicating pregnancy, third trimester CC M ♀

O98.419 Viral hepatitis complicating pregnancy, unspecified trimester M ♀

O98.42 Viral hepatitis complicating childbirth CC M ♀

O98.43 Viral hepatitis complicating the puerperium CC M ♀

5th **O98.5 Other viral diseases complicating pregnancy, childbirth and the puerperium**

Conditions in A80-B09, B25-B34, R87.81-, R87.82-

EXCLUDES 1 *human immunodeficiency virus [HIV] disease complicating pregnancy, childbirth and the puerperium (O98.7-)*

TIP: Assign a code from this subcategory as the principal or first-listed diagnosis for a patient admitted/presenting during pregnancy, childbirth, or the puerperium because of COVID-19; assign U07.1 and codes for associated manifestations as secondary codes.

6th **O98.51 Other viral diseases complicating pregnancy**

O98.511 Other viral diseases complicating pregnancy, first trimester CC M ♀

O98.512 Other viral diseases complicating pregnancy, second trimester CC M ♀

O98.513 Other viral diseases complicating pregnancy, third trimester CC M ♀

O98.519 Other viral diseases complicating pregnancy, unspecified trimester M ♀

O98.52 Other viral diseases complicating childbirth CC M ♀

O98.53 Other viral diseases complicating the puerperium CC M ♀

✓5th **O98.6 Protozoal diseases complicating pregnancy, childbirth and the puerperium**
Conditions in B5Ø-B64

✓6th **O98.61 Protozoal diseases complicating pregnancy**

O98.611 Protozoal diseases complicating pregnancy, first trimester CC M ♀

O98.612 Protozoal diseases complicating pregnancy, second trimester CC M ♀

O98.613 Protozoal diseases complicating pregnancy, third trimester CC M ♀

O98.619 Protozoal diseases complicating pregnancy, unspecified trimester M ♀

O98.62 Protozoal diseases complicating childbirth CC M ♀

O98.63 Protozoal diseases complicating the puerperium CC M ♀

✓5th **O98.7 Human immunodeficiency virus [HIV] disease complicating pregnancy, childbirth and the puerperium**
Use additional code to identify the type of HIV disease:
acquired immune deficiency syndrome (AIDS) (B2Ø)
asymptomatic HIV status (Z21)
HIV positive NOS (Z21)
symptomatic HIV disease (B2Ø)

✓6th **O98.71 Human immunodeficiency virus [HIV] disease complicating pregnancy**

O98.711 Human immunodeficiency virus [HIV] disease complicating pregnancy, first trimester CC M ♀

O98.712 Human immunodeficiency virus [HIV] disease complicating pregnancy, second trimester CC M ♀

O98.713 Human immunodeficiency virus [HIV] disease complicating pregnancy, third trimester CC M ♀

O98.719 Human immunodeficiency virus [HIV] disease complicating pregnancy, unspecified trimester M ♀

O98.72 Human immunodeficiency virus [HIV] disease complicating childbirth CC M ♀

O98.73 Human immunodeficiency virus [HIV] disease complicating the puerperium CC M ♀

✓5th **O98.8 Other maternal infectious and parasitic diseases complicating pregnancy, childbirth and the puerperium**
AHA: 2020,1Q,10

✓6th **O98.81 Other maternal infectious and parasitic diseases complicating pregnancy**

O98.811 Other maternal infectious and parasitic diseases complicating pregnancy, first trimester CC M ♀

O98.812 Other maternal infectious and parasitic diseases complicating pregnancy, second trimester CC M ♀

O98.813 Other maternal infectious and parasitic diseases complicating pregnancy, third trimester CC M ♀

O98.819 Other maternal infectious and parasitic diseases complicating pregnancy, unspecified trimester M ♀

O98.82 Other maternal infectious and parasitic diseases complicating childbirth CC M ♀

O98.83 Other maternal infectious and parasitic diseases complicating the puerperium CC M ♀
AHA: 2022,2Q,5

✓5th **O98.9 Unspecified maternal infectious and parasitic disease complicating pregnancy, childbirth and the puerperium**

✓6th **O98.91 Unspecified maternal infectious and parasitic disease complicating pregnancy**

O98.911 Unspecified maternal infectious and parasitic disease complicating pregnancy, first trimester CC M ♀

O98.912 Unspecified maternal infectious and parasitic disease complicating pregnancy, second trimester CC M ♀

O98.913 Unspecified maternal infectious and parasitic disease complicating pregnancy, third trimester CC M ♀

O98.919 Unspecified maternal infectious and parasitic disease complicating pregnancy, unspecified trimester M ♀

O98.92 Unspecified maternal infectious and parasitic disease complicating childbirth CC M ♀

O98.93 Unspecified maternal infectious and parasitic disease complicating the puerperium CC M ♀

✓4th **O99 Other maternal diseases classifiable elsewhere but complicating pregnancy, childbirth and the puerperium**
INCLUDES conditions which complicate the pregnant state, are aggravated by the pregnancy or are a main reason for obstetric care
Use additional code to identify specific condition
EXCLUDES 2 *when the reason for maternal care is that the condition is known or suspected to have affected the fetus (O35-O36)*

✓5th **O99.Ø Anemia complicating pregnancy, childbirth and the puerperium**
Conditions in D5Ø-D64
EXCLUDES 1 *anemia arising in the puerperium (O9Ø.81)*
postpartum anemia NOS (O9Ø.81)
AHA: 2019,3Q,11

✓6th **O99.Ø1 Anemia complicating pregnancy**
AHA: 2016,1Q,4

O99.Ø11 Anemia complicating pregnancy, first trimester M ♀

O99.Ø12 Anemia complicating pregnancy, second trimester M ♀

O99.Ø13 Anemia complicating pregnancy, third trimester M ♀

O99.Ø19 Anemia complicating pregnancy, unspecified trimester M ♀

O99.Ø2 Anemia complicating childbirth M ♀

O99.Ø3 Anemia complicating the puerperium M ♀
EXCLUDES 1 *postpartum anemia not pre-existing prior to delivery (O9Ø.81)*

✓5th **O99.1 Other diseases of the blood and blood-forming organs and certain disorders involving the immune mechanism complicating pregnancy, childbirth and the puerperium**
Conditions in D65-D89
EXCLUDES 1 *hemorrhage with coagulation defects (O45.-, O46.Ø-, O67.Ø, O72.3)*

✓6th **O99.11 Other diseases of the blood and blood-forming organs and certain disorders involving the immune mechanism complicating pregnancy**

O99.111 Other diseases of the blood and blood-forming organs and certain disorders involving the immune mechanism complicating pregnancy, first trimester CC M ♀

O99.112 Other diseases of the blood and blood-forming organs and certain disorders involving the immune mechanism complicating pregnancy, second trimester CC M ♀

O99.113 Other diseases of the blood and blood-forming organs and certain disorders involving the immune mechanism complicating pregnancy, third trimester CC M ♀

O99.119 Other diseases of the blood and blood-forming organs and certain disorders involving the immune mechanism complicating pregnancy, unspecified trimester CC M ♀

O99.12 Other diseases of the blood and blood-forming organs and certain disorders involving the immune mechanism complicating childbirth CC M ♀

O99.13 Other diseases of the blood and blood-forming organs and certain disorders involving the immune mechanism complicating the puerperium CC M ♀

O99.2 Endocrine, nutritional and metabolic diseases complicating pregnancy, childbirth and the puerperium
Conditions in E00-E89
EXCLUDES 2 *diabetes mellitus (O24.-)*
malnutrition (O25.-)
postpartum thyroiditis (O90.5)

O99.21 Obesity complicating pregnancy, childbirth, and the puerperium
Use additional code to identify the type of obesity (E66.-)
AHA: 2021,2Q,10; 2018,4Q,80
TIP: Do not assign a BMI code (Z68.-) for obese or overweight patients who are pregnant.

O99.210 Obesity complicating pregnancy, unspecified trimester M ♀
O99.211 Obesity complicating pregnancy, first trimester M ♀
O99.212 Obesity complicating pregnancy, second trimester M ♀
O99.213 Obesity complicating pregnancy, third trimester M ♀
O99.214 Obesity complicating childbirth M ♀
O99.215 Obesity complicating the puerperium M ♀

O99.28 Other endocrine, nutritional and metabolic diseases complicating pregnancy, childbirth and the puerperium
AHA: 2021,1Q,8

O99.280 Endocrine, nutritional and metabolic diseases complicating pregnancy, unspecified trimester M ♀
O99.281 Endocrine, nutritional and metabolic diseases complicating pregnancy, first trimester M ♀
O99.282 Endocrine, nutritional and metabolic diseases complicating pregnancy, second trimester M ♀
O99.283 Endocrine, nutritional and metabolic diseases complicating pregnancy, third trimester M ♀
O99.284 Endocrine, nutritional and metabolic diseases complicating childbirth M ♀
O99.285 Endocrine, nutritional and metabolic diseases complicating the puerperium M ♀

O99.3 Mental disorders and diseases of the nervous system complicating pregnancy, childbirth and the puerperium

O99.31 Alcohol use complicating pregnancy, childbirth, and the puerperium
Use additional code(s) from F10 to identify manifestations of the alcohol use

O99.310 Alcohol use complicating pregnancy, unspecified trimester M ♀
O99.311 Alcohol use complicating pregnancy, first trimester M ♀
O99.312 Alcohol use complicating pregnancy, second trimester M ♀
O99.313 Alcohol use complicating pregnancy, third trimester M ♀
O99.314 Alcohol use complicating childbirth M ♀
O99.315 Alcohol use complicating the puerperium M ♀

O99.32 Drug use complicating pregnancy, childbirth, and the puerperium
Use additional code(s) from F11-F16 and F18-F19 to identify manifestations of the drug use
AHA: 2018,4Q,69-70; 2018,2Q,10
TIP: When drug use is documented during pregnancy, assign first a code from this subcategory followed by an additional code from F11-F16 and F18-F19 identifying the specific drug use even if not documented as associated with a physical, mental, or behavioral disorder. According to chapter 15 guidelines, it is the provider's responsibility to state that the condition being treated is *not* affecting the pregnancy.

O99.320 Drug use complicating pregnancy, unspecified trimester M ♀
O99.321 Drug use complicating pregnancy, first trimester CC M ♀
O99.322 Drug use complicating pregnancy, second trimester CC M ♀
O99.323 Drug use complicating pregnancy, third trimester CC M ♀
O99.324 Drug use complicating childbirth CC M ♀
O99.325 Drug use complicating the puerperium CC M ♀

O99.33 Tobacco use disorder complicating pregnancy, childbirth, and the puerperium
Smoking complicating pregnancy, childbirth, and the puerperium
Use additional code from category F17 to identify type of tobacco nicotine dependence

O99.330 Smoking (tobacco) complicating pregnancy, unspecified trimester M ♀
O99.331 Smoking (tobacco) complicating pregnancy, first trimester M ♀
O99.332 Smoking (tobacco) complicating pregnancy, second trimester M ♀
O99.333 Smoking (tobacco) complicating pregnancy, third trimester M ♀
O99.334 Smoking (tobacco) complicating childbirth M ♀
O99.335 Smoking (tobacco) complicating the puerperium M ♀

O99.34 Other mental disorders complicating pregnancy, childbirth, and the puerperium
Conditions in F01-F09, F20-F52 and F54-F99
EXCLUDES 2 *postpartum mood disturbance (O90.6)*
postnatal psychosis (F53.1)
puerperal psychosis (F53.1)

O99.340 Other mental disorders complicating pregnancy, unspecified trimester M ♀
O99.341 Other mental disorders complicating pregnancy, first trimester M ♀
O99.342 Other mental disorders complicating pregnancy, second trimester M ♀
O99.343 Other mental disorders complicating pregnancy, third trimester M ♀
O99.344 Other mental disorders complicating childbirth M ♀
O99.345 Other mental disorders complicating the puerperium M ♀
AHA: 2018,4Q,8

O99.35 Diseases of the nervous system complicating pregnancy, childbirth, and the puerperium
Conditions in G00-G99
EXCLUDES 2 *pregnancy related peripheral neuritis (O26.8-)*

O99.350 Diseases of the nervous system complicating pregnancy, unspecified trimester M ♀
O99.351 Diseases of the nervous system complicating pregnancy, first trimester M ♀
O99.352 Diseases of the nervous system complicating pregnancy, second trimester M ♀
O99.353 Diseases of the nervous system complicating pregnancy, third trimester M ♀
O99.354 Diseases of the nervous system complicating childbirth CC M ♀
O99.355 Diseases of the nervous system complicating the puerperium CC M ♀

O99.4 Diseases of the circulatory system complicating pregnancy, childbirth and the puerperium
Conditions in I00-I99
EXCLUDES 1 *peripartum cardiomyopathy (O90.3)*
EXCLUDES 2 *hypertensive disorders (O10-O16)*
obstetric embolism (O88.-)
venous complications and cerebrovenous sinus thrombosis in labor, childbirth and the puerperium (O87.-)
venous complications and cerebrovenous sinus thrombosis in pregnancy (O22.-)
AHA: 2016,2Q,8

O99.41 Diseases of the circulatory system complicating pregnancy
O99.411 Diseases of the circulatory system complicating pregnancy, first trimester CC M ♀
O99.412 Diseases of the circulatory system complicating pregnancy, second trimester CC M ♀
O99.413 Diseases of the circulatory system complicating pregnancy, third trimester CC M ♀
O99.419 Diseases of the circulatory system complicating pregnancy, unspecified trimester M ♀
O99.42 Diseases of the circulatory system complicating childbirth MCC M ♀
O99.43 Diseases of the circulatory system complicating the puerperium CC M ♀

O99.5 Diseases of the respiratory system complicating pregnancy, childbirth and the puerperium
Conditions in J00-J99

O99.51 Diseases of the respiratory system complicating pregnancy
O99.511 Diseases of the respiratory system complicating pregnancy, first trimester M ♀
O99.512 Diseases of the respiratory system complicating pregnancy, second trimester M ♀
O99.513 Diseases of the respiratory system complicating pregnancy, third trimester M ♀
O99.519 Diseases of the respiratory system complicating pregnancy, unspecified trimester M ♀
O99.52 Diseases of the respiratory system complicating childbirth M ♀
O99.53 Diseases of the respiratory system complicating the puerperium M ♀

O99.6 Diseases of the digestive system complicating pregnancy, childbirth and the puerperium
Conditions in K00-K93
EXCLUDES 2 *hemorrhoids in pregnancy (O22.4-)*
liver and biliary tract disorders in pregnancy, childbirth and the puerperium (O26.6-)

O99.61 Diseases of the digestive system complicating pregnancy
AHA: 2016,1Q,4
O99.611 Diseases of the digestive system complicating pregnancy, first trimester M ♀
O99.612 Diseases of the digestive system complicating pregnancy, second trimester M ♀
O99.613 Diseases of the digestive system complicating pregnancy, third trimester M ♀
O99.619 Diseases of the digestive system complicating pregnancy, unspecified trimester M ♀
O99.62 Diseases of the digestive system complicating childbirth M ♀
O99.63 Diseases of the digestive system complicating the puerperium M ♀

O99.7 Diseases of the skin and subcutaneous tissue complicating pregnancy, childbirth and the puerperium
Conditions in L00-L99
EXCLUDES 2 *herpes gestationis (O26.4)*
pruritic urticarial papules and plaques of pregnancy (PUPPP) (O26.86)

O99.71 Diseases of the skin and subcutaneous tissue complicating pregnancy
O99.711 Diseases of the skin and subcutaneous tissue complicating pregnancy, first trimester M ♀
O99.712 Diseases of the skin and subcutaneous tissue complicating pregnancy, second trimester M ♀
O99.713 Diseases of the skin and subcutaneous tissue complicating pregnancy, third trimester M ♀
O99.719 Diseases of the skin and subcutaneous tissue complicating pregnancy, unspecified trimester M ♀
O99.72 Diseases of the skin and subcutaneous tissue complicating childbirth M ♀
O99.73 Diseases of the skin and subcutaneous tissue complicating the puerperium M ♀

O99.8 Other specified diseases and conditions complicating pregnancy, childbirth and the puerperium
Conditions in D00-D48, H00-H95, M00-N99, and Q00-Q99
Use additional code to identify condition
EXCLUDES 2 *genitourinary infections in pregnancy (O23.-)*
infection of genitourinary tract following delivery (O86.1-O86.4)
malignant neoplasm complicating pregnancy, childbirth and the puerperium (O9A.1-)
maternal care for known or suspected abnormality of maternal pelvic organs (O34.-)
postpartum acute kidney failure (O90.4)
traumatic injuries in pregnancy (O9A.2-)

O99.81 Abnormal glucose complicating pregnancy, childbirth and the puerperium
EXCLUDES 1 *gestational diabetes (O24.4-)*
O99.810 Abnormal glucose complicating pregnancy M ♀
O99.814 Abnormal glucose complicating childbirth M ♀
O99.815 Abnormal glucose complicating the puerperium M ♀

O99.82 Streptococcus B carrier state complicating pregnancy, childbirth and the puerperium
EXCLUDES 1 *carrier of streptococcus group B (GBS) in a nonpregnant woman (Z22.330)*
DEF: *Streptococcus* group B colonization: Bacteria normally found in the vagina or lower intestine of many healthy adult women that may infect the fetus during childbirth, causing mental or physical handicaps or death. Women who test positive for *Streptococcus* group B during pregnancy are considered a "colonized" status and are treated with IV antibiotics at the time of delivery and may also be treated with oral antibiotics during the pregnancy.
O99.820 Streptococcus B carrier state complicating pregnancy UPD M ♀
O99.824 Streptococcus B carrier state complicating childbirth M ♀
AHA: 2019,2Q,8
O99.825 Streptococcus B carrier state complicating the puerperium UPD M ♀

O99.83 Other infection carrier state complicating pregnancy, childbirth and the puerperium
Use additional code to identify the carrier state (Z22.-)
O99.830 Other infection carrier state complicating pregnancy CC M ♀
O99.834 Other infection carrier state complicating childbirth CC M ♀
O99.835 Other infection carrier state complicating the puerperium CC M ♀

✓6th **O99.84 Bariatric surgery status complicating pregnancy, childbirth and the puerperium**
Gastric banding status complicating pregnancy, childbirth and the puerperium
Gastric bypass status for obesity complicating pregnancy, childbirth and the puerperium
Obesity surgery status complicating pregnancy, childbirth and the puerperium

O99.840 Bariatric surgery status complicating pregnancy, unspecified trimester M ♀
O99.841 Bariatric surgery status complicating pregnancy, first trimester M ♀
O99.842 Bariatric surgery status complicating pregnancy, second trimester M ♀
O99.843 Bariatric surgery status complicating pregnancy, third trimester M ♀
O99.844 Bariatric surgery status complicating childbirth M ♀
O99.845 Bariatric surgery status complicating the puerperium M ♀

✓6th **O99.89 Other specified diseases and conditions complicating pregnancy, childbirth and the puerperium**
AHA: 2020,4Q,36-37

O99.891 Other specified diseases and conditions complicating pregnancy M ♀
O99.892 Other specified diseases and conditions complicating childbirth M ♀
O99.893 Other specified diseases and conditions complicating puerperium M ♀

✓4th **O9A Maternal malignant neoplasms, traumatic injuries and abuse classifiable elsewhere but complicating pregnancy, childbirth and the puerperium**

✓5th **O9A.1 Malignant neoplasm complicating pregnancy, childbirth and the puerperium**
Conditions in C00-C96
Use additional code to identify neoplasm
EXCLUDES 2 *maternal care for benign tumor of corpus uteri (O34.1-)*
maternal care for benign tumor of cervix (O34.4-)
AHA: 2015,3Q,19

✓6th **O9A.11 Malignant neoplasm complicating pregnancy**
O9A.111 Malignant neoplasm complicating pregnancy, first trimester M ♀
O9A.112 Malignant neoplasm complicating pregnancy, second trimester M ♀
O9A.113 Malignant neoplasm complicating pregnancy, third trimester M ♀
O9A.119 Malignant neoplasm complicating pregnancy, unspecified trimester M ♀
O9A.12 Malignant neoplasm complicating childbirth M ♀
O9A.13 Malignant neoplasm complicating the puerperium M ♀

✓5th **O9A.2 Injury, poisoning and certain other consequences of external causes complicating pregnancy, childbirth and the puerperium**
Conditions in S00-T88, except T74 and T76
Use additional code(s) to identify the injury or poisoning
EXCLUDES 2 *physical, sexual and psychological abuse complicating pregnancy, childbirth and the puerperium (O9A.3-, O9A.4-, O9A.5-)*

✓6th **O9A.21 Injury, poisoning and certain other consequences of external causes complicating pregnancy**
O9A.211 Injury, poisoning and certain other consequences of external causes complicating pregnancy, first trimester M ♀
O9A.212 Injury, poisoning and certain other consequences of external causes complicating pregnancy, second trimester M ♀
O9A.213 Injury, poisoning and certain other consequences of external causes complicating pregnancy, third trimester M ♀
O9A.219 Injury, poisoning and certain other consequences of external causes complicating pregnancy, unspecified trimester M ♀
O9A.22 Injury, poisoning and certain other consequences of external causes complicating childbirth M ♀
O9A.23 Injury, poisoning and certain other consequences of external causes complicating the puerperium M ♀

✓5th **O9A.3 Physical abuse complicating pregnancy, childbirth and the puerperium**
Conditions in T74.11 or T76.11
Use additional code (if applicable):
to identify any associated current injury due to physical abuse
to identify the perpetrator of abuse (Y07.-)
EXCLUDES 2 *sexual abuse complicating pregnancy, childbirth and the puerperium (O9A.4)*

✓6th **O9A.31 Physical abuse complicating pregnancy**
O9A.311 Physical abuse complicating pregnancy, first trimester M ♀
O9A.312 Physical abuse complicating pregnancy, second trimester M ♀
O9A.313 Physical abuse complicating pregnancy, third trimester M ♀
O9A.319 Physical abuse complicating pregnancy, unspecified trimester M ♀
O9A.32 Physical abuse complicating childbirth M ♀
O9A.33 Physical abuse complicating the puerperium M ♀

✓5th **O9A.4 Sexual abuse complicating pregnancy, childbirth and the puerperium**
Conditions in T74.21 or T76.21
Use additional code (if applicable):
to identify any associated current injury due to sexual abuse
to identify the perpetrator of abuse (Y07.-)

✓6th **O9A.41 Sexual abuse complicating pregnancy**
O9A.411 Sexual abuse complicating pregnancy, first trimester M ♀
O9A.412 Sexual abuse complicating pregnancy, second trimester M ♀
O9A.413 Sexual abuse complicating pregnancy, third trimester M ♀
O9A.419 Sexual abuse complicating pregnancy, unspecified trimester M ♀
O9A.42 Sexual abuse complicating childbirth M ♀
O9A.43 Sexual abuse complicating the puerperium M ♀

✓5th **O9A.5 Psychological abuse complicating pregnancy, childbirth and the puerperium**
Conditions in T74.31 or T76.31
Use additional code to identify the perpetrator of abuse (Y07.-)

✓6th **O9A.51 Psychological abuse complicating pregnancy**
O9A.511 Psychological abuse complicating pregnancy, first trimester M ♀
O9A.512 Psychological abuse complicating pregnancy, second trimester M ♀
O9A.513 Psychological abuse complicating pregnancy, third trimester M ♀
O9A.519 Psychological abuse complicating pregnancy, unspecified trimester M ♀
O9A.52 Psychological abuse complicating childbirth M ♀
O9A.53 Psychological abuse complicating the puerperium M ♀

Chapter 16. Certain Conditions Originating in the Perinatal Period (PØØ–P96)

Chapter-specific Guidelines with Coding Examples

The chapter-specific guidelines from the ICD-10-CM Official Guidelines for Coding and Reporting have been provided below. Along with these guidelines are coding examples, contained in the shaded boxes, that have been developed to help illustrate the coding and/or sequencing guidance found in these guidelines.

For coding and reporting purposes the perinatal period is defined as before birth through the 28th day following birth. The following guidelines are provided for reporting purposes

a. General perinatal rules

1) Use of Chapter 16 codes

Codes in this chapter are never for use on the maternal record. Codes from Chapter 15, the obstetric chapter, are never permitted on the newborn record. Chapter 16 codes may be used throughout the life of the patient if the condition is still present.

2) Principal diagnosis for birth record

When coding the birth episode in a newborn record, assign a code from category Z38, Liveborn infants according to place of birth and type of delivery, as the principal diagnosis. A code from category Z38 is assigned only once, to a newborn at the time of birth. If a newborn is transferred to another institution, a code from category Z38 should not be used at the receiving hospital.

A code from category Z38 is used only on the newborn record, not on the mother's record.

> Newborn delivered via vaginal delivery in Rural Hospital A, experienced meconium aspiration resulting in pneumonia. Rural Hospital A is not equipped to handle the extensive respiratory therapy this baby needs and transfers the patient to Metropolis Hospital B, where the pneumonia resolves and the newborn is eventually discharged.
>
> *Rural Hospital A*
>
> **Z38.ØØ Single liveborn infant, delivered vaginally**
>
> **P24.Ø1 Meconium aspiration with respiratory symptoms**
>
> *Metropolis Hospital B*
>
> **P24.Ø1 Meconium aspiration with respiratory symptoms**
>
> *Explanation:* A code from category Z38 is a one-time use only code. The hospital that actually delivered the newborn, in this case Rural Hospital A, can append a code from category Z38 but for the delivery admission only. Once the patient is transferred or discharged, the Z38 category no longer applies for that patient.
>
> The reason for the transfer to Metropolis Hospital B was for the respiratory symptoms (pneumonia) the newborn was exhibiting secondary to aspirating meconium.

3) Use of codes from other chapters with codes from Chapter 16

Codes from other chapters may be used with codes from chapter 16 if the codes from the other chapters provide more specific detail. Codes for signs and symptoms may be assigned when a definitive diagnosis has not been established. If the reason for the encounter is a perinatal condition, the code from chapter 16 should be sequenced first.

4) Use of Chapter 16 codes after the perinatal period

Should a condition originate in the perinatal period, and continue throughout the life of the patient, the perinatal code should continue to be used regardless of the patient's age.

> A 7-year-old patient with history of birth injury that resulted in Erb's palsy is seen for subscapularis release
>
> **P14.Ø Erb's paralysis due to birth injury**
>
> *Explanation:* Although in this instance Erb's palsy is specifically related to a birth injury, it has not resolved and continues to be a health concern. A perinatal code is appropriate even though this patient is beyond the perinatal period.

5) Birth process or community acquired conditions

If a newborn has a condition that may be either due to the birth process or community acquired and the documentation does not indicate which it is, the default is due to the birth process and the code from Chapter 16 should be used. If the condition is community-acquired, a code from Chapter 16 should not be assigned.

For COVID-19 infection in a newborn, see guideline I.C.16.h.

6) Code all clinically significant conditions

All clinically significant conditions noted on routine newborn examination should be coded. A condition is clinically significant if it requires:

clinical evaluation; or

therapeutic treatment; or

diagnostic procedures; or

extended length of hospital stay; or

increased nursing care and/or monitoring; or

has implications for future health care needs

Note: The perinatal guidelines listed above are the same as the general coding guidelines for "additional diagnoses", except for the final point regarding implications for future health care needs. Codes should be assigned for conditions that have been specified by the provider as having implications for future health care needs.

b. Observation and evaluation of newborns for suspected conditions not found

1) Use of ZØ5 codes

Assign a code from category ZØ5, Observation and evaluation of newborn for suspected **diseases and** conditions ruled out, to identify those instances when a healthy newborn is evaluated for a suspected condition/**disease** that is determined after study not to be present. Do not use a code from category ZØ5 when the patient **is documented to have** signs or symptoms of a suspected problem; in such cases code the sign or symptom.

2) ZØ5 on other than the birth record

A code from category ZØ5 may also be assigned as a principal or first-listed code for readmissions or encounters when the code from category Z38 code no longer applies. Codes from category ZØ5 are for use only for healthy newborns and infants for which no condition after study is found to be present.

3) ZØ5 on a birth record

A code from category ZØ5 is to be used as a secondary code after the code from category Z38, Liveborn infants according to place of birth and type of delivery.

> Newborn delivered via vaginal delivery; previous ultrasounds showed what appeared to be an abnormality of the right kidney. Kidney function tests were performed and ultrasounds taken and any genitourinary conditions ruled out.
>
> **Z38.ØØ Single liveborn infant, delivered vaginally**
>
> **ZØ5.6 Observation and evaluation of newborn for suspected genitourinary condition ruled out**
>
> Explanation: The newborn had no signs or symptoms of kidney or other genitourinary condition but was evaluated after delivery due to the abnormal prenatal ultrasound findings. A Z code describing the type and place of birth should be coded first, followed by a Z05 category code for the work performed to rule out a suspected genitourinary condition.

c. Coding additional perinatal diagnoses

1) Assigning codes for conditions that require treatment

Assign codes for conditions that require treatment or further investigation, prolong the length of stay, or require resource utilization.

2) **Codes for conditions specified as having implications for future health care needs**

Assign codes for conditions that have been specified by the provider as having implications for future health care needs.

Note: This guideline should not be used for adult patients.

An abnormal noise was heard in the left hip of a post-term newborn during a physical examination. The pediatrician would like to follow the patient after discharge as a hip click can be an early sign of hip dysplasia. The newborn was delivered via cesarean at 41 weeks.

Z38.01 Single liveborn infant, delivered by cesarean

P08.21 Post-term newborn

R29.4 Clicking hip

Explanation: The abnormal hip noise or click is appended as a secondary diagnosis not only because it is an abnormal finding upon examination, but also due to its potential to be part of a bigger health issue. The hip dysplasia has not yet been diagnosed and does not warrant a code at this time.

d. Prematurity and fetal growth retardation

Providers utilize different criteria in determining prematurity. A code for prematurity should not be assigned unless it is documented. Assignment of codes in categories P05, Disorders of newborn related to slow fetal growth and fetal malnutrition, and P07, Disorders of newborn related to short gestation and low birth weight, not elsewhere classified, should be based on the recorded birth weight and estimated gestational age.

When both birth weight and gestational age are available, two codes from category P07 should be assigned, with the code for birth weight sequenced before the code for gestational age.

e. Low birth weight and immaturity status

Codes from category P07, Disorders of newborn related to short gestation and low birth weight, not elsewhere classified, are for use for a child or adult who was premature or had a low birth weight as a newborn and this is affecting the patient's current health status.

See Section I.C.21. Factors influencing health status and contact with health services, Status.

A 35-year-old patient, who weighed 659 grams at birth, is seen for heart disease documented as being a consequence of the low birth weight

I51.9 Heart disease, unspecified

P07.02 Extremely low birth weight newborn, 500–749 grams

Explanation: A code from subcategories P07.0- and P07.1- is appropriate, regardless of the age of the patient, as long as the documentation provides a clear link between the patient's current illness and the low birth weight.

f. Bacterial sepsis of newborn

Category P36, Bacterial sepsis of newborn, includes congenital sepsis. If a perinate is documented as having sepsis without documentation of congenital or community acquired, the default is congenital and a code from category P36 should be assigned. If the P36 code includes the causal organism, an additional code from category B95, Streptococcus, Staphylococcus, and Enterococcus as the cause of diseases classified elsewhere, or B96, Other bacterial agents as the cause of diseases classified elsewhere, should not be assigned. If the P36 code does not include the causal organism, assign an additional code from category B96. If applicable, use additional codes to identify severe sepsis (R65.2-) and any associated acute organ dysfunction.

A full-term infant develops severe sepsis 24 hours after discharge from the hospital and is readmitted; cultures identified *E. coli* as the infective agent

P36.4 Sepsis of newborn due to Escherichia coli

R65.20 Severe sepsis without septic shock

Explanation: Even though this newborn was discharged and could have acquired *E. coli* from his/her external environment, due to the lack of documentation specifying specifically how this pathogen was acquired, the default is to code the *E. coli* sepsis as congenital. A code from chapter 1, "Certain Infectious and Parasitic Diseases," is not required because the perinatal sepsis code identifies both the sepsis and the bacteria causing the sepsis.

g. Stillbirth

Code P95, Stillbirth, is only for use in institutions that maintain separate records for stillbirths. No other code should be used with P95. Code P95 should not be used on the mother's record.

h. COVID-19 infection in newborn

For a newborn that tests positive for COVID-19, assign code U07.1, COVID-19, and the appropriate codes for associated manifestation(s) in neonates/newborns in the absence of documentation indicating a specific type of transmission. For a newborn that tests positive for COVID-19 and the provider documents the condition was contracted in utero or during the birth process, assign codes P35.8, Other congenital viral diseases, and U07.1, COVID-19. When coding the birth episode in a newborn record, the appropriate code from category Z38, Liveborn infants according to place of birth and type of delivery, should be assigned as the principal diagnosis.

Chapter 16. Certain Conditions Originating in the Perinatal Period (P00-P96)

NOTE Codes from this chapter are for use on newborn records only, never on maternal records

INCLUDES conditions that have their origin in the fetal or perinatal period (before birth through the first 28 days after birth) even if morbidity occurs later

EXCLUDES 2 *congenital malformations, deformations and chromosomal abnormalities (Q00-Q99)*
endocrine, nutritional and metabolic diseases (E00-E88)
injury, poisoning and certain other consequences of external causes (S00-T88)
neoplasms (C00-D49)
tetanus neonatorum (A33)

This chapter contains the following blocks:

- P00-P04 Newborn affected by maternal factors and by complications of pregnancy, labor, and delivery
- P05-P08 Disorders of newborn related to length of gestation and fetal growth
- P09 Abnormal findings on neonatal screening
- P10-P15 Birth trauma
- P19-P29 Respiratory and cardiovascular disorders specific to the perinatal period
- P35-P39 Infections specific to the perinatal period
- P50-P61 Hemorrhagic and hematological disorders of newborn
- P70-P74 Transitory endocrine and metabolic disorders specific to newborn
- P76-P78 Digestive system disorders of newborn
- P80-P83 Conditions involving the integument and temperature regulation of newborn
- P84 Other problems with newborn
- P90-P96 Other disorders originating in the perinatal period

Newborn affected by maternal factors and by complications of pregnancy, labor, and delivery (P00-P04)

NOTE These codes are for use when the listed maternal conditions are specified as the cause of confirmed morbidity or potential morbidity which have their origin in the perinatal period (before birth through the first 28 days after birth).

AHA: 2016,4Q,54-55

✓4th **P00 Newborn affected by maternal conditions that may be unrelated to present pregnancy**

Code first any current condition in newborn

EXCLUDES 2 *encounter for observation of newborn for suspected diseases and conditions ruled out (Z05.-)*
newborn affected by maternal complications of pregnancy (P01.-)
newborn affected by maternal endocrine and metabolic disorders (P70-P74)
newborn affected by noxious substances transmitted via placenta or breast milk (P04.-)

P00.0 Newborn affected by maternal hypertensive disorders
Newborn affected by maternal conditions classifiable to O10-O11, O13-O16

P00.1 Newborn affected by maternal renal and urinary tract diseases
Newborn affected by maternal conditions classifiable to N00-N39

P00.2 Newborn affected by maternal infectious and parasitic diseases
Newborn affected by maternal infectious disease classifiable to A00-B99, J09 and J10

EXCLUDES 1 *maternal genital tract or other localized infections (P00.8)*

EXCLUDES 2 *infections specific to the perinatal period (P35-P39)*
newborn affected by (positive) maternal group B streptococcus (GBS) colonization (P00.82)

AHA: 2019,2Q,10; 2015,3Q,20

P00.3 Newborn affected by other maternal circulatory and respiratory diseases
Newborn affected by maternal conditions classifiable to I00-I99, J00-J99, Q20-Q34 and not included in P00.0, P00.2

P00.4 Newborn affected by maternal nutritional disorders
Newborn affected by maternal disorders classifiable to E40-E64
Maternal malnutrition NOS

P00.5 Newborn affected by maternal injury
Newborn affected by maternal conditions classifiable to O9A.2-

P00.6 Newborn affected by surgical procedure on mother
Newborn affected by amniocentesis

EXCLUDES 1 *Cesarean delivery for present delivery (P03.4)*
damage to placenta from amniocentesis, Cesarean delivery or surgical induction (P02.1)
previous surgery to uterus or pelvic organs (P03.89)

EXCLUDES 2 *newborn affected by complication of (fetal) intrauterine procedure (P96.5)*

P00.7 Newborn affected by other medical procedures on mother, not elsewhere classified
Newborn affected by radiation to mother

EXCLUDES 1 *damage to placenta from amniocentesis, cesarean delivery or surgical induction (P02.1)*
newborn affected by other complications of labor and delivery (P03.-)

✓5th **P00.8 Newborn affected by other maternal conditions**

P00.81 Newborn affected by periodontal disease in mother

P00.82 Newborn affected by (positive) maternal group B streptococcus (GBS) colonization
Contact with positive maternal group B streptococcus
AHA: 2021,4Q,23

P00.89 Newborn affected by other maternal conditions
Newborn affected by conditions classifiable to T80-T88
Newborn affected by maternal genital tract or other localized infections
Newborn affected by maternal systemic lupus erythematosus
Use additional code to identify infectious agent, if known

EXCLUDES 2 *newborn affected by positive maternal group B streptococcus (GBS) colonization (P00.82)*

AHA: 2019,2Q,9

P00.9 Newborn affected by unspecified maternal condition

✓4th **P01 Newborn affected by maternal complications of pregnancy**

Code first any current condition in newborn

EXCLUDES 2 *encounter for observation of newborn for suspected diseases and conditions ruled out (Z05.-)*

P01.0 Newborn affected by incompetent cervix

P01.1 Newborn affected by premature rupture of membranes

P01.2 Newborn affected by oligohydramnios

EXCLUDES 1 *oligohydramnios due to premature rupture of membranes (P01.1)*

DEF: Low amniotic fluid level, resulting in underdeveloped organs in the fetus.

P01.3 Newborn affected by polyhydramnios
Newborn affected by hydramnios
DEF: Excess amniotic fluid surrounding the fetus, typically defined as a total fluid volume of greater than 24 cm.

P01.4 Newborn affected by ectopic pregnancy
Newborn affected by abdominal pregnancy

P01.5 Newborn affected by multiple pregnancy
Newborn affected by triplet (pregnancy)
Newborn affected by twin (pregnancy)

P01.6 Newborn affected by maternal death

P01.7 Newborn affected by malpresentation before labor
Newborn affected by breech presentation before labor
Newborn affected by external version before labor
Newborn affected by face presentation before labor
Newborn affected by transverse lie before labor
Newborn affected by unstable lie before labor

P01.8 Newborn affected by other maternal complications of pregnancy

P01.9 Newborn affected by maternal complication of pregnancy, unspecified

✓4th **P02 Newborn affected by complications of placenta, cord and membranes**

Code first any current condition in newborn

EXCLUDES 2 *encounter for observation of newborn for suspected diseases and conditions ruled out (Z05.-)*

P02.0 Newborn affected by placenta previa
DEF: Placenta developed in the lower segment of the uterus that can cause hemorrhaging leading to preterm delivery.

P02.1 Newborn affected by other forms of placental separation and hemorrhage
Newborn affected by abruptio placenta
Newborn affected by accidental hemorrhage
Newborn affected by antepartum hemorrhage
Newborn affected by damage to placenta from amniocentesis, cesarean delivery or surgical induction
Newborn affected by maternal blood loss
Newborn affected by premature separation of placenta

P02.2 Newborn affected by other and unspecified morphological and functional abnormalities of placenta

P02.20 Newborn affected by unspecified morphological and functional abnormalities of placenta

P02.29 Newborn affected by other morphological and functional abnormalities of placenta
Newborn affected by placental dysfunction
Newborn affected by placental infarction
Newborn affected by placental insufficiency

P02.3 Newborn affected by placental transfusion syndromes
Newborn affected by placental and cord abnormalities resulting in twin-to-twin or other transplacental transfusion

P02.4 Newborn affected by prolapsed cord

P02.5 Newborn affected by other compression of umbilical cord
Newborn affected by umbilical cord (tightly) around neck
Newborn affected by entanglement of umbilical cord
Newborn affected by knot in umbilical cord
AHA: 2022,1Q,22

P02.6 Newborn affected by other and unspecified conditions of umbilical cord

P02.60 Newborn affected by unspecified conditions of umbilical cord

P02.69 Newborn affected by other conditions of umbilical cord
Newborn affected by short umbilical cord
Newborn affected by vasa previa
EXCLUDES 1 *newborn affected by single umbilical artery (Q27.0)*

P02.7 Newborn affected by chorioamnionitis
AHA: 2018,4Q,23-24
DEF: Inflammation of the fetal membranes due to maternal infection characterized by fetal tachycardia, respiratory distress, apnea, weak cries, and poor sucking.

P02.70 Newborn affected by fetal inflammatory response syndrome HCC
Newborn affected by FIRS

P02.78 Newborn affected by other conditions from chorioamnionitis
Newborn affected by amnionitis
Newborn affected by membranitis
Newborn affected by placentitis

P02.8 Newborn affected by other abnormalities of membranes

P02.9 Newborn affected by abnormality of membranes, unspecified

P03 Newborn affected by other complications of labor and delivery
Code first any current condition in newborn
EXCLUDES 2 *encounter for observation of newborn for suspected diseases and conditions ruled out (Z05.-)*

P03.0 Newborn affected by breech delivery and extraction

P03.1 Newborn affected by other malpresentation, malposition and disproportion during labor and delivery
Newborn affected by contracted pelvis
Newborn affected by conditions classifiable to O64-O66
Newborn affected by persistent occipitoposterior
Newborn affected by transverse lie

P03.2 Newborn affected by forceps delivery

Forceps Assisted Birth

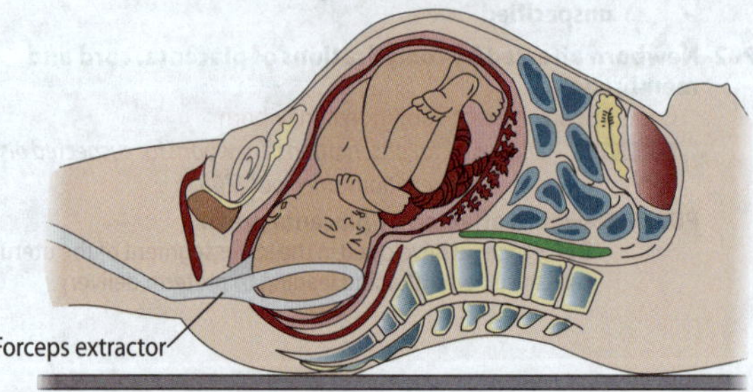

P03.3 Newborn affected by delivery by vacuum extractor [ventouse]

Vacuum Assisted Birth

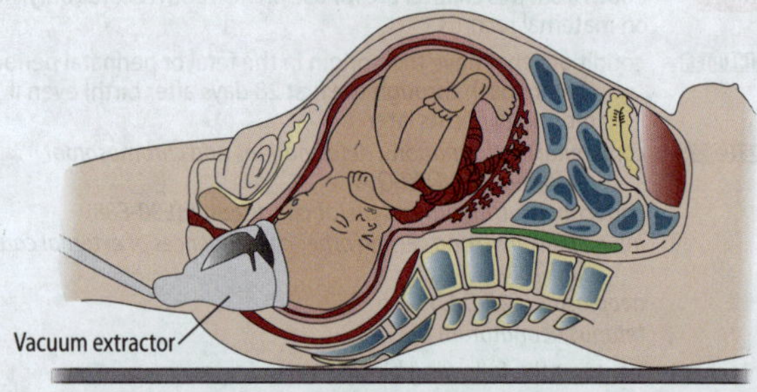

P03.4 Newborn affected by Cesarean delivery

P03.5 Newborn affected by precipitate delivery
Newborn affected by rapid second stage

P03.6 Newborn affected by abnormal uterine contractions
Newborn affected by conditions classifiable to O62.-, except O62.3
Newborn affected by hypertonic labor
Newborn affected by uterine inertia

P03.8 Newborn affected by other specified complications of labor and delivery

P03.81 Newborn affected by abnormality in fetal (intrauterine) heart rate or rhythm
EXCLUDES 1 *neonatal cardiac dysrhythmia (P29.1-)*

P03.810 Newborn affected by abnormality in fetal (intrauterine) heart rate or rhythm before the onset of labor

P03.811 Newborn affected by abnormality in fetal (intrauterine) heart rate or rhythm during labor

P03.819 Newborn affected by abnormality in fetal (intrauterine) heart rate or rhythm, unspecified as to time of onset

P03.82 Meconium passage during delivery
EXCLUDES 1 *meconium aspiration (P24.00, P24.01)*
meconium staining (P96.83)
DEF: Fetal intestinal activity that increases in response to a fetomaternal distressed state during delivery. The anal sphincter relaxes and meconium is passed into the amniotic fluid.

P03.89 Newborn affected by other specified complications of labor and delivery
Newborn affected by abnormality of maternal soft tissues
Newborn affected by conditions classifiable to O60-O75 and by procedures used in labor and delivery not included in P02.- and P03.0-P03.6
Newborn affected by induction of labor

P03.9 Newborn affected by complication of labor and delivery, unspecified

P04 Newborn affected by noxious substances transmitted via placenta or breast milk
INCLUDES nonteratogenic effects of substances transmitted via placenta
Code first any current condition in newborn, if applicable
EXCLUDES 2 *congenital malformations (Q00-Q99)*
encounter for observation of newborn for suspected diseases and conditions ruled out (Z05.-)
neonatal jaundice from excessive hemolysis due to drugs or toxins transmitted from mother (P58.4)
newborn in contact with and (suspected) exposures hazardous to health not transmitted via placenta or breast milk (Z77.-)

P04.0 Newborn affected by maternal anesthesia and analgesia in pregnancy, labor and delivery
Newborn affected by reactions and intoxications from maternal opiates and tranquilizers administered for procedures during pregnancy or labor and delivery
EXCLUDES 2 *newborn affected by other maternal medication (P04.1-)*

P04.1 Newborn affected by other maternal medication
Code first withdrawal symptoms from maternal use of drugs of addiction, if applicable (P96.1)
EXCLUDES 1 *dysmorphism due to warfarin (Q86.2)*
fetal hydantoin syndrome (Q86.1)
EXCLUDES 2 *maternal anesthesia and analgesia in pregnancy, labor and delivery (P04.0)*
maternal use of drugs of addiction (P04.4-)
AHA: 2018,4Q,24-25

P04.11 Newborn affected by maternal antineoplastic chemotherapy
P04.12 Newborn affected by maternal cytotoxic drugs
P04.13 Newborn affected by maternal use of anticonvulsants
P04.14 Newborn affected by maternal use of opiates
P04.15 Newborn affected by maternal use of antidepressants
P04.16 Newborn affected by maternal use of amphetamines
P04.17 Newborn affected by maternal use of sedative-hypnotics
P04.1A Newborn affected by maternal use of anxiolytics
P04.18 Newborn affected by other maternal medication
P04.19 Newborn affected by maternal use of unspecified medication

P04.2 Newborn affected by maternal use of tobacco
Newborn affected by exposure in utero to tobacco smoke
EXCLUDES 2 *newborn exposure to environmental tobacco smoke (P96.81)*

P04.3 Newborn affected by maternal use of alcohol
EXCLUDES 1 *fetal alcohol syndrome (Q86.0)*

P04.4 Newborn affected by maternal use of drugs of addiction
AHA: 2018,4Q,25

P04.40 Newborn affected by maternal use of unspecified drugs of addiction
P04.41 Newborn affected by maternal use of cocaine
P04.42 Newborn affected by maternal use of hallucinogens
EXCLUDES 2 *newborn affected by other maternal medication (P04.1-)*
P04.49 Newborn affected by maternal use of other drugs of addiction
EXCLUDES 2 *newborn affected by maternal anesthesia and analgesia (P04.0)*
withdrawal symptoms from maternal use of drugs of addiction (P96.1)

P04.5 Newborn affected by maternal use of nutritional chemical substances

P04.6 Newborn affected by maternal exposure to environmental chemical substances

P04.8 Newborn affected by other maternal noxious substances
AHA: 2018,4Q,25

P04.81 Newborn affected by maternal use of cannabis
P04.89 Newborn affected by other maternal noxious substances

P04.9 Newborn affected by maternal noxious substance, unspecified

Disorders of newborn related to length of gestation and fetal growth (P05-P08)

P05 Disorders of newborn related to slow fetal growth and fetal malnutrition
AHA: 2016,4Q,55-56

P05.0 Newborn light for gestational age
Newborn light-for-dates
Weight below but length above 10th percentile for gestational age

P05.00 Newborn light for gestational age, unspecified weight
P05.01 Newborn light for gestational age, less than 500 grams
P05.02 Newborn light for gestational age, 500-749 grams
P05.03 Newborn light for gestational age, 750-999 grams
P05.04 Newborn light for gestational age, 1000-1249 grams
P05.05 Newborn light for gestational age, 1250-1499 grams
P05.06 Newborn light for gestational age, 1500-1749 grams
P05.07 Newborn light for gestational age, 1750-1999 grams
P05.08 Newborn light for gestational age, 2000-2499 grams
P05.09 Newborn light for gestational age, 2500 grams and over
Newborn light for gestational age, other

P05.1 Newborn small for gestational age
Newborn small-and-light-for-dates
Newborn small-for-dates
Weight and length below 10th percentile for gestational age

P05.10 Newborn small for gestational age, unspecified weight
P05.11 Newborn small for gestational age, less than 500 grams
P05.12 Newborn small for gestational age, 500-749 grams
P05.13 Newborn small for gestational age, 750-999 grams
P05.14 Newborn small for gestational age, 1000-1249 grams
P05.15 Newborn small for gestational age, 1250-1499 grams
P05.16 Newborn small for gestational age, 1500-1749 grams
P05.17 Newborn small for gestational age, 1750-1999 grams
P05.18 Newborn small for gestational age, 2000-2499 grams
P05.19 Newborn small for gestational age, other
Newborn small for gestational age, 2500 grams and over

P05.2 Newborn affected by fetal (intrauterine) malnutrition not light or small for gestational age
Infant, not light or small for gestational age, showing signs of fetal malnutrition, such as dry, peeling skin and loss of subcutaneous tissue
EXCLUDES 1 *newborn affected by fetal malnutrition with light for gestational age (P05.0-)*
newborn affected by fetal malnutrition with small for gestational age (P05.1-)

P05.9 Newborn affected by slow intrauterine growth, unspecified
Newborn affected by fetal growth retardation NOS

P07 Disorders of newborn related to short gestation and low birth weight, not elsewhere classified
NOTE When both birth weight and gestational age of the newborn are available, both should be coded with birth weight sequenced before gestational age
INCLUDES the listed conditions, without further specification, as the cause of morbidity or additional care, in newborn

P07.0 Extremely low birth weight newborn
Newborn birth weight 999 g. or less
EXCLUDES 1 *low birth weight due to slow fetal growth and fetal malnutrition (P05.-)*

P07.00 Extremely low birth weight newborn, unspecified weight
P07.01 Extremely low birth weight newborn, less than 500 grams
P07.02 Extremely low birth weight newborn, 500-749 grams
P07.03 Extremely low birth weight newborn, 750-999 grams

P07.1 Other low birth weight newborn
Newborn birth weight 1000-2499 g.
EXCLUDES 1 *low birth weight due to slow fetal growth and fetal malnutrition (P05.-)*

P07.10 Other low birth weight newborn, unspecified weight
P07.14 Other low birth weight newborn, 1000-1249 grams
P07.15 Other low birth weight newborn, 1250-1499 grams
P07.16 Other low birth weight newborn, 1500-1749 grams
P07.17 Other low birth weight newborn, 1750-1999 grams
P07.18 Other low birth weight newborn, 2000-2499 grams

P07.2 Extreme immaturity of newborn
Less than 28 completed weeks (less than 196 completed days) of gestation.

P07.20 Extreme immaturity of newborn, unspecified weeks of gestation
Gestational age less than 28 completed weeks NOS

P07.21 Extreme immaturity of newborn, gestational age less than 23 completed weeks
Extreme immaturity of newborn, gestational age less than 23 weeks, 0 days

P07.22 Extreme immaturity of newborn, gestational age 23 completed weeks
Extreme immaturity of newborn, gestational age 23 weeks, 0 days through 23 weeks, 6 days

P07.23 Extreme immaturity of newborn, gestational age 24 completed weeks
Extreme immaturity of newborn, gestational age 24 weeks, 0 days through 24 weeks, 6 days

P07.24 Extreme immaturity of newborn, gestational age 25 completed weeks
Extreme immaturity of newborn, gestational age 25 weeks, 0 days through 25 weeks, 6 days

P07.25 Extreme immaturity of newborn, gestational age 26 completed weeks
Extreme immaturity of newborn, gestational age 26 weeks, 0 days through 26 weeks, 6 days

P07.26 Extreme immaturity of newborn, gestational age 27 completed weeks
Extreme immaturity of newborn, gestational age 27 weeks, 0 days through 27 weeks, 6 days

5th **P07.3 Preterm [premature] newborn [other]**
28 completed weeks or more but less than 37 completed weeks (196 completed days but less than 259 completed days) of gestation
Prematurity NOS
AHA: 2017,3Q,26

P07.30 Preterm newborn, unspecified weeks of gestation

P07.31 Preterm newborn, gestational age 28 completed weeks
Preterm newborn, gestational age 28 weeks, 0 days through 28 weeks, 6 days

P07.32 Preterm newborn, gestational age 29 completed weeks
Preterm newborn, gestational age 29 weeks, 0 days through 29 weeks, 6 days

P07.33 Preterm newborn, gestational age 30 completed weeks
Preterm newborn, gestational age 30 weeks, 0 days through 30 weeks, 6 days

P07.34 Preterm newborn, gestational age 31 completed weeks
Preterm newborn, gestational age 31 weeks, 0 days through 31 weeks, 6 days

P07.35 Preterm newborn, gestational age 32 completed weeks
Preterm newborn, gestational age 32 weeks, 0 days through 32 weeks, 6 days

P07.36 Preterm newborn, gestational age 33 completed weeks
Preterm newborn, gestational age 33 weeks, 0 days through 33 weeks, 6 days

P07.37 Preterm newborn, gestational age 34 completed weeks
Preterm newborn, gestational age 34 weeks, 0 days through 34 weeks, 6 days

P07.38 Preterm newborn, gestational age 35 completed weeks
Preterm newborn, gestational age 35 weeks, 0 days through 35 weeks, 6 days

P07.39 Preterm newborn, gestational age 36 completed weeks
Preterm newborn, gestational age 36 weeks, 0 days through 36 weeks, 6 days

4th **P08 Disorders of newborn related to long gestation and high birth weight**
NOTE When both birth weight and gestational age of the newborn are available, priority of assignment should be given to birth weight
INCLUDES the listed conditions, without further specification, as causes of morbidity or additional care, in newborn

P08.0 Exceptionally large newborn baby
Usually implies a birth weight of 4500 g. or more
EXCLUDES 1 *syndrome of infant of diabetic mother (P70.1)*
syndrome of infant of mother with gestational diabetes (P70.0)

P08.1 Other heavy for gestational age newborn
Other newborn heavy- or large-for-dates regardless of period of gestation
Usually implies a birth weight of 4000 g. to 4499 g.
EXCLUDES 1 *newborn with a birth weight of 4500 or more (P08.0)*
syndrome of infant of diabetic mother (P70.1)
syndrome of infant of mother with gestational diabetes (P70.0)

5th **P08.2 Late newborn, not heavy for gestational age**
AHA: 2014,1Q,14

P08.21 Post-term newborn
Newborn with gestation period over 40 completed weeks to 42 completed weeks

P08.22 Prolonged gestation of newborn
Newborn with gestation period over 42 completed weeks (294 days or more), not heavy- or large-for-dates.
Postmaturity NOS

Abnormal findings on neonatal screening (P09)

4th **P09 Abnormal findings on neonatal screening**
INCLUDES abnormal findings on state mandated newborn screens
failed newborn screening
EXCLUDES 2 *nonspecific serologic evidence of human immunodeficiency virus [HIV] (R75)*
AHA: 2021,4Q,24

P09.1 Abnormal findings on neonatal screening for inborn errors of metabolism

P09.2 Abnormal findings on neonatal screening for congenital endocrine disease
Abnormal findings on neonatal screening for congenital adrenal hyperplasia
Abnormal findings on neonatal screening for hypothyroidism screen

P09.3 Abnormal findings on neonatal screening for congenital hematologic disorders
Abnormal findings for hemoglobinothies screen
Abnormal findings on red cell membrane defects screen
Abnormal findings on sickle cell screen

P09.4 Abnormal findings on neonatal screening for cystic fibrosis

P09.5 Abnormal findings on neonatal screening for critical congenital heart disease
Neonatal congenital heart disease screening failure

P09.6 Abnormal findings on neonatal screening for neonatal hearing loss
EXCLUDES 2 *encounter for hearing examination following failed hearing screening (Z01.110)*

P09.8 Other abnormal findings on neonatal screening

P09.9 Abnormal findings on neonatal screening, unspecified

Birth trauma (P10-P15)

4th **P10 Intracranial laceration and hemorrhage due to birth injury**
EXCLUDES 1 *intracranial hemorrhage of newborn NOS (P52.9)*
intracranial hemorrhage of newborn due to anoxia or hypoxia (P52.-)
nontraumatic intracranial hemorrhage of newborn (P52.-)

P10.0 Subdural hemorrhage due to birth injury MCC
Subdural hematoma (localized) due to birth injury
EXCLUDES 1 *subdural hemorrhage accompanying tentorial tear (P10.4)*

P10.1 Cerebral hemorrhage due to birth injury MCC

P10.2 Intraventricular hemorrhage due to birth injury CC

P10.3 Subarachnoid hemorrhage due to birth injury MCC

P10.4 Tentorial tear due to birth injury MCC

P10.8 Other intracranial lacerations and hemorrhages due to birth injury MCC

P10.9 Unspecified intracranial laceration and hemorrhage due to birth injury MCC

P11 Other birth injuries to central nervous system

P11.0 Cerebral edema due to birth injury MCC

P11.1 Other specified brain damage due to birth injury

P11.2 Unspecified brain damage due to birth injury MCC

P11.3 Birth injury to facial nerve
Facial palsy due to birth injury

P11.4 Birth injury to other cranial nerves

P11.5 Birth injury to spine and spinal cord
Fracture of spine due to birth injury

P11.9 Birth injury to central nervous system, unspecified MCC

P12 Birth injury to scalp

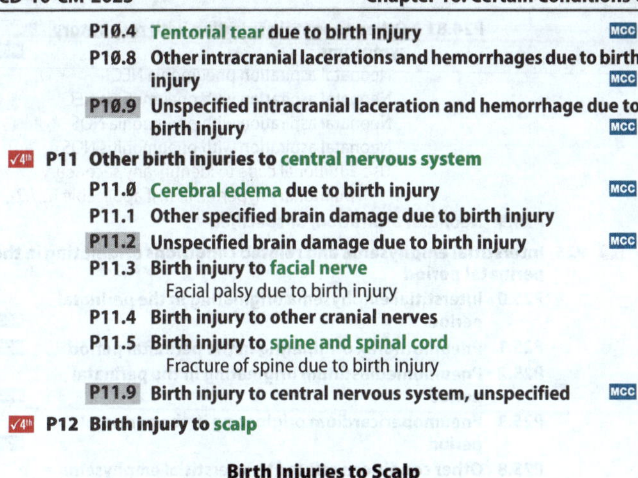

P12.0 Cephalhematoma due to birth injury
DEF: Condition that occurs in a neonate when blood vessels between the skull and periosteum rupture and blood collects in the subperiosteal space (below the periosteum). It is typically caused by prolonged labor or trauma due to instrument-assisted delivery (e.g., forceps, vacuum extraction), although in rare circumstances, it may indicate a linear skull fracture with intracranial hemorrhage.

P12.1 Chignon (from vacuum extraction) due to birth injury
DEF: Artificial swelling of the scalp that occurs when a collection of interstitial fluid and blood forms in the area of the scalp where the suction cup was applied during a vacuum-assisted delivery.

P12.2 Epicranial subaponeurotic hemorrhage due to birth injury CC
Subgaleal hemorrhage

P12.3 Bruising of scalp due to birth injury

P12.4 Injury of scalp of newborn due to monitoring equipment
Sampling incision of scalp of newborn
Scalp clip (electrode) injury of newborn

P12.8 Other birth injuries to scalp

P12.81 Caput succedaneum
DEF: Swelling of the scalp as a result of pressure being exerted on the head from the vaginal walls, uterus, or instrumentation used in assisting a delivery (e.g., vacuum).

P12.89 Other birth injuries to scalp

P12.9 Birth injury to scalp, unspecified

P13 Birth injury to skeleton
EXCLUDES 2 *birth injury to spine (P11.5)*

P13.0 Fracture of skull due to birth injury

P13.1 Other birth injuries to skull
EXCLUDES 1 *cephalhematoma (P12.0)*

P13.2 Birth injury to femur

P13.3 Birth injury to other long bones

P13.4 Fracture of clavicle due to birth injury

P13.8 Birth injuries to other parts of skeleton

P13.9 Birth injury to skeleton, unspecified

P14 Birth injury to peripheral nervous system

P14.0 Erb's paralysis due to birth injury
DEF: Erb's paralysis: Most common type of brachial plexus (peripheral nerve) injury in a neonate that involves nerve damage at the level of C5-C6. ***Synonym(s):*** *Erb's palsy*

P14.1 Klumpke's paralysis due to birth injury

P14.2 Phrenic nerve paralysis due to birth injury

P14.3 Other brachial plexus birth injuries

P14.8 Birth injuries to other parts of peripheral nervous system

P14.9 Birth injury to peripheral nervous system, unspecified

P15 Other birth injuries

P15.0 Birth injury to liver
Rupture of liver due to birth injury

P15.1 Birth injury to spleen
Rupture of spleen due to birth injury

P15.2 Sternomastoid injury due to birth injury

P15.3 Birth injury to eye
Subconjunctival hemorrhage due to birth injury
Traumatic glaucoma due to birth injury

P15.4 Birth injury to face
Facial congestion due to birth injury

P15.5 Birth injury to external genitalia

P15.6 Subcutaneous fat necrosis due to birth injury

P15.8 Other specified birth injuries

P15.9 Birth injury, unspecified

Respiratory and cardiovascular disorders specific to the perinatal period (P19-P29)

P19 Metabolic acidemia in newborn
INCLUDES metabolic acidemia in newborn

P19.0 Metabolic acidemia in newborn first noted before onset of labor

P19.1 Metabolic acidemia in newborn first noted during labor

P19.2 Metabolic acidemia noted at birth

P19.9 Metabolic acidemia, unspecified

P22 Respiratory distress of newborn
AHA: 2019,2Q,29

P22.0 Respiratory distress syndrome of newborn MCC
Cardiorespiratory distress syndrome of newborn
Hyaline membrane disease
Idiopathic respiratory distress syndrome [IRDS or RDS] of newborn
Pulmonary hypoperfusion syndrome
Respiratory distress syndrome, type I
EXCLUDES 2 *respiratory arrest of newborn (P28.81)*
respiratory failure of newborn NOS (P28.5)
AHA: 2019,2Q,29
DEF: Severe chest contractions upon air intake and expiratory grunting. The infant appears blue due to oxygen deficiency and has a rapid respiratory rate, formerly called hyaline membrane disease.

P22.1 Transient tachypnea of newborn
Idiopathic tachypnea of newborn
Respiratory distress syndrome, type II
Wet lung syndrome
DEF: Rapid, labored breathing of a newborn. It is a short-term problem that begins after birth and lasts about three days.

P22.8 Other respiratory distress of newborn
EXCLUDES 1 *respiratory arrest of newborn (P28.81)*
respiratory failure of newborn NOS (P28.5)

P22.9 Respiratory distress of newborn, unspecified
EXCLUDES 1 *respiratory arrest of newborn (P28.81)*
respiratory failure of newborn NOS (P28.5)

P23 Congenital pneumonia
INCLUDES infective pneumonia acquired in utero or during birth
EXCLUDES 1 *neonatal pneumonia resulting from aspiration (P24.-)*

P23.0 Congenital pneumonia due to viral agent MCC
Use additional code (B97) to identify organism
EXCLUDES 1 *congenital rubella pneumonitis (P35.0)*

P23.1 Congenital pneumonia due to Chlamydia MCC

P23.2 Congenital pneumonia due to staphylococcus MCC

P23.3 Congenital pneumonia due to streptococcus, group B MCC

P23.4 Congenital pneumonia due to Escherichia coli MCC

P23.5 Congenital pneumonia due to Pseudomonas MCC

Additional Character Required | Placeholder | Questionable PDx | Manifestation | Unspecified | UPD Unacceptable PDx | H1-H18 HAC | HCC CMS-HCC Dx | HIV HIV Dx

P23.6 Congenital pneumonia due to other bacterial agents MCC
Congenital pneumonia due to Hemophilus influenzae
Congenital pneumonia due to Klebsiella pneumoniae
Congenital pneumonia due to Mycoplasma
Congenital pneumonia due to Streptococcus, except group B
Use additional code (B95-B96) to identify organism

P23.8 Congenital pneumonia due to other organisms MCC

P23.9 Congenital pneumonia, unspecified MCC

P24 Neonatal aspiration
INCLUDES aspiration in utero and during delivery

P24.Ø Meconium aspiration
EXCLUDES 1 *meconium passage (without aspiration) during delivery (PØ3.82)*
meconium staining (P96.83)
DEF: Meconium in the trachea or seen on chest x-ray after birth.

P24.ØØ Meconium aspiration without respiratory symptoms
Meconium aspiration NOS

P24.Ø1 Meconium aspiration with respiratory symptoms MCC
Meconium aspiration pneumonia
Meconium aspiration pneumonitis
Meconium aspiration syndrome NOS
Use additional code to identify any secondary pulmonary hypertension, if applicable (I27.2-)
DEF: Aspiration of fetal intestinal material during or prior to delivery. It is usually a complication of placental insufficiency, causing pneumonitis and bronchial obstruction (inflammatory reaction of lungs).

P24.1 Neonatal aspiration of (clear) amniotic fluid and mucus
Neonatal aspiration of liquor (amnii)

P24.1Ø Neonatal aspiration of (clear) amniotic fluid and mucus without respiratory symptoms
Neonatal aspiration of amniotic fluid and mucus NOS

P24.11 Neonatal aspiration of (clear) amniotic fluid and mucus with respiratory symptoms MCC
Neonatal aspiration of amniotic fluid and mucus with pneumonia
Neonatal aspiration of amniotic fluid and mucus with pneumonitis
Use additional code to identify any secondary pulmonary hypertension, if applicable (I27.2-)

P24.2 Neonatal aspiration of blood

P24.2Ø Neonatal aspiration of blood without respiratory symptoms
Neonatal aspiration of blood NOS

P24.21 Neonatal aspiration of blood with respiratory symptoms MCC
Neonatal aspiration of blood with pneumonia
Neonatal aspiration of blood with pneumonitis
Use additional code to identify any secondary pulmonary hypertension, if applicable (I27.2-)

P24.3 Neonatal aspiration of milk and regurgitated food
Neonatal aspiration of stomach contents

P24.3Ø Neonatal aspiration of milk and regurgitated food without respiratory symptoms
Neonatal aspiration of milk and regurgitated food NOS

P24.31 Neonatal aspiration of milk and regurgitated food with respiratory symptoms MCC
Neonatal aspiration of milk and regurgitated food with pneumonia
Neonatal aspiration of milk and regurgitated food with pneumonitis
Use additional code to identify any secondary pulmonary hypertension, if applicable (I27.2-)

P24.8 Other neonatal aspiration

P24.8Ø Other neonatal aspiration without respiratory symptoms
Neonatal aspiration NEC

P24.81 Other neonatal aspiration with respiratory symptoms MCC
Neonatal aspiration pneumonia NEC
Neonatal aspiration with pneumonitis NEC
Neonatal aspiration with pneumonia NOS
Neonatal aspiration with pneumonitis NOS
Use additional code to identify any secondary pulmonary hypertension, if applicable (I27.2-)

P24.9 Neonatal aspiration, unspecified

P25 Interstitial emphysema and related conditions originating in the perinatal period

P25.Ø Interstitial emphysema originating in the perinatal period MCC

P25.1 Pneumothorax originating in the perinatal period MCC

P25.2 Pneumomediastinum originating in the perinatal period MCC

P25.3 Pneumopericardium originating in the perinatal period MCC

P25.8 Other conditions related to interstitial emphysema originating in the perinatal period MCC

P26 Pulmonary hemorrhage originating in the perinatal period
EXCLUDES 1 *acute idiopathic hemorrhage in infants over 28 days old (RØ4.81)*

P26.Ø Tracheobronchial hemorrhage originating in the perinatal period MCC

P26.1 Massive pulmonary hemorrhage originating in the perinatal period MCC

P26.8 Other pulmonary hemorrhages originating in the perinatal period MCC

P26.9 Unspecified pulmonary hemorrhage originating in the perinatal period MCC

P27 Chronic respiratory disease originating in the perinatal period
EXCLUDES 2 *respiratory distress of newborn (P22.Ø-P22.9)*

P27.Ø Wilson-Mikity syndrome MCC
Pulmonary dysmaturity
DEF: Pulmonary insufficiency in newborn babies, especially those with low birth weight. Rapid onset of hypercapnia and cyanosis occur during the first month of life frequently resulting in death.

P27.1 Bronchopulmonary dysplasia originating in the perinatal period MCC

P27.8 Other chronic respiratory diseases originating in the perinatal period MCC
Congenital pulmonary fibrosis
Ventilator lung in newborn

P27.9 Unspecified chronic respiratory disease originating in the perinatal period MCC

P28 Other respiratory conditions originating in the perinatal period
▶Code also, if applicable, congenital malformations of the respiratory system (Q3Ø-Q34)◀
EXCLUDES 1 *~~congenital malformations of the respiratory system (Q3Ø-Q34)~~*

P28.Ø Primary atelectasis of newborn CC
Primary failure to expand terminal respiratory units
Pulmonary hypoplasia associated with short gestation
Pulmonary immaturity NOS

P28.1 Other and unspecified atelectasis of newborn

P28.1Ø Unspecified atelectasis of newborn CC
Atelectasis of newborn NOS

P28.11 Resorption atelectasis without respiratory distress syndrome CC
EXCLUDES 1 *resorption atelectasis with respiratory distress syndrome (P22.Ø)*

P28.19 Other atelectasis of newborn CC
Partial atelectasis of newborn
Secondary atelectasis of newborn

P28.2 Cyanotic attacks of newborn CC
EXCLUDES 1 *apnea of newborn ▶(P28.3- - P28.4-)◀*

▲ ✓5th **P28.3 Primary sleep apnea of newborn**
~~Central sleep apnea of newborn~~
~~Obstructive sleep apnea of newborn~~
Sleep apnea of newborn NOS
EXCLUDES 2 ▶*other apnea of newborn (P28.4-)*◀
DEF: Unexplained cessation of breathing when a neonate makes no respiratory effort for 20 seconds or longer or when a neonate's breathing cessation is accompanied by cyanosis, bradycardia, or hypotonia.

● **P28.30 Primary sleep apnea of newborn, unspecified** CC
Transient oxygen desaturation spells of newborn during sleep

● **P28.31 Primary central sleep apnea of newborn** CC

● **P28.32 Primary obstructive sleep apnea of newborn** CC

● **P28.33 Primary mixed sleep apnea of newborn** CC

● **P28.39 Other primary sleep apnea of newborn** CC

▲ ✓5th **P28.4 Other apnea of newborn**
~~Apnea of prematurity~~
~~Obstructive apnea of newborn~~
EXCLUDES 1 ~~*obstructive sleep apnea of newborn (P28.3)*~~
EXCLUDES 2 ▶*primary sleep apnea of newborn (P28.3-)*◀

● **P28.40 Unspecified apnea of newborn** CC
Apnea of newborn, NOS
Transient oxygen desaturation spells of newborn

● **P28.41 Central neonatal apnea of newborn** CC

● **P28.42 Obstructive apnea of newborn** CC

● **P28.43 Mixed neonatal apnea of newborn** CC

● **P28.49 Other apnea of newborn** CC
Apnea of prematurity

P28.5 Respiratory failure of newborn MCC
EXCLUDES 1 *respiratory arrest of newborn (P28.81)*
respiratory distress of newborn (P22.0-)
AHA: 2019,2Q,29

✓5th **P28.8 Other specified respiratory conditions of newborn**

P28.81 Respiratory arrest of newborn MCC

P28.89 Other specified respiratory conditions of newborn
Congenital laryngeal stridor
Sniffles in newborn
Snuffles in newborn
EXCLUDES 1 *early congenital syphilitic rhinitis (A50.05)*

P28.9 Respiratory condition of newborn, unspecified
Respiratory depression in newborn

✓4th **P29 Cardiovascular disorders originating in the perinatal period**
EXCLUDES 2 *congenital malformations of the circulatory system (Q20-Q28)*

P29.0 Neonatal cardiac failure

✓5th **P29.1 Neonatal cardiac dysrhythmia**

P29.11 Neonatal tachycardia

P29.12 Neonatal bradycardia

P29.2 Neonatal hypertension

✓5th **P29.3 Persistent fetal circulation**
AHA: 2017,4Q,20-21

P29.30 Pulmonary hypertension of newborn MCC
Persistent pulmonary hypertension of newborn
DEF: Condition that occurs when pressure within the pulmonary artery is elevated and vascular resistance is observed in the lungs.

P29.38 Other persistent fetal circulation MCC
Delayed closure of ductus arteriosus

P29.4 Transient myocardial ischemia in newborn

✓5th **P29.8 Other cardiovascular disorders originating in the perinatal period**

P29.81 Cardiac arrest of newborn MCC

P29.89 Other cardiovascular disorders originating in the perinatal period
AHA: 2014,4Q,23

P29.9 Cardiovascular disorder originating in the perinatal period, unspecified

Infections specific to the perinatal period (P35-P39)

Infections acquired in utero, during birth via the umbilicus, or during the first 28 days after birth
EXCLUDES 2 *asymptomatic human immunodeficiency virus [HIV] infection status (Z21)*
congenital gonococcal infection (A54.-)
congenital pneumonia (P23.-)
congenital syphilis (A50.-)
human immunodeficiency virus [HIV] disease (B20)
infant botulism (A48.51)
infectious diseases not specific to the perinatal period (A00-B99, J09, J10.-)
intestinal infectious disease (A00-A09)
laboratory evidence of human immunodeficiency virus [HIV] (R75)
tetanus neonatorum (A33)

✓4th **P35 Congenital viral diseases**
INCLUDES infections acquired in utero or during birth

P35.0 Congenital rubella syndrome CC
Congenital rubella pneumonitis

P35.1 Congenital cytomegalovirus infection MCC

P35.2 Congenital herpesviral [herpes simplex] infection MCC

P35.3 Congenital viral hepatitis MCC

P35.4 Congenital Zika virus disease MCC
Use additional code to identify manifestations of congenital Zika virus disease
AHA: 2018,4Q,25-26

P35.8 Other congenital viral diseases MCC
Congenital varicella [chickenpox]
AHA: 2020,2Q,13

P35.9 Congenital viral disease, unspecified MCC

✓4th **P36 Bacterial sepsis of newborn**
INCLUDES congenital sepsis
Use additional code(s), if applicable, to identify severe sepsis (R65.2-) and associated acute organ dysfunction(s)

P36.0 Sepsis of newborn due to streptococcus, group B MCC HCC

✓5th **P36.1 Sepsis of newborn due to other and unspecified streptococci**

P36.10 Sepsis of newborn due to unspecified streptococci MCC HCC

P36.19 Sepsis of newborn due to other streptococci MCC HCC

P36.2 Sepsis of newborn due to Staphylococcus aureus MCC HCC

✓5th **P36.3 Sepsis of newborn due to other and unspecified staphylococci**

P36.30 Sepsis of newborn due to unspecified staphylococci MCC HCC

P36.39 Sepsis of newborn due to other staphylococci MCC HCC

P36.4 Sepsis of newborn due to Escherichia coli MCC HCC

P36.5 Sepsis of newborn due to anaerobes MCC HCC

P36.8 Other bacterial sepsis of newborn MCC HCC
Use additional code from category B96 to identify organism

P36.9 Bacterial sepsis of newborn, unspecified MCC HCC

✓4th **P37 Other congenital infectious and parasitic diseases**
EXCLUDES 2 *congenital syphilis (A50.-)*
infectious neonatal diarrhea (A00-A09)
necrotizing enterocolitis in newborn (P77.-)
noninfectious neonatal diarrhea (P78.3)
ophthalmia neonatorum due to gonococcus (A54.31)
tetanus neonatorum (A33)

P37.0 Congenital tuberculosis MCC

P37.1 Congenital toxoplasmosis MCC
Hydrocephalus due to congenital toxoplasmosis

P37.2 Neonatal (disseminated) listeriosis MCC

P37.3 Congenital falciparum malaria MCC

P37.4 Other congenital malaria MCC

P37.5 Neonatal candidiasis

P37.8 Other specified congenital infectious and parasitic diseases MCC

P37.9 Congenital infectious or parasitic disease, unspecified MCC

P38 Omphalitis of newborn
EXCLUDES 1 *omphalitis not of newborn (L08.82)*
tetanus omphalitis (A33)
umbilical hemorrhage of newborn (P51.-)
DEF: Omphalitis: Infection and inflammation of the umbilical stump, often due to bacteria that can spread beyond the umbilical stump to the fascia, muscle, or even the umbilical vessels.
P38.1 Omphalitis with mild hemorrhage CC
P38.9 Omphalitis without hemorrhage CC
Omphalitis of newborn NOS

P39 Other infections specific to the perinatal period
Use additional code to identify organism or specific infection
P39.0 Neonatal infective mastitis CC
EXCLUDES 1 *breast engorgement of newborn (P83.4)*
noninfective mastitis of newborn (P83.4)
P39.1 Neonatal conjunctivitis and dacryocystitis
Neonatal chlamydial conjunctivitis
Ophthalmia neonatorum NOS
EXCLUDES 1 *gonococcal conjunctivitis (A54.31)*
P39.2 Intra-amniotic infection affecting newborn, not elsewhere classified CC
P39.3 Neonatal urinary tract infection CC
P39.4 Neonatal skin infection CC
Neonatal pyoderma
EXCLUDES 1 *pemphigus neonatorum (L00)*
staphylococcal scalded skin syndrome (L00)
P39.8 Other specified infections specific to the perinatal period CC
P39.9 Infection specific to the perinatal period, unspecified CC

Hemorrhagic and hematological disorders of newborn (P50-P61)

EXCLUDES 1 *congenital stenosis and stricture of bile ducts (Q44.3)*
Crigler-Najjar syndrome (E80.5)
Dubin-Johnson syndrome (E80.6)
Gilbert syndrome (E80.4)
hereditary hemolytic anemias (D55-D58)

P50 Newborn affected by intrauterine (fetal) blood loss
EXCLUDES 1 *congenital anemia from intrauterine (fetal) blood loss (P61.3)*
P50.0 Newborn affected by intrauterine (fetal) blood loss from vasa previa
P50.1 Newborn affected by intrauterine (fetal) blood loss from ruptured cord
P50.2 Newborn affected by intrauterine (fetal) blood loss from placenta
P50.3 Newborn affected by hemorrhage into co-twin
P50.4 Newborn affected by hemorrhage into maternal circulation
P50.5 Newborn affected by intrauterine (fetal) blood loss from cut end of co-twin's cord
P50.8 Newborn affected by other intrauterine (fetal) blood loss
P50.9 Newborn affected by intrauterine (fetal) blood loss, unspecified
Newborn affected by fetal hemorrhage NOS

P51 Umbilical hemorrhage of newborn
EXCLUDES 1 *omphalitis with mild hemorrhage (P38.1)*
umbilical hemorrhage from cut end of co-twins cord (P50.5)
P51.0 Massive umbilical hemorrhage of newborn
P51.8 Other umbilical hemorrhages of newborn
Slipped umbilical ligature NOS
P51.9 Umbilical hemorrhage of newborn, unspecified

P52 Intracranial nontraumatic hemorrhage of newborn
INCLUDES intracranial hemorrhage due to anoxia or hypoxia
EXCLUDES 1 *intracranial hemorrhage due to birth injury (P10.-)*
intracranial hemorrhage due to other injury (S06.-)
P52.0 Intraventricular (nontraumatic) hemorrhage, grade 1, of newborn CC
Subependymal hemorrhage (without intraventricular extension)
Bleeding into germinal matrix
P52.1 Intraventricular (nontraumatic) hemorrhage, grade 2, of newborn CC
Subependymal hemorrhage with intraventricular extension
Bleeding into ventricle
P52.2 Intraventricular (nontraumatic) hemorrhage, grade 3 and grade 4, of newborn
P52.21 Intraventricular (nontraumatic) hemorrhage, grade 3, of newborn MCC
Subependymal hemorrhage with intraventricular extension with enlargement of ventricle
P52.22 Intraventricular (nontraumatic) hemorrhage, grade 4, of newborn MCC
Bleeding into cerebral cortex
Subependymal hemorrhage with intracerebral extension
P52.3 Unspecified intraventricular (nontraumatic) hemorrhage of newborn CC
P52.4 Intracerebral (nontraumatic) hemorrhage of newborn MCC
P52.5 Subarachnoid (nontraumatic) hemorrhage of newborn MCC
P52.6 Cerebellar (nontraumatic) and posterior fossa hemorrhage of newborn MCC
P52.8 Other intracranial (nontraumatic) hemorrhages of newborn MCC
P52.9 Intracranial (nontraumatic) hemorrhage of newborn, unspecified MCC

P53 Hemorrhagic disease of newborn CC
Vitamin K deficiency of newborn

P54 Other neonatal hemorrhages
EXCLUDES 1 *newborn affected by (intrauterine) blood loss (P50.-)*
pulmonary hemorrhage originating in the perinatal period (P26.-)
P54.0 Neonatal hematemesis
EXCLUDES 1 *neonatal hematemesis due to swallowed maternal blood (P78.2)*
P54.1 Neonatal melena MCC
EXCLUDES 1 *neonatal melena due to swallowed maternal blood (P78.2)*
P54.2 Neonatal rectal hemorrhage MCC
P54.3 Other neonatal gastrointestinal hemorrhage MCC
P54.4 Neonatal adrenal hemorrhage CC
P54.5 Neonatal cutaneous hemorrhage
Neonatal bruising
Neonatal ecchymoses
Neonatal petechiae
Neonatal superficial hematomata
EXCLUDES 2 *bruising of scalp due to birth injury (P12.3)*
cephalhematoma due to birth injury (P12.0)
P54.6 Neonatal vaginal hemorrhage ♀
Neonatal pseudomenses
P54.8 Other specified neonatal hemorrhages
P54.9 Neonatal hemorrhage, unspecified

P55 Hemolytic disease of newborn
P55.0 Rh isoimmunization of newborn
DEF: Incompatible Rh fetal-maternal blood grouping that prematurely destroys red blood cells. Symptoms include jaundice, asphyxia, pulmonary hypertension, edema, respiratory distress, kernicterus, and coagulopathies. It is detected by a Coombs test.
TIP: A positive Coombs test without documentation of associated Rh isoimmunization should be coded to R79.89 Other specified abnormal findings of blood chemistry.
P55.1 ABO isoimmunization of newborn
AHA: 2015,3Q,20
P55.8 Other hemolytic diseases of newborn
AHA: 2018,3Q,24
P55.9 Hemolytic disease of newborn, unspecified

P56 Hydrops fetalis due to hemolytic disease
EXCLUDES 1 *hydrops fetalis NOS (P83.2)*
P56.0 Hydrops fetalis due to isoimmunization MCC
P56.9 Hydrops fetalis due to other and unspecified hemolytic disease
P56.90 Hydrops fetalis due to unspecified hemolytic disease MCC
P56.99 Hydrops fetalis due to other hemolytic disease MCC

✓4th P57 Kernicterus

P57.Ø Kernicterus due to isoimmunization MCC

DEF: Complication of erythroblastosis fetalis associated with severe neural symptoms, high blood bilirubin levels, and nerve cell destruction. It results in bilirubin-pigmented gray matter of the central nervous system.

P57.8 Other specified kernicterus MCC

EXCLUDES 1 *Crigler-Najjar syndrome (E8Ø.5)*

P57.9 Kernicterus, unspecified MCC

✓4th P58 Neonatal jaundice due to other excessive hemolysis

EXCLUDES 1 *jaundice due to isoimmunization (P55-P57)*

P58.Ø Neonatal jaundice due to bruising

P58.1 Neonatal jaundice due to bleeding

P58.2 Neonatal jaundice due to infection

P58.3 Neonatal jaundice due to polycythemia

✓5th P58.4 Neonatal jaundice due to drugs or toxins transmitted from mother or given to newborn

Code first poisoning due to drug or toxin, if applicable (T36-T65 with fifth or sixth character 1-4 or 6)

Use additional code for adverse effect, if applicable, to identify drug (T36-T5Ø with fifth or sixth character 5)

P58.41 Neonatal jaundice due to drugs or toxins transmitted from mother

P58.42 Neonatal jaundice due to drugs or toxins given to newborn

P58.5 Neonatal jaundice due to swallowed maternal blood

P58.8 Neonatal jaundice due to other specified excessive hemolysis

P58.9 Neonatal jaundice due to excessive hemolysis, unspecified

✓4th P59 Neonatal jaundice from other and unspecified causes

EXCLUDES 1 *jaundice due to inborn errors of metabolism (E7Ø-E88)*
kernicterus (P57.-)

P59.Ø Neonatal jaundice associated with preterm delivery

Hyperbilirubinemia of prematurity

Jaundice due to delayed conjugation associated with preterm delivery

P59.1 Inspissated bile syndrome MCC

DEF: Biliary obstruction in newborn resulting from obstruction of outflow tract.

✓5th P59.2 Neonatal jaundice from other and unspecified hepatocellular damage

EXCLUDES 1 *congenital viral hepatitis (P35.3)*

P59.2Ø Neonatal jaundice from unspecified hepatocellular damage MCC

P59.29 Neonatal jaundice from other hepatocellular damage MCC

Neonatal giant cell hepatitis

Neonatal (idiopathic) hepatitis

P59.3 Neonatal jaundice from breast milk inhibitor

P59.8 Neonatal jaundice from other specified causes

P59.9 Neonatal jaundice, unspecified

Neonatal physiological jaundice (intense)(prolonged) NOS

AHA: 2015,3Q,20

P6Ø Disseminated intravascular coagulation of newborn MCC

Defibrination syndrome of newborn

✓4th P61 Other perinatal hematological disorders

EXCLUDES 1 *transient hypogammaglobulinemia of infancy (D8Ø.7)*

P61.Ø Transient neonatal thrombocytopenia MCC

Neonatal thrombocytopenia due to exchange transfusion

Neonatal thrombocytopenia due to idiopathic maternal thrombocytopenia

Neonatal thrombocytopenia due to isoimmunization

DEF: Temporary decrease in blood platelets of a newborn that is secondary to placental insufficiency.

P61.1 Polycythemia neonatorum

DEF: Abnormal increase of total red blood cells of a newborn that results in hyperviscosity, which slows the flow of blood through small blood vessels.

P61.2 Anemia of prematurity CC

P61.3 Congenital anemia from fetal blood loss CC

P61.4 Other congenital anemias, not elsewhere classified CC

Congenital anemia NOS

P61.5 Transient neonatal neutropenia MCC

EXCLUDES 1 *congenital neutropenia (nontransient) (D7Ø.Ø)*

DEF: Low blood neutrophil counts of newborn that occurs due to maternal hypertension, sepsis, twin-twin transfusion, alloimmunization, and hemolytic disease.

P61.6 Other transient neonatal disorders of coagulation CC

P61.8 Other specified perinatal hematological disorders

P61.9 Perinatal hematological disorder, unspecified

Transitory endocrine and metabolic disorders specific to newborn (P7Ø-P74)

INCLUDES transitory endocrine and metabolic disturbances caused by the infant's response to maternal endocrine and metabolic factors, or its adjustment to extrauterine environment

AHA: 2018,2Q,6

✓4th P7Ø Transitory disorders of carbohydrate metabolism specific to newborn

P7Ø.Ø Syndrome of infant of mother with gestational diabetes

Newborn (with hypoglycemia) affected by maternal gestational diabetes

EXCLUDES 1 *newborn (with hypoglycemia) affected by maternal (pre-existing) diabetes mellitus (P7Ø.1)*
syndrome of infant of a diabetic mother (P7Ø.1)

P7Ø.1 Syndrome of infant of a diabetic mother

Newborn (with hypoglycemia) affected by maternal (pre-existing) diabetes mellitus

EXCLUDES 1 *newborn (with hypoglycemia) affected by maternal gestational diabetes (P7Ø.Ø)*
syndrome of infant of mother with gestational diabetes (P7Ø.Ø)

P7Ø.2 Neonatal diabetes mellitus CC

P7Ø.3 Iatrogenic neonatal hypoglycemia

P7Ø.4 Other neonatal hypoglycemia

Transitory neonatal hypoglycemia

P7Ø.8 Other transitory disorders of carbohydrate metabolism of newborn CC

P7Ø.9 Transitory disorder of carbohydrate metabolism of newborn, unspecified

✓4th P71 Transitory neonatal disorders of calcium and magnesium metabolism

P71.Ø Cow's milk hypocalcemia in newborn CC

P71.1 Other neonatal hypocalcemia CC

EXCLUDES 1 *neonatal hypoparathyroidism (P71.4)*

P71.2 Neonatal hypomagnesemia CC

P71.3 Neonatal tetany without calcium or magnesium deficiency CC

Neonatal tetany NOS

P71.4 Transitory neonatal hypoparathyroidism CC

P71.8 Other transitory neonatal disorders of calcium and magnesium metabolism CC

AHA: 2016,4Q,54

P71.9 Transitory neonatal disorder of calcium and magnesium metabolism, unspecified CC

✓4th P72 Other transitory neonatal endocrine disorders

EXCLUDES 1 *congenital hypothyroidism with or without goiter (EØ3.Ø-EØ3.1)*
dyshormogenetic goiter (EØ7.1)
Pendred's syndrome (EØ7.1)

P72.Ø Neonatal goiter, not elsewhere classified CC

Transitory congenital goiter with normal functioning

P72.1 Transitory neonatal hyperthyroidism CC

Neonatal thyrotoxicosis

P72.2 Other transitory neonatal disorders of thyroid function, not elsewhere classified CC

Transitory neonatal hypothyroidism

P72.8 Other specified transitory neonatal endocrine disorders CC

P72.9 Transitory neonatal endocrine disorder, unspecified

✓4th P74 Other transitory neonatal electrolyte and metabolic disturbances

AHA: 2018,4Q,26-27

P74.Ø Late metabolic acidosis of newborn MCC

EXCLUDES 1 *(fetal) metabolic acidosis of newborn (P19)*

P74.1 Dehydration of newborn

✓5th P74.2 Disturbances of sodium balance of newborn

P74.21 Hypernatremia of newborn

P74.22 Hyponatremia of newborn

✓5th **P74.3 Disturbances of potassium balance of newborn**

P74.31 Hyperkalemia of newborn

P74.32 Hypokalemia of newborn

✓5th **P74.4 Other transitory electrolyte disturbances of newborn**

P74.41 Alkalosis of newborn CC

Hyperbicarbonatemia

✓6th **P74.42 Disturbances of chlorine balance of newborn**

P74.421 Hyperchloremia of newborn

Hyperchloremic metabolic acidosis

EXCLUDES 2 *late metabolic acidosis of the newborn (P74.Ø)*

P74.422 Hypochloremia of newborn

P74.49 Other transitory electrolyte disturbance of newborn

P74.5 Transitory tyrosinemia of newborn CC

P74.6 Transitory hyperammonemia of newborn CC

P74.8 Other transitory metabolic disturbances of newborn CC

Amino-acid metabolic disorders described as transitory

P74.9 Transitory metabolic disturbance of newborn, unspecified

Digestive system disorders of newborn (P76-P78)

✓4th **P76 Other intestinal obstruction of newborn**

P76.Ø Meconium plug syndrome

Meconium ileus NOS

EXCLUDES 1 *meconium ileus in cystic fibrosis (E84.11)*

DEF: Meconium obstruction of a newborn's intestines, resulting from unusually thick or hard meconium.

P76.1 Transitory ileus of newborn CC

EXCLUDES 1 *Hirschsprung's disease (Q43.1)*

P76.2 Intestinal obstruction due to inspissated milk

P76.8 Other specified intestinal obstruction of newborn

EXCLUDES 1 *intestinal obstruction classifiable to K56.-*

P76.9 Intestinal obstruction of newborn, unspecified

✓4th **P77 Necrotizing enterocolitis of newborn**

DEF: Serious intestinal infection and inflammation in preterm infants. Severity is measured by stages and may progress to life-threatening perforation or peritonitis. Resection surgical treatment may be necessary.

P77.1 Stage 1 necrotizing enterocolitis in newborn MCC

Necrotizing enterocolitis without pneumatosis, without perforation

DEF: Broad-spectrum symptoms with nonspecific signs, including feeding intolerance, abdominal distention, bradycardia, and metabolic abnormalities.

P77.2 Stage 2 necrotizing enterocolitis in newborn MCC

Necrotizing enterocolitis with pneumatosis, without perforation

DEF: Radiographic confirmation of necrotizing enterocolitis showing intestinal dilatation, fixed loops of bowels, pneumatosis intestinalis, metabolic acidosis, and thrombocytopenia.

P77.3 Stage 3 necrotizing enterocolitis in newborn MCC

Necrotizing enterocolitis with perforation

Necrotizing enterocolitis with pneumatosis and perforation

DEF: Advanced stage in which an infant demonstrates signs of bowel perforation, septic shock, metabolic acidosis, ascites, disseminated intravascular coagulopathy, and neutropenia.

P77.9 Necrotizing enterocolitis in newborn, unspecified MCC

Necrotizing enterocolitis in newborn, NOS

✓4th **P78 Other perinatal digestive system disorders**

EXCLUDES 1 *cystic fibrosis (E84.Ø-E84.9)*

neonatal gastrointestinal hemorrhages (P54.Ø-P54.3)

P78.Ø Perinatal intestinal perforation MCC

Meconium peritonitis

P78.1 Other neonatal peritonitis

Neonatal peritonitis NOS

P78.2 Neonatal hematemesis and melena due to swallowed maternal blood

P78.3 Noninfective neonatal diarrhea

Neonatal diarrhea NOS

✓5th **P78.8 Other specified perinatal digestive system disorders**

P78.81 Congenital cirrhosis (of liver)

P78.82 Peptic ulcer of newborn

P78.83 Newborn esophageal reflux

Neonatal esophageal reflux

P78.84 Gestational alloimmune liver disease

GALD

Neonatal hemochromatosis

EXCLUDES 1 *hemochromatosis (E83.11-)*

AHA: 2017,4Q,21

DEF: Severe hepatic injury with onset during fetal development with manifestations beginning during fetal life. It is due to maternal antibodies to fetal hepatic cells (hepatocytes) that cross the placenta into the fetal circulation, causing hepatic cell necrosis.

P78.89 Other specified perinatal digestive system disorders

P78.9 Perinatal digestive system disorder, unspecified

Conditions involving the integument and temperature regulation of newborn (P8Ø-P83)

✓4th **P8Ø Hypothermia of newborn**

DEF: Decrease in newborn body temperature due to their larger ratio of surface area to body weight, thin skin with blood vessels close to the surface, and a limited amount of subcutaneous fat.

P8Ø.Ø Cold injury syndrome

Severe and usually chronic hypothermia associated with a pink flushed appearance, edema and neurological and biochemical abnormalities.

EXCLUDES 1 *mild hypothermia of newborn (P8Ø.8)*

P8Ø.8 Other hypothermia of newborn

Mild hypothermia of newborn

P8Ø.9 Hypothermia of newborn, unspecified

✓4th **P81 Other disturbances of temperature regulation of newborn**

P81.Ø Environmental hyperthermia of newborn

P81.8 Other specified disturbances of temperature regulation of newborn

P81.9 Disturbance of temperature regulation of newborn, unspecified

Fever of newborn NOS

✓4th **P83 Other conditions of integument specific to newborn**

EXCLUDES 1 *congenital malformations of skin and integument (Q8Ø-Q84)*

hydrops fetalis due to hemolytic disease (P56.-)

neonatal skin infection (P39.4)

staphylococcal scalded skin syndrome (LØØ)

EXCLUDES 2 *cradle cap (L21.Ø)*

diaper [napkin] dermatitis (L22)

P83.Ø Sclerema neonatorum CC

DEF: Diffuse, rapidly progressing white, waxy, nonpitting hardening of tissue, usually of legs and feet that is life-threatening. It is found in preterm or debilitated infants. Etiology is unknown.

P83.1 Neonatal erythema toxicum

P83.2 Hydrops fetalis not due to hemolytic disease MCC

Hydrops fetalis NOS

DEF: Severe, life-threatening problem of a newborn characterized by severe edema of the entire body. It is unrelated to immune response.

✓5th **P83.3 Other and unspecified edema specific to newborn**

P83.3Ø Unspecified edema specific to newborn CC

P83.39 Other edema specific to newborn CC

P83.4 Breast engorgement of newborn

Noninfective mastitis of newborn

P83.5 Congenital hydrocele ♂

DEF: Hydrocele: Serous fluid that collects in the tunica vaginalis of the scrotum along the spermatic cord in males.

P83.6 Umbilical polyp of newborn

✓5th **P83.8 Other specified conditions of integument specific to newborn**

AHA: 2017,4Q,21-22

P83.81 Umbilical granuloma

EXCLUDES 2 *granulomatous disorder of the skin and subcutaneous tissue, unspecified (L92.9)*

P83.88 Other specified conditions of integument specific to newborn

Bronze baby syndrome

Neonatal scleroderma

Urticaria neonatorum

P83.9 Condition of the integument specific to newborn, unspecified

Other problems with newborn (P84)

P84 Other problems with newborn
Acidemia of newborn
Acidosis of newborn
Anoxia of newborn NOS
Asphyxia of newborn NOS
Hypercapnia of newborn
Hypoxemia of newborn
Hypoxia of newborn NOS
Mixed metabolic and respiratory acidosis of newborn
EXCLUDES 1 *intracranial hemorrhage due to anoxia or hypoxia (P52.-)*
hypoxic ischemic encephalopathy [HIE] (P91.6-)
late metabolic acidosis of newborn (P74.Ø)

Other disorders originating in the perinatal period (P9Ø-P96)

P9Ø Convulsions of newborn MCC
EXCLUDES 1 *benign myoclonic epilepsy in infancy (G4Ø.3-)*
benign neonatal convulsions (familial) (G4Ø.3-)

✓4th **P91 Other disturbances of cerebral status of newborn**
P91.Ø Neonatal cerebral ischemia MCC
EXCLUDES 1 *neonatal cerebral infarction (P91.82-)*
P91.1 Acquired periventricular cysts of newborn MCC
P91.2 Neonatal cerebral leukomalacia MCC
Periventricular leukomalacia
P91.3 Neonatal cerebral irritability MCC
P91.4 Neonatal cerebral depression MCC
P91.5 Neonatal coma MCC
✓5th **P91.6 Hypoxic ischemic encephalopathy [HIE]**
EXCLUDES 1 *neonatal cerebral depression (P91.4)*
neonatal cerebral irritability (P91.3)
neonatal coma (P91.5)
AHA: 2017,4Q,22
P91.6Ø Hypoxic ischemic encephalopathy [HIE], unspecified CC
P91.61 Mild hypoxic ischemic encephalopathy [HIE] CC
P91.62 Moderate hypoxic ischemic encephalopathy [HIE] CC
P91.63 Severe hypoxic ischemic encephalopathy [HIE] MCC
✓5th **P91.8 Other specified disturbances of cerebral status of newborn**
AHA: 2017,4Q,22
✓6th **P91.81 Neonatal encephalopathy**
P91.811 Neonatal encephalopathy in diseases classified elsewhere
Code first underlying condition, if known, such as:
congenital cirrhosis (of liver) (P78.81)
intracranial nontraumatic hemorrhage of newborn (P52.-)
kernicterus (P57.-)
P91.819 Neonatal encephalopathy, unspecified
✓6th **P91.82 Neonatal cerebral infarction**
Neonatal stroke
Perinatal arterial ischemic stroke
Perinatal cerebral infarction
EXCLUDES 1 *cerebral infarction (I63.-)*
EXCLUDES 2 *intracranial hemorrhage of newborn (P52.-)*
AHA: 2020,4Q,37-38
P91.821 Neonatal cerebral infarction, right side of brain MCC HCC
P91.822 Neonatal cerebral infarction, left side of brain MCC HCC
P91.823 Neonatal cerebral infarction, bilateral MCC HCC
P91.829 Neonatal cerebral infarction, unspecified side MCC HCC
P91.88 Other specified disturbances of cerebral status of newborn
P91.9 Disturbance of cerebral status of newborn, unspecified

✓4th **P92 Feeding problems of newborn**
EXCLUDES 1 *eating disorders (F5Ø.-)*
EXCLUDES 2 *feeding problems in child over 28 days old (R63.3)*
AHA: 2016,3Q,19
✓5th **P92.Ø Vomiting of newborn**
EXCLUDES 1 *vomiting of child over 28 days old (R11.-)*
P92.Ø1 Bilious vomiting of newborn MCC
EXCLUDES 1 *bilious vomiting in child over 28 days old (R11.14)*
P92.Ø9 Other vomiting of newborn
EXCLUDES 1 *regurgitation of food in newborn (P92.1)*
P92.1 Regurgitation and rumination of newborn
P92.2 Slow feeding of newborn
P92.3 Underfeeding of newborn
P92.4 Overfeeding of newborn
P92.5 Neonatal difficulty in feeding at breast
AHA: 2017,1Q,28
P92.6 Failure to thrive in newborn
EXCLUDES 1 *failure to thrive in child over 28 days old (R62.51)*
P92.8 Other feeding problems of newborn
P92.9 Feeding problem of newborn, unspecified

✓4th **P93 Reactions and intoxications due to drugs administered to newborn**
INCLUDES reactions and intoxications due to drugs administered to fetus affecting newborn
EXCLUDES 1 *jaundice due to drugs or toxins transmitted from mother or given to newborn (P58.4-)*
reactions and intoxications from maternal opiates, tranquilizers and other medication (PØ4.Ø-PØ4.1, PØ4.4-)
withdrawal symptoms from maternal use of drugs of addiction (P96.1)
withdrawal symptoms from therapeutic use of drugs in newborn (P96.2)
P93.Ø Grey baby syndrome CC
Grey syndrome from chloramphenicol administration in newborn
P93.8 Other reactions and intoxications due to drugs administered to newborn CC
Use additional code for adverse effect, if applicable, to identify drug (T36-T5Ø with fifth or sixth character 5)

✓4th **P94 Disorders of muscle tone of newborn**
P94.Ø Transient neonatal myasthenia gravis CC
EXCLUDES 1 *myasthenia gravis (G7Ø.Ø)*
P94.1 Congenital hypertonia
P94.2 Congenital hypotonia
Floppy baby syndrome, unspecified
P94.8 Other disorders of muscle tone of newborn
P94.9 Disorder of muscle tone of newborn, unspecified

P95 Stillbirth
Deadborn fetus NOS
Fetal death of unspecified cause
Stillbirth NOS
EXCLUDES 1 *maternal care for intrauterine death (O36.4)*
missed abortion (OØ2.1)
outcome of delivery, stillbirth (Z37.1, Z37.3, Z37.4, Z37.7)

✓4th **P96 Other conditions originating in the perinatal period**
P96.Ø Congenital renal failure
Uremia of newborn
P96.1 Neonatal withdrawal symptoms from maternal use of drugs of addiction CC
Drug withdrawal syndrome in infant of dependent mother
Neonatal abstinence syndrome
EXCLUDES 1 *reactions and intoxications from maternal opiates and tranquilizers administered during labor and delivery (PØ4.Ø)*
AHA: 2018,4Q,24-25
P96.2 Withdrawal symptoms from therapeutic use of drugs in newborn CC
P96.3 Wide cranial sutures of newborn
Neonatal craniotabes
P96.5 Complication to newborn due to (fetal) intrauterine procedure
EXCLUDES 2 *newborn affected by amniocentesis (PØØ.6)*

✓5th **P96.8 Other specified conditions originating in the perinatal period**

P96.81 Exposure to (parental) (environmental) tobacco smoke in the perinatal period

EXCLUDES 2 *newborn affected by in utero exposure to tobacco (PØ4.2)*
exposure to environmental tobacco smoke after the perinatal period (Z77.22)

P96.82 Delayed separation of umbilical cord

P96.83 Meconium staining

EXCLUDES 1 *meconium aspiration (P24.ØØ, P24.Ø1)*
meconium passage during delivery (PØ3.82)

DEF: Meconium passed in utero causing discoloration on the fetal skin and nails or on the umbilicus. This staining may be incidental or may be an indicator of significant fetal stress that could affect outcomes.

P96.89 Other specified conditions originating in the perinatal period

Use additional code to specify condition

P96.9 Condition originating in the perinatal period, unspecified

Congenital debility NOS

Chapter 17. Congenital Malformations, Deformations and Chromosomal Abnormalities (QØØ–Q99)

Chapter-specific Guidelines with Coding Examples

The chapter-specific guidelines from the ICD-10-CM Official Guidelines for Coding and Reporting have been provided below. Along with these guidelines are coding examples, contained in the shaded boxes, that have been developed to help illustrate the coding and/or sequencing guidance found in these guidelines.

Assign an appropriate code(s) from categories QØØ-Q99, Congenital malformations, deformations, and chromosomal abnormalities when a malformation/deformation or chromosomal abnormality is documented. A malformation/deformation/or chromosomal abnormality may be the principal/first-listed diagnosis on a record or a secondary diagnosis.

When a malformation/deformation/or chromosomal abnormality does not have a unique code assignment, assign additional code(s) for any manifestations that may be present.

When the code assignment specifically identifies the malformation/deformation/or chromosomal abnormality, manifestations that are an inherent component of the anomaly should not be coded separately. Additional codes should be assigned for manifestations that are not an inherent component.

8-day-old infant with tetralogy of Fallot and pulmonary stenosis

Q21.3 Tetralogy of Fallot

Explanation: Pulmonary stenosis is inherent in the disease process of tetralogy of Fallot. When the code assignment specifically identifies the malformation/deformation/or chromosomal abnormality, manifestations that are inherent components of the anomaly should not be coded separately.

7-month-old infant with Down syndrome and common atrioventricular canal

Q9Ø.9 Down syndrome, unspecified

Q21.23 Complete atrioventricular septal defect

Explanation: While a common atrioventricular canal is often associated with patients with Down syndrome, this manifestation is not an inherent component and may be reported separately. When the code assignment specifically identifies the anomaly, manifestations that are inherent components of the condition should not be coded separately. Additional codes should be assigned for manifestations that are not inherent components.

Codes from Chapter 17 may be used throughout the life of the patient. If a congenital malformation or deformity has been corrected, a personal history code should be used to identify the history of the malformation or deformity. Although present at birth, a malformation/deformation/or chromosomal abnormality may not be identified until later in life. Whenever the condition is diagnosed by the provider, it is appropriate to assign a code from codes QØØ-Q99. For the birth admission, the appropriate code from category Z38, Liveborn infants, according to place of birth and type of delivery, should be sequenced as the principal diagnosis, followed by any congenital anomaly codes, QØØ- Q99.

Three-year-old with history of corrected ventricular septal defect

Z87.74 Personal history of (corrected) congenital malformations of heart and circulatory system

Explanation: If a congenital malformation or deformity has been corrected, a personal history code should be used to identify the history of the malformation or deformity.

Forty-year-old man with headaches diagnosed with congenital arteriovenous malformation of cerebral vessels by brain scan

Q28.2 Arteriovenous malformation of cerebral vessels

Explanation: Although present at birth, malformations may not be identified until later in life. Whenever a congenital condition is diagnosed by the physician, it is appropriate to assign a code from the range QØØ–Q99.

Newborn with anencephaly delivered vaginally in hospital

Z38.ØØ Single liveborn infant, delivered vaginally

QØØ.Ø Anencephaly

Explanation: For the birth admission, the appropriate code from category Z38 Liveborn infants, according to place of birth and type of delivery, should be sequenced as the principal diagnosis, followed by any congenital anomaly codes, QØØ–Q99.

Chapter 17. Congenital Malformations, Deformations and Chromosomal Abnormalities (QØØ-Q99)

NOTE Codes from this chapter are not for use on maternal records

EXCLUDES 2 *inborn errors of metabolism (E7Ø-E88)*

This chapter contains the following blocks:

Congenital malformations of the nervous system (QØØ-QØ7)

✓4th **QØØ Anencephaly and similar malformations**

QØØ.Ø Anencephaly MCC HCC
- Acephaly
- Acrania
- Amyelencephaly
- Hemianencephaly
- Hemicephaly

QØØ.1 Craniorachischisis MCC HCC

QØØ.2 Iniencephaly MCC HCC

✓4th **QØ1 Encephalocele**

INCLUDES Arnold-Chiari syndrome, type III
- encephalocystocele
- encephalomyelocele
- hydroencephalocele
- hydromeningocele, cranial
- meningocele, cerebral
- meningoencephalocele

EXCLUDES 1 *Meckel-Gruber syndrome (Q61.9)*

DEF: Congenital protrusion of brain tissue through a defect in the skull.

QØ1.Ø Frontal encephalocele CC HCC

QØ1.1 Nasofrontal encephalocele CC HCC

QØ1.2 Occipital encephalocele CC HCC

QØ1.8 Encephalocele of other sites CC HCC

QØ1.9 Encephalocele, unspecified CC HCC

QØ2 Microcephaly HCC

INCLUDES hydromicrocephaly
- micrencephalon

Code first, if applicable, congenital Zika virus disease

EXCLUDES 1 *Meckel-Gruber syndrome (Q61.9)*

AHA: 2018,4Q,26

DEF: Congenital disorder in which the head circumference is more than two standard deviations below the mean for age, sex, race, and gestation and associated with a decreased life expectancy.

✓4th **QØ3 Congenital hydrocephalus**

INCLUDES hydrocephalus in newborn

EXCLUDES 1 *Arnold-Chiari syndrome, type II (QØ7.Ø-)*
- *acquired hydrocephalus (G91.-)*
- *hydrocephalus due to congenital toxoplasmosis (P37.1)*
- *hydrocephalus with spina bifida (QØ5.Ø-QØ5.4)*

DEF: Hydrocephalus: Abnormal buildup of cerebrospinal fluid in the brain causing dilation of the ventricles.

Congenital Hydrocephalus

Pressure

Normal ventricles Hydrocephalic ventricles

QØ3.Ø Malformations of aqueduct of Sylvius HCC
- Anomaly of aqueduct of Sylvius
- Obstruction of aqueduct of Sylvius, congenital
- Stenosis of aqueduct of Sylvius

QØ3.1 Atresia of foramina of Magendie and Luschka HCC
- Dandy-Walker syndrome

QØ3.8 Other congenital hydrocephalus HCC

QØ3.9 Congenital hydrocephalus, unspecified HCC

✓4th **QØ4 Other congenital malformations of brain**

EXCLUDES 1 *cyclopia (Q87.Ø)*
- *macrocephaly (Q75.3)*

QØ4.Ø Congenital malformations of corpus callosum MCC HCC
- Agenesis of corpus callosum

QØ4.1 Arhinencephaly MCC HCC

QØ4.2 Holoprosencephaly MCC HCC

QØ4.3 Other reduction deformities of brain MCC HCC
- Absence of part of brain
- Agenesis of part of brain
- Agyria
- Aplasia of part of brain
- Hydranencephaly
- Hypoplasia of part of brain
- Lissencephaly
- Microgyria
- Pachygyria

EXCLUDES 1 *congenital malformations of corpus callosum (QØ4.Ø)*

QØ4.4 Septo-optic dysplasia of brain CC HCC

QØ4.5 Megalencephaly CC HCC

QØ4.6 Congenital cerebral cysts CC HCC
- Porencephaly
- Schizencephaly

EXCLUDES 1 *acquired porencephalic cyst (G93.Ø)*

QØ4.8 Other specified congenital malformations of brain CC HCC
- Arnold-Chiari syndrome, type IV
- Macrogyria

QØ4.9 Congenital malformation of brain, unspecified HCC
- Congenital anomaly NOS of brain
- Congenital deformity NOS of brain
- Congenital disease or lesion NOS of brain
- Multiple anomalies NOS of brain, congenital

✓4th Q05 Spina bifida

INCLUDES hydromeningocele (spinal)
meningocele (spinal)
meningomyelocele
myelocele
myelomeningocele
rachischisis
spina bifida (aperta)(cystica)
syringomyelocele

Use additional code for any associated paraplegia (paraparesis) (G82.2-)

EXCLUDES 1 *Arnold-Chiari syndrome, type II (Q07.Ø-)*
spina bifida occulta (Q76.Ø)

DEF: Lack of closure in the vertebral column with protrusion of the spinal cord through the defect, often in the lumbosacral area. This condition can be recognized by the presence of alpha-fetoproteins in the amniotic fluid.

Spina Bifida

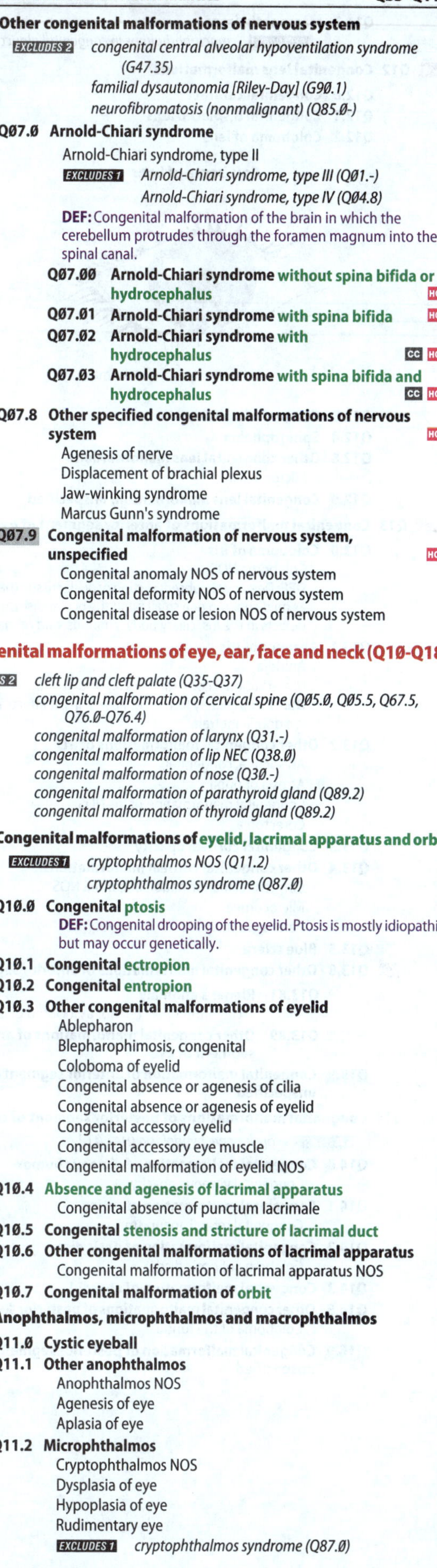

Q05.Ø Cervical spina bifida with hydrocephalus CC HCC

Q05.1 Thoracic spina bifida with hydrocephalus CC HCC
Dorsal spina bifida with hydrocephalus
Thoracolumbar spina bifida with hydrocephalus

Q05.2 Lumbar spina bifida with hydrocephalus CC HCC
Lumbosacral spina bifida with hydrocephalus

Q05.3 Sacral spina bifida with hydrocephalus CC HCC

Q05.4 Unspecified spina bifida with hydrocephalus CC HCC

Q05.5 Cervical spina bifida without hydrocephalus HCC

Q05.6 Thoracic spina bifida without hydrocephalus HCC
Dorsal spina bifida NOS
Thoracolumbar spina bifida NOS

Q05.7 Lumbar spina bifida without hydrocephalus HCC
Lumbosacral spina bifida NOS

Q05.8 Sacral spina bifida without hydrocephalus HCC

Q05.9 Spina bifida, unspecified HCC

✓4th Q06 Other congenital malformations of spinal cord

Q06.Ø Amyelia HCC

Q06.1 Hypoplasia and dysplasia of spinal cord HCC
Atelomyelia
Myelatelia
Myelodysplasia of spinal cord

Q06.2 Diastematomyelia HCC
DEF: Rare congenital anomaly often associated with spina bifida. The spinal cord is separated into longitudinal halves by a bony, cartilaginous or fibrous septum, each half surrounded by a dural sac.

Q06.3 Other congenital cauda equina malformations HCC

Q06.4 Hydromyelia HCC
Hydrorachis

Q06.8 Other specified congenital malformations of spinal cord HCC

Q06.9 Congenital malformation of spinal cord, unspecified HCC
Congenital anomaly NOS of spinal cord
Congenital deformity NOS of spinal cord
Congenital disease or lesion NOS of spinal cord

✓4th Q07 Other congenital malformations of nervous system

EXCLUDES 2 *congenital central alveolar hypoventilation syndrome (G47.35)*
familial dysautonomia [Riley-Day] (G9Ø.1)
neurofibromatosis (nonmalignant) (Q85.Ø-)

✓5th Q07.Ø Arnold-Chiari syndrome

Arnold-Chiari syndrome, type II

EXCLUDES 1 *Arnold-Chiari syndrome, type III (QØ1.-)*
Arnold-Chiari syndrome, type IV (QØ4.8)

DEF: Congenital malformation of the brain in which the cerebellum protrudes through the foramen magnum into the spinal canal.

Q07.ØØ Arnold-Chiari syndrome without spina bifida or hydrocephalus HCC

Q07.Ø1 Arnold-Chiari syndrome with spina bifida HCC

Q07.Ø2 Arnold-Chiari syndrome with hydrocephalus CC HCC

Q07.Ø3 Arnold-Chiari syndrome with spina bifida and hydrocephalus CC HCC

Q07.8 Other specified congenital malformations of nervous system HCC
Agenesis of nerve
Displacement of brachial plexus
Jaw-winking syndrome
Marcus Gunn's syndrome

Q07.9 Congenital malformation of nervous system, unspecified HCC
Congenital anomaly NOS of nervous system
Congenital deformity NOS of nervous system
Congenital disease or lesion NOS of nervous system

Congenital malformations of eye, ear, face and neck (Q1Ø-Q18)

EXCLUDES 2 *cleft lip and cleft palate (Q35-Q37)*
congenital malformation of cervical spine (QØ5.Ø, QØ5.5, Q67.5, Q76.Ø-Q76.4)
congenital malformation of larynx (Q31.-)
congenital malformation of lip NEC (Q38.Ø)
congenital malformation of nose (Q3Ø.-)
congenital malformation of parathyroid gland (Q89.2)
congenital malformation of thyroid gland (Q89.2)

✓4th Q1Ø Congenital malformations of eyelid, lacrimal apparatus and orbit

EXCLUDES 1 *cryptophthalmos NOS (Q11.2)*
cryptophthalmos syndrome (Q87.Ø)

Q1Ø.Ø Congenital ptosis
DEF: Congenital drooping of the eyelid. Ptosis is mostly idiopathic, but may occur genetically.

Q1Ø.1 Congenital ectropion

Q1Ø.2 Congenital entropion

Q1Ø.3 Other congenital malformations of eyelid
Ablepharon
Blepharophimosis, congenital
Coloboma of eyelid
Congenital absence or agenesis of cilia
Congenital absence or agenesis of eyelid
Congenital accessory eyelid
Congenital accessory eye muscle
Congenital malformation of eyelid NOS

Q1Ø.4 Absence and agenesis of lacrimal apparatus
Congenital absence of punctum lacrimale

Q1Ø.5 Congenital stenosis and stricture of lacrimal duct

Q1Ø.6 Other congenital malformations of lacrimal apparatus
Congenital malformation of lacrimal apparatus NOS

Q1Ø.7 Congenital malformation of orbit

✓4th Q11 Anophthalmos, microphthalmos and macrophthalmos

Q11.Ø Cystic eyeball

Q11.1 Other anophthalmos
Anophthalmos NOS
Agenesis of eye
Aplasia of eye

Q11.2 Microphthalmos
Cryptophthalmos NOS
Dysplasia of eye
Hypoplasia of eye
Rudimentary eye

EXCLUDES 1 *cryptophthalmos syndrome (Q87.Ø)*

Q11.3 Macrophthalmos
EXCLUDES 1 *macrophthalmos in congenital glaucoma (Q15.Ø)*

4th **Q12 Congenital lens malformations**

Q12.Ø Congenital cataract

Q12.1 Congenital displaced lens

Q12.2 Coloboma of lens

Coloboma of Lens

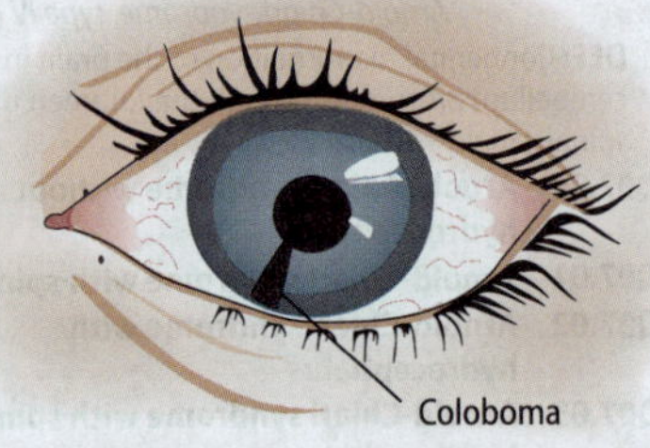

Q12.3 Congenital aphakia

Q12.4 Spherophakia

Q12.8 Other congenital lens malformations
Microphakia

Q12.9 Congenital lens malformation, unspecified

4th **Q13 Congenital malformations of anterior segment of eye**

Q13.Ø Coloboma of iris
Coloboma NOS
DEF: Defective or absent section of ocular tissue that may present as mild cupping or a small pit in the ocular disc due to extensive defects in the iris, ciliary body, choroids, and retina.

Q13.1 Absence of iris
Aniridia
Use additional code for associated glaucoma (H42)
DEF: Incompletely formed or absent iris. It affects both eyes and is a dominant trait.

Q13.2 Other congenital malformations of iris
Anisocoria, congenital
Atresia of pupil
Congenital malformation of iris NOS
Corectopia

Q13.3 Congenital corneal opacity

Q13.4 Other congenital corneal malformations
Congenital malformation of cornea NOS
Microcornea
Peter's anomaly

Q13.5 Blue sclera

5th **Q13.8 Other congenital malformations of anterior segment of eye**

Q13.81 Rieger's anomaly
Use additional code for associated glaucoma (H42)

Q13.89 Other congenital malformations of anterior segment of eye

Q13.9 Congenital malformation of anterior segment of eye, unspecified

4th **Q14 Congenital malformations of posterior segment of eye**
EXCLUDES 2 *optic nerve hypoplasia (H47.Ø3-)*

Q14.Ø Congenital malformation of vitreous humor
Congenital vitreous opacity

Q14.1 Congenital malformation of retina
Congenital retinal aneurysm

Q14.2 Congenital malformation of optic disc
Coloboma of optic disc

Q14.3 Congenital malformation of choroid

Q14.8 Other congenital malformations of posterior segment of eye
Coloboma of the fundus

Q14.9 Congenital malformation of posterior segment of eye, unspecified

4th **Q15 Other congenital malformations of eye**
EXCLUDES 1 *congenital nystagmus (H55.Ø1)*
ocular albinism (E7Ø.31-)
optic nerve hypoplasia (H47.Ø3-)
retinitis pigmentosa (H35.52)

Q15.Ø Congenital glaucoma
Axenfeld's anomaly
Buphthalmos
Glaucoma of childhood
Glaucoma of newborn
Hydrophthalmos
Keratoglobus, congenital, with glaucoma
Macrocornea with glaucoma
Macrophthalmos in congenital glaucoma
Megalocornea with glaucoma

Q15.8 Other specified congenital malformations of eye

Q15.9 Congenital malformation of eye, unspecified
Congenital anomaly of eye
Congenital deformity of eye

4th **Q16 Congenital malformations of ear causing impairment of hearing**
EXCLUDES 1 *congenital deafness (H9Ø.-)*

Q16.Ø Congenital absence of (ear) auricle

Q16.1 Congenital absence, atresia and stricture of auditory canal (external)
Congenital atresia or stricture of osseous meatus

Q16.2 Absence of eustachian tube

Q16.3 Congenital malformation of ear ossicles
Congenital fusion of ear ossicles

Q16.4 Other congenital malformations of middle ear
Congenital malformation of middle ear NOS

Q16.5 Congenital malformation of inner ear
Congenital anomaly of membranous labyrinth
Congenital anomaly of organ of Corti

Q16.9 Congenital malformation of ear causing impairment of hearing, unspecified
Congenital absence of ear NOS

4th **Q17 Other congenital malformations of ear**
EXCLUDES 1 *congenital malformations of ear with impairment of hearing (Q16.Ø-Q16.9)*
preauricular sinus (Q18.1)

Q17.Ø Accessory auricle
Accessory tragus
Polyotia
Preauricular appendage or tag
Supernumerary ear
Supernumerary lobule

Q17.1 Macrotia
DEF: Birth defect characterized by abnormal enlargement of the pinna of the ear.

Q17.2 Microtia

Q17.3 Other misshapen ear
Pointed ear

Q17.4 Misplaced ear
Low-set ears
EXCLUDES 1 *cervical auricle (Q18.2)*

Q17.5 Prominent ear
Bat ear

Q17.8 Other specified congenital malformations of ear
Congenital absence of lobe of ear

Q17.9 Congenital malformation of ear, unspecified
Congenital anomaly of ear NOS

4th **Q18 Other congenital malformations of face and neck**
EXCLUDES 1 *cleft lip and cleft palate (Q35-Q37)*
conditions classified to Q67.Ø-Q67.4
congenital malformations of skull and face bones (Q75.-)
cyclopia (Q87.Ø)
dentofacial anomalies [including malocclusion] (M26.-)
malformation syndromes affecting facial appearance (Q87.Ø)
persistent thyroglossal duct (Q89.2)

Q18.Ø Sinus, fistula and cyst of branchial cleft
Branchial vestige

Q18.1 Preauricular sinus and cyst
Fistula of auricle, congenital
Cervicoaural fistula

Q18.2 Other branchial cleft malformations
Branchial cleft malformation NOS
Cervical auricle
Otocephaly

Q18.3 Webbing of neck
Pterygium colli
DEF: Congenital malformation characterized by a thick, triangular skinfold that stretches from the lateral side of the neck across the shoulder. It is associated with genetic conditions such as Turner's and Noonan's syndromes.

Q18.4 Macrostomia
DEF: Rare congenital craniofacial bilateral or unilateral anomaly of the mouth due to malformed maxillary and mandibular processes. It results in an abnormally large mouth extending toward the ear.

Q18.5 Microstomia

Q18.6 Macrocheilia
Hypertrophy of lip, congenital

Q18.7 Microcheilia

Q18.8 Other specified congenital malformations of face and neck
Medial cyst of face and neck
Medial fistula of face and neck
Medial sinus of face and neck

Q18.9 Congenital malformation of face and neck, unspecified
Congenital anomaly NOS of face and neck

Congenital malformations of the circulatory system (Q2Ø-Q28)

✓4th Q2Ø Congenital malformations of cardiac chambers and connections
EXCLUDES 1 *dextrocardia with situs inversus (Q89.3)*
mirror-image atrial arrangement with situs inversus (Q89.3)

Q2Ø.Ø Common arterial trunk MCC
Persistent truncus arteriosus
EXCLUDES 1 *aortic septal defect (Q21.4)*

Q2Ø.1 Double outlet right ventricle MCC
Taussig-Bing syndrome

Q2Ø.2 Double outlet left ventricle MCC

Q2Ø.3 Discordant ventriculoarterial connection MCC
Dextrotransposition of aorta
Transposition of great vessels (complete)

Q2Ø.4 Double inlet ventricle MCC
Common ventricle
Cor triloculare biatriatum
Single ventricle

Q2Ø.5 Discordant atrioventricular connection CC
Corrected transposition
Levotransposition
Ventricular inversion

Q2Ø.6 Isomerism of atrial appendages
Isomerism of atrial appendages with asplenia or polysplenia

Q2Ø.8 Other congenital malformations of cardiac chambers and connections
Cor binoculare

Q2Ø.9 Congenital malformation of cardiac chambers and connections, unspecified

✓4th Q21 Congenital malformations of cardiac septa
EXCLUDES 1 *acquired cardiac septal defect (I51.Ø)*

Q21.Ø Ventricular septal defect CC
Roger's disease

Ventricular Septal Defect

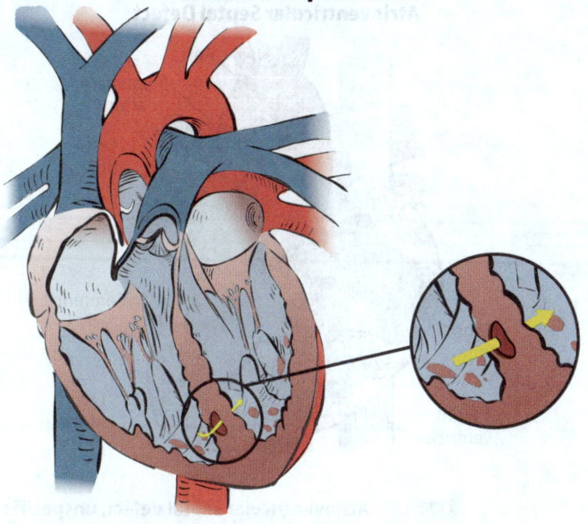

▲ **✓5th Q21.1 Atrial septal defect**
~~Coronary sinus defect~~
~~Patent or persistent foramen ovale~~
~~Patent or persistent ostium secundum defect (type II)~~
~~Patent or persistent sinus venosus defect~~
EXCLUDES 2 ▶*ostium primum atrial septal defect (type I) (Q21.2Ø)*◀

Atrial Septal Defect

Left atrium
Right atrium
Left ventricle
Right ventricle

● **Q21.1Ø Atrial septal defect, unspecified** CC

● **Q21.11 Secundum atrial septal defect** CC
Fenestrated atrial septum
Patent or persistent ostium secundum defect (type II)

● **Q21.12 Patent foramen ovale** CC
Persistent foramen ovale

● **Q21.13 Coronary sinus atrial septal defect** CC
Coronary sinus defect
Unroofed coronary sinus

● **Q21.14 Superior sinus venosus atrial septal defect** CC
Superior vena cava type atrial septal defect

● **Q21.15 Inferior sinus venosus atrial septal defect** CC
Inferior vena cava type atrial septal defect

● **Q21.16 Sinus venosus atrial septal defect, unspecified** CC
Sinus venosus defect, NOS

● **Q21.19 Other specified atrial septal defect** CC
Common atrium
Other specified atrial septal abnormality

▲ ✓5th **Q21.2 Atrioventricular septal defect**
▶Atrioventricular canal defect◀
~~Common atrioventricular canal~~
Endocardial cushion defect
Ostium primum atrial septal defect (type I)

Atrioventricular Septal Defect

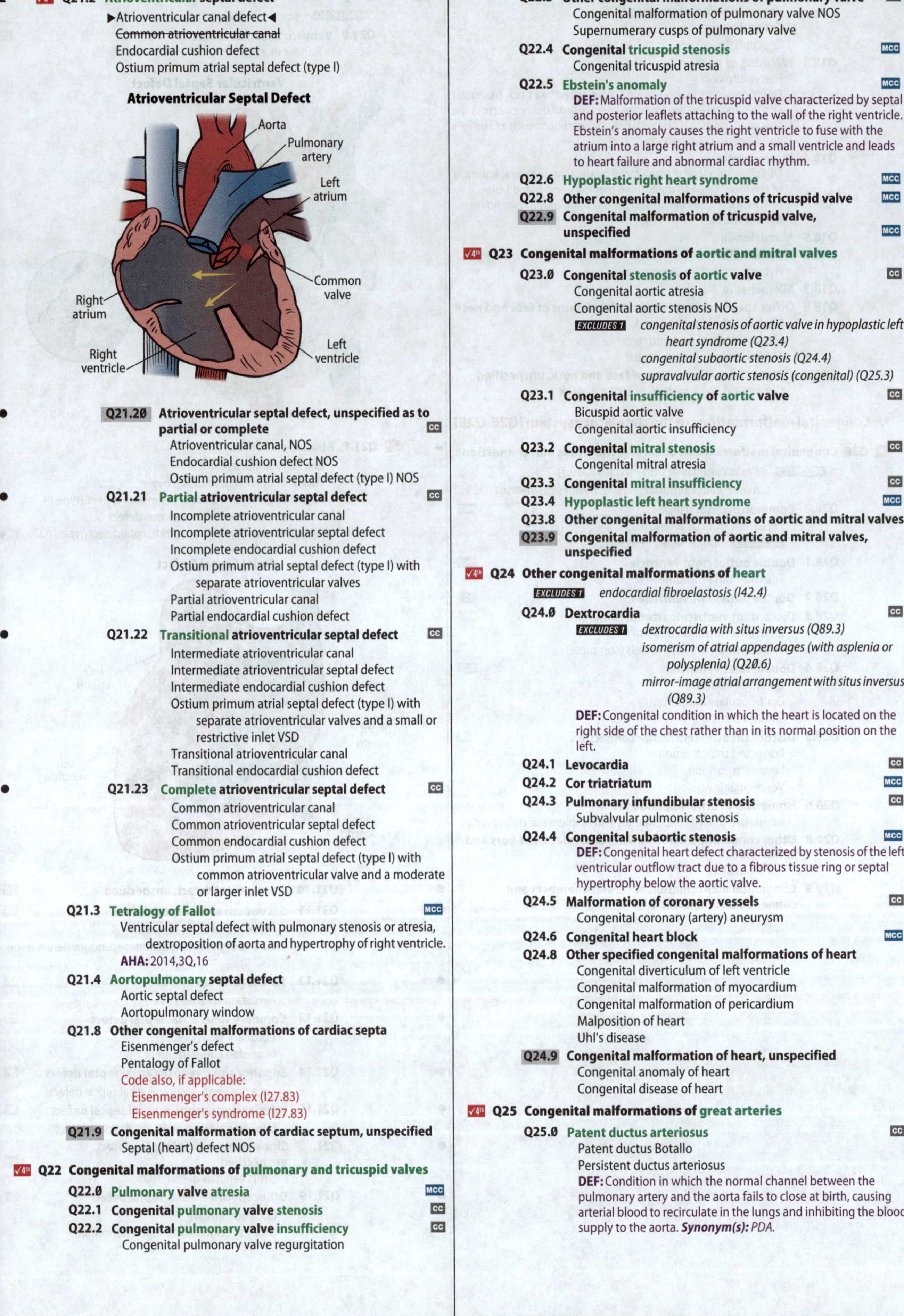

● **Q21.20 Atrioventricular septal defect, unspecified as to partial or complete** CC
Atrioventricular canal, NOS
Endocardial cushion defect NOS
Ostium primum atrial septal defect (type I) NOS

● **Q21.21 Partial atrioventricular septal defect** CC
Incomplete atrioventricular canal
Incomplete atrioventricular septal defect
Incomplete endocardial cushion defect
Ostium primum atrial septal defect (type I) with separate atrioventricular valves
Partial atrioventricular canal
Partial endocardial cushion defect

● **Q21.22 Transitional atrioventricular septal defect** CC
Intermediate atrioventricular canal
Intermediate atrioventricular septal defect
Intermediate endocardial cushion defect
Ostium primum atrial septal defect (type I) with separate atrioventricular valves and a small or restrictive inlet VSD
Transitional atrioventricular canal
Transitional endocardial cushion defect

● **Q21.23 Complete atrioventricular septal defect** CC
Common atrioventricular canal
Common atrioventricular septal defect
Common endocardial cushion defect
Ostium primum atrial septal defect (type I) with common atrioventricular valve and a moderate or larger inlet VSD

Q21.3 Tetralogy of Fallot MCC
Ventricular septal defect with pulmonary stenosis or atresia, dextroposition of aorta and hypertrophy of right ventricle.
AHA: 2014,3Q,16

Q21.4 Aortopulmonary septal defect
Aortic septal defect
Aortopulmonary window

Q21.8 Other congenital malformations of cardiac septa
Eisenmenger's defect
Pentalogy of Fallot
Code also, if applicable:
Eisenmenger's complex (I27.83)
Eisenmenger's syndrome (I27.83)

Q21.9 Congenital malformation of cardiac septum, unspecified
Septal (heart) defect NOS

✓4th **Q22 Congenital malformations of pulmonary and tricuspid valves**

Q22.Ø Pulmonary valve atresia MCC

Q22.1 Congenital pulmonary valve stenosis CC

Q22.2 Congenital pulmonary valve insufficiency CC
Congenital pulmonary valve regurgitation

Q22.3 Other congenital malformations of pulmonary valve CC
Congenital malformation of pulmonary valve NOS
Supernumerary cusps of pulmonary valve

Q22.4 Congenital tricuspid stenosis MCC
Congenital tricuspid atresia

Q22.5 Ebstein's anomaly MCC
DEF: Malformation of the tricuspid valve characterized by septal and posterior leaflets attaching to the wall of the right ventricle. Ebstein's anomaly causes the right ventricle to fuse with the atrium into a large right atrium and a small ventricle and leads to heart failure and abnormal cardiac rhythm.

Q22.6 Hypoplastic right heart syndrome MCC

Q22.8 Other congenital malformations of tricuspid valve MCC

Q22.9 Congenital malformation of tricuspid valve, unspecified MCC

✓4th **Q23 Congenital malformations of aortic and mitral valves**

Q23.Ø Congenital stenosis of aortic valve CC
Congenital aortic atresia
Congenital aortic stenosis NOS
EXCLUDES 1 *congenital stenosis of aortic valve in hypoplastic left heart syndrome (Q23.4)*
congenital subaortic stenosis (Q24.4)
supravalvular aortic stenosis (congenital) (Q25.3)

Q23.1 Congenital insufficiency of aortic valve CC
Bicuspid aortic valve
Congenital aortic insufficiency

Q23.2 Congenital mitral stenosis CC
Congenital mitral atresia

Q23.3 Congenital mitral insufficiency CC

Q23.4 Hypoplastic left heart syndrome MCC

Q23.8 Other congenital malformations of aortic and mitral valves

Q23.9 Congenital malformation of aortic and mitral valves, unspecified

✓4th **Q24 Other congenital malformations of heart**
EXCLUDES 1 *endocardial fibroelastosis (I42.4)*

Q24.Ø Dextrocardia CC
EXCLUDES 1 *dextrocardia with situs inversus (Q89.3)*
isomerism of atrial appendages (with asplenia or polysplenia) (Q2Ø.6)
mirror-image atrial arrangement with situs inversus (Q89.3)
DEF: Congenital condition in which the heart is located on the right side of the chest rather than in its normal position on the left.

Q24.1 Levocardia CC

Q24.2 Cor triatriatum MCC

Q24.3 Pulmonary infundibular stenosis CC
Subvalvular pulmonic stenosis

Q24.4 Congenital subaortic stenosis MCC
DEF: Congenital heart defect characterized by stenosis of the left ventricular outflow tract due to a fibrous tissue ring or septal hypertrophy below the aortic valve.

Q24.5 Malformation of coronary vessels CC
Congenital coronary (artery) aneurysm

Q24.6 Congenital heart block MCC

Q24.8 Other specified congenital malformations of heart
Congenital diverticulum of left ventricle
Congenital malformation of myocardium
Congenital malformation of pericardium
Malposition of heart
Uhl's disease

Q24.9 Congenital malformation of heart, unspecified
Congenital anomaly of heart
Congenital disease of heart

✓4th **Q25 Congenital malformations of great arteries**

Q25.Ø Patent ductus arteriosus CC
Patent ductus Botallo
Persistent ductus arteriosus
DEF: Condition in which the normal channel between the pulmonary artery and the aorta fails to close at birth, causing arterial blood to recirculate in the lungs and inhibiting the blood supply to the aorta. ***Synonym(s):*** *PDA.*

Q25.1 Coarctation of aorta CC
Coarctation of aorta (preductal) (postductal)
Stenosis of aorta
AHA: 2016,4Q,56-57

✓5th **Q25.2 Atresia of aorta**
AHA: 2016,4Q,56-57

Q25.21 Interruption of aortic arch CC
Atresia of aortic arch

Q25.29 Other atresia of aorta CC
Atresia of aorta

Q25.3 Supravalvular aortic stenosis CC
EXCLUDES 1 *congenital aortic stenosis NOS (Q23.0)*
congenital stenosis of aortic valve (Q23.0)

✓5th **Q25.4 Other congenital malformations of aorta**
EXCLUDES 1 *hypoplasia of aorta in hypoplastic left heart syndrome (Q23.4)*
AHA: 2016,4Q,57

Q25.40 Congenital malformation of aorta unspecified CC

Q25.41 Absence and aplasia of aorta CC

Q25.42 Hypoplasia of aorta CC

Q25.43 Congenital aneurysm of aorta CC
Congenital aneurysm of aortic root
Congenital aneurysm of aortic sinus

Q25.44 Congenital dilation of aorta CC

Q25.45 Double aortic arch CC
Vascular ring of aorta

Aortic Arch Anomalies

Q25.46 Tortuous aortic arch CC
Persistent convolutions of aortic arch

Q25.47 Right aortic arch CC
Persistent right aortic arch

Q25.48 Anomalous origin of subclavian artery CC

Q25.49 Other congenital malformations of aorta CC
Aortic arch
Bovine arch

Q25.5 Atresia of pulmonary artery MCC

Q25.6 Stenosis of pulmonary artery MCC
Supravalvular pulmonary stenosis

✓5th **Q25.7 Other congenital malformations of pulmonary artery**

Q25.71 Coarctation of pulmonary artery MCC

Q25.72 Congenital pulmonary arteriovenous malformation MCC
Congenital pulmonary arteriovenous aneurysm

Q25.79 Other congenital malformations of pulmonary artery MCC
Aberrant pulmonary artery
Agenesis of pulmonary artery
Congenital aneurysm of pulmonary artery
Congenital anomaly of pulmonary artery
Hypoplasia of pulmonary artery

Q25.8 Other congenital malformations of other great arteries CC

Q25.9 Congenital malformation of great arteries, unspecified CC

✓4th **Q26 Congenital malformations of great veins**

Q26.0 Congenital stenosis of vena cava CC
Congenital stenosis of vena cava (inferior)(superior)

Q26.1 Persistent left superior vena cava CC

Q26.2 Total anomalous pulmonary venous connection CC
Total anomalous pulmonary venous return [TAPVR], subdiaphragmatic
Total anomalous pulmonary venous return [TAPVR], supradiaphragmatic

Q26.3 Partial anomalous pulmonary venous connection CC
Partial anomalous pulmonary venous return

Q26.4 Anomalous pulmonary venous connection, unspecified CC

Q26.5 Anomalous portal venous connection

Q26.6 Portal vein-hepatic artery fistula

Q26.8 Other congenital malformations of great veins CC
Absence of vena cava (inferior) (superior)
Azygos continuation of inferior vena cava
Persistent left posterior cardinal vein
Scimitar syndrome

Q26.9 Congenital malformation of great vein, unspecified CC
Congenital anomaly of vena cava (inferior) (superior) NOS

✓4th **Q27 Other congenital malformations of peripheral vascular system**
EXCLUDES 2 *anomalies of cerebral and precerebral vessels (Q28.0-Q28.3)*
anomalies of coronary vessels (Q24.5)
anomalies of pulmonary artery (Q25.5-Q25.7)
congenital retinal aneurysm (Q14.1)
hemangioma and lymphangioma (D18.-)

Q27.0 Congenital absence and hypoplasia of umbilical artery
Single umbilical artery

Q27.1 Congenital renal artery stenosis

Q27.2 Other congenital malformations of renal artery
Congenital malformation of renal artery NOS
Multiple renal arteries

✓5th **Q27.3 Arteriovenous malformation (peripheral)**
Arteriovenous aneurysm
EXCLUDES 1 *acquired arteriovenous aneurysm (I77.0)*
EXCLUDES 2 *arteriovenous malformation of cerebral vessels (Q28.2)*
arteriovenous malformation of precerebral vessels (Q28.0)
DEF: Arteriovenous malformation: Connecting passage between an artery and a vein.

Q27.30 Arteriovenous malformation, site unspecified CC

Q27.31 Arteriovenous malformation of vessel of upper limb

Q27.32 Arteriovenous malformation of vessel of lower limb

Q27.33 Arteriovenous malformation of digestive system vessel
AHA: 2018,3Q,21

Q27.34 Arteriovenous malformation of renal vessel

Q27.39 Arteriovenous malformation, other site

Q27.4 Congenital phlebectasia CC

Q27.8 Other specified congenital malformations of peripheral vascular system
Absence of peripheral vascular system
Atresia of peripheral vascular system
Congenital aneurysm (peripheral)
Congenital stricture, artery
Congenital varix
EXCLUDES 1 *arteriovenous malformation (Q27.3-)*

Q27.9 Congenital malformation of peripheral vascular system, unspecified
Anomaly of artery or vein NOS

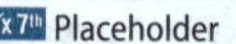

Q28 Other congenital malformations of circulatory system

EXCLUDES 1 *congenital aneurysm NOS (Q27.8)*
congenital coronary aneurysm (Q24.5)
ruptured cerebral arteriovenous malformation (I6Ø.8)
ruptured malformation of precerebral vessels (I72.Ø)

EXCLUDES 2 *congenital peripheral aneurysm (Q27.8)*
congenital pulmonary aneurysm (Q25.79)
congenital retinal aneurysm (Q14.1)

Q28.Ø Arteriovenous malformation of precerebral vessels CC
Congenital arteriovenous precerebral aneurysm (nonruptured)

Q28.1 Other malformations of precerebral vessels CC
Congenital malformation of precerebral vessels NOS
Congenital precerebral aneurysm (nonruptured)

Q28.2 Arteriovenous malformation of cerebral vessels MCC
Arteriovenous malformation of brain NOS
Congenital arteriovenous cerebral aneurysm (nonruptured)

Q28.3 Other malformations of cerebral vessels MCC
Congenital cerebral aneurysm (nonruptured)
Congenital malformation of cerebral vessels NOS
Developmental venous anomaly

Q28.8 Other specified congenital malformations of circulatory system CC
Congenital aneurysm, specified site NEC
Spinal vessel anomaly

Q28.9 Congenital malformation of circulatory system, unspecified CC

Congenital malformations of the respiratory system (Q3Ø-Q34)

Q3Ø Congenital malformations of nose

EXCLUDES 1 *congenital deviation of nasal septum (Q67.4)*

Q3Ø.Ø Choanal atresia
Atresia of nares (anterior) (posterior)
Congenital stenosis of nares (anterior) (posterior)

Q3Ø.1 Agenesis and underdevelopment of nose
Congenital absent of nose

Q3Ø.2 Fissured, notched and cleft nose

Q3Ø.3 Congenital perforated nasal septum

Q3Ø.8 Other congenital malformations of nose
Accessory nose
Congenital anomaly of nasal sinus wall
AHA: 2022,2Q,17

Q3Ø.9 Congenital malformation of nose, unspecified

Q31 Congenital malformations of larynx

EXCLUDES 1 *congenital laryngeal stridor NOS (P28.89)*

Q31.Ø Web of larynx
Glottic web of larynx
Subglottic web of larynx
Web of larynx NOS
DEF: Congenital malformation of the larynx marked by thin, translucent, or thick fibrotic membrane-like structure between the vocal folds. It is characterized by shortness of breath and stridor.

Q31.1 Congenital subglottic stenosis CC

Q31.2 Laryngeal hypoplasia CC

Q31.3 Laryngocele CC

Q31.5 Congenital laryngomalacia CC

Q31.8 Other congenital malformations of larynx CC
Absence of larynx
Agenesis of larynx
Atresia of larynx
Congenital cleft thyroid cartilage
Congenital fissure of epiglottis
Congenital stenosis of larynx NEC
Posterior cleft of cricoid cartilage

Q31.9 Congenital malformation of larynx, unspecified CC

Q32 Congenital malformations of trachea and bronchus

EXCLUDES 1 *congenital bronchiectasis (Q33.4)*

Q32.Ø Congenital tracheomalacia CC

Q32.1 Other congenital malformations of trachea CC
Atresia of trachea
Congenital anomaly of tracheal cartilage
Congenital dilatation of trachea
Congenital malformation of trachea
Congenital stenosis of trachea
Congenital tracheocele

Q32.2 Congenital bronchomalacia CC

Q32.3 Congenital stenosis of bronchus CC

Q32.4 Other congenital malformations of bronchus CC
Absence of bronchus
Agenesis of bronchus
Atresia of bronchus
Congenital diverticulum of bronchus
Congenital malformation of bronchus NOS

Q33 Congenital malformations of lung

Q33.Ø Congenital cystic lung CC
Congenital cystic lung disease
Congenital honeycomb lung
Congenital polycystic lung disease

EXCLUDES 1 *cystic fibrosis (E84.Ø)*
cystic lung disease, acquired or unspecified (J98.4)

Q33.1 Accessory lobe of lung
Azygos lobe (fissured), lung

Q33.2 Sequestration of lung MCC

Q33.3 Agenesis of lung MCC
Congenital absence of lung (lobe)

Q33.4 Congenital bronchiectasis CC

Q33.5 Ectopic tissue in lung

Q33.6 Congenital hypoplasia and dysplasia of lung MCC

EXCLUDES 1 *pulmonary hypoplasia associated with short gestation (P28.Ø)*

Q33.8 Other congenital malformations of lung

Q33.9 Congenital malformation of lung, unspecified

Q34 Other congenital malformations of respiratory system

EXCLUDES 2 *congenital central alveolar hypoventilation syndrome (G47.35)*

Q34.Ø Anomaly of pleura

Q34.1 Congenital cyst of mediastinum

Q34.8 Other specified congenital malformations of respiratory system
Atresia of nasopharynx

Q34.9 Congenital malformation of respiratory system, unspecified
Congenital absence of respiratory system
Congenital anomaly of respiratory system NOS

Cleft lip and cleft palate (Q35-Q37)

Use additional code to identify associated malformation of the nose (Q3Ø.2)

EXCLUDES 2 *Robin's syndrome (Q87.Ø)*

Q35 Cleft palate

INCLUDES fissure of palate
palatoschisis

EXCLUDES 1 *cleft palate with cleft lip (Q37.-)*

DEF: Congenital fissure or defect of the roof of the mouth opening to the nasal cavity due to failure of embryonic cells to fuse completely.

Cleft Palate

Q35.1 Cleft hard palate

Q35.3 Cleft soft palate

Q35.5 Cleft hard palate with cleft soft palate

Q35.7 Cleft uvula

Q35.9 Cleft palate, unspecified
Cleft palate NOS

Q36 Cleft lip

INCLUDES cheiloschisis
congenital fissure of lip
harelip
labium leporinum

EXCLUDES 1 *cleft lip with cleft palate (Q37.-)*

DEF: Congenital fissure or opening in the upper lip due to failure of embryonic cells to fuse completely.

Cleft Lip

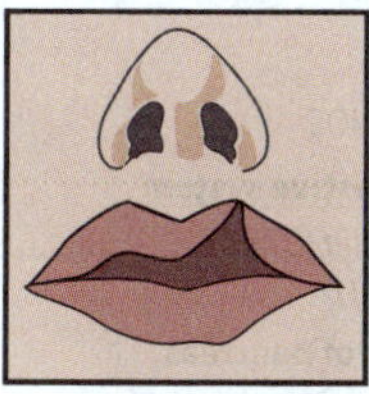
Unilateral incomplete

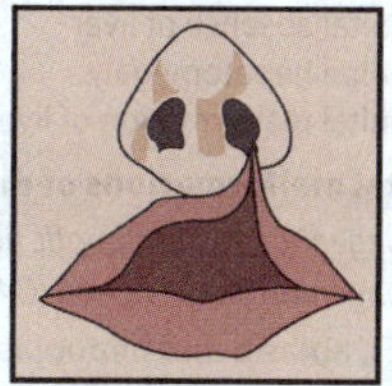
Unilateral complete

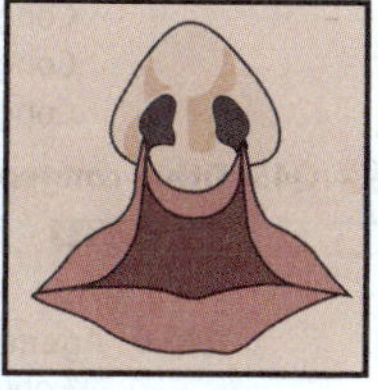
Bilateral complete

Q36.0 Cleft lip, bilateral

Q36.1 Cleft lip, median

Q36.9 Cleft lip, unilateral
Cleft lip NOS

Q37 Cleft palate with cleft lip

INCLUDES cheilopalatoschisis

Q37.0 Cleft hard palate with bilateral cleft lip

Q37.1 Cleft hard palate with unilateral cleft lip
Cleft hard palate with cleft lip NOS

Q37.2 Cleft soft palate with bilateral cleft lip

Q37.3 Cleft soft palate with unilateral cleft lip
Cleft soft palate with cleft lip NOS

Q37.4 Cleft hard and soft palate with bilateral cleft lip

Q37.5 Cleft hard and soft palate with unilateral cleft lip
Cleft hard and soft palate with cleft lip NOS

Q37.8 Unspecified cleft palate with bilateral cleft lip

Q37.9 Unspecified cleft palate with unilateral cleft lip
Cleft palate with cleft lip NOS

Other congenital malformations of the digestive system (Q38-Q45)

Q38 Other congenital malformations of tongue, mouth and pharynx

EXCLUDES 1 *dentofacial anomalies (M26.-)*
macrostomia (Q18.4)
microstomia (Q18.5)

Q38.0 Congenital malformations of lips, not elsewhere classified
Congenital fistula of lip
Congenital malformation of lip NOS
Van der Woude's syndrome

EXCLUDES 1 *cleft lip (Q36.-)*
cleft lip with cleft palate (Q37.-)
macrocheilia (Q18.6)
microcheilia (Q18.7)

Q38.1 Ankyloglossia
Tongue tie

Q38.2 Macroglossia
Congenital hypertrophy of tongue

Q38.3 Other congenital malformations of tongue
Aglossia
Bifid tongue
Congenital adhesion of tongue
Congenital fissure of tongue
Congenital malformation of tongue NOS
Double tongue
Hypoglossia
Hypoplasia of tongue
Microglossia

Q38.4 Congenital malformations of salivary glands and ducts
Atresia of salivary glands and ducts
Congenital absence of salivary glands and ducts
Congenital accessory salivary glands and ducts
Congenital fistula of salivary gland

Q38.5 Congenital malformations of palate, not elsewhere classified
Congenital absence of uvula
Congenital malformation of palate NOS
Congenital high arched palate

EXCLUDES 1 *cleft palate (Q35.-)*
cleft palate with cleft lip (Q37.-)

Q38.6 Other congenital malformations of mouth
Congenital malformation of mouth NOS

Q38.7 Congenital pharyngeal pouch
Congenital diverticulum of pharynx

EXCLUDES 1 *pharyngeal pouch syndrome (D82.1)*

Q38.8 Other congenital malformations of pharynx
Congenital malformation of pharynx NOS
Imperforate pharynx

Q39 Congenital malformations of esophagus

Q39.0 Atresia of esophagus without fistula MCC
Atresia of esophagus NOS

Q39.1 Atresia of esophagus with tracheo-esophageal fistula MCC
Atresia of esophagus with broncho-esophageal fistula

Q39.2 Congenital tracheo-esophageal fistula without atresia MCC
Congenital tracheo-esophageal fistula NOS

Q39.3 Congenital stenosis and stricture of esophagus MCC

Q39.4 Esophageal web MCC

Q39.5 Congenital dilatation of esophagus CC
Congenital cardiospasm

Q39.6 Congenital diverticulum of esophagus CC
Congenital esophageal pouch

Q39.8 Other congenital malformations of esophagus CC
Congenital absence of esophagus
Congenital displacement of esophagus
Congenital duplication of esophagus

Q39.9 Congenital malformation of esophagus, unspecified CC

Q40 Other congenital malformations of upper alimentary tract

Q40.0 Congenital hypertrophic pyloric stenosis
Congenital or infantile constriction
Congenital or infantile hypertrophy
Congenital or infantile spasm
Congenital or infantile stenosis
Congenital or infantile stricture

Q40.1 Congenital hiatus hernia
Congenital displacement of cardia through esophageal hiatus

EXCLUDES 1 *congenital diaphragmatic hernia (Q79.0)*

Q40.2 Other specified congenital malformations of stomach
Congenital displacement of stomach
Congenital diverticulum of stomach
Congenital hourglass stomach
Congenital duplication of stomach
Megalogastria
Microgastria

Q40.3 Congenital malformation of stomach, unspecified

Q40.8 Other specified congenital malformations of upper alimentary tract

Q40.9 Congenital malformation of upper alimentary tract, unspecified
Congenital anomaly of upper alimentary tract
Congenital deformity of upper alimentary tract

Q41 Congenital absence, atresia and stenosis of small intestine

INCLUDES congenital obstruction, occlusion or stricture of small intestine or intestine NOS

EXCLUDES 1 *cystic fibrosis with intestinal manifestation (E84.11)*
meconium ileus NOS (without cystic fibrosis) (P76.0)

Q41.0 Congenital absence, atresia and stenosis of duodenum CC

Q41.1 Congenital absence, atresia and stenosis of jejunum CC
Apple peel syndrome
Imperforate jejunum

Q41.2 Congenital absence, atresia and stenosis of ileum CC

Q41.8 Congenital absence, atresia and stenosis of other specified parts of small intestine CC

Q41.9 Congenital absence, atresia and stenosis of small intestine, part unspecified CC
Congenital absence, atresia and stenosis of intestine NOS

Q42 Congenital absence, atresia and stenosis of large intestine
INCLUDES congenital obstruction, occlusion and stricture of large intestine

Q42.Ø Congenital absence, atresia and stenosis of rectum with fistula CC

Q42.1 Congenital absence, atresia and stenosis of rectum without fistula CC
Imperforate rectum

Q42.2 Congenital absence, atresia and stenosis of anus with fistula CC

Q42.3 Congenital absence, atresia and stenosis of anus without fistula CC
Imperforate anus

Q42.8 Congenital absence, atresia and stenosis of other parts of large intestine CC

Q42.9 Congenital absence, atresia and stenosis of large intestine, part unspecified CC

Q43 Other congenital malformations of intestine

Q43.Ø Meckel's diverticulum (displaced) (hypertrophic)
Persistent omphalomesenteric duct
Persistent vitelline duct
DEF: Congenital, abnormal remnant of embryonic digestive system development that leaves a sacculation or outpouching from the wall of the small intestine near the terminal part of the ileum made of acid-secreting tissue as in the stomach.

Q43.1 Hirschsprung's disease CC
Aganglionosis
Congenital (aganglionic) megacolon
DEF: Congenital enlargement or dilation of the colon, with the absence of nerve cells in a segment of colon distally that causes the inability to defecate.

Q43.2 Other congenital functional disorders of colon CC
Congenital dilatation of colon

Q43.3 Congenital malformations of intestinal fixation CC
Congenital omental, anomalous adhesions [bands]
Congenital peritoneal adhesions [bands]
Incomplete rotation of cecum and colon
Insufficient rotation of cecum and colon
Jackson's membrane
Malrotation of colon
Rotation failure of cecum and colon
Universal mesentery

Q43.4 Duplication of intestine CC

Q43.5 Ectopic anus CC

Q43.6 Congenital fistula of rectum and anus CC
EXCLUDES 1 *congenital fistula of anus with absence, atresia and stenosis (Q42.2)*
congenital fistula of rectum with absence, atresia and stenosis (Q42.Ø)
congenital rectovaginal fistula (Q52.2)
congenital urethrorectal fistula (Q64.73)
pilonidal fistula or sinus (LØ5.-)

Q43.7 Persistent cloaca CC
Cloaca NOS

Q43.8 Other specified congenital malformations of intestine CC
Congenital blind loop syndrome
Congenital diverticulitis, colon
Congenital diverticulum, intestine
Dolichocolon
Megaloappendix
Megaloduodenum
Microcolon
Transposition of appendix
Transposition of colon
Transposition of intestine
AHA: 2013,2Q,31

Q43.9 Congenital malformation of intestine, unspecified CC

Q44 Congenital malformations of gallbladder, bile ducts and liver

Q44.Ø Agenesis, aplasia and hypoplasia of gallbladder CC
Congenital absence of gallbladder

Q44.1 Other congenital malformations of gallbladder CC
Congenital malformation of gallbladder NOS
Intrahepatic gallbladder

Q44.2 Atresia of bile ducts MCC

Q44.3 Congenital stenosis and stricture of bile ducts MCC

Q44.4 Choledochal cyst CC

Q44.5 Other congenital malformations of bile ducts CC
Accessory hepatic duct
Biliary duct duplication
Congenital malformation of bile duct NOS
Cystic duct duplication

Q44.6 Cystic disease of liver CC
Fibrocystic disease of liver

Q44.7 Other congenital malformations of liver CC
Accessory liver
Alagille's syndrome
Congenital absence of liver
Congenital hepatomegaly
Congenital malformation of liver NOS

Q45 Other congenital malformations of digestive system
EXCLUDES 2 *congenital diaphragmatic hernia (Q79.Ø)*
congenital hiatus hernia (Q4Ø.1)

Q45.Ø Agenesis, aplasia and hypoplasia of pancreas CC
Congenital absence of pancreas

Q45.1 Annular pancreas CC

Q45.2 Congenital pancreatic cyst CC

Q45.3 Other congenital malformations of pancreas and pancreatic duct CC
Accessory pancreas
Congenital malformation of pancreas or pancreatic duct NOS
EXCLUDES 1 *congenital diabetes mellitus (E1Ø.-)*
cystic fibrosis (E84.Ø-E84.9)
fibrocystic disease of pancreas (E84.-)
neonatal diabetes mellitus (P7Ø.2)

Q45.8 Other specified congenital malformations of digestive system
Absence (complete) (partial) of alimentary tract NOS
Duplication of digestive system
Malposition, congenital of digestive system

Q45.9 Congenital malformation of digestive system, unspecified
Congenital anomaly of digestive system
Congenital deformity of digestive system

Congenital malformations of genital organs (Q5Ø-Q56)

EXCLUDES 1 *androgen insensitivity syndrome (E34.5-)*
syndromes associated with anomalies in the number and form of chromosomes (Q9Ø-Q99)

Q5Ø Congenital malformations of ovaries, fallopian tubes and broad ligaments

Q5Ø.Ø Congenital absence of ovary
EXCLUDES 1 *Turner's syndrome (Q96.-)*

Q5Ø.Ø1 Congenital absence of ovary, unilateral ♀

Q5Ø.Ø2 Congenital absence of ovary, bilateral ♀

Q5Ø.1 Developmental ovarian cyst ♀

Q5Ø.2 Congenital torsion of ovary ♀

Q5Ø.3 Other congenital malformations of ovary

Q5Ø.31 Accessory ovary ♀

Q5Ø.32 Ovarian streak ♀
46, XX with streak gonads

Q5Ø.39 Other congenital malformation of ovary ♀
Congenital malformation of ovary NOS

Q5Ø.4 Embryonic cyst of fallopian tube ♀
Fimbrial cyst

Q5Ø.5 Embryonic cyst of broad ligament ♀
Epoophoron cyst
Parovarian cyst

Q5Ø.6 Other congenital malformations of fallopian tube and broad ligament ♀
Absence of fallopian tube and broad ligament
Accessory fallopian tube and broad ligament
Atresia of fallopian tube and broad ligament
Congenital malformation of fallopian tube or broad ligament NOS

Q51 Congenital malformations of uterus and cervix

Q51.Ø Agenesis and aplasia of uterus ♀
Congenital absence of uterus

√5th **Q51.1 Doubling of uterus with doubling of cervix and vagina**

Q51.10 Doubling of uterus with doubling of cervix and vagina without obstruction ♀
Doubling of uterus with doubling of cervix and vagina NOS

Q51.11 Doubling of uterus with doubling of cervix and vagina with obstruction ♀

√5th **Q51.2 Other doubling of uterus**
Doubling of uterus NOS
Septate uterus
AHA: 2018,4Q,27

Q51.21 Complete doubling of uterus ♀
Complete septate uterus

Q51.22 Partial doubling of uterus ♀
Partial septate uterus

Q51.28 Other and unspecified doubling of uterus ♀
Septate uterus NOS

Q51.3 Bicornate uterus ♀
Bicornate uterus, complete or partial

Q51.4 Unicornate uterus ♀
Unicornate uterus with or without a separate uterine horn
Uterus with only one functioning horn

Q51.5 Agenesis and aplasia of cervix ♀
Congenital absence of cervix

Q51.6 Embryonic cyst of cervix ♀

Q51.7 Congenital fistulae between uterus and digestive and urinary tracts ♀

√5th **Q51.8 Other congenital malformations of uterus and cervix**

√6th **Q51.81 Other congenital malformations of uterus**

Q51.810 Arcuate uterus ♀
Arcuatus uterus

Q51.811 Hypoplasia of uterus ♀

Q51.818 Other congenital malformations of uterus ♀
Müllerian anomaly of uterus NEC

√6th **Q51.82 Other congenital malformations of cervix**

Q51.820 Cervical duplication ♀

Q51.821 Hypoplasia of cervix ♀

Q51.828 Other congenital malformations of cervix ♀

Q51.9 Congenital malformation of uterus and cervix, unspecified ♀

√4th **Q52 Other congenital malformations of female genitalia**

Q52.0 Congenital absence of vagina ♀
Vaginal agenesis, total or partial

√5th **Q52.1 Doubling of vagina**

EXCLUDES 1 *doubling of vagina with doubling of uterus and cervix (Q51.1-)*

Q52.10 Doubling of vagina, unspecified ♀
Septate vagina NOS

Q52.11 Transverse vaginal septum ♀

√6th **Q52.12 Longitudinal vaginal septum**
AHA: 2016,4Q,58-59

Q52.120 Longitudinal vaginal septum, nonobstructing ♀

Q52.121 Longitudinal vaginal septum, obstructing, right side ♀

Q52.122 Longitudinal vaginal septum, obstructing, left side ♀

Q52.123 Longitudinal vaginal septum, microperforate, right side ♀

Q52.124 Longitudinal vaginal septum, microperforate, left side ♀

Q52.129 Other and unspecified longitudinal vaginal septum ♀

Q52.2 Congenital rectovaginal fistula ♀

EXCLUDES 1 *cloaca (Q43.7)*

Q52.3 Imperforate hymen ♀

DEF: Obstructive anomaly of vagina, characterized by complete closure of the membranous fold around the external opening of the vagina, obstructing the vaginal introitus.

Q52.4 Other congenital malformations of vagina ♀
Canal of Nuck cyst, congenital
Congenital malformation of vagina NOS
Embryonic vaginal cyst
Gartner's duct cyst
AHA: 2022,2Q,15

Q52.5 Fusion of labia ♀

Q52.6 Congenital malformation of clitoris ♀

√5th **Q52.7 Other and unspecified congenital malformations of vulva**

Q52.70 Unspecified congenital malformations of vulva ♀
Congenital malformation of vulva NOS

Q52.71 Congenital absence of vulva ♀

Q52.79 Other congenital malformations of vulva ♀
Congenital cyst of vulva

Q52.8 Other specified congenital malformations of female genitalia ♀

Q52.9 Congenital malformation of female genitalia, unspecified ♀

√4th **Q53 Undescended and ectopic testicle**

√5th **Q53.0 Ectopic testis**

Q53.00 Ectopic testis, unspecified ♂

Q53.01 Ectopic testis, unilateral ♂

Q53.02 Ectopic testes, bilateral ♂

√5th **Q53.1 Undescended testicle, unilateral**
AHA: 2017,4Q,22-23

Q53.10 Unspecified undescended testicle, unilateral ♂

√6th **Q53.11 Abdominal testis, unilateral**

Q53.111 Unilateral intraabdominal testis ♂

Q53.112 Unilateral inguinal testis ♂

Q53.12 Ectopic perineal testis, unilateral ♂

Q53.13 Unilateral high scrotal testis ♂

√5th **Q53.2 Undescended testicle, bilateral**
AHA: 2017,4Q,22-23

Q53.20 Undescended testicle, unspecified, bilateral ♂

√6th **Q53.21 Abdominal testis, bilateral**

Q53.211 Bilateral intraabdominal testes ♂

Q53.212 Bilateral inguinal testes ♂

Q53.22 Ectopic perineal testis, bilateral ♂

Q53.23 Bilateral high scrotal testes ♂

Q53.9 Undescended testicle, unspecified ♂
Cryptorchism NOS

√4th **Q54 Hypospadias**

EXCLUDES 1 *epispadias (Q64.0)*

DEF: Abnormal opening of the urethra on the ventral (underside) surface of the penis.

Hypospadias

Q54.0 Hypospadias, balanic ♂
Hypospadias, coronal
Hypospadias, glandular

Q54.1 Hypospadias, penile ♂

Q54.2 Hypospadias, penoscrotal ♂

Q54.3 Hypospadias, perineal ♂

Q54.4 Congenital chordee ♂
Chordee without hypospadias

Q54.8 Other hypospadias ♂
Hypospadias with intersex state

Q54.9 Hypospadias, unspecified ♂

Q55 Other congenital malformations of male genital organs

EXCLUDES 1 *congenital hydrocele (P83.5)*
hypospadias (Q54.-)

Q55.0 Absence and aplasia of testis ♂
Monorchism

Q55.1 Hypoplasia of testis and scrotum ♂
Fusion of testes

Q55.2 Other and unspecified congenital malformations of testis and scrotum

Q55.20 Unspecified congenital malformations of testis and scrotum ♂
Congenital malformation of testis or scrotum NOS

Q55.21 Polyorchism ♂
DEF: Congenital anomaly in which there are more than two testes.

Q55.22 Retractile testis ♂

Q55.23 Scrotal transposition ♂

Q55.29 Other congenital malformations of testis and scrotum ♂

Q55.3 Atresia of vas deferens ♂
Code first any associated cystic fibrosis (E84.-)

Q55.4 Other congenital malformations of vas deferens, epididymis, seminal vesicles and prostate ♂
Absence or aplasia of prostate
Absence or aplasia of spermatic cord
Congenital malformation of vas deferens, epididymis, seminal vesicles or prostate NOS

Q55.5 Congenital absence and aplasia of penis ♂

Q55.6 Other congenital malformations of penis

Q55.61 Curvature of penis (lateral) ♂

Q55.62 Hypoplasia of penis ♂
Micropenis

Q55.63 Congenital torsion of penis ♂
EXCLUDES 1 *acquired torsion of penis (N48.82)*

Q55.64 Hidden penis ♂
Buried penis
Concealed penis
EXCLUDES 1 *acquired buried penis (N48.83)*

Q55.69 Other congenital malformation of penis ♂
Congenital malformation of penis NOS

Q55.7 Congenital vasocutaneous fistula ♂

Q55.8 Other specified congenital malformations of male genital organs ♂

Q55.9 Congenital malformation of male genital organ, unspecified ♂
Congenital anomaly of male genital organ
Congenital deformity of male genital organ

Q56 Indeterminate sex and pseudohermaphroditism

EXCLUDES 1 *46, XX true hermaphrodite (Q99.1)*
androgen insensitivity syndrome (E34.5-)
chimera 46, XX/46, XY true hermaphrodite (Q99.0)
female pseudohermaphroditism with adrenocortical disorder (E25.-)
pseudohermaphroditism with specified chromosomal anomaly (Q96-Q99)
pure gonadal dysgenesis (Q99.1)

DEF: Indeterminate sex: External genitalia that is nondescript, lacking the physical appearance specific to either sex.
DEF: Pseudohermaphroditism: Presence of gonads of one sex and external genitalia of another sex.

Q56.0 Hermaphroditism, not elsewhere classified
Ovotestis

Q56.1 Male pseudohermaphroditism, not elsewhere classified ♂
46, XY with streak gonads
Male pseudohermaphroditism NOS

Q56.2 Female pseudohermaphroditism, not elsewhere classified ♀
Female pseudohermaphroditism NOS

Q56.3 Pseudohermaphroditism, unspecified

Q56.4 Indeterminate sex, unspecified
Ambiguous genitalia

Congenital malformations of the urinary system (Q60-Q64)

Q60 Renal agenesis and other reduction defects of kidney

INCLUDES congenital absence of kidney
congenital atrophy of kidney
infantile atrophy of kidney

Q60.0 Renal agenesis, unilateral CC
Q60.1 Renal agenesis, bilateral CC
Q60.2 Renal agenesis, unspecified CC
Q60.3 Renal hypoplasia, unilateral CC
Q60.4 Renal hypoplasia, bilateral CC
Q60.5 Renal hypoplasia, unspecified CC
Q60.6 Potter's syndrome CC

Q61 Cystic kidney disease

EXCLUDES 1 *acquired cyst of kidney (N28.1)*
Potter's syndrome (Q60.6)

Q61.0 Congenital renal cyst

Q61.00 Congenital renal cyst, unspecified CC
Cyst of kidney NOS (congenital)

Q61.01 Congenital single renal cyst CC

Q61.02 Congenital multiple renal cysts CC

Q61.1 Polycystic kidney, infantile type
Polycystic kidney, autosomal recessive

Q61.11 Cystic dilatation of collecting ducts CC

Q61.19 Other polycystic kidney, infantile type CC

Q61.2 Polycystic kidney, adult type CC
Polycystic kidney, autosomal dominant

Q61.3 Polycystic kidney, unspecified CC
AHA: 2016,3Q,22

Q61.4 Renal dysplasia CC
Multicystic dysplastic kidney
Multicystic kidney (development)
Multicystic kidney disease
Multicystic renal dysplasia
EXCLUDES 1 *polycystic kidney disease (Q61.11-Q61.3)*

Q61.5 Medullary cystic kidney CC
Nephronophthisis
Sponge kidney NOS
DEF: Sponge kidney: Dilated collecting tubules that are usually asymptomatic. Calcinosis in tubules may cause renal insufficiency.

Q61.8 Other cystic kidney diseases CC
Fibrocystic kidney
Fibrocystic renal degeneration or disease

Q61.9 Cystic kidney disease, unspecified CC
Meckel-Gruber syndrome

Q62 Congenital obstructive defects of renal pelvis and congenital malformations of ureter

Q62.0 Congenital hydronephrosis CC

Q62.1 Congenital occlusion of ureter
Atresia and stenosis of ureter

Q62.10 Congenital occlusion of ureter, unspecified CC

Q62.11 Congenital occlusion of ureteropelvic junction CC

Q62.12 Congenital occlusion of ureterovesical orifice CC

Q62.2 Congenital megaureter CC
Congenital dilatation of ureter

Q62.3 Other obstructive defects of renal pelvis and ureter

Q62.31 Congenital ureterocele, orthotopic CC

Q62.32 Cecoureterocele CC
Ectopic ureterocele

Q62.39 Other obstructive defects of renal pelvis and ureter CC
Ureteropelvic junction obstruction NOS

Q62.4 Agenesis of ureter
Congenital absence ureter

Q62.5 Duplication of ureter
Accessory ureter
Double ureter

Q62.6 Malposition of ureter

Q62.60 Malposition of ureter, unspecified

Q62.61 Deviation of ureter

Q62.62 Displacement of ureter

Q62.63 Anomalous implantation of ureter
Ectopia of ureter
Ectopic ureter

Q62.69 Other malposition of ureter

Q62.7 Congenital vesico-uretero-renal reflux

Q62.8 Other congenital malformations of ureter
Anomaly of ureter NOS

Q63 Other congenital malformations of kidney (4th)
EXCLUDES 1 *congenital nephrotic syndrome (NØ4.-)*

Q63.Ø Accessory kidney

Q63.1 Lobulated, fused and horseshoe kidney

Q63.2 Ectopic kidney
Congenital displaced kidney
Malrotation of kidney

Q63.3 Hyperplastic and giant kidney
Compensatory hypertrophy of kidney

Q63.8 Other specified congenital malformations of kidney
Congenital renal calculi

Q63.9 Congenital malformation of kidney, unspecified

Q64 Other congenital malformations of urinary system (4th)

Q64.Ø Epispadias
EXCLUDES 1 *hypospadias (Q54.-)*

Epispadias

Normal external urethral orifice
Glans penis
Foreskin (retracted)
Epispadias
Epispadias (dorsal view)

Q64.1 Exstrophy of urinary bladder (5th)

Q64.1Ø Exstrophy of urinary bladder, unspecified CC
Ectopia vesicae

Q64.11 Supravesical fissure of urinary bladder CC

Q64.12 Cloacal exstrophy of urinary bladder CC

Q64.19 Other exstrophy of urinary bladder CC
Extroversion of bladder

Q64.2 Congenital posterior urethral valves CC

Q64.3 Other atresia and stenosis of urethra and bladder neck (5th)

Q64.31 Congenital bladder neck obstruction CC
Congenital obstruction of vesicourethral orifice

Q64.32 Congenital stricture of urethra CC

Q64.33 Congenital stricture of urinary meatus CC

Q64.39 Other atresia and stenosis of urethra and bladder neck CC
Atresia and stenosis of urethra and bladder neck NOS

Q64.4 Malformation of urachus
Cyst of urachus
Patent urachus
Prolapse of urachus

Q64.5 Congenital absence of bladder and urethra

Q64.6 Congenital diverticulum of bladder

Q64.7 Other and unspecified congenital malformations of bladder and urethra (5th)
EXCLUDES 1 *congenital prolapse of bladder (mucosa) (Q79.4)*

Q64.7Ø Unspecified congenital malformation of bladder and urethra
Malformation of bladder or urethra NOS

Q64.71 Congenital prolapse of urethra

Q64.72 Congenital prolapse of urinary meatus

Q64.73 Congenital urethrorectal fistula

Q64.74 Double urethra

Q64.75 Double urinary meatus

Q64.79 Other congenital malformations of bladder and urethra

Q64.8 Other specified congenital malformations of urinary system

Q64.9 Congenital malformation of urinary system, unspecified
Congenital anomaly NOS of urinary system
Congenital deformity NOS of urinary system

Congenital malformations and deformations of the musculoskeletal system (Q65-Q79)

Q65 Congenital deformities of hip (4th)
EXCLUDES 1 *clicking hip (R29.4)*

Q65.Ø Congenital dislocation of hip, unilateral (5th)

Q65.ØØ Congenital dislocation of unspecified hip, unilateral

Q65.Ø1 Congenital dislocation of right hip, unilateral

Q65.Ø2 Congenital dislocation of left hip, unilateral

Q65.1 Congenital dislocation of hip, bilateral

Q65.2 Congenital dislocation of hip, unspecified

Q65.3 Congenital partial dislocation of hip, unilateral (5th)

Q65.3Ø Congenital partial dislocation of unspecified hip, unilateral

Q65.31 Congenital partial dislocation of right hip, unilateral

Q65.32 Congenital partial dislocation of left hip, unilateral

Q65.4 Congenital partial dislocation of hip, bilateral

Q65.5 Congenital partial dislocation of hip, unspecified

Q65.6 Congenital unstable hip
Congenital dislocatable hip

Q65.8 Other congenital deformities of hip (5th)

Q65.81 Congenital coxa valga

Q65.82 Congenital coxa vara

Q65.89 Other specified congenital deformities of hip
Anteversion of femoral neck
Congenital acetabular dysplasia

Q65.9 Congenital deformity of hip, unspecified

Q66 Congenital deformities of feet (4th)
EXCLUDES 1 *reduction defects of feet (Q72.-)*
valgus deformities (acquired) (M21.Ø-)
varus deformities (acquired) (M21.1-)

AHA: 2019,4Q,13

Q66.Ø Congenital talipes equinovarus (5th)

Q66.ØØ Congenital talipes equinovarus, unspecified foot

Q66.Ø1 Congenital talipes equinovarus, right foot

Q66.Ø2 Congenital talipes equinovarus, left foot

Q66.1 Congenital talipes calcaneovarus (5th)

Q66.1Ø Congenital talipes calcaneovarus, unspecified foot

Q66.11 Congenital talipes calcaneovarus, right foot

Q66.12 Congenital talipes calcaneovarus, left foot

Q66.2 Congenital metatarsus (primus) varus (5th)
AHA: 2016,4Q,59

Q66.21 Congenital metatarsus primus varus (6th)

Q66.211 Congenital metatarsus primus varus, right foot

Q66.212 Congenital metatarsus primus varus, left foot

Q66.219 Congenital metatarsus primus varus, unspecified foot

Q66.22 Congenital metatarsus adductus (6th)
Congenital metatarsus varus

Q66.221 Congenital metatarsus adductus, right foot

Q66.222 Congenital metatarsus adductus, left foot

Q66.229 Congenital metatarsus adductus, unspecified foot

Q66.3 Other congenital varus deformities of feet (5th)
Hallux varus, congenital

Q66.3Ø Other congenital varus deformities of feet, unspecified foot

Q66.31 Other congenital varus deformities of feet, right foot

Q66.32 Other congenital varus deformities of feet, left foot

Q66.4 Congenital talipes calcaneovalgus (5th)

Q66.4Ø Congenital talipes calcaneovalgus, unspecified foot

Q66.41 Congenital talipes calcaneovalgus, right foot

Q66.42 Congenital talipes calcaneovalgus, left foot

Q66.5 Congenital pes planus (5th)
Congenital flat foot
Congenital rigid flat foot
Congenital spastic (everted) flat foot
EXCLUDES 1 *pes planus, acquired (M21.4)*

Q66.5Ø Congenital pes planus, unspecified foot

Q66.51 **Congenital pes planus, right foot**
Q66.52 **Congenital pes planus, left foot**
Q66.6 **Other congenital valgus deformities of feet**
Congenital metatarsus valgus
Q66.7 **Congenital pes cavus**
Q66.70 **Congenital pes cavus, unspecified foot**
Q66.71 **Congenital pes cavus, right foot**
Q66.72 **Congenital pes cavus, left foot**
Q66.8 **Other congenital deformities of feet**
Q66.80 **Congenital vertical talus deformity, unspecified foot**
Q66.81 **Congenital vertical talus deformity, right foot**
Q66.82 **Congenital vertical talus deformity, left foot**
Q66.89 **Other specified congenital deformities of feet**
Congenital asymmetric talipes
Congenital clubfoot NOS
Congenital talipes NOS
Congenital tarsal coalition
Hammer toe, congenital
DEF: Clubfoot: Congenital anomaly of the foot with the heel elevated and rotated outward and the toes pointing inward.
Q66.9 **Congenital deformity of feet, unspecified**
Q66.90 **Congenital deformity of feet, unspecified, unspecified foot**
Q66.91 **Congenital deformity of feet, unspecified, right foot**
Q66.92 **Congenital deformity of feet, unspecified, left foot**

Q67 **Congenital musculoskeletal deformities of head, face, spine and chest**
EXCLUDES 1 *congenital malformation syndromes classified to Q87.-*
Potter's syndrome (Q60.6)
Q67.0 **Congenital facial asymmetry**
Q67.1 **Congenital compression facies**
Q67.2 **Dolichocephaly**
Q67.3 **Plagiocephaly**
Q67.4 **Other congenital deformities of skull, face and jaw**
Congenital depressions in skull
Congenital hemifacial atrophy or hypertrophy
Deviation of nasal septum, congenital
Squashed or bent nose, congenital
EXCLUDES 1 *dentofacial anomalies [including malocclusion] (M26.-)*
syphilitic saddle nose (A50.5)
DEF: Deviated septum: Condition in which the nasal septum, a thin wall composed of cartilage and bone that separates the two nostrils, is crooked or displaced from the midline.
Q67.5 **Congenital deformity of spine** CC
Congenital postural scoliosis
Congenital scoliosis NOS
EXCLUDES 1 *infantile idiopathic scoliosis (M41.0)*
scoliosis due to congenital bony malformation (Q76.3)
AHA: 2014,4Q,26
Q67.6 **Pectus excavatum**
Congenital funnel chest
Q67.7 **Pectus carinatum**
Congenital pigeon chest
Q67.8 **Other congenital deformities of chest** CC
Congenital deformity of chest wall NOS

Q68 **Other congenital musculoskeletal deformities**
EXCLUDES 1 *reduction defects of limb(s) (Q71-Q73)*
EXCLUDES 2 *congenital myotonic chondrodystrophy (G71.13)*
Q68.0 **Congenital deformity of sternocleidomastoid muscle**
Congenital contracture of sternocleidomastoid (muscle)
Congenital (sternomastoid) torticollis
Sternomastoid tumor (congenital)
Q68.1 **Congenital deformity of finger(s) and hand** CC
Congenital clubfinger
Spade-like hand (congenital)
Q68.2 **Congenital deformity of knee**
Congenital dislocation of knee
Congenital genu recurvatum
Q68.3 **Congenital bowing of femur**
EXCLUDES 1 *anteversion of femur (neck) (Q65.89)*
Q68.4 **Congenital bowing of tibia and fibula**
Q68.5 **Congenital bowing of long bones of leg, unspecified**
Q68.6 **Discoid meniscus**
Q68.8 **Other specified congenital musculoskeletal deformities**
Congenital deformity of clavicle
Congenital deformity of elbow
Congenital deformity of forearm
Congenital deformity of scapula
Congenital deformity of wrist
Congenital dislocation of elbow
Congenital dislocation of shoulder
Congenital dislocation of wrist

Q69 **Polydactyly**
Q69.0 **Accessory finger(s)**
Q69.1 **Accessory thumb(s)**
Q69.2 **Accessory toe(s)**
Accessory hallux
Q69.9 **Polydactyly, unspecified**
Supernumerary digit(s) NOS

Q70 **Syndactyly**
Q70.0 **Fused fingers**
Complex syndactyly of fingers with synostosis
Q70.00 **Fused fingers, unspecified hand**
Q70.01 **Fused fingers, right hand**
Q70.02 **Fused fingers, left hand**
Q70.03 **Fused fingers, bilateral**
Q70.1 **Webbed fingers**
Simple syndactyly of fingers without synostosis
Q70.10 **Webbed fingers, unspecified hand**
Q70.11 **Webbed fingers, right hand**
Q70.12 **Webbed fingers, left hand**
Q70.13 **Webbed fingers, bilateral**
Q70.2 **Fused toes**
Complex syndactyly of toes with synostosis
Q70.20 **Fused toes, unspecified foot**
Q70.21 **Fused toes, right foot**
Q70.22 **Fused toes, left foot**
Q70.23 **Fused toes, bilateral**
Q70.3 **Webbed toes**
Simple syndactyly of toes without synostosis
Q70.30 **Webbed toes, unspecified foot**
Q70.31 **Webbed toes, right foot**
Q70.32 **Webbed toes, left foot**
Q70.33 **Webbed toes, bilateral**
Q70.4 **Polysyndactyly, unspecified**
EXCLUDES 1 *specified syndactyly of hand and feet - code to specified conditions (Q70.0-Q70.3-)*
Q70.9 **Syndactyly, unspecified**
Symphalangy NOS

Q71 **Reduction defects of upper limb**
Q71.0 **Congenital complete absence of upper limb**
Q71.00 **Congenital complete absence of unspecified upper limb**
Q71.01 **Congenital complete absence of right upper limb**
Q71.02 **Congenital complete absence of left upper limb**
Q71.03 **Congenital complete absence of upper limb, bilateral**
Q71.1 **Congenital absence of upper arm and forearm with hand present**
Q71.10 **Congenital absence of unspecified upper arm and forearm with hand present**
Q71.11 **Congenital absence of right upper arm and forearm with hand present**
Q71.12 **Congenital absence of left upper arm and forearm with hand present**
Q71.13 **Congenital absence of upper arm and forearm with hand present, bilateral**
Q71.2 **Congenital absence of both forearm and hand**
Q71.20 **Congenital absence of both forearm and hand, unspecified upper limb**
Q71.21 **Congenital absence of both forearm and hand, right upper limb**
Q71.22 **Congenital absence of both forearm and hand, left upper limb**
Q71.23 **Congenital absence of both forearm and hand, bilateral**

Q71.3 Congenital absence of hand and finger
- Q71.3Ø Congenital absence of unspecified hand and finger
- Q71.31 Congenital absence of right hand and finger
- Q71.32 Congenital absence of left hand and finger
- Q71.33 Congenital absence of hand and finger, bilateral

Q71.4 Longitudinal reduction defect of radius
Clubhand (congenital)
Radial clubhand
- Q71.4Ø Longitudinal reduction defect of unspecified radius
- Q71.41 Longitudinal reduction defect of right radius
- Q71.42 Longitudinal reduction defect of left radius
- Q71.43 Longitudinal reduction defect of radius, bilateral

Q71.5 Longitudinal reduction defect of ulna
- Q71.5Ø Longitudinal reduction defect of unspecified ulna
- Q71.51 Longitudinal reduction defect of right ulna
- Q71.52 Longitudinal reduction defect of left ulna
- Q71.53 Longitudinal reduction defect of ulna, bilateral

Q71.6 Lobster-claw hand
- Q71.6Ø Lobster-claw hand, unspecified hand
- Q71.61 Lobster-claw right hand
- Q71.62 Lobster-claw left hand
- Q71.63 Lobster-claw hand, bilateral

Q71.8 Other reduction defects of upper limb

Q71.81 Congenital shortening of upper limb
- Q71.811 Congenital shortening of right upper limb
- Q71.812 Congenital shortening of left upper limb
- Q71.813 Congenital shortening of upper limb, bilateral
- Q71.819 Congenital shortening of unspecified upper limb

Q71.89 Other reduction defects of upper limb
- Q71.891 Other reduction defects of right upper limb
- Q71.892 Other reduction defects of left upper limb
- Q71.893 Other reduction defects of upper limb, bilateral
- Q71.899 Other reduction defects of unspecified upper limb

Q71.9 Unspecified reduction defect of upper limb
- Q71.9Ø Unspecified reduction defect of unspecified upper limb
- Q71.91 Unspecified reduction defect of right upper limb
- Q71.92 Unspecified reduction defect of left upper limb
- Q71.93 Unspecified reduction defect of upper limb, bilateral

Q72 Reduction defects of lower limb

Q72.Ø Congenital complete absence of lower limb
- Q72.ØØ Congenital complete absence of unspecified lower limb
- Q72.Ø1 Congenital complete absence of right lower limb
- Q72.Ø2 Congenital complete absence of left lower limb
- Q72.Ø3 Congenital complete absence of lower limb, bilateral

Q72.1 Congenital absence of thigh and lower leg with foot present
- Q72.1Ø Congenital absence of unspecified thigh and lower leg with foot present
- Q72.11 Congenital absence of right thigh and lower leg with foot present
- Q72.12 Congenital absence of left thigh and lower leg with foot present
- Q72.13 Congenital absence of thigh and lower leg with foot present, bilateral

Q72.2 Congenital absence of both lower leg and foot
- Q72.2Ø Congenital absence of both lower leg and foot, unspecified lower limb
- Q72.21 Congenital absence of both lower leg and foot, right lower limb
- Q72.22 Congenital absence of both lower leg and foot, left lower limb
- Q72.23 Congenital absence of both lower leg and foot, bilateral

Q72.3 Congenital absence of foot and toe(s)
- Q72.3Ø Congenital absence of unspecified foot and toe(s)
- Q72.31 Congenital absence of right foot and toe(s)
- Q72.32 Congenital absence of left foot and toe(s)
- Q72.33 Congenital absence of foot and toe(s), bilateral

Q72.4 Longitudinal reduction defect of femur
Proximal femoral focal deficiency
- Q72.4Ø Longitudinal reduction defect of unspecified femur
- Q72.41 Longitudinal reduction defect of right femur
- Q72.42 Longitudinal reduction defect of left femur
- Q72.43 Longitudinal reduction defect of femur, bilateral

Q72.5 Longitudinal reduction defect of tibia
- Q72.5Ø Longitudinal reduction defect of unspecified tibia
- Q72.51 Longitudinal reduction defect of right tibia
- Q72.52 Longitudinal reduction defect of left tibia
- Q72.53 Longitudinal reduction defect of tibia, bilateral

Q72.6 Longitudinal reduction defect of fibula
- Q72.6Ø Longitudinal reduction defect of unspecified fibula
- Q72.61 Longitudinal reduction defect of right fibula
- Q72.62 Longitudinal reduction defect of left fibula
- Q72.63 Longitudinal reduction defect of fibula, bilateral

Q72.7 Split foot
- Q72.7Ø Split foot, unspecified lower limb
- Q72.71 Split foot, right lower limb
- Q72.72 Split foot, left lower limb
- Q72.73 Split foot, bilateral

Q72.8 Other reduction defects of lower limb

Q72.81 Congenital shortening of lower limb
- Q72.811 Congenital shortening of right lower limb
- Q72.812 Congenital shortening of left lower limb
- Q72.813 Congenital shortening of lower limb, bilateral
- Q72.819 Congenital shortening of unspecified lower limb

Q72.89 Other reduction defects of lower limb
- Q72.891 Other reduction defects of right lower limb
- Q72.892 Other reduction defects of left lower limb
- Q72.893 Other reduction defects of lower limb, bilateral
- Q72.899 Other reduction defects of unspecified lower limb

Q72.9 Unspecified reduction defect of lower limb
- Q72.9Ø Unspecified reduction defect of unspecified lower limb
- Q72.91 Unspecified reduction defect of right lower limb
- Q72.92 Unspecified reduction defect of left lower limb
- Q72.93 Unspecified reduction defect of lower limb, bilateral

Q73 Reduction defects of unspecified limb

Q73.Ø Congenital absence of unspecified limb(s)
Amelia NOS

Q73.1 Phocomelia, unspecified limb(s)
Phocomelia NOS

Q73.8 Other reduction defects of unspecified limb(s)
Longitudinal reduction deformity of unspecified limb(s)
Ectromelia of limb NOS
Hemimelia of limb NOS
Reduction defect of limb NOS

Q74 Other congenital malformations of limb(s)

EXCLUDES 1 *polydactyly (Q69.-)*
reduction defect of limb (Q71-Q73)
syndactyly (Q7Ø.-)

Q74.Ø Other congenital malformations of upper limb(s), including shoulder girdle
Accessory carpal bones
Cleidocranial dysostosis
Congenital pseudarthrosis of clavicle
Macrodactylia (fingers)
Madelung's deformity
Radioulnar synostosis
Sprengel's deformity
Triphalangeal thumb

Q74.1 Congenital malformation of knee
Congenital absence of patella
Congenital dislocation of patella
Congenital genu valgum
Congenital genu varum
Rudimentary patella
EXCLUDES 1 *congenital dislocation of knee (Q68.2)*
congenital genu recurvatum (Q68.2)
nail patella syndrome (Q87.2)

Q74.2 Other congenital malformations of lower limb(s), including pelvic girdle
Congenital fusion of sacroiliac joint
Congenital malformation of ankle joint
Congenital malformation of sacroiliac joint
EXCLUDES 1 *anteversion of femur (neck) (Q65.89)*

Q74.3 Arthrogryposis multiplex congenita CC

Q74.8 Other specified congenital malformations of limb(s)

Q74.9 Unspecified congenital malformation of limb(s)
Congenital anomaly of limb(s) NOS

Q75 Other congenital malformations of skull and face bones
EXCLUDES 1 *congenital malformation of face NOS (Q18.-)*
congenital malformation syndromes classified to Q87.-
dentofacial anomalies [including malocclusion] (M26.-)
musculoskeletal deformities of head and face (Q67.Ø-Q67.4)
skull defects associated with congenital anomalies of brain such as:
anencephaly (QØØ.Ø)
encephalocele (QØ1.-)
hydrocephalus (QØ3.-)
microcephaly (QØ2)

Q75.Ø Craniosynostosis
Acrocephaly
Imperfect fusion of skull
Oxycephaly
Trigonocephaly
DEF: Congenital condition in which one or more of the cranial sutures fuse prematurely, creating a deformed or aberrant head shape.

Q75.1 Craniofacial dysostosis
Crouzon's disease

Q75.2 Hypertelorism

Q75.3 Macrocephaly

Q75.4 Mandibulofacial dysostosis
Franceschetti syndrome
Treacher Collins syndrome

Q75.5 Oculomandibular dysostosis

Q75.8 Other specified congenital malformations of skull and face bones
Absence of skull bone, congenital
Congenital deformity of forehead
Platybasia

Q75.9 Congenital malformation of skull and face bones, unspecified
Congenital anomaly of face bones NOS
Congenital anomaly of skull NOS

Q76 Congenital malformations of spine and bony thorax
EXCLUDES 1 *congenital musculoskeletal deformities of spine and chest (Q67.5-Q67.8)*

Q76.Ø Spina bifida occulta
EXCLUDES 1 *meningocele (spinal) (QØ5.-)*
spina bifida (aperta) (cystica) (QØ5.-)

Q76.1 Klippel-Feil syndrome
Cervical fusion syndrome

Q76.2 Congenital spondylolisthesis
Congenital spondylolysis
EXCLUDES 1 *spondylolisthesis (acquired) (M43.1-)*
spondylolysis (acquired) (M43.Ø-)

Q76.3 Congenital scoliosis due to congenital bony malformation CC
Hemivertebra fusion or failure of segmentation with scoliosis

Q76.4 Other congenital malformations of spine, not associated with scoliosis

Q76.41 Congenital kyphosis

Q76.411 Congenital kyphosis, occipito-atlanto-axial region

Q76.412 Congenital kyphosis, cervical region

Q76.413 Congenital kyphosis, cervicothoracic region

Q76.414 Congenital kyphosis, thoracic region

Q76.415 Congenital kyphosis, thoracolumbar region

Q76.419 Congenital kyphosis, unspecified region

Q76.42 Congenital lordosis

Q76.425 Congenital lordosis, thoracolumbar region CC

Q76.426 Congenital lordosis, lumbar region CC

Q76.427 Congenital lordosis, lumbosacral region CC

Q76.428 Congenital lordosis, sacral and sacrococcygeal region CC

Q76.429 Congenital lordosis, unspecified region CC

Q76.49 Other congenital malformations of spine, not associated with scoliosis
Congenital absence of vertebra NOS
Congenital fusion of spine NOS
Congenital malformation of lumbosacral (joint) (region) NOS
Congenital malformation of spine NOS
Hemivertebra NOS
Malformation of spine NOS
Platyspondylisis NOS
Supernumerary vertebra NOS

Q76.5 Cervical rib
Supernumerary rib in cervical region

Q76.6 Other congenital malformations of ribs CC
Accessory rib
Congenital absence of rib
Congenital fusion of ribs
Congenital malformation of ribs NOS
EXCLUDES 1 *short rib syndrome (Q77.2)*

Q76.7 Congenital malformation of sternum CC
Congenital absence of sternum
Sternum bifidum

Q76.8 Other congenital malformations of bony thorax CC

Q76.9 Congenital malformation of bony thorax, unspecified CC

Q77 Osteochondrodysplasia with defects of growth of tubular bones and spine
EXCLUDES 1 *mucopolysaccharidosis (E76.Ø-E76.3)*
EXCLUDES 2 *congenital myotonic chondrodystrophy (G71.13)*

Q77.Ø Achondrogenesis
Hypochondrogenesis

Q77.1 Thanatophoric short stature

Q77.2 Short rib syndrome CC
Asphyxiating thoracic dysplasia [Jeune]

Q77.3 Chondrodysplasia punctata
EXCLUDES 1 *Rhizomelic chondrodysplasia punctata (E71.43)*

Q77.4 Achondroplasia
Hypochondroplasia
Osteosclerosis congenita

Q77.5 Diastrophic dysplasia

Q77.6 Chondroectodermal dysplasia
Ellis-van Creveld syndrome

Q77.7 Spondyloepiphyseal dysplasia

Q77.8 Other osteochondrodysplasia with defects of growth of tubular bones and spine

Q77.9 Osteochondrodysplasia with defects of growth of tubular bones and spine, unspecified

Q78 Other osteochondrodysplasias
EXCLUDES 2 *congenital myotonic chondrodystrophy (G71.13)*

Q78.Ø Osteogenesis imperfecta CC
Fragilitas ossium
Osteopsathyrosis

Q78.1 Polyostotic fibrous dysplasia
Albright(-McCune)(-Sternberg) syndrome

Q78.2 Osteopetrosis CC
Albers-Schönberg syndrome
Osteosclerosis NOS
DEF: Rare congenital condition in which the bones are excessively dense, resulting from a discrepancy in the formation and breakdown of bone.

Q78.3 Progressive diaphyseal dysplasia
Camurati-Engelmann syndrome
Q78.4 Enchondromatosis
Maffucci's syndrome
Ollier's disease
Q78.5 Metaphyseal dysplasia
Pyle's syndrome
Q78.6 Multiple congenital exostoses
Diaphyseal aclasis
Q78.8 Other specified osteochondrodysplasias
Osteopoikilosis
Q78.9 Osteochondrodysplasia, unspecified
Chondrodystrophy NOS
Osteodystrophy NOS

Q79 Congenital malformations of musculoskeletal system, not elsewhere classified
EXCLUDES 2 *congenital (sternomastoid) torticollis (Q68.Ø)*

Q79.Ø Congenital diaphragmatic hernia MCC
EXCLUDES 1 *congenital hiatus hernia (Q4Ø.1)*

Q79.1 Other congenital malformations of diaphragm MCC
Absence of diaphragm
Congenital malformation of diaphragm NOS
Eventration of diaphragm

Q79.2 Exomphalos MCC
Omphalocele
EXCLUDES 1 *umbilical hernia (K42.-)*

Q79.3 Gastroschisis MCC

Gastroschisis

Q79.4 Prune belly syndrome MCC
Congenital prolapse of bladder mucosa
Eagle-Barrett syndrome

Q79.5 Other congenital malformations of abdominal wall
EXCLUDES 1 *umbilical hernia (K42.-)*
Q79.51 Congenital hernia of bladder MCC
Q79.59 Other congenital malformations of abdominal wall MCC

Q79.6 Ehlers-Danlos syndromes
AHA: 2019,4Q,13-14
DEF: Connective tissue disorder that causes hyperextended skin and joints and results in fragile blood vessels with bleeding, poor wound healing, and subcutaneous pseudotumors.
Q79.6Ø Ehlers-Danlos syndrome, unspecified CC
Q79.61 Classical Ehlers-Danlos syndrome CC
Classical EDS (cEDS)
Q79.62 Hypermobile Ehlers-Danlos syndrome CC
Hypermobile EDS (hEDS)
Q79.63 Vascular Ehlers-Danlos syndrome CC
Vascular EDS (vEDS)
Q79.69 Other Ehlers-Danlos syndromes CC

Q79.8 Other congenital malformations of musculoskeletal system
Absence of muscle
Absence of tendon
Accessory muscle
Amyotrophia congenita
Congenital constricting bands
Congenital shortening of tendon
Poland syndrome

Q79.9 Congenital malformation of musculoskeletal system, unspecified
Congenital anomaly of musculoskeletal system NOS
Congenital deformity of musculoskeletal system NOS

Other congenital malformations (Q8Ø-Q89)

Q8Ø Congenital ichthyosis
EXCLUDES 1 *Refsum's disease (G6Ø.1)*
DEF: Excessive production of skin cells resulting in red, dry, scaly skin.
Q8Ø.Ø Ichthyosis vulgaris
Q8Ø.1 X-linked ichthyosis
Q8Ø.2 Lamellar ichthyosis
Collodion baby
Q8Ø.3 Congenital bullous ichthyosiform erythroderma
Q8Ø.4 Harlequin fetus
Q8Ø.8 Other congenital ichthyosis
Q8Ø.9 Congenital ichthyosis, unspecified

Q81 Epidermolysis bullosa
Q81.Ø Epidermolysis bullosa simplex
EXCLUDES 1 *Cockayne's syndrome (Q87.19)*
Q81.1 Epidermolysis bullosa letalis
Herlitz' syndrome
Q81.2 Epidermolysis bullosa dystrophica
Q81.8 Other epidermolysis bullosa
Q81.9 Epidermolysis bullosa, unspecified

Q82 Other congenital malformations of skin
EXCLUDES 1 *acrodermatitis enteropathica (E83.2)*
congenital erythropoietic porphyria (E8Ø.Ø)
pilonidal cyst or sinus (LØ5.-)
Sturge-Weber (-Dimitri) syndrome ▶(Q85.89)◀
Q82.Ø Hereditary lymphedema
Q82.1 Xeroderma pigmentosum
Q82.2 Congenital cutaneous mastocytosis
Congenital diffuse cutaneous mastocytosis
Congenital maculopapular cutaneous mastocytosis
Congenital urticaria pigmentosa
EXCLUDES 1 *cutaneous mastocytosis NOS (D47.Ø1)*
diffuse cutaneous mastocytosis (with onset after newborn period) (D47.Ø1)
malignant mastocytosis (C96.2-)
systemic mastocytosis (D47.Ø2)
urticaria pigmentosa (non-congenital) (with onset after newborn period) (D47.Ø1)
AHA: 2017,4Q,5
Q82.3 Incontinentia pigmenti
Q82.4 Ectodermal dysplasia (anhidrotic)
EXCLUDES 1 *Ellis-van Creveld syndrome (Q77.6)*
Q82.5 Congenital non-neoplastic nevus
Birthmark NOS
Flammeus Nevus
Portwine Nevus
Sanguineous Nevus
Strawberry Nevus
Vascular Nevus NOS
Verrucous Nevus
EXCLUDES 2 *araneus nevus (I78.1)*
Café au lait spots (L81.3)
lentigo (L81.4)
melanocytic nevus (D22.-)
nevus NOS (D22.-)
pigmented nevus (D22.-)
spider nevus (I78.1)
stellar nevus (I78.1)
Q82.6 Congenital sacral dimple
Parasacral dimple
EXCLUDES 2 *pilonidal cyst with abscess (LØ5.Ø1)*
pilonidal cyst without abscess (LØ5.91)
AHA: 2016,4Q,60

Q82.8 Other specified congenital malformations of skin
Abnormal palmar creases
Accessory skin tags
Benign familial pemphigus [Hailey-Hailey]
Congenital poikiloderma
Cutis laxa (hyperelastica)
Dermatoglyphic anomalies
Inherited keratosis palmaris et plantaris
Keratosis follicularis [Darier-White]
EXCLUDES 1 *Ehlers-Danlos syndromes (Q79.6-)*
AHA: 2021,3Q,10; 2016,1Q,17

Q82.9 Congenital malformation of skin, unspecified

Q83 Congenital malformations of breast
EXCLUDES 2 *absence of pectoral muscle (Q79.8)*
hypoplasia of breast (N64.82)
micromastia (N64.82)

Q83.0 Congenital absence of breast with absent nipple
Q83.1 Accessory breast
Supernumerary breast
Q83.2 Absent nipple
Q83.3 Accessory nipple
Supernumerary nipple
Q83.8 Other congenital malformations of breast
Q83.9 Congenital malformation of breast, unspecified

Q84 Other congenital malformations of integument
Q84.0 Congenital alopecia
Congenital atrichosis
Q84.1 Congenital morphological disturbances of hair, not elsewhere classified
Beaded hair
Monilethrix
Pili annulati
EXCLUDES 1 *Menkes' kinky hair syndrome (E83.0)*
Q84.2 Other congenital malformations of hair
Congenital hypertrichosis
Congenital malformation of hair NOS
Persistent lanugo
Q84.3 Anonychia
EXCLUDES 1 *nail patella syndrome (Q87.2)*
Q84.4 Congenital leukonychia
Q84.5 Enlarged and hypertrophic nails
Congenital onychauxis
Pachyonychia
Q84.6 Other congenital malformations of nails
Congenital clubnail
Congenital koilonychia
Congenital malformation of nail NOS
Q84.8 Other specified congenital malformations of integument
Aplasia cutis congenita
Q84.9 Congenital malformation of integument, unspecified
Congenital anomaly of integument NOS
Congenital deformity of integument NOS

Q85 Phakomatoses, not elsewhere classified
EXCLUDES 1 *ataxia telangiectasia [Louis-Bar] (G11.3)*
familial dysautonomia [Riley-Day] (G90.1)

Q85.0 Neurofibromatosis (nonmalignant)
Q85.00 Neurofibromatosis, unspecified HCC
Q85.01 Neurofibromatosis, type 1 HCC
Von Recklinghausen disease
Q85.02 Neurofibromatosis, type 2 HCC
Acoustic neurofibromatosis
DEF: Inherited condition with cutaneous lesions, benign tumors of peripheral nerves, and bilateral 8th nerve masses.
Q85.03 Schwannomatosis HCC
DEF: Genetic mutation (SMARCB1/INI1) causing multiple benign tumors along the nerve pathways, except on the 8th cranial (vestibular) nerve.
Q85.09 Other neurofibromatosis HCC
Q85.1 Tuberous sclerosis CC HCC
Bourneville's disease
Epiloia

▲ **Q85.8 Other phakomatoses, not elsewhere classified**
~~Peutz-Jeghers Syndrome~~
~~Sturge-Weber(-Dimitri) syndrome~~
~~von Hippel-Lindau syndrome~~
EXCLUDES 1 *Meckel-Gruber syndrome (Q61.9)*
AHA: 2021,3Q,12

● **Q85.81 PTEN tumor syndrome** CC
PHTS
PTEN hamartoma tumor syndrome
PTEN related Cowden syndrome
Code also, if applicable, genetic susceptibility to malignant neoplasm (Z15.0-)

● **Q85.82 Other Cowden syndrome** CC

● **Q85.83 Von Hippel-Lindau syndrome** CC
Code also manifestations

● **Q85.89 Other phakomatoses, not elsewhere classified** CC
Peutz-Jeghers syndrome
Sturge-Weber(-Dimitri) syndrome

Q85.9 Phakomatosis, unspecified CC HCC
Hamartosis NOS

Q86 Congenital malformation syndromes due to known exogenous causes, not elsewhere classified
EXCLUDES 2 *iodine-deficiency-related hypothyroidism (E00-E02)*
nonteratogenic effects of substances transmitted via placenta or breast milk (P04.-)

Q86.0 Fetal alcohol syndrome (dysmorphic)
Q86.1 Fetal hydantoin syndrome
Meadow's syndrome
Q86.2 Dysmorphism due to warfarin
Q86.8 Other congenital malformation syndromes due to known exogenous causes

Q87 Other specified congenital malformation syndromes affecting multiple systems
Use additional code(s) to identify all associated manifestations

Q87.0 Congenital malformation syndromes predominantly affecting facial appearance
Acrocephalopolysyndactyly
Acrocephalosyndactyly [Apert]
Cryptophthalmos syndrome
Cyclopia
Goldenhar syndrome
Moebius syndrome
Oro-facial-digital syndrome
Robin syndrome
Whistling face

Q87.1 Congenital malformation syndromes predominantly associated with short stature
EXCLUDES 1 *Ellis-van Creveld syndrome (Q77.6)*
Smith-Lemli-Opitz syndrome (E78.72)
AHA: 2019,4Q,14-15

Q87.11 Prader-Willi syndrome CC
Q87.19 Other congenital malformation syndromes predominantly associated with short stature CC
Aarskog syndrome
Cockayne syndrome
De Lange syndrome
Dubowitz syndrome
Noonan syndrome
Robinow-Silverman-Smith syndrome
Russell-Silver syndrome
Seckel syndrome

Q87.2 Congenital malformation syndromes predominantly involving limbs CC
Holt-Oram syndrome
Klippel-Trenaunay-Weber syndrome
Nail patella syndrome
Rubinstein-Taybi syndrome
Sirenomelia syndrome
Thrombocytopenia with absent radius [TAR] syndrome
VATER syndrome

Q87.3 Congenital malformation syndromes involving early overgrowth CC
Beckwith-Wiedemann syndrome
Sotos syndrome
Weaver syndrome

Q87.4 Marfan's syndrome
DEF: Disorder that affects the connective tissue of multiple systems, including disproportionally long or abnormal bone structure and eye and cardiovascular complications.
Q87.40 Marfan's syndrome, unspecified CC
Q87.41 Marfan's syndrome with cardiovascular manifestations
Q87.410 Marfan's syndrome with aortic dilation CC
Q87.418 Marfan's syndrome with other cardiovascular manifestations CC
Q87.42 Marfan's syndrome with ocular manifestations CC
Q87.43 Marfan's syndrome with skeletal manifestation CC
Q87.5 Other congenital malformation syndromes with other skeletal changes CC
Q87.8 Other specified congenital malformation syndromes, not elsewhere classified
EXCLUDES 1 *Zellweger syndrome (E71.510)*
Q87.81 Alport syndrome CC
Use additional code to identify stage of chronic kidney disease (N18.1-N18.6)
Q87.82 Arterial tortuosity syndrome CC
AHA: 2016,4Q,60-61
Q87.89 Other specified congenital malformation syndromes, not elsewhere classified CC
Laurence-Moon (-Bardet)-Biedl syndrome

Q89 Other congenital malformations, not elsewhere classified
Q89.0 Congenital absence and malformations of spleen
EXCLUDES 1 *isomerism of atrial appendages (with asplenia or polysplenia) (Q20.6)*
Q89.01 Asplenia (congenital) CC
Q89.09 Congenital malformations of spleen CC
Congenital splenomegaly
Q89.1 Congenital malformations of adrenal gland
EXCLUDES 1 *adrenogenital disorders (E25.-)*
congenital adrenal hyperplasia (E25.0)
Q89.2 Congenital malformations of other endocrine glands
Congenital malformation of parathyroid or thyroid gland
Persistent thyroglossal duct
Thyroglossal cyst
EXCLUDES 1 *congenital goiter (E03.0)*
congenital hypothyroidism (E03.1)
Q89.3 Situs inversus CC
Dextrocardia with situs inversus
Mirror-image atrial arrangement with situs inversus
Situs inversus or transversus abdominalis
Situs inversus or transversus thoracis
Transposition of abdominal viscera
Transposition of thoracic viscera
EXCLUDES 1 *dextrocardia NOS (Q24.0)*
DEF: Congenital anomaly in which the internal thoracic and abdominal organs are transposed laterally and found on the opposite side from the normal position.
Q89.4 Conjoined twins MCC
Craniopagus
Dicephaly
Pygopagus
Thoracopagus
Q89.7 Multiple congenital malformations, not elsewhere classified CC
Multiple congenital anomalies NOS
Multiple congenital deformities NOS
EXCLUDES 1 *congenital malformation syndromes affecting multiple systems (Q87.-)*
Q89.8 Other specified congenital malformations CC
Use additional code(s) to identify all associated manifestations
AHA: 2021,3Q,12
Q89.9 Congenital malformation, unspecified
Congenital anomaly NOS
Congenital deformity NOS

Chromosomal abnormalities, not elsewhere classified (Q90-Q99)

EXCLUDES 2 *mitochondrial metabolic disorders (E88.4-)*

Q90 Down syndrome
Use additional code(s) to identify any associated physical conditions and degree of intellectual disabilities (F70-F79)
Q90.0 Trisomy 21, nonmosaicism (meiotic nondisjunction)
Q90.1 Trisomy 21, mosaicism (mitotic nondisjunction)
Q90.2 Trisomy 21, translocation
Q90.9 Down syndrome, unspecified
Trisomy 21 NOS

Q91 Trisomy 18 and Trisomy 13
Q91.0 Trisomy 18, nonmosaicism (meiotic nondisjunction) CC
Q91.1 Trisomy 18, mosaicism (mitotic nondisjunction) CC
Q91.2 Trisomy 18, translocation CC
Q91.3 Trisomy 18, unspecified CC
Q91.4 Trisomy 13, nonmosaicism (meiotic nondisjunction) CC
Q91.5 Trisomy 13, mosaicism (mitotic nondisjunction) CC
Q91.6 Trisomy 13, translocation CC
Q91.7 Trisomy 13, unspecified CC

Q92 Other trisomies and partial trisomies of the autosomes, not elsewhere classified
INCLUDES unbalanced translocations and insertions
EXCLUDES 1 *trisomies of chromosomes 13, 18, 21 (Q90-Q91)*
Q92.0 Whole chromosome trisomy, nonmosaicism (meiotic nondisjunction)
Q92.1 Whole chromosome trisomy, mosaicism (mitotic nondisjunction)
Q92.2 Partial trisomy
Less than whole arm duplicated
Whole arm or more duplicated
EXCLUDES 1 *partial trisomy due to unbalanced translocation (Q92.5)*
Q92.5 Duplications with other complex rearrangements
Partial trisomy due to unbalanced translocations
Code also any associated deletions due to unbalanced translocations, inversions and insertions (Q93.7)
Q92.6 Marker chromosomes
Trisomies due to dicentrics
Trisomies due to extra rings
Trisomies due to isochromosomes
Individual with marker heterochromatin
Q92.61 Marker chromosomes in normal individual
Q92.62 Marker chromosomes in abnormal individual
Q92.7 Triploidy and polyploidy
Q92.8 Other specified trisomies and partial trisomies of autosomes
Duplications identified by fluorescence in situ hybridization (FISH)
Duplications identified by in situ hybridization (ISH)
Duplications seen only at prometaphase
Q92.9 Trisomy and partial trisomy of autosomes, unspecified

Q93 Monosomies and deletions from the autosomes, not elsewhere classified
Q93.0 Whole chromosome monosomy, nonmosaicism (meiotic nondisjunction)
Q93.1 Whole chromosome monosomy, mosaicism (mitotic nondisjunction)
Q93.2 Chromosome replaced with ring, dicentric or isochromosome
Q93.3 Deletion of short arm of chromosome 4 CC
Wolff-Hirschorn syndrome
Q93.4 Deletion of short arm of chromosome 5 CC
Cri-du-chat syndrome
Q93.5 Other deletions of part of a chromosome
AHA: 2018,4Q,28
Q93.51 Angelman syndrome CC
Q93.59 Other deletions of part of a chromosome CC
Q93.7 Deletions with other complex rearrangements CC
Deletions due to unbalanced translocations, inversions and insertions
Code also any associated duplications due to unbalanced translocations, inversions and insertions (Q92.5)

✓5th **Q93.8 Other deletions from the autosomes**

Q93.81 Velo-cardio-facial syndrome MCC
Deletion 22q11.2
AHA: 2019,3Q,14
DEF: Microdeletion syndrome affecting multiple organs characterized by a cleft palate, heart defects, an elongated face with almond-shaped eyes, wide nose, small ears, weak immune system, weak musculature, hypothyroidism, short stature, and scoliosis. The deletion occurs at q11.2 on the long arm of the chromosome 22.

Q93.82 Williams syndrome CC
AHA: 2018,4Q,28-29

Q93.88 Other microdeletions CC
Miller-Dieker syndrome
Smith-Magenis syndrome

Q93.89 Other deletions from the autosomes CC
Deletions identified by fluorescence in situ hybridization (FISH)
Deletions identified by in situ hybridization (ISH)
Deletions seen only at prometaphase

Q93.9 Deletion from autosomes, unspecified CC

✓4th **Q95 Balanced rearrangements and structural markers, not elsewhere classified**

INCLUDES Robertsonian and balanced reciprocal translocations and insertions

Q95.0 Balanced translocation and insertion in normal individual
Q95.1 Chromosome inversion in normal individual
Q95.2 Balanced autosomal rearrangement in abnormal individual
Q95.3 Balanced sex/autosomal rearrangement in abnormal individual
Q95.5 Individual with autosomal fragile site
Q95.8 Other balanced rearrangements and structural markers
Q95.9 Balanced rearrangement and structural marker, unspecified

✓4th **Q96 Turner's syndrome**

EXCLUDES 1 *Noonan syndrome (Q87.19)*

Q96.0 Karyotype 45, X ♀
Q96.1 Karyotype 46, X iso (Xq) ♀
Karyotype 46, isochromosome Xq
Q96.2 Karyotype 46, X with abnormal sex chromosome, except iso (Xq) ♀
Karyotype 46, X with abnormal sex chromosome, except isochromosome Xq
Q96.3 Mosaicism, 45, X/46, XX or XY ♀
Q96.4 Mosaicism, 45, X/other cell line(s) with abnormal sex chromosome ♀
Q96.8 Other variants of Turner's syndrome ♀
Q96.9 Turner's syndrome, unspecified ♀

✓4th **Q97 Other sex chromosome abnormalities, female phenotype, not elsewhere classified**

EXCLUDES 1 *Turner's syndrome (Q96.-)*

Q97.0 Karyotype 47, XXX ♀
Q97.1 Female with more than three X chromosomes ♀
Q97.2 Mosaicism, lines with various numbers of X chromosomes ♀
Q97.3 Female with 46, XY karyotype ♀
Q97.8 Other specified sex chromosome abnormalities, female phenotype ♀
Q97.9 Sex chromosome abnormality, female phenotype, unspecified ♀

✓4th **Q98 Other sex chromosome abnormalities, male phenotype, not elsewhere classified**

Q98.0 Klinefelter syndrome karyotype 47, XXY ♂
Q98.1 Klinefelter syndrome, male with more than two X chromosomes ♂
Q98.3 Other male with 46, XX karyotype ♂
Q98.4 Klinefelter syndrome, unspecified ♂
Q98.5 Karyotype 47, XYY ♂
Q98.6 Male with structurally abnormal sex chromosome ♂
Q98.7 Male with sex chromosome mosaicism ♂
Q98.8 Other specified sex chromosome abnormalities, male phenotype ♂
Q98.9 Sex chromosome abnormality, male phenotype, unspecified ♂

✓4th **Q99 Other chromosome abnormalities, not elsewhere classified**

Q99.0 Chimera 46, XX/46, XY
Chimera 46, XX/46, XY true hermaphrodite

Q99.1 46, XX true hermaphrodite
46, XX with streak gonads
46, XY with streak gonads
Pure gonadal dysgenesis

Q99.2 Fragile X chromosome
Fragile X syndrome

Q99.8 Other specified chromosome abnormalities
Q99.9 Chromosomal abnormality, unspecified

Chapter 18. Symptoms, Signs and Abnormal Clinical and Laboratory Findings (RØØ–R99)

Chapter-specific Guidelines with Coding Examples

The chapter-specific guidelines from the ICD-10-CM Official Guidelines for Coding and Reporting have been provided below. Along with these guidelines are coding examples, contained in the shaded boxes, that have been developed to help illustrate the coding and/or sequencing guidance found in these guidelines.

Chapter 18 includes symptoms, signs, abnormal results of clinical or other investigative procedures, and ill-defined conditions regarding which no diagnosis classifiable elsewhere is recorded. Signs and symptoms that point to a specific diagnosis have been assigned to a category in other chapters of the classification.

a. Use of symptom codes

Codes that describe symptoms and signs are acceptable for reporting purposes when a related definitive diagnosis has not been established (confirmed) by the provider.

Chest pain of unknown origin

RØ7.9 Chest pain, unspecified

Explanation: Codes that describe symptoms such as chest pain are acceptable for reporting purposes when the provider has not established (confirmed) a related definitive diagnosis.

b. Use of a symptom code with a definitive diagnosis code

Codes for signs and symptoms may be reported in addition to a related definitive diagnosis when the sign or symptom is not routinely associated with that diagnosis, such as the various signs and symptoms associated with complex syndromes. The definitive diagnosis code should be sequenced before the symptom code.

Signs or symptoms that are associated routinely with a disease process should not be assigned as additional codes, unless otherwise instructed by the classification.

Pneumonia with hemoptysis

J18.9 Pneumonia, unspecified organism

RØ4.2 Hemoptysis

Explanation: Codes for signs and symptoms may be reported in addition to a related definitive diagnosis when the sign or symptom is not routinely associated with that diagnosis.

Abdominal pain due to acute appendicitis

K35.8Ø Unspecified acute appendicitis

Explanation: Codes for signs or symptoms routinely associated with a disease process should not be assigned unless the classification instructs otherwise.

c. Combination codes that include symptoms

ICD-10-CM contains a number of combination codes that identify both the definitive diagnosis and common symptoms of that diagnosis. When using one of these combination codes, an additional code should not be assigned for the symptom.

Acute gastritis with hemorrhage

K29.Ø1 Acute gastritis with bleeding

Explanation: When a combination code identifies both the definitive diagnosis and the symptom, an additional code should not be assigned for the symptom.

d. Repeated falls

Code R29.6, Repeated falls, is for use for encounters when a patient has recently fallen and the reason for the fall is being investigated.

Code Z91.81, History of falling, is for use when a patient has fallen in the past and is at risk for future falls. When appropriate, both codes R29.6 and Z91.81 may be assigned together.

e. Coma

Code R4Ø.2Ø, Unspecified coma, may be assigned in conjunction with codes for any medical condition.

Do not report codes for unspecified coma, individual or total Glasgow coma scale scores for a patient with a medically induced coma or a sedated patient.

1) Coma scale

The coma scale codes (R4Ø.21- to R4Ø.24-) can be used in conjunction with traumatic brain injury codes. These codes are primarily for use by trauma registries, but they may be used in any setting where this information is collected. The coma scale codes should be sequenced after the diagnosis code(s).

These codes, one from each subcategory, are needed to complete the scale. The 7th character indicates when the scale was recorded. The 7th character should match for all three codes.

At a minimum, report the initial score documented on presentation at your facility. This may be a score from the emergency medicine technician (EMT) or in the emergency department. If desired, a facility may choose to capture multiple coma scale scores.

Assign code R4Ø.24-, Glasgow coma scale, total score, when only the total score is documented in the medical record and not the individual score(s).

If multiple coma scores are captured within the first 24 hours after hospital admission, assign only the code for the score at the time of admission. ICD-1Ø-CM does not classify coma scores that are reported after admission but less than 24 hours later.

See Section I.B.14. for coma scale documentation by clinicians other than patient's provider

23-year-old man found down after unknown injury with skull fracture and with concussion and loss of consciousness of unknown duration. EMS evaluated the patient in the field and reported the individual Glasgow coma scores:

Eye opening response—3: eyes open to speech

Verbal response—4: confused but coherent speech

Motor response—6: obeys commands fully

SØ2.ØXXA Fracture of vault of skull, initial encounter for closed fracture

SØ6.ØX9A Concussion with loss of consciousness of unspecified duration, initial encounter

R4Ø.2131 Coma scale, eyes open, to sound, in the field [EMT or ambulance]

R4Ø.2241 Coma scale, best verbal response, confused conversation, in the field [EMT or ambulance]

R4Ø.2361 Coma scale, best motor response, obeys commands, in the field [EMT or ambulance]

Explanation: When individual scores for the Glasgow coma scale are documented, one code from each category is needed to complete the scale. The seventh character indicates when the scale was recorded and should match for all three codes. Assign a code from subcategory R4Ø.24- Glasgow coma scale, total score, when only the total and not the individual score(s) is documented.

f. Functional quadriplegia

GUIDELINE HAS BEEN DELETED EFFECTIVE OCTOBER 1, 2017

g. SIRS due to non-infectious process

The systemic inflammatory response syndrome (SIRS) can develop as a result of certain non-infectious disease processes, such as trauma, malignant neoplasm, or pancreatitis. When SIRS is documented with a noninfectious condition, and no subsequent infection is documented, the code for the underlying condition, such as an injury, should be assigned, followed by code R65.1Ø, Systemic inflammatory response syndrome (SIRS) of non-infectious origin without acute organ dysfunction, or code R65.11, Systemic inflammatory response syndrome (SIRS) of non-infectious origin with acute organ dysfunction. If an associated acute organ dysfunction is documented, the appropriate code(s) for the specific type of organ dysfunction(s) should be assigned in addition to code R65.11. If acute organ dysfunction is documented, but it cannot be determined if the acute organ dysfunction is associated with SIRS or due to another condition (e.g., directly due to the trauma), the provider should be queried.

Systemic inflammatory response syndrome (SIRS) due to acute gallstone pancreatitis

K85.1Ø **Biliary acute pancreatitis without necrosis or infection**

R65.1Ø **Systemic inflammatory response syndrome [SIRS] of non-infectious origin without acute organ dysfunction**

Explanation: When SIRS is documented with a non-infectious condition without subsequent infection documented, the code for the underlying condition such as pancreatitis should be assigned followed by the appropriate code for SIRS of noninfectious origin, either with or without associated organ dysfunction.

h. Death NOS

Code R99, Ill-defined and unknown cause of mortality, is only for use in the very limited circumstance when a patient who has already died is brought into an emergency department or other healthcare facility and is pronounced dead upon arrival. It does not represent the discharge disposition of death.

i. NIHSS stroke scale

The NIH stroke scale (NIHSS) codes (R29.7- -) can be used in conjunction with acute stroke codes (I63) to identify the patient's neurological status and the severity of the stroke. The stroke scale codes should be sequenced after the acute stroke diagnosis code(s).

At a minimum, report the initial score documented. If desired, a facility may choose to capture multiple stroke scale scores.

See Section I.B.14. for NIHSS stroke scale documentation by clinicians other than patient's provider

Patient admitted with CVA seen by neurology consult who documents moderate to severe stroke, 17 on NIHSS stroke scale.

I63.9 **Cerebral infarction, unspecified**

R29.717 **NIHSS score 17**

Explanation: Unspecified cerebral vascular accident (CVA) is sequenced before the NIHSS stroke scale score code. The stroke scale is an assessment tool to help measure stroke-related neurological deficits. Fifteen items are evaluated by trained observers and include such conditions as levels of consciousness, language, dysarthria, ataxia, and sensory loss. A facility may report multiple stroke scale scores if it wants to.

Chapter 18. Symptoms, Signs and Abnormal Clinical and Laboratory Findings, Not Elsewhere Classified (R00-R99)

NOTE This chapter includes symptoms, signs, abnormal results of clinical or other investigative procedures, and ill-defined conditions regarding which no diagnosis classifiable elsewhere is recorded.

Signs and symptoms that point rather definitely to a given diagnosis have been assigned to a category in other chapters of the classification. In general, categories in this chapter include the less well-defined conditions and symptoms that, without the necessary study of the case to establish a final diagnosis, point perhaps equally to two or more diseases or to two or more systems of the body. Practically all categories in the chapter could be designated 'not otherwise specified', 'unknown etiology' or 'transient'. The Alphabetical Index should be consulted to determine which symptoms and signs are to be allocated here and which to other chapters. The residual subcategories, numbered .8, are generally provided for other relevant symptoms that cannot be allocated elsewhere in the classification.

The conditions and signs or symptoms included in categories R00-R94 consist of:

(a) cases for which no more specific diagnosis can be made even after all the facts bearing on the case have been investigated;

(b) signs or symptoms existing at the time of initial encounter that proved to be transient and whose causes could not be determined;

(c) provisional diagnosis in a patient who failed to return for further investigation or care;

(d) cases referred elsewhere for investigation or treatment before the diagnosis was made;

(e) cases in which a more precise diagnosis was not available for any other reason;

(f) certain symptoms, for which supplementary information is provided, that represent important problems in medical care in their own right.

EXCLUDES 2 *abnormal findings on antenatal screening of mother (O28.-)*
certain conditions originating in the perinatal period (P04-P96)
signs and symptoms classified in the body system chapters
signs and symptoms of breast (N63, N64.5)

AHA: 2017,1Q,6,7

This chapter contains the following blocks:

R00-R09 Symptoms and signs involving the circulatory and respiratory systems
R10-R19 Symptoms and signs involving the digestive system and abdomen
R20-R23 Symptoms and signs involving the skin and subcutaneous tissue
R25-R29 Symptoms and signs involving the nervous and musculoskeletal systems
R30-R39 Symptoms and signs involving the genitourinary system
R40-R46 Symptoms and signs involving cognition, perception, emotional state and behavior
R47-R49 Symptoms and signs involving speech and voice
R50-R69 General symptoms and signs
R70-R79 Abnormal findings on examination of blood, without diagnosis
R80-R82 Abnormal findings on examination of urine, without diagnosis
R83-R89 Abnormal findings on examination of other body fluids, substances and tissues, without diagnosis
R90-R94 Abnormal findings on diagnostic imaging and in function studies, without diagnosis
R97 Abnormal tumor markers
R99 Ill-defined and unknown cause of mortality

Symptoms and signs involving the circulatory and respiratory systems (R00-R09)

R00 Abnormalities of heart beat

EXCLUDES 1 *abnormalities originating in the perinatal period (P29.1-)*
EXCLUDES 2 *specified arrhythmias (I47-I49)*

R00.0 Tachycardia, unspecified
Rapid heart beat
Sinoauricular tachycardia NOS
Sinus [sinusal] tachycardia NOS
EXCLUDES 1 *neonatal tachycardia (P29.11)*
paroxysmal tachycardia (I47.-)
DEF: Excessively rapid heart rate of more than 100 beats per minute.

R00.1 Bradycardia, unspecified
Sinoatrial bradycardia
Sinus bradycardia
Slow heart beat
Vagal bradycardia
Use additional code for adverse effect, if applicable, to identify drug (T36-T50 with fifth or sixth character 5)
EXCLUDES 1 *neonatal bradycardia (P29.12)*
AHA: 2020,2Q,23
DEF: Slowed heartbeat, usually defined as a rate fewer than 60 beats per minute. Heart rhythm may be slow as a result of a congenital defect or an acquired problem.

R00.2 Palpitations
Awareness of heart beat

R00.8 Other abnormalities of heart beat

R00.9 Unspecified abnormalities of heart beat

R01 Cardiac murmurs and other cardiac sounds

EXCLUDES 1 *cardiac murmurs and sounds originating in the perinatal period (P29.8)*

R01.0 Benign and innocent cardiac murmurs
Functional cardiac murmur

R01.1 Cardiac murmur, unspecified
Cardiac bruit NOS
Heart murmur NOS
Systolic murmur NOS

R01.2 Other cardiac sounds
Cardiac dullness, increased or decreased
Precordial friction

R03 Abnormal blood-pressure reading, without diagnosis

R03.0 Elevated blood-pressure reading, without diagnosis of hypertension
NOTE This category is to be used to record an episode of elevated blood pressure in a patient in whom no formal diagnosis of hypertension has been made, or as an isolated incidental finding.

R03.1 Nonspecific low blood-pressure reading
EXCLUDES 1 *hypotension (I95.-)*
maternal hypotension syndrome (O26.5-)
neurogenic orthostatic hypotension (G90.3)

R04 Hemorrhage from respiratory passages

R04.0 Epistaxis
Hemorrhage from nose
Nosebleed

R04.1 Hemorrhage from throat
EXCLUDES 2 *hemoptysis (R04.2)*

R04.2 Hemoptysis CC
Blood-stained sputum
Cough with hemorrhage
AHA: 2013,4Q,118

R04.8 Hemorrhage from other sites in respiratory passages

R04.81 Acute idiopathic pulmonary hemorrhage in infants CC P
AIPHI
Acute idiopathic hemorrhage in infants over 28 days old
EXCLUDES 1 *perinatal pulmonary hemorrhage (P26.-)*
▶von Willebrand disease (D68.0-)◀

R04.89 Hemorrhage from other sites in respiratory passages CC
Pulmonary hemorrhage NOS

R04.9 Hemorrhage from respiratory passages, unspecified CC

R05 Cough

EXCLUDES 1 *paroxysmal cough due to Bordetella pertussis (A37.0-)*
smoker's cough (J41.0)
EXCLUDES 2 *cough with hemorrhage (R04.2)*
AHA: 2021,4Q,24-25; 2016,2Q,33

R05.1 Acute cough

R05.2 Subacute cough

R05.3 Chronic cough
Persistent cough
Refractory cough
Unexplained cough

R05.4 Cough syncope UPD
Code first syncope and collapse (R55)

R05.8 Other specified cough

RØ5.9 Cough, unspecified

RØ6 Abnormalities of breathing
EXCLUDES 1 *acute respiratory distress syndrome (J8Ø)*
respiratory arrest (RØ9.2)
respiratory arrest of newborn (P28.81)
respiratory distress syndrome of newborn (P22.-)
respiratory failure (J96.-)
respiratory failure of newborn (P28.5)

RØ6.Ø Dyspnea
EXCLUDES 1 *tachypnea NOS (RØ6.82)*
transient tachypnea of newborn (P22.1)

RØ6.ØØ Dyspnea, unspecified
AHA: 2017,1Q,26

RØ6.Ø1 Orthopnea

RØ6.Ø2 Shortness of breath

RØ6.Ø3 Acute respiratory distress
AHA: 2017,4Q,23

RØ6.Ø9 Other forms of dyspnea

RØ6.1 Stridor
EXCLUDES 1 *congenital laryngeal stridor (P28.89)*
laryngismus (stridulus) (J38.5)

DEF: Certain type of wheezing described as a loud, constant, musical sound produced when breathing with an obstructed airway, like the inspiratory sound heard when laryngeal or esophageal obstruction is present.

RØ6.2 Wheezing
EXCLUDES 1 *asthma (J45.-)*
AHA: 2016,2Q,33
DEF: High-pitched whistling sound during breathing due to stenosis of the respiratory passageway. Wheezing is associated with asthma, sleep apnea, bronchiectasis, bronchiolitis, COPD, and pleural effusion.

RØ6.3 Periodic breathing CC
Cheyne-Stokes breathing

RØ6.4 Hyperventilation
EXCLUDES 1 *psychogenic hyperventilation (F45.8)*

RØ6.5 Mouth breathing
EXCLUDES 2 *dry mouth NOS (R68.2)*

RØ6.6 Hiccough
EXCLUDES 1 *psychogenic hiccough (F45.8)*

RØ6.7 Sneezing

RØ6.8 Other abnormalities of breathing

RØ6.81 Apnea, not elsewhere classified
Apnea NOS
EXCLUDES 1 *apnea (of) newborn ▶(P28.4-)◀*
sleep apnea (G47.3-)
sleep apnea of newborn (primary) ▶(P28.3-)◀

RØ6.82 Tachypnea, not elsewhere classified
Tachypnea NOS
EXCLUDES 1 *transitory tachypnea of newborn (P22.1)*

RØ6.83 Snoring

RØ6.89 Other abnormalities of breathing
Breath-holding (spells)
Sighing

RØ6.9 Unspecified abnormalities of breathing

RØ7 Pain in throat and chest
EXCLUDES 1 *epidemic myalgia (B33.Ø)*
EXCLUDES 2 *jaw pain R68.84*
pain in breast (N64.4)

RØ7.Ø Pain in throat
EXCLUDES 1 *chronic sore throat (J31.2)*
sore throat (acute) NOS (JØ2.9)
EXCLUDES 2 *dysphagia (R13.1-)*
pain in neck (M54.2)

RØ7.1 Chest pain on breathing
Painful respiration

RØ7.2 Precordial pain
DEF: Pain felt in the anterior (front) chest wall over the region of the heart. This type of pain is generally felt slightly to the left of the sternum, but may also extend into the surrounding chest wall region.

RØ7.8 Other chest pain

RØ7.81 Pleurodynia
Pleurodynia NOS
EXCLUDES 1 *epidemic pleurodynia (B33.Ø)*

RØ7.82 Intercostal pain

RØ7.89 Other chest pain
Anterior chest-wall pain NOS
AHA: 2021,1Q,42

RØ7.9 Chest pain, unspecified

RØ9 Other symptoms and signs involving the circulatory and respiratory system
EXCLUDES 1 *acute respiratory distress syndrome (J8Ø)*
respiratory arrest of newborn (P28.81)
respiratory distress syndrome of newborn (P22.Ø)
respiratory failure (J96.-)
respiratory failure of newborn (P28.5)

RØ9.Ø Asphyxia and hypoxemia
EXCLUDES 1 *asphyxia due to carbon monoxide (T58.-)*
asphyxia due to foreign body in respiratory tract (T17.-)
birth (intrauterine) asphyxia (P84)
hyperventilation (RØ6.4)
traumatic asphyxia (T71.-)
EXCLUDES 2 *hypercapnia (RØ6.89)*

RØ9.Ø1 Asphyxia CC
DEF: Interference of oxygen intake due to obstruction or injury of airways resulting in a lack of oxygen perfusion to the tissues or excessive carbon dioxide in the blood. Can cause unconsciousness or death.

RØ9.Ø2 Hypoxemia
AHA: 2019,3Q,15
DEF: Insufficient oxygen in the arterial blood resulting in inadequate delivery of oxygen to the body tissues.

RØ9.1 Pleurisy
EXCLUDES 1 *pleurisy with effusion (J9Ø)*

[1] **RØ9.2 Respiratory arrest** MCC HCC
Cardiorespiratory failure
EXCLUDES 1 *cardiac arrest (I46.-)*
respiratory arrest of newborn (P28.81)
respiratory distress of newborn (P22.Ø)
respiratory failure (J96.-)
respiratory failure of newborn (P28.5)
respiratory insufficiency (RØ6.89)
respiratory insufficiency of newborn (P28.5)

RØ9.3 Abnormal sputum
Abnormal amount of sputum
Abnormal color of sputum
Abnormal odor of sputum
Excessive sputum
EXCLUDES 1 *blood-stained sputum (RØ4.2)*

RØ9.8 Other specified symptoms and signs involving the circulatory and respiratory systems

RØ9.81 Nasal congestion

RØ9.82 Postnasal drip

RØ9.89 Other specified symptoms and signs involving the circulatory and respiratory systems
Abnormal chest percussion
Bruit (arterial)
Chest tympany
Choking sensation
Feeling of foreign body in throat
Friction sounds in chest
Rales
Weak pulse
EXCLUDES 2 *foreign body in throat (T17.2-)*
wheezing (RØ6.2)
AHA: 2021,1Q,42

Symptoms and signs involving the digestive system and abdomen (R1Ø-R19)

EXCLUDES 2 *congenital or infantile pylorospasm (Q4Ø.Ø)*
gastrointestinal hemorrhage (K92.Ø-K92.2)
intestinal obstruction (K56.-)
newborn gastrointestinal hemorrhage (P54.Ø-P54.3)
newborn intestinal obstruction (P76.-)
pylorospasm (K31.3)
signs and symptoms involving the urinary system (R3Ø-R39)
symptoms referable to female genital organs (N94.-)
symptoms referable to male genital organs (N48-N5Ø)

✓4th R1Ø Abdominal and pelvic pain
EXCLUDES 1 *renal colic (N23)*
EXCLUDES 2 *dorsalgia (M54.-)*
flatulence and related conditions (R14.-)

R1Ø.Ø Acute abdomen
Severe abdominal pain (generalized) (with abdominal rigidity)
EXCLUDES 1 *abdominal rigidity NOS (R19.3)*
generalized abdominal pain NOS (R1Ø.84)
localized abdominal pain (R1Ø.1-R1Ø.3-)

✓5th R1Ø.1 Pain localized to upper abdomen
R1Ø.1Ø Upper abdominal pain, unspecified
R1Ø.11 Right upper quadrant pain
R1Ø.12 Left upper quadrant pain
R1Ø.13 Epigastric pain
Dyspepsia
EXCLUDES 1 *functional dyspepsia (K3Ø)*

Abdominal Pain

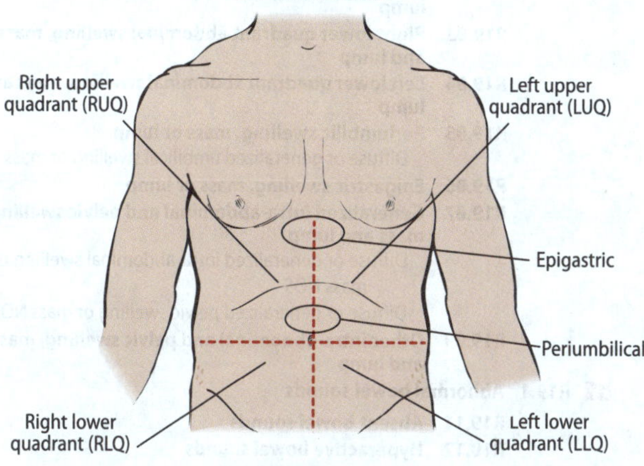

R1Ø.2 Pelvic and perineal pain
EXCLUDES 1 *vulvodynia (N94.81)*

✓5th R1Ø.3 Pain localized to other parts of lower abdomen
R1Ø.3Ø Lower abdominal pain, unspecified
R1Ø.31 Right lower quadrant pain
R1Ø.32 Left lower quadrant pain
R1Ø.33 Periumbilical pain

✓5th R1Ø.8 Other abdominal pain
✓6th R1Ø.81 Abdominal tenderness
Abdominal tenderness NOS
R1Ø.811 Right upper quadrant abdominal tenderness
R1Ø.812 Left upper quadrant abdominal tenderness
R1Ø.813 Right lower quadrant abdominal tenderness
R1Ø.814 Left lower quadrant abdominal tenderness
R1Ø.815 Periumbilic abdominal tenderness
R1Ø.816 Epigastric abdominal tenderness
R1Ø.817 Generalized abdominal tenderness
R1Ø.819 Abdominal tenderness, unspecified site
✓6th R1Ø.82 Rebound abdominal tenderness
R1Ø.821 Right upper quadrant rebound abdominal tenderness
R1Ø.822 Left upper quadrant rebound abdominal tenderness
R1Ø.823 Right lower quadrant rebound abdominal tenderness
R1Ø.824 Left lower quadrant rebound abdominal tenderness
R1Ø.825 Periumbilic rebound abdominal tenderness
R1Ø.826 Epigastric rebound abdominal tenderness
R1Ø.827 Generalized rebound abdominal tenderness
R1Ø.829 Rebound abdominal tenderness, unspecified site

R1Ø.83 Colic P
Colic NOS
Infantile colic
EXCLUDES 1 *colic in adult and child over 12 months old (R1Ø.84)*
DEF: Inconsolable crying in an otherwise well-fed and healthy infant for more than three hours a day, three days a week, for more than three weeks.

R1Ø.84 Generalized abdominal pain
EXCLUDES 1 *generalized abdominal pain associated with acute abdomen (R1Ø.Ø)*

R1Ø.9 Unspecified abdominal pain

✓4th R11 Nausea and vomiting
EXCLUDES 1 *cyclical vomiting associated with migraine (G43.A-)*
excessive vomiting in pregnancy (O21.-)
hematemesis (K92.Ø)
neonatal hematemesis (P54.Ø)
newborn vomiting (P92.Ø-)
psychogenic vomiting (F5Ø.89)
vomiting associated with bulimia nervosa (F5Ø.2)
vomiting following gastrointestinal surgery (K91.Ø)
AHA: 2017,1Q,28

R11.Ø Nausea
Nausea NOS
Nausea without vomiting

✓5th R11.1 Vomiting
R11.1Ø Vomiting, unspecified
Vomiting NOS
R11.11 Vomiting without nausea
R11.12 Projectile vomiting
R11.13 Vomiting of fecal matter
R11.14 Bilious vomiting
Bilious emesis
R11.15 Cyclical vomiting syndrome unrelated to migraine
Cyclic vomiting syndrome NOS
Persistent vomiting
EXCLUDES 1 *cyclical vomiting in migraine (G43.A-)*
EXCLUDES 2 *bulimia nervosa (F5Ø.2)*
diabetes mellitus due to underlying condition (EØ8.-)
AHA: 2019,4Q,15

R11.2 Nausea with vomiting, unspecified
Persistent nausea with vomiting NOS
AHA: 2020,1Q,8

R12 Heartburn
EXCLUDES 1 *dyspepsia NOS (R1Ø.13)*
functional dyspepsia (K3Ø)

✓4th R13 Aphagia and dysphagia
R13.Ø Aphagia
Inability to swallow
EXCLUDES 1 *psychogenic aphagia (F5Ø.9)*

R13.1 Dysphagia

Code first, if applicable, dysphagia following cerebrovascular disease (I69. with final characters -91)

EXCLUDES 1 *psychogenic dysphagia (F45.8)*

Swallowing Function

Oral phase **Oropharyngeal phase**

Pharyngeal phase **Pharyngoesophageal phase**

R13.10 Dysphagia, unspecified
Difficulty in swallowing NOS

R13.11 Dysphagia, oral phase

R13.12 Dysphagia, oropharyngeal phase

R13.13 Dysphagia, pharyngeal phase

R13.14 Dysphagia, pharyngoesophageal phase

R13.19 Other dysphagia
Cervical dysphagia
Neurogenic dysphagia

R14 Flatulence and related conditions

EXCLUDES 1 *psychogenic aerophagy (F45.8)*

R14.0 Abdominal distension (gaseous)
Bloating
Tympanites (abdominal) (intestinal)

R14.1 Gas pain

R14.2 Eructation

R14.3 Flatulence

R15 Fecal incontinence

INCLUDES encopresis NOS

EXCLUDES 1 *fecal incontinence of nonorganic origin (F98.1)*

R15.0 Incomplete defecation

EXCLUDES 1 *constipation (K59.0-)*
fecal impaction (K56.41)

R15.1 Fecal smearing
Fecal soiling

R15.2 Fecal urgency

R15.9 Full incontinence of feces
Fecal incontinence NOS

R16 Hepatomegaly and splenomegaly, not elsewhere classified

R16.0 Hepatomegaly, not elsewhere classified
Hepatomegaly NOS

R16.1 Splenomegaly, not elsewhere classified
Splenomegaly NOS

R16.2 Hepatomegaly with splenomegaly, not elsewhere classified
Hepatosplenomegaly NOS

R17 Unspecified jaundice CC

EXCLUDES 1 *neonatal jaundice (P55, P57-P59)*

R18 Ascites

INCLUDES fluid in peritoneal cavity

EXCLUDES 1 *ascites in alcoholic cirrhosis (K70.31)*
ascites in alcoholic hepatitis (K70.11)
ascites in toxic liver disease with chronic active hepatitis (K71.51)

DEF: Abnormal accumulation of free fluid in the abdominal cavity, causing distention and tightness in addition to shortness of breath as the fluid accumulates. Ascites is usually an underlying disorder and can be a manifestation of any number of diseases.

R18.0 Malignant ascites CC UPD

Code first malignancy, such as:
malignant neoplasm of ovary (C56.-)
secondary malignant neoplasm of retroperitoneum and peritoneum (C78.6)

R18.8 Other ascites CC
Ascites NOS
Peritoneal effusion (chronic)
AHA: 2018,1Q,4

R19 Other symptoms and signs involving the digestive system and abdomen

EXCLUDES 1 *acute abdomen (R10.0)*

R19.0 Intra-abdominal and pelvic swelling, mass and lump

EXCLUDES 1 *abdominal distension (gaseous) (R14.-)*
ascites (R18.-)

R19.00 Intra-abdominal and pelvic swelling, mass and lump, unspecified site

R19.01 Right upper quadrant abdominal swelling, mass and lump

R19.02 Left upper quadrant abdominal swelling, mass and lump

R19.03 Right lower quadrant abdominal swelling, mass and lump

R19.04 Left lower quadrant abdominal swelling, mass and lump

R19.05 Periumbilic swelling, mass or lump
Diffuse or generalized umbilical swelling or mass

R19.06 Epigastric swelling, mass or lump

R19.07 Generalized intra-abdominal and pelvic swelling, mass and lump
Diffuse or generalized intra-abdominal swelling or mass NOS
Diffuse or generalized pelvic swelling or mass NOS

R19.09 Other intra-abdominal and pelvic swelling, mass and lump

R19.1 Abnormal bowel sounds

R19.11 Absent bowel sounds

R19.12 Hyperactive bowel sounds

R19.15 Other abnormal bowel sounds
Abnormal bowel sounds NOS

R19.2 Visible peristalsis
Hyperperistalsis
DEF: Visible movements of muscular attempts to move food through the digestive tract due to pyloric obstruction, stomach obstruction, or intestinal obstruction.

R19.3 Abdominal rigidity

EXCLUDES 1 *abdominal rigidity with severe abdominal pain (R10.0)*

R19.30 Abdominal rigidity, unspecified site

R19.31 Right upper quadrant abdominal rigidity

R19.32 Left upper quadrant abdominal rigidity

R19.33 Right lower quadrant abdominal rigidity

R19.34 Left lower quadrant abdominal rigidity

R19.35 Periumbilic abdominal rigidity

R19.36 Epigastric abdominal rigidity

R19.37 Generalized abdominal rigidity

R19.4 Change in bowel habit

EXCLUDES 1 *constipation (K59.0-)*
functional diarrhea (K59.1)

R19.5 Other fecal abnormalities
Abnormal stool color
Bulky stools
Mucus in stools
Occult blood in feces
Occult blood in stools
EXCLUDES 1 *melena (K92.1)*
neonatal melena (P54.1)
AHA: 2021,1Q,9; 2019,1Q,32

R19.6 Halitosis

R19.7 Diarrhea, unspecified
Diarrhea NOS
EXCLUDES 1 *functional diarrhea (K59.1)*
neonatal diarrhea (P78.3)
psychogenic diarrhea (F45.8)
AHA: 2021,3Q,3

R19.8 Other specified symptoms and signs involving the digestive system and abdomen

Symptoms and signs involving the skin and subcutaneous tissue (R2Ø-R23)

EXCLUDES 2 *symptoms relating to breast (N64.4-N64.5)*

R2Ø Disturbances of skin sensation
EXCLUDES 1 *dissociative anesthesia and sensory loss (F44.6)*
psychogenic disturbances (F45.8)

R2Ø.Ø Anesthesia of skin
R2Ø.1 Hypoesthesia of skin
R2Ø.2 Paresthesia of skin
Formication
Pins and needles
Tingling skin
EXCLUDES 1 *acroparesthesia (I73.8)*
R2Ø.3 Hyperesthesia
R2Ø.8 Other disturbances of skin sensation
R2Ø.9 Unspecified disturbances of skin sensation

R21 Rash and other nonspecific skin eruption
INCLUDES rash NOS
EXCLUDES 1 *specified type of rash - code to condition*
vesicular eruption (R23.8)

R22 Localized swelling, mass and lump of skin and subcutaneous tissue
INCLUDES subcutaneous nodules (localized)(superficial)
EXCLUDES 1 *abnormal findings on diagnostic imaging (R9Ø-R93)*
edema (R6Ø.-)
enlarged lymph nodes (R59.-)
localized adiposity (E65)
swelling of joint (M25.4-)

R22.Ø Localized swelling, mass and lump, head
R22.1 Localized swelling, mass and lump, neck
R22.2 Localized swelling, mass and lump, trunk
EXCLUDES 1 *intra-abdominal or pelvic mass and lump (R19.Ø-)*
intra-abdominal or pelvic swelling (R19.Ø-)
EXCLUDES 2 *breast mass and lump (N63)*
R22.3 Localized swelling, mass and lump, upper limb
R22.3Ø Localized swelling, mass and lump, unspecified upper limb
R22.31 Localized swelling, mass and lump, right upper limb
R22.32 Localized swelling, mass and lump, left upper limb
R22.33 Localized swelling, mass and lump, upper limb, bilateral
R22.4 Localized swelling, mass and lump, lower limb
R22.4Ø Localized swelling, mass and lump, unspecified lower limb
R22.41 Localized swelling, mass and lump, right lower limb
R22.42 Localized swelling, mass and lump, left lower limb
R22.43 Localized swelling, mass and lump, lower limb, bilateral
R22.9 Localized swelling, mass and lump, unspecified

R23 Other skin changes
R23.Ø Cyanosis
EXCLUDES 1 *acrocyanosis (I73.8)*
cyanotic attacks of newborn (P28.2)
DEF: Bluish or purplish discoloration of the skin due to an inadequate oxygen blood level.
R23.1 Pallor
Clammy skin
R23.2 Flushing
Excessive blushing
Code first, if applicable, menopausal and female climacteric states (N95.1)
R23.3 Spontaneous ecchymoses
Petechiae
EXCLUDES 1 *ecchymoses of newborn (P54.5)*
purpura (D69.-)
R23.4 Changes in skin texture
Desquamation of skin
Induration of skin
Scaling of skin
EXCLUDES 1 *epidermal thickening NOS (L85.9)*
R23.8 Other skin changes
R23.9 Unspecified skin changes

Symptoms and signs involving the nervous and musculoskeletal systems (R25-R29)

R25 Abnormal involuntary movements
EXCLUDES 1 *specific movement disorders (G2Ø-G26)*
stereotyped movement disorders (F98.4)
tic disorders (F95.-)
R25.Ø Abnormal head movements
R25.1 Tremor, unspecified
EXCLUDES 1 *chorea NOS (G25.5)*
essential tremor (G25.Ø)
hysterical tremor (F44.4)
intention tremor (G25.2)
R25.2 Cramp and spasm
EXCLUDES 2 *carpopedal spasm (R29.Ø)*
charley-horse (M62.831)
infantile spasms (G4Ø.4-)
muscle spasm of back (M62.83Ø)
muscle spasm of calf (M62.831)
R25.3 Fasciculation
Twitching NOS
R25.8 Other abnormal involuntary movements
R25.9 Unspecified abnormal involuntary movements

R26 Abnormalities of gait and mobility
EXCLUDES 1 *ataxia NOS (R27.Ø)*
hereditary ataxia (G11.-)
locomotor (syphilitic) ataxia (A52.11)
immobility syndrome (paraplegic) (M62.3)
R26.Ø Ataxic gait
Staggering gait
AHA: 2022,2Q,12
R26.1 Paralytic gait
Spastic gait
R26.2 Difficulty in walking, not elsewhere classified
EXCLUDES 1 *falling (R29.6)*
unsteadiness on feet (R26.81)
AHA: 2016,2Q,7
R26.8 Other abnormalities of gait and mobility
R26.81 Unsteadiness on feet
R26.89 Other abnormalities of gait and mobility
AHA: 2020,2Q,29
R26.9 Unspecified abnormalities of gait and mobility

R27 Other lack of coordination
EXCLUDES 1 *ataxic gait (R26.Ø)*
hereditary ataxia (G11.-)
vertigo NOS (R42)
R27.Ø Ataxia, unspecified
EXCLUDES 1 *ataxia following cerebrovascular disease (I69. with final characters -93)*
R27.8 Other lack of coordination
R27.9 Unspecified lack of coordination

√4th **R29 Other symptoms and signs involving the nervous and musculoskeletal systems**

R29.Ø Tetany CC
Carpopedal spasm
EXCLUDES 1 *hysterical tetany (F44.5)*
neonatal tetany (P71.3)
parathyroid tetany (E2Ø.9)
post-thyroidectomy tetany (E89.2)
DEF: Calcium or other mineral imbalance causing voluntary muscles such as hands, feet, or larynx to spasm rhythmically.

R29.1 Meningismus CC

R29.2 Abnormal reflex
EXCLUDES 2 *abnormal pupillary reflex (H57.Ø)*
hyperactive gag reflex (J39.2)
vasovagal reaction or syncope (R55)

R29.3 Abnormal posture

R29.4 Clicking hip
EXCLUDES 1 *congenital deformities of hip (Q65.-)*

R29.5 Transient paralysis CC
Code first any associated spinal cord injury (S14.Ø, S14.1-, S24.Ø, S24.1-, S34.Ø-, S34.1-)
EXCLUDES 1 *transient ischemic attack (G45.9)*

R29.6 Repeated falls
Falling
Tendency to fall
EXCLUDES 2 *at risk for falling (Z91.81)*
history of falling (Z91.81)
AHA: 2016,2Q,6
TIP: Code in addition to Parkinson's disease (G20), when documented.

√5th **R29.7 National Institutes of Health Stroke Scale (NIHSS) score**
Code first the type of cerebral infarction (I63.-)
AHA: 2016,4Q,61-62
TIP: Codes from this subcategory may be assigned based on medical record documentation from clinicians who are not the patient's provider.

√6th **R29.7Ø NIHSS score Ø-9**
R29.7ØØ NIHSS score Ø UPD
R29.7Ø1 NIHSS score 1 UPD
R29.7Ø2 NIHSS score 2 UPD
R29.7Ø3 NIHSS score 3 UPD
R29.7Ø4 NIHSS score 4 UPD
R29.7Ø5 NIHSS score 5 UPD
R29.7Ø6 NIHSS score 6 UPD
R29.7Ø7 NIHSS score 7 UPD
R29.7Ø8 NIHSS score 8 UPD
R29.7Ø9 NIHSS score 9 UPD

√6th **R29.71 NIHSS score 1Ø-19**
R29.71Ø NIHSS score 1Ø UPD
R29.711 NIHSS score 11 UPD
R29.712 NIHSS score 12 UPD
R29.713 NIHSS score 13 UPD
R29.714 NIHSS score 14 UPD
R29.715 NIHSS score 15 UPD
R29.716 NIHSS score 16 UPD
R29.717 NIHSS score 17 UPD
R29.718 NIHSS score 18 UPD
R29.719 NIHSS score 19 UPD

√6th **R29.72 NIHSS score 2Ø-29**
R29.72Ø NIHSS score 2Ø UPD
R29.721 NIHSS score 21 UPD
R29.722 NIHSS score 22 UPD
R29.723 NIHSS score 23 UPD
R29.724 NIHSS score 24 UPD
R29.725 NIHSS score 25 UPD
R29.726 NIHSS score 26 UPD
R29.727 NIHSS score 27 UPD
R29.728 NIHSS score 28 UPD
R29.729 NIHSS score 29 UPD

√6th **R29.73 NIHSS score 3Ø-39**
R29.73Ø NIHSS score 3Ø UPD
R29.731 NIHSS score 31 UPD
R29.732 NIHSS score 32 UPD
R29.733 NIHSS score 33 UPD
R29.734 NIHSS score 34 UPD
R29.735 NIHSS score 35 UPD
R29.736 NIHSS score 36 UPD
R29.737 NIHSS score 37 UPD
R29.738 NIHSS score 38 UPD
R29.739 NIHSS score 39 UPD

√6th **R29.74 NIHSS score 4Ø-42**
R29.74Ø NIHSS score 4Ø UPD
R29.741 NIHSS score 41 UPD
R29.742 NIHSS score 42 UPD

√5th **R29.8 Other symptoms and signs involving the nervous and musculoskeletal systems**

√6th **R29.81 Other symptoms and signs involving the nervous system**

R29.81Ø Facial weakness
Facial droop
EXCLUDES 1 *Bell's palsy (G51.Ø)*
facial weakness following cerebrovascular disease (I69. with final characters -92)

R29.818 Other symptoms and signs involving the nervous system

√6th **R29.89 Other symptoms and signs involving the musculoskeletal system**
EXCLUDES 2 *pain in limb (M79.6-)*

R29.89Ø Loss of height
EXCLUDES 1 *osteoporosis (M8Ø-M81)*

R29.891 Ocular torticollis
EXCLUDES 1 *congenital (sternomastoid) torticollis Q68.Ø*
psychogenic torticollis (F45.8)
spasmodic torticollis (G24.3)
torticollis due to birth injury (P15.8)
torticollis NOS M43.6
DEF: Abnormal head posture as a result of a contracted state of cervical muscles to correct a visual disturbance, either double vision or a visual field defect.

R29.898 Other symptoms and signs involving the musculoskeletal system

√5th **R29.9 Unspecified symptoms and signs involving the nervous and musculoskeletal systems**

R29.9Ø Unspecified symptoms and signs involving the nervous system

R29.91 Unspecified symptoms and signs involving the musculoskeletal system

Symptoms and signs involving the genitourinary system (R3Ø-R39)

√4th **R3Ø Pain associated with micturition**
EXCLUDES 1 *psychogenic pain associated with micturition (F45.8)*

R3Ø.Ø Dysuria
Strangury

R3Ø.1 Vesical tenesmus
DEF: Feeling of a full bladder even when there is little or no urine in the bladder.

R3Ø.9 Painful micturition, unspecified
Painful urination NOS

√4th **R31 Hematuria**
EXCLUDES 1 *hematuria included with underlying conditions, such as:*
acute cystitis with hematuria (N3Ø.Ø1)
recurrent and persistent hematuria in glomerular diseases (NØ2.-)
AHA: 2017,1Q,17

R31.Ø Gross hematuria

R31.1 Benign essential microscopic hematuria

√5th **R31.2 Other microscopic hematuria**
AHA: 2016,4Q,62

R31.21 Asymptomatic microscopic hematuria
AMH

R31.29 Other microscopic hematuria

R31.9 Hematuria, unspecified

R32 Unspecified urinary incontinence
Enuresis NOS
EXCLUDES 1 *functional urinary incontinence (R39.81)*
nonorganic enuresis (F98.0)
stress incontinence and other specified urinary incontinence (N39.3-N39.4-)
urinary incontinence associated with cognitive impairment (R39.81)

R33 Retention of urine
EXCLUDES 1 *psychogenic retention of urine (F45.8)*

R33.0 Drug induced retention of urine
Use additional code for adverse effect, if applicable, to identify drug (T36-T50 with fifth or sixth character 5)

R33.8 Other retention of urine
Code first, if applicable, any causal condition, such as:
enlarged prostate (N40.1)
AHA: 2018,4Q,55

R33.9 Retention of urine, unspecified

R34 Anuria and oliguria
EXCLUDES 1 *anuria and oliguria complicating abortion or ectopic or molar pregnancy (O00-O07, O08.4)*
anuria and oliguria complicating pregnancy (O26.83-)
anuria and oliguria complicating the puerperium (O90.4)

R35 Polyuria
Code first, if applicable, any causal condition, such as:
enlarged prostate (N40.1)
EXCLUDES 1 *psychogenic polyuria (F45.8)*

R35.0 Frequency of micturition
R35.1 Nocturia
R35.8 Other polyuria
AHA: 2021,4Q,26

R35.81 Nocturnal polyuria
EXCLUDES 2 *nocturnal enuresis (N39.44)*

R35.89 Other polyuria
Polyuria NOS

R36 Urethral discharge
R36.0 Urethral discharge without blood
R36.1 Hematospermia ♂
R36.9 Urethral discharge, unspecified
Penile discharge NOS
Urethrorrhea

R37 Sexual dysfunction, unspecified

R39 Other and unspecified symptoms and signs involving the genitourinary system
R39.0 Extravasation of urine CC
R39.1 Other difficulties with micturition
Code first, if applicable, any causal condition, such as:
enlarged prostate (N40.1)

R39.11 Hesitancy of micturition
R39.12 Poor urinary stream
Weak urinary steam
R39.13 Splitting of urinary stream
R39.14 Feeling of incomplete bladder emptying
R39.15 Urgency of urination
EXCLUDES 1 *urge incontinence (N39.41, N39.46)*
R39.16 Straining to void
R39.19 Other difficulties with micturition
AHA: 2016,4Q,63
R39.191 Need to immediately re-void
R39.192 Position dependent micturition
R39.198 Other difficulties with micturition

R39.2 Extrarenal uremia
Prerenal uremia
EXCLUDES 1 *uremia NOS (N19)*

R39.8 Other symptoms and signs involving the genitourinary system
AHA: 2017,4Q,22-23

R39.81 Functional urinary incontinence
Urinary incontinence due to cognitive impairment, or severe physical disability or immobility
EXCLUDES 1 *stress incontinence and other specified urinary incontinence (N39.3-N39.4-)*
urinary incontinence NOS (R32)

R39.82 Chronic bladder pain
AHA: 2016,4Q,64
R39.83 Unilateral non-palpable testicle ♂
R39.84 Bilateral non-palpable testicles ♂
R39.89 Other symptoms and signs involving the genitourinary system

R39.9 Unspecified symptoms and signs involving the genitourinary system

Symptoms and signs involving cognition, perception, emotional state and behavior (R40-R46)

EXCLUDES 2 *symptoms and signs constituting part of a pattern of mental disorder (F01-F99)*

R40 Somnolence, stupor and coma
EXCLUDES 1 *neonatal coma (P91.5)*
somnolence, stupor and coma in diabetes (E08-E13)
somnolence, stupor and coma in hepatic failure (K72.-)
somnolence, stupor and coma in hypoglycemia (nondiabetic) (E15)

R40.0 Somnolence
Drowsiness
EXCLUDES 1 *coma (R40.2-)*

R40.1 Stupor
Catatonic stupor
Semicoma
EXCLUDES 1 *catatonic schizophrenia (F20.2)*
coma (R40.2-)
depressive stupor (F31-F33)
dissociative stupor (F44.2)
manic stupor (F30.2)

R40.2 Coma
Code first any associated:
fracture of skull (S02.-)
intracranial injury (S06.-)
NOTE One code from each subcategory, R40.21-R40.23, is required to complete the coma scale
AHA: 2020,3Q,46; 2019,2Q,12; 2018,4Q,70; 2017,4Q,23-25,95; 2015,2Q,17; 2014,1Q,19
TIP: The codes for individual (R40.21-, R40.22-, R40.23-) or total (R40.24-) coma scale scores are only assigned as secondary diagnoses with traumatic brain injury (TBI) codes (S06.2X-, S06.30-, S06.9X-). While individual or total coma scale scores may be useful to providers in their clinical decision making when trying to establish a diagnosis, the codes reflecting these scores may not be assigned in conjunction with conditions other than TBIs.
TIP: Codes for individual (R40.21-, R40.22-, R40.23-) or total (R40.24-) coma scale scores may be assigned based on medical record documentation from clinicians who are not the patient's provider.
TIP: It is not appropriate to assign individual (R40.21- , R40.22-, R40.23-) or total (R40.24-) coma scale score codes for patients who are sedated or in medically induced comas.

R40.20 Unspecified coma MCC HCC
Coma NOS
Unconsciousness NOS
AHA: 2021,4Q,112-113; 2021,2Q,5

R40.21 Coma scale, eyes open

The following appropriate 7th character is to be added to subcategory R40.21-, R40.22-, R40.23-, and R40.24-.
0 unspecified time
1 in the field [EMT or ambulance]
2 at arrival to emergency department
3 at hospital admission
4 24 hours or more after hospital admission

R40.211 Coma scale, eyes open, never MCC UPD HCC
Coma scale eye opening score of 1
R40.212 Coma scale, eyes open, to pain MCC UPD HCC
Coma scale eye opening score of 2
R40.213 Coma scale, eyes open, to sound UPD
Coma scale eye opening score of 3
R40.214 Coma scale, eyes open, spontaneous UPD
Coma scale eye opening score of 4

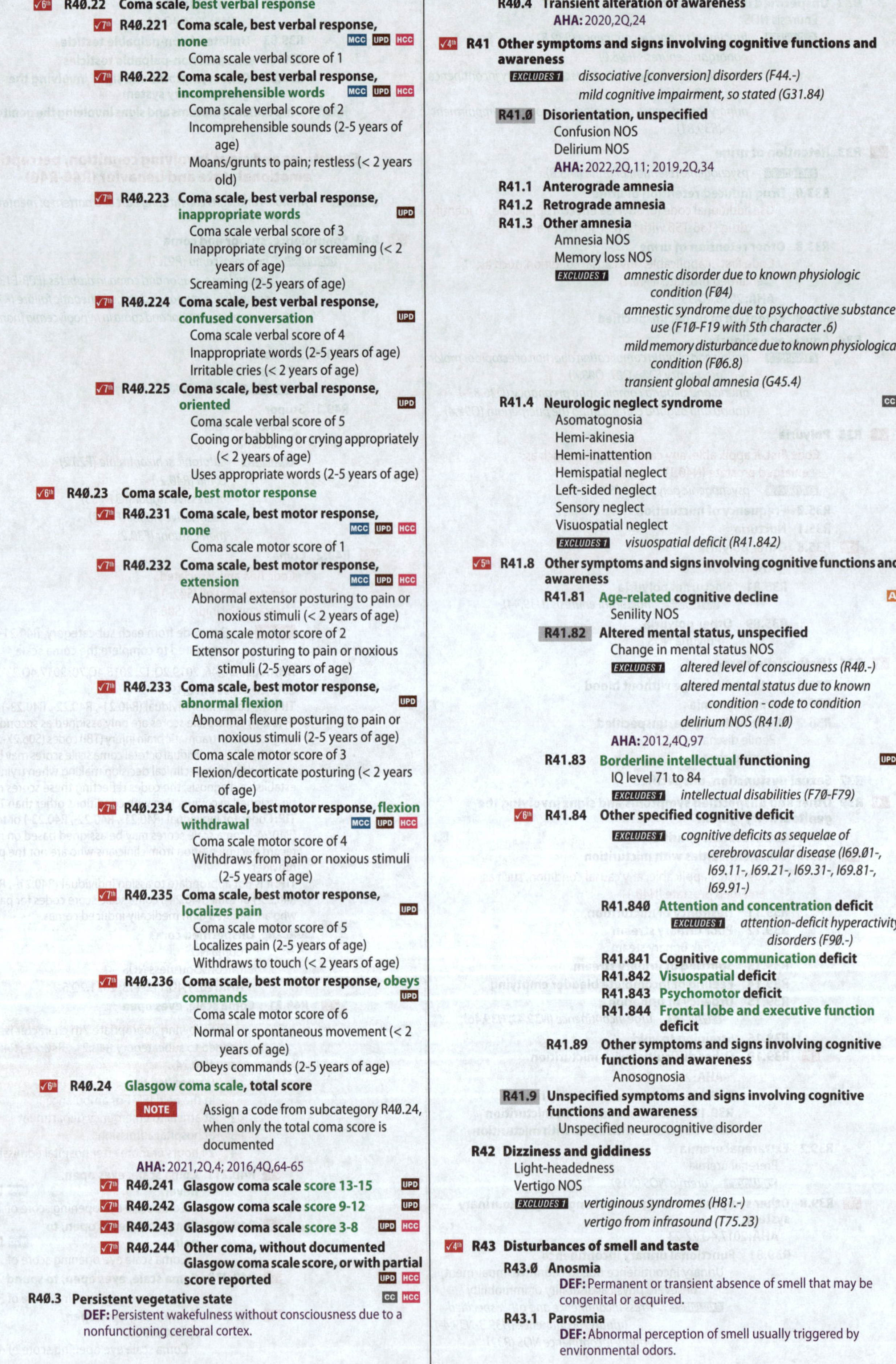

✓6th **R4Ø.22 Coma scale, best verbal response**

✓7th **R4Ø.221 Coma scale, best verbal response, none** MCC UPD HCC
Coma scale verbal score of 1

✓7th **R4Ø.222 Coma scale, best verbal response, incomprehensible words** MCC UPD HCC
Coma scale verbal score of 2
Incomprehensible sounds (2-5 years of age)
Moans/grunts to pain; restless (< 2 years old)

✓7th **R4Ø.223 Coma scale, best verbal response, inappropriate words** UPD
Coma scale verbal score of 3
Inappropriate crying or screaming (< 2 years of age)
Screaming (2-5 years of age)

✓7th **R4Ø.224 Coma scale, best verbal response, confused conversation** UPD
Coma scale verbal score of 4
Inappropriate words (2-5 years of age)
Irritable cries (< 2 years of age)

✓7th **R4Ø.225 Coma scale, best verbal response, oriented** UPD
Coma scale verbal score of 5
Cooing or babbling or crying appropriately (< 2 years of age)
Uses appropriate words (2-5 years of age)

✓6th **R4Ø.23 Coma scale, best motor response**

✓7th **R4Ø.231 Coma scale, best motor response, none** MCC UPD HCC
Coma scale motor score of 1

✓7th **R4Ø.232 Coma scale, best motor response, extension** MCC UPD HCC
Abnormal extensor posturing to pain or noxious stimuli (< 2 years of age)
Coma scale motor score of 2
Extensor posturing to pain or noxious stimuli (2-5 years of age)

✓7th **R4Ø.233 Coma scale, best motor response, abnormal flexion** UPD
Abnormal flexure posturing to pain or noxious stimuli (2-5 years of age)
Coma scale motor score of 3
Flexion/decorticate posturing (< 2 years of age)

✓7th **R4Ø.234 Coma scale, best motor response, flexion withdrawal** MCC UPD HCC
Coma scale motor score of 4
Withdraws from pain or noxious stimuli (2-5 years of age)

✓7th **R4Ø.235 Coma scale, best motor response, localizes pain** UPD
Coma scale motor score of 5
Localizes pain (2-5 years of age)
Withdraws to touch (< 2 years of age)

✓7th **R4Ø.236 Coma scale, best motor response, obeys commands** UPD
Coma scale motor score of 6
Normal or spontaneous movement (< 2 years of age)
Obeys commands (2-5 years of age)

✓6th **R4Ø.24 Glasgow coma scale, total score**
NOTE Assign a code from subcategory R4Ø.24, when only the total coma score is documented
AHA: 2021,2Q,4; 2016,4Q,64-65

✓7th **R4Ø.241 Glasgow coma scale score 13-15** UPD
✓7th **R4Ø.242 Glasgow coma scale score 9-12** UPD
✓7th **R4Ø.243 Glasgow coma scale score 3-8** UPD HCC
✓7th **R4Ø.244 Other coma, without documented Glasgow coma scale score, or with partial score reported** UPD HCC

R4Ø.3 Persistent vegetative state CC HCC
DEF: Persistent wakefulness without consciousness due to a nonfunctioning cerebral cortex.

R4Ø.4 Transient alteration of awareness
AHA: 2020,2Q,24

✓4th **R41 Other symptoms and signs involving cognitive functions and awareness**
EXCLUDES 1 *dissociative [conversion] disorders (F44.-)*
mild cognitive impairment, so stated (G31.84)

R41.Ø Disorientation, unspecified
Confusion NOS
Delirium NOS
AHA: 2022,2Q,11; 2019,2Q,34

R41.1 Anterograde amnesia

R41.2 Retrograde amnesia

R41.3 Other amnesia
Amnesia NOS
Memory loss NOS
EXCLUDES 1 *amnestic disorder due to known physiologic condition (FØ4)*
amnestic syndrome due to psychoactive substance use (F1Ø-F19 with 5th character .6)
mild memory disturbance due to known physiological condition (FØ6.8)
transient global amnesia (G45.4)

R41.4 Neurologic neglect syndrome CC
Asomatognosia
Hemi-akinesia
Hemi-inattention
Hemispatial neglect
Left-sided neglect
Sensory neglect
Visuospatial neglect
EXCLUDES 1 *visuospatial deficit (R41.842)*

✓5th **R41.8 Other symptoms and signs involving cognitive functions and awareness**

R41.81 Age-related cognitive decline A
Senility NOS

R41.82 Altered mental status, unspecified
Change in mental status NOS
EXCLUDES 1 *altered level of consciousness (R4Ø.-)*
altered mental status due to known condition - code to condition
delirium NOS (R41.Ø)
AHA: 2012,4Q,97

R41.83 Borderline intellectual functioning UPD
IQ level 71 to 84
EXCLUDES 1 *intellectual disabilities (F7Ø-F79)*

✓6th **R41.84 Other specified cognitive deficit**
EXCLUDES 1 *cognitive deficits as sequelae of cerebrovascular disease (I69.Ø1-, I69.11-, I69.21-, I69.31-, I69.81-, I69.91-)*

R41.84Ø Attention and concentration deficit
EXCLUDES 1 *attention-deficit hyperactivity disorders (F9Ø.-)*

R41.841 Cognitive communication deficit
R41.842 Visuospatial deficit
R41.843 Psychomotor deficit
R41.844 Frontal lobe and executive function deficit

R41.89 Other symptoms and signs involving cognitive functions and awareness
Anosognosia

R41.9 Unspecified symptoms and signs involving cognitive functions and awareness
Unspecified neurocognitive disorder

R42 Dizziness and giddiness
Light-headedness
Vertigo NOS
EXCLUDES 1 *vertiginous syndromes (H81.-)*
vertigo from infrasound (T75.23)

✓4th **R43 Disturbances of smell and taste**

R43.Ø Anosmia
DEF: Permanent or transient absence of smell that may be congenital or acquired.

R43.1 Parosmia
DEF: Abnormal perception of smell usually triggered by environmental odors.

R43.2 **Parageusia**
DEF: Abnormal perception of taste.

R43.8 **Other disturbances of smell and taste**
Mixed disturbance of smell and taste

R43.9 **Unspecified disturbances of smell and taste**

✓4th **R44 Other symptoms and signs involving general sensations and perceptions**
EXCLUDES 1 *alcoholic hallucinations (F1Ø.151, F1Ø.251, F1Ø.951)*
hallucinations in drug psychosis (F11-F19 with fifth to sixth characters 51)
hallucinations in mood disorders with psychotic symptoms (F3Ø.2, F31.5, F32.3, F33.3)
hallucinations in schizophrenia, schizotypal and delusional disorders (F2Ø-F29)
EXCLUDES 2 *disturbances of skin sensation (R2Ø.-)*

R44.Ø **Auditory hallucinations** CC
R44.1 **Visual hallucinations** CC
R44.2 **Other hallucinations** CC
R44.3 **Hallucinations, unspecified** CC
AHA: 2022,2Q,11
R44.8 **Other symptoms and signs involving general sensations and perceptions**
R44.9 **Unspecified symptoms and signs involving general sensations and perceptions**

✓4th **R45 Symptoms and signs involving emotional state**
R45.Ø **Nervousness**
Nervous tension
R45.1 **Restlessness and agitation**
R45.2 **Unhappiness**
R45.3 **Demoralization and apathy**
EXCLUDES 1 *anhedonia (R45.84)*
R45.4 **Irritability and anger**
R45.5 **Hostility**
R45.6 **Violent behavior**
R45.7 **State of emotional shock and stress, unspecified**
✓5th R45.8 **Other symptoms and signs involving emotional state**
R45.81 **Low self-esteem**
R45.82 **Worries**
R45.83 **Excessive crying of child, adolescent or adult**
EXCLUDES 1 *excessive crying of infant (baby) R68.11*
R45.84 **Anhedonia**
✓6th R45.85 **Homicidal and suicidal ideations**
EXCLUDES 1 *suicide attempt (T14.91)*
R45.85Ø **Homicidal ideations** UPD
R45.851 **Suicidal ideations** CC
AHA: 2022,1Q,29
DEF: Thoughts of committing suicide but no actual attempt of suicide has been made.
R45.86 **Emotional lability**
R45.87 **Impulsiveness**
R45.88 **Nonsuicidal self-harm** HCC
Nonsuicidal self-injury
Nonsuicidal self-mutilation
Self-inflicted injury without suicidal intent
Code also injury, if known
AHA: 2021,4Q,26-27
R45.89 **Other symptoms and signs involving emotional state**

✓4th **R46 Symptoms and signs involving appearance and behavior**
EXCLUDES 1 *appearance and behavior in schizophrenia, schizotypal and delusional disorders (F2Ø-F29)*
mental and behavioral disorders (FØ1-F99)
R46.Ø **Very low level of personal hygiene**
R46.1 **Bizarre personal appearance**
R46.2 **Strange and inexplicable behavior**
R46.3 **Overactivity**
R46.4 **Slowness and poor responsiveness**
EXCLUDES 1 *stupor (R4Ø.1)*
R46.5 **Suspiciousness and marked evasiveness**
R46.6 **Undue concern and preoccupation with stressful events**
R46.7 **Verbosity and circumstantial detail obscuring reason for contact**
✓5th R46.8 **Other symptoms and signs involving appearance and behavior**
R46.81 **Obsessive-compulsive behavior** UPD
EXCLUDES 1 *obsessive-compulsive disorder (F42.-)*
R46.89 **Other symptoms and signs involving appearance and behavior** UPD

Symptoms and signs involving speech and voice (R47-R49)

✓4th **R47 Speech disturbances, not elsewhere classified**
EXCLUDES 1 *autism (F84.Ø)*
cluttering (F8Ø.81)
specific developmental disorders of speech and language (F8Ø.-)
stuttering (F8Ø.81)
✓5th R47.Ø **Dysphasia and aphasia**
R47.Ø1 **Aphasia** CC
EXCLUDES 1 *aphasia following cerebrovascular disease (I69. with final characters -2Ø)*
progressive isolated aphasia (G31.Ø1)
R47.Ø2 **Dysphasia**
EXCLUDES 1 *dysphasia following cerebrovascular disease (I69. with final characters -21)*
R47.1 **Dysarthria and anarthria**
EXCLUDES 1 *dysarthria following cerebrovascular disease (I69. with final characters -22)*
✓5th R47.8 **Other speech disturbances**
EXCLUDES 1 *dysarthria following cerebrovascular disease (I69. with final characters -28)*
R47.81 **Slurred speech**
R47.82 ***Fluency disorder in conditions classified elsewhere***
Stuttering in conditions classified elsewhere
Code first underlying disease or condition, such as:
Parkinson's disease (G2Ø)
EXCLUDES 1 *adult onset fluency disorder (F98.5)*
childhood onset fluency disorder (F8Ø.81)
fluency disorder (stuttering) following cerebrovascular disease (I69. with final characters -23)
R47.89 **Other speech disturbances**
R47.9 **Unspecified speech disturbances**

✓4th **R48 Dyslexia and other symbolic dysfunctions, not elsewhere classified**
EXCLUDES 1 *specific developmental disorders of scholastic skills (F81.-)*
R48.Ø **Dyslexia and alexia**
R48.1 **Agnosia**
Astereognosia (astereognosis)
Autotopagnosia
EXCLUDES 1 *visual object agnosia (R48.3)*
DEF: Inability to recognize common things such as faces, objects, smells, or voices.
R48.2 **Apraxia**
EXCLUDES 1 *apraxia following cerebrovascular disease (I69. with final characters -9Ø)*
R48.3 **Visual agnosia**
Prosopagnosia
Simultanagnosia (asimultagnosia)
R48.8 **Other symbolic dysfunctions**
Acalculia
Agraphia
AHA: 2017,1Q,27
R48.9 **Unspecified symbolic dysfunctions**

✓4th **R49 Voice and resonance disorders**
EXCLUDES 1 *psychogenic voice and resonance disorders (F44.4)*
R49.Ø **Dysphonia**
Hoarseness
R49.1 **Aphonia**
Loss of voice
✓5th R49.2 **Hypernasality and hyponasality**
R49.21 **Hypernasality**
R49.22 **Hyponasality**
R49.8 **Other voice and resonance disorders**
R49.9 **Unspecified voice and resonance disorder**
Change in voice NOS
Resonance disorder NOS

General symptoms and signs (R5Ø-R69)

√4th R5Ø Fever of other and unknown origin

EXCLUDES 1 *chills without fever (R68.83)*
febrile convulsions (R56.Ø-)
fever of unknown origin during labor (O75.2)
fever of unknown origin in newborn (P81.9)
hypothermia due to illness (R68.Ø)
malignant hyperthermia due to anesthesia (T88.3)
puerperal pyrexia NOS (O86.4)

R5Ø.2 Drug induced fever
Use additional code for adverse effect, if applicable, to identify drug (T36-T5Ø with fifth or sixth character 5)
EXCLUDES 1 *postvaccination (postimmunization) fever (R5Ø.83)*

√5th R5Ø.8 Other specified fever

R5Ø.81 *Fever presenting with conditions classified elsewhere*
Code first underlying condition when associated fever is present, such as with:
leukemia (C91-C95)
neutropenia (D7Ø.-)
sickle-cell disease (D57.-)
AHA: 2020,3Q,22; 2014,4Q,22

R5Ø.82 Postprocedural fever
EXCLUDES 1 *postprocedural infection (T81.4-)*
posttransfusion fever (R5Ø.84)
postvaccination (postimmunization) fever (R5Ø.83)

R5Ø.83 Postvaccination fever
Postimmunization fever

R5Ø.84 Febrile nonhemolytic transfusion reaction
FNHTR
Posttransfusion fever

R5Ø.9 Fever, unspecified
Fever NOS
Fever of unknown origin [FUO]
Fever with chills
Fever with rigors
Hyperpyrexia NOS
Persistent fever
Pyrexia NOS

√4th R51 Headache

EXCLUDES 2 *atypical face pain (G5Ø.1)*
migraine and other headache syndromes (G43-G44)
trigeminal neuralgia (G5Ø.Ø)
AHA: 2020,4Q,38-39

R51.Ø Headache with orthostatic component, not elsewhere classified
Headache with positional component, not elsewhere classified

R51.9 Headache, unspecified
Facial pain NOS

R52 Pain, unspecified
Acute pain NOS
Generalized pain NOS
Pain NOS
EXCLUDES 1 *acute and chronic pain, not elsewhere classified (G89.-)*
localized pain, unspecified type - code to pain by site, such as:
abdomen pain (R1Ø.-)
back pain (M54.9)
breast pain (N64.4)
chest pain (RØ7.1-RØ7.9)
ear pain (H92.Ø-)
eye pain (H57.1)
headache (R51.9)
joint pain (M25.5-)
limb pain (M79.6-)
lumbar region pain (M54.5-)
pelvic and perineal pain (R1Ø.2)
renal colic (N23)
shoulder pain (M25.51-)
spine pain (M54.-)
throat pain (RØ7.Ø)
tongue pain (K14.6)
tooth pain (KØ8.8)
pain disorders exclusively related to psychological factors (F45.41)

√4th R53 Malaise and fatigue

R53.Ø Neoplastic (malignant) related fatigue
Code first associated neoplasm

R53.1 Weakness
Asthenia NOS
EXCLUDES 1 *age-related weakness (R54)*
muscle weakness (generalized) (M62.81)
sarcopenia (M62.84)
senile asthenia (R54)
AHA: 2017,1Q,7; 2015,1Q,25

R53.2 Functional quadriplegia MCC HCC
Complete immobility due to severe physical disability or frailty
EXCLUDES 1 *frailty NOS (R54)*
hysterical paralysis (F44.4)
immobility syndrome (M62.3)
neurologic quadriplegia (G82.5-)
quadriplegia (G82.5Ø)
AHA: 2016,2Q,6
DEF: Inability to move due to a nonphysiological condition, such as dementia. The patient has no mental ability to move independently.

√5th R53.8 Other malaise and fatigue
EXCLUDES 1 *combat exhaustion and fatigue (F43.Ø)*
congenital debility (P96.9)
exhaustion and fatigue due to excessive exertion (T73.3)
exhaustion and fatigue due to exposure (T73.2)
exhaustion and fatigue due to heat (T67.-)
exhaustion and fatigue due to pregnancy (O26.8-)
exhaustion and fatigue due to recurrent depressive episode (F33)
exhaustion and fatigue due to senile debility (R54)

R53.81 Other malaise
Chronic debility
Debility NOS
General physical deterioration
Malaise NOS
Nervous debility
EXCLUDES 1 *age-related physical debility (R54)*
AHA: 2021,1Q,43

R53.82 Chronic fatigue, unspecified
~~Chronic fatigue syndrome NOS~~
EXCLUDES 1 *►chronic fatigue syndrome (G93.32)◄*
►myalgic encephalomyelitis (G93.32)◄
►post infection and related fatigue syndromes (G93.39)◄
postviral fatigue syndrome ►(G93.31)◄

R53.83 Other fatigue
Fatigue NOS
Lack of energy
Lethargy
Tiredness
EXCLUDES 2 *exhaustion and fatigue due to depressive episode (F32.-)*

R54 Age-related physical debility A
Frailty
Old age
Senescence
Senile asthenia
Senile debility
EXCLUDES 1 *age-related cognitive decline (R41.81)*
sarcopenia (M62.84)
senile psychosis (FØ3)
senility NOS (R41.81)

R55 Syncope and collapse
Blackout
Fainting
Vasovagal attack
EXCLUDES 1 *cardiogenic shock (R57.Ø)*
carotid sinus syncope (G9Ø.Ø1)
heat syncope (T67.1)
neurocirculatory asthenia (F45.8)
neurogenic orthostatic hypotension (G9Ø.3)
orthostatic hypotension (I95.1)
postprocedural shock (T81.1-)
psychogenic syncope (F48.8)
shock NOS (R57.9)
shock complicating or following abortion or ectopic or molar pregnancy (OØØ-OØ7, OØ8.3)
shock complicating or following labor and delivery (O75.1)
Stokes-Adams attack (I45.9)
unconsciousness NOS (R4Ø.2-)

✓4th **R56 Convulsions, not elsewhere classified**
EXCLUDES 1 *dissociative convulsions and seizures (F44.5)*
epileptic convulsions and seizures (G4Ø.-)
newborn convulsions and seizures (P9Ø)

✓5th **R56.Ø Febrile convulsions**

R56.ØØ Simple febrile convulsions CC HCC
Febrile convulsion NOS
Febrile seizure NOS

R56.Ø1 Complex febrile convulsions CC HCC
Atypical febrile seizure
Complex febrile seizure
Complicated febrile seizure
EXCLUDES 1 *status epilepticus (G4Ø.9Ø1)*

R56.1 Post traumatic seizures CC HCC
EXCLUDES 1 *post traumatic epilepsy (G4Ø.-)*

R56.9 Unspecified convulsions HCC
Convulsion disorder
Fit NOS
Recurrent convulsions
Seizure(s) (convulsive) NOS
AHA: 2021,1Q,3; 2019,1Q,19

✓4th **R57 Shock, not elsewhere classified**
EXCLUDES 1 *anaphylactic shock NOS (T78.2)*
anaphylactic reaction or shock due to adverse food reaction (T78.Ø-)
anaphylactic shock due to adverse effect of correct drug or medicament properly administered (T88.6)
anaphylactic shock due to serum (T8Ø.5-)
electric shock (T75.4)
obstetric shock (O75.1)
postprocedural shock (T81.1-)
psychic shock (F43.Ø)
shock complicating or following ectopic or molar pregnancy (OØØ-OØ7, OØ8.3)
shock due to anesthesia (T88.2)
shock due to lightning (T75.Ø1)
toxic shock syndrome (A48.3)
traumatic shock (T79.4)

1 **R57.Ø Cardiogenic shock** MCC HCC
EXCLUDES 2 *septic shock (R65.21)*
AHA: 2020,3Q,26
DEF: Associated with myocardial infarction, cardiac tamponade, and massive pulmonary embolism. Symptoms include mental confusion, reduced blood pressure, tachycardia, pallor, and cold, clammy skin.

1 **R57.1 Hypovolemic shock** MCC HCC
AHA: 2019,2Q,7

1 **R57.8 Other shock** MCC HCC

R57.9 Shock, unspecified CC HCC
Failure of peripheral circulation NOS

R58 Hemorrhage, not elsewhere classified
Hemorrhage NOS
EXCLUDES 1 *hemorrhage included with underlying conditions, such as:*
acute duodenal ulcer with hemorrhage (K26.Ø)
acute gastritis with bleeding (K29.Ø1)
ulcerative enterocolitis with rectal bleeding (K51.Ø1)

✓4th **R59 Enlarged lymph nodes**
INCLUDES swollen glands
EXCLUDES 1 *acute lymphadenitis (LØ4.-)*
chronic lymphadenitis (I88.1)
lymphadenitis NOS (I88.9)
mesenteric (acute) (chronic) lymphadenitis (I88.Ø)

R59.Ø Localized enlarged lymph nodes

R59.1 Generalized enlarged lymph nodes
Lymphadenopathy NOS

R59.9 Enlarged lymph nodes, unspecified

✓4th **R6Ø Edema, not elsewhere classified**
EXCLUDES 1 *angioneurotic edema (T78.3)*
ascites (R18.-)
cerebral edema (G93.6)
cerebral edema due to birth injury (P11.Ø)
edema of larynx (J38.4)
edema of nasopharynx (J39.2)
edema of pharynx (J39.2)
gestational edema (O12.Ø-)
hereditary edema (Q82.Ø)
hydrops fetalis NOS (P83.2)
hydrothorax (J94.8)
newborn edema (P83.3)
pulmonary edema (J81.-)

R6Ø.Ø Localized edema

R6Ø.1 Generalized edema
EXCLUDES 2 *nutritional edema (E4Ø-E46)*

R6Ø.9 Edema, unspecified
Fluid retention NOS

R61 Generalized hyperhidrosis
Excessive sweating
Night sweats
Secondary hyperhidrosis
Code first, if applicable, menopausal and female climacteric states (N95.1)
EXCLUDES 1 *focal (primary) (secondary) hyperhidrosis (L74.5-)*
Frey's syndrome (L74.52)
localized (primary) (secondary) hyperhidrosis (L74.5-)

√4th R62 Lack of expected normal physiological development in childhood and adults

EXCLUDES 1 *delayed puberty (E30.0)*
gonadal dysgenesis (Q99.1)
hypopituitarism (E23.0)

R62.0 Delayed milestone in childhood P
Delayed attainment of expected physiological developmental stage
Late talker
Late walker

√5th R62.5 Other and unspecified lack of expected normal physiological development in childhood
EXCLUDES 1 *HIV disease resulting in failure to thrive (B20)*
physical retardation due to malnutrition (E45)

R62.50 Unspecified lack of expected normal physiological development in childhood
Infantilism NOS

R62.51 Failure to thrive (child) P
Failure to gain weight
EXCLUDES 1 *failure to thrive in child under 28 days old (P92.6)*
AHA: 2018,4Q,82
DEF: Organic failure to thrive (FTT): Acute or chronic illness that interferes with nutritional intake, absorption, metabolism excretion, and energy requirements.
DEF: Nonorganic failure to thrive (FTT): Symptom of neglect or abuse.

R62.52 Short stature (child)
Lack of growth
Physical retardation
Short stature NOS
EXCLUDES 1 *short stature due to endocrine disorder ►(E34.3-)◄*

R62.59 Other lack of expected normal physiological development in childhood

R62.7 Adult failure to thrive A

√4th R63 Symptoms and signs concerning food and fluid intake
EXCLUDES 1 *bulimia NOS (F50.2)*

R63.0 Anorexia
Loss of appetite
EXCLUDES 1 *anorexia nervosa (F50.0-)*
loss of appetite of nonorganic origin (F50.89)
AHA: 2018,4Q,82
TIP: Assign an additional code from category Z68 when BMI is documented. BMI can be based on documentation from clinicians who are not the patient's provider.

R63.1 Polydipsia
Excessive thirst

R63.2 Polyphagia
Excessive eating
Hyperalimentation NOS

√5th R63.3 Feeding difficulties
EXCLUDES 2 *eating disorders (F50.-)*
feeding problems of newborn (P92.-)
infant feeding disorder of nonorganic origin (F98.2-)
AHA: 2021,4Q,27-28; 2017,1Q,28; 2016,3Q,19

R63.30 Feeding difficulties, unspecified

R63.31 Pediatric feeding disorder, acute P
Pediatric feeding dysfunction, acute
Code also, if applicable, associated conditions such as:
aspiration pneumonia (J69.0)
dysphagia (R13.1-)
gastro-esophageal reflux disease (K21.-)
malnutrition (E40-E46)

R63.32 Pediatric feeding disorder, chronic P
Pediatric feeding dysfunction, chronic
Code also, if applicable, associated conditions such as:
aspiration pneumonia (J69.0)
dysphagia (R13.1-)
gastro-esophageal reflux disease (K21.-)
malnutrition (E40-E46)

R63.39 Other feeding difficulties
Feeding problem (elderly) (infant) NOS
Picky eater

R63.4 Abnormal weight loss
AHA: 2018,4Q,82
TIP: Assign an additional code from category Z68 when BMI is documented. BMI can be based on documentation from clinicians who are not the patient's provider.

R63.5 Abnormal weight gain
EXCLUDES 1 *excessive weight gain in pregnancy (O26.0-)*
obesity (E66.-)
AHA: 2018,4Q,82
TIP: Assign an additional code from category Z68 when BMI is documented. BMI can be based on documentation from clinicians who are not the patient's provider.

R63.6 Underweight
Use additional code to identify body mass index (BMI), if known (Z68.-)
EXCLUDES 1 *abnormal weight loss (R63.4)*
anorexia nervosa (F50.0-)
malnutrition (E40-E46)
AHA: 2018,4Q,82

R63.8 Other symptoms and signs concerning food and fluid intake

R64 Cachexia CC HCC
Wasting syndrome
Code first underlying condition, if known
EXCLUDES 1 *abnormal weight loss (R63.4)*
nutritional marasmus (E41)
AHA: 2018,4Q,82; 2017,3Q,24
TIP: Assign code E43 when emaciated or emaciation is documented in relation to malnutrition.

√4th R65 Symptoms and signs specifically associated with systemic inflammation and infection
AHA: 2019,2Q,38
TIP: When documentation states SIRS with an infection, assign only a code for the infection. ICD-10-CM does not offer a code for SIRS due to infectious process. If sepsis is suspected, query the provider.

√5th R65.1 Systemic inflammatory response syndrome [SIRS] of non-infectious origin
Code first underlying condition, such as:
heatstroke (T67.0-)
injury and trauma (S00-T88)
EXCLUDES 1 *sepsis - code to infection*
severe sepsis (R65.2)

R65.10 Systemic inflammatory response syndrome [SIRS] of non-infectious origin without acute organ dysfunction CC UPD HCC
Systemic inflammatory response syndrome (SIRS) NOS
AHA: 2019,2Q,24

R65.11 Systemic inflammatory response syndrome [SIRS] of non-infectious origin with acute organ dysfunction MCC UPD HCC
Use additional code to identify specific acute organ dysfunction, such as:
acute kidney failure (N17.-)
acute respiratory failure (J96.0-)
critical illness myopathy (G72.81)
critical illness polyneuropathy (G62.81)
disseminated intravascular coagulopathy [DIC] (D65)
encephalopathy (metabolic) (septic) (G93.41)
hepatic failure (K72.0-)

R65.2 Severe sepsis
Infection with associated acute organ dysfunction
Sepsis with acute organ dysfunction
Sepsis with multiple organ dysfunction
Systemic inflammatory response syndrome due to infectious process with acute organ dysfunction
Code first underlying infection, such as:
infection following a procedure (T81.4-)
infections following infusion, transfusion and therapeutic injection (T8Ø.2-)
puerperal sepsis (O85)
sepsis following complete or unspecified spontaneous abortion (OØ3.87)
sepsis following ectopic and molar pregnancy (OØ8.82)
sepsis following incomplete spontaneous abortion (OØ3.37)
sepsis following (induced) termination of pregnancy (OØ4.87)
sepsis NOS (A41.9)
Use additional code to identify specific acute organ dysfunction, such as:
acute kidney failure (N17.-)
acute respiratory failure (J96.Ø-)
critical illness myopathy (G72.81)
critical illness polyneuropathy (G62.81)
disseminated intravascular coagulopathy [DIC] (D65)
encephalopathy (metabolic) (septic) (G93.41)
hepatic failure (K72.Ø-)
AHA: 2020,2Q,17; 2018,4Q,62-63; 2017,4Q,98-99; 2016,3Q,8

R65.2Ø Severe sepsis without septic shock MCC UPD HCC
Severe sepsis NOS
AHA: 2020,2Q,17; 2016,3Q,14; 2013,4Q,119

R65.21 Severe sepsis with septic shock MCC UPD HCC
AHA: 2018,4Q,63

R68 Other general symptoms and signs

R68.Ø Hypothermia, not associated with low environmental temperature
EXCLUDES 1 *hypothermia NOS (accidental) (T68)*
hypothermia due to anesthesia (T88.51)
hypothermia due to low environmental temperature (T68)
newborn hypothermia (P8Ø.-)

R68.1 Nonspecific symptoms peculiar to infancy
EXCLUDES 1 *colic, infantile (R1Ø.83)*
neonatal cerebral irritability (P91.3)
teething syndrome (KØØ.7)

R68.11 Excessive crying of infant (baby) P
EXCLUDES 1 *excessive crying of child, adolescent, or adult (R45.83)*

R68.12 Fussy infant (baby) P
Irritable infant

R68.13 Apparent life threatening event in infant (ALTE) P
Apparent life threatening event in newborn
Brief resolved unexplained event (BRUE)
Code first confirmed diagnosis, if known
Use additional code(s) for associated signs and symptoms if no confirmed diagnosis established, or if signs and symptoms are not associated routinely with confirmed diagnosis, or provide additional information for cause of ALTE

R68.19 Other nonspecific symptoms peculiar to infancy P

R68.2 Dry mouth, unspecified
EXCLUDES 1 *dry mouth due to dehydration (E86.Ø)*
dry mouth due to Sjögren syndrome (M35.Ø-)
salivary gland hyposecretion (K11.7)

R68.3 Clubbing of fingers
Clubbing of nails
EXCLUDES 1 *congenital clubfinger (Q68.1)*
DEF: Enlarged soft tissue of the distal fingers that usually occurs in heart and lung diseases.

R68.8 Other general symptoms and signs

R68.81 Early satiety
DEF: Premature feeling of being full after eating only a small amount of food. The mechanism of satiety is multifactorial.

R68.82 Decreased libido A
Decreased sexual desire

R68.83 Chills (without fever)
Chills NOS
EXCLUDES 1 *chills with fever (R5Ø.9)*

R68.84 Jaw pain
Mandibular pain
Maxilla pain
EXCLUDES 1 *temporomandibular joint arthralgia (M26.62-)*

R68.89 Other general symptoms and signs

R69 Illness, unspecified
Unknown and unspecified cases of morbidity

Abnormal findings on examination of blood, without diagnosis (R7Ø-R79)

EXCLUDES 2 *abnormal findings on antenatal screening of mother (O28.-)*
abnormalities of lipids (E78.-)
abnormalities of platelets and thrombocytes (D69.-)
abnormalities of white blood cells classified elsewhere (D7Ø-D72)
coagulation hemorrhagic disorders (D65-D68)
diagnostic abnormal findings classified elsewhere - see Alphabetical Index
hemorrhagic and hematological disorders of newborn (P5Ø-P61)

R7Ø Elevated erythrocyte sedimentation rate and abnormality of plasma viscosity

R7Ø.Ø Elevated erythrocyte sedimentation rate

R7Ø.1 Abnormal plasma viscosity

R71 Abnormality of red blood cells
EXCLUDES 1 *anemias (D5Ø-D64)*
anemia of premature infant (P61.2)
benign (familial) polycythemia (D75.Ø)
congenital anemias (P61.2-P61.4)
newborn anemia due to isoimmunization (P55.-)
polycythemia neonatorum (P61.1)
polycythemia NOS (D75.1)
polycythemia vera (D45)
secondary polycythemia (D75.1)

R71.Ø Precipitous drop in hematocrit CC
Drop (precipitous) in hemoglobin
Drop in hematocrit

R71.8 Other abnormality of red blood cells
Abnormal red-cell morphology NOS
Abnormal red-cell volume NOS
Anisocytosis
Poikilocytosis

R73 Elevated blood glucose level
EXCLUDES 1 *diabetes mellitus (EØ8-E13)*
diabetes mellitus in pregnancy, childbirth and the puerperium (O24.-)
neonatal disorders (P7Ø.Ø-P7Ø.2)
postsurgical hypoinsulinemia (E89.1)

R73.Ø Abnormal glucose
EXCLUDES 1 *abnormal glucose in pregnancy (O99.81-)*
diabetes mellitus (EØ8-E13)
dysmetabolic syndrome X (E88.81)
gestational diabetes (O24.4-)
glycosuria (R81)
hypoglycemia (E16.2)

R73.Ø1 Impaired fasting glucose
Elevated fasting glucose

R73.Ø2 Impaired glucose tolerance (oral)
Elevated glucose tolerance

R73.Ø3 Prediabetes
Latent diabetes
AHA: 2016,4Q,65

R73.Ø9 Other abnormal glucose
Abnormal glucose NOS
Abnormal non-fasting glucose tolerance

R73.9 Hyperglycemia, unspecified

R74 Abnormal serum enzyme levels

R74.Ø Nonspecific elevation of levels of transaminase and lactic acid dehydrogenase [LDH]
AHA: 2020,4Q,39

R74.Ø1 Elevation of levels of liver transaminase levels
Elevation of levels of alanine transaminase (ALT)
Elevation of levels of aspartate transaminase (AST)

R74.Ø2 Elevation of levels of lactic acid dehydrogenase [LDH]

R74.8 Abnormal levels of other serum enzymes
Abnormal level of acid phosphatase
Abnormal level of alkaline phosphatase
Abnormal level of amylase
Abnormal level of lipase [triacylglycerol lipase]
AHA: 2019,2Q,6

R74.9 Abnormal serum enzyme level, unspecified

R75 Inconclusive laboratory evidence of human immunodeficiency virus [HIV]
Nonconclusive HIV-test finding in infants
EXCLUDES 1 *asymptomatic human immunodeficiency virus [HIV] infection status (Z21)*
human immunodeficiency virus [HIV] disease (B2Ø)

R76 Other abnormal immunological findings in serum

R76.Ø Raised antibody titer
EXCLUDES 1 *isoimmunization in pregnancy (O36.Ø-O36.1)*
isoimmunization affecting newborn (P55.-)
AHA: 2021,1Q,6

R76.1 Nonspecific reaction to test for tuberculosis

R76.11 Nonspecific reaction to tuberculin skin test without active tuberculosis
Abnormal result of Mantoux test
PPD positive
Tuberculin (skin test) positive
Tuberculin (skin test) reactor
EXCLUDES 1 *nonspecific reaction to cell mediated immunity measurement of gamma interferon antigen response without active tuberculosis (R76.12)*

R76.12 Nonspecific reaction to cell mediated immunity measurement of gamma interferon antigen response without active tuberculosis
Nonspecific reaction to QuantiFERON-TB test (QFT) without active tuberculosis
EXCLUDES 1 *nonspecific reaction to tuberculin skin test without active tuberculosis (R76.11)*
positive tuberculin skin test (R76.11)

R76.8 Other specified abnormal immunological findings in serum
Raised level of immunoglobulins NOS
AHA: 2021,1Q,6

R76.9 Abnormal immunological finding in serum, unspecified

R77 Other abnormalities of plasma proteins
EXCLUDES 1 *disorders of plasma-protein metabolism (E88.Ø-)*

R77.Ø Abnormality of albumin

R77.1 Abnormality of globulin
Hyperglobulinemia NOS

R77.2 Abnormality of alphafetoprotein

R77.8 Other specified abnormalities of plasma proteins

R77.9 Abnormality of plasma protein, unspecified
AHA: 2019,2Q,6

R78 Findings of drugs and other substances, not normally found in blood
Use additional code to identify the any retained foreign body, if applicable (Z18.-)
EXCLUDES 1 *mental or behavioral disorders due to psychoactive substance use (F1Ø-F19)*

R78.Ø Finding of alcohol in blood
Use additional external cause code (Y9Ø.-), for detail regarding alcohol level

R78.1 Finding of opiate drug in blood

R78.2 Finding of cocaine in blood

R78.3 Finding of hallucinogen in blood

R78.4 Finding of other drugs of addictive potential in blood

R78.5 Finding of other psychotropic drug in blood

R78.6 Finding of steroid agent in blood

R78.7 Finding of abnormal level of heavy metals in blood

R78.71 Abnormal lead level in blood
EXCLUDES 1 *lead poisoning (T56.Ø-)*

R78.79 Finding of abnormal level of heavy metals in blood

R78.8 Finding of other specified substances, not normally found in blood

R78.81 Bacteremia CC
EXCLUDES 1 *sepsis — code to specified infection*
DEF: Laboratory finding of bacteria in the blood in the absence of two or more signs of sepsis. Transient in nature, it can progress to septicemia with a severe infectious process.

R78.89 Finding of other specified substances, not normally found in blood
Finding of abnormal level of lithium in blood

R78.9 Finding of unspecified substance, not normally found in blood

R79 Other abnormal findings of blood chemistry
Use additional code to identify any retained foreign body, if applicable (Z18.-)
EXCLUDES 1 *asymptomatic hyperuricemia (E79.Ø)*
hyperglycemia NOS (R73.9)
hypoglycemia NOS (E16.2)
neonatal hypoglycemia (P7Ø.3-P7Ø.4)
specific findings indicating disorder of amino-acid metabolism (E7Ø-E72)
specific findings indicating disorder of carbohydrate metabolism (E73-E74)
specific findings indicating disorder of lipid metabolism (E75.-)

R79.Ø Abnormal level of blood mineral
Abnormal blood level of cobalt
Abnormal blood level of copper
Abnormal blood level of iron
Abnormal blood level of magnesium
Abnormal blood level of mineral NEC
Abnormal blood level of zinc
EXCLUDES 1 *abnormal level of lithium (R78.89)*
disorders of mineral metabolism (E83.-)
neonatal hypomagnesemia (P71.2)
nutritional mineral deficiency (E58-E61)

R79.1 Abnormal coagulation profile
Abnormal or prolonged bleeding time
Abnormal or prolonged coagulation time
Abnormal or prolonged partial thromboplastin time [PTT]
Abnormal or prolonged prothrombin time [PT]
▶Low von Willebrand factor◀
EXCLUDES 1 *coagulation defects (D68.-)*
EXCLUDES 2 *abnormality of fluid, electrolyte or acid-base balance (E86-E87)*

R79.8 Other specified abnormal findings of blood chemistry

R79.81 Abnormal blood-gas level

R79.82 Elevated C-reactive protein [CRP]

R79.83 Abnormal findings of blood amino-acid level
Homocysteinemia
EXCLUDES 1 *disorders of amino-acid metabolism (E7Ø-E72)*
AHA: 2021,4Q,28

R79.89 Other specified abnormal findings of blood chemistry
AHA: 2019,2Q,6
TIP: Assign for positive Coombs test when not further clarified in the documentation.

R79.9 Abnormal finding of blood chemistry, unspecified

Abnormal findings on examination of urine, without diagnosis (R80-R82)

EXCLUDES 1 *abnormal findings on antenatal screening of mother (O28.-)*
diagnostic abnormal findings classified elsewhere - see Alphabetical Index
specific findings indicating disorder of amino-acid metabolism (E70-E72)
specific findings indicating disorder of carbohydrate metabolism (E73-E74)

✓4th **R80 Proteinuria**
EXCLUDES 1 *gestational proteinuria (O12.1-)*
R80.0 Isolated proteinuria
Idiopathic proteinuria
EXCLUDES 1 *isolated proteinuria with specific morphological lesion (N06.-)*
R80.1 Persistent proteinuria, unspecified
R80.2 Orthostatic proteinuria, unspecified
Postural proteinuria
R80.3 Bence Jones proteinuria
R80.8 Other proteinuria
R80.9 Proteinuria, unspecified
Albuminuria NOS

R81 Glycosuria
EXCLUDES 1 *renal glycosuria (E74.818)*

✓4th **R82 Other and unspecified abnormal findings in urine**
INCLUDES chromoabnormalities in urine
Use additional code to identify any retained foreign body, if applicable (Z18.-)
EXCLUDES 2 *hematuria (R31.-)*
R82.0 Chyluria CC
EXCLUDES 1 *filarial chyluria (B74.-)*
R82.1 Myoglobinuria CC
R82.2 Biliuria
R82.3 Hemoglobinuria
EXCLUDES 1 *hemoglobinuria due to hemolysis from external causes NEC (D59.6)*
hemoglobinuria due to paroxysmal nocturnal [Marchiafava-Micheli] (D59.5)
DEF: Free hemoglobin in blood due to rapid hemolysis of red blood cells. Causes include burns, crushed injury, sickle cell anemia, thalassemia, parasitic infections, or kidney infections.
R82.4 Acetonuria
Ketonuria
DEF: Excessive excretion of acetone in urine that commonly occurs in diabetic acidosis.
R82.5 Elevated urine levels of drugs, medicaments and biological substances
Elevated urine levels of catecholamines
Elevated urine levels of indoleacetic acid
Elevated urine levels of 17-ketosteroids
Elevated urine levels of steroids
R82.6 Abnormal urine levels of substances chiefly nonmedicinal as to source
Abnormal urine level of heavy metals
✓5th **R82.7 Abnormal findings on microbiological examination of urine**
EXCLUDES 1 *colonization status (Z22.-)*
AHA: 2016,4Q,65
R82.71 Bacteriuria
R82.79 Other abnormal findings on microbiological examination of urine
Positive culture findings of urine
✓5th **R82.8 Abnormal findings on cytological and histological examination of urine**
AHA: 2019,4Q,16
R82.81 Pyuria
Sterile pyuria
R82.89 Other abnormal findings on cytological and histological examination of urine
✓5th **R82.9 Other and unspecified abnormal findings in urine**
R82.90 Unspecified abnormal findings in urine
R82.91 Other chromoabnormalities of urine
Chromoconversion (dipstick)
Idiopathic dipstick converts positive for blood with no cellular forms in sediment
EXCLUDES 1 *hemoglobinuria (R82.3)*
myoglobinuria (R82.1)
✓6th **R82.99 Other abnormal findings in urine**
AHA: 2018,4Q,29-30
R82.991 Hypocitraturia
R82.992 Hyperoxaluria
EXCLUDES 1 *primary hyperoxaluria (E72.53)*
R82.993 Hyperuricosuria
R82.994 Hypercalciuria
Idiopathic hypercalciuria
R82.998 Other abnormal findings in urine
Cells and casts in urine
Crystalluria
Melanuria

Abnormal findings on examination of other body fluids, substances and tissues, without diagnosis (R83-R89)

EXCLUDES 1 *abnormal findings on antenatal screening of mother (O28.-)*
diagnostic abnormal findings classified elsewhere - see Alphabetical Index
EXCLUDES 2 *abnormal findings on examination of blood, without diagnosis (R70-R79)*
abnormal findings on examination of urine, without diagnosis (R80-R82)
abnormal tumor markers (R97.-)

✓4th **R83 Abnormal findings in cerebrospinal fluid**
R83.0 Abnormal level of enzymes in cerebrospinal fluid
R83.1 Abnormal level of hormones in cerebrospinal fluid
R83.2 Abnormal level of other drugs, medicaments and biological substances in cerebrospinal fluid
R83.3 Abnormal level of substances chiefly nonmedicinal as to source in cerebrospinal fluid
R83.4 Abnormal immunological findings in cerebrospinal fluid
R83.5 Abnormal microbiological findings in cerebrospinal fluid
Positive culture findings in cerebrospinal fluid
EXCLUDES 1 *colonization status (Z22.-)*
R83.6 Abnormal cytological findings in cerebrospinal fluid
R83.8 Other abnormal findings in cerebrospinal fluid
Abnormal chromosomal findings in cerebrospinal fluid
R83.9 Unspecified abnormal finding in cerebrospinal fluid

✓4th **R84 Abnormal findings in specimens from respiratory organs and thorax**
INCLUDES abnormal findings in bronchial washings
abnormal findings in nasal secretions
abnormal findings in pleural fluid
abnormal findings in sputum
abnormal findings in throat scrapings
EXCLUDES 1 *blood-stained sputum (R04.2)*
R84.0 Abnormal level of enzymes in specimens from respiratory organs and thorax
R84.1 Abnormal level of hormones in specimens from respiratory organs and thorax
R84.2 Abnormal level of other drugs, medicaments and biological substances in specimens from respiratory organs and thorax
R84.3 Abnormal level of substances chiefly nonmedicinal as to source in specimens from respiratory organs and thorax
R84.4 Abnormal immunological findings in specimens from respiratory organs and thorax
R84.5 Abnormal microbiological findings in specimens from respiratory organs and thorax
Positive culture findings in specimens from respiratory organs and thorax
EXCLUDES 1 *colonization status (Z22.-)*
R84.6 Abnormal cytological findings in specimens from respiratory organs and thorax
R84.7 Abnormal histological findings in specimens from respiratory organs and thorax
R84.8 Other abnormal findings in specimens from respiratory organs and thorax
Abnormal chromosomal findings in specimens from respiratory organs and thorax
R84.9 Unspecified abnormal finding in specimens from respiratory organs and thorax

✓4th R85 Abnormal findings in specimens from digestive organs and abdominal cavity

INCLUDES abnormal findings in peritoneal fluid
abnormal findings in saliva

EXCLUDES 1 *cloudy peritoneal dialysis effluent (R88.Ø)*
fecal abnormalities (R19.5)

R85.Ø Abnormal level of enzymes in specimens from digestive organs and abdominal cavity

R85.1 Abnormal level of hormones in specimens from digestive organs and abdominal cavity

R85.2 Abnormal level of other drugs, medicaments and biological substances in specimens from digestive organs and abdominal cavity

R85.3 Abnormal level of substances chiefly nonmedicinal as to source in specimens from digestive organs and abdominal cavity

R85.4 Abnormal immunological findings in specimens from digestive organs and abdominal cavity

R85.5 Abnormal microbiological findings in specimens from digestive organs and abdominal cavity
Positive culture findings in specimens from digestive organs and abdominal cavity
EXCLUDES 1 *colonization status (Z22.-)*

✓5th R85.6 Abnormal cytological findings in specimens from digestive organs and abdominal cavity

✓6th R85.61 Abnormal cytologic smear of anus
EXCLUDES 1 *abnormal cytological findings in specimens from other digestive organs and abdominal cavity (R85.69)*
anal intraepithelial neoplasia I [AIN I] (K62.82)
anal intraepithelial neoplasia II [AIN II] (K62.82)
anal intraepithelial neoplasia III [AIN III] (DØ1.3)
carcinoma in situ of anus (histologically confirmed) (DØ1.3)
dysplasia (mild) (moderate) of anus (histologically confirmed) (K62.82)
severe dysplasia of anus (histologically confirmed) (DØ1.3)
EXCLUDES 2 *anal high risk human papillomavirus (HPV) DNA test positive (R85.81)*
anal low risk human papillomavirus (HPV) DNA test positive (R85.82)

R85.61Ø Atypical squamous cells of undetermined significance on cytologic smear of anus [ASC-US]

R85.611 Atypical squamous cells cannot exclude high grade squamous intraepithelial lesion on cytologic smear of anus [ASC-H]

R85.612 Low grade squamous intraepithelial lesion on cytologic smear of anus [LGSIL]

R85.613 High grade squamous intraepithelial lesion on cytologic smear of anus [HGSIL]

R85.614 Cytologic evidence of malignancy on smear of anus

R85.615 Unsatisfactory cytologic smear of anus
Inadequate sample of cytologic smear of anus

R85.616 Satisfactory anal smear but lacking transformation zone

R85.618 Other abnormal cytological findings on specimens from anus

R85.619 Unspecified abnormal cytological findings in specimens from anus
Abnormal anal cytology NOS
Atypical glandular cells of anus NOS

R85.69 Abnormal cytological findings in specimens from other digestive organs and abdominal cavity

R85.7 Abnormal histological findings in specimens from digestive organs and abdominal cavity

✓5th R85.8 Other abnormal findings in specimens from digestive organs and abdominal cavity

R85.81 Anal high risk human papillomavirus [HPV] DNA test positive
EXCLUDES 1 *anogenital warts due to human papillomavirus (HPV) (A63.Ø)*
condyloma acuminatum (A63.Ø)

R85.82 Anal low risk human papillomavirus [HPV] DNA test positive
Use additional code for associated human papillomavirus (B97.7)

R85.89 Other abnormal findings in specimens from digestive organs and abdominal cavity
Abnormal chromosomal findings in specimens from digestive organs and abdominal cavity

R85.9 Unspecified abnormal finding in specimens from digestive organs and abdominal cavity

✓4th R86 Abnormal findings in specimens from male genital organs

INCLUDES abnormal findings in prostatic secretions
abnormal findings in semen, seminal fluid
abnormal spermatozoa

EXCLUDES 1 *azoospermia (N46.Ø-)*
oligospermia (N46.1-)

R86.Ø Abnormal level of enzymes in specimens from male genital organs ♂

R86.1 Abnormal level of hormones in specimens from male genital organs ♂

R86.2 Abnormal level of other drugs, medicaments and biological substances in specimens from male genital organs ♂

R86.3 Abnormal level of substances chiefly nonmedicinal as to source in specimens from male genital organs ♂

R86.4 Abnormal immunological findings in specimens from male genital organs ♂

R86.5 Abnormal microbiological findings in specimens from male genital organs ♂
Positive culture findings in specimens from male genital organs
EXCLUDES 1 *colonization status (Z22.-)*

R86.6 Abnormal cytological findings in specimens from male genital organs ♂

R86.7 Abnormal histological findings in specimens from male genital organs ♂

R86.8 Other abnormal findings in specimens from male genital organs ♂
Abnormal chromosomal findings in specimens from male genital organs

R86.9 Unspecified abnormal finding in specimens from male genital organs ♂

✓4th R87 Abnormal findings in specimens from female genital organs

INCLUDES abnormal findings in secretion and smears from cervix uteri
abnormal findings in secretion and smears from vagina
abnormal findings in secretion and smears from vulva

R87.Ø Abnormal level of enzymes in specimens from female genital organs ♀

R87.1 Abnormal level of hormones in specimens from female genital organs ♀

R87.2 Abnormal level of other drugs, medicaments and biological substances in specimens from female genital organs ♀

R87.3 Abnormal level of substances chiefly nonmedicinal as to source in specimens from female genital organs ♀

R87.4 Abnormal immunological findings in specimens from female genital organs ♀

R87.5 Abnormal microbiological findings in specimens from female genital organs ♀
Positive culture findings in specimens from female genital organs
EXCLUDES 1 *colonization status (Z22.-)*

R87.6 Abnormal cytological findings in specimens from female genital organs

R87.61 Abnormal cytological findings in specimens from cervix uteri

EXCLUDES 1 *abnormal cytological findings in specimens from other female genital organs (R87.69)*
abnormal cytological findings in specimens from vagina (R87.62-)
carcinoma in situ of cervix uteri (histologically confirmed) (D06.-)
cervical intraepithelial neoplasia I [CIN I] (N87.0)
cervical intraepithelial neoplasia II [CIN II] (N87.1)
cervical intraepithelial neoplasia III [CIN III] (D06.-)
dysplasia (mild) (moderate) of cervix uteri (histologically confirmed) (N87.-)
severe dysplasia of cervix uteri (histologically confirmed) (D06.-)

EXCLUDES 2 *cervical high risk human papillomavirus (HPV) DNA test positive (R87.810)*
cervical low risk human papillomavirus (HPV) DNA test positive (R87.820)

R87.610 Atypical squamous cells of undetermined significance on cytologic smear of cervix [ASC-US] ♀

R87.611 Atypical squamous cells cannot exclude high grade squamous intraepithelial lesion on cytologic smear of cervix [ASC-H] ♀

R87.612 Low grade squamous intraepithelial lesion on cytologic smear of cervix [LGSIL] ♀

R87.613 High grade squamous intraepithelial lesion on cytologic smear of cervix [HGSIL] ♀

R87.614 Cytologic evidence of malignancy on smear of cervix ♀

R87.615 Unsatisfactory cytologic smear of cervix ♀
Inadequate sample of cytologic smear of cervix

R87.616 Satisfactory cervical smear but lacking transformation zone ♀

R87.618 Other abnormal cytological findings on specimens from cervix uteri ♀

R87.619 Unspecified abnormal cytological findings in specimens from cervix uteri ♀
Abnormal cervical cytology NOS
Abnormal Papanicolaou smear of cervix NOS
Abnormal thin preparation smear of cervix NOS
Atypical endocervial cells of cervix NOS
Atypical endometrial cells of cervix NOS
Atypical glandular cells of cervix NOS

R87.62 Abnormal cytological findings in specimens from vagina

Use additional code to identify acquired absence of uterus and cervix, if applicable (Z90.71-)

EXCLUDES 1 *abnormal cytological findings in specimens from cervix uteri (R87.61-)*
abnormal cytological findings in specimens from other female genital organs (R87.69)
carcinoma in situ of vagina (histologically confirmed) (D07.2)
dysplasia (mild) (moderate) of vagina (histologically confirmed) (N89.-)
severe dysplasia of vagina (histologically confirmed) (D07.2)
vaginal intraepithelial neoplasia I [VAIN I] (N89.0)
vaginal intraepithelial neoplasia II [VAIN II] (N89.1)
vaginal intraepithelial neoplasia III [VAIN III] (D07.2)

EXCLUDES 2 *vaginal high risk human papillomavirus (HPV) DNA test positive (R87.811)*
vaginal low risk human papillomavirus (HPV) DNA test positive (R87.821)

R87.620 Atypical squamous cells of undetermined significance on cytologic smear of vagina [ASC-US] ♀

R87.621 Atypical squamous cells cannot exclude high grade squamous intraepithelial lesion on cytologic smear of vagina [ASC-H] ♀

R87.622 Low grade squamous intraepithelial lesion on cytologic smear of vagina [LGSIL] ♀

R87.623 High grade squamous intraepithelial lesion on cytologic smear of vagina [HGSIL] ♀

R87.624 Cytologic evidence of malignancy on smear of vagina ♀

R87.625 Unsatisfactory cytologic smear of vagina ♀
Inadequate sample of cytologic smear of vagina

R87.628 Other abnormal cytological findings on specimens from vagina ♀

R87.629 Unspecified abnormal cytological findings in specimens from vagina ♀
Abnormal Papanicolaou smear of vagina NOS
Abnormal thin preparation smear of vagina NOS
Abnormal vaginal cytology NOS
Atypical endocervical cells of vagina NOS
Atypical endometrial cells of vagina NOS
Atypical glandular cells of vagina NOS

R87.69 Abnormal cytological findings in specimens from other female genital organs ♀
Abnormal cytological findings in specimens from female genital organs NOS

EXCLUDES 1 *dysplasia of vulva (histologically confirmed) (N90.0-N90.3)*

R87.7 Abnormal histological findings in specimens from female genital organs ♀

EXCLUDES 1 *carcinoma in situ (histologically confirmed) of female genital organs (D06-D07.3)*
cervical intraepithelial neoplasia I [CIN I] (N87.0)
cervical intraepithelial neoplasia II [CIN II] (N87.1)
cervical intraepithelial neoplasia III [CIN III] (D06.-)
dysplasia (mild) (moderate) of cervix uteri (histologically confirmed) (N87.-)
dysplasia (mild) (moderate) of vagina (histologically confirmed) (N89.-)
severe dysplasia of cervix uteri (histologically confirmed) (D06.-)
severe dysplasia of vagina (histologically confirmed) (D07.2)
vaginal intraepithelial neoplasia I [VAIN I] (N89.0)
vaginal intraepithelial neoplasia II [VAIN II] (N89.1)
vaginal intraepithelial neoplasia III [VAIN III] (D07.2)

✓5th **R87.8 Other abnormal findings in specimens from female genital organs**

✓6th **R87.81 High risk human papillomavirus [HPV] DNA test positive from female genital organs**

EXCLUDES 1 *anogenital warts due to human papillomavirus (HPV) (A63.0)*
condyloma acuminatum (A63.0)

R87.810 Cervical high risk human papillomavirus [HPV] DNA test positive ♀

R87.811 Vaginal high risk human papillomavirus [HPV] DNA test positive ♀

✓6th **R87.82 Low risk human papillomavirus [HPV] DNA test positive from female genital organs**

Use additional code for associated human papillomavirus (B97.7)

R87.820 Cervical low risk human papillomavirus [HPV] DNA test positive ♀

R87.821 Vaginal low risk human papillomavirus [HPV] DNA test positive ♀

R87.89 Other abnormal findings in specimens from female genital organs ♀

Abnormal chromosomal findings in specimens from female genital organs

UNS **R87.9 Unspecified abnormal finding in specimens from female genital organs** ♀

✓4th **R88 Abnormal findings in other body fluids and substances**

R88.0 Cloudy (hemodialysis) (peritoneal) dialysis effluent

R88.8 Abnormal findings in other body fluids and substances

✓4th **R89 Abnormal findings in specimens from other organs, systems and tissues**

INCLUDES abnormal findings in nipple discharge
abnormal findings in synovial fluid
abnormal findings in wound secretions

R89.0 Abnormal level of enzymes in specimens from other organs, systems and tissues

R89.1 Abnormal level of hormones in specimens from other organs, systems and tissues

R89.2 Abnormal level of other drugs, medicaments and biological substances in specimens from other organs, systems and tissues

R89.3 Abnormal level of substances chiefly nonmedicinal as to source in specimens from other organs, systems and tissues

R89.4 Abnormal immunological findings in specimens from other organs, systems and tissues

R89.5 Abnormal microbiological findings in specimens from other organs, systems and tissues

Positive culture findings in specimens from other organs, systems and tissues

EXCLUDES 1 *colonization status (Z22.-)*

R89.6 Abnormal cytological findings in specimens from other organs, systems and tissues

R89.7 Abnormal histological findings in specimens from other organs, systems and tissues

R89.8 Other abnormal findings in specimens from other organs, systems and tissues

Abnormal chromosomal findings in specimens from other organs, systems and tissues

UNS **R89.9 Unspecified abnormal finding in specimens from other organs, systems and tissues**

Abnormal findings on diagnostic imaging and in function studies, without diagnosis (R90-R94)

INCLUDES nonspecific abnormal findings on diagnostic imaging by computerized axial tomography [CAT scan]
nonspecific abnormal findings on diagnostic imaging by magnetic resonance imaging [MRI][NMR]
nonspecific abnormal findings on diagnostic imaging by positron emission tomography [PET scan]
nonspecific abnormal findings on diagnostic imaging by thermography
nonspecific abnormal findings on diagnostic imaging by ultrasound [echogram]
nonspecific abnormal findings on diagnostic imaging by X-ray examination

EXCLUDES 1 *abnormal findings on antenatal screening of mother (O28.-)*
diagnostic abnormal findings classified elsewhere - see Alphabetical Index

✓4th **R90 Abnormal findings on diagnostic imaging of central nervous system**

R90.0 Intracranial space-occupying lesion found on diagnostic imaging of central nervous system

✓5th **R90.8 Other abnormal findings on diagnostic imaging of central nervous system**

R90.81 Abnormal echoencephalogram

UNS **R90.82 White matter disease, unspecified**

R90.89 Other abnormal findings on diagnostic imaging of central nervous system

Other cerebrovascular abnormality found on diagnostic imaging of central nervous system

✓4th **R91 Abnormal findings on diagnostic imaging of lung**

R91.1 Solitary pulmonary nodule

Coin lesion lung
Solitary pulmonary nodule, subsegmental branch of the bronchial tree

R91.8 Other nonspecific abnormal finding of lung field

Lung mass NOS found on diagnostic imaging of lung
Pulmonary infiltrate NOS
Shadow, lung

✓4th **R92 Abnormal and inconclusive findings on diagnostic imaging of breast**

R92.0 Mammographic microcalcification found on diagnostic imaging of breast

EXCLUDES 2 *mammographic calcification (calculus) found on diagnostic imaging of breast (R92.1)*

DEF: Calcium and cellular debris deposits in the breast that cannot be felt but can be detected on a mammogram. The deposits can be a sign of cancer, benign conditions, or changes in the breast tissue as a result of inflammation, injury, or an obstructed duct.

R92.1 Mammographic calcification found on diagnostic imaging of breast

Mammographic calculus found on diagnostic imaging of breast

R92.2 Inconclusive mammogram

Dense breasts NOS
Inconclusive mammogram NEC
Inconclusive mammography due to dense breasts
Inconclusive mammography NEC

AHA: 2015,1Q,24

R92.8 Other abnormal and inconclusive findings on diagnostic imaging of breast

✓4th **R93 Abnormal findings on diagnostic imaging of other body structures**

R93.0 Abnormal findings on diagnostic imaging of skull and head, not elsewhere classified

EXCLUDES 1 *intracranial space-occupying lesion found on diagnostic imaging (R90.0)*

R93.1 Abnormal findings on diagnostic imaging of heart and coronary circulation

Abnormal echocardiogram NOS
Abnormal heart shadow

R93.2 Abnormal findings on diagnostic imaging of liver and biliary tract

Nonvisualization of gallbladder

R93.3 Abnormal findings on diagnostic imaging of other parts of digestive tract

R93.4 Abnormal findings on diagnostic imaging of urinary organs
EXCLUDES 2 *hypertrophy of kidney (N28.81)*
AHA: 2016,4Q,66

R93.41 Abnormal radiologic findings on diagnostic imaging of renal pelvis, ureter, or bladder
Filling defect of bladder found on diagnostic imaging
Filling defect of renal pelvis found on diagnostic imaging
Filling defect of ureter found on diagnostic imaging

R93.42 Abnormal radiologic findings on diagnostic imaging of kidney
R93.421 Abnormal radiologic findings on diagnostic imaging of right kidney
R93.422 Abnormal radiologic findings on diagnostic imaging of left kidney
R93.429 Abnormal radiologic findings on diagnostic imaging of unspecified kidney

R93.49 Abnormal radiologic findings on diagnostic imaging of other urinary organs

R93.5 Abnormal findings on diagnostic imaging of other abdominal regions, including retroperitoneum

R93.6 Abnormal findings on diagnostic imaging of limbs
EXCLUDES 2 *abnormal finding in skin and subcutaneous tissue (R93.8-)*
AHA: 2020,1Q,14

R93.7 Abnormal findings on diagnostic imaging of other parts of musculoskeletal system
EXCLUDES 2 *abnormal findings on diagnostic imaging of skull (R93.Ø)*

R93.8 Abnormal findings on diagnostic imaging of other specified body structures
AHA: 2018,4Q,30

R93.81 Abnormal radiologic findings on diagnostic imaging of testis
R93.811 Abnormal radiologic findings on diagnostic imaging of right testicle ♂
R93.812 Abnormal radiologic findings on diagnostic imaging of left testicle ♂
R93.813 Abnormal radiologic findings on diagnostic imaging of testicles, bilateral ♂
R93.819 Abnormal radiologic findings on diagnostic imaging of unspecified testicle ♂

R93.89 Abnormal findings on diagnostic imaging of other specified body structures
Abnormal finding by radioisotope localization of placenta
Abnormal radiological finding in skin and subcutaneous tissue
Mediastinal shift

R93.9 Diagnostic imaging inconclusive due to excess body fat of patient

R94 Abnormal results of function studies
INCLUDES abnormal results of radionuclide [radioisotope] uptake studies
abnormal results of scintigraphy

R94.Ø Abnormal results of function studies of central nervous system
R94.Ø1 Abnormal electroencephalogram [EEG]
R94.Ø2 Abnormal brain scan
R94.Ø9 Abnormal results of other function studies of central nervous system

R94.1 Abnormal results of function studies of peripheral nervous system and special senses

R94.11 Abnormal results of function studies of eye
R94.11Ø Abnormal electro-oculogram [EOG]
R94.111 Abnormal electroretinogram [ERG]
Abnormal retinal function study
R94.112 Abnormal visually evoked potential [VEP]
R94.113 Abnormal oculomotor study
R94.118 Abnormal results of other function studies of eye

R94.12 Abnormal results of function studies of ear and other special senses
AHA: 2016,3Q,17
R94.12Ø Abnormal auditory function study
R94.121 Abnormal vestibular function study
R94.128 Abnormal results of other function studies of ear and other special senses

R94.13 Abnormal results of function studies of peripheral nervous system
R94.13Ø Abnormal response to nerve stimulation, unspecified
R94.131 Abnormal electromyogram [EMG]
EXCLUDES 1 *electromyogram of eye (R94.113)*
R94.138 Abnormal results of other function studies of peripheral nervous system

R94.2 Abnormal results of pulmonary function studies
Reduced ventilatory capacity
Reduced vital capacity

R94.3 Abnormal results of cardiovascular function studies
R94.3Ø Abnormal result of cardiovascular function study, unspecified
R94.31 Abnormal electrocardiogram [ECG] [EKG]
EXCLUDES 1 *long QT syndrome (I45.81)*
R94.39 Abnormal result of other cardiovascular function study
Abnormal electrophysiological intracardiac studies
Abnormal phonocardiogram
Abnormal vectorcardiogram

R94.4 Abnormal results of kidney function studies
Abnormal renal function test

R94.5 Abnormal results of liver function studies

R94.6 Abnormal results of thyroid function studies

R94.7 Abnormal results of other endocrine function studies
EXCLUDES 2 *abnormal glucose (R73.Ø-)*

R94.8 Abnormal results of function studies of other organs and systems
Abnormal basal metabolic rate [BMR]
Abnormal bladder function test
Abnormal splenic function test

Abnormal tumor markers (R97)

R97 Abnormal tumor markers
Elevated tumor associated antigens [TAA]
Elevated tumor specific antigens [TSA]

R97.Ø Elevated carcinoembryonic antigen [CEA]

R97.1 Elevated cancer antigen 125 [CA 125]

R97.2 Elevated prostate specific antigen [PSA]
AHA: 2016,4Q,66
R97.2Ø Elevated prostate specific antigen [PSA] A ♂
R97.21 Rising PSA following treatment for malignant neoplasm of prostate A ♂

R97.8 Other abnormal tumor markers

Ill-defined and unknown cause of mortality (R99)

R99 Ill-defined and unknown cause of mortality
Death (unexplained) NOS
Unspecified cause of mortality

Chapter 19. Injury, Poisoning and Certain Other Consequences of External Causes (SØØ–T88)

Chapter-specific Guidelines with Coding Examples

The chapter-specific guidelines from the ICD-10-CM Official Guidelines for Coding and Reporting have been provided below. Along with these guidelines are coding examples, contained in the shaded boxes, that have been developed to help illustrate the coding and/or sequencing guidance found in these guidelines.

a. Application of 7th characters in Chapter 19

Most categories in chapter 19 have a 7th character requirement for each applicable code. Most categories in this chapter have three 7th character values (with the exception of fractures): A, initial encounter, D, subsequent encounter and S, sequela. Categories for traumatic fractures have additional 7th character values. While the patient may be seen by a new or different provider over the course of treatment for an injury, assignment of the 7th character is based on whether the patient is undergoing active treatment and not whether the provider is seeing the patient for the first time.

For complication codes, active treatment refers to treatment for the condition described by the code, even though it may be related to an earlier precipitating problem. For example, code T84.50XA, Infection and inflammatory reaction due to unspecified internal joint prosthesis, initial encounter, is used when active treatment is provided for the infection, even though the condition relates to the prosthetic device, implant or graft that was placed at a previous encounter.

7th character "A", initial encounter is used for each encounter where the patient is receiving active treatment for the condition.

Patient admitted after fall from a skateboard onto the sidewalk, x-rays identify a nondisplaced fracture to the distal pole of the right scaphoid bone. The patient is placed in a cast.

S62.Ø14A	**Nondisplaced fracture of distal pole of navicular [scaphoid] bone of right wrist, initial encounter for closed fracture**
VØØ.131A	**Fall from skateboard, initial encounter**
Y92.48Ø	**Sidewalk as the place of occurrence of the external cause**
Y93.51	**Activity, roller skating (inline) and skateboarding**
Y99.8	**Other external cause status**

Explanation: This fracture would be coded with a seventh character A for initial encounter because the patient received x-rays to identify the site of the fracture and treatment was rendered; this would be considered active treatment.

7th character "D" subsequent encounter is used for encounters after the patient has completed active treatment of the condition and is receiving routine care for the condition during the healing or recovery phase.

Patient admitted after fall from a skateboard onto the sidewalk resulted in casting of the right arm. X-rays are taken to evaluate how well the nondisplaced fracture to the distal pole of the right scaphoid bone is healing. The physician feels the fracture is healing appropriately; no adjustments to the cast are made.

S62.Ø14D	**Nondisplaced fracture of distal pole of navicular [scaphoid] bone of right wrist, subsequent encounter for fracture with routine healing**
VØØ.131D	**Fall from skateboard, subsequent encounter**

Explanation: This fracture would be coded with a seventh character D for subsequent encounter, whether the same physician who provided the initial cast application or a different physician is now seeing the patient. Although the patient received x-rays, the intent of the x-rays was to assess how the fracture was healing. There was no active treatment rendered and the visit is therefore considered a subsequent encounter.

The aftercare Z codes should not be used for aftercare for conditions such as injuries or poisonings, where 7th characters are provided to identify subsequent care. For example, for aftercare of an injury, assign the acute injury code with the 7th character "D" (subsequent encounter).

7th character "S", sequela, is for use for complications or conditions that arise as a direct result of a condition, such as scar formation after a burn. The scars are sequelae of the burn. When using 7th character "S", it is necessary to use both the injury code that precipitated the sequela and the code for the sequela itself. The "S" is added only to the injury code, not the sequela code. The 7th character "S" identifies the injury responsible for the sequela. The specific type of sequela (e.g. scar) is sequenced first, followed by the injury code.

See Section I.B.1Ø. Sequelae, (Late Effects)

Patient with a history of a nondisplaced fracture to the distal pole of the right scaphoid bone due to a fall from a skateboard is admitted for evaluation of arthritis to the right wrist that has developed as a consequence of the traumatic fracture.

M12.531	**Traumatic arthropathy, right wrist**
S62.Ø14S	**Nondisplaced fracture of distal pole of navicular [scaphoid] bone of right wrist, sequela**
VØØ.131S	**Fall from skateboard, sequela**

Explanation: The code identifying the specific sequela condition (traumatic arthritis) should be coded first followed by the injury that instigated the development of the sequela (fracture). The scaphoid fracture injury code is given a 7th character S for sequela to represent its role as the inciting injury. The fracture has healed and is not being managed or treated on this admit and therefore is not applicable as a first listed or principal diagnosis. However, it is directly related to the development of the arthritis and should be appended as a secondary code to signify this cause and effect relationship.

b. Coding of injuries

When coding injuries, assign separate codes for each injury unless a combination code is provided, in which case the combination code is assigned. Codes from category TØ7, Unspecified multiple injuries should not be assigned in the inpatient setting unless information for a more specific code is not available. Traumatic injury codes (SØØ-T14.9) are not to be used for normal, healing surgical wounds or to identify complications of surgical wounds.

The code for the most serious injury, as determined by the provider and the focus of treatment, is sequenced first.

1) Superficial injuries

Superficial injuries such as abrasions or contusions are not coded when associated with more severe injuries of the same site.

2) Primary injury with damage to nerves/blood vessels

When a primary injury results in minor damage to peripheral nerves or blood vessels, the primary injury is sequenced first with additional code(s) for injuries to nerves and spinal cord (such as category SØ4), and/or injury to blood vessels (such as category S15). When the primary injury is to the blood vessels or nerves, that injury should be sequenced first.

3) Iatrogenic injuries

Injury codes from Chapter 19 should not be assigned for injuries that occur during, or as a result of, a medical intervention. Assign the appropriate complication code(s).

c. Coding of traumatic fractures

The principles of multiple coding of injuries should be followed in coding fractures. Fractures of specified sites are coded individually by site in accordance with both the provisions within categories SØ2, S12, S22, S32, S42, S49, S52, S59, S62, S72, S79, S82, S89, S92 and the level of detail furnished by medical record content.

A fracture not indicated as open or closed should be coded to closed. A fracture not indicated whether displaced or not displaced should be coded to displaced.

More specific guidelines are as follows:

1) Initial vs. subsequent encounter for fractures

Traumatic fractures are coded using the appropriate 7th character for initial encounter (A, B, C) for each encounter where the patient is receiving active treatment for the fracture. The appropriate 7th character for initial encounter should also be assigned for a patient who delayed seeking treatment for the fracture or nonunion.

Fractures are coded using the appropriate 7th character for subsequent care for encounters after the patient has completed active treatment of the fracture and is receiving routine care for the fracture during the healing or recovery phase.

Care for complications of surgical treatment for fracture repairs during the healing or recovery phase should be coded with the appropriate complication codes.

Care of complications of fractures, such as malunion and nonunion, should be reported with the appropriate 7th character for subsequent care with nonunion (K, M, N,) or subsequent care with malunion (P, Q, R).

Malunion/nonunion: The appropriate 7th character for initial encounter should also be assigned for a patient who delayed seeking treatment for the fracture or nonunion.

Female patient fell during a forest hiking excursion almost six months ago and until recently did not feel she needed to seek medical attention for her left ankle pain; x-rays show nonunion of lateral malleolus and surgery has been scheduled

S82.62XA **Displaced fracture of lateral malleolus of left fibula, initial encounter for closed fracture**

WØ1.ØXXA **Fall on same level from slipping, tripping and stumbling without subsequent striking against object, initial encounter**

Y92.821 **Forest as place of occurrence of the external cause**

Y93.Ø1 **Activity, walking, marching and hiking**

Y99.8 **Other external cause status**

Explanation: A seventh character of A is used for the lateral malleolus nonunion fracture to signify that the fracture is receiving active treatment. The delayed care for the fracture has resulted in a nonunion, but capturing the nonunion in the seventh character is trumped by the provision of active care.

The open fracture designations in the assignment of the 7th character for fractures of the forearm, femur and lower leg, including ankle are based on the Gustilo open fracture classification. When the Gustilo classification type is not specified for an open fracture, the 7th character for open fracture type I or II should be assigned (B, E, H, M, Q).

A 17-year-old arrives at the trauma center with open, displaced right forearm fracture with extensive soft tissue damage. He fell while being tackled playing football for his high school team. On-call orthopaedic specialist documents segmental type IIIA fracture of radial shaft with no need for plastic consult.

S52.361C **Displaced segmental fracture of shaft of radius, right arm, initial encounter for open fracture type IIIA, IIIB, or IIIC**

WØ3.XXXA **Other fall on same level due to collision with another person, initial encounter**

Y92.321 **Football field as the place of occurrence of the external cause**

Y93.61 **Activity, American tackle football**

Explanation: The seventh character for forearm fractures capture the type of encounter and whether the fracture is open or closed; open fractures are broken down further by the type of fracture based on the Gustilo classification. The Gustilo classification describes the severity of open fracture and soft tissue injury. Type IIIA describes an open fracture with extensive soft tissue injury but adequate soft tissue remaining for wound coverage. A segmental fracture means that the bone is broken in two places, leaving at least one segment unattached to the bone. There is no need to report an additional code for the soft tissue injury as it is captured in the fracture code.

A code from category M8Ø, not a traumatic fracture code, should be used for any patient with known osteoporosis who suffers a fracture, even if the patient had a minor fall or trauma, if that fall or trauma would not usually break a normal, healthy bone.

See Section I.C.13. Osteoporosis.

The aftercare Z codes should not be used for aftercare for traumatic fractures. For aftercare of a traumatic fracture, assign the acute fracture code with the appropriate 7th character.

2) **Multiple fractures sequencing**

Multiple fractures are sequenced in accordance with the severity of the fracture.

3) **Physeal fractures**

For physeal fractures, assign only the code identifying the type of physeal fracture. Do not assign a separate code to identify the specific bone that is fractured.

d. **Coding of burns and corrosions**

The ICD-10-CM makes a distinction between burns and corrosions. The burn codes are for thermal burns, except sunburns, that come from a heat source, such as a fire or hot appliance. The burn codes are also for burns resulting from electricity and radiation. Corrosions are burns due to chemicals. The guidelines are the same for burns and corrosions.

Current burns (T2Ø-T25) are classified by depth, extent and by agent (X code). Burns are classified by depth as first degree (erythema), second degree (blistering), and third degree (full-thickness involvement). Burns of the eye and internal organs (T26-T28) are classified by site, but not by degree.

1) **Sequencing of burn and related condition codes**

Sequence first the code that reflects the highest degree of burn when more than one burn is present.

a. When the reason for the admission or encounter is for treatment of external multiple burns, sequence first the code that reflects the burn of the highest degree.

b. When a patient has both internal and external burns, the circumstances of admission govern the selection of the principal diagnosis or first-listed diagnosis.

c. When a patient is admitted for burn injuries and other related conditions such as smoke inhalation and/or respiratory failure, the circumstances of admission govern the selection of the principal or first-listed diagnosis.

Patient admitted with minor first-degree burns to multiple sites of her right and left hands as well as severe smoke inhalation. While she was sleeping at home, a candle on her dresser lit the bedroom curtains on fire.

T59.811A **Toxic effect of smoke, accidental (unintentional), initial encounter**

J7Ø.5 **Respiratory conditions due to smoke inhalation**

T23.191A **Burn of first degree of multiple sites of right wrist and hand, initial encounter**

T23.192A **Burn of first degree of multiple sites of left wrist and hand, initial encounter**

XØ8.8XXA **Exposure to other specified smoke, fire and flames, initial encounter**

Y92.ØØ3 **Bedroom of unspecified non-institutional (private) residence as the place of occurrence of the external cause**

Y93.84 **Activity, sleeping**

Explanation: Based on the documentation, the inhalation injury is more severe than the first-degree burns and is sequenced first. The burns to the hands are appended as secondary diagnoses.

2) **Burns of the same anatomic site**

Classify burns of the same anatomic site and on the same side but of different degrees to the subcategory identifying the highest degree recorded in the diagnosis (e.g., for second and third degree burns of right thigh, assign only code T24.311-).

3) **Non-healing burns**

Non-healing burns are coded as acute burns.

Necrosis of burned skin should be coded as a non-healed burn.

4) **Infected burn**

For any documented infected burn site, use an additional code for the infection.

5) **Assign separate codes for each burn site**

When coding burns, assign separate codes for each burn site. Category T3Ø, Burn and corrosion, body region unspecified is extremely vague and should rarely be used.

Codes for burns of "multiple sites" should only be assigned when the medical record documentation does not specify the individual sites.

Patient is admitted with third-degree burns of the scalp as well as second-degree burns to the back of the right hand

T2Ø.35XA **Burn of third degree of scalp [any part], initial encounter**

T23.261A **Burn of second degree of back of right hand, initial encounter**

Explanation: Two codes may be reported as the hand and face represent distinct burn sites.

6) **Burns and corrosions classified according to extent of body surface involved**

Assign codes from category T31, Burns classified according to extent of body surface involved, or T32, Corrosions classified according to extent of body surface involved, for acute burns or corrosions when the site of the burn or corrosion is not specified or when there is a need for additional data. It is advisable to use category T31 as additional coding when needed to provide data for evaluating burn mortality, such as that needed by burn units. It is also advisable to use category T31 as an additional code for reporting purposes when there is mention of a third-degree burn involving 20 percent or more of the body surface. Codes from categories T31 and T32 should not be used for sequelae of burns or corrosions.

Categories T31 and T32 are based on the classic "rule of nines" in estimating body surface involved: head and neck are assigned nine percent, each arm nine percent, each leg 18 percent, the anterior trunk 18 percent, posterior trunk 18 percent, and genitalia one percent. Providers may change these percentage assignments where necessary to accommodate infants and children who have proportionately larger heads than adults, and patients who have large buttocks, thighs, or abdomen that involve burns.

> Patient seen in burn unit for dressing change after he accidentally spilled acetic acid on himself two days ago. The second-degree burns to his right thigh, covering about 3 percent of his body surface, are healing appropriately.
>
> **T54.2X1D** **Toxic effect of corrosive acids and acid-like substances, accidental (unintentional), subsequent encounter**
>
> **T24.611D** **Corrosion of second degree of right thigh, subsequent encounter**
>
> **T32.Ø** **Corrosions involving less than 1Ø% of body surface**
>
> *Explanation:* Code T32.Ø provides additional information as to how much of the patient's body was affected by the corrosive substance.

7) Encounters for treatment of sequela of burns

Encounters for the treatment of the late effects of burns or corrosions (i.e., scars or joint contractures) should be coded with a burn or corrosion code with the 7th character "S" for sequela.

8) Sequelae with a late effect code and current burn

When appropriate, both a code for a current burn or corrosion with 7th character "A" or "D" and a burn or corrosion code with 7th character "S" may be assigned on the same record (when both a current burn and sequelae of an old burn exist). Burns and corrosions do not heal at the same rate and a current healing wound may still exist with sequela of a healed burn or corrosion.

See Section I.B.1Ø. Sequela (Late Effects)

> Female patient seen in ED for second-degree burn to the left ear; she also has significant scarring on her left elbow from a third-degree burn from childhood
>
> **T2Ø.212A** **Burn of second degree of left ear [any part, except ear drum], initial encounter**
>
> **L9Ø.5** **Scar conditions and fibrosis of skin**
>
> **T22.322S** **Burn of third degree of left elbow, sequela**
>
> *Explanation:* The patient is being seen for management of a current second-degree burn, which is reflected in the code by appending the seventh character of A, indicating active treatment or management of this burn. The elbow scarring is a sequela of a previous third-degree burn. The sequela condition precedes the original burn injury, which is appended with a seventh character of S.

9) Use of an external cause code with burns and corrosions

An external cause code should be used with burns and corrosions to identify the source and intent of the burn, as well as the place where it occurred.

e. Adverse effects, poisoning, underdosing and toxic effects

Codes in categories T36-T65 are combination codes that include the substance that was taken as well as the intent. No additional external cause code is required for poisonings, toxic effects, adverse effects and underdosing codes.

1) Do not code directly from the Table of Drugs

Do not code directly from the Table of Drugs and Chemicals. Always refer back to the Tabular List.

2) Use as many codes as necessary to describe

Use as many codes as necessary to describe completely all drugs, medicinal or biological substances.

3) If the same code would describe the causative agent

If the same code would describe the causative agent for more than one adverse reaction, poisoning, toxic effect or underdosing, assign the code only once.

4) If two or more drugs, medicinal or biological substances

If two or more drugs, medicinal or biological substances are taken, code each individually unless a combination code is listed in the Table of Drugs and Chemicals.

If multiple unspecified drugs, medicinal or biological substances were taken, assign the appropriate code from subcategory T5Ø.91, Poisoning by, adverse effect of and underdosing of multiple unspecified drugs, medicaments and biological substances.

5) The occurrence of drug toxicity is classified in ICD-10-CM as follows:

(a) Adverse effect

When coding an adverse effect of a drug that has been correctly prescribed and properly administered, assign the appropriate code for the nature of the adverse effect followed by the appropriate code for the adverse effect of the drug (T36-T5Ø). The code for the drug should have a 5th or 6th character "5" (for example T36.ØX5-) Examples of the nature of an adverse effect are tachycardia, delirium, gastrointestinal hemorrhaging, vomiting, hypokalemia, hepatitis, renal failure, or respiratory failure.

> Patient admitted for stomach pain and jaundice, indicated by physician as possible side-effects of Inderal, recently started for hypertension. Inderal was discontinued and the patient switched to Atenolol instead.
>
> **R1Ø.9** **Unspecified abdominal pain**
>
> **R17** **Unspecified jaundice**
>
> **T44.7X5A** **Adverse effect of beta-adrenoreceptor antagonists, initial encounter**
>
> **I1Ø** **Essential (primary) hypertension**
>
> *Explanation:* The side-effects caused by the drug are listed first, followed by the code for the adverse effect of the drug to capture the specific drug that was used.

(b) Poisoning

When coding a poisoning or reaction to the improper use of a medication (e.g., overdose, wrong substance given or taken in error, wrong route of administration), first assign the appropriate code from categories T36-T5Ø. The poisoning codes have an associated intent as their 5th or 6th character (accidental, intentional self-harm, assault and undetermined). If the intent of the poisoning is unknown or unspecified, code the intent as accidental intent. The undetermined intent is only for use if the documentation in the record specifies that the intent cannot be determined. Use additional code(s) for all manifestations of poisonings.

> A 55-year-old female status post recent left knee replacement is admitted due to confusion, dizziness, and nausea. Her spouse brought in her prescribed Xanax, Ambien, and Percocet bottles but has no idea how many she took. It is suspected that her symptoms are due to an overdose of these medications.
>
> **T42.4X1A** **Poisoning by benzodiazepines, accidental (unintentional), initial encounter**
>
> **T42.6X1A** **Poisoning by other antiepileptic and sedative-hypnotic drugs, accidental (unintentional), initial encounter**
>
> **T4Ø.2X1A** **Poisoning by other opioids, accidental (unintentional), initial encounter**
>
> **R41.Ø** **Disorientation, unspecified**
>
> **R42** **Dizziness and giddiness**
>
> **R11.Ø** **Nausea**
>
> *Explanation:* It was not documented whether the overdose of the drugs was accidental or intentional; therefore the correct reporting of the poisoning codes is accidental intent. The poisoning codes are sequenced first, followed by manifestations of the poisoning.

If there is also a diagnosis of abuse or dependence of the substance, the abuse or dependence is assigned as an additional code.

Examples of poisoning include:

(i) Error was made in drug prescription

Errors made in drug prescription or in the administration of the drug by provider, nurse, patient, or other person.

(ii Overdose of a drug intentionally taken

If an overdose of a drug was intentionally taken or administered and resulted in drug toxicity, it would be coded as a poisoning.

(iii) Nonprescribed drug taken with correctly prescribed and properly administered drug

If a nonprescribed drug or medicinal agent was taken in combination with a correctly prescribed and properly administered drug, any drug toxicity or other reaction resulting from the interaction of the two drugs would be classified as a poisoning.

(iv) Interaction of drug(s) and alcohol

When a reaction results from the interaction of a drug(s) and alcohol, this would be classified as poisoning.

See Section I.C.4. if poisoning is the result of insulin pump malfunctions.

(c) Underdosing

Underdosing refers to taking less of a medication than is prescribed by a provider or a manufacturer's instruction. Discontinuing the use of a prescribed medication on the patient's own initiative (not directed by the patient's provider) is also classified as an underdosing. For underdosing, assign the code from categories T36-T5Ø (fifth or sixth character "6"). **Documentation of a change in the patient's condition is not required in order to assign an underdosing code. Documentation that the patient is taking less of a medication than is prescribed or discontinued the prescribed medication is sufficient for code assignment.**

Codes for underdosing should never be assigned as principal or first-listed codes. If a patient has a relapse or exacerbation of the medical condition for which the drug is prescribed because of the reduction in dose, then the medical condition itself should be coded.

Noncompliance (Z91.12-, Z91.13- and Z91.14-) or complication of care (Y63.6-Y63.9) codes are to be used with an underdosing code to indicate intent, if known.

Patient admitted for atrial fibrillation with history of chronic atrial fibrillation for which she is prescribed amiodarone. Financial concerns have left the patient unable to pay for her prescriptions and she has been skipping her amiodarone dose every other day to offset the cost.

I48.2Ø	**Chronic atrial fibrillation, unspecified**
T46.2X6A	**Underdosing of other antidysrhythmic drugs, initial encounter**
Z91.12Ø	**Patient's intentional underdosing of medication regimen due to financial hardship**

Explanation: By skipping her amiodarone pill every other day, the patient's atrial fibrillation returned. The condition for which the drug was being taken is reported first, followed by an underdosing code to show that the patient was not adhering to her prescription regimen. The Z code helps elaborate on the patient's social and/or economic circumstances that led to the patient taking less then what she was prescribed.

(d) Toxic effects

When a harmful substance is ingested or comes in contact with a person, this is classified as a toxic effect. The toxic effect codes are in categories T51-T65.

Toxic effect codes have an associated intent: accidental, intentional self-harm, assault and undetermined.

f. Adult and child abuse, neglect and other maltreatment

Sequence first the appropriate code from categories T74.- (Adult and child abuse, neglect and other maltreatment, confirmed) or T76.- (Adult and child abuse, neglect and other maltreatment, suspected) for abuse, neglect and other maltreatment, followed by any accompanying mental health or injury code(s).

If the documentation in the medical record states abuse or neglect it is coded as confirmed (T74.-). It is coded as suspected if it is documented as suspected (T76.-).

For cases of confirmed abuse or neglect an external cause code from the assault section (X92-YØ9) should be added to identify the cause of any physical injuries. A perpetrator code (YØ7) should be added when the perpetrator of the abuse is known. For suspected cases of abuse or neglect, do not report external cause or perpetrator code.

If a suspected case of abuse, neglect or mistreatment is ruled out during an encounter code ZØ4.71, Encounter for examination and observation following alleged physical adult abuse, ruled out, or code ZØ4.72, Encounter for examination and observation following alleged child physical abuse, ruled out, should be used, not a code from T76.

If a suspected case of alleged rape or sexual abuse is ruled out during an encounter code ZØ4.41, Encounter for examination and observation following alleged adult rape or code ZØ4.42, Encounter for examination and observation following alleged child rape, should be used, not a code from T76.

If a suspected case of forced sexual exploitation or forced labor exploitation is ruled out during an encounter, code ZØ4.81, Encounter for examination and observation of victim following forced sexual exploitation, or code ZØ4.82, Encounter for examination and observation of victim following forced labor exploitation, should be used, not a code from T76.

See Section I.C.15. Abuse in a pregnant patient.

g. Complications of care

1) General guidelines for complications of care

(a) Documentation of complications of care

See Section I.B.16. for information on documentation of complications of care.

2) Pain due to medical devices

Pain associated with devices, implants or grafts left in a surgical site (for example painful hip prosthesis) is assigned to the appropriate code(s) found in Chapter 19, Injury, poisoning, and certain other consequences of external causes. Specific codes for pain due to medical devices are found in the T code section of the ICD-10-CM. Use additional code(s) from category G89 to identify acute or chronic pain due to presence of the device, implant or graft (G89.18 or G89.28).

3) Transplant complications

(a) Transplant complications other than kidney

Codes under category T86, Complications of transplanted organs and tissues, are for use for both complications and rejection of transplanted organs. A transplant complication code is only assigned if the complication affects the function of the transplanted organ. Two codes are required to fully describe a transplant complication: the appropriate code from category T86 and a secondary code that identifies the complication.

Pre-existing conditions or conditions that develop after the transplant are not coded as complications unless they affect the function of the transplanted organs.

See I.C.21. for transplant organ removal status

See I.C.2. for malignant neoplasm associated with transplanted organ.

(b) Kidney transplant complications

Patients who have undergone kidney transplant may still have some form of chronic kidney disease (CKD) because the kidney transplant may not fully restore kidney function. Code T86.1- should be assigned for documented complications of a kidney transplant, such as transplant failure or rejection or other transplant complication. Code T86.1- should not be assigned for post kidney transplant patients who have chronic kidney (CKD) unless a transplant complication such as transplant failure or rejection is documented. If the documentation is unclear as to whether the patient has a complication of the transplant, query the provider.

Conditions that affect the function of the transplanted kidney, other than CKD, should be assigned a code from subcategory T86.1, Complications of transplanted organ, Kidney, and a secondary code that identifies the complication.

For patients with CKD following a kidney transplant, but who do not have a complication such as failure or rejection, *see section I.C.14. Chronic kidney disease and kidney transplant status.*

Patient with chronic kidney disease stage 2; history of successful kidney transplant with no complications identified

N18.2	**Chronic kidney disease, stage 2 (mild)**
Z94.Ø	**Kidney transplant status**

Explanation: This patient's stage 2 CKD is not indicated as being due to the transplanted kidney but instead is just the residual disease the patient had prior to the transplant.

4) Complication codes that include the external cause

As with certain other T codes, some of the complications of care codes have the external cause included in the code. The code includes the nature of the complication as well as the type of procedure that caused the complication. No external cause code indicating the type of procedure is necessary for these codes.

5) Complications of care codes within the body system chapters

Intraoperative and postprocedural complication codes are found within the body system chapters with codes specific to the organs and structures of that body system. These codes should be sequenced first, followed by a code(s) for the specific complication, if applicable.

Complication codes from the body system chapters should be assigned for intraoperative and postprocedural complications (e.g., the appropriate complication code from chapter 9 would be assigned for a vascular intraoperative or postprocedural complication) unless the complication is specifically indexed to a T code in chapter 19.

During a spinal fusion procedure, the surgeon inadvertently punctured the dura. The midline durotomy was repaired, and the fusion procedure was completed.

G97.41	**Accidental puncture or laceration of dura during a procedure**

Explanation: The accidental durotomy is not coded to an injury code in chapter 19 but instead is categorized to the nervous system chapter.

Muscle/Tendon Table

ICD-10-CM categorizes certain muscles and tendons in the upper and lower extremities by their action (e.g., extension, flexion), their anatomical location (e.g., posterior, anterior), and/or whether they are intrinsic or extrinsic to a certain anatomical area. The Muscle/Tendon Table is provided at the beginning of chapters 13 and 19 as a resource to help users when code selection depends on one or more of these characteristics. Please note that this table is not all-inclusive, and proper code assignment should be based on the provider's documentation.

Body Region	Muscle	Extensor Tendon	Flexor Tendon	Other Tendon
Shoulder				
	Deltoid	Posterior deltoid	Anterior deltoid	
	Rotator cuff			
	Infraspinatus			Infraspinatus
	Subscapularis			Subscapularis
	Supraspinatus			Supraspinatus
	Teres minor			Teres minor
	Teres major	Teres major		
Upper arm				
	Anterior muscles			
	Biceps brachii — long head		Biceps brachii — long head	
	Biceps brachii — short head		Biceps brachii — short head	
	Brachialis		Brachialis	
	Coracobrachialis		Coracobrachialis	
	Posterior muscles			
	Triceps brachii	Triceps brachii		
Forearm				
	Anterior muscles			
	Flexors			
	Deep			
	Flexor digitorum profundus		Flexor digitorum profundus	
	Flexor pollicis longus		Flexor pollicis longus	
	Intermediate			
	Flexor digitorum superficialis		Flexor digitorum superficialis	
	Superficial			
	Flexor carpi radialis		Flexor carpi radialis	
	Flexor carpi ulnaris		Flexor carpi ulnaris	
	Palmaris longus		Palmaris longus	
	Pronators			
	Pronator quadratus			Pronator quadratus
	Pronator teres			Pronator teres
	Posterior muscles			
	Extensors			
	Deep			
	Abductor pollicis longus			Abductor pollicis longus
	Extensor indicis	Extensor indicis		
	Extensor pollicis brevis	Extensor pollicis brevis		
	Extensor pollicis longus	Extensor pollicis longus		
	Superficial			
	Brachioradialis			Brachioradialis
	Extensor carpi radialis brevis	Extensor carpi radialis brevis		
	Extensor carpi radialis longus	Extensor carpi radialis longus		
	Extensor carpi ulnaris	Extensor carpi ulnaris		
	Extensor digiti minimi	Extensor digiti minimi		
	Extensor digitorum	Extensor digitorum		
	Anconeus	Anconeus		
	Supinator			Supinator

Body Region	Muscle	Extensor Tendon	Flexor Tendon	Other Tendon
Hand				
Extrinsic — attach to a site in the forearm as well as a site in the hand with action related to hand movement at the wrist				
	Extensor carpi radialis brevis	Extensor carpi radialis brevis		
	Extensor carpi radialis longus	Extensor carpi radialis longus		
	Extensor carpi ulnaris	Extensor carpi ulnaris		
	Flexor carpi radialis		Flexor carpi radialis	
	Flexor carpi ulnaris		Flexor carpi ulnaris	
	Flexor digitorum superficialis		Flexor digitorum superficialis	
	Palmaris longus		Palmaris longus	
Extrinsic — attach to a site in the forearm as well as a site in the hand with action in the hand related to finger movement				
	Adductor pollicis longus			Adductor pollicis longus
	Extensor digiti minimi	Extensor digiti minimi		
	Extensor digitorum	Extensor digitorum		
	Extensor indicis	Extensor indicis		
	Flexor digitorum profundus		Flexor digitorum profundus	
	Flexor digitorum superficialis		Flexor digitorum superficialis	
Extrinsic — attach to a site in the forearm as well as a site in the hand with action in the hand related to thumb movement				
	Extensor pollicis brevis	Extensor pollicis brevis		
	Extensor pollicis longus	Extensor pollicis longus		
	Flexor pollicis longus		Flexor pollicis longus	
Intrinsic — found within the hand only				
	Adductor pollicis			Adductor pollicis
	Dorsal interossei	Dorsal interossei	Dorsal interossei	
	Lumbricals	Lumbricals	Lumbricals	
	Palmaris brevis			Palmaris brevis
	Palmar interossei	Palmar interossei	Palmar interossei	
	Hypothenar muscles			
	Abductor digiti minimi			Abductor digiti minimi
	Flexor digiti minimi brevis		Flexor digiti minimi brevis	
	Opponens digiti minimi		Opponens digiti minimi	
	Thenar muscles			
	Abductor pollicis brevis			Abductor pollicis brevis
	Flexor pollicis brevis		Flexor pollicis brevis	
	Opponens pollicis		Opponens pollicis	
Thigh				
	Anterior muscles			
	Iliopsoas		Iliopsoas	
	Pectineus		Pectineus	
	Quadriceps	Quadriceps		
	Rectus femoris	Rectus femoris — Extends knee	Rectus femoris — Flexes hip	
	Vastus intermedius	Vastus intermedius		
	Vastus lateralis	Vastus lateralis		
	Vastus medialis	Vastus medialis		
	Sartorius		Sartorius	
	Medial muscles			
	Adductor brevis			Adductor brevis
	Adductor longus			Adductor longus
	Adductor magnus			Adductor magnus
	Gracilis			Gracilis
	Obturator externus			Obturator externus
	Posterior muscles			
	Hamstring	Hamstring — Extends hip	Hamstring — Flexes knee	
	Biceps femoris	Biceps femoris	Biceps femoris	
	Semimembranosus	Semimembranosus	Semimembranosus	
	Semitendinosus	Semitendinosus	Semitendinosus	

Body Region	Muscle	Extensor Tendon	Flexor Tendon	Other Tendon
Lower leg				
	Anterior muscles			
	Extensor digitorum longus	Extensor digitorum longus		
	Extensor hallucis longus	Extensor hallucis longus		
	Fibularis (peroneus) tertius	Fibularis (peroneus) tertius		
	Tibialis anterior	Tibialis anterior		Tibialis anterior
	Lateral muscles			
	Fibularis (peroneus) brevis		Fibularis (peroneus) brevis	
	Fibularis (peroneus) longus		Fibularis (peroneus) longus	
	Posterior muscles			
	Deep			
	Flexor digitorum longus		Flexor digitorum longus	
	Flexor hallucis longus		Flexor hallucis longus	
	Popliteus		Popliteus	
	Tibialis posterior		Tibialis posterior	
	Superficial			
	Gastrocnemius		Gastrocnemius	
	Plantaris		Plantaris	
	Soleus		Soleus	
				Calcaneal (Achilles)
Ankle/Foot				
Extrinsic — attach to a site in the lower leg as well as a site in the foot with action related to foot movement at the ankle				
	Plantaris		Plantaris	
	Soleus		Soleus	
	Tibialis anterior	Tibialis anterior		
	Tibialis posterior		Tibialis posterior	
Extrinsic — attach to a site in the lower leg as well as a site in the foot with action in the foot related to toe movement				
	Extensor digitorum longus	Extensor digitorum longus		
	Extensor hallucis longus	Extensor hallucis longus		
	Flexor digitorum longus		Flexor digitorum longus	
	Flexor hallucis longus		Flexor hallucis longus	
Intrinsic — found within the ankle/foot only				
	Dorsal muscles			
	Extensor digitorum brevis	Extensor digitorum brevis		
	Extensor hallucis brevis	Extensor hallucis brevis		
	Plantar muscles			
	Abductor digiti minimi		Abductor digiti minimi	
	Abductor hallucis		Abductor hallucis	
	Dorsal interossei	Dorsal interossei	Dorsal interossei	
	Flexor digiti minimi brevis		Flexor digiti minimi brevis	
	Flexor digitorum brevis		Flexor digitorum brevis	
	Flexor hallucis brevis		Flexor hallucis brevis	
	Lumbricals	Lumbricals	Lumbricals	
	Quadratus plantae		Quadratus plantae	
	Plantar interossei	Plantar interossei	Plantar interossei	

Chapter 19. Injury, Poisoning and Certain Other Consequences of External Causes (S00-T88)

NOTE Use secondary code(s) from Chapter 20, External causes of morbidity, to indicate cause of injury. Codes within the T section that include the external cause do not require an additional external cause code.

Use additional code to identify any retained foreign body, if applicable (Z18.-)

EXCLUDES 1 *birth trauma (P10-P15)*
obstetric trauma (O70-O71)

NOTE The chapter uses the S-section for coding different types of injuries related to single body regions and the T-section to cover injuries to unspecified body regions as well as poisoning and certain other consequences of external causes.

AHA: 2016,2Q,3-7; 2015,4Q,35-38; 2015,3Q,37-39,40; 2015,2Q,6; 2015,1Q,3-21

TIP: The specific site of an injury can be determined from the radiology report when authenticated by a radiologist and available at the time of code assignment.

This chapter contains the following blocks:

- S00-S09 Injuries to the head
- S10-S19 Injuries to the neck
- S20-S29 Injuries to the thorax
- S30-S39 Injuries to the abdomen, lower back, lumbar spine, pelvis and external genitals
- S40-S49 Injuries to the shoulder and upper arm
- S50-S59 Injuries to the elbow and forearm
- S60-S69 Injuries to the wrist, hand and fingers
- S70-S79 Injuries to the hip and thigh
- S80-S89 Injuries to the knee and lower leg
- S90-S99 Injuries to the ankle and foot
- T07 Injuries involving multiple body regions
- T14 Injury of unspecified body region
- T15-T19 Effects of foreign body entering through natural orifice
- T20-T25 Burns and corrosions of external body surface, specified by site
- T26-T28 Burns and corrosions confined to eye and internal organs
- T30-T32 Burns and corrosions of multiple and unspecified body regions
- T33-T34 Frostbite
- T36-T50 Poisoning by, adverse effect of and underdosing of drugs, medicaments and biological substances
- T51-T65 Toxic effects of substances chiefly nonmedicinal as to source
- T66-T78 Other and unspecified effects of external causes
- T79 Certain early complications of trauma
- T80-T88 Complications of surgical and medical care, not elsewhere classified

Injuries to the head (S00-S09)

INCLUDES injuries of ear
injuries of eye
injuries of face [any part]
injuries of gum
injuries of jaw
injuries of oral cavity
injuries of palate
injuries of periocular area
injuries of scalp
injuries of temporomandibular joint area
injuries of tongue
injuries of tooth

Code also for any associated infection

EXCLUDES 2 *burns and corrosions (T20-T32)*
effects of foreign body in ear (T16)
effects of foreign body in larynx (T17.3)
effects of foreign body in mouth NOS (T18.0)
effects of foreign body in nose (T17.0-T17.1)
effects of foreign body in pharynx (T17.2)
effects of foreign body on external eye (T15.-)
frostbite (T33-T34)
insect bite or sting, venomous (T63.4)

4th **S00 Superficial injury of head**

EXCLUDES 1 *diffuse cerebral contusion (S06.2-)*
focal cerebral contusion (S06.3-)
injury of eye and orbit (S05.-)
open wound of head (S01.-)

The appropriate 7th character is to be added to each code from category S00.
A initial encounter
D subsequent encounter
S sequela

5th **S00.0 Superficial injury of scalp**
x7th **S00.00 Unspecified superficial injury of scalp**
x7th **S00.01 Abrasion of scalp**
x7th **S00.02 Blister (nonthermal) of scalp**
x7th **S00.03 Contusion of scalp**
Bruise of scalp
Hematoma of scalp
x7th **S00.04 External constriction of part of scalp**
x7th **S00.05 Superficial foreign body of scalp**
Splinter in the scalp
x7th **S00.06 Insect bite (nonvenomous) of scalp**
x7th **S00.07 Other superficial bite of scalp**
EXCLUDES 1 *open bite of scalp (S01.05)*

5th **S00.1 Contusion of eyelid and periocular area**
Black eye
EXCLUDES 2 *contusion of eyeball and orbital tissues (S05.1-)*
x7th **S00.10 Contusion of unspecified eyelid and periocular area**
x7th **S00.11 Contusion of right eyelid and periocular area**
x7th **S00.12 Contusion of left eyelid and periocular area**

5th **S00.2 Other and unspecified superficial injuries of eyelid and periocular area**
EXCLUDES 2 *superficial injury of conjunctiva and cornea (S05.0-)*
6th **S00.20 Unspecified superficial injury of eyelid and periocular area**
7th **S00.201 Unspecified superficial injury of right eyelid and periocular area**
7th **S00.202 Unspecified superficial injury of left eyelid and periocular area**
7th **S00.209 Unspecified superficial injury of unspecified eyelid and periocular area**
6th **S00.21 Abrasion of eyelid and periocular area**
7th **S00.211 Abrasion of right eyelid and periocular area**
7th **S00.212 Abrasion of left eyelid and periocular area**
7th **S00.219 Abrasion of unspecified eyelid and periocular area**
6th **S00.22 Blister (nonthermal) of eyelid and periocular area**
7th **S00.221 Blister (nonthermal) of right eyelid and periocular area**
7th **S00.222 Blister (nonthermal) of left eyelid and periocular area**
7th **S00.229 Blister (nonthermal) of unspecified eyelid and periocular area**
6th **S00.24 External constriction of eyelid and periocular area**
7th **S00.241 External constriction of right eyelid and periocular area**
7th **S00.242 External constriction of left eyelid and periocular area**
7th **S00.249 External constriction of unspecified eyelid and periocular area**
6th **S00.25 Superficial foreign body of eyelid and periocular area**
Splinter of eyelid and periocular area
EXCLUDES 2 *retained foreign body in eyelid (H02.81-)*
7th **S00.251 Superficial foreign body of right eyelid and periocular area**
7th **S00.252 Superficial foreign body of left eyelid and periocular area**
7th **S00.259 Superficial foreign body of unspecified eyelid and periocular area**
6th **S00.26 Insect bite (nonvenomous) of eyelid and periocular area**
7th **S00.261 Insect bite (nonvenomous) of right eyelid and periocular area**
7th **S00.262 Insect bite (nonvenomous) of left eyelid and periocular area**
7th **S00.269 Insect bite (nonvenomous) of unspecified eyelid and periocular area**
6th **S00.27 Other superficial bite of eyelid and periocular area**
EXCLUDES 1 *open bite of eyelid and periocular area (S01.15)*
7th **S00.271 Other superficial bite of right eyelid and periocular area**
7th **S00.272 Other superficial bite of left eyelid and periocular area**
7th **S00.279 Other superficial bite of unspecified eyelid and periocular area**

5th **S00.3 Superficial injury of nose**
x7th **S00.30 Unspecified superficial injury of nose**
x7th **S00.31 Abrasion of nose**
x7th **S00.32 Blister (nonthermal) of nose**

√x7th S00.33 Contusion of nose
Bruise of nose
Hematoma of nose
√x7th S00.34 External constriction of nose
√x7th S00.35 Superficial foreign body of nose
Splinter in the nose
√x7th S00.36 Insect bite (nonvenomous) of nose
√x7th S00.37 Other superficial bite of nose
EXCLUDES 1 *open bite of nose (S01.25)*

√5th S00.4 Superficial injury of ear
√6th S00.40 Unspecified superficial injury of ear
√7th S00.401 Unspecified superficial injury of right ear
√7th S00.402 Unspecified superficial injury of left ear
√7th S00.409 Unspecified superficial injury of unspecified ear
√6th S00.41 Abrasion of ear
√7th S00.411 Abrasion of right ear
√7th S00.412 Abrasion of left ear
√7th S00.419 Abrasion of unspecified ear
√6th S00.42 Blister (nonthermal) of ear
√7th S00.421 Blister (nonthermal) of right ear
√7th S00.422 Blister (nonthermal) of left ear
√7th S00.429 Blister (nonthermal) of unspecified ear
√6th S00.43 Contusion of ear
Bruise of ear
Hematoma of ear
√7th S00.431 Contusion of right ear
√7th S00.432 Contusion of left ear
√7th S00.439 Contusion of unspecified ear
√6th S00.44 External constriction of ear
√7th S00.441 External constriction of right ear
√7th S00.442 External constriction of left ear
√7th S00.449 External constriction of unspecified ear
√6th S00.45 Superficial foreign body of ear
Splinter in the ear
√7th S00.451 Superficial foreign body of right ear
√7th S00.452 Superficial foreign body of left ear
√7th S00.459 Superficial foreign body of unspecified ear
√6th S00.46 Insect bite (nonvenomous) of ear
√7th S00.461 Insect bite (nonvenomous) of right ear
√7th S00.462 Insect bite (nonvenomous) of left ear
√7th S00.469 Insect bite (nonvenomous) of unspecified ear
√6th S00.47 Other superficial bite of ear
EXCLUDES 1 *open bite of ear (S01.35)*
√7th S00.471 Other superficial bite of right ear
√7th S00.472 Other superficial bite of left ear
√7th S00.479 Other superficial bite of unspecified ear

√5th S00.5 Superficial injury of lip and oral cavity
√6th S00.50 Unspecified superficial injury of lip and oral cavity
√7th S00.501 Unspecified superficial injury of lip
√7th S00.502 Unspecified superficial injury of oral cavity
√6th S00.51 Abrasion of lip and oral cavity
√7th S00.511 Abrasion of lip
√7th S00.512 Abrasion of oral cavity
√6th S00.52 Blister (nonthermal) of lip and oral cavity
√7th S00.521 Blister (nonthermal) of lip
√7th S00.522 Blister (nonthermal) of oral cavity
√6th S00.53 Contusion of lip and oral cavity
√7th S00.531 Contusion of lip
Bruise of lip
Hematoma of lip
√7th S00.532 Contusion of oral cavity
Bruise of oral cavity
Hematoma of oral cavity
√6th S00.54 External constriction of lip and oral cavity
√7th S00.541 External constriction of lip
√7th S00.542 External constriction of oral cavity
√6th S00.55 Superficial foreign body of lip and oral cavity
√7th S00.551 Superficial foreign body of lip
Splinter of lip and oral cavity
√7th S00.552 Superficial foreign body of oral cavity
Splinter of lip and oral cavity
√6th S00.56 Insect bite (nonvenomous) of lip and oral cavity
√7th S00.561 Insect bite (nonvenomous) of lip
√7th S00.562 Insect bite (nonvenomous) of oral cavity
√6th S00.57 Other superficial bite of lip and oral cavity
√7th S00.571 Other superficial bite of lip
EXCLUDES 1 *open bite of lip (S01.551)*
√7th S00.572 Other superficial bite of oral cavity
EXCLUDES 1 *open bite of oral cavity (S01.552)*

√5th S00.8 Superficial injury of other parts of head
Superficial injuries of face [any part]
√x7th S00.80 Unspecified superficial injury of other part of head
√x7th S00.81 Abrasion of other part of head
√x7th S00.82 Blister (nonthermal) of other part of head
√x7th S00.83 Contusion of other part of head
Bruise of other part of head
Hematoma of other part of head
√x7th S00.84 External constriction of other part of head
√x7th S00.85 Superficial foreign body of other part of head
Splinter in other part of head
√x7th S00.86 Insect bite (nonvenomous) of other part of head
√x7th S00.87 Other superficial bite of other part of head
EXCLUDES 1 *open bite of other part of head (S01.85)*

√5th S00.9 Superficial injury of unspecified part of head
√x7th S00.90 Unspecified superficial injury of unspecified part of head
√x7th S00.91 Abrasion of unspecified part of head
√x7th S00.92 Blister (nonthermal) of unspecified part of head
√x7th S00.93 Contusion of unspecified part of head
Bruise of head
Hematoma of head
√x7th S00.94 External constriction of unspecified part of head
√x7th S00.95 Superficial foreign body of unspecified part of head
Splinter of head
√x7th S00.96 Insect bite (nonvenomous) of unspecified part of head
√x7th S00.97 Other superficial bite of unspecified part of head
EXCLUDES 1 *open bite of head (S01.95)*

√4th **S01 Open wound of head**
Code also any associated:
injury of cranial nerve (S04.-)
injury of muscle and tendon of head (S09.1-)
intracranial injury (S06.-)
wound infection
EXCLUDES 1 *open skull fracture (S02.- with 7th character B)*
EXCLUDES 2 *injury of eye and orbit (S05.-)*
traumatic amputation of part of head (S08.-)

The appropriate 7th character is to be added to each code from category S01.
A initial encounter
D subsequent encounter
S sequela

√5th S01.0 Open wound of scalp
EXCLUDES 1 *avulsion of scalp (S08.0-)*
√x7th S01.00 Unspecified open wound of scalp
√x7th S01.01 Laceration without foreign body of scalp
√x7th S01.02 Laceration with foreign body of scalp
√x7th S01.03 Puncture wound without foreign body of scalp
√x7th S01.04 Puncture wound with foreign body of scalp
√x7th S01.05 Open bite of scalp
Bite of scalp NOS
EXCLUDES 1 *superficial bite of scalp (S00.06, S00.07-)*

SØ1.1 Open wound of eyelid and periocular area
Open wound of eyelid and periocular area with or without involvement of lacrimal passages

SØ1.1Ø Unspecified open wound of eyelid and periocular area
- **SØ1.1Ø1 Unspecified open wound of right eyelid and periocular area** CC
- **SØ1.1Ø2 Unspecified open wound of left eyelid and periocular area** CC
- **SØ1.1Ø9 Unspecified open wound of unspecified eyelid and periocular area** CC UNS

SØ1.11 Laceration without foreign body of eyelid and periocular area
- **SØ1.111 Laceration without foreign body of right eyelid and periocular area**
- **SØ1.112 Laceration without foreign body of left eyelid and periocular area**
- **SØ1.119 Laceration without foreign body of unspecified eyelid and periocular area**

SØ1.12 Laceration with foreign body of eyelid and periocular area
- **SØ1.121 Laceration with foreign body of right eyelid and periocular area**
- **SØ1.122 Laceration with foreign body of left eyelid and periocular area**
- **SØ1.129 Laceration with foreign body of unspecified eyelid and periocular area**

SØ1.13 Puncture wound without foreign body of eyelid and periocular area
- **SØ1.131 Puncture wound without foreign body of right eyelid and periocular area**
- **SØ1.132 Puncture wound without foreign body of left eyelid and periocular area**
- **SØ1.139 Puncture wound without foreign body of unspecified eyelid and periocular area**

SØ1.14 Puncture wound with foreign body of eyelid and periocular area
- **SØ1.141 Puncture wound with foreign body of right eyelid and periocular area**
- **SØ1.142 Puncture wound with foreign body of left eyelid and periocular area**
- **SØ1.149 Puncture wound with foreign body of unspecified eyelid and periocular area**

SØ1.15 Open bite of eyelid and periocular area
Bite of eyelid and periocular area NOS
EXCLUDES 1 *superficial bite of eyelid and periocular area (SØØ.26, SØØ.27)*
- **SØ1.151 Open bite of right eyelid and periocular area**
- **SØ1.152 Open bite of left eyelid and periocular area**
- **SØ1.159 Open bite of unspecified eyelid and periocular area**

SØ1.2 Open wound of nose
- **SØ1.2Ø Unspecified open wound of nose**
- **SØ1.21 Laceration without foreign body of nose**
- **SØ1.22 Laceration with foreign body of nose**
- **SØ1.23 Puncture wound without foreign body of nose**
- **SØ1.24 Puncture wound with foreign body of nose**
- **SØ1.25 Open bite of nose**
  Bite of nose NOS
  EXCLUDES 1 *superficial bite of nose (SØØ.36, SØØ.37)*

SØ1.3 Open wound of ear

SØ1.3Ø Unspecified open wound of ear
- **SØ1.3Ø1 Unspecified open wound of right ear**
- **SØ1.3Ø2 Unspecified open wound of left ear**
- **SØ1.3Ø9 Unspecified open wound of unspecified ear**

SØ1.31 Laceration without foreign body of ear
- **SØ1.311 Laceration without foreign body of right ear**
- **SØ1.312 Laceration without foreign body of left ear**
- **SØ1.319 Laceration without foreign body of unspecified ear**

SØ1.32 Laceration with foreign body of ear
- **SØ1.321 Laceration with foreign body of right ear**
- **SØ1.322 Laceration with foreign body of left ear**
- **SØ1.329 Laceration with foreign body of unspecified ear**

SØ1.33 Puncture wound without foreign body of ear
- **SØ1.331 Puncture wound without foreign body of right ear**
- **SØ1.332 Puncture wound without foreign body of left ear**
- **SØ1.339 Puncture wound without foreign body of unspecified ear**

SØ1.34 Puncture wound with foreign body of ear
- **SØ1.341 Puncture wound with foreign body of right ear**
- **SØ1.342 Puncture wound with foreign body of left ear**
- **SØ1.349 Puncture wound with foreign body of unspecified ear**

SØ1.35 Open bite of ear
Bite of ear NOS
EXCLUDES 1 *superficial bite of ear (SØØ.46, SØØ.47)*
- **SØ1.351 Open bite of right ear**
- **SØ1.352 Open bite of left ear**
- **SØ1.359 Open bite of unspecified ear**

SØ1.4 Open wound of cheek and temporomandibular area

SØ1.4Ø Unspecified open wound of cheek and temporomandibular area
- **SØ1.4Ø1 Unspecified open wound of right cheek and temporomandibular area**
- **SØ1.4Ø2 Unspecified open wound of left cheek and temporomandibular area**
- **SØ1.4Ø9 Unspecified open wound of unspecified cheek and temporomandibular area**

SØ1.41 Laceration without foreign body of cheek and temporomandibular area
- **SØ1.411 Laceration without foreign body of right cheek and temporomandibular area**
- **SØ1.412 Laceration without foreign body of left cheek and temporomandibular area**
- **SØ1.419 Laceration without foreign body of unspecified cheek and temporomandibular area**

SØ1.42 Laceration with foreign body of cheek and temporomandibular area
- **SØ1.421 Laceration with foreign body of right cheek and temporomandibular area**
- **SØ1.422 Laceration with foreign body of left cheek and temporomandibular area**
- **SØ1.429 Laceration with foreign body of unspecified cheek and temporomandibular area**

SØ1.43 Puncture wound without foreign body of cheek and temporomandibular area
- **SØ1.431 Puncture wound without foreign body of right cheek and temporomandibular area**
- **SØ1.432 Puncture wound without foreign body of left cheek and temporomandibular area**
- **SØ1.439 Puncture wound without foreign body of unspecified cheek and temporomandibular area**

SØ1.44 Puncture wound with foreign body of cheek and temporomandibular area
- **SØ1.441 Puncture wound with foreign body of right cheek and temporomandibular area**
- **SØ1.442 Puncture wound with foreign body of left cheek and temporomandibular area**
- **SØ1.449 Puncture wound with foreign body of unspecified cheek and temporomandibular area**

SØ1.45 Open bite of cheek and temporomandibular area
Bite of cheek and temporomandibular area NOS
EXCLUDES 2 *superficial bite of cheek and temporomandibular area (SØØ.86, SØØ.87)*
- **SØ1.451 Open bite of right cheek and temporomandibular area**
- **SØ1.452 Open bite of left cheek and temporomandibular area**
- **SØ1.459 Open bite of unspecified cheek and temporomandibular area**

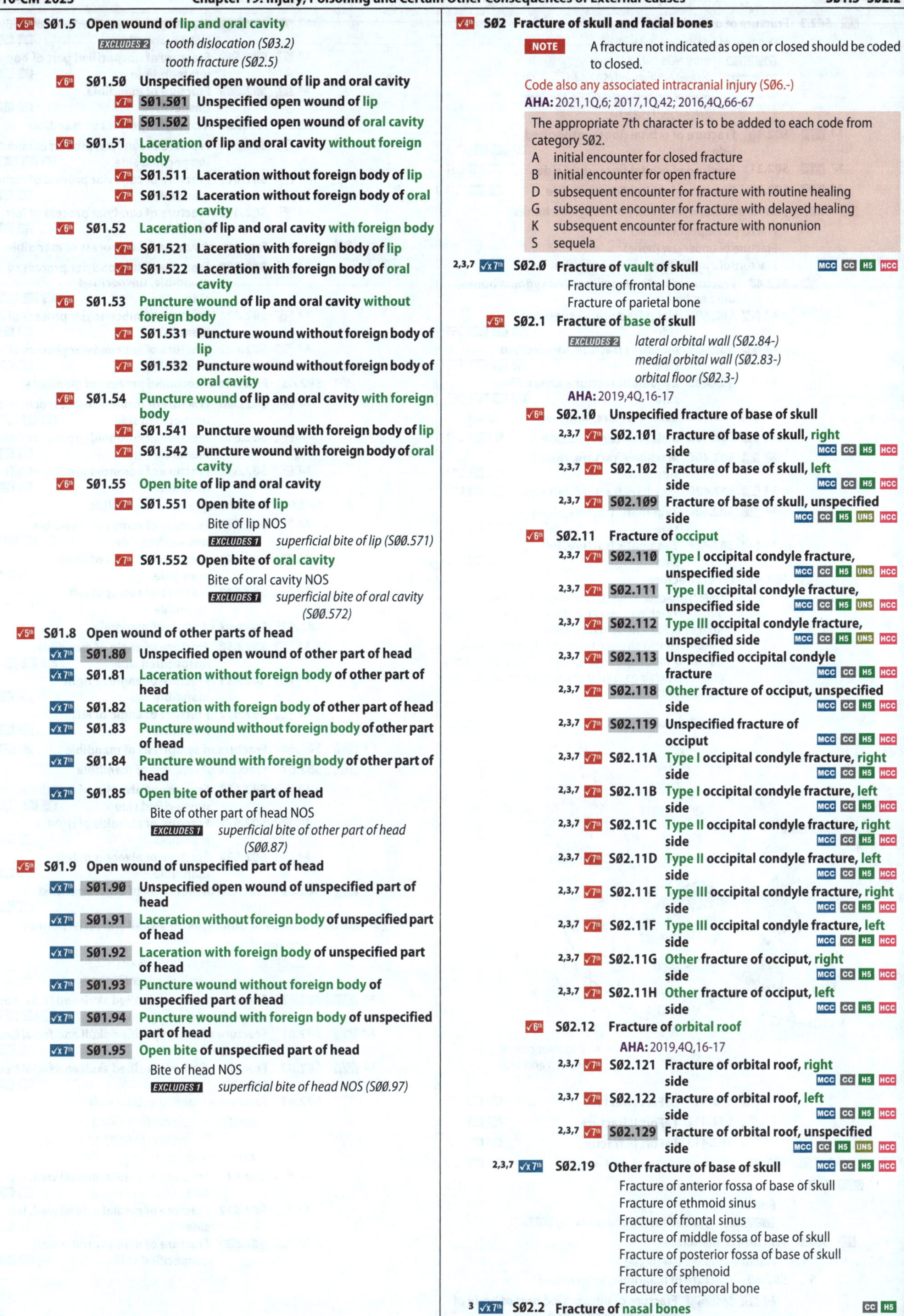

S01.5 Open wound of lip and oral cavity
EXCLUDES 2 *tooth dislocation (S03.2)*
tooth fracture (S02.5)

S01.50 Unspecified open wound of lip and oral cavity
S01.501 Unspecified open wound of lip
S01.502 Unspecified open wound of oral cavity
S01.51 Laceration of lip and oral cavity without foreign body
S01.511 Laceration without foreign body of lip
S01.512 Laceration without foreign body of oral cavity
S01.52 Laceration of lip and oral cavity with foreign body
S01.521 Laceration with foreign body of lip
S01.522 Laceration with foreign body of oral cavity
S01.53 Puncture wound of lip and oral cavity without foreign body
S01.531 Puncture wound without foreign body of lip
S01.532 Puncture wound without foreign body of oral cavity
S01.54 Puncture wound of lip and oral cavity with foreign body
S01.541 Puncture wound with foreign body of lip
S01.542 Puncture wound with foreign body of oral cavity
S01.55 Open bite of lip and oral cavity
S01.551 Open bite of lip
Bite of lip NOS
EXCLUDES 1 *superficial bite of lip (S00.571)*
S01.552 Open bite of oral cavity
Bite of oral cavity NOS
EXCLUDES 1 *superficial bite of oral cavity (S00.572)*

S01.8 Open wound of other parts of head
S01.80 Unspecified open wound of other part of head
S01.81 Laceration without foreign body of other part of head
S01.82 Laceration with foreign body of other part of head
S01.83 Puncture wound without foreign body of other part of head
S01.84 Puncture wound with foreign body of other part of head
S01.85 Open bite of other part of head
Bite of other part of head NOS
EXCLUDES 1 *superficial bite of other part of head (S00.87)*

S01.9 Open wound of unspecified part of head
S01.90 Unspecified open wound of unspecified part of head
S01.91 Laceration without foreign body of unspecified part of head
S01.92 Laceration with foreign body of unspecified part of head
S01.93 Puncture wound without foreign body of unspecified part of head
S01.94 Puncture wound with foreign body of unspecified part of head
S01.95 Open bite of unspecified part of head
Bite of head NOS
EXCLUDES 1 *superficial bite of head NOS (S00.97)*

S02 Fracture of skull and facial bones
NOTE A fracture not indicated as open or closed should be coded to closed.
Code also any associated intracranial injury (S06.-)
AHA: 2021,1Q,6; 2017,1Q,42; 2016,4Q,66-67

The appropriate 7th character is to be added to each code from category S02.
A initial encounter for closed fracture
B initial encounter for open fracture
D subsequent encounter for fracture with routine healing
G subsequent encounter for fracture with delayed healing
K subsequent encounter for fracture with nonunion
S sequela

2,3,7 **S02.0 Fracture of vault of skull** MCC CC H5 HCC
Fracture of frontal bone
Fracture of parietal bone

S02.1 Fracture of base of skull
EXCLUDES 2 *lateral orbital wall (S02.84-)*
medial orbital wall (S02.83-)
orbital floor (S02.3-)
AHA: 2019,4Q,16-17

S02.10 Unspecified fracture of base of skull
2,3,7 **S02.101 Fracture of base of skull, right side** MCC CC H5 HCC
2,3,7 **S02.102 Fracture of base of skull, left side** MCC CC H5 HCC
2,3,7 **S02.109 Fracture of base of skull, unspecified side** MCC CC H5 UNS HCC
S02.11 Fracture of occiput
2,3,7 **S02.110 Type I occipital condyle fracture, unspecified side** MCC CC H5 UNS HCC
2,3,7 **S02.111 Type II occipital condyle fracture, unspecified side** MCC CC H5 UNS HCC
2,3,7 **S02.112 Type III occipital condyle fracture, unspecified side** MCC CC H5 UNS HCC
2,3,7 **S02.113 Unspecified occipital condyle fracture** MCC CC H5 HCC
2,3,7 **S02.118 Other fracture of occiput, unspecified side** MCC CC H5 HCC
2,3,7 **S02.119 Unspecified fracture of occiput** MCC CC H5 HCC
2,3,7 **S02.11A Type I occipital condyle fracture, right side** MCC CC H5 HCC
2,3,7 **S02.11B Type I occipital condyle fracture, left side** MCC CC H5 HCC
2,3,7 **S02.11C Type II occipital condyle fracture, right side** MCC CC H5 HCC
2,3,7 **S02.11D Type II occipital condyle fracture, left side** MCC CC H5 HCC
2,3,7 **S02.11E Type III occipital condyle fracture, right side** MCC CC H5 HCC
2,3,7 **S02.11F Type III occipital condyle fracture, left side** MCC CC H5 HCC
2,3,7 **S02.11G Other fracture of occiput, right side** MCC CC H5 HCC
2,3,7 **S02.11H Other fracture of occiput, left side** MCC CC H5 HCC
S02.12 Fracture of orbital roof
AHA: 2019,4Q,16-17
2,3,7 **S02.121 Fracture of orbital roof, right side** MCC CC H5 HCC
2,3,7 **S02.122 Fracture of orbital roof, left side** MCC CC H5 HCC
2,3,7 **S02.129 Fracture of orbital roof, unspecified side** MCC CC H5 UNS HCC
2,3,7 **S02.19 Other fracture of base of skull** MCC CC H5 HCC
Fracture of anterior fossa of base of skull
Fracture of ethmoid sinus
Fracture of frontal sinus
Fracture of middle fossa of base of skull
Fracture of posterior fossa of base of skull
Fracture of sphenoid
Fracture of temporal bone

3 **S02.2 Fracture of nasal bones** CC H5

√5th **SØ2.3 Fracture of orbital floor**
Fracture of inferior orbital wall
EXCLUDES 1 *orbit NOS (SØ2.85)*
EXCLUDES 2 *lateral orbital wall (SØ2.84-)*
medial orbital wall (SØ2.83-)
orbital roof (SØ2.1-)

3,7 √x7th **SØ2.3Ø Fracture of orbital floor, unspecified side** CC HS UNS HCC

3,7 √x7th **SØ2.31 Fracture of orbital floor, right side** CC HS HCC

3,7 √x7th **SØ2.32 Fracture of orbital floor, left side** CC HS HCC

√5th **SØ2.4 Fracture of malar, maxillary and zygoma bones**
Fracture of superior maxilla
Fracture of upper jaw (bone)
Fracture of zygomatic process of temporal bone

√6th **SØ2.4Ø Fracture of malar, maxillary and zygoma bones, unspecified**

3,7 √7th **SØ2.4ØØ Malar fracture, unspecified side** CC HS UNS HCC

3,7 √7th **SØ2.4Ø1 Maxillary fracture, unspecified side** CC HS UNS HCC

3,7 √7th **SØ2.4Ø2 Zygomatic fracture, unspecified side** CC HS UNS HCC

3,7 √7th **SØ2.4ØA Malar fracture, right side** CC HS HCC

3,7 √7th **SØ2.4ØB Malar fracture, left side** CC HS HCC

3,7 √7th **SØ2.4ØC Maxillary fracture, right side** CC HS HCC

3,7 √7th **SØ2.4ØD Maxillary fracture, left side** CC HS HCC

3,7 √7th **SØ2.4ØE Zygomatic fracture, right side** CC HS HCC

3,7 √7th **SØ2.4ØF Zygomatic fracture, left side** CC HS HCC

√6th **SØ2.41 LeFort fracture**

DEF: Named for Rene Le Fort, these fractures describe different combinations of multiple fractures that occur from significant force to the midface. A common denominator in all three types of LeFort fractures is fracture of the pterygoid processes, which are two bony plates resembling wings that extend downward from the sphenoid bone.

LeFort Fracture Types

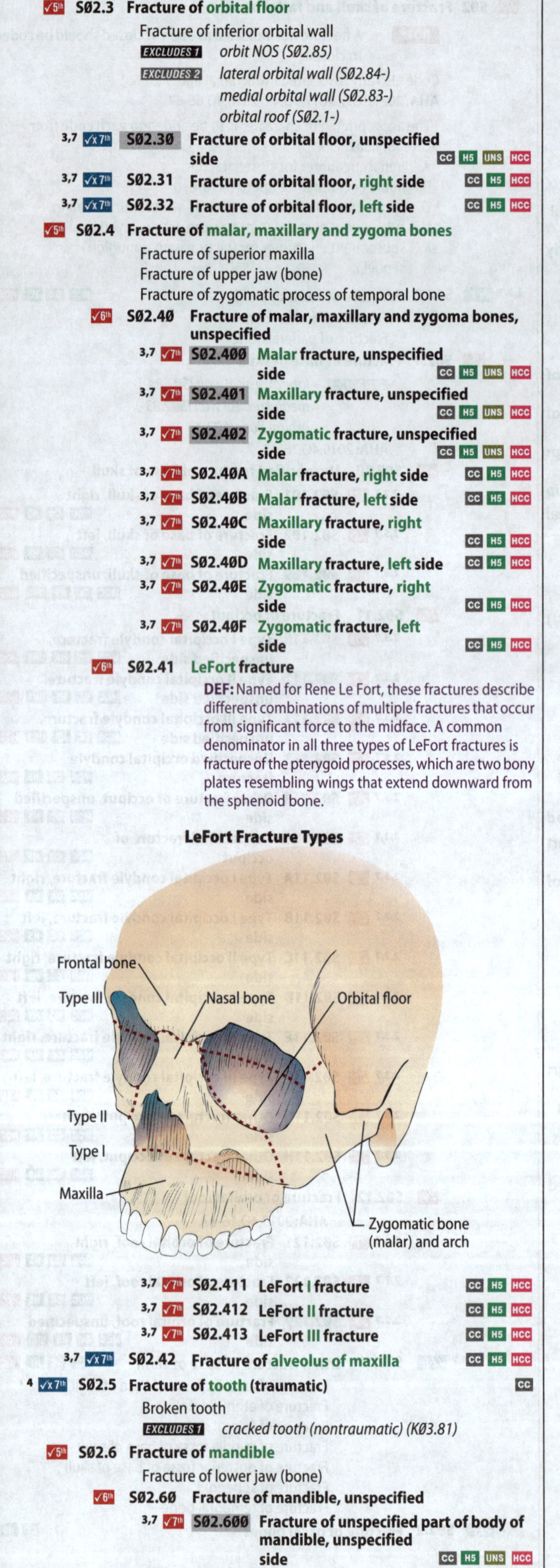

3,7 √7th **SØ2.411 LeFort I fracture** CC HS HCC

3,7 √7th **SØ2.412 LeFort II fracture** CC HS HCC

3,7 √7th **SØ2.413 LeFort III fracture** CC HS HCC

3,7 √x7th **SØ2.42 Fracture of alveolus of maxilla** CC HS HCC

4 √x7th **SØ2.5 Fracture of tooth (traumatic)** CC
Broken tooth
EXCLUDES 1 *cracked tooth (nontraumatic) (KØ3.81)*

√5th **SØ2.6 Fracture of mandible**
Fracture of lower jaw (bone)

√6th **SØ2.6Ø Fracture of mandible, unspecified**

3,7 √7th **SØ2.6ØØ Fracture of unspecified part of body of mandible, unspecified side** CC HS UNS HCC

3,7 √7th **SØ2.6Ø1 Fracture of unspecified part of body of right mandible** CC HS HCC

3,7 √7th **SØ2.6Ø2 Fracture of unspecified part of body of left mandible** CC HS HCC

3,7 √7th **SØ2.6Ø9 Fracture of mandible, unspecified** CC HS HCC

√6th **SØ2.61 Fracture of condylar process of mandible**

3,7 √7th **SØ2.61Ø Fracture of condylar process of mandible, unspecified side** CC HS UNS HCC

3,7 √7th **SØ2.611 Fracture of condylar process of right mandible** CC HS HCC

3,7 √7th **SØ2.612 Fracture of condylar process of left mandible** CC HS HCC

√6th **SØ2.62 Fracture of subcondylar process of mandible**

3,7 √7th **SØ2.62Ø Fracture of subcondylar process of mandible, unspecified side** CC HS UNS HCC

3,7 √7th **SØ2.621 Fracture of subcondylar process of right mandible** CC HS HCC

3,7 √7th **SØ2.622 Fracture of subcondylar process of left mandible** CC HS HCC

√6th **SØ2.63 Fracture of coronoid process of mandible**

3,7 √7th **SØ2.63Ø Fracture of coronoid process of mandible, unspecified side** CC HS UNS HCC

3,7 √7th **SØ2.631 Fracture of coronoid process of right mandible** CC HS HCC

3,7 √7th **SØ2.632 Fracture of coronoid process of left mandible** CC HS HCC

√6th **SØ2.64 Fracture of ramus of mandible**

3,7 √7th **SØ2.64Ø Fracture of ramus of mandible, unspecified side** CC HS UNS HCC

3,7 √7th **SØ2.641 Fracture of ramus of right mandible** CC HS HCC

3,7 √7th **SØ2.642 Fracture of ramus of left mandible** CC HS HCC

√6th **SØ2.65 Fracture of angle of mandible**

3,7 √7th **SØ2.65Ø Fracture of angle of mandible, unspecified side** CC HS UNS HCC

3,7 √7th **SØ2.651 Fracture of angle of right mandible** CC HS HCC

3,7 √7th **SØ2.652 Fracture of angle of left mandible** CC HS HCC

3,7 √x7th **SØ2.66 Fracture of symphysis of mandible** CC HS HCC

√6th **SØ2.67 Fracture of alveolus of mandible**

3,7 √7th **SØ2.67Ø Fracture of alveolus of mandible, unspecified side** CC HS UNS HCC

3,7 √7th **SØ2.671 Fracture of alveolus of right mandible** CC HS HCC

3,7 √7th **SØ2.672 Fracture of alveolus of left mandible** CC HS HCC

3,7 √x7th **SØ2.69 Fracture of mandible of other specified site** CC HS HCC

√5th **SØ2.8 Fractures of other specified skull and facial bones**
Fracture of palate
EXCLUDES 2 *fracture of orbital floor (SØ2.3-)*
fracture of orbital roof (SØ2.12-)

3,7 √x7th **SØ2.8Ø Fracture of other specified skull and facial bones, unspecified side** CC HS UNS HCC

3,7 √x7th **SØ2.81 Fracture of other specified skull and facial bones, right side** CC HS HCC

3,7 √x7th **SØ2.82 Fracture of other specified skull and facial bones, left side** CC HS HCC

√6th **SØ2.83 Fracture of medial orbital wall**
EXCLUDES 2 *orbital floor (SØ2.3-)*
orbital roof (SØ2.12-)
AHA: 2019,4Q,16-17

3,7 √7th **SØ2.831 Fracture of medial orbital wall, right side** CC HS HCC

3,7 √7th **SØ2.832 Fracture of medial orbital wall, left side** CC HS HCC

3,7 √7th **SØ2.839 Fracture of medial orbital wall, unspecified side** CC HS HCC

S02.84 Fracture of lateral orbital wall

EXCLUDES 2 *orbital floor (S02.3-)*
orbital roof (S02.12-)

AHA: 2019,4Q,16-17

3,7 **S02.841 Fracture of lateral orbital wall, right side** CC H5 HCC

3,7 **S02.842 Fracture of lateral orbital wall, left side** CC H5 HCC

3,7 **S02.849 Fracture of lateral orbital wall, unspecified side** CC H5 HCC

3,7 **S02.85 Fracture of orbit, unspecified** CC H5 HCC

Fracture of orbit NOS
Fracture of orbit wall NOS

EXCLUDES 1 *lateral orbital wall (S02.84-)*
medial orbital wall (S02.83-)
orbital floor (S02.3-)
orbital roof (S02.12-)

S02.9 Fracture of unspecified skull and facial bones

2,3,7 **S02.91 Unspecified fracture of skull** MCC CC H5 HCC

AHA: 2020,2Q,24

3,7 **S02.92 Unspecified fracture of facial bones** CC H5 HCC

S03 Dislocation and sprain of joints and ligaments of head

INCLUDES avulsion of joint (capsule) or ligament of head
laceration of cartilage, joint (capsule) or ligament of head
sprain of cartilage, joint (capsule) or ligament of head
traumatic hemarthrosis of joint or ligament of head
traumatic rupture of joint or ligament of head
traumatic subluxation of joint or ligament of head
traumatic tear of joint or ligament of head

Code also any associated open wound

EXCLUDES 2 *strain of muscle or tendon of head (S09.1)*

The appropriate 7th character is to be added to each code from category S03.
A initial encounter
D subsequent encounter
S sequela

S03.0 Dislocation of jaw

Dislocation of jaw (cartilage) (meniscus)
Dislocation of mandible
Dislocation of temporomandibular (joint)

AHA: 2016,4Q,67

S03.00 Dislocation of jaw, unspecified side

S03.01 Dislocation of jaw, right side

S03.02 Dislocation of jaw, left side

S03.03 Dislocation of jaw, bilateral

S03.1 Dislocation of septal cartilage of nose

S03.2 Dislocation of tooth

S03.4 Sprain of jaw

Sprain of temporomandibular (joint) (ligament)

AHA: 2016,4Q,67

S03.40 Sprain of jaw, unspecified side

S03.41 Sprain of jaw, right side

S03.42 Sprain of jaw, left side

S03.43 Sprain of jaw, bilateral

S03.8 Sprain of joints and ligaments of other parts of head

S03.9 Sprain of joints and ligaments of unspecified parts of head

S04 Injury of cranial nerve

The selection of side should be based on the side of the body being affected

Code first any associated intracranial injury (S06.-)

Code also any associated:
open wound of head (S01.-)
skull fracture (S02.-)

The appropriate 7th character is to be added to each code from category S04.
A initial encounter
D subsequent encounter
S sequela

S04.0 Injury of optic nerve and pathways

Use additional code to identify any visual field defect or blindness (H53.4-, H54.-)

S04.01 Injury of optic nerve

Injury of 2nd cranial nerve

S04.011 Injury of optic nerve, right eye CC

S04.012 Injury of optic nerve, left eye CC

S04.019 Injury of optic nerve, unspecified eye CC UNS

Injury of optic nerve NOS

S04.02 Injury of optic chiasm CC

S04.03 Injury of optic tract and pathways

Injury of optic radiation

S04.031 Injury of optic tract and pathways, right side CC

S04.032 Injury of optic tract and pathways, left side CC

S04.039 Injury of optic tract and pathways, unspecified side CC UNS

Injury of optic tract and pathways NOS

S04.04 Injury of visual cortex

S04.041 Injury of visual cortex, right side CC

S04.042 Injury of visual cortex, left side CC

S04.049 Injury of visual cortex, unspecified side CC UNS

Injury of visual cortex NOS

S04.1 Injury of oculomotor nerve

Injury of 3rd cranial nerve

S04.10 Injury of oculomotor nerve, unspecified side CC UNS

S04.11 Injury of oculomotor nerve, right side CC

S04.12 Injury of oculomotor nerve, left side CC

S04.2 Injury of trochlear nerve

Injury of 4th cranial nerve

S04.20 Injury of trochlear nerve, unspecified side CC UNS

S04.21 Injury of trochlear nerve, right side CC

S04.22 Injury of trochlear nerve, left side CC

S04.3 Injury of trigeminal nerve

Injury of 5th cranial nerve

S04.30 Injury of trigeminal nerve, unspecified side CC UNS

S04.31 Injury of trigeminal nerve, right side CC

S04.32 Injury of trigeminal nerve, left side CC

S04.4 Injury of abducent nerve

Injury of 6th cranial nerve

S04.40 Injury of abducent nerve, unspecified side CC UNS

S04.41 Injury of abducent nerve, right side CC

S04.42 Injury of abducent nerve, left side CC

S04.5 Injury of facial nerve

Injury of 7th cranial nerve

S04.50 Injury of facial nerve, unspecified side CC UNS

S04.51 Injury of facial nerve, right side CC

S04.52 Injury of facial nerve, left side CC

S04.6 Injury of acoustic nerve

Injury of auditory nerve
Injury of 8th cranial nerve

S04.60 Injury of acoustic nerve, unspecified side CC UNS

S04.61 Injury of acoustic nerve, right side CC

√x7th **S04.62 Injury of acoustic nerve, left side** CC

√5th **S04.7 Injury of accessory nerve**

Injury of 11th cranial nerve

√x7th **S04.70 Injury of accessory nerve, unspecified side** CC UNS

√x7th **S04.71 Injury of accessory nerve, right side** CC

√x7th **S04.72 Injury of accessory nerve, left side** CC

√5th **S04.8 Injury of other cranial nerves**

√6th **S04.81 Injury of olfactory [1st] nerve**

√7th **S04.811 Injury of olfactory [1st] nerve, right side** CC

√7th **S04.812 Injury of olfactory [1st] nerve, left side** CC

√7th **S04.819 Injury of olfactory [1st] nerve, unspecified side** CC

√6th **S04.89 Injury of other cranial nerves**

Injury of vagus [10th] nerve

√7th **S04.891 Injury of other cranial nerves, right side** CC

√7th **S04.892 Injury of other cranial nerves, left side** CC

√7th **S04.899 Injury of other cranial nerves, unspecified side** CC UNS

√x7th **S04.9 Injury of unspecified cranial nerve** CC

√4th **S05 Injury of eye and orbit**

INCLUDES open wound of eye and orbit

EXCLUDES 2 *2nd cranial [optic] nerve injury (S04.0-)*
3rd cranial [oculomotor] nerve injury (S04.1-)
open wound of eyelid and periocular area (S01.1-)
orbital bone fracture (S02.1-, S02.3-, S02.8-)
superficial injury of eyelid (S00.1-S00.2)

The appropriate 7th character is to be added to each code from category S05.
A initial encounter
D subsequent encounter
S sequela

√5th **S05.0 Injury of conjunctiva and corneal abrasion without foreign body**

EXCLUDES 1 *foreign body in conjunctival sac (T15.1)*
foreign body in cornea (T15.0)

√x7th **S05.00 Injury of conjunctiva and corneal abrasion without foreign body, unspecified eye**

√x7th **S05.01 Injury of conjunctiva and corneal abrasion without foreign body, right eye**

√x7th **S05.02 Injury of conjunctiva and corneal abrasion without foreign body, left eye**

√5th **S05.1 Contusion of eyeball and orbital tissues**

Traumatic hyphema

EXCLUDES 2 *black eye NOS (S00.1)*
contusion of eyelid and periocular area (S00.1)

√x7th **S05.10 Contusion of eyeball and orbital tissues, unspecified eye**

√x7th **S05.11 Contusion of eyeball and orbital tissues, right eye**

√x7th **S05.12 Contusion of eyeball and orbital tissues, left eye**

√5th **S05.2 Ocular laceration and rupture with prolapse or loss of intraocular tissue**

√x7th **S05.20 Ocular laceration and rupture with prolapse or loss of intraocular tissue, unspecified eye** CC UNS

√x7th **S05.21 Ocular laceration and rupture with prolapse or loss of intraocular tissue, right eye** CC

√x7th **S05.22 Ocular laceration and rupture with prolapse or loss of intraocular tissue, left eye** CC

√5th **S05.3 Ocular laceration without prolapse or loss of intraocular tissue**

Laceration of eye NOS

AHA: 2022,1Q,33

DEF: Tear in ocular tissue without displacing structures that is due to blunt trauma. It is characterized by pain, redness, and decreased vision.

√x7th **S05.30 Ocular laceration without prolapse or loss of intraocular tissue, unspecified eye** CC UNS

√x7th **S05.31 Ocular laceration without prolapse or loss of intraocular tissue, right eye** CC

√x7th **S05.32 Ocular laceration without prolapse or loss of intraocular tissue, left eye** CC

√5th **S05.4 Penetrating wound of orbit with or without foreign body**

EXCLUDES 2 *retained (old) foreign body following penetrating wound in orbit (H05.5-)*

√x7th **S05.40 Penetrating wound of orbit with or without foreign body, unspecified eye** CC UNS

√x7th **S05.41 Penetrating wound of orbit with or without foreign body, right eye** CC

√x7th **S05.42 Penetrating wound of orbit with or without foreign body, left eye** CC

√5th **S05.5 Penetrating wound with foreign body of eyeball**

EXCLUDES 2 *retained (old) intraocular foreign body (H44.6-, H44.7)*

√x7th **S05.50 Penetrating wound with foreign body of unspecified eyeball** CC UNS

√x7th **S05.51 Penetrating wound with foreign body of right eyeball** CC

√x7th **S05.52 Penetrating wound with foreign body of left eyeball** CC

√5th **S05.6 Penetrating wound without foreign body of eyeball**

Ocular penetration NOS

√x7th **S05.60 Penetrating wound without foreign body of unspecified eyeball**

√x7th **S05.61 Penetrating wound without foreign body of right eyeball**

√x7th **S05.62 Penetrating wound without foreign body of left eyeball**

√5th **S05.7 Avulsion of eye**

Traumatic enucleation

√x7th **S05.70 Avulsion of unspecified eye** CC UNS

√x7th **S05.71 Avulsion of right eye** CC

√x7th **S05.72 Avulsion of left eye** CC

√5th **S05.8 Other injuries of eye and orbit**

Lacrimal duct injury

√6th **S05.8X Other injuries of eye and orbit**

√7th **S05.8X1 Other injuries of right eye and orbit** CC

√7th **S05.8X2 Other injuries of left eye and orbit** CC

√7th **S05.8X9 Other injuries of unspecified eye and orbit** CC UNS

√5th **S05.9 Unspecified injury of eye and orbit**

Injury of eye NOS

√x7th **S05.90 Unspecified injury of unspecified eye and orbit**

√x7th **S05.91 Unspecified injury of right eye and orbit** CC

√x7th **S05.92 Unspecified injury of left eye and orbit** CC

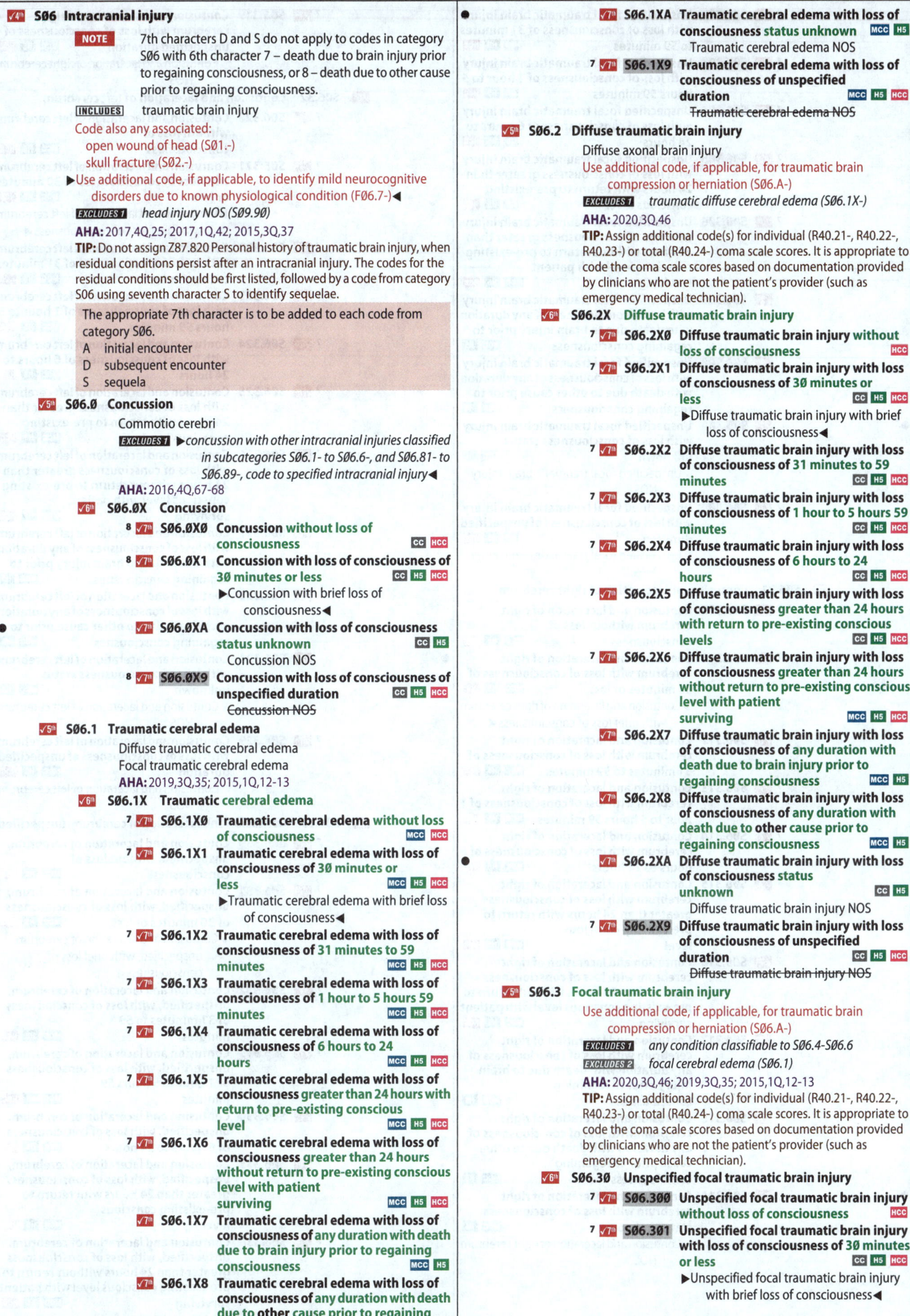

S06 Intracranial injury

NOTE 7th characters D and S do not apply to codes in category S06 with 6th character 7 – death due to brain injury prior to regaining consciousness, or 8 – death due to other cause prior to regaining consciousness.

INCLUDES traumatic brain injury

Code also any associated:
- open wound of head (S01.-)
- skull fracture (S02.-)

▶Use additional code, if applicable, to identify mild neurocognitive disorders due to known physiological condition (F06.7-)◀

EXCLUDES 1 *head injury NOS (S09.90)*

AHA: 2017,4Q,25; 2017,1Q,42; 2015,3Q,37

TIP: Do not assign Z87.820 Personal history of traumatic brain injury, when residual conditions persist after an intracranial injury. The codes for the residual conditions should be first listed, followed by a code from category S06 using seventh character S to identify sequelae.

The appropriate 7th character is to be added to each code from category S06.
- A initial encounter
- D subsequent encounter
- S sequela

S06.0 Concussion

Commotio cerebri

EXCLUDES 1 ▶*concussion with other intracranial injuries classified in subcategories S06.1- to S06.6-, and S06.81- to S06.89-, code to specified intracranial injury*◀

AHA: 2016,4Q,67-68

S06.0X Concussion

- **S06.0X0 Concussion without loss of consciousness** CC HCC
- **S06.0X1 Concussion with loss of consciousness of 30 minutes or less** CC H5 HCC
  - ▶Concussion with brief loss of consciousness◀
- ● **S06.0XA Concussion with loss of consciousness status unknown** CC H5
  - Concussion NOS
- **S06.0X9 Concussion with loss of consciousness of unspecified duration** CC H5 HCC
  - ~~Concussion NOS~~

S06.1 Traumatic cerebral edema

Diffuse traumatic cerebral edema
Focal traumatic cerebral edema

AHA: 2019,3Q,35; 2015,1Q,12-13

S06.1X Traumatic cerebral edema

- **S06.1X0 Traumatic cerebral edema without loss of consciousness** MCC HCC
- **S06.1X1 Traumatic cerebral edema with loss of consciousness of 30 minutes or less** MCC H5 HCC
  - ▶Traumatic cerebral edema with brief loss of consciousness◀
- **S06.1X2 Traumatic cerebral edema with loss of consciousness of 31 minutes to 59 minutes** MCC H5 HCC
- **S06.1X3 Traumatic cerebral edema with loss of consciousness of 1 hour to 5 hours 59 minutes** MCC H5 HCC
- **S06.1X4 Traumatic cerebral edema with loss of consciousness of 6 hours to 24 hours** MCC H5 HCC
- **S06.1X5 Traumatic cerebral edema with loss of consciousness greater than 24 hours with return to pre-existing conscious level** MCC H5 HCC
- **S06.1X6 Traumatic cerebral edema with loss of consciousness greater than 24 hours without return to pre-existing conscious level with patient surviving** MCC H5 HCC
- **S06.1X7 Traumatic cerebral edema with loss of consciousness of any duration with death due to brain injury prior to regaining consciousness** MCC H5
- **S06.1X8 Traumatic cerebral edema with loss of consciousness of any duration with death due to other cause prior to regaining consciousness** MCC H5
- ● **S06.1XA Traumatic cerebral edema with loss of consciousness status unknown** MCC H5
  - Traumatic cerebral edema NOS
- **S06.1X9 Traumatic cerebral edema with loss of consciousness of unspecified duration** MCC H5 HCC
  - ~~Traumatic cerebral edema NOS~~

S06.2 Diffuse traumatic brain injury

Diffuse axonal brain injury

Use additional code, if applicable, for traumatic brain compression or herniation (S06.A-)

EXCLUDES 1 *traumatic diffuse cerebral edema (S06.1X-)*

AHA: 2020,3Q,46

TIP: Assign additional code(s) for individual (R40.21-, R40.22-, R40.23-) or total (R40.24-) coma scale scores. It is appropriate to code the coma scale scores based on documentation provided by clinicians who are not the patient's provider (such as emergency medical technician).

S06.2X Diffuse traumatic brain injury

- **S06.2X0 Diffuse traumatic brain injury without loss of consciousness** HCC
- **S06.2X1 Diffuse traumatic brain injury with loss of consciousness of 30 minutes or less** CC H5 HCC
  - ▶Diffuse traumatic brain injury with brief loss of consciousness◀
- **S06.2X2 Diffuse traumatic brain injury with loss of consciousness of 31 minutes to 59 minutes** CC H5 HCC
- **S06.2X3 Diffuse traumatic brain injury with loss of consciousness of 1 hour to 5 hours 59 minutes** CC H5 HCC
- **S06.2X4 Diffuse traumatic brain injury with loss of consciousness of 6 hours to 24 hours** CC H5 HCC
- **S06.2X5 Diffuse traumatic brain injury with loss of consciousness greater than 24 hours with return to pre-existing conscious levels** CC H5 HCC
- **S06.2X6 Diffuse traumatic brain injury with loss of consciousness greater than 24 hours without return to pre-existing conscious level with patient surviving** MCC H5 HCC
- **S06.2X7 Diffuse traumatic brain injury with loss of consciousness of any duration with death due to brain injury prior to regaining consciousness** MCC H5
- **S06.2X8 Diffuse traumatic brain injury with loss of consciousness of any duration with death due to other cause prior to regaining consciousness** MCC H5
- ● **S06.2XA Diffuse traumatic brain injury with loss of consciousness status unknown** CC H5
  - Diffuse traumatic brain injury NOS
- **S06.2X9 Diffuse traumatic brain injury with loss of consciousness of unspecified duration** CC H5 HCC
  - ~~Diffuse traumatic brain injury NOS~~

S06.3 Focal traumatic brain injury

Use additional code, if applicable, for traumatic brain compression or herniation (S06.A-)

EXCLUDES 1 *any condition classifiable to S06.4-S06.6*

EXCLUDES 2 *focal cerebral edema (S06.1)*

AHA: 2020,3Q,46; 2019,3Q,35; 2015,1Q,12-13

TIP: Assign additional code(s) for individual (R40.21-, R40.22-, R40.23-) or total (R40.24-) coma scale scores. It is appropriate to code the coma scale scores based on documentation provided by clinicians who are not the patient's provider (such as emergency medical technician).

S06.30 Unspecified focal traumatic brain injury

- **S06.300 Unspecified focal traumatic brain injury without loss of consciousness** HCC
- **S06.301 Unspecified focal traumatic brain injury with loss of consciousness of 30 minutes or less** CC H5 HCC
  - ▶Unspecified focal traumatic brain injury with brief loss of consciousness◀

Additional Character Required — Placeholder — Questionable PDx — Manifestation — Unspecified — UPD Unacceptable PDx — H1-H14 HAC — HCC CMS-HCC Dx — HIV HIV Dx

7 ✓7th **SØ6.3Ø2 Unspecified focal traumatic brain injury with loss of consciousness of 31 minutes to 59 minutes** CC HS HCC

7 ✓7th **SØ6.3Ø3 Unspecified focal traumatic brain injury with loss of consciousness of 1 hour to 5 hours 59 minutes** CC HS HCC

7 ✓7th **SØ6.3Ø4 Unspecified focal traumatic brain injury with loss of consciousness of 6 hours to 24 hours** CC HS HCC

7 ✓7th **SØ6.3Ø5 Unspecified focal traumatic brain injury with loss of consciousness greater than 24 hours with return to pre-existing conscious level** CC HS HCC

7 ✓7th **SØ6.3Ø6 Unspecified focal traumatic brain injury with loss of consciousness greater than 24 hours without return to pre-existing conscious level with patient surviving** MCC HS HCC

✓7th **SØ6.3Ø7 Unspecified focal traumatic brain injury with loss of consciousness of any duration with death due to brain injury prior to regaining consciousness** MCC HS

✓7th **SØ6.3Ø8 Unspecified focal traumatic brain injury with loss of consciousness of any duration with death due to other cause prior to regaining consciousness** MCC HS

● ✓7th **SØ6.3ØA Unspecified focal traumatic brain injury with loss of consciousness status unknown** CC HS

Unspecified focal traumatic brain injury NOS

7 ✓7th **SØ6.3Ø9 Unspecified focal traumatic brain injury with loss of consciousness of unspecified duration** CC HS HCC

~~Unspecified focal traumatic brain injury NOS~~

✓6th **SØ6.31 Contusion and laceration of right cerebrum**

7 ✓7th **SØ6.31Ø Contusion and laceration of right cerebrum without loss of consciousness** MCC HS HCC

7 ✓7th **SØ6.311 Contusion and laceration of right cerebrum with loss of consciousness of 3Ø minutes or less** MCC HS HCC

▶Contusion and laceration of right cerebrum with brief loss of consciousness◀

7 ✓7th **SØ6.312 Contusion and laceration of right cerebrum with loss of consciousness of 31 minutes to 59 minutes** MCC HS HCC

7 ✓7th **SØ6.313 Contusion and laceration of right cerebrum with loss of consciousness of 1 hour to 5 hours 59 minutes** MCC HS HCC

7 ✓7th **SØ6.314 Contusion and laceration of right cerebrum with loss of consciousness of 6 hours to 24 hours** MCC HS HCC

7 ✓7th **SØ6.315 Contusion and laceration of right cerebrum with loss of consciousness greater than 24 hours with return to pre-existing conscious level** MCC HS HCC

7 ✓7th **SØ6.316 Contusion and laceration of right cerebrum with loss of consciousness greater than 24 hours without return to pre-existing conscious level with patient surviving** MCC HS HCC

✓7th **SØ6.317 Contusion and laceration of right cerebrum with loss of consciousness of any duration with death due to brain injury prior to regaining consciousness** MCC HS

✓7th **SØ6.318 Contusion and laceration of right cerebrum with loss of consciousness of any duration with death due to other cause prior to regaining consciousness** MCC HS

● ✓7th **SØ6.31A Contusion and laceration of right cerebrum with loss of consciousness status unknown** MCC HS

Contusion and laceration of right cerebrum NOS

7 ✓7th **SØ6.319 Contusion and laceration of right cerebrum with loss of consciousness of unspecified duration** MCC HS HCC

~~Contusion and laceration of right cerebrum NOS~~

✓6th **SØ6.32 Contusion and laceration of left cerebrum**

7 ✓7th **SØ6.32Ø Contusion and laceration of left cerebrum without loss of consciousness** MCC HS HCC

7 ✓7th **SØ6.321 Contusion and laceration of left cerebrum with loss of consciousness of 3Ø minutes or less** MCC HS HCC

▶Contusion and laceration of left cerebrum with brief loss of consciousness◀

7 ✓7th **SØ6.322 Contusion and laceration of left cerebrum with loss of consciousness of 31 minutes to 59 minutes** MCC HS HCC

7 ✓7th **SØ6.323 Contusion and laceration of left cerebrum with loss of consciousness of 1 hour to 5 hours 59 minutes** MCC HS HCC

7 ✓7th **SØ6.324 Contusion and laceration of left cerebrum with loss of consciousness of 6 hours to 24 hours** MCC HS HCC

7 ✓7th **SØ6.325 Contusion and laceration of left cerebrum with loss of consciousness greater than 24 hours with return to pre-existing conscious level** MCC HS HCC

7 ✓7th **SØ6.326 Contusion and laceration of left cerebrum with loss of consciousness greater than 24 hours without return to pre-existing conscious level with patient surviving** MCC HS HCC

✓7th **SØ6.327 Contusion and laceration of left cerebrum with loss of consciousness of any duration with death due to brain injury prior to regaining consciousness** MCC HS

✓7th **SØ6.328 Contusion and laceration of left cerebrum with loss of consciousness of any duration with death due to other cause prior to regaining consciousness** MCC HS

● ✓7th **SØ6.32A Contusion and laceration of left cerebrum with loss of consciousness status unknown** MCC HS

Contusion and laceration of left cerebrum NOS

7 ✓7th **SØ6.329 Contusion and laceration of left cerebrum with loss of consciousness of unspecified duration** MCC HS HCC

~~Contusion and laceration of left cerebrum NOS~~

✓6th **SØ6.33 Contusion and laceration of cerebrum, unspecified**

7 ✓7th **SØ6.33Ø Contusion and laceration of cerebrum, unspecified, without loss of consciousness** MCC HS HCC

7 ✓7th **SØ6.331 Contusion and laceration of cerebrum, unspecified, with loss of consciousness of 3Ø minutes or less** MCC HS HCC

▶Contusion and laceration of cerebrum, unspecified, with brief loss of consciousness◀

7 ✓7th **SØ6.332 Contusion and laceration of cerebrum, unspecified, with loss of consciousness of 31 minutes to 59 minutes** MCC HS HCC

7 ✓7th **SØ6.333 Contusion and laceration of cerebrum, unspecified, with loss of consciousness of 1 hour to 5 hours 59 minutes** MCC HS HCC

7 ✓7th **SØ6.334 Contusion and laceration of cerebrum, unspecified, with loss of consciousness of 6 hours to 24 hours** MCC HS HCC

7 ✓7th **SØ6.335 Contusion and laceration of cerebrum, unspecified, with loss of consciousness greater than 24 hours with return to pre-existing conscious level** MCC HS HCC

7 ✓7th **SØ6.336 Contusion and laceration of cerebrum, unspecified, with loss of consciousness greater than 24 hours without return to pre-existing conscious level with patient surviving** MCC HS HCC

S06.337 **Contusion and laceration of cerebrum, unspecified, with loss of consciousness of any duration with death due to brain injury prior to regaining consciousness** MCC H5

S06.338 **Contusion and laceration of cerebrum, unspecified, with loss of consciousness of any duration with death due to other cause prior to regaining consciousness** MCC H5

● S06.33A **Contusion and laceration of cerebrum, unspecified, with loss of consciousness status unknown** MCC H5
Contusion and laceration of cerebrum NOS

7 S06.339 **Contusion and laceration of cerebrum, unspecified, with loss of consciousness of unspecified duration** MCC H5 HCC
~~Contusion and laceration of cerebrum NOS~~

S06.34 **Traumatic hemorrhage of right cerebrum**
Traumatic intracerebral hemorrhage and hematoma of right cerebrum

7 S06.340 **Traumatic hemorrhage of right cerebrum without loss of consciousness** MCC H5 HCC

7 S06.341 **Traumatic hemorrhage of right cerebrum with loss of consciousness of 30 minutes or less** MCC H5 HCC
▶Traumatic hemorrhage of right cerebrum with loss of consciousness◀

7 S06.342 **Traumatic hemorrhage of right cerebrum with loss of consciousness of 31 minutes to 59 minutes** MCC H5 HCC

7 S06.343 **Traumatic hemorrhage of right cerebrum with loss of consciousness of 1 hours to 5 hours 59 minutes** MCC H5 HCC

7 S06.344 **Traumatic hemorrhage of right cerebrum with loss of consciousness of 6 hours to 24 hours** MCC H5 HCC

7 S06.345 **Traumatic hemorrhage of right cerebrum with loss of consciousness greater than 24 hours with return to pre-existing conscious level** MCC H5 HCC

7 S06.346 **Traumatic hemorrhage of right cerebrum with loss of consciousness greater than 24 hours without return to pre-existing conscious level with patient surviving** MCC H5 HCC

S06.347 **Traumatic hemorrhage of right cerebrum with loss of consciousness of any duration with death due to brain injury prior to regaining consciousness** MCC H5

S06.348 **Traumatic hemorrhage of right cerebrum with loss of consciousness of any duration with death due to other cause prior to regaining consciousness** MCC H5

● S06.34A **Traumatic hemorrhage of right cerebrum with loss of consciousness status unknown** MCC H5
Traumatic hemorrhage of right cerebrum NOS

7 S06.349 **Traumatic hemorrhage of right cerebrum with loss of consciousness of unspecified duration** MCC H5 HCC
~~Traumatic hemorrhage of right cerebrum NOS~~

S06.35 **Traumatic hemorrhage of left cerebrum**
Traumatic intracerebral hemorrhage and hematoma of left cerebrum

7 S06.350 **Traumatic hemorrhage of left cerebrum without loss of consciousness** MCC H5 HCC

7 S06.351 **Traumatic hemorrhage of left cerebrum with loss of consciousness of 30 minutes or less** MCC H5 HCC
▶Traumatic hemorrhage of left cerebrum with brief loss of consciousness◀

7 S06.352 **Traumatic hemorrhage of left cerebrum with loss of consciousness of 31 minutes to 59 minutes** MCC H5 HCC

7 S06.353 **Traumatic hemorrhage of left cerebrum with loss of consciousness of 1 hours to 5 hours 59 minutes** MCC H5 HCC

7 S06.354 **Traumatic hemorrhage of left cerebrum with loss of consciousness of 6 hours to 24 hours** MCC H5 HCC

7 S06.355 **Traumatic hemorrhage of left cerebrum with loss of consciousness greater than 24 hours with return to pre-existing conscious level** MCC H5 HCC

7 S06.356 **Traumatic hemorrhage of left cerebrum with loss of consciousness greater than 24 hours without return to pre-existing conscious level with patient surviving** MCC H5 HCC

S06.357 **Traumatic hemorrhage of left cerebrum with loss of consciousness of any duration with death due to brain injury prior to regaining consciousness** MCC H5

S06.358 **Traumatic hemorrhage of left cerebrum with loss of consciousness of any duration with death due to other cause prior to regaining consciousness** MCC H5

● S06.35A **Traumatic hemorrhage of left cerebrum with loss of consciousness status unknown** MCC H5
Traumatic hemorrhage of left cerebrum NOS

7 S06.359 **Traumatic hemorrhage of left cerebrum with loss of consciousness of unspecified duration** MCC H5 HCC
~~Traumatic hemorrhage of left cerebrum NOS~~

S06.36 **Traumatic hemorrhage of cerebrum, unspecified**
Traumatic intracerebral hemorrhage and hematoma, unspecified

7 S06.360 **Traumatic hemorrhage of cerebrum, unspecified, without loss of consciousness** MCC H5 HCC

7 S06.361 **Traumatic hemorrhage of cerebrum, unspecified, with loss of consciousness of 30 minutes or less** MCC H5 HCC
▶Traumatic hemorrhage of cerebrum, unspecified, with brief loss of consciousness◀

7 S06.362 **Traumatic hemorrhage of cerebrum, unspecified, with loss of consciousness of 31 minutes to 59 minutes** MCC H5 HCC

7 S06.363 **Traumatic hemorrhage of cerebrum, unspecified, with loss of consciousness of 1 hours to 5 hours 59 minutes** MCC H5 HCC

7 S06.364 **Traumatic hemorrhage of cerebrum, unspecified, with loss of consciousness of 6 hours to 24 hours** MCC H5 HCC

7 S06.365 **Traumatic hemorrhage of cerebrum, unspecified, with loss of consciousness greater than 24 hours with return to pre-existing conscious level** MCC H5 HCC

7 S06.366 **Traumatic hemorrhage of cerebrum, unspecified, with loss of consciousness greater than 24 hours without return to pre-existing conscious level with patient surviving** MCC H5 HCC

S06.367 **Traumatic hemorrhage of cerebrum, unspecified, with loss of consciousness of any duration with death due to brain injury prior to regaining consciousness** MCC H5

S06.368 **Traumatic hemorrhage of cerebrum, unspecified, with loss of consciousness of any duration with death due to other cause prior to regaining consciousness** MCC H5

● S06.36A **Traumatic hemorrhage of cerebrum, unspecified, with loss of consciousness status unknown** MCC H5
Traumatic hemorrhage of cerebrum NOS

7 S06.369 **Traumatic hemorrhage of cerebrum, unspecified, with loss of consciousness of unspecified duration** MCC H5 HCC
~~Traumatic hemorrhage of cerebrum NOS~~

S06.37 Contusion, laceration, and hemorrhage of cerebellum

S06.370 Contusion, laceration, and hemorrhage of cerebellum without loss of consciousness MCC HS HCC

S06.371 Contusion, laceration, and hemorrhage of cerebellum with loss of consciousness of 30 minutes or less CC HS HCC

▶Contusion, laceration, and hemorrhage of cerebellum with brief loss of consciousness◀

S06.372 Contusion, laceration, and hemorrhage of cerebellum with loss of consciousness of 31 minutes to 59 minutes CC HS HCC

S06.373 Contusion, laceration, and hemorrhage of cerebellum with loss of consciousness of 1 hour to 5 hours 59 minutes CC HS HCC

S06.374 Contusion, laceration, and hemorrhage of cerebellum with loss of consciousness of 6 hours to 24 hours CC HS HCC

S06.375 Contusion, laceration, and hemorrhage of cerebellum with loss of consciousness greater than 24 hours with return to pre-existing conscious level CC HS HCC

S06.376 Contusion, laceration, and hemorrhage of cerebellum with loss of consciousness greater than 24 hours without return to pre-existing conscious level with patient surviving MCC HS HCC

S06.377 Contusion, laceration, and hemorrhage of cerebellum with loss of consciousness of any duration with death due to brain injury prior to regaining consciousness MCC HS

S06.378 Contusion, laceration, and hemorrhage of cerebellum with loss of consciousness of any duration with death due to other cause prior to regaining consciousness MCC HS

● **S06.37A Contusion, laceration, and hemorrhage of cerebellum with loss of consciousness status unknown** MCC HS

Contusion, laceration, and hemorrhage of cerebellum NOS

S06.379 Contusion, laceration, and hemorrhage of cerebellum with loss of consciousness of unspecified duration CC HS HCC

~~Contusion, laceration, and hemorrhage of cerebellum NOS~~

S06.38 Contusion, laceration, and hemorrhage of brainstem

S06.380 Contusion, laceration, and hemorrhage of brainstem without loss of consciousness MCC HS HCC

S06.381 Contusion, laceration, and hemorrhage of brainstem with loss of consciousness of 30 minutes or less CC HS HCC

▶Contusion, laceration, and hemorrhage of brainstem with brief loss of consciousness◀

S06.382 Contusion, laceration, and hemorrhage of brainstem with loss of consciousness of 31 minutes to 59 minutes CC HS HCC

S06.383 Contusion, laceration, and hemorrhage of brainstem with loss of consciousness of 1 hour to 5 hours 59 minutes CC HS HCC

S06.384 Contusion, laceration, and hemorrhage of brainstem with loss of consciousness of 6 hours to 24 hours CC HS HCC

S06.385 Contusion, laceration, and hemorrhage of brainstem with loss of consciousness greater than 24 hours with return to pre-existing conscious level CC HS HCC

S06.386 Contusion, laceration, and hemorrhage of brainstem with loss of consciousness greater than 24 hours without return to pre-existing conscious level with patient surviving MCC HS HCC

S06.387 Contusion, laceration, and hemorrhage of brainstem with loss of consciousness of any duration with death due to brain injury prior to regaining consciousness MCC HS

S06.388 Contusion, laceration, and hemorrhage of brainstem with loss of consciousness of any duration with death due to other cause prior to regaining consciousness MCC HS

● **S06.38A Contusion, laceration, and hemorrhage of brainstem with loss of consciousness status unknown** MCC HS

Contusion, laceration, and hemorrhage of brainstem NOS

S06.389 Contusion, laceration, and hemorrhage of brainstem with loss of consciousness of unspecified duration CC HS HCC

~~Contusion, laceration, and hemorrhage of brainstem NOS~~

S06.4 Epidural hemorrhage

Extradural hemorrhage NOS

Extradural hemorrhage (traumatic)

DEF: Epidural space: Space between the endosteum of the cranium (skull) and the dura mater, the outermost layer of a three-layer membrane that covers the brain.

S06.4X Epidural hemorrhage

S06.4X0 Epidural hemorrhage without loss of consciousness MCC HS HCC

S06.4X1 Epidural hemorrhage with loss of consciousness of 30 minutes or less MCC HS HCC

▶Epidural hemorrhage with brief loss of consciousness◀

S06.4X2 Epidural hemorrhage with loss of consciousness of 31 minutes to 59 minutes MCC HS HCC

S06.4X3 Epidural hemorrhage with loss of consciousness of 1 hour to 5 hours 59 minutes MCC HS HCC

S06.4X4 Epidural hemorrhage with loss of consciousness of 6 hours to 24 hours MCC HS HCC

S06.4X5 Epidural hemorrhage with loss of consciousness greater than 24 hours with return to pre-existing conscious level MCC HS HCC

S06.4X6 Epidural hemorrhage with loss of consciousness greater than 24 hours without return to pre-existing conscious level with patient surviving MCC HS HCC

S06.4X7 Epidural hemorrhage with loss of consciousness of any duration with death due to brain injury prior to regaining consciousness MCC HS

S06.4X8 Epidural hemorrhage with loss of consciousness of any duration with death due to other causes prior to regaining consciousness MCC HS

● **S06.4XA Epidural hemorrhage with loss of consciousness status unknown** MCC HS

Epidural hemorrhage NOS

S06.4X9 Epidural hemorrhage with loss of consciousness of unspecified duration MCC HS HCC

~~Epidural hemorrhage NOS~~

S06.5 Traumatic subdural hemorrhage

Use additional code, if applicable, for traumatic brain compression or herniation (S06.A-)

AHA: 2021,2Q,5; 2021,1Q,4

DEF: Subdural: Potential space between the dura mater and arachnoid membrane around the brain.

S06.5X Traumatic subdural hemorrhage

S06.5X0 Traumatic subdural hemorrhage without loss of consciousness MCC HS HCC

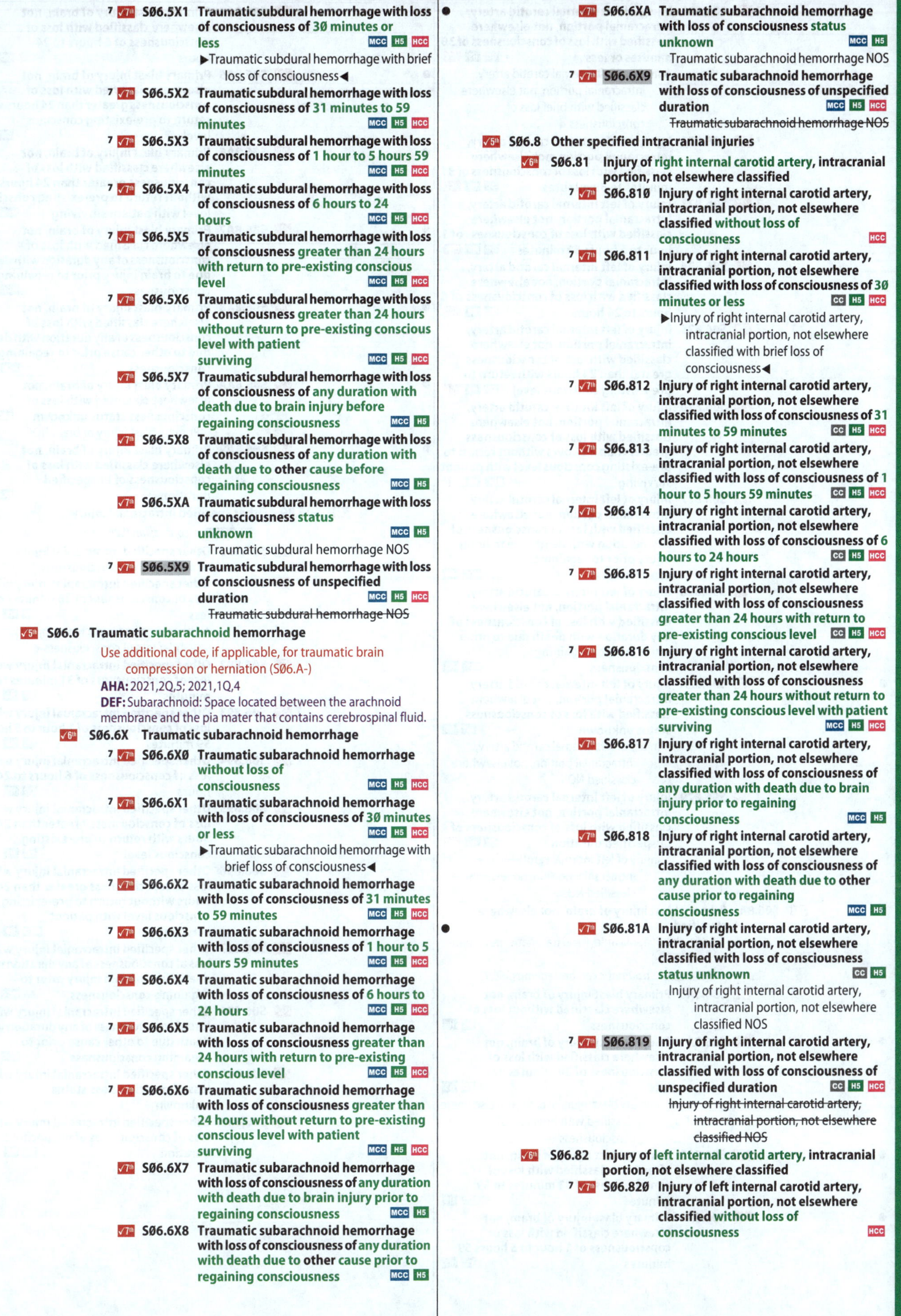

7 S06.5X1 Traumatic subdural hemorrhage with loss of consciousness of 30 minutes or less MCC H5 HCC
▶Traumatic subdural hemorrhage with brief loss of consciousness◀

7 S06.5X2 Traumatic subdural hemorrhage with loss of consciousness of 31 minutes to 59 minutes MCC H5 HCC

7 S06.5X3 Traumatic subdural hemorrhage with loss of consciousness of 1 hour to 5 hours 59 minutes MCC H5 HCC

7 S06.5X4 Traumatic subdural hemorrhage with loss of consciousness of 6 hours to 24 hours MCC H5 HCC

7 S06.5X5 Traumatic subdural hemorrhage with loss of consciousness greater than 24 hours with return to pre-existing conscious level MCC H5 HCC

7 S06.5X6 Traumatic subdural hemorrhage with loss of consciousness greater than 24 hours without return to pre-existing conscious level with patient surviving MCC H5 HCC

7 S06.5X7 Traumatic subdural hemorrhage with loss of consciousness of any duration with death due to brain injury before regaining consciousness MCC H5

7 S06.5X8 Traumatic subdural hemorrhage with loss of consciousness of any duration with death due to other cause before regaining consciousness MCC H5

● 7 S06.5XA Traumatic subdural hemorrhage with loss of consciousness status unknown MCC H5
Traumatic subdural hemorrhage NOS

7 S06.5X9 Traumatic subdural hemorrhage with loss of consciousness of unspecified duration MCC H5 HCC
~~Traumatic subdural hemorrhage NOS~~

5 S06.6 Traumatic subarachnoid hemorrhage
Use additional code, if applicable, for traumatic brain compression or herniation (S06.A-)
AHA: 2021,2Q,5; 2021,1Q,4
DEF: Subarachnoid: Space located between the arachnoid membrane and the pia mater that contains cerebrospinal fluid.

6 S06.6X Traumatic subarachnoid hemorrhage

7 S06.6X0 Traumatic subarachnoid hemorrhage without loss of consciousness MCC H5 HCC

7 S06.6X1 Traumatic subarachnoid hemorrhage with loss of consciousness of 30 minutes or less MCC H5 HCC
▶Traumatic subarachnoid hemorrhage with brief loss of consciousness◀

7 S06.6X2 Traumatic subarachnoid hemorrhage with loss of consciousness of 31 minutes to 59 minutes MCC H5 HCC

7 S06.6X3 Traumatic subarachnoid hemorrhage with loss of consciousness of 1 hour to 5 hours 59 minutes MCC H5 HCC

7 S06.6X4 Traumatic subarachnoid hemorrhage with loss of consciousness of 6 hours to 24 hours MCC H5 HCC

7 S06.6X5 Traumatic subarachnoid hemorrhage with loss of consciousness greater than 24 hours with return to pre-existing conscious level MCC H5 HCC

7 S06.6X6 Traumatic subarachnoid hemorrhage with loss of consciousness greater than 24 hours without return to pre-existing conscious level with patient surviving MCC H5 HCC

7 S06.6X7 Traumatic subarachnoid hemorrhage with loss of consciousness of any duration with death due to brain injury prior to regaining consciousness MCC H5

7 S06.6X8 Traumatic subarachnoid hemorrhage with loss of consciousness of any duration with death due to other cause prior to regaining consciousness MCC H5

● 7 S06.6XA Traumatic subarachnoid hemorrhage with loss of consciousness status unknown MCC H5
Traumatic subarachnoid hemorrhage NOS

7 S06.6X9 Traumatic subarachnoid hemorrhage with loss of consciousness of unspecified duration MCC H5 HCC
~~Traumatic subarachnoid hemorrhage NOS~~

5 S06.8 Other specified intracranial injuries

6 S06.81 Injury of right internal carotid artery, intracranial portion, not elsewhere classified

7 S06.810 Injury of right internal carotid artery, intracranial portion, not elsewhere classified without loss of consciousness HCC

7 S06.811 Injury of right internal carotid artery, intracranial portion, not elsewhere classified with loss of consciousness of 30 minutes or less CC H5 HCC
▶Injury of right internal carotid artery, intracranial portion, not elsewhere classified with brief loss of consciousness◀

7 S06.812 Injury of right internal carotid artery, intracranial portion, not elsewhere classified with loss of consciousness of 31 minutes to 59 minutes CC H5 HCC

7 S06.813 Injury of right internal carotid artery, intracranial portion, not elsewhere classified with loss of consciousness of 1 hour to 5 hours 59 minutes CC H5 HCC

7 S06.814 Injury of right internal carotid artery, intracranial portion, not elsewhere classified with loss of consciousness of 6 hours to 24 hours CC H5 HCC

7 S06.815 Injury of right internal carotid artery, intracranial portion, not elsewhere classified with loss of consciousness greater than 24 hours with return to pre-existing conscious level CC H5 HCC

7 S06.816 Injury of right internal carotid artery, intracranial portion, not elsewhere classified with loss of consciousness greater than 24 hours without return to pre-existing conscious level with patient surviving MCC H5 HCC

7 S06.817 Injury of right internal carotid artery, intracranial portion, not elsewhere classified with loss of consciousness of any duration with death due to brain injury prior to regaining consciousness MCC H5

7 S06.818 Injury of right internal carotid artery, intracranial portion, not elsewhere classified with loss of consciousness of any duration with death due to other cause prior to regaining consciousness MCC H5

● 7 S06.81A Injury of right internal carotid artery, intracranial portion, not elsewhere classified with loss of consciousness status unknown CC H5
Injury of right internal carotid artery, intracranial portion, not elsewhere classified NOS

7 S06.819 Injury of right internal carotid artery, intracranial portion, not elsewhere classified with loss of consciousness of unspecified duration CC H5 HCC
~~Injury of right internal carotid artery, intracranial portion, not elsewhere classified NOS~~

6 S06.82 Injury of left internal carotid artery, intracranial portion, not elsewhere classified

7 S06.820 Injury of left internal carotid artery, intracranial portion, not elsewhere classified without loss of consciousness HCC

7 ✓7th **SØ6.821 Injury of left internal carotid artery, intracranial portion, not elsewhere classified with loss of consciousness of 30 minutes or less** CC H5 HCC

▶Injury of left internal carotid artery, intracranial portion, not elsewhere classified with brief loss of consciousness◀

7 ✓7th **SØ6.822 Injury of left internal carotid artery, intracranial portion, not elsewhere classified with loss of consciousness of 31 minutes to 59 minutes** CC H5 HCC

7 ✓7th **SØ6.823 Injury of left internal carotid artery, intracranial portion, not elsewhere classified with loss of consciousness of 1 hour to 5 hours 59 minutes** CC H5 HCC

7 ✓7th **SØ6.824 Injury of left internal carotid artery, intracranial portion, not elsewhere classified with loss of consciousness of 6 hours to 24 hours** CC H5 HCC

7 ✓7th **SØ6.825 Injury of left internal carotid artery, intracranial portion, not elsewhere classified with loss of consciousness greater than 24 hours with return to pre-existing conscious level** CC H5 HCC

7 ✓7th **SØ6.826 Injury of left internal carotid artery, intracranial portion, not elsewhere classified with loss of consciousness greater than 24 hours without return to pre-existing conscious level with patient surviving** MCC H5 HCC

✓7th **SØ6.827 Injury of left internal carotid artery, intracranial portion, not elsewhere classified with loss of consciousness of any duration with death due to brain injury prior to regaining consciousness** MCC H5

✓7th **SØ6.828 Injury of left internal carotid artery, intracranial portion, not elsewhere classified with loss of consciousness of any duration with death due to other cause prior to regaining consciousness** MCC H5

● ✓7th **SØ6.82A Injury of left internal carotid artery, intracranial portion, not elsewhere classified with loss of consciousness status unknown** CC H5

Injury of left internal carotid artery, intracranial portion, not elsewhere classified NOS

7 ✓7th **SØ6.829 Injury of left internal carotid artery, intracranial portion, not elsewhere classified with loss of consciousness of unspecified duration** CC H5 HCC

~~Injury of left internal carotid artery, intracranial portion, not elsewhere classified NOS~~

● ✓6th **SØ6.8A Primary blast injury of brain, not elsewhere classified**

Code also, if applicable, focal traumatic brain injury (SØ6.3-)

EXCLUDES 2 *traumatic cerebral edema (SØ6.1)*

● ✓7th **SØ6.8AØ Primary blast injury of brain, not elsewhere classified without loss of consciousness** CC H5

● ✓7th **SØ6.8A1 Primary blast injury of brain, not elsewhere classified with loss of consciousness of 30 minutes or less** CC H5

Primary blast injury of brain, not elsewhere classified with brief loss of consciousness

● ✓7th **SØ6.8A2 Primary blast injury of brain, not elsewhere classified with loss of consciousness of 31 minutes to 59 minutes** CC H5

● ✓7th **SØ6.8A3 Primary blast injury of brain, not elsewhere classified with loss of consciousness of 1 hour to 5 hours 59 minutes** CC H5

● ✓7th **SØ6.8A4 Primary blast injury of brain, not elsewhere classified with loss of consciousness of 6 hours to 24 hours** CC H5

● ✓7th **SØ6.8A5 Primary blast injury of brain, not elsewhere classified with loss of consciousness greater than 24 hours with return to pre-existing conscious level** CC H5

● ✓7th **SØ6.8A6 Primary blast injury of brain, not elsewhere classified with loss of consciousness greater than 24 hours without return to pre-existing conscious level with patient surviving** MCC H5

● ✓7th **SØ6.8A7 Primary blast injury of brain, not elsewhere classified with loss of consciousness of any duration with death due to brain injury prior to regaining consciousness** MCC H5

● ✓7th **SØ6.8A8 Primary blast injury of brain, not elsewhere classified with loss of consciousness of any duration with death due to other cause prior to regaining consciousness** MCC H5

● ✓7th **SØ6.8AA Primary blast injury of brain, not elsewhere classified with loss of consciousness status unknown** CC H5

Primary blast injury of brain NOS

● ✓7th **SØ6.8A9 Primary blast injury of brain, not elsewhere classified with loss of consciousness of unspecified duration** CC H5

✓6th **SØ6.89 Other specified intracranial injury**

EXCLUDES 1 *concussion (SØ6.ØX-)*

7 ✓7th **SØ6.89Ø Other specified intracranial injury without loss of consciousness** HCC

7 ✓7th **SØ6.891 Other specified intracranial injury with loss of consciousness of 30 minutes or less** CC H5 HCC

▶Other specified intracranial injury with brief loss of consciousness◀

7 ✓7th **SØ6.892 Other specified intracranial injury with loss of consciousness of 31 minutes to 59 minutes** CC H5 HCC

7 ✓7th **SØ6.893 Other specified intracranial injury with loss of consciousness of 1 hour to 5 hours 59 minutes** CC H5 HCC

7 ✓7th **SØ6.894 Other specified intracranial injury with loss of consciousness of 6 hours to 24 hours** CC H5 HCC

7 ✓7th **SØ6.895 Other specified intracranial injury with loss of consciousness greater than 24 hours with return to pre-existing conscious level** CC H5 HCC

7 ✓7th **SØ6.896 Other specified intracranial injury with loss of consciousness greater than 24 hours without return to pre-existing conscious level with patient surviving** MCC H5 HCC

✓7th **SØ6.897 Other specified intracranial injury with loss of consciousness of any duration with death due to brain injury prior to regaining consciousness** MCC H5

✓7th **SØ6.898 Other specified intracranial injury with loss of consciousness of any duration with death due to other cause prior to regaining consciousness** MCC H5

● ✓7th **SØ6.89A Other specified intracranial injury with loss of consciousness status unknown** CC H5

7 ✓7th **SØ6.899 Other specified intracranial injury with loss of consciousness of unspecified duration** CC H5 HCC

S06.9 Unspecified intracranial injury

Brain injury NOS
Head injury NOS with loss of consciousness
Traumatic brain injury NOS

EXCLUDES 1 *conditions classifiable to S06.0- to S06.8- code to specified intracranial injury*
head injury NOS (S09.90)

AHA: 2020,3Q,46; 2020,2Q,31

TIP: Assign additional code(s) for individual (R40.21-, R40.22-, R40.23-) or total (R40.24-) coma scale scores. It is appropriate to code the coma scale scores based on documentation provided by clinicians who are not the patient's provider (such as emergency medical technician).

S06.9X Unspecified intracranial injury

S06.9X0 Unspecified intracranial injury without loss of consciousness HCC

S06.9X1 Unspecified intracranial injury with loss of consciousness of 30 minutes or less CC H5 HCC

▶Unspecified intracranial injury with brief loss of consciousness◀

S06.9X2 Unspecified intracranial injury with loss of consciousness of 31 minutes to 59 minutes CC H5 HCC

S06.9X3 Unspecified intracranial injury with loss of consciousness of 1 hour to 5 hours 59 minutes CC H5 HCC

S06.9X4 Unspecified intracranial injury with loss of consciousness of 6 hours to 24 hours CC H5 HCC

S06.9X5 Unspecified intracranial injury with loss of consciousness greater than 24 hours with return to pre-existing conscious level CC H5 HCC

S06.9X6 Unspecified intracranial injury with loss of consciousness greater than 24 hours without return to pre-existing conscious level with patient surviving MCC H5 HCC

S06.9X7 Unspecified intracranial injury with loss of consciousness of any duration with death due to brain injury prior to regaining consciousness MCC H5

S06.9X8 Unspecified intracranial injury with loss of consciousness of any duration with death due to other cause prior to regaining consciousness MCC H5

● **S06.9XA Unspecified intracranial injury with loss of consciousness status unknown** CC H5

S06.9X9 Unspecified intracranial injury with loss of consciousness of unspecified duration CC H5 HCC

S06.A Traumatic brain compression and herniation

Traumatic cerebral compression

Code first the underlying traumatic brain injury, such as:
diffuse traumatic brain injury (S06.2-)
focal traumatic brain injury (S06.3-)
traumatic subdural hemorrhage (S06.5-)
traumatic subarachnoid hemorrhage (S06.6-)

AHA: 2021,4Q,29

S06.A0 Traumatic brain compression without herniation MCC UPD HCC

Traumatic brain compression NOS
Traumatic cerebral compression NOS

S06.A1 Traumatic brain compression with herniation MCC UPD HCC

Traumatic brain herniation
Traumatic brainstem compression with herniation
Traumatic cerebellar compression with herniation
Traumatic cerebral compression with herniation

S07 Crushing injury of head

Use additional code for all associated injuries, such as:
intracranial injuries (S06.-)
skull fractures (S02.-)

The appropriate 7th character is to be added to each code from category S07.
A initial encounter
D subsequent encounter
S sequela

S07.0 Crushing injury of face CC H5

S07.1 Crushing injury of skull CC H5

S07.8 Crushing injury of other parts of head CC H5

S07.9 Crushing injury of head, part unspecified CC H5

S08 Avulsion and traumatic amputation of part of head

An amputation not identified as partial or complete should be coded to complete

The appropriate 7th character is to be added to each code from category S08.
A initial encounter
D subsequent encounter
S sequela

S08.0 Avulsion of scalp

S08.1 Traumatic amputation of ear

S08.11 Complete traumatic amputation of ear

S08.111 Complete traumatic amputation of right ear

S08.112 Complete traumatic amputation of left ear

S08.119 Complete traumatic amputation of unspecified ear

S08.12 Partial traumatic amputation of ear

S08.121 Partial traumatic amputation of right ear

S08.122 Partial traumatic amputation of left ear

S08.129 Partial traumatic amputation of unspecified ear

S08.8 Traumatic amputation of other parts of head

S08.81 Traumatic amputation of nose

S08.811 Complete traumatic amputation of nose

S08.812 Partial traumatic amputation of nose

S08.89 Traumatic amputation of other parts of head

S09 Other and unspecified injuries of head

The appropriate 7th character is to be added to each code from category S09.
A initial encounter
D subsequent encounter
S sequela

S09.0 Injury of blood vessels of head, not elsewhere classified CC

EXCLUDES 1 *injury of cerebral blood vessels (S06.-)*
injury of precerebral blood vessels (S15.-)

S09.1 Injury of muscle and tendon of head

Code also any associated open wound (S01.-)

EXCLUDES 2 *sprain to joints and ligament of head (S03.9)*

S09.10 Unspecified injury of muscle and tendon of head

Injury of muscle and tendon of head NOS

S09.11 Strain of muscle and tendon of head

S09.12 Laceration of muscle and tendon of head

S09.19 Other specified injury of muscle and tendon of head

S09.2 Traumatic rupture of ear drum

EXCLUDES 1 *traumatic rupture of ear drum due to blast injury (S09.31-)*

S09.20 Traumatic rupture of unspecified ear drum CC UNS

S09.21 Traumatic rupture of right ear drum CC

S09.22 Traumatic rupture of left ear drum CC

5th **SØ9.3 Other specified and unspecified injury of middle and inner ear**
EXCLUDES 1 *injury to ear NOS (SØ9.91-)*
EXCLUDES 2 *injury to external ear (SØØ.4-, SØ1.3-, SØ8.1-)*

6th **SØ9.30 Unspecified injury of middle and inner ear**
7th **SØ9.3Ø1 Unspecified injury of right middle and inner ear** CC
7th **SØ9.3Ø2 Unspecified injury of left middle and inner ear** CC
7th **SØ9.3Ø9 Unspecified injury of unspecified middle and inner ear** CC UNS

6th **SØ9.31 Primary blast injury of ear**
Blast injury of ear NOS
7th **SØ9.311 Primary blast injury of right ear** CC
7th **SØ9.312 Primary blast injury of left ear** CC
7th **SØ9.313 Primary blast injury of ear, bilateral** CC
7th **SØ9.319 Primary blast injury of unspecified ear** CC UNS

6th **SØ9.39 Other specified injury of middle and inner ear**
Secondary blast injury to ear
7th **SØ9.391 Other specified injury of right middle and inner ear** CC
7th **SØ9.392 Other specified injury of left middle and inner ear** CC
7th **SØ9.399 Other specified injury of unspecified middle and inner ear** CC UNS

x7th **SØ9.8 Other specified injuries of head**

5th **SØ9.9 Unspecified injury of face and head**
x7th **SØ9.9Ø Unspecified injury of head**
Head injury NOS
EXCLUDES 1 *brain injury NOS (SØ6.9-)*
head injury NOS with loss of consciousness (SØ6.9-)
intracranial injury NOS (SØ6.9-)
x7th **SØ9.91 Unspecified injury of ear**
Injury of ear NOS
x7th **SØ9.92 Unspecified injury of nose**
Injury of nose NOS
x7th **SØ9.93 Unspecified injury of face**
Injury of face NOS
AHA: 2019,2Q,23

Injuries to the neck (S1Ø-S19)

INCLUDES injuries of nape
injuries of supraclavicular region
injuries of throat

EXCLUDES 2 *burns and corrosions (T2Ø-T32)*
effects of foreign body in esophagus (T18.1)
effects of foreign body in larynx (T17.3)
effects of foreign body in pharynx (T17.2)
effects of foreign body in trachea (T17.4)
frostbite (T33-T34)
insect bite or sting, venomous (T63.4)

4th **S1Ø Superficial injury of neck**

The appropriate 7th character is to be added to each code from category S1Ø.
A initial encounter
D subsequent encounter
S sequela

x7th **S1Ø.Ø Contusion of throat**
Contusion of cervical esophagus
Contusion of larynx
Contusion of pharynx
Contusion of trachea

5th **S1Ø.1 Other and unspecified superficial injuries of throat**
x7th **S1Ø.1Ø Unspecified superficial injuries of throat**
x7th **S1Ø.11 Abrasion of throat**
x7th **S1Ø.12 Blister (nonthermal) of throat**
x7th **S1Ø.14 External constriction of part of throat**
x7th **S1Ø.15 Superficial foreign body of throat**
Splinter in the throat
x7th **S1Ø.16 Insect bite (nonvenomous) of throat**
x7th **S1Ø.17 Other superficial bite of throat**
EXCLUDES 1 *open bite of throat (S11.85)*

5th **S1Ø.8 Superficial injury of other specified parts of neck**
x7th **S1Ø.8Ø Unspecified superficial injury of other specified part of neck**
x7th **S1Ø.81 Abrasion of other specified part of neck**
x7th **S1Ø.82 Blister (nonthermal) of other specified part of neck**
x7th **S1Ø.83 Contusion of other specified part of neck**
x7th **S1Ø.84 External constriction of other specified part of neck**
x7th **S1Ø.85 Superficial foreign body of other specified part of neck**
Splinter in other specified part of neck
x7th **S1Ø.86 Insect bite of other specified part of neck**
x7th **S1Ø.87 Other superficial bite of other specified part of neck**
EXCLUDES 1 *open bite of other specified parts of neck (S11.85)*

5th **S1Ø.9 Superficial injury of unspecified part of neck**
x7th **S1Ø.9Ø Unspecified superficial injury of unspecified part of neck**
x7th **S1Ø.91 Abrasion of unspecified part of neck**
x7th **S1Ø.92 Blister (nonthermal) of unspecified part of neck**
x7th **S1Ø.93 Contusion of unspecified part of neck**
x7th **S1Ø.94 External constriction of unspecified part of neck**
x7th **S1Ø.95 Superficial foreign body of unspecified part of neck**
x7th **S1Ø.96 Insect bite of unspecified part of neck**
x7th **S1Ø.97 Other superficial bite of unspecified part of neck**

4th **S11 Open wound of neck**
Code also any associated:
spinal cord injury (S14.Ø, S14.1-)
wound infection
EXCLUDES 2 *open fracture of vertebra (S12.- with 7th character B)*

The appropriate 7th character is to be added to each code from category S11.
A initial encounter
D subsequent encounter
S sequela

5th **S11.Ø Open wound of larynx and trachea**
6th **S11.Ø1 Open wound of larynx**
EXCLUDES 2 *open wound of vocal cord (S11.Ø3)*
7th **S11.Ø11 Laceration without foreign body of larynx** MCC
7th **S11.Ø12 Laceration with foreign body of larynx** MCC
7th **S11.Ø13 Puncture wound without foreign body of larynx** MCC
7th **S11.Ø14 Puncture wound with foreign body of larynx** MCC
7th **S11.Ø15 Open bite of larynx** MCC
Bite of larynx NOS
7th **S11.Ø19 Unspecified open wound of larynx** MCC

6th **S11.Ø2 Open wound of trachea**
Open wound of cervical trachea
Open wound of trachea NOS
EXCLUDES 2 *open wound of thoracic trachea (S27.5-)*
7th **S11.Ø21 Laceration without foreign body of trachea** MCC
7th **S11.Ø22 Laceration with foreign body of trachea** MCC
7th **S11.Ø23 Puncture wound without foreign body of trachea** MCC
7th **S11.Ø24 Puncture wound with foreign body of trachea** MCC
7th **S11.Ø25 Open bite of trachea** MCC
Bite of trachea NOS
7th **S11.Ø29 Unspecified open wound of trachea** MCC

6th **S11.Ø3 Open wound of vocal cord**
7th **S11.Ø31 Laceration without foreign body of vocal cord** MCC
7th **S11.Ø32 Laceration with foreign body of vocal cord** MCC
7th **S11.Ø33 Puncture wound without foreign body of vocal cord** MCC

S11.034 Puncture wound with foreign body of vocal cord MCC

S11.035 Open bite of vocal cord MCC
Bite of vocal cord NOS

S11.039 Unspecified open wound of vocal cord MCC

S11.1 Open wound of thyroid gland

S11.10 Unspecified open wound of thyroid gland CC

S11.11 Laceration without foreign body of thyroid gland CC

S11.12 Laceration with foreign body of thyroid gland CC

S11.13 Puncture wound without foreign body of thyroid gland CC

S11.14 Puncture wound with foreign body of thyroid gland CC

S11.15 Open bite of thyroid gland CC
Bite of thyroid gland NOS

S11.2 Open wound of pharynx and cervical esophagus
EXCLUDES 1 *open wound of esophagus NOS (S27.8-)*

S11.20 Unspecified open wound of pharynx and cervical esophagus CC

S11.21 Laceration without foreign body of pharynx and cervical esophagus CC

S11.22 Laceration with foreign body of pharynx and cervical esophagus CC

S11.23 Puncture wound without foreign body of pharynx and cervical esophagus CC

S11.24 Puncture wound with foreign body of pharynx and cervical esophagus CC

S11.25 Open bite of pharynx and cervical esophagus CC
Bite of pharynx and cervical esophagus NOS

S11.8 Open wound of other specified parts of neck

S11.80 Unspecified open wound of other specified part of neck

S11.81 Laceration without foreign body of other specified part of neck

S11.82 Laceration with foreign body of other specified part of neck

S11.83 Puncture wound without foreign body of other specified part of neck

S11.84 Puncture wound with foreign body of other specified part of neck

S11.85 Open bite of other specified part of neck
Bite of other specified part of neck NOS
EXCLUDES 1 *superficial bite of other specified part of neck (S10.87)*

S11.89 Other open wound of other specified part of neck

S11.9 Open wound of unspecified part of neck

S11.90 Unspecified open wound of unspecified part of neck

S11.91 Laceration without foreign body of unspecified part of neck

S11.92 Laceration with foreign body of unspecified part of neck

S11.93 Puncture wound without foreign body of unspecified part of neck

S11.94 Puncture wound with foreign body of unspecified part of neck

S11.95 Open bite of unspecified part of neck
Bite of neck NOS
EXCLUDES 1 *superficial bite of neck (S10.97)*

S12 Fracture of cervical vertebra and other parts of neck

NOTE A fracture not indicated as displaced or nondisplaced should be coded to displaced.
A fracture not indicated as open or closed should be coded to closed.

INCLUDES fracture of cervical neural arch
fracture of cervical spine
fracture of cervical spinous process
fracture of cervical transverse process
fracture of cervical vertebral arch
fracture of neck

Code first any associated cervical spinal cord injury (S14.0, S14.1-)

AHA: 2021,1Q,6; 2018,2Q,12; 2015,3Q,37-39

The appropriate 7th character is to be added to all codes from subcategories S12.0-S12.6.
A initial encounter for closed fracture
B initial encounter for open fracture
D subsequent encounter for fracture with routine healing
G subsequent encounter for fracture with delayed healing
K subsequent encounter for fracture with nonunion
S sequela

S12.0 Fracture of first cervical vertebra
Atlas

S12.00 Unspecified fracture of first cervical vertebra

2,3,6 S12.000 Unspecified displaced fracture of first cervical vertebra MCC CC H5 HCC

2,3,6 S12.001 Unspecified nondisplaced fracture of first cervical vertebra MCC CC H5 HCC

2,3,6 S12.01 Stable burst fracture of first cervical vertebra MCC CC H5 HCC

2,3,6 S12.02 Unstable burst fracture of first cervical vertebra MCC CC H5 HCC

S12.03 Posterior arch fracture of first cervical vertebra

2,3,6 S12.030 Displaced posterior arch fracture of first cervical vertebra MCC CC H5 HCC

2,3,6 S12.031 Nondisplaced posterior arch fracture of first cervical vertebra MCC CC H5 HCC

S12.04 Lateral mass fracture of first cervical vertebra

2,3,6 S12.040 Displaced lateral mass fracture of first cervical vertebra MCC CC H5 HCC

2,3,6 S12.041 Nondisplaced lateral mass fracture of first cervical vertebra MCC CC H5 HCC

S12.09 Other fracture of first cervical vertebra

2,3,6 S12.090 Other displaced fracture of first cervical vertebra MCC CC H5 HCC

2,3,6 S12.091 Other nondisplaced fracture of first cervical vertebra MCC CC H5 HCC

S12.1 Fracture of second cervical vertebra
Axis

S12.10 Unspecified fracture of second cervical vertebra

2,3,6 S12.100 Unspecified displaced fracture of second cervical vertebra MCC CC H5 HCC

2,3,6 S12.101 Unspecified nondisplaced fracture of second cervical vertebra MCC CC H5 HCC

S12.11 Type II dens fracture

2,3,6 S12.110 Anterior displaced Type II dens fracture MCC CC H5 HCC

2,3,6 S12.111 Posterior displaced Type II dens fracture MCC CC H5 HCC

2,3,6 S12.112 Nondisplaced Type II dens fracture MCC CC H5 HCC

S12.12 Other dens fracture

2,3,6 S12.120 Other displaced dens fracture MCC CC H5 HCC

2,3,6 S12.121 Other nondisplaced dens fracture MCC CC H5 HCC

S12.13 Unspecified traumatic spondylolisthesis of second cervical vertebra

2,3,6 S12.130 Unspecified traumatic displaced spondylolisthesis of second cervical vertebra MCC CC H5 HCC

2,3,6 S12.131 Unspecified traumatic nondisplaced spondylolisthesis of second cervical vertebra MCC CC H5 HCC

2,3,6 √x7th **S12.14 Type III traumatic spondylolisthesis of second cervical vertebra** MCC CC HS HCC

√6th **S12.15 Other traumatic spondylolisthesis of second cervical vertebra**

2,3,6 √7th **S12.150 Other traumatic displaced spondylolisthesis of second cervical vertebra** MCC CC HS HCC

2,3,6 √7th **S12.151 Other traumatic nondisplaced spondylolisthesis of second cervical vertebra** MCC CC HS HCC

√6th **S12.19 Other fracture of second cervical vertebra**

2,3,6 √7th **S12.190 Other displaced fracture of second cervical vertebra** MCC CC HS HCC

2,3,6 √7th **S12.191 Other nondisplaced fracture of second cervical vertebra** MCC CC HS HCC

√5th **S12.2 Fracture of third cervical vertebra**

√6th **S12.20 Unspecified fracture of third cervical vertebra**

2,3,6 √7th **S12.200 Unspecified displaced fracture of third cervical vertebra** MCC CC HS HCC

2,3,6 √7th **S12.201 Unspecified nondisplaced fracture of third cervical vertebra** MCC CC HS HCC

√6th **S12.23 Unspecified traumatic spondylolisthesis of third cervical vertebra**

2,3,6 √7th **S12.230 Unspecified traumatic displaced spondylolisthesis of third cervical vertebra** MCC CC HS HCC

2,3,6 √7th **S12.231 Unspecified traumatic nondisplaced spondylolisthesis of third cervical vertebra** MCC CC HS HCC

2,3,6 √x7th **S12.24 Type III traumatic spondylolisthesis of third cervical vertebra** MCC CC HS HCC

√6th **S12.25 Other traumatic spondylolisthesis of third cervical vertebra**

2,3,6 √7th **S12.250 Other traumatic displaced spondylolisthesis of third cervical vertebra** MCC CC HS HCC

2,3,6 √7th **S12.251 Other traumatic nondisplaced spondylolisthesis of third cervical vertebra** MCC CC HS HCC

√6th **S12.29 Other fracture of third cervical vertebra**

2,3,6 √7th **S12.290 Other displaced fracture of third cervical vertebra** MCC CC HS HCC

2,3,6 √7th **S12.291 Other nondisplaced fracture of third cervical vertebra** MCC CC HS HCC

√5th **S12.3 Fracture of fourth cervical vertebra**

√6th **S12.30 Unspecified fracture of fourth cervical vertebra**

2,3,6 √7th **S12.300 Unspecified displaced fracture of fourth cervical vertebra** MCC CC HS HCC

2,3,6 √7th **S12.301 Unspecified nondisplaced fracture of fourth cervical vertebra** MCC CC HS HCC

√6th **S12.33 Unspecified traumatic spondylolisthesis of fourth cervical vertebra**

2,3,6 √7th **S12.330 Unspecified traumatic displaced spondylolisthesis of fourth cervical vertebra** MCC CC HS HCC

2,3,6 √7th **S12.331 Unspecified traumatic nondisplaced spondylolisthesis of fourth cervical vertebra** MCC CC HS HCC

2,3,6 √x7th **S12.34 Type III traumatic spondylolisthesis of fourth cervical vertebra** MCC CC HS HCC

√6th **S12.35 Other traumatic spondylolisthesis of fourth cervical vertebra**

2,3,6 √7th **S12.350 Other traumatic displaced spondylolisthesis of fourth cervical vertebra** MCC CC HS HCC

2,3,6 √7th **S12.351 Other traumatic nondisplaced spondylolisthesis of fourth cervical vertebra** MCC CC HS HCC

√6th **S12.39 Other fracture of fourth cervical vertebra**

2,3,6 √7th **S12.390 Other displaced fracture of fourth cervical vertebra** MCC CC HS HCC

2,3,6 √7th **S12.391 Other nondisplaced fracture of fourth cervical vertebra** MCC CC HS HCC

√5th **S12.4 Fracture of fifth cervical vertebra**

√6th **S12.40 Unspecified fracture of fifth cervical vertebra**

2,3,6 √7th **S12.400 Unspecified displaced fracture of fifth cervical vertebra** MCC CC HS HCC

2,3,6 √7th **S12.401 Unspecified nondisplaced fracture of fifth cervical vertebra** MCC CC HS HCC

√6th **S12.43 Unspecified traumatic spondylolisthesis of fifth cervical vertebra**

2,3,6 √7th **S12.430 Unspecified traumatic displaced spondylolisthesis of fifth cervical vertebra** MCC CC HS HCC

2,3,6 √7th **S12.431 Unspecified traumatic nondisplaced spondylolisthesis of fifth cervical vertebra** MCC CC HS HCC

2,3,6 √x7th **S12.44 Type III traumatic spondylolisthesis of fifth cervical vertebra** MCC CC HS HCC

√6th **S12.45 Other traumatic spondylolisthesis of fifth cervical vertebra**

2,3,6 √7th **S12.450 Other traumatic displaced spondylolisthesis of fifth cervical vertebra** MCC CC HS HCC

2,3,6 √7th **S12.451 Other traumatic nondisplaced spondylolisthesis of fifth cervical vertebra** MCC CC HS HCC

√6th **S12.49 Other fracture of fifth cervical vertebra**

2,3,6 √7th **S12.490 Other displaced fracture of fifth cervical vertebra** MCC CC HS HCC

2,3,6 √7th **S12.491 Other nondisplaced fracture of fifth cervical vertebra** MCC CC HS HCC

√5th **S12.5 Fracture of sixth cervical vertebra**

√6th **S12.50 Unspecified fracture of sixth cervical vertebra**

2,3,6 √7th **S12.500 Unspecified displaced fracture of sixth cervical vertebra** MCC CC HS HCC

2,3,6 √7th **S12.501 Unspecified nondisplaced fracture of sixth cervical vertebra** MCC CC HS HCC

√6th **S12.53 Unspecified traumatic spondylolisthesis of sixth cervical vertebra**

2,3,6 √7th **S12.530 Unspecified traumatic displaced spondylolisthesis of sixth cervical vertebra** MCC CC HS HCC

2,3,6 √7th **S12.531 Unspecified traumatic nondisplaced spondylolisthesis of sixth cervical vertebra** MCC CC HS HCC

2,3,6 √x7th **S12.54 Type III traumatic spondylolisthesis of sixth cervical vertebra** MCC CC HS HCC

√6th **S12.55 Other traumatic spondylolisthesis of sixth cervical vertebra**

2,3,6 √7th **S12.550 Other traumatic displaced spondylolisthesis of sixth cervical vertebra** MCC CC HS HCC

2,3,6 √7th **S12.551 Other traumatic nondisplaced spondylolisthesis of sixth cervical vertebra** MCC CC HS HCC

√6th **S12.59 Other fracture of sixth cervical vertebra**

2,3,6 √7th **S12.590 Other displaced fracture of sixth cervical vertebra** MCC CC HS HCC

2,3,6 √7th **S12.591 Other nondisplaced fracture of sixth cervical vertebra** MCC CC HS HCC

√5th **S12.6 Fracture of seventh cervical vertebra**

√6th **S12.60 Unspecified fracture of seventh cervical vertebra**

2,3,6 √7th **S12.600 Unspecified displaced fracture of seventh cervical vertebra** MCC CC HS HCC

2,3,6 √7th **S12.601 Unspecified nondisplaced fracture of seventh cervical vertebra** MCC CC HS HCC

√6th **S12.63 Unspecified traumatic spondylolisthesis of seventh cervical vertebra**

2,3,6 √7th **S12.630 Unspecified traumatic displaced spondylolisthesis of seventh cervical vertebra** MCC CC HS HCC

2,3,6 √7th **S12.631 Unspecified traumatic nondisplaced spondylolisthesis of seventh cervical vertebra** MCC CC HS HCC

2,3,6 √x7th **S12.64 Type III traumatic spondylolisthesis of seventh cervical vertebra** MCC CC HS HCC

√6th **S12.65 Other traumatic spondylolisthesis of seventh cervical vertebra**

2,3,6 √7th **S12.650 Other traumatic displaced spondylolisthesis of seventh cervical vertebra** MCC CC HS HCC

2,3,6 √7th **S12.651 Other traumatic nondisplaced spondylolisthesis of seventh cervical vertebra** MCC CC HS HCC

√6th **S12.69 Other fracture of seventh cervical vertebra**

2,3,6 √7th **S12.690 Other displaced fracture of seventh cervical vertebra** MCC CC HS HCC

2,3,6 S12.691 **Other nondisplaced fracture of seventh cervical vertebra** MCC CC H5 HCC

6 S12.8 **Fracture of other parts of neck** MCC H5 HCC
Hyoid bone
Larynx
Thyroid cartilage
Trachea

The appropriate 7th character is to be added to code S12.8.
A initial encounter
D subsequent encounter
S sequela

6 S12.9 **Fracture of neck, unspecified** CC H5 HCC
Fracture of neck NOS
Fracture of cervical spine NOS
Fracture of cervical vertebra NOS

The appropriate 7th character is to be added to code S12.9.
A initial encounter
D subsequent encounter
S sequela

S13 Dislocation and sprain of joints and ligaments at neck level

INCLUDES avulsion of joint or ligament at neck level
laceration of cartilage, joint or ligament at neck level
sprain of cartilage, joint or ligament at neck level
traumatic hemarthrosis of joint or ligament at neck level
traumatic rupture of joint or ligament at neck level
traumatic subluxation of joint or ligament at neck level
traumatic tear of joint or ligament at neck level

Code also any associated open wound

EXCLUDES 2 *strain of muscle or tendon at neck level (S16.1)*

The appropriate 7th character is to be added to each code from category S13.
A initial encounter
D subsequent encounter
S sequela

S13.Ø **Traumatic rupture of cervical intervertebral disc** CC H5
EXCLUDES 1 *rupture or displacement (nontraumatic) of cervical intervertebral disc NOS (M5Ø.-)*

S13.1 **Subluxation and dislocation of cervical vertebrae**
Code also any associated:
open wound of neck (S11.-)
spinal cord injury (S14.1-)
EXCLUDES 2 *fracture of cervical vertebrae (S12.Ø-S12.3-)*

S13.1Ø **Subluxation and dislocation of unspecified cervical vertebrae**
S13.1ØØ **Subluxation of unspecified cervical vertebrae** CC H5
S13.1Ø1 **Dislocation of unspecified cervical vertebrae** CC H5

S13.11 **Subluxation and dislocation of CØ/C1 cervical vertebrae**
Subluxation and dislocation of atlantooccipital joint
Subluxation and dislocation of atloidooccipital joint
Subluxation and dislocation of occipitoatloid joint
S13.11Ø **Subluxation of CØ/C1 cervical vertebrae** CC H5
S13.111 **Dislocation of CØ/C1 cervical vertebrae** CC H5

S13.12 **Subluxation and dislocation of C1/C2 cervical vertebrae**
Subluxation and dislocation of atlantoaxial joint
S13.12Ø **Subluxation of C1/C2 cervical vertebrae** CC H5
S13.121 **Dislocation of C1/C2 cervical vertebrae** CC H5

S13.13 **Subluxation and dislocation of C2/C3 cervical vertebrae**
S13.13Ø **Subluxation of C2/C3 cervical vertebrae** CC H5
S13.131 **Dislocation of C2/C3 cervical vertebrae** CC H5

S13.14 **Subluxation and dislocation of C3/C4 cervical vertebrae**
S13.14Ø **Subluxation of C3/C4 cervical vertebrae** CC H5
S13.141 **Dislocation of C3/C4 cervical vertebrae** CC H5

S13.15 **Subluxation and dislocation of C4/C5 cervical vertebrae**
S13.15Ø **Subluxation of C4/C5 cervical vertebrae** CC H5
S13.151 **Dislocation of C4/C5 cervical vertebrae** CC H5

S13.16 **Subluxation and dislocation of C5/C6 cervical vertebrae**
S13.16Ø **Subluxation of C5/C6 cervical vertebrae** CC H5
S13.161 **Dislocation of C5/C6 cervical vertebrae** CC H5

S13.17 **Subluxation and dislocation of C6/C7 cervical vertebrae**
S13.17Ø **Subluxation of C6/C7 cervical vertebrae** CC H5
S13.171 **Dislocation of C6/C7 cervical vertebrae** CC H5

S13.18 **Subluxation and dislocation of C7/T1 cervical vertebrae**
S13.18Ø **Subluxation of C7/T1 cervical vertebrae** CC H5
S13.181 **Dislocation of C7/T1 cervical vertebrae** CC H5

S13.2 **Dislocation of other and unspecified parts of neck**
S13.2Ø **Dislocation of unspecified parts of neck** CC H5
S13.29 **Dislocation of other parts of neck** CC H5

S13.4 **Sprain of ligaments of cervical spine**
Sprain of anterior longitudinal (ligament), cervical
Sprain of atlanto-axial (joints)
Sprain of atlanto-occipital (joints)
Whiplash injury of cervical spine

S13.5 **Sprain of thyroid region**
Sprain of cricoarytenoid (joint) (ligament)
Sprain of cricothyroid (joint) (ligament)
Sprain of thyroid cartilage

S13.8 **Sprain of joints and ligaments of other parts of neck**

S13.9 **Sprain of joints and ligaments of unspecified parts of neck**

S14 Injury of nerves and spinal cord at neck level

NOTE Code to highest level of cervical cord injury

Code also any associated:
fracture of cervical vertebra (S12.Ø- — S12.6.-)
open wound of neck (S11.-)
transient paralysis (R29.5)

The appropriate 7th character is to be added to each code from category S14.
A initial encounter
D subsequent encounter
S sequela

S14.Ø **Concussion and edema of cervical spinal cord** MCC HCC

S14.1 **Other and unspecified injuries of cervical spinal cord**

S14.1Ø **Unspecified injury of cervical spinal cord**
S14.1Ø1 **Unspecified injury at C1 level of cervical spinal cord** MCC H5 HCC
S14.1Ø2 **Unspecified injury at C2 level of cervical spinal cord** MCC H5 HCC
S14.1Ø3 **Unspecified injury at C3 level of cervical spinal cord** MCC H5 HCC
S14.1Ø4 **Unspecified injury at C4 level of cervical spinal cord** MCC H5 HCC
S14.1Ø5 **Unspecified injury at C5 level of cervical spinal cord** MCC H5 HCC
S14.1Ø6 **Unspecified injury at C6 level of cervical spinal cord** MCC H5 HCC
S14.1Ø7 **Unspecified injury at C7 level of cervical spinal cord** MCC H5 HCC
S14.1Ø8 **Unspecified injury at C8 level of cervical spinal cord** MCC HCC
S14.1Ø9 **Unspecified injury at unspecified level of cervical spinal cord** HCC
Injury of cervical spinal cord NOS

S14.11 **Complete lesion of cervical spinal cord**
S14.111 **Complete lesion at C1 level of cervical spinal cord** MCC H5 HCC
S14.112 **Complete lesion at C2 level of cervical spinal cord** MCC H5 HCC

S14.113 Complete lesion at C3 level of cervical spinal cord MCC HS HCC
S14.114 Complete lesion at C4 level of cervical spinal cord MCC HS HCC
S14.115 Complete lesion at C5 level of cervical spinal cord MCC HS HCC
S14.116 Complete lesion at C6 level of cervical spinal cord MCC HS HCC
S14.117 Complete lesion at C7 level of cervical spinal cord MCC HS HCC
S14.118 Complete lesion at C8 level of cervical spinal cord MCC HCC
S14.119 Complete lesion at unspecified level of cervical spinal cord HCC

S14.12 Central cord syndrome of cervical spinal cord
S14.121 Central cord syndrome at C1 level of cervical spinal cord MCC HS HCC
S14.122 Central cord syndrome at C2 level of cervical spinal cord MCC HS HCC
S14.123 Central cord syndrome at C3 level of cervical spinal cord MCC HS HCC
S14.124 Central cord syndrome at C4 level of cervical spinal cord MCC HS HCC
S14.125 Central cord syndrome at C5 level of cervical spinal cord MCC HS HCC
S14.126 Central cord syndrome at C6 level of cervical spinal cord MCC HS HCC
S14.127 Central cord syndrome at C7 level of cervical spinal cord MCC HS HCC
S14.128 Central cord syndrome at C8 level of cervical spinal cord MCC HCC
S14.129 Central cord syndrome at unspecified level of cervical spinal cord HCC

S14.13 Anterior cord syndrome of cervical spinal cord
S14.131 Anterior cord syndrome at C1 level of cervical spinal cord MCC HS HCC
S14.132 Anterior cord syndrome at C2 level of cervical spinal cord MCC HS HCC
S14.133 Anterior cord syndrome at C3 level of cervical spinal cord MCC HS HCC
S14.134 Anterior cord syndrome at C4 level of cervical spinal cord MCC HS HCC
S14.135 Anterior cord syndrome at C5 level of cervical spinal cord MCC HS HCC
S14.136 Anterior cord syndrome at C6 level of cervical spinal cord MCC HS HCC
S14.137 Anterior cord syndrome at C7 level of cervical spinal cord MCC HS HCC
S14.138 Anterior cord syndrome at C8 level of cervical spinal cord MCC HCC
S14.139 Anterior cord syndrome at unspecified level of cervical spinal cord HCC

S14.14 Brown-Séquard syndrome of cervical spinal cord
S14.141 Brown-Séquard syndrome at C1 level of cervical spinal cord MCC HCC
S14.142 Brown-Séquard syndrome at C2 level of cervical spinal cord MCC HCC
S14.143 Brown-Séquard syndrome at C3 level of cervical spinal cord MCC HCC
S14.144 Brown-Séquard syndrome at C4 level of cervical spinal cord MCC HCC
S14.145 Brown-Séquard syndrome at C5 level of cervical spinal cord MCC HCC
S14.146 Brown-Séquard syndrome at C6 level of cervical spinal cord MCC HCC
S14.147 Brown-Séquard syndrome at C7 level of cervical spinal cord MCC HCC
S14.148 Brown-Séquard syndrome at C8 level of cervical spinal cord MCC HCC
S14.149 Brown-Séquard syndrome at unspecified level of cervical spinal cord HCC

S14.15 Other incomplete lesions of cervical spinal cord
Incomplete lesion of cervical spinal cord NOS
Posterior cord syndrome of cervical spinal cord
S14.151 Other incomplete lesion at C1 level of cervical spinal cord MCC HS HCC
S14.152 Other incomplete lesion at C2 level of cervical spinal cord MCC HS HCC
S14.153 Other incomplete lesion at C3 level of cervical spinal cord MCC HS HCC
S14.154 Other incomplete lesion at C4 level of cervical spinal cord MCC HS HCC
S14.155 Other incomplete lesion at C5 level of cervical spinal cord MCC HS HCC
S14.156 Other incomplete lesion at C6 level of cervical spinal cord MCC HS HCC
S14.157 Other incomplete lesion at C7 level of cervical spinal cord MCC HS HCC
S14.158 Other incomplete lesion at C8 level of cervical spinal cord MCC HCC
S14.159 Other incomplete lesion at unspecified level of cervical spinal cord HCC

S14.2 Injury of nerve root of cervical spine
S14.3 Injury of brachial plexus
S14.4 Injury of peripheral nerves of neck
S14.5 Injury of cervical sympathetic nerves
S14.8 Injury of other specified nerves of neck
S14.9 Injury of unspecified nerves of neck

S15 Injury of blood vessels at neck level

Code also any associated open wound (S11.-)

The appropriate 7th character is to be added to each code from category S15.
A initial encounter
D subsequent encounter
S sequela

S15.0 Injury of carotid artery of neck
Injury of carotid artery (common) (external) (internal, extracranial portion)
Injury of carotid artery NOS
EXCLUDES 1 *injury of internal carotid artery, intracranial portion (S06.8)*

S15.00 Unspecified injury of carotid artery
S15.001 Unspecified injury of right carotid artery CC
S15.002 Unspecified injury of left carotid artery CC
S15.009 Unspecified injury of unspecified carotid artery CC UNS

S15.01 Minor laceration of carotid artery
Incomplete transection of carotid artery
Laceration of carotid artery NOS
Superficial laceration of carotid artery
S15.011 Minor laceration of right carotid artery CC
S15.012 Minor laceration of left carotid artery CC
S15.019 Minor laceration of unspecified carotid artery CC UNS

S15.02 Major laceration of carotid artery
Complete transection of carotid artery
Traumatic rupture of carotid artery
S15.021 Major laceration of right carotid artery CC
S15.022 Major laceration of left carotid artery CC
S15.029 Major laceration of unspecified carotid artery CC UNS

S15.09 Other specified injury of carotid artery
S15.091 Other specified injury of right carotid artery CC
S15.092 Other specified injury of left carotid artery CC
S15.099 Other specified injury of unspecified carotid artery CC UNS

S15.1 Injury of vertebral artery
S15.10 Unspecified injury of vertebral artery
S15.101 Unspecified injury of right vertebral artery CC
S15.102 Unspecified injury of left vertebral artery CC
S15.109 Unspecified injury of unspecified vertebral artery CC UNS

S15.11 Minor laceration of vertebral artery
Incomplete transection of vertebral artery
Laceration of vertebral artery NOS
Superficial laceration of vertebral artery
S15.111 Minor laceration of right vertebral artery CC
S15.112 Minor laceration of left vertebral artery CC
S15.119 Minor laceration of unspecified vertebral artery CC UNS
S15.12 Major laceration of vertebral artery
Complete transection of vertebral artery
Traumatic rupture of vertebral artery
S15.121 Major laceration of right vertebral artery CC
S15.122 Major laceration of left vertebral artery CC
S15.129 Major laceration of unspecified vertebral artery CC UNS
S15.19 Other specified injury of vertebral artery
S15.191 Other specified injury of right vertebral artery CC
S15.192 Other specified injury of left vertebral artery CC
S15.199 Other specified injury of unspecified vertebral artery CC UNS
S15.2 Injury of external jugular vein
S15.20 Unspecified injury of external jugular vein
S15.201 Unspecified injury of right external jugular vein CC
S15.202 Unspecified injury of left external jugular vein CC
S15.209 Unspecified injury of unspecified external jugular vein CC UNS
S15.21 Minor laceration of external jugular vein
Incomplete transection of external jugular vein
Laceration of external jugular vein NOS
Superficial laceration of external jugular vein
S15.211 Minor laceration of right external jugular vein CC
S15.212 Minor laceration of left external jugular vein CC
S15.219 Minor laceration of unspecified external jugular vein CC UNS
S15.22 Major laceration of external jugular vein
Complete transection of external jugular vein
Traumatic rupture of external jugular vein
S15.221 Major laceration of right external jugular vein CC
S15.222 Major laceration of left external jugular vein CC
S15.229 Major laceration of unspecified external jugular vein CC UNS
S15.29 Other specified injury of external jugular vein
S15.291 Other specified injury of right external jugular vein CC
S15.292 Other specified injury of left external jugular vein CC
S15.299 Other specified injury of unspecified external jugular vein CC UNS
S15.3 Injury of internal jugular vein
S15.30 Unspecified injury of internal jugular vein
S15.301 Unspecified injury of right internal jugular vein CC
S15.302 Unspecified injury of left internal jugular vein CC
S15.309 Unspecified injury of unspecified internal jugular vein CC UNS
S15.31 Minor laceration of internal jugular vein
Incomplete transection of internal jugular vein
Laceration of internal jugular vein NOS
Superficial laceration of internal jugular vein
S15.311 Minor laceration of right internal jugular vein CC
S15.312 Minor laceration of left internal jugular vein CC
S15.319 Minor laceration of unspecified internal jugular vein CC UNS
S15.32 Major laceration of internal jugular vein
Complete transection of internal jugular vein
Traumatic rupture of internal jugular vein
S15.321 Major laceration of right internal jugular vein CC
S15.322 Major laceration of left internal jugular vein CC
S15.329 Major laceration of unspecified internal jugular vein CC UNS
S15.39 Other specified injury of internal jugular vein
S15.391 Other specified injury of right internal jugular vein CC
S15.392 Other specified injury of left internal jugular vein CC
S15.399 Other specified injury of unspecified internal jugular vein CC UNS
S15.8 Injury of other specified blood vessels at neck level CC
S15.9 Injury of unspecified blood vessel at neck level CC

S16 Injury of muscle, fascia and tendon at neck level

Code also any associated open wound (S11.-)

EXCLUDES 2 *sprain of joint or ligament at neck level (S13.9)*

The appropriate 7th character is to be added to each code from category S16.
A initial encounter
D subsequent encounter
S sequela

S16.1 Strain of muscle, fascia and tendon at neck level
S16.2 Laceration of muscle, fascia and tendon at neck level
S16.8 Other specified injury of muscle, fascia and tendon at neck level
S16.9 Unspecified injury of muscle, fascia and tendon at neck level

S17 Crushing injury of neck

Use additional code for all associated injuries, such as:
injury of blood vessels (S15.-)
open wound of neck (S11.-)
spinal cord injury (S14.0, S14.1-)
vertebral fracture (S12.0- — S12.3-)

The appropriate 7th character is to be added to each code from category S17.
A initial encounter
D subsequent encounter
S sequela

S17.0 Crushing injury of larynx and trachea CC H5
S17.8 Crushing injury of other specified parts of neck CC H5
S17.9 Crushing injury of neck, part unspecified CC H5

S19 Other specified and unspecified injuries of neck

The appropriate 7th character is to be added to each code from category S19.
A initial encounter
D subsequent encounter
S sequela

S19.8 Other specified injuries of neck
S19.80 Other specified injuries of unspecified part of neck
S19.81 Other specified injuries of larynx
S19.82 Other specified injuries of cervical trachea
EXCLUDES 2 *other specified injury of thoracic trachea (S27.5-)*
S19.83 Other specified injuries of vocal cord
S19.84 Other specified injuries of thyroid gland
S19.85 Other specified injuries of pharynx and cervical esophagus
AHA: 2022,1Q,27
S19.89 Other specified injuries of other specified part of neck
S19.9 Unspecified injury of neck

Injuries to the thorax (S20-S29)

INCLUDES injuries of breast
injuries of chest (wall)
injuries of interscapular area

EXCLUDES 2 *burns and corrosions (T20-T32)*
effects of foreign body in bronchus (T17.5)
effects of foreign body in esophagus (T18.1)
effects of foreign body in lung (T17.8)
effects of foreign body in trachea (T17.4)
frostbite (T33-T34)
injuries of axilla
injuries of clavicle
injuries of scapular region
injuries of shoulder
insect bite or sting, venomous (T63.4)

S20 Superficial injury of thorax

AHA: 2020,4Q,39

The appropriate 7th character is to be added to each code from category S20.
A initial encounter
D subsequent encounter
S sequela

S20.0 Contusion of breast
- **S20.00 Contusion of breast, unspecified breast**
- **S20.01 Contusion of right breast**
- **S20.02 Contusion of left breast**

S20.1 Other and unspecified superficial injuries of breast
- **S20.10 Unspecified superficial injuries of breast**
  - **S20.101 Unspecified superficial injuries of breast, right breast**
  - **S20.102 Unspecified superficial injuries of breast, left breast**
  - **S20.109 Unspecified superficial injuries of breast, unspecified breast**
- **S20.11 Abrasion of breast**
  - **S20.111 Abrasion of breast, right breast**
  - **S20.112 Abrasion of breast, left breast**
  - **S20.119 Abrasion of breast, unspecified breast**
- **S20.12 Blister (nonthermal) of breast**
  - **S20.121 Blister (nonthermal) of breast, right breast**
  - **S20.122 Blister (nonthermal) of breast, left breast**
  - **S20.129 Blister (nonthermal) of breast, unspecified breast**
- **S20.14 External constriction of part of breast**
  - **S20.141 External constriction of part of breast, right breast**
  - **S20.142 External constriction of part of breast, left breast**
  - **S20.149 External constriction of part of breast, unspecified breast**
- **S20.15 Superficial foreign body of breast**
  Splinter in the breast
  - **S20.151 Superficial foreign body of breast, right breast**
  - **S20.152 Superficial foreign body of breast, left breast**
  - **S20.159 Superficial foreign body of breast, unspecified breast**
- **S20.16 Insect bite (nonvenomous) of breast**
  - **S20.161 Insect bite (nonvenomous) of breast, right breast**
  - **S20.162 Insect bite (nonvenomous) of breast, left breast**
  - **S20.169 Insect bite (nonvenomous) of breast, unspecified breast**
- **S20.17 Other superficial bite of breast**
  EXCLUDES 1 *open bite of breast (S21.05-)*
  - **S20.171 Other superficial bite of breast, right breast**
  - **S20.172 Other superficial bite of breast, left breast**
  - **S20.179 Other superficial bite of breast, unspecified breast**

S20.2 Contusion of thorax
- **S20.20 Contusion of thorax, unspecified**
- **S20.21 Contusion of front wall of thorax**
  - **S20.211 Contusion of right front wall of thorax**
  - **S20.212 Contusion of left front wall of thorax**
  - **S20.213 Contusion of bilateral front wall of thorax**
  - **S20.214 Contusion of middle front wall of thorax**
  - **S20.219 Contusion of unspecified front wall of thorax**
- **S20.22 Contusion of back wall of thorax**
  - **S20.221 Contusion of right back wall of thorax**
  - **S20.222 Contusion of left back wall of thorax**
  - **S20.223 Contusion of bilateral back wall of thorax**
  - **S20.224 Contusion of middle back wall of thorax**
  - **S20.229 Contusion of unspecified back wall of thorax**

S20.3 Other and unspecified superficial injuries of front wall of thorax
- **S20.30 Unspecified superficial injuries of front wall of thorax**
  - **S20.301 Unspecified superficial injuries of right front wall of thorax**
  - **S20.302 Unspecified superficial injuries of left front wall of thorax**
  - **S20.303 Unspecified superficial injuries of bilateral front wall of thorax**
  - **S20.304 Unspecified superficial injuries of middle front wall of thorax**
  - **S20.309 Unspecified superficial injuries of unspecified front wall of thorax**
- **S20.31 Abrasion of front wall of thorax**
  - **S20.311 Abrasion of right front wall of thorax**
  - **S20.312 Abrasion of left front wall of thorax**
  - **S20.313 Abrasion of bilateral front wall of thorax**
  - **S20.314 Abrasion of middle front wall of thorax**
  - **S20.319 Abrasion of unspecified front wall of thorax**
- **S20.32 Blister (nonthermal) of front wall of thorax**
  - **S20.321 Blister (nonthermal) of right front wall of thorax**
  - **S20.322 Blister (nonthermal) of left front wall of thorax**
  - **S20.323 Blister (nonthermal) of bilateral front wall of thorax**
  - **S20.324 Blister (nonthermal) of middle front wall of thorax**
  - **S20.329 Blister (nonthermal) of unspecified front wall of thorax**
- **S20.34 External constriction of front wall of thorax**
  - **S20.341 External constriction of right front wall of thorax**
  - **S20.342 External constriction of left front wall of thorax**
  - **S20.343 External constriction of bilateral front wall of thorax**
  - **S20.344 External constriction of middle front wall of thorax**
  - **S20.349 External constriction of unspecified front wall of thorax**
- **S20.35 Superficial foreign body of front wall of thorax**
  Splinter in front wall of thorax
  - **S20.351 Superficial foreign body of right front wall of thorax**
  - **S20.352 Superficial foreign body of left front wall of thorax**
  - **S20.353 Superficial foreign body of bilateral front wall of thorax**
  - **S20.354 Superficial foreign body of middle front wall of thorax**
  - **S20.359 Superficial foreign body of unspecified front wall of thorax**
- **S20.36 Insect bite (nonvenomous) of front wall of thorax**
  - **S20.361 Insect bite (nonvenomous) of right front wall of thorax**
  - **S20.362 Insect bite (nonvenomous) of left front wall of thorax**
  - **S20.363 Insect bite (nonvenomous) of bilateral front wall of thorax**
  - **S20.364 Insect bite (nonvenomous) of middle front wall of thorax**

S20.369 Insect bite (nonvenomous) of unspecified front wall of thorax

S20.37 Other superficial bite of front wall of thorax

EXCLUDES 1 *open bite of front wall of thorax (S21.15)*

S20.371 Other superficial bite of right front wall of thorax

S20.372 Other superficial bite of left front wall of thorax

S20.373 Other superficial bite of bilateral front wall of thorax

S20.374 Other superficial bite of middle front wall of thorax

S20.379 Other superficial bite of unspecified front wall of thorax

S20.4 Other and unspecified superficial injuries of back wall of thorax

S20.40 Unspecified superficial injuries of back wall of thorax

S20.401 Unspecified superficial injuries of right back wall of thorax

S20.402 Unspecified superficial injuries of left back wall of thorax

S20.409 Unspecified superficial injuries of unspecified back wall of thorax

S20.41 Abrasion of back wall of thorax

S20.411 Abrasion of right back wall of thorax

S20.412 Abrasion of left back wall of thorax

S20.419 Abrasion of unspecified back wall of thorax

S20.42 Blister (nonthermal) of back wall of thorax

S20.421 Blister (nonthermal) of right back wall of thorax

S20.422 Blister (nonthermal) of left back wall of thorax

S20.429 Blister (nonthermal) of unspecified back wall of thorax

S20.44 External constriction of back wall of thorax

S20.441 External constriction of right back wall of thorax

S20.442 External constriction of left back wall of thorax

S20.449 External constriction of unspecified back wall of thorax

S20.45 Superficial foreign body of back wall of thorax

Splinter of back wall of thorax

S20.451 Superficial foreign body of right back wall of thorax

S20.452 Superficial foreign body of left back wall of thorax

S20.459 Superficial foreign body of unspecified back wall of thorax

S20.46 Insect bite (nonvenomous) of back wall of thorax

S20.461 Insect bite (nonvenomous) of right back wall of thorax

S20.462 Insect bite (nonvenomous) of left back wall of thorax

S20.469 Insect bite (nonvenomous) of unspecified back wall of thorax

S20.47 Other superficial bite of back wall of thorax

EXCLUDES 1 *open bite of back wall of thorax (S21.25)*

S20.471 Other superficial bite of right back wall of thorax

S20.472 Other superficial bite of left back wall of thorax

S20.479 Other superficial bite of unspecified back wall of thorax

S20.9 Superficial injury of unspecified parts of thorax

EXCLUDES 1 *contusion of thorax NOS (S20.20)*

S20.90 Unspecified superficial injury of unspecified parts of thorax

Superficial injury of thoracic wall NOS

S20.91 Abrasion of unspecified parts of thorax

S20.92 Blister (nonthermal) of unspecified parts of thorax

S20.94 External constriction of unspecified parts of thorax

S20.95 Superficial foreign body of unspecified parts of thorax

Splinter in thorax NOS

S20.96 Insect bite (nonvenomous) of unspecified parts of thorax

S20.97 Other superficial bite of unspecified parts of thorax

EXCLUDES 1 *open bite of thorax NOS (S21.95)*

S21 Open wound of thorax

Code also any associated injury, such as:
- injury of heart (S26.-)
- injury of intrathoracic organs (S27.-)
- rib fracture (S22.3-, S22.4-)
- spinal cord injury (S24.0-, S24.1-)
- traumatic hemopneumothorax (S27.3)
- traumatic hemothorax (S27.1)
- traumatic pneumothorax (S27.0)
- wound infection

EXCLUDES 1 *traumatic amputation (partial) of thorax (S28.1)*

The appropriate 7th character is to be added to each code from category S21.
- A initial encounter
- D subsequent encounter
- S sequela

S21.0 Open wound of breast

S21.00 Unspecified open wound of breast

S21.001 Unspecified open wound of right breast

S21.002 Unspecified open wound of left breast

S21.009 Unspecified open wound of unspecified breast

S21.01 Laceration without foreign body of breast

S21.011 Laceration without foreign body of right breast

S21.012 Laceration without foreign body of left breast

S21.019 Laceration without foreign body of unspecified breast

S21.02 Laceration with foreign body of breast

S21.021 Laceration with foreign body of right breast

S21.022 Laceration with foreign body of left breast

S21.029 Laceration with foreign body of unspecified breast

S21.03 Puncture wound without foreign body of breast

S21.031 Puncture wound without foreign body of right breast

S21.032 Puncture wound without foreign body of left breast

S21.039 Puncture wound without foreign body of unspecified breast

S21.04 Puncture wound with foreign body of breast

S21.041 Puncture wound with foreign body of right breast

S21.042 Puncture wound with foreign body of left breast

S21.049 Puncture wound with foreign body of unspecified breast

S21.05 Open bite of breast

Bite of breast NOS

EXCLUDES 1 *superficial bite of breast (S20.17)*

S21.051 Open bite of right breast

S21.052 Open bite of left breast

S21.059 Open bite of unspecified breast

S21.1 Open wound of front wall of thorax without penetration into thoracic cavity

Open wound of chest without penetration into thoracic cavity

S21.10 Unspecified open wound of front wall of thorax without penetration into thoracic cavity

S21.101 Unspecified open wound of right front wall of thorax without penetration into thoracic cavity CC

S21.102 Unspecified open wound of left front wall of thorax without penetration into thoracic cavity CC

S21.109 Unspecified open wound of unspecified front wall of thorax without penetration into thoracic cavity CC UNS

S21.11 Laceration without foreign body of front wall of thorax without penetration into thoracic cavity

S21.111 Laceration without foreign body of right front wall of thorax without penetration into thoracic cavity CC

S21.112 Laceration without foreign body of left front wall of thorax without penetration into thoracic cavity CC

S21.119 Laceration without foreign body of unspecified front wall of thorax without penetration into thoracic cavity CC UNS

S21.12 Laceration with foreign body of front wall of thorax without penetration into thoracic cavity

S21.121 Laceration with foreign body of right front wall of thorax without penetration into thoracic cavity CC

S21.122 Laceration with foreign body of left front wall of thorax without penetration into thoracic cavity CC

S21.129 Laceration with foreign body of unspecified front wall of thorax without penetration into thoracic cavity CC UNS

S21.13 Puncture wound without foreign body of front wall of thorax without penetration into thoracic cavity

S21.131 Puncture wound without foreign body of right front wall of thorax without penetration into thoracic cavity CC

S21.132 Puncture wound without foreign body of left front wall of thorax without penetration into thoracic cavity CC

S21.139 Puncture wound without foreign body of unspecified front wall of thorax without penetration into thoracic cavity CC UNS

S21.14 Puncture wound with foreign body of front wall of thorax without penetration into thoracic cavity

S21.141 Puncture wound with foreign body of right front wall of thorax without penetration into thoracic cavity CC

S21.142 Puncture wound with foreign body of left front wall of thorax without penetration into thoracic cavity CC

S21.149 Puncture wound with foreign body of unspecified front wall of thorax without penetration into thoracic cavity CC UNS

S21.15 Open bite of front wall of thorax without penetration into thoracic cavity

Bite of front wall of thorax NOS

EXCLUDES 1 *superficial bite of front wall of thorax (S20.37)*

S21.151 Open bite of right front wall of thorax without penetration into thoracic cavity CC

S21.152 Open bite of left front wall of thorax without penetration into thoracic cavity CC

S21.159 Open bite of unspecified front wall of thorax without penetration into thoracic cavity CC UNS

S21.2 Open wound of back wall of thorax without penetration into thoracic cavity

S21.20 Unspecified open wound of back wall of thorax without penetration into thoracic cavity

S21.201 Unspecified open wound of right back wall of thorax without penetration into thoracic cavity

S21.202 Unspecified open wound of left back wall of thorax without penetration into thoracic cavity

S21.209 Unspecified open wound of unspecified back wall of thorax without penetration into thoracic cavity

S21.21 Laceration without foreign body of back wall of thorax without penetration into thoracic cavity

S21.211 Laceration without foreign body of right back wall of thorax without penetration into thoracic cavity

S21.212 Laceration without foreign body of left back wall of thorax without penetration into thoracic cavity

S21.219 Laceration without foreign body of unspecified back wall of thorax without penetration into thoracic cavity

S21.22 Laceration with foreign body of back wall of thorax without penetration into thoracic cavity

S21.221 Laceration with foreign body of right back wall of thorax without penetration into thoracic cavity

S21.222 Laceration with foreign body of left back wall of thorax without penetration into thoracic cavity

S21.229 Laceration with foreign body of unspecified back wall of thorax without penetration into thoracic cavity

S21.23 Puncture wound without foreign body of back wall of thorax without penetration into thoracic cavity

S21.231 Puncture wound without foreign body of right back wall of thorax without penetration into thoracic cavity

S21.232 Puncture wound without foreign body of left back wall of thorax without penetration into thoracic cavity

S21.239 Puncture wound without foreign body of unspecified back wall of thorax without penetration into thoracic cavity

S21.24 Puncture wound with foreign body of back wall of thorax without penetration into thoracic cavity

S21.241 Puncture wound with foreign body of right back wall of thorax without penetration into thoracic cavity

S21.242 Puncture wound with foreign body of left back wall of thorax without penetration into thoracic cavity

S21.249 Puncture wound with foreign body of unspecified back wall of thorax without penetration into thoracic cavity

S21.25 Open bite of back wall of thorax without penetration into thoracic cavity

Bite of back wall of thorax NOS

EXCLUDES 1 *superficial bite of back wall of thorax (S20.47)*

S21.251 Open bite of right back wall of thorax without penetration into thoracic cavity

S21.252 Open bite of left back wall of thorax without penetration into thoracic cavity

S21.259 Open bite of unspecified back wall of thorax without penetration into thoracic cavity

S21.3 Open wound of front wall of thorax with penetration into thoracic cavity

Open wound of chest with penetration into thoracic cavity

S21.30 Unspecified open wound of front wall of thorax with penetration into thoracic cavity

S21.301 Unspecified open wound of right front wall of thorax with penetration into thoracic cavity MCC

S21.302 Unspecified open wound of left front wall of thorax with penetration into thoracic cavity MCC

S21.309 Unspecified open wound of unspecified front wall of thorax with penetration into thoracic cavity MCC UNS

S21.31 Laceration without foreign body of front wall of thorax with penetration into thoracic cavity

S21.311 Laceration without foreign body of right front wall of thorax with penetration into thoracic cavity MCC

S21.312 Laceration without foreign body of left front wall of thorax with penetration into thoracic cavity MCC

S21.319 Laceration without foreign body of unspecified front wall of thorax with penetration into thoracic cavity MCC UNS

S21.32 Laceration with foreign body of front wall of thorax with penetration into thoracic cavity

S21.321 Laceration with foreign body of right front wall of thorax with penetration into thoracic cavity MCC

S21.322 Laceration with foreign body of left front wall of thorax with penetration into thoracic cavity MCC

S21.329 Laceration with foreign body of unspecified front wall of thorax with penetration into thoracic cavity MCC UNS

√6th S21.33 Puncture wound without foreign body of front wall of thorax with penetration into thoracic cavity
√7th S21.331 Puncture wound without foreign body of right front wall of thorax with penetration into thoracic cavity MCC
√7th S21.332 Puncture wound without foreign body of left front wall of thorax with penetration into thoracic cavity MCC
√7th S21.339 Puncture wound without foreign body of unspecified front wall of thorax with penetration into thoracic cavity MCC UNS
√6th S21.34 Puncture wound with foreign body of front wall of thorax with penetration into thoracic cavity
√7th S21.341 Puncture wound with foreign body of right front wall of thorax with penetration into thoracic cavity MCC
√7th S21.342 Puncture wound with foreign body of left front wall of thorax with penetration into thoracic cavity MCC
√7th S21.349 Puncture wound with foreign body of unspecified front wall of thorax with penetration into thoracic cavity MCC UNS
√6th S21.35 Open bite of front wall of thorax with penetration into thoracic cavity
EXCLUDES 1 *superficial bite of front wall of thorax (S20.37)*
√7th S21.351 Open bite of right front wall of thorax with penetration into thoracic cavity MCC
√7th S21.352 Open bite of left front wall of thorax with penetration into thoracic cavity MCC
√7th S21.359 Open bite of unspecified front wall of thorax with penetration into thoracic cavity MCC UNS
√5th S21.4 Open wound of back wall of thorax with penetration into thoracic cavity
√6th S21.40 Unspecified open wound of back wall of thorax with penetration into thoracic cavity
√7th S21.401 Unspecified open wound of right back wall of thorax with penetration into thoracic cavity MCC
√7th S21.402 Unspecified open wound of left back wall of thorax with penetration into thoracic cavity MCC
√7th S21.409 Unspecified open wound of unspecified back wall of thorax with penetration into thoracic cavity MCC UNS
√6th S21.41 Laceration without foreign body of back wall of thorax with penetration into thoracic cavity
√7th S21.411 Laceration without foreign body of right back wall of thorax with penetration into thoracic cavity MCC
√7th S21.412 Laceration without foreign body of left back wall of thorax with penetration into thoracic cavity MCC
√7th S21.419 Laceration without foreign body of unspecified back wall of thorax with penetration into thoracic cavity MCC UNS
√6th S21.42 Laceration with foreign body of back wall of thorax with penetration into thoracic cavity
√7th S21.421 Laceration with foreign body of right back wall of thorax with penetration into thoracic cavity MCC
√7th S21.422 Laceration with foreign body of left back wall of thorax with penetration into thoracic cavity MCC
√7th S21.429 Laceration with foreign body of unspecified back wall of thorax with penetration into thoracic cavity MCC UNS
√6th S21.43 Puncture wound without foreign body of back wall of thorax with penetration into thoracic cavity
√7th S21.431 Puncture wound without foreign body of right back wall of thorax with penetration into thoracic cavity MCC
√7th S21.432 Puncture wound without foreign body of left back wall of thorax with penetration into thoracic cavity MCC
√7th S21.439 Puncture wound without foreign body of unspecified back wall of thorax with penetration into thoracic cavity MCC UNS
√6th S21.44 Puncture wound with foreign body of back wall of thorax with penetration into thoracic cavity
√7th S21.441 Puncture wound with foreign body of right back wall of thorax with penetration into thoracic cavity MCC
√7th S21.442 Puncture wound with foreign body of left back wall of thorax with penetration into thoracic cavity MCC
√7th S21.449 Puncture wound with foreign body of unspecified back wall of thorax with penetration into thoracic cavity MCC UNS
√6th S21.45 Open bite of back wall of thorax with penetration into thoracic cavity
Bite of back wall of thorax NOS
EXCLUDES 1 *superficial bite of back wall of thorax (S20.47)*
√7th S21.451 Open bite of right back wall of thorax with penetration into thoracic cavity MCC
√7th S21.452 Open bite of left back wall of thorax with penetration into thoracic cavity MCC
√7th S21.459 Open bite of unspecified back wall of thorax with penetration into thoracic cavity MCC UNS
√5th S21.9 Open wound of unspecified part of thorax
Open wound of thoracic wall NOS
√x7th S21.90 Unspecified open wound of unspecified part of thorax CC UNS
√x7th S21.91 Laceration without foreign body of unspecified part of thorax CC UNS
√x7th S21.92 Laceration with foreign body of unspecified part of thorax CC UNS
√x7th S21.93 Puncture wound without foreign body of unspecified part of thorax CC UNS
√x7th S21.94 Puncture wound with foreign body of unspecified part of thorax CC UNS
√x7th S21.95 Open bite of unspecified part of thorax CC UNS
EXCLUDES 1 *superficial bite of thorax (S20.97)*

√4th **S22 Fracture of rib(s), sternum and thoracic spine**

NOTE A fracture not indicated as displaced or nondisplaced should be coded to displaced

A fracture not indicated as open or closed should be coded to closed

INCLUDES fracture of thoracic neural arch
fracture of thoracic spinous process
fracture of thoracic transverse process
fracture of thoracic vertebra
fracture of thoracic vertebral arch

Code first any associated:
injury of intrathoracic organ (S27.-)
spinal cord injury (S24.0-, S24.1-)

EXCLUDES 1 *transection of thorax (S28.1)*
EXCLUDES 2 *fracture of clavicle (S42.0-)*
fracture of scapula (S42.1-)

AHA: 2021,1Q,6; 2018,2Q,12; 2015,3Q,37-39

The appropriate 7th character is to be added to each code from category S22.
A initial encounter for closed fracture
B initial encounter for open fracture
D subsequent encounter for fracture with routine healing
G subsequent encounter for fracture with delayed healing
K subsequent encounter for fracture with nonunion
S sequela

√5th S22.0 Fracture of thoracic vertebra
√6th S22.00 Fracture of unspecified thoracic vertebra
2,3,6 √7th S22.000 Wedge compression fracture of unspecified thoracic vertebra MCC CC H5 HCC
2,3,6 √7th S22.001 Stable burst fracture of unspecified thoracic vertebra MCC CC H5 HCC
2,3,6 √7th S22.002 Unstable burst fracture of unspecified thoracic vertebra MCC CC H5 HCC

2,3,6 7th **S22.008** **Other fracture of unspecified thoracic vertebra** MCC CC H5 HCC

2,3,6 7th **S22.009** **Unspecified fracture of unspecified thoracic vertebra** MCC CC H5 HCC

6th **S22.01** **Fracture of first thoracic vertebra**

2,3,6 7th **S22.010** **Wedge compression fracture of first thoracic vertebra** MCC CC H5 HCC

2,3,6 7th **S22.011** **Stable burst fracture of first thoracic vertebra** MCC CC H5 HCC

2,3,6 7th **S22.012** **Unstable burst fracture of first thoracic vertebra** MCC CC H5 HCC

2,3,6 7th **S22.018** **Other fracture of first thoracic vertebra** MCC CC H5 HCC

2,3,6 7th **S22.019** **Unspecified fracture of first thoracic vertebra** MCC CC H5 HCC

6th **S22.02** **Fracture of second thoracic vertebra**

2,3,6 7th **S22.020** **Wedge compression fracture of second thoracic vertebra** MCC CC H5 HCC

2,3,6 7th **S22.021** **Stable burst fracture of second thoracic vertebra** MCC CC H5 HCC

2,3,6 7th **S22.022** **Unstable burst fracture of second thoracic vertebra** MCC CC H5 HCC

2,3,6 7th **S22.028** **Other fracture of second thoracic vertebra** MCC CC H5 HCC

2,3,6 7th **S22.029** **Unspecified fracture of second thoracic vertebra** MCC CC H5 HCC

6th **S22.03** **Fracture of third thoracic vertebra**

2,3,6 7th **S22.030** **Wedge compression fracture of third thoracic vertebra** MCC CC H5 HCC

2,3,6 7th **S22.031** **Stable burst fracture of third thoracic vertebra** MCC CC H5 HCC

2,3,6 7th **S22.032** **Unstable burst fracture of third thoracic vertebra** MCC CC H5 HCC

2,3,6 7th **S22.038** **Other fracture of third thoracic vertebra** MCC CC H5 HCC

2,3,6 7th **S22.039** **Unspecified fracture of third thoracic vertebra** MCC CC H5 HCC

6th **S22.04** **Fracture of fourth thoracic vertebra**

2,3,6 7th **S22.040** **Wedge compression fracture of fourth thoracic vertebra** MCC CC H5 HCC

2,3,6 7th **S22.041** **Stable burst fracture of fourth thoracic vertebra** MCC CC H5 HCC

2,3,6 7th **S22.042** **Unstable burst fracture of fourth thoracic vertebra** MCC CC H5 HCC

2,3,6 7th **S22.048** **Other fracture of fourth thoracic vertebra** MCC CC H5 HCC

2,3,6 7th **S22.049** **Unspecified fracture of fourth thoracic vertebra** MCC CC H5 HCC

6th **S22.05** **Fracture of T5-T6 vertebra**

2,3,6 7th **S22.050** **Wedge compression fracture of T5-T6 vertebra** MCC CC H5 HCC

2,3,6 7th **S22.051** **Stable burst fracture of T5-T6 vertebra** MCC CC H5 HCC

2,3,6 7th **S22.052** **Unstable burst fracture of T5-T6 vertebra** MCC CC H5 HCC

2,3,6 7th **S22.058** **Other fracture of T5-T6 vertebra** MCC CC H5 HCC

2,3,6 7th **S22.059** **Unspecified fracture of T5-T6 vertebra** MCC CC H5 HCC

6th **S22.06** **Fracture of T7-T8 vertebra**

2,3,6 7th **S22.060** **Wedge compression fracture of T7-T8 vertebra** MCC CC H5 HCC

2,3,6 7th **S22.061** **Stable burst fracture of T7-T8 vertebra** MCC CC H5 HCC

2,3,6 7th **S22.062** **Unstable burst fracture of T7-T8 vertebra** MCC CC H5 HCC

2,3,6 7th **S22.068** **Other fracture of T7-T8 thoracic vertebra** MCC CC H5 HCC

2,3,6 7th **S22.069** **Unspecified fracture of T7-T8 vertebra** MCC CC H5 HCC

6th **S22.07** **Fracture of T9-T10 vertebra**

2,3,6 7th **S22.070** **Wedge compression fracture of T9-T10 vertebra** MCC CC H5 HCC

2,3,6 7th **S22.071** **Stable burst fracture of T9-T10 vertebra** MCC CC H5 HCC

2,3,6 7th **S22.072** **Unstable burst fracture of T9-T10 vertebra** MCC CC H5 HCC

2,3,6 7th **S22.078** **Other fracture of T9-T10 vertebra** MCC CC H5 HCC

2,3,6 7th **S22.079** **Unspecified fracture of T9-T10 vertebra** MCC CC H5 HCC

6th **S22.08** **Fracture of T11-T12 vertebra**

2,3,6 7th **S22.080** **Wedge compression fracture of T11-T12 vertebra** MCC CC H5 HCC

2,3,6 7th **S22.081** **Stable burst fracture of T11-T12 vertebra** MCC CC H5 HCC

2,3,6 7th **S22.082** **Unstable burst fracture of T11-T12 vertebra** MCC CC H5 HCC

2,3,6 7th **S22.088** **Other fracture of T11-T12 vertebra** MCC CC H5 HCC

2,3,6 7th **S22.089** **Unspecified fracture of T11-T12 vertebra** MCC CC H5 HCC

5th **S22.2** **Fracture of sternum**

DEF: Break in flat bone (breast bone) in the anterior thorax caused by blunt trauma to the anterior chest.

2,3 x7th **S22.20** **Unspecified fracture of sternum** MCC CC H5

2,3 x7th **S22.21** **Fracture of manubrium** MCC CC H5

2,3 x7th **S22.22** **Fracture of body of sternum** MCC CC H5

2,3 x7th **S22.23** **Sternal manubrial dissociation** MCC CC H5

2,3 x7th **S22.24** **Fracture of xiphoid process** MCC CC H5

5th **S22.3** **Fracture of one rib**

AHA: 2021,1Q,5

2,3 x7th **S22.31** **Fracture of one rib, right side** MCC CC H5

2,3 x7th **S22.32** **Fracture of one rib, left side** MCC CC H5

2,3 x7th **S22.39** **Fracture of one rib, unspecified side** MCC CC H5 UNS

5th **S22.4** **Multiple fractures of ribs**

Fractures of two or more ribs

EXCLUDES 1 *flail chest (S22.5-)*

AHA: 2021,1Q,5

2,3 x7th **S22.41** **Multiple fractures of ribs, right side** MCC CC H5

2,3 x7th **S22.42** **Multiple fractures of ribs, left side** MCC CC H5

2,3 x7th **S22.43** **Multiple fractures of ribs, bilateral** MCC CC H5

2,3 x7th **S22.49** **Multiple fractures of ribs, unspecified side** MCC CC H5 UNS

4 x7th **S22.5** **Flail chest** MCC CC H5

2,3 x7th **S22.9** **Fracture of bony thorax, part unspecified** MCC CC H5

4th **S23** **Dislocation and sprain of joints and ligaments of thorax**

INCLUDES avulsion of joint or ligament of thorax
laceration of cartilage, joint or ligament of thorax
sprain of cartilage, joint or ligament of thorax
traumatic hemarthrosis of joint or ligament of thorax
traumatic rupture of joint or ligament of thorax
traumatic subluxation of joint or ligament of thorax
traumatic tear of joint or ligament of thorax

Code also any associated open wound

EXCLUDES 2 *dislocation, sprain of sternoclavicular joint (S43.2, S43.6)*
strain of muscle or tendon of thorax (S29.01-)

The appropriate 7th character is to be added to each code from category S23.
A initial encounter
D subsequent encounter
S sequela

x7th **S23.0** **Traumatic rupture of thoracic intervertebral disc**

EXCLUDES 1 *rupture or displacement (nontraumatic) of thoracic intervertebral disc NOS (M51.- with fifth character 4)*

5th **S23.1** **Subluxation and dislocation of thoracic vertebra**

Code also any associated:
open wound of thorax (S21.-)
spinal cord injury (S24.0-, S24.1-)

EXCLUDES 2 *fracture of thoracic vertebrae (S22.0-)*

6th **S23.10** **Subluxation and dislocation of unspecified thoracic vertebra**

7th **S23.100** **Subluxation of unspecified thoracic vertebra**

7th **S23.101** **Dislocation of unspecified thoracic vertebra**

S23.11 Subluxation and dislocation of T1/T2 thoracic vertebra
- S23.110 Subluxation of T1/T2 thoracic vertebra
- S23.111 Dislocation of T1/T2 thoracic vertebra

S23.12 Subluxation and dislocation of T2/T3-T3/T4 thoracic vertebra
- S23.120 Subluxation of T2/T3 thoracic vertebra
- S23.121 Dislocation of T2/T3 thoracic vertebra
- S23.122 Subluxation of T3/T4 thoracic vertebra
- S23.123 Dislocation of T3/T4 thoracic vertebra

S23.13 Subluxation and dislocation of T4/T5-T5/T6 thoracic vertebra
- S23.130 Subluxation of T4/T5 thoracic vertebra
- S23.131 Dislocation of T4/T5 thoracic vertebra
- S23.132 Subluxation of T5/T6 thoracic vertebra
- S23.133 Dislocation of T5/T6 thoracic vertebra

S23.14 Subluxation and dislocation of T6/T7-T7/T8 thoracic vertebra
- S23.140 Subluxation of T6/T7 thoracic vertebra
- S23.141 Dislocation of T6/T7 thoracic vertebra
- S23.142 Subluxation of T7/T8 thoracic vertebra
- S23.143 Dislocation of T7/T8 thoracic vertebra

S23.15 Subluxation and dislocation of T8/T9-T9/T10 thoracic vertebra
- S23.150 Subluxation of T8/T9 thoracic vertebra
- S23.151 Dislocation of T8/T9 thoracic vertebra
- S23.152 Subluxation of T9/T10 thoracic vertebra
- S23.153 Dislocation of T9/T10 thoracic vertebra

S23.16 Subluxation and dislocation of T10/T11-T11/T12 thoracic vertebra
- S23.160 Subluxation of T10/T11 thoracic vertebra
- S23.161 Dislocation of T10/T11 thoracic vertebra
- S23.162 Subluxation of T11/T12 thoracic vertebra
- S23.163 Dislocation of T11/T12 thoracic vertebra

S23.17 Subluxation and dislocation of T12/L1 thoracic vertebra
- S23.170 Subluxation of T12/L1 thoracic vertebra
- S23.171 Dislocation of T12/L1 thoracic vertebra

S23.2 Dislocation of other and unspecified parts of thorax
- S23.20 Dislocation of unspecified part of thorax
- S23.29 Dislocation of other parts of thorax

S23.3 Sprain of ligaments of thoracic spine

S23.4 Sprain of ribs and sternum
- S23.41 Sprain of ribs
- S23.42 Sprain of sternum
  - S23.420 Sprain of sternoclavicular (joint) (ligament)
  - S23.421 Sprain of chondrosternal joint
  - S23.428 Other sprain of sternum
  - S23.429 Unspecified sprain of sternum

S23.8 Sprain of other specified parts of thorax

S23.9 Sprain of unspecified parts of thorax

S24 Injury of nerves and spinal cord at thorax level

NOTE Code to highest level of thoracic spinal cord injury.
Injuries to the spinal cord (S24.0 and S24.1) refer to the cord level and not bone level injury, and can affect nerve roots at and below the level given.

Code also any associated:
- fracture of thoracic vertebra (S22.0-)
- open wound of thorax (S21.-)
- transient paralysis (R29.5)

EXCLUDES 2 *injury of brachial plexus (S14.3)*

The appropriate 7th character is to be added to each code from category S24.
- A initial encounter
- D subsequent encounter
- S sequela

S24.0 Concussion and edema of thoracic spinal cord MCC HCC

S24.1 Other and unspecified injuries of thoracic spinal cord

S24.10 Unspecified injury of thoracic spinal cord
- S24.101 Unspecified injury at T1 level of thoracic spinal cord MCC H5 HCC
- S24.102 Unspecified injury at T2-T6 level of thoracic spinal cord MCC H5 HCC
- S24.103 Unspecified injury at T7-T10 level of thoracic spinal cord MCC H5 HCC
- S24.104 Unspecified injury at T11-T12 level of thoracic spinal cord MCC H5 HCC
- S24.109 Unspecified injury at unspecified level of thoracic spinal cord HCC
  Injury of thoracic spinal cord NOS

S24.11 Complete lesion of thoracic spinal cord
- S24.111 Complete lesion at T1 level of thoracic spinal cord MCC H5 HCC
- S24.112 Complete lesion at T2-T6 level of thoracic spinal cord MCC H5 HCC
- S24.113 Complete lesion at T7-T10 level of thoracic spinal cord MCC H5 HCC
- S24.114 Complete lesion at T11-T12 level of thoracic spinal cord MCC H5 HCC
- S24.119 Complete lesion at unspecified level of thoracic spinal cord HCC

S24.13 Anterior cord syndrome of thoracic spinal cord
- S24.131 Anterior cord syndrome at T1 level of thoracic spinal cord MCC H5 HCC
- S24.132 Anterior cord syndrome at T2-T6 level of thoracic spinal cord MCC H5 HCC
- S24.133 Anterior cord syndrome at T7-T10 level of thoracic spinal cord MCC H5 HCC
- S24.134 Anterior cord syndrome at T11-T12 level of thoracic spinal cord MCC H5 HCC
- S24.139 Anterior cord syndrome at unspecified level of thoracic spinal cord HCC

S24.14 Brown-Séquard syndrome of thoracic spinal cord
- S24.141 Brown-Séquard syndrome at T1 level of thoracic spinal cord MCC HCC
- S24.142 Brown-Séquard syndrome at T2-T6 level of thoracic spinal cord MCC HCC
- S24.143 Brown-Séquard syndrome at T7-T10 level of thoracic spinal cord MCC HCC
- S24.144 Brown-Séquard syndrome at T11-T12 level of thoracic spinal cord MCC HCC
- S24.149 Brown-Séquard syndrome at unspecified level of thoracic spinal cord HCC

S24.15 Other incomplete lesions of thoracic spinal cord
Incomplete lesion of thoracic spinal cord NOS
Posterior cord syndrome of thoracic spinal cord
- S24.151 Other incomplete lesion at T1 level of thoracic spinal cord MCC H5 HCC
- S24.152 Other incomplete lesion at T2-T6 level of thoracic spinal cord MCC H5 HCC
- S24.153 Other incomplete lesion at T7-T10 level of thoracic spinal cord MCC H5 HCC
- S24.154 Other incomplete lesion at T11-T12 level of thoracic spinal cord MCC H5 HCC
- S24.159 Other incomplete lesion at unspecified level of thoracic spinal cord HCC

S24.2 Injury of nerve root of thoracic spine

S24.3 Injury of peripheral nerves of thorax

S24.4 Injury of thoracic sympathetic nervous system
Injury of cardiac plexus
Injury of esophageal plexus
Injury of pulmonary plexus
Injury of stellate ganglion
Injury of thoracic sympathetic ganglion

S24.8 Injury of other specified nerves of thorax

S24.9 Injury of unspecified nerve of thorax

4th **S25 Injury of blood vessels of thorax**

Code also any associated open wound (S21.-)

The appropriate 7th character is to be added to each code from category S25.
A initial encounter
D subsequent encounter
S sequela

5th **S25.Ø Injury of thoracic aorta**
  Injury of aorta NOS
  x7th **S25.ØØ Unspecified injury of thoracic aorta** MCC
  x7th **S25.Ø1 Minor laceration of thoracic aorta** MCC
    Incomplete transection of thoracic aorta
    Laceration of thoracic aorta NOS
    Superficial laceration of thoracic aorta
  x7th **S25.Ø2 Major laceration of thoracic aorta** MCC
    Complete transection of thoracic aorta
    Traumatic rupture of thoracic aorta
  x7th **S25.Ø9 Other specified injury of thoracic aorta** MCC

5th **S25.1 Injury of innominate or subclavian artery**
  6th **S25.1Ø Unspecified injury of innominate or subclavian artery**
    7th **S25.1Ø1 Unspecified injury of right innominate or subclavian artery** MCC
    7th **S25.1Ø2 Unspecified injury of left innominate or subclavian artery** MCC
    7th **S25.1Ø9 Unspecified injury of unspecified innominate or subclavian artery** MCC UNS
  6th **S25.11 Minor laceration of innominate or subclavian artery**
    Incomplete transection of innominate or subclavian artery
    Laceration of innominate or subclavian artery NOS
    Superficial laceration of innominate or subclavian artery
    7th **S25.111 Minor laceration of right innominate or subclavian artery** MCC
    7th **S25.112 Minor laceration of left innominate or subclavian artery** MCC
    7th **S25.119 Minor laceration of unspecified innominate or subclavian artery** MCC UNS
  6th **S25.12 Major laceration of innominate or subclavian artery**
    Complete transection of innominate or subclavian artery
    Traumatic rupture of innominate or subclavian artery
    7th **S25.121 Major laceration of right innominate or subclavian artery** MCC
    7th **S25.122 Major laceration of left innominate or subclavian artery** MCC
    7th **S25.129 Major laceration of unspecified innominate or subclavian artery** MCC UNS
  6th **S25.19 Other specified injury of innominate or subclavian artery**
    7th **S25.191 Other specified injury of right innominate or subclavian artery** MCC
    7th **S25.192 Other specified injury of left innominate or subclavian artery** MCC
    7th **S25.199 Other specified injury of unspecified innominate or subclavian artery** MCC UNS

5th **S25.2 Injury of superior vena cava**
  Injury of vena cava NOS
  x7th **S25.2Ø Unspecified injury of superior vena cava** MCC
  x7th **S25.21 Minor laceration of superior vena cava** MCC
    Incomplete transection of superior vena cava
    Laceration of superior vena cava NOS
    Superficial laceration of superior vena cava
  x7th **S25.22 Major laceration of superior vena cava** MCC
    Complete transection of superior vena cava
    Traumatic rupture of superior vena cava
  x7th **S25.29 Other specified injury of superior vena cava** MCC

5th **S25.3 Injury of innominate or subclavian vein**
  6th **S25.3Ø Unspecified injury of innominate or subclavian vein**
    7th **S25.3Ø1 Unspecified injury of right innominate or subclavian vein** MCC
    7th **S25.3Ø2 Unspecified injury of left innominate or subclavian vein** MCC
    7th **S25.3Ø9 Unspecified injury of unspecified innominate or subclavian vein** MCC UNS
  6th **S25.31 Minor laceration of innominate or subclavian vein**
    Incomplete transection of innominate or subclavian vein
    Laceration of innominate or subclavian vein NOS
    Superficial laceration of innominate or subclavian vein
    7th **S25.311 Minor laceration of right innominate or subclavian vein** MCC
    7th **S25.312 Minor laceration of left innominate or subclavian vein** MCC
    7th **S25.319 Minor laceration of unspecified innominate or subclavian vein** MCC UNS
  6th **S25.32 Major laceration of innominate or subclavian vein**
    Complete transection of innominate or subclavian vein
    Traumatic rupture of innominate or subclavian vein
    7th **S25.321 Major laceration of right innominate or subclavian vein** MCC
    7th **S25.322 Major laceration of left innominate or subclavian vein** MCC
    7th **S25.329 Major laceration of unspecified innominate or subclavian vein** MCC UNS
  6th **S25.39 Other specified injury of innominate or subclavian vein**
    7th **S25.391 Other specified injury of right innominate or subclavian vein** MCC
    7th **S25.392 Other specified injury of left innominate or subclavian vein** MCC
    7th **S25.399 Other specified injury of unspecified innominate or subclavian vein** MCC UNS

5th **S25.4 Injury of pulmonary blood vessels**
  6th **S25.4Ø Unspecified injury of pulmonary blood vessels**
    7th **S25.4Ø1 Unspecified injury of right pulmonary blood vessels** MCC
    7th **S25.4Ø2 Unspecified injury of left pulmonary blood vessels** MCC
    7th **S25.4Ø9 Unspecified injury of unspecified pulmonary blood vessels** MCC UNS
  6th **S25.41 Minor laceration of pulmonary blood vessels**
    Incomplete transection of pulmonary blood vessels
    Laceration of pulmonary blood vessels NOS
    Superficial laceration of pulmonary blood vessels
    7th **S25.411 Minor laceration of right pulmonary blood vessels** MCC
    7th **S25.412 Minor laceration of left pulmonary blood vessels** MCC
    7th **S25.419 Minor laceration of unspecified pulmonary blood vessels** MCC UNS
  6th **S25.42 Major laceration of pulmonary blood vessels**
    Complete transection of pulmonary blood vessels
    Traumatic rupture of pulmonary blood vessels
    7th **S25.421 Major laceration of right pulmonary blood vessels** MCC
    7th **S25.422 Major laceration of left pulmonary blood vessels** MCC
    7th **S25.429 Major laceration of unspecified pulmonary blood vessels** MCC UNS
  6th **S25.49 Other specified injury of pulmonary blood vessels**
    7th **S25.491 Other specified injury of right pulmonary blood vessels** MCC
    7th **S25.492 Other specified injury of left pulmonary blood vessels** MCC
    7th **S25.499 Other specified injury of unspecified pulmonary blood vessels** MCC UNS

5th **S25.5 Injury of intercostal blood vessels**
  6th **S25.5Ø Unspecified injury of intercostal blood vessels**
    7th **S25.5Ø1 Unspecified injury of intercostal blood vessels, right side** CC
    7th **S25.5Ø2 Unspecified injury of intercostal blood vessels, left side** CC

S25.509 Unspecified injury of intercostal blood vessels, unspecified side CC UNS

S25.51 Laceration of intercostal blood vessels

S25.511 Laceration of intercostal blood vessels, right side CC

S25.512 Laceration of intercostal blood vessels, left side CC

S25.519 Laceration of intercostal blood vessels, unspecified side CC UNS

S25.59 Other specified injury of intercostal blood vessels

S25.591 Other specified injury of intercostal blood vessels, right side CC

S25.592 Other specified injury of intercostal blood vessels, left side CC

S25.599 Other specified injury of intercostal blood vessels, unspecified side CC UNS

S25.8 Injury of other blood vessels of thorax

Injury of azygos vein

Injury of mammary artery or vein

S25.80 Unspecified injury of other blood vessels of thorax

S25.801 Unspecified injury of other blood vessels of thorax, right side CC

S25.802 Unspecified injury of other blood vessels of thorax, left side CC

S25.809 Unspecified injury of other blood vessels of thorax, unspecified side CC UNS

S25.81 Laceration of other blood vessels of thorax

S25.811 Laceration of other blood vessels of thorax, right side CC

S25.812 Laceration of other blood vessels of thorax, left side CC

S25.819 Laceration of other blood vessels of thorax, unspecified side CC UNS

S25.89 Other specified injury of other blood vessels of thorax

S25.891 Other specified injury of other blood vessels of thorax, right side CC

S25.892 Other specified injury of other blood vessels of thorax, left side CC

S25.899 Other specified injury of other blood vessels of thorax, unspecified side CC UNS

S25.9 Injury of unspecified blood vessel of thorax

S25.90 Unspecified injury of unspecified blood vessel of thorax CC UNS

S25.91 Laceration of unspecified blood vessel of thorax CC UNS

S25.99 Other specified injury of unspecified blood vessel of thorax CC UNS

S26 Injury of heart

Code also any associated:

open wound of thorax (S21.-)

traumatic hemopneumothorax (S27.2)

traumatic hemothorax (S27.1)

traumatic pneumothorax (S27.0)

The appropriate 7th character is to be added to each code from category S26.

A initial encounter

D subsequent encounter

S sequela

S26.0 Injury of heart with hemopericardium

S26.00 Unspecified injury of heart with hemopericardium CC

S26.01 Contusion of heart with hemopericardium CC

S26.02 Laceration of heart with hemopericardium

S26.020 Mild laceration of heart with hemopericardium MCC

Laceration of heart without penetration of heart chamber

S26.021 Moderate laceration of heart with hemopericardium MCC

Laceration of heart with penetration of heart chamber

S26.022 Major laceration of heart with hemopericardium MCC

Laceration of heart with penetration of multiple heart chambers

S26.09 Other injury of heart with hemopericardium CC

S26.1 Injury of heart without hemopericardium

S26.10 Unspecified injury of heart without hemopericardium CC

S26.11 Contusion of heart without hemopericardium CC

S26.12 Laceration of heart without hemopericardium MCC

S26.19 Other injury of heart without hemopericardium CC

S26.9 Injury of heart, unspecified with or without hemopericardium

S26.90 Unspecified injury of heart, unspecified with or without hemopericardium CC

S26.91 Contusion of heart, unspecified with or without hemopericardium CC

DEF: Bruising within the heart muscle, with no mention of an open wound, usually caused by blunt chest trauma in motor vehicle accidents, falling from great heights, or receiving CPR.

S26.92 Laceration of heart, unspecified with or without hemopericardium MCC

Laceration of heart NOS

AHA: 2019,2Q,24

S26.99 Other injury of heart, unspecified with or without hemopericardium CC

S27 Injury of other and unspecified intrathoracic organs

Code also any associated open wound of thorax (S21.-)

EXCLUDES 2 *injury of cervical esophagus (S10-S19)*

injury of trachea (cervical) (S10-S19)

The appropriate 7th character is to be added to each code from category S27.

A initial encounter

D subsequent encounter

S sequela

S27.0 Traumatic pneumothorax CC

EXCLUDES 1 *spontaneous pneumothorax (J93.-)*

S27.1 Traumatic hemothorax MCC

S27.2 Traumatic hemopneumothorax MCC

S27.3 Other and unspecified injuries of lung

S27.30 Unspecified injury of lung

S27.301 Unspecified injury of lung, unilateral CC

S27.302 Unspecified injury of lung, bilateral CC

S27.309 Unspecified injury of lung, unspecified CC UNS

S27.31 Primary blast injury of lung

Blast injury of lung NOS

S27.311 Primary blast injury of lung, unilateral CC

S27.312 Primary blast injury of lung, bilateral CC

S27.319 Primary blast injury of lung, unspecified CC UNS

S27.32 Contusion of lung

DEF: Bruising of the lung without mention of an open wound.

S27.321 Contusion of lung, unilateral CC

S27.322 Contusion of lung, bilateral CC

S27.329 Contusion of lung, unspecified CC UNS

S27.33 Laceration of lung

S27.331 Laceration of lung, unilateral MCC

S27.332 Laceration of lung, bilateral MCC

S27.339 Laceration of lung, unspecified MCC UNS

S27.39 Other injuries of lung

Secondary blast injury of lung

S27.391 Other injuries of lung, unilateral CC

S27.392 Other injuries of lung, bilateral CC

7th **S27.399** Other injuries of lung, unspecified CC UNS

5th **S27.4 Injury of bronchus**

6th **S27.40 Unspecified injury of bronchus**

7th **S27.401** Unspecified injury of bronchus, unilateral MCC

7th **S27.402** Unspecified injury of bronchus, bilateral MCC

7th **S27.409** Unspecified injury of bronchus, unspecified MCC UNS

6th **S27.41 Primary blast injury of bronchus**

Blast injury of bronchus NOS

7th **S27.411** Primary blast injury of bronchus, unilateral MCC

7th **S27.412** Primary blast injury of bronchus, bilateral MCC

7th **S27.419** Primary blast injury of bronchus, unspecified MCC UNS

6th **S27.42 Contusion of bronchus**

7th **S27.421** Contusion of bronchus, unilateral MCC

7th **S27.422** Contusion of bronchus, bilateral MCC

7th **S27.429** Contusion of bronchus, unspecified MCC UNS

6th **S27.43 Laceration of bronchus**

7th **S27.431** Laceration of bronchus, unilateral MCC

7th **S27.432** Laceration of bronchus, bilateral MCC

7th **S27.439** Laceration of bronchus, unspecified MCC UNS

6th **S27.49 Other injury of bronchus**

Secondary blast injury of bronchus

7th **S27.491** Other injury of bronchus, unilateral MCC

7th **S27.492** Other injury of bronchus, bilateral MCC

7th **S27.499** Other injury of bronchus, unspecified MCC UNS

5th **S27.5 Injury of thoracic trachea**

√x7th **S27.50** Unspecified injury of thoracic trachea CC

√x7th **S27.51** Primary blast injury of thoracic trachea CC

Blast injury of thoracic trachea NOS

√x7th **S27.52** Contusion of thoracic trachea CC

√x7th **S27.53** Laceration of thoracic trachea CC

√x7th **S27.59** Other injury of thoracic trachea CC

Secondary blast injury of thoracic trachea

5th **S27.6 Injury of pleura**

√x7th **S27.60** Unspecified injury of pleura CC

√x7th **S27.63** Laceration of pleura CC

√x7th **S27.69** Other injury of pleura CC

5th **S27.8 Injury of other specified intrathoracic organs**

6th **S27.80 Injury of diaphragm**

7th **S27.802** Contusion of diaphragm CC

7th **S27.803** Laceration of diaphragm CC

7th **S27.808** Other injury of diaphragm CC

7th **S27.809** Unspecified injury of diaphragm CC

6th **S27.81 Injury of esophagus (thoracic part)**

7th **S27.812** Contusion of esophagus (thoracic part) MCC

7th **S27.813** Laceration of esophagus (thoracic part) MCC

7th **S27.818** Other injury of esophagus (thoracic part) MCC

7th **S27.819** Unspecified injury of esophagus (thoracic part) MCC

6th **S27.89 Injury of other specified intrathoracic organs**

Injury of lymphatic thoracic duct

Injury of thymus gland

7th **S27.892** Contusion of other specified intrathoracic organs CC

7th **S27.893** Laceration of other specified intrathoracic organs CC

7th **S27.898** Other injury of other specified intrathoracic organs CC

7th **S27.899** Unspecified injury of other specified intrathoracic organs CC

√x7th **S27.9** Injury of unspecified intrathoracic organ CC

4th **S28 Crushing injury of thorax, and traumatic amputation of part of thorax**

The appropriate 7th character is to be added to each code from category S28.
A initial encounter
D subsequent encounter
S sequela

√x7th **S28.0 Crushed chest**

Use additional code for all associated injuries

EXCLUDES 1 *flail chest (S22.5)*

√x7th **S28.1** Traumatic amputation (partial) of part of thorax, except breast CC

5th **S28.2 Traumatic amputation of breast**

6th **S28.21 Complete traumatic amputation of breast**

Traumatic amputation of breast NOS

7th **S28.211** Complete traumatic amputation of right breast

7th **S28.212** Complete traumatic amputation of left breast

7th **S28.219** Complete traumatic amputation of unspecified breast

6th **S28.22 Partial traumatic amputation of breast**

7th **S28.221** Partial traumatic amputation of right breast

7th **S28.222** Partial traumatic amputation of left breast

7th **S28.229** Partial traumatic amputation of unspecified breast

4th **S29 Other and unspecified injuries of thorax**

Code also any associated open wound (S21.-)

The appropriate 7th character is to be added to each code from category S29.
A initial encounter
D subsequent encounter
S sequela

5th **S29.0 Injury of muscle and tendon at thorax level**

6th **S29.00 Unspecified injury of muscle and tendon of thorax**

7th **S29.001** Unspecified injury of muscle and tendon of front wall of thorax

7th **S29.002** Unspecified injury of muscle and tendon of back wall of thorax

7th **S29.009** Unspecified injury of muscle and tendon of unspecified wall of thorax

6th **S29.01 Strain of muscle and tendon of thorax**

7th **S29.011** Strain of muscle and tendon of front wall of thorax

7th **S29.012** Strain of muscle and tendon of back wall of thorax

7th **S29.019** Strain of muscle and tendon of unspecified wall of thorax

6th **S29.02 Laceration of muscle and tendon of thorax**

7th **S29.021** Laceration of muscle and tendon of front wall of thorax CC

7th **S29.022** Laceration of muscle and tendon of back wall of thorax

7th **S29.029** Laceration of muscle and tendon of unspecified wall of thorax CC UNS

6th **S29.09 Other injury of muscle and tendon of thorax**

7th **S29.091** Other injury of muscle and tendon of front wall of thorax

7th **S29.092** Other injury of muscle and tendon of back wall of thorax

7th **S29.099** Other injury of muscle and tendon of unspecified wall of thorax

√x7th **S29.8** Other specified injuries of thorax

√x7th **S29.9** Unspecified injury of thorax

Injuries to the abdomen, lower back, lumbar spine, pelvis and external genitals (S30-S39)

INCLUDES injuries to the abdominal wall
injuries to the anus
injuries to the buttock
injuries to the external genitalia
injuries to the flank
injuries to the groin

EXCLUDES 2 *burns and corrosions (T20-T32)*
effects of foreign body in anus and rectum (T18.5)
effects of foreign body in genitourinary tract (T19.-)
effects of foreign body in stomach, small intestine and colon (T18.2-T18.4)
frostbite (T33-T34)
insect bite or sting, venomous (T63.4)

S30 Superficial injury of abdomen, lower back, pelvis and external genitals

EXCLUDES 2 *superficial injury of hip (S70.-)*

The appropriate 7th character is to be added to each code from category S30.
A initial encounter
D subsequent encounter
S sequela

S30.0 Contusion of lower back and pelvis
Contusion of buttock

S30.1 Contusion of abdominal wall
Contusion of flank
Contusion of groin

S30.2 Contusion of external genital organs

S30.20 Contusion of unspecified external genital organ
S30.201 Contusion of unspecified external genital organ, male ♂
S30.202 Contusion of unspecified external genital organ, female ♀

S30.21 Contusion of penis ♂
S30.22 Contusion of scrotum and testes ♂
S30.23 Contusion of vagina and vulva ♀

S30.3 Contusion of anus

S30.8 Other superficial injuries of abdomen, lower back, pelvis and external genitals

S30.81 Abrasion of abdomen, lower back, pelvis and external genitals
S30.810 Abrasion of lower back and pelvis
S30.811 Abrasion of abdominal wall
S30.812 Abrasion of penis ♂
S30.813 Abrasion of scrotum and testes ♂
S30.814 Abrasion of vagina and vulva ♀
S30.815 Abrasion of unspecified external genital organs, male ♂
S30.816 Abrasion of unspecified external genital organs, female ♀
S30.817 Abrasion of anus

S30.82 Blister (nonthermal) of abdomen, lower back, pelvis and external genitals
S30.820 Blister (nonthermal) of lower back and pelvis
S30.821 Blister (nonthermal) of abdominal wall
S30.822 Blister (nonthermal) of penis ♂
S30.823 Blister (nonthermal) of scrotum and testes ♂
S30.824 Blister (nonthermal) of vagina and vulva ♀
S30.825 Blister (nonthermal) of unspecified external genital organs, male ♂
S30.826 Blister (nonthermal) of unspecified external genital organs, female ♀
S30.827 Blister (nonthermal) of anus

S30.84 External constriction of abdomen, lower back, pelvis and external genitals
S30.840 External constriction of lower back and pelvis
S30.841 External constriction of abdominal wall
S30.842 External constriction of penis ♂
Hair tourniquet syndrome of penis
Use additional cause code to identify the constricting item (W49.0-)
S30.843 External constriction of scrotum and testes ♂
S30.844 External constriction of vagina and vulva ♀
S30.845 External constriction of unspecified external genital organs, male ♂
S30.846 External constriction of unspecified external genital organs, female ♀

S30.85 Superficial foreign body of abdomen, lower back, pelvis and external genitals
Splinter in the abdomen, lower back, pelvis and external genitals
S30.850 Superficial foreign body of lower back and pelvis
S30.851 Superficial foreign body of abdominal wall
S30.852 Superficial foreign body of penis ♂
S30.853 Superficial foreign body of scrotum and testes ♂
S30.854 Superficial foreign body of vagina and vulva ♀
S30.855 Superficial foreign body of unspecified external genital organs, male ♂
S30.856 Superficial foreign body of unspecified external genital organs, female ♀
S30.857 Superficial foreign body of anus

S30.86 Insect bite (nonvenomous) of abdomen, lower back, pelvis and external genitals
S30.860 Insect bite (nonvenomous) of lower back and pelvis
S30.861 Insect bite (nonvenomous) of abdominal wall
S30.862 Insect bite (nonvenomous) of penis ♂
S30.863 Insect bite (nonvenomous) of scrotum and testes ♂
S30.864 Insect bite (nonvenomous) of vagina and vulva ♀
S30.865 Insect bite (nonvenomous) of unspecified external genital organs, male ♂
S30.866 Insect bite (nonvenomous) of unspecified external genital organs, female ♀
S30.867 Insect bite (nonvenomous) of anus

S30.87 Other superficial bite of abdomen, lower back, pelvis and external genitals

EXCLUDES 1 *open bite of abdomen, lower back, pelvis and external genitals (S31.05, S31.15, S31.25, S31.35, S31.45, S31.55)*

S30.870 Other superficial bite of lower back and pelvis
S30.871 Other superficial bite of abdominal wall
S30.872 Other superficial bite of penis ♂
S30.873 Other superficial bite of scrotum and testes ♂
S30.874 Other superficial bite of vagina and vulva ♀
S30.875 Other superficial bite of unspecified external genital organs, male ♂
S30.876 Other superficial bite of unspecified external genital organs, female ♀
S30.877 Other superficial bite of anus

S30.9 Unspecified superficial injury of abdomen, lower back, pelvis and external genitals
S30.91 Unspecified superficial injury of lower back and pelvis
S30.92 Unspecified superficial injury of abdominal wall
S30.93 Unspecified superficial injury of penis ♂
S30.94 Unspecified superficial injury of scrotum and testes ♂
S30.95 Unspecified superficial injury of vagina and vulva ♀
S30.96 Unspecified superficial injury of unspecified external genital organs, male ♂
S30.97 Unspecified superficial injury of unspecified external genital organs, female ♀
S30.98 Unspecified superficial injury of anus

S31 Open wound of abdomen, lower back, pelvis and external genitals

Code also any associated:
spinal cord injury (S24.0, S24.1-, S34.0-, S34.1-)
wound infection

EXCLUDES 1 *traumatic amputation of part of abdomen, lower back and pelvis (S38.2-, S38.3)*

EXCLUDES 2 *open wound of hip (S71.00-S71.02)*
open fracture of pelvis (S32.1- - S32.9 with 7th character B)

The appropriate 7th character is to be added to each code from category S31.
A initial encounter
D subsequent encounter
S sequela

S31.0 Open wound of lower back and pelvis

S31.00 Unspecified open wound of lower back and pelvis

S31.000 Unspecified open wound of lower back and pelvis without penetration into retroperitoneum
Unspecified open wound of lower back and pelvis NOS

S31.001 Unspecified open wound of lower back and pelvis with penetration into retroperitoneum MCC

S31.01 Laceration without foreign body of lower back and pelvis

S31.010 Laceration without foreign body of lower back and pelvis without penetration into retroperitoneum
Laceration without foreign body of lower back and pelvis NOS

S31.011 Laceration without foreign body of lower back and pelvis with penetration into retroperitoneum MCC

S31.02 Laceration with foreign body of lower back and pelvis

S31.020 Laceration with foreign body of lower back and pelvis without penetration into retroperitoneum
Laceration with foreign body of lower back and pelvis NOS

S31.021 Laceration with foreign body of lower back and pelvis with penetration into retroperitoneum MCC

S31.03 Puncture wound without foreign body of lower back and pelvis

S31.030 Puncture wound without foreign body of lower back and pelvis without penetration into retroperitoneum
Puncture wound without foreign body of lower back and pelvis NOS

S31.031 Puncture wound without foreign body of lower back and pelvis with penetration into retroperitoneum MCC

S31.04 Puncture wound with foreign body of lower back and pelvis

S31.040 Puncture wound with foreign body of lower back and pelvis without penetration into retroperitoneum
Puncture wound with foreign body of lower back and pelvis NOS

S31.041 Puncture wound with foreign body of lower back and pelvis with penetration into retroperitoneum MCC

S31.05 Open bite of lower back and pelvis
Bite of lower back and pelvis NOS

EXCLUDES 1 *superficial bite of lower back and pelvis (S30.860, S30.870)*

S31.050 Open bite of lower back and pelvis without penetration into retroperitoneum
Open bite of lower back and pelvis NOS

S31.051 Open bite of lower back and pelvis with penetration into retroperitoneum MCC

S31.1 Open wound of abdominal wall without penetration into peritoneal cavity
Open wound of abdominal wall NOS

EXCLUDES 2 *open wound of abdominal wall with penetration into peritoneal cavity (S31.6-)*

S31.10 Unspecified open wound of abdominal wall without penetration into peritoneal cavity

S31.100 Unspecified open wound of abdominal wall, right upper quadrant without penetration into peritoneal cavity

S31.101 Unspecified open wound of abdominal wall, left upper quadrant without penetration into peritoneal cavity

S31.102 Unspecified open wound of abdominal wall, epigastric region without penetration into peritoneal cavity

S31.103 Unspecified open wound of abdominal wall, right lower quadrant without penetration into peritoneal cavity

S31.104 Unspecified open wound of abdominal wall, left lower quadrant without penetration into peritoneal cavity

S31.105 Unspecified open wound of abdominal wall, periumbilic region without penetration into peritoneal cavity

S31.109 Unspecified open wound of abdominal wall, unspecified quadrant without penetration into peritoneal cavity
Unspecified open wound of abdominal wall NOS

S31.11 Laceration without foreign body of abdominal wall without penetration into peritoneal cavity

S31.110 Laceration without foreign body of abdominal wall, right upper quadrant without penetration into peritoneal cavity

S31.111 Laceration without foreign body of abdominal wall, left upper quadrant without penetration into peritoneal cavity

S31.112 Laceration without foreign body of abdominal wall, epigastric region without penetration into peritoneal cavity

S31.113 Laceration without foreign body of abdominal wall, right lower quadrant without penetration into peritoneal cavity

S31.114 Laceration without foreign body of abdominal wall, left lower quadrant without penetration into peritoneal cavity

S31.115 Laceration without foreign body of abdominal wall, periumbilic region without penetration into peritoneal cavity

S31.119 Laceration without foreign body of abdominal wall, unspecified quadrant without penetration into peritoneal cavity

S31.12 Laceration with foreign body of abdominal wall without penetration into peritoneal cavity

S31.120 Laceration of abdominal wall with foreign body, right upper quadrant without penetration into peritoneal cavity

S31.121 Laceration of abdominal wall with foreign body, left upper quadrant without penetration into peritoneal cavity

S31.122 Laceration of abdominal wall with foreign body, epigastric region without penetration into peritoneal cavity

S31.123 Laceration of abdominal wall with foreign body, right lower quadrant without penetration into peritoneal cavity

S31.124 Laceration of abdominal wall with foreign body, left lower quadrant without penetration into peritoneal cavity

S31.125 Laceration of abdominal wall with foreign body, periumbilic region without penetration into peritoneal cavity

S31.129 Laceration of abdominal wall with foreign body, unspecified quadrant without penetration into peritoneal cavity

S31.13 Puncture wound of abdominal wall without foreign body without penetration into peritoneal cavity
- S31.130 Puncture wound of abdominal wall without foreign body, right upper quadrant without penetration into peritoneal cavity
- S31.131 Puncture wound of abdominal wall without foreign body, left upper quadrant without penetration into peritoneal cavity
- S31.132 Puncture wound of abdominal wall without foreign body, epigastric region without penetration into peritoneal cavity
- S31.133 Puncture wound of abdominal wall without foreign body, right lower quadrant without penetration into peritoneal cavity
- S31.134 Puncture wound of abdominal wall without foreign body, left lower quadrant without penetration into peritoneal cavity
- S31.135 Puncture wound of abdominal wall without foreign body, periumbilic region without penetration into peritoneal cavity
- S31.139 Puncture wound of abdominal wall without foreign body, unspecified quadrant without penetration into peritoneal cavity

S31.14 Puncture wound of abdominal wall with foreign body without penetration into peritoneal cavity
- S31.140 Puncture wound of abdominal wall with foreign body, right upper quadrant without penetration into peritoneal cavity
- S31.141 Puncture wound of abdominal wall with foreign body, left upper quadrant without penetration into peritoneal cavity
- S31.142 Puncture wound of abdominal wall with foreign body, epigastric region without penetration into peritoneal cavity
- S31.143 Puncture wound of abdominal wall with foreign body, right lower quadrant without penetration into peritoneal cavity
- S31.144 Puncture wound of abdominal wall with foreign body, left lower quadrant without penetration into peritoneal cavity
- S31.145 Puncture wound of abdominal wall with foreign body, periumbilic region without penetration into peritoneal cavity
- S31.149 Puncture wound of abdominal wall with foreign body, unspecified quadrant without penetration into peritoneal cavity

S31.15 Open bite of abdominal wall without penetration into peritoneal cavity
Bite of abdominal wall NOS
EXCLUDES 1 *superficial bite of abdominal wall (S30.871)*
- S31.150 Open bite of abdominal wall, right upper quadrant without penetration into peritoneal cavity
- S31.151 Open bite of abdominal wall, left upper quadrant without penetration into peritoneal cavity
- S31.152 Open bite of abdominal wall, epigastric region without penetration into peritoneal cavity
- S31.153 Open bite of abdominal wall, right lower quadrant without penetration into peritoneal cavity
- S31.154 Open bite of abdominal wall, left lower quadrant without penetration into peritoneal cavity
- S31.155 Open bite of abdominal wall, periumbilic region without penetration into peritoneal cavity
- S31.159 Open bite of abdominal wall, unspecified quadrant without penetration into peritoneal cavity

S31.2 Open wound of penis
- S31.20 Unspecified open wound of penis ♂
- S31.21 Laceration without foreign body of penis ♂
- S31.22 Laceration with foreign body of penis ♂
- S31.23 Puncture wound without foreign body of penis ♂
- S31.24 Puncture wound with foreign body of penis ♂
- S31.25 Open bite of penis ♂
  Bite of penis NOS
  EXCLUDES 1 *superficial bite of penis (S30.862, S30.872)*

S31.3 Open wound of scrotum and testes
- S31.30 Unspecified open wound of scrotum and testes ♂
- S31.31 Laceration without foreign body of scrotum and testes ♂
- S31.32 Laceration with foreign body of scrotum and testes ♂
- S31.33 Puncture wound without foreign body of scrotum and testes ♂
- S31.34 Puncture wound with foreign body of scrotum and testes ♂
- S31.35 Open bite of scrotum and testes ♂
  Bite of scrotum and testes NOS
  EXCLUDES 1 *superficial bite of scrotum and testes (S30.863, S30.873)*

S31.4 Open wound of vagina and vulva
EXCLUDES 1 *injury to vagina and vulva during delivery (O70.-, O71.4)*
- S31.40 Unspecified open wound of vagina and vulva ♀
- S31.41 Laceration without foreign body of vagina and vulva ♀
- S31.42 Laceration with foreign body of vagina and vulva ♀
- S31.43 Puncture wound without foreign body of vagina and vulva ♀
- S31.44 Puncture wound with foreign body of vagina and vulva ♀
- S31.45 Open bite of vagina and vulva ♀
  Bite of vagina and vulva NOS
  EXCLUDES 1 *superficial bite of vagina and vulva (S30.864, S30.874)*

S31.5 Open wound of unspecified external genital organs
EXCLUDES 1 *traumatic amputation of external genital organs (S38.21, S38.22)*

S31.50 Unspecified open wound of unspecified external genital organs
- S31.501 Unspecified open wound of unspecified external genital organs, male ♂
- S31.502 Unspecified open wound of unspecified external genital organs, female ♀

S31.51 Laceration without foreign body of unspecified external genital organs
- S31.511 Laceration without foreign body of unspecified external genital organs, male ♂
- S31.512 Laceration without foreign body of unspecified external genital organs, female ♀

S31.52 Laceration with foreign body of unspecified external genital organs
- S31.521 Laceration with foreign body of unspecified external genital organs, male ♂
- S31.522 Laceration with foreign body of unspecified external genital organs, female ♀

S31.53 Puncture wound without foreign body of unspecified external genital organs
- S31.531 Puncture wound without foreign body of unspecified external genital organs, male ♂
- S31.532 Puncture wound without foreign body of unspecified external genital organs, female ♀

S31.54 Puncture wound with foreign body of unspecified external genital organs
- S31.541 Puncture wound with foreign body of unspecified external genital organs, male ♂

7th **S31.542** **Puncture wound with foreign body of unspecified external genital organs, female** ♀

6th **S31.55** **Open bite of unspecified external genital organs**

Bite of unspecified external genital organs NOS

EXCLUDES 1 *superficial bite of unspecified external genital organs (S30.865, S30.866, S30.875, S30.876)*

7th **S31.551** **Open bite of unspecified external genital organs, male** ♂

7th **S31.552** **Open bite of unspecified external genital organs, female** ♀

5th **S31.6** **Open wound of abdominal wall with penetration into peritoneal cavity**

6th **S31.60** **Unspecified open wound of abdominal wall with penetration into peritoneal cavity**

7th **S31.600** **Unspecified open wound of abdominal wall, right upper quadrant with penetration into peritoneal cavity** MCC

7th **S31.601** **Unspecified open wound of abdominal wall, left upper quadrant with penetration into peritoneal cavity** MCC

7th **S31.602** **Unspecified open wound of abdominal wall, epigastric region with penetration into peritoneal cavity** MCC

7th **S31.603** **Unspecified open wound of abdominal wall, right lower quadrant with penetration into peritoneal cavity** MCC

7th **S31.604** **Unspecified open wound of abdominal wall, left lower quadrant with penetration into peritoneal cavity** MCC

7th **S31.605** **Unspecified open wound of abdominal wall, periumbilic region with penetration into peritoneal cavity** MCC

7th **S31.609** **Unspecified open wound of abdominal wall, unspecified quadrant with penetration into peritoneal cavity** MCC UNS

6th **S31.61** **Laceration without foreign body of abdominal wall with penetration into peritoneal cavity**

7th **S31.610** **Laceration without foreign body of abdominal wall, right upper quadrant with penetration into peritoneal cavity** MCC

7th **S31.611** **Laceration without foreign body of abdominal wall, left upper quadrant with penetration into peritoneal cavity** MCC

7th **S31.612** **Laceration without foreign body of abdominal wall, epigastric region with penetration into peritoneal cavity** MCC

7th **S31.613** **Laceration without foreign body of abdominal wall, right lower quadrant with penetration into peritoneal cavity** MCC

7th **S31.614** **Laceration without foreign body of abdominal wall, left lower quadrant with penetration into peritoneal cavity** MCC

7th **S31.615** **Laceration without foreign body of abdominal wall, periumbilic region with penetration into peritoneal cavity** MCC

7th **S31.619** **Laceration without foreign body of abdominal wall, unspecified quadrant with penetration into peritoneal cavity** MCC UNS

6th **S31.62** **Laceration with foreign body of abdominal wall with penetration into peritoneal cavity**

7th **S31.620** **Laceration with foreign body of abdominal wall, right upper quadrant with penetration into peritoneal cavity** MCC

7th **S31.621** **Laceration with foreign body of abdominal wall, left upper quadrant with penetration into peritoneal cavity** MCC

7th **S31.622** **Laceration with foreign body of abdominal wall, epigastric region with penetration into peritoneal cavity** MCC

7th **S31.623** **Laceration with foreign body of abdominal wall, right lower quadrant with penetration into peritoneal cavity** MCC

7th **S31.624** **Laceration with foreign body of abdominal wall, left lower quadrant with penetration into peritoneal cavity** MCC

7th **S31.625** **Laceration with foreign body of abdominal wall, periumbilic region with penetration into peritoneal cavity** MCC

7th **S31.629** **Laceration with foreign body of abdominal wall, unspecified quadrant with penetration into peritoneal cavity** MCC UNS

6th **S31.63** **Puncture wound without foreign body of abdominal wall with penetration into peritoneal cavity**

7th **S31.630** **Puncture wound without foreign body of abdominal wall, right upper quadrant with penetration into peritoneal cavity** MCC

7th **S31.631** **Puncture wound without foreign body of abdominal wall, left upper quadrant with penetration into peritoneal cavity** MCC

7th **S31.632** **Puncture wound without foreign body of abdominal wall, epigastric region with penetration into peritoneal cavity** MCC

7th **S31.633** **Puncture wound without foreign body of abdominal wall, right lower quadrant with penetration into peritoneal cavity** MCC

7th **S31.634** **Puncture wound without foreign body of abdominal wall, left lower quadrant with penetration into peritoneal cavity** MCC

7th **S31.635** **Puncture wound without foreign body of abdominal wall, periumbilic region with penetration into peritoneal cavity** MCC

7th **S31.639** **Puncture wound without foreign body of abdominal wall, unspecified quadrant with penetration into peritoneal cavity** MCC UNS

6th **S31.64** **Puncture wound with foreign body of abdominal wall with penetration into peritoneal cavity**

7th **S31.640** **Puncture wound with foreign body of abdominal wall, right upper quadrant with penetration into peritoneal cavity** MCC

7th **S31.641** **Puncture wound with foreign body of abdominal wall, left upper quadrant with penetration into peritoneal cavity** MCC

7th **S31.642** **Puncture wound with foreign body of abdominal wall, epigastric region with penetration into peritoneal cavity** MCC

7th **S31.643** **Puncture wound with foreign body of abdominal wall, right lower quadrant with penetration into peritoneal cavity** MCC

7th **S31.644** **Puncture wound with foreign body of abdominal wall, left lower quadrant with penetration into peritoneal cavity** MCC

7th **S31.645** **Puncture wound with foreign body of abdominal wall, periumbilic region with penetration into peritoneal cavity** MCC

7th **S31.649** **Puncture wound with foreign body of abdominal wall, unspecified quadrant with penetration into peritoneal cavity** MCC UNS

6th **S31.65** **Open bite of abdominal wall with penetration into peritoneal cavity**

EXCLUDES 1 *superficial bite of abdominal wall (S30.861, S30.871)*

7th **S31.650** **Open bite of abdominal wall, right upper quadrant with penetration into peritoneal cavity** MCC

7th **S31.651** **Open bite of abdominal wall, left upper quadrant with penetration into peritoneal cavity** MCC

7th **S31.652** **Open bite of abdominal wall, epigastric region with penetration into peritoneal cavity** MCC

7th **S31.653** **Open bite of abdominal wall, right lower quadrant with penetration into peritoneal cavity** MCC

7th **S31.654** **Open bite of abdominal wall, left lower quadrant with penetration into peritoneal cavity** MCC

7th **S31.655** **Open bite of abdominal wall, periumbilic region with penetration into peritoneal cavity** MCC

7th **S31.659** **Open bite of abdominal wall, unspecified quadrant with penetration into peritoneal cavity** MCC UNS

S31.8 Open wound of other parts of abdomen, lower back and pelvis

S31.80 Open wound of unspecified buttock

S31.801 Laceration without foreign body of unspecified buttock

S31.802 Laceration with foreign body of unspecified buttock

S31.803 Puncture wound without foreign body of unspecified buttock

S31.804 Puncture wound with foreign body of unspecified buttock

S31.805 Open bite of unspecified buttock

Bite of buttock NOS

EXCLUDES 1 *superficial bite of buttock (S30.870)*

S31.809 Unspecified open wound of unspecified buttock

S31.81 Open wound of right buttock

S31.811 Laceration without foreign body of right buttock

S31.812 Laceration with foreign body of right buttock

S31.813 Puncture wound without foreign body of right buttock

S31.814 Puncture wound with foreign body of right buttock

S31.815 Open bite of right buttock

Bite of right buttock NOS

EXCLUDES 1 *superficial bite of buttock (S30.870)*

S31.819 Unspecified open wound of right buttock

S31.82 Open wound of left buttock

S31.821 Laceration without foreign body of left buttock

S31.822 Laceration with foreign body of left buttock

S31.823 Puncture wound without foreign body of left buttock

S31.824 Puncture wound with foreign body of left buttock

S31.825 Open bite of left buttock

Bite of left buttock NOS

EXCLUDES 1 *superficial bite of buttock (S30.870)*

S31.829 Unspecified open wound of left buttock

S31.83 Open wound of anus

S31.831 Laceration without foreign body of anus

S31.832 Laceration with foreign body of anus

S31.833 Puncture wound without foreign body of anus

S31.834 Puncture wound with foreign body of anus

S31.835 Open bite of anus

Bite of anus NOS

EXCLUDES 1 *superficial bite of anus (S30.877)*

S31.839 Unspecified open wound of anus

S32 Fracture of lumbar spine and pelvis

NOTE A fracture not indicated as displaced or nondisplaced should be coded to displaced.

A fracture not indicated as opened or closed should be coded to closed.

INCLUDES fracture of lumbosacral neural arch
fracture of lumbosacral spinous process
fracture of lumbosacral transverse process
fracture of lumbosacral vertebra
fracture of lumbosacral vertebral arch

Code first any associated spinal cord and spinal nerve injury (S34.-)

EXCLUDES 1 *transection of abdomen (S38.3)*

EXCLUDES 2 *fracture of hip NOS (S72.0-)*

AHA: 2021,1Q,6; 2018,2Q,12; 2015,3Q,37-39; 2012,4Q,93

The appropriate 7th character is to be added to each code from category S32.

- A initial encounter for closed fracture
- B initial encounter for open fracture
- D subsequent encounter for fracture with routine healing
- G subsequent encounter for fracture with delayed healing
- K subsequent encounter for fracture with nonunion
- S sequela

S32.0 Fracture of lumbar vertebra

Fracture of lumbar spine NOS

S32.00 Fracture of unspecified lumbar vertebra

2,3,6 **S32.000 Wedge compression fracture of unspecified lumbar vertebra** MCC CC H5 HCC

2,3,6 **S32.001 Stable burst fracture of unspecified lumbar vertebra** MCC CC H5 HCC

2,3,6 **S32.002 Unstable burst fracture of unspecified lumbar vertebra** MCC CC H5 HCC

2,3,6 **S32.008 Other fracture of unspecified lumbar vertebra** MCC CC H5 HCC

2,3,6 **S32.009 Unspecified fracture of unspecified lumbar vertebra** MCC CC H5 HCC

S32.01 Fracture of first lumbar vertebra

2,3,6 **S32.010 Wedge compression fracture of first lumbar vertebra** MCC CC H5 HCC

2,3,6 **S32.011 Stable burst fracture of first lumbar vertebra** MCC CC H5 HCC

2,3,6 **S32.012 Unstable burst fracture of first lumbar vertebra** MCC CC H5 HCC

2,3,6 **S32.018 Other fracture of first lumbar vertebra** MCC CC H5 HCC

2,3,6 **S32.019 Unspecified fracture of first lumbar vertebra** MCC CC H5 HCC

S32.02 Fracture of second lumbar vertebra

2,3,6 **S32.020 Wedge compression fracture of second lumbar vertebra** MCC CC H5 HCC

2,3,6 **S32.021 Stable burst fracture of second lumbar vertebra** MCC CC H5 HCC

2,3,6 **S32.022 Unstable burst fracture of second lumbar vertebra** MCC CC H5 HCC

2,3,6 **S32.028 Other fracture of second lumbar vertebra** MCC CC H5 HCC

2,3,6 **S32.029 Unspecified fracture of second lumbar vertebra** MCC CC H5 HCC

S32.03 Fracture of third lumbar vertebra

2,3,6 **S32.030 Wedge compression fracture of third lumbar vertebra** MCC CC H5 HCC

2,3,6 **S32.031 Stable burst fracture of third lumbar vertebra** MCC CC H5 HCC

2,3,6 **S32.032 Unstable burst fracture of third lumbar vertebra** MCC CC H5 HCC

2,3,6 **S32.038 Other fracture of third lumbar vertebra** MCC CC H5 HCC

2,3,6 **S32.039 Unspecified fracture of third lumbar vertebra** MCC CC H5 HCC

S32.04 Fracture of fourth lumbar vertebra

2,3,6 **S32.040 Wedge compression fracture of fourth lumbar vertebra** MCC CC H5 HCC

2,3,6 **S32.041 Stable burst fracture of fourth lumbar vertebra** MCC CC H5 HCC

2,3,6 **S32.042 Unstable burst fracture of fourth lumbar vertebra** MCC CC H5 HCC

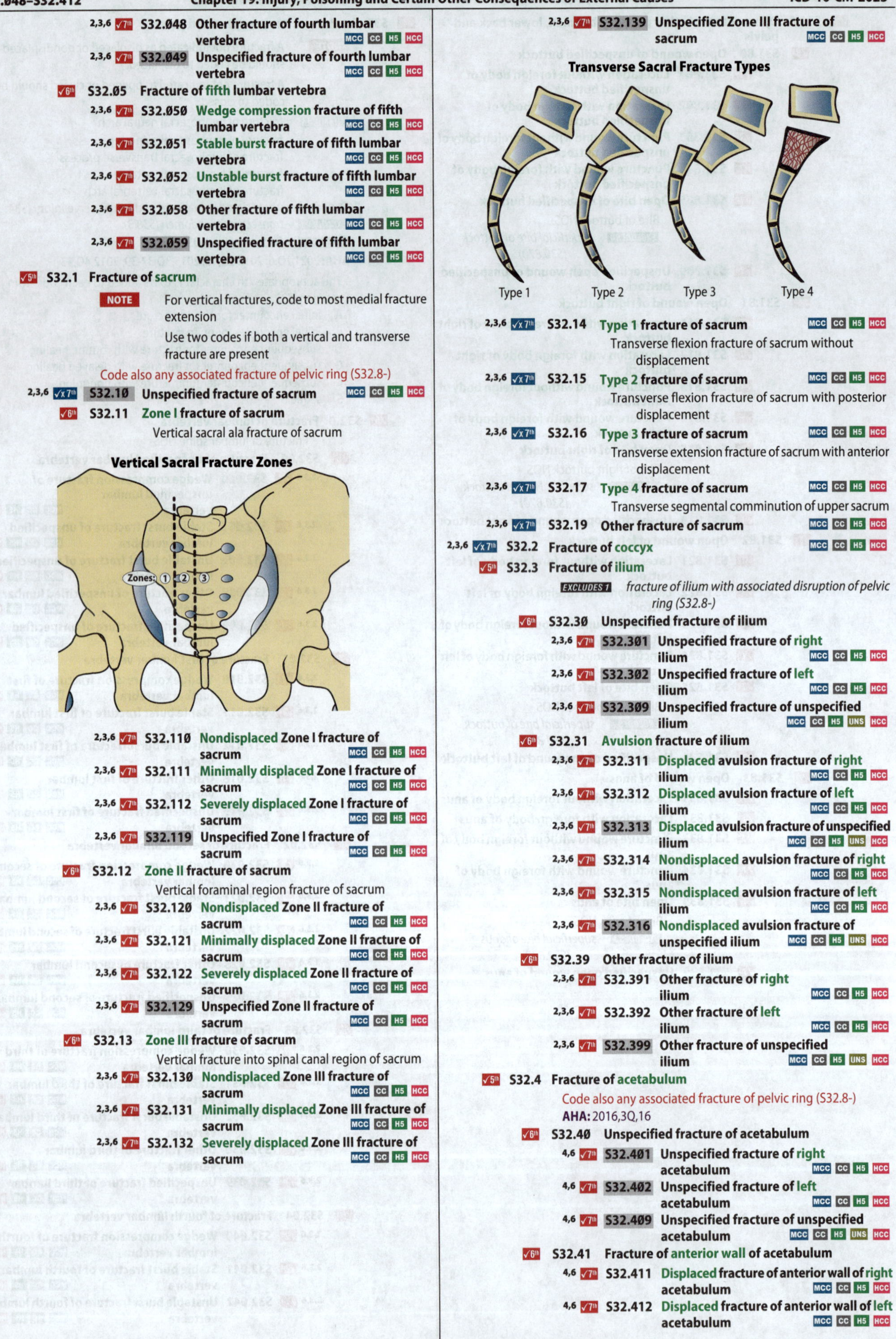

2,3,6 ✓7th **S32.048 Other fracture of fourth lumbar vertebra** MCC CC H5 HCC

2,3,6 ✓7th **S32.049 Unspecified fracture of fourth lumbar vertebra** MCC CC H5 HCC

✓6th **S32.05 Fracture of fifth lumbar vertebra**

2,3,6 ✓7th **S32.050 Wedge compression fracture of fifth lumbar vertebra** MCC CC H5 HCC

2,3,6 ✓7th **S32.051 Stable burst fracture of fifth lumbar vertebra** MCC CC H5 HCC

2,3,6 ✓7th **S32.052 Unstable burst fracture of fifth lumbar vertebra** MCC CC H5 HCC

2,3,6 ✓7th **S32.058 Other fracture of fifth lumbar vertebra** MCC CC H5 HCC

2,3,6 ✓7th **S32.059 Unspecified fracture of fifth lumbar vertebra** MCC CC H5 HCC

✓5th **S32.1 Fracture of sacrum**

NOTE For vertical fractures, code to most medial fracture extension

Use two codes if both a vertical and transverse fracture are present

Code also any associated fracture of pelvic ring (S32.8-)

2,3,6 ✓x7th **S32.10 Unspecified fracture of sacrum** MCC CC H5 HCC

✓6th **S32.11 Zone I fracture of sacrum**

Vertical sacral ala fracture of sacrum

Vertical Sacral Fracture Zones

2,3,6 ✓7th **S32.110 Nondisplaced Zone I fracture of sacrum** MCC CC H5 HCC

2,3,6 ✓7th **S32.111 Minimally displaced Zone I fracture of sacrum** MCC CC H5 HCC

2,3,6 ✓7th **S32.112 Severely displaced Zone I fracture of sacrum** MCC CC H5 HCC

2,3,6 ✓7th **S32.119 Unspecified Zone I fracture of sacrum** MCC CC H5 HCC

✓6th **S32.12 Zone II fracture of sacrum**

Vertical foraminal region fracture of sacrum

2,3,6 ✓7th **S32.120 Nondisplaced Zone II fracture of sacrum** MCC CC H5 HCC

2,3,6 ✓7th **S32.121 Minimally displaced Zone II fracture of sacrum** MCC CC H5 HCC

2,3,6 ✓7th **S32.122 Severely displaced Zone II fracture of sacrum** MCC CC H5 HCC

2,3,6 ✓7th **S32.129 Unspecified Zone II fracture of sacrum** MCC CC H5 HCC

✓6th **S32.13 Zone III fracture of sacrum**

Vertical fracture into spinal canal region of sacrum

2,3,6 ✓7th **S32.130 Nondisplaced Zone III fracture of sacrum** MCC CC H5 HCC

2,3,6 ✓7th **S32.131 Minimally displaced Zone III fracture of sacrum** MCC CC H5 HCC

2,3,6 ✓7th **S32.132 Severely displaced Zone III fracture of sacrum** MCC CC H5 HCC

2,3,6 ✓7th **S32.139 Unspecified Zone III fracture of sacrum** MCC CC H5 HCC

Transverse Sacral Fracture Types

2,3,6 ✓x7th **S32.14 Type 1 fracture of sacrum** MCC CC H5 HCC

Transverse flexion fracture of sacrum without displacement

2,3,6 ✓x7th **S32.15 Type 2 fracture of sacrum** MCC CC H5 HCC

Transverse flexion fracture of sacrum with posterior displacement

2,3,6 ✓x7th **S32.16 Type 3 fracture of sacrum** MCC CC H5 HCC

Transverse extension fracture of sacrum with anterior displacement

2,3,6 ✓x7th **S32.17 Type 4 fracture of sacrum** MCC CC H5 HCC

Transverse segmental comminution of upper sacrum

2,3,6 ✓x7th **S32.19 Other fracture of sacrum** MCC CC H5 HCC

2,3,6 ✓x7th **S32.2 Fracture of coccyx** MCC CC H5 HCC

✓5th **S32.3 Fracture of ilium**

EXCLUDES 1 *fracture of ilium with associated disruption of pelvic ring (S32.8-)*

✓6th **S32.30 Unspecified fracture of ilium**

2,3,6 ✓7th **S32.301 Unspecified fracture of right ilium** MCC CC H5 HCC

2,3,6 ✓7th **S32.302 Unspecified fracture of left ilium** MCC CC H5 HCC

2,3,6 ✓7th **S32.309 Unspecified fracture of unspecified ilium** MCC CC H5 UNS HCC

✓6th **S32.31 Avulsion fracture of ilium**

2,3,6 ✓7th **S32.311 Displaced avulsion fracture of right ilium** MCC CC H5 HCC

2,3,6 ✓7th **S32.312 Displaced avulsion fracture of left ilium** MCC CC H5 HCC

2,3,6 ✓7th **S32.313 Displaced avulsion fracture of unspecified ilium** MCC CC H5 UNS HCC

2,3,6 ✓7th **S32.314 Nondisplaced avulsion fracture of right ilium** MCC CC H5 HCC

2,3,6 ✓7th **S32.315 Nondisplaced avulsion fracture of left ilium** MCC CC H5 HCC

2,3,6 ✓7th **S32.316 Nondisplaced avulsion fracture of unspecified ilium** MCC CC H5 UNS HCC

✓6th **S32.39 Other fracture of ilium**

2,3,6 ✓7th **S32.391 Other fracture of right ilium** MCC CC H5 HCC

2,3,6 ✓7th **S32.392 Other fracture of left ilium** MCC CC H5 HCC

2,3,6 ✓7th **S32.399 Other fracture of unspecified ilium** MCC CC H5 UNS HCC

✓5th **S32.4 Fracture of acetabulum**

Code also any associated fracture of pelvic ring (S32.8-)

AHA: 2016,3Q,16

✓6th **S32.40 Unspecified fracture of acetabulum**

4,6 ✓7th **S32.401 Unspecified fracture of right acetabulum** MCC CC H5 HCC

4,6 ✓7th **S32.402 Unspecified fracture of left acetabulum** MCC CC H5 HCC

4,6 ✓7th **S32.409 Unspecified fracture of unspecified acetabulum** MCC CC H5 UNS HCC

✓6th **S32.41 Fracture of anterior wall of acetabulum**

4,6 ✓7th **S32.411 Displaced fracture of anterior wall of right acetabulum** MCC CC H5 HCC

4,6 ✓7th **S32.412 Displaced fracture of anterior wall of left acetabulum** MCC CC H5 HCC

4,6 ✓7th S32.413 Displaced fracture of anterior wall of unspecified acetabulum MCC CC H5 UNS HCC
4,6 ✓7th S32.414 Nondisplaced fracture of anterior wall of right acetabulum MCC CC H5 HCC
4,6 ✓7th S32.415 Nondisplaced fracture of anterior wall of left acetabulum MCC CC H5 HCC
4,6 ✓7th S32.416 Nondisplaced fracture of anterior wall of unspecified acetabulum MCC CC H5 UNS HCC
✓6th S32.42 Fracture of posterior wall of acetabulum
4,6 ✓7th S32.421 Displaced fracture of posterior wall of right acetabulum MCC CC H5 HCC
4,6 ✓7th S32.422 Displaced fracture of posterior wall of left acetabulum MCC CC H5 HCC
4,6 ✓7th S32.423 Displaced fracture of posterior wall of unspecified acetabulum MCC CC H5 UNS HCC
4,6 ✓7th S32.424 Nondisplaced fracture of posterior wall of right acetabulum MCC CC H5 HCC
4,6 ✓7th S32.425 Nondisplaced fracture of posterior wall of left acetabulum MCC CC H5 HCC
4,6 ✓7th S32.426 Nondisplaced fracture of posterior wall of unspecified acetabulum MCC CC H5 UNS HCC
✓6th S32.43 Fracture of anterior column [iliopubic] of acetabulum
4,6 ✓7th S32.431 Displaced fracture of anterior column [iliopubic] of right acetabulum MCC CC H5 HCC
4,6 ✓7th S32.432 Displaced fracture of anterior column [iliopubic] of left acetabulum MCC CC H5 HCC
4,6 ✓7th S32.433 Displaced fracture of anterior column [iliopubic] of unspecified acetabulum MCC CC H5 UNS HCC
4,6 ✓7th S32.434 Nondisplaced fracture of anterior column [iliopubic] of right acetabulum MCC CC H5 HCC
4,6 ✓7th S32.435 Nondisplaced fracture of anterior column [iliopubic] of left acetabulum MCC CC H5 HCC
4,6 ✓7th S32.436 Nondisplaced fracture of anterior column [iliopubic] of unspecified acetabulum MCC CC H5 UNS HCC
✓6th S32.44 Fracture of posterior column [ilioischial] of acetabulum
4,6 ✓7th S32.441 Displaced fracture of posterior column [ilioischial] of right acetabulum MCC CC H5 HCC
4,6 ✓7th S32.442 Displaced fracture of posterior column [ilioischial] of left acetabulum MCC CC H5 HCC
4,6 ✓7th S32.443 Displaced fracture of posterior column [ilioischial] of unspecified acetabulum MCC CC H5 UNS HCC
4,6 ✓7th S32.444 Nondisplaced fracture of posterior column [ilioischial] of right acetabulum MCC CC H5 HCC
4,6 ✓7th S32.445 Nondisplaced fracture of posterior column [ilioischial] of left acetabulum MCC CC H5 HCC
4,6 ✓7th S32.446 Nondisplaced fracture of posterior column [ilioischial] of unspecified acetabulum MCC CC H5 UNS HCC
✓6th S32.45 Transverse fracture of acetabulum
4,6 ✓7th S32.451 Displaced transverse fracture of right acetabulum MCC CC H5 HCC
4,6 ✓7th S32.452 Displaced transverse fracture of left acetabulum MCC CC H5 HCC
4,6 ✓7th S32.453 Displaced transverse fracture of unspecified acetabulum MCC CC H5 UNS HCC
4,6 ✓7th S32.454 Nondisplaced transverse fracture of right acetabulum MCC CC H5 HCC
4,6 ✓7th S32.455 Nondisplaced transverse fracture of left acetabulum MCC CC H5 HCC
4,6 ✓7th S32.456 Nondisplaced transverse fracture of unspecified acetabulum MCC CC H5 UNS HCC
✓6th S32.46 Associated transverse-posterior fracture of acetabulum
4,6 ✓7th S32.461 Displaced associated transverse-posterior fracture of right acetabulum MCC CC H5 HCC
4,6 ✓7th S32.462 Displaced associated transverse-posterior fracture of left acetabulum MCC CC H5 HCC
4,6 ✓7th S32.463 Displaced associated transverse-posterior fracture of unspecified acetabulum MCC CC H5 UNS HCC
4,6 ✓7th S32.464 Nondisplaced associated transverse-posterior fracture of right acetabulum MCC CC H5 HCC
4,6 ✓7th S32.465 Nondisplaced associated transverse-posterior fracture of left acetabulum MCC CC H5 HCC
4,6 ✓7th S32.466 Nondisplaced associated transverse-posterior fracture of unspecified acetabulum MCC CC H5 UNS HCC
✓6th S32.47 Fracture of medial wall of acetabulum
4,6 ✓7th S32.471 Displaced fracture of medial wall of right acetabulum MCC CC H5 HCC
4,6 ✓7th S32.472 Displaced fracture of medial wall of left acetabulum MCC CC H5 HCC
4,6 ✓7th S32.473 Displaced fracture of medial wall of unspecified acetabulum MCC CC H5 UNS HCC
4,6 ✓7th S32.474 Nondisplaced fracture of medial wall of right acetabulum MCC CC H5 HCC
4,6 ✓7th S32.475 Nondisplaced fracture of medial wall of left acetabulum MCC CC H5 HCC
4,6 ✓7th S32.476 Nondisplaced fracture of medial wall of unspecified acetabulum MCC CC H5 UNS HCC
✓6th S32.48 Dome fracture of acetabulum
4,6 ✓7th S32.481 Displaced dome fracture of right acetabulum MCC CC H5 HCC
4,6 ✓7th S32.482 Displaced dome fracture of left acetabulum MCC CC H5 HCC
4,6 ✓7th S32.483 Displaced dome fracture of unspecified acetabulum MCC CC H5 UNS HCC
4,6 ✓7th S32.484 Nondisplaced dome fracture of right acetabulum MCC CC H5 HCC
4,6 ✓7th S32.485 Nondisplaced dome fracture of left acetabulum MCC CC H5 HCC
4,6 ✓7th S32.486 Nondisplaced dome fracture of unspecified acetabulum MCC CC H5 UNS HCC
✓6th S32.49 Other specified fracture of acetabulum
4,6 ✓7th S32.491 Other specified fracture of right acetabulum MCC CC H5 HCC
4,6 ✓7th S32.492 Other specified fracture of left acetabulum MCC CC H5 HCC
4,6 ✓7th S32.499 Other specified fracture of unspecified acetabulum MCC CC H5 UNS HCC
✓5th S32.5 Fracture of pubis
EXCLUDES 1 *fracture of pubis with associated disruption of pelvic ring (S32.8-)*
✓6th S32.50 Unspecified fracture of pubis
2,3,6 ✓7th S32.501 Unspecified fracture of right pubis MCC CC H5 HCC
2,3,6 ✓7th S32.502 Unspecified fracture of left pubis MCC CC H5 HCC
2,3,6 ✓7th S32.509 Unspecified fracture of unspecified pubis MCC CC H5 UNS HCC
✓6th S32.51 Fracture of superior rim of pubis
2,3,6 ✓7th S32.511 Fracture of superior rim of right pubis MCC CC H5 HCC
2,3,6 ✓7th S32.512 Fracture of superior rim of left pubis MCC CC H5 HCC
2,3,6 ✓7th S32.519 Fracture of superior rim of unspecified pubis MCC CC H5 UNS HCC
✓6th S32.59 Other specified fracture of pubis
2,3,6 ✓7th S32.591 Other specified fracture of right pubis MCC CC H5 HCC
2,3,6 ✓7th S32.592 Other specified fracture of left pubis MCC CC H5 HCC

Chapter 19. Injury, Poisoning and Certain Other Consequences of External Causes

2,3,6 ✓7th **S32.599 Other specified fracture of unspecified pubis** MCC CC H5 UNS HCC

✓5th **S32.6 Fracture of ischium**

EXCLUDES 1 *fracture of ischium with associated disruption of pelvic ring (S32.8-)*

✓6th **S32.6Ø Unspecified fracture of ischium**

2,3,6 ✓7th **S32.6Ø1 Unspecified fracture of right ischium** MCC CC H5 HCC

2,3,6 ✓7th **S32.6Ø2 Unspecified fracture of left ischium** MCC CC H5 HCC

2,3,6 ✓7th **S32.6Ø9 Unspecified fracture of unspecified ischium** MCC CC H5 UNS HCC

✓6th **S32.61 Avulsion fracture of ischium**

2,3,6 ✓7th **S32.611 Displaced avulsion fracture of right ischium** MCC CC H5 HCC

2,3,6 ✓7th **S32.612 Displaced avulsion fracture of left ischium** MCC CC H5 HCC

2,3,6 ✓7th **S32.613 Displaced avulsion fracture of unspecified ischium** MCC CC H5 UNS HCC

2,3,6 ✓7th **S32.614 Nondisplaced avulsion fracture of right ischium** MCC CC H5 HCC

2,3,6 ✓7th **S32.615 Nondisplaced avulsion fracture of left ischium** MCC CC H5 HCC

2,3,6 ✓7th **S32.616 Nondisplaced avulsion fracture of unspecified ischium** MCC CC H5 UNS HCC

✓6th **S32.69 Other specified fracture of ischium**

2,3,6 ✓7th **S32.691 Other specified fracture of right ischium** MCC CC H5 HCC

2,3,6 ✓7th **S32.692 Other specified fracture of left ischium** MCC CC H5 HCC

2,3,6 ✓7th **S32.699 Other specified fracture of unspecified ischium** MCC CC H5 UNS HCC

✓5th **S32.8 Fracture of other parts of pelvis**

Code also any associated:
fracture of acetabulum (S32.4-)
sacral fracture (S32.1-)

Fractures Disrupting Pelvic Circle

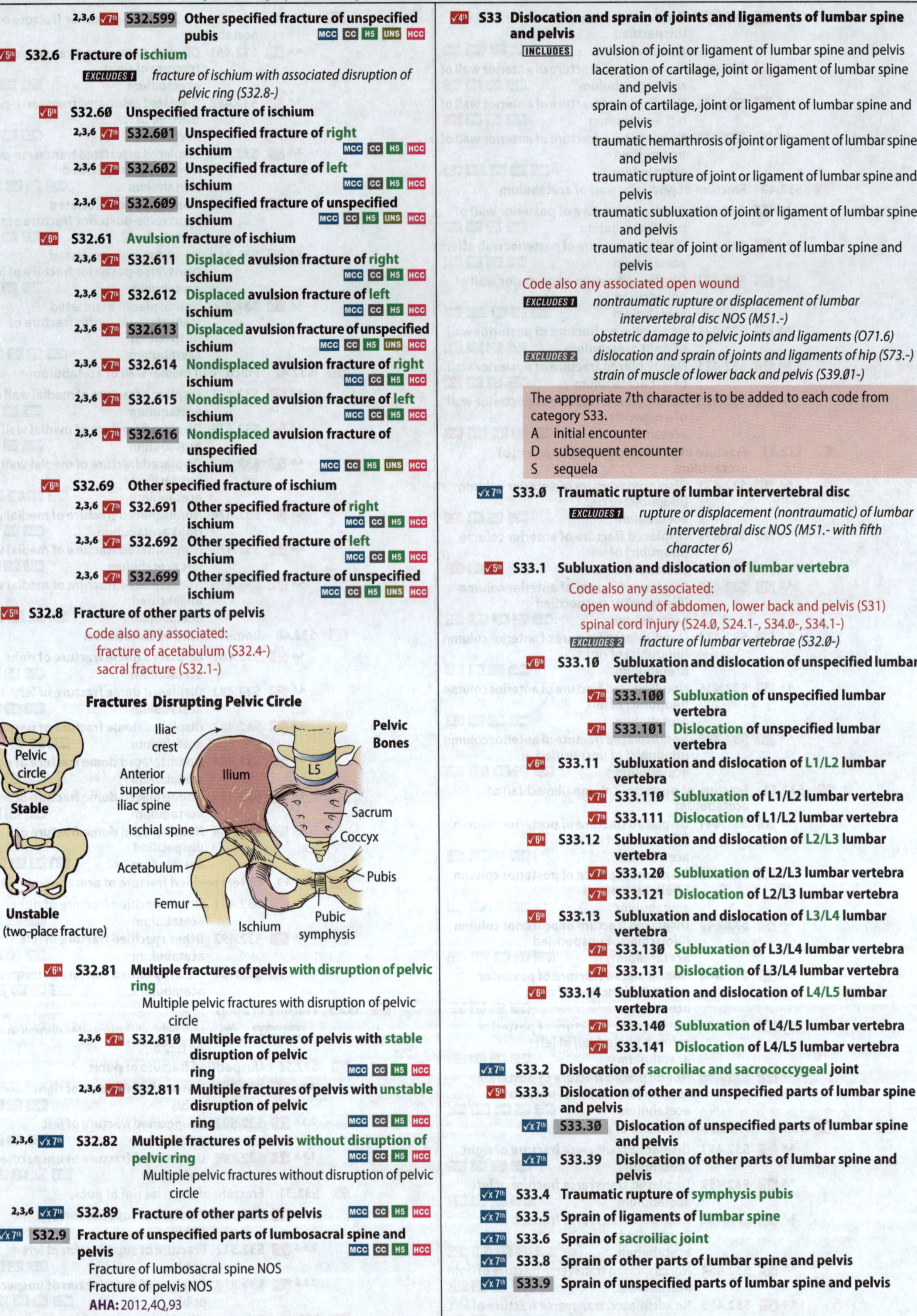

✓6th **S32.81 Multiple fractures of pelvis with disruption of pelvic ring**

Multiple pelvic fractures with disruption of pelvic circle

2,3,6 ✓7th **S32.81Ø Multiple fractures of pelvis with stable disruption of pelvic ring** MCC CC H5 HCC

2,3,6 ✓7th **S32.811 Multiple fractures of pelvis with unstable disruption of pelvic ring** MCC CC H5 HCC

2,3,6 ✓x7th **S32.82 Multiple fractures of pelvis without disruption of pelvic ring** MCC CC H5 HCC

Multiple pelvic fractures without disruption of pelvic circle

2,3,6 ✓x7th **S32.89 Fracture of other parts of pelvis** MCC CC H5 HCC

2,3,6 ✓x7th **S32.9 Fracture of unspecified parts of lumbosacral spine and pelvis** MCC CC H5 HCC

Fracture of lumbosacral spine NOS
Fracture of pelvis NOS
AHA: 2012,4Q,93

✓4th **S33 Dislocation and sprain of joints and ligaments of lumbar spine and pelvis**

INCLUDES avulsion of joint or ligament of lumbar spine and pelvis
laceration of cartilage, joint or ligament of lumbar spine and pelvis
sprain of cartilage, joint or ligament of lumbar spine and pelvis
traumatic hemarthrosis of joint or ligament of lumbar spine and pelvis
traumatic rupture of joint or ligament of lumbar spine and pelvis
traumatic subluxation of joint or ligament of lumbar spine and pelvis
traumatic tear of joint or ligament of lumbar spine and pelvis

Code also any associated open wound

EXCLUDES 1 *nontraumatic rupture or displacement of lumbar intervertebral disc NOS (M51.-)*
obstetric damage to pelvic joints and ligaments (O71.6)

EXCLUDES 2 *dislocation and sprain of joints and ligaments of hip (S73.-)*
strain of muscle of lower back and pelvis (S39.Ø1-)

The appropriate 7th character is to be added to each code from category S33.
A initial encounter
D subsequent encounter
S sequela

✓x7th **S33.Ø Traumatic rupture of lumbar intervertebral disc**

EXCLUDES 1 *rupture or displacement (nontraumatic) of lumbar intervertebral disc NOS (M51.- with fifth character 6)*

✓5th **S33.1 Subluxation and dislocation of lumbar vertebra**

Code also any associated:
open wound of abdomen, lower back and pelvis (S31)
spinal cord injury (S24.Ø, S24.1-, S34.Ø-, S34.1-)

EXCLUDES 2 *fracture of lumbar vertebrae (S32.Ø-)*

✓6th **S33.1Ø Subluxation and dislocation of unspecified lumbar vertebra**

✓7th **S33.1ØØ Subluxation of unspecified lumbar vertebra**

✓7th **S33.1Ø1 Dislocation of unspecified lumbar vertebra**

✓6th **S33.11 Subluxation and dislocation of L1/L2 lumbar vertebra**

✓7th **S33.11Ø Subluxation of L1/L2 lumbar vertebra**

✓7th **S33.111 Dislocation of L1/L2 lumbar vertebra**

✓6th **S33.12 Subluxation and dislocation of L2/L3 lumbar vertebra**

✓7th **S33.12Ø Subluxation of L2/L3 lumbar vertebra**

✓7th **S33.121 Dislocation of L2/L3 lumbar vertebra**

✓6th **S33.13 Subluxation and dislocation of L3/L4 lumbar vertebra**

✓7th **S33.13Ø Subluxation of L3/L4 lumbar vertebra**

✓7th **S33.131 Dislocation of L3/L4 lumbar vertebra**

✓6th **S33.14 Subluxation and dislocation of L4/L5 lumbar vertebra**

✓7th **S33.14Ø Subluxation of L4/L5 lumbar vertebra**

✓7th **S33.141 Dislocation of L4/L5 lumbar vertebra**

✓x7th **S33.2 Dislocation of sacroiliac and sacrococcygeal joint**

✓5th **S33.3 Dislocation of other and unspecified parts of lumbar spine and pelvis**

✓x7th **S33.3Ø Dislocation of unspecified parts of lumbar spine and pelvis**

✓x7th **S33.39 Dislocation of other parts of lumbar spine and pelvis**

✓x7th **S33.4 Traumatic rupture of symphysis pubis**

✓x7th **S33.5 Sprain of ligaments of lumbar spine**

✓x7th **S33.6 Sprain of sacroiliac joint**

✓x7th **S33.8 Sprain of other parts of lumbar spine and pelvis**

✓x7th **S33.9 Sprain of unspecified parts of lumbar spine and pelvis**

S34 Injury of lumbar and sacral spinal cord and nerves at abdomen, lower back and pelvis level

NOTE Code to highest level of lumbar cord injury.

Injuries to the spinal cord (S34.0 and S34.1) refer to the cord level and not bone level injury, and can affect nerve roots at and below the level given.

Code also any associated:
fracture of vertebra (S22.0-, S32.0-)
open wound of abdomen, lower back and pelvis (S31.-)
transient paralysis (R29.5)

The appropriate 7th character is to be added to each code from category S34.
A initial encounter
D subsequent encounter
S sequela

S34.0 Concussion and edema of lumbar and sacral spinal cord

S34.01 Concussion and edema of lumbar spinal cord MCC HCC

S34.02 Concussion and edema of sacral spinal cord MCC HCC
Concussion and edema of conus medullaris

S34.1 Other and unspecified injury of lumbar and sacral spinal cord

S34.10 Unspecified injury to lumbar spinal cord

S34.101 Unspecified injury to L1 level of lumbar spinal cord MCC H5 HCC
Unspecified injury to lumbar spinal cord level 1

S34.102 Unspecified injury to L2 level of lumbar spinal cord MCC H5 HCC
Unspecified injury to lumbar spinal cord level 2

S34.103 Unspecified injury to L3 level of lumbar spinal cord MCC H5 HCC
Unspecified injury to lumbar spinal cord level 3

S34.104 Unspecified injury to L4 level of lumbar spinal cord MCC H5 HCC
Unspecified injury to lumbar spinal cord level 4

S34.105 Unspecified injury to L5 level of lumbar spinal cord MCC H5 HCC
Unspecified injury to lumbar spinal cord level 5

S34.109 Unspecified injury to unspecified level of lumbar spinal cord MCC H5 HCC

S34.11 Complete lesion of lumbar spinal cord

S34.111 Complete lesion of L1 level of lumbar spinal cord MCC H5 HCC
Complete lesion of lumbar spinal cord level 1

S34.112 Complete lesion of L2 level of lumbar spinal cord MCC H5 HCC
Complete lesion of lumbar spinal cord level 2

S34.113 Complete lesion of L3 level of lumbar spinal cord MCC H5 HCC
Complete lesion of lumbar spinal cord level 3

S34.114 Complete lesion of L4 level of lumbar spinal cord MCC H5 HCC
Complete lesion of lumbar spinal cord level 4

S34.115 Complete lesion of L5 level of lumbar spinal cord MCC H5 HCC
Complete lesion of lumbar spinal cord level 5

S34.119 Complete lesion of unspecified level of lumbar spinal cord MCC H5 HCC

S34.12 Incomplete lesion of lumbar spinal cord

S34.121 Incomplete lesion of L1 level of lumbar spinal cord MCC H5 HCC
Incomplete lesion of lumbar spinal cord level 1

S34.122 Incomplete lesion of L2 level of lumbar spinal cord MCC H5 HCC
Incomplete lesion of lumbar spinal cord level 2

S34.123 Incomplete lesion of L3 level of lumbar spinal cord MCC H5 HCC
Incomplete lesion of lumbar spinal cord level 3

S34.124 Incomplete lesion of L4 level of lumbar spinal cord MCC H5 HCC
Incomplete lesion of lumbar spinal cord level 4

S34.125 Incomplete lesion of L5 level of lumbar spinal cord MCC H5 HCC
Incomplete lesion of lumbar spinal cord level 5

S34.129 Incomplete lesion of unspecified level of lumbar spinal cord MCC H5 HCC

S34.13 Other and unspecified injury to sacral spinal cord
Other injury to conus medullaris

S34.131 Complete lesion of sacral spinal cord MCC H5 HCC
Complete lesion of conus medullaris

S34.132 Incomplete lesion of sacral spinal cord MCC H5 HCC
Incomplete lesion of conus medullaris

S34.139 Unspecified injury to sacral spinal cord MCC H5 HCC
Unspecified injury of conus medullaris

S34.2 Injury of nerve root of lumbar and sacral spine

S34.21 Injury of nerve root of lumbar spine

S34.22 Injury of nerve root of sacral spine

S34.3 Injury of cauda equina MCC H5 HCC

S34.4 Injury of lumbosacral plexus

S34.5 Injury of lumbar, sacral and pelvic sympathetic nerves
Injury of celiac ganglion or plexus
Injury of hypogastric plexus
Injury of mesenteric plexus (inferior) (superior)
Injury of splanchnic nerve

S34.6 Injury of peripheral nerve(s) at abdomen, lower back and pelvis level

S34.8 Injury of other nerves at abdomen, lower back and pelvis level

S34.9 Injury of unspecified nerves at abdomen, lower back and pelvis level

S35 Injury of blood vessels at abdomen, lower back and pelvis level

Code also any associated open wound (S31.-)

The appropriate 7th character is to be added to each code from category S35.
A initial encounter
D subsequent encounter
S sequela

S35.0 Injury of abdominal aorta

EXCLUDES 1 *injury of aorta NOS (S25.0)*

S35.00 Unspecified injury of abdominal aorta MCC

S35.01 Minor laceration of abdominal aorta MCC
Incomplete transection of abdominal aorta
Laceration of abdominal aorta NOS
Superficial laceration of abdominal aorta

S35.02 Major laceration of abdominal aorta MCC
Complete transection of abdominal aorta
Traumatic rupture of abdominal aorta

S35.09 Other injury of abdominal aorta MCC

S35.1 Injury of inferior vena cava
Injury of hepatic vein

EXCLUDES 1 *injury of vena cava NOS (S25.2)*

S35.10 Unspecified injury of inferior vena cava MCC

S35.11 Minor laceration of inferior vena cava MCC
Incomplete transection of inferior vena cava
Laceration of inferior vena cava NOS
Superficial laceration of inferior vena cava

√x7th S35.12 **Major laceration of inferior vena cava** MCC
Complete transection of inferior vena cava
Traumatic rupture of inferior vena cava

√x7th S35.19 **Other injury of inferior vena cava** MCC

√5th S35.2 **Injury of celiac or mesenteric artery and branches**

√6th S35.21 **Injury of celiac artery**

√7th S35.211 **Minor laceration of celiac artery** MCC
Incomplete transection of celiac artery
Laceration of celiac artery NOS
Superficial laceration of celiac artery

√7th S35.212 **Major laceration of celiac artery** MCC
Complete transection of celiac artery
Traumatic rupture of celiac artery

√7th S35.218 **Other injury of celiac artery** MCC

√7th S35.219 **Unspecified injury of celiac artery** MCC

√6th S35.22 **Injury of superior mesenteric artery**

√7th S35.221 **Minor laceration of superior mesenteric artery** MCC
Incomplete transection of superior mesenteric artery
Laceration of superior mesenteric artery NOS
Superficial laceration of superior mesenteric artery

√7th S35.222 **Major laceration of superior mesenteric artery** MCC
Complete transection of superior mesenteric artery
Traumatic rupture of superior mesenteric artery

√7th S35.228 **Other injury of superior mesenteric artery** MCC

√7th S35.229 **Unspecified injury of superior mesenteric artery** MCC

√6th S35.23 **Injury of inferior mesenteric artery**

√7th S35.231 **Minor laceration of inferior mesenteric artery** MCC
Incomplete transection of inferior mesenteric artery
Laceration of inferior mesenteric artery NOS
Superficial laceration of inferior mesenteric artery

√7th S35.232 **Major laceration of inferior mesenteric artery** MCC
Complete transection of inferior mesenteric artery
Traumatic rupture of inferior mesenteric artery

√7th S35.238 **Other injury of inferior mesenteric artery** MCC

√7th S35.239 **Unspecified injury of inferior mesenteric artery** MCC

√6th S35.29 **Injury of branches of celiac and mesenteric artery**
Injury of gastric artery
Injury of gastroduodenal artery
Injury of hepatic artery
Injury of splenic artery

√7th S35.291 **Minor laceration of branches of celiac and mesenteric artery** MCC
Incomplete transection of branches of celiac and mesenteric artery
Laceration of branches of celiac and mesenteric artery NOS
Superficial laceration of branches of celiac and mesenteric artery

√7th S35.292 **Major laceration of branches of celiac and mesenteric artery** MCC
Complete transection of branches of celiac and mesenteric artery
Traumatic rupture of branches of celiac and mesenteric artery

√7th S35.298 **Other injury of branches of celiac and mesenteric artery** MCC

√7th S35.299 **Unspecified injury of branches of celiac and mesenteric artery** MCC

√5th S35.3 **Injury of portal or splenic vein and branches**

√6th S35.31 **Injury of portal vein**

√7th S35.311 **Laceration of portal vein** MCC

√7th S35.318 **Other specified injury of portal vein** MCC

√7th S35.319 **Unspecified injury of portal vein** MCC

√6th S35.32 **Injury of splenic vein**

√7th S35.321 **Laceration of splenic vein** MCC

√7th S35.328 **Other specified injury of splenic vein** MCC

√7th S35.329 **Unspecified injury of splenic vein** MCC

√6th S35.33 **Injury of superior mesenteric vein**

√7th S35.331 **Laceration of superior mesenteric vein** MCC

√7th S35.338 **Other specified injury of superior mesenteric vein** MCC

√7th S35.339 **Unspecified injury of superior mesenteric vein** MCC

√6th S35.34 **Injury of inferior mesenteric vein**

√7th S35.341 **Laceration of inferior mesenteric vein** MCC

√7th S35.348 **Other specified injury of inferior mesenteric vein** MCC

√7th S35.349 **Unspecified injury of inferior mesenteric vein** MCC

√5th S35.4 **Injury of renal blood vessels**

√6th S35.40 **Unspecified injury of renal blood vessel**

√7th S35.401 **Unspecified injury of right renal artery** MCC

√7th S35.402 **Unspecified injury of left renal artery** MCC

√7th S35.403 **Unspecified injury of unspecified renal artery** MCC UNS

√7th S35.404 **Unspecified injury of right renal vein** MCC

√7th S35.405 **Unspecified injury of left renal vein** MCC

√7th S35.406 **Unspecified injury of unspecified renal vein** MCC UNS

√6th S35.41 **Laceration of renal blood vessel**

√7th S35.411 **Laceration of right renal artery** MCC

√7th S35.412 **Laceration of left renal artery** MCC

√7th S35.413 **Laceration of unspecified renal artery** MCC UNS

√7th S35.414 **Laceration of right renal vein** MCC

√7th S35.415 **Laceration of left renal vein** MCC

√7th S35.416 **Laceration of unspecified renal vein** MCC UNS

√6th S35.49 **Other specified injury of renal blood vessel**

√7th S35.491 **Other specified injury of right renal artery** MCC

√7th S35.492 **Other specified injury of left renal artery** MCC

√7th S35.493 **Other specified injury of unspecified renal artery** MCC UNS

√7th S35.494 **Other specified injury of right renal vein** MCC

√7th S35.495 **Other specified injury of left renal vein** MCC

√7th S35.496 **Other specified injury of unspecified renal vein** MCC UNS

√5th S35.5 **Injury of iliac blood vessels**

√x7th S35.50 **Injury of unspecified iliac blood vessel(s)** MCC

√6th S35.51 **Injury of iliac artery or vein**
Injury of hypogastric artery or vein

√7th S35.511 **Injury of right iliac artery** MCC

√7th S35.512 **Injury of left iliac artery** MCC

√7th S35.513 **Injury of unspecified iliac artery** MCC UNS

√7th S35.514 **Injury of right iliac vein** MCC

√7th S35.515 **Injury of left iliac vein** MCC

√7th S35.516 **Injury of unspecified iliac vein** MCC UNS

√6th S35.53 **Injury of uterine artery or vein**

√7th S35.531 **Injury of right uterine artery** CC ♀

S35.532 Injury of left uterine artery CC ♀
S35.533 Injury of unspecified uterine artery CC UNS ♀
S35.534 Injury of right uterine vein CC ♀
S35.535 Injury of left uterine vein CC ♀
S35.536 Injury of unspecified uterine vein CC UNS ♀
S35.59 Injury of other iliac blood vessels MCC
S35.8 Injury of other blood vessels at abdomen, lower back and pelvis level
Injury of ovarian artery or vein
S35.8X Injury of other blood vessels at abdomen, lower back and pelvis level
S35.8X1 Laceration of other blood vessels at abdomen, lower back and pelvis level CC
S35.8X8 Other specified injury of other blood vessels at abdomen, lower back and pelvis level CC
S35.8X9 Unspecified injury of other blood vessels at abdomen, lower back and pelvis level CC
S35.9 Injury of unspecified blood vessel at abdomen, lower back and pelvis level
S35.90 Unspecified injury of unspecified blood vessel at abdomen, lower back and pelvis level CC
S35.91 Laceration of unspecified blood vessel at abdomen, lower back and pelvis level CC
S35.99 Other specified injury of unspecified blood vessel at abdomen, lower back and pelvis level CC

S36 Injury of intra-abdominal organs
Code also any associated open wound (S31.-)

The appropriate 7th character is to be added to each code from category S36.
A initial encounter
D subsequent encounter
S sequela

S36.0 Injury of spleen
AHA: 2015,2Q,36; 2015,1Q,10
S36.00 Unspecified injury of spleen CC
S36.02 Contusion of spleen
TIP: When both traumatic splenic laceration and contusion are documented in the same encounter, code only the laceration, as contusions are not coded when they occur with a more severe injury in the same body site.
S36.020 Minor contusion of spleen CC
Contusion of spleen less than 2 cm
S36.021 Major contusion of spleen CC
Contusion of spleen greater than 2 cm
S36.029 Unspecified contusion of spleen CC
S36.03 Laceration of spleen
TIP: When both traumatic splenic laceration and contusion are documented in the same encounter, code only the laceration, as contusions are not coded when they occur with a more severe injury in the same body site.
S36.030 Superficial (capsular) laceration of spleen CC
Laceration of spleen less than 1 cm
Minor laceration of spleen
S36.031 Moderate laceration of spleen MCC
Laceration of spleen 1 to 3 cm
S36.032 Major laceration of spleen MCC
Avulsion of spleen
Laceration of spleen greater than 3 cm
Massive laceration of spleen
Multiple moderate lacerations of spleen
Stellate laceration of spleen
S36.039 Unspecified laceration of spleen CC
S36.09 Other injury of spleen CC
S36.1 Injury of liver and gallbladder and bile duct
S36.11 Injury of liver
S36.112 Contusion of liver CC
S36.113 Laceration of liver, unspecified degree CC
S36.114 Minor laceration of liver CC
Laceration involving capsule only, or, without significant involvement of hepatic parenchyma [i.e., less than 1 cm deep]
S36.115 Moderate laceration of liver MCC
Laceration involving parenchyma but without major disruption of parenchyma [i.e., less than 10 cm long and less than 3 cm deep]
S36.116 Major laceration of liver MCC
Laceration with significant disruption of hepatic parenchyma [i.e., greater than 10 cm long and 3 cm deep]
Multiple moderate lacerations, with or without hematoma
Stellate laceration of liver
S36.118 Other injury of liver CC
S36.119 Unspecified injury of liver CC
S36.12 Injury of gallbladder
S36.122 Contusion of gallbladder CC
S36.123 Laceration of gallbladder CC
S36.128 Other injury of gallbladder CC
S36.129 Unspecified injury of gallbladder CC
S36.13 Injury of bile duct CC
S36.2 Injury of pancreas
S36.20 Unspecified injury of pancreas
S36.200 Unspecified injury of head of pancreas CC
S36.201 Unspecified injury of body of pancreas CC
S36.202 Unspecified injury of tail of pancreas CC
S36.209 Unspecified injury of unspecified part of pancreas CC
S36.22 Contusion of pancreas
S36.220 Contusion of head of pancreas CC
S36.221 Contusion of body of pancreas CC
S36.222 Contusion of tail of pancreas CC
S36.229 Contusion of unspecified part of pancreas CC
S36.23 Laceration of pancreas, unspecified degree
S36.230 Laceration of head of pancreas, unspecified degree CC
S36.231 Laceration of body of pancreas, unspecified degree CC
S36.232 Laceration of tail of pancreas, unspecified degree CC
S36.239 Laceration of unspecified part of pancreas, unspecified degree CC
S36.24 Minor laceration of pancreas
S36.240 Minor laceration of head of pancreas CC
S36.241 Minor laceration of body of pancreas CC
S36.242 Minor laceration of tail of pancreas CC
S36.249 Minor laceration of unspecified part of pancreas CC
S36.25 Moderate laceration of pancreas
S36.250 Moderate laceration of head of pancreas CC
S36.251 Moderate laceration of body of pancreas CC
S36.252 Moderate laceration of tail of pancreas CC
S36.259 Moderate laceration of unspecified part of pancreas CC
S36.26 Major laceration of pancreas
S36.260 Major laceration of head of pancreas CC
S36.261 Major laceration of body of pancreas CC
S36.262 Major laceration of tail of pancreas CC
S36.269 Major laceration of unspecified part of pancreas CC

S36.29 Other injury of pancreas
- **S36.290 Other injury of head of pancreas** CC
- **S36.291 Other injury of body of pancreas** CC
- **S36.292 Other injury of tail of pancreas** CC
- **S36.299 Other injury of unspecified part of pancreas** CC

S36.3 Injury of stomach
- **S36.30 Unspecified injury of stomach** CC
- **S36.32 Contusion of stomach** CC
- **S36.33 Laceration of stomach** CC
- **S36.39 Other injury of stomach** CC

S36.4 Injury of small intestine

S36.40 Unspecified injury of small intestine
- **S36.400 Unspecified injury of duodenum** CC
- **S36.408 Unspecified injury of other part of small intestine** CC
- **S36.409 Unspecified injury of unspecified part of small intestine** CC

S36.41 Primary blast injury of small intestine
Blast injury of small intestine NOS
- **S36.410 Primary blast injury of duodenum** CC
- **S36.418 Primary blast injury of other part of small intestine** CC
- **S36.419 Primary blast injury of unspecified part of small intestine** CC

S36.42 Contusion of small intestine
- **S36.420 Contusion of duodenum** CC
- **S36.428 Contusion of other part of small intestine** CC
- **S36.429 Contusion of unspecified part of small intestine** CC

S36.43 Laceration of small intestine
- **S36.430 Laceration of duodenum** CC
- **S36.438 Laceration of other part of small intestine** CC
- **S36.439 Laceration of unspecified part of small intestine** CC

S36.49 Other injury of small intestine
- **S36.490 Other injury of duodenum** CC
- **S36.498 Other injury of other part of small intestine** CC
- **S36.499 Other injury of unspecified part of small intestine** CC

S36.5 Injury of colon
EXCLUDES 2 *injury of rectum (S36.6-)*

S36.50 Unspecified injury of colon
- **S36.500 Unspecified injury of ascending [right] colon** CC
- **S36.501 Unspecified injury of transverse colon** CC
- **S36.502 Unspecified injury of descending [left] colon** CC
- **S36.503 Unspecified injury of sigmoid colon** CC
- **S36.508 Unspecified injury of other part of colon** CC
- **S36.509 Unspecified injury of unspecified part of colon** CC

S36.51 Primary blast injury of colon
Blast injury of colon NOS
- **S36.510 Primary blast injury of ascending [right] colon** CC
- **S36.511 Primary blast injury of transverse colon** CC
- **S36.512 Primary blast injury of descending [left] colon** CC
- **S36.513 Primary blast injury of sigmoid colon** CC
- **S36.518 Primary blast injury of other part of colon** CC
- **S36.519 Primary blast injury of unspecified part of colon** CC

S36.52 Contusion of colon
- **S36.520 Contusion of ascending [right] colon** CC
- **S36.521 Contusion of transverse colon** CC
- **S36.522 Contusion of descending [left] colon** CC
- **S36.523 Contusion of sigmoid colon** CC
- **S36.528 Contusion of other part of colon** CC
- **S36.529 Contusion of unspecified part of colon** CC

S36.53 Laceration of colon
- **S36.530 Laceration of ascending [right] colon** CC
- **S36.531 Laceration of transverse colon** CC
- **S36.532 Laceration of descending [left] colon** CC
- **S36.533 Laceration of sigmoid colon** CC
- **S36.538 Laceration of other part of colon** CC
- **S36.539 Laceration of unspecified part of colon** CC

S36.59 Other injury of colon
Secondary blast injury of colon
- **S36.590 Other injury of ascending [right] colon** CC
- **S36.591 Other injury of transverse colon** CC
- **S36.592 Other injury of descending [left] colon** CC
- **S36.593 Other injury of sigmoid colon** CC
- **S36.598 Other injury of other part of colon** CC
- **S36.599 Other injury of unspecified part of colon** CC

S36.6 Injury of rectum
- **S36.60 Unspecified injury of rectum** CC
- **S36.61 Primary blast injury of rectum** CC
  Blast injury of rectum NOS
- **S36.62 Contusion of rectum** CC
- **S36.63 Laceration of rectum** CC
- **S36.69 Other injury of rectum** CC
  Secondary blast injury of rectum

S36.8 Injury of other intra-abdominal organs
- **S36.81 Injury of peritoneum** CC

S36.89 Injury of other intra-abdominal organs
Injury of retroperitoneum
- **S36.892 Contusion of other intra-abdominal organs** CC
- **S36.893 Laceration of other intra-abdominal organs** CC
- **S36.898 Other injury of other intra-abdominal organs** CC
- **S36.899 Unspecified injury of other intra-abdominal organs** CC

S36.9 Injury of unspecified intra-abdominal organ
- **S36.90 Unspecified injury of unspecified intra-abdominal organ** CC
- **S36.92 Contusion of unspecified intra-abdominal organ** CC
- **S36.93 Laceration of unspecified intra-abdominal organ** CC
- **S36.99 Other injury of unspecified intra-abdominal organ** CC

S37 Injury of urinary and pelvic organs

Code also any associated open wound (S31.-)

EXCLUDES 1 *obstetric trauma to pelvic organs (O71.-)*

EXCLUDES 2 *injury of peritoneum (S36.81)*
injury of retroperitoneum (S36.89-)

The appropriate 7th character is to be added to each code from category S37.
- A initial encounter
- D subsequent encounter
- S sequela

S37.0 Injury of kidney
EXCLUDES 2 *acute kidney injury (nontraumatic) (N17.9)*

S37.00 Unspecified injury of kidney
- **S37.001 Unspecified injury of right kidney** CC
- **S37.002 Unspecified injury of left kidney** CC

S37.009 Unspecified injury of unspecified kidney CC UNS
S37.01 Minor contusion of kidney
Contusion of kidney less than 2 cm
Contusion of kidney NOS
S37.011 Minor contusion of right kidney CC
S37.012 Minor contusion of left kidney CC
S37.019 Minor contusion of unspecified kidney CC UNS
S37.02 Major contusion of kidney
Contusion of kidney greater than 2 cm
S37.021 Major contusion of right kidney CC
S37.022 Major contusion of left kidney CC
S37.029 Major contusion of unspecified kidney CC UNS
S37.03 Laceration of kidney, unspecified degree
S37.031 Laceration of right kidney, unspecified degree CC
S37.032 Laceration of left kidney, unspecified degree CC
S37.039 Laceration of unspecified kidney, unspecified degree CC UNS
S37.04 Minor laceration of kidney
Laceration of kidney less than 1 cm
S37.041 Minor laceration of right kidney CC
S37.042 Minor laceration of left kidney CC
S37.049 Minor laceration of unspecified kidney CC UNS
S37.05 Moderate laceration of kidney
Laceration of kidney 1 to 3 cm
S37.051 Moderate laceration of right kidney CC
S37.052 Moderate laceration of left kidney CC
S37.059 Moderate laceration of unspecified kidney CC UNS
S37.06 Major laceration of kidney
Avulsion of kidney
Laceration of kidney greater than 3 cm
Massive laceration of kidney
Multiple moderate lacerations of kidney
Stellate laceration of kidney
S37.061 Major laceration of right kidney MCC
S37.062 Major laceration of left kidney MCC
S37.069 Major laceration of unspecified kidney MCC UNS
S37.09 Other injury of kidney
S37.091 Other injury of right kidney MCC
S37.092 Other injury of left kidney MCC
S37.099 Other injury of unspecified kidney MCC UNS
S37.1 Injury of ureter
S37.10 Unspecified injury of ureter CC
S37.12 Contusion of ureter CC
S37.13 Laceration of ureter CC
S37.19 Other injury of ureter CC
S37.2 Injury of bladder
S37.20 Unspecified injury of bladder CC
S37.22 Contusion of bladder CC
S37.23 Laceration of bladder CC
S37.29 Other injury of bladder CC
S37.3 Injury of urethra
S37.30 Unspecified injury of urethra CC
S37.32 Contusion of urethra CC
S37.33 Laceration of urethra CC
S37.39 Other injury of urethra CC
S37.4 Injury of ovary
S37.40 Unspecified injury of ovary
S37.401 Unspecified injury of ovary, unilateral ♀
S37.402 Unspecified injury of ovary, bilateral ♀
S37.409 Unspecified injury of ovary, unspecified ♀
S37.42 Contusion of ovary
S37.421 Contusion of ovary, unilateral ♀
S37.422 Contusion of ovary, bilateral ♀
S37.429 Contusion of ovary, unspecified ♀
S37.43 Laceration of ovary
S37.431 Laceration of ovary, unilateral ♀
S37.432 Laceration of ovary, bilateral ♀
S37.439 Laceration of ovary, unspecified ♀
S37.49 Other injury of ovary
S37.491 Other injury of ovary, unilateral ♀
S37.492 Other injury of ovary, bilateral ♀
S37.499 Other injury of ovary, unspecified ♀
S37.5 Injury of fallopian tube
S37.50 Unspecified injury of fallopian tube
S37.501 Unspecified injury of fallopian tube, unilateral ♀
S37.502 Unspecified injury of fallopian tube, bilateral ♀
S37.509 Unspecified injury of fallopian tube, unspecified ♀
S37.51 Primary blast injury of fallopian tube
Blast injury of fallopian tube NOS
S37.511 Primary blast injury of fallopian tube, unilateral ♀
S37.512 Primary blast injury of fallopian tube, bilateral ♀
S37.519 Primary blast injury of fallopian tube, unspecified ♀
S37.52 Contusion of fallopian tube
S37.521 Contusion of fallopian tube, unilateral ♀
S37.522 Contusion of fallopian tube, bilateral ♀
S37.529 Contusion of fallopian tube, unspecified ♀
S37.53 Laceration of fallopian tube
S37.531 Laceration of fallopian tube, unilateral ♀
S37.532 Laceration of fallopian tube, bilateral ♀
S37.539 Laceration of fallopian tube, unspecified ♀
S37.59 Other injury of fallopian tube
Secondary blast injury of fallopian tube
S37.591 Other injury of fallopian tube, unilateral ♀
S37.592 Other injury of fallopian tube, bilateral ♀
S37.599 Other injury of fallopian tube, unspecified ♀
S37.6 Injury of uterus
EXCLUDES 1 *injury to gravid uterus (O9A.2-)*
injury to uterus during delivery (O71.-)
S37.60 Unspecified injury of uterus CC ♀
S37.62 Contusion of uterus CC ♀
S37.63 Laceration of uterus CC ♀
S37.69 Other injury of uterus CC ♀
S37.8 Injury of other urinary and pelvic organs
S37.81 Injury of adrenal gland
S37.812 Contusion of adrenal gland CC
S37.813 Laceration of adrenal gland CC
S37.818 Other injury of adrenal gland CC
S37.819 Unspecified injury of adrenal gland CC
S37.82 Injury of prostate
S37.822 Contusion of prostate ♂
S37.823 Laceration of prostate ♂
S37.828 Other injury of prostate ♂
S37.829 Unspecified injury of prostate ♂

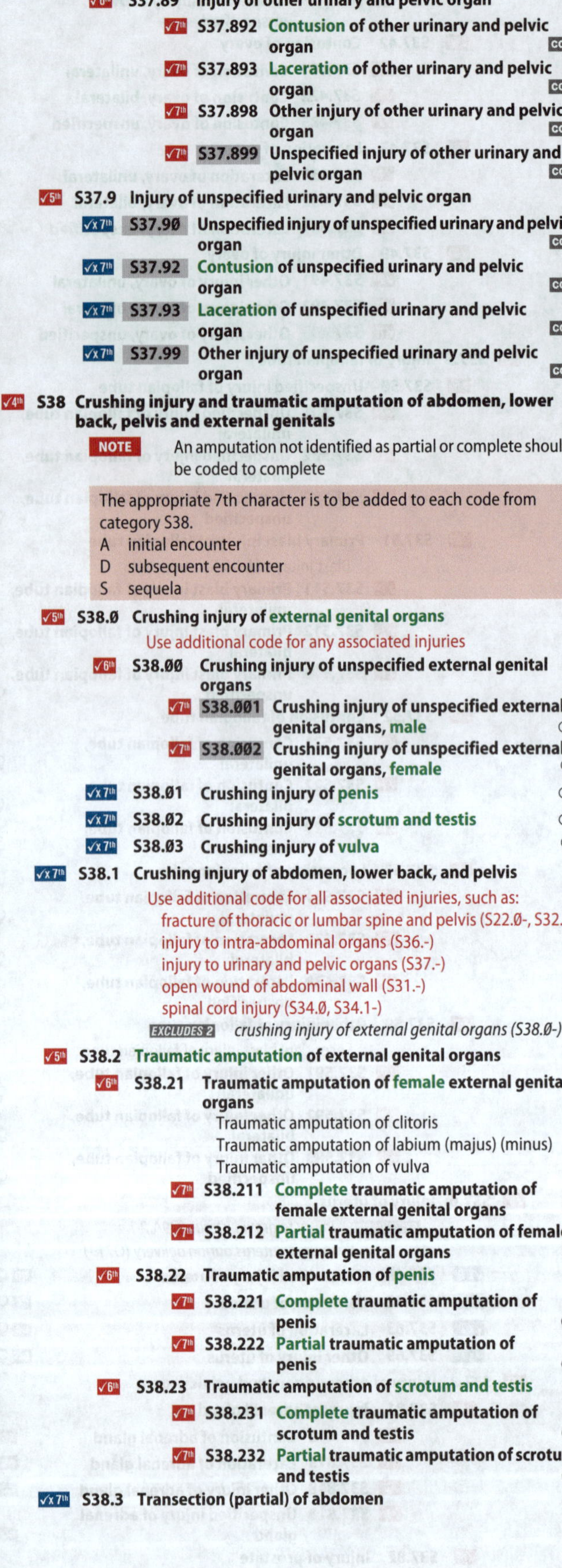

S37.89 Injury of other urinary and pelvic organ

- **S37.892 Contusion of other urinary and pelvic organ** CC
- **S37.893 Laceration of other urinary and pelvic organ** CC
- **S37.898 Other injury of other urinary and pelvic organ** CC
- **S37.899 Unspecified injury of other urinary and pelvic organ** CC

S37.9 Injury of unspecified urinary and pelvic organ

- **S37.90 Unspecified injury of unspecified urinary and pelvic organ** CC
- **S37.92 Contusion of unspecified urinary and pelvic organ** CC
- **S37.93 Laceration of unspecified urinary and pelvic organ** CC
- **S37.99 Other injury of unspecified urinary and pelvic organ** CC

S38 Crushing injury and traumatic amputation of abdomen, lower back, pelvis and external genitals

NOTE An amputation not identified as partial or complete should be coded to complete

The appropriate 7th character is to be added to each code from category S38.
A initial encounter
D subsequent encounter
S sequela

S38.0 Crushing injury of external genital organs

Use additional code for any associated injuries

S38.00 Crushing injury of unspecified external genital organs

- **S38.001 Crushing injury of unspecified external genital organs, male** ♂
- **S38.002 Crushing injury of unspecified external genital organs, female** ♀

- **S38.01 Crushing injury of penis** ♂
- **S38.02 Crushing injury of scrotum and testis** ♂
- **S38.03 Crushing injury of vulva** ♀

S38.1 Crushing injury of abdomen, lower back, and pelvis

Use additional code for all associated injuries, such as:
fracture of thoracic or lumbar spine and pelvis (S22.0-, S32.-)
injury to intra-abdominal organs (S36.-)
injury to urinary and pelvic organs (S37.-)
open wound of abdominal wall (S31.-)
spinal cord injury (S34.0, S34.1-)

EXCLUDES 2 *crushing injury of external genital organs (S38.0-)*

S38.2 Traumatic amputation of external genital organs

S38.21 Traumatic amputation of female external genital organs

Traumatic amputation of clitoris
Traumatic amputation of labium (majus) (minus)
Traumatic amputation of vulva

- **S38.211 Complete traumatic amputation of female external genital organs** ♀
- **S38.212 Partial traumatic amputation of female external genital organs** ♀

S38.22 Traumatic amputation of penis

- **S38.221 Complete traumatic amputation of penis** ♂
- **S38.222 Partial traumatic amputation of penis** ♂

S38.23 Traumatic amputation of scrotum and testis

- **S38.231 Complete traumatic amputation of scrotum and testis** ♂
- **S38.232 Partial traumatic amputation of scrotum and testis** ♂

S38.3 Transection (partial) of abdomen

S39 Other and unspecified injuries of abdomen, lower back, pelvis and external genitals

Code also any associated open wound (S31.-)

EXCLUDES 2 *sprain of joints and ligaments of lumbar spine and pelvis (S33.-)*

The appropriate 7th character is to be added to each code from category S39.
A initial encounter
D subsequent encounter
S sequela

S39.0 Injury of muscle, fascia and tendon of abdomen, lower back and pelvis

S39.00 Unspecified injury of muscle, fascia and tendon of abdomen, lower back and pelvis

- **S39.001 Unspecified injury of muscle, fascia and tendon of abdomen**
- **S39.002 Unspecified injury of muscle, fascia and tendon of lower back**
- **S39.003 Unspecified injury of muscle, fascia and tendon of pelvis**

S39.01 Strain of muscle, fascia and tendon of abdomen, lower back and pelvis

- **S39.011 Strain of muscle, fascia and tendon of abdomen**
- **S39.012 Strain of muscle, fascia and tendon of lower back**
- **S39.013 Strain of muscle, fascia and tendon of pelvis**

S39.02 Laceration of muscle, fascia and tendon of abdomen, lower back and pelvis

- **S39.021 Laceration of muscle, fascia and tendon of abdomen**
- **S39.022 Laceration of muscle, fascia and tendon of lower back**
- **S39.023 Laceration of muscle, fascia and tendon of pelvis**

S39.09 Other injury of muscle, fascia and tendon of abdomen, lower back and pelvis

- **S39.091 Other injury of muscle, fascia and tendon of abdomen**
- **S39.092 Other injury of muscle, fascia and tendon of lower back**
- **S39.093 Other injury of muscle, fascia and tendon of pelvis**

S39.8 Other specified injuries of abdomen, lower back, pelvis and external genitals

- **S39.81 Other specified injuries of abdomen**
- **S39.82 Other specified injuries of lower back**
- **S39.83 Other specified injuries of pelvis**

S39.84 Other specified injuries of external genitals

- **S39.840 Fracture of corpus cavernosum penis** ♂
- **S39.848 Other specified injuries of external genitals**

S39.9 Unspecified injury of abdomen, lower back, pelvis and external genitals

- **S39.91 Unspecified injury of abdomen**
- **S39.92 Unspecified injury of lower back**
- **S39.93 Unspecified injury of pelvis**
- **S39.94 Unspecified injury of external genitals**

Injuries to the shoulder and upper arm (S40-S49)

INCLUDES injuries of axilla
injuries of scapular region

EXCLUDES 2 *burns and corrosions (T20-T32)*
frostbite (T33-T34)
injuries of elbow (S50-S59)
insect bite or sting, venomous (T63.4)

S40 Superficial injury of shoulder and upper arm

The appropriate 7th character is to be added to each code from category S40.
A initial encounter
D subsequent encounter
S sequela

S40.0 Contusion of shoulder and upper arm

S40.01 Contusion of shoulder

- **S40.011 Contusion of right shoulder**

Chapter 19. Injury, Poisoning and Certain Other Consequences of External Causes
S37.89–S40.011

- S40.012 Contusion of left shoulder
- S40.019 Contusion of unspecified shoulder
- S40.02 Contusion of upper arm
  - S40.021 Contusion of right upper arm
  - S40.022 Contusion of left upper arm
  - S40.029 Contusion of unspecified upper arm

S40.2 Other superficial injuries of shoulder

- S40.21 Abrasion of shoulder
  - S40.211 Abrasion of right shoulder
  - S40.212 Abrasion of left shoulder
  - S40.219 Abrasion of unspecified shoulder
- S40.22 Blister (nonthermal) of shoulder
  - S40.221 Blister (nonthermal) of right shoulder
  - S40.222 Blister (nonthermal) of left shoulder
  - S40.229 Blister (nonthermal) of unspecified shoulder
- S40.24 External constriction of shoulder
  - S40.241 External constriction of right shoulder
  - S40.242 External constriction of left shoulder
  - S40.249 External constriction of unspecified shoulder
- S40.25 Superficial foreign body of shoulder
  - Splinter in the shoulder
  - S40.251 Superficial foreign body of right shoulder
  - S40.252 Superficial foreign body of left shoulder
  - S40.259 Superficial foreign body of unspecified shoulder
- S40.26 Insect bite (nonvenomous) of shoulder
  - S40.261 Insect bite (nonvenomous) of right shoulder
  - S40.262 Insect bite (nonvenomous) of left shoulder
  - S40.269 Insect bite (nonvenomous) of unspecified shoulder
- S40.27 Other superficial bite of shoulder
  - EXCLUDES 1 *open bite of shoulder (S41.05)*
  - S40.271 Other superficial bite of right shoulder
  - S40.272 Other superficial bite of left shoulder
  - S40.279 Other superficial bite of unspecified shoulder

S40.8 Other superficial injuries of upper arm

- S40.81 Abrasion of upper arm
  - S40.811 Abrasion of right upper arm
  - S40.812 Abrasion of left upper arm
  - S40.819 Abrasion of unspecified upper arm
- S40.82 Blister (nonthermal) of upper arm
  - S40.821 Blister (nonthermal) of right upper arm
  - S40.822 Blister (nonthermal) of left upper arm
  - S40.829 Blister (nonthermal) of unspecified upper arm
- S40.84 External constriction of upper arm
  - S40.841 External constriction of right upper arm
  - S40.842 External constriction of left upper arm
  - S40.849 External constriction of unspecified upper arm
- S40.85 Superficial foreign body of upper arm
  - Splinter in the upper arm
  - S40.851 Superficial foreign body of right upper arm
  - S40.852 Superficial foreign body of left upper arm
  - S40.859 Superficial foreign body of unspecified upper arm
- S40.86 Insect bite (nonvenomous) of upper arm
  - S40.861 Insect bite (nonvenomous) of right upper arm
  - S40.862 Insect bite (nonvenomous) of left upper arm
  - S40.869 Insect bite (nonvenomous) of unspecified upper arm
- S40.87 Other superficial bite of upper arm
  - EXCLUDES 1 *open bite of upper arm (S41.14)*
  - EXCLUDES 2 *other superficial bite of shoulder (S40.27-)*
  - S40.871 Other superficial bite of right upper arm
  - S40.872 Other superficial bite of left upper arm
  - S40.879 Other superficial bite of unspecified upper arm

S40.9 Unspecified superficial injury of shoulder and upper arm

- S40.91 Unspecified superficial injury of shoulder
  - S40.911 Unspecified superficial injury of right shoulder
  - S40.912 Unspecified superficial injury of left shoulder
  - S40.919 Unspecified superficial injury of unspecified shoulder
- S40.92 Unspecified superficial injury of upper arm
  - S40.921 Unspecified superficial injury of right upper arm
  - S40.922 Unspecified superficial injury of left upper arm
  - S40.929 Unspecified superficial injury of unspecified upper arm

S41 Open wound of shoulder and upper arm

Code also any associated wound infection

EXCLUDES 1 *traumatic amputation of shoulder and upper arm (S48.-)*

EXCLUDES 2 *open fracture of shoulder and upper arm (S42.- with 7th character B or C)*

The appropriate 7th character is to be added to each code from category S41.

- A initial encounter
- D subsequent encounter
- S sequela

S41.0 Open wound of shoulder

- S41.00 Unspecified open wound of shoulder
  - S41.001 Unspecified open wound of right shoulder
  - S41.002 Unspecified open wound of left shoulder
  - S41.009 Unspecified open wound of unspecified shoulder
- S41.01 Laceration without foreign body of shoulder
  - S41.011 Laceration without foreign body of right shoulder
  - S41.012 Laceration without foreign body of left shoulder
  - S41.019 Laceration without foreign body of unspecified shoulder
- S41.02 Laceration with foreign body of shoulder
  - S41.021 Laceration with foreign body of right shoulder
  - S41.022 Laceration with foreign body of left shoulder
  - S41.029 Laceration with foreign body of unspecified shoulder
- S41.03 Puncture wound without foreign body of shoulder
  - S41.031 Puncture wound without foreign body of right shoulder
  - S41.032 Puncture wound without foreign body of left shoulder
  - S41.039 Puncture wound without foreign body of unspecified shoulder
- S41.04 Puncture wound with foreign body of shoulder
  - S41.041 Puncture wound with foreign body of right shoulder
  - S41.042 Puncture wound with foreign body of left shoulder
  - S41.049 Puncture wound with foreign body of unspecified shoulder
- S41.05 Open bite of shoulder
  - Bite of shoulder NOS
  - EXCLUDES 1 *superficial bite of shoulder (S40.27)*
  - S41.051 Open bite of right shoulder
  - S41.052 Open bite of left shoulder
  - S41.059 Open bite of unspecified shoulder

5th S41.1 Open wound of upper arm
6th S41.10 Unspecified open wound of upper arm
AHA: 2016,3Q,24
7th S41.101 Unspecified open wound of right upper arm
7th S41.102 Unspecified open wound of left upper arm
7th S41.109 Unspecified open wound of unspecified upper arm
6th S41.11 Laceration without foreign body of upper arm
7th S41.111 Laceration without foreign body of right upper arm
7th S41.112 Laceration without foreign body of left upper arm
7th S41.119 Laceration without foreign body of unspecified upper arm
6th S41.12 Laceration with foreign body of upper arm
7th S41.121 Laceration with foreign body of right upper arm
7th S41.122 Laceration with foreign body of left upper arm
7th S41.129 Laceration with foreign body of unspecified upper arm
6th S41.13 Puncture wound without foreign body of upper arm
AHA: 2016,3Q,24
7th S41.131 Puncture wound without foreign body of right upper arm
7th S41.132 Puncture wound without foreign body of left upper arm
7th S41.139 Puncture wound without foreign body of unspecified upper arm
6th S41.14 Puncture wound with foreign body of upper arm
AHA: 2016,3Q,24
7th S41.141 Puncture wound with foreign body of right upper arm
7th S41.142 Puncture wound with foreign body of left upper arm
7th S41.149 Puncture wound with foreign body of unspecified upper arm
6th S41.15 Open bite of upper arm
Bite of upper arm NOS
EXCLUDES 1 *superficial bite of upper arm (S40.87)*
7th S41.151 Open bite of right upper arm
7th S41.152 Open bite of left upper arm
7th S41.159 Open bite of unspecified upper arm

4th S42 Fracture of shoulder and upper arm
NOTE A fracture not indicated as displaced or nondisplaced should be coded to displaced
A fracture not indicated as open or closed should be coded to closed
EXCLUDES 1 *traumatic amputation of shoulder and upper arm (S48.-)*
AHA: 2018,2Q,12; 2015,3Q,37-39
DEF: Diaphysis: Central shaft of a long bone.
DEF: Epiphysis: Proximal and distal rounded ends of a long bone, communicates with the joint.
DEF: Metaphysis: Section of a long bone located between the epiphysis and diaphysis at the proximal and distal ends.
DEF: Physis (growth plate): Narrow zone of cartilaginous tissue between the epiphysis and metaphysis at each end of a long bone. In childhood, proliferation of cells in this zone lengthens the bone. As the bone matures, this area thins, ossification eventually fusing into solid bone and growth stops. *Synonym(s): Epiphyseal plate.*

The appropriate 7th character is to be added to all codes from category S42 [unless otherwise indicated].
A initial encounter for closed fracture
B initial encounter for open fracture
D subsequent encounter for fracture with routine healing
G subsequent encounter for fracture with delayed healing
K subsequent encounter for fracture with nonunion
P subsequent encounter for fracture with malunion
S sequela

5th S42.0 Fracture of clavicle
6th S42.00 Fracture of unspecified part of clavicle
3 7th S42.001 Fracture of unspecified part of right clavicle CC HS
3 7th S42.002 Fracture of unspecified part of left clavicle CC HS
3 7th S42.009 Fracture of unspecified part of unspecified clavicle CC HS UNS
AHA: 2012,4Q,93
6th S42.01 Fracture of sternal end of clavicle
3 7th S42.011 Anterior displaced fracture of sternal end of right clavicle CC HS
3 7th S42.012 Anterior displaced fracture of sternal end of left clavicle CC HS
3 7th S42.013 Anterior displaced fracture of sternal end of unspecified clavicle CC HS UNS
Displaced fracture of sternal end of clavicle NOS
3 7th S42.014 Posterior displaced fracture of sternal end of right clavicle CC HS
3 7th S42.015 Posterior displaced fracture of sternal end of left clavicle CC HS
3 7th S42.016 Posterior displaced fracture of sternal end of unspecified clavicle CC HS UNS
3 7th S42.017 Nondisplaced fracture of sternal end of right clavicle CC HS
3 7th S42.018 Nondisplaced fracture of sternal end of left clavicle CC HS
3 7th S42.019 Nondisplaced fracture of sternal end of unspecified clavicle CC HS UNS
6th S42.02 Fracture of shaft of clavicle
3 7th S42.021 Displaced fracture of shaft of right clavicle CC HS
3 7th S42.022 Displaced fracture of shaft of left clavicle CC HS
3 7th S42.023 Displaced fracture of shaft of unspecified clavicle CC HS UNS
3 7th S42.024 Nondisplaced fracture of shaft of right clavicle CC HS
3 7th S42.025 Nondisplaced fracture of shaft of left clavicle CC HS
3 7th S42.026 Nondisplaced fracture of shaft of unspecified clavicle CC HS UNS
6th S42.03 Fracture of lateral end of clavicle
Fracture of acromial end of clavicle
3 7th S42.031 Displaced fracture of lateral end of right clavicle CC HS
3 7th S42.032 Displaced fracture of lateral end of left clavicle CC HS
3 7th S42.033 Displaced fracture of lateral end of unspecified clavicle CC HS UNS
3 7th S42.034 Nondisplaced fracture of lateral end of right clavicle CC HS
3 7th S42.035 Nondisplaced fracture of lateral end of left clavicle CC HS
3 7th S42.036 Nondisplaced fracture of lateral end of unspecified clavicle CC HS UNS
5th S42.1 Fracture of scapula
6th S42.10 Fracture of unspecified part of scapula
3 7th S42.101 Fracture of unspecified part of scapula, right shoulder CC HS
3 7th S42.102 Fracture of unspecified part of scapula, left shoulder CC HS
3 7th S42.109 Fracture of unspecified part of scapula, unspecified shoulder CC HS UNS
6th S42.11 Fracture of body of scapula
3 7th S42.111 Displaced fracture of body of scapula, right shoulder CC HS
3 7th S42.112 Displaced fracture of body of scapula, left shoulder CC HS
3 7th S42.113 Displaced fracture of body of scapula, unspecified shoulder CC HS UNS
3 7th S42.114 Nondisplaced fracture of body of scapula, right shoulder CC HS
3 7th S42.115 Nondisplaced fracture of body of scapula, left shoulder CC HS
3 7th S42.116 Nondisplaced fracture of body of scapula, unspecified shoulder CC HS UNS
6th S42.12 Fracture of acromial process
3 7th S42.121 Displaced fracture of acromial process, right shoulder CC HS

3 ✓7th S42.122 Displaced fracture of acromial process, left shoulder CC H5
3 ✓7th S42.123 Displaced fracture of acromial process, unspecified shoulder CC H5 UNS
3 ✓7th S42.124 Nondisplaced fracture of acromial process, right shoulder CC H5
3 ✓7th S42.125 Nondisplaced fracture of acromial process, left shoulder CC H5
3 ✓7th S42.126 Nondisplaced fracture of acromial process, unspecified shoulder CC H5 UNS

✓6th S42.13 Fracture of coracoid process
3 ✓7th S42.131 Displaced fracture of coracoid process, right shoulder CC H5
3 ✓7th S42.132 Displaced fracture of coracoid process, left shoulder CC H5
3 ✓7th S42.133 Displaced fracture of coracoid process, unspecified shoulder CC H5 UNS
3 ✓7th S42.134 Nondisplaced fracture of coracoid process, right shoulder CC H5
3 ✓7th S42.135 Nondisplaced fracture of coracoid process, left shoulder CC H5
3 ✓7th S42.136 Nondisplaced fracture of coracoid process, unspecified shoulder CC H5 UNS

✓6th S42.14 Fracture of glenoid cavity of scapula
3 ✓7th S42.141 Displaced fracture of glenoid cavity of scapula, right shoulder CC H5
3 ✓7th S42.142 Displaced fracture of glenoid cavity of scapula, left shoulder CC H5
3 ✓7th S42.143 Displaced fracture of glenoid cavity of scapula, unspecified shoulder CC H5 UNS
3 ✓7th S42.144 Nondisplaced fracture of glenoid cavity of scapula, right shoulder CC H5
3 ✓7th S42.145 Nondisplaced fracture of glenoid cavity of scapula, left shoulder CC H5
3 ✓7th S42.146 Nondisplaced fracture of glenoid cavity of scapula, unspecified shoulder CC H5 UNS

✓6th S42.15 Fracture of neck of scapula
3 ✓7th S42.151 Displaced fracture of neck of scapula, right shoulder CC H5
3 ✓7th S42.152 Displaced fracture of neck of scapula, left shoulder CC H5
3 ✓7th S42.153 Displaced fracture of neck of scapula, unspecified shoulder CC H5 UNS
3 ✓7th S42.154 Nondisplaced fracture of neck of scapula, right shoulder CC H5
3 ✓7th S42.155 Nondisplaced fracture of neck of scapula, left shoulder CC H5
3 ✓7th S42.156 Nondisplaced fracture of neck of scapula, unspecified shoulder CC H5 UNS

✓6th S42.19 Fracture of other part of scapula
3 ✓7th S42.191 Fracture of other part of scapula, right shoulder CC H5
3 ✓7th S42.192 Fracture of other part of scapula, left shoulder CC H5
3 ✓7th S42.199 Fracture of other part of scapula, unspecified shoulder CC H5 UNS

✓5th S42.2 Fracture of upper end of humerus

Fracture of proximal end of humerus

EXCLUDES 2 *fracture of shaft of humerus (S42.3-)*
physeal fracture of upper end of humerus (S49.Ø-)

✓6th S42.2Ø Unspecified fracture of upper end of humerus
2,3 ✓7th S42.2Ø1 Unspecified fracture of upper end of right humerus MCC CC H5
2,3 ✓7th S42.2Ø2 Unspecified fracture of upper end of left humerus MCC CC H5
2,3 ✓7th S42.2Ø9 Unspecified fracture of upper end of unspecified humerus MCC CC H5 UNS

✓6th S42.21 Unspecified fracture of surgical neck of humerus

Fracture of neck of humerus NOS

2,3 ✓7th S42.211 Unspecified displaced fracture of surgical neck of right humerus MCC CC H5
2,3 ✓7th S42.212 Unspecified displaced fracture of surgical neck of left humerus MCC CC H5
2,3 ✓7th S42.213 Unspecified displaced fracture of surgical neck of unspecified humerus MCC CC H5 UNS
2,3 ✓7th S42.214 Unspecified nondisplaced fracture of surgical neck of right humerus MCC CC H5
2,3 ✓7th S42.215 Unspecified nondisplaced fracture of surgical neck of left humerus MCC CC H5
2,3 ✓7th S42.216 Unspecified nondisplaced fracture of surgical neck of unspecified humerus MCC CC H5 UNS

✓6th S42.22 2-part fracture of surgical neck of humerus
2,3 ✓7th S42.221 2-part displaced fracture of surgical neck of right humerus MCC CC H5
2,3 ✓7th S42.222 2-part displaced fracture of surgical neck of left humerus MCC CC H5
2,3 ✓7th S42.223 2-part displaced fracture of surgical neck of unspecified humerus MCC CC H5 UNS
2,3 ✓7th S42.224 2-part nondisplaced fracture of surgical neck of right humerus MCC CC H5
2,3 ✓7th S42.225 2-part nondisplaced fracture of surgical neck of left humerus MCC CC H5
2,3 ✓7th S42.226 2-part nondisplaced fracture of surgical neck of unspecified humerus MCC CC H5 UNS

✓6th S42.23 3-part fracture of surgical neck of humerus
2,3 ✓7th S42.231 3-part fracture of surgical neck of right humerus MCC CC H5
2,3 ✓7th S42.232 3-part fracture of surgical neck of left humerus MCC CC H5
2,3 ✓7th S42.239 3-part fracture of surgical neck of unspecified humerus MCC CC H5 UNS

✓6th S42.24 4-part fracture of surgical neck of humerus
2,3 ✓7th S42.241 4-part fracture of surgical neck of right humerus MCC CC H5
2,3 ✓7th S42.242 4-part fracture of surgical neck of left humerus MCC CC H5
2,3 ✓7th S42.249 4-part fracture of surgical neck of unspecified humerus MCC CC H5 UNS

✓6th S42.25 Fracture of greater tuberosity of humerus
2,3 ✓7th S42.251 Displaced fracture of greater tuberosity of right humerus MCC CC H5
2,3 ✓7th S42.252 Displaced fracture of greater tuberosity of left humerus MCC CC H5
2,3 ✓7th S42.253 Displaced fracture of greater tuberosity of unspecified humerus MCC CC H5 UNS
2,3 ✓7th S42.254 Nondisplaced fracture of greater tuberosity of right humerus MCC CC H5
2,3 ✓7th S42.255 Nondisplaced fracture of greater tuberosity of left humerus MCC CC H5
2,3 ✓7th S42.256 Nondisplaced fracture of greater tuberosity of unspecified humerus MCC CC H5 UNS

✓6th S42.26 Fracture of lesser tuberosity of humerus
2,3 ✓7th S42.261 Displaced fracture of lesser tuberosity of right humerus MCC CC H5
2,3 ✓7th S42.262 Displaced fracture of lesser tuberosity of left humerus MCC CC H5
2,3 ✓7th S42.263 Displaced fracture of lesser tuberosity of unspecified humerus MCC CC H5 UNS
2,3 ✓7th S42.264 Nondisplaced fracture of lesser tuberosity of right humerus MCC CC H5
2,3 ✓7th S42.265 Nondisplaced fracture of lesser tuberosity of left humerus MCC CC H5
2,3 ✓7th S42.266 Nondisplaced fracture of lesser tuberosity of unspecified humerus MCC CC H5 UNS

√6th **S42.27 Torus fracture of upper end of humerus**

The appropriate 7th character is to be added to all codes in subcategory S42.27
- A initial encounter for closed fracture
- D subsequent encounter for fracture with routine healing
- G subsequent encounter for fracture with delayed healing
- K subsequent encounter for fracture with nonunion
- P subsequent encounter for fracture with malunion
- S sequela

3 √7th **S42.271 Torus fracture of upper end of right humerus** CC H5

3 √7th **S42.272 Torus fracture of upper end of left humerus** CC H5

3 √7th **S42.279 Torus fracture of upper end of unspecified humerus** CC H5 UNS

√6th **S42.29 Other fracture of upper end of humerus**

Fracture of anatomical neck of humerus

Fracture of articular head of humerus

AHA: 2019,1Q,18

2,3 √7th **S42.291 Other displaced fracture of upper end of right humerus** MCC CC H5

2,3 √7th **S42.292 Other displaced fracture of upper end of left humerus** MCC CC H5

2,3 √7th **S42.293 Other displaced fracture of upper end of unspecified humerus** MCC CC H5 UNS

2,3 √7th **S42.294 Other nondisplaced fracture of upper end of right humerus** MCC CC H5

2,3 √7th **S42.295 Other nondisplaced fracture of upper end of left humerus** MCC CC H5

2,3 √7th **S42.296 Other nondisplaced fracture of upper end of unspecified humerus** MCC CC H5 UNS

√5th **S42.3 Fracture of shaft of humerus**

Fracture of humerus NOS

Fracture of upper arm NOS

EXCLUDES 2 *physeal fractures of upper end of humerus (S49.Ø-)*

physeal fractures of lower end of humerus (S49.1-)

√6th **S42.3Ø Unspecified fracture of shaft of humerus**

2,3 √7th **S42.3Ø1 Unspecified fracture of shaft of humerus, right arm** MCC CC H5

2,3 √7th **S42.3Ø2 Unspecified fracture of shaft of humerus, left arm** MCC CC H5

2,3 √7th **S42.3Ø9 Unspecified fracture of shaft of humerus, unspecified arm** MCC CC H5 UNS

√6th **S42.31 Greenstick fracture of shaft of humerus**

The appropriate 7th character is to be added to all codes in subcategory S42.31
- A initial encounter for closed fracture
- D subsequent encounter for fracture with routine healing
- G subsequent encounter for fracture with delayed healing
- K subsequent encounter for fracture with nonunion
- P subsequent encounter for fracture with malunion
- S sequela

3 √7th **S42.311 Greenstick fracture of shaft of humerus, right arm** CC H5

3 √7th **S42.312 Greenstick fracture of shaft of humerus, left arm** CC H5

3 √7th **S42.319 Greenstick fracture of shaft of humerus, unspecified arm** CC H5 UNS

√6th **S42.32 Transverse fracture of shaft of humerus**

2,3 √7th **S42.321 Displaced transverse fracture of shaft of humerus, right arm** MCC CC H5

2,3 √7th **S42.322 Displaced transverse fracture of shaft of humerus, left arm** MCC CC H5

2,3 √7th **S42.323 Displaced transverse fracture of shaft of humerus, unspecified arm** MCC CC H5 UNS

2,3 √7th **S42.324 Nondisplaced transverse fracture of shaft of humerus, right arm** MCC CC H5

2,3 √7th **S42.325 Nondisplaced transverse fracture of shaft of humerus, left arm** MCC CC H5

2,3 √7th **S42.326 Nondisplaced transverse fracture of shaft of humerus, unspecified arm** MCC CC H5 UNS

√6th **S42.33 Oblique fracture of shaft of humerus**

2,3 √7th **S42.331 Displaced oblique fracture of shaft of humerus, right arm** MCC CC H5

2,3 √7th **S42.332 Displaced oblique fracture of shaft of humerus, left arm** MCC CC H5

2,3 √7th **S42.333 Displaced oblique fracture of shaft of humerus, unspecified arm** MCC CC H5 UNS

2,3 √7th **S42.334 Nondisplaced oblique fracture of shaft of humerus, right arm** MCC CC H5

2,3 √7th **S42.335 Nondisplaced oblique fracture of shaft of humerus, left arm** MCC CC H5

2,3 √7th **S42.336 Nondisplaced oblique fracture of shaft of humerus, unspecified arm** MCC CC H5 UNS

√6th **S42.34 Spiral fracture of shaft of humerus**

2,3 √7th **S42.341 Displaced spiral fracture of shaft of humerus, right arm** MCC CC H5

2,3 √7th **S42.342 Displaced spiral fracture of shaft of humerus, left arm** MCC CC H5

2,3 √7th **S42.343 Displaced spiral fracture of shaft of humerus, unspecified arm** MCC CC H5 UNS

2,3 √7th **S42.344 Nondisplaced spiral fracture of shaft of humerus, right arm** MCC CC H5

2,3 √7th **S42.345 Nondisplaced spiral fracture of shaft of humerus, left arm** MCC CC H5

2,3 √7th **S42.346 Nondisplaced spiral fracture of shaft of humerus, unspecified arm** MCC CC H5 UNS

√6th **S42.35 Comminuted fracture of shaft of humerus**

2,3 √7th **S42.351 Displaced comminuted fracture of shaft of humerus, right arm** MCC CC H5

2,3 √7th **S42.352 Displaced comminuted fracture of shaft of humerus, left arm** MCC CC H5

2,3 √7th **S42.353 Displaced comminuted fracture of shaft of humerus, unspecified arm** MCC CC H5 UNS

2,3 √7th **S42.354 Nondisplaced comminuted fracture of shaft of humerus, right arm** MCC CC H5

2,3 √7th **S42.355 Nondisplaced comminuted fracture of shaft of humerus, left arm** MCC CC H5

2,3 √7th **S42.356 Nondisplaced comminuted fracture of shaft of humerus, unspecified arm** MCC CC H5 UNS

√6th **S42.36 Segmental fracture of shaft of humerus**

2,3 √7th **S42.361 Displaced segmental fracture of shaft of humerus, right arm** MCC CC H5

2,3 √7th **S42.362 Displaced segmental fracture of shaft of humerus, left arm** MCC CC H5

2,3 √7th **S42.363 Displaced segmental fracture of shaft of humerus, unspecified arm** MCC CC H5 UNS

2,3 √7th **S42.364 Nondisplaced segmental fracture of shaft of humerus, right arm** MCC CC H5

2,3 √7th **S42.365 Nondisplaced segmental fracture of shaft of humerus, left arm** MCC CC H5

2,3 √7th **S42.366 Nondisplaced segmental fracture of shaft of humerus, unspecified arm** MCC CC H5 UNS

√6th **S42.39 Other fracture of shaft of humerus**

2,3 √7th **S42.391 Other fracture of shaft of right humerus** MCC CC H5

2,3 √7th **S42.392 Other fracture of shaft of left humerus** MCC CC H5

2,3 √7th **S42.399 Other fracture of shaft of unspecified humerus** MCC CC H5 UNS

S42.4 Fracture of lower end of humerus
Fracture of distal end of humerus
EXCLUDES 2 *fracture of shaft of humerus (S42.3-)*
physeal fracture of lower end of humerus (S49.1-)

S42.40 Unspecified fracture of lower end of humerus
Fracture of elbow NOS
2,3 **S42.401 Unspecified fracture of lower end of right humerus** MCC CC H5
2,3 **S42.402 Unspecified fracture of lower end of left humerus** MCC CC H5
2,3 **S42.409 Unspecified fracture of lower end of unspecified humerus** MCC CC H5 UNS

S42.41 Simple supracondylar fracture without intercondylar fracture of humerus
2,3 **S42.411 Displaced simple supracondylar fracture without intercondylar fracture of right humerus** MCC CC H5
2,3 **S42.412 Displaced simple supracondylar fracture without intercondylar fracture of left humerus** MCC CC H5
2,3 **S42.413 Displaced simple supracondylar fracture without intercondylar fracture of unspecified humerus** MCC CC H5 UNS
2,3 **S42.414 Nondisplaced simple supracondylar fracture without intercondylar fracture of right humerus** MCC CC H5
2,3 **S42.415 Nondisplaced simple supracondylar fracture without intercondylar fracture of left humerus** MCC CC H5
2,3 **S42.416 Nondisplaced simple supracondylar fracture without intercondylar fracture of unspecified humerus** MCC CC H5 UNS

S42.42 Comminuted supracondylar fracture without intercondylar fracture of humerus
2,3 **S42.421 Displaced comminuted supracondylar fracture without intercondylar fracture of right humerus** MCC CC H5
2,3 **S42.422 Displaced comminuted supracondylar fracture without intercondylar fracture of left humerus** MCC CC H5
2,3 **S42.423 Displaced comminuted supracondylar fracture without intercondylar fracture of unspecified humerus** MCC CC H5 UNS
2,3 **S42.424 Nondisplaced comminuted supracondylar fracture without intercondylar fracture of right humerus** MCC CC H5
2,3 **S42.425 Nondisplaced comminuted supracondylar fracture without intercondylar fracture of left humerus** MCC CC H5
2,3 **S42.426 Nondisplaced comminuted supracondylar fracture without intercondylar fracture of unspecified humerus** MCC CC H5 UNS

S42.43 Fracture (avulsion) of lateral epicondyle of humerus
2,3 **S42.431 Displaced fracture (avulsion) of lateral epicondyle of right humerus** MCC CC H5
2,3 **S42.432 Displaced fracture (avulsion) of lateral epicondyle of left humerus** MCC CC H5
2,3 **S42.433 Displaced fracture (avulsion) of lateral epicondyle of unspecified humerus** MCC CC H5 UNS
2,3 **S42.434 Nondisplaced fracture (avulsion) of lateral epicondyle of right humerus** MCC CC H5
2,3 **S42.435 Nondisplaced fracture (avulsion) of lateral epicondyle of left humerus** MCC CC H5
2,3 **S42.436 Nondisplaced fracture (avulsion) of lateral epicondyle of unspecified humerus** MCC CC H5 UNS

S42.44 Fracture (avulsion) of medial epicondyle of humerus
2,3 **S42.441 Displaced fracture (avulsion) of medial epicondyle of right humerus** MCC CC H5
2,3 **S42.442 Displaced fracture (avulsion) of medial epicondyle of left humerus** MCC CC H5
2,3 **S42.443 Displaced fracture (avulsion) of medial epicondyle of unspecified humerus** MCC CC H5 UNS
2,3 **S42.444 Nondisplaced fracture (avulsion) of medial epicondyle of right humerus** MCC CC H5
2,3 **S42.445 Nondisplaced fracture (avulsion) of medial epicondyle of left humerus** MCC CC H5
2,3 **S42.446 Nondisplaced fracture (avulsion) of medial epicondyle of unspecified humerus** MCC CC H5 UNS
2,3 **S42.447 Incarcerated fracture (avulsion) of medial epicondyle of right humerus** MCC CC H5
2,3 **S42.448 Incarcerated fracture (avulsion) of medial epicondyle of left humerus** MCC CC H5
2,3 **S42.449 Incarcerated fracture (avulsion) of medial epicondyle of unspecified humerus** MCC CC H5 UNS

S42.45 Fracture of lateral condyle of humerus
Fracture of capitellum of humerus
2,3 **S42.451 Displaced fracture of lateral condyle of right humerus** MCC CC H5
2,3 **S42.452 Displaced fracture of lateral condyle of left humerus** MCC CC H5
2,3 **S42.453 Displaced fracture of lateral condyle of unspecified humerus** MCC CC H5 UNS
2,3 **S42.454 Nondisplaced fracture of lateral condyle of right humerus** MCC CC H5
2,3 **S42.455 Nondisplaced fracture of lateral condyle of left humerus** MCC CC H5
2,3 **S42.456 Nondisplaced fracture of lateral condyle of unspecified humerus** MCC CC H5 UNS

S42.46 Fracture of medial condyle of humerus
Trochlea fracture of humerus
2,3 **S42.461 Displaced fracture of medial condyle of right humerus** MCC CC H5
2,3 **S42.462 Displaced fracture of medial condyle of left humerus** MCC CC H5
2,3 **S42.463 Displaced fracture of medial condyle of unspecified humerus** MCC CC H5 UNS
2,3 **S42.464 Nondisplaced fracture of medial condyle of right humerus** MCC CC H5
2,3 **S42.465 Nondisplaced fracture of medial condyle of left humerus** MCC CC H5
2,3 **S42.466 Nondisplaced fracture of medial condyle of unspecified humerus** MCC CC H5 UNS

S42.47 Transcondylar fracture of humerus
2,3 **S42.471 Displaced transcondylar fracture of right humerus** MCC CC H5
2,3 **S42.472 Displaced transcondylar fracture of left humerus** MCC CC H5
2,3 **S42.473 Displaced transcondylar fracture of unspecified humerus** MCC CC H5 UNS
2,3 **S42.474 Nondisplaced transcondylar fracture of right humerus** MCC CC H5
2,3 **S42.475 Nondisplaced transcondylar fracture of left humerus** MCC CC H5
2,3 **S42.476 Nondisplaced transcondylar fracture of unspecified humerus** MCC CC H5 UNS

S42.48 Torus fracture of lower end of humerus

The appropriate 7th character is to be added to all codes in subcategory S42.48.
A initial encounter for closed fracture
D subsequent encounter for fracture with routine healing
G subsequent encounter for fracture with delayed healing
K subsequent encounter for fracture with nonunion
P subsequent encounter for fracture with malunion
S sequela

3 **S42.481 Torus fracture of lower end of right humerus** CC H5
3 **S42.482 Torus fracture of lower end of left humerus** CC H5
3 **S42.489 Torus fracture of lower end of unspecified humerus** CC H5 UNS

Additional Character Required | Placeholder | Questionable PDx | Manifestation | Unspecified | UPD Unacceptable PDx | H1-H14 HAC | HCC CMS-HCC Dx | HIV HIV Dx

✓6th **S42.49 Other fracture of lower end of humerus**

2,3 ✓7th **S42.491 Other displaced fracture of lower end of right humerus** MCC CC H5

2,3 ✓7th **S42.492 Other displaced fracture of lower end of left humerus** MCC CC H5

2,3 ✓7th **S42.493 Other displaced fracture of lower end of unspecified humerus** MCC CC H5 UNS

2,3 ✓7th **S42.494 Other nondisplaced fracture of lower end of right humerus** MCC CC H5

2,3 ✓7th **S42.495 Other nondisplaced fracture of lower end of left humerus** MCC CC H5

2,3 ✓7th **S42.496 Other nondisplaced fracture of lower end of unspecified humerus** MCC CC H5 UNS

✓5th **S42.9 Fracture of shoulder girdle, part unspecified**

Fracture of shoulder NOS

2,3 ✓x7th **S42.9Ø Fracture of unspecified shoulder girdle, part unspecified** MCC CC H5 UNS

2,3 ✓x7th **S42.91 Fracture of right shoulder girdle, part unspecified** MCC CC H5

2,3 ✓x7th **S42.92 Fracture of left shoulder girdle, part unspecified** MCC CC H5

✓4th **S43 Dislocation and sprain of joints and ligaments of shoulder girdle**

INCLUDES avulsion of joint or ligament of shoulder girdle
laceration of cartilage, joint or ligament of shoulder girdle
sprain of cartilage, joint or ligament of shoulder girdle
traumatic hemarthrosis of joint or ligament of shoulder girdle
traumatic rupture of joint or ligament of shoulder girdle
traumatic subluxation of joint or ligament of shoulder girdle
traumatic tear of joint or ligament of shoulder girdle

Code also any associated open wound

EXCLUDES 2 *strain of muscle, fascia and tendon of shoulder and upper arm (S46.-)*

The appropriate 7th character is to be added to each code from category S43.
A initial encounter
D subsequent encounter
S sequela

✓5th **S43.Ø Subluxation and dislocation of shoulder joint**

Dislocation of glenohumeral joint
Subluxation of glenohumeral joint

✓6th **S43.ØØ Unspecified subluxation and dislocation of shoulder joint**

Dislocation of humerus NOS
Subluxation of humerus NOS

✓7th **S43.ØØ1 Unspecified subluxation of right shoulder joint**

✓7th **S43.ØØ2 Unspecified subluxation of left shoulder joint**

✓7th **S43.ØØ3 Unspecified subluxation of unspecified shoulder joint**

✓7th **S43.ØØ4 Unspecified dislocation of right shoulder joint**

✓7th **S43.ØØ5 Unspecified dislocation of left shoulder joint**

✓7th **S43.ØØ6 Unspecified dislocation of unspecified shoulder joint**

✓6th **S43.Ø1 Anterior subluxation and dislocation of humerus**

✓7th **S43.Ø11 Anterior subluxation of right humerus**

✓7th **S43.Ø12 Anterior subluxation of left humerus**

✓7th **S43.Ø13 Anterior subluxation of unspecified humerus**

✓7th **S43.Ø14 Anterior dislocation of right humerus**

✓7th **S43.Ø15 Anterior dislocation of left humerus**

✓7th **S43.Ø16 Anterior dislocation of unspecified humerus**

✓6th **S43.Ø2 Posterior subluxation and dislocation of humerus**

✓7th **S43.Ø21 Posterior subluxation of right humerus**

✓7th **S43.Ø22 Posterior subluxation of left humerus**

✓7th **S43.Ø23 Posterior subluxation of unspecified humerus**

✓7th **S43.Ø24 Posterior dislocation of right humerus**

✓7th **S43.Ø25 Posterior dislocation of left humerus**

✓7th **S43.Ø26 Posterior dislocation of unspecified humerus**

✓6th **S43.Ø3 Inferior subluxation and dislocation of humerus**

✓7th **S43.Ø31 Inferior subluxation of right humerus**

✓7th **S43.Ø32 Inferior subluxation of left humerus**

✓7th **S43.Ø33 Inferior subluxation of unspecified humerus**

✓7th **S43.Ø34 Inferior dislocation of right humerus**

✓7th **S43.Ø35 Inferior dislocation of left humerus**

✓7th **S43.Ø36 Inferior dislocation of unspecified humerus**

✓6th **S43.Ø8 Other subluxation and dislocation of shoulder joint**

✓7th **S43.Ø81 Other subluxation of right shoulder joint**

✓7th **S43.Ø82 Other subluxation of left shoulder joint**

✓7th **S43.Ø83 Other subluxation of unspecified shoulder joint**

✓7th **S43.Ø84 Other dislocation of right shoulder joint**

✓7th **S43.Ø85 Other dislocation of left shoulder joint**

✓7th **S43.Ø86 Other dislocation of unspecified shoulder joint**

✓5th **S43.1 Subluxation and dislocation of acromioclavicular joint**

✓6th **S43.1Ø Unspecified dislocation of acromioclavicular joint**

✓7th **S43.1Ø1 Unspecified dislocation of right acromioclavicular joint**

✓7th **S43.1Ø2 Unspecified dislocation of left acromioclavicular joint**

✓7th **S43.1Ø9 Unspecified dislocation of unspecified acromioclavicular joint**

✓6th **S43.11 Subluxation of acromioclavicular joint**

✓7th **S43.111 Subluxation of right acromioclavicular joint**

✓7th **S43.112 Subluxation of left acromioclavicular joint**

✓7th **S43.119 Subluxation of unspecified acromioclavicular joint**

✓6th **S43.12 Dislocation of acromioclavicular joint, 1ØØ%-2ØØ% displacement**

✓7th **S43.121 Dislocation of right acromioclavicular joint, 1ØØ%-2ØØ% displacement**

✓7th **S43.122 Dislocation of left acromioclavicular joint, 1ØØ%-2ØØ% displacement**

✓7th **S43.129 Dislocation of unspecified acromioclavicular joint, 1ØØ%-2ØØ% displacement**

✓6th **S43.13 Dislocation of acromioclavicular joint, greater than 2ØØ% displacement**

✓7th **S43.131 Dislocation of right acromioclavicular joint, greater than 2ØØ% displacement**

✓7th **S43.132 Dislocation of left acromioclavicular joint, greater than 2ØØ% displacement**

✓7th **S43.139 Dislocation of unspecified acromioclavicular joint, greater than 2ØØ% displacement**

✓6th **S43.14 Inferior dislocation of acromioclavicular joint**

✓7th **S43.141 Inferior dislocation of right acromioclavicular joint**

✓7th **S43.142 Inferior dislocation of left acromioclavicular joint**

✓7th **S43.149 Inferior dislocation of unspecified acromioclavicular joint**

✓6th **S43.15 Posterior dislocation of acromioclavicular joint**

✓7th **S43.151 Posterior dislocation of right acromioclavicular joint**

✓7th **S43.152 Posterior dislocation of left acromioclavicular joint**

✓7th **S43.159 Posterior dislocation of unspecified acromioclavicular joint**

✓5th **S43.2 Subluxation and dislocation of sternoclavicular joint**

✓6th **S43.2Ø Unspecified subluxation and dislocation of sternoclavicular joint**

✓7th **S43.2Ø1 Unspecified subluxation of right sternoclavicular joint** CC H5

✓7th **S43.2Ø2 Unspecified subluxation of left sternoclavicular joint** CC H5

✓7th **S43.2Ø3 Unspecified subluxation of unspecified sternoclavicular joint** CC H5 UNS

✓7th **S43.2Ø4 Unspecified dislocation of right sternoclavicular joint** CC H5

✓7th **S43.2Ø5 Unspecified dislocation of left sternoclavicular joint** CC H5

7th S43.206 Unspecified dislocation of unspecified sternoclavicular joint CC H5 UNS

6th S43.21 Anterior subluxation and dislocation of sternoclavicular joint

7th S43.211 Anterior subluxation of right sternoclavicular joint CC H5

7th S43.212 Anterior subluxation of left sternoclavicular joint CC H5

7th S43.213 Anterior subluxation of unspecified sternoclavicular joint CC H5 UNS

7th S43.214 Anterior dislocation of right sternoclavicular joint CC H5

7th S43.215 Anterior dislocation of left sternoclavicular joint CC H5

7th S43.216 Anterior dislocation of unspecified sternoclavicular joint CC H5 UNS

6th S43.22 Posterior subluxation and dislocation of sternoclavicular joint

7th S43.221 Posterior subluxation of right sternoclavicular joint CC H5

7th S43.222 Posterior subluxation of left sternoclavicular joint CC H5

7th S43.223 Posterior subluxation of unspecified sternoclavicular joint CC H5 UNS

7th S43.224 Posterior dislocation of right sternoclavicular joint CC H5

7th S43.225 Posterior dislocation of left sternoclavicular joint CC H5

7th S43.226 Posterior dislocation of unspecified sternoclavicular joint CC H5 UNS

5th S43.3 Subluxation and dislocation of other and unspecified parts of shoulder girdle

6th S43.30 Subluxation and dislocation of unspecified parts of shoulder girdle

Dislocation of shoulder girdle NOS

Subluxation of shoulder girdle NOS

7th S43.301 Subluxation of unspecified parts of right shoulder girdle

7th S43.302 Subluxation of unspecified parts of left shoulder girdle

7th S43.303 Subluxation of unspecified parts of unspecified shoulder girdle

7th S43.304 Dislocation of unspecified parts of right shoulder girdle

7th S43.305 Dislocation of unspecified parts of left shoulder girdle

7th S43.306 Dislocation of unspecified parts of unspecified shoulder girdle

6th S43.31 Subluxation and dislocation of scapula

7th S43.311 Subluxation of right scapula

7th S43.312 Subluxation of left scapula

7th S43.313 Subluxation of unspecified scapula

7th S43.314 Dislocation of right scapula

7th S43.315 Dislocation of left scapula

7th S43.316 Dislocation of unspecified scapula

6th S43.39 Subluxation and dislocation of other parts of shoulder girdle

7th S43.391 Subluxation of other parts of right shoulder girdle

7th S43.392 Subluxation of other parts of left shoulder girdle

7th S43.393 Subluxation of other parts of unspecified shoulder girdle

7th S43.394 Dislocation of other parts of right shoulder girdle

7th S43.395 Dislocation of other parts of left shoulder girdle

7th S43.396 Dislocation of other parts of unspecified shoulder girdle

5th S43.4 Sprain of shoulder joint

6th S43.40 Unspecified sprain of shoulder joint

7th S43.401 Unspecified sprain of right shoulder joint

7th S43.402 Unspecified sprain of left shoulder joint

7th S43.409 Unspecified sprain of unspecified shoulder joint

6th S43.41 Sprain of coracohumeral (ligament)

7th S43.411 Sprain of right coracohumeral (ligament)

7th S43.412 Sprain of left coracohumeral (ligament)

7th S43.419 Sprain of unspecified coracohumeral (ligament)

6th S43.42 Sprain of rotator cuff capsule

EXCLUDES 1 *rotator cuff syndrome (complete) (incomplete), not specified as traumatic (M75.1-)*

EXCLUDES 2 *injury of tendon of rotator cuff (S46.0-)*

7th S43.421 Sprain of right rotator cuff capsule

7th S43.422 Sprain of left rotator cuff capsule

7th S43.429 Sprain of unspecified rotator cuff capsule

6th S43.43 Superior glenoid labrum lesion

SLAP lesion

AHA: 2019,2Q,26

DEF: Detachment injury of the superior aspect of the glenoid labrum, which is the ring of fibrocartilage attached to the rim of the glenoid cavity of the scapula.

7th S43.431 Superior glenoid labrum lesion of right shoulder

7th S43.432 Superior glenoid labrum lesion of left shoulder

7th S43.439 Superior glenoid labrum lesion of unspecified shoulder

6th S43.49 Other sprain of shoulder joint

7th S43.491 Other sprain of right shoulder joint

7th S43.492 Other sprain of left shoulder joint

7th S43.499 Other sprain of unspecified shoulder joint

5th S43.5 Sprain of acromioclavicular joint

Sprain of acromioclavicular ligament

x7th S43.50 Sprain of unspecified acromioclavicular joint

x7th S43.51 Sprain of right acromioclavicular joint

x7th S43.52 Sprain of left acromioclavicular joint

5th S43.6 Sprain of sternoclavicular joint

x7th S43.60 Sprain of unspecified sternoclavicular joint

x7th S43.61 Sprain of right sternoclavicular joint

x7th S43.62 Sprain of left sternoclavicular joint

5th S43.8 Sprain of other specified parts of shoulder girdle

x7th S43.80 Sprain of other specified parts of unspecified shoulder girdle

x7th S43.81 Sprain of other specified parts of right shoulder girdle

x7th S43.82 Sprain of other specified parts of left shoulder girdle

5th S43.9 Sprain of unspecified parts of shoulder girdle

x7th S43.90 Sprain of unspecified parts of unspecified shoulder girdle

Sprain of shoulder girdle NOS

x7th S43.91 Sprain of unspecified parts of right shoulder girdle

x7th S43.92 Sprain of unspecified parts of left shoulder girdle

4th S44 Injury of nerves at shoulder and upper arm level

Code also any associated open wound (S41.-)

EXCLUDES 2 *injury of brachial plexus (S14.3-)*

The appropriate 7th character is to be added to each code from category S44.

A initial encounter

D subsequent encounter

S sequela

5th S44.0 Injury of ulnar nerve at upper arm level

EXCLUDES 1 *ulnar nerve NOS (S54.0)*

x7th S44.00 Injury of ulnar nerve at upper arm level, unspecified arm

x7th S44.01 Injury of ulnar nerve at upper arm level, right arm

x7th S44.02 Injury of ulnar nerve at upper arm level, left arm

5th S44.1 Injury of median nerve at upper arm level

EXCLUDES 1 *median nerve NOS (S54.1)*

x7th S44.10 Injury of median nerve at upper arm level, unspecified arm

x7th S44.11 Injury of median nerve at upper arm level, right arm

x7th S44.12 Injury of median nerve at upper arm level, left arm

5th S44.2 Injury of radial nerve at upper arm level

EXCLUDES 1 *radial nerve NOS (S54.2)*

x7th S44.20 Injury of radial nerve at upper arm level, unspecified arm

√x7th S44.21 Injury of radial nerve at upper arm level, right arm
√x7th S44.22 Injury of radial nerve at upper arm level, left arm
√5th S44.3 Injury of axillary nerve
√x7th S44.30 Injury of axillary nerve, unspecified arm
√x7th S44.31 Injury of axillary nerve, right arm
√x7th S44.32 Injury of axillary nerve, left arm
√5th S44.4 Injury of musculocutaneous nerve
√x7th S44.40 Injury of musculocutaneous nerve, unspecified arm
√x7th S44.41 Injury of musculocutaneous nerve, right arm
√x7th S44.42 Injury of musculocutaneous nerve, left arm
√5th S44.5 Injury of cutaneous sensory nerve at shoulder and upper arm level
√x7th S44.50 Injury of cutaneous sensory nerve at shoulder and upper arm level, unspecified arm
√x7th S44.51 Injury of cutaneous sensory nerve at shoulder and upper arm level, right arm
√x7th S44.52 Injury of cutaneous sensory nerve at shoulder and upper arm level, left arm
√5th S44.8 Injury of other nerves at shoulder and upper arm level
√6th S44.8X Injury of other nerves at shoulder and upper arm level
√7th S44.8X1 Injury of other nerves at shoulder and upper arm level, right arm
√7th S44.8X2 Injury of other nerves at shoulder and upper arm level, left arm
√7th S44.8X9 Injury of other nerves at shoulder and upper arm level, unspecified arm
√5th S44.9 Injury of unspecified nerve at shoulder and upper arm level
√x7th S44.90 Injury of unspecified nerve at shoulder and upper arm level, unspecified arm
√x7th S44.91 Injury of unspecified nerve at shoulder and upper arm level, right arm
√x7th S44.92 Injury of unspecified nerve at shoulder and upper arm level, left arm

√4th **S45 Injury of blood vessels at shoulder and upper arm level**

Code also any associated open wound (S41.-)

EXCLUDES 2 *injury of subclavian artery (S25.1)*
injury of subclavian vein (S25.3)

The appropriate 7th character is to be added to each code from category S45.
A initial encounter
D subsequent encounter
S sequela

√5th S45.0 Injury of axillary artery
√6th S45.00 Unspecified injury of axillary artery
√7th S45.001 Unspecified injury of axillary artery, right side MCC
√7th S45.002 Unspecified injury of axillary artery, left side MCC
√7th S45.009 Unspecified injury of axillary artery, unspecified side MCC UNS
√6th S45.01 Laceration of axillary artery
√7th S45.011 Laceration of axillary artery, right side MCC
√7th S45.012 Laceration of axillary artery, left side MCC
√7th S45.019 Laceration of axillary artery, unspecified side MCC UNS
√6th S45.09 Other specified injury of axillary artery
√7th S45.091 Other specified injury of axillary artery, right side MCC
√7th S45.092 Other specified injury of axillary artery, left side MCC
√7th S45.099 Other specified injury of axillary artery, unspecified side MCC UNS
√5th S45.1 Injury of brachial artery
√6th S45.10 Unspecified injury of brachial artery
√7th S45.101 Unspecified injury of brachial artery, right side CC
√7th S45.102 Unspecified injury of brachial artery, left side CC
√7th S45.109 Unspecified injury of brachial artery, unspecified side CC UNS
√6th S45.11 Laceration of brachial artery
√7th S45.111 Laceration of brachial artery, right side CC
√7th S45.112 Laceration of brachial artery, left side CC
√7th S45.119 Laceration of brachial artery, unspecified side CC UNS
√6th S45.19 Other specified injury of brachial artery
√7th S45.191 Other specified injury of brachial artery, right side CC
√7th S45.192 Other specified injury of brachial artery, left side CC
√7th S45.199 Other specified injury of brachial artery, unspecified side CC UNS
√5th S45.2 Injury of axillary or brachial vein
√6th S45.20 Unspecified injury of axillary or brachial vein
√7th S45.201 Unspecified injury of axillary or brachial vein, right side CC
√7th S45.202 Unspecified injury of axillary or brachial vein, left side CC
√7th S45.209 Unspecified injury of axillary or brachial vein, unspecified side CC UNS
√6th S45.21 Laceration of axillary or brachial vein
√7th S45.211 Laceration of axillary or brachial vein, right side CC
√7th S45.212 Laceration of axillary or brachial vein, left side CC
√7th S45.219 Laceration of axillary or brachial vein, unspecified side CC UNS
√6th S45.29 Other specified injury of axillary or brachial vein
√7th S45.291 Other specified injury of axillary or brachial vein, right side CC
√7th S45.292 Other specified injury of axillary or brachial vein, left side CC
√7th S45.299 Other specified injury of axillary or brachial vein, unspecified side CC UNS
√5th S45.3 Injury of superficial vein at shoulder and upper arm level
√6th S45.30 Unspecified injury of superficial vein at shoulder and upper arm level
√7th S45.301 Unspecified injury of superficial vein at shoulder and upper arm level, right arm CC
√7th S45.302 Unspecified injury of superficial vein at shoulder and upper arm level, left arm CC
√7th S45.309 Unspecified injury of superficial vein at shoulder and upper arm level, unspecified arm CC UNS
√6th S45.31 Laceration of superficial vein at shoulder and upper arm level
√7th S45.311 Laceration of superficial vein at shoulder and upper arm level, right arm CC
√7th S45.312 Laceration of superficial vein at shoulder and upper arm level, left arm CC
√7th S45.319 Laceration of superficial vein at shoulder and upper arm level, unspecified arm CC UNS
√6th S45.39 Other specified injury of superficial vein at shoulder and upper arm level
√7th S45.391 Other specified injury of superficial vein at shoulder and upper arm level, right arm CC
√7th S45.392 Other specified injury of superficial vein at shoulder and upper arm level, left arm CC
√7th S45.399 Other specified injury of superficial vein at shoulder and upper arm level, unspecified arm CC UNS
√5th S45.8 Injury of other specified blood vessels at shoulder and upper arm level
√6th S45.80 Unspecified injury of other specified blood vessels at shoulder and upper arm level
√7th S45.801 Unspecified injury of other specified blood vessels at shoulder and upper arm level, right arm CC
√7th S45.802 Unspecified injury of other specified blood vessels at shoulder and upper arm level, left arm CC

S45.809 Unspecified injury of other specified blood vessels at shoulder and upper arm level, unspecified arm CC UNS

S45.81 Laceration of other specified blood vessels at shoulder and upper arm level

S45.811 Laceration of other specified blood vessels at shoulder and upper arm level, right arm CC

S45.812 Laceration of other specified blood vessels at shoulder and upper arm level, left arm CC

S45.819 Laceration of other specified blood vessels at shoulder and upper arm level, unspecified arm CC UNS

S45.89 Other specified injury of other specified blood vessels at shoulder and upper arm level

S45.891 Other specified injury of other specified blood vessels at shoulder and upper arm level, right arm CC

S45.892 Other specified injury of other specified blood vessels at shoulder and upper arm level, left arm CC

S45.899 Other specified injury of other specified blood vessels at shoulder and upper arm level, unspecified arm CC UNS

S45.9 Injury of unspecified blood vessel at shoulder and upper arm level

S45.90 Unspecified injury of unspecified blood vessel at shoulder and upper arm level

S45.901 Unspecified injury of unspecified blood vessel at shoulder and upper arm level, right arm CC

S45.902 Unspecified injury of unspecified blood vessel at shoulder and upper arm level, left arm CC

S45.909 Unspecified injury of unspecified blood vessel at shoulder and upper arm level, unspecified arm CC UNS

S45.91 Laceration of unspecified blood vessel at shoulder and upper arm level

S45.911 Laceration of unspecified blood vessel at shoulder and upper arm level, right arm CC

S45.912 Laceration of unspecified blood vessel at shoulder and upper arm level, left arm CC

S45.919 Laceration of unspecified blood vessel at shoulder and upper arm level, unspecified arm CC UNS

S45.99 Other specified injury of unspecified blood vessel at shoulder and upper arm level

S45.991 Other specified injury of unspecified blood vessel at shoulder and upper arm level, right arm CC

S45.992 Other specified injury of unspecified blood vessel at shoulder and upper arm level, left arm CC

S45.999 Other specified injury of unspecified blood vessel at shoulder and upper arm level, unspecified arm CC UNS

S46 Injury of muscle, fascia and tendon at shoulder and upper arm level

Code also any associated open wound (S41.-)

EXCLUDES 2 *injury of muscle, fascia and tendon at elbow (S56.-)*
sprain of joints and ligaments of shoulder girdle (S43.9)

TIP: Refer to the Muscle/Tendon table at the beginning of this chapter.

The appropriate 7th character is to be added to each code from category S46.
A initial encounter
D subsequent encounter
S sequela

S46.0 Injury of muscle(s) and tendon(s) of the rotator cuff of shoulder

S46.00 Unspecified injury of muscle(s) and tendon(s) of the rotator cuff of shoulder

S46.001 Unspecified injury of muscle(s) and tendon(s) of the rotator cuff of right shoulder

S46.002 Unspecified injury of muscle(s) and tendon(s) of the rotator cuff of left shoulder

S46.009 Unspecified injury of muscle(s) and tendon(s) of the rotator cuff of unspecified shoulder

S46.01 Strain of muscle(s) and tendon(s) of the rotator cuff of shoulder

S46.011 Strain of muscle(s) and tendon(s) of the rotator cuff of right shoulder

S46.012 Strain of muscle(s) and tendon(s) of the rotator cuff of left shoulder

S46.019 Strain of muscle(s) and tendon(s) of the rotator cuff of unspecified shoulder

S46.02 Laceration of muscle(s) and tendon(s) of the rotator cuff of shoulder

S46.021 Laceration of muscle(s) and tendon(s) of the rotator cuff of right shoulder CC

S46.022 Laceration of muscle(s) and tendon(s) of the rotator cuff of left shoulder CC

S46.029 Laceration of muscle(s) and tendon(s) of the rotator cuff of unspecified shoulder CC UNS

S46.09 Other injury of muscle(s) and tendon(s) of the rotator cuff of shoulder

S46.091 Other injury of muscle(s) and tendon(s) of the rotator cuff of right shoulder

S46.092 Other injury of muscle(s) and tendon(s) of the rotator cuff of left shoulder

S46.099 Other injury of muscle(s) and tendon(s) of the rotator cuff of unspecified shoulder

S46.1 Injury of muscle, fascia and tendon of long head of biceps

S46.10 Unspecified injury of muscle, fascia and tendon of long head of biceps

S46.101 Unspecified injury of muscle, fascia and tendon of long head of biceps, right arm

S46.102 Unspecified injury of muscle, fascia and tendon of long head of biceps, left arm

S46.109 Unspecified injury of muscle, fascia and tendon of long head of biceps, unspecified arm

S46.11 Strain of muscle, fascia and tendon of long head of biceps

AHA: 2020,1Q,38; 2019,2Q,27

S46.111 Strain of muscle, fascia and tendon of long head of biceps, right arm

S46.112 Strain of muscle, fascia and tendon of long head of biceps, left arm

S46.119 Strain of muscle, fascia and tendon of long head of biceps, unspecified arm

S46.12 Laceration of muscle, fascia and tendon of long head of biceps

S46.121 Laceration of muscle, fascia and tendon of long head of biceps, right arm CC

S46.122 Laceration of muscle, fascia and tendon of long head of biceps, left arm CC

S46.129 Laceration of muscle, fascia and tendon of long head of biceps, unspecified arm CC UNS

S46.19 Other injury of muscle, fascia and tendon of long head of biceps

S46.191 Other injury of muscle, fascia and tendon of long head of biceps, right arm

S46.192 Other injury of muscle, fascia and tendon of long head of biceps, left arm

S46.199 Other injury of muscle, fascia and tendon of long head of biceps, unspecified arm

S46.2 Injury of muscle, fascia and tendon of other parts of biceps

S46.20 Unspecified injury of muscle, fascia and tendon of other parts of biceps

S46.201 Unspecified injury of muscle, fascia and tendon of other parts of biceps, right arm

S46.202 Unspecified injury of muscle, fascia and tendon of other parts of biceps, left arm

S46.209 Unspecified injury of muscle, fascia and tendon of other parts of biceps, unspecified arm

S46.21 Strain of muscle, fascia and tendon of other parts of biceps

S46.211 Strain of muscle, fascia and tendon of other parts of biceps, right arm

S46.212 Strain of muscle, fascia and tendon of other parts of biceps, left arm

S46.219 Strain of muscle, fascia and tendon of other parts of biceps, unspecified arm

S46.22 Laceration of muscle, fascia and tendon of other parts of biceps
S46.221 Laceration of muscle, fascia and tendon of other parts of biceps, right arm CC
S46.222 Laceration of muscle, fascia and tendon of other parts of biceps, left arm CC
S46.229 Laceration of muscle, fascia and tendon of other parts of biceps, unspecified arm CC UNS
S46.29 Other injury of muscle, fascia and tendon of other parts of biceps
S46.291 Other injury of muscle, fascia and tendon of other parts of biceps, right arm
S46.292 Other injury of muscle, fascia and tendon of other parts of biceps, left arm
S46.299 Other injury of muscle, fascia and tendon of other parts of biceps, unspecified arm
S46.3 Injury of muscle, fascia and tendon of triceps
S46.30 Unspecified injury of muscle, fascia and tendon of triceps
S46.301 Unspecified injury of muscle, fascia and tendon of triceps, right arm
S46.302 Unspecified injury of muscle, fascia and tendon of triceps, left arm
S46.309 Unspecified injury of muscle, fascia and tendon of triceps, unspecified arm
S46.31 Strain of muscle, fascia and tendon of triceps
S46.311 Strain of muscle, fascia and tendon of triceps, right arm
S46.312 Strain of muscle, fascia and tendon of triceps, left arm
S46.319 Strain of muscle, fascia and tendon of triceps, unspecified arm
S46.32 Laceration of muscle, fascia and tendon of triceps
S46.321 Laceration of muscle, fascia and tendon of triceps, right arm CC
S46.322 Laceration of muscle, fascia and tendon of triceps, left arm CC
S46.329 Laceration of muscle, fascia and tendon of triceps, unspecified arm CC UNS
S46.39 Other injury of muscle, fascia and tendon of triceps
S46.391 Other injury of muscle, fascia and tendon of triceps, right arm
S46.392 Other injury of muscle, fascia and tendon of triceps, left arm
S46.399 Other injury of muscle, fascia and tendon of triceps, unspecified arm
S46.8 Injury of other muscles, fascia and tendons at shoulder and upper arm level
S46.80 Unspecified injury of other muscles, fascia and tendons at shoulder and upper arm level
S46.801 Unspecified injury of other muscles, fascia and tendons at shoulder and upper arm level, right arm
S46.802 Unspecified injury of other muscles, fascia and tendons at shoulder and upper arm level, left arm
S46.809 Unspecified injury of other muscles, fascia and tendons at shoulder and upper arm level, unspecified arm
S46.81 Strain of other muscles, fascia and tendons at shoulder and upper arm level
S46.811 Strain of other muscles, fascia and tendons at shoulder and upper arm level, right arm
S46.812 Strain of other muscles, fascia and tendons at shoulder and upper arm level, left arm
S46.819 Strain of other muscles, fascia and tendons at shoulder and upper arm level, unspecified arm
S46.82 Laceration of other muscles, fascia and tendons at shoulder and upper arm level
S46.821 Laceration of other muscles, fascia and tendons at shoulder and upper arm level, right arm CC
S46.822 Laceration of other muscles, fascia and tendons at shoulder and upper arm level, left arm CC
S46.829 Laceration of other muscles, fascia and tendons at shoulder and upper arm level, unspecified arm CC UNS
S46.89 Other injury of other muscles, fascia and tendons at shoulder and upper arm level
S46.891 Other injury of other muscles, fascia and tendons at shoulder and upper arm level, right arm
S46.892 Other injury of other muscles, fascia and tendons at shoulder and upper arm level, left arm
S46.899 Other injury of other muscles, fascia and tendons at shoulder and upper arm level, unspecified arm
S46.9 Injury of unspecified muscle, fascia and tendon at shoulder and upper arm level
S46.90 Unspecified injury of unspecified muscle, fascia and tendon at shoulder and upper arm level
S46.901 Unspecified injury of unspecified muscle, fascia and tendon at shoulder and upper arm level, right arm
S46.902 Unspecified injury of unspecified muscle, fascia and tendon at shoulder and upper arm level, left arm
S46.909 Unspecified injury of unspecified muscle, fascia and tendon at shoulder and upper arm level, unspecified arm
S46.91 Strain of unspecified muscle, fascia and tendon at shoulder and upper arm level
S46.911 Strain of unspecified muscle, fascia and tendon at shoulder and upper arm level, right arm
S46.912 Strain of unspecified muscle, fascia and tendon at shoulder and upper arm level, left arm
S46.919 Strain of unspecified muscle, fascia and tendon at shoulder and upper arm level, unspecified arm
S46.92 Laceration of unspecified muscle, fascia and tendon at shoulder and upper arm level
S46.921 Laceration of unspecified muscle, fascia and tendon at shoulder and upper arm level, right arm CC
S46.922 Laceration of unspecified muscle, fascia and tendon at shoulder and upper arm level, left arm CC
S46.929 Laceration of unspecified muscle, fascia and tendon at shoulder and upper arm level, unspecified arm CC UNS
S46.99 Other injury of unspecified muscle, fascia and tendon at shoulder and upper arm level
S46.991 Other injury of unspecified muscle, fascia and tendon at shoulder and upper arm level, right arm
S46.992 Other injury of unspecified muscle, fascia and tendon at shoulder and upper arm level, left arm
S46.999 Other injury of unspecified muscle, fascia and tendon at shoulder and upper arm level, unspecified arm

S47 Crushing injury of shoulder and upper arm
Use additional code for all associated injuries
EXCLUDES 2 *crushing injury of elbow (S57.0-)*

The appropriate 7th character is to be added to each code from category S47.
A initial encounter
D subsequent encounter
S sequela

S47.1 Crushing injury of right shoulder and upper arm
S47.2 Crushing injury of left shoulder and upper arm
S47.9 Crushing injury of shoulder and upper arm, unspecified arm

S48 Traumatic amputation of shoulder and upper arm

An amputation not identified as partial or complete should be coded to complete

EXCLUDES 1 *traumatic amputation at elbow level (S58.0)*

The appropriate 7th character is to be added to each code from category S48.
A initial encounter
D subsequent encounter
S sequela

S48.0 Traumatic amputation at shoulder joint

S48.01 Complete traumatic amputation at shoulder joint

S48.011 Complete traumatic amputation at right shoulder joint CC HCC

S48.012 Complete traumatic amputation at left shoulder joint CC HCC

S48.019 Complete traumatic amputation at unspecified shoulder joint CC UNS HCC

S48.02 Partial traumatic amputation at shoulder joint

S48.021 Partial traumatic amputation at right shoulder joint CC HCC

S48.022 Partial traumatic amputation at left shoulder joint CC HCC

S48.029 Partial traumatic amputation at unspecified shoulder joint CC UNS HCC

S48.1 Traumatic amputation at level between shoulder and elbow

S48.11 Complete traumatic amputation at level between shoulder and elbow

S48.111 Complete traumatic amputation at level between right shoulder and elbow CC HCC

S48.112 Complete traumatic amputation at level between left shoulder and elbow CC HCC

S48.119 Complete traumatic amputation at level between unspecified shoulder and elbow CC UNS HCC

S48.12 Partial traumatic amputation at level between shoulder and elbow

S48.121 Partial traumatic amputation at level between right shoulder and elbow CC HCC

S48.122 Partial traumatic amputation at level between left shoulder and elbow CC HCC

S48.129 Partial traumatic amputation at level between unspecified shoulder and elbow CC UNS HCC

S48.9 Traumatic amputation of shoulder and upper arm, level unspecified

S48.91 Complete traumatic amputation of shoulder and upper arm, level unspecified

S48.911 Complete traumatic amputation of right shoulder and upper arm, level unspecified CC HCC

S48.912 Complete traumatic amputation of left shoulder and upper arm, level unspecified CC HCC

S48.919 Complete traumatic amputation of unspecified shoulder and upper arm, level unspecified CC UNS HCC

S48.92 Partial traumatic amputation of shoulder and upper arm, level unspecified

S48.921 Partial traumatic amputation of right shoulder and upper arm, level unspecified CC HCC

S48.922 Partial traumatic amputation of left shoulder and upper arm, level unspecified CC HCC

S48.929 Partial traumatic amputation of unspecified shoulder and upper arm, level unspecified CC UNS HCC

S49 Other and unspecified injuries of shoulder and upper arm

AHA: 2018,2Q,12; 2018,1Q,3

The appropriate 7th character is to be added to each code from subcategories S49.0 and S49.1.
A initial encounter for closed fracture
D subsequent encounter for fracture with routine healing
G subsequent encounter for fracture with delayed healing
K subsequent encounter for fracture with nonunion
P subsequent encounter for fracture with malunion
S sequela

S49.0 Physeal fracture of upper end of humerus

AHA: 2019,4Q,56

S49.00 Unspecified physeal fracture of upper end of humerus

S49.001 Unspecified physeal fracture of upper end of humerus, right arm CC H5

S49.002 Unspecified physeal fracture of upper end of humerus, left arm CC H5

S49.009 Unspecified physeal fracture of upper end of humerus, unspecified arm CC H5 UNS

S49.01 Salter-Harris Type I physeal fracture of upper end of humerus

S49.011 Salter-Harris Type I physeal fracture of upper end of humerus, right arm CC H5

S49.012 Salter-Harris Type I physeal fracture of upper end of humerus, left arm CC H5

S49.019 Salter-Harris Type I physeal fracture of upper end of humerus, unspecified arm CC H5 UNS

S49.02 Salter-Harris Type II physeal fracture of upper end of humerus

S49.021 Salter-Harris Type II physeal fracture of upper end of humerus, right arm CC H5

S49.022 Salter-Harris Type II physeal fracture of upper end of humerus, left arm CC H5

S49.029 Salter-Harris Type II physeal fracture of upper end of humerus, unspecified arm CC H5 UNS

S49.03 Salter-Harris Type III physeal fracture of upper end of humerus

S49.031 Salter-Harris Type III physeal fracture of upper end of humerus, right arm CC H5

S49.032 Salter-Harris Type III physeal fracture of upper end of humerus, left arm CC H5

S49.039 Salter-Harris Type III physeal fracture of upper end of humerus, unspecified arm CC H5 UNS

S49.04 Salter-Harris Type IV physeal fracture of upper end of humerus

S49.041 Salter-Harris Type IV physeal fracture of upper end of humerus, right arm CC H5

S49.042 Salter-Harris Type IV physeal fracture of upper end of humerus, left arm CC H5

S49.049 Salter-Harris Type IV physeal fracture of upper end of humerus, unspecified arm CC H5 UNS

S49.09 Other physeal fracture of upper end of humerus

S49.091 Other physeal fracture of upper end of humerus, right arm CC H5

S49.092 Other physeal fracture of upper end of humerus, left arm CC H5

S49.099 Other physeal fracture of upper end of humerus, unspecified arm CC H5 UNS

S49.1 Physeal fracture of lower end of humerus

AHA: 2019,4Q,56

S49.10 Unspecified physeal fracture of lower end of humerus

S49.101 Unspecified physeal fracture of lower end of humerus, right arm CC H5

S49.102 Unspecified physeal fracture of lower end of humerus, left arm CC H5

S49.109 Unspecified physeal fracture of lower end of humerus, unspecified arm CC H5 UNS

S49.11 **Salter-Harris Type I physeal fracture of lower end of humerus**

- **S49.111** **Salter-Harris Type I physeal fracture of lower end of humerus, right arm** CC H5
- **S49.112** **Salter-Harris Type I physeal fracture of lower end of humerus, left arm** CC H5
- **S49.119** **Salter-Harris Type I physeal fracture of lower end of humerus, unspecified arm** CC H5 UNS

S49.12 **Salter-Harris Type II physeal fracture of lower end of humerus**

- **S49.121** **Salter-Harris Type II physeal fracture of lower end of humerus, right arm** CC H5
- **S49.122** **Salter-Harris Type II physeal fracture of lower end of humerus, left arm** CC H5
- **S49.129** **Salter-Harris Type II physeal fracture of lower end of humerus, unspecified arm** CC H5 UNS

S49.13 **Salter-Harris Type III physeal fracture of lower end of humerus**

- **S49.131** **Salter-Harris Type III physeal fracture of lower end of humerus, right arm** CC H5
- **S49.132** **Salter-Harris Type III physeal fracture of lower end of humerus, left arm** CC H5
- **S49.139** **Salter-Harris Type III physeal fracture of lower end of humerus, unspecified arm** CC H5 UNS

S49.14 **Salter-Harris Type IV physeal fracture of lower end of humerus**

- **S49.141** **Salter-Harris Type IV physeal fracture of lower end of humerus, right arm** CC H5
- **S49.142** **Salter-Harris Type IV physeal fracture of lower end of humerus, left arm** CC H5
- **S49.149** **Salter-Harris Type IV physeal fracture of lower end of humerus, unspecified arm** CC H5 UNS

S49.19 **Other physeal fracture of lower end of humerus**

- **S49.191** **Other physeal fracture of lower end of humerus, right arm** CC H5
- **S49.192** **Other physeal fracture of lower end of humerus, left arm** CC H5
- **S49.199** **Other physeal fracture of lower end of humerus, unspecified arm** CC H5 UNS

S49.8 **Other specified injuries of shoulder and upper arm**

The appropriate 7th character is to be added to each code in subcategory S49.8.
A initial encounter
D subsequent encounter
S sequela

- **S49.8Ø** **Other specified injuries of shoulder and upper arm, unspecified arm**
- **S49.81** **Other specified injuries of right shoulder and upper arm**
- **S49.82** **Other specified injuries of left shoulder and upper arm**

S49.9 **Unspecified injury of shoulder and upper arm**

The appropriate 7th character is to be added to each code in subcategory S49.9.
A initial encounter
D subsequent encounter
S sequela

- **S49.9Ø** **Unspecified injury of shoulder and upper arm, unspecified arm**
- **S49.91** **Unspecified injury of right shoulder and upper arm**
- **S49.92** **Unspecified injury of left shoulder and upper arm**

Injuries to the elbow and forearm (S5Ø-S59)

EXCLUDES 2 *burns and corrosions (T2Ø-T32)*
frostbite (T33-T34)
injuries of wrist and hand (S6Ø-S69)
insect bite or sting, venomous (T63.4)

S5Ø **Superficial injury of elbow and forearm**

EXCLUDES 2 *superficial injury of wrist and hand (S6Ø.-)*

The appropriate 7th character is to be added to each code from category S5Ø.
A initial encounter
D subsequent encounter
S sequela

S5Ø.Ø **Contusion of elbow**

- **S5Ø.ØØ** **Contusion of unspecified elbow**
- **S5Ø.Ø1** **Contusion of right elbow**
- **S5Ø.Ø2** **Contusion of left elbow**

S5Ø.1 **Contusion of forearm**

- **S5Ø.1Ø** **Contusion of unspecified forearm**
- **S5Ø.11** **Contusion of right forearm**
- **S5Ø.12** **Contusion of left forearm**

S5Ø.3 **Other superficial injuries of elbow**

S5Ø.31 **Abrasion of elbow**

- **S5Ø.311** **Abrasion of right elbow**
- **S5Ø.312** **Abrasion of left elbow**
- **S5Ø.319** **Abrasion of unspecified elbow**

S5Ø.32 **Blister (nonthermal) of elbow**

- **S5Ø.321** **Blister (nonthermal) of right elbow**
- **S5Ø.322** **Blister (nonthermal) of left elbow**
- **S5Ø.329** **Blister (nonthermal) of unspecified elbow**

S5Ø.34 **External constriction of elbow**

- **S5Ø.341** **External constriction of right elbow**
- **S5Ø.342** **External constriction of left elbow**
- **S5Ø.349** **External constriction of unspecified elbow**

S5Ø.35 **Superficial foreign body of elbow**

Splinter in the elbow

- **S5Ø.351** **Superficial foreign body of right elbow**
- **S5Ø.352** **Superficial foreign body of left elbow**
- **S5Ø.359** **Superficial foreign body of unspecified elbow**

S5Ø.36 **Insect bite (nonvenomous) of elbow**

- **S5Ø.361** **Insect bite (nonvenomous) of right elbow**
- **S5Ø.362** **Insect bite (nonvenomous) of left elbow**
- **S5Ø.369** **Insect bite (nonvenomous) of unspecified elbow**

S5Ø.37 **Other superficial bite of elbow**

EXCLUDES 1 *open bite of elbow (S51.Ø5)*

- **S5Ø.371** **Other superficial bite of right elbow**
- **S5Ø.372** **Other superficial bite of left elbow**
- **S5Ø.379** **Other superficial bite of unspecified elbow**

S5Ø.8 **Other superficial injuries of forearm**

S5Ø.81 **Abrasion of forearm**

- **S5Ø.811** **Abrasion of right forearm**
- **S5Ø.812** **Abrasion of left forearm**
- **S5Ø.819** **Abrasion of unspecified forearm**

S5Ø.82 **Blister (nonthermal) of forearm**

- **S5Ø.821** **Blister (nonthermal) of right forearm**
- **S5Ø.822** **Blister (nonthermal) of left forearm**
- **S5Ø.829** **Blister (nonthermal) of unspecified forearm**

S5Ø.84 **External constriction of forearm**

- **S5Ø.841** **External constriction of right forearm**
- **S5Ø.842** **External constriction of left forearm**
- **S5Ø.849** **External constriction of unspecified forearm**

S50.85 **Superficial foreign body of forearm**
Splinter in the forearm
S50.851 **Superficial foreign body of right forearm**
S50.852 **Superficial foreign body of left forearm**
S50.859 **Superficial foreign body of unspecified forearm**
S50.86 **Insect bite (nonvenomous) of forearm**
S50.861 **Insect bite (nonvenomous) of right forearm**
S50.862 **Insect bite (nonvenomous) of left forearm**
S50.869 **Insect bite (nonvenomous) of unspecified forearm**
S50.87 **Other superficial bite of forearm**
EXCLUDES 1 *open bite of forearm (S51.85)*
S50.871 **Other superficial bite of right forearm**
S50.872 **Other superficial bite of left forearm**
S50.879 **Other superficial bite of unspecified forearm**
S50.9 **Unspecified superficial injury of elbow and forearm**
S50.90 **Unspecified superficial injury of elbow**
S50.901 **Unspecified superficial injury of right elbow**
S50.902 **Unspecified superficial injury of left elbow**
S50.909 **Unspecified superficial injury of unspecified elbow**
S50.91 **Unspecified superficial injury of forearm**
S50.911 **Unspecified superficial injury of right forearm**
S50.912 **Unspecified superficial injury of left forearm**
S50.919 **Unspecified superficial injury of unspecified forearm**

S51 **Open wound of elbow and forearm**
Code also any associated wound infection
EXCLUDES 1 *open fracture of elbow and forearm (S52.- with open fracture 7th character)*
traumatic amputation of elbow and forearm (S58.-)
EXCLUDES 2 *open wound of wrist and hand (S61.-)*

The appropriate 7th character is to be added to each code from category S51.
A initial encounter
D subsequent encounter
S sequela

S51.0 **Open wound of elbow**
S51.00 **Unspecified open wound of elbow**
S51.001 **Unspecified open wound of right elbow**
AHA: 2012,4Q,108
S51.002 **Unspecified open wound of left elbow**
S51.009 **Unspecified open wound of unspecified elbow**
Open wound of elbow NOS
S51.01 **Laceration without foreign body of elbow**
S51.011 **Laceration without foreign body of right elbow**
S51.012 **Laceration without foreign body of left elbow**
S51.019 **Laceration without foreign body of unspecified elbow**
S51.02 **Laceration with foreign body of elbow**
S51.021 **Laceration with foreign body of right elbow**
S51.022 **Laceration with foreign body of left elbow**
S51.029 **Laceration with foreign body of unspecified elbow**
S51.03 **Puncture wound without foreign body of elbow**
S51.031 **Puncture wound without foreign body of right elbow**
S51.032 **Puncture wound without foreign body of left elbow**
S51.039 **Puncture wound without foreign body of unspecified elbow**
S51.04 **Puncture wound with foreign body of elbow**
S51.041 **Puncture wound with foreign body of right elbow**
S51.042 **Puncture wound with foreign body of left elbow**
S51.049 **Puncture wound with foreign body of unspecified elbow**
S51.05 **Open bite of elbow**
Bite of elbow NOS
EXCLUDES 1 *superficial bite of elbow (S50.36, S50.37)*
S51.051 **Open bite, right elbow**
S51.052 **Open bite, left elbow**
S51.059 **Open bite, unspecified elbow**
S51.8 **Open wound of forearm**
EXCLUDES 2 *open wound of elbow (S51.0-)*
S51.80 **Unspecified open wound of forearm**
AHA: 2016,3Q,24
S51.801 **Unspecified open wound of right forearm**
S51.802 **Unspecified open wound of left forearm**
S51.809 **Unspecified open wound of unspecified forearm**
Open wound of forearm NOS
S51.81 **Laceration without foreign body of forearm**
S51.811 **Laceration without foreign body of right forearm**
S51.812 **Laceration without foreign body of left forearm**
S51.819 **Laceration without foreign body of unspecified forearm**
S51.82 **Laceration with foreign body of forearm**
S51.821 **Laceration with foreign body of right forearm**
S51.822 **Laceration with foreign body of left forearm**
S51.829 **Laceration with foreign body of unspecified forearm**
S51.83 **Puncture wound without foreign body of forearm**
AHA: 2016,3Q,24
S51.831 **Puncture wound without foreign body of right forearm**
S51.832 **Puncture wound without foreign body of left forearm**
S51.839 **Puncture wound without foreign body of unspecified forearm**
S51.84 **Puncture wound with foreign body of forearm**
AHA: 2016,3Q,24
S51.841 **Puncture wound with foreign body of right forearm**
S51.842 **Puncture wound with foreign body of left forearm**
S51.849 **Puncture wound with foreign body of unspecified forearm**
S51.85 **Open bite of forearm**
Bite of forearm NOS
EXCLUDES 1 *superficial bite of forearm (S50.86, S50.87)*
S51.851 **Open bite of right forearm**
S51.852 **Open bite of left forearm**
S51.859 **Open bite of unspecified forearm**

4th S52 Fracture of forearm

NOTE A fracture not indicated as displaced or nondisplaced should be coded to displaced.

A fracture not indicated as open or closed should be coded to closed.

The open fracture designations are based on the Gustilo open fracture classification.

EXCLUDES 1 *traumatic amputation of forearm (S58.-)*

EXCLUDES 2 *fracture at wrist and hand level (S62.-)*

AHA: 2018,2Q,12; 2016,1Q,33; 2015,3Q,37-39

DEF: Diaphysis: Central shaft of a long bone.

DEF: Epiphysis: Proximal and distal rounded ends of a long bone, communicates with the joint.

DEF: Metaphysis: Section of a long bone located between the epiphysis and diaphysis at the proximal and distal ends.

DEF: Physis (growth plate): Narrow zone of cartilaginous tissue between the epiphysis and metaphysis at each end of a long bone. In childhood, proliferation of cells in this zone lengthens the bone. As the bone matures, this area thins, ossification eventually fusing into solid bone and growth stops. ***Synonym(s):*** *Epiphyseal plate.*

The appropriate 7th character is to be added to all codes from category S52 [unless otherwise indicated].
- A initial encounter for closed fracture
- B initial encounter for open fracture type I or II; initial encounter for open fracture NOS
- C initial encounter for open fracture type IIIA, IIIB, or IIIC
- D subsequent encounter for closed fracture with routine healing
- E subsequent encounter for open fracture type I or II with routine healing
- F subsequent encounter for open fracture type IIIA, IIIB, or IIIC with routine healing
- G subsequent encounter for closed fracture with delayed healing
- H subsequent encounter for open fracture type I or II with delayed healing
- J subsequent encounter for open fracture type IIIA, IIIB, or IIIC with delayed healing
- K subsequent encounter for closed fracture with nonunion
- M subsequent encounter for open fracture type I or II with nonunion
- N subsequent encounter for open fracture type IIIA, IIIB, or IIIC with nonunion
- P subsequent encounter for closed fracture with malunion
- Q subsequent encounter for open fracture type I or II with malunion
- R subsequent encounter for open fracture type IIIA, IIIB, or IIIC with malunion
- S sequela

5th S52.0 Fracture of upper end of ulna

Fracture of proximal end of ulna

EXCLUDES 2 *fracture of elbow NOS (S42.40-)*
fractures of shaft of ulna (S52.2-)

6th S52.00 Unspecified fracture of upper end of ulna

- 2,4 7th **S52.001** Unspecified fracture of upper end of right ulna MCC CC HS
- 2,4 7th **S52.002** Unspecified fracture of upper end of left ulna MCC CC HS
- 2,4 7th **S52.009** Unspecified fracture of upper end of unspecified ulna MCC CC HS UNS

6th S52.01 Torus fracture of upper end of ulna

The appropriate 7th character is to be added to all codes in subcategory S52.01
- A initial encounter for closed fracture
- D subsequent encounter for fracture with routine healing
- G subsequent encounter for fracture with delayed healing
- K subsequent encounter for fracture with nonunion
- P subsequent encounter for fracture with malunion
- S sequela

- 3 7th **S52.011** Torus fracture of upper end of right ulna CC HS
- 3 7th **S52.012** Torus fracture of upper end of left ulna CC HS
- 3 7th **S52.019** Torus fracture of upper end of unspecified ulna CC HS UNS

6th S52.02 Fracture of olecranon process without intraarticular extension of ulna

- 2,4 7th **S52.021** Displaced fracture of olecranon process without intraarticular extension of right ulna MCC CC HS
- 2,4 7th **S52.022** Displaced fracture of olecranon process without intraarticular extension of left ulna MCC CC HS
- 2,4 7th **S52.023** Displaced fracture of olecranon process without intraarticular extension of unspecified ulna MCC CC HS UNS
- 2,4 7th **S52.024** Nondisplaced fracture of olecranon process without intraarticular extension of right ulna MCC CC HS
- 2,4 7th **S52.025** Nondisplaced fracture of olecranon process without intraarticular extension of left ulna MCC CC HS
- 2,4 7th **S52.026** Nondisplaced fracture of olecranon process without intraarticular extension of unspecified ulna MCC CC HS UNS

6th S52.03 Fracture of olecranon process with intraarticular extension of ulna

- 2,4 7th **S52.031** Displaced fracture of olecranon process with intraarticular extension of right ulna MCC CC HS
- 2,4 7th **S52.032** Displaced fracture of olecranon process with intraarticular extension of left ulna MCC CC HS
- 2,4 7th **S52.033** Displaced fracture of olecranon process with intraarticular extension of unspecified ulna MCC CC HS UNS
- 2,4 7th **S52.034** Nondisplaced fracture of olecranon process with intraarticular extension of right ulna MCC CC HS
- 2,4 7th **S52.035** Nondisplaced fracture of olecranon process with intraarticular extension of left ulna MCC CC HS
- 2,4 7th **S52.036** Nondisplaced fracture of olecranon process with intraarticular extension of unspecified ulna MCC CC HS UNS

6th S52.04 Fracture of coronoid process of ulna

- 2,4 7th **S52.041** Displaced fracture of coronoid process of right ulna MCC CC HS
- 2,4 7th **S52.042** Displaced fracture of coronoid process of left ulna MCC CC HS
- 2,4 7th **S52.043** Displaced fracture of coronoid process of unspecified ulna MCC CC HS UNS
- 2,4 7th **S52.044** Nondisplaced fracture of coronoid process of right ulna MCC CC HS
- 2,4 7th **S52.045** Nondisplaced fracture of coronoid process of left ulna MCC CC HS
- 2,4 7th **S52.046** Nondisplaced fracture of coronoid process of unspecified ulna MCC CC HS UNS

6th S52.09 Other fracture of upper end of ulna

- 2,4 7th **S52.091** Other fracture of upper end of right ulna MCC CC HS
- 2,4 7th **S52.092** Other fracture of upper end of left ulna MCC CC HS
- 2,4 7th **S52.099** Other fracture of upper end of unspecified ulna MCC CC HS UNS

5th S52.1 Fracture of upper end of radius

Fracture of proximal end of radius

EXCLUDES 2 *physeal fractures of upper end of radius (S59.2-)*
fracture of shaft of radius (S52.3-)

6th S52.10 Unspecified fracture of upper end of radius

- 2,4 7th **S52.101** Unspecified fracture of upper end of right radius MCC CC HS
- 2,4 7th **S52.102** Unspecified fracture of upper end of left radius MCC CC HS
- 2,4 7th **S52.109** Unspecified fracture of upper end of unspecified radius MCC CC HS UNS

S52.11 Torus fracture of upper end of radius

The appropriate 7th character is to be added to all codes in subcategory S52.11
A initial encounter for closed fracture
D subsequent encounter for fracture with routine healing
G subsequent encounter for fracture with delayed healing
K subsequent encounter for fracture with nonunion
P subsequent encounter for fracture with malunion
S sequela

S52.111 Torus fracture of upper end of right radius CC H5
S52.112 Torus fracture of upper end of left radius CC H5
S52.119 Torus fracture of upper end of unspecified radius CC H5 UNS

S52.12 Fracture of head of radius
S52.121 Displaced fracture of head of right radius MCC CC H5
S52.122 Displaced fracture of head of left radius MCC CC H5
S52.123 Displaced fracture of head of unspecified radius MCC CC H5 UNS
S52.124 Nondisplaced fracture of head of right radius MCC CC H5
S52.125 Nondisplaced fracture of head of left radius MCC CC H5
S52.126 Nondisplaced fracture of head of unspecified radius MCC CC H5 UNS

S52.13 Fracture of neck of radius
S52.131 Displaced fracture of neck of right radius MCC CC H5
S52.132 Displaced fracture of neck of left radius MCC CC H5
S52.133 Displaced fracture of neck of unspecified radius MCC CC H5 UNS
S52.134 Nondisplaced fracture of neck of right radius MCC CC H5
S52.135 Nondisplaced fracture of neck of left radius MCC CC H5
S52.136 Nondisplaced fracture of neck of unspecified radius MCC CC H5 UNS

S52.18 Other fracture of upper end of radius
S52.181 Other fracture of upper end of right radius MCC CC H5
S52.182 Other fracture of upper end of left radius MCC CC H5
S52.189 Other fracture of upper end of unspecified radius MCC CC H5 UNS

S52.2 Fracture of shaft of ulna

S52.20 Unspecified fracture of shaft of ulna
Fracture of ulna NOS
S52.201 Unspecified fracture of shaft of right ulna MCC CC H5
S52.202 Unspecified fracture of shaft of left ulna MCC CC H5
S52.209 Unspecified fracture of shaft of unspecified ulna MCC CC H5 UNS

S52.21 Greenstick fracture of shaft of ulna

The appropriate 7th character is to be added to all codes in subcategory S52.21
A initial encounter for closed fracture
D subsequent encounter for fracture with routine healing
G subsequent encounter for fracture with delayed healing
K subsequent encounter for fracture with nonunion
P subsequent encounter for fracture with malunion
S sequela

S52.211 Greenstick fracture of shaft of right ulna CC H5
S52.212 Greenstick fracture of shaft of left ulna CC H5
S52.219 Greenstick fracture of shaft of unspecified ulna CC H5 UNS

S52.22 Transverse fracture of shaft of ulna
S52.221 Displaced transverse fracture of shaft of right ulna MCC CC H5
S52.222 Displaced transverse fracture of shaft of left ulna MCC CC H5
S52.223 Displaced transverse fracture of shaft of unspecified ulna MCC CC H5 UNS
S52.224 Nondisplaced transverse fracture of shaft of right ulna MCC CC H5
S52.225 Nondisplaced transverse fracture of shaft of left ulna MCC CC H5
S52.226 Nondisplaced transverse fracture of shaft of unspecified ulna MCC CC H5 UNS

S52.23 Oblique fracture of shaft of ulna
S52.231 Displaced oblique fracture of shaft of right ulna MCC CC H5
S52.232 Displaced oblique fracture of shaft of left ulna MCC CC H5
S52.233 Displaced oblique fracture of shaft of unspecified ulna MCC CC H5 UNS
S52.234 Nondisplaced oblique fracture of shaft of right ulna MCC CC H5
S52.235 Nondisplaced oblique fracture of shaft of left ulna MCC CC H5
S52.236 Nondisplaced oblique fracture of shaft of unspecified ulna MCC CC H5 UNS

S52.24 Spiral fracture of shaft of ulna
S52.241 Displaced spiral fracture of shaft of ulna, right arm MCC CC H5
S52.242 Displaced spiral fracture of shaft of ulna, left arm MCC CC H5
S52.243 Displaced spiral fracture of shaft of ulna, unspecified arm MCC CC H5 UNS
S52.244 Nondisplaced spiral fracture of shaft of ulna, right arm MCC CC H5
S52.245 Nondisplaced spiral fracture of shaft of ulna, left arm MCC CC H5
S52.246 Nondisplaced spiral fracture of shaft of ulna, unspecified arm MCC CC H5 UNS

S52.25 Comminuted fracture of shaft of ulna
S52.251 Displaced comminuted fracture of shaft of ulna, right arm MCC CC H5
S52.252 Displaced comminuted fracture of shaft of ulna, left arm MCC CC H5
S52.253 Displaced comminuted fracture of shaft of ulna, unspecified arm MCC CC H5 UNS
S52.254 Nondisplaced comminuted fracture of shaft of ulna, right arm MCC CC H5
S52.255 Nondisplaced comminuted fracture of shaft of ulna, left arm MCC CC H5
S52.256 Nondisplaced comminuted fracture of shaft of ulna, unspecified arm MCC CC H5 UNS

S52.26 Segmental fracture of shaft of ulna
S52.261 Displaced segmental fracture of shaft of ulna, right arm MCC CC H5
S52.262 Displaced segmental fracture of shaft of ulna, left arm MCC CC H5
S52.263 Displaced segmental fracture of shaft of ulna, unspecified arm MCC CC H5 UNS
S52.264 Nondisplaced segmental fracture of shaft of ulna, right arm MCC CC H5
S52.265 Nondisplaced segmental fracture of shaft of ulna, left arm MCC CC H5
S52.266 Nondisplaced segmental fracture of shaft of ulna, unspecified arm MCC CC H5 UNS

S52.27 Monteggia's fracture of ulna
Fracture of upper shaft of ulna with dislocation of radial head
S52.271 Monteggia's fracture of right ulna MCC CC H5
S52.272 Monteggia's fracture of left ulna MCC CC H5

2,4 7th **S52.279 Monteggia's fracture of unspecified ulna** MCC CC H5 UNS

6th **S52.28 Bent bone of ulna**

2,3 7th **S52.281 Bent bone of right ulna** MCC CC H5

2,3 7th **S52.282 Bent bone of left ulna** MCC CC H5

2,3 7th **S52.283 Bent bone of unspecified ulna** MCC CC H5 UNS

6th **S52.29 Other fracture of shaft of ulna**

2,3 7th **S52.291 Other fracture of shaft of right ulna** MCC CC H5

2,3 7th **S52.292 Other fracture of shaft of left ulna** MCC CC H5

2,3 7th **S52.299 Other fracture of shaft of unspecified ulna** MCC CC H5 UNS

5th **S52.3 Fracture of shaft of radius**

6th **S52.30 Unspecified fracture of shaft of radius**

2,3 7th **S52.301 Unspecified fracture of shaft of right radius** MCC CC H5

2,3 7th **S52.302 Unspecified fracture of shaft of left radius** MCC CC H5

2,3 7th **S52.309 Unspecified fracture of shaft of unspecified radius** MCC CC H5 UNS

6th **S52.31 Greenstick fracture of shaft of radius**

The appropriate 7th character is to be added to all codes in subcategory S52.31.
- A initial encounter for closed fracture
- D subsequent encounter for fracture with routine healing
- G subsequent encounter for fracture with delayed healing
- K subsequent encounter for fracture with nonunion
- P subsequent encounter for fracture with malunion
- S sequela

3 7th **S52.311 Greenstick fracture of shaft of radius, right arm** CC H5

3 7th **S52.312 Greenstick fracture of shaft of radius, left arm** CC H5

3 7th **S52.319 Greenstick fracture of shaft of radius, unspecified arm** CC H5 UNS

6th **S52.32 Transverse fracture of shaft of radius**

2,3 7th **S52.321 Displaced transverse fracture of shaft of right radius** MCC CC H5

2,3 7th **S52.322 Displaced transverse fracture of shaft of left radius** MCC CC H5

2,3 7th **S52.323 Displaced transverse fracture of shaft of unspecified radius** MCC CC H5 UNS

2,3 7th **S52.324 Nondisplaced transverse fracture of shaft of right radius** MCC CC H5

2,3 7th **S52.325 Nondisplaced transverse fracture of shaft of left radius** MCC CC H5

2,3 7th **S52.326 Nondisplaced transverse fracture of shaft of unspecified radius** MCC CC H5 UNS

6th **S52.33 Oblique fracture of shaft of radius**

2,3 7th **S52.331 Displaced oblique fracture of shaft of right radius** MCC CC H5

2,3 7th **S52.332 Displaced oblique fracture of shaft of left radius** MCC CC H5

2,3 7th **S52.333 Displaced oblique fracture of shaft of unspecified radius** MCC CC H5 UNS

2,3 7th **S52.334 Nondisplaced oblique fracture of shaft of right radius** MCC CC H5

2,3 7th **S52.335 Nondisplaced oblique fracture of shaft of left radius** MCC CC H5

2,3 7th **S52.336 Nondisplaced oblique fracture of shaft of unspecified radius** MCC CC H5 UNS

6th **S52.34 Spiral fracture of shaft of radius**

2,3 7th **S52.341 Displaced spiral fracture of shaft of radius, right arm** MCC CC H5

2,3 7th **S52.342 Displaced spiral fracture of shaft of radius, left arm** MCC CC H5

2,3 7th **S52.343 Displaced spiral fracture of shaft of radius, unspecified arm** MCC CC H5 UNS

2,3 7th **S52.344 Nondisplaced spiral fracture of shaft of radius, right arm** MCC CC H5

2,3 7th **S52.345 Nondisplaced spiral fracture of shaft of radius, left arm** MCC CC H5

2,3 7th **S52.346 Nondisplaced spiral fracture of shaft of radius, unspecified arm** MCC CC H5 UNS

6th **S52.35 Comminuted fracture of shaft of radius**

2,3 7th **S52.351 Displaced comminuted fracture of shaft of radius, right arm** MCC CC H5

2,3 7th **S52.352 Displaced comminuted fracture of shaft of radius, left arm** MCC CC H5

2,3 7th **S52.353 Displaced comminuted fracture of shaft of radius, unspecified arm** MCC CC H5 UNS

2,3 7th **S52.354 Nondisplaced comminuted fracture of shaft of radius, right arm** MCC CC H5

2,3 7th **S52.355 Nondisplaced comminuted fracture of shaft of radius, left arm** MCC CC H5

2,3 7th **S52.356 Nondisplaced comminuted fracture of shaft of radius, unspecified arm** MCC CC H5 UNS

6th **S52.36 Segmental fracture of shaft of radius**

2,3 7th **S52.361 Displaced segmental fracture of shaft of radius, right arm** MCC CC H5

2,3 7th **S52.362 Displaced segmental fracture of shaft of radius, left arm** MCC CC H5

2,3 7th **S52.363 Displaced segmental fracture of shaft of radius, unspecified arm** MCC CC H5 UNS

2,3 7th **S52.364 Nondisplaced segmental fracture of shaft of radius, right arm** MCC CC H5

2,3 7th **S52.365 Nondisplaced segmental fracture of shaft of radius, left arm** MCC CC H5

2,3 7th **S52.366 Nondisplaced segmental fracture of shaft of radius, unspecified arm** MCC CC H5 UNS

6th **S52.37 Galeazzi's fracture**

Fracture of lower shaft of radius with radioulnar joint dislocation

2,3 7th **S52.371 Galeazzi's fracture of right radius** MCC CC H5

2,3 7th **S52.372 Galeazzi's fracture of left radius** MCC CC H5

2,3 7th **S52.379 Galeazzi's fracture of unspecified radius** MCC CC H5 UNS

6th **S52.38 Bent bone of radius**

2,3 7th **S52.381 Bent bone of right radius** MCC CC H5

2,3 7th **S52.382 Bent bone of left radius** MCC CC H5

2,3 7th **S52.389 Bent bone of unspecified radius** MCC CC H5 UNS

6th **S52.39 Other fracture of shaft of radius**

2,3 7th **S52.391 Other fracture of shaft of radius, right arm** MCC CC H5

2,3 7th **S52.392 Other fracture of shaft of radius, left arm** MCC CC H5

2,3 7th **S52.399 Other fracture of shaft of radius, unspecified arm** MCC CC H5 UNS

5th **S52.5 Fracture of lower end of radius**

Fracture of distal end of radius

EXCLUDES 2 *physeal fractures of lower end of radius (S59.2-)*

DEF: Fracture of the distal end of the radius above the wrist, most commonly caused by a fall onto an outstretched hand.

6th **S52.50 Unspecified fracture of the lower end of radius**

2,3 7th **S52.501 Unspecified fracture of the lower end of right radius** MCC CC H5

2,3 7th **S52.502 Unspecified fracture of the lower end of left radius** MCC CC H5

2,3 7th **S52.509 Unspecified fracture of the lower end of unspecified radius** MCC CC H5 UNS

6th **S52.51 Fracture of radial styloid process**

2,3 7th **S52.511 Displaced fracture of right radial styloid process** MCC CC H5

2,3 7th **S52.512 Displaced fracture of left radial styloid process** MCC CC H5

2,3 7th **S52.513 Displaced fracture of unspecified radial styloid process** MCC CC H5 UNS

2,3 7th **S52.514 Nondisplaced fracture of right radial styloid process** MCC CC H5

2,3 7th **S52.515 Nondisplaced fracture of left radial styloid process** MCC CC H5

2,3 ✓7th **S52.516** **Nondisplaced fracture of unspecified radial styloid process** MCC CC H5 UNS

✓6th **S52.52** **Torus fracture of lower end of radius**

The appropriate 7th character is to be added to all codes in subcategory S52.52.
- A initial encounter for closed fracture
- D subsequent encounter for fracture with routine healing
- G subsequent encounter for fracture with delayed healing
- K subsequent encounter for fracture with nonunion
- P subsequent encounter for fracture with malunion
- S sequela

3 ✓7th **S52.521** **Torus fracture of lower end of right radius** CC H5

3 ✓7th **S52.522** **Torus fracture of lower end of left radius** CC H5

3 ✓7th **S52.529** **Torus fracture of lower end of unspecified radius** CC H5 UNS

✓6th **S52.53** **Colles' fracture**

AHA: 2016,2Q,4

DEF: Fracture of the radius at the wrist in which the distal fragment is pushed posteriorly. The dorsal angulation of the fragment results in the wrist cocking up.

2,3 ✓7th **S52.531** **Colles' fracture of right radius** MCC CC H5

2,3 ✓7th **S52.532** **Colles' fracture of left radius** MCC CC H5

2,3 ✓7th **S52.539** **Colles' fracture of unspecified radius** MCC CC H5 UNS

✓6th **S52.54** **Smith's fracture**

2,3 ✓7th **S52.541** **Smith's fracture of right radius** MCC CC H5

2,3 ✓7th **S52.542** **Smith's fracture of left radius** MCC CC H5

2,3 ✓7th **S52.549** **Smith's fracture of unspecified radius** MCC CC H5 UNS

✓6th **S52.55** **Other extraarticular fracture of lower end of radius**

2,3 ✓7th **S52.551** **Other extraarticular fracture of lower end of right radius** MCC CC H5

2,3 ✓7th **S52.552** **Other extraarticular fracture of lower end of left radius** MCC CC H5

2,3 ✓7th **S52.559** **Other extraarticular fracture of lower end of unspecified radius** MCC CC H5 UNS

✓6th **S52.56** **Barton's fracture**

2,3 ✓7th **S52.561** **Barton's fracture of right radius** MCC CC H5

2,3 ✓7th **S52.562** **Barton's fracture of left radius** MCC CC H5

2,3 ✓7th **S52.569** **Barton's fracture of unspecified radius** MCC CC H5 UNS

✓6th **S52.57** **Other intraarticular fracture of lower end of radius**

2,3 ✓7th **S52.571** **Other intraarticular fracture of lower end of right radius** MCC CC H5

2,3 ✓7th **S52.572** **Other intraarticular fracture of lower end of left radius** MCC CC H5

2,3 ✓7th **S52.579** **Other intraarticular fracture of lower end of unspecified radius** MCC CC H5 UNS

✓6th **S52.59** **Other fractures of lower end of radius**

AHA: 2019,3Q,9

2,3 ✓7th **S52.591** **Other fractures of lower end of right radius** MCC CC H5

2,3 ✓7th **S52.592** **Other fractures of lower end of left radius** MCC CC H5

2,3 ✓7th **S52.599** **Other fractures of lower end of unspecified radius** MCC CC H5 UNS

✓5th **S52.6** **Fracture of lower end of ulna**

✓6th **S52.60** **Unspecified fracture of lower end of ulna**

2,3 ✓7th **S52.601** **Unspecified fracture of lower end of right ulna** MCC CC H5

2,3 ✓7th **S52.602** **Unspecified fracture of lower end of left ulna** MCC CC H5

2,3 ✓7th **S52.609** **Unspecified fracture of lower end of unspecified ulna** MCC CC H5 UNS

✓6th **S52.61** **Fracture of ulna styloid process**

2,3 ✓7th **S52.611** **Displaced fracture of right ulna styloid process** MCC CC H5

2,3 ✓7th **S52.612** **Displaced fracture of left ulna styloid process** MCC CC H5

2,3 ✓7th **S52.613** **Displaced fracture of unspecified ulna styloid process** MCC CC H5 UNS

2,3 ✓7th **S52.614** **Nondisplaced fracture of right ulna styloid process** MCC CC H5

2,3 ✓7th **S52.615** **Nondisplaced fracture of left ulna styloid process** MCC CC H5

2,3 ✓7th **S52.616** **Nondisplaced fracture of unspecified ulna styloid process** MCC CC H5 UNS

✓6th **S52.62** **Torus fracture of lower end of ulna**

The appropriate 7th character is to be added to all codes in subcategory S52.62.
- A initial encounter for closed fracture
- D subsequent encounter for fracture with routine healing
- G subsequent encounter for fracture with delayed healing
- K subsequent encounter for fracture with nonunion
- P subsequent encounter for fracture with malunion
- S sequela

3 ✓7th **S52.621** **Torus fracture of lower end of right ulna** CC H5

3 ✓7th **S52.622** **Torus fracture of lower end of left ulna** CC H5

3 ✓7th **S52.629** **Torus fracture of lower end of unspecified ulna** CC H5 UNS

✓6th **S52.69** **Other fracture of lower end of ulna**

AHA: 2019,3Q,9

2,3 ✓7th **S52.691** **Other fracture of lower end of right ulna** MCC CC H5

2,3 ✓7th **S52.692** **Other fracture of lower end of left ulna** MCC CC H5

2,3 ✓7th **S52.699** **Other fracture of lower end of unspecified ulna** MCC CC H5 UNS

✓5th **S52.9** **Unspecified fracture of forearm**

2,3 ✓x7th **S52.90** **Unspecified fracture of unspecified forearm** MCC CC H5 UNS

2,3 ✓x7th **S52.91** **Unspecified fracture of right forearm** MCC CC H5

2,3 ✓x7th **S52.92** **Unspecified fracture of left forearm** MCC CC H5

✓4th **S53** **Dislocation and sprain of joints and ligaments of elbow**

INCLUDES avulsion of joint or ligament of elbow
laceration of cartilage, joint or ligament of elbow
sprain of cartilage, joint or ligament of elbow
traumatic hemarthrosis of joint or ligament of elbow
traumatic rupture of joint or ligament of elbow
traumatic subluxation of joint or ligament of elbow
traumatic tear of joint or ligament of elbow

Code also any associated open wound

EXCLUDES 2 *strain of muscle, fascia and tendon at forearm level (S56.-)*

The appropriate 7th character is to be added to each code from category S53.
- A initial encounter
- D subsequent encounter
- S sequela

✓5th **S53.0** **Subluxation and dislocation of radial head**

Dislocation of radiohumeral joint
Subluxation of radiohumeral joint

EXCLUDES 1 *Monteggia's fracture-dislocation (S52.27-)*

✓6th **S53.00** **Unspecified subluxation and dislocation of radial head**

✓7th **S53.001** **Unspecified subluxation of right radial head**

✓7th **S53.002** **Unspecified subluxation of left radial head**

✓7th **S53.003** **Unspecified subluxation of unspecified radial head**

✓7th **S53.004** **Unspecified dislocation of right radial head**

✓7th **S53.005** **Unspecified dislocation of left radial head**

Chapter 19. Injury, Poisoning and Certain Other Consequences of External Causes

S52.516–S53.005

7th **S53.006 Unspecified dislocation of unspecified radial head**

6th **S53.01 Anterior subluxation and dislocation of radial head**
Anteriomedial subluxation and dislocation of radial head

7th **S53.011 Anterior subluxation of right radial head**
7th **S53.012 Anterior subluxation of left radial head**
7th **S53.013 Anterior subluxation of unspecified radial head**
7th **S53.014 Anterior dislocation of right radial head**
7th **S53.015 Anterior dislocation of left radial head**
7th **S53.016 Anterior dislocation of unspecified radial head**

6th **S53.02 Posterior subluxation and dislocation of radial head**
Posteriolateral subluxation and dislocation of radial head

7th **S53.021 Posterior subluxation of right radial head**
7th **S53.022 Posterior subluxation of left radial head**
7th **S53.023 Posterior subluxation of unspecified radial head**
7th **S53.024 Posterior dislocation of right radial head**
7th **S53.025 Posterior dislocation of left radial head**
7th **S53.026 Posterior dislocation of unspecified radial head**

6th **S53.03 Nursemaid's elbow**

7th **S53.031 Nursemaid's elbow, right elbow**
7th **S53.032 Nursemaid's elbow, left elbow**
7th **S53.033 Nursemaid's elbow, unspecified elbow**

6th **S53.09 Other subluxation and dislocation of radial head**

7th **S53.091 Other subluxation of right radial head**
7th **S53.092 Other subluxation of left radial head**
7th **S53.093 Other subluxation of unspecified radial head**
7th **S53.094 Other dislocation of right radial head**
7th **S53.095 Other dislocation of left radial head**
7th **S53.096 Other dislocation of unspecified radial head**

5th **S53.1 Subluxation and dislocation of ulnohumeral joint**
Subluxation and dislocation of elbow NOS
EXCLUDES 1 *dislocation of radial head alone (S53.0-)*

6th **S53.10 Unspecified subluxation and dislocation of ulnohumeral joint**

7th **S53.101 Unspecified subluxation of right ulnohumeral joint**
7th **S53.102 Unspecified subluxation of left ulnohumeral joint**
7th **S53.103 Unspecified subluxation of unspecified ulnohumeral joint**
7th **S53.104 Unspecified dislocation of right ulnohumeral joint**
7th **S53.105 Unspecified dislocation of left ulnohumeral joint**
7th **S53.106 Unspecified dislocation of unspecified ulnohumeral joint**

6th **S53.11 Anterior subluxation and dislocation of ulnohumeral joint**

7th **S53.111 Anterior subluxation of right ulnohumeral joint**
7th **S53.112 Anterior subluxation of left ulnohumeral joint**
7th **S53.113 Anterior subluxation of unspecified ulnohumeral joint**
7th **S53.114 Anterior dislocation of right ulnohumeral joint**
AHA: 2012,4Q,108
7th **S53.115 Anterior dislocation of left ulnohumeral joint**
7th **S53.116 Anterior dislocation of unspecified ulnohumeral joint**

6th **S53.12 Posterior subluxation and dislocation of ulnohumeral joint**

7th **S53.121 Posterior subluxation of right ulnohumeral joint**
7th **S53.122 Posterior subluxation of left ulnohumeral joint**
7th **S53.123 Posterior subluxation of unspecified ulnohumeral joint**
7th **S53.124 Posterior dislocation of right ulnohumeral joint**
7th **S53.125 Posterior dislocation of left ulnohumeral joint**
7th **S53.126 Posterior dislocation of unspecified ulnohumeral joint**

6th **S53.13 Medial subluxation and dislocation of ulnohumeral joint**

7th **S53.131 Medial subluxation of right ulnohumeral joint**
7th **S53.132 Medial subluxation of left ulnohumeral joint**
7th **S53.133 Medial subluxation of unspecified ulnohumeral joint**
7th **S53.134 Medial dislocation of right ulnohumeral joint**
7th **S53.135 Medial dislocation of left ulnohumeral joint**
7th **S53.136 Medial dislocation of unspecified ulnohumeral joint**

6th **S53.14 Lateral subluxation and dislocation of ulnohumeral joint**

7th **S53.141 Lateral subluxation of right ulnohumeral joint**
7th **S53.142 Lateral subluxation of left ulnohumeral joint**
7th **S53.143 Lateral subluxation of unspecified ulnohumeral joint**
7th **S53.144 Lateral dislocation of right ulnohumeral joint**
7th **S53.145 Lateral dislocation of left ulnohumeral joint**
7th **S53.146 Lateral dislocation of unspecified ulnohumeral joint**

6th **S53.19 Other subluxation and dislocation of ulnohumeral joint**

7th **S53.191 Other subluxation of right ulnohumeral joint**
7th **S53.192 Other subluxation of left ulnohumeral joint**
7th **S53.193 Other subluxation of unspecified ulnohumeral joint**
7th **S53.194 Other dislocation of right ulnohumeral joint**
7th **S53.195 Other dislocation of left ulnohumeral joint**
7th **S53.196 Other dislocation of unspecified ulnohumeral joint**

5th **S53.2 Traumatic rupture of radial collateral ligament**
EXCLUDES 1 *sprain of radial collateral ligament NOS (S53.43-)*

√x7th **S53.20 Traumatic rupture of unspecified radial collateral ligament**
√x7th **S53.21 Traumatic rupture of right radial collateral ligament**
√x7th **S53.22 Traumatic rupture of left radial collateral ligament**

5th **S53.3 Traumatic rupture of ulnar collateral ligament**
EXCLUDES 1 *sprain of ulnar collateral ligament (S53.44-)*

√x7th **S53.30 Traumatic rupture of unspecified ulnar collateral ligament**
√x7th **S53.31 Traumatic rupture of right ulnar collateral ligament**
√x7th **S53.32 Traumatic rupture of left ulnar collateral ligament**

5th **S53.4 Sprain of elbow**
EXCLUDES 2 *traumatic rupture of radial collateral ligament (S53.2-)*
traumatic rupture of ulnar collateral ligament (S53.3-)

6th **S53.40 Unspecified sprain of elbow**

7th **S53.401 Unspecified sprain of right elbow**
7th **S53.402 Unspecified sprain of left elbow**
7th **S53.409 Unspecified sprain of unspecified elbow**
Sprain of elbow NOS

6th **S53.41 Radiohumeral (joint) sprain**

7th **S53.411 Radiohumeral (joint) sprain of right elbow**
7th **S53.412 Radiohumeral (joint) sprain of left elbow**
7th **S53.419 Radiohumeral (joint) sprain of unspecified elbow**

6th **S53.42 Ulnohumeral (joint) sprain**

7th **S53.421 Ulnohumeral (joint) sprain of right elbow**

S53.422 Ulnohumeral (joint) sprain of left elbow
S53.429 Ulnohumeral (joint) sprain of unspecified elbow
S53.43 Radial collateral ligament sprain
S53.431 Radial collateral ligament sprain of right elbow
S53.432 Radial collateral ligament sprain of left elbow
S53.439 Radial collateral ligament sprain of unspecified elbow
S53.44 Ulnar collateral ligament sprain
S53.441 Ulnar collateral ligament sprain of right elbow
S53.442 Ulnar collateral ligament sprain of left elbow
S53.449 Ulnar collateral ligament sprain of unspecified elbow
S53.49 Other sprain of elbow
S53.491 Other sprain of right elbow
S53.492 Other sprain of left elbow
S53.499 Other sprain of unspecified elbow

S54 Injury of nerves at forearm level

Code also any associated open wound (S51.-)

EXCLUDES 2 *injury of nerves at wrist and hand level (S64.-)*

The appropriate 7th character is to be added to each code from category S54.
A initial encounter
D subsequent encounter
S sequela

S54.0 Injury of ulnar nerve at forearm level
Injury of ulnar nerve NOS
S54.00 Injury of ulnar nerve at forearm level, unspecified arm
S54.01 Injury of ulnar nerve at forearm level, right arm
S54.02 Injury of ulnar nerve at forearm level, left arm
S54.1 Injury of median nerve at forearm level
Injury of median nerve NOS
S54.10 Injury of median nerve at forearm level, unspecified arm
S54.11 Injury of median nerve at forearm level, right arm
S54.12 Injury of median nerve at forearm level, left arm
S54.2 Injury of radial nerve at forearm level
Injury of radial nerve NOS
S54.20 Injury of radial nerve at forearm level, unspecified arm
S54.21 Injury of radial nerve at forearm level, right arm
S54.22 Injury of radial nerve at forearm level, left arm
S54.3 Injury of cutaneous sensory nerve at forearm level
S54.30 Injury of cutaneous sensory nerve at forearm level, unspecified arm
S54.31 Injury of cutaneous sensory nerve at forearm level, right arm
S54.32 Injury of cutaneous sensory nerve at forearm level, left arm
S54.8 Injury of other nerves at forearm level
S54.8X Injury of other nerves at forearm level
S54.8X1 Injury of other nerves at forearm level, right arm
S54.8X2 Injury of other nerves at forearm level, left arm
S54.8X9 Injury of other nerves at forearm level, unspecified arm
S54.9 Injury of unspecified nerve at forearm level
S54.90 Injury of unspecified nerve at forearm level, unspecified arm
S54.91 Injury of unspecified nerve at forearm level, right arm
S54.92 Injury of unspecified nerve at forearm level, left arm

S55 Injury of blood vessels at forearm level

Code also any associated open wound (S51.-)

EXCLUDES 2 *injury of blood vessels at wrist and hand level (S65.-)*
injury of brachial vessels (S45.1-S45.2)

The appropriate 7th character is to be added to each code from category S55.
A initial encounter
D subsequent encounter
S sequela

S55.0 Injury of ulnar artery at forearm level
S55.00 Unspecified injury of ulnar artery at forearm level
S55.001 Unspecified injury of ulnar artery at forearm level, right arm CC
S55.002 Unspecified injury of ulnar artery at forearm level, left arm CC
S55.009 Unspecified injury of ulnar artery at forearm level, unspecified arm CC UNS
S55.01 Laceration of ulnar artery at forearm level
S55.011 Laceration of ulnar artery at forearm level, right arm CC
S55.012 Laceration of ulnar artery at forearm level, left arm CC
S55.019 Laceration of ulnar artery at forearm level, unspecified arm CC UNS
S55.09 Other specified injury of ulnar artery at forearm level
S55.091 Other specified injury of ulnar artery at forearm level, right arm CC
S55.092 Other specified injury of ulnar artery at forearm level, left arm CC
S55.099 Other specified injury of ulnar artery at forearm level, unspecified arm CC UNS
S55.1 Injury of radial artery at forearm level
S55.10 Unspecified injury of radial artery at forearm level
S55.101 Unspecified injury of radial artery at forearm level, right arm CC
S55.102 Unspecified injury of radial artery at forearm level, left arm CC
S55.109 Unspecified injury of radial artery at forearm level, unspecified arm CC UNS
S55.11 Laceration of radial artery at forearm level
S55.111 Laceration of radial artery at forearm level, right arm CC
S55.112 Laceration of radial artery at forearm level, left arm CC
S55.119 Laceration of radial artery at forearm level, unspecified arm CC UNS
S55.19 Other specified injury of radial artery at forearm level
S55.191 Other specified injury of radial artery at forearm level, right arm CC
S55.192 Other specified injury of radial artery at forearm level, left arm CC
S55.199 Other specified injury of radial artery at forearm level, unspecified arm CC UNS
S55.2 Injury of vein at forearm level
S55.20 Unspecified injury of vein at forearm level
S55.201 Unspecified injury of vein at forearm level, right arm CC
S55.202 Unspecified injury of vein at forearm level, left arm CC
S55.209 Unspecified injury of vein at forearm level, unspecified arm CC UNS
S55.21 Laceration of vein at forearm level
S55.211 Laceration of vein at forearm level, right arm CC
S55.212 Laceration of vein at forearm level, left arm CC
S55.219 Laceration of vein at forearm level, unspecified arm CC UNS
S55.29 Other specified injury of vein at forearm level
S55.291 Other specified injury of vein at forearm level, right arm CC
S55.292 Other specified injury of vein at forearm level, left arm CC
S55.299 Other specified injury of vein at forearm level, unspecified arm CC UNS

5th **S55.8 Injury of other blood vessels at forearm level**

6th **S55.80 Unspecified injury of other blood vessels at forearm level**

7th **S55.801 Unspecified injury of other blood vessels at forearm level, right arm** CC

7th **S55.802 Unspecified injury of other blood vessels at forearm level, left arm** CC

7th **S55.809 Unspecified injury of other blood vessels at forearm level, unspecified arm** CC UNS

6th **S55.81 Laceration of other blood vessels at forearm level**

7th **S55.811 Laceration of other blood vessels at forearm level, right arm** CC

7th **S55.812 Laceration of other blood vessels at forearm level, left arm** CC

7th **S55.819 Laceration of other blood vessels at forearm level, unspecified arm** CC UNS

6th **S55.89 Other specified injury of other blood vessels at forearm level**

7th **S55.891 Other specified injury of other blood vessels at forearm level, right arm** CC

7th **S55.892 Other specified injury of other blood vessels at forearm level, left arm** CC

7th **S55.899 Other specified injury of other blood vessels at forearm level, unspecified arm** CC UNS

5th **S55.9 Injury of unspecified blood vessel at forearm level**

6th **S55.90 Unspecified injury of unspecified blood vessel at forearm level**

7th **S55.901 Unspecified injury of unspecified blood vessel at forearm level, right arm** CC

7th **S55.902 Unspecified injury of unspecified blood vessel at forearm level, left arm** CC

7th **S55.909 Unspecified injury of unspecified blood vessel at forearm level, unspecified arm** CC UNS

6th **S55.91 Laceration of unspecified blood vessel at forearm level**

7th **S55.911 Laceration of unspecified blood vessel at forearm level, right arm** CC

7th **S55.912 Laceration of unspecified blood vessel at forearm level, left arm** CC

7th **S55.919 Laceration of unspecified blood vessel at forearm level, unspecified arm** CC UNS

6th **S55.99 Other specified injury of unspecified blood vessel at forearm level**

7th **S55.991 Other specified injury of unspecified blood vessel at forearm level, right arm** CC

7th **S55.992 Other specified injury of unspecified blood vessel at forearm level, left arm** CC

7th **S55.999 Other specified injury of unspecified blood vessel at forearm level, unspecified arm** CC UNS

4th **S56 Injury of muscle, fascia and tendon at forearm level**

Code also any associated open wound (S51.-)

EXCLUDES 2 *injury of muscle, fascia and tendon at or below wrist (S66.-)*
sprain of joints and ligaments of elbow (S53.4-)

TIP: Refer to the Muscle/Tendon table at the beginning of this chapter

The appropriate 7th character is to be added to each code from category S56.
A initial encounter
D subsequent encounter
S sequela

5th **S56.0 Injury of flexor muscle, fascia and tendon of thumb at forearm level**

6th **S56.00 Unspecified injury of flexor muscle, fascia and tendon of thumb at forearm level**

7th **S56.001 Unspecified injury of flexor muscle, fascia and tendon of right thumb at forearm level**

7th **S56.002 Unspecified injury of flexor muscle, fascia and tendon of left thumb at forearm level**

7th **S56.009 Unspecified injury of flexor muscle, fascia and tendon of unspecified thumb at forearm level**

6th **S56.01 Strain of flexor muscle, fascia and tendon of thumb at forearm level**

7th **S56.011 Strain of flexor muscle, fascia and tendon of right thumb at forearm level**

7th **S56.012 Strain of flexor muscle, fascia and tendon of left thumb at forearm level**

7th **S56.019 Strain of flexor muscle, fascia and tendon of unspecified thumb at forearm level**

6th **S56.02 Laceration of flexor muscle, fascia and tendon of thumb at forearm level**

7th **S56.021 Laceration of flexor muscle, fascia and tendon of right thumb at forearm level** CC

7th **S56.022 Laceration of flexor muscle, fascia and tendon of left thumb at forearm level** CC

7th **S56.029 Laceration of flexor muscle, fascia and tendon of unspecified thumb at forearm level** CC

6th **S56.09 Other injury of flexor muscle, fascia and tendon of thumb at forearm level**

7th **S56.091 Other injury of flexor muscle, fascia and tendon of right thumb at forearm level**

7th **S56.092 Other injury of flexor muscle, fascia and tendon of left thumb at forearm level**

7th **S56.099 Other injury of flexor muscle, fascia and tendon of unspecified thumb at forearm level**

5th **S56.1 Injury of flexor muscle, fascia and tendon of other and unspecified finger at forearm level**

6th **S56.10 Unspecified injury of flexor muscle, fascia and tendon of other and unspecified finger at forearm level**

7th **S56.101 Unspecified injury of flexor muscle, fascia and tendon of right index finger at forearm level**

7th **S56.102 Unspecified injury of flexor muscle, fascia and tendon of left index finger at forearm level**

7th **S56.103 Unspecified injury of flexor muscle, fascia and tendon of right middle finger at forearm level**

7th **S56.104 Unspecified injury of flexor muscle, fascia and tendon of left middle finger at forearm level**

7th **S56.105 Unspecified injury of flexor muscle, fascia and tendon of right ring finger at forearm level**

7th **S56.106 Unspecified injury of flexor muscle, fascia and tendon of left ring finger at forearm level**

7th **S56.107 Unspecified injury of flexor muscle, fascia and tendon of right little finger at forearm level**

7th **S56.108 Unspecified injury of flexor muscle, fascia and tendon of left little finger at forearm level**

7th **S56.109 Unspecified injury of flexor muscle, fascia and tendon of unspecified finger at forearm level**

6th **S56.11 Strain of flexor muscle, fascia and tendon of other and unspecified finger at forearm level**

7th **S56.111 Strain of flexor muscle, fascia and tendon of right index finger at forearm level**

7th **S56.112 Strain of flexor muscle, fascia and tendon of left index finger at forearm level**

7th **S56.113 Strain of flexor muscle, fascia and tendon of right middle finger at forearm level**

7th **S56.114 Strain of flexor muscle, fascia and tendon of left middle finger at forearm level**

7th **S56.115 Strain of flexor muscle, fascia and tendon of right ring finger at forearm level**

7th **S56.116 Strain of flexor muscle, fascia and tendon of left ring finger at forearm level**

7th **S56.117 Strain of flexor muscle, fascia and tendon of right little finger at forearm level**

7th **S56.118 Strain of flexor muscle, fascia and tendon of left little finger at forearm level**

7th **S56.119 Strain of flexor muscle, fascia and tendon of finger of unspecified finger at forearm level**

S56.12 Laceration of flexor muscle, fascia and tendon of other and unspecified finger at forearm level
- S56.121 Laceration of flexor muscle, fascia and tendon of right index finger at forearm level CC
- S56.122 Laceration of flexor muscle, fascia and tendon of left index finger at forearm level CC
- S56.123 Laceration of flexor muscle, fascia and tendon of right middle finger at forearm level CC
- S56.124 Laceration of flexor muscle, fascia and tendon of left middle finger at forearm level CC
- S56.125 Laceration of flexor muscle, fascia and tendon of right ring finger at forearm level CC
- S56.126 Laceration of flexor muscle, fascia and tendon of left ring finger at forearm level CC
- S56.127 Laceration of flexor muscle, fascia and tendon of right little finger at forearm level CC
- S56.128 Laceration of flexor muscle, fascia and tendon of left little finger at forearm level CC
- S56.129 Laceration of flexor muscle, fascia and tendon of unspecified finger at forearm level CC UNS

S56.19 Other injury of flexor muscle, fascia and tendon of other and unspecified finger at forearm level
- S56.191 Other injury of flexor muscle, fascia and tendon of right index finger at forearm level
- S56.192 Other injury of flexor muscle, fascia and tendon of left index finger at forearm level
- S56.193 Other injury of flexor muscle, fascia and tendon of right middle finger at forearm level
- S56.194 Other injury of flexor muscle, fascia and tendon of left middle finger at forearm level
- S56.195 Other injury of flexor muscle, fascia and tendon of right ring finger at forearm level
- S56.196 Other injury of flexor muscle, fascia and tendon of left ring finger at forearm level
- S56.197 Other injury of flexor muscle, fascia and tendon of right little finger at forearm level
- S56.198 Other injury of flexor muscle, fascia and tendon of left little finger at forearm level
- S56.199 Other injury of flexor muscle, fascia and tendon of unspecified finger at forearm level

S56.2 Injury of other flexor muscle, fascia and tendon at forearm level

S56.20 Unspecified injury of other flexor muscle, fascia and tendon at forearm level
- S56.201 Unspecified injury of other flexor muscle, fascia and tendon at forearm level, right arm
- S56.202 Unspecified injury of other flexor muscle, fascia and tendon at forearm level, left arm
- S56.209 Unspecified injury of other flexor muscle, fascia and tendon at forearm level, unspecified arm

S56.21 Strain of other flexor muscle, fascia and tendon at forearm level
- S56.211 Strain of other flexor muscle, fascia and tendon at forearm level, right arm
- S56.212 Strain of other flexor muscle, fascia and tendon at forearm level, left arm
- S56.219 Strain of other flexor muscle, fascia and tendon at forearm level, unspecified arm

S56.22 Laceration of other flexor muscle, fascia and tendon at forearm level
- S56.221 Laceration of other flexor muscle, fascia and tendon at forearm level, right arm CC
- S56.222 Laceration of other flexor muscle, fascia and tendon at forearm level, left arm CC
- S56.229 Laceration of other flexor muscle, fascia and tendon at forearm level, unspecified arm CC UNS

S56.29 Other injury of other flexor muscle, fascia and tendon at forearm level
- S56.291 Other injury of other flexor muscle, fascia and tendon at forearm level, right arm
- S56.292 Other injury of other flexor muscle, fascia and tendon at forearm level, left arm
- S56.299 Other injury of other flexor muscle, fascia and tendon at forearm level, unspecified arm

S56.3 Injury of extensor or abductor muscles, fascia and tendons of thumb at forearm level

S56.30 Unspecified injury of extensor or abductor muscles, fascia and tendons of thumb at forearm level
- S56.301 Unspecified injury of extensor or abductor muscles, fascia and tendons of right thumb at forearm level
- S56.302 Unspecified injury of extensor or abductor muscles, fascia and tendons of left thumb at forearm level
- S56.309 Unspecified injury of extensor or abductor muscles, fascia and tendons of unspecified thumb at forearm level

S56.31 Strain of extensor or abductor muscles, fascia and tendons of thumb at forearm level
- S56.311 Strain of extensor or abductor muscles, fascia and tendons of right thumb at forearm level
- S56.312 Strain of extensor or abductor muscles, fascia and tendons of left thumb at forearm level
- S56.319 Strain of extensor or abductor muscles, fascia and tendons of unspecified thumb at forearm level

S56.32 Laceration of extensor or abductor muscles, fascia and tendons of thumb at forearm level
- S56.321 Laceration of extensor or abductor muscles, fascia and tendons of right thumb at forearm level CC
- S56.322 Laceration of extensor or abductor muscles, fascia and tendons of left thumb at forearm level CC
- S56.329 Laceration of extensor or abductor muscles, fascia and tendons of unspecified thumb at forearm level CC

S56.39 Other injury of extensor or abductor muscles, fascia and tendons of thumb at forearm level
- S56.391 Other injury of extensor or abductor muscles, fascia and tendons of right thumb at forearm level
- S56.392 Other injury of extensor or abductor muscles, fascia and tendons of left thumb at forearm level
- S56.399 Other injury of extensor or abductor muscles, fascia and tendons of unspecified thumb at forearm level

S56.4 Injury of extensor muscle, fascia and tendon of other and unspecified finger at forearm level

S56.40 Unspecified injury of extensor muscle, fascia and tendon of other and unspecified finger at forearm level
- S56.401 Unspecified injury of extensor muscle, fascia and tendon of right index finger at forearm level
- S56.402 Unspecified injury of extensor muscle, fascia and tendon of left index finger at forearm level
- S56.403 Unspecified injury of extensor muscle, fascia and tendon of right middle finger at forearm level
- S56.404 Unspecified injury of extensor muscle, fascia and tendon of left middle finger at forearm level
- S56.405 Unspecified injury of extensor muscle, fascia and tendon of right ring finger at forearm level

7th **S56.406** **Unspecified injury of extensor muscle, fascia and tendon of left ring finger at forearm level**

7th **S56.407** **Unspecified injury of extensor muscle, fascia and tendon of right little finger at forearm level**

7th **S56.408** **Unspecified injury of extensor muscle, fascia and tendon of left little finger at forearm level**

7th **S56.409** **Unspecified injury of extensor muscle, fascia and tendon of unspecified finger at forearm level**

6th **S56.41** **Strain of extensor muscle, fascia and tendon of other and unspecified finger at forearm level**

7th **S56.411** **Strain of extensor muscle, fascia and tendon of right index finger at forearm level**

7th **S56.412** **Strain of extensor muscle, fascia and tendon of left index finger at forearm level**

7th **S56.413** **Strain of extensor muscle, fascia and tendon of right middle finger at forearm level**

7th **S56.414** **Strain of extensor muscle, fascia and tendon of left middle finger at forearm level**

7th **S56.415** **Strain of extensor muscle, fascia and tendon of right ring finger at forearm level**

7th **S56.416** **Strain of extensor muscle, fascia and tendon of left ring finger at forearm level**

7th **S56.417** **Strain of extensor muscle, fascia and tendon of right little finger at forearm level**

7th **S56.418** **Strain of extensor muscle, fascia and tendon of left little finger at forearm level**

7th **S56.419** **Strain of extensor muscle, fascia and tendon of finger, unspecified finger at forearm level**

6th **S56.42** **Laceration of extensor muscle, fascia and tendon of other and unspecified finger at forearm level**

7th **S56.421** **Laceration of extensor muscle, fascia and tendon of right index finger at forearm level** CC

7th **S56.422** **Laceration of extensor muscle, fascia and tendon of left index finger at forearm level** CC

7th **S56.423** **Laceration of extensor muscle, fascia and tendon of right middle finger at forearm level** CC

7th **S56.424** **Laceration of extensor muscle, fascia and tendon of left middle finger at forearm level** CC

7th **S56.425** **Laceration of extensor muscle, fascia and tendon of right ring finger at forearm level** CC

7th **S56.426** **Laceration of extensor muscle, fascia and tendon of left ring finger at forearm level** CC

7th **S56.427** **Laceration of extensor muscle, fascia and tendon of right little finger at forearm level** CC

7th **S56.428** **Laceration of extensor muscle, fascia and tendon of left little finger at forearm level** CC

7th **S56.429** **Laceration of extensor muscle, fascia and tendon of unspecified finger at forearm level** CC UNS

6th **S56.49** **Other injury of extensor muscle, fascia and tendon of other and unspecified finger at forearm level**

7th **S56.491** **Other injury of extensor muscle, fascia and tendon of right index finger at forearm level**

7th **S56.492** **Other injury of extensor muscle, fascia and tendon of left index finger at forearm level**

7th **S56.493** **Other injury of extensor muscle, fascia and tendon of right middle finger at forearm level**

7th **S56.494** **Other injury of extensor muscle, fascia and tendon of left middle finger at forearm level**

7th **S56.495** **Other injury of extensor muscle, fascia and tendon of right ring finger at forearm level**

7th **S56.496** **Other injury of extensor muscle, fascia and tendon of left ring finger at forearm level**

7th **S56.497** **Other injury of extensor muscle, fascia and tendon of right little finger at forearm level**

7th **S56.498** **Other injury of extensor muscle, fascia and tendon of left little finger at forearm level**

7th **S56.499** **Other injury of extensor muscle, fascia and tendon of unspecified finger at forearm level**

5th **S56.5** **Injury of other extensor muscle, fascia and tendon at forearm level**

6th **S56.50** **Unspecified injury of other extensor muscle, fascia and tendon at forearm level**

7th **S56.501** **Unspecified injury of other extensor muscle, fascia and tendon at forearm level, right arm**

7th **S56.502** **Unspecified injury of other extensor muscle, fascia and tendon at forearm level, left arm**

7th **S56.509** **Unspecified injury of other extensor muscle, fascia and tendon at forearm level, unspecified arm**

6th **S56.51** **Strain of other extensor muscle, fascia and tendon at forearm level**

7th **S56.511** **Strain of other extensor muscle, fascia and tendon at forearm level, right arm**

7th **S56.512** **Strain of other extensor muscle, fascia and tendon at forearm level, left arm**

7th **S56.519** **Strain of other extensor muscle, fascia and tendon at forearm level, unspecified arm**

6th **S56.52** **Laceration of other extensor muscle, fascia and tendon at forearm level**

7th **S56.521** **Laceration of other extensor muscle, fascia and tendon at forearm level, right arm** CC

7th **S56.522** **Laceration of other extensor muscle, fascia and tendon at forearm level, left arm** CC

7th **S56.529** **Laceration of other extensor muscle, fascia and tendon at forearm level, unspecified arm** CC UNS

6th **S56.59** **Other injury of other extensor muscle, fascia and tendon at forearm level**

7th **S56.591** **Other injury of other extensor muscle, fascia and tendon at forearm level, right arm**

7th **S56.592** **Other injury of other extensor muscle, fascia and tendon at forearm level, left arm**

7th **S56.599** **Other injury of other extensor muscle, fascia and tendon at forearm level, unspecified arm**

5th **S56.8** **Injury of other muscles, fascia and tendons at forearm level**

6th **S56.80** **Unspecified injury of other muscles, fascia and tendons at forearm level**

7th **S56.801** **Unspecified injury of other muscles, fascia and tendons at forearm level, right arm**

7th **S56.802** **Unspecified injury of other muscles, fascia and tendons at forearm level, left arm**

7th **S56.809** **Unspecified injury of other muscles, fascia and tendons at forearm level, unspecified arm**

6th **S56.81** **Strain of other muscles, fascia and tendons at forearm level**

7th **S56.811** **Strain of other muscles, fascia and tendons at forearm level, right arm**

7th **S56.812** **Strain of other muscles, fascia and tendons at forearm level, left arm**

7th **S56.819** **Strain of other muscles, fascia and tendons at forearm level, unspecified arm**

6th **S56.82** **Laceration of other muscles, fascia and tendons at forearm level**

7th **S56.821** **Laceration of other muscles, fascia and tendons at forearm level, right arm** CC

7th **S56.822** **Laceration of other muscles, fascia and tendons at forearm level, left arm** CC

S56.829 Laceration of other muscles, fascia and tendons at forearm level, unspecified arm CC UNS

S56.89 Other injury of other muscles, fascia and tendons at forearm level

S56.891 Other injury of other muscles, fascia and tendons at forearm level, right arm

S56.892 Other injury of other muscles, fascia and tendons at forearm level, left arm

S56.899 Other injury of other muscles, fascia and tendons at forearm level, unspecified arm

S56.9 Injury of unspecified muscles, fascia and tendons at forearm level

S56.90 Unspecified injury of unspecified muscles, fascia and tendons at forearm level

S56.901 Unspecified injury of unspecified muscles, fascia and tendons at forearm level, right arm

S56.902 Unspecified injury of unspecified muscles, fascia and tendons at forearm level, left arm

S56.909 Unspecified injury of unspecified muscles, fascia and tendons at forearm level, unspecified arm

S56.91 Strain of unspecified muscles, fascia and tendons at forearm level

S56.911 Strain of unspecified muscles, fascia and tendons at forearm level, right arm

S56.912 Strain of unspecified muscles, fascia and tendons at forearm level, left arm

S56.919 Strain of unspecified muscles, fascia and tendons at forearm level, unspecified arm

S56.92 Laceration of unspecified muscles, fascia and tendons at forearm level

S56.921 Laceration of unspecified muscles, fascia and tendons at forearm level, right arm CC

S56.922 Laceration of unspecified muscles, fascia and tendons at forearm level, left arm CC

S56.929 Laceration of unspecified muscles, fascia and tendons at forearm level, unspecified arm CC UNS

S56.99 Other injury of unspecified muscles, fascia and tendons at forearm level

S56.991 Other injury of unspecified muscles, fascia and tendons at forearm level, right arm

S56.992 Other injury of unspecified muscles, fascia and tendons at forearm level, left arm

S56.999 Other injury of unspecified muscles, fascia and tendons at forearm level, unspecified arm

S57 Crushing injury of elbow and forearm

Use additional code(s) for all associated injuries

EXCLUDES 2 *crushing injury of wrist and hand (S67.-)*

The appropriate 7th character is to be added to each code from category S57.
A initial encounter
D subsequent encounter
S sequela

S57.0 Crushing injury of elbow

S57.00 Crushing injury of unspecified elbow

S57.01 Crushing injury of right elbow

S57.02 Crushing injury of left elbow

S57.8 Crushing injury of forearm

S57.80 Crushing injury of unspecified forearm

S57.81 Crushing injury of right forearm

S57.82 Crushing injury of left forearm

S58 Traumatic amputation of elbow and forearm

An amputation not identified as partial or complete should be coded to complete

EXCLUDES 1 *traumatic amputation of wrist and hand (S68.-)*

The appropriate 7th character is to be added to each code from category S58.
A initial encounter
D subsequent encounter
S sequela

S58.0 Traumatic amputation at elbow level

S58.01 Complete traumatic amputation at elbow level

S58.011 Complete traumatic amputation at elbow level, right arm CC HCC

S58.012 Complete traumatic amputation at elbow level, left arm CC HCC

S58.019 Complete traumatic amputation at elbow level, unspecified arm CC UNS HCC

S58.02 Partial traumatic amputation at elbow level

S58.021 Partial traumatic amputation at elbow level, right arm CC HCC

S58.022 Partial traumatic amputation at elbow level, left arm CC HCC

S58.029 Partial traumatic amputation at elbow level, unspecified arm CC UNS HCC

S58.1 Traumatic amputation at level between elbow and wrist

S58.11 Complete traumatic amputation at level between elbow and wrist

S58.111 Complete traumatic amputation at level between elbow and wrist, right arm CC HCC

S58.112 Complete traumatic amputation at level between elbow and wrist, left arm CC HCC

S58.119 Complete traumatic amputation at level between elbow and wrist, unspecified arm CC UNS HCC

S58.12 Partial traumatic amputation at level between elbow and wrist

S58.121 Partial traumatic amputation at level between elbow and wrist, right arm CC HCC

S58.122 Partial traumatic amputation at level between elbow and wrist, left arm CC HCC

S58.129 Partial traumatic amputation at level between elbow and wrist, unspecified arm CC UNS HCC

S58.9 Traumatic amputation of forearm, level unspecified

EXCLUDES 1 *traumatic amputation of wrist (S68.-)*

S58.91 Complete traumatic amputation of forearm, level unspecified

S58.911 Complete traumatic amputation of right forearm, level unspecified CC HCC

S58.912 Complete traumatic amputation of left forearm, level unspecified CC HCC

S58.919 Complete traumatic amputation of unspecified forearm, level unspecified CC UNS HCC

S58.92 Partial traumatic amputation of forearm, level unspecified

S58.921 Partial traumatic amputation of right forearm, level unspecified CC HCC

S58.922 Partial traumatic amputation of left forearm, level unspecified CC HCC

S58.929 Partial traumatic amputation of unspecified forearm, level unspecified CC UNS HCC

✓4th S59 Other and unspecified injuries of elbow and forearm

EXCLUDES 2 *other and unspecified injuries of wrist and hand (S69.-)*

AHA: 2018,2Q,12; 2018,1Q,3; 2015,3Q,37-39

The appropriate 7th character is to be added to each code from subcategories S59.0, S59.1, and S59.2.
- A initial encounter for closed fracture
- D subsequent encounter for fracture with routine healing
- G subsequent encounter for fracture with delayed healing
- K subsequent encounter for fracture with nonunion
- P subsequent encounter for fracture with malunion
- S sequela

✓5th S59.0 Physeal fracture of lower end of ulna

AHA: 2019,4Q,56

✓6th S59.00 Unspecified physeal fracture of lower end of ulna
- 3 ✓7th **S59.001 Unspecified physeal fracture of lower end of ulna, right arm** CC H5
- 3 ✓7th **S59.002 Unspecified physeal fracture of lower end of ulna, left arm** CC H5
- 3 ✓7th **S59.009 Unspecified physeal fracture of lower end of ulna, unspecified arm** CC H5 UNS

✓6th S59.01 Salter-Harris Type I physeal fracture of lower end of ulna
- 3 ✓7th **S59.011 Salter-Harris Type I physeal fracture of lower end of ulna, right arm** CC H5
- 3 ✓7th **S59.012 Salter-Harris Type I physeal fracture of lower end of ulna, left arm** CC H5
- 3 ✓7th **S59.019 Salter-Harris Type I physeal fracture of lower end of ulna, unspecified arm** CC H5 UNS

✓6th S59.02 Salter-Harris Type II physeal fracture of lower end of ulna
- 3 ✓7th **S59.021 Salter-Harris Type II physeal fracture of lower end of ulna, right arm** CC H5
- 3 ✓7th **S59.022 Salter-Harris Type II physeal fracture of lower end of ulna, left arm** CC H5
- 3 ✓7th **S59.029 Salter-Harris Type II physeal fracture of lower end of ulna, unspecified arm** CC H5 UNS

✓6th S59.03 Salter-Harris Type III physeal fracture of lower end of ulna
- 3 ✓7th **S59.031 Salter-Harris Type III physeal fracture of lower end of ulna, right arm** CC H5
- 3 ✓7th **S59.032 Salter-Harris Type III physeal fracture of lower end of ulna, left arm** CC H5
- 3 ✓7th **S59.039 Salter-Harris Type III physeal fracture of lower end of ulna, unspecified arm** CC H5 UNS

✓6th S59.04 Salter-Harris Type IV physeal fracture of lower end of ulna
- 3 ✓7th **S59.041 Salter-Harris Type IV physeal fracture of lower end of ulna, right arm** CC H5
- 3 ✓7th **S59.042 Salter-Harris Type IV physeal fracture of lower end of ulna, left arm** CC H5
- 3 ✓7th **S59.049 Salter-Harris Type IV physeal fracture of lower end of ulna, unspecified arm** CC H5 UNS

✓6th S59.09 Other physeal fracture of lower end of ulna
- 3 ✓7th **S59.091 Other physeal fracture of lower end of ulna, right arm** CC H5
- 3 ✓7th **S59.092 Other physeal fracture of lower end of ulna, left arm** CC H5
- 3 ✓7th **S59.099 Other physeal fracture of lower end of ulna, unspecified arm** CC H5 UNS

✓5th S59.1 Physeal fracture of upper end of radius

AHA: 2019,4Q,56

✓6th S59.10 Unspecified physeal fracture of upper end of radius
- 4 ✓7th **S59.101 Unspecified physeal fracture of upper end of radius, right arm** CC
- 4 ✓7th **S59.102 Unspecified physeal fracture of upper end of radius, left arm** CC
- 4 ✓7th **S59.109 Unspecified physeal fracture of upper end of radius, unspecified arm** CC UNS

✓6th S59.11 Salter-Harris Type I physeal fracture of upper end of radius
- 4 ✓7th **S59.111 Salter-Harris Type I physeal fracture of upper end of radius, right arm** CC
- 4 ✓7th **S59.112 Salter-Harris Type I physeal fracture of upper end of radius, left arm** CC
- 4 ✓7th **S59.119 Salter-Harris Type I physeal fracture of upper end of radius, unspecified arm** CC UNS

✓6th S59.12 Salter-Harris Type II physeal fracture of upper end of radius
- 4 ✓7th **S59.121 Salter-Harris Type II physeal fracture of upper end of radius, right arm** CC
- 4 ✓7th **S59.122 Salter-Harris Type II physeal fracture of upper end of radius, left arm** CC
- 4 ✓7th **S59.129 Salter-Harris Type II physeal fracture of upper end of radius, unspecified arm** CC UNS

✓6th S59.13 Salter-Harris Type III physeal fracture of upper end of radius
- 4 ✓7th **S59.131 Salter-Harris Type III physeal fracture of upper end of radius, right arm** CC
- 4 ✓7th **S59.132 Salter-Harris Type III physeal fracture of upper end of radius, left arm** CC
- 4 ✓7th **S59.139 Salter-Harris Type III physeal fracture of upper end of radius, unspecified arm** CC UNS

✓6th S59.14 Salter-Harris Type IV physeal fracture of upper end of radius
- 4 ✓7th **S59.141 Salter-Harris Type IV physeal fracture of upper end of radius, right arm** CC
- 4 ✓7th **S59.142 Salter-Harris Type IV physeal fracture of upper end of radius, left arm** CC
- 4 ✓7th **S59.149 Salter-Harris Type IV physeal fracture of upper end of radius, unspecified arm** CC UNS

✓6th S59.19 Other physeal fracture of upper end of radius
- 4 ✓7th **S59.191 Other physeal fracture of upper end of radius, right arm** CC
- 4 ✓7th **S59.192 Other physeal fracture of upper end of radius, left arm** CC
- 4 ✓7th **S59.199 Other physeal fracture of upper end of radius, unspecified arm** CC UNS

✓5th S59.2 Physeal fracture of lower end of radius

AHA: 2019,4Q,56

✓6th S59.20 Unspecified physeal fracture of lower end of radius
- 3 ✓7th **S59.201 Unspecified physeal fracture of lower end of radius, right arm** CC H5
- 3 ✓7th **S59.202 Unspecified physeal fracture of lower end of radius, left arm** CC H5
- 3 ✓7th **S59.209 Unspecified physeal fracture of lower end of radius, unspecified arm** CC H5 UNS

✓6th S59.21 Salter-Harris Type I physeal fracture of lower end of radius
- 3 ✓7th **S59.211 Salter-Harris Type I physeal fracture of lower end of radius, right arm** CC H5
- 3 ✓7th **S59.212 Salter-Harris Type I physeal fracture of lower end of radius, left arm** CC H5
- 3 ✓7th **S59.219 Salter-Harris Type I physeal fracture of lower end of radius, unspecified arm** CC H5 UNS

✓6th S59.22 Salter-Harris Type II physeal fracture of lower end of radius
- 3 ✓7th **S59.221 Salter-Harris Type II physeal fracture of lower end of radius, right arm** CC H5
- 3 ✓7th **S59.222 Salter-Harris Type II physeal fracture of lower end of radius, left arm** CC H5
- 3 ✓7th **S59.229 Salter-Harris Type II physeal fracture of lower end of radius, unspecified arm** CC H5 UNS

✓6th S59.23 Salter-Harris Type III physeal fracture of lower end of radius
- 3 ✓7th **S59.231 Salter-Harris Type III physeal fracture of lower end of radius, right arm** CC H5
- 3 ✓7th **S59.232 Salter-Harris Type III physeal fracture of lower end of radius, left arm** CC H5
- 3 ✓7th **S59.239 Salter-Harris Type III physeal fracture of lower end of radius, unspecified arm** CC H5 UNS

✓6th S59.24 Salter-Harris Type IV physeal fracture of lower end of radius
- 3 ✓7th **S59.241 Salter-Harris Type IV physeal fracture of lower end of radius, right arm** CC H5
- 3 ✓7th **S59.242 Salter-Harris Type IV physeal fracture of lower end of radius, left arm** CC H5

3 ✓7th **S59.249** Salter-Harris Type IV physeal fracture of lower end of radius, unspecified arm CC HS UNS

✓6th **S59.29** Other physeal fracture of lower end of radius

3 ✓7th **S59.291** Other physeal fracture of lower end of radius, right arm CC HS

3 ✓7th **S59.292** Other physeal fracture of lower end of radius, left arm CC HS

3 ✓7th **S59.299** Other physeal fracture of lower end of radius, unspecified arm CC HS UNS

✓5th **S59.8** Other specified injuries of elbow and forearm

The appropriate 7th character is to be added to each code in subcategory S59.8.
A initial encounter
D subsequent encounter
S sequela

✓6th **S59.80** Other specified injuries of elbow

✓7th **S59.801** Other specified injuries of right elbow

✓7th **S59.802** Other specified injuries of left elbow

✓7th **S59.809** Other specified injuries of unspecified elbow

✓6th **S59.81** Other specified injuries of forearm

✓7th **S59.811** Other specified injuries right forearm

✓7th **S59.812** Other specified injuries left forearm

✓7th **S59.819** Other specified injuries unspecified forearm

✓5th **S59.9** Unspecified injury of elbow and forearm

The appropriate 7th character is to be added to each code in subcategory S59.9.
A initial encounter
D subsequent encounter
S sequela

✓6th **S59.90** Unspecified injury of elbow

✓7th **S59.901** Unspecified injury of right elbow

✓7th **S59.902** Unspecified injury of left elbow

✓7th **S59.909** Unspecified injury of unspecified elbow

✓6th **S59.91** Unspecified injury of forearm

✓7th **S59.911** Unspecified injury of right forearm

✓7th **S59.912** Unspecified injury of left forearm

✓7th **S59.919** Unspecified injury of unspecified forearm

Injuries to the wrist, hand and fingers (S60-S69)

EXCLUDES 2 *burns and corrosions (T20-T32)*
frostbite (T33-T34)
insect bite or sting, venomous (T63.4)

✓4th **S60** Superficial injury of wrist, hand and fingers

The appropriate 7th character is to be added to each code from category S60.
A initial encounter
D subsequent encounter
S sequela

✓5th **S60.0** Contusion of finger without damage to nail

EXCLUDES 1 *contusion involving nail (matrix) (S60.1)*

✓x7th **S60.00** Contusion of unspecified finger without damage to nail
Contusion of finger(s) NOS

✓6th **S60.01** Contusion of thumb without damage to nail

✓7th **S60.011** Contusion of right thumb without damage to nail

✓7th **S60.012** Contusion of left thumb without damage to nail

✓7th **S60.019** Contusion of unspecified thumb without damage to nail

✓6th **S60.02** Contusion of index finger without damage to nail

✓7th **S60.021** Contusion of right index finger without damage to nail

✓7th **S60.022** Contusion of left index finger without damage to nail

✓7th **S60.029** Contusion of unspecified index finger without damage to nail

✓6th **S60.03** Contusion of middle finger without damage to nail

✓7th **S60.031** Contusion of right middle finger without damage to nail

✓7th **S60.032** Contusion of left middle finger without damage to nail

✓7th **S60.039** Contusion of unspecified middle finger without damage to nail

✓6th **S60.04** Contusion of ring finger without damage to nail

✓7th **S60.041** Contusion of right ring finger without damage to nail

✓7th **S60.042** Contusion of left ring finger without damage to nail

✓7th **S60.049** Contusion of unspecified ring finger without damage to nail

✓6th **S60.05** Contusion of little finger without damage to nail

✓7th **S60.051** Contusion of right little finger without damage to nail

✓7th **S60.052** Contusion of left little finger without damage to nail

✓7th **S60.059** Contusion of unspecified little finger without damage to nail

✓5th **S60.1** Contusion of finger with damage to nail

✓x7th **S60.10** Contusion of unspecified finger with damage to nail

✓6th **S60.11** Contusion of thumb with damage to nail

✓7th **S60.111** Contusion of right thumb with damage to nail

✓7th **S60.112** Contusion of left thumb with damage to nail

✓7th **S60.119** Contusion of unspecified thumb with damage to nail

✓6th **S60.12** Contusion of index finger with damage to nail

✓7th **S60.121** Contusion of right index finger with damage to nail

✓7th **S60.122** Contusion of left index finger with damage to nail

✓7th **S60.129** Contusion of unspecified index finger with damage to nail

✓6th **S60.13** Contusion of middle finger with damage to nail

✓7th **S60.131** Contusion of right middle finger with damage to nail

✓7th **S60.132** Contusion of left middle finger with damage to nail

✓7th **S60.139** Contusion of unspecified middle finger with damage to nail

✓6th **S60.14** Contusion of ring finger with damage to nail

✓7th **S60.141** Contusion of right ring finger with damage to nail

✓7th **S60.142** Contusion of left ring finger with damage to nail

✓7th **S60.149** Contusion of unspecified ring finger with damage to nail

✓6th **S60.15** Contusion of little finger with damage to nail

✓7th **S60.151** Contusion of right little finger with damage to nail

✓7th **S60.152** Contusion of left little finger with damage to nail

✓7th **S60.159** Contusion of unspecified little finger with damage to nail

✓5th **S60.2** Contusion of wrist and hand

EXCLUDES 2 *contusion of fingers (S60.0-, S60.1-)*

✓6th **S60.21** Contusion of wrist

✓7th **S60.211** Contusion of right wrist

✓7th **S60.212** Contusion of left wrist

✓7th **S60.219** Contusion of unspecified wrist

✓6th **S60.22** Contusion of hand

✓7th **S60.221** Contusion of right hand

✓7th **S60.222** Contusion of left hand

✓7th **S60.229** Contusion of unspecified hand

✓5th **S60.3** Other superficial injuries of thumb

✓6th **S60.31** Abrasion of thumb

✓7th **S60.311** Abrasion of right thumb

✓7th **S60.312** Abrasion of left thumb

✓7th **S60.319** Abrasion of unspecified thumb

✓6th **S60.32** Blister (nonthermal) of thumb

✓7th **S60.321** Blister (nonthermal) of right thumb

✓7th **S60.322** Blister (nonthermal) of left thumb

✓7th **S60.329** Blister (nonthermal) of unspecified thumb

Chapter 19. Injury, Poisoning and Certain Other Consequences of External Causes
S59.249–S60.329

6th **S6Ø.34 External constriction of thumb**
Hair tourniquet syndrome of thumb
Use additional cause code to identify the constricting item (W49.Ø-)
7th **S6Ø.341 External constriction of right thumb**
7th **S6Ø.342 External constriction of left thumb**
7th **S6Ø.349 External constriction of unspecified thumb**

6th **S6Ø.35 Superficial foreign body of thumb**
Splinter in the thumb
7th **S6Ø.351 Superficial foreign body of right thumb**
7th **S6Ø.352 Superficial foreign body of left thumb**
7th **S6Ø.359 Superficial foreign body of unspecified thumb**

6th **S6Ø.36 Insect bite (nonvenomous) of thumb**
7th **S6Ø.361 Insect bite (nonvenomous) of right thumb**
7th **S6Ø.362 Insect bite (nonvenomous) of left thumb**
7th **S6Ø.369 Insect bite (nonvenomous) of unspecified thumb**

6th **S6Ø.37 Other superficial bite of thumb**
EXCLUDES 1 *open bite of thumb (S61.Ø5-, S61.15-)*
7th **S6Ø.371 Other superficial bite of right thumb**
7th **S6Ø.372 Other superficial bite of left thumb**
7th **S6Ø.379 Other superficial bite of unspecified thumb**

6th **S6Ø.39 Other superficial injuries of thumb**
7th **S6Ø.391 Other superficial injuries of right thumb**
7th **S6Ø.392 Other superficial injuries of left thumb**
7th **S6Ø.399 Other superficial injuries of unspecified thumb**

5th **S6Ø.4 Other superficial injuries of other fingers**

6th **S6Ø.41 Abrasion of fingers**
7th **S6Ø.41Ø Abrasion of right index finger**
7th **S6Ø.411 Abrasion of left index finger**
7th **S6Ø.412 Abrasion of right middle finger**
7th **S6Ø.413 Abrasion of left middle finger**
7th **S6Ø.414 Abrasion of right ring finger**
7th **S6Ø.415 Abrasion of left ring finger**
7th **S6Ø.416 Abrasion of right little finger**
7th **S6Ø.417 Abrasion of left little finger**
7th **S6Ø.418 Abrasion of other finger**
Abrasion of specified finger with unspecified laterality
7th **S6Ø.419 Abrasion of unspecified finger**

6th **S6Ø.42 Blister (nonthermal) of fingers**
7th **S6Ø.42Ø Blister (nonthermal) of right index finger**
7th **S6Ø.421 Blister (nonthermal) of left index finger**
7th **S6Ø.422 Blister (nonthermal) of right middle finger**
7th **S6Ø.423 Blister (nonthermal) of left middle finger**
7th **S6Ø.424 Blister (nonthermal) of right ring finger**
7th **S6Ø.425 Blister (nonthermal) of left ring finger**
7th **S6Ø.426 Blister (nonthermal) of right little finger**
7th **S6Ø.427 Blister (nonthermal) of left little finger**
7th **S6Ø.428 Blister (nonthermal) of other finger**
Blister (nonthermal) of specified finger with unspecified laterality
7th **S6Ø.429 Blister (nonthermal) of unspecified finger**

6th **S6Ø.44 External constriction of fingers**
Hair tourniquet syndrome of finger
Use additional cause code to identify the constricting item (W49.Ø-)
7th **S6Ø.44Ø External constriction of right index finger**
7th **S6Ø.441 External constriction of left index finger**
7th **S6Ø.442 External constriction of right middle finger**
7th **S6Ø.443 External constriction of left middle finger**
7th **S6Ø.444 External constriction of right ring finger**
7th **S6Ø.445 External constriction of left ring finger**
7th **S6Ø.446 External constriction of right little finger**
7th **S6Ø.447 External constriction of left little finger**
7th **S6Ø.448 External constriction of other finger**
External constriction of specified finger with unspecified laterality
7th **S6Ø.449 External constriction of unspecified finger**

6th **S6Ø.45 Superficial foreign body of fingers**
Splinter in the finger(s)
7th **S6Ø.45Ø Superficial foreign body of right index finger**
7th **S6Ø.451 Superficial foreign body of left index finger**
7th **S6Ø.452 Superficial foreign body of right middle finger**
7th **S6Ø.453 Superficial foreign body of left middle finger**
7th **S6Ø.454 Superficial foreign body of right ring finger**
7th **S6Ø.455 Superficial foreign body of left ring finger**
7th **S6Ø.456 Superficial foreign body of right little finger**
7th **S6Ø.457 Superficial foreign body of left little finger**
7th **S6Ø.458 Superficial foreign body of other finger**
Superficial foreign body of specified finger with unspecified laterality
7th **S6Ø.459 Superficial foreign body of unspecified finger**

6th **S6Ø.46 Insect bite (nonvenomous) of fingers**
7th **S6Ø.46Ø Insect bite (nonvenomous) of right index finger**
7th **S6Ø.461 Insect bite (nonvenomous) of left index finger**
7th **S6Ø.462 Insect bite (nonvenomous) of right middle finger**
7th **S6Ø.463 Insect bite (nonvenomous) of left middle finger**
7th **S6Ø.464 Insect bite (nonvenomous) of right ring finger**
7th **S6Ø.465 Insect bite (nonvenomous) of left ring finger**
7th **S6Ø.466 Insect bite (nonvenomous) of right little finger**
7th **S6Ø.467 Insect bite (nonvenomous) of left little finger**
7th **S6Ø.468 Insect bite (nonvenomous) of other finger**
Insect bite (nonvenomous) of specified finger with unspecified laterality
7th **S6Ø.469 Insect bite (nonvenomous) of unspecified finger**

6th **S6Ø.47 Other superficial bite of fingers**
EXCLUDES 1 *open bite of fingers (S61.25-, S61.35-)*
7th **S6Ø.47Ø Other superficial bite of right index finger**
7th **S6Ø.471 Other superficial bite of left index finger**
7th **S6Ø.472 Other superficial bite of right middle finger**
7th **S6Ø.473 Other superficial bite of left middle finger**
7th **S6Ø.474 Other superficial bite of right ring finger**
7th **S6Ø.475 Other superficial bite of left ring finger**
7th **S6Ø.476 Other superficial bite of right little finger**
7th **S6Ø.477 Other superficial bite of left little finger**
7th **S6Ø.478 Other superficial bite of other finger**
Other superficial bite of specified finger with unspecified laterality
7th **S6Ø.479 Other superficial bite of unspecified finger**

5th **S6Ø.5 Other superficial injuries of hand**
EXCLUDES 2 *superficial injuries of fingers (S6Ø.3-, S6Ø.4-)*

6th **S6Ø.51 Abrasion of hand**
7th **S6Ø.511 Abrasion of right hand**
7th **S6Ø.512 Abrasion of left hand**
7th **S6Ø.519 Abrasion of unspecified hand**

6th **S6Ø.52 Blister (nonthermal) of hand**
7th **S6Ø.521 Blister (nonthermal) of right hand**
7th **S6Ø.522 Blister (nonthermal) of left hand**
7th **S6Ø.529 Blister (nonthermal) of unspecified hand**

- S60.54 External constriction of hand
  - S60.541 External constriction of right hand
  - S60.542 External constriction of left hand
  - S60.549 External constriction of unspecified hand
- S60.55 Superficial foreign body of hand
  Splinter in the hand
  - S60.551 Superficial foreign body of right hand
  - S60.552 Superficial foreign body of left hand
  - S60.559 Superficial foreign body of unspecified hand
- S60.56 Insect bite (nonvenomous) of hand
  - S60.561 Insect bite (nonvenomous) of right hand
  - S60.562 Insect bite (nonvenomous) of left hand
  - S60.569 Insect bite (nonvenomous) of unspecified hand
- S60.57 Other superficial bite of hand
  EXCLUDES 1 *open bite of hand (S61.45-)*
  - S60.571 Other superficial bite of hand of right hand
  - S60.572 Other superficial bite of hand of left hand
  - S60.579 Other superficial bite of hand of unspecified hand

S60.8 Other superficial injuries of wrist

- S60.81 Abrasion of wrist
  - S60.811 Abrasion of right wrist
  - S60.812 Abrasion of left wrist
  - S60.819 Abrasion of unspecified wrist
- S60.82 Blister (nonthermal) of wrist
  - S60.821 Blister (nonthermal) of right wrist
  - S60.822 Blister (nonthermal) of left wrist
  - S60.829 Blister (nonthermal) of unspecified wrist
- S60.84 External constriction of wrist
  - S60.841 External constriction of right wrist
  - S60.842 External constriction of left wrist
  - S60.849 External constriction of unspecified wrist
- S60.85 Superficial foreign body of wrist
  Splinter in the wrist
  - S60.851 Superficial foreign body of right wrist
  - S60.852 Superficial foreign body of left wrist
  - S60.859 Superficial foreign body of unspecified wrist
- S60.86 Insect bite (nonvenomous) of wrist
  - S60.861 Insect bite (nonvenomous) of right wrist
  - S60.862 Insect bite (nonvenomous) of left wrist
  - S60.869 Insect bite (nonvenomous) of unspecified wrist
- S60.87 Other superficial bite of wrist
  EXCLUDES 1 *open bite of wrist (S61.55)*
  - S60.871 Other superficial bite of right wrist
  - S60.872 Other superficial bite of left wrist
  - S60.879 Other superficial bite of unspecified wrist

S60.9 Unspecified superficial injury of wrist, hand and fingers

- S60.91 Unspecified superficial injury of wrist
  - S60.911 Unspecified superficial injury of right wrist
  - S60.912 Unspecified superficial injury of left wrist
  - S60.919 Unspecified superficial injury of unspecified wrist
- S60.92 Unspecified superficial injury of hand
  - S60.921 Unspecified superficial injury of right hand
  - S60.922 Unspecified superficial injury of left hand
  - S60.929 Unspecified superficial injury of unspecified hand
- S60.93 Unspecified superficial injury of thumb
  - S60.931 Unspecified superficial injury of right thumb
  - S60.932 Unspecified superficial injury of left thumb
  - S60.939 Unspecified superficial injury of unspecified thumb
- S60.94 Unspecified superficial injury of other fingers
  - S60.940 Unspecified superficial injury of right index finger
  - S60.941 Unspecified superficial injury of left index finger
  - S60.942 Unspecified superficial injury of right middle finger
  - S60.943 Unspecified superficial injury of left middle finger
  - S60.944 Unspecified superficial injury of right ring finger
  - S60.945 Unspecified superficial injury of left ring finger
  - S60.946 Unspecified superficial injury of right little finger
  - S60.947 Unspecified superficial injury of left little finger
  - S60.948 Unspecified superficial injury of other finger
    Unspecified superficial injury of specified finger with unspecified laterality
  - S60.949 Unspecified superficial injury of unspecified finger

S61 Open wound of wrist, hand and fingers

Code also any associated wound infection

EXCLUDES 1 *open fracture of wrist, hand and finger (S62.- with 7th character B)*
traumatic amputation of wrist and hand (S68.-)

The appropriate 7th character is to be added to each code from category S61.
A initial encounter
D subsequent encounter
S sequela

S61.0 Open wound of thumb without damage to nail

EXCLUDES 1 *open wound of thumb with damage to nail (S61.1-)*

- S61.00 Unspecified open wound of thumb without damage to nail
  - S61.001 Unspecified open wound of right thumb without damage to nail
  - S61.002 Unspecified open wound of left thumb without damage to nail
  - S61.009 Unspecified open wound of unspecified thumb without damage to nail
- S61.01 Laceration without foreign body of thumb without damage to nail
  - S61.011 Laceration without foreign body of right thumb without damage to nail
  - S61.012 Laceration without foreign body of left thumb without damage to nail
  - S61.019 Laceration without foreign body of unspecified thumb without damage to nail
- S61.02 Laceration with foreign body of thumb without damage to nail
  - S61.021 Laceration with foreign body of right thumb without damage to nail
  - S61.022 Laceration with foreign body of left thumb without damage to nail
  - S61.029 Laceration with foreign body of unspecified thumb without damage to nail
- S61.03 Puncture wound without foreign body of thumb without damage to nail
  - S61.031 Puncture wound without foreign body of right thumb without damage to nail
  - S61.032 Puncture wound without foreign body of left thumb without damage to nail
  - S61.039 Puncture wound without foreign body of unspecified thumb without damage to nail
- S61.04 Puncture wound with foreign body of thumb without damage to nail
  - S61.041 Puncture wound with foreign body of right thumb without damage to nail
  - S61.042 Puncture wound with foreign body of left thumb without damage to nail
  - S61.049 Puncture wound with foreign body of unspecified thumb without damage to nail

S61.Ø5 Open bite of thumb without damage to nail

Bite of thumb NOS

EXCLUDES 1 *superficial bite of thumb (S6Ø.36-, S6Ø.37-)*

- **S61.Ø51** Open bite of right thumb without damage to nail
- **S61.Ø52** Open bite of left thumb without damage to nail
- **S61.Ø59** Open bite of unspecified thumb without damage to nail

S61.1 Open wound of thumb with damage to nail

S61.1Ø Unspecified open wound of thumb with damage to nail

- **S61.1Ø1** Unspecified open wound of right thumb with damage to nail
- **S61.1Ø2** Unspecified open wound of left thumb with damage to nail
- **S61.1Ø9** Unspecified open wound of unspecified thumb with damage to nail

S61.11 Laceration without foreign body of thumb with damage to nail

- **S61.111** Laceration without foreign body of right thumb with damage to nail
- **S61.112** Laceration without foreign body of left thumb with damage to nail
- **S61.119** Laceration without foreign body of unspecified thumb with damage to nail

S61.12 Laceration with foreign body of thumb with damage to nail

- **S61.121** Laceration with foreign body of right thumb with damage to nail
- **S61.122** Laceration with foreign body of left thumb with damage to nail
- **S61.129** Laceration with foreign body of unspecified thumb with damage to nail

S61.13 Puncture wound without foreign body of thumb with damage to nail

- **S61.131** Puncture wound without foreign body of right thumb with damage to nail
- **S61.132** Puncture wound without foreign body of left thumb with damage to nail
- **S61.139** Puncture wound without foreign body of unspecified thumb with damage to nail

S61.14 Puncture wound with foreign body of thumb with damage to nail

- **S61.141** Puncture wound with foreign body of right thumb with damage to nail
- **S61.142** Puncture wound with foreign body of left thumb with damage to nail
- **S61.149** Puncture wound with foreign body of unspecified thumb with damage to nail

S61.15 Open bite of thumb with damage to nail

Bite of thumb with damage to nail NOS

EXCLUDES 1 *superficial bite of thumb (S6Ø.36-, S6Ø.37-)*

- **S61.151** Open bite of right thumb with damage to nail
- **S61.152** Open bite of left thumb with damage to nail
- **S61.159** Open bite of unspecified thumb with damage to nail

S61.2 Open wound of other finger without damage to nail

EXCLUDES 1 *open wound of finger involving nail (matrix) (S61.3-)*

EXCLUDES 2 *open wound of thumb without damage to nail (S61.Ø-)*

S61.2Ø Unspecified open wound of other finger without damage to nail

- **S61.2ØØ** Unspecified open wound of right index finger without damage to nail
- **S61.2Ø1** Unspecified open wound of left index finger without damage to nail
- **S61.2Ø2** Unspecified open wound of right middle finger without damage to nail
- **S61.2Ø3** Unspecified open wound of left middle finger without damage to nail
- **S61.2Ø4** Unspecified open wound of right ring finger without damage to nail
- **S61.2Ø5** Unspecified open wound of left ring finger without damage to nail
- **S61.2Ø6** Unspecified open wound of right little finger without damage to nail
- **S61.2Ø7** Unspecified open wound of left little finger without damage to nail
- **S61.2Ø8** Unspecified open wound of other finger without damage to nail
  Unspecified open wound of specified finger with unspecified laterality without damage to nail
- **S61.2Ø9** Unspecified open wound of unspecified finger without damage to nail

S61.21 Laceration without foreign body of finger without damage to nail

- **S61.21Ø** Laceration without foreign body of right index finger without damage to nail
- **S61.211** Laceration without foreign body of left index finger without damage to nail
- **S61.212** Laceration without foreign body of right middle finger without damage to nail
- **S61.213** Laceration without foreign body of left middle finger without damage to nail
- **S61.214** Laceration without foreign body of right ring finger without damage to nail
- **S61.215** Laceration without foreign body of left ring finger without damage to nail
- **S61.216** Laceration without foreign body of right little finger without damage to nail
- **S61.217** Laceration without foreign body of left little finger without damage to nail
- **S61.218** Laceration without foreign body of other finger without damage to nail
  Laceration without foreign body of specified finger with unspecified laterality without damage to nail
- **S61.219** Laceration without foreign body of unspecified finger without damage to nail

S61.22 Laceration with foreign body of finger without damage to nail

- **S61.22Ø** Laceration with foreign body of right index finger without damage to nail
- **S61.221** Laceration with foreign body of left index finger without damage to nail
- **S61.222** Laceration with foreign body of right middle finger without damage to nail
- **S61.223** Laceration with foreign body of left middle finger without damage to nail
- **S61.224** Laceration with foreign body of right ring finger without damage to nail
- **S61.225** Laceration with foreign body of left ring finger without damage to nail
- **S61.226** Laceration with foreign body of right little finger without damage to nail
- **S61.227** Laceration with foreign body of left little finger without damage to nail
- **S61.228** Laceration with foreign body of other finger without damage to nail
  Laceration with foreign body of specified finger with unspecified laterality without damage to nail
- **S61.229** Laceration with foreign body of unspecified finger without damage to nail

S61.23 Puncture wound without foreign body of finger without damage to nail

- **S61.23Ø** Puncture wound without foreign body of right index finger without damage to nail
- **S61.231** Puncture wound without foreign body of left index finger without damage to nail
- **S61.232** Puncture wound without foreign body of right middle finger without damage to nail
- **S61.233** Puncture wound without foreign body of left middle finger without damage to nail
- **S61.234** Puncture wound without foreign body of right ring finger without damage to nail
- **S61.235** Puncture wound without foreign body of left ring finger without damage to nail
- **S61.236** Puncture wound without foreign body of right little finger without damage to nail
- **S61.237** Puncture wound without foreign body of left little finger without damage to nail

✓7th **S61.238 Puncture wound without foreign body of other finger without damage to nail**
Puncture wound without foreign body of specified finger with unspecified laterality without damage to nail

✓7th **S61.239 Puncture wound without foreign body of unspecified finger without damage to nail**

✓6th **S61.24 Puncture wound with foreign body of finger without damage to nail**

✓7th **S61.240 Puncture wound with foreign body of right index finger without damage to nail**

✓7th **S61.241 Puncture wound with foreign body of left index finger without damage to nail**

✓7th **S61.242 Puncture wound with foreign body of right middle finger without damage to nail**

✓7th **S61.243 Puncture wound with foreign body of left middle finger without damage to nail**

✓7th **S61.244 Puncture wound with foreign body of right ring finger without damage to nail**

✓7th **S61.245 Puncture wound with foreign body of left ring finger without damage to nail**

✓7th **S61.246 Puncture wound with foreign body of right little finger without damage to nail**

✓7th **S61.247 Puncture wound with foreign body of left little finger without damage to nail**

✓7th **S61.248 Puncture wound with foreign body of other finger without damage to nail**
Puncture wound with foreign body of specified finger with unspecified laterality without damage to nail

✓7th **S61.249 Puncture wound with foreign body of unspecified finger without damage to nail**

✓6th **S61.25 Open bite of finger without damage to nail**
Bite of finger without damage to nail NOS
EXCLUDES 1 *superficial bite of finger (S60.46-, S60.47-)*

✓7th **S61.250 Open bite of right index finger without damage to nail**

✓7th **S61.251 Open bite of left index finger without damage to nail**

✓7th **S61.252 Open bite of right middle finger without damage to nail**

✓7th **S61.253 Open bite of left middle finger without damage to nail**

✓7th **S61.254 Open bite of right ring finger without damage to nail**

✓7th **S61.255 Open bite of left ring finger without damage to nail**

✓7th **S61.256 Open bite of right little finger without damage to nail**

✓7th **S61.257 Open bite of left little finger without damage to nail**

✓7th **S61.258 Open bite of other finger without damage to nail**
Open bite of specified finger with unspecified laterality without damage to nail

✓7th **S61.259 Open bite of unspecified finger without damage to nail**

✓5th **S61.3 Open wound of other finger with damage to nail**

✓6th **S61.30 Unspecified open wound of finger with damage to nail**

✓7th **S61.300 Unspecified open wound of right index finger with damage to nail**

✓7th **S61.301 Unspecified open wound of left index finger with damage to nail**

✓7th **S61.302 Unspecified open wound of right middle finger with damage to nail**

✓7th **S61.303 Unspecified open wound of left middle finger with damage to nail**

✓7th **S61.304 Unspecified open wound of right ring finger with damage to nail**

✓7th **S61.305 Unspecified open wound of left ring finger with damage to nail**

✓7th **S61.306 Unspecified open wound of right little finger with damage to nail**

✓7th **S61.307 Unspecified open wound of left little finger with damage to nail**

✓7th **S61.308 Unspecified open wound of other finger with damage to nail**
Unspecified open wound of specified finger with unspecified laterality with damage to nail

✓7th **S61.309 Unspecified open wound of unspecified finger with damage to nail**

✓6th **S61.31 Laceration without foreign body of finger with damage to nail**

✓7th **S61.310 Laceration without foreign body of right index finger with damage to nail**

✓7th **S61.311 Laceration without foreign body of left index finger with damage to nail**

✓7th **S61.312 Laceration without foreign body of right middle finger with damage to nail**

✓7th **S61.313 Laceration without foreign body of left middle finger with damage to nail**

✓7th **S61.314 Laceration without foreign body of right ring finger with damage to nail**

✓7th **S61.315 Laceration without foreign body of left ring finger with damage to nail**

✓7th **S61.316 Laceration without foreign body of right little finger with damage to nail**

✓7th **S61.317 Laceration without foreign body of left little finger with damage to nail**

✓7th **S61.318 Laceration without foreign body of other finger with damage to nail**
Laceration without foreign body of specified finger with unspecified laterality with damage to nail

✓7th **S61.319 Laceration without foreign body of unspecified finger with damage to nail**

✓6th **S61.32 Laceration with foreign body of finger with damage to nail**

✓7th **S61.320 Laceration with foreign body of right index finger with damage to nail**

✓7th **S61.321 Laceration with foreign body of left index finger with damage to nail**

✓7th **S61.322 Laceration with foreign body of right middle finger with damage to nail**

✓7th **S61.323 Laceration with foreign body of left middle finger with damage to nail**

✓7th **S61.324 Laceration with foreign body of right ring finger with damage to nail**

✓7th **S61.325 Laceration with foreign body of left ring finger with damage to nail**

✓7th **S61.326 Laceration with foreign body of right little finger with damage to nail**

✓7th **S61.327 Laceration with foreign body of left little finger with damage to nail**

✓7th **S61.328 Laceration with foreign body of other finger with damage to nail**
Laceration with foreign body of specified finger with specified laterality with damage to nail

✓7th **S61.329 Laceration with foreign body of unspecified finger with damage to nail**

✓6th **S61.33 Puncture wound without foreign body of finger with damage to nail**

✓7th **S61.330 Puncture wound without foreign body of right index finger with damage to nail**

✓7th **S61.331 Puncture wound without foreign body of left index finger with damage to nail**

✓7th **S61.332 Puncture wound without foreign body of right middle finger with damage to nail**

✓7th **S61.333 Puncture wound without foreign body of left middle finger with damage to nail**

✓7th **S61.334 Puncture wound without foreign body of right ring finger with damage to nail**

✓7th **S61.335 Puncture wound without foreign body of left ring finger with damage to nail**

✓7th **S61.336 Puncture wound without foreign body of right little finger with damage to nail**

✓7th **S61.337 Puncture wound without foreign body of left little finger with damage to nail**

✓7th **S61.338 Puncture wound without foreign body of other finger with damage to nail**
Puncture wound without foreign body of specified finger with unspecified laterality with damage to nail

✓7th **S61.339 Puncture wound without foreign body of unspecified finger with damage to nail**

✓6th **S61.34 Puncture wound with foreign body of finger with damage to nail**
✓7th **S61.340 Puncture wound with foreign body of right index finger with damage to nail**
✓7th **S61.341 Puncture wound with foreign body of left index finger with damage to nail**
✓7th **S61.342 Puncture wound with foreign body of right middle finger with damage to nail**
✓7th **S61.343 Puncture wound with foreign body of left middle finger with damage to nail**
✓7th **S61.344 Puncture wound with foreign body of right ring finger with damage to nail**
✓7th **S61.345 Puncture wound with foreign body of left ring finger with damage to nail**
✓7th **S61.346 Puncture wound with foreign body of right little finger with damage to nail**
✓7th **S61.347 Puncture wound with foreign body of left little finger with damage to nail**
✓7th **S61.348 Puncture wound with foreign body of other finger with damage to nail**
Puncture wound with foreign body of specified finger with unspecified laterality with damage to nail
✓7th **S61.349 Puncture wound with foreign body of unspecified finger with damage to nail**
✓6th **S61.35 Open bite of finger with damage to nail**
Bite of finger with damage to nail NOS
EXCLUDES 1 *superficial bite of finger (S60.46-, S60.47-)*
✓7th **S61.350 Open bite of right index finger with damage to nail**
✓7th **S61.351 Open bite of left index finger with damage to nail**
✓7th **S61.352 Open bite of right middle finger with damage to nail**
✓7th **S61.353 Open bite of left middle finger with damage to nail**
✓7th **S61.354 Open bite of right ring finger with damage to nail**
✓7th **S61.355 Open bite of left ring finger with damage to nail**
✓7th **S61.356 Open bite of right little finger with damage to nail**
✓7th **S61.357 Open bite of left little finger with damage to nail**
✓7th **S61.358 Open bite of other finger with damage to nail**
Open bite of specified finger with unspecified laterality with damage to nail
✓7th **S61.359 Open bite of unspecified finger with damage to nail**
✓5th **S61.4 Open wound of hand**
✓6th **S61.40 Unspecified open wound of hand**
✓7th **S61.401 Unspecified open wound of right hand**
✓7th **S61.402 Unspecified open wound of left hand**
✓7th **S61.409 Unspecified open wound of unspecified hand**
✓6th **S61.41 Laceration without foreign body of hand**
✓7th **S61.411 Laceration without foreign body of right hand**
✓7th **S61.412 Laceration without foreign body of left hand**
✓7th **S61.419 Laceration without foreign body of unspecified hand**
✓6th **S61.42 Laceration with foreign body of hand**
✓7th **S61.421 Laceration with foreign body of right hand**
✓7th **S61.422 Laceration with foreign body of left hand**
✓7th **S61.429 Laceration with foreign body of unspecified hand**
✓6th **S61.43 Puncture wound without foreign body of hand**
✓7th **S61.431 Puncture wound without foreign body of right hand**
✓7th **S61.432 Puncture wound without foreign body of left hand**
✓7th **S61.439 Puncture wound without foreign body of unspecified hand**
✓6th **S61.44 Puncture wound with foreign body of hand**
✓7th **S61.441 Puncture wound with foreign body of right hand**
✓7th **S61.442 Puncture wound with foreign body of left hand**
✓7th **S61.449 Puncture wound with foreign body of unspecified hand**
✓6th **S61.45 Open bite of hand**
Bite of hand NOS
EXCLUDES 1 *superficial bite of hand (S60.56-, S60.57-)*
✓7th **S61.451 Open bite of right hand**
✓7th **S61.452 Open bite of left hand**
✓7th **S61.459 Open bite of unspecified hand**
✓5th **S61.5 Open wound of wrist**
✓6th **S61.50 Unspecified open wound of wrist**
✓7th **S61.501 Unspecified open wound of right wrist**
✓7th **S61.502 Unspecified open wound of left wrist**
✓7th **S61.509 Unspecified open wound of unspecified wrist**
✓6th **S61.51 Laceration without foreign body of wrist**
✓7th **S61.511 Laceration without foreign body of right wrist**
✓7th **S61.512 Laceration without foreign body of left wrist**
✓7th **S61.519 Laceration without foreign body of unspecified wrist**
✓6th **S61.52 Laceration with foreign body of wrist**
✓7th **S61.521 Laceration with foreign body of right wrist**
✓7th **S61.522 Laceration with foreign body of left wrist**
✓7th **S61.529 Laceration with foreign body of unspecified wrist**
✓6th **S61.53 Puncture wound without foreign body of wrist**
✓7th **S61.531 Puncture wound without foreign body of right wrist**
✓7th **S61.532 Puncture wound without foreign body of left wrist**
✓7th **S61.539 Puncture wound without foreign body of unspecified wrist**
✓6th **S61.54 Puncture wound with foreign body of wrist**
✓7th **S61.541 Puncture wound with foreign body of right wrist**
✓7th **S61.542 Puncture wound with foreign body of left wrist**
✓7th **S61.549 Puncture wound with foreign body of unspecified wrist**
✓6th **S61.55 Open bite of wrist**
Bite of wrist NOS
EXCLUDES 1 *superficial bite of wrist (S60.86-, S60.87-)*
✓7th **S61.551 Open bite of right wrist**
✓7th **S61.552 Open bite of left wrist**
✓7th **S61.559 Open bite of unspecified wrist**

✓4th **S62 Fracture at wrist and hand level**
NOTE A fracture not indicated as displaced or nondisplaced should be coded to displaced
A fracture not indicated as open or closed should be coded to closed
EXCLUDES 1 *traumatic amputation of wrist and hand (S68.-)*
EXCLUDES 2 *fracture of distal parts of ulna and radius (S52.-)*
AHA: 2018,2Q,12; 2015,3Q,37-39

The appropriate 7th character is to be added to each code from category S62.
A initial encounter for closed fracture
B initial encounter for open fracture
D subsequent encounter for fracture with routine healing
G subsequent encounter for fracture with delayed healing
K subsequent encounter for fracture with nonunion
P subsequent encounter for fracture with malunion
S sequela

✓5th **S62.0 Fracture of navicular [scaphoid] bone of wrist**
✓6th **S62.00 Unspecified fracture of navicular [scaphoid] bone of wrist**
3 ✓7th **S62.001 Unspecified fracture of navicular [scaphoid] bone of right wrist** CC HS
3 ✓7th **S62.002 Unspecified fracture of navicular [scaphoid] bone of left wrist** CC HS
AHA: 2012,4Q,106

S62.009 Unspecified fracture of navicular [scaphoid] bone of unspecified wrist CC H5 UNS

S62.01 Fracture of distal pole of navicular [scaphoid] bone of wrist
Fracture of volar tuberosity of navicular [scaphoid] bone of wrist

S62.011 Displaced fracture of distal pole of navicular [scaphoid] bone of right wrist CC H5

S62.012 Displaced fracture of distal pole of navicular [scaphoid] bone of left wrist CC H5

S62.013 Displaced fracture of distal pole of navicular [scaphoid] bone of unspecified wrist CC H5 UNS

S62.014 Nondisplaced fracture of distal pole of navicular [scaphoid] bone of right wrist CC H5

S62.015 Nondisplaced fracture of distal pole of navicular [scaphoid] bone of left wrist CC H5

S62.016 Nondisplaced fracture of distal pole of navicular [scaphoid] bone of unspecified wrist CC H5 UNS

S62.02 Fracture of middle third of navicular [scaphoid] bone of wrist

S62.021 Displaced fracture of middle third of navicular [scaphoid] bone of right wrist CC H5

S62.022 Displaced fracture of middle third of navicular [scaphoid] bone of left wrist CC H5

S62.023 Displaced fracture of middle third of navicular [scaphoid] bone of unspecified wrist CC H5 UNS

S62.024 Nondisplaced fracture of middle third of navicular [scaphoid] bone of right wrist CC H5

S62.025 Nondisplaced fracture of middle third of navicular [scaphoid] bone of left wrist CC H5

S62.026 Nondisplaced fracture of middle third of navicular [scaphoid] bone of unspecified wrist CC H5 UNS

S62.03 Fracture of proximal third of navicular [scaphoid] bone of wrist

S62.031 Displaced fracture of proximal third of navicular [scaphoid] bone of right wrist CC H5

S62.032 Displaced fracture of proximal third of navicular [scaphoid] bone of left wrist CC H5

S62.033 Displaced fracture of proximal third of navicular [scaphoid] bone of unspecified wrist CC H5 UNS

S62.034 Nondisplaced fracture of proximal third of navicular [scaphoid] bone of right wrist CC H5

S62.035 Nondisplaced fracture of proximal third of navicular [scaphoid] bone of left wrist CC H5

S62.036 Nondisplaced fracture of proximal third of navicular [scaphoid] bone of unspecified wrist CC H5 UNS

S62.1 Fracture of other and unspecified carpal bone(s)
EXCLUDES 2 *fracture of scaphoid of wrist (S62.0-)*

S62.10 Fracture of unspecified carpal bone
Fracture of wrist NOS

S62.101 Fracture of unspecified carpal bone, right wrist CC H5

S62.102 Fracture of unspecified carpal bone, left wrist CC H5
AHA: 2012,4Q,95

S62.109 Fracture of unspecified carpal bone, unspecified wrist CC H5 UNS

S62.11 Fracture of triquetrum [cuneiform] bone of wrist

S62.111 Displaced fracture of triquetrum [cuneiform] bone, right wrist CC H5

S62.112 Displaced fracture of triquetrum [cuneiform] bone, left wrist CC H5

S62.113 Displaced fracture of triquetrum [cuneiform] bone, unspecified wrist CC H5 UNS

S62.114 Nondisplaced fracture of triquetrum [cuneiform] bone, right wrist CC H5

S62.115 Nondisplaced fracture of triquetrum [cuneiform] bone, left wrist CC H5

S62.116 Nondisplaced fracture of triquetrum [cuneiform] bone, unspecified wrist CC H5 UNS

S62.12 Fracture of lunate [semilunar]

S62.121 Displaced fracture of lunate [semilunar], right wrist CC H5

S62.122 Displaced fracture of lunate [semilunar], left wrist CC H5

S62.123 Displaced fracture of lunate [semilunar], unspecified wrist CC H5 UNS

S62.124 Nondisplaced fracture of lunate [semilunar], right wrist CC H5

S62.125 Nondisplaced fracture of lunate [semilunar], left wrist CC H5

S62.126 Nondisplaced fracture of lunate [semilunar], unspecified wrist CC H5 UNS

S62.13 Fracture of capitate [os magnum] bone

S62.131 Displaced fracture of capitate [os magnum] bone, right wrist CC H5

S62.132 Displaced fracture of capitate [os magnum] bone, left wrist CC H5

S62.133 Displaced fracture of capitate [os magnum] bone, unspecified wrist CC H5 UNS

S62.134 Nondisplaced fracture of capitate [os magnum] bone, right wrist CC H5

S62.135 Nondisplaced fracture of capitate [os magnum] bone, left wrist CC H5

S62.136 Nondisplaced fracture of capitate [os magnum] bone, unspecified wrist CC H5 UNS

S62.14 Fracture of body of hamate [unciform] bone
Fracture of hamate [unciform] bone NOS

S62.141 Displaced fracture of body of hamate [unciform] bone, right wrist CC H5

S62.142 Displaced fracture of body of hamate [unciform] bone, left wrist CC H5

S62.143 Displaced fracture of body of hamate [unciform] bone, unspecified wrist CC H5 UNS

S62.144 Nondisplaced fracture of body of hamate [unciform] bone, right wrist CC H5

S62.145 Nondisplaced fracture of body of hamate [unciform] bone, left wrist CC H5

S62.146 Nondisplaced fracture of body of hamate [unciform] bone, unspecified wrist CC H5 UNS

S62.15 Fracture of hook process of hamate [unciform] bone
Fracture of unciform process of hamate [unciform] bone

S62.151 Displaced fracture of hook process of hamate [unciform] bone, right wrist CC H5

S62.152 Displaced fracture of hook process of hamate [unciform] bone, left wrist CC H5

S62.153 Displaced fracture of hook process of hamate [unciform] bone, unspecified wrist CC H5 UNS

S62.154 Nondisplaced fracture of hook process of hamate [unciform] bone, right wrist CC H5

S62.155 Nondisplaced fracture of hook process of hamate [unciform] bone, left wrist CC H5

S62.156 Nondisplaced fracture of hook process of hamate [unciform] bone, unspecified wrist CC H5 UNS

S62.16 Fracture of pisiform

S62.161 Displaced fracture of pisiform, right wrist CC H5

7th S62.162 Displaced fracture of pisiform, left wrist CC HS

7th S62.163 Displaced fracture of pisiform, unspecified wrist CC HS UNS

7th S62.164 Nondisplaced fracture of pisiform, right wrist CC HS

7th S62.165 Nondisplaced fracture of pisiform, left wrist CC HS

7th S62.166 Nondisplaced fracture of pisiform, unspecified wrist CC HS UNS

6th S62.17 Fracture of trapezium [larger multangular]

7th S62.171 Displaced fracture of trapezium [larger multangular], right wrist CC HS

7th S62.172 Displaced fracture of trapezium [larger multangular], left wrist CC HS

7th S62.173 Displaced fracture of trapezium [larger multangular], unspecified wrist CC HS UNS

7th S62.174 Nondisplaced fracture of trapezium [larger multangular], right wrist CC HS

7th S62.175 Nondisplaced fracture of trapezium [larger multangular], left wrist CC HS

7th S62.176 Nondisplaced fracture of trapezium [larger multangular], unspecified wrist CC HS UNS

6th S62.18 Fracture of trapezoid [smaller multangular]

7th S62.181 Displaced fracture of trapezoid [smaller multangular], right wrist CC HS

7th S62.182 Displaced fracture of trapezoid [smaller multangular], left wrist CC HS

7th S62.183 Displaced fracture of trapezoid [smaller multangular], unspecified wrist CC HS UNS

7th S62.184 Nondisplaced fracture of trapezoid [smaller multangular], right wrist CC HS

7th S62.185 Nondisplaced fracture of trapezoid [smaller multangular], left wrist CC HS

7th S62.186 Nondisplaced fracture of trapezoid [smaller multangular], unspecified wrist CC HS UNS

5th S62.2 Fracture of first metacarpal bone

6th S62.20 Unspecified fracture of first metacarpal bone

7th S62.201 Unspecified fracture of first metacarpal bone, right hand CC HS

7th S62.202 Unspecified fracture of first metacarpal bone, left hand CC HS

7th S62.209 Unspecified fracture of first metacarpal bone, unspecified hand CC HS UNS

6th S62.21 Bennett's fracture

DEF: Intra-articular, two-part fracture at the base of the first metacarpal bone (thumb) on the ulnar side at the carpometacarpal (CMC) joint.

7th S62.211 Bennett's fracture, right hand CC HS

7th S62.212 Bennett's fracture, left hand CC HS

7th S62.213 Bennett's fracture, unspecified hand CC HS UNS

6th S62.22 Rolando's fracture

DEF: Comminuted, three part intra-articular fracture at the base of the thumb metacarpal.

7th S62.221 Displaced Rolando's fracture, right hand CC HS

7th S62.222 Displaced Rolando's fracture, left hand CC HS

7th S62.223 Displaced Rolando's fracture, unspecified hand CC HS UNS

7th S62.224 Nondisplaced Rolando's fracture, right hand CC HS

7th S62.225 Nondisplaced Rolando's fracture, left hand CC HS

7th S62.226 Nondisplaced Rolando's fracture, unspecified hand CC HS UNS

6th S62.23 Other fracture of base of first metacarpal bone

7th S62.231 Other displaced fracture of base of first metacarpal bone, right hand CC HS

7th S62.232 Other displaced fracture of base of first metacarpal bone, left hand CC HS

7th S62.233 Other displaced fracture of base of first metacarpal bone, unspecified hand CC HS UNS

7th S62.234 Other nondisplaced fracture of base of first metacarpal bone, right hand CC HS

7th S62.235 Other nondisplaced fracture of base of first metacarpal bone, left hand CC HS

7th S62.236 Other nondisplaced fracture of base of first metacarpal bone, unspecified hand CC HS UNS

6th S62.24 Fracture of shaft of first metacarpal bone

7th S62.241 Displaced fracture of shaft of first metacarpal bone, right hand CC HS

7th S62.242 Displaced fracture of shaft of first metacarpal bone, left hand CC HS

7th S62.243 Displaced fracture of shaft of first metacarpal bone, unspecified hand CC HS UNS

7th S62.244 Nondisplaced fracture of shaft of first metacarpal bone, right hand CC HS

7th S62.245 Nondisplaced fracture of shaft of first metacarpal bone, left hand CC HS

7th S62.246 Nondisplaced fracture of shaft of first metacarpal bone, unspecified hand CC HS UNS

6th S62.25 Fracture of neck of first metacarpal bone

7th S62.251 Displaced fracture of neck of first metacarpal bone, right hand CC HS

7th S62.252 Displaced fracture of neck of first metacarpal bone, left hand CC HS

7th S62.253 Displaced fracture of neck of first metacarpal bone, unspecified hand CC HS UNS

7th S62.254 Nondisplaced fracture of neck of first metacarpal bone, right hand CC HS

7th S62.255 Nondisplaced fracture of neck of first metacarpal bone, left hand CC HS

7th S62.256 Nondisplaced fracture of neck of first metacarpal bone, unspecified hand CC HS UNS

6th S62.29 Other fracture of first metacarpal bone

7th S62.291 Other fracture of first metacarpal bone, right hand CC HS

7th S62.292 Other fracture of first metacarpal bone, left hand CC HS

7th S62.299 Other fracture of first metacarpal bone, unspecified hand CC HS UNS

5th S62.3 Fracture of other and unspecified metacarpal bone

EXCLUDES 2 *fracture of first metacarpal bone (S62.2-)*

6th S62.30 Unspecified fracture of other metacarpal bone

7th S62.300 Unspecified fracture of second metacarpal bone, right hand CC HS

7th S62.301 Unspecified fracture of second metacarpal bone, left hand CC HS

7th S62.302 Unspecified fracture of third metacarpal bone, right hand CC HS

7th S62.303 Unspecified fracture of third metacarpal bone, left hand CC HS

7th S62.304 Unspecified fracture of fourth metacarpal bone, right hand CC HS

7th S62.305 Unspecified fracture of fourth metacarpal bone, left hand CC HS

7th S62.306 Unspecified fracture of fifth metacarpal bone, right hand CC HS

7th S62.307 Unspecified fracture of fifth metacarpal bone, left hand CC HS

7th S62.308 Unspecified fracture of other metacarpal bone CC HS

Unspecified fracture of specified metacarpal bone with unspecified laterality

7th S62.309 Unspecified fracture of unspecified metacarpal bone CC HS UNS

6th S62.31 Displaced fracture of base of other metacarpal bone

7th S62.310 Displaced fracture of base of second metacarpal bone, right hand CC HS

7th S62.311 Displaced fracture of base of second metacarpal bone, left hand CC HS

S62.312 Displaced fracture of base of third metacarpal bone, right hand CC H5
S62.313 Displaced fracture of base of third metacarpal bone, left hand CC H5
S62.314 Displaced fracture of base of fourth metacarpal bone, right hand CC H5
S62.315 Displaced fracture of base of fourth metacarpal bone, left hand CC H5
S62.316 Displaced fracture of base of fifth metacarpal bone, right hand CC H5
S62.317 Displaced fracture of base of fifth metacarpal bone, left hand CC H5
S62.318 Displaced fracture of base of other metacarpal bone CC H5
Displaced fracture of base of specified metacarpal bone with unspecified laterality
S62.319 Displaced fracture of base of unspecified metacarpal bone CC H5 UNS

S62.32 Displaced fracture of shaft of other metacarpal bone
S62.320 Displaced fracture of shaft of second metacarpal bone, right hand CC H5
S62.321 Displaced fracture of shaft of second metacarpal bone, left hand CC H5
S62.322 Displaced fracture of shaft of third metacarpal bone, right hand CC H5
S62.323 Displaced fracture of shaft of third metacarpal bone, left hand CC H5
S62.324 Displaced fracture of shaft of fourth metacarpal bone, right hand CC H5
S62.325 Displaced fracture of shaft of fourth metacarpal bone, left hand CC H5
S62.326 Displaced fracture of shaft of fifth metacarpal bone, right hand CC H5
S62.327 Displaced fracture of shaft of fifth metacarpal bone, left hand CC H5
S62.328 Displaced fracture of shaft of other metacarpal bone CC H5
Displaced fracture of shaft of specified metacarpal bone with unspecified laterality
S62.329 Displaced fracture of shaft of unspecified metacarpal bone CC H5 UNS

S62.33 Displaced fracture of neck of other metacarpal bone
S62.330 Displaced fracture of neck of second metacarpal bone, right hand CC H5
S62.331 Displaced fracture of neck of second metacarpal bone, left hand CC H5
S62.332 Displaced fracture of neck of third metacarpal bone, right hand CC H5
S62.333 Displaced fracture of neck of third metacarpal bone, left hand CC H5
S62.334 Displaced fracture of neck of fourth metacarpal bone, right hand CC H5
S62.335 Displaced fracture of neck of fourth metacarpal bone, left hand CC H5
S62.336 Displaced fracture of neck of fifth metacarpal bone, right hand CC H5
S62.337 Displaced fracture of neck of fifth metacarpal bone, left hand CC H5
S62.338 Displaced fracture of neck of other metacarpal bone CC H5
Displaced fracture of neck of specified metacarpal bone with unspecified laterality
S62.339 Displaced fracture of neck of unspecified metacarpal bone CC H5 UNS

S62.34 Nondisplaced fracture of base of other metacarpal bone
S62.340 Nondisplaced fracture of base of second metacarpal bone, right hand CC H5
S62.341 Nondisplaced fracture of base of second metacarpal bone, left hand CC H5
S62.342 Nondisplaced fracture of base of third metacarpal bone, right hand CC H5
S62.343 Nondisplaced fracture of base of third metacarpal bone, left hand CC H5
S62.344 Nondisplaced fracture of base of fourth metacarpal bone, right hand CC H5
S62.345 Nondisplaced fracture of base of fourth metacarpal bone, left hand CC H5
S62.346 Nondisplaced fracture of base of fifth metacarpal bone, right hand CC H5
S62.347 Nondisplaced fracture of base of fifth metacarpal bone, left hand CC H5
S62.348 Nondisplaced fracture of base of other metacarpal bone CC H5
Nondisplaced fracture of base of specified metacarpal bone with unspecified laterality
S62.349 Nondisplaced fracture of base of unspecified metacarpal bone CC H5 UNS

S62.35 Nondisplaced fracture of shaft of other metacarpal bone
S62.350 Nondisplaced fracture of shaft of second metacarpal bone, right hand CC H5
S62.351 Nondisplaced fracture of shaft of second metacarpal bone, left hand CC H5
S62.352 Nondisplaced fracture of shaft of third metacarpal bone, right hand CC H5
S62.353 Nondisplaced fracture of shaft of third metacarpal bone, left hand CC H5
S62.354 Nondisplaced fracture of shaft of fourth metacarpal bone, right hand CC H5
S62.355 Nondisplaced fracture of shaft of fourth metacarpal bone, left hand CC H5
S62.356 Nondisplaced fracture of shaft of fifth metacarpal bone, right hand CC H5
S62.357 Nondisplaced fracture of shaft of fifth metacarpal bone, left hand CC H5
S62.358 Nondisplaced fracture of shaft of other metacarpal bone CC H5
Nondisplaced fracture of shaft of specified metacarpal bone with unspecified laterality
S62.359 Nondisplaced fracture of shaft of unspecified metacarpal bone CC H5 UNS

S62.36 Nondisplaced fracture of neck of other metacarpal bone
S62.360 Nondisplaced fracture of neck of second metacarpal bone, right hand CC H5
S62.361 Nondisplaced fracture of neck of second metacarpal bone, left hand CC H5
S62.362 Nondisplaced fracture of neck of third metacarpal bone, right hand CC H5
S62.363 Nondisplaced fracture of neck of third metacarpal bone, left hand CC H5
S62.364 Nondisplaced fracture of neck of fourth metacarpal bone, right hand CC H5
S62.365 Nondisplaced fracture of neck of fourth metacarpal bone, left hand CC H5
S62.366 Nondisplaced fracture of neck of fifth metacarpal bone, right hand CC H5
S62.367 Nondisplaced fracture of neck of fifth metacarpal bone, left hand CC H5
S62.368 Nondisplaced fracture of neck of other metacarpal bone CC H5
Nondisplaced fracture of neck of specified metacarpal bone with unspecified laterality
S62.369 Nondisplaced fracture of neck of unspecified metacarpal bone CC H5 UNS

S62.39 Other fracture of other metacarpal bone
S62.390 Other fracture of second metacarpal bone, right hand CC H5
S62.391 Other fracture of second metacarpal bone, left hand CC H5
S62.392 Other fracture of third metacarpal bone, right hand CC H5
S62.393 Other fracture of third metacarpal bone, left hand CC H5
S62.394 Other fracture of fourth metacarpal bone, right hand CC H5
S62.395 Other fracture of fourth metacarpal bone, left hand CC H5

- S62.396 Other fracture of fifth metacarpal bone, right hand CC HS
- S62.397 Other fracture of fifth metacarpal bone, left hand CC HS
- S62.398 Other fracture of other metacarpal bone CC HS
  Other fracture of specified metacarpal bone with unspecified laterality
- S62.399 Other fracture of unspecified metacarpal bone CC HS UNS

S62.5 Fracture of thumb

S62.50 Fracture of unspecified phalanx of thumb
- S62.501 Fracture of unspecified phalanx of right thumb CC HS
- S62.502 Fracture of unspecified phalanx of left thumb CC HS
- S62.509 Fracture of unspecified phalanx of unspecified thumb CC HS UNS

S62.51 Fracture of proximal phalanx of thumb
- S62.511 Displaced fracture of proximal phalanx of right thumb CC HS
- S62.512 Displaced fracture of proximal phalanx of left thumb CC HS
- S62.513 Displaced fracture of proximal phalanx of unspecified thumb CC HS UNS
- S62.514 Nondisplaced fracture of proximal phalanx of right thumb CC HS
- S62.515 Nondisplaced fracture of proximal phalanx of left thumb CC HS
- S62.516 Nondisplaced fracture of proximal phalanx of unspecified thumb CC HS

S62.52 Fracture of distal phalanx of thumb
- S62.521 Displaced fracture of distal phalanx of right thumb CC HS
- S62.522 Displaced fracture of distal phalanx of left thumb CC HS
- S62.523 Displaced fracture of distal phalanx of unspecified thumb CC HS UNS
- S62.524 Nondisplaced fracture of distal phalanx of right thumb CC HS
- S62.525 Nondisplaced fracture of distal phalanx of left thumb CC HS
- S62.526 Nondisplaced fracture of distal phalanx of unspecified thumb CC HS UNS

S62.6 Fracture of other and unspecified finger(s)

EXCLUDES 2 *fracture of thumb (S62.5-)*

S62.60 Fracture of unspecified phalanx of finger
- S62.600 Fracture of unspecified phalanx of right index finger CC HS
- S62.601 Fracture of unspecified phalanx of left index finger CC HS
- S62.602 Fracture of unspecified phalanx of right middle finger CC HS
- S62.603 Fracture of unspecified phalanx of left middle finger CC HS
- S62.604 Fracture of unspecified phalanx of right ring finger CC HS
- S62.605 Fracture of unspecified phalanx of left ring finger CC HS
- S62.606 Fracture of unspecified phalanx of right little finger CC HS
- S62.607 Fracture of unspecified phalanx of left little finger CC HS
- S62.608 Fracture of unspecified phalanx of other finger CC HS
  Fracture of unspecified phalanx of specified finger with unspecified laterality
- S62.609 Fracture of unspecified phalanx of unspecified finger CC HS UNS

S62.61 Displaced fracture of proximal phalanx of finger
- S62.610 Displaced fracture of proximal phalanx of right index finger CC HS
- S62.611 Displaced fracture of proximal phalanx of left index finger CC HS
- S62.612 Displaced fracture of proximal phalanx of right middle finger CC HS
- S62.613 Displaced fracture of proximal phalanx of left middle finger CC HS
- S62.614 Displaced fracture of proximal phalanx of right ring finger CC HS
- S62.615 Displaced fracture of proximal phalanx of left ring finger CC HS
- S62.616 Displaced fracture of proximal phalanx of right little finger CC HS
- S62.617 Displaced fracture of proximal phalanx of left little finger CC HS
- S62.618 Displaced fracture of proximal phalanx of other finger CC HS
  Displaced fracture of proximal phalanx of specified finger with unspecified laterality
- S62.619 Displaced fracture of proximal phalanx of unspecified finger CC HS UNS

S62.62 Displaced fracture of middle phalanx of finger
- S62.620 Displaced fracture of middle phalanx of right index finger CC HS
- S62.621 Displaced fracture of middle phalanx of left index finger CC HS
- S62.622 Displaced fracture of middle phalanx of right middle finger CC HS
- S62.623 Displaced fracture of middle phalanx of left middle finger CC HS
- S62.624 Displaced fracture of middle phalanx of right ring finger CC HS
- S62.625 Displaced fracture of middle phalanx of left ring finger CC HS
- S62.626 Displaced fracture of middle phalanx of right little finger CC HS
- S62.627 Displaced fracture of middle phalanx of left little finger CC HS
- S62.628 Displaced fracture of middle phalanx of other finger CC HS
  Displaced fracture of middle phalanx of specified finger with unspecified laterality
- S62.629 Displaced fracture of middle phalanx of unspecified finger CC HS UNS

S62.63 Displaced fracture of distal phalanx of finger
- S62.630 Displaced fracture of distal phalanx of right index finger CC HS
- S62.631 Displaced fracture of distal phalanx of left index finger CC HS
- S62.632 Displaced fracture of distal phalanx of right middle finger CC HS
- S62.633 Displaced fracture of distal phalanx of left middle finger CC HS
- S62.634 Displaced fracture of distal phalanx of right ring finger CC HS
- S62.635 Displaced fracture of distal phalanx of left ring finger CC HS
- S62.636 Displaced fracture of distal phalanx of right little finger CC HS
- S62.637 Displaced fracture of distal phalanx of left little finger CC HS
- S62.638 Displaced fracture of distal phalanx of other finger CC HS
  Displaced fracture of distal phalanx of specified finger with unspecified laterality
- S62.639 Displaced fracture of distal phalanx of unspecified finger CC HS UNS

S62.64 Nondisplaced fracture of proximal phalanx of finger
- S62.640 Nondisplaced fracture of proximal phalanx of right index finger CC HS
- S62.641 Nondisplaced fracture of proximal phalanx of left index finger CC HS
- S62.642 Nondisplaced fracture of proximal phalanx of right middle finger CC HS
- S62.643 Nondisplaced fracture of proximal phalanx of left middle finger CC HS
- S62.644 Nondisplaced fracture of proximal phalanx of right ring finger CC HS
- S62.645 Nondisplaced fracture of proximal phalanx of left ring finger CC HS

3 √7th **S62.646 Nondisplaced fracture of proximal phalanx of right little finger** CC H5

3 √7th **S62.647 Nondisplaced fracture of proximal phalanx of left little finger** CC H5

3 √7th **S62.648 Nondisplaced fracture of proximal phalanx of other finger** CC H5
Nondisplaced fracture of proximal phalanx of specified finger with unspecified laterality

3 √7th **S62.649 Nondisplaced fracture of proximal phalanx of unspecified finger** CC H5 UNS

√6th **S62.65 Nondisplaced fracture of middle phalanx of finger**

3 √7th **S62.650 Nondisplaced fracture of middle phalanx of right index finger** CC H5

3 √7th **S62.651 Nondisplaced fracture of middle phalanx of left index finger** CC H5

3 √7th **S62.652 Nondisplaced fracture of middle phalanx of right middle finger** CC H5

3 √7th **S62.653 Nondisplaced fracture of middle phalanx of left middle finger** CC H5

3 √7th **S62.654 Nondisplaced fracture of middle phalanx of right ring finger** CC H5

3 √7th **S62.655 Nondisplaced fracture of middle phalanx of left ring finger** CC H5

3 √7th **S62.656 Nondisplaced fracture of middle phalanx of right little finger** CC H5

3 √7th **S62.657 Nondisplaced fracture of middle phalanx of left little finger** CC H5

3 √7th **S62.658 Nondisplaced fracture of middle phalanx of other finger** CC H5
Nondisplaced fracture of middle phalanx of specified finger with unspecified laterality

3 √7th **S62.659 Nondisplaced fracture of middle phalanx of unspecified finger** CC H5 UNS

√6th **S62.66 Nondisplaced fracture of distal phalanx of finger**

3 √7th **S62.660 Nondisplaced fracture of distal phalanx of right index finger** CC H5

3 √7th **S62.661 Nondisplaced fracture of distal phalanx of left index finger** CC H5

3 √7th **S62.662 Nondisplaced fracture of distal phalanx of right middle finger** CC H5

3 √7th **S62.663 Nondisplaced fracture of distal phalanx of left middle finger** CC H5

3 √7th **S62.664 Nondisplaced fracture of distal phalanx of right ring finger** CC H5

3 √7th **S62.665 Nondisplaced fracture of distal phalanx of left ring finger** CC H5

3 √7th **S62.666 Nondisplaced fracture of distal phalanx of right little finger** CC H5

3 √7th **S62.667 Nondisplaced fracture of distal phalanx of left little finger** CC H5

3 √7th **S62.668 Nondisplaced fracture of distal phalanx of other finger** CC H5
Nondisplaced fracture of distal phalanx of specified finger with unspecified laterality

3 √7th **S62.669 Nondisplaced fracture of distal phalanx of unspecified finger** CC H5 UNS

√5th **S62.9 Unspecified fracture of wrist and hand**

3 √x7th **S62.90 Unspecified fracture of unspecified wrist and hand** CC H5 UNS

3 √x7th **S62.91 Unspecified fracture of right wrist and hand** CC H5

3 √x7th **S62.92 Unspecified fracture of left wrist and hand** CC H5

√4th **S63 Dislocation and sprain of joints and ligaments at wrist and hand level**

INCLUDES avulsion of joint or ligament at wrist and hand level
laceration of cartilage, joint or ligament at wrist and hand level
sprain of cartilage, joint or ligament at wrist and hand level
traumatic hemarthrosis of joint or ligament at wrist and hand level
traumatic rupture of joint or ligament at wrist and hand level
traumatic subluxation of joint or ligament at wrist and hand level
traumatic tear of joint or ligament at wrist and hand level

Code also any associated open wound

EXCLUDES 2 *strain of muscle, fascia and tendon of wrist and hand (S66.-)*

The appropriate 7th character is to be added to each code from category S63.
A initial encounter
D subsequent encounter
S sequela

√5th **S63.0 Subluxation and dislocation of wrist and hand joints**

√6th **S63.00 Unspecified subluxation and dislocation of wrist and hand**
Dislocation of carpal bone NOS
Dislocation of distal end of radius NOS
Subluxation of carpal bone NOS
Subluxation of distal end of radius NOS

√7th **S63.001 Unspecified subluxation of right wrist and hand**

√7th **S63.002 Unspecified subluxation of left wrist and hand**

√7th **S63.003 Unspecified subluxation of unspecified wrist and hand**

√7th **S63.004 Unspecified dislocation of right wrist and hand**

√7th **S63.005 Unspecified dislocation of left wrist and hand**

√7th **S63.006 Unspecified dislocation of unspecified wrist and hand**

√6th **S63.01 Subluxation and dislocation of distal radioulnar joint**

√7th **S63.011 Subluxation of distal radioulnar joint of right wrist**

√7th **S63.012 Subluxation of distal radioulnar joint of left wrist**

√7th **S63.013 Subluxation of distal radioulnar joint of unspecified wrist**

√7th **S63.014 Dislocation of distal radioulnar joint of right wrist**

√7th **S63.015 Dislocation of distal radioulnar joint of left wrist**

√7th **S63.016 Dislocation of distal radioulnar joint of unspecified wrist**

√6th **S63.02 Subluxation and dislocation of radiocarpal joint**

√7th **S63.021 Subluxation of radiocarpal joint of right wrist**

√7th **S63.022 Subluxation of radiocarpal joint of left wrist**

√7th **S63.023 Subluxation of radiocarpal joint of unspecified wrist**

√7th **S63.024 Dislocation of radiocarpal joint of right wrist**

√7th **S63.025 Dislocation of radiocarpal joint of left wrist**

√7th **S63.026 Dislocation of radiocarpal joint of unspecified wrist**

√6th **S63.03 Subluxation and dislocation of midcarpal joint**

√7th **S63.031 Subluxation of midcarpal joint of right wrist**

√7th **S63.032 Subluxation of midcarpal joint of left wrist**

√7th **S63.033 Subluxation of midcarpal joint of unspecified wrist**

√7th **S63.034 Dislocation of midcarpal joint of right wrist**

√7th **S63.035 Dislocation of midcarpal joint of left wrist**

√7th **S63.036 Dislocation of midcarpal joint of unspecified wrist**

6th **S63.04 Subluxation and dislocation of carpometacarpal joint of thumb**
EXCLUDES 2 *interphalangeal subluxation and dislocation of thumb (S63.1-)*
7th **S63.041 Subluxation of carpometacarpal joint of right thumb**
7th **S63.042 Subluxation of carpometacarpal joint of left thumb**
7th **S63.043 Subluxation of carpometacarpal joint of unspecified thumb**
7th **S63.044 Dislocation of carpometacarpal joint of right thumb**
7th **S63.045 Dislocation of carpometacarpal joint of left thumb**
7th **S63.046 Dislocation of carpometacarpal joint of unspecified thumb**
6th **S63.05 Subluxation and dislocation of other carpometacarpal joint**
EXCLUDES 2 *subluxation and dislocation of carpometacarpal joint of thumb (S63.04-)*
7th **S63.051 Subluxation of other carpometacarpal joint of right hand**
7th **S63.052 Subluxation of other carpometacarpal joint of left hand**
7th **S63.053 Subluxation of other carpometacarpal joint of unspecified hand**
7th **S63.054 Dislocation of other carpometacarpal joint of right hand**
7th **S63.055 Dislocation of other carpometacarpal joint of left hand**
7th **S63.056 Dislocation of other carpometacarpal joint of unspecified hand**
6th **S63.06 Subluxation and dislocation of metacarpal (bone), proximal end**
7th **S63.061 Subluxation of metacarpal (bone), proximal end of right hand**
7th **S63.062 Subluxation of metacarpal (bone), proximal end of left hand**
7th **S63.063 Subluxation of metacarpal (bone), proximal end of unspecified hand**
7th **S63.064 Dislocation of metacarpal (bone), proximal end of right hand**
7th **S63.065 Dislocation of metacarpal (bone), proximal end of left hand**
7th **S63.066 Dislocation of metacarpal (bone), proximal end of unspecified hand**
6th **S63.07 Subluxation and dislocation of distal end of ulna**
7th **S63.071 Subluxation of distal end of right ulna**
7th **S63.072 Subluxation of distal end of left ulna**
7th **S63.073 Subluxation of distal end of unspecified ulna**
7th **S63.074 Dislocation of distal end of right ulna**
7th **S63.075 Dislocation of distal end of left ulna**
7th **S63.076 Dislocation of distal end of unspecified ulna**
6th **S63.09 Other subluxation and dislocation of wrist and hand**
7th **S63.091 Other subluxation of right wrist and hand**
7th **S63.092 Other subluxation of left wrist and hand**
7th **S63.093 Other subluxation of unspecified wrist and hand**
7th **S63.094 Other dislocation of right wrist and hand**
7th **S63.095 Other dislocation of left wrist and hand**
7th **S63.096 Other dislocation of unspecified wrist and hand**
5th **S63.1 Subluxation and dislocation of thumb**
6th **S63.10 Unspecified subluxation and dislocation of thumb**
7th **S63.101 Unspecified subluxation of right thumb**
7th **S63.102 Unspecified subluxation of left thumb**
7th **S63.103 Unspecified subluxation of unspecified thumb**
7th **S63.104 Unspecified dislocation of right thumb**
7th **S63.105 Unspecified dislocation of left thumb**
7th **S63.106 Unspecified dislocation of unspecified thumb**
6th **S63.11 Subluxation and dislocation of metacarpophalangeal joint of thumb**
7th **S63.111 Subluxation of metacarpophalangeal joint of right thumb**
7th **S63.112 Subluxation of metacarpophalangeal joint of left thumb**
7th **S63.113 Subluxation of metacarpophalangeal joint of unspecified thumb**
7th **S63.114 Dislocation of metacarpophalangeal joint of right thumb**
7th **S63.115 Dislocation of metacarpophalangeal joint of left thumb**
7th **S63.116 Dislocation of metacarpophalangeal joint of unspecified thumb**
6th **S63.12 Subluxation and dislocation of interphalangeal joint of thumb**
7th **S63.121 Subluxation of interphalangeal joint of right thumb**
7th **S63.122 Subluxation of interphalangeal joint of left thumb**
7th **S63.123 Subluxation of interphalangeal joint of unspecified thumb**
7th **S63.124 Dislocation of interphalangeal joint of right thumb**
7th **S63.125 Dislocation of interphalangeal joint of left thumb**
7th **S63.126 Dislocation of interphalangeal joint of unspecified thumb**
5th **S63.2 Subluxation and dislocation of other finger(s)**
EXCLUDES 2 *subluxation and dislocation of thumb (S63.1-)*
6th **S63.20 Unspecified subluxation of other finger**
7th **S63.200 Unspecified subluxation of right index finger**
7th **S63.201 Unspecified subluxation of left index finger**
7th **S63.202 Unspecified subluxation of right middle finger**
7th **S63.203 Unspecified subluxation of left middle finger**
7th **S63.204 Unspecified subluxation of right ring finger**
7th **S63.205 Unspecified subluxation of left ring finger**
7th **S63.206 Unspecified subluxation of right little finger**
7th **S63.207 Unspecified subluxation of left little finger**
7th **S63.208 Unspecified subluxation of other finger**
Unspecified subluxation of specified finger with unspecified laterality
7th **S63.209 Unspecified subluxation of unspecified finger**
6th **S63.21 Subluxation of metacarpophalangeal joint of finger**
7th **S63.210 Subluxation of metacarpophalangeal joint of right index finger**
7th **S63.211 Subluxation of metacarpophalangeal joint of left index finger**
7th **S63.212 Subluxation of metacarpophalangeal joint of right middle finger**
7th **S63.213 Subluxation of metacarpophalangeal joint of left middle finger**
7th **S63.214 Subluxation of metacarpophalangeal joint of right ring finger**
7th **S63.215 Subluxation of metacarpophalangeal joint of left ring finger**
7th **S63.216 Subluxation of metacarpophalangeal joint of right little finger**
7th **S63.217 Subluxation of metacarpophalangeal joint of left little finger**
7th **S63.218 Subluxation of metacarpophalangeal joint of other finger**
Subluxation of metacarpophalangeal joint of specified finger with unspecified laterality
7th **S63.219 Subluxation of metacarpophalangeal joint of unspecified finger**
6th **S63.22 Subluxation of unspecified interphalangeal joint of finger**
7th **S63.220 Subluxation of unspecified interphalangeal joint of right index finger**
7th **S63.221 Subluxation of unspecified interphalangeal joint of left index finger**
7th **S63.222 Subluxation of unspecified interphalangeal joint of right middle finger**
7th **S63.223 Subluxation of unspecified interphalangeal joint of left middle finger**

7th **S63.224 Subluxation of unspecified interphalangeal joint of right ring finger**

7th **S63.225 Subluxation of unspecified interphalangeal joint of left ring finger**

7th **S63.226 Subluxation of unspecified interphalangeal joint of right little finger**

7th **S63.227 Subluxation of unspecified interphalangeal joint of left little finger**

7th **S63.228 Subluxation of unspecified interphalangeal joint of other finger**
Subluxation of unspecified interphalangeal joint of specified finger with unspecified laterality

7th **S63.229 Subluxation of unspecified interphalangeal joint of unspecified finger**

6th **S63.23 Subluxation of proximal interphalangeal joint of finger**

7th **S63.230 Subluxation of proximal interphalangeal joint of right index finger**

7th **S63.231 Subluxation of proximal interphalangeal joint of left index finger**

7th **S63.232 Subluxation of proximal interphalangeal joint of right middle finger**

7th **S63.233 Subluxation of proximal interphalangeal joint of left middle finger**

7th **S63.234 Subluxation of proximal interphalangeal joint of right ring finger**

7th **S63.235 Subluxation of proximal interphalangeal joint of left ring finger**

7th **S63.236 Subluxation of proximal interphalangeal joint of right little finger**

7th **S63.237 Subluxation of proximal interphalangeal joint of left little finger**

7th **S63.238 Subluxation of proximal interphalangeal joint of other finger**
Subluxation of proximal interphalangeal joint of specified finger with unspecified laterality

7th **S63.239 Subluxation of proximal interphalangeal joint of unspecified finger**

6th **S63.24 Subluxation of distal interphalangeal joint of finger**

7th **S63.240 Subluxation of distal interphalangeal joint of right index finger**

7th **S63.241 Subluxation of distal interphalangeal joint of left index finger**

7th **S63.242 Subluxation of distal interphalangeal joint of right middle finger**

7th **S63.243 Subluxation of distal interphalangeal joint of left middle finger**

7th **S63.244 Subluxation of distal interphalangeal joint of right ring finger**

7th **S63.245 Subluxation of distal interphalangeal joint of left ring finger**

7th **S63.246 Subluxation of distal interphalangeal joint of right little finger**

7th **S63.247 Subluxation of distal interphalangeal joint of left little finger**

7th **S63.248 Subluxation of distal interphalangeal joint of other finger**
Subluxation of distal interphalangeal joint of specified finger with unspecified laterality

7th **S63.249 Subluxation of distal interphalangeal joint of unspecified finger**

6th **S63.25 Unspecified dislocation of other finger**

7th **S63.250 Unspecified dislocation of right index finger**

7th **S63.251 Unspecified dislocation of left index finger**

7th **S63.252 Unspecified dislocation of right middle finger**

7th **S63.253 Unspecified dislocation of left middle finger**

7th **S63.254 Unspecified dislocation of right ring finger**

7th **S63.255 Unspecified dislocation of left ring finger**

7th **S63.256 Unspecified dislocation of right little finger**

7th **S63.257 Unspecified dislocation of left little finger**

7th **S63.258 Unspecified dislocation of other finger**
Unspecified dislocation of specified finger with unspecified laterality

7th **S63.259 Unspecified dislocation of unspecified finger**
Unspecified dislocation of unspecified finger with unspecified laterality

6th **S63.26 Dislocation of metacarpophalangeal joint of finger**

7th **S63.260 Dislocation of metacarpophalangeal joint of right index finger**

7th **S63.261 Dislocation of metacarpophalangeal joint of left index finger**

7th **S63.262 Dislocation of metacarpophalangeal joint of right middle finger**

7th **S63.263 Dislocation of metacarpophalangeal joint of left middle finger**

7th **S63.264 Dislocation of metacarpophalangeal joint of right ring finger**

7th **S63.265 Dislocation of metacarpophalangeal joint of left ring finger**

7th **S63.266 Dislocation of metacarpophalangeal joint of right little finger**

7th **S63.267 Dislocation of metacarpophalangeal joint of left little finger**

7th **S63.268 Dislocation of metacarpophalangeal joint of other finger**
Dislocation of metacarpophalangeal joint of specified finger with unspecified laterality

7th **S63.269 Dislocation of metacarpophalangeal joint of unspecified finger**

6th **S63.27 Dislocation of unspecified interphalangeal joint of finger**

7th **S63.270 Dislocation of unspecified interphalangeal joint of right index finger**

7th **S63.271 Dislocation of unspecified interphalangeal joint of left index finger**

7th **S63.272 Dislocation of unspecified interphalangeal joint of right middle finger**

7th **S63.273 Dislocation of unspecified interphalangeal joint of left middle finger**

7th **S63.274 Dislocation of unspecified interphalangeal joint of right ring finger**

7th **S63.275 Dislocation of unspecified interphalangeal joint of left ring finger**

7th **S63.276 Dislocation of unspecified interphalangeal joint of right little finger**

7th **S63.277 Dislocation of unspecified interphalangeal joint of left little finger**

7th **S63.278 Dislocation of unspecified interphalangeal joint of other finger**
Dislocation of unspecified interphalangeal joint of specified finger with unspecified laterality

7th **S63.279 Dislocation of unspecified interphalangeal joint of unspecified finger**
Dislocation of unspecified interphalangeal joint of unspecified finger without specified laterality

6th **S63.28 Dislocation of proximal interphalangeal joint of finger**

7th **S63.280 Dislocation of proximal interphalangeal joint of right index finger**

7th **S63.281 Dislocation of proximal interphalangeal joint of left index finger**

7th **S63.282 Dislocation of proximal interphalangeal joint of right middle finger**

7th **S63.283 Dislocation of proximal interphalangeal joint of left middle finger**

7th **S63.284 Dislocation of proximal interphalangeal joint of right ring finger**

7th **S63.285 Dislocation of proximal interphalangeal joint of left ring finger**

7th **S63.286 Dislocation of proximal interphalangeal joint of right little finger**

7th **S63.287 Dislocation of proximal interphalangeal joint of left little finger**

7th **S63.288 Dislocation of proximal interphalangeal joint of other finger**
Dislocation of proximal interphalangeal joint of specified finger with unspecified laterality

7th **S63.289 Dislocation of proximal interphalangeal joint of unspecified finger**

6th **S63.29 Dislocation of distal interphalangeal joint of finger**

7th **S63.290 Dislocation of distal interphalangeal joint of right index finger**

7th **S63.291 Dislocation of distal interphalangeal joint of left index finger**

7th **S63.292 Dislocation of distal interphalangeal joint of right middle finger**

7th **S63.293 Dislocation of distal interphalangeal joint of left middle finger**

7th **S63.294 Dislocation of distal interphalangeal joint of right ring finger**

7th **S63.295 Dislocation of distal interphalangeal joint of left ring finger**

7th **S63.296 Dislocation of distal interphalangeal joint of right little finger**

7th **S63.297 Dislocation of distal interphalangeal joint of left little finger**

7th **S63.298 Dislocation of distal interphalangeal joint of other finger**
Dislocation of distal interphalangeal joint of specified finger with unspecified laterality

7th **S63.299 Dislocation of distal interphalangeal joint of unspecified finger**

5th **S63.3 Traumatic rupture of ligament of wrist**

6th **S63.30 Traumatic rupture of unspecified ligament of wrist**

7th **S63.301 Traumatic rupture of unspecified ligament of right wrist**

7th **S63.302 Traumatic rupture of unspecified ligament of left wrist**

7th **S63.309 Traumatic rupture of unspecified ligament of unspecified wrist**

6th **S63.31 Traumatic rupture of collateral ligament of wrist**

7th **S63.311 Traumatic rupture of collateral ligament of right wrist**

7th **S63.312 Traumatic rupture of collateral ligament of left wrist**

7th **S63.319 Traumatic rupture of collateral ligament of unspecified wrist**

6th **S63.32 Traumatic rupture of radiocarpal ligament**

7th **S63.321 Traumatic rupture of right radiocarpal ligament**

7th **S63.322 Traumatic rupture of left radiocarpal ligament**

7th **S63.329 Traumatic rupture of unspecified radiocarpal ligament**

6th **S63.33 Traumatic rupture of ulnocarpal (palmar) ligament**

7th **S63.331 Traumatic rupture of right ulnocarpal (palmar) ligament**

7th **S63.332 Traumatic rupture of left ulnocarpal (palmar) ligament**

7th **S63.339 Traumatic rupture of unspecified ulnocarpal (palmar) ligament**

6th **S63.39 Traumatic rupture of other ligament of wrist**

7th **S63.391 Traumatic rupture of other ligament of right wrist**

7th **S63.392 Traumatic rupture of other ligament of left wrist**

7th **S63.399 Traumatic rupture of other ligament of unspecified wrist**

5th **S63.4 Traumatic rupture of ligament of finger at metacarpophalangeal and interphalangeal joint(s)**

6th **S63.40 Traumatic rupture of unspecified ligament of finger at metacarpophalangeal and interphalangeal joint**

7th **S63.400 Traumatic rupture of unspecified ligament of right index finger at metacarpophalangeal and interphalangeal joint**

7th **S63.401 Traumatic rupture of unspecified ligament of left index finger at metacarpophalangeal and interphalangeal joint**

7th **S63.402 Traumatic rupture of unspecified ligament of right middle finger at metacarpophalangeal and interphalangeal joint**

7th **S63.403 Traumatic rupture of unspecified ligament of left middle finger at metacarpophalangeal and interphalangeal joint**

7th **S63.404 Traumatic rupture of unspecified ligament of right ring finger at metacarpophalangeal and interphalangeal joint**

7th **S63.405 Traumatic rupture of unspecified ligament of left ring finger at metacarpophalangeal and interphalangeal joint**

7th **S63.406 Traumatic rupture of unspecified ligament of right little finger at metacarpophalangeal and interphalangeal joint**

7th **S63.407 Traumatic rupture of unspecified ligament of left little finger at metacarpophalangeal and interphalangeal joint**

7th **S63.408 Traumatic rupture of unspecified ligament of other finger at metacarpophalangeal and interphalangeal joint**
Traumatic rupture of unspecified ligament of specified finger with unspecified laterality at metacarpophalangeal and interphalangeal joint

7th **S63.409 Traumatic rupture of unspecified ligament of unspecified finger at metacarpophalangeal and interphalangeal joint**

6th **S63.41 Traumatic rupture of collateral ligament of finger at metacarpophalangeal and interphalangeal joint**

7th **S63.410 Traumatic rupture of collateral ligament of right index finger at metacarpophalangeal and interphalangeal joint**

7th **S63.411 Traumatic rupture of collateral ligament of left index finger at metacarpophalangeal and interphalangeal joint**

7th **S63.412 Traumatic rupture of collateral ligament of right middle finger at metacarpophalangeal and interphalangeal joint**

7th **S63.413 Traumatic rupture of collateral ligament of left middle finger at metacarpophalangeal and interphalangeal joint**

7th **S63.414 Traumatic rupture of collateral ligament of right ring finger at metacarpophalangeal and interphalangeal joint**

7th **S63.415 Traumatic rupture of collateral ligament of left ring finger at metacarpophalangeal and interphalangeal joint**

7th **S63.416 Traumatic rupture of collateral ligament of right little finger at metacarpophalangeal and interphalangeal joint**

7th **S63.417 Traumatic rupture of collateral ligament of left little finger at metacarpophalangeal and interphalangeal joint**

7th **S63.418 Traumatic rupture of collateral ligament of other finger at metacarpophalangeal and interphalangeal joint**
Traumatic rupture of collateral ligament of specified finger with unspecified laterality at metacarpophalangeal and interphalangeal joint

7th **S63.419 Traumatic rupture of collateral ligament of unspecified finger at metacarpophalangeal and interphalangeal joint**

N Newborn: 0 P Pediatric: 0-17 M Maternity: 9-64 A Adult: 15-124 UNS Unspecified Site MCC Major Complication/Comorbidity CC Complication/Comorbidity

S63.42 Traumatic rupture of palmar ligament of finger at metacarpophalangeal and interphalangeal joint

- **S63.420 Traumatic rupture of palmar ligament of right index finger at metacarpophalangeal and interphalangeal joint**
- **S63.421 Traumatic rupture of palmar ligament of left index finger at metacarpophalangeal and interphalangeal joint**
- **S63.422 Traumatic rupture of palmar ligament of right middle finger at metacarpophalangeal and interphalangeal joint**
- **S63.423 Traumatic rupture of palmar ligament of left middle finger at metacarpophalangeal and interphalangeal joint**
- **S63.424 Traumatic rupture of palmar ligament of right ring finger at metacarpophalangeal and interphalangeal joint**
- **S63.425 Traumatic rupture of palmar ligament of left ring finger at metacarpophalangeal and interphalangeal joint**
- **S63.426 Traumatic rupture of palmar ligament of right little finger at metacarpophalangeal and interphalangeal joint**
- **S63.427 Traumatic rupture of palmar ligament of left little finger at metacarpophalangeal and interphalangeal joint**
- **S63.428 Traumatic rupture of palmar ligament of other finger at metacarpophalangeal and interphalangeal joint**
  Traumatic rupture of palmar ligament of specified finger with unspecified laterality at metacarpophalangeal and interphalangeal joint
- **S63.429 Traumatic rupture of palmar ligament of unspecified finger at metacarpophalangeal and interphalangeal joint**

S63.43 Traumatic rupture of volar plate of finger at metacarpophalangeal and interphalangeal joint

- **S63.430 Traumatic rupture of volar plate of right index finger at metacarpophalangeal and interphalangeal joint**
- **S63.431 Traumatic rupture of volar plate of left index finger at metacarpophalangeal and interphalangeal joint**
- **S63.432 Traumatic rupture of volar plate of right middle finger at metacarpophalangeal and interphalangeal joint**
- **S63.433 Traumatic rupture of volar plate of left middle finger at metacarpophalangeal and interphalangeal joint**
- **S63.434 Traumatic rupture of volar plate of right ring finger at metacarpophalangeal and interphalangeal joint**
- **S63.435 Traumatic rupture of volar plate of left ring finger at metacarpophalangeal and interphalangeal joint**
- **S63.436 Traumatic rupture of volar plate of right little finger at metacarpophalangeal and interphalangeal joint**
- **S63.437 Traumatic rupture of volar plate of left little finger at metacarpophalangeal and interphalangeal joint**
- **S63.438 Traumatic rupture of volar plate of other finger at metacarpophalangeal and interphalangeal joint**
  Traumatic rupture of volar plate of specified finger with unspecified laterality at metacarpophalangeal and interphalangeal joint
- **S63.439 Traumatic rupture of volar plate of unspecified finger at metacarpophalangeal and interphalangeal joint**

S63.49 Traumatic rupture of other ligament of finger at metacarpophalangeal and interphalangeal joint

- **S63.490 Traumatic rupture of other ligament of right index finger at metacarpophalangeal and interphalangeal joint**
- **S63.491 Traumatic rupture of other ligament of left index finger at metacarpophalangeal and interphalangeal joint**
- **S63.492 Traumatic rupture of other ligament of right middle finger at metacarpophalangeal and interphalangeal joint**
- **S63.493 Traumatic rupture of other ligament of left middle finger at metacarpophalangeal and interphalangeal joint**
- **S63.494 Traumatic rupture of other ligament of right ring finger at metacarpophalangeal and interphalangeal joint**
- **S63.495 Traumatic rupture of other ligament of left ring finger at metacarpophalangeal and interphalangeal joint**
- **S63.496 Traumatic rupture of other ligament of right little finger at metacarpophalangeal and interphalangeal joint**
- **S63.497 Traumatic rupture of other ligament of left little finger at metacarpophalangeal and interphalangeal joint**
- **S63.498 Traumatic rupture of other ligament of other finger at metacarpophalangeal and interphalangeal joint**
  Traumatic rupture of ligament of specified finger with unspecified laterality at metacarpophalangeal and interphalangeal joint
- **S63.499 Traumatic rupture of other ligament of unspecified finger at metacarpophalangeal and interphalangeal joint**

S63.5 Other and unspecified sprain of wrist

S63.50 Unspecified sprain of wrist

- **S63.501 Unspecified sprain of right wrist**
- **S63.502 Unspecified sprain of left wrist**
- **S63.509 Unspecified sprain of unspecified wrist**

S63.51 Sprain of carpal (joint)

- **S63.511 Sprain of carpal joint of right wrist**
- **S63.512 Sprain of carpal joint of left wrist**
- **S63.519 Sprain of carpal joint of unspecified wrist**

S63.52 Sprain of radiocarpal joint

EXCLUDES 1 *traumatic rupture of radiocarpal ligament (S63.32-)*

- **S63.521 Sprain of radiocarpal joint of right wrist**
- **S63.522 Sprain of radiocarpal joint of left wrist**
- **S63.529 Sprain of radiocarpal joint of unspecified wrist**

S63.59 Other specified sprain of wrist

- **S63.591 Other specified sprain of right wrist**
- **S63.592 Other specified sprain of left wrist**
- **S63.599 Other specified sprain of unspecified wrist**

S63.6 Other and unspecified sprain of finger(s)

EXCLUDES 1 *traumatic rupture of ligament of finger at metacarpophalangeal and interphalangeal joint(s) (S63.4-)*

S63.60 Unspecified sprain of thumb

- **S63.601 Unspecified sprain of right thumb**
- **S63.602 Unspecified sprain of left thumb**
- **S63.609 Unspecified sprain of unspecified thumb**

S63.61 Unspecified sprain of other and unspecified finger(s)

- **S63.610 Unspecified sprain of right index finger**
- **S63.611 Unspecified sprain of left index finger**
- **S63.612 Unspecified sprain of right middle finger**
- **S63.613 Unspecified sprain of left middle finger**
- **S63.614 Unspecified sprain of right ring finger**
- **S63.615 Unspecified sprain of left ring finger**
- **S63.616 Unspecified sprain of right little finger**
- **S63.617 Unspecified sprain of left little finger**

√7th **S63.618 Unspecified sprain of other finger**
Unspecified sprain of specified finger with unspecified laterality
√7th **S63.619 Unspecified sprain of unspecified finger**

√6th **S63.62 Sprain of interphalangeal joint of thumb**
√7th **S63.621 Sprain of interphalangeal joint of right thumb**
√7th **S63.622 Sprain of interphalangeal joint of left thumb**
√7th **S63.629 Sprain of interphalangeal joint of unspecified thumb**

√6th **S63.63 Sprain of interphalangeal joint of other and unspecified finger(s)**
√7th **S63.630 Sprain of interphalangeal joint of right index finger**
√7th **S63.631 Sprain of interphalangeal joint of left index finger**
√7th **S63.632 Sprain of interphalangeal joint of right middle finger**
√7th **S63.633 Sprain of interphalangeal joint of left middle finger**
√7th **S63.634 Sprain of interphalangeal joint of right ring finger**
√7th **S63.635 Sprain of interphalangeal joint of left ring finger**
√7th **S63.636 Sprain of interphalangeal joint of right little finger**
√7th **S63.637 Sprain of interphalangeal joint of left little finger**
√7th **S63.638 Sprain of interphalangeal joint of other finger**
√7th **S63.639 Sprain of interphalangeal joint of unspecified finger**

√6th **S63.64 Sprain of metacarpophalangeal joint of thumb**
√7th **S63.641 Sprain of metacarpophalangeal joint of right thumb**
√7th **S63.642 Sprain of metacarpophalangeal joint of left thumb**
√7th **S63.649 Sprain of metacarpophalangeal joint of unspecified thumb**

√6th **S63.65 Sprain of metacarpophalangeal joint of other and unspecified finger(s)**
√7th **S63.650 Sprain of metacarpophalangeal joint of right index finger**
√7th **S63.651 Sprain of metacarpophalangeal joint of left index finger**
√7th **S63.652 Sprain of metacarpophalangeal joint of right middle finger**
√7th **S63.653 Sprain of metacarpophalangeal joint of left middle finger**
√7th **S63.654 Sprain of metacarpophalangeal joint of right ring finger**
√7th **S63.655 Sprain of metacarpophalangeal joint of left ring finger**
√7th **S63.656 Sprain of metacarpophalangeal joint of right little finger**
√7th **S63.657 Sprain of metacarpophalangeal joint of left little finger**
√7th **S63.658 Sprain of metacarpophalangeal joint of other finger**
Sprain of metacarpophalangeal joint of specified finger with unspecified laterality
√7th **S63.659 Sprain of metacarpophalangeal joint of unspecified finger**

√6th **S63.68 Other sprain of thumb**
√7th **S63.681 Other sprain of right thumb**
√7th **S63.682 Other sprain of left thumb**
√7th **S63.689 Other sprain of unspecified thumb**

√6th **S63.69 Other sprain of other and unspecified finger(s)**
√7th **S63.690 Other sprain of right index finger**
√7th **S63.691 Other sprain of left index finger**
√7th **S63.692 Other sprain of right middle finger**
√7th **S63.693 Other sprain of left middle finger**
√7th **S63.694 Other sprain of right ring finger**
√7th **S63.695 Other sprain of left ring finger**
√7th **S63.696 Other sprain of right little finger**
√7th **S63.697 Other sprain of left little finger**
√7th **S63.698 Other sprain of other finger**
Other sprain of specified finger with unspecified laterality
√7th **S63.699 Other sprain of unspecified finger**

√5th **S63.8 Sprain of other part of wrist and hand**
√6th **S63.8X Sprain of other part of wrist and hand**
√7th **S63.8X1 Sprain of other part of right wrist and hand**
√7th **S63.8X2 Sprain of other part of left wrist and hand**
√7th **S63.8X9 Sprain of other part of unspecified wrist and hand**

√5th **S63.9 Sprain of unspecified part of wrist and hand**
√x7th **S63.90 Sprain of unspecified part of unspecified wrist and hand**
√x7th **S63.91 Sprain of unspecified part of right wrist and hand**
√x7th **S63.92 Sprain of unspecified part of left wrist and hand**

√4th **S64 Injury of nerves at wrist and hand level**

Code also any associated open wound (S61.-)

The appropriate 7th character is to be added to each code from category S64.
A initial encounter
D subsequent encounter
S sequela

√5th **S64.0 Injury of ulnar nerve at wrist and hand level**
√x7th **S64.00 Injury of ulnar nerve at wrist and hand level of unspecified arm**
√x7th **S64.01 Injury of ulnar nerve at wrist and hand level of right arm**
√x7th **S64.02 Injury of ulnar nerve at wrist and hand level of left arm**

√5th **S64.1 Injury of median nerve at wrist and hand level**
√x7th **S64.10 Injury of median nerve at wrist and hand level of unspecified arm**
√x7th **S64.11 Injury of median nerve at wrist and hand level of right arm**
√x7th **S64.12 Injury of median nerve at wrist and hand level of left arm**

√5th **S64.2 Injury of radial nerve at wrist and hand level**
√x7th **S64.20 Injury of radial nerve at wrist and hand level of unspecified arm**
√x7th **S64.21 Injury of radial nerve at wrist and hand level of right arm**
√x7th **S64.22 Injury of radial nerve at wrist and hand level of left arm**

√5th **S64.3 Injury of digital nerve of thumb**
√x7th **S64.30 Injury of digital nerve of unspecified thumb**
√x7th **S64.31 Injury of digital nerve of right thumb**
√x7th **S64.32 Injury of digital nerve of left thumb**

√5th **S64.4 Injury of digital nerve of other and unspecified finger**
√x7th **S64.40 Injury of digital nerve of unspecified finger**
√6th **S64.49 Injury of digital nerve of other finger**
√7th **S64.490 Injury of digital nerve of right index finger**
√7th **S64.491 Injury of digital nerve of left index finger**
√7th **S64.492 Injury of digital nerve of right middle finger**
√7th **S64.493 Injury of digital nerve of left middle finger**
√7th **S64.494 Injury of digital nerve of right ring finger**
√7th **S64.495 Injury of digital nerve of left ring finger**
√7th **S64.496 Injury of digital nerve of right little finger**
√7th **S64.497 Injury of digital nerve of left little finger**
√7th **S64.498 Injury of digital nerve of other finger**
Injury of digital nerve of specified finger with unspecified laterality

√5th **S64.8 Injury of other nerves at wrist and hand level**
√6th **S64.8X Injury of other nerves at wrist and hand level**
√7th **S64.8X1 Injury of other nerves at wrist and hand level of right arm**
√7th **S64.8X2 Injury of other nerves at wrist and hand level of left arm**
√7th **S64.8X9 Injury of other nerves at wrist and hand level of unspecified arm**

S64.9 Injury of unspecified nerve at wrist and hand level
S64.90 Injury of unspecified nerve at wrist and hand level of unspecified arm
S64.91 Injury of unspecified nerve at wrist and hand level of right arm
S64.92 Injury of unspecified nerve at wrist and hand level of left arm

S65 Injury of blood vessels at wrist and hand level
Code also any associated open wound (S61.-)
The appropriate 7th character is to be added to each code from category S65.
A initial encounter
D subsequent encounter
S sequela

S65.0 Injury of ulnar artery at wrist and hand level
S65.00 Unspecified injury of ulnar artery at wrist and hand level
S65.001 Unspecified injury of ulnar artery at wrist and hand level of right arm CC
S65.002 Unspecified injury of ulnar artery at wrist and hand level of left arm CC
S65.009 Unspecified injury of ulnar artery at wrist and hand level of unspecified arm CC UNS
S65.01 Laceration of ulnar artery at wrist and hand level
S65.011 Laceration of ulnar artery at wrist and hand level of right arm CC
S65.012 Laceration of ulnar artery at wrist and hand level of left arm CC
S65.019 Laceration of ulnar artery at wrist and hand level of unspecified arm CC UNS
S65.09 Other specified injury of ulnar artery at wrist and hand level
S65.091 Other specified injury of ulnar artery at wrist and hand level of right arm CC
S65.092 Other specified injury of ulnar artery at wrist and hand level of left arm CC
S65.099 Other specified injury of ulnar artery at wrist and hand level of unspecified arm CC UNS

S65.1 Injury of radial artery at wrist and hand level
S65.10 Unspecified injury of radial artery at wrist and hand level
S65.101 Unspecified injury of radial artery at wrist and hand level of right arm CC
S65.102 Unspecified injury of radial artery at wrist and hand level of left arm CC
S65.109 Unspecified injury of radial artery at wrist and hand level of unspecified arm CC UNS
S65.11 Laceration of radial artery at wrist and hand level
S65.111 Laceration of radial artery at wrist and hand level of right arm CC
S65.112 Laceration of radial artery at wrist and hand level of left arm CC
S65.119 Laceration of radial artery at wrist and hand level of unspecified arm CC UNS
S65.19 Other specified injury of radial artery at wrist and hand level
S65.191 Other specified injury of radial artery at wrist and hand level of right arm CC
S65.192 Other specified injury of radial artery at wrist and hand level of left arm CC
S65.199 Other specified injury of radial artery at wrist and hand level of unspecified arm CC UNS

S65.2 Injury of superficial palmar arch
S65.20 Unspecified injury of superficial palmar arch
S65.201 Unspecified injury of superficial palmar arch of right hand CC
S65.202 Unspecified injury of superficial palmar arch of left hand CC
S65.209 Unspecified injury of superficial palmar arch of unspecified hand CC UNS
S65.21 Laceration of superficial palmar arch
S65.211 Laceration of superficial palmar arch of right hand CC
S65.212 Laceration of superficial palmar arch of left hand CC
S65.219 Laceration of superficial palmar arch of unspecified hand CC UNS
S65.29 Other specified injury of superficial palmar arch
S65.291 Other specified injury of superficial palmar arch of right hand CC
S65.292 Other specified injury of superficial palmar arch of left hand CC
S65.299 Other specified injury of superficial palmar arch of unspecified hand CC UNS

S65.3 Injury of deep palmar arch
S65.30 Unspecified injury of deep palmar arch
S65.301 Unspecified injury of deep palmar arch of right hand CC
S65.302 Unspecified injury of deep palmar arch of left hand CC
S65.309 Unspecified injury of deep palmar arch of unspecified hand CC UNS
S65.31 Laceration of deep palmar arch
S65.311 Laceration of deep palmar arch of right hand CC
S65.312 Laceration of deep palmar arch of left hand CC
S65.319 Laceration of deep palmar arch of unspecified hand CC UNS
S65.39 Other specified injury of deep palmar arch
S65.391 Other specified injury of deep palmar arch of right hand CC
S65.392 Other specified injury of deep palmar arch of left hand CC
S65.399 Other specified injury of deep palmar arch of unspecified hand CC UNS

S65.4 Injury of blood vessel of thumb
S65.40 Unspecified injury of blood vessel of thumb
S65.401 Unspecified injury of blood vessel of right thumb CC
S65.402 Unspecified injury of blood vessel of left thumb CC
S65.409 Unspecified injury of blood vessel of unspecified thumb CC UNS
S65.41 Laceration of blood vessel of thumb
S65.411 Laceration of blood vessel of right thumb CC
S65.412 Laceration of blood vessel of left thumb CC
S65.419 Laceration of blood vessel of unspecified thumb CC UNS
S65.49 Other specified injury of blood vessel of thumb
S65.491 Other specified injury of blood vessel of right thumb CC
S65.492 Other specified injury of blood vessel of left thumb CC
S65.499 Other specified injury of blood vessel of unspecified thumb CC UNS

S65.5 Injury of blood vessel of other and unspecified finger
S65.50 Unspecified injury of blood vessel of other and unspecified finger
S65.500 Unspecified injury of blood vessel of right index finger CC
S65.501 Unspecified injury of blood vessel of left index finger CC
S65.502 Unspecified injury of blood vessel of right middle finger CC
S65.503 Unspecified injury of blood vessel of left middle finger CC
S65.504 Unspecified injury of blood vessel of right ring finger CC
S65.505 Unspecified injury of blood vessel of left ring finger CC
S65.506 Unspecified injury of blood vessel of right little finger CC
S65.507 Unspecified injury of blood vessel of left little finger CC

S65.508 Unspecified injury of blood vessel of other finger CC UNS
Unspecified injury of blood vessel of specified finger with unspecified laterality
S65.509 Unspecified injury of blood vessel of unspecified finger CC UNS
S65.51 Laceration of blood vessel of other and unspecified finger
S65.510 Laceration of blood vessel of right index finger CC
S65.511 Laceration of blood vessel of left index finger CC
S65.512 Laceration of blood vessel of right middle finger CC
S65.513 Laceration of blood vessel of left middle finger CC
S65.514 Laceration of blood vessel of right ring finger CC
S65.515 Laceration of blood vessel of left ring finger CC
S65.516 Laceration of blood vessel of right little finger CC
S65.517 Laceration of blood vessel of left little finger CC
S65.518 Laceration of blood vessel of other finger CC
Laceration of blood vessel of specified finger with unspecified laterality
S65.519 Laceration of blood vessel of unspecified finger CC UNS
S65.59 Other specified injury of blood vessel of other and unspecified finger
S65.590 Other specified injury of blood vessel of right index finger CC
S65.591 Other specified injury of blood vessel of left index finger CC
S65.592 Other specified injury of blood vessel of right middle finger CC
S65.593 Other specified injury of blood vessel of left middle finger CC
S65.594 Other specified injury of blood vessel of right ring finger CC
S65.595 Other specified injury of blood vessel of left ring finger CC
S65.596 Other specified injury of blood vessel of right little finger CC
S65.597 Other specified injury of blood vessel of left little finger CC
S65.598 Other specified injury of blood vessel of other finger CC
Other specified injury of blood vessel of specified finger with unspecified laterality
S65.599 Other specified injury of blood vessel of unspecified finger CC UNS
S65.8 Injury of other blood vessels at wrist and hand level
S65.80 Unspecified injury of other blood vessels at wrist and hand level
S65.801 Unspecified injury of other blood vessels at wrist and hand level of right arm CC
S65.802 Unspecified injury of other blood vessels at wrist and hand level of left arm CC
S65.809 Unspecified injury of other blood vessels at wrist and hand level of unspecified arm CC UNS
S65.81 Laceration of other blood vessels at wrist and hand level
S65.811 Laceration of other blood vessels at wrist and hand level of right arm CC
S65.812 Laceration of other blood vessels at wrist and hand level of left arm CC
S65.819 Laceration of other blood vessels at wrist and hand level of unspecified arm CC UNS
S65.89 Other specified injury of other blood vessels at wrist and hand level
S65.891 Other specified injury of other blood vessels at wrist and hand level of right arm CC
S65.892 Other specified injury of other blood vessels at wrist and hand level of left arm CC
S65.899 Other specified injury of other blood vessels at wrist and hand level of unspecified arm CC UNS
S65.9 Injury of unspecified blood vessel at wrist and hand level
S65.90 Unspecified injury of unspecified blood vessel at wrist and hand level
S65.901 Unspecified injury of unspecified blood vessel at wrist and hand level of right arm CC
S65.902 Unspecified injury of unspecified blood vessel at wrist and hand level of left arm CC
S65.909 Unspecified injury of unspecified blood vessel at wrist and hand level of unspecified arm CC UNS
S65.91 Laceration of unspecified blood vessel at wrist and hand level
S65.911 Laceration of unspecified blood vessel at wrist and hand level of right arm CC
S65.912 Laceration of unspecified blood vessel at wrist and hand level of left arm CC
S65.919 Laceration of unspecified blood vessel at wrist and hand level of unspecified arm CC UNS
S65.99 Other specified injury of unspecified blood vessel at wrist and hand level
S65.991 Other specified injury of unspecified blood vessel at wrist and hand of right arm CC
S65.992 Other specified injury of unspecified blood vessel at wrist and hand of left arm CC
S65.999 Other specified injury of unspecified blood vessel at wrist and hand of unspecified arm CC UNS

S66 Injury of muscle, fascia and tendon at wrist and hand level
Code also any associated open wound (S61.-)
EXCLUDES 2 *sprain of joints and ligaments of wrist and hand (S63.-)*
TIP: Refer to the Muscle/Tendon table at the beginning of this chapter.

The appropriate 7th character is to be added to each code from category S66.
A initial encounter
D subsequent encounter
S sequela

S66.0 Injury of long flexor muscle, fascia and tendon of thumb at wrist and hand level
S66.00 Unspecified injury of long flexor muscle, fascia and tendon of thumb at wrist and hand level
S66.001 Unspecified injury of long flexor muscle, fascia and tendon of right thumb at wrist and hand level
S66.002 Unspecified injury of long flexor muscle, fascia and tendon of left thumb at wrist and hand level
S66.009 Unspecified injury of long flexor muscle, fascia and tendon of unspecified thumb at wrist and hand level
S66.01 Strain of long flexor muscle, fascia and tendon of thumb at wrist and hand level
S66.011 Strain of long flexor muscle, fascia and tendon of right thumb at wrist and hand level
S66.012 Strain of long flexor muscle, fascia and tendon of left thumb at wrist and hand level
S66.019 Strain of long flexor muscle, fascia and tendon of unspecified thumb at wrist and hand level
S66.02 Laceration of long flexor muscle, fascia and tendon of thumb at wrist and hand level
S66.021 Laceration of long flexor muscle, fascia and tendon of right thumb at wrist and hand level CC
S66.022 Laceration of long flexor muscle, fascia and tendon of left thumb at wrist and hand level CC
S66.029 Laceration of long flexor muscle, fascia and tendon of unspecified thumb at wrist and hand level CC

6th **S66.09 Other specified injury of long flexor muscle, fascia and tendon of thumb at wrist and hand level**

7th **S66.091 Other specified injury of long flexor muscle, fascia and tendon of right thumb at wrist and hand level**

7th **S66.092 Other specified injury of long flexor muscle, fascia and tendon of left thumb at wrist and hand level**

7th **S66.099 Other specified injury of long flexor muscle, fascia and tendon of unspecified thumb at wrist and hand level**

5th **S66.1 Injury of flexor muscle, fascia and tendon of other and unspecified finger at wrist and hand level**

EXCLUDES 2 *injury of long flexor muscle, fascia and tendon of thumb at wrist and hand level (S66.0-)*

6th **S66.10 Unspecified injury of flexor muscle, fascia and tendon of other and unspecified finger at wrist and hand level**

7th **S66.100 Unspecified injury of flexor muscle, fascia and tendon of right index finger at wrist and hand level**

7th **S66.101 Unspecified injury of flexor muscle, fascia and tendon of left index finger at wrist and hand level**

7th **S66.102 Unspecified injury of flexor muscle, fascia and tendon of right middle finger at wrist and hand level**

7th **S66.103 Unspecified injury of flexor muscle, fascia and tendon of left middle finger at wrist and hand level**

7th **S66.104 Unspecified injury of flexor muscle, fascia and tendon of right ring finger at wrist and hand level**

7th **S66.105 Unspecified injury of flexor muscle, fascia and tendon of left ring finger at wrist and hand level**

7th **S66.106 Unspecified injury of flexor muscle, fascia and tendon of right little finger at wrist and hand level**

7th **S66.107 Unspecified injury of flexor muscle, fascia and tendon of left little finger at wrist and hand level**

7th **S66.108 Unspecified injury of flexor muscle, fascia and tendon of other finger at wrist and hand level**

Unspecified injury of flexor muscle, fascia and tendon of specified finger with unspecified laterality at wrist and hand level

7th **S66.109 Unspecified injury of flexor muscle, fascia and tendon of unspecified finger at wrist and hand level**

6th **S66.11 Strain of flexor muscle, fascia and tendon of other and unspecified finger at wrist and hand level**

7th **S66.110 Strain of flexor muscle, fascia and tendon of right index finger at wrist and hand level**

7th **S66.111 Strain of flexor muscle, fascia and tendon of left index finger at wrist and hand level**

7th **S66.112 Strain of flexor muscle, fascia and tendon of right middle finger at wrist and hand level**

7th **S66.113 Strain of flexor muscle, fascia and tendon of left middle finger at wrist and hand level**

7th **S66.114 Strain of flexor muscle, fascia and tendon of right ring finger at wrist and hand level**

7th **S66.115 Strain of flexor muscle, fascia and tendon of left ring finger at wrist and hand level**

7th **S66.116 Strain of flexor muscle, fascia and tendon of right little finger at wrist and hand level**

7th **S66.117 Strain of flexor muscle, fascia and tendon of left little finger at wrist and hand level**

7th **S66.118 Strain of flexor muscle, fascia and tendon of other finger at wrist and hand level**

Strain of flexor muscle, fascia and tendon of specified finger with unspecified laterality at wrist and hand level

7th **S66.119 Strain of flexor muscle, fascia and tendon of unspecified finger at wrist and hand level**

6th **S66.12 Laceration of flexor muscle, fascia and tendon of other and unspecified finger at wrist and hand level**

7th **S66.120 Laceration of flexor muscle, fascia and tendon of right index finger at wrist and hand level** CC

7th **S66.121 Laceration of flexor muscle, fascia and tendon of left index finger at wrist and hand level** CC

7th **S66.122 Laceration of flexor muscle, fascia and tendon of right middle finger at wrist and hand level** CC

7th **S66.123 Laceration of flexor muscle, fascia and tendon of left middle finger at wrist and hand level** CC

7th **S66.124 Laceration of flexor muscle, fascia and tendon of right ring finger at wrist and hand level** CC

7th **S66.125 Laceration of flexor muscle, fascia and tendon of left ring finger at wrist and hand level** CC

7th **S66.126 Laceration of flexor muscle, fascia and tendon of right little finger at wrist and hand level** CC

7th **S66.127 Laceration of flexor muscle, fascia and tendon of left little finger at wrist and hand level** CC

7th **S66.128 Laceration of flexor muscle, fascia and tendon of other finger at wrist and hand level** CC

Laceration of flexor muscle, fascia and tendon of specified finger with unspecified laterality at wrist and hand level

7th **S66.129 Laceration of flexor muscle, fascia and tendon of unspecified finger at wrist and hand level** CC UNS

6th **S66.19 Other injury of flexor muscle, fascia and tendon of other and unspecified finger at wrist and hand level**

7th **S66.190 Other injury of flexor muscle, fascia and tendon of right index finger at wrist and hand level**

7th **S66.191 Other injury of flexor muscle, fascia and tendon of left index finger at wrist and hand level**

7th **S66.192 Other injury of flexor muscle, fascia and tendon of right middle finger at wrist and hand level**

7th **S66.193 Other injury of flexor muscle, fascia and tendon of left middle finger at wrist and hand level**

7th **S66.194 Other injury of flexor muscle, fascia and tendon of right ring finger at wrist and hand level**

7th **S66.195 Other injury of flexor muscle, fascia and tendon of left ring finger at wrist and hand level**

7th **S66.196 Other injury of flexor muscle, fascia and tendon of right little finger at wrist and hand level**

7th **S66.197 Other injury of flexor muscle, fascia and tendon of left little finger at wrist and hand level**

7th **S66.198 Other injury of flexor muscle, fascia and tendon of other finger at wrist and hand level**

Other injury of flexor muscle, fascia and tendon of specified finger with unspecified laterality at wrist and hand level

7th **S66.199 Other injury of flexor muscle, fascia and tendon of unspecified finger at wrist and hand level**

5th **S66.2 Injury of extensor muscle, fascia and tendon of thumb at wrist and hand level**

6th **S66.20 Unspecified injury of extensor muscle, fascia and tendon of thumb at wrist and hand level**

7th **S66.201 Unspecified injury of extensor muscle, fascia and tendon of right thumb at wrist and hand level**

7th **S66.202 Unspecified injury of extensor muscle, fascia and tendon of left thumb at wrist and hand level**

7th **S66.209** **Unspecified injury of extensor muscle, fascia and tendon of unspecified thumb at wrist and hand level**

6th **S66.21** **Strain of extensor muscle, fascia and tendon of thumb at wrist and hand level**

7th **S66.211** **Strain of extensor muscle, fascia and tendon of right thumb at wrist and hand level**

7th **S66.212** **Strain of extensor muscle, fascia and tendon of left thumb at wrist and hand level**

7th **S66.219** **Strain of extensor muscle, fascia and tendon of unspecified thumb at wrist and hand level**

6th **S66.22** **Laceration of extensor muscle, fascia and tendon of thumb at wrist and hand level**

7th **S66.221** **Laceration of extensor muscle, fascia and tendon of right thumb at wrist and hand level** CC

7th **S66.222** **Laceration of extensor muscle, fascia and tendon of left thumb at wrist and hand level** CC

7th **S66.229** **Laceration of extensor muscle, fascia and tendon of unspecified thumb at wrist and hand level** CC

6th **S66.29** **Other specified injury of extensor muscle, fascia and tendon of thumb at wrist and hand level**

7th **S66.291** **Other specified injury of extensor muscle, fascia and tendon of right thumb at wrist and hand level**

7th **S66.292** **Other specified injury of extensor muscle, fascia and tendon of left thumb at wrist and hand level**

7th **S66.299** **Other specified injury of extensor muscle, fascia and tendon of unspecified thumb at wrist and hand level**

5th **S66.3** **Injury of extensor muscle, fascia and tendon of other and unspecified finger at wrist and hand level**

EXCLUDES 2 *injury of extensor muscle, fascia and tendon of thumb at wrist and hand level (S66.2-)*

6th **S66.30** **Unspecified injury of extensor muscle, fascia and tendon of other and unspecified finger at wrist and hand level**

7th **S66.300** **Unspecified injury of extensor muscle, fascia and tendon of right index finger at wrist and hand level**

7th **S66.301** **Unspecified injury of extensor muscle, fascia and tendon of left index finger at wrist and hand level**

7th **S66.302** **Unspecified injury of extensor muscle, fascia and tendon of right middle finger at wrist and hand level**

7th **S66.303** **Unspecified injury of extensor muscle, fascia and tendon of left middle finger at wrist and hand level**

7th **S66.304** **Unspecified injury of extensor muscle, fascia and tendon of right ring finger at wrist and hand level**

7th **S66.305** **Unspecified injury of extensor muscle, fascia and tendon of left ring finger at wrist and hand level**

7th **S66.306** **Unspecified injury of extensor muscle, fascia and tendon of right little finger at wrist and hand level**

7th **S66.307** **Unspecified injury of extensor muscle, fascia and tendon of left little finger at wrist and hand level**

7th **S66.308** **Unspecified injury of extensor muscle, fascia and tendon of other finger at wrist and hand level**

Unspecified injury of extensor muscle, fascia and tendon of specified finger with unspecified laterality at wrist and hand level

7th **S66.309** **Unspecified injury of extensor muscle, fascia and tendon of unspecified finger at wrist and hand level**

6th **S66.31** **Strain of extensor muscle, fascia and tendon of other and unspecified finger at wrist and hand level**

7th **S66.310** **Strain of extensor muscle, fascia and tendon of right index finger at wrist and hand level**

7th **S66.311** **Strain of extensor muscle, fascia and tendon of left index finger at wrist and hand level**

7th **S66.312** **Strain of extensor muscle, fascia and tendon of right middle finger at wrist and hand level**

7th **S66.313** **Strain of extensor muscle, fascia and tendon of left middle finger at wrist and hand level**

7th **S66.314** **Strain of extensor muscle, fascia and tendon of right ring finger at wrist and hand level**

7th **S66.315** **Strain of extensor muscle, fascia and tendon of left ring finger at wrist and hand level**

7th **S66.316** **Strain of extensor muscle, fascia and tendon of right little finger at wrist and hand level**

7th **S66.317** **Strain of extensor muscle, fascia and tendon of left little finger at wrist and hand level**

7th **S66.318** **Strain of extensor muscle, fascia and tendon of other finger at wrist and hand level**

Strain of extensor muscle, fascia and tendon of specified finger with unspecified laterality at wrist and hand level

7th **S66.319** **Strain of extensor muscle, fascia and tendon of unspecified finger at wrist and hand level**

6th **S66.32** **Laceration of extensor muscle, fascia and tendon of other and unspecified finger at wrist and hand level**

7th **S66.320** **Laceration of extensor muscle, fascia and tendon of right index finger at wrist and hand level** CC

7th **S66.321** **Laceration of extensor muscle, fascia and tendon of left index finger at wrist and hand level** CC

7th **S66.322** **Laceration of extensor muscle, fascia and tendon of right middle finger at wrist and hand level** CC

7th **S66.323** **Laceration of extensor muscle, fascia and tendon of left middle finger at wrist and hand level** CC

7th **S66.324** **Laceration of extensor muscle, fascia and tendon of right ring finger at wrist and hand level** CC

7th **S66.325** **Laceration of extensor muscle, fascia and tendon of left ring finger at wrist and hand level** CC

7th **S66.326** **Laceration of extensor muscle, fascia and tendon of right little finger at wrist and hand level** CC

7th **S66.327** **Laceration of extensor muscle, fascia and tendon of left little finger at wrist and hand level** CC

7th **S66.328** **Laceration of extensor muscle, fascia and tendon of other finger at wrist and hand level** CC

Laceration of extensor muscle, fascia and tendon of specified finger with unspecified laterality at wrist and hand level

7th **S66.329** **Laceration of extensor muscle, fascia and tendon of unspecified finger at wrist and hand level** CC UNS

6th **S66.39** **Other injury of extensor muscle, fascia and tendon of other and unspecified finger at wrist and hand level**

7th **S66.390** **Other injury of extensor muscle, fascia and tendon of right index finger at wrist and hand level**

7th **S66.391** **Other injury of extensor muscle, fascia and tendon of left index finger at wrist and hand level**

7th **S66.392** **Other injury of extensor muscle, fascia and tendon of right middle finger at wrist and hand level**

7th **S66.393** **Other injury of extensor muscle, fascia and tendon of left middle finger at wrist and hand level**

S66.394 Other injury of extensor muscle, fascia and tendon of right ring finger at wrist and hand level

S66.395 Other injury of extensor muscle, fascia and tendon of left ring finger at wrist and hand level

S66.396 Other injury of extensor muscle, fascia and tendon of right little finger at wrist and hand level

S66.397 Other injury of extensor muscle, fascia and tendon of left little finger at wrist and hand level

S66.398 Other injury of extensor muscle, fascia and tendon of other finger at wrist and hand level

Other injury of extensor muscle, fascia and tendon of specified finger with unspecified laterality at wrist and hand level

S66.399 Other injury of extensor muscle, fascia and tendon of unspecified finger at wrist and hand level

S66.4 Injury of intrinsic muscle, fascia and tendon of thumb at wrist and hand level

S66.40 Unspecified injury of intrinsic muscle, fascia and tendon of thumb at wrist and hand level

S66.401 Unspecified injury of intrinsic muscle, fascia and tendon of right thumb at wrist and hand level

S66.402 Unspecified injury of intrinsic muscle, fascia and tendon of left thumb at wrist and hand level

S66.409 Unspecified injury of intrinsic muscle, fascia and tendon of unspecified thumb at wrist and hand level

S66.41 Strain of intrinsic muscle, fascia and tendon of thumb at wrist and hand level

S66.411 Strain of intrinsic muscle, fascia and tendon of right thumb at wrist and hand level

S66.412 Strain of intrinsic muscle, fascia and tendon of left thumb at wrist and hand level

S66.419 Strain of intrinsic muscle, fascia and tendon of unspecified thumb at wrist and hand level

S66.42 Laceration of intrinsic muscle, fascia and tendon of thumb at wrist and hand level

S66.421 Laceration of intrinsic muscle, fascia and tendon of right thumb at wrist and hand level CC

S66.422 Laceration of intrinsic muscle, fascia and tendon of left thumb at wrist and hand level CC

S66.429 Laceration of intrinsic muscle, fascia and tendon of unspecified thumb at wrist and hand level CC

S66.49 Other specified injury of intrinsic muscle, fascia and tendon of thumb at wrist and hand level

S66.491 Other specified injury of intrinsic muscle, fascia and tendon of right thumb at wrist and hand level

S66.492 Other specified injury of intrinsic muscle, fascia and tendon of left thumb at wrist and hand level

S66.499 Other specified injury of intrinsic muscle, fascia and tendon of unspecified thumb at wrist and hand level

S66.5 Injury of intrinsic muscle, fascia and tendon of other and unspecified finger at wrist and hand level

EXCLUDES 2 *injury of intrinsic muscle, fascia and tendon of thumb at wrist and hand level (S66.4-)*

S66.50 Unspecified injury of intrinsic muscle, fascia and tendon of other and unspecified finger at wrist and hand level

S66.500 Unspecified injury of intrinsic muscle, fascia and tendon of right index finger at wrist and hand level

S66.501 Unspecified injury of intrinsic muscle, fascia and tendon of left index finger at wrist and hand level

S66.502 Unspecified injury of intrinsic muscle, fascia and tendon of right middle finger at wrist and hand level

S66.503 Unspecified injury of intrinsic muscle, fascia and tendon of left middle finger at wrist and hand level

S66.504 Unspecified injury of intrinsic muscle, fascia and tendon of right ring finger at wrist and hand level

S66.505 Unspecified injury of intrinsic muscle, fascia and tendon of left ring finger at wrist and hand level

S66.506 Unspecified injury of intrinsic muscle, fascia and tendon of right little finger at wrist and hand level

S66.507 Unspecified injury of intrinsic muscle, fascia and tendon of left little finger at wrist and hand level

S66.508 Unspecified injury of intrinsic muscle, fascia and tendon of other finger at wrist and hand level

Unspecified injury of intrinsic muscle, fascia and tendon of specified finger with unspecified laterality at wrist and hand level

S66.509 Unspecified injury of intrinsic muscle, fascia and tendon of unspecified finger at wrist and hand level

S66.51 Strain of intrinsic muscle, fascia and tendon of other and unspecified finger at wrist and hand level

S66.510 Strain of intrinsic muscle, fascia and tendon of right index finger at wrist and hand level

S66.511 Strain of intrinsic muscle, fascia and tendon of left index finger at wrist and hand level

S66.512 Strain of intrinsic muscle, fascia and tendon of right middle finger at wrist and hand level

S66.513 Strain of intrinsic muscle, fascia and tendon of left middle finger at wrist and hand level

S66.514 Strain of intrinsic muscle, fascia and tendon of right ring finger at wrist and hand level

S66.515 Strain of intrinsic muscle, fascia and tendon of left ring finger at wrist and hand level

S66.516 Strain of intrinsic muscle, fascia and tendon of right little finger at wrist and hand level

S66.517 Strain of intrinsic muscle, fascia and tendon of left little finger at wrist and hand level

S66.518 Strain of intrinsic muscle, fascia and tendon of other finger at wrist and hand level

Strain of intrinsic muscle, fascia and tendon of specified finger with unspecified laterality at wrist and hand level

S66.519 Strain of intrinsic muscle, fascia and tendon of unspecified finger at wrist and hand level

S66.52 Laceration of intrinsic muscle, fascia and tendon of other and unspecified finger at wrist and hand level

S66.520 Laceration of intrinsic muscle, fascia and tendon of right index finger at wrist and hand level CC

S66.521 Laceration of intrinsic muscle, fascia and tendon of left index finger at wrist and hand level CC

S66.522 Laceration of intrinsic muscle, fascia and tendon of right middle finger at wrist and hand level CC

S66.523 Laceration of intrinsic muscle, fascia and tendon of left middle finger at wrist and hand level CC

S66.524 Laceration of intrinsic muscle, fascia and tendon of right ring finger at wrist and hand level CC

S66.525 Laceration of intrinsic muscle, fascia and tendon of left ring finger at wrist and hand level CC

S66.526 Laceration of intrinsic muscle, fascia and tendon of right little finger at wrist and hand level CC

7th **S66.527 Laceration of intrinsic muscle, fascia and tendon of left little finger at wrist and hand level** CC

7th **S66.528 Laceration of intrinsic muscle, fascia and tendon of other finger at wrist and hand level** CC

Laceration of intrinsic muscle, fascia and tendon of specified finger with unspecified laterality at wrist and hand level

7th **S66.529 Laceration of intrinsic muscle, fascia and tendon of unspecified finger at wrist and hand level** CC UNS

6th **S66.59 Other injury of intrinsic muscle, fascia and tendon of other and unspecified finger at wrist and hand level**

7th **S66.590 Other injury of intrinsic muscle, fascia and tendon of right index finger at wrist and hand level**

7th **S66.591 Other injury of intrinsic muscle, fascia and tendon of left index finger at wrist and hand level**

7th **S66.592 Other injury of intrinsic muscle, fascia and tendon of right middle finger at wrist and hand level**

7th **S66.593 Other injury of intrinsic muscle, fascia and tendon of left middle finger at wrist and hand level**

7th **S66.594 Other injury of intrinsic muscle, fascia and tendon of right ring finger at wrist and hand level**

7th **S66.595 Other injury of intrinsic muscle, fascia and tendon of left ring finger at wrist and hand level**

7th **S66.596 Other injury of intrinsic muscle, fascia and tendon of right little finger at wrist and hand level**

7th **S66.597 Other injury of intrinsic muscle, fascia and tendon of left little finger at wrist and hand level**

7th **S66.598 Other injury of intrinsic muscle, fascia and tendon of other finger at wrist and hand level**

Other injury of intrinsic muscle, fascia and tendon of specified finger with unspecified laterality at wrist and hand level

7th **S66.599 Other injury of intrinsic muscle, fascia and tendon of unspecified finger at wrist and hand level**

5th **S66.8 Injury of other specified muscles, fascia and tendons at wrist and hand level**

6th **S66.80 Unspecified injury of other specified muscles, fascia and tendons at wrist and hand level**

7th **S66.801 Unspecified injury of other specified muscles, fascia and tendons at wrist and hand level, right hand**

7th **S66.802 Unspecified injury of other specified muscles, fascia and tendons at wrist and hand level, left hand**

7th **S66.809 Unspecified injury of other specified muscles, fascia and tendons at wrist and hand level, unspecified hand**

6th **S66.81 Strain of other specified muscles, fascia and tendons at wrist and hand level**

7th **S66.811 Strain of other specified muscles, fascia and tendons at wrist and hand level, right hand**

7th **S66.812 Strain of other specified muscles, fascia and tendons at wrist and hand level, left hand**

7th **S66.819 Strain of other specified muscles, fascia and tendons at wrist and hand level, unspecified hand**

6th **S66.82 Laceration of other specified muscles, fascia and tendons at wrist and hand level**

7th **S66.821 Laceration of other specified muscles, fascia and tendons at wrist and hand level, right hand** CC

7th **S66.822 Laceration of other specified muscles, fascia and tendons at wrist and hand level, left hand** CC

7th **S66.829 Laceration of other specified muscles, fascia and tendons at wrist and hand level, unspecified hand** CC UNS

6th **S66.89 Other injury of other specified muscles, fascia and tendons at wrist and hand level**

7th **S66.891 Other injury of other specified muscles, fascia and tendons at wrist and hand level, right hand**

7th **S66.892 Other injury of other specified muscles, fascia and tendons at wrist and hand level, left hand**

7th **S66.899 Other injury of other specified muscles, fascia and tendons at wrist and hand level, unspecified hand**

5th **S66.9 Injury of unspecified muscle, fascia and tendon at wrist and hand level**

6th **S66.90 Unspecified injury of unspecified muscle, fascia and tendon at wrist and hand level**

7th **S66.901 Unspecified injury of unspecified muscle, fascia and tendon at wrist and hand level, right hand**

7th **S66.902 Unspecified injury of unspecified muscle, fascia and tendon at wrist and hand level, left hand**

7th **S66.909 Unspecified injury of unspecified muscle, fascia and tendon at wrist and hand level, unspecified hand**

6th **S66.91 Strain of unspecified muscle, fascia and tendon at wrist and hand level**

7th **S66.911 Strain of unspecified muscle, fascia and tendon at wrist and hand level, right hand**

7th **S66.912 Strain of unspecified muscle, fascia and tendon at wrist and hand level, left hand**

7th **S66.919 Strain of unspecified muscle, fascia and tendon at wrist and hand level, unspecified hand**

6th **S66.92 Laceration of unspecified muscle, fascia and tendon at wrist and hand level**

7th **S66.921 Laceration of unspecified muscle, fascia and tendon at wrist and hand level, right hand** CC

7th **S66.922 Laceration of unspecified muscle, fascia and tendon at wrist and hand level, left hand** CC

7th **S66.929 Laceration of unspecified muscle, fascia and tendon at wrist and hand level, unspecified hand** CC UNS

6th **S66.99 Other injury of unspecified muscle, fascia and tendon at wrist and hand level**

7th **S66.991 Other injury of unspecified muscle, fascia and tendon at wrist and hand level, right hand**

7th **S66.992 Other injury of unspecified muscle, fascia and tendon at wrist and hand level, left hand**

7th **S66.999 Other injury of unspecified muscle, fascia and tendon at wrist and hand level, unspecified hand**

4th **S67 Crushing injury of wrist, hand and fingers**

Use additional code for all associated injuries, such as:
fracture of wrist and hand (S62.-)
open wound of wrist and hand (S61.-)

The appropriate 7th character is to be added to each code from category S67.
A initial encounter
D subsequent encounter
S sequela

5th **S67.0 Crushing injury of thumb**

x7th **S67.00 Crushing injury of unspecified thumb**

x7th **S67.01 Crushing injury of right thumb**

x7th **S67.02 Crushing injury of left thumb**

5th **S67.1 Crushing injury of other and unspecified finger(s)**

EXCLUDES 2 *crushing injury of thumb (S67.0-)*

x7th **S67.10 Crushing injury of unspecified finger(s)**

6th **S67.19 Crushing injury of other finger(s)**

7th **S67.190 Crushing injury of right index finger**

7th **S67.191 Crushing injury of left index finger**

7th **S67.192 Crushing injury of right middle finger**

S67.193 Crushing injury of left middle finger
S67.194 Crushing injury of right ring finger
S67.195 Crushing injury of left ring finger
S67.196 Crushing injury of right little finger
S67.197 Crushing injury of left little finger
S67.198 Crushing injury of other finger
Crushing injury of specified finger with unspecified laterality

S67.2 Crushing injury of hand
EXCLUDES 2 *crushing injury of fingers (S67.1-)*
crushing injury of thumb (S67.Ø-)
S67.2Ø Crushing injury of unspecified hand
S67.21 Crushing injury of right hand
S67.22 Crushing injury of left hand

S67.3 Crushing injury of wrist
S67.3Ø Crushing injury of unspecified wrist
S67.31 Crushing injury of right wrist
S67.32 Crushing injury of left wrist

S67.4 Crushing injury of wrist and hand
EXCLUDES 1 *crushing injury of hand alone (S67.2-)*
crushing injury of wrist alone (S67.3-)
EXCLUDES 2 *crushing injury of fingers (S67.1-)*
crushing injury of thumb (S67.Ø-)
S67.4Ø Crushing injury of unspecified wrist and hand
S67.41 Crushing injury of right wrist and hand
S67.42 Crushing injury of left wrist and hand

S67.9 Crushing injury of unspecified part(s) of wrist, hand and fingers
S67.9Ø Crushing injury of unspecified part(s) of unspecified wrist, hand and fingers
S67.91 Crushing injury of unspecified part(s) of right wrist, hand and fingers
S67.92 Crushing injury of unspecified part(s) of left wrist, hand and fingers

S68 Traumatic amputation of wrist, hand and fingers

An amputation not identified as partial or complete should be coded to complete.

The appropriate 7th character is to be added to each code from category S68.
A initial encounter
D subsequent encounter
S sequela

S68.Ø Traumatic metacarpophalangeal amputation of thumb
Traumatic amputation of thumb NOS
S68.Ø1 Complete traumatic metacarpophalangeal amputation of thumb
S68.Ø11 Complete traumatic metacarpophalangeal amputation of right thumb HCC
S68.Ø12 Complete traumatic metacarpophalangeal amputation of left thumb HCC
S68.Ø19 Complete traumatic metacarpophalangeal amputation of unspecified thumb HCC
S68.Ø2 Partial traumatic metacarpophalangeal amputation of thumb
S68.Ø21 Partial traumatic metacarpophalangeal amputation of right thumb HCC
S68.Ø22 Partial traumatic metacarpophalangeal amputation of left thumb HCC
S68.Ø29 Partial traumatic metacarpophalangeal amputation of unspecified thumb HCC

S68.1 Traumatic metacarpophalangeal amputation of other and unspecified finger
Traumatic amputation of finger NOS
EXCLUDES 2 *traumatic metacarpophalangeal amputation of thumb (S68.Ø-)*
S68.11 Complete traumatic metacarpophalangeal amputation of other and unspecified finger
S68.11Ø Complete traumatic metacarpophalangeal amputation of right index finger HCC
S68.111 Complete traumatic metacarpophalangeal amputation of left index finger HCC
S68.112 Complete traumatic metacarpophalangeal amputation of right middle finger HCC
S68.113 Complete traumatic metacarpophalangeal amputation of left middle finger HCC
S68.114 Complete traumatic metacarpophalangeal amputation of right ring finger HCC
S68.115 Complete traumatic metacarpophalangeal amputation of left ring finger HCC
S68.116 Complete traumatic metacarpophalangeal amputation of right little finger HCC
S68.117 Complete traumatic metacarpophalangeal amputation of left little finger HCC
S68.118 Complete traumatic metacarpophalangeal amputation of other finger HCC
Complete traumatic metacarpophalangeal amputation of specified finger with unspecified laterality
S68.119 Complete traumatic metacarpophalangeal amputation of unspecified finger HCC
S68.12 Partial traumatic metacarpophalangeal amputation of other and unspecified finger
S68.12Ø Partial traumatic metacarpophalangeal amputation of right index finger HCC
S68.121 Partial traumatic metacarpophalangeal amputation of left index finger HCC
S68.122 Partial traumatic metacarpophalangeal amputation of right middle finger HCC
S68.123 Partial traumatic metacarpophalangeal amputation of left middle finger HCC
S68.124 Partial traumatic metacarpophalangeal amputation of right ring finger HCC
S68.125 Partial traumatic metacarpophalangeal amputation of left ring finger HCC
S68.126 Partial traumatic metacarpophalangeal amputation of right little finger HCC
S68.127 Partial traumatic metacarpophalangeal amputation of left little finger HCC
S68.128 Partial traumatic metacarpophalangeal amputation of other finger HCC
Partial traumatic metacarpophalangeal amputation of specified finger with unspecified laterality
S68.129 Partial traumatic metacarpophalangeal amputation of unspecified finger HCC

S68.4 Traumatic amputation of hand at wrist level
Traumatic amputation of hand NOS
Traumatic amputation of wrist
S68.41 Complete traumatic amputation of hand at wrist level
S68.411 Complete traumatic amputation of right hand at wrist level CC HCC
S68.412 Complete traumatic amputation of left hand at wrist level CC HCC
S68.419 Complete traumatic amputation of unspecified hand at wrist level CC UNS HCC
S68.42 Partial traumatic amputation of hand at wrist level
S68.421 Partial traumatic amputation of right hand at wrist level CC HCC
S68.422 Partial traumatic amputation of left hand at wrist level CC HCC
S68.429 Partial traumatic amputation of unspecified hand at wrist level CC UNS HCC

S68.5 Traumatic transphalangeal amputation of thumb
Traumatic interphalangeal joint amputation of thumb
S68.51 Complete traumatic transphalangeal amputation of thumb
S68.511 Complete traumatic transphalangeal amputation of right thumb HCC

8 ✓7th **S68.512 Complete traumatic transphalangeal amputation of left thumb** HCC

8 ✓7th **S68.519 Complete traumatic transphalangeal amputation of unspecified thumb** HCC

✓6th **S68.52 Partial traumatic transphalangeal amputation of thumb**

8 ✓7th **S68.521 Partial traumatic transphalangeal amputation of right thumb** HCC

8 ✓7th **S68.522 Partial traumatic transphalangeal amputation of left thumb** HCC

8 ✓7th **S68.529 Partial traumatic transphalangeal amputation of unspecified thumb** HCC

✓5th **S68.6 Traumatic transphalangeal amputation of other and unspecified finger**

✓6th **S68.61 Complete traumatic transphalangeal amputation of other and unspecified finger(s)**

8 ✓7th **S68.610 Complete traumatic transphalangeal amputation of right index finger** HCC

8 ✓7th **S68.611 Complete traumatic transphalangeal amputation of left index finger** HCC

8 ✓7th **S68.612 Complete traumatic transphalangeal amputation of right middle finger** HCC

8 ✓7th **S68.613 Complete traumatic transphalangeal amputation of left middle finger** HCC

8 ✓7th **S68.614 Complete traumatic transphalangeal amputation of right ring finger** HCC

8 ✓7th **S68.615 Complete traumatic transphalangeal amputation of left ring finger** HCC

8 ✓7th **S68.616 Complete traumatic transphalangeal amputation of right little finger** HCC

8 ✓7th **S68.617 Complete traumatic transphalangeal amputation of left little finger** HCC

8 ✓7th **S68.618 Complete traumatic transphalangeal amputation of other finger** HCC

Complete traumatic transphalangeal amputation of specified finger with unspecified laterality

8 ✓7th **S68.619 Complete traumatic transphalangeal amputation of unspecified finger** HCC

✓6th **S68.62 Partial traumatic transphalangeal amputation of other and unspecified finger**

8 ✓7th **S68.620 Partial traumatic transphalangeal amputation of right index finger** HCC

8 ✓7th **S68.621 Partial traumatic transphalangeal amputation of left index finger** HCC

8 ✓7th **S68.622 Partial traumatic transphalangeal amputation of right middle finger** HCC

8 ✓7th **S68.623 Partial traumatic transphalangeal amputation of left middle finger** HCC

8 ✓7th **S68.624 Partial traumatic transphalangeal amputation of right ring finger** HCC

8 ✓7th **S68.625 Partial traumatic transphalangeal amputation of left ring finger** HCC

8 ✓7th **S68.626 Partial traumatic transphalangeal amputation of right little finger** HCC

8 ✓7th **S68.627 Partial traumatic transphalangeal amputation of left little finger** HCC

8 ✓7th **S68.628 Partial traumatic transphalangeal amputation of other finger** HCC

Partial traumatic transphalangeal amputation of specified finger with unspecified laterality

8 ✓7th **S68.629 Partial traumatic transphalangeal amputation of unspecified finger** HCC

✓5th **S68.7 Traumatic transmetacarpal amputation of hand**

✓6th **S68.71 Complete traumatic transmetacarpal amputation of hand**

7 ✓7th **S68.711 Complete traumatic transmetacarpal amputation of right hand** CC HCC

7 ✓7th **S68.712 Complete traumatic transmetacarpal amputation of left hand** CC HCC

7 ✓7th **S68.719 Complete traumatic transmetacarpal amputation of unspecified hand** CC UNS HCC

✓6th **S68.72 Partial traumatic transmetacarpal amputation of hand**

7 ✓7th **S68.721 Partial traumatic transmetacarpal amputation of right hand** CC HCC

7 ✓7th **S68.722 Partial traumatic transmetacarpal amputation of left hand** CC HCC

7 ✓7th **S68.729 Partial traumatic transmetacarpal amputation of unspecified hand** CC UNS HCC

✓4th **S69 Other and unspecified injuries of wrist, hand and finger(s)**

The appropriate 7th character is to be added to each code from category S69.
- A initial encounter
- D subsequent encounter
- S sequela

✓5th **S69.8 Other specified injuries of wrist, hand and finger(s)**

✓x7th **S69.80 Other specified injuries of unspecified wrist, hand and finger(s)**

✓x7th **S69.81 Other specified injuries of right wrist, hand and finger(s)**

✓x7th **S69.82 Other specified injuries of left wrist, hand and finger(s)**

✓5th **S69.9 Unspecified injury of wrist, hand and finger(s)**

✓x7th **S69.90 Unspecified injury of unspecified wrist, hand and finger(s)**

✓x7th **S69.91 Unspecified injury of right wrist, hand and finger(s)**

✓x7th **S69.92 Unspecified injury of left wrist, hand and finger(s)**

Injuries to the hip and thigh (S70-S79)

EXCLUDES 2 *burns and corrosions (T20-T32)*
frostbite (T33-T34)
snake bite (T63.0-)
venomous insect bite or sting (T63.4-)

✓4th **S70 Superficial injury of hip and thigh**

The appropriate 7th character is to be added to each code from category S70.
- A initial encounter
- D subsequent encounter
- S sequela

✓5th **S70.0 Contusion of hip**

✓x7th **S70.00 Contusion of unspecified hip**

✓x7th **S70.01 Contusion of right hip**

✓x7th **S70.02 Contusion of left hip**

✓5th **S70.1 Contusion of thigh**

✓x7th **S70.10 Contusion of unspecified thigh**

✓x7th **S70.11 Contusion of right thigh**

✓x7th **S70.12 Contusion of left thigh**

✓5th **S70.2 Other superficial injuries of hip**

✓6th **S70.21 Abrasion of hip**

✓7th **S70.211 Abrasion, right hip**

✓7th **S70.212 Abrasion, left hip**

✓7th **S70.219 Abrasion, unspecified hip**

✓6th **S70.22 Blister (nonthermal) of hip**

✓7th **S70.221 Blister (nonthermal), right hip**

✓7th **S70.222 Blister (nonthermal), left hip**

✓7th **S70.229 Blister (nonthermal), unspecified hip**

✓6th **S70.24 External constriction of hip**

✓7th **S70.241 External constriction, right hip**

✓7th **S70.242 External constriction, left hip**

✓7th **S70.249 External constriction, unspecified hip**

✓6th **S70.25 Superficial foreign body of hip**

Splinter in the hip

✓7th **S70.251 Superficial foreign body, right hip**

✓7th **S70.252 Superficial foreign body, left hip**

✓7th **S70.259 Superficial foreign body, unspecified hip**

✓6th **S70.26 Insect bite (nonvenomous) of hip**

✓7th **S70.261 Insect bite (nonvenomous), right hip**

✓7th **S70.262 Insect bite (nonvenomous), left hip**

✓7th **S70.269 Insect bite (nonvenomous), unspecified hip**

✓6th **S70.27 Other superficial bite of hip**

EXCLUDES 1 *open bite of hip (S71.05-)*

✓7th **S70.271 Other superficial bite of hip, right hip**

✓7th **S70.272 Other superficial bite of hip, left hip**

✓7th **S70.279 Other superficial bite of hip, unspecified hip**

S70.3 Other superficial injuries of thigh

S70.31 Abrasion of thigh

S70.311 Abrasion, right thigh

S70.312 Abrasion, left thigh

S70.319 Abrasion, unspecified thigh

S70.32 Blister (nonthermal) of thigh

S70.321 Blister (nonthermal), right thigh

S70.322 Blister (nonthermal), left thigh

S70.329 Blister (nonthermal), unspecified thigh

S70.34 External constriction of thigh

S70.341 External constriction, right thigh

S70.342 External constriction, left thigh

S70.349 External constriction, unspecified thigh

S70.35 Superficial foreign body of thigh

Splinter in the thigh

S70.351 Superficial foreign body, right thigh

S70.352 Superficial foreign body, left thigh

S70.359 Superficial foreign body, unspecified thigh

S70.36 Insect bite (nonvenomous) of thigh

S70.361 Insect bite (nonvenomous), right thigh

S70.362 Insect bite (nonvenomous), left thigh

S70.369 Insect bite (nonvenomous), unspecified thigh

S70.37 Other superficial bite of thigh

EXCLUDES 1 *open bite of thigh (S71.15)*

S70.371 Other superficial bite of right thigh

S70.372 Other superficial bite of left thigh

S70.379 Other superficial bite of unspecified thigh

S70.9 Unspecified superficial injury of hip and thigh

S70.91 Unspecified superficial injury of hip

S70.911 Unspecified superficial injury of right hip

S70.912 Unspecified superficial injury of left hip

S70.919 Unspecified superficial injury of unspecified hip

S70.92 Unspecified superficial injury of thigh

S70.921 Unspecified superficial injury of right thigh

S70.922 Unspecified superficial injury of left thigh

S70.929 Unspecified superficial injury of unspecified thigh

S71 Open wound of hip and thigh

Code also any associated wound infection

EXCLUDES 1 *open fracture of hip and thigh (S72.-)*
traumatic amputation of hip and thigh (S78.-)

EXCLUDES 2 *bite of venomous animal (T63.-)*
open wound of ankle, foot and toes (S91.-)
open wound of knee and lower leg (S81.-)

The appropriate 7th character is to be added to each code from category S71.
A initial encounter
D subsequent encounter
S sequela

S71.0 Open wound of hip

S71.00 Unspecified open wound of hip

S71.001 Unspecified open wound, right hip

S71.002 Unspecified open wound, left hip

S71.009 Unspecified open wound, unspecified hip

S71.01 Laceration without foreign body of hip

S71.011 Laceration without foreign body, right hip

S71.012 Laceration without foreign body, left hip

S71.019 Laceration without foreign body, unspecified hip

S71.02 Laceration with foreign body of hip

S71.021 Laceration with foreign body, right hip

S71.022 Laceration with foreign body, left hip

S71.029 Laceration with foreign body, unspecified hip

S71.03 Puncture wound without foreign body of hip

S71.031 Puncture wound without foreign body, right hip

S71.032 Puncture wound without foreign body, left hip

S71.039 Puncture wound without foreign body, unspecified hip

S71.04 Puncture wound with foreign body of hip

S71.041 Puncture wound with foreign body, right hip

S71.042 Puncture wound with foreign body, left hip

S71.049 Puncture wound with foreign body, unspecified hip

S71.05 Open bite of hip

Bite of hip NOS

EXCLUDES 1 *superficial bite of hip (S70.26, S70.27)*

S71.051 Open bite, right hip

S71.052 Open bite, left hip

S71.059 Open bite, unspecified hip

S71.1 Open wound of thigh

S71.10 Unspecified open wound of thigh

AHA: 2016,3Q,24

S71.101 Unspecified open wound, right thigh

S71.102 Unspecified open wound, left thigh

S71.109 Unspecified open wound, unspecified thigh

S71.11 Laceration without foreign body of thigh

S71.111 Laceration without foreign body, right thigh

S71.112 Laceration without foreign body, left thigh

S71.119 Laceration without foreign body, unspecified thigh

S71.12 Laceration with foreign body of thigh

S71.121 Laceration with foreign body, right thigh

S71.122 Laceration with foreign body, left thigh

S71.129 Laceration with foreign body, unspecified thigh

S71.13 Puncture wound without foreign body of thigh

AHA: 2016,3Q,24

S71.131 Puncture wound without foreign body, right thigh

S71.132 Puncture wound without foreign body, left thigh

S71.139 Puncture wound without foreign body, unspecified thigh

S71.14 Puncture wound with foreign body of thigh

AHA: 2016,3Q,24

S71.141 Puncture wound with foreign body, right thigh

S71.142 Puncture wound with foreign body, left thigh

S71.149 Puncture wound with foreign body, unspecified thigh

S71.15 Open bite of thigh

Bite of thigh NOS

EXCLUDES 1 *superficial bite of thigh (S70.37-)*

S71.151 Open bite, right thigh

S71.152 Open bite, left thigh

S71.159 Open bite, unspecified thigh

✓4th S72 Fracture of femur

NOTE A fracture not indicated as displaced or nondisplaced should be coded to displaced.

A fracture not indicated as open or closed should be coded to closed.

The open fracture designations are based on the Gustilo open fracture classification.

EXCLUDES 1 *traumatic amputation of hip and thigh (S78.-)*

EXCLUDES 2 *fracture of lower leg and ankle (S82.-)*
fracture of foot (S92.-)
periprosthetic fracture of prosthetic implant of hip (M97.Ø-)

AHA: 2018,2Q,12; 2016,1Q,33; 2015,3Q,37-39; 2015,1Q,17; 2013,4Q,128

DEF: Diaphysis: Central shaft of a long bone.

DEF: Epiphysis: Proximal and distal rounded ends of a long bone communicates with the joint.

DEF: Metaphysis: Section of a long bone located between the epiphysis and diaphysis at the proximal and distal ends.

DEF: Physis (growth plate): Narrow zone of cartilaginous tissue between the epiphysis and metaphysis at each end of a long bone. In childhood, proliferation of cells in this zone lengthens the bone. As the bone matures, this area thins, ossification eventually fusing into solid bone and growth stops. ***Synonym(s):*** *Epiphyseal plate.*

The appropriate 7th character is to be added to all codes from category S72 [unless otherwise indicated].

- A initial encounter for closed fracture
- B initial encounter for open fracture type I or II
  initial encounter for open fracture NOS
- C initial encounter for open fracture type IIIA, IIIB, or IIIC
- D subsequent encounter for closed fracture with routine healing
- E subsequent encounter for open fracture type I or II with routine healing
- F subsequent encounter for open fracture type IIIA, IIIB, or IIIC with routine healing
- G subsequent encounter for closed fracture with delayed healing
- H subsequent encounter for open fracture type I or II with delayed healing
- J subsequent encounter for open fracture type IIIA, IIIB, or IIIC with delayed healing
- K subsequent encounter for closed fracture with nonunion
- M subsequent encounter for open fracture type I or II with nonunion
- N subsequent encounter for open fracture type IIIA, IIIB, or IIIC with nonunion
- P subsequent encounter for closed fracture with malunion
- Q subsequent encounter for open fracture type I or II with malunion
- R subsequent encounter for open fracture type IIIA, IIIB, or IIIC with malunion
- S sequela

✓5th S72.Ø Fracture of head and neck of femur

EXCLUDES 2 *physeal fracture of upper end of femur (S79.Ø-)*

AHA: 2016,3Q,16

✓6th S72.ØØ Fracture of unspecified part of neck of femur

Fracture of hip NOS
Fracture of neck of femur NOS

4,6 ✓7th **S72.ØØ1 Fracture of unspecified part of neck of right femur** MCC CC H5 HCC

4,6 ✓7th **S72.ØØ2 Fracture of unspecified part of neck of left femur** MCC CC H5 HCC

4,6 ✓7th **S72.ØØ9 Fracture of unspecified part of neck of unspecified femur** MCC CC H5 UNS HCC

✓6th S72.Ø1 Unspecified intracapsular fracture of femur

Subcapital fracture of femur

4,6 ✓7th **S72.Ø11 Unspecified intracapsular fracture of right femur** MCC CC H5 HCC

4,6 ✓7th **S72.Ø12 Unspecified intracapsular fracture of left femur** MCC CC H5 HCC

4,6 ✓7th **S72.Ø19 Unspecified intracapsular fracture of unspecified femur** MCC CC H5 UNS HCC

✓6th S72.Ø2 Fracture of epiphysis (separation) (upper) of femur

Transepiphyseal fracture of femur

EXCLUDES 1 *capital femoral epiphyseal fracture (pediatric) of femur (S79.Ø1-)*
Salter-Harris Type I physeal fracture of upper end of femur (S79.Ø1-)

4,6 ✓7th **S72.Ø21 Displaced fracture of epiphysis (separation) (upper) of right femur** MCC CC H5 HCC

4,6 ✓7th **S72.Ø22 Displaced fracture of epiphysis (separation) (upper) of left femur** MCC CC H5 HCC

4,6 ✓7th **S72.Ø23 Displaced fracture of epiphysis (separation) (upper) of unspecified femur** MCC CC H5 UNS HCC

4,6 ✓7th **S72.Ø24 Nondisplaced fracture of epiphysis (separation) (upper) of right femur** MCC CC H5 HCC

4,6 ✓7th **S72.Ø25 Nondisplaced fracture of epiphysis (separation) (upper) of left femur** MCC CC H5 HCC

4,6 ✓7th **S72.Ø26 Nondisplaced fracture of epiphysis (separation) (upper) of unspecified femur** MCC CC H5 UNS HCC

✓6th S72.Ø3 Midcervical fracture of femur

Transcervical fracture of femur NOS

4,6 ✓7th **S72.Ø31 Displaced midcervical fracture of right femur** MCC CC H5 HCC

4,6 ✓7th **S72.Ø32 Displaced midcervical fracture of left femur** MCC CC H5 HCC

4,6 ✓7th **S72.Ø33 Displaced midcervical fracture of unspecified femur** MCC CC H5 UNS HCC

4,6 ✓7th **S72.Ø34 Nondisplaced midcervical fracture of right femur** MCC CC H5 HCC

4,6 ✓7th **S72.Ø35 Nondisplaced midcervical fracture of left femur** MCC CC H5 HCC

4,6 ✓7th **S72.Ø36 Nondisplaced midcervical fracture of unspecified femur** MCC CC H5 UNS HCC

✓6th S72.Ø4 Fracture of base of neck of femur

Cervicotrochanteric fracture of femur

4,6 ✓7th **S72.Ø41 Displaced fracture of base of neck of right femur** MCC CC H5 HCC

4,6 ✓7th **S72.Ø42 Displaced fracture of base of neck of left femur** MCC CC H5 HCC

4,6 ✓7th **S72.Ø43 Displaced fracture of base of neck of unspecified femur** MCC CC H5 UNS HCC

4,6 ✓7th **S72.Ø44 Nondisplaced fracture of base of neck of right femur** MCC CC H5 HCC

4,6 ✓7th **S72.Ø45 Nondisplaced fracture of base of neck of left femur** MCC CC H5 HCC

4,6 ✓7th **S72.Ø46 Nondisplaced fracture of base of neck of unspecified femur** MCC CC H5 UNS HCC

✓6th S72.Ø5 Unspecified fracture of head of femur

Fracture of head of femur NOS

4,6 ✓7th **S72.Ø51 Unspecified fracture of head of right femur** MCC CC H5 HCC

4,6 ✓7th **S72.Ø52 Unspecified fracture of head of left femur** MCC CC H5 HCC

4,6 ✓7th **S72.Ø59 Unspecified fracture of head of unspecified femur** MCC CC H5 UNS HCC

✓6th S72.Ø6 Articular fracture of head of femur

4,6 ✓7th **S72.Ø61 Displaced articular fracture of head of right femur** MCC CC H5 HCC

4,6 ✓7th **S72.Ø62 Displaced articular fracture of head of left femur** MCC CC H5 HCC

4,6 ✓7th **S72.Ø63 Displaced articular fracture of head of unspecified femur** MCC CC H5 UNS HCC

4,6 ✓7th **S72.Ø64 Nondisplaced articular fracture of head of right femur** MCC CC H5 HCC

4,6 ✓7th **S72.Ø65 Nondisplaced articular fracture of head of left femur** MCC CC H5 HCC

4,6 ✓7th **S72.Ø66 Nondisplaced articular fracture of head of unspecified femur** MCC CC H5 UNS HCC

✓6th S72.Ø9 Other fracture of head and neck of femur

4,6 ✓7th **S72.Ø91 Other fracture of head and neck of right femur** MCC CC H5 HCC

4,6 ✓7th **S72.Ø92 Other fracture of head and neck of left femur** MCC CC H5 HCC

4,6 ✓7th **S72.Ø99 Other fracture of head and neck of unspecified femur** MCC CC H5 UNS HCC

✓5th S72.1 Pertrochanteric fracture

AHA: 2016,3Q,16

✓6th S72.1Ø Unspecified trochanteric fracture of femur

Fracture of trochanter NOS

4,6 ✓7th **S72.1Ø1 Unspecified trochanteric fracture of right femur** MCC CC H5 HCC

4,6 ✓7th **S72.102** Unspecified trochanteric fracture of left femur MCC CC H5 HCC

4,6 ✓7th **S72.109** Unspecified trochanteric fracture of unspecified femur MCC CC H5 UNS HCC

✓6th **S72.11** Fracture of greater trochanter of femur

4,6 ✓7th **S72.111** Displaced fracture of greater trochanter of right femur MCC CC H5 HCC

4,6 ✓7th **S72.112** Displaced fracture of greater trochanter of left femur MCC CC H5 HCC

4,6 ✓7th **S72.113** Displaced fracture of greater trochanter of unspecified femur MCC CC H5 UNS HCC

4,6 ✓7th **S72.114** Nondisplaced fracture of greater trochanter of right femur MCC CC H5 HCC

4,6 ✓7th **S72.115** Nondisplaced fracture of greater trochanter of left femur MCC CC H5 HCC

4,6 ✓7th **S72.116** Nondisplaced fracture of greater trochanter of unspecified femur MCC CC H5 UNS HCC

✓6th **S72.12** Fracture of lesser trochanter of femur

4,6 ✓7th **S72.121** Displaced fracture of lesser trochanter of right femur MCC CC H5 HCC

4,6 ✓7th **S72.122** Displaced fracture of lesser trochanter of left femur MCC CC H5 HCC

4,6 ✓7th **S72.123** Displaced fracture of lesser trochanter of unspecified femur MCC CC H5 UNS HCC

4,6 ✓7th **S72.124** Nondisplaced fracture of lesser trochanter of right femur MCC CC H5 HCC

4,6 ✓7th **S72.125** Nondisplaced fracture of lesser trochanter of left femur MCC CC H5 HCC

4,6 ✓7th **S72.126** Nondisplaced fracture of lesser trochanter of unspecified femur MCC CC H5 UNS HCC

✓6th **S72.13** Apophyseal fracture of femur

EXCLUDES 1 *chronic (nontraumatic) slipped upper femoral epiphysis (M93.Ø-)*

4,6 ✓7th **S72.131** Displaced apophyseal fracture of right femur MCC CC H5 HCC

4,6 ✓7th **S72.132** Displaced apophyseal fracture of left femur MCC CC H5 HCC

4,6 ✓7th **S72.133** Displaced apophyseal fracture of unspecified femur MCC CC H5 UNS HCC

4,6 ✓7th **S72.134** Nondisplaced apophyseal fracture of right femur MCC CC H5 HCC

4,6 ✓7th **S72.135** Nondisplaced apophyseal fracture of left femur MCC CC H5 HCC

4,6 ✓7th **S72.136** Nondisplaced apophyseal fracture of unspecified femur MCC CC H5 UNS HCC

✓6th **S72.14** Intertrochanteric fracture of femur

4,6 ✓7th **S72.141** Displaced intertrochanteric fracture of right femur MCC CC H5 HCC

4,6 ✓7th **S72.142** Displaced intertrochanteric fracture of left femur MCC CC H5 HCC

4,6 ✓7th **S72.143** Displaced intertrochanteric fracture of unspecified femur MCC CC H5 UNS HCC

4,6 ✓7th **S72.144** Nondisplaced intertrochanteric fracture of right femur MCC CC H5 HCC

4,6 ✓7th **S72.145** Nondisplaced intertrochanteric fracture of left femur MCC CC H5 HCC

4,6 ✓7th **S72.146** Nondisplaced intertrochanteric fracture of unspecified femur MCC CC H5 UNS HCC

✓5th **S72.2** Subtrochanteric fracture of femur

4,6 ✓x7th **S72.21** Displaced subtrochanteric fracture of right femur MCC CC H5 HCC

4,6 ✓x7th **S72.22** Displaced subtrochanteric fracture of left femur MCC CC H5 HCC

4,6 ✓x7th **S72.23** Displaced subtrochanteric fracture of unspecified femur MCC CC H5 UNS HCC

4,6 ✓x7th **S72.24** Nondisplaced subtrochanteric fracture of right femur MCC CC H5 HCC

4,6 ✓x7th **S72.25** Nondisplaced subtrochanteric fracture of left femur MCC CC H5 HCC

4,6 ✓x7th **S72.26** Nondisplaced subtrochanteric fracture of unspecified femur MCC CC H5 UNS HCC

✓5th **S72.3** Fracture of shaft of femur

✓6th **S72.3Ø** Unspecified fracture of shaft of femur

4,6 ✓7th **S72.3Ø1** Unspecified fracture of shaft of right femur MCC CC H5 HCC

4,6 ✓7th **S72.3Ø2** Unspecified fracture of shaft of left femur MCC CC H5 HCC

4,6 ✓7th **S72.3Ø9** Unspecified fracture of shaft of unspecified femur MCC CC H5 UNS HCC

✓6th **S72.32** Transverse fracture of shaft of femur

4,6 ✓7th **S72.321** Displaced transverse fracture of shaft of right femur MCC CC H5 HCC

4,6 ✓7th **S72.322** Displaced transverse fracture of shaft of left femur MCC CC H5 HCC

4,6 ✓7th **S72.323** Displaced transverse fracture of shaft of unspecified femur MCC CC H5 UNS HCC

4,6 ✓7th **S72.324** Nondisplaced transverse fracture of shaft of right femur MCC CC H5 HCC

4,6 ✓7th **S72.325** Nondisplaced transverse fracture of shaft of left femur MCC CC H5 HCC

4,6 ✓7th **S72.326** Nondisplaced transverse fracture of shaft of unspecified femur MCC CC H5 UNS HCC

✓6th **S72.33** Oblique fracture of shaft of femur

4,6 ✓7th **S72.331** Displaced oblique fracture of shaft of right femur MCC CC H5 HCC

4,6 ✓7th **S72.332** Displaced oblique fracture of shaft of left femur MCC CC H5 HCC

4,6 ✓7th **S72.333** Displaced oblique fracture of shaft of unspecified femur MCC CC H5 UNS HCC

4,6 ✓7th **S72.334** Nondisplaced oblique fracture of shaft of right femur MCC CC H5 HCC

4,6 ✓7th **S72.335** Nondisplaced oblique fracture of shaft of left femur MCC CC H5 HCC

4,6 ✓7th **S72.336** Nondisplaced oblique fracture of shaft of unspecified femur MCC CC H5 UNS HCC

✓6th **S72.34** Spiral fracture of shaft of femur

4,6 ✓7th **S72.341** Displaced spiral fracture of shaft of right femur MCC CC H5 HCC

4,6 ✓7th **S72.342** Displaced spiral fracture of shaft of left femur MCC CC H5 HCC

4,6 ✓7th **S72.343** Displaced spiral fracture of shaft of unspecified femur MCC CC H5 UNS HCC

4,6 ✓7th **S72.344** Nondisplaced spiral fracture of shaft of right femur MCC CC H5 HCC

4,6 ✓7th **S72.345** Nondisplaced spiral fracture of shaft of left femur MCC CC H5 HCC

4,6 ✓7th **S72.346** Nondisplaced spiral fracture of shaft of unspecified femur MCC CC H5 UNS HCC

✓6th **S72.35** Comminuted fracture of shaft of femur

4,6 ✓7th **S72.351** Displaced comminuted fracture of shaft of right femur MCC CC H5 HCC

4,6 ✓7th **S72.352** Displaced comminuted fracture of shaft of left femur MCC CC H5 HCC

4,6 ✓7th **S72.353** Displaced comminuted fracture of shaft of unspecified femur MCC CC H5 UNS HCC

4,6 ✓7th **S72.354** Nondisplaced comminuted fracture of shaft of right femur MCC CC H5 HCC

4,6 ✓7th **S72.355** Nondisplaced comminuted fracture of shaft of left femur MCC CC H5 HCC

4,6 ✓7th **S72.356** Nondisplaced comminuted fracture of shaft of unspecified femur MCC CC H5 UNS HCC

✓6th **S72.36** Segmental fracture of shaft of femur

4,6 ✓7th **S72.361** Displaced segmental fracture of shaft of right femur MCC CC H5 HCC

4,6 ✓7th **S72.362** Displaced segmental fracture of shaft of left femur MCC CC H5 HCC

4,6 ✓7th **S72.363** Displaced segmental fracture of shaft of unspecified femur MCC CC H5 UNS HCC

4,6 ✓7th **S72.364** Nondisplaced segmental fracture of shaft of right femur MCC CC H5 HCC

4,6 ✓7th **S72.365** Nondisplaced segmental fracture of shaft of left femur MCC CC H5 HCC

4,6 ✓7th **S72.366** Nondisplaced segmental fracture of shaft of unspecified femur MCC CC H5 UNS HCC

6th S72.39 Other fracture of shaft of femur
4,6 7th S72.391 Other fracture of shaft of right femur MCC CC H5 HCC
4,6 7th S72.392 Other fracture of shaft of left femur MCC CC H5 HCC
4,6 7th S72.399 Other fracture of shaft of unspecified femur MCC CC H5 UNS HCC

5th S72.4 Fracture of lower end of femur
Fracture of distal end of femur
EXCLUDES 2 *fracture of shaft of femur (S72.3-)*
physeal fracture of lower end of femur (S79.1-)
AHA: 2016,4Q,42

6th S72.40 Unspecified fracture of lower end of femur
AHA: 2018,1Q,21; 2016,4Q,42
2,3,6 7th S72.401 Unspecified fracture of lower end of right femur MCC CC H5 HCC
2,3,6 7th S72.402 Unspecified fracture of lower end of left femur MCC CC H5 HCC
2,3,6 7th S72.409 Unspecified fracture of lower end of unspecified femur MCC CC H5 UNS HCC

6th S72.41 Unspecified condyle fracture of lower end of femur
Condyle fracture of femur NOS
2,3,6 7th S72.411 Displaced unspecified condyle fracture of lower end of right femur MCC CC H5 HCC
2,3,6 7th S72.412 Displaced unspecified condyle fracture of lower end of left femur MCC CC H5 HCC
2,3,6 7th S72.413 Displaced unspecified condyle fracture of lower end of unspecified femur MCC CC H5 UNS HCC
2,3,6 7th S72.414 Nondisplaced unspecified condyle fracture of lower end of right femur MCC CC H5 HCC
2,3,6 7th S72.415 Nondisplaced unspecified condyle fracture of lower end of left femur MCC CC H5 HCC
2,3,6 7th S72.416 Nondisplaced unspecified condyle fracture of lower end of unspecified femur MCC CC H5 UNS HCC

6th S72.42 Fracture of lateral condyle of femur
2,3,6 7th S72.421 Displaced fracture of lateral condyle of right femur MCC CC H5 HCC
2,3,6 7th S72.422 Displaced fracture of lateral condyle of left femur MCC CC H5 HCC
2,3,6 7th S72.423 Displaced fracture of lateral condyle of unspecified femur MCC CC H5 UNS HCC
2,3,6 7th S72.424 Nondisplaced fracture of lateral condyle of right femur MCC CC H5 HCC
2,3,6 7th S72.425 Nondisplaced fracture of lateral condyle of left femur MCC CC H5 HCC
2,3,6 7th S72.426 Nondisplaced fracture of lateral condyle of unspecified femur MCC CC H5 UNS HCC

6th S72.43 Fracture of medial condyle of femur
2,3,6 7th S72.431 Displaced fracture of medial condyle of right femur MCC CC H5 HCC
2,3,6 7th S72.432 Displaced fracture of medial condyle of left femur MCC CC H5 HCC
2,3,6 7th S72.433 Displaced fracture of medial condyle of unspecified femur MCC CC H5 UNS HCC
2,3,6 7th S72.434 Nondisplaced fracture of medial condyle of right femur MCC CC H5 HCC
2,3,6 7th S72.435 Nondisplaced fracture of medial condyle of left femur MCC CC H5 HCC
2,3,6 7th S72.436 Nondisplaced fracture of medial condyle of unspecified femur MCC CC H5 UNS HCC

6th S72.44 Fracture of lower epiphysis (separation) of femur
EXCLUDES 1 *Salter-Harris Type I physeal fracture of lower end of femur (S79.11-)*
2,3,6 7th S72.441 Displaced fracture of lower epiphysis (separation) of right femur MCC CC H5 HCC
2,3,6 7th S72.442 Displaced fracture of lower epiphysis (separation) of left femur MCC CC H5 HCC
2,3,6 7th S72.443 Displaced fracture of lower epiphysis (separation) of unspecified femur MCC CC H5 UNS HCC
2,3,6 7th S72.444 Nondisplaced fracture of lower epiphysis (separation) of right femur MCC CC H5 HCC
2,3,6 7th S72.445 Nondisplaced fracture of lower epiphysis (separation) of left femur MCC CC H5 HCC
2,3,6 7th S72.446 Nondisplaced fracture of lower epiphysis (separation) of unspecified femur MCC CC H5 UNS HCC

6th S72.45 Supracondylar fracture without intracondylar extension of lower end of femur
Supracondylar fracture of lower end of femur NOS
EXCLUDES 1 *supracondylar fracture with intracondylar extension of lower end of femur (S72.46-)*
2,3,6 7th S72.451 Displaced supracondylar fracture without intracondylar extension of lower end of right femur MCC CC H5 HCC
2,3,6 7th S72.452 Displaced supracondylar fracture without intracondylar extension of lower end of left femur MCC CC H5 HCC
2,3,6 7th S72.453 Displaced supracondylar fracture without intracondylar extension of lower end of unspecified femur MCC CC H5 UNS HCC
2,3,6 7th S72.454 Nondisplaced supracondylar fracture without intracondylar extension of lower end of right femur MCC CC H5 HCC
2,3,6 7th S72.455 Nondisplaced supracondylar fracture without intracondylar extension of lower end of left femur MCC CC H5 HCC
2,3,6 7th S72.456 Nondisplaced supracondylar fracture without intracondylar extension of lower end of unspecified femur MCC CC H5 UNS HCC

6th S72.46 Supracondylar fracture with intracondylar extension of lower end of femur
EXCLUDES 1 *supracondylar fracture without intracondylar extension of lower end of femur (S72.45-)*
2,3,6 7th S72.461 Displaced supracondylar fracture with intracondylar extension of lower end of right femur MCC CC H5 HCC
2,3,6 7th S72.462 Displaced supracondylar fracture with intracondylar extension of lower end of left femur MCC CC H5 HCC
2,3,6 7th S72.463 Displaced supracondylar fracture with intracondylar extension of lower end of unspecified femur MCC CC H5 UNS HCC
2,3,6 7th S72.464 Nondisplaced supracondylar fracture with intracondylar extension of lower end of right femur MCC CC H5 HCC
2,3,6 7th S72.465 Nondisplaced supracondylar fracture with intracondylar extension of lower end of left femur MCC CC H5 HCC
2,3,6 7th S72.466 Nondisplaced supracondylar fracture with intracondylar extension of lower end of unspecified femur MCC CC H5 UNS HCC

6th S72.47 Torus fracture of lower end of femur

The appropriate 7th character is to be added to all codes in subcategory S72.47.
- A initial encounter for closed fracture
- D subsequent encounter for fracture with routine healing
- G subsequent encounter for fracture with delayed healing
- K subsequent encounter for fracture with nonunion
- P subsequent encounter for fracture with malunion
- S sequela

3,6 7th S72.471 Torus fracture of lower end of right femur CC H5 HCC
3,6 7th S72.472 Torus fracture of lower end of left femur CC H5 HCC
3,6 7th S72.479 Torus fracture of lower end of unspecified femur CC H5 UNS HCC

S72.49 Other fracture of lower end of femur

2,3,6 S72.491 Other fracture of lower end of right femur MCC CC H5 HCC

2,3,6 S72.492 Other fracture of lower end of left femur MCC CC H5 HCC

2,3,6 S72.499 Other fracture of lower end of unspecified femur MCC CC H5 UNS HCC

S72.8 Other fracture of femur

S72.8X Other fracture of femur

4,6 S72.8X1 Other fracture of right femur MCC CC H5 HCC

4,6 S72.8X2 Other fracture of left femur MCC CC H5 HCC

4,6 S72.8X9 Other fracture of unspecified femur MCC CC H5 UNS HCC

S72.9 Unspecified fracture of femur

Fracture of thigh NOS

Fracture of upper leg NOS

EXCLUDES 1 *fracture of hip NOS (S72.ØØ-, S72.Ø1-)*

4,6 S72.9Ø Unspecified fracture of unspecified femur MCC CC H5 UNS HCC

AHA: 2012,4Q,93

4,6 S72.91 Unspecified fracture of right femur MCC CC H5 HCC

4,6 S72.92 Unspecified fracture of left femur MCC CC H5 HCC

S73 Dislocation and sprain of joint and ligaments of hip

INCLUDES avulsion of joint or ligament of hip
laceration of cartilage, joint or ligament of hip
sprain of cartilage, joint or ligament of hip
traumatic hemarthrosis of joint or ligament of hip
traumatic rupture of joint or ligament of hip
traumatic subluxation of joint or ligament of hip
traumatic tear of joint or ligament of hip

Code also any associated open wound

EXCLUDES 2 *strain of muscle, fascia and tendon of hip and thigh (S76.-)*

The appropriate 7th character is to be added to each code from category S73.
A initial encounter
D subsequent encounter
S sequela

S73.Ø Subluxation and dislocation of hip

EXCLUDES 2 *dislocation and subluxation of hip prosthesis (T84.Ø2Ø, T84.Ø21)*

S73.ØØ Unspecified subluxation and dislocation of hip

Dislocation of hip NOS

Subluxation of hip NOS

6 S73.ØØ1 Unspecified subluxation of right hip CC H5 HCC

6 S73.ØØ2 Unspecified subluxation of left hip CC H5 HCC

6 S73.ØØ3 Unspecified subluxation of unspecified hip CC H5 UNS HCC

6 S73.ØØ4 Unspecified dislocation of right hip CC H5 HCC

6 S73.ØØ5 Unspecified dislocation of left hip CC H5 HCC

6 S73.ØØ6 Unspecified dislocation of unspecified hip CC H5 UNS HCC

S73.Ø1 Posterior subluxation and dislocation of hip

6 S73.Ø11 Posterior subluxation of right hip CC H5 HCC

6 S73.Ø12 Posterior subluxation of left hip CC H5 HCC

6 S73.Ø13 Posterior subluxation of unspecified hip CC H5 UNS HCC

6 S73.Ø14 Posterior dislocation of right hip CC H5 HCC

6 S73.Ø15 Posterior dislocation of left hip CC H5 HCC

6 S73.Ø16 Posterior dislocation of unspecified hip CC H5 UNS HCC

S73.Ø2 Obturator subluxation and dislocation of hip

6 S73.Ø21 Obturator subluxation of right hip CC H5 HCC

6 S73.Ø22 Obturator subluxation of left hip CC H5 HCC

6 S73.Ø23 Obturator subluxation of unspecified hip CC H5 UNS HCC

6 S73.Ø24 Obturator dislocation of right hip CC H5 HCC

6 S73.Ø25 Obturator dislocation of left hip CC H5 HCC

6 S73.Ø26 Obturator dislocation of unspecified hip CC H5 UNS HCC

S73.Ø3 Other anterior subluxation and dislocation of hip

6 S73.Ø31 Other anterior subluxation of right hip CC H5 HCC

6 S73.Ø32 Other anterior subluxation of left hip CC H5 HCC

6 S73.Ø33 Other anterior subluxation of unspecified hip CC H5 UNS HCC

6 S73.Ø34 Other anterior dislocation of right hip CC H5 HCC

6 S73.Ø35 Other anterior dislocation of left hip CC H5 HCC

6 S73.Ø36 Other anterior dislocation of unspecified hip CC H5 UNS HCC

S73.Ø4 Central subluxation and dislocation of hip

6 S73.Ø41 Central subluxation of right hip CC H5 HCC

6 S73.Ø42 Central subluxation of left hip CC H5 HCC

6 S73.Ø43 Central subluxation of unspecified hip CC H5 UNS HCC

6 S73.Ø44 Central dislocation of right hip CC H5 HCC

6 S73.Ø45 Central dislocation of left hip CC H5 HCC

6 S73.Ø46 Central dislocation of unspecified hip CC H5 UNS HCC

S73.1 Sprain of hip

AHA: 2014,4Q,25

S73.1Ø Unspecified sprain of hip

S73.1Ø1 Unspecified sprain of right hip

S73.1Ø2 Unspecified sprain of left hip

S73.1Ø9 Unspecified sprain of unspecified hip

S73.11 Iliofemoral ligament sprain of hip

S73.111 Iliofemoral ligament sprain of right hip

S73.112 Iliofemoral ligament sprain of left hip

S73.119 Iliofemoral ligament sprain of unspecified hip

S73.12 Ischiocapsular (ligament) sprain of hip

S73.121 Ischiocapsular ligament sprain of right hip

S73.122 Ischiocapsular ligament sprain of left hip

S73.129 Ischiocapsular ligament sprain of unspecified hip

S73.19 Other sprain of hip

S73.191 Other sprain of right hip

S73.192 Other sprain of left hip

S73.199 Other sprain of unspecified hip

S74 Injury of nerves at hip and thigh level

Code also any associated open wound (S71.-)

EXCLUDES 2 *injury of nerves at ankle and foot level (S94.-)*
injury of nerves at lower leg level (S84.-)

The appropriate 7th character is to be added to each code from category S74.
A initial encounter
D subsequent encounter
S sequela

S74.Ø Injury of sciatic nerve at hip and thigh level

S74.ØØ Injury of sciatic nerve at hip and thigh level, unspecified leg

S74.Ø1 Injury of sciatic nerve at hip and thigh level, right leg

S74.Ø2 Injury of sciatic nerve at hip and thigh level, left leg

S74.1 Injury of femoral nerve at hip and thigh level

S74.1Ø Injury of femoral nerve at hip and thigh level, unspecified leg

S74.11 Injury of femoral nerve at hip and thigh level, right leg

S74.12 Injury of femoral nerve at hip and thigh level, left leg

S74.2 Injury of cutaneous sensory nerve at hip and thigh level

S74.20 Injury of cutaneous sensory nerve at hip and thigh level, unspecified leg

S74.21 Injury of cutaneous sensory nerve at hip and high level, right leg

S74.22 Injury of cutaneous sensory nerve at hip and thigh level, left leg

S74.8 Injury of other nerves at hip and thigh level

S74.8X Injury of other nerves at hip and thigh level

S74.8X1 Injury of other nerves at hip and thigh level, right leg

S74.8X2 Injury of other nerves at hip and thigh level, left leg

S74.8X9 Injury of other nerves at hip and thigh level, unspecified leg

S74.9 Injury of unspecified nerve at hip and thigh level

S74.90 Injury of unspecified nerve at hip and thigh level, unspecified leg

S74.91 Injury of unspecified nerve at hip and thigh level, right leg

S74.92 Injury of unspecified nerve at hip and thigh level, left leg

S75 Injury of blood vessels at hip and thigh level

Code also any associated open wound (S71.-)

EXCLUDES 2 *injury of blood vessels at lower leg level (S85.-)*
injury of popliteal artery (S85.0)

The appropriate 7th character is to be added to each code from category S75.
- A initial encounter
- D subsequent encounter
- S sequela

S75.0 Injury of femoral artery

S75.00 Unspecified injury of femoral artery

S75.001 Unspecified injury of femoral artery, right leg MCC

S75.002 Unspecified injury of femoral artery, left leg MCC

S75.009 Unspecified injury of femoral artery, unspecified leg MCC UNS

S75.01 Minor laceration of femoral artery
Incomplete transection of femoral artery
Laceration of femoral artery NOS
Superficial laceration of femoral artery

S75.011 Minor laceration of femoral artery, right leg MCC

S75.012 Minor laceration of femoral artery, left leg MCC

S75.019 Minor laceration of femoral artery, unspecified leg MCC UNS

S75.02 Major laceration of femoral artery
Complete transection of femoral artery
Traumatic rupture of femoral artery

S75.021 Major laceration of femoral artery, right leg MCC

S75.022 Major laceration of femoral artery, left leg MCC

S75.029 Major laceration of femoral artery, unspecified leg MCC UNS

S75.09 Other specified injury of femoral artery

S75.091 Other specified injury of femoral artery, right leg MCC

S75.092 Other specified injury of femoral artery, left leg MCC

S75.099 Other specified injury of femoral artery, unspecified leg MCC UNS

S75.1 Injury of femoral vein at hip and thigh level

S75.10 Unspecified injury of femoral vein at hip and thigh level

S75.101 Unspecified injury of femoral vein at hip and thigh level, right leg MCC

S75.102 Unspecified injury of femoral vein at hip and thigh level, left leg MCC

S75.109 Unspecified injury of femoral vein at hip and thigh level, unspecified leg MCC UNS

S75.11 Minor laceration of femoral vein at hip and thigh level
Incomplete transection of femoral vein at hip and thigh level
Laceration of femoral vein at hip and thigh level NOS
Superficial laceration of femoral vein at hip and thigh level

S75.111 Minor laceration of femoral vein at hip and thigh level, right leg MCC

S75.112 Minor laceration of femoral vein at hip and thigh level, left leg MCC

S75.119 Minor laceration of femoral vein at hip and thigh level, unspecified leg MCC UNS

S75.12 Major laceration of femoral vein at hip and thigh level
Complete transection of femoral vein at hip and thigh level
Traumatic rupture of femoral vein at hip and thigh level

S75.121 Major laceration of femoral vein at hip and thigh level, right leg MCC

S75.122 Major laceration of femoral vein at hip and thigh level, left leg MCC

S75.129 Major laceration of femoral vein at hip and thigh level, unspecified leg MCC UNS

S75.19 Other specified injury of femoral vein at hip and thigh level

S75.191 Other specified injury of femoral vein at hip and thigh level, right leg MCC

S75.192 Other specified injury of femoral vein at hip and thigh level, left leg MCC

S75.199 Other specified injury of femoral vein at hip and thigh level, unspecified leg MCC UNS

S75.2 Injury of greater saphenous vein at hip and thigh level

EXCLUDES 1 *greater saphenous vein NOS (S85.3)*

S75.20 Unspecified injury of greater saphenous vein at hip and thigh level

S75.201 Unspecified injury of greater saphenous vein at hip and thigh level, right leg CC

S75.202 Unspecified injury of greater saphenous vein at hip and thigh level, left leg CC

S75.209 Unspecified injury of greater saphenous vein at hip and thigh level, unspecified leg CC UNS

S75.21 Minor laceration of greater saphenous vein at hip and thigh level
Incomplete transection of greater saphenous vein at hip and thigh level
Laceration of greater saphenous vein at hip and thigh level NOS
Superficial laceration of greater saphenous vein at hip and thigh level

S75.211 Minor laceration of greater saphenous vein at hip and thigh level, right leg CC

S75.212 Minor laceration of greater saphenous vein at hip and thigh level, left leg CC

S75.219 Minor laceration of greater saphenous vein at hip and thigh level, unspecified leg CC UNS

S75.22 Major laceration of greater saphenous vein at hip and thigh level
Complete transection of greater saphenous vein at hip and thigh level
Traumatic rupture of greater saphenous vein at hip and thigh level

S75.221 Major laceration of greater saphenous vein at hip and thigh level, right leg CC

S75.222 Major laceration of greater saphenous vein at hip and thigh level, left leg CC

S75.229 Major laceration of greater saphenous vein at hip and thigh level, unspecified leg CC UNS

S75.29 Other specified injury of greater saphenous vein at hip and thigh level
S75.291 Other specified injury of greater saphenous vein at hip and thigh level, right leg CC
S75.292 Other specified injury of greater saphenous vein at hip and thigh level, left leg CC
S75.299 Other specified injury of greater saphenous vein at hip and thigh level, unspecified leg CC UNS
S75.8 Injury of other blood vessels at hip and thigh level
S75.80 Unspecified injury of other blood vessels at hip and thigh level
S75.801 Unspecified injury of other blood vessels at hip and thigh level, right leg CC
S75.802 Unspecified injury of other blood vessels at hip and thigh level, left leg CC
S75.809 Unspecified injury of other blood vessels at hip and thigh level, unspecified leg CC UNS
S75.81 Laceration of other blood vessels at hip and thigh level
S75.811 Laceration of other blood vessels at hip and thigh level, right leg CC
S75.812 Laceration of other blood vessels at hip and thigh level, left leg CC
S75.819 Laceration of other blood vessels at hip and thigh level, unspecified leg CC UNS
S75.89 Other specified injury of other blood vessels at hip and thigh level
S75.891 Other specified injury of other blood vessels at hip and thigh level, right leg CC
S75.892 Other specified injury of other blood vessels at hip and thigh level, left leg CC
S75.899 Other specified injury of other blood vessels at hip and thigh level, unspecified leg CC UNS
S75.9 Injury of unspecified blood vessel at hip and thigh level
S75.90 Unspecified injury of unspecified blood vessel at hip and thigh level
S75.901 Unspecified injury of unspecified blood vessel at hip and thigh level, right leg CC
S75.902 Unspecified injury of unspecified blood vessel at hip and thigh level, left leg CC
S75.909 Unspecified injury of unspecified blood vessel at hip and thigh level, unspecified leg CC UNS
S75.91 Laceration of unspecified blood vessel at hip and thigh level
S75.911 Laceration of unspecified blood vessel at hip and thigh level, right leg CC
S75.912 Laceration of unspecified blood vessel at hip and thigh level, left leg CC
S75.919 Laceration of unspecified blood vessel at hip and thigh level, unspecified leg CC UNS
S75.99 Other specified injury of unspecified blood vessel at hip and thigh level
S75.991 Other specified injury of unspecified blood vessel at hip and thigh level, right leg CC
S75.992 Other specified injury of unspecified blood vessel at hip and thigh level, left leg CC
S75.999 Other specified injury of unspecified blood vessel at hip and thigh level, unspecified leg CC UNS

S76 Injury of muscle, fascia and tendon at hip and thigh level
Code also any associated open wound (S71.-)
EXCLUDES 2 *injury of muscle, fascia and tendon at lower leg level (S86)*
sprain of joint and ligament of hip (S73.1)
TIP: Refer to the Muscle/Tendon table at the beginning of this chapter.

The appropriate 7th character is to be added to each code from category S76.
A initial encounter
D subsequent encounter
S sequela

S76.0 Injury of muscle, fascia and tendon of hip
S76.00 Unspecified injury of muscle, fascia and tendon of hip
S76.001 Unspecified injury of muscle, fascia and tendon of right hip
S76.002 Unspecified injury of muscle, fascia and tendon of left hip
S76.009 Unspecified injury of muscle, fascia and tendon of unspecified hip
S76.01 Strain of muscle, fascia and tendon of hip
S76.011 Strain of muscle, fascia and tendon of right hip
S76.012 Strain of muscle, fascia and tendon of left hip
S76.019 Strain of muscle, fascia and tendon of unspecified hip
S76.02 Laceration of muscle, fascia and tendon of hip
S76.021 Laceration of muscle, fascia and tendon of right hip CC
S76.022 Laceration of muscle, fascia and tendon of left hip CC
S76.029 Laceration of muscle, fascia and tendon of unspecified hip CC UNS
S76.09 Other specified injury of muscle, fascia and tendon of hip
S76.091 Other specified injury of muscle, fascia and tendon of right hip
S76.092 Other specified injury of muscle, fascia and tendon of left hip
S76.099 Other specified injury of muscle, fascia and tendon of unspecified hip
S76.1 Injury of quadriceps muscle, fascia and tendon
Injury of patellar ligament (tendon)
S76.10 Unspecified injury of quadriceps muscle, fascia and tendon
S76.101 Unspecified injury of right quadriceps muscle, fascia and tendon
S76.102 Unspecified injury of left quadriceps muscle, fascia and tendon
S76.109 Unspecified injury of unspecified quadriceps muscle, fascia and tendon
S76.11 Strain of quadriceps muscle, fascia and tendon
S76.111 Strain of right quadriceps muscle, fascia and tendon
S76.112 Strain of left quadriceps muscle, fascia and tendon
S76.119 Strain of unspecified quadriceps muscle, fascia and tendon
S76.12 Laceration of quadriceps muscle, fascia and tendon
S76.121 Laceration of right quadriceps muscle, fascia and tendon CC
S76.122 Laceration of left quadriceps muscle, fascia and tendon CC
S76.129 Laceration of unspecified quadriceps muscle, fascia and tendon CC UNS
S76.19 Other specified injury of quadriceps muscle, fascia and tendon
S76.191 Other specified injury of right quadriceps muscle, fascia and tendon
S76.192 Other specified injury of left quadriceps muscle, fascia and tendon
S76.199 Other specified injury of unspecified quadriceps muscle, fascia and tendon
S76.2 Injury of adductor muscle, fascia and tendon of thigh
S76.20 Unspecified injury of adductor muscle, fascia and tendon of thigh
S76.201 Unspecified injury of adductor muscle, fascia and tendon of right thigh

√7th **S76.202** Unspecified injury of adductor muscle, fascia and tendon of left thigh

√7th **S76.209** Unspecified injury of adductor muscle, fascia and tendon of unspecified thigh

√6th **S76.21** Strain of adductor muscle, fascia and tendon of thigh

√7th **S76.211** Strain of adductor muscle, fascia and tendon of right thigh

√7th **S76.212** Strain of adductor muscle, fascia and tendon of left thigh

√7th **S76.219** Strain of adductor muscle, fascia and tendon of unspecified thigh

√6th **S76.22** Laceration of adductor muscle, fascia and tendon of thigh

√7th **S76.221** Laceration of adductor muscle, fascia and tendon of right thigh CC

√7th **S76.222** Laceration of adductor muscle, fascia and tendon of left thigh CC

√7th **S76.229** Laceration of adductor muscle, fascia and tendon of unspecified thigh CC UNS

√6th **S76.29** Other injury of adductor muscle, fascia and tendon of thigh

√7th **S76.291** Other injury of adductor muscle, fascia and tendon of right thigh

√7th **S76.292** Other injury of adductor muscle, fascia and tendon of left thigh

√7th **S76.299** Other injury of adductor muscle, fascia and tendon of unspecified thigh

√5th **S76.3** Injury of muscle, fascia and tendon of the posterior muscle group at thigh level

√6th **S76.30** Unspecified injury of muscle, fascia and tendon of the posterior muscle group at thigh level

√7th **S76.301** Unspecified injury of muscle, fascia and tendon of the posterior muscle group at thigh level, right thigh

√7th **S76.302** Unspecified injury of muscle, fascia and tendon of the posterior muscle group at thigh level, left thigh

√7th **S76.309** Unspecified injury of muscle, fascia and tendon of the posterior muscle group at thigh level, unspecified thigh

√6th **S76.31** Strain of muscle, fascia and tendon of the posterior muscle group at thigh level

√7th **S76.311** Strain of muscle, fascia and tendon of the posterior muscle group at thigh level, right thigh

√7th **S76.312** Strain of muscle, fascia and tendon of the posterior muscle group at thigh level, left thigh

√7th **S76.319** Strain of muscle, fascia and tendon of the posterior muscle group at thigh level, unspecified thigh

√6th **S76.32** Laceration of muscle, fascia and tendon of the posterior muscle group at thigh level

√7th **S76.321** Laceration of muscle, fascia and tendon of the posterior muscle group at thigh level, right thigh CC

√7th **S76.322** Laceration of muscle, fascia and tendon of the posterior muscle group at thigh level, left thigh CC

√7th **S76.329** Laceration of muscle, fascia and tendon of the posterior muscle group at thigh level, unspecified thigh CC UNS

√6th **S76.39** Other specified injury of muscle, fascia and tendon of the posterior muscle group at thigh level

√7th **S76.391** Other specified injury of muscle, fascia and tendon of the posterior muscle group at thigh level, right thigh

√7th **S76.392** Other specified injury of muscle, fascia and tendon of the posterior muscle group at thigh level, left thigh

√7th **S76.399** Other specified injury of muscle, fascia and tendon of the posterior muscle group at thigh level, unspecified thigh

√5th **S76.8** Injury of other specified muscles, fascia and tendons at thigh level

√6th **S76.80** Unspecified injury of other specified muscles, fascia and tendons at thigh level

√7th **S76.801** Unspecified injury of other specified muscles, fascia and tendons at thigh level, right thigh

√7th **S76.802** Unspecified injury of other specified muscles, fascia and tendons at thigh level, left thigh

√7th **S76.809** Unspecified injury of other specified muscles, fascia and tendons at thigh level, unspecified thigh

√6th **S76.81** Strain of other specified muscles, fascia and tendons at thigh level

√7th **S76.811** Strain of other specified muscles, fascia and tendons at thigh level, right thigh

√7th **S76.812** Strain of other specified muscles, fascia and tendons at thigh level, left thigh

√7th **S76.819** Strain of other specified muscles, fascia and tendons at thigh level, unspecified thigh

√6th **S76.82** Laceration of other specified muscles, fascia and tendons at thigh level

√7th **S76.821** Laceration of other specified muscles, fascia and tendons at thigh level, right thigh CC

√7th **S76.822** Laceration of other specified muscles, fascia and tendons at thigh level, left thigh CC

√7th **S76.829** Laceration of other specified muscles, fascia and tendons at thigh level, unspecified thigh CC UNS

√6th **S76.89** Other injury of other specified muscles, fascia and tendons at thigh level

√7th **S76.891** Other injury of other specified muscles, fascia and tendons at thigh level, right thigh

√7th **S76.892** Other injury of other specified muscles, fascia and tendons at thigh level, left thigh

√7th **S76.899** Other injury of other specified muscles, fascia and tendons at thigh level, unspecified thigh

√5th **S76.9** Injury of unspecified muscles, fascia and tendons at thigh level

√6th **S76.90** Unspecified injury of unspecified muscles, fascia and tendons at thigh level

√7th **S76.901** Unspecified injury of unspecified muscles, fascia and tendons at thigh level, right thigh

√7th **S76.902** Unspecified injury of unspecified muscles, fascia and tendons at thigh level, left thigh

√7th **S76.909** Unspecified injury of unspecified muscles, fascia and tendons at thigh level, unspecified thigh

√6th **S76.91** Strain of unspecified muscles, fascia and tendons at thigh level

√7th **S76.911** Strain of unspecified muscles, fascia and tendons at thigh level, right thigh

√7th **S76.912** Strain of unspecified muscles, fascia and tendons at thigh level, left thigh

√7th **S76.919** Strain of unspecified muscles, fascia and tendons at thigh level, unspecified thigh

√6th **S76.92** Laceration of unspecified muscles, fascia and tendons at thigh level

√7th **S76.921** Laceration of unspecified muscles, fascia and tendons at thigh level, right thigh CC

√7th **S76.922** Laceration of unspecified muscles, fascia and tendons at thigh level, left thigh CC

√7th **S76.929** Laceration of unspecified muscles, fascia and tendons at thigh level, unspecified thigh CC UNS

√6th **S76.99** Other specified injury of unspecified muscles, fascia and tendons at thigh level

√7th **S76.991** Other specified injury of unspecified muscles, fascia and tendons at thigh level, right thigh

√7th **S76.992** Other specified injury of unspecified muscles, fascia and tendons at thigh level, left thigh

√7th **S76.999** Other specified injury of unspecified muscles, fascia and tendons at thigh level, unspecified thigh

S77 Crushing injury of hip and thigh

Use additional code(s) for all associated injuries

EXCLUDES 2 *crushing injury of ankle and foot (S97.-)*
crushing injury of lower leg (S87.-)

The appropriate 7th character is to be added to each code from category S77.
A initial encounter
D subsequent encounter
S sequela

S77.0 Crushing injury of hip
- **S77.00 Crushing injury of unspecified hip** CC H5 UNS
- **S77.01 Crushing injury of right hip** CC H5
- **S77.02 Crushing injury of left hip** CC H5

S77.1 Crushing injury of thigh
- **S77.10 Crushing injury of unspecified thigh** CC H5 UNS
- **S77.11 Crushing injury of right thigh** CC H5
- **S77.12 Crushing injury of left thigh** CC H5

S77.2 Crushing injury of hip with thigh
- **S77.20 Crushing injury of unspecified hip with thigh**
- **S77.21 Crushing injury of right hip with thigh**
- **S77.22 Crushing injury of left hip with thigh**

S78 Traumatic amputation of hip and thigh

An amputation not identified as partial or complete should be coded to complete

EXCLUDES 1 *traumatic amputation of knee (S88.0-)*

The appropriate 7th character is to be added to each code from category S78.
A initial encounter
D subsequent encounter
S sequela

S78.0 Traumatic amputation at hip joint

S78.01 Complete traumatic amputation at hip joint
- **S78.011 Complete traumatic amputation at right hip joint** CC HCC
- **S78.012 Complete traumatic amputation at left hip joint** CC HCC
- **S78.019 Complete traumatic amputation at unspecified hip joint** CC UNS HCC

S78.02 Partial traumatic amputation at hip joint
- **S78.021 Partial traumatic amputation at right hip joint** CC HCC
- **S78.022 Partial traumatic amputation at left hip joint** CC HCC
- **S78.029 Partial traumatic amputation at unspecified hip joint** CC UNS HCC

S78.1 Traumatic amputation at level between hip and knee

EXCLUDES 1 *traumatic amputation of knee (S88.0-)*

S78.11 Complete traumatic amputation at level between hip and knee
- **S78.111 Complete traumatic amputation at level between right hip and knee** CC HCC
- **S78.112 Complete traumatic amputation at level between left hip and knee** CC HCC
- **S78.119 Complete traumatic amputation at level between unspecified hip and knee** CC UNS HCC

S78.12 Partial traumatic amputation at level between hip and knee
- **S78.121 Partial traumatic amputation at level between right hip and knee** CC HCC
- **S78.122 Partial traumatic amputation at level between left hip and knee** CC HCC
- **S78.129 Partial traumatic amputation at level between unspecified hip and knee** CC UNS HCC

S78.9 Traumatic amputation of hip and thigh, level unspecified

S78.91 Complete traumatic amputation of hip and thigh, level unspecified
- **S78.911 Complete traumatic amputation of right hip and thigh, level unspecified** CC HCC
- **S78.912 Complete traumatic amputation of left hip and thigh, level unspecified** CC HCC
- **S78.919 Complete traumatic amputation of unspecified hip and thigh, level unspecified** CC UNS HCC

S78.92 Partial traumatic amputation of hip and thigh, level unspecified
- **S78.921 Partial traumatic amputation of right hip and thigh, level unspecified** CC HCC
- **S78.922 Partial traumatic amputation of left hip and thigh, level unspecified** CC HCC
- **S78.929 Partial traumatic amputation of unspecified hip and thigh, level unspecified** CC UNS HCC

S79 Other and unspecified injuries of hip and thigh

NOTE A fracture not indicated as open or closed should be coded to closed

AHA: 2018,2Q,12; 2018,1Q,3; 2015,3Q,37-39

The appropriate 7th character is to be added to each code from subcategories S79.0 and S79.1.
A initial encounter for closed fracture
D subsequent encounter for fracture with routine healing
G subsequent encounter for fracture with delayed healing
K subsequent encounter for fracture with nonunion
P subsequent encounter for fracture with malunion
S sequela

S79.0 Physeal fracture of upper end of femur

EXCLUDES 1 *apophyseal fracture of upper end of femur (S72.13-)*
nontraumatic slipped upper femoral epiphysis (M93.0-)

AHA: 2019,4Q,56

S79.00 Unspecified physeal fracture of upper end of femur
- 4,6 **S79.001 Unspecified physeal fracture of upper end of right femur** MCC CC H5 HCC
- 4,6 **S79.002 Unspecified physeal fracture of upper end of left femur** MCC CC H5 HCC
- 4,6 **S79.009 Unspecified physeal fracture of upper end of unspecified femur** MCC CC H5 UNS HCC

S79.01 Salter-Harris Type I physeal fracture of upper end of femur

Acute on chronic slipped capital femoral epiphysis (traumatic)
Acute slipped capital femoral epiphysis (traumatic)
Capital femoral epiphyseal fracture

EXCLUDES 1 *chronic slipped upper femoral epiphysis (nontraumatic) (M93.02-)*

- 4,6 **S79.011 Salter-Harris Type I physeal fracture of upper end of right femur** MCC CC H5 HCC
- 4,6 **S79.012 Salter-Harris Type I physeal fracture of upper end of left femur** MCC CC H5 HCC
- 4,6 **S79.019 Salter-Harris Type I physeal fracture of upper end of unspecified femur** MCC CC H5 UNS HCC

S79.09 Other physeal fracture of upper end of femur
- 4,6 **S79.091 Other physeal fracture of upper end of right femur** MCC CC H5 HCC
- 4,6 **S79.092 Other physeal fracture of upper end of left femur** MCC CC H5 HCC
- 4,6 **S79.099 Other physeal fracture of upper end of unspecified femur** MCC CC H5 UNS HCC

S79.1 Physeal fracture of lower end of femur

AHA: 2019,4Q,56

S79.10 Unspecified physeal fracture of lower end of femur
- 3,6 **S79.101 Unspecified physeal fracture of lower end of right femur** CC H5 HCC
- 3,6 **S79.102 Unspecified physeal fracture of lower end of left femur** CC H5 HCC
- 3,6 **S79.109 Unspecified physeal fracture of lower end of unspecified femur** CC H5 UNS HCC

S79.11 Salter-Harris Type I physeal fracture of lower end of femur
- 3,6 **S79.111 Salter-Harris Type I physeal fracture of lower end of right femur** CC H5 HCC
- 3,6 **S79.112 Salter-Harris Type I physeal fracture of lower end of left femur** CC H5 HCC
- 3,6 **S79.119 Salter-Harris Type I physeal fracture of lower end of unspecified femur** CC H5 UNS HCC

S79.12 Salter-Harris Type II physeal fracture of lower end of femur
- 3,6 S79.121 Salter-Harris Type II physeal fracture of lower end of right femur CC HS HCC
- 3,6 S79.122 Salter-Harris Type II physeal fracture of lower end of left femur CC HS HCC
- 3,6 S79.129 Salter-Harris Type II physeal fracture of lower end of unspecified femur CC HS UNS HCC

S79.13 Salter-Harris Type III physeal fracture of lower end of femur
- 3,6 S79.131 Salter-Harris Type III physeal fracture of lower end of right femur CC HS HCC
- 3,6 S79.132 Salter-Harris Type III physeal fracture of lower end of left femur CC HS HCC
- 3,6 S79.139 Salter-Harris Type III physeal fracture of lower end of unspecified femur CC HS UNS HCC

S79.14 Salter-Harris Type IV physeal fracture of lower end of femur
- 3,6 S79.141 Salter-Harris Type IV physeal fracture of lower end of right femur CC HS HCC
- 3,6 S79.142 Salter-Harris Type IV physeal fracture of lower end of left femur CC HS HCC
- 3,6 S79.149 Salter-Harris Type IV physeal fracture of lower end of unspecified femur CC HS UNS HCC

S79.19 Other physeal fracture of lower end of femur
- 3,6 S79.191 Other physeal fracture of lower end of right femur CC HS HCC
- 3,6 S79.192 Other physeal fracture of lower end of left femur CC HS HCC
- 3,6 S79.199 Other physeal fracture of lower end of unspecified femur CC HS UNS HCC

S79.8 Other specified injuries of hip and thigh

The appropriate 7th character is to be added to each code in subcategory S79.8.
A initial encounter
D subsequent encounter
S sequela

S79.81 Other specified injuries of hip
- S79.811 Other specified injuries of right hip
- S79.812 Other specified injuries of left hip
- S79.819 Other specified injuries of unspecified hip

S79.82 Other specified injuries of thigh
- S79.821 Other specified injuries of right thigh
- S79.822 Other specified injuries of left thigh
- S79.829 Other specified injuries of unspecified thigh

S79.9 Unspecified injury of hip and thigh

The appropriate 7th character is to be added to each code in subcategory S79.9.
A initial encounter
D subsequent encounter
S sequela

S79.91 Unspecified injury of hip
- S79.911 Unspecified injury of right hip
- S79.912 Unspecified injury of left hip
- S79.919 Unspecified injury of unspecified hip

S79.92 Unspecified injury of thigh
- S79.921 Unspecified injury of right thigh
- S79.922 Unspecified injury of left thigh
- S79.929 Unspecified injury of unspecified thigh

Injuries to the knee and lower leg (S80-S89)

EXCLUDES 2 *burns and corrosions (T20-T32)*
frostbite (T33-T34)
injuries of ankle and foot, except fracture of ankle and malleolus (S90-S99)
insect bite or sting, venomous (T63.4)

S80 Superficial injury of knee and lower leg

EXCLUDES 2 *superficial injury of ankle and foot (S90.-)*

The appropriate 7th character is to be added to each code from category S80.
A initial encounter
D subsequent encounter
S sequela

S80.0 Contusion of knee
- S80.00 Contusion of unspecified knee
- S80.01 Contusion of right knee
- S80.02 Contusion of left knee

S80.1 Contusion of lower leg
- S80.10 Contusion of unspecified lower leg
- S80.11 Contusion of right lower leg
- S80.12 Contusion of left lower leg

S80.2 Other superficial injuries of knee

S80.21 Abrasion of knee
- S80.211 Abrasion, right knee
- S80.212 Abrasion, left knee
- S80.219 Abrasion, unspecified knee

S80.22 Blister (nonthermal) of knee
- S80.221 Blister (nonthermal), right knee
- S80.222 Blister (nonthermal), left knee
- S80.229 Blister (nonthermal), unspecified knee

S80.24 External constriction of knee
- S80.241 External constriction, right knee
- S80.242 External constriction, left knee
- S80.249 External constriction, unspecified knee

S80.25 Superficial foreign body of knee
Splinter in the knee
- S80.251 Superficial foreign body, right knee
- S80.252 Superficial foreign body, left knee
- S80.259 Superficial foreign body, unspecified knee

S80.26 Insect bite (nonvenomous) of knee
- S80.261 Insect bite (nonvenomous), right knee
- S80.262 Insect bite (nonvenomous), left knee
- S80.269 Insect bite (nonvenomous), unspecified knee

S80.27 Other superficial bite of knee
EXCLUDES 1 *open bite of knee (S81.05-)*
- S80.271 Other superficial bite of right knee
- S80.272 Other superficial bite of left knee
- S80.279 Other superficial bite of unspecified knee

S80.8 Other superficial injuries of lower leg

S80.81 Abrasion of lower leg
- S80.811 Abrasion, right lower leg
- S80.812 Abrasion, left lower leg
- S80.819 Abrasion, unspecified lower leg

S80.82 Blister (nonthermal) of lower leg
- S80.821 Blister (nonthermal), right lower leg
- S80.822 Blister (nonthermal), left lower leg
- S80.829 Blister (nonthermal), unspecified lower leg

S80.84 External constriction of lower leg
- S80.841 External constriction, right lower leg
- S80.842 External constriction, left lower leg
- S80.849 External constriction, unspecified lower leg

S80.85 Superficial foreign body of lower leg
Splinter in the lower leg
- S80.851 Superficial foreign body, right lower leg

S80.852 Superficial foreign body, left lower leg
S80.859 Superficial foreign body, unspecified lower leg
S80.86 Insect bite (nonvenomous) of lower leg
S80.861 Insect bite (nonvenomous), right lower leg
S80.862 Insect bite (nonvenomous), left lower leg
S80.869 Insect bite (nonvenomous), unspecified lower leg
S80.87 Other superficial bite of lower leg
EXCLUDES 1 *open bite of lower leg (S81.85-)*
S80.871 Other superficial bite, right lower leg
S80.872 Other superficial bite, left lower leg
S80.879 Other superficial bite, unspecified lower leg
S80.9 Unspecified superficial injury of knee and lower leg
S80.91 Unspecified superficial injury of knee
S80.911 Unspecified superficial injury of right knee
S80.912 Unspecified superficial injury of left knee
S80.919 Unspecified superficial injury of unspecified knee
S80.92 Unspecified superficial injury of lower leg
S80.921 Unspecified superficial injury of right lower leg
S80.922 Unspecified superficial injury of left lower leg
S80.929 Unspecified superficial injury of unspecified lower leg

S81 Open wound of knee and lower leg

Code also any associated wound infection

EXCLUDES 1 *open fracture of knee and lower leg (S82.-)*
traumatic amputation of lower leg (S88.-)

EXCLUDES 2 *open wound of ankle and foot (S91.-)*

The appropriate 7th character is to be added to each code from category S81.
A initial encounter
D subsequent encounter
S sequela

S81.0 Open wound of knee
S81.00 Unspecified open wound of knee
S81.001 Unspecified open wound, right knee
S81.002 Unspecified open wound, left knee
S81.009 Unspecified open wound, unspecified knee
S81.01 Laceration without foreign body of knee
S81.011 Laceration without foreign body, right knee
S81.012 Laceration without foreign body, left knee
S81.019 Laceration without foreign body, unspecified knee
S81.02 Laceration with foreign body of knee
S81.021 Laceration with foreign body, right knee
S81.022 Laceration with foreign body, left knee
S81.029 Laceration with foreign body, unspecified knee
S81.03 Puncture wound without foreign body of knee
S81.031 Puncture wound without foreign body, right knee
S81.032 Puncture wound without foreign body, left knee
S81.039 Puncture wound without foreign body, unspecified knee
S81.04 Puncture wound with foreign body of knee
S81.041 Puncture wound with foreign body, right knee
S81.042 Puncture wound with foreign body, left knee
S81.049 Puncture wound with foreign body, unspecified knee
S81.05 Open bite of knee
Bite of knee NOS
EXCLUDES 1 *superficial bite of knee (S80.27-)*
S81.051 Open bite, right knee
S81.052 Open bite, left knee
S81.059 Open bite, unspecified knee
S81.8 Open wound of lower leg
S81.80 Unspecified open wound of lower leg
AHA: 2016,3Q,24
S81.801 Unspecified open wound, right lower leg
S81.802 Unspecified open wound, left lower leg
S81.809 Unspecified open wound, unspecified lower leg
S81.81 Laceration without foreign body of lower leg
S81.811 Laceration without foreign body, right lower leg
S81.812 Laceration without foreign body, left lower leg
S81.819 Laceration without foreign body, unspecified lower leg
S81.82 Laceration with foreign body of lower leg
S81.821 Laceration with foreign body, right lower leg
S81.822 Laceration with foreign body, left lower leg
S81.829 Laceration with foreign body, unspecified lower leg
S81.83 Puncture wound without foreign body of lower leg
AHA: 2016,3Q,24
S81.831 Puncture wound without foreign body, right lower leg
S81.832 Puncture wound without foreign body, left lower leg
S81.839 Puncture wound without foreign body, unspecified lower leg
S81.84 Puncture wound with foreign body of lower leg
AHA: 2016,3Q,24
S81.841 Puncture wound with foreign body, right lower leg
S81.842 Puncture wound with foreign body, left lower leg
S81.849 Puncture wound with foreign body, unspecified lower leg
S81.85 Open bite of lower leg
Bite of lower leg NOS
EXCLUDES 1 *superficial bite of lower leg (S80.86-, S80.87-)*
S81.851 Open bite, right lower leg
S81.852 Open bite, left lower leg
S81.859 Open bite, unspecified lower leg

4th S82 Fracture of lower leg, including ankle

NOTE A fracture not indicated as displaced or nondisplaced should be coded to displaced

A fracture not indicated as open or closed should be coded to closed

The open fracture designations are based on the Gustilo open fracture classification.

INCLUDES fracture of malleolus

EXCLUDES 1 *traumatic amputation of lower leg (S88.-)*

EXCLUDES 2 *fracture of foot, except ankle (S92.-)*

periprosthetic fracture around internal prosthetic implant of knee joint (M97.1-)

AHA: 2018,2Q,12; 2016,1Q,33; 2015,3Q,37-39

DEF: Diaphysis: Central shaft of a long bone.

DEF: Epiphysis: Proximal and distal rounded ends of a long bone, communicates with the joint.

DEF: Metaphysis: Section of a long bone located between the epiphysis and diaphysis at the proximal and distal ends.

DEF: Physis (growth plate): Narrow zone of cartilaginous tissue between the epiphysis and metaphysis at each end of a long bone. In childhood, proliferation of cells in this zone lengthens the bone. As the bone matures, this area thins, ossification eventually fusing into solid bone and growth stops. ***Synonym(s):** Epiphyseal plate.*

The appropriate 7th character is to be added to all codes from category S82 [unless otherwise indicated].

A	initial encounter for closed fracture
B	initial encounter for open fracture type I or II
	initial encounter for open fracture NOS
C	initial encounter for open fracture type IIIA, IIIB, or IIIC
D	subsequent encounter for closed fracture with routine healing
E	subsequent encounter for open fracture type I or II with routine healing
F	subsequent encounter for open fracture type IIIA, IIIB, or IIIC with routine healing
G	subsequent encounter for closed fracture with delayed healing
H	subsequent encounter for open fracture type I or II with delayed healing
J	subsequent encounter for open fracture type IIIA, IIIB, or IIIC with delayed healing
K	subsequent encounter for closed fracture with nonunion
M	subsequent encounter for open fracture type I or II with nonunion
N	subsequent encounter for open fracture type IIIA, IIIB, or IIIC with nonunion
P	subsequent encounter for closed fracture with malunion
Q	subsequent encounter for open fracture type I or II with malunion
R	subsequent encounter for open fracture type IIIA, IIIB, or IIIC with malunion
S	sequela

5th S82.Ø Fracture of patella

Knee cap

6th S82.ØØ Unspecified fracture of patella

- 3 7th **S82.ØØ1 Unspecified fracture of right patella** CC HS
- 3 7th **S82.ØØ2 Unspecified fracture of left patella** CC HS
- 3 7th **S82.ØØ9 Unspecified fracture of unspecified patella** CC HS UNS

6th S82.Ø1 Osteochondral fracture of patella

- 3 7th **S82.Ø11 Displaced osteochondral fracture of right patella** CC HS
- 3 7th **S82.Ø12 Displaced osteochondral fracture of left patella** CC HS
- 3 7th **S82.Ø13 Displaced osteochondral fracture of unspecified patella** CC HS UNS
- 3 7th **S82.Ø14 Nondisplaced osteochondral fracture of right patella** CC HS
- 3 7th **S82.Ø15 Nondisplaced osteochondral fracture of left patella** CC HS
- 3 7th **S82.Ø16 Nondisplaced osteochondral fracture of unspecified patella** CC HS UNS

6th S82.Ø2 Longitudinal fracture of patella

- 3 7th **S82.Ø21 Displaced longitudinal fracture of right patella** CC HS
- 3 7th **S82.Ø22 Displaced longitudinal fracture of left patella** CC HS
- 3 7th **S82.Ø23 Displaced longitudinal fracture of unspecified patella** CC HS UNS
- 3 7th **S82.Ø24 Nondisplaced longitudinal fracture of right patella** CC HS
- 3 7th **S82.Ø25 Nondisplaced longitudinal fracture of left patella** CC HS
- 3 7th **S82.Ø26 Nondisplaced longitudinal fracture of unspecified patella** CC HS UNS

6th S82.Ø3 Transverse fracture of patella

- 3 7th **S82.Ø31 Displaced transverse fracture of right patella** CC HS
- 3 7th **S82.Ø32 Displaced transverse fracture of left patella** CC HS
- 3 7th **S82.Ø33 Displaced transverse fracture of unspecified patella** CC HS UNS
- 3 7th **S82.Ø34 Nondisplaced transverse fracture of right patella** CC HS
- 3 7th **S82.Ø35 Nondisplaced transverse fracture of left patella** CC HS
- 3 7th **S82.Ø36 Nondisplaced transverse fracture of unspecified patella** CC HS UNS

6th S82.Ø4 Comminuted fracture of patella

- 3 7th **S82.Ø41 Displaced comminuted fracture of right patella** CC HS
- 3 7th **S82.Ø42 Displaced comminuted fracture of left patella** CC HS
- 3 7th **S82.Ø43 Displaced comminuted fracture of unspecified patella** CC HS UNS
- 3 7th **S82.Ø44 Nondisplaced comminuted fracture of right patella** CC HS
- 3 7th **S82.Ø45 Nondisplaced comminuted fracture of left patella** CC HS
- 3 7th **S82.Ø46 Nondisplaced comminuted fracture of unspecified patella** CC HS UNS

6th S82.Ø9 Other fracture of patella

- 3 7th **S82.Ø91 Other fracture of right patella** CC HS
- 3 7th **S82.Ø92 Other fracture of left patella** CC HS
- 3 7th **S82.Ø99 Other fracture of unspecified patella** CC HS UNS

5th S82.1 Fracture of upper end of tibia

Fracture of proximal end of tibia

EXCLUDES 2 *fracture of shaft of tibia (S82.2-)*

physeal fracture of upper end of tibia (S89.Ø-)

6th S82.1Ø Unspecified fracture of upper end of tibia

- 2,3 7th **S82.1Ø1 Unspecified fracture of upper end of right tibia** MCC CC HS
- 2,3 7th **S82.1Ø2 Unspecified fracture of upper end of left tibia** MCC CC HS
- 2,3 7th **S82.1Ø9 Unspecified fracture of upper end of unspecified tibia** MCC CC HS UNS

6th S82.11 Fracture of tibial spine

- 2,3 7th **S82.111 Displaced fracture of right tibial spine** MCC CC HS
- 2,3 7th **S82.112 Displaced fracture of left tibial spine** MCC CC HS
- 2,3 7th **S82.113 Displaced fracture of unspecified tibial spine** MCC CC HS UNS
- 2,3 7th **S82.114 Nondisplaced fracture of right tibial spine** MCC CC HS
- 2,3 7th **S82.115 Nondisplaced fracture of left tibial spine** MCC CC HS
- 2,3 7th **S82.116 Nondisplaced fracture of unspecified tibial spine** MCC CC HS UNS

6th S82.12 Fracture of lateral condyle of tibia

- 2,3 7th **S82.121 Displaced fracture of lateral condyle of right tibia** MCC CC HS
- 2,3 7th **S82.122 Displaced fracture of lateral condyle of left tibia** MCC CC HS
- 2,3 7th **S82.123 Displaced fracture of lateral condyle of unspecified tibia** MCC CC HS UNS
- 2,3 7th **S82.124 Nondisplaced fracture of lateral condyle of right tibia** MCC CC HS
- 2,3 7th **S82.125 Nondisplaced fracture of lateral condyle of left tibia** MCC CC HS
- 2,3 7th **S82.126 Nondisplaced fracture of lateral condyle of unspecified tibia** MCC CC HS UNS

6th S82.13 Fracture of medial condyle of tibia

- 2,3 7th **S82.131 Displaced fracture of medial condyle of right tibia** MCC CC HS

2,3 ✓7th S82.132 Displaced fracture of medial condyle of left tibia MCC CC H5
2,3 ✓7th S82.133 Displaced fracture of medial condyle of unspecified tibia MCC CC H5 UNS
2,3 ✓7th S82.134 Nondisplaced fracture of medial condyle of right tibia MCC CC H5
2,3 ✓7th S82.135 Nondisplaced fracture of medial condyle of left tibia MCC CC H5
2,3 ✓7th S82.136 Nondisplaced fracture of medial condyle of unspecified tibia MCC CC H5 UNS
✓6th S82.14 Bicondylar fracture of tibia
Fracture of tibial plateau NOS
2,3 ✓7th S82.141 Displaced bicondylar fracture of right tibia MCC CC H5
2,3 ✓7th S82.142 Displaced bicondylar fracture of left tibia MCC CC H5
2,3 ✓7th S82.143 Displaced bicondylar fracture of unspecified tibia MCC CC H5 UNS
2,3 ✓7th S82.144 Nondisplaced bicondylar fracture of right tibia MCC CC H5
2,3 ✓7th S82.145 Nondisplaced bicondylar fracture of left tibia MCC CC H5
2,3 ✓7th S82.146 Nondisplaced bicondylar fracture of unspecified tibia MCC CC H5 UNS
✓6th S82.15 Fracture of tibial tuberosity
2,3 ✓7th S82.151 Displaced fracture of right tibial tuberosity MCC CC H5
2,3 ✓7th S82.152 Displaced fracture of left tibial tuberosity MCC CC H5
2,3 ✓7th S82.153 Displaced fracture of unspecified tibial tuberosity MCC CC H5 UNS
2,3 ✓7th S82.154 Nondisplaced fracture of right tibial tuberosity MCC CC H5
2,3 ✓7th S82.155 Nondisplaced fracture of left tibial tuberosity MCC CC H5
2,3 ✓7th S82.156 Nondisplaced fracture of unspecified tibial tuberosity MCC CC H5 UNS
✓6th S82.16 Torus fracture of upper end of tibia

The appropriate 7th character is to be added to all codes in subcategory S82.16.
A initial encounter for closed fracture
D subsequent encounter for fracture with routine healing
G subsequent encounter for fracture with delayed healing
K subsequent encounter for fracture with nonunion
P subsequent encounter for fracture with malunion
S sequela

3 ✓7th S82.161 Torus fracture of upper end of right tibia CC H5
3 ✓7th S82.162 Torus fracture of upper end of left tibia CC H5
3 ✓7th S82.169 Torus fracture of upper end of unspecified tibia CC H5 UNS
✓6th S82.19 Other fracture of upper end of tibia
2,3 ✓7th S82.191 Other fracture of upper end of right tibia MCC CC H5
2,3 ✓7th S82.192 Other fracture of upper end of left tibia MCC CC H5
2,3 ✓7th S82.199 Other fracture of upper end of unspecified tibia MCC CC H5 UNS
✓5th S82.2 Fracture of shaft of tibia
✓6th S82.20 Unspecified fracture of shaft of tibia
Fracture of tibia NOS
2,3 ✓7th S82.201 Unspecified fracture of shaft of right tibia MCC CC H5
2,3 ✓7th S82.202 Unspecified fracture of shaft of left tibia MCC CC H5
2,3 ✓7th S82.209 Unspecified fracture of shaft of unspecified tibia MCC CC H5 UNS
✓6th S82.22 Transverse fracture of shaft of tibia
2,3 ✓7th S82.221 Displaced transverse fracture of shaft of right tibia MCC CC H5
2,3 ✓7th S82.222 Displaced transverse fracture of shaft of left tibia MCC CC H5
2,3 ✓7th S82.223 Displaced transverse fracture of shaft of unspecified tibia MCC CC H5 UNS
2,3 ✓7th S82.224 Nondisplaced transverse fracture of shaft of right tibia MCC CC H5
2,3 ✓7th S82.225 Nondisplaced transverse fracture of shaft of left tibia MCC CC H5
2,3 ✓7th S82.226 Nondisplaced transverse fracture of shaft of unspecified tibia MCC CC H5 UNS
✓6th S82.23 Oblique fracture of shaft of tibia
2,3 ✓7th S82.231 Displaced oblique fracture of shaft of right tibia MCC CC H5
2,3 ✓7th S82.232 Displaced oblique fracture of shaft of left tibia MCC CC H5
2,3 ✓7th S82.233 Displaced oblique fracture of shaft of unspecified tibia MCC CC H5 UNS
2,3 ✓7th S82.234 Nondisplaced oblique fracture of shaft of right tibia MCC CC H5
2,3 ✓7th S82.235 Nondisplaced oblique fracture of shaft of left tibia MCC CC H5
2,3 ✓7th S82.236 Nondisplaced oblique fracture of shaft of unspecified tibia MCC CC H5 UNS
✓6th S82.24 Spiral fracture of shaft of tibia
Toddler fracture
2,3 ✓7th S82.241 Displaced spiral fracture of shaft of right tibia MCC CC H5
2,3 ✓7th S82.242 Displaced spiral fracture of shaft of left tibia MCC CC H5
2,3 ✓7th S82.243 Displaced spiral fracture of shaft of unspecified tibia MCC CC H5 UNS
2,3 ✓7th S82.244 Nondisplaced spiral fracture of shaft of right tibia MCC CC H5
2,3 ✓7th S82.245 Nondisplaced spiral fracture of shaft of left tibia MCC CC H5
2,3 ✓7th S82.246 Nondisplaced spiral fracture of shaft of unspecified tibia MCC CC H5 UNS
✓6th S82.25 Comminuted fracture of shaft of tibia
2,3 ✓7th S82.251 Displaced comminuted fracture of shaft of right tibia MCC CC H5
2,3 ✓7th S82.252 Displaced comminuted fracture of shaft of left tibia MCC CC H5
2,3 ✓7th S82.253 Displaced comminuted fracture of shaft of unspecified tibia MCC CC H5 UNS
2,3 ✓7th S82.254 Nondisplaced comminuted fracture of shaft of right tibia MCC CC H5
2,3 ✓7th S82.255 Nondisplaced comminuted fracture of shaft of left tibia MCC CC H5
2,3 ✓7th S82.256 Nondisplaced comminuted fracture of shaft of unspecified tibia MCC CC H5 UNS
✓6th S82.26 Segmental fracture of shaft of tibia
2,3 ✓7th S82.261 Displaced segmental fracture of shaft of right tibia MCC CC H5
2,3 ✓7th S82.262 Displaced segmental fracture of shaft of left tibia MCC CC H5
2,3 ✓7th S82.263 Displaced segmental fracture of shaft of unspecified tibia MCC CC H5 UNS
2,3 ✓7th S82.264 Nondisplaced segmental fracture of shaft of right tibia MCC CC H5
2,3 ✓7th S82.265 Nondisplaced segmental fracture of shaft of left tibia MCC CC H5
2,3 ✓7th S82.266 Nondisplaced segmental fracture of shaft of unspecified tibia MCC CC H5 UNS
✓6th S82.29 Other fracture of shaft of tibia
2,3 ✓7th S82.291 Other fracture of shaft of right tibia MCC CC H5
2,3 ✓7th S82.292 Other fracture of shaft of left tibia MCC CC H5
2,3 ✓7th S82.299 Other fracture of shaft of unspecified tibia MCC CC H5 UNS
✓5th S82.3 Fracture of lower end of tibia
EXCLUDES 1 *bimalleolar fracture of lower leg (S82.84-)*
fracture of medial malleolus alone (S82.5-)
Maisonneuve's fracture (S82.86-)
pilon fracture of distal tibia (S82.87-)
trimalleolar fractures of lower leg (S82.85-)
✓6th S82.30 Unspecified fracture of lower end of tibia
3 ✓7th S82.301 Unspecified fracture of lower end of right tibia CC H5

3 √7th **S82.302 Unspecified fracture of lower end of left tibia** CC H5

3 √7th **S82.309 Unspecified fracture of lower end of unspecified tibia** CC H5 UNS

√6th **S82.31 Torus fracture of lower end of tibia**

The appropriate 7th character is to be added to all codes in subcategory S82.31.
A initial encounter for closed fracture
D subsequent encounter for fracture with routine healing
G subsequent encounter for fracture with delayed healing
K subsequent encounter for fracture with nonunion
P subsequent encounter for fracture with malunion
S sequela

3 √7th **S82.311 Torus fracture of lower end of right tibia** CC H5

3 √7th **S82.312 Torus fracture of lower end of left tibia** CC H5

3 √7th **S82.319 Torus fracture of lower end of unspecified tibia** CC H5 UNS

√6th **S82.39 Other fracture of lower end of tibia**

AHA: 2015,1Q,25

3 √7th **S82.391 Other fracture of lower end of right tibia** CC H5

3 √7th **S82.392 Other fracture of lower end of left tibia** CC H5

3 √7th **S82.399 Other fracture of lower end of unspecified tibia** CC H5 UNS

√5th **S82.4 Fracture of shaft of fibula**

EXCLUDES 2 *fracture of lateral malleolus alone (S82.6-)*

√6th **S82.40 Unspecified fracture of shaft of fibula**

2,4 √7th **S82.401 Unspecified fracture of shaft of right fibula** MCC CC H5

2,4 √7th **S82.402 Unspecified fracture of shaft of left fibula** MCC CC H5

2,4 √7th **S82.409 Unspecified fracture of shaft of unspecified fibula** MCC CC H5 UNS

√6th **S82.42 Transverse fracture of shaft of fibula**

2,4 √7th **S82.421 Displaced transverse fracture of shaft of right fibula** MCC CC H5

2,4 √7th **S82.422 Displaced transverse fracture of shaft of left fibula** MCC CC H5

2,4 √7th **S82.423 Displaced transverse fracture of shaft of unspecified fibula** MCC CC H5 UNS

2,4 √7th **S82.424 Nondisplaced transverse fracture of shaft of right fibula** MCC CC H5

2,4 √7th **S82.425 Nondisplaced transverse fracture of shaft of left fibula** MCC CC H5

2,4 √7th **S82.426 Nondisplaced transverse fracture of shaft of unspecified fibula** MCC CC H5 UNS

√6th **S82.43 Oblique fracture of shaft of fibula**

2,4 √7th **S82.431 Displaced oblique fracture of shaft of right fibula** MCC CC H5

2,4 √7th **S82.432 Displaced oblique fracture of shaft of left fibula** MCC CC H5

2,4 √7th **S82.433 Displaced oblique fracture of shaft of unspecified fibula** MCC CC H5 UNS

2,4 √7th **S82.434 Nondisplaced oblique fracture of shaft of right fibula** MCC CC H5

2,4 √7th **S82.435 Nondisplaced oblique fracture of shaft of left fibula** MCC CC H5

2,4 √7th **S82.436 Nondisplaced oblique fracture of shaft of unspecified fibula** MCC CC H5 UNS

√6th **S82.44 Spiral fracture of shaft of fibula**

2,4 √7th **S82.441 Displaced spiral fracture of shaft of right fibula** MCC CC H5

2,4 √7th **S82.442 Displaced spiral fracture of shaft of left fibula** MCC CC H5

2,4 √7th **S82.443 Displaced spiral fracture of shaft of unspecified fibula** MCC CC H5 UNS

2,4 √7th **S82.444 Nondisplaced spiral fracture of shaft of right fibula** MCC CC H5

2,4 √7th **S82.445 Nondisplaced spiral fracture of shaft of left fibula** MCC CC H5

2,4 √7th **S82.446 Nondisplaced spiral fracture of shaft of unspecified fibula** MCC CC H5 UNS

√6th **S82.45 Comminuted fracture of shaft of fibula**

2,4 √7th **S82.451 Displaced comminuted fracture of shaft of right fibula** MCC CC H5

2,4 √7th **S82.452 Displaced comminuted fracture of shaft of left fibula** MCC CC H5

2,4 √7th **S82.453 Displaced comminuted fracture of shaft of unspecified fibula** MCC CC H5 UNS

2,4 √7th **S82.454 Nondisplaced comminuted fracture of shaft of right fibula** MCC CC H5

2,4 √7th **S82.455 Nondisplaced comminuted fracture of shaft of left fibula** MCC CC H5

2,4 √7th **S82.456 Nondisplaced comminuted fracture of shaft of unspecified fibula** MCC CC H5 UNS

√6th **S82.46 Segmental fracture of shaft of fibula**

2,4 √7th **S82.461 Displaced segmental fracture of shaft of right fibula** MCC CC H5

2,4 √7th **S82.462 Displaced segmental fracture of shaft of left fibula** MCC CC H5

2,4 √7th **S82.463 Displaced segmental fracture of shaft of unspecified fibula** MCC CC H5 UNS

2,4 √7th **S82.464 Nondisplaced segmental fracture of shaft of right fibula** MCC CC H5

2,4 √7th **S82.465 Nondisplaced segmental fracture of shaft of left fibula** MCC CC H5

2,4 √7th **S82.466 Nondisplaced segmental fracture of shaft of unspecified fibula** MCC CC H5 UNS

√6th **S82.49 Other fracture of shaft of fibula**

2,4 √7th **S82.491 Other fracture of shaft of right fibula** MCC CC H5

2,4 √7th **S82.492 Other fracture of shaft of left fibula** MCC CC H5

2,4 √7th **S82.499 Other fracture of shaft of unspecified fibula** MCC CC H5 UNS

√5th **S82.5 Fracture of medial malleolus**

EXCLUDES 1 *pilon fracture of distal tibia (S82.87-)*
Salter-Harris type III of lower end of tibia (S89.13-)
Salter-Harris type IV of lower end of tibia (S89.14-)

3 √x7th **S82.51 Displaced fracture of medial malleolus of right tibia** CC H5

3 √x7th **S82.52 Displaced fracture of medial malleolus of left tibia** CC H5

3 √x7th **S82.53 Displaced fracture of medial malleolus of unspecified tibia** CC H5 UNS

3 √x7th **S82.54 Nondisplaced fracture of medial malleolus of right tibia** CC H5

3 √x7th **S82.55 Nondisplaced fracture of medial malleolus of left tibia** CC H5

3 √x7th **S82.56 Nondisplaced fracture of medial malleolus of unspecified tibia** CC H5 UNS

√5th **S82.6 Fracture of lateral malleolus**

EXCLUDES 1 *pilon fracture of distal tibia (S82.87-)*

3 √x7th **S82.61 Displaced fracture of lateral malleolus of right fibula** CC H5

3 √x7th **S82.62 Displaced fracture of lateral malleolus of left fibula** CC H5

3 √x7th **S82.63 Displaced fracture of lateral malleolus of unspecified fibula** CC H5 UNS

3 √x7th **S82.64 Nondisplaced fracture of lateral malleolus of right fibula** CC H5

3 √x7th **S82.65 Nondisplaced fracture of lateral malleolus of left fibula** CC H5

3 √x7th **S82.66 Nondisplaced fracture of lateral malleolus of unspecified fibula** CC H5 UNS

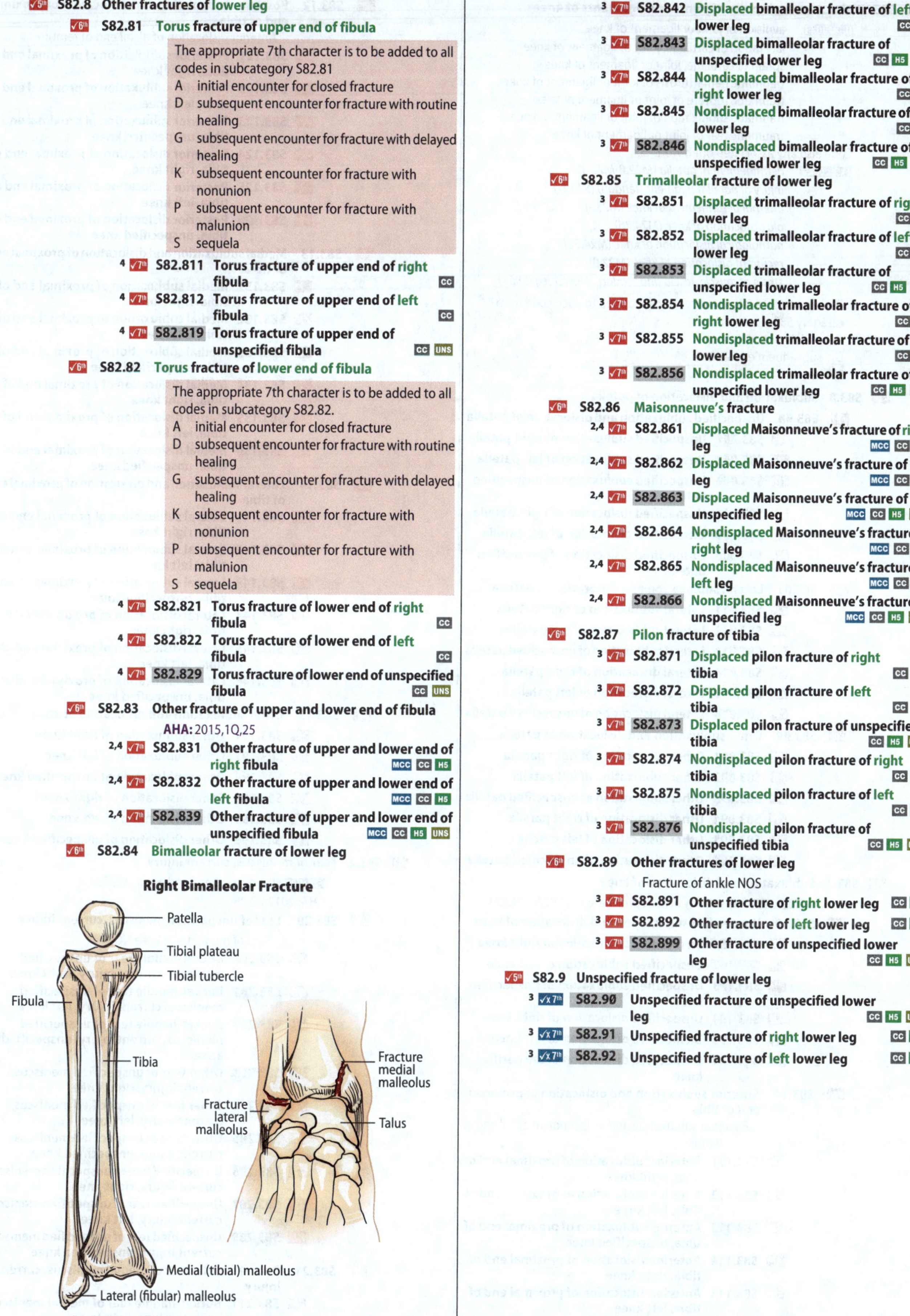

S82.8 Other fractures of lower leg (5th)

S82.81 Torus fracture of upper end of fibula (6th)

The appropriate 7th character is to be added to all codes in subcategory S82.81
- A initial encounter for closed fracture
- D subsequent encounter for fracture with routine healing
- G subsequent encounter for fracture with delayed healing
- K subsequent encounter for fracture with nonunion
- P subsequent encounter for fracture with malunion
- S sequela

- 4 (7th) **S82.811 Torus fracture of upper end of right fibula** CC
- 4 (7th) **S82.812 Torus fracture of upper end of left fibula** CC
- 4 (7th) **S82.819 Torus fracture of upper end of unspecified fibula** CC UNS

S82.82 Torus fracture of lower end of fibula (6th)

The appropriate 7th character is to be added to all codes in subcategory S82.82.
- A initial encounter for closed fracture
- D subsequent encounter for fracture with routine healing
- G subsequent encounter for fracture with delayed healing
- K subsequent encounter for fracture with nonunion
- P subsequent encounter for fracture with malunion
- S sequela

- 4 (7th) **S82.821 Torus fracture of lower end of right fibula** CC
- 4 (7th) **S82.822 Torus fracture of lower end of left fibula** CC
- 4 (7th) **S82.829 Torus fracture of lower end of unspecified fibula** CC UNS

S82.83 Other fracture of upper and lower end of fibula (6th)

AHA: 2015,1Q,25

- 2,4 (7th) **S82.831 Other fracture of upper and lower end of right fibula** MCC CC H5
- 2,4 (7th) **S82.832 Other fracture of upper and lower end of left fibula** MCC CC H5
- 2,4 (7th) **S82.839 Other fracture of upper and lower end of unspecified fibula** MCC CC H5 UNS

S82.84 Bimalleolar fracture of lower leg (6th)

Right Bimalleolar Fracture

- 3 (7th) **S82.841 Displaced bimalleolar fracture of right lower leg** CC H5
- 3 (7th) **S82.842 Displaced bimalleolar fracture of left lower leg** CC H5
- 3 (7th) **S82.843 Displaced bimalleolar fracture of unspecified lower leg** CC H5 UNS
- 3 (7th) **S82.844 Nondisplaced bimalleolar fracture of right lower leg** CC H5
- 3 (7th) **S82.845 Nondisplaced bimalleolar fracture of left lower leg** CC H5
- 3 (7th) **S82.846 Nondisplaced bimalleolar fracture of unspecified lower leg** CC H5 UNS

S82.85 Trimalleolar fracture of lower leg (6th)

- 3 (7th) **S82.851 Displaced trimalleolar fracture of right lower leg** CC H5
- 3 (7th) **S82.852 Displaced trimalleolar fracture of left lower leg** CC H5
- 3 (7th) **S82.853 Displaced trimalleolar fracture of unspecified lower leg** CC H5 UNS
- 3 (7th) **S82.854 Nondisplaced trimalleolar fracture of right lower leg** CC H5
- 3 (7th) **S82.855 Nondisplaced trimalleolar fracture of left lower leg** CC H5
- 3 (7th) **S82.856 Nondisplaced trimalleolar fracture of unspecified lower leg** CC H5 UNS

S82.86 Maisonneuve's fracture (6th)

- 2,4 (7th) **S82.861 Displaced Maisonneuve's fracture of right leg** MCC CC H5
- 2,4 (7th) **S82.862 Displaced Maisonneuve's fracture of left leg** MCC CC H5
- 2,4 (7th) **S82.863 Displaced Maisonneuve's fracture of unspecified leg** MCC CC H5 UNS
- 2,4 (7th) **S82.864 Nondisplaced Maisonneuve's fracture of right leg** MCC CC H5
- 2,4 (7th) **S82.865 Nondisplaced Maisonneuve's fracture of left leg** MCC CC H5
- 2,4 (7th) **S82.866 Nondisplaced Maisonneuve's fracture of unspecified leg** MCC CC H5 UNS

S82.87 Pilon fracture of tibia (6th)

- 3 (7th) **S82.871 Displaced pilon fracture of right tibia** CC H5
- 3 (7th) **S82.872 Displaced pilon fracture of left tibia** CC H5
- 3 (7th) **S82.873 Displaced pilon fracture of unspecified tibia** CC H5 UNS
- 3 (7th) **S82.874 Nondisplaced pilon fracture of right tibia** CC H5
- 3 (7th) **S82.875 Nondisplaced pilon fracture of left tibia** CC H5
- 3 (7th) **S82.876 Nondisplaced pilon fracture of unspecified tibia** CC H5 UNS

S82.89 Other fractures of lower leg (6th)

Fracture of ankle NOS

- 3 (7th) **S82.891 Other fracture of right lower leg** CC H5
- 3 (7th) **S82.892 Other fracture of left lower leg** CC H5
- 3 (7th) **S82.899 Other fracture of unspecified lower leg** CC H5 UNS

S82.9 Unspecified fracture of lower leg (5th)

- 3 (x7th) **S82.90 Unspecified fracture of unspecified lower leg** CC H5 UNS
- 3 (x7th) **S82.91 Unspecified fracture of right lower leg** CC H5
- 3 (x7th) **S82.92 Unspecified fracture of left lower leg** CC H5

S83 Dislocation and sprain of joints and ligaments of knee

INCLUDES
- avulsion of joint or ligament of knee
- laceration of cartilage, joint or ligament of knee
- sprain of cartilage, joint or ligament of knee
- traumatic hemarthrosis of joint or ligament of knee
- traumatic rupture of joint or ligament of knee
- traumatic subluxation of joint or ligament of knee
- traumatic tear of joint or ligament of knee

Code also any associated open wound

EXCLUDES 2
- *derangement of patella (M22.Ø-M22.3)*
- *injury of patellar ligament (tendon) (S76.1-)*
- *internal derangement of knee (M23.-)*
- *old dislocation of knee (M24.36)*
- *pathological dislocation of knee (M24.36)*
- *recurrent dislocation of knee (M22.Ø)*
- *strain of muscle, fascia and tendon of lower leg (S86.-)*

The appropriate 7th character is to be added to each code from category S83.
- A initial encounter
- D subsequent encounter
- S sequela

S83.Ø Subluxation and dislocation of patella

S83.ØØ Unspecified subluxation and dislocation of patella
- **S83.ØØ1 Unspecified subluxation of right patella**
- **S83.ØØ2 Unspecified subluxation of left patella**
- **S83.ØØ3 Unspecified subluxation of unspecified patella**
- **S83.ØØ4 Unspecified dislocation of right patella**
- **S83.ØØ5 Unspecified dislocation of left patella**
- **S83.ØØ6 Unspecified dislocation of unspecified patella**

S83.Ø1 Lateral subluxation and dislocation of patella
- **S83.Ø11 Lateral subluxation of right patella**
- **S83.Ø12 Lateral subluxation of left patella**
- **S83.Ø13 Lateral subluxation of unspecified patella**
- **S83.Ø14 Lateral dislocation of right patella**
- **S83.Ø15 Lateral dislocation of left patella**
- **S83.Ø16 Lateral dislocation of unspecified patella**

S83.Ø9 Other subluxation and dislocation of patella
- **S83.Ø91 Other subluxation of right patella**
- **S83.Ø92 Other subluxation of left patella**
- **S83.Ø93 Other subluxation of unspecified patella**
- **S83.Ø94 Other dislocation of right patella**
- **S83.Ø95 Other dislocation of left patella**
- **S83.Ø96 Other dislocation of unspecified patella**

S83.1 Subluxation and dislocation of knee

EXCLUDES 2 *instability of knee prosthesis (T84.Ø22, T84.Ø23)*

S83.1Ø Unspecified subluxation and dislocation of knee
- **S83.1Ø1 Unspecified subluxation of right knee**
- **S83.1Ø2 Unspecified subluxation of left knee**
- **S83.1Ø3 Unspecified subluxation of unspecified knee**
- **S83.1Ø4 Unspecified dislocation of right knee**
- **S83.1Ø5 Unspecified dislocation of left knee**
- **S83.1Ø6 Unspecified dislocation of unspecified knee**

S83.11 Anterior subluxation and dislocation of proximal end of tibia

Posterior subluxation and dislocation of distal end of femur
- **S83.111 Anterior subluxation of proximal end of tibia, right knee**
- **S83.112 Anterior subluxation of proximal end of tibia, left knee**
- **S83.113 Anterior subluxation of proximal end of tibia, unspecified knee**
- **S83.114 Anterior dislocation of proximal end of tibia, right knee**
- **S83.115 Anterior dislocation of proximal end of tibia, left knee**
- **S83.116 Anterior dislocation of proximal end of tibia, unspecified knee**

S83.12 Posterior subluxation and dislocation of proximal end of tibia

Anterior dislocation of distal end of femur
- **S83.121 Posterior subluxation of proximal end of tibia, right knee**
- **S83.122 Posterior subluxation of proximal end of tibia, left knee**
- **S83.123 Posterior subluxation of proximal end of tibia, unspecified knee**
- **S83.124 Posterior dislocation of proximal end of tibia, right knee**
- **S83.125 Posterior dislocation of proximal end of tibia, left knee**
- **S83.126 Posterior dislocation of proximal end of tibia, unspecified knee**

S83.13 Medial subluxation and dislocation of proximal end of tibia
- **S83.131 Medial subluxation of proximal end of tibia, right knee**
- **S83.132 Medial subluxation of proximal end of tibia, left knee**
- **S83.133 Medial subluxation of proximal end of tibia, unspecified knee**
- **S83.134 Medial dislocation of proximal end of tibia, right knee**
- **S83.135 Medial dislocation of proximal end of tibia, left knee**
- **S83.136 Medial dislocation of proximal end of tibia, unspecified knee**

S83.14 Lateral subluxation and dislocation of proximal end of tibia
- **S83.141 Lateral subluxation of proximal end of tibia, right knee**
- **S83.142 Lateral subluxation of proximal end of tibia, left knee**
- **S83.143 Lateral subluxation of proximal end of tibia, unspecified knee**
- **S83.144 Lateral dislocation of proximal end of tibia, right knee**
- **S83.145 Lateral dislocation of proximal end of tibia, left knee**
- **S83.146 Lateral dislocation of proximal end of tibia, unspecified knee**

S83.19 Other subluxation and dislocation of knee
- **S83.191 Other subluxation of right knee**
- **S83.192 Other subluxation of left knee**
- **S83.193 Other subluxation of unspecified knee**
- **S83.194 Other dislocation of right knee**
- **S83.195 Other dislocation of left knee**
- **S83.196 Other dislocation of unspecified knee**

S83.2 Tear of meniscus, current injury

EXCLUDES 1 *old bucket-handle tear (M23.2)*

AHA: 2019,2Q,26

S83.2Ø Tear of unspecified meniscus, current injury

Tear of meniscus of knee NOS
- **S83.2ØØ Bucket-handle tear of unspecified meniscus, current injury, right knee**
- **S83.2Ø1 Bucket-handle tear of unspecified meniscus, current injury, left knee**
- **S83.2Ø2 Bucket-handle tear of unspecified meniscus, current injury, unspecified knee**
- **S83.2Ø3 Other tear of unspecified meniscus, current injury, right knee**
- **S83.2Ø4 Other tear of unspecified meniscus, current injury, left knee**
- **S83.2Ø5 Other tear of unspecified meniscus, current injury, unspecified knee**
- **S83.2Ø6 Unspecified tear of unspecified meniscus, current injury, right knee**
- **S83.2Ø7 Unspecified tear of unspecified meniscus, current injury, left knee**
- **S83.2Ø9 Unspecified tear of unspecified meniscus, current injury, unspecified knee**

S83.21 Bucket-handle tear of medial meniscus, current injury
- **S83.211 Bucket-handle tear of medial meniscus, current injury, right knee**
- **S83.212 Bucket-handle tear of medial meniscus, current injury, left knee**

S83.219 Bucket-handle tear of medial meniscus, current injury, unspecified knee

S83.22 Peripheral tear of medial meniscus, current injury
- S83.221 Peripheral tear of medial meniscus, current injury, right knee
- S83.222 Peripheral tear of medial meniscus, current injury, left knee
- S83.229 Peripheral tear of medial meniscus, current injury, unspecified knee

S83.23 Complex tear of medial meniscus, current injury
- S83.231 Complex tear of medial meniscus, current injury, right knee
- S83.232 Complex tear of medial meniscus, current injury, left knee
- S83.239 Complex tear of medial meniscus, current injury, unspecified knee

S83.24 Other tear of medial meniscus, current injury
- S83.241 Other tear of medial meniscus, current injury, right knee
- S83.242 Other tear of medial meniscus, current injury, left knee
- S83.249 Other tear of medial meniscus, current injury, unspecified knee

S83.25 Bucket-handle tear of lateral meniscus, current injury
- S83.251 Bucket-handle tear of lateral meniscus, current injury, right knee
- S83.252 Bucket-handle tear of lateral meniscus, current injury, left knee
- S83.259 Bucket-handle tear of lateral meniscus, current injury, unspecified knee

S83.26 Peripheral tear of lateral meniscus, current injury
- S83.261 Peripheral tear of lateral meniscus, current injury, right knee
- S83.262 Peripheral tear of lateral meniscus, current injury, left knee
- S83.269 Peripheral tear of lateral meniscus, current injury, unspecified knee

S83.27 Complex tear of lateral meniscus, current injury
- S83.271 Complex tear of lateral meniscus, current injury, right knee
- S83.272 Complex tear of lateral meniscus, current injury, left knee
- S83.279 Complex tear of lateral meniscus, current injury, unspecified knee

S83.28 Other tear of lateral meniscus, current injury
- S83.281 Other tear of lateral meniscus, current injury, right knee
- S83.282 Other tear of lateral meniscus, current injury, left knee
- S83.289 Other tear of lateral meniscus, current injury, unspecified knee

S83.3 Tear of articular cartilage of knee, current
- S83.30 Tear of articular cartilage of unspecified knee, current
- S83.31 Tear of articular cartilage of right knee, current
- S83.32 Tear of articular cartilage of left knee, current

S83.4 Sprain of collateral ligament of knee

S83.40 Sprain of unspecified collateral ligament of knee
- S83.401 Sprain of unspecified collateral ligament of right knee
- S83.402 Sprain of unspecified collateral ligament of left knee
- S83.409 Sprain of unspecified collateral ligament of unspecified knee

S83.41 Sprain of medial collateral ligament of knee
Sprain of tibial collateral ligament
- S83.411 Sprain of medial collateral ligament of right knee
- S83.412 Sprain of medial collateral ligament of left knee
- S83.419 Sprain of medial collateral ligament of unspecified knee

S83.42 Sprain of lateral collateral ligament of knee
Sprain of fibular collateral ligament
- S83.421 Sprain of lateral collateral ligament of right knee
- S83.422 Sprain of lateral collateral ligament of left knee
- S83.429 Sprain of lateral collateral ligament of unspecified knee

S83.5 Sprain of cruciate ligament of knee
AHA: 2016,2Q,3

S83.50 Sprain of unspecified cruciate ligament of knee
- S83.501 Sprain of unspecified cruciate ligament of right knee
- S83.502 Sprain of unspecified cruciate ligament of left knee
- S83.509 Sprain of unspecified cruciate ligament of unspecified knee

S83.51 Sprain of anterior cruciate ligament of knee
- S83.511 Sprain of anterior cruciate ligament of right knee
- S83.512 Sprain of anterior cruciate ligament of left knee
- S83.519 Sprain of anterior cruciate ligament of unspecified knee

S83.52 Sprain of posterior cruciate ligament of knee
- S83.521 Sprain of posterior cruciate ligament of right knee
- S83.522 Sprain of posterior cruciate ligament of left knee
- S83.529 Sprain of posterior cruciate ligament of unspecified knee

S83.6 Sprain of the superior tibiofibular joint and ligament
- S83.60 Sprain of the superior tibiofibular joint and ligament, unspecified knee
- S83.61 Sprain of the superior tibiofibular joint and ligament, right knee
- S83.62 Sprain of the superior tibiofibular joint and ligament, left knee

S83.8 Sprain of other specified parts of knee

S83.8X Sprain of other specified parts of knee
- S83.8X1 Sprain of other specified parts of right knee
- S83.8X2 Sprain of other specified parts of left knee
- S83.8X9 Sprain of other specified parts of unspecified knee

S83.9 Sprain of unspecified site of knee
- S83.90 Sprain of unspecified site of unspecified knee
- S83.91 Sprain of unspecified site of right knee
- S83.92 Sprain of unspecified site of left knee

S84 Injury of nerves at lower leg level

Code also any associated open wound (S81.-)

EXCLUDES 2 *injury of nerves at ankle and foot level (S94.-)*

The appropriate 7th character is to be added to each code from category S84.
- A initial encounter
- D subsequent encounter
- S sequela

S84.0 Injury of tibial nerve at lower leg level
- S84.00 Injury of tibial nerve at lower leg level, unspecified leg
- S84.01 Injury of tibial nerve at lower leg level, right leg
- S84.02 Injury of tibial nerve at lower leg level, left leg

S84.1 Injury of peroneal nerve at lower leg level
- S84.10 Injury of peroneal nerve at lower leg level, unspecified leg
- S84.11 Injury of peroneal nerve at lower leg level, right leg
- S84.12 Injury of peroneal nerve at lower leg level, left leg

S84.2 Injury of cutaneous sensory nerve at lower leg level
- S84.20 Injury of cutaneous sensory nerve at lower leg level, unspecified leg
- S84.21 Injury of cutaneous sensory nerve at lower leg level, right leg
- S84.22 Injury of cutaneous sensory nerve at lower leg level, left leg

S84.8 Injury of other nerves at lower leg level

S84.80 Injury of other nerves at lower leg level
- S84.801 Injury of other nerves at lower leg level, right leg
- S84.802 Injury of other nerves at lower leg level, left leg

√7th **S84.809** **Injury of other nerves at lower leg level, unspecified leg**

√5th **S84.9** **Injury of unspecified nerve at lower leg level**

√x7th **S84.90** **Injury of unspecified nerve at lower leg level, unspecified leg**

√x7th **S84.91** **Injury of unspecified nerve at lower leg level, right leg**

√x7th **S84.92** **Injury of unspecified nerve at lower leg level, left leg**

√4th **S85** **Injury of blood vessels at lower leg level**

Code also any associated open wound (S81.-)

EXCLUDES 2 *injury of blood vessels at ankle and foot level (S95.-)*

The appropriate 7th character is to be added to each code from category S85.
A initial encounter
D subsequent encounter
S sequela

√5th **S85.0** **Injury of popliteal artery**

√6th **S85.00** **Unspecified injury of popliteal artery**

√7th **S85.001** **Unspecified injury of popliteal artery, right leg** MCC

√7th **S85.002** **Unspecified injury of popliteal artery, left leg** MCC

√7th **S85.009** **Unspecified injury of popliteal artery, unspecified leg** MCC UNS

√6th **S85.01** **Laceration of popliteal artery**

√7th **S85.011** **Laceration of popliteal artery, right leg** MCC

√7th **S85.012** **Laceration of popliteal artery, left leg** MCC

√7th **S85.019** **Laceration of popliteal artery, unspecified leg** MCC UNS

√6th **S85.09** **Other specified injury of popliteal artery**

√7th **S85.091** **Other specified injury of popliteal artery, right leg** MCC

√7th **S85.092** **Other specified injury of popliteal artery, left leg** MCC

√7th **S85.099** **Other specified injury of popliteal artery, unspecified leg** MCC UNS

√5th **S85.1** **Injury of tibial artery**

√6th **S85.10** **Unspecified injury of unspecified tibial artery**

Injury of tibial artery NOS

√7th **S85.101** **Unspecified injury of unspecified tibial artery, right leg** CC

√7th **S85.102** **Unspecified injury of unspecified tibial artery, left leg** CC

√7th **S85.109** **Unspecified injury of unspecified tibial artery, unspecified leg** CC UNS

√6th **S85.11** **Laceration of unspecified tibial artery**

√7th **S85.111** **Laceration of unspecified tibial artery, right leg** CC

√7th **S85.112** **Laceration of unspecified tibial artery, left leg** CC

√7th **S85.119** **Laceration of unspecified tibial artery, unspecified leg** CC UNS

√6th **S85.12** **Other specified injury of unspecified tibial artery**

√7th **S85.121** **Other specified injury of unspecified tibial artery, right leg** CC

√7th **S85.122** **Other specified injury of unspecified tibial artery, left leg** CC

√7th **S85.129** **Other specified injury of unspecified tibial artery, unspecified leg** CC UNS

√6th **S85.13** **Unspecified injury of anterior tibial artery**

√7th **S85.131** **Unspecified injury of anterior tibial artery, right leg** CC

√7th **S85.132** **Unspecified injury of anterior tibial artery, left leg** CC

√7th **S85.139** **Unspecified injury of anterior tibial artery, unspecified leg** CC UNS

√6th **S85.14** **Laceration of anterior tibial artery**

√7th **S85.141** **Laceration of anterior tibial artery, right leg** CC

√7th **S85.142** **Laceration of anterior tibial artery, left leg** CC

√7th **S85.149** **Laceration of anterior tibial artery, unspecified leg** CC UNS

√6th **S85.15** **Other specified injury of anterior tibial artery**

√7th **S85.151** **Other specified injury of anterior tibial artery, right leg** CC

√7th **S85.152** **Other specified injury of anterior tibial artery, left leg** CC

√7th **S85.159** **Other specified injury of anterior tibial artery, unspecified leg** CC UNS

√6th **S85.16** **Unspecified injury of posterior tibial artery**

√7th **S85.161** **Unspecified injury of posterior tibial artery, right leg** CC

√7th **S85.162** **Unspecified injury of posterior tibial artery, left leg** CC

√7th **S85.169** **Unspecified injury of posterior tibial artery, unspecified leg** CC UNS

√6th **S85.17** **Laceration of posterior tibial artery**

√7th **S85.171** **Laceration of posterior tibial artery, right leg** CC

√7th **S85.172** **Laceration of posterior tibial artery, left leg** CC

√7th **S85.179** **Laceration of posterior tibial artery, unspecified leg** CC UNS

√6th **S85.18** **Other specified injury of posterior tibial artery**

√7th **S85.181** **Other specified injury of posterior tibial artery, right leg** CC

√7th **S85.182** **Other specified injury of posterior tibial artery, left leg** CC

√7th **S85.189** **Other specified injury of posterior tibial artery, unspecified leg** CC UNS

√5th **S85.2** **Injury of peroneal artery**

√6th **S85.20** **Unspecified injury of peroneal artery**

√7th **S85.201** **Unspecified injury of peroneal artery, right leg** CC

√7th **S85.202** **Unspecified injury of peroneal artery, left leg** CC

√7th **S85.209** **Unspecified injury of peroneal artery, unspecified leg** CC UNS

√6th **S85.21** **Laceration of peroneal artery**

√7th **S85.211** **Laceration of peroneal artery, right leg** CC

√7th **S85.212** **Laceration of peroneal artery, left leg** CC

√7th **S85.219** **Laceration of peroneal artery, unspecified leg** CC UNS

√6th **S85.29** **Other specified injury of peroneal artery**

√7th **S85.291** **Other specified injury of peroneal artery, right leg** CC

√7th **S85.292** **Other specified injury of peroneal artery, left leg** CC

√7th **S85.299** **Other specified injury of peroneal artery, unspecified leg** CC UNS

√5th **S85.3** **Injury of greater saphenous vein at lower leg level**

Injury of greater saphenous vein NOS
Injury of saphenous vein NOS

√6th **S85.30** **Unspecified injury of greater saphenous vein at lower leg level**

√7th **S85.301** **Unspecified injury of greater saphenous vein at lower leg level, right leg** CC

√7th **S85.302** **Unspecified injury of greater saphenous vein at lower leg level, left leg** CC

√7th **S85.309** **Unspecified injury of greater saphenous vein at lower leg level, unspecified leg** CC UNS

√6th **S85.31** **Laceration of greater saphenous vein at lower leg level**

√7th **S85.311** **Laceration of greater saphenous vein at lower leg level, right leg** CC

√7th **S85.312** **Laceration of greater saphenous vein at lower leg level, left leg** CC

√7th **S85.319** **Laceration of greater saphenous vein at lower leg level, unspecified leg** CC UNS

√6th **S85.39** **Other specified injury of greater saphenous vein at lower leg level**

√7th **S85.391** **Other specified injury of greater saphenous vein at lower leg level, right leg** CC

√7th **S85.392** **Other specified injury of greater saphenous vein at lower leg level, left leg** CC

N Newborn: 0 P Pediatric: 0-17 M Maternity: 9-64 A Adult: 15-124 UNS Unspecified Site MCC Major Complication/Comorbidity CC Complication/Comorbidity

S85.399 Other specified injury of greater saphenous vein at lower leg level, unspecified leg CC UNS

S85.4 Injury of lesser saphenous vein at lower leg level

S85.40 Unspecified injury of lesser saphenous vein at lower leg level

S85.401 Unspecified injury of lesser saphenous vein at lower leg level, right leg CC

S85.402 Unspecified injury of lesser saphenous vein at lower leg level, left leg CC

S85.409 Unspecified injury of lesser saphenous vein at lower leg level, unspecified leg CC UNS

S85.41 Laceration of lesser saphenous vein at lower leg level

S85.411 Laceration of lesser saphenous vein at lower leg level, right leg CC

S85.412 Laceration of lesser saphenous vein at lower leg level, left leg CC

S85.419 Laceration of lesser saphenous vein at lower leg level, unspecified leg CC UNS

S85.49 Other specified injury of lesser saphenous vein at lower leg level

S85.491 Other specified injury of lesser saphenous vein at lower leg level, right leg CC

S85.492 Other specified injury of lesser saphenous vein at lower leg level, left leg CC

S85.499 Other specified injury of lesser saphenous vein at lower leg level, unspecified leg CC UNS

S85.5 Injury of popliteal vein

S85.50 Unspecified injury of popliteal vein

S85.501 Unspecified injury of popliteal vein, right leg MCC

S85.502 Unspecified injury of popliteal vein, left leg MCC

S85.509 Unspecified injury of popliteal vein, unspecified leg MCC UNS

S85.51 Laceration of popliteal vein

S85.511 Laceration of popliteal vein, right leg MCC

S85.512 Laceration of popliteal vein, left leg MCC

S85.519 Laceration of popliteal vein, unspecified leg MCC UNS

S85.59 Other specified injury of popliteal vein

S85.591 Other specified injury of popliteal vein, right leg MCC

S85.592 Other specified injury of popliteal vein, left leg MCC

S85.599 Other specified injury of popliteal vein, unspecified leg MCC UNS

S85.8 Injury of other blood vessels at lower leg level

S85.80 Unspecified injury of other blood vessels at lower leg level

S85.801 Unspecified injury of other blood vessels at lower leg level, right leg CC

S85.802 Unspecified injury of other blood vessels at lower leg level, left leg CC

S85.809 Unspecified injury of other blood vessels at lower leg level, unspecified leg CC UNS

S85.81 Laceration of other blood vessels at lower leg level

S85.811 Laceration of other blood vessels at lower leg level, right leg CC

S85.812 Laceration of other blood vessels at lower leg level, left leg CC

S85.819 Laceration of other blood vessels at lower leg level, unspecified leg CC UNS

S85.89 Other specified injury of other blood vessels at lower leg level

S85.891 Other specified injury of other blood vessels at lower leg level, right leg CC

S85.892 Other specified injury of other blood vessels at lower leg level, left leg CC

S85.899 Other specified injury of other blood vessels at lower leg level, unspecified leg CC UNS

S85.9 Injury of unspecified blood vessel at lower leg level

S85.90 Unspecified injury of unspecified blood vessel at lower leg level

S85.901 Unspecified injury of unspecified blood vessel at lower leg level, right leg CC

S85.902 Unspecified injury of unspecified blood vessel at lower leg level, left leg CC

S85.909 Unspecified injury of unspecified blood vessel at lower leg level, unspecified leg CC UNS

S85.91 Laceration of unspecified blood vessel at lower leg level

S85.911 Laceration of unspecified blood vessel at lower leg level, right leg CC

S85.912 Laceration of unspecified blood vessel at lower leg level, left leg CC

S85.919 Laceration of unspecified blood vessel at lower leg level, unspecified leg CC UNS

S85.99 Other specified injury of unspecified blood vessel at lower leg level

S85.991 Other specified injury of unspecified blood vessel at lower leg level, right leg CC

S85.992 Other specified injury of unspecified blood vessel at lower leg level, left leg CC

S85.999 Other specified injury of unspecified blood vessel at lower leg level, unspecified leg CC UNS

S86 Injury of muscle, fascia and tendon at lower leg level

Code also any associated open wound (S81.-)

EXCLUDES 2 *injury of muscle, fascia and tendon at ankle (S96.-)*
injury of patellar ligament (tendon) (S76.1-)
sprain of joints and ligaments of knee (S83.-)

TIP: Refer to the Muscle/Tendon table at the beginning of this chapter.

The appropriate 7th character is to be added to each code from category S86.
A initial encounter
D subsequent encounter
S sequela

S86.0 Injury of Achilles tendon

S86.00 Unspecified injury of Achilles tendon

S86.001 Unspecified injury of right Achilles tendon

S86.002 Unspecified injury of left Achilles tendon

S86.009 Unspecified injury of unspecified Achilles tendon

S86.01 Strain of Achilles tendon

S86.011 Strain of right Achilles tendon

S86.012 Strain of left Achilles tendon

S86.019 Strain of unspecified Achilles tendon

S86.02 Laceration of Achilles tendon

S86.021 Laceration of right Achilles tendon CC

S86.022 Laceration of left Achilles tendon CC

S86.029 Laceration of unspecified Achilles tendon CC UNS

S86.09 Other specified injury of Achilles tendon

S86.091 Other specified injury of right Achilles tendon

S86.092 Other specified injury of left Achilles tendon

S86.099 Other specified injury of unspecified Achilles tendon

S86.1 Injury of other muscle(s) and tendon(s) of posterior muscle group at lower leg level

S86.10 Unspecified injury of other muscle(s) and tendon(s) of posterior muscle group at lower leg level

S86.101 Unspecified injury of other muscle(s) and tendon(s) of posterior muscle group at lower leg level, right leg

S86.102 Unspecified injury of other muscle(s) and tendon(s) of posterior muscle group at lower leg level, left leg

S86.109 Unspecified injury of other muscle(s) and tendon(s) of posterior muscle group at lower leg level, unspecified leg

6th **S86.11** **Strain of other muscle(s) and tendon(s) of posterior muscle group at lower leg level**
- 7th **S86.111** Strain of other muscle(s) and tendon(s) of posterior muscle group at lower leg level, right leg
- 7th **S86.112** Strain of other muscle(s) and tendon(s) of posterior muscle group at lower leg level, left leg
- 7th **S86.119** Strain of other muscle(s) and tendon(s) of posterior muscle group at lower leg level, unspecified leg

6th **S86.12** **Laceration of other muscle(s) and tendon(s) of posterior muscle group at lower leg level**
- 7th **S86.121** Laceration of other muscle(s) and tendon(s) of posterior muscle group at lower leg level, right leg CC
- 7th **S86.122** Laceration of other muscle(s) and tendon(s) of posterior muscle group at lower leg level, left leg CC
- 7th **S86.129** Laceration of other muscle(s) and tendon(s) of posterior muscle group at lower leg level, unspecified leg CC UNS

6th **S86.19** **Other injury of other muscle(s) and tendon(s) of posterior muscle group at lower leg level**
- 7th **S86.191** Other injury of other muscle(s) and tendon(s) of posterior muscle group at lower leg level, right leg
- 7th **S86.192** Other injury of other muscle(s) and tendon(s) of posterior muscle group at lower leg level, left leg
- 7th **S86.199** Other injury of other muscle(s) and tendon(s) of posterior muscle group at lower leg level, unspecified leg

5th **S86.2** **Injury of muscle(s) and tendon(s) of anterior muscle group at lower leg level**

6th **S86.20** **Unspecified injury of muscle(s) and tendon(s) of anterior muscle group at lower leg level**
- 7th **S86.201** Unspecified injury of muscle(s) and tendon(s) of anterior muscle group at lower leg level, right leg
- 7th **S86.202** Unspecified injury of muscle(s) and tendon(s) of anterior muscle group at lower leg level, left leg
- 7th **S86.209** Unspecified injury of muscle(s) and tendon(s) of anterior muscle group at lower leg level, unspecified leg

6th **S86.21** **Strain of muscle(s) and tendon(s) of anterior muscle group at lower leg level**
- 7th **S86.211** Strain of muscle(s) and tendon(s) of anterior muscle group at lower leg level, right leg
- 7th **S86.212** Strain of muscle(s) and tendon(s) of anterior muscle group at lower leg level, left leg
- 7th **S86.219** Strain of muscle(s) and tendon(s) of anterior muscle group at lower leg level, unspecified leg

6th **S86.22** **Laceration of muscle(s) and tendon(s) of anterior muscle group at lower leg level**
- 7th **S86.221** Laceration of muscle(s) and tendon(s) of anterior muscle group at lower leg level, right leg CC
- 7th **S86.222** Laceration of muscle(s) and tendon(s) of anterior muscle group at lower leg level, left leg CC
- 7th **S86.229** Laceration of muscle(s) and tendon(s) of anterior muscle group at lower leg level, unspecified leg CC UNS

6th **S86.29** **Other injury of muscle(s) and tendon(s) of anterior muscle group at lower leg level**
- 7th **S86.291** Other injury of muscle(s) and tendon(s) of anterior muscle group at lower leg level, right leg
- 7th **S86.292** Other injury of muscle(s) and tendon(s) of anterior muscle group at lower leg level, left leg
- 7th **S86.299** Other injury of muscle(s) and tendon(s) of anterior muscle group at lower leg level, unspecified leg

5th **S86.3** **Injury of muscle(s) and tendon(s) of peroneal muscle group at lower leg level**

6th **S86.30** **Unspecified injury of muscle(s) and tendon(s) of peroneal muscle group at lower leg level**
- 7th **S86.301** Unspecified injury of muscle(s) and tendon(s) of peroneal muscle group at lower leg level, right leg
- 7th **S86.302** Unspecified injury of muscle(s) and tendon(s) of peroneal muscle group at lower leg level, left leg
- 7th **S86.309** Unspecified injury of muscle(s) and tendon(s) of peroneal muscle group at lower leg level, unspecified leg

6th **S86.31** **Strain of muscle(s) and tendon(s) of peroneal muscle group at lower leg level**
- 7th **S86.311** Strain of muscle(s) and tendon(s) of peroneal muscle group at lower leg level, right leg
- 7th **S86.312** Strain of muscle(s) and tendon(s) of peroneal muscle group at lower leg level, left leg
- 7th **S86.319** Strain of muscle(s) and tendon(s) of peroneal muscle group at lower leg level, unspecified leg

6th **S86.32** **Laceration of muscle(s) and tendon(s) of peroneal muscle group at lower leg level**
- 7th **S86.321** Laceration of muscle(s) and tendon(s) of peroneal muscle group at lower leg level, right leg CC
- 7th **S86.322** Laceration of muscle(s) and tendon(s) of peroneal muscle group at lower leg level, left leg CC
- 7th **S86.329** Laceration of muscle(s) and tendon(s) of peroneal muscle group at lower leg level, unspecified leg CC UNS

6th **S86.39** **Other injury of muscle(s) and tendon(s) of peroneal muscle group at lower leg level**
- 7th **S86.391** Other injury of muscle(s) and tendon(s) of peroneal muscle group at lower leg level, right leg
- 7th **S86.392** Other injury of muscle(s) and tendon(s) of peroneal muscle group at lower leg level, left leg
- 7th **S86.399** Other injury of muscle(s) and tendon(s) of peroneal muscle group at lower leg level, unspecified leg

5th **S86.8** **Injury of other muscles and tendons at lower leg level**

6th **S86.80** **Unspecified injury of other muscles and tendons at lower leg level**
- 7th **S86.801** Unspecified injury of other muscle(s) and tendon(s) at lower leg level, right leg
- 7th **S86.802** Unspecified injury of other muscle(s) and tendon(s) at lower leg level, left leg
- 7th **S86.809** Unspecified injury of other muscle(s) and tendon(s) at lower leg level, unspecified leg

6th **S86.81** **Strain of other muscles and tendons at lower leg level**
- 7th **S86.811** Strain of other muscle(s) and tendon(s) at lower leg level, right leg
- 7th **S86.812** Strain of other muscle(s) and tendon(s) at lower leg level, left leg
- 7th **S86.819** Strain of other muscle(s) and tendon(s) at lower leg level, unspecified leg

6th **S86.82** **Laceration of other muscles and tendons at lower leg level**
- 7th **S86.821** Laceration of other muscle(s) and tendon(s) at lower leg level, right leg CC
- 7th **S86.822** Laceration of other muscle(s) and tendon(s) at lower leg level, left leg CC
- 7th **S86.829** Laceration of other muscle(s) and tendon(s) at lower leg level, unspecified leg CC UNS

6th **S86.89** **Other injury of other muscles and tendons at lower leg level**
- 7th **S86.891** Other injury of other muscle(s) and tendon(s) at lower leg level, right leg
- 7th **S86.892** Other injury of other muscle(s) and tendon(s) at lower leg level, left leg
- 7th **S86.899** Other injury of other muscle(s) and tendon(s) at lower leg level, unspecified leg

S86.9 Injury of unspecified muscle and tendon at lower leg level
S86.9Ø Unspecified injury of unspecified muscle and tendon at lower leg level
S86.9Ø1 Unspecified injury of unspecified muscle(s) and tendon(s) at lower leg level, right leg
S86.9Ø2 Unspecified injury of unspecified muscle(s) and tendon(s) at lower leg level, left leg
S86.9Ø9 Unspecified injury of unspecified muscle(s) and tendon(s) at lower leg level, unspecified leg
S86.91 Strain of unspecified muscle and tendon at lower leg level
S86.911 Strain of unspecified muscle(s) and tendon(s) at lower leg level, right leg
S86.912 Strain of unspecified muscle(s) and tendon(s) at lower leg level, left leg
S86.919 Strain of unspecified muscle(s) and tendon(s) at lower leg level, unspecified leg
S86.92 Laceration of unspecified muscle and tendon at lower leg level
S86.921 Laceration of unspecified muscle(s) and tendon(s) at lower leg level, right leg CC
S86.922 Laceration of unspecified muscle(s) and tendon(s) at lower leg level, left leg CC
S86.929 Laceration of unspecified muscle(s) and tendon(s) at lower leg level, unspecified leg CC UNS
S86.99 Other injury of unspecified muscle and tendon at lower leg level
S86.991 Other injury of unspecified muscle(s) and tendon(s) at lower leg level, right leg
S86.992 Other injury of unspecified muscle(s) and tendon(s) at lower leg level, left leg
S86.999 Other injury of unspecified muscle(s) and tendon(s) at lower leg level, unspecified leg

S87 Crushing injury of lower leg

Use additional code(s) for all associated injuries

EXCLUDES 2 *crushing injury of ankle and foot (S97.-)*

The appropriate 7th character is to be added to each code from category S87.
A initial encounter
D subsequent encounter
S sequela

S87.Ø Crushing injury of knee
S87.ØØ Crushing injury of unspecified knee
S87.Ø1 Crushing injury of right knee
S87.Ø2 Crushing injury of left knee
S87.8 Crushing injury of lower leg
S87.8Ø Crushing injury of unspecified lower leg
S87.81 Crushing injury of right lower leg
S87.82 Crushing injury of left lower leg

S88 Traumatic amputation of lower leg

An amputation not identified as partial or complete should be coded to complete

EXCLUDES 1 *traumatic amputation of ankle and foot (S98.-)*

The appropriate 7th character is to be added to each code from category S88.
A initial encounter
D subsequent encounter
S sequela

S88.Ø Traumatic amputation at knee level
S88.Ø1 Complete traumatic amputation at knee level
S88.Ø11 Complete traumatic amputation at knee level, right lower leg CC HCC
S88.Ø12 Complete traumatic amputation at knee level, left lower leg CC HCC
S88.Ø19 Complete traumatic amputation at knee level, unspecified lower leg CC UNS HCC
S88.Ø2 Partial traumatic amputation at knee level
S88.Ø21 Partial traumatic amputation at knee level, right lower leg CC HCC
S88.Ø22 Partial traumatic amputation at knee level, left lower leg CC HCC
S88.Ø29 Partial traumatic amputation at knee level, unspecified lower leg CC UNS HCC
S88.1 Traumatic amputation at level between knee and ankle
S88.11 Complete traumatic amputation at level between knee and ankle
S88.111 Complete traumatic amputation at level between knee and ankle, right lower leg CC HCC
S88.112 Complete traumatic amputation at level between knee and ankle, left lower leg CC HCC
S88.119 Complete traumatic amputation at level between knee and ankle, unspecified lower leg CC UNS HCC
S88.12 Partial traumatic amputation at level between knee and ankle
S88.121 Partial traumatic amputation at level between knee and ankle, right lower leg CC HCC
S88.122 Partial traumatic amputation at level between knee and ankle, left lower leg CC HCC
S88.129 Partial traumatic amputation at level between knee and ankle, unspecified lower leg CC UNS HCC
S88.9 Traumatic amputation of lower leg, level unspecified
S88.91 Complete traumatic amputation of lower leg, level unspecified
S88.911 Complete traumatic amputation of right lower leg, level unspecified CC HCC
S88.912 Complete traumatic amputation of left lower leg, level unspecified CC HCC
S88.919 Complete traumatic amputation of unspecified lower leg, level unspecified CC HCC
S88.92 Partial traumatic amputation of lower leg, level unspecified
S88.921 Partial traumatic amputation of right lower leg, level unspecified CC HCC
S88.922 Partial traumatic amputation of left lower leg, level unspecified CC HCC
S88.929 Partial traumatic amputation of unspecified lower leg, level unspecified CC UNS HCC

S89 Other and unspecified injuries of lower leg

NOTE A fracture not indicated as open or closed should be coded to closed.

EXCLUDES 2 *other and unspecified injuries of ankle and foot (S99.-)*

AHA: 2018,2Q,12; 2018,1Q,3; 2015,3Q,37-39

The appropriate 7th character is to be added to each code from subcategories S89.Ø, S89.1, S89.2, and S89.3.
A initial encounter for closed fracture
D subsequent encounter for fracture with routine healing
G subsequent encounter for fracture with delayed healing
K subsequent encounter for fracture with nonunion
P subsequent encounter for fracture with malunion
S sequela

S89.Ø Physeal fracture of upper end of tibia

AHA: 2019,4Q,56

S89.ØØ Unspecified physeal fracture of upper end of tibia
3 S89.ØØ1 Unspecified physeal fracture of upper end of right tibia CC H5
3 S89.ØØ2 Unspecified physeal fracture of upper end of left tibia CC H5
3 S89.ØØ9 Unspecified physeal fracture of upper end of unspecified tibia CC H5 UNS
S89.Ø1 Salter-Harris Type I physeal fracture of upper end of tibia
3 S89.Ø11 Salter-Harris Type I physeal fracture of upper end of right tibia CC H5
3 S89.Ø12 Salter-Harris Type I physeal fracture of upper end of left tibia CC H5

Chapter 19. Injury, Poisoning and Certain Other Consequences of External Causes

S86.9–S89.Ø12

3 ✓7th S89.019 Salter-Harris Type I physeal fracture of upper end of unspecified tibia CC H5 UNS

✓6th S89.02 Salter-Harris Type II physeal fracture of upper end of tibia

3 ✓7th S89.021 Salter-Harris Type II physeal fracture of upper end of right tibia CC H5

3 ✓7th S89.022 Salter-Harris Type II physeal fracture of upper end of left tibia CC H5

3 ✓7th S89.029 Salter-Harris Type II physeal fracture of upper end of unspecified tibia CC H5 UNS

✓6th S89.03 Salter-Harris Type III physeal fracture of upper end of tibia

3 ✓7th S89.031 Salter-Harris Type III physeal fracture of upper end of right tibia CC H5

3 ✓7th S89.032 Salter-Harris Type III physeal fracture of upper end of left tibia CC H5

3 ✓7th S89.039 Salter-Harris Type III physeal fracture of upper end of unspecified tibia CC H5 UNS

✓6th S89.04 Salter-Harris Type IV physeal fracture of upper end of tibia

3 ✓7th S89.041 Salter-Harris Type IV physeal fracture of upper end of right tibia CC H5

3 ✓7th S89.042 Salter-Harris Type IV physeal fracture of upper end of left tibia CC H5

3 ✓7th S89.049 Salter-Harris Type IV physeal fracture of upper end of unspecified tibia CC H5 UNS

✓6th S89.09 Other physeal fracture of upper end of tibia

3 ✓7th S89.091 Other physeal fracture of upper end of right tibia CC H5

3 ✓7th S89.092 Other physeal fracture of upper end of left tibia CC H5

3 ✓7th S89.099 Other physeal fracture of upper end of unspecified tibia CC H5 UNS

✓5th S89.1 Physeal fracture of lower end of tibia

AHA: 2019,4Q,56

✓6th S89.10 Unspecified physeal fracture of lower end of tibia

4 ✓7th S89.101 Unspecified physeal fracture of lower end of right tibia CC

4 ✓7th S89.102 Unspecified physeal fracture of lower end of left tibia CC

4 ✓7th S89.109 Unspecified physeal fracture of lower end of unspecified tibia CC UNS

✓6th S89.11 Salter-Harris Type I physeal fracture of lower end of tibia

4 ✓7th S89.111 Salter-Harris Type I physeal fracture of lower end of right tibia CC

4 ✓7th S89.112 Salter-Harris Type I physeal fracture of lower end of left tibia CC

4 ✓7th S89.119 Salter-Harris Type I physeal fracture of lower end of unspecified tibia CC UNS

✓6th S89.12 Salter-Harris Type II physeal fracture of lower end of tibia

4 ✓7th S89.121 Salter-Harris Type II physeal fracture of lower end of right tibia CC

4 ✓7th S89.122 Salter-Harris Type II physeal fracture of lower end of left tibia CC

4 ✓7th S89.129 Salter-Harris Type II physeal fracture of lower end of unspecified tibia CC UNS

✓6th S89.13 Salter-Harris Type III physeal fracture of lower end of tibia

EXCLUDES 1 *fracture of medial malleolus (adult) (S82.5-)*

4 ✓7th S89.131 Salter-Harris Type III physeal fracture of lower end of right tibia CC

4 ✓7th S89.132 Salter-Harris Type III physeal fracture of lower end of left tibia CC

4 ✓7th S89.139 Salter-Harris Type III physeal fracture of lower end of unspecified tibia CC UNS

✓6th S89.14 Salter-Harris Type IV physeal fracture of lower end of tibia

EXCLUDES 1 *fracture of medial malleolus (adult) (S82.5-)*

4 ✓7th S89.141 Salter-Harris Type IV physeal fracture of lower end of right tibia CC

4 ✓7th S89.142 Salter-Harris Type IV physeal fracture of lower end of left tibia CC

4 ✓7th S89.149 Salter-Harris Type IV physeal fracture of lower end of unspecified tibia CC UNS

✓6th S89.19 Other physeal fracture of lower end of tibia

4 ✓7th S89.191 Other physeal fracture of lower end of right tibia CC

4 ✓7th S89.192 Other physeal fracture of lower end of left tibia CC

4 ✓7th S89.199 Other physeal fracture of lower end of unspecified tibia CC UNS

✓5th S89.2 Physeal fracture of upper end of fibula

AHA: 2019,4Q,56

✓6th S89.20 Unspecified physeal fracture of upper end of fibula

4 ✓7th S89.201 Unspecified physeal fracture of upper end of right fibula CC

4 ✓7th S89.202 Unspecified physeal fracture of upper end of left fibula CC

4 ✓7th S89.209 Unspecified physeal fracture of upper end of unspecified fibula CC UNS

✓6th S89.21 Salter-Harris Type I physeal fracture of upper end of fibula

4 ✓7th S89.211 Salter-Harris Type I physeal fracture of upper end of right fibula CC

4 ✓7th S89.212 Salter-Harris Type I physeal fracture of upper end of left fibula CC

4 ✓7th S89.219 Salter-Harris Type I physeal fracture of upper end of unspecified fibula CC UNS

✓6th S89.22 Salter-Harris Type II physeal fracture of upper end of fibula

4 ✓7th S89.221 Salter-Harris Type II physeal fracture of upper end of right fibula CC

4 ✓7th S89.222 Salter-Harris Type II physeal fracture of upper end of left fibula CC

4 ✓7th S89.229 Salter-Harris Type II physeal fracture of upper end of unspecified fibula CC UNS

✓6th S89.29 Other physeal fracture of upper end of fibula

4 ✓7th S89.291 Other physeal fracture of upper end of right fibula CC

4 ✓7th S89.292 Other physeal fracture of upper end of left fibula CC

4 ✓7th S89.299 Other physeal fracture of upper end of unspecified fibula CC UNS

✓5th S89.3 Physeal fracture of lower end of fibula

AHA: 2019,4Q,56

✓6th S89.30 Unspecified physeal fracture of lower end of fibula

4 ✓7th S89.301 Unspecified physeal fracture of lower end of right fibula CC

4 ✓7th S89.302 Unspecified physeal fracture of lower end of left fibula CC

4 ✓7th S89.309 Unspecified physeal fracture of lower end of unspecified fibula CC UNS

✓6th S89.31 Salter-Harris Type I physeal fracture of lower end of fibula

4 ✓7th S89.311 Salter-Harris Type I physeal fracture of lower end of right fibula CC

4 ✓7th S89.312 Salter-Harris Type I physeal fracture of lower end of left fibula CC

4 ✓7th S89.319 Salter-Harris Type I physeal fracture of lower end of unspecified fibula CC UNS

✓6th S89.32 Salter-Harris Type II physeal fracture of lower end of fibula

4 ✓7th S89.321 Salter-Harris Type II physeal fracture of lower end of right fibula CC

4 ✓7th S89.322 Salter-Harris Type II physeal fracture of lower end of left fibula CC

4 ✓7th S89.329 Salter-Harris Type II physeal fracture of lower end of unspecified fibula CC UNS

✓6th S89.39 Other physeal fracture of lower end of fibula

4 ✓7th S89.391 Other physeal fracture of lower end of right fibula CC

4 ✓7th S89.392 Other physeal fracture of lower end of left fibula CC

4 ✓7th S89.399 Other physeal fracture of lower end of unspecified fibula CC UNS

S89.8 Other specified injuries of lower leg

The appropriate 7th character is to be added to each code in subcategory S89.8.
A initial encounter
D subsequent encounter
S sequela

S89.80 Other specified injuries of unspecified lower leg
S89.81 Other specified injuries of right lower leg
S89.82 Other specified injuries of left lower leg

S89.9 Unspecified injury of lower leg

The appropriate 7th character is to be added to each code in subcategory S89.9.
A initial encounter
D subsequent encounter
S sequela

S89.90 Unspecified injury of unspecified lower leg
S89.91 Unspecified injury of right lower leg
S89.92 Unspecified injury of left lower leg

Injuries to the ankle and foot (S90-S99)

EXCLUDES 2 *burns and corrosions (T20-T32)*
fracture of ankle and malleolus (S82.-)
frostbite (T33-T34)
insect bite or sting, venomous (T63.4)

S90 Superficial injury of ankle, foot and toes

The appropriate 7th character is to be added to each code from category S90.
A initial encounter
D subsequent encounter
S sequela

S90.0 Contusion of ankle
S90.00 Contusion of unspecified ankle
S90.01 Contusion of right ankle
S90.02 Contusion of left ankle

S90.1 Contusion of toe without damage to nail
S90.11 Contusion of great toe without damage to nail
S90.111 Contusion of right great toe without damage to nail
S90.112 Contusion of left great toe without damage to nail
S90.119 Contusion of unspecified great toe without damage to nail
S90.12 Contusion of lesser toe without damage to nail
S90.121 Contusion of right lesser toe(s) without damage to nail
S90.122 Contusion of left lesser toe(s) without damage to nail
S90.129 Contusion of unspecified lesser toe(s) without damage to nail
Contusion of toe NOS

S90.2 Contusion of toe with damage to nail
S90.21 Contusion of great toe with damage to nail
S90.211 Contusion of right great toe with damage to nail
S90.212 Contusion of left great toe with damage to nail
S90.219 Contusion of unspecified great toe with damage to nail
S90.22 Contusion of lesser toe with damage to nail
S90.221 Contusion of right lesser toe(s) with damage to nail
S90.222 Contusion of left lesser toe(s) with damage to nail
S90.229 Contusion of unspecified lesser toe(s) with damage to nail

S90.3 Contusion of foot
EXCLUDES 2 *contusion of toes (S90.1-, S90.2-)*
S90.30 Contusion of unspecified foot
Contusion of foot NOS
S90.31 Contusion of right foot
S90.32 Contusion of left foot

S90.4 Other superficial injuries of toe
S90.41 Abrasion of toe
S90.411 Abrasion, right great toe
S90.412 Abrasion, left great toe
S90.413 Abrasion, unspecified great toe
S90.414 Abrasion, right lesser toe(s)
S90.415 Abrasion, left lesser toe(s)
S90.416 Abrasion, unspecified lesser toe(s)
S90.42 Blister (nonthermal) of toe
S90.421 Blister (nonthermal), right great toe
S90.422 Blister (nonthermal), left great toe
S90.423 Blister (nonthermal), unspecified great toe
S90.424 Blister (nonthermal), right lesser toe(s)
S90.425 Blister (nonthermal), left lesser toe(s)
S90.426 Blister (nonthermal), unspecified lesser toe(s)
S90.44 External constriction of toe
Hair tourniquet syndrome of toe
S90.441 External constriction, right great toe
S90.442 External constriction, left great toe
S90.443 External constriction, unspecified great toe
S90.444 External constriction, right lesser toe(s)
S90.445 External constriction, left lesser toe(s)
S90.446 External constriction, unspecified lesser toe(s)
S90.45 Superficial foreign body of toe
Splinter in the toe
S90.451 Superficial foreign body, right great toe
S90.452 Superficial foreign body, left great toe
S90.453 Superficial foreign body, unspecified great toe
S90.454 Superficial foreign body, right lesser toe(s)
S90.455 Superficial foreign body, left lesser toe(s)
S90.456 Superficial foreign body, unspecified lesser toe(s)
S90.46 Insect bite (nonvenomous) of toe
S90.461 Insect bite (nonvenomous), right great toe
S90.462 Insect bite (nonvenomous), left great toe
S90.463 Insect bite (nonvenomous), unspecified great toe
S90.464 Insect bite (nonvenomous), right lesser toe(s)
S90.465 Insect bite (nonvenomous), left lesser toe(s)
S90.466 Insect bite (nonvenomous), unspecified lesser toe(s)
S90.47 Other superficial bite of toe
EXCLUDES 1 *open bite of toe (S91.15-, S91.25-)*
S90.471 Other superficial bite of right great toe
S90.472 Other superficial bite of left great toe
S90.473 Other superficial bite of unspecified great toe
S90.474 Other superficial bite of right lesser toe(s)
S90.475 Other superficial bite of left lesser toe(s)
S90.476 Other superficial bite of unspecified lesser toe(s)

S90.5 Other superficial injuries of ankle
S90.51 Abrasion of ankle
S90.511 Abrasion, right ankle
S90.512 Abrasion, left ankle
S90.519 Abrasion, unspecified ankle
S90.52 Blister (nonthermal) of ankle
S90.521 Blister (nonthermal), right ankle
S90.522 Blister (nonthermal), left ankle
S90.529 Blister (nonthermal), unspecified ankle
S90.54 External constriction of ankle
S90.541 External constriction, right ankle
S90.542 External constriction, left ankle

√7th **S90.549 External constriction, unspecified ankle**

√6th **S90.55 Superficial foreign body of ankle**
Splinter in the ankle
√7th **S90.551 Superficial foreign body, right ankle**
√7th **S90.552 Superficial foreign body, left ankle**
√7th **S90.559 Superficial foreign body, unspecified ankle**

√6th **S90.56 Insect bite (nonvenomous) of ankle**
√7th **S90.561 Insect bite (nonvenomous), right ankle**
√7th **S90.562 Insect bite (nonvenomous), left ankle**
√7th **S90.569 Insect bite (nonvenomous), unspecified ankle**

√6th **S90.57 Other superficial bite of ankle**
EXCLUDES 1 *open bite of ankle (S91.05-)*
√7th **S90.571 Other superficial bite of ankle, right ankle**
√7th **S90.572 Other superficial bite of ankle, left ankle**
√7th **S90.579 Other superficial bite of ankle, unspecified ankle**

√5th **S90.8 Other superficial injuries of foot**

√6th **S90.81 Abrasion of foot**
√7th **S90.811 Abrasion, right foot**
√7th **S90.812 Abrasion, left foot**
√7th **S90.819 Abrasion, unspecified foot**

√6th **S90.82 Blister (nonthermal) of foot**
√7th **S90.821 Blister (nonthermal), right foot**
√7th **S90.822 Blister (nonthermal), left foot**
√7th **S90.829 Blister (nonthermal), unspecified foot**

√6th **S90.84 External constriction of foot**
√7th **S90.841 External constriction, right foot**
√7th **S90.842 External constriction, left foot**
√7th **S90.849 External constriction, unspecified foot**

√6th **S90.85 Superficial foreign body of foot**
Splinter in the foot
√7th **S90.851 Superficial foreign body, right foot**
√7th **S90.852 Superficial foreign body, left foot**
√7th **S90.859 Superficial foreign body, unspecified foot**

√6th **S90.86 Insect bite (nonvenomous) of foot**
√7th **S90.861 Insect bite (nonvenomous), right foot**
√7th **S90.862 Insect bite (nonvenomous), left foot**
√7th **S90.869 Insect bite (nonvenomous), unspecified foot**

√6th **S90.87 Other superficial bite of foot**
EXCLUDES 1 *open bite of foot (S91.35-)*
√7th **S90.871 Other superficial bite of right foot**
√7th **S90.872 Other superficial bite of left foot**
√7th **S90.879 Other superficial bite of unspecified foot**

√5th **S90.9 Unspecified superficial injury of ankle, foot and toe**

√6th **S90.91 Unspecified superficial injury of ankle**
√7th **S90.911 Unspecified superficial injury of right ankle**
√7th **S90.912 Unspecified superficial injury of left ankle**
√7th **S90.919 Unspecified superficial injury of unspecified ankle**

√6th **S90.92 Unspecified superficial injury of foot**
√7th **S90.921 Unspecified superficial injury of right foot**
√7th **S90.922 Unspecified superficial injury of left foot**
√7th **S90.929 Unspecified superficial injury of unspecified foot**

√6th **S90.93 Unspecified superficial injury of toes**
√7th **S90.931 Unspecified superficial injury of right great toe**
√7th **S90.932 Unspecified superficial injury of left great toe**
√7th **S90.933 Unspecified superficial injury of unspecified great toe**
√7th **S90.934 Unspecified superficial injury of right lesser toe(s)**
√7th **S90.935 Unspecified superficial injury of left lesser toe(s)**
√7th **S90.936 Unspecified superficial injury of unspecified lesser toe(s)**

√4th **S91 Open wound of ankle, foot and toes**
Code also any associated wound infection
EXCLUDES 1 *open fracture of ankle, foot and toes (S92.- with 7th character B)*
traumatic amputation of ankle and foot (S98.-)
AHA: 2021,1Q,7

The appropriate 7th character is to be added to each code from category S91.
A initial encounter
D subsequent encounter
S sequela

√5th **S91.0 Open wound of ankle**

√6th **S91.00 Unspecified open wound of ankle**
√7th **S91.001 Unspecified open wound, right ankle**
√7th **S91.002 Unspecified open wound, left ankle**
√7th **S91.009 Unspecified open wound, unspecified ankle**

√6th **S91.01 Laceration without foreign body of ankle**
√7th **S91.011 Laceration without foreign body, right ankle**
√7th **S91.012 Laceration without foreign body, left ankle**
√7th **S91.019 Laceration without foreign body, unspecified ankle**

√6th **S91.02 Laceration with foreign body of ankle**
√7th **S91.021 Laceration with foreign body, right ankle**
√7th **S91.022 Laceration with foreign body, left ankle**
√7th **S91.029 Laceration with foreign body, unspecified ankle**

√6th **S91.03 Puncture wound without foreign body of ankle**
√7th **S91.031 Puncture wound without foreign body, right ankle**
√7th **S91.032 Puncture wound without foreign body, left ankle**
√7th **S91.039 Puncture wound without foreign body, unspecified ankle**

√6th **S91.04 Puncture wound with foreign body of ankle**
√7th **S91.041 Puncture wound with foreign body, right ankle**
√7th **S91.042 Puncture wound with foreign body, left ankle**
√7th **S91.049 Puncture wound with foreign body, unspecified ankle**

√6th **S91.05 Open bite of ankle**
EXCLUDES 1 *superficial bite of ankle (S90.56-, S90.57-)*
√7th **S91.051 Open bite, right ankle**
√7th **S91.052 Open bite, left ankle**
√7th **S91.059 Open bite, unspecified ankle**

√5th **S91.1 Open wound of toe without damage to nail**

√6th **S91.10 Unspecified open wound of toe without damage to nail**
√7th **S91.101 Unspecified open wound of right great toe without damage to nail**
√7th **S91.102 Unspecified open wound of left great toe without damage to nail**
√7th **S91.103 Unspecified open wound of unspecified great toe without damage to nail**
√7th **S91.104 Unspecified open wound of right lesser toe(s) without damage to nail**
√7th **S91.105 Unspecified open wound of left lesser toe(s) without damage to nail**
√7th **S91.106 Unspecified open wound of unspecified lesser toe(s) without damage to nail**
√7th **S91.109 Unspecified open wound of unspecified toe(s) without damage to nail**

√6th **S91.11 Laceration without foreign body of toe without damage to nail**
√7th **S91.111 Laceration without foreign body of right great toe without damage to nail**
√7th **S91.112 Laceration without foreign body of left great toe without damage to nail**
√7th **S91.113 Laceration without foreign body of unspecified great toe without damage to nail**
√7th **S91.114 Laceration without foreign body of right lesser toe(s) without damage to nail**
√7th **S91.115 Laceration without foreign body of left lesser toe(s) without damage to nail**

S91.116 Laceration without foreign body of unspecified lesser toe(s) without damage to nail
S91.119 Laceration without foreign body of unspecified toe without damage to nail
S91.12 Laceration with foreign body of toe without damage to nail
S91.121 Laceration with foreign body of right great toe without damage to nail
S91.122 Laceration with foreign body of left great toe without damage to nail
S91.123 Laceration with foreign body of unspecified great toe without damage to nail
S91.124 Laceration with foreign body of right lesser toe(s) without damage to nail
S91.125 Laceration with foreign body of left lesser toe(s) without damage to nail
S91.126 Laceration with foreign body of unspecified lesser toe(s) without damage to nail
S91.129 Laceration with foreign body of unspecified toe(s) without damage to nail
S91.13 Puncture wound without foreign body of toe without damage to nail
S91.131 Puncture wound without foreign body of right great toe without damage to nail
S91.132 Puncture wound without foreign body of left great toe without damage to nail
S91.133 Puncture wound without foreign body of unspecified great toe without damage to nail
S91.134 Puncture wound without foreign body of right lesser toe(s) without damage to nail
S91.135 Puncture wound without foreign body of left lesser toe(s) without damage to nail
S91.136 Puncture wound without foreign body of unspecified lesser toe(s) without damage to nail
S91.139 Puncture wound without foreign body of unspecified toe(s) without damage to nail
S91.14 Puncture wound with foreign body of toe without damage to nail
S91.141 Puncture wound with foreign body of right great toe without damage to nail
S91.142 Puncture wound with foreign body of left great toe without damage to nail
S91.143 Puncture wound with foreign body of unspecified great toe without damage to nail
S91.144 Puncture wound with foreign body of right lesser toe(s) without damage to nail
S91.145 Puncture wound with foreign body of left lesser toe(s) without damage to nail
S91.146 Puncture wound with foreign body of unspecified lesser toe(s) without damage to nail
S91.149 Puncture wound with foreign body of unspecified toe(s) without damage to nail
S91.15 Open bite of toe without damage to nail
Bite of toe NOS
EXCLUDES 1 *superficial bite of toe (S90.46-, S90.47-)*
S91.151 Open bite of right great toe without damage to nail
S91.152 Open bite of left great toe without damage to nail
S91.153 Open bite of unspecified great toe without damage to nail
S91.154 Open bite of right lesser toe(s) without damage to nail
S91.155 Open bite of left lesser toe(s) without damage to nail
S91.156 Open bite of unspecified lesser toe(s) without damage to nail
S91.159 Open bite of unspecified toe(s) without damage to nail
S91.2 Open wound of toe with damage to nail
S91.20 Unspecified open wound of toe with damage to nail
S91.201 Unspecified open wound of right great toe with damage to nail
S91.202 Unspecified open wound of left great toe with damage to nail
S91.203 Unspecified open wound of unspecified great toe with damage to nail
S91.204 Unspecified open wound of right lesser toe(s) with damage to nail
S91.205 Unspecified open wound of left lesser toe(s) with damage to nail
S91.206 Unspecified open wound of unspecified lesser toe(s) with damage to nail
S91.209 Unspecified open wound of unspecified toe(s) with damage to nail
S91.21 Laceration without foreign body of toe with damage to nail
S91.211 Laceration without foreign body of right great toe with damage to nail
S91.212 Laceration without foreign body of left great toe with damage to nail
S91.213 Laceration without foreign body of unspecified great toe with damage to nail
S91.214 Laceration without foreign body of right lesser toe(s) with damage to nail
S91.215 Laceration without foreign body of left lesser toe(s) with damage to nail
S91.216 Laceration without foreign body of unspecified lesser toe(s) with damage to nail
S91.219 Laceration without foreign body of unspecified toe(s) with damage to nail
S91.22 Laceration with foreign body of toe with damage to nail
S91.221 Laceration with foreign body of right great toe with damage to nail
S91.222 Laceration with foreign body of left great toe with damage to nail
S91.223 Laceration with foreign body of unspecified great toe with damage to nail
S91.224 Laceration with foreign body of right lesser toe(s) with damage to nail
S91.225 Laceration with foreign body of left lesser toe(s) with damage to nail
S91.226 Laceration with foreign body of unspecified lesser toe(s) with damage to nail
S91.229 Laceration with foreign body of unspecified toe(s) with damage to nail
S91.23 Puncture wound without foreign body of toe with damage to nail
S91.231 Puncture wound without foreign body of right great toe with damage to nail
S91.232 Puncture wound without foreign body of left great toe with damage to nail
S91.233 Puncture wound without foreign body of unspecified great toe with damage to nail
S91.234 Puncture wound without foreign body of right lesser toe(s) with damage to nail
S91.235 Puncture wound without foreign body of left lesser toe(s) with damage to nail
S91.236 Puncture wound without foreign body of unspecified lesser toe(s) with damage to nail
S91.239 Puncture wound without foreign body of unspecified toe(s) with damage to nail
S91.24 Puncture wound with foreign body of toe with damage to nail
S91.241 Puncture wound with foreign body of right great toe with damage to nail
S91.242 Puncture wound with foreign body of left great toe with damage to nail
S91.243 Puncture wound with foreign body of unspecified great toe with damage to nail
S91.244 Puncture wound with foreign body of right lesser toe(s) with damage to nail
S91.245 Puncture wound with foreign body of left lesser toe(s) with damage to nail
S91.246 Puncture wound with foreign body of unspecified lesser toe(s) with damage to nail
S91.249 Puncture wound with foreign body of unspecified toe(s) with damage to nail
S91.25 Open bite of toe with damage to nail
Bite of toe with damage to nail NOS
EXCLUDES 1 *superficial bite of toe (S90.46-, S90.47-)*
S91.251 Open bite of right great toe with damage to nail

S91.252 Open bite of left great toe with damage to nail

S91.253 Open bite of unspecified great toe with damage to nail

S91.254 Open bite of right lesser toe(s) with damage to nail

S91.255 Open bite of left lesser toe(s) with damage to nail

S91.256 Open bite of unspecified lesser toe(s) with damage to nail

S91.259 Open bite of unspecified toe(s) with damage to nail

S91.3 Open wound of foot

S91.30 Unspecified open wound of foot

S91.301 Unspecified open wound, right foot

S91.302 Unspecified open wound, left foot

S91.309 Unspecified open wound, unspecified foot

S91.31 Laceration without foreign body of foot

S91.311 Laceration without foreign body, right foot

S91.312 Laceration without foreign body, left foot

S91.319 Laceration without foreign body, unspecified foot

S91.32 Laceration with foreign body of foot

S91.321 Laceration with foreign body, right foot

S91.322 Laceration with foreign body, left foot

S91.329 Laceration with foreign body, unspecified foot

S91.33 Puncture wound without foreign body of foot

S91.331 Puncture wound without foreign body, right foot

S91.332 Puncture wound without foreign body, left foot

S91.339 Puncture wound without foreign body, unspecified foot

S91.34 Puncture wound with foreign body of foot

S91.341 Puncture wound with foreign body, right foot

S91.342 Puncture wound with foreign body, left foot

S91.349 Puncture wound with foreign body, unspecified foot

S91.35 Open bite of foot

EXCLUDES 1 *superficial bite of foot (S90.86-, S90.87-)*

S91.351 Open bite, right foot

S91.352 Open bite, left foot

S91.359 Open bite, unspecified foot

S92 Fracture of foot and toe, except ankle

NOTE A fracture not indicated as displaced or nondisplaced should be coded to displaced

A fracture not indicated as open or closed should be coded to closed.

EXCLUDES 2 *fracture of ankle (S82.-)*

fracture of malleolus (S82.-)

traumatic amputation of ankle and foot (S98.-)

AHA: 2018,2Q,12; 2015,3Q,37-39

The appropriate 7th character is to be added to each code from category S92.

A initial encounter for closed fracture
B initial encounter for open fracture
D subsequent encounter for fracture with routine healing
G subsequent encounter for fracture with delayed healing
K subsequent encounter for fracture with nonunion
P subsequent encounter for fracture with malunion
S sequela

S92.0 Fracture of calcaneus

Heel bone

Os calcis

EXCLUDES 2 *physeal fracture of calcaneus (S99.0-)*

S92.00 Unspecified fracture of calcaneus

S92.001 Unspecified fracture of right calcaneus CC HS

S92.002 Unspecified fracture of left calcaneus CC HS

S92.009 Unspecified fracture of unspecified calcaneus CC HS UNS

S92.01 Fracture of body of calcaneus

S92.011 Displaced fracture of body of right calcaneus CC HS

S92.012 Displaced fracture of body of left calcaneus CC HS

S92.013 Displaced fracture of body of unspecified calcaneus CC HS UNS

S92.014 Nondisplaced fracture of body of right calcaneus CC HS

S92.015 Nondisplaced fracture of body of left calcaneus CC HS

S92.016 Nondisplaced fracture of body of unspecified calcaneus CC HS UNS

S92.02 Fracture of anterior process of calcaneus

S92.021 Displaced fracture of anterior process of right calcaneus CC HS

S92.022 Displaced fracture of anterior process of left calcaneus CC HS

S92.023 Displaced fracture of anterior process of unspecified calcaneus CC HS UNS

S92.024 Nondisplaced fracture of anterior process of right calcaneus CC HS

S92.025 Nondisplaced fracture of anterior process of left calcaneus CC HS

S92.026 Nondisplaced fracture of anterior process of unspecified calcaneus CC HS UNS

S92.03 Avulsion fracture of tuberosity of calcaneus

S92.031 Displaced avulsion fracture of tuberosity of right calcaneus CC HS

S92.032 Displaced avulsion fracture of tuberosity of left calcaneus CC HS

S92.033 Displaced avulsion fracture of tuberosity of unspecified calcaneus CC HS UNS

S92.034 Nondisplaced avulsion fracture of tuberosity of right calcaneus CC HS

S92.035 Nondisplaced avulsion fracture of tuberosity of left calcaneus CC HS

S92.036 Nondisplaced avulsion fracture of tuberosity of unspecified calcaneus CC HS UNS

S92.04 Other fracture of tuberosity of calcaneus

S92.041 Displaced other fracture of tuberosity of right calcaneus CC HS

S92.042 Displaced other fracture of tuberosity of left calcaneus CC HS

S92.043 Displaced other fracture of tuberosity of unspecified calcaneus CC HS UNS

S92.044 Nondisplaced other fracture of tuberosity of right calcaneus CC HS

S92.045 Nondisplaced other fracture of tuberosity of left calcaneus CC HS

S92.046 Nondisplaced other fracture of tuberosity of unspecified calcaneus CC HS UNS

S92.05 Other extraarticular fracture of calcaneus

S92.051 Displaced other extraarticular fracture of right calcaneus CC HS

S92.052 Displaced other extraarticular fracture of left calcaneus CC HS

S92.053 Displaced other extraarticular fracture of unspecified calcaneus CC HS UNS

S92.054 Nondisplaced other extraarticular fracture of right calcaneus CC HS

S92.055 Nondisplaced other extraarticular fracture of left calcaneus CC HS

S92.056 Nondisplaced other extraarticular fracture of unspecified calcaneus CC HS UNS

S92.06 Intraarticular fracture of calcaneus

S92.061 Displaced intraarticular fracture of right calcaneus CC HS

S92.062 Displaced intraarticular fracture of left calcaneus CC HS

S92.063 Displaced intraarticular fracture of unspecified calcaneus CC HS UNS

S92.064 Nondisplaced intraarticular fracture of right calcaneus CC HS

S92.065 Nondisplaced intraarticular fracture of left calcaneus CC HS
S92.066 Nondisplaced intraarticular fracture of unspecified calcaneus CC HS UNS

S92.1 Fracture of talus
Astragalus

S92.10 Unspecified fracture of talus
S92.101 Unspecified fracture of right talus CC HS
S92.102 Unspecified fracture of left talus CC HS
S92.109 Unspecified fracture of unspecified talus CC HS UNS

S92.11 Fracture of neck of talus
S92.111 Displaced fracture of neck of right talus CC HS
S92.112 Displaced fracture of neck of left talus CC HS
S92.113 Displaced fracture of neck of unspecified talus CC HS UNS
S92.114 Nondisplaced fracture of neck of right talus CC HS
S92.115 Nondisplaced fracture of neck of left talus CC HS
S92.116 Nondisplaced fracture of neck of unspecified talus CC HS UNS

S92.12 Fracture of body of talus
S92.121 Displaced fracture of body of right talus CC HS
S92.122 Displaced fracture of body of left talus CC HS
S92.123 Displaced fracture of body of unspecified talus CC HS UNS
S92.124 Nondisplaced fracture of body of right talus CC HS
S92.125 Nondisplaced fracture of body of left talus CC HS
S92.126 Nondisplaced fracture of body of unspecified talus CC HS UNS

S92.13 Fracture of posterior process of talus
S92.131 Displaced fracture of posterior process of right talus CC HS
S92.132 Displaced fracture of posterior process of left talus CC HS
S92.133 Displaced fracture of posterior process of unspecified talus CC HS UNS
S92.134 Nondisplaced fracture of posterior process of right talus CC HS
S92.135 Nondisplaced fracture of posterior process of left talus CC HS
S92.136 Nondisplaced fracture of posterior process of unspecified talus CC HS UNS

S92.14 Dome fracture of talus
EXCLUDES 1 *osteochondritis dissecans (M93.2)*
S92.141 Displaced dome fracture of right talus CC HS
S92.142 Displaced dome fracture of left talus CC HS
S92.143 Displaced dome fracture of unspecified talus CC HS UNS
S92.144 Nondisplaced dome fracture of right talus CC HS
S92.145 Nondisplaced dome fracture of left talus CC HS
S92.146 Nondisplaced dome fracture of unspecified talus CC HS UNS

S92.15 Avulsion fracture (chip fracture) of talus
S92.151 Displaced avulsion fracture (chip fracture) of right talus CC HS
S92.152 Displaced avulsion fracture (chip fracture) of left talus CC HS
S92.153 Displaced avulsion fracture (chip fracture) of unspecified talus CC HS UNS
S92.154 Nondisplaced avulsion fracture (chip fracture) of right talus CC HS
S92.155 Nondisplaced avulsion fracture (chip fracture) of left talus CC HS
S92.156 Nondisplaced avulsion fracture (chip fracture) of unspecified talus CC HS UNS

S92.19 Other fracture of talus
S92.191 Other fracture of right talus CC HS
S92.192 Other fracture of left talus CC HS
S92.199 Other fracture of unspecified talus CC HS UNS

S92.2 Fracture of other and unspecified tarsal bone(s)

S92.20 Fracture of unspecified tarsal bone(s)
S92.201 Fracture of unspecified tarsal bone(s) of right foot CC HS
S92.202 Fracture of unspecified tarsal bone(s) of left foot CC HS
S92.209 Fracture of unspecified tarsal bone(s) of unspecified foot CC HS UNS

S92.21 Fracture of cuboid bone
S92.211 Displaced fracture of cuboid bone of right foot CC HS
S92.212 Displaced fracture of cuboid bone of left foot CC HS
S92.213 Displaced fracture of cuboid bone of unspecified foot CC HS UNS
S92.214 Nondisplaced fracture of cuboid bone of right foot CC HS
S92.215 Nondisplaced fracture of cuboid bone of left foot CC HS
S92.216 Nondisplaced fracture of cuboid bone of unspecified foot CC HS UNS

S92.22 Fracture of lateral cuneiform
S92.221 Displaced fracture of lateral cuneiform of right foot CC HS
S92.222 Displaced fracture of lateral cuneiform of left foot CC HS
S92.223 Displaced fracture of lateral cuneiform of unspecified foot CC HS UNS
S92.224 Nondisplaced fracture of lateral cuneiform of right foot CC HS
S92.225 Nondisplaced fracture of lateral cuneiform of left foot CC HS
S92.226 Nondisplaced fracture of lateral cuneiform of unspecified foot CC HS UNS

S92.23 Fracture of intermediate cuneiform
S92.231 Displaced fracture of intermediate cuneiform of right foot CC HS
S92.232 Displaced fracture of intermediate cuneiform of left foot CC HS
S92.233 Displaced fracture of intermediate cuneiform of unspecified foot CC HS UNS
S92.234 Nondisplaced fracture of intermediate cuneiform of right foot CC HS
S92.235 Nondisplaced fracture of intermediate cuneiform of left foot CC HS
S92.236 Nondisplaced fracture of intermediate cuneiform of unspecified foot CC HS UNS

S92.24 Fracture of medial cuneiform
S92.241 Displaced fracture of medial cuneiform of right foot CC HS
S92.242 Displaced fracture of medial cuneiform of left foot CC HS
S92.243 Displaced fracture of medial cuneiform of unspecified foot CC HS UNS
S92.244 Nondisplaced fracture of medial cuneiform of right foot CC HS
S92.245 Nondisplaced fracture of medial cuneiform of left foot CC HS
S92.246 Nondisplaced fracture of medial cuneiform of unspecified foot CC HS UNS

S92.25 Fracture of navicular [scaphoid] of foot
S92.251 Displaced fracture of navicular [scaphoid] of right foot CC HS
S92.252 Displaced fracture of navicular [scaphoid] of left foot CC HS

3 7th S92.253 Displaced fracture of navicular [scaphoid] of unspecified foot CC HS UNS

3 7th S92.254 Nondisplaced fracture of navicular [scaphoid] of right foot CC HS

3 7th S92.255 Nondisplaced fracture of navicular [scaphoid] of left foot CC HS

3 7th S92.256 Nondisplaced fracture of navicular [scaphoid] of unspecified foot CC HS UNS

5th S92.3 Fracture of metatarsal bone(s)

EXCLUDES 2 *physeal fracture of metatarsal (S99.1-)*

AHA: 2018,1Q,3

6th S92.30 Fracture of unspecified metatarsal bone(s)

3 7th S92.301 Fracture of unspecified metatarsal bone(s), right foot CC HS

3 7th S92.302 Fracture of unspecified metatarsal bone(s), left foot CC HS

3 7th S92.309 Fracture of unspecified metatarsal bone(s), unspecified foot CC HS UNS

6th S92.31 Fracture of first metatarsal bone

3 7th S92.311 Displaced fracture of first metatarsal bone, right foot CC HS

3 7th S92.312 Displaced fracture of first metatarsal bone, left foot CC HS

3 7th S92.313 Displaced fracture of first metatarsal bone, unspecified foot CC HS UNS

3 7th S92.314 Nondisplaced fracture of first metatarsal bone, right foot CC HS

3 7th S92.315 Nondisplaced fracture of first metatarsal bone, left foot CC HS

3 7th S92.316 Nondisplaced fracture of first metatarsal bone, unspecified foot CC HS UNS

6th S92.32 Fracture of second metatarsal bone

3 7th S92.321 Displaced fracture of second metatarsal bone, right foot CC HS

3 7th S92.322 Displaced fracture of second metatarsal bone, left foot CC HS

3 7th S92.323 Displaced fracture of second metatarsal bone, unspecified foot CC HS UNS

3 7th S92.324 Nondisplaced fracture of second metatarsal bone, right foot CC HS

3 7th S92.325 Nondisplaced fracture of second metatarsal bone, left foot CC HS

3 7th S92.326 Nondisplaced fracture of second metatarsal bone, unspecified foot CC HS UNS

6th S92.33 Fracture of third metatarsal bone

3 7th S92.331 Displaced fracture of third metatarsal bone, right foot CC HS

3 7th S92.332 Displaced fracture of third metatarsal bone, left foot CC HS

3 7th S92.333 Displaced fracture of third metatarsal bone, unspecified foot CC HS UNS

3 7th S92.334 Nondisplaced fracture of third metatarsal bone, right foot CC HS

3 7th S92.335 Nondisplaced fracture of third metatarsal bone, left foot CC HS

3 7th S92.336 Nondisplaced fracture of third metatarsal bone, unspecified foot CC HS UNS

6th S92.34 Fracture of fourth metatarsal bone

3 7th S92.341 Displaced fracture of fourth metatarsal bone, right foot CC HS

3 7th S92.342 Displaced fracture of fourth metatarsal bone, left foot CC HS

3 7th S92.343 Displaced fracture of fourth metatarsal bone, unspecified foot CC HS UNS

3 7th S92.344 Nondisplaced fracture of fourth metatarsal bone, right foot CC HS

3 7th S92.345 Nondisplaced fracture of fourth metatarsal bone, left foot CC HS

3 7th S92.346 Nondisplaced fracture of fourth metatarsal bone, unspecified foot CC HS UNS

6th S92.35 Fracture of fifth metatarsal bone

3 7th S92.351 Displaced fracture of fifth metatarsal bone, right foot CC HS

3 7th S92.352 Displaced fracture of fifth metatarsal bone, left foot CC HS

3 7th S92.353 Displaced fracture of fifth metatarsal bone, unspecified foot CC HS UNS

3 7th S92.354 Nondisplaced fracture of fifth metatarsal bone, right foot CC HS

3 7th S92.355 Nondisplaced fracture of fifth metatarsal bone, left foot CC HS

3 7th S92.356 Nondisplaced fracture of fifth metatarsal bone, unspecified foot CC HS UNS

5th S92.4 Fracture of great toe

EXCLUDES 2 *physeal fracture of phalanx of toe (S99.2-)*

6th S92.40 Unspecified fracture of great toe

4 7th S92.401 Displaced unspecified fracture of right great toe CC

4 7th S92.402 Displaced unspecified fracture of left great toe CC

4 7th S92.403 Displaced unspecified fracture of unspecified great toe CC UNS

4 7th S92.404 Nondisplaced unspecified fracture of right great toe CC

4 7th S92.405 Nondisplaced unspecified fracture of left great toe CC

4 7th S92.406 Nondisplaced unspecified fracture of unspecified great toe CC UNS

6th S92.41 Fracture of proximal phalanx of great toe

4 7th S92.411 Displaced fracture of proximal phalanx of right great toe CC

4 7th S92.412 Displaced fracture of proximal phalanx of left great toe CC

4 7th S92.413 Displaced fracture of proximal phalanx of unspecified great toe CC UNS

4 7th S92.414 Nondisplaced fracture of proximal phalanx of right great toe CC

4 7th S92.415 Nondisplaced fracture of proximal phalanx of left great toe CC

4 7th S92.416 Nondisplaced fracture of proximal phalanx of unspecified great toe CC UNS

6th S92.42 Fracture of distal phalanx of great toe

4 7th S92.421 Displaced fracture of distal phalanx of right great toe CC

4 7th S92.422 Displaced fracture of distal phalanx of left great toe CC

4 7th S92.423 Displaced fracture of distal phalanx of unspecified great toe CC UNS

4 7th S92.424 Nondisplaced fracture of distal phalanx of right great toe CC

4 7th S92.425 Nondisplaced fracture of distal phalanx of left great toe CC

4 7th S92.426 Nondisplaced fracture of distal phalanx of unspecified great toe CC UNS

6th S92.49 Other fracture of great toe

4 7th S92.491 Other fracture of right great toe CC

4 7th S92.492 Other fracture of left great toe CC

4 7th S92.499 Other fracture of unspecified great toe CC UNS

5th S92.5 Fracture of lesser toe(s)

EXCLUDES 2 *physeal fracture of phalanx of toe (S99.2-)*

6th S92.50 Unspecified fracture of lesser toe(s)

4 7th S92.501 Displaced unspecified fracture of right lesser toe(s) CC

4 7th S92.502 Displaced unspecified fracture of left lesser toe(s) CC

4 7th S92.503 Displaced unspecified fracture of unspecified lesser toe(s) CC UNS

4 7th S92.504 Nondisplaced unspecified fracture of right lesser toe(s) CC

4 7th S92.505 Nondisplaced unspecified fracture of left lesser toe(s) CC

4 7th S92.506 Nondisplaced unspecified fracture of unspecified lesser toe(s) CC UNS

6th S92.51 Fracture of proximal phalanx of lesser toe(s)

4 7th S92.511 Displaced fracture of proximal phalanx of right lesser toe(s) CC

4 7th S92.512 Displaced fracture of proximal phalanx of left lesser toe(s) CC

4 7th S92.513 Displaced fracture of proximal phalanx of unspecified lesser toe(s) CC UNS

S92.514 Nondisplaced fracture of proximal phalanx of right lesser toe(s) CC

S92.515 Nondisplaced fracture of proximal phalanx of left lesser toe(s) CC

S92.516 Nondisplaced fracture of proximal phalanx of unspecified lesser toe(s) CC UNS

S92.52 Fracture of middle phalanx of lesser toe(s)

S92.521 Displaced fracture of middle phalanx of right lesser toe(s) CC

S92.522 Displaced fracture of middle phalanx of left lesser toe(s) CC

S92.523 Displaced fracture of middle phalanx of unspecified lesser toe(s) CC UNS

S92.524 Nondisplaced fracture of middle phalanx of right lesser toe(s) CC

S92.525 Nondisplaced fracture of middle phalanx of left lesser toe(s) CC

S92.526 Nondisplaced fracture of middle phalanx of unspecified lesser toe(s) CC UNS

S92.53 Fracture of distal phalanx of lesser toe(s)

S92.531 Displaced fracture of distal phalanx of right lesser toe(s) CC

S92.532 Displaced fracture of distal phalanx of left lesser toe(s) CC

S92.533 Displaced fracture of distal phalanx of unspecified lesser toe(s) CC UNS

S92.534 Nondisplaced fracture of distal phalanx of right lesser toe(s) CC

S92.535 Nondisplaced fracture of distal phalanx of left lesser toe(s) CC

S92.536 Nondisplaced fracture of distal phalanx of unspecified lesser toe(s) CC UNS

S92.59 Other fracture of lesser toe(s)

S92.591 Other fracture of right lesser toe(s) CC

S92.592 Other fracture of left lesser toe(s) CC

S92.599 Other fracture of unspecified lesser toe(s) CC UNS

S92.8 Other fracture of foot, except ankle

S92.81 Other fracture of foot

Sesamoid fracture of foot

AHA: 2016,4Q,68

S92.811 Other fracture of right foot CC H5

S92.812 Other fracture of left foot CC H5

S92.819 Other fracture of unspecified foot CC H5 UNS

S92.9 Unspecified fracture of foot and toe

S92.90 Unspecified fracture of foot

S92.901 Unspecified fracture of right foot CC H5

S92.902 Unspecified fracture of left foot CC H5

S92.909 Unspecified fracture of unspecified foot CC H5 UNS

S92.91 Unspecified fracture of toe

S92.911 Unspecified fracture of right toe(s) CC

S92.912 Unspecified fracture of left toe(s) CC

S92.919 Unspecified fracture of unspecified toe(s) CC UNS

S93 Dislocation and sprain of joints and ligaments at ankle, foot and toe level

INCLUDES avulsion of joint or ligament of ankle, foot and toe
laceration of cartilage, joint or ligament of ankle, foot and toe
sprain of cartilage, joint or ligament of ankle, foot and toe
traumatic hemarthrosis of joint or ligament of ankle, foot and toe
traumatic rupture of joint or ligament of ankle, foot and toe
traumatic subluxation of joint or ligament of ankle, foot and toe
traumatic tear of joint or ligament of ankle, foot and toe

Code also any associated open wound

EXCLUDES 2 *strain of muscle and tendon of ankle and foot (S96.-)*

The appropriate 7th character is to be added to each code from category S93.
A initial encounter
D subsequent encounter
S sequela

S93.0 Subluxation and dislocation of ankle joint

Subluxation and dislocation of astragalus
Subluxation and dislocation of fibula, lower end
Subluxation and dislocation of talus
Subluxation and dislocation of tibia, lower end

S93.01 Subluxation of right ankle joint

S93.02 Subluxation of left ankle joint

S93.03 Subluxation of unspecified ankle joint

S93.04 Dislocation of right ankle joint

S93.05 Dislocation of left ankle joint

S93.06 Dislocation of unspecified ankle joint

S93.1 Subluxation and dislocation of toe

S93.10 Unspecified subluxation and dislocation of toe

Dislocation of toe NOS
Subluxation of toe NOS

S93.101 Unspecified subluxation of right toe(s)

S93.102 Unspecified subluxation of left toe(s)

S93.103 Unspecified subluxation of unspecified toe(s)

S93.104 Unspecified dislocation of right toe(s)

S93.105 Unspecified dislocation of left toe(s)

S93.106 Unspecified dislocation of unspecified toe(s)

S93.11 Dislocation of interphalangeal joint

S93.111 Dislocation of interphalangeal joint of right great toe

S93.112 Dislocation of interphalangeal joint of left great toe

S93.113 Dislocation of interphalangeal joint of unspecified great toe

S93.114 Dislocation of interphalangeal joint of right lesser toe(s)

S93.115 Dislocation of interphalangeal joint of left lesser toe(s)

S93.116 Dislocation of interphalangeal joint of unspecified lesser toe(s)

S93.119 Dislocation of interphalangeal joint of unspecified toe(s)

S93.12 Dislocation of metatarsophalangeal joint

S93.121 Dislocation of metatarsophalangeal joint of right great toe

S93.122 Dislocation of metatarsophalangeal joint of left great toe

S93.123 Dislocation of metatarsophalangeal joint of unspecified great toe

S93.124 Dislocation of metatarsophalangeal joint of right lesser toe(s)

S93.125 Dislocation of metatarsophalangeal joint of left lesser toe(s)

S93.126 Dislocation of metatarsophalangeal joint of unspecified lesser toe(s)

S93.129 Dislocation of metatarsophalangeal joint of unspecified toe(s)

S93.13 Subluxation of interphalangeal joint

S93.131 Subluxation of interphalangeal joint of right great toe

7th S93.132 Subluxation of interphalangeal joint of left great toe
7th S93.133 Subluxation of interphalangeal joint of unspecified great toe
7th S93.134 Subluxation of interphalangeal joint of right lesser toe(s)
7th S93.135 Subluxation of interphalangeal joint of left lesser toe(s)
7th S93.136 Subluxation of interphalangeal joint of unspecified lesser toe(s)
7th S93.139 Subluxation of interphalangeal joint of unspecified toe(s)
6th S93.14 Subluxation of metatarsophalangeal joint
7th S93.141 Subluxation of metatarsophalangeal joint of right great toe
7th S93.142 Subluxation of metatarsophalangeal joint of left great toe
7th S93.143 Subluxation of metatarsophalangeal joint of unspecified great toe
7th S93.144 Subluxation of metatarsophalangeal joint of right lesser toe(s)
7th S93.145 Subluxation of metatarsophalangeal joint of left lesser toe(s)
7th S93.146 Subluxation of metatarsophalangeal joint of unspecified lesser toe(s)
7th S93.149 Subluxation of metatarsophalangeal joint of unspecified toe(s)
5th S93.3 Subluxation and dislocation of foot
EXCLUDES 2 *dislocation of toe (S93.1-)*
6th S93.30 Unspecified subluxation and dislocation of foot
Dislocation of foot NOS
Subluxation of foot NOS
7th S93.301 Unspecified subluxation of right foot
7th S93.302 Unspecified subluxation of left foot
7th S93.303 Unspecified subluxation of unspecified foot
7th S93.304 Unspecified dislocation of right foot
7th S93.305 Unspecified dislocation of left foot
7th S93.306 Unspecified dislocation of unspecified foot
6th S93.31 Subluxation and dislocation of tarsal joint
7th S93.311 Subluxation of tarsal joint of right foot
7th S93.312 Subluxation of tarsal joint of left foot
7th S93.313 Subluxation of tarsal joint of unspecified foot
7th S93.314 Dislocation of tarsal joint of right foot
7th S93.315 Dislocation of tarsal joint of left foot
7th S93.316 Dislocation of tarsal joint of unspecified foot
6th S93.32 Subluxation and dislocation of tarsometatarsal joint
7th S93.321 Subluxation of tarsometatarsal joint of right foot
7th S93.322 Subluxation of tarsometatarsal joint of left foot
7th S93.323 Subluxation of tarsometatarsal joint of unspecified foot
7th S93.324 Dislocation of tarsometatarsal joint of right foot
7th S93.325 Dislocation of tarsometatarsal joint of left foot
7th S93.326 Dislocation of tarsometatarsal joint of unspecified foot
6th S93.33 Other subluxation and dislocation of foot
7th S93.331 Other subluxation of right foot
7th S93.332 Other subluxation of left foot
7th S93.333 Other subluxation of unspecified foot
7th S93.334 Other dislocation of right foot
7th S93.335 Other dislocation of left foot
7th S93.336 Other dislocation of unspecified foot
5th S93.4 Sprain of ankle
EXCLUDES 2 *injury of Achilles tendon (S86.0-)*
6th S93.40 Sprain of unspecified ligament of ankle
Sprain of ankle NOS
Sprained ankle NOS
7th S93.401 Sprain of unspecified ligament of right ankle
7th S93.402 Sprain of unspecified ligament of left ankle
7th S93.409 Sprain of unspecified ligament of unspecified ankle
6th S93.41 Sprain of calcaneofibular ligament
7th S93.411 Sprain of calcaneofibular ligament of right ankle
7th S93.412 Sprain of calcaneofibular ligament of left ankle
7th S93.419 Sprain of calcaneofibular ligament of unspecified ankle
6th S93.42 Sprain of deltoid ligament
7th S93.421 Sprain of deltoid ligament of right ankle
7th S93.422 Sprain of deltoid ligament of left ankle
7th S93.429 Sprain of deltoid ligament of unspecified ankle
6th S93.43 Sprain of tibiofibular ligament
7th S93.431 Sprain of tibiofibular ligament of right ankle
7th S93.432 Sprain of tibiofibular ligament of left ankle
7th S93.439 Sprain of tibiofibular ligament of unspecified ankle
6th S93.49 Sprain of other ligament of ankle
Sprain of internal collateral ligament
Sprain of talofibular ligament
7th S93.491 Sprain of other ligament of right ankle
7th S93.492 Sprain of other ligament of left ankle
7th S93.499 Sprain of other ligament of unspecified ankle
5th S93.5 Sprain of toe
6th S93.50 Unspecified sprain of toe
7th S93.501 Unspecified sprain of right great toe
7th S93.502 Unspecified sprain of left great toe
7th S93.503 Unspecified sprain of unspecified great toe
7th S93.504 Unspecified sprain of right lesser toe(s)
7th S93.505 Unspecified sprain of left lesser toe(s)
7th S93.506 Unspecified sprain of unspecified lesser toe(s)
7th S93.509 Unspecified sprain of unspecified toe(s)
6th S93.51 Sprain of interphalangeal joint of toe
7th S93.511 Sprain of interphalangeal joint of right great toe
7th S93.512 Sprain of interphalangeal joint of left great toe
7th S93.513 Sprain of interphalangeal joint of unspecified great toe
7th S93.514 Sprain of interphalangeal joint of right lesser toe(s)
7th S93.515 Sprain of interphalangeal joint of left lesser toe(s)
7th S93.516 Sprain of interphalangeal joint of unspecified lesser toe(s)
7th S93.519 Sprain of interphalangeal joint of unspecified toe(s)
6th S93.52 Sprain of metatarsophalangeal joint of toe
7th S93.521 Sprain of metatarsophalangeal joint of right great toe
7th S93.522 Sprain of metatarsophalangeal joint of left great toe
7th S93.523 Sprain of metatarsophalangeal joint of unspecified great toe
7th S93.524 Sprain of metatarsophalangeal joint of right lesser toe(s)
7th S93.525 Sprain of metatarsophalangeal joint of left lesser toe(s)
7th S93.526 Sprain of metatarsophalangeal joint of unspecified lesser toe(s)
7th S93.529 Sprain of metatarsophalangeal joint of unspecified toe(s)
5th S93.6 Sprain of foot
EXCLUDES 2 *sprain of metatarsophalangeal joint of toe (S93.52-)*
sprain of toe (S93.5-)
6th S93.60 Unspecified sprain of foot
7th S93.601 Unspecified sprain of right foot
7th S93.602 Unspecified sprain of left foot

S93.609 Unspecified sprain of unspecified foot

S93.61 Sprain of tarsal ligament of foot

S93.611 Sprain of tarsal ligament of right foot

S93.612 Sprain of tarsal ligament of left foot

S93.619 Sprain of tarsal ligament of unspecified foot

S93.62 Sprain of tarsometatarsal ligament of foot

S93.621 Sprain of tarsometatarsal ligament of right foot

S93.622 Sprain of tarsometatarsal ligament of left foot

S93.629 Sprain of tarsometatarsal ligament of unspecified foot

S93.69 Other sprain of foot

S93.691 Other sprain of right foot

S93.692 Other sprain of left foot

S93.699 Other sprain of unspecified foot

S94 Injury of nerves at ankle and foot level

Code also any associated open wound (S91.-)

The appropriate 7th character is to be added to each code from category S94.
- A initial encounter
- D subsequent encounter
- S sequela

S94.0 Injury of lateral plantar nerve

S94.00 Injury of lateral plantar nerve, unspecified leg

S94.01 Injury of lateral plantar nerve, right leg

S94.02 Injury of lateral plantar nerve, left leg

S94.1 Injury of medial plantar nerve

S94.10 Injury of medial plantar nerve, unspecified leg

S94.11 Injury of medial plantar nerve, right leg

S94.12 Injury of medial plantar nerve, left leg

S94.2 Injury of deep peroneal nerve at ankle and foot level

Injury of terminal, lateral branch of deep peroneal nerve

S94.20 Injury of deep peroneal nerve at ankle and foot level, unspecified leg

S94.21 Injury of deep peroneal nerve at ankle and foot level, right leg

S94.22 Injury of deep peroneal nerve at ankle and foot level, left leg

S94.3 Injury of cutaneous sensory nerve at ankle and foot level

S94.30 Injury of cutaneous sensory nerve at ankle and foot level, unspecified leg

S94.31 Injury of cutaneous sensory nerve at ankle and foot level, right leg

S94.32 Injury of cutaneous sensory nerve at ankle and foot level, left leg

S94.8 Injury of other nerves at ankle and foot level

S94.8X Injury of other nerves at ankle and foot level

S94.8X1 Injury of other nerves at ankle and foot level, right leg

S94.8X2 Injury of other nerves at ankle and foot level, left leg

S94.8X9 Injury of other nerves at ankle and foot level, unspecified leg

S94.9 Injury of unspecified nerve at ankle and foot level

S94.90 Injury of unspecified nerve at ankle and foot level, unspecified leg

S94.91 Injury of unspecified nerve at ankle and foot level, right leg

S94.92 Injury of unspecified nerve at ankle and foot level, left leg

S95 Injury of blood vessels at ankle and foot level

Code also any associated open wound (S91.-)

EXCLUDES 2 *injury of posterior tibial artery and vein (S85.1-, S85.8-)*

The appropriate 7th character is to be added to each code from category S95.
- A initial encounter
- D subsequent encounter
- S sequela

S95.0 Injury of dorsal artery of foot

S95.00 Unspecified injury of dorsal artery of foot

S95.001 Unspecified injury of dorsal artery of right foot CC

S95.002 Unspecified injury of dorsal artery of left foot CC

S95.009 Unspecified injury of dorsal artery of unspecified foot CC UNS

S95.01 Laceration of dorsal artery of foot

S95.011 Laceration of dorsal artery of right foot CC

S95.012 Laceration of dorsal artery of left foot CC

S95.019 Laceration of dorsal artery of unspecified foot CC UNS

S95.09 Other specified injury of dorsal artery of foot

S95.091 Other specified injury of dorsal artery of right foot CC

S95.092 Other specified injury of dorsal artery of left foot CC

S95.099 Other specified injury of dorsal artery of unspecified foot CC UNS

S95.1 Injury of plantar artery of foot

S95.10 Unspecified injury of plantar artery of foot

S95.101 Unspecified injury of plantar artery of right foot CC

S95.102 Unspecified injury of plantar artery of left foot CC

S95.109 Unspecified injury of plantar artery of unspecified foot CC UNS

S95.11 Laceration of plantar artery of foot

S95.111 Laceration of plantar artery of right foot CC

S95.112 Laceration of plantar artery of left foot CC

S95.119 Laceration of plantar artery of unspecified foot CC UNS

S95.19 Other specified injury of plantar artery of foot

S95.191 Other specified injury of plantar artery of right foot CC

S95.192 Other specified injury of plantar artery of left foot CC

S95.199 Other specified injury of plantar artery of unspecified foot CC UNS

S95.2 Injury of dorsal vein of foot

S95.20 Unspecified injury of dorsal vein of foot

S95.201 Unspecified injury of dorsal vein of right foot CC

S95.202 Unspecified injury of dorsal vein of left foot CC

S95.209 Unspecified injury of dorsal vein of unspecified foot CC UNS

S95.21 Laceration of dorsal vein of foot

S95.211 Laceration of dorsal vein of right foot CC

S95.212 Laceration of dorsal vein of left foot CC

S95.219 Laceration of dorsal vein of unspecified foot CC UNS

S95.29 Other specified injury of dorsal vein of foot

S95.291 Other specified injury of dorsal vein of right foot CC

S95.292 Other specified injury of dorsal vein of left foot CC

S95.299 Other specified injury of dorsal vein of unspecified foot CC UNS

5th **S95.8 Injury of other blood vessels at ankle and foot level**

6th **S95.80 Unspecified injury of other blood vessels at ankle and foot level**

7th **S95.801 Unspecified injury of other blood vessels at ankle and foot level, right leg** CC

7th **S95.802 Unspecified injury of other blood vessels at ankle and foot level, left leg** CC

7th **S95.809 Unspecified injury of other blood vessels at ankle and foot level, unspecified leg** CC UNS

6th **S95.81 Laceration of other blood vessels at ankle and foot level**

7th **S95.811 Laceration of other blood vessels at ankle and foot level, right leg** CC

7th **S95.812 Laceration of other blood vessels at ankle and foot level, left leg** CC

7th **S95.819 Laceration of other blood vessels at ankle and foot level, unspecified leg** CC UNS

6th **S95.89 Other specified injury of other blood vessels at ankle and foot level**

7th **S95.891 Other specified injury of other blood vessels at ankle and foot level, right leg** CC

7th **S95.892 Other specified injury of other blood vessels at ankle and foot level, left leg** CC

7th **S95.899 Other specified injury of other blood vessels at ankle and foot level, unspecified leg** CC UNS

5th **S95.9 Injury of unspecified blood vessel at ankle and foot level**

6th **S95.90 Unspecified injury of unspecified blood vessel at ankle and foot level**

7th **S95.901 Unspecified injury of unspecified blood vessel at ankle and foot level, right leg** CC

7th **S95.902 Unspecified injury of unspecified blood vessel at ankle and foot level, left leg** CC

7th **S95.909 Unspecified injury of unspecified blood vessel at ankle and foot level, unspecified leg** CC UNS

6th **S95.91 Laceration of unspecified blood vessel at ankle and foot level**

7th **S95.911 Laceration of unspecified blood vessel at ankle and foot level, right leg** CC

7th **S95.912 Laceration of unspecified blood vessel at ankle and foot level, left leg** CC

7th **S95.919 Laceration of unspecified blood vessel at ankle and foot level, unspecified leg** CC UNS

6th **S95.99 Other specified injury of unspecified blood vessel at ankle and foot level**

7th **S95.991 Other specified injury of unspecified blood vessel at ankle and foot level, right leg** CC

7th **S95.992 Other specified injury of unspecified blood vessel at ankle and foot level, left leg** CC

7th **S95.999 Other specified injury of unspecified blood vessel at ankle and foot level, unspecified leg** CC UNS

4th **S96 Injury of muscle and tendon at ankle and foot level**

Code also any associated open wound (S91.-)

EXCLUDES 2 *injury of Achilles tendon (S86.0-)*

sprain of joints and ligaments of ankle and foot (S93.-)

TIP: Refer to the Muscle/Tendon table at the beginning of this chapter.

The appropriate 7th character is to be added to each code from category S96.

A initial encounter

D subsequent encounter

S sequela

5th **S96.0 Injury of muscle and tendon of long flexor muscle of toe at ankle and foot level**

6th **S96.00 Unspecified injury of muscle and tendon of long flexor muscle of toe at ankle and foot level**

7th **S96.001 Unspecified injury of muscle and tendon of long flexor muscle of toe at ankle and foot level, right foot**

7th **S96.002 Unspecified injury of muscle and tendon of long flexor muscle of toe at ankle and foot level, left foot**

7th **S96.009 Unspecified injury of muscle and tendon of long flexor muscle of toe at ankle and foot level, unspecified foot**

6th **S96.01 Strain of muscle and tendon of long flexor muscle of toe at ankle and foot level**

7th **S96.011 Strain of muscle and tendon of long flexor muscle of toe at ankle and foot level, right foot**

7th **S96.012 Strain of muscle and tendon of long flexor muscle of toe at ankle and foot level, left foot**

7th **S96.019 Strain of muscle and tendon of long flexor muscle of toe at ankle and foot level, unspecified foot**

6th **S96.02 Laceration of muscle and tendon of long flexor muscle of toe at ankle and foot level**

7th **S96.021 Laceration of muscle and tendon of long flexor muscle of toe at ankle and foot level, right foot** CC

7th **S96.022 Laceration of muscle and tendon of long flexor muscle of toe at ankle and foot level, left foot** CC

7th **S96.029 Laceration of muscle and tendon of long flexor muscle of toe at ankle and foot level, unspecified foot** CC UNS

6th **S96.09 Other injury of muscle and tendon of long flexor muscle of toe at ankle and foot level**

7th **S96.091 Other injury of muscle and tendon of long flexor muscle of toe at ankle and foot level, right foot**

7th **S96.092 Other injury of muscle and tendon of long flexor muscle of toe at ankle and foot level, left foot**

7th **S96.099 Other injury of muscle and tendon of long flexor muscle of toe at ankle and foot level, unspecified foot**

5th **S96.1 Injury of muscle and tendon of long extensor muscle of toe at ankle and foot level**

6th **S96.10 Unspecified injury of muscle and tendon of long extensor muscle of toe at ankle and foot level**

7th **S96.101 Unspecified injury of muscle and tendon of long extensor muscle of toe at ankle and foot level, right foot**

7th **S96.102 Unspecified injury of muscle and tendon of long extensor muscle of toe at ankle and foot level, left foot**

7th **S96.109 Unspecified injury of muscle and tendon of long extensor muscle of toe at ankle and foot level, unspecified foot**

6th **S96.11 Strain of muscle and tendon of long extensor muscle of toe at ankle and foot level**

7th **S96.111 Strain of muscle and tendon of long extensor muscle of toe at ankle and foot level, right foot**

7th **S96.112 Strain of muscle and tendon of long extensor muscle of toe at ankle and foot level, left foot**

7th **S96.119 Strain of muscle and tendon of long extensor muscle of toe at ankle and foot level, unspecified foot**

6th **S96.12 Laceration of muscle and tendon of long extensor muscle of toe at ankle and foot level**

7th **S96.121 Laceration of muscle and tendon of long extensor muscle of toe at ankle and foot level, right foot** CC

7th **S96.122 Laceration of muscle and tendon of long extensor muscle of toe at ankle and foot level, left foot** CC

7th **S96.129 Laceration of muscle and tendon of long extensor muscle of toe at ankle and foot level, unspecified foot** CC UNS

6th **S96.19 Other specified injury of muscle and tendon of long extensor muscle of toe at ankle and foot level**

7th **S96.191 Other specified injury of muscle and tendon of long extensor muscle of toe at ankle and foot level, right foot**

7th **S96.192 Other specified injury of muscle and tendon of long extensor muscle of toe at ankle and foot level, left foot**

7th **S96.199 Other specified injury of muscle and tendon of long extensor muscle of toe at ankle and foot level, unspecified foot**

S96.2 Injury of intrinsic muscle and tendon at ankle and foot level
- S96.20 Unspecified injury of intrinsic muscle and tendon at ankle and foot level
  - S96.201 Unspecified injury of intrinsic muscle and tendon at ankle and foot level, right foot
  - S96.202 Unspecified injury of intrinsic muscle and tendon at ankle and foot level, left foot
  - S96.209 Unspecified injury of intrinsic muscle and tendon at ankle and foot level, unspecified foot
- S96.21 Strain of intrinsic muscle and tendon at ankle and foot level
  - S96.211 Strain of intrinsic muscle and tendon at ankle and foot level, right foot
  - S96.212 Strain of intrinsic muscle and tendon at ankle and foot level, left foot
  - S96.219 Strain of intrinsic muscle and tendon at ankle and foot level, unspecified foot
- S96.22 Laceration of intrinsic muscle and tendon at ankle and foot level
  - S96.221 Laceration of intrinsic muscle and tendon at ankle and foot level, right foot CC
  - S96.222 Laceration of intrinsic muscle and tendon at ankle and foot level, left foot CC
  - S96.229 Laceration of intrinsic muscle and tendon at ankle and foot level, unspecified foot CC UNS
- S96.29 Other specified injury of intrinsic muscle and tendon at ankle and foot level
  - S96.291 Other specified injury of intrinsic muscle and tendon at ankle and foot level, right foot
  - S96.292 Other specified injury of intrinsic muscle and tendon at ankle and foot level, left foot
  - S96.299 Other specified injury of intrinsic muscle and tendon at ankle and foot level, unspecified foot

S96.8 Injury of other specified muscles and tendons at ankle and foot level
- S96.80 Unspecified injury of other specified muscles and tendons at ankle and foot level
  - S96.801 Unspecified injury of other specified muscles and tendons at ankle and foot level, right foot
  - S96.802 Unspecified injury of other specified muscles and tendons at ankle and foot level, left foot
  - S96.809 Unspecified injury of other specified muscles and tendons at ankle and foot level, unspecified foot
- S96.81 Strain of other specified muscles and tendons at ankle and foot level
  - S96.811 Strain of other specified muscles and tendons at ankle and foot level, right foot
  - S96.812 Strain of other specified muscles and tendons at ankle and foot level, left foot
  - S96.819 Strain of other specified muscles and tendons at ankle and foot level, unspecified foot
- S96.82 Laceration of other specified muscles and tendons at ankle and foot level
  - S96.821 Laceration of other specified muscles and tendons at ankle and foot level, right foot CC
  - S96.822 Laceration of other specified muscles and tendons at ankle and foot level, left foot CC
  - S96.829 Laceration of other specified muscles and tendons at ankle and foot level, unspecified foot CC UNS
- S96.89 Other specified injury of other specified muscles and tendons at ankle and foot level
  - S96.891 Other specified injury of other specified muscles and tendons at ankle and foot level, right foot
  - S96.892 Other specified injury of other specified muscles and tendons at ankle and foot level, left foot
  - S96.899 Other specified injury of other specified muscles and tendons at ankle and foot level, unspecified foot

S96.9 Injury of unspecified muscle and tendon at ankle and foot level
- S96.90 Unspecified injury of unspecified muscle and tendon at ankle and foot level
  - S96.901 Unspecified injury of unspecified muscle and tendon at ankle and foot level, right foot
  - S96.902 Unspecified injury of unspecified muscle and tendon at ankle and foot level, left foot
  - S96.909 Unspecified injury of unspecified muscle and tendon at ankle and foot level, unspecified foot
- S96.91 Strain of unspecified muscle and tendon at ankle and foot level
  - S96.911 Strain of unspecified muscle and tendon at ankle and foot level, right foot
  - S96.912 Strain of unspecified muscle and tendon at ankle and foot level, left foot
  - S96.919 Strain of unspecified muscle and tendon at ankle and foot level, unspecified foot
- S96.92 Laceration of unspecified muscle and tendon at ankle and foot level
  - S96.921 Laceration of unspecified muscle and tendon at ankle and foot level, right foot CC
  - S96.922 Laceration of unspecified muscle and tendon at ankle and foot level, left foot CC
  - S96.929 Laceration of unspecified muscle and tendon at ankle and foot level, unspecified foot CC UNS
- S96.99 Other specified injury of unspecified muscle and tendon at ankle and foot level
  - S96.991 Other specified injury of unspecified muscle and tendon at ankle and foot level, right foot
  - S96.992 Other specified injury of unspecified muscle and tendon at ankle and foot level, left foot
  - S96.999 Other specified injury of unspecified muscle and tendon at ankle and foot level, unspecified foot

S97 Crushing injury of ankle and foot

Use additional code(s) for all associated injuries

The appropriate 7th character is to be added to each code from category S97.
- A initial encounter
- D subsequent encounter
- S sequela

S97.0 Crushing injury of ankle
- S97.00 Crushing injury of unspecified ankle
- S97.01 Crushing injury of right ankle
- S97.02 Crushing injury of left ankle

S97.1 Crushing injury of toe
- S97.10 Crushing injury of unspecified toe(s)
  - S97.101 Crushing injury of unspecified right toe(s)
  - S97.102 Crushing injury of unspecified left toe(s)
  - S97.109 Crushing injury of unspecified toe(s)
    - Crushing injury of toe NOS
- S97.11 Crushing injury of great toe
  - S97.111 Crushing injury of right great toe
  - S97.112 Crushing injury of left great toe
  - S97.119 Crushing injury of unspecified great toe
- S97.12 Crushing injury of lesser toe(s)
  - S97.121 Crushing injury of right lesser toe(s)
  - S97.122 Crushing injury of left lesser toe(s)
  - S97.129 Crushing injury of unspecified lesser toe(s)

S97.8 Crushing injury of foot
- S97.80 Crushing injury of unspecified foot
  - Crushing injury of foot NOS
- S97.81 Crushing injury of right foot
- S97.82 Crushing injury of left foot

S98 Traumatic amputation of ankle and foot

An amputation not identified as partial or complete should be coded to complete

The appropriate 7th character is to be added to each code from category S98.
A initial encounter
D subsequent encounter
S sequela

S98.Ø Traumatic amputation of foot at ankle level
S98.Ø1 Complete traumatic amputation of foot at ankle level
S98.Ø11 Complete traumatic amputation of right foot at ankle level CC HCC
S98.Ø12 Complete traumatic amputation of left foot at ankle level CC HCC
S98.Ø19 Complete traumatic amputation of unspecified foot at ankle level CC UNS HCC
S98.Ø2 Partial traumatic amputation of foot at ankle level
S98.Ø21 Partial traumatic amputation of right foot at ankle level CC HCC
S98.Ø22 Partial traumatic amputation of left foot at ankle level CC HCC
S98.Ø29 Partial traumatic amputation of unspecified foot at ankle level CC UNS HCC
S98.1 Traumatic amputation of one toe
S98.11 Complete traumatic amputation of great toe
S98.111 Complete traumatic amputation of right great toe HCC
S98.112 Complete traumatic amputation of left great toe HCC
S98.119 Complete traumatic amputation of unspecified great toe HCC
S98.12 Partial traumatic amputation of great toe
S98.121 Partial traumatic amputation of right great toe HCC
S98.122 Partial traumatic amputation of left great toe HCC
S98.129 Partial traumatic amputation of unspecified great toe HCC
S98.13 Complete traumatic amputation of one lesser toe
Traumatic amputation of toe NOS
S98.131 Complete traumatic amputation of one right lesser toe HCC
S98.132 Complete traumatic amputation of one left lesser toe HCC
S98.139 Complete traumatic amputation of one unspecified lesser toe HCC
S98.14 Partial traumatic amputation of one lesser toe
S98.141 Partial traumatic amputation of one right lesser toe HCC
S98.142 Partial traumatic amputation of one left lesser toe HCC
S98.149 Partial traumatic amputation of one unspecified lesser toe HCC
S98.2 Traumatic amputation of two or more lesser toes
S98.21 Complete traumatic amputation of two or more lesser toes
S98.211 Complete traumatic amputation of two or more right lesser toes HCC
S98.212 Complete traumatic amputation of two or more left lesser toes HCC
S98.219 Complete traumatic amputation of two or more unspecified lesser toes HCC
S98.22 Partial traumatic amputation of two or more lesser toes
S98.221 Partial traumatic amputation of two or more right lesser toes HCC
S98.222 Partial traumatic amputation of two or more left lesser toes HCC
S98.229 Partial traumatic amputation of two or more unspecified lesser toes HCC
S98.3 Traumatic amputation of midfoot
S98.31 Complete traumatic amputation of midfoot
S98.311 Complete traumatic amputation of right midfoot CC HCC
S98.312 Complete traumatic amputation of left midfoot CC HCC
S98.319 Complete traumatic amputation of unspecified midfoot CC UNS HCC
S98.32 Partial traumatic amputation of midfoot
S98.321 Partial traumatic amputation of right midfoot CC HCC
S98.322 Partial traumatic amputation of left midfoot CC HCC
S98.329 Partial traumatic amputation of unspecified midfoot CC UNS HCC
S98.9 Traumatic amputation of foot, level unspecified
S98.91 Complete traumatic amputation of foot, level unspecified
S98.911 Complete traumatic amputation of right foot, level unspecified CC HCC
S98.912 Complete traumatic amputation of left foot, level unspecified CC HCC
S98.919 Complete traumatic amputation of unspecified foot, level unspecified CC UNS HCC
S98.92 Partial traumatic amputation of foot, level unspecified
S98.921 Partial traumatic amputation of right foot, level unspecified CC HCC
S98.922 Partial traumatic amputation of left foot, level unspecified CC HCC
S98.929 Partial traumatic amputation of unspecified foot, level unspecified CC UNS HCC

S99 Other and unspecified injuries of ankle and foot

AHA: 2018,2Q,12; 2018,1Q,3; 2016,4Q,68-69

S99.Ø Physeal fracture of calcaneus

AHA: 2019,4Q,56

The appropriate 7th character is to be added to each code from subcategory S99.Ø.
A initial encounter for closed fracture
B initial encounter for open fracture
D subsequent encounter for fracture with routine healing
G subsequent encounter for fracture with delayed healing
K subsequent encounter for fracture with nonunion
P subsequent encounter for fracture with malunion
S sequela

S99.ØØ Unspecified physeal fracture of calcaneus
S99.ØØ1 Unspecified physeal fracture of right calcaneus
S99.ØØ2 Unspecified physeal fracture of left calcaneus
S99.ØØ9 Unspecified physeal fracture of unspecified calcaneus
S99.Ø1 Salter-Harris Type I physeal fracture of calcaneus
S99.Ø11 Salter-Harris Type I physeal fracture of right calcaneus
S99.Ø12 Salter-Harris Type I physeal fracture of left calcaneus
S99.Ø19 Salter-Harris Type I physeal fracture of unspecified calcaneus
S99.Ø2 Salter-Harris Type II physeal fracture of calcaneus
S99.Ø21 Salter-Harris Type II physeal fracture of right calcaneus
S99.Ø22 Salter-Harris Type II physeal fracture of left calcaneus
S99.Ø29 Salter-Harris Type II physeal fracture of unspecified calcaneus
S99.Ø3 Salter-Harris Type III physeal fracture of calcaneus
S99.Ø31 Salter-Harris Type III physeal fracture of right calcaneus
S99.Ø32 Salter-Harris Type III physeal fracture of left calcaneus
S99.Ø39 Salter-Harris Type III physeal fracture of unspecified calcaneus
S99.Ø4 Salter-Harris Type IV physeal fracture of calcaneus
S99.Ø41 Salter-Harris Type IV physeal fracture of right calcaneus
S99.Ø42 Salter-Harris Type IV physeal fracture of left calcaneus
S99.Ø49 Salter-Harris Type IV physeal fracture of unspecified calcaneus

S99.09 Other physeal fracture of calcaneus
- S99.091 Other physeal fracture of right calcaneus
- S99.092 Other physeal fracture of left calcaneus
- S99.099 Other physeal fracture of unspecified calcaneus

S99.1 Physeal fracture of metatarsal

AHA: 2019,4Q,56

The appropriate 7th character is to be added to each code from subcategory S99.1
- A initial encounter for closed fracture
- B initial encounter for open fracture
- D subsequent encounter for fracture with routine healing
- G subsequent encounter for fracture with delayed healing
- K subsequent encounter for fracture with nonunion
- P subsequent encounter for fracture with malunion
- S sequela

S99.10 Unspecified physeal fracture of metatarsal
- S99.101 Unspecified physeal fracture of right metatarsal
- S99.102 Unspecified physeal fracture of left metatarsal
- S99.109 Unspecified physeal fracture of unspecified metatarsal

S99.11 Salter-Harris Type I physeal fracture of metatarsal
- S99.111 Salter-Harris Type I physeal fracture of right metatarsal
- S99.112 Salter-Harris Type I physeal fracture of left metatarsal
- S99.119 Salter-Harris Type I physeal fracture of unspecified metatarsal

S99.12 Salter-Harris Type II physeal fracture of metatarsal
- S99.121 Salter-Harris Type II physeal fracture of right metatarsal
- S99.122 Salter-Harris Type II physeal fracture of left metatarsal
- S99.129 Salter-Harris Type II physeal fracture of unspecified metatarsal

S99.13 Salter-Harris Type III physeal fracture of metatarsal
- S99.131 Salter-Harris Type III physeal fracture of right metatarsal
- S99.132 Salter-Harris Type III physeal fracture of left metatarsal
- S99.139 Salter-Harris Type III physeal fracture of unspecified metatarsal

S99.14 Salter-Harris Type IV physeal fracture of metatarsal
- S99.141 Salter-Harris Type IV physeal fracture of right metatarsal
- S99.142 Salter-Harris Type IV physeal fracture of left metatarsal
- S99.149 Salter-Harris Type IV physeal fracture of unspecified metatarsal

S99.19 Other physeal fracture of metatarsal
- S99.191 Other physeal fracture of right metatarsal
- S99.192 Other physeal fracture of left metatarsal
- S99.199 Other physeal fracture of unspecified metatarsal

S99.2 Physeal fracture of phalanx of toe

AHA: 2019,4Q,56

The appropriate 7th character is to be added to each code from subcategories S99.2.
- A initial encounter for closed fracture
- B initial encounter for open fracture
- D subsequent encounter for fracture with routine healing
- G subsequent encounter for fracture with delayed healing
- K subsequent encounter for fracture with nonunion
- P subsequent encounter for fracture with malunion
- S sequela

S99.20 Unspecified physeal fracture of phalanx of toe
- S99.201 Unspecified physeal fracture of phalanx of right toe
- S99.202 Unspecified physeal fracture of phalanx of left toe
- S99.209 Unspecified physeal fracture of phalanx of unspecified toe

S99.21 Salter-Harris Type I physeal fracture of phalanx of toe
- S99.211 Salter-Harris Type I physeal fracture of phalanx of right toe
- S99.212 Salter-Harris Type I physeal fracture of phalanx of left toe
- S99.219 Salter-Harris Type I physeal fracture of phalanx of unspecified toe

S99.22 Salter-Harris Type II physeal fracture of phalanx of toe
- S99.221 Salter-Harris Type II physeal fracture of phalanx of right toe
- S99.222 Salter-Harris Type II physeal fracture of phalanx of left toe
- S99.229 Salter-Harris Type II physeal fracture of phalanx of unspecified toe

S99.23 Salter-Harris Type III physeal fracture of phalanx of toe
- S99.231 Salter-Harris Type III physeal fracture of phalanx of right toe
- S99.232 Salter-Harris Type III physeal fracture of phalanx of left toe
- S99.239 Salter-Harris Type III physeal fracture of phalanx of unspecified toe

S99.24 Salter-Harris Type IV physeal fracture of phalanx of toe
- S99.241 Salter-Harris Type IV physeal fracture of phalanx of right toe
- S99.242 Salter-Harris Type IV physeal fracture of phalanx of left toe
- S99.249 Salter-Harris Type IV physeal fracture of phalanx of unspecified toe

S99.29 Other physeal fracture of phalanx of toe
- S99.291 Other physeal fracture of phalanx of right toe
- S99.292 Other physeal fracture of phalanx of left toe
- S99.299 Other physeal fracture of phalanx of unspecified toe

S99.8 Other specified injuries of ankle and foot

The appropriate 7th character is to be added to each code from subcategory S99.8.
- A initial encounter
- D subsequent encounter
- S sequela

S99.81 Other specified injuries of ankle
- S99.811 Other specified injuries of right ankle
- S99.812 Other specified injuries of left ankle
- S99.819 Other specified injuries of unspecified ankle

S99.82 Other specified injuries of foot
- S99.821 Other specified injuries of right foot
- S99.822 Other specified injuries of left foot
- S99.829 Other specified injuries of unspecified foot

S99.9 Unspecified injury of ankle and foot

The appropriate 7th character is to be added to each code from subcategory S99.9.
- A initial encounter
- D subsequent encounter
- S sequela

S99.91 Unspecified injury of ankle
- S99.911 Unspecified injury of right ankle
- S99.912 Unspecified injury of left ankle
- S99.919 Unspecified injury of unspecified ankle

S99.92 Unspecified injury of foot
- S99.921 Unspecified injury of right foot
- S99.922 Unspecified injury of left foot
- S99.929 Unspecified injury of unspecified foot

INJURY, POISONING AND CERTAIN OTHER CONSEQUENCES OF EXTERNAL CAUSES (T07-T88)

Injuries involving multiple body regions (T07)

EXCLUDES 1 *burns and corrosions (T20-T32)*
frostbite (T33-T34)
insect bite or sting, venomous (T63.4)
sunburn (L55.-)

T07 Unspecified multiple injuries

EXCLUDES 1 injury NOS (T14.90)

AHA: 2017,4Q,26

The appropriate 7th character is to be added to code T07.
A initial encounter
D subsequent encounter
S sequela

Injury of unspecified body region (T14)

T14 Injury of unspecified body region

EXCLUDES 1 *multiple unspecified injuries (T07)*

AHA: 2017,4Q,26

The appropriate 7th character is to be added to each code from category T14.
A initial encounter
D subsequent encounter
S sequela

T14.8 Other injury of unspecified body region
Abrasion NOS
Contusion NOS
Crush injury NOS
Fracture NOS
Skin injury NOS
Vascular injury NOS
Wound NOS

T14.9 Unspecified injury

T14.90 Injury, unspecified
Injury NOS

T14.91 Suicide attempt HCC
Attempted suicide NOS

Effects of foreign body entering through natural orifice (T15-T19)

EXCLUDES 2 *foreign body accidentally left in operation wound (T81.5-)*
foreign body in penetrating wound - see open wound by body region
residual foreign body in soft tissue (M79.5)
splinter, without open wound - see superficial injury by body region

T15 Foreign body on external eye

EXCLUDES 2 *foreign body in penetrating wound of orbit and eye ball (S05.4-, S05.5-)*
open wound of eyelid and periocular area (S01.1-)
retained foreign body in eyelid (H02.8-)
retained (old) foreign body in penetrating wound of orbit and eye ball (H05.5-, H44.6-, H44.7-)
superficial foreign body of eyelid and periocular area (S00.25-)

The appropriate 7th character is to be added to each code from category T15.
A initial encounter
D subsequent encounter
S sequela

T15.0 Foreign body in cornea

T15.00 Foreign body in cornea, unspecified eye

T15.01 Foreign body in cornea, right eye

T15.02 Foreign body in cornea, left eye

T15.1 Foreign body in conjunctival sac

T15.10 Foreign body in conjunctival sac, unspecified eye

T15.11 Foreign body in conjunctival sac, right eye

T15.12 Foreign body in conjunctival sac, left eye

T15.8 Foreign body in other and multiple parts of external eye
Foreign body in lacrimal punctum

T15.80 Foreign body in other and multiple parts of external eye, unspecified eye

T15.81 Foreign body in other and multiple parts of external eye, right eye

T15.82 Foreign body in other and multiple parts of external eye, left eye

T15.9 Foreign body on external eye, part unspecified

T15.90 Foreign body on external eye, part unspecified, unspecified eye

T15.91 Foreign body on external eye, part unspecified, right eye

T15.92 Foreign body on external eye, part unspecified, left eye

T16 Foreign body in ear

INCLUDES foreign body in auditory canal

The appropriate 7th character is to be added to each code from category T16.
A initial encounter
D subsequent encounter
S sequela

T16.1 Foreign body in right ear

T16.2 Foreign body in left ear

T16.9 Foreign body in ear, unspecified ear

T17 Foreign body in respiratory tract

The appropriate 7th character is to be added to each code from category T17.
A initial encounter
D subsequent encounter
S sequela

T17.0 Foreign body in nasal sinus

T17.1 Foreign body in nostril
Foreign body in nose NOS

T17.2 Foreign body in pharynx
Foreign body in nasopharynx
Foreign body in throat NOS

T17.20 Unspecified foreign body in pharynx

T17.200 Unspecified foreign body in pharynx causing asphyxiation

T17.208 Unspecified foreign body in pharynx causing other injury

T17.21 Gastric contents in pharynx
Aspiration of gastric contents into pharynx
Vomitus in pharynx

T17.210 Gastric contents in pharynx causing asphyxiation

T17.218 Gastric contents in pharynx causing other injury

T17.22 Food in pharynx
Bones in pharynx
Seeds in pharynx

T17.220 Food in pharynx causing asphyxiation

T17.228 Food in pharynx causing other injury

T17.29 Other foreign object in pharynx

T17.290 Other foreign object in pharynx causing asphyxiation

T17.298 Other foreign object in pharynx causing other injury

T17.3 Foreign body in larynx

T17.30 Unspecified foreign body in larynx

T17.300 Unspecified foreign body in larynx causing asphyxiation

T17.308 Unspecified foreign body in larynx causing other injury

T17.31 Gastric contents in larynx
Aspiration of gastric contents into larynx
Vomitus in larynx

T17.310 Gastric contents in larynx causing asphyxiation

T17.318 Gastric contents in larynx causing other injury

T17.32 Food in larynx
Bones in larynx
Seeds in larynx

T17.320 Food in larynx causing asphyxiation

T17.328 Food in larynx causing other injury

T17.39 Other foreign object in larynx
T17.390 Other foreign object in larynx causing asphyxiation
T17.398 Other foreign object in larynx causing other injury
T17.4 Foreign body in trachea
T17.40 Unspecified foreign body in trachea
T17.400 Unspecified foreign body in trachea causing asphyxiation CC
T17.408 Unspecified foreign body in trachea causing other injury CC
T17.41 Gastric contents in trachea
Aspiration of gastric contents into trachea
Vomitus in trachea
T17.410 Gastric contents in trachea causing asphyxiation CC
T17.418 Gastric contents in trachea causing other injury CC
T17.42 Food in trachea
Bones in trachea
Seeds in trachea
T17.420 Food in trachea causing asphyxiation CC
T17.428 Food in trachea causing other injury CC
T17.49 Other foreign object in trachea
T17.490 Other foreign object in trachea causing asphyxiation CC
T17.498 Other foreign object in trachea causing other injury CC
T17.5 Foreign body in bronchus
T17.50 Unspecified foreign body in bronchus
T17.500 Unspecified foreign body in bronchus causing asphyxiation CC
T17.508 Unspecified foreign body in bronchus causing other injury CC
T17.51 Gastric contents in bronchus
Aspiration of gastric contents into bronchus
Vomitus in bronchus
T17.510 Gastric contents in bronchus causing asphyxiation CC
T17.518 Gastric contents in bronchus causing other injury CC
T17.52 Food in bronchus
Bones in bronchus
Seeds in bronchus
T17.520 Food in bronchus causing asphyxiation CC
T17.528 Food in bronchus causing other injury CC
T17.59 Other foreign object in bronchus
T17.590 Other foreign object in bronchus causing asphyxiation CC
T17.598 Other foreign object in bronchus causing other injury CC
T17.8 Foreign body in other parts of respiratory tract
Foreign body in bronchioles
Foreign body in lung
T17.80 Unspecified foreign body in other parts of respiratory tract
T17.800 Unspecified foreign body in other parts of respiratory tract causing asphyxiation CC
T17.808 Unspecified foreign body in other parts of respiratory tract causing other injury CC
T17.81 Gastric contents in other parts of respiratory tract
Aspiration of gastric contents into other parts of respiratory tract
Vomitus in other parts of respiratory tract
T17.810 Gastric contents in other parts of respiratory tract causing asphyxiation CC
T17.818 Gastric contents in other parts of respiratory tract causing other injury CC
T17.82 Food in other parts of respiratory tract
Bones in other parts of respiratory tract
Seeds in other parts of respiratory tract
T17.820 Food in other parts of respiratory tract causing asphyxiation CC
T17.828 Food in other parts of respiratory tract causing other injury CC
T17.89 Other foreign object in other parts of respiratory tract
T17.890 Other foreign object in other parts of respiratory tract causing asphyxiation CC
T17.898 Other foreign object in other parts of respiratory tract causing other injury CC
T17.9 Foreign body in respiratory tract, part unspecified
T17.90 Unspecified foreign body in respiratory tract, part unspecified
T17.900 Unspecified foreign body in respiratory tract, part unspecified causing asphyxiation
T17.908 Unspecified foreign body in respiratory tract, part unspecified causing other injury
T17.91 Gastric contents in respiratory tract, part unspecified
Aspiration of gastric contents into respiratory tract, part unspecified
Vomitus in trachea respiratory tract, part unspecified
T17.910 Gastric contents in respiratory tract, part unspecified causing asphyxiation
T17.918 Gastric contents in respiratory tract, part unspecified causing other injury
T17.92 Food in respiratory tract, part unspecified
Bones in respiratory tract, part unspecified
Seeds in respiratory tract, part unspecified
T17.920 Food in respiratory tract, part unspecified causing asphyxiation
T17.928 Food in respiratory tract, part unspecified causing other injury
T17.99 Other foreign object in respiratory tract, part unspecified
T17.990 Other foreign object in respiratory tract, part unspecified in causing asphyxiation
AHA: 2019,3Q,15
T17.998 Other foreign object in respiratory tract, part unspecified causing other injury

T18 Foreign body in alimentary tract
EXCLUDES 2 *foreign body in pharynx (T17.2-)*

The appropriate 7th character is to be added to each code from category T18.
A initial encounter
D subsequent encounter
S sequela

T18.0 Foreign body in mouth
T18.1 Foreign body in esophagus
EXCLUDES 2 *foreign body in respiratory tract (T17.-)*
T18.10 Unspecified foreign body in esophagus
T18.100 Unspecified foreign body in esophagus causing compression of trachea
Unspecified foreign body in esophagus causing obstruction of respiration
T18.108 Unspecified foreign body in esophagus causing other injury
T18.11 Gastric contents in esophagus
Vomitus in esophagus
T18.110 Gastric contents in esophagus causing compression of trachea
Gastric contents in esophagus causing obstruction of respiration
T18.118 Gastric contents in esophagus causing other injury

6th **T18.12 Food in esophagus**
Bones in esophagus
Seeds in esophagus

7th **T18.120 Food in esophagus causing compression of trachea**
Food in esophagus causing obstruction of respiration

7th **T18.128 Food in esophagus causing other injury**

6th **T18.19 Other foreign object in esophagus**
AHA: 2022,1Q,27; 2015,1Q,23

7th **T18.190 Other foreign object in esophagus causing compression of trachea**
Other foreign body in esophagus causing obstruction of respiration
TIP: Any foreign object lodged in the esophagus requires immediate treatment and is considered an injury. Assign this code when there is respiratory compromise or compression. If no respiratory compromise or compression is documented, assign code T18.198-.

7th **T18.198 Other foreign object in esophagus causing other injury**
TIP: Any foreign object lodged in the esophagus requires immediate treatment and is considered an injury. Assign this code when there is no respiratory compromise or compression. If respiratory compromise or compression is documented, assign code T18.190-.

x7th **T18.2 Foreign body in stomach**

x7th **T18.3 Foreign body in small intestine**

x7th **T18.4 Foreign body in colon**

x7th **T18.5 Foreign body in anus and rectum**
Foreign body in rectosigmoid (junction)

x7th **T18.8 Foreign body in other parts of alimentary tract**

x7th **T18.9 Foreign body of alimentary tract, part unspecified**
Foreign body in digestive system NOS
Swallowed foreign body NOS

4th **T19 Foreign body in genitourinary tract**

EXCLUDES 2 *complications due to implanted mesh (T83.7-)*
mechanical complications of contraceptive device (intrauterine) (vaginal) (T83.3-)
presence of contraceptive device (intrauterine) (vaginal) (Z97.5)

The appropriate 7th character is to be added to each code from category T19.
A initial encounter
D subsequent encounter
S sequela

x7th **T19.0 Foreign body in urethra**

x7th **T19.1 Foreign body in bladder**

x7th **T19.2 Foreign body in vulva and vagina** ♀

x7th **T19.3 Foreign body in uterus** ♀

x7th **T19.4 Foreign body in penis** ♂

x7th **T19.8 Foreign body in other parts of genitourinary tract**

x7th **T19.9 Foreign body in genitourinary tract, part unspecified**

BURNS AND CORROSIONS (T20-T32)

INCLUDES burns (thermal) from electrical heating appliances
burns (thermal) from electricity
burns (thermal) from flame
burns (thermal) from friction
burns (thermal) from hot air and hot gases
burns (thermal) from hot objects
burns (thermal) from lightning
burns (thermal) from radiation
chemical burn [corrosion] (external) (internal)
scalds

EXCLUDES 2 *erythema [dermatitis] ab igne (L59.0)*
radiation-related disorders of the skin and subcutaneous tissue (L55-L59)
sunburn (L55.-)

AHA: 2016,2Q,4

Burns and corrosions of external body surface, specified by site (T20-T25)

INCLUDES burns and corrosions of first degree [erythema]
burns and corrosions of second degree [blisters] [epidermal loss]
burns and corrosions of third degree [deep necrosis of underlying tissue] [full-thickness skin loss]

Use additional code from category T31 or T32 to identify extent of body surface involved

4th **T20 Burn and corrosion of head, face, and neck**

EXCLUDES 2 *burn and corrosion of ear drum (T28.41, T28.91)*
burn and corrosion of eye and adnexa (T26.-)
burn and corrosion of mouth and pharynx (T28.0)

AHA: 2015,1Q,18-19

The appropriate 7th character is to be added to each code from category T20.
A initial encounter
D subsequent encounter
S sequela

5th **T20.0 Burn of unspecified degree of head, face, and neck**
Use additional external cause code to identify the source, place and intent of the burn (X00-X19, X75-X77, X96-X98, Y92)

x7th **T20.00 Burn of unspecified degree of head, face, and neck, unspecified site**

6th **T20.01 Burn of unspecified degree of ear [any part, except ear drum]**
EXCLUDES 2 *burn of ear drum (T28.41-)*

7th **T20.011 Burn of unspecified degree of right ear [any part, except ear drum]**

7th **T20.012 Burn of unspecified degree of left ear [any part, except ear drum]**

7th **T20.019 Burn of unspecified degree of unspecified ear [any part, except ear drum]**

x7th **T20.02 Burn of unspecified degree of lip(s)**

x7th **T20.03 Burn of unspecified degree of chin**

x7th **T20.04 Burn of unspecified degree of nose (septum)**

x7th **T20.05 Burn of unspecified degree of scalp [any part]**

x7th **T20.06 Burn of unspecified degree of forehead and cheek**

x7th **T20.07 Burn of unspecified degree of neck**

x7th **T20.09 Burn of unspecified degree of multiple sites of head, face, and neck**

5th **T20.1 Burn of first degree of head, face, and neck**
Use additional external cause code to identify the source, place and intent of the burn (X00-X19, X75-X77, X96-X98, Y92)

x7th **T20.10 Burn of first degree of head, face, and neck, unspecified site**

6th **T20.11 Burn of first degree of ear [any part, except ear drum]**
EXCLUDES 2 *burn of ear drum (T28.41-)*

7th **T20.111 Burn of first degree of right ear [any part, except ear drum]**

7th **T20.112 Burn of first degree of left ear [any part, except ear drum]**

7th **T20.119 Burn of first degree of unspecified ear [any part, except ear drum]**

x7th **T20.12 Burn of first degree of lip(s)**

x7th **T20.13 Burn of first degree of chin**

x7th **T20.14 Burn of first degree of nose (septum)**

x7th **T20.15 Burn of first degree of scalp [any part]**

x7th **T20.16 Burn of first degree of forehead and cheek**

T20.17 Burn of first degree of neck

T20.19 Burn of first degree of multiple sites of head, face, and neck

Degree of Burns

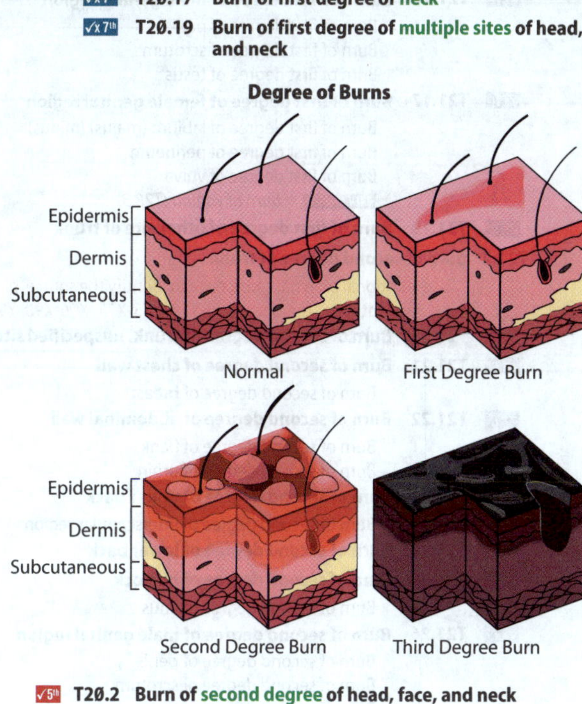

T20.2 Burn of second degree of head, face, and neck

Use additional external cause code to identify the source, place and intent of the burn (X00-X19, X75-X77, X96-X98, Y92)

T20.20 Burn of second degree of head, face, and neck, unspecified site

T20.21 Burn of second degree of ear [any part, except ear drum]

EXCLUDES 2 burn of ear drum (T28.41-)

T20.211 Burn of second degree of right ear [any part, except ear drum]

T20.212 Burn of second degree of left ear [any part, except ear drum]

T20.219 Burn of second degree of unspecified ear [any part, except ear drum]

T20.22 Burn of second degree of lip(s)

T20.23 Burn of second degree of chin

T20.24 Burn of second degree of nose (septum)

T20.25 Burn of second degree of scalp [any part]

T20.26 Burn of second degree of forehead and cheek

T20.27 Burn of second degree of neck

T20.29 Burn of second degree of multiple sites of head, face, and neck

T20.3 Burn of third degree of head, face, and neck

Use additional external cause code to identify the source, place and intent of the burn (X00-X19, X75-X77, X96-X98, Y92)

T20.30 Burn of third degree of head, face, and neck, unspecified site CC H5

T20.31 Burn of third degree of ear [any part, except ear drum]

EXCLUDES 2 burn of ear drum (T28.41-)

AHA: 2015,1Q,18

T20.311 Burn of third degree of right ear [any part, except ear drum] CC H5

T20.312 Burn of third degree of left ear [any part, except ear drum] CC H5

T20.319 Burn of third degree of unspecified ear [any part, except ear drum] CC H5 UNS

T20.32 Burn of third degree of lip(s) CC H5

T20.33 Burn of third degree of chin CC H5

T20.34 Burn of third degree of nose (septum) CC H5

T20.35 Burn of third degree of scalp [any part] CC H5

T20.36 Burn of third degree of forehead and cheek CC H5

T20.37 Burn of third degree of neck CC H5

T20.39 Burn of third degree of multiple sites of head, face, and neck CC H5

T20.4 Corrosion of unspecified degree of head, face, and neck

Code first (T51-T65) to identify chemical and intent
Use additional external cause code to identify place (Y92)

T20.40 Corrosion of unspecified degree of head, face, and neck, unspecified site

T20.41 Corrosion of unspecified degree of ear [any part, except ear drum]

EXCLUDES 2 corrosion of ear drum (T28.91-)

T20.411 Corrosion of unspecified degree of right ear [any part, except ear drum]

T20.412 Corrosion of unspecified degree of left ear [any part, except ear drum]

T20.419 Corrosion of unspecified degree of unspecified ear [any part, except ear drum]

T20.42 Corrosion of unspecified degree of lip(s)

T20.43 Corrosion of unspecified degree of chin

T20.44 Corrosion of unspecified degree of nose (septum)

T20.45 Corrosion of unspecified degree of scalp [any part]

T20.46 Corrosion of unspecified degree of forehead and cheek

T20.47 Corrosion of unspecified degree of neck

T20.49 Corrosion of unspecified degree of multiple sites of head, face, and neck

T20.5 Corrosion of first degree of head, face, and neck

Code first (T51-T65) to identify chemical and intent
Use additional external cause code to identify place (Y92)

T20.50 Corrosion of first degree of head, face, and neck, unspecified site

T20.51 Corrosion of first degree of ear [any part, except ear drum]

EXCLUDES 2 corrosion of ear drum (T28.91-)

T20.511 Corrosion of first degree of right ear [any part, except ear drum]

T20.512 Corrosion of first degree of left ear [any part, except ear drum]

T20.519 Corrosion of first degree of unspecified ear [any part, except ear drum]

T20.52 Corrosion of first degree of lip(s)

T20.53 Corrosion of first degree of chin

T20.54 Corrosion of first degree of nose (septum)

T20.55 Corrosion of first degree of scalp [any part]

T20.56 Corrosion of first degree of forehead and cheek

T20.57 Corrosion of first degree of neck

T20.59 Corrosion of first degree of multiple sites of head, face, and neck

T20.6 Corrosion of second degree of head, face, and neck

Code first (T51-T65) to identify chemical and intent
Use additional external cause code to identify place (Y92)

T20.60 Corrosion of second degree of head, face, and neck, unspecified site

T20.61 Corrosion of second degree of ear [any part, except ear drum]

EXCLUDES 2 corrosion of ear drum (T28.91-)

T20.611 Corrosion of second degree of right ear [any part, except ear drum]

T20.612 Corrosion of second degree of left ear [any part, except ear drum]

T20.619 Corrosion of second degree of unspecified ear [any part, except ear drum]

T20.62 Corrosion of second degree of lip(s)

T20.63 Corrosion of second degree of chin

T20.64 Corrosion of second degree of nose (septum)

T20.65 Corrosion of second degree of scalp [any part]

T20.66 Corrosion of second degree of forehead and cheek

T20.67 Corrosion of second degree of neck

T20.69 Corrosion of second degree of multiple sites of head, face, and neck

T20.7 Corrosion of third degree of head, face, and neck

Code first (T51-T65) to identify chemical and intent
Use additional external cause code to identify place (Y92)

T20.70 Corrosion of third degree of head, face, and neck, unspecified site CC H5

√6th **T20.71 Corrosion of third degree of ear [any part, except ear drum]**
EXCLUDES 2 *corrosion of ear drum (T28.91-)*

√7th **T20.711 Corrosion of third degree of right ear [any part, except ear drum]** CC H5

√7th **T20.712 Corrosion of third degree of left ear [any part, except ear drum]** CC H5

√7th **T20.719 Corrosion of third degree of unspecified ear [any part, except ear drum]** CC H5 UNS

√x7th **T20.72 Corrosion of third degree of lip(s)** CC H5

√x7th **T20.73 Corrosion of third degree of chin** CC H5

√x7th **T20.74 Corrosion of third degree of nose (septum)** CC H5

√x7th **T20.75 Corrosion of third degree of scalp [any part]** CC H5

√x7th **T20.76 Corrosion of third degree of forehead and cheek** CC H5

√x7th **T20.77 Corrosion of third degree of neck** CC H5

√x7th **T20.79 Corrosion of third degree of multiple sites of head, face, and neck** CC H5

√4th **T21 Burn and corrosion of trunk**

INCLUDES burns and corrosion of hip region

EXCLUDES 2 *burns and corrosion of axilla (T22.- with fifth character 4)*
burns and corrosion of scapular region (T22.- with fifth character 6)
burns and corrosion of shoulder (T22.- with fifth character 5)

The appropriate 7th character is to be added to each code from category T21.
A initial encounter
D subsequent encounter
S sequela

√5th **T21.0 Burn of unspecified degree of trunk**
Use additional external cause code to identify the source, place and intent of the burn (X00-X19, X75-X77, X96-X98, Y92)

√x7th **T21.00 Burn of unspecified degree of trunk, unspecified site**

√x7th **T21.01 Burn of unspecified degree of chest wall**
Burn of unspecified degree of breast

√x7th **T21.02 Burn of unspecified degree of abdominal wall**
Burn of unspecified degree of flank
Burn of unspecified degree of groin

√x7th **T21.03 Burn of unspecified degree of upper back**
Burn of unspecified degree of interscapular region

√x7th **T21.04 Burn of unspecified degree of lower back**

√x7th **T21.05 Burn of unspecified degree of buttock**
Burn of unspecified degree of anus

√x7th **T21.06 Burn of unspecified degree of male genital region** ♂
Burn of unspecified degree of penis
Burn of unspecified degree of scrotum
Burn of unspecified degree of testis

√x7th **T21.07 Burn of unspecified degree of female genital region** ♀
Burn of unspecified degree of labium (majus) (minus)
Burn of unspecified degree of perineum
Burn of unspecified degree of vulva
EXCLUDES 2 *burn of vagina (T28.3)*

√x7th **T21.09 Burn of unspecified degree of other site of trunk**

√5th **T21.1 Burn of first degree of trunk**
Use additional external cause code to identify the source, place and intent of the burn (X00-X19, X75-X77, X96-X98, Y92)

√x7th **T21.10 Burn of first degree of trunk, unspecified site**

√x7th **T21.11 Burn of first degree of chest wall**
Burn of first degree of breast

√x7th **T21.12 Burn of first degree of abdominal wall**
Burn of first degree of flank
Burn of first degree of groin

√x7th **T21.13 Burn of first degree of upper back**
Burn of first degree of interscapular region

√x7th **T21.14 Burn of first degree of lower back**

√x7th **T21.15 Burn of first degree of buttock**
Burn of first degree of anus

√x7th **T21.16 Burn of first degree of male genital region** ♂
Burn of first degree of penis
Burn of first degree of scrotum
Burn of first degree of testis

√x7th **T21.17 Burn of first degree of female genital region** ♀
Burn of first degree of labium (majus) (minus)
Burn of first degree of perineum
Burn of first degree of vulva
EXCLUDES 2 *burn of vagina (T28.3)*

√x7th **T21.19 Burn of first degree of other site of trunk**

√5th **T21.2 Burn of second degree of trunk**
Use additional external cause code to identify the source, place and intent of the burn (X00-X19, X75-X77, X96-X98, Y92)

√x7th **T21.20 Burn of second degree of trunk, unspecified site**

√x7th **T21.21 Burn of second degree of chest wall**
Burn of second degree of breast

√x7th **T21.22 Burn of second degree of abdominal wall**
Burn of second degree of flank
Burn of second degree of groin

√x7th **T21.23 Burn of second degree of upper back**
Burn of second degree of interscapular region

√x7th **T21.24 Burn of second degree of lower back**

√x7th **T21.25 Burn of second degree of buttock**
Burn of second degree of anus

√x7th **T21.26 Burn of second degree of male genital region** ♂
Burn of second degree of penis
Burn of second degree of scrotum
Burn of second degree of testis

√x7th **T21.27 Burn of second degree of female genital region** ♀
Burn of second degree of labium (majus) (minus)
Burn of second degree of perineum
Burn of second degree of vulva
EXCLUDES 2 *burn of vagina (T28.3)*

√x7th **T21.29 Burn of second degree of other site of trunk**

√5th **T21.3 Burn of third degree of trunk**
Use additional external cause code to identify the source, place and intent of the burn (X00-X19, X75-X77, X96-X98, Y92)

√x7th **T21.30 Burn of third degree of trunk, unspecified site** CC H5

√x7th **T21.31 Burn of third degree of chest wall** CC H5
Burn of third degree of breast
AHA: 2016,2Q,5

√x7th **T21.32 Burn of third degree of abdominal wall** CC H5
Burn of third degree of flank
Burn of third degree of groin

√x7th **T21.33 Burn of third degree of upper back** CC H5
Burn of third degree of interscapular region

√x7th **T21.34 Burn of third degree of lower back** CC H5

√x7th **T21.35 Burn of third degree of buttock** CC H5
Burn of third degree of anus

√x7th **T21.36 Burn of third degree of male genital region** CC H5 ♂
Burn of third degree of penis
Burn of third degree of scrotum
Burn of third degree of testis

√x7th **T21.37 Burn of third degree of female genital region** CC H5 ♀
Burn of third degree of labium (majus) (minus)
Burn of third degree of perineum
Burn of third degree of vulva
EXCLUDES 2 *burn of vagina (T28.3)*

√x7th **T21.39 Burn of third degree of other site of trunk** CC H5

√5th **T21.4 Corrosion of unspecified degree of trunk**
Code first (T51-T65) to identify chemical and intent
Use additional external cause code to identify place (Y92)

√x7th **T21.40 Corrosion of unspecified degree of trunk, unspecified site**

√x7th **T21.41 Corrosion of unspecified degree of chest wall**
Corrosion of unspecified degree of breast

T21.42 **Corrosion of unspecified degree of abdominal wall**
Corrosion of unspecified degree of flank
Corrosion of unspecified degree of groin

T21.43 **Corrosion of unspecified degree of upper back**
Corrosion of unspecified degree of interscapular region

T21.44 **Corrosion of unspecified degree of lower back**

T21.45 **Corrosion of unspecified degree of buttock**
Corrosion of unspecified degree of anus

T21.46 **Corrosion of unspecified degree of male genital region** ♂
Corrosion of unspecified degree of penis
Corrosion of unspecified degree of scrotum
Corrosion of unspecified degree of testis

T21.47 **Corrosion of unspecified degree of female genital region** ♀
Corrosion of unspecified degree of labium (majus) (minus)
Corrosion of unspecified degree of perineum
Corrosion of unspecified degree of vulva
EXCLUDES 2 *corrosion of vagina (T28.8)*

T21.49 **Corrosion of unspecified degree of other site of trunk**

T21.5 **Corrosion of first degree of trunk**
Code first (T51-T65) to identify chemical and intent
Use additional external cause code to identify place (Y92)

T21.5Ø **Corrosion of first degree of trunk, unspecified site**

T21.51 **Corrosion of first degree of chest wall**
Corrosion of first degree of breast

T21.52 **Corrosion of first degree of abdominal wall**
Corrosion of first degree of flank
Corrosion of first degree of groin

T21.53 **Corrosion of first degree of upper back**
Corrosion of first degree of interscapular region

T21.54 **Corrosion of first degree of lower back**

T21.55 **Corrosion of first degree of buttock**
Corrosion of first degree of anus

T21.56 **Corrosion of first degree of male genital region** ♂
Corrosion of first degree of penis
Corrosion of first degree of scrotum
Corrosion of first degree of testis

T21.57 **Corrosion of first degree of female genital region** ♀
Corrosion of first degree of labium (majus) (minus)
Corrosion of first degree of perineum
Corrosion of first degree of vulva
EXCLUDES 2 *corrosion of vagina (T28.8)*

T21.59 **Corrosion of first degree of other site of trunk**

T21.6 **Corrosion of second degree of trunk**
Code first (T51-T65) to identify chemical and intent
Use additional external cause code to identify place (Y92)

T21.6Ø **Corrosion of second degree of trunk, unspecified site**

T21.61 **Corrosion of second degree of chest wall**
Corrosion of second degree of breast

T21.62 **Corrosion of second degree of abdominal wall**
Corrosion of second degree of flank
Corrosion of second degree of groin

T21.63 **Corrosion of second degree of upper back**
Corrosion of second degree of interscapular region

T21.64 **Corrosion of second degree of lower back**

T21.65 **Corrosion of second degree of buttock**
Corrosion of second degree of anus

T21.66 **Corrosion of second degree of male genital region** ♂
Corrosion of second degree of penis
Corrosion of second degree of scrotum
Corrosion of second degree of testis

T21.67 **Corrosion of second degree of female genital region** ♀
Corrosion of second degree of labium (majus) (minus)
Corrosion of second degree of perineum
Corrosion of second degree of vulva
EXCLUDES 2 *corrosion of vagina (T28.8)*

T21.69 **Corrosion of second degree of other site of trunk**

T21.7 **Corrosion of third degree of trunk**
Code first (T51-T65) to identify chemical and intent
Use additional external cause code to identify place (Y92)

T21.7Ø **Corrosion of third degree of trunk, unspecified site** CC HS

T21.71 **Corrosion of third degree of chest wall** CC HS
Corrosion of third degree of breast

T21.72 **Corrosion of third degree of abdominal wall** CC HS
Corrosion of third degree of flank
Corrosion of third degree of groin

T21.73 **Corrosion of third degree of upper back** CC HS
Corrosion of third degree of interscapular region

T21.74 **Corrosion of third degree of lower back** CC HS

T21.75 **Corrosion of third degree of buttock** CC HS
Corrosion of third degree of anus

T21.76 **Corrosion of third degree of male genital region** CC HS ♂
Corrosion of third degree of penis
Corrosion of third degree of scrotum
Corrosion of third degree of testis

T21.77 **Corrosion of third degree of female genital region** CC HS ♀
Corrosion of third degree of labium (majus) (minus)
Corrosion of third degree of perineum
Corrosion of third degree of vulva
EXCLUDES 2 *corrosion of vagina (T28.8)*

T21.79 **Corrosion of third degree of other site of trunk** CC HS

T22 Burn and corrosion of shoulder and upper limb, except wrist and hand

EXCLUDES 2 *burn and corrosion of interscapular region (T21.-)*
burn and corrosion of wrist and hand (T23.-)

The appropriate 7th character is to be added to each code from category T22.
A initial encounter
D subsequent encounter
S sequela

T22.Ø **Burn of unspecified degree of shoulder and upper limb, except wrist and hand**
Use additional external cause code to identify the source, place and intent of the burn (XØØ-X19, X75-X77, X96-X98, Y92)

T22.ØØ **Burn of unspecified degree of shoulder and upper limb, except wrist and hand, unspecified site**

T22.Ø1 **Burn of unspecified degree of forearm**
T22.Ø11 **Burn of unspecified degree of right forearm**
T22.Ø12 **Burn of unspecified degree of left forearm**
T22.Ø19 **Burn of unspecified degree of unspecified forearm**

T22.Ø2 **Burn of unspecified degree of elbow**
T22.Ø21 **Burn of unspecified degree of right elbow**
T22.Ø22 **Burn of unspecified degree of left elbow**
T22.Ø29 **Burn of unspecified degree of unspecified elbow**

T22.Ø3 **Burn of unspecified degree of upper arm**
T22.Ø31 **Burn of unspecified degree of right upper arm**
T22.Ø32 **Burn of unspecified degree of left upper arm**
T22.Ø39 **Burn of unspecified degree of unspecified upper arm**

T22.Ø4 **Burn of unspecified degree of axilla**
T22.Ø41 **Burn of unspecified degree of right axilla**
T22.Ø42 **Burn of unspecified degree of left axilla**
T22.Ø49 **Burn of unspecified degree of unspecified axilla**

- T22.05 Burn of unspecified degree of shoulder
  - T22.051 Burn of unspecified degree of right shoulder
  - T22.052 Burn of unspecified degree of left shoulder
  - T22.059 Burn of unspecified degree of unspecified shoulder
- T22.06 Burn of unspecified degree of scapular region
  - T22.061 Burn of unspecified degree of right scapular region
  - T22.062 Burn of unspecified degree of left scapular region
  - T22.069 Burn of unspecified degree of unspecified scapular region
- T22.09 Burn of unspecified degree of multiple sites of shoulder and upper limb, except wrist and hand
  - T22.091 Burn of unspecified degree of multiple sites of right shoulder and upper limb, except wrist and hand
  - T22.092 Burn of unspecified degree of multiple sites of left shoulder and upper limb, except wrist and hand
  - T22.099 Burn of unspecified degree of multiple sites of unspecified shoulder and upper limb, except wrist and hand

T22.1 Burn of first degree of shoulder and upper limb, except wrist and hand

Use additional external cause code to identify the source, place and intent of the burn (X00-X19, X75-X77, X96-X98, Y92)

- T22.10 Burn of first degree of shoulder and upper limb, except wrist and hand, unspecified site
- T22.11 Burn of first degree of forearm
  - T22.111 Burn of first degree of right forearm
  - T22.112 Burn of first degree of left forearm
  - T22.119 Burn of first degree of unspecified forearm
- T22.12 Burn of first degree of elbow
  - T22.121 Burn of first degree of right elbow
  - T22.122 Burn of first degree of left elbow
  - T22.129 Burn of first degree of unspecified elbow
- T22.13 Burn of first degree of upper arm
  - T22.131 Burn of first degree of right upper arm
  - T22.132 Burn of first degree of left upper arm
  - T22.139 Burn of first degree of unspecified upper arm
- T22.14 Burn of first degree of axilla
  - T22.141 Burn of first degree of right axilla
  - T22.142 Burn of first degree of left axilla
  - T22.149 Burn of first degree of unspecified axilla
- T22.15 Burn of first degree of shoulder
  - T22.151 Burn of first degree of right shoulder
  - T22.152 Burn of first degree of left shoulder
  - T22.159 Burn of first degree of unspecified shoulder
- T22.16 Burn of first degree of scapular region
  - T22.161 Burn of first degree of right scapular region
  - T22.162 Burn of first degree of left scapular region
  - T22.169 Burn of first degree of unspecified scapular region
- T22.19 Burn of first degree of multiple sites of shoulder and upper limb, except wrist and hand
  - T22.191 Burn of first degree of multiple sites of right shoulder and upper limb, except wrist and hand
  - T22.192 Burn of first degree of multiple sites of left shoulder and upper limb, except wrist and hand
  - T22.199 Burn of first degree of multiple sites of unspecified shoulder and upper limb, except wrist and hand

T22.2 Burn of second degree of shoulder and upper limb, except wrist and hand

Use additional external cause code to identify the source, place and intent of the burn (X00-X19, X75-X77, X96-X98, Y92)

- T22.20 Burn of second degree of shoulder and upper limb, except wrist and hand, unspecified site
- T22.21 Burn of second degree of forearm
  - T22.211 Burn of second degree of right forearm
  - T22.212 Burn of second degree of left forearm
  - T22.219 Burn of second degree of unspecified forearm
- T22.22 Burn of second degree of elbow
  - T22.221 Burn of second degree of right elbow
  - T22.222 Burn of second degree of left elbow
  - T22.229 Burn of second degree of unspecified elbow
- T22.23 Burn of second degree of upper arm
  - T22.231 Burn of second degree of right upper arm
  - T22.232 Burn of second degree of left upper arm
  - T22.239 Burn of second degree of unspecified upper arm
- T22.24 Burn of second degree of axilla
  - T22.241 Burn of second degree of right axilla
  - T22.242 Burn of second degree of left axilla
  - T22.249 Burn of second degree of unspecified axilla
- T22.25 Burn of second degree of shoulder
  - T22.251 Burn of second degree of right shoulder
  - T22.252 Burn of second degree of left shoulder
  - T22.259 Burn of second degree of unspecified shoulder
- T22.26 Burn of second degree of scapular region
  - T22.261 Burn of second degree of right scapular region
  - T22.262 Burn of second degree of left scapular region
  - T22.269 Burn of second degree of unspecified scapular region
- T22.29 Burn of second degree of multiple sites of shoulder and upper limb, except wrist and hand
  - T22.291 Burn of second degree of multiple sites of right shoulder and upper limb, except wrist and hand
  - T22.292 Burn of second degree of multiple sites of left shoulder and upper limb, except wrist and hand
  - T22.299 Burn of second degree of multiple sites of unspecified shoulder and upper limb, except wrist and hand

T22.3 Burn of third degree of shoulder and upper limb, except wrist and hand

Use additional external cause code to identify the source, place and intent of the burn (X00-X19, X75-X77, X96-X98, Y92)

- T22.30 Burn of third degree of shoulder and upper limb, except wrist and hand, unspecified site CC H5 UNS
- T22.31 Burn of third degree of forearm
  - T22.311 Burn of third degree of right forearm CC H5
  - T22.312 Burn of third degree of left forearm CC H5
  - T22.319 Burn of third degree of unspecified forearm CC H5 UNS
- T22.32 Burn of third degree of elbow
  - T22.321 Burn of third degree of right elbow CC H5
  - T22.322 Burn of third degree of left elbow CC H5
  - T22.329 Burn of third degree of unspecified elbow CC H5 UNS
- T22.33 Burn of third degree of upper arm
  - T22.331 Burn of third degree of right upper arm CC H5
  - T22.332 Burn of third degree of left upper arm CC H5
  - T22.339 Burn of third degree of unspecified upper arm CC H5 UNS
- T22.34 Burn of third degree of axilla
  - T22.341 Burn of third degree of right axilla CC H5
  - T22.342 Burn of third degree of left axilla CC H5

✓7th **T22.349** Burn of third degree of unspecified axilla CC H5 UNS

✓6th **T22.35** Burn of third degree of shoulder

✓7th **T22.351** Burn of third degree of right shoulder CC H5

✓7th **T22.352** Burn of third degree of left shoulder CC H5

✓7th **T22.359** Burn of third degree of unspecified shoulder CC H5 UNS

✓6th **T22.36** Burn of third degree of scapular region

✓7th **T22.361** Burn of third degree of right scapular region CC H5

✓7th **T22.362** Burn of third degree of left scapular region CC H5

✓7th **T22.369** Burn of third degree of unspecified scapular region CC H5 UNS

✓6th **T22.39** Burn of third degree of multiple sites of shoulder and upper limb, except wrist and hand

✓7th **T22.391** Burn of third degree of multiple sites of right shoulder and upper limb, except wrist and hand CC H5

✓7th **T22.392** Burn of third degree of multiple sites of left shoulder and upper limb, except wrist and hand CC H5

✓7th **T22.399** Burn of third degree of multiple sites of unspecified shoulder and upper limb, except wrist and hand CC H5

✓5th **T22.4** Corrosion of unspecified degree of shoulder and upper limb, except wrist and hand

Code first (T51-T65) to identify chemical and intent

Use additional external cause code to identify place (Y92)

✓x7th **T22.40** Corrosion of unspecified degree of shoulder and upper limb, except wrist and hand, unspecified site

✓6th **T22.41** Corrosion of unspecified degree of forearm

✓7th **T22.411** Corrosion of unspecified degree of right forearm

✓7th **T22.412** Corrosion of unspecified degree of left forearm

✓7th **T22.419** Corrosion of unspecified degree of unspecified forearm

✓6th **T22.42** Corrosion of unspecified degree of elbow

✓7th **T22.421** Corrosion of unspecified degree of right elbow

✓7th **T22.422** Corrosion of unspecified degree of left elbow

✓7th **T22.429** Corrosion of unspecified degree of unspecified elbow

✓6th **T22.43** Corrosion of unspecified degree of upper arm

✓7th **T22.431** Corrosion of unspecified degree of right upper arm

✓7th **T22.432** Corrosion of unspecified degree of left upper arm

✓7th **T22.439** Corrosion of unspecified degree of unspecified upper arm

✓6th **T22.44** Corrosion of unspecified degree of axilla

✓7th **T22.441** Corrosion of unspecified degree of right axilla

✓7th **T22.442** Corrosion of unspecified degree of left axilla

✓7th **T22.449** Corrosion of unspecified degree of unspecified axilla

✓6th **T22.45** Corrosion of unspecified degree of shoulder

✓7th **T22.451** Corrosion of unspecified degree of right shoulder

✓7th **T22.452** Corrosion of unspecified degree of left shoulder

✓7th **T22.459** Corrosion of unspecified degree of unspecified shoulder

✓6th **T22.46** Corrosion of unspecified degree of scapular region

✓7th **T22.461** Corrosion of unspecified degree of right scapular region

✓7th **T22.462** Corrosion of unspecified degree of left scapular region

✓7th **T22.469** Corrosion of unspecified degree of unspecified scapular region

✓6th **T22.49** Corrosion of unspecified degree of multiple sites of shoulder and upper limb, except wrist and hand

✓7th **T22.491** Corrosion of unspecified degree of multiple sites of right shoulder and upper limb, except wrist and hand

✓7th **T22.492** Corrosion of unspecified degree of multiple sites of left shoulder and upper limb, except wrist and hand

✓7th **T22.499** Corrosion of unspecified degree of multiple sites of unspecified shoulder and upper limb, except wrist and hand

✓5th **T22.5** Corrosion of first degree of shoulder and upper limb, except wrist and hand

Code first (T51-T65) to identify chemical and intent

Use additional external cause code to identify place (Y92)

✓x7th **T22.50** Corrosion of first degree of shoulder and upper limb, except wrist and hand unspecified site

✓6th **T22.51** Corrosion of first degree of forearm

✓7th **T22.511** Corrosion of first degree of right forearm

✓7th **T22.512** Corrosion of first degree of left forearm

✓7th **T22.519** Corrosion of first degree of unspecified forearm

✓6th **T22.52** Corrosion of first degree of elbow

✓7th **T22.521** Corrosion of first degree of right elbow

✓7th **T22.522** Corrosion of first degree of left elbow

✓7th **T22.529** Corrosion of first degree of unspecified elbow

✓6th **T22.53** Corrosion of first degree of upper arm

✓7th **T22.531** Corrosion of first degree of right upper arm

✓7th **T22.532** Corrosion of first degree of left upper arm

✓7th **T22.539** Corrosion of first degree of unspecified upper arm

✓6th **T22.54** Corrosion of first degree of axilla

✓7th **T22.541** Corrosion of first degree of right axilla

✓7th **T22.542** Corrosion of first degree of left axilla

✓7th **T22.549** Corrosion of first degree of unspecified axilla

✓6th **T22.55** Corrosion of first degree of shoulder

✓7th **T22.551** Corrosion of first degree of right shoulder

✓7th **T22.552** Corrosion of first degree of left shoulder

✓7th **T22.559** Corrosion of first degree of unspecified shoulder

✓6th **T22.56** Corrosion of first degree of scapular region

✓7th **T22.561** Corrosion of first degree of right scapular region

✓7th **T22.562** Corrosion of first degree of left scapular region

✓7th **T22.569** Corrosion of first degree of unspecified scapular region

✓6th **T22.59** Corrosion of first degree of multiple sites of shoulder and upper limb, except wrist and hand

✓7th **T22.591** Corrosion of first degree of multiple sites of right shoulder and upper limb, except wrist and hand

✓7th **T22.592** Corrosion of first degree of multiple sites of left shoulder and upper limb, except wrist and hand

✓7th **T22.599** Corrosion of first degree of multiple sites of unspecified shoulder and upper limb, except wrist and hand

✓5th **T22.6** Corrosion of second degree of shoulder and upper limb, except wrist and hand

Code first (T51-T65) to identify chemical and intent

Use additional external cause code to identify place (Y92)

✓x7th **T22.60** Corrosion of second degree of shoulder and upper limb, except wrist and hand, unspecified site

✓6th **T22.61** Corrosion of second degree of forearm

✓7th **T22.611** Corrosion of second degree of right forearm

✓7th **T22.612** Corrosion of second degree of left forearm

✓7th **T22.619** Corrosion of second degree of unspecified forearm

✓6th **T22.62** Corrosion of second degree of elbow

✓7th **T22.621** Corrosion of second degree of right elbow

✓7th **T22.622** Corrosion of second degree of left elbow

✓7th **T22.629** Corrosion of second degree of unspecified elbow

✓6th **T22.63** Corrosion of second degree of upper arm

✓7th **T22.631** Corrosion of second degree of right upper arm

7th **T22.632 Corrosion of second degree of left upper arm**

7th **T22.639 Corrosion of second degree of unspecified upper arm**

6th **T22.64 Corrosion of second degree of axilla**

7th **T22.641 Corrosion of second degree of right axilla**

7th **T22.642 Corrosion of second degree of left axilla**

7th **T22.649 Corrosion of second degree of unspecified axilla**

6th **T22.65 Corrosion of second degree of shoulder**

7th **T22.651 Corrosion of second degree of right shoulder**

7th **T22.652 Corrosion of second degree of left shoulder**

7th **T22.659 Corrosion of second degree of unspecified shoulder**

6th **T22.66 Corrosion of second degree of scapular region**

7th **T22.661 Corrosion of second degree of right scapular region**

7th **T22.662 Corrosion of second degree of left scapular region**

7th **T22.669 Corrosion of second degree of unspecified scapular region**

6th **T22.69 Corrosion of second degree of multiple sites of shoulder and upper limb, except wrist and hand**

7th **T22.691 Corrosion of second degree of multiple sites of right shoulder and upper limb, except wrist and hand**

7th **T22.692 Corrosion of second degree of multiple sites of left shoulder and upper limb, except wrist and hand**

7th **T22.699 Corrosion of second degree of multiple sites of unspecified shoulder and upper limb, except wrist and hand**

5th **T22.7 Corrosion of third degree of shoulder and upper limb, except wrist and hand**

Code first (T51-T65) to identify chemical and intent

Use additional external cause code to identify place (Y92)

x7th **T22.70 Corrosion of third degree of shoulder and upper limb, except wrist and hand, unspecified site** CC H5 UNS

6th **T22.71 Corrosion of third degree of forearm**

7th **T22.711 Corrosion of third degree of right forearm** CC H5

7th **T22.712 Corrosion of third degree of left forearm** CC H5

7th **T22.719 Corrosion of third degree of unspecified forearm** CC H5 UNS

6th **T22.72 Corrosion of third degree of elbow**

7th **T22.721 Corrosion of third degree of right elbow** CC H5

7th **T22.722 Corrosion of third degree of left elbow** CC H5

7th **T22.729 Corrosion of third degree of unspecified elbow** CC H5 UNS

6th **T22.73 Corrosion of third degree of upper arm**

7th **T22.731 Corrosion of third degree of right upper arm** CC H5

7th **T22.732 Corrosion of third degree of left upper arm** CC H5

7th **T22.739 Corrosion of third degree of unspecified upper arm** CC H5 UNS

6th **T22.74 Corrosion of third degree of axilla**

7th **T22.741 Corrosion of third degree of right axilla** CC H5

7th **T22.742 Corrosion of third degree of left axilla** CC H5

7th **T22.749 Corrosion of third degree of unspecified axilla** CC H5 UNS

6th **T22.75 Corrosion of third degree of shoulder**

7th **T22.751 Corrosion of third degree of right shoulder** CC H5

7th **T22.752 Corrosion of third degree of left shoulder** CC H5

7th **T22.759 Corrosion of third degree of unspecified shoulder** CC H5 UNS

6th **T22.76 Corrosion of third degree of scapular region**

7th **T22.761 Corrosion of third degree of right scapular region** CC H5

7th **T22.762 Corrosion of third degree of left scapular region** CC H5

7th **T22.769 Corrosion of third degree of unspecified scapular region** CC H5 UNS

6th **T22.79 Corrosion of third degree of multiple sites of shoulder and upper limb, except wrist and hand**

7th **T22.791 Corrosion of third degree of multiple sites of right shoulder and upper limb, except wrist and hand** CC H5

7th **T22.792 Corrosion of third degree of multiple sites of left shoulder and upper limb, except wrist and hand** CC H5

7th **T22.799 Corrosion of third degree of multiple sites of unspecified shoulder and upper limb, except wrist and hand** CC H5

4th **T23 Burn and corrosion of wrist and hand**

AHA: 2015,1Q,19

The appropriate 7th character is to be added to each code from category T23.

A initial encounter

D subsequent encounter

S sequela

5th **T23.0 Burn of unspecified degree of wrist and hand**

Use additional external cause code to identify the source, place and intent of the burn (X00-X19, X75-X77, X96-X98, Y92)

6th **T23.00 Burn of unspecified degree of hand, unspecified site**

7th **T23.001 Burn of unspecified degree of right hand, unspecified site**

7th **T23.002 Burn of unspecified degree of left hand, unspecified site**

7th **T23.009 Burn of unspecified degree of unspecified hand, unspecified site**

6th **T23.01 Burn of unspecified degree of thumb (nail)**

7th **T23.011 Burn of unspecified degree of right thumb (nail)**

7th **T23.012 Burn of unspecified degree of left thumb (nail)**

7th **T23.019 Burn of unspecified degree of unspecified thumb (nail)**

6th **T23.02 Burn of unspecified degree of single finger (nail) except thumb**

7th **T23.021 Burn of unspecified degree of single right finger (nail) except thumb**

7th **T23.022 Burn of unspecified degree of single left finger (nail) except thumb**

7th **T23.029 Burn of unspecified degree of unspecified single finger (nail) except thumb**

6th **T23.03 Burn of unspecified degree of multiple fingers (nail), not including thumb**

7th **T23.031 Burn of unspecified degree of multiple right fingers (nail), not including thumb**

7th **T23.032 Burn of unspecified degree of multiple left fingers (nail), not including thumb**

7th **T23.039 Burn of unspecified degree of unspecified multiple fingers (nail), not including thumb**

6th **T23.04 Burn of unspecified degree of multiple fingers (nail), including thumb**

7th **T23.041 Burn of unspecified degree of multiple right fingers (nail), including thumb**

7th **T23.042 Burn of unspecified degree of multiple left fingers (nail), including thumb**

7th **T23.049 Burn of unspecified degree of unspecified multiple fingers (nail), including thumb**

6th **T23.05 Burn of unspecified degree of palm**

7th **T23.051 Burn of unspecified degree of right palm**

7th **T23.052 Burn of unspecified degree of left palm**

7th **T23.059 Burn of unspecified degree of unspecified palm**

6th **T23.06 Burn of unspecified degree of back of hand**

7th **T23.061 Burn of unspecified degree of back of right hand**

7th **T23.062 Burn of unspecified degree of back of left hand**

7th **T23.069 Burn of unspecified degree of back of unspecified hand**

6th **T23.07 Burn of unspecified degree of wrist**

7th **T23.071 Burn of unspecified degree of right wrist**

T23.072 Burn of unspecified degree of left wrist
T23.079 Burn of unspecified degree of unspecified wrist
T23.09 Burn of unspecified degree of multiple sites of wrist and hand
T23.091 Burn of unspecified degree of multiple sites of right wrist and hand
T23.092 Burn of unspecified degree of multiple sites of left wrist and hand
T23.099 Burn of unspecified degree of multiple sites of unspecified wrist and hand
T23.1 Burn of first degree of wrist and hand
Use additional external cause code to identify the source, place and intent of the burn (X00-X19, X75-X77, X96-X98, Y92)
T23.10 Burn of first degree of hand, unspecified site
T23.101 Burn of first degree of right hand, unspecified site
T23.102 Burn of first degree of left hand, unspecified site
T23.109 Burn of first degree of unspecified hand, unspecified site
T23.11 Burn of first degree of thumb (nail)
T23.111 Burn of first degree of right thumb (nail)
T23.112 Burn of first degree of left thumb (nail)
T23.119 Burn of first degree of unspecified thumb (nail)
T23.12 Burn of first degree of single finger (nail) except thumb
T23.121 Burn of first degree of single right finger (nail) except thumb
T23.122 Burn of first degree of single left finger (nail) except thumb
T23.129 Burn of first degree of unspecified single finger (nail) except thumb
T23.13 Burn of first degree of multiple fingers (nail), not including thumb
T23.131 Burn of first degree of multiple right fingers (nail), not including thumb
T23.132 Burn of first degree of multiple left fingers (nail), not including thumb
T23.139 Burn of first degree of unspecified multiple fingers (nail), not including thumb
T23.14 Burn of first degree of multiple fingers (nail), including thumb
T23.141 Burn of first degree of multiple right fingers (nail), including thumb
T23.142 Burn of first degree of multiple left fingers (nail), including thumb
T23.149 Burn of first degree of unspecified multiple fingers (nail), including thumb
T23.15 Burn of first degree of palm
T23.151 Burn of first degree of right palm
T23.152 Burn of first degree of left palm
T23.159 Burn of first degree of unspecified palm
T23.16 Burn of first degree of back of hand
T23.161 Burn of first degree of back of right hand
T23.162 Burn of first degree of back of left hand
T23.169 Burn of first degree of back of unspecified hand
T23.17 Burn of first degree of wrist
T23.171 Burn of first degree of right wrist
T23.172 Burn of first degree of left wrist
T23.179 Burn of first degree of unspecified wrist
T23.19 Burn of first degree of multiple sites of wrist and hand
T23.191 Burn of first degree of multiple sites of right wrist and hand
T23.192 Burn of first degree of multiple sites of left wrist and hand
T23.199 Burn of first degree of multiple sites of unspecified wrist and hand
T23.2 Burn of second degree of wrist and hand
Use additional external cause code to identify the source, place and intent of the burn (X00-X19, X75-X77, X96-X98, Y92)
T23.20 Burn of second degree of hand, unspecified site
T23.201 Burn of second degree of right hand, unspecified site
T23.202 Burn of second degree of left hand, unspecified site
T23.209 Burn of second degree of unspecified hand, unspecified site
T23.21 Burn of second degree of thumb (nail)
T23.211 Burn of second degree of right thumb (nail)
T23.212 Burn of second degree of left thumb (nail)
T23.219 Burn of second degree of unspecified thumb (nail)
T23.22 Burn of second degree of single finger (nail) except thumb
T23.221 Burn of second degree of single right finger (nail) except thumb
T23.222 Burn of second degree of single left finger (nail) except thumb
T23.229 Burn of second degree of unspecified single finger (nail) except thumb
T23.23 Burn of second degree of multiple fingers (nail), not including thumb
T23.231 Burn of second degree of multiple right fingers (nail), not including thumb
T23.232 Burn of second degree of multiple left fingers (nail), not including thumb
T23.239 Burn of second degree of unspecified multiple fingers (nail), not including thumb
T23.24 Burn of second degree of multiple fingers (nail), including thumb
T23.241 Burn of second degree of multiple right fingers (nail), including thumb
T23.242 Burn of second degree of multiple left fingers (nail), including thumb
T23.249 Burn of second degree of unspecified multiple fingers (nail), including thumb
T23.25 Burn of second degree of palm
T23.251 Burn of second degree of right palm
T23.252 Burn of second degree of left palm
T23.259 Burn of second degree of unspecified palm
T23.26 Burn of second degree of back of hand
T23.261 Burn of second degree of back of right hand
T23.262 Burn of second degree of back of left hand
T23.269 Burn of second degree of back of unspecified hand
T23.27 Burn of second degree of wrist
T23.271 Burn of second degree of right wrist
T23.272 Burn of second degree of left wrist
T23.279 Burn of second degree of unspecified wrist
T23.29 Burn of second degree of multiple sites of wrist and hand
T23.291 Burn of second degree of multiple sites of right wrist and hand
T23.292 Burn of second degree of multiple sites of left wrist and hand
T23.299 Burn of second degree of multiple sites of unspecified wrist and hand
T23.3 Burn of third degree of wrist and hand
Use additional external cause code to identify the source, place and intent of the burn (X00-X19, X75-X77, X96-X98, Y92)
T23.30 Burn of third degree of hand, unspecified site
AHA: 2016,2Q,5
T23.301 Burn of third degree of right hand, unspecified site CC H5
T23.302 Burn of third degree of left hand, unspecified site CC H5
T23.309 Burn of third degree of unspecified hand, unspecified site CC H5 UNS
T23.31 Burn of third degree of thumb (nail)
T23.311 Burn of third degree of right thumb (nail) CC H5
T23.312 Burn of third degree of left thumb (nail) CC H5
T23.319 Burn of third degree of unspecified thumb (nail) CC H5 UNS

6th T23.32 Burn of third degree of single finger (nail) except thumb

7th T23.321 Burn of third degree of single right finger (nail) except thumb CC H5

7th T23.322 Burn of third degree of single left finger (nail) except thumb CC H5

7th T23.329 Burn of third degree of unspecified single finger (nail) except thumb CC H5 UNS

6th T23.33 Burn of third degree of multiple fingers (nail), not including thumb

7th T23.331 Burn of third degree of multiple right fingers (nail), not including thumb CC H5

7th T23.332 Burn of third degree of multiple left fingers (nail), not including thumb CC H5

7th T23.339 Burn of third degree of unspecified multiple fingers (nail), not including thumb CC H5 UNS

6th T23.34 Burn of third degree of multiple fingers (nail), including thumb

7th T23.341 Burn of third degree of multiple right fingers (nail), including thumb CC H5

7th T23.342 Burn of third degree of multiple left fingers (nail), including thumb CC H5

7th T23.349 Burn of third degree of unspecified multiple fingers (nail), including thumb CC H5 UNS

6th T23.35 Burn of third degree of palm

7th T23.351 Burn of third degree of right palm CC H5

7th T23.352 Burn of third degree of left palm CC H5

7th T23.359 Burn of third degree of unspecified palm CC H5 UNS

6th T23.36 Burn of third degree of back of hand

7th T23.361 Burn of third degree of back of right hand CC H5

7th T23.362 Burn of third degree of back of left hand CC H5

7th T23.369 Burn of third degree of back of unspecified hand CC H5 UNS

6th T23.37 Burn of third degree of wrist

7th T23.371 Burn of third degree of right wrist CC H5

7th T23.372 Burn of third degree of left wrist CC H5

7th T23.379 Burn of third degree of unspecified wrist CC H5 UNS

6th T23.39 Burn of third degree of multiple sites of wrist and hand

7th T23.391 Burn of third degree of multiple sites of right wrist and hand CC H5

7th T23.392 Burn of third degree of multiple sites of left wrist and hand CC H5

7th T23.399 Burn of third degree of multiple sites of unspecified wrist and hand CC H5 UNS

5th T23.4 Corrosion of unspecified degree of wrist and hand

Code first (T51-T65) to identify chemical and intent

Use additional external cause code to identify place (Y92)

6th T23.40 Corrosion of unspecified degree of hand, unspecified site

7th T23.401 Corrosion of unspecified degree of right hand, unspecified site

7th T23.402 Corrosion of unspecified degree of left hand, unspecified site

7th T23.409 Corrosion of unspecified degree of unspecified hand, unspecified site

6th T23.41 Corrosion of unspecified degree of thumb (nail)

7th T23.411 Corrosion of unspecified degree of right thumb (nail)

7th T23.412 Corrosion of unspecified degree of left thumb (nail)

7th T23.419 Corrosion of unspecified degree of unspecified thumb (nail)

6th T23.42 Corrosion of unspecified degree of single finger (nail) except thumb

7th T23.421 Corrosion of unspecified degree of single right finger (nail) except thumb

7th T23.422 Corrosion of unspecified degree of single left finger (nail) except thumb

7th T23.429 Corrosion of unspecified degree of unspecified single finger (nail) except thumb

6th T23.43 Corrosion of unspecified degree of multiple fingers (nail), not including thumb

7th T23.431 Corrosion of unspecified degree of multiple right fingers (nail), not including thumb

7th T23.432 Corrosion of unspecified degree of multiple left fingers (nail), not including thumb

7th T23.439 Corrosion of unspecified degree of unspecified multiple fingers (nail), not including thumb

6th T23.44 Corrosion of unspecified degree of multiple fingers (nail), including thumb

7th T23.441 Corrosion of unspecified degree of multiple right fingers (nail), including thumb

7th T23.442 Corrosion of unspecified degree of multiple left fingers (nail), including thumb

7th T23.449 Corrosion of unspecified degree of unspecified multiple fingers (nail), including thumb

6th T23.45 Corrosion of unspecified degree of palm

7th T23.451 Corrosion of unspecified degree of right palm

7th T23.452 Corrosion of unspecified degree of left palm

7th T23.459 Corrosion of unspecified degree of unspecified palm

6th T23.46 Corrosion of unspecified degree of back of hand

7th T23.461 Corrosion of unspecified degree of back of right hand

7th T23.462 Corrosion of unspecified degree of back of left hand

7th T23.469 Corrosion of unspecified degree of back of unspecified hand

6th T23.47 Corrosion of unspecified degree of wrist

7th T23.471 Corrosion of unspecified degree of right wrist

7th T23.472 Corrosion of unspecified degree of left wrist

7th T23.479 Corrosion of unspecified degree of unspecified wrist

6th T23.49 Corrosion of unspecified degree of multiple sites of wrist and hand

7th T23.491 Corrosion of unspecified degree of multiple sites of right wrist and hand

7th T23.492 Corrosion of unspecified degree of multiple sites of left wrist and hand

7th T23.499 Corrosion of unspecified degree of multiple sites of unspecified wrist and hand

5th T23.5 Corrosion of first degree of wrist and hand

Code first (T51-T65) to identify chemical and intent

Use additional external cause code to identify place (Y92)

6th T23.50 Corrosion of first degree of hand, unspecified site

7th T23.501 Corrosion of first degree of right hand, unspecified site

7th T23.502 Corrosion of first degree of left hand, unspecified site

7th T23.509 Corrosion of first degree of unspecified hand, unspecified site

6th T23.51 Corrosion of first degree of thumb (nail)

7th T23.511 Corrosion of first degree of right thumb (nail)

7th T23.512 Corrosion of first degree of left thumb (nail)

7th T23.519 Corrosion of first degree of unspecified thumb (nail)

6th T23.52 Corrosion of first degree of single finger (nail) except thumb

7th T23.521 Corrosion of first degree of single right finger (nail) except thumb

7th T23.522 Corrosion of first degree of single left finger (nail) except thumb

7th T23.529 Corrosion of first degree of unspecified single finger (nail) except thumb

T23.53 Corrosion of first degree of multiple fingers (nail), not including thumb
T23.531 Corrosion of first degree of multiple right fingers (nail), not including thumb
T23.532 Corrosion of first degree of multiple left fingers (nail), not including thumb
T23.539 Corrosion of first degree of unspecified multiple fingers (nail), not including thumb
T23.54 Corrosion of first degree of multiple fingers (nail), including thumb
T23.541 Corrosion of first degree of multiple right fingers (nail), including thumb
T23.542 Corrosion of first degree of multiple left fingers (nail), including thumb
T23.549 Corrosion of first degree of unspecified multiple fingers (nail), including thumb
T23.55 Corrosion of first degree of palm
T23.551 Corrosion of first degree of right palm
T23.552 Corrosion of first degree of left palm
T23.559 Corrosion of first degree of unspecified palm
T23.56 Corrosion of first degree of back of hand
T23.561 Corrosion of first degree of back of right hand
T23.562 Corrosion of first degree of back of left hand
T23.569 Corrosion of first degree of back of unspecified hand
T23.57 Corrosion of first degree of wrist
T23.571 Corrosion of first degree of right wrist
T23.572 Corrosion of first degree of left wrist
T23.579 Corrosion of first degree of unspecified wrist
T23.59 Corrosion of first degree of multiple sites of wrist and hand
T23.591 Corrosion of first degree of multiple sites of right wrist and hand
T23.592 Corrosion of first degree of multiple sites of left wrist and hand
T23.599 Corrosion of first degree of multiple sites of unspecified wrist and hand
T23.6 Corrosion of second degree of wrist and hand
Code first (T51-T65) to identify chemical and intent
Use additional external cause code to identify place (Y92)
T23.60 Corrosion of second degree of hand, unspecified site
T23.601 Corrosion of second degree of right hand, unspecified site
T23.602 Corrosion of second degree of left hand, unspecified site
T23.609 Corrosion of second degree of unspecified hand, unspecified site
T23.61 Corrosion of second degree of thumb (nail)
T23.611 Corrosion of second degree of right thumb (nail)
T23.612 Corrosion of second degree of left thumb (nail)
T23.619 Corrosion of second degree of unspecified thumb (nail)
T23.62 Corrosion of second degree of single finger (nail) except thumb
T23.621 Corrosion of second degree of single right finger (nail) except thumb
T23.622 Corrosion of second degree of single left finger (nail) except thumb
T23.629 Corrosion of second degree of unspecified single finger (nail) except thumb
T23.63 Corrosion of second degree of multiple fingers (nail), not including thumb
T23.631 Corrosion of second degree of multiple right fingers (nail), not including thumb
T23.632 Corrosion of second degree of multiple left fingers (nail), not including thumb
T23.639 Corrosion of second degree of unspecified multiple fingers (nail), not including thumb
T23.64 Corrosion of second degree of multiple fingers (nail), including thumb
T23.641 Corrosion of second degree of multiple right fingers (nail), including thumb
T23.642 Corrosion of second degree of multiple left fingers (nail), including thumb
T23.649 Corrosion of second degree of unspecified multiple fingers (nail), including thumb
T23.65 Corrosion of second degree of palm
T23.651 Corrosion of second degree of right palm
T23.652 Corrosion of second degree of left palm
T23.659 Corrosion of second degree of unspecified palm
T23.66 Corrosion of second degree of back of hand
T23.661 Corrosion of second degree back of right hand
T23.662 Corrosion of second degree back of left hand
T23.669 Corrosion of second degree back of unspecified hand
T23.67 Corrosion of second degree of wrist
T23.671 Corrosion of second degree of right wrist
T23.672 Corrosion of second degree of left wrist
T23.679 Corrosion of second degree of unspecified wrist
T23.69 Corrosion of second degree of multiple sites of wrist and hand
T23.691 Corrosion of second degree of multiple sites of right wrist and hand
T23.692 Corrosion of second degree of multiple sites of left wrist and hand
T23.699 Corrosion of second degree of multiple sites of unspecified wrist and hand
T23.7 Corrosion of third degree of wrist and hand
Code first (T51-T65) to identify chemical and intent
Use additional external cause code to identify place (Y92)
T23.70 Corrosion of third degree of hand, unspecified site
T23.701 Corrosion of third degree of right hand, unspecified site CC H5
T23.702 Corrosion of third degree of left hand, unspecified site CC H5
T23.709 Corrosion of third degree of unspecified hand, unspecified site CC H5 UNS
T23.71 Corrosion of third degree of thumb (nail)
T23.711 Corrosion of third degree of right thumb (nail) CC H5
T23.712 Corrosion of third degree of left thumb (nail) CC H5
T23.719 Corrosion of third degree of unspecified thumb (nail) CC H5 UNS
T23.72 Corrosion of third degree of single finger (nail) except thumb
T23.721 Corrosion of third degree of single right finger (nail) except thumb CC H5
T23.722 Corrosion of third degree of single left finger (nail) except thumb CC H5
T23.729 Corrosion of third degree of unspecified single finger (nail) except thumb CC H5 UNS
T23.73 Corrosion of third degree of multiple fingers (nail), not including thumb
T23.731 Corrosion of third degree of multiple right fingers (nail), not including thumb CC H5
T23.732 Corrosion of third degree of multiple left fingers (nail), not including thumb CC H5
T23.739 Corrosion of third degree of unspecified multiple fingers (nail), not including thumb CC H5 UNS
T23.74 Corrosion of third degree of multiple fingers (nail), including thumb
T23.741 Corrosion of third degree of multiple right fingers (nail), including thumb CC H5
T23.742 Corrosion of third degree of multiple left fingers (nail), including thumb CC H5
T23.749 Corrosion of third degree of unspecified multiple fingers (nail), including thumb CC H5 UNS
T23.75 Corrosion of third degree of palm
T23.751 Corrosion of third degree of right palm CC H5

7th T23.752 Corrosion of third degree of left palm CC HS

7th T23.759 Corrosion of third degree of unspecified palm CC HS UNS

6th T23.76 Corrosion of third degree of back of hand

7th T23.761 Corrosion of third degree of back of right hand CC HS

7th T23.762 Corrosion of third degree of back of left hand CC HS

7th T23.769 Corrosion of third degree back of unspecified hand CC HS UNS

6th T23.77 Corrosion of third degree of wrist

7th T23.771 Corrosion of third degree of right wrist CC HS

7th T23.772 Corrosion of third degree of left wrist CC HS

7th T23.779 Corrosion of third degree of unspecified wrist CC HS UNS

6th T23.79 Corrosion of third degree of multiple sites of wrist and hand

7th T23.791 Corrosion of third degree of multiple sites of right wrist and hand CC HS

7th T23.792 Corrosion of third degree of multiple sites of left wrist and hand CC HS

7th T23.799 Corrosion of third degree of multiple sites of unspecified wrist and hand CC HS UNS

4th **T24 Burn and corrosion of lower limb, except ankle and foot**

EXCLUDES 2 *burn and corrosion of ankle and foot (T25.-)*
burn and corrosion of hip region (T21.-)

The appropriate 7th character is to be added to each code from category T24.
A initial encounter
D subsequent encounter
S sequela

5th T24.0 Burn of unspecified degree of lower limb, except ankle and foot

Use additional external cause code to identify the source, place and intent of the burn (X00-X19, X75-X77, X96-X98, Y92)

6th T24.00 Burn of unspecified degree of unspecified site of lower limb, except ankle and foot

7th T24.001 Burn of unspecified degree of unspecified site of right lower limb, except ankle and foot

7th T24.002 Burn of unspecified degree of unspecified site of left lower limb, except ankle and foot

7th T24.009 Burn of unspecified degree of unspecified site of unspecified lower limb, except ankle and foot

6th T24.01 Burn of unspecified degree of thigh

7th T24.011 Burn of unspecified degree of right thigh

7th T24.012 Burn of unspecified degree of left thigh

7th T24.019 Burn of unspecified degree of unspecified thigh

6th T24.02 Burn of unspecified degree of knee

7th T24.021 Burn of unspecified degree of right knee

7th T24.022 Burn of unspecified degree of left knee

7th T24.029 Burn of unspecified degree of unspecified knee

6th T24.03 Burn of unspecified degree of lower leg

7th T24.031 Burn of unspecified degree of right lower leg

7th T24.032 Burn of unspecified degree of left lower leg

7th T24.039 Burn of unspecified degree of unspecified lower leg

6th T24.09 Burn of unspecified degree of multiple sites of lower limb, except ankle and foot

7th T24.091 Burn of unspecified degree of multiple sites of right lower limb, except ankle and foot

7th T24.092 Burn of unspecified degree of multiple sites of left lower limb, except ankle and foot

7th T24.099 Burn of unspecified degree of multiple sites of unspecified lower limb, except ankle and foot

5th T24.1 Burn of first degree of lower limb, except ankle and foot

Use additional external cause code to identify the source, place and intent of the burn (X00-X19, X75-X77, X96-X98, Y92)

6th T24.10 Burn of first degree of unspecified site of lower limb, except ankle and foot

7th T24.101 Burn of first degree of unspecified site of right lower limb, except ankle and foot

7th T24.102 Burn of first degree of unspecified site of left lower limb, except ankle and foot

7th T24.109 Burn of first degree of unspecified site of unspecified lower limb, except ankle and foot

6th T24.11 Burn of first degree of thigh

7th T24.111 Burn of first degree of right thigh

7th T24.112 Burn of first degree of left thigh

7th T24.119 Burn of first degree of unspecified thigh

6th T24.12 Burn of first degree of knee

7th T24.121 Burn of first degree of right knee

7th T24.122 Burn of first degree of left knee

7th T24.129 Burn of first degree of unspecified knee

6th T24.13 Burn of first degree of lower leg

7th T24.131 Burn of first degree of right lower leg

7th T24.132 Burn of first degree of left lower leg

7th T24.139 Burn of first degree of unspecified lower leg

6th T24.19 Burn of first degree of multiple sites of lower limb, except ankle and foot

7th T24.191 Burn of first degree of multiple sites of right lower limb, except ankle and foot

7th T24.192 Burn of first degree of multiple sites of left lower limb, except ankle and foot

7th T24.199 Burn of first degree of multiple sites of unspecified lower limb, except ankle and foot

5th T24.2 Burn of second degree of lower limb, except ankle and foot

Use additional external cause code to identify the source, place and intent of the burn (X00-X19, X75-X77, X96-X98, Y92)

6th T24.20 Burn of second degree of unspecified site of lower limb, except ankle and foot

7th T24.201 Burn of second degree of unspecified site of right lower limb, except ankle and foot

7th T24.202 Burn of second degree of unspecified site of left lower limb, except ankle and foot

7th T24.209 Burn of second degree of unspecified site of unspecified lower limb, except ankle and foot

6th T24.21 Burn of second degree of thigh

7th T24.211 Burn of second degree of right thigh

7th T24.212 Burn of second degree of left thigh

7th T24.219 Burn of second degree of unspecified thigh

6th T24.22 Burn of second degree of knee

7th T24.221 Burn of second degree of right knee

7th T24.222 Burn of second degree of left knee

7th T24.229 Burn of second degree of unspecified knee

6th T24.23 Burn of second degree of lower leg

7th T24.231 Burn of second degree of right lower leg

7th T24.232 Burn of second degree of left lower leg

7th T24.239 Burn of second degree of unspecified lower leg

6th T24.29 Burn of second degree of multiple sites of lower limb, except ankle and foot

7th T24.291 Burn of second degree of multiple sites of right lower limb, except ankle and foot

7th T24.292 Burn of second degree of multiple sites of left lower limb, except ankle and foot

7th T24.299 Burn of second degree of multiple sites of unspecified lower limb, except ankle and foot

T24.3 Burn of third degree of lower limb, except ankle and foot
Use additional external cause code to identify the source, place and intent of the burn (X00-X19, X75-X77, X96-X98, Y92)
T24.30 Burn of third degree of unspecified site of lower limb, except ankle and foot
T24.301 Burn of third degree of unspecified site of right lower limb, except ankle and foot CC H5
T24.302 Burn of third degree of unspecified site of left lower limb, except ankle and foot CC H5
T24.309 Burn of third degree of unspecified site of unspecified lower limb, except ankle and foot CC H5 UNS
T24.31 Burn of third degree of thigh
T24.311 Burn of third degree of right thigh CC H5
T24.312 Burn of third degree of left thigh CC H5
T24.319 Burn of third degree of unspecified thigh CC H5 UNS
T24.32 Burn of third degree of knee
T24.321 Burn of third degree of right knee CC H5
T24.322 Burn of third degree of left knee CC H5
T24.329 Burn of third degree of unspecified knee CC H5 UNS
T24.33 Burn of third degree of lower leg
T24.331 Burn of third degree of right lower leg CC H5
T24.332 Burn of third degree of left lower leg CC H5
T24.339 Burn of third degree of unspecified lower leg CC H5 UNS
T24.39 Burn of third degree of multiple sites of lower limb, except ankle and foot
AHA: 2016,2Q,4
T24.391 Burn of third degree of multiple sites of right lower limb, except ankle and foot CC H5
T24.392 Burn of third degree of multiple sites of left lower limb, except ankle and foot CC H5
T24.399 Burn of third degree of multiple sites of unspecified lower limb, except ankle and foot CC H5 UNS
T24.4 Corrosion of unspecified degree of lower limb, except ankle and foot
Code first (T51-T65) to identify chemical and intent
Use additional external cause code to identify place (Y92)
T24.40 Corrosion of unspecified degree of unspecified site of lower limb, except ankle and foot
T24.401 Corrosion of unspecified degree of unspecified site of right lower limb, except ankle and foot
T24.402 Corrosion of unspecified degree of unspecified site of left lower limb, except ankle and foot
T24.409 Corrosion of unspecified degree of unspecified site of unspecified lower limb, except ankle and foot
T24.41 Corrosion of unspecified degree of thigh
T24.411 Corrosion of unspecified degree of right thigh
T24.412 Corrosion of unspecified degree of left thigh
T24.419 Corrosion of unspecified degree of unspecified thigh
T24.42 Corrosion of unspecified degree of knee
T24.421 Corrosion of unspecified degree of right knee
T24.422 Corrosion of unspecified degree of left knee
T24.429 Corrosion of unspecified degree of unspecified knee
T24.43 Corrosion of unspecified degree of lower leg
T24.431 Corrosion of unspecified degree of right lower leg
T24.432 Corrosion of unspecified degree of left lower leg
T24.439 Corrosion of unspecified degree of unspecified lower leg
T24.49 Corrosion of unspecified degree of multiple sites of lower limb, except ankle and foot
T24.491 Corrosion of unspecified degree of multiple sites of right lower limb, except ankle and foot
T24.492 Corrosion of unspecified degree of multiple sites of left lower limb, except ankle and foot
T24.499 Corrosion of unspecified degree of multiple sites of unspecified lower limb, except ankle and foot
T24.5 Corrosion of first degree of lower limb, except ankle and foot
Code first (T51-T65) to identify chemical and intent
Use additional external cause code to identify place (Y92)
T24.50 Corrosion of first degree of unspecified site of lower limb, except ankle and foot
T24.501 Corrosion of first degree of unspecified site of right lower limb, except ankle and foot
T24.502 Corrosion of first degree of unspecified site of left lower limb, except ankle and foot
T24.509 Corrosion of first degree of unspecified site of unspecified lower limb, except ankle and foot
T24.51 Corrosion of first degree of thigh
T24.511 Corrosion of first degree of right thigh
T24.512 Corrosion of first degree of left thigh
T24.519 Corrosion of first degree of unspecified thigh
T24.52 Corrosion of first degree of knee
T24.521 Corrosion of first degree of right knee
T24.522 Corrosion of first degree of left knee
T24.529 Corrosion of first degree of unspecified knee
T24.53 Corrosion of first degree of lower leg
T24.531 Corrosion of first degree of right lower leg
T24.532 Corrosion of first degree of left lower leg
T24.539 Corrosion of first degree of unspecified lower leg
T24.59 Corrosion of first degree of multiple sites of lower limb, except ankle and foot
T24.591 Corrosion of first degree of multiple sites of right lower limb, except ankle and foot
T24.592 Corrosion of first degree of multiple sites of left lower limb, except ankle and foot
T24.599 Corrosion of first degree of multiple sites of unspecified lower limb, except ankle and foot
T24.6 Corrosion of second degree of lower limb, except ankle and foot
Code first (T51-T65) to identify chemical and intent
Use additional external cause code to identify place (Y92)
T24.60 Corrosion of second degree of unspecified site of lower limb, except ankle and foot
T24.601 Corrosion of second degree of unspecified site of right lower limb, except ankle and foot
T24.602 Corrosion of second degree of unspecified site of left lower limb, except ankle and foot
T24.609 Corrosion of second degree of unspecified site of unspecified lower limb, except ankle and foot
T24.61 Corrosion of second degree of thigh
T24.611 Corrosion of second degree of right thigh
T24.612 Corrosion of second degree of left thigh
T24.619 Corrosion of second degree of unspecified thigh
T24.62 Corrosion of second degree of knee
T24.621 Corrosion of second degree of right knee
T24.622 Corrosion of second degree of left knee
T24.629 Corrosion of second degree of unspecified knee

T24.63 Corrosion of second degree of lower leg
T24.631 Corrosion of second degree of right lower leg
T24.632 Corrosion of second degree of left lower leg
T24.639 Corrosion of second degree of unspecified lower leg
T24.69 Corrosion of second degree of multiple sites of lower limb, except ankle and foot
T24.691 Corrosion of second degree of multiple sites of right lower limb, except ankle and foot
T24.692 Corrosion of second degree of multiple sites of left lower limb, except ankle and foot
T24.699 Corrosion of second degree of multiple sites of unspecified lower limb, except ankle and foot
T24.7 Corrosion of third degree of lower limb, except ankle and foot
Code first (T51-T65) to identify chemical and intent
Use additional external cause code to identify place (Y92)
T24.70 Corrosion of third degree of unspecified site of lower limb, except ankle and foot
T24.701 Corrosion of third degree of unspecified site of right lower limb, except ankle and foot CC HS
T24.702 Corrosion of third degree of unspecified site of left lower limb, except ankle and foot CC HS
T24.709 Corrosion of third degree of unspecified site of unspecified lower limb, except ankle and foot CC HS UNS
T24.71 Corrosion of third degree of thigh
T24.711 Corrosion of third degree of right thigh CC HS
T24.712 Corrosion of third degree of left thigh CC HS
T24.719 Corrosion of third degree of unspecified thigh CC HS UNS
T24.72 Corrosion of third degree of knee
T24.721 Corrosion of third degree of right knee CC HS
T24.722 Corrosion of third degree of left knee CC HS
T24.729 Corrosion of third degree of unspecified knee CC HS UNS
T24.73 Corrosion of third degree of lower leg
T24.731 Corrosion of third degree of right lower leg CC HS
T24.732 Corrosion of third degree of left lower leg CC HS
T24.739 Corrosion of third degree of unspecified lower leg CC HS UNS
T24.79 Corrosion of third degree of multiple sites of lower limb, except ankle and foot
T24.791 Corrosion of third degree of multiple sites of right lower limb, except ankle and foot CC HS
T24.792 Corrosion of third degree of multiple sites of left lower limb, except ankle and foot CC HS
T24.799 Corrosion of third degree of multiple sites of unspecified lower limb, except ankle and foot CC HS UNS

T25 Burn and corrosion of ankle and foot

The appropriate 7th character is to be added to each code from category T25.
A initial encounter
D subsequent encounter
S sequela

T25.0 Burn of unspecified degree of ankle and foot
Use additional external cause code to identify the source, place and intent of the burn (X00-X19, X75-X77, X96-X98, Y92)
T25.01 Burn of unspecified degree of ankle
T25.011 Burn of unspecified degree of right ankle
T25.012 Burn of unspecified degree of left ankle
T25.019 Burn of unspecified degree of unspecified ankle
T25.02 Burn of unspecified degree of foot
EXCLUDES 2 *burn of unspecified degree of toe(s) (nail) (T25.03-)*
T25.021 Burn of unspecified degree of right foot
T25.022 Burn of unspecified degree of left foot
T25.029 Burn of unspecified degree of unspecified foot
T25.03 Burn of unspecified degree of toe(s) (nail)
T25.031 Burn of unspecified degree of right toe(s) (nail)
T25.032 Burn of unspecified degree of left toe(s) (nail)
T25.039 Burn of unspecified degree of unspecified toe(s) (nail)
T25.09 Burn of unspecified degree of multiple sites of ankle and foot
T25.091 Burn of unspecified degree of multiple sites of right ankle and foot
T25.092 Burn of unspecified degree of multiple sites of left ankle and foot
T25.099 Burn of unspecified degree of multiple sites of unspecified ankle and foot
T25.1 Burn of first degree of ankle and foot
Use additional external cause code to identify the source, place and intent of the burn (X00-X19, X75-X77, X96-X98, Y92)
T25.11 Burn of first degree of ankle
T25.111 Burn of first degree of right ankle
T25.112 Burn of first degree of left ankle
T25.119 Burn of first degree of unspecified ankle
T25.12 Burn of first degree of foot
EXCLUDES 2 *burn of first degree of toe(s) (nail) (T25.13-)*
T25.121 Burn of first degree of right foot
T25.122 Burn of first degree of left foot
T25.129 Burn of first degree of unspecified foot
T25.13 Burn of first degree of toe(s) (nail)
T25.131 Burn of first degree of right toe(s) (nail)
T25.132 Burn of first degree of left toe(s) (nail)
T25.139 Burn of first degree of unspecified toe(s) (nail)
T25.19 Burn of first degree of multiple sites of ankle and foot
T25.191 Burn of first degree of multiple sites of right ankle and foot
T25.192 Burn of first degree of multiple sites of left ankle and foot
T25.199 Burn of first degree of multiple sites of unspecified ankle and foot
T25.2 Burn of second degree of ankle and foot
Use additional external cause code to identify the source, place and intent of the burn (X00-X19, X75-X77, X96-X98, Y92)
T25.21 Burn of second degree of ankle
T25.211 Burn of second degree of right ankle
T25.212 Burn of second degree of left ankle
T25.219 Burn of second degree of unspecified ankle
T25.22 Burn of second degree of foot
EXCLUDES 2 *burn of second degree of toe(s) (nail) (T25.23-)*
T25.221 Burn of second degree of right foot
T25.222 Burn of second degree of left foot
T25.229 Burn of second degree of unspecified foot
T25.23 Burn of second degree of toe(s) (nail)
T25.231 Burn of second degree of right toe(s) (nail)
T25.232 Burn of second degree of left toe(s) (nail)
T25.239 Burn of second degree of unspecified toe(s) (nail)
T25.29 Burn of second degree of multiple sites of ankle and foot
T25.291 Burn of second degree of multiple sites of right ankle and foot
T25.292 Burn of second degree of multiple sites of left ankle and foot
T25.299 Burn of second degree of multiple sites of unspecified ankle and foot

√5th **T25.3 Burn of third degree of ankle and foot**
Use additional external cause code to identify the source, place and intent of the burn (X00-X19, X75-X77, X96-X98, Y92)
√6th **T25.31 Burn of third degree of ankle**
√7th **T25.311 Burn of third degree of right ankle** CC H5
√7th **T25.312 Burn of third degree of left ankle** CC H5
√7th **T25.319 Burn of third degree of unspecified ankle** CC H5 UNS
√6th **T25.32 Burn of third degree of foot**
EXCLUDES 2 *burn of third degree of toe(s) (nail) (T25.33-)*
√7th **T25.321 Burn of third degree of right foot** CC H5
√7th **T25.322 Burn of third degree of left foot** CC H5
√7th **T25.329 Burn of third degree of unspecified foot** CC H5 UNS
√6th **T25.33 Burn of third degree of toe(s) (nail)**
√7th **T25.331 Burn of third degree of right toe(s) (nail)** CC H5
√7th **T25.332 Burn of third degree of left toe(s) (nail)** CC H5
√7th **T25.339 Burn of third degree of unspecified toe(s) (nail)** CC H5 UNS
√6th **T25.39 Burn of third degree of multiple sites of ankle and foot**
√7th **T25.391 Burn of third degree of multiple sites of right ankle and foot** CC H5
√7th **T25.392 Burn of third degree of multiple sites of left ankle and foot** CC H5
√7th **T25.399 Burn of third degree of multiple sites of unspecified ankle and foot** CC H5 UNS
√5th **T25.4 Corrosion of unspecified degree of ankle and foot**
Code first (T51-T65) to identify chemical and intent
Use additional external cause code to identify place (Y92)
√6th **T25.41 Corrosion of unspecified degree of ankle**
√7th **T25.411 Corrosion of unspecified degree of right ankle**
√7th **T25.412 Corrosion of unspecified degree of left ankle**
√7th **T25.419 Corrosion of unspecified degree of unspecified ankle**
√6th **T25.42 Corrosion of unspecified degree of foot**
EXCLUDES 2 *corrosion of unspecified degree of toe(s) (nail) (T25.43-)*
√7th **T25.421 Corrosion of unspecified degree of right foot**
√7th **T25.422 Corrosion of unspecified degree of left foot**
√7th **T25.429 Corrosion of unspecified degree of unspecified foot**
√6th **T25.43 Corrosion of unspecified degree of toe(s) (nail)**
√7th **T25.431 Corrosion of unspecified degree of right toe(s) (nail)**
√7th **T25.432 Corrosion of unspecified degree of left toe(s) (nail)**
√7th **T25.439 Corrosion of unspecified degree of unspecified toe(s) (nail)**
√6th **T25.49 Corrosion of unspecified degree of multiple sites of ankle and foot**
√7th **T25.491 Corrosion of unspecified degree of multiple sites of right ankle and foot**
√7th **T25.492 Corrosion of unspecified degree of multiple sites of left ankle and foot**
√7th **T25.499 Corrosion of unspecified degree of multiple sites of unspecified ankle and foot**
√5th **T25.5 Corrosion of first degree of ankle and foot**
Code first (T51-T65) to identify chemical and intent
Use additional external cause code to identify place (Y92)
√6th **T25.51 Corrosion of first degree of ankle**
√7th **T25.511 Corrosion of first degree of right ankle**
√7th **T25.512 Corrosion of first degree of left ankle**
√7th **T25.519 Corrosion of first degree of unspecified ankle**
√6th **T25.52 Corrosion of first degree of foot**
EXCLUDES 2 *corrosion of first degree of toe(s) (nail) (T25.53-)*
√7th **T25.521 Corrosion of first degree of right foot**
√7th **T25.522 Corrosion of first degree of left foot**
√7th **T25.529 Corrosion of first degree of unspecified foot**
√6th **T25.53 Corrosion of first degree of toe(s) (nail)**
√7th **T25.531 Corrosion of first degree of right toe(s) (nail)**
√7th **T25.532 Corrosion of first degree of left toe(s) (nail)**
√7th **T25.539 Corrosion of first degree of unspecified toe(s) (nail)**
√6th **T25.59 Corrosion of first degree of multiple sites of ankle and foot**
√7th **T25.591 Corrosion of first degree of multiple sites of right ankle and foot**
√7th **T25.592 Corrosion of first degree of multiple sites of left ankle and foot**
√7th **T25.599 Corrosion of first degree of multiple sites of unspecified ankle and foot**
√5th **T25.6 Corrosion of second degree of ankle and foot**
Code first (T51-T65) to identify chemical and intent
Use additional external cause code to identify place (Y92)
√6th **T25.61 Corrosion of second degree of ankle**
√7th **T25.611 Corrosion of second degree of right ankle**
√7th **T25.612 Corrosion of second degree of left ankle**
√7th **T25.619 Corrosion of second degree of unspecified ankle**
√6th **T25.62 Corrosion of second degree of foot**
EXCLUDES 2 *corrosion of second degree of toe(s) (nail) (T25.63-)*
√7th **T25.621 Corrosion of second degree of right foot**
√7th **T25.622 Corrosion of second degree of left foot**
√7th **T25.629 Corrosion of second degree of unspecified foot**
√6th **T25.63 Corrosion of second degree of toe(s) (nail)**
√7th **T25.631 Corrosion of second degree of right toe(s) (nail)**
√7th **T25.632 Corrosion of second degree of left toe(s) (nail)**
√7th **T25.639 Corrosion of second degree of unspecified toe(s) (nail)**
√6th **T25.69 Corrosion of second degree of multiple sites of ankle and foot**
√7th **T25.691 Corrosion of second degree of right ankle and foot**
√7th **T25.692 Corrosion of second degree of left ankle and foot**
√7th **T25.699 Corrosion of second degree of unspecified ankle and foot**
√5th **T25.7 Corrosion of third degree of ankle and foot**
Code first (T51-T65) to identify chemical and intent
Use additional external cause code to identify place (Y92)
√6th **T25.71 Corrosion of third degree of ankle**
√7th **T25.711 Corrosion of third degree of right ankle** CC H5
√7th **T25.712 Corrosion of third degree of left ankle** CC H5
√7th **T25.719 Corrosion of third degree of unspecified ankle** CC H5 UNS
√6th **T25.72 Corrosion of third degree of foot**
EXCLUDES 2 *corrosion of third degree of toe(s) (nail) (T25.73-)*
√7th **T25.721 Corrosion of third degree of right foot** CC H5
√7th **T25.722 Corrosion of third degree of left foot** CC H5
√7th **T25.729 Corrosion of third degree of unspecified foot** CC H5 UNS
√6th **T25.73 Corrosion of third degree of toe(s) (nail)**
√7th **T25.731 Corrosion of third degree of right toe(s) (nail)** CC H5
√7th **T25.732 Corrosion of third degree of left toe(s) (nail)** CC H5

7th **T25.739 Corrosion of third degree of unspecified toe(s) (nail)** CC H5 UNS

6th **T25.79 Corrosion of third degree of multiple sites of ankle and foot**

7th **T25.791 Corrosion of third degree of multiple sites of right ankle and foot** CC H5

7th **T25.792 Corrosion of third degree of multiple sites of left ankle and foot** CC H5

7th **T25.799 Corrosion of third degree of multiple sites of unspecified ankle and foot** CC H5 UNS

Burns and corrosions confined to eye and internal organs (T26-T28)

4th **T26 Burn and corrosion confined to eye and adnexa**

The appropriate 7th character is to be added to each code from category T26.
A initial encounter
D subsequent encounter
S sequela

5th **T26.Ø Burn of eyelid and periocular area**
Use additional external cause code to identify the source, place and intent of the burn (XØØ-X19, X75-X77, X96-X98, Y92)

x7th **T26.ØØ Burn of unspecified eyelid and periocular area**

x7th **T26.Ø1 Burn of right eyelid and periocular area**

x7th **T26.Ø2 Burn of left eyelid and periocular area**

5th **T26.1 Burn of cornea and conjunctival sac**
Use additional external cause code to identify the source, place and intent of the burn (XØØ-X19, X75-X77, X96-X98, Y92)

x7th **T26.1Ø Burn of cornea and conjunctival sac, unspecified eye**

x7th **T26.11 Burn of cornea and conjunctival sac, right eye**

x7th **T26.12 Burn of cornea and conjunctival sac, left eye**

5th **T26.2 Burn with resulting rupture and destruction of eyeball**
Use additional external cause code to identify the source, place and intent of the burn (XØØ-X19, X75-X77, X96-X98, Y92)

x7th **T26.2Ø Burn with resulting rupture and destruction of unspecified eyeball** CC H5 UNS

x7th **T26.21 Burn with resulting rupture and destruction of right eyeball** CC H5

x7th **T26.22 Burn with resulting rupture and destruction of left eyeball** CC H5

5th **T26.3 Burns of other specified parts of eye and adnexa**
Use additional external cause code to identify the source, place and intent of the burn (XØØ-X19, X75-X77, X96-X98, Y92)

x7th **T26.3Ø Burns of other specified parts of unspecified eye and adnexa**

x7th **T26.31 Burns of other specified parts of right eye and adnexa**

x7th **T26.32 Burns of other specified parts of left eye and adnexa**

5th **T26.4 Burn of eye and adnexa, part unspecified**
Use additional external cause code to identify the source, place and intent of the burn (XØØ-X19, X75-X77, X96-X98, Y92)

x7th **T26.4Ø Burn of unspecified eye and adnexa, part unspecified**

x7th **T26.41 Burn of right eye and adnexa, part unspecified**

x7th **T26.42 Burn of left eye and adnexa, part unspecified**

5th **T26.5 Corrosion of eyelid and periocular area**
Code first (T51-T65) to identify chemical and intent
Use additional external cause code to identify place (Y92)

x7th **T26.5Ø Corrosion of unspecified eyelid and periocular area**

x7th **T26.51 Corrosion of right eyelid and periocular area**

x7th **T26.52 Corrosion of left eyelid and periocular area**

5th **T26.6 Corrosion of cornea and conjunctival sac**
Code first (T51-T65) to identify chemical and intent
Use additional external cause code to identify place (Y92)

x7th **T26.6Ø Corrosion of cornea and conjunctival sac, unspecified eye**

x7th **T26.61 Corrosion of cornea and conjunctival sac, right eye**

x7th **T26.62 Corrosion of cornea and conjunctival sac, left eye**

5th **T26.7 Corrosion with resulting rupture and destruction of eyeball**
Code first (T51-T65) to identify chemical and intent
Use additional external cause code to identify place (Y92)

x7th **T26.7Ø Corrosion with resulting rupture and destruction of unspecified eyeball** CC H5 UNS

x7th **T26.71 Corrosion with resulting rupture and destruction of right eyeball** CC H5

x7th **T26.72 Corrosion with resulting rupture and destruction of left eyeball** CC H5

5th **T26.8 Corrosions of other specified parts of eye and adnexa**
Code first (T51-T65) to identify chemical and intent
Use additional external cause code to identify place (Y92)

x7th **T26.8Ø Corrosions of other specified parts of unspecified eye and adnexa**

x7th **T26.81 Corrosions of other specified parts of right eye and adnexa**

x7th **T26.82 Corrosions of other specified parts of left eye and adnexa**

5th **T26.9 Corrosion of eye and adnexa, part unspecified**
Code first (T51-T65) to identify chemical and intent
Use additional external cause code to identify place (Y92)

x7th **T26.9Ø Corrosion of unspecified eye and adnexa, part unspecified**

x7th **T26.91 Corrosion of right eye and adnexa, part unspecified**

x7th **T26.92 Corrosion of left eye and adnexa, part unspecified**

4th **T27 Burn and corrosion of respiratory tract**
Use additional external cause code to identify the source and intent of the burn (XØØ-X19, X75-X77, X96-X98)
Use additional external cause code to identify place (Y92)

The appropriate 7th character is to be added to each code from category T27.
A initial encounter
D subsequent encounter
S sequela

x7th **T27.Ø Burn of larynx and trachea** CC H5

x7th **T27.1 Burn involving larynx and trachea with lung** CC H5

x7th **T27.2 Burn of other parts of respiratory tract** CC H5
Burn of thoracic cavity

x7th **T27.3 Burn of respiratory tract, part unspecified** CC H5

x7th **T27.4 Corrosion of larynx and trachea** CC H5
Code first (T51-T65) to identify chemical and intent

x7th **T27.5 Corrosion involving larynx and trachea with lung** CC H5
Code first (T51-T65) to identify chemical and intent

x7th **T27.6 Corrosion of other parts of respiratory tract** CC H5
Code first (T51-T65) to identify chemical and intent

x7th **T27.7 Corrosion of respiratory tract, part unspecified** CC H5
Code first (T51-T65) to identify chemical and intent

4th **T28 Burn and corrosion of other internal organs**
Use additional external cause code to identify the source and intent of the burn (XØØ-X19, X75-X77, X96-X98)
Use additional external cause code to identify place (Y92)

The appropriate 7th character is to be added to each code from category T28.
A initial encounter
D subsequent encounter
S sequela

x7th **T28.Ø Burn of mouth and pharynx**

x7th **T28.1 Burn of esophagus** CC H5

x7th **T28.2 Burn of other parts of alimentary tract** CC H5

x7th **T28.3 Burn of internal genitourinary organs**

5th **T28.4 Burns of other and unspecified internal organs**

x7th **T28.4Ø Burn of unspecified internal organ**

6th **T28.41 Burn of ear drum**

7th **T28.411 Burn of right ear drum**

7th **T28.412 Burn of left ear drum**

7th **T28.419 Burn of unspecified ear drum**

x7th **T28.49 Burn of other internal organ**

x7th **T28.5 Corrosion of mouth and pharynx**
Code first (T51-T65) to identify chemical and intent

T28.6 Corrosion of esophagus
Code first (T51-T65) to identify chemical and intent

T28.7 Corrosion of other parts of alimentary tract
Code first (T51-T65) to identify chemical and intent

T28.8 Corrosion of internal genitourinary organs
Code first (T51-T65) to identify chemical and intent

T28.9 Corrosions of other and unspecified internal organs
Code first (T51-T65) to identify chemical and intent

T28.90 Corrosions of unspecified internal organs

T28.91 Corrosions of ear drum

T28.911 Corrosions of right ear drum

T28.912 Corrosions of left ear drum

T28.919 Corrosions of unspecified ear drum

T28.99 Corrosions of other internal organs

Burns and corrosions of multiple and unspecified body regions (T30-T32)

T30 Burn and corrosion, body region unspecified

T30.0 Burn of unspecified body region, unspecified degree
This code is not for inpatient use. Code to specified site and degree of burns
Burn NOS
Multiple burns NOS

T30.4 Corrosion of unspecified body region, unspecified degree
This code is not for inpatient use. Code to specified site and degree of corrosion
Corrosion NOS
Multiple corrosion NOS

T31 Burns classified according to extent of body surface involved

NOTE This category is to be used as the primary code only when the site of the burn is unspecified. It should be used as a supplementary code with categories T20-T25 when the site is specified.

T31.0 Burns involving less than 10% of body surface

T31.1 Burns involving 10-19% of body surface

T31.10 Burns involving 10-19% of body surface with 0% to 9% third degree burns CC H5
Burns involving 10-19% of body surface NOS

T31.11 Burns involving 10-19% of body surface with 10-19% third degree burns CC H5 HCC

T31.2 Burns involving 20-29% of body surface

T31.20 Burns involving 20-29% of body surface with 0% to 9% third degree burns CC H5
Burns involving 20-29% of body surface NOS

T31.21 Burns involving 20-29% of body surface with 10-19% third degree burns MCC H5 HCC

T31.22 Burns involving 20-29% of body surface with 20-29% third degree burns MCC H5 HCC

T31.3 Burns involving 30-39% of body surface

T31.30 Burns involving 30-39% of body surface with 0% to 9% third degree burns CC H5
Burns involving 30-39% of body surface NOS

T31.31 Burns involving 30-39% of body surface with 10-19% third degree burns MCC H5 HCC

T31.32 Burns involving 30-39% of body surface with 20-29% third degree burns MCC H5 HCC

T31.33 Burns involving 30-39% of body surface with 30-39% third degree burns MCC H5 HCC

T31.4 Burns involving 40-49% of body surface

T31.40 Burns involving 40-49% of body surface with 0% to 9% third degree burns CC H5
Burns involving 40-49% of body surface NOS

T31.41 Burns involving 40-49% of body surface with 10-19% third degree burns MCC H5 HCC

T31.42 Burns involving 40-49% of body surface with 20-29% third degree burns MCC H5 HCC

T31.43 Burns involving 40-49% of body surface with 30-39% third degree burns MCC H5 HCC

T31.44 Burns involving 40-49% of body surface with 40-49% third degree burns MCC H5 HCC

T31.5 Burns involving 50-59% of body surface

T31.50 Burns involving 50-59% of body surface with 0% to 9% third degree burns CC H5
Burns involving 50-59% of body surface NOS

T31.51 Burns involving 50-59% of body surface with 10-19% third degree burns MCC H5 HCC

T31.52 Burns involving 50-59% of body surface with 20-29% third degree burns MCC H5 HCC

T31.53 Burns involving 50-59% of body surface with 30-39% third degree burns MCC H5 HCC

T31.54 Burns involving 50-59% of body surface with 40-49% third degree burns MCC H5 HCC

T31.55 Burns involving 50-59% of body surface with 50-59% third degree burns MCC H5 HCC

T31.6 Burns involving 60-69% of body surface

T31.60 Burns involving 60-69% of body surface with 0% to 9% third degree burns CC H5
Burns involving 60-69% of body surface NOS

T31.61 Burns involving 60-69% of body surface with 10-19% third degree burns MCC H5 HCC

T31.62 Burns involving 60-69% of body surface with 20-29% third degree burns MCC H5 HCC

T31.63 Burns involving 60-69% of body surface with 30-39% third degree burns MCC H5 HCC

T31.64 Burns involving 60-69% of body surface with 40-49% third degree burns MCC H5 HCC

T31.65 Burns involving 60-69% of body surface with 50-59% third degree burns MCC H5 HCC

T31.66 Burns involving 60-69% of body surface with 60-69% third degree burns MCC H5 HCC

T31.7 Burns involving 70-79% of body surface

T31.70 Burns involving 70-79% of body surface with 0% to 9% third degree burns CC H5
Burns involving 70-79% of body surface NOS

T31.71 Burns involving 70-79% of body surface with 10-19% third degree burns MCC H5 HCC

T31.72 Burns involving 70-79% of body surface with 20-29% third degree burns MCC H5 HCC

T31.73 Burns involving 70-79% of body surface with 30-39% third degree burns MCC H5 HCC

T31.74 Burns involving 70-79% of body surface with 40-49% third degree burns MCC H5 HCC

T31.75 Burns involving 70-79% of body surface with 50-59% third degree burns MCC H5 HCC

T31.76 Burns involving 70-79% of body surface with 60-69% third degree burns MCC H5 HCC

T31.77 Burns involving 70-79% of body surface with 70-79% third degree burns MCC H5 HCC

T31.8 Burns involving 80-89% of body surface

T31.80 Burns involving 80-89% of body surface with 0% to 9% third degree burns CC H5
Burns involving 80-89% of body surface NOS

T31.81 Burns involving 80-89% of body surface with 10-19% third degree burns MCC H5 HCC

T31.82 Burns involving 80-89% of body surface with 20-29% third degree burns MCC H5 HCC

T31.83 Burns involving 80-89% of body surface with 30-39% third degree burns MCC H5 HCC

T31.84 Burns involving 80-89% of body surface with 40-49% third degree burns MCC H5 HCC

T31.85 Burns involving 80-89% of body surface with 50-59% third degree burns MCC H5 HCC

T31.86 Burns involving 80-89% of body surface with 60-69% third degree burns MCC H5 HCC

T31.87 Burns involving 80-89% of body surface with 70-79% third degree burns MCC H5 HCC

T31.88 Burns involving 80-89% of body surface with 80-89% third degree burns MCC H5 HCC

T31.9 Burns involving 90% or more of body surface

T31.90 Burns involving 90% or more of body surface with 0% to 9% third degree burns CC H5
Burns involving 90% or more of body surface NOS

T31.91 Burns involving 90% or more of body surface with 10-19% third degree burns MCC H5 HCC

T31.92 Burns involving 90% or more of body surface with 20-29% third degree burns MCC H5 HCC

T31.93 Burns involving 90% or more of body surface with 30-39% third degree burns MCC H5 HCC

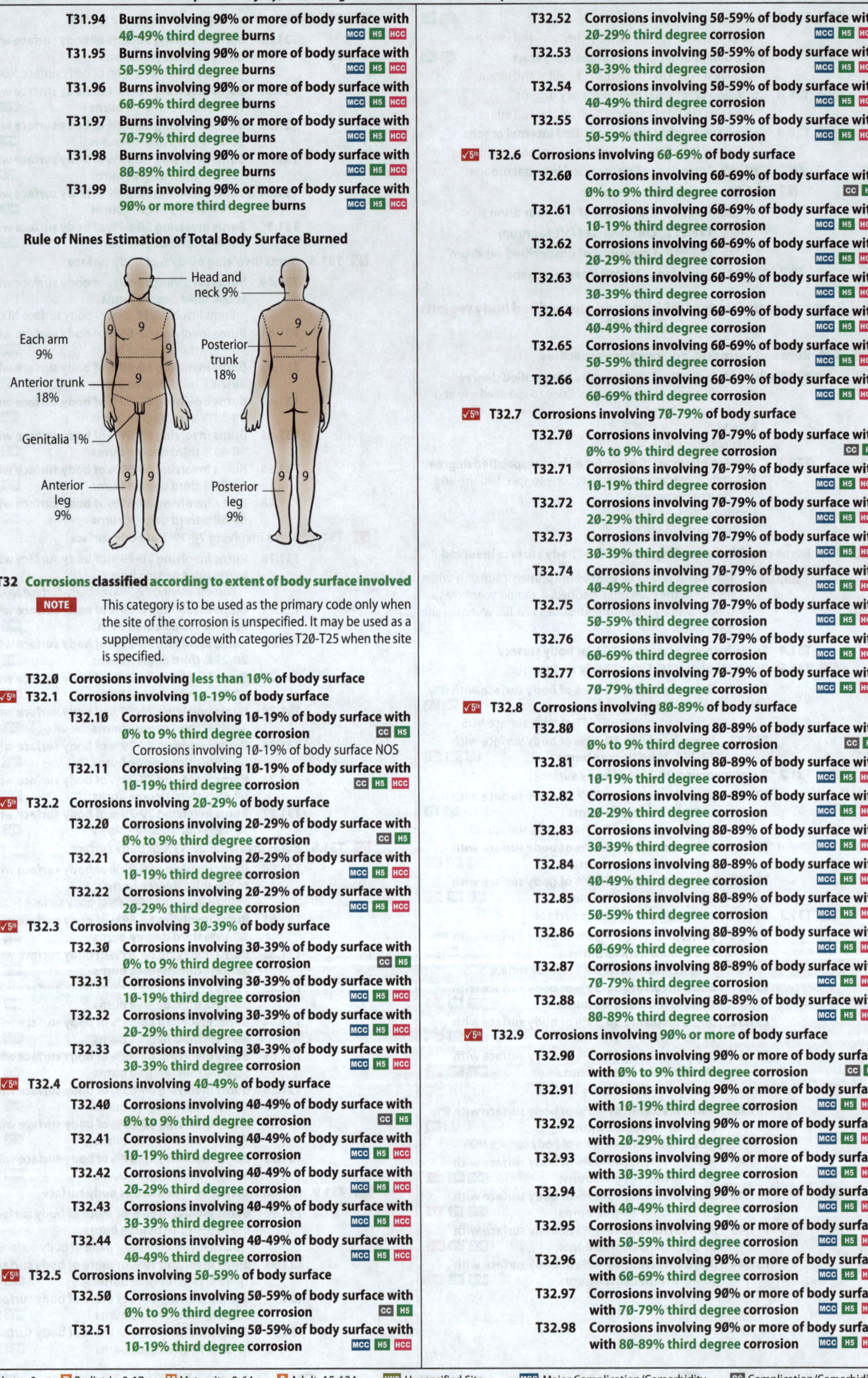

T31.94 **Burns involving 9Ø% or more of body surface with 4Ø-49% third degree burns** MCC HS HCC

T31.95 **Burns involving 9Ø% or more of body surface with 5Ø-59% third degree burns** MCC HS HCC

T31.96 **Burns involving 9Ø% or more of body surface with 6Ø-69% third degree burns** MCC HS HCC

T31.97 **Burns involving 9Ø% or more of body surface with 7Ø-79% third degree burns** MCC HS HCC

T31.98 **Burns involving 9Ø% or more of body surface with 8Ø-89% third degree burns** MCC HS HCC

T31.99 **Burns involving 9Ø% or more of body surface with 9Ø% or more third degree burns** MCC HS HCC

Rule of Nines Estimation of Total Body Surface Burned

√4th **T32** **Corrosions classified according to extent of body surface involved**

NOTE This category is to be used as the primary code only when the site of the corrosion is unspecified. It may be used as a supplementary code with categories T2Ø-T25 when the site is specified.

T32.Ø **Corrosions involving less than 1Ø% of body surface**

√5th **T32.1** **Corrosions involving 1Ø-19% of body surface**

T32.1Ø **Corrosions involving 1Ø-19% of body surface with Ø% to 9% third degree corrosion** CC HS
Corrosions involving 1Ø-19% of body surface NOS

T32.11 **Corrosions involving 1Ø-19% of body surface with 1Ø-19% third degree corrosion** CC HS HCC

√5th **T32.2** **Corrosions involving 2Ø-29% of body surface**

T32.2Ø **Corrosions involving 2Ø-29% of body surface with Ø% to 9% third degree corrosion** CC HS

T32.21 **Corrosions involving 2Ø-29% of body surface with 1Ø-19% third degree corrosion** MCC HS HCC

T32.22 **Corrosions involving 2Ø-29% of body surface with 2Ø-29% third degree corrosion** MCC HS HCC

√5th **T32.3** **Corrosions involving 3Ø-39% of body surface**

T32.3Ø **Corrosions involving 3Ø-39% of body surface with Ø% to 9% third degree corrosion** CC HS

T32.31 **Corrosions involving 3Ø-39% of body surface with 1Ø-19% third degree corrosion** MCC HS HCC

T32.32 **Corrosions involving 3Ø-39% of body surface with 2Ø-29% third degree corrosion** MCC HS HCC

T32.33 **Corrosions involving 3Ø-39% of body surface with 3Ø-39% third degree corrosion** MCC HS HCC

√5th **T32.4** **Corrosions involving 4Ø-49% of body surface**

T32.4Ø **Corrosions involving 4Ø-49% of body surface with Ø% to 9% third degree corrosion** CC HS

T32.41 **Corrosions involving 4Ø-49% of body surface with 1Ø-19% third degree corrosion** MCC HS HCC

T32.42 **Corrosions involving 4Ø-49% of body surface with 2Ø-29% third degree corrosion** MCC HS HCC

T32.43 **Corrosions involving 4Ø-49% of body surface with 3Ø-39% third degree corrosion** MCC HS HCC

T32.44 **Corrosions involving 4Ø-49% of body surface with 4Ø-49% third degree corrosion** MCC HS HCC

√5th **T32.5** **Corrosions involving 5Ø-59% of body surface**

T32.5Ø **Corrosions involving 5Ø-59% of body surface with Ø% to 9% third degree corrosion** CC HS

T32.51 **Corrosions involving 5Ø-59% of body surface with 1Ø-19% third degree corrosion** MCC HS HCC

T32.52 **Corrosions involving 5Ø-59% of body surface with 2Ø-29% third degree corrosion** MCC HS HCC

T32.53 **Corrosions involving 5Ø-59% of body surface with 3Ø-39% third degree corrosion** MCC HS HCC

T32.54 **Corrosions involving 5Ø-59% of body surface with 4Ø-49% third degree corrosion** MCC HS HCC

T32.55 **Corrosions involving 5Ø-59% of body surface with 5Ø-59% third degree corrosion** MCC HS HCC

√5th **T32.6** **Corrosions involving 6Ø-69% of body surface**

T32.6Ø **Corrosions involving 6Ø-69% of body surface with Ø% to 9% third degree corrosion** CC HS

T32.61 **Corrosions involving 6Ø-69% of body surface with 1Ø-19% third degree corrosion** MCC HS HCC

T32.62 **Corrosions involving 6Ø-69% of body surface with 2Ø-29% third degree corrosion** MCC HS HCC

T32.63 **Corrosions involving 6Ø-69% of body surface with 3Ø-39% third degree corrosion** MCC HS HCC

T32.64 **Corrosions involving 6Ø-69% of body surface with 4Ø-49% third degree corrosion** MCC HS HCC

T32.65 **Corrosions involving 6Ø-69% of body surface with 5Ø-59% third degree corrosion** MCC HS HCC

T32.66 **Corrosions involving 6Ø-69% of body surface with 6Ø-69% third degree corrosion** MCC HS HCC

√5th **T32.7** **Corrosions involving 7Ø-79% of body surface**

T32.7Ø **Corrosions involving 7Ø-79% of body surface with Ø% to 9% third degree corrosion** CC HS

T32.71 **Corrosions involving 7Ø-79% of body surface with 1Ø-19% third degree corrosion** MCC HS HCC

T32.72 **Corrosions involving 7Ø-79% of body surface with 2Ø-29% third degree corrosion** MCC HS HCC

T32.73 **Corrosions involving 7Ø-79% of body surface with 3Ø-39% third degree corrosion** MCC HS HCC

T32.74 **Corrosions involving 7Ø-79% of body surface with 4Ø-49% third degree corrosion** MCC HS HCC

T32.75 **Corrosions involving 7Ø-79% of body surface with 5Ø-59% third degree corrosion** MCC HS HCC

T32.76 **Corrosions involving 7Ø-79% of body surface with 6Ø-69% third degree corrosion** MCC HS HCC

T32.77 **Corrosions involving 7Ø-79% of body surface with 7Ø-79% third degree corrosion** MCC HS HCC

√5th **T32.8** **Corrosions involving 8Ø-89% of body surface**

T32.8Ø **Corrosions involving 8Ø-89% of body surface with Ø% to 9% third degree corrosion** CC HS

T32.81 **Corrosions involving 8Ø-89% of body surface with 1Ø-19% third degree corrosion** MCC HS HCC

T32.82 **Corrosions involving 8Ø-89% of body surface with 2Ø-29% third degree corrosion** MCC HS HCC

T32.83 **Corrosions involving 8Ø-89% of body surface with 3Ø-39% third degree corrosion** MCC HS HCC

T32.84 **Corrosions involving 8Ø-89% of body surface with 4Ø-49% third degree corrosion** MCC HS HCC

T32.85 **Corrosions involving 8Ø-89% of body surface with 5Ø-59% third degree corrosion** MCC HS HCC

T32.86 **Corrosions involving 8Ø-89% of body surface with 6Ø-69% third degree corrosion** MCC HS HCC

T32.87 **Corrosions involving 8Ø-89% of body surface with 7Ø-79% third degree corrosion** MCC HS HCC

T32.88 **Corrosions involving 8Ø-89% of body surface with 8Ø-89% third degree corrosion** MCC HS HCC

√5th **T32.9** **Corrosions involving 9Ø% or more of body surface**

T32.9Ø **Corrosions involving 9Ø% or more of body surface with Ø% to 9% third degree corrosion** CC HS

T32.91 **Corrosions involving 9Ø% or more of body surface with 1Ø-19% third degree corrosion** MCC HS HCC

T32.92 **Corrosions involving 9Ø% or more of body surface with 2Ø-29% third degree corrosion** MCC HS HCC

T32.93 **Corrosions involving 9Ø% or more of body surface with 3Ø-39% third degree corrosion** MCC HS HCC

T32.94 **Corrosions involving 9Ø% or more of body surface with 4Ø-49% third degree corrosion** MCC HS HCC

T32.95 **Corrosions involving 9Ø% or more of body surface with 5Ø-59% third degree corrosion** MCC HS HCC

T32.96 **Corrosions involving 9Ø% or more of body surface with 6Ø-69% third degree corrosion** MCC HS HCC

T32.97 **Corrosions involving 9Ø% or more of body surface with 7Ø-79% third degree corrosion** MCC HS HCC

T32.98 **Corrosions involving 9Ø% or more of body surface with 8Ø-89% third degree corrosion** MCC HS HCC

T32.99 Corrosions involving 90% or more of body surface with 90% or more third degree corrosion MCC H5 HCC

Frostbite (T33-T34)

EXCLUDES 2 hypothermia and other effects of reduced temperature (T68, T69.-)

T33 Superficial frostbite

INCLUDES frostbite with partial thickness skin loss

The appropriate 7th character is to be added to each code from category T33.
A initial encounter
D subsequent encounter
S sequela

T33.0 Superficial frostbite of head
T33.01 Superficial frostbite of ear
T33.011 Superficial frostbite of right ear CC H5
T33.012 Superficial frostbite of left ear CC H5
T33.019 Superficial frostbite of unspecified ear CC H5 UNS
T33.02 Superficial frostbite of nose CC H5
T33.09 Superficial frostbite of other part of head CC H5
T33.1 Superficial frostbite of neck CC H5
T33.2 Superficial frostbite of thorax CC H5
T33.3 Superficial frostbite of abdominal wall, lower back and pelvis CC H5
T33.4 Superficial frostbite of arm
EXCLUDES 2 superficial frostbite of wrist and hand (T33.5-)
T33.40 Superficial frostbite of unspecified arm CC H5 UNS
T33.41 Superficial frostbite of right arm CC H5
T33.42 Superficial frostbite of left arm CC H5
T33.5 Superficial frostbite of wrist, hand, and fingers
T33.51 Superficial frostbite of wrist
T33.511 Superficial frostbite of right wrist CC H5
T33.512 Superficial frostbite of left wrist CC H5
T33.519 Superficial frostbite of unspecified wrist CC H5 UNS
T33.52 Superficial frostbite of hand
EXCLUDES 2 superficial frostbite of fingers (T33.53-)
T33.521 Superficial frostbite of right hand CC H5
T33.522 Superficial frostbite of left hand CC H5
T33.529 Superficial frostbite of unspecified hand CC H5 UNS
T33.53 Superficial frostbite of finger(s)
T33.531 Superficial frostbite of right finger(s) CC H5
T33.532 Superficial frostbite of left finger(s) CC H5
T33.539 Superficial frostbite of unspecified finger(s) CC H5 UNS
T33.6 Superficial frostbite of hip and thigh
T33.60 Superficial frostbite of unspecified hip and thigh CC H5 UNS
T33.61 Superficial frostbite of right hip and thigh CC H5
T33.62 Superficial frostbite of left hip and thigh CC H5
T33.7 Superficial frostbite of knee and lower leg
EXCLUDES 2 superficial frostbite of ankle and foot (T33.8-)
T33.70 Superficial frostbite of unspecified knee and lower leg CC H5 UNS
T33.71 Superficial frostbite of right knee and lower leg CC H5
T33.72 Superficial frostbite of left knee and lower leg CC H5
T33.8 Superficial frostbite of ankle, foot, and toe(s)
T33.81 Superficial frostbite of ankle
T33.811 Superficial frostbite of right ankle CC H5
T33.812 Superficial frostbite of left ankle CC H5
T33.819 Superficial frostbite of unspecified ankle CC H5 UNS
T33.82 Superficial frostbite of foot
T33.821 Superficial frostbite of right foot CC H5
T33.822 Superficial frostbite of left foot CC H5
T33.829 Superficial frostbite of unspecified foot CC H5 UNS
T33.83 Superficial frostbite of toe(s)
T33.831 Superficial frostbite of right toe(s) CC H5
T33.832 Superficial frostbite of left toe(s) CC H5
T33.839 Superficial frostbite of unspecified toe(s) CC H5 UNS
T33.9 Superficial frostbite of other and unspecified sites
T33.90 Superficial frostbite of unspecified sites CC H5 UNS
Superficial frostbite NOS
T33.99 Superficial frostbite of other sites CC H5
Superficial frostbite of leg NOS
Superficial frostbite of trunk NOS

T34 Frostbite with tissue necrosis

The appropriate 7th character is to be added to each code from category T34.
A initial encounter
D subsequent encounter
S sequela

T34.0 Frostbite with tissue necrosis of head
T34.01 Frostbite with tissue necrosis of ear
T34.011 Frostbite with tissue necrosis of right ear CC H5
T34.012 Frostbite with tissue necrosis of left ear CC H5
T34.019 Frostbite with tissue necrosis of unspecified ear CC H5 UNS
T34.02 Frostbite with tissue necrosis of nose CC H5
T34.09 Frostbite with tissue necrosis of other part of head CC H5
T34.1 Frostbite with tissue necrosis of neck CC H5
T34.2 Frostbite with tissue necrosis of thorax CC H5
T34.3 Frostbite with tissue necrosis of abdominal wall, lower back and pelvis CC H5
T34.4 Frostbite with tissue necrosis of arm
EXCLUDES 2 frostbite with tissue necrosis of wrist and hand (T34.5-)
T34.40 Frostbite with tissue necrosis of unspecified arm CC H5 UNS
T34.41 Frostbite with tissue necrosis of right arm CC H5
T34.42 Frostbite with tissue necrosis of left arm CC H5
T34.5 Frostbite with tissue necrosis of wrist, hand, and finger(s)
T34.51 Frostbite with tissue necrosis of wrist
T34.511 Frostbite with tissue necrosis of right wrist CC H5
T34.512 Frostbite with tissue necrosis of left wrist CC H5
T34.519 Frostbite with tissue necrosis of unspecified wrist CC H5 UNS
T34.52 Frostbite with tissue necrosis of hand
EXCLUDES 2 frostbite with tissue necrosis of finger(s) (T34.53-)
T34.521 Frostbite with tissue necrosis of right hand CC H5
T34.522 Frostbite with tissue necrosis of left hand CC H5
T34.529 Frostbite with tissue necrosis of unspecified hand CC H5 UNS
T34.53 Frostbite with tissue necrosis of finger(s)
T34.531 Frostbite with tissue necrosis of right finger(s) CC H5
T34.532 Frostbite with tissue necrosis of left finger(s) CC H5
T34.539 Frostbite with tissue necrosis of unspecified finger(s) CC H5 UNS

T34.6 Frostbite with tissue necrosis of hip and thigh

T34.60 Frostbite with tissue necrosis of unspecified hip and thigh CC H5 UNS

T34.61 Frostbite with tissue necrosis of right hip and thigh CC H5

T34.62 Frostbite with tissue necrosis of left hip and thigh CC H5

T34.7 Frostbite with tissue necrosis of knee and lower leg

EXCLUDES 2 *frostbite with tissue necrosis of ankle and foot (T34.8-)*

T34.70 Frostbite with tissue necrosis of unspecified knee and lower leg CC H5 UNS

T34.71 Frostbite with tissue necrosis of right knee and lower leg CC H5

T34.72 Frostbite with tissue necrosis of left knee and lower leg CC H5

T34.8 Frostbite with tissue necrosis of ankle, foot, and toe(s)

T34.81 Frostbite with tissue necrosis of ankle

T34.811 Frostbite with tissue necrosis of right ankle CC H5

T34.812 Frostbite with tissue necrosis of left ankle CC H5

T34.819 Frostbite with tissue necrosis of unspecified ankle CC H5 UNS

T34.82 Frostbite with tissue necrosis of foot

T34.821 Frostbite with tissue necrosis of right foot CC H5

T34.822 Frostbite with tissue necrosis of left foot CC H5

T34.829 Frostbite with tissue necrosis of unspecified foot CC H5 UNS

T34.83 Frostbite with tissue necrosis of toe(s)

T34.831 Frostbite with tissue necrosis of right toe(s) CC H5

T34.832 Frostbite with tissue necrosis of left toe(s) CC H5

T34.839 Frostbite with tissue necrosis of unspecified toe(s) CC H5 UNS

T34.9 Frostbite with tissue necrosis of other and unspecified sites

T34.90 Frostbite with tissue necrosis of unspecified sites CC H5 UNS

Frostbite with tissue necrosis NOS

T34.99 Frostbite with tissue necrosis of other sites CC H5

Frostbite with tissue necrosis of leg NOS

Frostbite with tissue necrosis of trunk NOS

Poisoning by, adverse effects of and underdosing of drugs, medicaments and biological substances (T36-T5Ø)

INCLUDES adverse effect of correct substance properly administered
poisoning by overdose of substance
poisoning by wrong substance given or taken in error
underdosing by (inadvertently) (deliberately) taking less substance than prescribed or instructed

Code first, for adverse effects, the nature of the adverse effect, such as:
adverse effect NOS (T88.7)
aspirin gastritis (K29.-)
blood disorders (D56-D76)
contact dermatitis (L23-L25)
dermatitis due to substances taken internally (L27.-)
nephropathy (N14.Ø-N14.2)

NOTE The drug giving rise to the adverse effect should be identified by use of codes from categories T36-T5Ø with fifth or sixth character 5.

Use additional code(s) to specify:
manifestations of poisoning
underdosing or failure in dosage during medical and surgical care (Y63.6, Y63.8-Y63.9)
underdosing of medication regimen (Z91.12-, Z91.13-)

EXCLUDES 1 *toxic reaction to local anesthesia in pregnancy (O29.3-)*

EXCLUDES 2 *abuse and dependence of psychoactive substances (F1Ø-F19)*
abuse of non-dependence-producing substances (F55.-)
drug reaction and poisoning affecting newborn (PØØ-P96)
immunodeficiency due to drugs (D84.821)
pathological drug intoxication (inebriation) (F1Ø-F19)

AHA: 2018,4Q,71; 2016,2Q,8; 2015,3Q,22

T36 Poisoning by, adverse effect of and underdosing of systemic antibiotics

EXCLUDES 1 *antineoplastic antibiotics (T45.1-)*
locally applied antibiotic NEC (T49.Ø)
topically used antibiotic for ear, nose and throat (T49.6)
topically used antibiotic for eye (T49.5)

The appropriate 7th character is to be added to each code from category T36.
A initial encounter
D subsequent encounter
S sequela

T36.Ø Poisoning by, adverse effect of and underdosing of penicillins

T36.ØX Poisoning by, adverse effect of and underdosing of penicillins

T36.ØX1 Poisoning by penicillins, accidental (unintentional)

Poisoning by penicillins NOS

T36.ØX2 Poisoning by penicillins, intentional self-harm HCC

T36.ØX3 Poisoning by penicillins, assault

T36.ØX4 Poisoning by penicillins, undetermined

T36.ØX5 Adverse effect of penicillins UPD

T36.ØX6 Underdosing of penicillins UPD

T36.1 Poisoning by, adverse effect of and underdosing of cephalosporins and other beta-lactam antibiotics

T36.1X Poisoning by, adverse effect of and underdosing of cephalosporins and other beta-lactam antibiotics

T36.1X1 Poisoning by cephalosporins and other beta-lactam antibiotics, accidental (unintentional)

Poisoning by cephalosporins and other beta-lactam antibiotics NOS

T36.1X2 Poisoning by cephalosporins and other beta-lactam antibiotics, intentional self-harm HCC

T36.1X3 Poisoning by cephalosporins and other beta-lactam antibiotics, assault

T36.1X4 Poisoning by cephalosporins and other beta-lactam antibiotics, undetermined

T36.1X5 Adverse effect of cephalosporins and other beta-lactam antibiotics UPD

T36.1X6 Underdosing of cephalosporins and other beta-lactam antibiotics UPD

T36.2 Poisoning by, adverse effect of and underdosing of chloramphenicol group

T36.2X Poisoning by, adverse effect of and underdosing of chloramphenicol group

T36.2X1 Poisoning by chloramphenicol group, accidental (unintentional)

Poisoning by chloramphenicol group NOS

7 T36.2X2 Poisoning by chloramphenicol group, intentional self-harm HCC
T36.2X3 Poisoning by chloramphenicol group, assault
T36.2X4 Poisoning by chloramphenicol group, undetermined
T36.2X5 Adverse effect of chloramphenicol group UPD
T36.2X6 Underdosing of chloramphenicol group UPD

T36.3 Poisoning by, adverse effect of and underdosing of macrolides
T36.3X Poisoning by, adverse effect of and underdosing of macrolides
T36.3X1 Poisoning by macrolides, accidental (unintentional)
Poisoning by macrolides NOS
7 T36.3X2 Poisoning by macrolides, intentional self-harm HCC
T36.3X3 Poisoning by macrolides, assault
T36.3X4 Poisoning by macrolides, undetermined
T36.3X5 Adverse effect of macrolides UPD
T36.3X6 Underdosing of macrolides UPD

T36.4 Poisoning by, adverse effect of and underdosing of tetracyclines
T36.4X Poisoning by, adverse effect of and underdosing of tetracyclines
T36.4X1 Poisoning by tetracyclines, accidental (unintentional)
Poisoning by tetracyclines NOS
7 T36.4X2 Poisoning by tetracyclines, intentional self-harm HCC
T36.4X3 Poisoning by tetracyclines, assault
T36.4X4 Poisoning by tetracyclines, undetermined
T36.4X5 Adverse effect of tetracyclines UPD
T36.4X6 Underdosing of tetracyclines UPD

T36.5 Poisoning by, adverse effect of and underdosing of aminoglycosides
Poisoning by, adverse effect of and underdosing of streptomycin
T36.5X Poisoning by, adverse effect of and underdosing of aminoglycosides
T36.5X1 Poisoning by aminoglycosides, accidental (unintentional)
Poisoning by aminoglycosides NOS
7 T36.5X2 Poisoning by aminoglycosides, intentional self-harm HCC
T36.5X3 Poisoning by aminoglycosides, assault
T36.5X4 Poisoning by aminoglycosides, undetermined
T36.5X5 Adverse effect of aminoglycosides UPD
T36.5X6 Underdosing of aminoglycosides UPD

T36.6 Poisoning by, adverse effect of and underdosing of rifampicins
T36.6X Poisoning by, adverse effect of and underdosing of rifampicins
T36.6X1 Poisoning by rifampicins, accidental (unintentional)
Poisoning by rifampicins NOS
7 T36.6X2 Poisoning by rifampicins, intentional self-harm HCC
T36.6X3 Poisoning by rifampicins, assault
T36.6X4 Poisoning by rifampicins, undetermined
T36.6X5 Adverse effect of rifampicins UPD
T36.6X6 Underdosing of rifampicins UPD

T36.7 Poisoning by, adverse effect of and underdosing of antifungal antibiotics, systemically used
T36.7X Poisoning by, adverse effect of and underdosing of antifungal antibiotics, systemically used
T36.7X1 Poisoning by antifungal antibiotics, systemically used, accidental (unintentional)
Poisoning by antifungal antibiotics, systemically used NOS
7 T36.7X2 Poisoning by antifungal antibiotics, systemically used, intentional self-harm HCC
T36.7X3 Poisoning by antifungal antibiotics, systemically used, assault
T36.7X4 Poisoning by antifungal antibiotics, systemically used, undetermined
T36.7X5 Adverse effect of antifungal antibiotics, systemically used UPD
T36.7X6 Underdosing of antifungal antibiotics, systemically used UPD

T36.8 Poisoning by, adverse effect of and underdosing of other systemic antibiotics
T36.8X Poisoning by, adverse effect of and underdosing of other systemic antibiotics
AHA: 2017,1Q,39
T36.8X1 Poisoning by other systemic antibiotics, accidental (unintentional)
Poisoning by other systemic antibiotics NOS
7 T36.8X2 Poisoning by other systemic antibiotics, intentional self-harm HCC
T36.8X3 Poisoning by other systemic antibiotics, assault
T36.8X4 Poisoning by other systemic antibiotics, undetermined
T36.8X5 Adverse effect of other systemic antibiotics UPD
T36.8X6 Underdosing of other systemic antibiotics UPD

T36.9 Poisoning by, adverse effect of and underdosing of unspecified systemic antibiotic
T36.91 Poisoning by unspecified systemic antibiotic, accidental (unintentional)
Poisoning by systemic antibiotic NOS
7 T36.92 Poisoning by unspecified systemic antibiotic, intentional self-harm HCC
T36.93 Poisoning by unspecified systemic antibiotic, assault
T36.94 Poisoning by unspecified systemic antibiotic, undetermined
T36.95 Adverse effect of unspecified systemic antibiotic UPD
T36.96 Underdosing of unspecified systemic antibiotic UPD

T37 Poisoning by, adverse effect of and underdosing of other systemic anti-infectives and antiparasitics
EXCLUDES 1 *anti-infectives topically used for ear, nose and throat (T49.6-)*
anti-infectives topically used for eye (T49.5-)
locally applied anti-infectives NEC (T49.Ø-)

The appropriate 7th character is to be added to each code from category T37.
A initial encounter
D subsequent encounter
S sequela

T37.Ø Poisoning by, adverse effect of and underdosing of sulfonamides
T37.ØX Poisoning by, adverse effect of and underdosing of sulfonamides
T37.ØX1 Poisoning by sulfonamides, accidental (unintentional)
Poisoning by sulfonamides NOS
7 T37.ØX2 Poisoning by sulfonamides, intentional self-harm HCC
T37.ØX3 Poisoning by sulfonamides, assault
T37.ØX4 Poisoning by sulfonamides, undetermined
T37.ØX5 Adverse effect of sulfonamides UPD
T37.ØX6 Underdosing of sulfonamides UPD

T37.1 Poisoning by, adverse effect of and underdosing of antimycobacterial drugs
EXCLUDES 1 *rifampicins (T36.6-)*
streptomycin (T36.5-)
T37.1X Poisoning by, adverse effect of and underdosing of antimycobacterial drugs
T37.1X1 Poisoning by antimycobacterial drugs, accidental (unintentional)
Poisoning by antimycobacterial drugs NOS
7 T37.1X2 Poisoning by antimycobacterial drugs, intentional self-harm HCC
T37.1X3 Poisoning by antimycobacterial drugs, assault
T37.1X4 Poisoning by antimycobacterial drugs, undetermined

7th **T37.1X5** **Adverse effect of antimycobacterial drugs** UPD

7th **T37.1X6** **Underdosing of antimycobacterial drugs** UPD

5th **T37.2** **Poisoning by, adverse effect of and underdosing of antimalarials and drugs acting on other blood protozoa**

EXCLUDES 1 *hydroxyquinoline derivatives (T37.8-)*

6th **T37.2X** **Poisoning by, adverse effect of and underdosing of antimalarials and drugs acting on other blood protozoa**

7th **T37.2X1** **Poisoning by antimalarials and drugs acting on other blood protozoa, accidental (unintentional)**

Poisoning by antimalarials and drugs acting on other blood protozoa NOS

7 7th **T37.2X2** **Poisoning by antimalarials and drugs acting on other blood protozoa, intentional self-harm** HCC

7th **T37.2X3** **Poisoning by antimalarials and drugs acting on other blood protozoa, assault**

7th **T37.2X4** **Poisoning by antimalarials and drugs acting on other blood protozoa, undetermined**

7th **T37.2X5** **Adverse effect of antimalarials and drugs acting on other blood protozoa** UPD

7th **T37.2X6** **Underdosing of antimalarials and drugs acting on other blood protozoa** UPD

5th **T37.3** **Poisoning by, adverse effect of and underdosing of other antiprotozoal drugs**

6th **T37.3X** **Poisoning by, adverse effect of and underdosing of other antiprotozoal drugs**

7th **T37.3X1** **Poisoning by other antiprotozoal drugs, accidental (unintentional)**

Poisoning by other antiprotozoal drugs NOS

7 7th **T37.3X2** **Poisoning by other antiprotozoal drugs, intentional self-harm** HCC

7th **T37.3X3** **Poisoning by other antiprotozoal drugs, assault**

7th **T37.3X4** **Poisoning by other antiprotozoal drugs, undetermined**

7th **T37.3X5** **Adverse effect of other antiprotozoal drugs** UPD

7th **T37.3X6** **Underdosing of other antiprotozoal drugs** UPD

5th **T37.4** **Poisoning by, adverse effect of and underdosing of anthelminthics**

6th **T37.4X** **Poisoning by, adverse effect of and underdosing of anthelminthics**

7th **T37.4X1** **Poisoning by anthelminthics, accidental (unintentional)**

Poisoning by anthelminthics NOS

7 7th **T37.4X2** **Poisoning by anthelminthics, intentional self-harm** HCC

7th **T37.4X3** **Poisoning by anthelminthics, assault**

7th **T37.4X4** **Poisoning by anthelminthics, undetermined**

7th **T37.4X5** **Adverse effect of anthelminthics** UPD

7th **T37.4X6** **Underdosing of anthelminthics** UPD

5th **T37.5** **Poisoning by, adverse effect of and underdosing of antiviral drugs**

EXCLUDES 1 *amantadine (T42.8-)*
cytarabine (T45.1-)

6th **T37.5X** **Poisoning by, adverse effect of and underdosing of antiviral drugs**

7th **T37.5X1** **Poisoning by antiviral drugs, accidental (unintentional)**

Poisoning by antiviral drugs NOS

7 7th **T37.5X2** **Poisoning by antiviral drugs, intentional self-harm** HCC

7th **T37.5X3** **Poisoning by antiviral drugs, assault**

7th **T37.5X4** **Poisoning by antiviral drugs, undetermined**

7th **T37.5X5** **Adverse effect of antiviral drugs** UPD

7th **T37.5X6** **Underdosing of antiviral drugs** UPD

5th **T37.8** **Poisoning by, adverse effect of and underdosing of other specified systemic anti-infectives and antiparasitics**

Poisoning by, adverse effect of and underdosing of hydroxyquinoline derivatives

EXCLUDES 1 *antimalarial drugs (T37.2-)*

6th **T37.8X** **Poisoning by, adverse effect of and underdosing of other specified systemic anti-infectives and antiparasitics**

7th **T37.8X1** **Poisoning by other specified systemic anti-infectives and antiparasitics, accidental (unintentional)**

Poisoning by other specified systemic anti-infectives and antiparasitics NOS

7 7th **T37.8X2** **Poisoning by other specified systemic anti-infectives and antiparasitics, intentional self-harm** HCC

7th **T37.8X3** **Poisoning by other specified systemic anti-infectives and antiparasitics, assault**

7th **T37.8X4** **Poisoning by other specified systemic anti-infectives and antiparasitics, undetermined**

7th **T37.8X5** **Adverse effect of other specified systemic anti-infectives and antiparasitics** UPD

7th **T37.8X6** **Underdosing of other specified systemic anti-infectives and antiparasitics** UPD

5th **T37.9** **Poisoning by, adverse effect of and underdosing of unspecified systemic anti-infective and antiparasitics**

x7th **T37.91** **Poisoning by unspecified systemic anti-infective and antiparasitics, accidental (unintentional)**

Poisoning by, adverse effect of and underdosing of systemic anti-infective and antiparasitics NOS

7 x7th **T37.92** **Poisoning by unspecified systemic anti-infective and antiparasitics, intentional self-harm** HCC

x7th **T37.93** **Poisoning by unspecified systemic anti-infective and antiparasitics, assault**

x7th **T37.94** **Poisoning by unspecified systemic anti-infective and antiparasitics, undetermined**

x7th **T37.95** **Adverse effect of unspecified systemic anti-infective and antiparasitic** UPD

x7th **T37.96** **Underdosing of unspecified systemic anti-infectives and antiparasitics** UPD

4th **T38** **Poisoning by, adverse effect of and underdosing of hormones and their synthetic substitutes and antagonists, not elsewhere classified**

EXCLUDES 1 *mineralocorticoids and their antagonists (T5Ø.Ø-)*
oxytocic hormones (T48.Ø-)
parathyroid hormones and derivatives (T5Ø.9-)

The appropriate 7th character is to be added to each code from category T38.
A initial encounter
D subsequent encounter
S sequela

5th **T38.Ø** **Poisoning by, adverse effect of and underdosing of glucocorticoids and synthetic analogues**

EXCLUDES 1 *glucocorticoids, topically used (T49.-)*

6th **T38.ØX** **Poisoning by, adverse effect of and underdosing of glucocorticoids and synthetic analogues**

7th **T38.ØX1** **Poisoning by glucocorticoids and synthetic analogues, accidental (unintentional)**

Poisoning by glucocorticoids and synthetic analogues NOS

7 7th **T38.ØX2** **Poisoning by glucocorticoids and synthetic analogues, intentional self-harm** HCC

7th **T38.ØX3** **Poisoning by glucocorticoids and synthetic analogues, assault**

7th **T38.ØX4** **Poisoning by glucocorticoids and synthetic analogues, undetermined**

7th **T38.ØX5** **Adverse effect of glucocorticoids and synthetic analogues** UPD

7th **T38.ØX6** **Underdosing of glucocorticoids and synthetic analogues** UPD

T38.1 Poisoning by, adverse effect of and underdosing of thyroid hormones and substitutes

T38.1X Poisoning by, adverse effect of and underdosing of thyroid hormones and substitutes

T38.1X1 Poisoning by thyroid hormones and substitutes, accidental (unintentional)
Poisoning by thyroid hormones and substitutes NOS

7 **T38.1X2 Poisoning by thyroid hormones and substitutes, intentional self-harm** HCC

T38.1X3 Poisoning by thyroid hormones and substitutes, assault

T38.1X4 Poisoning by thyroid hormones and substitutes, undetermined

T38.1X5 Adverse effect of thyroid hormones and substitutes UPD

T38.1X6 Underdosing of thyroid hormones and substitutes UPD

T38.2 Poisoning by, adverse effect of and underdosing of antithyroid drugs

T38.2X Poisoning by, adverse effect of and underdosing of antithyroid drugs

T38.2X1 Poisoning by antithyroid drugs, accidental (unintentional)
Poisoning by antithyroid drugs NOS

7 **T38.2X2 Poisoning by antithyroid drugs, intentional self-harm** HCC

T38.2X3 Poisoning by antithyroid drugs, assault

T38.2X4 Poisoning by antithyroid drugs, undetermined

T38.2X5 Adverse effect of antithyroid drugs UPD

T38.2X6 Underdosing of antithyroid drugs UPD

T38.3 Poisoning by, adverse effect of and underdosing of insulin and oral hypoglycemic [antidiabetic] drugs

T38.3X Poisoning by, adverse effect of and underdosing of insulin and oral hypoglycemic [antidiabetic] drugs

T38.3X1 Poisoning by insulin and oral hypoglycemic [antidiabetic] drugs, accidental (unintentional)
Poisoning by insulin and oral hypoglycemic [antidiabetic] drugs NOS

7 **T38.3X2 Poisoning by insulin and oral hypoglycemic [antidiabetic] drugs, intentional self-harm** HCC

T38.3X3 Poisoning by insulin and oral hypoglycemic [antidiabetic] drugs, assault

T38.3X4 Poisoning by insulin and oral hypoglycemic [antidiabetic] drugs, undetermined

T38.3X5 Adverse effect of insulin and oral hypoglycemic [antidiabetic] drugs UPD

T38.3X6 Underdosing of insulin and oral hypoglycemic [antidiabetic] drugs UPD

T38.4 Poisoning by, adverse effect of and underdosing of oral contraceptives
Poisoning by, adverse effect of and underdosing of multiple- and single-ingredient oral contraceptive preparations

T38.4X Poisoning by, adverse effect of and underdosing of oral contraceptives

T38.4X1 Poisoning by oral contraceptives, accidental (unintentional)
Poisoning by oral contraceptives NOS

7 **T38.4X2 Poisoning by oral contraceptives, intentional self-harm** HCC

T38.4X3 Poisoning by oral contraceptives, assault

T38.4X4 Poisoning by oral contraceptives, undetermined

T38.4X5 Adverse effect of oral contraceptives UPD

T38.4X6 Underdosing of oral contraceptives UPD

T38.5 Poisoning by, adverse effect of and underdosing of other estrogens and progestogens
Poisoning by, adverse effect of and underdosing of estrogens and progestogens mixtures and substitutes

T38.5X Poisoning by, adverse effect of and underdosing of other estrogens and progestogens

T38.5X1 Poisoning by other estrogens and progestogens, accidental (unintentional)
Poisoning by other estrogens and progestogens NOS

7 **T38.5X2 Poisoning by other estrogens and progestogens, intentional self-harm** HCC

T38.5X3 Poisoning by other estrogens and progestogens, assault

T38.5X4 Poisoning by other estrogens and progestogens, undetermined

T38.5X5 Adverse effect of other estrogens and progestogens UPD

T38.5X6 Underdosing of other estrogens and progestogens UPD

T38.6 Poisoning by, adverse effect of and underdosing of antigonadotrophins, antiestrogens, antiandrogens, not elsewhere classified
Poisoning by, adverse effect of and underdosing of tamoxifen

T38.6X Poisoning by, adverse effect of and underdosing of antigonadotrophins, antiestrogens, antiandrogens, not elsewhere classified

T38.6X1 Poisoning by antigonadotrophins, antiestrogens, antiandrogens, not elsewhere classified, accidental (unintentional)
Poisoning by antigonadotrophins, antiestrogens, antiandrogens, not elsewhere classified NOS

7 **T38.6X2 Poisoning by antigonadotrophins, antiestrogens, antiandrogens, not elsewhere classified, intentional self-harm** HCC

T38.6X3 Poisoning by antigonadotrophins, antiestrogens, antiandrogens, not elsewhere classified, assault

T38.6X4 Poisoning by antigonadotrophins, antiestrogens, antiandrogens, not elsewhere classified, undetermined

T38.6X5 Adverse effect of antigonadotrophins, antiestrogens, antiandrogens, not elsewhere classified UPD

T38.6X6 Underdosing of antigonadotrophins, antiestrogens, antiandrogens, not elsewhere classified UPD

T38.7 Poisoning by, adverse effect of and underdosing of androgens and anabolic congeners

T38.7X Poisoning by, adverse effect of and underdosing of androgens and anabolic congeners

T38.7X1 Poisoning by androgens and anabolic congeners, accidental (unintentional)
Poisoning by androgens and anabolic congeners NOS

7 **T38.7X2 Poisoning by androgens and anabolic congeners, intentional self-harm** HCC

T38.7X3 Poisoning by androgens and anabolic congeners, assault

T38.7X4 Poisoning by androgens and anabolic congeners, undetermined

T38.7X5 Adverse effect of androgens and anabolic congeners UPD

T38.7X6 Underdosing of androgens and anabolic congeners UPD

T38.8 Poisoning by, adverse effect of and underdosing of other and unspecified hormones and synthetic substitutes

T38.80 Poisoning by, adverse effect of and underdosing of unspecified hormones and synthetic substitutes

T38.801 Poisoning by unspecified hormones and synthetic substitutes, accidental (unintentional)
Poisoning by unspecified hormones and synthetic substitutes NOS

7 **T38.802 Poisoning by unspecified hormones and synthetic substitutes, intentional self-harm** HCC

T38.803 Poisoning by unspecified hormones and synthetic substitutes, assault

Additional Character Required | Placeholder | Questionable PDx | Manifestation | Unspecified | UPD Unacceptable PDx | H1-H14 HAC | HCC CMS-HCC Dx | HIV HIV Dx

√7th **T38.804** **Poisoning by unspecified hormones and synthetic substitutes, undetermined**
√7th **T38.805** **Adverse effect of unspecified hormones and synthetic substitutes** UPD
√7th **T38.806** **Underdosing of unspecified hormones and synthetic substitutes** UPD
√6th **T38.81** **Poisoning by, adverse effect of and underdosing of anterior pituitary [adenohypophyseal] hormones**
√7th **T38.811** **Poisoning by anterior pituitary [adenohypophyseal] hormones, accidental (unintentional)**
Poisoning by anterior pituitary [adenohypophyseal] hormones NOS
7 √7th **T38.812** **Poisoning by anterior pituitary [adenohypophyseal] hormones, intentional self-harm** HCC
√7th **T38.813** **Poisoning by anterior pituitary [adenohypophyseal] hormones, assault**
√7th **T38.814** **Poisoning by anterior pituitary [adenohypophyseal] hormones, undetermined**
√7th **T38.815** **Adverse effect of anterior pituitary [adenohypophyseal] hormones** UPD
√7th **T38.816** **Underdosing of anterior pituitary [adenohypophyseal] hormones** UPD
√6th **T38.89** **Poisoning by, adverse effect of and underdosing of other hormones and synthetic substitutes**
√7th **T38.891** **Poisoning by other hormones and synthetic substitutes, accidental (unintentional)**
Poisoning by other hormones and synthetic substitutes NOS
7 √7th **T38.892** **Poisoning by other hormones and synthetic substitutes, intentional self-harm** HCC
√7th **T38.893** **Poisoning by other hormones and synthetic substitutes, assault**
√7th **T38.894** **Poisoning by other hormones and synthetic substitutes, undetermined**
√7th **T38.895** **Adverse effect of other hormones and synthetic substitutes** UPD
√7th **T38.896** **Underdosing of other hormones and synthetic substitutes** UPD
√5th **T38.9** **Poisoning by, adverse effect of and underdosing of other and unspecified hormone antagonists**
√6th **T38.90** **Poisoning by, adverse effect of and underdosing of unspecified hormone antagonists**
√7th **T38.901** **Poisoning by unspecified hormone antagonists, accidental (unintentional)**
Poisoning by unspecified hormone antagonists NOS
7 √7th **T38.902** **Poisoning by unspecified hormone antagonists, intentional self-harm** HCC
√7th **T38.903** **Poisoning by unspecified hormone antagonists, assault**
√7th **T38.904** **Poisoning by unspecified hormone antagonists, undetermined**
√7th **T38.905** **Adverse effect of unspecified hormone antagonists** UPD
√7th **T38.906** **Underdosing of unspecified hormone antagonists** UPD
√6th **T38.99** **Poisoning by, adverse effect of and underdosing of other hormone antagonists**
√7th **T38.991** **Poisoning by other hormone antagonists, accidental (unintentional)**
Poisoning by other hormone antagonists NOS
7 √7th **T38.992** **Poisoning by other hormone antagonists, intentional self-harm** HCC
√7th **T38.993** **Poisoning by other hormone antagonists, assault**
√7th **T38.994** **Poisoning by other hormone antagonists, undetermined**
√7th **T38.995** **Adverse effect of other hormone antagonists** UPD
√7th **T38.996** **Underdosing of other hormone antagonists** UPD

√4th **T39** **Poisoning by, adverse effect of and underdosing of nonopioid analgesics, antipyretics and antirheumatics**

The appropriate 7th character is to be added to each code from category T39.
A initial encounter
D subsequent encounter
S sequela

√5th **T39.0** **Poisoning by, adverse effect of and underdosing of salicylates**
√6th **T39.01** **Poisoning by, adverse effect of and underdosing of aspirin**
Poisoning by, adverse effect of and underdosing of acetylsalicylic acid
√7th **T39.011** **Poisoning by aspirin, accidental (unintentional)**
7 √7th **T39.012** **Poisoning by aspirin, intentional self-harm** HCC
√7th **T39.013** **Poisoning by aspirin, assault**
√7th **T39.014** **Poisoning by aspirin, undetermined**
√7th **T39.015** **Adverse effect of aspirin** UPD
AHA: 2016,1Q,15
√7th **T39.016** **Underdosing of aspirin** UPD
√6th **T39.09** **Poisoning by, adverse effect of and underdosing of other salicylates**
√7th **T39.091** **Poisoning by salicylates, accidental (unintentional)**
Poisoning by salicylates NOS
7 √7th **T39.092** **Poisoning by salicylates, intentional self-harm** HCC
√7th **T39.093** **Poisoning by salicylates, assault**
√7th **T39.094** **Poisoning by salicylates, undetermined**
√7th **T39.095** **Adverse effect of salicylates** UPD
√7th **T39.096** **Underdosing of salicylates** UPD
√5th **T39.1** **Poisoning by, adverse effect of and underdosing of 4-Aminophenol derivatives**
√6th **T39.1X** **Poisoning by, adverse effect of and underdosing of 4-Aminophenol derivatives**
√7th **T39.1X1** **Poisoning by 4-Aminophenol derivatives, accidental (unintentional)**
Poisoning by 4-Aminophenol derivatives NOS
7 √7th **T39.1X2** **Poisoning by 4-Aminophenol derivatives, intentional self-harm** HCC
√7th **T39.1X3** **Poisoning by 4-Aminophenol derivatives, assault**
√7th **T39.1X4** **Poisoning by 4-Aminophenol derivatives, undetermined**
√7th **T39.1X5** **Adverse effect of 4-Aminophenol derivatives** UPD
√7th **T39.1X6** **Underdosing of 4-Aminophenol derivatives** UPD
√5th **T39.2** **Poisoning by, adverse effect of and underdosing of pyrazolone derivatives**
√6th **T39.2X** **Poisoning by, adverse effect of and underdosing of pyrazolone derivatives**
√7th **T39.2X1** **Poisoning by pyrazolone derivatives, accidental (unintentional)**
Poisoning by pyrazolone derivatives NOS
7 √7th **T39.2X2** **Poisoning by pyrazolone derivatives, intentional self-harm** HCC
√7th **T39.2X3** **Poisoning by pyrazolone derivatives, assault**
√7th **T39.2X4** **Poisoning by pyrazolone derivatives, undetermined**
√7th **T39.2X5** **Adverse effect of pyrazolone derivatives** UPD
√7th **T39.2X6** **Underdosing of pyrazolone derivatives** UPD

T39.3 Poisoning by, adverse effect of and underdosing of other nonsteroidal anti-inflammatory drugs [NSAID]

T39.31 Poisoning by, adverse effect of and underdosing of propionic acid derivatives

Poisoning by, adverse effect of and underdosing of fenoprofen

Poisoning by, adverse effect of and underdosing of flurbiprofen

Poisoning by, adverse effect of and underdosing of ibuprofen

Poisoning by, adverse effect of and underdosing of ketoprofen

Poisoning by, adverse effect of and underdosing of naproxen

Poisoning by, adverse effect of and underdosing of oxaprozin

T39.311 Poisoning by propionic acid derivatives, accidental (unintentional)

T39.312 Poisoning by propionic acid derivatives, intentional self-harm HCC

T39.313 Poisoning by propionic acid derivatives, assault

T39.314 Poisoning by propionic acid derivatives, undetermined

T39.315 Adverse effect of propionic acid derivatives UPD

T39.316 Underdosing of propionic acid derivatives UPD

T39.39 Poisoning by, adverse effect of and underdosing of other nonsteroidal anti-inflammatory drugs [NSAID]

T39.391 Poisoning by other nonsteroidal anti-inflammatory drugs [NSAID], accidental (unintentional)

Poisoning by other nonsteroidal anti-inflammatory drugs NOS

T39.392 Poisoning by other nonsteroidal anti-inflammatory drugs [NSAID], intentional self-harm HCC

T39.393 Poisoning by other nonsteroidal anti-inflammatory drugs [NSAID], assault

T39.394 Poisoning by other nonsteroidal anti-inflammatory drugs [NSAID], undetermined

T39.395 Adverse effect of other nonsteroidal anti-inflammatory drugs [NSAID] UPD

T39.396 Underdosing of other nonsteroidal anti-inflammatory drugs [NSAID] UPD

T39.4 Poisoning by, adverse effect of and underdosing of antirheumatics, not elsewhere classified

EXCLUDES 1 *poisoning by, adverse effect of and underdosing of glucocorticoids (T38.Ø-)*

poisoning by, adverse effect of and underdosing of salicylates (T39.Ø-)

T39.4X Poisoning by, adverse effect of and underdosing of antirheumatics, not elsewhere classified

T39.4X1 Poisoning by antirheumatics, not elsewhere classified, accidental (unintentional)

Poisoning by antirheumatics, not elsewhere classified NOS

T39.4X2 Poisoning by antirheumatics, not elsewhere classified, intentional self-harm HCC

T39.4X3 Poisoning by antirheumatics, not elsewhere classified, assault

T39.4X4 Poisoning by antirheumatics, not elsewhere classified, undetermined

T39.4X5 Adverse effect of antirheumatics, not elsewhere classified UPD

T39.4X6 Underdosing of antirheumatics, not elsewhere classified UPD

T39.8 Poisoning by, adverse effect of and underdosing of other nonopioid analgesics and antipyretics, not elsewhere classified

T39.8X Poisoning by, adverse effect of and underdosing of other nonopioid analgesics and antipyretics, not elsewhere classified

T39.8X1 Poisoning by other nonopioid analgesics and antipyretics, not elsewhere classified, accidental (unintentional)

Poisoning by other nonopioid analgesics and antipyretics, not elsewhere classified NOS

T39.8X2 Poisoning by other nonopioid analgesics and antipyretics, not elsewhere classified, intentional self-harm HCC

T39.8X3 Poisoning by other nonopioid analgesics and antipyretics, not elsewhere classified, assault

T39.8X4 Poisoning by other nonopioid analgesics and antipyretics, not elsewhere classified, undetermined

T39.8X5 Adverse effect of other nonopioid analgesics and antipyretics, not elsewhere classified UPD

T39.8X6 Underdosing of other nonopioid analgesics and antipyretics, not elsewhere classified UPD

T39.9 Poisoning by, adverse effect of and underdosing of unspecified nonopioid analgesic, antipyretic and antirheumatic

T39.91 Poisoning by unspecified nonopioid analgesic, antipyretic and antirheumatic, accidental (unintentional)

Poisoning by nonopioid analgesic, antipyretic and antirheumatic NOS

T39.92 Poisoning by unspecified nonopioid analgesic, antipyretic and antirheumatic, intentional self-harm HCC

T39.93 Poisoning by unspecified nonopioid analgesic, antipyretic and antirheumatic, assault

T39.94 Poisoning by unspecified nonopioid analgesic, antipyretic and antirheumatic, undetermined

T39.95 Adverse effect of unspecified nonopioid analgesic, antipyretic and antirheumatic UPD

T39.96 Underdosing of unspecified nonopioid analgesic, antipyretic and antirheumatic UPD

T4Ø Poisoning by, adverse effect of and underdosing of narcotics and psychodysleptics [hallucinogens]

EXCLUDES 2 *drug dependence and related mental and behavioral disorders due to psychoactive substance use (F1Ø.-F19.-)*

The appropriate 7th character is to be added to each code from category T4Ø.

A initial encounter
D subsequent encounter
S sequela

T4Ø.Ø Poisoning by, adverse effect of and underdosing of opium

T4Ø.ØX Poisoning by, adverse effect of and underdosing of opium

T4Ø.ØX1 Poisoning by opium, accidental (unintentional) HCC

Poisoning by opium NOS

T4Ø.ØX2 Poisoning by opium, intentional self-harm HCC

T4Ø.ØX3 Poisoning by opium, assault

T4Ø.ØX4 Poisoning by opium, undetermined HCC

T4Ø.ØX5 Adverse effect of opium UPD

T4Ø.ØX6 Underdosing of opium UPD

T4Ø.1 Poisoning by and adverse effect of heroin

T4Ø.1X Poisoning by and adverse effect of heroin

T4Ø.1X1 Poisoning by heroin, accidental (unintentional) HCC

Poisoning by heroin NOS

T4Ø.1X2 Poisoning by heroin, intentional self-harm HCC

T4Ø.1X3 Poisoning by heroin, assault

T4Ø.1X4 Poisoning by heroin, undetermined HCC

5th **T40.2 Poisoning by, adverse effect of and underdosing of other opioids**

6th **T40.2X Poisoning by, adverse effect of and underdosing of other opioids**

6 7th **T40.2X1 Poisoning by other opioids, accidental (unintentional)** HCC
Poisoning by other opioids NOS

7 7th **T40.2X2 Poisoning by other opioids, intentional self-harm** HCC

7th **T40.2X3 Poisoning by other opioids, assault**

6 7th **T40.2X4 Poisoning by other opioids, undetermined** HCC

7th **T40.2X5 Adverse effect of other opioids** UPD
AHA: 2020,2Q,24

7th **T40.2X6 Underdosing of other opioids** UPD

5th **T40.3 Poisoning by, adverse effect of and underdosing of methadone**

6th **T40.3X Poisoning by, adverse effect of and underdosing of methadone**

6 7th **T40.3X1 Poisoning by methadone, accidental (unintentional)** HCC
Poisoning by methadone NOS

7 7th **T40.3X2 Poisoning by methadone, intentional self-harm** HCC

7th **T40.3X3 Poisoning by methadone, assault**

6 7th **T40.3X4 Poisoning by methadone, undetermined** HCC

7th **T40.3X5 Adverse effect of methadone** UPD

7th **T40.3X6 Underdosing of methadone** UPD

5th **T40.4 Poisoning by, adverse effect of and underdosing of other synthetic narcotics**
AHA: 2020,4Q,40

6th **T40.41 Poisoning by, adverse effect of and underdosing of fentanyl or fentanyl analogs**

7th **T40.411 Poisoning by fentanyl or fentanyl analogs, accidental (unintentional)** HCC

7th **T40.412 Poisoning by fentanyl or fentanyl analogs, intentional self-harm** HCC

7th **T40.413 Poisoning by fentanyl or fentanyl analogs, assault**

7th **T40.414 Poisoning by fentanyl or fentanyl analogs, undetermined** HCC

7th **T40.415 Adverse effect of fentanyl or fentanyl analogs** UPD

7th **T40.416 Underdosing of fentanyl or fentanyl analogs** UPD

6th **T40.42 Poisoning by, adverse effect of and underdosing of tramadol**

7th **T40.421 Poisoning by tramadol, accidental (unintentional)** HCC

7th **T40.422 Poisoning by tramadol, intentional self-harm** HCC

7th **T40.423 Poisoning by tramadol, assault**

7th **T40.424 Poisoning by tramadol, undetermined** HCC

7th **T40.425 Adverse effect of tramadol** UPD

7th **T40.426 Underdosing of tramadol** UPD

6th **T40.49 Poisoning by, adverse effect of and underdosing of other synthetic narcotics**

7th **T40.491 Poisoning by other synthetic narcotics, accidental (unintentional)** HCC

7th **T40.492 Poisoning by other synthetic narcotics, intentional self-harm** HCC

7th **T40.493 Poisoning by other synthetic narcotics, assault**

7th **T40.494 Poisoning by other synthetic narcotics, undetermined** HCC

7th **T40.495 Adverse effect of other synthetic narcotics** UPD

7th **T40.496 Underdosing of other synthetic narcotics** UPD

5th **T40.5 Poisoning by, adverse effect of and underdosing of cocaine**

6th **T40.5X Poisoning by, adverse effect of and underdosing of cocaine**

6 7th **T40.5X1 Poisoning by cocaine, accidental (unintentional)** HCC
Poisoning by cocaine NOS
AHA: 2016,2Q,8

7 7th **T40.5X2 Poisoning by cocaine, intentional self-harm** HCC

7th **T40.5X3 Poisoning by cocaine, assault**

6 7th **T40.5X4 Poisoning by cocaine, undetermined** HCC

7th **T40.5X5 Adverse effect of cocaine** UPD

7th **T40.5X6 Underdosing of cocaine** UPD

5th **T40.6 Poisoning by, adverse effect of and underdosing of other and unspecified narcotics**

6th **T40.60 Poisoning by, adverse effect of and underdosing of unspecified narcotics**

6 7th **T40.601 Poisoning by unspecified narcotics, accidental (unintentional)** HCC
Poisoning by narcotics NOS

7 7th **T40.602 Poisoning by unspecified narcotics, intentional self-harm** HCC

7th **T40.603 Poisoning by unspecified narcotics, assault**

6 7th **T40.604 Poisoning by unspecified narcotics, undetermined** HCC

7th **T40.605 Adverse effect of unspecified narcotics** UPD

7th **T40.606 Underdosing of unspecified narcotics** UPD

6th **T40.69 Poisoning by, adverse effect of and underdosing of other narcotics**

6 7th **T40.691 Poisoning by other narcotics, accidental (unintentional)** HCC
Poisoning by other narcotics NOS

7 7th **T40.692 Poisoning by other narcotics, intentional self-harm** HCC

7th **T40.693 Poisoning by other narcotics, assault**

6 7th **T40.694 Poisoning by other narcotics, undetermined** HCC

7th **T40.695 Adverse effect of other narcotics** UPD

7th **T40.696 Underdosing of other narcotics** UPD

5th **T40.7 Poisoning by, adverse effect of and underdosing of cannabis (derivatives)**

6th **T40.71 Poisoning by, adverse effect of and underdosing of cannabis (derivatives)**
AHA: 2021,4Q,30

7th **T40.711 Poisoning by cannabis, accidental (unintentional)**

7th **T40.712 Poisoning by cannabis, intentional self-harm** HCC

7th **T40.713 Poisoning by cannabis, assault**

7th **T40.714 Poisoning by cannabis, undetermined**

7th **T40.715 Adverse effect of cannabis** UPD

7th **T40.716 Underdosing of cannabis** UPD

6th **T40.72 Poisoning by, adverse effect of and underdosing of synthetic cannabinoids**
AHA: 2021,4Q,30

7th **T40.721 Poisoning by synthetic cannabinoids, accidental (unintentional)**

7th **T40.722 Poisoning by synthetic cannabinoids, intentional self-harm** HCC

7th **T40.723 Poisoning by synthetic cannabinoids, assault**

7th **T40.724 Poisoning by synthetic cannabinoids, undetermined**

7th **T40.725 Adverse effect of synthetic cannabinoids** UPD

7th **T40.726 Underdosing of synthetic cannabinoids** UPD

5th **T40.8 Poisoning by and adverse effect of lysergide [LSD]**

6th **T40.8X Poisoning by and adverse effect of lysergide [LSD]**

6 7th **T40.8X1 Poisoning by lysergide [LSD], accidental (unintentional)** HCC
Poisoning by lysergide [LSD] NOS

7 7th **T40.8X2 Poisoning by lysergide [LSD], intentional self-harm** HCC

N Newborn: 0 P Pediatric: 0-17 M Maternity: 9-64 A Adult: 15-124 UNS Unspecified Site MCC Major Complication/Comorbidity CC Complication/Comorbidity

T40.8X3 Poisoning by lysergide [LSD], assault
T40.8X4 Poisoning by lysergide [LSD], undetermined HCC

T40.9 Poisoning by, adverse effect of and underdosing of other and unspecified psychodysleptics [hallucinogens]

T40.90 Poisoning by, adverse effect of and underdosing of unspecified psychodysleptics [hallucinogens]

T40.901 Poisoning by unspecified psychodysleptics [hallucinogens], accidental (unintentional) HCC
T40.902 Poisoning by unspecified psychodysleptics [hallucinogens], intentional self-harm HCC
T40.903 Poisoning by unspecified psychodysleptics [hallucinogens], assault
T40.904 Poisoning by unspecified psychodysleptics [hallucinogens], undetermined HCC
T40.905 Adverse effect of unspecified psychodysleptics [hallucinogens] UPD
T40.906 Underdosing of unspecified psychodysleptics [hallucinogens] UPD

T40.99 Poisoning by, adverse effect of and underdosing of other psychodysleptics [hallucinogens]

T40.991 Poisoning by other psychodysleptics [hallucinogens], accidental (unintentional) HCC
Poisoning by other psychodysleptics [hallucinogens] NOS
T40.992 Poisoning by other psychodysleptics [hallucinogens], intentional self-harm HCC
T40.993 Poisoning by other psychodysleptics [hallucinogens], assault
T40.994 Poisoning by other psychodysleptics [hallucinogens], undetermined HCC
T40.995 Adverse effect of other psychodysleptics [hallucinogens] UPD
T40.996 Underdosing of other psychodysleptics [hallucinogens] UPD

T41 Poisoning by, adverse effect of and underdosing of anesthetics and therapeutic gases

EXCLUDES 1 *benzodiazepines (T42.4-)*
cocaine (T40.5-)
complications of anesthesia during labor and delivery (O74.-)
complications of anesthesia during pregnancy (O29.-)
complications of anesthesia during the puerperium (O89.-)
opioids (T40.0-T40.2-)

The appropriate 7th character is to be added to each code from category T41.
A initial encounter
D subsequent encounter
S sequela

T41.0 Poisoning by, adverse effect of and underdosing of inhaled anesthetics

EXCLUDES 1 *oxygen (T41.5-)*

T41.0X Poisoning by, adverse effect of and underdosing of inhaled anesthetics

T41.0X1 Poisoning by inhaled anesthetics, accidental (unintentional)
Poisoning by inhaled anesthetics NOS
T41.0X2 Poisoning by inhaled anesthetics, intentional self-harm HCC
T41.0X3 Poisoning by inhaled anesthetics, assault
T41.0X4 Poisoning by inhaled anesthetics, undetermined
T41.0X5 Adverse effect of inhaled anesthetics UPD
T41.0X6 Underdosing of inhaled anesthetics UPD

T41.1 Poisoning by, adverse effect of and underdosing of intravenous anesthetics

Poisoning by, adverse effect of and underdosing of thiobarbiturates

T41.1X Poisoning by, adverse effect of and underdosing of intravenous anesthetics

T41.1X1 Poisoning by intravenous anesthetics, accidental (unintentional)
Poisoning by intravenous anesthetics NOS
T41.1X2 Poisoning by intravenous anesthetics, intentional self-harm HCC
T41.1X3 Poisoning by intravenous anesthetics, assault
T41.1X4 Poisoning by intravenous anesthetics, undetermined
T41.1X5 Adverse effect of intravenous anesthetics UPD
T41.1X6 Underdosing of intravenous anesthetics UPD

T41.2 Poisoning by, adverse effect of and underdosing of other and unspecified general anesthetics

T41.20 Poisoning by, adverse effect of and underdosing of unspecified general anesthetics

T41.201 Poisoning by unspecified general anesthetics, accidental (unintentional)
Poisoning by general anesthetics NOS
T41.202 Poisoning by unspecified general anesthetics, intentional self-harm HCC
T41.203 Poisoning by unspecified general anesthetics, assault
T41.204 Poisoning by unspecified general anesthetics, undetermined
T41.205 Adverse effect of unspecified general anesthetics UPD
AHA: 2016,4Q,73
T41.206 Underdosing of unspecified general anesthetics UPD

T41.29 Poisoning by, adverse effect of and underdosing of other general anesthetics

T41.291 Poisoning by other general anesthetics, accidental (unintentional)
Poisoning by other general anesthetics NOS
T41.292 Poisoning by other general anesthetics, intentional self-harm HCC
T41.293 Poisoning by other general anesthetics, assault
T41.294 Poisoning by other general anesthetics, undetermined
T41.295 Adverse effect of other general anesthetics UPD
T41.296 Underdosing of other general anesthetics UPD

T41.3 Poisoning by, adverse effect of and underdosing of local anesthetics

Cocaine (topical)
EXCLUDES 2 *poisoning by cocaine used as a central nervous system stimulant (T40.5X1-T40.5X4)*

T41.3X Poisoning by, adverse effect of and underdosing of local anesthetics

T41.3X1 Poisoning by local anesthetics, accidental (unintentional)
Poisoning by local anesthetics NOS
T41.3X2 Poisoning by local anesthetics, intentional self-harm HCC
T41.3X3 Poisoning by local anesthetics, assault
T41.3X4 Poisoning by local anesthetics, undetermined
T41.3X5 Adverse effect of local anesthetics UPD
T41.3X6 Underdosing of local anesthetics UPD

T41.4 Poisoning by, adverse effect of and underdosing of unspecified anesthetic

T41.41 Poisoning by unspecified anesthetic, accidental (unintentional)
Poisoning by anesthetic NOS
T41.42 Poisoning by unspecified anesthetic, intentional self-harm HCC
T41.43 Poisoning by unspecified anesthetic, assault
T41.44 Poisoning by unspecified anesthetic, undetermined
T41.45 Adverse effect of unspecified anesthetic UPD
T41.46 Underdosing of unspecified anesthetics UPD

T41.5 Poisoning by, adverse effect of and underdosing of therapeutic gases

T41.5X Poisoning by, adverse effect of and underdosing of therapeutic gases

T41.5X1 Poisoning by therapeutic gases, accidental (unintentional)
Poisoning by therapeutic gases NOS

7 ✓7th T41.5X2 **Poisoning by therapeutic gases, intentional self-harm** HCC
✓7th T41.5X3 **Poisoning by therapeutic gases, assault**
✓7th T41.5X4 **Poisoning by therapeutic gases, undetermined**
✓7th T41.5X5 **Adverse effect of therapeutic gases** UPD
✓7th T41.5X6 **Underdosing of therapeutic gases** UPD

✓4th **T42 Poisoning by, adverse effect of and underdosing of antiepileptic, sedative- hypnotic and antiparkinsonism drugs**

EXCLUDES 2 *drug dependence and related mental and behavioral disorders due to psychoactive substance use (F10.- - F19.-)*

The appropriate 7th character is to be added to each code from category T42.
A initial encounter
D subsequent encounter
S sequela

✓5th **T42.0 Poisoning by, adverse effect of and underdosing of hydantoin derivatives**
✓6th **T42.0X Poisoning by, adverse effect of and underdosing of hydantoin derivatives**
✓7th T42.0X1 **Poisoning by hydantoin derivatives, accidental (unintentional)**
Poisoning by hydantoin derivatives NOS
7 ✓7th T42.0X2 **Poisoning by hydantoin derivatives, intentional self-harm** HCC
✓7th T42.0X3 **Poisoning by hydantoin derivatives, assault**
✓7th T42.0X4 **Poisoning by hydantoin derivatives, undetermined**
✓7th T42.0X5 **Adverse effect of hydantoin derivatives** UPD
✓7th T42.0X6 **Underdosing of hydantoin derivatives** UPD

✓5th **T42.1 Poisoning by, adverse effect of and underdosing of iminostilbenes**
Poisoning by, adverse effect of and underdosing of carbamazepine
✓6th **T42.1X Poisoning by, adverse effect of and underdosing of iminostilbenes**
✓7th T42.1X1 **Poisoning by iminostilbenes, accidental (unintentional)**
Poisoning by iminostilbenes NOS
7 ✓7th T42.1X2 **Poisoning by iminostilbenes, intentional self-harm** HCC
✓7th T42.1X3 **Poisoning by iminostilbenes, assault**
✓7th T42.1X4 **Poisoning by iminostilbenes, undetermined**
✓7th T42.1X5 **Adverse effect of iminostilbenes** UPD
✓7th T42.1X6 **Underdosing of iminostilbenes** UPD

✓5th **T42.2 Poisoning by, adverse effect of and underdosing of succinimides and oxazolidinediones**
✓6th **T42.2X Poisoning by, adverse effect of and underdosing of succinimides and oxazolidinediones**
✓7th T42.2X1 **Poisoning by succinimides and oxazolidinediones, accidental (unintentional)**
Poisoning by succinimides and oxazolidinediones NOS
7 ✓7th T42.2X2 **Poisoning by succinimides and oxazolidinediones, intentional self-harm** HCC
✓7th T42.2X3 **Poisoning by succinimides and oxazolidinediones, assault**
✓7th T42.2X4 **Poisoning by succinimides and oxazolidinediones, undetermined**
✓7th T42.2X5 **Adverse effect of succinimides and oxazolidinediones** UPD
✓7th T42.2X6 **Underdosing of succinimides and oxazolidinediones** UPD

✓5th **T42.3 Poisoning by, adverse effect of and underdosing of barbiturates**
EXCLUDES 1 *poisoning by, adverse effect of and underdosing of thiobarbiturates (T41.1-)*
✓6th **T42.3X Poisoning by, adverse effect of and underdosing of barbiturates**
✓7th T42.3X1 **Poisoning by barbiturates, accidental (unintentional)**
Poisoning by barbiturates NOS
7 ✓7th T42.3X2 **Poisoning by barbiturates, intentional self-harm** HCC
✓7th T42.3X3 **Poisoning by barbiturates, assault**
✓7th T42.3X4 **Poisoning by barbiturates, undetermined**
✓7th T42.3X5 **Adverse effect of barbiturates** UPD
✓7th T42.3X6 **Underdosing of barbiturates** UPD

✓5th **T42.4 Poisoning by, adverse effect of and underdosing of benzodiazepines**
✓6th **T42.4X Poisoning by, adverse effect of and underdosing of benzodiazepines**
✓7th T42.4X1 **Poisoning by benzodiazepines, accidental (unintentional)**
Poisoning by benzodiazepines NOS
7 ✓7th T42.4X2 **Poisoning by benzodiazepines, intentional self-harm** HCC
✓7th T42.4X3 **Poisoning by benzodiazepines, assault**
✓7th T42.4X4 **Poisoning by benzodiazepines, undetermined**
✓7th T42.4X5 **Adverse effect of benzodiazepines** UPD
✓7th T42.4X6 **Underdosing of benzodiazepines** UPD

✓5th **T42.5 Poisoning by, adverse effect of and underdosing of mixed antiepileptics**
✓6th **T42.5X Poisoning by, adverse effect of and underdosing of antiepileptics**
✓7th T42.5X1 **Poisoning by mixed antiepileptics, accidental (unintentional)**
Poisoning by mixed antiepileptics NOS
7 ✓7th T42.5X2 **Poisoning by mixed antiepileptics, intentional self-harm** HCC
✓7th T42.5X3 **Poisoning by mixed antiepileptics, assault**
✓7th T42.5X4 **Poisoning by mixed antiepileptics, undetermined**
✓7th T42.5X5 **Adverse effect of mixed antiepileptics** UPD
✓7th T42.5X6 **Underdosing of mixed antiepileptics** UPD

✓5th **T42.6 Poisoning by, adverse effect of and underdosing of other antiepileptic and sedative-hypnotic drugs**
Poisoning by, adverse effect of and underdosing of methaqualone
Poisoning by, adverse effect of and underdosing of valproic acid
EXCLUDES 1 *poisoning by, adverse effect of and underdosing of carbamazepine (T42.1-)*
✓6th **T42.6X Poisoning by, adverse effect of and underdosing of other antiepileptic and sedative-hypnotic drugs**
✓7th T42.6X1 **Poisoning by other antiepileptic and sedative-hypnotic drugs, accidental (unintentional)**
Poisoning by other antiepileptic and sedative-hypnotic drugs NOS
7 ✓7th T42.6X2 **Poisoning by other antiepileptic and sedative-hypnotic drugs, intentional self-harm** HCC
✓7th T42.6X3 **Poisoning by other antiepileptic and sedative-hypnotic drugs, assault**
✓7th T42.6X4 **Poisoning by other antiepileptic and sedative-hypnotic drugs, undetermined**
✓7th T42.6X5 **Adverse effect of other antiepileptic and sedative-hypnotic drugs** UPD
✓7th T42.6X6 **Underdosing of other antiepileptic and sedative-hypnotic drugs** UPD

✓5th **T42.7 Poisoning by, adverse effect of and underdosing of unspecified antiepileptic and sedative-hypnotic drugs**
✓x7th T42.71 **Poisoning by unspecified antiepileptic and sedative-hypnotic drugs, accidental (unintentional)**
Poisoning by antiepileptic and sedative-hypnotic drugs NOS
7 ✓x7th T42.72 **Poisoning by unspecified antiepileptic and sedative-hypnotic drugs, intentional self-harm** HCC
✓x7th T42.73 **Poisoning by unspecified antiepileptic and sedative-hypnotic drugs, assault**
✓x7th T42.74 **Poisoning by unspecified antiepileptic and sedative-hypnotic drugs, undetermined**
✓x7th T42.75 **Adverse effect of unspecified antiepileptic and sedative-hypnotic drugs** UPD
✓x7th T42.76 **Underdosing of unspecified antiepileptic and sedative-hypnotic drugs** UPD

T42.8 Poisoning by, adverse effect of and underdosing of antiparkinsonism drugs and other central muscle-tone depressants
Poisoning by, adverse effect of and underdosing of amantadine

T42.8X Poisoning by, adverse effect of and underdosing of antiparkinsonism drugs and other central muscle-tone depressants

T42.8X1 Poisoning by antiparkinsonism drugs and other central muscle-tone depressants, accidental (unintentional)
Poisoning by antiparkinsonism drugs and other central muscle-tone depressants NOS

T42.8X2 Poisoning by antiparkinsonism drugs and other central muscle-tone depressants, intentional self-harm HCC

T42.8X3 Poisoning by antiparkinsonism drugs and other central muscle-tone depressants, assault

T42.8X4 Poisoning by antiparkinsonism drugs and other central muscle-tone depressants, undetermined

T42.8X5 Adverse effect of antiparkinsonism drugs and other central muscle-tone depressants UPD

T42.8X6 Underdosing of antiparkinsonism drugs and other central muscle-tone depressants UPD

T43 Poisoning by, adverse effect of and underdosing of psychotropic drugs, not elsewhere classified

EXCLUDES 1 *appetite depressants (T50.5-)*
barbiturates (T42.3-)
benzodiazepines (T42.4-)
methaqualone (T42.6-)
psychodysleptics [hallucinogens] (T40.7-T40.9-)

EXCLUDES 2 *drug dependence and related mental and behavioral disorders due to psychoactive substance use (F10.- – F19.-)*

The appropriate 7th character is to be added to each code from category T43.
A initial encounter
D subsequent encounter
S sequela

T43.0 Poisoning by, adverse effect of and underdosing of tricyclic and tetracyclic antidepressants

T43.01 Poisoning by, adverse effect of and underdosing of tricyclic antidepressants

T43.011 Poisoning by tricyclic antidepressants, accidental (unintentional)
Poisoning by tricyclic antidepressants NOS

T43.012 Poisoning by tricyclic antidepressants, intentional self-harm HCC

T43.013 Poisoning by tricyclic antidepressants, assault

T43.014 Poisoning by tricyclic antidepressants, undetermined

T43.015 Adverse effect of tricyclic antidepressants UPD

T43.016 Underdosing of tricyclic antidepressants UPD

T43.02 Poisoning by, adverse effect of and underdosing of tetracyclic antidepressants

T43.021 Poisoning by tetracyclic antidepressants, accidental (unintentional)
Poisoning by tetracyclic antidepressants NOS

T43.022 Poisoning by tetracyclic antidepressants, intentional self-harm HCC

T43.023 Poisoning by tetracyclic antidepressants, assault

T43.024 Poisoning by tetracyclic antidepressants, undetermined

T43.025 Adverse effect of tetracyclic antidepressants UPD

T43.026 Underdosing of tetracyclic antidepressants UPD

T43.1 Poisoning by, adverse effect of and underdosing of monoamine-oxidase-inhibitor antidepressants

T43.1X Poisoning by, adverse effect of and underdosing of monoamine-oxidase-inhibitor antidepressants

T43.1X1 Poisoning by monoamine-oxidase-inhibitor antidepressants, accidental (unintentional)
Poisoning by monoamine-oxidase-inhibitor antidepressants NOS

T43.1X2 Poisoning by monoamine-oxidase-inhibitor antidepressants, intentional self-harm HCC

T43.1X3 Poisoning by monoamine-oxidase-inhibitor antidepressants, assault

T43.1X4 Poisoning by monoamine-oxidase-inhibitor antidepressants, undetermined

T43.1X5 Adverse effect of monoamine-oxidase-inhibitor antidepressants UPD

T43.1X6 Underdosing of monoamine-oxidase-inhibitor antidepressants UPD

T43.2 Poisoning by, adverse effect of and underdosing of other and unspecified antidepressants

T43.20 Poisoning by, adverse effect of and underdosing of unspecified antidepressants

T43.201 Poisoning by unspecified antidepressants, accidental (unintentional)
Poisoning by antidepressants NOS

T43.202 Poisoning by unspecified antidepressants, intentional self-harm HCC

T43.203 Poisoning by unspecified antidepressants, assault

T43.204 Poisoning by unspecified antidepressants, undetermined

T43.205 Adverse effect of unspecified antidepressants UPD
Antidepressant discontinuation syndrome

T43.206 Underdosing of unspecified antidepressants UPD

T43.21 Poisoning by, adverse effect of and underdosing of selective serotonin and norepinephrine reuptake inhibitors
Poisoning by, adverse effect of and underdosing of SSNRI antidepressants

T43.211 Poisoning by selective serotonin and norepinephrine reuptake inhibitors, accidental (unintentional)

T43.212 Poisoning by selective serotonin and norepinephrine reuptake inhibitors, intentional self-harm HCC

T43.213 Poisoning by selective serotonin and norepinephrine reuptake inhibitors, assault

T43.214 Poisoning by selective serotonin and norepinephrine reuptake inhibitors, undetermined

T43.215 Adverse effect of selective serotonin and norepinephrine reuptake inhibitors UPD

T43.216 Underdosing of selective serotonin and norepinephrine reuptake inhibitors UPD

T43.22 Poisoning by, adverse effect of and underdosing of selective serotonin reuptake inhibitors
Poisoning by, adverse effect of and underdosing of SSRI antidepressants

T43.221 Poisoning by selective serotonin reuptake inhibitors, accidental (unintentional)

T43.222 Poisoning by selective serotonin reuptake inhibitors, intentional self-harm HCC

T43.223 Poisoning by selective serotonin reuptake inhibitors, assault

T43.224 Poisoning by selective serotonin reuptake inhibitors, undetermined

7th **T43.225** Adverse effect of selective serotonin reuptake inhibitors UPD
AHA: 2022,2Q,11

7th **T43.226** Underdosing of selective serotonin reuptake inhibitors UPD

6th **T43.29** Poisoning by, adverse effect of and underdosing of other antidepressants

7th **T43.291** Poisoning by other antidepressants, accidental (unintentional)
Poisoning by other antidepressants NOS

7 7th **T43.292** Poisoning by other antidepressants, intentional self-harm HCC

7th **T43.293** Poisoning by other antidepressants, assault

7th **T43.294** Poisoning by other antidepressants, undetermined

7th **T43.295** Adverse effect of other antidepressants UPD

7th **T43.296** Underdosing of other antidepressants UPD

5th **T43.3** Poisoning by, adverse effect of and underdosing of phenothiazine antipsychotics and neuroleptics

6th **T43.3X** Poisoning by, adverse effect of and underdosing of phenothiazine antipsychotics and neuroleptics

7th **T43.3X1** Poisoning by phenothiazine antipsychotics and neuroleptics, accidental (unintentional)
Poisoning by phenothiazine antipsychotics and neuroleptics NOS

7 7th **T43.3X2** Poisoning by phenothiazine antipsychotics and neuroleptics, intentional self-harm HCC

7th **T43.3X3** Poisoning by phenothiazine antipsychotics and neuroleptics, assault

7th **T43.3X4** Poisoning by phenothiazine antipsychotics and neuroleptics, undetermined

7th **T43.3X5** Adverse effect of phenothiazine antipsychotics and neuroleptics UPD

7th **T43.3X6** Underdosing of phenothiazine antipsychotics and neuroleptics UPD

5th **T43.4** Poisoning by, adverse effect of and underdosing of butyrophenone and thiothixene neuroleptics

6th **T43.4X** Poisoning by, adverse effect of and underdosing of butyrophenone and thiothixene neuroleptics

7th **T43.4X1** Poisoning by butyrophenone and thiothixene neuroleptics, accidental (unintentional)
Poisoning by butyrophenone and thiothixene neuroleptics NOS

7 7th **T43.4X2** Poisoning by butyrophenone and thiothixene neuroleptics, intentional self-harm HCC

7th **T43.4X3** Poisoning by butyrophenone and thiothixene neuroleptics, assault

7th **T43.4X4** Poisoning by butyrophenone and thiothixene neuroleptics, undetermined

7th **T43.4X5** Adverse effect of butyrophenone and thiothixene neuroleptics UPD

7th **T43.4X6** Underdosing of butyrophenone and thiothixene neuroleptics UPD

5th **T43.5** Poisoning by, adverse effect of and underdosing of other and unspecified antipsychotics and neuroleptics
EXCLUDES 1 *poisoning by, adverse effect of and underdosing of rauwolfia (T46.5-)*

6th **T43.50** Poisoning by, adverse effect of and underdosing of unspecified antipsychotics and neuroleptics

7th **T43.501** Poisoning by unspecified antipsychotics and neuroleptics, accidental (unintentional)
Poisoning by antipsychotics and neuroleptics NOS

7 7th **T43.502** Poisoning by unspecified antipsychotics and neuroleptics, intentional self-harm HCC

7th **T43.503** Poisoning by unspecified antipsychotics and neuroleptics, assault

7th **T43.504** Poisoning by unspecified antipsychotics and neuroleptics, undetermined

7th **T43.505** Adverse effect of unspecified antipsychotics and neuroleptics UPD

7th **T43.506** Underdosing of unspecified antipsychotics and neuroleptics UPD

6th **T43.59** Poisoning by, adverse effect of and underdosing of other antipsychotics and neuroleptics
AHA: 2017,1Q,40

7th **T43.591** Poisoning by other antipsychotics and neuroleptics, accidental (unintentional)
Poisoning by other antipsychotics and neuroleptics NOS

7 7th **T43.592** Poisoning by other antipsychotics and neuroleptics, intentional self-harm HCC

7th **T43.593** Poisoning by other antipsychotics and neuroleptics, assault

7th **T43.594** Poisoning by other antipsychotics and neuroleptics, undetermined

7th **T43.595** Adverse effect of other antipsychotics and neuroleptics UPD
AHA: 2022,2Q,11

7th **T43.596** Underdosing of other antipsychotics and neuroleptics UPD

5th **T43.6** Poisoning by, adverse effect of and underdosing of psychostimulants
EXCLUDES 1 *poisoning by, adverse effect of and underdosing of cocaine (T40.5-)*

6th **T43.60** Poisoning by, adverse effect of and underdosing of unspecified psychostimulant

6 7th **T43.601** Poisoning by unspecified psychostimulants, accidental (unintentional) HCC
Poisoning by psychostimulants NOS

7 7th **T43.602** Poisoning by unspecified psychostimulants, intentional self-harm HCC

7th **T43.603** Poisoning by unspecified psychostimulants, assault

6 7th **T43.604** Poisoning by unspecified psychostimulants, undetermined HCC

7th **T43.605** Adverse effect of unspecified psychostimulants UPD

7th **T43.606** Underdosing of unspecified psychostimulants UPD

6th **T43.61** Poisoning by, adverse effect of and underdosing of caffeine

6 7th **T43.611** Poisoning by caffeine, accidental (unintentional) HCC
Poisoning by caffeine NOS

7 7th **T43.612** Poisoning by caffeine, intentional self-harm HCC

7th **T43.613** Poisoning by caffeine, assault

6 7th **T43.614** Poisoning by caffeine, undetermined HCC

7th **T43.615** Adverse effect of caffeine UPD

7th **T43.616** Underdosing of caffeine UPD

6th **T43.62** Poisoning by, adverse effect of and underdosing of amphetamines
~~Poisoning by, adverse effect of and underdosing of methamphetamines~~

6 7th **T43.621** Poisoning by amphetamines, accidental (unintentional) HCC
Poisoning by amphetamines NOS
AHA: 2021,3Q,8

7 7th **T43.622** Poisoning by amphetamines, intentional self-harm HCC

7th **T43.623** Poisoning by amphetamines, assault

6 7th **T43.624** Poisoning by amphetamines, undetermined HCC

7th **T43.625** Adverse effect of amphetamines UPD

7th **T43.626** Underdosing of amphetamines UPD

6th **T43.63** Poisoning by, adverse effect of and underdosing of methylphenidate

6 7th **T43.631** Poisoning by methylphenidate, accidental (unintentional) HCC
Poisoning by methylphenidate NOS

7 7th **T43.632** Poisoning by methylphenidate, intentional self-harm HCC

7th **T43.633** Poisoning by methylphenidate, assault

6 7th **T43.634** Poisoning by methylphenidate, undetermined HCC

T43.635 Adverse effect of methylphenidate UPD

T43.636 Underdosing of methylphenidate UPD

T43.64 Poisoning by ecstasy
Poisoning by MDMA
Poisoning by 3,4-methylenedioxymethamphetamine
AHA: 2018,4Q,30-31

T43.641 Poisoning by ecstasy, accidental (unintentional) HCC
Poisoning by ecstasy NOS

T43.642 Poisoning by ecstasy, intentional self-harm HCC

T43.643 Poisoning by ecstasy, assault

T43.644 Poisoning by ecstasy, undetermined HCC

● T43.65 Poisoning by, adverse effect of and underdosing of methamphetamines

● T43.651 Poisoning by methamphetamines accidental (unintentional)
Poisoning by methamphetamines NOS

● T43.652 Poisoning by methamphetamines intentional self-harm

● T43.653 Poisoning by methamphetamines, assault

● T43.654 Poisoning by methamphetamines, undetermined

● T43.655 Adverse effect of methamphetamines UPD

● T43.656 Underdosing of methamphetamines UPD

T43.69 Poisoning by, adverse effect of and underdosing of other psychostimulants

T43.691 Poisoning by other psychostimulants, accidental (unintentional) HCC
Poisoning by other psychostimulants NOS

T43.692 Poisoning by other psychostimulants, intentional self-harm HCC

T43.693 Poisoning by other psychostimulants, assault

T43.694 Poisoning by other psychostimulants, undetermined HCC

T43.695 Adverse effect of other psychostimulants UPD

T43.696 Underdosing of other psychostimulants UPD

T43.8 Poisoning by, adverse effect of and underdosing of other psychotropic drugs

T43.8X Poisoning by, adverse effect of and underdosing of other psychotropic drugs

T43.8X1 Poisoning by other psychotropic drugs, accidental (unintentional)
Poisoning by other psychotropic drugs NOS

T43.8X2 Poisoning by other psychotropic drugs, intentional self-harm HCC

T43.8X3 Poisoning by other psychotropic drugs, assault

T43.8X4 Poisoning by other psychotropic drugs, undetermined

T43.8X5 Adverse effect of other psychotropic drugs UPD

T43.8X6 Underdosing of other psychotropic drugs UPD

T43.9 Poisoning by, adverse effect of and underdosing of unspecified psychotropic drug

T43.91 Poisoning by unspecified psychotropic drug, accidental (unintentional)
Poisoning by psychotropic drug NOS

T43.92 Poisoning by unspecified psychotropic drug, intentional self-harm HCC

T43.93 Poisoning by unspecified psychotropic drug, assault

T43.94 Poisoning by unspecified psychotropic drug, undetermined

T43.95 Adverse effect of unspecified psychotropic drug UPD

T43.96 Underdosing of unspecified psychotropic drug UPD

T44 Poisoning by, adverse effect of and underdosing of drugs primarily affecting the autonomic nervous system

The appropriate 7th character is to be added to each code from category T44.
A initial encounter
D subsequent encounter
S sequela

T44.0 Poisoning by, adverse effect of and underdosing of anticholinesterase agents

T44.0X Poisoning by, adverse effect of and underdosing of anticholinesterase agents

T44.0X1 Poisoning by anticholinesterase agents, accidental (unintentional)
Poisoning by anticholinesterase agents NOS

T44.0X2 Poisoning by anticholinesterase agents, intentional self-harm HCC

T44.0X3 Poisoning by anticholinesterase agents, assault

T44.0X4 Poisoning by anticholinesterase agents, undetermined

T44.0X5 Adverse effect of anticholinesterase agents UPD

T44.0X6 Underdosing of anticholinesterase agents UPD

T44.1 Poisoning by, adverse effect of and underdosing of other parasympathomimetics [cholinergics]

T44.1X Poisoning by, adverse effect of and underdosing of other parasympathomimetics [cholinergics]

T44.1X1 Poisoning by other parasympathomimetics [cholinergics], accidental (unintentional)
Poisoning by other parasympathomimetics [cholinergics] NOS

T44.1X2 Poisoning by other parasympathomimetics [cholinergics], intentional self-harm HCC

T44.1X3 Poisoning by other parasympathomimetics [cholinergics], assault

T44.1X4 Poisoning by other parasympathomimetics [cholinergics], undetermined

T44.1X5 Adverse effect of other parasympathomimetics [cholinergics] UPD

T44.1X6 Underdosing of other parasympathomimetics [cholinergics] UPD

T44.2 Poisoning by, adverse effect of and underdosing of ganglionic blocking drugs

T44.2X Poisoning by, adverse effect of and underdosing of ganglionic blocking drugs

T44.2X1 Poisoning by ganglionic blocking drugs, accidental (unintentional)
Poisoning by ganglionic blocking drugs NOS

T44.2X2 Poisoning by ganglionic blocking drugs, intentional self-harm HCC

T44.2X3 Poisoning by ganglionic blocking drugs, assault

T44.2X4 Poisoning by ganglionic blocking drugs, undetermined

T44.2X5 Adverse effect of ganglionic blocking drugs UPD

T44.2X6 Underdosing of ganglionic blocking drugs UPD

T44.3 Poisoning by, adverse effect of and underdosing of other parasympatholytics [anticholinergics and antimuscarinics] and spasmolytics
Poisoning by, adverse effect of and underdosing of papaverine

T44.3X Poisoning by, adverse effect of and underdosing of other parasympatholytics [anticholinergics and antimuscarinics] and spasmolytics

T44.3X1 Poisoning by other parasympatholytics [anticholinergics and antimuscarinics] and spasmolytics, accidental (unintentional)
Poisoning by other parasympatholytics [anticholinergics and antimuscarinics] and spasmolytics NOS

7 7th **T44.3X2 Poisoning by other parasympatholytics [anticholinergics and antimuscarinics] and spasmolytics, intentional self-harm** HCC

7th **T44.3X3 Poisoning by other parasympatholytics [anticholinergics and antimuscarinics] and spasmolytics, assault**

7th **T44.3X4 Poisoning by other parasympatholytics [anticholinergics and antimuscarinics] and spasmolytics, undetermined**

7th **T44.3X5 Adverse effect of other parasympatholytics [anticholinergics and antimuscarinics] and spasmolytics** UPD

7th **T44.3X6 Underdosing of other parasympatholytics [anticholinergics and antimuscarinics] and spasmolytics** UPD

5th **T44.4 Poisoning by, adverse effect of and underdosing of predominantly alpha-adrenoreceptor agonists**

Poisoning by, adverse effect of and underdosing of metaraminol

6th **T44.4X Poisoning by, adverse effect of and underdosing of predominantly alpha-adrenoreceptor agonists**

7th **T44.4X1 Poisoning by predominantly alpha-adrenoreceptor agonists, accidental (unintentional)**

Poisoning by predominantly alpha-adrenoreceptor agonists NOS

7 7th **T44.4X2 Poisoning by predominantly alpha-adrenoreceptor agonists, intentional self-harm** HCC

7th **T44.4X3 Poisoning by predominantly alpha-adrenoreceptor agonists, assault**

7th **T44.4X4 Poisoning by predominantly alpha-adrenoreceptor agonists, undetermined**

7th **T44.4X5 Adverse effect of predominantly alpha-adrenoreceptor agonists** UPD

7th **T44.4X6 Underdosing of predominantly alpha-adrenoreceptor agonists** UPD

5th **T44.5 Poisoning by, adverse effect of and underdosing of predominantly beta-adrenoreceptor agonists**

EXCLUDES 1 *poisoning by, adverse effect of and underdosing of beta-adrenoreceptor agonists used in asthma therapy (T48.6-)*

6th **T44.5X Poisoning by, adverse effect of and underdosing of predominantly beta-adrenoreceptor agonists**

7th **T44.5X1 Poisoning by predominantly beta-adrenoreceptor agonists, accidental (unintentional)**

Poisoning by predominantly beta-adrenoreceptor agonists NOS

7 7th **T44.5X2 Poisoning by predominantly beta-adrenoreceptor agonists, intentional self-harm** HCC

7th **T44.5X3 Poisoning by predominantly beta-adrenoreceptor agonists, assault**

7th **T44.5X4 Poisoning by predominantly beta-adrenoreceptor agonists, undetermined**

7th **T44.5X5 Adverse effect of predominantly beta-adrenoreceptor agonists** UPD

7th **T44.5X6 Underdosing of predominantly beta-adrenoreceptor agonists** UPD

5th **T44.6 Poisoning by, adverse effect of and underdosing of alpha-adrenoreceptor antagonists**

EXCLUDES 1 *poisoning by, adverse effect of and underdosing of ergot alkaloids (T48.0)*

6th **T44.6X Poisoning by, adverse effect of and underdosing of alpha-adrenoreceptor antagonists**

7th **T44.6X1 Poisoning by alpha-adrenoreceptor antagonists, accidental (unintentional)**

Poisoning by alpha-adrenoreceptor antagonists NOS

7 7th **T44.6X2 Poisoning by alpha-adrenoreceptor antagonists, intentional self-harm** HCC

7th **T44.6X3 Poisoning by alpha-adrenoreceptor antagonists, assault**

7th **T44.6X4 Poisoning by alpha-adrenoreceptor antagonists, undetermined**

7th **T44.6X5 Adverse effect of alpha-adrenoreceptor antagonists** UPD

7th **T44.6X6 Underdosing of alpha-adrenoreceptor antagonists** UPD

5th **T44.7 Poisoning by, adverse effect of and underdosing of beta-adrenoreceptor antagonists**

6th **T44.7X Poisoning by, adverse effect of and underdosing of beta-adrenoreceptor antagonists**

7th **T44.7X1 Poisoning by beta-adrenoreceptor antagonists, accidental (unintentional)**

Poisoning by beta-adrenoreceptor antagonists NOS

7 7th **T44.7X2 Poisoning by beta-adrenoreceptor antagonists, intentional self-harm** HCC

7th **T44.7X3 Poisoning by beta-adrenoreceptor antagonists, assault**

7th **T44.7X4 Poisoning by beta-adrenoreceptor antagonists, undetermined**

7th **T44.7X5 Adverse effect of beta-adrenoreceptor antagonists** UPD

7th **T44.7X6 Underdosing of beta-adrenoreceptor antagonists** UPD

5th **T44.8 Poisoning by, adverse effect of and underdosing of centrally-acting and adrenergic-neuron- blocking agents**

EXCLUDES 2 *poisoning by, adverse effect of and underdosing of clonidine (T46.5)*

poisoning by, adverse effect of and underdosing of guanethidine (T46.5)

6th **T44.8X Poisoning by, adverse effect of and underdosing of centrally-acting and adrenergic- neuron-blocking agents**

7th **T44.8X1 Poisoning by centrally-acting and adrenergic-neuron-blocking agents, accidental (unintentional)**

Poisoning by centrally-acting and adrenergic-neuron-blocking agents NOS

7 7th **T44.8X2 Poisoning by centrally-acting and adrenergic-neuron-blocking agents, intentional self-harm** HCC

7th **T44.8X3 Poisoning by centrally-acting and adrenergic-neuron-blocking agents, assault**

7th **T44.8X4 Poisoning by centrally-acting and adrenergic-neuron-blocking agents, undetermined**

7th **T44.8X5 Adverse effect of centrally-acting and adrenergic-neuron-blocking agents** UPD

7th **T44.8X6 Underdosing of centrally-acting and adrenergic-neuron-blocking agents** UPD

5th **T44.9 Poisoning by, adverse effect of and underdosing of other and unspecified drugs primarily affecting the autonomic nervous system**

Poisoning by, adverse effect of and underdosing of drug stimulating both alpha and beta-adrenoreceptors

6th **T44.90 Poisoning by, adverse effect of and underdosing of unspecified drugs primarily affecting the autonomic nervous system**

7th **T44.901 Poisoning by unspecified drugs primarily affecting the autonomic nervous system, accidental (unintentional)**

Poisoning by unspecified drugs primarily affecting the autonomic nervous system NOS

7 7th **T44.902 Poisoning by unspecified drugs primarily affecting the autonomic nervous system, intentional self-harm** HCC

7th **T44.903 Poisoning by unspecified drugs primarily affecting the autonomic nervous system, assault**

7th **T44.904 Poisoning by unspecified drugs primarily affecting the autonomic nervous system, undetermined**

7th **T44.905 Adverse effect of unspecified drugs primarily affecting the autonomic nervous system** UPD

7th **T44.906 Underdosing of unspecified drugs primarily affecting the autonomic nervous system** UPD

T44.99 Poisoning by, adverse effect of and underdosing of other drugs primarily affecting the autonomic nervous system

T44.991 Poisoning by other drug primarily affecting the autonomic nervous system, accidental (unintentional)
Poisoning by other drugs primarily affecting the autonomic nervous system NOS

T44.992 Poisoning by other drug primarily affecting the autonomic nervous system, intentional self-harm HCC

T44.993 Poisoning by other drug primarily affecting the autonomic nervous system, assault

T44.994 Poisoning by other drug primarily affecting the autonomic nervous system, undetermined

T44.995 Adverse effect of other drug primarily affecting the autonomic nervous system UPD

T44.996 Underdosing of other drug primarily affecting the autonomic nervous system UPD

T45 Poisoning by, adverse effect of and underdosing of primarily systemic and hematological agents, not elsewhere classified

The appropriate 7th character is to be added to each code from category T45.
A initial encounter
D subsequent encounter
S sequela

T45.Ø Poisoning by, adverse effect of and underdosing of antiallergic and antiemetic drugs
EXCLUDES 1 *poisoning by, adverse effect of and underdosing of phenothiazine-based neuroleptics (T43.3)*

T45.ØX Poisoning by, adverse effect of and underdosing of antiallergic and antiemetic drugs

T45.ØX1 Poisoning by antiallergic and antiemetic drugs, accidental (unintentional)
Poisoning by antiallergic and antiemetic drugs NOS

T45.ØX2 Poisoning by antiallergic and antiemetic drugs, intentional self-harm HCC

T45.ØX3 Poisoning by antiallergic and antiemetic drugs, assault

T45.ØX4 Poisoning by antiallergic and antiemetic drugs, undetermined

T45.ØX5 Adverse effect of antiallergic and antiemetic drugs UPD

T45.ØX6 Underdosing of antiallergic and antiemetic drugs UPD

T45.1 Poisoning by, adverse effect of and underdosing of antineoplastic and immunosuppressive drugs
EXCLUDES 1 *poisoning by, adverse effect of and underdosing of tamoxifen (T38.6)*
AHA: 2019,1Q,17,20; 2014,4Q,22

T45.1X Poisoning by, adverse effect of and underdosing of antineoplastic and immunosuppressive drugs

T45.1X1 Poisoning by antineoplastic and immunosuppressive drugs, accidental (unintentional)
Poisoning by antineoplastic and immunosuppressive drugs NOS

T45.1X2 Poisoning by antineoplastic and immunosuppressive drugs, intentional self-harm HCC

T45.1X3 Poisoning by antineoplastic and immunosuppressive drugs, assault

T45.1X4 Poisoning by antineoplastic and immunosuppressive drugs, undetermined

T45.1X5 Adverse effect of antineoplastic and immunosuppressive drugs UPD
AHA: 2021,3Q,4; 2020,4Q,11; 2020,3Q,22; 2019,2Q,24,28

T45.1X6 Underdosing of antineoplastic and immunosuppressive drugs UPD

T45.2 Poisoning by, adverse effect of and underdosing of vitamins
EXCLUDES 2 *poisoning by, adverse effect of and underdosing of iron (T45.4)*
poisoning by, adverse effect of and underdosing of nicotinic acid (derivatives) (T46.7)
poisoning by, adverse effect of and underdosing of vitamin K (T45.7)

T45.2X Poisoning by, adverse effect of and underdosing of vitamins

T45.2X1 Poisoning by vitamins, accidental (unintentional)
Poisoning by vitamins NOS

T45.2X2 Poisoning by vitamins, intentional self-harm HCC

T45.2X3 Poisoning by vitamins, assault

T45.2X4 Poisoning by vitamins, undetermined

T45.2X5 Adverse effect of vitamins UPD

T45.2X6 Underdosing of vitamins UPD
EXCLUDES 1 *vitamin deficiencies (E5Ø-E56)*

T45.3 Poisoning by, adverse effect of and underdosing of enzymes

T45.3X Poisoning by, adverse effect of and underdosing of enzymes

T45.3X1 Poisoning by enzymes, accidental (unintentional)
Poisoning by enzymes NOS

T45.3X2 Poisoning by enzymes, intentional self-harm HCC

T45.3X3 Poisoning by enzymes, assault

T45.3X4 Poisoning by enzymes, undetermined

T45.3X5 Adverse effect of enzymes UPD

T45.3X6 Underdosing of enzymes UPD

T45.4 Poisoning by, adverse effect of and underdosing of iron and its compounds

T45.4X Poisoning by, adverse effect of and underdosing of iron and its compounds

T45.4X1 Poisoning by iron and its compounds, accidental (unintentional)
Poisoning by iron and its compounds NOS

T45.4X2 Poisoning by iron and its compounds, intentional self-harm HCC

T45.4X3 Poisoning by iron and its compounds, assault

T45.4X4 Poisoning by iron and its compounds, undetermined

T45.4X5 Adverse effect of iron and its compounds UPD

T45.4X6 Underdosing of iron and its compounds UPD
EXCLUDES 1 *iron deficiency (E61.1)*

T45.5 Poisoning by, adverse effect of and underdosing of anticoagulants and antithrombotic drugs

T45.51 Poisoning by, adverse effect of and underdosing of anticoagulants

T45.511 Poisoning by anticoagulants, accidental (unintentional)
Poisoning by anticoagulants NOS

T45.512 Poisoning by anticoagulants, intentional self-harm HCC

T45.513 Poisoning by anticoagulants, assault

T45.514 Poisoning by anticoagulants, undetermined

T45.515 Adverse effect of anticoagulants UPD
AHA: 2021,1Q,4; 2016,1Q,14; 2013,2Q,34

T45.516 Underdosing of anticoagulants UPD

T45.52 Poisoning by, adverse effect of and underdosing of antithrombotic drugs
Poisoning by, adverse effect of and underdosing of antiplatelet drugs
EXCLUDES 2 *poisoning by, adverse effect of and underdosing of aspirin (T39.Ø1-)*
poisoning by, adverse effect of and underdosing of acetylsalicylic acid (T39.Ø1-)

T45.521 Poisoning by antithrombotic drugs, accidental (unintentional)
Poisoning by antithrombotic drug NOS

T45.522 Poisoning by antithrombotic drugs, intentional self-harm HCC

✓7th T45.523 **Poisoning by antithrombotic drugs, assault**

✓7th T45.524 **Poisoning by antithrombotic drugs, undetermined**

✓7th T45.525 **Adverse effect of antithrombotic drugs** UPD
AHA: 2016,1Q,15

✓7th T45.526 **Underdosing of antithrombotic drugs** UPD

✓5th T45.6 **Poisoning by, adverse effect of and underdosing of fibrinolysis-affecting drugs**

✓6th T45.60 **Poisoning by, adverse effect of and underdosing of unspecified fibrinolysis-affecting drugs**

✓7th T45.601 **Poisoning by unspecified fibrinolysis-affecting drugs, accidental (unintentional)**
Poisoning by fibrinolysis-affecting drug NOS

7 ✓7th T45.602 **Poisoning by unspecified fibrinolysis-affecting drugs, intentional self-harm** HCC

✓7th T45.603 **Poisoning by unspecified fibrinolysis-affecting drugs, assault**

✓7th T45.604 **Poisoning by unspecified fibrinolysis-affecting drugs, undetermined**

✓7th T45.605 **Adverse effect of unspecified fibrinolysis-affecting drugs** UPD

✓7th T45.606 **Underdosing of unspecified fibrinolysis-affecting drugs** UPD

✓6th T45.61 **Poisoning by, adverse effect of and underdosing of thrombolytic drugs**

✓7th T45.611 **Poisoning by thrombolytic drug, accidental (unintentional)**
Poisoning by thrombolytic drug NOS

7 ✓7th T45.612 **Poisoning by thrombolytic drug, intentional self-harm** HCC

✓7th T45.613 **Poisoning by thrombolytic drug, assault**

✓7th T45.614 **Poisoning by thrombolytic drug, undetermined**

✓7th T45.615 **Adverse effect of thrombolytic drugs** UPD
AHA: 2017,2Q,9

✓7th T45.616 **Underdosing of thrombolytic drugs** UPD

✓6th T45.62 **Poisoning by, adverse effect of and underdosing of hemostatic drugs**

✓7th T45.621 **Poisoning by hemostatic drug, accidental (unintentional)**
Poisoning by hemostatic drug NOS

7 ✓7th T45.622 **Poisoning by hemostatic drug, intentional self-harm** HCC

✓7th T45.623 **Poisoning by hemostatic drug, assault**

✓7th T45.624 **Poisoning by hemostatic drug, undetermined**

✓7th T45.625 **Adverse effect of hemostatic drug** UPD

✓7th T45.626 **Underdosing of hemostatic drugs** UPD

✓6th T45.69 **Poisoning by, adverse effect of and underdosing of other fibrinolysis-affecting drugs**

✓7th T45.691 **Poisoning by other fibrinolysis-affecting drugs, accidental (unintentional)**
Poisoning by other fibrinolysis-affecting drug NOS

7 ✓7th T45.692 **Poisoning by other fibrinolysis-affecting drugs, intentional self-harm** HCC

✓7th T45.693 **Poisoning by other fibrinolysis-affecting drugs, assault**

✓7th T45.694 **Poisoning by other fibrinolysis-affecting drugs, undetermined**

✓7th T45.695 **Adverse effect of other fibrinolysis-affecting drugs** UPD

✓7th T45.696 **Underdosing of other fibrinolysis-affecting drugs** UPD

✓5th T45.7 **Poisoning by, adverse effect of and underdosing of anticoagulant antagonists, vitamin K and other coagulants**

✓6th T45.7X **Poisoning by, adverse effect of and underdosing of anticoagulant antagonists, vitamin K and other coagulants**

✓7th T45.7X1 **Poisoning by anticoagulant antagonists, vitamin K and other coagulants, accidental (unintentional)**
Poisoning by anticoagulant antagonists, vitamin K and other coagulants NOS

7 ✓7th T45.7X2 **Poisoning by anticoagulant antagonists, vitamin K and other coagulants, intentional self-harm** HCC

✓7th T45.7X3 **Poisoning by anticoagulant antagonists, vitamin K and other coagulants, assault**

✓7th T45.7X4 **Poisoning by anticoagulant antagonists, vitamin K and other coagulants, undetermined**

✓7th T45.7X5 **Adverse effect of anticoagulant antagonists, vitamin K and other coagulants** UPD

✓7th T45.7X6 **Underdosing of anticoagulant antagonist, vitamin K and other coagulants** UPD
EXCLUDES 1 *vitamin K deficiency (E56.1)*

✓5th T45.8 **Poisoning by, adverse effect of and underdosing of other primarily systemic and hematological agents**
Poisoning by, adverse effect of and underdosing of liver preparations and other antianemic agents
Poisoning by, adverse effect of and underdosing of natural blood and blood products
Poisoning by, adverse effect of and underdosing of plasma substitute
EXCLUDES 2 *poisoning by, adverse effect of and underdosing of immunoglobulin (T50.Z1)*
poisoning by, adverse effect of and underdosing of iron (T45.4)
transfusion reactions (T80.-)

✓6th T45.8X **Poisoning by, adverse effect of and underdosing of other primarily systemic and hematological agents**

✓7th T45.8X1 **Poisoning by other primarily systemic and hematological agents, accidental (unintentional)**
Poisoning by other primarily systemic and hematological agents NOS

7 ✓7th T45.8X2 **Poisoning by other primarily systemic and hematological agents, intentional self-harm** HCC

✓7th T45.8X3 **Poisoning by other primarily systemic and hematological agents, assault**

✓7th T45.8X4 **Poisoning by other primarily systemic and hematological agents, undetermined**

✓7th T45.8X5 **Adverse effect of other primarily systemic and hematological agents** UPD
AHA: 2016,4Q,42

✓7th T45.8X6 **Underdosing of other primarily systemic and hematological agents** UPD

✓5th T45.9 **Poisoning by, adverse effect of and underdosing of unspecified primarily systemic and hematological agent**

✓x7th T45.91 **Poisoning by unspecified primarily systemic and hematological agent, accidental (unintentional)**
Poisoning by primarily systemic and hematological agent NOS

7 ✓x7th T45.92 **Poisoning by unspecified primarily systemic and hematological agent, intentional self-harm** HCC

✓x7th T45.93 **Poisoning by unspecified primarily systemic and hematological agent, assault**

✓x7th T45.94 **Poisoning by unspecified primarily systemic and hematological agent, undetermined**

✓x7th T45.95 **Adverse effect of unspecified primarily systemic and hematological agent** UPD

✓x7th T45.96 **Underdosing of unspecified primarily systemic and hematological agent** UPD

T46 Poisoning by, adverse effect of and underdosing of agents primarily affecting the cardiovascular system

EXCLUDES 1 *poisoning by, adverse effect of and underdosing of metaraminol (T44.4)*

The appropriate 7th character is to be added to each code from category T46.
A initial encounter
D subsequent encounter
S sequela

T46.Ø Poisoning by, adverse effect of and underdosing of cardiac-stimulant glycosides and drugs of similar action

T46.ØX Poisoning by, adverse effect of and underdosing of cardiac-stimulant glycosides and drugs of similar action

T46.ØX1 Poisoning by cardiac-stimulant glycosides and drugs of similar action, accidental (unintentional)
Poisoning by cardiac-stimulant glycosides and drugs of similar action NOS

T46.ØX2 Poisoning by cardiac-stimulant glycosides and drugs of similar action, intentional self-harm HCC

T46.ØX3 Poisoning by cardiac-stimulant glycosides and drugs of similar action, assault

T46.ØX4 Poisoning by cardiac-stimulant glycosides and drugs of similar action, undetermined

T46.ØX5 Adverse effect of cardiac-stimulant glycosides and drugs of similar action UPD

T46.ØX6 Underdosing of cardiac-stimulant glycosides and drugs of similar action UPD

T46.1 Poisoning by, adverse effect of and underdosing of calcium-channel blockers

T46.1X Poisoning by, adverse effect of and underdosing of calcium-channel blockers

T46.1X1 Poisoning by calcium-channel blockers, accidental (unintentional)
Poisoning by calcium-channel blockers NOS

T46.1X2 Poisoning by calcium-channel blockers, intentional self-harm HCC

T46.1X3 Poisoning by calcium-channel blockers, assault

T46.1X4 Poisoning by calcium-channel blockers, undetermined

T46.1X5 Adverse effect of calcium-channel blockers UPD

T46.1X6 Underdosing of calcium-channel blockers UPD

T46.2 Poisoning by, adverse effect of and underdosing of other antidysrhythmic drugs, not elsewhere classified

EXCLUDES 1 *poisoning by, adverse effect of and underdosing of beta-adrenoreceptor antagonists (T44.7-)*

T46.2X Poisoning by, adverse effect of and underdosing of other antidysrhythmic drugs

T46.2X1 Poisoning by other antidysrhythmic drugs, accidental (unintentional)
Poisoning by other antidysrhythmic drugs NOS

T46.2X2 Poisoning by other antidysrhythmic drugs, intentional self-harm HCC

T46.2X3 Poisoning by other antidysrhythmic drugs, assault

T46.2X4 Poisoning by other antidysrhythmic drugs, undetermined

T46.2X5 Adverse effect of other antidysrhythmic drugs UPD

T46.2X6 Underdosing of other antidysrhythmic drugs UPD

T46.3 Poisoning by, adverse effect of and underdosing of coronary vasodilators
Poisoning by, adverse effect of and underdosing of dipyridamole

EXCLUDES 1 *poisoning by, adverse effect of and underdosing of calcium-channel blockers (T46.1)*

T46.3X Poisoning by, adverse effect of and underdosing of coronary vasodilators

T46.3X1 Poisoning by coronary vasodilators, accidental (unintentional)
Poisoning by coronary vasodilators NOS

T46.3X2 Poisoning by coronary vasodilators, intentional self-harm HCC

T46.3X3 Poisoning by coronary vasodilators, assault

T46.3X4 Poisoning by coronary vasodilators, undetermined

T46.3X5 Adverse effect of coronary vasodilators UPD

T46.3X6 Underdosing of coronary vasodilators UPD

T46.4 Poisoning by, adverse effect of and underdosing of angiotensin-converting-enzyme inhibitors

T46.4X Poisoning by, adverse effect of and underdosing of angiotensin-converting-enzyme inhibitors

T46.4X1 Poisoning by angiotensin-converting-enzyme inhibitors, accidental (unintentional)
Poisoning by angiotensin-converting-enzyme inhibitors NOS

T46.4X2 Poisoning by angiotensin-converting-enzyme inhibitors, intentional self-harm HCC

T46.4X3 Poisoning by angiotensin-converting-enzyme inhibitors, assault

T46.4X4 Poisoning by angiotensin-converting-enzyme inhibitors, undetermined

T46.4X5 Adverse effect of angiotensin-converting-enzyme inhibitors UPD

T46.4X6 Underdosing of angiotensin-converting-enzyme inhibitors UPD

T46.5 Poisoning by, adverse effect of and underdosing of other antihypertensive drugs

EXCLUDES 2 *poisoning by, adverse effect of and underdosing of beta-adrenoreceptor antagonists (T44.7)*
poisoning by, adverse effect of and underdosing of calcium-channel blockers (T46.1)
poisoning by, adverse effect of and underdosing of diuretics (T5Ø.Ø-T5Ø.2)

T46.5X Poisoning by, adverse effect of and underdosing of other antihypertensive drugs

T46.5X1 Poisoning by other antihypertensive drugs, accidental (unintentional)
Poisoning by other antihypertensive drugs NOS

T46.5X2 Poisoning by other antihypertensive drugs, intentional self-harm HCC

T46.5X3 Poisoning by other antihypertensive drugs, assault

T46.5X4 Poisoning by other antihypertensive drugs, undetermined

T46.5X5 Adverse effect of other antihypertensive drugs UPD

T46.5X6 Underdosing of other antihypertensive drugs UPD
AHA: 2022,1Q,36

T46.6 Poisoning by, adverse effect of and underdosing of antihyperlipidemic and antiarteriosclerotic drugs

T46.6X Poisoning by, adverse effect of and underdosing of antihyperlipidemic and antiarteriosclerotic drugs

T46.6X1 Poisoning by antihyperlipidemic and antiarteriosclerotic drugs, accidental (unintentional)
Poisoning by antihyperlipidemic and antiarteriosclerotic drugs NOS

T46.6X2 Poisoning by antihyperlipidemic and antiarteriosclerotic drugs, intentional self-harm HCC

7th **T46.6X3** **Poisoning by antihyperlipidemic and antiarteriosclerotic drugs, assault**

7th **T46.6X4** **Poisoning by antihyperlipidemic and antiarteriosclerotic drugs, undetermined**

7th **T46.6X5** **Adverse effect of antihyperlipidemic and antiarteriosclerotic drugs** UPD

7th **T46.6X6** **Underdosing of antihyperlipidemic and antiarteriosclerotic drugs** UPD

5th **T46.7** **Poisoning by, adverse effect of and underdosing of peripheral vasodilators**

Poisoning by, adverse effect of and underdosing of nicotinic acid (derivatives)

EXCLUDES 1 *poisoning by, adverse effect of and underdosing of papaverine (T44.3)*

6th **T46.7X** **Poisoning by, adverse effect of and underdosing of peripheral vasodilators**

7th **T46.7X1** **Poisoning by peripheral vasodilators, accidental (unintentional)**

Poisoning by peripheral vasodilators NOS

7 7th **T46.7X2** **Poisoning by peripheral vasodilators, intentional self-harm** HCC

7th **T46.7X3** **Poisoning by peripheral vasodilators, assault**

7th **T46.7X4** **Poisoning by peripheral vasodilators, undetermined**

7th **T46.7X5** **Adverse effect of peripheral vasodilators** UPD

7th **T46.7X6** **Underdosing of peripheral vasodilators** UPD

5th **T46.8** **Poisoning by, adverse effect of and underdosing of antivaricose drugs, including sclerosing agents**

6th **T46.8X** **Poisoning by, adverse effect of and underdosing of antivaricose drugs, including sclerosing agents**

7th **T46.8X1** **Poisoning by antivaricose drugs, including sclerosing agents, accidental (unintentional)**

Poisoning by antivaricose drugs, including sclerosing agents NOS

7 7th **T46.8X2** **Poisoning by antivaricose drugs, including sclerosing agents, intentional self-harm** HCC

7th **T46.8X3** **Poisoning by antivaricose drugs, including sclerosing agents, assault**

7th **T46.8X4** **Poisoning by antivaricose drugs, including sclerosing agents, undetermined**

7th **T46.8X5** **Adverse effect of antivaricose drugs, including sclerosing agents** UPD

7th **T46.8X6** **Underdosing of antivaricose drugs, including sclerosing agents** UPD

5th **T46.9** **Poisoning by, adverse effect of and underdosing of other and unspecified agents primarily affecting the cardiovascular system**

6th **T46.90** **Poisoning by, adverse effect of and underdosing of unspecified agents primarily affecting the cardiovascular system**

7th **T46.901** **Poisoning by unspecified agents primarily affecting the cardiovascular system, accidental (unintentional)**

7 7th **T46.902** **Poisoning by unspecified agents primarily affecting the cardiovascular system, intentional self-harm** HCC

7th **T46.903** **Poisoning by unspecified agents primarily affecting the cardiovascular system, assault**

7th **T46.904** **Poisoning by unspecified agents primarily affecting the cardiovascular system, undetermined**

7th **T46.905** **Adverse effect of unspecified agents primarily affecting the cardiovascular system** UPD

7th **T46.906** **Underdosing of unspecified agents primarily affecting the cardiovascular system** UPD

6th **T46.99** **Poisoning by, adverse effect of and underdosing of other agents primarily affecting the cardiovascular system**

7th **T46.991** **Poisoning by other agents primarily affecting the cardiovascular system, accidental (unintentional)**

7 7th **T46.992** **Poisoning by other agents primarily affecting the cardiovascular system, intentional self-harm** HCC

7th **T46.993** **Poisoning by other agents primarily affecting the cardiovascular system, assault**

7th **T46.994** **Poisoning by other agents primarily affecting the cardiovascular system, undetermined**

7th **T46.995** **Adverse effect of other agents primarily affecting the cardiovascular system** UPD

7th **T46.996** **Underdosing of other agents primarily affecting the cardiovascular system** UPD

4th **T47** **Poisoning by, adverse effect of and underdosing of agents primarily affecting the gastrointestinal system**

The appropriate 7th character is to be added to each code from category T47.
- A initial encounter
- D subsequent encounter
- S sequela

5th **T47.0** **Poisoning by, adverse effect of and underdosing of histamine H2-receptor blockers**

6th **T47.0X** **Poisoning by, adverse effect of and underdosing of histamine H2-receptor blockers**

7th **T47.0X1** **Poisoning by histamine H2-receptor blockers, accidental (unintentional)**

Poisoning by histamine H2-receptor blockers NOS

7 7th **T47.0X2** **Poisoning by histamine H2-receptor blockers, intentional self-harm** HCC

7th **T47.0X3** **Poisoning by histamine H2-receptor blockers, assault**

7th **T47.0X4** **Poisoning by histamine H2-receptor blockers, undetermined**

7th **T47.0X5** **Adverse effect of histamine H2-receptor blockers** UPD

7th **T47.0X6** **Underdosing of histamine H2-receptor blockers** UPD

5th **T47.1** **Poisoning by, adverse effect of and underdosing of other antacids and anti-gastric-secretion drugs**

6th **T47.1X** **Poisoning by, adverse effect of and underdosing of other antacids and anti-gastric-secretion drugs**

7th **T47.1X1** **Poisoning by other antacids and anti-gastric-secretion drugs, accidental (unintentional)**

Poisoning by other antacids and anti-gastric-secretion drugs NOS

7 7th **T47.1X2** **Poisoning by other antacids and anti-gastric-secretion drugs, intentional self-harm** HCC

7th **T47.1X3** **Poisoning by other antacids and anti-gastric-secretion drugs, assault**

7th **T47.1X4** **Poisoning by other antacids and anti-gastric-secretion drugs, undetermined**

7th **T47.1X5** **Adverse effect of other antacids and anti-gastric-secretion drugs** UPD

7th **T47.1X6** **Underdosing of other antacids and anti-gastric-secretion drugs** UPD

5th **T47.2** **Poisoning by, adverse effect of and underdosing of stimulant laxatives**

6th **T47.2X** **Poisoning by, adverse effect of and underdosing of stimulant laxatives**

7th **T47.2X1** **Poisoning by stimulant laxatives, accidental (unintentional)**

Poisoning by stimulant laxatives NOS

7 7th **T47.2X2** **Poisoning by stimulant laxatives, intentional self-harm** HCC

7th **T47.2X3** **Poisoning by stimulant laxatives, assault**

7th **T47.2X4** **Poisoning by stimulant laxatives, undetermined**

7th **T47.2X5** **Adverse effect of stimulant laxatives** UPD

7th **T47.2X6** **Underdosing of stimulant laxatives** UPD

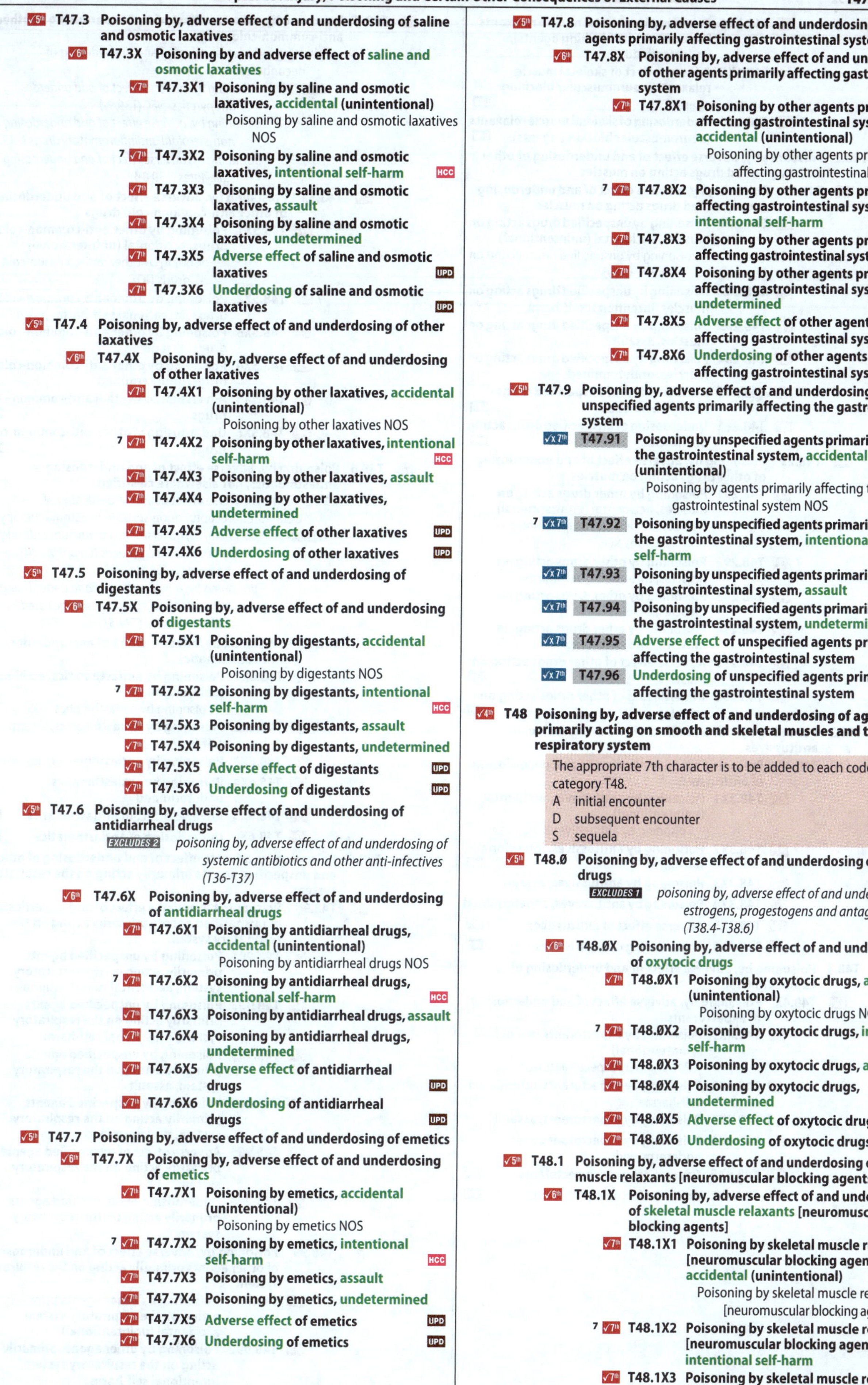

T47.3 Poisoning by, adverse effect of and underdosing of saline and osmotic laxatives
T47.3X Poisoning by and adverse effect of saline and osmotic laxatives
T47.3X1 Poisoning by saline and osmotic laxatives, accidental (unintentional)
Poisoning by saline and osmotic laxatives NOS
T47.3X2 Poisoning by saline and osmotic laxatives, intentional self-harm HCC
T47.3X3 Poisoning by saline and osmotic laxatives, assault
T47.3X4 Poisoning by saline and osmotic laxatives, undetermined
T47.3X5 Adverse effect of saline and osmotic laxatives UPD
T47.3X6 Underdosing of saline and osmotic laxatives UPD
T47.4 Poisoning by, adverse effect of and underdosing of other laxatives
T47.4X Poisoning by, adverse effect of and underdosing of other laxatives
T47.4X1 Poisoning by other laxatives, accidental (unintentional)
Poisoning by other laxatives NOS
T47.4X2 Poisoning by other laxatives, intentional self-harm HCC
T47.4X3 Poisoning by other laxatives, assault
T47.4X4 Poisoning by other laxatives, undetermined
T47.4X5 Adverse effect of other laxatives UPD
T47.4X6 Underdosing of other laxatives UPD
T47.5 Poisoning by, adverse effect of and underdosing of digestants
T47.5X Poisoning by, adverse effect of and underdosing of digestants
T47.5X1 Poisoning by digestants, accidental (unintentional)
Poisoning by digestants NOS
T47.5X2 Poisoning by digestants, intentional self-harm HCC
T47.5X3 Poisoning by digestants, assault
T47.5X4 Poisoning by digestants, undetermined
T47.5X5 Adverse effect of digestants UPD
T47.5X6 Underdosing of digestants UPD
T47.6 Poisoning by, adverse effect of and underdosing of antidiarrheal drugs
EXCLUDES 2 *poisoning by, adverse effect of and underdosing of systemic antibiotics and other anti-infectives (T36-T37)*
T47.6X Poisoning by, adverse effect of and underdosing of antidiarrheal drugs
T47.6X1 Poisoning by antidiarrheal drugs, accidental (unintentional)
Poisoning by antidiarrheal drugs NOS
T47.6X2 Poisoning by antidiarrheal drugs, intentional self-harm HCC
T47.6X3 Poisoning by antidiarrheal drugs, assault
T47.6X4 Poisoning by antidiarrheal drugs, undetermined
T47.6X5 Adverse effect of antidiarrheal drugs UPD
T47.6X6 Underdosing of antidiarrheal drugs UPD
T47.7 Poisoning by, adverse effect of and underdosing of emetics
T47.7X Poisoning by, adverse effect of and underdosing of emetics
T47.7X1 Poisoning by emetics, accidental (unintentional)
Poisoning by emetics NOS
T47.7X2 Poisoning by emetics, intentional self-harm HCC
T47.7X3 Poisoning by emetics, assault
T47.7X4 Poisoning by emetics, undetermined
T47.7X5 Adverse effect of emetics UPD
T47.7X6 Underdosing of emetics UPD
T47.8 Poisoning by, adverse effect of and underdosing of other agents primarily affecting gastrointestinal system
T47.8X Poisoning by, adverse effect of and underdosing of other agents primarily affecting gastrointestinal system
T47.8X1 Poisoning by other agents primarily affecting gastrointestinal system, accidental (unintentional)
Poisoning by other agents primarily affecting gastrointestinal system NOS
T47.8X2 Poisoning by other agents primarily affecting gastrointestinal system, intentional self-harm HCC
T47.8X3 Poisoning by other agents primarily affecting gastrointestinal system, assault
T47.8X4 Poisoning by other agents primarily affecting gastrointestinal system, undetermined
T47.8X5 Adverse effect of other agents primarily affecting gastrointestinal system UPD
T47.8X6 Underdosing of other agents primarily affecting gastrointestinal system UPD
T47.9 Poisoning by, adverse effect of and underdosing of unspecified agents primarily affecting the gastrointestinal system
T47.91 Poisoning by unspecified agents primarily affecting the gastrointestinal system, accidental (unintentional)
Poisoning by agents primarily affecting the gastrointestinal system NOS
T47.92 Poisoning by unspecified agents primarily affecting the gastrointestinal system, intentional self-harm HCC
T47.93 Poisoning by unspecified agents primarily affecting the gastrointestinal system, assault
T47.94 Poisoning by unspecified agents primarily affecting the gastrointestinal system, undetermined
T47.95 Adverse effect of unspecified agents primarily affecting the gastrointestinal system UPD
T47.96 Underdosing of unspecified agents primarily affecting the gastrointestinal system UPD
T48 Poisoning by, adverse effect of and underdosing of agents primarily acting on smooth and skeletal muscles and the respiratory system

The appropriate 7th character is to be added to each code from category T48.
A initial encounter
D subsequent encounter
S sequela

T48.Ø Poisoning by, adverse effect of and underdosing of oxytocic drugs
EXCLUDES 1 *poisoning by, adverse effect of and underdosing of estrogens, progestogens and antagonists (T38.4-T38.6)*
T48.ØX Poisoning by, adverse effect of and underdosing of oxytocic drugs
T48.ØX1 Poisoning by oxytocic drugs, accidental (unintentional)
Poisoning by oxytocic drugs NOS
T48.ØX2 Poisoning by oxytocic drugs, intentional self-harm HCC
T48.ØX3 Poisoning by oxytocic drugs, assault
T48.ØX4 Poisoning by oxytocic drugs, undetermined
T48.ØX5 Adverse effect of oxytocic drugs UPD
T48.ØX6 Underdosing of oxytocic drugs UPD
T48.1 Poisoning by, adverse effect of and underdosing of skeletal muscle relaxants [neuromuscular blocking agents]
T48.1X Poisoning by, adverse effect of and underdosing of skeletal muscle relaxants [neuromuscular blocking agents]
T48.1X1 Poisoning by skeletal muscle relaxants [neuromuscular blocking agents], accidental (unintentional)
Poisoning by skeletal muscle relaxants [neuromuscular blocking agents] NOS
T48.1X2 Poisoning by skeletal muscle relaxants [neuromuscular blocking agents], intentional self-harm HCC
T48.1X3 Poisoning by skeletal muscle relaxants [neuromuscular blocking agents], assault

Additional Character Required | Placeholder | Questionable PDx | Manifestation | Unspecified | UPD Unacceptable PDx | H1-H14 HAC | HCC CMS-HCC Dx | HIV HIV Dx

7th **T48.1X4 Poisoning by skeletal muscle relaxants [neuromuscular blocking agents], undetermined**

7th **T48.1X5 Adverse effect of skeletal muscle relaxants [neuromuscular blocking agents]** UPD

7th **T48.1X6 Underdosing of skeletal muscle relaxants [neuromuscular blocking agents]** UPD

5th **T48.2 Poisoning by, adverse effect of and underdosing of other and unspecified drugs acting on muscles**

6th **T48.20 Poisoning by, adverse effect of and underdosing of unspecified drugs acting on muscles**

7th **T48.201 Poisoning by unspecified drugs acting on muscles, accidental (unintentional)**
Poisoning by unspecified drugs acting on muscles NOS

7 7th **T48.202 Poisoning by unspecified drugs acting on muscles, intentional self-harm** HCC

7th **T48.203 Poisoning by unspecified drugs acting on muscles, assault**

7th **T48.204 Poisoning by unspecified drugs acting on muscles, undetermined**

7th **T48.205 Adverse effect of unspecified drugs acting on muscles** UPD

7th **T48.206 Underdosing of unspecified drugs acting on muscles** UPD

6th **T48.29 Poisoning by, adverse effect of and underdosing of other drugs acting on muscles**

7th **T48.291 Poisoning by other drugs acting on muscles, accidental (unintentional)**
Poisoning by other drugs acting on muscles NOS

7 7th **T48.292 Poisoning by other drugs acting on muscles, intentional self-harm** HCC

7th **T48.293 Poisoning by other drugs acting on muscles, assault**

7th **T48.294 Poisoning by other drugs acting on muscles, undetermined**

7th **T48.295 Adverse effect of other drugs acting on muscles** UPD

7th **T48.296 Underdosing of other drugs acting on muscles** UPD

5th **T48.3 Poisoning by, adverse effect of and underdosing of antitussives**

6th **T48.3X Poisoning by, adverse effect of and underdosing of antitussives**

7th **T48.3X1 Poisoning by antitussives, accidental (unintentional)**
Poisoning by antitussives NOS

7 7th **T48.3X2 Poisoning by antitussives, intentional self-harm** HCC

7th **T48.3X3 Poisoning by antitussives, assault**

7th **T48.3X4 Poisoning by antitussives, undetermined**

7th **T48.3X5 Adverse effect of antitussives** UPD

7th **T48.3X6 Underdosing of antitussives** UPD

5th **T48.4 Poisoning by, adverse effect of and underdosing of expectorants**

6th **T48.4X Poisoning by, adverse effect of and underdosing of expectorants**

7th **T48.4X1 Poisoning by expectorants, accidental (unintentional)**
Poisoning by expectorants NOS

7 7th **T48.4X2 Poisoning by expectorants, intentional self-harm** HCC

7th **T48.4X3 Poisoning by expectorants, assault**

7th **T48.4X4 Poisoning by expectorants, undetermined**

7th **T48.4X5 Adverse effect of expectorants** UPD

7th **T48.4X6 Underdosing of expectorants** UPD

5th **T48.5 Poisoning by, adverse effect of and underdosing of other anti-common-cold drugs**
Poisoning by, adverse effect of and underdosing of decongestants

EXCLUDES 2 *poisoning by, adverse effect of and underdosing of antipyretics, NEC (T39.9-)*
poisoning by, adverse effect of and underdosing of non-steroidal antiinflammatory drugs (T39.3-)
poisoning by, adverse effect of and underdosing of salicylates (T39.0-)

6th **T48.5X Poisoning by, adverse effect of and underdosing of other anti-common-cold drugs**

7th **T48.5X1 Poisoning by other anti-common-cold drugs, accidental (unintentional)**
Poisoning by other anti-common-cold drugs NOS

7 7th **T48.5X2 Poisoning by other anti-common-cold drugs, intentional self-harm** HCC

7th **T48.5X3 Poisoning by other anti-common-cold drugs, assault**

7th **T48.5X4 Poisoning by other anti-common-cold drugs, undetermined**

7th **T48.5X5 Adverse effect of other anti-common-cold drugs** UPD

7th **T48.5X6 Underdosing of other anti-common-cold drugs** UPD

5th **T48.6 Poisoning by, adverse effect of and underdosing of antiasthmatics, not elsewhere classified**
Poisoning by, adverse effect of and underdosing of beta-adrenoreceptor agonists used in asthma therapy

EXCLUDES 1 *poisoning by, adverse effect of and underdosing of anterior pituitary [adenohypophyseal] hormones (T38.8)*
poisoning by, adverse effect of and underdosing of beta-adrenoreceptor agonists not used in asthma therapy (T44.5)

6th **T48.6X Poisoning by, adverse effect of and underdosing of antiasthmatics**

7th **T48.6X1 Poisoning by antiasthmatics, accidental (unintentional)**
Poisoning by antiasthmatics NOS

7th **T48.6X2 Poisoning by antiasthmatics, intentional self-harm** HCC

7th **T48.6X3 Poisoning by antiasthmatics, assault**

7th **T48.6X4 Poisoning by antiasthmatics, undetermined**

7th **T48.6X5 Adverse effect of antiasthmatics** UPD

7th **T48.6X6 Underdosing of antiasthmatics** UPD

5th **T48.9 Poisoning by, adverse effect of and underdosing of other and unspecified agents primarily acting on the respiratory system**

6th **T48.90 Poisoning by, adverse effect of and underdosing of unspecified agents primarily acting on the respiratory system**

7th **T48.901 Poisoning by unspecified agents primarily acting on the respiratory system, accidental (unintentional)**

7 7th **T48.902 Poisoning by unspecified agents primarily acting on the respiratory system, intentional self-harm** HCC

7th **T48.903 Poisoning by unspecified agents primarily acting on the respiratory system, assault**

7th **T48.904 Poisoning by unspecified agents primarily acting on the respiratory system, undetermined**

7th **T48.905 Adverse effect of unspecified agents primarily acting on the respiratory system** UPD

7th **T48.906 Underdosing of unspecified agents primarily acting on the respiratory system** UPD

6th **T48.99 Poisoning by, adverse effect of and underdosing of other agents primarily acting on the respiratory system**

7th **T48.991 Poisoning by other agents primarily acting on the respiratory system, accidental (unintentional)**

7 7th **T48.992 Poisoning by other agents primarily acting on the respiratory system, intentional self-harm** HCC

T48.993 Poisoning by other agents primarily acting on the respiratory system, assault

T48.994 Poisoning by other agents primarily acting on the respiratory system, undetermined

T48.995 Adverse effect of other agents primarily acting on the respiratory system UPD

T48.996 Underdosing of other agents primarily acting on the respiratory system UPD

T49 Poisoning by, adverse effect of and underdosing of topical agents primarily affecting skin and mucous membrane and by ophthalmological, otorhinolaryngological and dental drugs

INCLUDES poisoning by, adverse effect of and underdosing of glucocorticoids, topically used

The appropriate 7th character is to be added to each code from category T49.
A initial encounter
D subsequent encounter
S sequela

T49.0 Poisoning by, adverse effect of and underdosing of local antifungal, anti-infective and anti-inflammatory drugs

T49.0X Poisoning by, adverse effect of and underdosing of local antifungal, anti-infective and anti-inflammatory drugs

T49.0X1 Poisoning by local antifungal, anti-infective and anti-inflammatory drugs, accidental (unintentional)
Poisoning by local antifungal, anti-infective and anti-inflammatory drugs NOS

7 **T49.0X2 Poisoning by local antifungal, anti-infective and anti-inflammatory drugs, intentional self-harm** HCC

T49.0X3 Poisoning by local antifungal, anti-infective and anti-inflammatory drugs, assault

T49.0X4 Poisoning by local antifungal, anti-infective and anti-inflammatory drugs, undetermined

T49.0X5 Adverse effect of local antifungal, anti-infective and anti-inflammatory drugs UPD

T49.0X6 Underdosing of local antifungal, anti-infective and anti-inflammatory drugs UPD

T49.1 Poisoning by, adverse effect of and underdosing of antipruritics

T49.1X Poisoning by, adverse effect of and underdosing of antipruritics

T49.1X1 Poisoning by antipruritics, accidental (unintentional)
Poisoning by antipruritics NOS

7 **T49.1X2 Poisoning by antipruritics, intentional self-harm** HCC

T49.1X3 Poisoning by antipruritics, assault

T49.1X4 Poisoning by antipruritics, undetermined

T49.1X5 Adverse effect of antipruritics UPD

T49.1X6 Underdosing of antipruritics UPD

T49.2 Poisoning by, adverse effect of and underdosing of local astringents and local detergents

T49.2X Poisoning by, adverse effect of and underdosing of local astringents and local detergents

T49.2X1 Poisoning by local astringents and local detergents, accidental (unintentional)
Poisoning by local astringents and local detergents NOS

7 **T49.2X2 Poisoning by local astringents and local detergents, intentional self-harm** HCC

T49.2X3 Poisoning by local astringents and local detergents, assault

T49.2X4 Poisoning by local astringents and local detergents, undetermined

T49.2X5 Adverse effect of local astringents and local detergents UPD

T49.2X6 Underdosing of local astringents and local detergents UPD

T49.3 Poisoning by, adverse effect of and underdosing of emollients, demulcents and protectants

T49.3X Poisoning by, adverse effect of and underdosing of emollients, demulcents and protectants

T49.3X1 Poisoning by emollients, demulcents and protectants, accidental (unintentional)
Poisoning by emollients, demulcents and protectants NOS

7 **T49.3X2 Poisoning by emollients, demulcents and protectants, intentional self-harm** HCC

T49.3X3 Poisoning by emollients, demulcents and protectants, assault

T49.3X4 Poisoning by emollients, demulcents and protectants, undetermined

T49.3X5 Adverse effect of emollients, demulcents and protectants UPD

T49.3X6 Underdosing of emollients, demulcents and protectants UPD

T49.4 Poisoning by, adverse effect of and underdosing of keratolytics, keratoplastics, and other hair treatment drugs and preparations

T49.4X Poisoning by, adverse effect of and underdosing of keratolytics, keratoplastics, and other hair treatment drugs and preparations

T49.4X1 Poisoning by keratolytics, keratoplastics, and other hair treatment drugs and preparations, accidental (unintentional)
Poisoning by keratolytics, keratoplastics, and other hair treatment drugs and preparations NOS

7 **T49.4X2 Poisoning by keratolytics, keratoplastics, and other hair treatment drugs and preparations, intentional self-harm** HCC

T49.4X3 Poisoning by keratolytics, keratoplastics, and other hair treatment drugs and preparations, assault

T49.4X4 Poisoning by keratolytics, keratoplastics, and other hair treatment drugs and preparations, undetermined

T49.4X5 Adverse effect of keratolytics, keratoplastics, and other hair treatment drugs and preparations UPD

T49.4X6 Underdosing of keratolytics, keratoplastics, and other hair treatment drugs and preparations UPD

T49.5 Poisoning by, adverse effect of and underdosing of ophthalmological drugs and preparations

T49.5X Poisoning by, adverse effect of and underdosing of ophthalmological drugs and preparations

T49.5X1 Poisoning by ophthalmological drugs and preparations, accidental (unintentional)
Poisoning by ophthalmological drugs and preparations NOS

7 **T49.5X2 Poisoning by ophthalmological drugs and preparations, intentional self-harm** HCC

T49.5X3 Poisoning by ophthalmological drugs and preparations, assault

T49.5X4 Poisoning by ophthalmological drugs and preparations, undetermined

T49.5X5 Adverse effect of ophthalmological drugs and preparations UPD

T49.5X6 Underdosing of ophthalmological drugs and preparations UPD

T49.6 Poisoning by, adverse effect of and underdosing of otorhinolaryngological drugs and preparations

T49.6X Poisoning by, adverse effect of and underdosing of otorhinolaryngological drugs and preparations

T49.6X1 Poisoning by otorhinolaryngological drugs and preparations, accidental (unintentional)
Poisoning by otorhinolaryngological drugs and preparations NOS

7 **T49.6X2 Poisoning by otorhinolaryngological drugs and preparations, intentional self-harm** HCC

T49.6X3 Poisoning by otorhinolaryngological drugs and preparations, assault

T49.6X4 Poisoning by otorhinolaryngological drugs and preparations, undetermined

T49.6X5 Adverse effect of otorhinolaryngological drugs and preparations UPD

√7th **T49.6X6 Underdosing of otorhinolaryngological drugs and preparations** UPD

√5th **T49.7 Poisoning by, adverse effect of and underdosing of dental drugs, topically applied**

√6th **T49.7X Poisoning by, adverse effect of and underdosing of dental drugs, topically applied**

√7th **T49.7X1 Poisoning by dental drugs, topically applied, accidental (unintentional)**
Poisoning by dental drugs, topically applied NOS

7 √7th **T49.7X2 Poisoning by dental drugs, topically applied, intentional self-harm** HCC

√7th **T49.7X3 Poisoning by dental drugs, topically applied, assault**

√7th **T49.7X4 Poisoning by dental drugs, topically applied, undetermined**

√7th **T49.7X5 Adverse effect of dental drugs, topically applied** UPD

√7th **T49.7X6 Underdosing of dental drugs, topically applied** UPD

√5th **T49.8 Poisoning by, adverse effect of and underdosing of other topical agents**
Poisoning by, adverse effect of and underdosing of spermicides

√6th **T49.8X Poisoning by, adverse effect of and underdosing of other topical agents**

√7th **T49.8X1 Poisoning by other topical agents, accidental (unintentional)**
Poisoning by other topical agents NOS

7 √7th **T49.8X2 Poisoning by other topical agents, intentional self-harm** HCC

√7th **T49.8X3 Poisoning by other topical agents, assault**

√7th **T49.8X4 Poisoning by other topical agents, undetermined**

√7th **T49.8X5 Adverse effect of other topical agents** UPD

√7th **T49.8X6 Underdosing of other topical agents** UPD

√5th **T49.9 Poisoning by, adverse effect of and underdosing of unspecified topical agent**

√x7th **T49.91 Poisoning by unspecified topical agent, accidental (unintentional)**

7 √x7th **T49.92 Poisoning by unspecified topical agent, intentional self-harm** HCC

√x7th **T49.93 Poisoning by unspecified topical agent, assault**

√x7th **T49.94 Poisoning by unspecified topical agent, undetermined**

√x7th **T49.95 Adverse effect of unspecified topical agent** UPD

√x7th **T49.96 Underdosing of unspecified topical agent** UPD

√4th **T5Ø Poisoning by, adverse effect of and underdosing of diuretics and other and unspecified drugs, medicaments and biological substances**

The appropriate 7th character is to be added to each code from category T5Ø.
- A initial encounter
- D subsequent encounter
- S sequela

√5th **T5Ø.Ø Poisoning by, adverse effect of and underdosing of mineralocorticoids and their antagonists**

√6th **T5Ø.ØX Poisoning by, adverse effect of and underdosing of mineralocorticoids and their antagonists**

√7th **T5Ø.ØX1 Poisoning by mineralocorticoids and their antagonists, accidental (unintentional)**
Poisoning by mineralocorticoids and their antagonists NOS

7 √7th **T5Ø.ØX2 Poisoning by mineralocorticoids and their antagonists, intentional self-harm** HCC

√7th **T5Ø.ØX3 Poisoning by mineralocorticoids and their antagonists, assault**

√7th **T5Ø.ØX4 Poisoning by mineralocorticoids and their antagonists, undetermined**

√7th **T5Ø.ØX5 Adverse effect of mineralocorticoids and their antagonists** UPD

√7th **T5Ø.ØX6 Underdosing of mineralocorticoids and their antagonists** UPD

√5th **T5Ø.1 Poisoning by, adverse effect of and underdosing of loop [high-ceiling] diuretics**

√6th **T5Ø.1X Poisoning by, adverse effect of and underdosing of loop [high-ceiling] diuretics**

√7th **T5Ø.1X1 Poisoning by loop [high-ceiling] diuretics, accidental (unintentional)**
Poisoning by loop [high-ceiling] diuretics NOS

7 √7th **T5Ø.1X2 Poisoning by loop [high-ceiling] diuretics, intentional self-harm** HCC

√7th **T5Ø.1X3 Poisoning by loop [high-ceiling] diuretics, assault**

√7th **T5Ø.1X4 Poisoning by loop [high-ceiling] diuretics, undetermined**

√7th **T5Ø.1X5 Adverse effect of loop [high-ceiling] diuretics** UPD

√7th **T5Ø.1X6 Underdosing of loop [high-ceiling] diuretics** UPD

√5th **T5Ø.2 Poisoning by, adverse effect of and underdosing of carbonic-anhydrase inhibitors, benzothiadiazides and other diuretics**
Poisoning by, adverse effect of and underdosing of acetazolamide

√6th **T5Ø.2X Poisoning by, adverse effect of and underdosing of carbonic-anhydrase inhibitors, benzothiadiazides and other diuretics**

√7th **T5Ø.2X1 Poisoning by carbonic-anhydrase inhibitors, benzothiadiazides and other diuretics, accidental (unintentional)**
Poisoning by carbonic-anhydrase inhibitors, benzothiadiazides and other diuretics NOS

7 √7th **T5Ø.2X2 Poisoning by carbonic-anhydrase inhibitors, benzothiadiazides and other diuretics, intentional self-harm** HCC

√7th **T5Ø.2X3 Poisoning by carbonic-anhydrase inhibitors, benzothiadiazides and other diuretics, assault**

√7th **T5Ø.2X4 Poisoning by carbonic-anhydrase inhibitors, benzothiadiazides and other diuretics, undetermined**

√7th **T5Ø.2X5 Adverse effect of carbonic-anhydrase inhibitors, benzothiadiazides and other diuretics** UPD

√7th **T5Ø.2X6 Underdosing of carbonic-anhydrase inhibitors, benzothiadiazides and other diuretics** UPD

√5th **T5Ø.3 Poisoning by, adverse effect of and underdosing of electrolytic, caloric and water-balance agents**
Poisoning by, adverse effect of and underdosing of oral rehydration salts

√6th **T5Ø.3X Poisoning by, adverse effect of and underdosing of electrolytic, caloric and water-balance agents**

√7th **T5Ø.3X1 Poisoning by electrolytic, caloric and water-balance agents, accidental (unintentional)**
Poisoning by electrolytic, caloric and water-balance agents NOS

7 √7th **T5Ø.3X2 Poisoning by electrolytic, caloric and water-balance agents, intentional self-harm** HCC

√7th **T5Ø.3X3 Poisoning by electrolytic, caloric and water-balance agents, assault**

√7th **T5Ø.3X4 Poisoning by electrolytic, caloric and water-balance agents, undetermined**

√7th **T5Ø.3X5 Adverse effect of electrolytic, caloric and water-balance agents** UPD
AHA: 2022,2Q,10

√7th **T5Ø.3X6 Underdosing of electrolytic, caloric and water-balance agents** UPD

√5th **T5Ø.4 Poisoning by, adverse effect of and underdosing of drugs affecting uric acid metabolism**

√6th **T5Ø.4X Poisoning by, adverse effect of and underdosing of drugs affecting uric acid metabolism**

√7th **T5Ø.4X1 Poisoning by drugs affecting uric acid metabolism, accidental (unintentional)**
Poisoning by drugs affecting uric acid metabolism NOS

7 √7th **T5Ø.4X2 Poisoning by drugs affecting uric acid metabolism, intentional self-harm** HCC

√7th **T5Ø.4X3 Poisoning by drugs affecting uric acid metabolism, assault**

T50.4X4 Poisoning by drugs affecting uric acid metabolism, undetermined

T50.4X5 Adverse effect of drugs affecting uric acid metabolism UPD

T50.4X6 Underdosing of drugs affecting uric acid metabolism UPD

T50.5 Poisoning by, adverse effect of and underdosing of appetite depressants

T50.5X Poisoning by, adverse effect of and underdosing of appetite depressants

T50.5X1 Poisoning by appetite depressants, accidental (unintentional)
Poisoning by appetite depressants NOS

7 T50.5X2 Poisoning by appetite depressants, intentional self-harm HCC

T50.5X3 Poisoning by appetite depressants, assault

T50.5X4 Poisoning by appetite depressants, undetermined

T50.5X5 Adverse effect of appetite depressants UPD

T50.5X6 Underdosing of appetite depressants UPD

T50.6 Poisoning by, adverse effect of and underdosing of antidotes and chelating agents
Poisoning by, adverse effect of and underdosing of alcohol deterrents

T50.6X Poisoning by, adverse effect of and underdosing of antidotes and chelating agents

T50.6X1 Poisoning by antidotes and chelating agents, accidental (unintentional)
Poisoning by antidotes and chelating agents NOS

7 T50.6X2 Poisoning by antidotes and chelating agents, intentional self-harm HCC

T50.6X3 Poisoning by antidotes and chelating agents, assault

T50.6X4 Poisoning by antidotes and chelating agents, undetermined

T50.6X5 Adverse effect of antidotes and chelating agents UPD

T50.6X6 Underdosing of antidotes and chelating agents UPD

T50.7 Poisoning by, adverse effect of and underdosing of analeptics and opioid receptor antagonists

T50.7X Poisoning by, adverse effect of and underdosing of analeptics and opioid receptor antagonists

T50.7X1 Poisoning by analeptics and opioid receptor antagonists, accidental (unintentional)
Poisoning by analeptics and opioid receptor antagonists NOS

7 T50.7X2 Poisoning by analeptics and opioid receptor antagonists, intentional self-harm HCC

T50.7X3 Poisoning by analeptics and opioid receptor antagonists, assault

T50.7X4 Poisoning by analeptics and opioid receptor antagonists, undetermined

T50.7X5 Adverse effect of analeptics and opioid receptor antagonists UPD

T50.7X6 Underdosing of analeptics and opioid receptor antagonists UPD

T50.8 Poisoning by, adverse effect of and underdosing of diagnostic agents

T50.8X Poisoning by, adverse effect of and underdosing of diagnostic agents

T50.8X1 Poisoning by diagnostic agents, accidental (unintentional)
Poisoning by diagnostic agents NOS

7 T50.8X2 Poisoning by diagnostic agents, intentional self-harm HCC

T50.8X3 Poisoning by diagnostic agents, assault

T50.8X4 Poisoning by diagnostic agents, undetermined

T50.8X5 Adverse effect of diagnostic agents UPD
AHA: 2021,3Q,9-10

T50.8X6 Underdosing of diagnostic agents UPD

T50.A Poisoning by, adverse effect of and underdosing of bacterial vaccines

T50.A1 Poisoning by, adverse effect of and underdosing of pertussis vaccine, including combinations with a pertussis component

T50.A11 Poisoning by pertussis vaccine, including combinations with a pertussis component, accidental (unintentional)

7 T50.A12 Poisoning by pertussis vaccine, including combinations with a pertussis component, intentional self-harm HCC

T50.A13 Poisoning by pertussis vaccine, including combinations with a pertussis component, assault

T50.A14 Poisoning by pertussis vaccine, including combinations with a pertussis component, undetermined

T50.A15 Adverse effect of pertussis vaccine, including combinations with a pertussis component UPD

T50.A16 Underdosing of pertussis vaccine, including combinations with a pertussis component UPD

T50.A2 Poisoning by, adverse effect of and underdosing of mixed bacterial vaccines without a pertussis component

T50.A21 Poisoning by mixed bacterial vaccines without a pertussis component, accidental (unintentional)

7 T50.A22 Poisoning by mixed bacterial vaccines without a pertussis component, intentional self-harm HCC

T50.A23 Poisoning by mixed bacterial vaccines without a pertussis component, assault

T50.A24 Poisoning by mixed bacterial vaccines without a pertussis component, undetermined

T50.A25 Adverse effect of mixed bacterial vaccines without a pertussis component UPD

T50.A26 Underdosing of mixed bacterial vaccines without a pertussis component UPD

T50.A9 Poisoning by, adverse effect of and underdosing of other bacterial vaccines

T50.A91 Poisoning by other bacterial vaccines, accidental (unintentional)

7 T50.A92 Poisoning by other bacterial vaccines, intentional self-harm HCC

T50.A93 Poisoning by other bacterial vaccines, assault

T50.A94 Poisoning by other bacterial vaccines, undetermined

T50.A95 Adverse effect of other bacterial vaccines UPD

T50.A96 Underdosing of other bacterial vaccines UPD

T50.B Poisoning by, adverse effect of and underdosing of viral vaccines

T50.B1 Poisoning by, adverse effect of and underdosing of smallpox vaccines

T50.B11 Poisoning by smallpox vaccines, accidental (unintentional)

7 T50.B12 Poisoning by smallpox vaccines, intentional self-harm HCC

T50.B13 Poisoning by smallpox vaccines, assault

T50.B14 Poisoning by smallpox vaccines, undetermined

T50.B15 Adverse effect of smallpox vaccines UPD

T50.B16 Underdosing of smallpox vaccines UPD

T50.B9 Poisoning by, adverse effect of and underdosing of other viral vaccines

T50.B91 Poisoning by other viral vaccines, accidental (unintentional)

7 T50.B92 Poisoning by other viral vaccines, intentional self-harm HCC

T50.B93 Poisoning by other viral vaccines, assault

T50.B94 Poisoning by other viral vaccines, undetermined

T50.B95 Adverse effect of other viral vaccines UPD
AHA: 2021,1Q,43

7th T50.B96 Underdosing of other viral vaccines UPD

5th T50.Z Poisoning by, adverse effect of and underdosing of other vaccines and biological substances

6th T50.Z1 Poisoning by, adverse effect of and underdosing of immunoglobulin

7th T50.Z11 Poisoning by immunoglobulin, accidental (unintentional)

7 7th T50.Z12 Poisoning by immunoglobulin, intentional self-harm HCC

7th T50.Z13 Poisoning by immunoglobulin, assault

7th T50.Z14 Poisoning by immunoglobulin, undetermined

7th T50.Z15 Adverse effect of immunoglobulin UPD

7th T50.Z16 Underdosing of immunoglobulin UPD

6th T50.Z9 Poisoning by, adverse effect of and underdosing of other vaccines and biological substances

7th T50.Z91 Poisoning by other vaccines and biological substances, accidental (unintentional)

7 7th T50.Z92 Poisoning by other vaccines and biological substances, intentional self-harm HCC

7th T50.Z93 Poisoning by other vaccines and biological substances, assault

7th T50.Z94 Poisoning by other vaccines and biological substances, undetermined

7th T50.Z95 Adverse effect of other vaccines and biological substances UPD
AHA: 2020,1Q,18

7th T50.Z96 Underdosing of other vaccines and biological substances UPD

5th T50.9 Poisoning by, adverse effect of and underdosing of other and unspecified drugs, medicaments and biological substances

6th T50.90 Poisoning by, adverse effect of and underdosing of unspecified drugs, medicaments and biological substances

7th T50.901 Poisoning by unspecified drugs, medicaments and biological substances, accidental (unintentional)

7 7th T50.902 Poisoning by unspecified drugs, medicaments and biological substances, intentional self-harm HCC

7th T50.903 Poisoning by unspecified drugs, medicaments and biological substances, assault

7th T50.904 Poisoning by unspecified drugs, medicaments and biological substances, undetermined

7th T50.905 Adverse effect of unspecified drugs, medicaments and biological substances

7th T50.906 Underdosing of unspecified drugs, medicaments and biological substances

6th T50.91 Poisoning by, adverse effect of and underdosing of multiple unspecified drugs, medicaments and biological substances
Multiple drug ingestion NOS
Code also any specific drugs, medicaments and biological substances

7th T50.911 Poisoning by multiple unspecified drugs, medicaments and biological substances, accidental (unintentional)

7 7th T50.912 Poisoning by multiple unspecified drugs, medicaments and biological substances, intentional self-harm HCC

7th T50.913 Poisoning by multiple unspecified drugs, medicaments and biological substances, assault

7th T50.914 Poisoning by multiple unspecified drugs, medicaments and biological substances, undetermined

7th T50.915 Adverse effect of multiple unspecified drugs, medicaments and biological substances UPD

7th T50.916 Underdosing of multiple unspecified drugs, medicaments and biological substances UPD

6th T50.99 Poisoning by, adverse effect of and underdosing of other drugs, medicaments and biological substances

7th T50.991 Poisoning by other drugs, medicaments and biological substances, accidental (unintentional)

7 7th T50.992 Poisoning by other drugs, medicaments and biological substances, intentional self-harm HCC

7th T50.993 Poisoning by other drugs, medicaments and biological substances, assault

7th T50.994 Poisoning by other drugs, medicaments and biological substances, undetermined

7th T50.995 Adverse effect of other drugs, medicaments and biological substances

7th T50.996 Underdosing of other drugs, medicaments and biological substances

Toxic effects of substances chiefly nonmedicinal as to source (T51-T65)

NOTE When no intent is indicated code to accidental. Undetermined intent is only for use when there is specific documentation in the record that the intent of the toxic effect cannot be determined.

Use additional code(s) for all associated manifestations of toxic effect, such as:
personal history of foreign body fully removed (Z87.821)
respiratory conditions due to external agents (J60-J70)
to identify any retained foreign body, if applicable (Z18.-)

EXCLUDES 1 *contact with and (suspected) exposure to toxic substances (Z77.-)*

AHA: 2017,1Q,39-40

4th T51 Toxic effect of alcohol

The appropriate 7th character is to be added to each code from category T51.
A initial encounter
D subsequent encounter
S sequela

5th T51.0 Toxic effect of ethanol
Toxic effect of ethyl alcohol
EXCLUDES 2 *acute alcohol intoxication or "hangover" effects (F10.129, F10.229, F10.929)*
drunkenness (F10.129, F10.229, F10.929)
pathological alcohol intoxication (F10.129, F10.229, F10.929)

6th T51.0X Toxic effect of ethanol

6 7th T51.0X1 Toxic effect of ethanol, accidental (unintentional) HCC
Toxic effect of ethanol NOS

7 7th T51.0X2 Toxic effect of ethanol, intentional self-harm HCC

7th T51.0X3 Toxic effect of ethanol, assault

6 7th T51.0X4 Toxic effect of ethanol, undetermined HCC

5th T51.1 Toxic effect of methanol
Toxic effect of methyl alcohol

6th T51.1X Toxic effect of methanol

7th T51.1X1 Toxic effect of methanol, accidental (unintentional)
Toxic effect of methanol NOS

7 7th T51.1X2 Toxic effect of methanol, intentional self-harm HCC

7th T51.1X3 Toxic effect of methanol, assault

7th T51.1X4 Toxic effect of methanol, undetermined

5th T51.2 Toxic effect of 2-Propanol
Toxic effect of isopropyl alcohol

6th T51.2X Toxic effect of 2-Propanol

7th T51.2X1 Toxic effect of 2-Propanol, accidental (unintentional)
Toxic effect of 2-Propanol NOS

7 7th T51.2X2 Toxic effect of 2-Propanol, intentional self-harm HCC

7th T51.2X3 Toxic effect of 2-Propanol, assault

7th T51.2X4 Toxic effect of 2-Propanol, undetermined

T51.3 Toxic effect of fusel oil
Toxic effect of amyl alcohol
Toxic effect of butyl [1-butanol] alcohol
Toxic effect of propyl [1-propanol] alcohol
T51.3X Toxic effect of fusel oil
T51.3X1 Toxic effect of fusel oil, accidental (unintentional)
Toxic effect of fusel oil NOS
T51.3X2 Toxic effect of fusel oil, intentional self-harm HCC
T51.3X3 Toxic effect of fusel oil, assault
T51.3X4 Toxic effect of fusel oil, undetermined
T51.8 Toxic effect of other alcohols
T51.8X Toxic effect of other alcohols
T51.8X1 Toxic effect of other alcohols, accidental (unintentional)
Toxic effect of other alcohols NOS
T51.8X2 Toxic effect of other alcohols, intentional self-harm HCC
T51.8X3 Toxic effect of other alcohols, assault
T51.8X4 Toxic effect of other alcohols, undetermined
T51.9 Toxic effect of unspecified alcohol
T51.91 Toxic effect of unspecified alcohol, accidental (unintentional)
T51.92 Toxic effect of unspecified alcohol, intentional self-harm HCC
T51.93 Toxic effect of unspecified alcohol, assault
T51.94 Toxic effect of unspecified alcohol, undetermined

T52 Toxic effect of organic solvents

EXCLUDES 1 *halogen derivatives of aliphatic and aromatic hydrocarbons (T53.-)*

The appropriate 7th character is to be added to each code from category T52.
A initial encounter
D subsequent encounter
S sequela

T52.0 Toxic effects of petroleum products
Toxic effects of ether petroleum
Toxic effects of gasoline [petrol]
Toxic effects of kerosene [paraffin oil]
Toxic effects of naphtha petroleum
Toxic effects of paraffin wax
Toxic effects of spirit petroleum
T52.0X Toxic effects of petroleum products
T52.0X1 Toxic effect of petroleum products, accidental (unintentional)
Toxic effects of petroleum products NOS
T52.0X2 Toxic effect of petroleum products, intentional self-harm HCC
T52.0X3 Toxic effect of petroleum products, assault
T52.0X4 Toxic effect of petroleum products, undetermined
T52.1 Toxic effects of benzene
EXCLUDES 1 *homologues of benzene (T52.2)*
nitroderivatives and aminoderivatives of benzene and its homologues (T65.3)
T52.1X Toxic effects of benzene
T52.1X1 Toxic effect of benzene, accidental (unintentional)
Toxic effects of benzene NOS
T52.1X2 Toxic effect of benzene, intentional self-harm HCC
T52.1X3 Toxic effect of benzene, assault
T52.1X4 Toxic effect of benzene, undetermined
T52.2 Toxic effects of homologues of benzene
Toxic effects of toluene [methylbenzene]
Toxic effects of xylene [dimethylbenzene]
T52.2X Toxic effects of homologues of benzene
T52.2X1 Toxic effect of homologues of benzene, accidental (unintentional)
Toxic effects of homologues of benzene NOS
T52.2X2 Toxic effect of homologues of benzene, intentional self-harm HCC
T52.2X3 Toxic effect of homologues of benzene, assault
T52.2X4 Toxic effect of homologues of benzene, undetermined
T52.3 Toxic effects of glycols
T52.3X Toxic effects of glycols
T52.3X1 Toxic effect of glycols, accidental (unintentional)
Toxic effects of glycols NOS
T52.3X2 Toxic effect of glycols, intentional self-harm HCC
T52.3X3 Toxic effect of glycols, assault
T52.3X4 Toxic effect of glycols, undetermined
T52.4 Toxic effects of ketones
T52.4X Toxic effects of ketones
T52.4X1 Toxic effect of ketones, accidental (unintentional)
Toxic effects of ketones NOS
T52.4X2 Toxic effect of ketones, intentional self-harm HCC
T52.4X3 Toxic effect of ketones, assault
T52.4X4 Toxic effect of ketones, undetermined
T52.8 Toxic effects of other organic solvents
T52.8X Toxic effects of other organic solvents
T52.8X1 Toxic effect of other organic solvents, accidental (unintentional)
Toxic effects of other organic solvents NOS
T52.8X2 Toxic effect of other organic solvents, intentional self-harm HCC
T52.8X3 Toxic effect of other organic solvents, assault
T52.8X4 Toxic effect of other organic solvents, undetermined
T52.9 Toxic effects of unspecified organic solvent
T52.91 Toxic effect of unspecified organic solvent, accidental (unintentional)
T52.92 Toxic effect of unspecified organic solvent, intentional self-harm HCC
T52.93 Toxic effect of unspecified organic solvent, assault
T52.94 Toxic effect of unspecified organic solvent, undetermined

T53 Toxic effect of halogen derivatives of aliphatic and aromatic hydrocarbons

The appropriate 7th character is to be added to each code from category T53.
A initial encounter
D subsequent encounter
S sequela

T53.0 Toxic effects of carbon tetrachloride
Toxic effects of tetrachloromethane
T53.0X Toxic effects of carbon tetrachloride
T53.0X1 Toxic effect of carbon tetrachloride, accidental (unintentional)
Toxic effects of carbon tetrachloride NOS
T53.0X2 Toxic effect of carbon tetrachloride, intentional self-harm HCC
T53.0X3 Toxic effect of carbon tetrachloride, assault
T53.0X4 Toxic effect of carbon tetrachloride, undetermined
T53.1 Toxic effects of chloroform
Toxic effects of trichloromethane
T53.1X Toxic effects of chloroform
T53.1X1 Toxic effect of chloroform, accidental (unintentional)
Toxic effects of chloroform NOS
T53.1X2 Toxic effect of chloroform, intentional self-harm HCC
T53.1X3 Toxic effect of chloroform, assault
T53.1X4 Toxic effect of chloroform, undetermined

T53.2 Toxic effects of trichloroethylene
Toxic effects of trichloroethene
T53.2X Toxic effects of trichloroethylene
T53.2X1 Toxic effect of trichloroethylene, accidental (unintentional)
Toxic effects of trichloroethylene NOS
T53.2X2 Toxic effect of trichloroethylene, intentional self-harm HCC
T53.2X3 Toxic effect of trichloroethylene, assault
T53.2X4 Toxic effect of trichloroethylene, undetermined

T53.3 Toxic effects of tetrachloroethylene
Toxic effects of perchloroethylene
Toxic effect of tetrachloroethene
T53.3X Toxic effects of tetrachloroethylene
T53.3X1 Toxic effect of tetrachloroethylene, accidental (unintentional)
Toxic effects of tetrachloroethylene NOS
T53.3X2 Toxic effect of tetrachloroethylene, intentional self-harm HCC
T53.3X3 Toxic effect of tetrachloroethylene, assault
T53.3X4 Toxic effect of tetrachloroethylene, undetermined

T53.4 Toxic effects of dichloromethane
Toxic effects of methylene chloride
T53.4X Toxic effects of dichloromethane
T53.4X1 Toxic effect of dichloromethane, accidental (unintentional)
Toxic effects of dichloromethane NOS
T53.4X2 Toxic effect of dichloromethane, intentional self-harm HCC
T53.4X3 Toxic effect of dichloromethane, assault
T53.4X4 Toxic effect of dichloromethane, undetermined

T53.5 Toxic effects of chlorofluorocarbons
T53.5X Toxic effects of chlorofluorocarbons
T53.5X1 Toxic effect of chlorofluorocarbons, accidental (unintentional)
Toxic effects of chlorofluorocarbons NOS
T53.5X2 Toxic effect of chlorofluorocarbons, intentional self-harm HCC
T53.5X3 Toxic effect of chlorofluorocarbons, assault
T53.5X4 Toxic effect of chlorofluorocarbons, undetermined

T53.6 Toxic effects of other halogen derivatives of aliphatic hydrocarbons
T53.6X Toxic effects of other halogen derivatives of aliphatic hydrocarbons
T53.6X1 Toxic effect of other halogen derivatives of aliphatic hydrocarbons, accidental (unintentional)
Toxic effects of other halogen derivatives of aliphatic hydrocarbons NOS
T53.6X2 Toxic effect of other halogen derivatives of aliphatic hydrocarbons, intentional self-harm HCC
T53.6X3 Toxic effect of other halogen derivatives of aliphatic hydrocarbons, assault
T53.6X4 Toxic effect of other halogen derivatives of aliphatic hydrocarbons, undetermined

T53.7 Toxic effects of other halogen derivatives of aromatic hydrocarbons
T53.7X Toxic effects of other halogen derivatives of aromatic hydrocarbons
T53.7X1 Toxic effect of other halogen derivatives of aromatic hydrocarbons, accidental (unintentional)
Toxic effects of other halogen derivatives of aromatic hydrocarbons NOS
T53.7X2 Toxic effect of other halogen derivatives of aromatic hydrocarbons, intentional self-harm HCC
T53.7X3 Toxic effect of other halogen derivatives of aromatic hydrocarbons, assault
T53.7X4 Toxic effect of other halogen derivatives of aromatic hydrocarbons, undetermined

T53.9 Toxic effects of unspecified halogen derivatives of aliphatic and aromatic hydrocarbons
T53.91 Toxic effect of unspecified halogen derivatives of aliphatic and aromatic hydrocarbons, accidental (unintentional)
T53.92 Toxic effect of unspecified halogen derivatives of aliphatic and aromatic hydrocarbons, intentional self-harm HCC
T53.93 Toxic effect of unspecified halogen derivatives of aliphatic and aromatic hydrocarbons, assault
T53.94 Toxic effect of unspecified halogen derivatives of aliphatic and aromatic hydrocarbons, undetermined

T54 Toxic effect of corrosive substances

The appropriate 7th character is to be added to each code from category T54.
A initial encounter
D subsequent encounter
S sequela

T54.0 Toxic effects of phenol and phenol homologues
T54.0X Toxic effects of phenol and phenol homologues
T54.0X1 Toxic effect of phenol and phenol homologues, accidental (unintentional)
Toxic effects of phenol and phenol homologues NOS
T54.0X2 Toxic effect of phenol and phenol homologues, intentional self-harm HCC
T54.0X3 Toxic effect of phenol and phenol homologues, assault
T54.0X4 Toxic effect of phenol and phenol homologues, undetermined

T54.1 Toxic effects of other corrosive organic compounds
T54.1X Toxic effects of other corrosive organic compounds
T54.1X1 Toxic effect of other corrosive organic compounds, accidental (unintentional)
Toxic effects of other corrosive organic compounds NOS
T54.1X2 Toxic effect of other corrosive organic compounds, intentional self-harm HCC
T54.1X3 Toxic effect of other corrosive organic compounds, assault
T54.1X4 Toxic effect of other corrosive organic compounds, undetermined

T54.2 Toxic effects of corrosive acids and acid-like substances
Toxic effects of hydrochloric acid
Toxic effects of sulfuric acid
T54.2X Toxic effects of corrosive acids and acid-like substances
T54.2X1 Toxic effect of corrosive acids and acid-like substances, accidental (unintentional)
Toxic effects of corrosive acids and acid-like substances NOS
T54.2X2 Toxic effect of corrosive acids and acid-like substances, intentional self-harm HCC
T54.2X3 Toxic effect of corrosive acids and acid-like substances, assault
T54.2X4 Toxic effect of corrosive acids and acid-like substances, undetermined

T54.3 Toxic effects of corrosive alkalis and alkali-like substances
Toxic effects of potassium hydroxide
Toxic effects of sodium hydroxide
T54.3X Toxic effects of corrosive alkalis and alkali-like substances
T54.3X1 Toxic effect of corrosive alkalis and alkali-like substances, accidental (unintentional)
Toxic effects of corrosive alkalis and alkali-like substances NOS
T54.3X2 Toxic effect of corrosive alkalis and alkali-like substances, intentional self-harm HCC
T54.3X3 Toxic effect of corrosive alkalis and alkali-like substances, assault
T54.3X4 Toxic effect of corrosive alkalis and alkali-like substances, undetermined

T54.9 Toxic effects of unspecified corrosive substance
- **T54.91 Toxic effect of unspecified corrosive substance, accidental (unintentional)**
- **T54.92 Toxic effect of unspecified corrosive substance, intentional self-harm** HCC
- **T54.93 Toxic effect of unspecified corrosive substance, assault**
- **T54.94 Toxic effect of unspecified corrosive substance, undetermined**

T55 Toxic effect of soaps and detergents

The appropriate 7th character is to be added to each code from category T55.
A initial encounter
D subsequent encounter
S sequela

T55.Ø Toxic effect of soaps
- **T55.ØX Toxic effect of soaps**
  - **T55.ØX1 Toxic effect of soaps, accidental (unintentional)**
    Toxic effect of soaps NOS
  - **T55.ØX2 Toxic effect of soaps, intentional self-harm** HCC
  - **T55.ØX3 Toxic effect of soaps, assault**
  - **T55.ØX4 Toxic effect of soaps, undetermined**

T55.1 Toxic effect of detergents
- **T55.1X Toxic effect of detergents**
  - **T55.1X1 Toxic effect of detergents, accidental (unintentional)**
    Toxic effect of detergents NOS
  - **T55.1X2 Toxic effect of detergents, intentional self-harm** HCC
  - **T55.1X3 Toxic effect of detergents, assault**
  - **T55.1X4 Toxic effect of detergents, undetermined**

T56 Toxic effect of metals

INCLUDES toxic effects of fumes and vapors of metals
toxic effects of metals from all sources, except medicinal substances

Use additional code to identify any retained metal foreign body, if applicable (Z18.Ø-, T18.1-)

EXCLUDES 1 *arsenic and its compounds (T57.Ø)*
manganese and its compounds (T57.2)

The appropriate 7th character is to be added to each code from category T56.
A initial encounter
D subsequent encounter
S sequela

T56.Ø Toxic effects of lead and its compounds
- **T56.ØX Toxic effects of lead and its compounds**
  - **T56.ØX1 Toxic effect of lead and its compounds, accidental (unintentional)**
    Toxic effects of lead and its compounds NOS
  - **T56.ØX2 Toxic effect of lead and its compounds, intentional self-harm** HCC
  - **T56.ØX3 Toxic effect of lead and its compounds, assault**
  - **T56.ØX4 Toxic effect of lead and its compounds, undetermined**

T56.1 Toxic effects of mercury and its compounds
- **T56.1X Toxic effects of mercury and its compounds**
  - **T56.1X1 Toxic effect of mercury and its compounds, accidental (unintentional)**
    Toxic effects of mercury and its compounds NOS
  - **T56.1X2 Toxic effect of mercury and its compounds, intentional self-harm** HCC
  - **T56.1X3 Toxic effect of mercury and its compounds, assault**
  - **T56.1X4 Toxic effect of mercury and its compounds, undetermined**

T56.2 Toxic effects of chromium and its compounds
- **T56.2X Toxic effects of chromium and its compounds**
  - **T56.2X1 Toxic effect of chromium and its compounds, accidental (unintentional)**
    Toxic effects of chromium and its compounds NOS
  - **T56.2X2 Toxic effect of chromium and its compounds, intentional self-harm** HCC
  - **T56.2X3 Toxic effect of chromium and its compounds, assault**
  - **T56.2X4 Toxic effect of chromium and its compounds, undetermined**

T56.3 Toxic effects of cadmium and its compounds
- **T56.3X Toxic effects of cadmium and its compounds**
  - **T56.3X1 Toxic effect of cadmium and its compounds, accidental (unintentional)**
    Toxic effects of cadmium and its compounds NOS
  - **T56.3X2 Toxic effect of cadmium and its compounds, intentional self-harm** HCC
  - **T56.3X3 Toxic effect of cadmium and its compounds, assault**
  - **T56.3X4 Toxic effect of cadmium and its compounds, undetermined**

T56.4 Toxic effects of copper and its compounds
- **T56.4X Toxic effects of copper and its compounds**
  - **T56.4X1 Toxic effect of copper and its compounds, accidental (unintentional)**
    Toxic effects of copper and its compounds NOS
  - **T56.4X2 Toxic effect of copper and its compounds, intentional self-harm** HCC
  - **T56.4X3 Toxic effect of copper and its compounds, assault**
  - **T56.4X4 Toxic effect of copper and its compounds, undetermined**

T56.5 Toxic effects of zinc and its compounds
- **T56.5X Toxic effects of zinc and its compounds**
  - **T56.5X1 Toxic effect of zinc and its compounds, accidental (unintentional)**
    Toxic effects of zinc and its compounds NOS
  - **T56.5X2 Toxic effect of zinc and its compounds, intentional self-harm** HCC
  - **T56.5X3 Toxic effect of zinc and its compounds, assault**
  - **T56.5X4 Toxic effect of zinc and its compounds, undetermined**

T56.6 Toxic effects of tin and its compounds
- **T56.6X Toxic effects of tin and its compounds**
  - **T56.6X1 Toxic effect of tin and its compounds, accidental (unintentional)**
    Toxic effects of tin and its compounds NOS
  - **T56.6X2 Toxic effect of tin and its compounds, intentional self-harm** HCC
  - **T56.6X3 Toxic effect of tin and its compounds, assault**
  - **T56.6X4 Toxic effect of tin and its compounds, undetermined**

T56.7 Toxic effects of beryllium and its compounds
- **T56.7X Toxic effects of beryllium and its compounds**
  - **T56.7X1 Toxic effect of beryllium and its compounds, accidental (unintentional)**
    Toxic effects of beryllium and its compounds NOS
  - **T56.7X2 Toxic effect of beryllium and its compounds, intentional self-harm** HCC
  - **T56.7X3 Toxic effect of beryllium and its compounds, assault**
  - **T56.7X4 Toxic effect of beryllium and its compounds, undetermined**

T56.8 Toxic effects of other metals
- **T56.81 Toxic effect of thallium**
  - **T56.811 Toxic effect of thallium, accidental (unintentional)**
    Toxic effect of thallium NOS
  - **T56.812 Toxic effect of thallium, intentional self-harm** HCC

T56.813 Toxic effect of thallium, assault
T56.814 Toxic effect of thallium, undetermined
T56.89 Toxic effects of other metals
T56.891 Toxic effect of other metals, accidental (unintentional)
Toxic effects of other metals NOS
T56.892 Toxic effect of other metals, intentional self-harm HCC
T56.893 Toxic effect of other metals, assault
T56.894 Toxic effect of other metals, undetermined
T56.9 Toxic effects of unspecified metal
T56.91 Toxic effect of unspecified metal, accidental (unintentional)
T56.92 Toxic effect of unspecified metal, intentional self-harm HCC
T56.93 Toxic effect of unspecified metal, assault
T56.94 Toxic effect of unspecified metal, undetermined

T57 Toxic effect of other inorganic substances

The appropriate 7th character is to be added to each code from category T57.
A initial encounter
D subsequent encounter
S sequela

T57.0 Toxic effect of arsenic and its compounds
T57.0X Toxic effect of arsenic and its compounds
T57.0X1 Toxic effect of arsenic and its compounds, accidental (unintentional)
Toxic effect of arsenic and its compounds NOS
T57.0X2 Toxic effect of arsenic and its compounds, intentional self-harm HCC
T57.0X3 Toxic effect of arsenic and its compounds, assault
T57.0X4 Toxic effect of arsenic and its compounds, undetermined
T57.1 Toxic effect of phosphorus and its compounds
EXCLUDES 1 *organophosphate insecticides (T60.0)*
T57.1X Toxic effect of phosphorus and its compounds
T57.1X1 Toxic effect of phosphorus and its compounds, accidental (unintentional)
Toxic effect of phosphorus and its compounds NOS
T57.1X2 Toxic effect of phosphorus and its compounds, intentional self-harm HCC
T57.1X3 Toxic effect of phosphorus and its compounds, assault
T57.1X4 Toxic effect of phosphorus and its compounds, undetermined
T57.2 Toxic effect of manganese and its compounds
T57.2X Toxic effect of manganese and its compounds
T57.2X1 Toxic effect of manganese and its compounds, accidental (unintentional)
Toxic effect of manganese and its compounds NOS
T57.2X2 Toxic effect of manganese and its compounds, intentional self-harm HCC
T57.2X3 Toxic effect of manganese and its compounds, assault
T57.2X4 Toxic effect of manganese and its compounds, undetermined
T57.3 Toxic effect of hydrogen cyanide
T57.3X Toxic effect of hydrogen cyanide
T57.3X1 Toxic effect of hydrogen cyanide, accidental (unintentional)
Toxic effect of hydrogen cyanide NOS
T57.3X2 Toxic effect of hydrogen cyanide, intentional self-harm HCC
T57.3X3 Toxic effect of hydrogen cyanide, assault
T57.3X4 Toxic effect of hydrogen cyanide, undetermined
T57.8 Toxic effect of other specified inorganic substances
T57.8X Toxic effect of other specified inorganic substances
T57.8X1 Toxic effect of other specified inorganic substances, accidental (unintentional)
Toxic effect of other specified inorganic substances NOS
T57.8X2 Toxic effect of other specified inorganic substances, intentional self-harm HCC
T57.8X3 Toxic effect of other specified inorganic substances, assault
T57.8X4 Toxic effect of other specified inorganic substances, undetermined
T57.9 Toxic effect of unspecified inorganic substance
T57.91 Toxic effect of unspecified inorganic substance, accidental (unintentional)
T57.92 Toxic effect of unspecified inorganic substance, intentional self-harm HCC
T57.93 Toxic effect of unspecified inorganic substance, assault
T57.94 Toxic effect of unspecified inorganic substance, undetermined

T58 Toxic effect of carbon monoxide

INCLUDES asphyxiation from carbon monoxide
toxic effect of carbon monoxide from all sources

The appropriate 7th character is to be added to each code from category T58.
A initial encounter
D subsequent encounter
S sequela

T58.0 Toxic effect of carbon monoxide from motor vehicle exhaust
Toxic effect of exhaust gas from gas engine
Toxic effect of exhaust gas from motor pump
T58.01 Toxic effect of carbon monoxide from motor vehicle exhaust, accidental (unintentional)
T58.02 Toxic effect of carbon monoxide from motor vehicle exhaust, intentional self-harm HCC
T58.03 Toxic effect of carbon monoxide from motor vehicle exhaust, assault
T58.04 Toxic effect of carbon monoxide from motor vehicle exhaust, undetermined
T58.1 Toxic effect of carbon monoxide from utility gas
Toxic effect of acetylene
Toxic effect of gas NOS used for lighting, heating, cooking
Toxic effect of water gas
T58.11 Toxic effect of carbon monoxide from utility gas, accidental (unintentional)
T58.12 Toxic effect of carbon monoxide from utility gas, intentional self-harm HCC
T58.13 Toxic effect of carbon monoxide from utility gas, assault
T58.14 Toxic effect of carbon monoxide from utility gas, undetermined
T58.2 Toxic effect of carbon monoxide from incomplete combustion of other domestic fuels
Toxic effect of carbon monoxide from incomplete combustion of coal, coke, kerosene, wood
T58.2X Toxic effect of carbon monoxide from incomplete combustion of other domestic fuels
T58.2X1 Toxic effect of carbon monoxide from incomplete combustion of other domestic fuels, accidental (unintentional)
T58.2X2 Toxic effect of carbon monoxide from incomplete combustion of other domestic fuels, intentional self-harm HCC
T58.2X3 Toxic effect of carbon monoxide from incomplete combustion of other domestic fuels, assault
T58.2X4 Toxic effect of carbon monoxide from incomplete combustion of other domestic fuels, undetermined
T58.8 Toxic effect of carbon monoxide from other source
Toxic effect of carbon monoxide from blast furnace gas
Toxic effect of carbon monoxide from fuels in industrial use
Toxic effect of carbon monoxide from kiln vapor
T58.8X Toxic effect of carbon monoxide from other source
T58.8X1 Toxic effect of carbon monoxide from other source, accidental (unintentional)

7 T58.8X2 Toxic effect of carbon monoxide from other source, intentional self-harm HCC

T58.8X3 Toxic effect of carbon monoxide from other source, assault

T58.8X4 Toxic effect of carbon monoxide from other source, undetermined

T58.9 Toxic effect of carbon monoxide from unspecified source

T58.91 Toxic effect of carbon monoxide from unspecified source, accidental (unintentional)

7 T58.92 Toxic effect of carbon monoxide from unspecified source, intentional self-harm HCC

T58.93 Toxic effect of carbon monoxide from unspecified source, assault

T58.94 Toxic effect of carbon monoxide from unspecified source, undetermined

T59 Toxic effect of other gases, fumes and vapors

INCLUDES aerosol propellants

EXCLUDES 1 *chlorofluorocarbons (T53.5)*

The appropriate 7th character is to be added to each code from category T59.
A initial encounter
D subsequent encounter
S sequela

T59.Ø Toxic effect of nitrogen oxides

T59.ØX Toxic effect of nitrogen oxides

T59.ØX1 Toxic effect of nitrogen oxides, accidental (unintentional)
Toxic effect of nitrogen oxides NOS

7 T59.ØX2 Toxic effect of nitrogen oxides, intentional self-harm HCC

T59.ØX3 Toxic effect of nitrogen oxides, assault

T59.ØX4 Toxic effect of nitrogen oxides, undetermined

T59.1 Toxic effect of sulfur dioxide

T59.1X Toxic effect of sulfur dioxide

T59.1X1 Toxic effect of sulfur dioxide, accidental (unintentional)
Toxic effect of sulfur dioxide NOS

7 T59.1X2 Toxic effect of sulfur dioxide, intentional self-harm HCC

T59.1X3 Toxic effect of sulfur dioxide, assault

T59.1X4 Toxic effect of sulfur dioxide, undetermined

T59.2 Toxic effect of formaldehyde

T59.2X Toxic effect of formaldehyde

T59.2X1 Toxic effect of formaldehyde, accidental (unintentional)
Toxic effect of formaldehyde NOS

7 T59.2X2 Toxic effect of formaldehyde, intentional self-harm HCC

T59.2X3 Toxic effect of formaldehyde, assault

T59.2X4 Toxic effect of formaldehyde, undetermined

T59.3 Toxic effect of lacrimogenic gas
Toxic effect of tear gas

T59.3X Toxic effect of lacrimogenic gas

T59.3X1 Toxic effect of lacrimogenic gas, accidental (unintentional)
Toxic effect of lacrimogenic gas NOS

7 T59.3X2 Toxic effect of lacrimogenic gas, intentional self-harm HCC

T59.3X3 Toxic effect of lacrimogenic gas, assault

T59.3X4 Toxic effect of lacrimogenic gas, undetermined

T59.4 Toxic effect of chlorine gas

T59.4X Toxic effect of chlorine gas

T59.4X1 Toxic effect of chlorine gas, accidental (unintentional)
Toxic effect of chlorine gas NOS

7 T59.4X2 Toxic effect of chlorine gas, intentional self-harm HCC

T59.4X3 Toxic effect of chlorine gas, assault

T59.4X4 Toxic effect of chlorine gas, undetermined

T59.5 Toxic effect of fluorine gas and hydrogen fluoride

T59.5X Toxic effect of fluorine gas and hydrogen fluoride

T59.5X1 Toxic effect of fluorine gas and hydrogen fluoride, accidental (unintentional)
Toxic effect of fluorine gas and hydrogen fluoride NOS

7 T59.5X2 Toxic effect of fluorine gas and hydrogen fluoride, intentional self-harm HCC

T59.5X3 Toxic effect of fluorine gas and hydrogen fluoride, assault

T59.5X4 Toxic effect of fluorine gas and hydrogen fluoride, undetermined

T59.6 Toxic effect of hydrogen sulfide

T59.6X Toxic effect of hydrogen sulfide

T59.6X1 Toxic effect of hydrogen sulfide, accidental (unintentional)
Toxic effect of hydrogen sulfide NOS

7 T59.6X2 Toxic effect of hydrogen sulfide, intentional self-harm HCC

T59.6X3 Toxic effect of hydrogen sulfide, assault

T59.6X4 Toxic effect of hydrogen sulfide, undetermined

T59.7 Toxic effect of carbon dioxide

T59.7X Toxic effect of carbon dioxide

T59.7X1 Toxic effect of carbon dioxide, accidental (unintentional)
Toxic effect of carbon dioxide NOS

7 T59.7X2 Toxic effect of carbon dioxide, intentional self-harm HCC

T59.7X3 Toxic effect of carbon dioxide, assault

T59.7X4 Toxic effect of carbon dioxide, undetermined

T59.8 Toxic effect of other specified gases, fumes and vapors

T59.81 Toxic effect of smoke
Smoke inhalation
EXCLUDES 2 *toxic effect of cigarette (tobacco) smoke (T65.22-)*

T59.811 Toxic effect of smoke, accidental (unintentional)
Toxic effect of smoke NOS
AHA: 2013,4Q,121

7 T59.812 Toxic effect of smoke, intentional self-harm HCC

T59.813 Toxic effect of smoke, assault

T59.814 Toxic effect of smoke, undetermined

T59.89 Toxic effect of other specified gases, fumes and vapors

T59.891 Toxic effect of other specified gases, fumes and vapors, accidental (unintentional)

7 T59.892 Toxic effect of other specified gases, fumes and vapors, intentional self-harm HCC

T59.893 Toxic effect of other specified gases, fumes and vapors, assault

T59.894 Toxic effect of other specified gases, fumes and vapors, undetermined

T59.9 Toxic effect of unspecified gases, fumes and vapors

T59.91 Toxic effect of unspecified gases, fumes and vapors, accidental (unintentional)

7 T59.92 Toxic effect of unspecified gases, fumes and vapors, intentional self-harm HCC

T59.93 Toxic effect of unspecified gases, fumes and vapors, assault

T59.94 Toxic effect of unspecified gases, fumes and vapors, undetermined

T60 Toxic effect of pesticides

INCLUDES toxic effect of wood preservatives

The appropriate 7th character is to be added to each code from category T60.
A initial encounter
D subsequent encounter
S sequela

T60.0 Toxic effect of organophosphate and carbamate insecticides

T60.0X Toxic effect of organophosphate and carbamate insecticides

T60.0X1 Toxic effect of organophosphate and carbamate insecticides, accidental (unintentional)
Toxic effect of organophosphate and carbamate insecticides NOS

T60.0X2 Toxic effect of organophosphate and carbamate insecticides, intentional self-harm HCC

T60.0X3 Toxic effect of organophosphate and carbamate insecticides, assault

T60.0X4 Toxic effect of organophosphate and carbamate insecticides, undetermined

T60.1 Toxic effect of halogenated insecticides

EXCLUDES 1 *chlorinated hydrocarbon (T53.-)*

T60.1X Toxic effect of halogenated insecticides

T60.1X1 Toxic effect of halogenated insecticides, accidental (unintentional)
Toxic effect of halogenated insecticides NOS

T60.1X2 Toxic effect of halogenated insecticides, intentional self-harm HCC

T60.1X3 Toxic effect of halogenated insecticides, assault

T60.1X4 Toxic effect of halogenated insecticides, undetermined

T60.2 Toxic effect of other insecticides

T60.2X Toxic effect of other insecticides

T60.2X1 Toxic effect of other insecticides, accidental (unintentional)
Toxic effect of other insecticides NOS

T60.2X2 Toxic effect of other insecticides, intentional self-harm HCC

T60.2X3 Toxic effect of other insecticides, assault

T60.2X4 Toxic effect of other insecticides, undetermined

T60.3 Toxic effect of herbicides and fungicides

T60.3X Toxic effect of herbicides and fungicides

T60.3X1 Toxic effect of herbicides and fungicides, accidental (unintentional)
Toxic effect of herbicides and fungicides NOS

T60.3X2 Toxic effect of herbicides and fungicides, intentional self-harm HCC

T60.3X3 Toxic effect of herbicides and fungicides, assault

T60.3X4 Toxic effect of herbicides and fungicides, undetermined

T60.4 Toxic effect of rodenticides

EXCLUDES 1 *strychnine and its salts (T65.1)*
thallium (T56.81-)

T60.4X Toxic effect of rodenticides

T60.4X1 Toxic effect of rodenticides, accidental (unintentional)
Toxic effect of rodenticides NOS

T60.4X2 Toxic effect of rodenticides, intentional self-harm HCC

T60.4X3 Toxic effect of rodenticides, assault

T60.4X4 Toxic effect of rodenticides, undetermined

T60.8 Toxic effect of other pesticides

T60.8X Toxic effect of other pesticides

T60.8X1 Toxic effect of other pesticides, accidental (unintentional)
Toxic effect of other pesticides NOS

T60.8X2 Toxic effect of other pesticides, intentional self-harm HCC

T60.8X3 Toxic effect of other pesticides, assault

T60.8X4 Toxic effect of other pesticides, undetermined

T60.9 Toxic effect of unspecified pesticide

T60.91 Toxic effect of unspecified pesticide, accidental (unintentional)

T60.92 Toxic effect of unspecified pesticide, intentional self-harm HCC

T60.93 Toxic effect of unspecified pesticide, assault

T60.94 Toxic effect of unspecified pesticide, undetermined

T61 Toxic effect of noxious substances eaten as seafood

EXCLUDES 1 *allergic reaction to food, such as:*
anaphylactic reaction or shock due to adverse food reaction (T78.0-)
bacterial foodborne intoxications (A05.-)
dermatitis (L23.6, L25.4, L27.2)
food protein-induced enterocolitis syndrome (K52.21)
food protein-induced enteropathy (K52.22)
gastroenteritis (noninfective) (K52.29)
toxic effect of aflatoxin and other mycotoxins (T64)
toxic effect of cyanides (T65.0-)
toxic effect of harmful algae bloom (T65.82-)
toxic effect of hydrogen cyanide (T57.3-)
toxic effect of mercury (T56.1-)
toxic effect of red tide (T65.82-)

The appropriate 7th character is to be added to each code from category T61.
A initial encounter
D subsequent encounter
S sequela

T61.0 Ciguatera fish poisoning

T61.01 Ciguatera fish poisoning, accidental (unintentional)

T61.02 Ciguatera fish poisoning, intentional self-harm HCC

T61.03 Ciguatera fish poisoning, assault

T61.04 Ciguatera fish poisoning, undetermined

T61.1 Scombroid fish poisoning
Histamine-like syndrome

T61.11 Scombroid fish poisoning, accidental (unintentional)

T61.12 Scombroid fish poisoning, intentional self-harm HCC

T61.13 Scombroid fish poisoning, assault

T61.14 Scombroid fish poisoning, undetermined

T61.7 Other fish and shellfish poisoning

T61.77 Other fish poisoning

T61.771 Other fish poisoning, accidental (unintentional)

T61.772 Other fish poisoning, intentional self-harm HCC

T61.773 Other fish poisoning, assault

T61.774 Other fish poisoning, undetermined

T61.78 Other shellfish poisoning

T61.781 Other shellfish poisoning, accidental (unintentional)

T61.782 Other shellfish poisoning, intentional self-harm HCC

T61.783 Other shellfish poisoning, assault

T61.784 Other shellfish poisoning, undetermined

T61.8 Toxic effect of other seafood

T61.8X Toxic effect of other seafood

T61.8X1 Toxic effect of other seafood, accidental (unintentional)

T61.8X2 Toxic effect of other seafood, intentional self-harm HCC

T61.8X3 Toxic effect of other seafood, assault

T61.8X4 Toxic effect of other seafood, undetermined

T61.9 Toxic effect of unspecified seafood

T61.91 Toxic effect of unspecified seafood, accidental (unintentional)

T61.92 Toxic effect of unspecified seafood, intentional self-harm HCC

T61.93 Toxic effect of unspecified seafood, assault

T61.94 Toxic effect of unspecified seafood, undetermined

T62 Toxic effect of other noxious substances eaten as food

EXCLUDES 1 allergic reaction to food, such as:
- anaphylactic shock (reaction) due to adverse food reaction (T78.0-)
- bacterial food borne intoxications (A05.-)
- dermatitis (L23.6, L25.4, L27.2)
- food protein-induced enterocolitis syndrome (K52.21)
- food protein-induced enteropathy (K52.22)
- gastroenteritis (noninfective) (K52.29)

toxic effect of aflatoxin and other mycotoxins (T64)
toxic effect of cyanides (T65.0-)
toxic effect of hydrogen cyanide (T57.3-)
toxic effect of mercury (T56.1-)

The appropriate 7th character is to be added to each code from category T62.
A initial encounter
D subsequent encounter
S sequela

T62.0 Toxic effect of ingested mushrooms
T62.0X Toxic effect of ingested mushrooms
T62.0X1 Toxic effect of ingested mushrooms, accidental (unintentional)
Toxic effect of ingested mushrooms NOS
T62.0X2 Toxic effect of ingested mushrooms, intentional self-harm HCC
T62.0X3 Toxic effect of ingested mushrooms, assault
T62.0X4 Toxic effect of ingested mushrooms, undetermined

T62.1 Toxic effect of ingested berries
T62.1X Toxic effect of ingested berries
T62.1X1 Toxic effect of ingested berries, accidental (unintentional)
Toxic effect of ingested berries NOS
T62.1X2 Toxic effect of ingested berries, intentional self-harm HCC
T62.1X3 Toxic effect of ingested berries, assault
T62.1X4 Toxic effect of ingested berries, undetermined

T62.2 Toxic effect of other ingested (parts of) plant(s)
T62.2X Toxic effect of other ingested (parts of) plant(s)
T62.2X1 Toxic effect of other ingested (parts of) plant(s), accidental (unintentional)
Toxic effect of other ingested (parts of) plant(s) NOS
T62.2X2 Toxic effect of other ingested (parts of) plant(s), intentional self-harm HCC
T62.2X3 Toxic effect of other ingested (parts of) plant(s), assault
T62.2X4 Toxic effect of other ingested (parts of) plant(s), undetermined

T62.8 Toxic effect of other specified noxious substances eaten as food
T62.8X Toxic effect of other specified noxious substances eaten as food
T62.8X1 Toxic effect of other specified noxious substances eaten as food, accidental (unintentional)
Toxic effect of other specified noxious substances eaten as food NOS
T62.8X2 Toxic effect of other specified noxious substances eaten as food, intentional self-harm HCC
T62.8X3 Toxic effect of other specified noxious substances eaten as food, assault
T62.8X4 Toxic effect of other specified noxious substances eaten as food, undetermined

T62.9 Toxic effect of unspecified noxious substance eaten as food
T62.91 Toxic effect of unspecified noxious substance eaten as food, accidental (unintentional)
Toxic effect of unspecified noxious substance eaten as food NOS
T62.92 Toxic effect of unspecified noxious substance eaten as food, intentional self-harm HCC
T62.93 Toxic effect of unspecified noxious substance eaten as food, assault
T62.94 Toxic effect of unspecified noxious substance eaten as food, undetermined

T63 Toxic effect of contact with venomous animals and plants

INCLUDES bite or touch of venomous animal
pricked or stuck by thorn or leaf

EXCLUDES 2 ingestion of toxic animal or plant (T61.-, T62.-)

The appropriate 7th character is to be added to each code from category T63.
A initial encounter
D subsequent encounter
S sequela

T63.0 Toxic effect of snake venom
T63.00 Toxic effect of unspecified snake venom
T63.001 Toxic effect of unspecified snake venom, accidental (unintentional)
Toxic effect of unspecified snake venom NOS
T63.002 Toxic effect of unspecified snake venom, intentional self-harm HCC
T63.003 Toxic effect of unspecified snake venom, assault
T63.004 Toxic effect of unspecified snake venom, undetermined

T63.01 Toxic effect of rattlesnake venom
T63.011 Toxic effect of rattlesnake venom, accidental (unintentional)
Toxic effect of rattlesnake venom NOS
T63.012 Toxic effect of rattlesnake venom, intentional self-harm HCC
T63.013 Toxic effect of rattlesnake venom, assault
T63.014 Toxic effect of rattlesnake venom, undetermined

T63.02 Toxic effect of coral snake venom
T63.021 Toxic effect of coral snake venom, accidental (unintentional)
Toxic effect of coral snake venom NOS
T63.022 Toxic effect of coral snake venom, intentional self-harm HCC
T63.023 Toxic effect of coral snake venom, assault
T63.024 Toxic effect of coral snake venom, undetermined

T63.03 Toxic effect of taipan venom
T63.031 Toxic effect of taipan venom, accidental (unintentional)
Toxic effect of taipan venom NOS
T63.032 Toxic effect of taipan venom, intentional self-harm HCC
T63.033 Toxic effect of taipan venom, assault
T63.034 Toxic effect of taipan venom, undetermined

T63.04 Toxic effect of cobra venom
T63.041 Toxic effect of cobra venom, accidental (unintentional)
Toxic effect of cobra venom NOS
T63.042 Toxic effect of cobra venom, intentional self-harm HCC
T63.043 Toxic effect of cobra venom, assault
T63.044 Toxic effect of cobra venom, undetermined

T63.06 Toxic effect of venom of other North and South American snake
T63.061 Toxic effect of venom of other North and South American snake, accidental (unintentional)
Toxic effect of venom of other North and South American snake NOS
T63.062 Toxic effect of venom of other North and South American snake, intentional self-harm HCC
T63.063 Toxic effect of venom of other North and South American snake, assault
T63.064 Toxic effect of venom of other North and South American snake, undetermined

✓6th **T63.07 Toxic effect of venom of other Australian snake**

✓7th **T63.071 Toxic effect of venom of other Australian snake, accidental (unintentional)**
Toxic effect of venom of other Australian snake NOS

7 ✓7th **T63.072 Toxic effect of venom of other Australian snake, intentional self-harm** HCC

✓7th **T63.073 Toxic effect of venom of other Australian snake, assault**

✓7th **T63.074 Toxic effect of venom of other Australian snake, undetermined**

✓6th **T63.08 Toxic effect of venom of other African and Asian snake**

✓7th **T63.081 Toxic effect of venom of other African and Asian snake, accidental (unintentional)**
Toxic effect of venom of other African and Asian snake NOS

7 ✓7th **T63.082 Toxic effect of venom of other African and Asian snake, intentional self-harm** HCC

✓7th **T63.083 Toxic effect of venom of other African and Asian snake, assault**

✓7th **T63.084 Toxic effect of venom of other African and Asian snake, undetermined**

✓6th **T63.09 Toxic effect of venom of other snake**

✓7th **T63.091 Toxic effect of venom of other snake, accidental (unintentional)**
Toxic effect of venom of other snake NOS

7 ✓7th **T63.092 Toxic effect of venom of other snake, intentional self-harm** HCC

✓7th **T63.093 Toxic effect of venom of other snake, assault**

✓7th **T63.094 Toxic effect of venom of other snake, undetermined**

✓5th **T63.1 Toxic effect of venom of other reptiles**

✓6th **T63.11 Toxic effect of venom of gila monster**

✓7th **T63.111 Toxic effect of venom of gila monster, accidental (unintentional)**
Toxic effect of venom of gila monster NOS

7 ✓7th **T63.112 Toxic effect of venom of gila monster, intentional self-harm** HCC

✓7th **T63.113 Toxic effect of venom of gila monster, assault**

✓7th **T63.114 Toxic effect of venom of gila monster, undetermined**

✓6th **T63.12 Toxic effect of venom of other venomous lizard**

✓7th **T63.121 Toxic effect of venom of other venomous lizard, accidental (unintentional)**
Toxic effect of venom of other venomous lizard NOS

7 ✓7th **T63.122 Toxic effect of venom of other venomous lizard, intentional self-harm** HCC

✓7th **T63.123 Toxic effect of venom of other venomous lizard, assault**

✓7th **T63.124 Toxic effect of venom of other venomous lizard, undetermined**

✓6th **T63.19 Toxic effect of venom of other reptiles**

✓7th **T63.191 Toxic effect of venom of other reptiles, accidental (unintentional)**
Toxic effect of venom of other reptiles NOS

7 ✓7th **T63.192 Toxic effect of venom of other reptiles, intentional self-harm** HCC

✓7th **T63.193 Toxic effect of venom of other reptiles, assault**

✓7th **T63.194 Toxic effect of venom of other reptiles, undetermined**

✓5th **T63.2 Toxic effect of venom of scorpion**

✓6th **T63.2X Toxic effect of venom of scorpion**

✓7th **T63.2X1 Toxic effect of venom of scorpion, accidental (unintentional)**
Toxic effect of venom of scorpion NOS

7 ✓7th **T63.2X2 Toxic effect of venom of scorpion, intentional self-harm** HCC

✓7th **T63.2X3 Toxic effect of venom of scorpion, assault**

✓7th **T63.2X4 Toxic effect of venom of scorpion, undetermined**

✓5th **T63.3 Toxic effect of venom of spider**

✓6th **T63.30 Toxic effect of unspecified spider venom**

✓7th **T63.301 Toxic effect of unspecified spider venom, accidental (unintentional)**

7 ✓7th **T63.302 Toxic effect of unspecified spider venom, intentional self-harm** HCC

✓7th **T63.303 Toxic effect of unspecified spider venom, assault**

✓7th **T63.304 Toxic effect of unspecified spider venom, undetermined**

✓6th **T63.31 Toxic effect of venom of black widow spider**

✓7th **T63.311 Toxic effect of venom of black widow spider, accidental (unintentional)**

7 ✓7th **T63.312 Toxic effect of venom of black widow spider, intentional self-harm** HCC

✓7th **T63.313 Toxic effect of venom of black widow spider, assault**

✓7th **T63.314 Toxic effect of venom of black widow spider, undetermined**

✓6th **T63.32 Toxic effect of venom of tarantula**

✓7th **T63.321 Toxic effect of venom of tarantula, accidental (unintentional)**

7 ✓7th **T63.322 Toxic effect of venom of tarantula, intentional self-harm** HCC

✓7th **T63.323 Toxic effect of venom of tarantula, assault**

✓7th **T63.324 Toxic effect of venom of tarantula, undetermined**

✓6th **T63.33 Toxic effect of venom of brown recluse spider**

✓7th **T63.331 Toxic effect of venom of brown recluse spider, accidental (unintentional)**

7 ✓7th **T63.332 Toxic effect of venom of brown recluse spider, intentional self-harm** HCC

✓7th **T63.333 Toxic effect of venom of brown recluse spider, assault**

✓7th **T63.334 Toxic effect of venom of brown recluse spider, undetermined**

✓6th **T63.39 Toxic effect of venom of other spider**

✓7th **T63.391 Toxic effect of venom of other spider, accidental (unintentional)**

7 ✓7th **T63.392 Toxic effect of venom of other spider, intentional self-harm** HCC

✓7th **T63.393 Toxic effect of venom of other spider, assault**

✓7th **T63.394 Toxic effect of venom of other spider, undetermined**

✓5th **T63.4 Toxic effect of venom of other arthropods**

✓6th **T63.41 Toxic effect of venom of centipedes and venomous millipedes**

✓7th **T63.411 Toxic effect of venom of centipedes and venomous millipedes, accidental (unintentional)**

7 ✓7th **T63.412 Toxic effect of venom of centipedes and venomous millipedes, intentional self-harm** HCC

✓7th **T63.413 Toxic effect of venom of centipedes and venomous millipedes, assault**

✓7th **T63.414 Toxic effect of venom of centipedes and venomous millipedes, undetermined**

✓6th **T63.42 Toxic effect of venom of ants**

✓7th **T63.421 Toxic effect of venom of ants, accidental (unintentional)**

7 ✓7th **T63.422 Toxic effect of venom of ants, intentional self-harm** HCC

✓7th **T63.423 Toxic effect of venom of ants, assault**

✓7th **T63.424 Toxic effect of venom of ants, undetermined**

✓6th **T63.43 Toxic effect of venom of caterpillars**

✓7th **T63.431 Toxic effect of venom of caterpillars, accidental (unintentional)**

7 ✓7th **T63.432 Toxic effect of venom of caterpillars, intentional self-harm** HCC

✓7th **T63.433 Toxic effect of venom of caterpillars, assault**

✓7th **T63.434 Toxic effect of venom of caterpillars, undetermined**

✓6th **T63.44 Toxic effect of venom of bees**

✓7th **T63.441 Toxic effect of venom of bees, accidental (unintentional)**

7 ✓7th **T63.442 Toxic effect of venom of bees, intentional self-harm** HCC

✓7th **T63.443 Toxic effect of venom of bees, assault**

✓7th **T63.444 Toxic effect of venom of bees, undetermined**

T63.45 Toxic effect of venom of hornets
T63.451 Toxic effect of venom of hornets, accidental (unintentional)
T63.452 Toxic effect of venom of hornets, intentional self-harm HCC
T63.453 Toxic effect of venom of hornets, assault
T63.454 Toxic effect of venom of hornets, undetermined
T63.46 Toxic effect of venom of wasps
Toxic effect of yellow jacket
T63.461 Toxic effect of venom of wasps, accidental (unintentional)
T63.462 Toxic effect of venom of wasps, intentional self-harm HCC
T63.463 Toxic effect of venom of wasps, assault
T63.464 Toxic effect of venom of wasps, undetermined
T63.48 Toxic effect of venom of other arthropod
T63.481 Toxic effect of venom of other arthropod, accidental (unintentional)
T63.482 Toxic effect of venom of other arthropod, intentional self-harm HCC
T63.483 Toxic effect of venom of other arthropod, assault
T63.484 Toxic effect of venom of other arthropod, undetermined
T63.5 Toxic effect of contact with venomous fish
EXCLUDES 2 *poisoning by ingestion of fish (T61.-)*
T63.51 Toxic effect of contact with stingray
T63.511 Toxic effect of contact with stingray, accidental (unintentional)
T63.512 Toxic effect of contact with stingray, intentional self-harm HCC
T63.513 Toxic effect of contact with stingray, assault
T63.514 Toxic effect of contact with stingray, undetermined
T63.59 Toxic effect of contact with other venomous fish
T63.591 Toxic effect of contact with other venomous fish, accidental (unintentional)
T63.592 Toxic effect of contact with other venomous fish, intentional self-harm HCC
T63.593 Toxic effect of contact with other venomous fish, assault
T63.594 Toxic effect of contact with other venomous fish, undetermined
T63.6 Toxic effect of contact with other venomous marine animals
EXCLUDES 1 *sea-snake venom (T63.Ø9)*
EXCLUDES 2 *poisoning by ingestion of shellfish (T61.78-)*
T63.61 Toxic effect of contact with Portuguese Man-o-war
Toxic effect of contact with bluebottle
T63.611 Toxic effect of contact with Portuguese Man-o-war, accidental (unintentional)
T63.612 Toxic effect of contact with Portuguese Man-o-war, intentional self-harm HCC
T63.613 Toxic effect of contact with Portuguese Man-o-war, assault
T63.614 Toxic effect of contact with Portuguese Man-o-war, undetermined
T63.62 Toxic effect of contact with other jellyfish
T63.621 Toxic effect of contact with other jellyfish, accidental (unintentional)
T63.622 Toxic effect of contact with other jellyfish, intentional self-harm HCC
T63.623 Toxic effect of contact with other jellyfish, assault
T63.624 Toxic effect of contact with other jellyfish, undetermined
T63.63 Toxic effect of contact with sea anemone
T63.631 Toxic effect of contact with sea anemone, accidental (unintentional)
T63.632 Toxic effect of contact with sea anemone, intentional self-harm HCC
T63.633 Toxic effect of contact with sea anemone, assault
T63.634 Toxic effect of contact with sea anemone, undetermined
T63.69 Toxic effect of contact with other venomous marine animals
T63.691 Toxic effect of contact with other venomous marine animals, accidental (unintentional)
T63.692 Toxic effect of contact with other venomous marine animals, intentional self-harm HCC
T63.693 Toxic effect of contact with other venomous marine animals, assault
T63.694 Toxic effect of contact with other venomous marine animals, undetermined
T63.7 Toxic effect of contact with venomous plant
T63.71 Toxic effect of contact with venomous marine plant
T63.711 Toxic effect of contact with venomous marine plant, accidental (unintentional)
T63.712 Toxic effect of contact with venomous marine plant, intentional self-harm HCC
T63.713 Toxic effect of contact with venomous marine plant, assault
T63.714 Toxic effect of contact with venomous marine plant, undetermined
T63.79 Toxic effect of contact with other venomous plant
T63.791 Toxic effect of contact with other venomous plant, accidental (unintentional)
T63.792 Toxic effect of contact with other venomous plant, intentional self-harm HCC
T63.793 Toxic effect of contact with other venomous plant, assault
T63.794 Toxic effect of contact with other venomous plant, undetermined
T63.8 Toxic effect of contact with other venomous animals
T63.81 Toxic effect of contact with venomous frog
EXCLUDES 1 *contact with nonvenomous frog (W62.Ø)*
T63.811 Toxic effect of contact with venomous frog, accidental (unintentional)
T63.812 Toxic effect of contact with venomous frog, intentional self-harm HCC
T63.813 Toxic effect of contact with venomous frog, assault
T63.814 Toxic effect of contact with venomous frog, undetermined
T63.82 Toxic effect of contact with venomous toad
EXCLUDES 1 *contact with nonvenomous toad (W62.1)*
T63.821 Toxic effect of contact with venomous toad, accidental (unintentional)
T63.822 Toxic effect of contact with venomous toad, intentional self-harm HCC
T63.823 Toxic effect of contact with venomous toad, assault
T63.824 Toxic effect of contact with venomous toad, undetermined
T63.83 Toxic effect of contact with other venomous amphibian
EXCLUDES 1 *contact with nonvenomous amphibian (W62.9)*
T63.831 Toxic effect of contact with other venomous amphibian, accidental (unintentional)
T63.832 Toxic effect of contact with other venomous amphibian, intentional self-harm HCC
T63.833 Toxic effect of contact with other venomous amphibian, assault
T63.834 Toxic effect of contact with other venomous amphibian, undetermined
T63.89 Toxic effect of contact with other venomous animals
T63.891 Toxic effect of contact with other venomous animals, accidental (unintentional)
T63.892 Toxic effect of contact with other venomous animals, intentional self-harm HCC
T63.893 Toxic effect of contact with other venomous animals, assault
T63.894 Toxic effect of contact with other venomous animals, undetermined

T63.9 Toxic effect of contact with unspecified venomous animal

T63.91 Toxic effect of contact with unspecified venomous animal, accidental (unintentional)

T63.92 Toxic effect of contact with unspecified venomous animal, intentional self-harm HCC

T63.93 Toxic effect of contact with unspecified venomous animal, assault

T63.94 Toxic effect of contact with unspecified venomous animal, undetermined

T64 Toxic effect of aflatoxin and other mycotoxin food contaminants

The appropriate 7th character is to be added to each code from category T64.
A initial encounter
D subsequent encounter
S sequela

T64.Ø Toxic effect of aflatoxin

T64.Ø1 Toxic effect of aflatoxin, accidental (unintentional)

T64.Ø2 Toxic effect of aflatoxin, intentional self-harm HCC

T64.Ø3 Toxic effect of aflatoxin, assault

T64.Ø4 Toxic effect of aflatoxin, undetermined

T64.8 Toxic effect of other mycotoxin food contaminants

T64.81 Toxic effect of other mycotoxin food contaminants, accidental (unintentional)

T64.82 Toxic effect of other mycotoxin food contaminants, intentional self-harm HCC

T64.83 Toxic effect of other mycotoxin food contaminants, assault

T64.84 Toxic effect of other mycotoxin food contaminants, undetermined

T65 Toxic effect of other and unspecified substances

The appropriate 7th character is to be added to each code from category T65.
A initial encounter
D subsequent encounter
S sequela

T65.Ø Toxic effect of cyanides

EXCLUDES 1 *hydrogen cyanide (T57.3-)*

T65.ØX Toxic effect of cyanides

T65.ØX1 Toxic effect of cyanides, accidental (unintentional)
Toxic effect of cyanides NOS

T65.ØX2 Toxic effect of cyanides, intentional self-harm HCC

T65.ØX3 Toxic effect of cyanides, assault

T65.ØX4 Toxic effect of cyanides, undetermined

T65.1 Toxic effect of strychnine and its salts

T65.1X Toxic effect of strychnine and its salts

T65.1X1 Toxic effect of strychnine and its salts, accidental (unintentional)
Toxic effect of strychnine and its salts NOS

T65.1X2 Toxic effect of strychnine and its salts, intentional self-harm HCC

T65.1X3 Toxic effect of strychnine and its salts, assault

T65.1X4 Toxic effect of strychnine and its salts, undetermined

T65.2 Toxic effect of tobacco and nicotine

EXCLUDES 2 *nicotine dependence (F17.-)*

T65.21 Toxic effect of chewing tobacco

T65.211 Toxic effect of chewing tobacco, accidental (unintentional)
Toxic effect of chewing tobacco NOS

T65.212 Toxic effect of chewing tobacco, intentional self-harm HCC

T65.213 Toxic effect of chewing tobacco, assault

T65.214 Toxic effect of chewing tobacco, undetermined

T65.22 Toxic effect of tobacco cigarettes
Toxic effect of tobacco smoke
Use additional code for exposure to second hand tobacco smoke (Z57.31, Z77.22)

T65.221 Toxic effect of tobacco cigarettes, accidental (unintentional)
Toxic effect of tobacco cigarettes NOS

T65.222 Toxic effect of tobacco cigarettes, intentional self-harm HCC

T65.223 Toxic effect of tobacco cigarettes, assault

T65.224 Toxic effect of tobacco cigarettes, undetermined

T65.29 Toxic effect of other tobacco and nicotine

T65.291 Toxic effect of other tobacco and nicotine, accidental (unintentional)
Toxic effect of other tobacco and nicotine NOS

T65.292 Toxic effect of other tobacco and nicotine, intentional self-harm HCC

T65.293 Toxic effect of other tobacco and nicotine, assault

T65.294 Toxic effect of other tobacco and nicotine, undetermined

T65.3 Toxic effect of nitroderivatives and aminoderivatives of benzene and its homologues
Toxic effect of anilin [benzenamine]
Toxic effect of nitrobenzene
Toxic effect of trinitrotoluene

T65.3X Toxic effect of nitroderivatives and aminoderivatives of benzene and its homologues

T65.3X1 Toxic effect of nitroderivatives and aminoderivatives of benzene and its homologues, accidental (unintentional)
Toxic effect of nitroderivatives and aminoderivatives of benzene and its homologues NOS

T65.3X2 Toxic effect of nitroderivatives and aminoderivatives of benzene and its homologues, intentional self-harm HCC

T65.3X3 Toxic effect of nitroderivatives and aminoderivatives of benzene and its homologues, assault

T65.3X4 Toxic effect of nitroderivatives and aminoderivatives of benzene and its homologues, undetermined

T65.4 Toxic effect of carbon disulfide

T65.4X Toxic effect of carbon disulfide

T65.4X1 Toxic effect of carbon disulfide, accidental (unintentional)
Toxic effect of carbon disulfide NOS

T65.4X2 Toxic effect of carbon disulfide, intentional self-harm HCC

T65.4X3 Toxic effect of carbon disulfide, assault

T65.4X4 Toxic effect of carbon disulfide, undetermined

T65.5 Toxic effect of nitroglycerin and other nitric acids and esters
Toxic effect of 1,2,3-Propanetriol trinitrate

T65.5X Toxic effect of nitroglycerin and other nitric acids and esters

T65.5X1 Toxic effect of nitroglycerin and other nitric acids and esters, accidental (unintentional)
Toxic effect of nitroglycerin and other nitric acids and esters NOS

T65.5X2 Toxic effect of nitroglycerin and other nitric acids and esters, intentional self-harm HCC

T65.5X3 Toxic effect of nitroglycerin and other nitric acids and esters, assault

T65.5X4 Toxic effect of nitroglycerin and other nitric acids and esters, undetermined

T65.6 Toxic effect of paints and dyes, not elsewhere classified

T65.6X Toxic effect of paints and dyes, not elsewhere classified

T65.6X1 Toxic effect of paints and dyes, not elsewhere classified, accidental (unintentional)
Toxic effect of paints and dyes NOS

7 T65.6X2 **Toxic effect of paints and dyes, not elsewhere classified, intentional self-harm** HCC

T65.6X3 **Toxic effect of paints and dyes, not elsewhere classified, assault**

T65.6X4 **Toxic effect of paints and dyes, not elsewhere classified, undetermined**

T65.8 **Toxic effect of other specified substances**

T65.81 **Toxic effect of latex**

T65.811 **Toxic effect of latex, accidental (unintentional)**
Toxic effect of latex NOS

7 T65.812 **Toxic effect of latex, intentional self-harm** HCC

T65.813 **Toxic effect of latex, assault**

T65.814 **Toxic effect of latex, undetermined**

T65.82 **Toxic effect of harmful algae and algae toxins**
Toxic effect of (harmful) algae bloom NOS
Toxic effect of blue-green algae bloom
Toxic effect of brown tide
Toxic effect of cyanobacteria bloom
Toxic effect of Florida red tide
Toxic effect of pfiesteria piscicida
Toxic effect of red tide

T65.821 **Toxic effect of harmful algae and algae toxins, accidental (unintentional)**
Toxic effect of harmful algae and algae toxins NOS

7 T65.822 **Toxic effect of harmful algae and algae toxins, intentional self-harm** HCC

T65.823 **Toxic effect of harmful algae and algae toxins, assault**

T65.824 **Toxic effect of harmful algae and algae toxins, undetermined**

T65.83 **Toxic effect of fiberglass**

T65.831 **Toxic effect of fiberglass, accidental (unintentional)**
Toxic effect of fiberglass NOS

7 T65.832 **Toxic effect of fiberglass, intentional self-harm** HCC

T65.833 **Toxic effect of fiberglass, assault**

T65.834 **Toxic effect of fiberglass, undetermined**

T65.89 **Toxic effect of other specified substances**

T65.891 **Toxic effect of other specified substances, accidental (unintentional)**
Toxic effect of other specified substances NOS
AHA: 2018,1Q,5

7 T65.892 **Toxic effect of other specified substances, intentional self-harm** HCC

T65.893 **Toxic effect of other specified substances, assault**

T65.894 **Toxic effect of other specified substances, undetermined**

T65.9 **Toxic effect of unspecified substance**

T65.91 **Toxic effect of unspecified substance, accidental (unintentional)**
Poisoning NOS

7 T65.92 **Toxic effect of unspecified substance, intentional self-harm** HCC

T65.93 **Toxic effect of unspecified substance, assault**

T65.94 **Toxic effect of unspecified substance, undetermined**

Other and unspecified effects of external causes (T66-T78)

T66 **Radiation sickness, unspecified**

EXCLUDES 1 *specified adverse effects of radiation, such as:*
burns (T2Ø-T31)
leukemia (C91-C95)
radiation gastroenteritis and colitis (K52.Ø)
radiation pneumonitis (J7Ø.Ø)
radiation related disorders of the skin and subcutaneous tissue (L55-L59)
radiation sunburn (L55.-)

The appropriate 7th character is to be added to code T66.
A initial encounter
D subsequent encounter
S sequela

T67 **Effects of heat and light**

EXCLUDES 1 *erythema [dermatitis] ab igne (L59.Ø)*
malignant hyperpyrexia due to anesthesia (T88.3)
radiation-related disorders of the skin and subcutaneous tissue (L55-L59)

EXCLUDES 2 *burns (T2Ø-T31)*
sunburn (L55.-)
sweat disorder due to heat (L74-L75)

The appropriate 7th character is to be added to each code from category T67.
A initial encounter
D subsequent encounter
S sequela

T67.Ø **Heatstroke and sunstroke**
Use additional code(s) to identify any associated complications of heatstroke, such as:
coma and stupor (R4Ø.-)
rhabdomyolysis (M62.82)
systemic inflammatory response syndrome (R65.1-)
AHA: 2019,4Q,17-18
DEF: Headache, vertigo, cramps, and elevated body temperature due to prolonged exposure to high environmental temperatures that requires emergency intervention.

T67.Ø1 **Heatstroke and sunstroke** CC H5
Heat apoplexy
Heat pyrexia
Siriasis
Thermoplegia

T67.Ø2 **Exertional heatstroke** CC H5

T67.Ø9 **Other heatstroke and sunstroke** CC H5

T67.1 **Heat syncope**
Heat collapse

T67.2 **Heat cramp**

T67.3 **Heat exhaustion, anhydrotic**
Heat prostration due to water depletion
EXCLUDES 1 *heat exhaustion due to salt depletion (T67.4)*

T67.4 **Heat exhaustion due to salt depletion**
Heat prostration due to salt (and water) depletion

T67.5 **Heat exhaustion, unspecified**
Heat prostration NOS

T67.6 **Heat fatigue, transient**

T67.7 **Heat edema**

T67.8 **Other effects of heat and light**

T67.9 **Effect of heat and light, unspecified**

T68 Hypothermia

Accidental hypothermia

Hypothermia NOS

Use additional code to identify source of exposure:

exposure to excessive cold of man-made origin (W93)

exposure to excessive cold of natural origin (X31)

EXCLUDES 1 *hypothermia following anesthesia (T88.51)*

hypothermia not associated with low environmental temperature (R68.Ø)

hypothermia of newborn (P8Ø.-)

EXCLUDES 2 *frostbite (T33-T34)*

The appropriate 7th character is to be added to code T68.
A initial encounter
D subsequent encounter
S sequela

T69 Other effects of reduced temperature

Use additional code to identify source of exposure:

exposure to excessive cold of man-made origin (W93)

exposure to excessive cold of natural origin (X31)

EXCLUDES 2 *frostbite (T33-T34)*

The appropriate 7th character is to be added to each code from category T69.
A initial encounter
D subsequent encounter
S sequela

T69.Ø Immersion hand and foot

T69.Ø1 Immersion hand

T69.Ø11 Immersion hand, right hand

T69.Ø12 Immersion hand, left hand

T69.Ø19 Immersion hand, unspecified hand

T69.Ø2 Immersion foot

Trench foot

T69.Ø21 Immersion foot, right foot CC HS

T69.Ø22 Immersion foot, left foot CC HS

T69.Ø29 Immersion foot, unspecified foot CC HS UNS

T69.1 Chilblains

DEF: Red, swollen, itchy skin primarily affecting the fingers and toes, nose and ears, and legs. Chilblains follows damp-cold exposure, and can also be associated with pruritus and a burning feeling.

T69.8 Other specified effects of reduced temperature

T69.9 Effect of reduced temperature, unspecified

T7Ø Effects of air pressure and water pressure

The appropriate 7th character is to be added to each code from category T7Ø.
A initial encounter
D subsequent encounter
S sequela

T7Ø.Ø Otitic barotrauma

Aero-otitis media

Effects of change in ambient atmospheric pressure or water pressure on ears

T7Ø.1 Sinus barotrauma

Aerosinusitis

Effects of change in ambient atmospheric pressure on sinuses

T7Ø.2 Other and unspecified effects of high altitude

EXCLUDES 2 *polycythemia due to high altitude (D75.1)*

T7Ø.2Ø Unspecified effects of high altitude

T7Ø.29 Other effects of high altitude

Alpine sickness

Anoxia due to high altitude

Barotrauma NOS

Hypobaropathy

Mountain sickness

T7Ø.3 Caisson disease [decompression sickness] CC HS

Compressed-air disease

Diver's palsy or paralysis

DEF: Rapid reduction in air pressure while breathing compressed air. Symptoms include skin lesions, joint pains, and respiratory and neurological problems.

T7Ø.4 Effects of high-pressure fluids

Hydraulic jet injection (industrial)

Pneumatic jet injection (industrial)

Traumatic jet injection (industrial)

T7Ø.8 Other effects of air pressure and water pressure

T7Ø.9 Effect of air pressure and water pressure, unspecified

T71 Asphyxiation

Mechanical suffocation

Traumatic suffocation

EXCLUDES 1 *acute respiratory distress (syndrome) (J8Ø)*

anoxia due to high altitude (T7Ø.2)

asphyxia NOS (RØ9.Ø1)

asphyxia from carbon monoxide (T58.-)

asphyxia from inhalation of food or foreign body (T17.-)

asphyxia from other gases, fumes and vapors (T59.-)

respiratory distress (syndrome) in newborn (P22.-)

The appropriate 7th character is to be added to each code from category T71.
A initial encounter
D subsequent encounter
S sequela

T71.1 Asphyxiation due to mechanical threat to breathing

Suffocation due to mechanical threat to breathing

T71.11 Asphyxiation due to smothering under pillow

T71.111 Asphyxiation due to smothering under pillow, accidental CC HS

Asphyxiation due to smothering under pillow NOS

7 **T71.112 Asphyxiation due to smothering under pillow, intentional self-harm** CC HS HCC

T71.113 Asphyxiation due to smothering under pillow, assault CC HS

T71.114 Asphyxiation due to smothering under pillow, undetermined CC HS

T71.12 Asphyxiation due to plastic bag

T71.121 Asphyxiation due to plastic bag, accidental CC HS

Asphyxiation due to plastic bag NOS

7 **T71.122 Asphyxiation due to plastic bag, intentional self-harm** CC HS HCC

T71.123 Asphyxiation due to plastic bag, assault CC HS

T71.124 Asphyxiation due to plastic bag, undetermined CC HS

T71.13 Asphyxiation due to being trapped in bed linens

T71.131 Asphyxiation due to being trapped in bed linens, accidental CC HS

Asphyxiation due to being trapped in bed linens NOS

7 **T71.132 Asphyxiation due to being trapped in bed linens, intentional self-harm** CC HS HCC

T71.133 Asphyxiation due to being trapped in bed linens, assault CC HS

T71.134 Asphyxiation due to being trapped in bed linens, undetermined CC HS

T71.14 Asphyxiation due to smothering under another person's body (in bed)

T71.141 Asphyxiation due to smothering under another person's body (in bed), accidental CC HS

Asphyxiation due to smothering under another person's body (in bed) NOS

T71.143 Asphyxiation due to smothering under another person's body (in bed), assault CC HS

T71.144 Asphyxiation due to smothering under another person's body (in bed), undetermined CC HS

T71.15 Asphyxiation due to smothering in furniture

T71.151 Asphyxiation due to smothering in furniture, accidental CC HS

Asphyxiation due to smothering in furniture NOS

7 T71.152 **Asphyxiation due to smothering in furniture, intentional self-harm** CC H5 HCC

T71.153 **Asphyxiation due to smothering in furniture, assault** CC H5

T71.154 **Asphyxiation due to smothering in furniture, undetermined** CC H5

T71.16 **Asphyxiation due to hanging**

Hanging by window shade cord

Use additional code for any associated injuries, such as:
- crushing injury of neck (S17.-)
- fracture of cervical vertebrae (S12.Ø-S12.2-)
- open wound of neck (S11.-)

T71.161 **Asphyxiation due to hanging, accidental** CC H5

Asphyxiation due to hanging NOS

Hanging NOS

7 T71.162 **Asphyxiation due to hanging, intentional self-harm** CC H5 HCC

T71.163 **Asphyxiation due to hanging, assault** CC H5

T71.164 **Asphyxiation due to hanging, undetermined** CC H5

T71.19 **Asphyxiation due to mechanical threat to breathing due to other causes**

T71.191 **Asphyxiation due to mechanical threat to breathing due to other causes, accidental** CC H5

Asphyxiation due to other causes NOS

7 T71.192 **Asphyxiation due to mechanical threat to breathing due to other causes, intentional self-harm** CC H5 HCC

T71.193 **Asphyxiation due to mechanical threat to breathing due to other causes, assault** CC H5

T71.194 **Asphyxiation due to mechanical threat to breathing due to other causes, undetermined** CC H5

T71.2 **Asphyxiation due to systemic oxygen deficiency due to low oxygen content in ambient air**

Suffocation due to systemic oxygen deficiency due to low oxygen content in ambient air

T71.2Ø **Asphyxiation due to systemic oxygen deficiency due to low oxygen content in ambient air due to unspecified cause** CC H5

T71.21 **Asphyxiation due to cave-in or falling earth** CC H5

Use additional code for any associated cataclysm (X34-X38)

T71.22 **Asphyxiation due to being trapped in a car trunk**

T71.221 **Asphyxiation due to being trapped in a car trunk, accidental** CC

7 T71.222 **Asphyxiation due to being trapped in a car trunk, intentional self-harm** CC HCC

T71.223 **Asphyxiation due to being trapped in a car trunk, assault** CC

T71.224 **Asphyxiation due to being trapped in a car trunk, undetermined** CC

T71.23 **Asphyxiation due to being trapped in a (discarded) refrigerator**

T71.231 **Asphyxiation due to being trapped in a (discarded) refrigerator, accidental** CC

7 T71.232 **Asphyxiation due to being trapped in a (discarded) refrigerator, intentional self-harm** CC HCC

T71.233 **Asphyxiation due to being trapped in a (discarded) refrigerator, assault** CC

T71.234 **Asphyxiation due to being trapped in a (discarded) refrigerator, undetermined** CC

T71.29 **Asphyxiation due to being trapped in other low oxygen environment** CC H5

T71.9 **Asphyxiation due to unspecified cause** CC H5

Suffocation (by strangulation) due to unspecified cause

Suffocation NOS

Systemic oxygen deficiency due to low oxygen content in ambient air due to unspecified cause

Systemic oxygen deficiency due to mechanical threat to breathing due to unspecified cause

Traumatic asphyxia NOS

T73 Effects of other deprivation

The appropriate 7th character is to be added to each code from category T73.
- A initial encounter
- D subsequent encounter
- S sequela

T73.Ø **Starvation**

Deprivation of food

T73.1 **Deprivation of water**

T73.2 **Exhaustion due to exposure**

T73.3 **Exhaustion due to excessive exertion**

Exhaustion due to overexertion

T73.8 **Other effects of deprivation**

T73.9 **Effect of deprivation, unspecified**

T74 Adult and child abuse, neglect and other maltreatment, confirmed

Use additional code, if applicable, to identify any associated current injury

Use additional external cause code to identify perpetrator, if known (YØ7.-)

EXCLUDES 1 *abuse and maltreatment in pregnancy (O9A.3-, O9A.4-, O9A.5-)*
adult and child maltreatment, suspected (T76.-)

The appropriate 7th character is to be added to each code from category T74.
- A initial encounter
- D subsequent encounter
- S sequela

T74.Ø **Neglect or abandonment, confirmed**

T74.Ø1 **Adult neglect or abandonment, confirmed** CC A

T74.Ø2 **Child neglect or abandonment, confirmed** CC P

T74.1 **Physical abuse, confirmed**

EXCLUDES 2 *sexual abuse (T74.2-)*

T74.11 **Adult physical abuse, confirmed** CC A

T74.12 **Child physical abuse, confirmed** CC P

EXCLUDES 2 *shaken infant syndrome (T74.4)*

T74.2 **Sexual abuse, confirmed**

Rape, confirmed

Sexual assault, confirmed

T74.21 **Adult sexual abuse, confirmed** CC A

T74.22 **Child sexual abuse, confirmed** CC P

T74.3 **Psychological abuse, confirmed**

Bullying and intimidation, confirmed

Intimidation through social media, confirmed

T74.31 **Adult psychological abuse, confirmed** A

T74.32 **Child psychological abuse, confirmed** CC P

T74.4 **Shaken infant syndrome** CC P

T74.5 **Forced sexual exploitation, confirmed**

AHA: 2018,4Q,32-33,65

T74.51 **Adult forced sexual exploitation, confirmed** CC A

T74.52 **Child sexual exploitation, confirmed** CC P

T74.6 **Forced labor exploitation, confirmed**

AHA: 2018,4Q,32-33,65

T74.61 **Adult forced labor exploitation, confirmed** CC A

T74.62 **Child forced labor exploitation, confirmed** CC P

T74.9 **Unspecified maltreatment, confirmed**

T74.91 **Unspecified adult maltreatment, confirmed** CC A

T74.92 **Unspecified child maltreatment, confirmed** CC P

✓4th T75 Other and unspecified effects of other external causes

EXCLUDES 1 *adverse effects NEC (T78.-)*

EXCLUDES 2 *burns (electric) (T2Ø-T31)*

The appropriate 7th character is to be added to each code from category T75.
A initial encounter
D subsequent encounter
S sequela

✓5th T75.Ø Effects of lightning
Struck by lightning

✓x7th T75.ØØ Unspecified effects of lightning
Struck by lightning NOS

✓x7th T75.Ø1 Shock due to being struck by lightning

✓x7th T75.Ø9 Other effects of lightning
Use additional code for other effects of lightning

✓x7th T75.1 Unspecified effects of drowning and nonfatal submersion CC HS
Immersion
EXCLUDES 1 *specified effects of drowning - code to effects*

✓5th T75.2 Effects of vibration

✓x7th T75.2Ø Unspecified effects of vibration

✓x7th T75.21 Pneumatic hammer syndrome

✓x7th T75.22 Traumatic vasospastic syndrome

✓x7th T75.23 Vertigo from infrasound
EXCLUDES 1 *vertigo NOS (R42)*

✓x7th T75.29 Other effects of vibration

✓x7th T75.3 Motion sickness
Airsickness
Seasickness
Travel sickness
Use additional external cause code to identify vehicle or type of motion (Y92.81-, Y93.5-)

✓x7th T75.4 Electrocution
Shock from electric current
Shock from electroshock gun (taser)

✓5th T75.8 Other specified effects of external causes

✓x7th T75.81 Effects of abnormal gravitation [G] forces

✓x7th T75.82 Effects of weightlessness

✓x7th T75.89 Other specified effects of external causes

✓4th T76 Adult and child abuse, neglect and other maltreatment, suspected
Use additional code, if applicable, to identify any associated current injury
EXCLUDES 1 *adult and child maltreatment, confirmed (T74.-)*
suspected abuse and maltreatment in pregnancy (O9A.3-, O9A.4-, O9A.5-)
suspected adult physical abuse, ruled out (ZØ4.71)
suspected adult sexual abuse, ruled out (ZØ4.41)
suspected child physical abuse, ruled out (ZØ4.72)
suspected child sexual abuse, ruled out (ZØ4.42)
AHA: 2018,4Q,72

The appropriate 7th character is to be added to each code from category T76.
A initial encounter
D subsequent encounter
S sequela

✓5th T76.Ø Neglect or abandonment, suspected

✓x7th T76.Ø1 Adult neglect or abandonment, suspected CC A

✓x7th T76.Ø2 Child neglect or abandonment, suspected CC P

✓5th T76.1 Physical abuse, suspected

✓x7th T76.11 Adult physical abuse, suspected CC A

✓x7th T76.12 Child physical abuse, suspected CC P
AHA: 2019,2Q,12

✓5th T76.2 Sexual abuse, suspected
Rape, suspected
EXCLUDES 1 *alleged abuse, ruled out (ZØ4.7)*

✓x7th T76.21 Adult sexual abuse, suspected CC A

✓x7th T76.22 Child sexual abuse, suspected CC P

✓5th T76.3 Psychological abuse, suspected
Bullying and intimidation, suspected
Intimidation through social media, suspected

✓x7th T76.31 Adult psychological abuse, suspected A

✓x7th T76.32 Child psychological abuse, suspected CC P

✓5th T76.5 Forced sexual exploitation, suspected
AHA: 2018,4Q,32-33,65

✓x7th T76.51 Adult forced sexual exploitation, suspected CC A

✓x7th T76.52 Child sexual exploitation, suspected CC P

✓5th T76.6 Forced labor exploitation, suspected
AHA: 2018,4Q,32-33,65

✓x7th T76.61 Adult forced labor exploitation, suspected CC A

✓x7th T76.62 Child forced labor exploitation, suspected CC P

✓5th T76.9 Unspecified maltreatment, suspected

✓x7th T76.91 Unspecified adult maltreatment, suspected CC A

✓x7th T76.92 Unspecified child maltreatment, suspected CC P

✓4th T78 Adverse effects, not elsewhere classified
EXCLUDES 2 *complications of surgical and medical care NEC (T8Ø-T88)*

The appropriate 7th character is to be added to each code from category T78.
A initial encounter
D subsequent encounter
S sequela

✓5th T78.Ø Anaphylactic reaction due to food
Anaphylactic reaction due to adverse food reaction
Anaphylactic shock or reaction due to nonpoisonous foods
Anaphylactoid reaction due to food

✓x7th T78.ØØ Anaphylactic reaction due to unspecified food CC

✓x7th T78.Ø1 Anaphylactic reaction due to peanuts CC

✓x7th T78.Ø2 Anaphylactic reaction due to shellfish (crustaceans) CC

✓x7th T78.Ø3 Anaphylactic reaction due to other fish CC

✓x7th T78.Ø4 Anaphylactic reaction due to fruits and vegetables CC

✓x7th T78.Ø5 Anaphylactic reaction due to tree nuts and seeds CC
EXCLUDES 2 *anaphylactic reaction due to peanuts (T78.Ø1)*

✓x7th T78.Ø6 Anaphylactic reaction due to food additives CC

✓x7th T78.Ø7 Anaphylactic reaction due to milk and dairy products CC

✓x7th T78.Ø8 Anaphylactic reaction due to eggs CC

✓x7th T78.Ø9 Anaphylactic reaction due to other food products CC

✓x7th T78.1 Other adverse food reactions, not elsewhere classified
Use additional code to identify the type of reaction, if applicable
EXCLUDES 1 *anaphylactic reaction or shock due to adverse food reaction (T78.Ø-)*
anaphylactic reaction due to food (T78.Ø-)
bacterial food borne intoxications (AØ5.-)
EXCLUDES 2 *allergic and dietetic gastroenteritis and colitis (K52.29)*
allergic rhinitis due to food (J3Ø.5)
dermatitis due to food in contact with skin (L23.6, L24.6, L25.4)
dermatitis due to ingested food (L27.2)
food protein-induced enterocolitis syndrome (K52.21)
food protein-induced enteropathy (K52.22)

✓x7th T78.2 Anaphylactic shock, unspecified CC
Allergic shock
Anaphylactic reaction
Anaphylaxis
EXCLUDES 1 *anaphylactic reaction or shock due to adverse effect of correct medicinal substance properly administered (T88.6)*
anaphylactic reaction or shock due to adverse food reaction (T78.Ø-)
anaphylactic reaction or shock due to serum (T8Ø.5-)

N Newborn: 0 P Pediatric: 0-17 M Maternity: 9-64 A Adult: 15-124 UNS Unspecified Site MCC Major Complication/Comorbidity CC Complication/Comorbidity

√x7th **T78.3 Angioneurotic edema**
Allergic angioedema
Giant urticaria
Quincke's edema
EXCLUDES 1 *serum urticaria (T8Ø.6-)*
urticaria (L5Ø.-)

√5th **T78.4 Other and unspecified allergy**
EXCLUDES 1 *specified types of allergic reaction such as:*
allergic diarrhea (K52.29)
allergic gastroenteritis and colitis (K52.29)
dermatitis (L23-L25, L27.-)
food protein-induced enterocolitis syndrome (K52.21)
food protein-induced enteropathy (K52.22)
hay fever (J3Ø.1)

√x7th **T78.4Ø Allergy, unspecified**
Allergic reaction NOS
Hypersensitivity NOS

√x7th **T78.41 Arthus phenomenon**
Arthus reaction

√x7th **T78.49 Other allergy**
AHA: 2021,1Q,42

√x7th **T78.8 Other adverse effects, not elsewhere classified**

Certain early complications of trauma (T79)

√4th **T79 Certain early complications of trauma, not elsewhere classified**
EXCLUDES 2 *acute respiratory distress syndrome (J8Ø)*
complications occurring during or following medical procedures (T8Ø-T88)
complications of surgical and medical care NEC (T8Ø-T88)
newborn respiratory distress syndrome (P22.Ø)

The appropriate 7th character is to be added to each code from category T79.
A initial encounter
D subsequent encounter
S sequela

6 √x7th **T79.Ø Air embolism (traumatic)** MCC HCC
EXCLUDES 1 *air embolism complicating abortion or ectopic or molar pregnancy (OØØ-OØ7, OØ8.2)*
air embolism complicating pregnancy, childbirth and the puerperium (O88.Ø)
air embolism following infusion, transfusion, and therapeutic injection (T8Ø.Ø)
air embolism following procedure NEC (T81.7-)
DEF: Arterial or venous obstruction due to the introduction of air bubbles into the blood vessels following surgery or trauma.

6 √x7th **T79.1 Fat embolism (traumatic)** MCC HCC
EXCLUDES 1 *fat embolism complicating:*
abortion or ectopic or molar pregnancy (OØØ-OØ7, OØ8.2)
pregnancy, childbirth and the puerperium (O88.8)
DEF: Arterial blockage due to the entrance of fat into the circulatory system after a fracture of the large bones or administration of corticosteroids.

6 √x7th **T79.2 Traumatic secondary and recurrent hemorrhage and seroma** CC HCC

6 √x7th **T79.4 Traumatic shock** MCC HCC
Shock (immediate) (delayed) following injury
EXCLUDES 1 *anaphylactic shock due to adverse food reaction (T78.Ø-)*
anaphylactic shock due to correct medicinal substance properly administered (T88.6)
anaphylactic shock due to serum (T8Ø.5-)
anaphylactic shock NOS (T78.2)
electric shock (T75.4)
nontraumatic shock NEC (R57.-)
obstetric shock (O75.1)
postprocedural shock (T81.1-)
septic shock (R65.21)
shock complicating abortion or ectopic or molar pregnancy (OØØ-OØ7, OØ8.3)
shock due to anesthesia (T88.2)
shock due to lightning (T75.Ø1)
shock NOS (R57.9)

6 √x7th **T79.5 Traumatic anuria** MCC HCC
Crush syndrome
Renal failure following crushing

6 √x7th **T79.6 Traumatic ischemia of muscle** HCC
Traumatic rhabdomyolysis
Volkmann's ischemic contracture
EXCLUDES 2 *anterior tibial syndrome (M76.8)*
compartment syndrome (traumatic) (T79.A-)
nontraumatic ischemia of muscle (M62.2-)
AHA: 2019,2Q,12

6 √x7th **T79.7 Traumatic subcutaneous emphysema** CC HCC
EXCLUDES 2 *emphysema NOS (J43)*
emphysema (subcutaneous) resulting from a procedure (T81.82)

√5th **T79.A Traumatic compartment syndrome**
EXCLUDES 1 *fibromyalgia (M79.7)*
nontraumatic compartment syndrome (M79.A-)
EXCLUDES 2 *traumatic ischemic infarction of muscle (T79.6)*
DEF: Compression of nerves and blood vessels within an enclosed muscle space due to previous trauma, which leads to impaired blood flow and muscle and nerve damage.

6 √x7th **T79.AØ Compartment syndrome, unspecified** CC HCC
Compartment syndrome NOS

√6th **T79.A1 Traumatic compartment syndrome of upper extremity**
Traumatic compartment syndrome of shoulder, arm, forearm, wrist, hand, and fingers

6 √7th **T79.A11 Traumatic compartment syndrome of right upper extremity** CC HCC
6 √7th **T79.A12 Traumatic compartment syndrome of left upper extremity** CC HCC
6 √7th **T79.A19 Traumatic compartment syndrome of unspecified upper extremity** CC UNS HCC

√6th **T79.A2 Traumatic compartment syndrome of lower extremity**
Traumatic compartment syndrome of hip, buttock, thigh, leg, foot, and toes

6 √7th **T79.A21 Traumatic compartment syndrome of right lower extremity** CC HCC
6 √7th **T79.A22 Traumatic compartment syndrome of left lower extremity** CC HCC
6 √7th **T79.A29 Traumatic compartment syndrome of unspecified lower extremity** CC UNS HCC

6 √x7th **T79.A3 Traumatic compartment syndrome of abdomen** CC HCC

6 √x7th **T79.A9 Traumatic compartment syndrome of other sites** CC HCC

6 √x7th **T79.8 Other early complications of trauma** HCC

6 √x7th **T79.9 Unspecified early complication of trauma** HCC

Complications of surgical and medical care, not elsewhere classified (T8Ø-T88)

Use additional code for adverse effect, if applicable, to identify drug (T36-T5Ø with fifth or sixth character 5)
Use additional code(s) to identify the specified condition resulting from the complication
Use additional code to identify devices involved and details of circumstances (Y62-Y82)

EXCLUDES 2 *any encounters with medical care for postprocedural conditions in which no complications are present, such as:*
artificial opening status (Z93.-)
closure of external stoma (Z43.-)
fitting and adjustment of external prosthetic device (Z44.-)
burns and corrosions from local applications and irradiation (T2Ø-T32)
complications of surgical procedures during pregnancy, childbirth and the puerperium (OØØ-O9A)
mechanical complication of respirator [ventilator] (J95.85Ø)
poisoning and toxic effects of drugs and chemicals (T36-T65 with fifth or sixth character 1-4 or 6)
postprocedural fever (R5Ø.82)
specified complications classified elsewhere, such as:
cerebrospinal fluid leak from spinal puncture (G97.Ø)
colostomy malfunction (K94.Ø-)
disorders of fluid and electrolyte imbalance (E86-E87)
functional disturbances following cardiac surgery (I97.Ø-I97.1)
intraoperative and postprocedural complications of specified body systems (D78.-, E36.-, E89.-, G97.3-, G97.4, H59.3-, H59.-, H95.2-, H95.3, I97.4-, I97.5, J95.6-, J95.7, K91.6-, L76.-, M96.-, N99.-)
ostomy complications (J95.Ø-, K94.-, N99.5-)
postgastric surgery syndromes (K91.1)
postlaminectomy syndrome NEC (M96.1)
postmastectomy lymphedema syndrome (I97.2)
postsurgical blind-loop syndrome (K91.2)
ventilator associated pneumonia (J95.851)

AHA: 2015,1Q,15

✓4th T8Ø Complications following infusion, transfusion and therapeutic injection

INCLUDES complications following perfusion

EXCLUDES 2 *bone marrow transplant rejection (T86.Ø1)*
febrile nonhemolytic transfusion reaction (R5Ø.84)
fluid overload due to transfusion (E87.71)
posttransfusion purpura (D69.51)
transfusion associated circulatory overload (TACO) (E87.71)
transfusion (red blood cell) associated hemochromatosis (E83.111)
transfusion related acute lung injury (TRALI) (J95.84)

The appropriate 7th character is to be added to each code from category T8Ø.
A initial encounter
D subsequent encounter
S sequela

✓x7th T8Ø.Ø Air embolism following infusion, transfusion and therapeutic injection MCC H2

✓x7th T8Ø.1 Vascular complications following infusion, transfusion and therapeutic injection CC

Use additional code to identify the vascular complication

EXCLUDES 2 *extravasation of vesicant agent (T8Ø.81-)*
infiltration of vesicant agent (T8Ø.81-)
postprocedural vascular complications (T81.7-)
vascular complications specified as due to prosthetic devices, implants and grafts (T82.8-, T83.8-, T84.8-, T85.8-)

✓5th T8Ø.2 Infections following infusion, transfusion and therapeutic injection

Use additional code to identify the specific infection, such as: sepsis (A41.9)
Use additional code (R65.2-) to identify severe sepsis, if applicable

EXCLUDES 2 *infections specified as due to prosthetic devices, implants and grafts (T82.6-T82.7, T83.5-T83.6, T84.5-T84.7, T85.7)*
postprocedural infections (T81.4-)

AHA: 2018,4Q,62

✓6th T8Ø.21 Infection due to central venous catheter

Infection due to pulmonary artery catheter (Swan-Ganz catheter)

AHA: 2019,1Q,13-14

DEF: Central venous catheter: Catheter positioned in the superior vena cava or right atrium and introduced through a large vein, such as the jugular or subclavian, and used to measure venous pressure or administer fluids or medication.

TIP: Code assignment is based on the location of the catheter and not how the catheter is being used; for example, for hemodialysis. Infections resulting from catheters that are not central lines should be coded to T82.7-.

✓7th T8Ø.211 Bloodstream infection due to central venous catheter CC H7

Catheter-related bloodstream infection (CRBSI) NOS
Central line-associated bloodstream infection (CLABSI)
Bloodstream infection due to Hickman catheter
Bloodstream infection due to peripherally inserted central catheter (PICC)
Bloodstream infection due to portacath (port-a-cath)
Bloodstream infection due to pulmonary artery catheter
Bloodstream infection due to triple lumen catheter
Bloodstream infection due to umbilical venous catheter

AHA: 2019,1Q,13,14; 2018,4Q,89

✓7th T8Ø.212 Local infection due to central venous catheter CC H7

Exit or insertion site infection
Local infection due to Hickman catheter
Local infection due to peripherally inserted central catheter (PICC)
Local infection due to portacath (port-a-cath)
Local infection due to pulmonary artery catheter
Local infection due to triple lumen catheter
Local infection due to umbilical venous catheter
Port or reservoir infection
Tunnel infection

✓7th T8Ø.218 Other infection due to central venous catheter CC H7

Other central line-associated infection
Other infection due to Hickman catheter
Other infection due to peripherally inserted central catheter (PICC)
Other infection due to portacath (port-a-cath)
Other infection due to pulmonary artery catheter
Other infection due to triple lumen catheter
Other infection due to umbilical venous catheter

T80.219 **Unspecified infection due to central venous catheter** CC H7
Central line-associated infection NOS
Unspecified infection due to Hickman catheter
Unspecified infection due to peripherally inserted central catheter (PICC)
Unspecified infection due to portacath (port-a-cath)
Unspecified infection due to pulmonary artery catheter
Unspecified infection due to triple lumen catheter
Unspecified infection due to umbilical venous catheter

T80.22 **Acute infection following transfusion, infusion, or injection of blood and blood products** CC

T80.29 **Infection following other infusion, transfusion and therapeutic injection** CC

T80.3 **ABO incompatibility reaction due to transfusion of blood or blood products**
EXCLUDES 1 *minor blood group antigens reactions (Duffy) (E) (K) (Kell) (Kidd) (Lewis) (M) (N) (P) (S) (T80.A-)*

T80.30 **ABO incompatibility reaction due to transfusion of blood or blood products, unspecified** CC H3
ABO incompatibility blood transfusion NOS
Reaction to ABO incompatibility from transfusion NOS

T80.31 **ABO incompatibility with hemolytic transfusion reaction**

T80.310 **ABO incompatibility with acute hemolytic transfusion reaction** CC H3
ABO incompatibility with hemolytic transfusion reaction less than 24 hours after transfusion
Acute hemolytic transfusion reaction (AHTR) due to ABO incompatibility

T80.311 **ABO incompatibility with delayed hemolytic transfusion reaction** CC H3
ABO incompatibility with hemolytic transfusion reaction 24 hours or more after transfusion
Delayed hemolytic transfusion reaction (DHTR) due to ABO incompatibility

T80.319 **ABO incompatibility with hemolytic transfusion reaction, unspecified** CC H3
ABO incompatibility with hemolytic transfusion reaction at unspecified time after transfusion
Hemolytic transfusion reaction (HTR) due to ABO incompatibility NOS

T80.39 **Other ABO incompatibility reaction due to transfusion of blood or blood products** CC H3
Delayed serologic transfusion reaction (DSTR) from ABO incompatibility
Other ABO incompatible blood transfusion
Other reaction to ABO incompatible blood transfusion

T80.4 **Rh incompatibility reaction due to transfusion of blood or blood products**
Reaction due to incompatibility of Rh antigens (C) (c) (D) (E) (e)

T80.40 **Rh incompatibility reaction due to transfusion of blood or blood products, unspecified** CC
Reaction due to Rh factor in transfusion NOS
Rh incompatible blood transfusion NOS

T80.41 **Rh incompatibility with hemolytic transfusion reaction**

T80.410 **Rh incompatibility with acute hemolytic transfusion reaction** CC
Acute hemolytic transfusion reaction (AHTR) due to Rh incompatibility
Rh incompatibility with hemolytic transfusion reaction less than 24 hours after transfusion

T80.411 **Rh incompatibility with delayed hemolytic transfusion reaction** CC
Delayed hemolytic transfusion reaction (DHTR) due to Rh incompatibility
Rh incompatibility with hemolytic transfusion reaction 24 hours or more after transfusion

T80.419 **Rh incompatibility with hemolytic transfusion reaction, unspecified** CC
Rh incompatibility with hemolytic transfusion reaction at unspecified time after transfusion
Hemolytic transfusion reaction (HTR) due to Rh incompatibility NOS

T80.49 **Other Rh incompatibility reaction due to transfusion of blood or blood products** CC
Delayed serologic transfusion reaction (DSTR) from Rh incompatibility
Other reaction to Rh incompatible blood transfusion

T80.A **Non-ABO incompatibility reaction due to transfusion of blood or blood products**
Reaction due to incompatibility of minor antigens (Duffy) (Kell) (Kidd) (Lewis) (M) (N) (P) (S)

T80.A0 **Non-ABO incompatibility reaction due to transfusion of blood or blood products, unspecified** CC
Non-ABO antigen incompatibility reaction from transfusion NOS

T80.A1 **Non-ABO incompatibility with hemolytic transfusion reaction**

T80.A10 **Non-ABO incompatibility with acute hemolytic transfusion reaction** CC
Acute hemolytic transfusion reaction (AHTR) due to non-ABO incompatibility
Non-ABO incompatibility with hemolytic transfusion reaction less than 24 hours after transfusion

T80.A11 **Non-ABO incompatibility with delayed hemolytic transfusion reaction** CC
Delayed hemolytic transfusion reaction (DHTR) due to non-ABO incompatibility
Non-ABO incompatibility with hemolytic transfusion reaction 24 or more hours after transfusion

T80.A19 **Non-ABO incompatibility with hemolytic transfusion reaction, unspecified** CC
Hemolytic transfusion reaction (HTR) due to non-ABO incompatibility NOS
Non-ABO incompatibility with hemolytic transfusion reaction at unspecified time after transfusion

T80.A9 **Other non-ABO incompatibility reaction due to transfusion of blood or blood products** CC
Delayed serologic transfusion reaction (DSTR) from non-ABO incompatibility
Other reaction to non-ABO incompatible blood transfusion

T80.5 **Anaphylactic reaction due to serum**
Allergic shock due to serum
Anaphylactic shock due to serum
Anaphylactoid reaction due to serum
Anaphylaxis due to serum
EXCLUDES 1 *ABO incompatibility reaction due to transfusion of blood or blood products (T80.3-)*
allergic reaction or shock NOS (T78.2)
anaphylactic reaction or shock NOS (T78.2)
anaphylactic reaction or shock due to adverse effect of correct medicinal substance properly administered (T88.6)
other serum reaction (T80.6-)
DEF: Life-threatening hypersensitivity to a foreign serum causing respiratory distress, vascular collapse, and shock.

T80.51 **Anaphylactic reaction due to administration of blood and blood products** CC

T80.52 **Anaphylactic reaction due to vaccination** CC
AHA: 2021,1Q,43

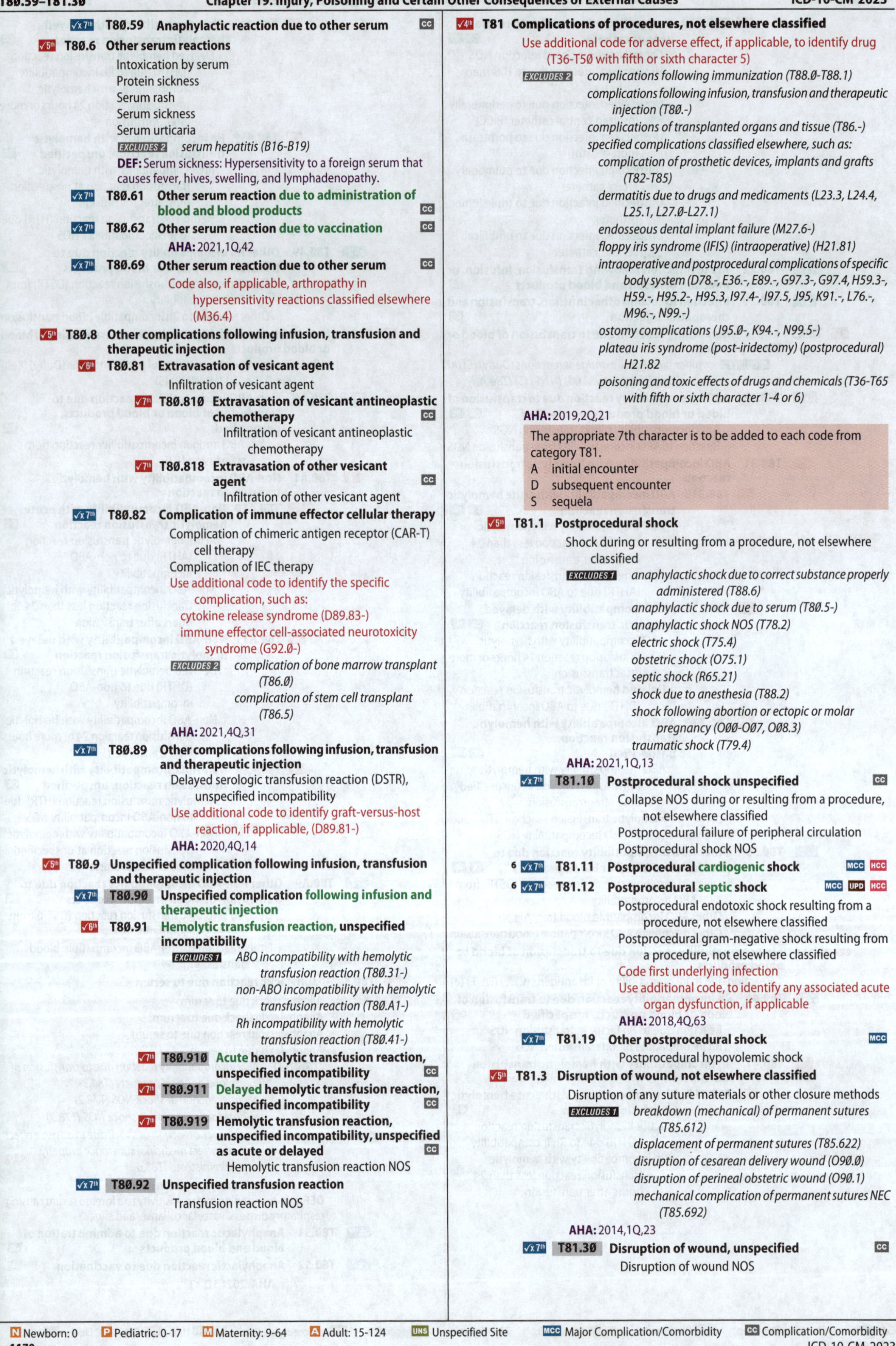

T80.59 Anaphylactic reaction due to other serum CC

T80.6 Other serum reactions
Intoxication by serum
Protein sickness
Serum rash
Serum sickness
Serum urticaria
EXCLUDES 2 *serum hepatitis (B16-B19)*
DEF: Serum sickness: Hypersensitivity to a foreign serum that causes fever, hives, swelling, and lymphadenopathy.

T80.61 Other serum reaction due to administration of blood and blood products CC

T80.62 Other serum reaction due to vaccination CC
AHA: 2021,1Q,42

T80.69 Other serum reaction due to other serum CC
Code also, if applicable, arthropathy in hypersensitivity reactions classified elsewhere (M36.4)

T80.8 Other complications following infusion, transfusion and therapeutic injection

T80.81 Extravasation of vesicant agent
Infiltration of vesicant agent

T80.810 Extravasation of vesicant antineoplastic chemotherapy CC
Infiltration of vesicant antineoplastic chemotherapy

T80.818 Extravasation of other vesicant agent CC
Infiltration of other vesicant agent

T80.82 Complication of immune effector cellular therapy
Complication of chimeric antigen receptor (CAR-T) cell therapy
Complication of IEC therapy
Use additional code to identify the specific complication, such as:
cytokine release syndrome (D89.83-)
immune effector cell-associated neurotoxicity syndrome (G92.0-)
EXCLUDES 2 *complication of bone marrow transplant (T86.0)*
complication of stem cell transplant (T86.5)
AHA: 2021,4Q,31

T80.89 Other complications following infusion, transfusion and therapeutic injection
Delayed serologic transfusion reaction (DSTR), unspecified incompatibility
Use additional code to identify graft-versus-host reaction, if applicable, (D89.81-)
AHA: 2020,4Q,14

T80.9 Unspecified complication following infusion, transfusion and therapeutic injection

T80.90 Unspecified complication following infusion and therapeutic injection

T80.91 Hemolytic transfusion reaction, unspecified incompatibility
EXCLUDES 1 *ABO incompatibility with hemolytic transfusion reaction (T80.31-)*
non-ABO incompatibility with hemolytic transfusion reaction (T80.A1-)
Rh incompatibility with hemolytic transfusion reaction (T80.41-)

T80.910 Acute hemolytic transfusion reaction, unspecified incompatibility CC

T80.911 Delayed hemolytic transfusion reaction, unspecified incompatibility CC

T80.919 Hemolytic transfusion reaction, unspecified incompatibility, unspecified as acute or delayed CC
Hemolytic transfusion reaction NOS

T80.92 Unspecified transfusion reaction
Transfusion reaction NOS

T81 Complications of procedures, not elsewhere classified
Use additional code for adverse effect, if applicable, to identify drug (T36-T50 with fifth or sixth character 5)
EXCLUDES 2 *complications following immunization (T88.0-T88.1)*
complications following infusion, transfusion and therapeutic injection (T80.-)
complications of transplanted organs and tissue (T86.-)
specified complications classified elsewhere, such as:
complication of prosthetic devices, implants and grafts (T82-T85)
dermatitis due to drugs and medicaments (L23.3, L24.4, L25.1, L27.0-L27.1)
endosseous dental implant failure (M27.6-)
floppy iris syndrome (IFIS) (intraoperative) (H21.81)
intraoperative and postprocedural complications of specific body system (D78.-, E36.-, E89.-, G97.3-, G97.4, H59.3-, H59.-, H95.2-, H95.3, I97.4-, I97.5, J95, K91.-, L76.-, M96.-, N99.-)
ostomy complications (J95.0-, K94.-, N99.5-)
plateau iris syndrome (post-iridectomy) (postprocedural) H21.82
poisoning and toxic effects of drugs and chemicals (T36-T65 with fifth or sixth character 1-4 or 6)
AHA: 2019,2Q,21

The appropriate 7th character is to be added to each code from category T81.
A initial encounter
D subsequent encounter
S sequela

T81.1 Postprocedural shock
Shock during or resulting from a procedure, not elsewhere classified
EXCLUDES 1 *anaphylactic shock due to correct substance properly administered (T88.6)*
anaphylactic shock due to serum (T80.5-)
anaphylactic shock NOS (T78.2)
electric shock (T75.4)
obstetric shock (O75.1)
septic shock (R65.21)
shock due to anesthesia (T88.2)
shock following abortion or ectopic or molar pregnancy (O00-O07, O08.3)
traumatic shock (T79.4)
AHA: 2021,1Q,13

T81.10 Postprocedural shock unspecified CC
Collapse NOS during or resulting from a procedure, not elsewhere classified
Postprocedural failure of peripheral circulation
Postprocedural shock NOS

6 **T81.11 Postprocedural cardiogenic shock** MCC HCC

6 **T81.12 Postprocedural septic shock** MCC UPD HCC
Postprocedural endotoxic shock resulting from a procedure, not elsewhere classified
Postprocedural gram-negative shock resulting from a procedure, not elsewhere classified
Code first underlying infection
Use additional code, to identify any associated acute organ dysfunction, if applicable
AHA: 2018,4Q,63

T81.19 Other postprocedural shock MCC
Postprocedural hypovolemic shock

T81.3 Disruption of wound, not elsewhere classified
Disruption of any suture materials or other closure methods
EXCLUDES 1 *breakdown (mechanical) of permanent sutures (T85.612)*
displacement of permanent sutures (T85.622)
disruption of cesarean delivery wound (O90.0)
disruption of perineal obstetric wound (O90.1)
mechanical complication of permanent sutures NEC (T85.692)
AHA: 2014,1Q,23

T81.30 Disruption of wound, unspecified CC
Disruption of wound NOS

√x7th **T81.31 Disruption of external operation (surgical) wound, not elsewhere classified** CC
Dehiscence of operation wound NOS
Disruption of operation wound NOS
Disruption or dehiscence of closure of cornea
Disruption or dehiscence of closure of mucosa
Disruption or dehiscence of closure of skin and subcutaneous tissue
Full-thickness skin disruption or dehiscence
Superficial disruption or dehiscence of operation wound
EXCLUDES 1 *dehiscence of amputation stump (T87.81)*

√x7th **T81.32 Disruption of internal operation (surgical) wound, not elsewhere classified** CC
Deep disruption or dehiscence of operation wound NOS
Disruption or dehiscence of closure of internal organ or other internal tissue
Disruption or dehiscence of closure of muscle or muscle flap
Disruption or dehiscence of closure of ribs or rib cage
Disruption or dehiscence of closure of skull or craniotomy
Disruption or dehiscence of closure of sternum or sternotomy
Disruption or dehiscence of closure of tendon or ligament
Disruption or dehiscence of closure of superficial or muscular fascia
AHA: 2020,2Q,22; 2017,3Q,4

√x7th **T81.33 Disruption of traumatic injury wound repair** CC
Disruption or dehiscence of closure of traumatic laceration (external) (internal)

√5th **T81.4 Infection following a procedure**
Wound abscess following a procedure
Use additional code to identify infection
Use additional code (R65.2-) to identify severe sepsis, if applicable
EXCLUDES 2 *bleb associated endophthalmitis (H59.4-)*
infection due to infusion, transfusion and therapeutic injection (T80.2-)
infection due to prosthetic devices, implants and grafts (T82.6-T82.7, T83.5-T83.6, T84.5-T84.7, T85.7)
obstetric surgical wound infection (O86.0-)
postprocedural fever NOS (R50.82)
postprocedural retroperitoneal abscess (K68.11)
AHA: 2018,4Q,33-34,62; 2014,1Q,23

√x7th **T81.40 Infection following a procedure, unspecified** CC H11 H12 H13

√x7th **T81.41 Infection following a procedure, superficial incisional surgical site** CC H11 H12 H13
Subcutaneous abscess following a procedure
Stitch abscess following a procedure

√x7th **T81.42 Infection following a procedure, deep incisional surgical site** CC H11 H12 H13
Intra-muscular abscess following a procedure

√x7th **T81.43 Infection following a procedure, organ and space surgical site** CC H11 H12 H13
Intra-abdominal abscess following a procedure
Subphrenic abscess following a procedure

6 √x7th **T81.44 Sepsis following a procedure** CC H11 H12 H13 HCC
Use additional code to identify the sepsis

√x7th **T81.49 Infection following a procedure, other surgical site** CC H11 H12 H13

√5th **T81.5 Complications of foreign body accidentally left in body following procedure**
AHA: 2014,4Q,24

√6th **T81.50 Unspecified complication of foreign body accidentally left in body following procedure**

√7th **T81.500 Unspecified complication of foreign body accidentally left in body following surgical operation** CC H1

√7th **T81.501 Unspecified complication of foreign body accidentally left in body following infusion or transfusion** CC H1

√7th **T81.502 Unspecified complication of foreign body accidentally left in body following kidney dialysis** CC H1 HCC

√7th **T81.503 Unspecified complication of foreign body accidentally left in body following injection or immunization** CC H1

√7th **T81.504 Unspecified complication of foreign body accidentally left in body following endoscopic examination** CC H1

√7th **T81.505 Unspecified complication of foreign body accidentally left in body following heart catheterization** CC H1

√7th **T81.506 Unspecified complication of foreign body accidentally left in body following aspiration, puncture or other catheterization** CC H1

√7th **T81.507 Unspecified complication of foreign body accidentally left in body following removal of catheter or packing** CC H1

√7th **T81.508 Unspecified complication of foreign body accidentally left in body following other procedure** CC H1

√7th **T81.509 Unspecified complication of foreign body accidentally left in body following unspecified procedure** CC H1

√6th **T81.51 Adhesions due to foreign body accidentally left in body following procedure**

√7th **T81.510 Adhesions due to foreign body accidentally left in body following surgical operation** CC H1

√7th **T81.511 Adhesions due to foreign body accidentally left in body following infusion or transfusion** CC H1

√7th **T81.512 Adhesions due to foreign body accidentally left in body following kidney dialysis** CC H1 HCC

√7th **T81.513 Adhesions due to foreign body accidentally left in body following injection or immunization** CC H1

√7th **T81.514 Adhesions due to foreign body accidentally left in body following endoscopic examination** CC H1

√7th **T81.515 Adhesions due to foreign body accidentally left in body following heart catheterization** CC H1

√7th **T81.516 Adhesions due to foreign body accidentally left in body following aspiration, puncture or other catheterization** CC H1

√7th **T81.517 Adhesions due to foreign body accidentally left in body following removal of catheter or packing** CC H1

√7th **T81.518 Adhesions due to foreign body accidentally left in body following other procedure** CC H1

√7th **T81.519 Adhesions due to foreign body accidentally left in body following unspecified procedure** CC H1

√6th **T81.52 Obstruction due to foreign body accidentally left in body following procedure**

√7th **T81.520 Obstruction due to foreign body accidentally left in body following surgical operation** CC H1

√7th **T81.521 Obstruction due to foreign body accidentally left in body following infusion or transfusion** CC H1

√7th **T81.522 Obstruction due to foreign body accidentally left in body following kidney dialysis** CC H1 HCC

√7th **T81.523 Obstruction due to foreign body accidentally left in body following injection or immunization** CC H1

√7th **T81.524 Obstruction due to foreign body accidentally left in body following endoscopic examination** CC H1

√7th **T81.525 Obstruction due to foreign body accidentally left in body following heart catheterization** CC H1

√7th **T81.526 Obstruction due to foreign body accidentally left in body following aspiration, puncture or other catheterization** CC H1

T81.527 Obstruction due to foreign body accidentally left in body following removal of catheter or packing CC H1

T81.528 Obstruction due to foreign body accidentally left in body following other procedure CC H1

T81.529 Obstruction due to foreign body accidentally left in body following unspecified procedure CC H1

T81.53 Perforation due to foreign body accidentally left in body following procedure

T81.530 Perforation due to foreign body accidentally left in body following surgical operation CC H1

T81.531 Perforation due to foreign body accidentally left in body following infusion or transfusion CC H1

T81.532 Perforation due to foreign body accidentally left in body following kidney dialysis CC H1 HCC

T81.533 Perforation due to foreign body accidentally left in body following injection or immunization CC H1

T81.534 Perforation due to foreign body accidentally left in body following endoscopic examination CC H1

T81.535 Perforation due to foreign body accidentally left in body following heart catheterization CC H1

T81.536 Perforation due to foreign body accidentally left in body following aspiration, puncture or other catheterization CC H1

T81.537 Perforation due to foreign body accidentally left in body following removal of catheter or packing CC H1

T81.538 Perforation due to foreign body accidentally left in body following other procedure CC H1

T81.539 Perforation due to foreign body accidentally left in body following unspecified procedure CC H1

T81.59 Other complications of foreign body accidentally left in body following procedure

EXCLUDES 2 *obstruction or perforation due to prosthetic devices and implants intentionally left in body (T82.0-T82.5, T83.0-T83.4, T83.7, T84.0-T84.4, T85.0-T85.6)*

T81.590 Other complications of foreign body accidentally left in body following surgical operation CC H1

T81.591 Other complications of foreign body accidentally left in body following infusion or transfusion CC H1

T81.592 Other complications of foreign body accidentally left in body following kidney dialysis CC H1 HCC

T81.593 Other complications of foreign body accidentally left in body following injection or immunization CC H1

T81.594 Other complications of foreign body accidentally left in body following endoscopic examination CC H1

T81.595 Other complications of foreign body accidentally left in body following heart catheterization CC H1

T81.596 Other complications of foreign body accidentally left in body following aspiration, puncture or other catheterization CC H1

T81.597 Other complications of foreign body accidentally left in body following removal of catheter or packing CC H1

T81.598 Other complications of foreign body accidentally left in body following other procedure CC H1

T81.599 Other complications of foreign body accidentally left in body following unspecified procedure CC H1

T81.6 Acute reaction to foreign substance accidentally left during a procedure

EXCLUDES 2 *complications of foreign body accidentally left in body cavity or operation wound following procedure (T81.5-)*

T81.60 Unspecified acute reaction to foreign substance accidentally left during a procedure CC H1

T81.61 Aseptic peritonitis due to foreign substance accidentally left during a procedure CC H1

Chemical peritonitis

T81.69 Other acute reaction to foreign substance accidentally left during a procedure CC H1

T81.7 Vascular complications following a procedure, not elsewhere classified

Air embolism following procedure NEC

Phlebitis or thrombophlebitis resulting from a procedure

EXCLUDES 1 *embolism complicating abortion or ectopic or molar pregnancy (O00-O07, O08.2)*

embolism complicating pregnancy, childbirth and the puerperium (O88.-)

traumatic embolism (T79.0)

EXCLUDES 2 *embolism due to prosthetic devices, implants and grafts (T82.8-, T83.81, T84.8-, T85.81-)*

embolism following infusion, transfusion and therapeutic injection (T80.0)

AHA: 2019,2Q,22

T81.71 Complication of artery following a procedure, not elsewhere classified

T81.710 Complication of mesenteric artery following a procedure, not elsewhere classified CC

T81.711 Complication of renal artery following a procedure, not elsewhere classified CC

T81.718 Complication of other artery following a procedure, not elsewhere classified CC

AHA: 2019,2Q,21-22

T81.719 Complication of unspecified artery following a procedure, not elsewhere classified CC

T81.72 Complication of vein following a procedure, not elsewhere classified CC

T81.8 Other complications of procedures, not elsewhere classified

EXCLUDES 2 *hypothermia following anesthesia (T88.51)*

malignant hyperpyrexia due to anesthesia (T88.3)

T81.81 Complication of inhalation therapy

T81.82 Emphysema (subcutaneous) resulting from a procedure

T81.83 Persistent postprocedural fistula CC

AHA: 2017,3Q,3-4

T81.89 Other complications of procedures, not elsewhere classified

Use additional code to specify complication, such as: postprocedural delirium (F05)

AHA: 2014,1Q,23

T81.9 Unspecified complication of procedure

T82 Complications of cardiac and vascular prosthetic devices, implants and grafts

EXCLUDES 2 *failure and rejection of transplanted organs and tissue (T86.-)*

AHA: 2020,3Q,36-37

The appropriate 7th character is to be added to each code from category T82.

A initial encounter

D subsequent encounter

S sequela

T82.0 Mechanical complication of heart valve prosthesis

Mechanical complication of artificial heart valve

EXCLUDES 1 *mechanical complication of biological heart valve graft (T82.22-)*

T82.01 Breakdown (mechanical) of heart valve prosthesis CC

T82.02 Displacement of heart valve prosthesis CC

Malposition of heart valve prosthesis

T82.03 Leakage of heart valve prosthesis CC

T82.09 Other mechanical complication of heart valve prosthesis CC
Obstruction (mechanical) of heart valve prosthesis
Perforation of heart valve prosthesis
Protrusion of heart valve prosthesis

T82.1 Mechanical complication of cardiac electronic device

T82.11 Breakdown (mechanical) of cardiac electronic device
- **T82.110 Breakdown (mechanical) of cardiac electrode** CC
- **T82.111 Breakdown (mechanical) of cardiac pulse generator (battery)** CC
- **T82.118 Breakdown (mechanical) of other cardiac electronic device** CC
- **T82.119 Breakdown (mechanical) of unspecified cardiac electronic device** CC

T82.12 Displacement of cardiac electronic device
Malposition of cardiac electronic device
- **T82.120 Displacement of cardiac electrode** CC
- **T82.121 Displacement of cardiac pulse generator (battery)** CC
- **T82.128 Displacement of other cardiac electronic device** CC
- **T82.129 Displacement of unspecified cardiac electronic device** CC

T82.19 Other mechanical complication of cardiac electronic device
Leakage of cardiac electronic device
Obstruction of cardiac electronic device
Perforation of cardiac electronic device
Protrusion of cardiac electronic device
- **T82.190 Other mechanical complication of cardiac electrode** CC
- **T82.191 Other mechanical complication of cardiac pulse generator (battery)** CC
- **T82.198 Other mechanical complication of other cardiac electronic device** CC
- **T82.199 Other mechanical complication of unspecified cardiac device** CC

T82.2 Mechanical complication of coronary artery bypass graft and biological heart valve graft
EXCLUDES 1 *mechanical complication of artificial heart valve prosthesis (T82.0-)*

T82.21 Mechanical complication of coronary artery bypass graft
- **T82.211 Breakdown (mechanical) of coronary artery bypass graft** CC
- **T82.212 Displacement of coronary artery bypass graft** CC
  Malposition of coronary artery bypass graft
- **T82.213 Leakage of coronary artery bypass graft** CC
- **T82.218 Other mechanical complication of coronary artery bypass graft** CC
  Obstruction, mechanical of coronary artery bypass graft
  Perforation of coronary artery bypass graft
  Protrusion of coronary artery bypass graft

T82.22 Mechanical complication of biological heart valve graft
- **T82.221 Breakdown (mechanical) of biological heart valve graft** CC
- **T82.222 Displacement of biological heart valve graft** CC
  Malposition of biological heart valve graft
- **T82.223 Leakage of biological heart valve graft** CC
- **T82.228 Other mechanical complication of biological heart valve graft** CC
  Obstruction of biological heart valve graft
  Perforation of biological heart valve graft
  Protrusion of biological heart valve graft

T82.3 Mechanical complication of other vascular grafts

T82.31 Breakdown (mechanical) of other vascular grafts
- 6 **T82.310 Breakdown (mechanical) of aortic (bifurcation) graft (replacement)** CC HCC
  AHA: 2020,3Q,3-8
- 6 **T82.311 Breakdown (mechanical) of carotid arterial graft (bypass)** CC HCC
- 6 **T82.312 Breakdown (mechanical) of femoral arterial graft (bypass)** CC HCC
- 6 **T82.318 Breakdown (mechanical) of other vascular grafts** CC HCC
- 6 **T82.319 Breakdown (mechanical) of unspecified vascular grafts** CC HCC

T82.32 Displacement of other vascular grafts
Malposition of other vascular grafts
- 6 **T82.320 Displacement of aortic (bifurcation) graft (replacement)** CC HCC
- 6 **T82.321 Displacement of carotid arterial graft (bypass)** CC HCC
- 6 **T82.322 Displacement of femoral arterial graft (bypass)** CC HCC
- 6 **T82.328 Displacement of other vascular grafts** CC HCC
- 6 **T82.329 Displacement of unspecified vascular grafts** CC HCC

T82.33 Leakage of other vascular grafts
- 6 **T82.330 Leakage of aortic (bifurcation) graft (replacement)** CC HCC
  AHA: 2020,3Q,3-8
- 6 **T82.331 Leakage of carotid arterial graft (bypass)** CC HCC
- 6 **T82.332 Leakage of femoral arterial graft (bypass)** CC HCC
- 6 **T82.338 Leakage of other vascular grafts** CC HCC
- 6 **T82.339 Leakage of unspecified vascular graft** CC HCC

T82.39 Other mechanical complication of other vascular grafts
Obstruction (mechanical) of other vascular grafts
Perforation of other vascular grafts
Protrusion of other vascular grafts
- 6 **T82.390 Other mechanical complication of aortic (bifurcation) graft (replacement)** CC HCC
  AHA: 2020,3Q,3-5
- 6 **T82.391 Other mechanical complication of carotid arterial graft (bypass)** CC HCC
- 6 **T82.392 Other mechanical complication of femoral arterial graft (bypass)** CC HCC
- 6 **T82.398 Other mechanical complication of other vascular grafts** CC HCC
- 6 **T82.399 Other mechanical complication of unspecified vascular grafts** CC HCC

T82.4 Mechanical complication of vascular dialysis catheter
Mechanical complication of hemodialysis catheter
EXCLUDES 1 *mechanical complication of intraperitoneal dialysis catheter (T85.62)*
- **T82.41 Breakdown (mechanical) of vascular dialysis catheter** CC HCC
- **T82.42 Displacement of vascular dialysis catheter** CC HCC
  Malposition of vascular dialysis catheter
- **T82.43 Leakage of vascular dialysis catheter** CC HCC
- **T82.49 Other complication of vascular dialysis catheter** CC HCC
  Obstruction (mechanical) of vascular dialysis catheter
  Perforation of vascular dialysis catheter
  Protrusion of vascular dialysis catheter

T82.5 Mechanical complication of other cardiac and vascular devices and implants
EXCLUDES 2 *mechanical complication of epidural and subdural infusion catheter (T85.61)*

T82.51 Breakdown (mechanical) of other cardiac and vascular devices and implants
- 6 **T82.510 Breakdown (mechanical) of surgically created arteriovenous fistula** CC HCC
  AHA: 2020,3Q,36
- 6 **T82.511 Breakdown (mechanical) of surgically created arteriovenous shunt** CC HCC
  AHA: 2020,3Q,37
- **T82.512 Breakdown (mechanical) of artificial heart** CC

Chapter 19. Injury, Poisoning and Certain Other Consequences of External Causes

6 ✓7th **T82.513 Breakdown (mechanical) of balloon (counterpulsation) device** CC HCC

6 ✓7th **T82.514 Breakdown (mechanical) of infusion catheter** CC HCC

6 ✓7th **T82.515 Breakdown (mechanical) of umbrella device** CC HCC

6 ✓7th **T82.518 Breakdown (mechanical) of other cardiac and vascular devices and implants** CC HCC

✓7th **T82.519 Breakdown (mechanical) of unspecified cardiac and vascular devices and implants** CC

✓6th **T82.52 Displacement of other cardiac and vascular devices and implants**

Malposition of other cardiac and vascular devices and implants

6 ✓7th **T82.520 Displacement of surgically created arteriovenous fistula** CC HCC

AHA: 2020,3Q,36

6 ✓7th **T82.521 Displacement of surgically created arteriovenous shunt** CC HCC

✓7th **T82.522 Displacement of artificial heart** CC

6 ✓7th **T82.523 Displacement of balloon (counterpulsation) device** CC HCC

6 ✓7th **T82.524 Displacement of infusion catheter** CC HCC

AHA: 2020,2Q,21; 2019,3Q,15

6 ✓7th **T82.525 Displacement of umbrella device** CC HCC

6 ✓7th **T82.528 Displacement of other cardiac and vascular devices and implants** CC HCC

✓7th **T82.529 Displacement of unspecified cardiac and vascular devices and implants** CC

✓6th **T82.53 Leakage of other cardiac and vascular devices and implants**

6 ✓7th **T82.530 Leakage of surgically created arteriovenous fistula** CC HCC

AHA: 2020,3Q,36

6 ✓7th **T82.531 Leakage of surgically created arteriovenous shunt** CC HCC

✓7th **T82.532 Leakage of artificial heart** CC

6 ✓7th **T82.533 Leakage of balloon (counterpulsation) device** CC HCC

6 ✓7th **T82.534 Leakage of infusion catheter** CC HCC

6 ✓7th **T82.535 Leakage of umbrella device** CC HCC

6 ✓7th **T82.538 Leakage of other cardiac and vascular devices and implants** CC HCC

✓7th **T82.539 Leakage of unspecified cardiac and vascular devices and implants** CC

✓6th **T82.59 Other mechanical complication of other cardiac and vascular devices and implants**

Obstruction (mechanical) of other cardiac and vascular devices and implants

Perforation of other cardiac and vascular devices and implants

Protrusion of other cardiac and vascular devices and implants

6 ✓7th **T82.590 Other mechanical complication of surgically created arteriovenous fistula** CC HCC

AHA: 2020,3Q,36

6 ✓7th **T82.591 Other mechanical complication of surgically created arteriovenous shunt** CC HCC

✓7th **T82.592 Other mechanical complication of artificial heart** CC

6 ✓7th **T82.593 Other mechanical complication of balloon (counterpulsation) device** CC HCC

6 ✓7th **T82.594 Other mechanical complication of infusion catheter** CC HCC

6 ✓7th **T82.595 Other mechanical complication of umbrella device** CC HCC

6 ✓7th **T82.598 Other mechanical complication of other cardiac and vascular devices and implants** CC HCC

✓7th **T82.599 Other mechanical complication of unspecified cardiac and vascular devices and implants** CC

6 ✓x7th **T82.6 Infection and inflammatory reaction due to cardiac valve prosthesis** CC HCC

Use additional code to identify infection

6 ✓x7th **T82.7 Infection and inflammatory reaction due to other cardiac and vascular devices, implants and grafts** CC H13 HCC

Use additional code to identify infection

AHA: 2019,1Q,13-14

DEF: Midline catheter: Long peripheral catheter introduced via the cephalic, basilic, brachial, or median cubital veins in the upper arm and positioned so that the tip is level or near the level of the axilla and distal to the shoulder. Midline catheters are typically used for IV access, fluid replacement, and medication administration.

TIP: Assign this code for infections and/or cellulitis resulting from catheters that are not centrally placed (e.g., midline catheters).

✓5th **T82.8 Other specified complications of cardiac and vascular prosthetic devices, implants and grafts**

AHA: 2016,4Q,70

✓6th **T82.81 Embolism due to cardiac and vascular prosthetic devices, implants and grafts**

✓7th **T82.817 Embolism due to cardiac prosthetic devices, implants and grafts** CC

6 ✓7th **T82.818 Embolism due to vascular prosthetic devices, implants and grafts** CC HCC

✓6th **T82.82 Fibrosis due to cardiac and vascular prosthetic devices, implants and grafts**

✓7th **T82.827 Fibrosis due to cardiac prosthetic devices, implants and grafts** CC

6 ✓7th **T82.828 Fibrosis due vascular prosthetic devices, implants and grafts** CC HCC

✓6th **T82.83 Hemorrhage due to cardiac and vascular prosthetic devices, implants and grafts**

✓7th **T82.837 Hemorrhage due to cardiac prosthetic devices, implants and grafts** CC

6 ✓7th **T82.838 Hemorrhage due to vascular prosthetic devices, implants and grafts** CC HCC

AHA: 2020,3Q,36-37

✓6th **T82.84 Pain due to cardiac and vascular prosthetic devices, implants and grafts**

✓7th **T82.847 Pain due to cardiac prosthetic devices, implants and grafts** CC

6 ✓7th **T82.848 Pain due to vascular prosthetic devices, implants and grafts** CC HCC

✓6th **T82.85 Stenosis due to cardiac and vascular prosthetic devices, implants and grafts**

✓7th **T82.855 Stenosis of coronary artery stent** CC

In-stent stenosis (restenosis) of coronary artery stent

Restenosis of coronary artery stent

AHA: 2021,3Q,6-7

6 ✓7th **T82.856 Stenosis of peripheral vascular stent** CC HCC

In-stent stenosis (restenosis) of peripheral vascular stent

Restenosis of peripheral vascular stent

✓7th **T82.857 Stenosis of other cardiac prosthetic devices, implants and grafts** CC

6 ✓7th **T82.858 Stenosis of other vascular prosthetic devices, implants and grafts** CC HCC

✓6th **T82.86 Thrombosis of cardiac and vascular prosthetic devices, implants and grafts**

✓7th **T82.867 Thrombosis due to cardiac prosthetic devices, implants and grafts** CC

6 ✓7th **T82.868 Thrombosis due to vascular prosthetic devices, implants and grafts** CC HCC

✓6th **T82.89 Other specified complication of cardiac and vascular prosthetic devices, implants and grafts**

✓7th **T82.897 Other specified complication of cardiac prosthetic devices, implants and grafts** CC

AHA: 2019,2Q,33

6 ✓7th **T82.898 Other specified complication of vascular prosthetic devices, implants and grafts** CC HCC

AHA: 2020,3Q,3-5

✓x7th **T82.9 Unspecified complication of cardiac and vascular prosthetic device, implant and graft** CC

T83 Complications of genitourinary prosthetic devices, implants and grafts

EXCLUDES 2 *failure and rejection of transplanted organs and tissue (T86.-)*

AHA: 2016,4Q,70-71

The appropriate 7th character is to be added to each code from category T83.
A initial encounter
D subsequent encounter
S sequela

T83.0 Mechanical complication of urinary catheter

EXCLUDES 2 *complications of stoma of urinary tract (N99.5-)*

T83.01 Breakdown (mechanical) of urinary catheter

T83.010 Breakdown (mechanical) of cystostomy catheter CC HCC

T83.011 Breakdown (mechanical) of indwelling urethral catheter HCC

T83.012 Breakdown (mechanical) of nephrostomy catheter HCC

T83.018 Breakdown (mechanical) of other urinary catheter HCC
Breakdown (mechanical) of Hopkins catheter
Breakdown (mechanical) of ileostomy catheter
Breakdown (mechanical) urostomy catheter

T83.02 Displacement of urinary catheter
Malposition of urinary catheter

T83.020 Displacement of cystostomy catheter CC HCC

T83.021 Displacement of indwelling urethral catheter HCC

T83.022 Displacement of nephrostomy catheter HCC

T83.028 Displacement of other urinary catheter HCC
Displacement of Hopkins catheter
Displacement of ileostomy catheter
Displacement of urostomy catheter

T83.03 Leakage of urinary catheter

T83.030 Leakage of cystostomy catheter CC HCC
AHA: 2021,4Q,18

T83.031 Leakage of indwelling urethral catheter HCC

T83.032 Leakage of nephrostomy catheter HCC

T83.038 Leakage of other urinary catheter HCC
Leakage of Hopkins catheter
Leakage of ileostomy catheter
Leakage of urostomy catheter

T83.09 Other mechanical complication of urinary catheter
Obstruction (mechanical) of urinary catheter
Perforation of urinary catheter
Protrusion of urinary catheter

T83.090 Other mechanical complication of cystostomy catheter CC HCC

T83.091 Other mechanical complication of indwelling urethral catheter HCC

T83.092 Other mechanical complication of nephrostomy catheter HCC

T83.098 Other mechanical complication of other urinary catheter HCC
Other mechanical complication of Hopkins catheter
Other mechanical complication of ileostomy catheter
Other mechanical complication of urostomy catheter

T83.1 Mechanical complication of other urinary devices and implants

T83.11 Breakdown (mechanical) of other urinary devices and implants

T83.110 Breakdown (mechanical) of urinary electronic stimulator device CC HCC

EXCLUDES 2 *breakdown (mechanical) of electrode (lead) for sacral nerve neurostimulator (T85.111)*
breakdown (mechanical) of implanted electronic sacral neurostimulator, pulse generator or receiver (T85.113)

T83.111 Breakdown (mechanical) of implanted urinary sphincter CC HCC

T83.112 Breakdown (mechanical) of indwelling ureteral stent CC HCC

T83.113 Breakdown (mechanical) of other urinary stents CC HCC
Breakdown (mechanical) of ileal conduit stent
Breakdown (mechanical) of nephroureteral stent

T83.118 Breakdown (mechanical) of other urinary devices and implants CC HCC

T83.12 Displacement of other urinary devices and implants
Malposition of other urinary devices and implants

T83.120 Displacement of urinary electronic stimulator device CC HCC

EXCLUDES 2 *displacement of electrode (lead) for sacral nerve neurostimulator (T85.121)*
displacement of implanted electronic sacral neurostimulator, pulse generator or receiver (T85.123)

T83.121 Displacement of implanted urinary sphincter CC HCC

T83.122 Displacement of indwelling ureteral stent CC HCC

T83.123 Displacement of other urinary stents CC HCC
Displacement of ileal conduit stent
Displacement of nephroureteral stent

T83.128 Displacement of other urinary devices and implants CC HCC

T83.19 Other mechanical complication of other urinary devices and implants
Leakage of other urinary devices and implants
Obstruction (mechanical) of other urinary devices and implants
Perforation of other urinary devices and implants
Protrusion of other urinary devices and implants

T83.190 Other mechanical complication of urinary electronic stimulator device CC HCC

EXCLUDES 2 *other mechanical complication of electrode (lead) for sacral nerve neurostimulator (T85.191)*
other mechanical complication of implanted electronic sacral neurostimulator, pulse generator or receiver (T85.193)

T83.191 Other mechanical complication of implanted urinary sphincter CC HCC

T83.192 Other mechanical complication of indwelling ureteral stent CC HCC

T83.193 Other mechanical complication of other urinary stent CC HCC
Other mechanical complication of ileal conduit stent
Other mechanical complication of nephroureteral stent

T83.198 Other mechanical complication of other urinary devices and implants CC HCC

√5th **T83.2 Mechanical complication of graft of urinary organ**

6 √x7th **T83.21 Breakdown (mechanical) of graft of urinary organ** CC HCC

6 √x7th **T83.22 Displacement of graft of urinary organ** CC HCC
Malposition of graft of urinary organ

6 √x7th **T83.23 Leakage of graft of urinary organ** CC HCC

6 √x7th **T83.24 Erosion of graft of urinary organ** CC HCC

6 √x7th **T83.25 Exposure of graft of urinary organ** CC HCC

6 √x7th **T83.29 Other mechanical complication of graft of urinary organ** CC HCC
Obstruction (mechanical) of graft of urinary organ
Perforation of graft of urinary organ
Protrusion of graft of urinary organ

√5th **T83.3 Mechanical complication of intrauterine contraceptive device**

√x7th **T83.31 Breakdown (mechanical) of intrauterine contraceptive device** ♀

√x7th **T83.32 Displacement of intrauterine contraceptive device** ♀
Malposition of intrauterine contraceptive device
Missing string of intrauterine contraceptive device
AHA: 2018,1Q,5

√x7th **T83.39 Other mechanical complication of intrauterine contraceptive device** ♀
Leakage of intrauterine contraceptive device
Obstruction (mechanical) of intrauterine contraceptive device
Perforation of intrauterine contraceptive device
Protrusion of intrauterine contraceptive device

√5th **T83.4 Mechanical complication of other prosthetic devices, implants and grafts of genital tract**

√6th **T83.41 Breakdown (mechanical) of other prosthetic devices, implants and grafts of genital tract**

6 √7th **T83.410 Breakdown (mechanical) of implanted penile prosthesis** CC HCC ♂
Breakdown (mechanical) of penile prosthesis cylinder
Breakdown (mechanical) of penile prosthesis pump
Breakdown (mechanical) of penile prosthesis reservoir

6 √7th **T83.411 Breakdown (mechanical) of implanted testicular prosthesis** CC HCC

6 √7th **T83.418 Breakdown (mechanical) of other prosthetic devices, implants and grafts of genital tract** CC HCC

√6th **T83.42 Displacement of other prosthetic devices, implants and grafts of genital tract**
Malposition of other prosthetic devices, implants and grafts of genital tract

6 √7th **T83.420 Displacement of implanted penile prosthesis** CC HCC ♂
Displacement of penile prosthesis cylinder
Displacement of penile prosthesis pump
Displacement of penile prosthesis reservoir

6 √7th **T83.421 Displacement of implanted testicular prosthesis** CC HCC

6 √7th **T83.428 Displacement of other prosthetic devices, implants and grafts of genital tract** CC HCC
AHA: 2018,1Q,5

√6th **T83.49 Other mechanical complication of other prosthetic devices, implants and grafts of genital tract**
Leakage of other prosthetic devices, implants and grafts of genital tract
Obstruction, mechanical of other prosthetic devices, implants and grafts of genital tract
Perforation of other prosthetic devices, implants and grafts of genital tract
Protrusion of other prosthetic devices, implants and grafts of genital tract

6 √7th **T83.490 Other mechanical complication of implanted penile prosthesis** CC HCC ♂
Other mechanical complication of penile prosthesis cylinder
Other mechanical complication of penile prosthesis pump
Other mechanical complication of penile prosthesis reservoir

6 √7th **T83.491 Other mechanical complication of implanted testicular prosthesis** CC HCC

6 √7th **T83.498 Other mechanical complication of other prosthetic devices, implants and grafts of genital tract** CC HCC

√5th **T83.5 Infection and inflammatory reaction due to prosthetic device, implant and graft in urinary system**
Use additional code to identify infection

√6th **T83.51 Infection and inflammatory reaction due to urinary catheter**
EXCLUDES 2 *complications of stoma of urinary tract (N99.5-)*
AHA: 2019,3Q,17

6 √7th **T83.510 Infection and inflammatory reaction due to cystostomy catheter** CC HCC

6 √7th **T83.511 Infection and inflammatory reaction due to indwelling urethral catheter** CC H6 HCC
AHA: 2022,2Q,7

6 √7th **T83.512 Infection and inflammatory reaction due to nephrostomy catheter** CC HCC

6 √7th **T83.518 Infection and inflammatory reaction due to other urinary catheter** CC H6 HCC
Infection and inflammatory reaction due to Hopkins catheter
Infection and inflammatory reaction due to ileostomy catheter
Infection and inflammatory reaction due to urostomy catheter

√6th **T83.59 Infection and inflammatory reaction due to prosthetic device, implant and graft in urinary system**

6 √7th **T83.590 Infection and inflammatory reaction due to implanted urinary neurostimulation device** CC HCC
EXCLUDES 2 *infection and inflammatory reaction due to electrode lead of sacral nerve neurostimulator (T85.732)*
infection and inflammatory reaction due to pulse generator or receiver of sacral nerve neurostimulator (T85.734)

6 √7th **T83.591 Infection and inflammatory reaction due to implanted urinary sphincter** CC HCC

6 √7th **T83.592 Infection and inflammatory reaction due to indwelling ureteral stent** CC HCC

6 √7th **T83.593 Infection and inflammatory reaction due to other urinary stents** CC HCC
Infection and inflammatory reaction due to ileal conduit stents
Infection and inflammatory reaction due to nephroureteral stent

6 √7th **T83.598 Infection and inflammatory reaction due to other prosthetic device, implant and graft in urinary system** CC HCC
AHA: 2020,3Q,25

T83.6 Infection and inflammatory reaction due to prosthetic device, implant and graft in genital tract
Use additional code to identify infection

T83.61 Infection and inflammatory reaction due to implanted penile prosthesis CC HCC
Infection and inflammatory reaction due to penile prosthesis cylinder
Infection and inflammatory reaction due to penile prosthesis pump
Infection and inflammatory reaction due to penile prosthesis reservoir

T83.62 Infection and inflammatory reaction due to implanted testicular prosthesis CC HCC

T83.69 Infection and inflammatory reaction due to other prosthetic device, implant and graft in genital tract CC HCC

T83.7 Complications due to implanted mesh and other prosthetic materials

T83.71 Erosion of implanted mesh and other prosthetic materials

T83.711 Erosion of implanted vaginal mesh to surrounding organ or tissue HCC ♀
Erosion of implanted vaginal mesh into pelvic floor muscles

T83.712 Erosion of implanted urethral mesh to surrounding organ or tissue CC HCC
Erosion of implanted female urethral sling
Erosion of implanted male urethral sling
Erosion of implanted urethral mesh into pelvic floor muscles

T83.713 Erosion of implanted urethral bulking agent to surrounding organ or tissue CC HCC

T83.714 Erosion of implanted ureteral bulking agent to surrounding organ or tissue CC HCC

T83.718 Erosion of other implanted mesh to organ or tissue CC HCC

T83.719 Erosion of other prosthetic materials to surrounding organ or tissue CC HCC

T83.72 Exposure of implanted mesh and other prosthetic materials into surrounding organ or tissue
Extrusion of implanted mesh

T83.721 Exposure of implanted vaginal mesh into vagina HCC ♀
Exposure of implanted vaginal mesh through vaginal wall

T83.722 Exposure of implanted urethral mesh into urethra CC HCC
Exposure of implanted female urethral sling
Exposure of implanted male urethral sling
Exposure of implanted urethral mesh through urethral wall

T83.723 Exposure of implanted urethral bulking agent into urethra CC HCC

T83.724 Exposure of implanted ureteral bulking agent into ureter CC HCC

T83.728 Exposure of other implanted mesh into organ or tissue CC HCC

T83.729 Exposure of other prosthetic materials into organ or tissue CC HCC

T83.79 Other specified complications due to other genitourinary prosthetic materials CC HCC

T83.8 Other specified complications of genitourinary prosthetic devices, implants and grafts

T83.81 Embolism due to genitourinary prosthetic devices, implants and grafts CC HCC

T83.82 Fibrosis due to genitourinary prosthetic devices, implants and grafts CC HCC

T83.83 Hemorrhage due to genitourinary prosthetic devices, implants and grafts CC HCC

T83.84 Pain due to genitourinary prosthetic devices, implants and grafts CC HCC

T83.85 Stenosis due to genitourinary prosthetic devices, implants and grafts CC HCC

T83.86 Thrombosis due to genitourinary prosthetic devices, implants and grafts CC HCC

T83.89 Other specified complication of genitourinary prosthetic devices, implants and grafts CC HCC
AHA: 2016,1Q,19

T83.9 Unspecified complication of genitourinary prosthetic device, implant and graft CC HCC

T84 Complications of internal orthopedic prosthetic devices, implants and grafts
EXCLUDES 2 *failure and rejection of transplanted organs and tissues (T86.-)*
fracture of bone following insertion of orthopedic implant, joint prosthesis or bone plate (M96.6)

The appropriate 7th character is to be added to each code from category T84.
A initial encounter
D subsequent encounter
S sequela

T84.0 Mechanical complication of internal joint prosthesis

T84.01 Broken internal joint prosthesis
Breakage (fracture) of prosthetic joint
Broken prosthetic joint implant
EXCLUDES 1 *periprosthetic joint implant fracture (M97.-)*
AHA: 2016,4Q,42

T84.010 Broken internal right hip prosthesis CC HCC

T84.011 Broken internal left hip prosthesis CC HCC

T84.012 Broken internal right knee prosthesis CC HCC

T84.013 Broken internal left knee prosthesis CC HCC

T84.018 Broken internal joint prosthesis, other site CC HCC
Use additional code to identify the joint (Z96.6-)

T84.019 Broken internal joint prosthesis, unspecified site CC UNS HCC

T84.02 Dislocation of internal joint prosthesis
Instability of internal joint prosthesis
Subluxation of internal joint prosthesis
AHA: 2019,2Q,27

T84.020 Dislocation of internal right hip prosthesis CC HCC

T84.021 Dislocation of internal left hip prosthesis CC HCC

T84.022 Instability of internal right knee prosthesis CC HCC

T84.023 Instability of internal left knee prosthesis CC HCC

T84.028 Dislocation of other internal joint prosthesis CC HCC
Use additional code to identify the joint (Z96.6-)

T84.029 Dislocation of unspecified internal joint prosthesis CC UNS HCC

T84.03 Mechanical loosening of internal prosthetic joint
Aseptic loosening of prosthetic joint

T84.030 Mechanical loosening of internal right hip prosthetic joint CC HCC

T84.031 Mechanical loosening of internal left hip prosthetic joint CC HCC

T84.032 Mechanical loosening of internal right knee prosthetic joint CC HCC

T84.033 Mechanical loosening of internal left knee prosthetic joint CC HCC

T84.038 Mechanical loosening of other internal prosthetic joint CC HCC
Use additional code to identify the joint (Z96.6-)

T84.039 Mechanical loosening of unspecified internal prosthetic joint CC UNS HCC

T84.05 Periprosthetic osteolysis of internal prosthetic joint
Use additional code to identify major osseous defect, if applicable (M89.7-)

T84.050 Periprosthetic osteolysis of internal prosthetic right hip joint CC HCC

T84.051 Periprosthetic osteolysis of internal prosthetic left hip joint CC HCC

6 ✓7th **T84.052 Periprosthetic osteolysis of internal prosthetic right knee joint** CC HCC

6 ✓7th **T84.053 Periprosthetic osteolysis of internal prosthetic left knee joint** CC HCC

6 ✓7th **T84.058 Periprosthetic osteolysis of other internal prosthetic joint** CC HCC

Use additional code to identify the joint (Z96.6-)

6 ✓7th **T84.059 Periprosthetic osteolysis of unspecified internal prosthetic joint** CC UNS HCC

✓6th **T84.06 Wear of articular bearing surface of internal prosthetic joint**

6 ✓7th **T84.060 Wear of articular bearing surface of internal prosthetic right hip joint** CC HCC

6 ✓7th **T84.061 Wear of articular bearing surface of internal prosthetic left hip joint** CC HCC

6 ✓7th **T84.062 Wear of articular bearing surface of internal prosthetic right knee joint** CC HCC

6 ✓7th **T84.063 Wear of articular bearing surface of internal prosthetic left knee joint** CC HCC

6 ✓7th **T84.068 Wear of articular bearing surface of other internal prosthetic joint** CC HCC

Use additional code to identify the joint (Z96.6-)

6 ✓7th **T84.069 Wear of articular bearing surface of unspecified internal prosthetic joint** CC UNS HCC

✓6th **T84.09 Other mechanical complication of internal joint prosthesis**

Prosthetic joint implant failure NOS

AHA: 2019,1Q,20

6 ✓7th **T84.090 Other mechanical complication of internal right hip prosthesis** CC HCC

6 ✓7th **T84.091 Other mechanical complication of internal left hip prosthesis** CC HCC

6 ✓7th **T84.092 Other mechanical complication of internal right knee prosthesis** CC HCC

6 ✓7th **T84.093 Other mechanical complication of internal left knee prosthesis** CC HCC

6 ✓7th **T84.098 Other mechanical complication of other internal joint prosthesis** CC HCC

Use additional code to identify the joint (Z96.6-)

6 ✓7th **T84.099 Other mechanical complication of unspecified internal joint prosthesis** CC UNS HCC

✓5th **T84.1 Mechanical complication of internal fixation device of bones of limb**

EXCLUDES 2 *mechanical complication of internal fixation device of bones of feet (T84.2-)*
mechanical complication of internal fixation device of bones of fingers (T84.2-)
mechanical complication of internal fixation device of bones of hands (T84.2-)
mechanical complication of internal fixation device of bones of toes (T84.2-)

✓6th **T84.11 Breakdown (mechanical) of internal fixation device of bones of limb**

6 ✓7th **T84.110 Breakdown (mechanical) of internal fixation device of right humerus** CC HCC

6 ✓7th **T84.111 Breakdown (mechanical) of internal fixation device of left humerus** CC HCC

6 ✓7th **T84.112 Breakdown (mechanical) of internal fixation device of bone of right forearm** CC HCC

6 ✓7th **T84.113 Breakdown (mechanical) of internal fixation device of bone of left forearm** CC HCC

6 ✓7th **T84.114 Breakdown (mechanical) of internal fixation device of right femur** CC HCC

6 ✓7th **T84.115 Breakdown (mechanical) of internal fixation device of left femur** CC HCC

6 ✓7th **T84.116 Breakdown (mechanical) of internal fixation device of bone of right lower leg** CC HCC

6 ✓7th **T84.117 Breakdown (mechanical) of internal fixation device of bone of left lower leg** CC HCC

6 ✓7th **T84.119 Breakdown (mechanical) of internal fixation device of unspecified bone of limb** CC UNS HCC

✓6th **T84.12 Displacement of internal fixation device of bones of limb**

Malposition of internal fixation device of bones of limb

6 ✓7th **T84.120 Displacement of internal fixation device of right humerus** CC HCC

6 ✓7th **T84.121 Displacement of internal fixation device of left humerus** CC HCC

6 ✓7th **T84.122 Displacement of internal fixation device of bone of right forearm** CC HCC

6 ✓7th **T84.123 Displacement of internal fixation device of bone of left forearm** CC HCC

6 ✓7th **T84.124 Displacement of internal fixation device of right femur** CC HCC

6 ✓7th **T84.125 Displacement of internal fixation device of left femur** CC HCC

6 ✓7th **T84.126 Displacement of internal fixation device of bone of right lower leg** CC HCC

6 ✓7th **T84.127 Displacement of internal fixation device of bone of left lower leg** CC HCC

6 ✓7th **T84.129 Displacement of internal fixation device of unspecified bone of limb** CC UNS HCC

✓6th **T84.19 Other mechanical complication of internal fixation device of bones of limb**

Obstruction (mechanical) of internal fixation device of bones of limb
Perforation of internal fixation device of bones of limb
Protrusion of internal fixation device of bones of limb

6 ✓7th **T84.190 Other mechanical complication of internal fixation device of right humerus** CC HCC

6 ✓7th **T84.191 Other mechanical complication of internal fixation device of left humerus** CC HCC

6 ✓7th **T84.192 Other mechanical complication of internal fixation device of bone of right forearm** CC HCC

6 ✓7th **T84.193 Other mechanical complication of internal fixation device of bone of left forearm** CC HCC

6 ✓7th **T84.194 Other mechanical complication of internal fixation device of right femur** CC HCC

6 ✓7th **T84.195 Other mechanical complication of internal fixation device of left femur** CC HCC

6 ✓7th **T84.196 Other mechanical complication of internal fixation device of bone of right lower leg** CC HCC

6 ✓7th **T84.197 Other mechanical complication of internal fixation device of bone of left lower leg** CC HCC

6 ✓7th **T84.199 Other mechanical complication of internal fixation device of unspecified bone of limb** CC UNS HCC

✓5th **T84.2 Mechanical complication of internal fixation device of other bones**

✓6th **T84.21 Breakdown (mechanical) of internal fixation device of other bones**

6 ✓7th **T84.210 Breakdown (mechanical) of internal fixation device of bones of hand and fingers** CC HCC

6 ✓7th **T84.213 Breakdown (mechanical) of internal fixation device of bones of foot and toes** CC HCC

6 ✓7th **T84.216 Breakdown (mechanical) of internal fixation device of vertebrae** CC HCC

6 ✓7th **T84.218 Breakdown (mechanical) of internal fixation device of other bones** CC HCC

✓6th **T84.22 Displacement of internal fixation device of other bones**

Malposition of internal fixation device of other bones

6 ✓7th **T84.220 Displacement of internal fixation device of bones of hand and fingers** CC HCC

6 T84.223 **Displacement of internal fixation device of bones of foot and toes** CC HCC

6 T84.226 **Displacement of internal fixation device of vertebrae** CC HCC

6 T84.228 **Displacement of internal fixation device of other bones** CC HCC

T84.29 **Other mechanical complication of internal fixation device of other bones**
Obstruction (mechanical) of internal fixation device of other bones
Perforation of internal fixation device of other bones
Protrusion of internal fixation device of other bones

6 T84.290 **Other mechanical complication of internal fixation device of bones of hand and fingers** CC HCC

6 T84.293 **Other mechanical complication of internal fixation device of bones of foot and toes** CC HCC

6 T84.296 **Other mechanical complication of internal fixation device of vertebrae** CC HCC

6 T84.298 **Other mechanical complication of internal fixation device of other bones** CC HCC

T84.3 **Mechanical complication of other bone devices, implants and grafts**
EXCLUDES 2 *other complications of bone graft (T86.83-)*

T84.31 **Breakdown (mechanical) of other bone devices, implants and grafts**

6 T84.310 **Breakdown (mechanical) of electronic bone stimulator** CC HCC

6 T84.318 **Breakdown (mechanical) of other bone devices, implants and grafts** CC HCC

T84.32 **Displacement of other bone devices, implants and grafts**
Malposition of other bone devices, implants and grafts

6 T84.320 **Displacement of electronic bone stimulator** CC HCC

6 T84.328 **Displacement of other bone devices, implants and grafts** CC HCC
AHA: 2014,4Q,28

T84.39 **Other mechanical complication of other bone devices, implants and grafts**
Obstruction (mechanical) of other bone devices, implants and grafts
Perforation of other bone devices, implants and grafts
Protrusion of other bone devices, implants and grafts

6 T84.390 **Other mechanical complication of electronic bone stimulator** CC HCC

6 T84.398 **Other mechanical complication of other bone devices, implants and grafts** CC HCC

T84.4 **Mechanical complication of other internal orthopedic devices, implants and grafts**

T84.41 **Breakdown (mechanical) of other internal orthopedic devices, implants and grafts**

6 T84.410 **Breakdown (mechanical) of muscle and tendon graft** CC HCC

6 T84.418 **Breakdown (mechanical) of other internal orthopedic devices, implants and grafts** CC HCC

T84.42 **Displacement of other internal orthopedic devices, implants and grafts**
Malposition of other internal orthopedic devices, implants and grafts

6 T84.420 **Displacement of muscle and tendon graft** CC HCC

6 T84.428 **Displacement of other internal orthopedic devices, implants and grafts** CC HCC

T84.49 **Other mechanical complication of other internal orthopedic devices, implants and grafts**
Mechanical complication of other internal orthopedic devices, implants and grafts NOS
Obstruction (mechanical) of other internal orthopedic devices, implants and grafts
Perforation of other internal orthopedic devices, implants and grafts
Protrusion of other internal orthopedic devices, implants and grafts

6 T84.490 **Other mechanical complication of muscle and tendon graft** CC HCC

6 T84.498 **Other mechanical complication of other internal orthopedic devices, implants and grafts** CC HCC

T84.5 **Infection and inflammatory reaction due to internal joint prosthesis**
Use additional code to identify infection
AHA: 2019,3Q,16; 2015,1Q,16

6 T84.50 **Infection and inflammatory reaction due to unspecified internal joint prosthesis** CC UNS HCC

6 T84.51 **Infection and inflammatory reaction due to internal right hip prosthesis** CC HCC

6 T84.52 **Infection and inflammatory reaction due to internal left hip prosthesis** CC HCC

6 T84.53 **Infection and inflammatory reaction due to internal right knee prosthesis** CC HCC

6 T84.54 **Infection and inflammatory reaction due to internal left knee prosthesis** CC HCC

6 T84.59 **Infection and inflammatory reaction due to other internal joint prosthesis** CC HCC

T84.6 **Infection and inflammatory reaction due to internal fixation device**
Use additional code to identify infection

6 T84.60 **Infection and inflammatory reaction due to internal fixation device of unspecified site** CC H12 UNS HCC

T84.61 **Infection and inflammatory reaction due to internal fixation device of arm**

6 T84.610 **Infection and inflammatory reaction due to internal fixation device of right humerus** CC H12 HCC

6 T84.611 **Infection and inflammatory reaction due to internal fixation device of left humerus** CC H12 HCC

6 T84.612 **Infection and inflammatory reaction due to internal fixation device of right radius** CC H12 HCC

6 T84.613 **Infection and inflammatory reaction due to internal fixation device of left radius** CC H12 HCC

6 T84.614 **Infection and inflammatory reaction due to internal fixation device of right ulna** CC H12 HCC

6 T84.615 **Infection and inflammatory reaction due to internal fixation device of left ulna** CC H12 HCC

6 T84.619 **Infection and inflammatory reaction due to internal fixation device of unspecified bone of arm** CC H12 UNS HCC

T84.62 **Infection and inflammatory reaction due to internal fixation device of leg**

6 T84.620 **Infection and inflammatory reaction due to internal fixation device of right femur** CC HCC

6 T84.621 **Infection and inflammatory reaction due to internal fixation device of left femur** CC HCC

6 T84.622 **Infection and inflammatory reaction due to internal fixation device of right tibia** CC HCC

6 T84.623 **Infection and inflammatory reaction due to internal fixation device of left tibia** CC HCC

6 T84.624 **Infection and inflammatory reaction due to internal fixation device of right fibula** CC HCC

6 T84.625 **Infection and inflammatory reaction due to internal fixation device of left fibula** CC HCC

6 T84.629 **Infection and inflammatory reaction due to internal fixation device of unspecified bone of leg** CC UNS HCC

6 ✓x7th **T84.63 Infection and inflammatory reaction due to internal fixation device of spine** CC H12 HCC

6 ✓x7th **T84.69 Infection and inflammatory reaction due to internal fixation device of other site** CC H12 HCC

6 ✓x7th **T84.7 Infection and inflammatory reaction due to other internal orthopedic prosthetic devices, implants and grafts** CC H12 HCC
Use additional code to identify infection

✓5th **T84.8 Other specified complications of internal orthopedic prosthetic devices, implants and grafts**

6 ✓x7th **T84.81 Embolism due to internal orthopedic prosthetic devices, implants and grafts** CC HCC

6 ✓x7th **T84.82 Fibrosis due to internal orthopedic prosthetic devices, implants and grafts** CC HCC

6 ✓x7th **T84.83 Hemorrhage due to internal orthopedic prosthetic devices, implants and grafts** CC HCC

6 ✓x7th **T84.84 Pain due to internal orthopedic prosthetic devices, implants and grafts** CC HCC

6 ✓x7th **T84.85 Stenosis due to internal orthopedic prosthetic devices, implants and grafts** CC HCC

6 ✓x7th **T84.86 Thrombosis due to internal orthopedic prosthetic devices, implants and grafts** CC HCC

6 ✓x7th **T84.89 Other specified complication of internal orthopedic prosthetic devices, implants and grafts** CC HCC

6 ✓x7th **T84.9 Unspecified complication of internal orthopedic prosthetic device, implant and graft** CC HCC

✓4th **T85 Complications of other internal prosthetic devices, implants and grafts**

EXCLUDES 2 *failure and rejection of transplanted organs and tissue (T86.-)*

AHA: 2016,4Q,71-72

The appropriate 7th character is to be added to each code from category T85.
A initial encounter
D subsequent encounter
S sequela

✓5th **T85.0 Mechanical complication of ventricular intracranial (communicating) shunt**

6 ✓x7th **T85.01 Breakdown (mechanical) of ventricular intracranial (communicating) shunt** CC HCC

6 ✓x7th **T85.02 Displacement of ventricular intracranial (communicating) shunt** CC HCC
Malposition of ventricular intracranial (communicating) shunt

6 ✓x7th **T85.03 Leakage of ventricular intracranial (communicating) shunt** CC HCC

6 ✓x7th **T85.09 Other mechanical complication of ventricular intracranial (communicating) shunt** CC HCC
Obstruction (mechanical) of ventricular intracranial (communicating) shunt
Perforation of ventricular intracranial (communicating) shunt
Protrusion of ventricular intracranial (communicating) shunt

✓5th **T85.1 Mechanical complication of implanted electronic stimulator of nervous system**

✓6th **T85.11 Breakdown (mechanical) of implanted electronic stimulator of nervous system**

6 ✓7th **T85.110 Breakdown (mechanical) of implanted electronic neurostimulator of brain electrode (lead)** CC HCC

6 ✓7th **T85.111 Breakdown (mechanical) of implanted electronic neurostimulator of peripheral nerve electrode (lead)** CC HCC
Breakdown of electrode (lead) for cranial nerve neurostimulators
Breakdown of electrode (lead) for gastric neurostimulator
Breakdown of electrode (lead) for sacral nerve neurostimulator
Breakdown of electrode (lead) for vagal nerve neurostimulators

6 ✓7th **T85.112 Breakdown (mechanical) of implanted electronic neurostimulator of spinal cord electrode (lead)** CC HCC

6 ✓7th **T85.113 Breakdown (mechanical) of implanted electronic neurostimulator, generator** CC HCC
Breakdown (mechanical) of implanted electronic neurostimulator generator, brain, peripheral, gastric, spinal
Breakdown (mechanical) of implanted electronic sacral neurostimulator, pulse generator or receiver

6 ✓7th **T85.118 Breakdown (mechanical) of other implanted electronic stimulator of nervous system** CC HCC

✓6th **T85.12 Displacement of implanted electronic stimulator of nervous system**
Malposition of implanted electronic stimulator of nervous system

6 ✓7th **T85.120 Displacement of implanted electronic neurostimulator of brain electrode (lead)** CC HCC

6 ✓7th **T85.121 Displacement of implanted electronic neurostimulator of peripheral nerve electrode (lead)** CC HCC
Displacement of electrode (lead) for cranial nerve neurostimulators
Displacement of electrode (lead) for gastric neurostimulator
Displacement of electrode (lead) for sacral nerve neurostimulator
Displacement of electrode (lead) for vagal nerve neurostimulators

6 ✓7th **T85.122 Displacement of implanted electronic neurostimulator of spinal cord electrode (lead)** CC HCC

6 ✓7th **T85.123 Displacement of implanted electronic neurostimulator, generator** CC HCC
Displacement of implanted electronic neurostimulator generator, brain, peripheral, gastric, spinal
Displacement of implanted electronic sacral neurostimulator, pulse generator or receiver

6 ✓7th **T85.128 Displacement of other implanted electronic stimulator of nervous system** CC HCC

✓6th **T85.19 Other mechanical complication of implanted electronic stimulator of nervous system**
Leakage of implanted electronic stimulator of nervous system
Obstruction (mechanical) of implanted electronic stimulator of nervous system
Perforation of implanted electronic stimulator of nervous system
Protrusion of implanted electronic stimulator of nervous system

6 ✓7th **T85.190 Other mechanical complication of implanted electronic neurostimulator of brain electrode (lead)** CC HCC

6 ✓7th **T85.191 Other mechanical complication of implanted electronic neurostimulator of peripheral nerve electrode (lead)** CC HCC
Other mechanical complication of electrode (lead) for cranial nerve neurostimulators
Other mechanical complication of electrode (lead) for gastric neurostimulator
Other mechanical complication of electrode (lead) for sacral nerve neurostimulator
Other mechanical complication of electrode (lead) for vagal nerve neurostimulators

6 ✓7th **T85.192 Other mechanical complication of implanted electronic neurostimulator of spinal cord electrode (lead)** CC HCC

6 ✓7th **T85.193 Other mechanical complication of implanted electronic neurostimulator, generator** CC HCC
Other mechanical complication of implanted electronic neurostimulator generator, brain, peripheral, gastric, spinal
Other mechanical complication of implanted electronic sacral neurostimulator, pulse generator or receiver

6 ✓7th **T85.199 Other mechanical complication of other implanted electronic stimulator of nervous system** CC HCC

✓5th **T85.2 Mechanical complication of intraocular lens**

✓x7th **T85.21 Breakdown (mechanical) of intraocular lens** CC

✓x7th **T85.22 Displacement of intraocular lens** CC
Malposition of intraocular lens

✓x7th **T85.29 Other mechanical complication of intraocular lens** CC
Obstruction (mechanical) of intraocular lens
Perforation of intraocular lens
Protrusion of intraocular lens

✓5th **T85.3 Mechanical complication of other ocular prosthetic devices, implants and grafts**
EXCLUDES 2 *other complications of corneal graft (T86.84-)*

✓6th **T85.31 Breakdown (mechanical) of other ocular prosthetic devices, implants and grafts**

✓7th **T85.310 Breakdown (mechanical) of prosthetic orbit of right eye** CC

✓7th **T85.311 Breakdown (mechanical) of prosthetic orbit of left eye** CC

✓7th **T85.318 Breakdown (mechanical) of other ocular prosthetic devices, implants and grafts**

✓6th **T85.32 Displacement of other ocular prosthetic devices, implants and grafts**
Malposition of other ocular prosthetic devices, implants and grafts

✓7th **T85.320 Displacement of prosthetic orbit of right eye** CC

✓7th **T85.321 Displacement of prosthetic orbit of left eye** CC

✓7th **T85.328 Displacement of other ocular prosthetic devices, implants and grafts**

✓6th **T85.39 Other mechanical complication of other ocular prosthetic devices, implants and grafts**
Obstruction (mechanical) of other ocular prosthetic devices, implants and grafts
Perforation of other ocular prosthetic devices, implants and grafts
Protrusion of other ocular prosthetic devices, implants and grafts

✓7th **T85.390 Other mechanical complication of prosthetic orbit of right eye** CC

✓7th **T85.391 Other mechanical complication of prosthetic orbit of left eye** CC

✓7th **T85.398 Other mechanical complication of other ocular prosthetic devices, implants and grafts**

✓5th **T85.4 Mechanical complication of breast prosthesis and implant**

✓x7th **T85.41 Breakdown (mechanical) of breast prosthesis and implant** CC

✓x7th **T85.42 Displacement of breast prosthesis and implant** CC
Malposition of breast prosthesis and implant

✓x7th **T85.43 Leakage of breast prosthesis and implant** CC

✓x7th **T85.44 Capsular contracture of breast implant** CC

✓x7th **T85.49 Other mechanical complication of breast prosthesis and implant** CC
Obstruction (mechanical) of breast prosthesis and implant
Perforation of breast prosthesis and implant
Protrusion of breast prosthesis and implant

✓5th **T85.5 Mechanical complication of gastrointestinal prosthetic devices, implants and grafts**

✓6th **T85.51 Breakdown (mechanical) of gastrointestinal prosthetic devices, implants and grafts**

✓7th **T85.510 Breakdown (mechanical) of bile duct prosthesis** CC

✓7th **T85.511 Breakdown (mechanical) of esophageal anti-reflux device** CC

✓7th **T85.518 Breakdown (mechanical) of other gastrointestinal prosthetic devices, implants and grafts** CC

✓6th **T85.52 Displacement of gastrointestinal prosthetic devices, implants and grafts**
Malposition of gastrointestinal prosthetic devices, implants and grafts

✓7th **T85.520 Displacement of bile duct prosthesis** CC

✓7th **T85.521 Displacement of esophageal anti-reflux device** CC

✓7th **T85.528 Displacement of other gastrointestinal prosthetic devices, implants and grafts** CC

✓6th **T85.59 Other mechanical complication of gastrointestinal prosthetic devices, implants and**
Obstruction, mechanical of gastrointestinal prosthetic devices, implants and grafts
Perforation of gastrointestinal prosthetic devices, implants and grafts
Protrusion of gastrointestinal prosthetic devices, implants and grafts

✓7th **T85.590 Other mechanical complication of bile duct prosthesis** CC

✓7th **T85.591 Other mechanical complication of esophageal anti-reflux device** CC

✓7th **T85.598 Other mechanical complication of other gastrointestinal prosthetic devices, implants and grafts** CC

✓5th **T85.6 Mechanical complication of other specified internal and external prosthetic devices, implants and grafts**

✓6th **T85.61 Breakdown (mechanical) of other specified internal prosthetic devices, implants and grafts**

✓7th **T85.610 Breakdown (mechanical) of cranial or spinal infusion catheter** CC
Breakdown (mechanical) of epidural infusion catheter
Breakdown (mechanical) of intrathecal infusion catheter
Breakdown (mechanical) of subarachnoid infusion catheter
Breakdown (mechanical) of subdural infusion catheter

✓7th **T85.611 Breakdown (mechanical) of intraperitoneal dialysis catheter** CC HCC
EXCLUDES 1 *mechanical complication of vascular dialysis catheter (T82.4-)*

✓7th **T85.612 Breakdown (mechanical) of permanent sutures** CC
EXCLUDES 1 *mechanical complication of permanent (wire) suture used in bone repair (T84.1-T84.2)*

✓7th **T85.613 Breakdown (mechanical) of artificial skin graft and decellularized allodermis** CC
Failure of artificial skin graft and decellularized allodermis
Non-adherence of artificial skin graft and decellularized allodermis
Poor incorporation of artificial skin graft and decellularized allodermis
Shearing of artificial skin graft and decellularized allodermis

✓7th **T85.614 Breakdown (mechanical) of insulin pump** CC

6 ✓7th **T85.615 Breakdown (mechanical) of other nervous system device, implant or graft** CC HCC
Breakdown (mechanical) of intrathecal infusion pump

✓7th **T85.618 Breakdown (mechanical) of other specified internal prosthetic devices, implants and grafts** CC

T85.62 Displacement of other specified internal prosthetic devices, implants and grafts
Malposition of other specified internal prosthetic devices, implants and grafts

T85.620 Displacement of cranial or spinal infusion catheter CC
Displacement of epidural infusion catheter
Displacement of intrathecal infusion catheter
Displacement of subarachnoid infusion catheter
Displacement of subdural infusion catheter

T85.621 Displacement of intraperitoneal dialysis catheter CC HCC
EXCLUDES 1 *mechanical complication of vascular dialysis catheter (T82.4-)*

T85.622 Displacement of permanent sutures CC
EXCLUDES 1 *mechanical complication of permanent (wire) suture used in bone repair (T84.1-T84.2)*

T85.623 Displacement of artificial skin graft and decellularized allodermis CC
Dislodgement of artificial skin graft and decellularized allodermis

T85.624 Displacement of insulin pump CC

6 **T85.625 Displacement of other nervous system device, implant or graft** CC HCC
Displacement of intrathecal infusion pump

T85.628 Displacement of other specified internal prosthetic devices, implants and grafts CC

T85.63 Leakage of other specified internal prosthetic devices, implants and grafts

T85.630 Leakage of cranial or spinal infusion catheter CC
Leakage of epidural infusion catheter
Leakage of intrathecal infusion catheter
Leakage of subdural infusion catheter
Leakage of subarachnoid infusion catheter

T85.631 Leakage of intraperitoneal dialysis catheter CC HCC
EXCLUDES 1 *mechanical complication of vascular dialysis catheter (T82.4)*

T85.633 Leakage of insulin pump CC

6 **T85.635 Leakage of other nervous system device, implant or graft** CC HCC
Leakage of intrathecal infusion pump

T85.638 Leakage of other specified internal prosthetic devices, implants and grafts CC

T85.69 Other mechanical complication of other specified internal prosthetic devices, implants and grafts
Obstruction, mechanical of other specified internal prosthetic devices, implants and grafts
Perforation of other specified internal prosthetic devices, implants and grafts
Protrusion of other specified internal prosthetic devices, implants and grafts

T85.690 Other mechanical complication of cranial or spinal infusion catheter CC
Other mechanical complication of epidural infusion catheter
Other mechanical complication of intrathecal infusion catheter
Other mechanical complication of subarachnoid infusion catheter
Other mechanical complication of subdural infusion catheter

T85.691 Other mechanical complication of intraperitoneal dialysis catheter CC HCC
EXCLUDES 1 *mechanical complication of vascular dialysis catheter (T82.4)*

T85.692 Other mechanical complication of permanent sutures CC
EXCLUDES 1 *mechanical complication of permanent (wire) suture used in bone repair (T84.1-T84.2)*

T85.693 Other mechanical complication of artificial skin graft and decellularized allodermis CC

T85.694 Other mechanical complication of insulin pump CC

6 **T85.695 Other mechanical complication of other nervous system device, implant or graft** CC HCC
Other mechanical complication of intrathecal infusion pump

T85.698 Other mechanical complication of other specified internal prosthetic devices, implants and grafts CC
Mechanical complication of nonabsorbable surgical material NOS

T85.7 Infection and inflammatory reaction due to other internal prosthetic devices, implants and grafts
Use additional code to identify infection

T85.71 Infection and inflammatory reaction due to peritoneal dialysis catheter CC HCC

6 **T85.72 Infection and inflammatory reaction due to insulin pump** CC HCC

T85.73 Infection and inflammatory reaction due to nervous system devices, implants and graft

6 **T85.730 Infection and inflammatory reaction due to ventricular intracranial (communicating) shunt** CC HCC

6 **T85.731 Infection and inflammatory reaction due to implanted electronic neurostimulator of brain, electrode (lead)** CC HCC

6 **T85.732 Infection and inflammatory reaction due to implanted electronic neurostimulator of peripheral nerve, electrode (lead)** CC HCC
Infection and inflammatory reaction due to electrode (lead) for cranial nerve neurostimulators
Infection and inflammatory reaction due to electrode (lead) for gastric neurostimulator
Infection and inflammatory reaction due to electrode (lead) for sacral nerve neurostimulator
Infection and inflammatory reaction due to electrode (lead) for vagal nerve neurostimulators

6 **T85.733 Infection and inflammatory reaction due to implanted electronic neurostimulator of spinal cord, electrode (lead)** CC HCC

6 **T85.734 Infection and inflammatory reaction due to implanted electronic neurostimulator, generator** CC HCC
Generator pocket infection

6 **T85.735 Infection and inflammatory reaction due to cranial or spinal infusion catheter** CC HCC
Infection and inflammatory reaction due to epidural catheter
Infection and inflammatory reaction due to intrathecal infusion catheter
Infection and inflammatory reaction due to subarachnoid catheter
Infection and inflammatory reaction due to subdural catheter

6 7th **T85.738 Infection and inflammatory reaction due to other nervous system device, implant or graft** CC HCC
Infection and inflammatory reaction due to intrathecal infusion pump

6 x7th **T85.79 Infection and inflammatory reaction due to other internal prosthetic devices, implants and grafts** CC HCC
AHA: 2022,2Q,7

5th **T85.8 Other specified complications of internal prosthetic devices, implants and grafts, not elsewhere classified**

6th **T85.81 Embolism due to internal prosthetic devices, implants and grafts, not elsewhere classified**

5,6 7th **T85.810 Embolism due to nervous system prosthetic devices, implants and grafts** CC HCC

7th **T85.818 Embolism due to other internal prosthetic devices, implants and grafts**

6th **T85.82 Fibrosis due to internal prosthetic devices, implants and grafts, not elsewhere classified**

5,6 7th **T85.820 Fibrosis due to nervous system prosthetic devices, implants and grafts** CC HCC

7th **T85.828 Fibrosis due to other internal prosthetic devices, implants and grafts**

6th **T85.83 Hemorrhage due to internal prosthetic devices, implants and grafts, not elsewhere classified**

5,6 7th **T85.830 Hemorrhage due to nervous system prosthetic devices, implants and grafts** CC HCC

7th **T85.838 Hemorrhage due to other internal prosthetic devices, implants and grafts**

6th **T85.84 Pain due to internal prosthetic devices, implants and grafts, not elsewhere classified**

5,6 7th **T85.840 Pain due to nervous system prosthetic devices, implants and grafts** CC HCC

7th **T85.848 Pain due to other internal prosthetic devices, implants and grafts**

6th **T85.85 Stenosis due to internal prosthetic devices, implants and grafts, not elsewhere classified**

5,6 7th **T85.850 Stenosis due to nervous system prosthetic devices, implants and grafts** CC HCC

7th **T85.858 Stenosis due to other internal prosthetic devices, implants and grafts**

6th **T85.86 Thrombosis due to internal prosthetic devices, implants and grafts, not elsewhere classified**

5,6 7th **T85.860 Thrombosis due to nervous system prosthetic devices, implants and grafts** CC HCC

7th **T85.868 Thrombosis due to other internal prosthetic devices, implants and grafts**

6th **T85.89 Other specified complication of internal prosthetic devices, implants and grafts, not elsewhere classified**
Erosion or breakdown of subcutaneous device pocket

5,6 7th **T85.890 Other specified complication of nervous system prosthetic devices, implants and grafts** CC HCC

7th **T85.898 Other specified complication of other internal prosthetic devices, implants and grafts**

x7th **T85.9 Unspecified complication of internal prosthetic device, implant and graft**
Complication of internal prosthetic device, implant and graft NOS

4th **T86 Complications of transplanted organs and tissue**
Use additional code to identify other transplant complications, such as:
graft-versus-host disease (D89.81-)
malignancy associated with organ transplant (C80.2)
post-transplant lymphoproliferative disorders (PTLD) (D47.Z1)
AHA: 2020,1Q,18

5th **T86.0 Complications of bone marrow transplant**

T86.00 Unspecified complication of bone marrow transplant CC HCC

T86.01 Bone marrow transplant rejection CC HCC

T86.02 Bone marrow transplant failure CC HCC

T86.03 Bone marrow transplant infection CC HCC

T86.09 Other complications of bone marrow transplant CC HCC

5th **T86.1 Complications of kidney transplant**

T86.10 Unspecified complication of kidney transplant CC

T86.11 Kidney transplant rejection CC

T86.12 Kidney transplant failure CC
AHA: 2013,1Q,24

T86.13 Kidney transplant infection CC
Use additional code to specify infection

T86.19 Other complication of kidney transplant CC
AHA: 2019,2Q,7

5th **T86.2 Complications of heart transplant**
EXCLUDES 1 *complication of:*
artificial heart device (T82.5-)
heart-lung transplant (T86.3-)

T86.20 Unspecified complication of heart transplant CC HCC

T86.21 Heart transplant rejection CC HCC

T86.22 Heart transplant failure CC HCC

T86.23 Heart transplant infection CC HCC
Use additional code to specify infection

6th **T86.29 Other complications of heart transplant**

T86.290 Cardiac allograft vasculopathy CC HCC
EXCLUDES 1 *atherosclerosis of coronary arteries (I25.75-, I25.76-, I25.81-)*

T86.298 Other complications of heart transplant CC HCC

5th **T86.3 Complications of heart-lung transplant**

T86.30 Unspecified complication of heart-lung transplant CC HCC

T86.31 Heart-lung transplant rejection CC HCC

T86.32 Heart-lung transplant failure CC HCC

T86.33 Heart-lung transplant infection CC HCC
Use additional code to specify infection

T86.39 Other complications of heart-lung transplant CC HCC

5th **T86.4 Complications of liver transplant**

T86.40 Unspecified complication of liver transplant CC HCC

T86.41 Liver transplant rejection CC HCC

T86.42 Liver transplant failure CC HCC

T86.43 Liver transplant infection CC HCC
Use additional code to identify infection, such as:
cytomegalovirus (CMV) infection (B25.-)

T86.49 Other complications of liver transplant CC HCC

T86.5 Complications of stem cell transplant CC HCC
Complications from stem cells from peripheral blood
Complications from stem cells from umbilical cord
AHA: 2020,4Q,14

5th **T86.8 Complications of other transplanted organs and tissues**

6th **T86.81 Complications of lung transplant**
EXCLUDES 1 *complication of heart-lung transplant (T86.3-)*

T86.810 Lung transplant rejection CC HCC

T86.811 Lung transplant failure CC HCC

T86.812 Lung transplant infection CC HCC
Use additional code to specify infection

T86.818 Other complications of lung transplant CC HCC
AHA: 2019,2Q,6

T86.819 Unspecified complication of lung transplant CC HCC

6th **T86.82 Complications of skin graft (allograft) (autograft)**
EXCLUDES 2 *complication of artificial skin graft (T85.693)*

T86.820 Skin graft (allograft) rejection CC

T86.821 Skin graft (allograft) (autograft) failure CC

T86.822 Skin graft (allograft) (autograft) infection CC
Use additional code to specify infection

T86.828 Other complications of skin graft (allograft) (autograft) CC

T86.829 Unspecified complication of skin graft (allograft) (autograft) CC

T86.83 Complications of bone graft
EXCLUDES 2 mechanical complications of bone graft (T84.3-)
T86.830 Bone graft rejection CC
T86.831 Bone graft failure CC
T86.832 Bone graft infection CC
Use additional code to specify infection
T86.838 Other complications of bone graft CC
T86.839 Unspecified complication of bone graft CC

T86.84 Complications of corneal transplant
EXCLUDES 2 mechanical complications of corneal graft (T85.3-)
AHA: 2020,4Q,40
T86.840 Corneal transplant rejection
T86.8401 Corneal transplant rejection, right eye CC
T86.8402 Corneal transplant rejection, left eye CC
T86.8403 Corneal transplant rejection, bilateral CC
T86.8409 Corneal transplant rejection, unspecified eye CC UNS
T86.841 Corneal transplant failure
T86.8411 Corneal transplant failure, right eye CC
T86.8412 Corneal transplant failure, left eye CC
T86.8413 Corneal transplant failure, bilateral CC
T86.8419 Corneal transplant failure, unspecified eye CC UNS
T86.842 Corneal transplant infection
Use additional code to specify infection
T86.8421 Corneal transplant infection, right eye CC HCC
T86.8422 Corneal transplant infection, left eye CC HCC
T86.8423 Corneal transplant infection, bilateral CC HCC
T86.8429 Corneal transplant infection, unspecified eye CC UNS HCC
T86.848 Other complications of corneal transplant
T86.8481 Other complications of corneal transplant, right eye CC
T86.8482 Other complications of corneal transplant, left eye CC
T86.8483 Other complications of corneal transplant, bilateral CC
T86.8489 Other complications of corneal transplant, unspecified eye CC UNS
T86.849 Unspecified complication of corneal transplant
T86.8491 Unspecified complication of corneal transplant, right eye CC
T86.8492 Unspecified complication of corneal transplant, left eye CC
T86.8493 Unspecified complication of corneal transplant, bilateral CC
T86.8499 Unspecified complication of corneal transplant, unspecified eye CC UNS

T86.85 Complication of intestine transplant
T86.850 Intestine transplant rejection CC HCC
T86.851 Intestine transplant failure CC HCC
T86.852 Intestine transplant infection CC HCC
Use additional code to specify infection
T86.858 Other complications of intestine transplant CC HCC
T86.859 Unspecified complication of intestine transplant CC HCC

T86.89 Complications of other transplanted tissue
Transplant failure or rejection of pancreas
AHA: 2020,1Q,18
T86.890 Other transplanted tissue rejection CC
T86.891 Other transplanted tissue failure CC
T86.892 Other transplanted tissue infection CC
Use additional code to specify infection
T86.898 Other complications of other transplanted tissue CC
T86.899 Unspecified complication of other transplanted tissue CC

T86.9 Complication of unspecified transplanted organ and tissue
T86.90 Unspecified complication of unspecified transplanted organ and tissue CC
T86.91 Unspecified transplanted organ and tissue rejection CC
T86.92 Unspecified transplanted organ and tissue failure CC
T86.93 Unspecified transplanted organ and tissue infection CC
Use additional code to specify infection
T86.99 Other complications of unspecified transplanted organ and tissue CC

T87 Complications peculiar to reattachment and amputation

T87.0 Complications of reattached (part of) upper extremity
T87.0X Complications of reattached (part of) upper extremity
T87.0X1 Complications of reattached (part of) right upper extremity CC HCC
T87.0X2 Complications of reattached (part of) left upper extremity CC HCC
T87.0X9 Complications of reattached (part of) unspecified upper extremity CC UNS HCC

T87.1 Complications of reattached (part of) lower extremity
T87.1X Complications of reattached (part of) lower extremity
T87.1X1 Complications of reattached (part of) right lower extremity CC HCC
T87.1X2 Complications of reattached (part of) left lower extremity CC HCC
T87.1X9 Complications of reattached (part of) unspecified lower extremity CC UNS HCC

T87.2 Complications of other reattached body part CC HCC

T87.3 Neuroma of amputation stump
DEF: Non-neoplastic tumor generated at the proximal end of severed, partially transected, or injured nerve following amputation.
T87.30 Neuroma of amputation stump, unspecified extremity HCC
T87.31 Neuroma of amputation stump, right upper extremity HCC
T87.32 Neuroma of amputation stump, left upper extremity HCC
T87.33 Neuroma of amputation stump, right lower extremity HCC
T87.34 Neuroma of amputation stump, left lower extremity HCC

T87.4 Infection of amputation stump
T87.40 Infection of amputation stump, unspecified extremity CC UNS HCC
T87.41 Infection of amputation stump, right upper extremity CC HCC
T87.42 Infection of amputation stump, left upper extremity CC HCC
T87.43 Infection of amputation stump, right lower extremity CC HCC
T87.44 Infection of amputation stump, left lower extremity CC HCC

T87.5 Necrosis of amputation stump
T87.50 Necrosis of amputation stump, unspecified extremity HCC
T87.51 Necrosis of amputation stump, right upper extremity HCC
T87.52 Necrosis of amputation stump, left upper extremity HCC

N Newborn: 0 P Pediatric: 0-17 M Maternity: 9-64 A Adult: 15-124 UNS Unspecified Site MCC Major Complication/Comorbidity CC Complication/Comorbidity

T87.53 Necrosis of amputation stump, right lower extremity HCC

T87.54 Necrosis of amputation stump, left lower extremity HCC

✓5th **T87.8 Other complications of amputation stump**

T87.81 Dehiscence of amputation stump HCC

T87.89 Other complications of amputation stump HCC

Amputation stump contracture

Amputation stump contracture of next proximal joint

Amputation stump flexion

Amputation stump edema

Amputation stump hematoma

EXCLUDES 2 *phantom limb syndrome (G54.6-G54.7)*

T87.9 Unspecified complications of amputation stump HCC

✓4th **T88 Other complications of surgical and medical care, not elsewhere classified**

EXCLUDES 2 *complication following infusion, transfusion and therapeutic injection (T8Ø.-)*

complication following procedure NEC (T81.-)

complications of anesthesia in labor and delivery (O74.-)

complications of anesthesia in pregnancy (O29.-)

complications of anesthesia in puerperium (O89.-)

complications of devices, implants and grafts (T82-T85)

complications of obstetric surgery and procedure (O75.4)

dermatitis due to drugs and medicaments (L23.3, L24.4, L25.1, L27.Ø-L27.1)

poisoning and toxic effects of drugs and chemicals (T36-T65 with fifth or sixth character 1-4 or 6)

specified complications classified elsewhere

The appropriate 7th character is to be added to each code from category T88.

A initial encounter

D subsequent encounter

S sequela

√x7th **T88.Ø Infection following immunization** CC

Sepsis following immunization

AHA: 2018,4Q,62-63

√x7th **T88.1 Other complications following immunization, not elsewhere classified** CC

Generalized vaccinia

Rash following immunization

EXCLUDES 1 *vaccinia not from vaccine (BØ8.Ø11)*

EXCLUDES 2 *anaphylactic shock due to serum (T8Ø.5-)*

other serum reactions (T8Ø.6-)

postimmunization arthropathy (MØ2.2)

postimmunization encephalitis (GØ4.Ø2)

postimmunization fever (R5Ø.83)

√x7th **T88.2 Shock due to anesthesia** CC

Use additional code for adverse effect, if applicable, to identify drug (T41.- with fifth or sixth character 5)

EXCLUDES 1 *complications of anesthesia (in):*

labor and delivery (O74.-)

postprocedural shock NOS (T81.1-)

pregnancy (O29.-)

puerperium (O89.-)

√x7th **T88.3 Malignant hyperthermia due to anesthesia** CC

Use additional code for adverse effect, if applicable, to identify drug (T41.- with fifth or sixth character 5)

√x7th **T88.4 Failed or difficult intubation**

✓5th **T88.5 Other complications of anesthesia**

Use additional code for adverse effect, if applicable, to identify drug (T41.- with fifth or sixth character 5)

√x7th **T88.51 Hypothermia following anesthesia**

√x7th **T88.52 Failed moderate sedation during procedure**

Failed conscious sedation during procedure

EXCLUDES 2 *personal history of failed moderate sedation (Z92.83)*

√x7th **T88.53 Unintended awareness under general anesthesia during procedure**

EXCLUDES 2 *personal history of unintended awareness under general anesthesia (Z92.84)*

AHA: 2016,4Q,72-73

√x7th **T88.59 Other complications of anesthesia**

√x7th **T88.6 Anaphylactic reaction due to adverse effect of correct drug or medicament properly administered** CC

Anaphylactic shock due to adverse effect of correct drug or medicament properly administered

Anaphylactoid reaction NOS

Use additional code for adverse effect, if applicable, to identify drug (T36-T5Ø with fifth or sixth character 5)

EXCLUDES 1 *anaphylactic reaction due to serum (T8Ø.5-)*

anaphylactic shock or reaction due to adverse food reaction (T78.Ø-)

AHA: 2020,1Q,18

√x7th **T88.7 Unspecified adverse effect of drug or medicament**

Drug hypersensitivity NOS

Drug reaction NOS

Use additional code for adverse effect, if applicable, to identify drug (T36-T5Ø with fifth or sixth character 5)

EXCLUDES 1 *specified adverse effects of drugs and medicaments (AØØ-R94 and T8Ø-T88.6, T88.8)*

√x7th **T88.8 Other specified complications of surgical and medical care, not elsewhere classified**

Use additional code to identify the complication

AHA: 2022,2Q,7

√x7th **T88.9 Complication of surgical and medical care, unspecified**

Chapter 20. External Causes of Morbidity (VØØ–Y99)

Chapter-specific Guidelines with Coding Examples

The chapter-specific guidelines from the ICD-10-CM Official Guidelines for Coding and Reporting have been provided below. Along with these guidelines are coding examples, contained in the shaded boxes, that have been developed to help illustrate the coding and/or sequencing guidance found in these guidelines.

The external causes of morbidity codes should never be sequenced as the first-listed or principal diagnosis.

External cause codes are intended to provide data for injury research and evaluation of injury prevention strategies. These codes capture how the injury or health condition happened (cause), the intent (unintentional or accidental; or intentional, such as suicide or assault), the place where the event occurred the activity of the patient at the time of the event, and the person's status (e.g., civilian, military).

There is no national requirement for mandatory ICD-10-CM external cause code reporting. Unless a provider is subject to a state-based external cause code reporting mandate or these codes are required by a particular payer, reporting of ICD-10-CM codes in Chapter 20, External Causes of Morbidity, is not required. In the absence of a mandatory reporting requirement, providers are encouraged to voluntarily report external cause codes, as they provide valuable data for injury research and evaluation of injury prevention strategies.

a. General external cause coding guidelines

1) Used with any code in the range of AØØ.Ø–T88.9, ZØØ–Z99

An external cause code may be used with any code in the range of AØØ.Ø-T88.9, ZØØ-Z99, classification that represents a health condition due to an external cause. Though they are most applicable to injuries, they are also valid for use with such things as infections or diseases due to an external source, and other health conditions, such as a heart attack that occurs during strenuous physical activity.

Actinic reticuloid due to tanning bed use

L57.1	**Actinic reticuloid**
W89.1XXA	**Exposure to tanning bed, initial encounter**

Explanation: An external cause code may be used with any code in the range of AØØ.Ø–T88.9, ZØØ–Z99, classifications that describe health conditions due to an external cause. Code W89.1 Exposure to tanning bed requires a seventh character of A to report this initial encounter, with a placeholder X for the fifth and sixth characters.

2) External cause code used for length of treatment

Assign the external cause code, with the appropriate 7th character (initial encounter, subsequent encounter or sequela) for each encounter for which the injury or condition is being treated.

Most categories in chapter 20 have a 7th character requirement for each applicable code. Most categories in this chapter have three 7th character values: A, initial encounter, D, subsequent encounter and S, sequela. While the patient may be seen by a new or different provider over the course of treatment for an injury or condition, assignment of the 7th character for external cause should match the 7th character of the code assigned for the associated injury or condition for the encounter.

3) Use the full range of external cause codes

Use the full range of external cause codes to completely describe the cause, the intent, the place of occurrence, and if applicable, the activity of the patient at the time of the event, and the patient's status, for all injuries, and other health conditions due to an external cause.

4) Assign as many external cause codes as necessary

Assign as many external cause codes as necessary to fully explain each cause. If only one external code can be recorded, assign the code most related to the principal diagnosis.

5) The selection of the appropriate external cause code

The selection of the appropriate external cause code is guided by the Alphabetic Index of External Causes and by Inclusion and Exclusion notes in the Tabular List.

6) External cause code can never be a principal diagnosis

An external cause code can never be a principal (first-listed) diagnosis.

7) Combination external cause codes

Certain of the external cause codes are combination codes that identify sequential events that result in an injury, such as a fall which results in striking against an object. The injury may be due to either event or both. The combination external cause code used should correspond to the sequence of events regardless of which caused the most serious injury.

Toddler tripped and fell while walking and struck his head on an end table, sustaining a scalp contusion

SØØ.Ø3XA	**Contusion of scalp, initial encounter**
WØ1.19ØA	**Fall on same level from slipping, tripping and stumbling with subsequent striking against furniture, initial encounter**

Explanation: Combination external cause codes identify sequential events that result in an injury, such as a fall resulting in striking against an object. The injury may be due to either or both events.

8) No external cause code needed in certain circumstances

No external cause code from Chapter 20 is needed if the external cause and intent are included in a code from another chapter (e.g., T36.ØX1-, Poisoning by penicillins, accidental (unintentional)).

b. Place of occurrence guideline

Codes from category Y92, Place of occurrence of the external cause, are secondary codes for use after other external cause codes to identify the location of the patient at the time of injury or other condition.

Generally, a place of occurrence code is assigned only once, at the initial encounter for treatment. However, in the rare instance that a new injury occurs during hospitalization, an additional place of occurrence code may be assigned. No 7th characters are used for Y92.

Do not use place of occurrence code Y92.9 if the place is not stated or is not applicable.

A farmer was working in his barn and sustained a foot contusion when the horse stepped on his left foot

S9Ø.32XA	**Contusion of left foot, initial encounter**
W55.19XA	**Other contact with horse, initial encounter**
Y92.71	**Barn as the place of occurrence of the external cause**

Explanation: A place-of-occurrence code from category Y92 is assigned at the initial encounter to identify the location of the patient at the time the injury occurred.

c. Activity code

Assign a code from category Y93, Activity code, to describe the activity of the patient at the time the injury or other health condition occurred.

An activity code is used only once, at the initial encounter for treatment. Only one code from Y93 should be recorded on a medical record.

The activity codes are not applicable to poisonings, adverse effects, misadventures or sequela.

Do not assign Y93.9, Unspecified activity, if the activity is not stated.

A code from category Y93 is appropriate for use with external cause and intent codes if identifying the activity provides additional information about the event.

Ranch hand who was grooming a horse sustained a foot contusion when the horse stepped on his left foot

S9Ø.32XA	**Contusion of left foot, initial encounter**
W55.19XA	**Other contact with horse, initial encounter**
Y93.K3	**Activity, grooming and shearing an animal**

Explanation: One activity code from category Y93 is assigned at the initial encounter only to describe the activity of the patient at the time the injury occurred.

d. Place of occurrence, activity, and status codes used with other external cause code

When applicable, place of occurrence, activity, and external cause status codes are sequenced after the main external cause code(s). Regardless of the number of external cause codes assigned, generally there should be only one place of occurrence code, one activity code, and one external cause status code assigned to an encounter. However, in the rare instance that a new injury occurs during hospitalization, an additional place of occurrence code may be assigned.

e. If the reporting format limits the number of external cause codes

If the reporting format limits the number of external cause codes that can be used in reporting clinical data, report the code for the cause/intent most related to the principal diagnosis. If the format permits capture of additional external cause codes, the cause/intent, including medical misadventures, of the additional events should be reported rather than the codes for place, activity, or external status.

f. Multiple external cause coding guidelines

More than one external cause code is required to fully describe the external cause of an illness or injury. The assignment of external cause codes should be sequenced in the following priority:

If two or more events cause separate injuries, an external cause code should be assigned for each cause. The first-listed external cause code will be selected in the following order:

External codes for child and adult abuse take priority over all other external cause codes.

See Section I.C.19., Child and Adult abuse guidelines.

External cause codes for terrorism events take priority over all other external cause codes except child and adult abuse.

External cause codes for cataclysmic events take priority over all other external cause codes except child and adult abuse and terrorism.

External cause codes for transport accidents take priority over all other external cause codes except cataclysmic events, child and adult abuse and terrorism.

Activity and external cause status codes are assigned following all causal (intent) external cause codes.

The first-listed external cause code should correspond to the cause of the most serious diagnosis due to an assault, accident, or self-harm, following the order of hierarchy listed above..

30-year-old man accidentally discharged his hunting rifle, sustaining an open gunshot wound to the right thigh, which caused him to fall down the stairs, resulting in closed displaced comminuted fracture of his left radial shaft

S71.131A	**Puncture wound without foreign body, right thigh, initial encounter**
W33.02XA	**Accidental discharge of hunting rifle, initial encounter**
S52.352A	**Displaced comminuted fracture of shaft of radius, left arm, initial encounter for closed fracture**
W10.9XXA	**Fall (on) (from) unspecified stairs and steps, initial encounter**

Explanation: If two or more events cause separate injuries, an external cause code should be assigned for each cause.

g. Child and adult abuse guideline

Adult and child abuse, neglect and maltreatment are classified as assault. Any of the assault codes may be used to indicate the external cause of any injury resulting from the confirmed abuse.

For confirmed cases of abuse, neglect and maltreatment, when the perpetrator is known, a code from Y07, Perpetrator of maltreatment and neglect, should accompany any other assault codes.

See Section I.C.19. Adult and child abuse, neglect and other maltreatment

h. Unknown or undetermined intent guideline

If the intent (accident, self-harm, assault) of the cause of an injury or other condition is unknown or unspecified, code the intent as accidental intent. All transport accident categories assume accidental intent.

1) Use of undetermined intent

External cause codes for events of undetermined intent are only for use if the documentation in the record specifies that the intent cannot be determined.

i. Sequelae (late effects) of external cause guidelines

1) Sequelae external cause codes

Sequela are reported using the external cause code with the 7th character "S" for sequela. These codes should be used with any report of a late effect or sequela resulting from a previous injury.

See Section I.B.10. Sequela (Late Effects)

2) Sequela external cause code with a related current injury

A sequela external cause code should never be used with a related current nature of injury code.

3) Use of sequela external cause codes for subsequent visits

Use a late effect external cause code for subsequent visits when a late effect of the initial injury is being treated. Do not use a late effect external cause code for subsequent visits for follow-up care (e.g., to assess healing, to receive rehabilitative therapy) of the injury when no late effect of the injury has been documented.

j. Terrorism guidelines

1) Cause of injury identified by the Federal Government (FBI) as terrorism

When the cause of an injury is identified by the Federal Government (FBI) as terrorism, the first-listed external cause code should be a code from category Y38, Terrorism. The definition of terrorism employed by the FBI is found at the inclusion note at the beginning of category Y38. Use additional code for place of occurrence (Y92.-). More than one Y38 code may be assigned if the injury is the result of more than one mechanism of terrorism.

2) Cause of an injury is suspected to be the result of terrorism

When the cause of an injury is suspected to be the result of terrorism a code from category Y38 should not be assigned. Suspected cases should be classified as assault.

3) Code Y38.9, Terrorism, secondary effects

Assign code Y38.9, Terrorism, secondary effects, for conditions occurring subsequent to the terrorist event. This code should not be assigned for conditions that are due to the initial terrorist act.

It is acceptable to assign code Y38.9 with another code from Y38 if there is an injury due to the initial terrorist event and an injury that is a subsequent result of the terrorist event.

k. External cause status

A code from category Y99, External cause status, should be assigned whenever any other external cause code is assigned for an encounter, including an Activity code, except for the events noted below. Assign a code from category Y99, External cause status, to indicate the work status of the person at the time the event occurred. The status code indicates whether the event occurred during military activity, whether a non-military person was at work, whether an individual including a student or volunteer was involved in a non-work activity at the time of the causal event.

A code from Y99, External cause status, should be assigned, when applicable, with other external cause codes, such as transport accidents and falls. The external cause status codes are not applicable to poisonings, adverse effects, misadventures or late effects.

Do not assign a code from category Y99 if no other external cause codes (cause, activity) are applicable for the encounter.

An external cause status code is used only once, at the initial encounter for treatment. Only one code from Y99 should be recorded on a medical record.

Do not assign code Y99.9, Unspecified external cause status, if the status is not stated.

Chapter 20. External Causes of Morbidity (V00-Y99)

NOTE This chapter permits the classification of environmental events and circumstances as the cause of injury, and other adverse effects. Where a code from this section is applicable, it is intended that it shall be used secondary to a code from another chapter of the Classification indicating the nature of the condition. Most often, the condition will be classifiable to Chapter 19, Injury, poisoning and certain other consequences of external causes (S00-T88). Other conditions that may be stated to be due to external causes are classified in Chapters I to XVIII. For these conditions, codes from Chapter 20 should be used to provide additional information as to the cause of the condition.

AHA: 2018,4Q,58-60

This chapter contains the following blocks:

V00-X58 Accidents
V00-V99 Transport accidents
V00-V09 Pedestrian injured in transport accident
V10-V19 Pedal cycle rider injured in transport accident
V20-V29 Motorcycle rider injured in transport accident
V30-V39 Occupant of three-wheeled motor vehicle injured in transport accident
V40-V49 Car occupant injured in transport accident
V50-V59 Occupant of pick-up truck or van injured in transport accident
V60-V69 Occupant of heavy transport vehicle injured in transport accident
V70-V79 Bus occupant injured in transport accident
V80-V89 Other land transport accidents
V90-V94 Water transport accidents
V95-V97 Air and space transport accidents
V98-V99 Other and unspecified transport accidents
W00-X58 Other external causes of accidental injury
W00-W19 Slipping, tripping, stumbling and falls
W20-W49 Exposure to inanimate mechanical forces
W50-W64 Exposure to animate mechanical forces
W65-W74 Accidental non-transport drowning and submersion
W85-W99 Exposure to electric current, radiation and extreme ambient air temperature and pressure
X00-X08 Exposure to smoke, fire and flames
X10-X19 Contact with heat and hot substances
X30-X39 Exposure to forces of nature
X50 Overexertion and strenuous or repetitive movements
X52-X58 Accidental exposure to other specified factors
X71-X83 Intentional self-harm
X92-Y09 Assault
Y21-Y33 Event of undetermined intent
Y35-Y38 Legal intervention, operations of war, military operations, and terrorism
Y62-Y84 Complications of medical and surgical care
Y62-Y69 Misadventures to patients during surgical and medical care
Y70-Y82 Medical devices associated with adverse incidents in diagnostic and therapeutic use
Y83-Y84 Surgical and other medical procedures as the cause of abnormal reaction of the patient, or of later complication, without mention of misadventure at the time of the procedure
Y90-Y99 Supplementary factors related to causes of morbidity classified elsewhere

ACCIDENTS (V00-X58)

AHA: 2018,2Q,7-8

Transport accidents (V00-V99)

NOTE This section is structured in 12 groups. Those relating to land transport accidents (V00-V89) reflect the victim's mode of transport and are subdivided to identify the victim's 'counterpart' or the type of event. The vehicle of which the injured person is an occupant is identified in the first two characters since it is seen as the most important factor to identify for prevention purposes. A transport accident is one in which the vehicle involved must be moving or running or in use for transport purposes at the time of the accident.

Use additional code to identify:
- airbag injury (W22.1)
- type of street or road (Y92.4-)
- use of cellular telephone and other electronic equipment at the time of the transport accident (Y93.C-)

EXCLUDES 1
agricultural vehicles in stationary use or maintenance (W31.-)
assault by crashing of motor vehicle (Y03.-)
automobile or motor cycle in stationary use or maintenance - code to type of accident
crashing of motor vehicle, undetermined intent (Y32)
intentional self-harm by crashing of motor vehicle (X82)

EXCLUDES 2
transport accidents due to cataclysm (X34-X38)

NOTE Definitions related to transport accidents:

(a) A transport accident (V00-V99) is any accident involving a device designed primarily for, or used at the time primarily for, conveying persons or good from one place to another.

(b) A public highway [trafficway] or street is the entire width between property lines (or other boundary lines) of land open to the public as a matter of right or custom for purposes of moving persons or property from one place to another. A roadway is that part of the public highway designed, improved and customarily used for vehicular traffic.

(c) A traffic accident is any vehicle accident occurring on the public highway [i.e. originating on, terminating on, or involving a vehicle partially on the highway]. A vehicle accident is assumed to have occurred on the public highway unless another place is specified, except in the case of accidents involving only off-road motor vehicles, which are classified as nontraffic accidents unless the contrary is stated.

(d) A nontraffic accident is any vehicle accident that occurs entirely in any place other than a public highway.

(e) A pedestrian is any person involved in an accident who was not at the time of the accident riding in or on a motor vehicle, railway train, streetcar or animal-drawn or other vehicle, or on a pedal cycle or animal. This includes, a person changing a tire, working on a parked car, or a person on foot. It also includes the user of a pedestrian conveyance such as a baby stroller, ice-skates, skis, sled, roller skates, a skateboard, nonmotorized or motorized wheelchair, motorized mobility scooter, or nonmotorized scooter.

(f) A driver is an occupant of a transport vehicle who is operating or intending to operate it.

(g) A passenger is any occupant of a transport vehicle other than the driver, except a person traveling on the outside of the vehicle.

(h) A person on the outside of a vehicle is any person being transported by a vehicle but not occupying the space normally reserved for the driver or passengers, or the space intended for the transport of property. This includes a person travelling on the bodywork, bumper, fender, roof, running board or step of a vehicle, as well as, hanging on the outside of the vehicle.

(i) A pedal cycle is any land transport vehicle operated solely by nonmotorized pedals including a bicycle or tricycle.

(j) A pedal cyclist is any person riding a pedal cycle or in a sidecar or trailer attached to a pedal cycle.

(k) A motorcycle is a two-wheeled motor vehicle with one or two riding saddles and sometimes with a third wheel for the support of a sidecar. The sidecar is considered part of the motorcycle. This includes a moped, motor scooter, or motorized bicycle.

(l) A motorcycle rider is any person riding a motorcycle or in a sidecar or trailer attached to the motorcycle.

(m) A three-wheeled motor vehicle is a motorized tricycle designed primarily for on-road use. This includes a motor-driven tricycle, a motorized rickshaw, or a three-wheeled motor car.

(n) A car [automobile] is a four-wheeled motor vehicle designed primarily for carrying up to 7 persons. A trailer being towed by the car is considered part of the car. It does not include a van or minivan — see definition (o).

(o) A pick-up truck or van is a four or six-wheeled motor vehicle designed for carrying passengers as well as property or cargo weighing less than the local limit for classification as a heavy goods vehicle, and not requiring a special driver's license. This includes a minivan and a sport-utility vehicle (SUV).

(p) A heavy transport vehicle is a motor vehicle designed primarily for carrying property, meeting local criteria for classification as a heavy goods vehicle in terms of weight and requiring a special driver's license.

(q) A bus (coach) is a motor vehicle designed or adapted primarily for carrying more than 10 passengers, and requiring a special driver's license.

(r) A railway train or railway vehicle is any device, with or without freight or passenger cars couple to it, designed for traffic on a railway track. This includes subterranean (subways) or elevated trains.

(s) A streetcar, is a device designed and used primarily for transporting passengers within a municipality, running on rails, usually subject to normal traffic control signals, and operated principally on a right-of-way that forms part of the roadway. This includes a tram or trolley that runs on rails. A trailer being towed by a streetcar is considered part of the streetcar.

(t) A special vehicle mainly used on industrial premises is a motor vehicle designed primarily for use within the buildings and premises of industrial or commercial establishments. This includes battery-powered airport passenger vehicles or baggage/mail trucks, forklifts, coal-cars in a coal mine, logging cars and trucks used in mines or quarries.

(u) A special vehicle mainly used in agriculture is a motor vehicle designed specifically for use in farming and agriculture (horticulture), to work the land, tend and harvest crops and transport materials on the farm. This includes harvesters, farm machinery and tractor and trailers.

(v) A special construction vehicle is a motor vehicle designed specifically for use on construction and demolition sites. This includes bulldozers, diggers, earth levellers, dump trucks. backhoes, front-end loaders, pavers, and mechanical shovels.

(w) A special all-terrain vehicle is a motor vehicle of special design to enable it to negotiate over rough or soft terrain, snow or sand. Examples of special design are high construction, special wheels and tires, tracks, and support on a cushion of air. This includes snow mobiles, All-terrain vehicles (ATV), and dune buggies. It does not include passenger vehicle designated as Sport Utility Vehicles. (SUV)

(x) A watercraft is any device designed for transporting passengers or goods on water. This includes motor or sailboats, ships, and hovercraft.

(y) An aircraft is any device for transporting passengers or goods in the air. This includes hot-air balloons, gliders, helicopters and airplanes.

(z) A military vehicle is any motorized vehicle operating on a public roadway owned by the military and being operated by a member of the military.

Pedestrian injured in transport accident (V00-V09)

INCLUDES person changing tire on transport vehicle
person examining engine of vehicle broken down in (on side of) road

EXCLUDES 1 *fall due to non-transport collision with other person (W03)*
pedestrian on foot falling (slipping) on ice and snow (W00.-)
struck or bumped by another person (W51)

The appropriate 7th character is to be added to each code from categories V00-V09.
A initial encounter
D subsequent encounter
S sequela

V00 Pedestrian conveyance accident

Use additional place of occurrence and activity external cause codes, if known (Y92.-, Y93.-)

EXCLUDES 1 *collision with another person without fall (W51)*
fall due to person on foot colliding with another person on foot (W03)
fall from non-moving wheelchair, nonmotorized scooter and motorized mobility scooter without collision (W05.-)
pedestrian (conveyance) collision with other land transport vehicle (V01-V09)
pedestrian on foot falling (slipping) on ice and snow (W00.-)

V00.0 Pedestrian on foot injured in collision with pedestrian conveyance

V00.01 Pedestrian on foot injured in collision with roller-skater

V00.02 Pedestrian on foot injured in collision with skateboarder

V00.03 Pedestrian on foot injured in collision with standing micro-mobility pedestrian conveyance

V00.031 Pedestrian on foot injured in collision with rider of standing electric scooter

V00.038 Pedestrian on foot injured in collision with rider of other standing micro-mobility pedestrian conveyance
Pedestrian on foot injured in collision with rider of hoverboard
Pedestrian on foot injured in collision with rider of segway

V00.09 Pedestrian on foot injured in collision with other pedestrian conveyance

V00.1 Rolling-type pedestrian conveyance accident

EXCLUDES 1 *accident with baby stroller (V00.82-)*
accident with motorized mobility scooter (V00.83-)
accident with wheelchair (powered) (V00.81-)

V00.11 In-line roller-skate accident

V00.111 Fall from in-line roller-skates

V00.112 In-line roller-skater colliding with stationary object

V00.118 Other in-line roller-skate accident

EXCLUDES 1 *roller-skater collision with other land transport vehicle (V01-V09 with 5th character 1)*

V00.12 Non-in-line roller-skate accident

V00.121 Fall from non-in-line roller-skates

V00.122 Non-in-line roller-skater colliding with stationary object

V00.128 Other non-in-line roller-skating accident

EXCLUDES 1 *roller-skater collision with other land transport vehicle (V01-V09 with 5th character 1)*

V00.13 Skateboard accident

V00.131 Fall from skateboard

V00.132 Skateboarder colliding with stationary object

V00.138 Other skateboard accident

EXCLUDES 1 *skateboarder collision with other land transport vehicle (V01-V09 with 5th character 2)*

V00.14 Scooter (nonmotorized) accident

EXCLUDES 1 *motor scooter accident (V20-V29)*

V00.141 Fall from scooter (nonmotorized)

V00.142 Scooter (nonmotorized) colliding with stationary object

V00.148 Other scooter (nonmotorized) accident

EXCLUDES 1 *scooter (nonmotorized) collision with other land transport vehicle (V01-V09 with fifth character 9)*

V00.15 Heelies accident
Rolling shoe
Wheeled shoe
Wheelies accident

V00.151 Fall from heelies

V00.152 Heelies colliding with stationary object

V00.158 Other heelies accident

V00.18 Accident on other rolling-type pedestrian conveyance

V00.181 Fall from other rolling-type pedestrian conveyance

V00.182 Pedestrian on other rolling-type pedestrian conveyance colliding with stationary object

V00.188 Other accident on other rolling-type pedestrian conveyance

V00.2 Gliding-type pedestrian conveyance accident

V00.21 Ice-skates accident

V00.211 Fall from ice-skates

V00.212 Ice-skater colliding with stationary object

V00.218 Other ice-skates accident

EXCLUDES 1 *ice-skater collision with other land transport vehicle (V01-V09 with 5th character 9)*

V00.22 Sled accident

V00.221 Fall from sled

V00.222 Sledder colliding with stationary object

V00.228 Other sled accident

EXCLUDES 1 *sled collision with other land transport vehicle (V01-V09 with 5th character 9)*

V00.28 Other gliding-type pedestrian conveyance accident

V00.281 Fall from other gliding-type pedestrian conveyance

V00.282 Pedestrian on other gliding-type pedestrian conveyance colliding with stationary object

7th **V00.288 Other accident on other gliding-type pedestrian conveyance**
EXCLUDES 1 *gliding-type pedestrian conveyance collision with other land transport vehicle (V01-V09 with 5th character 9)*

5th **V00.3 Flat-bottomed pedestrian conveyance accident**
6th **V00.31 Snowboard accident**
7th **V00.311 Fall from snowboard**
7th **V00.312 Snowboarder colliding with stationary object**
7th **V00.318 Other snowboard accident**
EXCLUDES 1 *snowboarder collision with other land transport vehicle (V01-V09 with 5th character 9)*

6th **V00.32 Snow-ski accident**
7th **V00.321 Fall from snow-skis**
7th **V00.322 Snow-skier colliding with stationary object**
7th **V00.328 Other snow-ski accident**
EXCLUDES 1 *snow-skier collision with other land transport vehicle (V01-V09 with 5th character 9)*

6th **V00.38 Other flat-bottomed pedestrian conveyance accident**
7th **V00.381 Fall from other flat-bottomed pedestrian conveyance**
7th **V00.382 Pedestrian on other flat-bottomed pedestrian conveyance colliding with stationary object**
7th **V00.388 Other accident on other flat-bottomed pedestrian conveyance**

5th **V00.8 Accident on other pedestrian conveyance**
6th **V00.81 Accident with wheelchair (powered)**
7th **V00.811 Fall from moving wheelchair (powered)**
EXCLUDES 1 *fall from non-moving wheelchair (W05.0)*
7th **V00.812 Wheelchair (powered) colliding with stationary object**
7th **V00.818 Other accident with wheelchair (powered)**
6th **V00.82 Accident with baby stroller**
7th **V00.821 Fall from baby stroller**
7th **V00.822 Baby stroller colliding with stationary object**
7th **V00.828 Other accident with baby stroller**
6th **V00.83 Accident with motorized mobility scooter**
7th **V00.831 Fall from motorized mobility scooter**
EXCLUDES 1 *fall from non-moving motorized mobility scooter (W05.2)*
7th **V00.832 Motorized mobility scooter colliding with stationary object**
7th **V00.838 Other accident with motorized mobility scooter**
6th **V00.84 Accident with standing micro-mobility pedestrian conveyance**
7th **V00.841 Fall from standing electric scooter**
7th **V00.842 Pedestrian on standing electric scooter colliding with stationary object**
7th **V00.848 Other accident with standing micro-mobility pedestrian conveyance**
Accident with hoverboard
Accident with segway
6th **V00.89 Accident on other pedestrian conveyance**
7th **V00.891 Fall from other pedestrian conveyance**
7th **V00.892 Pedestrian on other pedestrian conveyance colliding with stationary object**
7th **V00.898 Other accident on other pedestrian conveyance**
EXCLUDES 1 *other pedestrian (conveyance) collision with other land transport vehicle (V01-V09 with 5th character 9)*

4th **V01 Pedestrian injured in collision with pedal cycle**
5th **V01.0 Pedestrian injured in collision with pedal cycle in nontraffic accident**
x7th **V01.00 Pedestrian on foot injured in collision with pedal cycle in nontraffic accident**
Pedestrian NOS injured in collision with pedal cycle in nontraffic accident
x7th **V01.01 Pedestrian on roller-skates injured in collision with pedal cycle in nontraffic accident**
x7th **V01.02 Pedestrian on skateboard injured in collision with pedal cycle in nontraffic accident**
6th **V01.03 Pedestrian on standing micro-mobility pedestrian conveyance injured in collision with pedal cycle in nontraffic accident**
7th **V01.031 Pedestrian on standing electric scooter injured in collision with pedal cycle in nontraffic accident**
7th **V01.038 Pedestrian on other standing micro-mobility pedestrian conveyance injured in collision with pedal cycle in nontraffic accident**
Pedestrian on hoverboard injured in collision with pedal cycle in nontraffic accident
Pedestrian on segway injured in collision with pedal cycle in nontraffic accident
x7th **V01.09 Pedestrian with other conveyance injured in collision with pedal cycle in nontraffic accident**
Pedestrian with baby stroller injured in collision with pedal cycle in nontraffic accident
Pedestrian on ice-skates injured in collision with pedal cycle in nontraffic accident
Pedestrian on nonmotorized scooter injured in collision with pedal cycle in nontraffic accident
Pedestrian on sled injured in collision with pedal cycle in nontraffic accident
Pedestrian on snowboard injured in collision with pedal cycle in nontraffic accident
Pedestrian on snow-skis injured in collision with pedal cycle in nontraffic accident
Pedestrian in wheelchair (powered) injured in collision with pedal cycle in nontraffic accident
Pedestrian in motorized mobility scooter injured in collision with pedal cycle in nontraffic accident
5th **V01.1 Pedestrian injured in collision with pedal cycle in traffic accident**
x7th **V01.10 Pedestrian on foot injured in collision with pedal cycle in traffic accident**
Pedestrian NOS injured in collision with pedal cycle in traffic accident
x7th **V01.11 Pedestrian on roller-skates injured in collision with pedal cycle in traffic accident**
x7th **V01.12 Pedestrian on skateboard injured in collision with pedal cycle in traffic accident**
6th **V01.13 Pedestrian on standing micro-mobility pedestrian conveyance injured in collision with pedal cycle in traffic accident**
7th **V01.131 Pedestrian on standing electric scooter injured in collision with pedal cycle in traffic accident**
7th **V01.138 Pedestrian on other standing micro-mobility pedestrian conveyance injured in collision with pedal cycle in traffic accident**
Pedestrian on hoverboard injured in collision with pedal cycle in traffic accident
Pedestrian on segway injured in collision with pedal cycle in traffic accident

√x7th **V01.19 Pedestrian with other conveyance injured in collision with pedal cycle in traffic accident**
Pedestrian with baby stroller injured in collision with pedal cycle in traffic accident
Pedestrian on ice-skates injured in collision with pedal cycle in traffic accident
Pedestrian on nonmotorized scooter injured in collision with pedal cycle in traffic accident
Pedestrian on sled injured in collision with pedal cycle in traffic accident
Pedestrian on snowboard injured in collision with pedal cycle in traffic accident
Pedestrian on snow-skis injured in collision with pedal cycle in traffic accident
Pedestrian in wheelchair (powered) injured in collision with pedal cycle in traffic accident
Pedestrian in motorized mobility scooter injured in collision with pedal cycle in traffic accident

√5th **V01.9 Pedestrian injured in collision with pedal cycle, unspecified whether traffic or nontraffic accident**

√x7th **V01.90 Pedestrian on foot injured in collision with pedal cycle, unspecified whether traffic or nontraffic accident**
Pedestrian NOS injured in collision with pedal cycle, unspecified whether traffic or nontraffic accident

√x7th **V01.91 Pedestrian on roller-skates injured in collision with pedal cycle, unspecified whether traffic or nontraffic accident**

√x7th **V01.92 Pedestrian on skateboard injured in collision with pedal cycle, unspecified whether traffic or nontraffic accident**

√6th **V01.93 Pedestrian on standing micro-mobility pedestrian conveyance injured in collision with pedal cycle, unspecified whether traffic or nontraffic accident**

√7th **V01.931 Pedestrian on standing electric scooter injured in collision with pedal cycle, unspecified whether traffic or nontraffic accident**

√7th **V01.938 Pedestrian on other standing micro-mobility pedestrian conveyance injured in collision with pedal cycle, unspecified whether traffic or nontraffic accident**
Pedestrian on hoverboard injured in collision with pedal cycle, unspecified whether traffic or nontraffic accident
Pedestrian on segway injured in collision with pedal cycle, unspecified whether traffic or nontraffic accident

√x7th **V01.99 Pedestrian with other conveyance injured in collision with pedal cycle, unspecified whether traffic or nontraffic accident**
Pedestrian with baby stroller injured in collision with pedal cycle, unspecified whether traffic or nontraffic accident
Pedestrian on ice-skates injured in collision with pedal cycle unspecified, whether traffic or nontraffic accident
Pedestrian on nonmotorized scooter injured in collision with pedal cycle, unspecified whether traffic or nontraffic accident
Pedestrian on sled injured in collision with pedal cycle unspecified, whether traffic or nontraffic accident
Pedestrian on snowboard injured in collision with pedal cycle, unspecified whether traffic or nontraffic accident
Pedestrian on snow-skis injured in collision with pedal cycle, unspecified whether traffic or nontraffic accident
Pedestrian in wheelchair (powered) injured in collision with pedal cycle, unspecified whether traffic or nontraffic accident
Pedestrian in motorized mobility scooter injured in collision with pedal cycle, unspecified whether traffic or nontraffic accident

√4th **V02 Pedestrian injured in collision with two- or three-wheeled motor vehicle**

√5th **V02.0 Pedestrian injured in collision with two- or three-wheeled motor vehicle in nontraffic accident**

√x7th **V02.00 Pedestrian on foot injured in collision with two- or three-wheeled motor vehicle in nontraffic accident**
Pedestrian NOS injured in collision with two- or three-wheeled motor vehicle in nontraffic accident

√x7th **V02.01 Pedestrian on roller-skates injured in collision with two- or three-wheeled motor vehicle in nontraffic accident**

√x7th **V02.02 Pedestrian on skateboard injured in collision with two- or three-wheeled motor vehicle in nontraffic accident**

√6th **V02.03 Pedestrian on standing micro-mobility pedestrian conveyance injured in collision with two- or three-wheeled motor vehicle in nontraffic accident**

√7th **V02.031 Pedestrian on standing electric scooter injured in collision with two- or three-wheeled motor vehicle in nontraffic accident**

√7th **V02.038 Pedestrian on other standing micro-mobility pedestrian conveyance injured in collision with two- or three-wheeled motor vehicle in nontraffic accident**
Pedestrian on hoverboard injured in collision with two-or three wheeled motor vehicle in nontraffic accident
Pedestrian on segway injured in collision with two- or three-wheeled motor vehicle in nontraffic accident

√x7th **V02.09 Pedestrian with other conveyance injured in collision with two- or three-wheeled motor vehicle in nontraffic accident**
Pedestrian with baby stroller injured in collision with two- or three-wheeled motor vehicle in nontraffic accident
Pedestrian on ice-skates injured in collision with two- or three-wheeled motor vehicle in nontraffic accident
Pedestrian on nonmotorized scooter injured in collision with two- or three-wheeled motor vehicle in nontraffic accident
Pedestrian on sled injured in collision with two- or three-wheeled motor vehicle in nontraffic accident
Pedestrian on snowboard injured in collision with two- or three-wheeled motor vehicle in nontraffic accident
Pedestrian on snow-skis injured in collision with two- or three-wheeled motor vehicle in nontraffic accident
Pedestrian in wheelchair (powered) injured in collision with two- or three-wheeled motor vehicle in nontraffic accident
Pedestrian in motorized mobility scooter injured in collision with two- or three-wheeled motor vehicle in nontraffic accident

√5th **V02.1 Pedestrian injured in collision with two- or three-wheeled motor vehicle in traffic accident**

√x7th **V02.10 Pedestrian on foot injured in collision with two- or three-wheeled motor vehicle in traffic accident**
Pedestrian NOS injured in collision with two- or three-wheeled motor vehicle in traffic accident

√x7th **V02.11 Pedestrian on roller-skates injured in collision with two- or three-wheeled motor vehicle in traffic accident**

√x7th **V02.12 Pedestrian on skateboard injured in collision with two- or three-wheeled motor vehicle in traffic accident**

√6th **V02.13 Pedestrian on standing micro-mobility pedestrian conveyance injured in collision with two- or three-wheeled motor vehicle in traffic accident**

√7th **V02.131 Pedestrian on standing electric scooter injured in collision with two- or three-wheeled motor vehicle in traffic accident**

V02.138 **Pedestrian on other standing micro-mobility pedestrian conveyance injured in collision with two- or three-wheeled motor vehicle in traffic accident**
Pedestrian on hoverboard injured in collision with two-or three wheeled motor vehicle in traffic accident
Pedestrian on segway injured in collision with two- or three-wheeled motor vehicle in traffic accident

V02.19 **Pedestrian with other conveyance injured in collision with two- or three-wheeled motor vehicle in traffic accident**
Pedestrian with baby stroller injured in collision with two- or three-wheeled motor vehicle in traffic accident
Pedestrian on ice-skates injured in collision with two- or three-wheeled motor vehicle in traffic accident
Pedestrian on nonmotorized scooter injured in collision with two- or three-wheeled motor vehicle in traffic accident
Pedestrian on sled injured in collision with two- or three-wheeled motor vehicle in traffic accident
Pedestrian on snowboard injured in collision with two- or three-wheeled motor vehicle in traffic accident
Pedestrian on snow-skis injured in collision with two- or three-wheeled motor vehicle in traffic accident
Pedestrian in wheelchair (powered) injured in collision with two- or three-wheeled motor vehicle in traffic accident
Pedestrian in motorized mobility scooter injued in collision with two- or three-wheeled motor vehicle in traffic accident

V02.9 **Pedestrian injured in collision with two- or three-wheeled motor vehicle, unspecified whether traffic or nontraffic accident**

V02.90 **Pedestrian on foot injured in collision with two- or three-wheeled motor vehicle, unspecified whether traffic or nontraffic accident**
Pedestrian NOS injured in collision with two- or three-wheeled motor vehicle, unspecified whether traffic or nontraffic accident

V02.91 **Pedestrian on roller-skates injured in collision with two- or three-wheeled motor vehicle, unspecified whether traffic or nontraffic accident**

V02.92 **Pedestrian on skateboard injured in collision with two- or three-wheeled motor vehicle, unspecified whether traffic or nontraffic accident**

V02.93 **Pedestrian on standing micro-mobility pedestrian conveyance injured in collision with two- or three-wheeled motor vehicle, unspecified whether traffic or nontraffic accident**

V02.931 **Pedestrian on standing electric scooter injured in collision with two- or three wheeled motor vehicle, unspecified whether traffic or nontraffic accident**

V02.938 **Pedestrian on other standing micro-mobility pedestrian conveyance injured in collision with two- or three wheeled motor vehicle, unspecified whether traffic or nontraffic accident**
Pedestrian on hoverboard injured in collision with two-three-wheeled motor vehicle, unspecified whether traffic or nontraffic accident
Pedestrian on segway injured in collision with two- or three wheeled motor vehicle, unspecified whether traffic or nontraffic accident

V02.99 **Pedestrian with other conveyance injured in collision with two- or three-wheeled motor vehicle, unspecified whether traffic or nontraffic accident**
Pedestrian with baby stroller injured in collision with two- or three-wheeled motor vehicle, unspecified whether traffic or nontraffic accident
Pedestrian on ice-skates injured in collision with two- or three-wheeled motor vehicle, unspecified whether traffic or nontraffic accident
Pedestrian on nonmotorized scooter injured in collision with two- or three-wheeled motor vehicle, unspecified whether traffic or nontraffic accident
Pedestrian on sled injured in collision with two- or three-wheeled motor vehicle, unspecified whether traffic or nontraffic accident
Pedestrian on snowboard injured in collision with two- or three-wheeled motor vehicle, unspecified whether traffic or nontraffic accident
Pedestrian on snow-skis injured in collision with two- or three-wheeled motor vehicle, unspecified whether traffic or nontraffic accident
Pedestrian in wheelchair (powered) injured in collision with two- or three-wheeled motor vehicle, unspecified whether traffic or nontraffic accident
Pedestrian in motorized mobility scooter injured in collision with two- or three wheeled motor vehicle, unspecified whether traffic or nontraffic accident

V03 **Pedestrian injured in collision with car, pick-up truck or van**

V03.0 **Pedestrian injured in collision with car, pick-up truck or van in nontraffic accident**

V03.00 **Pedestrian on foot injured in collision with car, pick-up truck or van in nontraffic accident**
Pedestrian NOS injured in collision with car, pick-up truck or van in nontraffic accident

V03.01 **Pedestrian on roller-skates injured in collision with car, pick-up truck or van in nontraffic accident**

V03.02 **Pedestrian on skateboard injured in collision with car, pick-up truck or van in nontraffic accident**

V03.03 **Pedestrian on standing micro-mobility pedestrian conveyance injured in collision with car, pick-up or van in nontraffic accident**

V03.031 **Pedestrian on standing electric scooter injured in collision with car, pick-up or van in nontraffic accident**

V03.038 **Pedestrian on other standing micro-mobility pedestrian conveyance injured in collision with car, pick-up or van in nontraffic accident**
Pedestrian on hoverboard injured in collision with car, pick-up or van in nontraffic accident
Pedestrian on segway injured in collision with car, pick-up or van in nontraffic accident

V03.09 **Pedestrian with other conveyance injured in collision with car, pick-up truck or van in nontraffic accident**
Pedestrian with baby stroller injured in collision with car, pick-up truck or van in nontraffic accident
Pedestrian on ice-skates injured in collision with car, pick-up truck or van in nontraffic accident
Pedestrian on nonmotorized scooter injured in collision with car, pick-up truck or van in nontraffic accident
Pedestrian on sled injured in collision with car, pick-up truck or van in nontraffic accident
Pedestrian on snowboard injured in collision with car, pick-up truck or van in nontraffic accident
Pedestrian on snow-skis injured in collision with car, pick-up truck or van in nontraffic accident
Pedestrian in wheelchair (powered) injured in collision with car, pick-up truck or van in nontraffic accident
Pedestrian in motorized mobility scooter injured in collision with car, pick-up truck or van in nontraffic accident

✓5th **V03.1 Pedestrian injured in collision with car, pick-up truck or van in traffic accident**

✓x7th **V03.10 Pedestrian on foot injured in collision with car, pick-up truck or van in traffic accident**
Pedestrian NOS injured in collision with car, pick-up truck or van in traffic accident

✓x7th **V03.11 Pedestrian on roller-skates injured in collision with car, pick-up truck or van in traffic accident**

✓x7th **V03.12 Pedestrian on skateboard injured in collision with car, pick-up truck or van in traffic accident**

✓6th **V03.13 Pedestrian on standing micro-mobility pedestrian conveyance injured in collision with car, pick-up or van in traffic accident**

✓7th **V03.131 Pedestrian on standing electric scooter injured in collision with car, pick-up or van in traffic accident**

✓7th **V03.138 Pedestrian on other standing micro-mobility pedestrian conveyance injured in collision with car, pick-up or van in traffic accident**
Pedestrian on hoverboard injured in collision with car, pick-up or van in traffic accident
Pedestrian on segway injured in collision with car, pick-up or van in traffic accident

✓x7th **V03.19 Pedestrian with other conveyance injured in collision with car, pick-up truck or van in traffic accident**
Pedestrian with baby stroller injured in collision with car, pick-up truck or van in traffic accident
Pedestrian on ice-skates injured in collision with car, pick-up truck or van in traffic accident
Pedestrian on nonmotorized scooter injured in collision with car, pick-up truck or van in nontraffic accident
Pedestrian on sled injured in collision with car, pick-up truck or van in traffic accident
Pedestrian on snowboard injured in collision with car, pick-up truck or van in traffic accident
Pedestrian on snow-skis injured in collision with car, pick-up truck or van in traffic accident
Pedestrian in wheelchair (powered) injured in collision with car, pick-up truck or van in traffic accident
Pedestrian in motorized mobility scooter injured in collision with car, pick-up truck or van in nontraffic accident

✓5th **V03.9 Pedestrian injured in collision with car, pick-up truck or van, unspecified whether traffic or nontraffic accident**

✓x7th **V03.90 Pedestrian on foot injured in collision with car, pick-up truck or van, unspecified whether traffic or nontraffic accident**
Pedestrian NOS injured in collision with car, pick-up truck or van, unspecified whether traffic or nontraffic accident

✓x7th **V03.91 Pedestrian on roller-skates injured in collision with car, pick-up truck or van, unspecified whether traffic or nontraffic accident**

✓x7th **V03.92 Pedestrian on skateboard injured in collision with car, pick-up truck or van, unspecified whether traffic or nontraffic accident**

✓6th **V03.93 Pedestrian on standing micro-mobility pedestrian conveyance injured in collision with car, pick-up or van, unspecified whether traffic or nontraffic accident**

✓7th **V03.931 Pedestrian on standing electric scooter injured in collision with car, pick-up or van, unspecified whether traffic or nontraffic accident**

✓7th **V03.938 Pedestrian on other standing micro-mobility pedestrian conveyance injured in collision with car, pick-up or van, unspecified whether traffic or nontraffic accident**
Pedestrian on hoverboard injured in collision with car, pick-up or van, unspecified whether traffic or nontraffic accident
Pedestrian on segway injured in collision with car, pick-up or van, unspecified whether traffic or nontraffic accident

✓x7th **V03.99 Pedestrian with other conveyance injured in collision with car, pick-up truck or van, unspecified whether traffic or nontraffic accident**
Pedestrian with baby stroller injured in collision with car, pick-up truck or van, unspecified whether traffic or nontraffic accident
Pedestrian on ice-skates injured in collision with car, pick-up truck or van, unspecified whether traffic or nontraffic accident
Pedestrian on nonmotorized scooter injured in collision with car, pick-up truck or van, unspecified whether traffic or nontraffic accident
Pedestrian on sled injured in collision with car, pick-up truck or van in nontraffic accident
Pedestrian on snowboard injured in collision with car, pick-up truck or van, unspecified whether traffic or nontraffic accident
Pedestrian on snow-skis injured in collision with car, pick-up truck or van, unspecified whether traffic or nontraffic accident
Pedestrian in wheelchair (powered) injured in collision with car, pick-up truck or van, unspecified whether traffic or nontraffic accident
Pedestrian in motorized mobility scooter injured in collision with car, pick-up truck or van, unspecified whether traffic or nontraffic accident

✓4th **V04 Pedestrian injured in collision with heavy transport vehicle or bus**
EXCLUDES 1 *pedestrian injured in collision with military vehicle (V09.01, V09.21)*

✓5th **V04.0 Pedestrian injured in collision with heavy transport vehicle or bus in nontraffic accident**

✓x7th **V04.00 Pedestrian on foot injured in collision with heavy transport vehicle or bus in nontraffic accident**
Pedestrian NOS injured in collision with heavy transport vehicle or bus in nontraffic accident

✓x7th **V04.01 Pedestrian on roller-skates injured in collision with heavy transport vehicle or bus in nontraffic accident**

✓x7th **V04.02 Pedestrian on skateboard injured in collision with heavy transport vehicle or bus in nontraffic accident**

✓6th **V04.03 Pedestrian on standing micro-mobility pedestrian conveyance injured in collision with heavy transport vehicle or bus in nontraffic accident**

✓7th **V04.031 Pedestrian on standing electric scooter injured in collision with heavy transport vehicle or bus in nontraffic accident**

✓7th **V04.038 Pedestrian on other standing micro-mobility pedestrian conveyance injured in collision with heavy transport vehicle or bus in nontraffic accident**
Pedestrian on hoverboard injured in collision with heavy transport vehicle or bus in nontraffic accident
Pedestrian on segway injured in collision with heavy transport vehicle or bus in nontraffic accident

V04.09 Pedestrian with other conveyance injured in collision with heavy transport vehicle or bus in nontraffic accident
Pedestrian with baby stroller injured in collision with heavy transport vehicle or bus in nontraffic accident
Pedestrian on ice-skates injured in collision with heavy transport vehicle or bus in nontraffic accident
Pedestrian on nonmotorized scooter injured in collision with heavy transport vehicle or bus in nontraffic accident
Pedestrian on sled injured in collision with heavy transport vehicle or bus in nontraffic accident
Pedestrian on snowboard injured in collision with heavy transport vehicle or bus in nontraffic accident
Pedestrian on snow-skis injured in collision with heavy transport vehicle or bus in nontraffic accident
Pedestrian in wheelchair (powered) injured in collision with heavy transport vehicle or bus in nontraffic accident
Pedestrian in motorized mobility scooter injured in collision with heavy transport vehicle or bus in nontraffic accident

V04.1 Pedestrian injured in collision with heavy transport vehicle or bus in traffic accident

V04.10 Pedestrian on foot injured in collision with heavy transport vehicle or bus in traffic accident
Pedestrian NOS injured in collision with heavy transport vehicle or bus in traffic accident

V04.11 Pedestrian on roller-skates injured in collision with heavy transport vehicle or bus in traffic accident

V04.12 Pedestrian on skateboard injured in collision with heavy transport vehicle or bus in traffic accident

V04.13 Pedestrian on standing micro-mobility pedestrian conveyance injured in collision with heavy transport vehicle or bus in traffic accident

V04.131 Pedestrian on standing electric scooter injured in collision with heavy transport vehicle or bus in traffic accident

V04.138 Pedestrian on other standing micro-mobility pedestrian conveyance injured in collision with heavy transport vehicle or bus in traffic accident
Pedestrian on hoverboard injured in collision with heavy transport vehicle or bus in traffic accident
Pedestrian on segway injured in collision with heavy transport vehicle or bus in traffic accident

V04.19 Pedestrian with other conveyance injured in collision with heavy transport vehicle or bus in traffic accident
Pedestrian with baby stroller injured in collision with heavy transport vehicle or bus in traffic accident
Pedestrian on ice-skates injured in collision with heavy transport vehicle or bus in traffic accident
Pedestrian on nonmotorized scooter injured in collision with heavy transport vehicle or bus in traffic accident
Pedestrian on sled injured in collision with heavy transport vehicle or bus in traffic accident
Pedestrian on snowboard injured in collision with heavy transport vehicle or bus in traffic accident
Pedestrian on snow-skis injured in collision with heavy transport vehicle or bus in traffic accident
Pedestrian in wheelchair (powered) injured in collision with heavy transport vehicle or bus in traffic accident
Pedestrian in motorized mobility scooter injured in collision with heavy transport vehicle or bus in traffic accident

V04.9 Pedestrian injured in collision with heavy transport vehicle or bus, unspecified whether traffic or nontraffic accident

V04.90 Pedestrian on foot injured in collision with heavy transport vehicle or bus, unspecified whether traffic or nontraffic accident
Pedestrian NOS injured in collision with heavy transport vehicle or bus, unspecified whether traffic or nontraffic accident

V04.91 Pedestrian on roller-skates injured in collision with heavy transport vehicle or bus, unspecified whether traffic or nontraffic accident

V04.92 Pedestrian on skateboard injured in collision with heavy transport vehicle or bus, unspecified whether traffic or nontraffic accident

V04.93 Pedestrian on standing micro-mobility pedestrian conveyance injured in collision with heavy transport vehicle or bus, unspecified whether traffic or nontraffic accident

V04.931 Pedestrian on standing electric scooter injured in collision with heavy transport vehicle or bus, unspecified whether traffic or nontraffic accident

V04.938 Pedestrian on other standing micro-mobility pedestrian conveyance injured in collision with heavy transport vehicle or bus, unspecified whether traffic or nontraffic accident
Pedestrian on hoverboard injured in collision with heavy transport vehicle or bus, unspecified whether traffic or nontraffic accident
Pedestrian on segway injured in collision with heavy transport vehicle or bus, unspecified whether traffic or nontraffic accident

V04.99 Pedestrian with other conveyance injured in collision with heavy transport vehicle or bus, unspecified whether traffic or nontraffic accident
Pedestrian with baby stroller injured in collision with heavy transport vehicle or bus, unspecified whether traffic or nontraffic accident
Pedestrian on ice-skates injured in collision with heavy transport vehicle or bus, unspecified whether traffic or nontraffic accident
Pedestrian on nonmotorized scooter injured in collision with heavy transport vehicle or bus, unspecified whether traffic or nontraffic accident
Pedestrian on sled injured in collision with heavy transport vehicle or bus, unspecified whether traffic or nontraffic accident
Pedestrian on snowboard injured in collision with heavy transport vehicle or bus, unspecified whether traffic or nontraffic accident
Pedestrian on snow-skis injured in collision with heavy transport vehicle or bus, unspecified whether traffic or nontraffic accident
Pedestrian in wheelchair (powered) injured in collision with heavy transport vehicle or bus, unspecified whether traffic or nontraffic accident
Pedestrian in motorized mobility scooter injured in collision with heavy transport vehicle or bus, unspecified whether traffic or nontraffic accident

V05 Pedestrian injured in collision with railway train or railway vehicle

V05.0 Pedestrian injured in collision with railway train or railway vehicle in nontraffic accident

V05.00 Pedestrian on foot injured in collision with railway train or railway vehicle in nontraffic accident
Pedestrian NOS injured in collision with railway train or railway vehicle in nontraffic accident

V05.01 Pedestrian on roller-skates injured in collision with railway train or railway vehicle in nontraffic accident

V05.02 Pedestrian on skateboard injured in collision with railway train or railway vehicle in nontraffic accident

V05.03 Pedestrian on standing micro-mobility pedestrian conveyance injured in collision with railway train or railway vehicle in nontraffic accident

V05.031 Pedestrian on standing electric scooter injured in collision with railway train or railway vehicle in nontraffic accident

VØ5.Ø38 Pedestrian on other standing micro-mobility pedestrian conveyance injured in collision with railway train or railway vehicle in nontraffic accident

Pedestrian on hoverboard injured in collision with railway train or railway vehicle in nontraffic accident

Pedestrian on segway injured in collision with railway train or railway vehicle in nontraffic accident

VØ5.Ø9 Pedestrian with other conveyance injured in collision with railway train or railway vehicle in nontraffic accident

Pedestrian with baby stroller injured in collision with railway train or railway vehicle in nontraffic accident

Pedestrian on ice-skates injured in collision with railway train or railway vehicle in nontraffic accident

Pedestrian on nonmotorized scooter injured in collision with railway train or railway vehicle in nontraffic accident

Pedestrian on sled injured in collision with railway train or railway vehicle in nontraffic accident

Pedestrian on snowboard injured in collision with railway train or railway vehicle in nontraffic accident

Pedestrian on snow-skis injured in collision with railway train or railway vehicle in nontraffic accident

Pedestrian in wheelchair (powered) injured in collision with railway train or railway vehicle in nontraffic accident

Pedestrian in motorized mobility scooter injured in collision with railway train or railway vehicle in nontraffic accident

VØ5.1 Pedestrian injured in collision with railway train or railway vehicle in traffic accident

VØ5.1Ø Pedestrian on foot injured in collision with railway train or railway vehicle in traffic accident

Pedestrian NOS injured in collision with railway train or railway vehicle in traffic accident

VØ5.11 Pedestrian on roller-skates injured in collision with railway train or railway vehicle in traffic accident

VØ5.12 Pedestrian on skateboard injured in collision with railway train or railway vehicle in traffic accident

VØ5.13 Pedestrian on standing micro-mobility pedestrian conveyance injured in collision with railway train or railway vehicle in traffic accident

VØ5.131 Pedestrian on standing electric scooter injured in collision with railway train or railway vehicle in traffic accident

VØ5.138 Pedestrian on other standing micro-mobility pedestrian conveyance injured in collision with railway train or railway vehicle in traffic accident

Pedestrian on hoverboard injured in collision with railway train or railway vehicle in traffic accident

Pedestrian on segway injured in collision with railway train or railway vehicle in traffic accident

VØ5.19 Pedestrian with other conveyance injured in collision with railway train or railway vehicle in traffic accident

Pedestrian with baby stroller injured in collision with railway train or railway vehicle in traffic accident

Pedestrian on ice-skates injured in collision with railway train or railway vehicle in traffic accident

Pedestrian on nonmotorized scooter injured in collision with railway train or railway vehicle in traffic accident

Pedestrian on sled injured in collision with railway train or railway vehicle in traffic accident

Pedestrian on snowboard injured in collision with railway train or railway vehicle in traffic accident

Pedestrian on snow-skis injured in collision with railway train or railway vehicle in traffic accident

Pedestrian in wheelchair (powered) injured in collision with railway train or railway vehicle in traffic accident

Pedestrian in motorized mobility scooter injured in collision with railway train or railway vehicle in traffic accident

VØ5.9 Pedestrian injured in collision with railway train or railway vehicle, unspecified whether traffic or nontraffic accident

VØ5.9Ø Pedestrian on foot injured in collision with railway train or railway vehicle, unspecified whether traffic or nontraffic accident

Pedestrian NOS injured in collision with railway train or railway vehicle, unspecified whether traffic or nontraffic accident

VØ5.91 Pedestrian on roller-skates injured in collision with railway train or railway vehicle, unspecified whether traffic or nontraffic accident

VØ5.92 Pedestrian on skateboard injured in collision with railway train or railway vehicle, unspecified whether traffic or nontraffic accident

VØ5.93 Pedestrian on standing micro-mobility pedestrian conveyance injured in collision with railway train or railway vehicle, unspecified whether traffic or nontraffic accident

VØ5.931 Pedestrian on standing electric scooter injured in collision with railway train or railway vehicle, unspecified whether traffic or nontraffic accident

VØ5.938 Pedestrian on other standing micro-mobility pedestrian conveyance injured in collision with railway train or railway vehicle, unspecified whether traffic or nontraffic accident

Pedestrian on hoverboard injured in collision with railway train or railway vehicle, unspecified whether traffic or nontraffic accident

Pedestrian on segway injured in collision with railway train or railway vehicle, unspecified whether traffic or nontraffic accident

√x7th **V05.99 Pedestrian with other conveyance injured in collision with railway train or railway vehicle, unspecified whether traffic or nontraffic accident**
Pedestrian with baby stroller injured in collision with railway train or railway vehicle, unspecified whether traffic or nontraffic
Pedestrian on ice-skates injured in collision with railway train or railway vehicle, unspecified whether traffic or nontraffic
Pedestrian on nonmotorized scooter injured in collision with railway train or railway vehicle, unspecified whether traffic or nontraffic
Pedestrian on sled injured in collision with railway train or railway vehicle, unspecified whether traffic or nontraffic
Pedestrian on snowboard injured in collision with railway train or railway vehicle, unspecified whether traffic or nontraffic
Pedestrian on snow-skis injured in collision with railway train or railway vehicle, unspecified whether traffic or nontraffic
Pedestrian in wheelchair (powered) injured in collision with railway train or railway vehicle, unspecified whether traffic or nontraffic
Pedestrian in motorized mobility scooter injured in collision with railway train or railway vehicle, unspecified whether traffic or nontraffic

√4th **V06 Pedestrian injured in collision with other nonmotor vehicle**
INCLUDES collision with animal-drawn vehicle, animal being ridden, nonpowered streetcar
EXCLUDES 1 *pedestrian injured in collision with pedestrian conveyance (V00.0-)*

√5th **V06.0 Pedestrian injured in collision with other nonmotor vehicle in nontraffic accident**

√x7th **V06.00 Pedestrian on foot injured in collision with other nonmotor vehicle in nontraffic accident**
Pedestrian NOS injured in collision with other nonmotor vehicle in nontraffic accident

√x7th **V06.01 Pedestrian on roller-skates injured in collision with other nonmotor vehicle in nontraffic accident**

√x7th **V06.02 Pedestrian on skateboard injured in collision with other nonmotor vehicle in nontraffic accident**

√6th **V06.03 Pedestrian on standing micro-mobility pedestrian conveyance injured in collision with other nonmotor vehicle in nontraffic accident**

√7th **V06.031 Pedestrian on standing electric scooter injured in collision with other nonmotor vehicle in nontraffic accident**

√7th **V06.038 Pedestrian on other standing micro-mobility pedestrian conveyance injured in collision with other nonmotor vehicle in nontraffic accident**
Pedestrian on hoverboard injured in collision with other nonmotor vehicle in nontraffic accident
Pedestrian on segway injured in collision with other nonmotor vehicle in nontraffic accident

√x7th **V06.09 Pedestrian with other conveyance injured in collision with other nonmotor vehicle in nontraffic accident**
Pedestrian with baby stroller injured in collision with other nonmotor vehicle in nontraffic accident
Pedestrian on ice-skates injured in collision with other nonmotor vehicle in nontraffic accident
Pedestrian on nonmotorized scooter injured in collision with other nonmotor vehicle in nontraffic accident
Pedestrian on sled injured in collision with other nonmotor vehicle in nontraffic accident
Pedestrian on snowboard injured in collision with other nonmotor vehicle in nontraffic accident
Pedestrian on snow-skis injured in collision with other nonmotor vehicle in nontraffic accident
Pedestrian in wheelchair (powered) injured in collision with other nonmotor vehicle in nontraffic accident
Pedestrian in motorized mobility scooter injured in collision with other nonmotor vehicle in nontraffic accident

√5th **V06.1 Pedestrian injured in collision with other nonmotor vehicle in traffic accident**

√x7th **V06.10 Pedestrian on foot injured in collision with other nonmotor vehicle in traffic accident**
Pedestrian NOS injured in collision with other nonmotor vehicle in traffic accident

√x7th **V06.11 Pedestrian on roller-skates injured in collision with other nonmotor vehicle in traffic accident**

√x7th **V06.12 Pedestrian on skateboard injured in collision with other nonmotor vehicle in traffic accident**

√6th **V06.13 Pedestrian on standing micro-mobility pedestrian conveyance injured in collision with other nonmotor vehicle in traffic accident**

√7th **V06.131 Pedestrian on standing electric scooter injured in collision with other nonmotor vehicle in traffic accident**

√7th **V06.138 Pedestrian on other standing micro-mobility pedestrian conveyance injured in collision with other nonmotor vehicle in traffic accident**
Pedestrian on hoverboard injured in collision with other nonmotor vehicle in traffic accident
Pedestrian on segway injured in collision with other nonmotor vehicle in traffic accident

√x7th **V06.19 Pedestrian with other conveyance injured in collision with other nonmotor vehicle in traffic accident**
Pedestrian with baby stroller injured in collision with other nonmotor vehicle in nontraffic accident
Pedestrian on ice-skates injured in collision with other nonmotor vehicle in traffic accident
Pedestrian on nonmotorized scooter injured in collision with other nonmotor vehicle in traffic accident
Pedestrian on sled injured in collision with other nonmotor vehicle in traffic accident
Pedestrian on snowboard injured in collision with other nonmotor vehicle in traffic accident
Pedestrian on snow-skis injured in collision with other nonmotor vehicle in traffic accident
Pedestrian in wheelchair (powered) injured in collision with other nonmotor vehicle in traffic accident
Pedestrian in motorized mobility scooter injured in collision with other nonmotor vehicle in traffic accident

√5th **V06.9 Pedestrian injured in collision with other nonmotor vehicle, unspecified whether traffic or nontraffic accident**

√x7th **V06.90 Pedestrian on foot injured in collision with other nonmotor vehicle, unspecified whether traffic or nontraffic accident**
Pedestrian NOS injured in collision with other nonmotor vehicle, unspecified whether traffic or nontraffic accident

√x7th **V06.91 Pedestrian on roller-skates injured in collision with other nonmotor vehicle, unspecified whether traffic or nontraffic accident**

√x7th V06.92 Pedestrian on skateboard injured in collision with other nonmotor vehicle, unspecified whether traffic or nontraffic accident

√6th V06.93 Pedestrian on standing micro-mobility pedestrian conveyance injured in collision with other nonmotor vehicle, unspecified whether traffic or nontraffic accident

√7th V06.931 Pedestrian on standing electric scooter injured in collision with other nonmotor vehicle, unspecified whether traffic or nontraffic accident

√7th V06.938 Pedestrian on other standing micro-mobility pedestrian conveyance injured in collision with other nonmotor vehicle, unspecified whether traffic or nontraffic accident
Pedestrian on hoverboard injured in collision with other nonmotor, unspecified whether traffic or nontraffic accident
Pedestrian on segway injured in collision with other nonmotor vehicle, unspecified whether traffic or nontraffic accident

√x7th V06.99 Pedestrian with other conveyance injured in collision with other nonmotor vehicle, unspecified whether traffic or nontraffic accident
Pedestrian with baby stroller injured in collision with other nonmotor vehicle, unspecified whether traffic or nontraffic accident
Pedestrian on ice-skates injured in collision with other nonmotor vehicle, unspecified whether traffic or nontraffic accident
Pedestrian on nonmotorized scooter injured in collision with other nonmotor vehicle, unspecified whether traffic or nontraffic accident
Pedestrian on sled injured in collision with other nonmotor vehicle, unspecified whether traffic or nontraffic accident
Pedestrian on snowboard injured in collision with other nonmotor vehicle, unspecified whether traffic or nontraffic accident
Pedestrian on snow-skis injured in collision with other nonmotor vehicle, unspecified whether traffic or nontraffic accident
Pedestrian in wheelchair (powered) injured in collision with other nonmotor vehicle, unspecified whether traffic or nontraffic accident
Pedestrian in motorized mobility scooter injured in collision with other nonmotorized vehicle, unspecified whether traffic or nontraffic accident

√4th V09 Pedestrian injured in other and unspecified transport accidents

√5th V09.0 Pedestrian injured in nontraffic accident involving other and unspecified motor vehicles

√x7th V09.00 Pedestrian injured in nontraffic accident involving unspecified motor vehicles

√x7th V09.01 Pedestrian injured in nontraffic accident involving military vehicle

√x7th V09.09 Pedestrian injured in nontraffic accident involving other motor vehicles
Pedestrian injured in nontraffic accident by special vehicle

√x7th V09.1 Pedestrian injured in unspecified nontraffic accident

√5th V09.2 Pedestrian injured in traffic accident involving other and unspecified motor vehicles

√x7th V09.20 Pedestrian injured in traffic accident involving unspecified motor vehicles

√x7th V09.21 Pedestrian injured in traffic accident involving military vehicle

√x7th V09.29 Pedestrian injured in traffic accident involving other motor vehicles

√x7th V09.3 Pedestrian injured in unspecified traffic accident

√x7th V09.9 Pedestrian injured in unspecified transport accident

Pedal cycle rider injured in transport accident (V10-V19)

INCLUDES any non-motorized vehicle, excluding an animal-drawn vehicle, or a sidecar or trailer attached to the pedal cycle

EXCLUDES 2 *rupture of pedal cycle tire (W37.0)*

The appropriate 7th character is to be added to each code from categories V10-V19.
A initial encounter
D subsequent encounter
S sequela

√4th V10 Pedal cycle rider injured in collision with pedestrian or animal

EXCLUDES 1 *pedal cycle rider collision with animal-drawn vehicle or animal being ridden (V16.-)*

√x7th V10.0 Pedal cycle driver injured in collision with pedestrian or animal in nontraffic accident

√x7th V10.1 Pedal cycle passenger injured in collision with pedestrian or animal in nontraffic accident

√x7th V10.2 Unspecified pedal cyclist injured in collision with pedestrian or animal in nontraffic accident

√x7th V10.3 Person boarding or alighting a pedal cycle injured in collision with pedestrian or animal

√x7th V10.4 Pedal cycle driver injured in collision with pedestrian or animal in traffic accident

√x7th V10.5 Pedal cycle passenger injured in collision with pedestrian or animal in traffic accident

√x7th V10.9 Unspecified pedal cyclist injured in collision with pedestrian or animal in traffic accident

√4th V11 Pedal cycle rider injured in collision with other pedal cycle

√x7th V11.0 Pedal cycle driver injured in collision with other pedal cycle in nontraffic accident

√x7th V11.1 Pedal cycle passenger injured in collision with other pedal cycle in nontraffic accident

√x7th V11.2 Unspecified pedal cyclist injured in collision with other pedal cycle in nontraffic accident

√x7th V11.3 Person boarding or alighting a pedal cycle injured in collision with other pedal cycle

√x7th V11.4 Pedal cycle driver injured in collision with other pedal cycle in traffic accident

√x7th V11.5 Pedal cycle passenger injured in collision with other pedal cycle in traffic accident

√x7th V11.9 Unspecified pedal cyclist injured in collision with other pedal cycle in traffic accident

√4th V12 Pedal cycle rider injured in collision with two- or three-wheeled motor vehicle

√x7th V12.0 Pedal cycle driver injured in collision with two- or three-wheeled motor vehicle in nontraffic accident

√x7th V12.1 Pedal cycle passenger injured in collision with two- or three-wheeled motor vehicle in nontraffic accident

√x7th V12.2 Unspecified pedal cyclist injured in collision with two- or three-wheeled motor vehicle in nontraffic accident

√x7th V12.3 Person boarding or alighting a pedal cycle injured in collision with two- or three-wheeled motor vehicle

√x7th V12.4 Pedal cycle driver injured in collision with two- or three-wheeled motor vehicle in traffic accident

√x7th V12.5 Pedal cycle passenger injured in collision with two- or three-wheeled motor vehicle in traffic accident

√x7th V12.9 Unspecified pedal cyclist injured in collision with two- or three-wheeled motor vehicle in traffic accident

√4th V13 Pedal cycle rider injured in collision with car, pick-up truck or van

√x7th V13.0 Pedal cycle driver injured in collision with car, pick-up truck or van in nontraffic accident

√x7th V13.1 Pedal cycle passenger injured in collision with car, pick-up truck or van in nontraffic accident

√x7th V13.2 Unspecified pedal cyclist injured in collision with car, pick-up truck or van in nontraffic accident

√x7th V13.3 Person boarding or alighting a pedal cycle injured in collision with car, pick-up truck or van

√x7th V13.4 Pedal cycle driver injured in collision with car, pick-up truck or van in traffic accident

√x7th V13.5 Pedal cycle passenger injured in collision with car, pick-up truck or van in traffic accident

√x7th V13.9 Unspecified pedal cyclist injured in collision with car, pick-up truck or van in traffic accident

√4th V14 Pedal cycle rider injured in collision with heavy transport vehicle or bus

EXCLUDES 1 *pedal cycle rider injured in collision with military vehicle (V19.81)*

√x7th V14.0 Pedal cycle driver injured in collision with heavy transport vehicle or bus in nontraffic accident

V14.1 **Pedal cycle passenger injured in collision with heavy transport vehicle or bus in nontraffic accident**

V14.2 **Unspecified pedal cyclist injured in collision with heavy transport vehicle or bus in nontraffic accident**

V14.3 **Person boarding or alighting a pedal cycle injured in collision with heavy transport vehicle or bus**

V14.4 **Pedal cycle driver injured in collision with heavy transport vehicle or bus in traffic accident**

V14.5 **Pedal cycle passenger injured in collision with heavy transport vehicle or bus in traffic accident**

V14.9 **Unspecified pedal cyclist injured in collision with heavy transport vehicle or bus in traffic accident**

V15 Pedal cycle rider injured in collision with railway train or railway vehicle

V15.0 **Pedal cycle driver injured in collision with railway train or railway vehicle in nontraffic accident**

V15.1 **Pedal cycle passenger injured in collision with railway train or railway vehicle in nontraffic accident**

V15.2 **Unspecified pedal cyclist injured in collision with railway train or railway vehicle in nontraffic accident**

V15.3 **Person boarding or alighting a pedal cycle injured in collision with railway train or railway vehicle**

V15.4 **Pedal cycle driver injured in collision with railway train or railway vehicle in traffic accident**

V15.5 **Pedal cycle passenger injured in collision with railway train or railway vehicle in traffic accident**

V15.9 **Unspecified pedal cyclist injured in collision with railway train or railway vehicle in traffic accident**

V16 Pedal cycle rider injured in collision with other nonmotor vehicle

INCLUDES collision with animal-drawn vehicle, animal being ridden, streetcar

V16.0 **Pedal cycle driver injured in collision with other nonmotor vehicle in nontraffic accident**

V16.1 **Pedal cycle passenger injured in collision with other nonmotor vehicle in nontraffic accident**

V16.2 **Unspecified pedal cyclist injured in collision with other nonmotor vehicle in nontraffic accident**

V16.3 **Person boarding or alighting a pedal cycle injured in collision with other nonmotor vehicle in nontraffic accident**

V16.4 **Pedal cycle driver injured in collision with other nonmotor vehicle in traffic accident**

V16.5 **Pedal cycle passenger injured in collision with other nonmotor vehicle in traffic accident**

V16.9 **Unspecified pedal cyclist injured in collision with other nonmotor vehicle in traffic accident**

V17 Pedal cycle rider injured in collision with fixed or stationary object

V17.0 **Pedal cycle driver injured in collision with fixed or stationary object in nontraffic accident**

V17.1 **Pedal cycle passenger injured in collision with fixed or stationary object in nontraffic accident**

V17.2 **Unspecified pedal cyclist injured in collision with fixed or stationary object in nontraffic accident**

V17.3 **Person boarding or alighting a pedal cycle injured in collision with fixed or stationary object**

V17.4 **Pedal cycle driver injured in collision with fixed or stationary object in traffic accident**

V17.5 **Pedal cycle passenger injured in collision with fixed or stationary object in traffic accident**

V17.9 **Unspecified pedal cyclist injured in collision with fixed or stationary object in traffic accident**

V18 Pedal cycle rider injured in noncollision transport accident

INCLUDES fall or thrown from pedal cycle (without antecedent collision)
overturning pedal cycle NOS
overturning pedal cycle without collision

V18.0 **Pedal cycle driver injured in noncollision transport accident in nontraffic accident**

V18.1 **Pedal cycle passenger injured in noncollision transport accident in nontraffic accident**

V18.2 **Unspecified pedal cyclist injured in noncollision transport accident in nontraffic accident**

V18.3 **Person boarding or alighting a pedal cycle injured in noncollision transport accident**

V18.4 **Pedal cycle driver injured in noncollision transport accident in traffic accident**

V18.5 **Pedal cycle passenger injured in noncollision transport accident in traffic accident**

V18.9 **Unspecified pedal cyclist injured in noncollision transport accident in traffic accident**

V19 Pedal cycle rider injured in other and unspecified transport accidents

V19.0 **Pedal cycle driver injured in collision with other and unspecified motor vehicles in nontraffic accident**

V19.00 **Pedal cycle driver injured in collision with unspecified motor vehicles in nontraffic accident**

V19.09 **Pedal cycle driver injured in collision with other motor vehicles in nontraffic accident**

V19.1 **Pedal cycle passenger injured in collision with other and unspecified motor vehicles in nontraffic accident**

V19.10 **Pedal cycle passenger injured in collision with unspecified motor vehicles in nontraffic accident**

V19.19 **Pedal cycle passenger injured in collision with other motor vehicles in nontraffic accident**

V19.2 **Unspecified pedal cyclist injured in collision with other and unspecified motor vehicles in nontraffic accident**

V19.20 **Unspecified pedal cyclist injured in collision with unspecified motor vehicles in nontraffic accident**
Pedal cycle collision NOS, nontraffic

V19.29 **Unspecified pedal cyclist injured in collision with other motor vehicles in nontraffic accident**

V19.3 **Pedal cyclist (driver) (passenger) injured in unspecified nontraffic accident**
Pedal cycle accident NOS, nontraffic
Pedal cyclist injured in nontraffic accident NOS

V19.4 **Pedal cycle driver injured in collision with other and unspecified motor vehicles in traffic accident**

V19.40 **Pedal cycle driver injured in collision with unspecified motor vehicles in traffic accident**

V19.49 **Pedal cycle driver injured in collision with other motor vehicles in traffic accident**

V19.5 **Pedal cycle passenger injured in collision with other and unspecified motor vehicles in traffic accident**

V19.50 **Pedal cycle passenger injured in collision with unspecified motor vehicles in traffic accident**

V19.59 **Pedal cycle passenger injured in collision with other motor vehicles in traffic accident**

V19.6 **Unspecified pedal cyclist injured in collision with other and unspecified motor vehicles in traffic accident**

V19.60 **Unspecified pedal cyclist injured in collision with unspecified motor vehicles in traffic accident**
Pedal cycle collision NOS (traffic)

V19.69 **Unspecified pedal cyclist injured in collision with other motor vehicles in traffic accident**

V19.8 **Pedal cyclist (driver) (passenger) injured in other specified transport accidents**

V19.81 **Pedal cyclist (driver) (passenger) injured in transport accident with military vehicle**

V19.88 **Pedal cyclist (driver) (passenger) injured in other specified transport accidents**

V19.9 **Pedal cyclist (driver) (passenger) injured in unspecified traffic accident**
Pedal cycle accident NOS

Motorcycle rider injured in transport accident (V20-V29)

INCLUDES ▶electric bicycle◀
▶e-bike◀
▶e-bicycle◀
moped
motorcycle with sidecar
motorized bicycle
motor scooter

EXCLUDES 1 *three-wheeled motor vehicle (V30-V39)*

The appropriate 7th character is to be added to each code from categories V20-V29.
A initial encounter
D subsequent encounter
S sequela

V20 Motorcycle rider injured in collision with pedestrian or animal

EXCLUDES 1 *motorcycle rider collision with animal-drawn vehicle or animal being ridden (V26.-)*

V20.0 **Motorcycle driver injured in collision with pedestrian or animal in nontraffic accident**

● V20.01 **Electric (assisted) bicycle driver injured in collision with pedestrian or animal in nontraffic accident**

● V20.09 **Other motorcycle driver injured in collision with pedestrian or animal in nontraffic accident**

- ✓5th **V20.1** Motorcycle passenger injured in collision with pedestrian or animal in nontraffic accident
  - ● ✓x7th **V20.11** Electric (assisted) bicycle passenger injured in collision with pedestrian or animal in nontraffic accident
  - ● ✓x7th **V20.19** Other motorcycle passenger injured in collision with pedestrian or animal in nontraffic accident
- ✓5th **V20.2** Unspecified motorcycle rider injured in collision with pedestrian or animal in nontraffic accident
  - ● ✓x7th **V20.21** Unspecified electric (assisted) bicycle rider injured in collision with pedestrian or animal in nontraffic accident
  - ● ✓x7th **V20.29** Unspecified rider of other motorcycle injured in collision with pedestrian or animal in nontraffic accident
- ✓5th **V20.3** Person boarding or alighting a motorcycle injured in collision with pedestrian or animal
  - ● ✓x7th **V20.31** Person boarding or alighting an electric (assisted) bicycle injured in collision with pedestrian or animal
  - ● ✓x7th **V20.39** Person boarding or alighting other motorcycle injured in collision with pedestrian or animal
- ✓5th **V20.4** Motorcycle driver injured in collision with pedestrian or animal in traffic accident
  - ● ✓x7th **V20.41** Electric (assisted) bicycle driver injured in collision with pedestrian or animal in traffic accident
  - ● ✓x7th **V20.49** Other motorcycle driver injured in collision with pedestrian or animal in traffic accident
- ✓5th **V20.5** Motorcycle passenger injured in collision with pedestrian or animal in traffic accident
  - ● ✓x7th **V20.51** Electric (assisted) bicycle passenger injured in collision with pedestrian or animal in traffic accident
  - ● ✓x7th **V20.59** Other motorcycle passenger injured in collision with pedestrian or animal in traffic accident
- ✓5th **V20.9** Unspecified motorcycle rider injured in collision with pedestrian or animal in traffic accident
  - ● ✓x7th **V20.91** Unspecified electric (assisted) bicycle rider injured in collision with pedestrian or animal in traffic accident
  - ● ✓x7th **V20.99** Unspecified rider of other motorcycle injured in collision with pedestrian or animal in traffic accident

✓4th **V21 Motorcycle rider injured in collision with pedal cycle**

- ✓5th **V21.0** Motorcycle driver injured in collision with pedal cycle in nontraffic accident
  - ● ✓x7th **V21.01** Electric (assisted) bicycle driver injured in collision with pedal cycle in nontraffic accident
  - ● ✓x7th **V21.09** Other motorcycle driver injured in collision with pedal cycle in nontraffic accident
- ✓5th **V21.1** Motorcycle passenger injured in collision with pedal cycle in nontraffic accident
  - ● ✓x7th **V21.11** Electric (assisted) bicycle passenger injured in collision with pedal cycle in nontraffic accident
  - ● ✓x7th **V21.19** Other motorcycle passenger injured in collision with pedal cycle nontraffic accident
- ✓5th **V21.2** Unspecified motorcycle rider injured in collision with pedal cycle in nontraffic accident
  - ● ✓x7th **V21.21** Unspecified electric (assisted) bicycle rider injured in collision with pedal cycle in nontraffic accident
  - ● ✓x7th **V21.29** Unspecified rider of other motorcycle injured in collision with pedal cycle in nontraffic accident
- ✓5th **V21.3** Person boarding or alighting a motorcycle injured in collision with pedal cycle
  - ● ✓x7th **V21.31** Person boarding or alighting an electric (assisted) bicycle injured in collision with pedal cycle
  - ● ✓x7th **V21.39** Person boarding or alighting other motorcycle injured in collision with pedal cycle
- ✓5th **V21.4** Motorcycle driver injured in collision with pedal cycle in traffic accident
  - ● ✓x7th **V21.41** Electric (assisted) bicycle driver injured in collision with pedal cycle in traffic accident
  - ● ✓x7th **V21.49** Other motorcycle driver injured in collision with pedal cycle in traffic accident
- ✓5th **V21.5** Motorcycle passenger injured in collision with pedal cycle in traffic accident
  - ● ✓x7th **V21.51** Electric (assisted) bicycle passenger injured in collision with pedal cycle in traffic accident
  - ● ✓x7th **V21.59** Other motorcycle passenger injured in collision with pedal cycle in traffic accident
- ✓5th **V21.9** Unspecified motorcycle rider injured in collision with pedal cycle in traffic accident
  - ● ✓x7th **V21.91** Unspecified electric (assisted) bicycle rider injured in collision with pedal cycle in traffic accident
  - ● ✓x7th **V21.99** Unspecified rider of other motorcycle injured in collision with pedal cycle in traffic accident

✓4th **V22 Motorcycle rider injured in collision with two- or three-wheeled motor vehicle**

- ✓5th **V22.0** Motorcycle driver injured in collision with two- or three-wheeled motor vehicle in nontraffic accident
  - ● ✓x7th **V22.01** Electric (assisted) bicycle driver injured in collision with two- or three-wheeled motor vehicle in nontraffic accident
  - ● ✓x7th **V22.09** Other motorcycle driver injured in collision with two- or three-wheeled motor vehicle in nontraffic accident
- ✓5th **V22.1** Motorcycle passenger injured in collision with two- or three-wheeled motor vehicle in nontraffic accident
  - ● ✓x7th **V22.11** Electric (assisted) bicycle passenger injured in collision with two- or three-wheeled motor vehicle in nontraffic accident
  - ● ✓x7th **V22.19** Other motorcycle passenger injured in collision with two- or three-wheeled motor vehicle in nontraffic accident
- ✓5th **V22.2** Unspecified motorcycle rider injured in collision with two- or three-wheeled motor vehicle in nontraffic accident
  - ● ✓x7th **V22.21** Unspecified electric (assisted) bicycle rider injured in collision with two- or three-wheeled motor vehicle in nontraffic accident
  - ● ✓x7th **V22.29** Unspecified rider of other motorcycle injured in collision with two- or three-wheeled motor vehicle in nontraffic accident
- ✓5th **V22.3** Person boarding or alighting a motorcycle injured in collision with two- or three-wheeled motor vehicle
  - ● ✓x7th **V22.31** Person boarding or alighting an electric (assisted) bicycle injured in collision with two- or three-wheeled motor vehicle
  - ● ✓x7th **V22.39** Person boarding or alighting other motorcycle injured in collision with two- or three-wheeled motor vehicle
- ✓5th **V22.4** Motorcycle driver injured in collision with two- or three-wheeled motor vehicle in traffic accident
  - ● ✓x7th **V22.41** Electric (assisted) bicycle driver injured in collision with two- or three-wheeled motor vehicle in traffic accident
  - ● ✓x7th **V22.49** Other motorcycle driver injured in collision with two- or three-wheeled motor vehicle in traffic accident
- ✓5th **V22.5** Motorcycle passenger injured in collision with two- or three-wheeled motor vehicle in traffic accident
  - ● ✓x7th **V22.51** Electric (assisted) bicycle passenger injured in collision with two- or three-wheeled motor vehicle in traffic accident
  - ● ✓x7th **V22.59** Other motorcycle passenger injured in collision with two- or three-wheeled motor vehicle in traffic accident
- ✓5th **V22.9** Unspecified motorcycle rider injured in collision with two- or three-wheeled motor vehicle in traffic accident
  - ● ✓x7th **V22.91** Unspecified electric (assisted) bicycle rider injured in collision with two- or three-wheeled motor vehicle in traffic accident
  - ● ✓x7th **V22.99** Unspecified rider of other motorcycle injured in collision with two- or three-wheeled motor vehicle in traffic accident

✓4th **V23 Motorcycle rider injured in collision with car, pick-up truck or van**

- ✓5th **V23.0** Motorcycle driver injured in collision with car, pick-up truck or van in nontraffic accident
  - ● ✓x7th **V23.01** Electric (assisted) bicycle driver injured in collision with car, pick-up truck or van in nontraffic accident
  - ● ✓x7th **V23.09** Other motorcycle driver injured in collision with car, pick-up truck or van in nontraffic accident
- ✓5th **V23.1** Motorcycle passenger injured in collision with car, pick-up truck or van in nontraffic accident
  - ● ✓x7th **V23.11** Electric (assisted) bicycle passenger injured in collision with car, pick-up truck or van in nontraffic accident
  - ● ✓x7th **V23.19** Other motorcycle passenger injured in collision with car, pick-up truck or van in nontraffic accident

V23.2 Unspecified motorcycle rider injured in collision with car, pick-up truck or van in nontraffic accident
- V23.21 Unspecified electric (assisted) bicycle rider injured in collision with car, pick-up truck or van in nontraffic accident
- V23.29 Unspecified rider of other motorcycle injured in collision with car, pick-up truck or van in nontraffic accident

V23.3 Person boarding or alighting a motorcycle injured in collision with car, pick-up truck or van
- V23.31 Person boarding or alighting an electric (assisted) bicycle injured in collision with car, pick-up truck or van
- V23.39 Person boarding or alighting other motorcycle injured in collision with car, pick-up truck or van

V23.4 Motorcycle driver injured in collision with car, pick-up truck or van in traffic accident
- V23.41 Electric (assisted) bicycle driver injured in collision with car, pick-up truck or van in traffic accident
- V23.49 Other motorcycle driver injured in collision with car, pick-up truck or van in traffic accident

V23.5 Motorcycle passenger injured in collision with car, pick-up truck or van in traffic accident
- V23.51 Electric (assisted) bicycle passenger injured in collision with car, pick-up truck or van in traffic accident
- V23.59 Other motorcycle passenger injured in collision with car, pick-up truck or van in traffic accident

V23.9 Unspecified motorcycle rider injured in collision with car, pick-up truck or van in traffic accident
- V23.91 Unspecified electric (assisted) bicycle rider injured in collision with car, pick-up truck or van in traffic accident
- V23.99 Unspecified rider of other motorcycle injured in collision with car, pick-up truck or van in traffic accident

V24 Motorcycle rider injured in collision with heavy transport vehicle or bus

EXCLUDES1 *motorcycle rider injured in collision with military vehicle ▶(V29.818)◀*

V24.0 Motorcycle driver injured in collision with heavy transport vehicle or bus in nontraffic accident
- V24.01 Electric (assisted) bicycle driver injured in collision with heavy transport vehicle or bus in nontraffic accident
- V24.09 Other motorcycle driver injured in collision with heavy transport vehicle or bus in nontraffic accident

V24.1 Motorcycle passenger injured in collision with heavy transport vehicle or bus in nontraffic accident
- V24.11 Electric (assisted) bicycle passenger injured in collision with heavy transport vehicle or bus in nontraffic accident
- V24.19 Other motorcycle passenger injured in collision with heavy transport vehicle or bus in nontraffic accident

V24.2 Unspecified motorcycle rider injured in collision with heavy transport vehicle or bus in nontraffic accident
- V24.21 Unspecified electric (assisted) bicycle rider injured in collision with heavy transport vehicle or bus in nontraffic accident
- V24.29 Unspecified rider of other motorcycle injured in collision with heavy transport vehicle or bus in nontraffic accident

V24.3 Person boarding or alighting a motorcycle injured in collision with heavy transport vehicle or bus
- V24.31 Person boarding or alighting an electric (assisted) bicycle injured in collision with heavy transport vehicle or bus
- V24.39 Person boarding or alighting other motorcycle injured in collision with heavy transport vehicle or bus

V24.4 Motorcycle driver injured in collision with heavy transport vehicle or bus in traffic accident
- V24.41 Electric (assisted) bicycle driver injured in collision with heavy transport vehicle or bus in traffic accident
- V24.49 Other motorcycle driver injured in collision with heavy transport vehicle or bus in traffic accident

V24.5 Motorcycle passenger injured in collision with heavy transport vehicle or bus in traffic accident
- V24.51 Electric (assisted) bicycle passenger injured in collision with heavy transport vehicle or bus in traffic accident
- V24.59 Other motorcycle passenger injured in collision with heavy transport vehicle or bus in traffic accident

V24.9 Unspecified motorcycle rider injured in collision with heavy transport vehicle or bus in traffic accident
- V24.91 Unspecified electric (assisted) bicycle rider injured in collision with heavy transport vehicle or bus in traffic accident
- V24.99 Unspecified rider of other motorcycle injured in collision with heavy transport vehicle or bus in traffic accident

V25 Motorcycle rider injured in collision with railway train or railway vehicle

V25.0 Motorcycle driver injured in collision with railway train or railway vehicle in nontraffic accident
- V25.01 Electric (assisted) bicycle driver injured in collision with railway train or railway vehicle in nontraffic accident
- V25.09 Other motorcycle driver injured in collision with railway train or railway vehicle in nontraffic accident

V25.1 Motorcycle passenger injured in collision with railway train or railway vehicle in nontraffic accident
- V25.11 Electric (assisted) bicycle passenger injured in collision with railway train or railway vehicle in nontraffic accident
- V25.19 Other motorcycle passenger injured in collision with railway train or railway vehicle in nontraffic accident

V25.2 Unspecified motorcycle rider injured in collision with railway train or railway vehicle in nontraffic accident
- V25.21 Unspecified electric (assisted) bicycle rider injured in collision with railway train or railway vehicle in nontraffic accident
- V25.29 Unspecified rider of other motorcycle injured in collision with railway train or railway vehicle in nontraffic accident

V25.3 Person boarding or alighting a motorcycle injured in collision with railway train or railway vehicle
- V25.31 Person boarding or alighting an electric (assisted) bicycle injured in collision with railway train or railway vehicle
- V25.39 Person boarding or alighting other motorcycle injured in collision with railway train or railway vehicle

V25.4 Motorcycle driver injured in collision with railway train or railway vehicle in traffic accident
- V25.41 Electric (assisted) bicycle driver injured in collision with railway train or railway vehicle in traffic accident
- V25.49 Other motorcycle driver injured in collision with railway train or railway vehicle in traffic accident

V25.5 Motorcycle passenger injured in collision with railway train or railway vehicle in traffic accident
- V25.51 Electric (assisted) bicycle passenger injured in collision with railway train or railway vehicle in traffic accident
- V25.59 Other motorcycle passenger injured in collision with railway train or railway vehicle in traffic accident

V25.9 Unspecified motorcycle rider injured in collision with railway train or railway vehicle in traffic accident
- V25.91 Unspecified electric (assisted) bicycle rider injured in collision with railway train or railway vehicle in traffic accident
- V25.99 Unspecified rider of other motorcycle injured in collision with railway train or railway vehicle in traffic accident

V26 Motorcycle rider injured in collision with other nonmotor vehicle

INCLUDES collision with animal-drawn vehicle, animal being ridden, streetcar

V26.0 Motorcycle driver injured in collision with other nonmotor vehicle in nontraffic accident
- V26.01 Electric (assisted) bicycle driver injured in collision with other nonmotor vehicle in nontraffic accident
- V26.09 Other motorcycle driver injured in collision with other nonmotor vehicle in nontraffic accident

V26.1 Motorcycle passenger injured in collision with other nonmotor vehicle in nontraffic accident
- V26.11 Electric (assisted) bicycle passenger injured in collision with other nonmotor vehicle in nontraffic accident

- ● √x7th V26.19 Other motorcycle passenger injured in collision with other nonmotor vehicle in nontraffic accident
- √5th V26.2 Unspecified motorcycle rider injured in collision with other nonmotor vehicle in nontraffic accident
  - ● √x7th V26.21 Unspecified electric (assisted) bicycle rider injured in collision with other nonmotor vehicle in nontraffic accident
  - ● √x7th V26.29 Unspecified rider of other motorcycle injured in collision with other nonmotor vehicle in nontraffic accident
- √5th V26.3 Person boarding or alighting a motorcycle injured in collision with other nonmotor vehicle
  - ● √x7th V26.31 Person boarding or alighting an electric (assisted) bicycle injured in collision with other nonmotor vehicle
  - ● √x7th V26.39 Person boarding or alighting other motorcycle injured in collision with other nonmotor vehicle
- √5th V26.4 Motorcycle driver injured in collision with other nonmotor vehicle in traffic accident
  - ● √x7th V26.41 Electric (assisted) bicycle driver injured in collision with other nonmotor vehicle in traffic accident
  - ● √x7th V26.49 Other motorcycle driver injured in collision with other nonmotor vehicle in traffic accident
- √5th V26.5 Motorcycle passenger injured in collision with other nonmotor vehicle in traffic accident
  - ● √x7th V26.51 Electric (assisted) bicycle passenger injured in collision with other nonmotor vehicle in traffic accident
  - ● √x7th V26.59 Other motorcycle passenger injured in collision with other nonmotor vehicle in traffic accident
- √5th V26.9 Unspecified motorcycle rider injured in collision with other nonmotor vehicle in traffic accident
  - ● √x7th V26.91 Unspecified electric (assisted) bicycle rider injured in collision with other nonmotor vehicle in traffic accident
  - ● √x7th V26.99 Unspecified rider of other motorcycle injured in collision with other nonmotor vehicle in traffic accident

√4th V27 Motorcycle rider injured in collision with fixed or stationary object

- √5th V27.Ø Motorcycle driver injured in collision with fixed or stationary object in nontraffic accident
  - ● √x7th V27.Ø1 Electric (assisted) bicycle driver injured in collision with fixed or stationary object in nontraffic accident
  - ● √x7th V27.Ø9 Other motorcycle driver injured in collision with fixed or stationary object in nontraffic accident
- √5th V27.1 Motorcycle passenger injured in collision with fixed or stationary object in nontraffic accident
  - ● √x7th V27.11 Electric (assisted) bicycle passenger injured in collision with fixed or stationary object in nontraffic accident
  - ● √x7th V27.19 Other motorcycle passenger injured in collision with fixed or stationary object in nontraffic accident
- √5th V27.2 Unspecified motorcycle rider injured in collision with fixed or stationary object in nontraffic accident
  - ● √x7th V27.21 Unspecified electric (assisted) bicycle rider injured in collision with fixed or stationary object in nontraffic accident
  - ● √x7th V27.29 Unspecified rider of other motorcycle injured in collision with fixed or stationary object in nontraffic accident
- √5th V27.3 Person boarding or alighting a motorcycle injured in collision with fixed or stationary object
  - ● √x7th V27.31 Person boarding or alighting an electric (assisted) bicycle injured in collision with fixed or stationary object
  - ● √x7th V27.39 Person boarding or alighting other motorcycle injured in collision with fixed or stationary object
- √5th V27.4 Motorcycle driver injured in collision with fixed or stationary object in traffic accident
  - ● √x7th V27.41 Electric (assisted) bicycle driver injured in collision with fixed or stationary object in traffic accident
  - ● √x7th V27.49 Other motorcycle driver injured in collision with fixed or stationary object in traffic accident
- √5th V27.5 Motorcycle passenger injured in collision with fixed or stationary object in traffic accident
  - ● √x7th V27.51 Electric (assisted) bicycle passenger injured in collision with fixed or stationary object in traffic accident
  - ● √x7th V27.59 Other motorcycle passenger injured in collision with fixed or stationary object in traffic accident
- √5th V27.9 Unspecified motorcycle rider injured in collision with fixed or stationary object in traffic accident
  - ● √x7th V27.91 Unspecified electric (assisted) bicycle rider injured in collision with fixed or stationary object in traffic accident
  - ● √x7th V27.99 Unspecified rider of other motorcycle injured in collision with fixed or stationary object in traffic accident

√4th V28 Motorcycle rider injured in noncollision transport accident

INCLUDES fall or thrown from motorcycle (without antecedent collision)
overturning motorcycle NOS
overturning motorcycle without collision

- √5th V28.Ø Motorcycle driver injured in noncollision transport accident in nontraffic accident
  - ● √x7th V28.Ø1 Electric (assisted) bicycle driver injured in noncollision transport accident in nontraffic accident
  - ● √x7th V28.Ø9 Other motorcycle driver injured in noncollision transport accident in nontraffic accident
- √5th V28.1 Motorcycle passenger injured in noncollision transport accident in nontraffic accident
  - ● √x7th V28.11 Electric (assisted) bicycle passenger injured in noncollision transport accident in nontraffic accident
  - ● √x7th V28.19 Other motorcycle passenger injured in noncollision transport accident in nontraffic accident
- √5th V28.2 Unspecified motorcycle rider injured in noncollision transport accident in nontraffic accident
  - ● √x7th V28.21 Unspecified electric (assisted) bicycle rider injured in noncollision transport accident in nontraffic accident
  - ● √x7th V28.29 Unspecified rider of other motorcycle injured in noncollision transport accident in nontraffic accident
- √5th V28.3 Person boarding or alighting a motorcycle injured in noncollision transport accident
  - ● √x7th V28.31 Person boarding or alighting an electric (assisted) bicycle injured in noncollision transport accident
  - ● √x7th V28.39 Person boarding or alighting other motorcycle injured in noncollision transport accident
- √5th V28.4 Motorcycle driver injured in noncollision transport accident in traffic accident
  - ● √x7th V28.41 Electric (assisted) bicycle driver injured in noncollision transport accident in traffic accident
  - ● √x7th V28.49 Other motorcycle driver injured in noncollision transport accident in traffic accident
- √5th V28.5 Motorcycle passenger injured in noncollision transport accident in traffic accident
  - ● √x7th V28.51 Electric (assisted) bicycle passenger injured in noncollision transport accident in traffic accident
  - ● √x7th V28.59 Other motorcycle passenger injured in noncollision transport accident in traffic accident
- √5th V28.9 Unspecified motorcycle rider injured in noncollision transport accident in traffic accident
  - ● √x7th V28.91 Unspecified electric (assisted) bicycle rider injured in noncollision transport accident in traffic accident
  - ● √x7th V28.99 Unspecified rider of other motorcycle injured in noncollision transport accident in traffic accident

√4th V29 Motorcycle rider injured in other and unspecified transport accidents

- √5th V29.Ø Motorcycle driver injured in collision with other and unspecified motor vehicles in nontraffic accident
  - √6th V29.ØØ Motorcycle driver injured in collision with unspecified motor vehicles in nontraffic accident
    - ● √7th V29.ØØ1 Electric (assisted) bicycle driver injured in collision with unspecified motor vehicles in nontraffic accident
    - ● √7th V29.ØØ8 Other motorcycle driver injured in collision with unspecified motor vehicles in nontraffic accident
  - √6th V29.Ø9 Motorcycle driver injured in collision with other motor vehicles in nontraffic accident
    - ● √7th V29.Ø91 Electric (assisted) bicycle driver injured in collision with other motor vehicles in nontraffic accident
    - ● √7th V29.Ø98 Other motorcycle driver injured in collision with other motor vehicles in nontraffic accident

V29.1 Motorcycle passenger injured in collision with other and unspecified motor vehicles in nontraffic accident

V29.1Ø Motorcycle passenger injured in collision with unspecified motor vehicles in nontraffic accident

● **V29.1Ø1** Electric (assisted) bicycle passenger injured in collision with unspecified motor vehicles in nontraffic accident

● **V29.1Ø8** Other motorcycle passenger injured in collision with unspecified motor vehicles in nontraffic accident

V29.19 Motorcycle passenger injured in collision with other motor vehicles in nontraffic accident

● **V29.191** Electric (assisted) bicycle passenger injured in collision with other motor vehicles in nontraffic accident

● **V29.198** Other motorcycle passenger injured in collision with other motor vehicles in nontraffic accident

V29.2 Unspecified motorcycle rider injured in collision with other and unspecified motor vehicles in nontraffic accident

V29.2Ø Unspecified motorcycle rider injured in collision with unspecified motor vehicles in nontraffic accident

~~Motorcycle collision NOS, nontraffic~~

● **V29.2Ø1** Unspecified electric (assisted) bicycle rider injured in collision with unspecified motor vehicles in nontraffic accident

● **V29.2Ø8** Unspecified rider of other motorcycle injured in collision with unspecified motor vehicles in nontraffic accident

Motorcycle collision NOS, nontraffic

V29.29 Unspecified motorcycle rider injured in collision with other motor vehicles in nontraffic accident

● **V29.291** Unspecified electric (assisted) bicycle rider injured in collision with other motor vehicles in nontraffic accident

● **V29.298** Unspecified rider of other motorcycle injured in collision with other motor vehicles in nontraffic accident

V29.3 Motorcycle rider (driver) (passenger) injured in unspecified nontraffic accident

~~Motorcycle accident NOS, nontraffic~~

~~Motorcycle rider injured in nontraffic accident NOS~~

● **V29.31** Electric (assisted) bicycle (driver) (passenger) injured in unspecified nontraffic accident

● **V29.39** Other motorcycle (driver) (passenger) injured in unspecified nontraffic accident

Motorcycle accident NOS, nontraffic

Motorcycle rider injured in nontraffic accident NOS

V29.4 Motorcycle driver injured in collision with other and unspecified motor vehicles in traffic accident

V29.4Ø Motorcycle driver injured in collision with unspecified motor vehicles in traffic accident

● **V29.4Ø1** Electric (assisted) bicycle driver injured in collision with unspecified motor vehicles in traffic accident

● **V29.4Ø8** Other motorcycle driver injured in collision with unspecified motor vehicles in traffic accident

V29.49 Motorcycle driver injured in collision with other motor vehicles in traffic accident

● **V29.491** Electric (assisted) bicycle driver injured in collision with other motor vehicles in traffic accident

● **V29.498** Other motorcycle driver injured in collision with other motor vehicles in traffic accident

V29.5 Motorcycle passenger injured in collision with other and unspecified motor vehicles in traffic accident

V29.5Ø Motorcycle passenger injured in collision with unspecified motor vehicles in traffic accident

● **V29.5Ø1** Electric (assisted) bicycle passenger injured in collision with unspecified motor vehicles in traffic accident

● **V29.5Ø8** Other motorcycle passenger injured in collision with unspecified motor vehicles in traffic accident

V29.59 Motorcycle passenger injured in collision with other motor vehicles in traffic accident

● **V29.591** Electric (assisted) bicycle passenger injured in collision with other motor vehicles in traffic accident

● **V29.598** Other motorcycle passenger injured in collision with other motor vehicles in traffic accident

V29.6 Unspecified motorcycle rider injured in collision with other and unspecified motor vehicles in traffic accident

V29.6Ø Unspecified motorcycle rider injured in collision with unspecified motor vehicles in traffic accident

~~Motorcycle collision NOS (traffic)~~

● **V29.6Ø1** Unspecified electric (assisted) bicycle rider injured in collision with unspecified motor vehicles in traffic accident

● **V29.6Ø8** Unspecified rider of other motorcycle injured in collision with unspecified motor vehicles in traffic accident

Motorcycle collision NOS (traffic)

V29.69 Unspecified motorcycle rider injured in collision with other motor vehicles in traffic accident

● **V29.691** Unspecified electric (assisted) bicycle rider injured in collision with other motor vehicles in traffic accident

● **V29.698** Unspecified rider of other motorcycle injured in collision with other motor vehicles in traffic accident

V29.8 Motorcycle rider (driver) (passenger) injured in other specified transport accidents

V29.81 Motorcycle rider (driver) (passenger) injured in transport accident with military vehicle

● **V29.811** Electric (assisted) bicycle rider (driver) (passenger) injured in transport accident with military vehicle

● **V29.818** Rider (driver) (passenger) of other motorcycle injured in transport accident with military vehicle

V29.88 Motorcycle rider (driver) (passenger) injured in other specified transport accidents

● **V29.881** Electric (assisted) bicycle rider (driver) (passenger) injured in other specified transport accidents

● **V29.888** Rider (driver) (passenger) of other motorcycle injured in other specified transport accidents

V29.9 Motorcycle rider (driver) (passenger) injured in unspecified traffic accident

~~Motorcycle accident NOS~~

● **V29.91** Electric (assisted) bicycle rider (driver) (passenger) injured in unspecified traffic accident

● **V29.99** Rider (driver) (passenger) of other motorcycle injured in unspecified traffic accident

Motorcycle accident NOS

Occupant of three-wheeled motor vehicle injured in transport accident (V3Ø-V39)

INCLUDES motorized tricycle
motorized rickshaw
three-wheeled motor car

EXCLUDES 1 *all-terrain vehicles (V86.-)*
motorcycle with sidecar (V2Ø-V29)
vehicle designed primarily for off-road use (V86.-)

The appropriate 7th character is to be added to each code from categories V3Ø-V39.
A initial encounter
D subsequent encounter
S sequela

V3Ø Occupant of three-wheeled motor vehicle injured in collision with pedestrian or animal

EXCLUDES 1 *three-wheeled motor vehicle collision with animal-drawn vehicle or animal being ridden (V36.-)*

V3Ø.Ø Driver of three-wheeled motor vehicle injured in collision with pedestrian or animal in nontraffic accident

V3Ø.1 Passenger in three-wheeled motor vehicle injured in collision with pedestrian or animal in nontraffic accident

V3Ø.2 Person on outside of three-wheeled motor vehicle injured in collision with pedestrian or animal in nontraffic accident

V3Ø.3 Unspecified occupant of three-wheeled motor vehicle injured in collision with pedestrian or animal in nontraffic accident

V3Ø.4 Person boarding or alighting a three-wheeled motor vehicle injured in collision with pedestrian or animal

V3Ø.5 Driver of three-wheeled motor vehicle injured in collision with pedestrian or animal in traffic accident

V3Ø.6 Passenger in three-wheeled motor vehicle injured in collision with pedestrian or animal in traffic accident

√7th V30.7 Person on outside of three-wheeled motor vehicle injured in collision with pedestrian or animal in traffic accident

√7th V30.9 Unspecified occupant of three-wheeled motor vehicle injured in collision with pedestrian or animal in traffic accident

√4th **V31 Occupant of three-wheeled motor vehicle injured in collision with pedal cycle**

√7th V31.0 Driver of three-wheeled motor vehicle injured in collision with pedal cycle in nontraffic accident

√7th V31.1 Passenger in three-wheeled motor vehicle injured in collision with pedal cycle in nontraffic accident

√7th V31.2 Person on outside of three-wheeled motor vehicle injured in collision with pedal cycle in nontraffic accident

√7th V31.3 Unspecified occupant of three-wheeled motor vehicle injured in collision with pedal cycle in nontraffic accident

√7th V31.4 Person boarding or alighting a three-wheeled motor vehicle injured in collision with pedal cycle

√7th V31.5 Driver of three-wheeled motor vehicle injured in collision with pedal cycle in traffic accident

√7th V31.6 Passenger in three-wheeled motor vehicle injured in collision with pedal cycle in traffic accident

√7th V31.7 Person on outside of three-wheeled motor vehicle injured in collision with pedal cycle in traffic accident

√7th V31.9 Unspecified occupant of three-wheeled motor vehicle injured in collision with pedal cycle in traffic accident

√4th **V32 Occupant of three-wheeled motor vehicle injured in collision with two- or three-wheeled motor vehicle**

√7th V32.0 Driver of three-wheeled motor vehicle injured in collision with two- or three-wheeled motor vehicle in nontraffic accident

√7th V32.1 Passenger in three-wheeled motor vehicle injured in collision with two- or three-wheeled motor vehicle in nontraffic accident

√7th V32.2 Person on outside of three-wheeled motor vehicle injured in collision with two- or three-wheeled motor vehicle in nontraffic accident

√7th V32.3 Unspecified occupant of three-wheeled motor vehicle injured in collision with two- or three-wheeled motor vehicle in nontraffic accident

√7th V32.4 Person boarding or alighting a three-wheeled motor vehicle injured in collision with two- or three-wheeled motor vehicle

√7th V32.5 Driver of three-wheeled motor vehicle injured in collision with two- or three-wheeled motor vehicle in traffic accident

√7th V32.6 Passenger in three-wheeled motor vehicle injured in collision with two- or three-wheeled motor vehicle in traffic accident

√7th V32.7 Person on outside of three-wheeled motor vehicle injured in collision with two- or three-wheeled motor vehicle in traffic accident

√7th V32.9 Unspecified occupant of three-wheeled motor vehicle injured in collision with two- or three-wheeled motor vehicle in traffic accident

√4th **V33 Occupant of three-wheeled motor vehicle injured in collision with car, pick-up truck or van**

√7th V33.0 Driver of three-wheeled motor vehicle injured in collision with car, pick-up truck or van in nontraffic accident

√7th V33.1 Passenger in three-wheeled motor vehicle injured in collision with car, pick-up truck or van in nontraffic accident

√7th V33.2 Person on outside of three-wheeled motor vehicle injured in collision with car, pick-up truck or van in nontraffic accident

√7th V33.3 Unspecified occupant of three-wheeled motor vehicle injured in collision with car, pick-up truck or van in nontraffic accident

√7th V33.4 Person boarding or alighting a three-wheeled motor vehicle injured in collision with car, pick-up truck or van

√7th V33.5 Driver of three-wheeled motor vehicle injured in collision with car, pick-up truck or van in traffic accident

√7th V33.6 Passenger in three-wheeled motor vehicle injured in collision with car, pick-up truck or van in traffic accident

√7th V33.7 Person on outside of three-wheeled motor vehicle injured in collision with car, pick-up truck or van in traffic accident

√7th V33.9 Unspecified occupant of three-wheeled motor vehicle injured in collision with car, pick-up truck or van in traffic accident

√4th **V34 Occupant of three-wheeled motor vehicle injured in collision with heavy transport vehicle or bus**

EXCLUDES1 *occupant of three-wheeled motor vehicle injured in collision with military vehicle (V39.81)*

√7th V34.0 Driver of three-wheeled motor vehicle injured in collision with heavy transport vehicle or bus in nontraffic accident

√7th V34.1 Passenger in three-wheeled motor vehicle injured in collision with heavy transport vehicle or bus in nontraffic accident

√7th V34.2 Person on outside of three-wheeled motor vehicle injured in collision with heavy transport vehicle or bus in nontraffic accident

√7th V34.3 Unspecified occupant of three-wheeled motor vehicle injured in collision with heavy transport vehicle or bus in nontraffic accident

√7th V34.4 Person boarding or alighting a three-wheeled motor vehicle injured in collision with heavy transport vehicle or bus

√7th V34.5 Driver of three-wheeled motor vehicle injured in collision with heavy transport vehicle or bus in traffic accident

√7th V34.6 Passenger in three-wheeled motor vehicle injured in collision with heavy transport vehicle or bus in traffic accident

√7th V34.7 Person on outside of three-wheeled motor vehicle injured in collision with heavy transport vehicle or bus in traffic accident

√7th V34.9 Unspecified occupant of three-wheeled motor vehicle injured in collision with heavy transport vehicle or bus in traffic accident

√4th **V35 Occupant of three-wheeled motor vehicle injured in collision with railway train or railway vehicle**

√7th V35.0 Driver of three-wheeled motor vehicle injured in collision with railway train or railway vehicle in nontraffic accident

√7th V35.1 Passenger in three-wheeled motor vehicle injured in collision with railway train or railway vehicle in nontraffic accident

√7th V35.2 Person on outside of three-wheeled motor vehicle injured in collision with railway train or railway vehicle in nontraffic accident

√7th V35.3 Unspecified occupant of three-wheeled motor vehicle injured in collision with railway train or railway vehicle in nontraffic accident

√7th V35.4 Person boarding or alighting a three-wheeled motor vehicle injured in collision with railway train or railway vehicle

√7th V35.5 Driver of three-wheeled motor vehicle injured in collision with railway train or railway vehicle in traffic accident

√7th V35.6 Passenger in three-wheeled motor vehicle injured in collision with railway train or railway vehicle in traffic accident

√7th V35.7 Person on outside of three-wheeled motor vehicle injured in collision with railway train or railway vehicle in traffic accident

√7th V35.9 Unspecified occupant of three-wheeled motor vehicle injured in collision with railway train or railway vehicle in traffic accident

√4th **V36 Occupant of three-wheeled motor vehicle injured in collision with other nonmotor vehicle**

INCLUDES collision with animal-drawn vehicle, animal being ridden, streetcar

√7th V36.0 Driver of three-wheeled motor vehicle injured in collision with other nonmotor vehicle in nontraffic accident

√7th V36.1 Passenger in three-wheeled motor vehicle injured in collision with other nonmotor vehicle in nontraffic accident

√7th V36.2 Person on outside of three-wheeled motor vehicle injured in collision with other nonmotor vehicle in nontraffic accident

√7th V36.3 Unspecified occupant of three-wheeled motor vehicle injured in collision with other nonmotor vehicle in nontraffic accident

√7th V36.4 Person boarding or alighting a three-wheeled motor vehicle injured in collision with other nonmotor vehicle

√7th V36.5 Driver of three-wheeled motor vehicle injured in collision with other nonmotor vehicle in traffic accident

√7th V36.6 Passenger in three-wheeled motor vehicle injured in collision with other nonmotor vehicle in traffic accident

√7th V36.7 Person on outside of three-wheeled motor vehicle injured in collision with other nonmotor vehicle in traffic accident

√7th V36.9 Unspecified occupant of three-wheeled motor vehicle injured in collision with other nonmotor vehicle in traffic accident

√4th **V37 Occupant of three-wheeled motor vehicle injured in collision with fixed or stationary object**

√7th V37.0 Driver of three-wheeled motor vehicle injured in collision with fixed or stationary object in nontraffic accident

√7th V37.1 Passenger in three-wheeled motor vehicle injured in collision with fixed or stationary object in nontraffic accident

√7th V37.2 Person on outside of three-wheeled motor vehicle injured in collision with fixed or stationary object in nontraffic accident

√7th V37.3 Unspecified occupant of three-wheeled motor vehicle injured in collision with fixed or stationary object in nontraffic accident

√7th V37.4 Person boarding or alighting a three-wheeled motor vehicle injured in collision with fixed or stationary object

√7th V37.5 Driver of three-wheeled motor vehicle injured in collision with fixed or stationary object in traffic accident

√x7th **V37.6 Passenger in three-wheeled motor vehicle injured in collision with fixed or stationary object in traffic accident**

√x7th **V37.7 Person on outside of three-wheeled motor vehicle injured in collision with fixed or stationary object in traffic accident**

√x7th **V37.9 Unspecified occupant of three-wheeled motor vehicle injured in collision with fixed or stationary object in traffic accident**

√4th **V38 Occupant of three-wheeled motor vehicle injured in noncollision transport accident**

INCLUDES fall or thrown from three-wheeled motor vehicle
overturning of three-wheeled motor vehicle NOS
overturning of three-wheeled motor vehicle without collision

√x7th **V38.Ø Driver of three-wheeled motor vehicle injured in noncollision transport accident in nontraffic accident**

√x7th **V38.1 Passenger in three-wheeled motor vehicle injured in noncollision transport accident in nontraffic accident**

√x7th **V38.2 Person on outside of three-wheeled motor vehicle injured in noncollision transport accident in nontraffic accident**

√x7th **V38.3 Unspecified occupant of three-wheeled motor vehicle injured in noncollision transport accident in nontraffic accident**

√x7th **V38.4 Person boarding or alighting a three-wheeled motor vehicle injured in noncollision transport accident**

√x7th **V38.5 Driver of three-wheeled motor vehicle injured in noncollision transport accident in traffic accident**

√x7th **V38.6 Passenger in three-wheeled motor vehicle injured in noncollision transport accident in traffic accident**

√x7th **V38.7 Person on outside of three-wheeled motor vehicle injured in noncollision transport accident in traffic accident**

√x7th **V38.9 Unspecified occupant of three-wheeled motor vehicle injured in noncollision transport accident in traffic accident**

√4th **V39 Occupant of three-wheeled motor vehicle injured in other and unspecified transport accidents**

√5th **V39.Ø Driver of three-wheeled motor vehicle injured in collision with other and unspecified motor vehicles in nontraffic accident**

√x7th **V39.ØØ Driver of three-wheeled motor vehicle injured in collision with unspecified motor vehicles in nontraffic accident**

√x7th **V39.Ø9 Driver of three-wheeled motor vehicle injured in collision with other motor vehicles in nontraffic accident**

√5th **V39.1 Passenger in three-wheeled motor vehicle injured in collision with other and unspecified motor vehicles in nontraffic accident**

√x7th **V39.1Ø Passenger in three-wheeled motor vehicle injured in collision with unspecified motor vehicles in nontraffic accident**

√x7th **V39.19 Passenger in three-wheeled motor vehicle injured in collision with other motor vehicles in nontraffic accident**

√5th **V39.2 Unspecified occupant of three-wheeled motor vehicle injured in collision with other and unspecified motor vehicles in nontraffic accident**

√x7th **V39.2Ø Unspecified occupant of three-wheeled motor vehicle injured in collision with unspecified motor vehicles in nontraffic accident**
Collision NOS involving three-wheeled motor vehicle, nontraffic

√x7th **V39.29 Unspecified occupant of three-wheeled motor vehicle injured in collision with other motor vehicles in nontraffic accident**

√x7th **V39.3 Occupant (driver) (passenger) of three-wheeled motor vehicle injured in unspecified nontraffic accident**
Accident NOS involving three-wheeled motor vehicle, nontraffic
Occupant of three-wheeled motor vehicle injured in nontraffic accident NOS

√5th **V39.4 Driver of three-wheeled motor vehicle injured in collision with other and unspecified motor vehicles in traffic accident**

√x7th **V39.4Ø Driver of three-wheeled motor vehicle injured in collision with unspecified motor vehicles in traffic accident**

√x7th **V39.49 Driver of three-wheeled motor vehicle injured in collision with other motor vehicles in traffic accident**

√5th **V39.5 Passenger in three-wheeled motor vehicle injured in collision with other and unspecified motor vehicles in traffic accident**

√x7th **V39.5Ø Passenger in three-wheeled motor vehicle injured in collision with unspecified motor vehicles in traffic accident**

√x7th **V39.59 Passenger in three-wheeled motor vehicle injured in collision with other motor vehicles in traffic accident**

√5th **V39.6 Unspecified occupant of three-wheeled motor vehicle injured in collision with other and unspecified motor vehicles in traffic accident**

√x7th **V39.6Ø Unspecified occupant of three-wheeled motor vehicle injured in collision with unspecified motor vehicles in traffic accident**
Collision NOS involving three-wheeled motor vehicle (traffic)

√x7th **V39.69 Unspecified occupant of three-wheeled motor vehicle injured in collision with other motor vehicles in traffic accident**

√5th **V39.8 Occupant (driver) (passenger) of three-wheeled motor vehicle injured in other specified transport accidents**

√x7th **V39.81 Occupant (driver) (passenger) of three-wheeled motor vehicle injured in transport accident with military vehicle**

√x7th **V39.89 Occupant (driver) (passenger) of three-wheeled motor vehicle injured in other specified transport accidents**

√x7th **V39.9 Occupant (driver) (passenger) of three-wheeled motor vehicle injured in unspecified traffic accident**
Accident NOS involving three-wheeled motor vehicle

Car occupant injured in transport accident (V4Ø-V49)

INCLUDES a four-wheeled motor vehicle designed primarily for carrying passengers
automobile (pulling a trailer or camper)

EXCLUDES 1 *bus (V5Ø-V59)*
minibus (V5Ø-V59)
minivan (V5Ø-V59)
motorcoach (V7Ø-V79)
pick-up truck (V5Ø-V59)
sport utility vehicle (SUV) (V5Ø-V59)

The appropriate 7th character is to be added to each code from categories V4Ø-V49.
A initial encounter
D subsequent encounter
S sequela

√4th **V4Ø Car occupant injured in collision with pedestrian or animal**

EXCLUDES 1 *car collision with animal-drawn vehicle or animal being ridden (V46.-)*

√x7th **V4Ø.Ø Car driver injured in collision with pedestrian or animal in nontraffic accident**

√x7th **V4Ø.1 Car passenger injured in collision with pedestrian or animal in nontraffic accident**

√x7th **V4Ø.2 Person on outside of car injured in collision with pedestrian or animal in nontraffic accident**

√x7th **V4Ø.3 Unspecified car occupant injured in collision with pedestrian or animal in nontraffic accident**

√x7th **V4Ø.4 Person boarding or alighting a car injured in collision with pedestrian or animal**

√x7th **V4Ø.5 Car driver injured in collision with pedestrian or animal in traffic accident**

√x7th **V4Ø.6 Car passenger injured in collision with pedestrian or animal in traffic accident**

√x7th **V4Ø.7 Person on outside of car injured in collision with pedestrian or animal in traffic accident**

√x7th **V4Ø.9 Unspecified car occupant injured in collision with pedestrian or animal in traffic accident**

√4th **V41 Car occupant injured in collision with pedal cycle**

√x7th **V41.Ø Car driver injured in collision with pedal cycle in nontraffic accident**

√x7th **V41.1 Car passenger injured in collision with pedal cycle in nontraffic accident**

√x7th **V41.2 Person on outside of car injured in collision with pedal cycle in nontraffic accident**

√x7th **V41.3 Unspecified car occupant injured in collision with pedal cycle in nontraffic accident**

√x7th **V41.4 Person boarding or alighting a car injured in collision with pedal cycle**

√x7th **V41.5 Car driver injured in collision with pedal cycle in traffic accident**

√x7th **V41.6 Car passenger injured in collision with pedal cycle in traffic accident**

√x7th **V41.7 Person on outside of car injured in collision with pedal cycle in traffic accident**

√x7th **V41.9 Unspecified car occupant injured in collision with pedal cycle in traffic accident**

V42 Car occupant injured in collision with two- or three-wheeled motor vehicle
- **V42.0** Car driver injured in collision with two- or three-wheeled motor vehicle in nontraffic accident
- **V42.1** Car passenger injured in collision with two- or three-wheeled motor vehicle in nontraffic accident
- **V42.2** Person on outside of car injured in collision with two- or three-wheeled motor vehicle in nontraffic accident
- **V42.3** Unspecified car occupant injured in collision with two- or three-wheeled motor vehicle in nontraffic accident
- **V42.4** Person boarding or alighting a car injured in collision with two- or three-wheeled motor vehicle
- **V42.5** Car driver injured in collision with two- or three-wheeled motor vehicle in traffic accident
- **V42.6** Car passenger injured in collision with two- or three-wheeled motor vehicle in traffic accident
- **V42.7** Person on outside of car injured in collision with two- or three-wheeled motor vehicle in traffic accident
- **V42.9** Unspecified car occupant injured in collision with two- or three-wheeled motor vehicle in traffic accident

V43 Car occupant injured in collision with car, pick-up truck or van
- **V43.0** Car driver injured in collision with car, pick-up truck or van in nontraffic accident
  - **V43.01** Car driver injured in collision with sport utility vehicle in nontraffic accident
  - **V43.02** Car driver injured in collision with other type car in nontraffic accident
  - **V43.03** Car driver injured in collision with pick-up truck in nontraffic accident
  - **V43.04** Car driver injured in collision with van in nontraffic accident
- **V43.1** Car passenger injured in collision with car, pick-up truck or van in nontraffic accident
  - **V43.11** Car passenger injured in collision with sport utility vehicle in nontraffic accident
  - **V43.12** Car passenger injured in collision with other type car in nontraffic accident
  - **V43.13** Car passenger injured in collision with pick-up truck in nontraffic accident
  - **V43.14** Car passenger injured in collision with van in nontraffic accident
- **V43.2** Person on outside of car injured in collision with car, pick-up truck or van in nontraffic accident
  - **V43.21** Person on outside of car injured in collision with sport utility vehicle in nontraffic accident
  - **V43.22** Person on outside of car injured in collision with other type car in nontraffic accident
  - **V43.23** Person on outside of car injured in collision with pick-up truck in nontraffic accident
  - **V43.24** Person on outside of car injured in collision with van in nontraffic accident
- **V43.3** Unspecified car occupant injured in collision with car, pick-up truck or van in nontraffic accident
  - **V43.31** Unspecified car occupant injured in collision with sport utility vehicle in nontraffic accident
  - **V43.32** Unspecified car occupant injured in collision with other type car in nontraffic accident
  - **V43.33** Unspecified car occupant injured in collision with pick-up truck in nontraffic accident
  - **V43.34** Unspecified car occupant injured in collision with van in nontraffic accident
- **V43.4** Person boarding or alighting a car injured in collision with car, pick-up truck or van
  - **V43.41** Person boarding or alighting a car injured in collision with sport utility vehicle
  - **V43.42** Person boarding or alighting a car injured in collision with other type car
  - **V43.43** Person boarding or alighting a car injured in collision with pick-up truck
  - **V43.44** Person boarding or alighting a car injured in collision with van
- **V43.5** Car driver injured in collision with car, pick-up truck or van in traffic accident
  - **V43.51** Car driver injured in collision with sport utility vehicle in traffic accident
  - **V43.52** Car driver injured in collision with other type car in traffic accident
  - **V43.53** Car driver injured in collision with pick-up truck in traffic accident
  - **V43.54** Car driver injured in collision with van in traffic accident
- **V43.6** Car passenger injured in collision with car, pick-up truck or van in traffic accident
  - **V43.61** Car passenger injured in collision with sport utility vehicle in traffic accident
  - **V43.62** Car passenger injured in collision with other type car in traffic accident
  - **V43.63** Car passenger injured in collision with pick-up truck in traffic accident
  - **V43.64** Car passenger injured in collision with van in traffic accident
- **V43.7** Person on outside of car injured in collision with car, pick-up truck or van in traffic accident
  - **V43.71** Person on outside of car injured in collision with sport utility vehicle in traffic accident
  - **V43.72** Person on outside of car injured in collision with other type car in traffic accident
  - **V43.73** Person on outside of car injured in collision with pick-up truck in traffic accident
  - **V43.74** Person on outside of car injured in collision with van in traffic accident
- **V43.9** Unspecified car occupant injured in collision with car, pick-up truck or van in traffic accident
  - **V43.91** Unspecified car occupant injured in collision with sport utility vehicle in traffic accident
  - **V43.92** Unspecified car occupant injured in collision with other type car in traffic accident
  - **V43.93** Unspecified car occupant injured in collision with pick-up truck in traffic accident
  - **V43.94** Unspecified car occupant injured in collision with van in traffic accident

V44 Car occupant injured in collision with heavy transport vehicle or bus

EXCLUDES 1 *car occupant injured in collision with military vehicle (V49.81)*

- **V44.0** Car driver injured in collision with heavy transport vehicle or bus in nontraffic accident
- **V44.1** Car passenger injured in collision with heavy transport vehicle or bus in nontraffic accident
- **V44.2** Person on outside of car injured in collision with heavy transport vehicle or bus in nontraffic accident
- **V44.3** Unspecified car occupant injured in collision with heavy transport vehicle or bus in nontraffic accident
- **V44.4** Person boarding or alighting a car injured in collision with heavy transport vehicle or bus
- **V44.5** Car driver injured in collision with heavy transport vehicle or bus in traffic accident
- **V44.6** Car passenger injured in collision with heavy transport vehicle or bus in traffic accident
- **V44.7** Person on outside of car injured in collision with heavy transport vehicle or bus in traffic accident
- **V44.9** Unspecified car occupant injured in collision with heavy transport vehicle or bus in traffic accident

V45 Car occupant injured in collision with railway train or railway vehicle
- **V45.0** Car driver injured in collision with railway train or railway vehicle in nontraffic accident
- **V45.1** Car passenger injured in collision with railway train or railway vehicle in nontraffic accident
- **V45.2** Person on outside of car injured in collision with railway train or railway vehicle in nontraffic accident
- **V45.3** Unspecified car occupant injured in collision with railway train or railway vehicle in nontraffic accident
- **V45.4** Person boarding or alighting a car injured in collision with railway train or railway vehicle
- **V45.5** Car driver injured in collision with railway train or railway vehicle in traffic accident
- **V45.6** Car passenger injured in collision with railway train or railway vehicle in traffic accident
- **V45.7** Person on outside of car injured in collision with railway train or railway vehicle in traffic accident
- **V45.9** Unspecified car occupant injured in collision with railway train or railway vehicle in traffic accident

V46 Car occupant injured in collision with other nonmotor vehicle

INCLUDES collision with animal-drawn vehicle, animal being ridden, streetcar

- **V46.0** Car driver injured in collision with other nonmotor vehicle in nontraffic accident
- **V46.1** Car passenger injured in collision with other nonmotor vehicle in nontraffic accident
- **V46.2** Person on outside of car injured in collision with other nonmotor vehicle in nontraffic accident

Chapter 20. External Causes of Morbidity
V42–V46.2

√x7th **V46.3** **Unspecified car occupant injured in collision with other nonmotor vehicle in nontraffic accident**
√x7th **V46.4** **Person boarding or alighting a car injured in collision with other nonmotor vehicle**
√x7th **V46.5** **Car driver injured in collision with other nonmotor vehicle in traffic accident**
√x7th **V46.6** **Car passenger injured in collision with other nonmotor vehicle in traffic accident**
√x7th **V46.7** **Person on outside of car injured in collision with other nonmotor vehicle in traffic accident**
√x7th **V46.9** **Unspecified car occupant injured in collision with other nonmotor vehicle in traffic accident**

√4th **V47** **Car occupant injured in collision with fixed or stationary object**
AHA: 2016,4Q,73
√x7th **V47.0** **Car driver injured in collision with fixed or stationary object in nontraffic accident**
√x7th **V47.1** **Car passenger injured in collision with fixed or stationary object in nontraffic accident**
√x7th **V47.2** **Person on outside of car injured in collision with fixed or stationary object in nontraffic accident**
√x7th **V47.3** **Unspecified car occupant injured in collision with fixed or stationary object in nontraffic accident**
√x7th **V47.4** **Person boarding or alighting a car injured in collision with fixed or stationary object**
√x7th **V47.5** **Car driver injured in collision with fixed or stationary object in traffic accident**
√x7th **V47.6** **Car passenger injured in collision with fixed or stationary object in traffic accident**
√x7th **V47.7** **Person on outside of car injured in collision with fixed or stationary object in traffic accident**
√x7th **V47.9** **Unspecified car occupant injured in collision with fixed or stationary object in traffic accident**

√4th **V48** **Car occupant injured in noncollision transport accident**
INCLUDES overturning car NOS
overturning car without collision
√x7th **V48.0** **Car driver injured in noncollision transport accident in nontraffic accident**
√x7th **V48.1** **Car passenger injured in noncollision transport accident in nontraffic accident**
√x7th **V48.2** **Person on outside of car injured in noncollision transport accident in nontraffic accident**
√x7th **V48.3** **Unspecified car occupant injured in noncollision transport accident in nontraffic accident**
√x7th **V48.4** **Person boarding or alighting a car injured in noncollision transport accident**
√x7th **V48.5** **Car driver injured in noncollision transport accident in traffic accident**
√x7th **V48.6** **Car passenger injured in noncollision transport accident in traffic accident**
√x7th **V48.7** **Person on outside of car injured in noncollision transport accident in traffic accident**
√x7th **V48.9** **Unspecified car occupant injured in noncollision transport accident in traffic accident**

√4th **V49** **Car occupant injured in other and unspecified transport accidents**
√5th **V49.0** **Driver injured in collision with other and unspecified motor vehicles in nontraffic accident**
√x7th **V49.00** **Driver injured in collision with unspecified motor vehicles in nontraffic accident**
√x7th **V49.09** **Driver injured in collision with other motor vehicles in nontraffic accident**
√5th **V49.1** **Passenger injured in collision with other and unspecified motor vehicles in nontraffic accident**
√x7th **V49.10** **Passenger injured in collision with unspecified motor vehicles in nontraffic accident**
√x7th **V49.19** **Passenger injured in collision with other motor vehicles in nontraffic accident**
√5th **V49.2** **Unspecified car occupant injured in collision with other and unspecified motor vehicles in nontraffic accident**
√x7th **V49.20** **Unspecified car occupant injured in collision with unspecified motor vehicles in nontraffic accident**
Car collision NOS, nontraffic
√x7th **V49.29** **Unspecified car occupant injured in collision with other motor vehicles in nontraffic accident**
√x7th **V49.3** **Car occupant (driver) (passenger) injured in unspecified nontraffic accident**
Car accident NOS, nontraffic
Car occupant injured in nontraffic accident NOS

√5th **V49.4** **Driver injured in collision with other and unspecified motor vehicles in traffic accident**
√x7th **V49.40** **Driver injured in collision with unspecified motor vehicles in traffic accident**
√x7th **V49.49** **Driver injured in collision with other motor vehicles in traffic accident**
√5th **V49.5** **Passenger injured in collision with other and unspecified motor vehicles in traffic accident**
√x7th **V49.50** **Passenger injured in collision with unspecified motor vehicles in traffic accident**
√x7th **V49.59** **Passenger injured in collision with other motor vehicles in traffic accident**
√5th **V49.6** **Unspecified car occupant injured in collision with other and unspecified motor vehicles in traffic accident**
√x7th **V49.60** **Unspecified car occupant injured in collision with unspecified motor vehicles in traffic accident**
Car collision NOS (traffic)
√x7th **V49.69** **Unspecified car occupant injured in collision with other motor vehicles in traffic accident**
√5th **V49.8** **Car occupant (driver) (passenger) injured in other specified transport accidents**
√x7th **V49.81** **Car occupant (driver) (passenger) injured in transport accident with military vehicle**
√x7th **V49.88** **Car occupant (driver) (passenger) injured in other specified transport accidents**
√x7th **V49.9** **Car occupant (driver) (passenger) injured in unspecified traffic accident**
Car accident NOS

Occupant of pick-up truck or van injured in transport accident (V50-V59)

INCLUDES a four or six wheel motor vehicle designed primarily for carrying passengers and property but weighing less than the local limit for classification as a heavy goods vehicle
minibus
minivan
sport utility vehicle (SUV)
truck
van

EXCLUDES 1 *heavy transport vehicle (V60-V69)*

The appropriate 7th character is to be added to each code from categories V50-V59.
A initial encounter
D subsequent encounter
S sequela

√4th **V50** **Occupant of pick-up truck or van injured in collision with pedestrian or animal**
EXCLUDES 1 *pick-up truck or van collision with animal-drawn vehicle or animal being ridden (V56.-)*
√x7th **V50.0** **Driver of pick-up truck or van injured in collision with pedestrian or animal in nontraffic accident**
√x7th **V50.1** **Passenger in pick-up truck or van injured in collision with pedestrian or animal in nontraffic accident**
√x7th **V50.2** **Person on outside of pick-up truck or van injured in collision with pedestrian or animal in nontraffic accident**
√x7th **V50.3** **Unspecified occupant of pick-up truck or van injured in collision with pedestrian or animal in nontraffic accident**
√x7th **V50.4** **Person boarding or alighting a pick-up truck or van injured in collision with pedestrian or animal**
√x7th **V50.5** **Driver of pick-up truck or van injured in collision with pedestrian or animal in traffic accident**
√x7th **V50.6** **Passenger in pick-up truck or van injured in collision with pedestrian or animal in traffic accident**
√x7th **V50.7** **Person on outside of pick-up truck or van injured in collision with pedestrian or animal in traffic accident**
√x7th **V50.9** **Unspecified occupant of pick-up truck or van injured in collision with pedestrian or animal in traffic accident**

√4th **V51** **Occupant of pick-up truck or van injured in collision with pedal cycle**
√x7th **V51.0** **Driver of pick-up truck or van injured in collision with pedal cycle in nontraffic accident**
√x7th **V51.1** **Passenger in pick-up truck or van injured in collision with pedal cycle in nontraffic accident**
√x7th **V51.2** **Person on outside of pick-up truck or van injured in collision with pedal cycle in nontraffic accident**
√x7th **V51.3** **Unspecified occupant of pick-up truck or van injured in collision with pedal cycle in nontraffic accident**
√x7th **V51.4** **Person boarding or alighting a pick-up truck or van injured in collision with pedal cycle**
√x7th **V51.5** **Driver of pick-up truck or van injured in collision with pedal cycle in traffic accident**

√x7th V51.6 Passenger in pick-up truck or van injured in collision with pedal cycle in traffic accident

√x7th V51.7 Person on outside of pick-up truck or van injured in collision with pedal cycle in traffic accident

√x7th V51.9 Unspecified occupant of pick-up truck or van injured in collision with pedal cycle in traffic accident

√4th V52 Occupant of pick-up truck or van injured in collision with two- or three-wheeled motor vehicle

√x7th V52.0 Driver of pick-up truck or van injured in collision with two- or three-wheeled motor vehicle in nontraffic accident

√x7th V52.1 Passenger in pick-up truck or van injured in collision with two- or three-wheeled motor vehicle in nontraffic accident

√x7th V52.2 Person on outside of pick-up truck or van injured in collision with two- or three-wheeled motor vehicle in nontraffic accident

√x7th V52.3 Unspecified occupant of pick-up truck or van injured in collision with two- or three-wheeled motor vehicle in nontraffic accident

√x7th V52.4 Person boarding or alighting a pick-up truck or van injured in collision with two- or three-wheeled motor vehicle

√x7th V52.5 Driver of pick-up truck or van injured in collision with two- or three-wheeled motor vehicle in traffic accident

√x7th V52.6 Passenger in pick-up truck or van injured in collision with two- or three-wheeled motor vehicle in traffic accident

√x7th V52.7 Person on outside of pick-up truck or van injured in collision with two- or three-wheeled motor vehicle in traffic accident

√x7th V52.9 Unspecified occupant of pick-up truck or van injured in collision with two- or three-wheeled motor vehicle in traffic accident

√4th V53 Occupant of pick-up truck or van injured in collision with car, pick-up truck or van

√x7th V53.0 Driver of pick-up truck or van injured in collision with car, pick-up truck or van in nontraffic accident

√x7th V53.1 Passenger in pick-up truck or van injured in collision with car, pick-up truck or van in nontraffic accident

√x7th V53.2 Person on outside of pick-up truck or van injured in collision with car, pick-up truck or van in nontraffic accident

√x7th V53.3 Unspecified occupant of pick-up truck or van injured in collision with car, pick-up truck or van in nontraffic accident

√x7th V53.4 Person boarding or alighting a pick-up truck or van injured in collision with car, pick-up truck or van

√x7th V53.5 Driver of pick-up truck or van injured in collision with car, pick-up truck or van in traffic accident

√x7th V53.6 Passenger in pick-up truck or van injured in collision with car, pick-up truck or van in traffic accident

√x7th V53.7 Person on outside of pick-up truck or van injured in collision with car, pick-up truck or van in traffic accident

√x7th V53.9 Unspecified occupant of pick-up truck or van injured in collision with car, pick-up truck or van in traffic accident

√4th V54 Occupant of pick-up truck or van injured in collision with heavy transport vehicle or bus

EXCLUDES 1 *occupant of pick-up truck or van injured in collision with military vehicle (V59.81)*

√x7th V54.0 Driver of pick-up truck or van injured in collision with heavy transport vehicle or bus in nontraffic accident

√x7th V54.1 Passenger in pick-up truck or van injured in collision with heavy transport vehicle or bus in nontraffic accident

√x7th V54.2 Person on outside of pick-up truck or van injured in collision with heavy transport vehicle or bus in nontraffic accident

√x7th V54.3 Unspecified occupant of pick-up truck or van injured in collision with heavy transport vehicle or bus in nontraffic accident

√x7th V54.4 Person boarding or alighting a pick-up truck or van injured in collision with heavy transport vehicle or bus

√x7th V54.5 Driver of pick-up truck or van injured in collision with heavy transport vehicle or bus in traffic accident

√x7th V54.6 Passenger in pick-up truck or van injured in collision with heavy transport vehicle or bus in traffic accident

√x7th V54.7 Person on outside of pick-up truck or van injured in collision with heavy transport vehicle or bus in traffic accident

√x7th V54.9 Unspecified occupant of pick-up truck or van injured in collision with heavy transport vehicle or bus in traffic accident

√4th V55 Occupant of pick-up truck or van injured in collision with railway train or railway vehicle

√x7th V55.0 Driver of pick-up truck or van injured in collision with railway train or railway vehicle in nontraffic accident

√x7th V55.1 Passenger in pick-up truck or van injured in collision with railway train or railway vehicle in nontraffic accident

√x7th V55.2 Person on outside of pick-up truck or van injured in collision with railway train or railway vehicle in nontraffic accident

√x7th V55.3 Unspecified occupant of pick-up truck or van injured in collision with railway train or railway vehicle in nontraffic accident

√x7th V55.4 Person boarding or alighting a pick-up truck or van injured in collision with railway train or railway vehicle

√x7th V55.5 Driver of pick-up truck or van injured in collision with railway train or railway vehicle in traffic accident

√x7th V55.6 Passenger in pick-up truck or van injured in collision with railway train or railway vehicle in traffic accident

√x7th V55.7 Person on outside of pick-up truck or van injured in collision with railway train or railway vehicle in traffic accident

√x7th V55.9 Unspecified occupant of pick-up truck or van injured in collision with railway train or railway vehicle in traffic accident

√4th V56 Occupant of pick-up truck or van injured in collision with other nonmotor vehicle

INCLUDES collision with animal-drawn vehicle, animal being ridden, streetcar

√x7th V56.0 Driver of pick-up truck or van injured in collision with other nonmotor vehicle in nontraffic accident

√x7th V56.1 Passenger in pick-up truck or van injured in collision with other nonmotor vehicle in nontraffic accident

√x7th V56.2 Person on outside of pick-up truck or van injured in collision with other nonmotor vehicle in nontraffic accident

√x7th V56.3 Unspecified occupant of pick-up truck or van injured in collision with other nonmotor vehicle in nontraffic accident

√x7th V56.4 Person boarding or alighting a pick-up truck or van injured in collision with other nonmotor vehicle

√x7th V56.5 Driver of pick-up truck or van injured in collision with other nonmotor vehicle in traffic accident

√x7th V56.6 Passenger in pick-up truck or van injured in collision with other nonmotor vehicle in traffic accident

√x7th V56.7 Person on outside of pick-up truck or van injured in collision with other nonmotor vehicle in traffic accident

√x7th V56.9 Unspecified occupant of pick-up truck or van injured in collision with other nonmotor vehicle in traffic accident

√4th V57 Occupant of pick-up truck or van injured in collision with fixed or stationary object

√x7th V57.0 Driver of pick-up truck or van injured in collision with fixed or stationary object in nontraffic accident

√x7th V57.1 Passenger in pick-up truck or van injured in collision with fixed or stationary object in nontraffic accident

√x7th V57.2 Person on outside of pick-up truck or van injured in collision with fixed or stationary object in nontraffic accident

√x7th V57.3 Unspecified occupant of pick-up truck or van injured in collision with fixed or stationary object in nontraffic accident

√x7th V57.4 Person boarding or alighting a pick-up truck or van injured in collision with fixed or stationary object

√x7th V57.5 Driver of pick-up truck or van injured in collision with fixed or stationary object in traffic accident

√x7th V57.6 Passenger in pick-up truck or van injured in collision with fixed or stationary object in traffic accident

√x7th V57.7 Person on outside of pick-up truck or van injured in collision with fixed or stationary object in traffic accident

√x7th V57.9 Unspecified occupant of pick-up truck or van injured in collision with fixed or stationary object in traffic accident

√4th V58 Occupant of pick-up truck or van injured in noncollision transport accident

INCLUDES overturning pick-up truck or van NOS
overturning pick-up truck or van without collision

√x7th V58.0 Driver of pick-up truck or van injured in noncollision transport accident in nontraffic accident

√x7th V58.1 Passenger in pick-up truck or van injured in noncollision transport accident in nontraffic accident

√x7th V58.2 Person on outside of pick-up truck or van injured in noncollision transport accident in nontraffic accident

√x7th V58.3 Unspecified occupant of pick-up truck or van injured in noncollision transport accident in nontraffic accident

√x7th V58.4 Person boarding or alighting a pick-up truck or van injured in noncollision transport accident

√x7th V58.5 Driver of pick-up truck or van injured in noncollision transport accident in traffic accident

√x7th V58.6 Passenger in pick-up truck or van injured in noncollision transport accident in traffic accident

√x7th V58.7 Person on outside of pick-up truck or van injured in noncollision transport accident in traffic accident

√x7th V58.9 Unspecified occupant of pick-up truck or van injured in noncollision transport accident in traffic accident

V59 Occupant of pick-up truck or van injured in other and unspecified transport accidents

V59.0 Driver of pick-up truck or van injured in collision with other and unspecified motor vehicles in nontraffic accident

V59.00 Driver of pick-up truck or van injured in collision with unspecified motor vehicles in nontraffic accident

V59.09 Driver of pick-up truck or van injured in collision with other motor vehicles in nontraffic accident

V59.1 Passenger in pick-up truck or van injured in collision with other and unspecified motor vehicles in nontraffic accident

V59.10 Passenger in pick-up truck or van injured in collision with unspecified motor vehicles in nontraffic accident

V59.19 Passenger in pick-up truck or van injured in collision with other motor vehicles in nontraffic accident

V59.2 Unspecified occupant of pick-up truck or van injured in collision with other and unspecified motor vehicles in nontraffic accident

V59.20 Unspecified occupant of pick-up truck or van injured in collision with unspecified motor vehicles in nontraffic accident

Collision NOS involving pick-up truck or van, nontraffic

V59.29 Unspecified occupant of pick-up truck or van injured in collision with other motor vehicles in nontraffic accident

V59.3 Occupant (driver) (passenger) of pick-up truck or van injured in unspecified nontraffic accident

Accident NOS involving pick-up truck or van, nontraffic

Occupant of pick-up truck or van injured in nontraffic accident NOS

V59.4 Driver of pick-up truck or van injured in collision with other and unspecified motor vehicles in traffic accident

V59.40 Driver of pick-up truck or van injured in collision with unspecified motor vehicles in traffic accident

V59.49 Driver of pick-up truck or van injured in collision with other motor vehicles in traffic accident

V59.5 Passenger in pick-up truck or van injured in collision with other and unspecified motor vehicles in traffic accident

V59.50 Passenger in pick-up truck or van injured in collision with unspecified motor vehicles in traffic accident

V59.59 Passenger in pick-up truck or van injured in collision with other motor vehicles in traffic accident

V59.6 Unspecified occupant of pick-up truck or van injured in collision with other and unspecified motor vehicles in traffic accident

V59.60 Unspecified occupant of pick-up truck or van injured in collision with unspecified motor vehicles in traffic accident

Collision NOS involving pick-up truck or van (traffic)

V59.69 Unspecified occupant of pick-up truck or van injured in collision with other motor vehicles in traffic accident

V59.8 Occupant (driver) (passenger) of pick-up truck or van injured in other specified transport accidents

V59.81 Occupant (driver) (passenger) of pick-up truck or van injured in transport accident with military vehicle

V59.88 Occupant (driver) (passenger) of pick-up truck or van injured in other specified transport accidents

V59.9 Occupant (driver) (passenger) of pick-up truck or van injured in unspecified traffic accident

Accident NOS involving pick-up truck or van

Occupant of heavy transport vehicle injured in transport accident (V60-V69)

INCLUDES 18 wheeler
armored car
panel truck

EXCLUDES 1 *bus*
motorcoach

The appropriate 7th character is to be added to each code from categories V60-V69.
A initial encounter
D subsequent encounter
S sequela

V60 Occupant of heavy transport vehicle injured in collision with pedestrian or animal

EXCLUDES 1 *heavy transport vehicle collision with animal-drawn vehicle or animal being ridden (V66.-)*

V60.0 Driver of heavy transport vehicle injured in collision with pedestrian or animal in nontraffic accident

V60.1 Passenger in heavy transport vehicle injured in collision with pedestrian or animal in nontraffic accident

V60.2 Person on outside of heavy transport vehicle injured in collision with pedestrian or animal in nontraffic accident

V60.3 Unspecified occupant of heavy transport vehicle injured in collision with pedestrian or animal in nontraffic accident

V60.4 Person boarding or alighting a heavy transport vehicle injured in collision with pedestrian or animal

V60.5 Driver of heavy transport vehicle injured in collision with pedestrian or animal in traffic accident

V60.6 Passenger in heavy transport vehicle injured in collision with pedestrian or animal in traffic accident

V60.7 Person on outside of heavy transport vehicle injured in collision with pedestrian or animal in traffic accident

V60.9 Unspecified occupant of heavy transport vehicle injured in collision with pedestrian or animal in traffic accident

V61 Occupant of heavy transport vehicle injured in collision with pedal cycle

V61.0 Driver of heavy transport vehicle injured in collision with pedal cycle in nontraffic accident

V61.1 Passenger in heavy transport vehicle injured in collision with pedal cycle in nontraffic accident

V61.2 Person on outside of heavy transport vehicle injured in collision with pedal cycle in nontraffic accident

V61.3 Unspecified occupant of heavy transport vehicle injured in collision with pedal cycle in nontraffic accident

V61.4 Person boarding or alighting a heavy transport vehicle injured in collision with pedal cycle while boarding or alighting

V61.5 Driver of heavy transport vehicle injured in collision with pedal cycle in traffic accident

V61.6 Passenger in heavy transport vehicle injured in collision with pedal cycle in traffic accident

V61.7 Person on outside of heavy transport vehicle injured in collision with pedal cycle in traffic accident

V61.9 Unspecified occupant of heavy transport vehicle injured in collision with pedal cycle in traffic accident

V62 Occupant of heavy transport vehicle injured in collision with two- or three-wheeled motor vehicle

V62.0 Driver of heavy transport vehicle injured in collision with two- or three-wheeled motor vehicle in nontraffic accident

V62.1 Passenger in heavy transport vehicle injured in collision with two- or three-wheeled motor vehicle in nontraffic accident

V62.2 Person on outside of heavy transport vehicle injured in collision with two- or three-wheeled motor vehicle in nontraffic accident

V62.3 Unspecified occupant of heavy transport vehicle injured in collision with two- or three-wheeled motor vehicle in nontraffic accident

V62.4 Person boarding or alighting a heavy transport vehicle injured in collision with two- or three-wheeled motor vehicle

V62.5 Driver of heavy transport vehicle injured in collision with two- or three-wheeled motor vehicle in traffic accident

V62.6 Passenger in heavy transport vehicle injured in collision with two- or three-wheeled motor vehicle in traffic accident

V62.7 Person on outside of heavy transport vehicle injured in collision with two- or three-wheeled motor vehicle in traffic accident

V62.9 Unspecified occupant of heavy transport vehicle injured in collision with two- or three-wheeled motor vehicle in traffic accident

V63 Occupant of heavy transport vehicle injured in collision with car, pick-up truck or van

- **V63.0** Driver of heavy transport vehicle injured in collision with car, pick-up truck or van in nontraffic accident
- **V63.1** Passenger in heavy transport vehicle injured in collision with car, pick-up truck or van in nontraffic accident
- **V63.2** Person on outside of heavy transport vehicle injured in collision with car, pick-up truck or van in nontraffic accident
- **V63.3** Unspecified occupant of heavy transport vehicle injured in collision with car, pick-up truck or van in nontraffic accident
- **V63.4** Person boarding or alighting a heavy transport vehicle injured in collision with car, pick-up truck or van
- **V63.5** Driver of heavy transport vehicle injured in collision with car, pick-up truck or van in traffic accident
- **V63.6** Passenger in heavy transport vehicle injured in collision with car, pick-up truck or van in traffic accident
- **V63.7** Person on outside of heavy transport vehicle injured in collision with car, pick-up truck or van in traffic accident
- **V63.9** Unspecified occupant of heavy transport vehicle injured in collision with car, pick-up truck or van in traffic accident

V64 Occupant of heavy transport vehicle injured in collision with heavy transport vehicle or bus

EXCLUDES 1 *occupant of heavy transport vehicle injured in collision with military vehicle (V69.81)*

- **V64.0** Driver of heavy transport vehicle injured in collision with heavy transport vehicle or bus in nontraffic accident
- **V64.1** Passenger in heavy transport vehicle injured in collision with heavy transport vehicle or bus in nontraffic accident
- **V64.2** Person on outside of heavy transport vehicle injured in collision with heavy transport vehicle or bus in nontraffic accident
- **V64.3** Unspecified occupant of heavy transport vehicle injured in collision with heavy transport vehicle or bus in nontraffic accident
- **V64.4** Person boarding or alighting a heavy transport vehicle injured in collision with heavy transport vehicle or bus while boarding or alighting
- **V64.5** Driver of heavy transport vehicle injured in collision with heavy transport vehicle or bus in traffic accident
- **V64.6** Passenger in heavy transport vehicle injured in collision with heavy transport vehicle or bus in traffic accident
- **V64.7** Person on outside of heavy transport vehicle injured in collision with heavy transport vehicle or bus in traffic accident
- **V64.9** Unspecified occupant of heavy transport vehicle injured in collision with heavy transport vehicle or bus in traffic accident

V65 Occupant of heavy transport vehicle injured in collision with railway train or railway vehicle

- **V65.0** Driver of heavy transport vehicle injured in collision with railway train or railway vehicle in nontraffic accident
- **V65.1** Passenger in heavy transport vehicle injured in collision with railway train or railway vehicle in nontraffic accident
- **V65.2** Person on outside of heavy transport vehicle injured in collision with railway train or railway vehicle in nontraffic accident
- **V65.3** Unspecified occupant of heavy transport vehicle injured in collision with railway train or railway vehicle in nontraffic accident
- **V65.4** Person boarding or alighting a heavy transport vehicle injured in collision with railway train or railway vehicle
- **V65.5** Driver of heavy transport vehicle injured in collision with railway train or railway vehicle in traffic accident
- **V65.6** Passenger in heavy transport vehicle injured in collision with railway train or railway vehicle in traffic accident
- **V65.7** Person on outside of heavy transport vehicle injured in collision with railway train or railway vehicle in traffic accident
- **V65.9** Unspecified occupant of heavy transport vehicle injured in collision with railway train or railway vehicle in traffic accident

V66 Occupant of heavy transport vehicle injured in collision with other nonmotor vehicle

INCLUDES collision with animal-drawn vehicle, animal being ridden, streetcar

- **V66.0** Driver of heavy transport vehicle injured in collision with other nonmotor vehicle in nontraffic accident
- **V66.1** Passenger in heavy transport vehicle injured in collision with other nonmotor vehicle in nontraffic accident
- **V66.2** Person on outside of heavy transport vehicle injured in collision with other nonmotor vehicle in nontraffic accident
- **V66.3** Unspecified occupant of heavy transport vehicle injured in collision with other nonmotor vehicle in nontraffic accident
- **V66.4** Person boarding or alighting a heavy transport vehicle injured in collision with other nonmotor vehicle
- **V66.5** Driver of heavy transport vehicle injured in collision with other nonmotor vehicle in traffic accident
- **V66.6** Passenger in heavy transport vehicle injured in collision with other nonmotor vehicle in traffic accident
- **V66.7** Person on outside of heavy transport vehicle injured in collision with other nonmotor vehicle in traffic accident
- **V66.9** Unspecified occupant of heavy transport vehicle injured in collision with other nonmotor vehicle in traffic accident

V67 Occupant of heavy transport vehicle injured in collision with fixed or stationary object

- **V67.0** Driver of heavy transport vehicle injured in collision with fixed or stationary object in nontraffic accident
- **V67.1** Passenger in heavy transport vehicle injured in collision with fixed or stationary object in nontraffic accident
- **V67.2** Person on outside of heavy transport vehicle injured in collision with fixed or stationary object in nontraffic accident
- **V67.3** Unspecified occupant of heavy transport vehicle injured in collision with fixed or stationary object in nontraffic accident
- **V67.4** Person boarding or alighting a heavy transport vehicle injured in collision with fixed or stationary object
- **V67.5** Driver of heavy transport vehicle injured in collision with fixed or stationary object in traffic accident
- **V67.6** Passenger in heavy transport vehicle injured in collision with fixed or stationary object in traffic accident
- **V67.7** Person on outside of heavy transport vehicle injured in collision with fixed or stationary object in traffic accident
- **V67.9** Unspecified occupant of heavy transport vehicle injured in collision with fixed or stationary object in traffic accident

V68 Occupant of heavy transport vehicle injured in noncollision transport accident

INCLUDES overturning heavy transport vehicle NOS
overturning heavy transport vehicle without collision

- **V68.0** Driver of heavy transport vehicle injured in noncollision transport accident in nontraffic accident
- **V68.1** Passenger in heavy transport vehicle injured in noncollision transport accident in nontraffic accident
- **V68.2** Person on outside of heavy transport vehicle injured in noncollision transport accident in nontraffic accident
- **V68.3** Unspecified occupant of heavy transport vehicle injured in noncollision transport accident in nontraffic accident
- **V68.4** Person boarding or alighting a heavy transport vehicle injured in noncollision transport accident
- **V68.5** Driver of heavy transport vehicle injured in noncollision transport accident in traffic accident
- **V68.6** Passenger in heavy transport vehicle injured in noncollision transport accident in traffic accident
- **V68.7** Person on outside of heavy transport vehicle injured in noncollision transport accident in traffic accident
- **V68.9** Unspecified occupant of heavy transport vehicle injured in noncollision transport accident in traffic accident

V69 Occupant of heavy transport vehicle injured in other and unspecified transport accidents

- **V69.0** Driver of heavy transport vehicle injured in collision with other and unspecified motor vehicles in nontraffic accident
  - **V69.00** Driver of heavy transport vehicle injured in collision with unspecified motor vehicles in nontraffic accident
  - **V69.09** Driver of heavy transport vehicle injured in collision with other motor vehicles in nontraffic accident
- **V69.1** Passenger in heavy transport vehicle injured in collision with other and unspecified motor vehicles in nontraffic accident
  - **V69.10** Passenger in heavy transport vehicle injured in collision with unspecified motor vehicles in nontraffic accident
  - **V69.19** Passenger in heavy transport vehicle injured in collision with other motor vehicles in nontraffic accident
- **V69.2** Unspecified occupant of heavy transport vehicle injured in collision with other and unspecified motor vehicles in nontraffic accident
  - **V69.20** Unspecified occupant of heavy transport vehicle injured in collision with unspecified motor vehicles in nontraffic accident
    Collision NOS involving heavy transport vehicle, nontraffic

√x7th **V69.29** **Unspecified occupant of heavy transport vehicle injured in collision with other motor vehicles in nontraffic accident**

√x7th **V69.3** **Occupant (driver) (passenger) of heavy transport vehicle injured in unspecified nontraffic accident**
Accident NOS involving heavy transport vehicle, nontraffic
Occupant of heavy transport vehicle injured in nontraffic accident NOS

√5th **V69.4** **Driver of heavy transport vehicle injured in collision with other and unspecified motor vehicles in traffic accident**

√x7th **V69.40** **Driver of heavy transport vehicle injured in collision with unspecified motor vehicles in traffic accident**

√x7th **V69.49** **Driver of heavy transport vehicle injured in collision with other motor vehicles in traffic accident**

√5th **V69.5** **Passenger in heavy transport vehicle injured in collision with other and unspecified motor vehicles in traffic accident**

√x7th **V69.50** **Passenger in heavy transport vehicle injured in collision with unspecified motor vehicles in traffic accident**

√x7th **V69.59** **Passenger in heavy transport vehicle injured in collision with other motor vehicles in traffic accident**

√5th **V69.6** **Unspecified occupant of heavy transport vehicle injured in collision with other and unspecified motor vehicles in traffic accident**

√x7th **V69.60** **Unspecified occupant of heavy transport vehicle injured in collision with unspecified motor vehicles in traffic accident**
Collision NOS involving heavy transport vehicle (traffic)

√x7th **V69.69** **Unspecified occupant of heavy transport vehicle injured in collision with other motor vehicles in traffic accident**

√5th **V69.8** **Occupant (driver) (passenger) of heavy transport vehicle injured in other specified transport accidents**

√x7th **V69.81** **Occupant (driver) (passenger) of heavy transport vehicle injured in transport accidents with military vehicle**

√x7th **V69.88** **Occupant (driver) (passenger) of heavy transport vehicle injured in other specified transport accidents**

√x7th **V69.9** **Occupant (driver) (passenger) of heavy transport vehicle injured in unspecified traffic accident**
Accident NOS involving heavy transport vehicle

Bus occupant injured in transport accident (V70-V79)

INCLUDES motorcoach
EXCLUDES 1 *minibus (V50-V59)*

The appropriate 7th character is to be added to each code from categories V70-V79.
A initial encounter
D subsequent encounter
S sequela

√4th **V70** **Bus occupant injured in collision with pedestrian or animal**
EXCLUDES 1 *bus collision with animal-drawn vehicle or animal being ridden (V76.-)*

√x7th **V70.0** **Driver of bus injured in collision with pedestrian or animal in nontraffic accident**

√x7th **V70.1** **Passenger on bus injured in collision with pedestrian or animal in nontraffic accident**

√x7th **V70.2** **Person on outside of bus injured in collision with pedestrian or animal in nontraffic accident**

√x7th **V70.3** **Unspecified occupant of bus injured in collision with pedestrian or animal in nontraffic accident**

√x7th **V70.4** **Person boarding or alighting from bus injured in collision with pedestrian or animal**

√x7th **V70.5** **Driver of bus injured in collision with pedestrian or animal in traffic accident**

√x7th **V70.6** **Passenger on bus injured in collision with pedestrian or animal in traffic accident**

√x7th **V70.7** **Person on outside of bus injured in collision with pedestrian or animal in traffic accident**

√x7th **V70.9** **Unspecified occupant of bus injured in collision with pedestrian or animal in traffic accident**

√4th **V71** **Bus occupant injured in collision with pedal cycle**

√x7th **V71.0** **Driver of bus injured in collision with pedal cycle in nontraffic accident**

√x7th **V71.1** **Passenger on bus injured in collision with pedal cycle in nontraffic accident**

√x7th **V71.2** **Person on outside of bus injured in collision with pedal cycle in nontraffic accident**

√x7th **V71.3** **Unspecified occupant of bus injured in collision with pedal cycle in nontraffic accident**

√x7th **V71.4** **Person boarding or alighting from bus injured in collision with pedal cycle**

√x7th **V71.5** **Driver of bus injured in collision with pedal cycle in traffic accident**

√x7th **V71.6** **Passenger on bus injured in collision with pedal cycle in traffic accident**

√x7th **V71.7** **Person on outside of bus injured in collision with pedal cycle in traffic accident**

√x7th **V71.9** **Unspecified occupant of bus injured in collision with pedal cycle in traffic accident**

√4th **V72** **Bus occupant injured in collision with two- or three-wheeled motor vehicle**

√x7th **V72.0** **Driver of bus injured in collision with two- or three-wheeled motor vehicle in nontraffic accident**

√x7th **V72.1** **Passenger on bus injured in collision with two- or three-wheeled motor vehicle in nontraffic accident**

√x7th **V72.2** **Person on outside of bus injured in collision with two- or three-wheeled motor vehicle in nontraffic accident**

√x7th **V72.3** **Unspecified occupant of bus injured in collision with two- or three-wheeled motor vehicle in nontraffic accident**

√x7th **V72.4** **Person boarding or alighting from bus injured in collision with two- or three-wheeled motor vehicle**

√x7th **V72.5** **Driver of bus injured in collision with two- or three-wheeled motor vehicle in traffic accident**

√x7th **V72.6** **Passenger on bus injured in collision with two- or three-wheeled motor vehicle in traffic accident**

√x7th **V72.7** **Person on outside of bus injured in collision with two- or three-wheeled motor vehicle in traffic accident**

√x7th **V72.9** **Unspecified occupant of bus injured in collision with two- or three-wheeled motor vehicle in traffic accident**

√4th **V73** **Bus occupant injured in collision with car, pick-up truck or van**

√x7th **V73.0** **Driver of bus injured in collision with car, pick-up truck or van in nontraffic accident**

√x7th **V73.1** **Passenger on bus injured in collision with car, pick-up truck or van in nontraffic accident**

√x7th **V73.2** **Person on outside of bus injured in collision with car, pick-up truck or van in nontraffic accident**

√x7th **V73.3** **Unspecified occupant of bus injured in collision with car, pick-up truck or van in nontraffic accident**

√x7th **V73.4** **Person boarding or alighting from bus injured in collision with car, pick-up truck or van**

√x7th **V73.5** **Driver of bus injured in collision with car, pick-up truck or van in traffic accident**

√x7th **V73.6** **Passenger on bus injured in collision with car, pick-up truck or van in traffic accident**

√x7th **V73.7** **Person on outside of bus injured in collision with car, pick-up truck or van in traffic accident**

√x7th **V73.9** **Unspecified occupant of bus injured in collision with car, pick-up truck or van in traffic accident**

√4th **V74** **Bus occupant injured in collision with heavy transport vehicle or bus**
EXCLUDES 1 *bus occupant injured in collision with military vehicle (V79.81)*

√x7th **V74.0** **Driver of bus injured in collision with heavy transport vehicle or bus in nontraffic accident**

√x7th **V74.1** **Passenger on bus injured in collision with heavy transport vehicle or bus in nontraffic accident**

√x7th **V74.2** **Person on outside of bus injured in collision with heavy transport vehicle or bus in nontraffic accident**

√x7th **V74.3** **Unspecified occupant of bus injured in collision with heavy transport vehicle or bus in nontraffic accident**

√x7th **V74.4** **Person boarding or alighting from bus injured in collision with heavy transport vehicle or bus**

√x7th **V74.5** **Driver of bus injured in collision with heavy transport vehicle or bus in traffic accident**

√x7th **V74.6** **Passenger on bus injured in collision with heavy transport vehicle or bus in traffic accident**

√x7th **V74.7** **Person on outside of bus injured in collision with heavy transport vehicle or bus in traffic accident**

√x7th **V74.9** **Unspecified occupant of bus injured in collision with heavy transport vehicle or bus in traffic accident**

√4th **V75** **Bus occupant injured in collision with railway train or railway vehicle**

√x7th **V75.0** **Driver of bus injured in collision with railway train or railway vehicle in nontraffic accident**

√x7th **V75.1** **Passenger on bus injured in collision with railway train or railway vehicle in nontraffic accident**

√x7th **V75.2** **Person on outside of bus injured in collision with railway train or railway vehicle in nontraffic accident**

✓x7th **V75.3** **Unspecified occupant of bus injured in collision with railway train or railway vehicle in nontraffic accident**

✓x7th **V75.4** **Person boarding or alighting from bus injured in collision with railway train or railway vehicle**

✓x7th **V75.5** **Driver of bus injured in collision with railway train or railway vehicle in traffic accident**

✓x7th **V75.6** **Passenger on bus injured in collision with railway train or railway vehicle in traffic accident**

✓x7th **V75.7** **Person on outside of bus injured in collision with railway train or railway vehicle in traffic accident**

✓x7th **V75.9** **Unspecified occupant of bus injured in collision with railway train or railway vehicle in traffic accident**

✓4th **V76 Bus occupant injured in collision with other nonmotor vehicle**

INCLUDES collision with animal-drawn vehicle, animal being ridden, streetcar

✓x7th **V76.0** **Driver of bus injured in collision with other nonmotor vehicle in nontraffic accident**

✓x7th **V76.1** **Passenger on bus injured in collision with other nonmotor vehicle in nontraffic accident**

✓x7th **V76.2** **Person on outside of bus injured in collision with other nonmotor vehicle in nontraffic accident**

✓x7th **V76.3** **Unspecified occupant of bus injured in collision with other nonmotor vehicle in nontraffic accident**

✓x7th **V76.4** **Person boarding or alighting from bus injured in collision with other nonmotor vehicle**

✓x7th **V76.5** **Driver of bus injured in collision with other nonmotor vehicle in traffic accident**

✓x7th **V76.6** **Passenger on bus injured in collision with other nonmotor vehicle in traffic accident**

✓x7th **V76.7** **Person on outside of bus injured in collision with other nonmotor vehicle in traffic accident**

✓x7th **V76.9** **Unspecified occupant of bus injured in collision with other nonmotor vehicle in traffic accident**

✓4th **V77 Bus occupant injured in collision with fixed or stationary object**

✓x7th **V77.0** **Driver of bus injured in collision with fixed or stationary object in nontraffic accident**

✓x7th **V77.1** **Passenger on bus injured in collision with fixed or stationary object in nontraffic accident**

✓x7th **V77.2** **Person on outside of bus injured in collision with fixed or stationary object in nontraffic accident**

✓x7th **V77.3** **Unspecified occupant of bus injured in collision with fixed or stationary object in nontraffic accident**

✓x7th **V77.4** **Person boarding or alighting from bus injured in collision with fixed or stationary object**

✓x7th **V77.5** **Driver of bus injured in collision with fixed or stationary object in traffic accident**

✓x7th **V77.6** **Passenger on bus injured in collision with fixed or stationary object in traffic accident**

✓x7th **V77.7** **Person on outside of bus injured in collision with fixed or stationary object in traffic accident**

✓x7th **V77.9** **Unspecified occupant of bus injured in collision with fixed or stationary object in traffic accident**

✓4th **V78 Bus occupant injured in noncollision transport accident**

INCLUDES overturning bus NOS
overturning bus without collision

✓x7th **V78.0** **Driver of bus injured in noncollision transport accident in nontraffic accident**

✓x7th **V78.1** **Passenger on bus injured in noncollision transport accident in nontraffic accident**

✓x7th **V78.2** **Person on outside of bus injured in noncollision transport accident in nontraffic accident**

✓x7th **V78.3** **Unspecified occupant of bus injured in noncollision transport accident in nontraffic accident**

✓x7th **V78.4** **Person boarding or alighting from bus injured in noncollision transport accident**

✓x7th **V78.5** **Driver of bus injured in noncollision transport accident in traffic accident**

✓x7th **V78.6** **Passenger on bus injured in noncollision transport accident in traffic accident**

✓x7th **V78.7** **Person on outside of bus injured in noncollision transport accident in traffic accident**

✓x7th **V78.9** **Unspecified occupant of bus injured in noncollision transport accident in traffic accident**

✓4th **V79 Bus occupant injured in other and unspecified transport accidents**

✓5th **V79.0** **Driver of bus injured in collision with other and unspecified motor vehicles in nontraffic accident**

✓x7th **V79.00** **Driver of bus injured in collision with unspecified motor vehicles in nontraffic accident**

✓x7th **V79.09** **Driver of bus injured in collision with other motor vehicles in nontraffic accident**

✓5th **V79.1** **Passenger on bus injured in collision with other and unspecified motor vehicles in nontraffic accident**

✓x7th **V79.10** **Passenger on bus injured in collision with unspecified motor vehicles in nontraffic accident**

✓x7th **V79.19** **Passenger on bus injured in collision with other motor vehicles in nontraffic accident**

✓5th **V79.2** **Unspecified bus occupant injured in collision with other and unspecified motor vehicles in nontraffic accident**

✓x7th **V79.20** **Unspecified bus occupant injured in collision with unspecified motor vehicles in nontraffic accident**
Bus collision NOS, nontraffic

✓x7th **V79.29** **Unspecified bus occupant injured in collision with other motor vehicles in nontraffic accident**

✓x7th **V79.3** **Bus occupant (driver) (passenger) injured in unspecified nontraffic accident**
Bus accident NOS, nontraffic
Bus occupant injured in nontraffic accident NOS

✓5th **V79.4** **Driver of bus injured in collision with other and unspecified motor vehicles in traffic accident**

✓x7th **V79.40** **Driver of bus injured in collision with unspecified motor vehicles in traffic accident**

✓x7th **V79.49** **Driver of bus injured in collision with other motor vehicles in traffic accident**

✓5th **V79.5** **Passenger on bus injured in collision with other and unspecified motor vehicles in traffic accident**

✓x7th **V79.50** **Passenger on bus injured in collision with unspecified motor vehicles in traffic accident**

✓x7th **V79.59** **Passenger on bus injured in collision with other motor vehicles in traffic accident**

✓5th **V79.6** **Unspecified bus occupant injured in collision with other and unspecified motor vehicles in traffic accident**

✓x7th **V79.60** **Unspecified bus occupant injured in collision with unspecified motor vehicles in traffic accident**
Bus collision NOS (traffic)

✓x7th **V79.69** **Unspecified bus occupant injured in collision with other motor vehicles in traffic accident**

✓5th **V79.8** **Bus occupant (driver) (passenger) injured in other specified transport accidents**

✓x7th **V79.81** **Bus occupant (driver) (passenger) injured in transport accidents with military vehicle**

✓x7th **V79.88** **Bus occupant (driver) (passenger) injured in other specified transport accidents**

✓x7th **V79.9** **Bus occupant (driver) (passenger) injured in unspecified traffic accident**
Bus accident NOS

Other land transport accidents (V80-V89)

The appropriate 7th character is to be added to each code from categories V80-V89.
A initial encounter
D subsequent encounter
S sequela

✓4th **V80 Animal-rider or occupant of animal-drawn vehicle injured in transport accident**

✓5th **V80.0** **Animal-rider or occupant of animal drawn vehicle injured by fall from or being thrown from animal or animal-drawn vehicle in noncollision accident**

✓6th **V80.01** **Animal-rider injured by fall from or being thrown from animal in noncollision accident**

✓7th **V80.010** **Animal-rider injured by fall from or being thrown from horse in noncollision accident**

✓7th **V80.018** **Animal-rider injured by fall from or being thrown from other animal in noncollision accident**

✓x7th **V80.02** **Occupant of animal-drawn vehicle injured by fall from or being thrown from animal-drawn vehicle in noncollision accident**
Overturning animal-drawn vehicle NOS
Overturning animal-drawn vehicle without collision

✓5th **V80.1** **Animal-rider or occupant of animal-drawn vehicle injured in collision with pedestrian or animal**

EXCLUDES 1 *animal-rider or animal-drawn vehicle collision with animal-drawn vehicle or animal being ridden (V80.7)*

✓x7th **V80.11** **Animal-rider injured in collision with pedestrian or animal**

✓x7th **V80.12** **Occupant of animal-drawn vehicle injured in collision with pedestrian or animal**

✓5th **V8Ø.2 Animal-rider or occupant of animal-drawn vehicle injured in collision with pedal cycle**

✓x7th **V8Ø.21 Animal-rider injured in collision with pedal cycle**

✓x7th **V8Ø.22 Occupant of animal-drawn vehicle injured in collision with pedal cycle**

✓5th **V8Ø.3 Animal-rider or occupant of animal-drawn vehicle injured in collision with two- or three-wheeled motor vehicle**

✓x7th **V8Ø.31 Animal-rider injured in collision with two- or three-wheeled motor vehicle**

✓x7th **V8Ø.32 Occupant of animal-drawn vehicle injured in collision with two- or three-wheeled motor vehicle**

✓5th **V8Ø.4 Animal-rider or occupant of animal-drawn vehicle injured in collision with car, pick-up truck, van, heavy transport vehicle or bus**

EXCLUDES 1 *animal-rider injured in collision with military vehicle (V8Ø.91Ø)*

occupant of animal-drawn vehicle injured in collision with military vehicle (V8Ø.92Ø)

✓x7th **V8Ø.41 Animal-rider injured in collision with car, pick-up truck, van, heavy transport vehicle or bus**

✓x7th **V8Ø.42 Occupant of animal-drawn vehicle injured in collision with car, pick-up truck, van, heavy transport vehicle or bus**

✓5th **V8Ø.5 Animal-rider or occupant of animal-drawn vehicle injured in collision with other specified motor vehicle**

✓x7th **V8Ø.51 Animal-rider injured in collision with other specified motor vehicle**

✓x7th **V8Ø.52 Occupant of animal-drawn vehicle injured in collision with other specified motor vehicle**

✓5th **V8Ø.6 Animal-rider or occupant of animal-drawn vehicle injured in collision with railway train or railway vehicle**

✓x7th **V8Ø.61 Animal-rider injured in collision with railway train or railway vehicle**

✓x7th **V8Ø.62 Occupant of animal-drawn vehicle injured in collision with railway train or railway vehicle**

✓5th **V8Ø.7 Animal-rider or occupant of animal-drawn vehicle injured in collision with other nonmotor vehicles**

✓6th **V8Ø.71 Animal-rider or occupant of animal-drawn vehicle injured in collision with animal being ridden**

✓7th **V8Ø.71Ø Animal-rider injured in collision with other animal being ridden**

✓7th **V8Ø.711 Occupant of animal-drawn vehicle injured in collision with animal being ridden**

✓6th **V8Ø.72 Animal-rider or occupant of animal-drawn vehicle injured in collision with other animal-drawn vehicle**

✓7th **V8Ø.72Ø Animal-rider injured in collision with animal-drawn vehicle**

✓7th **V8Ø.721 Occupant of animal-drawn vehicle injured in collision with other animal-drawn vehicle**

✓6th **V8Ø.73 Animal-rider or occupant of animal-drawn vehicle injured in collision with streetcar**

✓7th **V8Ø.73Ø Animal-rider injured in collision with streetcar**

✓7th **V8Ø.731 Occupant of animal-drawn vehicle injured in collision with streetcar**

✓6th **V8Ø.79 Animal-rider or occupant of animal-drawn vehicle injured in collision with other nonmotor vehicles**

✓7th **V8Ø.79Ø Animal-rider injured in collision with other nonmotor vehicles**

✓7th **V8Ø.791 Occupant of animal-drawn vehicle injured in collision with other nonmotor vehicles**

✓5th **V8Ø.8 Animal-rider or occupant of animal-drawn vehicle injured in collision with fixed or stationary object**

✓x7th **V8Ø.81 Animal-rider injured in collision with fixed or stationary object**

✓x7th **V8Ø.82 Occupant of animal-drawn vehicle injured in collision with fixed or stationary object**

✓5th **V8Ø.9 Animal-rider or occupant of animal-drawn vehicle injured in other and unspecified transport accidents**

✓6th **V8Ø.91 Animal-rider injured in other and unspecified transport accidents**

✓7th **V8Ø.91Ø Animal-rider injured in transport accident with military vehicle**

✓7th **V8Ø.918 Animal-rider injured in other transport accident**

✓7th **V8Ø.919 Animal-rider injured in unspecified transport accident**

Animal rider accident NOS

✓6th **V8Ø.92 Occupant of animal-drawn vehicle injured in other and unspecified transport accidents**

✓7th **V8Ø.92Ø Occupant of animal-drawn vehicle injured in transport accident with military vehicle**

✓7th **V8Ø.928 Occupant of animal-drawn vehicle injured in other transport accident**

✓7th **V8Ø.929 Occupant of animal-drawn vehicle injured in unspecified transport accident**

Animal-drawn vehicle accident NOS

✓4th **V81 Occupant of railway train or railway vehicle injured in transport accident**

INCLUDES derailment of railway train or railway vehicle

person on outside of train

EXCLUDES 1 *streetcar (V82.-)*

✓x7th **V81.Ø Occupant of railway train or railway vehicle injured in collision with motor vehicle in nontraffic accident**

EXCLUDES 1 *occupant of railway train or railway vehicle injured due to collision with military vehicle (V81.83)*

✓x7th **V81.1 Occupant of railway train or railway vehicle injured in collision with motor vehicle in traffic accident**

EXCLUDES 1 *occupant of railway train or railway vehicle injured due to collision with military vehicle (V81.83)*

✓x7th **V81.2 Occupant of railway train or railway vehicle injured in collision with or hit by rolling stock**

✓x7th **V81.3 Occupant of railway train or railway vehicle injured in collision with other object**

Railway collision NOS

✓x7th **V81.4 Person injured while boarding or alighting from railway train or railway vehicle**

✓x7th **V81.5 Occupant of railway train or railway vehicle injured by fall in railway train or railway vehicle**

✓x7th **V81.6 Occupant of railway train or railway vehicle injured by fall from railway train or railway vehicle**

✓x7th **V81.7 Occupant of railway train or railway vehicle injured in derailment without antecedent collision**

✓5th **V81.8 Occupant of railway train or railway vehicle injured in other specified railway accidents**

✓x7th **V81.81 Occupant of railway train or railway vehicle injured due to explosion or fire on train**

✓x7th **V81.82 Occupant of railway train or railway vehicle injured due to object falling onto train**

Occupant of railway train or railway vehicle injured due to falling earth onto train

Occupant of railway train or railway vehicle injured due to falling rocks onto train

Occupant of railway train or railway vehicle injured due to falling snow onto train

Occupant of railway train or railway vehicle injured due to falling trees onto train

✓x7th **V81.83 Occupant of railway train or railway vehicle injured due to collision with military vehicle**

✓x7th **V81.89 Occupant of railway train or railway vehicle injured due to other specified railway accident**

✓x7th **V81.9 Occupant of railway train or railway vehicle injured in unspecified railway accident**

Railway accident NOS

✓4th **V82 Occupant of powered streetcar injured in transport accident**

INCLUDES interurban electric car

person on outside of streetcar

tram (car)

trolley (car)

EXCLUDES 1 *bus (V7Ø-V79)*

motorcoach (V7Ø-V79)

nonpowered streetcar (V76.-)

train (V81.-)

✓x7th **V82.Ø Occupant of streetcar injured in collision with motor vehicle in nontraffic accident**

✓x7th **V82.1 Occupant of streetcar injured in collision with motor vehicle in traffic accident**

✓x7th **V82.2 Occupant of streetcar injured in collision with or hit by rolling stock**

✓x7th **V82.3 Occupant of streetcar injured in collision with other object**

EXCLUDES 1 *collision with animal-drawn vehicle or animal being ridden (V82.8)*

✓x7th **V82.4 Person injured while boarding or alighting from streetcar**

√x7th **V82.5 Occupant of streetcar injured by fall in streetcar**
EXCLUDES 1 *fall in streetcar:*
while boarding or alighting (V82.4)
with antecedent collision (V82.Ø-V82.3)

√x7th **V82.6 Occupant of streetcar injured by fall from streetcar**
EXCLUDES 1 *fall from streetcar:*
while boarding or alighting (V82.4)
with antecedent collision (V82.Ø-V82.3)

√x7th **V82.7 Occupant of streetcar injured in derailment without antecedent collision**
EXCLUDES 1 *occupant of streetcar injured in derailment with antecedent collision (V82.Ø-V82.3)*

√x7th **V82.8 Occupant of streetcar injured in other specified transport accidents**
Streetcar collision with military vehicle
Streetcar collision with train or nonmotor vehicles

√x7th **V82.9 Occupant of streetcar injured in unspecified traffic accident**
Streetcar accident NOS

√4th **V83 Occupant of special vehicle mainly used on industrial premises injured in transport accident**
INCLUDES battery-powered airport passenger vehicle
battery-powered truck (baggage) (mail)
coal-car in mine
forklift (truck)
logging car
self-propelled industrial truck
station baggage truck (powered)
tram, truck, or tub (powered) in mine or quarry
EXCLUDES 1 *special construction vehicles (V85.-)*
special industrial vehicle in stationary use or maintenance (W31.-)

√x7th **V83.Ø Driver of special industrial vehicle injured in traffic accident**

√x7th **V83.1 Passenger of special industrial vehicle injured in traffic accident**

√x7th **V83.2 Person on outside of special industrial vehicle injured in traffic accident**

√x7th **V83.3 Unspecified occupant of special industrial vehicle injured in traffic accident**

√x7th **V83.4 Person injured while boarding or alighting from special industrial vehicle**

√x7th **V83.5 Driver of special industrial vehicle injured in nontraffic accident**

√x7th **V83.6 Passenger of special industrial vehicle injured in nontraffic accident**

√x7th **V83.7 Person on outside of special industrial vehicle injured in nontraffic accident**

√x7th **V83.9 Unspecified occupant of special industrial vehicle injured in nontraffic accident**
Special-industrial-vehicle accident NOS

√4th **V84 Occupant of special vehicle mainly used in agriculture injured in transport accident**
INCLUDES self-propelled farm machinery
tractor (and trailer)
EXCLUDES 1 *animal-powered farm machinery accident (W3Ø.8-)*
contact with combine harvester (W3Ø.Ø)
special agricultural vehicle in stationary use or maintenance (W3Ø.-)

√x7th **V84.Ø Driver of special agricultural vehicle injured in traffic accident**

√x7th **V84.1 Passenger of special agricultural vehicle injured in traffic accident**

√x7th **V84.2 Person on outside of special agricultural vehicle injured in traffic accident**

√x7th **V84.3 Unspecified occupant of special agricultural vehicle injured in traffic accident**

√x7th **V84.4 Person injured while boarding or alighting from special agricultural vehicle**

√x7th **V84.5 Driver of special agricultural vehicle injured in nontraffic accident**

√x7th **V84.6 Passenger of special agricultural vehicle injured in nontraffic accident**

√x7th **V84.7 Person on outside of special agricultural vehicle injured in nontraffic accident**

√x7th **V84.9 Unspecified occupant of special agricultural vehicle injured in nontraffic accident**
Special-agricultural vehicle accident NOS

√4th **V85 Occupant of special construction vehicle injured in transport accident**
INCLUDES bulldozer
digger
dump truck
earth-leveller
mechanical shovel
road-roller
EXCLUDES 1 *special industrial vehicle (V83.-)*
special construction vehicle in stationary use or maintenance (W31.-)

√x7th **V85.Ø Driver of special construction vehicle injured in traffic accident**

√x7th **V85.1 Passenger of special construction vehicle injured in traffic accident**

√x7th **V85.2 Person on outside of special construction vehicle injured in traffic accident**

√x7th **V85.3 Unspecified occupant of special construction vehicle injured in traffic accident**

√x7th **V85.4 Person injured while boarding or alighting from special construction vehicle**

√x7th **V85.5 Driver of special construction vehicle injured in nontraffic accident**

√x7th **V85.6 Passenger of special construction vehicle injured in nontraffic accident**

√x7th **V85.7 Person on outside of special construction vehicle injured in nontraffic accident**

√x7th **V85.9 Unspecified occupant of special construction vehicle injured in nontraffic accident**
Special-construction-vehicle accident NOS

√4th **V86 Occupant of special all-terrain or other off-road motor vehicle, injured in transport accident**
EXCLUDES 1 *special all-terrain vehicle in stationary use or maintenance (W31.-)*
sport-utility vehicle (V5Ø-V59)
three-wheeled motor vehicle designed for on-road use (V3Ø-V39)

AHA: 2017,4Q,26

√5th **V86.Ø Driver of special all-terrain or other off-road motor vehicle injured in traffic accident**

√x7th **V86.Ø1 Driver of ambulance or fire engine injured in traffic accident**

√x7th **V86.Ø2 Driver of snowmobile injured in traffic accident**

√x7th **V86.Ø3 Driver of dune buggy injured in traffic accident**

√x7th **V86.Ø4 Driver of military vehicle injured in traffic accident**

√x7th **V86.Ø5 Driver of 3- or 4- wheeled all-terrain vehicle (ATV) injured in traffic accident**

√x7th **V86.Ø6 Driver of dirt bike or motor/cross bike injured in traffic accident**

√x7th **V86.Ø9 Driver of other special all-terrain or other off-road motor vehicle injured in traffic accident**
Driver of go cart injured in traffic accident
Driver of golf cart injured in traffic accident

√5th **V86.1 Passenger of special all-terrain or other off-road motor vehicle injured in traffic accident**

√x7th **V86.11 Passenger of ambulance or fire engine injured in traffic accident**

√x7th **V86.12 Passenger of snowmobile injured in traffic accident**

√x7th **V86.13 Passenger of dune buggy injured in traffic accident**

√x7th **V86.14 Passenger of military vehicle injured in traffic accident**

√x7th **V86.15 Passenger of 3- or 4- wheeled all-terrain vehicle (ATV) injured in traffic accident**

√x7th **V86.16 Passenger of dirt bike or motor/cross bike injured in traffic accident**

√x7th **V86.19 Passenger of other special all-terrain or other off-road motor vehicle injured in traffic accident**
Passenger of go cart injured in traffic accident
Passenger of golf cart injured in traffic accident

√5th **V86.2 Person on outside of special all-terrain or other off-road motor vehicle injured in traffic accident**

√x7th **V86.21 Person on outside of ambulance or fire engine injured in traffic accident**

√x7th **V86.22 Person on outside of snowmobile injured in traffic accident**

√x7th **V86.23 Person on outside of dune buggy injured in traffic accident**

√x7th **V86.24 Person on outside of military vehicle injured in traffic accident**

√x7th **V86.25 Person on outside of 3- or 4- wheeled all-terrain vehicle (ATV) injured in traffic accident**

√x7th **V86.26 Person on outside of dirt bike or motor/cross bike injured in traffic accident**

√x7th **V86.29 Person on outside of other special all-terrain or other off-road motor vehicle injured in traffic accident**

Person on outside of go cart in traffic accident

Person on outside of golf cart injured in traffic accident

√5th **V86.3 Unspecified occupant of special all-terrain or other off-road motor vehicle injured in traffic accident**

√x7th **V86.31 Unspecified occupant of ambulance or fire engine injured in traffic accident**

√x7th **V86.32 Unspecified occupant of snowmobile injured in traffic accident**

√x7th **V86.33 Unspecified occupant of dune buggy injured in traffic accident**

√x7th **V86.34 Unspecified occupant of military vehicle injured in traffic accident**

√x7th **V86.35 Unspecified occupant of 3- or 4- wheeled all-terrain vehicle (ATV) injured in traffic accident**

√x7th **V86.36 Unspecified occupant of dirt bike or motor/cross bike injured in traffic accident**

√x7th **V86.39 Unspecified occupant of other special all-terrain or other off-road motor vehicle injured in traffic accident**

Unspecified occupant of go cart injured in traffic accident

Unspecified occupant of golf cart injured in traffic accident

√5th **V86.4 Person injured while boarding or alighting from special all-terrain or other off-road motor vehicle**

√x7th **V86.41 Person injured while boarding or alighting from ambulance or fire engine**

√x7th **V86.42 Person injured while boarding or alighting from snowmobile**

√x7th **V86.43 Person injured while boarding or alighting from dune buggy**

√x7th **V86.44 Person injured while boarding or alighting from military vehicle**

√x7th **V86.45 Person injured while boarding or alighting from a 3- or 4- wheeled all-terrain vehicle (ATV)**

√x7th **V86.46 Person injured while boarding or alighting from a dirt bike or motor/cross bike**

√x7th **V86.49 Person injured while boarding or alighting from other special all-terrain or other off-road motor vehicle**

Person injured while boarding or alighting from go cart

Person injured while boarding or alighting from golf cart

√5th **V86.5 Driver of special all-terrain or other off-road motor vehicle injured in nontraffic accident**

√x7th **V86.51 Driver of ambulance or fire engine injured in nontraffic accident**

√x7th **V86.52 Driver of snowmobile injured in nontraffic accident**

√x7th **V86.53 Driver of dune buggy injured in nontraffic accident**

√x7th **V86.54 Driver of military vehicle injured in nontraffic accident**

√x7th **V86.55 Driver of 3- or 4- wheeled all-terrain vehicle (ATV) injured in nontraffic accident**

√x7th **V86.56 Driver of dirt bike or motor/cross bike injured in nontraffic accident**

√x7th **V86.59 Driver of other special all-terrain or other off-road motor vehicle injured in nontraffic accident**

Driver of go cart injured in nontraffic accident

Driver of golf cart injured in nontraffic accident

√5th **V86.6 Passenger of special all-terrain or other off-road motor vehicle injured in nontraffic accident**

√x7th **V86.61 Passenger of ambulance or fire engine injured in nontraffic accident**

√x7th **V86.62 Passenger of snowmobile injured in nontraffic accident**

√x7th **V86.63 Passenger of dune buggy injured in nontraffic accident**

√x7th **V86.64 Passenger of military vehicle injured in nontraffic accident**

√x7th **V86.65 Passenger of 3- or 4- wheeled all-terrain vehicle (ATV) injured in nontraffic accident**

√x7th **V86.66 Passenger of dirt bike or motor/cross bike injured in nontraffic accident**

√x7th **V86.69 Passenger of other special all-terrain or other off-road motor vehicle injured in nontraffic accident**

Passenger of go cart injured in nontraffic accident

Passenger of golf cart injured in nontraffic accident

√5th **V86.7 Person on outside of special all-terrain or other off-road motor vehicle injured in nontraffic accident**

√x7th **V86.71 Person on outside of ambulance or fire engine injured in nontraffic accident**

√x7th **V86.72 Person on outside of snowmobile injured in nontraffic accident**

√x7th **V86.73 Person on outside of dune buggy injured in nontraffic accident**

√x7th **V86.74 Person on outside of military vehicle injured in nontraffic accident**

√x7th **V86.75 Person on outside of 3- or 4- wheeled all-terrain vehicle (ATV) injured in nontraffic accident**

√x7th **V86.76 Person on outside of dirt bike or motor/cross bike injured in nontraffic accident**

√x7th **V86.79 Person on outside of other special all-terrain or other off-road motor vehicles injured in nontraffic accident**

Person on outside of go cart injured in nontraffic accident

Person on outside of golf cart injured in nontraffic accident

√5th **V86.9 Unspecified occupant of special all-terrain or other off-road motor vehicle injured in nontraffic accident**

√x7th **V86.91 Unspecified occupant of ambulance or fire engine injured in nontraffic accident**

√x7th **V86.92 Unspecified occupant of snowmobile injured in nontraffic accident**

√x7th **V86.93 Unspecified occupant of dune buggy injured in nontraffic accident**

√x7th **V86.94 Unspecified occupant of military vehicle injured in nontraffic accident**

√x7th **V86.95 Unspecified occupant of 3- or 4- wheeled all-terrain vehicle (ATV) injured in nontraffic accident**

√x7th **V86.96 Unspecified occupant of dirt bike or motor/cross bike injured in nontraffic accident**

√x7th **V86.99 Unspecified occupant of other special all-terrain or other off-road motor vehicle injured in nontraffic accident**

Off-road motor-vehicle accident NOS

Other motor-vehicle accident NOS

Unspecified occupant of go cart injured in nontraffic accident

Unspecified occupant of golf cart injured in nontraffic accident

√4th **V87 Traffic accident of specified type but victim's mode of transport unknown**

EXCLUDES 1 *collision involving:*

pedal cycle (V1Ø-V19)

pedestrian (VØ1-VØ9)

√x7th **V87.Ø Person injured in collision between car and two- or three-wheeled powered vehicle (traffic)**

√x7th **V87.1 Person injured in collision between other motor vehicle and two- or three-wheeled motor vehicle (traffic)**

√x7th **V87.2 Person injured in collision between car and pick-up truck or van (traffic)**

√x7th **V87.3 Person injured in collision between car and bus (traffic)**

√x7th **V87.4 Person injured in collision between car and heavy transport vehicle (traffic)**

√x7th **V87.5 Person injured in collision between heavy transport vehicle and bus (traffic)**

√x7th **V87.6 Person injured in collision between railway train or railway vehicle and car (traffic)**

√x7th **V87.7 Person injured in collision between other specified motor vehicles (traffic)**

√x7th **V87.8 Person injured in other specified noncollision transport accidents involving motor vehicle (traffic)**

√x7th **V87.9 Person injured in other specified (collision)(noncollision) transport accidents involving nonmotor vehicle (traffic)**

V88 Nontraffic accident of specified type but victim's mode of transport unknown

EXCLUDES 1 *collision involving:*
pedal cycle (V10-V19)
pedestrian (V01-V09)

V88.0 Person injured in collision between car and two- or three-wheeled motor vehicle, nontraffic

V88.1 Person injured in collision between other motor vehicle and two- or three-wheeled motor vehicle, nontraffic

V88.2 Person injured in collision between car and pick-up truck or van, nontraffic

V88.3 Person injured in collision between car and bus, nontraffic

V88.4 Person injured in collision between car and heavy transport vehicle, nontraffic

V88.5 Person injured in collision between heavy transport vehicle and bus, nontraffic

V88.6 Person injured in collision between railway train or railway vehicle and car, nontraffic

V88.7 Person injured in collision between other specified motor vehicle, nontraffic

V88.8 Person injured in other specified noncollision transport accidents involving motor vehicle, nontraffic

V88.9 Person injured in other specified (collision)(noncollision) transport accidents involving nonmotor vehicle, nontraffic

V89 Motor- or nonmotor-vehicle accident, type of vehicle unspecified

V89.0 Person injured in unspecified motor-vehicle accident, nontraffic
Motor-vehicle accident NOS, nontraffic

V89.1 Person injured in unspecified nonmotor-vehicle accident, nontraffic
Nonmotor-vehicle accident NOS (nontraffic)

V89.2 Person injured in unspecified motor-vehicle accident, traffic
Motor-vehicle accident [MVA] NOS
Road (traffic) accident [RTA] NOS

V89.3 Person injured in unspecified nonmotor-vehicle accident, traffic
Nonmotor-vehicle traffic accident NOS

V89.9 Person injured in unspecified vehicle accident
Collision NOS

Water transport accidents (V90-V94)

The appropriate 7th character is to be added to each code from categories V90-V94.
A initial encounter
D subsequent encounter
S sequela

V90 Drowning and submersion due to accident to watercraft

EXCLUDES 1 *civilian water transport accident involving military watercraft (V94.81-)*
fall into water not from watercraft (W16.-)
military watercraft accident in military or war operations (Y36.0-, Y37.0-)
water-transport-related drowning or submersion without accident to watercraft (V92.-)

V90.0 Drowning and submersion due to watercraft overturning

V90.00 Drowning and submersion due to merchant ship overturning

V90.01 Drowning and submersion due to passenger ship overturning
Drowning and submersion due to Ferry-boat overturning
Drowning and submersion due to Liner overturning

V90.02 Drowning and submersion due to fishing boat overturning

V90.03 Drowning and submersion due to other powered watercraft overturning
Drowning and submersion due to Hovercraft (on open water) overturning
Drowning and submersion due to Jet ski overturning

V90.04 Drowning and submersion due to sailboat overturning

V90.05 Drowning and submersion due to canoe or kayak overturning

V90.06 Drowning and submersion due to (nonpowered) inflatable craft overturning

V90.08 Drowning and submersion due to other unpowered watercraft overturning
Drowning and submersion due to windsurfer overturning

V90.09 Drowning and submersion due to unspecified watercraft overturning
Drowning and submersion due to boat NOS overturning
Drowning and submersion due to ship NOS overturning
Drowning and submersion due to watercraft NOS overturning

V90.1 Drowning and submersion due to watercraft sinking

V90.10 Drowning and submersion due to merchant ship sinking

V90.11 Drowning and submersion due to passenger ship sinking
Drowning and submersion due to Ferry-boat sinking
Drowning and submersion due to Liner sinking

V90.12 Drowning and submersion due to fishing boat sinking

V90.13 Drowning and submersion due to other powered watercraft sinking
Drowning and submersion due to Hovercraft (on open water) sinking
Drowning and submersion due to Jet ski sinking

V90.14 Drowning and submersion due to sailboat sinking

V90.15 Drowning and submersion due to canoe or kayak sinking

V90.16 Drowning and submersion due to (nonpowered) inflatable craft sinking

V90.18 Drowning and submersion due to other unpowered watercraft sinking

V90.19 Drowning and submersion due to unspecified watercraft sinking
Drowning and submersion due to boat NOS sinking
Drowning and submersion due to ship NOS sinking
Drowning and submersion due to watercraft NOS sinking

V90.2 Drowning and submersion due to falling or jumping from burning watercraft

V90.20 Drowning and submersion due to falling or jumping from burning merchant ship

V90.21 Drowning and submersion due to falling or jumping from burning passenger ship
Drowning and submersion due to falling or jumping from burning Ferry-boat
Drowning and submersion due to falling or jumping from burning Liner

V90.22 Drowning and submersion due to falling or jumping from burning fishing boat

V90.23 Drowning and submersion due to falling or jumping from other burning powered watercraft
Drowning and submersion due to falling and jumping from burning Hovercraft (on open water)
Drowning and submersion due to falling and jumping from burning Jet ski

V90.24 Drowning and submersion due to falling or jumping from burning sailboat

V90.25 Drowning and submersion due to falling or jumping from burning canoe or kayak

V90.26 Drowning and submersion due to falling or jumping from burning (nonpowered) inflatable craft

V90.27 Drowning and submersion due to falling or jumping from burning water-skis

V90.28 Drowning and submersion due to falling or jumping from other burning unpowered watercraft
Drowning and submersion due to falling and jumping from burning surf-board
Drowning and submersion due to falling and jumping from burning windsurfer

V90.29 Drowning and submersion due to falling or jumping from unspecified burning watercraft
Drowning and submersion due to falling or jumping from burning boat NOS
Drowning and submersion due to falling or jumping from burning ship NOS
Drowning and submersion due to falling or jumping from burning watercraft NOS

V90.3 Drowning and submersion due to falling or jumping from crushed watercraft

V90.30 Drowning and submersion due to falling or jumping from crushed merchant ship

V90.31 Drowning and submersion due to falling or jumping from crushed passenger ship
Drowning and submersion due to falling and jumping from crushed Ferry boat
Drowning and submersion due to falling and jumping from crushed Liner

V90.32 Drowning and submersion due to falling or jumping from crushed fishing boat

V90.33 Drowning and submersion due to falling or jumping from other crushed powered watercraft
Drowning and submersion due to falling and jumping from crushed Hovercraft
Drowning and submersion due to falling and jumping from crushed Jet ski

V90.34 Drowning and submersion due to falling or jumping from crushed sailboat

V90.35 Drowning and submersion due to falling or jumping from crushed canoe or kayak

V90.36 Drowning and submersion due to falling or jumping from crushed (nonpowered) inflatable craft

V90.37 Drowning and submersion due to falling or jumping from crushed water-skis

V90.38 Drowning and submersion due to falling or jumping from other crushed unpowered watercraft
Drowning and submersion due to falling and jumping from crushed surf-board
Drowning and submersion due to falling and jumping from crushed windsurfer

V90.39 Drowning and submersion due to falling or jumping from crushed unspecified watercraft
Drowning and submersion due to falling and jumping from crushed boat NOS
Drowning and submersion due to falling and jumping from crushed ship NOS
Drowning and submersion due to falling and jumping from crushed watercraft NOS

V90.8 Drowning and submersion due to other accident to watercraft

V90.80 Drowning and submersion due to other accident to merchant ship

V90.81 Drowning and submersion due to other accident to passenger ship
Drowning and submersion due to other accident to Ferry-boat
Drowning and submersion due to other accident to Liner

V90.82 Drowning and submersion due to other accident to fishing boat

V90.83 Drowning and submersion due to other accident to other powered watercraft
Drowning and submersion due to other accident to Hovercraft (on open water)
Drowning and submersion due to other accident to Jet ski

V90.84 Drowning and submersion due to other accident to sailboat

V90.85 Drowning and submersion due to other accident to canoe or kayak

V90.86 Drowning and submersion due to other accident to (nonpowered) inflatable craft

V90.87 Drowning and submersion due to other accident to water-skis

V90.88 Drowning and submersion due to other accident to other unpowered watercraft
Drowning and submersion due to other accident to surf-board
Drowning and submersion due to other accident to windsurfer

V90.89 Drowning and submersion due to other accident to unspecified watercraft
Drowning and submersion due to other accident to boat NOS
Drowning and submersion due to other accident to ship NOS
Drowning and submersion due to other accident to watercraft NOS

V91 Other injury due to accident to watercraft

INCLUDES any injury except drowning and submersion as a result of an accident to watercraft

EXCLUDES 1 *civilian water transport accident involving military watercraft (V94.81-)*
military watercraft accident in military or war operations (Y36, Y37.-)

EXCLUDES 2 *drowning and submersion due to accident to watercraft (V90.-)*

V91.0 Burn due to watercraft on fire

EXCLUDES 1 *burn from localized fire or explosion on board ship without accident to watercraft (V93.-)*

V91.00 Burn due to merchant ship on fire

V91.01 Burn due to passenger ship on fire
Burn due to Ferry-boat on fire
Burn due to Liner on fire

V91.02 Burn due to fishing boat on fire

V91.03 Burn due to other powered watercraft on fire
Burn due to Hovercraft (on open water) on fire
Burn due to Jet ski on fire

V91.04 Burn due to sailboat on fire

V91.05 Burn due to canoe or kayak on fire

V91.06 Burn due to (nonpowered) inflatable craft on fire

V91.07 Burn due to water-skis on fire

V91.08 Burn due to other unpowered watercraft on fire

V91.09 Burn due to unspecified watercraft on fire
Burn due to boat NOS on fire
Burn due to ship NOS on fire
Burn due to watercraft NOS on fire

V91.1 Crushed between watercraft and other watercraft or other object due to collision
Crushed by lifeboat after abandoning ship in a collision

NOTE Select the specified type of watercraft that the victim was on at the time of the collision

V91.10 Crushed between merchant ship and other watercraft or other object due to collision

V91.11 Crushed between passenger ship and other watercraft or other object due to collision
Crushed between Ferry-boat and other watercraft or other object due to collision
Crushed between Liner and other watercraft or other object due to collision

V91.12 Crushed between fishing boat and other watercraft or other object due to collision

V91.13 Crushed between other powered watercraft and other watercraft or other object due to collision
Crushed between Hovercraft (on open water) and other watercraft or other object due to collision
Crushed between Jet ski and other watercraft or other object due to collision

V91.14 Crushed between sailboat and other watercraft or other object due to collision

V91.15 Crushed between canoe or kayak and other watercraft or other object due to collision

V91.16 Crushed between (nonpowered) inflatable craft and other watercraft or other object due to collision

V91.18 Crushed between other unpowered watercraft and other watercraft or other object due to collision
Crushed between surfboard and other watercraft or other object due to collision
Crushed between windsurfer and other watercraft or other object due to collision

✓x7th **V91.19 Crushed between unspecified watercraft and other watercraft or other object due to collision**
Crushed between boat NOS and other watercraft or other object due to collision
Crushed between ship NOS and other watercraft or other object due to collision
Crushed between watercraft NOS and other watercraft or other object due to collision

✓5th **V91.2 Fall due to collision between watercraft and other watercraft or other object**
Fall while remaining on watercraft after collision
NOTE Select the specified type of watercraft that the victim was on at the time of the collision
EXCLUDES 1 *crushed between watercraft and other watercraft and other object due to collision (V91.1-)*
drowning and submersion due to falling from crushed watercraft (V9Ø.3-)

✓x7th **V91.2Ø Fall due to collision between merchant ship and other watercraft or other object**

✓x7th **V91.21 Fall due to collision between passenger ship and other watercraft or other object**
Fall due to collision between Ferry-boat and other watercraft or other object
Fall due to collision between Liner and other watercraft or other object

✓x7th **V91.22 Fall due to collision between fishing boat and other watercraft or other object**

✓x7th **V91.23 Fall due to collision between other powered watercraft and other watercraft or other object**
Fall due to collision between Hovercraft (on open water) and other watercraft or other object
Fall due to collision between Jet ski and other watercraft or other object

✓x7th **V91.24 Fall due to collision between sailboat and other watercraft or other object**

✓x7th **V91.25 Fall due to collision between canoe or kayak and other watercraft or other object**

✓x7th **V91.26 Fall due to collision between (nonpowered) inflatable craft and other watercraft or other object**

✓x7th **V91.29 Fall due to collision between unspecified watercraft and other watercraft or other object**
Fall due to collision between boat NOS and other watercraft or other object
Fall due to collision between ship NOS and other watercraft or other object
Fall due to collision between watercraft NOS and other watercraft or other object

✓5th **V91.3 Hit or struck by falling object due to accident to watercraft**
Hit or struck by falling object (part of damaged watercraft or other object) after falling or jumping from damaged watercraft
EXCLUDES 2 *drowning or submersion due to fall or jumping from damaged watercraft (V9Ø.2-, V9Ø.3-)*

✓x7th **V91.3Ø Hit or struck by falling object due to accident to merchant ship**

✓x7th **V91.31 Hit or struck by falling object due to accident to passenger ship**
Hit or struck by falling object due to accident to Ferry-boat
Hit or struck by falling object due to accident to Liner

✓x7th **V91.32 Hit or struck by falling object due to accident to fishing boat**

✓x7th **V91.33 Hit or struck by falling object due to accident to other powered watercraft**
Hit or struck by falling object due to accident to Hovercraft (on open water)
Hit or struck by falling object due to accident to Jet ski

✓x7th **V91.34 Hit or struck by falling object due to accident to sailboat**

✓x7th **V91.35 Hit or struck by falling object due to accident to canoe or kayak**

✓x7th **V91.36 Hit or struck by falling object due to accident to (nonpowered) inflatable craft**

✓x7th **V91.37 Hit or struck by falling object due to accident to water-skis**
Hit by water-skis after jumping off of waterskis

✓x7th **V91.38 Hit or struck by falling object due to accident to other unpowered watercraft**
Hit or struck by surf-board after falling off damaged surf-board
Hit or struck by object after falling off damaged windsurfer

✓x7th **V91.39 Hit or struck by falling object due to accident to unspecified watercraft**
Hit or struck by falling object due to accident to boat NOS
Hit or struck by falling object due to accident to ship NOS
Hit or struck by falling object due to accident to watercraft NOS

✓5th **V91.8 Other injury due to other accident to watercraft**

✓x7th **V91.8Ø Other injury due to other accident to merchant ship**

✓x7th **V91.81 Other injury due to other accident to passenger ship**
Other injury due to other accident to Ferry-boat
Other injury due to other accident to Liner

✓x7th **V91.82 Other injury due to other accident to fishing boat**

✓x7th **V91.83 Other injury due to other accident to other powered watercraft**
Other injury due to other accident to Hovercraft (on open water)
Other injury due to other accident to Jet ski

✓x7th **V91.84 Other injury due to other accident to sailboat**

✓x7th **V91.85 Other injury due to other accident to canoe or kayak**

✓x7th **V91.86 Other injury due to other accident to (nonpowered) inflatable craft**

✓x7th **V91.87 Other injury due to other accident to water-skis**

✓x7th **V91.88 Other injury due to other accident to other unpowered watercraft**
Other injury due to other accident to surf-board
Other injury due to other accident to windsurfer

✓x7th **V91.89 Other injury due to other accident to unspecified watercraft**
Other injury due to other accident to boat NOS
Other injury due to other accident to ship NOS
Other injury due to other accident to watercraft NOS

✓4th **V92 Drowning and submersion due to accident on board watercraft, without accident to watercraft**
EXCLUDES 1 *civilian water transport accident involving military watercraft (V94.81-)*
drowning or submersion due to accident to watercraft (V9Ø-V91)
drowning or submersion of diver who voluntarily jumps from boat not involved in an accident (W16.711, W16.721)
fall into water without watercraft (W16.-)
military watercraft accident in military or war operations (Y36, Y37)

✓5th **V92.Ø Drowning and submersion due to fall off watercraft**
Drowning and submersion due to fall from gangplank of watercraft
Drowning and submersion due to fall overboard watercraft
EXCLUDES 2 *hitting head on object or bottom of body of water due to fall from watercraft (V94.Ø-)*

✓x7th **V92.ØØ Drowning and submersion due to fall off merchant ship**

✓x7th **V92.Ø1 Drowning and submersion due to fall off passenger ship**
Drowning and submersion due to fall off Ferry-boat
Drowning and submersion due to fall off Liner

✓x7th **V92.Ø2 Drowning and submersion due to fall off fishing boat**

✓x7th **V92.Ø3 Drowning and submersion due to fall off other powered watercraft**
Drowning and submersion due to fall off Hovercraft (on open water)
Drowning and submersion due to fall off Jet ski

✓x7th **V92.Ø4 Drowning and submersion due to fall off sailboat**

✓x7th **V92.Ø5 Drowning and submersion due to fall off canoe or kayak**

✓x7th **V92.Ø6 Drowning and submersion due to fall off (nonpowered) inflatable craft**

V92.07 Drowning and submersion due to fall off water-skis
EXCLUDES 1 *drowning and submersion due to falling off burning water-skis (V90.27)*
drowning and submersion due to falling off crushed water-skis (V90.37)
hit by boat while water-skiing NOS (V94.X)

V92.08 Drowning and submersion due to fall off other unpowered watercraft
Drowning and submersion due to fall off surf-board
Drowning and submersion due to fall off windsurfer
EXCLUDES 1 *drowning and submersion due to fall off burning unpowered watercraft (V90.28)*
drowning and submersion due to fall off crushed unpowered watercraft (V90.38)
drowning and submersion due to fall off damaged unpowered watercraft (V90.88)
drowning and submersion due to rider of nonpowered watercraft being hit by other watercraft (V94.-)
other injury due to rider of nonpowered watercraft being hit by other watercraft (V94.-)

V92.09 Drowning and submersion due to fall off unspecified watercraft
Drowning and submersion due to fall off boat NOS
Drowning and submersion due to fall off ship
Drowning and submersion due to fall off watercraft NOS

V92.1 Drowning and submersion due to being thrown overboard by motion of watercraft
EXCLUDES 1 *drowning and submersion due to fall off surf-board (V92.08)*
drowning and submersion due to fall off water-skis (V92.07)
drowning and submersion due to fall off windsurfer (V92.08)

V92.10 Drowning and submersion due to being thrown overboard by motion of merchant ship

V92.11 Drowning and submersion due to being thrown overboard by motion of passenger ship
Drowning and submersion due to being thrown overboard by motion of Ferry-boat
Drowning and submersion due to being thrown overboard by motion of Liner

V92.12 Drowning and submersion due to being thrown overboard by motion of fishing boat

V92.13 Drowning and submersion due to being thrown overboard by motion of other powered watercraft
Drowning and submersion due to being thrown overboard by motion of Hovercraft

V92.14 Drowning and submersion due to being thrown overboard by motion of sailboat

V92.15 Drowning and submersion due to being thrown overboard by motion of canoe or kayak

V92.16 Drowning and submersion due to being thrown overboard by motion of (nonpowered) inflatable craft

V92.19 Drowning and submersion due to being thrown overboard by motion of unspecified watercraft
Drowning and submersion due to being thrown overboard by motion of boat NOS
Drowning and submersion due to being thrown overboard by motion of ship NOS
Drowning and submersion due to being thrown overboard by motion of watercraft NOS

V92.2 Drowning and submersion due to being washed overboard from watercraft
Code first any associated cataclysm (X37.0-)

V92.20 Drowning and submersion due to being washed overboard from merchant ship

V92.21 Drowning and submersion due to being washed overboard from passenger ship
Drowning and submersion due to being washed overboard from Ferry-boat
Drowning and submersion due to being washed overboard from Liner

V92.22 Drowning and submersion due to being washed overboard from fishing boat

V92.23 Drowning and submersion due to being washed overboard from other powered watercraft
Drowning and submersion due to being washed overboard from Hovercraft (on open water)
Drowning and submersion due to being washed overboard from Jet ski

V92.24 Drowning and submersion due to being washed overboard from sailboat

V92.25 Drowning and submersion due to being washed overboard from canoe or kayak

V92.26 Drowning and submersion due to being washed overboard from (nonpowered) inflatable craft

V92.27 Drowning and submersion due to being washed overboard from water-skis
EXCLUDES 1 *drowning and submersion due to fall off water-skis (V92.07)*

V92.28 Drowning and submersion due to being washed overboard from other unpowered watercraft
Drowning and submersion due to being washed overboard from surf-board
Drowning and submersion due to being washed overboard from windsurfer

V92.29 Drowning and submersion due to being washed overboard from unspecified watercraft
Drowning and submersion due to being washed overboard from boat NOS
Drowning and submersion due to being washed overboard from ship NOS
Drowning and submersion due to being washed overboard from watercraft NOS

V93 Other injury due to accident on board watercraft, without accident to watercraft
EXCLUDES 1 *civilian water transport accident involving military watercraft (V94.81-)*
other injury due to accident to watercraft (V91.-)
military watercraft accident in military or war operations (Y36, Y37.-)
EXCLUDES 2 *drowning and submersion due to accident on board watercraft, without accident to watercraft (V92.-)*

V93.0 Burn due to localized fire on board watercraft
EXCLUDES 1 *burn due to watercraft on fire (V91.0-)*

V93.00 Burn due to localized fire on board merchant vessel

V93.01 Burn due to localized fire on board passenger vessel
Burn due to localized fire on board Ferry-boat
Burn due to localized fire on board Liner

V93.02 Burn due to localized fire on board fishing boat

V93.03 Burn due to localized fire on board other powered watercraft
Burn due to localized fire on board Hovercraft
Burn due to localized fire on board Jet ski

V93.04 Burn due to localized fire on board sailboat

V93.09 Burn due to localized fire on board unspecified watercraft
Burn due to localized fire on board boat NOS
Burn due to localized fire on board ship NOS
Burn due to localized fire on board watercraft NOS

V93.1 Other burn on board watercraft
Burn due to source other than fire on board watercraft
EXCLUDES 1 *burn due to watercraft on fire (V91.0-)*

V93.10 Other burn on board merchant vessel

V93.11 Other burn on board passenger vessel
Other burn on board Ferry-boat
Other burn on board Liner

V93.12 Other burn on board fishing boat

V93.13 Other burn on board other powered watercraft
Other burn on board Hovercraft
Other burn on board Jet ski

V93.14 Other burn on board sailboat

√7th **V93.19 Other burn on board unspecified watercraft**
Other burn on board boat NOS
Other burn on board ship NOS
Other burn on board watercraft NOS

√5th **V93.2 Heat exposure on board watercraft**
EXCLUDES 1 *exposure to man-made heat not aboard watercraft (W92)*
exposure to natural heat while on board watercraft (X30)
exposure to sunlight while on board watercraft (X32)
EXCLUDES 2 *burn due to fire on board watercraft (V93.0-)*

√7th **V93.20 Heat exposure on board merchant ship**
√7th **V93.21 Heat exposure on board passenger ship**
Heat exposure on board Ferry-boat
Heat exposure on board Liner
√7th **V93.22 Heat exposure on board fishing boat**
√7th **V93.23 Heat exposure on board other powered watercraft**
Heat exposure on board hovercraft
√7th **V93.24 Heat exposure on board sailboat**
√7th **V93.29 Heat exposure on board unspecified watercraft**
Heat exposure on board boat NOS
Heat exposure on board ship NOS
Heat exposure on board watercraft NOS

√5th **V93.3 Fall on board watercraft**
EXCLUDES 1 *fall due to collision of watercraft (V91.2-)*

√7th **V93.30 Fall on board merchant ship**
√7th **V93.31 Fall on board passenger ship**
Fall on board Ferry-boat
Fall on board Liner
√7th **V93.32 Fall on board fishing boat**
√7th **V93.33 Fall on board other powered watercraft**
Fall on board Hovercraft (on open water)
Fall on board Jet ski
√7th **V93.34 Fall on board sailboat**
√7th **V93.35 Fall on board canoe or kayak**
√7th **V93.36 Fall on board (nonpowered) inflatable craft**
√7th **V93.38 Fall on board other unpowered watercraft**
√7th **V93.39 Fall on board unspecified watercraft**
Fall on board boat NOS
Fall on board ship NOS
Fall on board watercraft NOS

√5th **V93.4 Struck by falling object on board watercraft**
Hit by falling object on board watercraft
EXCLUDES 1 *struck by falling object due to accident to watercraft (V91.3)*

√7th **V93.40 Struck by falling object on merchant ship**
√7th **V93.41 Struck by falling object on passenger ship**
Struck by falling object on Ferry-boat
Struck by falling object on Liner
√7th **V93.42 Struck by falling object on fishing boat**
√7th **V93.43 Struck by falling object on other powered watercraft**
Struck by falling object on Hovercraft
√7th **V93.44 Struck by falling object on sailboat**
√7th **V93.48 Struck by falling object on other unpowered watercraft**
√7th **V93.49 Struck by falling object on unspecified watercraft**

√5th **V93.5 Explosion on board watercraft**
Boiler explosion on steamship
EXCLUDES 2 *fire on board watercraft (V93.0-)*

√7th **V93.50 Explosion on board merchant ship**
√7th **V93.51 Explosion on board passenger ship**
Explosion on board Ferry-boat
Explosion on board Liner
√7th **V93.52 Explosion on board fishing boat**
√7th **V93.53 Explosion on board other powered watercraft**
Explosion on board Hovercraft
Explosion on board Jet ski
√7th **V93.54 Explosion on board sailboat**
√7th **V93.59 Explosion on board unspecified watercraft**
Explosion on board boat NOS
Explosion on board ship NOS
Explosion on board watercraft NOS

√5th **V93.6 Machinery accident on board watercraft**
EXCLUDES 1 *machinery explosion on board watercraft (V93.4-)*
machinery fire on board watercraft (V93.0-)

√7th **V93.60 Machinery accident on board merchant ship**
√7th **V93.61 Machinery accident on board passenger ship**
Machinery accident on board Ferry-boat
Machinery accident on board Liner
√7th **V93.62 Machinery accident on board fishing boat**
√7th **V93.63 Machinery accident on board other powered watercraft**
Machinery accident on board Hovercraft
√7th **V93.64 Machinery accident on board sailboat**
√7th **V93.69 Machinery accident on board unspecified watercraft**
Machinery accident on board boat NOS
Machinery accident on board ship NOS
Machinery accident on board watercraft NOS

√5th **V93.8 Other injury due to other accident on board watercraft**
Accidental poisoning by gases or fumes on watercraft

√7th **V93.80 Other injury due to other accident on board merchant ship**
√7th **V93.81 Other injury due to other accident on board passenger ship**
Other injury due to other accident on board Ferry-boat
Other injury due to other accident on board Liner
√7th **V93.82 Other injury due to other accident on board fishing boat**
√7th **V93.83 Other injury due to other accident on board other powered watercraft**
Other injury due to other accident on board Hovercraft
Other injury due to other accident on board Jet ski
√7th **V93.84 Other injury due to other accident on board sailboat**
√7th **V93.85 Other injury due to other accident on board canoe or kayak**
√7th **V93.86 Other injury due to other accident on board (nonpowered) inflatable craft**
√7th **V93.87 Other injury due to other accident on board water-skis**
Hit or struck by object while waterskiing
√7th **V93.88 Other injury due to other accident on board other unpowered watercraft**
Hit or struck by object while surfing
Hit or struck by object while on board windsurfer
√7th **V93.89 Other injury due to other accident on board unspecified watercraft**
Other injury due to other accident on board boat NOS
Other injury due to other accident on board ship NOS
Other injury due to other accident on board watercraft NOS

√4th **V94 Other and unspecified water transport accidents**
EXCLUDES 1 *military watercraft accidents in military or war operations (Y36, Y37)*

√7th **V94.0 Hitting object or bottom of body of water due to fall from watercraft**
EXCLUDES 2 *drowning and submersion due to fall from watercraft (V92.0-)*

√5th **V94.1 Bather struck by watercraft**
Swimmer hit by watercraft

√7th **V94.11 Bather struck by powered watercraft**
√7th **V94.12 Bather struck by nonpowered watercraft**

√5th **V94.2 Rider of nonpowered watercraft struck by other watercraft**

√7th **V94.21 Rider of nonpowered watercraft struck by other nonpowered watercraft**
Canoer hit by other nonpowered watercraft
Surfer hit by other nonpowered watercraft
Windsurfer hit by other nonpowered watercraft

✓x7th **V94.22 Rider of nonpowered watercraft struck by powered watercraft**
Canoer hit by motorboat
Surfer hit by motorboat
Windsurfer hit by motorboat

✓5th **V94.3 Injury to rider of (inflatable) watercraft being pulled behind other watercraft**

✓x7th **V94.31 Injury to rider of (inflatable) recreational watercraft being pulled behind other watercraft**
Injury to rider of inner-tube pulled behind motor boat

✓x7th **V94.32 Injury to rider of non-recreational watercraft being pulled behind other watercraft**
Injury to occupant of dingy being pulled behind boat or ship
Injury to occupant of life-raft being pulled behind boat or ship

✓x7th **V94.4 Injury to barefoot water-skier**
Injury to person being pulled behind boat or ship

✓5th **V94.8 Other water transport accident**

✓6th **V94.81 Water transport accident involving military watercraft**

✓7th **V94.810 Civilian watercraft involved in water transport accident with military watercraft**
Passenger on civilian watercraft injured due to accident with military watercraft

✓7th **V94.811 Civilian in water injured by military watercraft**

✓7th **V94.818 Other water transport accident involving military watercraft**

✓x7th **V94.89 Other water transport accident**

✓x7th **V94.9 Unspecified water transport accident**
Water transport accident NOS

Air and space transport accidents (V95-V97)

EXCLUDES 1 *military aircraft accidents in military or war operations (Y36, Y37)*

The appropriate 7th character is to be added to each code from categories V95-V97.
A initial encounter
D subsequent encounter
S sequela

✓4th **V95 Accident to powered aircraft causing injury to occupant**

✓5th **V95.0 Helicopter accident injuring occupant**

✓x7th **V95.00 Unspecified helicopter accident injuring occupant**

✓x7th **V95.01 Helicopter crash injuring occupant**

✓x7th **V95.02 Forced landing of helicopter injuring occupant**

✓x7th **V95.03 Helicopter collision injuring occupant**
Helicopter collision with any object, fixed, movable or moving

✓x7th **V95.04 Helicopter fire injuring occupant**

✓x7th **V95.05 Helicopter explosion injuring occupant**

✓x7th **V95.09 Other helicopter accident injuring occupant**

✓5th **V95.1 Ultralight, microlight or powered-glider accident injuring occupant**

✓x7th **V95.10 Unspecified ultralight, microlight or powered-glider accident injuring occupant**

✓x7th **V95.11 Ultralight, microlight or powered-glider crash injuring occupant**

✓x7th **V95.12 Forced landing of ultralight, microlight or powered-glider injuring occupant**

✓x7th **V95.13 Ultralight, microlight or powered-glider collision injuring occupant**
Ultralight, microlight or powered-glider collision with any object, fixed, movable or moving

✓x7th **V95.14 Ultralight, microlight or powered-glider fire injuring occupant**

✓x7th **V95.15 Ultralight, microlight or powered-glider explosion injuring occupant**

✓x7th **V95.19 Other ultralight, microlight or powered-glider accident injuring occupant**

✓5th **V95.2 Other private fixed-wing aircraft accident injuring occupant**

✓x7th **V95.20 Unspecified accident to other private fixed-wing aircraft, injuring occupant**

✓x7th **V95.21 Other private fixed-wing aircraft crash injuring occupant**

✓x7th **V95.22 Forced landing of other private fixed-wing aircraft injuring occupant**

✓x7th **V95.23 Other private fixed-wing aircraft collision injuring occupant**
Other private fixed-wing aircraft collision with any object, fixed, movable or moving

✓x7th **V95.24 Other private fixed-wing aircraft fire injuring occupant**

✓x7th **V95.25 Other private fixed-wing aircraft explosion injuring occupant**

✓x7th **V95.29 Other accident to other private fixed-wing aircraft injuring occupant**

✓5th **V95.3 Commercial fixed-wing aircraft accident injuring occupant**

✓x7th **V95.30 Unspecified accident to commercial fixed-wing aircraft injuring occupant**

✓x7th **V95.31 Commercial fixed-wing aircraft crash injuring occupant**

✓x7th **V95.32 Forced landing of commercial fixed-wing aircraft injuring occupant**

✓x7th **V95.33 Commercial fixed-wing aircraft collision injuring occupant**
Commercial fixed-wing aircraft collision with any object, fixed, movable or moving

✓x7th **V95.34 Commercial fixed-wing aircraft fire injuring occupant**

✓x7th **V95.35 Commercial fixed-wing aircraft explosion injuring occupant**

✓x7th **V95.39 Other accident to commercial fixed-wing aircraft injuring occupant**

✓5th **V95.4 Spacecraft accident injuring occupant**

✓x7th **V95.40 Unspecified spacecraft accident injuring occupant**

✓x7th **V95.41 Spacecraft crash injuring occupant**

✓x7th **V95.42 Forced landing of spacecraft injuring occupant**

✓x7th **V95.43 Spacecraft collision injuring occupant**
Spacecraft collision with any object, fixed, moveable or moving

✓x7th **V95.44 Spacecraft fire injuring occupant**

✓x7th **V95.45 Spacecraft explosion injuring occupant**

✓x7th **V95.49 Other spacecraft accident injuring occupant**

✓x7th **V95.8 Other powered aircraft accidents injuring occupant**

✓x7th **V95.9 Unspecified aircraft accident injuring occupant**
Aircraft accident NOS
Air transport accident NOS

✓4th **V96 Accident to nonpowered aircraft causing injury to occupant**

✓5th **V96.0 Balloon accident injuring occupant**

✓x7th **V96.00 Unspecified balloon accident injuring occupant**

✓x7th **V96.01 Balloon crash injuring occupant**

✓x7th **V96.02 Forced landing of balloon injuring occupant**

✓x7th **V96.03 Balloon collision injuring occupant**
Balloon collision with any object, fixed, moveable or moving

✓x7th **V96.04 Balloon fire injuring occupant**

✓x7th **V96.05 Balloon explosion injuring occupant**

✓x7th **V96.09 Other balloon accident injuring occupant**

✓5th **V96.1 Hang-glider accident injuring occupant**

✓x7th **V96.10 Unspecified hang-glider accident injuring occupant**

✓x7th **V96.11 Hang-glider crash injuring occupant**

✓x7th **V96.12 Forced landing of hang-glider injuring occupant**

✓x7th **V96.13 Hang-glider collision injuring occupant**
Hang-glider collision with any object, fixed, moveable or moving

✓x7th **V96.14 Hang-glider fire injuring occupant**

✓x7th **V96.15 Hang-glider explosion injuring occupant**

✓x7th **V96.19 Other hang-glider accident injuring occupant**

✓5th **V96.2 Glider (nonpowered) accident injuring occupant**

✓x7th **V96.20 Unspecified glider (nonpowered) accident injuring occupant**

✓x7th **V96.21 Glider (nonpowered) crash injuring occupant**

✓x7th **V96.22 Forced landing of glider (nonpowered) injuring occupant**

√7th **V96.23 Glider (nonpowered) collision injuring occupant**
Glider (nonpowered) collision with any object, fixed, moveable or moving

√7th **V96.24 Glider (nonpowered) fire injuring occupant**

√7th **V96.25 Glider (nonpowered) explosion injuring occupant**

√7th **V96.29 Other glider (nonpowered) accident injuring occupant**

√7th **V96.8 Other nonpowered-aircraft accidents injuring occupant**
Kite carrying a person accident injuring occupant

√7th **V96.9 Unspecified nonpowered-aircraft accident injuring occupant**
Nonpowered-aircraft accident NOS

√4th **V97 Other specified air transport accidents**

√7th **V97.0 Occupant of aircraft injured in other specified air transport accidents**
Fall in, on or from aircraft in air transport accident
EXCLUDES 1 *accident while boarding or alighting aircraft (V97.1)*

√7th **V97.1 Person injured while boarding or alighting from aircraft**

√5th **V97.2 Parachutist accident**

√7th **V97.21 Parachutist entangled in object**
Parachutist landing in tree

√7th **V97.22 Parachutist injured on landing**

√7th **V97.29 Other parachutist accident**

√5th **V97.3 Person on ground injured in air transport accident**

√7th **V97.31 Hit by object falling from aircraft**
Hit by crashing aircraft
Injured by aircraft hitting house
Injured by aircraft hitting car

√7th **V97.32 Injured by rotating propeller**

√7th **V97.33 Sucked into jet engine**

√7th **V97.39 Other injury to person on ground due to air transport accident**

√5th **V97.8 Other air transport accidents, not elsewhere classified**
EXCLUDES 1 *aircraft accident NOS (V95.9)*
exposure to changes in air pressure during ascent or descent (W94.-)

√6th **V97.81 Air transport accident involving military aircraft**

√7th **V97.810 Civilian aircraft involved in air transport accident with military aircraft**
Passenger in civilian aircraft injured due to accident with military aircraft

√7th **V97.811 Civilian injured by military aircraft**

√7th **V97.818 Other air transport accident involving military aircraft**

√7th **V97.89 Other air transport accidents, not elsewhere classified**
Injury from machinery on aircraft

Other and unspecified transport accidents (V98-V99)

EXCLUDES 1 *vehicle accident, type of vehicle unspecified (V89.-)*

The appropriate 7th character is to be added to each code from categories V98-V99.
A initial encounter
D subsequent encounter
S sequela

√4th **V98 Other specified transport accidents**

√7th **V98.0 Accident to, on or involving cable-car, not on rails**
Caught or dragged by cable-car, not on rails
Fall or jump from cable-car, not on rails
Object thrown from or in cable-car, not on rails

√7th **V98.1 Accident to, on or involving land-yacht**

√7th **V98.2 Accident to, on or involving ice yacht**

√7th **V98.3 Accident to, on or involving ski lift**
Accident to, on or involving ski chair-lift
Accident to, on or involving ski-lift with gondola

√7th **V98.8 Other specified transport accidents**

√7th **V99 Unspecified transport accident**

OTHER EXTERNAL CAUSES OF ACCIDENTAL INJURY (W00-X58)

Slipping, tripping, stumbling and falls (W00-W19)

EXCLUDES 1 *assault involving a fall (Y01-Y02)*
fall from animal (V80.-)
fall (in) (from) machinery (in operation) (W28-W31)
fall (in) (from) transport vehicle (V01-V99)
intentional self-harm involving a fall (X80-X81)
EXCLUDES 2 *at risk for fall (history of fall) Z91.81*
fall (in) (from) burning building (X00.-)
fall into fire (X00-X04, X08)

The appropriate 7th character is to be added to each code from categories W00-W19.
A initial encounter
D subsequent encounter
S sequela

√4th **W00 Fall due to ice and snow**
INCLUDES pedestrian on foot falling (slipping) on ice and snow
EXCLUDES 1 *fall on (from) ice and snow involving pedestrian conveyance (V00.-)*
fall from stairs and steps not due to ice and snow (W10.-)
AHA: 2016,2Q,4

√7th **W00.0 Fall on same level due to ice and snow**

√7th **W00.1 Fall from stairs and steps due to ice and snow**

√7th **W00.2 Other fall from one level to another due to ice and snow**

√7th **W00.9 Unspecified fall due to ice and snow**

√4th **W01 Fall on same level from slipping, tripping and stumbling**
INCLUDES fall on moving sidewalk
EXCLUDES 1 *fall due to bumping (striking) against object (W18.0-)*
fall in shower or bathtub (W18.2-)
fall on same level NOS (W18.30)
fall on same level from slipping, tripping and stumbling due to ice or snow (W00.0)
fall off or from toilet (W18.1-)
slipping, tripping and stumbling NOS (W18.40)
slipping, tripping and stumbling without falling (W18.4-)

√7th **W01.0 Fall on same level from slipping, tripping and stumbling without subsequent striking against object**
Falling over animal

√5th **W01.1 Fall on same level from slipping, tripping and stumbling with subsequent striking against object**

√7th **W01.10 Fall on same level from slipping, tripping and stumbling with subsequent striking against unspecified object**

√6th **W01.11 Fall on same level from slipping, tripping and stumbling with subsequent striking against sharp object**

√7th **W01.110 Fall on same level from slipping, tripping and stumbling with subsequent striking against sharp glass**

√7th **W01.111 Fall on same level from slipping, tripping and stumbling with subsequent striking against power tool or machine**

√7th **W01.118 Fall on same level from slipping, tripping and stumbling with subsequent striking against other sharp object**

√7th **W01.119 Fall on same level from slipping, tripping and stumbling with subsequent striking against unspecified sharp object**

√6th **W01.19 Fall on same level from slipping, tripping and stumbling with subsequent striking against other object**

√7th **W01.190 Fall on same level from slipping, tripping and stumbling with subsequent striking against furniture**

√7th **W01.198 Fall on same level from slipping, tripping and stumbling with subsequent striking against other object**

W03 Other fall on same level due to collision with another person
Fall due to non-transport collision with other person
EXCLUDES 1 *collision with another person without fall (W51)*
crushed or pushed by a crowd or human stampede (W52)
fall involving pedestrian conveyance (V00-V09)
fall due to ice or snow (W00)
fall on same level NOS (W18.30)
AHA: 2012,4Q,108

W04 Fall while being carried or supported by other persons
Accidentally dropped while being carried

W05 Fall from non-moving wheelchair, nonmotorized scooter and motorized mobility scooter
EXCLUDES 1 *fall from moving wheelchair (powered) (V00.811)*
fall from moving motorized mobility scooter (V00.831)
fall from nonmotorized scooter (V00.141)

W05.0 Fall from non-moving wheelchair
AHA: 2019,2Q,27

W05.1 Fall from non-moving nonmotorized scooter

W05.2 Fall from non-moving motorized mobility scooter

W06 Fall from bed

W07 Fall from chair

W08 Fall from other furniture
▶Fall from stool◀

W09 Fall on and from playground equipment
EXCLUDES 1 *fall involving recreational machinery (W31)*

W09.0 Fall on or from playground slide

W09.1 Fall from playground swing

W09.2 Fall on or from jungle gym

W09.8 Fall on or from other playground equipment

W10 Fall on and from stairs and steps
EXCLUDES 1 *Fall from stairs and steps due to ice and snow (W00.1)*

W10.0 Fall (on)(from) escalator

W10.1 Fall (on)(from) sidewalk curb

W10.2 Fall (on)(from) incline
Fall (on) (from) ramp

W10.8 Fall (on) (from) other stairs and steps

W10.9 Fall (on) (from) unspecified stairs and steps

W11 Fall on and from ladder

W12 Fall on and from scaffolding

W13 Fall from, out of or through building or structure

W13.0 Fall from, out of or through balcony
Fall from, out of or through railing

W13.1 Fall from, out of or through bridge

W13.2 Fall from, out of or through roof

W13.3 Fall through floor

W13.4 Fall from, out of or through window
EXCLUDES 2 *fall with subsequent striking against sharp glass (W01.110-)*

W13.8 Fall from, out of or through other building or structure
Fall from, out of or through viaduct
Fall from, out of or through wall
Fall from, out of or through flag-pole

W13.9 Fall from, out of or through building, not otherwise specified
EXCLUDES 1 *collapse of a building or structure (W20.-)*
fall or jump from burning building or structure (X00.-)

W14 Fall from tree

W15 Fall from cliff

W16 Fall, jump or diving into water
EXCLUDES 1 *accidental non-watercraft drowning and submersion not involving fall (W65-W74)*
effects of air pressure from diving (W94.-)
fall into water from watercraft (V90-V94)
hitting an object or against bottom when falling from watercraft (V94.0)
EXCLUDES 2 *striking or hitting diving board (W21.4)*

W16.0 Fall into swimming pool
Fall into swimming pool NOS
EXCLUDES 1 *fall into empty swimming pool (W17.3)*

W16.01 Fall into swimming pool striking water surface

W16.011 Fall into swimming pool striking water surface causing drowning and submersion
EXCLUDES 1 *drowning and submersion while in swimming pool without fall (W67)*

W16.012 Fall into swimming pool striking water surface causing other injury

W16.02 Fall into swimming pool striking bottom

W16.021 Fall into swimming pool striking bottom causing drowning and submersion
EXCLUDES 1 *drowning and submersion while in swimming pool without fall (W67)*

W16.022 Fall into swimming pool striking bottom causing other injury

W16.03 Fall into swimming pool striking wall

W16.031 Fall into swimming pool striking wall causing drowning and submersion
EXCLUDES 1 *drowning and submersion while in swimming pool without fall (W67)*

W16.032 Fall into swimming pool striking wall causing other injury

W16.1 Fall into natural body of water
Fall into lake
Fall into open sea
Fall into river
Fall into stream

W16.11 Fall into natural body of water striking water surface

W16.111 Fall into natural body of water striking water surface causing drowning and submersion
EXCLUDES 1 *drowning and submersion while in natural body of water without fall (W69)*

W16.112 Fall into natural body of water striking water surface causing other injury

W16.12 Fall into natural body of water striking bottom

W16.121 Fall into natural body of water striking bottom causing drowning and submersion
EXCLUDES 1 *drowning and submersion while in natural body of water without fall (W69)*

W16.122 Fall into natural body of water striking bottom causing other injury

W16.13 Fall into natural body of water striking side

W16.131 Fall into natural body of water striking side causing drowning and submersion
EXCLUDES 1 *drowning and submersion while in natural body of water without fall (W69)*

W16.132 Fall into natural body of water striking side causing other injury

W16.2 Fall in (into) filled bathtub or bucket of water

W16.21 Fall in (into) filled bathtub
EXCLUDES 1 *fall into empty bathtub (W18.2)*

W16.211 Fall in (into) filled bathtub causing drowning and submersion
EXCLUDES 1 *drowning and submersion while in filled bathtub without fall (W65)*

W16.212 Fall in (into) filled bathtub causing other injury

6th **W16.22 Fall in (into) bucket of water**

7th **W16.221 Fall in (into) bucket of water causing drowning and submersion**

7th **W16.222 Fall in (into) bucket of water causing other injury**

5th **W16.3 Fall into other water**

Fall into fountain

Fall into reservoir

6th **W16.31 Fall into other water striking water surface**

7th **W16.311 Fall into other water striking water surface causing drowning and submersion**

EXCLUDES 1 *drowning and submersion while in other water without fall (W73)*

7th **W16.312 Fall into other water striking water surface causing other injury**

6th **W16.32 Fall into other water striking bottom**

7th **W16.321 Fall into other water striking bottom causing drowning and submersion**

EXCLUDES 1 *drowning and submersion while in other water without fall (W73)*

7th **W16.322 Fall into other water striking bottom causing other injury**

6th **W16.33 Fall into other water striking wall**

7th **W16.331 Fall into other water striking wall causing drowning and submersion**

EXCLUDES 1 *drowning and submersion while in other water without fall (W73)*

7th **W16.332 Fall into other water striking wall causing other injury**

5th **W16.4 Fall into unspecified water**

x7th **W16.41 Fall into unspecified water causing drowning and submersion**

x7th **W16.42 Fall into unspecified water causing other injury**

5th **W16.5 Jumping or diving into swimming pool**

6th **W16.51 Jumping or diving into swimming pool striking water surface**

7th **W16.511 Jumping or diving into swimming pool striking water surface causing drowning and submersion**

EXCLUDES 1 *drowning and submersion while in swimming pool without jumping or diving (W67)*

7th **W16.512 Jumping or diving into swimming pool striking water surface causing other injury**

6th **W16.52 Jumping or diving into swimming pool striking bottom**

7th **W16.521 Jumping or diving into swimming pool striking bottom causing drowning and submersion**

EXCLUDES 1 *drowning and submersion while in swimming pool without jumping or diving (W67)*

7th **W16.522 Jumping or diving into swimming pool striking bottom causing other injury**

6th **W16.53 Jumping or diving into swimming pool striking wall**

7th **W16.531 Jumping or diving into swimming pool striking wall causing drowning and submersion**

EXCLUDES 1 *drowning and submersion while in swimming pool without jumping or diving (W67)*

7th **W16.532 Jumping or diving into swimming pool striking wall causing other injury**

5th **W16.6 Jumping or diving into natural body of water**

Jumping or diving into lake

Jumping or diving into open sea

Jumping or diving into river

Jumping or diving into stream

6th **W16.61 Jumping or diving into natural body of water striking water surface**

7th **W16.611 Jumping or diving into natural body of water striking water surface causing drowning and submersion**

EXCLUDES 1 *drowning and submersion while in natural body of water without jumping or diving (W69)*

7th **W16.612 Jumping or diving into natural body of water striking water surface causing other injury**

6th **W16.62 Jumping or diving into natural body of water striking bottom**

7th **W16.621 Jumping or diving into natural body of water striking bottom causing drowning and submersion**

EXCLUDES 1 *drowning and submersion while in natural body of water without jumping or diving (W69)*

7th **W16.622 Jumping or diving into natural body of water striking bottom causing other injury**

5th **W16.7 Jumping or diving from boat**

EXCLUDES 1 *fall from boat into water - see watercraft accident (V90-V94)*

6th **W16.71 Jumping or diving from boat striking water surface**

7th **W16.711 Jumping or diving from boat striking water surface causing drowning and submersion**

7th **W16.712 Jumping or diving from boat striking water surface causing other injury**

6th **W16.72 Jumping or diving from boat striking bottom**

7th **W16.721 Jumping or diving from boat striking bottom causing drowning and submersion**

7th **W16.722 Jumping or diving from boat striking bottom causing other injury**

5th **W16.8 Jumping or diving into other water**

Jumping or diving into fountain

Jumping or diving into reservoir

6th **W16.81 Jumping or diving into other water striking water surface**

7th **W16.811 Jumping or diving into other water striking water surface causing drowning and submersion**

EXCLUDES 1 *drowning and submersion while in other water without jumping or diving (W73)*

7th **W16.812 Jumping or diving into other water striking water surface causing other injury**

6th **W16.82 Jumping or diving into other water striking bottom**

7th **W16.821 Jumping or diving into other water striking bottom causing drowning and submersion**

EXCLUDES 1 *drowning and submersion while in other water without jumping or diving (W73)*

7th **W16.822 Jumping or diving into other water striking bottom causing other injury**

6th **W16.83 Jumping or diving into other water striking wall**

7th **W16.831 Jumping or diving into other water striking wall causing drowning and submersion**

EXCLUDES 1 *drowning and submersion while in other water without jumping or diving (W73)*

7th **W16.832 Jumping or diving into other water striking wall causing other injury**

W16.9 Jumping or diving into unspecified water
- W16.91 Jumping or diving into unspecified water causing drowning and submersion
- W16.92 Jumping or diving into unspecified water causing other injury

W17 Other fall from one level to another
- W17.0 Fall into well
- W17.1 Fall into storm drain or manhole
- W17.2 Fall into hole
  - Fall into pit
- W17.3 Fall into empty swimming pool
  - EXCLUDES 1 *fall into filled swimming pool (W16.0-)*
- W17.4 Fall from dock
- W17.8 Other fall from one level to another
  - W17.81 Fall down embankment (hill)
  - W17.82 Fall from (out of) grocery cart
    - Fall due to grocery cart tipping over
  - W17.89 Other fall from one level to another
    - Fall from cherry picker
    - Fall from lifting device
    - Fall from mobile elevated work platform [MEWP]
    - Fall from sky lift
    - AHA: 2015,2Q,6

W18 Other slipping, tripping and stumbling and falls
- W18.0 Fall due to bumping against object
  - Striking against object with subsequent fall
  - EXCLUDES 1 *fall on same level due to slipping, tripping, or stumbling with subsequent striking against object (W01.1-)*
  - W18.00 Striking against unspecified object with subsequent fall
  - W18.01 Striking against sports equipment with subsequent fall
  - W18.02 Striking against glass with subsequent fall
  - W18.09 Striking against other object with subsequent fall
- W18.1 Fall from or off toilet
  - W18.11 Fall from or off toilet without subsequent striking against object
    - Fall from (off) toilet NOS
  - W18.12 Fall from or off toilet with subsequent striking against object
- W18.2 Fall in (into) shower or empty bathtub
  - EXCLUDES 1 *fall in full bathtub causing drowning or submersion (W16.21-)*
- W18.3 Other and unspecified fall on same level
  - W18.30 Fall on same level, unspecified
  - W18.31 Fall on same level due to stepping on an object
    - Fall on same level due to stepping on an animal
    - EXCLUDES 1 *slipping, tripping and stumbling without fall due to stepping on animal (W18.41)*
  - W18.39 Other fall on same level
- W18.4 Slipping, tripping and stumbling without falling
  - EXCLUDES 1 *collision with another person without fall (W51)*
  - W18.40 Slipping, tripping and stumbling without falling, unspecified
  - W18.41 Slipping, tripping and stumbling without falling due to stepping on object
    - Slipping, tripping and stumbling without falling due to stepping on animal
    - EXCLUDES 1 *slipping, tripping and stumbling with fall due to stepping on animal (W18.31)*
  - W18.42 Slipping, tripping and stumbling without falling due to stepping into hole or opening
  - W18.43 Slipping, tripping and stumbling without falling due to stepping from one level to another
  - W18.49 Other slipping, tripping and stumbling without falling

W19 Unspecified fall
- Accidental fall NOS
- AHA: 2012,4Q,95

Exposure to inanimate mechanical forces (W20-W49)

EXCLUDES 1
- *assault (X92-Y09)*
- *contact or collision with animals or persons (W50-W64)*
- *exposure to inanimate mechanical forces involving military or war operations (Y36.-, Y37.-)*
- *intentional self-harm (X71-X83)*

The appropriate 7th character is to be added to each code from categories W20-W49.
- A initial encounter
- D subsequent encounter
- S sequela

W20 Struck by thrown, projected or falling object
- Code first any associated:
  - cataclysm (X34-X39)
  - lightning strike (T75.00)
- EXCLUDES 1
  - *falling object in machinery accident (W24, W28-W31)*
  - *falling object in transport accident (V01-V99)*
  - *object set in motion by explosion (W35-W40)*
  - *object set in motion by firearm (W32-W34)*
  - *struck by thrown sports equipment (W21.-)*
- W20.0 Struck by falling object in cave-in
  - EXCLUDES 2 *asphyxiation due to cave-in (T71.21)*
- W20.1 Struck by object due to collapse of building
  - EXCLUDES 1 *struck by object due to collapse of burning building (X00.2, X02.2)*
- W20.8 Other cause of strike by thrown, projected or falling object
  - EXCLUDES 1 *struck by thrown sports equipment (W21.-)*

W21 Striking against or struck by sports equipment
- EXCLUDES 1
  - *assault with sports equipment (Y08.0-)*
  - *striking against or struck by sports equipment with subsequent fall (W18.01)*
- W21.0 Struck by hit or thrown ball
  - W21.00 Struck by hit or thrown ball, unspecified type
  - W21.01 Struck by football
  - W21.02 Struck by soccer ball
  - W21.03 Struck by baseball
  - W21.04 Struck by golf ball
  - W21.05 Struck by basketball
  - W21.06 Struck by volleyball
  - W21.07 Struck by softball
  - W21.09 Struck by other hit or thrown ball
- W21.1 Struck by bat, racquet or club
  - W21.11 Struck by baseball bat
  - W21.12 Struck by tennis racquet
  - W21.13 Struck by golf club
  - W21.19 Struck by other bat, racquet or club
- W21.2 Struck by hockey stick or puck
  - W21.21 Struck by hockey stick
    - W21.210 Struck by ice hockey stick
    - W21.211 Struck by field hockey stick
  - W21.22 Struck by hockey puck
    - W21.220 Struck by ice hockey puck
    - W21.221 Struck by field hockey puck
- W21.3 Struck by sports foot wear
  - W21.31 Struck by shoe cleats
    - Stepped on by shoe cleats
  - W21.32 Struck by skate blades
    - Skated over by skate blades
  - W21.39 Struck by other sports foot wear
- W21.4 Striking against diving board
  - Use additional code for subsequent falling into water, if applicable (W16.-)
- W21.8 Striking against or struck by other sports equipment
  - W21.81 Striking against or struck by football helmet
  - W21.89 Striking against or struck by other sports equipment
- W21.9 Striking against or struck by unspecified sports equipment

W22 Striking against or struck by other objects
EXCLUDES 1 *striking against or struck by object with subsequent fall (W18.09)*

W22.0 Striking against stationary object
EXCLUDES 1 *striking against stationary sports equipment (W21.8)*

W22.01 Walked into wall

W22.02 Walked into lamppost

W22.03 Walked into furniture

W22.04 Striking against wall of swimming pool

W22.041 Striking against wall of swimming pool causing drowning and submersion
EXCLUDES 1 *drowning and submersion while swimming without striking against wall (W67)*

W22.042 Striking against wall of swimming pool causing other injury

W22.09 Striking against other stationary object

W22.1 Striking against or struck by automobile airbag

W22.10 Striking against or struck by unspecified automobile airbag

W22.11 Striking against or struck by driver side automobile airbag

W22.12 Striking against or struck by front passenger side automobile airbag

W22.19 Striking against or struck by other automobile airbag

W22.8 Striking against or struck by other objects
Striking against or struck by object NOS
EXCLUDES 1 *struck by thrown, projected or falling object (W20.-)*

W23 Caught, crushed, jammed or pinched in or between objects
EXCLUDES 1 *injury caused by cutting or piercing instruments (W25-W27)*
injury caused by firearms malfunction (W32.1, W33.1-, W34.1-)
injury caused by lifting and transmission devices (W24.-)
injury caused by machinery (W28-W31)
injury caused by nonpowered hand tools (W27.-)
injury caused by transport vehicle being used as a means of transportation (V01-V99)
injury caused by struck by thrown, projected or falling object (W20.-)

W23.0 Caught, crushed, jammed, or pinched between moving objects

W23.1 Caught, crushed, jammed, or pinched between stationary objects

● **W23.2 Caught, crushed, jammed or pinched between a moving and stationary object**

W24 Contact with lifting and transmission devices, not elsewhere classified
EXCLUDES 1 *transport accidents (V01-V99)*

W24.0 Contact with lifting devices, not elsewhere classified
Contact with chain hoist
Contact with drive belt
Contact with pulley (block)

W24.1 Contact with transmission devices, not elsewhere classified
Contact with transmission belt or cable

W25 Contact with sharp glass
Code first any associated:
injury due to flying glass from explosion or firearm discharge (W32-W40)
transport accident (V00-V99)
EXCLUDES 1 *fall on same level due to slipping, tripping and stumbling with subsequent striking against sharp glass (W01.110-)*
striking against sharp glass with subsequent fall (W18.02-)
EXCLUDES 2 *glass embedded in skin (W45.-)*

W26 Contact with other sharp objects
EXCLUDES 2 *sharp object(s) embedded in skin (W45.-)*
AHA: 2016,4Q,73

W26.0 Contact with knife
EXCLUDES 1 *contact with electric knife (W29.1)*

W26.1 Contact with sword or dagger

W26.2 Contact with edge of stiff paper
Paper cut

W26.8 Contact with other sharp object(s), not elsewhere classified
Contact with tin can lid

W26.9 Contact with unspecified sharp object(s)

W27 Contact with nonpowered hand tool

W27.0 Contact with workbench tool
Contact with auger
Contact with axe
Contact with chisel
Contact with handsaw
Contact with screwdriver

W27.1 Contact with garden tool
Contact with hoe
Contact with nonpowered lawn mower
Contact with pitchfork
Contact with rake

W27.2 Contact with scissors

W27.3 Contact with needle (sewing)
EXCLUDES 1 *contact with hypodermic needle (W46.-)*

W27.4 Contact with kitchen utensil
Contact with fork
Contact with ice-pick
Contact with can-opener NOS

W27.5 Contact with paper-cutter

W27.8 Contact with other nonpowered hand tool
Contact with nonpowered sewing machine
Contact with shovel

W28 Contact with powered lawn mower
Powered lawn mower (commercial) (residential)
EXCLUDES 1 *contact with nonpowered lawn mower (W27.1)*
EXCLUDES 2 *exposure to electric current (W86.-)*

W29 Contact with other powered hand tools and household machinery
EXCLUDES 1 *contact with commercial machinery (W31.82)*
contact with hot household appliance (X15)
contact with nonpowered hand tool (W27.-)
exposure to electric current (W86)

W29.0 Contact with powered kitchen appliance
Contact with blender
Contact with can-opener
Contact with garbage disposal
Contact with mixer

W29.1 Contact with electric knife

W29.2 Contact with other powered household machinery
Contact with electric fan
Contact with powered dryer (clothes) (powered) (spin)
Contact with washing-machine
Contact with sewing machine

W29.3 Contact with powered garden and outdoor hand tools and machinery
Contact with chainsaw
Contact with edger
Contact with garden cultivator (tiller)
Contact with hedge trimmer
Contact with other powered garden tool
EXCLUDES 1 *contact with powered lawn mower (W28)*

W29.4 Contact with nail gun

W29.8 Contact with other powered hand tools and household machinery
Contact with do-it-yourself tool NOS

W30 Contact with agricultural machinery
INCLUDES animal-powered farm machine
EXCLUDES 1 *agricultural transport vehicle accident (V01-V99)*
explosion of grain store (W40.8)
exposure to electric current (W86.-)

W30.0 Contact with combine harvester
Contact with reaper
Contact with thresher

W30.1 Contact with power take-off devices (PTO)

W30.2 Contact with hay derrick

W30.3 Contact with grain storage elevator
EXCLUDES 1 *explosion of grain store (W40.8)*

W30.8 Contact with other specified agricultural machinery

W30.81 Contact with agricultural transport vehicle in stationary use
Contact with agricultural transport vehicle under repair, not on public roadway
EXCLUDES 1 *agricultural transport vehicle accident (V01-V99)*

W30.89 Contact with other specified agricultural machinery

W30.9 Contact with unspecified agricultural machinery
Contact with farm machinery NOS

W31 Contact with other and unspecified machinery
EXCLUDES 1 *contact with agricultural machinery (W30.-)*
contact with machinery in transport under own power or being towed by a vehicle (V01-V99)
exposure to electric current (W86)

W31.0 Contact with mining and earth-drilling machinery
Contact with bore or drill (land) (seabed)
Contact with shaft hoist
Contact with shaft lift
Contact with undercutter

W31.1 Contact with metalworking machines
Contact with abrasive wheel
Contact with forging machine
Contact with lathe
Contact with mechanical shears
Contact with metal drilling machine
Contact with milling machine
Contact with power press
Contact with rolling-mill
Contact with metal sawing machine

W31.2 Contact with powered woodworking and forming machines
Contact with band saw
Contact with bench saw
Contact with circular saw
Contact with molding machine
Contact with overhead plane
Contact with powered saw
Contact with radial saw
Contact with sander
EXCLUDES 1 *nonpowered woodworking tools (W27.0)*

W31.3 Contact with prime movers
Contact with gas turbine
Contact with internal combustion engine
Contact with steam engine
Contact with water driven turbine

W31.8 Contact with other specified machinery

W31.81 Contact with recreational machinery
Contact with roller coaster

W31.82 Contact with other commercial machinery
Contact with commercial electric fan
Contact with commercial kitchen appliances
Contact with commercial powered dryer (clothes) (powered) (spin)
Contact with commercial washing-machine
Contact with commercial sewing machine
EXCLUDES 1 *contact with household machinery (W29.-)*
contact with powered lawn mower (W28)

W31.83 Contact with special construction vehicle in stationary use
Contact with special construction vehicle under repair, not on public roadway
EXCLUDES 1 *special construction vehicle accident (V01-V99)*

W31.89 Contact with other specified machinery

W31.9 Contact with unspecified machinery
Contact with machinery NOS

W32 Accidental handgun discharge and malfunction
INCLUDES accidental discharge and malfunction of gun for single hand use
accidental discharge and malfunction of pistol
accidental discharge and malfunction of revolver
handgun discharge and malfunction NOS
EXCLUDES 1 *accidental airgun discharge and malfunction (W34.010, W34.110)*
accidental BB gun discharge and malfunction (W34.010, W34.110)
accidental pellet gun discharge and malfunction (W34.010, W34.110)
accidental shotgun discharge and malfunction (W33.01, W33.11)
assault by handgun discharge (X93)
handgun discharge involving legal intervention (Y35.0-)
handgun discharge involving military or war operations (Y36.4-)
intentional self-harm by handgun discharge (X72)
Very pistol discharge and malfunction (W34.09, W34.19)

W32.0 Accidental handgun discharge

W32.1 Accidental handgun malfunction
Injury due to explosion of handgun (parts)
Injury due to malfunction of mechanism or component of handgun
Injury due to recoil of handgun
Powder burn from handgun

W33 Accidental rifle, shotgun and larger firearm discharge and malfunction
INCLUDES rifle, shotgun and larger firearm discharge and malfunction NOS
EXCLUDES 1 *accidental airgun discharge and malfunction (W34.010, W34.110)*
accidental BB gun discharge and malfunction (W34.010, W34.110)
accidental handgun discharge and malfunction (W32.-)
accidental pellet gun discharge and malfunction (W34.010, W34.110)
assault by rifle, shotgun and larger firearm discharge (X94)
firearm discharge involving legal intervention (Y35.0-)
firearm discharge involving military or war operations (Y36.4-)
intentional self-harm by rifle, shotgun and larger firearm discharge (X73)

W33.0 Accidental rifle, shotgun and larger firearm discharge

W33.00 Accidental discharge of unspecified larger firearm
Discharge of unspecified larger firearm NOS

W33.01 Accidental discharge of shotgun
Discharge of shotgun NOS

W33.02 Accidental discharge of hunting rifle
Discharge of hunting rifle NOS

W33.03 Accidental discharge of machine gun
Discharge of machine gun NOS

W33.09 Accidental discharge of other larger firearm
Discharge of other larger firearm NOS

W33.1 Accidental rifle, shotgun and larger firearm malfunction
Injury due to explosion of rifle, shotgun and larger firearm (parts)
Injury due to malfunction of mechanism or component of rifle, shotgun and larger firearm
Injury due to piercing, cutting, crushing or pinching due to (by) slide trigger mechanism, scope or other gun part
Injury due to recoil of rifle, shotgun and larger firearm
Powder burn from rifle, shotgun and larger firearm

W33.10 Accidental malfunction of unspecified larger firearm
Malfunction of unspecified larger firearm NOS

W33.11 Accidental malfunction of shotgun
Malfunction of shotgun NOS

W33.12 Accidental malfunction of hunting rifle
Malfunction of hunting rifle NOS

W33.13 Accidental malfunction of machine gun
Malfunction of machine gun NOS

W33.19 Accidental malfunction of other larger firearm
Malfunction of other larger firearm NOS

W34 Accidental discharge and malfunction from other and unspecified firearms and guns

W34.0 Accidental discharge from other and unspecified firearms and guns

W34.00 Accidental discharge from unspecified firearms or gun
Discharge from firearm NOS
Gunshot wound NOS
Shot NOS

W34.01 Accidental discharge of gas, air or spring-operated guns

W34.010 Accidental discharge of airgun
Accidental discharge of BB gun
Accidental discharge of pellet gun

W34.011 Accidental discharge of paintball gun
Accidental injury due to paintball discharge

W34.018 Accidental discharge of other gas, air or spring-operated gun

W34.09 Accidental discharge from other specified firearms
Accidental discharge from Very pistol [flare]

W34.1 Accidental malfunction from other and unspecified firearms and guns

W34.10 Accidental malfunction from unspecified firearms or gun
Firearm malfunction NOS

W34.11 Accidental malfunction of gas, air or spring-operated guns

W34.110 Accidental malfunction of airgun
Accidental malfunction of BB gun
Accidental malfunction of pellet gun

W34.111 Accidental malfunction of paintball gun
Accidental injury due to paintball gun malfunction

W34.118 Accidental malfunction of other gas, air or spring-operated gun

W34.19 Accidental malfunction from other specified firearms
Accidental malfunction from Very pistol [flare]

W35 Explosion and rupture of boiler
EXCLUDES 1 *explosion and rupture of boiler on watercraft (V93.4)*

W36 Explosion and rupture of gas cylinder

W36.1 Explosion and rupture of aerosol can

W36.2 Explosion and rupture of air tank

W36.3 Explosion and rupture of pressurized-gas tank

W36.8 Explosion and rupture of other gas cylinder

W36.9 Explosion and rupture of unspecified gas cylinder

W37 Explosion and rupture of pressurized tire, pipe or hose

W37.0 Explosion of bicycle tire

W37.8 Explosion and rupture of other pressurized tire, pipe or hose

W38 Explosion and rupture of other specified pressurized devices

W39 Discharge of firework

W40 Explosion of other materials
EXCLUDES 1 *assault by explosive material (X96)*
explosion involving legal intervention (Y35.1-)
explosion involving military or war operations (Y36.0-, Y36.2-)
intentional self-harm by explosive material (X75)

W40.0 Explosion of blasting material
Explosion of blasting cap
Explosion of detonator
Explosion of dynamite
Explosion of explosive (any) used in blasting operations

W40.1 Explosion of explosive gases
Explosion of acetylene
Explosion of butane
Explosion of coal gas
Explosion in mine NOS
Explosion of explosive gas
Explosion of fire damp
Explosion of gasoline fumes
Explosion of methane
Explosion of propane

W40.8 Explosion of other specified explosive materials
Explosion in dump NOS
Explosion in factory NOS
Explosion in grain store
Explosion in munitions
EXCLUDES 1 *explosion involving legal intervention (Y35.1-)*
explosion involving military or war operations (Y36.0-, Y36.2-)

W40.9 Explosion of unspecified explosive materials
Explosion NOS

W42 Exposure to noise

W42.0 Exposure to supersonic waves

W42.9 Exposure to other noise
Exposure to sound waves NOS

W45 Foreign body or object entering through skin
INCLUDES foreign body or object embedded in skin
nail embedded in skin
EXCLUDES 2 *contact with hand tools (nonpowered) (powered) (W27-W29)*
contact with other sharp objects (W26.-)
contact with sharp glass (W25.-)
struck by objects (W20-W22)

W45.0 Nail entering through skin

W45.8 Other foreign body or object entering through skin
Splinter in skin NOS

W46 Contact with hypodermic needle

W46.0 Contact with hypodermic needle
Hypodermic needle stick NOS

W46.1 Contact with contaminated hypodermic needle

W49 Exposure to other inanimate mechanical forces
INCLUDES exposure to abnormal gravitational [G] forces
exposure to inanimate mechanical forces NEC
EXCLUDES 1 *exposure to inanimate mechanical forces involving military or war operations (Y36.-, Y37.-)*

W49.0 Item causing external constriction

W49.01 Hair causing external constriction

W49.02 String or thread causing external constriction

W49.03 Rubber band causing external constriction

W49.04 Ring or other jewelry causing external constriction

W49.09 Other specified item causing external constriction

W49.9 Exposure to other inanimate mechanical forces

Exposure to animate mechanical forces (W50-W64)

EXCLUDES 1 *toxic effect of contact with venomous animals and plants (T63.-)*

The appropriate 7th character is to be added to each code from categories W50-W64.
A initial encounter
D subsequent encounter
S sequela

W50 Accidental hit, strike, kick, twist, bite or scratch by another person
INCLUDES hit, strike, kick, twist, bite, or scratch by another person NOS
EXCLUDES 1 *assault by bodily force (Y04)*
struck by objects (W20-W22)

W50.0 Accidental hit or strike by another person
Hit or strike by another person NOS

W50.1 Accidental kick by another person
Kick by another person NOS

W50.2 Accidental twist by another person
Twist by another person NOS

W50.3 Accidental bite by another person
Human bite
Bite by another person NOS

W50.4 Accidental scratch by another person
Scratch by another person NOS

W51 Accidental striking against or bumped into by another person
EXCLUDES 1 *assault by striking against or bumping into by another person (Y04.2)*
fall due to collision with another person (W03)

W52 Crushed, pushed or stepped on by crowd or human stampede
Crushed, pushed or stepped on by crowd or human stampede with or without fall

W53 Contact with rodent
INCLUDES contact with saliva, feces or urine of rodent

W53.0 Contact with mouse
W53.01 Bitten by mouse
W53.09 Other contact with mouse

W53.1 Contact with rat
W53.11 Bitten by rat
W53.19 Other contact with rat

W53.2 Contact with squirrel
W53.21 Bitten by squirrel
W53.29 Other contact with squirrel

W53.8 Contact with other rodent
W53.81 Bitten by other rodent
W53.89 Other contact with other rodent

W54 Contact with dog
INCLUDES contact with saliva, feces or urine of dog

W54.0 Bitten by dog
W54.1 Struck by dog
Knocked over by dog
W54.8 Other contact with dog

W55 Contact with other mammals
INCLUDES contact with saliva, feces or urine of mammal
EXCLUDES 1 *animal being ridden - see transport accidents*
bitten or struck by dog (W54)
bitten or struck by rodent (W53.-)
contact with marine mammals (W56.-)

W55.0 Contact with cat
W55.01 Bitten by cat
W55.03 Scratched by cat
W55.09 Other contact with cat

W55.1 Contact with horse
W55.11 Bitten by horse
W55.12 Struck by horse
W55.19 Other contact with horse

W55.2 Contact with cow
Contact with bull
W55.21 Bitten by cow
W55.22 Struck by cow
Gored by bull
W55.29 Other contact with cow

W55.3 Contact with other hoof stock
Contact with goats
Contact with sheep
W55.31 Bitten by other hoof stock
W55.32 Struck by other hoof stock
Gored by goat
Gored by ram
W55.39 Other contact with other hoof stock

W55.4 Contact with pig
W55.41 Bitten by pig
W55.42 Struck by pig
W55.49 Other contact with pig

W55.5 Contact with raccoon
W55.51 Bitten by raccoon
W55.52 Struck by raccoon
W55.59 Other contact with raccoon

W55.8 Contact with other mammals
W55.81 Bitten by other mammals
W55.82 Struck by other mammals
W55.89 Other contact with other mammals

W56 Contact with nonvenomous marine animal
EXCLUDES 1 *contact with venomous marine animal (T63.-)*

W56.0 Contact with dolphin
W56.01 Bitten by dolphin
W56.02 Struck by dolphin
W56.09 Other contact with dolphin

W56.1 Contact with sea lion
W56.11 Bitten by sea lion
W56.12 Struck by sea lion
W56.19 Other contact with sea lion

W56.2 Contact with orca
Contact with killer whale
W56.21 Bitten by orca
W56.22 Struck by orca
W56.29 Other contact with orca

W56.3 Contact with other marine mammals
W56.31 Bitten by other marine mammals
W56.32 Struck by other marine mammals
W56.39 Other contact with other marine mammals

W56.4 Contact with shark
W56.41 Bitten by shark
W56.42 Struck by shark
W56.49 Other contact with shark

W56.5 Contact with other fish
W56.51 Bitten by other fish
W56.52 Struck by other fish
W56.59 Other contact with other fish

W56.8 Contact with other nonvenomous marine animals
W56.81 Bitten by other nonvenomous marine animals
W56.82 Struck by other nonvenomous marine animals
W56.89 Other contact with other nonvenomous marine animals

W57 Bitten or stung by nonvenomous insect and other nonvenomous arthropods
EXCLUDES 1 *contact with venomous insects and arthropods (T63.2-, T63.3-, T63.4-)*

W58 Contact with crocodile or alligator

W58.0 Contact with alligator
W58.01 Bitten by alligator
W58.02 Struck by alligator
W58.03 Crushed by alligator
W58.09 Other contact with alligator

W58.1 Contact with crocodile
W58.11 Bitten by crocodile
W58.12 Struck by crocodile
W58.13 Crushed by crocodile
W58.19 Other contact with crocodile

W59 Contact with other nonvenomous reptiles
EXCLUDES 1 *contact with venomous reptile (T63.0-, T63.1-)*

W59.0 Contact with nonvenomous lizards
W59.01 Bitten by nonvenomous lizards
W59.02 Struck by nonvenomous lizards
W59.09 Other contact with nonvenomous lizards
Exposure to nonvenomous lizards

W59.1 Contact with nonvenomous snakes
W59.11 Bitten by nonvenomous snake
W59.12 Struck by nonvenomous snake
W59.13 Crushed by nonvenomous snake
W59.19 Other contact with nonvenomous snake

5th **W59.2 Contact with turtles**
EXCLUDES 1 *contact with tortoises (W59.8-)*
√x7th **W59.21 Bitten by turtle**
√x7th **W59.22 Struck by turtle**
√x7th **W59.29 Other contact with turtle**
Exposure to turtles
5th **W59.8 Contact with other nonvenomous reptiles**
√x7th **W59.81 Bitten by other nonvenomous reptiles**
√x7th **W59.82 Struck by other nonvenomous reptiles**
√x7th **W59.83 Crushed by other nonvenomous reptiles**
√x7th **W59.89 Other contact with other nonvenomous reptiles**

√x7th **W60 Contact with nonvenomous plant thorns and spines and sharp leaves**
EXCLUDES 1 *contact with venomous plants (T63.7-)*

4th **W61 Contact with birds (domestic) (wild)**
INCLUDES contact with excreta of birds
5th **W61.0 Contact with parrot**
√x7th **W61.01 Bitten by parrot**
√x7th **W61.02 Struck by parrot**
√x7th **W61.09 Other contact with parrot**
Exposure to parrots
5th **W61.1 Contact with macaw**
√x7th **W61.11 Bitten by macaw**
√x7th **W61.12 Struck by macaw**
√x7th **W61.19 Other contact with macaw**
Exposure to macaws
5th **W61.2 Contact with other psittacines**
√x7th **W61.21 Bitten by other psittacines**
√x7th **W61.22 Struck by other psittacines**
√x7th **W61.29 Other contact with other psittacines**
Exposure to other psittacines
5th **W61.3 Contact with chicken**
√x7th **W61.32 Struck by chicken**
√x7th **W61.33 Pecked by chicken**
√x7th **W61.39 Other contact with chicken**
Exposure to chickens
5th **W61.4 Contact with turkey**
√x7th **W61.42 Struck by turkey**
√x7th **W61.43 Pecked by turkey**
√x7th **W61.49 Other contact with turkey**
5th **W61.5 Contact with goose**
√x7th **W61.51 Bitten by goose**
√x7th **W61.52 Struck by goose**
√x7th **W61.59 Other contact with goose**
5th **W61.6 Contact with duck**
√x7th **W61.61 Bitten by duck**
√x7th **W61.62 Struck by duck**
√x7th **W61.69 Other contact with duck**
5th **W61.9 Contact with other birds**
√x7th **W61.91 Bitten by other birds**
√x7th **W61.92 Struck by other birds**
√x7th **W61.99 Other contact with other birds**
Contact with bird NOS

4th **W62 Contact with nonvenomous amphibians**
EXCLUDES 1 *contact with venomous amphibians (T63.81-R63.83)*
√x7th **W62.0 Contact with nonvenomous frogs**
√x7th **W62.1 Contact with nonvenomous toads**
√x7th **W62.9 Contact with other nonvenomous amphibians**

√x7th **W64 Exposure to other animate mechanical forces**
INCLUDES exposure to nonvenomous animal NOS
EXCLUDES 1 *contact with venomous animal (T63.-)*

Accidental non-transport drowning and submersion (W65-W74)

EXCLUDES 1 *accidental drowning and submersion due to fall into water (W16.-)*
accidental drowning and submersion due to water transport accident (V90.-, V92.-)
EXCLUDES 2 *accidental drowning and submersion due to cataclysm (X34-X39)*

The appropriate 7th character is to be added to each code from categories W65-W74.
A initial encounter
D subsequent encounter
S sequela

√x7th **W65 Accidental drowning and submersion while in bath-tub**
EXCLUDES 1 *accidental drowning and submersion due to fall in (into) bathtub (W16.211)*

√x7th **W67 Accidental drowning and submersion while in swimming-pool**
EXCLUDES 1 *accidental drowning and submersion due to fall into swimming pool (W16.011, W16.021, W16.031)*
accidental drowning and submersion due to striking into wall of swimming pool (W22.041)

√x7th **W69 Accidental drowning and submersion while in natural water**
Accidental drowning and submersion while in lake
Accidental drowning and submersion while in open sea
Accidental drowning and submersion while in river
Accidental drowning and submersion while in stream
EXCLUDES 1 *accidental drowning and submersion due to fall into natural body of water (W16.111, W16.121, W16.131)*

√x7th **W73 Other specified cause of accidental non-transport drowning and submersion**
Accidental drowning and submersion while in quenching tank
Accidental drowning and submersion while in reservoir
EXCLUDES 1 *accidental drowning and submersion due to fall into other water (W16.311, W16.321, W16.331)*

√x7th **W74 Unspecified cause of accidental drowning and submersion**
Drowning NOS

Exposure to electric current, radiation and extreme ambient air temperature and pressure (W85-W99)

EXCLUDES 1 *exposure to:*
failure in dosage of radiation or temperature during surgical and medical care (Y63.2-Y63.5)
lightning (T75.0-)
natural cold (X31)
natural heat (X30)
natural radiation NOS (X39)
radiological procedure and radiotherapy (Y84.2)
sunlight (X32)

AHA: 2018,2Q,7-8

The appropriate 7th character is to be added to each code from categories W85-W99.
A initial encounter
D subsequent encounter
S sequela

√x7th **W85 Exposure to electric transmission lines**
Broken power line

4th **W86 Exposure to other specified electric current**
√x7th **W86.0 Exposure to domestic wiring and appliances**
√x7th **W86.1 Exposure to industrial wiring, appliances and electrical machinery**
Exposure to conductors
Exposure to control apparatus
Exposure to electrical equipment and machinery
Exposure to transformers
√x7th **W86.8 Exposure to other electric current**
Exposure to wiring and appliances in or on farm (not farmhouse)
Exposure to wiring and appliances outdoors
Exposure to wiring and appliances in or on public building
Exposure to wiring and appliances in or on residential institutions
Exposure to wiring and appliances in or on schools

4th **W88 Exposure to ionizing radiation**
EXCLUDES 1 *exposure to sunlight (X32)*
√x7th **W88.0 Exposure to X-rays**
√x7th **W88.1 Exposure to radioactive isotopes**

√x7th W88.8 **Exposure to other ionizing radiation**

√4th **W89 Exposure to man-made visible and ultraviolet light**

INCLUDES exposure to welding light (arc)

EXCLUDES 2 *exposure to sunlight (X32)*

√x7th W89.Ø **Exposure to welding light (arc)**

√x7th W89.1 **Exposure to tanning bed**

√x7th W89.8 **Exposure to other man-made visible and ultraviolet light**

√x7th W89.9 **Exposure to unspecified man-made visible and ultraviolet light**

√4th **W9Ø Exposure to other nonionizing radiation**

EXCLUDES 2 *exposure to sunlight (X32)*

AHA: 2019,1Q,21

√x7th W9Ø.Ø **Exposure to radiofrequency**

√x7th W9Ø.1 **Exposure to infrared radiation**

√x7th W9Ø.2 **Exposure to laser radiation**

√x7th W9Ø.8 **Exposure to other nonionizing radiation**

√x7th **W92 Exposure to excessive heat of man-made origin**

√4th **W93 Exposure to excessive cold of man-made origin**

√5th W93.Ø **Contact with or inhalation of dry ice**

√x7th W93.Ø1 **Contact with dry ice**

√x7th W93.Ø2 **Inhalation of dry ice**

√5th W93.1 **Contact with or inhalation of liquid air**

√x7th W93.11 **Contact with liquid air**

Contact with liquid hydrogen
Contact with liquid nitrogen

√x7th W93.12 **Inhalation of liquid air**

Inhalation of liquid hydrogen
Inhalation of liquid nitrogen

√x7th W93.2 **Prolonged exposure in deep freeze unit or refrigerator**

√x7th W93.8 **Exposure to other excessive cold of man-made origin**

√4th **W94 Exposure to high and low air pressure and changes in air pressure**

√x7th W94.Ø **Exposure to prolonged high air pressure**

√5th W94.1 **Exposure to prolonged low air pressure**

√x7th W94.11 **Exposure to residence or prolonged visit at high altitude**

√x7th W94.12 **Exposure to other prolonged low air pressure**

√5th W94.2 **Exposure to rapid changes in air pressure during ascent**

√x7th W94.21 **Exposure to reduction in atmospheric pressure while surfacing from deep-water diving**

√x7th W94.22 **Exposure to reduction in atmospheric pressure while surfacing from underground**

√x7th W94.23 **Exposure to sudden change in air pressure in aircraft during ascent**

√x7th W94.29 **Exposure to other rapid changes in air pressure during ascent**

√5th W94.3 **Exposure to rapid changes in air pressure during descent**

√x7th W94.31 **Exposure to sudden change in air pressure in aircraft during descent**

√x7th W94.32 **Exposure to high air pressure from rapid descent in water**

√x7th W94.39 **Exposure to other rapid changes in air pressure during descent**

√x7th **W99 Exposure to other man-made environmental factors**

Exposure to smoke, fire and flames (XØØ-XØ8)

EXCLUDES 1 *arson (X97)*

EXCLUDES 2 *explosions (W35-W4Ø)*
lightning (T75.Ø-)
transport accident (VØ1-V99)

AHA: 2018,2Q,7-8

The appropriate 7th character is to be added to each code from categories XØØ-XØ8.
A initial encounter
D subsequent encounter
S sequela

√4th **XØØ Exposure to uncontrolled fire in building or structure**

INCLUDES conflagration in building or structure

Code first any associated cataclysm

EXCLUDES 2 *exposure to ignition or melting of nightwear (XØ5)*
exposure to ignition or melting of other clothing and apparel (XØ6.-)
exposure to other specified smoke, fire and flames (XØ8.-)

AHA: 2016,2Q,5

√x7th XØØ.Ø **Exposure to flames in uncontrolled fire in building or structure**

√x7th XØØ.1 **Exposure to smoke in uncontrolled fire in building or structure**

√x7th XØØ.2 **Injury due to collapse of burning building or structure in uncontrolled fire**

EXCLUDES 1 *injury due to collapse of building not on fire (W2Ø.1)*

√x7th XØØ.3 **Fall from burning building or structure in uncontrolled fire**

√x7th XØØ.4 **Hit by object from burning building or structure in uncontrolled fire**

AHA: 2016,2Q,4

√x7th XØØ.5 **Jump from burning building or structure in uncontrolled fire**

√x7th XØØ.8 **Other exposure to uncontrolled fire in building or structure**

√4th **XØ1 Exposure to uncontrolled fire, not in building or structure**

INCLUDES exposure to forest fire

√x7th XØ1.Ø **Exposure to flames in uncontrolled fire, not in building or structure**

√x7th XØ1.1 **Exposure to smoke in uncontrolled fire, not in building or structure**

√x7th XØ1.3 **Fall due to uncontrolled fire, not in building or structure**

√x7th XØ1.4 **Hit by object due to uncontrolled fire, not in building or structure**

√x7th XØ1.8 **Other exposure to uncontrolled fire, not in building or structure**

√4th **XØ2 Exposure to controlled fire in building or structure**

INCLUDES exposure to fire in fireplace
exposure to fire in stove

√x7th XØ2.Ø **Exposure to flames in controlled fire in building or structure**

√x7th XØ2.1 **Exposure to smoke in controlled fire in building or structure**

√x7th XØ2.2 **Injury due to collapse of burning building or structure in controlled fire**

EXCLUDES 1 *injury due to collapse of building not on fire (W2Ø.1)*

√x7th XØ2.3 **Fall from burning building or structure in controlled fire**

√x7th XØ2.4 **Hit by object from burning building or structure in controlled fire**

√x7th XØ2.5 **Jump from burning building or structure in controlled fire**

√x7th XØ2.8 **Other exposure to controlled fire in building or structure**

√4th **XØ3 Exposure to controlled fire, not in building or structure**

INCLUDES exposure to bon fire
exposure to camp-fire
exposure to trash fire

√x7th XØ3.Ø **Exposure to flames in controlled fire, not in building or structure**

√x7th XØ3.1 **Exposure to smoke in controlled fire, not in building or structure**

√x7th XØ3.3 **Fall due to controlled fire, not in building or structure**

√x7th XØ3.4 **Hit by object due to controlled fire, not in building or structure**

√x7th XØ3.8 **Other exposure to controlled fire, not in building or structure**

X04 Exposure to ignition of highly flammable material
Exposure to ignition of gasoline
Exposure to ignition of kerosene
Exposure to ignition of petrol
EXCLUDES 2 *exposure to ignition or melting of nightwear (X05)*
exposure to ignition or melting of other clothing and apparel (X06)
AHA: 2016,2Q,4

X05 Exposure to ignition or melting of nightwear
EXCLUDES 2 *exposure to uncontrolled fire in building or structure (X00.-)*
exposure to uncontrolled fire, not in building or structure (X01.-)
exposure to controlled fire in building or structure (X02.-)
exposure to controlled fire, not in building or structure (X03.-)
exposure to ignition of highly flammable materials (X04.-)

X06 Exposure to ignition or melting of other clothing and apparel
EXCLUDES 2 *exposure to uncontrolled fire in building or structure (X00.-)*
exposure to uncontrolled fire, not in building or structure (X01.-)
exposure to controlled fire in building or structure (X02.-)
exposure to controlled fire, not in building or structure (X03.-)
exposure to ignition of highly flammable materials (X04.-)

X06.0 Exposure to ignition of plastic jewelry
X06.1 Exposure to melting of plastic jewelry
X06.2 Exposure to ignition of other clothing and apparel
X06.3 Exposure to melting of other clothing and apparel

X08 Exposure to other specified smoke, fire and flames
X08.0 Exposure to bed fire
Exposure to mattress fire
X08.00 Exposure to bed fire due to unspecified burning material
X08.01 Exposure to bed fire due to burning cigarette
X08.09 Exposure to bed fire due to other burning material
X08.1 Exposure to sofa fire
X08.10 Exposure to sofa fire due to unspecified burning material
X08.11 Exposure to sofa fire due to burning cigarette
X08.19 Exposure to sofa fire due to other burning material
X08.2 Exposure to other furniture fire
X08.20 Exposure to other furniture fire due to unspecified burning material
X08.21 Exposure to other furniture fire due to burning cigarette
X08.29 Exposure to other furniture fire due to other burning material
X08.8 Exposure to other specified smoke, fire and flames

Contact with heat and hot substances (X10-X19)

EXCLUDES 1 *exposure to excessive natural heat (X30)*
exposure to fire and flames (X00-X08)
AHA: 2018,2Q,7-8

The appropriate 7th character is to be added to each code from categories X10-X19.
A initial encounter
D subsequent encounter
S sequela

X10 Contact with hot drinks, food, fats and cooking oils
X10.0 Contact with hot drinks
X10.1 Contact with hot food
X10.2 Contact with fats and cooking oils

X11 Contact with hot tap-water
INCLUDES contact with boiling tap-water
contact with boiling water NOS
EXCLUDES 1 *contact with water heated on stove (X12)*
X11.0 Contact with hot water in bath or tub
EXCLUDES 1 *contact with running hot water in bath or tub (X11.1)*
X11.1 Contact with running hot water
Contact with hot water running out of hose
Contact with hot water running out of tap
X11.8 Contact with other hot tap-water
Contact with hot water in bucket
Contact with hot tap-water NOS

X12 Contact with other hot fluids
Contact with water heated on stove
EXCLUDES 1 *hot (liquid) metals (X18)*

X13 Contact with steam and other hot vapors
X13.0 Inhalation of steam and other hot vapors
X13.1 Other contact with steam and other hot vapors

X14 Contact with hot air and other hot gases
X14.0 Inhalation of hot air and gases
X14.1 Other contact with hot air and other hot gases

X15 Contact with hot household appliances
EXCLUDES 1 *contact with heating appliances (X16)*
contact with powered household appliances (W29.-)
exposure to controlled fire in building or structure due to household appliance (X02.8)
exposure to household appliances electrical current (W86.0)
X15.0 Contact with hot stove (kitchen)
X15.1 Contact with hot toaster
X15.2 Contact with hotplate
X15.3 Contact with hot saucepan or skillet
▶Contact with hot cooking pan◀
▶Contact with hot cooking pot◀
X15.8 Contact with other hot household appliances
Contact with cooker
Contact with kettle
Contact with light bulbs

X16 Contact with hot heating appliances, radiators and pipes
EXCLUDES 1 *contact with powered appliances (W29.-)*
exposure to controlled fire in building or structure due to appliance (X02.8)
exposure to industrial appliances electrical current (W86.1)

X17 Contact with hot engines, machinery and tools
EXCLUDES 1 *contact with hot heating appliances, radiators and pipes (X16)*
contact with hot household appliances (X15)

X18 Contact with other hot metals
Contact with liquid metal

X19 Contact with other heat and hot substances
EXCLUDES 1 *objects that are not normally hot, e.g., an object made hot by a house fire (X00-X08)*

Exposure to forces of nature (X30-X39)

AHA: 2018,2Q,7-8

The appropriate 7th character is to be added to each code from categories X30-X39.
A initial encounter
D subsequent encounter
S sequela

X30 Exposure to excessive natural heat
Exposure to excessive heat as the cause of sunstroke
Exposure to heat NOS
EXCLUDES 1 *excessive heat of man-made origin (W92)*
exposure to man-made radiation (W89)
exposure to sunlight (X32)
exposure to tanning bed (W89)

X31 Exposure to excessive natural cold
Excessive cold as the cause of chilblains NOS
Excessive cold as the cause of immersion foot or hand
Exposure to cold NOS
Exposure to weather conditions
EXCLUDES 1 *cold of man-made origin (W93.-)*
contact with or inhalation of dry ice (W93.-)
contact with or inhalation of liquefied gas (W93.-)

X32 Exposure to sunlight
EXCLUDES 1 *man-made radiation (tanning bed) (W89)*
EXCLUDES 2 *radiation-related disorders of the skin and subcutaneous tissue (L55-L59)*

X34 Earthquake

EXCLUDES 2 *tidal wave (tsunami) due to earthquake (X37.41)*

X35 Volcanic eruption

EXCLUDES 2 *tidal wave (tsunami) due to volcanic eruption (X37.41)*

X36 Avalanche, landslide and other earth movements

INCLUDES victim of mudslide of cataclysmic nature

EXCLUDES 1 *earthquake (X34)*

EXCLUDES 2 *transport accident involving collision with avalanche or landslide not in motion (V01-V99)*

X36.0 Collapse of dam or man-made structure causing earth movement

X36.1 Avalanche, landslide, or mudslide

X37 Cataclysmic storm

X37.0 Hurricane

Storm surge
Typhoon

X37.1 Tornado

Cyclone
Twister

X37.2 Blizzard (snow)(ice)

X37.3 Dust storm

X37.4 Tidalwave

X37.41 Tidal wave due to earthquake or volcanic eruption

Tidal wave NOS
Tsunami

X37.42 Tidal wave due to storm

X37.43 Tidal wave due to landslide

X37.8 Other cataclysmic storms

Cloudburst
Torrential rain

EXCLUDES 2 *flood (X38)*

X37.9 Unspecified cataclysmic storm

Storm NOS

EXCLUDES 1 *collapse of dam or man-made structure causing earth movement (X36.0)*

X38 Flood

Flood arising from remote storm
Flood of cataclysmic nature arising from melting snow
Flood resulting directly from storm

EXCLUDES 1 *collapse of dam or man-made structure causing earth movement (X36.0)*
tidal wave NOS (X37.41)
tidal wave caused by storm (X37.42)

X39 Exposure to other forces of nature

X39.0 Exposure to natural radiation

EXCLUDES 1 *contact with and (suspected) exposure to radon and other naturally occurring radiation (Z77.123)*
exposure to man-made radiation (W88-W90)
exposure to sunlight (X32)

X39.01 Exposure to radon

X39.08 Exposure to other natural radiation

X39.8 Other exposure to forces of nature

Overexertion and strenuous or repetitive movements (X50)

X50 Overexertion and strenuous or repetitive movements

AHA: 2018,2Q,7-8; 2016,4Q,73-74

The appropriate 7th character is to be added to each code from category X50.
A initial encounter
D subsequent encounter
S sequela

X50.0 Overexertion from strenuous movement or load

Lifting heavy objects
Lifting weights

X50.1 Overexertion from prolonged static or awkward postures

Prolonged bending
Prolonged kneeling
Prolonged reaching
Prolonged sitting
Prolonged standing
Prolonged twisting
Static bending
Static kneeling
Static reaching
Static sitting
Static standing
Static twisting

X50.3 Overexertion from repetitive movements

Use of hand as hammer

EXCLUDES 2 *overuse from prolonged static or awkward postures (X50.1)*

X50.9 Other and unspecified overexertion or strenuous movements or postures

Contact pressure
Contact stress

Accidental exposure to other specified factors (X52-X58)

AHA: 2018,2Q,7-8

The appropriate 7th character is to be added to each code from categories X52-X58.
A initial encounter
D subsequent encounter
S sequela

X52 Prolonged stay in weightless environment

Weightlessness in spacecraft (simulator)

X58 Exposure to other specified factors

Accident NOS
Exposure NOS

Intentional self-harm (X71-X83)

Purposely self-inflicted injury
Suicide (attempted)

The appropriate 7th character is to be added to each code from categories X71-X83.
A initial encounter
D subsequent encounter
S sequela

X71 Intentional self-harm by drowning and submersion

X71.0 Intentional self-harm by drowning and submersion while in bathtub HCC

X71.1 Intentional self-harm by drowning and submersion while in swimming pool HCC

X71.2 Intentional self-harm by drowning and submersion after jump into swimming pool HCC

X71.3 Intentional self-harm by drowning and submersion in natural water HCC

X71.8 Other intentional self-harm by drowning and submersion HCC

X71.9 Intentional self-harm by drowning and submersion, unspecified HCC

X72 Intentional self-harm by handgun discharge HCC

Intentional self-harm by gun for single hand use
Intentional self-harm by pistol
Intentional self-harm by revolver

EXCLUDES 1 *Very pistol (X74.8)*

X73 Intentional self-harm by rifle, shotgun and larger firearm discharge

EXCLUDES 1 *airgun (X74.01)*

X73.0 Intentional self-harm by shotgun discharge HCC

X73.1 Intentional self-harm by hunting rifle discharge HCC

X73.2 Intentional self-harm by machine gun discharge HCC

X73.8 Intentional self-harm by other larger firearm discharge HCC

X73.9 Intentional self-harm by unspecified larger firearm discharge HCC

X74 Intentional self-harm by other and unspecified firearm and gun discharge

X74.0 Intentional self-harm by gas, air or spring-operated guns

X74.01 Intentional self-harm by airgun HCC
Intentional self-harm by BB gun discharge
Intentional self-harm by pellet gun discharge

X74.02 Intentional self-harm by paintball gun HCC

X74.09 Intentional self-harm by other gas, air or spring-operated gun HCC

X74.8 Intentional self-harm by other firearm discharge HCC
Intentional self-harm by Very pistol [flare] discharge

X74.9 Intentional self-harm by unspecified firearm discharge HCC

X75 Intentional self-harm by explosive material HCC

X76 Intentional self-harm by smoke, fire and flames HCC

X77 Intentional self-harm by steam, hot vapors and hot objects

X77.0 Intentional self-harm by steam or hot vapors HCC

X77.1 Intentional self-harm by hot tap water HCC

X77.2 Intentional self-harm by other hot fluids HCC

X77.3 Intentional self-harm by hot household appliances HCC

X77.8 Intentional self-harm by other hot objects HCC

X77.9 Intentional self-harm by unspecified hot objects HCC

X78 Intentional self-harm by sharp object

X78.0 Intentional self-harm by sharp glass HCC

X78.1 Intentional self-harm by knife HCC

X78.2 Intentional self-harm by sword or dagger HCC

X78.8 Intentional self-harm by other sharp object HCC
AHA: 2022,1Q,27

X78.9 Intentional self-harm by unspecified sharp object HCC

X79 Intentional self-harm by blunt object HCC

X80 Intentional self-harm by jumping from a high place HCC
Intentional fall from one level to another

X81 Intentional self-harm by jumping or lying in front of moving object

X81.0 Intentional self-harm by jumping or lying in front of motor vehicle HCC

X81.1 Intentional self-harm by jumping or lying in front of (subway) train HCC

X81.8 Intentional self-harm by jumping or lying in front of other moving object HCC

X82 Intentional self-harm by crashing of motor vehicle

X82.0 Intentional collision of motor vehicle with other motor vehicle HCC

X82.1 Intentional collision of motor vehicle with train HCC

X82.2 Intentional collision of motor vehicle with tree HCC

X82.8 Other intentional self-harm by crashing of motor vehicle HCC

X83 Intentional self-harm by other specified means
EXCLUDES 1 *intentional self-harm by poisoning or contact with toxic substance - see Table of Drugs and Chemicals*

X83.0 Intentional self-harm by crashing of aircraft HCC

X83.1 Intentional self-harm by electrocution HCC

X83.2 Intentional self-harm by exposure to extremes of cold HCC

X83.8 Intentional self-harm by other specified means HCC

Assault (X92-Y09)

INCLUDES homicide
injuries inflicted by another person with intent to injure or kill, by any means

EXCLUDES 1 *injuries due to legal intervention (Y35.-)*
injuries due to operations of war (Y36.-)
injuries due to terrorism (Y38.-)

The appropriate 7th character is to be added to each code from categories X92-Y04 and Y08.
A initial encounter
D subsequent encounter
S sequela

X92 Assault by drowning and submersion

X92.0 Assault by drowning and submersion while in bathtub

X92.1 Assault by drowning and submersion while in swimming pool

X92.2 Assault by drowning and submersion after push into swimming pool

X92.3 Assault by drowning and submersion in natural water

X92.8 Other assault by drowning and submersion

X92.9 Assault by drowning and submersion, unspecified

X93 Assault by handgun discharge
Assault by discharge of gun for single hand use
Assault by discharge of pistol
Assault by discharge of revolver
EXCLUDES 1 *Very pistol (X95.8)*

X94 Assault by rifle, shotgun and larger firearm discharge
EXCLUDES 1 *airgun (X95.01)*

X94.0 Assault by shotgun

X94.1 Assault by hunting rifle

X94.2 Assault by machine gun

X94.8 Assault by other larger firearm discharge

X94.9 Assault by unspecified larger firearm discharge

X95 Assault by other and unspecified firearm and gun discharge

X95.0 Assault by gas, air or spring-operated guns

X95.01 Assault by airgun discharge
Assault by BB gun discharge
Assault by pellet gun discharge

X95.02 Assault by paintball gun discharge

X95.09 Assault by other gas, air or spring-operated gun

X95.8 Assault by other firearm discharge
Assault by Very pistol [flare] discharge

X95.9 Assault by unspecified firearm discharge

X96 Assault by explosive material
EXCLUDES 1 *incendiary device (X97)*
terrorism involving explosive material (Y38.2-)

X96.0 Assault by antipersonnel bomb
EXCLUDES 1 *antipersonnel bomb use in military or war (Y36.2-)*

X96.1 Assault by gasoline bomb

X96.2 Assault by letter bomb

X96.3 Assault by fertilizer bomb

X96.4 Assault by pipe bomb

X96.8 Assault by other specified explosive

X96.9 Assault by unspecified explosive

X97 Assault by smoke, fire and flames
Assault by arson
Assault by cigarettes
Assault by incendiary device

X98 Assault by steam, hot vapors and hot objects

X98.0 Assault by steam or hot vapors

X98.1 Assault by hot tap water

X98.2 Assault by hot fluids

X98.3 Assault by hot household appliances

X98.8 Assault by other hot objects

X98.9 Assault by unspecified hot objects

X99 Assault by sharp object
EXCLUDES 1 *assault by strike by sports equipment (Y08.0-)*

X99.0 Assault by sharp glass

X99.1 Assault by knife

X99.2 Assault by sword or dagger

X99.8 Assault by other sharp object

X99.9 Assault by unspecified sharp object
Assault by stabbing NOS

Y00 Assault by blunt object
EXCLUDES 1 *assault by strike by sports equipment (Y08.0-)*

Y01 Assault by pushing from high place

Y02 Assault by pushing or placing victim in front of moving object

Y02.0 Assault by pushing or placing victim in front of motor vehicle

Y02.1 Assault by pushing or placing victim in front of (subway) train

Y02.8 Assault by pushing or placing victim in front of other moving object

Y03 Assault by crashing of motor vehicle

Y03.0 Assault by being hit or run over by motor vehicle

Y03.8 Other assault by crashing of motor vehicle

Y04 Assault by bodily force

EXCLUDES 1 *assault by:*
submersion (X92.-)
use of weapon (X93-X95, X99, Y00)

Y04.0 Assault by unarmed brawl or fight

Y04.1 Assault by human bite

Y04.2 Assault by strike against or bumped into by another person

Y04.8 Assault by other bodily force

Assault by bodily force NOS

Y07 Perpetrator of assault, maltreatment and neglect

NOTE Codes from this category are for use only in cases of confirmed abuse (T74.-)

Selection of the correct perpetrator code is based on the relationship between the perpetrator and the victim

INCLUDES perpetrator of abandonment
perpetrator of emotional neglect
perpetrator of mental cruelty
perpetrator of physical abuse
perpetrator of physical neglect
perpetrator of sexual abuse
perpetrator of torture

Y07.0 Spouse or partner, perpetrator of maltreatment and neglect

Spouse or partner, perpetrator of maltreatment and neglect against spouse or partner

Y07.01 Husband, perpetrator of maltreatment and neglect

Y07.02 Wife, perpetrator of maltreatment and neglect

Y07.03 Male partner, perpetrator of maltreatment and neglect

Y07.04 Female partner, perpetrator of maltreatment and neglect

Y07.1 Parent (adoptive) (biological), perpetrator of maltreatment and neglect

Y07.11 Biological father, perpetrator of maltreatment and neglect

Y07.12 Biological mother, perpetrator of maltreatment and neglect

Y07.13 Adoptive father, perpetrator of maltreatment and neglect

Y07.14 Adoptive mother, perpetrator of maltreatment and neglect

Y07.4 Other family member, perpetrator of maltreatment and neglect

Y07.41 Sibling, perpetrator of maltreatment and neglect

EXCLUDES 1 *stepsibling, perpetrator of maltreatment and neglect (Y07.435, Y07.436)*

Y07.410 Brother, perpetrator of maltreatment and neglect

Y07.411 Sister, perpetrator of maltreatment and neglect

Y07.42 Foster parent, perpetrator of maltreatment and neglect

Y07.420 Foster father, perpetrator of maltreatment and neglect

Y07.421 Foster mother, perpetrator of maltreatment and neglect

Y07.43 Stepparent or stepsibling, perpetrator of maltreatment and neglect

Y07.430 Stepfather, perpetrator of maltreatment and neglect

Y07.432 Male friend of parent (co-residing in household), perpetrator of maltreatment and neglect

Y07.433 Stepmother, perpetrator of maltreatment and neglect

Y07.434 Female friend of parent (co-residing in household), perpetrator of maltreatment and neglect

Y07.435 Stepbrother, perpetrator or maltreatment and neglect

Y07.436 Stepsister, perpetrator of maltreatment and neglect

Y07.49 Other family member, perpetrator of maltreatment and neglect

Y07.490 Male cousin, perpetrator of maltreatment and neglect

Y07.491 Female cousin, perpetrator of maltreatment and neglect

Y07.499 Other family member, perpetrator of maltreatment and neglect

Y07.5 Non-family member, perpetrator of maltreatment and neglect

Y07.50 Unspecified non-family member, perpetrator of maltreatment and neglect

Y07.51 Daycare provider, perpetrator of maltreatment and neglect

Y07.510 At-home childcare provider, perpetrator of maltreatment and neglect

Y07.511 Daycare center childcare provider, perpetrator of maltreatment and neglect

Y07.512 At-home adultcare provider, perpetrator of maltreatment and neglect

Y07.513 Adultcare center provider, perpetrator of maltreatment and neglect

Y07.519 Unspecified daycare provider, perpetrator of maltreatment and neglect

Y07.52 Healthcare provider, perpetrator of maltreatment and neglect

Y07.521 Mental health provider, perpetrator of maltreatment and neglect

Y07.528 Other therapist or healthcare provider, perpetrator of maltreatment and neglect

Nurse perpetrator of maltreatment and neglect
Occupational therapist perpetrator of maltreatment and neglect
Physical therapist perpetrator of maltreatment and neglect
Speech therapist perpetrator of maltreatment and neglect

Y07.529 Unspecified healthcare provider, perpetrator of maltreatment and neglect

Y07.53 Teacher or instructor, perpetrator of maltreatment and neglect

Coach, perpetrator of maltreatment and neglect

Y07.59 Other non-family member, perpetrator of maltreatment and neglect

Y07.6 Multiple perpetrators of maltreatment and neglect

AHA: 2018,4Q,32

Y07.9 Unspecified perpetrator of maltreatment and neglect

Y08 Assault by other specified means

Y08.0 Assault by strike by sport equipment

Y08.01 Assault by strike by hockey stick

Y08.02 Assault by strike by baseball bat

Y08.09 Assault by strike by other specified type of sport equipment

Y08.8 Assault by other specified means

Y08.81 Assault by crashing of aircraft

Y08.89 Assault by other specified means

Y09 Assault by unspecified means

Assassination (attempted) NOS
Homicide (attempted) NOS
Manslaughter (attempted) NOS
Murder (attempted) NOS

Event of undetermined intent (Y21-Y33)

Undetermined intent is only for use when there is specific documentation in the record that the intent of the injury cannot be determined. If no such documentation is present, code to accidental (unintentional).

The appropriate 7th character is to be added to each code from categories Y21-Y33.
A initial encounter
D subsequent encounter
S sequela

Y21 Drowning and submersion, undetermined intent

Y21.0 Drowning and submersion while in bathtub, undetermined intent

Y21.1 Drowning and submersion after fall into bathtub, undetermined intent

Y21.2 Drowning and submersion while in swimming pool, undetermined intent

Y21.3 Drowning and submersion after fall into swimming pool, undetermined intent

Y21.4 Drowning and submersion in natural water, undetermined intent

Y21.8 Other drowning and submersion, undetermined intent

Y21.9 Unspecified drowning and submersion, undetermined intent

Y22 Handgun discharge, undetermined intent

Discharge of gun for single hand use, undetermined intent
Discharge of pistol, undetermined intent
Discharge of revolver, undetermined intent

EXCLUDES 2 *Very pistol (Y24.8)*

Y23 Rifle, shotgun and larger firearm discharge, undetermined intent

EXCLUDES 2 *airgun (Y24.0)*

Y23.0 Shotgun discharge, undetermined intent

Y23.1 Hunting rifle discharge, undetermined intent

Y23.2 Military firearm discharge, undetermined intent

Y23.3 Machine gun discharge, undetermined intent

Y23.8 Other larger firearm discharge, undetermined intent

Y23.9 Unspecified larger firearm discharge, undetermined intent

Y24 Other and unspecified firearm discharge, undetermined intent

Y24.0 Airgun discharge, undetermined intent

BB gun discharge, undetermined intent
Pellet gun discharge, undetermined intent

Y24.8 Other firearm discharge, undetermined intent

Paintball gun discharge, undetermined intent
Very pistol [flare] discharge, undetermined intent

Y24.9 Unspecified firearm discharge, undetermined intent

Y25 Contact with explosive material, undetermined intent

Y26 Exposure to smoke, fire and flames, undetermined intent

Y27 Contact with steam, hot vapors and hot objects, undetermined intent

Y27.0 Contact with steam and hot vapors, undetermined intent

Y27.1 Contact with hot tap water, undetermined intent

Y27.2 Contact with hot fluids, undetermined intent

Y27.3 Contact with hot household appliance, undetermined intent

Y27.8 Contact with other hot objects, undetermined intent

Y27.9 Contact with unspecified hot objects, undetermined intent

Y28 Contact with sharp object, undetermined intent

Y28.0 Contact with sharp glass, undetermined intent

Y28.1 Contact with knife, undetermined intent

Y28.2 Contact with sword or dagger, undetermined intent

Y28.8 Contact with other sharp object, undetermined intent

Y28.9 Contact with unspecified sharp object, undetermined intent

Y29 Contact with blunt object, undetermined intent

Y30 Falling, jumping or pushed from a high place, undetermined intent

Victim falling from one level to another, undetermined intent

Y31 Falling, lying or running before or into moving object, undetermined intent

Y32 Crashing of motor vehicle, undetermined intent

Y33 Other specified events, undetermined intent

Legal intervention, operations of war, military operations, and terrorism (Y35-Y38)

The appropriate 7th character is to be added to each code from categories Y35-Y38.
A initial encounter
D subsequent encounter
S sequela

Y35 Legal intervention

INCLUDES any injury sustained as a result of an encounter with any law enforcement official, serving in any capacity at the time of the encounter, whether on-duty or off-duty. Includes injury to law enforcement official, suspect and bystander

AHA: 2019,4Q,18-19

Y35.0 Legal intervention involving firearm discharge

Y35.00 Legal intervention involving unspecified firearm discharge

Legal intervention involving gunshot wound
Legal intervention involving shot NOS

Y35.001 Legal intervention involving unspecified firearm discharge, law enforcement official injured

Y35.002 Legal intervention involving unspecified firearm discharge, bystander injured

Y35.003 Legal intervention involving unspecified firearm discharge, suspect injured

Y35.009 Legal intervention involving unspecified firearm discharge, unspecified person injured

Y35.01 Legal intervention involving injury by machine gun

Y35.011 Legal intervention involving injury by machine gun, law enforcement official injured

Y35.012 Legal intervention involving injury by machine gun, bystander injured

Y35.013 Legal intervention involving injury by machine gun, suspect injured

Y35.019 Legal intervention involving injury by machine gun, unspecified person injured

Y35.02 Legal intervention involving injury by handgun

Y35.021 Legal intervention involving injury by handgun, law enforcement official injured

Y35.022 Legal intervention involving injury by handgun, bystander injured

Y35.023 Legal intervention involving injury by handgun, suspect injured

Y35.029 Legal intervention involving injury by handgun, unspecified person injured

Y35.03 Legal intervention involving injury by rifle pellet

Y35.031 Legal intervention involving injury by rifle pellet, law enforcement official injured

Y35.032 Legal intervention involving injury by rifle pellet, bystander injured

Y35.033 Legal intervention involving injury by rifle pellet, suspect injured

Y35.039 Legal intervention involving injury by rifle pellet, unspecified person injured

Y35.04 Legal intervention involving injury by rubber bullet

Y35.041 Legal intervention involving injury by rubber bullet, law enforcement official injured

Y35.042 Legal intervention involving injury by rubber bullet, bystander injured

Y35.043 Legal intervention involving injury by rubber bullet, suspect injured

Y35.049 Legal intervention involving injury by rubber bullet, unspecified person injured

Y35.09 Legal intervention involving other firearm discharge

Y35.091 Legal intervention involving other firearm discharge, law enforcement official injured

Y35.092 Legal intervention involving other firearm discharge, bystander injured

Y35.093 Legal intervention involving other firearm discharge, suspect injured

Y35.099 Legal intervention involving other firearm discharge, unspecified person injured

Y35.1 Legal intervention involving explosives

Y35.10 Legal intervention involving unspecified explosives

Y35.101 Legal intervention involving unspecified explosives, law enforcement official injured

Y35.102 Legal intervention involving unspecified explosives, bystander injured

Y35.103 Legal intervention involving unspecified explosives, suspect injured

Y35.109 Legal intervention involving unspecified explosives, unspecified person injured

Y35.11 Legal intervention involving injury by dynamite

Y35.111 Legal intervention involving injury by dynamite, law enforcement official injured

Y35.112 Legal intervention involving injury by dynamite, bystander injured

Y35.113 Legal intervention involving injury by dynamite, suspect injured

Y35.119 Legal intervention involving injury by dynamite, unspecified person injured

Y35.12 Legal intervention involving injury by explosive shell

Y35.121 Legal intervention involving injury by explosive shell, law enforcement official injured

Y35.122 Legal intervention involving injury by explosive shell, bystander injured

Y35.123 Legal intervention involving injury by explosive shell, suspect injured

Y35.129 Legal intervention involving injury by explosive shell, unspecified person injured

Y35.19 Legal intervention involving other explosives

Legal intervention involving injury by grenade

Legal intervention involving injury by mortar bomb

Y35.191 Legal intervention involving other explosives, law enforcement official injured

Y35.192 Legal intervention involving other explosives, bystander injured

Y35.193 Legal intervention involving other explosives, suspect injured

Y35.199 Legal intervention involving other explosives, unspecified person injured

Y35.2 Legal intervention involving gas

Legal intervention involving asphyxiation by gas

Legal intervention involving poisoning by gas

Y35.20 Legal intervention involving unspecified gas

Y35.201 Legal intervention involving unspecified gas, law enforcement official injured

Y35.202 Legal intervention involving unspecified gas, bystander injured

Y35.203 Legal intervention involving unspecified gas, suspect injured

Y35.209 Legal intervention involving unspecified gas, unspecified person injured

Y35.21 Legal intervention involving injury by tear gas

Y35.211 Legal intervention involving injury by tear gas, law enforcement official injured

Y35.212 Legal intervention involving injury by tear gas, bystander injured

Y35.213 Legal intervention involving injury by tear gas, suspect injured

Y35.219 Legal intervention involving injury by tear gas, unspecified person injured

Y35.29 Legal intervention involving other gas

Y35.291 Legal intervention involving other gas, law enforcement official injured

Y35.292 Legal intervention involving other gas, bystander injured

Y35.293 Legal intervention involving other gas, suspect injured

Y35.299 Legal intervention involving other gas, unspecified person injured

Y35.3 Legal intervention involving blunt objects

Legal intervention involving being hit or struck by blunt object

Y35.30 Legal intervention involving unspecified blunt objects

Y35.301 Legal intervention involving unspecified blunt objects, law enforcement official injured

Y35.302 Legal intervention involving unspecified blunt objects, bystander injured

Y35.303 Legal intervention involving unspecified blunt objects, suspect injured

Y35.309 Legal intervention involving unspecified blunt objects, unspecified person injured

Y35.31 Legal intervention involving baton

Y35.311 Legal intervention involving baton, law enforcement official injured

Y35.312 Legal intervention involving baton, bystander injured

Y35.313 Legal intervention involving baton, suspect injured

Y35.319 Legal intervention involving baton, unspecified person injured

Y35.39 Legal intervention involving other blunt objects

Y35.391 Legal intervention involving other blunt objects, law enforcement official injured

Y35.392 Legal intervention involving other blunt objects, bystander injured

Y35.393 Legal intervention involving other blunt objects, suspect injured

Y35.399 Legal intervention involving other blunt objects, unspecified person injured

Y35.4 Legal intervention involving sharp objects

Legal intervention involving being cut by sharp objects

Legal intervention involving being stabbed by sharp objects

Y35.40 Legal intervention involving unspecified sharp objects

Y35.401 Legal intervention involving unspecified sharp objects, law enforcement official injured

Y35.402 Legal intervention involving unspecified sharp objects, bystander injured

Y35.403 Legal intervention involving unspecified sharp objects, suspect injured

Y35.409 Legal intervention involving unspecified sharp objects, unspecified person injured

Y35.41 Legal intervention involving bayonet

Y35.411 Legal intervention involving bayonet, law enforcement official injured

Y35.412 Legal intervention involving bayonet, bystander injured

Y35.413 Legal intervention involving bayonet, suspect injured

Y35.419 Legal intervention involving bayonet, unspecified person injured

Y35.49 Legal intervention involving other sharp objects

Y35.491 Legal intervention involving other sharp objects, law enforcement official injured

Y35.492 Legal intervention involving other sharp objects, bystander injured

Y35.493 Legal intervention involving other sharp objects, suspect injured

Y35.499 Legal intervention involving other sharp objects, unspecified person injured

Y35.8 Legal intervention involving other specified means

AHA: 2019,4Q,19

Y35.81 Legal intervention involving manhandling

Y35.811 Legal intervention involving manhandling, law enforcement official injured

Y35.812 Legal intervention involving manhandling, bystander injured

Y35.813 Legal intervention involving manhandling, suspect injured

Y35.819 Legal intervention involving manhandling, unspecified person injured

✓6th **Y35.83 Legal intervention involving a conducted energy device**
Electroshock device (taser)
Stun gun
✓7th **Y35.831 Legal intervention involving a conducted energy device, law enforcement official injured**
✓7th **Y35.832 Legal intervention involving a conducted energy device, bystander injured**
✓7th **Y35.833 Legal intervention involving a conducted energy device, suspect injured**
✓7th **Y35.839 Legal intervention involving a conducted energy device, unspecified person injured**
✓6th **Y35.89 Legal intervention involving other specified means**
✓7th **Y35.891 Legal intervention involving other specified means, law enforcement official injured**
✓7th **Y35.892 Legal intervention involving other specified means, bystander injured**
✓7th **Y35.893 Legal intervention involving other specified means, suspect injured**
AHA: 2018,1Q,5
✓7th **Y35.899 Legal intervention involving other specified means, unspecified person injured**
✓5th **Y35.9 Legal intervention, means unspecified**
✓x7th **Y35.91 Legal intervention, means unspecified, law enforcement official injured**
✓x7th **Y35.92 Legal intervention, means unspecified, bystander injured**
✓x7th **Y35.93 Legal intervention, means unspecified, suspect injured**
✓x7th **Y35.99 Legal intervention, means unspecified, unspecified person injured**

✓4th **Y36 Operations of war**
INCLUDES injuries to military personnel and civilians caused by war, civil insurrection, and peacekeeping missions
EXCLUDES 1 *injury to military personnel occurring during peacetime military operations (Y37.-)*
military vehicles involved in transport accidents with non-military vehicle during peacetime ▶(V09.01, V09.21, V19.81, V29.818, V39.81, V49.81, V59.81, V69.81, V79.81)◀
AHA: 2014,3Q,4
✓5th **Y36.0 War operations involving explosion of marine weapons**
✓6th **Y36.00 War operations involving explosion of unspecified marine weapon**
War operations involving underwater blast NOS
✓7th **Y36.000 War operations involving explosion of unspecified marine weapon, military personnel**
✓7th **Y36.001 War operations involving explosion of unspecified marine weapon, civilian**
✓6th **Y36.01 War operations involving explosion of depth-charge**
✓7th **Y36.010 War operations involving explosion of depth-charge, military personnel**
✓7th **Y36.011 War operations involving explosion of depth-charge, civilian**
✓6th **Y36.02 War operations involving explosion of marine mine**
War operations involving explosion of marine mine, at sea or in harbor
✓7th **Y36.020 War operations involving explosion of marine mine, military personnel**
✓7th **Y36.021 War operations involving explosion of marine mine, civilian**
✓6th **Y36.03 War operations involving explosion of sea-based artillery shell**
✓7th **Y36.030 War operations involving explosion of sea-based artillery shell, military personnel**
✓7th **Y36.031 War operations involving explosion of sea-based artillery shell, civilian**
✓6th **Y36.04 War operations involving explosion of torpedo**
✓7th **Y36.040 War operations involving explosion of torpedo, military personnel**
✓7th **Y36.041 War operations involving explosion of torpedo, civilian**
✓6th **Y36.05 War operations involving accidental detonation of onboard marine weapons**
✓7th **Y36.050 War operations involving accidental detonation of onboard marine weapons, military personnel**
✓7th **Y36.051 War operations involving accidental detonation of onboard marine weapons, civilian**
✓6th **Y36.09 War operations involving explosion of other marine weapons**
✓7th **Y36.090 War operations involving explosion of other marine weapons, military personnel**
✓7th **Y36.091 War operations involving explosion of other marine weapons, civilian**
✓5th **Y36.1 War operations involving destruction of aircraft**
✓6th **Y36.10 War operations involving unspecified destruction of aircraft**
✓7th **Y36.100 War operations involving unspecified destruction of aircraft, military personnel**
✓7th **Y36.101 War operations involving unspecified destruction of aircraft, civilian**
✓6th **Y36.11 War operations involving destruction of aircraft due to enemy fire or explosives**
War operations involving destruction of aircraft due to air to air missile
War operations involving destruction of aircraft due to explosive placed on aircraft
War operations involving destruction of aircraft due to rocket propelled grenade [RPG]
War operations involving destruction of aircraft due to small arms fire
War operations involving destruction of aircraft due to surface to air missile
✓7th **Y36.110 War operations involving destruction of aircraft due to enemy fire or explosives, military personnel**
✓7th **Y36.111 War operations involving destruction of aircraft due to enemy fire or explosives, civilian**
✓6th **Y36.12 War operations involving destruction of aircraft due to collision with other aircraft**
✓7th **Y36.120 War operations involving destruction of aircraft due to collision with other aircraft, military personnel**
✓7th **Y36.121 War operations involving destruction of aircraft due to collision with other aircraft, civilian**
✓6th **Y36.13 War operations involving destruction of aircraft due to onboard fire**
✓7th **Y36.130 War operations involving destruction of aircraft due to onboard fire, military personnel**
✓7th **Y36.131 War operations involving destruction of aircraft due to onboard fire, civilian**
✓6th **Y36.14 War operations involving destruction of aircraft due to accidental detonation of onboard munitions and explosives**
✓7th **Y36.140 War operations involving destruction of aircraft due to accidental detonation of onboard munitions and explosives, military personnel**
✓7th **Y36.141 War operations involving destruction of aircraft due to accidental detonation of onboard munitions and explosives, civilian**
✓6th **Y36.19 War operations involving other destruction of aircraft**
✓7th **Y36.190 War operations involving other destruction of aircraft, military personnel**
✓7th **Y36.191 War operations involving other destruction of aircraft, civilian**

Y36.2 War operations involving other explosions and fragments

EXCLUDES 1 *war operations involving explosion of aircraft (Y36.1-)*
war operations involving explosion of marine weapons (Y36.Ø-)
war operations involving explosion of nuclear weapons (Y36.5-)
war operations involving explosion occurring after cessation of hostilities (Y36.8-)

Y36.2Ø War operations involving unspecified explosion and fragments

War operations involving air blast NOS
War operations involving blast NOS
War operations involving blast fragments NOS
War operations involving blast wave NOS
War operations involving blast wind NOS
War operations involving explosion NOS
War operations involving explosion of bomb NOS

Y36.2ØØ War operations involving unspecified explosion and fragments, military personnel

Y36.2Ø1 War operations involving unspecified explosion and fragments, civilian

Y36.21 War operations involving explosion of aerial bomb

Y36.21Ø War operations involving explosion of aerial bomb, military personnel

Y36.211 War operations involving explosion of aerial bomb, civilian

Y36.22 War operations involving explosion of guided missile

Y36.22Ø War operations involving explosion of guided missile, military personnel

Y36.221 War operations involving explosion of guided missile, civilian

Y36.23 War operations involving explosion of improvised explosive device [IED]

War operations involving explosion of person-borne improvised explosive device [IED]
War operations involving explosion of vehicle-borne improvised explosive device [IED]
War operations involving explosion of roadside improvised explosive device [IED]

Y36.23Ø War operations involving explosion of improvised explosive device [IED], military personnel

Y36.231 War operations involving explosion of improvised explosive device [IED], civilian

Y36.24 War operations involving explosion due to accidental detonation and discharge of own munitions or munitions launch device

Y36.24Ø War operations involving explosion due to accidental detonation and discharge of own munitions or munitions launch device, military personnel

Y36.241 War operations involving explosion due to accidental detonation and discharge of own munitions or munitions launch device, civilian

Y36.25 War operations involving fragments from munitions

Y36.25Ø War operations involving fragments from munitions, military personnel

Y36.251 War operations involving fragments from munitions, civilian

Y36.26 War operations involving fragments of improvised explosive device [IED]

War operations involving fragments of person-borne improvised explosive device [IED]
War operations involving fragments of vehicle-borne improvised explosive device [IED]
War operations involving fragments of roadside improvised explosive device [IED]

Y36.26Ø War operations involving fragments of improvised explosive device [IED], military personnel

Y36.261 War operations involving fragments of improvised explosive device [IED], civilian

Y36.27 War operations involving fragments from weapons

Y36.27Ø War operations involving fragments from weapons, military personnel

Y36.271 War operations involving fragments from weapons, civilian

Y36.29 War operations involving other explosions and fragments

War operations involving explosion of grenade
War operations involving explosions of land mine
War operations involving shrapnel NOS

Y36.29Ø War operations involving other explosions and fragments, military personnel

Y36.291 War operations involving other explosions and fragments, civilian

Y36.3 War operations involving fires, conflagrations and hot substances

War operations involving smoke, fumes, and heat from fires, conflagrations and hot substances

EXCLUDES 1 *war operations involving fires and conflagrations aboard military aircraft (Y36.1-)*
war operations involving fires and conflagrations aboard military watercraft (Y36.Ø-)
war operations involving fires and conflagrations caused indirectly by conventional weapons (Y36.2-)
war operations involving fires and thermal effects of nuclear weapons (Y36.53-)

Y36.3Ø War operations involving unspecified fire, conflagration and hot substance

Y36.3ØØ War operations involving unspecified fire, conflagration and hot substance, military personnel

Y36.3Ø1 War operations involving unspecified fire, conflagration and hot substance, civilian

Y36.31 War operations involving gasoline bomb

War operations involving incendiary bomb
War operations involving petrol bomb

Y36.31Ø War operations involving gasoline bomb, military personnel

Y36.311 War operations involving gasoline bomb, civilian

Y36.32 War operations involving incendiary bullet

Y36.32Ø War operations involving incendiary bullet, military personnel

Y36.321 War operations involving incendiary bullet, civilian

Y36.33 War operations involving flamethrower

Y36.33Ø War operations involving flamethrower, military personnel

Y36.331 War operations involving flamethrower, civilian

Y36.39 War operations involving other fires, conflagrations and hot substances

Y36.39Ø War operations involving other fires, conflagrations and hot substances, military personnel

Y36.391 War operations involving other fires, conflagrations and hot substances, civilian

Y36.4 War operations involving firearm discharge and other forms of conventional warfare

Y36.41 War operations involving rubber bullets

Y36.41Ø War operations involving rubber bullets, military personnel

Y36.411 War operations involving rubber bullets, civilian

Y36.42 War operations involving firearms pellets

Y36.42Ø War operations involving firearms pellets, military personnel

Y36.421 War operations involving firearms pellets, civilian

Y36.43 War operations involving other firearms discharge

War operations involving bullets NOS

EXCLUDES 1 *war operations involving munitions fragments (Y36.25-)*
war operations involving incendiary bullets (Y36.32-)

Y36.43Ø War operations involving other firearms discharge, military personnel

Y36.431 War operations involving other firearms discharge, civilian

Y36.44 War operations involving unarmed hand to hand combat

EXCLUDES 1 *war operations involving combat using blunt or piercing object (Y36.45-)*
war operations involving intentional restriction of air and airway (Y36.46-)
war operations involving unintentional restriction of air and airway (Y36.47-)

Y36.440 War operations involving unarmed hand to hand combat, military personnel

Y36.441 War operations involving unarmed hand to hand combat, civilian

Y36.45 War operations involving combat using blunt or piercing object

Y36.450 War operations involving combat using blunt or piercing object, military personnel

Y36.451 War operations involving combat using blunt or piercing object, civilian

Y36.46 War operations involving intentional restriction of air and airway

Y36.460 War operations involving intentional restriction of air and airway, military personnel

Y36.461 War operations involving intentional restriction of air and airway, civilian

Y36.47 War operations involving unintentional restriction of air and airway

Y36.470 War operations involving unintentional restriction of air and airway, military personnel

Y36.471 War operations involving unintentional restriction of air and airway, civilian

Y36.49 War operations involving other forms of conventional warfare

Y36.490 War operations involving other forms of conventional warfare, military personnel

Y36.491 War operations involving other forms of conventional warfare, civilian

Y36.5 War operations involving nuclear weapons

War operations involving dirty bomb NOS

Y36.50 War operations involving unspecified effect of nuclear weapon

Y36.500 War operations involving unspecified effect of nuclear weapon, military personnel

Y36.501 War operations involving unspecified effect of nuclear weapon, civilian

Y36.51 War operations involving direct blast effect of nuclear weapon

War operations involving blast pressure of nuclear weapon

Y36.510 War operations involving direct blast effect of nuclear weapon, military personnel

Y36.511 War operations involving direct blast effect of nuclear weapon, civilian

Y36.52 War operations involving indirect blast effect of nuclear weapon

War operations involving being thrown by blast of nuclear weapon
War operations involving being struck or crushed by blast debris of nuclear weapon

Y36.520 War operations involving indirect blast effect of nuclear weapon, military personnel

Y36.521 War operations involving indirect blast effect of nuclear weapon, civilian

Y36.53 War operations involving thermal radiation effect of nuclear weapon

War operations involving direct heat from nuclear weapon
War operation involving fireball effects from nuclear weapon

Y36.530 War operations involving thermal radiation effect of nuclear weapon, military personnel

Y36.531 War operations involving thermal radiation effect of nuclear weapon, civilian

Y36.54 War operation involving nuclear radiation effects of nuclear weapon

War operation involving acute radiation exposure from nuclear weapon
War operation involving exposure to immediate ionizing radiation from nuclear weapon
War operation involving fallout exposure from nuclear weapon
War operation involving secondary effects of nuclear weapons

Y36.540 War operation involving nuclear radiation effects of nuclear weapon, military personnel

Y36.541 War operation involving nuclear radiation effects of nuclear weapon, civilian

Y36.59 War operation involving other effects of nuclear weapons

Y36.590 War operation involving other effects of nuclear weapons, military personnel

Y36.591 War operation involving other effects of nuclear weapons, civilian

Y36.6 War operations involving biological weapons

Y36.6X War operations involving biological weapons

Y36.6X0 War operations involving biological weapons, military personnel

Y36.6X1 War operations involving biological weapons, civilian

Y36.7 War operations involving chemical weapons and other forms of unconventional warfare

EXCLUDES 1 *war operations involving incendiary devices (Y36.3-, Y36.5-)*

Y36.7X War operations involving chemical weapons and other forms of unconventional warfare

Y36.7X0 War operations involving chemical weapons and other forms of unconventional warfare, military personnel

Y36.7X1 War operations involving chemical weapons and other forms of unconventional warfare, civilian

Y36.8 War operations occurring after cessation of hostilities

War operations classifiable to categories Y36.0-Y36.8 but occurring after cessation of hostilities

Y36.81 Explosion of mine placed during war operations but exploding after cessation of hostilities

Y36.810 Explosion of mine placed during war operations but exploding after cessation of hostilities, military personnel

Y36.811 Explosion of mine placed during war operations but exploding after cessation of hostilities, civilian

Y36.82 Explosion of bomb placed during war operations but exploding after cessation of hostilities

Y36.820 Explosion of bomb placed during war operations but exploding after cessation of hostilities, military personnel

Y36.821 Explosion of bomb placed during war operations but exploding after cessation of hostilities, civilian

Y36.88 Other war operations occurring after cessation of hostilities

Y36.880 Other war operations occurring after cessation of hostilities, military personnel

Y36.881 Other war operations occurring after cessation of hostilities, civilian

Y36.89 Unspecified war operations occurring after cessation of hostilities

Y36.890 Unspecified war operations occurring after cessation of hostilities, military personnel

Y36.891 Unspecified war operations occurring after cessation of hostilities, civilian

Y36.9 Other and unspecified war operations

Y36.90 War operations, unspecified

Y36.91 War operations involving unspecified weapon of mass destruction [WMD]

Y36.92 War operations involving friendly fire

Y37 Military operations

INCLUDES injuries to military personnel and civilians occurring during peacetime on military property and during routine military exercises and operations

EXCLUDES 1 *military aircraft involved in aircraft accident with civilian aircraft (V97.81-)*

military vehicles involved in transport accident with civilian vehicle ►(V09.01, V09.21, V19.81, V29.818, V39.81, V49.81, V59.81, V69.81, V79.81)◄

military watercraft involved in water transport accident with civilian watercraft (V94.81-)

war operations (Y36.-)

Y37.0 Military operations involving explosion of marine weapons

Y37.00 Military operations involving explosion of unspecified marine weapon

Military operations involving underwater blast NOS

Y37.000 Military operations involving explosion of unspecified marine weapon, military personnel

Y37.001 Military operations involving explosion of unspecified marine weapon, civilian

Y37.01 Military operations involving explosion of depth-charge

Y37.010 Military operations involving explosion of depth-charge, military personnel

Y37.011 Military operations involving explosion of depth-charge, civilian

Y37.02 Military operations involving explosion of marine mine

Military operations involving explosion of marine mine, at sea or in harbor

Y37.020 Military operations involving explosion of marine mine, military personnel

Y37.021 Military operations involving explosion of marine mine, civilian

Y37.03 Military operations involving explosion of sea-based artillery shell

Y37.030 Military operations involving explosion of sea-based artillery shell, military personnel

Y37.031 Military operations involving explosion of sea-based artillery shell, civilian

Y37.04 Military operations involving explosion of torpedo

Y37.040 Military operations involving explosion of torpedo, military personnel

Y37.041 Military operations involving explosion of torpedo, civilian

Y37.05 Military operations involving accidental detonation of onboard marine weapons

Y37.050 Military operations involving accidental detonation of onboard marine weapons, military personnel

Y37.051 Military operations involving accidental detonation of onboard marine weapons, civilian

Y37.09 Military operations involving explosion of other marine weapons

Y37.090 Military operations involving explosion of other marine weapons, military personnel

Y37.091 Military operations involving explosion of other marine weapons, civilian

Y37.1 Military operations involving destruction of aircraft

Y37.10 Military operations involving unspecified destruction of aircraft

Y37.100 Military operations involving unspecified destruction of aircraft, military personnel

Y37.101 Military operations involving unspecified destruction of aircraft, civilian

Y37.11 Military operations involving destruction of aircraft due to enemy fire or explosives

Military operations involving destruction of aircraft due to air to air missile

Military operations involving destruction of aircraft due to explosive placed on aircraft

Military operations involving destruction of aircraft due to rocket propelled grenade [RPG]

Military operations involving destruction of aircraft due to small arms fire

Military operations involving destruction of aircraft due to surface to air missile

Y37.110 Military operations involving destruction of aircraft due to enemy fire or explosives, military personnel

Y37.111 Military operations involving destruction of aircraft due to enemy fire or explosives, civilian

Y37.12 Military operations involving destruction of aircraft due to collision with other aircraft

Y37.120 Military operations involving destruction of aircraft due to collision with other aircraft, military personnel

Y37.121 Military operations involving destruction of aircraft due to collision with other aircraft, civilian

Y37.13 Military operations involving destruction of aircraft due to onboard fire

Y37.130 Military operations involving destruction of aircraft due to onboard fire, military personnel

Y37.131 Military operations involving destruction of aircraft due to onboard fire, civilian

Y37.14 Military operations involving destruction of aircraft due to accidental detonation of onboard munitions and explosives

Y37.140 Military operations involving destruction of aircraft due to accidental detonation of onboard munitions and explosives, military personnel

Y37.141 Military operations involving destruction of aircraft due to accidental detonation of onboard munitions and explosives, civilian

Y37.19 Military operations involving other destruction of aircraft

Y37.190 Military operations involving other destruction of aircraft, military personnel

Y37.191 Military operations involving other destruction of aircraft, civilian

Y37.2 Military operations involving other explosions and fragments

EXCLUDES 1 *military operations involving explosion of aircraft (Y37.1-)*

military operations involving explosion of marine weapons (Y37.0-)

military operations involving explosion of nuclear weapons (Y37.5-)

Y37.20 Military operations involving unspecified explosion and fragments

Military operations involving air blast NOS

Military operations involving blast NOS

Military operations involving blast fragments NOS

Military operations involving blast wave NOS

Military operations involving blast wind NOS

Military operations involving explosion NOS

Military operations involving explosion of bomb NOS

Y37.200 Military operations involving unspecified explosion and fragments, military personnel

Y37.201 Military operations involving unspecified explosion and fragments, civilian

Y37.21 Military operations involving explosion of aerial bomb

Y37.210 Military operations involving explosion of aerial bomb, military personnel

Y37.211 Military operations involving explosion of aerial bomb, civilian

Y37.22 Military operations involving explosion of guided missile

Y37.220 Military operations involving explosion of guided missile, military personnel

7th **Y37.221 Military operations involving explosion of guided missile, civilian**

6th **Y37.23 Military operations involving explosion of improvised explosive device [IED]**
Military operations involving explosion of person-borne improvised explosive device [IED]
Military operations involving explosion of vehicle-borne improvised explosive device [IED]
Military operations involving explosion of roadside improvised explosive device [IED]

7th **Y37.230 Military operations involving explosion of improvised explosive device [IED], military personnel**

7th **Y37.231 Military operations involving explosion of improvised explosive device [IED], civilian**

6th **Y37.24 Military operations involving explosion due to accidental detonation and discharge of own munitions or munitions launch device**

7th **Y37.240 Military operations involving explosion due to accidental detonation and discharge of own munitions or munitions launch device, military personnel**

7th **Y37.241 Military operations involving explosion due to accidental detonation and discharge of own munitions or munitions launch device, civilian**

6th **Y37.25 Military operations involving fragments from munitions**

7th **Y37.250 Military operations involving fragments from munitions, military personnel**

7th **Y37.251 Military operations involving fragments from munitions, civilian**

6th **Y37.26 Military operations involving fragments of improvised explosive device [IED]**
Military operations involving fragments of person-borne improvised explosive device [IED]
Military operations involving fragments of vehicle-borne improvised explosive device [IED]
Military operations involving fragments of roadside improvised explosive device [IED]

7th **Y37.260 Military operations involving fragments of improvised explosive device [IED], military personnel**

7th **Y37.261 Military operations involving fragments of improvised explosive device [IED], civilian**

6th **Y37.27 Military operations involving fragments from weapons**

7th **Y37.270 Military operations involving fragments from weapons, military personnel**

7th **Y37.271 Military operations involving fragments from weapons, civilian**

6th **Y37.29 Military operations involving other explosions and fragments**
Military operations involving explosion of grenade
Military operations involving explosions of land mine
Military operations involving shrapnel NOS

7th **Y37.290 Military operations involving other explosions and fragments, military personnel**

7th **Y37.291 Military operations involving other explosions and fragments, civilian**

5th **Y37.3 Military operations involving fires, conflagrations and hot substances**
Military operations involving smoke, fumes, and heat from fires, conflagrations and hot substances

EXCLUDES 1 *military operations involving fires and conflagrations aboard military aircraft (Y37.1-)*
military operations involving fires and conflagrations aboard military watercraft (Y37.0-)
military operations involving fires and conflagrations caused indirectly by conventional weapons (Y37.2-)
military operations involving fires and thermal effects of nuclear weapons (Y36.53-)

6th **Y37.30 Military operations involving unspecified fire, conflagration and hot substance**

7th **Y37.300 Military operations involving unspecified fire, conflagration and hot substance, military personnel**

7th **Y37.301 Military operations involving unspecified fire, conflagration and hot substance, civilian**

6th **Y37.31 Military operations involving gasoline bomb**
Military operations involving incendiary bomb
Military operations involving petrol bomb

7th **Y37.310 Military operations involving gasoline bomb, military personnel**

7th **Y37.311 Military operations involving gasoline bomb, civilian**

6th **Y37.32 Military operations involving incendiary bullet**

7th **Y37.320 Military operations involving incendiary bullet, military personnel**

7th **Y37.321 Military operations involving incendiary bullet, civilian**

6th **Y37.33 Military operations involving flamethrower**

7th **Y37.330 Military operations involving flamethrower, military personnel**

7th **Y37.331 Military operations involving flamethrower, civilian**

6th **Y37.39 Military operations involving other fires, conflagrations and hot substances**

7th **Y37.390 Military operations involving other fires, conflagrations and hot substances, military personnel**

7th **Y37.391 Military operations involving other fires, conflagrations and hot substances, civilian**

5th **Y37.4 Military operations involving firearm discharge and other forms of conventional warfare**

6th **Y37.41 Military operations involving rubber bullets**

7th **Y37.410 Military operations involving rubber bullets, military personnel**

7th **Y37.411 Military operations involving rubber bullets, civilian**

6th **Y37.42 Military operations involving firearms pellets**

7th **Y37.420 Military operations involving firearms pellets, military personnel**

7th **Y37.421 Military operations involving firearms pellets, civilian**

6th **Y37.43 Military operations involving other firearms discharge**
Military operations involving bullets NOS

EXCLUDES 1 *military operations involving munitions fragments (Y37.25-)*
military operations involving incendiary bullets (Y37.32-)

7th **Y37.430 Military operations involving other firearms discharge, military personnel**

7th **Y37.431 Military operations involving other firearms discharge, civilian**

6th **Y37.44 Military operations involving unarmed hand to hand combat**

EXCLUDES 1 *military operations involving combat using blunt or piercing object (Y37.45-)*
military operations involving intentional restriction of air and airway (Y37.46-)
military operations involving unintentional restriction of air and airway (Y37.47-)

7th **Y37.440 Military operations involving unarmed hand to hand combat, military personnel**

7th **Y37.441 Military operations involving unarmed hand to hand combat, civilian**

6th **Y37.45 Military operations involving combat using blunt or piercing object**

7th **Y37.450 Military operations involving combat using blunt or piercing object, military personnel**

7th **Y37.451 Military operations involving combat using blunt or piercing object, civilian**

6th **Y37.46 Military operations involving intentional restriction of air and airway**

7th **Y37.460 Military operations involving intentional restriction of air and airway, military personnel**

7th **Y37.461 Military operations involving intentional restriction of air and airway, civilian**

Y37.47 Military operations involving unintentional restriction of air and airway

Y37.470 Military operations involving unintentional restriction of air and airway, military personnel

Y37.471 Military operations involving unintentional restriction of air and airway, civilian

Y37.49 Military operations involving other forms of conventional warfare

Y37.490 Military operations involving other forms of conventional warfare, military personnel

Y37.491 Military operations involving other forms of conventional warfare, civilian

Y37.5 Military operations involving nuclear weapons

Military operation involving dirty bomb NOS

Y37.50 Military operations involving unspecified effect of nuclear weapon

Y37.500 Military operations involving unspecified effect of nuclear weapon, military personnel

Y37.501 Military operations involving unspecified effect of nuclear weapon, civilian

Y37.51 Military operations involving direct blast effect of nuclear weapon

Military operations involving blast pressure of nuclear weapon

Y37.510 Military operations involving direct blast effect of nuclear weapon, military personnel

Y37.511 Military operations involving direct blast effect of nuclear weapon, civilian

Y37.52 Military operations involving indirect blast effect of nuclear weapon

Military operations involving being thrown by blast of nuclear weapon

Military operations involving being struck or crushed by blast debris of nuclear weapon

Y37.520 Military operations involving indirect blast effect of nuclear weapon, military personnel

Y37.521 Military operations involving indirect blast effect of nuclear weapon, civilian

Y37.53 Military operations involving thermal radiation effect of nuclear weapon

Military operations involving direct heat from nuclear weapon

Military operation involving fireball effects from nuclear weapon

Y37.530 Military operations involving thermal radiation effect of nuclear weapon, military personnel

Y37.531 Military operations involving thermal radiation effect of nuclear weapon, civilian

Y37.54 Military operation involving nuclear radiation effects of nuclear weapon

Military operation involving acute radiation exposure from nuclear weapon

Military operation involving exposure to immediate ionizing radiation from nuclear weapon

Military operation involving fallout exposure from nuclear weapon

Military operation involving secondary effects of nuclear weapons

Y37.540 Military operation involving nuclear radiation effects of nuclear weapon, military personnel

Y37.541 Military operation involving nuclear radiation effects of nuclear weapon, civilian

Y37.59 Military operation involving other effects of nuclear weapons

Y37.590 Military operation involving other effects of nuclear weapons, military personnel

Y37.591 Military operation involving other effects of nuclear weapons, civilian

Y37.6 Military operations involving biological weapons

Y37.6X Military operations involving biological weapons

Y37.6X0 Military operations involving biological weapons, military personnel

Y37.6X1 Military operations involving biological weapons, civilian

Y37.7 Military operations involving chemical weapons and other forms of unconventional warfare

EXCLUDES 1 *military operations involving incendiary devices (Y36.3-, Y36.5-)*

Y37.7X Military operations involving chemical weapons and other forms of unconventional warfare

Y37.7X0 Military operations involving chemical weapons and other forms of unconventional warfare, military personnel

Y37.7X1 Military operations involving chemical weapons and other forms of unconventional warfare, civilian

Y37.9 Other and unspecified military operations

Y37.90 Military operations, unspecified

Y37.91 Military operations involving unspecified weapon of mass destruction [WMD]

Y37.92 Military operations involving friendly fire

Y38 Terrorism

NOTE These codes are for use to identify injuries resulting from the unlawful use of force or violence against persons or property to intimidate or coerce a Government, the civilian population, or any segment thereof, in furtherance of political or social objective

Use additional code for place of occurrence (Y92.-)

Y38.0 Terrorism involving explosion of marine weapons

Terrorism involving depth-charge
Terrorism involving marine mine
Terrorism involving mine NOS, at sea or in harbor
Terrorism involving sea-based artillery shell
Terrorism involving torpedo
Terrorism involving underwater blast

Y38.0X Terrorism involving explosion of marine weapons

Y38.0X1 Terrorism involving explosion of marine weapons, public safety official injured

Y38.0X2 Terrorism involving explosion of marine weapons, civilian injured

Y38.0X3 Terrorism involving explosion of marine weapons, terrorist injured

Y38.1 Terrorism involving destruction of aircraft

Terrorism involving aircraft burned
Terrorism involving aircraft exploded
Terrorism involving aircraft being shot down
Terrorism involving aircraft used as a weapon

Y38.1X Terrorism involving destruction of aircraft

Y38.1X1 Terrorism involving destruction of aircraft, public safety official injured

Y38.1X2 Terrorism involving destruction of aircraft, civilian injured

Y38.1X3 Terrorism involving destruction of aircraft, terrorist injured

Y38.2 Terrorism involving other explosions and fragments

Terrorism involving antipersonnel (fragments) bomb
Terrorism involving blast NOS
Terrorism involving explosion NOS
Terrorism involving explosion of breech block
Terrorism involving explosion of cannon block
Terrorism involving explosion (fragments) of artillery shell
Terrorism involving explosion (fragments) of bomb
Terrorism involving explosion (fragments) of grenade
Terrorism involving explosion (fragments) of guided missile
Terrorism involving explosion (fragments) of land mine
Terrorism involving explosion of mortar bomb
Terrorism involving explosion of munitions
Terrorism involving explosion (fragments) of rocket
Terrorism involving explosion (fragments) of shell
Terrorism involving shrapnel
Terrorism involving mine NOS, on land

EXCLUDES 1 *terrorism involving explosion of nuclear weapon (Y38.5)*
terrorism involving suicide bomber (Y38.81)

Y38.2X Terrorism involving other explosions and fragments

Y38.2X1 Terrorism involving other explosions and fragments, public safety official injured

Y38.2X2 Terrorism involving other explosions and fragments, civilian injured

Y38.2X3 Terrorism involving other explosions and fragments, terrorist injured

Y38.3 Terrorism involving fires, conflagration and hot substances

Terrorism involving conflagration NOS

Terrorism involving fire NOS

Terrorism involving petrol bomb

EXCLUDES 1 *terrorism involving fire or heat of nuclear weapon (Y38.5)*

Y38.3X Terrorism involving fires, conflagration and hot substances

Y38.3X1 Terrorism involving fires, conflagration and hot substances, public safety official injured

Y38.3X2 Terrorism involving fires, conflagration and hot substances, civilian injured

Y38.3X3 Terrorism involving fires, conflagration and hot substances, terrorist injured

Y38.4 Terrorism involving firearms

Terrorism involving carbine bullet

Terrorism involving machine gun bullet

Terrorism involving pellets (shotgun)

Terrorism involving pistol bullet

Terrorism involving rifle bullet

Terrorism involving rubber (rifle) bullet

Y38.4X Terrorism involving firearms

Y38.4X1 Terrorism involving firearms, public safety official injured

Y38.4X2 Terrorism involving firearms, civilian injured

Y38.4X3 Terrorism involving firearms, terrorist injured

Y38.5 Terrorism involving nuclear weapons

Terrorism involving blast effects of nuclear weapon

Terrorism involving exposure to ionizing radiation from nuclear weapon

Terrorism involving fireball effect of nuclear weapon

Terrorism involving heat from nuclear weapon

Y38.5X Terrorism involving nuclear weapons

Y38.5X1 Terrorism involving nuclear weapons, public safety official injured

Y38.5X2 Terrorism involving nuclear weapons, civilian injured

Y38.5X3 Terrorism involving nuclear weapons, terrorist injured

Y38.6 Terrorism involving biological weapons

Terrorism involving anthrax

Terrorism involving cholera

Terrorism involving smallpox

Y38.6X Terrorism involving biological weapons

Y38.6X1 Terrorism involving biological weapons, public safety official injured

Y38.6X2 Terrorism involving biological weapons, civilian injured

Y38.6X3 Terrorism involving biological weapons, terrorist injured

Y38.7 Terrorism involving chemical weapons

Terrorism involving gases, fumes, chemicals

Terrorism involving hydrogen cyanide

Terrorism involving phosgene

Terrorism involving sarin

Y38.7X Terrorism involving chemical weapons

Y38.7X1 Terrorism involving chemical weapons, public safety official injured

Y38.7X2 Terrorism involving chemical weapons, civilian injured

Y38.7X3 Terrorism involving chemical weapons, terrorist injured

Y38.8 Terrorism involving other and unspecified means

Y38.80 Terrorism involving unspecified means

Terrorism NOS

Y38.81 Terrorism involving suicide bomber

Y38.811 Terrorism involving suicide bomber, public safety official injured

Y38.812 Terrorism involving suicide bomber, civilian injured

Y38.89 Terrorism involving other means

Terrorism involving drowning and submersion

Terrorism involving lasers

Terrorism involving piercing or stabbing instruments

Y38.891 Terrorism involving other means, public safety official injured

Y38.892 Terrorism involving other means, civilian injured

Y38.893 Terrorism involving other means, terrorist injured

Y38.9 Terrorism, secondary effects

NOTE This code is for use to identify conditions occurring subsequent to a terrorist attack not those that are due to the initial terrorist attack

Y38.9X Terrorism, secondary effects

Y38.9X1 Terrorism, secondary effects, public safety official injured

Y38.9X2 Terrorism, secondary effects, civilian injured

COMPLICATIONS OF MEDICAL AND SURGICAL CARE (Y62-Y84)

INCLUDES complications of medical devices

surgical and medical procedures as the cause of abnormal reaction of the patient, or of later complication, without mention of misadventure at the time of the procedure

Misadventures to patients during surgical and medical care (Y62-Y69)

EXCLUDES 1 *surgical and medical procedures as the cause of abnormal reaction of the patient, without mention of misadventure at the time of the procedure (Y83-Y84)*

EXCLUDES 2 *breakdown or malfunctioning of medical device (during procedure) (after implantation) (ongoing use) (Y70-Y82)*

Y62 Failure of sterile precautions during surgical and medical care

Y62.0 Failure of sterile precautions during surgical operation

Y62.1 Failure of sterile precautions during infusion or transfusion

Y62.2 Failure of sterile precautions during kidney dialysis and other perfusion HCC

Y62.3 Failure of sterile precautions during injection or immunization

Y62.4 Failure of sterile precautions during endoscopic examination

Y62.5 Failure of sterile precautions during heart catheterization

Y62.6 Failure of sterile precautions during aspiration, puncture and other catheterization

Y62.8 Failure of sterile precautions during other surgical and medical care

Y62.9 Failure of sterile precautions during unspecified surgical and medical care

Y63 Failure in dosage during surgical and medical care

EXCLUDES 2 *accidental overdose of drug or wrong drug given in error (T36-T50)*

Y63.0 Excessive amount of blood or other fluid given during transfusion or infusion

Y63.1 Incorrect dilution of fluid used during infusion

Y63.2 Overdose of radiation given during therapy

Y63.3 Inadvertent exposure of patient to radiation during medical care

Y63.4 Failure in dosage in electroshock or insulin-shock therapy

Y63.5 Inappropriate temperature in local application and packing

Y63.6 Underdosing and nonadministration of necessary drug, medicament or biological substance

AHA: 2018,4Q,72

Y63.8 Failure in dosage during other surgical and medical care

AHA: 2018,4Q,72

Y63.9 Failure in dosage during unspecified surgical and medical care

AHA: 2018,4Q,72

Y64 Contaminated medical or biological substances

Y64.0 Contaminated medical or biological substance, transfused or infused

Y64.1 Contaminated medical or biological substance, injected or used for immunization

Y64.8 Contaminated medical or biological substance administered by other means

Y64.9 Contaminated medical or biological substance administered by unspecified means
Administered contaminated medical or biological substance NOS

Y65 Other misadventures during surgical and medical care
- **Y65.0 Mismatched blood in transfusion**
- **Y65.1 Wrong fluid used in infusion**
- **Y65.2 Failure in suture or ligature during surgical operation**
- **Y65.3 Endotracheal tube wrongly placed during anesthetic procedure**
- **Y65.4 Failure to introduce or to remove other tube or instrument**
- **Y65.5 Performance of wrong procedure (operation)**
  - **Y65.51 Performance of wrong procedure (operation) on correct patient**
    Wrong device implanted into correct surgical site
    EXCLUDES 1 *performance of correct procedure (operation) on wrong side or body part (Y65.53)*
  - **Y65.52 Performance of procedure (operation) on patient not scheduled for surgery**
    Performance of procedure (operation) intended for another patient
    Performance of procedure (operation) on wrong patient
  - **Y65.53 Performance of correct procedure (operation) on wrong side or body part**
    Performance of correct procedure (operation) on wrong side
    Performance of correct procedure (operation) on wrong site
- **Y65.8 Other specified misadventures during surgical and medical care**
  AHA: 2022,1Q,22; 2019,2Q,23-24

Y66 Nonadministration of surgical and medical care
Premature cessation of surgical and medical care
EXCLUDES 1 *DNR status (Z66)*
palliative care (Z51.5)

Y69 Unspecified misadventure during surgical and medical care

Medical devices associated with adverse incidents in diagnostic and therapeutic use (Y70-Y82)

INCLUDES breakdown or malfunction of medical devices (during use) (after implantation) (ongoing use)

EXCLUDES 2 *later complications following use of medical devices without breakdown or malfunctioning of device (Y83-Y84)*
misadventure to patients during surgical and medical care, classifiable to (Y62-Y69)
surgical and other medical procedures as the cause of abnormal reaction of the patient, or of later complication, without mention of misadventure at the time of the procedure (Y83-Y84)

Y70 Anesthesiology devices associated with adverse incidents
- **Y70.0 Diagnostic and monitoring anesthesiology devices associated with adverse incidents**
- **Y70.1 Therapeutic (nonsurgical) and rehabilitative anesthesiology devices associated with adverse incidents**
- **Y70.2 Prosthetic and other implants, materials and accessory anesthesiology devices associated with adverse incidents**
- **Y70.3 Surgical instruments, materials and anesthesiology devices (including sutures) associated with adverse incidents**
- **Y70.8 Miscellaneous anesthesiology devices associated with adverse incidents, not elsewhere classified**

Y71 Cardiovascular devices associated with adverse incidents
- **Y71.0 Diagnostic and monitoring cardiovascular devices associated with adverse incidents**
- **Y71.1 Therapeutic (nonsurgical) and rehabilitative cardiovascular devices associated with adverse incidents**
- **Y71.2 Prosthetic and other implants, materials and accessory cardiovascular devices associated with adverse incidents**
- **Y71.3 Surgical instruments, materials and cardiovascular devices (including sutures) associated with adverse incidents**
- **Y71.8 Miscellaneous cardiovascular devices associated with adverse incidents, not elsewhere classified**

Y72 Otorhinolaryngological devices associated with adverse incidents
- **Y72.0 Diagnostic and monitoring otorhinolaryngological devices associated with adverse incidents**
- **Y72.1 Therapeutic (nonsurgical) and rehabilitative otorhinolaryngological devices associated with adverse incidents**
- **Y72.2 Prosthetic and other implants, materials and accessory otorhinolaryngological devices associated with adverse incidents**
- **Y72.3 Surgical instruments, materials and otorhinolaryngological devices (including sutures) associated with adverse incidents**
- **Y72.8 Miscellaneous otorhinolaryngological devices associated with adverse incidents, not elsewhere classified**

Y73 Gastroenterology and urology devices associated with adverse incidents
- **Y73.0 Diagnostic and monitoring gastroenterology and urology devices associated with adverse incidents**
- **Y73.1 Therapeutic (nonsurgical) and rehabilitative gastroenterology and urology devices associated with adverse incidents**
- **Y73.2 Prosthetic and other implants, materials and accessory gastroenterology and urology devices associated with adverse incidents**
- **Y73.3 Surgical instruments, materials and gastroenterology and urology devices (including sutures) associated with adverse incidents**
- **Y73.8 Miscellaneous gastroenterology and urology devices associated with adverse incidents, not elsewhere classified**

Y74 General hospital and personal-use devices associated with adverse incidents
- **Y74.0 Diagnostic and monitoring general hospital and personal-use devices associated with adverse incidents**
- **Y74.1 Therapeutic (nonsurgical) and rehabilitative general hospital and personal-use devices associated with adverse incidents**
- **Y74.2 Prosthetic and other implants, materials and accessory general hospital and personal-use devices associated with adverse incidents**
- **Y74.3 Surgical instruments, materials and general hospital and personal-use devices (including sutures) associated with adverse incidents**
- **Y74.8 Miscellaneous general hospital and personal-use devices associated with adverse incidents, not elsewhere classified**

Y75 Neurological devices associated with adverse incidents
- **Y75.0 Diagnostic and monitoring neurological devices associated with adverse incidents**
- **Y75.1 Therapeutic (nonsurgical) and rehabilitative neurological devices associated with adverse incidents**
- **Y75.2 Prosthetic and other implants, materials and neurological devices associated with adverse incidents**
- **Y75.3 Surgical instruments, materials and neurological devices (including sutures) associated with adverse incidents**
- **Y75.8 Miscellaneous neurological devices associated with adverse incidents, not elsewhere classified**

Y76 Obstetric and gynecological devices associated with adverse incidents
- **Y76.0 Diagnostic and monitoring obstetric and gynecological devices associated with adverse incidents** ♀
- **Y76.1 Therapeutic (nonsurgical) and rehabilitative obstetric and gynecological devices associated with adverse incidents** ♀
- **Y76.2 Prosthetic and other implants, materials and accessory obstetric and gynecological devices associated with adverse incidents** ♀
- **Y76.3 Surgical instruments, materials and obstetric and gynecological devices (including sutures) associated with adverse incidents** ♀
- **Y76.8 Miscellaneous obstetric and gynecological devices associated with adverse incidents, not elsewhere classified** ♀

Y77 Ophthalmic devices associated with adverse incidents
- **Y77.0 Diagnostic and monitoring ophthalmic devices associated with adverse incidents**
- **Y77.1 Therapeutic (nonsurgical) and rehabilitative ophthalmic devices associated with adverse incidents**
  AHA: 2020,4Q,41
  - **Y77.11 Contact lens associated with adverse incidents**
    Rigid gas permeable contact lens associated with adverse incidents
    Soft (hydrophilic) contact lens associated with adverse incidents
  - **Y77.19 Other therapeutic (nonsurgical) and rehabilitative ophthalmic devices associated with adverse incidents**
- **Y77.2 Prosthetic and other implants, materials and accessory ophthalmic devices associated with adverse incidents**
- **Y77.3 Surgical instruments, materials and ophthalmic devices (including sutures) associated with adverse incidents**

Y77.8 Miscellaneous ophthalmic devices associated with adverse incidents, not elsewhere classified

Y78 Radiological devices associated with adverse incidents

Y78.0 Diagnostic and monitoring radiological devices associated with adverse incidents

Y78.1 Therapeutic (nonsurgical) and rehabilitative radiological devices associated with adverse incidents

Y78.2 Prosthetic and other implants, materials and accessory radiological devices associated with adverse incidents

Y78.3 Surgical instruments, materials and radiological devices (including sutures) associated with adverse incidents

Y78.8 Miscellaneous radiological devices associated with adverse incidents, not elsewhere classified

Y79 Orthopedic devices associated with adverse incidents

Y79.0 Diagnostic and monitoring orthopedic devices associated with adverse incidents

Y79.1 Therapeutic (nonsurgical) and rehabilitative orthopedic devices associated with adverse incidents

Y79.2 Prosthetic and other implants, materials and accessory orthopedic devices associated with adverse incidents

Y79.3 Surgical instruments, materials and orthopedic devices (including sutures) associated with adverse incidents

Y79.8 Miscellaneous orthopedic devices associated with adverse incidents, not elsewhere classified

Y80 Physical medicine devices associated with adverse incidents

Y80.0 Diagnostic and monitoring physical medicine devices associated with adverse incidents

Y80.1 Therapeutic (nonsurgical) and rehabilitative physical medicine devices associated with adverse incidents

Y80.2 Prosthetic and other implants, materials and accessory physical medicine devices associated with adverse incidents

Y80.3 Surgical instruments, materials and physical medicine devices (including sutures) associated with adverse incidents

Y80.8 Miscellaneous physical medicine devices associated with adverse incidents, not elsewhere classified

Y81 General- and plastic-surgery devices associated with adverse incidents

Y81.0 Diagnostic and monitoring general- and plastic-surgery devices associated with adverse incidents

Y81.1 Therapeutic (nonsurgical) and rehabilitative general- and plastic-surgery devices associated with adverse incidents

Y81.2 Prosthetic and other implants, materials and accessory general- and plastic-surgery devices associated with adverse incidents

Y81.3 Surgical instruments, materials and general- and plastic-surgery devices (including sutures) associated with adverse incidents

Y81.8 Miscellaneous general- and plastic-surgery devices associated with adverse incidents, not elsewhere classified

Y82 Other and unspecified medical devices associated with adverse incidents

Y82.8 Other medical devices associated with adverse incidents

Y82.9 Unspecified medical devices associated with adverse incidents

Surgical and other medical procedures as the cause of abnormal reaction of the patient, or of later complication, without mention of misadventure at the time of the procedure (Y83-Y84)

EXCLUDES 1 *misadventures to patients during surgical and medical care, classifiable to (Y62-Y69)*

EXCLUDES 2 *breakdown or malfunctioning of medical device (during procedure) (after implantation) (ongoing use) (Y70-Y82)*

Y83 Surgical operation and other surgical procedures as the cause of abnormal reaction of the patient, or of later complication, without mention of misadventure at the time of the procedure

Y83.0 Surgical operation with transplant of whole organ as the cause of abnormal reaction of the patient, or of later complication, without mention of misadventure at the time of the procedure

Y83.1 Surgical operation with implant of artificial internal device as the cause of abnormal reaction of the patient, or of later complication, without mention of misadventure at the time of the procedure

Y83.2 Surgical operation with anastomosis, bypass or graft as the cause of abnormal reaction of the patient, or of later complication, without mention of misadventure at the time of the procedure

Y83.3 Surgical operation with formation of external stoma as the cause of abnormal reaction of the patient, or of later complication, without mention of misadventure at the time of the procedure

Y83.4 Other reconstructive surgery as the cause of abnormal reaction of the patient, or of later complication, without mention of misadventure at the time of the procedure

Y83.5 Amputation of limb(s) as the cause of abnormal reaction of the patient, or of later complication, without mention of misadventure at the time of the procedure

Y83.6 Removal of other organ (partial) (total) as the cause of abnormal reaction of the patient, or of later complication, without mention of misadventure at the time of the procedure

Y83.8 Other surgical procedures as the cause of abnormal reaction of the patient, or of later complication, without mention of misadventure at the time of the procedure

Y83.9 Surgical procedure, unspecified as the cause of abnormal reaction of the patient, or of later complication, without mention of misadventure at the time of the procedure

Y84 Other medical procedures as the cause of abnormal reaction of the patient, or of later complication, without mention of misadventure at the time of the procedure

Y84.0 Cardiac catheterization as the cause of abnormal reaction of the patient, or of later complication, without mention of misadventure at the time of the procedure

Y84.1 Kidney dialysis as the cause of abnormal reaction of the patient, or of later complication, without mention of misadventure at the time of the procedure

Y84.2 Radiological procedure and radiotherapy as the cause of abnormal reaction of the patient, or of later complication, without mention of misadventure at the time of the procedure

AHA: 2019,1Q,21; 2017,1Q,33

Y84.3 Shock therapy as the cause of abnormal reaction of the patient, or of later complication, without mention of misadventure at the time of the procedure

Y84.4 Aspiration of fluid as the cause of abnormal reaction of the patient, or of later complication, without mention of misadventure at the time of the procedure

Y84.5 Insertion of gastric or duodenal sound as the cause of abnormal reaction of the patient, or of later complication, without mention of misadventure at the time of the procedure

Y84.6 Urinary catheterization as the cause of abnormal reaction of the patient, or of later complication, without mention of misadventure at the time of the procedure

Y84.7 Blood-sampling as the cause of abnormal reaction of the patient, or of later complication, without mention of misadventure at the time of the procedure

Y84.8 Other medical procedures as the cause of abnormal reaction of the patient, or of later complication, without mention of misadventure at the time of the procedure

AHA: 2021,1Q,5; 2014,4Q,24

Y84.9 Medical procedure, unspecified as the cause of abnormal reaction of the patient, or of later complication, without mention of misadventure at the time of the procedure

Supplementary factors related to causes of morbidity classified elsewhere (Y90-Y99)

NOTE These categories may be used to provide supplementary information concerning causes of morbidity. They are not to be used for single-condition coding.

Y90 Evidence of alcohol involvement determined by blood alcohol level

Code first any associated alcohol related disorders (F10)

Y90.0 Blood alcohol level of less than 20 mg/100 ml

Y90.1 Blood alcohol level of 20-39 mg/100 ml

Y90.2 Blood alcohol level of 40-59 mg/100 ml

Y90.3 Blood alcohol level of 60-79 mg/100 ml

Y90.4 Blood alcohol level of 80-99 mg/100 ml

Y90.5 Blood alcohol level of 100-119 mg/100 ml

Y90.6 Blood alcohol level of 120-199 mg/100 ml

Y90.7 Blood alcohol level of 200-239 mg/100 ml

Y90.8 Blood alcohol level of 240 mg/100 ml or more

Y90.9 Presence of alcohol in blood, level not specified

Y92 Place of occurrence of the external cause

The following category is for use, when relevant, to identify the place of occurrence of the external cause. Use in conjunction with an activity code.

Place of occurrence should be recorded only at the initial encounter for treatment

Y92.0 Non-institutional (private) residence as the place of occurrence of the external cause

EXCLUDES 1 *abandoned or derelict house (Y92.89)*
home under construction but not yet occupied (Y92.6-)
institutional place of residence (Y92.1-)

Y92.00 Unspecified non-institutional (private) residence as the place of occurrence of the external cause

Y92.000 Kitchen of unspecified non-institutional (private) residence as the place of occurrence of the external cause

Y92.001 Dining room of unspecified non-institutional (private) residence as the place of occurrence of the external cause

Y92.002 Bathroom of unspecified non-institutional (private) residence as the place of occurrence of the external cause

Y92.003 Bedroom of unspecified non-institutional (private) residence as the place of occurrence of the external cause

Y92.007 Garden or yard of unspecified non-institutional (private) residence as the place of occurrence of the external cause

Y92.008 Other place in unspecified non-institutional (private) residence as the place of occurrence of the external cause

Y92.009 Unspecified place in unspecified non-institutional (private) residence as the place of occurrence of the external cause

Home (NOS) as the place of occurrence of the external cause

Y92.01 Single-family non-institutional (private) house as the place of occurrence of the external cause

Farmhouse as the place of occurrence of the external cause

EXCLUDES 1 *barn (Y92.71)*
chicken coop or hen house (Y92.72)
farm field (Y92.73)
orchard (Y92.74)
single family mobile home or trailer (Y92.02-)
slaughter house (Y92.86)

Y92.010 Kitchen of single-family (private) house as the place of occurrence of the external cause

Y92.011 Dining room of single-family (private) house as the place of occurrence of the external cause

Y92.012 Bathroom of single-family (private) house as the place of occurrence of the external cause

Y92.013 Bedroom of single-family (private) house as the place of occurrence of the external cause

Y92.014 Private driveway to single-family (private) house as the place of occurrence of the external cause

Y92.015 Private garage of single-family (private) house as the place of occurrence of the external cause

Y92.016 Swimming-pool in single-family (private) house or garden as the place of occurrence of the external cause

Y92.017 Garden or yard in single-family (private) house as the place of occurrence of the external cause

Y92.018 Other place in single-family (private) house as the place of occurrence of the external cause

Y92.019 Unspecified place in single-family (private) house as the place of occurrence of the external cause

Y92.02 Mobile home as the place of occurrence of the external cause

Y92.020 Kitchen in mobile home as the place of occurrence of the external cause

Y92.021 Dining room in mobile home as the place of occurrence of the external cause

Y92.022 Bathroom in mobile home as the place of occurrence of the external cause

Y92.023 Bedroom in mobile home as the place of occurrence of the external cause

Y92.024 Driveway of mobile home as the place of occurrence of the external cause

Y92.025 Garage of mobile home as the place of occurrence of the external cause

Y92.026 Swimming-pool of mobile home as the place of occurrence of the external cause

Y92.027 Garden or yard of mobile home as the place of occurrence of the external cause

Y92.028 Other place in mobile home as the place of occurrence of the external cause

Y92.029 Unspecified place in mobile home as the place of occurrence of the external cause

Y92.03 Apartment as the place of occurrence of the external cause

Condominium as the place of occurrence of the external cause

Co-op apartment as the place of occurrence of the external cause

Y92.030 Kitchen in apartment as the place of occurrence of the external cause

Y92.031 Bathroom in apartment as the place of occurrence of the external cause

Y92.032 Bedroom in apartment as the place of occurrence of the external cause

Y92.038 Other place in apartment as the place of occurrence of the external cause

Y92.039 Unspecified place in apartment as the place of occurrence of the external cause

Y92.04 Boarding-house as the place of occurrence of the external cause

Y92.040 Kitchen in boarding-house as the place of occurrence of the external cause

Y92.041 Bathroom in boarding-house as the place of occurrence of the external cause

Y92.042 Bedroom in boarding-house as the place of occurrence of the external cause

Y92.043 Driveway of boarding-house as the place of occurrence of the external cause

Y92.044 Garage of boarding-house as the place of occurrence of the external cause

Y92.045 Swimming-pool of boarding-house as the place of occurrence of the external cause

Y92.046 Garden or yard of boarding-house as the place of occurrence of the external cause

Y92.048 Other place in boarding-house as the place of occurrence of the external cause

Y92.049 Unspecified place in boarding-house as the place of occurrence of the external cause

Y92.09 Other non-institutional residence as the place of occurrence of the external cause

AHA: 2017,2Q,10

Y92.090 Kitchen in other non-institutional residence as the place of occurrence of the external cause

Y92.091 Bathroom in other non-institutional residence as the place of occurrence of the external cause

Y92.092 Bedroom in other non-institutional residence as the place of occurrence of the external cause

Y92.093 Driveway of other non-institutional residence as the place of occurrence of the external cause

Y92.094 Garage of other non-institutional residence as the place of occurrence of the external cause

Y92.095 Swimming-pool of other non-institutional residence as the place of occurrence of the external cause

Y92.096 Garden or yard of other non-institutional residence as the place of occurrence of the external cause

Y92.098 Other place in other non-institutional residence as the place of occurrence of the external cause

Y92.099 Unspecified place in other non-institutional residence as the place of occurrence of the external cause

Y92.1 Institutional (nonprivate) residence as the place of occurrence of the external cause

Y92.10 Unspecified residential institution as the place of occurrence of the external cause

Y92.11 Children's home and orphanage as the place of occurrence of the external cause

Y92.110 Kitchen in children's home and orphanage as the place of occurrence of the external cause

Y92.111 Bathroom in children's home and orphanage as the place of occurrence of the external cause

Y92.112 Bedroom in children's home and orphanage as the place of occurrence of the external cause

Y92.113 Driveway of children's home and orphanage as the place of occurrence of the external cause

Y92.114 Garage of children's home and orphanage as the place of occurrence of the external cause

Y92.115 Swimming-pool of children's home and orphanage as the place of occurrence of the external cause

Y92.116 Garden or yard of children's home and orphanage as the place of occurrence of the external cause

Y92.118 Other place in children's home and orphanage as the place of occurrence of the external cause

Y92.119 Unspecified place in children's home and orphanage as the place of occurrence of the external cause

Y92.12 Nursing home as the place of occurrence of the external cause

Home for the sick as the place of occurrence of the external cause

Hospice as the place of occurrence of the external cause

AHA: 2017,2Q,10

Y92.120 Kitchen in nursing home as the place of occurrence of the external cause

Y92.121 Bathroom in nursing home as the place of occurrence of the external cause

Y92.122 Bedroom in nursing home as the place of occurrence of the external cause

Y92.123 Driveway of nursing home as the place of occurrence of the external cause

Y92.124 Garage of nursing home as the place of occurrence of the external cause

Y92.125 Swimming-pool of nursing home as the place of occurrence of the external cause

Y92.126 Garden or yard of nursing home as the place of occurrence of the external cause

Y92.128 Other place in nursing home as the place of occurrence of the external cause

Y92.129 Unspecified place in nursing home as the place of occurrence of the external cause

Y92.13 Military base as the place of occurrence of the external cause

EXCLUDES 1 *military training grounds (Y92.84)*

Y92.130 Kitchen on military base as the place of occurrence of the external cause

Y92.131 Mess hall on military base as the place of occurrence of the external cause

Y92.133 Barracks on military base as the place of occurrence of the external cause

Y92.135 Garage on military base as the place of occurrence of the external cause

Y92.136 Swimming-pool on military base as the place of occurrence of the external cause

Y92.137 Garden or yard on military base as the place of occurrence of the external cause

Y92.138 Other place on military base as the place of occurrence of the external cause

Y92.139 Unspecified place military base as the place of occurrence of the external cause

Y92.14 Prison as the place of occurrence of the external cause

Y92.140 Kitchen in prison as the place of occurrence of the external cause

Y92.141 Dining room in prison as the place of occurrence of the external cause

Y92.142 Bathroom in prison as the place of occurrence of the external cause

Y92.143 Cell of prison as the place of occurrence of the external cause

Y92.146 Swimming-pool of prison as the place of occurrence of the external cause

Y92.147 Courtyard of prison as the place of occurrence of the external cause

Y92.148 Other place in prison as the place of occurrence of the external cause

Y92.149 Unspecified place in prison as the place of occurrence of the external cause

Y92.15 Reform school as the place of occurrence of the external cause

Y92.150 Kitchen in reform school as the place of occurrence of the external cause

Y92.151 Dining room in reform school as the place of occurrence of the external cause

Y92.152 Bathroom in reform school as the place of occurrence of the external cause

Y92.153 Bedroom in reform school as the place of occurrence of the external cause

Y92.154 Driveway of reform school as the place of occurrence of the external cause

Y92.155 Garage of reform school as the place of occurrence of the external cause

Y92.156 Swimming-pool of reform school as the place of occurrence of the external cause

Y92.157 Garden or yard of reform school as the place of occurrence of the external cause

Y92.158 Other place in reform school as the place of occurrence of the external cause

Y92.159 Unspecified place in reform school as the place of occurrence of the external cause

Y92.16 School dormitory as the place of occurrence of the external cause

EXCLUDES 1 *reform school as the place of occurrence of the external cause (Y92.15-)*

school buildings and grounds as the place of occurrence of the external cause (Y92.2-)

school sports and athletic areas as the place of occurrence of the external cause (Y92.3-)

Y92.160 Kitchen in school dormitory as the place of occurrence of the external cause

Y92.161 Dining room in school dormitory as the place of occurrence of the external cause

Y92.162 Bathroom in school dormitory as the place of occurrence of the external cause

Y92.163 Bedroom in school dormitory as the place of occurrence of the external cause

Y92.168 Other place in school dormitory as the place of occurrence of the external cause

Y92.169 Unspecified place in school dormitory as the place of occurrence of the external cause

Y92.19 Other specified residential institution as the place of occurrence of the external cause

AHA: 2017,2Q,10

Y92.190 Kitchen in other specified residential institution as the place of occurrence of the external cause

Y92.191 Dining room in other specified residential institution as the place of occurrence of the external cause

Y92.192 Bathroom in other specified residential institution as the place of occurrence of the external cause

Y92.193 Bedroom in other specified residential institution as the place of occurrence of the external cause

Y92.194 Driveway of other specified residential institution as the place of occurrence of the external cause

Y92.195 Garage of other specified residential institution as the place of occurrence of the external cause

Y92.196 Pool of other specified residential institution as the place of occurrence of the external cause

Y92.197 Garden or yard of other specified residential institution as the place of occurrence of the external cause

Y92.198 Other place in other specified residential institution as the place of occurrence of the external cause

Y92.199 Unspecified place in other specified residential institution as the place of occurrence of the external cause

5th **Y92.2 School, other institution and public administrative area as the place of occurrence of the external cause**

Building and adjacent grounds used by the general public or by a particular group of the public

EXCLUDES 1 *building under construction as the place of occurrence of the external cause (Y92.6)*

residential institution as the place of occurrence of the external cause (Y92.1)

school dormitory as the place of occurrence of the external cause (Y92.16-)

sports and athletics area of schools as the place of occurrence of the external cause (Y92.3-)

6th **Y92.21 School (private) (public) (state) as the place of occurrence of the external cause**

Y92.210 Daycare center as the place of occurrence of the external cause

Y92.211 Elementary school as the place of occurrence of the external cause

Kindergarten as the place of occurrence of the external cause

Y92.212 Middle school as the place of occurrence of the external cause

Y92.213 High school as the place of occurrence of the external cause

AHA: 2012,4Q,108

Y92.214 College as the place of occurrence of the external cause

University as the place of occurrence of the external cause

Y92.215 Trade school as the place of occurrence of the external cause

Y92.218 Other school as the place of occurrence of the external cause

Y92.219 Unspecified school as the place of occurrence of the external cause

Y92.22 Religious institution as the place of occurrence of the external cause

Church as the place of occurrence of the external cause

Mosque as the place of occurrence of the external cause

Synagogue as the place of occurrence of the external cause

6th **Y92.23 Hospital as the place of occurrence of the external cause**

EXCLUDES 1 *ambulatory (outpatient) health services establishments (Y92.53-)*

home for the sick as the place of occurrence of the external cause (Y92.12-)

hospice as the place of occurrence of the external cause (Y92.12-)

nursing home as the place of occurrence of the external cause (Y92.12-)

Y92.230 Patient room in hospital as the place of occurrence of the external cause

Y92.231 Patient bathroom in hospital as the place of occurrence of the external cause

Y92.232 Corridor of hospital as the place of occurrence of the external cause

Y92.233 Cafeteria of hospital as the place of occurrence of the external cause

Y92.234 Operating room of hospital as the place of occurrence of the external cause

Y92.238 Other place in hospital as the place of occurrence of the external cause

Y92.239 Unspecified place in hospital as the place of occurrence of the external cause

6th **Y92.24 Public administrative building as the place of occurrence of the external cause**

Y92.240 Courthouse as the place of occurrence of the external cause

Y92.241 Library as the place of occurrence of the external cause

Y92.242 Post office as the place of occurrence of the external cause

Y92.243 City hall as the place of occurrence of the external cause

Y92.248 Other public administrative building as the place of occurrence of the external cause

6th **Y92.25 Cultural building as the place of occurrence of the external cause**

Y92.250 Art Gallery as the place of occurrence of the external cause

Y92.251 Museum as the place of occurrence of the external cause

Y92.252 Music hall as the place of occurrence of the external cause

Y92.253 Opera house as the place of occurrence of the external cause

Y92.254 Theater (live) as the place of occurrence of the external cause

Y92.258 Other cultural public building as the place of occurrence of the external cause

Y92.26 Movie house or cinema as the place of occurrence of the external cause

Y92.29 Other specified public building as the place of occurrence of the external cause

Assembly hall as the place of occurrence of the external cause

Clubhouse as the place of occurrence of the external cause

5th **Y92.3 Sports and athletics area as the place of occurrence of the external cause**

6th **Y92.31 Athletic court as the place of occurrence of the external cause**

EXCLUDES 1 *tennis court in private home or garden (Y92.09)*

Y92.310 Basketball court as the place of occurrence of the external cause

Y92.311 Squash court as the place of occurrence of the external cause

Y92.312 Tennis court as the place of occurrence of the external cause

Y92.318 Other athletic court as the place of occurrence of the external cause

6th **Y92.32 Athletic field as the place of occurrence of the external cause**

Y92.320 Baseball field as the place of occurrence of the external cause

Y92.321 Football field as the place of occurrence of the external cause

Y92.322 Soccer field as the place of occurrence of the external cause

Y92.328 Other athletic field as the place of occurrence of the external cause

Cricket field as the place of occurrence of the external cause

Hockey field as the place of occurrence of the external cause

6th **Y92.33 Skating rink as the place of occurrence of the external cause**

Y92.330 Ice skating rink (indoor) (outdoor) as the place of occurrence of the external cause

Y92.331 Roller skating rink as the place of occurrence of the external cause

Y92.34 Swimming pool (public) as the place of occurrence of the external cause

EXCLUDES 1 *swimming pool in private home or garden (Y92.016)*

Y92.39 Other specified sports and athletic area as the place of occurrence of the external cause

Golf-course as the place of occurrence of the external cause

Gymnasium as the place of occurrence of the external cause

Riding-school as the place of occurrence of the external cause

Stadium as the place of occurrence of the external cause

✓5th **Y92.4 Street, highway and other paved roadways as the place of occurrence of the external cause**

EXCLUDES 1 *private driveway of residence (Y92.014, Y92.024, Y92.043, Y92.093, Y92.113, Y92.123, Y92.154, Y92.194)*

✓6th **Y92.41 Street and highway as the place of occurrence of the external cause**

Y92.410 Unspecified street and highway as the place of occurrence of the external cause

Road NOS as the place of occurrence of the external cause

Y92.411 Interstate highway as the place of occurrence of the external cause

Freeway as the place of occurrence of the external cause

Motorway as the place of occurrence of the external cause

Y92.412 Parkway as the place of occurrence of the external cause

Y92.413 State road as the place of occurrence of the external cause

Y92.414 Local residential or business street as the place of occurrence of the external cause

Y92.415 Exit ramp or entrance ramp of street or highway as the place of occurrence of the external cause

✓6th **Y92.48 Other paved roadways as the place of occurrence of the external cause**

Y92.480 Sidewalk as the place of occurrence of the external cause

Y92.481 Parking lot as the place of occurrence of the external cause

Y92.482 Bike path as the place of occurrence of the external cause

Y92.488 Other paved roadways as the place of occurrence of the external cause

✓5th **Y92.5 Trade and service area as the place of occurrence of the external cause**

EXCLUDES 1 *garage in private home (Y92.015)*
schools and other public administration buildings (Y92.2-)

✓6th **Y92.51 Private commercial establishments as the place of occurrence of the external cause**

Y92.510 Bank as the place of occurrence of the external cause

Y92.511 Restaurant or café as the place of occurrence of the external cause

Y92.512 Supermarket, store or market as the place of occurrence of the external cause

Y92.513 Shop (commercial) as the place of occurrence of the external cause

✓6th **Y92.52 Service areas as the place of occurrence of the external cause**

Y92.520 Airport as the place of occurrence of the external cause

Y92.521 Bus station as the place of occurrence of the external cause

Y92.522 Railway station as the place of occurrence of the external cause

Y92.523 Highway rest stop as the place of occurrence of the external cause

Y92.524 Gas station as the place of occurrence of the external cause

Petroleum station as the place of occurrence of the external cause

Service station as the place of occurrence of the external cause

✓6th **Y92.53 Ambulatory health services establishments as the place of occurrence of the external cause**

Y92.530 Ambulatory surgery center as the place of occurrence of the external cause

Outpatient surgery center, including that connected with a hospital as the place of occurrence of the external cause

Same day surgery center, including that connected with a hospital as the place of occurrence of the external cause

Y92.531 Health care provider office as the place of occurrence of the external cause

Physician office as the place of occurrence of the external cause

Y92.532 Urgent care center as the place of occurrence of the external cause

Y92.538 Other ambulatory health services establishments as the place of occurrence of the external cause

AHA: 2019,1Q,21

Y92.59 Other trade areas as the place of occurrence of the external cause

Office building as the place of occurrence of the external cause

Casino as the place of occurrence of the external cause

Garage (commercial) as the place of occurrence of the external cause

Hotel as the place of occurrence of the external cause

Radio or television station as the place of occurrence of the external cause

Shopping mall as the place of occurrence of the external cause

Warehouse as the place of occurrence of the external cause

✓5th **Y92.6 Industrial and construction area as the place of occurrence of the external cause**

Y92.61 Building [any] under construction as the place of occurrence of the external cause

Y92.62 Dock or shipyard as the place of occurrence of the external cause

Dockyard as the place of occurrence of the external cause

Dry dock as the place of occurrence of the external cause

Shipyard as the place of occurrence of the external cause

Y92.63 Factory as the place of occurrence of the external cause

Factory building as the place of occurrence of the external cause

Factory premises as the place of occurrence of the external cause

Industrial yard as the place of occurrence of the external cause

Y92.64 Mine or pit as the place of occurrence of the external cause

Mine as the place of occurrence of the external cause

Y92.65 Oil rig as the place of occurrence of the external cause

Pit (coal) (gravel) (sand) as the place of occurrence of the external cause

Y92.69 Other specified industrial and construction area as the place of occurrence of the external cause

Gasworks as the place of occurrence of the external cause

Power-station (coal) (nuclear) (oil) as the place of occurrence of the external cause

Tunnel under construction as the place of occurrence of the external cause

Workshop as the place of occurrence of the external cause

✓5th **Y92.7 Farm as the place of occurrence of the external cause**

Ranch as the place of occurrence of the external cause

EXCLUDES 1 *farmhouse and home premises of farm (Y92.01-)*

Y92.71 Barn as the place of occurrence of the external cause

Y92.72 Chicken coop as the place of occurrence of the external cause
Hen house as the place of occurrence of the external cause

Y92.73 Farm field as the place of occurrence of the external cause

Y92.74 Orchard as the place of occurrence of the external cause

Y92.79 Other farm location as the place of occurrence of the external cause

√5th **Y92.8 Other places as the place of occurrence of the external cause**

√6th **Y92.81 Transport vehicle as the place of occurrence of the external cause**
EXCLUDES 1 *transport accidents (VØØ-V99)*

Y92.81Ø Car as the place of occurrence of the external cause

Y92.811 Bus as the place of occurrence of the external cause

Y92.812 Truck as the place of occurrence of the external cause

Y92.813 Airplane as the place of occurrence of the external cause

Y92.814 Boat as the place of occurrence of the external cause

Y92.815 Train as the place of occurrence of the external cause

Y92.816 Subway car as the place of occurrence of the external cause

Y92.818 Other transport vehicle as the place of occurrence of the external cause

√6th **Y92.82 Wilderness area**

Y92.82Ø Desert as the place of occurrence of the external cause

Y92.821 Forest as the place of occurrence of the external cause

Y92.828 Other wilderness area as the place of occurrence of the external cause
Swamp as the place of occurrence of the external cause
Mountain as the place of occurrence of the external cause
Marsh as the place of occurrence of the external cause
Prairie as the place of occurrence of the external cause

√6th **Y92.83 Recreation area as the place of occurrence of the external cause**

Y92.83Ø Public park as the place of occurrence of the external cause

Y92.831 Amusement park as the place of occurrence of the external cause

Y92.832 Beach as the place of occurrence of the external cause
Seashore as the place of occurrence of the external cause

Y92.833 Campsite as the place of occurrence of the external cause

Y92.834 Zoological garden (Zoo) as the place of occurrence of the external cause

Y92.838 Other recreation area as the place of occurrence of the external cause

Y92.84 Military training ground as the place of occurrence of the external cause

Y92.85 Railroad track as the place of occurrence of the external cause

Y92.86 Slaughter house as the place of occurrence of the external cause

Y92.89 Other specified places as the place of occurrence of the external cause
Derelict house as the place of occurrence of the external cause

Y92.9 Unspecified place or not applicable

√4th **Y93 Activity codes**

NOTE Category Y93 is provided for use to indicate the activity of the person seeking healthcare for an injury or health condition, such as a heart attack while shoveling snow, which resulted from, or was contributed to, by the activity. These codes are appropriate for use for both acute injuries, such as those from chapter 19, and conditions that are due to the long-term, cumulative effects of an activity, such as those from chapter 13. They are also appropriate for use with external cause codes for cause and intent if identifying the activity provides additional information on the event. These codes should be used in conjunction with codes for external cause status (Y99) and place of occurrence (Y92).

This section contains the following broad activity categories:

Y93.Ø	Activities involving walking and running
Y93.1	Activities involving water and water craft
Y93.2	Activities involving ice and snow
Y93.3	Activities involving climbing, rappelling, and jumping off
Y93.4	Activities involving dancing and other rhythmic movement
Y93.5	Activities involving other sports and athletics played individually
Y93.6	Activities involving other sports and athletics played as a team or group
Y93.7	Activities involving other specified sports and athletics
Y93.A	Activities involving other cardiorespiratory exercise
Y93.B	Activities involving other muscle strengthening exercises
Y93.C	Activities involving computer technology and electronic devices
Y93.D	Activities involving arts and handcrafts
Y93.E	Activities involving personal hygiene and interior property and clothing maintenance
Y93.F	Activities involving caregiving
Y93.G	Activities involving food preparation, cooking and grilling
Y93.H	Activities involving exterior property and land maintenance, building and construction
Y93.I	Activities involving roller coasters and other types of external motion
Y93.J	Activities involving playing musical instrument
Y93.K	Activities involving animal care
Y93.8	Activities, other specified
Y93.9	Activity, unspecified

√5th **Y93.Ø Activities involving walking and running**
EXCLUDES 1 *activity, walking an animal (Y93.K1)*
activity, walking or running on a treadmill (Y93.A1)

Y93.Ø1 Activity, walking, marching and hiking
Activity, walking, marching and hiking on level or elevated terrain
EXCLUDES 1 *activity, mountain climbing (Y93.31)*

Y93.Ø2 Activity, running

√5th **Y93.1 Activities involving water and water craft**
EXCLUDES 1 *activities involving ice (Y93.2-)*

Y93.11 Activity, swimming

Y93.12 Activity, springboard and platform diving

Y93.13 Activity, water polo

Y93.14 Activity, water aerobics and water exercise

Y93.15 Activity, underwater diving and snorkeling
Activity, SCUBA diving

Y93.16 Activity, rowing, canoeing, kayaking, rafting and tubing
Activity, canoeing, kayaking, rafting and tubing in calm and turbulent water

Y93.17 Activity, water skiing and wake boarding

Y93.18 Activity, surfing, windsurfing and boogie boarding
Activity, water sliding

Y93.19 Activity, other involving water and watercraft
Activity involving water NOS
Activity, parasailing
Activity, water survival training and testing

Y93.2 Activities involving ice and snow
EXCLUDES 1 *activity, shoveling ice and snow (Y93.H1)*

Y93.21 Activity, ice skating
Activity, figure skating (singles) (pairs)
Activity, ice dancing
EXCLUDES 1 *activity, ice hockey (Y93.22)*

Y93.22 Activity, ice hockey

Y93.23 Activity, snow (alpine) (downhill) skiing, snowboarding, sledding, tobogganing and snow tubing
EXCLUDES 1 *activity, cross country skiing (Y93.24)*

Y93.24 Activity, cross country skiing
Activity, nordic skiing

Y93.29 Activity, other involving ice and snow
Activity involving ice and snow NOS

Y93.3 Activities involving climbing, rappelling and jumping off
EXCLUDES 1 *activity, hiking on level or elevated terrain (Y93.Ø1)*
activity, jumping rope (Y93.56)
activity, trampoline jumping (Y93.44)

Y93.31 Activity, mountain climbing, rock climbing and wall climbing

Y93.32 Activity, rappelling

Y93.33 Activity, BASE jumping
Activity, Building, Antenna, Span, Earth jumping

Y93.34 Activity, bungee jumping

Y93.35 Activity, hang gliding

Y93.39 Activity, other involving climbing, rappelling and jumping off

Y93.4 Activities involving dancing and other rhythmic movement
EXCLUDES 1 *activity, martial arts (Y93.75)*

Y93.41 Activity, dancing
AHA: 2012,4Q,108

Y93.42 Activity, yoga

Y93.43 Activity, gymnastics
Activity, rhythmic gymnastics
EXCLUDES 1 *activity, trampolining (Y93.44)*

Y93.44 Activity, trampolining

Y93.45 Activity, cheerleading

Y93.49 Activity, other involving dancing and other rhythmic movements

Y93.5 Activities involving other sports and athletics played individually
EXCLUDES 1 *activity, dancing (Y93.41)*
activity, gymnastic (Y93.43)
activity, trampolining (Y93.44)
activity, yoga (Y93.42)

Y93.51 Activity, roller skating (inline) and skateboarding

Y93.52 Activity, horseback riding

Y93.53 Activity, golf

Y93.54 Activity, bowling

Y93.55 Activity, bike riding

Y93.56 Activity, jumping rope

Y93.57 Activity, non-running track and field events
EXCLUDES 1 *activity, running (any form) (Y93.Ø2)*

Y93.59 Activity, other involving other sports and athletics played individually
EXCLUDES 1 *activities involving climbing, rappelling, and jumping (Y93.3-)*
activities involving ice and snow (Y93.2-)
activities involving walking and running (Y93.Ø-)
activities involving water and watercraft (Y93.1-)

Y93.6 Activities involving other sports and athletics played as a team or group
EXCLUDES 1 *activity, ice hockey (Y93.22)*
activity, water polo (Y93.13)

Y93.61 Activity, American tackle football
Activity, football NOS

Y93.62 Activity, American flag or touch football

Y93.63 Activity, rugby

Y93.64 Activity, baseball
Activity, softball

Y93.65 Activity, lacrosse and field hockey

Y93.66 Activity, soccer

Y93.67 Activity, basketball

Y93.68 Activity, volleyball (beach) (court)

Y93.6A Activity, physical games generally associated with school recess, summer camp and children
Activity, capture the flag
Activity, dodge ball
Activity, four square
Activity, kickball

Y93.69 Activity, other involving other sports and athletics played as a team or group
Activity, cricket

Y93.7 Activities involving other specified sports and athletics

Y93.71 Activity, boxing

Y93.72 Activity, wrestling

Y93.73 Activity, racquet and hand sports
Activity, handball
Activity, racquetball
Activity, squash
Activity, tennis

Y93.74 Activity, frisbee
Activity, ultimate frisbee

Y93.75 Activity, martial arts
Activity, combatives

Y93.79 Activity, other specified sports and athletics
EXCLUDES 1 *sports and athletics activities specified in categories Y93.Ø-Y93.6*

Y93.A Activities involving other cardiorespiratory exercise
Activities involving physical training

Y93.A1 Activity, exercise machines primarily for cardiorespiratory conditioning
Activity, elliptical and stepper machines
Activity, stationary bike
Activity, treadmill

Y93.A2 Activity, calisthenics
Activity, jumping jacks
Activity, warm up and cool down

Y93.A3 Activity, aerobic and step exercise

Y93.A4 Activity, circuit training

Y93.A5 Activity, obstacle course
Activity, challenge course
Activity, confidence course

Y93.A6 Activity, grass drills
Activity, guerilla drills

Y93.A9 Activity, other involving cardiorespiratory exercise
EXCLUDES 1 *activities involving cardiorespiratory exercise specified in categories Y93.Ø-Y93.7*

Y93.B Activities involving other muscle strengthening exercises

Y93.B1 Activity, exercise machines primarily for muscle strengthening

Y93.B2 Activity, push-ups, pull-ups, sit-ups

Y93.B3 Activity, free weights
Activity, barbells
Activity, dumbbells

Y93.B4 Activity, pilates

Y93.B9 Activity, other involving muscle strengthening exercises
EXCLUDES 1 *activities involving muscle strengthening specified in categories Y93.Ø-Y93.A*

Y93.C Activities involving computer technology and electronic devices
EXCLUDES 1 *activity, electronic musical keyboard or instruments (Y93.J-)*

Y93.C1 Activity, computer keyboarding
Activity, electronic game playing using keyboard or other stationary device

Y93.C2 Activity, hand held interactive electronic device
Activity, cellular telephone and communication device
Activity, electronic game playing using interactive device
EXCLUDES 1 *activity, electronic game playing using keyboard or other stationary device (Y93.C1)*

Y93.C9 Activity, other involving computer technology and electronic devices

Y93.D Activities involving arts and handcrafts
EXCLUDES 1 *activities involving playing musical instrument (Y93.J-)*

Y93.D1 Activity, knitting and crocheting

Y93.D2 Activity, sewing

Y93.D3 Activity, furniture building and finishing
Activity, furniture repair

Y93.D9 Activity, other involving arts and handcrafts

Y93.E Activities involving personal hygiene and interior property and clothing maintenance

EXCLUDES 1 *activities involving cooking and grilling (Y93.G-)*
activities involving exterior property and land maintenance, building and construction (Y93.H-)
activities involving caregiving (Y93.F-)
activity, dishwashing (Y93.G1)
activity, food preparation (Y93.G1)
activity, gardening (Y93.H2)

Y93.E1 Activity, personal bathing and showering

Y93.E2 Activity, laundry

Y93.E3 Activity, vacuuming

Y93.E4 Activity, ironing

Y93.E5 Activity, floor mopping and cleaning

Y93.E6 Activity, residential relocation
Activity, packing up and unpacking involved in moving to a new residence

Y93.E8 Activity, other personal hygiene

Y93.E9 Activity, other interior property and clothing maintenance

Y93.F Activities involving caregiving
Activity involving the provider of caregiving

Y93.F1 Activity, caregiving, bathing

Y93.F2 Activity, caregiving, lifting

Y93.F9 Activity, other caregiving

Y93.G Activities involving food preparation, cooking and grilling

Y93.G1 Activity, food preparation and clean up
Activity, dishwashing

Y93.G2 Activity, grilling and smoking food

Y93.G3 Activity, cooking and baking
Activity, use of stove, oven and microwave oven

Y93.G9 Activity, other involving cooking and grilling

Y93.H Activities involving exterior property and land maintenance, building and construction

Y93.H1 Activity, digging, shoveling and raking
Activity, dirt digging
Activity, raking leaves
Activity, snow shoveling

Y93.H2 Activity, gardening and landscaping
Activity, pruning, trimming shrubs, weeding

Y93.H3 Activity, building and construction

Y93.H9 Activity, other involving exterior property and land maintenance, building and construction

Y93.I Activities involving roller coasters and other types of external motion

Y93.I1 Activity, rollercoaster riding

Y93.I9 Activity, other involving external motion

Y93.J Activities involving playing musical instrument
Activity involving playing electric musical instrument

Y93.J1 Activity, piano playing
Activity, musical keyboard (electronic) playing

Y93.J2 Activity, drum and other percussion instrument playing

Y93.J3 Activity, string instrument playing

Y93.J4 Activity, winds and brass instrument playing

Y93.K Activities involving animal care

EXCLUDES 1 *activity, horseback riding (Y93.52)*

Y93.K1 Activity, walking an animal

Y93.K2 Activity, milking an animal

Y93.K3 Activity, grooming and shearing an animal

Y93.K9 Activity, other involving animal care

Y93.8 Activities, other specified

Y93.81 Activity, refereeing a sports activity

Y93.82 Activity, spectator at an event

Y93.83 Activity, rough housing and horseplay

Y93.84 Activity, sleeping

Y93.85 Activity, choking game
Activity, blackout game
Activity, fainting game
Activity, pass out game
AHA: 2016,4Q,74-76

Y93.89 Activity, other specified

Y93.9 Activity, unspecified

Y95 Nosocomial condition
AHA: 2013,4Q,119

Y99 External cause status

NOTE A single code from category Y99 should be used in conjunction with the external cause code(s) assigned to a record to indicate the status of the person at the time the event occurred.

Y99.Ø Civilian activity done for income or pay
Civilian activity done for financial or other compensation

EXCLUDES 1 *military activity (Y99.1)*
volunteer activity (Y99.2)

Y99.1 Military activity

EXCLUDES 1 *activity of off duty military personnel (Y99.8)*

Y99.2 Volunteer activity

EXCLUDES 1 *activity of child or other family member assisting in compensated work of other family member (Y99.8)*

Y99.8 Other external cause status
Activity NEC
Activity of child or other family member assisting in compensated work of other family member
Hobby not done for income
Leisure activity
Off-duty activity of military personnel
Recreation or sport not for income or while a student
Student activity

EXCLUDES 1 *civilian activity done for income or compensation (Y99.Ø)*
military activity (Y99.1)

AHA: 2012,4Q,108

Y99.9 Unspecified external cause status

Chapter 21. Factors Influencing Health Status and Contact with Health Services (ZØØ–Z99)

Chapter-specific Guidelines with Coding Examples

The chapter-specific guidelines from the ICD-10-CM Official Guidelines for Coding and Reporting have been provided below. Along with these guidelines are coding examples, contained in the shaded boxes, that have been developed to help illustrate the coding and/or sequencing guidance found in these guidelines.

Note: The chapter-specific guidelines provide additional information about the use of Z codes for specified encounters.

a. Use of Z Codes in any healthcare setting

Z codes are for use in any healthcare setting. Z codes may be used as either a first-listed (principal diagnosis code in the inpatient setting) or secondary code, depending on the circumstances of the encounter. Certain Z codes may only be used as first-listed or principal diagnosis.

Patient with middle lobe lung cancer admitted for initiation of chemotherapy

Z51.11	**Encounter for antineoplastic chemotherapy**
C34.2	**Malignant neoplasm of middle lobe, bronchus or lung**

Explanation: A Z code can be used as first-listed in this situation based on guidelines in this chapter as well as chapter 2, "Neoplasms."

b. Z Codes indicate a reason for an encounter or provide additional information about a patient encounter

Z codes are not procedure codes. A corresponding procedure code must accompany a Z code to describe any procedure performed.

c. Categories of Z Codes

1) Contact/exposure

Category Z2Ø indicates contact with, and suspected exposure to, communicable diseases. These codes are for patients who are suspected to have been exposed to a disease by close personal contact with an infected individual or are in an area where a disease is epidemic.

Category Z77, Other contact with and (suspected) exposures hazardous to health, indicates contact with and suspected exposures hazardous to health.

Contact/exposure codes may be used as a first-listed code to explain an encounter for testing, or, more commonly, as a secondary code to identify a potential risk.

2) Inoculations and vaccinations

Code Z23 is for encounters for inoculations and vaccinations. It indicates that a patient is being seen to receive a prophylactic inoculation against a disease. Procedure codes are required to identify the actual administration of the injection and the type(s) of immunizations given. Code Z23 may be used as a secondary code if the inoculation is given as a routine part of preventive health care, such as a well-baby visit.

3) Status

Status codes indicate that a patient is either a carrier of a disease or has the sequelae or residual of a past disease or condition. This includes such things as the presence of prosthetic or mechanical devices resulting from past treatment. A status code is informative, because the status may affect the course of treatment and its outcome. A status code is distinct from a history code. The history code indicates that the patient no longer has the condition.

A status code should not be used with a diagnosis code from one of the body system chapters, if the diagnosis code includes the information provided by the status code. For example, code Z94.1, Heart transplant status, should not be used with a code from subcategory T86.2, Complications of heart transplant. The status code does not provide additional information. The complication code indicates that the patient is a heart transplant patient.

For encounters for weaning from a mechanical ventilator, assign a code from subcategory J96.1, Chronic respiratory failure, followed by code Z99.11, Dependence on respirator [ventilator] status.

The status Z codes/categories are:

Z14 Genetic carrier

Genetic carrier status indicates that a person carries a gene, associated with a particular disease, which may be passed to offspring who may develop that disease. The person does not have the disease and is not at risk of developing the disease.

Z15 Genetic susceptibility to disease

Genetic susceptibility indicates that a person has a gene that increases the risk of that person developing the disease.

Codes from category Z15 should not be used as principal or first-listed codes. If the patient has the condition to which he/she is susceptible, and that condition is the reason for the encounter, the code for the current condition should be sequenced first. If the patient is being seen for follow-up after completed treatment for this condition, and the condition no longer exists, a follow-up code should be sequenced first, followed by the appropriate personal history and genetic susceptibility codes. If the purpose of the encounter is genetic counseling associated with procreative management, code Z31.5, Encounter for genetic counseling, should be assigned as the first-listed code, followed by a code from category Z15. Additional codes should be assigned for any applicable family or personal history.

Z16 Resistance to antimicrobial drugs

This code indicates that a patient has a condition that is resistant to antimicrobial drug treatment. Sequence the infection code first.

Penicillin resistant streptococcus pneumoniae meningitis

GØØ.1	**Pneumococcal meningitis**
Z16.11	**Resistance to penicillins**

Explanation: The status Z code is used to describe the presence of a drug-resistant organism that most likely altered how the meningitis was treated.

Z17 Estrogen receptor status

Z18 Retained foreign body fragments

Z19 Hormone sensitivity malignancy status

Z21 Asymptomatic HIV infection status

This code indicates that a patient has tested positive for HIV but has manifested no signs or symptoms of the disease.

Z22 Carrier of infectious disease

Carrier status indicates that a person harbors the specific organisms of a disease without manifest symptoms and is capable of transmitting the infection.

Z28.3 Underimmunization status

See Section I.B.14. for underimmunization documentation by clinicians other than the patient's provider.

Z33.1 Pregnant state, incidental

This code is a secondary code only for use when the pregnancy is in no way complicating the reason for visit. Otherwise, a code from the obstetric chapter is required.

Z66 Do not resuscitate

This code may be used when it is documented by the provider that a patient is on do not resuscitate status at any time during the stay.

Z67 Blood type

Z68 Body mass index (BMI)

BMI codes should only be assigned when there is an associated, reportable diagnosis (such as obesity). Do not assign BMI codes during pregnancy.

See Section I.B.14. for BMI documentation by clinicians other than the patient's provider.

Z74.Ø1 Bed confinement status

Z76.82 Awaiting organ transplant status

Z78 Other specified health status

Code Z78.1, Physical restraint status, may be used when it is documented by the provider that a patient has been put in restraints during the current encounter. Please note that this code should not be reported when it is documented by the provider that a patient is temporarily restrained during a procedure.

Z79 Long-term (current) drug therapy

Codes from this category indicate a patient's continuous use of a prescribed drug (including such things as aspirin therapy) for the long-term treatment of a condition or for prophylactic use. It is not for use for patients who have addictions to drugs. This subcategory is not for use of medications for detoxification or maintenance programs to prevent withdrawal symptoms (e.g., methadone maintenance for opiate dependence). Assign the appropriate code for the drug use, abuse, or dependence instead.

Assign a code from Z79 if the patient is receiving a medication for an extended period as a prophylactic measure (such as for the prevention of deep vein thrombosis) or as treatment of a chronic condition (such as arthritis) or a disease requiring a lengthy course of treatment (such as cancer). Do not assign a code from category Z79 for medication being administered for a brief period of time to treat an acute illness or injury (such as a course of antibiotics to treat acute bronchitis).

Z88 Allergy status to drugs, medicaments and biological substances

Except: Z88.9, Allergy status to unspecified drugs, medicaments and biological substances status

Z89 Acquired absence of limb

Z90 Acquired absence of organs, not elsewhere classified

Z91.0- Allergy status, other than to drugs and biological substances

Z92.82 Status post administration of tPA (rtPA) in a different facility within the last 24 hours prior to admission to a current facility

Assign code Z92.82, Status post administration of tPA (rtPA) in a different facility within the last 24 hours prior to admission to current facility, as a secondary diagnosis when a patient is received by transfer into a facility and documentation indicates they were administered tissue plasminogen activator (tPA) within the last 24 hours prior to admission to the current facility.

This guideline applies even if the patient is still receiving the tPA at the time they are received into the current facility.

The appropriate code for the condition for which the tPA was administered (such as cerebrovascular disease or myocardial infarction) should be assigned first.

Code Z92.82 is only applicable to the receiving facility record and not to the transferring facility record.

Z93 Artificial opening status

Z94 Transplanted organ and tissue status

Z95 Presence of cardiac and vascular implants and grafts

Z96 Presence of other functional implants

Z97 Presence of other devices

Z98 Other postprocedural states

Assign code Z98.85, Transplanted organ removal status, to indicate that a transplanted organ has been previously removed. This code should not be assigned for the encounter in which the transplanted organ is removed. The complication necessitating removal of the transplant organ should be assigned for that encounter.

See section I.C.19. for information on the coding of organ transplant complications.

Z99 Dependence on enabling machines and devices, not elsewhere classified

Note: Categories Z89-Z90 and Z93-Z99 are for use only if there are no complications or malfunctions of the organ or tissue replaced, the amputation site or the equipment on which the patient is dependent.

4) History (of)

There are two types of history Z codes, personal and family. Personal history codes explain a patient's past medical condition that no longer exists and is not receiving any treatment, but that has the potential for recurrence, and therefore may require continued monitoring.

Family history codes are for use when a patient has a family member(s) who has had a particular disease that causes the patient to be at higher risk of also contracting the disease.

Personal history codes may be used in conjunction with follow-up codes and family history codes may be used in conjunction with screening codes to explain the need for a test or procedure. History codes are also acceptable on any medical record regardless of the reason for visit. A history of an illness, even if no longer present, is important information that may alter the type of treatment ordered.

The reason for the encounter (for example, screening or counseling) should be sequenced first and the appropriate personal and/or family history code(s) should be assigned as additional diagnos(es).

The history Z code categories are:

Z80 Family history of primary malignant neoplasm

Z81 Family history of mental and behavioral disorders

Z82 Family history of certain disabilities and chronic diseases (leading to disablement)

Z83 Family history of other specific disorders

Z84 Family history of other conditions

Z85 Personal history of malignant neoplasm

Z86 Personal history of certain other diseases

Z87 Personal history of other diseases and conditions

Z91.4- Personal history of psychological trauma, not elsewhere classified

Z91.5- Personal history of self-harm

Z91.81 History of falling

Z91.82 Personal history of military deployment

Z92 Personal history of medical treatment

Except: Z92.0, Personal history of contraception

Except: Z92.82, Status post administration of tPA (rtPA) in a different facility within the last 24 hours prior to admission to a current facility

Patient has chronic lymphocytic leukemia for which the patient had previous chemotherapy and is now in remission

C91.11 Chronic lymphocytic leukemia of B-cell type in remission

Z92.21 Personal history of antineoplastic chemotherapy

Explanation: The personal history Z code is used to describe a secondary (supplementary) diagnosis to identify that this patient has had chemotherapy in the past.

5) Screening

Screening is the testing for disease or disease precursors in seemingly well individuals so that early detection and treatment can be provided for those who test positive for the disease (e.g., screening mammogram).

The testing of a person to rule out or confirm a suspected diagnosis because the patient has some sign or symptom is a diagnostic examination, not a screening. In these cases, the sign or symptom is used to explain the reason for the test.

A screening code may be a first-listed code if the reason for the visit is specifically the screening exam. It may also be used as an additional code if the screening is done during an office visit for other health problems. A screening code is not necessary if the screening is inherent to a routine examination, such as a pap smear done during a routine pelvic examination.

Should a condition be discovered during the screening then the code for the condition may be assigned as an additional diagnosis.

The Z code indicates that a screening exam is planned. A procedure code is required to confirm that the screening was performed.

The screening Z codes/categories:

Z11 Encounter for screening for infectious and parasitic diseases

Z12 Encounter for screening for malignant neoplasms

Z13 Encounter for screening for other diseases and disorders

Except: Z13.9, Encounter for screening, unspecified

Z36 Encounter for antenatal screening for mother

6) Observation

There are three observation Z code categories. They are for use in very limited circumstances when a person is being observed for a suspected condition that is ruled out. The observation codes are not for use if an injury or illness or any signs or symptoms related to the suspected condition are present. In such cases the diagnosis/symptom code is used with the corresponding external cause code.

The observation codes are primarily to be used as a principal/first-listed diagnosis. An observation code may be assigned as a secondary diagnosis code when the patient is being observed for a condition that is ruled out and is unrelated to the principal/first-listed diagnosis Also, when the principal diagnosis is required to be a code from category Z38, Liveborn infants according to place of birth and type of delivery, then a code from category Z05, Encounter for observation and evaluation of newborn for suspected diseases and conditions ruled out, is sequenced after the Z38 code. Additional codes may be used in addition to the observation code, but only if they are unrelated to the suspected condition being observed.

Codes from subcategory Z03.7, Encounter for suspected maternal and fetal conditions ruled out, may either be used as a first-listed or as an additional code assignment depending on the case. They are for use in very limited circumstances on a maternal record when an encounter is for a suspected maternal or fetal condition that is ruled out during that encounter (for example, a maternal or fetal condition may be suspected due to an abnormal test result). These codes should not be used when the condition is confirmed. In those cases, the confirmed condition should be coded. In addition, these codes are not for use if an illness or any signs or symptoms related to the suspected condition or problem are present. In such cases the diagnosis/symptom code is used.

Additional codes may be used in addition to the code from subcategory Z03.7, but only if they are unrelated to the suspected condition being evaluated.

Codes from subcategory Z03.7 may not be used for encounters for antenatal screening of mother. *See Section I.C.21. Screening.*

For encounters for suspected fetal condition that are inconclusive following testing and evaluation, assign the appropriate code from category O35, O36, O40 or O41.

The observation Z code categories:

Z03	Encounter for medical observation for suspected diseases and conditions ruled out
Z04	Encounter for examination and observation for other reasons
	Except: Z04.9, Encounter for examination and observation for unspecified reason
Z05	Encounter for observation and evaluation of newborn for suspected diseases and conditions ruled out

Upon initial examination, a heart murmur was heard in a newborn infant delivered vaginally in the hospital; however, after further observation, any serious cardiac conditions were ruled out.

Z38.00 Single liveborn infant, delivered vaginally

Z05.0 Observation and evaluation of newborn for suspected cardiac condition ruled out

Explanation: Normally an observation code is used as the principal diagnosis except when the patient is a newborn. A code from category Z38 Liveborn infants according to place of birth and type of delivery code would be sequenced first, followed by the encounter for observation and evaluation of newborn for suspected diseases and conditions ruled out.

7) Aftercare

Aftercare visit codes cover situations when the initial treatment of a disease has been performed and the patient requires continued care during the healing or recovery phase, or for the long-term consequences of the disease. The aftercare Z code should not be used if treatment is directed at a current, acute disease. The diagnosis code is to be used in these cases. Exceptions to this rule are codes Z51.0, Encounter for antineoplastic radiation therapy, and codes from subcategory Z51.1, Encounter for antineoplastic chemotherapy and immunotherapy. These codes are to be first listed, followed by the diagnosis code when a patient's encounter is solely to receive radiation therapy, chemotherapy, or immunotherapy for the treatment of a neoplasm. If the reason for the encounter is more than one type of antineoplastic therapy, code Z51.0 and a code from subcategory Z51.1 may be assigned together, in which case one of these codes would be reported as a secondary diagnosis.

The aftercare Z codes should also not be used for aftercare for injuries. For aftercare of an injury, assign the acute injury code with the appropriate 7th character (for subsequent encounter).

The aftercare codes are generally first listed to explain the specific reason for the encounter. An aftercare code may be used as an additional code when some type of aftercare is provided in addition to the reason for admission and no diagnosis code is applicable. An example of this would be the closure of a colostomy during an encounter for treatment of another condition.

Aftercare codes should be used in conjunction with other aftercare codes or diagnosis codes to provide better detail on the specifics of an aftercare encounter visit, unless otherwise directed by the classification. The sequencing of multiple aftercare codes depends on the circumstances of the encounter.

Certain aftercare Z code categories need a secondary diagnosis code to describe the resolving condition or sequelae. For others, the condition is included in the code title.

Additional Z code aftercare category terms include fitting and adjustment, and attention to artificial openings.

Status Z codes may be used with aftercare Z codes to indicate the nature of the aftercare. For example code Z95.1, Presence of aortocoronary bypass graft, may be used with code Z48.812, Encounter for surgical aftercare following surgery on the circulatory system, to indicate the surgery for which the aftercare is being performed. A status code should not be used when the aftercare code indicates the type of status, such as using Z43.0, Encounter for attention to tracheostomy, with Z93.0, Tracheostomy status.

The aftercare Z category/codes:

Z42	Encounter for plastic and reconstructive surgery following medical procedure or healed injury
Z43	Encounter for attention to artificial openings
Z44	Encounter for fitting and adjustment of external prosthetic device
Z45	Encounter for adjustment and management of implanted device
Z46	Encounter for fitting and adjustment of other devices
Z47	Orthopedic aftercare
Z48	Encounter for other postprocedural aftercare
Z49	Encounter for care involving renal dialysis
Z51	Encounter for other aftercare and medical care

8) Follow-up

The follow-up codes are used to explain continuing surveillance following completed treatment of a disease, condition, or injury. They imply that the condition has been fully treated and no longer exists. They should not be confused with aftercare codes, or injury codes with a 7th character for subsequent encounter, that explain ongoing care of a healing condition or its sequelae. Follow-up codes may be used in conjunction with history codes to provide the full picture of the healed condition and its treatment. The follow-up code is sequenced first, followed by the history code.

A follow-up code may be used to explain multiple visits. Should a condition be found to have recurred on the follow-up visit, then the diagnosis code for the condition should be assigned in place of the follow-up code.

The follow-up Z code categories:

Z08	Encounter for follow-up examination after completed treatment for malignant neoplasm
Z09	Encounter for follow-up examination after completed treatment for conditions other than malignant neoplasm
Z39	Encounter for maternal postpartum care and examination

9) Donor

Codes in category Z52, Donors of organs and tissues, are used for living individuals who are donating blood or other body tissue. These codes are for individuals donating for others, as well as for self-donations. They are not used to identify cadaveric donations.

10) Counseling

Counseling Z codes are used when a patient or family member receives assistance in the aftermath of an illness or injury, or when support is required in coping with family or social problems.

The counseling Z codes/categories:

Z30.0-	Encounter for general counseling and advice on contraception
Z31.5	Encounter for procreative genetic counseling
Z31.6-	Encounter for general counseling and advice on procreation
Z32.2	Encounter for childbirth instruction
Z32.3	Encounter for childcare instruction
Z69	Encounter for mental health services for victim and perpetrator of abuse
Z70	Counseling related to sexual attitude, behavior and orientation
Z71	Persons encountering health services for other counseling and medical advice, not elsewhere classified

Note: Code Z71.84, Encounter for health counseling related to travel, is to be used for health risk and safety counseling for future travel purposes.

Code Z71.85, Encounter for immunization safety counseling, is to be used for counseling of the patient or caregiver regarding the safety of a vaccine. This code should not be used for the provision of general information regarding risks and potential side effects during routine encounters for the administration of vaccines.

Code Z71.87, Encounter for pediatric-to-adult transition counseling, should be assigned when pediatric-to-adult transition counseling is the sole reason for the encounter or when this counseling is provided in addition to other services, such as treatment of a chronic condition. If both

transition counseling and treatment of a medical condition are provided during the same encounter, the code(s) for the medical condition(s) treated and code Z71.87 should be assigned, with sequencing depending on the circumstances of the encounter.

Z76.81 Expectant mother prebirth pediatrician visit

11) Encounters for obstetrical and reproductive services

See Section I.C.15. Pregnancy, Childbirth, and the Puerperium, for further instruction on the use of these codes.

Z codes for pregnancy are for use in those circumstances when none of the problems or complications included in the codes from the Obstetrics chapter exist (a routine prenatal visit or postpartum care). Codes in category Z34, Encounter for supervision of normal pregnancy, are always first listed and are not to be used with any other code from the OB chapter.

Codes in category Z3A, Weeks of gestation, may be assigned to provide additional information about the pregnancy. Category Z3A codes should not be assigned for pregnancies with abortive outcomes (categories O00-O08), elective termination of pregnancy (code Z33.2), nor for postpartum conditions, as category Z3A is not applicable to these conditions. The date of the admission should be used to determine weeks of gestation for inpatient admissions that encompass more than one gestational week.

The outcome of delivery, category Z37, should be included on all maternal delivery records. It is always a secondary code.

Codes in category Z37 should not be used on the newborn record.

Z codes for family planning (contraceptive) or procreative management and counseling should be included on an obstetric record either during the pregnancy or the postpartum stage, if applicable.

Z codes/categories for obstetrical and reproductive services:

Z30	Encounter for contraceptive management
Z31	Encounter for procreative management
Z32.2	Encounter for childbirth instruction
Z32.3	Encounter for childcare instruction
Z33	Pregnant state
Z34	Encounter for supervision of normal pregnancy
Z36	Encounter for antenatal screening of mother
Z3A	Weeks of gestation
Z37	Outcome of delivery
Z39	Encounter for maternal postpartum care and examination
Z76.81	Expectant mother prebirth pediatrician visit

12) Newborns and infants

See Section I.C.16. Newborn (Perinatal) Guidelines, for further instruction on the use of these codes.

Newborn Z codes/categories:

Z76.1	Encounter for health supervision and care of foundling
Z00.1-	Encounter for routine child health examination
Z38	Liveborn infants according to place of birth and type of delivery

13) Routine and administrative examinations

The Z codes allow for the description of encounters for routine examinations, such as, a general check-up, or, examinations for administrative purposes, such as, a pre-employment physical. The codes are not to be used if the examination is for diagnosis of a suspected condition or for treatment purposes. In such cases the diagnosis code is used. During a routine exam, should a diagnosis or condition be discovered, it should be coded as an additional code. Pre-existing and chronic conditions and history codes may also be included as additional codes as long as the examination is for administrative purposes and not focused on any particular condition.

Some of the codes for routine health examinations distinguish between "with" and "without" abnormal findings. Code assignment depends on the information that is known at the time the encounter is being coded. For example, if no abnormal findings were found during the examination, but the encounter is being coded before test results are back, it is acceptable to assign the code for "without abnormal findings." When assigning a code for "with abnormal findings," additional code(s) should be assigned to identify the specific abnormal finding(s).

Pre-operative examination and pre-procedural laboratory examination Z codes are for use only in those situations when a patient is being cleared for a procedure or surgery and no treatment is given.

The Z codes/categories for routine and administrative examinations:

Z00	Encounter for general examination without complaint, suspected or reported diagnosis
Z01	Encounter for other special examination without complaint, suspected or reported diagnosis
Z02	Encounter for administrative examination Except: Z02.9, Encounter for administrative examinations, unspecified
Z32.0-	Encounter for pregnancy test

14) Miscellaneous Z codes

The miscellaneous Z codes capture a number of other health care encounters that do not fall into one of the other categories. Some of these codes identify the reason for the encounter; others are for use as additional codes that provide useful information on circumstances that may affect a patient's care and treatment.

Prophylactic organ removal

For encounters specifically for prophylactic removal of an organ (such as prophylactic removal of breasts due to a genetic susceptibility to cancer or a family history of cancer), the principal or first-listed code should be a code from category Z40, Encounter for prophylactic surgery, followed by the appropriate codes to identify the associated risk factor (such as genetic susceptibility or family history).

If the patient has a malignancy of one site and is having prophylactic removal at another site to prevent either a new primary malignancy or metastatic disease, a code for the malignancy should also be assigned in addition to a code from subcategory Z40.0, Encounter for prophylactic surgery for risk factors related to malignant neoplasms. A Z40.0 code should not be assigned if the patient is having organ removal for treatment of a malignancy, such as the removal of the testes for the treatment of prostate cancer.

Female patient with cancer in lower inner quadrant of right breast and positive BRCA 1 noted on testing is admitted for mastectomy of right breast and prophylactic removal of left breast

C50.311	**Malignant neoplasm of lower-inner quadrant of right female breast**
Z40.01	**Encounter for prophylactic removal of breast**
Z15.01	**Genetic susceptibility to malignant neoplasm of breast**

Explanation: Removal of the current neoplastic disease in the right breast was the focus of treatment for this admission and is sequenced first. The removal of the left breast was not required to treat a current disease process but as a means of prevention. The two Z codes are informational; they capture the reason behind the removal of what is currently a healthy left breast.

Miscellaneous Z codes/categories:

Z28	Immunization not carried out Except: Z28.3-, Underimmunization status
Z29	Encounter for other prophylactic measures
Z40	Encounter for prophylactic surgery
Z41	Encounter for procedures for purposes other than remedying health state Except: Z41.9, Encounter for procedure for purposes other than remedying health state, unspecified
Z53	Persons encountering health services for specific procedures and treatment, not carried out
Z72	Problems related to lifestyle **Note:** These codes should be assigned only when the documentation specifies that the patient has an associated problem
Z73	Problems related to life management difficulty **Note: These codes should be assigned only when the documentation specifies that the patient has an associated problem.**
Z74	Problems related to care provider dependency Except: Z74.01, Bed confinement status
Z75	Problems related to medical facilities and other health care
Z76.0	Encounter for issue of repeat prescription
Z76.3	Healthy person accompanying sick person
Z76.4	Other boarder to healthcare facility
Z76.5	Malingerer [conscious simulation]
Z91.1-	Patient's noncompliance with medical treatment and regimen
Z91.83	Wandering in diseases classified elsewhere
Z91.84-	Oral health risk factors
Z91.89	Other specified personal risk factors, not elsewhere classified

See Section I.B.14. for Z55-Z65 Persons with potential health hazards related to socioeconomic and psychosocial circumstances, documentation by clinicians other than the patient's provider

15)Nonspecific Z codes

Certain Z codes are so non-specific, or potentially redundant with other codes in the classification, that there can be little justification for their use in the inpatient setting. Their use in the outpatient setting should be limited to those instances when there is no further documentation to permit more precise coding. Otherwise, any sign or symptom or any other reason for visit that is captured in another code should be used.

Nonspecific Z codes/categories:

Z02.9	Encounter for administrative examinations, unspecified
Z04.9	Encounter for examination and observation for unspecified reason
Z13.9	Encounter for screening, unspecified
Z41.9	Encounter for procedure for purposes other than remedying health state, unspecified
Z52.9	Donor of unspecified organ or tissue
Z86.59	Personal history of other mental and behavioral disorders
Z88.9	Allergy status to unspecified drugs, medicaments and biological substances status
Z92.0	Personal history of contraception

16) Z codes that may only be principal/first-listed diagnosis

The following Z codes/categories may only be reported as the principal/first-listed diagnosis, except when there are multiple encounters on the same day and the medical records for the encounters are combined:

Z00	Encounter for general examination without complaint, suspected or reported diagnosis Except: Z00.6
Z01	Encounter for other special examination without complaint, suspected or reported diagnosis
Z02	Encounter for administrative examination
Z04	Encounter for examination and observation for other reasons
Z33.2	Encounter for elective termination of pregnancy
Z31.81	Encounter for male factor infertility in female patient
Z31.83	Encounter for assisted reproductive fertility procedure cycle
Z31.84	Encounter for fertility preservation procedure
Z34	Encounter for supervision of normal pregnancy
Z39	Encounter for maternal postpartum care and examination
Z38	Liveborn infants according to place of birth and type of delivery
Z40	Encounter for prophylactic surgery
Z42	Encounter for plastic and reconstructive surgery following medical procedure or healed injury
Z51.0	Encounter for antineoplastic radiation therapy
Z51.1-	Encounter for antineoplastic chemotherapy and immunotherapy
Z52	Donors of organs and tissues Except: Z52.9, Donor of unspecified organ or tissue
Z76.1	Encounter for health supervision and care of foundling
Z76.2	Encounter for health supervision and care of other healthy infant and child
Z99.12	Encounter for respirator [ventilator] dependence during power failure

17)Social determinants of health

Codes describing **problems or risk factors related to** social determinants of health (SDOH) should be assigned when this information is documented. **Assign as many SDOH codes as are necessary to describe all of the problems or risk factors. These codes should be assigned only when the documentation specifies that the patient has an associated problem or risk factor. For example, not every individual living alone would be assigned code Z60.2, Problems related to living alone.**

For social determinants of health, such as information found in categories Z55-Z65, Persons with potential health hazards related to socioeconomic and psychosocial circumstances, code assignment may be based on medical record documentation from clinicians involved in the care of the patient who are not the patient's provider since this information represents social information, rather than medical diagnoses.

For example, coding professionals may utilize documentation of social information from social workers, community health workers, case managers, or nurses, if their documentation is included in the official medical record.

Patient self-reported documentation may be used to assign codes for social determinants of health, as long as the patient self-reported information is signed-off by and incorporated into the medical record by either a clinician or provider.

Social determinants of health codes are located primarily in these Z code categories:

Z55	Problems related to education and literacy
Z56	Problems related to employment and unemployment
Z57	Occupational exposure to risk factors
Z58	Problems related to physical environment
Z59	Problems related to housing and economic circumstances
Z60	Problems related to social environment
Z62	Problems related to upbringing
Z63	Other problems related to primary support group, including family circumstances
Z64	Problems related to certain psychosocial circumstances
Z65	Problems related to other psychosocial circumstances

See Section I.B.14. Documentation by Clinicians Other than the Patient's Provider.

Chapter 21. Factors Influencing Health Status and Contact With Health Services (Z00-Z99)

NOTE Z codes represent reasons for encounters. A corresponding procedure code must accompany a Z code if a procedure is performed. Categories Z00-Z99 are provided for occasions when circumstances other than a disease, injury or external cause classifiable to categories A00-Y89 are recorded as "diagnoses" or "problems." This can arise in two main ways:

(a) When a person who may or may not be sick encounters the health services for some specific purpose, such as to receive limited care or service for a current condition, to donate an organ or tissue, to receive prophylactic vaccination (immunization), or to discuss a problem which is in itself not a disease or injury.

(b) When some circumstance or problem is present which influences the person's health status but is not in itself a current illness or injury.

AHA: 2018,4Q,60-61

This chapter contains the following blocks:

- Z00-Z13 Persons encountering health services for examinations
- Z14-Z15 Genetic carrier and genetic susceptibility to disease
- Z16 Resistance to antimicrobial drugs
- Z17 Estrogen receptor status
- Z18 Retained foreign body fragments
- Z19 Hormone sensitivity malignancy status
- Z20-Z29 Persons with potential health hazards related to communicable diseases
- Z30-Z39 Persons encountering health services in circumstances related to reproduction
- Z40-Z53 Encounters for other specific health care
- Z55-Z65 Persons with potential health hazards related to socioeconomic and psychosocial circumstances
- Z66 Do not resuscitate status
- Z67 Blood type
- Z68 Body mass index (BMI)
- Z69-Z76 Persons encountering health services in other circumstances
- Z77-Z99 Persons with potential health hazards related to family and personal history and certain conditions influencing health status

Persons encountering health services for examinations (Z00-Z13)

NOTE Nonspecific abnormal findings disclosed at the time of these examinations are classified to categories R70-R94.

EXCLUDES 1 *examinations related to pregnancy and reproduction (Z30-Z36, Z39.-)*

√4th **Z00 Encounter for general examination without complaint, suspected or reported diagnosis**

EXCLUDES 1 *encounter for examination for administrative purposes (Z02.-)*

EXCLUDES 2 *encounter for pre-procedural examinations (Z01.81-)*
special screening examinations (Z11-Z13)

AHA: 2017,4Q,95

√5th **Z00.0 Encounter for general adult medical examination**

Encounter for adult periodic examination (annual) (physical) and any associated laboratory and radiologic examinations

EXCLUDES 1 *encounter for examination of sign or symptom - code to sign or symptom*
general health check-up of infant or child (Z00.12.-)

Z00.00 Encounter for general adult medical examination without abnormal findings UPD A

Encounter for adult health check-up NOS

AHA: 2016,1Q,36

Z00.01 Encounter for general adult medical examination with abnormal findings UPD A

Use additional code to identify abnormal findings

AHA: 2016,1Q,35-36

√5th **Z00.1 Encounter for newborn, infant and child health examinations**

√6th **Z00.11 Newborn health examination**

Health check for child under 29 days old

Use additional code to identify any abnormal findings

EXCLUDES 1 *health check for child over 28 days old (Z00.12-)*

Z00.110 Health examination for newborn under 8 days old UPD N

Health check for newborn under 8 days old

Z00.111 Health examination for newborn 8 to 28 days old UPD N

Health check for newborn 8 to 28 days old
Newborn weight check

√6th **Z00.12 Encounter for routine child health examination**

Health check (routine) for child over 28 days old
Immunizations appropriate for age
Routine developmental screening of infant or child
Routine vison and hearing testing

EXCLUDES 1 *health check for child under 29 days old (Z00.11-)*
health supervision of foundling or other healthy infant or child (Z76.1-Z76.2)
newborn health examination (Z00.11-)

AHA: 2018,4Q,36

Z00.121 Encounter for routine child health examination with abnormal findings UPD P

Use additional code to identify abnormal findings

AHA: 2016,1Q,34-35

Z00.129 Encounter for routine child health examination without abnormal findings UPD P

Encounter for routine child health examination NOS

AHA: 2016,1Q,34

Z00.2 Encounter for examination for period of rapid growth in childhood UPD P

Z00.3 Encounter for examination for adolescent development state UPD P

Encounter for puberty development state

Z00.5 Encounter for examination of potential donor of organ and tissue UPD

Z00.6 Encounter for examination for normal comparison and control in clinical research program

Examination of participant or control in clinical research program

√5th **Z00.7 Encounter for examination for period of delayed growth in childhood**

Z00.70 Encounter for examination for period of delayed growth in childhood without abnormal findings UPD P

Z00.71 Encounter for examination for period of delayed growth in childhood with abnormal findings UPD P

Use additional code to identify abnormal findings

Z00.8 Encounter for other general examination UPD

Encounter for health examination in population surveys

√4th **Z01 Encounter for other special examination without complaint, suspected or reported diagnosis**

INCLUDES routine examination of specific system

NOTE Codes from category Z01 represent the reason for the encounter. A separate procedure code is required to identify any examinations or procedures performed

EXCLUDES 1 *encounter for examination for administrative purposes (Z02.-)*
encounter for examination for suspected conditions, proven not to exist (Z03.-)
encounter for laboratory and radiologic examinations as a component of general medical examinations (Z00.0-)
encounter for laboratory, radiologic and imaging examinations for sign(s) and symptom(s) - code to the sign(s) or symptom(s)

EXCLUDES 2 *screening examinations (Z11-Z13)*

√5th **Z01.0 Encounter for examination of eyes and vision**

EXCLUDES 1 *examination for driving license (Z02.4)*

Z01.00 Encounter for examination of eyes and vision without abnormal findings

Encounter for examination of eyes and vision NOS

Z01.01 Encounter for examination of eyes and vision with abnormal findings

Use additional code to identify abnormal findings

AHA: 2016,4Q,21

Z01.02 Encounter for examination of eyes and vision following failed vision screening

EXCLUDES 1 *encounter for examination of eyes and vision with abnormal findings (Z01.01)*

encounter for examination of eyes and vision without abnormal findings (Z01.00)

AHA: 2019,4Q,20

Z01.020 Encounter for examination of eyes and vision following failed vision screening without abnormal findings

Z01.021 Encounter for examination of eyes and vision following failed vision screening with abnormal findings

Use additional code to identify abnormal findings

Z01.1 Encounter for examination of ears and hearing

Z01.10 Encounter for examination of ears and hearing without abnormal findings UPD

Encounter for examination of ears and hearing NOS

AHA: 2016,4Q,24

Z01.11 Encounter for examination of ears and hearing with abnormal findings

AHA: 2016,3Q,17-18

Z01.110 Encounter for hearing examination following failed hearing screening UPD

Z01.118 Encounter for examination of ears and hearing with other abnormal findings UPD

Use additional code to identify abnormal findings

Z01.12 Encounter for hearing conservation and treatment UPD

Z01.2 Encounter for dental examination and cleaning

Z01.20 Encounter for dental examination and cleaning without abnormal findings UPD

Encounter for dental examination and cleaning NOS

Z01.21 Encounter for dental examination and cleaning with abnormal findings UPD

Use additional code to identify abnormal findings

Z01.3 Encounter for examination of blood pressure

Z01.30 Encounter for examination of blood pressure without abnormal findings UPD

Encounter for examination of blood pressure NOS

Z01.31 Encounter for examination of blood pressure with abnormal findings UPD

Use additional code to identify abnormal findings

Z01.4 Encounter for gynecological examination

EXCLUDES 2 *pregnancy examination or test (Z32.0-)*

routine examination for contraceptive maintenance (Z30.4-)

Z01.41 Encounter for routine gynecological examination

Encounter for general gynecological examination with or without cervical smear

Encounter for gynecological examination (general) (routine) NOS

Encounter for pelvic examination (annual) (periodic)

Use additional code:

for screening for human papillomavirus, if applicable, (Z11.51)

for screening vaginal pap smear, if applicable (Z12.72)

to identify acquired absence of uterus, if applicable (Z90.71-)

EXCLUDES 1 *gynecologic examination status-post hysterectomy for malignant condition (Z08)*

screening cervical pap smear not a part of a routine gynecological examination (Z12.4)

Z01.411 Encounter for gynecological examination (general) (routine) with abnormal findings ♀

Use additional code to identify abnormal findings

Z01.419 Encounter for gynecological examination (general) (routine) without abnormal findings ♀

Z01.42 Encounter for cervical smear to confirm findings of recent normal smear following initial abnormal smear ♀

Z01.8 Encounter for other specified special examinations

Z01.81 Encounter for preprocedural examinations

Encounter for preoperative examinations

Encounter for radiological and imaging examinations as part of preprocedural examination

Z01.810 Encounter for preprocedural cardiovascular examination

Z01.811 Encounter for preprocedural respiratory examination

Z01.812 Encounter for preprocedural laboratory examination UPD

Blood and urine tests prior to treatment or procedure

AHA: 2020,3Q,14

Z01.818 Encounter for other preprocedural examination UPD

Encounter for preprocedural examination NOS

Encounter for examinations prior to antineoplastic chemotherapy

Z01.82 Encounter for allergy testing UPD

EXCLUDES 1 *encounter for antibody response examination (Z01.84)*

Z01.83 Encounter for blood typing UPD

Encounter for Rh typing

Z01.84 Encounter for antibody response examination UPD

Encounter for immunity status testing

EXCLUDES 1 *encounter for allergy testing (Z01.82)*

AHA: 2020,2Q,11

Z01.89 Encounter for other specified special examinations UPD

Z02 Encounter for administrative examination

Z02.0 Encounter for examination for admission to educational institution UPD

Encounter for examination for admission to preschool (education)

Encounter for examination for re-admission to school following illness or medical treatment

Z02.1 Encounter for pre-employment examination

Z02.2 Encounter for examination for admission to residential institution UPD

EXCLUDES 1 *examination for admission to prison (Z02.89)*

Z02.3 Encounter for examination for recruitment to armed forces

Z02.4 Encounter for examination for driving license UPD

Z02.5 Encounter for examination for participation in sport UPD

EXCLUDES 1 *blood-alcohol and blood-drug test (Z02.83)*

Z02.6 Encounter for examination for insurance purposes UPD

Z02.7 Encounter for issue of medical certificate

EXCLUDES 1 *encounter for general medical examination (Z00-Z01, Z02.0-Z02.6, Z02.8-Z02.9)*

Z02.71 Encounter for disability determination UPD

Encounter for issue of medical certificate of incapacity

Encounter for issue of medical certificate of invalidity

Z02.79 Encounter for issue of other medical certificate UPD

Z02.8 Encounter for other administrative examinations

Z02.81 Encounter for paternity testing

Z02.82 Encounter for adoption services UPD

Z02.83 Encounter for blood-alcohol and blood-drug test

Use additional code for findings of alcohol or drugs in blood (R78.-)

Z02.89 Encounter for other administrative examinations UPD

Encounter for examination for admission to prison
Encounter for examination for admission to summer camp
Encounter for immigration examination
Encounter for naturalization examination
Encounter for premarital examination

EXCLUDES 1 *health supervision of foundling or other healthy infant or child (Z76.1-Z76.2)*

Z02.9 Encounter for administrative examinations, unspecified UPD

✓4th **Z03 Encounter for medical observation for suspected diseases and conditions ruled out**

This category is to be used when a person without a diagnosis is suspected of having an abnormal condition, without signs or symptoms, which requires study, but after examination and observation, is ruled out. This category is also for use for administrative and legal observation status.

EXCLUDES 1 *contact with and (suspected) exposures hazardous to health (Z77.-)*
encounter for observation and evaluation of newborn for suspected diseases and conditions ruled out (Z05.-)
person with feared complaint in whom no diagnosis is made (Z71.1)
signs or symptoms under study - code to signs or symptoms

AHA: 2020,2Q,8; 2018,2Q,7-8; 2017,4Q,27

Z03.6 Encounter for observation for suspected toxic effect from ingested substance ruled out

Encounter for observation for suspected adverse effect from drug
Encounter for observation for suspected poisoning

✓5th **Z03.7 Encounter for suspected maternal and fetal conditions ruled out**

Encounter for suspected maternal and fetal conditions not found

EXCLUDES 1 *known or suspected fetal anomalies affecting management of mother, not ruled out (O26.-, O35.-, O36.-, O40.-, O41.-)*

Z03.71 Encounter for suspected problem with amniotic cavity and membrane ruled out UPD M ♀

Encounter for suspected oligohydramnios ruled out
Encounter for suspected polyhydramnios ruled out

Z03.72 Encounter for suspected placental problem ruled out UPD M ♀

Z03.73 Encounter for suspected fetal anomaly ruled out UPD M ♀

Z03.74 Encounter for suspected problem with fetal growth ruled out UPD M ♀

Z03.75 Encounter for suspected cervical shortening ruled out UPD M ♀

Z03.79 Encounter for other suspected maternal and fetal conditions ruled out UPD M ♀

✓5th **Z03.8 Encounter for observation for other suspected diseases and conditions ruled out**

✓6th **Z03.81 Encounter for observation for suspected exposure to biological agents ruled out**

Z03.810 Encounter for observation for suspected exposure to anthrax ruled out

Z03.818 Encounter for observation for suspected exposure to other biological agents ruled out

AHA: 2020,2Q,8; 2020,1Q,34-36

TIP: During the COVID-19 pandemic, possible exposure to COVID-19 should be coded using Z20.822 Contact with and (suspected) exposure to COVID-19, even when the COVID-19 infection has been ruled out.

✓6th **Z03.82 Encounter for observation for suspected foreign body ruled out**

EXCLUDES 1 *retained foreign body (Z18.-)*
retained foreign body in eyelid (H02.81)
residual foreign body in soft tissue (M79.5)

EXCLUDES 2 *confirmed foreign body ingestion or aspiration including:*
foreign body in alimentary tract (T18)
foreign body in ear (T16)
foreign body on external eye (T15)
foreign body in respiratory tract (T17)

AHA: 2020,4Q,42

Z03.821 Encounter for observation for suspected ingested foreign body ruled out UPD

Z03.822 Encounter for observation for suspected aspirated (inhaled) foreign body ruled out UPD

Z03.823 Encounter for observation for suspected inserted (injected) foreign body ruled out UPD

Encounter for observation for suspected inserted (injected) foreign body in eye ruled out
Encounter for observation for suspected inserted (injected) foreign body in orifice ruled out
Encounter for observation for suspected inserted (injected) foreign body in skin ruled out

● **Z03.83 Encounter for observation for suspected conditions related to home physiologic monitoring device ruled out** UPD

Encounter for observation for apnea alarm without findings
Encounter for observation for bradycardia alarm without findings
Encounter for observation for malfunction of home cardiorespiratory monitor
Encounter for observation for non-specific findings home physiologic monitoring device
Encounter for observation for pulse oximeter alarm without findings

EXCLUDES 1 *apnea NOS (R06.81)*
neonatal bradycardia (P29.12)
newborn apnea (P28.4-)
primary sleep apnea of newborn (P28.3-)
sleep apnea (G47.3-)

Z03.89 Encounter for observation for other suspected diseases and conditions ruled out

✓4th **Z04 Encounter for examination and observation for other reasons**

INCLUDES encounter for examination for medicolegal reasons

This category is to be used when a person without a diagnosis is suspected of having an abnormal condition, without signs or symptoms, which requires study, but after examination and observation, is ruled-out. This category is also for use for administrative and legal observation status.

AHA: 2018,2Q,7-8

Z04.1 Encounter for examination and observation following transport accident

EXCLUDES 1 *encounter for examination and observation following work accident (Z04.2)*

AHA: 2019,2Q,11; 2018,2Q,8

Z04.2 Encounter for examination and observation following work accident

Z04.3 Encounter for examination and observation following other accident

✓5th **Z04.4 Encounter for examination and observation following alleged rape**

Encounter for examination and observation of victim following alleged rape
Encounter for examination and observation of victim following alleged sexual abuse

Z04.41 Encounter for examination and observation following alleged adult rape A

Suspected adult rape, ruled out
Suspected adult sexual abuse, ruled out

Z04.42 Encounter for examination and observation following alleged child rape P
Suspected child rape, ruled out
Suspected child sexual abuse, ruled out

Z04.6 Encounter for general psychiatric examination, requested by authority

✓5th **Z04.7 Encounter for examination and observation following alleged physical abuse**

Z04.71 Encounter for examination and observation following alleged adult physical abuse A
Suspected adult physical abuse, ruled out
EXCLUDES 1 *confirmed case of adult physical abuse (T74.-)*
encounter for examination and observation following alleged adult sexual abuse (Z04.41)
suspected case of adult physical abuse, not ruled out (T76.-)

Z04.72 Encounter for examination and observation following alleged child physical abuse P
Suspected child physical abuse, ruled out
EXCLUDES 1 *confirmed case of child physical abuse (T74.-)*
encounter for examination and observation following alleged child sexual abuse (Z04.42)
suspected case of child physical abuse, not ruled out (T76.-)

✓5th **Z04.8 Encounter for examination and observation for other specified reasons**
Encounter for examination and observation for request for expert evidence
AHA: 2018,4Q,32,35,72

Z04.81 Encounter for examination and observation of victim following forced sexual exploitation

Z04.82 Encounter for examination and observation of victim following forced labor exploitation

Z04.89 Encounter for examination and observation for other specified reasons

Z04.9 Encounter for examination and observation for unspecified reason UPD
Encounter for observation NOS

✓4th **Z05 Encounter for observation and evaluation of newborn for suspected diseases and conditions ruled out**
This category is to be used for newborns, within the neonatal period (the first 28 days of life), who are suspected of having an abnormal condition, but without signs or symptoms, and which, after examination and observation, is ruled out.
AHA: 2022,1Q,17-18; 2017,4Q,27; 2016,4Q,77

Z05.0 Observation and evaluation of newborn for suspected cardiac condition ruled out N

Z05.1 Observation and evaluation of newborn for suspected infectious condition ruled out N
AHA: 2019,2Q,10

Z05.2 Observation and evaluation of newborn for suspected neurological condition ruled out N

Z05.3 Observation and evaluation of newborn for suspected respiratory condition ruled out N

✓5th **Z05.4 Observation and evaluation of newborn for suspected genetic, metabolic or immunologic condition ruled out**

Z05.41 Observation and evaluation of newborn for suspected genetic condition ruled out N
AHA: 2016,4Q,55

Z05.42 Observation and evaluation of newborn for suspected metabolic condition ruled out N

Z05.43 Observation and evaluation of newborn for suspected immunologic condition ruled out N

Z05.5 Observation and evaluation of newborn for suspected gastrointestinal condition ruled out N

Z05.6 Observation and evaluation of newborn for suspected genitourinary condition ruled out N

✓5th **Z05.7 Observation and evaluation of newborn for suspected skin, subcutaneous, musculoskeletal and connective tissue condition ruled out**

Z05.71 Observation and evaluation of newborn for suspected skin and subcutaneous tissue condition ruled out N

Z05.72 Observation and evaluation of newborn for suspected musculoskeletal condition ruled out N

Z05.73 Observation and evaluation of newborn for suspected connective tissue condition ruled out N

Z05.8 Observation and evaluation of newborn for other specified suspected condition ruled out N
AHA: 2022,1Q,17-18

Z05.9 Observation and evaluation of newborn for unspecified suspected condition ruled out N

Z08 Encounter for follow-up examination after completed treatment for malignant neoplasm UPD
Medical surveillance following completed treatment
Use additional code to identify any acquired absence of organs (Z90.-)
Use additional code to identify the personal history of malignant neoplasm (Z85.-)
EXCLUDES 1 *aftercare following medical care (Z43-Z49, Z51)*
AHA: 2020,3Q,30

Z09 Encounter for follow-up examination after completed treatment for conditions other than malignant neoplasm UPD
Medical surveillance following completed treatment
Use additional code to identify any applicable history of disease code (Z86.-, Z87.-)
EXCLUDES 1 *aftercare following medical care (Z43-Z49, Z51)*
surveillance of contraception (Z30.4-)
surveillance of prosthetic and other medical devices (Z44-Z46)
AHA: 2021,1Q,33; 2020,2Q,10; 2017,1Q,9; 2015,1Q,8

✓4th **Z11 Encounter for screening for infectious and parasitic diseases**
Screening is the testing for disease or disease precursors in asymptomatic individuals so that early detection and treatment can be provided for those who test positive for the disease.
EXCLUDES 1 *encounter for diagnostic examination - code to sign or symptom*

Z11.0 Encounter for screening for intestinal infectious diseases UPD

Z11.1 Encounter for screening for respiratory tuberculosis UPD
Encounter for screening for active tuberculosis disease

Z11.2 Encounter for screening for other bacterial diseases UPD

Z11.3 Encounter for screening for infections with a predominantly sexual mode of transmission UPD
EXCLUDES 2 *encounter for screening for human immunodeficiency virus [HIV] (Z11.4)*
encounter for screening for human papillomavirus (Z11.51)

Z11.4 Encounter for screening for human immunodeficiency virus [HIV] UPD

✓5th **Z11.5 Encounter for screening for other viral diseases**
EXCLUDES 2 *encounter for screening for viral intestinal disease (Z11.0)*

Z11.51 Encounter for screening for human papillomavirus (HPV) UPD

Z11.52 Encounter for screening for COVID-19 UPD
AHA: 2021,1Q,27,37,41
TIP: This code is not appropriate for use during the pandemic phase of COVID-19. Use Z20.822 Contact with or (suspected) exposure to COVID-19, instead.

Z11.59 Encounter for screening for other viral diseases UPD
AHA: 2020,3Q,14

Z11.6 Encounter for screening for other protozoal diseases and helminthiases UPD
EXCLUDES 2 *encounter for screening for protozoal intestinal disease (Z11.0)*

Z11.7 Encounter for testing for latent tuberculosis infection UPD
AHA: 2019,4Q,20

Z11.8 Encounter for screening for other infectious and parasitic diseases UPD
Encounter for screening for chlamydia
Encounter for screening for rickettsial
Encounter for screening for spirochetal
Encounter for screening for mycoses

Z11.9 Encounter for screening for infectious and parasitic diseases, unspecified UPD

Z12 Encounter for screening for malignant neoplasms

Screening is the testing for disease or disease precursors in asymptomatic individuals so that early detection and treatment can be provided for those who test positive for the disease.

Use additional code to identify any family history of malignant neoplasm (Z80.-)

EXCLUDES 1 *encounter for diagnostic examination - code to sign or symptom*

Z12.0 Encounter for screening for malignant neoplasm of stomach UPD

Z12.1 Encounter for screening for malignant neoplasm of intestinal tract

AHA: 2017,1Q,8,9

Z12.10 Encounter for screening for malignant neoplasm of intestinal tract, unspecified UPD

Z12.11 Encounter for screening for malignant neoplasm of colon UPD

Encounter for screening colonoscopy NOS

AHA: 2019,1Q,32-33; 2018,1Q,6

Z12.12 Encounter for screening for malignant neoplasm of rectum UPD

AHA: 2018,1Q,6

Z12.13 Encounter for screening for malignant neoplasm of small intestine UPD

Z12.2 Encounter for screening for malignant neoplasm of respiratory organs UPD

Z12.3 Encounter for screening for malignant neoplasm of breast

Z12.31 Encounter for screening mammogram for malignant neoplasm of breast UPD

EXCLUDES 1 *inconclusive mammogram (R92.2)*

AHA: 2015,1Q,24

Z12.39 Encounter for other screening for malignant neoplasm of breast UPD

Z12.4 Encounter for screening for malignant neoplasm of cervix UPD ♀

Encounter for screening pap smear for malignant neoplasm of cervix

EXCLUDES 1 *when screening is part of general gynecological examination (Z01.4-)*

EXCLUDES 2 *encounter for screening for human papillomavirus (Z11.51)*

Z12.5 Encounter for screening for malignant neoplasm of prostate ♂

Z12.6 Encounter for screening for malignant neoplasm of bladder UPD

Z12.7 Encounter for screening for malignant neoplasm of other genitourinary organs

Z12.71 Encounter for screening for malignant neoplasm of testis UPD ♂

Z12.72 Encounter for screening for malignant neoplasm of vagina UPD ♀

Vaginal pap smear status-post hysterectomy for non-malignant condition

Use additional code to identify acquired absence of uterus (Z90.71-)

EXCLUDES 1 *vaginal pap smear status-post hysterectomy for malignant conditions (Z08)*

Z12.73 Encounter for screening for malignant neoplasm of ovary UPD ♀

Z12.79 Encounter for screening for malignant neoplasm of other genitourinary organs UPD

Z12.8 Encounter for screening for malignant neoplasm of other sites

Z12.81 Encounter for screening for malignant neoplasm of oral cavity UPD

Z12.82 Encounter for screening for malignant neoplasm of nervous system UPD

Z12.83 Encounter for screening for malignant neoplasm of skin UPD

Z12.89 Encounter for screening for malignant neoplasm of other sites UPD

AHA: 2021,1Q,14

Z12.9 Encounter for screening for malignant neoplasm, site unspecified UPD

Z13 Encounter for screening for other diseases and disorders

Screening is the testing for disease or disease precursors in asymptomatic individuals so that early detection and treatment can be provided for those who test positive for the disease.

EXCLUDES 1 *encounter for diagnostic examination - code to sign or symptom*

Z13.0 Encounter for screening for diseases of the blood and blood-forming organs and certain disorders involving the immune mechanism UPD

Z13.1 Encounter for screening for diabetes mellitus UPD

Z13.2 Encounter for screening for nutritional, metabolic and other endocrine disorders

Z13.21 Encounter for screening for nutritional disorder UPD

Z13.22 Encounter for screening for metabolic disorder

Z13.220 Encounter for screening for lipoid disorders UPD

Encounter for screening for cholesterol level

Encounter for screening for hypercholesterolemia

Encounter for screening for hyperlipidemia

Z13.228 Encounter for screening for other metabolic disorders UPD

Z13.29 Encounter for screening for other suspected endocrine disorder UPD

EXCLUDES 2 *encounter for screening for diabetes mellitus (Z13.1)*

Z13.3 Encounter for screening examination for mental health and behavioral disorders

AHA: 2018,4Q,35-36

Z13.30 Encounter for screening examination for mental health and behavioral disorders, unspecified UPD

Z13.31 Encounter for screening for depression UPD

Encounter for screening for depression, adult

Encounter for screening for depression for child or adolescent

Z13.32 Encounter for screening for maternal depression UPD ♀

Encounter for screening for perinatal depression

Z13.39 Encounter for screening examination for other mental health and behavioral disorders UPD

Encounter for screening for alcoholism

Encounter for screening for intellectual disabilities

Z13.4 Encounter for screening for certain developmental disorders in childhood

Encounter for development testing of infant or child

Encounter for screening for developmental handicaps in early childhood

EXCLUDES 2 *encounter for routine child health examination (Z00.12-)*

AHA: 2018,4Q,36

Z13.40 Encounter for screening for unspecified developmental delays UPD

Z13.41 Encounter for autism screening UPD

Z13.42 Encounter for screening for global developmental delays (milestones) UPD

Encounter for screening for developmental handicaps in early childhood

Z13.49 Encounter for screening for other developmental delays UPD

Z13.5 Encounter for screening for eye and ear disorders UPD

EXCLUDES 2 *encounter for general hearing examination (Z01.1-)*

encounter for general vision examination (Z01.0-)

AHA: 2016,3Q,17

Z13.6 Encounter for screening for cardiovascular disorders UPD

Z13.7 Encounter for screening for genetic and chromosomal anomalies

EXCLUDES 1 *genetic testing for procreative management (Z31.4-)*

Z13.71 Encounter for nonprocreative screening for genetic disease carrier status UPD

Z13.79 Encounter for other screening for genetic and chromosomal anomalies UPD

Z13.8 Encounter for screening for other specified diseases and disorders
EXCLUDES 2 *screening for malignant neoplasms (Z12.-)*

Z13.81 Encounter for screening for digestive system disorders
Z13.810 Encounter for screening for upper gastrointestinal disorder UPD
Z13.811 Encounter for screening for lower gastrointestinal disorder UPD
EXCLUDES 1 *encounter for screening for intestinal infectious disease (Z11.0)*
Z13.818 Encounter for screening for other digestive system disorders UPD

Z13.82 Encounter for screening for musculoskeletal disorder
Z13.820 Encounter for screening for osteoporosis UPD
Z13.828 Encounter for screening for other musculoskeletal disorder UPD

Z13.83 Encounter for screening for respiratory disorder NEC UPD
EXCLUDES 1 *encounter for screening for respiratory tuberculosis (Z11.1)*

Z13.84 Encounter for screening for dental disorders UPD

Z13.85 Encounter for screening for nervous system disorders
Z13.850 Encounter for screening for traumatic brain injury UPD
Z13.858 Encounter for screening for other nervous system disorders UPD

Z13.88 Encounter for screening for disorder due to exposure to contaminants UPD
EXCLUDES 1 *those exposed to contaminants without suspected disorders (Z57.-, Z77.-)*

Z13.89 Encounter for screening for other disorder UPD
Encounter for screening for genitourinary disorders

Z13.9 Encounter for screening, unspecified UPD

Genetic carrier and genetic susceptibility to disease (Z14-Z15)

Z14 Genetic carrier
DEF: Individuals carrying a gene mutation associated with a certain disease that typically do not develop the disease but are able to pass the mutated genes to offspring.

Z14.0 Hemophilia A carrier
Z14.01 Asymptomatic hemophilia A carrier UPD
Z14.02 Symptomatic hemophilia A carrier UPD
Z14.1 Cystic fibrosis carrier UPD
Z14.8 Genetic carrier of other disease UPD

Z15 Genetic susceptibility to disease
INCLUDES confirmed abnormal gene
Use additional code, if applicable, for any associated family history of the disease (Z80-Z84)
EXCLUDES 1 *chromosomal anomalies (Q90-Q99)*

Z15.0 Genetic susceptibility to malignant neoplasm
Code first, if applicable, any current malignant neoplasm (C00-C75, C81-C96)
Use additional code, if applicable, for any personal history of malignant neoplasm (Z85.-)
Z15.01 Genetic susceptibility to malignant neoplasm of breast UPD
Z15.02 Genetic susceptibility to malignant neoplasm of ovary UPD ♀
Z15.03 Genetic susceptibility to malignant neoplasm of prostate UPD ♂
Z15.04 Genetic susceptibility to malignant neoplasm of endometrium UPD ♀
Z15.09 Genetic susceptibility to other malignant neoplasm UPD
AHA: 2021,1Q,14

Z15.8 Genetic susceptibility to other disease
Z15.81 Genetic susceptibility to multiple endocrine neoplasia [MEN] UPD
EXCLUDES 1 *multiple endocrine neoplasia [MEN] syndromes (E31.2-)*
DEF: Group of conditions in which several endocrine glands grow excessively (such as in adenomatous hyperplasia) and/or develop benign or malignant tumors. Tumors and hyperplasia associated with MEN often produce excess hormones, which impede normal physiology. There is no comprehensive cure known for MEN syndrome. Treatment is directed at the hyperplasia or tumors in each individual gland. Tumors are usually surgically removed and oral medications or hormonal injections are used to correct hormone imbalances.
Z15.89 Genetic susceptibility to other disease UPD

Resistance to antimicrobial drugs (Z16)

Z16 Resistance to antimicrobial drugs
NOTE The codes in this category are provided for use as additional codes to identify the resistance and non-responsiveness of a condition to antimicrobial drugs.
Code first the infection
EXCLUDES 1 *Methicillin resistant Staphylococcus aureus infection (A49.02)*
Methicillin resistant Staphylococcus aureus pneumonia (J15.212)
sepsis due to Methicillin resistant Staphylococcus aureus (A41.02)

Z16.1 Resistance to beta lactam antibiotics
Z16.10 Resistance to unspecified beta lactam antibiotics CC UPD
Z16.11 Resistance to penicillins CC UPD
Resistance to amoxicillin
Resistance to ampicillin
Z16.12 Extended spectrum beta lactamase (ESBL) resistance CC UPD
EXCLUDES 2 *Methicillin resistant Staphylococcus aureus infection in diseases classified elsewhere (B95.62)*
Z16.19 Resistance to other specified beta lactam antibiotics CC UPD
Resistance to cephalosporins

Z16.2 Resistance to other antibiotics
Z16.20 Resistance to unspecified antibiotic CC UPD
Resistance to antibiotics NOS
Z16.21 Resistance to vancomycin CC UPD
Z16.22 Resistance to vancomycin related antibiotics CC UPD
Z16.23 Resistance to quinolones and fluoroquinolones CC UPD
Z16.24 Resistance to multiple antibiotics CC UPD
Z16.29 Resistance to other single specified antibiotic CC UPD
Resistance to aminoglycosides
Resistance to macrolides
Resistance to sulfonamides
Resistance to tetracyclines

Z16.3 Resistance to other antimicrobial drugs
EXCLUDES 1 *resistance to antibiotics (Z16.1-, Z16.2-)*
Z16.30 Resistance to unspecified antimicrobial drugs CC UPD
Drug resistance NOS
Z16.31 Resistance to antiparasitic drug(s) CC UPD
Resistance to quinine and related compounds
Z16.32 Resistance to antifungal drug(s) CC UPD
Z16.33 Resistance to antiviral drug(s) CC UPD
Z16.34 Resistance to antimycobacterial drug(s)
Resistance to tuberculostatics
Z16.341 Resistance to single antimycobacterial drug CC UPD
Resistance to antimycobacterial drug NOS
Z16.342 Resistance to multiple antimycobacterial drugs CC UPD

Z16.35 Resistance to multiple antimicrobial drugs CC UPD

EXCLUDES 1 *resistance to multiple antibiotics only (Z16.24)*

Z16.39 Resistance to other specified antimicrobial drug CC UPD

Estrogen receptor status (Z17)

Z17 Estrogen receptor status

Code first malignant neoplasm of breast (C50.-)

DEF: Receptor status of breast cancer cells for the hormone estrogen that is used to help determine treatment and evaluate prognosis. ER+ breast cancer responds to hormone therapies while ER- breast cancer does not.

Z17.0 Estrogen receptor positive status [ER+] UPD

Z17.1 Estrogen receptor negative status [ER-] UPD

Retained foreign body fragments (Z18)

Z18 Retained foreign body fragments

INCLUDES embedded fragment (status)
embedded splinter (status)
retained foreign body status

EXCLUDES 1 *artificial joint prosthesis status (Z96.6-)*
foreign body accidentally left during a procedure (T81.5-)
foreign body entering through orifice (T15-T19)
in situ cardiac device (Z95.-)
organ or tissue replaced by means other than transplant (Z96.-, Z97.-)
organ or tissue replaced by transplant (Z94.-)
personal history of retained foreign body fully removed Z87.821
superficial foreign body (non-embedded splinter) - code to superficial foreign body, by site

DEF: Embedded or retained fragment, splinter, or foreign body, natural or synthetic that can cause infection.

Z18.0 Retained radioactive fragments

Z18.01 Retained depleted uranium fragments UPD

Z18.09 Other retained radioactive fragments UPD

Other retained depleted isotope fragments
Retained nontherapeutic radioactive fragments

Z18.1 Retained metal fragments

EXCLUDES 1 *retained radioactive metal fragments (Z18.01-Z18.09)*

Z18.10 Retained metal fragments, unspecified UPD

Retained metal fragment NOS

Z18.11 Retained magnetic metal fragments UPD

Z18.12 Retained nonmagnetic metal fragments UPD

Z18.2 Retained plastic fragments UPD

Acrylics fragments
Diethylhexyl phthalates fragments
Isocyanate fragments

Z18.3 Retained organic fragments

Z18.31 Retained animal quills or spines UPD

Z18.32 Retained tooth UPD

Z18.33 Retained wood fragments UPD

Z18.39 Other retained organic fragments UPD

Z18.8 Other specified retained foreign body

Z18.81 Retained glass fragments UPD

Z18.83 Retained stone or crystalline fragments UPD

Retained concrete or cement fragments

Z18.89 Other specified retained foreign body fragments UPD

Z18.9 Retained foreign body fragments, unspecified material UPD

Hormone sensitivity malignancy status (Z19)

Z19 Hormone sensitivity malignancy status

Code first malignant neoplasm — see Table of Neoplasms, by site, malignant

AHA: 2016,4Q,76

Z19.1 Hormone sensitive malignancy status UPD

Z19.2 Hormone resistant malignancy status UPD

Castrate resistant prostate malignancy status

Persons with potential health hazards related to communicable diseases (Z20-Z29)

Z20 Contact with and (suspected) exposure to communicable diseases

EXCLUDES 1 *carrier of infectious disease (Z22.-)*
diagnosed current infectious or parasitic disease - see Alphabetic Index

EXCLUDES 2 *personal history of infectious and parasitic diseases (Z86.1-)*

Z20.0 Contact with and (suspected) exposure to intestinal infectious diseases

Z20.01 Contact with and (suspected) exposure to intestinal infectious diseases due to Escherichia coli (E. coli)

Z20.09 Contact with and (suspected) exposure to other intestinal infectious diseases UPD

Z20.1 Contact with and (suspected) exposure to tuberculosis UPD

Z20.2 Contact with and (suspected) exposure to infections with a predominantly sexual mode of transmission UPD

Z20.3 Contact with and (suspected) exposure to rabies UPD

Z20.4 Contact with and (suspected) exposure to rubella UPD

Z20.5 Contact with and (suspected) exposure to viral hepatitis

Z20.6 Contact with and (suspected) exposure to human immunodeficiency virus [HIV]

EXCLUDES 1 *asymptomatic human immunodeficiency virus [HIV] HIV infection status (Z21)*

Z20.7 Contact with and (suspected) exposure to pediculosis, acariasis and other infestations UPD

Z20.8 Contact with and (suspected) exposure to other communicable diseases

Z20.81 Contact with and (suspected) exposure to other bacterial communicable diseases

Z20.810 Contact with and (suspected) exposure to anthrax UPD

Z20.811 Contact with and (suspected) exposure to meningococcus

Z20.818 Contact with and (suspected) exposure to other bacterial communicable diseases UPD

AHA: 2019,2Q,10

Z20.82 Contact with and (suspected) exposure to other viral communicable diseases

Z20.820 Contact with and (suspected) exposure to varicella

Z20.821 Contact with and (suspected) exposure to Zika virus UPD

AHA: 2018,4Q,35,64

Z20.822 Contact with and (suspected) exposure to COVID-19 UPD

Contact with and (suspected) exposure to SARS-CoV-2

AHA: 2022,2Q,28-29; 2021,4Q,109; 2021,1Q,27-29,37-38,41

TIP: During the COVID-19 pandemic, this code should be used for any individual being tested due to actual or suspected COVID-19 exposure. This is true regardless of whether the patient is asymptomatic or has symptoms and the infection has been ruled out, is inconclusive, or unknown.

Z20.828 Contact with and (suspected) exposure to other viral communicable diseases

AHA: 2021,1Q,37-38; 2020,4Q,99; 2020,3Q,14-15; 2020,2Q,4,8; 2020,1Q,34-36

Z20.89 Contact with and (suspected) exposure to other communicable diseases UPD

Z20.9 Contact with and (suspected) exposure to unspecified communicable disease UPD

Z21 Asymptomatic human immunodeficiency virus [HIV] infection status HCC

HIV positive NOS

Code first human immunodeficiency virus [HIV] disease complicating pregnancy, childbirth and the puerperium, if applicable (O98.7-)

EXCLUDES 1 *acquired immunodeficiency syndrome (B2Ø)*
contact with human immunodeficiency virus [HIV] (Z2Ø.6)
exposure to human immunodeficiency virus [HIV] (Z2Ø.6)
human immunodeficiency virus [HIV] disease (B2Ø)
inconclusive laboratory evidence of human immunodeficiency virus [HIV] (R75)

AHA: 2022,1Q,36; 2019,1Q,8-11

DEF: Phase of human immunodeficiency virus (HIV) infection with no clinical symptoms. This phase may last for 10 years or more.

Z22 Carrier of infectious disease

INCLUDES colonization status
suspected carrier

EXCLUDES 2 *carrier of viral hepatitis (B18.-)*

Z22.Ø Carrier of typhoid UPD

Z22.1 Carrier of other intestinal infectious diseases UPD

Z22.2 Carrier of diphtheria UPD

Z22.3 Carrier of other specified bacterial diseases

Z22.31 Carrier of bacterial disease due to meningococci UPD

Z22.32 Carrier of bacterial disease due to staphylococci

Z22.321 Carrier or suspected carrier of Methicillin susceptible Staphylococcus aureus UPD

MSSA colonization

Z22.322 Carrier or suspected carrier of Methicillin resistant Staphylococcus aureus UPD

MRSA colonization

DEF: Carriers (colonization) of methicillin resistant *Staphylococcus aureus* (MRSA) have MRSA on their skin or in their body but do not exhibit signs of infection. These individuals are able to pass MRSA on to others who may develop an infection.

Z22.33 Carrier of bacterial disease due to streptococci

Z22.33Ø Carrier of Group B streptococcus UPD

EXCLUDES 1 *carrier of streptococcus group B (GBS) complicating pregnancy, childbirth and the puerperium (O99.82-)*

Z22.338 Carrier of other streptococcus UPD

Z22.39 Carrier of other specified bacterial diseases UPD

Z22.4 Carrier of infections with a predominantly sexual mode of transmission UPD

Z22.6 Carrier of human T-lymphotropic virus type-1 [HTLV-1] infection UPD

Z22.7 Latent tuberculosis UPD

Latent tuberculosis infection (LTBI)

EXCLUDES 1 *nonspecific reaction to cell mediated immunity measurement of gamma interferon antigen response without active tuberculosis (R76.12)*
nonspecific reaction to tuberculin skin test without active tuberculosis (R76.11)

AHA: 2019,4Q,19

Z22.8 Carrier of other infectious diseases UPD

Z22.9 Carrier of infectious disease, unspecified UPD

Z23 Encounter for immunization UPD

NOTE Procedure codes are required to identify the types of immunizations given

Code first any routine childhood examination

Code also, if applicable, encounter for immunization safety counseling (Z71.85)

Z28 Immunization not carried out and underimmunization status

INCLUDES vaccination not carried out

Code also, if applicable, encounter for immunization safety counseling (Z71.85)

Z28.Ø Immunization not carried out because of contraindication

DEF: Contraindication: Situation where a drug, surgery, or other procedure may negatively affect or cause harm to a patient.

Z28.Ø1 Immunization not carried out because of acute illness of patient UPD

Z28.Ø2 Immunization not carried out because of chronic illness or condition of patient UPD

Z28.Ø3 Immunization not carried out because of immune compromised state of patient UPD

Z28.Ø4 Immunization not carried out because of patient allergy to vaccine or component UPD

Z28.Ø9 Immunization not carried out because of other contraindication UPD

Z28.1 Immunization not carried out because of patient decision for reasons of belief or group pressure UPD

Immunization not carried out because of religious belief

Z28.2 Immunization not carried out because of patient decision for other and unspecified reason

Z28.2Ø Immunization not carried out because of patient decision for unspecified reason UPD

Z28.21 Immunization not carried out because of patient refusal UPD

Z28.29 Immunization not carried out because of patient decision for other reason UPD

Z28.3 Underimmunization status

~~Delinquent immunization status~~
~~Lapsed immunization schedule status~~

▶Use additional code, if applicable, to identify:◀
▶immunization not carried out because of contraindication (Z28.Ø-)◀
▶immunization not carried out because of patient decision for other and unspecified reason (Z28.2-)◀
▶immunization not carried out because of patient decision for reasons of belief or group pressure (Z28.1)◀
▶immunization not carried out for other reason (Z28.8-)◀

AHA: 2022,1Q,4-5

Z28.31 Underimmunization for COVID-19 status

NOTE These codes should not be used for individuals who are not eligible for the COVID-19 vaccines, as determined by the healthcare provider.

Z28.31Ø Unvaccinated for COVID-19 UPD

Z28.311 Partially vaccinated for COVID-19 UPD

Z28.39 Other underimmunization status UPD

Delinquent immunization status
Lapsed immunization schedule status

Z28.8 Immunization not carried out for other reason

Z28.81 Immunization not carried out due to patient having had the disease UPD

Z28.82 Immunization not carried out because of caregiver refusal UPD

Immunization not carried out because of guardian refusal
Immunization not carried out because of parent refusal

EXCLUDES 1 *immunization not carried out because of caregiver refusal because of religious belief (Z28.1)*

Z28.83 Immunization not carried out due to unavailability of vaccine UPD

Delay in delivery of vaccine
Lack of availability of vaccine
Manufacturer delay of vaccine

AHA: 2018,4Q,36

Z28.89 Immunization not carried out for other reason UPD

Z28.9 Immunization not carried out for unspecified reason UPD

Z29 Encounter for other prophylactic measures

EXCLUDES 1 *desensitization to allergens (Z51.6)*
prophylactic surgery (Z4Ø.-)

AHA: 2016,4Q,78-79

Z29.1 Encounter for prophylactic immunotherapy

Encounter for administration of immunoglobulin

Z29.11 Encounter for prophylactic immunotherapy for respiratory syncytial virus (RSV) UPD

Z29.12 Encounter for prophylactic antivenin UPD

Z29.13 Encounter for prophylactic Rho(D) immune globulin UPD

AHA: 2019,3Q,5

Z29.14 Encounter for prophylactic rabies immune globulin UPD

Z29.3 Encounter for prophylactic fluoride administration UPD

Z29.8 **Encounter for other specified prophylactic measures** UPD
AHA: 2022,2Q,27

Z29.9 **Encounter for prophylactic measures, unspecified** UPD

Persons encountering health services in circumstances related to reproduction (Z30-Z39)

✓4th Z30 **Encounter for contraceptive management**
AHA: 2016,4Q,78
DEF: Contraceptive management to prevent pregnancy. Methods include oral medications, intrauterine devices, and surgical procedures for males and females (sterilization).

✓5th Z30.0 **Encounter for general counseling and advice on contraception**

✓6th Z30.01 **Encounter for initial prescription of contraceptives**
EXCLUDES 1 *encounter for surveillance of contraceptives (Z30.4-)*

Z30.011 **Encounter for initial prescription of contraceptive pills** UPD ♀

Z30.012 **Encounter for prescription of emergency contraception** UPD ♀
Encounter for postcoital contraception

Z30.013 **Encounter for initial prescription of injectable contraceptive** UPD ♀

Z30.014 **Encounter for initial prescription of intrauterine contraceptive device** UPD ♀
EXCLUDES 1 *encounter for insertion of intrauterine contraceptive device (Z30.430, Z30.432)*

Z30.015 **Encounter for initial prescription of vaginal ring hormonal contraceptive** UPD ♀

Z30.016 **Encounter for initial prescription of transdermal patch hormonal contraceptive device** UPD

Z30.017 **Encounter for initial prescription of implantable subdermal contraceptive** UPD

Z30.018 **Encounter for initial prescription of other contraceptives** UPD ♀
Encounter for initial prescription of barrier contraception
Encounter for initial prescription of diaphragm

Z30.019 **Encounter for initial prescription of contraceptives, unspecified** UPD ♀

Z30.02 **Counseling and instruction in natural family planning to avoid pregnancy** UPD

Z30.09 **Encounter for other general counseling and advice on contraception** UPD
Encounter for family planning advice NOS

Z30.2 **Encounter for sterilization**
AHA: 2021,3Q,13

✓5th Z30.4 **Encounter for surveillance of contraceptives**

Z30.40 **Encounter for surveillance of contraceptives, unspecified** UPD

Z30.41 **Encounter for surveillance of contraceptive pills** UPD ♀
Encounter for repeat prescription for contraceptive pill

Z30.42 **Encounter for surveillance of injectable contraceptive** UPD ♀

✓6th Z30.43 **Encounter for surveillance of intrauterine contraceptive device**

Z30.430 **Encounter for insertion of intrauterine contraceptive device** UPD ♀

Z30.431 **Encounter for routine checking of intrauterine contraceptive device** UPD ♀

Z30.432 **Encounter for removal of intrauterine contraceptive device** UPD ♀

Z30.433 **Encounter for removal and reinsertion of intrauterine contraceptive device** UPD ♀
Encounter for replacement of intrauterine contraceptive device

Z30.44 **Encounter for surveillance of vaginal ring hormonal contraceptive device** UPD ♀

Z30.45 **Encounter for surveillance of transdermal patch hormonal contraceptive device** UPD ♀

Z30.46 **Encounter for surveillance of implantable subdermal contraceptive** UPD ♀
Encounter for checking, reinsertion or removal of implantable subdermal contraceptive

Z30.49 **Encounter for surveillance of other contraceptives** UPD ♀
Encounter for surveillance of barrier contraception
Encounter for surveillance of diaphragm

Z30.8 **Encounter for other contraceptive management** UPD
Encounter for postvasectomy sperm count
Encounter for routine examination for contraceptive maintenance
EXCLUDES 1 *sperm count following sterilization reversal (Z31.42)*
sperm count for fertility testing (Z31.41)

Z30.9 **Encounter for contraceptive management, unspecified** UPD

✓4th Z31 **Encounter for procreative management**
EXCLUDES 2 *complications associated with artificial fertilization (N98.-)*
female infertility (N97.-)
male infertility (N46.-)

Z31.0 **Encounter for reversal of previous sterilization**

✓5th Z31.4 **Encounter for procreative investigation and testing**
EXCLUDES 1 *postvasectomy sperm count (Z30.8)*

Z31.41 **Encounter for fertility testing** UPD
Encounter for fallopian tube patency testing
Encounter for sperm count for fertility testing

Z31.42 **Aftercare following sterilization reversal** UPD
Sperm count following sterilization reversal

✓6th Z31.43 **Encounter for genetic testing of female for procreative management**
Use additional code for recurrent pregnancy loss, if applicable (N96, O26.2-)
EXCLUDES 1 *nonprocreative genetic testing (Z13.7-)*

Z31.430 **Encounter of female for testing for genetic disease carrier status for procreative management** UPD ♀

Z31.438 **Encounter for other genetic testing of female for procreative management** UPD ♀

✓6th Z31.44 **Encounter for genetic testing of male for procreative management**
EXCLUDES 1 *nonprocreative genetic testing (Z13.7-)*

Z31.440 **Encounter of male for testing for genetic disease carrier status for procreative management** UPD ♂

Z31.441 **Encounter for testing of male partner of patient with recurrent pregnancy loss** UPD A ♂

Z31.448 **Encounter for other genetic testing of male for procreative management** UPD A ♂

Z31.49 **Encounter for other procreative investigation and testing** UPD

Z31.5 **Encounter for procreative genetic counseling** UPD
AHA: 2017,4Q,27

✓5th Z31.6 **Encounter for general counseling and advice on procreation**

Z31.61 **Procreative counseling and advice using natural family planning** UPD

Z31.62 **Encounter for fertility preservation counseling** UPD
Encounter for fertility preservation counseling prior to cancer therapy
Encounter for fertility preservation counseling prior to surgical removal of gonads

Z31.69 **Encounter for other general counseling and advice on procreation** UPD

Z31.7 **Encounter for procreative management and counseling for gestational carrier** UPD ♀
EXCLUDES 1 *pregnant state, gestational carrier (Z33.3)*
AHA: 2016,4Q,78

✓5th Z31.8 **Encounter for other procreative management**

Z31.81 **Encounter for male factor infertility in female patient** UPD ♀

Z31.82 Encounter for Rh incompatibility status UPD ♀
AHA: 2015,3Q,40; 2014,4Q,17

Z31.83 Encounter for assisted reproductive fertility procedure cycle UPD ♀
Patient undergoing in vitro fertilization cycle
Use additional code to identify the type of infertility
EXCLUDES 1 *pre-cycle diagnosis and testing - code to reason for encounter*
AHA: 2022,2Q,15-16

Z31.84 Encounter for fertility preservation procedure UPD
Encounter for fertility preservation procedure prior to cancer therapy
Encounter for fertility preservation procedure prior to surgical removal of gonads

Z31.89 Encounter for other procreative management UPD

Z31.9 Encounter for procreative management, unspecified UPD

Z32 Encounter for pregnancy test and childbirth and childcare instruction

Z32.0 Encounter for pregnancy test

Z32.00 Encounter for pregnancy test, result unknown ♀
Encounter for pregnancy test NOS

Z32.01 Encounter for pregnancy test, result positive M ♀

Z32.02 Encounter for pregnancy test, result negative ♀

Z32.2 Encounter for childbirth instruction UPD

Z32.3 Encounter for childcare instruction UPD
Encounter for prenatal or postpartum childcare instruction

Z33 Pregnant state

Z33.1 Pregnant state, incidental UPD M ♀
Pregnancy NOS
Pregnant state NOS
EXCLUDES 1 *complications of pregnancy (O00-O9A)*
pregnant state, gestational carrier (Z33.3)

Z33.2 Encounter for elective termination of pregnancy M ♀
EXCLUDES 1 *early fetal death with retention of dead fetus (O02.1)*
late fetal death (O36.4)
spontaneous abortion (O03)
AHA: 2022,1Q,20
TIP: Do not assign a code from category Z3A with this code.

Z33.3 Pregnant state, gestational carrier UPD M ♀
EXCLUDES 1 *encounter for procreative management and counseling for gestational carrier (Z31.7)*
AHA: 2016,4Q,78

Z34 Encounter for supervision of normal pregnancy
EXCLUDES 1 *any complication of pregnancy (O00-O9A)*
encounter for pregnancy test (Z32.0-)
encounter for supervision of high risk pregnancy (O09.-)
AHA: 2019,3Q,5; 2014,4Q,17

Z34.0 Encounter for supervision of normal first pregnancy

Z34.00 Encounter for supervision of normal first pregnancy, unspecified trimester UPD M ♀

Z34.01 Encounter for supervision of normal first pregnancy, first trimester UPD M ♀

Z34.02 Encounter for supervision of normal first pregnancy, second trimester UPD M ♀

Z34.03 Encounter for supervision of normal first pregnancy, third trimester UPD M ♀

Z34.8 Encounter for supervision of other normal pregnancy

Z34.80 Encounter for supervision of other normal pregnancy, unspecified trimester UPD M ♀

Z34.81 Encounter for supervision of other normal pregnancy, first trimester UPD M ♀

Z34.82 Encounter for supervision of other normal pregnancy, second trimester UPD M ♀

Z34.83 Encounter for supervision of other normal pregnancy, third trimester UPD M ♀

Z34.9 Encounter for supervision of normal pregnancy, unspecified

Z34.90 Encounter for supervision of normal pregnancy, unspecified, unspecified trimester UPD M ♀

Z34.91 Encounter for supervision of normal pregnancy, unspecified, first trimester UPD M ♀

Z34.92 Encounter for supervision of normal pregnancy, unspecified, second trimester UPD M ♀

Z34.93 Encounter for supervision of normal pregnancy, unspecified, third trimester UPD M ♀

Z36 Encounter for antenatal screening of mother
INCLUDES encounter for placental sample (taken vaginally)
screening is the testing for disease or disease precursors in asymptomatic individuals so that early detection and treatment can be provided for those who test positive for the disease.
EXCLUDES 1 *diagnostic examination - code to sign or symptom*
encounter for suspected maternal and fetal conditions ruled out (Z03.7-)
suspected fetal condition affecting management of pregnancy - code to condition in Chapter 15
EXCLUDES 2 *abnormal findings on antenatal screening of mother (O28.-)*
genetic counseling and testing (Z31.43-, Z31.5)
routine prenatal care (Z34)
AHA: 2017,4Q,28

Z36.0 Encounter for antenatal screening for chromosomal anomalies M ♀

Z36.1 Encounter for antenatal screening for raised alphafetoprotein level M ♀
Encounter for antenatal screening for elevated maternal serum alphafetoprotein level
DEF: High levels of alpha-fetoprotein (AFP) that may indicate a possibility of spina bifida and other neural tube defects, anencephaly, or omphalocele in the fetus.

Z36.2 Encounter for other antenatal screening follow-up M ♀
Non-visualized anatomy on a previous scan

Z36.3 Encounter for antenatal screening for malformations M ♀
Screening for a suspected anomaly

Z36.4 Encounter for antenatal screening for fetal growth retardation M ♀
Intrauterine growth restriction (IUGR)/small-for-dates

Z36.5 Encounter for antenatal screening for isoimmunization M ♀

Z36.8 Encounter for other antenatal screening

Z36.81 Encounter for antenatal screening for hydrops fetalis M ♀
DEF: Hydrops fetalis: Abnormal accumulation of fluid in two or more parts of the fetus, such as ascites, effusion of the pleural or pericardial tissues, or edema.

Z36.82 Encounter for antenatal screening for nuchal translucency M ♀

Z36.83 Encounter for fetal screening for congenital cardiac abnormalities M ♀

Z36.84 Encounter for antenatal screening for fetal lung maturity M ♀

Z36.85 Encounter for antenatal screening for Streptococcus B M ♀

Z36.86 Encounter for antenatal screening for cervical length M ♀
Screening for risk of pre-term labor

Z36.87 Encounter for antenatal screening for uncertain dates M ♀

Z36.88 Encounter for antenatal screening for fetal macrosomia M ♀
Screening for large-for-dates

Z36.89 Encounter for other specified antenatal screening M ♀

Z36.8A Encounter for antenatal screening for other genetic defects M ♀

Z36.9 Encounter for antenatal screening, unspecified M ♀

Z3A Weeks of gestation
NOTE Codes from category Z3A are for use, only on the maternal record, to indicate the weeks of gestation of the pregnancy, if known.
Code first obstetric condition or encounter for delivery (O09-O60, O80-O82)
AHA: 2022,2Q,3; 2019,2Q,11; 2016,2Q,34; 2014,3Q,17; 2014,2Q,9; 2013,2Q,33
TIP: Do not assign a code from this category with codes from categories O00-O08 or code Z33.2.

Z3A.0 Weeks of gestation of pregnancy, unspecified or less than 10 weeks

Z3A.00 Weeks of gestation of pregnancy not specified UPD M ♀

Chapter 21. Factors Influencing Health Status and Contact With Health Services

Z3A.01 Less than 8 weeks gestation of pregnancy UPD M ♀
Z3A.08 8 weeks gestation of pregnancy UPD M ♀
Z3A.09 9 weeks gestation of pregnancy UPD M ♀

Z3A.1 Weeks of gestation of pregnancy, weeks 10-19
Z3A.10 10 weeks gestation of pregnancy UPD M ♀
Z3A.11 11 weeks gestation of pregnancy UPD M ♀
Z3A.12 12 weeks gestation of pregnancy UPD M ♀
Z3A.13 13 weeks gestation of pregnancy UPD M ♀
Z3A.14 14 weeks gestation of pregnancy UPD M ♀
Z3A.15 15 weeks gestation of pregnancy UPD M ♀
Z3A.16 16 weeks gestation of pregnancy UPD M ♀
Z3A.17 17 weeks gestation of pregnancy UPD M ♀
Z3A.18 18 weeks gestation of pregnancy UPD M ♀
Z3A.19 19 weeks gestation of pregnancy UPD M ♀

Z3A.2 Weeks of gestation of pregnancy, weeks 20-29
Z3A.20 20 weeks gestation of pregnancy UPD M ♀
Z3A.21 21 weeks gestation of pregnancy UPD M ♀
Z3A.22 22 weeks gestation of pregnancy UPD M ♀
Z3A.23 23 weeks gestation of pregnancy UPD M ♀
Z3A.24 24 weeks gestation of pregnancy UPD M ♀
Z3A.25 25 weeks gestation of pregnancy UPD M ♀
Z3A.26 26 weeks gestation of pregnancy UPD M ♀
Z3A.27 27 weeks gestation of pregnancy UPD M ♀
Z3A.28 28 weeks gestation of pregnancy UPD M ♀
Z3A.29 29 weeks gestation of pregnancy UPD M ♀

Z3A.3 Weeks of gestation of pregnancy, weeks 30-39
Z3A.30 30 weeks gestation of pregnancy UPD M ♀
Z3A.31 31 weeks gestation of pregnancy UPD M ♀
Z3A.32 32 weeks gestation of pregnancy UPD M ♀
Z3A.33 33 weeks gestation of pregnancy UPD M ♀
Z3A.34 34 weeks gestation of pregnancy UPD M ♀
Z3A.35 35 weeks gestation of pregnancy UPD M ♀
Z3A.36 36 weeks gestation of pregnancy UPD M ♀
Z3A.37 37 weeks gestation of pregnancy UPD M ♀
Z3A.38 38 weeks gestation of pregnancy UPD M ♀
Z3A.39 39 weeks gestation of pregnancy UPD M ♀

Z3A.4 Weeks of gestation of pregnancy, weeks 40 or greater
AHA: 2014,4Q,23
Z3A.40 40 weeks gestation of pregnancy UPD M ♀
Z3A.41 41 weeks gestation of pregnancy UPD M ♀
Z3A.42 42 weeks gestation of pregnancy UPD M ♀
Z3A.49 Greater than 42 weeks gestation of pregnancy UPD M ♀

Z37 Outcome of delivery

This category is intended for use as an additional code to identify the outcome of delivery on the mother's record. It is not for use on the newborn record.

EXCLUDES 1 *stillbirth (P95)*

Z37.0 Single live birth UPD M ♀
AHA: 2016,2Q,34; 2014,2Q,9
Z37.1 Single stillbirth UPD M ♀
Z37.2 Twins, both liveborn UPD M ♀
Z37.3 Twins, one liveborn and one stillborn UPD M ♀
Z37.4 Twins, both stillborn UPD M ♀

Z37.5 Other multiple births, all liveborn
Z37.50 Multiple births, unspecified, all liveborn UPD M ♀
Z37.51 Triplets, all liveborn UPD M ♀
Z37.52 Quadruplets, all liveborn UPD M ♀
Z37.53 Quintuplets, all liveborn UPD M ♀
Z37.54 Sextuplets, all liveborn UPD M ♀
Z37.59 Other multiple births, all liveborn UPD M ♀

Z37.6 Other multiple births, some liveborn
Z37.60 Multiple births, unspecified, some liveborn UPD M ♀
Z37.61 Triplets, some liveborn UPD M ♀
Z37.62 Quadruplets, some liveborn UPD M ♀
Z37.63 Quintuplets, some liveborn UPD M ♀
Z37.64 Sextuplets, some liveborn UPD M ♀
Z37.69 Other multiple births, some liveborn UPD M ♀
Z37.7 Other multiple births, all stillborn UPD M ♀
Z37.9 Outcome of delivery, unspecified UPD M ♀
Multiple birth NOS
Single birth NOS

Z38 Liveborn infants according to place of birth and type of delivery

This category is for use as the principal code on the initial record of a newborn baby. It is to be used for the initial birth record only. It is not to be used on the mother's record.

AHA: 2020,2Q,13; 2017,2Q,5-7; 2016,3Q,18; 2015,2Q,15

Z38.0 Single liveborn infant, born in hospital
Single liveborn infant, born in birthing center or other health care facility
Z38.00 Single liveborn infant, delivered vaginally N
Z38.01 Single liveborn infant, delivered by cesarean N
Z38.1 Single liveborn infant, born outside hospital N
Z38.2 Single liveborn infant, unspecified as to place of birth N
Single liveborn infant NOS

Z38.3 Twin liveborn infant, born in hospital
Z38.30 Twin liveborn infant, delivered vaginally N
Z38.31 Twin liveborn infant, delivered by cesarean N
Z38.4 Twin liveborn infant, born outside hospital N
Z38.5 Twin liveborn infant, unspecified as to place of birth N

Z38.6 Other multiple liveborn infant, born in hospital
Z38.61 Triplet liveborn infant, delivered vaginally N
Z38.62 Triplet liveborn infant, delivered by cesarean N
Z38.63 Quadruplet liveborn infant, delivered vaginally N
Z38.64 Quadruplet liveborn infant, delivered by cesarean N
Z38.65 Quintuplet liveborn infant, delivered vaginally N
Z38.66 Quintuplet liveborn infant, delivered by cesarean N
Z38.68 Other multiple liveborn infant, delivered vaginally N
Z38.69 Other multiple liveborn infant, delivered by cesarean N
Z38.7 Other multiple liveborn infant, born outside hospital N
Z38.8 Other multiple liveborn infant, unspecified as to place of birth N

Z39 Encounter for maternal postpartum care and examination

Z39.0 Encounter for care and examination of mother immediately after delivery M ♀
Care and observation in uncomplicated cases when the delivery occurs outside a healthcare facility
EXCLUDES 1 *care for postpartum complication - see Alphabetic Index*
AHA: 2021,3Q,13
Z39.1 Encounter for care and examination of lactating mother UPD M ♀
Encounter for supervision of lactation
EXCLUDES 1 *disorders of lactation (O92.-)*
Z39.2 Encounter for routine postpartum follow-up UPD M ♀

Encounters for other specific health care (Z40-Z53)

Categories Z40-Z53 are intended for use to indicate a reason for care. They may be used for patients who have already been treated for a disease or injury, but who are receiving aftercare or prophylactic care, or care to consolidate the treatment, or to deal with a residual state

EXCLUDES 2 *follow-up examination for medical surveillance after treatment (Z08-Z09)*

Z40 Encounter for prophylactic surgery

EXCLUDES 1 *organ donations (Z52.-)*
therapeutic organ removal - code to condition

DEF: Treatment measure intended to prevent or ward off a disease or condition.

Z40.0 Encounter for prophylactic surgery for risk factors related to malignant neoplasms
Admission for prophylactic organ removal
Use additional code to identify risk factor
AHA: 2017,4Q,28-29
Z40.00 Encounter for prophylactic removal of unspecified organ
Z40.01 Encounter for prophylactic removal of breast

Z40.02 **Encounter for prophylactic removal of ovary(s)** ♀
Encounter for prophylactic removal of ovary(s) and fallopian tube(s)

Z40.03 **Encounter for prophylactic removal of fallopian tube(s)** ♀

Z40.09 **Encounter for prophylactic removal of other organ**

Z40.8 **Encounter for other prophylactic surgery** UPD

Z40.9 **Encounter for prophylactic surgery, unspecified** UPD

Z41 Encounter for procedures for purposes other than remedying health state

Z41.1 **Encounter for cosmetic surgery**
Encounter for cosmetic breast implant
Encounter for cosmetic procedure
EXCLUDES 1 *encounter for plastic and reconstructive surgery following medical procedure or healed injury (Z42.-)*
encounter for post-mastectomy breast implantation (Z42.1)

Z41.2 **Encounter for routine and ritual male circumcision** ♂
AHA: 2018,3Q,15
TIP: Do not report this code when circumcision is performed during the birth admission.

Z41.3 **Encounter for ear piercing** UPD

Z41.8 **Encounter for other procedures for purposes other than remedying health state**

Z41.9 **Encounter for procedure for purposes other than remedying health state, unspecified** UPD

Z42 Encounter for plastic and reconstructive surgery following medical procedure or healed injury
EXCLUDES 1 *encounter for cosmetic plastic surgery (Z41.1)*
encounter for plastic surgery for treatment of current injury - code to relevent injury

Z42.1 **Encounter for breast reconstruction following mastectomy** A
EXCLUDES 1 *deformity and disproportion of reconstructed breast (N65.1-)*

Z42.8 **Encounter for other plastic and reconstructive surgery following medical procedure or healed injury**
AHA: 2017,1Q,42

Z43 Encounter for attention to artificial openings
INCLUDES closure of artificial openings
passage of sounds or bougies through artificial openings
reforming artificial openings
removal of catheter from artificial openings
toilet or cleansing of artificial openings
EXCLUDES 1 *complications of external stoma (J95.0-, K94.-, N99.5-)*
EXCLUDES 2 *fitting and adjustment of prosthetic and other devices (Z44-Z46)*
AHA: 2019,2Q,33

Z43.0 **Encounter for attention to tracheostomy** HCC

Z43.1 **Encounter for attention to gastrostomy** CC HCC
EXCLUDES 2 *artificial opening status only, without need for care (Z93.-)*

Z43.2 **Encounter for attention to ileostomy** HCC

Z43.3 **Encounter for attention to colostomy** HCC

Z43.4 **Encounter for attention to other artificial openings of digestive tract** HCC

Z43.5 **Encounter for attention to cystostomy** HCC

Z43.6 **Encounter for attention to other artificial openings of urinary tract** HCC
Encounter for attention to nephrostomy
Encounter for attention to ureterostomy
Encounter for attention to urethrostomy

Z43.7 **Encounter for attention to artificial vagina**

Z43.8 **Encounter for attention to other artificial openings** HCC

Z43.9 **Encounter for attention to unspecified artificial opening** UPD HCC

Z44 Encounter for fitting and adjustment of external prosthetic device
INCLUDES removal or replacement of external prosthetic device
EXCLUDES 1 *malfunction or other complications of device - see Alphabetical Index*
presence of prosthetic device (Z97.-)

Z44.0 **Encounter for fitting and adjustment of artificial arm**

Z44.00 **Encounter for fitting and adjustment of unspecified artificial arm**

Z44.001 **Encounter for fitting and adjustment of unspecified right artificial arm**

Z44.002 **Encounter for fitting and adjustment of unspecified left artificial arm**

Z44.009 **Encounter for fitting and adjustment of unspecified artificial arm, unspecified arm**

Z44.01 **Encounter for fitting and adjustment of complete artificial arm**

Z44.011 **Encounter for fitting and adjustment of complete right artificial arm**

Z44.012 **Encounter for fitting and adjustment of complete left artificial arm**

Z44.019 **Encounter for fitting and adjustment of complete artificial arm, unspecified arm**

Z44.02 **Encounter for fitting and adjustment of partial artificial arm**

Z44.021 **Encounter for fitting and adjustment of partial artificial right arm**

Z44.022 **Encounter for fitting and adjustment of partial artificial left arm**

Z44.029 **Encounter for fitting and adjustment of partial artificial arm, unspecified arm**

Z44.1 **Encounter for fitting and adjustment of artificial leg**

Z44.10 **Encounter for fitting and adjustment of unspecified artificial leg**

Z44.101 **Encounter for fitting and adjustment of unspecified right artificial leg** HCC

Z44.102 **Encounter for fitting and adjustment of unspecified left artificial leg** HCC

Z44.109 **Encounter for fitting and adjustment of unspecified artificial leg, unspecified leg** HCC

Z44.11 **Encounter for fitting and adjustment of complete artificial leg**

Z44.111 **Encounter for fitting and adjustment of complete right artificial leg** HCC

Z44.112 **Encounter for fitting and adjustment of complete left artificial leg** HCC

Z44.119 **Encounter for fitting and adjustment of complete artificial leg, unspecified leg** HCC

Z44.12 **Encounter for fitting and adjustment of partial artificial leg**

Z44.121 **Encounter for fitting and adjustment of partial artificial right leg** HCC

Z44.122 **Encounter for fitting and adjustment of partial artificial left leg** HCC

Z44.129 **Encounter for fitting and adjustment of partial artificial leg, unspecified leg** HCC

Z44.2 **Encounter for fitting and adjustment of artificial eye**
EXCLUDES 1 *mechanical complication of ocular prosthesis (T85.3)*

Z44.20 **Encounter for fitting and adjustment of artificial eye, unspecified**

Z44.21 **Encounter for fitting and adjustment of artificial right eye**

Z44.22 **Encounter for fitting and adjustment of artificial left eye**

Z44.3 **Encounter for fitting and adjustment of external breast prosthesis**
EXCLUDES 1 *complications of breast implant (T85.4-)*
encounter for adjustment or removal of breast implant (Z45.81-)
encounter for initial breast implant insertion for cosmetic breast augmentation (Z41.1)
encounter for breast reconstruction following mastectomy (Z42.1)

Z44.30 **Encounter for fitting and adjustment of external breast prosthesis, unspecified breast**

Z44.31 **Encounter for fitting and adjustment of external right breast prosthesis**

Z44.32 Encounter for fitting and adjustment of external left breast prosthesis

Z44.8 Encounter for fitting and adjustment of other external prosthetic devices

Z44.9 Encounter for fitting and adjustment of unspecified external prosthetic device UPD

Z45 Encounter for adjustment and management of implanted device

INCLUDES removal or replacement of implanted device

EXCLUDES 1 *malfunction or other complications of device - see Alphabetical Index*

EXCLUDES 2 *encounter for fitting and adjustment of non-implanted device (Z46.-)*

Z45.Ø Encounter for adjustment and management of cardiac device

TIP: Assign an additional code for the associated condition if that condition requires constant intervention from the device, as in cases of sick sinus syndrome. For conditions that do not require constant intervention from the device, as in cases of ventricular fibrillation, an additional code for the associated condition should be assigned only if the patient is experiencing the condition and the device is firing during the current admission.

Z45.Ø1 Encounter for adjustment and management of cardiac pacemaker

Encounter for adjustment and management of cardiac resynchronization therapy pacemaker (CRT-P)

EXCLUDES 1 *encounter for adjustment and management of automatic implantable cardiac defibrillator with synchronous cardiac pacemaker (Z45.Ø2)*

Z45.Ø1Ø Encounter for checking and testing of cardiac pacemaker pulse generator [battery]

Encounter for replacing cardiac pacemaker pulse generator [battery]

Z45.Ø18 Encounter for adjustment and management of other part of cardiac pacemaker

EXCLUDES 1 *presence of other part of cardiac pacemaker (Z95.Ø)*

EXCLUDES 2 *presence of prosthetic and other devices (Z95.1-Z95.5, Z95.811-Z97)*

Z45.Ø2 Encounter for adjustment and management of automatic implantable cardiac defibrillator

Encounter for adjustment and management of automatic implantable cardiac defibrillator with synchronous cardiac pacemaker

Encounter for adjustment and management of cardiac resynchronization therapy defibrillator (CRT-D)

Z45.Ø9 Encounter for adjustment and management of other cardiac device

Z45.1 Encounter for adjustment and management of infusion pump

Z45.2 Encounter for adjustment and management of vascular access device

Encounter for adjustment and management of vascular catheters

EXCLUDES 1 *encounter for adjustment and management of renal dialysis catheter (Z49.Ø1)*

AHA: 2020,2Q,21; 2018,3Q,20

Z45.3 Encounter for adjustment and management of implanted devices of the special senses

Z45.31 Encounter for adjustment and management of implanted visual substitution device

Z45.32 Encounter for adjustment and management of implanted hearing device

EXCLUDES 1 *encounter for fitting and adjustment of hearing aide (Z46.1)*

Z45.32Ø Encounter for adjustment and management of bone conduction device

Z45.321 Encounter for adjustment and management of cochlear device

Z45.328 Encounter for adjustment and management of other implanted hearing device

Z45.4 Encounter for adjustment and management of implanted nervous system device

Z45.41 Encounter for adjustment and management of cerebrospinal fluid drainage device

Encounter for adjustment and management of cerebral ventricular (communicating) shunt

Z45.42 Encounter for adjustment and management of neurostimulator

Encounter for adjustment and management of brain neurostimulator

Encounter for adjustment and management of gastric neurostimulator

Encounter for adjustment and management of peripheral nerve neurostimulator

Encounter for adjustment and management of sacral nerve neurostimulator

Encounter for adjustment and management of spinal cord neurostimulator

Encounter for adjustment and management of vagus nerve neurostimulator

Z45.49 Encounter for adjustment and management of other implanted nervous system device

AHA: 2014,3Q,19

Z45.8 Encounter for adjustment and management of other implanted devices

Z45.81 Encounter for adjustment or removal of breast implant

Encounter for elective implant exchange (different material) (different size)

Encounter for removal of tissue expander with or without synchronous insertion of permanent implant

EXCLUDES 1 *complications of breast implant (T85.4-)*

encounter for initial breast implant insertion for cosmetic breast augmentation (Z41.1)

encounter for breast reconstruction following mastectomy (Z42.1)

Z45.811 Encounter for adjustment or removal of right breast implant

Z45.812 Encounter for adjustment or removal of left breast implant

Z45.819 Encounter for adjustment or removal of unspecified breast implant

Z45.82 Encounter for adjustment or removal of myringotomy device (stent) (tube) UPD

Z45.89 Encounter for adjustment and management of other implanted devices UPD

AHA: 2014,4Q,26-28

Z45.9 Encounter for adjustment and management of unspecified implanted device UPD

Z46 Encounter for fitting and adjustment of other devices

INCLUDES removal or replacement of other device

EXCLUDES 1 *malfunction or other complications of device - see Alphabetical Index*

EXCLUDES 2 *encounter for fitting and management of implanted devices (Z45.-)*

issue of repeat prescription only (Z76.Ø)

presence of prosthetic and other devices (Z95-Z97)

Z46.Ø Encounter for fitting and adjustment of spectacles and contact lenses UPD

Z46.1 Encounter for fitting and adjustment of hearing aid UPD

EXCLUDES 1 *encounter for adjustment and management of implanted hearing device (Z45.32-)*

Z46.2 Encounter for fitting and adjustment of other devices related to nervous system and special senses

EXCLUDES 2 *encounter for adjustment and management of implanted nervous system device (Z45.4-)*

encounter for adjustment and management of implanted visual substitution device (Z45.31)

Z46.3 Encounter for fitting and adjustment of dental prosthetic device

Encounter for fitting and adjustment of dentures

Z46.4 Encounter for fitting and adjustment of orthodontic device UPD

✓5th **Z46.5 Encounter for fitting and adjustment of other gastrointestinal appliance and device**
EXCLUDES 1 *encounter for attention to artificial openings of digestive tract (Z43.1-Z43.4)*

Z46.51 Encounter for fitting and adjustment of gastric lap band UPD

Z46.59 Encounter for fitting and adjustment of other gastrointestinal appliance and device UPD

Z46.6 Encounter for fitting and adjustment of urinary device UPD
EXCLUDES 2 *attention to artificial openings of urinary tract (Z43.5, Z43.6)*

✓5th **Z46.8 Encounter for fitting and adjustment of other specified devices**

Z46.81 Encounter for fitting and adjustment of insulin pump UPD
Encounter for insulin pump instruction and training
Encounter for insulin pump titration

Z46.82 Encounter for fitting and adjustment of non-vascular catheter

Z46.89 Encounter for fitting and adjustment of other specified devices UPD
Encounter for fitting and adjustment of wheelchair

Z46.9 Encounter for fitting and adjustment of unspecified device UPD

✓4th **Z47 Orthopedic aftercare**
EXCLUDES 1 *aftercare for healing fracture - code to fracture with 7th character D*

Z47.1 Aftercare following joint replacement surgery
Use additional code to identify the joint (Z96.6-)
AHA: 2020,1Q,23

Z47.2 Encounter for removal of internal fixation device
EXCLUDES 1 *encounter for adjustment of internal fixation device for fracture treatment - code to fracture with appropriate 7th character*
encounter for removal of external fixation device - code to fracture with 7th character D
infection or inflammatory reaction to internal fixation device (T84.6-)
mechanical complication of internal fixation device (T84.1-)

✓5th **Z47.3 Aftercare following explantation of joint prosthesis**
Aftercare following explantation of joint prosthesis, staged procedure
Encounter for joint prosthesis insertion following prior explantation of joint prosthesis
AHA: 2020,1Q,23; 2015,1Q,16
TIP: For staged removal of elbow joint prosthesis, assign code Z47.1.

Z47.31 Aftercare following explantation of shoulder joint prosthesis
EXCLUDES 1 *acquired absence of shoulder joint following prior explantation of shoulder joint prosthesis (Z89.23-)*
shoulder joint prosthesis explantation status (Z89.23-)

Z47.32 Aftercare following explantation of hip joint prosthesis
EXCLUDES 1 *acquired absence of hip joint following prior explantation of hip joint prosthesis (Z89.62-)*
hip joint prosthesis explantation status (Z89.62-)

Z47.33 Aftercare following explantation of knee joint prosthesis
EXCLUDES 1 *acquired absence of knee joint following prior explantation of knee prosthesis (Z89.52-)*
knee joint prosthesis explantation status (Z89.52-)

✓5th **Z47.8 Encounter for other orthopedic aftercare**

Z47.81 Encounter for orthopedic aftercare following surgical amputation
Use additional code to identify the limb amputated (Z89.-)

Z47.82 Encounter for orthopedic aftercare following scoliosis surgery

Z47.89 Encounter for other orthopedic aftercare
AHA: 2015,1Q,8

✓4th **Z48 Encounter for other postprocedural aftercare**
EXCLUDES 1 *encounter for aftercare following injury - code to Injury, by site, with appropriate 7th character for subsequent encounter*
encounter for follow-up examination after completed treatment (Z08-Z09)
EXCLUDES 2 *encounter for attention to artificial openings (Z43.-)*
encounter for fitting and adjustment of prosthetic and other devices (Z44-Z46)
AHA: 2015,4Q,38; 2015,1Q,6-7

✓5th **Z48.0 Encounter for attention to dressings, sutures and drains**
EXCLUDES 1 *encounter for planned postprocedural wound closure (Z48.1)*

Z48.00 Encounter for change or removal of nonsurgical wound dressing UPD
Encounter for change or removal of wound dressing NOS

Z48.01 Encounter for change or removal of surgical wound dressing UPD
AHA: 2019,2Q,33

Z48.02 Encounter for removal of sutures UPD
Encounter for removal of staples

Z48.03 Encounter for change or removal of drains
AHA: 2019,2Q,33

Z48.1 Encounter for planned postprocedural wound closure
EXCLUDES 1 *encounter for attention to dressings and sutures (Z48.0-)*

✓5th **Z48.2 Encounter for aftercare following organ transplant**

Z48.21 Encounter for aftercare following heart transplant CC HCC

Z48.22 Encounter for aftercare following kidney transplant CC

Z48.23 Encounter for aftercare following liver transplant CC HCC

Z48.24 Encounter for aftercare following lung transplant CC HCC

✓6th **Z48.28 Encounter for aftercare following multiple organ transplant**

Z48.280 Encounter for aftercare following heart-lung transplant CC HCC

Z48.288 Encounter for aftercare following multiple organ transplant

✓6th **Z48.29 Encounter for aftercare following other organ transplant**

Z48.290 Encounter for aftercare following bone marrow transplant CC HCC

Z48.298 Encounter for aftercare following other organ transplant

Z48.3 Aftercare following surgery for neoplasm
Use additional code to identify the neoplasm

✓5th **Z48.8 Encounter for other specified postprocedural aftercare**

✓6th **Z48.81 Encounter for surgical aftercare following surgery on specified body systems**
These codes identify the body system requiring aftercare. They are for use in conjunction with other aftercare codes to fully explain the aftercare encounter. The condition treated should also be coded if still present.
EXCLUDES 1 *aftercare for injury - code the injury with 7th character D*
aftercare following surgery for neoplasm (Z48.3)
EXCLUDES 2 *aftercare following organ transplant (Z48.2-)*
orthopedic aftercare (Z47.-)
AHA: 2015,4Q,38

Z48.810 Encounter for surgical aftercare following surgery on the sense organs

Z48.811 Encounter for surgical aftercare following surgery on the nervous system
EXCLUDES 2 *encounter for surgical aftercare following surgery on the sense organs (Z48.810)*

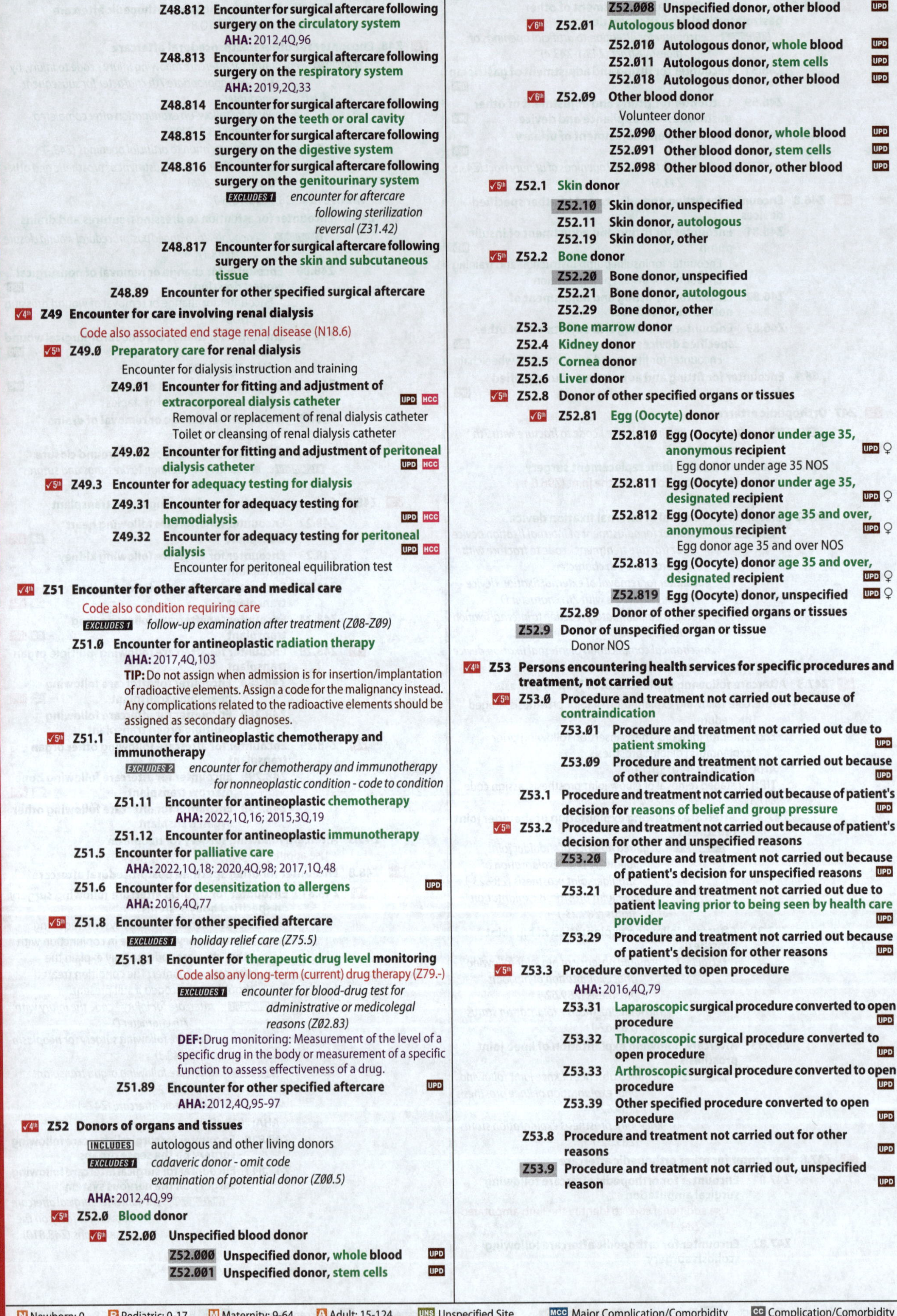

Z48.812 Encounter for surgical aftercare following surgery on the circulatory system
AHA: 2012,4Q,96

Z48.813 Encounter for surgical aftercare following surgery on the respiratory system
AHA: 2019,2Q,33

Z48.814 Encounter for surgical aftercare following surgery on the teeth or oral cavity

Z48.815 Encounter for surgical aftercare following surgery on the digestive system

Z48.816 Encounter for surgical aftercare following surgery on the genitourinary system
EXCLUDES 1 *encounter for aftercare following sterilization reversal (Z31.42)*

Z48.817 Encounter for surgical aftercare following surgery on the skin and subcutaneous tissue

Z48.89 Encounter for other specified surgical aftercare

Z49 Encounter for care involving renal dialysis
Code also associated end stage renal disease (N18.6)

Z49.0 Preparatory care for renal dialysis
Encounter for dialysis instruction and training

Z49.01 Encounter for fitting and adjustment of extracorporeal dialysis catheter UPD HCC
Removal or replacement of renal dialysis catheter
Toilet or cleansing of renal dialysis catheter

Z49.02 Encounter for fitting and adjustment of peritoneal dialysis catheter UPD HCC

Z49.3 Encounter for adequacy testing for dialysis

Z49.31 Encounter for adequacy testing for hemodialysis UPD HCC

Z49.32 Encounter for adequacy testing for peritoneal dialysis UPD HCC
Encounter for peritoneal equilibration test

Z51 Encounter for other aftercare and medical care
Code also condition requiring care
EXCLUDES 1 *follow-up examination after treatment (Z08-Z09)*

Z51.0 Encounter for antineoplastic radiation therapy
AHA: 2017,4Q,103
TIP: Do not assign when admission is for insertion/implantation of radioactive elements. Assign a code for the malignancy instead. Any complications related to the radioactive elements should be assigned as secondary diagnoses.

Z51.1 Encounter for antineoplastic chemotherapy and immunotherapy
EXCLUDES 2 *encounter for chemotherapy and immunotherapy for nonneoplastic condition - code to condition*

Z51.11 Encounter for antineoplastic chemotherapy
AHA: 2022,1Q,16; 2015,3Q,19

Z51.12 Encounter for antineoplastic immunotherapy

Z51.5 Encounter for palliative care
AHA: 2022,1Q,18; 2020,4Q,98; 2017,1Q,48

Z51.6 Encounter for desensitization to allergens UPD
AHA: 2016,4Q,77

Z51.8 Encounter for other specified aftercare
EXCLUDES 1 *holiday relief care (Z75.5)*

Z51.81 Encounter for therapeutic drug level monitoring
Code also any long-term (current) drug therapy (Z79.-)
EXCLUDES 1 *encounter for blood-drug test for administrative or medicolegal reasons (Z02.83)*
DEF: Drug monitoring: Measurement of the level of a specific drug in the body or measurement of a specific function to assess effectiveness of a drug.

Z51.89 Encounter for other specified aftercare UPD
AHA: 2012,4Q,95-97

Z52 Donors of organs and tissues
INCLUDES autologous and other living donors
EXCLUDES 1 *cadaveric donor - omit code*
examination of potential donor (Z00.5)
AHA: 2012,4Q,99

Z52.0 Blood donor

Z52.00 Unspecified blood donor

Z52.000 Unspecified donor, whole blood UPD

Z52.001 Unspecified donor, stem cells UPD

Z52.008 Unspecified donor, other blood UPD

Z52.01 Autologous blood donor

Z52.010 Autologous donor, whole blood UPD

Z52.011 Autologous donor, stem cells UPD

Z52.018 Autologous donor, other blood UPD

Z52.09 Other blood donor
Volunteer donor

Z52.090 Other blood donor, whole blood UPD

Z52.091 Other blood donor, stem cells UPD

Z52.098 Other blood donor, other blood UPD

Z52.1 Skin donor

Z52.10 Skin donor, unspecified

Z52.11 Skin donor, autologous

Z52.19 Skin donor, other

Z52.2 Bone donor

Z52.20 Bone donor, unspecified

Z52.21 Bone donor, autologous

Z52.29 Bone donor, other

Z52.3 Bone marrow donor

Z52.4 Kidney donor

Z52.5 Cornea donor

Z52.6 Liver donor

Z52.8 Donor of other specified organs or tissues

Z52.81 Egg (Oocyte) donor

Z52.810 Egg (Oocyte) donor under age 35, anonymous recipient UPD ♀
Egg donor under age 35 NOS

Z52.811 Egg (Oocyte) donor under age 35, designated recipient UPD ♀

Z52.812 Egg (Oocyte) donor age 35 and over, anonymous recipient UPD ♀
Egg donor age 35 and over NOS

Z52.813 Egg (Oocyte) donor age 35 and over, designated recipient UPD ♀

Z52.819 Egg (Oocyte) donor, unspecified UPD ♀

Z52.89 Donor of other specified organs or tissues

Z52.9 Donor of unspecified organ or tissue
Donor NOS

Z53 Persons encountering health services for specific procedures and treatment, not carried out

Z53.0 Procedure and treatment not carried out because of contraindication

Z53.01 Procedure and treatment not carried out due to patient smoking UPD

Z53.09 Procedure and treatment not carried out because of other contraindication UPD

Z53.1 Procedure and treatment not carried out because of patient's decision for reasons of belief and group pressure UPD

Z53.2 Procedure and treatment not carried out because of patient's decision for other and unspecified reasons

Z53.20 Procedure and treatment not carried out because of patient's decision for unspecified reasons UPD

Z53.21 Procedure and treatment not carried out due to patient leaving prior to being seen by health care provider UPD

Z53.29 Procedure and treatment not carried out because of patient's decision for other reasons UPD

Z53.3 Procedure converted to open procedure
AHA: 2016,4Q,79

Z53.31 Laparoscopic surgical procedure converted to open procedure UPD

Z53.32 Thoracoscopic surgical procedure converted to open procedure UPD

Z53.33 Arthroscopic surgical procedure converted to open procedure UPD

Z53.39 Other specified procedure converted to open procedure UPD

Z53.8 Procedure and treatment not carried out for other reasons UPD

Z53.9 Procedure and treatment not carried out, unspecified reason UPD

Persons with potential health hazards related to socioeconomic and psychosocial circumstances (Z55-Z65)

AHA: 2021,4Q,34-37; 2019,4Q,66; 2018,4Q,58,73; 2018,1Q,18

DEF: Social determinants of health: Socioeconomic factors that can affect a person's health, including both environmental and societal conditions such as education and literacy, employment, health behaviors, housing, lack of adequate food or water, occupational exposure to risk factors, social support, transportation, and violence. Tracking social needs that impact patients allows providers to identify population health trends and to promote the personalized care that addresses the medical and social needs of individual patients. ***Synonym(s):*** *SDOH.*

TIP: Because codes in these categories represent social information rather than medical diagnoses, they can be assigned based on documentation by nonphysician clinicians involved in the care of these patients as well as self-reported documentation from the patient, as long as the information is approved and incorporated into the medical record by a clinician or provider.

Z55 Problems related to education and literacy (4th)

EXCLUDES 1 *disorders of psychological development (F8Ø-F89)*

- **Z55.Ø Illiteracy and low-level literacy** UPD
- **Z55.1 Schooling unavailable and unattainable** UPD
- **Z55.2 Failed school examinations** UPD
- **Z55.3 Underachievement in school** UPD
- **Z55.4 Educational maladjustment and discord with teachers and classmates** UPD
- **Z55.5 Less than a high school diploma** UPD
  - No general equivalence degree (GED)
- **Z55.8 Other problems related to education and literacy** UPD
  - Problems related to inadequate teaching
- **Z55.9 Problems related to education and literacy, unspecified** UPD
  - Academic problems NOS

Z56 Problems related to employment and unemployment (4th)

EXCLUDES 2 *occupational exposure to risk factors (Z57.-)*
problems related to housing and economic circumstances (Z59.-)

- **Z56.Ø Unemployment, unspecified** UPD
- **Z56.1 Change of job** UPD A
- **Z56.2 Threat of job loss** UPD
- **Z56.3 Stressful work schedule** UPD
- **Z56.4 Discord with boss and workmates** UPD
- **Z56.5 Uncongenial work environment** UPD
  - Difficult conditions at work
- **Z56.6 Other physical and mental strain related to work** UPD
- **Z56.8 Other problems related to employment** (5th)
  - **Z56.81 Sexual harassment on the job** UPD
  - **Z56.82 Military deployment status** UPD
    - Individual (civilian or military) currently deployed in theater or in support of military war, peacekeeping and humanitarian operations
  - **Z56.89 Other problems related to employment** UPD
- **Z56.9 Unspecified problems related to employment** UPD
  - Occupational problems NOS

Z57 Occupational exposure to risk factors (4th)

- **Z57.Ø Occupational exposure to noise** UPD
- **Z57.1 Occupational exposure to radiation** UPD
- **Z57.2 Occupational exposure to dust** UPD
- **Z57.3 Occupational exposure to other air contaminants** (5th)
  - **Z57.31 Occupational exposure to environmental tobacco smoke** UPD
    - EXCLUDES 2 *exposure to environmental tobacco smoke (Z77.22)*
  - **Z57.39 Occupational exposure to other air contaminants** UPD
- **Z57.4 Occupational exposure to toxic agents in agriculture** UPD
  - Occupational exposure to solids, liquids, gases or vapors in agriculture
- **Z57.5 Occupational exposure to toxic agents in other industries** UPD
  - Occupational exposure to solids, liquids, gases or vapors in other industries
- **Z57.6 Occupational exposure to extreme temperature** UPD
- **Z57.7 Occupational exposure to vibration** UPD
- **Z57.8 Occupational exposure to other risk factors** UPD
- **Z57.9 Occupational exposure to unspecified risk factor** UPD

Z58 Problems related to physical environment (4th)

EXCLUDES 2 *occupational exposure (Z57.-)*

- **Z58.6 Inadequate drinking-water supply** UPD
  - Lack of safe drinking water
  - EXCLUDES 2 *deprivation of water (T73.1)*

Z59 Problems related to housing and economic circumstances (4th)

EXCLUDES 2 *problems related to upbringing (Z62.-)*

- **Z59.Ø Homelessness** (5th)
  - **Z59.ØØ Homelessness unspecified** UPD
  - **Z59.Ø1 Sheltered homelessness** UPD
    - Doubled up
    - Living in a shelter such as: motel, scattered site housing, temporary or transitional living situation
  - **Z59.Ø2 Unsheltered homelessness** UPD
    - Residing in place not meant for human habitation such as: abandoned buildings, cars, parks, sidewalk
    - Residing on the street
- **Z59.1 Inadequate housing** UPD
  - Lack of heating
  - Restriction of space
  - Technical defects in home preventing adequate care
  - Unsatisfactory surroundings
  - EXCLUDES 1 *problems related to the natural and physical environment (Z77.1-)*
- **Z59.2 Discord with neighbors, lodgers and landlord** UPD
- **Z59.3 Problems related to living in residential institution** UPD
  - Boarding-school resident
  - EXCLUDES 1 *institutional upbringing (Z62.2)*
- **Z59.4 Lack of adequate food** (5th)
  - EXCLUDES 2 *deprivation of food (T73.Ø)*
    effects of hunger (T73.Ø)
    inappropriate diet or eating habits (Z72.4)
    malnutrition (E4Ø-E46)
  - **Z59.41 Food insecurity** UPD
  - **Z59.48 Other specified lack of adequate food** UPD
    - Inadequate food
    - Lack of food
- **Z59.5 Extreme poverty** UPD
- **Z59.6 Low income** UPD
- **Z59.7 Insufficient social insurance and welfare support** UPD
- **Z59.8 Other problems related to housing and economic circumstances** (5th)
  - **Z59.81 Housing instability, housed** (6th)
    - Foreclosure on home loan
    - Past due on rent or mortgage
    - Unwanted multiple moves in the last 12 months
    - **Z59.811 Housing instability, housed, with risk of homelessness** UPD
      - Imminent risk of homelessness
    - **Z59.812 Housing instability, housed, homelessness in past 12 months** UPD
    - **Z59.819 Housing instability, housed unspecified** UPD
  - ● **Z59.82 Transportation insecurity** UPD
    - Excessive transportation time
    - Inaccessible transportation
    - Inadequate transportation
    - Lack of transportation
    - Unaffordable transportation
    - Unreliable transportation
    - Unsafe transportation

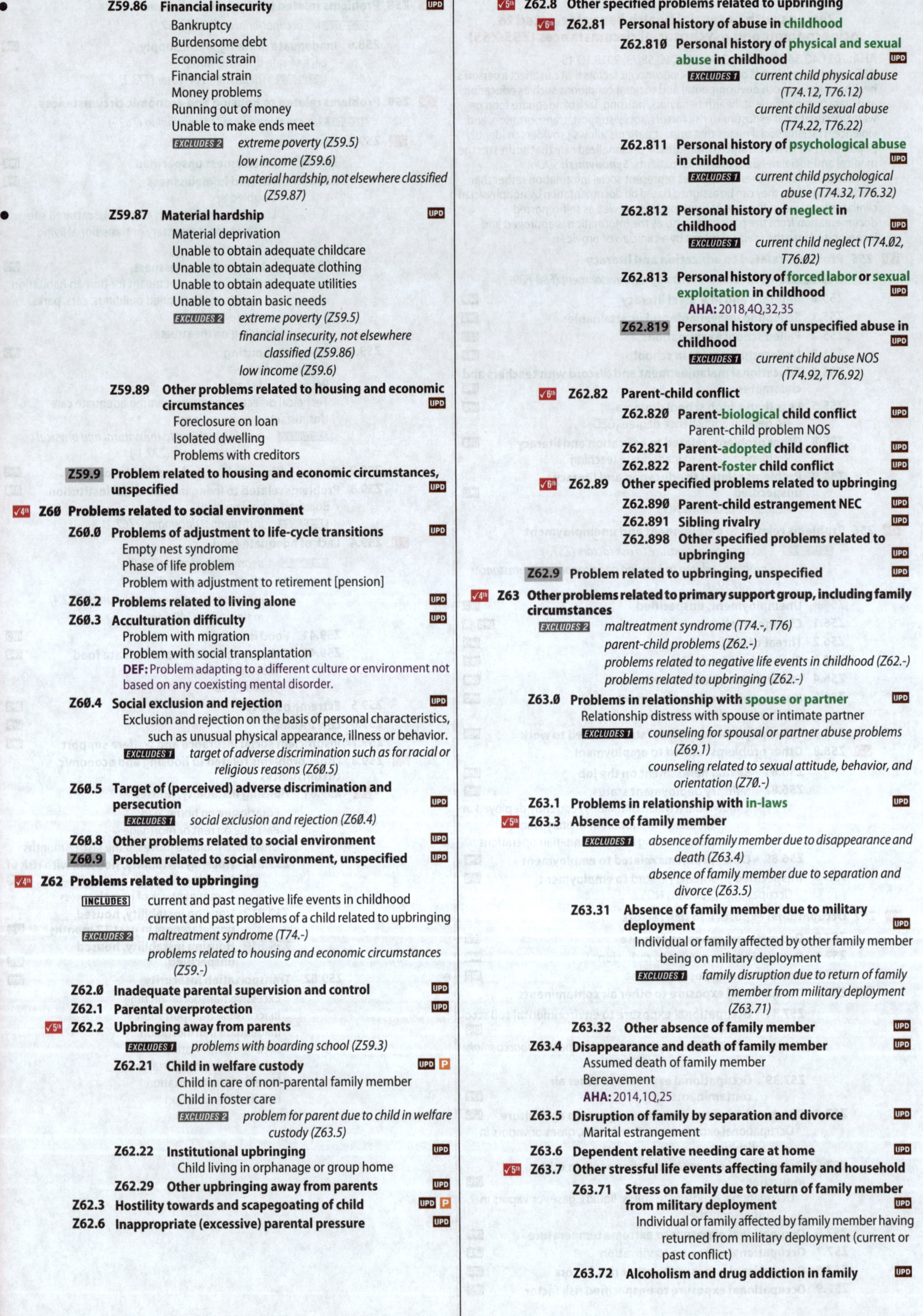

● **Z59.86 Financial insecurity** UPD
Bankruptcy
Burdensome debt
Economic strain
Financial strain
Money problems
Running out of money
Unable to make ends meet
EXCLUDES 2 *extreme poverty (Z59.5)*
low income (Z59.6)
material hardship, not elsewhere classified (Z59.87)

● **Z59.87 Material hardship** UPD
Material deprivation
Unable to obtain adequate childcare
Unable to obtain adequate clothing
Unable to obtain adequate utilities
Unable to obtain basic needs
EXCLUDES 2 *extreme poverty (Z59.5)*
financial insecurity, not elsewhere classified (Z59.86)
low income (Z59.6)

Z59.89 Other problems related to housing and economic circumstances UPD
Foreclosure on loan
Isolated dwelling
Problems with creditors

Z59.9 Problem related to housing and economic circumstances, unspecified UPD

✓4th **Z60 Problems related to social environment**

Z60.0 Problems of adjustment to life-cycle transitions UPD
Empty nest syndrome
Phase of life problem
Problem with adjustment to retirement [pension]

Z60.2 Problems related to living alone UPD

Z60.3 Acculturation difficulty UPD
Problem with migration
Problem with social transplantation
DEF: Problem adapting to a different culture or environment not based on any coexisting mental disorder.

Z60.4 Social exclusion and rejection UPD
Exclusion and rejection on the basis of personal characteristics, such as unusual physical appearance, illness or behavior.
EXCLUDES 1 *target of adverse discrimination such as for racial or religious reasons (Z60.5)*

Z60.5 Target of (perceived) adverse discrimination and persecution UPD
EXCLUDES 1 *social exclusion and rejection (Z60.4)*

Z60.8 Other problems related to social environment UPD

Z60.9 Problem related to social environment, unspecified UPD

✓4th **Z62 Problems related to upbringing**
INCLUDES current and past negative life events in childhood
current and past problems of a child related to upbringing
EXCLUDES 2 *maltreatment syndrome (T74.-)*
problems related to housing and economic circumstances (Z59.-)

Z62.0 Inadequate parental supervision and control UPD

Z62.1 Parental overprotection UPD

✓5th **Z62.2 Upbringing away from parents**
EXCLUDES 1 *problems with boarding school (Z59.3)*

Z62.21 Child in welfare custody UPD P
Child in care of non-parental family member
Child in foster care
EXCLUDES 2 *problem for parent due to child in welfare custody (Z63.5)*

Z62.22 Institutional upbringing UPD
Child living in orphanage or group home

Z62.29 Other upbringing away from parents UPD

Z62.3 Hostility towards and scapegoating of child UPD P

Z62.6 Inappropriate (excessive) parental pressure UPD

✓5th **Z62.8 Other specified problems related to upbringing**

✓6th **Z62.81 Personal history of abuse in childhood**

Z62.810 Personal history of physical and sexual abuse in childhood UPD
EXCLUDES 1 *current child physical abuse (T74.12, T76.12)*
current child sexual abuse (T74.22, T76.22)

Z62.811 Personal history of psychological abuse in childhood UPD
EXCLUDES 1 *current child psychological abuse (T74.32, T76.32)*

Z62.812 Personal history of neglect in childhood UPD
EXCLUDES 1 *current child neglect (T74.02, T76.02)*

Z62.813 Personal history of forced labor or sexual exploitation in childhood UPD
AHA: 2018,4Q,32,35

Z62.819 Personal history of unspecified abuse in childhood UPD
EXCLUDES 1 *current child abuse NOS (T74.92, T76.92)*

✓6th **Z62.82 Parent-child conflict**

Z62.820 Parent-biological child conflict UPD
Parent-child problem NOS

Z62.821 Parent-adopted child conflict UPD

Z62.822 Parent-foster child conflict UPD

✓6th **Z62.89 Other specified problems related to upbringing**

Z62.890 Parent-child estrangement NEC UPD

Z62.891 Sibling rivalry UPD

Z62.898 Other specified problems related to upbringing UPD

Z62.9 Problem related to upbringing, unspecified UPD

✓4th **Z63 Other problems related to primary support group, including family circumstances**
EXCLUDES 2 *maltreatment syndrome (T74.-, T76)*
parent-child problems (Z62.-)
problems related to negative life events in childhood (Z62.-)
problems related to upbringing (Z62.-)

Z63.0 Problems in relationship with spouse or partner UPD
Relationship distress with spouse or intimate partner
EXCLUDES 1 *counseling for spousal or partner abuse problems (Z69.1)*
counseling related to sexual attitude, behavior, and orientation (Z70.-)

Z63.1 Problems in relationship with in-laws UPD

✓5th **Z63.3 Absence of family member**
EXCLUDES 1 *absence of family member due to disappearance and death (Z63.4)*
absence of family member due to separation and divorce (Z63.5)

Z63.31 Absence of family member due to military deployment UPD
Individual or family affected by other family member being on military deployment
EXCLUDES 1 *family disruption due to return of family member from military deployment (Z63.71)*

Z63.32 Other absence of family member UPD

Z63.4 Disappearance and death of family member UPD
Assumed death of family member
Bereavement
AHA: 2014,1Q,25

Z63.5 Disruption of family by separation and divorce UPD
Marital estrangement

Z63.6 Dependent relative needing care at home UPD

✓5th **Z63.7 Other stressful life events affecting family and household**

Z63.71 Stress on family due to return of family member from military deployment UPD
Individual or family affected by family member having returned from military deployment (current or past conflict)

Z63.72 Alcoholism and drug addiction in family UPD

N Newborn: 0 P Pediatric: 0-17 M Maternity: 9-64 A Adult: 15-124 UNS Unspecified Site MCC Major Complication/Comorbidity CC Complication/Comorbidity

Z63.79 **Other stressful life events affecting family and household** UPD
Anxiety (normal) about sick person in family
Health problems within family
Ill or disturbed family member
Isolated family

Z63.8 **Other specified problems related to primary support group** UPD
Family discord NOS
Family estrangement NOS
High expressed emotional level within family
Inadequate family support NOS
Inadequate or distorted communication within family

Z63.9 **Problem related to primary support group, unspecified** UPD
Relationship disorder NOS

✓4th **Z64 Problems related to certain psychosocial circumstances**

Z64.0 **Problems related to unwanted pregnancy** UPD ♀
Z64.1 **Problems related to multiparity** UPD ♀
Z64.4 **Discord with counselors** UPD
Discord with probation officer
Discord with social worker

✓4th **Z65 Problems related to other psychosocial circumstances**

Z65.0 **Conviction in civil and criminal proceedings without imprisonment** UPD
Z65.1 **Imprisonment and other incarceration** UPD
Z65.2 **Problems related to release from prison** UPD
Z65.3 **Problems related to other legal circumstances** UPD
Arrest
Child custody or support proceedings
Litigation
Prosecution
Z65.4 **Victim of crime and terrorism** UPD
Victim of torture
Z65.5 **Exposure to disaster, war and other hostilities** UPD
EXCLUDES 1 *target of perceived discrimination or persecution (Z60.5)*
Z65.8 **Other specified problems related to psychosocial circumstances** UPD
Religious or spiritual problem
Z65.9 **Problem related to unspecified psychosocial circumstances** UPD

Do not resuscitate status (Z66)

Z66 Do not resuscitate UPD
DNR status
DEF: Medical order written by a physician that instructs others not to perform cardiopulmonary resuscitation (CPR), intubation, or advanced cardiac life support (ACLS). It prevents unnecessary invasive treatment to prolong life should breathing stop or cardiac arrest occur.

Blood type (Z67)

✓4th **Z67 Blood type**
AHA: 2015,3Q,40

✓5th Z67.1 **Type A blood**
Z67.10 **Type A blood, Rh positive** UPD
Z67.11 **Type A blood, Rh negative** UPD
✓5th Z67.2 **Type B blood**
Z67.20 **Type B blood, Rh positive** UPD
Z67.21 **Type B blood, Rh negative** UPD
✓5th Z67.3 **Type AB blood**
Z67.30 **Type AB blood, Rh positive** UPD
Z67.31 **Type AB blood, Rh negative** UPD
✓5th Z67.4 **Type O blood**
Z67.40 **Type O blood, Rh positive** UPD
Z67.41 **Type O blood, Rh negative** UPD
✓5th Z67.9 **Unspecified blood type**
Z67.90 **Unspecified blood type, Rh positive** UPD
Z67.91 **Unspecified blood type, Rh negative** UPD

Body mass index [BMI] (Z68)

✓4th **Z68 Body mass index [BMI]**
Kilograms per meters squared
NOTE BMI adult codes are for use for persons 20 years of age or older
BMI pediatric codes are for use for persons 2-19 years of age.
These percentiles are based on the growth charts published by the Centers for Disease Control and Prevention (CDC)
AHA: 2019,4Q,19,57; 2018,4Q,73,77-83; 2017,1Q,39
DEF: Index used to help determine whether an individual is underweight, a healthy weight, overweight, or obese.
TIP: A BMI code may be assigned to support an associated condition based on medical record documentation from clinicians who are not the patient's provider.
TIP: Do not assign when used in association with fluctuations in body fluid during an encounter, such as fluid overload or fluid retention, or during pregnancy.
TIP: In order to assign a BMI code, the associated condition must meet the definition of a reportable diagnosis for nonoutpatient encounters, per section III of the *ICD-10-CM Official Guidelines for Coding and Reporting*.

Z68.1 **Body mass index [BMI] 19.9 or less, adult** CC UPD A
✓5th Z68.2 **Body mass index [BMI] 20-29, adult**
Z68.20 **Body mass index [BMI] 20.0-20.9, adult** UPD A
Z68.21 **Body mass index [BMI] 21.0-21.9, adult** UPD A
Z68.22 **Body mass index [BMI] 22.0-22.9, adult** UPD A
Z68.23 **Body mass index [BMI] 23.0-23.9, adult** UPD A
Z68.24 **Body mass index [BMI] 24.0-24.9, adult** UPD A
Z68.25 **Body mass index [BMI] 25.0-25.9, adult** UPD A
Z68.26 **Body mass index [BMI] 26.0-26.9, adult** UPD A
Z68.27 **Body mass index [BMI] 27.0-27.9, adult** UPD A
Z68.28 **Body mass index [BMI] 28.0-28.9, adult** UPD A
Z68.29 **Body mass index [BMI] 29.0-29.9, adult** UPD A
✓5th Z68.3 **Body mass index [BMI] 30-39, adult**
Z68.30 **Body mass index [BMI] 30.0-30.9, adult** UPD A
Z68.31 **Body mass index [BMI] 31.0-31.9, adult** UPD A
Z68.32 **Body mass index [BMI] 32.0-32.9, adult** UPD A
Z68.33 **Body mass index [BMI] 33.0-33.9, adult** UPD A
Z68.34 **Body mass index [BMI] 34.0-34.9, adult** UPD A
Z68.35 **Body mass index [BMI] 35.0-35.9, adult** UPD A
Z68.36 **Body mass index [BMI] 36.0-36.9, adult** UPD A
Z68.37 **Body mass index [BMI] 37.0-37.9, adult** UPD A
Z68.38 **Body mass index [BMI] 38.0-38.9, adult** UPD A
Z68.39 **Body mass index [BMI] 39.0-39.9, adult** UPD A
✓5th Z68.4 **Body mass index [BMI] 40 or greater, adult**
Z68.41 **Body mass index [BMI] 40.0-44.9, adult** CC UPD HCC A
Z68.42 **Body mass index [BMI] 45.0-49.9, adult** CC UPD HCC A
Z68.43 **Body mass index [BMI] 50.0-59.9, adult** CC UPD HCC A
Z68.44 **Body mass index [BMI] 60.0-69.9, adult** CC UPD HCC A
Z68.45 **Body mass index [BMI] 70 or greater, adult** CC UPD HCC A
✓5th Z68.5 **Body mass index [BMI] pediatric**
AHA: 2018,4Q,81-82
Z68.51 **Body mass index [BMI] pediatric, less than 5th percentile for age** UPD
Z68.52 **Body mass index [BMI] pediatric, 5th percentile to less than 85th percentile for age** UPD
Z68.53 **Body mass index [BMI] pediatric, 85th percentile to less than 95th percentile for age** UPD
Z68.54 **Body mass index [BMI] pediatric, greater than or equal to 95th percentile for age** UPD

Persons encountering health services in other circumstances (Z69-Z76)

Z69 Encounter for mental health services for victim and perpetrator of abuse
INCLUDES counseling for victims and perpetrators of abuse

Z69.0 Encounter for mental health services for child abuse problems

Z69.01 Encounter for mental health services for parental child abuse

Z69.010 Encounter for mental health services for victim of parental child abuse P
Encounter for mental health services for victim of child abuse by parent
Encounter for mental health services for victim of child neglect by parent
Encounter for mental health services for victim of child psychological abuse by parent
Encounter for mental health services for victim of child sexual abuse by parent

Z69.011 Encounter for mental health services for perpetrator of parental child abuse UPD
Encounter for mental health services for perpetrator of parental child neglect
Encounter for mental health services for perpetrator of parental child psychological abuse
Encounter for mental health services for perpetrator of parental child sexual abuse
EXCLUDES 1 *encounter for mental health services for non-parental child abuse (Z69.02-)*

Z69.02 Encounter for mental health services for non-parental child abuse

Z69.020 Encounter for mental health services for victim of non-parental child abuse P
Encounter for mental health services for victim of non-parental child neglect
Encounter for mental health services for victim of non-parental child psychological abuse
Encounter for mental health services for victim of non-parental child sexual abuse

Z69.021 Encounter for mental health services for perpetrator of non-parental child abuse UPD
Encounter for mental health services for perpetrator of non-parental child neglect
Encounter for mental health services for perpetrator of non-parental child psychological abuse
Encounter for mental health services for perpetrator of non-parental child sexual abuse

Z69.1 Encounter for mental health services for spousal or partner abuse problems

Z69.11 Encounter for mental health services for victim of spousal or partner abuse UPD
Encounter for mental health services for victim of spouse or partner neglect
Encounter for mental health services for victim of spouse or partner psychological abuse
Encounter for mental health services for victim of spouse or partner violence, physical

Z69.12 Encounter for mental health services for perpetrator of spousal or partner abuse UPD
Encounter for mental health services for perpetrator of spouse or partner neglect
Encounter for mental health services for perpetrator of spouse or partner psychological abuse
Encounter for mental health services for perpetrator of spouse or partner violence, physical
Encounter for mental health services for perpetrator of spouse or partner violence, sexual

Z69.8 Encounter for mental health services for victim or perpetrator of other abuse

Z69.81 Encounter for mental health services for victim of other abuse UPD
Encounter for mental health services for victim of non-spousal adult abuse
Encounter for mental health services for victim of spouse or partner violence, sexual
Encounter for rape victim counseling

Z69.82 Encounter for mental health services for perpetrator of other abuse UPD
Encounter for mental health services for perpetrator of non-spousal adult abuse

Z70 Counseling related to sexual attitude, behavior and orientation
INCLUDES encounter for mental health services for sexual attitude, behavior and orientation
EXCLUDES 2 *contraceptive or procreative counseling (Z30-Z31)*

Z70.0 Counseling related to sexual attitude UPD

Z70.1 Counseling related to patient's sexual behavior and orientation UPD
Patient concerned regarding impotence
Patient concerned regarding non-responsiveness
Patient concerned regarding promiscuity
Patient concerned regarding sexual orientation

Z70.2 Counseling related to sexual behavior and orientation of third party UPD
Advice sought regarding sexual behavior and orientation of child
Advice sought regarding sexual behavior and orientation of partner
Advice sought regarding sexual behavior and orientation of spouse

Z70.3 Counseling related to combined concerns regarding sexual attitude, behavior and orientation UPD

Z70.8 Other sex counseling UPD
Encounter for sex education

Z70.9 Sex counseling, unspecified UPD

Z71 Persons encountering health services for other counseling and medical advice, not elsewhere classified
EXCLUDES 2 *contraceptive or procreation counseling (Z30-Z31)*
sex counseling (Z70.-)

Z71.0 Person encountering health services to consult on behalf of another person UPD
Person encountering health services to seek advice or treatment for non-attending third party
EXCLUDES 2 *anxiety (normal) about sick person in family (Z63.7)*
expectant (adoptive) parent(s) pre-birth pediatrician visit (Z76.81)

Z71.1 Person with feared health complaint in whom no diagnosis is made UPD
Person encountering health services with feared condition which was not demonstrated
Person encountering health services in which problem was normal state
"Worried well"
EXCLUDES 1 *medical observation for suspected diseases and conditions proven not to exist (Z03.-)*

Z71.2 Person consulting for explanation of examination or test findings UPD

Z71.3 Dietary counseling and surveillance UPD
Use additional code for any associated underlying medical condition
Use additional code to identify body mass index (BMI), if known (Z68.-)

Z71.4 Alcohol abuse counseling and surveillance
Use additional code for alcohol abuse or dependence (F10.-)

Z71.41 Alcohol abuse counseling and surveillance of alcoholic UPD

Z71.42 Counseling for family member of alcoholic UPD
Counseling for significant other, partner, or friend of alcoholic

Z71.5 Drug abuse counseling and surveillance
Use additional code for drug abuse or dependence (F11-F16, F18-F19)

Z71.51 Drug abuse counseling and surveillance of drug abuser UPD

Z71.52 Counseling for family member of drug abuser UPD
Counseling for significant other, partner, or friend of drug abuser

Z71.6 Tobacco abuse counseling UPD
Use additional code for nicotine dependence (F17.-)

Z71.7 Human immunodeficiency virus [HIV] counseling UPD

Z71.8 Other specified counseling
EXCLUDES 2 *counseling for contraception (Z30.0-)*
AHA: 2017,4Q,27

Z71.81 Spiritual or religious counseling UPD

Z71.82 Exercise counseling UPD

Z71.83 Encounter for nonprocreative genetic counseling
EXCLUDES 1 *counseling for procreative genetics (Z31.5)*
counseling for procreative management (Z31.6)

Z71.84 Encounter for health counseling related to travel UPD
Encounter for health risk and safety counseling for (international) travel
Code also, if applicable, encounter for immunization (Z23)
EXCLUDES 2 *encounter for administrative examination (Z02.-)*
encounter for other special examination without complaint, suspected or reported diagnosis (Z01.-)
AHA: 2019,4Q,20,57

Z71.85 Encounter for immunization safety counseling UPD
Encounter for vaccine product safety counseling
Code also, if applicable, encounter for immunization (Z23)
Code also, if applicable, immunization not carried out (Z28.-)
EXCLUDES 1 *encounter for health counseling related to travel (Z71.84)*
AHA: 2021,4Q,34

● **Z71.87 Encounter for pediatric-to-adult transition counseling** UPD
Code also chronic condition, if applicable, such as:
autism spectrum disorder (F84.0)
congenital malformations of the circulatory system (Q20-Q28)
cystic fibrosis (E84-)
sickle-cell disorder (D57-)

● **Z71.88 Encounter for counseling for socioeconomic factors** UPD

Z71.89 Other specified counseling UPD

Z71.9 Counseling, unspecified UPD
Encounter for medical advice NOS

Z72 Problems related to lifestyle
EXCLUDES 2 *problems related to life-management difficulty (Z73.-)*
problems related to socioeconomic and psychosocial circumstances (Z55-Z65)

Z72.0 Tobacco use UPD
Tobacco use NOS
EXCLUDES 1 *history of tobacco dependence (Z87.891)*
nicotine dependence (F17.2-)
tobacco dependence (F17.2-)
tobacco use during pregnancy (O99.33-)

Z72.3 Lack of physical exercise UPD

Z72.4 Inappropriate diet and eating habits UPD
EXCLUDES 1 *behavioral eating disorders of infancy or childhood (F98.2-F98.3)*
eating disorders (F50.-)
lack of adequate food (Z59.48)
malnutrition and other nutritional deficiencies (E40-E64)

Z72.5 High risk sexual behavior
Promiscuity
EXCLUDES 1 *paraphilias (F65)*

Z72.51 High risk heterosexual behavior UPD

Z72.52 High risk homosexual behavior UPD

Z72.53 High risk bisexual behavior UPD

Z72.6 Gambling and betting UPD
EXCLUDES 1 *compulsive or pathological gambling (F63.0)*

Z72.8 Other problems related to lifestyle

Z72.81 Antisocial behavior
EXCLUDES 1 *conduct disorders (F91.-)*

Z72.810 Child and adolescent antisocial behavior P
Antisocial behavior (child) (adolescent) without manifest psychiatric disorder
Delinquency NOS
Group delinquency
Offenses in the context of gang membership
Stealing in company with others
Truancy from school

Z72.811 Adult antisocial behavior A
Adult antisocial behavior without manifest psychiatric disorder

Z72.82 Problems related to sleep

Z72.820 Sleep deprivation
Lack of adequate sleep
EXCLUDES 1 *insomnia (G47.0-)*

Z72.821 Inadequate sleep hygiene UPD
Bad sleep habits
Irregular sleep habits
Unhealthy sleep wake schedule
EXCLUDES 1 *insomnia (F51.0-, G47.0-)*

● **Z72.823 Risk of suffocation (smothering) under another while sleeping** UPD
Child-caregiver co-sleeping
Infant bed-sharing

Z72.89 Other problems related to lifestyle UPD
Self-damaging behavior

Z72.9 Problem related to lifestyle, unspecified UPD

Z73 Problems related to life management difficulty
EXCLUDES 2 *problems related to socioeconomic and psychosocial circumstances (Z55-Z65)*
DEF: State of emotional, and physical exhaustion causing difficulties in managing personal, school, or work circumstances. It is usually due to prolonged stress or poor interpersonal relationship skills or parenting skills.

Z73.0 Burn-out UPD

Z73.1 Type A behavior pattern UPD

Z73.2 Lack of relaxation and leisure UPD

Z73.3 Stress, not elsewhere classified UPD
Physical and mental strain NOS
EXCLUDES 1 *stress related to employment or unemployment (Z56.-)*

Z73.4 Inadequate social skills, not elsewhere classified UPD

Z73.5 Social role conflict, not elsewhere classified UPD

Z73.6 Limitation of activities due to disability UPD
EXCLUDES 1 *care-provider dependency (Z74.-)*

Z73.8 Other problems related to life management difficulty

Z73.81 Behavioral insomnia of childhood
DEF: Behaviors on the part of the child or caregivers that cause negative compliance with a child's sleep schedule resulting in lack of adequate sleep.

Z73.810 Behavioral insomnia of childhood, sleep-onset association type UPD P

Z73.811 Behavioral insomnia of childhood, limit setting type UPD P

Z73.812 Behavioral insomnia of childhood, combined type UPD P

Z73.819 Behavioral insomnia of childhood, unspecified type UPD P

Z73.82 Dual sensory impairment UPD

Z73.89 Other problems related to life management difficulty UPD

Z73.9 Problem related to life management difficulty, unspecified UPD

Z74 Problems related to care provider dependency

EXCLUDES 2 *dependence on enabling machines or devices NEC (Z99.-)*

Z74.Ø Reduced mobility

Z74.Ø1 Bed confinement status UPD

Bedridden

Z74.Ø9 Other reduced mobility UPD

Chair ridden

Reduced mobility NOS

EXCLUDES 2 *wheelchair dependence (Z99.3)*

Z74.1 Need for assistance with personal care UPD

Z74.2 Need for assistance at home and no other household member able to render care UPD

Z74.3 Need for continuous supervision UPD

Z74.8 Other problems related to care provider dependency UPD

Z74.9 Problem related to care provider dependency, unspecified UPD

Z75 Problems related to medical facilities and other health care

Z75.Ø Medical services not available in home UPD

EXCLUDES 1 *no other household member able to render care (Z74.2)*

Z75.1 Person awaiting admission to adequate facility elsewhere UPD

Z75.2 Other waiting period for investigation and treatment UPD

Z75.3 Unavailability and inaccessibility of health-care facilities UPD

EXCLUDES 1 *bed unavailable (Z75.1)*

Z75.4 Unavailability and inaccessibility of other helping agencies UPD

Z75.5 Holiday relief care UPD

Z75.8 Other problems related to medical facilities and other health care UPD

Z75.9 Unspecified problem related to medical facilities and other health care UPD

Z76 Persons encountering health services in other circumstances

Z76.Ø Encounter for issue of repeat prescription UPD

Encounter for issue of repeat prescription for appliance

Encounter for issue of repeat prescription for medicaments

Encounter for issue of repeat prescription for spectacles

EXCLUDES 2 *issue of medical certificate (ZØ2.7)*

repeat prescription for contraceptive (Z3Ø.4-)

Z76.1 Encounter for health supervision and care of foundling

Z76.2 Encounter for health supervision and care of other healthy infant and child UPD P

Encounter for medical or nursing care or supervision of healthy infant under circumstances such as adverse socioeconomic conditions at home

Encounter for medical or nursing care or supervision of healthy infant under circumstances such as awaiting foster or adoptive placement

Encounter for medical or nursing care or supervision of healthy infant under circumstances such as maternal illness

Encounter for medical or nursing care or supervision of healthy infant under circumstances such as number of children at home preventing or interfering with normal care

Z76.3 Healthy person accompanying sick person

Z76.4 Other boarder to healthcare facility

EXCLUDES 1 *homelessness (Z59.Ø-)*

Z76.5 Malingerer [conscious simulation]

Person feigning illness (with obvious motivation)

EXCLUDES 1 *factitious disorder (F68.1-, F68.A)*

peregrinating patient (F68.1-)

DEF: Act of intentionally exaggerating an illness or disability in order to receive personal gain or to avoid punishment or responsibility.

Z76.8 Persons encountering health services in other specified circumstances

Z76.81 Expectant parent(s) prebirth pediatrician visit UPD

Pre-adoption pediatrician visit for adoptive parent(s)

Z76.82 Awaiting organ transplant status UPD

Patient waiting for organ availability

Z76.89 Persons encountering health services in other specified circumstances UPD

Persons encountering health services NOS

AHA: 2014,2Q,10

Persons with potential health hazards related to family and personal history and certain conditions influencing health status (Z77-Z99)

Code also any follow-up examination (ZØ8-ZØ9)

Z77 Other contact with and (suspected) exposures hazardous to health

INCLUDES contact with and (suspected) exposures to potential hazards to health

EXCLUDES 2 *contact with and (suspected) exposure to communicable diseases (Z2Ø.-)*

exposure to (parental) (environmental) tobacco smoke in the perinatal period (P96.81)

newborn affected by noxious substances transmitted via placenta or breast milk (PØ4.-)

occupational exposure to risk factors (Z57.-)

retained foreign body (Z18.-)

retained foreign body fully removed (Z87.821)

toxic effects of substances chiefly nonmedicinal as to source (T51-T65)

Z77.Ø Contact with and (suspected) exposure to hazardous, chiefly nonmedicinal, chemicals

Z77.Ø1 Contact with and (suspected) exposure to hazardous metals

Z77.Ø1Ø Contact with and (suspected) exposure to arsenic UPD

Z77.Ø11 Contact with and (suspected) exposure to lead UPD

Z77.Ø12 Contact with and (suspected) exposure to uranium UPD

EXCLUDES 1 *retained depleted uranium fragments (Z18.Ø1)*

Z77.Ø18 Contact with and (suspected) exposure to other hazardous metals UPD

Contact with and (suspected) exposure to chromium compounds

Contact with and (suspected) exposure to nickel dust

Z77.Ø2 Contact with and (suspected) exposure to hazardous aromatic compounds

Z77.Ø2Ø Contact with and (suspected) exposure to aromatic amines UPD

Z77.Ø21 Contact with and (suspected) exposure to benzene UPD

Z77.Ø28 Contact with and (suspected) exposure to other hazardous aromatic compounds UPD

Aromatic dyes NOS

Polycyclic aromatic hydrocarbons

Z77.Ø9 Contact with and (suspected) exposure to other hazardous, chiefly nonmedicinal, chemicals

Z77.Ø9Ø Contact with and (suspected) exposure to asbestos UPD

Z77.Ø98 Contact with and (suspected) exposure to other hazardous, chiefly nonmedicinal, chemicals UPD

Dyes NOS

Z77.1 Contact with and (suspected) exposure to environmental pollution and hazards in the physical environment

Z77.11 Contact with and (suspected) exposure to environmental pollution

Z77.11Ø Contact with and (suspected) exposure to air pollution UPD

Z77.111 Contact with and (suspected) exposure to water pollution UPD

Z77.112 Contact with and (suspected) exposure to soil pollution UPD

Z77.118 Contact with and (suspected) exposure to other environmental pollution UPD

Z77.12 Contact with and (suspected) exposure to hazards in the physical environment

Z77.120 Contact with and (suspected) exposure to mold (toxic) UPD

Z77.121 Contact with and (suspected) exposure to harmful algae and algae toxins UPD

Contact with and (suspected) exposure to (harmful) algae bloom NOS

Contact with and (suspected) exposure to blue-green algae bloom

Contact with and (suspected) exposure to brown tide

Contact with and (suspected) exposure to cyanobacteria bloom

Contact with and (suspected) exposure to Florida red tide

Contact with and (suspected) exposure to pfiesteria piscicida

Contact with and (suspected) exposure to red tide

Z77.122 Contact with and (suspected) exposure to noise UPD

Z77.123 Contact with and (suspected) exposure to radon and other naturally occurring radiation UPD

EXCLUDES 2 *radiation exposure as the cause of a confirmed condition (W88-W90, X39.0-)*

radiation sickness NOS (T66)

Z77.128 Contact with and (suspected) exposure to other hazards in the physical environment UPD

Z77.2 Contact with and (suspected) exposure to other hazardous substances

Z77.21 Contact with and (suspected) exposure to potentially hazardous body fluids UPD

Z77.22 Contact with and (suspected) exposure to environmental tobacco smoke (acute) (chronic) UPD

Exposure to second hand tobacco smoke (acute) (chronic)

Passive smoking (acute) (chronic)

EXCLUDES 1 *nicotine dependence (F17.-)*

tobacco use (Z72.0)

EXCLUDES 2 *occupational exposure to environmental tobacco smoke (Z57.31)*

Z77.29 Contact with and (suspected) exposure to other hazardous substances UPD

AHA: 2016,2Q,33

Z77.9 Other contact with and (suspected) exposures hazardous to health UPD

Z78 Other specified health status

EXCLUDES 2 *asymptomatic human immunodeficiency virus [HIV] infection status (Z21)*

postprocedural status (Z93-Z99)

sex reassignment status (Z87.890)

Z78.0 Asymptomatic menopausal state UPD A ♀

Menopausal state NOS

Postmenopausal status NOS

EXCLUDES 2 *symptomatic menopausal state (N95.1)*

Z78.1 Physical restraint status UPD

EXCLUDES 1 *physical restraint due to a procedure - omit code*

DEF: Application of mechanical restraining devices or manual restraints to limit physical mobility of a patient.

Z78.9 Other specified health status UPD

Z79 Long term (current) drug therapy

INCLUDES long term (current) drug use for prophylactic purposes

Code also any therapeutic drug level monitoring (Z51.81)

EXCLUDES 2 *drug abuse and dependence (F11-F19)*

drug use complicating pregnancy, childbirth, and the puerperium (O99.32-)

AHA: 2021,1Q,12

Z79.0 Long term (current) use of anticoagulants and antithrombotics/antiplatelets

EXCLUDES 2 *long term (current) use of aspirin (Z79.82)*

Z79.01 Long term (current) use of anticoagulants

AHA: 2022,2Q,17; 2021,1Q,4; 2020,2Q,20

Z79.02 Long term (current) use of antithrombotics/antiplatelets UPD

Z79.1 Long term (current) use of non-steroidal anti-inflammatories (NSAID) UPD

EXCLUDES 2 *long term (current) use of aspirin (Z79.82)*

Z79.2 Long term (current) use of antibiotics UPD

Z79.3 Long term (current) use of hormonal contraceptives

Long term (current) use of birth control pill or patch

Z79.4 Long term (current) use of insulin HCC

EXCLUDES 2 ▶*long-term (current) use of injectable non-insulin antidiabetic drugs (Z79.85)*◀

long term (current) use of oral antidiabetic drugs (Z79.84)

long term (current) use of oral hypoglycemic drugs (Z79.84)

AHA: 2020,3Q,31

Z79.5 Long term (current) use of steroids

Z79.51 Long term (current) use of inhaled steroids UPD

Z79.52 Long term (current) use of systemic steroids UPD

● **Z79.6 Long term (current) use of immunomodulators and immunosuppressants**

EXCLUDES 2 *long term (current) use of steroids (Z79.5-)*

long term (current) use of agents affecting estrogen receptors and estrogen levels (Z79.81-)

● **Z79.60 Long term (current) use of unspecified immunomodulators and immunosuppressants** UPD

● **Z79.61 Long term (current) use of immunomodulator** UPD

Long term (current) use of apremilast

Long term (current) use of immunomodulatory imide drug

Long term (current) use of lenalidomide

Long term (current) use of pomalidomide

● **Z79.62 Long term (current) use of immunosuppressant**

● **Z79.620 Long term (current) use of immunosuppressive biologic** UPD

Long term (current) use of adalimumab

Long term (current) use of etanercept

Long term (current) use of infliximab

Long term (current) use of monoclonal antibodies

● **Z79.621 Long term (current) use of calcineurin inhibitor** UPD

Long term (current) use of cyclosporine

Long term (current) use of tacrolimus

● **Z79.622 Long term (current) use of Janus kinase inhibitor** UPD

Long term (current) use of tofacitinib

● **Z79.623 Long term (current) use of mammalian target of rapamycin (mTOR) inhibitor** UPD

Long term (current) use of sirolimus

● **Z79.624 Long term (current) use of inhibitors of nucleotide synthesis** UPD

Long term (current) use of azathioprine

Long term (current) use omycophenolate

Long term (current) use of purine synthesis (IMDH) inhibitors

● **Z79.63 Long term (current) use of chemotherapeutic agent**

● **Z79.630 Long term (current) use of alkylating agent** UPD

Long term (current) use of chlorambucil

Long term (current) use of cisplatin

Long term (current) use of cyclophosphamide

● **Z79.631 Long term (current) use of antimetabolite agent** UPD

Long term (current) use of 5-fluorouracil

Long term (current) use of 6-mercaptopurine

Long term (current) use of cytarabine

Long term (current) use of methotrexate

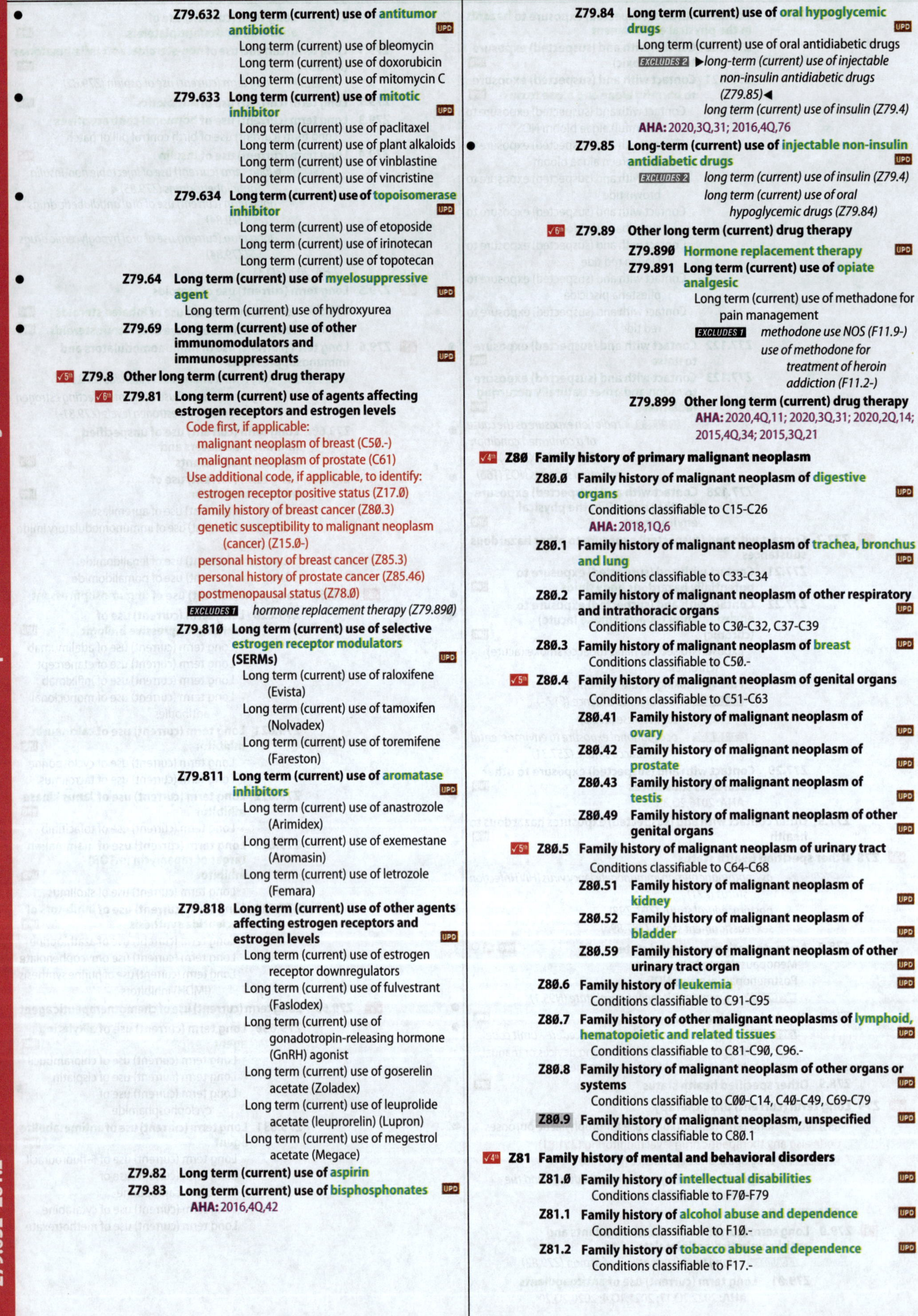

● **Z79.632 Long term (current) use of antitumor antibiotic** UPD
Long term (current) use of bleomycin
Long term (current) use of doxorubicin
Long term (current) use of mitomycin C

● **Z79.633 Long term (current) use of mitotic inhibitor** UPD
Long term (current) use of paclitaxel
Long term (current) use of plant alkaloids
Long term (current) use of vinblastine
Long term (current) use of vincristine

● **Z79.634 Long term (current) use of topoisomerase inhibitor** UPD
Long term (current) use of etoposide
Long term (current) use of irinotecan
Long term (current) use of topotecan

● **Z79.64 Long term (current) use of myelosuppressive agent** UPD
Long term (current) use of hydroxyurea

● **Z79.69 Long term (current) use of other immunomodulators and immunosuppressants** UPD

5th **Z79.8 Other long term (current) drug therapy**

6th **Z79.81 Long term (current) use of agents affecting estrogen receptors and estrogen levels**
Code first, if applicable:
malignant neoplasm of breast (C5Ø.-)
malignant neoplasm of prostate (C61)
Use additional code, if applicable, to identify:
estrogen receptor positive status (Z17.Ø)
family history of breast cancer (Z8Ø.3)
genetic susceptibility to malignant neoplasm (cancer) (Z15.Ø-)
personal history of breast cancer (Z85.3)
personal history of prostate cancer (Z85.46)
postmenopausal status (Z78.Ø)
EXCLUDES 1 *hormone replacement therapy (Z79.89Ø)*

Z79.81Ø Long term (current) use of selective estrogen receptor modulators (SERMs) UPD
Long term (current) use of raloxifene (Evista)
Long term (current) use of tamoxifen (Nolvadex)
Long term (current) use of toremifene (Fareston)

Z79.811 Long term (current) use of aromatase inhibitors UPD
Long term (current) use of anastrozole (Arimidex)
Long term (current) use of exemestane (Aromasin)
Long term (current) use of letrozole (Femara)

Z79.818 Long term (current) use of other agents affecting estrogen receptors and estrogen levels UPD
Long term (current) use of estrogen receptor downregulators
Long term (current) use of fulvestrant (Faslodex)
Long term (current) use of gonadotropin-releasing hormone (GnRH) agonist
Long term (current) use of goserelin acetate (Zoladex)
Long term (current) use of leuprolide acetate (leuprorelin) (Lupron)
Long term (current) use of megestrol acetate (Megace)

Z79.82 Long term (current) use of aspirin

Z79.83 Long term (current) use of bisphosphonates UPD
AHA: 2016,4Q,42

Z79.84 Long term (current) use of oral hypoglycemic drugs UPD
Long term (current) use of oral antidiabetic drugs
EXCLUDES 2 ▶*long-term (current) use of injectable non-insulin antidiabetic drugs (Z79.85)*◀
long term (current) use of insulin (Z79.4)
AHA: 2020,3Q,31; 2016,4Q,76

● **Z79.85 Long-term (current) use of injectable non-insulin antidiabetic drugs** UPD
EXCLUDES 2 *long term (current) use of insulin (Z79.4)*
long term (current) use of oral hypoglycemic drugs (Z79.84)

6th **Z79.89 Other long term (current) drug therapy**

Z79.89Ø Hormone replacement therapy UPD

Z79.891 Long term (current) use of opiate analgesic
Long term (current) use of methadone for pain management
EXCLUDES 1 *methadone use NOS (F11.9-)*
use of methadone for treatment of heroin addiction (F11.2-)

Z79.899 Other long term (current) drug therapy
AHA: 2020,4Q,11; 2020,3Q,31; 2020,2Q,14; 2015,4Q,34; 2015,3Q,21

4th **Z8Ø Family history of primary malignant neoplasm**

Z8Ø.Ø Family history of malignant neoplasm of digestive organs UPD
Conditions classifiable to C15-C26
AHA: 2018,1Q,6

Z8Ø.1 Family history of malignant neoplasm of trachea, bronchus and lung UPD
Conditions classifiable to C33-C34

Z8Ø.2 Family history of malignant neoplasm of other respiratory and intrathoracic organs UPD
Conditions classifiable to C3Ø-C32, C37-C39

Z8Ø.3 Family history of malignant neoplasm of breast UPD
Conditions classifiable to C5Ø.-

5th **Z8Ø.4 Family history of malignant neoplasm of genital organs**
Conditions classifiable to C51-C63

Z8Ø.41 Family history of malignant neoplasm of ovary UPD

Z8Ø.42 Family history of malignant neoplasm of prostate UPD

Z8Ø.43 Family history of malignant neoplasm of testis UPD

Z8Ø.49 Family history of malignant neoplasm of other genital organs UPD

5th **Z8Ø.5 Family history of malignant neoplasm of urinary tract**
Conditions classifiable to C64-C68

Z8Ø.51 Family history of malignant neoplasm of kidney UPD

Z8Ø.52 Family history of malignant neoplasm of bladder UPD

Z8Ø.59 Family history of malignant neoplasm of other urinary tract organ UPD

Z8Ø.6 Family history of leukemia UPD
Conditions classifiable to C91-C95

Z8Ø.7 Family history of other malignant neoplasms of lymphoid, hematopoietic and related tissues UPD
Conditions classifiable to C81-C9Ø, C96.-

Z8Ø.8 Family history of malignant neoplasm of other organs or systems UPD
Conditions classifiable to CØØ-C14, C4Ø-C49, C69-C79

Z8Ø.9 Family history of malignant neoplasm, unspecified UPD
Conditions classifiable to C8Ø.1

4th **Z81 Family history of mental and behavioral disorders**

Z81.Ø Family history of intellectual disabilities UPD
Conditions classifiable to F7Ø-F79

Z81.1 Family history of alcohol abuse and dependence UPD
Conditions classifiable to F1Ø.-

Z81.2 Family history of tobacco abuse and dependence UPD
Conditions classifiable to F17.-

Z81.3 Family history of other psychoactive substance abuse and dependence UPD
Conditions classifiable to F11-F16, F18-F19

Z81.4 Family history of other substance abuse and dependence UPD
Conditions classifiable to F55

Z81.8 Family history of other mental and behavioral disorders UPD
Conditions classifiable elsewhere in F01-F99

Z82 Family history of certain disabilities and chronic diseases (leading to disablement)

Z82.0 Family history of epilepsy and other diseases of the nervous system UPD
Conditions classifiable to G00-G99

Z82.1 Family history of blindness and visual loss UPD
Conditions classifiable to H54.-

Z82.2 Family history of deafness and hearing loss UPD
Conditions classifiable to H90-H91

Z82.3 Family history of stroke UPD
Conditions classifiable to I60-I64

Z82.4 Family history of ischemic heart disease and other diseases of the circulatory system
Conditions classifiable to I00-I5A, I65-I99

Z82.41 Family history of sudden cardiac death UPD

Z82.49 Family history of ischemic heart disease and other diseases of the circulatory system UPD

Z82.5 Family history of asthma and other chronic lower respiratory diseases UPD
Conditions classifiable to J40-J47
EXCLUDES 2 *family history of other diseases of the respiratory system (Z83.6)*

Z82.6 Family history of arthritis and other diseases of the musculoskeletal system and connective tissue
Conditions classifiable to M00-M99

Z82.61 Family history of arthritis UPD

Z82.62 Family history of osteoporosis UPD

Z82.69 Family history of other diseases of the musculoskeletal system and connective tissue UPD

Z82.7 Family history of congenital malformations, deformations and chromosomal abnormalities
Conditions classifiable to Q00-Q99

Z82.71 Family history of polycystic kidney UPD

Z82.79 Family history of other congenital malformations, deformations and chromosomal abnormalities UPD

Z82.8 Family history of other disabilities and chronic diseases leading to disablement, not elsewhere classified UPD

Z83 Family history of other specific disorders
EXCLUDES 2 *contact with and (suspected) exposure to communicable disease in the family (Z20.-)*

Z83.0 Family history of human immunodeficiency virus [HIV] disease UPD
Conditions classifiable to B20

Z83.1 Family history of other infectious and parasitic diseases UPD
Conditions classifiable to A00-B19, B25-B94, B99

Z83.2 Family history of diseases of the blood and blood-forming organs and certain disorders involving the immune mechanism UPD
Conditions classifiable to D50-D89

Z83.3 Family history of diabetes mellitus UPD
Conditions classifiable to E08-E13

Z83.4 Family history of other endocrine, nutritional and metabolic diseases
Conditions classifiable to E00-E07, E15-E88

Z83.41 Family history of multiple endocrine neoplasia [MEN] syndrome UPD

Z83.42 Family history of familial hypercholesterolemia UPD
AHA: 2016,4Q,77

Z83.43 Family history of other disorder of lipoprotein metabolism and other lipidemias
AHA: 2018,4Q,6,35

Z83.430 Family history of elevated lipoprotein(a) UPD
Family history of elevated Lp(a)

Z83.438 Family history of other disorder of lipoprotein metabolism and other lipidemia UPD
Family history of familial combined hyperlipidemia

Z83.49 Family history of other endocrine, nutritional and metabolic diseases UPD

Z83.5 Family history of eye and ear disorders

Z83.51 Family history of eye disorders
Conditions classifiable to H00-H53, H55-H59
EXCLUDES 2 *family history of blindness and visual loss (Z82.1)*

Z83.511 Family history of glaucoma UPD

Z83.518 Family history of other specified eye disorder UPD

Z83.52 Family history of ear disorders UPD
Conditions classifiable to H60-H83, H92-H95
EXCLUDES 2 *family history of deafness and hearing loss (Z82.2)*

Z83.6 Family history of other diseases of the respiratory system UPD
Conditions classifiable to J00-J39, J60-J99
EXCLUDES 2 *family history of asthma and other chronic lower respiratory diseases (Z82.5)*

Z83.7 Family history of diseases of the digestive system
Conditions classifiable to K00-K93

Z83.71 Family history of colonic polyps UPD
EXCLUDES 2 *family history of malignant neoplasm of digestive organs (Z80.0)*
AHA: 2021,1Q,14

Z83.79 Family history of other diseases of the digestive system UPD

Z84 Family history of other conditions

Z84.0 Family history of diseases of the skin and subcutaneous tissue UPD
Conditions classifiable to L00-L99

Z84.1 Family history of disorders of kidney and ureter UPD
Conditions classifiable to N00-N29

Z84.2 Family history of other diseases of the genitourinary system UPD
Conditions classifiable to N30-N99

Z84.3 Family history of consanguinity UPD

Z84.8 Family history of other specified conditions

Z84.81 Family history of carrier of genetic disease UPD
AHA: 2021,1Q,14

Z84.82 Family history of sudden infant death syndrome UPD
Family history of SIDS
AHA: 2016,4Q,77

Z84.89 Family history of other specified conditions UPD

Z85 Personal history of malignant neoplasm
Code first any follow-up examination after treatment of malignant neoplasm (Z08)
Use additional code to identify:
- alcohol use and dependence (F10.-)
- exposure to environmental tobacco smoke (Z77.22)
- history of tobacco dependence (Z87.891)
- occupational exposure to environmental tobacco smoke (Z57.31)
- tobacco dependence (F17.-)
- tobacco use (Z72.0)

EXCLUDES 2 *personal history of benign neoplasm (Z86.01-)*
personal history of carcinoma-in-situ (Z86.00-)
AHA: 2020,3Q,30; 2018,4Q,64

Z85.0 Personal history of malignant neoplasm of digestive organs
AHA: 2017,1Q,9

Z85.00 Personal history of malignant neoplasm of unspecified digestive organ UPD

Z85.01 Personal history of malignant neoplasm of esophagus UPD
Conditions classifiable to C15

Z85.02 Personal history of malignant neoplasm of stomach

Z85.020 Personal history of malignant carcinoid tumor of stomach UPD
Conditions classifiable to C7A.092

Z85.028 **Personal history of other malignant neoplasm of stomach** UPD
Conditions classifiable to C16

✓6th Z85.03 **Personal history of malignant neoplasm of large intestine**

Z85.030 **Personal history of malignant carcinoid tumor of large intestine** UPD
Conditions classifiable to C7A.022-C7A.025, C7A.029

Z85.038 **Personal history of other malignant neoplasm of large intestine** UPD
Conditions classifiable to C18

✓6th Z85.04 **Personal history of malignant neoplasm of rectum, rectosigmoid junction, and anus**

Z85.040 **Personal history of malignant carcinoid tumor of rectum** UPD
Conditions classifiable to C7A.026

Z85.048 **Personal history of other malignant neoplasm of rectum, rectosigmoid junction, and anus** UPD
Conditions classifiable to C19-C21

Z85.05 **Personal history of malignant neoplasm of liver** UPD
Conditions classifiable to C22

✓6th Z85.06 **Personal history of malignant neoplasm of small intestine**

Z85.060 **Personal history of malignant carcinoid tumor of small intestine** UPD
Conditions classifiable to C7A.01-

Z85.068 **Personal history of other malignant neoplasm of small intestine** UPD
Conditions classifiable to C17

Z85.07 **Personal history of malignant neoplasm of pancreas** UPD
Conditions classifiable to C25

Z85.09 **Personal history of malignant neoplasm of other digestive organs** UPD

✓5th Z85.1 **Personal history of malignant neoplasm of trachea, bronchus and lung**

✓6th Z85.11 **Personal history of malignant neoplasm of bronchus and lung**

Z85.110 **Personal history of malignant carcinoid tumor of bronchus and lung** UPD
Conditions classifiable to C7A.090

Z85.118 **Personal history of other malignant neoplasm of bronchus and lung** UPD
Conditions classifiable to C34

Z85.12 **Personal history of malignant neoplasm of trachea** UPD
Conditions classifiable to C33

✓5th Z85.2 **Personal history of malignant neoplasm of other respiratory and intrathoracic organs**

Z85.20 **Personal history of malignant neoplasm of unspecified respiratory organ** UPD

Z85.21 **Personal history of malignant neoplasm of larynx** UPD
Conditions classifiable to C32

Z85.22 **Personal history of malignant neoplasm of nasal cavities, middle ear, and accessory sinuses** UPD
Conditions classifiable to C30-C31

✓6th Z85.23 **Personal history of malignant neoplasm of thymus**

Z85.230 **Personal history of malignant carcinoid tumor of thymus** UPD
Conditions classifiable to C7A.091

Z85.238 **Personal history of other malignant neoplasm of thymus** UPD
Conditions classifiable to C37

Z85.29 **Personal history of malignant neoplasm of other respiratory and intrathoracic organs** UPD

Z85.3 **Personal history of malignant neoplasm of breast** UPD
Conditions classifiable to C50.-

✓5th Z85.4 **Personal history of malignant neoplasm of genital organs**
Conditions classifiable to C51-C63

Z85.40 **Personal history of malignant neoplasm of unspecified female genital organ** UPD ♀

Z85.41 **Personal history of malignant neoplasm of cervix uteri** UPD ♀

Z85.42 **Personal history of malignant neoplasm of other parts of uterus** UPD ♀

Z85.43 **Personal history of malignant neoplasm of ovary** UPD ♀

Z85.44 **Personal history of malignant neoplasm of other female genital organs** UPD ♀

Z85.45 **Personal history of malignant neoplasm of unspecified male genital organ** UPD ♂

Z85.46 **Personal history of malignant neoplasm of prostate** UPD ♂

Z85.47 **Personal history of malignant neoplasm of testis** UPD ♂

Z85.48 **Personal history of malignant neoplasm of epididymis** UPD ♂

Z85.49 **Personal history of malignant neoplasm of other male genital organs** UPD ♂

✓5th Z85.5 **Personal history of malignant neoplasm of urinary tract**
Conditions classifiable to C64-C68

Z85.50 **Personal history of malignant neoplasm of unspecified urinary tract organ** UPD

Z85.51 **Personal history of malignant neoplasm of bladder** UPD

✓6th Z85.52 **Personal history of malignant neoplasm of kidney**
EXCLUDES 1 *personal history of malignant neoplasm of renal pelvis (Z85.53)*

Z85.520 **Personal history of malignant carcinoid tumor of kidney** UPD
Conditions classifiable to C7A.093

Z85.528 **Personal history of other malignant neoplasm of kidney** UPD
Conditions classifiable to C64

Z85.53 **Personal history of malignant neoplasm of renal pelvis** UPD

Z85.54 **Personal history of malignant neoplasm of ureter** UPD

Z85.59 **Personal history of malignant neoplasm of other urinary tract organ** UPD

Z85.6 **Personal history of leukemia** UPD
Conditions classifiable to C91-C95
EXCLUDES 1 *leukemia in remission C91.0-C95.9 with 5th character 1*

✓5th Z85.7 **Personal history of other malignant neoplasms of lymphoid, hematopoietic and related tissues**

Z85.71 **Personal history of Hodgkin lymphoma** UPD
Conditions classifiable to C81

Z85.72 **Personal history of non-Hodgkin lymphomas** UPD
Conditions classifiable to C82-C85

Z85.79 **Personal history of other malignant neoplasms of lymphoid, hematopoietic and related tissues** UPD
Conditions classifiable to C88-C90, C96
EXCLUDES 1 *multiple myeloma in remission (C90.01)*
plasma cell leukemia in remission (C90.11)
plasmacytoma in remission (C90.21)

✓5th Z85.8 **Personal history of malignant neoplasms of other organs and systems**
Conditions classifiable to C00-C14, C40-C49, C69-C75, C7A.098, C76-C79

✓6th Z85.81 **Personal history of malignant neoplasm of lip, oral cavity, and pharynx**
Conditions classifiable to C00-C14

Z85.810 **Personal history of malignant neoplasm of tongue** UPD

Z85.818 **Personal history of malignant neoplasm of other sites of lip, oral cavity, and pharynx** UPD

Z85.819 **Personal history of malignant neoplasm of unspecified site of lip, oral cavity, and pharynx** UPD

✓6th Z85.82 **Personal history of malignant neoplasm of skin**

Z85.820 **Personal history of malignant melanoma of skin** UPD
Conditions classifiable to C43

Z85.821 **Personal history of Merkel cell carcinoma** UPD
Conditions classifiable to C4A

Z85.828 **Personal history of other malignant neoplasm of skin** UPD
Conditions classifiable to C44

Z85.83 Personal history of malignant neoplasm of bone and soft tissue
Conditions classifiable to C40-C41; C45-C49

Z85.830 Personal history of malignant neoplasm of bone UPD

Z85.831 Personal history of malignant neoplasm of soft tissue UPD
EXCLUDES 2 *personal history of malignant neoplasm of skin (Z85.82-)*

Z85.84 Personal history of malignant neoplasm of eye and nervous tissue
Conditions classifiable to C69-C72

Z85.840 Personal history of malignant neoplasm of eye UPD

Z85.841 Personal history of malignant neoplasm of brain UPD

Z85.848 Personal history of malignant neoplasm of other parts of nervous tissue UPD

Z85.85 Personal history of malignant neoplasm of endocrine glands
Conditions classifiable to C73-C75

Z85.850 Personal history of malignant neoplasm of thyroid UPD

Z85.858 Personal history of malignant neoplasm of other endocrine glands UPD

Z85.89 Personal history of malignant neoplasm of other organs and systems UPD
Conditions classifiable to C7A.098, C76, C77-C79

Z85.9 Personal history of malignant neoplasm, unspecified UPD
Conditions classifiable to C7A.00, C80.1

Z86 Personal history of certain other diseases
Code first any follow-up examination after treatment (Z09)

Z86.0 Personal history of in-situ and benign neoplasms and neoplasms of uncertain behavior
EXCLUDES 2 *personal history of malignant neoplasms (Z85.-)*
AHA: 2017,1Q,9

Z86.00 Personal history of in-situ neoplasm
Conditions classifiable to D00-D09
AHA: 2019,4Q,20

Z86.000 Personal history of in-situ neoplasm of breast UPD
Conditions classifiable to D05

Z86.001 Personal history of in-situ neoplasm of cervix uteri UPD ♀
Conditions classifiable to D06
Personal history of cervical intraepithelial neoplasia III [CIN III]

Z86.002 Personal history of in-situ neoplasm of other and unspecified genital organs UPD
Conditions classifiable to D07
Personal history of high-grade prostatic intraepithelial neoplasia III [HGPIN III]
Personal history of vaginal intraepithelial neoplasia III [VAIN III]
Personal history of vulvar intraepithelial neoplasia III [VIN III]

Z86.003 Personal history of in-situ neoplasm of oral cavity, esophagus and stomach UPD
Conditions classifiable to D00

Z86.004 Personal history of in-situ neoplasm of other and unspecified digestive organs UPD
Conditions classifiable to D01
Personal history of anal intraepithelial neoplasia (AIN III)

Z86.005 Personal history of in-situ neoplasm of middle ear and respiratory system UPD
Conditions classifiable to D02

Z86.006 Personal history of melanoma in-situ UPD
Conditions classifiable to D03
EXCLUDES 2 *sites other than skin - code to personal history of in-situ neoplasm of the site*

Z86.007 Personal history of in-situ neoplasm of skin UPD
Conditions classifiable to D04
Personal history of carcinoma in situ of skin

Z86.008 Personal history of in-situ neoplasm of other site UPD
Conditions classifiable to D09

Z86.01 Personal history of benign neoplasm

Z86.010 Personal history of colonic polyps UPD
AHA: 2021,1Q,14; 2017,1Q,14

Z86.011 Personal history of benign neoplasm of the brain UPD

Z86.012 Personal history of benign carcinoid tumor UPD

Z86.018 Personal history of other benign neoplasm UPD
AHA: 2017,1Q,14

Z86.03 Personal history of neoplasm of uncertain behavior UPD

Z86.1 Personal history of infectious and parasitic diseases
Conditions classifiable to A00-B89, B99
EXCLUDES 1 *personal history of infectious diseases specific to a body system*
sequelae of infectious and parasitic diseases (B90-B94)

Z86.11 Personal history of tuberculosis UPD

Z86.12 Personal history of poliomyelitis UPD

Z86.13 Personal history of malaria UPD

Z86.14 Personal history of Methicillin resistant Staphylococcus aureus infection UPD
Personal history of MRSA infection

Z86.15 Personal history of latent tuberculosis infection UPD

Z86.16 Personal history of COVID-19 UPD
EXCLUDES 1 *post COVID-19 condition (U09.9)*
AHA: 2021,4Q,107-108; 2021,1Q,28-29,33-35,40-41,44-45

Z86.19 Personal history of other infectious and parasitic diseases UPD
AHA: 2021,1Q,33-34,40; 2020,3Q,13; 2020,2Q,10,12

Z86.2 Personal history of diseases of the blood and blood-forming organs and certain disorders involving the immune mechanism UPD
Conditions classifiable to D50-D89

Z86.3 Personal history of endocrine, nutritional and metabolic diseases
Conditions classifiable to E00-E88

Z86.31 Personal history of diabetic foot ulcer UPD
EXCLUDES 2 *current diabetic foot ulcer (E08.621, E09.621, E10.621, E11.621, E13.621)*

Z86.32 Personal history of gestational diabetes UPD ♀
Personal history of conditions classifiable to O24.4-
EXCLUDES 1 *gestational diabetes mellitus in current pregnancy (O24.4-)*

Z86.39 Personal history of other endocrine, nutritional and metabolic disease UPD
AHA: 2020,1Q,12

Z86.5 Personal history of mental and behavioral disorders
Conditions classifiable to F40-F59

Z86.51 Personal history of combat and operational stress reaction UPD A

Z86.59 Personal history of other mental and behavioral disorders UPD

Z86.6 Personal history of diseases of the nervous system and sense organs
Conditions classifiable to G00-G99, H00-H95

Z86.61 Personal history of infections of the central nervous system UPD
Personal history of encephalitis
Personal history of meningitis

Z86.69 Personal history of other diseases of the nervous system and sense organs UPD
AHA: 2016,4Q,24

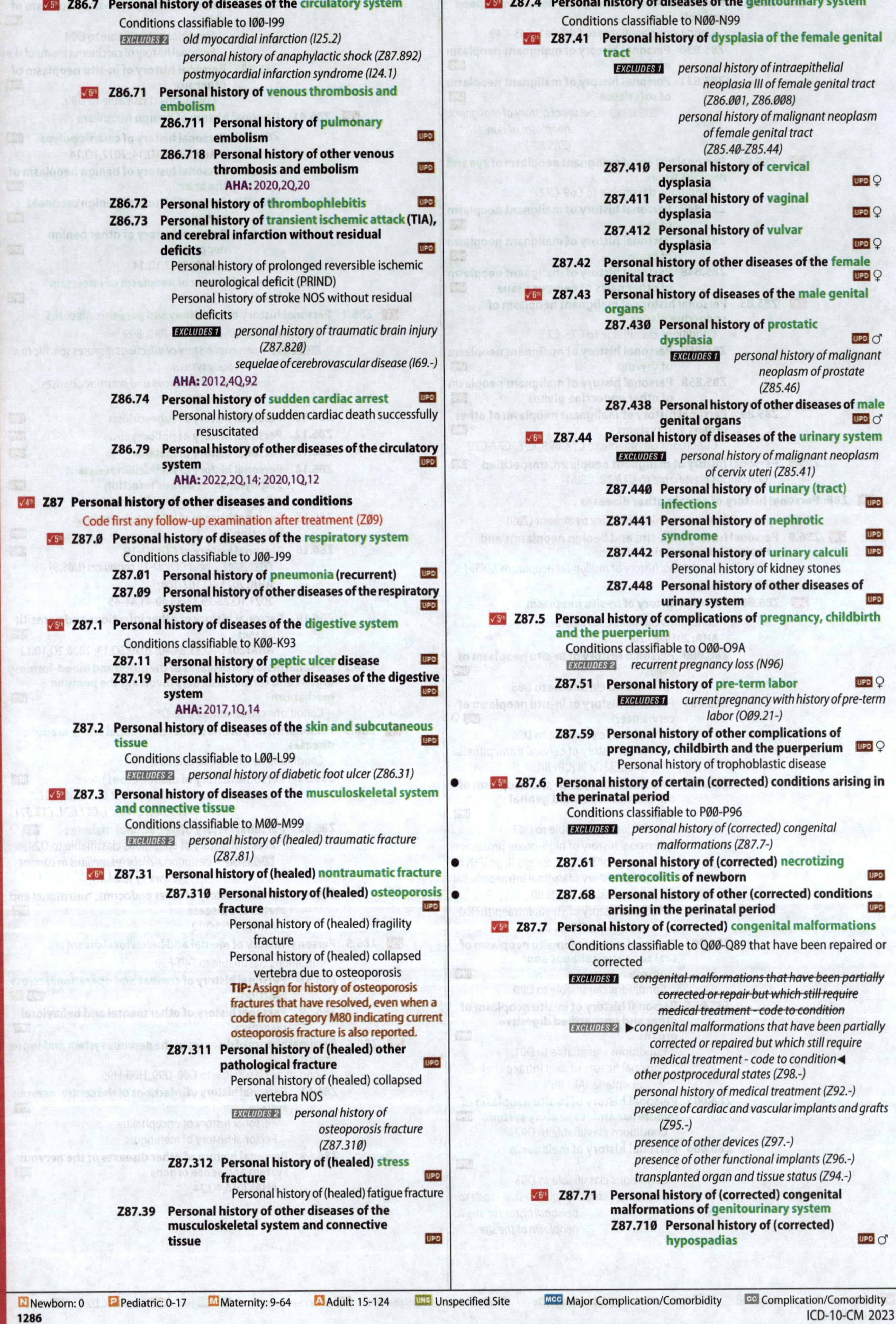

Z86.7 Personal history of diseases of the circulatory system
Conditions classifiable to IØØ-I99
EXCLUDES 2 *old myocardial infarction (I25.2)*
personal history of anaphylactic shock (Z87.892)
postmyocardial infarction syndrome (I24.1)

Z86.71 Personal history of venous thrombosis and embolism

Z86.711 Personal history of pulmonary embolism

Z86.718 Personal history of other venous thrombosis and embolism
AHA: 2020,2Q,20

Z86.72 Personal history of thrombophlebitis

Z86.73 Personal history of transient ischemic attack (TIA), and cerebral infarction without residual deficits
Personal history of prolonged reversible ischemic neurological deficit (PRIND)
Personal history of stroke NOS without residual deficits
EXCLUDES 1 *personal history of traumatic brain injury (Z87.82Ø)*
sequelae of cerebrovascular disease (I69.-)
AHA: 2012,4Q,92

Z86.74 Personal history of sudden cardiac arrest
Personal history of sudden cardiac death successfully resuscitated

Z86.79 Personal history of other diseases of the circulatory system
AHA: 2022,2Q,14; 2020,1Q,12

Z87 Personal history of other diseases and conditions
Code first any follow-up examination after treatment (ZØ9)

Z87.Ø Personal history of diseases of the respiratory system
Conditions classifiable to JØØ-J99

Z87.Ø1 Personal history of pneumonia (recurrent)

Z87.Ø9 Personal history of other diseases of the respiratory system

Z87.1 Personal history of diseases of the digestive system
Conditions classifiable to KØØ-K93

Z87.11 Personal history of peptic ulcer disease

Z87.19 Personal history of other diseases of the digestive system
AHA: 2017,1Q,14

Z87.2 Personal history of diseases of the skin and subcutaneous tissue
Conditions classifiable to LØØ-L99
EXCLUDES 2 *personal history of diabetic foot ulcer (Z86.31)*

Z87.3 Personal history of diseases of the musculoskeletal system and connective tissue
Conditions classifiable to MØØ-M99
EXCLUDES 2 *personal history of (healed) traumatic fracture (Z87.81)*

Z87.31 Personal history of (healed) nontraumatic fracture

Z87.31Ø Personal history of (healed) osteoporosis fracture
Personal history of (healed) fragility fracture
Personal history of (healed) collapsed vertebra due to osteoporosis
TIP: Assign for history of osteoporosis fractures that have resolved, even when a code from category M80 indicating current osteoporosis fracture is also reported.

Z87.311 Personal history of (healed) other pathological fracture
Personal history of (healed) collapsed vertebra NOS
EXCLUDES 2 *personal history of osteoporosis fracture (Z87.31Ø)*

Z87.312 Personal history of (healed) stress fracture
Personal history of (healed) fatigue fracture

Z87.39 Personal history of other diseases of the musculoskeletal system and connective tissue

Z87.4 Personal history of diseases of the genitourinary system
Conditions classifiable to NØØ-N99

Z87.41 Personal history of dysplasia of the female genital tract
EXCLUDES 1 *personal history of intraepithelial neoplasia III of female genital tract (Z86.ØØ1, Z86.ØØ8)*
personal history of malignant neoplasm of female genital tract (Z85.4Ø-Z85.44)

Z87.41Ø Personal history of cervical dysplasia ♀

Z87.411 Personal history of vaginal dysplasia ♀

Z87.412 Personal history of vulvar dysplasia ♀

Z87.42 Personal history of other diseases of the female genital tract ♀

Z87.43 Personal history of diseases of the male genital organs

Z87.43Ø Personal history of prostatic dysplasia ♂
EXCLUDES 1 *personal history of malignant neoplasm of prostate (Z85.46)*

Z87.438 Personal history of other diseases of male genital organs ♂

Z87.44 Personal history of diseases of the urinary system
EXCLUDES 1 *personal history of malignant neoplasm of cervix uteri (Z85.41)*

Z87.44Ø Personal history of urinary (tract) infections

Z87.441 Personal history of nephrotic syndrome

Z87.442 Personal history of urinary calculi
Personal history of kidney stones

Z87.448 Personal history of other diseases of urinary system

Z87.5 Personal history of complications of pregnancy, childbirth and the puerperium
Conditions classifiable to OØØ-O9A
EXCLUDES 2 *recurrent pregnancy loss (N96)*

Z87.51 Personal history of pre-term labor ♀
EXCLUDES 1 *current pregnancy with history of pre-term labor (OØ9.21-)*

Z87.59 Personal history of other complications of pregnancy, childbirth and the puerperium ♀
Personal history of trophoblastic disease

● **Z87.6 Personal history of certain (corrected) conditions arising in the perinatal period**
Conditions classifiable to PØØ-P96
EXCLUDES 1 *personal history of (corrected) congenital malformations (Z87.7-)*

● **Z87.61 Personal history of (corrected) necrotizing enterocolitis of newborn**

● **Z87.68 Personal history of other (corrected) conditions arising in the perinatal period**

Z87.7 Personal history of (corrected) congenital malformations
Conditions classifiable to QØØ-Q89 that have been repaired or corrected
EXCLUDES 1 ~~*congenital malformations that have been partially corrected or repair but which still require medical treatment - code to condition*~~
EXCLUDES 2 ▶*congenital malformations that have been partially corrected or repaired but which still require medical treatment - code to condition*◀
other postprocedural states (Z98.-)
personal history of medical treatment (Z92.-)
presence of cardiac and vascular implants and grafts (Z95.-)
presence of other devices (Z97.-)
presence of other functional implants (Z96.-)
transplanted organ and tissue status (Z94.-)

Z87.71 Personal history of (corrected) congenital malformations of genitourinary system

Z87.71Ø Personal history of (corrected) hypospadias ♂

Z87.718 Personal history of other specified (corrected) congenital malformations of genitourinary system UPD

Z87.72 Personal history of (corrected) congenital malformations of nervous system and sense organs

Z87.720 Personal history of (corrected) congenital malformations of eye UPD

Z87.721 Personal history of (corrected) congenital malformations of ear UPD

Z87.728 Personal history of other specified (corrected) congenital malformations of nervous system and sense organs UPD

Z87.73 Personal history of (corrected) congenital malformations of digestive system

Z87.730 Personal history of (corrected) cleft lip and palate UPD

● Z87.731 Personal history of (corrected) tracheoesophageal fistula or atresia UPD

● Z87.732 Personal history of (corrected) persistent cloaca or cloacal malformations UPD

Z87.738 Personal history of other specified (corrected) congenital malformations of digestive system UPD

Z87.74 Personal history of (corrected) congenital malformations of heart and circulatory system UPD

Z87.75 Personal history of (corrected) congenital malformations of respiratory system UPD

▲ Z87.76 Personal history of (corrected) congenital malformations of integument, limbs and musculoskeletal system

● Z87.760 Personal history of (corrected) congenital diaphragmatic hernia or other congenital diaphragm malformations UPD

● Z87.761 Personal history of (corrected) gastroschisis UPD

● Z87.762 Personal history of (corrected) prune belly malformation UPD

● Z87.763 Personal history of other (corrected) congenital abdominal wall malformations UPD

● Z87.768 Personal history of other specified (corrected) congenital malformations of integument, limbs and musculoskeletal system UPD

Z87.79 Personal history of other (corrected) congenital malformations

Z87.790 Personal history of (corrected) congenital malformations of face and neck UPD

Z87.798 Personal history of other (corrected) congenital malformations UPD

Z87.8 Personal history of other specified conditions

EXCLUDES 2 *personal history of self harm (Z91.5-)*

Z87.81 Personal history of (healed) traumatic fracture UPD

EXCLUDES 2 *personal history of (healed) nontraumatic fracture (Z87.31-)*

Z87.82 Personal history of other (healed) physical injury and trauma

Conditions classifiable to SØØ-T88, except traumatic fractures

Z87.82Ø Personal history of traumatic brain injury UPD

EXCLUDES 1 *personal history of transient ischemic attack (TIA), and cerebral infarction without residual deficits (Z86.73)*

Z87.821 Personal history of retained foreign body fully removed UPD

Z87.828 Personal history of other (healed) physical injury and trauma UPD

Z87.89 Personal history of other specified conditions

Z87.89Ø Personal history of sex reassignment

Z87.891 Personal history of nicotine dependence UPD

EXCLUDES 1 *current nicotine dependence (F17.2-)*

AHA: 2017,2Q,27

Z87.892 Personal history of anaphylaxis UPD

Code also allergy status such as:

allergy status to drugs, medicaments and biological substances (Z88.-)

allergy status, other than to drugs and biological substances (Z91.Ø-)

Z87.898 Personal history of other specified conditions UPD

AHA: 2013,1Q,21

Z88 Allergy status to drugs, medicaments and biological substances

EXCLUDES 2 *allergy status, other than to drugs and biological substances (Z91.Ø-)*

AHA: 2015,3Q,23

Z88.Ø Allergy status to penicillin UPD

Z88.1 Allergy status to other antibiotic agents UPD

Z88.2 Allergy status to sulfonamides UPD

Z88.3 Allergy status to other anti-infective agents UPD

Z88.4 Allergy status to anesthetic agent UPD

Z88.5 Allergy status to narcotic agent UPD

Z88.6 Allergy status to analgesic agent UPD

Z88.7 Allergy status to serum and vaccine UPD

Z88.8 Allergy status to other drugs, medicaments and biological substances UPD

Z88.9 Allergy status to unspecified drugs, medicaments and biological substances UPD

Z89 Acquired absence of limb

INCLUDES amputation status

postprocedural loss of limb

post-traumatic loss of limb

EXCLUDES 1 *acquired deformities of limbs (M2Ø-M21)*

congenital absence of limbs (Q71-Q73)

Z89.Ø Acquired absence of thumb and other finger(s)

Z89.Ø1 Acquired absence of thumb

Z89.Ø11 Acquired absence of right thumb UPD

Z89.Ø12 Acquired absence of left thumb UPD

Z89.Ø19 Acquired absence of unspecified thumb UPD

Z89.Ø2 Acquired absence of other finger(s)

EXCLUDES 2 *acquired absence of thumb (Z89.Ø1-)*

Z89.Ø21 Acquired absence of right finger(s) UPD

Z89.Ø22 Acquired absence of left finger(s) UPD

Z89.Ø29 Acquired absence of unspecified finger(s) UPD

Z89.1 Acquired absence of hand and wrist

Z89.11 Acquired absence of hand

Z89.111 Acquired absence of right hand UPD

Z89.112 Acquired absence of left hand UPD

Z89.119 Acquired absence of unspecified hand UPD

Z89.12 Acquired absence of wrist

Disarticulation at wrist

Z89.121 Acquired absence of right wrist UPD

Z89.122 Acquired absence of left wrist UPD

Z89.129 Acquired absence of unspecified wrist UPD

Z89.2 Acquired absence of upper limb above wrist

Z89.2Ø Acquired absence of upper limb, unspecified level

Z89.2Ø1 Acquired absence of right upper limb, unspecified level UPD

Z89.2Ø2 Acquired absence of left upper limb, unspecified level UPD

Z89.2Ø9 Acquired absence of unspecified upper limb, unspecified level UPD

Acquired absence of arm NOS

Z89.21 Acquired absence of upper limb below elbow

Z89.211 Acquired absence of right upper limb below elbow UPD

Z89.212 Acquired absence of left upper limb below elbow UPD

Z89.219 Acquired absence of unspecified upper limb below elbow UPD

Chapter 21. Factors Influencing Health Status and Contact With Health Services

Z89.22 Acquired absence of upper limb above elbow
Disarticulation at elbow
Z89.221 Acquired absence of right upper limb above elbow UPD
Z89.222 Acquired absence of left upper limb above elbow UPD
Z89.229 Acquired absence of unspecified upper limb above elbow UPD

Z89.23 Acquired absence of shoulder
Acquired absence of shoulder joint following explantation of shoulder joint prosthesis, with or without presence of antibiotic-impregnated cement spacer
Z89.231 Acquired absence of right shoulder UPD
Z89.232 Acquired absence of left shoulder UPD
Z89.239 Acquired absence of unspecified shoulder UPD

Z89.4 Acquired absence of toe(s), foot, and ankle

Z89.41 Acquired absence of great toe
Z89.411 Acquired absence of right great toe UPD HCC
Z89.412 Acquired absence of left great toe UPD HCC
Z89.419 Acquired absence of unspecified great toe UPD HCC

Z89.42 Acquired absence of other toe(s)
EXCLUDES 2 *acquired absence of great toe (Z89.41-)*
Z89.421 Acquired absence of other right toe(s) UPD HCC
Z89.422 Acquired absence of other left toe(s) UPD HCC
Z89.429 Acquired absence of other toe(s), unspecified side UPD HCC

Z89.43 Acquired absence of foot
Z89.431 Acquired absence of right foot UPD HCC
Z89.432 Acquired absence of left foot UPD HCC
Z89.439 Acquired absence of unspecified foot UPD HCC

Z89.44 Acquired absence of ankle
Disarticulation of ankle
Z89.441 Acquired absence of right ankle UPD HCC
Z89.442 Acquired absence of left ankle UPD HCC
Z89.449 Acquired absence of unspecified ankle UPD HCC

Z89.5 Acquired absence of leg below knee

Z89.51 Acquired absence of leg below knee
Z89.511 Acquired absence of right leg below knee UPD HCC
Z89.512 Acquired absence of left leg below knee UPD HCC
Z89.519 Acquired absence of unspecified leg below knee UPD HCC

Z89.52 Acquired absence of knee
Acquired absence of knee joint following explantation of knee joint prosthesis, with or without presence of antibiotic-impregnated cement spacer
Z89.521 Acquired absence of right knee UPD
Z89.522 Acquired absence of left knee UPD
Z89.529 Acquired absence of unspecified knee UPD

Z89.6 Acquired absence of leg above knee

Z89.61 Acquired absence of leg above knee
Acquired absence of leg NOS
Disarticulation at knee
Z89.611 Acquired absence of right leg above knee UPD HCC
Z89.612 Acquired absence of left leg above knee UPD HCC
Z89.619 Acquired absence of unspecified leg above knee UPD HCC

Z89.62 Acquired absence of hip
Acquired absence of hip joint following explantation of hip joint prosthesis, with or without presence of antibiotic-impregnated cement spacer
Disarticulation at hip
Z89.621 Acquired absence of right hip joint UPD
Z89.622 Acquired absence of left hip joint UPD
Z89.629 Acquired absence of unspecified hip joint UPD

Z89.9 Acquired absence of limb, unspecified UPD

Z90 Acquired absence of organs, not elsewhere classified
INCLUDES postprocedural or post-traumatic loss of body part NEC
EXCLUDES 1 *congenital absence - see Alphabetical Index*
EXCLUDES 2 *postprocedural absence of endocrine glands (E89.-)*

Z90.0 Acquired absence of part of head and neck
Z90.01 Acquired absence of eye UPD
Z90.02 Acquired absence of larynx UPD
Z90.09 Acquired absence of other part of head and neck UPD
Acquired absence of nose
EXCLUDES 2 *teeth (K08.1)*

Z90.1 Acquired absence of breast and nipple
Z90.10 Acquired absence of unspecified breast and nipple
Z90.11 Acquired absence of right breast and nipple
Z90.12 Acquired absence of left breast and nipple
Z90.13 Acquired absence of bilateral breasts and nipples

Z90.2 Acquired absence of lung [part of] UPD
Z90.3 Acquired absence of stomach [part of] UPD

Z90.4 Acquired absence of other specified parts of digestive tract

Z90.41 Acquired absence of pancreas
Code also exocrine pancreatic insufficiency (K86.81)
Use additional code to identify any associated:
diabetes mellitus, postpancreatectomy (E13.-)
insulin use (Z79.4)
Z90.410 Acquired total absence of pancreas UPD
Acquired absence of pancreas NOS
Z90.411 Acquired partial absence of pancreas UPD
Z90.49 Acquired absence of other specified parts of digestive tract UPD

Z90.5 Acquired absence of kidney UPD
Z90.6 Acquired absence of other parts of urinary tract UPD
Acquired absence of bladder

Z90.7 Acquired absence of genital organ(s)
EXCLUDES 1 *personal history of sex reassignment (Z87.890)*
EXCLUDES 2 *female genital mutilation status (N90.81-)*

Z90.71 Acquired absence of cervix and uterus
Z90.710 Acquired absence of both cervix and uterus UPD ♀
Acquired absence of uterus NOS
Status post total hysterectomy
Z90.711 Acquired absence of uterus with remaining cervical stump UPD ♀
Status post partial hysterectomy with remaining cervical stump
Z90.712 Acquired absence of cervix with remaining uterus UPD ♀

Z90.72 Acquired absence of ovaries
Z90.721 Acquired absence of ovaries, unilateral UPD ♀
Z90.722 Acquired absence of ovaries, bilateral UPD ♀
Z90.79 Acquired absence of other genital organ(s) UPD

Z90.8 Acquired absence of other organs
Z90.81 Acquired absence of spleen UPD
Z90.89 Acquired absence of other organs UPD

Z91 Personal risk factors, not elsewhere classified

EXCLUDES 2 *contact with and (suspected) exposures hazardous to health (Z77.-)*
exposure to pollution and other problems related to physical environment (Z77.1-)
female genital mutilation status (N90.81-)
personal history of physical injury and trauma (Z87.81, Z87.82-)
occupational exposure to risk factors (Z57.-)

Z91.0 Allergy status, other than to drugs and biological substances

EXCLUDES 2 *allergy status to drugs, medicaments, and biological substances (Z88.-)*

Z91.01 Food allergy status

EXCLUDES 2 *food additives allergy status (Z91.02)*

Z91.010 Allergy to peanuts UPD

Z91.011 Allergy to milk products UPD

EXCLUDES 1 *lactose intolerance (E73.-)*

Z91.012 Allergy to eggs UPD

Z91.013 Allergy to seafood UPD

Allergy to shellfish
Allergy to octopus or squid ink

Z91.014 Allergy to mammalian meats UPD

Allergy to beef
Allergy to lamb
Allergy to pork
Allergy to red meats

AHA: 2021,4Q,33

Z91.018 Allergy to other foods UPD

Allergy to nuts other than peanuts

Z91.02 Food additives allergy status UPD

Z91.03 Insect allergy status

Z91.030 Bee allergy status UPD

Z91.038 Other insect allergy status UPD

Z91.04 Nonmedicinal substance allergy status

Z91.040 Latex allergy status UPD

Latex sensitivity status

Z91.041 Radiographic dye allergy status UPD

Allergy status to contrast media used for diagnostic X-ray procedure

Z91.048 Other nonmedicinal substance allergy status UPD

Z91.09 Other allergy status, other than to drugs and biological substances UPD

Z91.1 Patient's noncompliance with medical treatment and regimen

EXCLUDES 2 ▶*caregiver noncompliance with patient's medical treatment and regimen (Z91.A-)*◀

▲ **Z91.11 Patient's noncompliance with dietary regimen**

▶Code also, if applicable, food insecurity (Z59.4-)◀

● **Z91.110 Patient's noncompliance with dietary regimen due to financial hardship** UPD

● **Z91.118 Patient's noncompliance with dietary regimen for other reason** UPD

Inability to comply with dietary regimen

● **Z91.119 Patient's noncompliance with dietary regimen due to unspecified reason** UPD

Z91.12 Patient's intentional underdosing of medication regimen

Code first underdosing of medication (T36-T50) with fifth or sixth character 6

EXCLUDES 1 *adverse effect of prescribed drug taken as directed - code to adverse effect*
poisoning (overdose) - code to poisoning

AHA: 2018,4Q,72

Z91.120 Patient's intentional underdosing of medication regimen due to financial hardship UPD

Z91.128 Patient's intentional underdosing of medication regimen for other reason UPD

Z91.13 Patient's unintentional underdosing of medication regimen

Code first underdosing of medication (T36-T50) with fifth or sixth character 6

EXCLUDES 1 *adverse effect of prescribed drug taken as directed - code to adverse effect*
poisoning (overdose) - code to poisoning

AHA: 2018,4Q,72

Z91.130 Patient's unintentional underdosing of medication regimen due to age-related debility UPD

Z91.138 Patient's unintentional underdosing of medication regimen for other reason UPD

Z91.14 Patient's other noncompliance with medication regimen UPD

Patient's underdosing of medication NOS

AHA: 2022,1Q,36; 2018,4Q,72

Z91.15 Patient's noncompliance with renal dialysis UPD HCC

▲ **Z91.19 Patient's noncompliance with other medical treatment and regimen**

▶Patient's nonadherence to medical treatment◀

● **Z91.190 Patient's noncompliance with other medical treatment and regimen due to financial hardship** UPD

● **Z91.198 Patient's noncompliance with other medical treatment and regimen for other reason** UPD

● **Z91.199 Patient's noncompliance with other medical treatment and regimen due to unspecified reason** UPD

● **Z91.A Caregiver's noncompliance with patient's medical treatment and regimen**

● **Z91.A1 Caregiver's noncompliance with patient's dietary regimen**

Caregiver's inability to comply with patient's dietary regimen

Code also, if applicable, food insecurity (Z59.4-)

● **Z91.A10 Caregiver's noncompliance with patient's dietary regimen due to financial hardship** UPD

● **Z91.A18 Caregiver's noncompliance with patient's dietary regimen for other reason** UPD

● **Z91.A2 Caregiver's intentional underdosing of patient's medication regimen**

Code first underdosing of medication (T36-T50) with fifth or sixth character 6

● **Z91.A20 Caregiver's intentional underdosing of patient's medication regimen due to financial hardship** UPD

● **Z91.A28 Caregiver's intentional underdosing of medication regimen for other reason** UPD

● **Z91.A3 Caregiver's unintentional underdosing of patient's medication regimen** UPD

Code first underdosing of medication (T36-T50) with fifth or sixth character 6

● **Z91.A4 Caregiver's other noncompliance with patient's medication regimen** UPD

Caregiver's underdosing of patient's medication NOS

● **Z91.A5 Caregiver's noncompliance with patient's renal dialysis** UPD

● **Z91.A9 Caregiver's noncompliance with patient's other medical treatment and regimen** UPD

Caregiver's nonadherence to patient's medical treatment

Z91.4 Personal history of psychological trauma, not elsewhere classified

Z91.41 Personal history of adult abuse

EXCLUDES 2 *personal history of abuse in childhood (Z62.81-)*

Z91.410 Personal history of adult physical and sexual abuse UPD A

EXCLUDES 1 *current adult physical abuse (T74.11, T76.11)*
current adult sexual abuse (T74.21, T76.11)

Z91.411 Personal history of adult psychological abuse UPD A

Z91.412 Personal history of adult neglect UPD A
EXCLUDES 1 *current adult neglect (T74.01, T76.01)*

Z91.419 Personal history of unspecified adult abuse UPD A

Z91.42 Personal history of forced labor or sexual exploitation UPD
AHA: 2018,4Q,32,35

Z91.49 Other personal history of psychological trauma, not elsewhere classified UPD

5th **Z91.5 Personal history of self-harm**
Code also mental health disorder, if known
AHA: 2021,4Q,33

Z91.51 Personal history of suicidal behavior UPD
Personal history of parasuicide
Personal history of self-poisoning
Personal history of suicide attempt

Z91.52 Personal history of nonsuicidal self-harm UPD
Personal history of nonsuicidal self-injury
Personal history of self-inflicted injury without suicidal intent
Personal history of self-mutilation

5th **Z91.8 Other specified personal risk factors, not elsewhere classified**

Z91.81 History of falling UPD
At risk for falling

Z91.82 Personal history of military deployment UPD A
Individual (civilian or military) with past history of military war, peacekeeping and humanitarian deployment (current or past conflict)
Returned from military deployment

Z91.83 Wandering in diseases classified elsewhere
Code first underlying disorder such as:
Alzheimer's disease (G30.-)
autism or pervasive developmental disorder (F84.-)
intellectual disabilities (F70-F79)
unspecified dementia with behavioral disturbance ►(F03.9-, F03.A-, F03.B-, F03.C-)◄

6th **Z91.84 Oral health risk factors**
AHA: 2017,4Q,29

Z91.841 Risk for dental caries, low UPD
Z91.842 Risk for dental caries, moderate UPD
Z91.843 Risk for dental caries, high UPD
Z91.849 Unspecified risk for dental caries UPD

Z91.89 Other specified personal risk factors, not elsewhere classified UPD
AHA: 2017,1Q,45

4th **Z92 Personal history of medical treatment**
EXCLUDES 2 *postprocedural states (Z98.-)*

Z92.0 Personal history of contraception UPD
EXCLUDES 1 *counseling or management of current contraceptive practices (Z30.-)*
long term (current) use of contraception (Z79.3)
presence of (intrauterine) contraceptive device (Z97.5)

5th **Z92.2 Personal history of drug therapy**
EXCLUDES 2 *long term (current) drug therapy (Z79.-)*

Z92.21 Personal history of antineoplastic chemotherapy UPD
Z92.22 Personal history of monoclonal drug therapy UPD
Z92.23 Personal history of estrogen therapy UPD

6th **Z92.24 Personal history of steroid therapy**

Z92.240 Personal history of inhaled steroid therapy UPD
Z92.241 Personal history of systemic steroid therapy UPD
Personal history of steroid therapy NOS

Z92.25 Personal history of immunosuppression therapy UPD
EXCLUDES 2 *personal history of steroid therapy (Z92.24)*

Z92.29 Personal history of other drug therapy UPD

Z92.3 Personal history of irradiation UPD
Personal history of exposure to therapeutic radiation
EXCLUDES 1 *exposure to radiation in the physical environment (Z77.12)*
occupational exposure to radiation (Z57.1)

5th **Z92.8 Personal history of other medical treatment**

Z92.81 Personal history of extracorporeal membrane oxygenation (ECMO) UPD

Z92.82 Status post administration of tPA (rtPA) in a different facility within the last 24 hours prior to admission to current facility UPD
Code first condition requiring tPA administration, such as:
acute cerebral infarction (I63.-)
acute myocardial infarction (I21.-, I22.-)
AHA: 2013,4Q,124

Z92.83 Personal history of failed moderate sedation UPD
Personal history of failed conscious sedation
EXCLUDES 2 *failed moderate sedation during procedure (T88.52)*

Z92.84 Personal history of unintended awareness under general anesthesia UPD
EXCLUDES 2 *unintended awareness under general anesthesia during procedure (T88.53)*
AHA: 2016,4Q,72-73,77

6th **Z92.85 Personal history of cellular therapy**
AHA: 2021,4Q,33-34

Z92.850 Personal history of Chimeric Antigen Receptor T-cell therapy UPD
Personal history of CAR T-cell therapy

Z92.858 Personal history of other cellular therapy UPD

Z92.859 Personal history of cellular therapy, unspecified UPD

Z92.86 Personal history of gene therapy UPD
AHA: 2021,4Q,33-34

Z92.89 Personal history of other medical treatment UPD
AHA: 2020,1Q,18

4th **Z93 Artificial opening status**
EXCLUDES 1 *artificial openings requiring attention or management (Z43.-)*
complications of external stoma (J95.0-, K94.-, N99.5-)

Z93.0 Tracheostomy status UPD HCC
AHA: 2013,4Q,129

Z93.1 Gastrostomy status UPD HCC
Z93.2 Ileostomy status UPD HCC
Z93.3 Colostomy status UPD HCC
Z93.4 Other artificial openings of gastrointestinal tract status UPD HCC

5th **Z93.5 Cystostomy status**

Z93.50 Unspecified cystostomy status UPD HCC
Z93.51 Cutaneous-vesicostomy status UPD HCC
Z93.52 Appendico-vesicostomy status UPD HCC
Z93.59 Other cystostomy status UPD HCC

Z93.6 Other artificial openings of urinary tract status UPD HCC
Nephrostomy status
Ureterostomy status
Urethrostomy status

Z93.8 Other artificial opening status UPD HCC
Z93.9 Artificial opening status, unspecified UPD HCC

4th **Z94 Transplanted organ and tissue status**
INCLUDES organ or tissue replaced by heterogenous or homogenous transplant
EXCLUDES 1 *complications of transplanted organ or tissue - see Alphabetical Index*
EXCLUDES 2 *presence of vascular grafts (Z95.-)*

Z94.0 Kidney transplant status CC UPD
Z94.1 Heart transplant status CC UPD HCC
EXCLUDES 1 *artificial heart status (Z95.812)*
heart-valve replacement status (Z95.2-Z95.4)

Z94.2 Lung transplant status CC UPD HCC
Z94.3 Heart and lungs transplant status CC UPD HCC
Z94.4 Liver transplant status CC UPD HCC
Z94.5 Skin transplant status UPD
Autogenous skin transplant status

Z94.6 Bone transplant status UPD

N Newborn: 0 P Pediatric: 0-17 M Maternity: 9-64 A Adult: 15-124 UNS Unspecified Site MCC Major Complication/Comorbidity CC Complication/Comorbidity

Z94.7 Corneal transplant status UPD

5th Z94.8 Other transplanted organ and tissue status

Z94.81 Bone marrow transplant status CC UPD HCC

Z94.82 Intestine transplant status CC UPD HCC

Z94.83 Pancreas transplant status CC UPD HCC

Z94.84 Stem cells transplant status CC UPD HCC

Z94.89 Other transplanted organ and tissue status UPD

Z94.9 Transplanted organ and tissue status, unspecified UPD

4th **Z95 Presence of cardiac and vascular implants and grafts**

EXCLUDES 2 *complications of cardiac and vascular devices, implants and grafts (T82.-)*

Z95.0 Presence of cardiac pacemaker UPD

Presence of cardiac resynchronization therapy (CRT-P) pacemaker

EXCLUDES 1 *adjustment or management of cardiac device (Z45.0-)*

adjustment or management of cardiac pacemaker (Z45.0)

presence of automatic (implantable) cardiac defibrillator with synchronous cardiac pacemaker (Z95.810)

AHA: 2022,2Q,14; 2019,1Q,33

TIP: Assign an additional code for the associated condition if that condition requires constant intervention from the device, as in cases of sick sinus syndrome. For conditions that do not require constant intervention from the device, as in cases of ventricular fibrillation, an additional code for the associated condition should be assigned only if the patient is experiencing the condition and the device is firing during the current admission.

Z95.1 Presence of aortocoronary bypass graft UPD

Presence of coronary artery bypass graft

Z95.2 Presence of prosthetic heart valve UPD

Presence of heart valve NOS

Z95.3 Presence of xenogenic heart valve UPD

Z95.4 Presence of other heart-valve replacement UPD

Z95.5 Presence of coronary angioplasty implant and graft UPD

EXCLUDES 1 *coronary angioplasty status without implant and graft (Z98.61)*

5th Z95.8 Presence of other cardiac and vascular implants and grafts

6th Z95.81 Presence of other cardiac implants and grafts

Z95.810 Presence of automatic (implantable) cardiac defibrillator UPD

Presence of automatic (implantable) cardiac defibrillator with synchronous cardiac pacemaker

Presence of cardiac resynchronization therapy defibrillator (CRT-D)

Presence of cardioverter-defibrillator (ICD)

AHA: 2022,2Q,14; 2019,1Q,33

TIP: Assign an additional code for the associated condition if that condition requires constant intervention from the device, as in cases of sick sinus syndrome. For conditions that do not require constant intervention from the device, as in cases of ventricular fibrillation, an additional code for the associated condition should be assigned only if the patient is experiencing the condition and the device is firing during the current admission.

Z95.811 Presence of heart assist device CC UPD HCC

Z95.812 Presence of fully implantable artificial heart CC UPD HCC

Z95.818 Presence of other cardiac implants and grafts UPD

6th Z95.82 Presence of other vascular implants and grafts

Z95.820 Peripheral vascular angioplasty status with implants and grafts UPD

EXCLUDES 1 *peripheral vascular angioplasty without implant and graft (Z98.62)*

Z95.828 Presence of other vascular implants and grafts UPD

Presence of intravascular prosthesis NEC

Z95.9 Presence of cardiac and vascular implant and graft, unspecified UPD

4th **Z96 Presence of other functional implants**

EXCLUDES 2 *complications of internal prosthetic devices, implants and grafts (T82-T85)*

fitting and adjustment of prosthetic and other devices (Z44-Z46)

Z96.0 Presence of urogenital implants UPD

Z96.1 Presence of intraocular lens UPD

Presence of pseudophakia

5th Z96.2 Presence of otological and audiological implants

Z96.20 Presence of otological and audiological implant, unspecified UPD

Z96.21 Cochlear implant status UPD

Z96.22 Myringotomy tube(s) status UPD

Z96.29 Presence of other otological and audiological implants UPD

Presence of bone-conduction hearing device

Presence of eustachian tube stent

Stapes replacement

Z96.3 Presence of artificial larynx UPD

5th Z96.4 Presence of endocrine implants

Z96.41 Presence of insulin pump (external) (internal) UPD

Z96.49 Presence of other endocrine implants UPD

Z96.5 Presence of tooth-root and mandibular implants UPD

5th Z96.6 Presence of orthopedic joint implants

AHA: 2019,3Q,16

Z96.60 Presence of unspecified orthopedic joint implant UPD

6th Z96.61 Presence of artificial shoulder joint

Z96.611 Presence of right artificial shoulder joint UPD

Z96.612 Presence of left artificial shoulder joint UPD

Z96.619 Presence of unspecified artificial shoulder joint UPD

6th Z96.62 Presence of artificial elbow joint

Z96.621 Presence of right artificial elbow joint UPD

Z96.622 Presence of left artificial elbow joint UPD

Z96.629 Presence of unspecified artificial elbow joint UPD

6th Z96.63 Presence of artificial wrist joint

Z96.631 Presence of right artificial wrist joint UPD

Z96.632 Presence of left artificial wrist joint UPD

Z96.639 Presence of unspecified artificial wrist joint UPD

6th Z96.64 Presence of artificial hip joint

Hip-joint replacement (partial) (total)

Z96.641 Presence of right artificial hip joint UPD

Z96.642 Presence of left artificial hip joint UPD

Z96.643 Presence of artificial hip joint, bilateral UPD

Z96.649 Presence of unspecified artificial hip joint UPD

6th Z96.65 Presence of artificial knee joint

Z96.651 Presence of right artificial knee joint UPD

Z96.652 Presence of left artificial knee joint UPD

Z96.653 Presence of artificial knee joint, bilateral UPD

Z96.659 Presence of unspecified artificial knee joint UPD

6th Z96.66 Presence of artificial ankle joint

Z96.661 Presence of right artificial ankle joint UPD

Z96.662 Presence of left artificial ankle joint UPD

Z96.669 Presence of unspecified artificial ankle joint UPD

6th Z96.69 Presence of other orthopedic joint implants

Z96.691 Finger-joint replacement of right hand UPD

Chapter 21. Factors Influencing Health Status and Contact With Health Services

Z94.7–Z96.691

Z96.692 Finger-joint replacement of left hand UPD

Z96.693 Finger-joint replacement, bilateral UPD

Z96.698 Presence of other orthopedic joint implants UPD

Z96.7 Presence of other bone and tendon implants UPD
Presence of skull plate

Z96.8 Presence of other specified functional implants

Z96.81 Presence of artificial skin UPD

Z96.82 Presence of neurostimulator UPD
Presence of brain neurostimulator
Presence of gastric neurostimulator
Presence of peripheral nerve neurostimulator
Presence of sacral nerve neurostimulator
Presence of spinal cord neurostimulator
Presence of vagus nerve neurostimulator
AHA: 2019,4Q,19

Z96.89 Presence of other specified functional implants UPD

Z96.9 Presence of functional implant, unspecified UPD

Z97 Presence of other devices
EXCLUDES 1 *complications of internal prosthetic devices, implants and grafts (T82-T85)*
EXCLUDES 2 *fitting and adjustment of prosthetic and other devices (Z44-Z46)*
presence of cerebrospinal fluid drainage device (Z98.2)

Z97.Ø Presence of artificial eye UPD

Z97.1 Presence of artificial limb (complete) (partial)

Z97.1Ø Presence of artificial limb (complete) (partial), unspecified UPD

Z97.11 Presence of artificial right arm (complete) (partial) UPD

Z97.12 Presence of artificial left arm (complete) (partial) UPD

Z97.13 Presence of artificial right leg (complete) (partial) UPD

Z97.14 Presence of artificial left leg (complete) (partial) UPD

Z97.15 Presence of artificial arms, bilateral (complete) (partial) UPD

Z97.16 Presence of artificial legs, bilateral (complete) (partial) UPD

Z97.2 Presence of dental prosthetic device (complete) (partial) UPD
Presence of dentures (complete) (partial)

Z97.3 Presence of spectacles and contact lenses UPD

Z97.4 Presence of external hearing-aid UPD

Z97.5 Presence of (intrauterine) contraceptive device UPD ♀
EXCLUDES 1 *checking, reinsertion or removal of implantable subdermal contraceptive (Z3Ø.46)*
checking, reinsertion or removal of intrauterine contraceptive device (Z3Ø.43-)

Z97.8 Presence of other specified devices UPD

Z98 Other postprocedural states
EXCLUDES 2 *aftercare (Z43-Z49, Z51)*
follow-up medical care (ZØ8-ZØ9)
postprocedural complication - see Alphabetical Index

Z98.Ø Intestinal bypass and anastomosis status UPD
EXCLUDES 2 *bariatric surgery status (Z98.84)*
gastric bypass status (Z98.84)
obesity surgery status (Z98.84)

Z98.1 Arthrodesis status UPD

Z98.2 Presence of cerebrospinal fluid drainage device UPD
Presence of CSF shunt

Z98.3 Post therapeutic collapse of lung status UPD
Code first underlying disease

Z98.4 Cataract extraction status
Use additional code to identify intraocular lens implant status (Z96.1)
EXCLUDES 1 *aphakia (H27.Ø)*

Z98.41 Cataract extraction status, right eye UPD

Z98.42 Cataract extraction status, left eye UPD

Z98.49 Cataract extraction status, unspecified eye UPD

Z98.5 Sterilization status
EXCLUDES 1 *female infertility (N97.-)*
male infertility (N46.-)

Z98.51 Tubal ligation status UPD ♀

Z98.52 Vasectomy status UPD A ♂

Z98.6 Angioplasty status

Z98.61 Coronary angioplasty status UPD
EXCLUDES 1 *coronary angioplasty status with implant and graft (Z95.5)*

Z98.62 Peripheral vascular angioplasty status UPD
EXCLUDES 1 *peripheral vascular angioplasty status with implant and graft (Z95.82Ø)*

Z98.8 Other specified postprocedural states

Z98.81 Dental procedure status

Z98.81Ø Dental sealant status UPD

Z98.811 Dental restoration status UPD
Dental crown status
Dental fillings status

Z98.818 Other dental procedure status UPD

Z98.82 Breast implant status UPD
EXCLUDES 1 *breast implant removal status (Z98.86)*

Z98.83 Filtering (vitreous) bleb after glaucoma surgery status UPD
EXCLUDES 1 *inflammation (infection) of postprocedural bleb (H59.4-)*
AHA: 2020,3Q,29

Z98.84 Bariatric surgery status UPD
Gastric banding status
Gastric bypass status for obesity
Obesity surgery status
EXCLUDES 1 *bariatric surgery status complicating pregnancy, childbirth, or the puerperium (O99.84)*
EXCLUDES 2 *intestinal bypass and anastomosis status (Z98.Ø)*
AHA: 2020,1Q,12

Z98.85 Transplanted organ removal status UPD
Transplanted organ previously removed due to complication, failure, rejection or infection
EXCLUDES 1 *encounter for removal of transplanted organ - code to complication of transplanted organ (T86.-)*

Z98.86 Personal history of breast implant removal UPD

Z98.87 Personal history of in utero procedure

Z98.87Ø Personal history of in utero procedure during pregnancy UPD ♀
EXCLUDES 2 *complications from in utero procedure for current pregnancy (O35.7)*
supervision of current pregnancy with history of in utero procedure during previous pregnancy (OØ9.82-)

Z98.871 Personal history of in utero procedure while a fetus UPD

Z98.89 Other specified postprocedural states

Z98.89Ø Other specified postprocedural states UPD
Personal history of surgery, not elsewhere classified

Z98.891 History of uterine scar from previous surgery UPD ♀
EXCLUDES 1 *maternal care due to uterine scar from previous surgery (O34.2-)*
AHA: 2016,4Q,51-52,76

Z99 Dependence on enabling machines and devices, not elsewhere classified
AHA: 2020,1Q,11

Z99.Ø Dependence on aspirator UPD

✓5th **Z99.1 Dependence on respirator**
Dependence on ventilator

Z99.11 Dependence on respirator [ventilator] status CC HCC
AHA: 2015,1Q,21

Z99.12 Encounter for respirator [ventilator] dependence during power failure CC HCC
EXCLUDES 1 *mechanical complication of respirator [ventilator] (J95.85Ø)*

Z99.2 Dependence on renal dialysis UPD HCC
Hemodialysis status
Peritoneal dialysis status
Presence of arteriovenous shunt for dialysis
Renal dialysis status NOS
EXCLUDES 1 *encounter for fitting and adjustment of dialysis catheter (Z49.Ø-)*
EXCLUDES 2 *noncompliance with renal dialysis (Z91.15)*
AHA: 2016,1Q,12; 2013,4Q,125

Z99.3 Dependence on wheelchair UPD
Wheelchair confinement status
Code first cause of dependence, such as:
muscular dystrophy (G71.Ø-)
obesity (E66.-)

✓5th **Z99.8 Dependence on other enabling machines and devices**

Z99.81 Dependence on supplemental oxygen UPD
Dependence on long-term oxygen
AHA: 2013,4Q,129

Z99.89 Dependence on other enabling machines and devices UPD
Dependence on machine or device NOS
AHA: 2020,1Q,11

Chapter 22. Codes for Special Purposes (UØØ–U85)

Chapter-specific Guidelines

UØ7.Ø Vaping-related disorder (see Section I.C.1Ø.e., Vaping-related disorders)

UØ7.1 COVID-19 (see Section I.C.1.g.1., COVID-19 infection)

UØ9.9 Post COVID-19 condition, unspecified (see Section I.C.1.g.1.m.)

Chapter 22. Codes for Special Purposes

Chapter 22. Codes for Special Purposes (U00-U85)

This chapter contains the following blocks:

U00-U49 Provisional assignment of new diseases of uncertain etiology or emergency use

Provisional assignment of new diseases of uncertain etiology or emergency use (U00-U49)

4th U07 Emergency use of U07

U07.0 Vaping-related disorder

Dabbing related lung damage
Dabbing related lung injury
E-cigarette, or vaping, product use associated lung injury [EVALI]
Electronic cigarette related lung damage
Electronic cigarette related lung injury

Use additional code, to identify manifestations, such as:
- abdominal pain (R10.84)
- acute respiratory distress syndrome (J80)
- diarrhea (R19.7)
- drug-induced interstitial lung disorder (J70.4)
- lipoid pneumonia (J69.1)
- weight loss (R63.4)

DEF: Respiratory illness or injury caused by harmful aerosolized substances and chemicals produced by electronic cigarettes, vapes, e-pipes, and other battery-powered vaping devices. Symptoms may include shortness of breath and fever, while some patients experience severe, sometimes fatal, lung damage. ***Synonym(s):*** *e-cigarette and vaping product use-associated lung injury, EVALI.*

U07.1 COVID-19 HIV MCC

Use additional code to identify pneumonia or other manifestations, such as:
- pneumonia due to COVID-19 (J12.82)

EXCLUDES 2 *coronavirus as the cause of diseases classified elsewhere (B97.2-)*
coronavirus infection, unspecified (B34.2)
pneumonia due to SARS-associated coronavirus (J12.81)

AHA: 2022,2Q,28; 2021,4Q,101,107-108; 2021,1Q,25-30,31-49; 2020,4Q,14,99; 2020,3Q,9-16; 2020,2Q,3-13

DEF: First diagnosed in December 2019 in China, coronavirus disease 2019 (COVID-19) is a respiratory infection caused by a newly identified (novel) virus not previously seen in humans, known as severe acute respiratory syndrome coronavirus 2 (SARS-CoV-2). Symptoms of this lower respiratory illness include fever, dry cough, and tiredness that may progress to include difficulty breathing. Older patients and those with high blood pressure, heart problems, and diabetes are more likely to develop serious symptoms of the illness. ***Synonym(s):*** *SARS-CoV-2, coronavirus disease 2019.*

TIP: Only a confirmed diagnosis of COVID-19, either through a positive test result documented in the medical record or documentation by the provider, can be coded to U07.1.

TIP: Assign for asymptomatic individuals who test positive for COVID-19. Even though asymptomatic, the individual is considered to have the COVID-19 infection due to the positive test result.

TIP: Assign appropriate codes for presenting signs/symptoms associated with COVID-19 (cough, fever, shortness of breath), instead of U07.1, if a definitive diagnosis has not been established.

4th U09 Post COVID-19 condition

U09.9 Post COVID-19 condition, unspecified

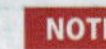
NOTE This code enables establishment of a link with COVID-19.

This code is not to be used in cases that are still presenting with active COVID-19. However, an exception is made in cases of re-infection with COVID-19, occurring with a condition related to prior COVID-19.

~~Post-acute sequela of COVID-19~~

▶Post-acute sequela of COVID-19◀

Code first the specific condition related to COVID-19 if known, such as:
- chronic respiratory failure (J96.1-)
- loss of smell (R43.8)
- loss of taste (R43.8)
- multisystem inflammatory syndrome (M35.81)
- pulmonary embolism (I26.-)
- pulmonary fibrosis (J84.10)

AHA: 2021,4Q,31-32,102-106

U07–U09.9

Notes

Notes

Notes

Notes

Notes

Notes

Illustrations

Chapter 3. Diseases of the Blood and Blood-forming Organs and Certain Disorders Involving the Immune Mechanism (D5Ø–D89)

Red Blood Cells

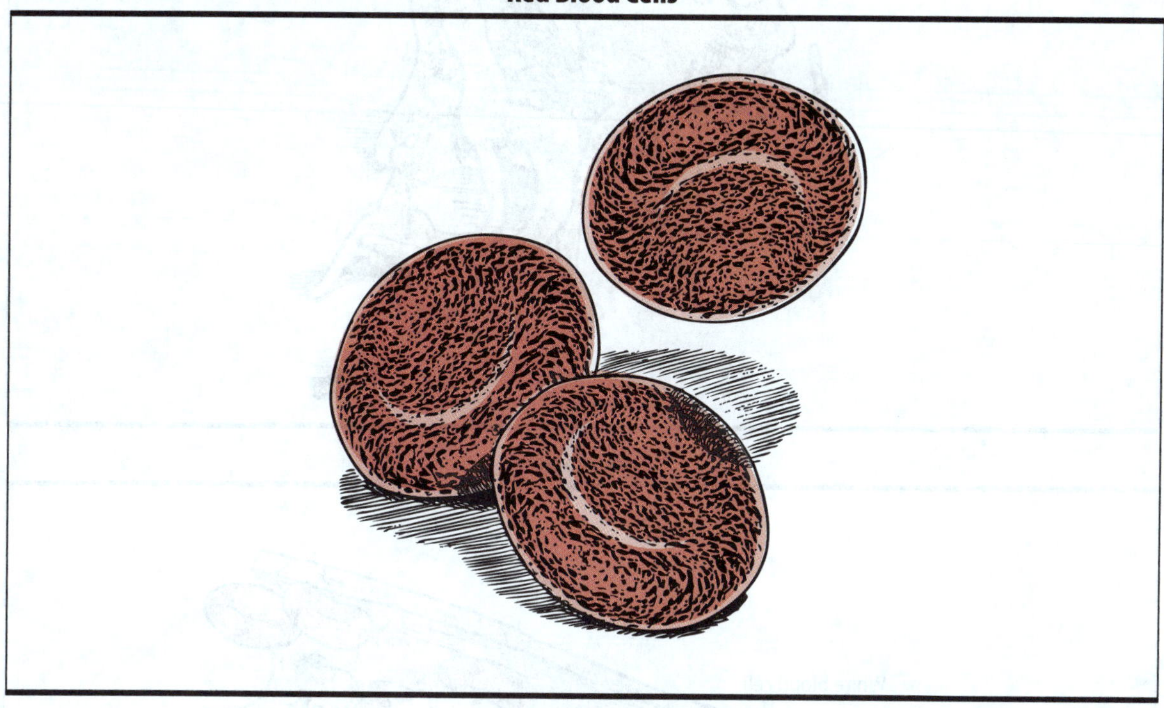

White Blood Cell

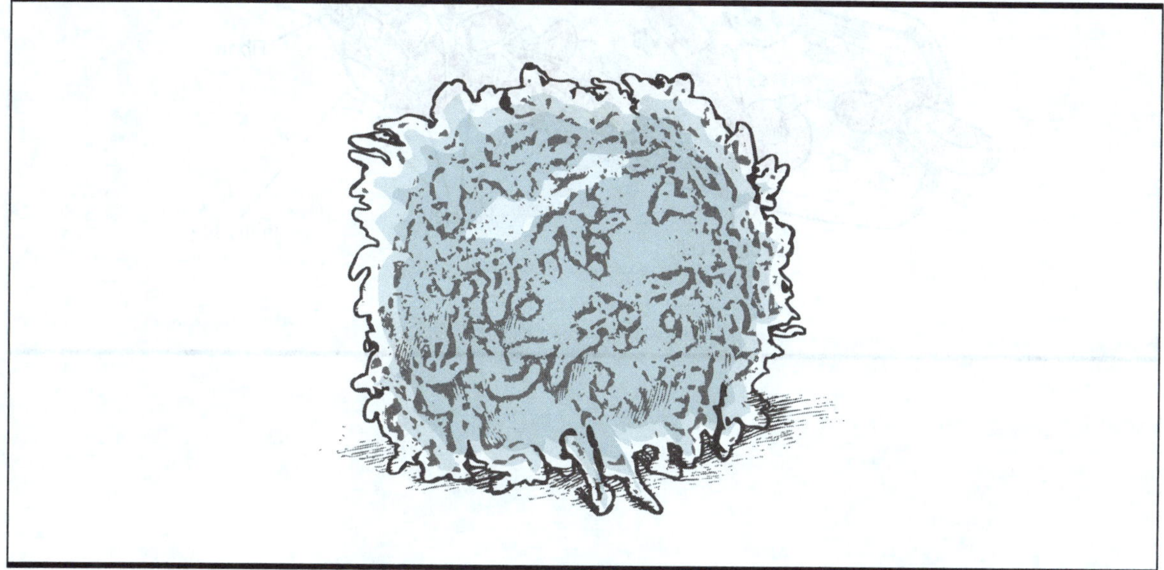

Platelet

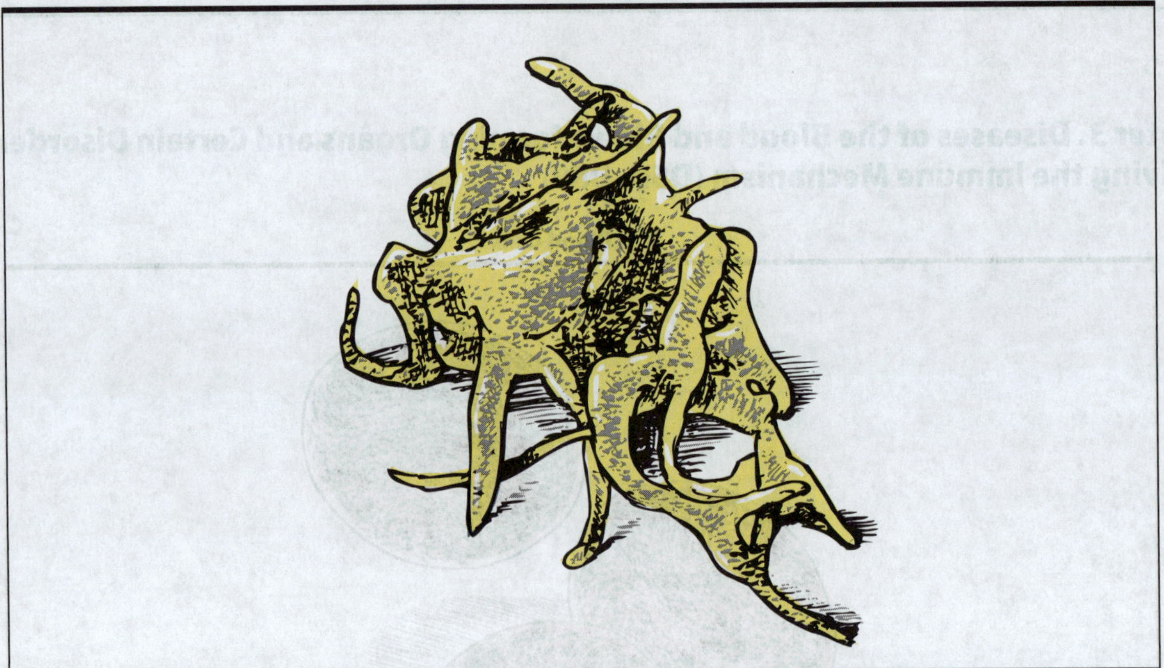

Coagulation

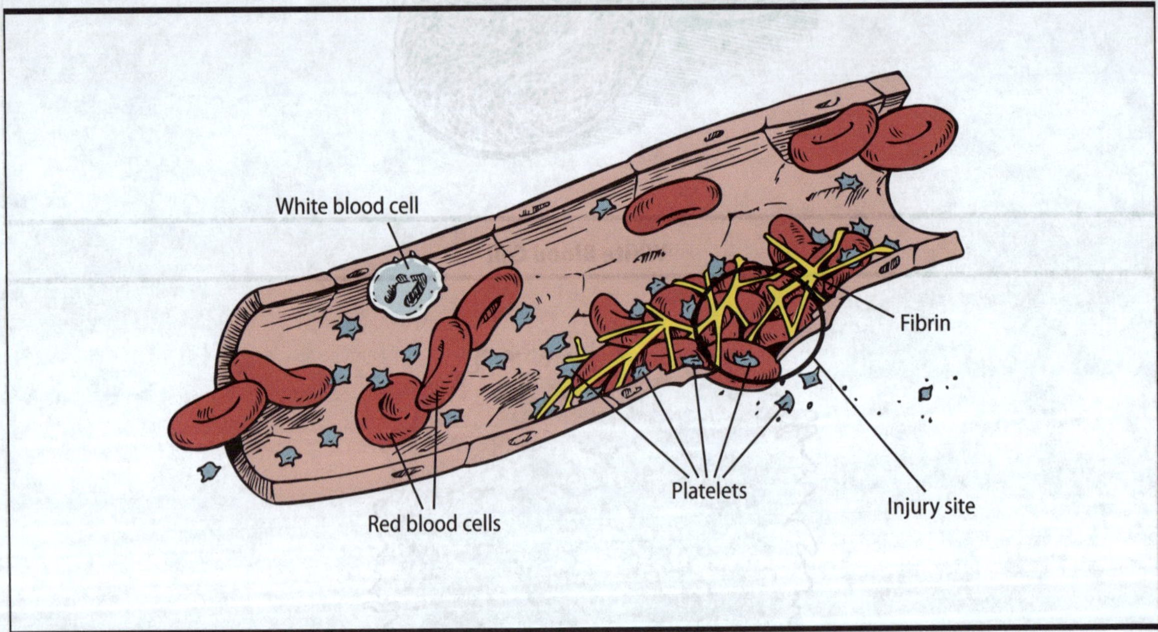

Spleen Anatomical Location and External Structures

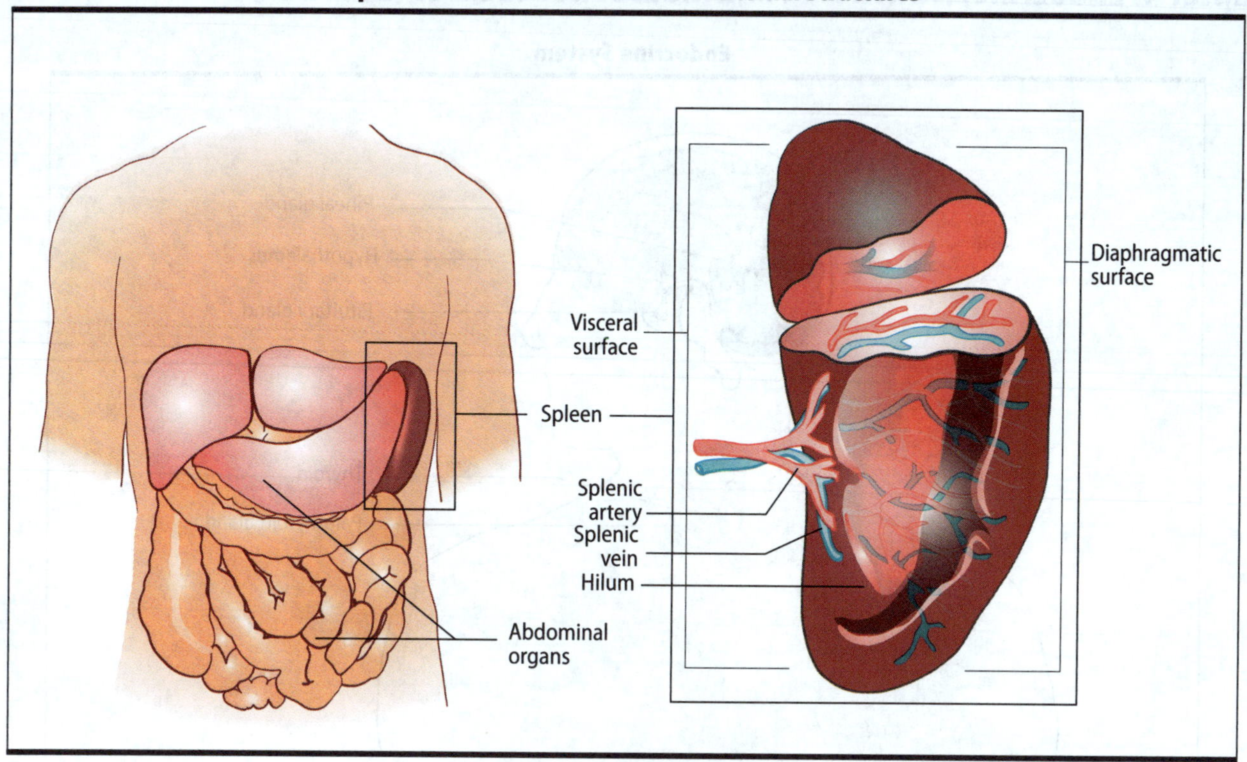

Spleen Interior Structures

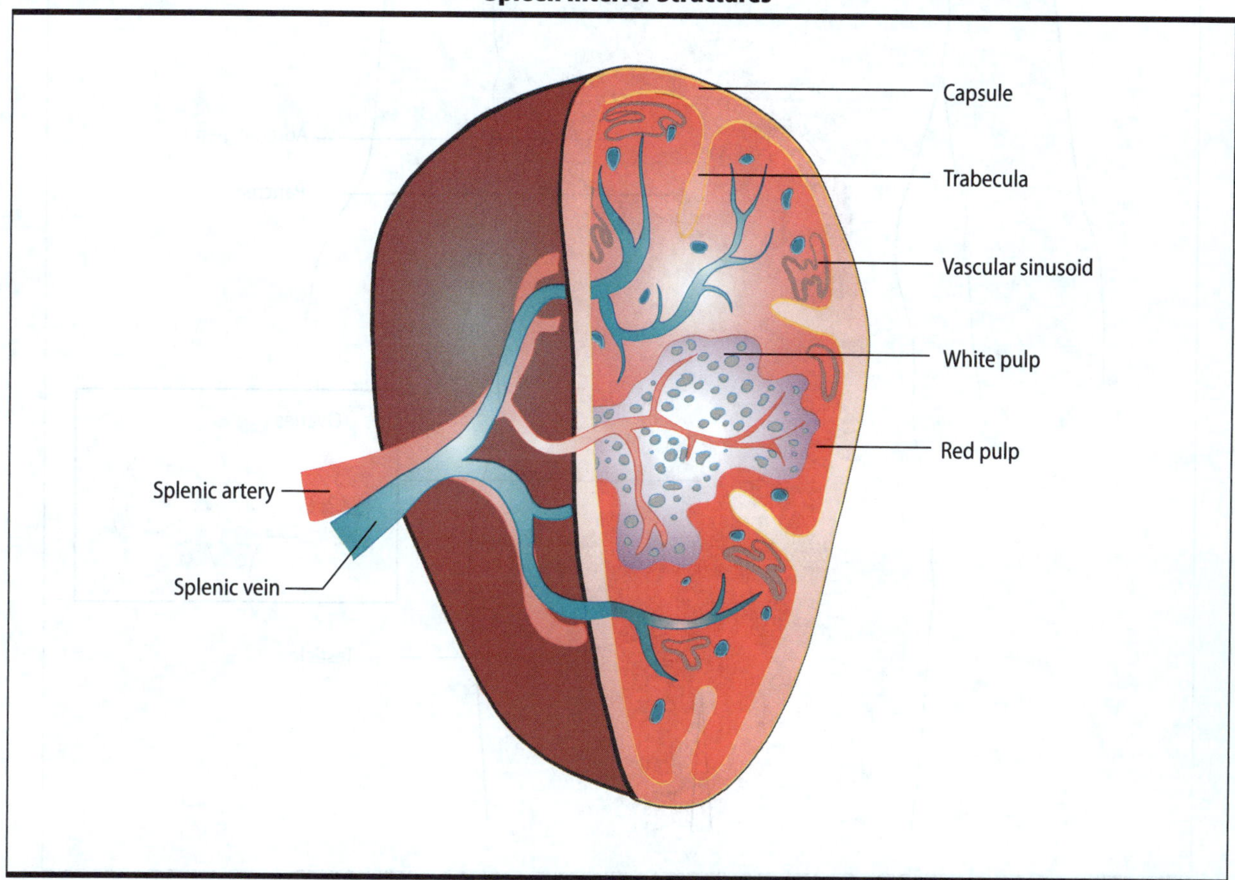

Chapter 4. Endocrine, Nutritional and Metabolic Diseases (EØØ–E89)

Endocrine System

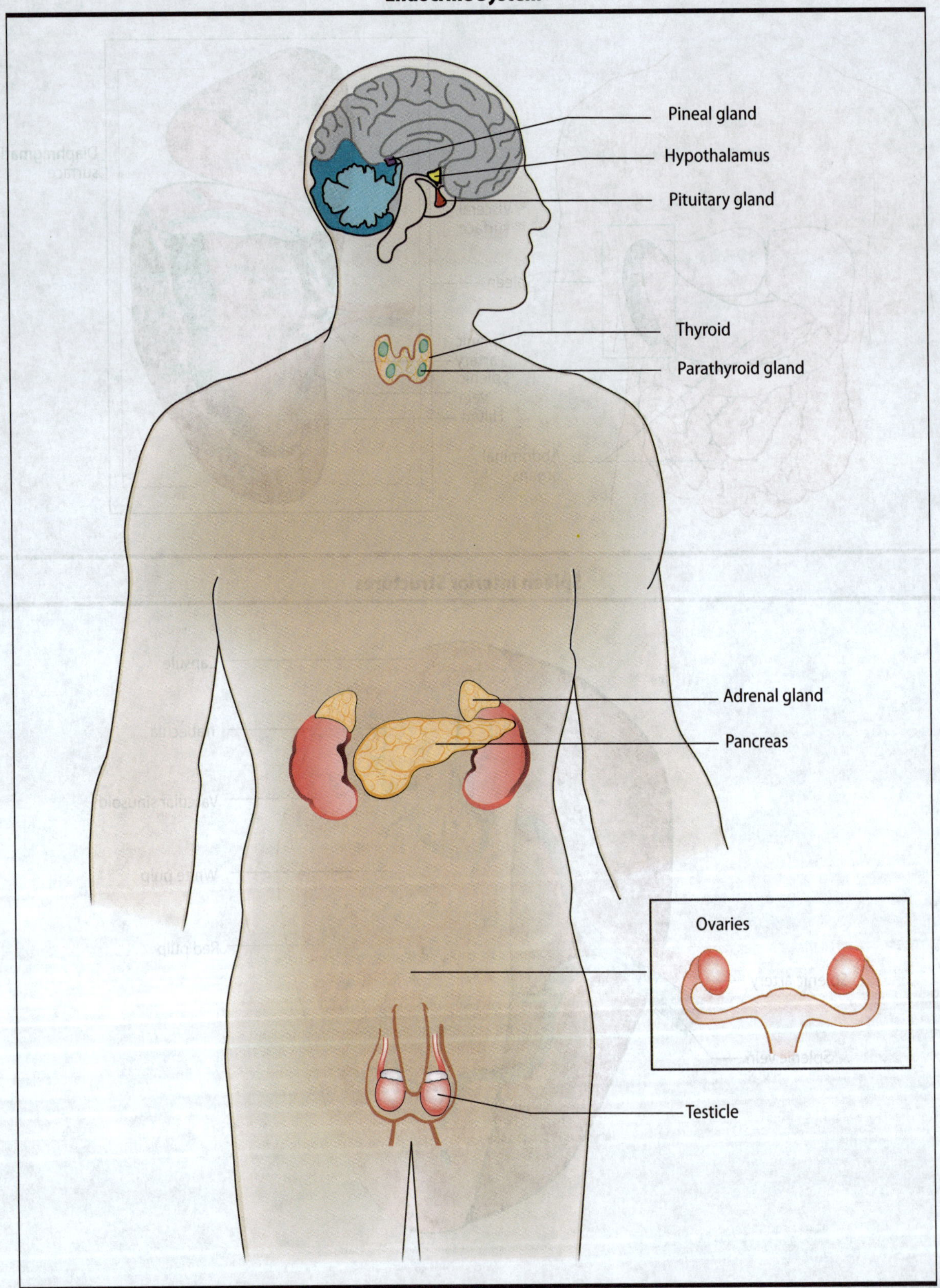

Thyroid

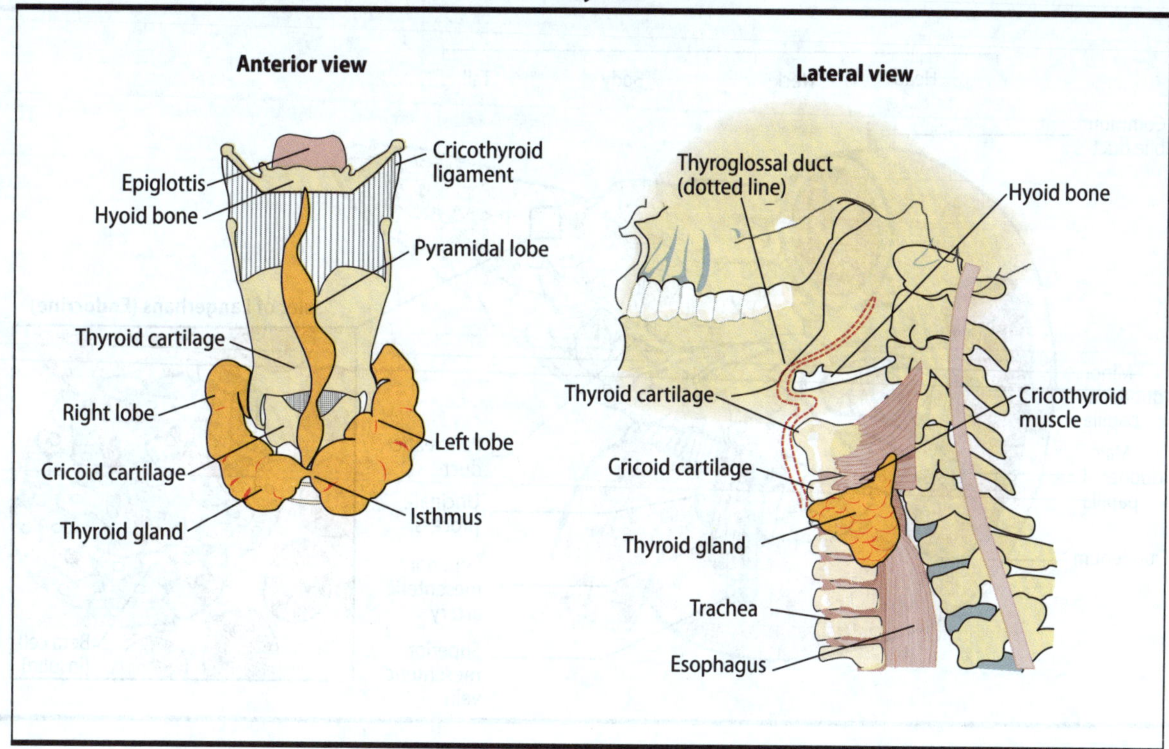

Thyroid and Parathyroid Glands

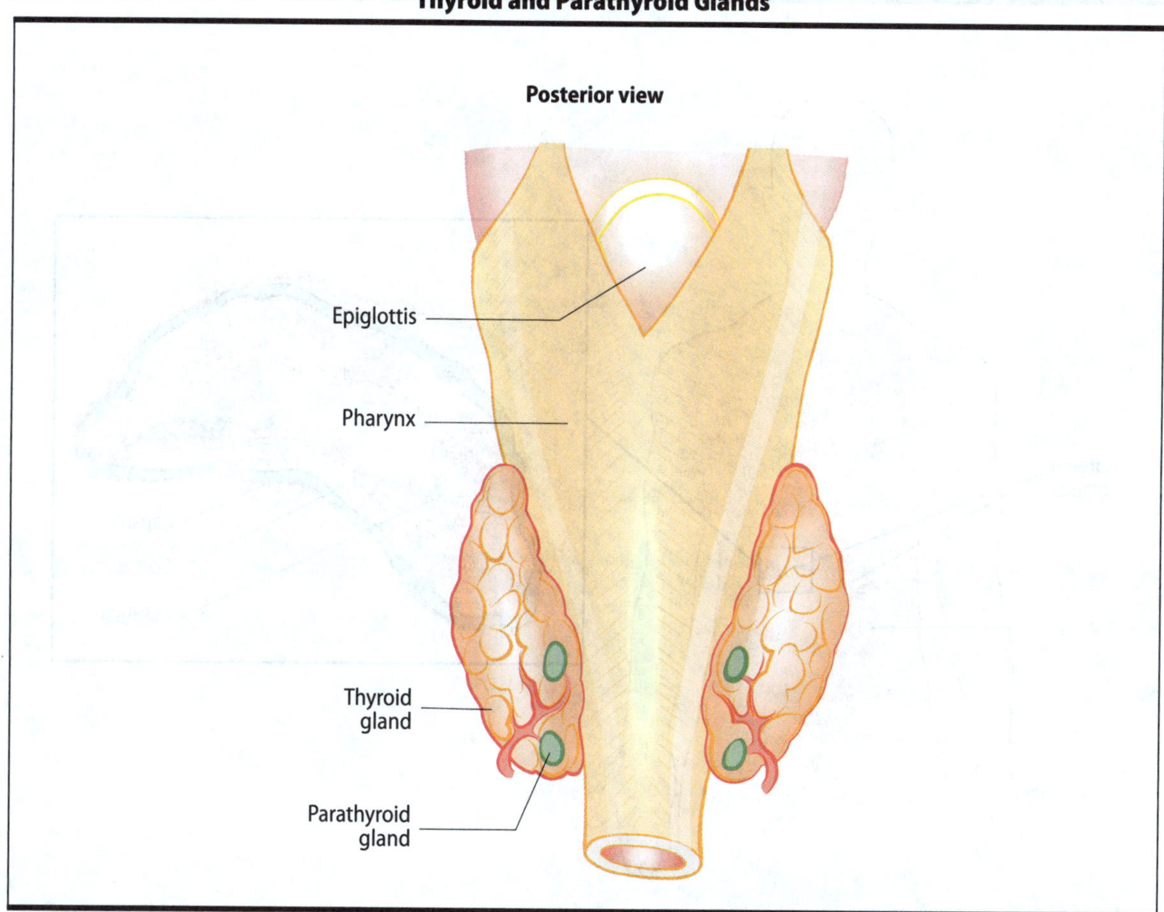

Pancreas

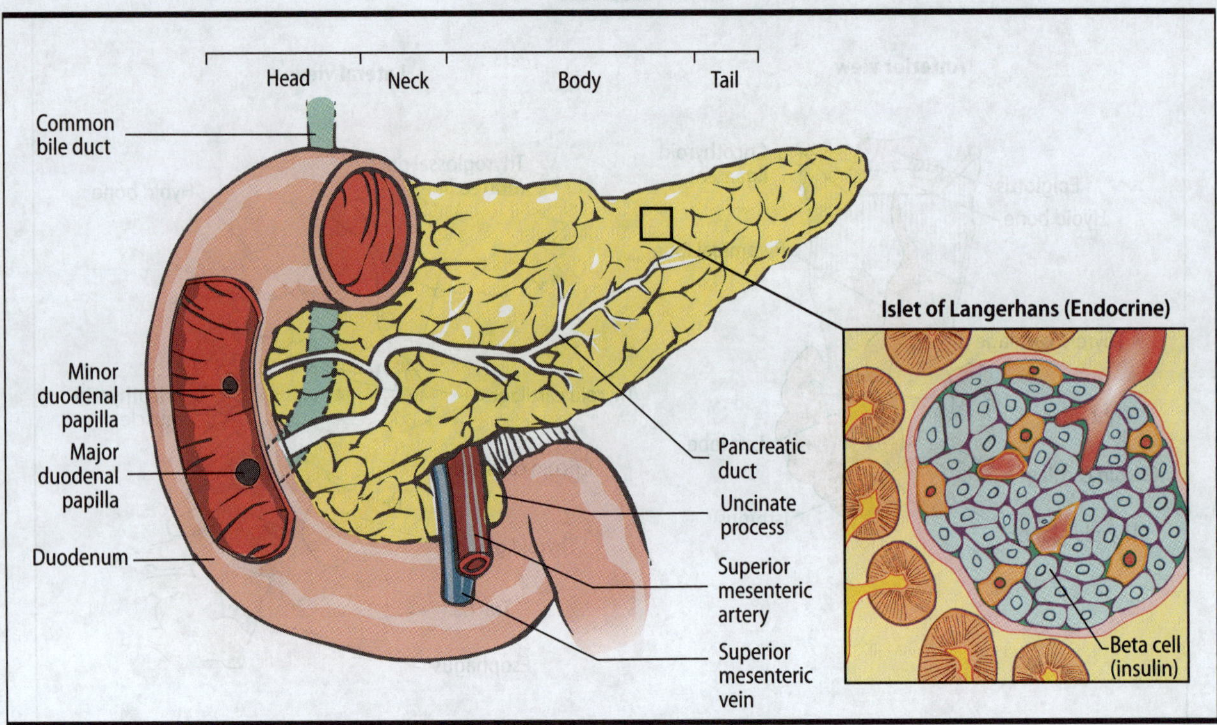

Anatomy of the Adrenal Gland

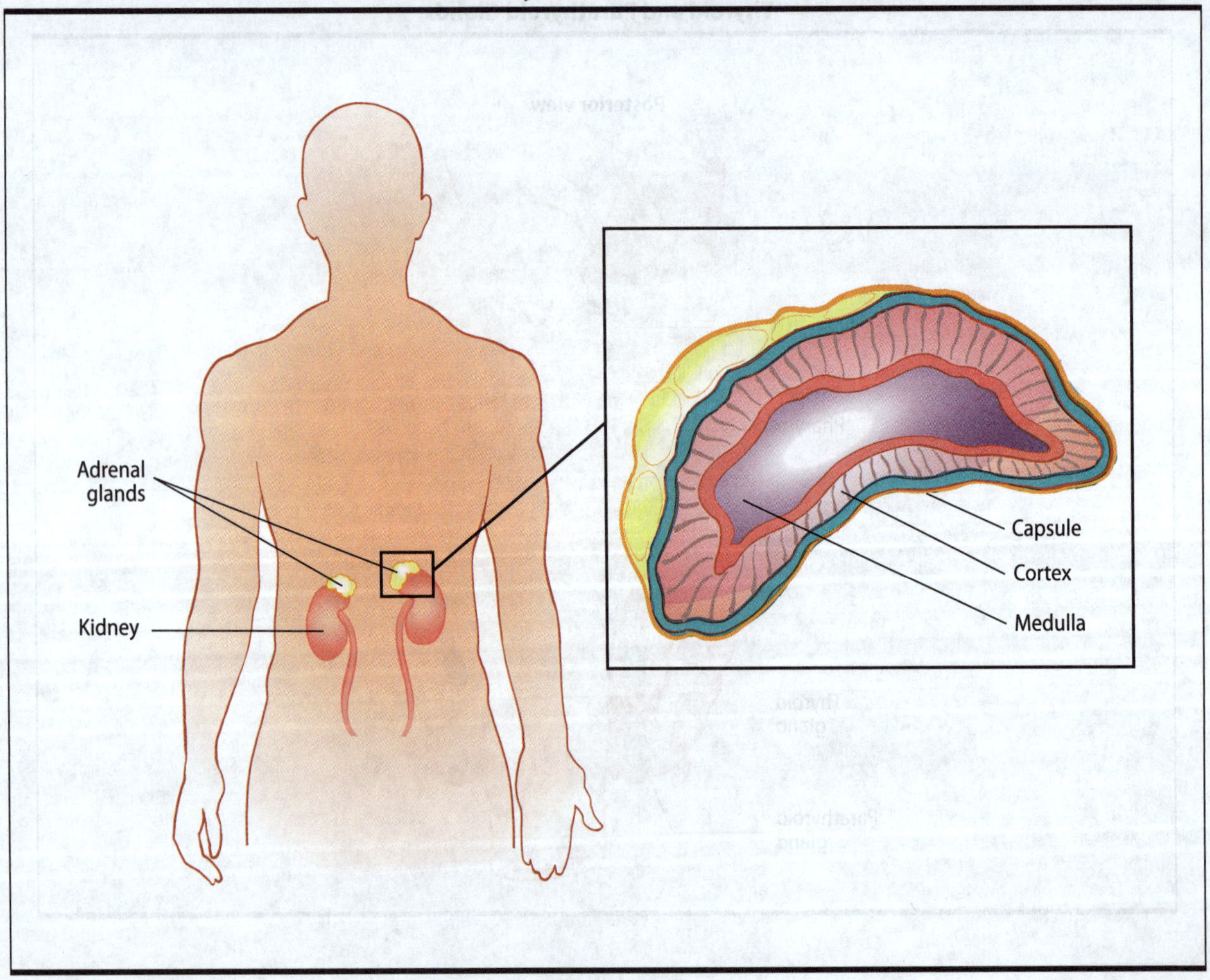

Adrenal glands
Kidney
Capsule
Cortex
Medulla

Structure of an Ovary

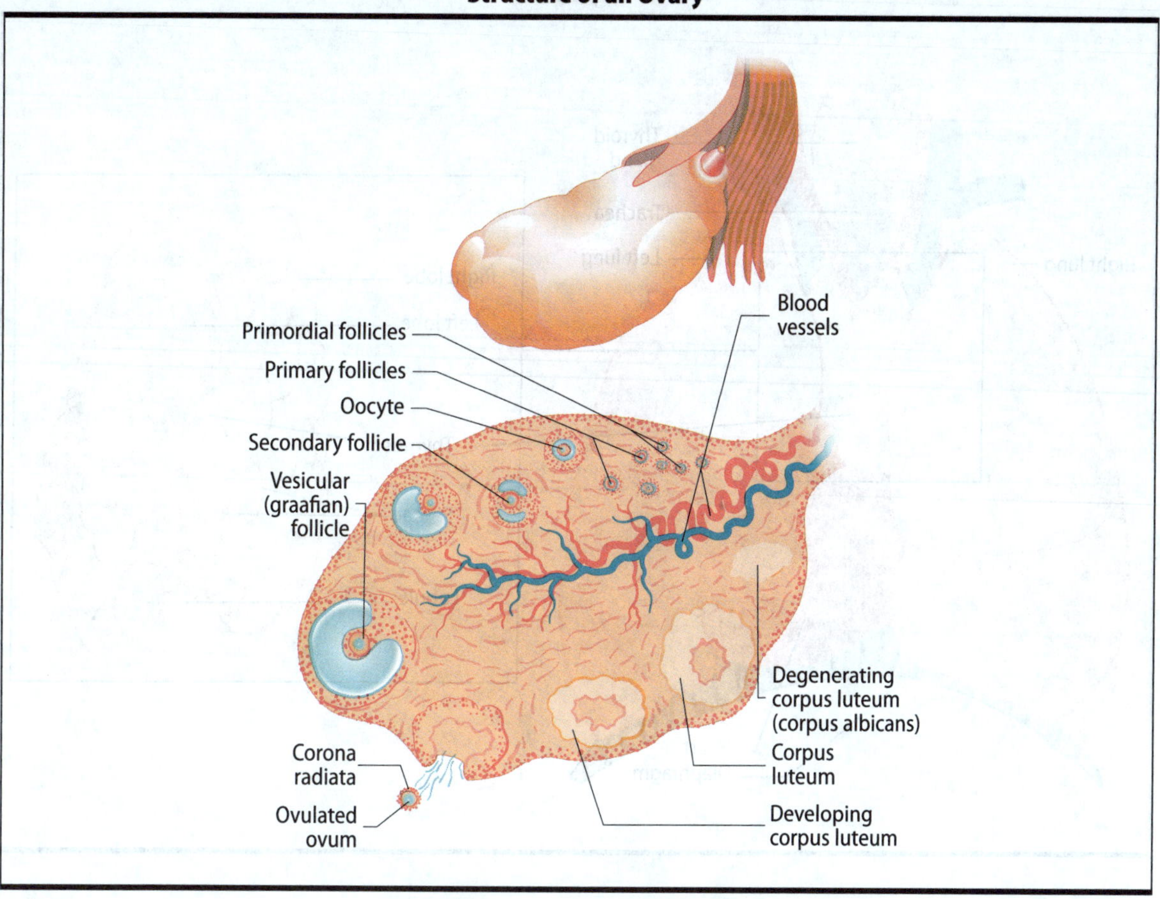

Testis and Associated Structures

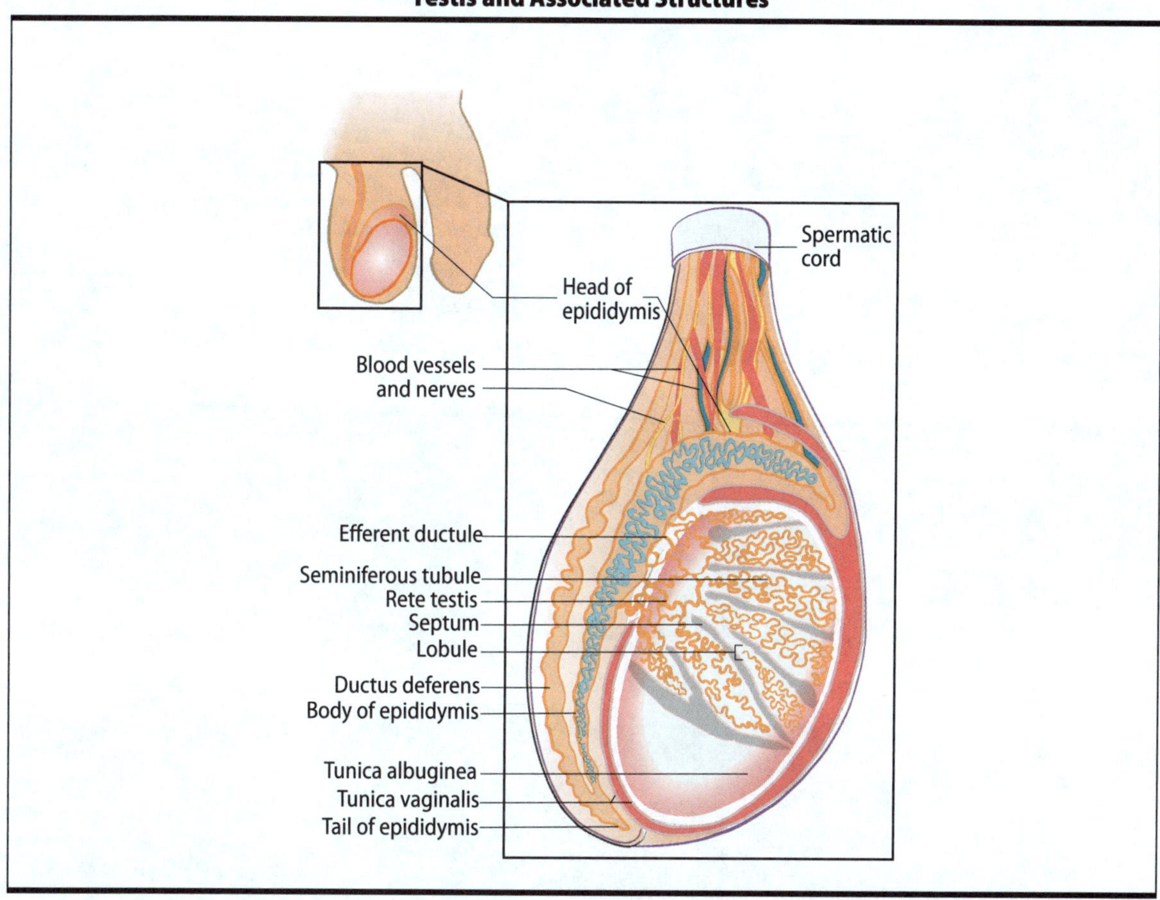

Thymus

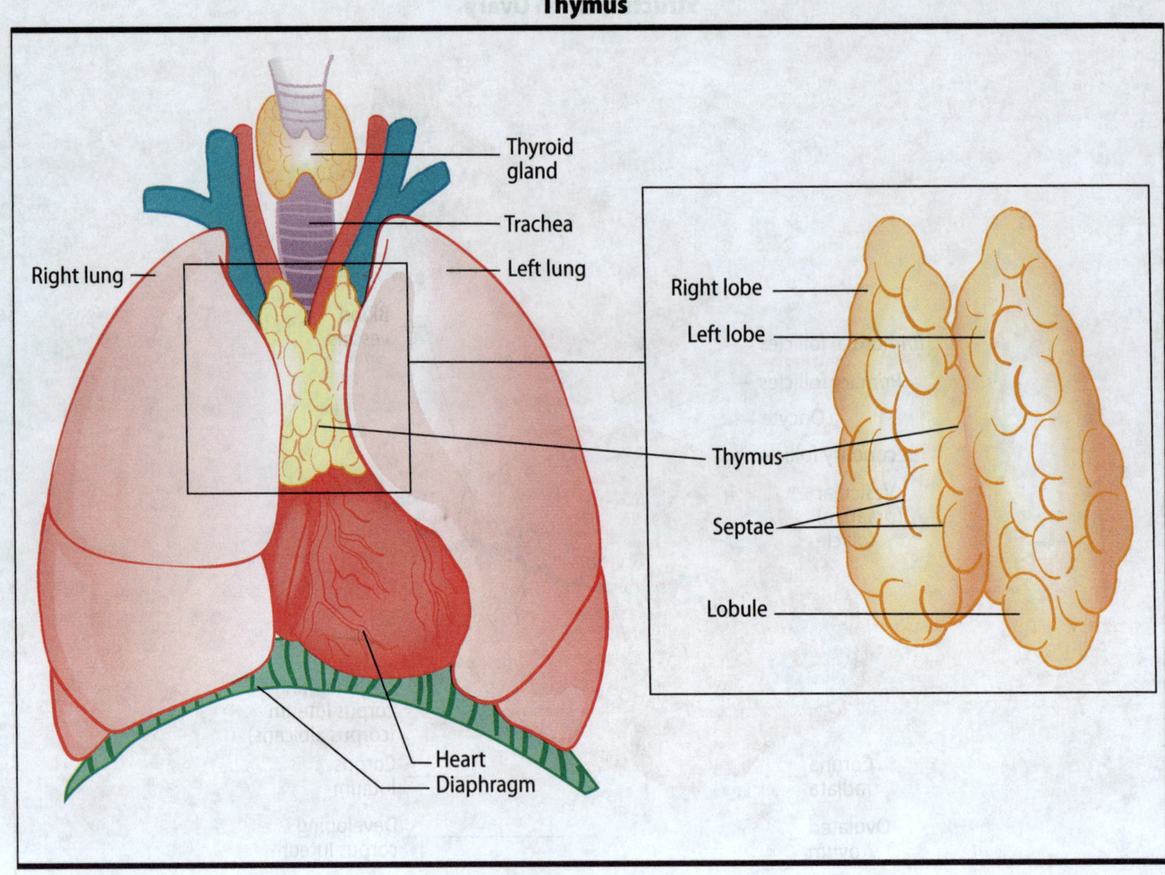

Thyroid gland
Trachea
Right lung
Left lung
Heart
Diaphragm
Right lobe
Left lobe
Thymus
Septae
Lobule

Chapter 6. Diseases of the Nervous System (GØØ–G99)

Brain

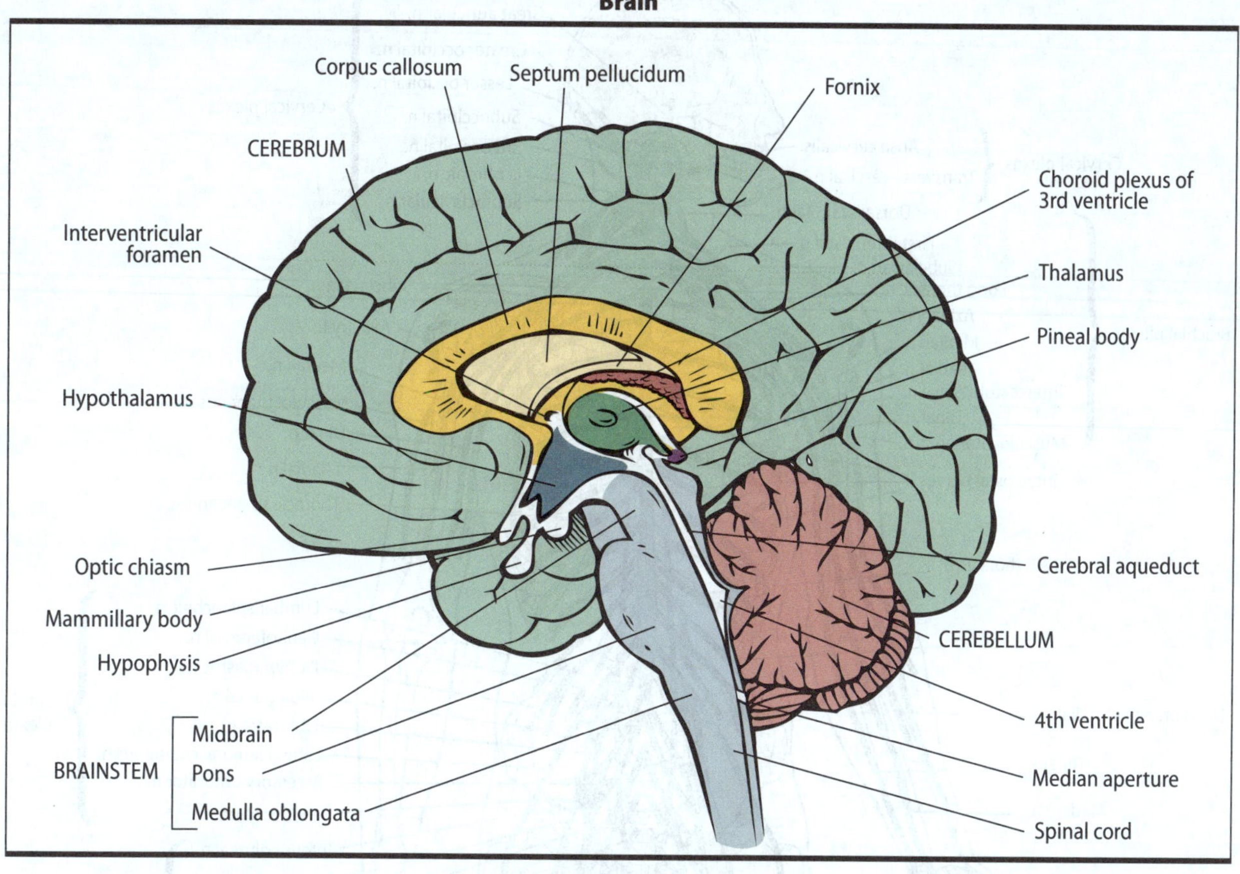

Cranial Nerves

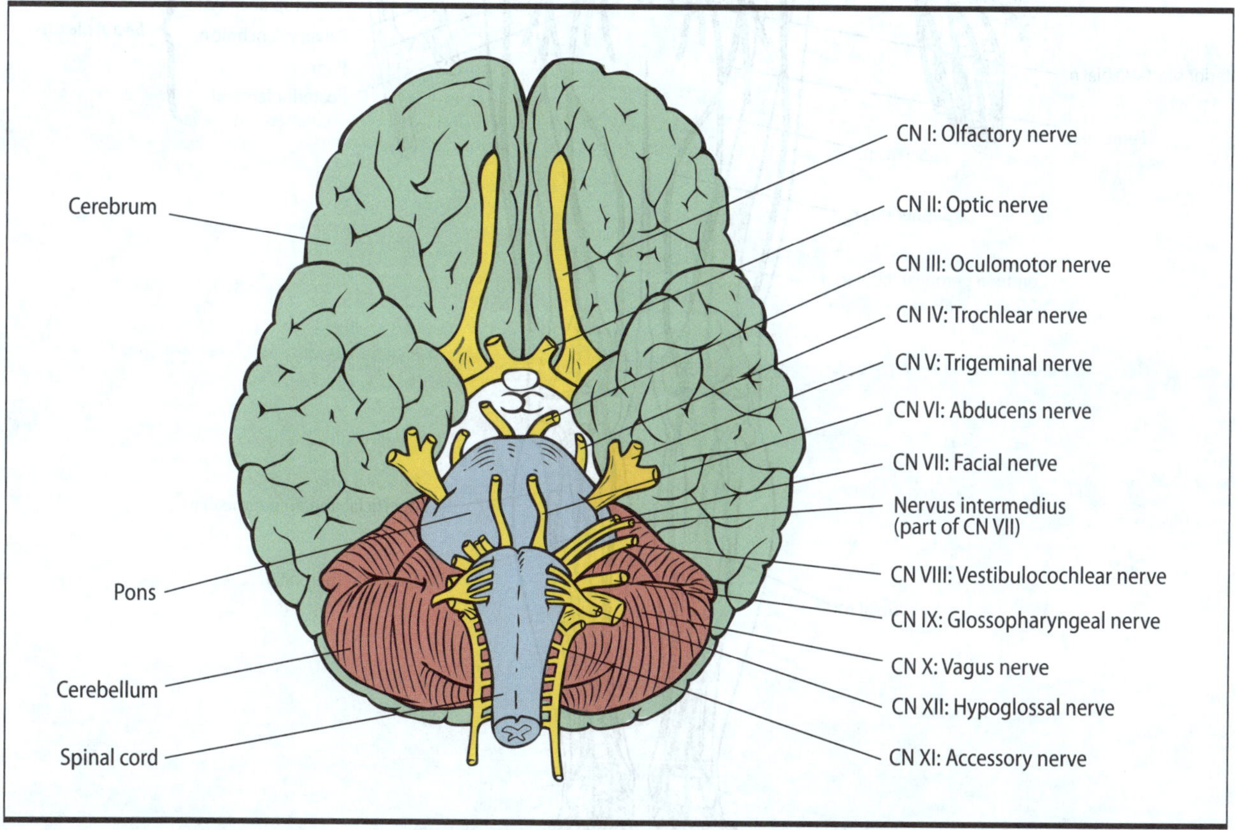

Peripheral Nervous System

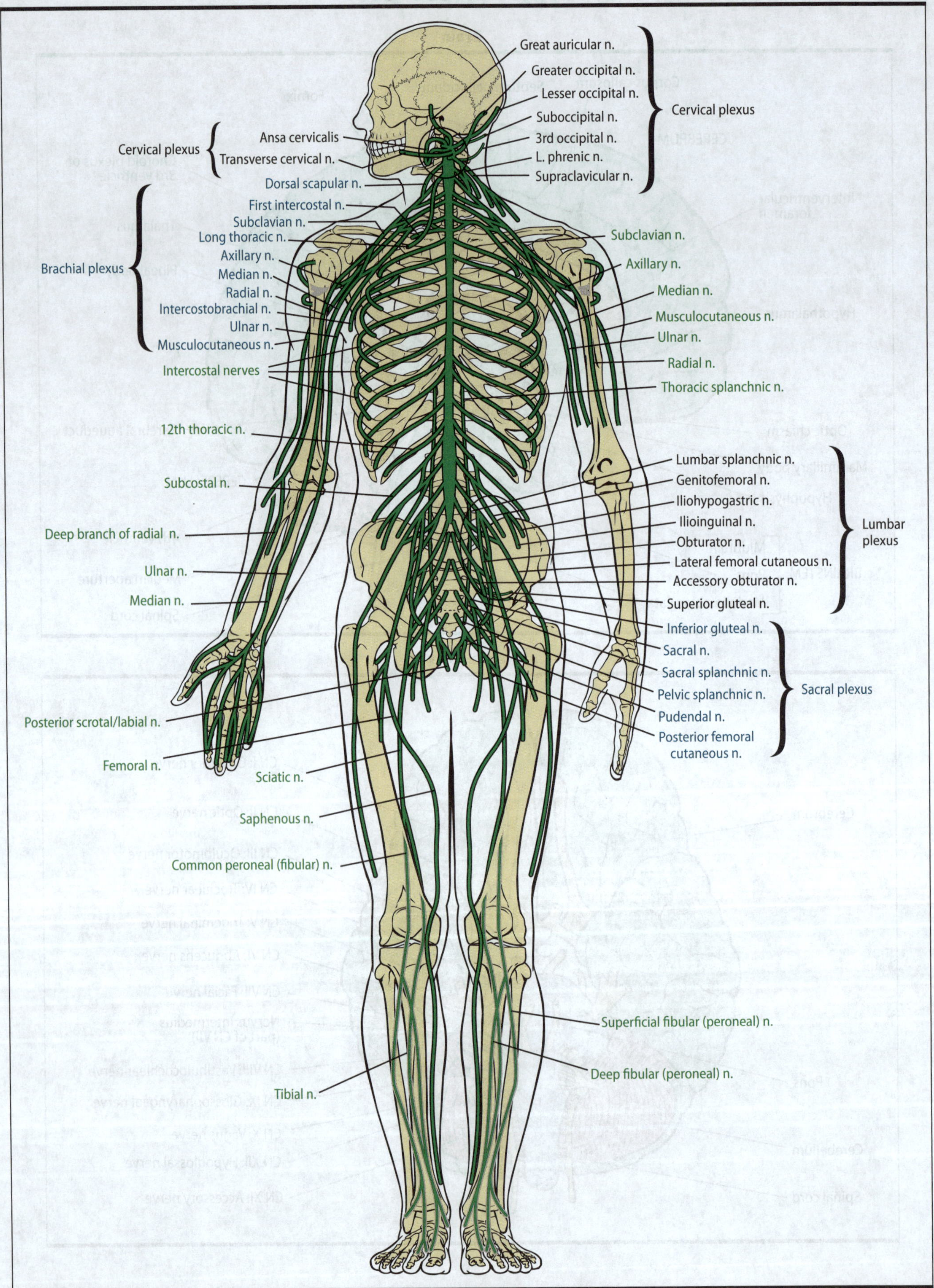

Spinal Cord and Spinal Nerves

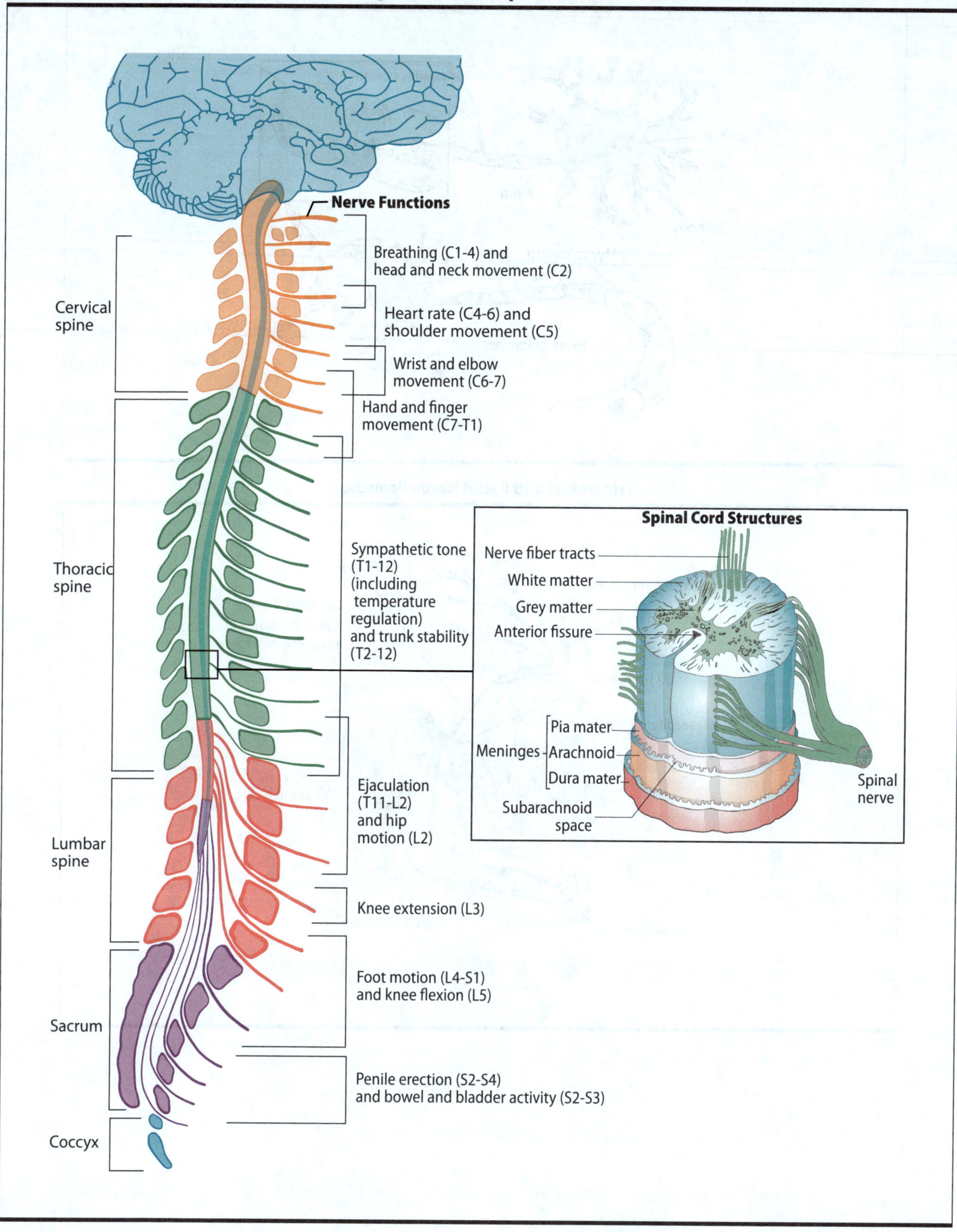

Nerve Cell

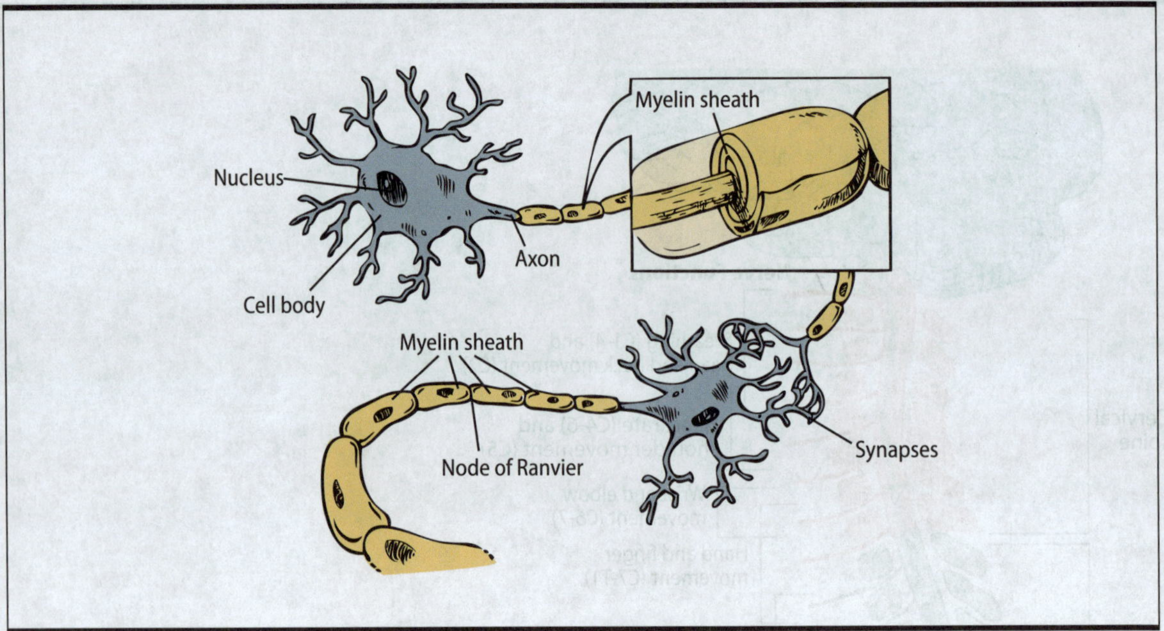

Trigeminal and Facial Nerve Branches

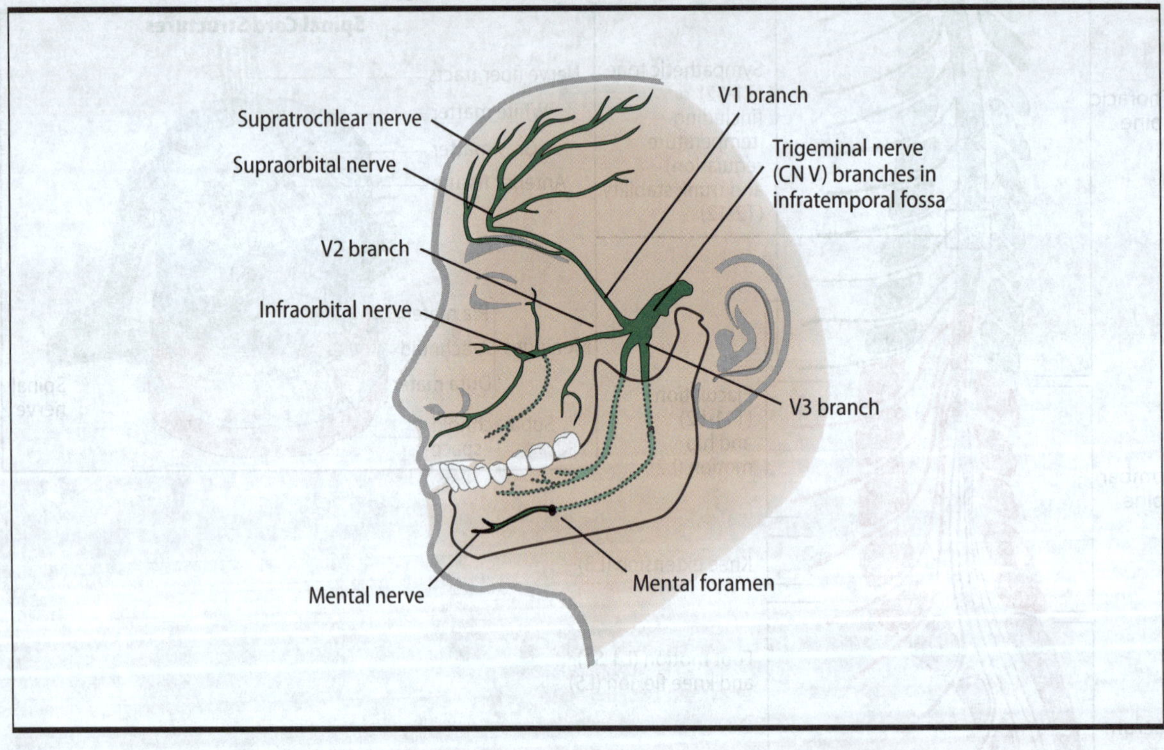

Chapter 7. Diseases of the Eye and Adnexa (HØØ–H59)

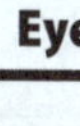

Eye

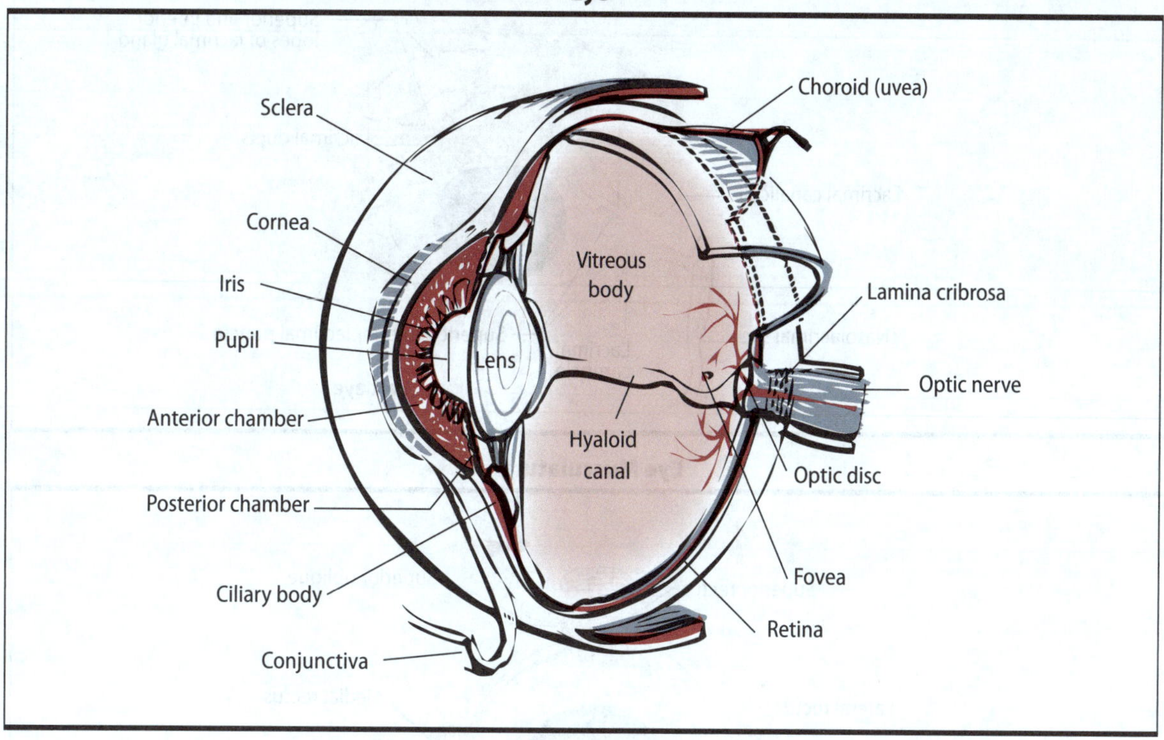

Posterior Pole of Globe/Flow of Aqueous Humor

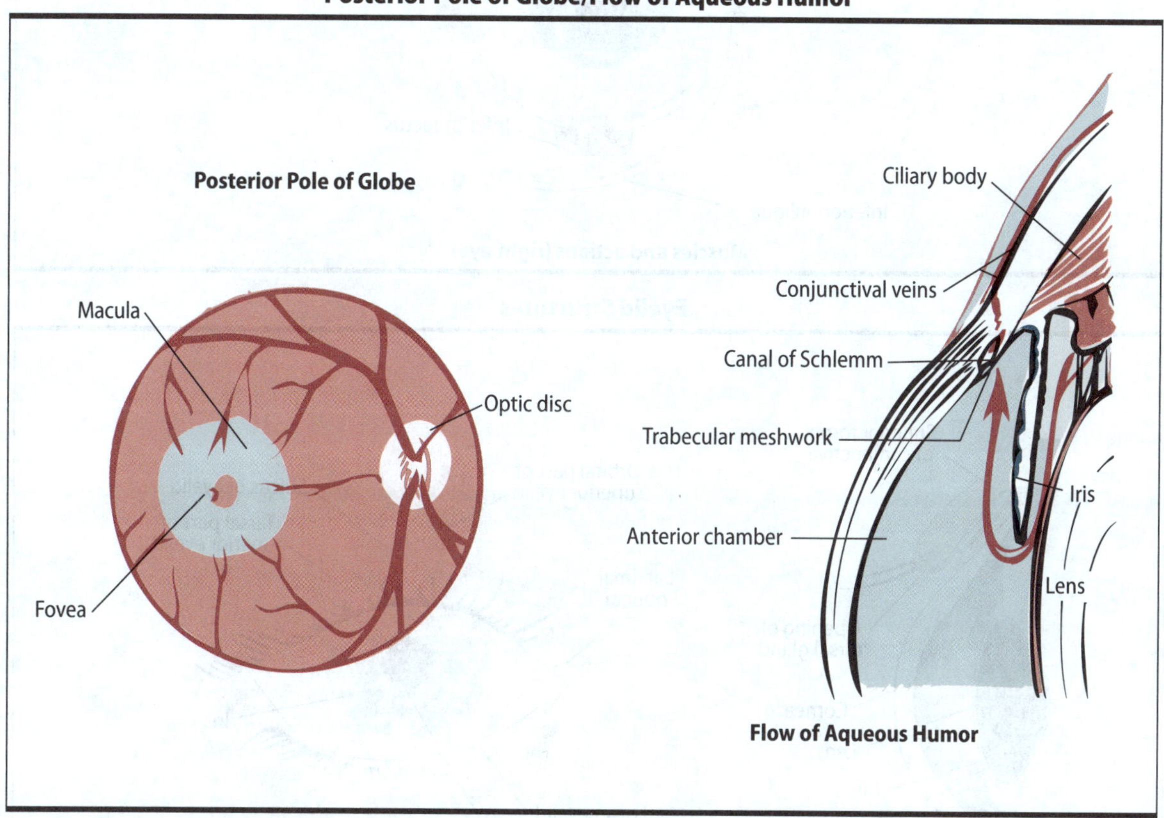

Lacrimal System

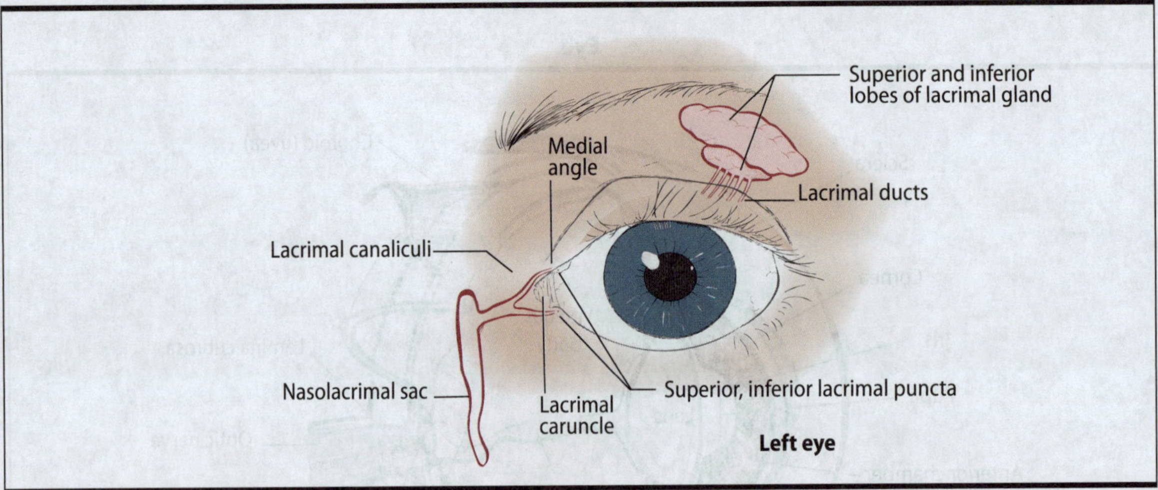

Eye Musculature

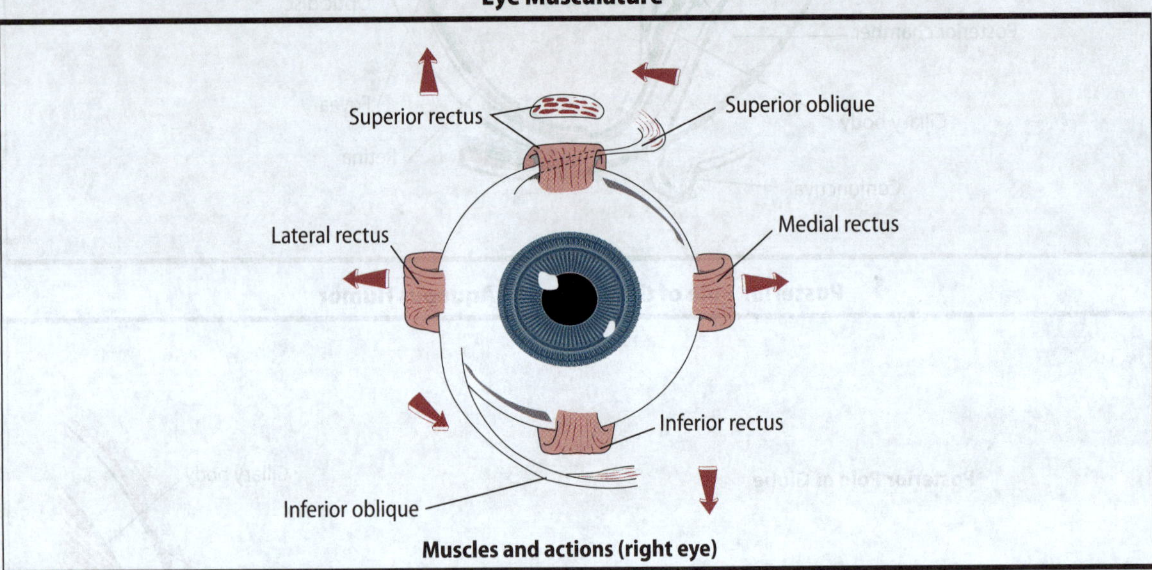

Eyelid Structures

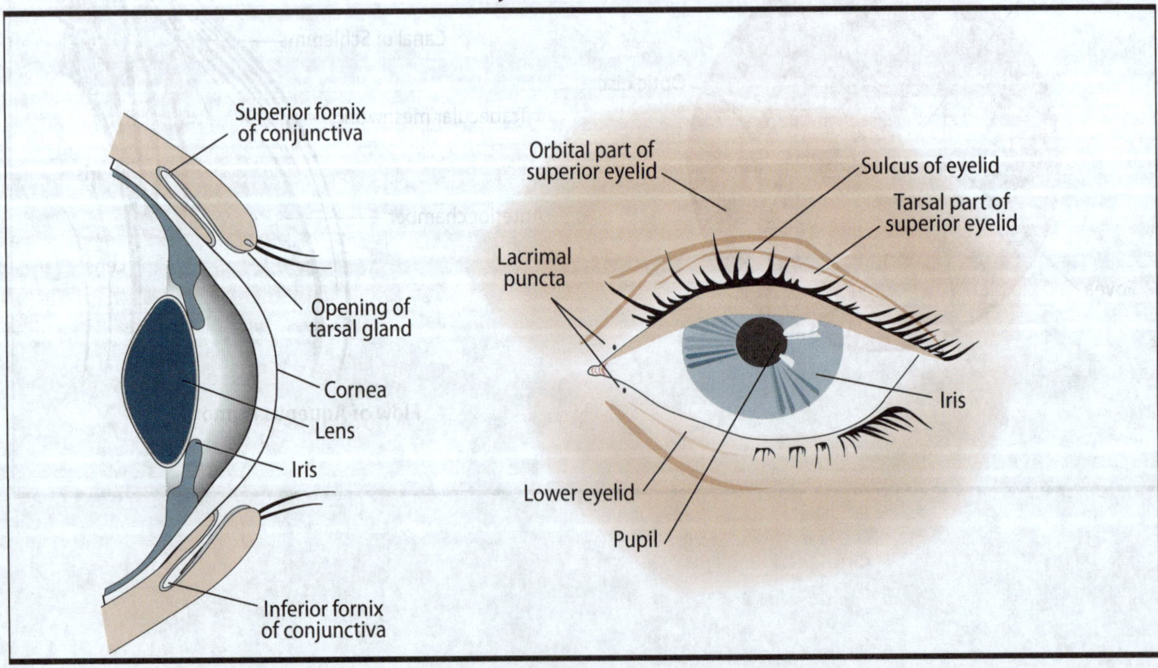

Chapter 8. Diseases of the Ear and Mastoid Process (H60–H95)

Ear Anatomy

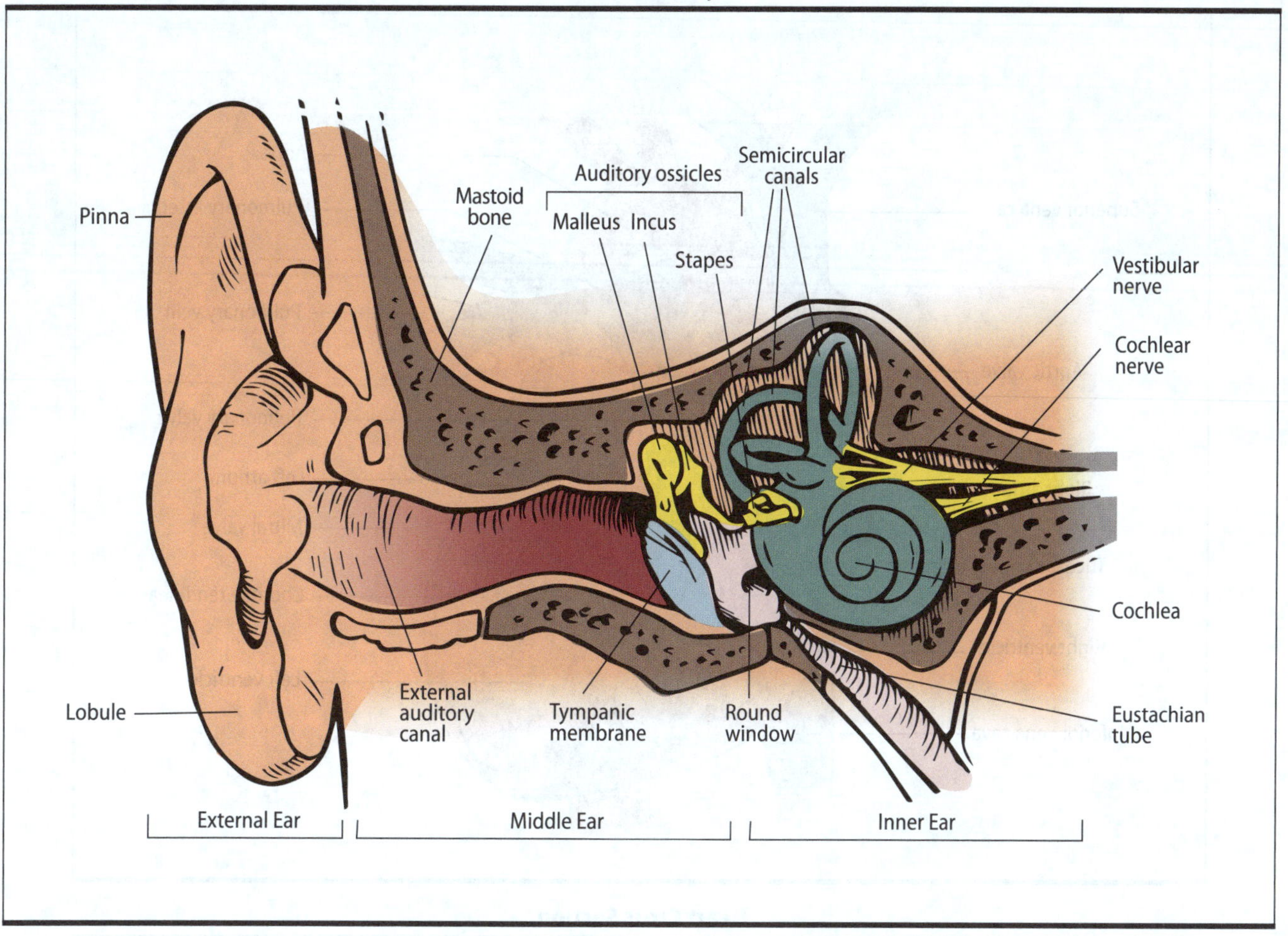

Chapter 9. Diseases of the Circulatory System (IØØ–I99)

Anatomy of the Heart

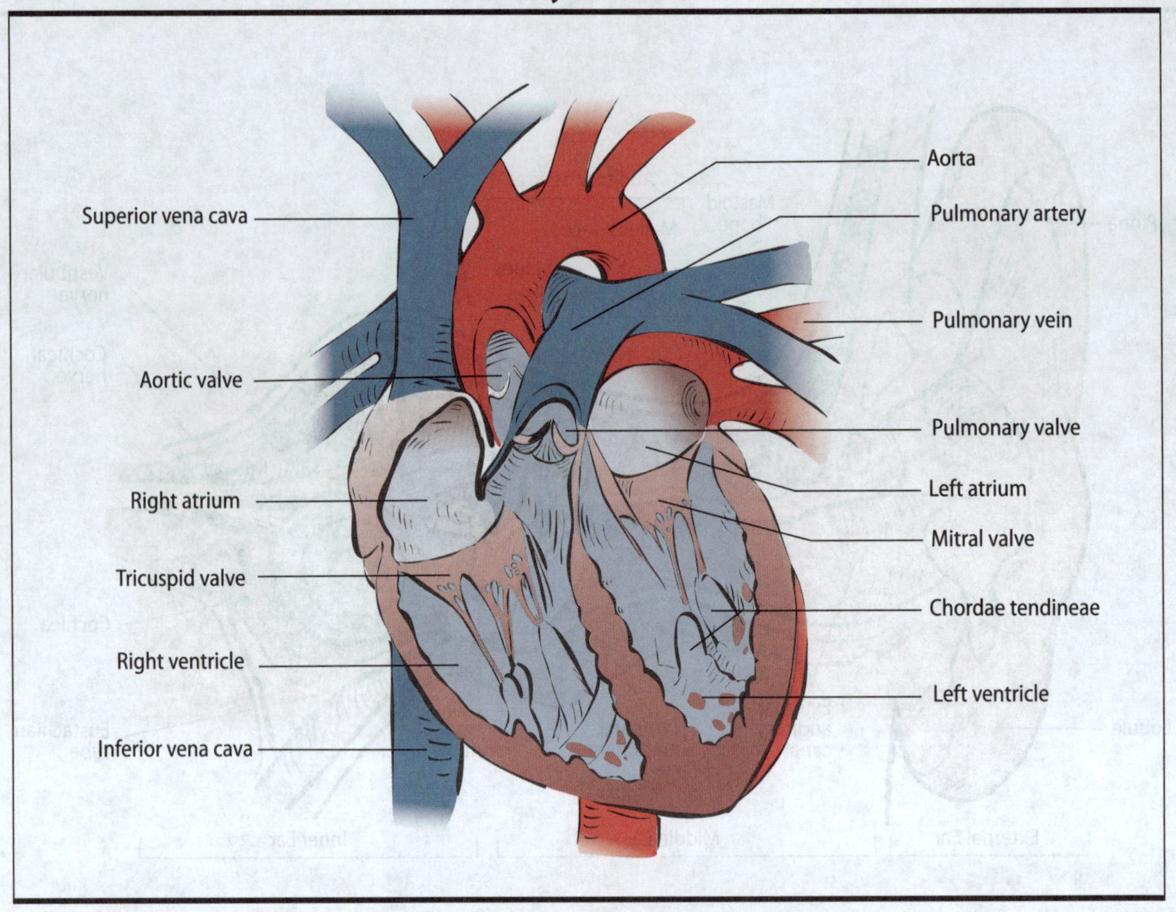

Heart Cross Section

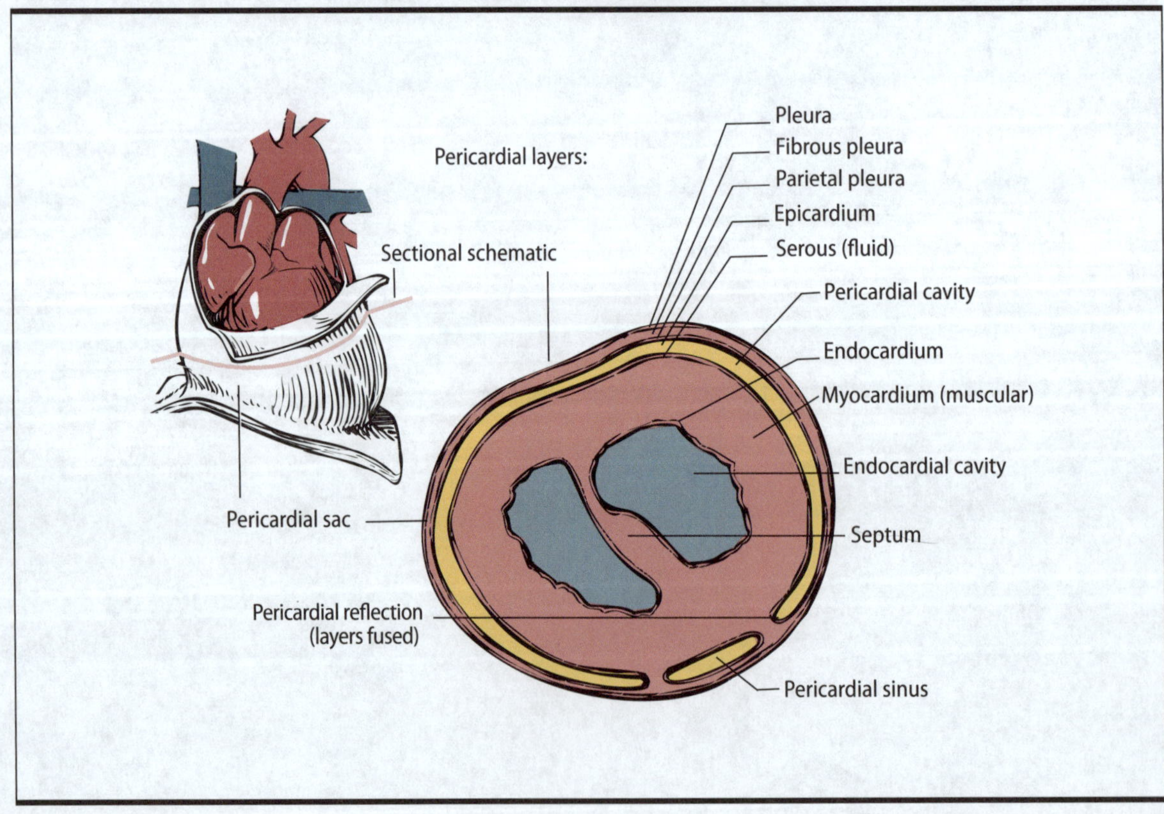

Heart Valves

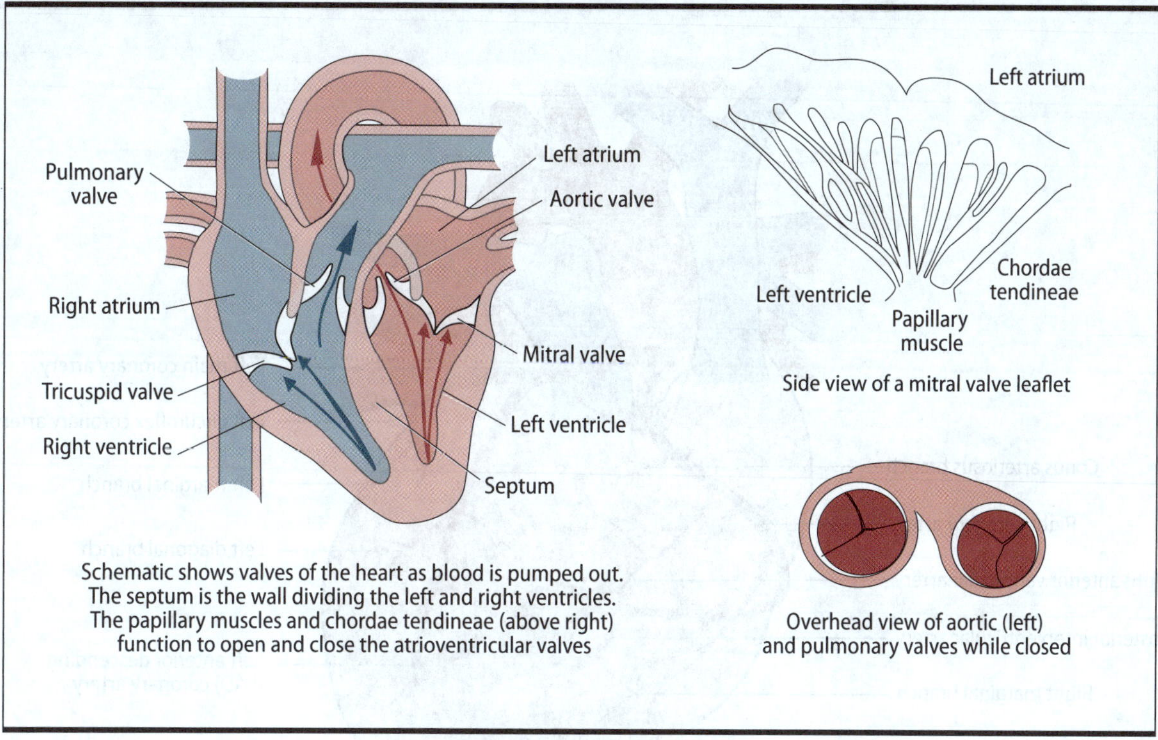

Schematic shows valves of the heart as blood is pumped out. The septum is the wall dividing the left and right ventricles. The papillary muscles and chordae tendineae (above right) function to open and close the atrioventricular valves

Heart Conduction System

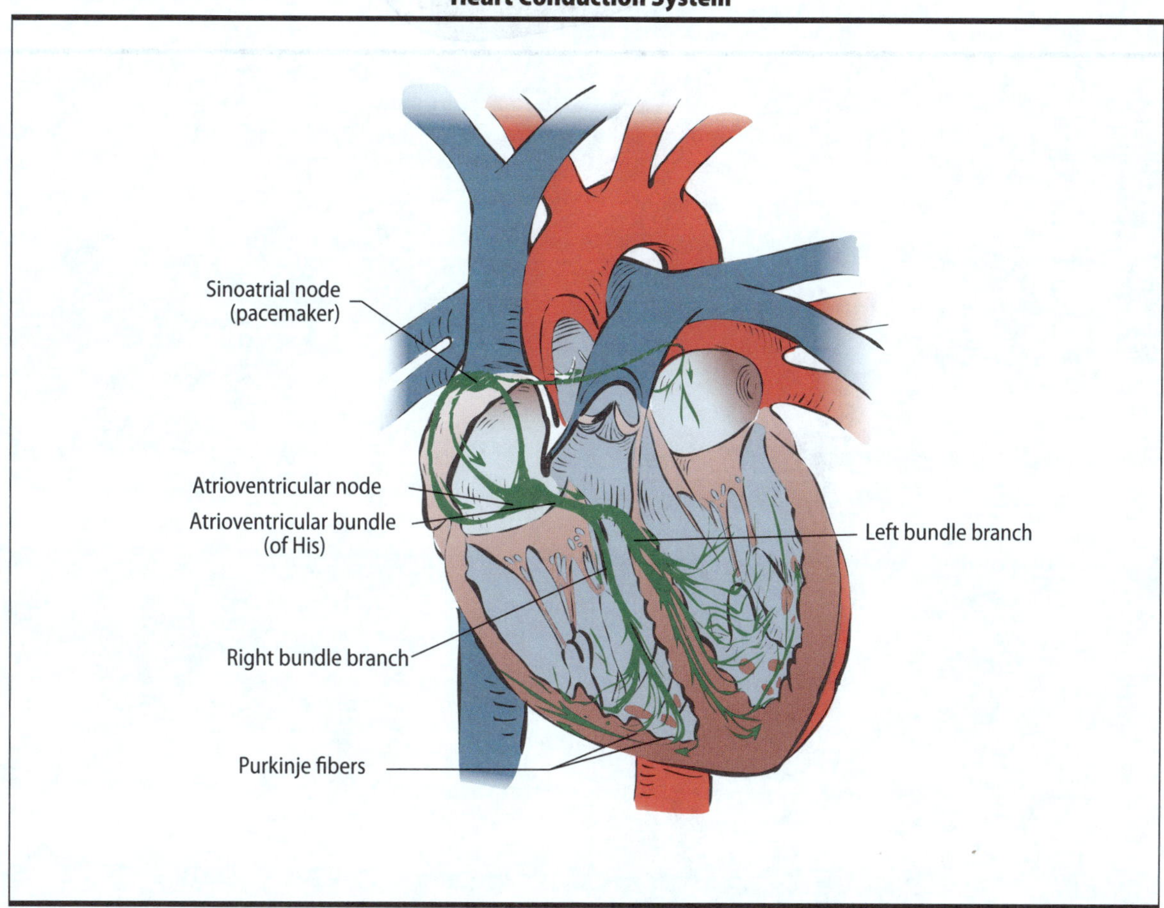

Coronary Arteries

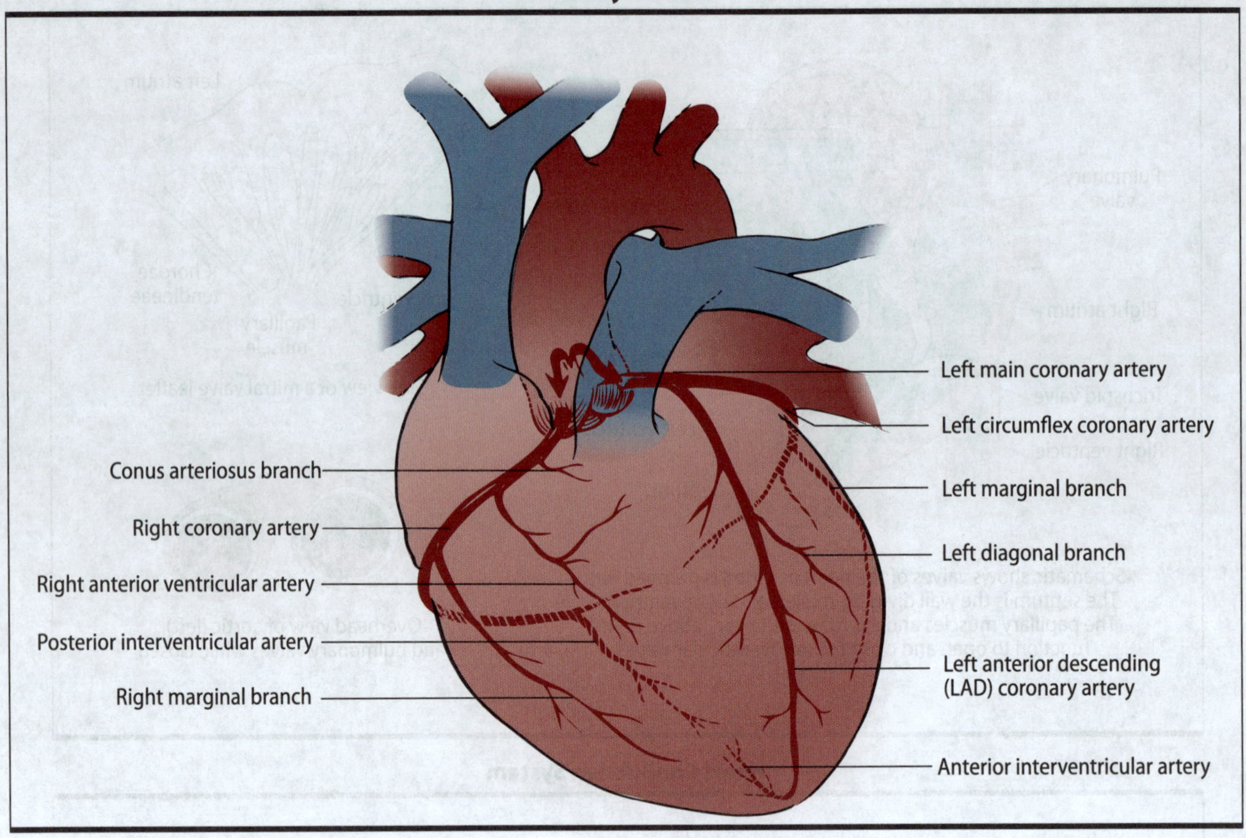

Arteries

Middle temporal a.
Transverse facial a.
Superficial temporal a.
External carotid a.
Internal carotid a.
Common carotid a.
Superior thyroid a.
Vertebral a.
Inferior thyroid a.
Subclavian a.
Innominate a.
Arch of aorta
Ascending aorta
Pulmonary a.
Axillary a.
Internal thoracic a. (mammary)
Descending aorta
Brachial a.
Common hepatic a.
L. gastric a.
Celiac trunk (artery)
Splenic a.
R. gastric a.
Renal a.
Superior mesenteric a.
R. colic a.
Abdominal aorta
L. colic a.
Radial a.
Inferior mesenteric a.
Ulnar a.
Common iliac a.
Internal iliac a.
External iliac a.
Uterine a.
Femoral a.
Popliteal a.
Anterior tibial a.
Peroneal a.
Posterior tibial a.

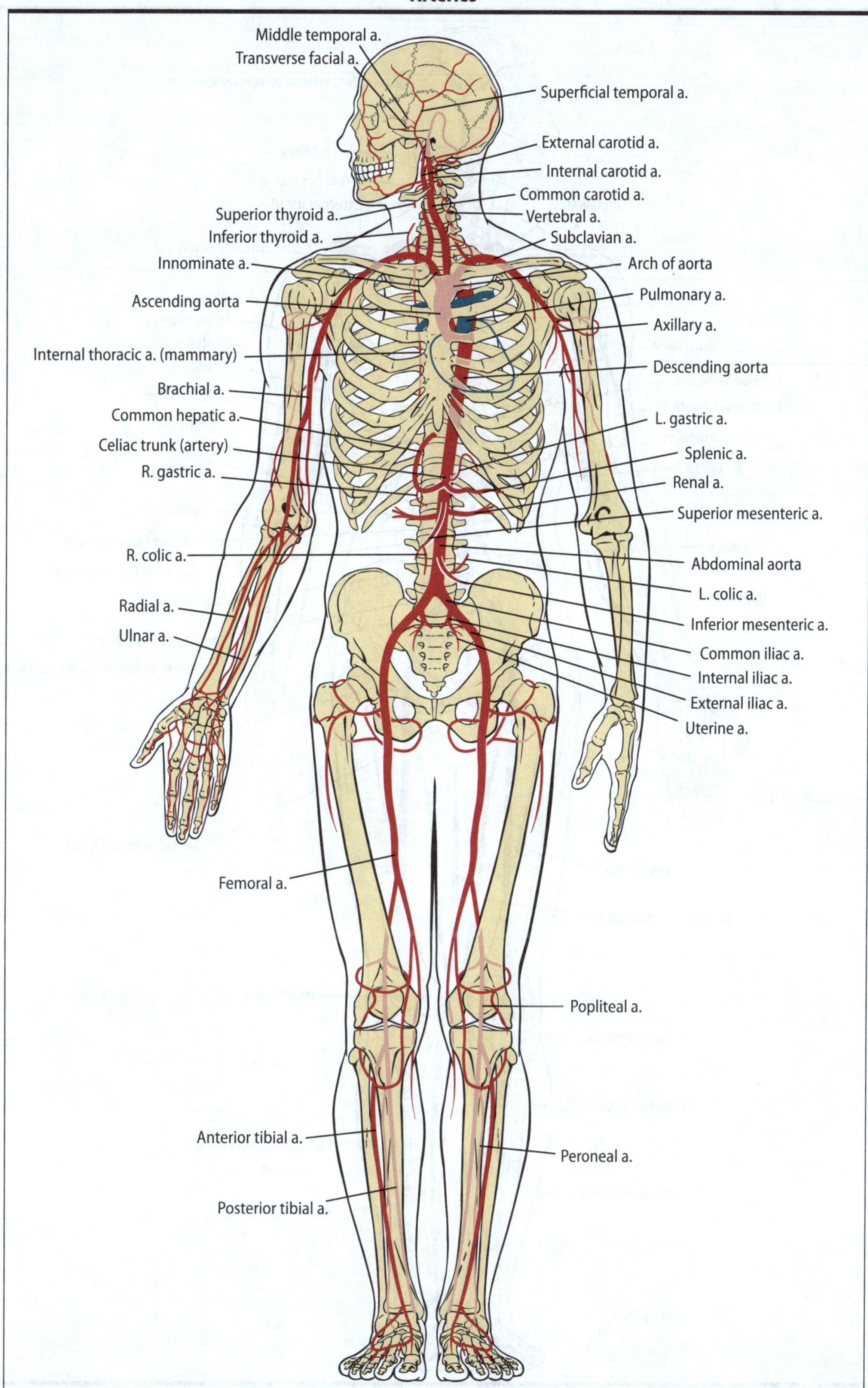

Veins

Superficial temporal v.
Vertebral v.
Internal jugular v.
Subclavian v.
External jugular v.
Innominate v.
Azygos v.
Axillary v.
Hemiazygos v.
Brachial v.
Cephalic v.
Inferior vena cava
Basilic v.
Esophageal v.
Common hepatic v.
L. gastric v.
Portal v.
R. gastric v.
Splenic v.
Renal v.
Inferior mesenteric v.
R. colic v.
Superior mesenteric v.
Radial v.
L. colic v.
Ulnar v.
Common iliac v.
Internal iliac v. (Hypogastric v.)
External iliac v.
Internal pudendal v.
Rectal venous plexus
Femoral v.
Greater saphenous v.
Popliteal v.
Lesser saphenous v.
Anterior tibial v.
Lesser saphenous v.
Posterior tibial v.
Greater saphenous v.

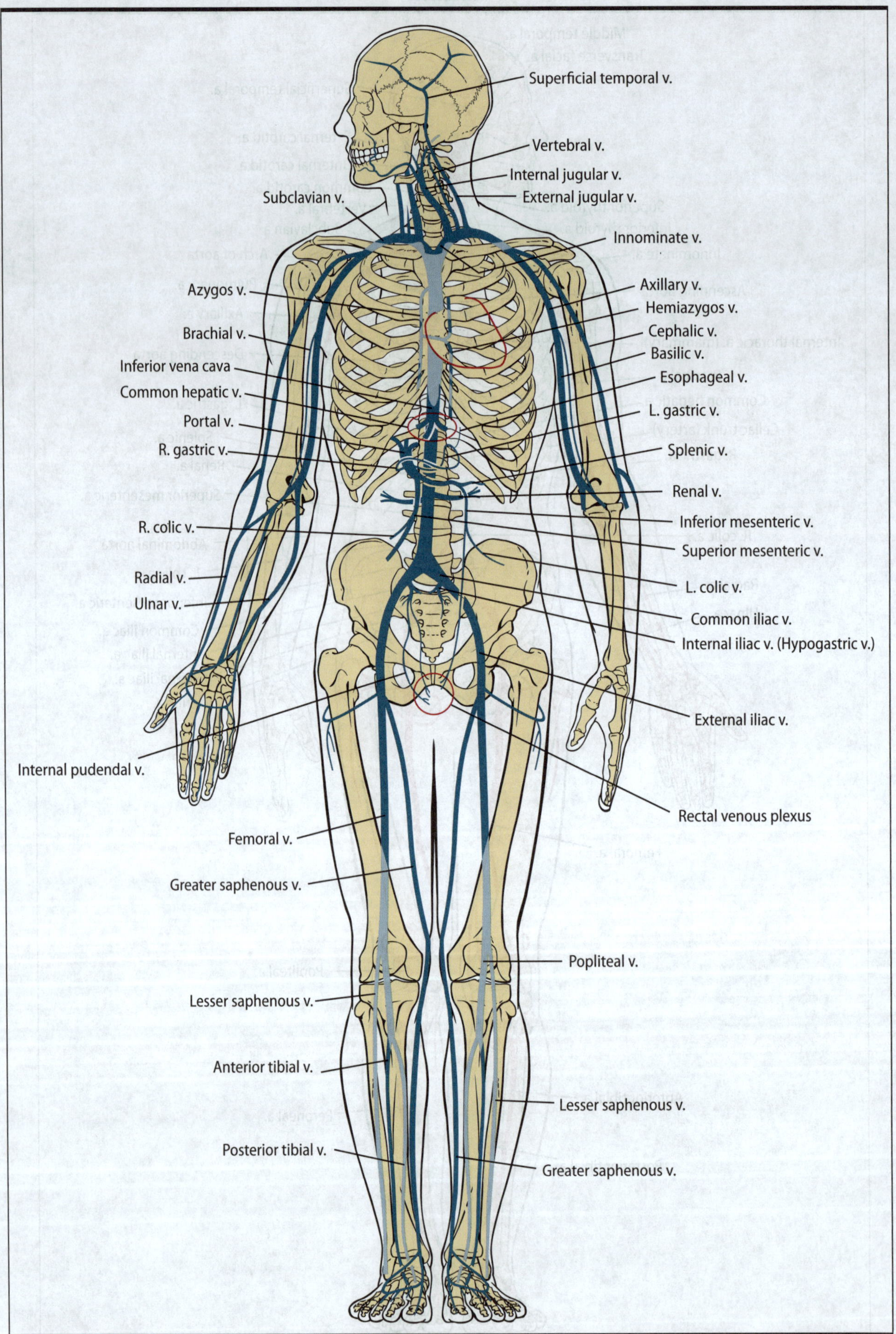

Internal Carotid and Vertebral Arteries and Branches

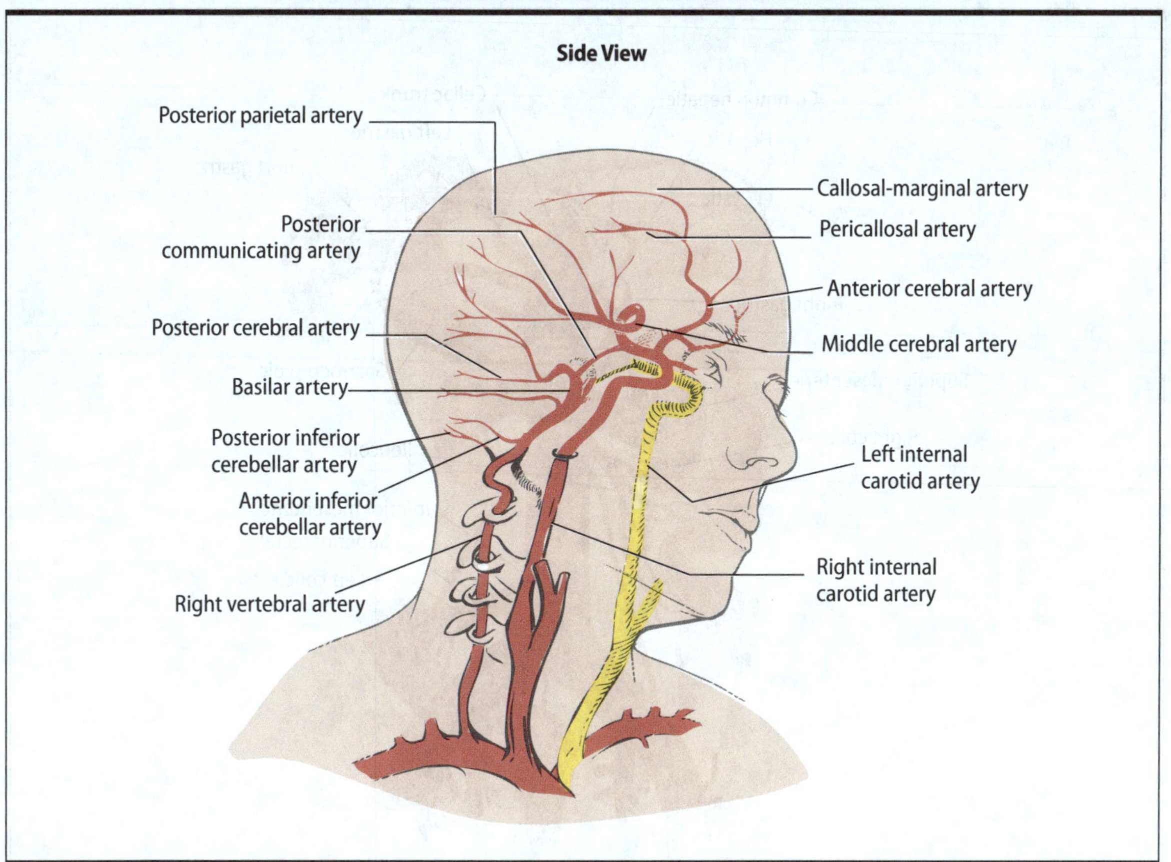

External Carotid Artery and Branches

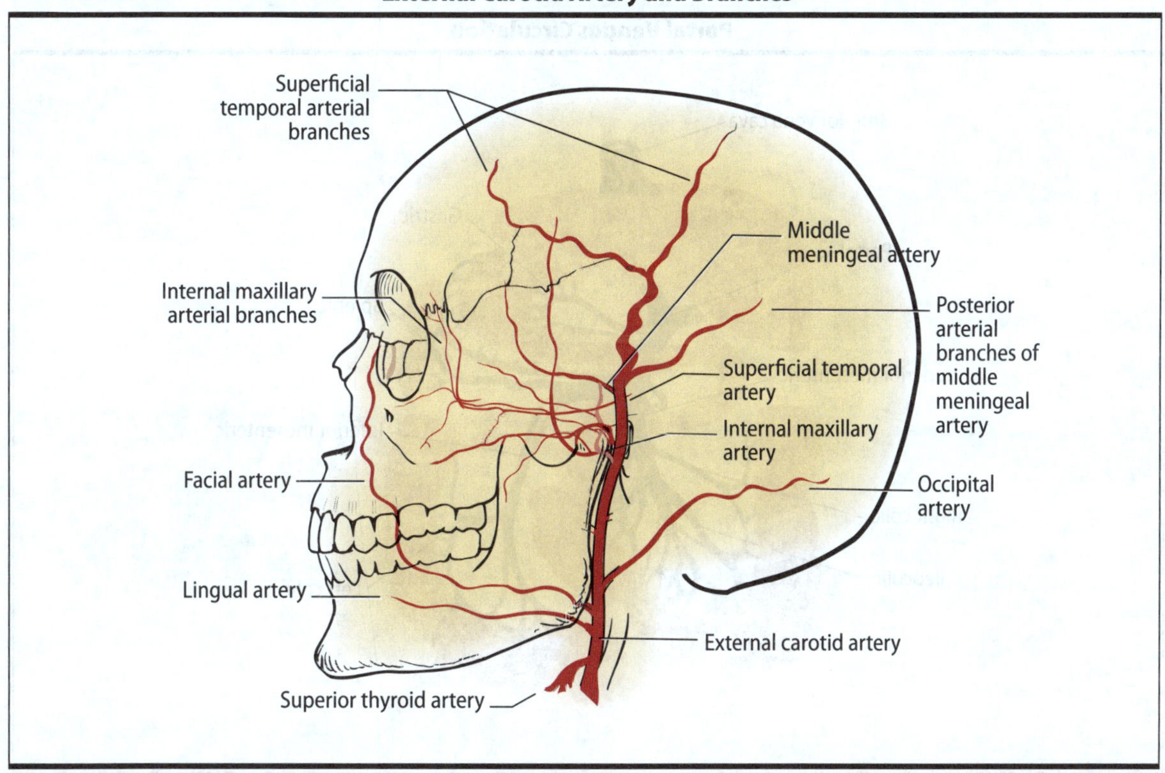

Branches of Abdominal Aorta

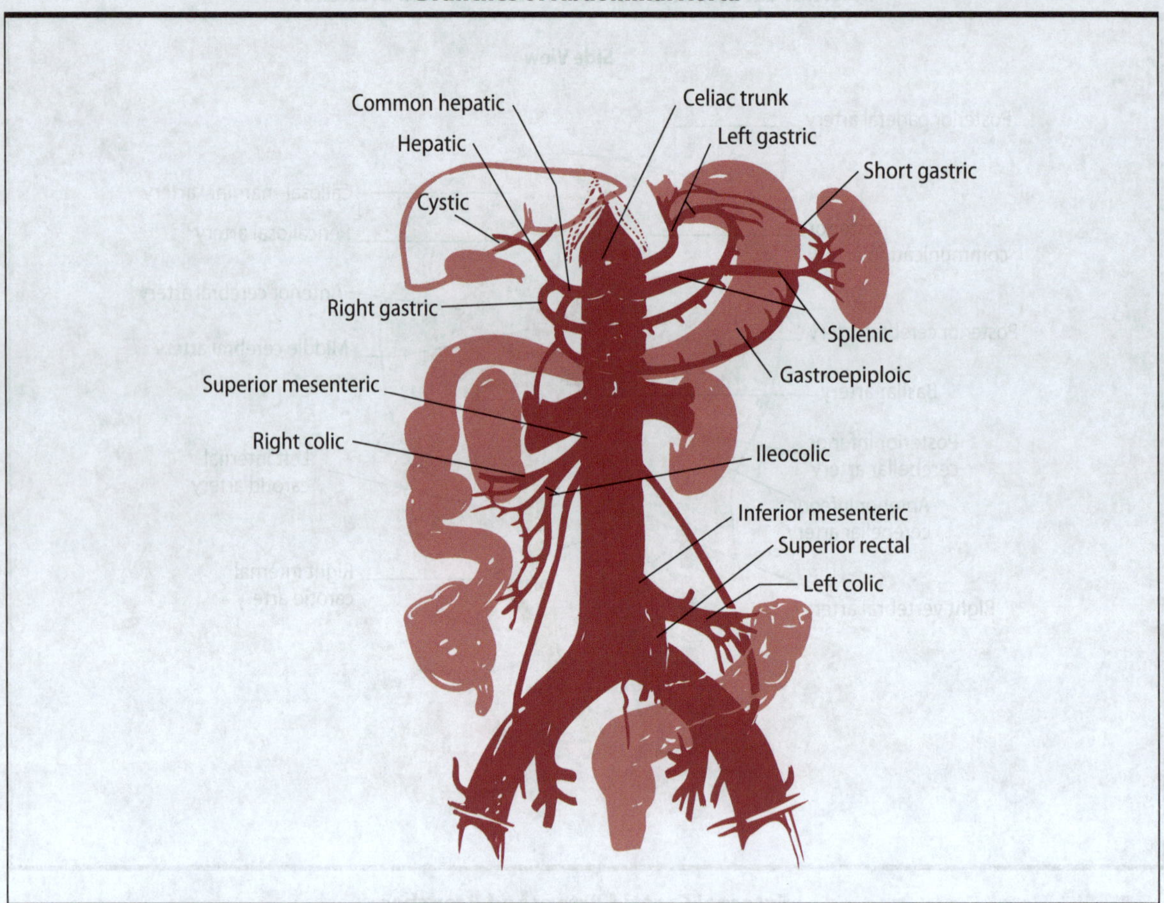

Portal Venous Circulation

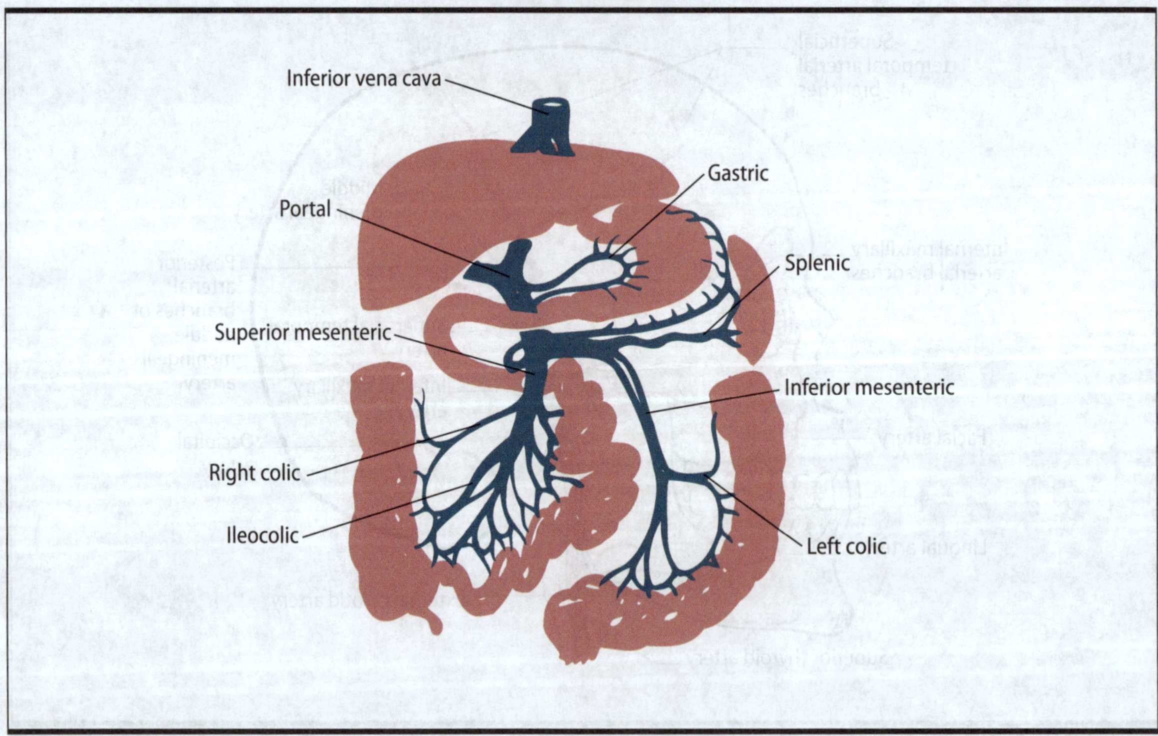

Lymphatic System

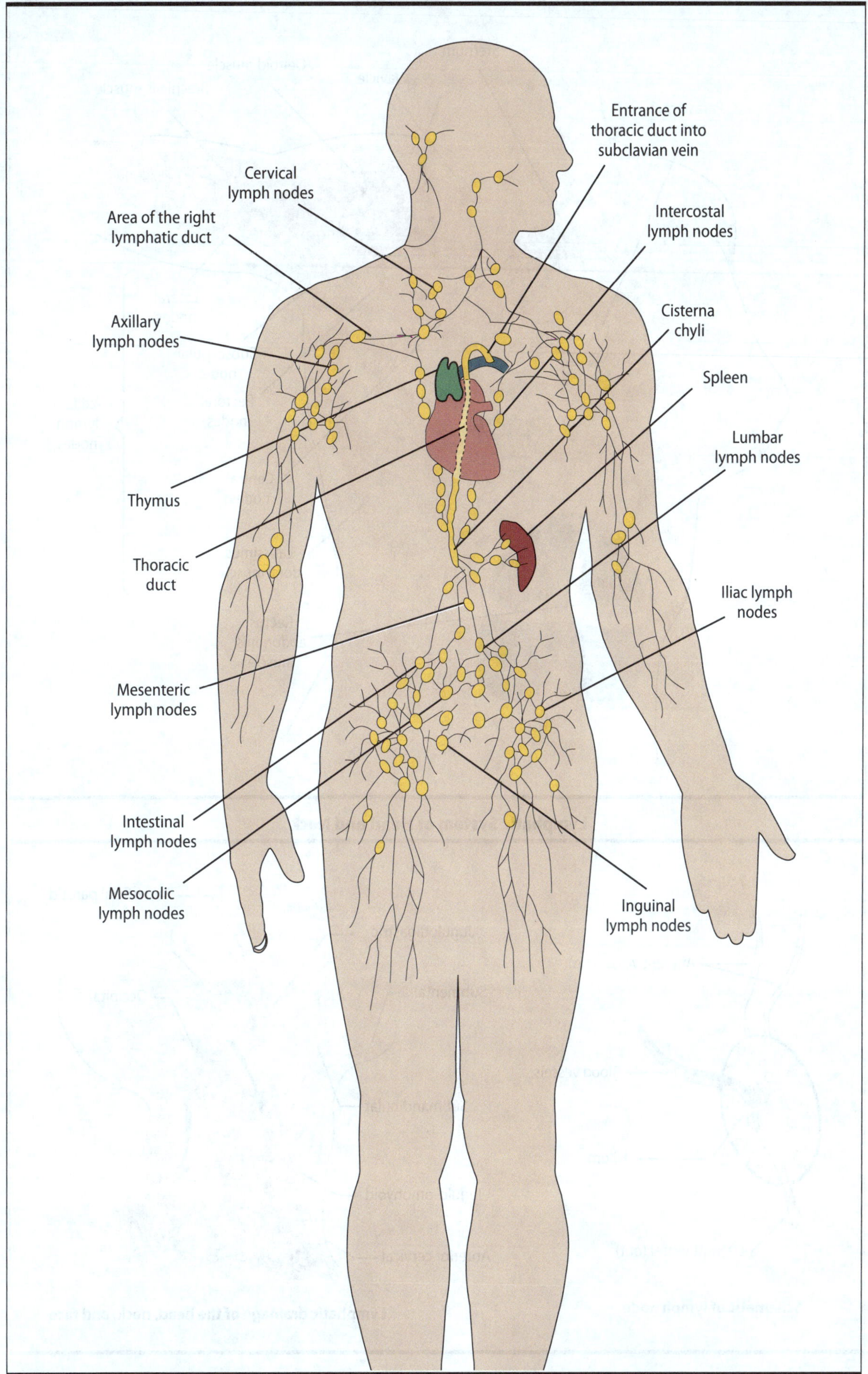

Axillary Lymph Nodes

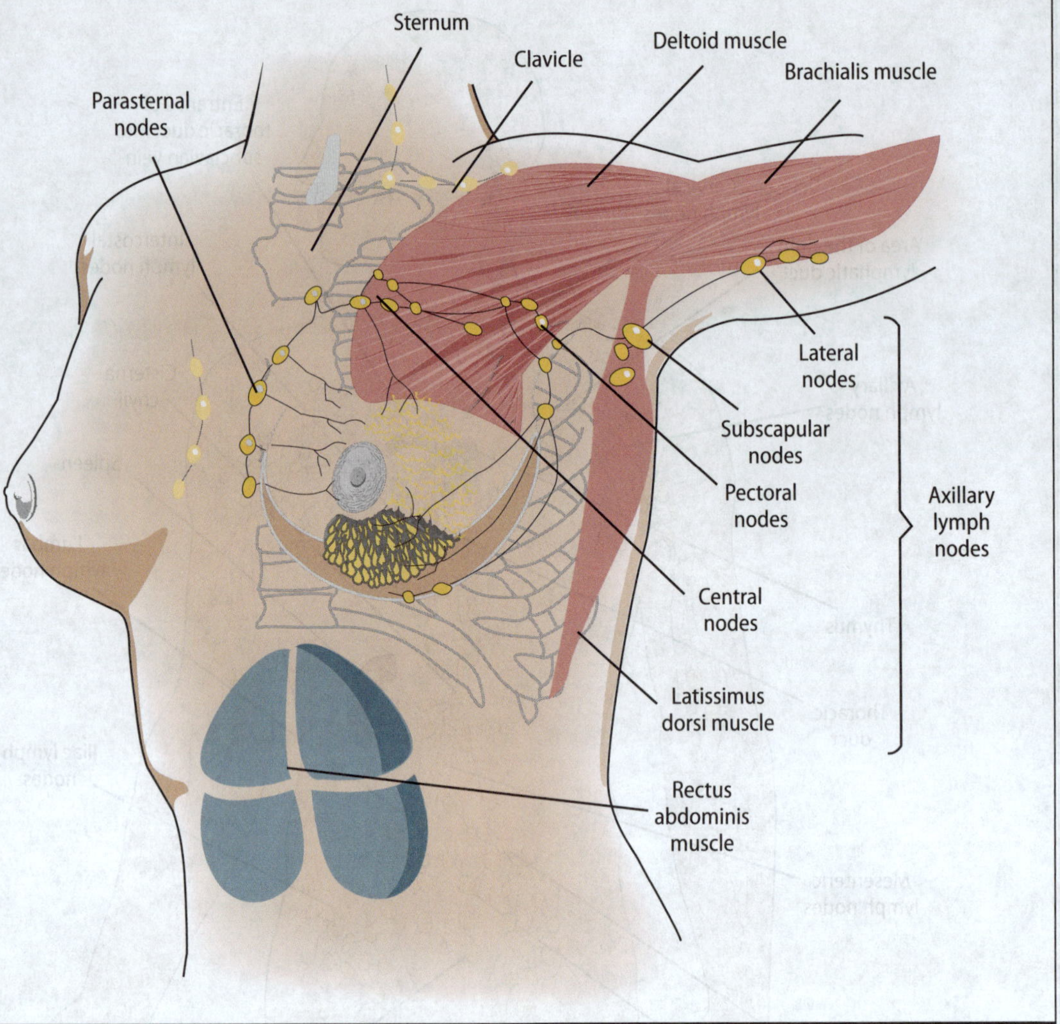

Sternum
Clavicle
Deltoid muscle
Brachialis muscle
Parasternal nodes
Lateral nodes
Subscapular nodes
Pectoral nodes
Axillary lymph nodes
Central nodes
Latissimus dorsi muscle
Rectus abdominis muscle

Lymphatic System of Head and Neck

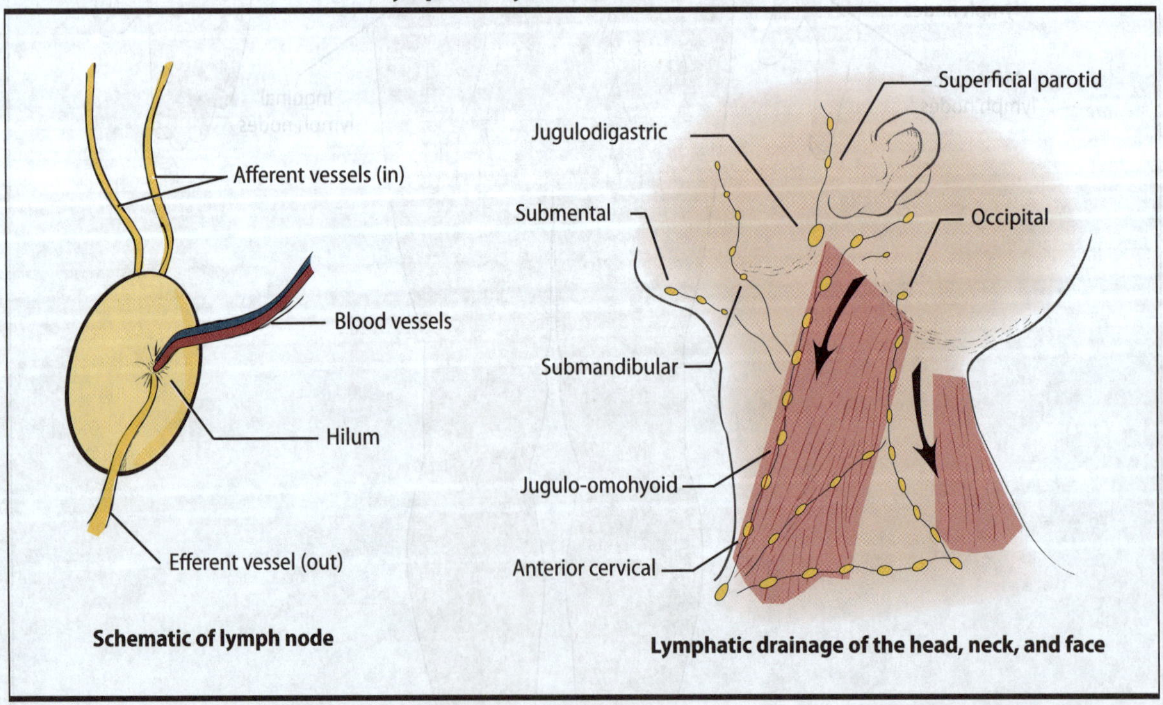

Schematic of lymph node

Lymphatic drainage of the head, neck, and face

Lymphatic Capillaries

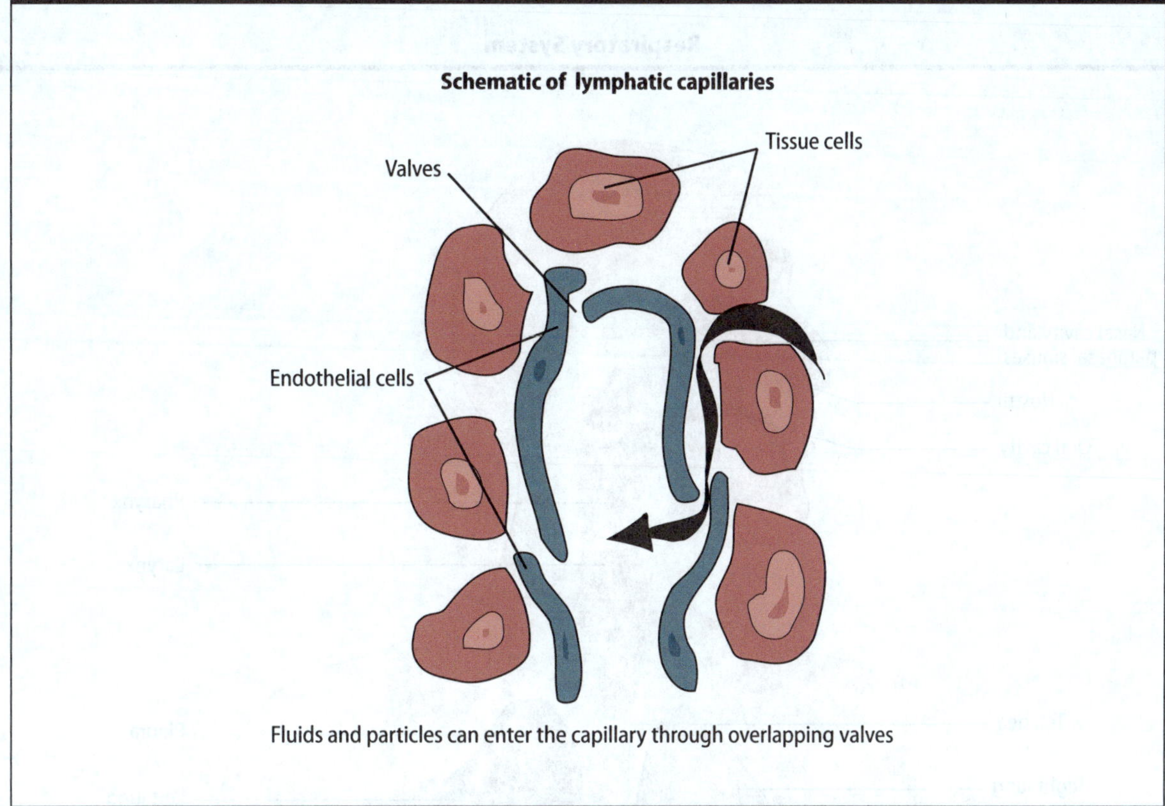

Schematic of lymphatic capillaries
Tissue cells
Valves
Endothelial cells
Fluids and particles can enter the capillary through overlapping valves

Lymphatic Drainage

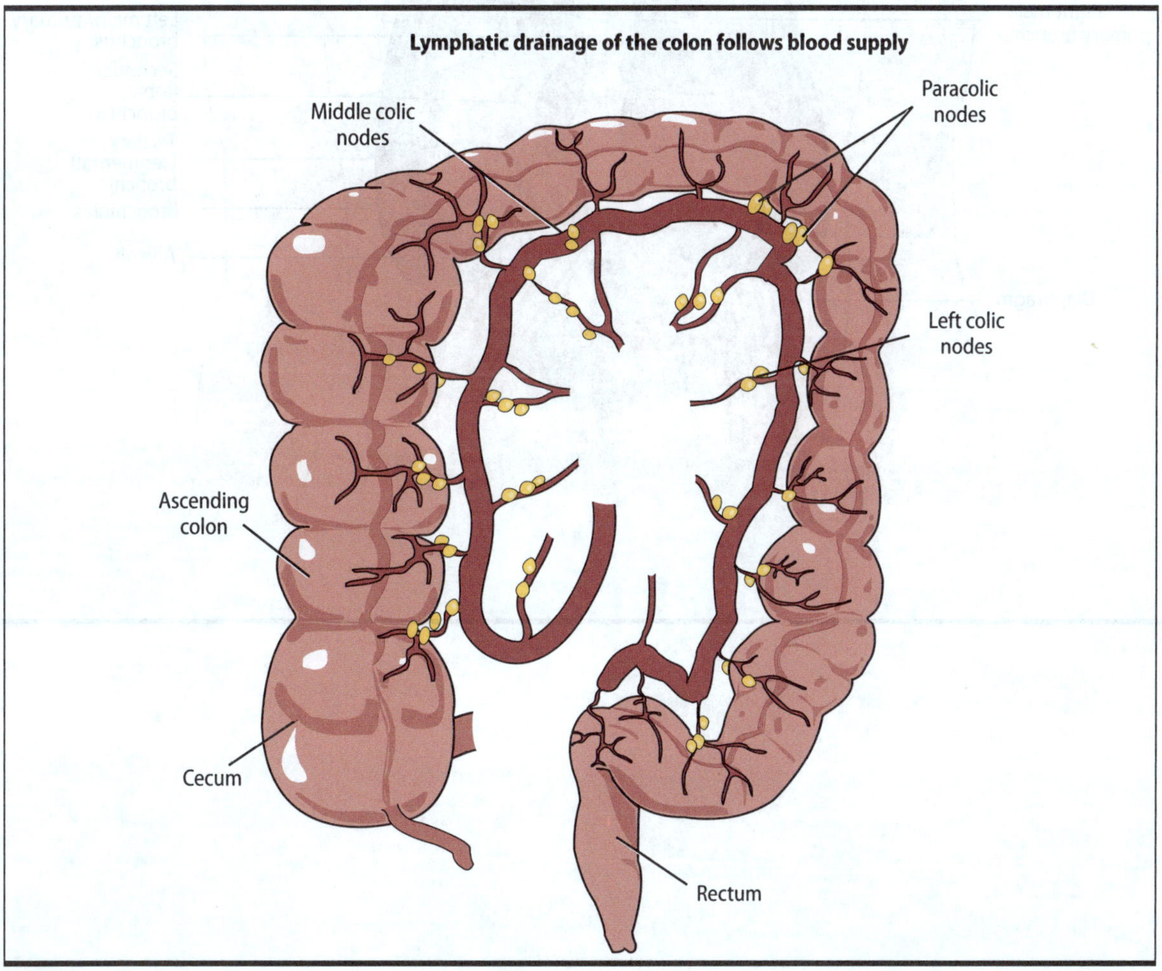

Lymphatic drainage of the colon follows blood supply
Middle colic nodes
Paracolic nodes
Left colic nodes
Ascending colon
Cecum
Rectum

Chapter 10. Diseases of the Respiratory System (JØØ–J99)

Respiratory System

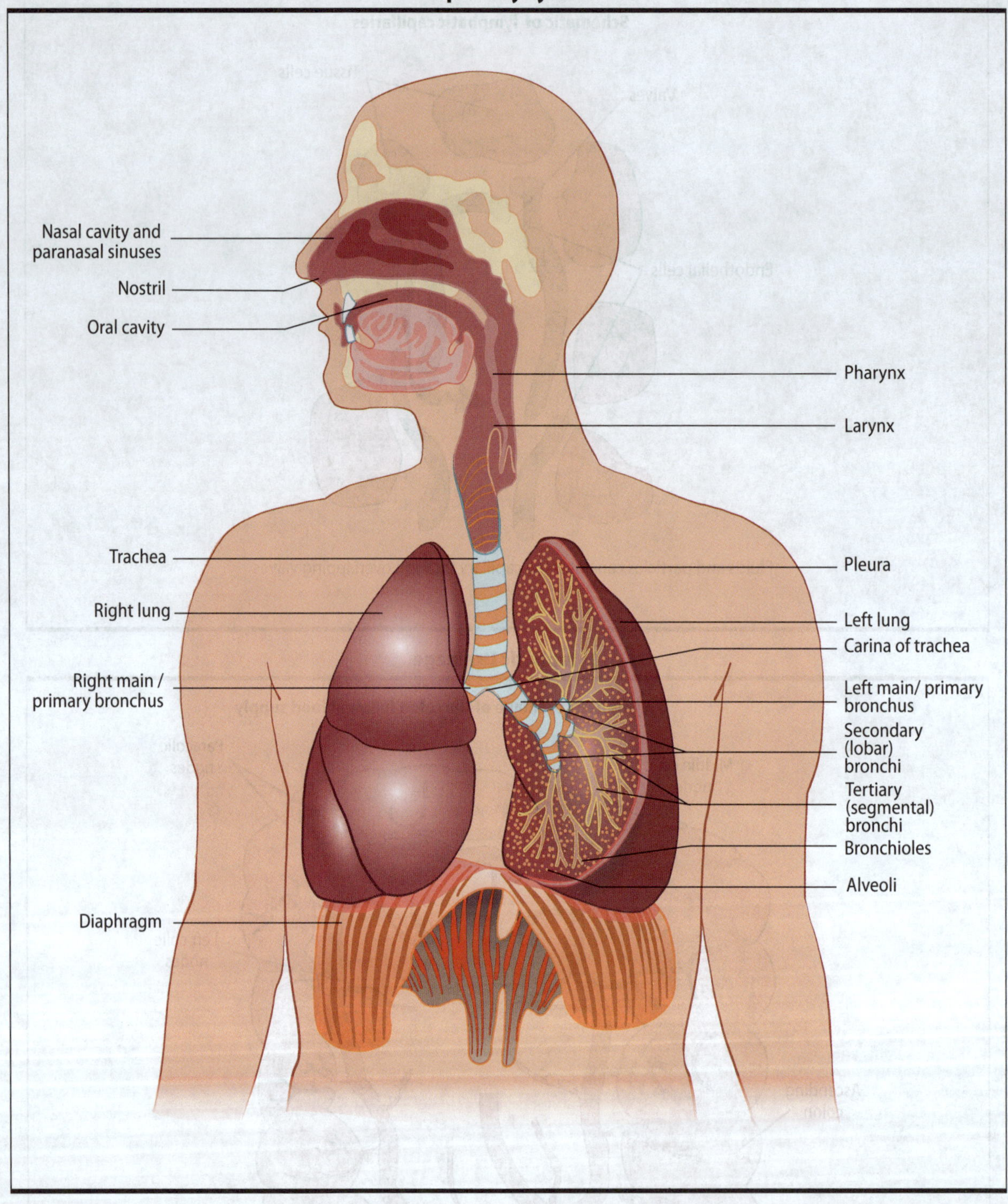

Upper Respiratory System

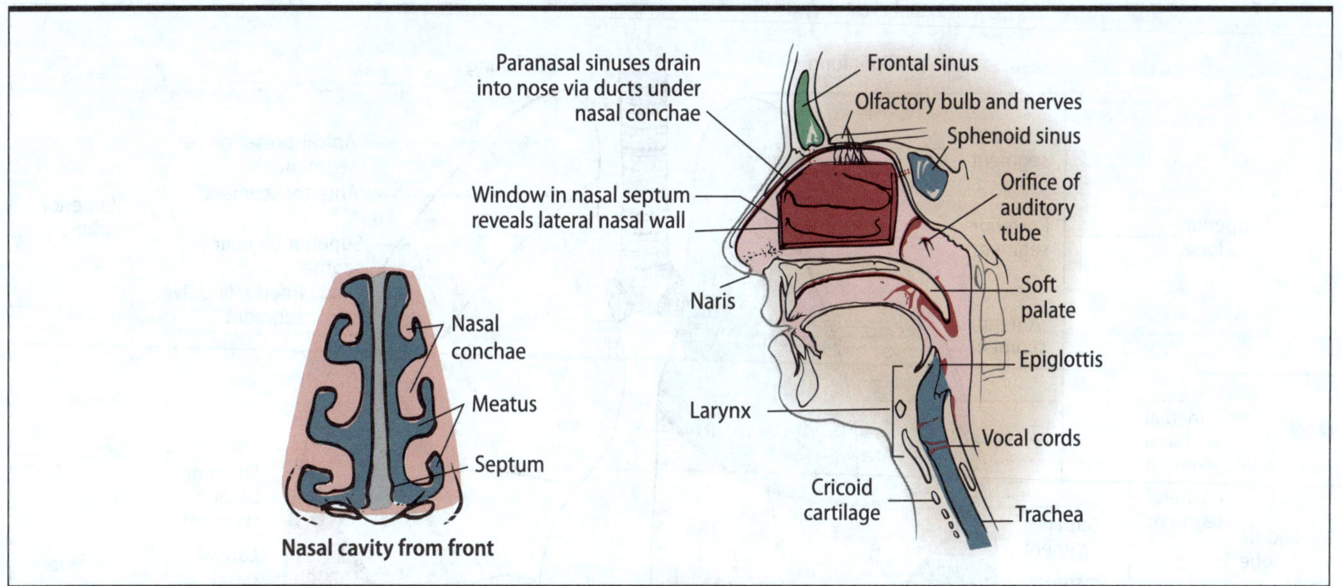

Lower Respiratory System

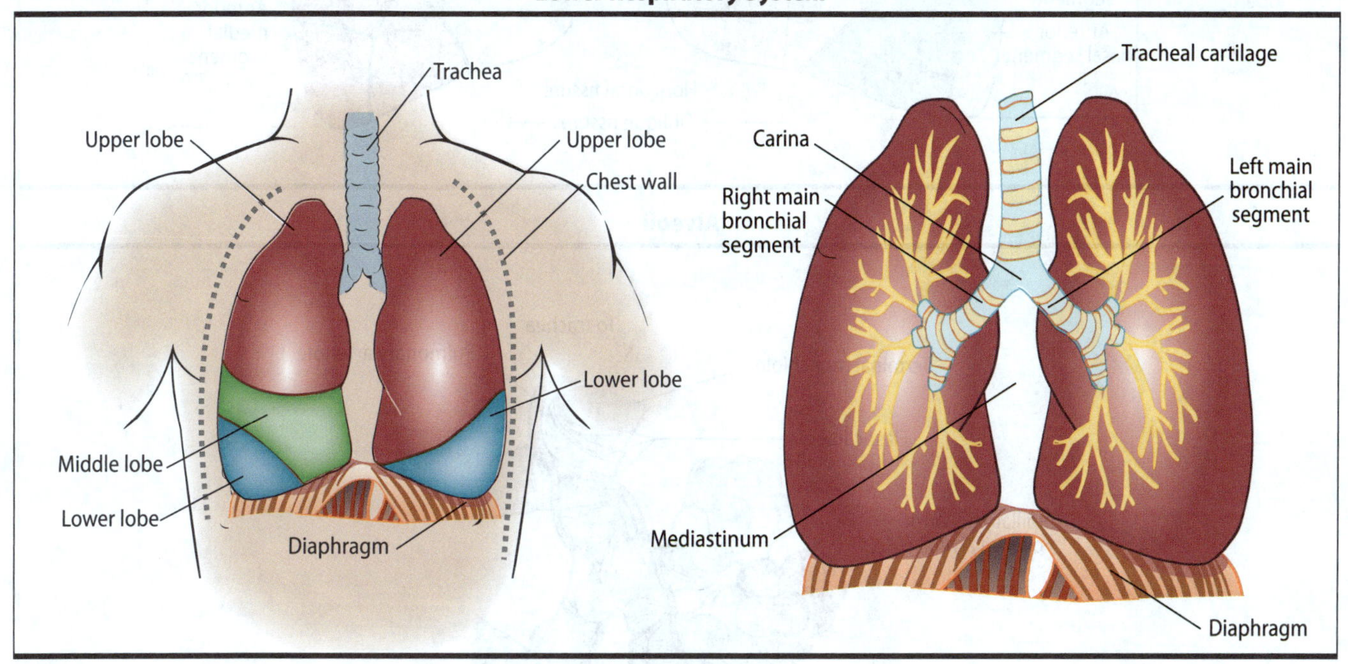

Paranasal Sinuses

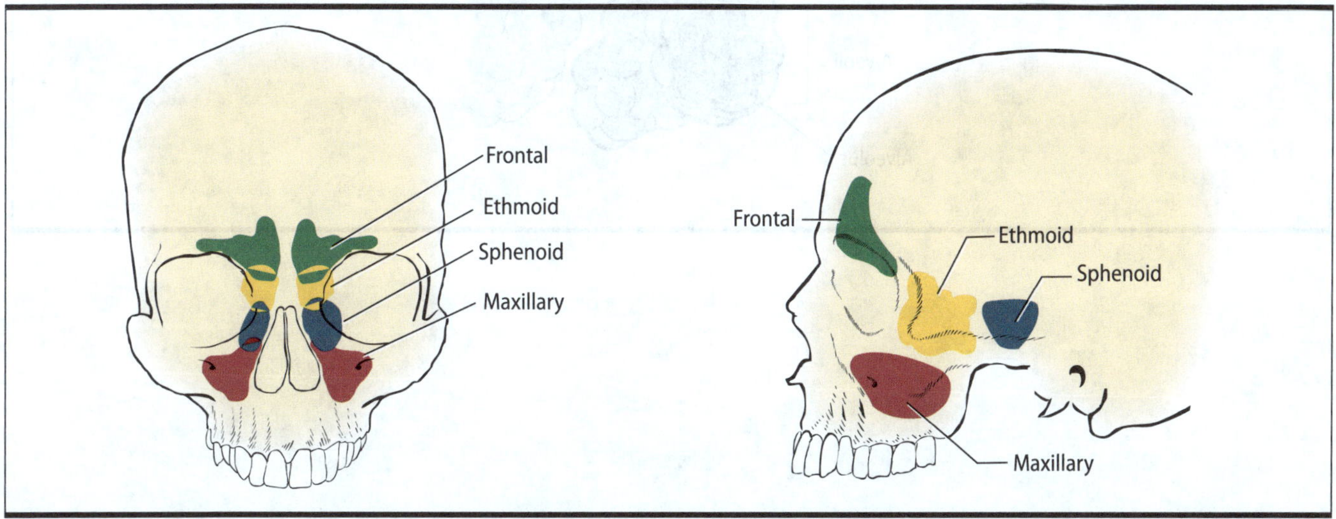

Lung Segments

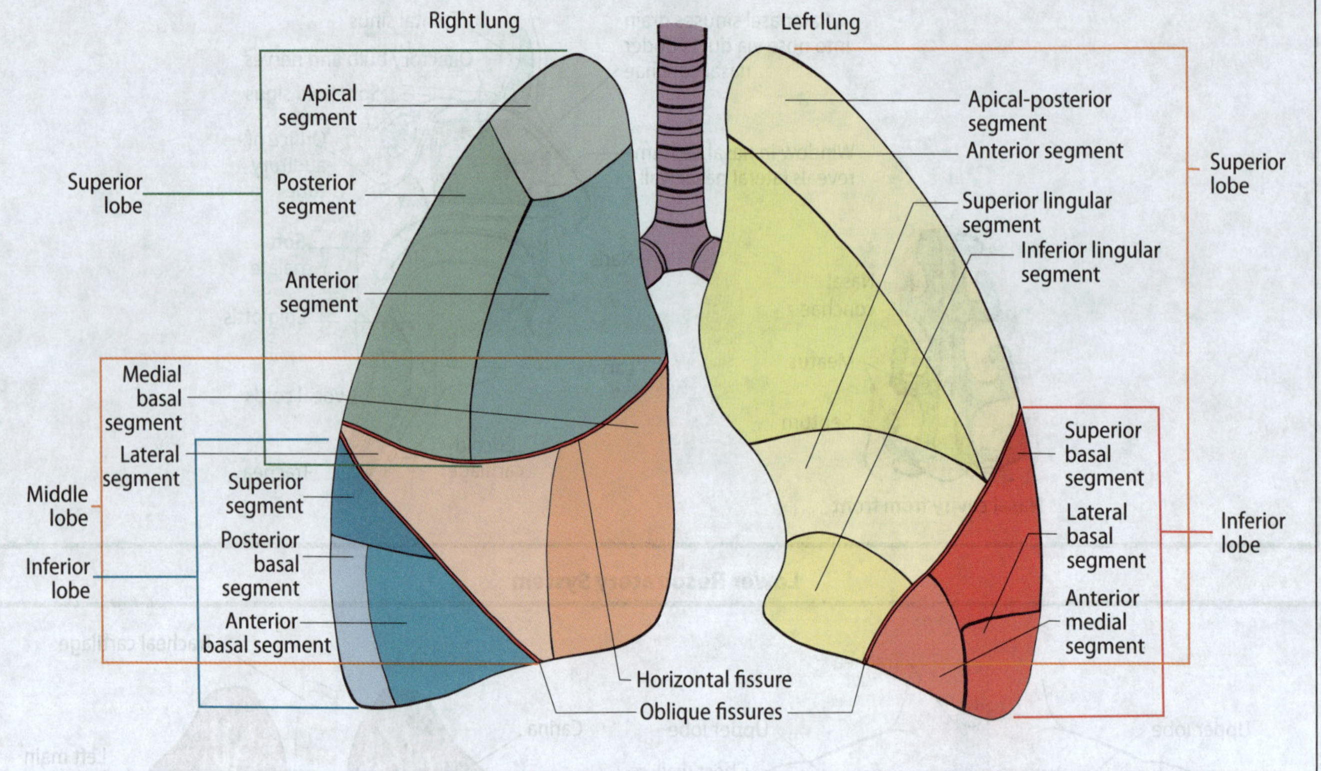

Right lung
Left lung
Superior lobe
Apical segment
Posterior segment
Anterior segment
Medial basal segment
Lateral segment
Middle lobe
Superior segment
Posterior basal segment
Inferior lobe
Anterior basal segment
Apical-posterior segment
Anterior segment
Superior lingular segment
Inferior lingular segment
Superior lobe
Superior basal segment
Lateral basal segment
Inferior lobe
Anterior medial segment
Horizontal fissure
Oblique fissures

Alveoli

To trachea
Terminal bronchiole
Pulmonary arteriole
Elastic fibers
Capillary network over all alveoli
Alveoli
Alveolus

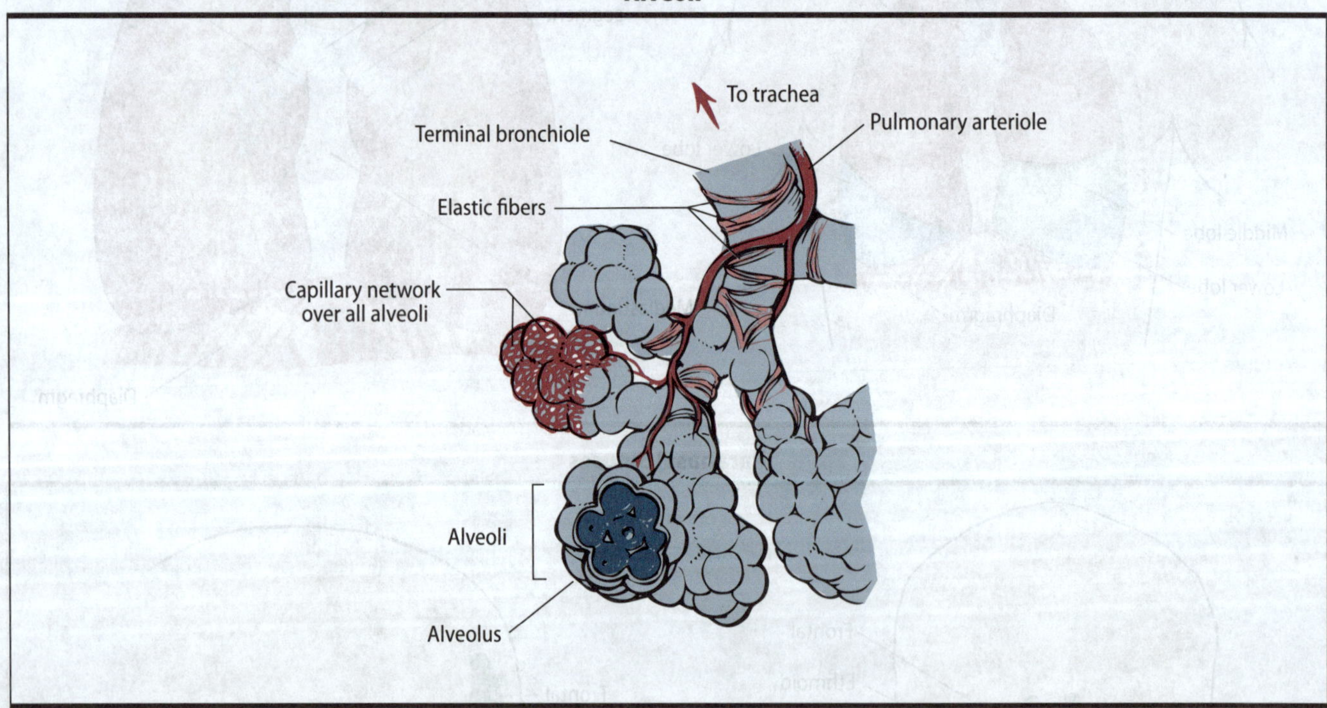

Chapter 11. Diseases of the Digestive System (KØØ–K95)

Digestive System

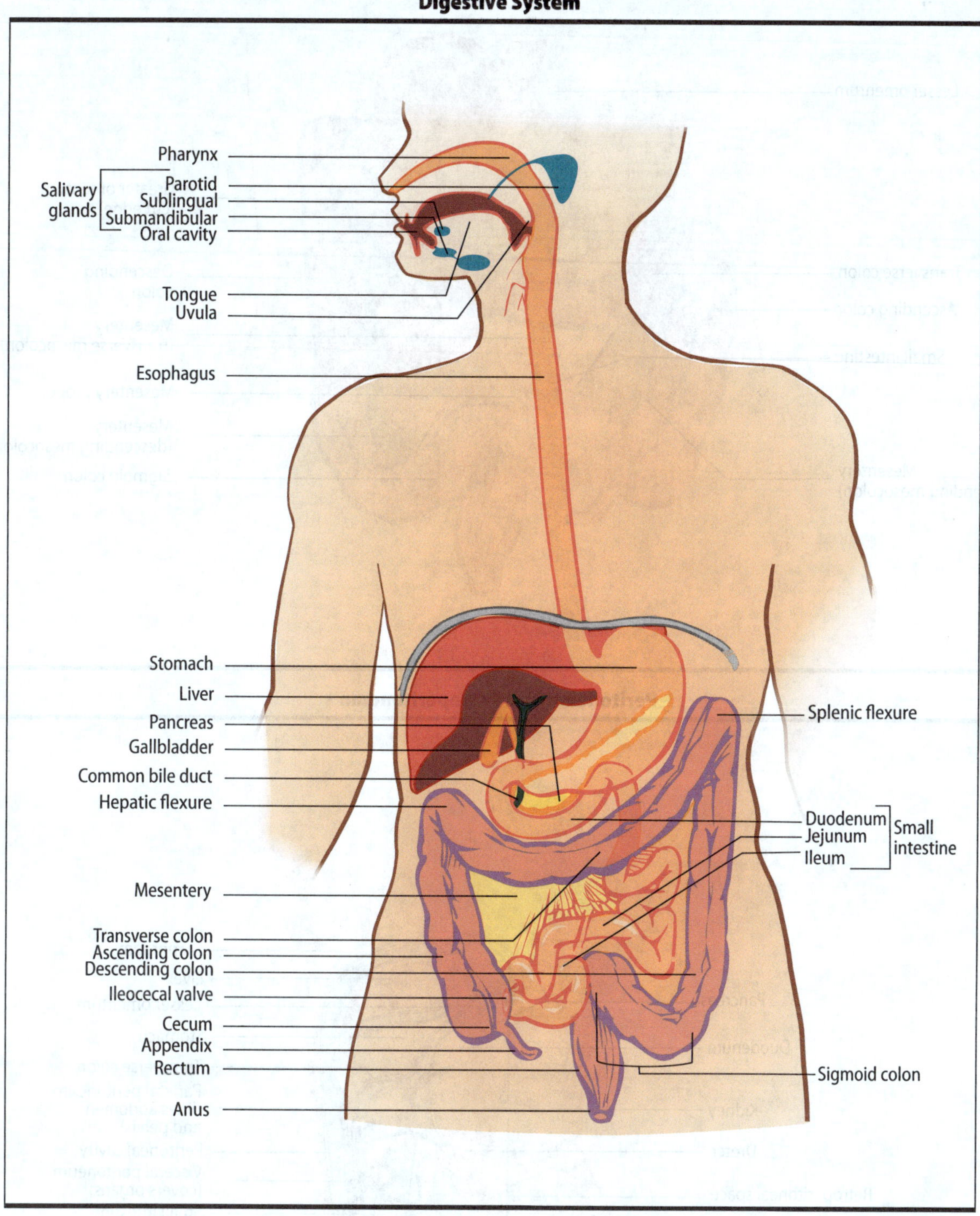

Omentum and Mesentery

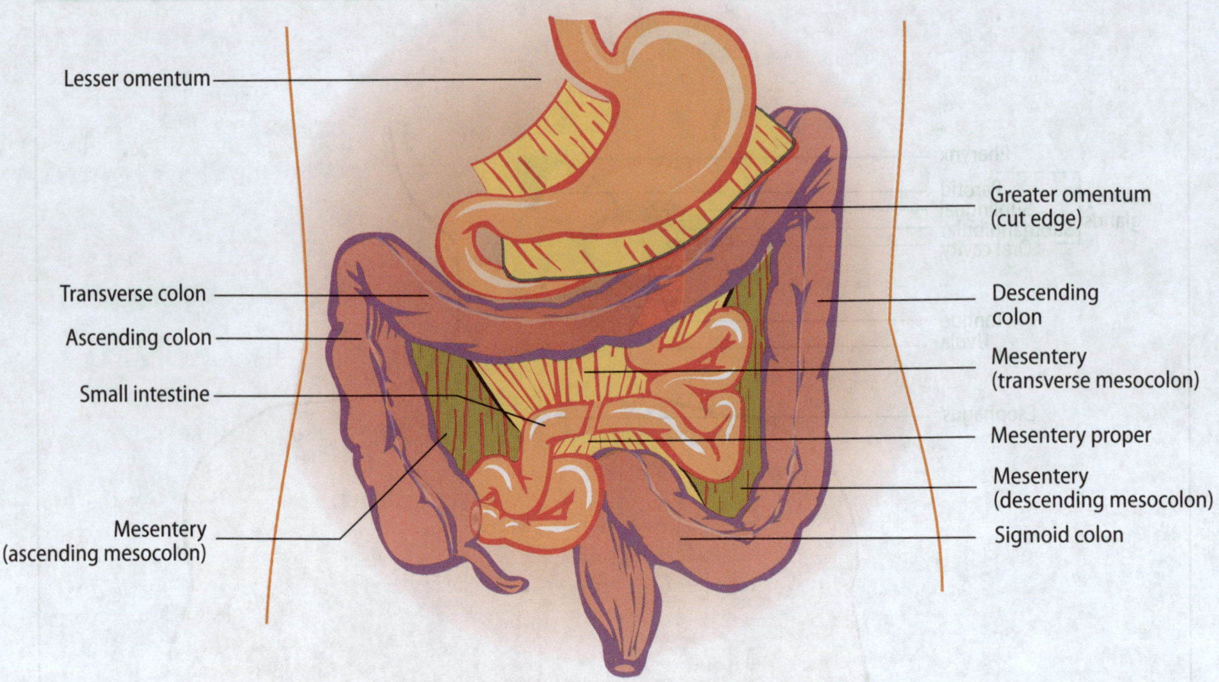

Lesser omentum
Greater omentum (cut edge)
Transverse colon
Descending colon
Ascending colon
Mesentery (transverse mesocolon)
Small intestine
Mesentery proper
Mesentery (descending mesocolon)
Mesentery (ascending mesocolon)
Sigmoid colon

Peritoneum and Retroperitoneum

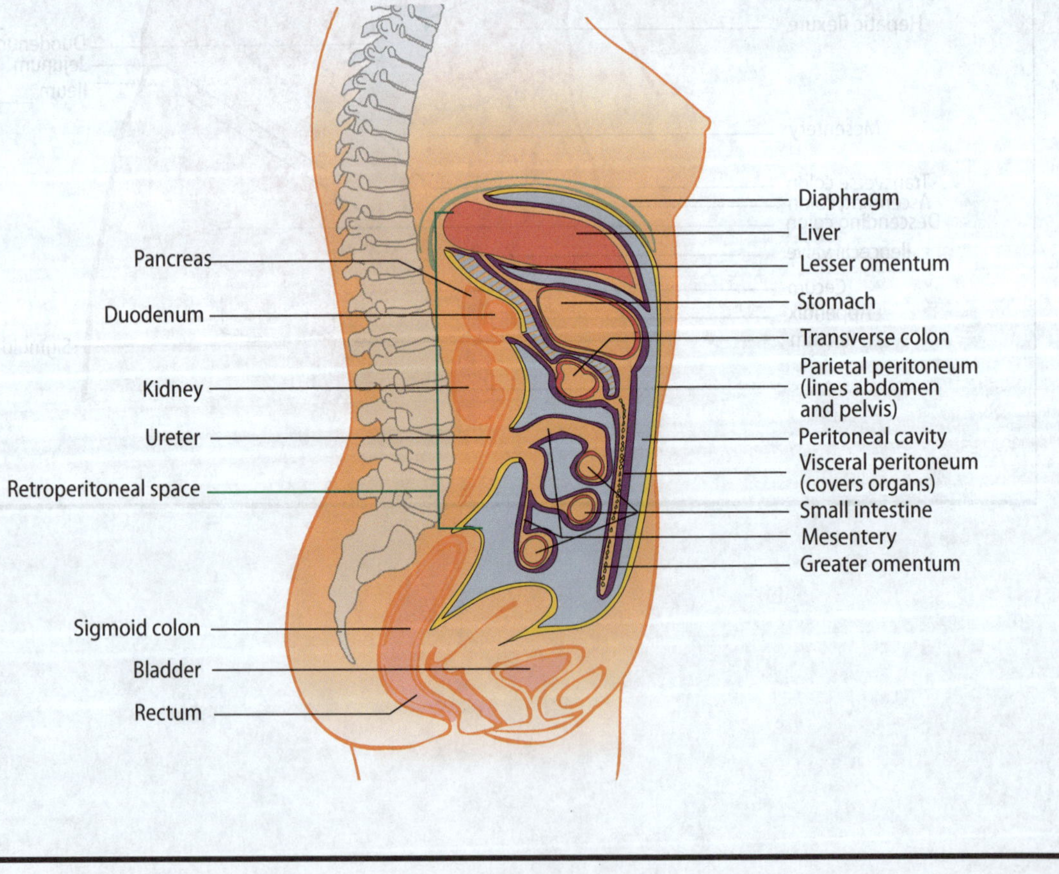

Diaphragm
Liver
Pancreas
Lesser omentum
Stomach
Duodenum
Transverse colon
Parietal peritoneum (lines abdomen and pelvis)
Kidney
Ureter
Peritoneal cavity
Visceral peritoneum (covers organs)
Retroperitoneal space
Small intestine
Mesentery
Greater omentum
Sigmoid colon
Bladder
Rectum

Chapter 12. Diseases of the Skin and Subcutaneous Tissue (LØØ–L99)

Nail Anatomy

Hyponychium
Cuticle
Nail plate
Nail fold
Nail bed
Nail root
Hyponychium
Matrix
Skin
Distal phalanx bone

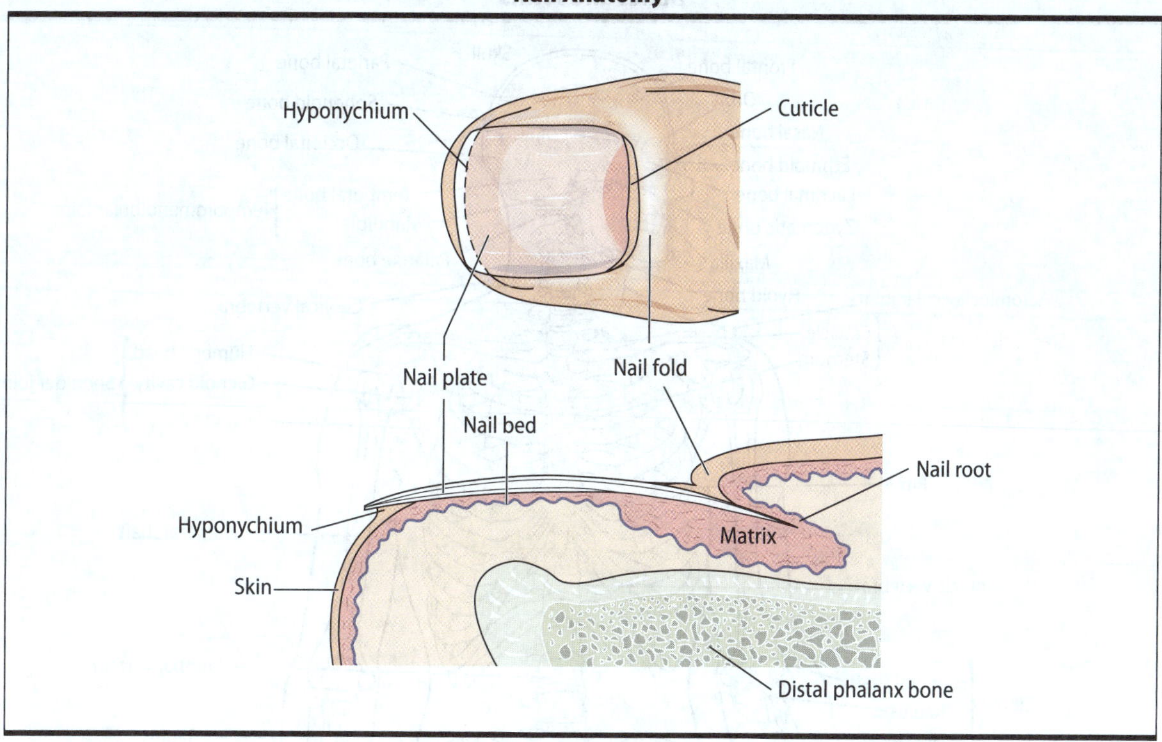

Skin and Subcutaneous Tissue

Hair
Basal layer
Corneal layer (corneum)
Epidermis
Hair shaft
Dermis
Sebaceous gland
Bulb
Hypodermis (subcutaneous layer)
Hair follicles
Sweat (eccrine gland)
Sensory nerve
Adipose tissue
Blood vessels

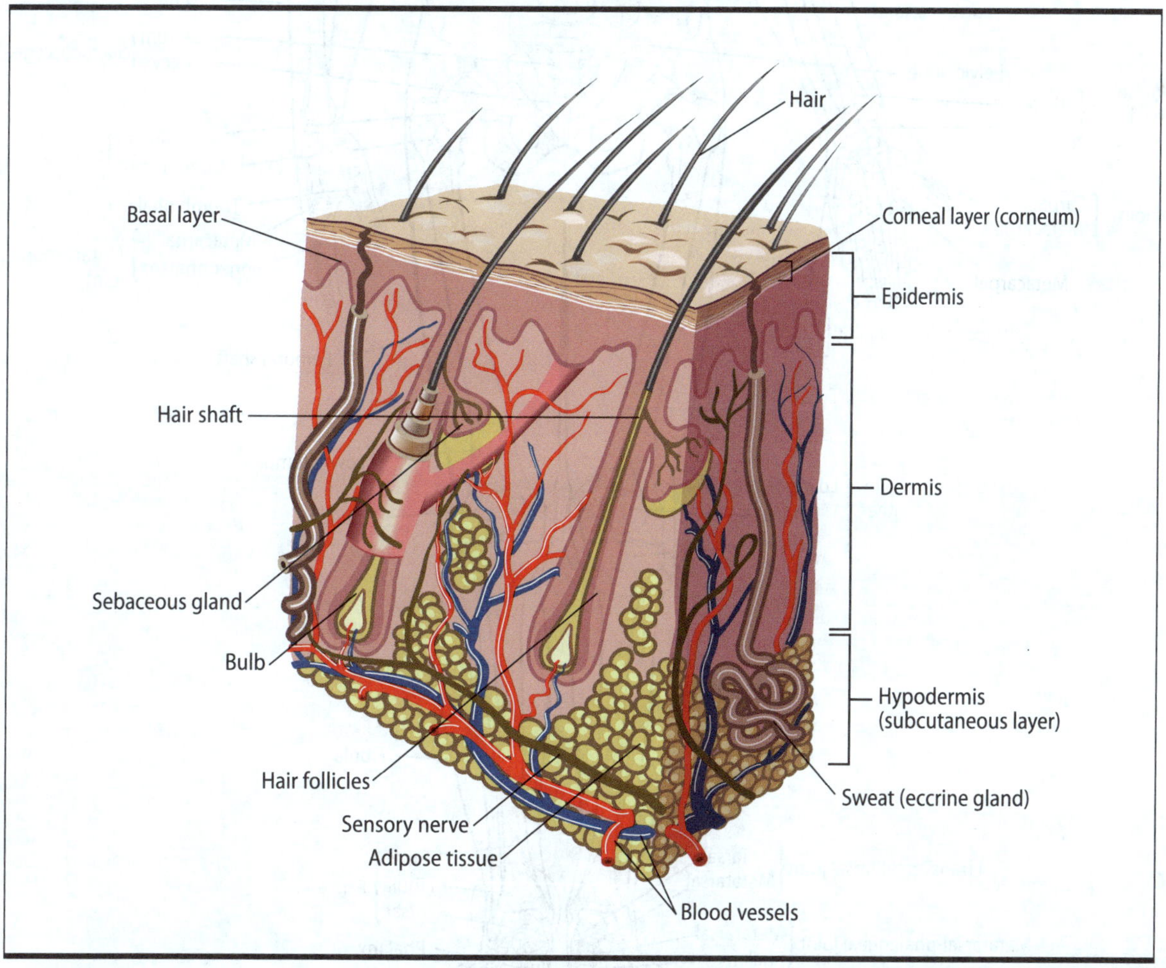

Chapter 13. Diseases of the Musculoskeletal System and Connective Tissue (MØØ–M99)

Bones and Joints

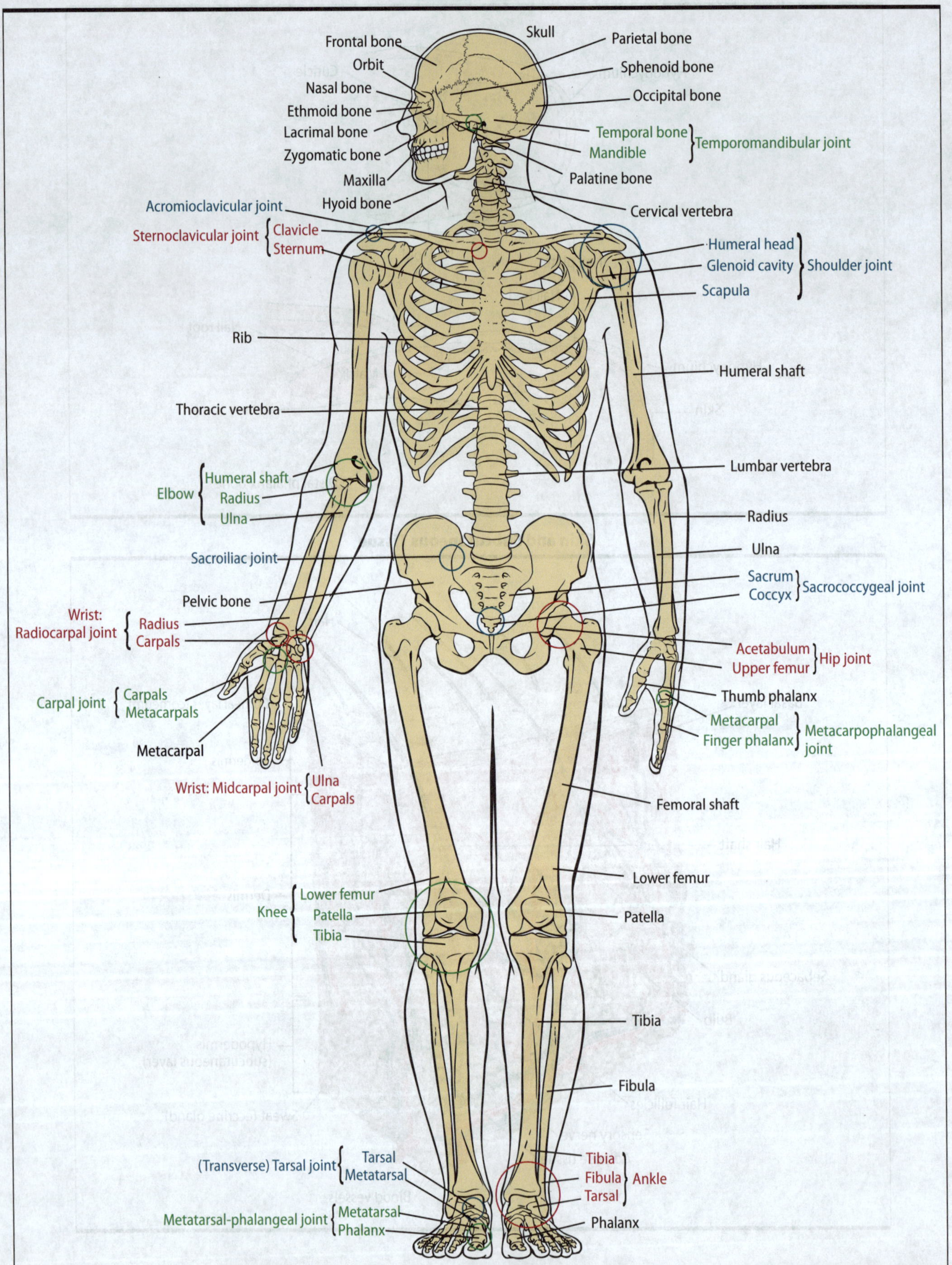

Shoulder Anterior View

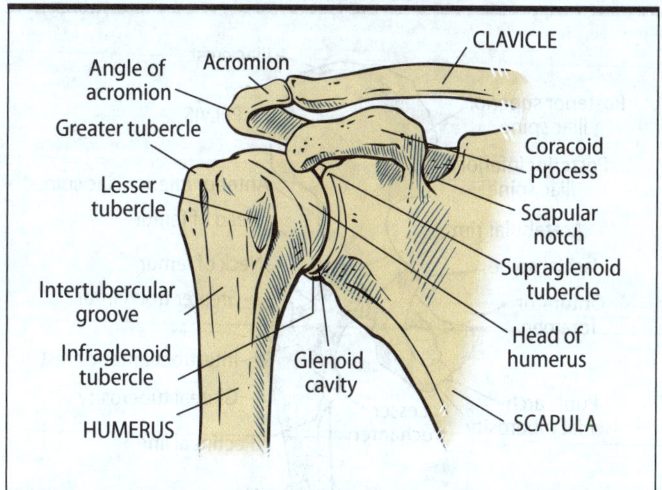

Shoulder Posterior View

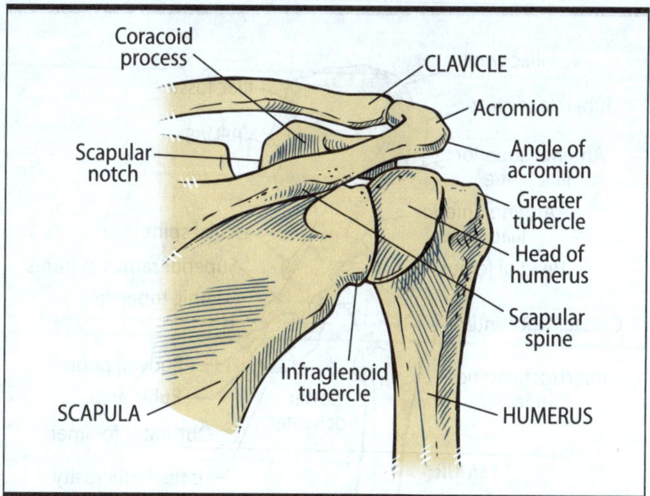

Elbow Anterior View

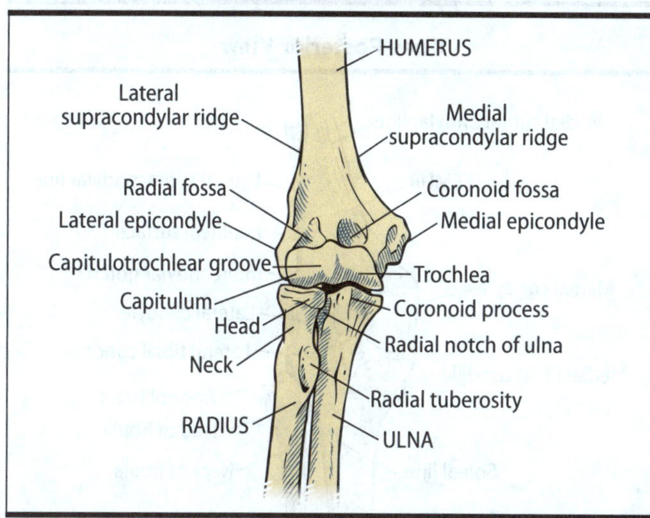

Elbow Posterior View

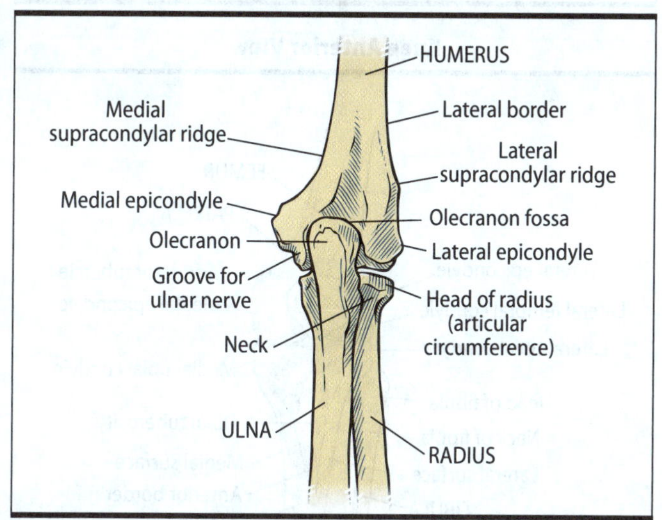

Hand

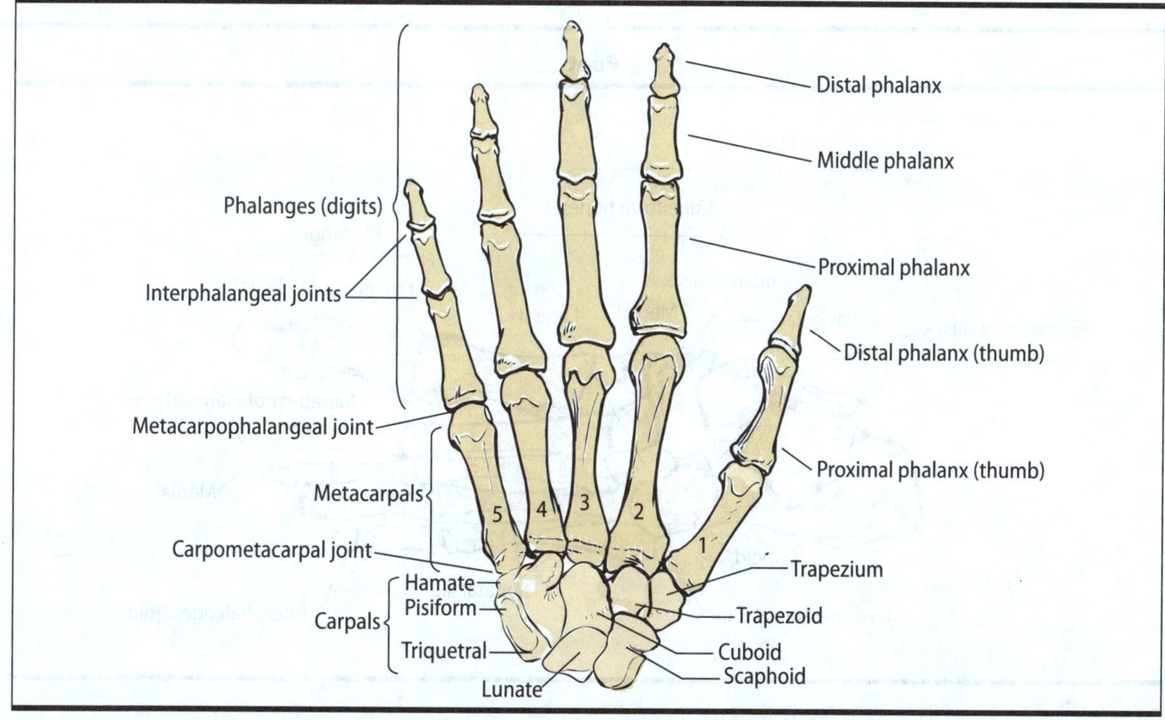

Hip Anterior View

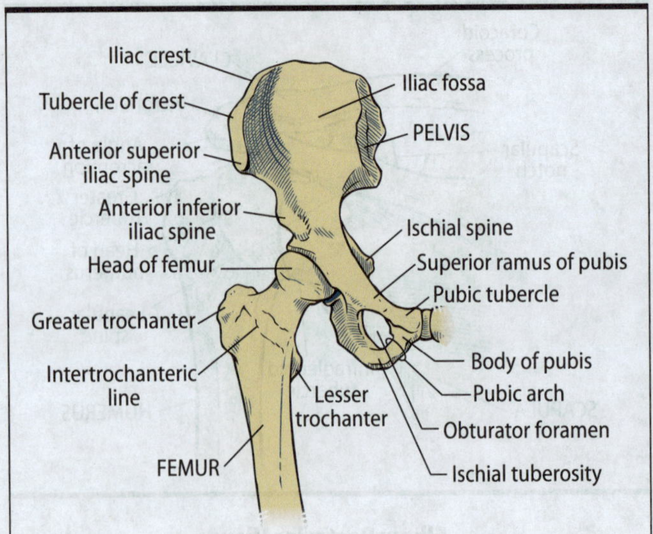

Hip Posterior View

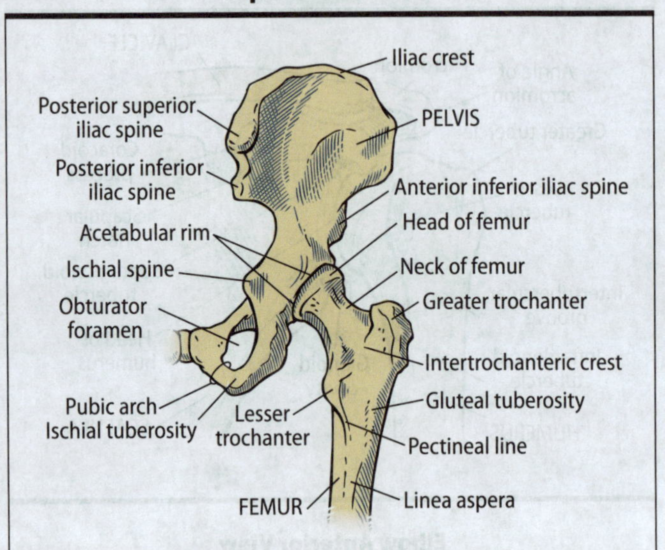

Knee Anterior View

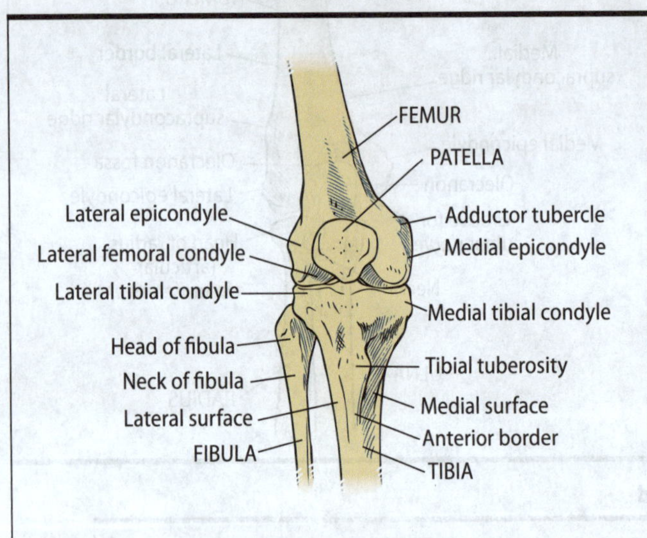

Knee Posterior View

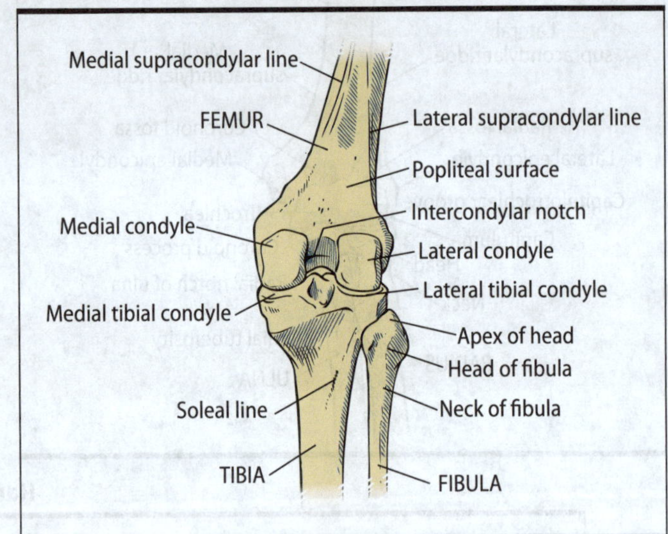

Foot

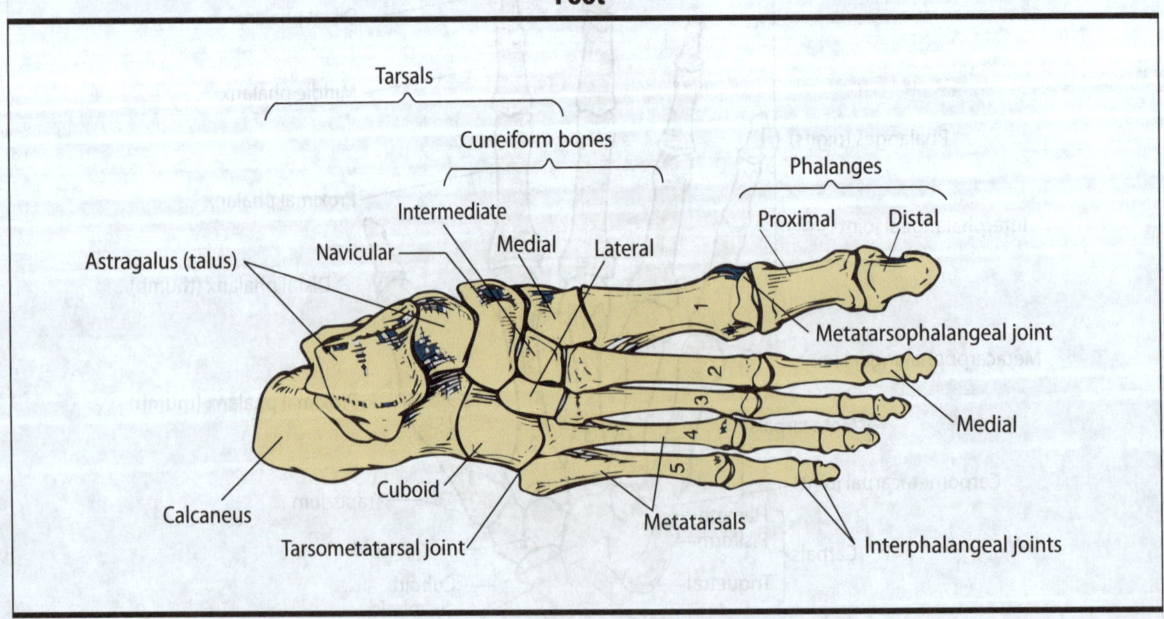

Muscles

Temporalis m.
Frontalis m.
Orbicularis oculi m.
Orbicularis oris m.
Depressor labii inferioris m.
Mentalis m.
Sternocleidomastoid m. (clavicular head)
Sternocleidomastoid m. (sternal head)
Masseter m.
Zygomaticus major m.
Splenius m.
Omohyoid m.
Levator scapulae m.
Platysma m.
Deltoid m.
Pectoralis major m.
Latissimus dorsi m.
Coracobrachialis m.
Serratus anterior m.
Biceps brachii m.
Biceps brachii m. (short head)
Biceps brachii m. (long head)
Triceps m.
Brachialis m.
Linea alba
Rectus abdominis m.
Brachioradialis m.
Extensor carpi radialis longus m.
Bicipital aponeurosis
External oblique m.
Flexor carpi radialis m.
Palmaris longus m.
Flexor carpi ulnaris m.
Flexor digitorum superficialis m.
Brachioradialis m.
Pronator teres m.
Flexor carpi radialis m.
Extensor carpi radialis longus m.
Extensor carpi radialis brevis m.
Extensor digitorum m.
Extensor digiti minimi m.
Extensor retinaculum
Extensor retinaculum
Anterior superior iliac spine
Pubic tubercle
Iliopsoas m.
Pectineus m.
Adductor longus m.
Sartorius m.
Gracilis m.
Tensor fascia latae m.
Vastus lateralis m.
Vastus medialis m.
Rectus femoris m.
Tensor fascia latae m.
Patella
Gastrocnemius m.
Tibia
Tibialis anterior m.
Soleus m.
Peroneus longus m.
Extensor digitorum longus m.
Superior extensor retinaculum
Medial malleolus
Lateral malleolus

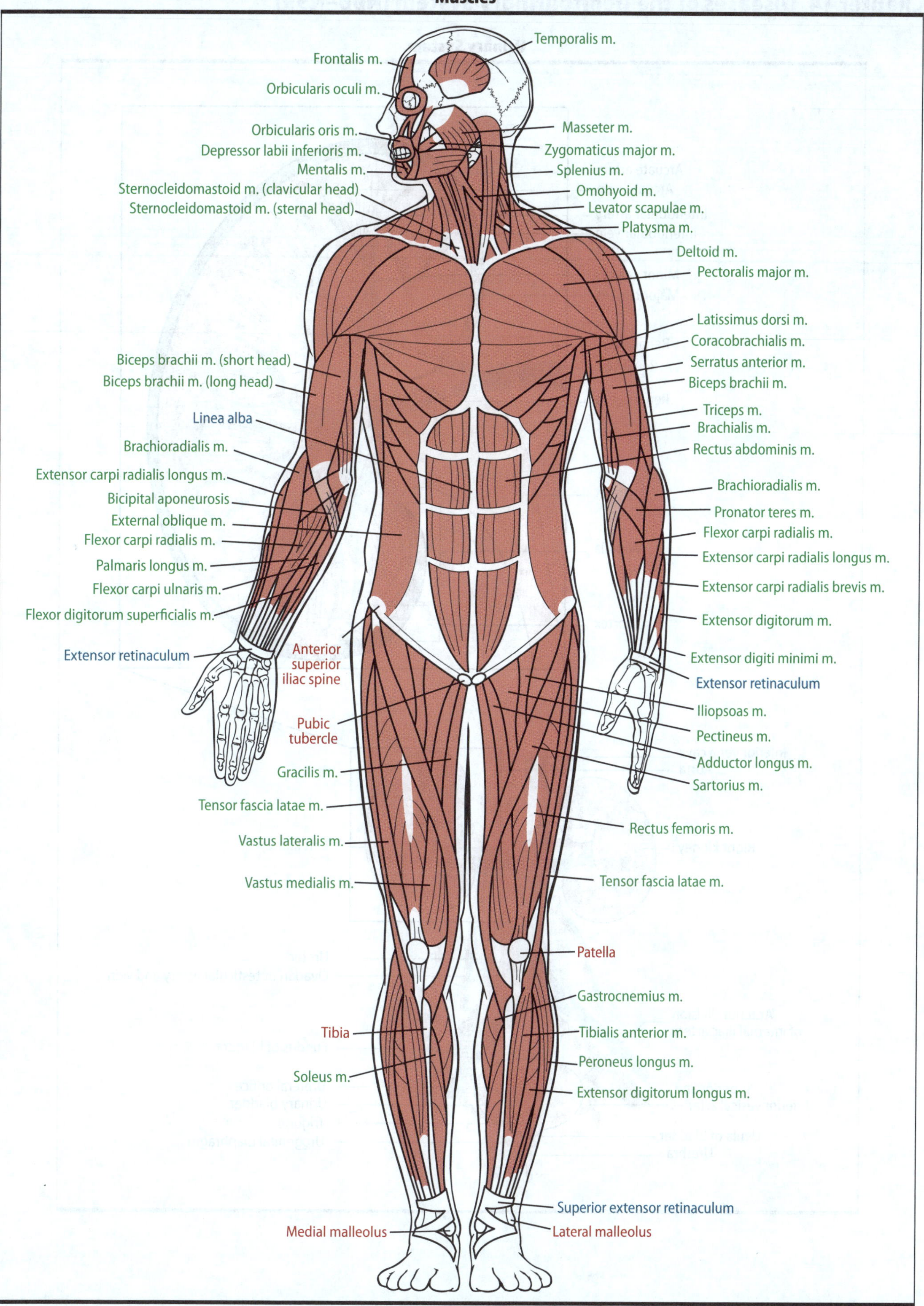

Chapter 14. Diseases of the Genitourinary System (NØØ–N99)

Urinary System

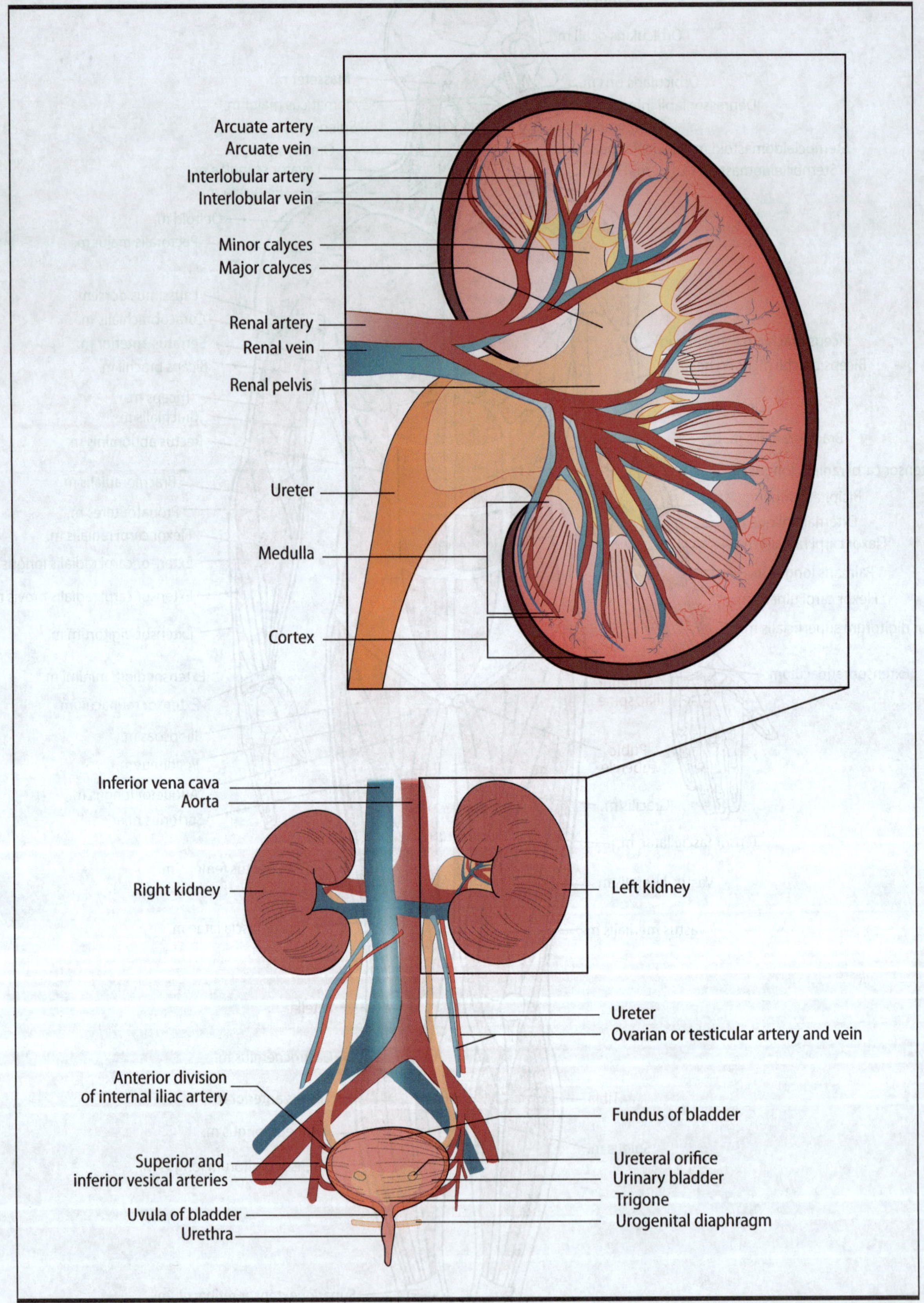

Male Genitourinary System

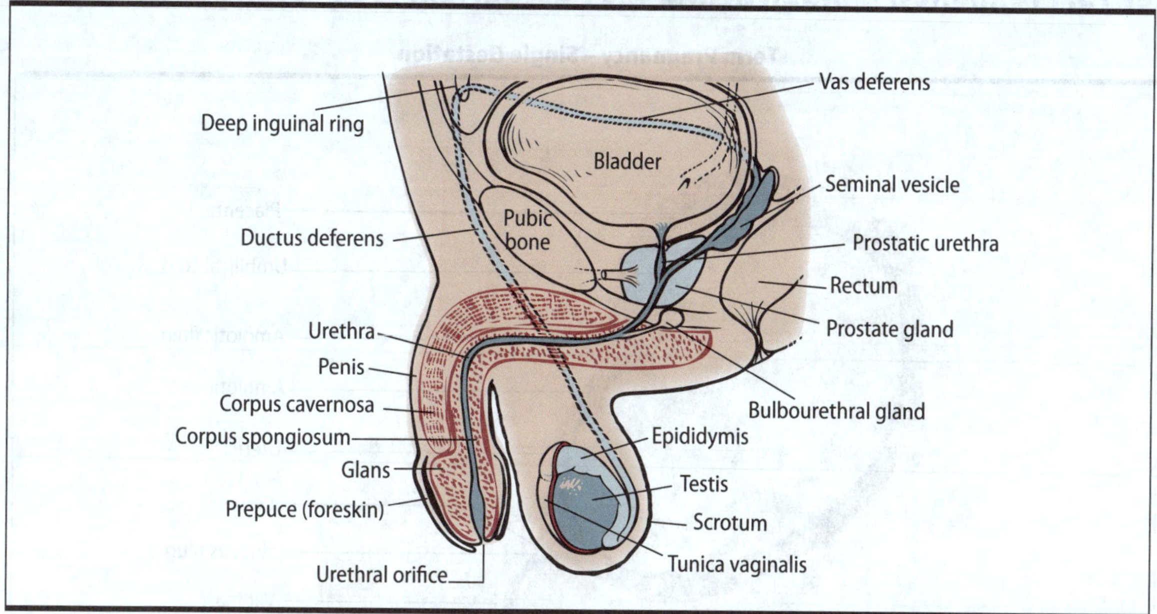

Female Internal Genitalia

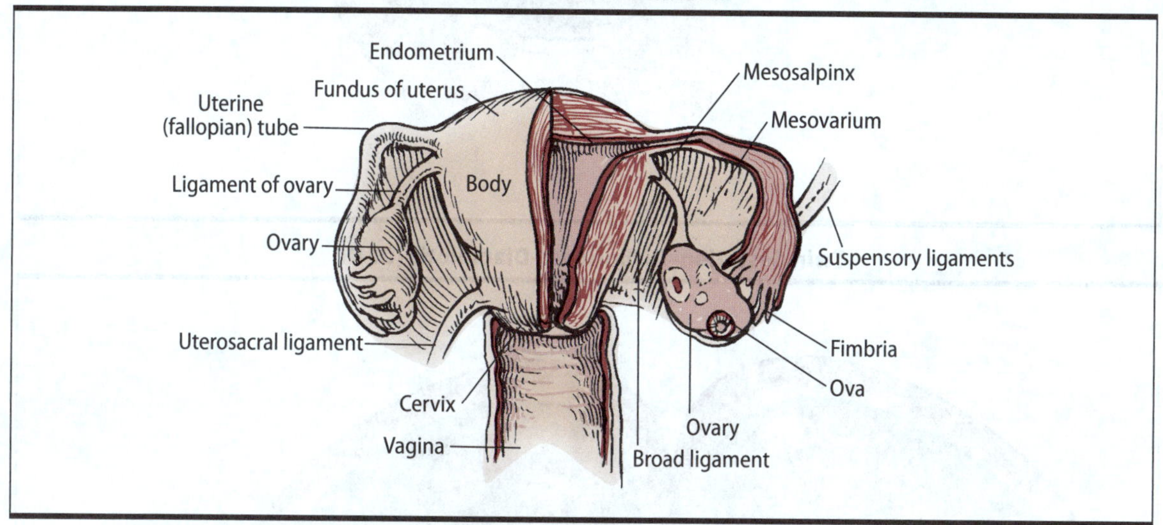

Female Genitourinary Tract Lateral View

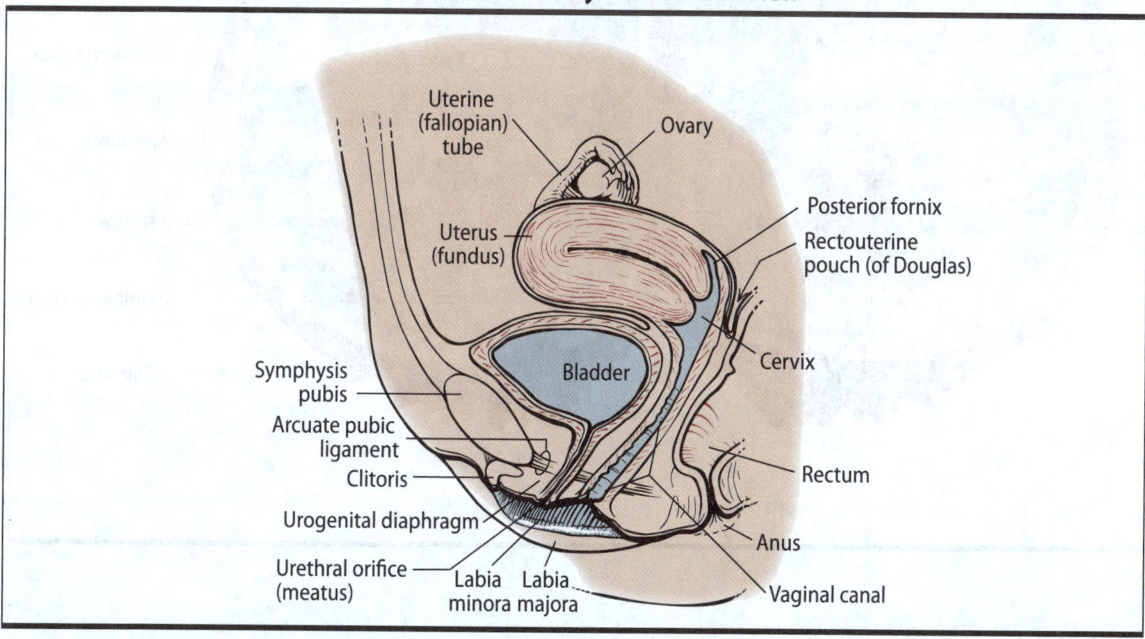

Chapter 15. Pregnancy, Childbirth and the Puerperium (OØØ–O9A)

Term Pregnancy – Single Gestation

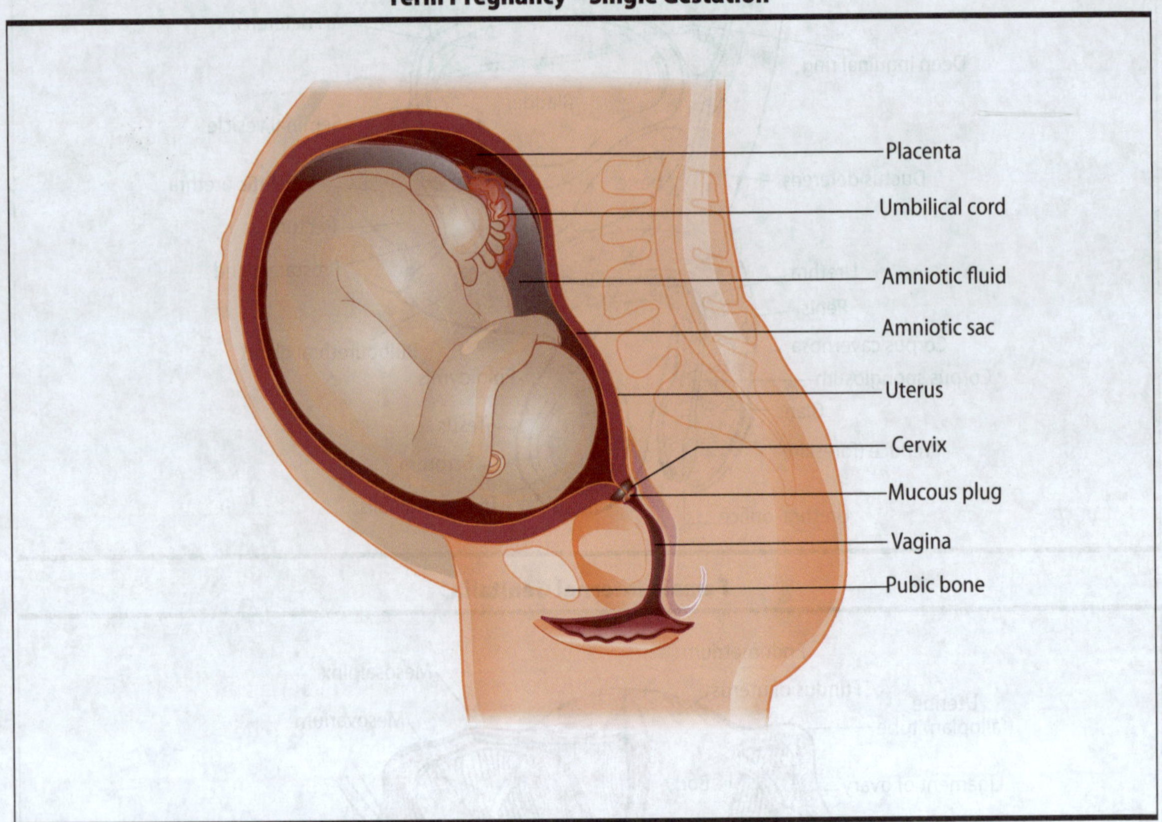

Twin Gestation–Dichorionic–Diamniotic (DI-DI)

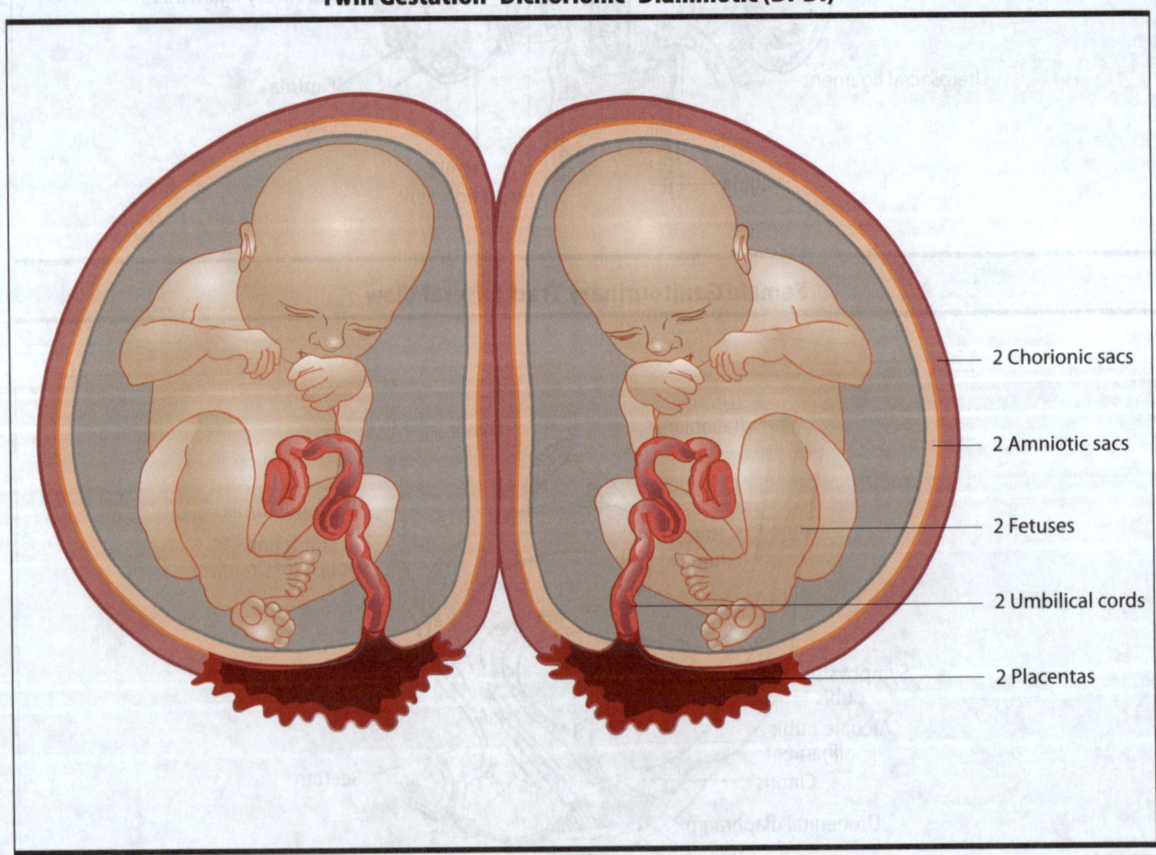

Twin Gestation–Monochorionic–Diamniotic (MO-DI)

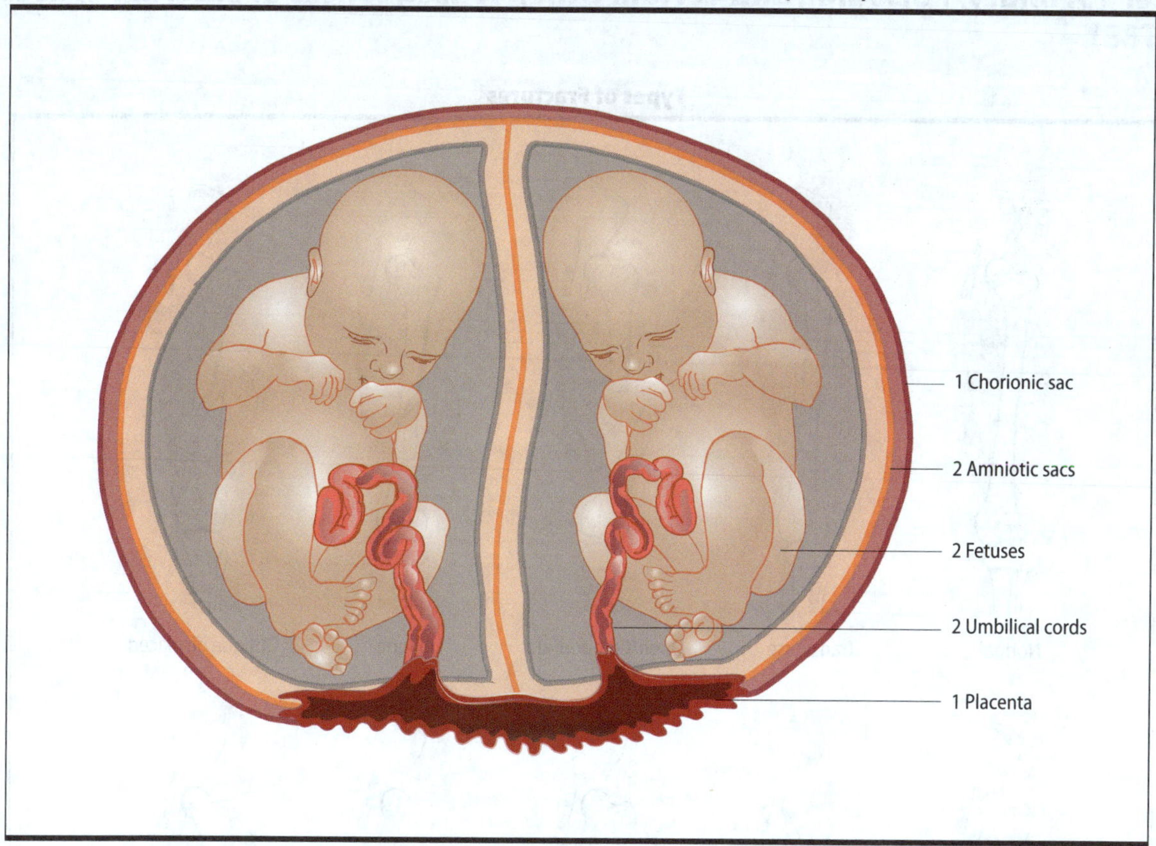

Twin Gestation–Monochorionic–Monoamniotic (MO-MO)

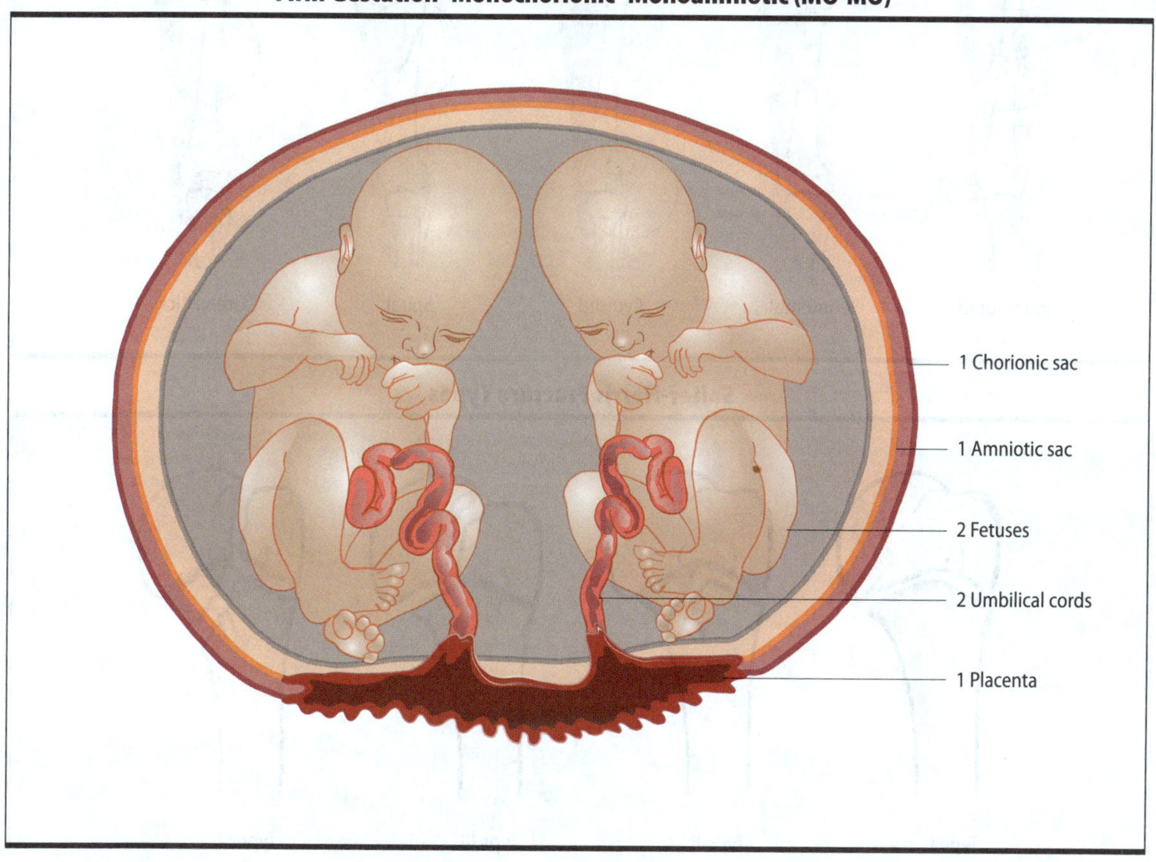

Chapter 19. Injury, Poisoning and Certain Other Consequences of External Causes (SØØ–T88)

Types of Fractures

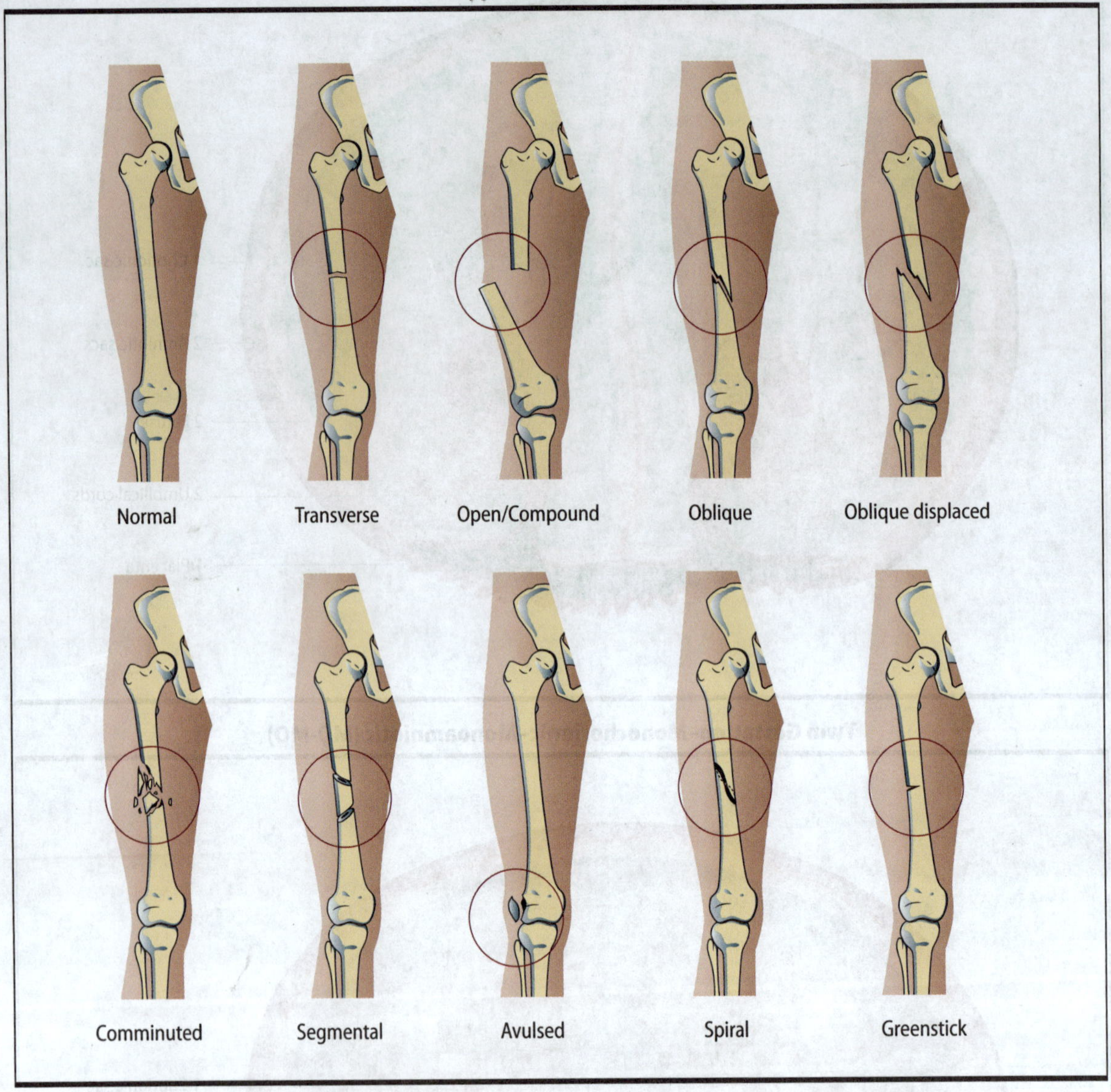

Normal
Transverse
Open/Compound
Oblique
Oblique displaced
Comminuted
Segmental
Avulsed
Spiral
Greenstick

Salter-Harris Fracture Types

Type I
Type II
Type III
Type IV

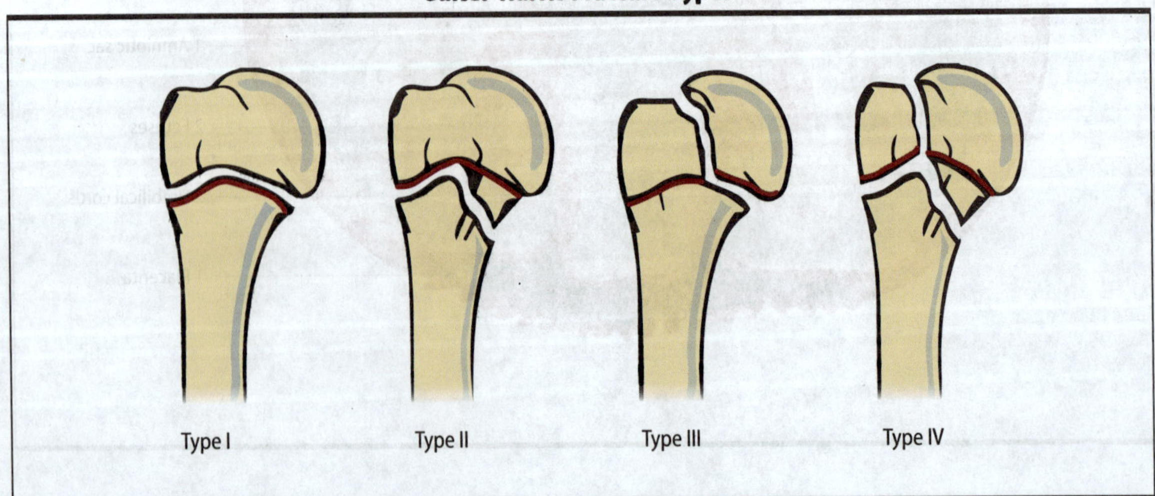